Mark frequently used sections in your code book with these color-coded flags.

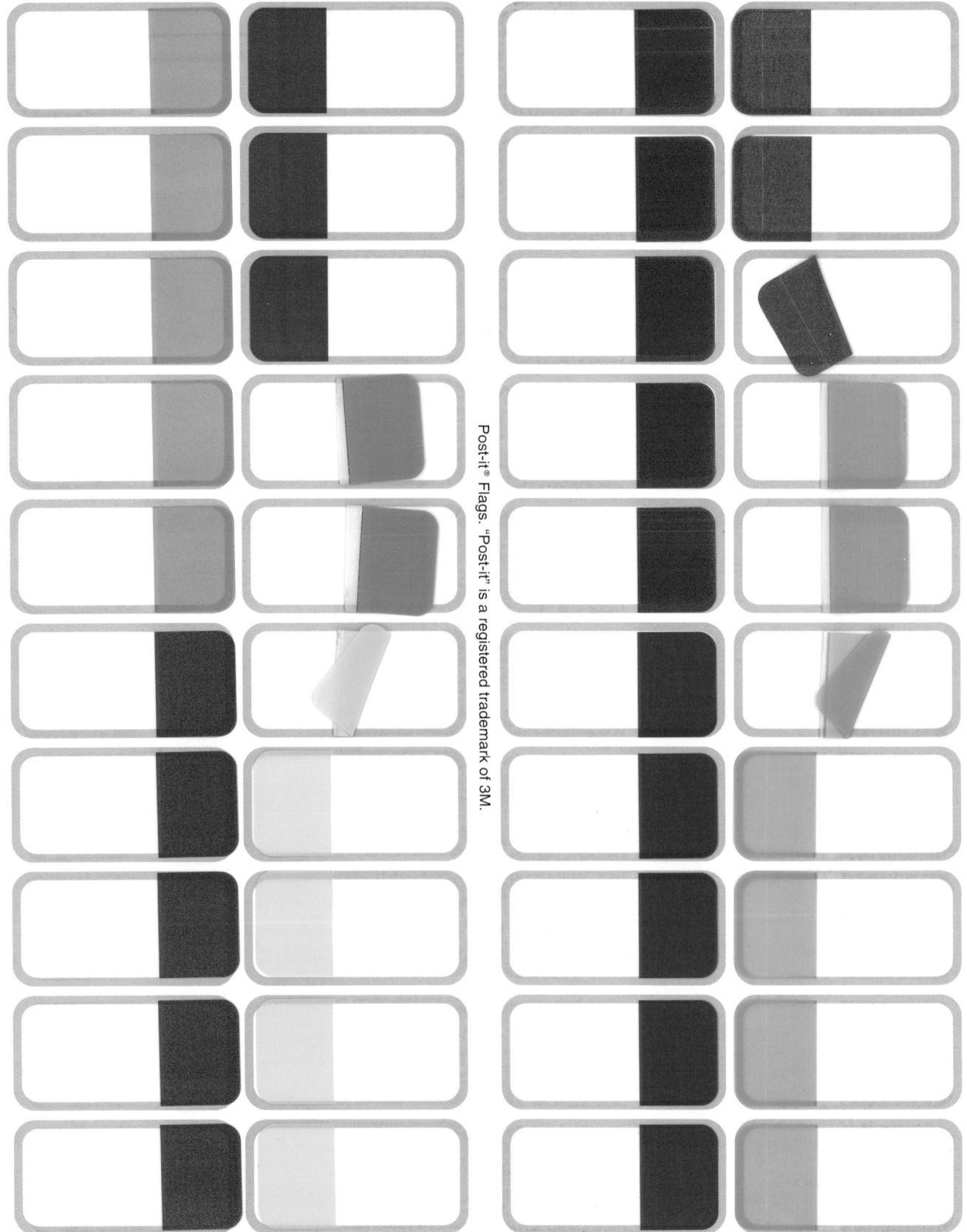

ICD-10-CM **Code Book** 2021

Anne B. Casto, RHIA, CCS
Consulting Editor

AHIMA
American Health Information
Management Association®

Softbound
ISBN: 978-1-58426-810-9
AHIMA Product No.: AC221020

Spiralbound
ISBN: 978-1-58426-811-6
AHIMA Product No.: AC221120

AHIMA Staff:
Colton Gigot, MA, Production Development Editor
Megan Grennan, Director, Content Production and AHIMA Press
James Pinnick, Vice President, Content and Product Development
Rachel Schratz, MA, Assistant Editor

Cover image: © knikola, Shutterstock

The Centers for Medicare and Medicaid Services (CMS) and the National Center for Health Statistics (NCHS), two departments within the US Federal Government's Department of Health and Human Services (HHS) provide the *International Classification of Diseases, Tenth Revision, Clinical Modification* (ICD-10-CM) for coding and reporting. ICD-10-CM is the US modification to the World Health Organization's (WHO) International Classification of Diseases, Tenth Revision (ICD-10).

Coding Clinic for ICD-10-CM and ICD-10-PCS is a publication of the American Hospital Association (AHA).

Unless otherwise noted, art pieces were created by Jason Isley and Cognition Studio, Inc, and are all copyright of the American Health Information Management Association.

The websites listed in this book were current and valid as of the date of publication. However, webpage addresses and the information on them may change at any time. The user is encouraged to perform his or her own general web searches to locate any site addresses listed here that are no longer valid.

For more information about AHIMA Press publications, including updates, visit **http://www.ahima.org/education/press**.

American Health Information Management Association
233 North Michigan Avenue, 21st Floor
Chicago, Illinois 60601-5809
ahima.org

Contents

About the Consulting Editor

Anne B. Casto, RHIA, CCS, is the president of Casto Consulting, LLC. Casto Consulting, LLC is a consulting firm that provides services to hospitals and other healthcare stakeholders primarily in the areas of reimbursement and coding. Casto Consulting, LLC specializes in linking coding and billing practices to positive revenue cycle outcomes. Additionally, the firm provides guidance to consulting firms, healthcare organizations and healthcare insurers regarding reimbursement methodologies and Medicare regulations.

Additionally, Ms. Casto is a lecturer in the HIMS department at The Ohio State University, School of Health and Rehabilitation Sciences. Over the past 18 years, Ms. Casto has taught numerous courses in the areas of healthcare reimbursement, coding, healthcare data trending, and coding analytics.

Prior to her current roles, Ms. Casto was the vice president of clinical information for Cleverley & Associates where she worked very closely with APC regulations and guidelines, preparing hospitals for the implementation of the Medicare OPPS. Ms. Casto was also the clinical information product manager for CHIPS/Ingenix. She joined CHIPS/Ingenix in 1998 and spent the majority of her time developing coding compliance products for the inpatient and outpatient settings.

Ms. Casto has been responsible for inpatient and outpatient coding activities in several large hospitals including Mt. Sinai Medical Center (NYC), Beth Israel Medical Center (NYC), and The Ohio State University. She has worked extensively with CMI, quality measures, physician documentation, and coding accuracy efforts at these facilities.

Ms. Casto received her degree in Health Information Management at The Ohio State University in 1995. She received her Certified Coding Specialist credential in 1998 from the American Health Information Management Association. In 2009 Ms. Casto received her ICD-10-CM/PCS Trainer certificate from AHIMA. Ms. Casto is the co-author of an AHIMA published text book entitled *Principles of Healthcare Reimbursement*. Additionally, Ms. Casto was a contributing author to the published AHIMA books: *Severity DRGs and Reimbursement; A MS-DRG Primer* and *Effective Management of Coding Services*.

Ms. Casto received the AHIMA Legacy Award, part of the FORE Triumph Awards, in 2007 which honors a significant contribution to the knowledge base of the HIM field through an insightful publication. Additionally, Ms. Casto was honored with the Ohio Health Information Management Association's Distinguished Member Award in 2008 and the Ohio Health Information Management Association's Professional Achievement Award in 2011.

Acknowledgments

Many thanks to my family for their support during this project. Thanks to Dr. Susan White, The Ohio State University; your data manipulation skills are second to none. Thanks to Drew Beverick for providing valuable insight from the student perspective. Many thanks to Linda Hyde, RHIA, and Rachael D'Andrea, MS, RHIA, CDIP, CHTS-TR, CPHQ, for their very thorough technical review of the book.

ICD-10-CM History and Background

The International Classification of Diseases, Tenth Revision, Clinical Modification (ICD-10-CM) is the United Stated modification to the World Health Organization's (WHO) International Classification of Diseases, Tenth Revision (ICD-10). The WHO adopted the tenth revision in 1990. Since that time, several countries, including Australia and Canada, have developed their own modification to ICD-10 and have implemented it for use.

In 1994, the National Center for Health Statistics (NCHS) began the process of determining the viability of ICD-10 and the applicability of a clinical modification of the code set for the United States. The NCHS has made draft versions of ICD-10-CM available since 2002. NCHS continued to refine and update the code set for use in the United States while the healthcare community waited for adoption of the code set by Congress. On August 22, 2008, the long-awaited official Notice of Proposed Rule Making (NPRM) regarding the adopting of the ICD-10-CM and ICD-10-PCS classifications was published in the *Federal Register*. On January 16, 2009, the Centers for Medicare and Medicaid Services (CMS) published the Final Rule for adoption of the ICD-10-CM and ICD-10-PCS code sets udders rules, 45 CFR Parts 160 and 162 of the Health Insurance Portability and Accountability Act of 1996 (HIPAA). Within this rule, a compliance (implementation) date of October 1, 2013 was released. The compliance date was revised and ICD-10-CM was successfully implemented on October 1, 2015.

Characteristics of ICD-10-CM

ICD-10-CM far exceeds its predecessors in the number of codes provided. The disease classification has been expanded to include health-related conditions and to provide greater specificity at the seventh-character level of detail. When available, these seventh characters are not optional; they are intended for use in recording the information substantiated in the clinical record.

The ICD-10-CM/PCS Coordination and Maintenance Committee

Annual modifications are made to ICD-10-CM through the ICD-10-CM Coordination and Maintenance Committee (C&M). The Committee is made up of representatives from two US federal government agencies, the National Center for Health Statistics, and the Centers for Medicare and Medicaid Services (CMS). C&M holds meetings twice a year, which are open to the public. Modification proposals submitted to C&M for consideration are presented at the meetings for public discussion. An open comment period follows each of these meetings. Those modification proposals which are approved are incorporated into the official government version of ICD-10-CM and become effective for use on October 1 of each year.

Guidance in the Use of ICD10-CM

To code accurately, it is necessary to have a working knowledge of medical terminology and to understand the characteristics, code book terminology, and conventions of ICD-10-CM. Transforming verbal descriptions of diseases, injuries, and conditions into numerical designations (coding) is a complex activity and should not be undertaken without proper training.

Originally, coding was accomplished to provide access to health records by diagnoses and operations through retrieval for medical research education and administration. Today, medical codes are utilized to facilitate payment of health services, evaluate utilization patterns, and study the appropriateness of healthcare costs. Coding also provides the basis for epidemiological studies and research into the quality of healthcare.

Coding must be performed correctly and consistently to produce meaningful statics to aid in planning for the health needs of the nation.

Official Conventions

ICD-10-CM Official Guidelines for Coding and Reporting 2021
(October 1, 2020 - September 30, 2021)

Narrative changes appear in bold text

Items <u>underlined</u> have been moved within the guidelines since the 2020 version

Italics **are used to indicate revisions to heading changes**

The Centers for Medicare and Medicaid Services (CMS) and the National Center for Health Statistics (NCHS), two departments within the US Federal Government's Department of Health and Human Services (HHS) provide the following guidelines for coding and reporting using the International Classification of Diseases, Tenth Revision, Clinical Modification (ICD-10-CM). These guidelines should be used as a companion document to the official version of the ICD-10-CM as published on the NCHS website. The ICD-10-CM is a morbidity classification published by the United States for classifying diagnoses and reason for visits in all healthcare settings. The ICD-10-CM is based on the ICD-10, the statistical classification of disease published by the World Health Organization (WHO).

These guidelines have been approved by the four organizations that make up the Cooperating Parties for the ICD-10-CM: the American Hospital Association (AHA), the American Health Information Management Association (AHIMA), CMS, and NCHS.

These guidelines are a set of rules that have been developed to accompany and complement the official conventions and instructions provided within the ICD-10-CM itself. The instructions and conventions of the classification take precedence over guidelines. These guidelines are based on the coding and sequencing instructions in the Tabular List and Alphabetic Index of ICD-10-CM, but provide additional instruction. Adherence to these guidelines when assigning ICD-10-CM diagnosis codes is required under the Health Insurance Portability and Accountability Act (HIPAA). The diagnosis codes (Tabular List and Alphabetic Index) have been adopted under HIPAA for all healthcare settings. A joint effort between the healthcare provider and the coder is essential to achieve complete and accurate documentation, code assignment, and reporting of diagnoses and procedures. These guidelines have been developed to assist both the healthcare provider and the coder in identifying those diagnoses that are to be reported. The importance of consistent, complete documentation in the medical record cannot be overemphasized. Without such documentation accurate coding cannot be achieved. The entire record should be reviewed to determine the specific reason for the encounter and the conditions treated.

The term encounter is used for all settings, including hospital admissions. In the context of these guidelines, the term provider is used throughout the guidelines to mean physician or any qualified healthcare practitioner who is legally accountable for establishing the patient's diagnosis. Only this set of guidelines, approved by the Cooperating Parties, is official.

The guidelines are organized into sections. Section I includes the structure and conventions of the classification and general guidelines that apply to the entire classification, and chapter-specific guidelines that correspond to the chapters as they are arranged in the classification. Section II includes guidelines for selection of principal diagnosis for non-outpatient settings. Section III includes guidelines for reporting additional diagnoses in non-outpatient settings. Section IV is for outpatient coding and reporting. It is necessary to review all sections of the guidelines to fully understand all of the rules and instructions needed to code properly.

Section I. Conventions, General Coding Guidelines and Chapter Specific Guidelines

The conventions, general guidelines and chapter-specific guidelines are applicable to all healthcare settings unless otherwise indicated. The conventions and instructions of the classification take precedence over guidelines.

A. Conventions for the ICD-10-CM

The conventions for the ICD-10-CM are the general rules for use of the classification independent of the guidelines. These conventions are incorporated within the Alphabetic Index and Tabular List of the ICD-10-CM as instructional notes.

1. The Alphabetic Index and Tabular List

The ICD-10-CM is divided into the Alphabetic Index, an alphabetical list of terms and their corresponding code, and the Tabular List, a structured list of codes divided into chapters based on body system or condition. The Alphabetic Index consists of the following parts: the Index of Diseases and Injury, the Index of External Causes of Injury, the Table of Neoplasms, and the Table of Drugs and Chemicals.

See Section I.C2. General guidelines

See Section I.C.19. Adverse effects, poisoning, underdosing and toxic effects

2. Format and Structure

The ICD-10-CM Tabular List contains categories, subcategories and codes. Characters for categories, subcategories and codes may be either a letter or a number. All categories are 3 characters. A three-character category that has no further subdivision is equivalent to a code. Subcategories are either 4 or 5 characters. Codes may be 3, 4, 5, 6, or 7 characters. That is, each level of subdivision after a category is a subcategory. The final level of subdivision is a code. Codes that have applicable 7th characters are still referred to as codes, not subcategories. A code that has an applicable 7th character is considered invalid without the 7th character.

The ICD-10-CM uses an indented format for ease in reference.

3. Use of Codes for Reporting Purposes

For reporting purposes only codes are permissible, not categories or subcategories, and any applicable 7th character is required.

4. Placeholder Character

The ICD-10-CM utilizes a placeholder character X. The X is used as a placeholder at certain codes to allow for future expansion. An example of this is at the poisoning, adverse effect and underdosing codes, categories T36–T50. Where a placeholder exists, the X must be used in order for the code to be considered a valid code.

5. 7th Characters

Certain ICD-10-CM categories have applicable 7th characters. The applicable 7th character is required for all codes within the category, or as the notes in the Tabular List instruct. The 7th character must always be the 7th character in the data field. If a code that requires a 7th character is not 6 characters, a placeholder X must be used to fill in the empty characters.

6. Abbreviations

a. Alphabetic Index Abbreviations

NEC "Not elsewhere classifiable"
This abbreviation in the Alphabetic Index represents "other specified". When a specific code is not available for a condition, the Alphabetic Index directs the coder to the "other specified" code in the Tabular List.

NOS "Not otherwise specified"
This abbreviation is the equivalent of unspecified.

b. Tabular List Abbreviations

NEC "Not elsewhere classifiable"
This abbreviation in the Tabular List represents "other specified". When a specific code is not available for a condition the Tabular List includes an NEC entry under a code to identify the code as the "other specified" code.

NOS "Not otherwise specified"
This abbreviation is the equivalent of unspecified.

7. Punctuation

[ ] Brackets are used in the Tabular List to enclose synonyms, alternative wording or explanatory phrases. Brackets are used in the Alphabetic Index to identify manifestation codes.

( ) Parentheses are used in both the Alphabetic Index and Tabular List to enclose supplementary words that may be present or absent in the statement of a disease or procedure without affecting the code number to which it is assigned. The terms within the parentheses are referred to as nonessential modifiers. The nonessential modifiers in the Alphabetic Index to Diseases apply to subterms following a main term except when a nonessential modifier and a subentry are mutually exclusive, the subentry takes precedence. For example, in the ICD-10-CM Alphabetic Index under the main term Enteritis, "acute" is a nonessential modifier and "chronic" is a subentry. In this case, the nonessential modifier "acute" does not apply to the subentry "chronic".

: Colons are used in the Tabular List after an incomplete term which needs one or more of the modifiers following the colon to make it assignable to a given category.

8. Use of "and"

See Section I.A.14. Use of the term "And"

9. Other and Unspecified Codes

a. "Other" Codes

Codes titled "other" or "other specified" are for use when the information in the medical record provides detail for which a specific code does not exist. Alphabetic Index entries with NEC in the line designate "other" codes in the Tabular List. These Alphabetic Index entries represent specific disease entities for which no specific code exists so the term is included within an "other" code.

b. "Unspecified" Codes

Codes titled "unspecified" are for use when the information in the medical record is insufficient to assign a more specific code. For those categories for which an unspecified code is not provided, the "other specified" code may represent both other and unspecified.

See Section I.B.18 Use of Signs/Symptom/Unspecified Codes

10. Includes Notes

This note appears immediately under a three character code title to further define, or give examples of, the content of the category.

11. Inclusion Terms

List of terms is included under some codes. These terms are the conditions for which that code is to be used. The terms may be synonyms of the code title, or, in the case of "other specified" codes, the terms are a list of the various conditions assigned to that code. The inclusion terms are not necessarily exhaustive. Additional terms found only in the Alphabetic Index may also be assigned to a code.

12. Excludes Notes

The ICD-10-CM has two types of excludes notes. Each type of note has a different definition for use but they are all similar in that they indicate that codes excluded from each other are independent of each other.

a. Excludes1

A type 1 Excludes note is a pure excludes note. It means "NOT CODED HERE!" An Excludes1 note indicates that the code excluded should never be used at the same time as the code above the Excludes1 note. An Excludes1 is used when two conditions cannot occur together, such as a congenital form versus an acquired form of the same condition.

An exception to the Excludes1 definition is the circumstance when the two conditions are unrelated to each other. If it is not clear whether the two conditions involving an Excludes1 note are related or not, query the provider. For example, code F45.8, Other somatoform disorders, has an Exlcudes1 note for "sleep related teeth grinding (G47.63)," because "teeth grinding" is an inclusion term under F45.8. Only one of these two codes should be assigned for teeth grinding. However, psychogenic dysmenorrhea is also an inclusion term under F45.8, and a patient could have both this conditions and sleep related teeth grinding. In this case, the two conditions are clearly unrelated to each other, and do it would be appropriate to report F45.8 and G47.63 together.

b. Excludes2

A type 2 Excludes note represents "Not included here". An Excludes2 note indicates that the condition excluded is not part of the condition represented by the code, but a patient may have both conditions at the same time. When an Excludes2 note appears under a code, it is acceptable to use both the code and the excluded code together, when appropriate.

13. Etiology/Manifestation Convention ("Code first", "Use additional code" and "In Diseases Classified Elsewhere" Notes)

Certain conditions have both an underlying etiology and multiple body system manifestations due to the underlying etiology. For such conditions, the ICD-10-CM has a coding convention that requires the underlying condition be sequenced first, if applicable, followed by the manifestation. Wherever such a combination exists, there is a "use additional code" note at the etiology code, and a "code first" note at the manifestation code. These instructional notes indicate the proper sequencing order of the codes, etiology followed by manifestation.

In most cases the manifestation codes will have in the code title, "in diseases classified elsewhere." Codes with this title are a component of the etiology/manifestation convention. The code title indicates that it is a manifestation code. "In diseases classified elsewhere" codes are never permitted to be used as first-listed or principal diagnosis codes. They must be used in conjunction with an underlying condition code and they must be listed following the underlying condition. See category F02, Dementia in other diseases classified elsewhere, for an example of this convention.

There are manifestation codes that do not have "in diseases classified elsewhere" in the title. For such codes, there is a "use additional code" note at the etiology code and a "code first" note at the manifestation code and the rules for sequencing apply.

In addition to the notes in the Tabular List, these conditions also have a specific Alphabetic Index entry structure. In the Alphabetic Index both conditions are listed together with the etiology code first followed by the manifestation codes in brackets. The code in brackets is always to be sequenced second.

An example of the etiology/manifestation convention is dementia in Parkinson's disease. In the Alphabetic Index, code G20 is listed first, followed by code F02.80 or F02.81 in brackets. Code G20 represents the underlying etiology, Parkinson's disease, and must be sequenced first, whereas codes F02.80 and F02.81 represent the manifestation of dementia in diseases classified elsewhere, with or without behavioral disturbance.

"Code first" and "Use additional code" notes are also used as sequencing rules in the classification for certain codes that are not part of an etiology/ manifestation combination.

See Section I.B. 7. Multiple coding for a single condition.

14. "And"

The word "and" should be interpreted to mean either "and" or "or" when it appears in a title.

For example, cases of "tuberculosis of bones", "tuberculosis of joints" and "tuberculosis of bones and joints" are classified to subcategory A18.0, Tuberculosis of bones and joints.

15. "With"

The word "with" or "in" should be interpreted to mean "associated with" or "due to" when it appears in a code title, the Alphabetic Index (either under a main term or subterm), or an instructional note in the Tabular List. The classification presumes a causal relationship between the two conditions linked by these terms in the Alphabetic Index or Tabular List. These conditions should be coded as related even in the absence of provider documentation explicitly linking them, unless the documentation clearly states the conditions are unrelated or when another guideline exists that specifically requires a documented linkage between two conditions (e.g., sepsis guideline for "acute organ dysfunction that is not clearly associated with the sepsis"). For conditions not specifically linked by these relational terms in the classification or when a guideline requires that a linkage between two conditions be explicitly documented, provider documentation must link the conditions in order to code them as related.

The word "with" in the Alphabetic Index is sequenced immediately following the main term or subterm, not in alphabetical order.

16. "See" and "See Also"

The "see" instruction following a main term in the Alphabetic Index indicates that another term should be referenced. It is necessary to go to the main term referenced with the "see" note to locate the correct code.

A "see also" instruction following a main term in the Alphabetic Index instructs that there is another main term that may also be referenced that may provide additional Alphabetic Index entries that may be useful. It is not necessary to follow the "see also" note when the original main term provides the necessary code.

17. "Code Also Note"

A "code also" note instructs that two codes may be required to fully describe a condition, but this note does not provide sequencing direction. The sequencing depends on the circumstances of the encounter.

18. **Default Codes**

A code listed next to a main term in the ICD-10-CM Alphabetic Index is referred to as a default code. The default code represents that condition that is most commonly associated with the main term, or is the unspecified code for the condition. If a condition is documented in a medical record (for example, appendicitis) without any additional information, such as acute or chronic, the default code should be assigned.

19. **Code Assignment and Clinical Criteria**

The assignment of a diagnosis code is based on the provider's diagnostic statement that the condition exists. The provider's statement that the patient has a particular condition is sufficient. Code assignment is not based on clinical criteria used by the provider to establish the diagnosis.

B. General Coding Guidelines

1. **Locating a Code in the ICD-10-CM**

To select a code in the classification that corresponds to a diagnosis or reason for visit documented in a medical record, first locate the term in the Alphabetic Index, and then verify the code in the Tabular List. Read and be guided by instructional notations that appear in both the Alphabetic Index and the Tabular List.

It is essential to use both the Alphabetic Index and Tabular List when locating and assigning a code. The Alphabetic Index does not always provide the full code. Selection of the full code, including laterality and any applicable 7th character can only be done in the Tabular List. A dash (-) at the end of an Alphabetic Index entry indicates that additional characters are required. Even if a dash is not included at the Alphabetic Index entry, it is necessary to refer to the Tabular List to verify that no 7th character is required.

2. **Level of Detail in Coding**

Diagnosis codes are to be used and reported at their highest number of characters available.

ICD-10-CM diagnosis codes are composed of codes with 3, 4, 5, 6, or 7 characters. Codes with three characters are included in ICD-10-CM as the heading of a category of codes that may be further subdivided by the use of fourth and/or fifth characters and/or sixth characters, which provide greater detail.

A three-character code is to be used only if it is not further subdivided. A code is invalid if it has not been coded to the full number of characters required for that code, including the 7th character, if applicable.

3. **Code or Codes from A00.0–T88.9, Z00–Z99.8**

The appropriate code or codes from A00.0–T88.9, Z00–Z99.8 must be used to identify diagnoses, symptoms, conditions, problems, complaints or other reason(s) for the encounter/visit.

4. **Signs and Symptoms**

Codes that describe symptoms and signs, as opposed to diagnoses, are acceptable for reporting purposes when a related definitive diagnosis has not been established (confirmed) by the provider. Chapter 18 of ICD-10-CM, Symptoms, Signs, and Abnormal Clinical and Laboratory Findings, Not Elsewhere Classified (codes R00.0–R99) contains many, but not all codes for symptoms.

See Section I.B.18 Use of Signs/Symptom/Unspecified Codes

5. **Conditions that are an Integral Part of a Disease Process**

Signs and symptoms that are associated routinely with a disease process should not be assigned as additional codes, unless otherwise instructed by the classification.

6. **Conditions that are not an Integral Part of a Disease Process**

Additional signs and symptoms that may not be associated routinely with a disease process should be coded when present.

7. **Multiple Coding for a Single Condition**

In addition to the etiology/manifestation convention that requires two codes to fully describe a single condition that affects multiple body systems, there are other single conditions that also require more than one code. "Use additional code" notes are found in the Tabular List at codes that are not part of an etiology/manifestation pair where a secondary code is useful to fully describe a condition. The sequencing rule is the same as the etiology/manifestation pair, "use additional code" indicates that a secondary code should be added, if known.

For example, for bacterial infections that are not included in chapter 1, a secondary code from category B95, Streptococcus, Staphylococcus, and Enterococcus, as the cause of diseases classified elsewhere, or B96, Other bacterial agents as the cause of diseases classified elsewhere, may be required to identify the bacterial organism causing the infection. A "use additional code" note will normally be found at the infectious disease code, indicating a need for the organism code to be added as a secondary code.

"Code first" notes are also under certain codes that are not specifically manifestation codes but may be due to an underlying cause. When there is a "code first" note and an underlying condition is present, the underlying condition should be sequenced first, if known.

"Code, if applicable, any causal condition first", notes indicate that this code may be assigned as a principal diagnosis when the causal condition is unknown or not applicable. If a causal condition is known, the code for that condition should be sequenced as the principal or first-listed diagnosis.

Multiple codes may be needed for sequela, complication codes and obstetric codes to more fully describe a condition. See the specific guidelines for these conditions for further instruction.

8. Acute and Chronic Conditions

If the same condition is described as both acute (subacute) and chronic, and separate subentries exist in the Alphabetic Index at the same indentation level, code both and sequence the acute (subacute) code first.

9. Combination Code

A combination code is a single code used to classify:

- Two diagnoses, or
- A diagnosis with an associated secondary process (manifestation)
- A diagnosis with an associated complication

Combination codes are identified by referring to subterm entries in the Alphabetic Index and by reading the inclusion and exclusion notes in the Tabular List.

Assign only the combination code when that code fully identifies the diagnostic conditions involved or when the Alphabetic Index so directs. Multiple coding should not be used when the classification provides a combination code that clearly identifies all of the elements documented in the diagnosis. When the combination code lacks necessary specificity in describing the manifestation or complication, an additional code should be used as a secondary code.

10. Sequela (Late Effects)

A sequela is the residual effect (condition produced) after the acute phase of an illness or injury has terminated. There is no time limit on when a sequela code can be used. The residual may be apparent early, such as in cerebral infarction, or it may occur months or years later, such as that due to a previous injury. Examples of sequela include: scar formation resulting from a burn, deviated septum due to a nasal fracture, and infertility due to tubal occlusion from old tuberculosis. Coding of sequela generally requires two codes sequenced in the following order: The condition or nature of the sequela is sequenced first. The sequela code is sequenced second.

An exception to the above guidelines are those instances where the code for the sequela is followed by a manifestation code identified in the Tabular List and title, or the sequela code has been expanded (at the fourth, fifth or sixth, character levels) to include the manifestation(s). The code for the acute phase of an illness or injury that led to the sequela is never used with a code for the late effect.

- *See Section I.C.9. Sequelae of cerebrovascular disease*
- *See Section I.C.15. Sequelae of complication of pregnancy, childbirth and the puerperium*
- *See Section I.C.19. Application of 7th characters for Chapter 19*

11. Impending or Threatened Condition

Code any condition described at the time of discharge as "impending" or "threatened" as follows:

- If it did occur, code as confirmed diagnosis.
- If it did not occur, reference the Alphabetic Index to determine if the condition has a subentry term for "impending" or "threatened" and also reference main term entries for "Impending" and for "Threatened."
- If the subterms are listed, assign the given code.
- If the subterms are not listed, code the existing underlying condition(s) and not the condition described as impending or threatened.

12. Reporting Same Diagnosis Code More than Once

Each unique ICD-10-CM diagnosis code may be reported only once for an encounter. This applies to bilateral conditions when there are no distinct codes identifying laterality or two different conditions classified to the same ICD-10-CM diagnosis code.

13. Laterality

Some ICD-10-CM codes indicate laterality, specifying whether the condition occurs on the left, right or is bilateral. If no bilateral code is provided and the condition is bilateral, assign separate codes for both the left and right side. If the side is not identified in the medical record, assign the code for the unspecified side.

When a patient has a bilateral condition and each side is treated during separate encounters, assign the "bilateral" code (as the conditions still exists on both sides), including for the encounter to treat the first side. For the second encounter for treatment after one side has previously been treated and the condition no longer exists on that side, assign the appropriate unilateral code for the side where the conditions still exists (e.g., cataract surgery performed on each eye in separate encounters). The bilateral code would not be assigned for the subsequent encounter, as the patient no longer has the condition in the previously-treated site. If the treatment on the first side did not completely resolve the condition, then the bilateral code would still be appropriate.

14. Documentation by Clinicians Other than the Patient's Provider

Code assignment is based on the documentation by the patient's provider (i.e., physician or other qualified healthcare practitioner legally accountable for establishing the patient's diagnosis). There are a few exceptions, such as codes for the body mass index (BMI), depth of non-pressure chronic ulcers, pressure ulcer stage, coma scale, and NIH stroke scale (NIHSS) codes, code assignment may be based on medical record documentation from clinicians who are not the patient's provider (i.e., physician or other qualified healthcare practitioner legally accountable for establishing the patient's diagnosis), since this information is typically documented by other clinicians involved in the care of the patient (e.g., a dietitian often documents the BMI, a nurse often documents the pressure ulcer stages, and an emergency medical technician often documents the coma scale). However, the associated diagnosis (such as overweight, obesity, acute stroke or pressure ulcer) must be documented by the patient's provider. If there is conflicting medical record documentation, either from the same clinician or different clinicians, the patient's attending provider should be queried for clarification.

For social determinants of health, such as information found in categories Z55-Z65, Persons with potential health hazards related to socioeconomic and psychosocial circumstances, code assignment may be based on medical record documentation from clinicians involved in the care of the patient who are not the patient's provider since this information represents social information, rather than medical diagnoses. **Patient self-reported documentation may also be used to assign codes for social determinants of health, as long as the patient self-reported information is signed-off by and incorporated into the health record by either a clinician or provider.**

The BMI, coma scale, and NIHSS codes and categories Z55-Z65 should only be reported as secondary diagnoses.

15. Syndromes

Follow the Alphabetic Index guidance when coding syndromes. In the absence of Alphabetic Index guidance, assign codes for the documented manifestations of the syndrome. Additional codes for manifestations that are not an integral part of the disease process may also be assigned when the condition does not have a unique code.

16. Documentation of Complications of Care

Code assignment is based on the provider's documentation of the relationship between the condition and the care or procedure, unless otherwise instructed by the classification. The guideline extends to any complications of care, regardless of the chapter the code is located in. It is important to note that not all conditions that occur during or following medical care or surgery are classified as complications. There must be a cause-and-effect relationship between the care provided and the condition, and an indication in the documentation that it is a complication. Query the provider for clarification, if the complication is not clearly documented.

17. Borderline Diagnosis

If the provider documents a "borderline" diagnosis at the time of discharge, the diagnosis is coded as confirmed, unless the classification provides a specific entry (e.g., borderline diabetes). If a borderline condition has a specific index entry in ICD-10-CM, it should be coded as such. Since borderline conditions are not uncertain diagnoses, no distinction is made between the care setting (inpatient versus outpatient). Whenever the documentation is unclear regarding a borderline condition, coders are encouraged to query for clarification.

18. Use of Sign/Symptom/Unspecified Codes

Sign/symptom and "unspecified" codes have acceptable, even necessary, uses. While specific diagnosis codes should be reported when they are supported by the available medical record documentation and clinical knowledge of the patient's health condition, there are instances when signs/symptoms or unspecified codes are the best choices for accurately reflecting the healthcare encounter. Each healthcare encounter should be coded to the level of certainty known for that encounter.

If a definitive diagnosis has not been established by the end of the encounter, it is appropriate to report codes for sign(s) and/or symptom(s) in lieu of a definitive diagnosis. When sufficient clinical information isn't known or available about a particular health condition to assign a more specific code, it is acceptable to report the appropriate "unspecified" code (e.g., a diagnosis of pneumonia has been determined, but not the specific type). Unspecified codes should be reported when they are the codes that most accurately reflects what is known about the patient's condition at the time of that particular encounter. It would be inappropriate to select a specific code that is not supported by the medical record documentation or conduct medically unnecessary diagnostic testing in order to determine a more specific code.

19. Coding for Healthcare Encounters in Hurricane Aftermath

a. Use of External Cause of Morbidity Codes

An external cause of morbidity code should be assigned to identify the cause of the injury(ies) incurred as a result of the hurricane. The use of external cause of morbidity codes is supplemental to the application of ICD-10-CM codes. External cause of morbidity codes are never to be recorded as a principal diagnosis (first-listed in non-inpatient settings). The appropriate injury code should be sequenced before any external cause codes. The external cause of morbidity codes capture how the injury or health condition happened (cause), the intent (unintentional or accidental; or intentional, such as suicide or assault), the place where the event occurred, the activity of the patient at the time of the event, and the person's status (e.g., civilian, military). They should not be assigned for encounters to treat hurricane victims' medical conditions when no injury, adverse effect or poisoning is involved. External cause of morbidity codes should be assigned for each encounter for care and treatment of the injury. External cause of morbidity codes may be assigned in all health care settings. For the purpose of capturing complete and accurate ICD-10-CM data in the aftermath of the hurricane, a healthcare setting should be considered as any location where medical care is provided by licensed healthcare professionals.

b. **Sequencing of External Causes of Morbidity Codes**

Codes for cataclysmic events, such as hurricane, take priority over all other external cause codes except child and adult abuse and terrorism and should be sequenced before other external cause of injury codes. Assign as many external cause of morbidity codes as necessary to fully explain each cause. For example, if an injury occurs as a result of a building collapse during the hurricane, external cause codes for both the hurricane and the building collapse should be assigned with the external causes code for hurricane being sequenced as the first external cause code. For injuries incurred as a direct result of the hurricane, assign the appropriate code(s) for the injuries, followed by the code X37.0-, Hurricane (with the appropriate 7th character), and any other applicable external cause of injury codes. Code X37.0- also should be assigned when an injury is incurred as a result of flooding caused by a levee breaking related to the hurricane. Code X38.-, Flood (with appropriate 7th character), should be assigned when an injury is from flooding resulting directly from the storm. Code X36.0-, Collapse of dam or man-made structure, should not be assigned when the cause of the collapse is due to the hurricane. Use of code X36.0- is limited to collapses of man-made structures due to earth surface movements, not due to storm surges directly from a hurricane.

c. **Other External Causes of Morbidity Code Issues**

For injuries that are not a direct result of the hurricane, such as an evacuee that has incurred an injury as a result of a motor vehicle accident, assign the appropriate external cause of morbidity code(s) to describe the cause of the injury, but do not assign code X37.0-, Hurricane. If it is not clear whether the injury was a direct result of the hurricane, assume the injury is due to the hurricane and assign code X37.0-, Hurricane, as well as any other applicable external cause of morbidity codes. In addition to code X37.0-, Hurricane, other possible applicable external cause of morbidity codes include:

- W54.0-, Bitten by dog
- X30-, Exposure to excessive natural heat
- X31-, Exposure to excessive natural cold
- X38-, Flood

d. **Use of Z codes**

Z codes (other reasons for healthcare encounters) may be assigned as appropriate to further explain the reasons for presenting for healthcare services, including transfers between healthcare facilities. The ICD-10-CM Official Guidelines for Coding and Reporting identify which codes may be assigned as principal or first-listed diagnosis only, secondary diagnosis only, or principal/first-listed or secondary (depending on the circumstances). Possible applicable Z codes include:

- Z59.0. Homelessness
- Z59.1, Inadequate housing
- Z59.5, Extreme poverty
- Z75.1, Person awaiting admission to adequate facility elsewhere
- Z75.3, Unavailability and inaccessibility of health-care facilities
- Z74.4, Unavailability and inaccessibility of other helping agencies
- Z76.2, Encounter for health supervision and care of other healthy infant and child
- Z99.12, Encounter for respirator [ventilator] dependence during power failure

The external cause of morbidity codes and the Z codes listed above are not an all-inclusive list. Other codes may be applicable to the encounter based upon the documentation. Assign as many codes as necessary to fully explain each healthcare encounter. Since patient history information may be very limited, use any available documentation to assign the appropriate external cause of morbidity and Z codes.

C. Chapter-Specific Coding Guidelines

Consulting Editor Note

In this book the Chapter-Specific Coding Guidelines are included here and in the Tabular List of Diseases and Injuries at the beginning of the chapter for which they are applicable.

Additionally, notes have been added throughout the Diagnosis and Procedure Tabular to alert the coder when the code under review is included in a chapter specific coding guideline. The user can then reference the coding guideline prior to making their final code selection. For example:

A41 Other sepsis

Review coding guideline C.1.d

This note alerts the coder to reference the chapter specific coding guidelines (C), chapter 1, guideline d, before making the final code selection. The guidelines for chapter 1, Certain Infectious and Parasitic Diseases, is located at the beginning of Chapter 1 in the Diagnosis Tabular. Please note that the coding guideline notes may be provided at the category, sub-category, or sub-classification level, whichever is applicable to the coding guidance.

In addition to general coding guidelines, there are guidelines for specific diagnoses and/or conditions in the classification. Unless otherwise indicated, these guidelines apply to all health care settings. Please refer to Section II for guidelines on the selection of principal diagnosis.

1. Chapter 1: Certain Infectious and Parasitic Diseases (A00-B99), *U07.1*

a. Human Immunodeficiency Virus (HIV) Infections

1) Code only confirmed cases

Code only confirmed cases of HIV infection/illness. This is an exception to the hospital inpatient guideline Section II, H.

In this context, "confirmation" does not require documentation of positive serology or culture for HIV; the provider's diagnostic statement that the patient is HIV positive, or has an HIV-related illness is sufficient.

2) Selection and sequencing of HIV codes

(a) Patient admitted for HIV-related condition

If a patient is admitted for an HIV-related condition, the principal diagnosis should be B20, Human immunodeficiency virus [HIV] disease followed by additional diagnosis codes for all reported HIV-related conditions.

(b) Patient with HIV disease admitted for unrelated condition

If a patient with HIV disease is admitted for an unrelated condition (such as a traumatic injury), the code for the unrelated condition (e.g., the nature of injury code) should be the principal diagnosis. Other diagnoses would be B20 followed by additional diagnosis codes for all reported HIV-related conditions.

(c) Whether the patient is newly diagnosed

Whether the patient is newly diagnosed or has had previous admissions/encounters for HIV conditions is irrelevant to the sequencing decision.

(d) Asymptomatic human immunodeficiency virus

Z21, Asymptomatic human immunodeficiency virus [HIV] infection status, is to be applied when the patient without any documentation of symptoms is listed as being "HIV positive," "known HIV," "HIV test positive," or similar terminology. Do not use this code if the term "AIDS" is used or if the patient is treated for any HIV-related illness or is described as having any condition(s) resulting from his/her HIV positive status; use B20 in these cases.

(e) Patients with inconclusive HIV serology

Patients with inconclusive HIV serology, but no definitive diagnosis or manifestations of the illness, may be assigned code R75, Inconclusive laboratory evidence of human immunodeficiency virus [HIV].

(f) Previously diagnosed HIV-related illness

Patients with any known prior diagnosis of an HIV-related illness should be coded to B20. Once a patient has developed an HIV-related illness, the patient should always be assigned code B20 on every subsequent admission/encounter. Patients previously diagnosed with any HIV illness (B20) should never be assigned to R75 or Z21, Asymptomatic human immunodeficiency virus [HIV] infection status.

(g) HIV Infection in Pregnancy, Childbirth and the Puerperium

During pregnancy, childbirth or the puerperium, a patient admitted (or presenting for a health care encounter) because of an HIV-related illness should receive a principal diagnosis code of O98.7-, Human immunodeficiency [HIV] disease complicating pregnancy, childbirth and the puerperium, followed by B20 and the code(s) for the HIV-related illness(es). Codes from Chapter 15 always take sequencing priority. Patients with asymptomatic HIV infection status admitted (or presenting for a health care encounter) during pregnancy, childbirth, or the puerperium should receive codes of O98.7- and Z21.

(h) Encounters for testing for HIV

If a patient is being seen to determine his/her HIV status, use code Z11.4, Encounter for screening for human immunodeficiency virus [HIV]. Use additional codes for any associated high risk behavior.

If a patient with signs or symptoms is being seen for HIV testing, code the signs and symptoms. An additional counseling code Z71.7, Human immunodeficiency virus [HIV] counseling, may be used if counseling is provided during the encounter for the test.

When a patient returns to be informed of his/her HIV test results and the test result is negative, use code Z71.7, Human immunodeficiency virus [HIV] counseling.

If the results are positive, see previous guidelines and assign codes as appropriate.

b. Infectious agents as the cause of diseases classified to other chapters

Certain infections are classified in chapters other than Chapter 1 and no organism is identified as part of the infection code. In these instances, it is necessary to use an additional code from Chapter 1 to identify the organism. A code from category B95, Streptococcus, Staphylococcus, and Enterococcus as the cause of diseases classified to other chapters, B96, Other bacterial agents as the cause of diseases classified to other chapters, or B97, Viral agents as the cause of diseases classified to other chapters, is to be used as an additional code to identify the organism. An instructional note will be found at the infection code advising that an additional organism code is required.

c. Infections resistant to antibiotics

Many bacterial infections are resistant to current antibiotics. It is necessary to identify all infections documented as antibiotic resistant. Assign a code from category Z16, Resistance to antimicrobial drugs, following the infection code only if the infection code does not identify drug resistance.

d. Sepsis, Severe Sepsis, and Septic Shock

1) Coding of Sepsis and Severe Sepsis

(a) Sepsis

For a diagnosis of sepsis, assign the appropriate code for the underlying systemic infection. If the type of infection or causal organism is not further specified, assign code A41.9, Sepsis, unspecified organism.

A code from subcategory R65.2, Severe sepsis, should not be assigned unless severe sepsis or an associated acute organ dysfunction is documented.

(i) Negative or inconclusive blood cultures and sepsis

Negative or inconclusive blood cultures do not preclude a diagnosis of sepsis in patients with clinical evidence of the condition, however, the provider should be queried.

(ii) Urosepsis

The term urosepsis is a nonspecific term. It is not to be considered synonymous with sepsis. It has no default code in the Alphabetic Index. Should a provider use this term, he/she must be queried for clarification.

(iii) Sepsis with organ dysfunction

If a patient has sepsis and associated acute organ dysfunction or multiple organ dysfunction (MOD), follow the instructions for coding severe sepsis.

(iv) Acute organ dysfunction that is not clearly associated with the sepsis

If a patient has sepsis and an acute organ dysfunction, but the medical record documentation indicates that the acute organ dysfunction is related to a medical condition other than the sepsis, do not assign a code from subcategory R65.2, Severe sepsis. An acute organ dysfunction must be associated with the sepsis in order to assign the severe sepsis code. If the documentation is not clear as to whether an acute organ dysfunction is related to the sepsis or another medical condition, query the provider.

(b) Severe sepsis

The coding of severe sepsis requires a minimum of 2 codes: first a code for the underlying systemic infection, followed by a code from subcategory R65.2, Severe sepsis. If the causal organism is not documented, assign code A41.9, Sepsis, unspecified organism, for the infection. Additional code(s) for the associated acute organ dysfunction are also required.

Due to the complex nature of severe sepsis, some cases may require querying the provider prior to assignment of the codes.

2) Septic shock

(a) Septic shock generally refers to circulatory failure associated with severe sepsis, and therefore, it represents a type of acute organ dysfunction.

For cases of septic shock, the code for the systemic infection should be sequenced first, followed by code R65.21, Severe sepsis with septic shock or code T81.12, Postprocedural septic shock. Any additional codes for the other acute organ dysfunctions should also be assigned. As noted in the sequencing instructions in the Tabular List, the code for septic shock cannot be assigned as a principal diagnosis.

3) Sequencing of severe sepsis

If severe sepsis is present on admission, and meets the definition of principal diagnosis, the underlying systemic infection should be assigned as principal diagnosis followed by the appropriate code from subcategory R65.2 as required by the sequencing rules in the Tabular List. A code from subcategory R65.2 can never be assigned as a principal diagnosis.

When severe sepsis develops during an encounter (it was not present on admission) the underlying systemic infection and the appropriate code from subcategory R65.2 should be assigned as secondary diagnoses.

Severe sepsis may be present on admission but the diagnosis may not be confirmed until sometime after admission. If the documentation is not clear whether severe sepsis was present on admission, the provider should be queried.

4) Sepsis or severe sepsis with a localized infection

If the reason for admission is both sepsis or severe sepsis and a localized infection, such as pneumonia or cellulitis, a code(s) for the underlying systemic infection should be assigned first and the code for the localized infection should be assigned as a secondary diagnosis. If the patient has severe sepsis, a code from subcategory R65.2 should also be assigned as a secondary diagnosis. If the patient is admitted with a localized infection, such as pneumonia, and sepsis/severe sepsis doesn't develop until after admission, the localized infection should be assigned first, followed by the appropriate sepsis/severe sepsis codes.

5) Sepsis due to a postprocedural infection

(a) Documentation of causal relationship

As with all postprocedural complications, code assignment is based on the provider's documentation of the relationship between the infection and the procedure.

(b) Sepsis due to a postprocedural infection

For infections following a procedure, a code from T81.40, to T81.43, Infection following a procedure, or a code from O86.00 to O86.03, Infection of obstetric surgical wound, that identifies the site of the infection should be coded first, if known. Assign an additional code for sepsis following a procedure (T81.44) or sepsis following an obstetrical procedure (O86.04). Use an additional code to identify the infectious agent. If the patient has severe sepsis the appropriate code from subcategory R65.2 should also be assigned with the additional code(s) for any acute organ dysfunction.

For infections following infusion, transfusion, therapeutic injection, or immunization, a code from subcategory T80.2, Infections following infusion, transfusion, and therapeutic injection, or code T88.0-, Infection following immunization, should be coded first, followed by the code for the specific infection. If the patient has severe sepsis, the appropriate code from subcategory R65.2 should also be assigned, with the additional code(s) for any acute organ dysfunction.

(c) Postprocedural infection and postprocedural septic shock

If a postprocedural infection has resulted in postprocedural septic shock, assign the codes indicated above for sepsis due to a postprocedural infection, followed by code T81.12-, Postprocedural septic shock. Do not assign code R65.21, Severe sepsis with septic shock. Additional code(s) should be assigned for any acute organ dysfunction.

6) Sepsis and severe sepsis associated with a noninfectious process (condition)

In some cases a noninfectious process (condition), such as trauma, may lead to an infection which can result in sepsis or severe sepsis. If sepsis or severe sepsis is documented as associated with a noninfectious condition, such as a burn or serious injury, and this condition meets the definition for principal diagnosis, the code for the noninfectious condition should be sequenced first, followed by the code for the resulting infection. If severe sepsis, is present a code from subcategory R65.2 should also be assigned with any associated organ dysfunction(s) codes. It is not necessary to assign a code from subcategory R65.1, Systemic inflammatory response syndrome (SIRS) of non-infectious origin, for these cases.

If the infection meets the definition of principal diagnosis it should be sequenced before the non-infectious condition. When both the associated non-infectious condition and the infection meet the definition of principal diagnosis either may be assigned as principal diagnosis.

Only one code from category R65, Symptoms and signs specifically associated with systemic inflammation and infection, should be assigned. Therefore, when a non-infectious condition leads to an infection resulting in severe sepsis, assign the appropriate code from subcategory R65.2, Severe sepsis. Do not additionally assign a code from subcategory R65.1, Systemic inflammatory response syndrome (SIRS) of non-infectious origin.

See Section I.C.18. SIRS due to non-infectious process

7) Sepsis and septic shock complicating abortion, pregnancy, childbirth, and the puerperium

See Section I.C.15. Sepsis and septic shock complicating abortion, pregnancy, childbirth and the puerperium

8) Newborn sepsis

See Section I.C.16. f. Bacterial sepsis of Newborn

e. Methicillin Resistant Staphylococcus aureus (MRSA) Conditions

1) Selection and sequencing of MRSA codes

(a) Combination codes for MRSA infection

When a patient is diagnosed with an infection that is due to methicillin resistant Staphylococcus aureus (MRSA), and that infection has a combination code that includes the causal organism (e.g., sepsis, pneumonia) assign the appropriate combination code for the condition (e.g., code A41.02, Sepsis due to Methicillin resistant Staphylococcus aureus or code J15.212, Pneumonia due to Methicillin resistant Staphylococcus aureus). Do not assign code B95.62, Methicillin resistant Staphylococcus aureus infection as the cause of diseases classified elsewhere, as an additional code because the combination code includes the type of infection and the MRSA organism. Do not assign a code from subcategory Z16.11, Resistance to penicillins, as an additional diagnosis.

See Section C.1. for instructions on coding and sequencing of sepsis and severe sepsis.

(b) Other codes for MRSA infection

When there is documentation of a current infection (e.g., wound infection, stitch abscess, urinary tract infection) due to MRSA, and that infection does not have a combination code that includes the causal organism, assign the appropriate code to identify the condition along with code B95.62, Methicillin resistant Staphylococcus aureus infection as the cause of diseases classified elsewhere for the MRSA infection. Do not assign a code from subcategory Z16.11, Resistance to penicillins.

(c) Methicillin susceptible Staphylococcus aureus (MSSA) and MRSA colonization

The condition or state of being colonized or carrying MSSA or MRSA is called colonization or carriage, while an individual person is described as being colonized or being a carrier. Colonization means that MSSA or MSRA is present on or in the body without necessarily causing illness. A positive MRSA colonization test might be documented by the provider as "MRSA screen positive" or "MRSA nasal swab positive".

Assign code Z22.322, Carrier or suspected carrier of Methicillin resistant Staphylococcus aureus, for patients documented as having MRSA colonization. Assign code Z22.321, Carrier or suspected carrier of Methicillin susceptible Staphylococcus aureus, for patient documented as having MSSA colonization. Colonization is not necessarily indicative of a disease process or as the cause of a specific condition the patient may have unless documented as such by the provider.

(d) MRSA colonization and infection

If a patient is documented as having both MRSA colonization and infection during a hospital admission, code Z22.322, Carrier or suspected carrier of Methicillin resistant Staphylococcus aureus, and a code for the MRSA infection may both be assigned.

f. Zika virus infections

1) Code only confirmed cases

Code only a confirmed diagnosis of Zika virus (A92.5, Zika virus disease) as documented by the provider. This is an exception to the hospital inpatient guideline Section II, H. In this context, "confirmation" does not require documentation of the type of test performed; the provider's diagnostic statement that the condition is confirmed is sufficient. This code should be assigned regardless of the stated mode of transmission.

If the provider documents "suspected", "possible" or "provable" Zika, do not assign code A92.5. Assign a code(s) explaining the reason for encounter (such as fever, rash, or joint pain) or Z20.821, Contact with and (suspected) exposure to Zika virus.

g. Coronavirus infections

1) COVID-19 infection (infection due to SARS-CoV-2)

(a) Code only confirmed cases

Code only a confirmed diagnosis of the 2019 novel coronavirus disease (COVID-19) as documented by the provider or documentation of a positive COVID-19 test result. For a confirmed diagnosis, assign code U07.1, COVID-19. This is an exception to the hospital inpatient guideline Section II, H. In this context, "confirmation" does not require documentation of a positive test result for COVID-19; the provider's documentation that the individual has COVID-19 is sufficient.

If the provider documents "suspected," "possible," "probable," or "inconclusive" COVID-19, do not assign code U07.1. Instead, code the signs and symptoms reported.

See guideline I.C.1.g.1.g.

(b) Sequencing of codes

When COVID-19 meets the definition of principle diagnosis, code U07.1, COVID-19, should be sequenced first, followed by the appropriate codes for associated manifestations, except when another guideline requires that certain codes be sequenced first, such as obstetrics, sepsis, or transplant complications.

For a COVID-19 infection that progresses to sepsis, see Section I.C.1.d Sepsis, Severe Sepsis, and Septic Shock

See Section I.C.15.s. for COVID-19 infection in pregnancy, childbirth, and the puerperium

See Section I.C.16.h. for COVID-19 infection in newborn

For a COVID-19 infection in a lung transplant patient, see Section I.C.19.g.3.a. Transplant complications other than kidney

(c) Acute respiratory manifestations of COVID-19

When the reason for the encounter/admission is a respiratory manifestation of COVID-19, assign code U07.1, COVID-19, as the principal/first-listed diagnosis and assign code(s) for the respiratory manifestation(s) as additional diagnoses.

The following conditions are examples of common respiratory manifestations of COVID-19.

(i) Pneumonia

For a patient with pneumonia confirmed as due to COVID-19, assign codes U07.1, COVID-19, and J12.89, Other viral pneumonia.

(ii) Acute bronchitis

For a patient with acute bronchitis confirmed as due to COVID-19, assign codes U07.1, and J20.8, Acute bronchitis due to other specified organisms.

Bronchitis not otherwise specified (NOS) due to COVID-19 should be coded using code U07.1 and J40, Bronchitis, not specified as acute or chronic.

(iii) **Lower respiratory infection**

If the COVID-19 is documented as being associated with lower respiratory infection, not otherwise specified (NOS), or an acute respiratory infection, NOS, codes U07.1 and J22, Unspecified acute lower respiratory infection, should be assigned.

If the COVID-19 is documented as being associated with a respiratory infection, NOS, codes U07.1 and J98.8, Other specified respiratory disorders, should be assigned.

(iv) **Acute respiratory distress syndrome**

For acute respiratory distress syndrome (ARDS) due to COVID-19, assign codes U07.1 and J80, Acute respiratory distress syndrome

(v) **Acute respiratory failure**

For acute respiratory failure due to COVID-19, assign code U07.1 and code J96.0-, Acute respiratory failure.

(d) **Non-respiratory manifestations of COVID-19**

When the reason for the encounter/admission is a non-respiratory manifestation (e.g., viral enteritis) of COVID-19, assign code U07.1, COVID-19, as the principal/first-listed diagnosis and assign code(s) for the manifestation(s) as additional diagnoses.

(e) **Exposure to COVID-19**

For asymptomatic individuals with actual or suspected exposure to COVID-19, assign code Z20.828, Contact with and (suspected) exposure to other viral communicable diseases.

For symptomatic individuals with actual or suspected exposure to COVID-19 and the infection has been ruled out, or test results are inconclusive or unknown, assign code Z20.828, Contact with and (suspected) exposure to other viral communicable diseases.

See guidelines I.C.21.c.1, Contact/Exposure, for additional guidance regarding the use of category Z20 codes.

If COVID-19 is confirmed, see guidelines I.C.1.g.1.a.

(f) **Screening for COVID-19**

During the COVID-19 pandemic, a screening code is generally not appropriate. For encounters for COVID-19 testing, including preoperative testing, code as exposure to COVID-19 (guideline I.C.1.g.1.e).

Coding guidance will be updated as new information concerning any changes in the pandemic status becomes available.

(g) **Signs and symptoms without definitive diagnosis of COVID-19**

For patient presenting with any signs/symptoms associated with COVID-19 (such as fever, etc.) but a definitive diagnosis has not been established, assign the appropriate code(s) for each of the presenting signs and symptoms such as:

- R05 Cough
- R06.02 Shortness of breath
- R50.9 Fever, unspecified

If a patient with signs/symptoms associated with COVID-19 also has an actual or suspected contact with or exposure to COVID-19, assign Z20.828, Contact with and (suspected) exposure to other viral communicable diseases, as an additional code.

(h) **Asymptomatic individuals who test positive for COVID-19**

For asymptomatic individuals who test positive for COVID-19, *see guideline I.C.1.g.1.a.* Although the individual is asymptomatic, the individual has tested positive and is considered to have a COVID-19 infection.

(i) **Personal history of COVID-19**

For patients with a history of COVID-19, assign code Z86.19, Personal history of other infectious and parasitic diseases.

(j) **Follow-up visits after COVID-19 infection has resolved**

For individuals who previously had COVID-19 and are being seen for follow-up evaluation, and COVID-19 test results are negative, assign codes Z09, Encounter for follow-up examination after completed treatment for conditions other than malignant neoplasm, and Z86.19, Personal history of other infections and parasitic diseases.

(k) **Encounter for antibody testing**

For an encounter for antibody testing that is not being performed to confirm a current COVID-19 infection, nor is a follow-up test after resolution of COVID-19, assign Z01.84, Encounter for antibody response examination.

Follow the applicable guidelines above if the individual is being tested to confirm a current COVID-19 infection.

For follow-up testing after a COVID-19 infection, see guideline I.C.1.g.1.j.

2. Chapter 2: Neoplasms (C00-D49)

General guidelines

Chapter 2 of the ICD-10-CM contains the codes for most benign and all malignant neoplasms. Certain benign neoplasms, such as prostatic adenomas, may be found in the specific body system chapters. To properly code a neoplasm it is necessary to determine from the record if the neoplasm is benign, in-situ, malignant, or of uncertain histologic behavior. If malignant, any secondary (metastatic) sites should also be determined.

Primary malignant neoplasms overlapping site boundaries

A primary malignant neoplasm that overlaps two or more contiguous (next to each other) sites should be classified to the subcategory/code .8 ('overlapping lesion'), unless the combination is specifically indexed elsewhere. For multiple neoplasms of the same site that are not contiguous such as tumors in different quadrants of the same breast, codes for each site should be assigned.

Malignant neoplasm of ectopic tissue

Malignant neoplasms of ectopic tissue are to be coded to the site of origin mentioned, e.g., ectopic pancreatic malignant neoplasms involving the stomach are coded to malignant neoplasm of pancreas, unspecified (C25.9).

The neoplasm table in the Alphabetic Index should be referenced first. However, if the histological term is documented, that term should be referenced first, rather than going immediately to the Neoplasm Table, in order to determine which column in the Neoplasm Table is appropriate. For example, if the documentation indicates "adenoma," refer to the term in the Alphabetic Index to review the entries under this term and the instructional note to "see also neoplasm, by site, benign." The table provides the proper code based on the type of neoplasm and the site. It is important to select the proper column in the table that corresponds to the type of neoplasm. The Tabular List should then be referenced to verify that the correct code has been selected from the table and that a more specific site code does not exist.

See Section I.C.21. Factors influencing health status and contact with health services, Status, for information regarding Z15.0, codes for genetic susceptibility to cancer.

a. Treatment directed at the malignancy

If the treatment is directed at the malignancy, designate the malignancy as the principal diagnosis.

The only exception to this guideline is if a patient admission/encounter is solely for the administration of chemotherapy, immunotherapy or external beam radiation therapy, assign the appropriate Z51.-- code as the first-listed or principal diagnosis, and the diagnosis or problem for which the service is being performed as a secondary diagnosis.

b. Treatment of secondary site

When a patient is admitted because of a primary neoplasm with metastasis and treatment is directed toward the secondary site only, the secondary neoplasm is designated as the principal diagnosis even though the primary malignancy is still present.

c. Coding and sequencing of complications

Coding and sequencing of complications associated with the malignancies or with the therapy thereof are subject to the following guidelines:

1) Anemia associated with malignancy

When admission/encounter is for management of an anemia associated with the malignancy, and the treatment is only for anemia, the appropriate code for the malignancy is sequenced as the principal or first-listed diagnosis followed by the appropriate code for the anemia (such as code D63.0, Anemia in neoplastic disease).

2) Anemia associated with chemotherapy, immunotherapy and radiation therapy

When the admission/encounter is for management of an anemia associated with an adverse effect of the administration of chemotherapy or immunotherapy and the only treatment is for the anemia, the anemia code is sequenced first followed by the appropriate codes for the neoplasm and the adverse effect (T45.1X5, Adverse effect of antineoplastic and immunosuppressive drugs).

When the admission/encounter is for management of an anemia associated with an adverse effect of radiotherapy, the anemia code should be sequenced first, followed by the appropriate neoplasm code and code Y84.2, Radiological procedure and radiotherapy as the cause of abnormal reaction of the patient, or of later complication, without mention of misadventure at the time of the procedure.

3) Management of dehydration due to the malignancy

When the admission/encounter is for management of dehydration due to the malignancy and only the dehydration is being treated (intravenous rehydration), the dehydration is sequenced first, followed by the code(s) for the malignancy.

4) Treatment of a complication resulting from a surgical procedure

When the admission/encounter is for treatment of a complication resulting from a surgical procedure, designate the complication as the principal or first-listed diagnosis if treatment is directed at resolving the complication.

d. Primary malignancy previously excised

When a primary malignancy has been previously excised or eradicated from its site and there is no further treatment directed to that site and there is no evidence of any existing primary malignancy at that site, a code from category Z85, Personal history of malignant neoplasm, should be used to indicate the former site of the malignancy. Any mention of extension, invasion, or metastasis to another site is coded as a secondary malignant neoplasm to that site. The secondary site may be the principal or first-listed **diagnosis** with the Z85 code used as a secondary code.

e. Admissions/Encounters involving chemotherapy, immunotherapy and radiation therapy

1) Episode of care involves surgical removal of neoplasm

When an episode of care involves the surgical removal of a neoplasm, primary or secondary site, followed by adjunct chemotherapy or radiation treatment during the same episode of care, the code for the neoplasm should be assigned as principal or first-listed diagnosis.

2) Patient admission/encounter solely for administration of chemotherapy, immunotherapy and radiation therapy

If a patient admission/encounter is solely for the administration of chemotherapy, immunotherapy or external beam radiation therapy assign code Z51.0, Encounter for antineoplastic radiation therapy, or Z51.11, Encounter for antineoplastic chemotherapy, or Z51.12, Encounter for antineoplastic immunotherapy as the first-listed or principal diagnosis. If a patient receives more than one of these therapies during the same admission more than one of these codes may be assigned, in any sequence.

The malignancy for which the therapy is being administered should be assigned as a secondary diagnosis.

If a patient admission/encounter is for the insertion or implantation of radioactive elements (e.g., brachytherapy) the appropriate code for the malignancy is sequenced as the principal or first-listed diagnosis. Code Z51.0 should not be assigned.

3) Patient admitted for radiation therapy, chemotherapy or immunotherapy and develops complications

When a patient is admitted for the purpose of external beam radiotherapy, immunotherapy or chemotherapy and develops complications such as uncontrolled nausea and vomiting or dehydration, the principal or first-listed diagnosis is Z51.0, Encounter for antineoplastic radiation therapy, or Z51.11, Encounter for antineoplastic chemotherapy, or Z51.12, Encounter for antineoplastic immunotherapy followed by any codes for the complications.

When a patient is admitted for the purpose of insertion or implantation of radioactive elements (e.g., brachytherapy) and develops complications such as uncontrolled nausea and vomiting or dehydration, the principal or first-listed diagnosis is the appropriate code for the malignancy followed by any codes for the complications.

f. Admission/encounter to determine extent of malignancy

When the reason for admission/encounter is to determine the extent of the malignancy, or for a procedure such as paracentesis or thoracentesis, the primary malignancy or appropriate metastatic site is designated as the principal or first-listed diagnosis, even though chemotherapy or radiotherapy is administered.

g. Symptoms, signs, and abnormal findings listed in Chapter 18 associated with neoplasms

Symptoms, signs, and ill-defined conditions listed in Chapter 18 characteristic of, or associated with, an existing primary or secondary site malignancy cannot be used to replace the malignancy as principal or first-listed diagnosis, regardless of the number of admissions or encounters for treatment and care of the neoplasm.

See section I.C.21. Factors influencing health status and contact with health services, Encounter for prophylactic organ removal.

h. Admission/encounter for pain control/management

See Section I.C.6. for information on coding admission/encounter for pain control/management.

i. Malignancy in two or more noncontiguous sites

A patient may have more than one malignant tumor in the same organ. These tumors may represent different primaries or metastatic disease, depending on the site. Should the documentation be unclear, the provider should be queried as to the status of each tumor so that the correct codes can be assigned.

j. Disseminated malignant neoplasm, unspecified

Code C80.0, Disseminated malignant neoplasm, unspecified, is for use only in those cases where the patient has advanced metastatic disease and no known primary or secondary sites are specified. It should not be used in place of assigning codes for the primary site and all known secondary sites.

k. Malignant neoplasm without specification of site

Code C80.1, Malignant (primary) neoplasm, unspecified, equates to Cancer, unspecified. This code should only be used when no determination can be made as to the primary site of a malignancy. This code should rarely be used in the inpatient setting.

l. Sequencing of neoplasm codes

1) Encounter for treatment of primary malignancy

If the reason for the encounter is for treatment of a primary malignancy, assign the malignancy as the principal/first-listed diagnosis. The primary site is to be sequenced first, followed by any metastatic sites.

2) Encounter for treatment of secondary malignancy

When an encounter is for a primary malignancy with metastasis and treatment is directed toward the metastatic (secondary) site(s) only, the metastatic site(s) is designated as the principal/first-listed diagnosis. The primary malignancy is coded as an additional code.

3) Malignant neoplasm in a pregnant patient

When a pregnant woman has a malignant neoplasm, a code from subcategory O9A.1-, Malignant neoplasm complicating pregnancy, childbirth, and the puerperium, should be sequenced first, followed by the appropriate code from Chapter 2 to indicate the type of neoplasm.

4) Encounter for complication associated with a neoplasm

When an encounter is for management of a complication associated with a neoplasm, such as dehydration, and the treatment is only for the complication, the complication is coded first, followed by the appropriate code(s) for the neoplasm.

The exception to this guideline is anemia. When the admission/encounter is for management of an anemia associated with the malignancy, and the treatment is only for anemia, the appropriate code for the malignancy is sequenced as the principal or first-listed diagnosis followed by code D63.0, Anemia in neoplastic disease.

5) Complication from surgical procedure for treatment of a neoplasm

When an encounter is for treatment of a complication resulting from a surgical procedure performed for the treatment of the neoplasm, designate the complication as the principal/first-listed diagnosis. See the guideline regarding the coding of a current malignancy versus personal history to determine if the code for the neoplasm should also be assigned.

6) Pathologic fracture due to a neoplasm

When an encounter is for a pathological fracture due to a neoplasm, and the focus of treatment is the fracture, a code from subcategory M84.5, Pathological fracture in neoplastic disease, should be sequenced first, followed by the code for the neoplasm.

If the focus of treatment is the neoplasm with an associated pathological fracture, the neoplasm code should be sequenced first, followed by a code from M84.5 for the pathological fracture.

m. Current malignancy versus personal history of malignancy

When a primary malignancy has been excised but further treatment, such as an additional surgery for the malignancy, radiation therapy or chemotherapy is directed to that site, the primary malignancy code should be used until treatment is completed.

When a primary malignancy has been previously excised or eradicated from its site, there is no further treatment (of the malignancy) directed to that site, and there is no evidence of any existing primary malignancy at that site, a code from category Z85, Personal history of malignant neoplasm, should be used to indicate the former site of the malignancy.

Subcategories Z85.0-Z85.7 should only be assigned for the former site of a primary malignancy, not the site of a secondary malignancy. Codes from subcategory Z85.8-, may be assigned for the former site(s) of either a primary or secondary malignancy included in this subcategory.

See Section I.C.21. Factors influencing health status and contact with health services, History (of)

n. Leukemia, Multiple Myeloma, and Malignant Plasma Cell Neoplasms in remission versus personal history

The categories for leukemia, and category C90, Multiple myeloma and malignant plasma cell neoplasms, have codes indicating whether or not the leukemia has achieved remission. There are also codes Z85.6, Personal history of leukemia, and Z85.79, Personal history of other malignant neoplasms of lymphoid, hematopoietic and related tissues. If the documentation is unclear, as to whether the leukemia has achieved remission, the provider should be queried.

See Section I.C.21. Factors influencing health status and contact with health services, History (of)

o. Aftercare following surgery for neoplasm

See Section I.C.21. Factors influencing health status and contact with health services, Aftercare

p. Follow-up care for completed treatment of a malignancy

See Section I.C.21. Factors influencing health status and contact with health services, Follow-up

q. Prophylactic organ removal for prevention of malignancy

See Section I.C. 21, Factors influencing health status and contact with health services, Prophylactic organ removal

r. Malignant neoplasm associated with transplanted organ

A malignant neoplasm of a transplanted organ should be coded as a transplant complication. Assign first the appropriate code from category T86.-, Complications of transplanted organs and tissue, followed by code C80.2, Malignant neoplasm associated with transplanted organ. Use an additional code for the specific malignancy.

3. Chapter 3: Diseases of the Blood and Blood-Forming Organs and Certain Disorders Involving the Immune Mechanism (D50-D89)

Reserved for future guideline expansion

4. Chapter 4: Endocrine, Nutritional and Metabolic Diseases (E00-E89)

a. Diabetes mellitus

The diabetes mellitus codes are combination codes that include the type of diabetes mellitus, the body system affected, and the complications affecting that body system. As many codes within a particular category as are necessary to describe all of the complications of the disease may be used. They should be sequenced based on the reason for a particular encounter. Assign as many codes from categories E08 – E13 as needed to identify all of the associated conditions that the patient has.

1) Type of diabetes

The age of a patient is not the sole determining factor, though most type 1 diabetics develop the condition before reaching puberty. For this reason type 1 diabetes mellitus is also referred to as juvenile diabetes.

2) **Type of diabetes mellitus not documented**

If the type of diabetes mellitus is not documented in the medical record the default is E11.-, Type 2 diabetes mellitus.

3) **Diabetes mellitus and the use of insulin and oral hypoglycemics**

If the documentation in a medical record does not indicate the type of diabetes but does indicate that the patient uses insulin, code E11-, Type 2 diabetes mellitus, should be assigned. An additional code should be assigned from category Z79 to identify the long-term (current) use of insulin or oral hypoglycemic drugs. If the patient is treated with both oral medications and insulin, only the code for long-term (current) use of insulin should be assigned. **If the patient is treated with both insulin and an injectable non-insulin antidiabetic drug, assign codes Z79.4, Long-term (current) use of insulin, and Z79.899, Other long term (current) drug therapy. If the patient is treated with both oral hypoglycemic drugs and an injectable non-insulin antidiabetic drug, assign codes Z79.84, Long-term (current) use of oral hypoglycemic drugs, and Z79.899, Other long-term (current) drug therapy.** Code Z79.4 should not be assigned if insulin is given temporarily to bring a type 2 patient's blood sugar under control during an encounter.

4) **Diabetes mellitus in pregnancy and gestational diabetes**

See Section I.C.15. Diabetes mellitus in pregnancy.

See Section I.C.15. Gestational (pregnancy induced) diabetes

5) **Complications due to insulin pump malfunction**

   (a) **Underdose of insulin due to insulin pump failure**

   An underdose of insulin due to an insulin pump failure should be assigned to a code from subcategory T85.6, Mechanical complication of other specified internal and external prosthetic devices, implants and grafts, that specifies the type of pump malfunction, as the principal or first-listed code, followed by code T38.3x6-, Underdosing of insulin and oral hypoglycemic [antidiabetic] drugs. Additional codes for the type of diabetes mellitus and any associated complications due to the underdosing should also be assigned.

   (b) **Overdose of insulin due to insulin pump failure**

   The principal or first-listed code for an encounter due to an insulin pump malfunction resulting in an overdose of insulin, should also be T85.6-, Mechanical complication of other specified internal and external prosthetic devices, implants and grafts, followed by code T38.3x1-, Poisoning by insulin and oral hypoglycemic [antidiabetic] drugs, accidental (unintentional).

6) **Secondary diabetes mellitus**

Codes under categories E08, Diabetes mellitus due to underlying condition, E09, Drug or chemical induced diabetes mellitus, and E13, Other specified diabetes mellitus, identify complications/manifestations associated with secondary diabetes mellitus. Secondary diabetes is always caused by another condition or event (e.g., cystic fibrosis, malignant neoplasm of pancreas, pancreatectomy, adverse effect of drug, or poisoning).

   (a) **Secondary diabetes mellitus and the use of insulin or *oral* hypoglycemic drugs**

   For patients with secondary diabetes mellitus who routinely use insulin or oral hypoglycemic drugs, an additional code from category Z79 should be assigned to identify the long-term (current) use of insulin or oral hypoglycemic drugs. If the patient is treated with both oral medications and insulin, only the code for long-term (current) use of insulin should be assigned. **If the patient is treated with both insulin and an injectable non-insulin antidiabetic drug, assign codes Z79.4, Long-term (current) use of insulin, and Z79.899, Other long term (current) drug therapy. If the patient is treated with both oral hypoglycemic drugs and an injectable non-insulin antidiabetic drug, assign codes Z79.84, Long-term (current) use of oral hypoglycemic drugs, and Z79.899, Other long-term (current) drug therapy.** Code Z79.4 should not be assigned if insulin is given temporarily to bring a secondary diabetic patient's blood sugar under control during an encounter.

   (b) **Assigning and sequencing secondary diabetes codes and its causes**

   The sequencing of the secondary diabetes codes in relationship to codes for the cause of the diabetes is based on the Tabular List instructions for categories E08, E09 and E13.

      (i) **Secondary diabetes mellitus due to pancreatectomy**

      For postpancreatectomy diabetes mellitus (lack of insulin due to the surgical removal of all or part of the pancreas), assign code E89.1, Postprocedural hypoinsulinemia. Assign a code from category E13 and a code from subcategory Z90.41-, Acquired absence of pancreas, as additional codes.

      (ii) **Secondary diabetes due to drugs**

      Secondary diabetes may be caused by an adverse effect of correctly administered medications, poisoning or sequela of poisoning.

      See section I.C.19.e for coding of adverse effects and poisoning, and section I.C.20 for external cause code reporting.

5. **Chapter 5: Mental, Behavioral and Neurodevelopmental Disorders (F01-F99)**

   a. **Pain disorders related to psychological factors**

   Assign code F45.41, for pain that is exclusively related to psychological disorders. As indicated by the Excludes 1 note under category G89, a code from category G89 should not be assigned with code F45.41

Code F45.42, Pain disorders with related psychological factors, should be used with a code from category G89, Pain, not elsewhere classified, if there is documentation of a psychological component for a patient with acute or chronic pain.

See Section I.C.6. Pain

b. Mental and behavioral disorders due to psychoactive substance use

1) In Remission

Selection of codes for "in remission" for categories F10-F19, Mental and behavioral disorders due to psychoactive substance use (categories F10-F19 with -.11, -.21) requires the provider's clinical judgment. The appropriate codes for "in remission" are assigned only on the basis of provider documentation (as defined in the Official Guidelines for Coding and Reporting), unless otherwise instructed by the classification.

Mild substance use disorders in early or sustained remission are classified to the appropriate codes for substance abuse in remission, and moderate or severe substance use disorders in early or sustained remission are classified to the appropriate codes for substance dependence in remission.

2) Psychoactive Substance Use, Abuse And Dependence

When the provider documentation refers to use, abuse and dependence of the same substance (e.g. alcohol, opioid, cannabis, etc.), only one code should be assigned to identify the pattern of use based on the following hierarchy:

- If both use and abuse are documented, assign only the code for abuse
- If both abuse and dependence are documented, assign only the code for dependence
- If use, abuse and dependence are all documented, assign only the code for dependence
- If both use and dependence are documented, assign only the code for dependence.

3) Psychoactive Substance Use Unspecified

As with all other unspecified diagnoses, the codes for unspecified psychoactive substance use disorders (F10.9-, F11.9-, F12.9-, F13.9-, F14.9-, F15.9-, F16.9-, F18.9-, F19.9-) should only be assigned based on provider documentation and when they meet the definition of a reportable diagnosis (see Section III, Reporting Additional Diagnoses). These codes are to be used only when the psychoactive substance use is associated with a physical **disorder included in chapter 5 (such as sexual dysfunction and sleep disorder),** mental or behavioral disorder, and such a relationship is documented by the provider.

c. Factitious Disorder

Factitious disorder imposed on self or Munchausen's syndrome is a disorder in which a person falsely reports or causes his or her own physical or psychological signs or symptoms. For patients with documented factitious disorder on self or Munchausen's syndrome, assign the appropriate code from subcategory F68.1-, Factitious disorder imposed on self.

Munchausen's syndrome by proxy (MSBP) is a disorder in which a caregiver (perpetrator) falsely reports or causes an illness or injury in another person (victim) under his or her care, such as a child, an elderly adult, or a person who has a disability. The conditions is also referred to as "factitious disorder imposed on another" or "factitious disorder by proxy." The perpetrator, not the victim, receives this diagnosis. Assign code F68.A, Factitious disorder imposed on another, to the perpetrator's record. For the victim of a patient suffering from MSBP, assign the appropriate code from categories T74, Adult and child abuse, neglect and other maltreatment, confirmed, or T76, Adult and child abuse, neglect and other maltreatment, suspected.

See Section I.C.19.f. Adult and child abuse, neglect and other maltreatment

6. Chapter 6: Diseases of the Nervous System (G00-G99)

a. Dominant/nondominant side

Codes from category G81, Hemiplegia and hemiparesis, and subcategories, G83.1, Monoplegia of lower limb, G83.2, Monoplegia of upper limb, and G83.3, Monoplegia, unspecified, identify whether the dominant or nondominant side is affected. Should the affected side be documented, but not specified as dominant or nondominant, and the classification system does not indicate a default, code selection is as follows:

- For ambidextrous patients, the default should be dominant.
- If the left side is affected, the default is non-dominant.
- If the right side is affected, the default is dominant.

b. Pain-Category G89

1) General coding information

Codes in category G89, Pain, not elsewhere classified, may be used in conjunction with codes from other categories and chapters to provide more detail about acute or chronic pain and neoplasm-related pain, unless otherwise indicated below.

If the pain is not specified as acute or chronic, post- thoracotomy, post procedural, or neoplasm-related, do not assign codes from category G89.

A code from category G89 should not be assigned if the underlying (definitive) diagnosis is known, unless the reason for the encounter is pain control/management and not management of the underlying condition.

When an admission or encounter is for a procedure aimed at treating the underlying condition (e.g., spinal fusion, kyphoplasty), a code for the underlying condition (e.g., vertebral fracture, spinal stenosis) should be assigned as the principal diagnosis. No code from category G89 should be assigned.

(a) Category G89 Codes as Principal or First-Listed Diagnosis

Category G89 codes are acceptable as principal diagnosis or the first-listed code:

- When pain control or pain management is the reason for the admission/encounter (e.g., a patient with displaced intervertebral disc, nerve impingement and severe back pain presents for injection of steroid into the spinal canal). The underlying cause of the pain should be reported as an additional diagnosis, if known.

- When a patient is admitted for the insertion of a neurostimulator for pain control, assign the appropriate pain code as the principal or first-listed diagnosis. When an admission or encounter is for a procedure aimed at treating the underlying condition and a neurostimulator is inserted for pain control during the same admission/encounter, a code for the underlying condition should be assigned as the principal diagnosis and the appropriate pain code should be assigned as a secondary diagnosis.

(b) Use of Category G89 Codes in Conjunction with Site Specific Pain Codes

(i) Assigning Category G89 and Site-Specific Pain Codes

Codes from category G89 may be used in conjunction with codes that identify the site of pain (including codes from chapter 18) if the category G89 code provides additional information. For example, if the code describes the site of the pain, but does not fully describe whether the pain is acute or chronic, then both codes should be assigned.

(ii) Sequencing of Category G89 Codes with Site- Specific Pain Codes

The sequencing of category G89 codes with site-specific pain codes (including chapter 18 codes), is dependent on the circumstances of the encounter/admission as follows:

- If the encounter is for pain control or pain management, assign the code from category G89 followed by the code identifying the specific site of pain (e.g., encounter for pain management for acute neck pain from trauma is assigned code G89.11, Acute pain due to trauma, followed by code M54.2, Cervicalgia, to identify the site of pain).

- If the encounter is for any other reason except pain control or pain management, and a related definitive diagnosis has not been established (confirmed) by the provider, assign the code for the specific site of pain first, followed by the appropriate code from category G89.

2) Pain due to devices, implants and grafts

See Section I.C.19. Pain due to medical devices

3) Postoperative Pain

The provider's documentation should be used to guide the coding of postoperative pain, as well as *Section III. Reporting Additional Diagnoses and Section IV. Diagnostic Coding* and *Reporting in the Outpatient Setting.*

The default for post-thoracotomy and other postoperative pain not specified as acute or chronic is the code for the acute form.

Routine or expected postoperative pain immediately after surgery should not be coded.

(a) Postoperative pain not associated with specific postoperative complication

Postoperative pain not associated with a specific postoperative complication is assigned to the appropriate postoperative pain code in category G89.

(b) Postoperative pain associated with specific postoperative complication

Postoperative pain associated with a specific postoperative complication (such as painful wire sutures) is assigned to the appropriate code(s) found in Chapter 19, Injury, poisoning, and certain other consequences of external causes. If appropriate, use additional code(s) from category G89 to identify acute or chronic pain (G89.18 or G89.28).

4) Chronic pain

Chronic pain is classified to subcategory G89.2. There is no time frame defining when pain becomes chronic pain. The provider's documentation should be used to guide use of these codes.

5) Neoplasm Related Pain

Code G89.3 is assigned to pain documented as being related, associated or due to cancer, primary or secondary malignancy, or tumor. This code is assigned regardless of whether the pain is acute or chronic.

This code may be assigned as the principal or first- listed code when the stated reason for the admission/encounter is documented as pain control/pain management. The underlying neoplasm should be reported as an additional diagnosis.

When the reason for the admission/encounter is management of the neoplasm and the pain associated with the neoplasm is also documented, code G89.3 may be assigned as an additional diagnosis. It is not necessary to assign an additional code for the site of the pain.

See Section I.C.2 for instructions on the sequencing of neoplasms for all other stated reasons for the admission/encounter (except for pain control/pain management).

6) Chronic pain syndrome

Central pain syndrome (G89.0) and chronic pain syndrome (G89.4) are different than the term "chronic pain," and therefore codes should only be used when the provider has specifically documented this condition.

See Section I.C.5. Pain disorders related to psychological factors

7. Chapter 7: Diseases of the Eye and Adnexa (H00-H59)

a. Glaucoma

1) Assigning Glaucoma Codes

Assign as many codes from category H40, Glaucoma, as needed to identify the type of glaucoma, the affected eye, and the glaucoma stage.

2) Bilateral glaucoma with same type and stage

When a patient has bilateral glaucoma and both eyes are documented as being the same type and stage, and there is a code for bilateral glaucoma, report only the code for the type of glaucoma, bilateral, with the seventh character for the stage.

When a patient has bilateral glaucoma and both eyes are documented as being the same type and stage, and the classification does not provide a code for bilateral glaucoma (i.e. subcategories H40.10, H40.11 and H40.20) report only one code for the type of glaucoma with the appropriate seventh character for the stage.

3) Bilateral glaucoma stage with different types or stages

When a patient has bilateral glaucoma and each eye is documented as having a different type or stage, and the classification distinguishes laterality, assign the appropriatecode for each eye rather than the code for bilateral glaucoma.

When a patient has bilateral glaucoma and each eye is documented as having a different type, and the classification does not distinguish laterality (i.e. subcategories H40.10, H40.11 and H40.20), assign one code for each type of glaucoma with the appropriate seventh character for the stage.

When a patient has bilateral glaucoma and each eye is documented as having the same type, but different stage, and the classification does not distinguish laterality (i.e. subcategories H40.10, H40.11 and H40.20), assign a code for the type of glaucoma for each eye with the seventh character for the specific glaucoma stage documented for each eye.

4) Patient admitted with glaucoma and stage evolves during the admission

If a patient is admitted with glaucoma and the stage progresses during the admission, assign the code for highest stage documented.

5) Indeterminate stage glaucoma

Assignment of the seventh character "4" for "indeterminate stage" should be based on the clinical documentation. The seventh character "4" is used for glaucomas whose stage cannot be clinically determined. This seventh character should not be confused with the seventh character "0", unspecified, which should be assigned when there is no documentation regarding the stage of the glaucoma.

b. Blindness

If "blindness" or "low vision" of both eyes is documented but the visual impairment category is not documented, assign code H54.3, Unqualified visual loss, both eyes. If "blindness" or "low vision" in one eye is documented but the visual impairment category is not documented, assign a code from H54.6-, Unqualified visual loss, one eye. If "blindness" or "visual loss" is documented without any information about whether one or both eyes are affected, assign code H54.7, Unspecified visual loss.

8. Chapter 8: Diseases of the Ear and Mastoid Process (H60-H95)

Reserved for future guideline expansion

9. Chapter 9: Diseases of the Circulatory System (I00-I99)

a. Hypertension

The classification presumes a causal relationship between hypertension and heart involvement and between hypertension and kidney involvement, as the two conditions are linked by the term "with" in the Alphabetic Index. These conditions should be coded as related even in the absence of provider documentation explicitly linking them, unless the documentation clearly states the conditions are unrelated.

For hypertension and conditions not specifically linked by relational terms such as "with," "associated with" or "due to" in the classification, provider documentation must link the conditions in order to code them as related.

1) Hypertension with Heart Disease

Hypertension with heart conditions classified to I50.- or I51.4-I51.7, I51.89, I51.9, are assigned to, a code from category I11, Hypertensive heart disease. Use an additional code(s) from category I50, Heart failure, to identify the type(s) of heart failure in those patients with heart failure.

The same heart conditions (I50.-, I51.4-I51.7, I51.89, I51.9) with hypertension are coded separately if the provider has documented they are unrelated to the hypertension. Sequence according to the circumstances of the admission/encounter.

2) Hypertensive Chronic Kidney Disease

Assign codes from category I12, Hypertensive chronic kidney disease, when both hypertension and a condition classifiable to category N18, Chronic kidney disease (CKD), are present. CKD should not be coded as hypertensive if the provider indicates the CKD is not related to the hypertension.

The appropriate code from category N18 should be used as a secondary code with a code from category I12 to identify the stage of chronic kidney disease.

See Section I.C.14. Chronic kidney disease.

If a patient has hypertensive chronic kidney disease and acute renal failure, **the acute renal failure should also be coded. Sequence according to the circumstances of the admission/encounter.**

3) Hypertensive Heart and Chronic Kidney Disease

Assign codes from combination category I13, Hypertensive heart and chronic kidney disease, when there is hypertension with both heart and kidney involvement. If heart failure is present, assign an additional code from category I50 to identify the type of heart failure.

The appropriate code from category N18, Chronic kidney disease, should be used as a secondary code with a code from category I13 to identify the stage of chronic kidney disease.

See Section I.C.14. Chronic kidney disease.

The codes in category I13, Hypertensive heart and chronic kidney disease, are combination codes that include hypertension, heart disease and chronic kidney disease. The Includes note at I13 specifies that the conditions included at I11 and I12 are included together in I13. If a patient has hypertension, heart disease and chronic kidney disease then a code from I13 should be used, not individual codes for hypertension, heart disease and chronic kidney disease, or codes from I11 or I12.

For patients with both acute renal failure and chronic kidney disease the acute renal failure **should also be coded. Sequence according to the circumstances of the admission/encounter.**

4) Hypertensive Cerebrovascular Disease

For hypertensive cerebrovascular disease, first assign the appropriate code from categories I60-I69, followed by the appropriate hypertension code.

5) Hypertensive Retinopathy

Subcategory H35.0, Background retinopathy and retinal vascular changes, should be used with a code from category I10 – I15, Hypertensive disease to include the systemic hypertension. The sequencing is based on the reason for the encounter.

6) Hypertension, Secondary

Secondary hypertension is due to an underlying condition. Two codes are required: one to identify the underlying etiology and one from category I15 to identify the hypertension. Sequencing of codes is determined by the reason for admission/encounter.

7) Hypertension, Transient

Assign code R03.0, Elevated blood pressure reading without diagnosis of hypertension, unless patient has an established diagnosis of hypertension. Assign code O13.-, Gestational [pregnancy-induced] hypertension without significant proteinuria, or O14.-, Pre-eclampsia, for transient hypertension of pregnancy.

8) Hypertension, Controlled

This diagnostic statement usually refers to an existing state of hypertension under control by therapy. Assign the appropriate code from categories I10-I15, Hypertensive diseases.

9) Hypertension, Uncontrolled

Uncontrolled hypertension may refer to untreated hypertension or hypertension not responding to current therapeutic regimen. In either case, assign the appropriate code from categories I10-I15, Hypertensive diseases.

10) Hypertensive Crisis

Assign a code from category I16, Hypertensive crisis, for documented hypertensive urgency, hypertensive emergency or unspecified hypertensive crisis. Code also any identified hypertensive disease (I10-I15). The sequencing is based on the reason for the encounter.

11) Pulmonary Hypertension

Pulmonary hypertension is classified to category I27, Other pulmonary heart diseases. For secondary pulmonary hypertension (I27.1, I27.2-), code also any associated conditions or adverse effects of drugs or toxins. The sequencing is based on the reason for the encounter, except for adverse effects of drugs (See Section I.C.19.e).

b. Atherosclerotic Coronary Artery Disease and Angina

ICD-10-CM has combination codes for atherosclerotic heart disease with angina pectoris. The subcategories for these codes are I25.11, Atherosclerotic heart disease of native coronary artery with angina pectoris and I25.7, Atherosclerosis of coronary artery bypass graft(s) and coronary artery of transplanted heart with angina pectoris.

When using one of these combination codes it is not necessary to use an additional code for angina pectoris. A causal relationship can be assumed in a patient with both atherosclerosis and angina pectoris, unless the documentation indicates the angina is due to something other than the atherosclerosis.

If a patient with coronary artery disease is admitted due to an acute myocardial infarction (AMI), the AMI should be sequenced before the coronary artery disease.

See Section I.C.9. Acute myocardial infarction (AMI)

c. Intraoperative and Postprocedural Cerebrovascular Accident

Medical record documentation should clearly specify the cause- and-effect relationship between the medical intervention and the cerebrovascular accident in order to assign a code for intraoperative or postprocedural cerebrovascular accident.

Proper code assignment depends on whether it was an infarction or hemorrhage and whether it occurred intraoperatively or postoperatively. If it was a cerebral hemorrhage, code assignment depends on the type of procedure performed.

d. Sequelae of Cerebrovascular Disease

1) Category I69, Sequelae of Cerebrovascular disease

Category I69 is used to indicate conditions classifiable to categories I60-I67 as the causes of sequela (neurologic deficits), themselves classified elsewhere. These "late effects" include neurologic deficits that persist after initial onset of conditions classifiable to categories I60-I67. The neurologic deficits caused by cerebrovascular disease may be present from the onset or may arise at any time after the onset of the condition classifiable to categories I60-I67.

Codes from category I69, Sequelae of cerebrovascular disease, that specify hemiplegia, hemiparesis and monoplegia identify whether the dominant or nondominant side is affected. Should the affected side be documented, but not specified as dominant or nondominant, and the classification system does not indicate a default, code selection is as follows:

- For ambidextrous patients, the default should be dominant.
- If the left side is affected, the default is non-dominant.
- If the right side is affected, the default is dominant.

2) Codes from category I69 with codes from I60-I67

Codes from category I69 may be assigned on a health care record with codes from I60-I67, if the patient has a current cerebrovascular disease and deficits from an old cerebrovascular disease.

3) Codes from category I69 and Personal history of transient ischemic attack (TIA) and cerebral infarction (Z86.73)

Codes from category I69 should not be assigned if the patient does not have neurologic deficits.

See Section I.C.21. 4. History (of) for use of personal history codes

e. Acute myocardial infarction (AMI)

1) ST elevation myocardial infarction (STEMI) and non ST elevation myocardial infarction (NSTEMI)

The ICD-10-CM codes for type 1 acute myocardial infarction (AMI) identify the site, such as anterolateral wall or true posterior wall. Subcategories I21.0-I21.2 and code I21.3 are used for type 1 ST elevation myocardial infarction (STEMI). Code I21.4, Non-ST elevation (NSTEMI) myocardial infarction, is used for type 1 non ST elevation myocardial infarction (NSTEMI) and nontransmural MIs.

If a type 1 NSTEMI evolves to STEMI, assign the STEMI code. If a type 1 STEMI converts to NSTEMI due to thrombolytic therapy, it is still coded as STEMI.

For encounters occurring while the myocardial infarction is equal to, or less than, four weeks old, including transfers to another acute setting or a postacute setting, and the myocardial infarction meets the definition for "other diagnoses" (see Section III, Reporting Additional Diagnoses), codes from category I21 may continue to be reported. For encounters after the 4 week time frame and the patient is still receiving care related to the myocardial infarction, the appropriate aftercare code should be assigned, rather than a code from category I21. For old or healed myocardial infarctions not requiring further care, code I25.2, Old myocardial infarction, may be assigned.

2) Acute myocardial infarction, unspecified

Code I21.9, Acute myocardial infarction, unspecified, is the default for unspecified acute myocardial infarction or unspecified type. If only type 1 STEMI or transmural MI without the site is documented, assign code I21.3, ST elevation (STEMI) myocardial infarction of unspecified site.

3) AMI documented as nontransmural or subendocardial but site provided

If an AMI is documented as nontransmural or subendocardial, but the site is provided, it is still coded as a subendocardial AMI.

See Section I.C.21.3 for information on coding status post administration of tPA in a different facility within the last 24 hours.

4) Subsequent acute myocardial infarction

A code from category I22, Subsequent ST elevation (STEMI) and non-ST elevation (NSTEMI) myocardial infarction, is to be used when a patient who has suffered a type 1 or unspecified AMI has a new AMI within the 4 week time frame of the initial

AMI. A code from category I22 must be used in conjunction with a code from category I21. The sequencing of the I22 and I21 codes depends on the circumstances of the encounter.

Do not assign code I22 for subsequent myocardial infarctions other than type 1 or unspecified. For subsequent type 2 AMI assign only code I21.A1. For subsequent type 4 or type 5 AMI, assign only code I21.A9.

If a subsequent myocardial infarction of one type occurs within 4 weeks of a myocardial infarction of a different type, assign the appropriate codes from category I21 to identify each type. Do not assign a code from I22. Codes from category I22 should only be assigned if both the initial and subsequent myocardial infarctions are type 1 or unspecified.

5) Other Types of Myocardial Infarction

The ICD-10-CM provides codes for different types of myocardial infarction. Type 1 myocardial infarctions are assigned to codes I21.0-I21.4.

Type 2 myocardial infarction (myocardial infarction due to demand ischemia or secondary to ischemic imbalance) is assigned to code I21.A1, Myocardial infarction type 2 with the underlying cause coded first. Do not assign code I24.8, Other forms of acute ischemic heart disease, for the demand ischemia. If a type 2 AMI is described as NSTEMI or STEMI, only assign code I21.A1. Codes I21.0-I21.4 should only be assigned for type 1 AMIs.

Acute myocardial infarctions type 3, 4a, 4b, 4c and 5 are assigned to code I21.A9, Other myocardial infarction type.

The "Code also" and "Code first" notes should be followed related to complications, and for coding of postprocedural myocardial infarctions during or following cardiac surgery.

10. Chapter 10: Diseases of the Respiratory System (J00-J99), *U07.0*

a. Chronic Obstructive Pulmonary Disease [COPD] and Asthma

1) Acute exacerbation of chronic obstructive bronchitis and asthma

The codes in categories J44 and J45 distinguish between uncomplicated cases and those in acute exacerbation. An acute exacerbation is a worsening or a decompensation of a chronic condition. An acute exacerbation is not equivalent to an infection superimposed on a chronic condition, though an exacerbation may be triggered by an infection.

b. Acute Respiratory Failure

1) Acute respiratory failure as principal diagnosis

A code from subcategory J96.0, Acute respiratory failure, or subcategory J96.2, Acute and chronic respiratory failure, may be assigned as a principal diagnosis when it is the condition established after study to be chiefly responsible for occasioning the admission to the hospital, and the selection is supported by the Alphabetic Index and Tabular List. However, chapter- specific coding guidelines (such as obstetrics, poisoning, HIV, newborn) that provide sequencing direction take precedence.

2) Acute respiratory failure as secondary diagnosis

Respiratory failure may be listed as a secondary diagnosis if it occurs after admission, or if it is present on admission, but does not meet the definition of principal diagnosis.

3) Sequencing of acute respiratory failure and another acute condition

When a patient is admitted with respiratory failure and another acute condition, (e.g., myocardial infarction, cerebrovascular accident, aspiration pneumonia), the principal diagnosis will not be the same in every situation. This applies whether the other acute condition is a respiratory or nonrespiratory condition. Selection of the principal diagnosis will be dependent on the circumstances of admission. If both the respiratory failure and the other acute condition are equally responsible for occasioning the admission to the hospital, and there are no chapter-specific sequencing rules, the guideline regarding two or more diagnoses that equally meet the definition for principal diagnosis *(Section II, C.)* may be applied in these situations.

If the documentation is not clear as to whether acute respiratory failure and another condition are equally responsible for occasioning the admission, query the provider for clarification.

c. Influenza due to certain identified influenza viruses

Code only confirmed cases of influenza due to certain identified influenza viruses (category J09), and due to other identified influenza virus (category J10). This is an exception to the hospital inpatient guideline Section II, H. (Uncertain Diagnosis).

In this context, "confirmation" does not require documentation of positive laboratory testing specific for avian or other novel influenza A or other identified influenza virus. However, coding should be based on the provider's diagnostic statement that the patient has avian influenza, or other novel influenza A, for category J09, or has another particular identified strain of influenza, such as H1N1 or H3N2, but not identified as novel or variant, for category J10.

If the provider records "suspected" or "possible" or "probable" avian influenza, or novel influenza, or other identified influenza, then the appropriate influenza code from category J11, Influenza due to unidentified influenza virus, should be assigned. A code from category J09, Influenza due to certain identified influenza viruses, should not be assigned nor should a code from category J10, Influenza due to other identified influenza virus.

d. Ventilator associated Pneumonia

1) Documentation of Ventilator associated Pneumonia

As with all procedural or postprocedural complications, code assignment is based on the provider's documentation of the relationship between the condition and the procedure.

Code J95.851, Ventilator associated pneumonia, should be assigned only when the provider has documented ventilator associated pneumonia (VAP). An additional code to identify the organism (e.g., Pseudomonas aeruginosa, code B96.5) should also be assigned. Do not assign an additional code from categories J12-J18 to identify the type of pneumonia.

Code J95.851 should not be assigned for cases where the patient has pneumonia and is on a mechanical ventilator and the provider has not specifically stated that the pneumonia is ventilator-associated pneumonia. If the documentation is unclear as to whether the patient has a pneumonia that is a complication attributable to the mechanical ventilator, query the provider.

2) Ventilator associated Pneumonia Develops after Admission

A patient may be admitted with one type of pneumonia (e.g., code J13, Pneumonia due to Streptococcus pneumonia) and subsequently develop VAP. In this instance, the principal diagnosis would be the appropriate code from categories J12- J18 for the pneumonia diagnosed at the time of admission. Code J95.851, Ventilator associated pneumonia, would be assigned as an additional diagnosis when the provider has also documented the presence of ventilator associated pneumonia.

e. Vaping-related disorders

For patients presenting with condition(s) related to vaping, assign code U07.0, Vaping-related disorder, as the principal diagnosis. For lung injury due to vaping, assign only code U07.0. Assign additional codes for other manifestations, such as acute respiratory failure (subcategory J96.0-) or pneumonitis (code J68.0).

Associated respiratory signs and symptoms due to vaping, such as cough, shortness of breath, etc., are not coded separately, when a definitive diagnosis has been established. However, it would be appropriate to code separately any gastrointestinal symptoms, such as diarrhea and abdominal pain.

11. Chapter 11: Diseases of the Digestive System (K00-K95)

Reserved for future guideline expansion

12. Chapter 12: Diseases of the Skin and Subcutaneous Tissue (L00-L99)

a. Pressure ulcer stage codes

1) Pressure ulcer stages

Codes **in** category L89, Pressure ulcer, identify the site **and stage** of the pressure ulcer.

The ICD-10-CM classifies pressure ulcer stages based on severity, which is designated by stages 1-4, **deep tissue pressure injury**, unspecified stage and unstageable.

Assign as many codes from category L89 as needed to identify all the pressure ulcers the patient has, if applicable.

See Section I.B.14 for pressure ulcer stage documentation by clinicians other than patient's provider.

2) Unstageable pressure ulcers

Assignment of the code for unstageable pressure ulcer (L89.--0) should be based on the clinical documentation. These codes are used for pressure ulcers whose stage cannot be clinically determined (e.g., the ulcer is covered by eschar or has been treated with a skin or muscle graft) and pressure ulcers that are documented as deep tissue injury but not documented as due to trauma. This code should not be confused with the codes for unspecified stage (L89.--9). When there is no documentation regarding the stage of the pressure ulcer, assign the appropriate code for unspecified stage (L89.--9).

3) Documented pressure ulcer stage

Assignment of the pressure ulcer stage code should be guided by clinical documentation of the stage or documentation of the terms found in the Alphabetic Index. For clinical terms describing the stage that are not found in the Alphabetic Index, and there is no documentation of the stage, the provider should be queried.

4) Patients admitted with pressure ulcers documented as healed

No code is assigned if the documentation states that the pressure ulcer is completely healed at the time of admission.

5) Patients admitted with pressure ulcers documented as healing

Pressure ulcers described as healing should be assigned the appropriate pressure ulcer stage code based on the documentation in the medical record. If the documentation does not provide information about the stage of the healing pressure ulcer, assign the appropriate code for unspecified stage.

If the documentation is unclear as to whether the patient has a current (new) pressure ulcer or if the patient is being treated for a healing pressure ulcer, query the provider.

For ulcers that were present on admission but healed at the time of discharge, assign the code for the site and stage of the pressure ulcer at the time of admission.

6) Patient admitted with pressure ulcer evolving into another stage during the admission

If a patient is admitted to an inpatient hospital with a pressure ulcer at one stage and it progresses to a higher stage, two separate codes should be assigned: one code for the site and stage of the ulcer on admission and a second code for the same ulcer site and the highest stage reported during the stay.

7) Pressure-induced deep tissue damage

For pressure-induced deep tissue damage or deep tissue pressure injury, assign only the appropriate code for pressure-induced deep tissue damage (L89.--6).

b. Non-Pressure Chronic Ulcers

1) Patients admitted with non-pressure ulcers documented as healed

No code is assigned if the documentation states that the non-pressure ulcer is completely healed at the time of admission.

2) Patients admitted with non-pressure ulcers documented as healing

Non-pressure ulcers described as healing should be assigned the appropriate non-pressure ulcer code based on the documentation in the medical record. If the documentation does not provide information about the severity of the healing non-pressure ulcer, assign the appropriate code unspecified severity.

If the documentation is unclear as to whether the patient has a current (new) non-pressure ulcer or if the patient is being treated for a healing non-pressure ulcer, query the provider.

For ulcers that were present on admission but healed at the time of discharge, assign the code for the site and severity of the non-pressure ulcer at the time of admission.

3) Patient admitted with non-pressure ulcer that progresses to another severity level during the admission

If a patient is admitted to an inpatient hospital with a non-pressure ulcer at one severity level and it progresses to a higher severity level, two separate codes should be assigned; one code for the site and severity level of the ulcer on admission and a second code for the same ulcer site and the highest severity level reported during the stay.

See Section I.B.14 for pressure ulcer stage documentation by clinicians other than patient's provider.

13. Chapter 13: Diseases of the Musculoskeletal System and Connective Tissue (M00-M99)

a. Site and laterality

Most of the codes within Chapter 13 have site and laterality designations. The site represents the bone, joint or the muscle involved. For some conditions where more than one bone, joint or muscle is usually involved, such as osteoarthritis, there is a "multiple sites" code available. For categories where no multiple site code is provided and more than one bone, joint or muscle is involved, multiple codes should be used to indicate the different sites involved.

1) Bone versus joint

For certain conditions, the bone may be affected at the upper or lower end, (e.g., avascular necrosis of bone, M87, Osteoporosis, M80, M81). Though the portion of the bone affected may be at the joint, the site designation will be the bone, not the joint.

b. Acute traumatic versus chronic or recurrent musculoskeletal conditions

Many musculoskeletal conditions are a result of previous injury or trauma to a site, or are recurrent conditions. Bone, joint or muscle conditions that are the result of a healed injury are usually found in chapter 13. Recurrent bone, joint or muscle conditions are also usually found in chapter 13. Any current, acute injury should be coded to the appropriate injury code from chapter 19. Chronic or recurrent conditions should generally be coded with a code from chapter 13. If it is difficult to determine from the documentation in the record which code is best to describe a condition, query the provider.

c. Coding of Pathologic Fractures

7th character A is for use as long as the patient is receiving active treatment for the fracture. While the patient may be seen by a new or different provider over the course of treatment for a pathological fracture, assignment of the 7th character is based on whether the patient is undergoing active treatment and not whether the provider is seeing the patient for the first time.

7th character, D is to be used for encounters after the patient has completed active treatment for the fracture and is receiving routine care for the fracture during the healing or recovery phase. The other 7th characters, listed under each subcategory in the Tabular List, are to be used for subsequent encounters for routine care of fractures during the healing and recovery phase as well as treatment of problems associated with the healing, such as malunions, nonunions, and sequelae.

Care for complications of surgical treatment for fracture repairs during the healing or recovery phase should be coded with the appropriate complication codes.

See Section I.C.19. Coding of traumatic fractures.

d. Osteoporosis

Osteoporosis is a systemic condition, meaning that all bones of the musculoskeletal system are affected. Therefore, site is not a component of the codes under category M81, Osteoporosis without current pathological fracture. The site codes under category M80, Osteoporosis with current pathological fracture, identify the site of the fracture, not the osteoporosis.

1) Osteoporosis without pathological fracture

Category M81, Osteoporosis without current pathological fracture, is for use for patients with osteoporosis who do not currently have a pathologic fracture due to the osteoporosis, even if they have had a fracture in the past. For patients with a history of osteoporosis fractures, status code Z87.310, Personal history of (healed) osteoporosis fracture, should follow the code from M81.

2) Osteoporosis with current pathological fracture

Category M80, Osteoporosis with current pathological fracture, is for patients who have a current pathologic fracture at the time of an encounter. The codes under M80 identify the site of the fracture. A code from category M80, not a traumatic fracture code, should be used for any patient with known osteoporosis who suffers a fracture, even if the patient had a minor fall or trauma, if that fall or trauma would not usually break a normal, healthy bone.

14. Chapter 14: Diseases of the Genitourinary System (N00-N99)

a. Chronic kidney disease

1) Stages of chronic kidney disease (CKD)

The ICD-10-CM classifies CKD based on severity. The severity of CKD is designated by stages 1-5. Stage 2, code N18.2, equates to mild CKD; stage 3, code N18.3, equates to moderate CKD; and stage 4, code N18.4, equates to severe CKD. Code N18.6, End stage renal disease (ESRD), is assigned when the provider has documented end-stage-renal disease (ESRD).

If both a stage of CKD and ESRD are documented, assign code N18.6 only.

2) Chronic kidney disease and kidney transplant status

Patients who have undergone kidney transplant may still have some form of chronic kidney disease (CKD) because the kidney transplant may not fully restore kidney function. Therefore, the presence of CKD alone does not constitute a transplant complication. Assign the appropriate N18 code for the patient's stage of CKD and code Z94.0, Kidney transplant status. If a transplant complication such as failure or rejection or other transplant complication is documented, see section I.C.19.g for information on coding complications of a kidney transplant. If the documentation is unclear as to whether the patient has a complication of the transplant, query the provider.

3) Chronic kidney disease with other conditions

Patients with CKD may also suffer from other serious conditions, most commonly diabetes mellitus and hypertension. The sequencing of the CKD code in relationship to codes for other contributing conditions is based on the conventions in the Tabular List.

See I.C.9. Hypertensive chronic kidney disease.

See I.C.19. Chronic kidney disease and kidney transplant complications.

15. Chapter 15: Pregnancy, Childbirth and the Puerperium (O00-O9A)

a. General Rules for Obstetric Cases

1) Codes from chapter 15 and sequencing priority

Obstetric cases require codes from chapter 15, codes in the range O00-O9A, Pregnancy, Childbirth, and the Puerperium. Chapter 15 codes have sequencing priority over codes from other chapters. Additional codes from other chapters may be used in conjunction with chapter 15 codes to further specify conditions. Should the provider document that the pregnancy is incidental to the encounter, then code Z33.1, Pregnant state, incidental, should be used in place of any chapter 15 codes. It is the provider's responsibility to state that the condition being treated is not affecting the pregnancy.

2) Chapter 15 codes used only on the maternal record

Chapter 15 codes are to be used only on the maternal record, never on the record of the newborn.

3) Final character for trimester

The majority of codes in Chapter 15 have a final character indicating the trimester of pregnancy. The timeframes for the trimesters are indicated at the beginning of the chapter. If trimester is not a component of a code it is because the condition always occurs in a specific trimester, or the concept of trimester of pregnancy is not applicable. Certain codes have characters for only certain trimesters because the condition does not occur in all trimesters, but it may occur in more than just one.

Assignment of the final character for trimester should be based on the provider's documentation of the trimester (or number of weeks) for the current admission/encounter. This applies to the assignment of trimester for pre-existing conditions as well as those that develop during or are due to the pregnancy. The provider's documentation of the number of weeks may be used to assign the appropriate code identifying the trimester.

Whenever delivery occurs during the current admission, and there is an "in childbirth" option for the obstetric complication being coded, the "in childbirth" code should be assigned.

4) Selection of trimester for inpatient admissions that encompass more than one trimester

In instances when a patient is admitted to a hospital for complications of pregnancy during one trimester and remains in the hospital into a subsequent trimester, the trimester character for the antepartum complication code should be assigned on the basis of the trimester when the complication developed, not the trimester of the discharge. If the condition developed prior to the current admission/encounter or represents a pre-existing condition, the trimester character for the trimester at the time of the admission/encounter should be assigned.

5) **Unspecified trimester**

Each category that includes codes for trimester has a code for "unspecified trimester." The "unspecified trimester" code should rarely be used, such as when the documentation in the record is insufficient to determine the trimester and it is not possible to obtain clarification.

6) **7ᵗʰ character for Fetus Identification**

Where applicable, a 7ᵗʰ character is to be assigned for certain categories (O31, O32, O33.3 - O33.6, O35, O36, O40, O41, O60.1, O60.2, O64, and O69) to identify the fetus for which the complication code applies.

Assign 7ᵗʰ character "0":

- For single gestations
- When the documentation in the record is insufficient to determine the fetus affected and it is not possible to obtain clarification.
- When it is not possible to clinically determine which fetus is affected.

b. **Selection of OB Principal or First-listed Diagnosis**

1) **Routine outpatient prenatal visits**

For routine outpatient prenatal visits when no complications are present, a code from category Z34, Encounter for supervision of normal pregnancy, should be used as the first-listed diagnosis. These codes should not be used in conjunction with chapter 15 codes.

2) **Supervision of High-Risk Pregnancy**

Codes from category O09, Supervision of high-risk pregnancy, are intended for use only during the prenatal period. For complications during the labor or delivery episode as a result of a high-risk pregnancy, assign the applicable complication codes from Chapter 15. If there are no complications during the labor or delivery episode, assign code O80, Encounter for full-term uncomplicated delivery.

For routine prenatal outpatient visits for patients with high-risk pregnancies, a code from category O09, Supervision of high-risk pregnancy, should be used as the first-listed diagnosis. Secondary chapter 15 codes may be used in conjunction with these codes if appropriate.

3) **Episodes when no delivery occurs**

In episodes when no delivery occurs, the principal diagnosis should correspond to the principal complication of the pregnancy which necessitated the encounter. Should more than one complication exist, all of which are treated or monitored, any of the complications codes may be sequenced first.

4) **When a delivery occurs**

When an obstetric patient is admitted and delivers during that admission, the condition that prompted the admission should be sequenced as the principal diagnosis. If multiple conditions prompted the admission, sequence the one most related to the delivery as the principal diagnosis. A code for any complication of the delivery should be assigned as an additional diagnosis. In cases of cesarean delivery, if the patient was admitted with a condition that resulted in the performance of a cesarean procedure, that condition should be selected as the principal diagnosis. If the reason for the admission was unrelated to the condition resulting in the cesarean delivery, the condition related to the reason for the admission should be selected as the principal diagnosis.

5) **Outcome of delivery**

A code from category Z37, Outcome of delivery, should be included on every maternal record when a delivery has occurred. These codes are not to be used on subsequent records or on the newborn record.

c. **Pre-existing conditions versus conditions due to the pregnancy**

Certain categories in Chapter 15 distinguish between conditions of the mother that existed prior to pregnancy (pre-existing) and those that are a direct result of pregnancy. When assigning codes from Chapter 15, it is important to assess if a condition was pre-existing prior to pregnancy or developed during or due to the pregnancy in order to assign the correct code.

Categories that do not distinguish between pre-existing and pregnancy- related conditions may be used for either. It is acceptable to use codes specifically for the puerperium with codes complicating pregnancy and childbirth if a condition arises postpartum during the delivery encounter.

d. **Pre-existing hypertension in pregnancy**

Category O10, Pre-existing hypertension complicating pregnancy, childbirth and the puerperium, includes codes for hypertensive heart and hypertensive chronic kidney disease. When assigning one of the O10 codes that includes hypertensive heart disease or hypertensive chronic kidney disease, it is necessary to add a secondary code from the appropriate hypertension category to specify the type of heart failure or chronic kidney disease.

See Section I.C.9. Hypertension.

e. Fetal Conditions Affecting the Management of the Mother

1) Codes from categories O35 and O36

Codes from categories O35, Maternal care for known or suspected fetal abnormality and damage, and O36, Maternal care for other fetal problems, are assigned only when the fetal condition is actually responsible for modifying the management of the mother, i.e., by requiring diagnostic studies, additional observation, special care, or termination of pregnancy. The fact that the fetal condition exists does not justify assigning a code from this series to the mother's record.

2) In utero surgery

In cases when surgery is performed on the fetus, a diagnosis code from category O35, Maternal care for known or suspected fetal abnormality and damage, should be assigned identifying the fetal condition. Assign the appropriate procedure code for the procedure performed.

No code from Chapter 16, the perinatal codes, should be used on the mother's record to identify fetal conditions. Surgery performed in utero on a fetus is still to be coded as an obstetric encounter.

f. HIV Infection in Pregnancy, Childbirth and the Puerperium

During pregnancy, childbirth or the puerperium, a patient admitted because of an HIV-related illness should receive a principal diagnosis from subcategory O98.7-, Human immunodeficiency [HIV] disease complicating pregnancy, childbirth and the puerperium, followed by the code(s) for the HIV-related illness(es).

Patients with asymptomatic HIV infection status admitted during pregnancy, childbirth, or the puerperium should receive codes of O98.7- and Z21, Asymptomatic human immunodeficiency virus [HIV] infection status.

g. Diabetes mellitus in pregnancy

Diabetes mellitus is a significant complicating factor in pregnancy. Pregnant women who are diabetic should be assigned a code from category O24, Diabetes mellitus in pregnancy, childbirth, and the puerperium, first, followed by the appropriate diabetes code(s) (E08- E13) from Chapter 4.

h. Long term use of insulin and oral hypoglycemics

See section I.C.4.a.3 for information on the long term use of insulin and oral hypoglycemic.

i. Gestational (pregnancy induced) diabetes

Gestational (pregnancy induced) diabetes can occur during the second and third trimester of pregnancy in women who were not diabetic prior to pregnancy. Gestational diabetes can cause complications in the pregnancy similar to those of pre-existing diabetes mellitus. It also puts the woman at greater risk of developing diabetes after the pregnancy. Codes for gestational diabetes are in subcategory O24.4, Gestational diabetes mellitus. No other code from category O24, Diabetes mellitus in pregnancy, childbirth, and the puerperium, should be used with a code from O24.4

The codes under subcategory O24.4 include diet controlled, insulin controlled, and controlled by oral hypoglycemic drugs. If a patient with gestational diabetes is treated with both diet and insulin, only the code for insulin-controlled is required. If a patient with gestational diabetes is treated with both diet and oral hypoglycemic medications, only the code for "controlled by oral hypoglycemic drugs" is required. Code Z79.4, Long-term (current) use of insulin or code Z79.84, Long-term (current) use of oral hypoglycemic drugs, should not be assigned with codes from subcategory O24.4.

An abnormal glucose tolerance in pregnancy is assigned a code from subcategory O99.81, Abnormal glucose complicating pregnancy, childbirth, and the puerperium.

j. Sepsis and septic shock complicating abortion, pregnancy, childbirth and the puerperium

When assigning a chapter 15 code for sepsis complicating abortion, pregnancy, childbirth, and the puerperium, a code for the specific type of infection should be assigned as an additional diagnosis. If severe sepsis is present, a code from subcategory R65.2, Severe sepsis, and code(s) for associated organ dysfunction(s) should also be assigned as additional diagnoses.

k. Puerperal sepsis

Code O85, Puerperal sepsis, should be assigned with a secondary code to identify the causal organism (e.g., for a bacterial infection, assign a code from category B95-B96, Bacterial infections in conditions classified elsewhere). A code from category A40, Streptococcal sepsis, or A41, Other sepsis, should not be used for puerperal sepsis. If applicable, use additional codes to identify severe sepsis (R65.2-) and any associated acute organ dysfunction.

Code O85 should not be assigned for sepsis following an obstetrical procedure (*See Section I.C.1.d.5b., Sepsis due to a postprocedural infection*).

l. Alcohol, tobacco and drug use during pregnancy, childbirth and the puerperium

1) Alcohol use during pregnancy, childbirth and the puerperium

Codes under subcategory O99.31, Alcohol use complicating pregnancy, childbirth, and the puerperium, should be assigned for any pregnancy case when a mother uses alcohol during the pregnancy or postpartum. A secondary code from category F10, Alcohol related disorders, should also be assigned to identify manifestations of the alcohol use.

2) Tobacco use during pregnancy, childbirth and the puerperium

Codes under subcategory O99.33, Smoking (tobacco) complicating pregnancy, childbirth, and the puerperium, should be assigned for any pregnancy case when a mother uses any type of tobacco product during the pregnancy or postpartum. A secondary code from category F17, Nicotine dependence, should also be assigned to identify the type of nicotine dependence.

3) Drug use during pregnancy, childbirth and the puerperium

Codes under subcategory O99.32, Drug use complicating pregnancy, childbirth, and the puerperium, should be assigned for any pregnancy case when a mother uses drugs during the pregnancy or postpartum. This can involve illegal drugs, or inappropriate use or abuse of prescription drugs. Secondary code(s) from categories F11-F16 and F18-F19 should also be assigned to identify manifestations of the drug use.

m. Poisoning, toxic effects, adverse effects and underdosing in a pregnant patient

A code from subcategory O9A.2, Injury, poisoning and certain other consequences of external causes complicating pregnancy, childbirth, and the puerperium, should be sequenced first, followed by the appropriate injury, poisoning, toxic effect, adverse effect or underdosing code, and then the additional code(s) that specifies the condition caused by the poisoning, toxic effect, adverse effect or underdosing.

See Section I.C.19. Adverse effects, poisoning, underdosing and toxic effects.

n. Normal Delivery, Code O80

1) Encounter for full term uncomplicated delivery

Code O80 should be assigned when a woman is admitted for a full-term normal delivery and delivers a single, healthy infant without any complications antepartum, during the delivery, or postpartum during the delivery episode. Code O80 is always a principal diagnosis. It is not to be used if any other code from chapter 15 is needed to describe a current complication of the antenatal, delivery, or postnatal period. Additional codes from other chapters may be used with code O80 if they are not related to or are in any way complicating the pregnancy.

2) Uncomplicated delivery with resolved antepartum complication

Code O80 may be used if the patient had a complication at some point during the pregnancy, but the complication is not present at the time of the admission for delivery.

3) Outcome of delivery for O80

Z37.0, Single live birth, is the only outcome of delivery code appropriate for use with O80.

o. The Peripartum and Postpartum Periods

1) Peripartum and Postpartum periods

The postpartum period begins immediately after delivery and continues for six weeks following delivery. The peripartum period is defined as the last month of pregnancy to five months postpartum.

2) Peripartum and postpartum complication

A postpartum complication is any complication occurring within the six-week period.

3) Pregnancy-related complications after 6 week period

Chapter 15 codes may also be used to describe pregnancy-related complications after the peripartum or postpartum period if the provider documents that a condition is pregnancy related.

4) Admission for routine postpartum care following delivery outside hospital

When the mother delivers outside the hospital prior to admission and is admitted for routine postpartum care and no complications are noted, code Z39.0, Encounter for care and examination of mother immediately after delivery, should be assigned as the principal diagnosis.

5) Pregnancy associated cardiomyopathy

Pregnancy associated cardiomyopathy, code O90.3, is unique in that it may be diagnosed in the third trimester of pregnancy but may continue to progress months after delivery. For this reason, it is referred to as peripartum cardiomyopathy. Code O90.3 is only for use when the cardiomyopathy develops as a result of pregnancy in a woman who did not have pre-existing heart disease.

p. Code O94, Sequelae of complication of pregnancy, childbirth, and the puerperium

1) Code O94

Code O94, Sequelae of complication of pregnancy, childbirth, and the puerperium, is for use in those cases when an initial complication of a pregnancy develops a sequelae requiring care or treatment at a future date.

2) After the initial postpartum period

This code may be used at any time after the initial postpartum period.

3) Sequencing of Code O94

This code, like all sequela codes, is to be sequenced following the code describing the sequelae of the complication.

Official Coding Guidelines

q. **Termination of Pregnancy and Spontaneous abortions**

1) **Abortion with Liveborn Fetus**

When an attempted termination of pregnancy results in a liveborn fetus, assign code Z33.2, Encounter for elective termination of pregnancy and a code from category Z37, Outcome of Delivery.

2) **Retained Products of Conception following an abortion**

Subsequent encounters for retained products of conception following a spontaneous abortion or elective termination of pregnancy, without complications are assigned O03.4, Incomplete spontaneous, abortion without complication, or codes O07.4, Failed attempted termination of pregnancy without complication. This advice is appropriate even when the patient was discharged previously with a discharge diagnosis of complete abortion. If the patient has a specific complication associated with the spontaneous abortion or elective termination of pregnancy in addition to retained products of conception, assign the appropriate complication code (e.g., O03.-, O04.-, O07.-) instead of code O03.4 or O07.4.

3) **Complications leading to abortion**

Codes from Chapter 15 may be used as additional codes to identify any documented complications of the pregnancy in conjunction with codes in categories in O04, O07 and O08.

r. **Abuse in a pregnant patient**

For suspected or confirmed cases of abuse of a pregnant patient, a code(s) from subcategories O9A.3, Physical abuse complicating pregnancy, childbirth, and the puerperium, O9A.4, Sexual abuse complicating pregnancy, childbirth, and the puerperium, and O9A.5, Psychological abuse complicating pregnancy, childbirth, and the puerperium, should be sequenced first, followed by the appropriate codes (if applicable) to identify any associated current injury due to physical abuse, sexual abuse, and the perpetrator of abuse.

See Section I.C.19. Adult and child abuse, neglect and other maltreatment.

s. **COVID-19 infection in pregnancy, childbirth, and the puerperium**

During pregnancy, childbirth or the puerperium, when COVID-19 is the reason for admission/encounter, code O98.5-, Other viral diseases complicating pregnancy, childbirth and the puerperium, should be sequenced as the principal/first-listed diagnosis, and code U07.1, COVID-19, and the appropriate codes for associated manifestation(s) should be assigned as additional diagnoses. Codes from Chapter 15 always take sequencing priority.

If the reason for admission/encounter is unrelated to COVID-19 but the patient tests positive for COVID-19 during the admission/encounter, the appropriate code for the reason for admission/encounter should be sequenced as the principal/first-listed diagnosis, and code O98.5- and U07.1, as well as the appropriate codes for associated COVID-19 manifestations, should be assigned as additional diagnoses.

16. Chapter 16: Certain Conditions Originating in the Perinatal Period (P00-P96)

For coding and reporting purposes the perinatal period is defined as before birth through the 28th day following birth. The following guidelines are provided for reporting purposes

a. **General Perinatal Rules**

1) **Use of Chapter 16 Codes**

Codes in this chapter are <u>never</u> for use on the maternal record. Codes from Chapter 15, the obstetric chapter, are never permitted on the newborn record. Chapter 16 codes may be used throughout the life of the patient if the condition is still present.

2) **Principal Diagnosis for Birth Record**

When coding the birth episode in a newborn record, assign a code from category Z38, Liveborn infants according to place of birth and type of delivery, as the principal diagnosis. A code from category Z38 is assigned only once, to a newborn at the time of birth. If a newborn is transferred to another institution, a code from category Z38 should not be used at the receiving hospital.

A code from category Z38 is used only on the newborn record, not on the mother's record.

3) **Use of Codes from other Chapters with Codes from Chapter 16**

Codes from other chapters may be used with codes from chapter 16 if the codes from the other chapters provide more specific detail. Codes for signs and symptoms may be assigned when a definitive diagnosis has not been established. If the reason for the encounter is a perinatal condition, the code from chapter 16 should be sequenced first.

4) **Use of Chapter 16 Codes after the Perinatal Period**

Should a condition originate in the perinatal period, and continue throughout the life of the patient, the perinatal code should continue to be used regardless of the patient's age.

5) **Birth process or community acquired conditions**

If a newborn has a condition that may be either due to the birth process or community acquired and the documentation does not indicate which it is, the default is due to the birth process and the code from Chapter 16 should be used. If the condition is community-acquired, a code from Chapter 16 should not be assigned.

For COVID-19 infection in a newborn, see guideline I.C.16.h

6) **Code all clinically significant conditions**

All clinically significant conditions noted on routine newborn examination should be coded. A condition is clinically significant if it requires:

- clinical evaluation; or
- therapeutic treatment; or
- diagnostic procedures; or
- extended length of hospital stay; or
- increased nursing care and/or monitoring; or
- has implications for future health care needs

Note: The perinatal guidelines listed above are the same as the general coding guidelines for "additional diagnoses", except for the final point regarding implications for future health care needs. Codes should be assigned for conditions that have been specified by the provider as having implications for future health care needs.

b. Observation and Evaluation of Newborns for Suspected Conditions not Found

1) **Use of Z05 codes**

Assign a code from category Z05, Observation and evaluation of newborns and infants for suspected conditions ruled out, to identify those instances when a healthy newborn is evaluated for a suspected condition that is determined after study not to be present. Do not use a code from category Z05 when the patient has identified signs or symptoms of a suspected problem; in such cases code the sign or symptom.

2) **Z05 on Other than the Birth Record**

A code from category Z05 may also be assigned as a principal or first-listed code for readmissions or encounters when the code from category Z38 code no longer applies. Codes from category Z05 are fur use only for healthy newborns and infants for which no condition after study is found to be present.

3) **Z05 on a birth record**

A code from category Z05 is to be used as a secondary code after the code from category Z38, Liveborn infants according to place of birth and type of delivery.

c. Coding Additional Perinatal Diagnoses

1) **Assigning codes for conditions that require treatment**

Assign codes for conditions that require treatment or further investigation, prolong the length of stay, or require resource utilization.

2) **Codes for conditions specified as having implications for future health care needs**

Assign codes for conditions that have been specified by the provider as having implications for future health care needs.

Note: This guideline should not be used for adult patients.

d. Prematurity and Fetal Growth Retardation

Providers utilize different criteria in determining prematurity. A code for prematurity should not be assigned unless it is documented. Assignment of codes in categories P05, Disorders of newborn related to slow fetal growth and fetal malnutrition, and P07, Disorders of newborn related to short gestation and low birth weight, not elsewhere classified, should be based on the recorded birth weight and estimated gestational age.

When both birth weight and gestational age are available, two codes from category P07 should be assigned, with the code for birth weight sequenced before the code for gestational age.

e. Low birth weight and immaturity status

Codes from category P07, Disorders of newborn related to short gestation and low birth weight, not elsewhere classified, are for use for a child or adult who was premature or had a low birth weight as a newborn and this is affecting the patient's current health status.

See Section I.C.21. Factors influencing health status and contact with health services, Status.

f. Bacterial Sepsis of Newborn

Category P36, Bacterial sepsis of newborn, includes congenital sepsis. If a perinate is documented as having sepsis without documentation of congenital or community acquired, the default is congenital and a code from category P36 should be assigned. If the P36 code includes the causal organism, an additional code from category B95, Streptococcus, Staphylococcus, and Enterococcus as the cause of diseases classified elsewhere, or B96, Other bacterial agents as the cause of diseases classified elsewhere, should not be assigned. If the P36 code does not include the causal organism, assign an additional code from category B96. If applicable, use additional codes to identify severe sepsis (R65.2-) and any associated acute organ dysfunction.

g. Stillbirth

Code P95, Stillbirth, is only for use in institutions that maintain separate records for stillbirths. No other code should be used with P95. Code P95 should not be used on the mother's record.

h. COVID-19 Infection in Newborn

For a newborn that tests positive for COVID-19, assign code U07.1, COVID-19, and the appropriate codes for associated manifestation(s) in neonates/newborns in the absence of documentation indicating a specific type of transmission. For a newborn that tests positive for COVID-19 and the provider documents the condition was contracted in utero or during the birth process, assign codes P35.8, Other congenital viral diseases, and U07.1, COVID-19. When coding the birth episode in a newborn record, the appropriate code from category Z38, Liveborn infants according to place of birth and type of delivery, should be assigned as the principal diagnosis.

17. Chapter 17: Congenital Malformations, Deformations and Chromosomal Abnormalities (Q00-Q99)

Assign an appropriate code(s) from categories Q00-Q99, Congenital malformations, deformations, and chromosomal abnormalities when a malformation/deformation or chromosomal abnormality is documented. A malformation/deformation or chromosomal abnormality may be the principal/first-listed diagnosis on a record or a secondary diagnosis.

When a malformation/deformation or chromosomal abnormality does not have a unique code assignment, assign additional code(s) for any manifestations that may be present.

When the code assignment specifically identifies the malformation/deformation or chromosomal abnormality, manifestations that are an inherent component of the anomaly should not be coded separately. Additional codes should be assigned for manifestations that are not an inherent component.

Codes from Chapter 17 may be used throughout the life of the patient. If a congenital malformation or deformity has been corrected, a personal history code should be used to identify the history of the malformation or deformity. Although present at birth, a malformation/deformation or chromosomal abnormality may not be identified until later in life. Whenever the condition is diagnosed by the provider, it is appropriate to assign a code from codes Q00-Q99. For the birth admission, the appropriate code from category Z38, Liveborn infants, according to place of birth and type of delivery, should be sequenced as the principal diagnosis, followed by any congenital anomaly codes, Q00-Q99.

18. Chapter 18: Symptoms, Signs, and Abnormal Clinical and Laboratory Findings, Not Elsewhere Classified (R00-R99)

Chapter 18 includes symptoms, signs, abnormal results of clinical or other investigative procedures, and ill-defined conditions regarding which no diagnosis classifiable elsewhere is recorded. Signs and symptoms that point to a specific diagnosis have been assigned to a category in other chapters of the classification.

a. Use of symptom codes

Codes that describe symptoms and signs are acceptable for reporting purposes when a related definitive diagnosis has not been established (confirmed) by the provider.

b. Use of a symptom code with a definitive diagnosis code

Codes for signs and symptoms may be reported in addition to a related definitive diagnosis when the sign or symptom is not routinely associated with that diagnosis, such as the various signs and symptoms associated with complex syndromes. The definitive diagnosis code should be sequenced before the symptom code.

Signs or symptoms that are associated routinely with a disease process should not be assigned as additional codes, unless otherwise instructed by the classification.

c. Combination codes that include symptoms

ICD-10-CM contains a number of combination codes that identify both the definitive diagnosis and common symptoms of that diagnosis. When using one of these combination codes, an additional code should not be assigned for the symptom.

d. Repeated falls

Code R29.6, Repeated falls, is for use for encounters when a patient has recently fallen and the reason for the fall is being investigated.

Code Z91.81, History of falling, is for use when a patient has fallen in the past and is at risk for future falls. When appropriate, both codes R29.6 and Z91.81 may be assigned together.

e. Coma scale

The coma scale codes (R40.2-) can be used in conjunction with traumatic brain injury codes, acute cerebrovascular disease or sequelae of cerebrovascular disease codes. These codes are primarily for use by trauma registries, but they may be used in any setting where this information is collected. The coma scale codes should be sequenced after the diagnosis code(s).

These codes, one from each subcategory, are needed to complete the scale. The 7th character indicates when the scale was recorded. The 7th character should match for all three codes.

At a minimum, report the initial score documented on presentation at your facility. This may be a score from the emergency medicine technician (EMT) or in the emergency department. If desired, a facility may choose to capture multiple coma scale scores.

Assign code R40.24, Glasgow coma scale, total score, when only the total score is documented in the medical record and not the individual score(s).

Do not report codes for individual or total Glasgow coma scale scores for a patient with a medically induced coma or a sedated patient.

See Section I.B.14 for coma scale documentation by clinicians other than the patient's provider.

f. Functional quadriplegia

GUIDELINE HAS BEEN DELETED EFFECTIVE OCTOBER 1, 2017

g. SIRS due to Non-Infectious Process

The systemic inflammatory response syndrome (SIRS) can develop as a result of certain non-infectious disease processes, such as trauma, malignant neoplasm, or pancreatitis. When SIRS is documented with a noninfectious condition, and no subsequent infection is documented, the code for the underlying condition, such as an injury, should be assigned, followed by code R65.10, Systemic inflammatory response syndrome (SIRS) of non-infectious origin without acute organ dysfunction, or code R65.11, Systemic inflammatory response syndrome (SIRS) of non-infectious origin with acute organ dysfunction. If an associated acute organ dysfunction is documented, the appropriate code(s) for the specific type of organ dysfunction(s) should be assigned in addition to code R65.11. If acute organ dysfunction is documented, but it cannot be determined if the acute organ dysfunction is associated with SIRS or due to another condition (e.g., directly due to the trauma), the provider should be queried.

h. Death NOS

Code R99, Ill-defined and unknown cause of mortality, is only for use in the very limited circumstance when a patient who has already died is brought into an emergency department or other healthcare facility and is pronounced dead upon arrival. It does not represent the discharge disposition of death.

i. NIHSS Stroke Scale

The NIH stroke scale (NIHSS) codes (R29.7--) can be used in conjunction with acute stroke codes (I63) to identify the patient's neurological status and the severity of the stroke. The stroke scale codes should be sequenced after the acute stroke diagnosis code(s).

At a minimum, report the initial score documented. If desired, a facility may choose to capture multiple stroke scale scores.

See Section I.B.14 for NIHSS stroke scale documentation by clinicians other than patient's provider.

19. Chapter 19: Injury, Poisoning and Certain Other Consequences of External Causes (S00-T88)

a. Application of 7th Characters in Chapter 19

Most categories in chapter 19 have a 7th character requirement for each applicable code. Most categories in this chapter have three 7th character values (with the exception of fractures): A, initial encounter, D, subsequent encounter and S, sequela. Categories for traumatic fractures have additional 7th character values. While the patient may be seen by a new or different provider over the course of treatment for an injury, assignment of the 7th character is based on whether the patient is undergoing active treatment and not whether the provider is seeing the patient for the first time.

For complication codes, active treatment refers to treatment for the condition described by the code, even though it may be related to an earlier precipitating problem. For example, code T84.50XA, Infection and inflammatory reaction due to unspecified internal joint prosthesis, initial encounter, is used when active treatment is provided for the infection, even though the condition relates to the prosthetic device, implant or graft that was placed at a previous encounter.

7th character "A", initial encounter is used for each encounter where the patient is receiving active treatment for the condition.

7th character "D" subsequent encounter is used for encounters after the patient has completed active treatment of the condition and is receiving routine care for the condition during the healing or recovery phase.

The aftercare Z codes should not be used for aftercare for conditions such as injuries or poisonings, where 7th characters are provided to identify subsequent care. For example, for aftercare of an injury, assign the acute injury code with the 7th character "D" (subsequent encounter).

7th character "S", sequela, is for use for complications or conditions that arise as a direct result of a condition, such as scar formation after a burn. The scars are sequelae of the burn. When using 7th character "S", it is necessary to use both the injury code that precipitated the sequela and the code for the sequela itself. The "S" is added only to the injury code, not the sequela code. The 7th character "S" identifies the injury responsible for the sequela. The specific type of sequela (e.g. scar) is sequenced first, followed by the injury code.

See Section I.B.10 Sequela (Late Effects)

b. Coding of Injuries

When coding injuries, assign separate codes for each injury unless a combination code is provided, in which case the combination code is assigned. Codes from category T07, Unspecified multiple injuries should not be assigned in the inpatient setting unless information for a more specific code is not available. Traumatic injury codes (S00-T14.9) are not to be used for normal, healing surgical wounds or to identify complications of surgical wounds.

The code for the most serious injury, as determined by the provider and the focus of treatment, is sequenced first.

1) Superficial injuries

Superficial injuries such as abrasions or contusions are not coded when associated with more severe injuries of the same site.

2) Primary injury with damage to nerves/blood vessels

When a primary injury results in minor damage to peripheral nerves or blood vessels, the primary injury is sequenced first with additional code(s) for injuries to nerves and spinal cord (such as category S04), and/or injury to blood vessels (such as category S15). When the primary injury is to the blood vessels or nerves, that injury should be sequenced first.

3) Iatrogenic injuries

Injury codes from Chapter 19 should not be assigned for injuries that occur during, or as a result of, a medical intervention. Assign the appropriate complication code(s).

c. Coding of Traumatic Fractures

The principles of multiple coding of injuries should be followed in coding fractures. Fractures of specified sites are coded individually by site in accordance with both the provisions within categories S02, S12, S22, S32, S42, S49, S52, S59, S62, S72, S79, S82, S89, S92 and the level of detail furnished by medical record content.

A fracture not indicated as open or closed should be coded to closed. A fracture not indicated whether displaced or not displaced should be coded to displaced.

More specific guidelines are as follows:

1) Initial vs. Subsequent Encounter for Fractures

Traumatic fractures are coded using the appropriate 7th character for initial encounter (A, B, C) for each encounter where the patient is receiving active treatment for the fracture. The appropriate 7th character for initial encounter should also be assigned for a patient who delayed seeking treatment for the fracture or nonunion.

Fractures are coded using the appropriate 7th character for subsequent care for encounters after the patient has completed active treatment of the fracture and is receiving routine care for the fracture during the healing or recovery phase.

Care for complications of surgical treatment for fracture repairs during the healing or recovery phase should be coded with the appropriate complication codes.

Care of complications of fractures, such as malunion and nonunion, should be reported with the appropriate 7th character for subsequent care with nonunion (K, M, N,) or subsequent care with malunion (P, Q, R).

Malunion/nonunion: The appropriate 7th character for initial encounter should also be assigned for a patient who delayed seeking treatment for the fracture or nonunion.

The open fracture designations in the assignment of the 7th character for fractures of the forearm, femur and lower leg, including ankle are based on the Gustilo open fracture classification. When the Gustilo classification type is not specified for an open fracture, the 7th character for open fracture type I or II should be assigned (B, E, H, M, Q).

A code from category M80, not a traumatic fracture code, should be used for any patient with known osteoporosis who suffers a fracture, even if the patient had a minor fall or trauma, if that fall or trauma would not usually break a normal, healthy bone.

See Section I.C.13. Osteoporosis.

The aftercare Z codes should not be used for aftercare for traumatic fractures. For aftercare of a traumatic fracture, assign the acute fracture code with the appropriate 7th character.

2) Multiple fractures sequencing

Multiple fractures are sequenced in accordance with the severity of the fracture.

3) Physeal fractures

For physeal fractures, assign only the code identifying the type of physeal fracture. Do not assign a separate code to identify the specific bone that is fractured.

d. Coding of Burns and Corrosions

The ICD-10-CM makes a distinction between burns and corrosions. The burn codes are for thermal burns, except sunburns, that come from a heat source, such as a fire or hot appliance. The burn codes are also for burns resulting from electricity and radiation. Corrosions are burns due to chemicals. The guidelines are the same for burns and corrosions.

Current burns (T20-T25) are classified by depth, extent and by agent (X code). Burns are classified by depth as first degree (erythema), second degree (blistering), and third degree (full-thickness involvement). Burns of the eye and internal organs (T26-T28) are classified by site, but not by degree.

1) Sequencing of burn and related condition codes

Sequence first the code that reflects the highest degree of burn when more than one burn is present.

a. When the reason for the admission or encounter is for treatment of external multiple burns, sequence first the code that reflects the burn of the highest degree.

b. When a patient has both internal and external burns, the circumstances of admission govern the selection of the principal diagnosis or first-listed diagnosis.

c. When a patient is admitted for burn injuries and other related conditions such as smoke inhalation and/or respiratory failure, the circumstances of admission govern the selection of the principal or first-listed diagnosis.

2) Burns of the same anatomic site

Classify burns of the same anatomic site and on the same side but of different degrees to the subcategory identifying the highest degree recorded in the diagnosis (e.g., for second and third degree burns of right thigh, assign only code T24.311-).

3) Non-healing burns

Non-healing burns are coded as acute burns.

Necrosis of burned skin should be coded as a non-healed burn.

4) Infected Burn

For any documented infected burn site, use an additional code for the infection.

5) Assign separate codes for each burn site

When coding burns, assign separate codes for each burn site. Category T30, Burn and corrosion, body region unspecified is extremely vague and should rarely be used.

Codes for burns of "multiple sites" should only be assigned when the medical record documentation does not specify the individual sites.

6) Burns and Corrosions Classified According to Extent of Body Surface Involved

Assign codes from category T31, Burns classified according to extent of body surface involved, or T32, Corrosions classified according to extent of body surface involved, when the site of the burn is not specified or when there is a need for additional data. It is advisable to use category T31 as additional coding when needed to provide data for evaluating burn mortality, such as that needed by burn units. It is also advisable to use category T31 as an additional code for reporting purposes when there is mention of a third-degree burn involving 20 percent or more of the body surface.

Categories T31 and T32 are based on the classic "rule of nines" in estimating body surface involved: head and neck are assigned nine percent, each arm nine percent, each leg 18 percent, the anterior trunk 18 percent, posterior trunk 18 percent, and genitalia one percent. Providers may change these percentage assignments where necessary to accommodate infants and children who have proportionately larger heads than adults, and patients who have large buttocks, thighs, or abdomen that involve burns.

7) Encounters for treatment of sequela of burns

Encounters for the treatment of the late effects of burns or corrosions (i.e., scars or joint contractures) should be coded with a burn or corrosion code with the 7th character "S" for sequela.

8) Sequelae with a late effect code and current burn

When appropriate, both a code for a current burn or corrosion with 7th character "A" or "D" and a burn or corrosion code with 7th character "S" may be assigned on the same record (when both a current burn and sequelae of an old burn exist). Burns and corrosions do not heal at the same rate and a current healing wound may still exist with sequela of a healed burn or corrosion.

See Section I.B.10 Sequela (Late Effects)

9) Use of an external cause code with burns and corrosions

An external cause code should be used with burns and corrosions to identify the source and intent of the burn, as well as the place where it occurred.

e. Adverse Effects, Poisoning, Underdosing and Toxic Effects

Codes in categories T36-T65 are combination codes that include the substance that was taken as well as the intent. No additional external cause code is required for poisonings, toxic effects, adverse effects and underdosing codes.

1) Do not code directly from the Table of Drugs

Do not code directly from the Table of Drugs and Chemicals. Always refer back to the Tabular List.

2) Use as many codes as necessary to describe

Use as many codes as necessary to describe completely all drugs, medicinal or biological substances.

3) If the same code would describe the causative agent

If the same code would describe the causative agent for more than one adverse reaction, poisoning, toxic effect or underdosing, assign the code only once.

4) If two or more drugs, medicinal or biological substances

If two or more drugs, medicinal or biological substances are taken, code each individually unless a combination code is listed in the Table of Drugs and Chemicals.

If multiple unspecified drugs, medicinal or biological substances were taken, assign the appropriate code from subcategory T50.91, Poisoning by, adverse effect of and underdosing of multiple unspecified drugs, medicaments and biological substances.

5) **The occurrence of drug toxicity is classified in ICD-10-CM as follows:**

(a) **Adverse Effect**

When coding an adverse effect of a drug that has been correctly prescribed and properly administered, assign the appropriate code for the nature of the adverse effect followed by the appropriate code for the adverse effect of the drug (T36-T50). The code for the drug should have a 5th or 6th character "5" (for example T36.0X5-) Examples of the nature of an adverse effect are tachycardia, delirium, gastrointestinal hemorrhaging, vomiting, hypokalemia, hepatitis, renal failure, or respiratory failure.

(b) **Poisoning**

When coding a poisoning or reaction to the improper use of a medication (e.g., overdose, wrong substance given or taken in error, wrong route of administration), first assign the appropriate code from categories T36-T50. The poisoning codes have an associated intent as their 5th or 6th character (accidental, intentional self-harm, assault and undetermined.) If the intent of the poisoning is unknown or unspecified, code the intent as accidental intent. The undetermined intent is only for use if the documentation in the record specifies that the intent cannot be determined. Use additional code(s) for all manifestations of poisonings.

If there is also a diagnosis of abuse or dependence of the substance, the abuse or dependence is assigned as an additional code.

Examples of poisoning include:

(i) Error was made in drug prescription

Errors made in drug prescription or in the administration of the drug by provider, nurse, patient, or other person.

(ii) Overdose of a drug intentionally taken

If an overdose of a drug was intentionally taken or administered and resulted in drug toxicity, it would be coded as a poisoning.

(iii) Nonprescribed drug taken with correctly prescribed and properly administered drug

If a nonprescribed drug or medicinal agent was taken in combination with a correctly prescribed and properly administered drug, any drug toxicity or other reaction resulting from the interaction of the two drugs would be classified as a poisoning.

(iv) Interaction of drug(s) and alcohol

When a reaction results from the interaction of a drug(s) and alcohol, this would be classified as poisoning.

See Section I.C.4. if poisoning is the result of insulin pump malfunctions.

(c) **Underdosing**

Underdosing refers to taking less of a medication than is prescribed by a provider or a manufacturer's instruction. Discontinuing the use of a prescribed medication on the patient's own initiative (not directed by the patient's provider) is also classified as an underdosing. For underdosing, assign the code from categories T36-T50 (fifth or sixth character "6").

Codes for underdosing should never be assigned as principal or first-listed codes. If a patient has a relapse or exacerbation of the medical condition for which the drug is prescribed because of the reduction in dose, then the medical condition itself should be coded.

Noncompliance (Z91.12-, Z91.13- and Z91.14-) or complication of care (Y63.6-Y63.9) codes are to be used with an underdosing code to indicate intent, if known.

(d) **Toxic Effects**

When a harmful substance is ingested or comes in contact with a person, this is classified as a toxic effect. The toxic effect codes are in categories T51-T65.

Toxic effect codes have an associated intent: accidental, intentional self-harm, assault and undetermined.

f. **Adult and child abuse, neglect and other maltreatment**

Sequence first the appropriate code from categories T74.- (Adult and child abuse, neglect and other maltreatment, confirmed) or T76.- (Adult and child abuse, neglect and other maltreatment, suspected) for abuse, neglect and other maltreatment, followed by any accompanying mental health or injury code(s).

If the documentation in the medical record states abuse or neglect it is coded as confirmed (T74.-). It is coded as suspected if it is documented as suspected (T76.-).

For cases of confirmed abuse or neglect an external cause code from the assault section (X92-Y09) should be added to identify the cause of any physical injuries. A perpetrator code (Y07) should be added when the perpetrator of the abuse is known. For suspected cases of abuse or neglect, do not report external cause or perpetrator code.

If a suspected case of abuse, neglect or mistreatment is ruled out during an encounter code Z04.71, Encounter for examination and observation following alleged physical adult abuse, ruled out, or code Z04.72, Encounter for examination and observation following alleged child physical abuse, ruled out, should be used, not a code from T76.

If a suspected case of alleged rape or sexual abuse is ruled out during an encounter code Z04.41, Encounter for examination and observation following alleged adult rape or code Z04.42, Encounter for examination and observation following alleged child rape, should be used, not a code from T76.

If a suspected case of forced sexual exploitation or forced labor exploitation is ruled out during an encounter, code Z04.81, Encounter for examination and observation of victim following forced sexual exploitation, or code Z04.82, Encounter for examination and observation of victim following forced labor exploitation, should be used, not a code from T76.

See Section I.C.15. Abuse in a pregnant patient.

g. Complications of care

1) General guidelines for complications of care

(a) Documentation of complications of care

See Section I.B.16. for information on documentation of complications of care.

2) Pain due to medical devices

Pain associated with devices, implants or grafts left in a surgical site (for example painful hip prosthesis) is assigned to the appropriate code(s) found in Chapter 19, Injury, poisoning, and certain other consequences of external causes. Specific codes for pain due to medical devices are found in the T code section of the ICD-10-CM. Use additional code(s) from category G89 to identify acute or chronic pain due to presence of the device, implant or graft (G89.18 or G89.28).

3) Transplant complications

(a) Transplant complications other than kidney

Codes under category T86, Complications of transplanted organs and tissues, are for use for both complications and rejection of transplanted organs. A transplant complication code is only assigned if the complication affects the function of the transplanted organ. Two codes are required to fully describe a transplant complication: the appropriate code from category T86 and a secondary code that identifies the complication.

Pre-existing conditions or conditions that develop after the transplant are not coded as complications unless they affect the function of the transplanted organs.

See I.C.21. for transplant organ removal status.

See I.C.2. for malignant neoplasm associated with transplanted organ.

(b) Kidney transplant complications

Patients who have undergone kidney transplant may still have some form of chronic kidney disease (CKD) because the kidney transplant may not fully restore kidney function. Code T86.1- should be assigned for documented complications of a kidney transplant, such as transplant failure or rejection or other transplant complication. Code T86.1- should not be assigned for post kidney transplant patients who have chronic kidney (CKD) unless a transplant complication such as transplant failure or rejection is documented. If the documentation is unclear as to whether the patient has a complication of the transplant, query the provider.

Conditions that affect the function of the transplanted kidney, other than CKD, should be assigned a code from subcategory T86.1, Complications of transplanted organ, Kidney, and a secondary code that identifies the complication.

For patients with CKD following a kidney transplant, but who do not have a complication such as failure or rejection, *see section I.C.14. Chronic kidney disease and kidney transplant status.*

4) Complication codes that include the external cause

As with certain other T codes, some of the complications of care codes have the external cause included in the code. The code includes the nature of the complication as well as the type of procedure that caused the complication. No external cause code indicating the type of procedure is necessary for these codes.

5) Complications of care codes within the body system chapters

Intraoperative and postprocedural complication codes are found within the body system chapters with codes specific to the organs and structures of that body system. These codes should be sequenced first, followed by a code(s) for the specific complication, if applicable.

Complication codes from the body system chapters should be assigned for intraoperative and postprocedural complications (e.g., the appropriate complication code from chapter 9 would be assigned for a vascular intraoperative or postprocedural complication) unless the complication is specifically indexed to a T code in chapter 19.

20. Chapter 20: External Causes of Morbidity (V00-Y99)

The external causes of morbidity codes should never be sequenced as the first-listed or principal diagnosis.

External cause codes are intended to provide data for injury research and evaluation of injury prevention strategies. These codes capture how the injury or health condition happened (cause), the intent (unintentional or accidental; or intentional, such as suicide or assault), the place where the event occurred the activity of the patient at the time of the event, and the person's status (e.g., civilian, military).

There is no national requirement for mandatory ICD-10-CM external cause code reporting. Unless a provider is subject to a state-based external cause code reporting mandate or these codes are required by a particular payer, reporting of ICD-10-CM codes in Chapter 20, External Causes of Morbidity, is not required. In the absence of a mandatory reporting requirement, providers are encouraged to voluntarily report external cause codes, as they provide valuable data for injury research and evaluation of injury prevention strategies.

a. General External Cause Coding Guidelines

1) Used with any code in the range of A00.0-T88.9, Z00-Z99

An external cause code may be used with any code in the range of A00.0-T88.9, Z00-Z99, classification that represents a health condition due to an external cause. Though they are most applicable to injuries, they are also valid for use with such things as infections or diseases due to an external source, and other health conditions, such as a heart attack that occurs during strenuous physical activity.

2) External cause code used for length of treatment

Assign the external cause code, with the appropriate 7th character (initial encounter, subsequent encounter or sequela) for each encounter for which the injury or condition is being treated.

Most categories in chapter 20 have a 7th character requirement for each applicable code. Most categories in this chapter have three 7th character values: A, initial encounter, D, subsequent encounter and S, sequela. While the patient may be seen by a new or different provider over the course of treatment for an injury or condition, assignment of the 7th character for external cause should match the 7th character of the code assigned for the associated injury or condition for the encounter.

3) Use the full range of external cause codes

Use the full range of external cause codes to completely describe the cause, the intent, the place of occurrence, and if applicable, the activity of the patient at the time of the event, and the patient's status, for all injuries, and other health conditions due to an external cause.

4) Assign as many external cause codes as necessary

Assign as many external cause codes as necessary to fully explain each cause. If only one external code can be recorded, assign the code most related to the principal diagnosis.

5) The selection of the appropriate external cause code

The selection of the appropriate external cause code is guided by the Alphabetic Index of External Causes and by Inclusion and Exclusion notes in the Tabular List.

6) External cause code can never be a principal diagnosis

An external cause code can never be a principal (first-listed) diagnosis.

7) Combination external cause codes

Certain of the external cause codes are combination codes that identify sequential events that result in an injury, such as a fall which results in striking against an object. The injury may be due to either event or both. The combination external cause code used should correspond to the sequence of events regardless of which caused the most serious injury.

8) No external cause code needed in certain circumstances

No external cause code from Chapter 20 is needed if the external cause and intent are included in a code from another chapter (e.g. T36.0X1- Poisoning by penicillins, accidental (unintentional)).

b. Place of Occurrence Guideline

Codes from category Y92, Place of occurrence of the external cause, are secondary codes for use after other external cause codes to identify the location of the patient at the time of injury or other condition.

Generally, a place of occurrent code is assigned only once, at the initial encounter for treatment. However, in the rare instance that a new injury occurs during hospitalization, an additional place of occurrence code may be assigned. No 7th characters are used for Y92.

Do not use place of occurrence code Y92.9 if the place is not stated or is not applicable.

c. Activity Code

Assign a code from category Y93, Activity code, to describe the activity of the patient at the time the injury or other health condition occurred.

An activity code is used only once, at the initial encounter for treatment. Only one code from Y93 should be recorded on a medical record.

The activity codes are not applicable to poisonings, adverse effects, misadventures or sequela.

Do not assign Y93.9, Unspecified activity, if the activity is not stated.

A code from category Y93 is appropriate for use with external cause and intent codes if identifying the activity provides additional information about the event.

d. Place of Occurrence, Activity, and Status Codes Used with other External Cause Code

When applicable, place of occurrence, activity, and external cause status codes are sequenced after the main external cause code(s). Regardless of the number of external cause codes assigned, generally there should be only one place of occurrence code, one activity code, and one external cause status code assigned to an encounter. However, in the rare instance that a new injury occurs during hospitalization, an additional place of occurrence code may be assigned.

e. If the Reporting Format Limits the Number of External Cause Codes

If the reporting format limits the number of external cause codes that can be used in reporting clinical data, report the code for the cause/intent most related to the principal diagnosis. If the format permits capture of additional external cause codes, the cause/intent, including medical misadventures, of the additional events should be reported rather than the codes for place, activity, or external status.

f. Multiple External Cause Coding Guidelines

More than one external cause code is required to fully describe the external cause of an illness or injury. The assignment of external cause codes should be sequenced in the following priority:

If two or more events cause separate injuries, an external cause code should be assigned for each cause. The first-listed external cause code will be selected in the following order:

External codes for child and adult abuse take priority over all other external cause codes.

See Section I.C.19., Child and Adult abuse guidelines.

External cause codes for terrorism events take priority over all other external cause codes except child and adult abuse.

External cause codes for cataclysmic events take priority over all other external cause codes except child and adult abuse and terrorism.

External cause codes for transport accidents take priority over all other external cause codes except cataclysmic events, child and adult abuse and terrorism.

Activity and external cause status codes are assigned following all causal (intent) external cause codes.

The first-listed external cause code should correspond to the cause of the most serious diagnosis due to an assault, accident, or self-harm, following the order of hierarchy listed above.

g. Child and Adult Abuse Guideline

Adult and child abuse, neglect and maltreatment are classified as assault. Any of the assault codes may be used to indicate the external cause of any injury resulting from the confirmed abuse.

For confirmed cases of abuse, neglect and maltreatment, when the perpetrator is known, a code from Y07, Perpetrator of maltreatment and neglect, should accompany any other assault codes.

See Section I.C.19. Adult and child abuse, neglect and other maltreatment

h. Unknown or Undetermined Intent Guideline

If the intent (accident, self-harm, assault) of the cause of an injury or other condition is unknown or unspecified, code the intent as accidental intent. All transport accident categories assume accidental intent.

1) Use of undetermined intent

External cause codes for events of undetermined intent are only for use if the documentation in the record specifies that the intent cannot be determined.

i. Sequelae (Late Effects) of External Cause Guidelines

1) Sequelae external cause codes

Sequela are reported using the external cause code with the 7th character "S" for sequela. These codes should be used with any report of a late effect or sequela resulting from a previous injury.

See Section I.B.10 Sequela (Late Effects)

2) Sequela external cause code with a related current injury

A sequela external cause code should never be used with a related current nature of injury code.

3) Use of sequela external cause codes for subsequent visits

Use a late effect external cause code for subsequent visits when a late effect of the initial injury is being treated. Do not use a late effect external cause code for subsequent visits for follow-up care (e.g., to assess healing, to receive rehabilitative therapy) of the injury when no late effect of the injury has been documented.

j. Terrorism Guidelines

1) Cause of injury identified by the Federal Government (FBI) as terrorism

When the cause of an injury is identified by the Federal Government (FBI) as terrorism, the first-listed external cause code should be a code from category Y38, Terrorism. The definition of terrorism employed by the FBI is found at the inclusion note at the beginning of category Y38. Use additional code for place of occurrence (Y92.-). More than one Y38 code may be assigned if the injury is the result of more than one mechanism of terrorism.

2) Cause of an injury is suspected to be the result of terrorism

When the cause of an injury is suspected to be the result of terrorism a code from category Y38 should not be assigned. Suspected cases should be classified as assault.

3) Code Y38.9, Terrorism, secondary effects

Assign code Y38.9, Terrorism, secondary effects, for conditions occurring subsequent to the terrorist event. This code should not be assigned for conditions that are due to the initial terrorist act.

It is acceptable to assign code Y38.9 with another code from Y38 if there is an injury due to the initial terrorist event and an injury that is a subsequent result of the terrorist event.

k. External cause status

A code from category Y99, External cause status, should be assigned whenever any other external cause code is assigned for an encounter, including an Activity code, except for the events noted below. Assign a code from category Y99, External cause status, to indicate the work status of the person at the time the event occurred. The status code indicates whether the event occurred during military activity, whether a non-military person was at work, whether an individual including a student or volunteer was involved in a non-work activity at the time of the causal event.

A code from Y99, External cause status, should be assigned, when applicable, with other external cause codes, such as transport accidents and falls. The external cause status codes are not applicable to poisonings, adverse effects, misadventures or late effects. Do not assign a code from category Y99 if no other external cause codes (cause, activity) are applicable for the encounter.

An external cause status code is used only once, at the initial encounter for treatment. Only one code from Y99 should be recorded on a medical record.

Do not assign code Y99.9, Unspecified external cause status, if the status is not stated.

21. Chapter 21: Factors Influencing Health Status and Contact with Health Services (Z00-Z99)

NOTE The chapter specific guidelines provide additional information about the use of Z codes for specified encounters.

a. Use of Z codes in any healthcare setting

Z codes are for use in any healthcare setting. Z codes may be used as either a first-listed (principal diagnosis code in the inpatient setting) or secondary code, depending on the circumstances of the encounter. Certain Z codes may only be used as first-listed or principal diagnosis.

b. Z Codes indicate a reason for an encounter

Z codes are not procedure codes. A corresponding procedure code must accompany a Z code to describe any procedure performed.

c. Categories of Z Codes

1) Contact/Exposure

Category Z20 indicates contact with, and suspected exposure to, communicable diseases. These codes are for patients who do not show any sign or symptom of a disease but are suspected to have been exposed to it by close personal contact with an infected individual or are in an area where a disease is epidemic.

Category Z77, Other contact with and (suspected) exposures hazardous to health, indicates contact with and suspected exposures hazardous to health.

Contact/exposure codes may be used as a first-listed code to explain an encounter for testing, or, more commonly, as a secondary code to identify a potential risk.

2) Inoculations and vaccinations

Code Z23 is for encounters for inoculations and vaccinations. It indicates that a patient is being seen to receive a prophylactic inoculation against a disease. Procedure codes are required to identify the actual administration of the injection and the type(s) of immunizations given. Code Z23 may be used as a secondary code if the inoculation is given as a routine part of preventive health care, such as a well-baby visit.

3) Status

Status codes indicate that a patient is either a carrier of a disease or has the sequelae or residual of a past disease or condition. This includes such things as the presence of prosthetic or mechanical devices resulting from past treatment. A status code is informative, because the status may affect the course of treatment and its outcome. A status code is distinct from a history code. The history code indicates that the patient no longer has the condition.

A status code should not be used with a diagnosis code from one of the body system chapters, if the diagnosis code includes the information provided by the status code. For example, code Z94.1, Heart transplant status, should not be used with a code from subcategory T86.2, Complications of heart transplant. The status code does not provide additional information. The complication code indicates that the patient is a heart transplant patient.

For encounters for weaning from a mechanical ventilator, assign a code from subcategory J96.1, Chronic respiratory failure, followed by code Z99.11, Dependence on respirator [ventilator] status.

The status Z codes/categories are:

Z14 Genetic carrier

   Genetic carrier status indicates that a person carries a gene, associated with a particular disease, which may be passed to offspring who may develop that disease. The person does not have the disease and is not at risk of developing the disease.

Z15 Genetic susceptibility to disease

   Genetic susceptibility indicates that a person has a gene that increases the risk of that person developing the disease.

Codes from category Z15 should not be used as principal or first-listed codes. If the patient has the condition to which he/she is susceptible, and that condition is the reason for the encounter, the code for the current condition should be sequenced first. If the patient is being seen for follow-up after completed treatment for this condition, and the condition no longer exists, a follow-up code should be sequenced first, followed by the appropriate personal history and genetic susceptibility codes. If the purpose of the encounter is genetic counseling associated with procreative management, code Z31.5, Encounter for genetic counseling, should be assigned as the first-listed code, followed by a code from category Z15. Additional codes should be assigned for any applicable family or personal history.

Z16   Resistance to antimicrobial drugs

This code indicates that a patient has a condition that is resistant to antimicrobial drug treatment. Sequence the infection code first.

Z17   Estrogen receptor status

Z18   Retained foreign body fragments

Z19   Hormone sensitivity malignancy status

Z21   Asymptomatic HIV infection status

This code indicates that a patient has tested positive for HIV but has manifested no signs or symptoms of the disease.

Z22   Carrier of infectious disease

Carrier status indicates that a person harbors the specific organisms of a disease without manifest symptoms and is capable of transmitting the infection.

Z28.3   Underimmunization status

Z33.1   Pregnant state, incidental

This code is a secondary code only for use when the pregnancy is in no way complicating the reason for visit. Otherwise, a code from the obstetric chapter is required.

Z66   Do not resuscitate

This code may be used when it is documented by the provider that a patient is on do not resuscitate status at any time during the stay.

Z67   Blood type

Z68   Body mass index (BMI)

BMI codes should only be assigned when **there is an associated, reportable diagnosis (such as obesity).** Do not assign BMI codes during pregnancy.

See Section I.B.14 for BMI documentation by clinicians other than the patient's provider.

Z74.01   Bed confinement status

Z76.82   Awaiting organ transplant status

Z78   Other specified health status

Code Z78.1, Physical restraint status, may be used when it is documented by the provider that a patient has been put in restraints during the current encounter. Please note that this code should not be reported when it is documented by the provider that a patient is temporarily restrained during a procedure.

Z79   Long-term (current) drug therapy

Codes from this category indicate a patient's continuous use of a prescribed drug (including such things as aspirin therapy) for the long-term treatment of a condition or for prophylactic use. It is not for use for patients who have addictions to drugs. This subcategory is not for use of medications for detoxification or maintenance programs to prevent withdrawal symptoms in patients with drug dependence (e.g., methadone maintenance for opiate dependence). Assign the appropriate code for the drug dependence instead.

Assign a code from Z79 if the patient is receiving a medication for an extended period as a prophylactic measure (such as for the prevention of deep vein thrombosis) or as treatment of a chronic condition (such as arthritis) or a disease requiring a lengthy course of treatment (such as cancer). Do not assign a code from category Z79 for medication being administered for a brief period of time to treat an acute illness or injury (such as a course of antibiotics to treat acute bronchitis).

Z88   Allergy status to drugs, medicaments and biological substances

Except: Z88.9, Allergy status to unspecified drugs, medicaments and biological substances status

Z89   Acquired absence of limb

Z90   Acquired absence of organs, not elsewhere classified

Z91.0-   Allergy status, other than to drugs and biological substances

Z92.82   Status post administration of tPA (rtPA) in a different facility within the last 24 hours prior to admission to a current facility

Assign code Z92.82, Status post administration of tPA (rtPA) in a different facility within the last 24 hours prior to admission to current facility, as a secondary diagnosis when a patient is received by transfer into a facility and documentation indicates they were administered tissue plasminogen activator (tPA) within the last 24 hours prior to admission to the current facility.

This guideline applies even if the patient is still receiving the tPA at the time they are received into the current facility.

The appropriate code for the condition for which the tPA was administered (such as cerebrovascular disease or myocardial infarction) should be assigned first.

Code Z92.82 is only applicable to the receiving facility record and not to the transferring facility record.

Z93   Artificial opening status

Z94   Transplanted organ and tissue status

Z95   Presence of cardiac and vascular implants and grafts

Z96   Presence of other functional implants

Z97   Presence of other devices

Z98   Other postprocedural states

Assign code Z98.85, Transplanted organ removal status, to indicate that a transplanted organ has been previously removed. This code should not be assigned for the encounter in which the transplanted organ is removed. The complication necessitating removal of the transplant organ should be assigned for that encounter.

See section I.C19. for information on the coding of organ transplant complications.

Z99   Dependence on enabling machines and devices, not elsewhere classified

NOTE Categories Z89-Z90 and Z93-Z99 are for use only if there are no complications or malfunctions of the organ or tissue replaced, the amputation site or the equipment on which the patient is dependent.

4) History (of)

There are two types of history Z codes, personal and family. Personal history codes explain a patient's past medical condition that no longer exists and is not receiving any treatment, but that has the potential for recurrence, and therefore may require continued monitoring.

Family history codes are for use when a patient has a family member(s) who has had a particular disease that causes the patient to be at higher risk of also contracting the disease.

Personal history codes may be used in conjunction with follow-up codes and family history codes may be used in conjunction with screening codes to explain the need for a test or procedure. History codes are also acceptable on any medical record regardless of the reason for visit. A history of an illness, even if no longer present, is important information that may alter the type of treatment ordered.

The history Z code categories are:

Z80   Family history of primary malignant neoplasm

Z81   Family history of mental and behavioral disorders

Z82   Family history of certain disabilities and chronic diseases (leading to disablement)

Z83   Family history of other specific disorders

Z84   Family history of other conditions

Z85   Personal history of malignant neoplasm

Z86   Personal history of certain other diseases

Z87   Personal history of other diseases and conditions

Z91.4-   Personal history of psychological trauma, not elsewhere classified

Z91.5   Personal history of self-harm

Z91.81   History of falling

Z91.82   Personal history of military deployment

Z92   Personal history of medical treatment

Except: Z92.0, Personal history of contraception Except: Z92.82, Status post administration of tPA (rtPA) in a different facility within the last 24 hours prior to admission to a current facility

5) Screening

Screening is the testing for disease or disease precursors in seemingly well individuals so that early detection and treatment can be provided for those who test positive for the disease (e.g., screening mammogram).

The testing of a person to rule out or confirm a suspected diagnosis because the patient has some sign or symptom is a diagnostic examination, not a screening. In these cases, the sign or symptom is used to explain the reason for the test.

A screening code may be a first-listed code if the reason for the visit is specifically the screening exam. It may also be used as an additional code if the screening is done during an office visit for other health problems. A screening code is not necessary if the screening is inherent to a routine examination, such as a pap smear done during a routine pelvic examination.

Should a condition be discovered during the screening then the code for the condition may be assigned as an additional diagnosis.

The Z code indicates that a screening exam is planned. A procedure code is required to confirm that the screening was performed.

The screening Z codes/categories:

Z11	Encounter for screening for infectious and parasitic diseases
Z12	Encounter for screening for malignant neoplasms
Z13	Encounter for screening for other diseases and disorders
	Except: Z13.9, Encounter for screening, unspecified
Z36	Encounter for antenatal screening for mother

6) Observation

There are three observation Z code categories. They are for use in very limited circumstances when a person is being observed for a suspected condition that is ruled out. The observation codes are not for use if an injury or illness or any signs or symptoms related to the suspected condition are present. In such cases the diagnosis/symptom code is used with the corresponding external cause code.

The observation codes are **primarily** to be used as principal/**first-listed** diagnosis. **An observation code may be assigned as a secondary diagnosis code when the patient is being observed for a condition that is ruled out and is unrelated to the principal/first-listed diagnosis (e.g., patient presents for treatment following injuries sustained in a motor vehicle accident and is also observed for suspected COVID-19 infection that is subsequently ruled out). Also,** when the principal diagnosis is required to be a code from category Z38, Liveborn infants according to place of birth and type of delivery, **then** a code form category Z05, Encounter for observation and evaluation of newborn for suspected diseases and conditions ruled out, is sequenced after the Z38 code. Additional codes may be used in addition to the observation code but only if they are unrelated to the suspected condition being observed.

Codes from subcategory Z03.7, Encounter for suspected maternal and fetal conditions ruled out, may either be used as a first-listed or as an additional code assignment depending on the case. They are for use in very limited circumstances on a maternal record when an encounter is for a suspected maternal or fetal condition that is ruled out during that encounter (for example, a maternal or fetal condition may be suspected due to an abnormal test result). These codes should not be used when the condition is confirmed. In those cases, the confirmed condition should be coded. In addition, these codes are not for use if an illness or any signs or symptoms related to the suspected condition or problem are present. In such cases the diagnosis/symptom code is used.

Additional codes may be used in addition to the code from subcategory Z03.7, but only if they are unrelated to the suspected condition being evaluated.

Codes from subcategory Z03.7 may not be used for encounters for antenatal screening of mother. *See Section I.C.21. Screening.*

For encounters for suspected fetal condition that are inconclusive following testing and evaluation, assign the appropriate code from category O35, O36, O40 or O41.

The observation Z code categories:

Z03	Encounter for medical observation for suspected diseases and conditions ruled out
Z04	Encounter for examination and observation for other reasons
	Except: Z04.9, Encounter for examination and observation for unspecified reason
Z05	Encounter for observation and evaluation of newborn for suspected diseases and conditions ruled out

7) Aftercare

Aftercare visit codes cover situations when the initial treatment of a disease has been performed and the patient requires continued care during the healing or recovery phase, or for the long-term consequences of the disease. The aftercare Z code should not be used if treatment is directed at a current, acute disease. The diagnosis code is to be used in these cases. Exceptions to this rule are codes Z51.0, Encounter for antineoplastic radiation therapy, and codes from subcategory Z51.1, Encounter for antineoplastic chemotherapy and immunotherapy. These codes are to be first-listed, followed by the diagnosis code when a patient's encounter is solely to receive radiation therapy, chemotherapy, or immunotherapy for the treatment of a neoplasm. If the reason for the encounter is more than one type of antineoplastic therapy, code Z51.0 and a code from subcategory Z51.1 may be assigned together, in which case one of these codes would be reported as a secondary diagnosis.

The aftercare Z codes should also not be used for aftercare for injuries. For aftercare of an injury, assign the acute injury code with the appropriate 7th character (for subsequent encounter).

The aftercare codes are generally first-listed to explain the specific reason for the encounter. An aftercare code may be used as an additional code when some type of aftercare is provided in addition to the reason for admission and no diagnosis code is applicable. An example of this would be the closure of a colostomy during an encounter for treatment of another condition.

Aftercare codes should be used in conjunction with other aftercare codes or diagnosis codes to provide better detail on the specifics of an aftercare encounter visit, unless otherwise directed by the classification. Should a patient receive multiple types of antineoplastic therapy during the same encounter, code Z51.0, Encounter for antineoplastic radiation therapy, and codes from subcategory Z51.1, Encounter for antineoplastic chemotherapy and immunotherapy, may be used together on a record. The sequencing of multiple aftercare codes depends on the circumstances of the encounter.

Certain aftercare Z code categories need a secondary diagnosis code to describe the resolving condition or sequelae. For others, the condition is included in the code title.

Additional Z code aftercare category terms include fitting and adjustment, and attention to artificial openings.

Status Z codes may be used with aftercare Z codes to indicate the nature of the aftercare. For example code Z95.1, Presence of aortocoronary bypass graft, may be used with code Z48.812, Encounter for surgical aftercare following surgery on the circulatory system, to indicate the surgery for which the aftercare is being performed. A status code should not be used when the aftercare code indicates the type of status, such as using Z43.0, Encounter for attention to tracheostomy, with Z93.0, Tracheostomy status.

The aftercare Z category/codes:

Z42	Encounter for plastic and reconstructive surgery following medical procedure or healed injury
Z43	Encounter for attention to artificial openings
Z44	Encounter for fitting and adjustment of external prosthetic device
Z45	Encounter for adjustment and management of implanted device
Z46	Encounter for fitting and adjustment of other devices
Z47	Orthopedic aftercare
Z48	Encounter for other postprocedural aftercare
Z49	Encounter for care involving renal dialysis
Z51	Encounter for other aftercare and medical care

8) Follow-up

The follow-up codes are used to explain continuing surveillance following completed treatment of a disease, condition, or injury. They imply that the condition has been fully treated and no longer exists. They should not be confused with aftercare codes, or injury codes with a 7th character for subsequent encounter, that explain ongoing care of a healing condition or its sequelae. Follow-up codes may be used in conjunction with history codes to provide the full picture of the healed condition and its treatment. The follow-up code is sequenced first, followed by the history code.

A follow-up code may be used to explain multiple visits. Should a condition be found to have recurred on the follow-up visit, then the diagnosis code for the condition should be assigned in place of the follow-up code.

The follow-up Z code categories:

Z08	Encounter for follow-up examination after completed treatment for malignant neoplasm
Z09	Encounter for follow-up examination after completed treatment for conditions other than malignant neoplasm
Z39	Encounter for maternal postpartum care and examination

9) Donor

Codes in category Z52, Donors of organs and tissues, are used for living individuals who are donating blood or other body tissue. These codes are only for individuals donating for others, not for self-donations. They are not used to identify cadaveric donations.

10) Counseling

Counseling Z codes are used when a patient or family member receives assistance in the aftermath of an illness or injury, or when support is required in coping with family or social problems.

The counseling Z codes/categories:

Z30.0-	Encounter for general counseling and advice on contraception
Z31.5	Encounter for procreative genetic counseling
Z31.6-	Encounter for general counseling and advice on procreation
Z32.2	Encounter for childbirth instruction
Z32.3	Encounter for childcare instruction
Z69	Encounter for mental health services for victim and perpetrator of abuse
Z70	Counseling related to sexual attitude, behavior and orientation

Z71   Persons encountering health services for other counseling and medical advice, not elsewhere classified

NOTE **Code Z71.84, Encounter for health counseling related to travel, is to be used for health risk and safety counseling for future travel purposes.**

Z76.81   Expectant mother prebirth pediatrician visit

11) Encounters for Obstetrical and Reproductive Services

See Section I.C.15. Pregnancy, Childbirth, and the Puerperium, for further instruction on the use of these codes.

Z codes for pregnancy are for use in those circumstances when none of the problems or complications included in the codes from the Obstetrics chapter exist (a routine prenatal visit or postpartum care). Codes in category Z34, Encounter for supervision of normal pregnancy, are always first-listed and are not to be used with any other code from the OB chapter.

Codes in category Z3A, Weeks of gestation, may be assigned to provide additional information about the pregnancy. Category Z3A codes should not be assigned for pregnancies with abortive outcomes (categories O00-O08), elective termination of pregnancy (code Z33.2), nor for postpartum conditions, as category Z3A is not applicable to these conditions. The date of the admission should be used to determine weeks of gestation for inpatient admissions that encompass more than one gestational week.

The outcome of delivery, category Z37, should be included on all maternal delivery records. It is always a secondary code. Codes in category Z37 should not be used on the newborn record.

Z codes for family planning (contraceptive) or procreative management and counseling should be included on an obstetric record either during the pregnancy or the postpartum stage, if applicable.

Z codes/categories for obstetrical and reproductive services:

Z30   Encounter for contraceptive management

Z31   Encounter for procreative management

Z32.2   Encounter for childbirth instruction

Z32.3   Encounter for childcare instruction

Z33   Pregnant state

Z34   Encounter for supervision of normal pregnancy

Z36   Encounter for antenatal screening of mother

Z3A   Weeks of gestation

Z37   Outcome of delivery

Z39   Encounter for maternal postpartum care and examination

Z76.81   Expectant mother prebirth pediatrician visit

12) Newborns and Infants

See Section I.C.16. Newborn (Perinatal) Guidelines, for further instruction on the use of these codes.

Newborn Z codes/categories:

Z76.1   Encounter for health supervision and care of foundling

Z00.1-   Encounter for routine child health examination

Z38   Liveborn infants according to place of birth and type of delivery

13) Routine and administrative examinations

The Z codes allow for the description of encounters for routine examinations, such as, a general check-up, or, examinations for administrative purposes, such as, a pre-employment physical. The codes are not to be used if the examination is for diagnosis of a suspected condition or for treatment purposes. In such cases the diagnosis code is used. During a routine exam, should a diagnosis or condition be discovered, it should be coded as an additional code. Pre-existing and chronic conditions and history codes may also be included as additional codes as long as the examination is for administrative purposes and not focused on any particular condition.

Some of the codes for routine health examinations distinguish between "with" and "without" abnormal findings. Code assignment depends on the information that is known at the time the encounter is being coded. For example, if no abnormal findings were found during the examination, but the encounter is being coded before test results are back, it is acceptable to assign the code for "without abnormal findings." When assigning a code for "with abnormal findings," additional code(s) should be assigned to identify the specific abnormal finding(s).

Pre-operative examination and pre-procedural laboratory examination Z codes are for use only in those situations when a patient is being cleared for a procedure or surgery and no treatment is given.

The Z codes/categories for routine and administrative examinations:

Z00   Encounter for general examination without complaint, suspected or reported diagnosis

Z01   Encounter for other special examination without complaint, suspected or reported diagnosis

Z02   Encounter for administrative examination

Except: Z02.9, Encounter for administrative examinations, unspecified

Z32.0-   Encounter for pregnancy test

14) Miscellaneous Z codes

The miscellaneous Z codes capture a number of other health care encounters that do not fall into one of the other categories. Certain of these codes identify the reason for the encounter; others are for use as additional codes that provide useful information on circumstances that may affect a patient's care and treatment.

Prophylactic Organ Removal

For encounters specifically for prophylactic removal of an organ (such as prophylactic removal of breasts due to a genetic susceptibility to cancer or a family history of cancer), the principal or first-listed code should be a code from category Z40, Encounter for prophylactic surgery, followed by the appropriate codes to identify the associated risk factor (such as genetic susceptibility or family history).

If the patient has a malignancy of one site and is having prophylactic removal at another site to prevent either a new primary malignancy or metastatic disease, a code for the malignancy should also be assigned in addition to a code from subcategory Z40.0, Encounter for prophylactic surgery for risk factors related to malignant neoplasms. A Z40.0 code should not be assigned if the patient is having organ removal for treatment of a malignancy, such as the removal of the testes for the treatment of prostate cancer.

Miscellaneous Z codes/categories:

Z28   Immunization not carried out

Except: Z28.3, Underimmunization status

Z29   Encounter for other prophylactic measures

Z40   Encounter for prophylactic surgery

Z41   Encounter for procedures for purposes other than remedying health state

Except: Z41.9, Encounter for procedure for purposes other than remedying health state, unspecified

Z53   Persons encountering health services for specific procedures and treatment, not carried out

Z55   Problems related to education and literacy

Z56   Problems related to employment and unemployment

Z57   Occupational exposure to risk factors

Z58   Problems related to physical environment

Z59   Problems related to housing and economic circumstances

Z60   Problems related to social environment

Z62   Problems related to upbringing

Z63   Other problems related to primary support group, including family circumstances

Z64   Problems related to certain psychosocial circumstances

Z65   Problems related to other psychosocial circumstances

Z72   Problems related to lifestyle

Note: These codes should be assigned only when the documentation specifies that the patient has an associated problem.

Z73   Problems related to life management difficulty

Z74   Problems related to care provider dependency

Except: Z74.01, Bed confinement status

Z75   Problems related to medical facilities and other health care

Z76.0   Encounter for issue of repeat prescription

Z76.3   Healthy person accompanying sick person

Z76.4   Other boarder to healthcare facility

Z76.5   Malingerer [conscious simulation]

Z91.1-   Patient's noncompliance with medical treatment and regimen

Z91.83   Wandering in diseases classified elsewhere

Z91.84-   Oral health risk factors

Z91.89   Other specified personal risk factors, not elsewhere classified

See Section I.B.14 for Z55-Z65 Persons with potential health hazards related to socioeconomic and psychosocial circumstances, documentation by clinicians other than the patient's provider.

15) Nonspecific Z codes

Certain Z codes are so non-specific, or potentially redundant with other codes in the classification, that there can be little justification for their use in the inpatient setting. Their use in the outpatient setting should be limited to those instances when there is no further documentation to permit more precise coding. Otherwise, any sign or symptom or any other reason for visit that is captured in another code should be used.

Nonspecific Z codes/categories:

Z02.9	Encounter for administrative examinations, unspecified
Z04.9	Encounter for examination and observation for unspecified reason
Z13.9	Encounter for screening, unspecified
Z41.9	Encounter for procedure for purposes other than remedying health state, unspecified
Z52.9	Donor of unspecified organ or tissue
Z86.59	Personal history of other mental and behavioral disorders
Z88.9	Allergy status to unspecified drugs, medicaments and biological substances status
Z92.0	Personal history of contraception

16) Z Codes That May Only be Principal/First-Listed Diagnosis

The following Z codes/categories may only be reported as the principal/first-listed diagnosis, except when there are multiple encounters on the same day and the medical records for the encounters are combined:

Z00	Encounter for general examination without complaint, suspected or reported diagnosis
	Except: Z00.6
Z01	Encounter for other special examination without complaint, suspected or reported diagnosis
Z02	Encounter for administrative examination
Z03	Encounter for medical observation for suspected diseases and conditions ruled out
Z04	Encounter for examination and observation for other reasons
Z33.2	Encounter for elective termination of pregnancy
Z31.81	Encounter for male factor infertility in female patient
Z31.83	Encounter for assisted reproductive fertility procedure cycle
Z31.84	Encounter for fertility preservation procedure
Z34	Encounter for supervision of normal pregnancy
Z39	Encounter for maternal postpartum care and examination
Z38	Liveborn infants according to place of birth and type of delivery
Z40	Encounter for prophylactic surgery
Z42	Encounter for plastic and reconstructive surgery following medical procedure or healed injury
Z51.0	Encounter for antineoplastic radiation therapy
Z51.1-	Encounter for antineoplastic chemotherapy and immunotherapy
Z52	Donors of organs and tissues
	Except: Z52.9, Donor of unspecified organ or tissue
Z76.1	Encounter for health supervision and care of foundling
Z76.2	Encounter for health supervision and care of other healthy infant and child
Z99.12	Encounter for respirator [ventilator] dependence during power failure

22. Chapter 22: Codes for Special Purposes (U00-U85)

U07.0   **Vaping-related disorder** (*see Section I.C.10.e, Vaping-related disorders*)

U07.1   **COVID-19** (*see Section I.C.1.g.1., COVID-19 infection*)

Section II. Selection of Principal Diagnosis

The circumstances of inpatient admission always govern the selection of principal diagnosis. The principal diagnosis is defined in the Uniform Hospital Discharge Data Set (UHDDS) as "that condition established after study to be chiefly responsible for occasioning the admission of the patient to the hospital for care."

The UHDDS definitions are used by hospitals to report inpatient data elements in a standardized manner. These data elements and their definitions can be found in the July 31, 1985, Federal Register (Vol. 50, No, 147), pp. 31038–40.

Since that time the application of the UHDDS definitions has been expanded to include all non-outpatient settings (acute care, short term, long term care and psychiatric hospitals; home health agencies; rehab facilities; nursing homes, etc). The UHDDS definitions also apply to hospice services (all levels of care).

In determining principal diagnosis, coding conventions in the ICD-10-CM, the Tabular List and Alphabetic Index take precedence over these official coding guidelines.

(See Section I.A., Conventions for the ICD-10-CM)

The importance of consistent, complete documentation in the medical record cannot be overemphasized. Without such documentation the application of all coding guidelines is a difficult, if not impossible, task.

A. Codes for Symptoms, Signs, and Ill-Defined Conditions

Codes for symptoms, signs, and ill-defined conditions from Chapter 18 are not to be used as principal diagnosis when a related definitive diagnosis has been established.

B. Two or More Interrelated Conditions, Each Potentially Meeting the Definition for Principal Diagnosis

When there are two or more interrelated conditions (such as diseases in the same ICD-10-CM chapter or manifestations characteristically associated with a certain disease) potentially meeting the definition of principal diagnosis, either condition may be sequenced first, unless the circumstances of the admission, the therapy provided, the Tabular List, or the Alphabetic Index indicate otherwise.

C. Two or More Diagnoses that Equally Meet the Definition for Principal Diagnosis

In the unusual instance when two or more diagnoses equally meet the criteria for principal diagnosis as determined by the circumstances of admission, diagnostic workup and/or therapy provided, and the Alphabetic Index, Tabular List, or another coding guidelines does not provide sequencing direction, any one of the diagnoses may be sequenced first.

D. Two or More Comparative or Contrasting Conditions

In those rare instances when two or more contrasting or comparative diagnoses are documented as "either/or" (or similar terminology), they are coded as if the diagnoses were confirmed and the diagnoses are sequenced according to the circumstances of the admission. If no further determination can be made as to which diagnosis should be principal, either diagnosis may be sequenced first.

E. A Symptom(s) Followed by Contrasting/Comparative Diagnoses

GUIDELINE HAS BEEN DELETED EFFECTIVE OCTOBER 1, 2014.

F. Original Treatment Plan not Carried out

Sequence as the principal diagnosis the condition, which after study occasioned the admission to the hospital, even though treatment may not have been carried out due to unforeseen circumstances.

G. Complications of Surgery and Other Medical Care

When the admission is for treatment of a complication resulting from surgery or other medical care, the complication code is sequenced as the principal diagnosis. If the complication is classified to the T80–T88 series and the code lacks the necessary specificity in describing the complication, an additional code for the specific complication should be assigned.

H. Uncertain Diagnosis

If the diagnosis documented at the time of discharge is qualified as "probable", "suspected", "likely", "questionable", "possible", or "still to be ruled out," "compatible with," "consistent with," or other similar terms indicating uncertainty, code the condition as if it existed or was established. The bases for these guidelines are the diagnostic workup, arrangements for further workup or observation, and initial therapeutic approach that correspond most closely with the established diagnosis.

Note: This guideline is applicable only to inpatient admissions to short-term, acute, long-term care and psychiatric hospitals.

I. Admission from Observation Unit

1. Admission Following Medical Observation

When a patient is admitted to an observation unit for a medical condition, which either worsens or does not improve, and is subsequently admitted as an inpatient of the same hospital for this same medical condition, the principal diagnosis would be the medical condition which led to the hospital admission.

2. Admission Following Post-Operative Observation

When a patient is admitted to an observation unit to monitor a condition (or complication) that develops following outpatient surgery, and then is subsequently admitted as an inpatient of the same hospital, hospitals should apply the Uniform Hospital Discharge Data Set (UHDDS) definition of principal diagnosis as "that condition established after study to be chiefly responsible for occasioning the admission of the patient to the hospital for care."

J. Admission from Outpatient Surgery

When a patient receives surgery in the hospital's outpatient surgery department and is subsequently admitted for continuing inpatient care at the same hospital, the following guidelines should be followed in selecting the principal diagnosis for the inpatient admission:

- If the reason for the inpatient admission is a complication, assign the complication as the principal diagnosis.

- If no complication, or other condition, is documented as the reason for the inpatient admission, assign the reason for the outpatient surgery as the principal diagnosis.

- If the reason for the inpatient admission is another condition unrelated to the surgery, assign the unrelated condition as the principal diagnosis.

K. Admissions/Encounters for Rehabilitation

When the purpose for the admission/encounter is rehabilitation, sequence first the code for the condition for which the service is being performed. For example, for an admission/encounter for rehabilitation for rightsided dominant hemiplegia following a cerebrovascular infarction, report code I69.351, Hemiplegia and hemiparesis following cerebral infarction affecting right dominant side, as the first-listed or principal diagnosis.

If the condition for which the rehabilitation service is being provided is no longer present, report the appropriate aftercare code as the first-listed or principal diagnosis, unless the rehabilitation service is being provided following an injury. For rehabilitation services following active treatment of an injury, assign the injury code with the appropriate seventh character for subsequent encounter as the first-listed or principal diagnosis. For example, if a patient with severe degenerative osteoarthritis of the hip, underwent hip replacement and the current encounter/admission is for rehabilitation, report code Z47.1, Aftercare following joint replacement surgery, as the first-listed or principal diagnosis. If the patient requires rehabilitation post hip replacement for right intertrochanteric femur fracture, report code S72.141D, Displaced intertrochanteric fracture of right femur, subsequent encounter for closed fracture with routine healing, as the first-listed or principal diagnosis.

See Section I.C.21.c.7, Factors influencing health states and contact with health services, Aftercare.
See Section I.C.19.a for additional information about the use of 7th characters for injury codes.

Section III. Reporting Additional Diagnoses

GENERAL RULES FOR OTHER (ADDITIONAL) DIAGNOSES

For reporting purposes the definition for "other diagnoses" is interpreted as additional conditions that affect patient care in terms of requiring:

- clinical evaluation; or
- therapeutic treatment; or
- diagnostic procedures; or
- extended length of hospital stay; or
- increased nursing care and/or
- monitoring

The UHDDS item #11-b defines Other Diagnoses as "all conditions that coexist at the time of admission, that develop subsequently, or that affect the treatment received and/or the length of stay. Diagnoses that relate to an earlier episode which have no bearing on the current hospital stay are to be excluded." UHDDS definitions apply to inpatients in acute-care, short-term, long term care and psychiatric hospital setting. The UHDDS definitions are used by acute-care shortterm hospitals to report inpatient data elements in a standardized manner. These data elements and their definitions can be found in the July 31, 1985, *Federal Register* (Vol. 50, No, 147), pp. 31038–40.

Since that time the application of the UHDDS definitions has been expanded to include all nonoutpatient settings (acute-care, short-term, long-term care and psychiatric hospitals; home health agencies; rehab facilities; nursing homes, etc). The UHDDS definitions also apply to hospice services (all levels of care).

The following guidelines are to be applied in designating "other diagnoses" when neither the Alphabetic Index nor the Tabular List in ICD-10-CM provide direction. The listing of the diagnoses in the patient record is the responsibility of the attending provider.

A. Previous Conditions

If the provider has included a diagnosis in the final diagnostic statement, such as the discharge summary or the face sheet, it should ordinarily be coded. Some providers include in the diagnostic statement resolved conditions or diagnoses and status-post procedures from previous admission that have no bearing on the current stay. Such conditions are not to be reported and are coded only if required by hospital policy.

However, history codes (categories Z80–Z87) may be used as secondary codes if the historical condition or family history has an impact on current care or influences treatment.

B. Abnormal Findings

Abnormal findings (laboratory, x-ray, pathologic, and other diagnostic results) are not coded and reported unless the provider indicates their clinical significance. If the findings are outside the normal range and the attending provider has ordered other tests to evaluate the condition or prescribed treatment, it is appropriate to ask the provider whether the abnormal finding should be added.

Please note: This differs from the coding practices in the outpatient setting for coding encounters for diagnostic tests that have been interpreted by a provider.

C. Uncertain Diagnosis

If the diagnosis documented at the time of discharge is qualified as "probable", "suspected", "likely", "questionable", "possible", or "still to be ruled out," "compatible with," "consistent with," or other similar terms indicating uncertainty, code the condition as if it existed or was established. The bases for these guidelines are the diagnostic workup, arrangements for further workup or observation, and initial therapeutic approach that correspond most closely with the established diagnosis.

Note: This guideline is applicable only to inpatient admissions to short-term, acute-care, long-term care and psychiatric hospitals.

Section IV. Diagnostic Coding and Reporting Guidelines for Outpatient Services

These coding guidelines for outpatient diagnoses have been approved for use by hospitals/ providers in coding and reporting hospital-based outpatient services and provider-based office visits. Guidelines in Section I, Conventions, general coding guidelines and chapter-specific guidelines, should also be applied for outpatient services and office visits.

Information about the use of certain abbreviations, punctuation, symbols, and other conventions used in the ICD-10-CM Tabular List (code numbers and titles), can be found in Section IA of these guidelines, under "Conventions Used in the Tabular List." Section I.B. contains general guidelines that apply to the entire classification. Section I.C. contains chapter-specific guidelines that correspond to the chapters as they are arranged in the classification. Information about the correct sequence to use in finding a code is also described in Section I.

The terms encounter and visit are often used interchangeably in describing outpatient service contacts and, therefore, appear together in these guidelines without distinguishing one from the other.

Though the conventions and general guidelines apply to all settings, coding guidelines for outpatient and provider reporting of diagnoses will vary in a number of instances from those for inpatient diagnoses, recognizing that:

The Uniform Hospital Discharge Data Set (UHDDS) definition of principal diagnosis does not apply to hospital-based outpatient services and provider-based office visits.

Coding guidelines for inconclusive diagnoses (probable, suspected, rule out, etc.) were developed for inpatient reporting and do not apply to outpatients.

A. Selection of First-Listed Condition

In the outpatient setting, the term first-listed diagnosis is used in lieu of principal diagnosis.

In determining the first-listed diagnosis the coding conventions of ICD-10-CM, as well as the general and disease specific guidelines take precedence over the outpatient guidelines.

Diagnoses often are not established at the time of the initial encounter/visit. It may take two or more visits before the diagnosis is confirmed.

The most critical rule involves beginning the search for the correct code assignment through the Alphabetic Index. Never begin searching initially in the Tabular List as this will lead to coding errors.

1. Outpatient Surgery

When a patient presents for outpatient surgery (same day surgery), code the reason for the surgery as the first-listed diagnosis (reason for the encounter), even if the surgery is not performed due to a contraindication.

2. Observation Stay

When a patient is admitted for observation for a medical condition, assign a code for the medical condition as the first-listed diagnosis.

When a patient presents for outpatient surgery and develops complications requiring admission to observation, code the reason for the surgery as the first reported diagnosis (reason for the encounter), followed by codes for the complications as secondary diagnoses.

B. Codes from A00.0–T88.9, Z00–Z99

The appropriate code(s) from A00.0–T88.9, Z00–Z99 must be used to identify diagnoses, symptoms, conditions, problems, complaints, or other reason(s) for the encounter/visit.

C. Accurate Reporting of ICD-10-CM Diagnosis Codes

For accurate reporting of ICD-10-CM diagnosis codes, the documentation should describe the patient's condition, using terminology which includes specific diagnoses as well as symptoms, problems, or reasons for the encounter. There are ICD-10-CM codes to describe all of these.

D. Codes that Describe Symptoms and Signs

Codes that describe symptoms and signs, as opposed to diagnoses, are acceptable for reporting purposes when a diagnosis has not been established (confirmed) by the provider. Chapter 18 of ICD-10-CM, Symptoms, Signs, and Abnormal Clinical, and Laboratory Findings Not Elsewhere Classified (codes R00–R99) contain many, but not all codes for symptoms.

E. Encounters for Circumstances Other than a Disease or Injury

ICD-10-CM provides codes to deal with encounters for circumstances other than a disease or injury. The Factors Influencing Health Status and Contact with Health Services codes (Z00–Z99) are provided to deal with occasions when circumstances other than a disease or injury are recorded as diagnosis or problems.
See Section I.C.21. Factors influencing health status and contact with health services.

F. Level of Detail in Coding

1. ICD-10-CM Codes with 3, 4, 5, 6, Or 7 Characters
ICD-10-CM is composed of codes with 3, 4, 5, 6, or 7 characters. Codes with three characters are included in ICD-10-CM as the heading of a category of codes that may be further subdivided by the use of fourth, fifth, sixth, or seventh characters to provide greater specificity.

2. Use of Full Number of Characters Required for a Code
A three-character code is to be used only if it is not further subdivided. A code is invalid if it has not been coded to the full number of characters required for that code, including the 7th character, if applicable.

G. ICD-10-CM Code for the Diagnosis, Condition, Problem, or Other Reason for Encounter/Visit

List first the ICD-10-CM code for the diagnosis, condition, problem, or other reason for encounter/visit shown in the medical record to be chiefly responsible for the services provided. List additional codes that describe any coexisting conditions. In some cases the first-listed diagnosis may be a symptom when a diagnosis has not been established (confirmed) by the provider.

H. Uncertain Diagnosis

Do not code diagnoses documented as "probable", "suspected," "questionable," "rule out," "compatible with," "consistent with," or "working diagnosis" or other similar terms indicating uncertainty. Rather, code the condition(s) to the highest degree of certainty for that encounter/visit, such as symptoms, signs, abnormal test results, or other reason for the visit.

Please note: This differs from the coding practices used by short-term, acute-care, long-term care and psychiatric hospitals.

I. Chronic Diseases

Chronic diseases treated on an ongoing basis may be coded and reported as many times as the patient receives treatment and care for the condition(s).

J. Code All Documented Conditions that Coexist

Code all documented conditions that coexist at the time of the encounter/visit, and require or affect patient care treatment or management. Do not code conditions that were previously treated and no longer exist. However, history codes (categories Z80–Z87) may be used as secondary codes if the historical condition or family history has an impact on current care or influences treatment.

K. Patients Receiving Diagnostic Services Only

For patients receiving diagnostic services only during an encounter/visit, sequence first the diagnosis, condition, problem, or other reason for encounter/visit shown in the medical record to be chiefly responsible for the outpatient services provided during the encounter/visit. Codes for other diagnoses (e.g., chronic conditions) may be sequenced as additional diagnoses.

For encounters for routine laboratory/radiology testing in the absence of any signs, symptoms, or associated diagnosis, assign Z01.89, Encounter for other specified special examinations. If routine testing is performed during the same encounter as a test to evaluate a sign, symptom, or diagnosis, it is appropriate to assign both the Z code and the code describing the reason for the non-routine test.

For outpatient encounters for diagnostic tests that have been interpreted by a physician, and the final report is available at the time of coding, code any confirmed or definitive diagnosis(es) documented in the interpretation. Do not code related signs and symptoms as additional diagnoses.

Please note: This differs from the coding practice in the hospital inpatient setting regarding abnormal findings on test results.

L. Patients Receiving Therapeutic Services Only

For patients receiving therapeutic services only during an encounter/visit, sequence first the diagnosis, condition, problem, or other reason for encounter/visit shown in the medical record to be chiefly responsible for the outpatient services provided during the encounter/visit. Codes for other diagnoses (e.g., chronic conditions) may be sequenced as additional diagnoses.

The only exception to this rule is that when the primary reason for the admission/encounter is chemotherapy or radiation therapy, the appropriate Z code for the service is listed first, and the diagnosis or problem for which the service is being performed listed second.

M. Patients Receiving Preoperative Evaluations Only

For patients receiving preoperative evaluations only, sequence first a code from subcategory Z01.81, Encounter for pre-procedural examinations, to describe the pre-op consultations. Assign a code for the condition to describe the reason for the surgery as an additional diagnosis. Code also any findings related to the pre-op evaluation.

N. Ambulatory Surgery

For ambulatory surgery, code the diagnosis for which the surgery was performed. If the postoperative diagnosis is known to be different from the preoperative diagnosis at the time the diagnosis is confirmed, select the postoperative diagnosis for coding, since it is the most definitive.

O. Routine Outpatient Prenatal Visits

See Section I.C.15. Routine outpatient prenatal visits.

P. Encounters for General Medical Examinations with Abnormal Findings

The subcategories for encounters for general medical examinations, Z00.0- and encounter for routine child health examination, Z00.12-, provide codes for with and without abnormal findings. Should a general medical examination result in an abnormal finding, the code for general medical examination with abnormal finding should be assigned as the first-listed diagnosis. An examination with abnormal findings refers to a condition/diagnosis that is newly identified or a change in severity of a chronic condition (such as uncontrolled hypertension, or an acute exacerbation of chronic obstructive pulmonary disease) during a routine physical examination. A secondary code for the abnormal finding should also be coded.

Q. Encounters for Routine Health Screenings

See Section I.C.21. Factors influencing health status and contact with health services, Screening

Appendix I. Present on Admission Reporting Guidelines

Introduction

These guidelines are to be used as a supplement to the *ICD-10-CM Official Guidelines for Coding and Reporting* to facilitate the assignment of the Present on Admission (POA) indicator for each diagnosis and external cause of injury code reported on claim forms (UB-04 and 837 Institutional).

These guidelines are not intended to replace any guidelines in the main body of the *ICD-10-CM Official Guidelines for Coding and Reporting*. The POA guidelines are not intended to provide guidance on when a condition should be coded, but rather, how to apply the POA indicator to the final set of diagnosis codes that have been assigned in accordance with Sections I, II, and III of the official coding guidelines. Subsequent to the assignment of the ICD-10-CM codes, the POA indicator should then be assigned to those conditions that have been coded.

As stated in the Introduction to the ICD-10-CM Official Guidelines for Coding and Reporting, a joint effort between the healthcare provider and the coder is essential to achieve complete and accurate documentation, code assignment, and reporting of diagnoses and procedures. The importance of consistent, complete documentation in the medical record cannot be overemphasized. Medical record documentation from any provider involved in the care and treatment of the patient may be used to support the determination of whether a condition was present on admission or not. In the context of the official coding guidelines, the term "provider" means a physician or any qualified healthcare practitioner who is legally accountable for establishing the patient's diagnosis.

These guidelines are not a substitute for the provider's clinical judgment as to the determination of whether a condition was or was not present on admission. The provider should be queried regarding issues related to the linking of signs/symptoms, timing of test results, and the timing of findings.

Please see the CDC website for the detailed list of ICD-10-CM codes that do not require the use of a POA indicator (https://www.cdc.gov/nchs/icd/icd10cm.htm). The codes and categories on this exempt list are for circumstances regarding the healthcare encounter or factors influencing health status that do not represent a current disease or injury or that describe conditions that are always present on admission.

General Reporting Requirements

All claims involving inpatient admissions to general acute-care hospitals or other facilities that are subject to a law or regulation mandating collection of present on admission information.

Present on admission is defined as present at the time the order for inpatient admission occurs—conditions that develop during an outpatient encounter, including emergency department, observation, or outpatient surgery, are considered as present on admission.

POA indicator is assigned to principal and secondary diagnoses (as defined in Section II of the Official Guidelines for Coding and Reporting) and the external cause of injury codes.

Issues related to inconsistent, missing, conflicting or unclear documentation must still be resolved by the provider.

If a condition would not be coded and reported based on UHDDS definitions and current official coding guidelines, then the POA indicator would not be reported.

Reporting Options

    Y—Yes
    N—No
    U—Unknown
    W—Clinically undetermined
    Unreported/Not used—(Exempt from POA reporting)

Reporting Definitions

    Y = present at the time of inpatient admission
    N = not present at the time of inpatient admission
    U = documentation is insufficient to determine if condition is present on admission
    W = provider is unable to clinically determine whether condition was present on admission or not

Timeframe for POA Identification and Documentation

There is no required timeframe as to when a provider (per the definition of "provider" used in these guidelines) must identify or document a condition to be present on admission. In some clinical situations, it may not be possible for a provider to make a definitive diagnosis (or a condition may not be recognized or reported by the patient) for a period of time after admission. In some cases it may be several days before the provider arrives at a definitive diagnosis. This does not mean that the condition was not present on admission. Determination of whether the condition was present on admission or not will be based on the applicable POA guideline as identified in this document, or on the provider's best clinical judgment.

If at the time of code assignment the documentation is unclear as to whether a condition was present on admission or not, it is appropriate to query the provider for clarification.

Assigning the POA Indicator

Condition is on the "Exempt from Reporting" list
Leave the "present on admission" field blank if the condition is on the list of ICD-10-CM codes for which this field is not applicable. This is the only circumstance in which the field may be left blank.

POA Explicitly Documented
Assign "Y" for any condition the provider explicitly documents as being present on admission.

Assign "N" for any condition the provider explicitly documents as not present at the time of admission.

Conditions diagnosed prior to inpatient admission
Assign "Y" for conditions that were diagnosed prior to admission (example: hypertension, diabetes mellitus, asthma)

Conditions diagnosed during the admission but clearly present before admission
Assign "Y" for conditions diagnosed during the admission that were clearly present but not diagnosed until after admission occurred.

Diagnoses subsequently confirmed after admission are considered present on admission if at the time of admission they are documented as suspected, possible, rule out, differential diagnosis, or constitute an underlying cause of a symptom that is present at the time of admission.

Condition develops during outpatient encounter prior to inpatient admission
Assign "Y" for any condition that develops during an outpatient encounter prior to a written order for inpatient admission.

Documentation does not indicate whether condition was present on admission
Assign "U" when the medical record documentation is unclear as to whether the condition was present on admission. "U" should not be routinely assigned and used only in very limited circumstances. Coders are encouraged to query the providers when the documentation is unclear.

Documentation states that it cannot be determined whether the condition was or was not present on admission
Assign "W" when the medical record documentation indicates that it cannot be clinically determined whether or not the condition was present on admission.

Chronic condition with acute exacerbation during the admission
If a single code identifies both the chronic condition and the acute exacerbation, see POA guidelines pertaining to codes that contain multiple clinical concepts.

If a single code only identifies the chronic condition and not the acute exacerbation (e.g., acute exacerbation of chronic leukemia), assign "Y."

Conditions documented as possible, probable, suspected, or rule out at the time of discharge

If the final diagnosis contains a possible, probable, suspected, or rule out diagnosis, and this diagnosis was based on signs, symptoms or clinical findings suspected at the time of inpatient admission, assign "Y."

If the final diagnosis contains a possible, probable, suspected, or rule out diagnosis, and this diagnosis was based on signs, symptoms or clinical findings that were not present on admission, assign "N".

Conditions documented as impending or threatened at the time of discharge

If the final diagnosis contains an impending or threatened diagnosis, and this diagnosis is based on symptoms or clinical findings that were present on admission, assign "Y".

If the final diagnosis contains an impending or threatened diagnosis, and this diagnosis is based on symptoms or clinical findings that were not present on admission, assign "N".

Acute and Chronic Conditions

Assign "Y" for acute conditions that are present at time of admission and N for acute conditions that are not present at time of admission.

Assign "Y" for chronic conditions, even though the condition may not be diagnosed until after admission.

If a single code identifies both an acute and chronic condition, see the POA guidelines for codes that contain multiple clinical concepts.

Codes That Contain Multiple Clinical Concepts

Assign "N" if at least one of the clinical concepts included in the code was not present on admission (e.g., COPD with acute exacerbation and the exacerbation was not present on admission; gastric ulcer that does not start bleeding until after admission; asthma patient develops status asthmaticus after admission)

Assign "Y" if all parts of the clinical concepts included in the code were present on admission (e.g., duodenal ulcer that perforates prior to admission)

For infection codes that include the causal organism, assign "Y" if the infection (or signs of the infection) were present on admission, even though the culture results may not be known until after admission (e.g., patient is admitted with pneumonia and the provider documents pseudomonas as the causal organism a few days later).

Same Diagnosis Code for Two or More Conditions

When the same ICD-10-CM diagnosis code applies to two or more conditions during the same encounter (e.g. two separate conditions classified to the same ICD-10-CM diagnosis code):

Assign "Y" if all conditions represented by the single ICD-10-CM code were present on admission (e.g. bilateral unspecified age-related cataracts).

Assign "N" if any of the conditions represented by the single ICD-10-CM code was not present on admission (e.g. traumatic secondary and recurrent hemorrhage and seroma is assigned to a single code T79.2, but only one of the conditions was present on admission).

Obstetrical Conditions

Whether or not the patient delivers during the current hospitalization does not affect assignment of the POA indicator.
The determining factor for POA assignment is whether the pregnancy complication or obstetrical condition described by the code was present at the time of admission or not.

If the pregnancy complication or obstetrical condition was present on admission (e.g., patient admitted in preterm labor), assign "Y".

If the pregnancy complication or obstetrical condition was not present on admission (e.g., 2nd degree laceration during delivery, postpartum hemorrhage that occurred during current hospitalization, fetal distress develops after admission), assign "N".

If the obstetrical code includes more than one diagnosis and any of the diagnoses identified by the code were not present on admission assign "N" (e.g., Category O11, Pre-existing hypertension with pre-eclampsia).

Perinatal Conditions

Newborns are not considered to be admitted until after birth. Therefore, any condition present at birth or that developed in utero is considered present at admission and should be assigned "Y". This includes conditions that occur during delivery (e.g., injury during delivery, meconium aspiration, exposure to streptococcus B in the vaginal canal).

Congenital Conditions and Anomalies

Assign "Y" for congenital conditions and anomalies except for categories Q00–Q99, Congenital anomalies, which are on the exempt list. Congenital conditions are always considered present on admission.

External Cause of Injury Codes

Assign "Y" for any external cause code representing an external cause of morbidity that occurred prior to inpatient admission (e.g., patient fell out of bed at home, patient fell out of bed in emergency room prior to admission).

Assign "N" for any external cause code representing an external cause of morbidity that occurred during inpatient hospitalization (e.g., patient fell out of hospital bed during hospital stay, patient experienced an adverse reaction to a medication administered after inpatient admission).

> **Consulting Editor's Note**
>
> The Official Coding Guidelines Appendix I, Present on Admission Reporting Guidelines, no longer provides a listing of Present on Admission (POA) exempt codes by category/sub-category. Instead interested parties can view a full list of the POA exempt code list via the National Center for Health Statistics webpage.
>
> Here we are providing an updated 2021 POA exempt code list by category/sub-category to be used as a reference guide for the users of this code book. Users, including educators, can use this list to provide examples of the types of codes included on the POA exempt code list.

B90–B94	Sequelae of infectious and parasitic diseases
E64	Sequelae of malnutrition and other nutritional deficiencies
I25.2	Old myocardial infarction
I69	Sequelae of cerebrovascular disease
M84.7	Nontraumatic fracture, NEC (excluding codes ending in 7th character A)
M97	Periprosthetic fracture around internal prosthetic joint (excluding codes ending in 7th character A)
O09	Supervision of high risk pregnancy
O66.5	Attempted application of vacuum extractor and forceps
O80	Encounter for full-term uncomplicated delivery
O94	Sequelae of complication of pregnancy, childbirth, and the puerperium
P00	Newborn affected by maternal conditions that may be unrelated to present pregnancy
P29.3	Persistent fetal circulation
P78.84	Gestational alloimmune liver disease
P83.8	Other specified conditions of integument specific to newborn
P91.81	Neonatal encephalopathy
P91.82-	Neonatal cerebral infarction
P91.88	Other specified disturbances of cerebral status of newborn
Q00–Q99	Congenital malformations, deformations and chromosomal abnormalities
S00–T88.9	Injury, poisoning and certain other consequences of external causes with 7th character representing subsequent encounter or sequela
V00–V09	Pedestrian injured in transport accident
	Except V00.81-, Accident with wheelchair (powered)
	V00.83-, Accident with motorized mobility scooter
V10–V19	Pedal cycle rider injured in transport accident
V20–V29	Motorcycle rider injured in transport accident
V30–V39	Occupant of three-wheeled motor vehicle injured in transport accident
V40–V49	Car occupant injured in transport accident
V50–V59	Occupant of pick-up truck or van injured in transport accident
V60–V69	Occupant of heavy transport vehicle injured in transport accident
V70–V79	Bus occupant injured in transport accident
V80–V89	Other land transport accidents
V90–V94	Water transport accidents
V95–V97	Air and space transport accidents
V98–V99	Other and unspecified transport accidents
W09	Fall on and from playground equipment (except codes ending in 7th character A)
W14	Fall from tree
W15	Fall from cliff
W16	Fall, jump or diving into water (excluding codes that end in 7th character A)

W17.0	Fall into well
W17.1	Fall into storm drain or manhole
W17.3	Fall into empty swimming pool
W17.4	Fall from dock
W17.8	Other fall from one level to another
W18.00	Striking against unspecified object with subsequent fall (excluding codes ending in 7th character A)
W18.01	Striking against sports equipment with subsequent fall
W18.02	Striking against glass with subsequent fall (except codes ending in 7th character A)
W18.09	Striking against other object with subsequent fall (except codes ending in 7th character A)
W18.1	Fall from or off toilet (except codes ending in 7th character A)
W18.2	Fall in (into) shower or empty bathtub (except codes ending in 7th character A)
W18.3	Other and unspecified fall on same level (except codes ending in 7th character A)
W18.4	Slipping, tripping and stumbling without falling (except codes ending in 7th character A)
W21	Striking against or struck by sports equipment
W22.01	Walked into wall (except codes ending in 7th character A)
W22.02	Walked into lamppost
W22.03	Walked into furniture (except codes ending in 7th character A)
W22.04	Striking against wall of swimming pool (except codes ending in 7th character A)
W22.09	Striking against other stationary object (except codes ending in 7th character A)
W22.1	Striking against or struck by automobile airbag
W22.8	Striking against or struck by other objects
W24.0	Contact with lifting devices, not elsewhere classified (except codes ending in 7th character A)
W24.1	Contact with transmission devices, NEC
W26.1–W26.9	Contact with knife, sword or dagger
W27.0	Contact with workbench
W27.1	Contact with garden tool
W27.2	Contact with scissors (except codes ending in 7th character A)
W27.3	Contact with needle (except codes ending in 7th character A)
W27.4	Contact with kitchen utensil (except codes ending in 7th character A)
W27.5	Contact with paper-cutter (except codes ending in 7th character A)
W27.8	Contact with other nonpowered hand tool
W28	Contact with powered lawn mower
W29	Contact with other powered hand tools and household machinery
W30	Contact with agricultural machinery
W31	Contact with other and unspecified machinery
W32–W34	Accidental handgun discharge and malfunction
W35–W40	Exposure to inanimate mechanical forces
W42.0	Exposure to supersonic waves
W42.9	Exposure to other noise (except codes ending in 7th character A)
W45.0	Nail entering through skin
W49	Exposure to other inanimate mechanical forces (except codes ending in 7th character A)
W52	Crushed, pushed or stepped on by crowd or human stampede
W53	Contact with rodent
W54	Contact with dog
W55	Contact with other mammals
W56	Contact with nonvenomous marine animal

W57	Bitten or stung by nonvenomous insect and other nonvenomous arthropods (except codes ending in 7th character A)
W58	Contact with crocodile or alligator
W59.01	Bitten by nonvenomous lizards (except codes ending in 7th character A)
W59.02–W59.8	Contact with other nonvenomous reptiles
W60	Contact with nonvenomous plant thorns and spines and sharp leaves
W61	Contact with birds (domestic) (wild)
W62	Contact with nonvenomous amphibians
W64	Exposure to other animate mechanical forces
W65	Accidental drowning and submersion while in bath-tub (except codes ending in 7th character A)
W67	Accidental drowning and submersion while in swimming pool (except codes ending in 7th character A)
W69	Accidental drowning and submersion while in natural water
W73	Other specified cause of accidental non-transport drowning and submersion
W74	Unspecified cause of accidental drowning and submersion
W85	Exposure to electric transmission lines (except codes ending in 7th character A)
W86	Exposure to other specified electric current (except codes ending in 7th character A)
W88	Exposure to ionizing radiation (except codes ending in 7th character A)
W89	Exposure to man-made visible and ultraviolet light
W90	Exposure to other nonionizing radiation (except codes ending in 7th character A)
W92	Exposure to excessive heat of man-made origin
W93	Exposure to excessive cold of man-made origin
W94	Exposure to high and low air pressure and changes in air pressure
W99	Exposure to other man-made environmental factors
X02	Exposure to controlled fire in building or structure (except codes ending in 7th character A)
X03	Exposure to controlled fire, not in building or structure (except codes ending in 7th character A)
X04	Exposure to ignition of highly flammable material
X30	Exposure to excessive natural heat
X31	Exposure to excessive natural cold
X32	Exposure to sunlight
X34	Earthquake (except codes ending in 7th character A)
X35	Volcanic eruption
X36	Avalanche, landslide and other earth movements (except codes ending in 7th character A)
X37	Cataclysmic storm (except codes ending in 7th character A)
X38	Flood (except codes ending in 7th character A)
X39	Exposure to other forces of nature
X50	Overexertion and strenuous or repetitive movements
X52	Prolonged stay in weightless environment
X71	Intentional self-harm by drowning and submersion (except codes ending in 7th character A)
	Except X71.0-, Intentional self-harm by drowning and submersion while in bath tub
X72	Intentional self-harm by handgun discharge
X73	Intentional self-harm by rifle, shotgun and larger firearm discharge
X74	Intentional self-harm by other and unspecified firearm and gun discharge
X75	Intentional self-harm by explosive material
X76	Intentional self-harm by smoke, fire and flames
X77	Intentional self-harm by steam, hot vapors and hot objects
X81	Intentional self-harm by jumping or lying in front of moving object
X82	Intentional self-harm by crashing of motor vehicle

X83	Intentional self-harm by other specified means
X92	Assault by drowning and submersion (except codes ending in 7th character A)
X93	Assault by handgun discharge (except codes ending in 7th character A)
X94	Assault by rifle, shotgun and larger firearm discharge (except codes ending in 7th character A)
X95	Assault by other and unspecified firearm and gun discharge (except codes ending in 7th character A)
X96	Assault by explosive material (except codes ending in 7th character A)
X97	Assault by smoke, fire and flames (except codes ending in 7th character A)
X98	Assault by steam, hot vapors and hot objects (except codes ending in 7th character A)
X99	Assault by sharp object (except codes ending in 7th character A)
Y00	Assault by blunt object (except codes ending in 7th character A)
Y01	Assault by pushing from high place (except codes ending in 7th character A)
Y02	Assault by pushing or placing victim in front of moving object
Y03	Assault by crashing of motor vehicle
Y04	Assault by bodily force (except codes ending in 7th character A)
Y07	Perpetrator of assault, maltreatment and neglect
Y08	Assault by other specified means
Y21	Drowning and submersion, undetermined intent
Y22	Handgun discharge, undetermined intent (except codes ending in 7th character A)
Y23	Rifle, shotgun and larger firearm discharge, undetermined intent (except codes ending in 7th character A)
Y24	Other and unspecified firearm discharge, undetermined intent (except Y24.9, Unspecified firearm discharge, undetermined intent, initial encounter)
Y30	Falling, jumping or pushed from a high place, undetermined intent
Y32	Assault by crashing of motor vehicle, undetermined intent
Y35	Legal intervention (except codes ending in 7th character A)
Y36	Operations of war
Y37	Military operations
Y38	Terrorism (except codes ending in 7th character A)
Y92	Place of occurrence of the external cause (except Y92.23-, Y92.530 and Y92.538)
Y93.12–Y93.9	Activity code
Y99	External cause status
Z00	Encounter for general examination without complaint, suspected or reported diagnosis
Z01	Encounter for other special examination without complaint, suspected or reported diagnosis
Z02	Encounter for administrative examination
Z03	Encounter for medical observation for suspected diseases and conditions ruled out
Z04.8-	Encounter for examination and observation for other specified reasons
Z05	Encounter for observation and evaluation of newborn for suspected diseases and conditions ruled out
Z08	Encounter for follow-up examination following completed treatment for malignant neoplasm
Z09	Encounter for follow-up examination after completed treatment for conditions other than malignant neoplasm
Z11	Encounter for screening for infectious and parasitic diseases
Z11.8	Encounter for screening for other infectious and parasitic diseases
Z12	Encounter for screening for malignant neoplasms
Z13	Encounter for screening for other diseases and disorders
Z14	Genetic carrier
Z15	Genetic susceptibility to disease
Z17	Estrogen receptor status
Z18	Retained foreign body fragments
Z19	Hormone sensitivity malignancy status

Z20.821	Contact with and (suspected) exposure to Zika virus
Z22	Carrier of infectious disease
Z23	Encounter for immunization
Z28	Immunization not carried out and underimmunization status
Z29	Encounter for prophylactic measures
Z30	Encounter for contraceptive management
Z31	Encounter for procreative management
Z34	Encounter for supervision of normal pregnancy
Z3A	Weeks of gestation
Z36	Encounter for antenatal screening of mother
Z37	Outcome of delivery
Z38	Liveborn infants according to place of birth and type of delivery
Z39	Encounter for maternal postpartum care and examination
Z40.3	Encounter for prophylactic removal of fallopian tube(s)
Z41	Encounter for procedures for purposes other than remedying health state
Z42	Encounter for plastic and reconstructive surgery following medical procedure or healed injury
Z43	Encounter for attention to artificial openings
Z44	Encounter for fitting and adjustment of external prosthetic device
Z45	Encounter for adjustment and management of implanted device
Z46	Encounter for fitting and adjustment of other devices
Z47	Orthopedic aftercare
Z48	Encounter for other postprocedural aftercare
Z49	Encounter for care involving renal dialysis
Z51	Encounter for other aftercare (except Z51.5, Encounter for palliative care)
Z52	Donors of organs and tissues
Z53.3	Procedure converted to open procedure
Z55	Problems related to education and literacy
Z56	Problems related to employment and unemployment
Z57	Occupational exposure to risk factors
Z59	Problems related to housing and economic circumstances
Z62.813	Personal history of forced labor or sexual exploitation in childhood
Z63	Other problems related to primary support group, including family circumstances
Z64	Problems related to certain psychosocial circumstances
Z65	Problems related to other psychosocial circumstances
Z65.8	Other specified problems related to psychosocial circumstances
Z67.1–Z67.9	Blood type
Z68	Body mass index (BMI)
Z69	Encounter for mental health services for victim and perpetrator of abuse
Z70	Counseling related to sexual attitude, behavior and orientation
Z71	Persons encountering health services for other counseling and medical advice, NEC
Z72	Problems related to lifestyle
Z73	Problems related to life management difficulty
Z74.01	Bed confinement status
Z75	Problems related to medical facilities and other health care
Z76	Persons encountering health services in other circumstances
Z77.110–Z77.128	Environmental pollution and hazards in the physical environment
Z78	Other specified health status
Z79	Long-term (current) drug therapy

Z80	Family history of primary malignant neoplasm
Z81	Family history of mental and behavioral disorders
Z82	Family history of certain disabilities and chronic diseases (leading to disablement)
Z83	Family history of other specific disorders
Z84	Family history of other conditions
Z85	Personal history of primary malignant neoplasm
Z86	Personal history of certain other diseases
Z87	Personal history of other diseases and conditions
Z87.828	Personal history of other (healed) physical injury and trauma
Z87.891	Personal history of nicotine dependence
Z88	Allergy status to drugs, medicaments and biological substances
Z89	Acquired absence of limb
Z90	Acquired absence of organs, NEC
Z91	Personal risk factors, NEC
Z92	Personal history of medical treatment
Z93	Artificial opening status
Z94	Transplanted organ and tissue status
Z95	Presence of cardiac and vascular implants and grafts
Z96.82	Presence of neurostimulator
Z97	Presence of other devices
Z98	Other postprocedural states
Z99	Dependence on enabling machines and devices, not elsewhere classified

Additional Conventions

The use of symbols and color-coding has been added to this code book to alert the user to Medicare reimbursement logic and edits that are impacted by diagnosis coding. Although some third-party payers have adopted Medicare's reimbursement methodology, others have not. Therefore, it is important to review your facilities payer reporting requirements for non-Medicare payers prior to diagnosis coding.

Some codes may be included in multiple reimbursement issues and, therefore, may have more than one symbol or color-coding feature. For a quick reference review, the legend at the bottom of each page of the Tabular as well as the inside cover of the code book. The symbols and color-coding features are described in detail here.

Tabular Enhancements

In an effort to make the Tabular more user-friendly, the following symbols and color-coding features have been added. These features are indented to help the user in selecting a complete and accurate diagnosis code.

Final Character Indicator

ICD-10-CM codes range in length from 3 to 7 characters. In order for a code to be "valid" it must be listed to the fullest character length available. For example, if a fourth character is available, a three-character code is considered invalid.

To help users comply with this convention, a red plus sign (+) is listed to the left of any subcategory or subclassification code that requires an additional character. For example:

+ J45.2 Mild intermittent asthma

The assignment of the seventh character can, at times, be tricky. There are designated categories of codes that require a seventh character even though the code may not already have six characters present. For these codes, the user must insert the placeholder character of X after the code to fill any open characters prior to the seventh character.

To help users comply with this convention, in this book, the phrase **X+7th** is in red and is located to the left of the code that requires the placeholder of X and/or the seventh character. For example:

X+7th M80.00 Age-related osteoporosis with current pathological fracture

Additionally, there are six character codes that require the application of a seventh character. For these codes a placeholder X is not required. To help users differentiate these codes, in this book, the phrase **+7th** is in red and is located to the left of the code that requires the seventh character. For example:

+7th S72.021 Displaced fracture of epiphysis (separation) (upper) of right femur

Lastly, there are some codes that have only three characters. They require no further specification with additional characters and are therefore valid codes. The following note: Valid 3-character code, no further characters required is located below the code description in this book. This note alerts the coder that the three-character code is valid and can be used for reporting.

Color Identification

The Tabular section of this code book contains many instructional notes for the user. In order to help navigate the various types of instructional notes, a color-coding system has been applied:

- Category block headers are presented in dark green font.
- Category codes (three characters) are presented in blue font.
- Includes notes have a gray color bar over the **Includes**
- Excludes1 notes have a yellow color bar over the *Excludes1*
- Excludes2 notes have a bright green color bar over the *Excludes2*
- Notes have a maroon color bar over the **NOTE**
- *Use additional code* notes are presented in orange font
- *Code also* notes are presented in orange font
- *Code first* notes are presented in orange font
- Seventh character options are presented in a box and are highlighted in gray

The following excerpt from the Tabular illustrates the color-coding applied in this code book.

Disorders of bone density and structure (M80–M85)
M80 Osteoporosis with current pathological fracture

Includes: osteoporosis with current fragility fracture

Use additional code to identify major osseous defect, if applicable (M89.7-)

Excludes1: *collapsed vertebra NOS (M48.5)*
pathological fracture NOS (M84.4)
wedging of vertebra NOS (M48.5)

Excludes2: *personal history of (healed) osteoporosis fracture (Z87.310)*

The appropriate 7th character is to be added to each code from category M80:
A   initial encounter for fracture
D   subsequent encounter for fracture with routine healing
G   subsequent encounter for fracture with delayed healing
K   subsequent encounter for fracture with nonunion
P   subsequent encounter for fracture with malunion
S   sequela

Medicare Code Edits

Hospital inpatient Medicare claims paid under the Inpatient Prospective payment System (IPPS) are processed through the Medicare Code Editor (MCE) prior to payment by the Medicare administrative contractor (MAC). The code edits are intended to ensure that all claims processed by the MAC are accurate and complete. The information in this manual is based on the MCE v38.

Several of the MCE edits pertain to diagnoses. We have identified the codes included in these edits throughout the Tabular section this manual to assist users with preparing accurate and complete claims. The MCE edits included in this manual:

- Age conflict
- Sex Conflict Edit
- Manifestation codes not allowed as principal diagnosis
- Unacceptable principal diagnoses

Note: It is important to remember these edits are Medicare edits and may not apply to other third-party payers claim processing.

Age Conflict

The age conflict edit is activated when the age of the patient and the type diagnosis code reported does not match. The following symbols are used to identify the four age conflict categories.

- Newborn diagnosis age 0: This symbol appears to the left of the applicable code in the Tabular.
- Pediatric diagnosis age 0–17: This symbol appears to the left of the applicable code in the Tabular.
- Maternity diagnosis age 12–55: This symbol appears to the left of the applicable code in the Tabular.
- Adult diagnosis age 15–124: This symbol appears to the left of the applicable code in the Tabular.

Sex Conflict Edit

The sex conflict edit is activated when the sex of the patient and the diagnosis reported does not match. The following symbols are used to identify female-only and male-only diagnoses.

♀ Female-only diagnosis: This symbol appears to the left of the applicable code in the Tabular.

♂ Male-only diagnosis: This symbol appears to the left of the applicable code in the Tabular.

Manifestation Code Not Allowed as Principal Diagnosis

Manifestation codes are used to report the manifestation of an underlying disease, not to report the disease itself. Therefore, within ICD-10-CM the manifestation should not be reported as the principal diagnosis; rather it should always be reported as a secondary diagnosis.

Manifestation codes are identified with a light green color bar over the code in the Tabular. For example:

D63.0 Anemia in neoplastic disease

Unacceptable Principal Diagnosis

There are specified codes that describe a circumstance which influences an individual's health status but not a current illness or injury, or codes that are not specific manifestations but may be due to an underlying cause. These codes are considered unacceptable as a principal diagnosis.

Unacceptable principal diagnosis codes are identified with a light blue color bar over the code in the Tabular:

B60.13 Keratoconjunctivitis due to Acanthamoeba

MS-DRG Diagnosis Designations

The MS-DRG system is utilized within the IPPS to determine the unadjusted reimbursement amount for Medicare hospital inpatient claims. The MS-DRG Definitions Manual includes the logic for MS-DRG refinement and selection as well as logic based on the IPPS final rules released each August. The information in this book is based on the MS-DRG v38. *Note:* It is important to remember that these edits are Medicare edits and may not apply to other third-party payers claim processing.

CC and MCC Codes

Within the MS-DRG system, one of the refinement pathways is whether there is a complication/comorbidity (CC) or major complication/comorbidity (MCC) code reported as a secondary diagnosis. For some of the MS-DRG families, the presence of a CC or MCC allows for an MS-DRG assignment that has a higher relative weight and, therefore, a higher reimbursement amount. There are exceptions to the application of the CC or MCC codes and the exceptions are referred to as *CC Exclusions* or *MCC Exclusions*. If exclusions apply, the CC/MCC code is assigned a principal diagnosis collection. Within this collection are the codes that, when reported as principal diagnosis, excludes the CC/MCC status from the secondary diagnosis code under review. Essentially, it takes away the CC/MCC code's ability to influence the MS-DRG assignment.

Codes that are considered CC codes have a purple **CC** to the left of the code in the Tabular. The principal diagnosis collection for each CC code is provided in Appendix A. Coding professionals may review the principal diagnosis collection identified if required for the task at hand. If the code requires a seventh character, the characters that are eligible for CC status are included within Appendix A.

Codes that are considered MCC codes have a purple **MCC** to the left of the code in the Tabular. The principal diagnosis collection for each MCC code is provided in Appendix A. Coding professionals may review the principal diagnosis collection identified if required for the task at hand. If the code requires a seventh character, the characters that are eligible for MCC status are included within Appendix A.

Hospital-Acquired Conditions Related Diagnoses

As part of the Medicare Value-Based Purchasing program, CMS has implemented a Paying for Value program entitled Hospital-Acquired Conditions (HACs) Present on Admission Indicator Program. This program is designed to reduce reimbursements to facilities where the value of the medical or surgical services have been comprised due to preventable conditions. Reimbursement for admissions that meet the HAC Present on Admission Indicator Program criteria will be reduced. In this manual, the HAC-associated procedures are identified with an orange rectangle **HAC** with HAC. The orange rectangle is located below the code description in the code listing. If there is conditional logic for the diagnosis code, it is included in Appendix B.

AHA *Coding Clinic for ICD-10-CM and ICD-10-PCS*

The American Hospital Association began publishing coding guidance for ICD-10-CM and ICD-10-PCS in the fourth quarter of 2012. In this code book we identify diagnosis codes that are discussed in the *Coding Clinic* guidance fourth quarter 2012 through second quarter 2020. Within the Tabular the following sky-blue note alerts the coder to review the AHA *Coding Clinic* prior to assignment of the code to ensure appropriate and accurate reporting. The quarter of publication, year, and page number(s) are provided in the note.

AHA CC: 4Q; 2012; pg#-pg#

CMS Hierarchical Condition Categories Risk Adjustment System

Since 2004, Medicare has utilized the CMS Hierarchical Condition Categories (CMS-HCC) model to risk adjust within the Medicare Advantage capitation payment system. Using the CMS-HCC model Medicare uses large pools of data to predict average costs for a predetermined set of factors; one of the factors is individual disease groups. The HCC diagnosis code listing is utilized to determine the individual disease groups from Medicare claims data. Additionally, CMS-HCC model is utilized in accountable care organizations payment methodologies (inpatient and outpatient settings) and in Medicare's inpatient acute care (IPPS) value-based purchasing program. The use of the CMS-HCC model for risk adjustment within payment systems continues to grow. Therefore, it is imperative that coding professionals in all settings are familiar with the reporting of HCC diagnosis codes. The most current list of CMS-HCC model diagnosis codes are identified in this code book. The CMS-HCC model is updated each year with an effective date of January 1.

CMS-HCC diagnosis codes are identified with a lavender color bar over the code in the Tabular:

E11.21 Type 2 diabetes mellitus with diabetic nephropathy

Basic Steps in ICD-10-CM Coding

To code each disease or condition completely and accurately, the coder should:

1. Identify all main terms included in the diagnostic statement.
2. Locate each main term in the Alphabetic Index.
3. Refer to any subterms indented under the main term. The subterms form individual line entries and describe essential differences by site, etiology, or clinical type.
4. Follow the instructions (see, see also) provided in the Alphabetic Index if the needed code is not located under the first main entry consulted.
5. Verify the code selected in the Tabular List.
6. Read and be guided by any instructional terms in the Tabular List.
7. Assign codes to their highest level of specificity, up to a total of seven characters if applicable.
8. Continue coding the diagnostic statement until all the component elements are fully identified.

(*Source:* Schraffenberger, L.A. *Basic ICD-10-CM/PCS Coding*, 2020 Edition, pp. 43–44. AHIMA.)

A

Aarskog's syndrome Q87.19

Abandonment —*see* Maltreatment

Abasia (-astasia) (hysterical) F44.4

Abderhalden-Kaufmann-Lignac syndrome (cystinosis) E72.04

Abdomen, abdominal —*see also*
condition
acute R10.0
angina K55.1
muscle deficiency syndrome Q79.4

Abdominalgia —*see* Pain, abdominal

Abduction contracture, hip or other joint —*see* Contraction, joint

Aberrant (congenital) —*see also*
Malposition, congenital
adrenal gland Q89.1
artery (peripheral) Q27.8
basilar NEC Q28.1
cerebral Q28.3
coronary Q24.5
digestive system Q27.8
eye Q15.8
lower limb Q27.8
precerebral Q28.1
pulmonary Q25.79
renal Q27.2
retina Q14.1
specified site NEC Q27.8
subclavian Q27.8
upper limb Q27.8
vertebral Q28.1
breast Q83.8
endocrine gland NEC Q89.2
hepatic duct Q44.5
pancreas Q45.3
parathyroid gland Q89.2
pituitary gland Q89.2
sebaceous glands, mucous
membrane, mouth, congenital
Q38.6
spleen Q89.09
subclavian artery Q27.8
thymus (gland) Q89.2
thyroid gland Q89.2
vein (peripheral) NEC Q27.8
cerebral Q28.3
digestive system Q27.8
lower limb Q27.8
precerebral Q28.1
specified site NEC Q27.8
upper limb Q27.8

Aberration
distantial —*see* Disturbance, visual
mental F99

Abetalipoproteinemia E78.6

Abiotrophy R68.89

Ablatio, ablation
retinae —*see* Detachment, retina

Ablepharia, ablepharon Q10.3

Abnormal, abnormality, abnormalities —*see also* Anomaly
acid-base balance (mixed) E87.4
albumin R77.0
alphafetoprotein R77.2
alveolar ridge K08.9
anatomical relationship Q89.9
apertures, congenital, diaphragm
Q79.1
auditory perception H93.29-

Abnormal, abnormality, abnormalities *(continued)*
auditory perception *(continued)*
diplacusis —*see* Diplacusis
hyperacusis —*see* Hyperacusis
recruitment —*see* Recruitment, auditory
threshold shift —*see* Shift, auditory threshold
autosomes Q99.9
fragile site Q95.5
basal metabolic rate R94.8
biosynthesis, testicular androgen
E29.1
bleeding time R79.1
blood-gas level R79.81
blood level (of)
cobalt R79.0
copper R79.0
iron R79.0
lithium R78.89
magnesium R79.0
mineral NEC R79.0
zinc R79.0
blood pressure
elevated R03.0
low reading (nonspecific) R03.1
blood sugar R73.09
bowel sounds R19.15
absent R19.11
hyperactive R19.12
brain scan R94.02
breathing R06.9
caloric test R94.138
cerebrospinal fluid R83.9
cytology R83.6
drug level R83.2
enzyme level R83.0
hormones R83.1
immunology R83.4
microbiology R83.5
nonmedicinal level R83.3
specified type NEC R83.8
chemistry, blood R79.9
C-reactive protein R79.82
drugs —*see* Findings, abnormal, in blood
gas level R79.81
minerals R79.0
pancytopenia D61.818
PTT R79.1
specified NEC R79.89
toxins —*see* Findings, abnormal, in blood
chest sounds (friction) (rales) R09.89
chromosome, chromosomal Q99.9
with more than three X
chromosomes, female Q97.1
analysis result R89.8
bronchial washings R84.8
cerebrospinal fluid R83.8
cervix uteri NEC R87.89
nasal secretions R84.8
nipple discharge R89.8
peritoneal fluid R85.89
pleural fluid R84.8
prostatic secretions R86.8
saliva R85.89
seminal fluid R86.8
sputum R84.8
synovial fluid R89.8
throat scrapings R84.8
vagina R87.89
vulva R87.89
wound secretions R89.8

Abnormal, abnormality, abnormalities *(continued)*
chromosome *(continued)*
dicentric replacement Q93.2
ring replacement Q93.2
sex Q99.8
female phenotype Q97.9
specified NEC Q97.8
male phenotype Q98.9
specified NEC Q98.8
structural male Q98.6
specified NEC Q99.8
clinical findings NEC R68.89
coagulation D68.9
newborn, transient P61.6
profile R79.1
time R79.1
communication —*see* Fistula
conjunctiva, vascular H11.41-
coronary artery Q24.5
cortisol-binding globulin E27.8
course, eustachian tube Q17.8
creatinine clearance R94.4
cytology R85.619
anus R85.619
atypical squamous cells
cannot exclude high grade
squamous intraepithelial
lesion (ASC-H) R85.611
atypical squamous cells of
undetermined significance
(ASC-US) R85.610
cytologic evidence of
malignancy R85.614
high grade squamous
intraepithelial lesion
(HGSIL) R85.613
human papillomavirus (HPV)
DNA test
high risk positive R85.81
low risk postive R85.82
inadequate smear R85.615
low grade squamous
intraepithelial lesion
(LGSIL) R85.612
satisfactory anal smear but
lacking transformation zone
R85.616
specified NEC R85.618
unsatisfactory smear R85.615
female genital organs —*see*
Abnormal, Papanicolaou
(smear)
dark adaptation curve H53.61
dentofacial NEC —*see* Anomaly,
dentofacial
development, developmental Q89.9
central nervous system Q07.9
diagnostic imaging
abdomen, abdominal region
NEC R93.5
biliary tract R93.2
bladder R93.41
breast R92.8
central nervous system NEC
R90.89
cerebrovascular NEC R90.89
coronary circulation R93.1
digestive tract NEC R93.3
gastrointestinal (tract) R93.3
genitourinary organs R93.89
head R93.0
heart R93.1
intrathoracic organ NEC R93.89
kidney R93.42-

Abnormal, abnormality, abnormalities *(continued)*
diagnostic imaging *(continued)*
limbs R93.6
liver R93.2
lung (field) R91.8
musculoskeletal system NEC
R93.7
renal pelvis R93.41
retroperitoneum R93.5
site specified NEC R93.89
skin and subcutaneous tissue
R93.89
skull R93.0
testis R93.81-
urinary organs specified NEC
R93.49
ureter R93.41
direction, teeth, fully erupted
M26.30
ear ossicles, acquired NEC H74.39-
ankylosis —*see* Ankylosis, ear
ossicles
discontinuity —*see*
Discontinuity, ossicles, ear
partial loss —*see* Loss, ossicles,
ear (partial)
Ebstein Q22.5
echocardiogram R93.1
echoencephalogram R90.81
echogram —*see* Abnormal,
diagnostic imaging
electrocardiogram [ECG] [EKG]
R94.31
electroencephalogram [EEG]
R94.01
electrolyte —*see* Imbalance,
electrolyte
electromyogram [EMG] R94.131
electro-oculogram [EOG] R94.110
electrophysiological intracardiac
studies R94.39
electroretinogram [ERG] R94.111
erythrocytes
congenital, with perinatal
jaundice D58.9
feces (color) (contents) (mucus)
R19.5
finding —*see* Findings, abnormal,
without diagnosis
fluid
amniotic —*see* Abnormal,
specimen, specified
cerebrospinal —*see* Abnormal,
cerebrospinal fluid
peritoneal —*see* Abnormal,
specimen, digestive organs
pleural —*see* Abnormal,
specimen, respiratory organs
synovial —*see* Abnormal,
specimen, specified
thorax (bronchial washings)
(pleural fluid) —*see*
Abnormal, specimen,
respiratory organs
vaginal —*see* Abnormal,
specimen, female genital
organs
form
teeth K00.2
uterus —*see* Anomaly, uterus
function studies
auditory R94.120
bladder R94.8
brain R94.09

Abnormal, abnormality, abnormalities (*continued*)
  function studies (*continued*)
    cardiovascular R94.30
    ear R94.128
    endocrine NEC R94.7
    eye NEC R94.118
    kidney R94.4
    liver R94.5
    nervous system
      central NEC R94.09
      peripheral NEC R94.138
    pancreas R94.8
    placenta R94.8
    pulmonary R94.2
    special senses NEC R94.128
    spleen R94.8
    thyroid R94.6
    vestibular R94.121
  gait —*see* Gait
    hysterical F44.4
  gastrin secretion E16.4
  globulin R77.1
    cortisol-binding E27.8
    thyroid-binding E07.89
  glomerular, minor (*see also* N00-N07 with fourth character .0) N05.0
  glucagon secretion E16.3
  glucose tolerance (test) (non-fasting) R73.09
  gravitational (G) forces or states (effect of) T75.81
  hair (color) (shaft) L67.9
    specified NEC L67.8
  hard tissue formation in pulp (dental) K04.3
  head movement R25.0
  heart
    rate R00.9
      specified NEC R00.8
    shadow R93.1
    sounds NEC R01.2
  hemoglobin (disease) —*see also* Disease, hemoglobin D58.2
    trait —*see* Trait, hemoglobin, abnormal
  histology NEC R89.7
  immunological findings R89.4
    in serum R76.9
      specified NEC R76.8
  increase in appetite R63.2
  involuntary movement —*see* Abnormal, movement, involuntary
  jaw closure M26.51
  karyotype R89.8
  kidney function test R94.4
  knee jerk R29.2
  leukocyte (cell) (differential) NEC D72.9
  liver function test R94.5
  loss of
    height R29.890
    weight R63.4
  mammogram NEC R92.8
    calcification (calculus) R92.1
    microcalcification R92.0
  Mantoux test R76.11
  movement (disorder) —*see also* Disorder, movement
    head R25.0
    involuntary R25.9
      fasciculation R25.3
      of head R25.0
      spasm R25.2
      specified type NEC R25.8
      tremor R25.1
  myoglobin (Aberdeen) (Annapolis) R89.7
  neonatal screening P09

  oculomotor study R94.113
  palmar creases Q82.8
  Papanicolaou (smear)
    anus R85.619
      atypical squamous cells cannot exclude high grade squamous intraepithelial lesion (ASC-H) R85.611
      atypical squamous cells of undetermined significance (ASC-US) R85.610
      cytologic evidence of malignancy R85.614
      high grade squamous intraepithelial lesion (HGSIL) R85.613
      human papillomavirus (HPV) DNA test
        high risk positive R85.81
        low risk postive R85.82
      inadequate smear R85.615
      low grade squamous intraepithelial lesion (LGSIL) R85.612
      satisfactory anal smear but lacking transformation zone R85.616
      specified NEC R85.618
      unsatisfactory smear R85.615
    bronchial washings R84.6
    cerebrospinal fluid R83.6
    cervix R87.619
      atypical squamous cells cannot exclude high grade squamous intraepithelial lesion (ASC-H) R87.611
      atypical squamous cells of undetermined significance (ASC-US) R87.610
      cytologic evidence of malignancy R87.614
      high grade squamous intraepithelial lesion (HGSIL) R87.613
      inadequate smear R87.615
      low grade squamous intraepithelial lesion (LGSIL) R87.612
      non-atypical endometrial cells R87.618
      satisfactory cervical smear but lacking transformation zone R87.616
      specified NEC R87.618
      thin preparaton R87.619
      unsatisfactory smear R87.615
    nasal secretions R84.6
    nipple discharge R89.6
    peritoneal fluid R85.69
    pleural fluid R84.6
    prostatic secretions R86.6
    saliva R85.69
    seminal fluid R86.6
    sites NEC R89.6
    sputum R84.6
    synovial fluid R89.6
    throat scrapings R84.6
    vagina R87.629
      atypical squamous cells cannot exclude high grade squamous intraepithelial lesion (ASC-H) R87.621
      atypical squamous cells of undetermined significance (ASC-US) R87.620
      cytologic evidence of malignancy R87.624

    Papanicolaou (*continued*)
      vagina (*continued*)
        high grade squamous intraepithelial lesion (HGSIL) R87.623
        inadequate smear R87.625
        low grade squamous intraepithelial lesion (LGSIL) R87.622
        specified NEC R87.628
        thin preparation R87.629
        unsatisfactory smear R87.625
      vulva R87.69
      wound secretions R89.6
  partial thromboplastin time (PTT) R79.1
  pelvis (bony) —*see* Deformity, pelvis
  percussion, chest (tympany) R09.89
  periods (grossly) —*see* Menstruation
  phonocardiogram R94.39
  plantar reflex R29.2
  plasma
    protein R77.9
      specified NEC R77.8
    viscosity R70.1
  pleural (folds) Q34.0
  posture R29.3
  product of conception O02.9
    specified type NEC O02.89
  prothrombin time (PT) R79.1
  pulmonary
    artery, congenital Q25.79
    function, newborn P28.89
    test results R94.2
  pulsations in neck R00.2
  pupillary H21.56-
    function (reaction) (reflex) —*see* Anomaly, pupil, function
  radiological examination —*see* Abnormal, diagnostic imaging
  red blood cell(s) (morphology) (volume) R71.8
  reflex —*see* Reflex
  renal function test R94.4
  response to nerve stimulation R94.130
  retinal correspondence H53.31
  retinal function study R94.111
  rhythm, heart —*see also* Arrhythmia
  saliva —*see* Abnormal, specimen, digestive organs
  scan
    kidney R94.4
    liver R93.2
    thyroid R94.6
  secretion
    gastrin E16.4
    glucagon E16.3
  semen, seminal fluid —*see* Abnormal, specimen, male genital organs
  serum level (of)
    acid phosphatase R74.8
    alkaline phosphatase R74.8
    amylase R74.8
    enzymes R74.9
      specified NEC R74.8
    lipase R74.8
    triacylglycerol lipase R74.8
  shape
    gravid uterus —*see* Anomaly, uterus
  sinus venosus Q21.1
  size, tooth, teeth K00.2
  spacing, tooth, teeth, fully erupted M26.30

  specimen
    digestive organs (peritoneal fluid) (saliva) R85.9
      cytology R85.69
      drug level R85.2
      enzyme level R85.0
      histology R85.7
      hormones R85.1
      immunology R85.4
      microbiology R85.5
      nonmedicinal level R85.3
      specified type NEC R85.89
    female genital organs (secretions) (smears) R87.9
      cytology R87.69
        cervix R87.619
          human papillomavirus (HPV) DNA test
            high risk positive R87.810
            low risk positive R87.820
          inadequate (unsatisfactory) smear R87.615
          non-atypical endometrial cells R87.618
          specified NEC R87.618
        vagina R87.629
          human papillomavirus (HPV) DNA test
            high risk positive R87.811
            low risk positive R87.821
          inadequate (unsatisfactory) smear R87.625
        vulva R87.69
      drug level R87.2
      enzyme level R87.0
      histological R87.7
      hormones R87.1
      immunology R87.4
      microbiology R87.5
      nonmedicinal level R87.3
      specified type NEC R87.89
    male genital organs (prostatic secretions) (semen) R86.9
      cytology R86.6
      drug level R86.2
      enzyme level R86.0
      histological R86.7
      hormones R86.1
      immunology R86.4
      microbiology R86.5
      nonmedicinal level R86.3
      specified type NEC R86.8
    nipple discharge —*see* Abnormal, specimen, specified
    respiratory organs (bronchial washings) (nasal secretions) (pleural fluid) (sputum) R84.9
      cytology R84.6
      drug level R84.2
      enzyme level R84.0
      histology R84.7
      hormones R84.1
      immunology R84.4
      microbiology R84.5
      nonmedicinal level R84.3
      specified type NEC R84.8
    specified organ, system and tissue NOS R89.9
      cytology R89.6
      drug level R89.2
      enzyme level R89.0
      histology R89.7
      hormones R89.1

Abnormal, abnormality, abnormalities *(continued)*
  specimen *(continued)*
    specified organ, system and
      tissue NOS *(continued)*
        immunology R89.4
        microbiology R89.5
        nonmedicinal level R89.3
        specified type NEC R89.8
      synovial fluid —*see* Abnormal,
        specimen, specified
      thorax (bronchial washings)
        (pleural fluids) —*see*
        Abnormal, specimen,
        respiratory organs
      vagina (secretion) (smear) R87.629
      vulva (secretion) (smear) R87.69
      wound secretion —*see*
        Abnormal, specimen, specified
    spermatozoa —*see* Abnormal,
      specimen, male genital organs
    sputum (amount) (color) (odor) R09.3
    stool (color) (contents) (mucus)
      R19.5
      bloody K92.1
      guaiac positive R19.5
  synchondrosis Q78.8
  thermography —*see also*
    Abnormal, diagnostic imaging
    R93.89
  thyroid-binding globulin E07.89
  tooth, teeth (form) (size) K00.2
  toxicology (findings) R78.9
  transport protein E88.09
  tumor marker NEC R97.8
  ultrasound results —*see* Abnormal,
    diagnostic imaging
  umbilical cord complicating
    delivery O69.9
  urination NFC R39.198
  urine (constituents) R82.90
    bile R82.2
    cytological examination R82.89
    drugs R82.5
    fat R82.0
    glucose R81
    heavy metals R82.6
    hemoglobin R82.3
    histological examination R82.89
    ketones R82.4
    microbiological examination
      (culture) R82.79
    myoglobin R82.1
    positive culture R82.79
    protein —*see* Proteinuria
    specified substance NEC R82.998
      chromoabnormality NEC
        R82.91
    substances nonmedical R82.6
  uterine hemorrhage —*see*
    Hemorrhage, uterus
  vectorcardiogram R94.39
  visually evoked potential (VEP)
    R94.112
  white blood cells D72.9
    specified NEC D72.89
  X-ray examination —*see*
    Abnormal, diagnostic imaging
Abnormity (any organ or part) —*see*
  Anomaly
Abocclusion M26.29
  hemolytic disease (newborn) P55.1
  incompatibility reaction ABO
    —*see* Complication(s),
    transfusion, incompatibility
    reaction, ABO
Abolition, language R48.8
Aborter, habitual or recurrent
  —*see* Loss (of), pregnancy,
  recurrent

Abortion (complete) (spontaneous)
  O03.9
  with
    retained products of conception
      —*see* Abortion, incomplete
  attempted (elective) (failed) O07.4
    complicated by O07.30
      afibrinogenemia O07.1
      cardiac arrest O07.36
      chemical damage of pelvic
        organ(s) O07.34
      circulatory collapse O07.31
      cystitis O07.38
      defibrination syndrome
        O07.1
      electrolyte imbalance O07.33
      embolism (air) (amniotic
        fluid) (blood clot) (fat)
        (pulmonary) (septic) (soap)
        O07.2
      endometritis O07.0
      genital tract and pelvic
        infection O07.0
      hemolysis O07.1
      hemorrhage (delayed)
        (excessive) O07.1
      infection
        genital tract or pelvic O07.0
        urinary tract tract O07.38
      intravascular coagulation
        O07.1
      laceration of pelvic organ(s)
        O07.34
      metabolic disorder O07.33
      oliguria O07.32
      oophoritis O07.0
      parametritis O07.0
      pelvic peritonitis O07.0
      perforation of pelvic organ(s)
        O07.34
      renal failure or shutdown
        O07.32
      salpingitis or salpingo-
        oophoritis O07.0
      sepsis O07.37
      shock O07.31
      specified condition NEC
        O07.39
      tubular necrosis (renal)
        O07.32
      uremia O07.32
      urinary tract infection O07.38
      venous complication NEC
        O07.35
        embolism (air) (amniotic
          fluid) (blood clot) (fat)
          (pulmonary) (septic)
          (soap) O07.2
  complicated (by) (following)
    O03.80
    afibrinogenemia O03.6
    cardiac arrest O03.86
    chemical damage of pelvic
      organ(s) O03.84
    circulatory collapse O03.81
    cystitis O03.88
    defibrination syndrome O03.6
    electrolyte imbalance O03.83
    embolism (air) (amniotic fluid)
      (blood clot) (fat) (pulmonary)
      (septic) (soap) O03.7
    endometritis O03.5
    genital tract and pelvic infection
      O03.5
    hemolysis O03.6
    hemorrhage (delayed)
      (excessive) O03.6
    infection
      genital tract or pelvic O03.5
      urinary tract O03.88
    intravascular coagulation O03.6

Abortion *(continued)*
  complicated *(continued)*
    laceration of pelvic organ(s)
      O03.84
    metabolic disorder O03.83
    oliguria O03.82
    oophoritis O03.5
    parametritis O03.5
    pelvic peritonitis O03.5
    perforation of pelvic organ(s)
      O03.84
    renal failure or shutdown
      O03.82
    salpingitis or salpingo-oophoritis
      O03.5
    sepsis O03.87
    shock O03.81
    specified condition NEC O03.89
    tubular necrosis (renal) O03.82
    uremia O03.82
    urinary tract infection O03.88
    venous complication NEC
      O03.85
      embolism (air) (amniotic
        fluid) (blood clot) (fat)
        (pulmonary) (septic) (soap)
        O03.7
  failed —*see* Abortion, attempted
  habitual or recurrent N96
    with current abortion —*see*
      categories O03-O04
    without current pregnancy N96
    care in current pregnancy O26.2-
  incomplete (spontaneous) O03.4
    complicated (by) (following)
      O03.30
      afibrinogenemia O03.1
      cardiac arrest O03.36
      chemical damage of pelvic
        organ(s) O03.34
      circulatory collapse O03.31
      cystitis O03.38
      defibrination syndrome O03.1
      electrolyte imbalance O03.33
      embolism (air) (amniotic
        fluid) (blood clot) (fat)
        (pulmonary) (septic) (soap)
        O03.2
      endometritis O03.0
      genital tract and pelvic
        infection O03.0
      hemolysis O03.1
      hemorrhage (delayed)
        (excessive) O03.1
      infection
        genital tract or pelvic O03.0
        urinary tract O03.38
      intravascular coagulation
        O03.1
      laceration of pelvic organ(s)
        O03.34
      metabolic disorder O03.33
      oliguria O03.32
      oophoritis O03.0
      parametritis O03.0
      pelvic peritonitis O03.0
      perforation of pelvic organ(s)
        O03.34
      renal failure or shutdown
        O03.32
      salpingitis or salpingo-
        oophoritis O03.0
      sepsis O03.37
      shock O03.31
      specified condition NEC
        O03.39
      tubular necrosis (renal) O03.32
      uremia O03.32
      urinary infection O03.38
      venous complication NEC
        O03.35

Abortion *(continued)*
  incomplete *(continued)*
    complicated *(continued)*
      venous complication
        (continued)
        embolism (air) (amniotic
          fluid) (blood clot) (fat)
          (pulmonary) (septic)
          (soap) O03.2
  induced (encounter for) Z33.2
    complicated by O04.80
      afibrinogenemia O04.6
      cardiac arrest O04.86
      chemical damage of pelvic
        organ(s) O04.84
      circulatory collapse O04.81
      cystitis O04.88
      defibrination syndrome O04.6
      electrolyte imbalance O04.83
      embolism (air) (amniotic fluid)
        (blood clot) (fat) (pulmonary)
        (septic) (soap) O04.7
      endometritis O04.5
      genital tract and pelvic
        infection O04.5
      hemolysis O04.6
      hemorrhage (delayed)
        (excessive) O04.6
      infection
        genital tract or pelvic O04.5
        urinary tract O04.88
      intravascular coagulation
        O04.6
      laceration of pelvic organ(s)
        O04.84
      metabolic disorder O04.83
      oliguria O04.82
      oophoritis O04.5
      parametritis O04.5
      pelvic peritonitis O04.5
      perforation of pelvic organ(s)
        O04.84
      renal failure or shutdown
        O04.82
      salpingitis or salpingo-
        oophoritis O04.5
      sepsis O04.87
      shock O04.81
      specified condition NEC
        O04.89
      tubular necrosis (renal) O04.82
      uremia O04.82
      urinary tract infection O04.88
      venous complication NEC
        O04.85
        embolism (air) (amniotic
          fluid) (blood clot) (fat)
          (pulmonary) (septic)
          (soap) O04.7
  inevitable O03.4
  missed O02.1
  spontaneous —*see* Abortion
    (complete) (spontaneous)
    threatened O20.0
  threatened (spontaneous) O20.0
  tubal O00.10-
    with intrauterine pregnancy
      O00.11-

Abortus fever A23.1

Aboulomania F60.7

Abrami's disease D59.8

Abramov-Fiedler myocarditis (acute
  isolated myocarditis) I40.1

Abrasion T14.8
  abdomen, abdominal (wall) S30.811
  alveolar process S00.512
  ankle S90.51-
  antecubital space —*see* Abrasion,
    elbow

Abrasion *(continued)*
anus S30.817
arm (upper) S40.81-
auditory canal —*see* Abrasion, ear
auricle —*see* Abrasion, ear
axilla —*see* Abrasion, arm
back, lower S30.810
breast S20.11-
brow S00.81
buttock S30.810
calf —*see* Abrasion, leg
canthus —*see* Abrasion, eyelid
cheek S00.81
   internal S00.512
chest wall —*see* Abrasion, thorax
chin S00.81
clitoris S30.814
cornea S05.0-
costal region —*see* Abrasion,
   thorax
dental K03.1
digit(s)
   foot —*see* Abrasion, toe
   hand —*see* Abrasion, finger
ear S00.41-
elbow S50.31-
epididymis S30.813
epigastric region S30.811
epiglottis S10.11
esophagus (thoracic) S27.818
   cervical S10.11
eyebrow —*see* Abrasion, eyelid
eyelid S00.21-
face S00.81
finger(s) S60.41-
   index S60.41-
   little S60.41-
   middle S60.41-
   ring S60.41-
flank S30.811
foot (except toe(s) alone) S90.81-
   toe —*see* Abrasion, toe
forearm S50.81-
   elbow only —*see* Abrasion,
      elbow
forehead S00.81
genital organs, external
   female S30.816
   male S30.815
groin S30.811
gum S00.512
hand S60.51-
head S00.91
   ear —*see* Abrasion, ear
   eyelid —*see* Abrasion, eyelid
   lip S00.511
   nose S00.31
   oral cavity S00.512
   scalp S00.01
   specified site NEC S00.81
heel —*see* Abrasion, foot
hip S70.21-
inguinal region S30.811
interscapular region S20.419
jaw S00.81
knee S80.21-
labium (majus) (minus) S30.814
larynx S10.11
leg (lower) S80.81-
   knee —*see* Abrasion, knee
   upper —*see* Abrasion, thigh
lip S00.511
lower back S30.810
lumbar region S30.810
malar region S00.81
mammary —*see* Abrasion, breast
mastoid region S00.81
mouth S00.512
nail
   finger —*see* Abrasion, finger
   toe —*see* Abrasion, toe

Abrasion *(continued)*
nape S10.81
nasal S00.31
neck S10.91
   specified site NEC S10.81
   throat S10.11
nose S00.31
occipital region S00.01
oral cavity S00.512
orbital region —*see* Abrasion,
   eyelid
palate S00.512
palm —*see* Abrasion, hand
parietal region S00.01
pelvis S30.810
penis S30.812
perineum
   female S30.814
   male S30.810
periocular area —*see* Abrasion,
   eyelid
phalanges
   finger —*see* Abrasion, finger
   toe —*see* Abrasion, toe
pharynx S10.11
pinna —*see* Abrasion, ear
popliteal space —*see* Abrasion,
   knee
prepuce S30.812
pubic region S30.810
pudendum
   female S30.816
   male S30.815
sacral region S30.810
scalp S00.01
scapular region —*see* Abrasion,
   shoulder
scrotum S30.813
shin —*see* Abrasion, leg
shoulder S40.21-
skin NEC T14.8
sternal region S20.319
submaxillary region S00.81
submental region S00.81
subungual
   finger(s) —*see* Abrasion, finger
   toe(s) —*see* Abrasion, toe
supraclavicular fossa S10.81
supraorbital S00.81
temple S00.81
temporal region S00.81
testis S30.813
thigh S70.31-
thorax, thoracic (wall) S20.91
   back S20.41-
   front S20.31-
   throat S10.11
thumb S60.31-
toe(s) (lesser) S90.416
   great S90.41-
tongue S00.512
tooth, teeth (dentifrice) (habitual)
   (hard tissues) (occupational)
   (ritual) (traditional) K03.1
trachea S10.11
tunica vaginalis S30.813
tympanum, tympanic membrane
   —*see* Abrasion, ear
uvula S00.512
vagina S30.814
vocal cords S10.11
vulva S30.814
wrist S60.81-

Abrism —*see* Poisoning, food,
   noxious, plant

Abruptio placentae O45.9-
with
   afibrinogenemia O45.01-
   coagulation defect O45.00-
      specified NEC O45.09-

Abruptio placentae *(continued)*
with *(continued)*
   disseminated intravascular
      coagulation O45.02-
   hypofibrinogenemia O45.01-
specified NEC O45.8-

Abruption, placenta —*see* Abruptio
   placentae

Abscess (connective tissue) (embolic)
   (fistulous) (infective) (metastatic)
   (multiple) (pernicious) (pyogenic)
   (septic) L02.91
with
   diverticular disease (intestine)
      K57.80
      with bleeding K57.81
      large intestine K57.20
         with
            bleeding K57.21
            small intestine K57.40
               with bleeding K57.41
      small intestine K57.00
         with
            bleeding K57.01
            large intestine K57.40
               with bleeding K57.41
   lymphangitis - code by site under
      Abscess
abdomen, abdominal
   cavity K65.1
   wall L02.211
abdominopelvic K65.1
accessory sinus —*see* Sinusitis
adrenal (capsule) (gland) E27.8
alveolar K04.7
   with sinus K04.6
amebic A06.4
   brain (and liver or lung abscess)
      A06.6
   genitourinary tract A06.82
   liver (without mention of brain
      or lung abscess) A06.4
   lung (and liver) (without mention
      of brain abscess) A06.5
   specified site NEC A06.89
   spleen A06.89
anerobic A48.0
ankle —*see* Abscess, lower limb
anorectal K61.2
antecubital space —*see* Abscess,
   upper limb
antrum (chronic) (Highmore) —*see*
   Sinusitis, maxillary
anus K61.0
apical (tooth) K04.7
   with sinus (alveolar) K04.6
appendix K35.33
areola (acute) (chronic)
   (nonpuerperal) N61.1
   puerperal, postpartum or
      gestational —*see* Infection,
      nipple
arm (any part) —*see* Abscess,
   upper limb
artery (wall) I77.89
atheromatous I77.2
auricle, ear —*see* Abscess, ear,
   external
axilla (region) L02.41-
   lymph gland or node L04.2
back (any part, except buttock)
   L02.212
Bartholin's gland N75.1
with
   abortion —*see* Abortion, by
      type complicated by, sepsis
   ectopic or molar pregnancy
      O08.0
   following ectopic or molar
      pregnancy O08.0

Abscess *(continued)*
Bezold's —*see* Mastoiditis, acute
bilharziasis B65.1
bladder (wall) —*see* Cystitis,
   specified type NEC
bone (subperiosteal) —*see also*
   Osteomyelitis, specified type
   NEC
   accessory sinus (chronic) —*see*
      Sinusitis
   chronic or old —*see*
      Osteomyelitis, chronic
   jaw (lower) (upper) M27.2
   mastoid —*see* Mastoiditis, acute,
      subperiosteal
   petrous —*see* Petrositis
   spinal (tuberculous) A18.01
      nontuberculous —*see*
         Osteomyelitis, vertebra
bowel K63.0
brain (any part) (cystic) (otogenic)
   G06.0
   amebic (with abscess of any
      other site) A06.6
   gonococcal A54.82
   pheomycotic (chromomycotic)
      B43.1
   tuberculous A17.81
breast (acute) (chronic)
   (nonpuerperal) N61.1
   newborn P39.0
   puerperal, postpartum,
      gestational —*see* Mastitis,
      obstetric, purulent
broad ligament N73.2
   acute N73.0
   chronic N73.1
Brodie's (localized) (chronic)
   M86.8X-
bronchi J98.09
buccal cavity K12.2
bulbourethral gland N34.0
bursa M71.00
   ankle M71.07-
   elbow M71.02-
   foot M71.07-
   hand M71.04-
   hip M71.05-
   knee M71.06-
   multiple sites M71.09
   pharyngeal J39.1
   shoulder M71.01-
   specified site NEC M71.08
   wrist M71.03-
buttock L02.31
canthus —*see*
   Blepharoconjunctivitis
cartilage —*see* Disorder, cartilage,
   specified type NEC
cecum K35.33
cerebellum, cerebellar G06.0
   sequelae G09
cerebral (embolic) G06.0
   sequelae G09
cervical (meaning neck) L02.11
   lymph gland or node L04.0
cervix (stump) (uteri) —*see*
   Cervicitis
cheek (external) L02.01
   inner K12.2
chest J86.9
   with fistula J86.0
   wall L02.213
chin L02.01
choroid —*see* Inflammation,
   chorioretinal
circumtonsillar J36
cold (lung) (tuberculous) —*see*
   also Tuberculosis, abscess, lung
   articular —*see* Tuberculosis,
      joint

Abscess (*continued*)

colon (wall) K63.0
colostomy K94.02
conjunctiva —*see* Conjunctivitis, acute
cornea H16.31-
corpus
  cavernosum N48.21
  luteum —*see* Oophoritis
Cowper's gland N34.0
cranium G06.0
cul-de-sac (Douglas') (posterior) —*see* Peritonitis, pelvic, female
cutaneous —*see* Abscess, by site
dental K04.7
  with sinus (alveolar) K04.6
dentoalveolar K04.7
  with sinus K04.6
diaphragm, diaphragmatic K65.1
Douglas' cul-de-sac or pouch —*see* Peritonitis, pelvic, female
Dubois A50.59
ear (middle) —*see also* Otitis, media, suppurative
  acute —*see* Otitis, media, suppurative, acute
  external H60.0-
entamebic —*see* Abscess, amebic
enterostomy K94.12
epididymis N45.4
epidural G06.2
  brain G06.0
  spinal cord G06.1
epiglottis J38.7
epiploon, epiploic K65.1
erysipelatous —*see* Erysipelas
esophagus K20.80
ethmoid (bone) (chronic) (sinus) J32.2
external auditory canal —*see* Abscess, ear, external
extradural G06.2
  brain G06.0
    sequelae G09
  spinal cord G06.1
extraperitoneal K68.19
eye —*see* Endophthalmitis, purulent
eyelid H00.03-
face (any part, except ear, eye and nose) L02.01
fallopian tube —*see* Salpingitis
fascia M72.8
fauces J39.1
fecal K63.0
femoral (region) —*see* Abscess, lower limb
filaria, filarial —*see* Infestation, filarial
finger (any) —*see also* Abscess, hand
  nail —*see* Cellulitis, finger
foot L02.61-
forehead L02.01
frontal sinus (chronic) J32.1
gallbladder K81.0
genital organ or tract
  female (external) N76.4
  male N49.9
    multiple sites N49.8
    specified NEC N49.8
gestational mammary O91.11-
gestational subareolar O91.11-
gingival — *see* Periodontitis, localized
gland, glandular (lymph) (acute) —*see* Lymphadenitis, acute
gluteal (region) L02.31
gonorrheal —*see* Gonococcus
groin L02.214
gum — *see* Periodontitis, localized

Abscess (*continued*)

hand L02.51-
head NEC L02.811
  face (any part, except ear, eye and nose) L02.01
heart —*see* Carditis
heel —*see* Abscess, foot
helminthic —*see* Infestation, helminth
hepatic (cholangitic) (hematogenic) (lymphogenic) (pylephlebitic) K75.0
  amebic A06.4
horseshoe K61.31
hip (region) —*see* Abscess, lower limb
ileocecal K35.33
ileostomy (bud) K94.12
iliac (region) L02.214
  fossa K35.33
infraclavicular (fossa) —*see* Abscess, upper limb
inguinal (region) L02.214
  lymph gland or node L04.1
intersphincteric K61.4
intestine, intestinal NEC K63.0
  rectal K61.1
intra-abdominal (*see also* Abscess, peritoneum) K65.1
  following procedure T81.43
    obstetrical O86.03
  postprocedural T81.43
    retroperitoneal K68.11
intracranial G06.0
intramammary —*see* Abscess, breast
intramuscular, following procedure T81.42
  obstetrical O86.02
intraorbital —*see* Abscess, orbit
intraperitoneal K65.1
intrasphincteric (anus) K61.4
intraspinal G06.1
intratonsillar J36
ischiorectal (fossa) (specified NEC) K61.39
jaw (bone) (lower) (upper) M27.2
joint —*see* Arthritis, pyogenic or pyemic
  spine (tuberculous) A18.01
    nontuberculous —*see* Spondylopathy, infective
kidney N15.1
  with calculus N20.0
    with hydronephrosis N13.6
  puerperal (postpartum) O86.21
knee —*see also* Abscess, lower limb
  joint M00.9
labium (majus) (minus) N76.4
lacrimal
  caruncle —*see* Inflammation, lacrimal, passages, acute
  gland —*see* Dacryoadenitis
  passages (duct) (sac) —*see* Inflammation, lacrimal, passages, acute
lacunar N34.0
larynx J38.7
lateral (alveolar) K04.7
  with sinus K04.6
leg (any part) —*see* Abscess, lower limb
lens H27.8
lingual K14.0
  tonsil J36
lip K13.0
Littre's gland N34.0
liver (cholangitic) (hematogenic) (lymphogenic) (pylephlebitic) (pyogenic) K75.0

Abscess (*continued*)

liver (*continued*)
  amebic (due to Entamoeba histolytica) (dysenteric) (tropical) A06.4
    with
      brain abscess (and liver or lung abscess) A06.6
      lung abscess A06.5
loin (region) L02.211
lower limb L02.41-
lumbar (tuberculous) A18.01
  nontuberculous L02.212
lung (miliary) (putrid) J85.2
  with pneumonia J85.1
    due to specified organism (*see* Pneumonia, in (due to))
  amebic (with liver abscess) A06.5
    with
      brain abscess A06.6
      pneumonia A06.5
lymph, lymphatic, gland or node (acute) —*see also* Lymphadenitis, acute
  mesentery I88.0
malar M27.2
mammary gland —*see* Abscess, breast
marginal, anus K61.0
mastoid —*see* Mastoiditis, acute
maxilla, maxillary M27.2
  molar (tooth) K04.7
    with sinus K04.6
  premolar K04.7
  sinus (chronic) J32.0
mediastinum J85.3
meibomian gland —*see* Hordeolum
meninges G06.2
mesentery, mesenteric K65.1
mesosalpinx —*see* Salpingitis
mons pubis L02.215
mouth (floor) K12.2
muscle —*see* Myositis, infective
myocardium I40.0
nabothian (follicle) —*see* Cervicitis
nasal J32.9
nasopharyngeal J39.1
navel L02.216
  newborn P38.9
    with mild hemorrhage P38.1
    without hemorrhage P38.9
neck (region) L02.11
  lymph gland or node L04.0
nephritic —*see* Abscess, kidney
nipple N61.1
  associated with
    lactation —*see* Pregnancy, complicated by
    pregnancy —*see* Pregnancy, complicated by
nose (external) (fossa) (septum) J34.0
  sinus (chronic) —*see* Sinusitis
omentum K65.1
operative wound T81.49
orbit, orbital —*see* Cellulitis, orbit
otogenic G06.0
ovary, ovarian (corpus luteum) —*see* Oophoritis
oviduct —*see* Oophoritis
palate (soft) K12.2
  hard M27.2
palmar (space) —*see* Abscess, hand
pancreas (duct) —*see* Pancreatitis, acute
parafrenal N48.21
parametric, parametrium N73.2
  acute N73.0
  chronic N73.1

Abscess (*continued*)

paranephric N15.1
parapancreatic —*see* Pancreatitis, acute
parapharyngeal J39.0
pararectal K61.1
parasinus —*see* Sinusitis
parauterine —*see also* Disease, pelvis, inflammatory N73.2
paravaginal —*see* Vaginitis
parietal region (scalp) L02.811
parodontal —*see* Periodontitis, aggressive, localized
parotid (duct) (gland) K11.3
  region K12.2
pectoral (region) L02.213
pelvis, pelvic
  female —*see* Disease, pelvis, inflammatory
  male, peritoneal K65.1
penis N48.21
  gonococcal (accessory gland) (periurethral) A54.1
perianal K61.0
periapical K04.7
  with sinus (alveolar) K04.6
periappendicular K35.33
pericardial I30.1
pericecal K35.33
pericemental —*see* Periodontitis, aggressive, localized
pericholecystic —*see* Cholecystitis, acute
pericoronal —*see* Periodontitis, aggressive, localized
peridental —*see* Periodontitis, aggressive, localized
perimetric —*see also* Disease, pelvis, inflammatory N73.2
perinephric, perinephritic —*see* Abscess, kidney
perineum, perineal (superficial) L02.215
  urethra N34.0
periodontal (parietal) —*see* Periodontitis, aggressive, localized
  apical K04.7
periosteum, periosteal —*see also* Osteomyelitis, specified type NEC
  with osteomyelitis —*see also* Osteomyelitis, specified type NEC
    acute —*see* Osteomyelitis, acute
    chronic —*see* Osteomyelitis, chronic
peripharyngeal J39.0
peripleuritic J86.9
  with fistula J86.0
periprostatic N41.2
perirectal K61.1
perirenal (tissue) —*see* Abscess, kidney
perisinuous (nose) —*see* Sinusitis
peritoneum, peritoneal (perforated) K66.0 (ruptured) K65.1
  with appendicitis (*see also* Appendicitis) K35.33
  pelvic
    female —*see* Peritonitis, pelvic, female
    male K65.1
  postoperative T81.49
  puerperal, postpartum, childbirth O85
  tuberculous A18.31
peritonsillar J36
perityphlic K35.33
periureteral N28.89

Abscess *(continued)*

pechurethral N34.0
 gonococcal (accessory gland)
  (periurethral) A54.1
periuterine —*see also* Disease,
 pelvis, inflammatory N73.2
perivesical —*see* Cystitis, specified
 type NEC
petrous bone —*see* Petrositis
phagedenic NOS L02.91
 chancroid A57
pharynx, pharyngeal (lateral)
 J39.1
pilonidal L05.01
pituitary (gland) E23.6
pleura J86.9
 with fistula J86.0
popliteal —*see* Abscess, lower
 limb
postcecal K35.33
postlaryngeal J38.7
postnasal J34.0
postoperative (any site) (*see also*
 Infection, postoperative wound)
 T81.49
 retroperitoneal K68.11
postpharyngeal J39.0
posttonsillar J36
post-typhoid A01.09
pouch of Douglas —*see* Peritonitis,
 pelvic, female
premammary —*see* Abscess, breast
prepatellar —*see* Abscess, lower
 limb
prostate N41.2
 gonococcal (acute) (chronic)
  A54.22
psoas muscle K68.12
puerperal - code by site under
 Puerperal, abscess
pulmonary —*see* Abscess, lung
pulp, pulpal (dental) K04.01
 irreversible K04.02
 reversible K04.01
rectovaginal septum K63.0
rectovesical —*see* Cystitis,
 specified type NEC
rectum K61.1
renal —*see* Abscess, kidney
retina —*see* Inflammation,
 chorioretinal
retrobulbar —*see* Abscess, orbit
retrocecal K65.1
retrolaryngeal J38.7
retromammary —*see* Abscess,
 breast
retroperitoneal NEC K68.19
 postprocedural K68.11
retropharyngeal J39.0
retrouterine —*see* Peritonitis,
 pelvic, female
retrovesical —*see* Cystitis,
 specified type NEC
root, tooth K04.7
 with sinus (alveolar) K04.6
round ligament —*see also* Disease,
 pelvis, inflammatory N73.2
rupture (spontaneous) NOS L02.91
sacrum (tuberculous) A18.01
 nontuberculous M46.28
salivary (duct) (gland) K11.3
scalp (any part) L02.811
scapular —*see* Osteomyelitis,
 specified type NEC
sclera —*see* Scleritis
scrofulous (tuberculous) A18.2
scrotum N49.2
seminal vesicle N49.0
septal, dental K04.7
 with sinus (alveolar) K04.6
serous —*see* Periostitis

Abscess *(continued)*

shoulder (region) —*see* Abscess,
 upper limb
sigmoid K63.0
sinus (accessory) (chronic) (nasal)
 —*see also* Sinusitis
 intracranial venous (any) G06.0
Skene's duct or gland N34.0
skin —*see* Abscess, by site
specified site NEC L02.818
spermatic cord N49.1
sphenoidal (sinus) (chronic) J32.3
spinal cord (any part)
 (staphylococcal) G06.1
 tuberculous A17.81
spine (column) (tuberculous) A18.01
 epidural G06.1
 nontuberculous —*see*
  Osteomyelitis, vertebra
spleen D73.3
 amebic A06.89
stitch T81.41
 following an obstetrical
  procedure O86.01
subarachnoid G06.2
 brain G06.0
 spinal cord G06.1
subareolar —*see* Abscess, breast
subcecal K35.33
subcutaneous —*see also* Abscess,
 by site
 following procedure T81.41
  obstetrical O86.01
 pheomycotic (chromomycotic)
  B43.2
subdiaphragmatic K65.1
subdural G06.2
 brain G06.0
  sequelae G09
 spinal cord G06.1
sub-fascial, following an obstetrical
 procedure O86.02
subgaleal L02.811
subhepatic K65.1
sublingual K12.2
 gland K11.3
submammary —*see* Abscess, breast
submandibular (region) (space)
 (triangle) K12.2
 gland K11.3
submaxillary (region) L02.01
 gland K11.3
submental L02.01
 gland K11.3
subperiosteal —*see* Osteomyelitis,
 specified type NEC
subphrenic K65.1
 following an obstetrical
  procedure O86.03
 postoperative T81.43
suburethral N34.0
sudoriparous L75.8
supraclavicular (fossa) —*see*
 Abscess, upper limb
supralevator K61.5
suprapelvic, acute N73.0
suprarenal (capsule) (gland) E27.8
sweat gland L74.8
tear duct —*see* Inflammation,
 lacrimal, passages, acute
temple L02.01
temporal region L02.01
temporosphenoidal G06.0
tendon (sheath) M65.00
 ankle M65.07-
 foot M65.07-
 forearm M65.03-
 hand M65.04-
 lower leg M65.06-
 pelvic region M65.05-
 shoulder region M65.01-

Abscess *(continued)*

tendon *(continued)*
 specified site NEC M65.08
 thigh M65.05-
 upper arm M65.02-
testis N45.4
thigh —*see* Abscess, lower limb
thorax J86.9
 with fistula J86.0
throat J39.1
thumb —*see also* Abscess, hand
 nail —*see* Cellulitis, finger
thymus (gland) E32.1
thyroid (gland) E06.0
toe (any) —*see also* Abscess, foot
 nail —*see* Cellulitis, toe
tongue (staphylococcal) K14.0
tonsil(s) (lingual) J36
tonsillopharyngeal J36
tooth, teeth (root) K04.7
 with sinus (alveolar) K04.6
 supporting structures NEC
  — *see* Periodontitis,
  aggressive, localized
trachea J39.8
trunk L02.219
 abdominal wall L02.211
 back L02.212
 chest wall L02.213
 groin L02.214
 perineum L02.215
 umbilicus L02.216
tubal —*see* Salpingitis
tuberculous —*see* Tuberculosis,
 abscess
tubo-ovarian —*see* Salpingo-
 oophoritis
tunica vaginalis N49.1
umbilicus L02.216
upper
 limb L02.41-
 respiratory J39.8
urethral (gland) N34.0
urinary N34.0
uterus, uterine (wall) —*see also*
 Endometritis
 ligament —*see also* Disease,
  pelvis, inflammatory N73.2
 neck —*see* Cervicitis
uvula K12.2
vagina (wall) —*see* Vaginitis
vaginorectal —*see* Vaginitis
vas deferens N49.1
vermiform appendix K35.33
vertebra (column) (tuberculous)
 A18.01
 nontuberculous —*see*
  Osteomyelitis, vertebra
vesical —*see* Cystitis, specified
 type NEC
vesico-uterine pouch —*see*
 Peritonitis, pelvic, female
vitreous (humor) —*see*
 Endophthalmitis, purulent
vocal cord J38.3
von Bezold's —*see* Mastoiditis, acute
vulva N76.4
vulvovaginal gland N75.1
web space —*see* Abscess, hand
wound T81.49
wrist —*see* Abscess, upper limb

Absence (of) (organ or part)
 (complete or partial)
 adrenal (gland) (congenital) Q89.1
  acquired E89.6
 albumin in blood E88.09
 alimentary tract (congenital) Q45.8
  upper Q40.8
 alveolar process (acquired) —*see*
  Anomaly, alveolar
 ankle (acquired) Z89.44-

Absence *(continued)*

anus (congenital) Q42.3
 with fistula Q42.2
aorta (congenital) Q25.41
appendix, congenital Q42.8
arm (acquired) Z89.20-
 above elbow Z89.22-
  congenital (with hand present)
   —*see* Agenesis, arm, with
   hand present
   and hand —*see* Agenesis,
   forearm, and hand
 below elbow Z89.21-
  congenital (with hand present)
   —*see* Agenesis, arm, with
   hand present
   and hand —*see* Agenesis,
   forearm, and hand
 congenital —*see* Defect,
  reduction, upper limb
 shoulder (following explantation
  of shoulder joint prosthesis)
  (joint) (with or without
  presence of antibiotic-
  impregnated cement spacer)
  Z89.23-
  congenital (with hand present)
   —*see* Agenesis, arm, with
   hand present
artery (congenital) (peripheral)
 Q27.8
 brain Q28.3
 coronary Q24.5
 pulmonary Q25.79
 specified NEC Q27.8
 umbilical Q27.0
atrial septum (congenital) Q21.1
auditory canal (congenital)
 (external) Q16.1
auricle (ear), congenital Q16.0
bile, biliary duct, congenital
 Q44.5
bladder (acquired) Z90.6
 congenital Q64.5
bowel sounds R19.11
brain Q00.0
 part of Q04.3
breast(s) (and nipple(s)) (acquired)
 Z90.1-
 congenital Q83.8
broad ligament Q50.6
bronchus (congenital) Q32.4
canaliculus lacrimalis, congenital
 Q10.4
cerebellum (vermis) Q04.3
cervix (acquired) (with uterus)
 Z90.710
 with remaining uterus Z90.712
 congenital Q51.5
chin, congenital Q18.8
cilia (congenital) Q10.3
 acquired —*see* Madarosis
clitoris (congenital) Q52.6
coccyx, congenital Q76.49
cold sense R20.8
congenital
 lumen —*see* Atresia
 organ or site NEC —*see*
  Agenesis
 septum —*see* Imperfect, closure
corpus callosum Q04.0
cricoid cartilage, congenital Q31.8
diaphragm (with hernia), congenital
 Q79.1
digestive organ(s) or tract,
 congenital Q45.8
 acquired NEC Z90.49
 upper Q40.8
ductus arteriosus Q28.8
duodenum (acquired) Z90.49
 congenital Q41.0

Absence *(continued)*
ear, congenital Q16.9
  acquired H93.8-
  auricle Q16.0
  external Q16.0
  inner Q16.5
  lobe, lobule Q17.8
  middle, except ossicles Q16.4
    ossicles Q16.3
  ossicles Q16.3
ejaculatory duct (congenital) Q55.4
endocrine gland (congenital) NEC
  Q89.2
  acquired E89.89
epididymis (congenital) Q55.4
  acquired Z90.79
epiglottis, congenital Q31.8
esophagus (congenital) Q39.8
  acquired (partial) Z90.49
eustachian tube (congenital) Q16.2
extremity (acquired) Z89.9
  congenital Q73.0
  knee (following explantation of
    knee joint prosthesis) (joint)
    (with or without presence of
    antibiotic-impregnated cement
    spacer) Z89.52-
  lower (above knee) Z89.619
    below knee Z89.51-
  upper —*see* Absence, arm
eye (acquired) Z90.01
  congenital Q11.1
  muscle (congenital) Q10.3
eyeball (acquired) Z90.01
eyelid (fold) (congenital) Q10.3
  acquired Z90.01
face, specified part NEC Q18.8
fallopian tube(s) (acquired) Z90.79
  congenital Q50.6
family member (causing problem
  in home) NEC —*see also*
  Disruption, family Z63.32
femur, congenital —*see* Defect,
  reduction, lower limb,
  longitudinal, femur
fibrinogen (congenital) D68.2
  acquired D65
finger(s) (acquired) Z89.02-
  congenital —*see* Agenesis, hand
foot (acquired) Z89.43-
  congenital —*see* Agenesis, foot
forearm (acquired) —*see* Absence,
  arm, below elbow
gallbladder (acquired) Z90.49
  congenital Q44.0
gamma globulin in blood D80.1
  hereditary D80.0
genital organs
  acquired (female) (male)
    Z90.79
  female, congenital Q52.8
    external Q52.71
    internal NEC Q52.8
  male, congenital Q55.8
genitourinary organs, congenital
  NEC
  female Q52.8
  male Q55.8
globe (acquired) Z90.01
  congenital Q11.1
glottis, congenital Q31.8
hand and wrist (acquired) Z89.11-
  congenital —*see* Agenesis, hand
head, part (acquired) NEC Z90.09
heat sense R20.8
hip (following explantation of hip
  joint prosthesis) (joint) (with or
  without presence of antibiotic-
  impregnated cement spacer)
  Z89.62-
hymen (congenital) Q52.4

Absence *(continued)*
ileum (acquired) Z90.49
  congenital Q41.2
immunoglobulin, isolated NEC
  D80.3
  IgA D80.2
  IgG D80.3
  IgM D80.4
incus (acquired) —*see* Loss,
  ossicles, ear
  congenital Q16.3
inner ear, congenital Q16.5
intestine (acquired) (small) Z90.49
  congenital Q41.9
    specified NEC Q41.8
  large Z90.49
    congenital Q42.9
      specified NEC Q42.8
iris, congenital Q13.1
jejunum (acquired) Z90.49
  congenital Q41.1
joint
  acquired
    hip (following explantation
      of hip joint prosthesis)
      (with or without presence
      of antibiotic-impregnated
      cement spacer) Z89.62-
    knee (following explantation
      of knee joint prosthesis)
      (with or without presence
      of antibiotic-impregnated
      cement spacer) Z89.52-
    shoulder (following
      explantation of shoulder
      joint prosthesis) (with
      or without presence of
      antibiotic-impregnated
      cement spacer) Z89.23-
  congenital NEC Q74.8
kidney(s) (acquired) Z90.5
  congenital Q60.2
    bilateral Q60.1
    unilateral Q60.0
knee (following explantation of
  knee joint prosthesis) (joint)
  (with or without presence of
  antibiotic-impregnated cement
  spacer) Z89.52-
labyrinth, membranous Q16.5
larynx (congenital) Q31.8
  acquired Z90.02
leg (acquired) (above knee) Z89.61-
  below knee (acquired) Z89.51-
  congenital —*see* Defect,
    reduction, lower limb
lens (acquired) —*see also* Aphakia
  congenital Q12.3
  post cataract extraction Z98.4-
limb (acquired) —*see* Absence,
  extremity
lip Q38.6
liver (congenital) Q44.7
lung (fissure) (lobe) (bilateral)
  (unilateral) (congenital) Q33.3
  acquired (any part) Z90.2
menstruation —*see* Amenorrhea
muscle (congenital) (pectoral)
  Q79.8
  ocular Q10.3
neck, part Q18.8
neutrophil —*see* Agranulocytosis
nipple(s) (with breast(s)) (acquired)
  Z90.1-
  congenital Q83.2
nose (congenital) Q30.1
  acquired Z90.09
organ
  of Corti, congenital Q16.5
  or site, congenital NEC Q89.8
    acquired NEC Z90.89

Absence *(continued)*
osseous meatus (ear) Q16.4
ovary (acquired)
  bilateral Z90.722
  congenital
    bilateral Q50.02
    unilateral Q50.01
  unilateral Z90.721
oviduct (acquired)
  bilateral Z90.722
  congenital Q50.6
  unilateral Z90.721
pancreas (congenital) Q45.0
  acquired Z90.410
  complete Z90.410
  partial Z90.411
  total Z90.410
parathyroid gland (acquired) E89.2
  congenital Q89.2
patella, congenital Q74.1
penis (congenital) Q55.5
  acquired Z90.79
pericardium (congenital) Q24.8
pituitary gland (congenital) Q89.2
  acquired E89.3
prostate (acquired) Z90.79
  congenital Q55.4
pulmonary valve Q22.0
punctum lacrimale (congenital)
  Q10.4
radius, congenital —*see* Defect,
  reduction, upper limb,
  longitudinal, radius
rectum (congenital) Q42.1
  with fistula Q42.0
  acquired Z90.49
respiratory organ NOS Q34.9
rib (acquired) Z90.89
  congenital Q76.6
sacrum, congenital Q76.49
salivary gland(s), congenital Q38.4
scrotum, congenital Q55.29
seminal vesicles (congenital) Q55.4
  acquired Z90.79
septum
  atrial (congenital) Q21.1
  between aorta and pulmonary
    artery Q21.4
  ventricular (congenital) Q20.4
sex chromosome
  female phenotype Q97.8
  male phenotype Q98.8
skull bone (congenital) Q75.8
  with
    anencephaly Q00.0
    encephalocele —*see*
      Encephalocele
    hydrocephalus Q03.9
      with spina bifida —*see*
        Spina bifida, by site, with
        hydrocephalus
    microcephaly Q02
spermatic cord, congenital Q55.4
spine, congenital Q76.49
spleen (congenital) Q89.01
  acquired Z90.81
sternum, congenital Q76.7
stomach (acquired) (partial) Z90.3
  congenital Q40.2
superior vena cava, congenital
  Q26.8
teeth, tooth (congenital) K00.0
  acquired (complete) K08.109
    class I K08.101
    class II K08.102
    class III K08.103
    class IV K08.104
    due to
      caries K08.139
        class I K08.131
        class II K08.132

Absence *(continued)*
teeth, tooth *(continued)*
  acquired *(continued)*
    due to *(continued)*
      caries *(continued)*
        class III K08.133
        class IV K08.134
      periodontal disease K08.129
        class I K08.121
        class II K08.122
        class III K08.123
        class IV K08.124
      specified NEC K08.199
        class I K08.191
        class II K08.192
        class III K08.193
        class IV K08.194
      trauma K08.119
        class I K08.111
        class II K08.112
        class III K08.113
        class IV K08.114
    partial K08.409
      class I K08.401
      class II K08.402
      class III K08.403
      class IV K08.404
      due to
        caries K08.439
          class I K08.431
          class II K08.432
          class III K08.433
          class IV K08.434
        periodontal disease
          K08.429
          class I K08.421
          class II K08.422
          class III K08.423
          class IV K08.424
        specified NEC K08.499
          class I K08.491
          class II K08.492
          class III K08.493
          class IV K08.494
        trauma K08.419
          class I K08.411
          class II K08.412
          class III K08.413
          class IV K08.414
tendon (congenital) Q79.8
testis (congenital) Q55.0
  acquired Z90.79
thumb (acquired) Z89.01-
  congenital —*see* Agenesis, hand
thymus gland Q89.2
thyroid (gland) (acquired) E89.0
  cartilage, congenital Q31.8
  congenital E03.1
toe(s) (acquired) Z89.42-
  with foot —*see* Absence, foot
    and ankle
  congenital —*see* Agenesis, foot
  great Z89.41-
tongue, congenital Q38.3
trachea (cartilage), congenital
  Q32.1
transverse aortic arch, congenital
  Q25.49
tricuspid valve Q22.4
umbilical artery, congenital Q27.0
upper arm and forearm with
  hand present, congenital —*see*
  Agenesis, arm, with hand present
ureter (congenital) Q62.4
  acquired Z90.6
urethra, congenital Q64.5
uterus (acquired) Z90.710
  with cervix Z90.710
  with remaining cervical stump
    Z90.711
  congenital Q51.0

Absence–Abuse

8

Abuse (*continued*)
  drug NEC (*continued*)
    sedative, hypnotic or anxiolytic
    (*continued*)
      with
        anxiety disorder F13.180
        intoxication F13.129
          with delirium F13.121
          uncomplicated F13.120
        mood disorder F13.14
        other specified disorder
          F13.188
        psychosis F13.159
          delusions F13.150
          hallucinations F13.151
        sexual dysfunction F13.181
        sleep disorder F13.182
        unspecified disorder F13.19
        withdrawal F13.139
        with
          perceptual disturbance
            F13.132
          delirium F13.131
          uncomplicated F13.130
      in remission (early)
        (sustained) F13.11
    solvent —*see* Abuse, drug,
      inhalant
    steroids F55.3
    stimulant NEC F15.10
      with
        anxiety disorder F15.180
        intoxication F15.129
          with
            delirium F15.121
            perceptual disturbance
              F15.122
          uncomplicated F15.120
        mood disorder F15.14
        other specified disorder
          F15.188
        psychosis F15.159
          delusions F15.150
          hallucinations F15.151
        sexual dysfunction F15.181
        sleep disorder F15.182
        unspecified disorder F15.19
        withdrawal F15.13
      in remission (early)
        (sustained) F15.11
    tranquilizers —*see* Abuse, drug,
      sedative
    vitamins F55.4
  hallucinogens —*see* Abuse, drug,
    hallucinogen
  hashish —*see* Abuse, drug,
    cannabis
  herbal or folk remedies F55.1
  hormones F55.3
  hypnotic —*see* Abuse, drug,
    sedative
  inhalant —*see* Abuse, drug,
    inhalant
  laxatives F55.2
  LSD —*see* Abuse, drug,
    hallucinogen
  marihuana —*see* Abuse, drug,
    cannabis
  morphine type (opioids) —*see*
    Abuse, drug, opioid
  non-psychoactive substance NEC
    F55.8
    antacids F55.0
    folk remedies F55.1
    herbal remedies F55.1
    hormones F55.3
    laxatives F55.2
    steroids F55.3
    vitamins F55.4
  opioids —*see* Abuse,
    drug, opioid

Abuse (*continued*)
  PCP (phencyclidine) (or related
    substance) —*see* Abuse, drug,
    hallucinogen
  physical (adult) (child) —*see*
    Maltreatment
  psychoactive substance —*see*
    Abuse, drug, psychoactive NEC
  psychological (adult) (child) —*see*
    Maltreatment
  sedative —*see* Abuse, drug, sedative
  sexual —*see* Maltreatment
  solvent —*see* Abuse, drug, inhalant
  steroids F55.3
  vitamins F55.4

Acalculia R48.8
  developmental F81.2

Acanthamebiasis (with) B60.10
  conjunctiva B60.12
  keratoconjunctivitis B60.13
  meningoencephalitis B60.11
  other specified B60.19

Acanthocephaliasis B83.8

Acanthocheilonemiasis B74.4

Acanthocytosis E78.6

Acantholysis L11.9

Acanthosis (acquired) (nigricans) L83
  benign Q82.8
  congenital Q82.8
  seborrheic L82.1
    inflamed L82.0
  tongue K14.3

Acapnia E87.3

Acarbia E87.2

Acardia, acardius Q89.8

Acardiacus amorphus Q89.8

Acardiotrophia I51.4

Acariasis B88.0
  scabies B86

Acarodermatitis (urticarioides) B88.0

Acarophobia F40.218

Acatalasemia, acatalasia E80.3

Acathisia (drug induced) G25.71

**Accelerated atrioventricular
conduction** I45.6

Accentuation of personality traits
(type A) Z73.1

Accessory (congenital)
  adrenal gland Q89.1
  anus Q43.4
  appendix Q43.4
  atrioventricular conduction I45.6
  auditory ossicles Q16.3
  auricle (ear) Q17.0
  biliary duct or passage Q44.5
  bladder Q64.79
  blood vessels NEC Q27.9
    coronary Q24.5
  bone NEC Q79.8
  breast tissue, axilla Q83.1
  carpal bones Q74.0
  cecum Q43.4
  chromosome(s) NEC (nonsex) Q92.9
    with complex rearrangements
      NEC Q92.5
      seen only at prometaphase Q92.8
    partial Q92.9
    sex
      female phenotype Q97.8
    13 —*see* Trisomy, 13
    18 —*see* Trisomy, 18
    21 —*see* Trisomy, 21
  coronary artery Q24.5
  cusp(s), heart valve NEC Q24.8
    pulmonary Q22.3

Accessory (*continued*)
  cystic duct Q44.5
  digit(s) Q69.9
  ear (auricle) (lobe) Q17.0
  endocrine gland NEC Q89.2
  eye muscle Q10.3
  eyelid Q10.3
  face bone(s) Q75.8
  fallopian tube (fimbria) (ostium)
    Q50.6
  finger(s) Q69.0
  foreskin N47.8
  frontonasal process Q75.8
  gallbladder Q44.1
  genital organ(s)
    female Q52.8
      external Q52.79
      internal NEC Q52.8
    male Q55.8
  genitourinary organs NEC Q89.8
    female Q52.8
    male Q55.8
  hallux Q69.2
  heart Q24.8
    valve NEC Q24.8
      pulmonary Q22.3
  hepatic ducts Q44.5
  hymen Q52.4
  intestine (large) (small) Q43.4
  kidney Q63.0
  lacrimal canal Q10.6
  leaflet, heart valve NEC Q24.8
  ligament, broad Q50.6
  liver Q44.7
    duct Q44.5
  lobule (ear) Q17.0
  lung (lobe) Q33.1
  muscle Q79.8
  navicular of carpus Q74.0
  nervous system, part NEC Q07.8
  nipple Q83.3
  nose Q30.8
  organ or site not listed —*see*
    Anomaly, by site
  ovary Q50.31
  oviduct Q50.6
  pancreas Q45.3
  parathyroid gland Q89.2
  parotid gland (and duct) Q38.4
  pituitary gland Q89.2
  preauricular appendage Q17.0
  prepuce N47.8
  renal arteries (multiple) Q27.2
  rib Q76.6
    cervical Q76.5
  roots (teeth) K00.2
  salivary gland Q38.4
  sesamoid bones Q74.8
    foot Q74.2
    hand Q74.0
  skin tags Q82.8
  spleen Q89.09
  sternum Q76.7
  submaxillary gland Q38.4
  tarsal bones Q74.2
  teeth, tooth K00.1
  tendon Q79.8
  thumb Q69.1
  thymus gland Q89.2
  thyroid gland Q89.2
  toes Q69.2
  tongue Q38.3
  tooth, teeth K00.1
  tragus Q17.0
  ureter Q62.5
  urethra Q64.79
  urinary organ or tract NEC Q64.8
  uterus Q51.28
  vagina Q52.10
  valve, heart NEC Q24.8
    pulmonary Q22.3

Accessory (*continued*)
  vertebra Q76.49
  vocal cords Q31.8
  vulva Q52.79

Accident
  birth —*see* Birth, injury
  cardiac —*see* Infarct, myocardium
  cerebral I63.9
  cerebrovascular (embolic)
    (ischemic) (thrombotic) I63.9
    aborted I63.9
    hemorrhagic —*see* Hemorrhage,
      intracranial, intracerebral
    old (without sequelae) Z86.73
      with sequelae (of) —*see*
        Sequelae, infarction, cerebral
    coronary —*see* Infarct, myocardium
  craniovascular I63.9
  vascular, brain I63.9

Accidental —*see* condition

Accommodation (disorder) —*see
also* condition
  hysterical paralysis of F44.89
  insufficiency of H52.4
  paresis —*see* Paresis, of
    accommodation
  spasm —*see* Spasm, of
    accommodation

Accouchement —*see* Delivery

Accreta placenta O43.21-

Accretio cordis (nonrheumatic) I31.0

Accretions, tooth, teeth K03.6

Acculturation difficulty Z60.3

Accumulation secretion, prostate
N42.89

**Acephalia, acephalism, acephalus,
acephaly** Q00.0

Acephalobrachia monster Q89.8

Acephalochirus monster Q89.8

Acephalogaster Q89.8

Acephalostomus monster Q89.8

Acephalothorax Q89.8

Acerophobia F40.298

Acetonemia R79.89
  in Type 1 diabetes E10.10
    with coma E10.11

Acetonuria R82.4

Achalasia (cardia) (esophagus) K22.0
  congenital Q39.5
  pylorus Q40.0
  sphincteral NEC K59.89

Ache(s) —*see* Pain

Acheilia Q38.6

Achillobursitis —*see* Tendinitis, Achilles

Achillodynia —*see* Tendinitis, Achilles

Achlorhydria, achlorhydric
(neurogenic) K31.83
  anemia D50.8
  diarrhea K31.83
  psychogenic F45.8
  secondary to vagotomy K91.1

Achluophobia F40.228

Acholia K82.8

Acholuric jaundice (familial)
(splenomegalic) —*see also*
Spherocytosis
  acquired D59.8

Achondrogenesis Q77.0

Achondroplasia (osteosclerosis
congenita) Q77.4

Achroma, cutis L80

Achromat (ism), achromatopsia
(acquired) (congenital) H53.51

Achromia, congenital —*see* Albinism

Achromia parasitica B36.0

Achylia gastrica K31.89
  psychogenic F45.8

Acid
  burn —*see* Corrosion
  deficiency
    amide nicotinic E52
    ascorbic E54
    folic E53.8
    nicotinic E52
    pantothenic E53.8
  intoxication E87.2
  peptic disease K30
  phosphatase deficiency E83.39
  stomach K30
    psychogenic F45.8

Acidemia E87.2
  argininosuccinic E72.22
  isovaleric E71.110
  metabolic (newborn) P19.9
    first noted before onset of labor P19.0
    first noted during labor P19.1
    noted at birth P19.2
  methylmalonic E71.120
  pipecolic E72.3
  propionic E71.121

Acidity, gastric (high) K30
  psychogenic F45.8

Acidocytopenia —*see* Agranulocytosis

Acidocytosis D72.10

Acidopenia —*see* Agranulocytosis

Acidosis (lactic) (respiratory) E87.2
  in Type 1 diabetes E10.10
    with coma E10.11
  kidney, tubular N25.89
  lactic E87.2
  metabolic NEC E87.2
    with respiratory acidosis E87.4
    hyperchloremic, of newborn P74.421
    late, of newborn P74.0
  mixed metabolic and respiratory, newborn P84
  newborn P84
  renal (hyperchloremic) (tubular) N25.89
  respiratory E87.2
    complicated by
      metabolic
        acidosis E87.4
        alkalosis E87.4

Aciduria
  4-hydroxybutyric E72.81
  argininosuccinic E72.22
  gamma-hydroxybutyric E72.81
  glutaric (type I) E72.3
    type II E71.313
    type III E71.5-
  orotic (congenital) (hereditary) (pyrimidine deficiency) E79.8
    anemia D53.0

Acladiosis (skin) B36.0

Aclasis, diaphyseal Q78.6

Acleistocardia Q21.1

Aclusion —*see* Anomaly, dentofacial, malocclusion

Acne L70.9
  artificialis L70.8
  atrophica L70.2
  cachecticorum (Hebra) L70.8
  conglobata L70.1
  cystic L70.0
  decalvans L66.2
  excoriée (des jeunes filles) L70.5

Acne (continued)
  frontalis L70.2
  indurata L70.0
  infantile L70.4
  keloid L73.0
  lupoid L70.2
  necrotic, necrotica (miliaris) L70.2
  neonatal L70.4
  nodular L70.0
  occupational L70.8
  picker's L70.5
  pustular L70.0
  rodens L70.2
  rosacea L71.9
  specified NEC L70.8
  tropica L70.3
  varioliformis L70.2
  vulgaris L70.0

Acnitis (primary) A18.4

Acosta's disease T70.29

Acoustic —*see* condition

Acousticophobia F40.298

ACPO (acute colonic pseudo-obstruction) K59.81

Acquired —*see also* condition
  immunodeficiency syndrome (AIDS) B20

Acrania Q00.0

Acroangiodermatitis I78.9

Acroasphyxia, chronic I73.89

Acrobystitis N47.7

Acrocephalopolysyndactyly Q87.0

Acrocephalosyndactyly Q87.0

Acrocephaly Q75.0

Acrochondrohyperplasia —*see* Syndrome, Marfan's

Acrocyanosis I73.89
  newborn P28.2
    meaning transient blue hands and feet - omit code

Acrodermatitis L30.8
  atrophicans (chronica) L90.4
  continua (Hallopeau) L40.2
  enteropathica (hereditary) E83.2
  Hallopeau's L40.2
  infantile papular L44.4
  perstans L40.2
  pustulosa continua L40.2
  recalcitrant pustular L40.2

Acrodynia —*see* Poisoning, mercury

Acromegaly, acromegalia E22.0

Acromelalgia I73.81

Acromicria, acromikria Q79.8

Acronyx L60.0

Acropachy, thyroid —*see* Thyrotoxicosis

Acroparesthesia (simple) (vasomotor) I73.89

Acropathy, thyroid —*see* Thyrotoxicosis

Acrophobia F40.241

Acroposthitis N47.7

Acroscleriasis, acroscleroderma, acrosclerosis —*see* Sclerosis, systemic

Acrosphacelus I96

Acrospiroma, eccrine —*see* Neoplasm, skin, benign

Acrostealgia —*see* Osteochondropathy

Acrotrophodynia —*see* Immersion

ACTH ectopic syndrome E24.3

Actinic —*see* condition

Actinobacillosis, actinobacillus A28.8
  mallei A24.0
  muris A25.1

Actinomyces israelii (infection) —*see* Actinomycosis

Actinomycetoma (foot) B47.1

Actinomycosis, actinomycotic A42.9
  with pneumonia A42.0
  abdominal A42.1
  cervicofacial A42.2
  cutaneous A42.89
  gastrointestinal A42.1
  pulmonary A42.0
  sepsis A42.7
  specified site NEC A42.89

Actinoneuritis G62.82

Action, heart
  disorder I49.9
  irregular I49.9
    psychogenic F45.8

Activated protein C resistance D68.51

Activation
  mast cell (disorder) (syndrom) D89.40
    idiopathic D89.42
    monoclonal D89.41
    secondary D89.43
    specified type NEC D89.49

Active —*see* condition

Acute —*see also* condition
  abdomen R10.0
  gallbladder —*see* Cholecystitis, acute

Acyanotic heart disease (congenital) Q24.9

Acystia Q64.5

Adair-Dighton syndrome (brittle bones and blue sclera, deafness) Q78.0

Adamantinoblastoma —*see* Ameloblastoma

Adamantinoma —*see also* Cyst, calcifying odontogenic
  long bones C40.90
    lower limb C40.2-
    upper limb C40.0-
  malignant C41.1
    jaw (bone) (lower) C41.1
      upper C41.0
  tibial C40.2-

Adamantoblastoma —*see* Ameloblastoma

Adams-Stokes (-Morgagni) disease or syndrome I45.9

Adaption reaction —*see* Disorder, adjustment

Addiction —*see also* Dependence F19.20
  alcohol, alcoholic (ethyl) (methyl) (wood) (without remission) F10.20
    with remission F10.21
  drug —*see* Dependence, drug
  ethyl alcohol (without remission) F10.20
    with remission F10.21
  heroin —*see* Dependence, drug, opioid
  methyl alcohol (without remission) F10.20
    with remission F10.21
  methylated spirit (without remission) F10.20
    with remission F10.21

Addiction (continued)
  morphine(-like substances) —*see* Dependence, drug, opioid
  nicotine —*see* Dependence, drug, nicotine
  opium and opioids —*see* Dependence, drug, opioid
  tobacco —*see* Dependence, drug, nicotine

Addisonian crisis E27.2

Addison's
  anemia (pernicious) D51.0
  disease (bronze) or syndrome E27.1
    tuberculous A18.7
  keloid L94.0

Addison-Biermer anemia (pernicious) D51.0

Addison-Schilder complex E71.528

Additional —*see also* Accessory
  chromosome(s) Q99.8
    sex —*see* Abnormal, chromosome, sex
    21 —*see* Trisomy, 21

Adduction contracture, hip or other joint —*see* Contraction, joint

Adenitis —*see also* Lymphadenitis
  acute, unspecified site L04.9
  axillary I88.9
    acute L04.2
    chronic or subacute I88.1
  Bartholin's gland N75.8
  bulbourethral gland —*see* Urethritis
  cervical I88.9
    acute L04.0
    chronic or subacute I88.1
  chancroid (Hemophilus ducreyi) A57
  chronic, unspecified site I88.1
  Cowper's gland —*see* Urethritis
  due to Pasteurella multocida (P. septica) A28.0
  epidemic, acute B27.09
  gangrenous L04.9
  gonorrheal NEC A54.89
  groin I88.9
    acute L04.1
    chronic or subacute I88.1
  infectious (acute) (epidemic) B27.09
  inguinal I88.9
    acute L04.1
    chronic or subacute I88.1
  lymph gland or node, except mesenteric I88.9
    acute —*see* Lymphadenitis, acute
    chronic or subacute I88.1
  mesenteric (acute) (chronic) (nonspecific) (subacute) I88.0
  parotid gland (suppurative) —*see* Sialoadenitis
  salivary gland (any) (suppurative) —*see* Sialoadenitis
  scrofulous (tuberculous) A18.2
  Skene's duct or gland —*see* Urethritis
  strumous, tuberculous A18.2
  subacute, unspecified site I88.1
  sublingual gland (suppurative) —*see* Sialoadenitis
  submandibular gland (suppurative) —*see* Sialoadenitis
  submaxillary gland (suppurative) —*see* Sialoadenitis
  tuberculous —*see* Tuberculosis, lymph gland
  urethral gland —*see* Urethritis
  Wharton's duct (suppurative) —*see* Sialoadenitis

Adenoacanthoma —see Neoplasm, malignant, by site

Adenoameloblastoma —see Cyst, calcifying odontogenic

Adenocarcinoid (tumor) —see Neoplasm, malignant, by site

Adenocarcinoma —see also
Neoplasm, malignant, by site
    acidophil
        specified site —see Neoplasm, malignant, by site
        unspecified site C75.1
    adrenal cortical C74.0-
    alveolar —see Neoplasm, lung, malignant
    apocrine
        breast —see Neoplasm, breast, malignant
        in situ
            breast D05.8-
            specified site NEC —see Neoplasm, skin, in situ
            unspecified site D04.9
        specified site NEC —see Neoplasm, skin, malignant
        unspecified site C44.99
    basal cell
        specified site —see Neoplasm, skin, malignant
        unspecified site C08.9
    basophil
        specified site —see Neoplasm, malignant, by site
        unspecified site C75.1
    bile duct type C22.1
        liver C22.1
        specified site NEC —see Neoplasm, malignant, by site
        unspecified site C22.1
    bronchiolar —see Neoplasm, lung, malignant
    bronchioloalveolar —see Neoplasm, lung, malignant
    ceruminous C44.29-
    cervix, in situ —see also
        Carcinoma, cervix uteri, in situ D06.9
    chromophobe
        specified site —see Neoplasm, malignant, by site
        unspecified site C75.1
    diffuse type
        specified site —see Neoplasm, malignant, by site
        unspecified site C16.9
    duct
        infiltrating
            with Paget's disease —see Neoplasm, breast, malignant
            specified site —see Neoplasm, malignant, by site
            unspecified site (female) 50.91-
                male C50.92-
        specified site —see Neoplasm, malignant, by site
        unspecified site
            female C56.9
            male C61
    eosinophil
        specified site —see Neoplasm, malignant, by site
        unspecified site C75.1
    follicular
        with papillary C73
        moderately differentiated C73
        specified site —see Neoplasm, malignant, by site
        trabecular C73

Adenocarcinoma (continued)
    follicular (continued)
        unspecified site C73
        well differentiated C73
    Hurthle cell C73
    in
        adenomatous
            polyposis coli C18.9
    infiltrating duct
        with Paget's disease —see Neoplasm, breast, malignant
        specified site —see Neoplasm, by site, malignant
        unspecified site (female) C50.91-
            male C50.92-
    inflammatory
        specified site —see Neoplasm, by site, malignant
        unspecified site (female) C50.91-
            male C50.92-
    intestinal type
        specified site —see Neoplasm, by site, malignant
        unspecified site C16.9
    intracystic papillary
    intraductal
        breast D05.1-
        noninfiltrating
            breast D05.1-
            papillary
                with invasion
                    specified site —see Neoplasm, by site, malignant
                    unspecified site (female) C50.91-
                        male C50.92-
                breast D05.1-
                specified site NEC —see Neoplasm, in situ, by site
                unspecified site D05.1-
            specified site NEC —see Neoplasm, in situ, by site
            unspecified site D05.1-
        papillary
            with invasion
                specified site —see Neoplasm, malignant, by site
                unspecified site (female) C50.91-
                    male C50.92-
            breast D05.1-
            specified site —see Neoplasm, in situ, by site
            unspecified site D05.1-
        specified site NEC —see Neoplasm, in situ, by site
        unspecified site D05.1-
    islet cell
        with exocrine, mixed
            specified site —see Neoplasm, malignant, by site
            unspecified site C25.9
        pancreas C25.4
        specified site NEC —see Neoplasm, malignant, by site
        unspecified site C25.4
    lobular
        in situ
            breast D05.0-
            specified site NEC —see Neoplasm, in situ, by site
            unspecified site D05.0-
        specified site —see Neoplasm, malignant, by site
        unspecified site (female) C50.91-
            male C50.92-

Adenocarcinoma (continued)
    mucoid —see also Neoplasm, malignant, by site
        cell
            specified site —see Neoplasm, malignant, by site
            unspecified site C75.1
    nonencapsulated sclerosing C73
    papillary
        with follicular C73
        follicular variant C73
        intraductal (noninfiltrating)
            with invasion
                specified site —see Neoplasm, malignant, by site
                unspecified site (female) C50.91-
                    male C50.92-
            breast D05.1-
            specified site NEC —see Neoplasm, in situ, by site
            unspecified site D05.1-
    serous
        specified site —see Neoplasm, malignant, by site
        unspecified site C56.9
    papillocystic
        specified site —see Neoplasm, malignant, by site
        unspecified site C56.9
    pseudomucinous
        specified site —see Neoplasm, malignant, by site
        unspecified site C56.9
    renal cell C64-
    sebaceous —see Neoplasm, skin, malignant
    serous —see also Neoplasm, malignant, by site
        papillary
            specified site —see Neoplasm, malignant, by site
            unspecified site C56.9
    sweat gland —see Neoplasm, skin, malignant
    water-clear cell C75.0

Adenocarcinoma-in-situ —see also
Neoplasm, in situ, by site
    breast D05.9-

Adenofibroma
    clear cell —see Neoplasm, benign, by site
    endometrioid D27.9
        borderline malignancy D39.10
        malignant C56-
    mucinous
        specified site —see Neoplasm, benign, by site
        unspecified site D27.9
    papillary
        specified site —see Neoplasm, benign, by site
        unspecified site D27.9
    prostate —see Enlargement, enlarged, prostate
    serous
        specified site —see Neoplasm, benign, by site
        unspecified site D27.9
    specified site —see Neoplasm, benign, by site
    unspecified site D27.9

Adenofibrosis
    breast —see Fibroadenosis, breast
    endometrioid N80.0

Adenoiditis (chronic) J35.02
    with tonsillitis J35.03
    acute J03.90

Adenoiditis (continued)
    acute (continued)
        recurrent J03.91
        specified organism NEC J03.80
            recurrent J03.81
        staphylococcal J03.80
            recurrent J03.81
        streptococcal J03.00
            recurrent J03.01

Adenoids —see condition

Adenolipoma —see Neoplasm, benign, by site

Adenolipomatosis, Launois-Bensaude E88.89

Adenolymphoma
    specified site —see Neoplasm, benign, by site
    unspecified site D11.9

Adenoma —see also Neoplasm, benign, by site
    acidophil
        specified site —see Neoplasm, benign, by site
        unspecified site D35.2
    acidophil-basophil, mixed
        specified site —see Neoplasm, benign, by site
        unspecified site D35.2
    adrenal (cortical) D35.00
        clear cell D35.00
        compact cell D35.00
        glomerulosa cell D35.00
        heavily pigmented variant D35.00
        mixed cell D35.00
    alpha-cell
        pancreas D13.7
        specified site NEC —see Neoplasm, benign, by site
        unspecified site D13.7
    alveolar D14.30
    apocrine
        breast D24-
        specified site NEC —see Neoplasm, skin, benign, by site
        unspecified site D23.9
    basal cell D11.9
    basophil
        specified site —see Neoplasm, benign, by site
        unspecified site D35.2
    basophil-acidophil, mixed
        specified site —see Neoplasm, benign, by site
        unspecified site D35.2
    beta-cell
        pancreas D13.7
        specified site NEC —see Neoplasm, benign, by site
        unspecified site D13.7
    bile duct D13.4
        common D13.5
        extrahepatic D13.5
        intrahepatic D13.4
        specified site NEC —see Neoplasm, benign, by site
        unspecified site D13.4
    black D35.00
    bronchial D38.1
        cylindroid type —see Neoplasm, lung, malignant
    ceruminous D23.2-
    chief cell D35.1
    chromophobe
        specified site —see Neoplasm, benign, by site
        unspecified site D35.2
    colloid
        specified site —see Neoplasm, benign, by site
        unspecified site D34

Adenoma (continued)
  duct
  eccrine, papillary —see Neoplasm,
    skin, benign
  endocrine, multiple
    single specified site —see
      Neoplasm, uncertain behavior,
      by site
    two or more specified sites
      D44-
    unspecified site D44.9
  endometrioid —see also Neoplasm,
    benign
    borderline malignancy —see
      Neoplasm, uncertain behavior,
      by site
  eosinophil
    specified site —see Neoplasm,
      benign, by site
    unspecified site D35.2
  fetal
    specified site —see Neoplasm,
      benign, by site
    unspecified site D34
  follicular
    specified site —see Neoplasm,
      benign, by site
    unspecified site D34
  hepatocellular D13.4
  Hurthle cell D34
  islet cell
    pancreas D13.7
    specified site NEC —see
      Neoplasm, benign, by site
    unspecified site D13.7
  liver cell D13.4
  macrofollicular
    specified site —see Neoplasm,
      benign, by site
    unspecified site D34
  malignant, malignum —see
    Neoplasm, malignant, by site
  microcystic
    pancreas D13.6
    specified site NEC —see
      Neoplasm, benign, by site
    unspecified site D13.6
  microfollicular
    specified site —see Neoplasm,
      benign, by site
    unspecified site D34
  mucoid cell
    specified site —see Neoplasm,
      benign, by site
    unspecified site D35.2
  multiple endocrine
    single specified site —see
      Neoplasm, uncertain behavior,
      by site
    two or more specified sites
      D44-
    unspecified site D44.9
  nipple D24-
  papillary —see also Neoplasm,
    benign, by site
    eccrine —see Neoplasm, skin,
      benign, by site
  Pick's tubular
    specified site —see Neoplasm,
      benign, by site
    unspecified site
      female D27.9
      male D29.20
  pleomorphic
    carcinoma in —see Neoplasm,
      salivary gland, malignant
    specified site —see Neoplasm,
      malignant, by site
    unspecified site C08.9
  polypoid —see also Neoplasm,
    benign

Adenoma (continued)
  polypoid (continued)
    adenocarcinoma in —see
      Neoplasm, malignant, by site
    adenocarcinoma in situ —see
      Neoplasm, in situ, by site
    prostate —see Neoplasm, benign,
      prostate
  rete cell D29.20
  sebaceous —see Neoplasm, skin,
    benign
  Sertoli cell
    specified site —see Neoplasm,
      benign, by site
    unspecified site
      female D27.9
      male D29.20
  skin appendage —see Neoplasm,
    skin, benign
  sudoriferous gland —see
    Neoplasm, skin, benign
  sweat gland —see Neoplasm, skin,
    benign
  testicular
    specified site —see Neoplasm,
      benign, by site
    unspecified site
      female D27.9
      male D29.20
  tubular —see also Neoplasm,
    benign, by site
    adenocarcinoma in —see
      Neoplasm, malignant, by site
    adenocarcinoma in situ —see
      Neoplasm, in situ, by site
    Pick's
      specified site —see Neoplasm,
        benign, by site
      unspecified site
        female D27.9
        male D29.20
  tubulovillous —see also Neoplasm,
    benign, by site
    adenocarcinoma in —see
      Neoplasm, malignant,
      by site
    adenocarcinoma in situ —see
      Neoplasm, in situ, by site
  villous —see Neoplasm, uncertain
    behavior, by site
    adenocarcinoma in —see
      Neoplasm, malignant, by site
    adenocarcinoma in situ —see
      Neoplasm, in situ, by site
  water-clear cell D35.1

Adenomatosis
  endocrine (multiple) E31.20
    single specified site —see
      Neoplasm, uncertain behavior,
      by site
  erosive of nipple D24-
  pluriendocrine —see
    Adenomatosis, endocrine
  pulmonary D38.1
    malignant —see Neoplasm, lung,
      malignant
  specified site —see Neoplasm,
    benign, by site
  unspecified site D12.6

Adenomatous
  goiter (nontoxic) E04.9
    with hyperthyroidism —see
      Hyperthyroidism, with, goiter,
      nodular
    toxic —see Hyperthyroidism,
      with, goiter, nodular

Adenomyoma —see also Neoplasm,
  benign, by site
  prostate —see Enlarged, prostate

Adenomyometritis N80.0

Adenomyosis N80.0

Adenopathy (lymph gland) R59.9
  generalized R59.1
  inguinal R59.0
  localized R59.0
  mediastinal R59.0
  mesentery R59.0
  syphilitic (secondary) A51.49
  tracheobronchial R59.0
    tuberculous A15.4
      primary (progressive) A15.7
  tuberculous —see also
    Tuberculosis, lymph gland
    tracheobronchial A15.4
      primary (progressive) A15.7

Adenosalpingitis —see Salpingitis

Adenosarcoma —see Neoplasm,
  malignant, by site

Adenosclerosis I88.8

Adenosis (sclerosing) breast —see
  Fibroadenosis, breast

**Adenovirus, as cause of disease
classified elsewhere** B97.0

Adentia (complete) (partial) —see
  Absence, teeth

Adherent —see also Adhesions
  labia (minora) N90.89
  pericardium (nonrheumatic) I31.0
    rheumatic I09.2
  placenta (with hemorrhage) O72.0
    without hemorrhage O73.0
  prepuce, newborn N47.0
  scar (skin) L90.5
  tendon in scar L90.5

Adhesions, adhesive (postinfective)
  with intestinal obstruction K56.50
    complete K56.52
    incomplete K56.51
    partial K56.51
  abdominal (wall) —see Adhesions,
    peritoneum
  appendix K38.8
  bile duct (common) (hepatic) K83.8
  bladder (sphincter) N32.89
  bowel —see also Adhesions,
    peritoneum
  cardiac I31.0
    rheumatic I09.2
  cecum —see Adhesions,
    peritoneum
  cervicovaginal N88.1
    congenital Q52.8
    postpartal O90.89
    old N88.1
  cervix N88.1
  ciliary body NEC —see Adhesions,
    iris
  clitoris N90.89
  colon —see Adhesions, peritoneum
  common duct K83.8
  congenital —see also Anomaly,
    by site
    fingers —see Syndactylism,
      complex, fingers
    omental, anomalous Q43.3
    peritoneal Q43.3
    tongue (to gum or roof of mouth)
      Q38.3
  conjunctiva (acquired) H11.21-
    congenital Q15.8
  cystic duct K82.8
  diaphragm —see Adhesions,
    peritoneum
  due to foreign body —see Foreign
    body
  duodenum —see Adhesions,
    peritoneum
  ear
    middle H74.1-

Adhesions, adhesive (continued)
  epididymis N50.89
  epidural —see Adhesions,
    meninges
  epiglottis J38.7
  eyelid H02.59
  female pelvis N73.6
  gallbladder K82.8
  globe H44.89
  heart I31.0
    rheumatic I09.2
  ileocecal (coil) —see Adhesions,
    peritoneum
  ileum —see Adhesions, peritoneum
  intestine —see also Adhesions,
    peritoneum
    with obstruction K56.50
      complete K56.52
      incomplete K56.51
      partial K56.51
  intra-abdominal —see Adhesions,
    peritoneum
  iris H21.50-
    anterior H21.51-
    goniosynechiae H21.52-
    posterior H21.54-
    to corneal graft T85.898
  joint —see Ankylosis
    knee M23.8X
    temporomandibular M26.61-
  labium (majus) (minus), congenital
    Q52.5
  liver —see Adhesions, peritoneum
  lung J98.4
  mediastinum J98.59
  meninges (cerebral) (spinal) G96.12
    congenital Q07.8
    tuberculous (cerebral) (spinal)
      A17.0
  mesenteric —see Adhesions,
    peritoneum
  nasal (septum) (to turbinates)
    J34.89
  ocular muscle —see Strabismus,
    mechanical
  omentum —see Adhesions,
    peritoneum
  ovary N73.6
    congenital (to cecum, kidney or
      omentum) Q50.39
  paraovarian N73.6
  pelvic (peritoneal)
    female N73.6
      postprocedural N99.4
    male —see Adhesions,
      peritoneum
    postpartal (old) N73.6
    tuberculous A18.17
  penis to scrotum (congenital)
    Q55.8
  periappendiceal —see also
    Adhesions, peritoneum
  pericardium (nonrheumatic) I31.0
    focal I31.8
    rheumatic I09.2
    tuberculous A18.84
  pericholecystic K82.8
  perigastric —see Adhesions,
    peritoneum
  periovarian N73.6
  periprostatic N42.89
  perirectal —see Adhesions,
    peritoneum
  perirenal N28.89
  peritoneum, peritoneal
    (postinfective) K66.0
    with obstruction (intestinal)
      K56.50
      complete K56.52
      incomplete K56.51
      partial K56.51

Adhesions, adhesive *(continued)*

peritoneum, peritoneal *(continued)*
  congenital Q43.3
  pelvic, female N73.6
    postprocedural N99.4
  postpartal, pelvic N73.6
  postprocedural K66.0
  to uterus N73.6
peritubal N73.6
periureteral N28.89
periuterine N73.6
perivesical N32.89
perivesicular (seminal vesicle)
  N50.89
pleura, pleuritic J94.8
  tuberculous NEC A15.6
pleuropericardial J94.8
postoperative (gastrointestinal
  tract) K66.0
  with obstruction *(see also*
    Obstruction, intestine,
    postoperative) K91.30
  due to foreign body accidentally
    left in wound —*see* Foreign
    body, accidentally left during
    a procedure
  pelvic peritoneal N99.4
  urethra —*see* Stricture, urethra,
    postprocedural
  vagina N99.2
postpartal, old (vulva or perineum)
  N90.89
preputial, prepuce N47.5
pulmonary J98.4
pylorus —*see* Adhesions,
  peritoneum
sciatic nerve —*see* Lesion, nerve,
  sciatic
seminal vesicle N50.89
shoulder (joint) —*see* Capsulitis,
  adhesive
sigmoid flexure —*see* Adhesions,
  peritoneum
spermatic cord (acquired) N50.89
  congenital Q55.4
spinal canal G96.12
stomach —*see* Adhesions,
  peritoneum
subscapular —*see* Capsulitis,
  adhesive
temporomandibular M26.61-
tendinitis —*see also* Tenosynovitis,
  specified type NEC
  shoulder —*see* Capsulitis, adhesive
testis N44.8
tongue, congenital (to gum or roof
  of mouth) Q38.3
  acquired K14.8
trachea J39.8
tubo-ovarian N73.6
tunica vaginalis N44.8
uterus N73.6
  internal N85.6
  to abdominal wall N73.6
vagina (chronic) N89.5
  postoperative N99.2
vitreomacular H43.82-
vitreous H43.89
vulva N90.89

Adiaspiromycosis B48.88

Adie (-Holmes) **pupil or syndrome**
—*see* Anomaly, pupil, function,
tonic pupil

Adiponecrosis neonatorum P83.88

Adiposis —*see also* Obesity
cerebralis E23.6
dolorosa E88.2

Adiposity —*see also* Obesity
heart —*see* Degeneration, myocardial
localized E65

Adiposogenital dystrophy E23.6

Adjustment

disorder —*see* Disorder, adjustment
implanted device —*see* Encounter
  (for), adjustment (of)
prosthesis, external —*see* Fitting
reaction —*see* Disorder, adjustment

Administration of tPA (rtPA) in a
**different facility within the last
24 hours prior to admission to
current facility** Z92.82

Admission (for) —*see also* Encounter
(for)
adjustment (of)
  artificial
    arm Z44.00-
      complete Z44.01-
      partial Z44.02-
    eye Z44.2
    leg Z44.10-
      complete Z44.11-
      partial Z44.12-
  brain neuropacemaker Z46.2
    implanted Z45.42
  breast
    implant Z45.81
    prosthesis (external) Z44.3
  colostomy belt Z46.89
  contact lenses Z46.0
  cystostomy device Z46.6
  dental prosthesis Z46.3
  device NEC
    abdominal Z46.89
    implanted Z45.89
      cardiac Z45.09
        defibrillator (with
          synchronous cardiac
          pacemaker) Z45.02
        pacemaker (cardiac
          resynchronization
          therapy (CRT-P))
          Z45.018
          pulse generator
          Z45.010
        resynchronization
          therapy defibrillator
          (CRT-D) Z45.02
      hearing device Z45.328
        bone conduction Z45.320
        cochlear Z45.321
      infusion pump Z45.1
      nervous system Z45.49
        CSF drainage Z45.41
        hearing device —*see*
          Admission, adjustment,
          device, implanted,
          hearing device
        neuropacemaker Z45.42
        visual substitution
          Z45.31
      specified NEC Z45.89
      vascular access Z45.2
      visual substitution Z45.31
    nervous system Z46.2
      implanted —*see* Admission,
        adjustment, device,
        implanted, nervous
        system
    orthodontic Z46.4
    prosthetic Z44.9
      arm —*see* Admission,
        adjustment, artificial, arm
      breast Z44.3
      dental Z46.3
      eye Z44.2
      leg —*see* Admission,
        adjustment, artificial, leg
      specified type NEC Z44.8
  substitution
    auditory Z46.2

Admission *(continued)*

adjustment *(continued)*
  device NEC *(continued)*
    substitution *(continued)*
      auditory *(continued)*
        implanted —*see*
          Admission, adjustment,
          device, implanted,
          hearing device
      nervous system Z46.2
        implanted —*see*
          Admission, adjustment,
          device, implanted,
          nervous system
      visual Z46.2
        implanted Z45.31
      urinary Z46.6
  hearing aid Z46.1
    implanted —*see* Admission,
      adjustment, device,
      implanted, hearing device
  ileostomy device Z46.89
  intestinal appliance or device
    NEC Z46.89
  neuropacemaker (brain) (peripheral
    nerve) (spinal cord) Z46.2
    implanted Z45.42
  orthodontic device Z46.4
  orthopedic (brace) (cast) (device)
    (shoes) Z46.89
  pacemaker (cardiac
    resynchronization therapy
    (CRT-P))
    cardiac Z45.018
      pulse generator Z45.010
    nervous system Z46.2
      implanted Z45.42
  portacath (port-a-cath) Z45.2
  prosthesis Z44.9
    arm —*see* Admission,
      adjustment, artificial, arm
    breast Z44.3
    dental Z46.3
    eye Z44.2
    leg —*see* Admission,
      adjustment, artificial, leg
    specified NEC Z44.8
  spectacles Z46.0
aftercare —*see also* Aftercare Z51.89
  postpartum
    immediately after delivery Z39.0
    routine follow-up Z39.2
  radiation therapy (antineoplastic)
    Z51.0
attention to artificial opening (of)
  Z43.9
  artificial vagina Z43.7
  colostomy Z43.3
  cystostomy Z43.5
  enterostomy Z43.4
  gastrostomy Z43.1
  ileostomy Z43.2
  jejunostomy Z43.4
  nephrostomy Z43.6
  specified site NEC Z43.8
    intestinal tract Z43.4
    urinary tract Z43.6
  tracheostomy Z43.0
  ureterostomy Z43.6
  urethrostomy Z43.6
breast augmentation or reduction
  Z41.1
breast reconstruction following
  mastectomy Z42.1
change of
  dressing (nonsurgical) Z48.00
  neuropacemaker device (brain)
    (peripheral nerve) (spinal
    cord) Z46.2
    implanted Z45.42
  surgical dressing Z48.01

Admission *(continued)*

circumcision, ritual or routine
  (in absence of diagnosis) Z41.2
clinical research investigation
  (control) (normal comparison)
  (participant) Z00.6
contraceptive management Z30.9
cosmetic surgery NEC Z41.1
counseling —*see also* Counseling
  dietary Z71.3
  gestational carrier Z31.7
  HIV Z71.7
  human immunodeficiency virus
    Z71.7
  nonattending third party Z71.0
  procreative management NEC
    Z31.69
delivery, full-term, uncomplicated
  O80
  cesarean, without indication O82
desensitization to allergens Z51.6
dietary surveillance and counseling
  Z71.3
ear piercing Z41.3
examination at health care facility
  (adult) *(see also* Examination)
  Z00.00
  with abnormal findings Z00.01
  clinical research investigation
    (control) (normal comparison)
    (participant) Z00.6
  dental Z01.20
    with abnormal findings Z01.21
  donor (potential) Z00.5
  ear Z01.10
    with abnormal findings NEC
      Z01.118
  eye Z01.00
    with abnormal findings
      Z01.01
    following failed vision
      screening Z01.020
      with abnormal findings
        Z01.021
  general, specified reason NEC
    Z00.8
  hearing Z01.10
    with abnormal findings NEC
      Z01.118
  infant or child (over 28 days
    old) Z00.129
    with abnormal findings
      Z00.121
  postpartum checkup Z39.2
  psychiatric (general) Z00.8
    requested by authority Z04.6
  vision Z01.00
    with abnormal findings Z01.01
    following failed vision
      screening Z01.020
      with abnormal findings
        Z01.021
    infant or child (over 28 days
      old) Z00.129
      with abnormal findings
        Z00.121
fitting (of)
  artificial
    arm —*see* Admission,
      adjustment, artificial, arm
    eye Z44.2
    leg —*see* Admission,
      adjustment, artificial, leg
  brain neuropacemaker Z46.2
    implanted Z45.42
  breast prosthesis (external) Z44.3
  colostomy belt Z46.89
  contact lenses Z46.0
  cystostomy device Z46.6
  dental prosthesis Z46.3
  dentures Z46.3

13

Admission *(continued)*
  fitting *(continued)*
    device NEC
      abdominal Z46.89
      nervous system Z46.2
        implanted —*see* Admission,
          adjustment, device,
          implanted, nervous system
      orthodontic Z46.4
      prosthetic Z44.9
        breast Z44.3
        dental Z46.3
        eye Z44.2
      substitution
        auditory Z46.2
          implanted —*see*
            Admission, adjustment,
            device, implanted,
            hearing device
        nervous system Z46.2
          implanted —*see*
            Admission, adjustment,
            device, implanted,
            nervous system
        visual Z46.2
          implanted Z45.31
    hearing aid Z46.1
    ileostomy device Z46.89
    intestinal appliance or device
      NEC Z46.89
    neuropacemaker (brain)
      (peripheral nerve) (spinal cord)
      Z46.2
      implanted Z45.42
    orthodontic device Z46.4
    orthopedic device (brace) (cast)
      (shoes) Z46.89
    prosthesis Z44.9
      arm —*see* Admission,
        adjustment, artificial, arm
      breast Z44.3
      dental Z46.3
      eye Z44.2
      leg —*see* Admission,
        adjustment, artificial, leg
      specified type NEC Z44.8
    spectacles Z46.0
  follow-up examination Z09
  intrauterine device management
    Z30.431
    initial prescription Z30.014
  mental health evaluation Z00.8
    requested by authority Z04.6
  observation —*see* Observation
  Papanicolaou smear, cervix Z12.4
    for suspected malignant
      neoplasm Z12.4
  plastic and reconstructive surgery
    following medical procedure or
    healed injury NEC Z42.8
  plastic surgery, cosmetic NEC Z41.1
  postpartum observation
    immediately after delivery Z39.0
    routine follow-up Z39.2
  poststerilization (for restoration)
    Z31.0
    aftercare Z31.42
  procreative management Z31.9
  prophylactic (measure) —*see also*
    Encounter, prophylactic measures
    organ removal Z40.00
      breast Z40.01
      fallopian tube(s) Z40.03
        with ovary(s) Z40.02
      ovary(s) Z40.02
      specified organ NEC Z40.09
      testes Z40.09
  vaccination Z23
  psychiatric examination (general)
    Z00.8
    requested by authority Z04.6

Admission *(continued)*
  radiation therapy (antineoplastic)
    Z51.0
  reconstructive surgery following
    medical procedure or healed
    injury NEC Z42.8
  removal of
    cystostomy catheter Z43.5
    drains Z48.03
    dressing (nonsurgical) Z48.00
    implantable subdermal
      contraceptive Z30.46
    intrauterine contraceptive device
      Z30.432
    neuropacemaker (brain) (peripheral
      nerve) (spinal cord) Z46.2
      implanted Z45.42
    staples Z48.02
    surgical dressing Z48.01
    sutures Z48.02
    ureteral stent Z46.6
  respirator [ventilator] use during
    power failure Z99.12
  restoration of organ continuity
    (poststerilization) Z31.0
    aftercare Z31.42
  sensitivity test —*see also* Test, skin
    allergy NEC Z01.82
    Mantoux Z11.1
  tuboplasty following previous
    sterilization Z31.0
    aftercare Z31.42
  vasoplasty following previous
    sterilization Z31.0
    aftercare Z31.42
  vision examination Z01.00
    with abnormal findings Z01.01
    following failed vision screening
      Z01.020
      with abnormal findings
        Z01.021
    infant or child (over 28 days old)
      Z00.129
      with abnormal findings Z00.121
  waiting period for admission to
    other facility Z75.1

Adnexitis (suppurative) —*see*
  Salpingo-oophoritis

**Adolescent X-linked
  adrenoleukodystrophy** E71.521

Adrenal (gland) —*see* condition

Adrenalism, tuberculous A18.7

Adrenalitis, adrenitis E27.8
  autoimmune E27.1
  meningococcal, hemorrhagic A39.1

Adrenarche, premature E27.0

Adrenocortical syndrome —*see*
  Cushing's, syndrome

Adrenogenital syndrome E25.9
  acquired E25.8
  congenital E25.0
  salt loss E25.0

Adrenogenitalism, congenital E25.0

Adrenoleukodystrophy E71.529
  neonatal E71.511
  X-linked E71.529
    Addison only phenotype E71.528
    Addison-Schilder E71.528
    adolescent E71.521
    adrenomyeloneuropathy E71.522
    childhood cerebral E71.520
    other specified E71.528

Adrenomyeloneuropathy E71.522

Adventitious bursa —*see*
  Bursopathy, specified type NEC

Adverse effect —*see* Table of
  Drugs and Chemicals, categories
  T36-T50, with 6th character 5

Advice —*see* Counseling

Adynamia (episodica) (hereditary)
  (periodic) G72.3

Aeration lung imperfect, newborn
  —*see* Atelectasis

Aerobullosis T70.3

Aerocele —*see* Embolism, air

Aerodermectasia
  subcutaneous (traumatic) T79.7

Aerodontalgia T70.29

Aeroembolism T70.3

Aerogenes capsulatus infection A48.0

Aero-otitis media T70.0

Aerophagy, aerophagia
  (psychogenic) F45.8

Aerophobia F40.228

Aerosinusitis T70.1

Aerotitis T70.0

Affection —*see* Disease

Afibrinogenemia (*see also* Defect,
  coagulation) D68.8
  acquired D65
  congenital D68.2
  following ectopic or molar
    pregnancy O08.1
  in abortion —*see* Abortion,
    by type, complicated by,
    afibrinogenemia
  puerperal O72.3

African
  sleeping sickness B56.9
  tick fever A68.1
  trypanosomiasis B56.9
    gambian B56.0
    rhodesian B56.1

Aftercare (*see also* Care) Z51.89
  following surgery (for) (on)
    amputation Z47.81
    attention to
      drains Z48.03
      dressings (nonsurgical) Z48.00
        surgical Z48.01
      sutures Z48.02
    circulatory system Z48.812
    delayed (planned) wound closure
      Z48.1
    digestive system Z48.815
    explantation of joint prosthesis
      (staged procedure)
      hip Z47.32
      knee Z47.33
      shoulder Z47.31
    genitourinary system Z48.816
    joint replacement Z47.1
    neoplasm Z48.3
    nervous system Z48.811
    oral cavity Z48.814
    organ transplant
      bone marrow Z48.290
      heart Z48.21
      heart-lung Z48.280
      kidney Z48.22
      liver Z48.23
      lung Z48.24
      multiple organs NEC Z48.288
      specified NEC Z48.298
    orthopedic NEC Z47.89
    planned wound closure Z48.1
    removal of internal fixation
      device Z47.2
    respiratory system Z48.813
    scoliosis Z47.82
    sense organs Z48.810
    skin and subcutaneous tissue
      Z48.817
    specified body system
      circulatory Z48.812

Aftercare *(continued)*
  following surgery *(continued)*
    specified body system *(continued)*
      digestive Z48.815
      genitourinary Z48.816
      nervous Z48.811
      oral cavity Z48.814
      respiratory Z48.813
      sense organs Z48.810
      skin and subcutaneous tissue
        Z48.817
      teeth Z48.814
    specified NEC Z48.89
    spinal Z47.89
    teeth Z48.814
  fracture - code to fracture with
    seventh character D
  involving
    removal of
      drains Z48.03
      dressings (nonsurgical)
        Z48.00
      staples Z48.02
      surgical dressings Z48.01
      sutures Z48.02
  neuropacemaker (brain)
    (peripheral nerve) (spinal cord)
    Z46.2
    implanted Z45.42
  orthopedic NEC Z47.89
  postprocedural —*see* Aftercare,
    following surgery

After-cataract —*see* Cataract,
  secondary

Agalactia (primary) O92.3
  elective, secondary or therapeutic
    O92.5

Agammaglobulinemia (acquired
  (secondary)) (nonfamilial) D80.1
  with
    immunoglobulin-bearing
      B-lymphocytes D80.1
    lymphopenia D81.9
  autosomal recessive (Swiss type)
    D80.0
  Bruton's X-linked D80.0
  common variable (CVAgamma)
    D80.1
  congenital sex-linked D80.0
  hereditary D80.0
  lymphopenic D81.9
  Swiss type (autosomal recessive)
    D80.0
  X-linked (with growth hormone
    deficiency) (Bruton) D80.0

Aganglionosis (bowel) (colon) Q43.1

Age (old) —*see* Senility

Agenesis
  adrenal (gland) Q89.1
  alimentary tract (complete) (partial)
    NEC Q45.8
    upper Q40.8
  anus, anal (canal) Q42.3
    with fistula Q42.2
  aorta Q25.41
  appendix Q42.8
  arm (complete) Q71.0-
    with hand present Q71.1-
  artery (peripheral) Q27.9
    brain Q28.3
    coronary Q24.5
    pulmonary Q25.79
    specified NEC Q27.8
    umbilical Q27.0
  auditory (canal) (external) Q16.1
  auricle (ear) Q16.0
  bile duct or passage Q44.5
  bladder Q64.5
  bone Q79.9

Agenesis *(continued)*
brain Q00.0
  part of Q04.3
breast (with nipple present) Q83.8
  with absent nipple Q83.0
bronchus Q32.4
canaliculus lacrimalis Q10.4
carpus —*see* Agenesis, hand
cartilage Q79.9
cecum Q42.8
cerebellum Q04.3
cervix Q51.5
chin Q18.8
cilia Q10.3
circulatory system, part
  NOS Q28.9
clavicle Q74.0
clitoris Q52.6
coccyx Q76.49
colon Q42.9
  specified NEC Q42.8
corpus callosum Q04.0
cricoid cartilage Q31.8
diaphragm (with hernia) Q79.1
digestive organ(s) or tract
  (complete) (partial) NEC Q45.8
  upper Q40.8
ductus arteriosus Q28.8
duodenum Q41.0
ear Q16.9
  auricle Q16.0
  lobe Q17.8
ejaculatory duct Q55.4
endocrine (gland) NEC Q89.2
epiglottis Q31.8
esophagus Q39.8
eustachian tube Q16.2
eye Q11.1
  adnexa Q15.8
eyelid (fold) Q10.3
face
  bones NEC Q75.8
  specified part NEC Q18.8
fallopian tube Q50.6
femur —*see* Defect, reduction,
  lower limb, longitudinal, femur
fibula —*see* Defect, reduction,
  lower limb, longitudinal, fibula
finger (complete) (partial) —*see*
  Agenesis, hand
foot (and toes) (complete) (partial)
  Q72.3-
forearm (with hand present) —*see*
  Agenesis, arm, with hand present
  and hand Q71.2-
gallbladder Q44.0
gastric Q40.2
genitalia, genital (organ(s))
  female Q52.8
    external Q52.71
    internal NEC Q52.8
  male Q55.8
glottis Q31.8
hair Q84.0
hand(and fingers) (complete)
  (partial) Q71.3-
heart Q24.8
  valve NEC Q24.8
    pulmonary Q22.0
hepatic Q44.7
humerus —*see* Defect, reduction,
  upper limb
hymen Q52.4
ileum Q41.2
incus Q16.3
intestine (small) Q41.9
  large Q42.9
    specified NEC Q42.8
iris (dilator fibers) Q13.1
jaw M26.09
jejunum Q41.1

Agenesis *(continued)*
kidney(s) (partial) Q60.2
  bilateral Q60.1
  unilateral Q60.0
labium (majus) (minus) Q52.71
labyrinth, membranous Q16.5
lacrimal apparatus Q10.4
larynx Q31.8
leg (complete) Q72.0-
  with foot present Q72.1-
  lower leg (with foot present)
    —*see* Agenesis, leg, with foot
    present and foot Q72.2-
lens Q12.3
limb (complete) Q73.0
  lower —*see* Agenesis, leg
  upper —*see* Agenesis, arm
lip Q38.0
liver Q44.7
lung (fissure) (lobe) (bilateral)
  (unilateral) Q33.3
mandible, maxilla M26.09
metacarpus —*see* Agenesis, hand
metatarsus —*see* Agenesis, foot
muscle Q79.8
  eyelid Q10.3
  ocular Q15.8
musculoskeletal system
  NEC Q79.8
nail(s) Q84.3
neck, part Q18.8
nerve Q07.8
nervous system, part NEC Q07.8
nipple Q83.2
nose Q30.1
nuclear Q07.8
organ
  of Corti Q16.5
  or site not listed —*see* Anomaly,
    by site
osseous meatus (ear) Q16.1
ovary
  bilateral Q50.02
  unilateral Q50.01
oviduct Q50.6
pancreas Q45.0
parathyroid (gland) Q89.2
parotid gland(s) Q38.4
patella Q74.1
pelvic girdle (complete) (partial)
  Q74.2
penis Q55.5
pericardium Q24.8
pituitary (gland) Q89.2
prostate Q55.4
punctum lacrimale Q10.4
radioulnar —*see* Defect, reduction,
  upper limb
radius —*see* Defect, reduction,
  upper limb, longitudinal, radius
rectum Q42.1
  with fistula Q42.0
renal Q60.2
  bilateral Q60.1
  unilateral Q60.0
respiratory organ NEC Q34.8
rib Q76.6
roof of orbit Q75.8
round ligament Q52.8
sacrum Q76.49
salivary gland Q38.4
scapula Q74.0
scrotum Q55.29
seminal vesicles Q55.4
septum
  atrial Q21.1
  between aorta and pulmonary
    artery Q21.4
  ventricular Q20.4
shoulder girdle (complete) (partial)
  Q74.0

Agenesis *(continued)*
skull (bone) Q75.8
  with
    anencephaly Q00.0
    encephalocele —*see*
      Encephalocele
    hydrocephalus Q03.9
      with spina bifida —*see*
        Spina bifida, by site, with
        hydrocephalus
    microcephaly Q02
spermatic cord Q55.4
spinal cord Q06.0
spine Q76.49
spleen Q89.01
sternum Q76.7
stomach Q40.2
submaxillary gland(s) (congenital)
  Q38.4
tarsus —*see* Agenesis, foot
tendon Q79.8
testicle Q55.0
thymus (gland) Q89.2
thyroid (gland) E03.1
  cartilage Q31.8
tibia —*see* Defect, reduction, lower
  limb, longitudinal, tibia
tibiofibular —*see* Defect, reduction,
  lower limb, specified type NEC
toe (and foot) (complete) (partial)
  —*see* Agenesis, foot
tongue Q38.3
trachea (cartilage) Q32.1
ulna —*see* Defect, reduction, upper
  limb, longitudinal, ulna
upper limb —*see* Agenesis, arm
ureter Q62.4
urethra Q64.5
urinary tract NEC Q64.8
uterus Q51.0
uvula Q38.5
vagina Q52.0
vas deferens Q55.4
vein(s) (peripheral) Q27.9
  brain Q28.3
  great NEC Q26.8
  portal Q26.5
vena cava (inferior) (superior) Q26.8
vermis of cerebellum Q04.3
vertebra Q76.49
vulva Q52.71

Ageusia R43.2

Agitated —*see* condition

Agitation R45.1

Aglossia (congenital) Q38.3

Aglossia-adactylia syndrome Q87.0

Aglycogenosis E74.00

Agnosia (body image) (other senses)
(tactile) R48.1
  developmental F88
  verbal R48.1
    auditory R48.1
      developmental F80.2
    developmental F80.2
  visual (object) R48.3

Agoraphobia F40.00
  with panic disorder F40.01
  without panic disorder F40.02

Agrammatism R48.8

Agranulocytopenia —*see*
Agranulocytosis

Agranulocytosis (chronic)
(cyclical) (genetic) (infantile)
(periodic) (pernicious) —*see also*
Neutropenia D70.9
  congenital D70.0
  cytoreductive cancer chemotherapy
    sequela D70.1

Agranulocytosis *(continued)*
drug-induced D70.2
  due to cytoreductive cancer
    chemotherapy D70.1
due to infection D70.3
secondary D70.4
  drug-induced D70.2
    due to cytoreductive cancer
      chemotherapy D70.1

Agraphia (absolute) R48.8
  with alexia R48.0
  developmental F81.81

Ague (dumb) —*see* Malaria

Agyria Q04.3

Ahumada-del Castillo syndrome
E23.0

Aichomophobia F40.298

AIDS (related complex) B20

Ailment heart —*see* Disease, heart

Ailurophobia F40.218

AIN —*see* Neoplasia, intraepithelial,
anal

Ainhum (disease) L94.6

AIPHI (acute idiopathic pulmonary
hemorrhage in infants (over 28
days old)) R04.81

Air
anterior mediastinum J98.2
compressed, disease T70.3
conditioner lung or pneumonitis
  J67.7
embolism (artery) (cerebral) (any
  site) T79.0
  with ectopic or molar pregnancy
    O08.2
  due to implanted device NEC
    —*see* Complications, by site
    and type, specified NEC
  following
    abortion —*see* Abortion
      by type, complicated by,
      embolism
    ectopic or molar pregnancy
      O08.2
  infusion, therapeutic injection
    or transfusion T80.0
  in pregnancy, childbirth or
    puerperium —*see* Embolism,
    obstetric
  traumatic T79.0
hunger, psychogenic F45.8
rarefied, effects of —*see* Effect,
  adverse, high altitude
sickness T75.3

Airplane sickness T75.3

Akathisia (drug-induced) (treatment-
induced) G25.71
  neuroleptic induced (acute) G25.71
  tardive G25.71

Akinesia R29.898

Akinetic mutism R41.89

Akureyri's disease G93.3

Alactasia, congenital E73.0

Alagille's syndrome Q44.7

Alastrim B03

Albers-Schönberg syndrome Q78.2

Albert's syndrome —*see* Tendinitis,
Achilles

Albinism, albino E70.30
  with hematologic abnormality
    E70.339
    Chédiak-Higashi syndrome
      E70.330

Albinism, albino *(continued)*
  with hematologic abnormality
    (continued)
      Hermansky-Pudlak syndrome
        E70.331
      other specified E70.338
      I E70.320
      II E70.321
      ocular E70.319
        autosomal recessive E70.311
        other specified E70.318
        X-linked E70.310
      oculocutaneous E70.329
        other specified E70.328
        tyrosinase (ty) negative E70.320
        tyrosinase (ty) positive E70.321
      other specified E70.39

Albinismus E70.30

Albright (-McCune) (-Sternberg)
  syndrome Q78.1

Albuminous —*see* condition

Albuminuria, albuminuric (acute)
  (chronic) (subacute) (*see also*
  Proteinuria) R80.9
  complicating pregnancy —*see*
    Proteinuria, gestational
    with
      gestational hypertension —*see*
        Pre-eclampsia
      pre-existing hypertension
        —*see* Hypertension,
        complicating pregnancy,
        pre-existing, with,
        pre-eclampsia
  gestational —*see* Proteinuria,
    gestational
    with
      gestational hypertension —*see*
        Pre-eclampsia
      pre-existing hypertension
        —*see* Hypertension,
        complicating pregnancy,
        pre-existing, with,
        pre-eclampsia
  orthostatic R80.2
  postural R80.2
  pre-eclamptic —*see* Pre-eclampsia
  scarlatinal A38.8

Albuminurophobia F40.298

Alcaptonuria E70.29

Alcohol, alcoholic, alcohol-induced
  addiction (without remission)
    F10.20
    with remission F10.21
  amnestic disorder, persisting F10.96
    with dependence F10.26
  anxiety disorder F10.980
  bipolar and related disorder F10.94
  brain syndrome, chronic F10.97
    with dependence F10.27
  cardiopathy I42.6
  counseling and surveillance Z71.41
    family member Z71.42
  delirium (acute) (tremens)
    (withdrawal) F10.231
    with intoxication F10.921
      in
        abuse F10.121
        dependence F10.221
  dementia F10.97
    with dependence F10.27
  depressive disorder F10.94
    with dependence F10.27
  deterioration F10.97
  hallucinosis (acute) F10.951
    in
      abuse F10.151
      dependence F10.251
  insanity F10.959

Alcohol, alcoholic, alcohol-induced
  (continued)
  intoxication (acute) (without
    dependence) F10.129
    with
      delirium F10.121
      dependence F10.229
        with delirium F10.221
        uncomplicated F10.220
    uncomplicated F10.120
  jealousy F10.988
  Korsakoff's, Korsakov's,
    Korsakow's F10.26
  liver K70.9
    acute —*see* Disease, liver,
      alcoholic, hepatitis
  major neurocognitive disorder,
    amnestic-confabulatory type
    F10.96
  major neurocognitive disorder,
    nonamnestic-confabulatory type
    F10.97
  mania (acute) (chronic) F10.959
  mild neurocognitive disorder
    F10.988
  paranoia, paranoid (type) psychosis
    F10.950
  pellagra E52
  poisoning, accidental (acute)
    NEC —*see* Table of Drugs and
    Chemicals, alcohol, poisoning
  psychosis —*see* Psychosis,
    alcoholic
  psychotic disorder F10.959
  sexual dysfunction F10.981
  sleep disorder F10.982
  withdrawal (without convulsions)
    F10.239
    with delirium F10.231

Alcoholism (chronic) (without
  remission) F10.20
  with
    psychosis —*see* Psychosis,
      alcoholic
    remission F10.21
  Korsakov's F10.96
    with dependence F10.26

Alder (-Reilly) anomaly or syndrome
  (leukocyte granulation) D72.0

Aldosteronism E26.9
  familial (type I) E26.02
  glucocorticoid-remediable E26.02
  primary (due to (bilateral) adrenal
    hyperplasia) E26.09
  primary NEC E26.09
  secondary E26.1
  specified NEC E26.89

Aldosteronoma D44.10

Aldrich (-Wiskott) syndrome
  (eczema-thrombocytopenia) D82.0

Alektorophobia F40.218

Aleppo boil B55.1

Aleukemic —*see* condition

Aleukia
  congenital D70.0
  hemorrhagica D61.9
    congenital D61.09
  splenica D73.1

Alexia R48.0
  developmental F81.0
  secondary to organic lesion R48.0

Algoneurodystrophy M89.00
  ankle M89.07-
  foot M89.07-
  forearm M89.03-
  hand M89.04-
  lower leg M89.06-

Algoneurodystrophy *(continued)*
  multiple sites M89.0-
  shoulder M89.01-
  specified site NEC M89.08
  thigh M89.05-
  upper arm M89.02-

Algophobia F40.298

Alienation, mental —*see* Psychosis

Alkalemia E87.3

Alkalosis E87.3
  metabolic E87.3
    with respiratory acidosis E87.4
    of newborn P74.41
  respiratory E87.3

Alkaptonuria E70.29

Allen-Masters syndrome N83.8

Allergy, allergic (reaction) (to)
  T78.40
  air-borne substance NEC (rhinitis)
    J30.89
  alveolitis (extrinsic) J67.9
    due to
      Aspergillus clavatus J67.4
      Cryptostroma corticale J67.6
      organisms (fungal,
        thermophilic actinomycete)
        growing in ventilation (air
        conditioning) systems J67.7
    specified type NEC J67.8
  anaphylactic reaction or shock T78.2
  angioneurotic edema T78.3
  animal (dander) (epidermal) (hair)
    (rhinitis) J30.81
  bee sting (anaphylactic shock) —*see*
    Toxicity, venom, arthropod, bee
  biological —*see* Allergy, drug
  colitis (*see also* Colitis, allergic)
    K52.29
  dander (animal) (rhinitis) J30.81
  dandruff (rhinitis) J30.81
  dental restorative material
    (existing) K08.55
  dermatitis —*see* Dermatitis,
    contact, allergic
  diathesis —*see* History, allergy
  drug, medicament & biological
    (any) (external) (internal) T78.40
    correct substance properly
      administered —*see* Table
      of Drugs and Chemicals, by
      drug, adverse effect
    wrong substance given or taken
      NEC (by accident) —*see*
      Table of Drugs and Chemicals,
      by drug, poisoning
  due to pollen J30.1
  dust (house) (stock) (rhinitis) J30.89
    with asthma —*see* Asthma,
      allergic extrinsic
  eczema —*see* Dermatitis, contact,
    allergic
  epidermal (animal) (rhinitis) J30.81
  feathers (rhinitis) J30.89
  food (any) (ingested) NEC T78.1
    anaphylactic shock —*see* Shock,
      anaphylactic, due to food
    dermatitis —*see* Dermatitis, due
      to, food
    dietary counseling and
      surveillance Z71.3
    in contact with skin L23.6
    rhinitis J30.5
    status (without reaction) Z91.018
      eggs Z91.012
      milk products Z91.011
      peanuts Z91.010
      seafood Z91.013
      specified NEC Z91.018

Allergy, allergic *(continued)*
  gastrointestinal —*see also* specific
    type of allergic reaction
    meaning colitis (*see also* Colitis,
      allergic) K52.29
    meaning gastroenteritis (*see*
      also Gastroenteritis, allergic)
      K52.29
    meaning other adverse food
      reaction not elsewhere
      classified T78.1
  grain J30.1
  grass (hay fever) (pollen) J30.1
    asthma —*see* Asthma, allergic
      extrinsic
  hair (animal) (rhinitis) J30.81
  history (of) —*see* History, allergy
  horse serum —*see* Allergy, serum
  inhalant (rhinitis) J30.89
    pollen J30.1
  kapok (rhinitis) J30.89
  medicine —*see* Allergy, drug
  milk protein (*see also* Allergy,
    food) Z91.011
    anaphylactic reaction T78.07
    dematitis L27.2
    entercolitis syndrome K52.21
    enteropathy K52.22
    gastroenteritis K52.29
    gastroesophageal reflux (*see*
      also Reaction, adverse, food)
      K21.9
      with esophagitis (without
        bleeding) K21.00
        with bleeding K21.01
    proctocolitis K52.82
  nasal, seasonal due to
    pollen J30.1
  pneumonia J82.89
  pollen (any) (hay fever) J30.1
    asthma —*see* Asthma, allergic
      extrinsic
  primrose J30.1
  primula J30.1
  proctocolitis K52.82
  purpura D69.0
  ragweed (hay fever) (pollen) J30.1
    asthma —*see* Asthma, allergic
      extrinsic
  rose (pollen) J30.1
  seasonal NEC J30.2
  Senecio jacobae (pollen) J30.1
  serum (*see also* Reaction, serum)
    T80.69
    anaphylactic shock T80.59
  shock (anaphylactic) T78.2
    due to
      administration of blood and
        blood products T80.51
      adverse effect of correct
        medicinal substance
        properly administered
        T88.6
      immunization T80.52
      serum NEC T80.59
      vaccination T80.52
  specific NEC T78.49
  tree (any) (hay fever) (pollen) J30.1
    asthma —*see* Asthma, allergic
      extrinsic
  upper respiratory J30.9
  urticaria L50.0
  vaccine —*see* Allergy, serum
  wheat —*see* Allergy, food

Allescheriasis B48.2

Alligator skin disease Q80.9

Allocheiria, allochiria R20.8

Almeida's disease —*see*
  Paracoccidioidomycosis

Alopecia (hereditaria) (seborrheica) L65.9
  androgenic L64.9
    drug-induced L64.0
    specified NEC L64.8
  areata L63.9
    ophiasis L63.2
    specified NEC L63.8
    totalis L63.0
    universalis L63.1
  cicatricial L66.9
    specified NEC L66.8
  circumscripta L63.9
  congenital, congenitalis Q84.0
  due to cytotoxic drugs NEC L65.8
  mucinosa L65.2
  postinfective NEC L65.8
  postpartum L65.0
  premature L64.8
  specific (syphilitic) A51.32
  specified NEC L65.8
  syphilitic (secondary) A51.32
  totalis (capitis) L63.0
  universalis (entire body) L63.1
  X-ray L58.1

Alpers' disease G31.81

Alpine sickness T70.29

Alport syndrome Q87.81

ALTE (apparent life threatening event) in newborn and infant R68.13

Alteration (of), **Altered**
  awareness
    transient R40.4
    unintended under general anesthesia, during procedure T88.53
  mental status R41.82
  pattern of family relationships affecting child Z62.898
  sensation
    following
      cerebrovascular disease I69.998
        cerebral infarction I69.398
        intracerebral hemorrhage I69.198
        nontraumatic intracranial hemorrhage NEC I69.298
        specified disease NEC I69.898
        subarachnoid hemorrhage I69.098

Alternating —*see* condition

Altitude, high (effects) —*see* Effect, adverse, high altitude

Aluminosis (of lung) J63.0

Alveolitis
  allergic (extrinsic) —*see* Pneumonitis, hypersensitivity
  due to
    Aspergillus clavatus J67.4
    Cryptostroma corticale J67.6
  fibrosing (cryptogenic) (idiopathic) J84.112
  jaw M27.3
  sicca dolorosa M27.3

Alveolus, alveolar —*see* condition

Alymphocytosis D72.810
  thymic (with immunodeficiency) D82.1

Alymphoplasia, thymic D82.1

Alzheimer's disease or sclerosis — *see* Disease, Alzheimer's

Amastia (with nipple present) Q83.8
  with absent nipple Q83.0

Amathophobia F40.228

Amaurosis (acquired) (congenital) — *see also* Blindness
  fugax G45.3
  hysterical F44.6
  Leber's congenital H35.50
  uremic —*see* Uremia

Amaurotic idiocy (infantile) (juvenile) (late) E75.4

Amaxophobia F40.248

Ambiguous genitalia Q56.4

Amblyopia (congenital) (ex anopsia) (partial) (suppression) H53.00-
  anisometropic —*see* Amblyopia, refractive
  deprivation H53.01-
  hysterical F44.6
  nocturnal —*see also* Blindness, night
    vitamin A deficiency E50.5
  refractive H53.02-
  strabismic H53.03-
  suspect H53.04-
  tobacco H53.8
  toxic NEC H53.8
  uremic —*see* Uremia

Ameba, amebic (histolytica) —*see also* Amebiasis
  abscess (liver) A06.4

Amebiasis A06.9
  with abscess —*see* Abscess, amebic
  acute A06.0
  chronic (intestine) A06.1
    with abscess —*see* Abscess, amebic
  cutaneous A06.7
  cutis A06.7
  cystitis A06.81
  genitourinary tract NEC A06.82
  hepatic —*see* Abscess, liver, amebic
  intestine A06.0
  nondysenteric colitis A06.2
  skin A06.7
  specified site NEC A06.89

Ameboma (of intestine) A06.3

Amelia Q73.0
  lower limb —*see* Agenesis, leg
  upper limb —*see* Agenesis, arm

Ameloblastoma —*see also* Cyst, calcifying odontogenic
  long bones C40.9-
    lower limb C40.2-
    upper limb C40.0-
  malignant C41.1
    jaw (bone) (lower) C41.1
      upper C41.0
  tibial C40.2-

Amelogenesis imperfecta K00.5
  nonhereditaria (segmentalis) K00.4

Amenorrhea N91.2
  hyperhormonal E28.8
  primary N91.0
  secondary N91.1

Amentia —*see* Disability, intellectual
  Meynert's (nonalcoholic) F04

American
  leishmaniasis B55.2
  mountain tick fever A93.2

Ametropia —*see* Disorder, refraction

AMH (asymptomatic microscopic hematuria) R31.21

Amianthosis J61

Amimia R48.8

Amino-acid disorder E72.9
  anemia D53.0

Aminoacidopathy E72.9

Aminoaciduria E72.9

Amnes(t)ic syndrome (post-traumatic) F04
  induced by
    alcohol F10.96
      with dependence F10.26
    psychoactive NEC F19.96
      with
        abuse F19.16
        dependence F19.26
    sedative F13.96
      with dependence F13.26

Amnesia R41.3
  anterograde R41.1
  auditory R48.8
  dissociative F44.0
    with dissociative fugue F44.1
  hysterical F44.0
  postictal in epilepsy —*see* Epilepsy
  psychogenic F44.0
  retrograde R41.2
  transient global G45.4

Amnion, amniotic —*see* condition

Amnionitis —*see* Pregnancy, complicated by

Amok F68.8

Amoral traits F60.89

Amphetamine (or other stimulant)-induced
  anxiety disorder F15.980
  bipolar and related disorder F15.94
  delirium F15.921
  depressive disorder F15.94
  obsessive-compulsive and related disorder F15.988
  psychotic disorder F15.959
  sexual dysfunction F15.981
  sleep disorder F15.982
  stimulant withdrawal F15.23

Ampulla
  lower esophagus K22.8
  phrenic K22.8

Amputation —*see also* Absence, by site, acquired
  neuroma (postoperative) (traumatic) —*see* Complications, amputation stump, neuroma
  stump (surgical)
    abnormal, painful, or with complication (late) —*see* Complications, amputation stump
    healed or old NOS Z89.9
  traumatic (complete) (partial)
    arm (upper) (complete) S48.91- at
      elbow S58.01-
        partial S58.02-
      shoulder joint (complete) S48.01-
        partial S48.02-
      between
        elbow and wrist (complete) S58.11-
          partial S58.12-
        shoulder and elbow (complete) S48.11-
          partial S48.12-
      partial S48.92-
    breast (complete) S28.21-
      partial S28.22-
    clitoris (complete) S38.211
      partial S38.212
    ear (complete) S08.11-
      partial S08.12-

Amputation (*continued*)
  traumatic (*continued*)
    finger (complete)
      (metacarpophalangeal) S68.11-
        index S68.11-
        little S68.11-
        middle S68.11-
        partial S68.12-
          index S68.12-
          little S68.12-
          middle S68.12-
          ring S68.12-
        ring S68.11-
      thumb —*see* Amputation, traumatic, thumb
      transphalangeal (complete) S68.61-
        index S68.61-
        little S68.61-
        middle S68.61-
        partial S68.62-
          index S68.62-
          little S68.62-
          middle S68.62-
          ring S68.62-
        ring S68.61-
    foot (complete) S98.91-
      at ankle level S98.01-
        partial S98.02-
      midfoot S98.31-
        partial S98.32-
      partial S98.92-
    forearm (complete) S58.91-
      at elbow level (complete) S58.01-
        partial S58.02-
      between elbow and wrist (complete) S58.11-
        partial S58.12-
      partial S58.92-
    genital organ(s) (external)
      female (complete) S38.211
        partial S38.212
      male
        penis (complete) S38.221
          partial S38.222
        scrotum (complete) S38.231
          partial S38.232
        testes (complete) S38.231
          partial S38.232
    hand (complete) (wrist level) S68.41-
      finger(s) alone —*see* Amputation, traumatic, finger
      partial S68.42-
      thumb alone —*see* Amputation, traumatic, thumb
      transmetacarpal (complete) S68.71-
        partial S68.72-
    head
      ear —*see* Amputation, traumatic, ear
      nose (partial) S08.812
        complete S08.811
      part S08.89
      scalp S08.0
    hip (and thigh) (complete) S78.91-
      at hip joint (complete) S78.01-
        partial S78.02-
      between hip and knee (complete) S78.11-
        partial S78.12-
      partial S78.92-
    labium (majus) (minus) (complete) S38.21-
      partial S38.21-

Amputation *(continued)*
  traumatic *(continued)*
    leg (lower) S88.91-
      at knee level S88.01-
        partial S88.02-
      between knee and ankle
        S88.11-
        partial S88.12-
      partial S88.92-
    nose (partial) S08.812
      complete S08.811
    penis (complete) S38.221
      partial S38.222
    scrotum (complete) S38.231
      partial S38.232
    shoulder —*see* Amputation,
      traumatic, arm
      at shoulder joint —*see*
        Amputation, traumatic, arm,
        at shoulder joint
    testes (complete) S38.231
      partial S38.232
    thigh —*see* Amputation,
      traumatic, hip
    thorax, part of S28.1
      breast —*see* Amputation,
        traumatic, breast
    thumb (complete)
      (metacarpophalangeal) S68.01-
      partial S68.02-
      transphalangeal (complete)
        S68.51-
        partial S68.52-
    toe (lesser) S98.13-
      great S98.11-
        partial S98.12-
      more than one S98.21-
        partial S98.22-
      partial S98.14-
    vulva (complete) S38.211
      partial S38.212
Amputee (bilateral) (old) Z89.9
Amsterdam dwarfism Q87.19
Amusia R48.8
  developmental F80.89
Amyelencephalus, amyelencephaly
  Q00.0
Amyelia Q06.0
Amygdalitis —*see* Tonsillitis
Amygdalolith J35.8
Amyloid heart (disease) E85.4 *[I43]*
Amyloidosis (generalized) (primary)
  E85.9
  with lung involvement E85.4 *[J99]*
  familial E85.2
  genetic E85.2
  heart E85.4 *[I43]*
  hemodialysis-associated E85.3
  liver E85.4 *[K77]*
  light chain (AL) E85.81
  localized E85.4
  neuropathic heredofamilial E85.1
  non-neuropathic heredofamilial E85.0
  organ limited E85.4
  Portuguese E85.1
  pulmonary E85.4 *[J99]*
  secondary systemic E85.3
  senile systemic (SSA) E85.82
  skin (lichen) (macular) E85.4 *[L99]*
  specified NEC E85.89
  subglottic E85.4 *[J99]*
  wild-type transthyretin-related
    (ATTR) E85.82
Amylopectinosis (brancher enzyme
  deficiency) E74.03
Amylophagia —*see* Pica
Amyoplasia congenita Q79.8

Amyotonia M62.89
  congenita G70.2
Amyotrophia, amyotrophy,
  amyotrophic G71.8
  congenita Q79.8
  diabetic —*see* Diabetes, amyotrophy
  lateral sclerosis G12.21
  neuralgic G54.5
  spinal progressive G12.25
Anacidity, gastric K31.83
  psychogenic F45.8
Anaerosis of newborn P28.89
Analbuminemia E88.09
Analgesia —*see* Anesthesia
Analphalipoproteinemia E78.6
Anaphylactic
  purpura D69.0
  shock or reaction —*see* Shock,
    anaphylactic
Anaphylactoid shock or reaction
  —*see* Shock, anaphylactic
Anaphylactoid syndrome of
  pregnancy O88.01-
Anaphylaxis —*see* Shock, anaphylactic
Anaplasia cervix —*see also*
  Dysplasia, cervix N87.9
Anaplasmosis, human A77.49
Anarthria R47.1
Anasarca R60.1
  cardiac —*see* Failure, heart,
    congestive
  lung J18.2
  newborn P83.2
  nutritional E43
  pulmonary J18.2
  renal N04.9
Anastomosis
  aneurysmal —*see* Aneurysm
  arteriovenous ruptured brain I60.8
    intracerebral I61.8
    intraparenchymal I61.8
    intraventricular I61.5
    subarachnoid I60.8
  intestinal K63.89
    complicated NEC K91.89
      involving urinary tract N99.89
  retinal and choroidal vessels
    (congenital) Q14.8
Anatomical narrow angle H40.03-
Ancylostoma, ancylostomiasis
  (braziliense) (caninum)
  (ceylanicum) (duodenale) B76.0
  Necator americanus B76.1
Andersen's disease (glycogen
  storage) E74.09
Anderson-Fabry disease E75.21
Andes disease T70.29
Andrews' disease (bacterid) L08.89
Androblastoma
  benign
    specified site —*see* Neoplasm,
      benign, by site
    unspecified site
      female D27.9
      male D29.20
  malignant
    specified site —*see* Neoplasm,
      malignant, by site
    unspecified site
      female C56.9
      male C62.90
  specified site —*see* Neoplasm,
    uncertain behavior, by site

Androblastoma *(continued)*
  tubular
    with lipid storage
      specified site —*see* Neoplasm,
        benign, by site
      unspecified site
        female D27.9
        male D29.20
    specified site —*see* Neoplasm,
      benign, by site
    unspecified site
      female D27.9
      male D29.20
  unspecified site
    female D39.10
    male D40.10
Androgen insensitivity syndrome
  —*see also* Syndrome, androgen
  insensitivity E34.50
Androgen resistance syndrome
  —*see also* Syndrome, androgen
  insensitivity E34.50
Android pelvis Q74.2
  with disproportion (fetopelvic) O33.3
    causing obstructed labor O65.3
Androphobia F40.290
Anectasis, pulmonary (newborn)
  —*see* Atelectasis
Anemia (essential) (general)
  (hemoglobin deficiency) (infantile)
  (primary) (profound) D64.9
  with (due to) (in)
    disorder of
      anaerobic glycolysis D55.2
      pentose phosphate pathway
        D55.1
    koilonychia D50.9
  achlorhydric D50.8
  achrestic D53.1
  Addison (-Biermer) (pernicious)
    D51.0
  agranulocytic —*see*
    Agranulocytosis
  amino-acid-deficiency D53.0
  aplastic D61.9
    congenital D61.09
    drug-induced D61.1
    due to
      drugs D61.1
      external agents NEC D61.2
      infection D61.2
      radiation D61.2
    idiopathic D61.3
    red cell (pure) D60.9
      chronic D60.0
      congenital D61.01
      specified type NEC D60.8
      transient D60.1
    specified type NEC D61.89
    toxic D61.2
  aregenerative
    congenital D61.09
  asiderotic D50.9
  atypical (primary) D64.9
  Baghdad spring D55.0
  Balantidium coli A07.0
  Biermer's (pernicious) D51.0
  blood loss (chronic) D50.0
    acute D62
  bothriocephalus B70.0 *[D63.8]*
  brickmaker's B76.9 *[D63.8]*
  cerebral I67.89
  childhood D58.9
  chlorotic D50.8
  chronic
    blood loss D50.0
    hemolytic D58.9
      idiopathic D59.9
    simple D53.9

Anemia *(continued)*
  chronica congenita aregenerativa
    D61.09
  combined system disease NEC
    D51.0 *[G32.0]*
    due to dietary vitamin B12
      deficiency D51.3 *[G32.0]*
  complicating pregnancy, childbirth
    or puerperium —*see* Pregnancy,
    complicated by (management
    affected by), anemia
  congenital P61.4
    aplastic D61.09
    due to isoimmunization NOS
      P55.9
    dyserythropoietic,
      dyshematopoietic D64.4
    following fetal blood loss P61.3
    Heinz body D58.2
    hereditary hemolytic NOS D58.9
    pernicious D51.0
    spherocytic D58.0
  Cooley's (erythroblastic) D56.1
  cytogenic D51.0
  deficiency D53.9
    2, 3 diphosphoglycurate mutase
      D55.2
    2, 3 PG D55.2
    6 phosphogluconate
      dehydrogenase D55.1
    6-PGD D55.1
    amino-acid D53.0
    combined B12 and folate
      D53.1
    enzyme D55.9
      drug-induced (hemolytic)
        D59.2
      glucose-6-phosphate
        dehydrogenase (G6PD)
        D55.0
      glycolytic D55.2
      nucleotide metabolism D55.3
      related to hexose
        monophosphate (HMP)
        shunt pathway NEC D55.1
      specified type NEC D55.8
    erythrocytic glutathione D55.1
    folate D52.9
      dietary D52.0
      drug-induced D52.1
    folic acid D52.9
      dietary D52.0
      drug-induced D52.1
    G SH D55.1
    GGS-R D55.1
    glucose-6-phosphate
      dehydrogenase D55.0
    glutathione reductase D55.1
    glyceraldehyde phosphate
      dehydrogenase D55.2
    G6PD D55.0
    hexokinase D55.2
    iron D50.9
      secondary to blood loss
        (chronic) D50.0
    nutritional D53.9
      with
        poor iron absorption D50.8
        specified deficiency NEC
          D53.8
    phosphofructo-aldolase D55.2
    phosphoglycerate kinase D55.2
    PK D55.2
    protein D53.0
    pyruvate kinase D55.2
    transcobalamin II D51.2
    triose-phosphate isomerase
      D55.2
    vitamin B12 NOS D51.9
      dietary D51.3

Anemia *(continued)*
refractory *(continued)*
sideroblastic D46.1
sideropenic D50.9
without ring sideroblasts, so
stated D46.0
without sideroblasts without
excess of blasts D46.0
Rietti-Greppi-Micheli D56.9
scorbutic D53.2
secondary to
blood loss (chronic) D50.0
acute D62
hemorrhage (chronic) D50.0
acute D62
semiplastic D61.89
sickle-cell —*see* Disease, sickle-cell
sideroblastic D64.3
hereditary D64.0
hypochromic, sex-linked D64.0
pyridoxine-responsive NEC
D64.3
refractory D46.1
secondary (due to)
disease D64.1
drugs and toxins D64.2
specified type NEC D64.3
sideropenic (refractory) D50.9
due to blood loss (chronic) D50.0
acute D62
simple chronic D53.9
specified type NEC D64.89
spherocytic (hereditary) —*see*
Spherocytosis
splenic D64.89
splenomegalic D64.89
stomatocytosis D58.8
syphilitic (acquired) (late) A52.79
[D63.8]
target cell D64.89
thalassemia D56.9
thrombocytopenic —*see*
Thrombocytopenia
toxic D61.2
tropical B76.9 *[D63.8]*
macrocytic D52.8
tuberculous A18.89 *[D63.8]*
vegan D51.3
vitamin
B6-responsive D64.3
B12 deficiency (dietary)
pernicious D51.0
von Jaksch's D64.89
Witts'(achlorhydric anemia) D50.8

Anemophobia F40.228

Anencephalus, anencephaly Q00.0

Anergasia —*see* Psychosis, organic

Anesthesia, anesthetic R20.0
complication or reaction NEC (*see
also* Complications, anesthesia)
T88.59
due to
correct substance properly
administered —*see* Table
of Drugs and Chemicals, by
drug, adverse effect
overdose or wrong substance
given —*see* Table of Drugs
and Chemicals, by drug,
poisoning
unintended awareness under
general anesthesia during
procedure T88.53
personal history of Z92.84
cornea H18.81-
dissociative F44.6
functional (hysterical) F44.6
hyperesthetic, thalamic G89.0
hysterical F44.6
local skin lesion R20.0

Anesthesia, anesthetic *(continued)*
sexual (psychogenic) F52.1
shock (due to) T88.2
skin R20.0
testicular N50.9

Anetoderma (maculosum) (of) L90.8
Jadassohn-Pellizzari L90.2
Schweniger-Buzzi L90.1

Aneurin deficiency E51.9

Aneurysm (anastomotic) (artery)
(cirsoid) (diffuse) (false) (fusiform)
(multiple) (saccular) I72.9
abdominal (aorta) I71.4
ruptured I71.3
syphilitic A52.01
aorta, aortic (nonsyphilitic) I71.9
abdominal I71.4
ruptured I71.3
arch I71.2
ruptured I71.1
arteriosclerotic I71.9
ruptured I71.8
ascending I71.2
ruptured I71.1
congenital Q25.43
descending I71.9
abdominal I71.4
ruptured I71.3
ruptured I71.8
thoracic I71.2
ruptured I71.1
congenital Q25.43
root Q25.43
ruptured I71.8
sinus, congenital Q25.43
syphilitic A52.01
thoracic I71.2
ruptured I71.1
thoracoabdominal I71.6
ruptured I71.5
thorax, thoracic (arch) I71.2
ruptured I71.1
root Q25.43
transverse I71.2
ruptured I71.1
valve (heart) (*see also*
Endocarditis, aortic) I35.8
arteriosclerotic I72.9
cerebral I67.1
ruptured —*see* Hemorrhage,
intracranial, subarachnoid
arteriovenous (congenital)
—*see also* Malformation,
arteriovenous
acquired I77.0
brain I67.1
ruptured —*see* Aneurysm,
arteriovenous, brain,
ruptured
coronary I25.41
pulmonary I28.0
brain Q28.2
ruptured I60.8
intracerebral I61.8
intraparenchymal I61.8
intraventricular I61.5
subarachnoid I60.8
peripheral —*see* Malformation,
arteriovenous, peripheral
precerebral vessels Q28.0
specified site NEC —*see also*
Malformation, arteriovenous
acquired I77.0
basal —*see* Aneurysm, brain
basilar (trunk) I72.5
berry (congenital) (nonruptured) I67.1
ruptured I60.7
brain I67.1
arteriosclerotic I67.1
ruptured —*see* Hemorrhage,
intracranial, subarachnoid

Aneurysm *(continued)*
brain *(continued)*
arteriovenous (congenital)
(nonruptured) Q28.2
acquired I67.1
ruptured —*see* Aneurysm,
arteriovenous, brain,
ruptured I60.8-
ruptured —*see* Aneurysm,
arteriovenous, brain,
ruptured I60.8-
berry (congenital) (nonruptured)
I67.1
ruptured (*see also*
Hemorrhage, intracranial,
subarachnoid) I60.7
congenital Q28.3
ruptured I60.7
meninges I67.1
ruptured I60.8
miliary (congenital)
(nonruptured) I67.1
ruptured (*see also*
Hemorrhage, intracranial,
subarachnoid) I60.7
mycotic I33.0
ruptured —*see* Hemorrhage,
intracranial, subarachnoid
syphilitic (hemorrhage) A52.05
cardiac (false) (*see also* Aneurysm,
heart) I25.3
carotid artery (common) (external)
I72.0
internal (intracranial) I67.1
extracranial portion I72.0
ruptured into brain I60.0-
syphilitic A52.09
intracranial A52.05
cavernous sinus I67.1
arteriovenous (congenital)
(nonruptured) Q28.3
ruptured I60.8
celiac I72.8
central nervous system, syphilitic
A52.05
cerebral —*see* Aneurysm, brain
chest —*see* Aneurysm, thorax
circle of Willis I67.1
congenital Q28.3
ruptured I60.6
ruptured I60.6
common iliac artery I72.3
congenital (peripheral) Q27.8
aorta (root) (sinus) Q25.43
brain Q28.3
ruptured I60.7
coronary Q24.5
digestive system Q27.8
lower limb Q27.8
pulmonary Q25.79
retina Q14.1
specified site NEC Q27.8
upper limb Q27.8
conjunctiva —*see* Abnormality,
conjunctiva, vascular
conus arteriosus —*see* Aneurysm,
heart
coronary (arteriosclerotic) (artery)
I25.41
arteriovenous, congenital Q24.5
congenital Q24.5
ruptured —*see* Infarct,
myocardium
syphilitic A52.06
vein I25.89
cylindroid (aorta) I71.9
ruptured I71.8
syphilitic A52.01
ductus arteriosus Q25.0
endocardial, infective (any valve)
I33.0

Aneurysm *(continued)*
femoral (artery) (ruptured) I72.4
gastroduodenal I72.8
gastroepiploic I72.8
heart (wall) (chronic or with a stated
duration of over 4 weeks) I25.3
valve —*see* Endocarditis
hepatic I72.8
iliac (common) (artery) (ruptured)
I72.3
infective I72.9
endocardial (any valve) I33.0
innominate (nonsyphilitic) I72.8
syphilitic A52.09
interauricular septum —*see*
Aneurysm, heart
interventricular septum —*see*
Aneurysm, heart
intrathoracic (nonsyphilitic) I71.2
ruptured I71.1
syphilitic A52.01
lower limb I72.4
lung (pulmonary artery) I28.1
mediastinal (nonsyphilitic) I72.8
syphilitic A52.09
miliary (congenital) I67.1
ruptured —*see* Hemorrhage,
intracerebral, subarachnoid,
intracranial
mitral (heart) (valve) I34.8
mural —*see* Aneurysm, heart
mycotic I72.9
endocardial (any valve) I33.0
ruptured, brain —*see* Hemorrhage,
intracerebral, subarachnoid
myocardium —*see* Aneurysm, heart
neck I72.0
pancreaticoduodenal I72.8
patent ductus arteriosus Q25.0
peripheral NEC I72.8
congenital Q27.8
digestive system Q27.8
lower limb Q27.8
specified site NEC Q27.8
upper limb Q27.8
popliteal (artery) (ruptured) I72.4
precerebral
congenital (nonruptured) Q28.1
specified site, NEC I72.5
pulmonary I28.1
arteriovenous Q25.72
acquired I28.0
syphilitic A52.09
valve (heart) —*see* Endocarditis,
pulmonary
racemose (peripheral) I72.9
congenital —*see* Aneurysm,
congenital
radial I72.1
Rasmussen NEC A15.0
renal (artery) I72.2
retina —*see also* Disorder, retina,
microaneurysms
congenital Q14.1
diabetic —*see* E08-E13 with .3-
sinus of Valsalva Q25.49
specified NEC I72.8
spinal (cord) I72.8
syphilitic (hemorrhage) A52.09
splenic I72.8
subclavian (artery) (ruptured)
I72.8
syphilitic A52.09
superior mesenteric I72.8
syphilitic (aorta) A52.01
central nervous system A52.05
congenital (late) A50.54 *[I79.0]*
spine, spinal A52.09
thoracoabdominal (aorta) I71.6
ruptured I71.5
syphilitic A52.01

Aneurysm *(continued)*
 thorax, thoracic (aorta) (arch)
   (nonsyphilitic) I71.2
   ruptured I71.1
   syphilitic A52.01
  traumatic (complication) (early),
   specified site —*see* Injury, blood
   vessel
  tricuspid (heart) (valve) I07.8
  ulnar I72.1
  upper limb (ruptured) I72.1
  valve, valvular —*see* Endocarditis
  venous (*see also* Varix) I86.8
   congenital Q27.8
    digestive system Q27.8
    lower limb Q27.8
    specified site NEC Q27.8
    upper limb Q27.8
  ventricle —*see* Aneurysm, heart
  vertebral artery I72.6
  visceral NEC I72.8

Angelman syndrome Q93.51

Anger R45.4

Angiectasis, angiectopia I99.8

Angiitis I77.6
 allergic granulomatous M30.1
 hypersensitivity M31.0
 necrotizing M31.9
   specified NEC M31.8
 nervous system, granulomatous I67.7

Angina (attack) (cardiac) (chest)
  (heart) (pectoris) (syndrome)
  (vasomotor) I20.9
 with
   atherosclerotic heart disease
    —*see* Arteriosclerosis,
    coronary (artery),
    documented spasm I20.1
 abdominal K55.1
 accelerated —*see* Angina, unstable
 agranulocytic —*see* Agranulocytosis
 angiospastic —*see* Angina, with
   documented spasm
 aphthous B08.5
 crescendo —*see* Angina, unstable
 croupous J05.0
 cruris I73.9
 de novo effort —*see* Angina,
   unstable
 diphtheritic, membranous A36.0
 equivalent I20.8
 exudative, chronic J37.0
 following acute myocardial
   infarction I23.7
 gangrenous diphtheritic A36.0
 intestinal K55.1
 Ludovici K12.2
 Ludwig's K12.2
 malignant diphtheritic A36.0
 membranous J05.0
   diphtheritic A36.0
   Vincent's A69.1
 mesenteric K55.1
 monocytic —*see* Mononucleosis,
   infectious
 of effort —*see* Angina, specified
   NEC
 phlegmonous J36
   diphtheritic A36.0
 post-infarctional I23.7
 pre-infarctional —*see* Angina,
   unstable
 Prinzmetal —*see* Angina, with
   documented spasm
 progressive —*see* Angina, unstable
 pseudomembranous A69.1
 pultaceous, diphtheritic A36.0
 spasm-induced —*see* Angina, with
   documented spasm

Angina *(continued)*
 specified NEC I20.8
 stable I20.8
 stenocardia —*see* Angina, specified
   NEC
 stridulous, diphtheritic A36.2
 tonsil J36
 trachealis J05.0
 unstable I20.0
 variant —*see* Angina, with
   documented spasm
 Vincent's A69.1
 worsening effort —*see* Angina,
   unstable

Angioblastoma —*see* Neoplasm,
 connective tissue, uncertain behavior

Angiocholecystitis —*see*
 Cholecystitis, acute

Angiocholitis —*see also*
 Cholecystitis, acute K83.09

Angiodysgenesis spinalis G95.19

Angiodysplasia (cecum) (colon)
  K55.20
 with bleeding K55.21
 duodenum (and stomach)
   K31.819
   with bleeding K31.811
 stomach (and duodenum) K31.819
   with bleeding K31.811

Angioedema (allergic) (any site)
  (with urticaria) T78.3
 episodic, with eosinophilia
   D72.118
 hereditary D84.1

Angioendothelioma —*see*
 Neoplasm, uncertain behavior, by
 site
 benign D18.00
   intra-abdominal D18.03
   intracranial D18.02
   skin D18.01
   specified site NEC D18.09
 bone —*see* Neoplasm, bone,
   malignant
 Ewing's —*see* Neoplasm, bone,
   malignant

Angioendotheliomatosis C85.8-

Angiofibroma —*see also* Neoplasm,
 benign, by site
 juvenile
   specified site —*see* Neoplasm,
    benign, by site
   unspecified site D10.6

Angiohemophilia (A) (B) D68.0

Angioid streaks (choroid) (macula)
  (retina) H35.33

Angiokeratoma —*see* Neoplasm,
 skin, benign
 corporis diffusum E75.21

Angioleiomyoma —*see* Neoplasm,
 connective tissue, benign

Angiolipoma —*see also* Lipoma
 infiltrating —*see* Lipoma

Angioma —*see also* Hemangioma,
 by site
 capillary I78.1
 hemorrhagicum hereditaria I78.0
 intra-abdominal D18.03
 intracranial D18.02
 malignant —*see* Neoplasm,
   connective tissue, malignant
 plexiform D18.00
   intra-abdominal D18.03
   intracranial D18.02
   skin D18.01
   specified site NEC D18.09

Angioma *(continued)*
 senile I78.1
 serpiginosum L81.7
 skin D18.01
 specified site NEC D18.09
 spider I78.1
 stellate I78.1
 venous Q28.3

Angiomatosis Q82.8
 bacillary A79.89
 encephalotrigeminal Q85.8
 hemorrhagic familial I78.0
 hereditary familial I78.0
 liver K76.4

Angiomyolipoma —*see* Lipoma

Angiomyoliposarcoma —*see*
 Neoplasm, connective tissue,
 malignant

Angiomyoma —*see* Neoplasm,
 connective tissue, benign

Angiomyosarcoma —*see* Neoplasm,
 connective tissue, malignant

Angiomyxoma —*see* Neoplasm,
 connective tissue, uncertain behavior

Angioneurosis F45.8

Angioneurotic edema (allergic) (any
 site) (with urticaria) T78.3
 hereditary D84.1

Angiopathia, angiopathy I99.9
 cerebral I67.9
   amyloid E85.4 *[I68.0]*
 diabetic (peripheral) —*see*
   Diabetes, angiopathy
 peripheral I73.9
   diabetic —*see* Diabetes,
    angiopathy
   specified type NEC I73.89
 retinae syphilitica A52.05
 retinalis (juvenilis)
   diabetic —*see* Diabetes,
    retinopathy
   proliferative —*see* Retinopathy,
    proliferative

Angiosarcoma —*see also* Neoplasm,
 connective tissue, malignant
 liver C22.3

Angiosclerosis —*see*
 Arteriosclerosis

Angiospasm (peripheral) (traumatic)
  (vessel) I73.9
 brachial plexus G54.0
 cerebral G45.9
 cervical plexus G54.2
 nerve
   arm —*see* Mononeuropathy,
    upper limb
    axillary G54.0
    median —*see* Lesion, nerve,
     median
    ulnar —*see* Lesion, nerve,
     ulnar
   axillary G54.0
   leg —*see* Mononeuropathy,
    lower limb
   median —*see* Lesion, nerve,
    median
   plantar —*see* Lesion, nerve,
    plantar
   ulnar —*see* Lesion, nerve, ulnar

Angiospastic disease or edema I73.9

Angiostrongyliasis
 due to
   Parastrongylus
    cantonensis B83.2
    costaricensis B81.3
 intestinal B81.3

Anguillulosis —*see* Strongyloidiasis

Angulation
 cecum —*see* Obstruction, intestine
 coccyx (acquired) (*see also*
   subcategory) M43.8
   congenital NEC Q76.49
 femur (acquired) —*see also*
   Deformity, limb, specified type
   NEC, thigh
   congenital Q74.2
 intestine (large) (small) —*see*
   Obstruction, intestine
 sacrum (acquired) (*see also*
   subcategory) M43.8
   congenital NEC Q76.49
 sigmoid (flexure) —*see*
   Obstruction, intestine
 spine —*see* Dorsopathy, deforming,
   specified NEC
 tibia (acquired) —*see also*
   Deformity, limb, specified type
   NEC, lower leg
   congenital Q74.2
 ureter N13.5
   with infection N13.6
 wrist (acquired) —*see also*
   Deformity, limb, specified type
   NEC, forearm
   congenital Q74.0

Angulus infectiosus (lips) K13.0

Anhedonia R45.84
 sexual F52.0

Anhidrosis L74.4

Anhydration E86.0

Anhydremia E86.0

Anidrosis L74.4

Aniridia (congenital) Q13.1

Anisakiasis (infection) (infestation)
  B81.0

Anisakis larvae infestation B81.0

Aniseikonia H52.32

Anisocoria (pupil) H57.02
 congenital Q13.2

Anisocytosis R71.8

Anisometropia (congenital)
  H52.31

Ankle —*see* condition

Ankyloblepharon (eyelid) (acquired)
 —*see also* Blepharophimosis
 filiforme (adnatum) (congenital)
   Q10.3
 total Q10.3

Ankyloglossia Q38.1

Ankylosis (fibrous) (osseous) (joint)
  M24.60
 ankle M24.67-
 arthrodesis status Z98.1
 cricoarytenoid (cartilage) (joint)
   (larynx) J38.7
 dental K03.5
 ear ossicles H74.31-
 elbow M24.62-
 foot M24.67-
 hand M24.64-
 hip M24.65-
 incostapedial joint (infectional)
   —*see* Ankylosis, ear ossicles
 jaw (temporomandibular)
   M26.61-
 knee M24.66-
 lumbosacral (joint) M43.27
 postoperative (status) Z98.1
 produced by surgical fusion, status
   Z98.1
 sacro-iliac (joint) M43.28

Ankylosis *(continued)*
   shoulder M24.61-
   specified site NEC M24.69
   spine (joint) —*see also* Fusion, spine
      spondylitic —*see* Spondylitis,
         ankylosing
   surgical Z98.1
   temporomandibular M26.61-
   tooth, teeth (hard tissues) K03.5
   wrist M24.63-

Ankylostoma —*see* Ancylostoma

Ankylostomiasis —*see*
   Ancylostomiasis

Ankylurethria —*see* Stricture,
   urethra

Annular —*see also* condition
   detachment, cervix N88.8
   organ or site, congenital NEC
      —*see* Distortion
   pancreas (congenital) Q45.1

Anodontia (complete) (partial) (vera)
   K00.0
   acquired K08.10

Anomaly, anomalous (congenital)
   (unspecified type) Q89.9
   abdominal wall NEC Q79.59
   acoustic nerve Q07.8
   adrenal (gland) Q89.1
   Alder (-Reilly) (leukocyte
      granulation) D72.0
   alimentary tract Q45.9
      upper Q40.9
   alveolar M26.70
      hyperplasia M26.79
         mandibular M26.72
         maxillary M26.71
      hypoplasia M26.79
         mandibular M26.74
         maxillary M26.73
      ridge (process) M26.79
      specified NEC M26.79
   ankle (joint) Q74.2
   anus Q43.9
   aorta (arch) NEC Q25.40
      coarctation (preductal)
         (postductal) Q25.1
   aortic cusp or valve Q23.9
   appendix Q43.8
   apple peel syndrome Q41.1
   aqueduct of Sylvius Q03.0
      with spina bifida —*see* Spina
         bifida, with hydrocephalus
   arm Q74.0
   arteriovenous NEC
      coronary Q24.5
      gastrointestinal Q27.33
         acquired —*see*
            Angiodysplasia
   artery (peripheral) Q27.9
      basilar NEC Q28.1
      cerebral Q28.3
      coronary Q24.5
      digestive system Q27.8
      eye Q15.8
      great Q25.9
         specified NEC Q25.8
      lower limb Q27.8
      peripheral Q27.9
         specified NEC Q27.8
      pulmonary NEC Q25.79
      renal Q27.2
      retina Q14.1
      specified site NEC Q27.8
      subclavian Q27.8
         origin Q25.48
      umbilical Q27.0
      upper limb Q27.8
      vertebral NEC Q28.1
   aryteno-epiglottic folds Q31.8

Anomaly, anomalous *(continued)*
   atrial
      bands or folds Q20.8
      septa Q21.1
   atrioventricular
      excitation I45.6
      septum Q21.0
   auditory canal Q17.8
   auricle
      ear Q17.8
         causing impairment of hearing
            Q16.9
      heart Q20.8
   Axenfeld's Q15.0
   back Q89.9
   band
      atrial Q20.8
      heart Q24.8
      ventricular Q24.8
   Bartholin's duct Q38.4
   biliary duct or passage Q44.5
   bladder Q64.70
      absence Q64.5
      diverticulum Q64.6
      exstrophy Q64.10
         cloacal Q64.12
         extroversion Q64.19
            specified type NEC Q64.19
         supravesical fissure Q64.11
      neck obstruction Q64.31
      specified type NEC Q64.79
   bone Q79.9
      arm Q74.0
      face Q75.9
      leg Q74.2
      pelvic girdle Q74.2
      shoulder girdle Q74.0
      skull Q75.9
         with
            anencephaly Q00.0
            encephalocele —*see*
               Encephalocele
            hydrocephalus Q03.9
               with spina bifida —*see*
                  Spina bifida, by site,
                  with hydrocephalus
            microcephaly Q02
   brain (multiple) Q04.9
      vessel Q28.3
   breast Q83.9
   broad ligament Q50.6
   bronchus Q32.4
   bulbus cordis Q21.9
   bursa Q79.9
   canal of Nuck Q52.4
   canthus Q10.3
   capillary Q27.9
   cardiac Q24.9
      chambers Q20.9
         specified NEC Q20.8
      septal closure Q21.9
         specified NEC Q21.8
      valve NEC Q24.8
         pulmonary Q22.3
   cardiovascular system Q28.8
   carpus Q74.0
   caruncle, lacrimal Q10.6
   cascade stomach Q40.2
   cauda equina Q06.3
   cecum Q43.9
   cerebral Q04.9
      vessels Q28.3
   cervix Q51.9
   Chédiak-Higashi (-Steinbrinck)
      (congenital gigantism of
      peroxidase granules) E70.330
   cheek Q18.9
   chest wall Q67.8
      bones Q76.9
   chin Q18.9
   chordae tendineae Q24.8

Anomaly, anomalous *(continued)*
   choroid Q14.3
      plexus Q07.8
   chromosomes, chromosomal Q99.9
      D (1) —*see* condition,
         chromosome 13
      E (3) —*see* condition,
         chromosome 18
      G —*see* condition, chromosome 21
      sex
         female phenotype Q97.8
         gonadal dysgenesis (pure) Q99.1
         Klinefelter's Q98.4
         male phenotype Q98.9
         Turner's Q96.9
      specified NEC Q99.8
   cilia Q10.3
   circulatory system Q28.9
   clavicle Q74.0
   clitoris Q52.6
   coccyx Q76.49
   colon Q43.9
   common duct Q44.5
   communication
      coronary artery Q24.5
      left ventricle with right atrium
         Q21.0
      pulmonary venous Q26.4
         partial Q26.3
         total Q26.2
      renal artery with kidney Q27.2
   cornea (shape) Q13.4
   coronary artery or vein Q24.5
   cranium —*see* Anomaly, skull
   cricoid cartilage Q31.8
   cystic duct Q44.5
   dental
      alveolar —*see* Anomaly, alveolar
      arch relationship M26.20
         specified NEC M26.29
   dentofacial M26.9
      alveolar —*see* Anomaly, alveolar
      dental arch relationship M26.20
         specified NEC M26.29
      functional M26.50
         specified NEC M26.59
      jaw-cranial base relationship
         M26.10
         asymmetry M26.12
            maxillary M26.11
         specified type NEC M26.19
      jaw size M26.00
         macrogenia M26.05
         mandibular
            hyperplasia M26.03
            hypoplasia M26.04
         maxillary
            hyperplasia M26.01
            hypoplasia M26.02
         microgenia M26.06
         specified type NEC M26.09
      malocclusion M26.4
         dental arch relationship NEC
            M26.29
         jaw-cranial base relationship
            —*see* Anomaly, dentofacial,
            jaw-cranial base
            relationship
         jaw size —*see* Anomaly,
            dentofacial, jaw size
      specified type NEC M26.89
   temporomandibular joint
      M26.60 -
      adhesions M26.61 -
      ankylosis M26.61 -
      arthralgia M26.62 -
      articular disc M26.63 -
      specified type NEC M26.69

Anomaly, anomalous *(continued)*
   temporomandibular joint
      (continued)
      tooth position, fully erupted
         M26.30
         specified NEC M26.39
   dermatoglyphic Q82.8
   diaphragm (apertures) NEC Q79.1
   digestive organ(s) or tract Q45.9
      lower Q43.9
      upper Q40.9
   distance, interarch (excessive)
      (inadequate) M26.25
   distribution, coronary artery Q24.5
   ductus
      arteriosus Q25.0
      botalli Q25.0
   duodenum Q43.9
   dura (brain) Q04.9
      spinal cord Q06.9
   ear (external) Q17.9
      causing impairment of hearing
         Q16.9
      inner Q16.5
      middle (causing impairment of
         hearing) Q16.4
         ossicles Q16.3
   Ebstein's (heart) (tricuspid valve)
      Q22.5
   ectodermal Q82.9
   Eisenmenger's (ventricular septal
      defect) Q21.8
   ejaculatory duct Q55.4
   elbow Q74.0
   endocrine gland NEC Q89.2
   epididymis Q55.4
   epiglottis Q31.8
   esophagus Q39.9
   eustachian tube Q17.8
   eye Q15.9
      anterior segment Q13.9
         specified NEC Q13.89
      posterior segment Q14.9
         specified NEC Q14.8
      ptosis (eyelid) Q10.0
      specified NEC Q15.8
   eyebrow Q18.8
   eyelid Q10.3
      ptosis Q10.0
   face Q18.9
      bone(s) Q75.9
   fallopian tube Q50.6
   fascia Q79.9
   femur NEC Q74.2
   fibula NEC Q74.2
   finger Q74.0
   fixation, intestine Q43.3
   flexion (joint) NOS Q74.9
      hip or thigh Q65.89
   foot NEC Q74.2
      varus (congenital) Q66.3-
   foramen
      Botalli Q21.1
      ovale Q21.1
   forearm Q74.0
   forehead Q75.8
   form, teeth K00.2
   fovea centralis Q14.1
   frontal bone —*see* Anomaly, skull
   gallbladder (position) (shape) (size)
      Q44.1
   Gartner's duct Q52.4
   gastrointestinal tract Q45.9
   genitalia, genital organ(s)
      or system
      female Q52.9
         external Q52.70
         internal NOS Q52.9
      male Q55.9
         hydrocele P83.5
         specified NEC Q55.8

Anomaly, anomalous *(continued)*
genitourinary NEC
  female Q52.9
  male Q55.9
Gerbode Q21.0
glottis Q31.8
granulation or granulocyte, genetic
  (constitutional) (leukocyte)
  D72.0
gum Q38.6
gyri Q07.9
hair Q84.2
hand Q74.0
hard tissue formation in pulp K04.3
head —*see* Anomaly, skull
heart Q24.9
  auricle Q20.8
  bands or folds Q24.8
  fibroelastosis cordis I42.4
  obstructive NEC Q22.6
  patent ductus arteriosus (Botalli)
    Q25.0
  septum Q21.9
    auricular Q21.1
    interatrial Q21.1
    interventricular Q21.0
      with pulmonary stenosis or
        atresia, dextraposition of
        aorta and hypertrophy of
        right ventricle Q21.3
    specified NEC Q21.8
    ventricular Q21.0
      with pulmonary stenosis or
        atresia, dextraposition of
        aorta and hypertrophy of
        right ventricle Q21.3
  tetralogy of Fallot Q21.3
  valve NEC Q24.8
    aortic
      bicuspid valve Q23.1
      insufficiency Q23.1
      stenosis Q23.0
        subaortic Q24.4
    mitral
      insufficiency Q23.3
      stenosis Q23.2
    pulmonary Q22.3
      atresia Q22.0
      insufficiency Q22.2
      stenosis Q22.1
        infundibular Q24.3
        subvalvular Q24.3
    tricuspid
      atresia Q22.4
      stenosis Q22.4
  ventricle Q20.8
heel NEC Q74.2
Hegglin's D72.0
hemianencephaly Q00.0
hemicephaly Q00.0
hemicrania Q00.0
hepatic duct Q44.5
hip NEC Q74.2
hourglass stomach Q40.2
humerus Q74.0
hydatid of Morgagni
  female Q50.5
  male (epididymal) Q55.4
    testicular Q55.29
hymen Q52.4
hypersegmentation of neutrophils,
  hereditary D72.0
hypophyseal Q89.2
ileocecal (coil) (valve) Q43.9
ileum Q43.9
ilium NEC Q74.2
integument Q84.9
  specified NEC Q84.8
interarch distance (excessive)
  (inadequate) M26.25
intervertebral cartilage or disc Q76.49

Anomaly, anomalous *(continued)*
intestine (large) (small) Q43.9
  with anomalous adhesions,
    fixation or malrotation Q43.3
iris Q13.2
ischium NEC Q74.2
jaw —*see* Anomaly, dentofacial
  alveolar —*see* Anomaly, alveolar
jaw-cranial base relationship —*see*
  Anomaly, dentofacial, jaw-
  cranial base relationship
jejunum Q43.8
joint Q74.9
  specified NEC Q74.8
Jordan's D72.0
kidney(s) (calyx) (pelvis) Q63.9
  artery Q27.2
  specified NEC Q63.8
Klippel-Feil (brevicollis) Q76.1
knee Q74.1
labium (majus) (minus) Q52.70
labyrinth, membranous Q16.5
lacrimal apparatus or duct Q10.6
larynx, laryngeal (muscle) Q31.9
  web (bed) Q31.0
lens Q12.9
leukocytes, genetic D72.0
  granulation (constitutional)
    D72.0
lid (fold) Q10.3
ligament Q79.9
  broad Q50.6
  round Q52.8
limb Q74.9
  lower NEC Q74.2
    reduction deformity —*see*
      Defect, reduction, lower limb
  upper Q74.0
lip Q38.0
liver Q44.7
  duct Q44.5
lower limb NEC Q74.2
lumbosacral (joint) (region) Q76.49
  kyphosis —*see* Kyphosis,
    congenital
  lordosis —*see* Lordosis,
    congenital
lung (fissure) (lobe) Q33.9
mandible —*see* Anomaly,
  dentofacial
maxilla —*see* Anomaly, dentofacial
May (-Hegglin) D72.0
meatus urinarius NEC Q64.79
meningeal bands or folds Q07.9
  constriction of Q07.8
  spinal Q06.9
meninges Q07.9
  cerebral Q04.8
  spinal Q06.9
meningocele Q05.9
mesentery Q45.9
metacarpus Q74.0
metatarsus NEC Q74.2
middle ear Q16.4
  ossicles Q16.3
mitral (leaflets) (valve) Q23.9
  insufficiency Q23.3
  specified NEC Q23.8
  stenosis Q23.2
mouth Q38.6
Müllerian —*see also* Anomaly,
  by site
  uterus NEC Q51.818
multiple NEC Q89.7
muscle Q79.9
  eyelid Q10.3
musculoskeletal system, except
  limbs Q79.9
myocardium Q24.8
nail Q84.6
narrowness, eyelid Q10.3

Anomaly, anomalous *(continued)*
nasal sinus (wall) Q30.8
neck (any part) Q18.9
nerve Q07.9
  acoustic Q07.8
  optic Q07.8
nervous system (central) Q07.9
nipple Q83.9
nose, nasal (bones) (cartilage)
  (septum) (sinus) Q30.9
  specified NEC Q30.8
ocular muscle Q15.8
omphalomesenteric duct Q43.0
opening, pulmonary veins Q26.4
optic
  disc Q14.2
  nerve Q07.8
opticociliary vessels Q13.2
orbit (eye) Q10.7
organ Q89.9
  of Corti Q16.5
origin
  artery
    innominate Q25.48
    pulmonary Q25.79
    renal Q27.2
    subclavian Q25.48
osseous meatus (ear) Q16.1
ovary Q50.39
oviduct Q50.6
palate (hard) (soft) NEC Q38.5
pancreas or pancreatic duct Q45.3
papillary muscles Q24.8
parathyroid gland Q89.2
paraurethral ducts Q64.79
parotid (gland) Q38.4
patella Q74.1
Pelger-Huët (hereditary
  hyposegmentation) D72.0
pelvic girdle NEC Q74.2
pelvis (bony) NEC Q74.2
  rachitic E64.3
penis (glans) Q55.69
pericardium Q24.8
peripheral vascular system Q27.9
Peter's Q13.4
pharynx Q38.8
pigmentation L81.9
  congenital Q82.8
pituitary (gland) Q89.2
pleural (folds) Q34.0
portal vein Q26.5
  connection Q26.5
position, tooth, teeth, fully erupted
  M26.30
  specified NEC M26.39
precerebral vessel Q28.1
prepuce Q55.69
prostate Q55.4
pulmonary Q33.9
  artery NEC Q25.79
  valve Q22.3
    atresia Q22.0
    insufficiency Q22.2
    specified type NEC Q22.3
    stenosis Q22.1
      infundibular Q24.3
      subvalvular Q24.3
  venous connection Q26.4
    partial Q26.3
    total Q26.2
pupil Q13.2
  function H57.00
    anisocoria H57.02
    Argyll Robertson pupil
      H57.01
    miosis H57.03
    mydriasis H57.04
    specified type NEC H57.09
    tonic pupil H57.05-
pylorus Q40.3

Anomaly, anomalous *(continued)*
radius Q74.0
rectum Q43.9
reduction (extremity) (limb)
  femur (longitudinal) —*see*
    Defect, reduction, lower limb,
    longitudinal, femur
  fibula (longitudinal) —*see*
    Defect, reduction, lower limb,
    longitudinal, fibula
  lower limb —*see* Defect,
    reduction, lower limb
  radius (longitudinal) —*see*
    Defect, reduction, upper limb,
    longitudinal, radius
  tibia (longitudinal) —*see*
    Defect, reduction, lower limb,
    longitudinal, tibia
  ulna (longitudinal) —*see*
    Defect, reduction, upper limb,
    longitudinal, ulna
  upper limb —*see* Defect,
    reduction, upper limb
refraction —*see* Disorder, refraction
renal Q63.9
  artery Q27.2
  pelvis Q63.9
    specified NEC Q63.8
respiratory system Q34.9
  specified NEC Q34.8
retina Q14.1
rib Q76.6
  cervical Q76.5
Rieger's Q13.81
rotation —*see* Malrotation
  hip or thigh Q65.89
round ligament Q52.8
sacroiliac (joint) NEC Q74.2
sacrum NEC Q76.49
  kyphosis —*see* Kyphosis,
    congenital
  lordosis —*see* Lordosis,
    congenital
saddle nose, syphilitic A50.57
salivary duct or gland Q38.4
scapula Q74.0
scrotum —*see* Malformation, testis
  and scrotum
sebaceous gland Q82.9
seminal vesicles Q55.4
sense organs NEC Q07.8
sex chromosomes NEC —*see also*
  Anomaly, chromosomes
  female phenotype Q97.8
  male phenotype Q98.9
shoulder (girdle) (joint) Q74.0
sigmoid (flexure) Q43.9
simian crease Q82.8
sinus of Valsalva Q25.49
skeleton generalized Q78.9
skin (appendage) Q82.9
skull Q75.9
  with
    anencephaly Q00.0
    encephalocele —*see*
      Encephalocele
    hydrocephalus Q03.9
      with spina bifida —*see*
        Spina bifida, by site, with
        hydrocephalus
    microcephaly Q02
specified organ or site NEC Q89.8
spermatic cord Q55.4
spine, spinal NEC Q76.49
  column NEC Q76.49
    kyphosis —*see* Kyphosis,
      congenital
    lordosis —*see* Lordosis,
      congenital
  cord Q06.9
  nerve root Q07.8

Anomaly, anomalous (*continued*)
spleen Q89.09
    agenesis Q89.01
stenonian duct Q38.4
sternum NEC Q76.7
stomach Q40.3
submaxillary gland Q38.4
tarsus NEC Q74.2
tendon Q79.9
testis —*see* Malformation, testis
    and scrotum
thigh NEC Q74.2
thorax (wall) Q67.8
    bony Q76.9
throat Q38.8
thumb Q74.0
thymus gland Q89.2
thyroid (gland) Q89.2
    cartilage Q31.8
tibia NEC Q74.2
    saber A50.56
toe Q74.2
tongue Q38.3
tooth, teeth K00.9
    eruption K00.6
    position, fully erupted M26.30
    spacing, fully erupted M26.30
trachea (cartilage) Q32.1
tragus Q17.9
tricuspid (leaflet) (valve) Q22.9
    atresia or stenosis Q22.4
    Ebstein's Q22.5
Uhl's (hypoplasia of myocardium,
    right ventricle) Q24.8
ulna Q74.0
umbilical artery Q27.0
union
    cricoid cartilage and thyroid
        cartilage Q31.8
    thyroid cartilage and hyoid bone
        Q31.8
    trachea with larynx Q31.8
upper limb Q74.0
urachus Q64.4
ureter Q62.8
    obstructive NEC Q62.39
        cecoureterocele Q62.32
        orthotopic ureterocele
            Q62.31
urethra Q64.70
    absence Q64.5
    double Q64.74
    fistula to rectum Q64.73
    obstructive Q64.39
        stricture Q64.32
    prolapse Q64.71
    specified type NEC Q64.79
urinary tract Q64.9
uterus Q51.9
    with only one functioning horn
        Q51.4
uvula Q38.5
vagina Q52.4
valleculae Q31.8
valve (heart) NEC Q24.8
    coronary sinus Q24.5
    inferior vena cava Q24.8
    pulmonary Q22.3
    sinus coronario Q24.5
    venae cavae inferioris Q24.8
vas deferens Q55.4
vascular Q27.9
    brain Q28.3
    ring Q25.45
vein(s) (peripheral) Q27.9
    brain Q28.3
    cerebral Q28.3
    coronary Q24.5
    developmental Q28.3
    great Q26.9
        specified NEC Q26.8

Anomaly, anomalous (*continued*)
vena cava (inferior) (superior)
    Q26.9
venous —*see* Anomaly, vein(s)
venous return Q26.8
ventricular
    bands or folds Q24.8
    septa Q21.0
vertebra Q76.49
    kyphosis —*see* Kyphosis,
        congenital
    lordosis —*see* Lordosis,
        congenital
vesicourethral orifice Q64.79
vessel(s) Q27.9
    optic papilla Q14.2
    precerebral Q28.1
vitelline duct Q43.0
vitreous body or humor Q14.0
vulva Q52.70
wrist (joint) Q74.0

Anomia R48.8

Anonychia (congenital) Q84.3
acquired L60.8

Anophthalmos, anophthalmus
(congenital) (globe) Q11.1
acquired Z90.01

Anopia, anopsia H53.46-
quadrant H53.46-

Anorchia, anorchism, anorchidism
Q55.0

Anorexia R63.0
hysterical F44.89
nervosa F50.00
    atypical F50.9
    binge-eating type F50.2
        with purging F50.02
    restricting type F50.01

Anorgasmy, psychogenic (female)
F52.31
male F52.32

Anosmia R43.0
hysterical F44.6
postinfectional J39.8

Anosognosia R41.89

Anosteoplasia Q78.9

Anovulatory cycle N97.0

Anoxemia R09.02
newborn P84

Anoxia (pathological) R09.02
altitude T70.29
cerebral G93.1
    complicating
        anesthesia (general) (local) or
            other sedation T88.59
        in labor and delivery O74.3
        in pregnancy O29.21-
            postpartum, puerperal
            O89.2
        delivery (cesarean)
            (instrumental) O75.4
    during a procedure G97.81
    newborn P84
    resulting from a procedure G97.82
due to
    drowning T75.1
    high altitude T70.29
heart —*see* Insufficiency, coronary
intrauterine P84
myocardial —*see* Insufficiency,
    coronary
newborn P84
spinal cord G95.11
systemic (by suffocation) (low
    content in atmosphere) —*see*
    Asphyxia, traumatic

Anteflexion —*see* Anteversion

Antenatal
care (normal pregnancy) Z34.90
screening (encounter for) of mother
    (*see also* Encounter, antenatal
    screening) Z36.9

Antepartum —*see* condition

Anterior —*see* condition

Antero-occlusion M26.220

Anteversion
cervix —*see* Anteversion, uterus
femur (neck), congenital Q65.89
uterus, uterine (cervix)
    (postinfectional) (postpartal, old)
    N85.4
    congenital Q51.818
    in pregnancy or childbirth —*see*
        Pregnancy, complicated by

Anthophobia F40.228

Anthracosilicosis J60

Anthracosis (lung) (occupational)
J60
lingua K14.3

Anthrax A22.9
with pneumonia A22.1
cerebral A22.8
colitis A22.2
cutaneous A22.0
gastrointestinal A22.2
inhalation A22.1
intestinal A22.2
meningitis A22.8
pulmonary A22.1
respiratory A22.1
sepsis A22.7
specified manifestation NEC A22.8

Anthropoid pelvis Q74.2
with disproportion (fetopelvic) O33.0

Anthropophobia F40.10
generalized F40.11

Antibodies, maternal (blood group)
—*see* Isoimmunization, affecting
management of pregnancy
anti-D —*see* Isoimmunization,
    affecting management of
    pregnancy, Rh
newborn P55.0

Antibody
anticardiolipin R76.0
    with
        hemorrhagic disorder D68.312
        hypercoagulable state D68.61
antiphosphatidylglycerol R76.0
    with
        hemorrhagic disorder D68.312
        hypercoagulable state D68.61
antiphosphatidylinositol R76.0
    with
        hemorrhagic disorder D68.312
        hypercoagulable state D68.61
antiphosphatidylserine R76.0
    with
        hemorrhagic disorder D68.312
        hypercoagulable state D68.61
antiphospholipid R76.0
    with
        hemorrhagic disorder D68.312
        hypercoagulable state D68.61

Anticardiolipin syndrome D68.61

Anticoagulant, circulating (intrinsic)
(*see also* Disorder, hemorrhagic)
D68.318
drug-induced (extrinsic) (*see also*
    Disorder, hemorrhagic) D68.32
iatrogenic D68.32

Antidiuretic hormone syndrome
E22.2

Antimonial cholera —*see* Poisoning,
antimony

Antiphospholipid
antibody
    with hemorrhagic disorder
        D68.312
    syndrome D68.61

Antisocial personality F60.2

Antithrombinemia —*see* Circulating
anticoagulants

Antithromboplastinemia D68.318

Antithromboplastinogenemia
D68.318

Antitoxin complication or reaction
—*see* Complications, vaccination

Antlophobia F40.228

Antritis J32.0
maxilla J32.0
    acute J01.00
        recurrent J01.01
stomach K29.60
    with bleeding K29.61

Antrum, antral —*see* condition

Anuria R34
calculous (impacted) (recurrent) (*see
    also* Calculus, urinary) N20.9
following
    abortion —*see* Abortion by type
        complicated by, renal failure
    ectopic or molar pregnancy O08.4
newborn P96.0
postprocedural N99.0
postrenal N13.8
traumatic (following crushing)
    T79.5

Anus, anal —*see* condition

Anusitis K62.89

Anxiety F41.9
depression F41.8
episodic paroxysmal F41.0
generalized F41.1
hysteria F41.8
neurosis F41.1
panic type F41.0
reaction F41.1
separation, abnormal (of childhood)
    F93.0
specified NEC F41.8
state F41.1

Aorta, aortic —*see* condition

Aortectasia —*see* Ectasia, aorta
with aneurysm —*see* Aneurysm,
    aorta

Aortitis (nonsyphilitic) (calcific) I77.6
arteriosclerotic I70.0
Doehle-Heller A52.02
luetic A52.02
rheumatic —*see* Endocarditis,
    acute, rheumatic
specific (syphilitic) A52.02
syphilitic A52.02
    congenital A50.54 *[179.1]*

Apathetic thyroid storm —*see*
Thyrotoxicosis

Apathy R45.3

Apeirophobia F40.228

Apepsia K30
psychogenic F45.8

Aperistalsis, esophagus K22.0

Apertognathia M26.29

Apert's syndrome Q87.0

Aphagia R13.0
psychogenic F50.9

Aphakia (acquired) (postoperative) H27.0-
congenital Q12.3

Aphasia (amnestic) (global) (nominal) (semantic) (syntactic) R47.01
acquired, with epilepsy (Landau-Kleffner syndrome) —see Epilepsy, specified NEC
auditory (developmental) F80.2
developmental (receptive type) F80.2
expressive type F80.1
Wernicke's F80.2
following
cerebrovascular disease I69.920
cerebral infarction I69.320
intracerebral hemorrhage I69.120
nontraumatic intracranial hemorrhage NEC I69.220
specified disease NEC I69.820
subarachnoid hemorrhage I69.020
primary progressive G31.01 *[F02.80]*
with behavioral disturbance G31.01 *[F02.81]*
progressive isolated G31.01 *[F02.80]*
with behavioral disturbance G31.01 *[F02.81]*
sensory F80.2
syphilis, tertiary A52.19
Wernicke's (developmental) F80.2

Aphonia (organic) R49.1
hysterical F44.4
psychogenic F44.4

Aphthae, aphthous —see also condition
Bednar's K12.0
cachectic K14.0
epizootic B08.8
fever B08.8
oral (recurrent) K12.0
stomatitis (major) (minor) K12.0
thrush B37.0
ulcer (oral) (recurrent) K12.0
genital organ(s) NEC
female N76.6
male N50.89
larynx J38.7

Apical —see condition

Apiphobia F40.218

Aplasia —see also Agenesis
abdominal muscle syndrome Q79.4
alveolar process (acquired) —see Anomaly, alveolar
congenital Q38.6
aorta (congenital) Q25.41
axialis extracorticalis (congenita) E75.29
bone marrow (myeloid) D61.9
congenital D61.01
brain Q00.0
part of Q04.3
bronchus Q32.4
cementum K00.4
cerebellum Q04.3
cervix (congenital) Q51.5
congenital pure red cell D61.01
corpus callosum Q04.0
cutis congenita Q84.8
erythrocyte congenital D61.01
extracortical axial E75.29
eye Q11.1
fovea centralis (congenital) Q14.1
gallbladder, congenital Q44.0
iris Q13.1
labyrinth, membranous Q16.5

Aplasia *(continued)*
limb (congenital) Q73.8
lower —see Defect, reduction, lower limb
upper —see Agenesis, arm
lung, congenital (bilateral) (unilateral) Q33.3
pancreas Q45.0
parathyroid-thymic D82.1
Pelizaeus-Merzbacher E75.29
penis Q55.5
prostate Q55.4
red cell (with thymoma) D60.9
acquired D60.9
due to drugs D60.9
adult D60.9
chronic D60.0
congenital D61.01
constitutional D61.01
due to drugs D60.9
hereditary D61.01
of infants D61.01
primary D61.01
pure D61.01
due to drugs D60.9
specified type NEC D60.8
transient D60.1
round ligament Q52.8
skin Q84.8
spermatic cord Q55.4
spleen Q89.01
testicle Q55.0
thymic, with immunodeficiency D82.1
thyroid (congenital) (with myxedema) E03.1
uterus Q51.0
ventral horn cell Q06.1

Apnea, apneic (of) (spells) R06.81
newborn NEC P28.4
obstructive P28.4
sleep (central) (obstructive) (primary) P28.3
prematurity P28.4
sleep G47.30
central (primary) G47.31
idiopathic G47.31
in conditions classified elsewhere G47.37
obstructive (adult) (pediatric) G47.33
hypopnea G47.33
primary central G47.31
specified NEC G47.39

Apneumatosis, newborn P28.0

Apocrine metaplasia (breast) —see Dysplasia, mammary, specified type NEC

Apophysitis (bone) —see also Osteochondropathy
calcaneus M92.8
juvenile M92.9

Apoplectiform convulsions (cerebral ischemia) I67.82

Apoplexia, apoplexy, apoplectic
adrenal A39.1
heart (auricle) (ventricle) —see Infarct, myocardium
heat T67.01
hemorrhagic (stroke) —see Hemorrhage, intracranial
meninges, hemorrhagic —see Hemorrhage, intracranial, subarachnoid
uremic N18.9 *[I68.8]*

Appearance
bizarre R46.1
specified NEC R46.89
very low level of personal hygiene R46.0

Appendage
epididymal (organ of Morgagni) Q55.4
intestine (epiploic) Q43.8
preauricular Q17.0
testicular (organ of Morgagni) Q55.29

Appendicitis (pneumococcal) (retrocecal) K37
with
gangrene K35.891
perforation NOS K35.32
peritoneal abscess K35.33
peritonitis NEC K35.33
generalized (with perforation or rupture) K35.20
with abscess K35.21
localized K35.30
with
gangrene K35.31
perforation K35.32
and abscess K35.33
rupture (with localized peritonitis) K35.32
acute (catarrhal) (fulminating) (gangrenous) (obstructive) (retrocecal) (suppurative) K35.80
with
gangrene K35.891
peritoneal abscess K35.33
peritonitis NEC K35.33
generalized (with perforation or rupture) K35.20
with abscess K35.21
localized K35.30
with
gangrene K35.31
perforation K35.32
and abscess K35.33
specified NEC K35.890
with gangrene K35.891
amebic A06.89
chronic (recurrent) K36
exacerbation —see Appendicitis, acute
gangrenous —see Appendicitis, acute
healed (obliterative) K36
interval K36
neurogenic K36
obstructive K36
recurrent K36
relapsing K36
ruptured NOS (with localized peritonitis) K35.32
subacute (adhesive) K36
subsiding K36
suppurative —see Appendicitis, acute
tuberculous A18.32

Appendicopathia oxyurica B80

Appendix, appendicular —see also condition
epididymis Q55.4
Morgagni
female Q50.5
male (epididymal) Q55.4
testicular Q55.29
testis Q55.29

Appetite
depraved —see Pica
excessive R63.2
lack or loss (see also Anorexia) R63.0
nonorganic origin F50.89
psychogenic F50.89
perverted (hysterical) —see Pica

Apple peel syndrome Q41.1

Apprehension state F41.1

Apprehensiveness, abnormal F41.9

Approximal wear K03.0

Apraxia (classic) (ideational) (ideokinetic) (ideomotor) (motor) (verbal) R48.2
following
cerebrovascular disease I69.990
cerebral infarction I69.390
intracerebral hemorrhage I69.190
nontraumatic intracranial hemorrhage NEC I69.290
specified disease NEC I69.890
subarachnoid hemorrhage I69.090
oculomotor, congenital H51.8

Aptyalism K11.7

Apudoma —see Neoplasm, uncertain behavior, by site

Aqueous misdirection H40.83-

Arabicum elephantiasis —see Infestation, filarial

Arachnitis —see Meningitis

Arachnodactyly —see Syndrome, Marfan's

Arachnoiditis (acute) (adhesive) (basal) (brain) (cerebrospinal) —see Meningitis

Arachnophobia F40.210

Arboencephalitis, Australian A83.4

Arborization block (heart) I45.5

ARC (AIDS-related complex) B20

Arch
aortic Q25.49
bovine Q25.49

Arches —see condition

Arcuate uterus Q51.810

Arcuatus uterus Q51.810

Arcus (cornea) **senilis** —see Degeneration, cornea, senile

Arc-welder's lung J63.4

Areflexia R29.2

Areola —see condition

Argentaffinoma —see also Neoplasm, uncertain behavior, by site
malignant —see Neoplasm, malignant, by site
syndrome E34.0

Argininemia E72.21

Arginosuccinic aciduria E72.22

Argyll Robertson phenomenon, pupil or syndrome (syphilitic) A52.19
atypical H57.09
nonsyphilitic H57.09

Argyria, argyriasis
conjunctival H11.13-
from drug or medicament —see Table of Drugs and Chemicals, by substance

Argyrosis, conjunctival H11.13-

Arhinencephaly Q04.1

Ariboflavinosis E53.0

Arm —see condition

Arnold-Chiari disease, obstruction or syndrome (type II) Q07.00
with
hydrocephalus Q07.02
with spina bifida Q07.03

Arnold-Chiari disease, obstruction or syndrome *(continued)*
with *(continued)*
spina bifida Q07.01
with hydrocephalus Q07.03
type III —*see* Encephalocele
type IV Q04.8

Aromatic amino-acid metabolism disorder E70.9
specified NEC E70.89

Arousals, confusional G47.51

Arrest, arrested
cardiac I46.9
complicating
abortion —*see* Abortion, by type, complicated by, cardiac arrest
anesthesia (general) (local) or other sedation —*see* Table of Drugs and Chemicals, by drug,
in labor and delivery O74.2
in pregnancy O29.11-
postpartum, puerperal O89.1
delivery (cesarean) (instrumental) O75.4
due to
cardiac condition I46.2
specified condition NEC I46.8
intraoperative I97.71-
newborn P29.81
personal history, successfully resuscitated Z86.74
postprocedural I97.12-
obstetric procedure O75.4
cardiorespiratory —*see* Arrest, cardiac
circulatory —*see* Arrest, cardiac
deep transverse O64.0
development or growth
bone —*see* Disorder, bone, development or growth
child R62.50
tracheal rings Q32.1
epiphyseal
complete
femur M89.15-
humerus M89.12-
tibia M89.16-
ulna M89.13-
forearm M89.13-
specified NEC M89.13-
ulna —*see* Arrest, epiphyseal, by type, ulna
lower leg M89.16-
specified NEC M89.168
tibia —*see* Arrest, epiphyseal, by type, tibia
partial
femur M89.15-
humerus M89.12-
tibia M89.16-
ulna M89.13-
specified NEC M89.18
granulopoiesis —*see* Agranulocytosis
growth plate —*see* Arrest, epiphyseal
heart —*see* Arrest, cardiac
legal, anxiety concerning Z65.3
physeal —*see* Arrest, epiphyseal
respiratory R09.2
newborn P28.81
sinus I45.5
spermatogenesis (complete) —*see* Azoospermia
incomplete —*see* Oligospermia
transverse (deep) O64.0

Arrhenoblastoma
benign
specified site —*see* Neoplasm, benign, by site
unspecified site
female D27.9
male D29.20
malignant
specified site —*see* Neoplasm, malignant, by site
unspecified site
female C56.9
male C62.90
specified site —*see* Neoplasm, uncertain behavior, by site
unspecified site
female D39.10
male D40.10

Arrhythmia (auricle)(cardiac)(juvenile) (nodal) (reflex)(supraventricular) (transitory)(ventricle) I49.9
block I45.9
extrasystolic I49.49
newborn
bradycardia P29.12
occurring before birth P03.819
before onset of labor P03.810
during labor P03.811
tachycardia P29.11
psychogenic F45.8
sinus I49.8
specified NEC I49.8
vagal R55
ventricular re-entry I47.0

Arrillaga-Ayerza syndrome (pulmonary sclerosis with pulmonary hypertension) I27.0

Arsenical pigmentation L81.8
from drug or medicament —*see* Table of Drugs and Chemicals

Arsenism —*see* Poisoning, arsenic

Arterial —*see* condition

Arteriofibrosis — *see* Arteriosclerosis

Arteriolar sclerosis —*see* Arteriosclerosis

Arteriolith —*see* Arteriosclerosis

Arteriolitis I77.6
necrotizing, kidney I77.5
renal —*see* Hypertension, kidney

Arteriolosclerosis —*see* Arteriosclerosis

Arterionephrosclerosis —*see* Hypertension, kidney

Arteriopathy I77.9
cerebral autosomal dominant, with subcortical infarcts and leukoencephalopathy (CADASIL) I67.850

Arteriosclerosis, arteriosclerotic (diffuse) (obliterans) (of) (senile) (with calcification) I70.90
with
chronic limb-threatening ischemia —*see* Arteriosclerosis, with critical limb ischemia
critical limb ischemia
bypass graft I70.329
autologous vein graft I70.429
leg I70.429
with
gangrene (and intermittent claudication, rest pain, and ulcer) I70.469

Arteriosclerosis, arteriosclerotic
(continued)
with *(continued)*
critical limb ischemia *(continued)*
bypass graft *(continued)*
autologous vein graft *(continued)*
leg *(continued)*
with *(continued)*
rest pain (and intermittent claudication) I70.429
bilateral I70.423
with
gangrene (and intermittent claudication, rest pain, and ulcer) I70.463
rest pain (and intermittent claudication) I70.423
left I70.422
with
gangrene (and intermittent claudication, rest pain, and ulcer) I70.462
rest pain (and intermittent claudication) I70.422
ulceration (and intermittent claudication and rest pain) I70.449
ankle I70.443
calf I70.442
foot site NEC I70.445
heel I70.444
lower leg NEC I70.448
mid foot I70.444
thigh I70.441
right I70.421
with
gangrene (and intermittent claudication, rest pain, and ulcer) I70.461
rest pain (and intermittent claudication) I70.421
ulceration (and intermittent claudication and rest pain) I70.439
ankle I70.433
calf I70.432
foot site NEC I70.435
heel I70.434
lower leg NEC I70.438
mid foot I70.434
thigh I70.431
leg I70.329
with

Arteriosclerosis, arteriosclerotic
(continued)
with *(continued)*
critical limb ischemia *(continued)*
bypass graft *(continued)*
leg *(continued)*
with *(continued)*
gangrene (and intermittent claudication, rest pain, and ulcer) I70.369
rest pain (and intermittent claudication) I70.329
bilateral I70.323
with
gangrene (and intermittent claudication, rest pain, and ulcer) I70.363
rest pain (and intermittent claudication) I70.323
left I70.322
with
gangrene (and intermittent claudication, rest pain, and ulcer) I70.362
rest pain (and intermittent claudication) I70.322
ulceration (and intermittent claudication and rest pain) I70.349
ankle I70.343
calf I70.342
foot site NEC I70.345
heel I70.344
lower leg NEC I70.348
mid foot I70.344
thigh I70.341
right I70.321
with
gangrene (and intermittent claudication, rest pain, and ulcer) I70.361
rest pain (and intermittent claudication) I70.321
ulceration (and intermittent claudication and rest pain) I70.339
ankle I70.333
calf I70.332
foot site NEC I70.335
heel I70.334
lower leg NEC I70.338
mid foot I70.334
thigh I70.331
nonautologous biological graft I70.529
leg I70.529
with

Arteriosclerosis, arteriosclerotic
(continued)
  with *(continued)*
    critical limb ischemia *(continued)*
      bypass graft *(continued)*
        nonautologous biological
          graft *(continued)*
          leg *(continued)*
            with *(continued)*
              gangrene (and
                intermittent
                claudication, rest
                pain, and ulcer)
                I70.569
              rest pain (and
                intermittent
                claudication)
                I70.529
            bilateral I70.523
              with
                gangrene (and
                  intermittent
                  claudication,
                  rest pain, and
                  ulcer) I70.563
                rest pain (and
                  intermittent
                  claudication)
                  I70.523
            left I70.522
              with
                gangrene (and
                  intermittent
                  claudication,
                  rest pain, and
                  ulcer) I70.562
                rest pain (and
                  intermittent
                  claudication)
                  I70.522
              ulceration (and
                intermittent
                claudication
                and rest pain)
                I70.549
                ankle I70.543
                calf I70.542
                foot site NEC
                  I70.545
                heel I70.544
                lower leg NEC
                  I70.548
                mid foot
                  I70.544
                thigh I70.541
            right I70.521
              with
                gangrene (and
                  intermittent
                  claudication,
                  rest pain, and
                  ulcer) I70.561
                rest pain (and
                  intermittent
                  claudication)
                  I70.521
              ulceration (and
                intermittent
                claudication
                and rest pain)
                I70.539
                ankle I70.533
                calf I70.532
                foot site NEC
                  I70.535
                heel I70.534
                lower leg NEC
                  I70.538
                mid foot
                  I70.534
                thigh I70.531

Arteriosclerosis, arteriosclerotic
(continued)
  with *(continued)*
    critical limb ischemia
      (continued)
      bypass graft *(continued)*
        nonbiological graft I70.629
        leg I70.629
          with
            gangrene (and
              intermittent
              claudication, rest
              pain, and ulcer)
              I70.669
            rest pain (and
              intermittent
              claudication)
              I70.629
          bilateral I70.623
            with
              gangrene (and
                intermittent
                claudication,
                rest pain, and
                ulcer) I70.663
              rest pain (and
                intermittent
                claudication)
                I70.623
          left I70.622
            with
              gangrene (and
                intermittent
                claudication,
                rest pain, and
                ulcer) I70.662
              rest pain (and
                intermittent
                claudication)
                I70.622
              ulceration (and
                intermittent
                claudication
                and rest pain)
                I70.649
              ankle I70.643
              calf I70.642
              foot site NEC
                I70.645
              heel I70.644
              lower leg NEC
                I70.648
              mid foot
                I70.644
              thigh I70.641
          right I70.621
            with
              gangrene (and
                intermittent
                claudication,
                rest pain, and
                ulcer) I70.661
              rest pain (and
                intermittent
                claudication)
                I70.621
              ulceration (and
                intermittent
                claudication
                and rest pain)
                I70.639
              ankle I70.633
              calf I70.632
              foot site NEC
                I70.635
              heel I70.634
              lower leg NEC
                I70.638
              mid foot
                I70.634
              thigh I70.631

Arteriosclerosis, arteriosclerotic
(continued)
  with *(continued)*
    critical limb ischemia
      (continued)
      bypass graft *(continued)*
        specified graft NEC I70.729
        leg I70.729
          with
            gangrene (and
              intermittent
              claudication, rest
              pain, and ulcer)
              I70.769
            rest pain (and
              intermittent
              claudication)
              I70.729
          bilateral I70.723
            with
              gangrene (and
                intermittent
                claudication,
                rest pain, and
                ulcer) I70.763
              rest pain (and
                intermittent
                claudication)
                I70.723
          left I70.722
            with
              gangrene (and
                intermittent
                claudication,
                rest pain, and
                ulcer) I70.762
              rest pain (and
                intermittent
                claudication)
                I70.722
              ulceration (and
                intermittent
                claudication
                and rest pain)
                I70.749
              ankle I70.743
              calf I70.742
              foot site NEC
                I70.745
              heel I70.744
              lower leg NEC
                I70.748
              mid foot
                I70.744
              thigh I70.741
          right I70.721
            with
              gangrene (and
                intermittent
                claudication,
                rest pain, and
                ulcer) I70.761
              rest pain (and
                intermittent
                claudication)
                I70.721
              ulceration (and
                intermittent
                claudication
                and rest pain)
                I70.739
              ankle I70.733
              calf I70.732
              foot site NEC
                I70.735
              heel I70.734
              lower leg NEC
                I70.738
              mid foot
                I70.734
              thigh I70.731

Arteriosclerosis, arteriosclerotic
(continued)
  with *(continued)*
    critical limb ischemia *(continued)*
      leg I70.229
        with
          gangrene (and
            intermittent
            claudication, rest
            pain, and ulcer)
            I70.269
          rest pain (and
            intermittent
            claudication) I70.229
        bilateral I70.223
          with
            gangrene (and
              intermittent
              claudication, rest
              pain, and ulcer)
              I70.263
            rest pain (and
              intermittent
              claudication)
              I70.223
        left I70.222
          with
            gangrene (and
              intermittent
              claudication, rest
              pain, and ulcer)
              I70.262
            rest pain (and
              intermittent
              claudication)
              I70.222
            ulceration (and
              intermittent
              claudication and
              rest pain) I70.249
              ankle I70.243
              calf I70.242
              foot site NEC
                I70.245
              heel I70.244
              lower leg NEC
                I70.248
              mid foot I70.244
              thigh I70.241
        right I70.221
          with
            gangrene (and
              intermittent
              claudication, rest
              pain, and ulcer)
              I70.261
            rest pain (and
              intermittent
              claudication)
              I70.221
            ulceration (and
              intermittent
              claudication and
              rest pain) I70.239
              ankle I70.233
              calf I70.232
              foot site NEC
                I70.235
              heel I70.234
              lower leg NEC
                I70.238
              mid foot I70.234
              thigh I70.231
    aorta I70.0
    arteries of extremities —*see*
      Arteriosclerosis, extremities
    with
      chronic limb-threatening
        ischemia —*see*
        Arteriosclerosis, with
        critical limb ischemia

Arteriosclerosis, arteriosclerotic
(continued)
arteries of extremities
  (continued)
    with *(continued)*
      critical limb ischemia —*see*
        Arteriosclerosis, with
        clinical limb ischemia
  brain I67.2
  bypass graft
    with
      chronic limb-threatening
        ischemia —*see*
        Arteriosclerosis, with
        critical limb ischemia
      critical limb ischemia —*see*
        Arteriosclerosis, with
        clinical limb ischemia
  coronary —*see* Arteriosclerosis,
    coronary, bypass graft
  extremities —*see* Arteriosclerosis,
    extremities, bypass graft
  cardiac —*see* Disease, heart,
    ischemic, atherosclerotic
  cardiopathy —*see* Disease, heart,
    ischemic, atherosclerotic
  cardiorenal —*see* Hypertension,
    cardiorenal
  cardiovascular —*see* Disease,
    heart, ischemic, atherosclerotic
  carotid (*see also* Occlusion, artery,
    carotid) I65.2-
  central nervous system I67.2
  cerebral I67.2
  cerebrovascular I67.2
  coronary (artery) I25.10
    due to
      calcified coronary lesion
        (severely) I25.84
      lipid rich plaque I25.83
    bypass graft I25.810
      with
        angina pectoris I25.709
          with documented spasm
            I25.701
          specified type NEC
            I25.708
          unstable I25.700
        ischemic chest pain
          I25.709
      autologous artery I25.810
        with
          angina pectoris I25.729
            with documented
              spasm I25.721
            specified type I25.728
            unstable I25.720
          ischemic chest pain
            I25.729
      autologous vein I25.810
        with
          angina pectoris I25.719
            with documented
              spasm I25.711
            specified type I25.718
            unstable I25.710
          ischemic chest pain
            I25.719
      nonautologous biological
        I25.810
        with
          angina pectoris I25.739
            with documented
              spasm I25.731
            specified type I25.738
            unstable I25.730
          ischemic chest pain
            I25.739
      specified type NEC I25.810
        with
          angina pectoris I25.799

Arteriosclerosis, arteriosclerotic
(continued)
coronary *(continued)*
  bypass graft *(continued)*
    specified type NEC *(continued)*
      with *(continued)*
        angina pectoris *(continued)*
          with documented
            spasm I25.791
          specified type I25.798
          unstable I25.790
        ischemic chest pain
          I25.799
  native vessel
    with
      angina pectoris I25.119
        with documented spasm
          I25.111
        specified type NEC I25.118
        unstable I25.110
      ischemic chest pain I25.119
  transplanted heart I25.811
    bypass graft I25.812
      with
        angina pectoris I25.769
          with documented
            spasm I25.761
          specified type I25.768
          unstable I25.760
        ischemic chest pain I25.769
    native coronary artery I25.811
      with
        angina pectoris I25.759
          with documented
            spasm I25.751
          specified type I25.758
          unstable I25.750
        ischemic chest pain I25.759
extremities (native arteries) I70.209
  with
    chronic limb-threatening
      ischemia —*see*
      Arteriosclerosis, with
      critical limb ischemia
    critical limb ischemia —*see*
      Arteriosclerosis, with
      clinical limb ischemia
  bypass graft I70.309
    with
      chronic limb-threatening
        ischemia —*see*
        Arteriosclerosis, with
        critical limb ischemia
      critical limb ischemia —*see*
        Arteriosclerosis, with
        clinical limb ischemia
    autologous vein graft I70.409
      leg I70.409
        with
          gangrene (and
            intermittent
            claudication, rest pain
            and ulcer) I70.469
          intermittent
            claudication I70.419
          rest pain (and
            intermittent
            claudication) I70.429
        bilateral I70.403
          with
            gangrene (and
              intermittent
              claudication, rest
              pain and ulcer)
              I70.463
            intermittent
              claudication I70.413
            rest pain (and
             intermittent
             claudication)
             I70.423

Arteriosclerosis, arteriosclerotic
(continued)
extremities *(continued)*
  bypass graft *(continued)*
    autologous vein graft *(continued)*
      leg *(continued)*
        bilateral *(continued)*
          specified type NEC
            I70.493
        left I70.402
          with
            gangrene (and
              intermittent
              claudication, rest
              pain and ulcer)
              I70.462
            intermittent
              claudication
              I70.412
            rest pain (and
             intermittent
             claudication)
             I70.422
            ulceration (and
             intermittent
             claudication and
             rest pain) I70.449
            ankle I70.443
            calf I70.442
            foot site NEC
             I70.445
            heel I70.444
            lower leg NEC
             I70.448
            midfoot I70.444
            thigh I70.441
          specified type NEC
            I70.492
        right I70.401
          with
            gangrene (and
              intermittent
              claudication, rest
              pain and ulcer)
              I70.461
            intermittent
              claudication
              I70.411
            rest pain (and
             intermittent
             claudication)
             I70.421
            ulceration (and
             intermittent
             claudication and
             rest pain) I70.439
            ankle I70.433
            calf I70.432
            foot site NEC
             I70.435
            heel I70.434
            lower leg NEC
             I70.438
            midfoot I70.434
            thigh I70.431
          specified type NEC
            I70.491
        specified type NEC
          I70.499
      specified NEC I70.408
        with
          gangrene (and
            intermittent
            claudication, rest pain
            and ulcer) I70.468
          intermittent
            claudication I70.418
          rest pain (and
            intermittent
            claudication)
            I70.428

Arteriosclerosis, arteriosclerotic
(continued)
extremities *(continued)*
  bypass graft *(continued)*
    autologous vein graft
      (continued)
      specified NEC *(continued)*
        with *(continued)*
          ulceration (and
            intermittent
            claudication and rest
            pain) I70.45
        specified type NEC
          I70.498
    leg I70.309
      with
        gangrene (and
          intermittent
          claudication, rest pain
          and ulcer) I70.369
        intermittent claudication
          I70.319
        rest pain (and intermittent
          claudication) I70.329
      bilateral I70.303
        with
          gangrene (and
           intermittent
           claudication, rest pain
           and ulcer) I70.363
          intermittent
           claudication I70.313
          rest pain (and
           intermittent
           claudication) I70.323
        specified type NEC
          I70.393
      left I70.302
        with
          gangrene (and
           intermittent
           claudication, rest
           pain and ulcer)
           I70.362
          intermittent
           claudication I70.312
          rest pain (and
           intermittent
           claudication)
           I70.322
          ulceration (and
           intermittent
           claudication and rest
           pain) I70.349
          ankle I70.343
          calf I70.342
          foot site NEC
           I70.345
          heel I70.344
          lower leg NEC
           I70.348
          midfoot I70.344
          thigh I70.341
        specified type NEC
         I70.392
      right I70.301
        with
          gangrene (and
           intermittent
           claudication, rest pain
           and ulcer) I70.361
          intermittent
           claudication I70.311
          rest pain (and
           intermittent
           claudication) I70.321
          ulceration (and
           intermittent
           claudication and rest
           pain) I70.339
          ankle I70.333

(continued)
extremities *(continued)*
bypass graft *(continued)*
leg *(continued)*
right *(continued)*
with *(continued)*
ulceration *(continued)*
calf I70.332
foot site NEC
I70.335
heel I70.334
lower leg NEC
I70.338
midfoot I70.334
thigh I70.331
specified type NEC
I70.391
specified type NEC I70.399
nonautologous biological graft
I70.509
leg I70.509
with
gangrene (and
intermittent
claudication, rest
pain and ulcer)
I70.569
intermittent
claudication
I70.519
rest pain (and
intermittent
claudication)
I70.529
bilateral I70.503
with
gangrene (and
intermittent
claudication, rest
pain and ulcer)
I70.563
intermittent
claudication
I70.513
rest pain (and
intermittent
claudication)
I70.523
specified type NEC
I70.593
left I70.502
with
gangrene (and
intermittent
claudication, rest
pain and ulcer)
I70.562
intermittent
claudication
I70.512
rest pain (and
intermittent
claudication)
I70.522
ulceration (and
intermittent
claudication and
rest pain) I70.549
ankle I70.543
calf I70.542
foot site NEC
I70.545
heel I70.544
lower leg NEC
I70.548
midfoot I70.544
thigh I70.541
specified type NEC
I70.592
right I70.501

(continued)
extremities *(continued)*
bypass graft *(continued)*
nonautologous biological graft
(continued)
leg *(continued)*
right *(continued)*
with
gangrene (and
intermittent
claudication, rest
pain and ulcer)
I70.561
intermittent
claudication
I70.511
rest pain (and
intermittent
claudication)
I70.521
ulceration (and
intermittent
claudication and
rest pain) I70.539
ankle I70.533
calf I70.532
foot site NEC
I70.535
heel I70.534
lower leg NEC
I70.538
midfoot I70.534
thigh I70.531
specified type NEC
I70.591
specified type NEC
I70.599
specified NEC I70.508
with
gangrene (and
intermittent
claudication, rest pain
and ulcer) I70.568
intermittent
claudication I70.518
rest pain (and
intermittent
claudication)
I70.528
ulceration (and
intermittent
claudication and rest
pain) I70.55
specified type NEC
I70.598
nonbiological graft I70.609
leg I70.609
with
gangrene (and
intermittent
claudication, rest
pain and ulcer)
I70.669
intermittent
claudication
I70.619
rest pain (and
intermittent
claudication)
I70.629
bilateral I70.603
with
gangrene (and
intermittent
claudication, rest
pain and ulcer)
I70.663
intermittent
claudication
I70.613

(continued)
extremities *(continued)*
bypass graft *(continued)*
nonbiological graft *(continued)*
leg *(continued)*
bilateral *(continued)*
with *(continued)*
rest pain(and
intermittent
claudication)
I70.623
specified type NEC
I70.693
left I70.602
with
gangrene (and
intermittent
claudication, rest
pain and ulcer)
I70.662
intermittent
claudication
I70.612
rest pain (and
intermittent
claudication)
I70.622
ulceration (and
intermittent
claudication and
rest pain) I70.649
ankle I70.643
calf I70.642
foot site NEC
I70.645
heel I70.644
lower leg NEC
I70.648
midfoot I70.644
thigh I70.641
specified type NEC
I70.692
right I70.601
with
gangrene (and
intermittent
claudication, rest
pain and ulcer)
I70.661
intermittent
claudication
I70.611
rest pain (and
intermittent
claudication)
I70.621
ulceration (and
intermittent
claudication and
rest pain) I70.639
ankle I70.633
calf I70.632
foot site NEC
I70.635
heel I70.634
lower leg NEC
I70.638
midfoot I70.634
thigh I70.631
specified type NEC
I70.691
specified type NEC
I70.699
specified NEC I70.608
with
gangrene (and
intermittent
claudication, rest
pain and ulcer)
I70.668

(continued)
extremities *(continued)*
bypass graft *(continued)*
nonbiological graft *(continued)*
specified NEC *(continued)*
with *(continued)*
intermittent
claudication
I70.618
rest pain (and
intermittent
claudication)
I70.628
ulceration (and
intermittent
claudication and rest
pain) I70.65
specified type NEC
I70.698
specified graft NEC I70.709
leg I70.709
with
gangrene (and
intermittent
claudication, rest
pain and ulcer)
I70.769
intermittent
claudication I70.719
rest pain (and
intermittent
claudication)
I70.729
bilateral I70.703
with
gangrene (and
intermittent
claudication, rest
pain and ulcer)
I70.763
intermittent
claudication
I70.713
rest pain (and
intermittent
claudication)
I70.723
specified type NEC
I70.793
left I70.702
with
gangrene (and
intermittent
claudication, rest
pain and ulcer)
I70.762
intermittent
claudication
I70.712
rest pain (and
intermittent
claudication)
I70.722
ulceration (and
intermittent
claudication
and rest pain)
I70.749
ankle I70.743
calf I70.742
foot site NEC
I70.745
heel I70.744
lower leg NEC
I70.748
midfoot I70.744
thigh I70.741
specified type NEC
I70.792
right I70.701

Arteriosclerosis, arteriosclerotic
(continued)
extremities *(continued)*
bypass graft *(continued)*
specified grafft NEC *(continued)*
leg *(continued)*
right *(continued)*
with
gangrene (and intermittent claudication, rest pain and ulcer) I70.761
intermittent claudication I70.711
rest pain (and intermittent claudication) I70.721
ulceration (and intermittent claudication and rest pain) I70.739
ankle I70.733
calf I70.732
foot site NEC I70.735
heel I70.734
lower leg NEC I70.738
midfoot I70.734
thigh I70.731
specified type NEC I70.791
specified type NEC I70.799
specified NEC I70.708
with
gangrene (and intermittent claudication, rest pain and ulcer) I70.768
intermittent claudication I70.718
rest pain (and intermittent claudication) I70.728
ulceration (and intermittent claudication and rest pain) I70.75
specified type NEC I70.798
spcified NEC I70.308
with
gangrene (and intermittent claudication, rest pain and ulcer) I70.368
intermittent claudication I70.318
rest pain (and intermittent claudication) I70.328
ulceration (and intermittent claudication and rest pain) I70.35
specified type NEC I70.398
leg I70.209
with
gangrene (and intermittent claudication, rest pain and ulcer) I70.269
intermittent claudication I70.219
rest pain (and intermittent claudication) I70.229

Arteriosclerosis, arteriosclerotic
(continued)
extremities *(continued)*
leg *(continued)*
bilateral I70.203
with
gangrene (and intermittent claudication, rest pain and ulcer) I70.263
intermittent claudication I70.213
rest pain (and intermittent claudication) I70.223
specified type NEC I70.293
left I70.202
with
gangrene (and intermittent claudication, rest pain and ulcer) I70.262
intermittent claudication I70.212
rest pain (and intermittent claudication) I70.222
ulceration (and intermittent claudication and rest pain) I70.249
ankle I70.243
calf I70.242
foot site NEC I70.245
heel I70.244
lower leg NEC I70.248
midfoot I70.244
thigh I70.241
specified type NEC I70.292
right I70.201
with
gangrene (and intermittent claudication, rest pain and ulcer) I70.261
intermittent claudication I70.211
rest pain (and intermittent claudication) I70.221
ulceration (and intermittent claudication and rest pain) I70.239
ankle I70.233
calf I70.232
foot site NEC I70.235
heel I70.234
lower leg NEC I70.238
midfoot I70.234
thigh I70.231
specified type NEC I70.291
specified type NEC I70.299
specified site NEC I70.208
with
gangrene (and intermittent claudication, rest pain and ulcer) I70.268
intermittent claudication I70.218
rest pain (and intermittent claudication) I70.228
ulceration (and intermittent claudication and rest pain) I70.25
specified type NEC I70.298
generalized I70.91
heart (disease) —*see* Arteriosclerosis, coronary (artery),
kidney —*see* Hypertension, kidney
medial —*see* Arteriosclerosis, extremities
mesenteric (artery) K55.1
Mönckeberg's —*see* Arteriosclerosis, extremities
myocarditis I51.4
peripheral (of extremities) —*see* Arteriosclerosis, extremities
pulmonary (idiopathic) I27.0

Arteriosclerosis, arteriosclerotic
(continued)
renal (arterioles) —*see also* Hypertension, kidney
artery I70.1
retina (vascular) I70.8 *[H35.0]-*
specified artery NEC I70.8
spinal (cord) G95.19
vertebral (artery) I67.2

Arteriospasm I73.9

Arteriovenous —*see* condition

Arteritis I77.6
allergic M31.0
aorta (nonsyphilitic) I77.6
syphilitic A52.02
aortic arch M31.4
brachiocephalic M31.4
brain I67.7
syphilitic A52.04
cerebral I67.7
in
diseases classified elsewhere I68.2
systemic lupus erythematosus M32.19
listerial A32.89
syphilitic A52.04
tuberculous A18.89
coronary (artery) I25.89
rheumatic I01.8
chronic I09.89
syphilitic A52.06
cranial (left) (right), giant cell M31.6
deformans —*see* Arteriosclerosis
giant cell NEC M31.6
with polymyalgia rheumatica M31.5
necrosing or necrotizing M31.9
specified NEC M31.8
nodosa M30.0
obliterans —*see* Arteriosclerosis
pulmonary I28.8
rheumatic —*see* Fever, rheumatic
senile —*see* Arteriosclerosis
suppurative I77.2
syphilitic (general) A52.09
brain A52.04
coronary A52.06
spinal A52.09
temporal, giant cell M31.6
young female aortic arch syndrome M31.4

Artery, arterial —*see also* condition
abscess I77.89
single umbilical Q27.0

Arthralgia (allergic) —*see also* Pain, joint
in caisson disease T70.3
temporomandibular M26.62-

Arthritis, arthritic (acute) (chronic) (nonpyogenic) (subacute) M19.90
allergic —*see* Arthritis, specified form NEC
ankylosing (crippling) (spine) —*see also* Spondylitis, ankylosing
sites other than spine —*see* Arthritis, specified form NEC
atrophic —*see* Osteoarthritis
spine —*see* Spondylitis, ankylosing
back —*see* Spondylopathy, inflammatory
blennorrhagic (gonococcal) A54.42
Charcot's —*see* Arthropathy, neuropathic
diabetic —*see* Diabetes, arthropathy, neuropathic
syringomyelic G95.0

Arthritis, arthritic *(continued)*
chylous (filarial) (*see also* category M01) B74.9
climacteric (any site) NEC —*see* Arthritis, specified form NEC
crystal (-induced) —*see* Arthritis, in, crystals
deformans —*see* Osteoarthritis
degenerative —*see* Osteoarthritis
due to or associated with
acromegaly E22.0
brucellosis —*see* Brucellosis
caisson disease T70.3
diabetes —*see* Diabetes, arthropathy
dracontiasis (*see also* category M01) B72
enteritis NEC
regional —*see* Enteritis, regional
erysipelas (*see also* category M01) A46
erythema
epidemic A25.1
nodosum L52
filariasis NOS B74.9
glanders A24.0
helminthiasis (*see also* category M01) B83.9
hemophilia D66 *[M36.2]*
Henoch-(Schönlein) purpura D69.0 *[M36.4]*
human parvovirus (*see also* category M01) B97.6
infectious disease NEC M01
leprosy (*see also* category M01) —*see also* Leprosy A30.9
Lyme disease A69.23
mycobacteria (*see also* category M01) A31.8
parasitic disease NEC (*see also* category M01) B89
paratyphoid fever (*see also* category M01) (*see also* Fever, paratyphoid) A01.4
rat bite fever (*see also* category M01) A25.1
regional enteritis —*see* Enteritis, regional
respiratory disorder NOS J98.9
serum sickness (*see also* Reaction, serum) T80.69
syringomyelia G95.0
typhoid fever A01.04
epidemic erythema A25.1
febrile —*see* Fever, rheumatic
gonococcal A54.42
gouty (acute) —*see* Gout
in (due to)
acromegaly (*see also* subcategory M14.8-) E22.0
amyloidosis (*see also* subcategory M14.8-) E85.4
bacterial disease (*see also* subcategory M01) A49.9
Behçet's syndrome M35.2
caisson disease (*see also* subcategory M14.8-) T70.3
coliform bacilli (Escherichia coli) —*see* Arthritis, in, pyogenic organism NEC
crystals M11.9
dicalcium phosphate —*see* Arthritis, in, crystals, specified type NEC
hydroxyapatite M11.0-
pyrophosphate —*see* Arthritis, in, crystals, specified type NEC
specified type NEC M11.80
ankle M11.87-

in *(continued)*
 crystals *(continued)*
  specified type *(continued)*
   elbow M11.82-
   foot joint M11.87-
   hand joint M11.84-
   hip M11.85-
   knee M11.86-
   multiple sites M11.8-
   shoulder M11.81-
   vertebrae M11.88
   wrist M11.83-
 dermatoarthritis, lipoid E78.81
 dracontiasis (dracunculiasis) *(see also* category M01) B72
 endocrine disorder NEC *(see also* subcategory M14.8-) E34.9
 enteritis, infectious NEC *(see also* category M01) A09
  specified organism NEC *(see also* category M01) A08.8
 erythema
  multiforme *(see also* subcategory M14.8-) L51.9
  nodosum *(see also* subcategory M14.8-) L52
 gout —*see* Gout
 helminthiasis NEC *(see also* category M01) B83.9
 hemochromatosis *(see also* subcategory M14.8-) E83.118
 hemoglobinopathy NEC D58.2 *[M36.3]*
 hemophilia NEC D66 *[M36.2]*
 Hemophilus influenzae M00.8- *[B96.2]*
 Henoch (-Schönlein) purpura D69.0 *[M36.4]*
 hyperparathyroidism NEC *(see also* subcategory M14.8-) E21.3
 hypersensitivity reaction NEC T78.49 *[M36.4]*
 hypogammaglobulinemia *(see also* subcategory M14.8-) D80.1
 hypothyroidism NEC *(see also* subcategory M14.8-) E03.9
 infection —*see* Arthritis, pyogenic or pyemic
  spine —*see* Spondylopathy, infective
 infectious disease NEC M01
 leprosy *(see also* category M01) A30.9
 leukemia NEC C95.9- *[M36.1]*
 lipoid dermatoarthritis E78.81
 Lyme disease A69.23
 Mediterranean fever, familial *(see also* subcategory M14.8-) M04.1
 Meningococcus A39.83
 metabolic disorder NEC *(see also* subcategory M14.8-) E88.9
 multiple myelomatosis C90.0- *[M36.1]*
 mumps B26.85
 mycosis NEC *(see also* category M01) B49
 myelomatosis (multiple) C90.0- *[M36.1]*
 neurological disorder NEC G98.0
 ochronosis *(see also* subcategory M14.8-) E70.29
 O'nyong-nyong *(see also* category M01) A92.1
 parasitic disease NEC *(see also* category M01) B89
 paratyphoid fever *(see also* category M01) A01.4

in *(continued)*
 Pseudomonas —*see* Arthritis, pyogenic, bacterial NEC
 psoriasis L40.50
 pyogenic organism NEC —*see* Arthritis, pyogenic, bacterial NEC
 Reiter's disease —*see* Reiter's disease
 respiratory disorder NEC *(see also* subcategory M14.8-) J98.9
 reticulosis, malignant *(see also* subcategory M14.8-) C86.0
 rubella B06.82
 Salmonella (arizonae) (cholerae-suis) (enteritidis) (typhimurium) A02.23
 sarcoidosis D86.86
 specified bacteria NEC —*see* Arthritis, pyogenic, bacterial NEC
 sporotrichosis B42.82
 syringomyelia G95.0
 thalassemia NEC D56.9 *[M36.3]*
 tuberculosis —*see* Tuberculosis, arthritis
 typhoid fever A01.04
 urethritis, Reiter's —*see* Reiter's disease
 viral disease NEC *(see also* category M01) B34.9
infectious or infective —*see also* Arthritis, pyogenic or pyemic
 spine —*see* Spondylopathy, infective
juvenile M08.90
 with systemic onset —*see* Still's disease
 ankle M08.97-
 elbow M08.92-
 foot joint M08.97-
 hand joint M08.94-
 hip M08.95-
 knee M08.96-
 multiple site M08.99
 pauciarticular M08.40
  ankle M08.47-
  elbow M08.42-
  foot joint M08.47-
  hand joint M08.44-
  hip M08.45-
  knee M08.46-
  shoulder M08.41-
  specified site NEC M08.4A
  vertebrae M08.48
  wrist M08.43-
 psoriatic L40.54
 rheumatoid —*see* Arthritis, rheumatoid, juvenile
 shoulder M08.91-
 specified site NEC M08.9A
 specified type NEC M08.80
  ankle M08.87-
  elbow M08.82-
  foot joint M08.87-
  hand joint M08.84-
  hip M08.85-
  knee M08.86-
  multiple site M08.89
  shoulder M08.81-
  specified joint NEC M08.88
  vertebrae M08.88
  wrist M08.83-
 vertebra M08.98
 wrist M08.93-
meaning osteoarthritis —*see* Osteoarthritis
meningococcal A39.83

menopausal (any site) NEC —*see* Arthritis, specified form NEC
mutilans (psoriatic) L40.52
mycotic NEC *(see also* category M01) B49
neuropathic (Charcot) —*see* Arthropathy, neuropathic
 diabetic —*see* Diabetes, arthropathy, neuropathic
 nonsyphilitic NEC G98.0
 syringomyelic G95.0
ochronotic *(see also* subcategory M14.8-) E70.29
palindromic (any site) —*see* Rheumatism, palindromic
pneumococcal M00.10
 ankle M00.17-
 elbow M00.12-
 foot joint —*see* Arthritis, pneumococcal, ankle
 hand joint M00.14-
 hip M00.15-
 knee M00.16-
 multiple site M00.19
 shoulder M00.11-
 vertebra M00.18
 wrist M00.13-
postdysenteric —*see* Arthropathy, postdysenteric
postmeningococcal A39.84
postrheumatic, chronic —*see* Arthropathy, postrheumatic, chronic
primary progressive —*see also* Arthritis, specified form NEC
 spine —*see* Spondylitis, ankylosing
psoriatic L40.50
purulent (any site except spine) — *see* Arthritis, pyogenic or pyemic
 spine —*see* Spondylopathy, infective
pyogenic or pyemic (any site except spine) M00.9
 bacterial NEC M00.80
  ankle M00.87-
  elbow M00.82-
  foot joint —*see* Arthritis, pyogenic, bacterial NEC, ankle
  hand joint M00.84-
  hip M00.85-
  knee M00.86-
  multiple site M00.89
  shoulder M00.81-
  vertebra M00.88
  wrist M00.83-
 pneumococcal —*see* Arthritis, pneumococcal
 spine —*see* Spondylopathy, infective
 staphylococcal —*see* Arthritis, staphylococcal
 streptococcal —*see* Arthritis, streptococcal NEC
 pneumococcal —*see* Arthritis, pneumococcal
reactive —*see* Reiter's disease
rheumatic —*see also* Arthritis, rheumatoid
 acute or subacute —*see* Fever, rheumatic
rheumatoid M06.9
 with
  carditis —*see* Rheumatoid, carditis
  endocarditis —*see* Rheumatoid, carditis
  heart involvement NEC —*see* Rheumatoid, carditis

rheumatoid M06.9 *(continued)*
 with *(continued)*
  lung involvement —*see* Rheumatoid, lung
  myocarditis —*see* Rheumatoid, carditis
  myopathy —*see* Rheumatoid, myopathy
  pericarditis —*see* Rheumatoid, carditis
  polyneuropathy —*see* Rheumatoid, polyneuropathy
  rheumatoid factor —*see* Arthritis, rheumatoid, seropositive
  splenoadenomegaly and leukopenia —*see* Felty's syndrome
  vasculitis —*see* Rheumatoid, vasculitis
  visceral involvement NEC —*see* Rheumatoid, arthritis, with involvement of organs NEC
 juvenile (with or without rheumatoid factor) M08.00
  with systemic onset —*see* Still's disease
  ankle M08.07-
  elbow M08.02-
  foot joint M08.07-
  hand joint M08.04-
  hip M08.05-
  knee M08.06-
  multiple site M08.09
  shoulder M08.01-
  specified site NEC M08.0A
  vertebra M08.08
  wrist M08.03-
 seronegative M06.00
  ankle M06.07-
  elbow M06.02-
  foot joint M06.07-
  hand joint M06.04-
  hip M06.05-
  knee M06.06-
  multiple site M06.09
  shoulder M06.01-
  specified site NEC M06.0A
  vertebra M06.08
  wrist M06.03-
 seropositive M05.9
  specified NEC M05.80
   ankle M05.87-
   elbow M05.82-
   foot joint M05.87-
   hand joint M05.84-
   hip M05.85-
   knee M05.86-
   multiple sites M05.89
   shoulder M05.81-
   specified site NEC M05.8A
   vertebra —*see* Spondylitis, ankylosing
   wrist M05.83-
  without organ involvement M05.70
   ankle M05.77-
   elbow M05.72-
   foot joint M05.77-
   hand joint M05.74-
   hip M05.75-
   knee M05.76-
   multiple sites M05.79
   shoulder M05.71-
   specified site NEC M05.7A
   vertebra —*see* Spondylitis, ankylosing
   wrist M05.73-

Arthritis, arthritic *(continued)*
 rheumatoid *(continued)*
  specified type NEC M06.80
   ankle M06.87-
   elbow M06.82-
   foot joint M06.87-
   hand joint M06.84-
   hip M06.85-
   knee M06.86-
   multiple site M06.89
   shoulder M06.81-
   specified site NEC M06.8A
   vertebra M06.88
   wrist M06.83-
  spine —*see* Spondylitis,
   ankylosing
 rubella B06.82
 scorbutic (*see also* subcategory
  M14.8-) E54
 senile or senescent —*see*
  Osteoarthritis
 septic (any site except spine) —*see*
  Arthritis, pyogenic or pyemic
  spine —*see* Spondylopathy,
   infective
 serum (nontherapeutic)
  (therapeutic) —*see* Arthropathy,
  postimmunization
 specified form NEC M13.80
  ankle M13.87-
  elbow M13.82-
  foot joint M13.87-
  hand joint M13.84-
  hip M13.85-
  knee M13.86-
  multiple site M13.89
  shoulder M13.81-
  specified joint NEC M13.88
  wrist M13.83-
 spine —*see also* Spondylosis
  infectious or infective NEC —
   see Spondylopathy, infective
  Marie-Strümpell —*see*
   Spondylitis, ankylosing
  pyogenic —*see* Spondylopathy,
   infective
  rheumatoid —*see* Spondylitis,
   ankylosing
  traumatic (old) —*see*
   Spondylopathy, traumatic
  tuberculous A18.01
 staphylococcal M00.00
  ankle M00.07-
  elbow M00.02-
  foot joint —*see* Arthritis,
   staphylococcal, ankle
  hand joint M00.04-
  hip M00.05-
  knee M00.06-
  multiple site M00.09
  shoulder M00.01-
  vertebra M00.08
  wrist M00.03-
 streptococcal NEC M00.20
  ankle M00.27-
  elbow M00.22-
  foot joint —*see* Arthritis,
   streptococcal, ankle
  hand joint M00.24-
  hip M00.25-
  knee M00.26-
  multiple site M00.29
  shoulder M00.21-
  vertebra M00.28
  wrist M00.23-
 suppurative —*see* Arthritis,
  pyogenic or pyemic
 syphilitic (late) A52.16
  congenital A50.55 *[M12.80]*
 syphilitica deformans (Charcot)
  A52.16

Arthritis, arthritic *(continued)*
 temporomandibular M26.64-
 toxic of menopause (any site) —*see*
  Arthritis, specified form NEC
 transient —*see* Arthropathy,
  specified form NEC
 traumatic (chronic) —*see*
  Arthropathy, traumatic
 tuberculous A18.02
  spine A18.01
 uratic —*see* Gout
 urethritica (Reiter's) —*see* Reiter's
  disease
 vertebral —*see* Spondylopathy,
  inflammatory
 villous (any site) —*see*
  Arthropathy, specified form NEC

Arthrocele —*see* Effusion, joint

Arthrodesis status Z98.1

Arthrodynia —*see also* Pain, joint

Arthrodysplasia Q74.9

Arthrofibrosis, joint —*see* Ankylosis

Arthrogryposis (congenital) Q68.8
 multiplex congenita Q74.3

Arthrokatadysis M24.7

Arthropathy —*see also* Arthritis
 M12.9
 Charcot's —*see* Arthropathy,
  neuropathic
  diabetic —*see* Diabetes,
   arthropathy, neuropathic
  syringomyelic G95.0
 cricoarytenoid J38.7
 crystal (-induced) —*see* Arthritis,
  in, crystals
 diabetic NEC —*see* Diabetes,
  arthropathy
 distal interphalangeal, psoriatic
  L40.51
 enteropathic M07.60
  ankle M07.67-
  elbow M07.62-
  foot joint M07.67-
  hand joint M07.64-
  hip M07.65-
  knee M07.66-
  multiple site M07.69
  shoulder M07.61-
  vertebra M07.68
  wrist M07.63-
 following intestinal bypass M02.00
  ankle M02.07-
  elbow M02.02-
  foot joint M02.07-
  hand joint M02.04-
  hip M02.05-
  knee M02.06-
  multiple site M02.09
  shoulder M02.01-
  vertebra M02.08
  wrist M02.03-
 gouty —*see also* Gout
  in (due to)
   Lesch-Nyhan syndrome E79.1
    [M14.8-]
   sickle-cell disorders D57-
    [M14.8-]
 hemophilic NEC D66 *[M36.2]*
  in (due to)
   hyperparathyroidism NEC
    E21.3 *[M14.8-]*
   metabolic disease NOS E88.9
    [M14.8-]
 in (due to)
  acromegaly E22.0 *[M14.8-]*
  amyloidosis E85.4 *[M14.8-]*
  blood disorder NOS D75.9
   [M36.3]

Arthropathy *(continued)*
 in *(continued)*
  diabetes —*see* Diabetes,
   arthropathy
  endocrine disease NOS E34.9
   [M14.8-]
  erythema
   multiforme L51.9 *[M14.8-]*
   nodosum L52 *[M14.8-]*
  hemochromatosis E83.118
   [M14.8-]
  hemoglobinopathy NEC D58.2
   [M36.3]
  hemophilia NEC D66 *[M36.2]*
  Henoch-Schönlein purpura
   D69.0 *[M36.4]*
  hyperthyroidism E05.90 *[M14.8-]*
  hypothyroidism E03.9 *[M14.8-]*
  infective endocarditis I33.0
   [M12.80]
  leukemia NEC C95.9- *[M36.1]*
  malignant histiocytosis C96.A
   [M36.1]
  metabolic disease NOS E88.9
   [M14.8-]
  multiple myeloma C90.0- *[M36.1]*
  neoplastic disease NOS (*see also*
   Neoplasm) D49.9 *[M36.1]*
  nutritional deficiency (*see also*
   subcategory M14.8-) E63.9
  psoriasis NOS L40.50
  sarcoidosis D86.86
  syphilis (late) A52.77
   congenital A50.55 *[M12.80]*
  thyrotoxicosis (*see also*
   subcategory M14.8-) E05.90
  ulcerative colitis K51.90 *[M07.60]*
  viral hepatitis (postinfectious)
   NEC B19.9 *[M12.80]*
  Whipple's disease (*see also*
   subcategory M14.8-) K90.81
 Jaccoud —*see* Arthropathy,
  postrheumatic, chronic
 juvenile —*see* Arthritis, juvenile
  psoriatic L40.54
 mutilans (psoriatic) L40.52
 neuropathic (Charcot) M14.60
  ankle M14.67-
  diabetic —*see* Diabetes,
   arthropathy, neuropathic
  elbow M14.62-
  foot joint M14.67-
  hand joint M14.64-
  hip M14.65-
  knee M14.66-
  multiple site M14.69
  nonsyphilitic NEC G98.0
  shoulder M14.61-
  syringomyelic G95.0
  vertebra M14.68
  wrist M14.63-
 osteopulmonary —*see*
  Osteoarthropathy, hypertrophic,
  specified NEC
 postdysenteric M02.10
  ankle M02.17-
  elbow M02.12-
  foot joint M02.17-
  hand joint M02.14-
  hip M02.15-
  knee M02.16-
  multiple site M02.19
  shoulder M02.11-
  vertebra M02.18
  wrist M02.13-
 postimmunization M02.20
  ankle M02.27-
  elbow M02.22-
  foot joint M02.27-
  hand joint M02.24-
  hip M02.25-

Arthropathy *(continued)*
 postimmunization *(continued)*
  knee M02.26-
  multiple site M02.29
  shoulder M02.21-
  vertebra M02.28
  wrist M02.23-
 postinfectious NEC B99 *[M12.80]*
  in (due to)
   enteritis due to Yersinia
    enterocolitica A04.6 *[M12.80]*
   syphilis A52.77
   viral hepatitis NEC B19.9
    [M12.80]
 postrheumatic, chronic (Jaccoud)
  M12.00
  ankle M12.07-
  elbow M12.02-
  foot joint M12.07-
  hand joint M12.04-
  hip M12.05-
  knee M12.06-
  multiple site M12.09
  shoulder M12.01-
  specified joint NEC M12.08
  vertebrae M12.08
  wrist M12.03-
 psoriatic NEC L40.59
  interphalangeal, distal L40.51
 reactive M02.9
  in (due to)
   infective endocarditis I33.0
    [M02.9]
  specified type NEC M02.80
   ankle M02.87-
   elbow M02.82-
   foot joint M02.87-
   hand joint M02.84-
   hip M02.85-
   knee M02.86-
   multiple site M02.89
   shoulder M02.81-
   vertebra M02.88
   wrist M02.83-
 specified form NEC M12.80
  ankle M12.87-
  elbow M12.82-
  foot joint M12.87-
  hand joint M12.84-
  hip M12.85-
  knee M12.86-
  multiple site M12.89
  shoulder M12.81-
  specified joint NEC M12.88
  vertebrae M12.88
  wrist M12.83-
 syringomyelic G95.0
 tabes dorsalis A52.16
 tabetic A52.16
 temporomandibular joint M26.65-
 transient —*see* Arthropathy,
  specified form NEC
 traumatic M12.50
  ankle M12.57-
  elbow M12.52-
  foot joint M12.57-
  hand joint M12.54-
  hip M12.55-
  knee M12.56-
  multiple site M12.59
  shoulder M12.51-
  specified joint NEC M12.58
  vertebrae M12.58
  wrist M12.53-

Arthropyosis —*see* Arthritis,
 pyogenic or pyemic

Arthrosis (deformans) (degenerative)
 (localized) —*see also*
 Osteoarthritis M19.90
 spine —*see* Spondylosis

Arthus' phenomenon or reaction
T78.41
due to
drug —*see* Table of Drugs and Chemicals, by drug

Articular —*see* condition

Articulation, reverse (teeth) M26.24

Artificial
insemination complication —*see* Complications, artificial, fertilization
opening status (functioning) (without complication) Z93.9
anus (colostomy) Z93.3
colostomy Z93.3
cystostomy Z93.50
appendico-vesicostomy Z93.52
cutaneous Z93.51
specified NEC Z93.59
enterostomy Z93.4
gastrostomy Z93.1
ileostomy Z93.2
intestinal tract NEC Z93.4
jejunostomy Z93.4
nephrostomy Z93.6
specified site NEC Z93.8
tracheostomy Z93.0
ureterostomy Z93.6
urethrostomy Z93.6
urinary tract NEC Z93.6
vagina Z93.8
vagina status Z93.8

Arytenoid —*see* condition

Asbestosis (occupational) J61

ASC-H (atypical squamous cells cannot exclude high grade squamous intraepithelial lesion on cytologic smear)
anus R85.611
cervix R87.611
vagina R87.621

ASC-US (atypical squamous cells of undetermined significance on cytologic smear)
anus R85.610
cervix R87.610
vagina R87.620

Ascariasis B77.9
with
complications NEC B77.89
intestinal complications B77.0
pneumonia, pneumonitis B77.81

Ascaridosis, ascaridiasis —*see* Ascariasis

Ascaris (infection) (infestation) (lumbricoides) —*see* Ascariasis

Ascending —*see* condition

Aschoff's bodies —*see* Myocarditis, rheumatic

Ascites (abdominal) R18.8
cardiac (*see also* Failure, heart, right) I50.810
chylous (nonfilarial) I89.8
filarial —*see* Infestation, filarial
due to
cirrhosis, alcoholic K70.31
hepatitis
alcoholic K70.11
chronic active K71.51
S. japonicum B65.2
heart (*see also* Failure, heart, right) I50.810
malignant R18.0
pseudochylous R18.8
syphilitic A52.74
tuberculous A18.31

Aseptic —*see* condition

Asherman's syndrome N85.6

Asialia K11.7

Asiatic cholera —*see* Cholera

Asimultagnosia (simultanagnosia) R48.3

Askin's tumor —*see* Neoplasm, connective tissue, malignant

Asocial personality F60.2

Asomatognosia R41.4

Aspartylglucosaminuria E77.1

Asperger's disease or syndrome F84.5

Aspergilloma —*see* Aspergillosis

Aspergillosis (with pneumonia) B44.9
bronchopulmonary, allergic B44.81
disseminated B44.7
generalized B44.7
pulmonary NEC B44.1
allergic B44.81
invasive B44.0
specified NEC B44.89
tonsillar B44.2

Aspergillus (flavus) (fumigatus) (infection) (terreus) —*see* Aspergillosis

Aspermatogenesis —*see* Azoospermia

Aspermia (testis) —*see* Azoospermia

Asphyxia, asphyxiation (by) R09.01
antenatal P84
birth P84
bunny bag —*see* Asphyxia, due to, mechanical threat to breathing, trapped in bed clothes
crushing S28.0
drowning T75.1
gas, fumes, or vapor —*see* Table of Drugs and Chemicals
inhalation —*see* Inhalation
intrauterine P84
local I73.00
with gangrene I73.01
mucus —*see also* Foreign body, respiratory tract, causing asphyxia
newborn P84
pathological R09.01
postnatal P84
mechanical —*see* Asphyxia, due to, mechanical threat to breathing
prenatal P84
reticularis R23.1
strangulation —*see* Asphyxia, due to, mechanical threat to breathing
submersion T75.1
traumatic T71.9
due to
crushed chest S28.0
foreign body (in) —*see* Foreign body, respiratory tract, causing asphyxia
low oxygen content of ambient air T71.20
due to
being trapped in low oxygen environment T71.29
in car trunk T71.221
circumstances undetermined T71.224

Asphyxia, asphyxiation (*continued*)
traumatic (*continued*)
due to (*continued*)
low oxygen content of ambient air (*continued*)
due to (*continued*)
being trapped in (*continued*)
low oxygen environment (*continued*)
in car trunk (*continued*)
done with intent to harm by another person T71.223
self T71.222
in refrigerator T71.231
circumstances undetermined T71.234
done with intent to harm by another person T71.233
self T71.232
cave-in T71.21
mechanical threat to breathing (accidental) T71.191
circumstances undetermined T71.194
done with intent to harm by another person T71.193
self T71.192
hanging T71.161
circumstances undetermined T71.164
done with intent to harm by another person T71.163
self T71.162
plastic bag T71.121
circumstances undetermined T71.124
done with intent to harm by another person T71.123
self T71.122
smothering
in furniture T71.151
circumstances undetermined T71.154
done with intent to harm by another person T71.153
self T71.152
under another person's body T71.141
circumstances undetermined T71.144
done with intent to harm T71.143
pillow T71.111
circumstances undetermined T71.114
done with intent to harm by another person T71.113
self T71.112
trapped in bed clothes T71.131
circumstances undetermined T71.134

Asphyxia, asphyxiation (*continued*)
traumatic (*continued*)
due to (*continued*)
mechanical threat to breathing (*continued*)
trapped in bed clothes (*continued*)
done with intent to harm by another person T71.133
self T71.132
vomiting, vomitus —*see* Foreign body, respiratory tract, causing asphyxia

Aspiration
amniotic (clear) fluid (newborn) P24.10
with
pneumonia (pneumonitis) P24.11
respiratory symptoms P24.11
blood
newborn (without respiratory symptoms) P24.20
with
pneumonia (pneumonitis) P24.21
respiratory symptoms P24.21
specified age NEC —*see* Foreign body, respiratory tract
bronchitis J69.0
food or foreign body (with asphyxiation) —*see* Asphyxia, food
liquor (amnii) (newborn) P24.10
with
pneumonia (pneumonitis) P24.11
respiratory symptoms P24.11
meconium (newborn) (without respiratory symptoms) P24.00
with
pneumonitis (pneumonitis) P24.01
respiratory symptoms P24.01
milk (newborn) (without respiratory symptoms) P24.30
with
pneumonia (pneumonitis) P24.31
respiratory symptoms P24.31
specified age NEC —*see* Foreign body, respiratory tract
mucus —*see also* Foreign body, by site, causing asphyxia
newborn P24.10
with
pneumonia (pneumonitis) P24.11
respiratory symptoms P24.11
neonatal P24.9
specific NEC (without respiratory symptoms) P24.80
with
pneumonia (pneumonitis) P24.81
respiratory symptoms P24.81
newborn P24.9
specific NEC (without respiratory symptoms) P24.80
with
pneumonia (pneumonitis) P24.81
respiratory symptoms P24.81
pneumonia J69.0
pneumonitis J69.0
syndrome of newborn —*see* Aspiration, by substance, with pneumonia
vernix caseosa (newborn) P24.80
with
pneumonia (pneumonitis) P24.81

Aspiration *(continued)*
  vernix caseosa *(continued)*
    with *(continued)*
      respiratory symptoms P24.81
  vomitus —*see also* Foreign body,
    respiratory tract
  newborn (without respiratory
    symptoms) P24.30
    with
      pneumonia (pneumonitis)
        P24.31
      respiratory symptoms P24.31

Asplenia (congenital) Q89.01
  postsurgical Z90.81

Assam fever B55.0

Assault, sexual —*see* Maltreatment

Assmann's focus NEC A15.0

Astasia(-abasia) (hysterical) F44.4

Asteatosis cutis L85.3

Astereognosia, astereognosis R48.1

Asterixis R27.8
  in liver disease K71.3

Asteroid hyalitis —*see* Deposit,
  crystalline

Asthenia, asthenic R53.1
  cardiac (*see also* Failure, heart) I50.9
    psychogenic F45.8
  cardiovascular (*see also* Failure,
    heart) I50.9
    psychogenic F45.8
  heart (*see also* Failure, heart) I50.9
    psychogenic F45.8
  hysterical F44.4
  myocardial (*see also* Failure, heart)
    I50.9
    psychogenic F45.8
  nervous F48.8
  neurocirculatory F45.8
  neurotic F48.8
  psychogenic F48.8
  psychoneurotic F48.8
  psychophysiologic F48.8
  reaction (psychophysiologic) F48.8
  senile R54

Asthenopia —*see also* Discomfort,
  visual
  hysterical F44.6
  psychogenic F44.6

Asthenospermia —*see* Abnormal,
  specimen, male genital organs

Asthma, asthmatic (bronchial)
  (catarrh) (spasmodic) J45.909
  with
    chronic obstructive bronchitis J44.9
      with
        acute lower respiratory
          infection J44.0
        exacerbation (acute) J44.1
    chronic obstructive pulmonary
      disease J44.9
      with
        acute lower respiratory
          infection J44.0
        exacerbation (acute) J44.1
    exacerbation (acute) J45.901
    hay fever —*see* Asthma, allergic
      extrinsic
    rhinitis, allergic —*see* Asthma,
      allergic extrinsic
    status asthmaticus J45.902
  allergic extrinsic J45.909
    with
      exacerbation (acute) J45.901
      status asthmaticus J45.902
  atopic —*see* Asthma, allergic
    extrinsic
  cardiac —*see* Failure, ventricular,
    left

Asthenia, asthenic *(continued)*
  cardiobronchial I50.1
  childhood J45.909
    with
      exacerbation (acute) J45.901
      status asthmaticus J45.902
  chronic obstructive J44.9
    with
      acute lower respiratory
        infection J44.0
      exacerbation (acute) J44.1
  collier's J60
  cough variant J45.991
  detergent J69.8
  due to
    detergent J69.8
    inhalation of fumes J68.3
  eosinophilic J82.83
  extrinsic, allergic —*see* Asthma,
    allergic extrinsic
  grinder's J62.8
  hay —*see* Asthma, allergic extrinsic
  heart I50.1
  idiosyncratic —*see* Asthma,
    nonallergic
  intermittent (mild) J45.20
    with
      exacerbation (acute) J45.21
      status asthmaticus J45.22
  intrinsic, nonallergic —*see* Asthma,
    nonallergic
  Kopp's E32.8
  late-onset J45.909
    with
      exacerbation (acute) J45.901
      status asthmaticus J45.902
  mild intermittent J45.20
    with
      exacerbation (acute) J45.21
      status asthmaticus J45.22
  mild persistent J45.30
    with
      exacerbation (acute) J45.31
      status asthmaticus J45.32
  Millar's (laryngismus stridulus) J38.5
  miner's J60
  mixed J45.909
    with
      exacerbation (acute) J45.901
      status asthmaticus J45.902
  moderate persistent J45.40
    with
      exacerbation (acute) J45.41
      status asthmaticus J45.42
  nervous —*see* Asthma, nonallergic
  nonallergic (intrinsic) J45.909
    with
      exacerbation (acute) J45.901
      status asthmaticus J45.902
  persistent
    mild J45.30
      with
        exacerbation (acute) J45.31
        status asthmaticus J45.32
    moderate J45.40
      with
        exacerbation (acute) J45.41
        status asthmaticus J45.42
    severe J45.50
      with
        exacerbation (acute) J45.51
        status asthmaticus J45.52
  platinum J45.998
  pneumoconiotic NEC J64
  potter's J62.8
  predominantly allergic J45.909
  psychogenic F54
  pulmonary eosinophilic J82.83
  red cedar J67.8
  Rostan's I50.1
  sandblaster's J62.8

Asthma, asthmatic *(continued)*
  sequoiosis J67.8
  severe persistent J45.50
    with
      exacerbation (acute) J45.51
      status asthmaticus J45.52
  specified NEC J45.998
  stonemason's J62.8
  thymic E32.8
  tuberculous —*see* Tuberculosis,
    pulmonary
  Wichmann's (laryngismus
    stridulus) J38.5
  wood J67.8

Astigmatism (compound)
  (congenital) H52.20-
  irregular H52.21-
  regular H52.22-

Astraphobia F40.220

Astroblastoma
  specified site —*see* Neoplasm,
    malignant, by site
  unspecified site C71.9

Astrocytoma (cystic)
  anaplastic
    specified site —*see* Neoplasm,
      malignant, by site
    unspecified site C71.9
  fibrillary
    specified site —*see* Neoplasm,
      malignant, by site
    unspecified site C71.9
  fibrous
    specified site —*see* Neoplasm,
      malignant, by site
    unspecified site C71.9
  gemistocytic
    specified site —*see* Neoplasm,
      malignant, by site
    unspecified site C71.9
  juvenile
    specified site —*see* Neoplasm,
      malignant, by site
    unspecified site C71.9
  pilocytic
    specified site —*see* Neoplasm,
      malignant, by site
    unspecified site C71.9
  piloid
    specified site —*see* Neoplasm,
      malignant, by site
    unspecified site C71.9
  protoplasmic
    specified site —*see* Neoplasm,
      malignant, by site
    unspecified site C71.9
  specified site NEC —*see*
    Neoplasm, malignant, by site
  subependymal D43.2
    giant cell
      specified site —*see* Neoplasm,
        uncertain behavior, by site
      unspecified site D43.2
    specified site —*see* Neoplasm,
      uncertain behavior, by site
    unspecified site D43.2
  unspecified site C71.9

Astroglioma
  specified site —*see* Neoplasm,
    malignant, by site
  unspecified site C71.9

Asymbolia R48.8

Asymmetry —*see also* Distortion
  between native and reconstructed
    breast N65.1
  face Q67.0
  jaw (lower) —*see* Anomaly,
    dentofacial, jaw-cranial base
    relationship, asymmetry

Asynergia, asynergy R27.8
  ventricular I51.89

Asystole (heart) —*see* Arrest, cardiac

At risk
  for
    dental caries Z91.849
      high Z91.843
      low Z91.841
      moderate Z91.842
  falling Z91.81

Ataxia, ataxy, ataxic R27.0
  acute R27.8
  autosomal recessive Friedreich
    G11.11
  brain (hereditary) G11.9
  cerebellar (hereditary) G11.9
    with defective DNA repair G11.3
    alcoholic G31.2
    early-onset G11.10
      with
        essential tremor G11.19
        myoclonus [Hunt's ataxia]
          G11.19
        retained tendon reflexes G11.19
      in
        alcoholism G31.2
        myxedema E03.9 *[G13.2]*
        neoplastic disease (*see also*
          Neoplasm) D49.9 *[G32.81]*
        specified disease NEC G32.81
    late-onset (Marie's) G11.2
  cerebral (hereditary) G11.9
  congenital nonprogressive G11.0
  family, familial —*see* Ataxia,
    hereditary
  following
    cerebrovascular disease I69.993
      cerebral infarction I69.393
      intracerebral hemorrhage
        I69.193
      nontraumatic intracranial
        hemorrhage NEC I69.293
      specified disease NEC I69.893
      subarachnoid hemorrhage
        I69.093
  Friedreich's (heredofamilial)
    (cerebellar) (spinal) (with
    retained reflexes) G11.11
  gait R26.0
    hysterical F44.4
  general R27.8
  gluten M35.9 *[G32.81]*
    with celiac disease K90.0 *[G32.81]*
  hereditary G11.9
    with neuropathy G60.2
    cerebellar —*see* Ataxia, cerebellar
    spastic G11.4
    specified NEC G11.8
    spinal (Friedreich's) G11.11
  heredofamilial —*see* Ataxia,
    hereditary
  Hunt's G11.19
  hysterical F44.4
  locomotor (progressive) (syphilitic)
    (partial) (spastic) A52.11
    diabetic —*see* Diabetes, ataxia
  Marie's (cerebellar) (heredofamilial)
    (late- onset) G11.2
  nonorganic origin F44.4
  nonprogressive, congenital G11.0
  psychogenic F44.4
  Roussy-Lévy G60.0
  Sanger-Brown's (hereditary) G11.2
  spastic hereditary G11.4
  spinal
    hereditary (Friedreich's) G11.11
    progressive (syphilitic) A52.11
  spinocerebellar, X-linked recessive
    G11.19
  telangiectasia (Louis-Bar) G11.3

Ataxia-telangiectasia (Louis-Bar)
G11.3

Atelectasis (massive) (partial)
(pressure) (pulmonary) J98.11
newborn P28.10
due to resorption P28.11
partial P28.19
primary P28.0
secondary P28.19
primary (newborn) P28.0
tuberculous —see Tuberculosis,
pulmonary

Atelocardia Q24.9

Atelomyelia Q06.1

Atheroembolism
of
extremities
lower I75.02-
upper I75.01-
kidney I75.81
specified NEC I75.89

Atheroma, atheromatous —see also
Arteriosclerosis I70.90
aorta, aortic I70.0
valve —see also Endocarditis,
aortic I35.8
aorto-iliac I70.0
artery —see Arteriosclerosis
basilar (artery) I67.2
carotid (artery) (common)
(internal) I67.2
cerebral (arteries) I67.2
coronary (artery) I25.10
with angina pectoris —see
Arteriosclerosis, coronary
(artery),
degeneration —see Arteriosclerosis
heart, cardiac —see Disease, heart,
ischemic, atherosclerotic
mitral (valve) I34.8
myocardium, myocardial —see
Disease, heart, ischemic,
atherosclerotic
pulmonary valve (heart) (see also
Endocarditis, pulmonary) I37.8
tricuspid (heart) (valve) I36.8
valve, valvular —see Endocarditis
vertebral (artery) I67.2

Atheromatosis —see Arteriosclerosis

Atherosclerosis —see also
Arteriosclerosis
coronary
artery I25.10
with angina pectoris —see
Arteriosclerosis, coronary
(artery),
due to
calcified coronary lesion
(severely) I25.84
lipid rich plaque I25.83
transplanted heart I25.811
bypass graft I25.812
with angina pectoris —see
Arteriosclerosis, coronary
(artery),
native coronary artery I25.811
with angina pectoris —see
Arteriosclerosis, coronary
(artery),

Athetosis (acquired) R25.8
bilateral (congenital) G80.3
congenital (bilateral) (double) G80.3
double (congenital) G80.3
unilateral R25.8

Athlete's
foot B35.3
heart I51.7

Athrepsia E41

Athyrea (acquired) —see also
Hypothyroidism
congenital E03.1

Atonia, atony, atonic
bladder (sphincter) (neurogenic)
N31.2
capillary I78.8
cecum K59.89
psychogenic F45.8
colon —see Atony, intestine
congenital P94.2
esophagus K22.8
intestine K59.89
psychogenic F45.8
stomach K31.89
neurotic or psychogenic F45.8
uterus (during labor) O62.2
with hemorrhage (postpartum)
O72.1
postpartum (with hemorrhage)
O72.1
without hemorrhage O75.89

Atopy —see History, allergy

Atransferrinemia, congenital
E88.09

Atresia, atretic
alimentary organ or tract NEC
Q45.8
upper Q40.8
ani, anus, anal (canal) Q42.3
with fistula Q42.2
aorta (ring) Q25.29
aortic (orifice) (valve) Q23.0
arch Q25.21
congenital with hypoplasia of
ascending aorta and defective
development of left ventricle
(with mitral stenosis) Q23.4
in hypoplastic left heart
syndrome Q23.4
aqueduct of Sylvius Q03.0
with spina bifida —see Spina
bifida, with hydrocephalus
artery NEC Q27.8
cerebral Q28.3
coronary Q24.5
digestive system Q27.8
eye Q15.8
lower limb Q27.8
pulmonary Q25.5
specified site NEC Q27.8
umbilical Q27.0
upper limb Q27.8
auditory canal (external) Q16.1
bile duct (common) (congenital)
(hepatic) Q44.2
acquired —see Obstruction, bile
duct
bladder (neck) Q64.39
obstruction Q64.31
bronchus Q32.4
cecum Q42.8
cervix (acquired) N88.2
congenital Q51.828
in pregnancy or childbirth —see
Anomaly, cervix, in pregnancy
or childbirth
causing obstructed labor
O65.5
choana Q30.0
colon Q42.9
specified NEC Q42.8
common duct Q44.2
cricoid cartilage Q31.8
cystic duct Q44.2
acquired K82.8
with obstruction K82.0
digestive organs NEC Q45.8

Atresia, atretic (continued)
duodenum Q41.0
ear canal Q16.1
ejaculatory duct Q55.4
epiglottis Q31.8
esophagus Q39.0
with tracheoesophageal fistula
Q39.1
eustachian tube Q17.8
fallopian tube (congenital) Q50.6
acquired N97.1
follicular cyst N83.0-
foramen of
Luschka Q03.1
with spina bifida —see Spina
bifida, with hydrocephalus
Magendie Q03.1
with spina bifida —see Spina
bifida, with hydrocephalus
gallbladder Q44.1
genital organ
external
female Q52.79
male Q55.8
internal
female Q52.8
male Q55.8
glottis Q31.8
gullet Q39.0
with tracheoesophageal fistula
Q39.1
heart valve NEC Q24.8
pulmonary Q22.0
tricuspid Q22.4
hymen Q52.3
acquired (postinfective) N89.6
ileum Q41.2
intestine (small) Q41.9
large Q42.9
specified NEC Q42.8
iris, filtration angle Q15.0
jejunum Q41.1
lacrimal apparatus Q10.4
larynx Q31.8
meatus urinarius Q64.33
mitral valve Q23.2
in hypoplastic left heart
syndrome Q23.4
nares (anterior) (posterior) Q30.0
nasopharynx Q34.8
nose, nostril Q30.0
acquired J34.89
organ or site NEC Q89.8
osseous meatus (ear) Q16.1
oviduct (congenital) Q50.6
acquired N97.1
parotid duct Q38.4
acquired K11.8
pulmonary (artery) Q25.5
valve Q22.0
pulmonic Q22.0
pupil Q13.2
rectum Q42.1
with fistula Q42.0
salivary duct Q38.4
acquired K11.8
sublingual duct Q38.4
acquired K11.8
submandibular duct Q38.4
acquired K11.8
submaxillary duct Q38.4
acquired K11.8
thyroid cartilage Q31.8
trachea Q32.1
tricuspid valve Q22.4
ureter Q62.10
pelvic junction Q62.11
vesical orifice Q62.12
ureteropelvic junction Q62.11
ureterovesical orifice Q62.12

Atresia, atretic (continued)
urethra (valvular) Q64.39
stricture Q64.32
urinary tract NEC Q64.8
uterus Q51.818
acquired N85.8
vagina (congenital) Q52.4
acquired (postinfectional)
(senile) N89.5
vas deferens Q55.3
vascular NEC Q27.8
cerebral Q28.3
digestive system Q27.8
lower limb Q27.8
specified site NEC Q27.8
upper limb Q27.8
vein NEC Q27.8
digestive system Q27.8
great Q26.8
lower limb Q27.8
portal Q26.5
pulmonary Q26.4
partial Q26.3
total Q26.2
specified site NEC Q27.8
upper limb Q27.8
vena cava (inferior) (superior) Q26.8
vesicourethral orifice Q64.31
vulva Q52.79
acquired N90.5

Atrichia, atrichosis —see Alopecia

Atrophia —see also Atrophy
cutis senilis L90.8
due to radiation L57.8
gyrata of choroid and retina H31.23
senilis R54
dermatological L90.8
due to radiation (nonionizing)
(solar) L57.8
unguium L60.3
congenita Q84.6

Atrophie blanche (en plaque)
(de Milian) L95.0

Atrophoderma, atrophodermia (of)
L90.9
diffusum (idiopathic) L90.4
maculatum L90.8
et striatum L90.8
due to syphilis A52.79
syphilitic A51.39
neuriticum L90.8
Pasini and Pierini L90.3
pigmentosum Q82.1
reticulatum symmetricum faciei
L66.4
senile L90.8
due to radiation (nonionizing)
(solar) L57.8
vermiculata (cheeks) L66.4

Atrophy, atrophic (of)
adrenal (capsule) (gland) E27.49
primary (autoimmune) E27.1
alveolar process or ridge
(edentulous) K08.20
anal sphincter (disuse) N81.84
appendix K38.8
arteriosclerotic —see
Arteriosclerosis
bile duct (common) (hepatic) K83.8
bladder N32.89
neurogenic N31.8
blanche (en plaque) (of Milian)
L95.0
bone (senile) NEC —see also
Disorder, bone, specified type
NEC
due to
tabes dorsalis (neurogenic)
A52.11

brain (cortex) (progressive) G31.9
  frontotemporal circumscribed
    G31.01 *[F02.80]*
    with behavioral disturbance
      G31.01 *[F02.81]*
  senile NEC G31.1
breast N64.2
  obstetric —*see* Disorder, breast,
    specified type NEC
buccal cavity K13.79
cardiac —*see* Degeneration,
  myocardial
cartilage (infectional) (joint) —*see*
  Disorder, cartilage, specified
  NEC
cerebellar —*see* Atrophy, brain
cerebral —*see* Atrophy, brain
cervix (mucosa) (senile) (uteri)
  N88.8
  menopausal N95.8
Charcot-Marie-Tooth G60.0
choroid (central) (macular)
  (myopic) (retina) H31.10-
  diffuse secondary H31.12-
  gyrate H31.23
  senile H31.11-
ciliary body —*see* Atrophy, iris
conjunctiva (senile) H11.89
corpus cavernosum N48.89
cortical —*see* Atrophy, brain
cystic duct K82.8
Déjérine-Thomas G23.8
disuse NEC —*see* Atrophy, muscle
Duchenne-Aran G12.21
ear H93.8-
edentulous alveolar ridge K08.20
endometrium (senile) N85.8
  cervix N88.8
enteric K63.89
epididymis N50.89
eyeball —*see* Disorder, globe,
  degenerated condition, atrophy
eyelid (senile) —*see* Disorder,
  eyelid, degenerative
facial (skin) L90.9
fallopian tube (senile) N83.32-
  with ovary N83.33-
fascioscapulohumeral (Landouzy-
  Déjérine) G71.02
fatty, thymus (gland) E32.8
gallbladder K82.8
gastric K29.40
  with bleeding K29.41
gastrointestinal K63.89
glandular I89.8
globe H44.52-
gum -*see* Recession, gingival
hair L67.8
heart (brown) —*see* Degeneration,
  myocardial
hemifacial Q67.4
  Romberg G51.8
infantile E41
  paralysis, acute —*see*
    Poliomyelitis, paralytic
intestine K63.89
iris (essential) (progressive)
  H21.26-
  specified NEC H21.29
kidney (senile) (terminal) (*see also*
  Sclerosis, renal) N26.1
  congenital or infantile Q60.5
    bilateral Q60.4
    unilateral Q60.3
  hydronephrotic —*see*
    Hydronephrosis
lacrimal gland (primary) H04.14-
  secondary H04.15-
Landouzy-Déjérine G71.02

laryngitis, infective J37.0
larynx J38.7
Leber's optic (hereditary) H47.22
lip K13.0
liver (yellow) K72.90
  with coma K72.91
  acute, subacute K72.00
    with coma K72.01
  chronic K72.10
    with coma K72.11
lung (senile) J98.4
macular (dermatological) L90.8
  syphilitic, skin A51.39
    striated A52.79
mandible (edentulous) K08.20
  minimal K08.21
  moderate K08.22
  severe K08.23
maxilla K08.20
  minimal K08.24
  moderate K08.25
  severe K08.26
muscle, muscular (diffuse)
  (general) (idiopathic) (primary)
  M62.50
  ankle M62.57-
  Duchenne-Aran G12.21
  foot M62.57-
  forearm M62.53-
  hand M62.54-
  infantile spinal G12.0
  lower leg M62.56-
  multiple sites M62.59
  myelopathic —*see* Atrophy,
    muscle, spinal
  myotonic G71.11
  neuritic G58.9
  neuropathic (peroneal)
    (progressive) G60.0
  pelvic (disuse) N81.84
  peroneal G60.0
  progressive (bulbar) G12.21
    adult G12.1
    infantile (spinal) G12.0
    spinal G12.25
      adult G12.1
      infantile G12.0
  pseudohypertrophic G71.02
  shoulder region M62.51-
  specified site NEC M62.58
  spinal G12.9
    adult form G12.1
    Aran-Duchenne G12.21
    childhood form, type II G12.1
    distal G12.1
    hereditary NEC G12.1
    infantile, type I (Werdnig-
      Hoffmann) G12.0
    juvenile form, type III
      (Kugelberg- Welander)
      G12.1
    progressive G12.25
    scapuloperoneal form G12.1
    specified NEC G12.8
  syphilitic A52.78
  thigh M62.55-
  upper arm M62.52-
myocardium —*see* Degeneration,
  myocardial
myometrium (senile) N85.8
  cervix N88.8
myopathic NEC —*see* Atrophy,
  muscle
myotonia G71.11
nail L60.3
nasopharynx J31.1
nerve —*see also* Disorder, nerve
  abducens —*see* Strabismus,
    paralytic, sixth nerve
  accessory G52.8

nerve *(continued)*
  acoustic or auditory H93.3
  cranial G52.9
    eighth (auditory) H93.3
    eleventh (accessory) G52.8
    fifth (trigeminal) G50.8
    first (olfactory) G52.0
    fourth (trochlear) —*see*
      Strabismus, paralytic,
      fourth nerve
    second (optic) H47.20
    sixth (abducens) —*see*
      Strabismus, paralytic, sixth
      nerve
    tenth (pneumogastric) (vagus)
      G52.2
    third (oculomotor) —*see*
      Strabismus, paralytic, third
      nerve
    twelfth (hypoglossal) G52.3
  hypoglossal G52.3
  oculomotor —*see* Strabismus,
    paralytic, third nerve
  olfactory G52.0
  optic (papillomacular bundle)
    syphilitic (late) A52.15
      congenital A50.44
  pneumogastric G52.2
  trigeminal G50.8
  trochlear —*see* Strabismus,
    paralytic, fourth nerve
  vagus (pneumogastric) G52.2
neurogenic, bone, tabetic A52.11
nutritional E41
old age R54
olivopontocerebellar G23.8
optic (nerve) H47.20
  glaucomatous H47.23-
  hereditary H47.22
  primary H47.21-
  specified type NEC H47.29-
  syphilitic (late) A52.15
    congenital A50.44
orbit H05.31-
ovary (senile) N83.31-
  with fallopian tube N83.33-
oviduct (senile) —*see* Atrophy,
  fallopian tube
palsy, diffuse (progressive) G12.22
pancreas (duct) (senile) K86.89
parotid gland K11.0
pelvic muscle N81.84
penis N48.89
pharynx J39.2
pluriglandular E31.8
  autoimmune E31.0
polyarthritis M15.9
prostate N42.89
pseudohypertrophic (muscle)
  G71.02
renal (*see also* Sclerosis, renal)
  N26.1
retina, retinal (postinfectional) H35.89
rhinitis J31.0
salivary gland K11.0
scar L90.5
sclerosis, lobar (of brain) G31.09
  [F02.80]
  with behavioral disturbance
    G31.09 *[F02.81]*
scrotum N50.89
seminal vesicle N50.89
senile R54
  due to radiation (nonionizing)
    (solar) L57.8
skin (patches) (spots) L90.9
  degenerative (senile) L90.8
  due to radiation (nonionizing)
    (solar) L57.8
  senile L90.8

spermatic cord N50.89
spinal (acute) (cord) G95.89
  muscular —*see* Atrophy, muscle,
    spinal
  paralysis G12.20
    acute —*see* Poliomyelitis,
      paralytic
    meaning progressive muscular
      atrophy G12.25
spine (column) —*see*
  Spondylopathy, specified NEC
spleen (senile) D73.0
stomach K29.40
  with bleeding K29.41
striate (skin) L90.6
  syphilitic A52.79
subcutaneous L90.9
sublingual gland K11.0
submandibular gland K11.0
submaxillary gland K11.0
Sudeck's —*see*
  Algoneurodystrophy
suprarenal (capsule) (gland) E27.49
  primary E27.1
systemic affecting central nervous
  system
  in
    myxedema E03.9 *[G13.2]*
    neoplastic disease (*see also*
      Neoplasm) D49.9 *[G13.1]*
    specified disease NEC G13.8
tarso-orbital fascia, congenital
  Q10.3
testis N50.0
thenar, partial —*see* Syndrome,
  carpal tunnel
thymus (fatty) E32.8
thyroid (gland) (acquired)
  E03.4
  with cretinism E03.1
  congenital (with myxedema)
    E03.1
tongue (senile) K14.8
  papillae K14.4
trachea J39.8
tunica vaginalis N50.89
turbinate J34.89
tympanic membrane (nonflaccid)
  H73.82-
  flaccid H73.81-
upper respiratory tract J39.8
uterus, uterine (senile) N85.8
  cervix N88.8
  due to radiation (intended effect)
    N85.8
    adverse effect or misadventure
      N99.89
vagina (senile) N95.2
vas deferens N50.89
vascular I99.8
vertebra (senile) —*see*
  Spondylopathy, specified NEC
vulva (senile) N90.5
Werdnig-Hoffmann G12.0
yellow —*see* Failure, hepatic

Attack, attacks
  with alteration of consciousness
    (with automatisms) —*see*
    Epilepsy, localization-related,
    symptomatic, with complex
    partial seizures
  Adams-Stokes I45.9
  akinetic —*see* Epilepsy,
    generalized, specified NEC
  angina —*see* Angina
  atonic —*see* Epilepsy, generalized,
    specified NEC
  benign shuddering G25.83
  cataleptic —*see* Catalepsy

Attack, attacks (continued)
  sp
    coronary —*see* Infarct,
      myocardium
    cyanotic, newborn P28.2
    drop NEC R55
    epileptic —*see* Epilepsy
    heart —*see* infarct, myocardium
    hysterical F44.9
    jacksonian —*see* Epilepsy,
      localization-related,
      symptomatic, with simple partial
      seizures
    myocardium, myocardial —*see*
      Infarct, myocardium
    myoclonic —*see* Epilepsy,
      generalized, specified NEC
    panic F41.0
    psychomotor —*see* Epilepsy,
      localization-related,
      symptomatic, with complex
      partial seizures
    salaam —*see* Epilepsy, spasms
    schizophreniform, brief F23
    shuddering, benign G25.83
    Stokes-Adams I45.9
    syncope R55
    transient ischemic (TIA) G45.9
      specified NEC G45.8
    unconsciousness R55
      hysterical F44.89
    vasomotor R55
    vasovagal (paroxysmal)
      (idiopathic) R55
    without alteration of consciousness
      —*see* Epilepsy, localization-
      related, symptomatic, with
      simple partial seizures

Attention (to)
  artificial
    opening (of) Z43.9
      digestive tract NEC Z43.4
        colon Z43.3
        ilium Z43.2
        stomach Z43.1
      specified NEC Z43.8
      trachea Z43.0
      urinary tract NEC Z43.6
        cystostomy Z43.5
        nephrostomy Z43.6
        ureterostomy Z43.6
        urethrostomy Z43.6
      vagina Z43.7
    colostomy Z43.3
    cystostomy Z43.5
    deficit disorder or syndrome
      F98.8
      with hyperactivity —*see*
        Disorder, attention-deficit
        hyperactivity
    gastrostomy Z43.1
    ileostomy Z43.2
    jejunostomy Z43.4
    nephrostomy Z43.6
    surgical dressings Z48.01
    sutures Z48.02
    tracheostomy Z43.0
    ureterostomy Z43.6
    urethrostomy Z43.6

Attrition
  gum -*see* Recession, gingival
  tooth, teeth (excessive) (hard
    tissues) K03.0

Atypical, atypism —*see also*
  condition
  cells (on cytological smear)
    (endocervical) (endometrial)
    (glandular)
      cervix R87.619
      vagina R87.629

Atypical, atypism (continued)
  cervical N87.9
  endometrium N85.9
    hyperplasia N85.00
  parenting situation Z62.9

Auditory —*see* condition

Aujeszky's disease B33.8

Aurantiasis, cutis E67.1

Auricle, auricular —*see also*
  condition
  cervical Q18.2

Auriculotemporal syndrome
  G50.8

Austin Flint murmur (aortic
  insufficiency) I35.1

Australian
  Q fever A78
  X disease A83.4

Autism, autistic (childhood)
  (infantile) F84.0
  atypical F84.9
  spectrum disorder F84.0

Autodigestion R68.89

Autoerythrocyte sensitization
  (syndrome) D69.2

Autographism L50.3

Autoimmune
  disease (systemic)
    M35.9
  inhibitors to clotting factors
    D68.311
  lymphoproliferative syndrome
    [ALPS] D89.82
  thyroiditis E06.3

Autointoxication R68.89

Automatism G93.89
  with temporal sclerosis
    G93.81
  epileptic —*see* Epilepsy,
    localization-related,
    symptomatic, with complex
    partial seizures
  paroxysmal, idiopathic —*see*
    Epilepsy, localization-related,
    symptomatic, with complex
    partial seizures

Autonomic, autonomous
  bladder (neurogenic) N31.2
  hysteria seizure F44.5

Autosensitivity, erythrocyte
  D69.2

Autosensitization, cutaneous
  L30.2

Autosome —*see* condition by
  chromosome involved

Autotopagnosia R48.1

Autotoxemia R68.89

Autumn —*see* condition

Avellis' syndrome G46.8

Aversion
  oral R63.3
    newborn P92.-
    nonorganic origin F98.2
  sexual F52.1

Aviator's
  disease or sickness —*see* Effect,
    adverse, high altitude
  ear T70.0

Avitaminosis (multiple) (*see also*
  Deficiency, vitamin) E56.9
  B E53.9

Avitaminosis (continued)
  B (continued)
    with
      beriberi E51.11
      pellagra E52
  B2 E53.0
  B6 E53.1
  B12 E53.8
  D E55.9
    with rickets E55.0
  G E53.0
  K E56.1
  nicotinic acid E52

AVNRT (atrioventricular nodal
  re-entrant tachycardia) I47.1

AVRT (atrioventricular nodal
  re-entrant tachycardia) I47.1

Avulsion (traumatic)
  blood vessel —*see* Injury, blood
    vessel
  bone —*see* Fracture, by site
  cartilage —*see also* Dislocation,
    by site
    symphyseal (inner), complicating
      delivery O71.6
  external site other than limb —*see*
    Wound, open, by site
  eye S05.7-
  head (intracranial)
    external site NEC S08.89
    scalp S08.0
  internal organ or site —*see* Injury,
    by site
  joint —*see also* Dislocation, by
    site
    capsule —*see* Sprain, by site
  kidney S37.06-
  ligament —*see* Sprain, by site
  limb —*see also* Amputation,
    traumatic, by site
    skin and subcutaneous tissue
      —*see* Wound, open, by site
  muscle —*see* Injury, muscle
  nerve (root) —*see* Injury, nerve
  scalp S08.0
  skin and subcutaneous tissue —*see*
    Wound, open, by site
  spleen S36.032
  symphyseal cartilage (inner),
    complicating delivery O71.6
  tendon —*see* Injury, muscle
  tooth S03.2

Awareness of heart beat R00.2

Axenfeld's
  anomaly or syndrome Q15.0
  degeneration (calcareous) Q13.4

Axilla, axillary —*see also* condition
  breast Q83.1

Axonotmesis —*see* Injury, nerve

Ayerza's disease or syndrome
  (pulmonary artery sclerosis with
  pulmonary hypertension) I27.0

Azoospermia (organic) N46.01
  due to
    drug therapy N46.021
    efferent duct obstruction N46.023
    infection N46.022
    radiation N46.024
    specified cause NEC N46.029
    systemic disease N46.025

Azotemia R79.89
  meaning uremia N19

Aztec ear Q17.3

Azygos
  continuation inferior vena cava
    Q26.8
  lobe (lung) Q33.1

B

Baastrup's disease —*see* Kissing
  spine

Babesiosis B60.00
  due to
    Babesia
      divergens B60.03
      duncani B60.02
      KO-1 B60.09
      microti B60.01
      MO-1 B60.03
      species
        unspecified B60.00
      venatorum B60.09
    specified NEC B60.09

Babington's disease (familial
  hemorrhagic telangiectasia) I78.0

Babinski's syndrome A52.79

Baby
  crying constantly R68.11
  floppy (syndrome) P94.2

Bacillary —*see* condition

Bacilluria R82.71

Bacillus —*see also* Infection, bacillus
  abortus infection A23.1
  anthracis infection A22.9
  coli infection —*see also*
    Escherichia coli B96.20
  Flexner's A03.1
  mallei infection A24.0
  Shiga's A03.0
  suipestifer infection —*see*
    Infection, salmonella

Back —*see* condition

Backache (postural) M54.9
  sacroiliac M53.3
  specified NEC M54.89

Backflow —*see* Reflux

Backward reading (dyslexia) F81.0

Bacteremia R78.81
  with sepsis —*see* Sepsis

Bactericholia —*see* Cholecystitis,
  acute

Bacterid, bacteride (pustular) L40.3

Bacterium, bacteria, bacterial
  agent NEC, as cause of disease
    classified elsewhere B96.89
  in blood —*see* Bacteremia
  in urine —*see* Bacteriuria

Bacteriuria, bacteruria R82.71
  asymptomatic R82.71

Bacteroides
  fragilis, as cause of disease
    classified elsewhere B96.6

Bad
  heart —*see* Disease, heart
  trip
    due to drug abuse —*see* Abuse,
      drug, hallucinogen
    due to drug dependence
      —*see* Dependence, drug,
      hallucinogen

Baelz's disease (cheilitis glandularis
  apostematosa) K13.0

Baerensprung's disease (eczema
  marginatum) B35.6

Bagasse disease or pneumonitis J67.1

Bagassosis J67.1

Baker's cyst —*see* Cyst, Baker's

Bakwin-Krida syndrome
  (metaphyseal dysplasia) Q78.5

Balancing side interference M26.56

Balanitis (circinata) (erosiva) (gangrenosa) (phagedenic) (vulgaris) N48.1
amebic A06.82
candidal B37.42
due to Haemophilus ducreyi A57
gonococcal (acute) (chronic) A54.23
xerotica obliterans N48.0

Balanoposthitis N47.6
gonococcal (acute) (chronic) A54.23
ulcerative (specific) A63.8

Balanorrhagia —see Balanitis

Balantidiasis, balantidiosis A07.0

Bald tongue K14.4

Baldness —see also Alopecia
male-pattern —see Alopecia, androgenic

Balkan grippe A78

Balloon disease —see Effect, adverse, high altitude

Balo's disease (concentric sclerosis) G37.5

Bamberger-Marie disease —see Osteoarthropathy, hypertrophic, specified type NEC

Bancroft's filariasis B74.0

Band(s)
adhesive —see Adhesions, peritoneum
anomalous or congenital —see also Anomaly, by site
heart (atrial) (ventricular) Q24.8
intestine Q43.3
omentum Q43.3
cervix N88.1
constricting, congenital Q79.8
gallbladder (congenital) Q44.1
intestinal (adhesive) —see Adhesions, peritoneum
obstructive
intestine K56.50
complete K56.52
incomplete K56.51
partial K56.51
peritoneum K56.50
complete K56.52
incomplete K56.51
partial K56.51
periappendiceal, congenital Q43.3
peritoneal (adhesive) —see Adhesions, peritoneum
uterus N73.6
internal N85.6
vagina N89.5

Bandemia D72.825

Bandl's ring (contraction), **complicating delivery** O62.4

Bangkok hemorrhagic fever A91

Bang's disease (brucella abortus) A23.1

Bankruptcy, anxiety concerning Z59.8

Bannister's disease T78.3
hereditary D84.1

Banti's disease or syndrome (with cirrhosis) (with portal hypertension) K76.6

Bar, median, prostate —see Enlargement, enlarged, prostate

Barcoo disease or rot —see Ulcer, skin

Barlow's disease E54

Barodontalgia T70.29

Baron Münchausen syndrome —see Disorder, factitious

Barosinusitis T70.1

Barotitis T70.0

Barotrauma T70.29
odontalgia T70.29
otitic T70.0
sinus T70.1

Barraquer (-Simons) **disease or syndrome** (progressive lipodystrophy) E88.1

Barré-Guillain disease or syndrome G61.0

Barré-Liéou syndrome (posterior cervical sympathetic) M53.0

Barrel chest M95.4

Barrett's
disease —see Barrett's, esophagus
esophagus K22.70
with dysplasia K22.719
high grade K22.711
low grade K22.710
without dysplasia K22.70
syndrome —see Barrett's, esophagus
ulcer K22.10
with bleeding K22.11
without bleeding K22.10

Bársony (-Polgár) (-Teschendorf) **syndrome** (corkscrew esophagus) K22.4

Bartholinitis (suppurating) N75.8
gonococcal (acute) (chronic) (with abscess) A54.1

Barth syndrome E78.71

Bartonellosis A44.9
cutaneous A44.1
mucocutaneous A44.1
specified NEC A44.8
systemic A44.0

Barton's fracture S52.56-

Bartter's syndrome E26.81

Basal —see condition

Basan's (hidrotic) **ectodermal dysplasia** Q82.4

Baseball finger —see Dislocation, finger

Basedow's disease (exophthalmic goiter) —see Hyperthyroidism, with, goiter

Basic —see condition

Basilar —see condition

Bason's (hidrotic) **ectodermal dysplasia** Q82.4

Basopenia —see Agranulocytosis

Basophilia D72.824

Basophilism (cortico-adrenal) (Cushing's) (pituitary) E24.0

Bassen-Kornzweig disease or syndrome E78.6

Bat ear Q17.5

Bateman's
disease B08.1
purpura (senile) D69.2

Bathing cramp T75.1

Bathophobia F40.248

Batten (-Mayou) **disease** E75.4
retina E75.4 [H36]

Batten-Steinert syndrome G71.11

Battered —see Maltreatment

Battey Mycobacterium infection A31.0

Battle exhaustion F43.0

Battledore placenta O43.19-

Baumgarten-Cruveilhier cirrhosis, disease or syndrome K74.69

Bauxite fibrosis (of lung) J63.1

Bayle's disease (general paresis) A52.17

Bazin's disease (primary) (tuberculous) A18.4

Beach ear —see Swimmer's, ear

Beaded hair (congenital) Q84.1

Béal conjunctivitis or syndrome B30.2

Beard's disease (neurasthenia) F48.8

Beat(s)
atrial, premature I49.1
ectopic I49.49
elbow —see Bursitis, elbow
escaped, heart I49.49
hand —see Bursitis, hand
knee —see Bursitis, knee
premature I49.40
atrial I49.1
auricular I49.1
supraventricular I49.1

Beau's
disease or syndrome —see Degeneration, myocardial
lines (transverse furrows on fingernails) L60.4

Bechterev's syndrome —see Spondylitis, ankylosing

Beck's syndrome (anterior spinal artery occlusion) I65.8

Becker's
cardiomyopathy I42.8
disease
idiopathic mural endomyocardial disease I42.3
myotonia congenita, recessive form G71.12
dystrophy G71.01
pigmented hairy nevus D22.5

Beckwith-Wiedemann syndrome Q87.3

Bed confinement status Z74.01

Bed sore —see Ulcer, pressure, by site

Bedbug bite(s) —see Bite(s), by site, superficial, insect

Bedclothes, asphyxiation or suffocation by —see Asphyxia, traumatic, due to, mechanical, trapped

Bednar's
aphthae K12.0
tumor —see Neoplasm, malignant, by site

Bedridden Z74.01

Bedsore —see Ulcer, pressure, by site

Bedwetting —see Enuresis

Bee sting (with allergic or anaphylactic shock) —see Toxicity, venom, arthropod, bee

Beer drinker's heart (disease) I42.6

Begbie's disease (exophthalmic goiter) —see Hyperthyroidism, with, goiter

Behavior
antisocial
adult Z72.811
child or adolescent Z72.810
disorder, disturbance —see Disorder, conduct
disruptive —see Disorder, conduct
drug seeking Z76.5
inexplicable R46.2
marked evasiveness R46.5
obsessive-compulsive R46.81
overactivity R46.3
poor responsiveness R46.4
self-damaging(life-style) Z72.89
sleep-incompatible Z72.821
slowness R46.4
specified NEC R46.89
strange (and inexplicable) R46.2
suspiciousness R46.5
type A pattern Z73.1
undue concern or preoccupation with stressful events R46.6
verbosity and circumstantial detail obscuring reason for contact R46.7

Behçet's disease or syndrome M35.2

Behr's disease —see Degeneration, macula

Beigel's disease or morbus (white piedra) B36.2

Bejel A65

Bekhterev's syndrome —see Spondylitis, ankylosing

Belching —see Eructation

Bell's
mania F30.8
palsy, paralysis G51.0
infant or newborn P11.3
spasm G51.3-

Bence Jones albuminuria or proteinuria NEC R80.3

Bends T70.3

Benedikt's paralysis or syndrome G46.3

Benign —see also condition
prostatic hyperplasia —see Hyperplasia, prostate

Bennett's fracture (displaced) S62.21-

Benson's disease —see Deposit, crystalline

Bent
back (hysterical) F44.4
nose M95.0
congenital Q67.4

Bereavement (uncomplicated) Z63.4

Bergeron's disease (hysterical chorea) F44.4

Berger's disease —see Nephropathy, IgA

Beriberi (dry) E51.11
heart (disease) E51.12
polyneuropathy E51.11
wet E51.12
involving circulatory system E51.11

Berlin's disease or edema (traumatic) S05.8X-

Berlock (berloque) **dermatitis** L56.2

Bernard-Horner syndrome G90.2

Bernard-Soulier disease or thrombopathia D69.1

Bernhardt (-Roth) **disease** —*see* Mononeuropathy, lower limb, meralgia paresthetica

Bernheim's syndrome —*see* Failure, heart, right

Bertielliasis B71.8

Berylliosis (lung) J63.2

Besnier-Boeck (-Schaumann) **disease** —*see* Sarcoidosis

Besnier's
lupus pernio D86.3
prurigo L20.0

Bestiality F65.89

Best's disease H35.50

Beta-mercaptolactate-cysteine disulfiduria E72.09

Betalipoproteinemia, broad or floating E78.2

Betting and gambling Z72.6
pathological (compulsive) F63.0

Bezoar T18.9
intestine T18.3
stomach T18.2

Bezold's abscess —*see* Mastoiditis, acute

Bianchi's syndrome R48.8

Bicornate or bicornis uterus Q51.3
in pregnancy or childbirth O34.00
causing obstructed labor O65.5

Bicuspid aortic valve Q23.1

Biedl-Bardet syndrome Q87.89

Bielschowsky (-Jansky) **disease** E75.4

Biermer's (pernicious) **anemia or disease** D51.0

Biett's disease L93.0

Bifid (congenital)
apex, heart Q24.8
clitoris Q52.6
kidney Q63.8
nose Q30.2
patella Q74.1
scrotum Q55.29
toe NEC Q74.2
tongue Q38.3
ureter Q62.8
uterus Q51.3
uvula Q35.7

Biforis uterus (suprasimplex) Q51.3

Bifurcation (congenital)
gallbladder Q44.1
kidney pelvis Q63.8
renal pelvis Q63.8
rib Q76.6
tongue, congenital Q38.3
trachea Q32.1
ureter Q62.8
urethra Q64.74
vertebra Q76.49

Big spleen syndrome D73.1

Bigeminal pulse R00.8

Bilateral —*see* condition

Bile
duct —*see* condition
pigments in urine R82.2

Bilharziasis —*see also* Schistosomiasis
chyluria B65.0
cutaneous B65.3
galacturia B65.0

Bilharziasis (continued)
hematochyluria B65.0
intestinal B65.1
lipemia B65.9
lipuria B65.0
oriental B65.2
piarhemia B65.9
pulmonary NOS B65.9 [J99]
pneumonia B65.9 [J17]
tropical hematuria B65.0
vesical B65.0

Biliary —*see* condition

Bilirubin metabolism disorder E80.7
specified NEC E80.6

Bilirubinemia, familial nonhemolytic E80.4

Bilirubinuria R82.2

Biliuria R82.2

Bilocular stomach K31.2

Binswanger's disease I67.3

Biparta, bipartite
carpal scaphoid Q74.0
patella Q74.1
vagina Q52.10

Bird
face Q75.8
fancier's disease or lung J67.2

Birt-Hogg-Dube syndrome Q87.89

Birth
complications in mother —*see* Delivery, complicated
compression during NOS P15.9
defect —*see* Anomaly

Birth
immature (less than 37 completed weeks) —*see* Preterm, newborn
extremely (less than 28 completed weeks) —*see* Immaturity, extreme
inattention, at or after —*see* Maltreatment, child, neglect
injury NOS P15.9
basal ganglia P11.1
brachial plexus NEC P14.3
brain (compression) (pressure) P11.2
central nervous system NOS P11.9
cerebellum P11.1
cerebral hemorrhage P10.1
external genitalia P15.5
eye P15.3
face P15.4
fracture
bone P13.9
specified NEC P13.8
clavicle P13.4
femur P13.2
humerus P13.3
long bone, except femur P13.3
radius and ulna P13.3
skull P13.0
spine P11.5
tibia and fibula P13.3
intracranial P11.2
laceration or hemorrhage P10.9
specified NEC P10.8
intraventricular hemorrhage P10.2
laceration
brain P10.1
by scalpel P15.8
peripheral nerve P14.9
liver P15.0
meninges
brain P11.1
spinal cord P11.5

Birth (continued)
injury (continued)
nerve
brachial plexus P14.3
cranial NEC (except facial) P11.4
facial P11.3
peripheral P14.9
phrenic (paralysis) P14.2
paralysis
facial nerve P11.3
spinal P11.5
penis P15.5
rupture
spinal cord P11.5
scalp P12.9
scalpel wound P15.8
scrotum P15.5
skull NEC P13.1
fracture P13.0
specified type NEC P15.8
spinal cord P11.5
spine P11.5
spleen P15.1
sternomastoid (hematoma) P15.2
subarachnoid hemorrhage P10.3
subcutaneous fat necrosis P15.6
subdural hemorrhage P10.0
tentorial tear P10.4
testes P15.5
vulva P15.5
lack of care, at or after —*see* Maltreatment, child, neglect
neglect, at or after —*see* Maltreatment, child, neglect
palsy or paralysis, newborn, NOS (birth injury) P14.9
premature (infant) —*see* Preterm, newborn
shock, newborn P96.89
trauma —*see* Birth, injury
weight
low (2499 grams or less) —*see* Low, birthweight
extremely (999 grams or less) —*see* Low, birthweight, extreme
4000 grams to 4499 grams P08.1
4500 grams or more P08.0

Birthmark Q82.5

Bisalbuminemia E88.09

Biskra's button B55.1

Bite(s) (animal) (human)
abdomen, abdominal
wall S31.159
with penetration into peritoneal cavity S31.659
epigastric region S31.152
with penetration into peritoneal cavity S31.652
left
lower quadrant S31.154
with penetration into peritoneal cavity S31.654
upper quadrant S31.151
with penetration into peritoneal cavity S31.651
periumbilic region S31.155
with penetration into peritoneal cavity S31.655
right
lower quadrant S31.153
with penetration into peritoneal cavity S31.653
upper quadrant S31.150
with penetration into peritoneal cavity S31.650

Bite (continued)
abdomen, abdominal (continued)
wall (continued)
superficial NEC S30.871
insect S30.861
alveolar (process) —*see* Bite, oral cavity
amphibian (venomous) —*see* Venom, bite, amphibian
animal —*see also* Bite, by site
venomous —*see* Venom
ankle S91.05-
superficial NEC S90.57-
insect S90.56-
antecubital space —*see* Bite, elbow
anus S31.835
superficial NEC S30.877
insect S30.867
arm (upper) S41.15-
lower —*see* Bite, forearm
superficial NEC S40.87-
insect S40.86-
arthropod NEC —*see* Venom, bite, arthropod
auditory canal (external) (meatus) —*see* Bite, ear
auricle, ear —*see* Bite, ear
axilla —*see* Bite, arm
back —*see also* Bite, thorax, back
lower S31.050
with penetration into retroperitoneal space S31.051
superficial NEC S30.870
insect S30.860
bedbug —*see* Bite(s), by site, superficial, insect
breast S21.05-
superficial NEC S20.17-
insect S20.16-
brow —*see* Bite, head, specified site NEC
buttock S31.805
left S31.825
right S31.815
superficial NEC S30.870
insect S30.860
calf —*see* Bite, leg
canaliculus lacrimalis —*see* Bite, eyelid
canthus, eye —*see* Bite, eyelid
centipede —*see* Toxicity, venom, arthropod, centipede
cheek (external) S01.45-
superficial NEC S00.87
insect S00.86
internal —*see* Bite, oral cavity
chest wall —*see* Bite, thorax
chigger B88.0
chin —*see* Bite, head, specified site NEC
clitoris —*see* Bite, vulva
costal region —*see* Bite, thorax
digit(s)
hand —*see* Bite, finger
toe —*see* Bite, toe
ear (canal) (external) S01.35-
superficial NEC S00.47-
insect S00.46-
elbow S51.05-
superficial NEC S50.37-
insect S50.36-
epididymis —*see* Bite, testis
epigastric region —*see* Bite, abdomen
epiglottis —*see* Bite, neck, specified site NEC
esophagus, cervical S11.25
superficial NEC S10.17
insect S10.16
eyebrow —*see* Bite, eyelid

Black
death A20.9
eye S00.1-
hairy tongue K14.3
heel (foot) S90.3-
lung (disease) J60
palm (hand) S60.22-

Blackfan-Diamond anemia or syndrome (congenital hypoplastic anemia) D61.01

Blackhead L70.0

Blackout R55

Bladder —see condition

Blast (air) (hydraulic) (immersion) (underwater)
blindness S05.8X-
injury
abdomen or thorax —see Injury, by site
ear (acoustic nerve trauma)
—see Injury, nerve, acoustic, specified type NEC
syndrome NEC T70.8

Blastoma —see Neoplasm, malignant, by site
pulmonary —see Neoplasm, lung, malignant

Blastomycosis, blastomycotic B40.9
Brazilian —see Paracoccidioidomycosis
cutaneous B40.3
disseminated B40.7
European —see Cryptococcosis
generalized B40.7
keloidal B48.0
North American B40.9
primary pulmonary B40.0
pulmonary B40.2
acute B40.0
chronic B40.1
skin B40.3
South American —see Paracoccidioidomycosis
specified NEC B40.89

Bleb(s) R23.8
emphysematous (lung) (solitary) J43.9
endophthalmitis H59.43
filtering (vitreous), after glaucoma surgery Z98.83
inflamed (infected), postprocedural H59.40
stage 1 H59.41
stage 2 H59.42
stage 3 H59.43
lung (ruptured) J43.9
congenital —see Atelectasis
newborn P25.8
subpleural (emphysematous) J43.9

Blebitis, postprocedural H59.40
stage 1 H59.41
stage 2 H59.42
stage 3 H59.43

Bleeder (familial) (hereditary) —see Hemophilia

Bleeding —see also Hemorrhage
anal K62.5
anovulatory N97.0
atonic, following delivery O72.1
capillary I78.8
puerperal O72.2
contact (postcoital) N93.0
due to uterine subinvolution N85.3

Bleeding (continued)
ear —see Otorrhagia
excessive, associated with menopausal onset N92.4
familial —see Defect, coagulation
following intercourse N93.0
gastrointestinal K92.2
hemorrhoids —see Hemorrhoids
intermenstrual (regular) N92.3
irregular N92.1
intraoperative —see Complication, intraoperative, hemorrhage
irregular N92.6
menopausal N92.4
newborn, intraventricular
—see Newborn, affected by, hemorrhage, intraventricular
nipple N64.59
nose R04.0
ovulation N92.3
perimenopausal N92.4
pre-pubertal vaginal N93.1
postclimacteric N95.0
postcoital N93.0
postmenopausal N95.0
postoperative —see Complication, postprocedural, hemorrhage
preclimacteric N92.4
puberty (excessive, with onset of menstrual periods) N92.2
rectum, rectal K62.5
newborn P54.2
tendencies —see Defect, coagulation
throat R04.1
tooth socket (post-extraction) K91.840
umbilical stump P51.9
uterus, uterine NEC N93.9
climacteric N92.4
dysfunctional or functional N93.8
menopausal N92.4
preclimacteric or premenopausal N92.4
unrelated to menstrual cycle N93.9
vagina, vaginal (abnormal) N93.9
dysfunctional or functional N93.8
newborn P54.6
pre-pubertal N93.1
vicarious N94.89

Blennorrhagia, blennorrhagic —see Gonorrhea

Blennorrhea (acute) (chronic) —see also Gonorrhea
inclusion (neonatal) (newborn) P39.1
lower genitourinary tract (gonococcal) A54.00
neonatorum (gonococcal ophthalmia) A54.31

Blepharelosis —see Entropion

Blepharitis (angularis) (ciliaris) (eyelid) (marginal) (nonulcerative) H01.009
herpes zoster B02.39
left H01.006
lower H01.005
upper H01.004
upper and lower H01.00B
right H01.003
lower H01.002
upper H01.001
upper and lower H01.00A
squamous H01.029
left H01.026
lower H01.025
upper H01.024
upper and lower H01.02B

Blepharitis (continued)
squamous (continued)
right H01.023
lower H01.022
upper H01.021
upper and lower H01.02A
ulcerative H01.019
left H01.016
lower H01.015
upper H01.014
upper and lower H01.01B
right H01.013
lower H01.012
upper H01.011
upper and lower H01.01A

Blepharochalasis H02.30
congenital Q10.0
left H02.36
lower H02.35
upper H02.34
right H02.33
lower H02.32
upper H02.31

Blepharoclonus H02.59

Blepharoconjunctivitis H10.50-
angular H10.52-
contact H10.53-
ligneous H10.51-

Blepharophimosis (eyelid) H02.529
congenital Q10.3
left H02.526
lower H02.525
upper H02.524
right H02.523
lower H02.522
upper H02.521

Blepharoptosis H02.40-
congenital Q10.0
mechanical H02.41-
myogenic H02.42-
neurogenic H02.43-
paralytic H02.43-

Blepharopyorrhea, gonococcal A54.39

Blepharospasm G24.5
drug induced G24.01

Blighted ovum O02.0

Blind —see also Blindness
bronchus (congenital) Q32.4
loop syndrome K90.2
congenital Q43.8
sac, fallopian tube (congenital) Q50.6
spot, enlarged —see Defect, visual field, localized, scotoma, blind spot area
tract or tube, congenital NEC —see Atresia, by site

Blindness (acquired) (congenital) (both eyes) H54.0X-
blast S05.8X-
color —see Deficiency, color vision
concussion S05.8X-
cortical H47.619
left brain H47.612
right brain H47.611
day H53.11
due to injury (current episode) S05.9-
sequelae -- code to injury with seventh character S
eclipse (total) —see Retinopathy, solar
emotional (hysterical) F44.6
face H53.16
hysterical F44.6
legal (both eyes) (USA definition) H54.8
mind R48.8

Blindness (continued)
night H53.60
abnormal dark adaptation curve H53.61
acquired H53.62
congenital H53.63
specified type NEC H53.69
vitamin A deficiency E50.5
one eye (other eye normal) H54.40
left (normal vision on right) H54.42-
low vision on right H54.12-
low vision, other eye H54.10
right (normal vision on left) H54.41-
low vision on left H54.11-
psychic R48.8
river B73.01
snow —see Photokeratitis
sun, solar —see Retinopathy, solar
transient —see Disturbance, vision, subjective, loss, transient
traumatic (current episode) S05.9-
word (developmental) F81.0
acquired R48.0
secondary to organic lesion R48.0

Blister (nonthermal)
abdominal wall S30.821
alveolar process S00.522
ankle S90.52-
antecubital space —see Blister, elbow
anus S30.827
arm (upper) S40.82-
auditory canal —see Blister, ear
auricle —see Blister, ear
axilla —see Blister, arm
back, lower S30.820
beetle dermatitis L24.89
breast S20.12-
brow S00.82
calf —see Blister, leg
canthus —see Blister, eyelid
cheek S00.82
internal S00.522
chest wall —see Blister, thorax
chin S00.82
costal region —see Blister, thorax
digit(s)
foot —see Blister, toe
hand —see Blister, finger
due to burn —see Burn, by site, second degree
ear S00.42-
elbow S50.32-
epiglottis S10.12
esophagus, cervical S10.12
eyebrow —see Blister, eyelid
eyelid S00.22-
face S00.82
fever B00.1
finger(s) S60.429
index S60.42-
little S60.42-
middle S60.42-
ring S60.42-
foot (except toe(s) alone) S90.82-
toe —see Blister, toe
forearm S50.82-
elbow only —see Blister, elbow
forehead S00.82
fracture - omit code
genital organ
female S30.826
male S30.825
gum S00.522
hand S60.52-
head S00.92
ear —see Blister, ear
eyelid —see Blister, eyelid

Blister (continued)
  lip S00.521
  nose S00.32
  oral cavity S00.522
  scalp S00.02
  specified site NEC S00.82
  heel —see Blister, foot
  hip S70.22-
  interscapular region S20.429
  jaw S00.82
  knee S80.22-
  larynx S10.12
  leg (lower) S80.82-
    knee —see Blister, knee
    upper —see Blister, thigh
  lip S00.521
  malar region S00.82
  mammary —see Blister, breast
  mastoid region S00.82
  mouth S00.522
  multiple, skin, nontraumatic R23.8
  nail
    finger —see Blister, finger
    toe —see Blister, toe
  nasal S00.32
  neck S10.92
    specified site NEC S10.82
    throat S10.12
  nose S00.32
  occipital region S00.02
  oral cavity S00.522
  orbital region —see Blister, eyelid
  palate S00.522
  palm —see Blister, hand
  parietal region S00.02
  pelvis S30.820
  penis S30.822
  periocular area —see Blister, eyelid
  phalanges
    finger —see Blister, finger
    toe —see Blister, toe
  pharynx S10.12
  pinna —see Blister, ear
  popliteal space —see Blister, knee
  scalp S00.02
  scapular region —see Blister, shoulder
  scrotum S30.823
  shin —see Blister, leg
  shoulder S40.22-
  sternal region S20.329
  submaxillary region S00.82
  submental region S00.82
  subungual
    finger(s) —see Blister, finger
    toe(s) —see Blister, toe
  supraclavicular fossa S10.82
  supraorbital S00.82
  temple S00.82
  temporal region S00.82
  testis S30.823
  thermal —see Burn, second degree, by site
  thigh S70.32-
  thorax, thoracic (wall) S20.92
    back S20.42-
    front S20.32-
  throat S10.12
  thumb S60.32-
  toe(s) S90.42-
    great S90.42-
  tongue S00.522
  trachea S10.12
  tympanum, tympanic membrane —see Blister, ear
  upper arm —see Blister, arm (upper)
  uvula S00.522
  vagina S30.824
  vocal cords S10.12
  vulva S30.824
  wrist S60.82-

Bloating R14.0

Bloch-Sulzberger disease or syndrome Q82.3

Block, blocked
  alveolocapillary J84.10
  arborization (heart) I45.5
  arrhythmic I45.9
  atrioventricular (incomplete) (partial) I44.30
    with atrioventricular dissociation I44.2
    complete I44.2
      congenital Q24.6
    congenital Q24.6
    first degree I44.0
    second degree (types I and II) I44.1
    specified NEC I44.39
    third degree I44.2
    types I and II I44.1
  auriculoventricular —see Block, atrioventricular
  bifascicular (cardiac) I45.2
  bundle-branch (complete) (false) (incomplete) I45.4
    bilateral I45.2
    left I44.7
      with right bundle branch block I45.2
      hemiblock I44.60
        anterior I44.4
        posterior I44.5
      incomplete I44.7
        with right bundle branch block I45.2
    right I45.10
      with
        left bundle branch block I45.2
        left fascicular block I45.2
      specified NEC I45.19
    Wilson's type I45.19
  cardiac I45.9
  conduction I45.9
    complete I44.2
  fascicular (left) I44.60
    anterior I44.4
    posterior I44.5
    right I45.0
    specified NEC I44.69
  foramen Magendie (acquired) G91.1
    congenital Q03.1
      with spina bifida —see Spina bifida, by site, with hydrocephalus
  heart I45.9
    bundle branch I45.4
      bilateral I45.2
    complete (atrioventricular) I44.2
    congenital Q24.6
    first degree (atrioventricular) I44.0
    second degree (atrioventricular) I44.1
    specified type NEC I45.5
    third degree (atrioventricular) I44.2
  hepatic vein I82.0
  intraventricular (nonspecific) I45.4
    bundle branch
      bilateral I45.2
  kidney N28.9
    postcystoscopic or postprocedural N99.0
  Mobitz (types I and II) I44.1
  myocardial —see Block, heart
  nodal I45.5
  organ or site, congenital NEC —see Atresia, by site
  portal (vein) I81

Block, blocked (continued)
  second degree (types I and II) I44.1
  sinoatrial I45.5
  sinoauricular I45.5
  third degree I44.2
  trifascicular I45.3
  tubal N97.1
  vein NOS I82.90
  Wenckebach (types I and II) I44.1

Blockage —see Obstruction

Blocq's disease F44.4

Blood
  constituents, abnormal R78.9
  disease D75.9
  donor —see Donor, blood
  dyscrasia D75.9
    with
      abortion —see Abortion, by type, complicated by, hemorrhage
      ectopic pregnancy O08.1
      molar pregnancy O08.1
    following ectopic or molar pregnancy O08.1
    newborn P61.9
    puerperal, postpartum O72.3
  flukes NEC —see Schistosomiasis
  in
    feces K92.1
      occult R19.5
    urine —see Hematuria
  mole O02.0
  occult in feces R19.5
  pressure
    decreased, due to shock following injury T79.4
    examination only Z01.30
    fluctuating I99.8
    high —see Hypertension
      borderline R03.0
      incidental reading, without diagnosis of hypertension R03.0
    low —see also Hypotension
      incidental reading, without diagnosis of hypotension R03.1
  spitting —see Hemoptysis
  staining cornea —see Pigmentation, cornea, stromal
  transfusion
    reaction or complication —see Complications, transfusion
  type
    A (Rh positive) Z67.10
      Rh negative Z67.11
    AB (Rh positive) Z67.30
      Rh negative Z67.31
    B (Rh positive) Z67.20
      Rh negative Z67.21
    O (Rh positive) Z67.40
      Rh negative Z67.41
    Rh (positive) Z67.90
      negative Z67.91
  vessel rupture —see Hemorrhage
  vomiting —see Hematemesis

Blood-forming organs, disease D75.9

Bloodgood's disease —see Mastopathy, cystic

Bloom (-Machacek) (-Torre) syndrome Q82.8

Blount disease or osteochondrosis M92.51-

Blue
  baby Q24.9
  diaper syndrome E72.09

Blue (continued)
  dome cyst (breast) —see Cyst, breast
  dot cataract Q12.0
  nevus D22.9
  sclera Q13.5
    with fragility of bone and deafness Q78.0
  toe syndrome I75.02-

Blueness —see Cyanosis

Blues, postpartal O90.6
  baby O90.6

Blurring, visual H53.8

Blushing (abnormal) (excessive) R23.2

BMI —see Body, mass index

Boarder, hospital NEC Z76.4
  accompanying sick person Z76.3
  healthy infant or child Z76.2
    foundling Z76.1

Bockhart's impetigo L01.02

Bodechtel-Guttman disease (subacute sclerosing panencephalitis) A81.1

Boder-Sedgwick syndrome (ataxia-telangiectasia) G11.3

Body, bodies
  Aschoff's —see Myocarditis, rheumatic
  asteroid, vitreous —see Deposit, crystalline
  cytoid (retina) —see Occlusion, artery, retina
  drusen (degenerative) (macula) (retinal) —see also Degeneration, macula, drusen
    optic disc —see Drusen, optic disc
  foreign —see Foreign body
  loose
    joint, except knee —see Loose, body, joint
      knee M23.4-
    sheath, tendon —see Disorder, tendon, specified type NEC
  mass index (BMI)
    adult
      19.9 or less Z68.1
      20.0-20.9 Z68.20
      21.0-21.9 Z68.21
      22.0-22.9 Z68.22
      23.0-23.9 Z68.23
      24.0-24.9 Z68.24
      25.0-25.9 Z68.25
      26.0-26.9 Z68.26
      27.0-27.9 Z68.27
      28.0-28.9 Z68.28
      29.0-29.9 Z68.29
      30.0-30.9 Z68.30
      31.0-31.9 Z68.31
      32.0-32.9 Z68.32
      33.0-33.9 Z68.33
      34.0-34.9 Z68.34
      35.0-35.9 Z68.35
      36.0-36.9 Z68.36
      37.0-37.9 Z68.37
      38.0-38.9 Z68.38
      39.0-39.9 Z68.39
      40.0-44.9 Z68.41
      45.0-49.9 Z68.42
      50.0-59.9 Z68.43
      60.0-69.9 Z68.44
      70 and over Z68.45
    pediatric
      5th percentile to less than 85th percentile for age Z68.52
      85th percentile to less than 95th percentile for age Z68.53

Body, bodies (continued)
  mass index (continued)
    pediatric (continued)
      greater than or equal to ninety-
        fifth percentile for age
        Z68.54
      less than fifth percentile for
        age Z68.51
    Mooser's A75.2
    rice —see also Loose, body, joint
      knee M23.4-
    rocking F98.4

Boeck's
  disease or sarcoid —see
    Sarcoidosis
  lupoid (miliary) D86.3

Boerhaave's syndrome (spontaneous
  esophageal rupture) K22.3

Boggy
  cervix N88.8
  uterus N85.8

Boil —see also Furuncle, by site
  Aleppo B55.1
  Baghdad B55.1
  Delhi B55.1
  lacrimal
    gland —see Dacryoadenitis
    passages (duct) (sac) —see
      Inflammation, lacrimal,
      passages, acute
  Natal B55.1
  orbit, orbital —see Abscess, orbit
  tropical B55.1

Bold hives —see Urticaria

Bombé, iris —see Membrane,
  pupillary

Bone —see condition

Bonnevie-Ullrich syndrome
  (see also Turner's syndrome)
  Q87.19

Bonnier's syndrome —see
  subcategory H81.8

Bonvale dam fever T73.3

Bony block of joint —see Ankylosis

BOOP (bronchiolitis obliterans
  organized pneumonia) J84.89

Borderline
  diabetes mellitus R73.03
  hypertension R03.0
  osteopenia M85.8-
  pelvis, with obstruction during
    labor O65.1
  personality F60.3

Borna disease A83.9

Bornholm disease B33.0

Boston exanthem A88.0

Botalli, ductus (patent) (persistent)
  Q25.0

Bothriocephalus latus infestation
  B70.0

Botulism (foodborne intoxication)
  A05.1
  infant A48.51
  non-foodborne A48.52
  wound A48.52

Bouba —see Yaws

Bouchard's nodes (with arthropathy)
  M15.2

Bouffée délirante F23

Bouillaud's disease or syndrome
  (rheumatic heart disease) I01.9

Bourneville's disease Q85.1

Boutonniere deformity (finger)
  —see Deformity, finger,
  boutonniere

Bouveret (-Hoffmann) syndrome
  (paroxysmal tachycardia) I47.9

Bovine heart —see Hypertrophy,
  cardiac

Bowel —see condition

Bowen's
  dermatosis (precancerous) —see
    Neoplasm, skin, in situ
  disease —see Neoplasm, skin, in
    situ
  epithelioma —see Neoplasm, skin,
    in situ
  type
    epidermoid carcinoma-in-situ
      —see Neoplasm, skin, in situ
    intraepidermal squamous cell
      carcinoma —see Neoplasm,
      skin, in situ

Bowing
  femur —see also Deformity, limb,
    specified type NEC, thigh
    congenital Q68.3
  fibula —see also Deformity, limb,
    specified type NEC, lower leg
    congenital Q68.4
  forearm —see Deformity, limb,
    specified type NEC, forearm
  leg(s), long bones, congenital Q68.5
  radius —see Deformity, limb,
    specified type NEC, forearm
  tibia —see also Deformity, limb,
    specified type NEC, lower leg
    congenital Q68.4

Bowleg(s) (acquired) M21.16-
  congenital Q68.5
  rachitic E64.3

Boyd's dysentery A03.2

Brachial —see condition

Brachycardia R00.1

Brachycephaly Q75.0

Bradley's disease A08.19

Bradyarrhythmia, cardiac I49.8

Bradycardia (sinoatrial) (sinus)
  (vagal) R00.1
  neonatal P29.12
  reflex G90.09
  tachycardia syndrome I49.5

Bradykinesia R25.8

Bradypnea R06.89

Bradytachycardia I49.5

**Brailsford's disease or
  osteochondrosis** —see
  Osteochondrosis, juvenile, radius

Brain —see also condition
  death G93.82
  syndrome —see Syndrome, brain

**Branched-chain amino-acid
  disorder** E71.2

Branchial —see condition
  cartilage, congenital Q18.2

Branchiogenic remnant (in neck)
  Q18.0

Brandt's syndrome (acrodermatitis
  enteropathica) E83.2

Brash (water) R12

Bravais-jacksonian epilepsy —see
  Epilepsy, localization-related,
  symptomatic, with simple partial
  seizures

Braxton Hicks contractions —see
  False, labor

Brazilian leishmaniasis B55.2

BRBPR K62.5

Break, retina (without detachment)
  H33.30-
  with retinal detachment —see
    Detachment, retina
  horseshoe tear H33.31-
  multiple H33.33-
  round hole H33.32-

Breakdown
  device, graft or implant —see also
    Complications, by site and type,
    mechanical T85.618
    arterial graft NEC —see
      Complication, cardiovascular
      device, mechanical, vascular
    breast (implant) T85.41
    catheter NEC T85.618
      cystostomy T83.010
      dialysis (renal) T82.41
        intraperitoneal T85.611
      Hopkins T83.018
      ileostomy T83.018
      infusion NEC T82.514
        cranial T85.610
        epidural T85.610
        intrathecal T85.610
        spinal T85.610
        subarachnoid T85.610
        subdural T85.610
      nephrostomy T83.012
      urethral indwelling T83.011
      urinary NEC T83.018
      urostomy T83.018
    electronic (electrode) (pulse
      generator) (stimulator)
      bone T84.310
      cardiac T82.119
        electrode T82.110
        pulse generator T82.111
        specified type NEC T82.118
      nervous system —see
        Complication, prosthetic
        device, mechanical,
        electronic nervous system
        stimulator
      urinary —see Complication,
        genitourinary, device,
        urinary, mechanical
    fixation, internal (orthopedic)
      NEC —see Complication,
      fixation device, mechanical
    gastrointestinal —see
      Complications, prosthetic
      device, mechanical,
      gastrointestinal device
    genital NEC T83.418
      intrauterine contraceptive
        device T83.31
      penile prosthesis (cylinder)
        (implanted) (pump)
        (resevoir) T83.410
      testicular prosthesis T83.411
    heart NEC —see Complication,
      cardiovascular device,
      mechanical
    intrathecal infusion pump
      T85.615
    joint prosthesis —see
      Complications..., joint
      prosthesis,internal,
      mechanical, by site
    nervous system, specified device
      NEC T85.615
    ocular NEC —see Complications,
      prosthetic device, mechanical,
      ocular device

Breakdown (continued)
  device, graft or implant (continued)
    orthopedic NEC —see
      Complication, orthopedic,
      device, mechanical
    specified NEC T85.618
    subcutaneous device pocket
      nervous system prosthetic
      device, implant, or graft
      T85.890
    other internal prosthetic
      device, implant or graft
      T85.898
    sutures, permanent T85.612
      used in bone repair —see
        Complications, fixation
        device, internal
        (orthopedic), mechanical
    urinary NEC T83.118
      graft T83.21
      sphincter, implanted T83.111
      stent (ileal conduit)
        (nephroureteral) T83.113
      ureteral indwelling T83.112
    vascular NEC —see
      Complication, cardiovascular
      device, mechanical
    ventricular intracranial shunt
      T85.01
  nervous F48.8
  perineum O90.1
  respirator J95.850
    specified NEC J95.859
    ventilator J95.850
    specified NEC J95.859

Breast —see also condition
  buds E30.1
    in newborn P96.89
  dense R92.2
  nodule (see also Lump, breast)
    N63.0

Breath
  foul R19.6
  holder, child R06.89
  holding spell R06.89
  shortness R06.02

Breathing
  labored —see Hyperventilation
  mouth R06.5
    causing malocclusion M26.5
  periodic R06.3
    high altitude G47.32

Breathlessness R06.81

Breda's disease —see Yaws

Breech presentation (mother) O32.1
  causing obstructed labor O64.1
  footling O32.8
    causing obstructed labor O64.8
  incomplete O32.8
    causing obstructed labor O64.8

Breisky's disease N90.4

Brennemann's syndrome I88.0

Brenner
  tumor (benign) D27.9
    borderline malignancy D39.1-
    malignant C56
    proliferating D39.1-

Bretonneau's disease or angina
  A36.0

Breus' mole O02.0

Brevicollis Q76.49

Brickmakers' anemia B76.9 [D63.8]

Bridge, myocardial Q24.5

Bright red blood per rectum
  (BRBPR) K62.5

Bright's disease —*see also*
  Nephritis
  arteriosclerotic —*see* Hypertension,
    kidney

Brill (-Zinsser) disease (recrudescent
  typhus) A75.1

Brill-Symmers' disease C82.90

Brion-Kayser disease —*see* Fever,
  parathyroid

Briquet's disorder or syndrome
  F45.0

Brissaud's
  infantilism or dwarfism E23.0
  motor-verbal tic F95.2

Brittle
  bones disease Q78.0
  nails L60.3
    congenital Q84.6

Broad —*see also* condition
  beta disease E78.2
  ligament laceration syndrome
    N83.8

**Broad- or floating-
  betalipoproteinemia** E78.2

Brock's syndrome (atelectasis due to
  enlarged lymph nodes) J98.19

Brocq-Duhring disease (dermatitis
  herpetiformis) L13.0

Brodie's abscess or disease
  M86.8X-

Broken
  arches —*see also* Deformity, limb,
    flat foot
  arm (meaning upper limb) —*see*
    Fracture, arm
  back —*see* Fracture, vertebra
  bone —*see* Fracture
  implant or internal device —*see*
    Complications, by site and type,
    mechanical
  leg (meaning lower limb) —*see*
    Fracture, leg
  nose S02.2
  tooth, teeth —*see* Fracture, tooth

Bromhidrosis, bromidrosis L75.0

Bromidism, bromism G92
  due to
    correct substance properly
      administered —*see* Table
      of Drugs and Chemicals, by
      drug, adverse effect
    overdose or wrong substance
      given or taken —*see* Table
      of Drugs and Chemicals, by
      drug, poisoning
  chronic (dependence) F13.20

Bromidrosiphobia F40.298

Bronchi, bronchial
  —*see* condition

Bronchiectasis (cylindrical) (diffuse)
  (fusiform) (localized) (saccular)
  J47.9
  with
    acute
      bronchitis J47.0
      lower respiratory infection
        J47.0
    exacerbation (acute) J47.1
  congenital Q33.4
  tuberculous NEC —*see*
    Tuberculosis, pulmonary

Bronchiolectasis —*see*
  Bronchiectasis

Bronchiolitis (acute) (infective)
  (subacute) J21.9

Bronchiolitis *(continued)*
  with
    bronchospasm or obstruction
      J21.9
    influenza, flu or grippe —*see*
      Influenza, with, respiratory
      manifestations NEC
  chemical (chronic) J68.4
    acute J68.0
  chronic (fibrosing) (obliterative)
    J44.9
  due to
    external agent —*see* Bronchitis,
      acute, due to
    human metapneumovirus
      J21.1
    respiratory syncytial virus (RSV)
      J21.0
    specified organism NEC J21.8
  fibrosa obliterans J44.9
  influenzal —*see* Influenza, with,
    respiratory manifestations NEC
  obliterans J42
    with organizing pneumonia
      (BOOP) J84.89
  obliterative (chronic) (subacute)
    J44.9
    due to fumes or vapors J68.4
    due to chemicals, gases, fumes
      or vapors (inhalation) J68.4
  respiratory, interstitial lung disease
    J84.115

Bronchitis (diffuse) (fibrinous)
  (hypostatic) (infective)
  (membranous) J40
  with
    influenza, flu or grippe —*see*
      Influenza, with, respiratory
      manifestations NEC
    obstruction (airway) (lung) J44.9
    tracheitis (15 years of age and
      above) J40
      acute or subacute J20.9
      chronic J42
      under 15 years of age J20.9
  acute or subacute (with bronchos-
    pasm or obstruction) J20.9
    with
      bronchiectasis J47.0
      chronic obstructive pulmonary
        disease J44.0
    chemical (due to gases, fumes or
      vapors) J68.0
    due to
      fumes or vapors J68.0
      Haemophilus influenzae J20.1
      Mycoplasma pneumoniae J20.0
      radiation J70.0
      specified organism NEC J20.8
      Streptococcus J20.2
      virus
        coxsackie J20.3
        echovirus J20.7
        parainfluenzae J20.4
        respiratory syncytial (RSV)
          J20.5
        rhinovirus J20.6
    viral NEC J20.8
  allergic (acute) J45.909
    with
      exacerbation (acute) J45.901
      status asthmaticus J45.902
  arachidic T17.528
  aspiration (due to food and vomit)
    J69.0
  asthmatic J45.9
    chronic J44.9
      with
        acute lower respiratory
          infection J44.0
        exacerbation (acute) J44.1

Bronchitis *(continued)*
  capillary —*see* Pneumonia, broncho
  caseous (tuberculous) A15.5
  Castellani's A69.8
  catarrhal (15 years of age and
    above) J40
    acute —*see* Bronchitis, acute
    chronic J41.0
    under 15 years of age J20.9
  chemical (acute) (subacute) J68.0
    chronic J68.4
    due to fumes or vapors J68.0
      chronic J68.4
  chronic J42
    with
      airways obstruction J44.9
      tracheitis (chronic) J42
    asthmatic (obstructive) J44.9
    catarrhal J41.0
    chemical (due to fumes or
      vapors) J68.4
    due to
      chemicals, gases, fumes or
        vapors (inhalation) J68.4
      radiation J70.1
      tobacco smoking J41.0
    emphysematous J44.9
    mucopurulent J41.1
    non-obstructive J41.0
    obliterans J44.9
    obstructive J44.9
    purulent J41.1
    simple J41.0
  croupous —*see* Bronchitis, acute
  due to gases, fumes or vapors
    (chemical) J68.0
  emphysematous (obstructive) J44.9
  exudative —*see* Bronchitis, acute
  fetid J41.1
  grippal —*see* Influenza, with,
    respiratory manifestations NEC
  in those under 15 years age —*see*
    Bronchitis, acute
    chronic —*see* Bronchitis, chronic
  influenzal —*see* Influenza, with,
    respiratory manifestations NEC
  mixed simple and mucopurulent
    J41.8
  moulder's J62.8
  mucopurulent (chronic) (recurrent)
    J41.1
    acute or subacute J20.9
    simple (mixed) J41.8
  obliterans (chronic) J44.9
  obstructive (chronic) (diffuse)
    J443.9
  pituitous J41.1
  pneumococcal, acute or subacute
    J20.2
  pseudomembranous, acute or
    subacute —*see* Bronchitis,
    acute
  purulent (chronic) (recurrent) J41.1
    acute or subacute —*see*
      Bronchitis, acute
  putrid J41.1
  senile (chronic) J42
  simple and mucopurulent (mixed)
    J41.8
  smokers' J41.0
  spirochetal NEC A69.8
  subacute —*see* Bronchitis, acute
  suppurative (chronic) J41.1
    acute or subacute —*see*
      Bronchitis, acute
  tuberculous A15.5
  under 15 years of age —*see*
    Bronchitis, acute
    chronic —*see* Bronchitis, chronic
  viral NEC, acute or subacute —*see
    also* Bronchitis, acute J20.8

Bronchoalveolitis J18.0

Bronchoaspergillosis B44.1

Bronchocele meaning goiter E04.0

Broncholithiasis J98.09
  tuberculous NEC A15.5

Bronchomalacia J98.09
  congenital Q32.2

Bronchomycosis NOS B49 *[J99]*
  candidal B37.1

Bronchopleuropneumonia —*see*
  Pneumonia, broncho

Bronchopneumonia —*see*
  Pneumonia, broncho

Bronchopneumonitis —*see*
  Pneumonia, broncho

Bronchopulmonary —*see* condition

Bronchopulmonitis —*see*
  Pneumonia, broncho

Bronchorrhagia (*see* Hemoptysis)

Bronchorrhea J98.09
  acute J20.9
  chronic (infective) (purulent) J42

Bronchospasm (acute) J98.01
  with
    bronchiolitis, acute J21.9
    bronchitis, acute (conditions in
      J20) —*see* Bronchitis, acute
  due to external agent —*see* condition,
    respiratory, acute, due to
  exercise induced J45.990

Bronchospirochetosis A69.8
  Castellani A69.8

Bronchostenosis J98.09

Bronchus —*see* condition

Brontophobia F40.220

Bronze baby syndrome P83.88

Brooke's tumor —*see* Neoplasm,
  skin, benign

Brown enamel of teeth (hereditary)
  K00.5

Brown's sheath syndrome H50.61-

**Brown-Séquard disease, paralysis
  or syndrome** G83.81

Bruce sepsis A23.0

Brucellosis (infection) A23.9
  abortus A23.1
  canis A23.3
  dermatitis A23.9
  melitensis A23.0
  mixed A23.8
  sepsis A23.9
    melitensis A23.0
    specified NEC A23.8
  suis A23.2

Bruck-de Lange disease Q87.19

Bruck's disease —*see* Deformity,
  limb

**BRUE (brief resolved unexplained
  event)** R68.13

Brugsch's syndrome Q82.8

Bruise (skin surface intact) —*see
  also* Contusion
  with
    open wound —*see* Wound, open
  internal organ —*see* Injury, by site
  newborn P54.5
  scalp, due to birth injury, newborn
    P12.3
  umbilical cord O69.5

Bruit (arterial) R09.89
  cardiac R01.1

Brush burn —*see* Abrasion,
  by site

Bruton's X-linked agammaglobulinemia D80.0

Bruxism
psychogenic F45.8
sleep related G47.63

Bubbly lung syndrome P27.0

Bubo I88.8
blennorrhagic (gonococcal) A54.89
chancroidal A57
climatic A55
due to Haemophilus ducreyi A57
gonococcal A54.89
indolent (nonspecific) I88.8
inguinal (nonspecific) I88.8
chancroidal A57
climatic A55
due to H. ducreyi A57
infective I88.8
scrofulous (tuberculous) A18.2
soft chancre A57
suppurating —see Lymphadenitis, acute
syphilitic (primary) A51.0
congenital A50.07
tropical A55
virulent (chancroidal) A57

Bubonic plague A20.0

Bubonocele —see Hernia, inguinal

Buccal —see condition

Buchanan's disease or osteochondrosis M91.0

Buchem's syndrome (hyperostosis corticalis) M85.2

Bucket-handle fracture or tear (semilunar cartilage) —see Tear, meniscus

Budd-Chiari syndrome (hepatic vein thrombosis) I82.0

Budgerigar fancier's disease or lung J67.2

Buds
breast E30.1
in newborn P96.89

Buerger's disease (thromboangiitis obliterans) I73.1

Bulbar —see condition

Bulbus cordis (left ventricle) (persistent) Q21.8

Bulimia (nervosa) F50.2
atypical F50.9
normal weight F50.9

Bulky
stools R19.5
uterus N85.2

Bulla (e) R23.8
lung (emphysematous) (solitary) J43.9
newborn P25.8

Bullet wound —see also Wound, open
fracture - code as Fracture, by site
internal organ —see Injury, by site

Bundle
branch block (complete) (false) (incomplete) —see Block, bundle-branch
of His —see condition

Bunion M21.61-
tailor's M21.62-

Bunionette M21.62-

Buphthalmia, buphthalmos (congenital) Q15.0

Burdwan fever B55.0

Bürger-Grütz disease or syndrome E78.3

Buried
penis (congenital) Q55.64
acquired N48.83
roots K08.3

Burke's syndrome K86.89

Burkitt
cell leukemia C91.0-
lymphoma (malignant) C83.7-
small noncleaved, diffuse C83.7-
spleen C83.77
undifferentiated C83.7-
tumor C83.7-
type
acute lymphoblastic leukemia C91.0-
undifferentiated C83.7-

Burn (electricity) (flame) (hot gas, liquid or hot object) (radiation) (steam) (thermal) T30.0
abdomen, abdominal (muscle) (wall) T21.02
first degree T21.12
second degree T21.22
third degree T21.32
above elbow T22.039
first degree T22.139
left T22.032
first degree T22.132
second degree T22.232
third degree T22.332
right T22.031
first degree T22.131
second degree T22.231
third degree T22.331
second degree T22.239
third degree T22.339
acid (caustic) (external) (internal) —see Corrosion, by site
alimentary tract NEC T28.2
esophagus T28.1
mouth T28.0
pharynx T28.0
alkaline (caustic) (external) (internal) —see Corrosion, by site
ankle T25.019
first degree T25.119
left T25.012
first degree T25.112
second degree T25.212
third degree T25.312
multiple with foot —see Burn, lower, limb, multiple, ankle and foot
right T25.011
first degree T25.111
second degree T25.211
third degree T25.311
second degree T25.219
third degree T25.319
anus —see Burn, buttock
arm (lower) (upper) —see Burn, upper, limb
axilla T22.049
first degree T22.149
left T22.042
first degree T22.142
second degree T22.242
third degree T22.342
right T22.041
first degree T22.141
second degree T22.241
third degree T22.341
second degree T22.249
third degree T22.349
back (lower) T21.04
first degree T21.14

Burn (continued)
back (continued)
second degree T21.24
third degree T21.34
upper T21.03
first degree T21.13
second degree T21.23
third degree T21.33
blisters - code as Burn, second degree, by site
breast(s) —see Burn, chest wall
buttock(s) T21.05
first degree T21.15
second degree T21.25
third degree T21.35
calf T24.039
first degree T24.139
left T24.032
first degree T24.132
second degree T24.232
third degree T24.332
right T24.031
first degree T24.131
second degree T24.231
third degree T24.331
second degree T24.239
third degree T24.339
canthus (eye) —see Burn, eyelid
caustic acid or alkaline —see Corrosion, by site
cervix T28.3
cheek T20.06
first degree T20.16
second degree T20.26
third degree T20.36
chemical (acids) (alkalines) (caustics) (external) (internal) —see Corrosion, by site
chest wall T21.01
first degree T21.11
second degree T21.21
third degree T21.31
chin T20.03
first degree T20.13
second degree T20.23
third degree T20.33
colon T28.2
conjunctiva (and cornea) —see Burn, cornea
cornea (and conjunctiva) T26.1-
chemical —see Corrosion, cornea
corrosion (external) (internal) —see Corrosion, by site
deep necrosis of underlying tissue - code as Burn, third degree, by site
dorsum of hand T23.069
first degree T23.169
left T23.062
first degree T23.162
second degree T23.262
third degree T23.362
right T23.061
first degree T23.161
second degree T23.261
third degree T23.361
second degree T23.269
third degree T23.369
due to ingested chemical agent —see Corrosion, by site
ear (auricle) (external) (canal) T20.01
first degree T20.11
second degree T20.21
third degree T20.31
elbow T22.029
first degree T22.129
left T22.022
first degree T22.122
second degree T22.222
third degree T22.322

Burn (continued)
elbow (continued)
right T22.021
first degree T22.121
second degree T22.221
third degree T22.321
second degree T22.229
third degree T22.329
epidermal loss - code as Burn, second degree, by site
erythema, erythematous - code as Burn, first degree, by site
esophagus T28.1
extent (percentage of body surface)
less than 10 percent T31.0
10-19 percent T31.10
with 0-9 percent third degree burns T31.10
with 10-19 percent third degree burns T31.11
20-29 percent T31.20
with 0-9 percent third degree burns T31.20
with 10-19 percent third degree burns T31.21
with 20-29 percent third degree burns T31.22
30-39 percent T31.30
with 0-9 percent third degree burns T31.30
with 10-19 percent third degree burns T31.31
with 20-29 percent third degree burns T31.32
with 30-39 percent third degree burns T31.33
40-49 percent T31.40
with 0-9 percent third degree burns T31.40
with 10-19 percent third degree burns T31.41
with 20-29 percent third degree burns T31.42
with 30-39 percent third degree burns T31.43
with 40-49 percent third degree burns T31.44
50-59 percent T31.50
with 0-9 percent third degree burns T31.50
with 10-19 percent third degree burns T31.51
with 20-29 percent third degree burns T31.52
with 30-39 percent third degree burns T31.53
with 40-49 percent third degree burns T31.54
with 50-59 percent third degree burns T31.55
60-69 percent T31.60
with 0-9 percent third degree burns T31.60
with 10-19 percent third degree burns T31.61
with 20-29 percent third degree burns T31.62
with 30-39 percent third degree burns T31.63
with 40-49 percent third degree burns T31.64
with 50-59 percent third degree burns T31.65
with 60-69 percent third degree burns T31.66
70-79 percent T31.70
with 0-9 percent third degree burns T31.70

45

Burn *(continued)*
 extent *(continued)*
  70-79 percent *(continued)*
   with 10-19 percent third
    degree burns T31.71
   with 20-29 percent third
    degree burns T31.72
   with 30-39 percent third
    degree burns T31.73
   with 40-49 percent third
    degree burns T31.74
   with 50-59 percent third
    degree burns T31.75
   with 60-69 percent third
    degree burns T31.76
   with 70-79 percent third
    degree burns T31.77
  80-89 percent T31.80
   with 0-9 percent
    third degree burns
    T31.80
   with 10-19 percent third
    degree burns T31.81
   with 20-29 percent third
    degree burns T31.82
   with 30-39 percent third
    degree burns T31.83
   with 40-49 percent third
    degree burns T31.84
   with 50-59 percent third
    degree burns T31.85
   with 60-69 percent third
    degree burns T31.86
   with 70-79 percent third
    degree burns T31.87
   with 80-89 percent third
    degree burns T31.88
  90 percent or more T31.90
   with 0-9 percent third degree
    burns T31.90
   with 10-19 percent third
    degree burns T31.91
   with 20-29 percent third
    degree burns T31.92
   with 30-39 percent third
    degree burns T31.93
   with 40-49 percent third
    degree burns T31.94
   with 50-59 percent third
    degree burns T31.95
   with 60-69 percent third
    degree burns T31.96
   with 70-79 percent third
    degree burns T31.97
   with 80-89 percent third
    degree burns T31.98
   with 90 percent or more third
    degree burns T31.99
 extremity —*see* Burn, limb
 eye(s) and adnexa T26.4-
  with resulting rupture and
   destruction of eyeball T26.2-
  conjunctival sac —*see* Burn,
   cornea
  cornea —*see* Burn, cornea
  lid —*see* Burn, eyelid
  periocular area —*see* Burn, eyelid
  specified site NEC T26.3-
 eyeball —*see* Burn, eye
 eyelid(s) T26.0-
  chemical —*see* Corrosion, eyelid
 face —*see* Burn, head
 finger T23.029
  first degree T23.129
  left T23.022
   first degree T23.122
   second degree T23.222
   third degree T23.322
  multiple sites (without thumb)
   T23.039
   with thumb T23.049

Burn *(continued)*
 finger *(continued)*
  multiple sites *(continued)*
   with thumb *(continued)*
    first degree T23.149
    left T23.042
     first degree T23.142
     second degree T23.242
     third degree T23.342
    right T23.041
     first degree T23.141
     second degree T23.241
     third degree T23.341
    second degree T23.249
    third degree T23.349
   first degree T23.139
   left T23.032
    first degree T23.132
    second degree T23.232
    third degree T23.332
   right T23.031
    first degree T23.131
    second degree T23.231
    third degree T23.331
   second degree T23.239
   third degree T23.339
  right T23.021
   first degree T23.121
   second degree T23.221
   third degree T23.321
  second degree T23.229
  third degree T23.329
 flank —*see* Burn, abdominal wall
 foot T25.029
  first degree T25.129
  left T25.022
   first degree T25.122
   second degree T25.222
   third degree T25.322
  multiple with ankle —*see* Burn,
   lower, limb, multiple, ankle
   and foot
  right T25.021
   first degree T25.121
   second degree T25.221
   third degree T25.321
  second degree T25.229
  third degree T25.329
 forearm T22.019
  first degree T22.119
  left T22.012
   first degree T22.112
   second degree T22.212
   third degree T22.312
  right T22.011
   first degree T22.111
   second degree T22.211
   third degree T22.311
  second degree T22.219
  third degree T22.319
 forehead T20.06
  first degree T20.16
  second degree T20.26
  third degree T20.36
 fourth degree - code as Burn, third
  degree, by site
 friction —*see* Burn, by site
 from swallowing caustic or
  corrosive substance NEC —*see*
  Corrosion, by site
 full thickness skin loss - code as
  Burn, third degree, by site
 gastrointestinal tract NEC T28.2
  from swallowing caustic or
   corrosive substance T28.7
 genital organs
  external
   female T21.07
    first degree T21.17
    second degree T21.27
    third degree T21.37

Burn *(continued)*
 genital organs *(continued)*
  external *(continued)*
   male T21.06
    first degree T21.16
    second degree T21.26
    third degree T21.36
  internal T28.3
   from caustic or corrosive
    substance T28.8
 groin —*see* Burn, abdominal wall
 hand(s) T23.009
  back —*see* Burn, dorsum of hand
  finger —*see* Burn, finger
  first degree T23.109
  left T23.002
   first degree T23.102
   second degree T23.202
   third degree T23.302
  multiple sites with wrist T23.099
   first degree T23.199
   left T23.092
    first degree T23.192
    second degree T23.292
    third degree T23.392
   right T23.091
    first degree T23.191
    second degree T23.291
    third degree T23.391
   second degree T23.299
   third degree T23.399
  palm —*see* Burn, palm
  right T23.001
   first degree T23.101
   second degree T23.201
   third degree T23.301
  second degree T23.209
  third degree T23.309
  thumb —*see* Burn, thumb
 head (and face) (and neck) T20.00
  cheek —*see* Burn, cheek
  chin —*see* Burn, chin
  ear —*see* Burn, ear
  eye(s) only —*see* Burn, eye
  first degree T20.10
  forehead —*see* Burn, forehead
  lip —*see* Burn, lip
  multiple sites T20.09
   first degree T20.19
   second degree T20.29
   third degree T20.39
  neck —*see* Burn, neck
  nose —*see* Burn, nose
  scalp —*see* Burn, scalp
  second degree T20.20
  third degree T20.30
 hip(s) —*see* Burn, thigh
 inhalation —*see* Burn, respiratory
  tract
  caustic or corrosive substance
   (fumes) —*see* Corrosion,
   respiratory tract
 internal organ(s) T28.40
  alimentary tract T28.2
   esophagus T28.1
  eardrum T28.41
  esophagus T28.1
  from caustic or corrosive
   substance (swallowing) NEC
   —*see* Corrosion, by site
  genitourinary T28.3
  mouth T28.0
  pharynx T28.0
  respiratory tract —*see* Burn,
   respiratory tract
  specified organ NEC T28.49
  interscapular region —*see* Burn,
   back, upper
  intestine (large) (small) T28.2
 knee T24.029
  first degree T24.129

Burn *(continued)*
 knee *(continued)*
  left T24.022
   first degree T24.122
   second degree T24.222
   third degree T24.322
  right T24.021
   first degree T24.121
   second degree T24.221
   third degree T24.321
  second degree T24.229
  third degree T24.329
 labium (majus) (minus) —*see*
  Burn, genital organs, external,
  female
 lacrimal apparatus, duct, gland or
  sac —*see* Burn, eye, specified
  site NEC
 larynx T27.0
  with lung T27.1
 leg(s) (lower) (upper) —*see* Burn,
  lower, limb
 lightning —*see* Burn, by site
 limb(s)
  lower (except ankle or foot
   alone) —*see* Burn, lower,
   limb
  upper —*see* Burn, upper limb
 lip(s) T20.02
  first degree T20.12
  second degree T20.22
  third degree T20.32
 lower
  back —*see* Burn, back
  limb T24.009
   ankle —*see* Burn, ankle
   calf —*see* Burn, calf
   first degree T24.109
   foot —*see* Burn, foot
   hip —*see* Burn, thigh
   knee —*see* Burn, knee
   left T24.002
    first degree T24.102
    second degree T24.202
    third degree T24.302
   multiple sites, except ankle
    and foot T24.099
    ankle and foot T25.099
     first degree T25.199
     left T25.092
      first degree T25.192
      second degree T25.292
      third degree T25.392
     right T25.091
      first degree T25.191
      second degree T25.291
      third degree T25.391
     second degree T25.299
     third degree T25.399
    first degree T24.199
    left T24.092
     first degree T24.192
     second degree T24.292
     third degree T24.392
    right T24.091
     first degree T24.191
     second degree T24.291
     third degree T24.391
    second degree T24.299
    third degree T24.399
   right T24.001
    first degree T24.101
    second degree T24.201
    third degree T24.301
   second degree T24.209
   thigh —*see* Burn, thigh
   third degree T24.309
   toe —*see* Burn, toe
 lung (with larynx and trachea)
  T27.1
 mouth T28.0

Burn (continued)

upper limb (continued)
  multiple sites (continued)
    left (continued)
      first degree T22.192
      second degree T22.292
      third degree T22.392
      right T22.091
        first degree T22.191
        second degree T22.291
        third degree T22.391
      second degree T22.299
      third degree T22.399
    scapular region —see Burn, scapular region
    second degree T22.20
    shoulder —see Burn, shoulder
    third degree T22.30
    wrist —see Burn, wrist
uterus T28.3
vagina T28.3
vulva —see Burn, genital organs, external, female
wrist T23.079
  first degree T23.179
  left T23.072
    first degree T23.172
    second degree T23.272
    third degree T23.372
  multiple sites with hand T23.099
    first degree T23.199
    left T23.092
      first degree T23.192
      second degree T23.292
      third degree T23.392
    right T23.091
      first degree T23.191
      second degree T23.291
      third degree T23.391
    second degree T23.299
    third degree T23.399
  right T23.071
    first degree T23.171
    second degree T23.271
    third degree T23.371
  second degree T23.279
  third degree T23.379

Burnett's syndrome E83.52

Burning
  feet syndrome E53.9
  sensation R20.8
  tongue K14.6

Burn-out (state) Z73.0

Burns' disease or osteochondrosis —see Osteochondrosis, juvenile, ulna

Bursa —see condition

Bursitis M71.9
  Achilles —see Tendinitis, Achilles
  adhesive —see Bursitis, specified NEC
  ankle —see Enthesopathy, lower limb, ankle, specified type NEC
  calcaneal —see Enthesopathy, foot, specified type NEC
  collateral ligament, tibial —see Bursitis, tibial collateral
  due to use, overuse, pressure —see also Disorder, soft tissue, due to use, specified type NEC
  specified NEC —see Disorder, soft tissue, due to use, specified NEC
  Duplay's M75.0
  elbow NEC M70.3-
    olecranon M70.2-
  finger —see Disorder, soft tissue, due to use, specified type NEC, hand
  foot —see Enthesopathy, foot, specified type NEC

Burn (continued)

gonococcal A54.49
gouty —see Gout
hand M70.1-
hip NEC M70.7-
  trochanteric M70.6-
infective NEC M71.10
  abscess —see Abscess, bursa
  ankle M71.17-
  elbow M71.12-
  foot M71.17-
  hand M71.14-
  hip M71.15-
  knee M71.16-
  multiple sites M71.19
  shoulder M71.11-
  specified site NEC M71.18
  wrist M71.13-
ischial —see Bursitis, hip
knee NEC M70.5-
  prepatellar M70.4-
occupational NEC —see also Disorder, soft tissue, due to, use
olecranon —see Bursitis, elbow, olecranon
pharyngeal J39.1
popliteal —see Bursitis, knee
prepatellar M70.4-
radiohumeral M77.8
rheumatoid M06.20
  ankle M06.27-
  elbow M06.22-
  foot joint M06.27-
  hand joint M06.24-
  hip M06.25-
  knee M06.26-
  multiple site M06.29
  shoulder M06.21-
  vertebra M06.28
  wrist M06.23-
scapulohumeral —see Bursitis, shoulder
semimembranous muscle (knee) —see Bursitis, knee
shoulder M75.5-
  adhesive —see Capsulitis, adhesive

Bursitis M71.9
specified NEC M71.50
  ankle M71.57-
  due to use, overuse or pressure —see Disorder, soft tissue, due to, use
  elbow M71.52-
  foot M71.57-
  hand M71.54-
  hip M71.55-
  knee M71.56-
  shoulder —see Bursitis, shoulder
  specified site NEC M71.58
  tibial collateral M76.4-
  wrist M71.53-
subacromial —see Bursitis, shoulder
subcoracoid —see Bursitis, shoulder
subdeltoid —see Bursitis, shoulder
syphilitic A52.78
Thornwaldt, Tornwaldt J39.2
tibial collateral M76.4-
toe —see Enthesopathy, foot, specified type NEC
trochanteric (area) —see Bursitis, hip, trochanteric
wrist —see Bursitis, hand

Bursopathy M71.9
specified type NEC M71.80
  ankle M71.87-
  elbow M71.82-
  foot M71.87-

Bursopathy (continued)

specified type NEC (continued)
  hand M71.84-
  hip M71.85-
  knee M71.86-
  multiple sites M71.89
  shoulder M71.81-
  specified site NEC M71.88
  wrist M71.83-

Burst stitches or sutures
  (complication of surgery) T81.31
  external operation wound T81.31
  internal operation wound T81.32

Buruli ulcer A31.1

Bury's disease L95.1

Buschke's
  disease —see Cryptococcosis by site
  scleredema —see Sclerosis, systemic

Busse-Buschke disease —see Cryptococcosis by site

Buttock —see condition

Button
  Biskra B55.1
  Delhi B55.1
  oriental B55.1

Buttonhole deformity (finger) —see Deformity, finger, boutonniere

Bwamba fever A92.8

Byssinosis J66.0

Bywaters' syndrome T79.5

C

Cachexia R64
  cancerous R64
  cardiac —see Disease, heart
  dehydration E86.0
  due to malnutrition R64
  exophthalmic —see Hyperthyroidism
  heart —see Disease, heart
  hypophyseal E23.0
  hypopituitary E23.0
  lead —see Poisoning, lead
  malignant R64
  marsh —see Malaria
  nervous F48.8
  old age R54
  paludal —see Malaria
  pituitary E23.0
  renal N28.9
  saturnine —see Poisoning, lead
  senile R54
  Simmonds' E23.0
  splenica D73.0
  strumipriva E03.4
  tuberculous NEC —see Tuberculosis

CADASIL (cerebral autosomal dominant arteriopathy with subcortical infarcts and leukoencephalopathy) I67.850

Café, au lait spots L81.3

Caffeine-induced
  anxiety disorder F15.980
  sleep disorder F15.982

Caffey's syndrome Q78.8

Caisson disease T70.3

Cake kidney Q63.1

Caked breast (puerperal, postpartum) O92.79

Calabar swelling B74.3

Calcaneal spur —see Spur, bone, calcaneal

Calcaneo-apophysitis M92.8

Calcareous —see condition

Calcicosis J62.8

Calciferol (vitamin D) **deficiency** E55.9
  with rickets E55.0

Calcification
  adrenal (capsule) (gland) E27.49
    tuberculous E35 [B90.8]
  aorta I70.0
  artery (annular) —see Arteriosclerosis
  auricle (ear) —see Disorder, pinna, specified type NEC
  basal ganglia G23.8
  bladder N32.89
    due to Schistosoma hematobium B65.0
  brain (cortex) —see Calcification, cerebral
  bronchus J98.09
  bursa M71.40
    ankle M71.47-
    elbow M71.42-
    foot M71.47-
    hand M71.44-
    hip M71.45-
    knee M71.46-
    multiple sites M71.49
    shoulder M75.3-
    specified site NEC M71.48
    wrist M71.43-
  cardiac —see Degeneration, myocardial
  cerebral (cortex) G93.89
    artery I67.2
  cervix (uteri) N88.8
  choroid plexus G93.89
  conjunctiva —see Concretion, conjunctiva
  corpora cavernosa (penis) N48.89
  cortex (brain) —see Calcification, cerebral
  dental pulp (nodular) K04.2
  dentinal papilla K00.4
  fallopian tube N83.8
  falx cerebri G96.198
  gallbladder K82.8
  general E83.59
  heart —see also Degeneration, myocardial
    valve —see Endocarditis
  idiopathic infantile arterial (IIAC) Q28.8
  intervertebral cartilage or disc (postinfective) —see Disorder, disc, specified NEC
  intracranial —see Calcification, cerebral
  joint —see Disorder, joint, specified type NEC
  kidney N28.89
    tuberculous N29 [B90.1]
  larynx (senile) J38.7
  lens —see Cataract, specified NEC
  lung (active) (postinfectional) J98.4
    tuberculous B90.9
  lymph gland or node (postinfectional) I89.8
    tuberculous (see also Tuberculosis, lymph gland) B90.8
  mammographic R92.1
  massive (paraplegic) —see Myositis, ossificans, in, quadriplegia
  medial —see Arteriosclerosis, extremities

Calcification (continued)

meninges (cerebral) (spinal) G96.198
metastatic E83.59
Mönckeberg's —see Arteriosclerosis, extremities
muscle M61.9
  due to burns —see Myositis, ossificans, in, burns
  paralytic —see Myositis, ossificans, in, quadriplegia
  specified type NEC M61.40
    ankle M61.47-
    foot M61.47-
    forearm M61.43-
    hand M61.44-
    lower leg M61.46-
    multiple sites M61.49
    pelvic region M61.45-
    shoulder region M61.41-
    specified site NEC M61.48
    thigh M61.45-
    upper arm M61.42-
myocardium, myocardial —see Degeneration, myocardial
ovary N83.8
pancreas K86.89
penis N48.89
periarticular —see Disorder, joint, specified type NEC
pericardium —see also Pericarditis I31.1
pineal gland E34.8
pleura J94.8
  postinfectional J94.8
  tuberculous NEC B90.9
pulpal (dental) (nodular) K04.2
sclera H15.89
spleen D73.89
subcutaneous L94.2
suprarenal (capsule) (gland) E27.49
tendon (sheath) —see also Tenosynovitis, specified type NEC
  with bursitis, synovitis or tenosynovitis —see Tendinitis, calcific
trachea J39.8
ureter N28.89
uterus N85.8
vitreous —see Deposit, crystalline

Calcified —see Calcification

Calcinosis (interstitial) (tumoral) (universalis) E83.59
with Raynaud's phenomenon, esophageal dysfunction, sclerodactyly, telangiectasia (CREST syndrome) M34.1
circumscripta (skin) L94.2
cutis L94.2

Calciphylaxis —see also Calcification, by site E83.59

Calcium
deposits —see Calcification, by site
metabolism disorder E83.50
salts or soaps in vitreous —see Deposit, crystalline

Calciuria R82.994

Calculi —see Calculus

Calculosis, intrahepatic —see Calculus, bile duct

Calculus, calculi, calculous
ampulla of Vater —see Calculus, bile duct
anuria (impacted) (recurrent) —see also Calculus, urinary N20.9
appendix K38.1
bile duct (common) (hepatic) K80.50

Calculus, calculi, calculous (continued)

bile duct (continued)
  with
    calculus of gallbladder —see Calculus, gallbladder and bile duct
    cholangitis K80.30
      with
        cholecystitis —see Calculus, bile duct, with cholecystitis
        obstruction K80.31
      acute K80.32
        with
          chronic cholangitis K80.36
            with obstruction K80.37
          obstruction K80.33
      chronic K80.34
        with
          acute cholangitis K80.36
            with obstruction K80.37
          obstruction K80.35
    cholecystitis (with cholangitis) K80.40
      with obstruction K80.41
      acute K80.42
        with
          chronic cholecystitis K80.46
            with obstruction K80.47
          obstruction K80.43
      chronic K80.44
        with
          acute cholecystitis K80.46
            with obstruction K80.47
          obstruction K80.45
    obstruction K80.51
biliary —see also Calculus, gallbladder
  specified NEC K80.80
    with obstruction K80.81
bilirubin, multiple —see Calculus, gallbladder
bladder (encysted) (impacted) (urinary) (diverticulum) N21.0
bronchus J98.09
calyx (kidney) (renal) —see Calculus, kidney
cholesterol (pure) (solitary) —see Calculus, gallbladder
common duct (bile) —see Calculus, bile duct
conjunctiva —see Concretion, conjunctiva
cystic N21.0
  duct —see Calculus, gallbladder
dental (subgingival) (supragingival) K03.6
diverticulum
  bladder N21.0
  kidney N20.0
epididymis N50.89
gallbladder K80.20
  with
    bile duct calculus —see Calculus, gallbladder and bile duct
    cholecystitis K80.10
      with obstruction K80.11
      acute K80.00
        with
          chronic cholecystitis K80.12
            with obstruction K80.13
          obstruction K80.01

Calculus, calculi, calculous (continued)

gallbladder (continued)
  with (continued)
    cholecystitis (continued)
      chronic K80.10
        with
          acute cholecystitis K80.12
            with obstruction K80.13
          obstruction K80.11
      specified NEC K80.18
        with obstruction K80.19
      obstruction K80.21
gallbladder and bile duct K80.70
  with
    cholecystitis K80.60
      with obstruction K80.61
      acute K80.62
        with
          chronic cholecystitis K80.66
            with obstruction K80.67
          obstruction K80.63
      chronic K80.64
        with
          acute cholecystitis K80.66
            with obstruction K80.67
          obstruction K80.65
    obstruction K80.71
hepatic (duct) —see Calculus, bile duct
hepatobiliary K80.80
  with obstruction K80.81
ileal conduit N21.8
intestinal (impaction) (obstruction) K56.49
kidney (impacted) (multiple) (pelvis) (recurrent) (staghorn) N20.0
  with calculus, ureter N20.2
  congenital Q63.8
lacrimal passages —see Dacryolith
liver (impacted) —see Calculus, bile duct
lung J98.4
mammographic R92.1
nephritic (impacted) (recurrent) —see Calculus, kidney
nose J34.89
pancreas (duct) K86.89
parotid duct or gland K11.5
pelvis, encysted —see Calculus, kidney
prostate N42.0
pulmonary J98.4
pyelitis (impacted) (recurrent) N20.0
  with hydronephrosis N13.6
pyelonephritis (impacted) (recurrent) N20
  with hydronephrosis N13.6
renal (impacted) (recurrent) —see Calculus, kidney
salivary (duct) (gland) K11.5
seminal vesicle N50.89
staghorn —see Calculus, kidney
Stensen's duct K11.5
stomach K31.89
sublingual duct or gland K11.5
  congenital Q38.4
submandibular duct, gland or region K11.5
submaxillary duct, gland or region K11.5
suburethral N21.8
tonsil J35.8
tooth, teeth (subgingival) (supragingival) K03.6

Calculus, calculi, calculous (continued)

tunica vaginalis N50.89
ureter (impacted) (recurrent) N20.1
  with calculus, kidney N20.2
    with hydronephrosis N13.2
      with infection N13.6
ureteropelvic junction N20.1
urethra (impacted) N21.1
urinary (duct) (impacted) (passage) (tract) N20.9
  with hydronephrosis N13.2
    with infection N13.6
  in (due to)
  lower N21.9
    specified NEC N21.8
vagina N89.8
vesical (impacted) N21.0
Wharton's duct K11.5
xanthine E79.8 [N22]

Calicectasis N28.89

Caliectasis N28.89

California
disease B38.9
encephalitis A83.5

Caligo cornea —see Opacity, cornea, central

Callositas, callosity (infected) L84

Callus (infected) L84
bone —see Osteophyte
excessive, following fracture - code as Sequelae of fracture

CALME (childhood asymmetric labium majus enlargement) N90.61

Calorie deficiency or malnutrition (see also Malnutrition) E46

Calvé-Perthes disease —see Legg-Calvé-Perthes disease

Calvé's disease —see Osteochondrosis, juvenile, spine

Calvities —see Alopecia, androgenic

Cameroon fever —see Malaria

Camptocormia (hysterical) F44.4

Camurati-Engelmann syndrome Q78.3

Canal —see also condition
atrioventricular common Q21.2

Canaliculitis (lacrimal) (acute) (subacute) H04.33-
Actinomyces A42.89
chronic H04.42-

Canavan's disease E75.29

Canceled procedure (surgical) Z53.9
because of
  contraindication Z53.09
    smoking Z53.01
  left against medical advice (AMA) Z53.29
  patient's decision Z53.20
    for reasons of belief or group pressure Z53.1
    specified reason NEC Z53.29
  specified reason NEC Z53.8

Cancer —see also Neoplasm, by site, malignant
bile duct type liver C22.1
blood —see Leukemia
breast (see also Neoplasm, breast, malignant) C50.91-
hepatocellular C22.0
lung (see also Neoplasm, lung, malignant) C34.90-
ovarian (see also Neoplasm, ovary, malignant) C56.9-
unspecified site (primary) C80.1

Cancer (o)phobia F45.29

Cancerous —*see* Neoplasm, malignant, by site

Cancrum oris A69.0

Candidiasis, candidal B37.9
balanitis B37.42
bronchitis B37.1
cheilitis B37.83
congenital P37.5
cystitis B37.41
disseminated B37.7
endocarditis B37.6
enteritis B37.82
esophagitis B37.81
intertrigo B37.2
lung B37.1
meningitis B37.5
mouth B37.0
nails B37.2
neonatal P37.5
onychia B37.2
oral B37.0
osteomyelitis B37.89
otitis externa B37.84
paronychia B37.2
perionyxis B37.2
pneumonia B37.1
proctitis B37.82
pulmonary B37.1
pyelonephritis B37.49
sepsis B37.7
skin B37.2
specified site NEC B37.89
stomatitis B37.0
systemic B37.7
urethritis B37.41
urogenital site NEC B37.49
vagina B37.3
vulva B37.3
vulvovaginitis B37.3

Candidid L30.2

Candidosis —*see* Candidiasis

Candiru infection or infestation B88.8

Canities (premature) L67.1
congenital Q84.2

Canker (mouth) (sore) K12.0
rash A38.9

Cannabinosis J66.2

Cannabis induced
anxiety disorder F12.980
psychotic disorder F12.959
sleep disorder F12.988

Canton fever A75.9

Cantrell's syndrome Q87.89

Capillariasis (intestinal) B81.1
hepatic B83.8

Capillary —*see* condition

Caplan's syndrome —*see* Rheumatoid, lung

Capsule —*see* condition

Capsulitis (joint) —*see also* Enthesopathy
adhesive (shoulder) M75.0-
hepatic K65.8
labyrinthine —*see* Otosclerosis, specified NEC
thyroid E06.9

Caput
crepitus Q75.8
medusae I86.8
succedaneum P12.81

Car sickness T75.3

Carapata (disease) A68.0

Carate —*see* Pinta

Carbon lung J60

Carbuncle L02.93
abdominal wall L02.231
anus K61.0
auditory canal, external —*see* Abscess, ear, external
auricle ear —*see* Abscess, ear, external
axilla L02.43-
back (any part) L02.232
breast N61.1
buttock L02.33
cheek (external) L02.03
chest wall L02.233
chin L02.03
corpus cavernosum N48.21
ear (any part) (external) (middle) —*see* Abscess, ear, external
external auditory canal —*see* Abscess, ear, external
eyelid —*see* Abscess, eyelid
face NEC L02.03
femoral (region) —*see* Carbuncle, lower limb
finger —*see* Carbuncle, hand
flank L02.231
foot L02.63-
forehead L02.03
genital —*see* Abscess, genital
gluteal (region) L02.33
groin L02.234
hand L02.53-
head NEC L02.831
heel —*see* Carbuncle, foot
hip —*see* Carbuncle, lower limb
kidney —*see* Abscess, kidney
knee —*see* Carbuncle, lower limb
labium (majus) (minus) N76.4
lacrimal
gland —*see* Dacryoadenitis
passages (duct) (sac) —*see* Inflammation, lacrimal, passages, acute
leg —*see* Carbuncle, lower limb
lower limb L02.43-
malignant A22.0
navel L02.236
neck L02.13
nose (external) (septum) J34.0
orbit, orbital —*see* Abscess, orbit
palmar (space) —*see* Carbuncle, hand
partes posteriores L02.33
pectoral region L02.233
penis N48.21
perineum L02.235
pinna —*see* Abscess, ear, external
popliteal —*see* Carbuncle, lower limb
scalp L02.831
seminal vesicle N49.0
shoulder —*see* Carbuncle, upper limb
specified site NEC L02.838
temple (region) L02.03
thumb —*see* Carbuncle, hand
toe —*see* Carbuncle, foot
trunk L02.239
abdominal wall L02.231
back L02.232
chest wall L02.233
groin L02.234
perineum L02.235
umbilicus L02.236
umbilicus L02.236
upper limb L02.43-
urethra N34.0
vulva N76.4

Carbunculus —*see* Carbuncle

Carcinoid (tumor) —*see* Tumor, carcinoid

Carcinoidosis E34.0

Carcinoma (malignant) —*see also* Neoplasm, by site, malignant
acidophil
specified site —*see* Neoplasm, malignant, by site
unspecified site C75.1
acidophil-basophil, mixed
specified site —*see* Neoplasm, malignant, by site
unspecified site C75.1
adnexal (skin) —*see* Neoplasm, skin, malignant
adrenal cortical C74.0-
alveolar —*see* Neoplasm, lung, malignant
cell —*see* Neoplasm, lung, malignant
ameloblastic C41.1
upper jaw (bone) C41.0
apocrine
breast —*see* Neoplasm, breast, malignant
specified site NEC —*see* Neoplasm, skin, malignant
unspecified site C44.99
basal cell (pigmented) (*see also* Neoplasm, skin, malignant) C44.91
fibro-epithelial —*see* Neoplasm, skin, malignant
morphea —*see* Neoplasm, skin, malignant
multicentric —*see* Neoplasm, skin, malignant
basaloid
basal-squamous cell, mixed —*see* Neoplasm, skin, malignant
basophil
specified site —*see* Neoplasm, malignant, by site
unspecified site C75.1
basophil-acidophil, mixed
specified site —*see* Neoplasm, malignant, by site
unspecified site C75.1
basosquamous —*see* Neoplasm, skin, malignant
bile duct
with hepatocellular, mixed C22.0
liver C22.1
specified site NEC —*see* Neoplasm, malignant, by site
unspecified site C22.1
branchial or branchiogenic C10.4
bronchial or bronchogenic —*see* Neoplasm, lung, malignant
bronchiolar —*see* Neoplasm, lung, malignant
bronchioloalveolar —*see* Neoplasm, lung, malignant
C cell
specified site —*see* Neoplasm, malignant, by site
unspecified site C73
ceruminous C44.29-
cervix uteri
in situ D06.9
endocervix D06.0
exocervix D06.1
specified site NEC D06.7
chorionic
specified site —*see* Neoplasm, malignant, by site
unspecified site
female C58
male C62.90

Carcinoma (*continued*)
chromophobe
specified site —*see* Neoplasm, malignant, by site
unspecified site C75.1
cloacogenic
specified site —*see* Neoplasm, malignant, by site
unspecified site C21.2
diffuse type
specified site —*see* Neoplasm, malignant, by site
unspecified site C16.9
duct (cell)
with Paget's disease —*see* Neoplasm, breast, malignant
infiltrating
with lobular carcinoma (in situ)
specified site —*see* Neoplasm, malignant, by site
unspecified site (female) C50.91-
male C50.92-
specified site —*see* Neoplasm, malignant, by site
unspecified site (female) C50.91-
male C50.92-
ductal
with lobular
specified site —*see* Neoplasm, malignant, by site
unspecified site (female) C50.91-
male C50.92-
ductular, infiltrating
specified site —*see* Neoplasm, malignant, by site
unspecified site (female) C50.91-
male C50.92-
embryonal
liver C22.7
endometrioid
specified site —*see* Neoplasm, malignant, by site
unspecified site
female C56.9
male C61
eosinophil
specified site —*see* Neoplasm, malignant, by site
unspecified site C75.1
epidermoid —*see also* Neoplasm, skin malignant
in situ, Bowen's type —*see* Neoplasm, skin, in situ
fibroepithelial, basal cell —*see* Neoplasm, skin, malignant
follicular
with papillary (mixed) C73
moderately differentiated C73
pure follicle C73
specified site —*see* Neoplasm, malignant, by site
trabecular C73
unspecified site C73
well differentiated C73
generalized, with unspecified primary site C80.0
glycogen-rich —*see* Neoplasm, breast, malignant
granulosa cell C56-
hepatic cell C22.0
hepatocellular C22.0
with bile duct, mixed C22.0
fibrolamellar C22.0
hepatocholangiolitic C22.0
Hurthle cell C73

Carcinoma (*continued*)

in
  adenomatous
    polyposis coli C18.9
  pleomorphic adenoma —*see*
    Neoplasm, salivary glands,
    malignant
  situ —*see* Carcinoma-in-situ
infiltrating
  duct
    with lobular
      specified site —*see*
        Neoplasm, malignant,
        by site
      unspecified site (female)
        C50.91-
        male C50.92-
    with Paget's disease —*see*
      Neoplasm, breast,
      malignant
    specified site —*see* Neoplasm,
      malignant
    unspecified site (female)
      C50.91-
      male C50.92-
  ductular
    specified site —*see* Neoplasm,
      malignant
    unspecified site (female)
      C50.91-
      male C50.92-
  lobular
    specified site —*see* Neoplasm,
      malignant
    unspecified site (female)
      C50.91-
      male C50.92-
inflammatory
  specified site —*see* Neoplasm,
    malignant
  unspecified site (female) C50.91-
    male C50.92-
intestinal type
  specified site —*see* Neoplasm,
    malignant, by site
  unspecified site C16.9
intracystic
  noninfiltrating —*see* Neoplasm,
    in situ, by site
intraductal (noninfiltrating)
  with Paget's disease —*see*
    Neoplasm, breast, malignant
  breast D05.1-
  papillary
    with invasion
      specified site —*see*
        Neoplasm, malignant,
        by site
      unspecified site (female)
        C50.91-
        male C50.92-
    breast D05.1-
    specified site NEC —*see*
      Neoplasm, in situ, by site
    unspecified site (female)
      D05.1-
  specified site NEC —*see*
    Neoplasm, in situ, by site
  unspecified site (female)
    D05.1-
intraepidermal —*see* Neoplasm,
  in situ
  squamous cell, Bowen's type
    —*see* Neoplasm, skin,
    in situ
intraepithelial —*see* Neoplasm, in
  situ, by site
  squamous cell —*see* Neoplasm,
    in situ, by site
intraosseous C41.1
  upper jaw (bone) C41.0

Carcinoma (*continued*)

islet cell
  with exocrine, mixed
    specified site —*see* Neoplasm,
      malignant, by site
    unspecified site C25.9
  pancreas C25.4
  specified site NEC —*see*
    Neoplasm, malignant, by site
  unspecified site C25.4
juvenile, breast —*see* Neoplasm,
  breast, malignant
large cell
  small cell
    specified site —*see* Neoplasm,
      malignant, by site
    unspecified site C34.90
Leydig cell (testis)
  specified site —*see* Neoplasm,
    malignant, by site
  unspecified site
    female C56.9
    male C62.90
lipid-rich (female) C50.91-
  male C50.92-
liver cell C22.0
liver NEC C22.7
lobular (infiltrating)
  with intraductal
    specified site —*see* Neoplasm,
      malignant, by site
    unspecified site (female)
      C50.91-
      male C50.92-
  noninfiltrating
    breast D05.0-
    specified site NEC —*see*
      Neoplasm, in situ, by site
    unspecified site D05.0-
  specified site —*see* Neoplasm,
    malignant, by site
  unspecified site (female) C50.91-
    male C50.92-
medullary
  with
    amyloid stroma
      specified site —*see*
        Neoplasm, malignant,
        by site
      unspecified site C73
    lymphoid stroma
      specified site —*see*
        Neoplasm, malignant,
        by site
      unspecified site (female)
        C50.91-
        male C50.92-
Merkel cell C4A.9
  anal margin C4A.51
  anal skin C4A.51
  canthus C4A.1-
  ear and external auricular canal
    C4A.2-
  external auricular canal C4A.2-
  eyelid, including canthus C4A.1-
  face C4A.30
    specified NEC C4A.39
  hip C4A.7-
  lip C4A.0
  lower limb, including hip
    C4A.7-
  neck C4A.4
  nodal presentation C7B.1
  nose C4A.31
  overlapping sites C4A.8
  perianal skin C4A.51
  scalp C4A.4
  secondary C7B.1
  shoulder C4A.6-
  skin of breast C4A.52
  trunk NEC C4A.59

Carcinoma (*continued*)

Merkel cell (*continued*)
  upper limb, including shoulder
    C4A.6-
  visceral metastatic C7B.1
metastatic —*see* Neoplasm,
  secondary, by site
metatypical —*see* Neoplasm, skin,
  malignant
morphea, basal cell —*see*
  Neoplasm, skin, malignant
mucoid
  cell
    specified site —*see* Neoplasm,
      malignant, by site
    unspecified site C75.1
neuroendocrine —*see also* Tumor,
  neuroendocrine
  high grade, any site C7A.1
  poorly differentiated, any site
    C7A.1
nonencapsulated sclerosing C73
noninfiltrating
  intracystic —*see* Neoplasm, in
    situ, by site
  intraductal
    breast D05.1-
    papillary
      breast D05.1-
      specified site NEC —*see*
        Neoplasm, in situ, by
        site
      unspecified site D05.1-
    specified site —*see* Neoplasm,
      in situ, by site
    unspecified site D05.1-
  lobular
    breast D05.0-
    specified site NEC —*see*
      Neoplasm, in situ, by site
    unspecified site (female)
      D05.0-
oat cell
  specified site —*see* Neoplasm,
    malignant, by site
  unspecified site C34.90
odontogenic C41.1
  upper jaw (bone) C41.0
papillary
  with follicular
    (mixed) C73
  follicular variant C73
  intraductal (noninfiltrating)
    with invasion
      specified site —*see*
        Neoplasm, malignant,
        by site
      unspecified site (female)
        C50.91-
        male C50.92-
    breast D05.1-
    specified site NEC —*see*
      Neoplasm, in situ, by site
    unspecified site D05.1-
  serous
    specified site —*see* Neoplasm,
      malignant, by site
    surface
      specified site —*see*
        Neoplasm, malignant,
        by site
      unspecified site C56.9
    unspecified site C56.9
papillocystic
  specified site —*see* Neoplasm,
    malignant, by site
  unspecified site C56.9
parafollicular cell
  specified site —*see* Neoplasm,
    malignant, by site
  unspecified site C73

Carcinoma (*continued*)

pilomatrix —*see* Neoplasm, skin,
  malignant
pseudomucinous
  specified site —*see* Neoplasm,
    malignant, by site
  unspecified site C56.9
renal cell C64-
Schmincke —*see* Neoplasm,
  nasopharynx, malignant
Schneiderian
  specified site —*see* Neoplasm,
    malignant, by site
  unspecified site C30.0
sebaceous —*see* Neoplasm, skin,
  malignant
secondary —*see also* Neoplasm,
  secondary, by site
  Merkel cell C7B.1
secretory, breast —*see* Neoplasm,
  breast, malignant
serous
  papillary
    specified site —*see* Neoplasm,
      malignant, by site
    unspecified site C56.9
  surface, papillary
    specified site —*see* Neoplasm,
      malignant, by site
    unspecified site C56.9
Sertoli cell
  specified site —*see* Neoplasm,
    malignant, by site
  unspecified site C62.90
    female C56.9
    male C62.90
skin appendage —*see* Neoplasm,
  skin, malignant
small cell
  fusiform cell
    specified site —*see* Neoplasm,
      malignant, by site
    unspecified site C34.90
  intermediate cell
    specified site —*see* Neoplasm,
      malignant, by site
    unspecified site C34.90
  large cell
    specified site —*see* Neoplasm,
      malignant, by site
    unspecified site C34.90
solid
  with amyloid stroma
    specified site —*see* Neoplasm,
      malignant, by site
    unspecified site C73
  microinvasive
    specified site —*see* Neoplasm,
      malignant, by site
    unspecified site C53.9
sweat gland —*see* Neoplasm, skin,
  malignant
theca cell C56.-
thymic C37
unspecified site (primary) C80.1
water-clear cell C75.0

Carcinoma-in-situ —*see also*
  Neoplasm, in situ, by site
breast NOS D05.9-
  specified type NEC D05.8-
epidermoid —*see also* Neoplasm,
  in situ, by site
  with questionable stromal
    invasion
    cervix D06.9
    specified site NEC —*see*
      Neoplasm, in situ, by site
    unspecified site D06.9
  Bowen's type —*see* Neoplasm,
    skin, in situ

Carcinoma-in-situ (continued)
intraductal
  breast D05.1-
    specified site NEC —see
      Neoplasm, in situ, by site
    unspecified site D05.1-
lobular
  with
    infiltrating duct
      breast (female) C50.91-
        male C50.92-
      specified site NEC —see
        Neoplasm, malignant
      unspecified site (female)
        C50.91-
        male C50.92-
    intraductal
      breast D05.8-
      specified site NEC —see
        Neoplasm, in situ, by site
      unspecified site (female)
        D05.8-
  breast D05.0-
  specified site NEC —see
    Neoplasm, in situ, by site
  unspecified site D05.0-
squamous cell —see also
  Neoplasm, in situ, by site
  with questionable stromal
    invasion
    cervix D06.9
    specified site NEC —see
      Neoplasm, in situ, by site
    unspecified site D06.9

Carcinomaphobia F45.29

Carcinomatosis C80.0
peritonei C78.6
unspecified site (primary)
  (secondary) C80.0

Carcinosarcoma —see Neoplasm,
malignant, by site
embryonal —see Neoplasm,
malignant, by site

Cardia, cardial —see condition

Cardiac —see also condition
death, sudden —see Arrest, cardiac
pacemaker
  in situ Z95.0
  management or adjustment Z45.018
tamponade I31.4

Cardialgia —see Pain, precordial

Cardiectasis —see Hypertrophy,
cardiac

Cardiochalasia K21.9

Cardiomalacia I51.5

Cardiomegalia glycogenica diffusa
E74.02 [I43]

Cardiomegaly —see also
Hypertrophy, cardiac
congenital Q24.8
glycogen E74.02 [I43]
idiopathic I51.7

Cardiomyoliposis I51.5

Cardiomyopathy (familial)
(idiopathic) I42.9
alcoholic I42.6
amyloid E85.4 [I43]
  transthyretin-related (ATTR)
    familial E85.4 [I43]
arteriosclerotic —see Disease,
  heart, ischemic, atherosclerotic
beriberi E51.12
cobalt-beer I42.6
congenital I42.4
congestive I42.0
constrictive NOS I42.5
dilated I42.0

Cardiomyopathy (continued)
due to
  alcohol I42.6
  beriberi E51.12
  cardiac glycogenosis E74.02 [I43]
  drugs I42.7
  external agents NEC I42.7
  Friedreich's ataxia G11.11
  myotonia atrophica G71.11 [I43]
  progressive muscular dystrophy
    G71.09 [I43]
glycogen storage E74.02 [I43]
hypertensive —see Hypertension,
  heart
hypertrophic (nonobstructive) I42.2
  obstructive I42.1
    congenital Q24.8
in
  Chagas' disease (chronic) B57.2
    acute B57.0
  sarcoidosis D86.85
ischemic I25.5
metabolic E88.9 [I43]
  thyrotoxic E05.90 [I43]
    with thyroid storm E05.91 [I43]
newborn I42.8
  congenital I42.4
non-ischemic (see also by cause)
  I42.8
nutritional E63.9 [I43]
  beriberi E51.12
obscure of Africa I42.8
peripartum O90.3
postpartum O90.3
restrictive NEC I42.5
rheumatic I09.0
secondary I42.9
specified NEC I42.8
stress induced I51.81
takotsubo I51.81
thyrotoxic E05.90 [I43]
  with thyroid storm E05.91 [I43]
toxic NEC I42.7
transthyretin-related (ATTR)
  familial amyloid E85.4
tuberculous A18.84
viral B33.24

Cardionephritis —see Hypertension,
cardiorenal

Cardionephropathy —see
Hypertension, cardiorenal

Cardionephrosis —see
Hypertension, cardiorenal

Cardiopathia nigra I27.0

Cardiopathy —see also Disease,
heart I51.9
idiopathic I42.9
mucopolysaccharidosis E76.3 [I52]

Cardiopericarditis —see Pericarditis

Cardiophobia F45.29

Cardiorenal —see condition

Cardiorrhexis —see Infarct,
myocardium

Cardiosclerosis —see Disease, heart,
ischemic, atherosclerotic

Cardiosis —see Disease, heart

Cardiospasm (esophagus) (reflex)
(stomach) K22.0
congenital Q39.5
  with megaesophagus Q39.5

Cardiostenosis —see Disease, heart

Cardiosymphysis I31.0

Cardiovascular —see condition

Carditis (acute) (bacterial) (chronic)
(subacute) I51.89

Carditis (continued)
meningococcal A39.50
rheumatic —see Disease, heart,
  rheumatic
rheumatoid —see Rheumatoid,
  carditis
viral B33.20

Care (of) (for) (following)
child (routine) Z76.2
family member (handicapped) (sick)
  creating problem for family
    Z63.6
  provided away from home for
    holiday relief Z75.5
  unavailable, due to
    absence (person rendering
      care) (sufferer) Z74.2
    inability (any reason) of
      person rendering care
      Z74.2
foundling Z76.1
holiday relief Z75.5
improper —see Maltreatment
lack of (at or after birth) (infant)
  —see Maltreatment, child,
  neglect
lactating mother Z39.1
palliative Z51.5
postpartum
  immediately after delivery Z39.0
  routine follow-up Z39.2
respite Z75.5
unavailable, due to
  absence of person rendering care
    Z74.2
  inability (any reason) of person
    rendering care Z74.2
well-baby Z76.2

Caries
bone NEC A18.03
dental (dentino enamel junction)
  (early in childhood) (of dentine)
  (pre-eruptive) (recurrent) (to the
  pulp) K02.9
  arrested (coronal) (root) K02.3
  chewing surface
    limited to enamel K02.51
    penetrating into dentin
      K02.52
    penetrating into pulp K02.53
  coronal surface
    chewing surface
      limited to enamel K02.51
      penetrating into dentin
        K02.52
      penetrating into pulp
        K02.53
    pit and fissure surface
      limited to enamel K02.51
      penetrating into dentin
        K02.52
      penetrating into pulp
        K02.53
    smooth surface
      limited to enamel K02.61
      penetrating into dentin
        K02.62
      penetrating into pulp
        K02.63
  pit and fissure surface
    limited to enamel K02.51
    penetrating into dentin
      K02.52
    penetrating into pulp K02.53
  primary, cervical origin K02.52
  root K02.7
  smooth surface
    limited to enamel K02.61
    penetrating into dentin K02.62
    penetrating into pulp K02.63

Caries (continued)
external meatus —see Disorder,
  ear, external, specified type NEC
hip (tuberculous) A18.02
initial (tooth)
  chewing surface K02.51
  pit and fissure surface K02.51
  smooth surface K02.61
knee (tuberculous) A18.02
labyrinth —see subcategory H83.8
limb NEC (tuberculous) A18.03
mastoid process (chronic) —see
  Mastoiditis, chronic
  tuberculous A18.03
middle ear —see subcategory
  H74.8
nose (tuberculous) A18.03
orbit (tuberculous) A18.03
ossicles, ear —see Abnormal, ear
  ossicles
petrous bone —see Petrositis
root (dental) (tooth) K02.7
sacrum (tuberculous) A18.01
spine, spinal (column)
  (tuberculous) A18.01
syphilitic A52.77
  congenital (early) A50.02
    [M90.80]
tooth, teeth —see Caries, dental
tuberculous A18.03
vertebra (column) (tuberculous)
  A18.01

Carious teeth —see Caries, dental

Carneous mole O02.0

Carnitine insufficiency E71.40

Carotenemia (dietary) E67.1

Carotenosis (cutis) (skin) E67.1

Carotid body or sinus syndrome
G90.01

Carotidynia G90.01

Carpal tunnel syndrome —see
Syndrome, carpal tunnel

Carpenter's syndrome Q87.0

Carpopedal spasm —see Tetany

Carr-Barr-Plunkett syndrome
Q97.1

Carrier (suspected) of
amebiasis Z22.1
bacterial disease NEC Z22.39
  diphtheria Z22.2
  intestinal infectious NEC Z22.1
    typhoid Z22.0
  meningococcal Z22.31
  sexually transmitted Z22.4
  specified NEC Z22.39
  staphylococcal (Methicillin
    susceptible) Z22.321
    Methicillin resistant Z22.322
  streptococcal Z22.338
    group B Z22.330
      complicating pregnancy or
        delivery O99.82-
  typhoid Z22.0
cholera Z22.1
diphtheria Z22.2
gastrointestinal pathogens NEC
  Z22.1
genetic Z14.8
  cystic fibrosis Z14.1
  hemophilia A (asymptomatic)
    Z14.01
    symptomatic Z14.02
gestational, pregnant Z33.1
gonorrhea Z22.4
HAA (hepatitis Australian-antigen)
  B18.8
HB (c)(s)-AG B18.1

Cellulitis *(continued)*
chronic L03.90
clostridial A48.0
corpus cavernosum N48.22
digit
  finger —*see* Cellulitis, finger
  toe —*see* Cellulitis, toe
Douglas' cul-de-sac or pouch
  acute N73.0
drainage site (following operation) T81.49
ear (external) H60.1-
eosinophilic (granulomatous) L98.3
erysipelatous —*see* Erysipelas
external auditory canal —*see* Cellulitis, ear
eyelid —*see* Abscess, eyelid
face NEC L03.211
finger (intrathecal) (periosteal) (subcutaneous) (subcuticular) L03.01-
foot —*see* Cellulitis, lower limb
gangrenous —*see* Gangrene
genital organ NEC
  female (external) N76.4
  male N49.9
    multiple sites N49.8
    specified NEC N49.8
gluteal (region) L03.317
gonococcal A54.89
groin L03.314
hand —*see* Cellulitis, upper limb
head NEC L03.811
  face (any part, except ear, eye and nose) L03.211
heel —*see* Cellulitis, lower limb
hip —*see* Cellulitis, lower limb
jaw (region) L03.211
knee —*see* Cellulitis, lower limb
labium (majus) (minus) —*see* Vulvitis
lacrimal passages —*see* Inflammation, lacrimal, passages
larynx J38.7
leg —*see* Cellulitis, lower limb
lip K13.0
lower limb L03.11-
  toe —*see* Cellulitis, toe
mouth (floor) K12.2
multiple sites, so stated L03.90
nasopharynx J39.1
navel L03.316
  newborn P38.9
    with mild hemorrhage P38.1
    without hemorrhage P38.9
neck (region) L03.221
nipple (acute) (nonpuerperal) (subacute) N61.0
nose (septum) (external) J34.0
orbit, orbital H05.01-
palate (soft) K12.2
pectoral (region) L03.313
pelvis, pelvic (chronic)
  female —*see also* Disease, pelvis, inflammatory N73.2
    acute N73.0
    following ectopic or molar pregnancy O08.0
  male K65.0
penis N48.22
perineal, perineum L03.315
periorbital L03.213
perirectal K61.1
peritonsillar J36
periuterine (*see also* Disease pelvis, inflammatory) N73.2
  acute N73.0
pharynx J39.1
preseptal L03.213
rectum K61.1

Cellulitis *(continued)*
retroperitoneal K68.9
round ligament
  acute N73.0
scalp (any part) L03.811
scrotum N49.2
seminal vesicle N49.0
shoulder —*see* Cellulitis, upper limb
specified site NEC L03.818
submandibular (region) (space) (triangle) K12.2
  gland K11.3
submaxillary (region) K12.2
  gland K11.3
thigh —*see* Cellulitis, lower limb
thumb (intrathecal) (periosteal) (subcutaneous) (subcuticular) —*see* Cellulitis, finger
toe (intrathecal) (periosteal) (subcutaneous) (subcuticular) L03.03-
tonsil J36
trunk L03.319
  abdominal wall L03.311
  back (any part) L03.312
  buttock L03.317
  chest wall L03.313
  groin L03.314
  perineal, perineum L03.315
  umbilicus L03.316
tuberculous (primary) A18.4
umbilicus L03.316
upper limb L03.11-
  axilla —*see* Cellulitis, axilla
  finger —*see* Cellulitis, finger
  thumb —*see* Cellulitis, finger
vaccinal T88.0
vocal cord J38.3
vulva —*see* Vulvitis
wrist —*see* Cellulitis, upper limb

Cementoblastoma, benign —*see* Cyst, calcifying odontogenic

Cementoma —*see* Cyst, calcifying odontogenic

Cementoperiostitis —*see* Periodontitis

Cementosis K03.4

Central auditory processing disorder H93.25

Central pain syndrome G89.0

Cephalematocele, cephalhematocele
newborn P52.8
  birth injury P10.8
traumatic —*see* Hematoma, brain

Cephalematoma, cephalhematoma (calcified)
newborn (birth injury) P12.0
traumatic —*see* Hematoma, brain

Cephalgia, cephalalgia —*see also* Headache
histamine G44.009
  intractable G44.001
  not intractable G44.009
trigeminal autonomic (TAC) NEC G44.099
  intractable G44.091
  not intractable G44.099

Cephalic —*see* condition

Cephalitis —*see* Encephalitis

Cephalocele —*see* Encephalocele

Cephalomenia N94.89

Cephalopelvic —*see* condition

Cerclage (with cervical incompetence) **in pregnancy** —*see* Incompetence, cervix, in pregnancy

Cerebellitis —*see* Encephalitis

Cerebellum, cerebellar —*see* condition

Cerebral —*see* condition

Cerebritis —*see* Encephalitis

Cerebro-hepato-renal syndrome Q87.89

Cerebromalacia —*see* Softening, brain
sequelae of cerebrovascular disease I69.398

Cerebroside lipidosis E75.22

Cerebrospasticity (congenital) G80.1

Cerebrospinal —*see* condition

Cerebrum —*see* condition

Ceroid-lipofuscinosis, neuronal E75.4

Cerumen (accumulation) (impacted) H61.2-

Cervical —*see also* condition
auricle Q18.2
dysplasia in pregnancy —*see* Abnormal, cervix, in pregnancy or childbirth
erosion in pregnancy —*see* Abnormal, cervix, in pregnancy or childbirth
fibrosis in pregnancy —*see* Abnormal, cervix, in pregnancy or childbirth
fusion syndrome Q76.1
rib Q76.5
shortening (complicating pregnancy) O26.87-

Cervicalgia M54.2

Cervicitis (acute) (chronic) (nonvenereal) (senile (atrophic)) (subacute) (with ulceration) N72
with
  abortion —*see* Abortion, by type complicated by genital tract and pelvic infection
  ectopic pregnancy O08.0
  molar pregnancy O08.0
chlamydial A56.09
gonococcal A54.03
herpesviral A60.03
puerperal (postpartum) O86.11
syphilitic A52.76
trichomonal A59.09
tuberculous A18.16

Cervicocolpitis (emphysematosa) (*see also* Cervicitis) N72

Cervix —*see* condition

Cesarean delivery, previous, affecting management of pregnancy O34.219
classical (vertical) scar O34.212
isthmocele O34.22
low transverse scar O34.211
mid-transverse T incision O34.218
scar
  defect (isthmocele) O34.22
  specified type NEC O34.218

Céstan (-Chenais) **paralysis or syndrome** G46.3

Céstan-Raymond syndrome I65.8

Cestode infestation B71.9
specified type NEC B71.8

Cestodiasis B71.9

Chabert's disease A22.9

Chacaleh E53.8

Chafing L30.4

Chagas' (-Mazza) **disease** (chronic) B57.2
with
  cardiovascular involvement NEC B57.2
  digestive system involvement B57.30
    megacolon B57.32
    megaesophagus B57.31
    other specified B57.39
  megacolon B57.32
  megaesophagus B57.31
  myocarditis B57.2
  nervous system involvement B57.40
    meningitis B57.41
    meningoencephalitis B57.42
    other specified B57.49
  specified organ involvement NEC B57.5
acute (with) B57.1
  cardiovascular NEC B57.0
  myocarditis B57.0

Chagres fever B50.9

Chairridden Z74.09

Chalasia (cardiac sphincter) K21.9

Chalazion H00.19
left H00.16
  lower H00.15
  upper H00.14
right H00.13
  lower H00.12
  upper H00.11

Chalcosis —*see also* Disorder, globe, degenerative, chalcosis
cornea —*see* Deposit, cornea
crystalline lens —*see* Cataract, complicated
retina H35.89

Chalicosis (pulmonum) J62.8

Chancre (any genital site) (hard) (hunterian) (mixed) (primary) (seronegative) (seropositive) (syphilitic) A51.0
congenital A50.07
conjunctiva NEC A51.2
Ducrey's A57
extragenital A51.2
eyelid A51.2
lip A51.2
nipple A51.2
Nisbet's A57
of
  carate A67.0
  pinta A67.0
  yaws A66.0
palate, soft A51.2
phagedenic A57
simple A57
soft A57
  bubo A57
  palate A51.2
urethra A51.0
yaws A66.0

Chancroid (anus) (genital) (penis) (perineum) (rectum) (urethra) (vulva) A57

Chandler's disease (osteochondritis dissecans, hip) —*see* Osteochondritis, dissecans, hip

Change(s) (in) (of) —*see also* Removal
arteriosclerotic —*see* Arteriosclerosis
bone —*see also* Disorder, bone
  diabetic —*see* Diabetes, bone change

Change *(continued)*
  bowel habit R19.4
  cardiorenal (vascular) —*see*
    Hypertension, cardiorenal
  cardiovascular —*see* Disease,
    cardiovascular
  circulatory I99.9
  cognitive (mild) (organic) R41.89
  color, tooth, teeth
    during formation K00.8
    posteruptive K03.7
  contraceptive device Z30.433
  corneal membrane H18.30
    Bowman's membrane fold or
      rupture H18.31-
    Descemet's membrane
      fold H18.32-
      rupture H18.33-
  coronary —*see* Disease, heart,
    ischemic
  degenerative, spine or vertebra
    —*see* Spondylosis
  dental pulp, regressive K04.2
  dressing (nonsurgical) Z48.00
    surgical Z48.01
  heart —*see* Disease, heart
  hip joint —*see* Derangement, joint, hip
  hyperplastic larynx J38.7
  hypertrophic
    nasal sinus J34.89
    turbinate, nasal J34.3
    upper respiratory tract J39.8
  indwelling catheter Z46.6
  inflammatory —*see also*
    Inflammation
    sacroiliac M46.1
  job, anxiety concerning Z56.1
  joint —*see* Derangement, joint
  life —*see* Menopause
  mental status R41.82
  minimal (glomerular) (*see also*
    N00-N07 with fourth character .0)
    N05.0
  myocardium, myocardial —*see*
    Degeneration, myocardial
  of life —*see* Menopause
  pacemaker Z45.018
    pulse generator Z45.010
  personality (enduring) F68.8
    due to (secondary to)
      general medical condition F07.0
      secondary (nonspecific) F60.89
  regressive, dental pulp K04.2
  renal —*see* Disease, renal
  retina H35.9
    myopic (*see also* Myopia,
      degenerative) H44.2-
  sacroiliac joint M53.3
  senile (*see also* condition) R54
  sensory R20.8
  skin R23.9
    acute, due to ultraviolet radiation
      L56.9
      specified NEC L56.8
    chronic, due to nonionizing
      radiation L57.9
      specified NEC L57.8
    cyanosis R23.0
    flushing R23.2
    pallor R23.1
    petechiae R23.3
    specified change NEC R23.8
    swelling —*see* Mass, localized
    texture R23.4
  trophic
    arm —*see* Mononeuropathy,
      upper limb
    leg —*see* Mononeuropathy,
      lower limb
  vascular I99.9
  vasomotor I73.9

Change *(continued)*
  voice R49.9
    psychogenic F44.4
    specified NEC R49.8
Changing sleep-work schedule,
  affecting sleep G47.26
Changuinola fever A93.1
Chapping skin T69.8
Charcot-Marie-Tooth disease,
  paralysis or syndrome G60.0
Charcot's
  arthropathy —*see* Arthropathy,
    neuropathic
  cirrhosis K74.3
  disease (tabetic arthropathy) A52.16
  joint (disease) (tabetic) A52.16
    diabetic —*see* Diabetes, with,
      arthropathy
    syringomyelic G95.0
  syndrome (intermittent
    claudication) I73.9
CHARGE association Q89.8
Charley-horse (quadriceps) M62.831
  traumatic (quadriceps) S76.11-
Charlouis' disease —*see* Yaws
Cheadle's disease E54
Checking (of)
  cardiac pacemaker (battery)
    (electrode(s)) Z45.018
    pulse generator Z45.010
  implantable subdermal
    contraceptive Z30.46
  intrauterine contraceptive device
    Z30.431
  wound Z48.0-
    due to injury - code to Injury, by
      site, using appropriate seventh
      character for subsequent
      encounter
Check-up —*see* Examination
Chédiak-Higashi (-Steinbrinck)
  syndrome (congenital gigantism of
    peroxidase granules) E70.330
Cheek —*see* condition
Cheese itch B88.0
Cheese-washer's lung J67.8
Cheese-worker's lung J67.8
Cheilitis (acute) (angular) (catarrhal)
  (chronic) (exfoliative) (gangrenous)
  (glandular) (infectional)
  (suppurative) (ulcerative)
  (vesicular) K13.0
  actinic (due to sun) L56.8
    other than from sun L59.8
  candidal B37.83
Cheilodynia K13.0
Cheiloschisis —*see* Cleft, lip
Cheilosis (angular) K13.0
  with pellagra E52
  due to
    vitamin B2(riboflavin) deficiency
      E53.0
Cheiromegaly M79.89
Cheiropompholyx L30.1
Cheloid —*see* Keloid
Chemical burn —*see* Corrosion, by site
Chemodectoma —*see*
  Paraganglioma, nonchromaffin
Chemosis, conjunctiva —*see*
  Edema, conjunctiva
Chemotherapy (session) (for)
  cancer Z51.11
  neoplasm Z51.11

Cherubism M27.8
Chest —*see* condition
Cheyne-Stokes breathing
  (respiration) R06.3
Chiari's
  disease or syndrome (hepatic vein
    thrombosis) I82.0
  malformation
    type I G93.5
    type II —*see* Spina bifida
    net Q24.3
Chicago disease B40.9
Chickenpox —*see* Varicella
Chiclero ulcer or sore B55.1
Chigger (infestation) B88.0
Chignon (disease) B36.8
  newborn (from vacuum extraction)
    (birth injury) P12.1
Chilaiditi's syndrome (subphrenic
  displacement, colon) Q43.3
Chilblain(s) (lupus) T69.1
Child
  custody dispute Z65.3
Childbirth —*see* Delivery
Childhood
  cerebral X-linked
    adrenoleukodystrophy E71.520
  period of rapid growth Z00.2
Chill(s) R68.83
  with fever R50.9
  congestive in malarial regions B54
  without fever R68.83
Chilomastigiasis A07.8
Chimera 46,XX/46,XY Q99.0
Chin —*see* condition
Chinese dysentery A03.9
Chionophobia F40.228
Chitral fever A93.1
Chlamydia, chlamydial A74.9
  cervicitis A56.09
  conjunctivitis A74.0
  cystitis A56.01
  endometritis A56.11
  epididymitis A56.19
  female
    pelvic inflammatory disease A56.11
    pelviperitonitis A56.11
  orchitis A56.19
  peritonitis A74.81
  pharyngitis A56.4
  proctitis A56.3
  psittaci (infection) A70
  salpingitis A56.11
  sexually-transmitted infection NEC
    A56.8
  specified NEC A74.89
  urethritis A56.01
  vulvovaginitis A56.02
Chlamydiosis —*see* Chlamydia
Chloasma (skin) (idiopathic)
  (symptomatic) L81.1
  eyelid H02.719
    hyperthyroid E05.90 *[H02.719]*
      with thyroid storm E05.91
        [H02.719]
    left H02.716
      lower H02.715
      upper H02.714
    right H02.713
      lower H02.712
      upper H02.711
Chloroma C92.3-
Chlorosis D50.9
  Egyptian B76.9 *[D63.8]*
  miner's B76.9 *[D63.8]*

Chlorotic anemia D50.8
Chocolate cyst (ovary) N80.1
Choked
  disc or disk —*see* Papilledema
  on food, phlegm, or vomitus NOS
    —*see* Foreign body, by site
  while vomiting NOS —*see* Foreign
    body, by site
Chokes (resulting from bends) T70.3
Choking sensation R09.89
Cholangiectasis K83.8
Cholangiocarcinoma
  with hepatocellular carcinoma,
    combined C22.0
  liver C22.1
  specified site NEC —*see*
    Neoplasm, malignant, by site
  unspecified site C22.1
Cholangiohepatitis K83.8
  due to fluke infestation B66.1
Cholangiohepatoma C22.0
Cholangiolitis (acute) (chronic)
  (extrahepatic) (gangrenous)
  (intrahepatic) K83.09
  paratyphoidal —*see* Fever,
    paratyphoid
  typhoidal A01.09
Cholangioma D13.4
  malignant —*see*
    Cholangiocarcinoma
Cholangitis (ascending) (primary)
  (recurrent) (sclerosing) (secondary)
  (stenosing) (suppurative) K83.09
  with calculus, bile duct —*see*
    Calculus, bile duct, with cholangitis
  chronic nonsuppurative destructive
    K74.3
  primary K83.09
    sclerosing K83.01
  sclerosing K83.09
Cholecystectasia K82.8
Cholecystitis K81.9
  with
    calculus, stones in
      bile duct (common) (hepatic)
        —*see* Calculus, bile duct,
          with cholecystitis
      cystic duct —*see* Calculus,
        gallbladder, with
        cholecystitis
      gallbladder —*see* Calculus,
        gallbladder, with
        cholecystitis
    choledocholithiasis —*see*
      Calculus, bile duct, with
      cholecystitis
    cholelithiasis —*see* Calculus,
      gallbladder, with cholecystitis
    gangrene of gallbladder K82.A1
    perforation of gallbladder K82.A2
  acute (emphysematous)
    (gangrenous) (suppurative)
    K81.0
    with
      calculus, stones in
        cystic duct —*see* Calculus,
          gallbladder, with
          cholecystitis, acute
        gallbladder —*see* Calculus,
          gallbladder, with
          cholecystitis, acute
      choledocholithiasis —*see*
        Calculus, bile duct, with
        cholecystitis, acute
      cholelithiasis —*see*
        Calculus, gallbladder, with
        cholecystitis, acute
    chronic cholecystitis K81.2

Cholecystitis *(continued)*
  acute *(continued)*
    with *(continued)*
      chronic cholecystitis
        (continued)
        with gallbladder calculus
          K80.12
          with obstruction K80.13
  chronic K81.1
    with acute cholecystitis K81.2
      with gallbladder calculus
        K80.12
        with obstruction K80.13
  emphysematous (acute) —*see*
    Cholecystitis, acute
  gangrenous —*see* Cholecystitis,
    acute
  paratyphoidal, current A01.4
  suppurative —*see* Cholecystitis,
    acute
  typhoidal A01.09
Cholecystolithiasis —*see* Calculus,
  gallbladder
Choledochitis (suppurative) K83.09
Choledocholith —*see* Calculus, bile
  duct
Choledocholithiasis (common duct)
  (hepatic duct) —*see* Calculus, bile
  duct
  cystic —*see* Calculus, gallbladder
  typhoidal A01.09
Cholelithiasis (cystic duct)
  (gallbladder) (impacted) (multiple)
  —*see* Calculus, gallbladder
  bile duct (common) (hepatic) —*see*
    Calculus, bile duct
  hepatic duct —*see* Calculus, bile duct
  specified NEC K80.80
    with obstruction K80.81
Cholemia —*see also* Jaundice
  familial (simple) (congenital) E80.4
  Gilbert's E80.4
Choleperitoneum, choleperitonitis
  K65.3
Cholera (Asiatic) (epidemic)
  (malignant) A00.9
  antimonial —*see* Poisoning,
    antimony
  classical A00.0
  due to Vibrio cholerae 01 A00.9
    biovar cholerae A00.0
    biovar eltor A00.1
    el tor A00.1
  el tor A00.1
Cholerine —*see* Cholera
Cholestasis NEC K83.1
  with hepatocyte injury K71.0
  due to total parenteral nutrition
    (TPN) K76.89
  pure K71.0
Cholesteatoma (ear) (middle) (with
  reaction) H71.9-
  attic H71.0-
  external ear (canal) H60.4-
  mastoid H71.2-
  postmastoidectomy cavity
    (recurrent) —*see* Complications,
    postmastoidectomy, recurrent
    cholesteatoma
  recurrent (postmastoidectomy)
    —*see* Complications,
    postmastoidectomy, recurrent
    cholesteatoma
  tympanum H71.1-
Cholesteatosis, diffuse H71.3-
Cholesteremia E78.00

Cholesterin in vitreous —*see*
  Deposit, crystalline
Cholesterol
  deposit
    retina H35.89
    vitreous —*see* Deposit,
      crystalline
  elevated (high) E78.00
    with elevated (high) triglycerides
      E78.2
  screening for Z13.220
  imbibition of gallbladder K82.4
Cholesterolemia (essential) (pure)
  E78.00
  familial E78.01
  hereditary E78.01
Cholesterolosis, cholesterosis
  (gallbladder) K82.4
  cerebrotendinous E75.5
Cholocolic fistula K82.3
Choluria R82.2
Chondritis M94.8X9
  aurical H61.03-
  costal (Tietze's) M94.0
  external ear H61.03-
  patella, posttraumatic —*see*
    Chondromalacia, patella
  pinna H61.03-
  purulent M94.8X-
  tuberculous NEC A18.02
    intervertebral A18.01
Chondroblastoma —*see also*
  Neoplasm, bone, benign
  malignant —*see* Neoplasm, bone,
    malignant
Chondrocalcinosis M11.20
  ankle M11.27-
  elbow M11.22-
  familial M11.10
    ankle M11.17-
    elbow M11.12-
    foot joint M11.17
    hand joint M11.14-
    hip M11.15-
    knee M11.16-
    multiple site M11.19
    shoulder M11.11-
    vertebrae M11.18
    wrist M11.13-
  foot joint M11.27-
  hand joint M11.24-
  hip M11.25-
  knee M11.26-
  multiple site M11.29
  shoulder M11.21-
  vertebrae M11.28
  specified type NEC M11.20
    ankle M11.27-
    elbow M11.22-
    foot joint M11.27-
    hand joint M11.24-
    hip M11.25-
    knee M11.26-
    multiple site M11.29
    shoulder M11.21-
    vertebrae M11.28
    wrist M11.23-
  wrist M11.23-
Chondrodermatitis nodularis
  helicis or anthelicis —*see*
  Perichondritis, ear
Chondrodysplasia Q78.9
  with hemangioma Q78.4
  calcificans congenita Q77.3
  fetalis Q77.4
  metaphyseal (Jansen's)
    (McKusick's) (Schmid's) Q78.8
  punctata Q77.3

Chondrodystrophy,
  chondrodystrophia (familial)
  (fetalis) (hypoplastic) Q78.9
  calcificans congenita Q77.3
  myotonic (congenital) G71.13
  punctata Q77.3
Chondroectodermal dysplasia
  Q77.6
Chondrogenesis imperfecta
  Q77.4
Chondrolysis M94.35-
Chondroma —*see also* Neoplasm,
  cartilage, benign
  juxtacortical —*see* Neoplasm,
    bone, benign
  periosteal —*see* Neoplasm, bone,
    benign
Chondromalacia (systemic) M94.20
  acromioclavicular joint M94.21-
  ankle M94.27-
  elbow M94.22-
  foot joint M94.27-
  glenohumeral joint M94.21-
  hand joint M94.24-
  hip M94.25-
  knee M94.26-
    patella M22.4-
  multiple sites M94.29
  patella M22.4-
  rib M94.28
  sacroiliac joint M94.259
  shoulder M94.21-
  sternoclavicular joint M94.21-
  vertebral joint M94.28
  wrist M94.23-
Chondromatosis —*see also* Neoplasm,
  cartilage, uncertain behavior
  internal Q78.4
Chondromyxosarcoma —*see*
  Neoplasm, cartilage, malignant
Chondro-osteodysplasia
  (Morquio-Brailsford type)
  E76.219
Chondro-osteodystrophy E76.29
Chondro-osteoma —*see* Neoplasm,
  bone, benign
Chondropathia tuberosa M94.0
Chondrosarcoma —*see* Neoplasm,
  cartilage, malignant
  juxtacortical —*see* Neoplasm,
    bone, malignant
  mesenchymal —*see* Neoplasm,
    connective tissue, malignant
  myxoid —*see* Neoplasm, cartilage,
    malignant
Chordee (nonvenereal) N48.89
  congenital Q54.4
  gonococcal A54.09
Chorditis (fibrinous) (nodosa)
  (tuberosa) J38.2
Chordoma —*see* Neoplasm,
  vertebral (column), malignant
Chorea (chronic) (gravis)
  (posthemiplegic) (senile)
  (spasmodic) G25.5
  with
    heart involvement I02.0
      active or acute (conditions in
        I01-) I02.0
      rheumatic I02.9
        with valvular disorder I02.0
    rheumatic heart disease
      (chronic) (inactive) (quiescent)
      - code to rheumatic heart
      condition involved

Chorea *(continued)*
  drug-induced G25.4
  habit F95.8
  hereditary G10
  Huntington's G10
  hysterical F44.4
  minor I02.9
    with heart involvement I02.0
  progressive G25.5
    hereditary G10
  rheumatic (chronic) I02.9
    with heart involvement I02.0
  Sydenham's I02.9
    with heart involvement —*see*
      Chorea, with rheumatic heart
      disease
  nonrheumatic G25.5
Choreoathetosis (paroxysmal)
  G25.5
Chorioadenoma (destruens) D39.2
Chorioamnionitis O41.12-
Chorioangioma D26.7
Choriocarcinoma —*see* Neoplasm,
  malignant, by site
  combined with
    embryonal carcinoma —*see*
      Neoplasm, malignant, by site
    other germ cell elements —*see*
      Neoplasm, malignant, by site
    teratoma —*see* Neoplasm,
      malignant, by site
  specified site —*see* Neoplasm,
    malignant, by site
  unspecified site
    female C58
    male C62.90
Chorioencephalitis (acute)
  (lymphocytic) (serous) A87.2
Chorioepithelioma —*see*
  Choriocarcinoma
Choriomeningitis (acute)
  (lymphocytic) (serous) A87.2
Chorionepithelioma —*see*
  Choriocarcinoma
Chorioretinitis —*see also*
  Inflammation, chorioretinal
  disseminated —*see also*
    Inflammation, chorioretinal,
    disseminated
  in neurosyphilis A52.19
  Egyptian B76.9 *[D63.8]*
  focal —*see also* Inflammation,
    chorioretinal, focal
  histoplasmic B39.9 *[H32]*
  in (due to)
    histoplasmosis B39.9 *[H32]*
    syphilis (secondary) A51.43
      late A52.71
    toxoplasmosis (acquired)
      B58.01
      congenital (active) P37.1
      [H32]
    tuberculosis A18.53
  juxtapapillary, juxtapapillaris —*see*
    Inflammation, chorioretinal,
    focal, juxtapapillary
  leprous A30.9 *[H32]*
  miner's B76.9 *[D63.8]*
  progressive myopia (degeneration)
    (*see also* Myopia, degenerative)
    H44.2-
  syphilitic (secondary) A51.43
    congenital (early) A50.01
    [H32]
    late A50.32
    late A52.71
  tuberculous A18.53

Chorioretinopathy, central serous
H35.71-

Choroid —*see* condition

Choroideremia H31.21

Choroiditis —*see* Chorioretinitis

Choroidopathy —*see* Disorder,
choroid

Choroidoretinitis —*see*
Chorioretinitis

**Choroidoretinopathy, central
serous** —*see* Chorioretinopathy,
central serous

Christian-Weber disease M35.6

Christmas disease D67

Chromaffinoma —*see also*
Neoplasm, benign, by site
malignant —*see* Neoplasm,
malignant, by site

Chromatopsia —*see* Deficiency,
color vision

Chromhidrosis, chromidrosis L75.1

Chromoblastomycosis —*see*
Chromomycosis

Chromoconversion R82.91

Chromomycosis B43.9
brain abscess B43.1
cerebral B43.1
cutaneous B43.0
skin B43.0
specified NEC B43.8
subcutaneous abscess or cyst
B43.2

Chromophytosis B36.0

Chromosome —*see* condition by
chromosome involved
D (1) —*see* condition, chromosome
13
E (3) —*see* condition, chromosome
18
G —*see* condition, chromosome 21

Chromotrichomycosis B36.8

Chronic —*see* condition
fracture —*see* Fracture,
pathological

Churg-Strauss syndrome M30.1

Chyle cyst, mesentery I89.8

Chylocele (nonfilarial) I89.8
filarial (*see also* Infestation, filarial)
B74.9 *[N51]*
tunica vaginalis N50.89
filarial (*see also* Infestation,
filarial) B74.9 *[N51]*

Chylomicronemia (fasting) (with
hyperprebetalipoproteinemia)
E78.3

Chylopericardium I31.3
acute I30.9

Chylothorax (nonfilarial) I89.8
filarial (*see also* Infestation, filarial)
B74.9 *[J91.8]*

Chylous —*see* condition

Chyluria (nonfilarial) R82.0
due to
bilharziasis B65.0
Brugia (malayi) B74.1
timori B74.2
schistosomiasis (bilharziasis)
B65.0
Wuchereria (bancrofti) B74.0
filarial —*see* Infestation,
filarial

Cicatricial (deformity) —*see* Cicatrix

Cicatrix (adherent) (contracted)
(painful) (vicious) (*see also* Scar)
L90.5
adenoid (and tonsil) J35.8
alveolar process M26.79
anus K62.89
auricle —*see* Disorder, pinna,
specified type NEC
bile duct (common) (hepatic)
K83.8
bladder N32.89
bone —*see* Disorder, bone,
specified type NEC
brain G93.89
cervix (postoperative) (postpartal)
N88.1
common duct K83.8
cornea H17.9
tuberculous A18.59
duodenum (bulb), obstructive
K31.5
esophagus K22.2
eyelid —*see* Disorder, eyelid
function
hypopharynx J39.2
lacrimal passages —*see*
Obstruction, lacrimal
larynx J38.7
lung J98.4
middle ear H74.8
mouth K13.79
muscle M62.89
with contracture —*see*
Contraction, muscle NEC
nasopharynx J39.2
palate (soft) K13.79
penis N48.89
pharynx J39.2
prostate N42.89
rectum K62.89
retina —*see* Scar, chorioretinal
semilunar cartilage —*see*
Derangement, meniscus
seminal vesicle N50.89
skin L90.5
infected L08.89
postinfective L90.5
tuberculous B90.8
specified site NEC L90.5
throat J39.2
tongue K14.8
tonsil (and adenoid) J35.8
trachea J39.8
tuberculous NEC B90.9
urethra N36.8
uterus N85.8
postoperative N99.2
vagina N89.8
postoperative N99.2
vocal cord J38.3
wrist, constricting (annular) L90.5

CIDP (chronic inflammatory
demyelinating polyneuropathy)
G61.81

CIN —*see* Neoplasia, intraepithelial,
cervix

**CINCA (chronic infantile
neurological, cutaneous and
articular syndrome)** M04.2

Cinchonism —*see* Deafness, ototoxic
correct substance properly
administered —*see* Table of
Drugs and Chemicals, by drug,
adverse effect
overdose or wrong substance
given or taken —*see* Table of
Drugs and Chemicals, by drug,
poisoning

Circle of Willis —*see* condition

Circular —*see* condition

Circulating anticoagulants
(*see also* Disorder, hemorrhagic)
D68.318
due to drugs (*see also* Disorder,
hemorrhagic) D68.32
following childbirth O72.3

Circulation
collateral, any site I99.8
defective (lower extremity) I99.9
congenital Q28.9
embryonic Q28.9
failure (peripheral) R57.9
newborn P29.89
fetal, persistent P29.38
heart, incomplete Q28.9

Circulatory system —*see* condition

Circulus senilis (cornea) —*see*
Degeneration, cornea, senile

Circumcision (in absence of medical
indication) (ritual) (routine) Z41.2

Circumscribed —*see* condition

Circumvallate placenta O43.11-

Cirrhosis, cirrhotic (hepatic) (liver)
K74.60
alcoholic K70.30
with ascites K70.31
atrophic —*see* Cirrhosis, liver
Baumgarten-Cruveilhier K74.69
biliary (cholangiolitic) (cholangitic)
(hypertrophic) (obstructive)
(pericholangiolitic) K74.5
due to
Clonorchiasis B66.1
flukes B66.3
primary K74.3
secondary K74.4
cardiac (of liver) K76.1
Charcot's K74.3
cholangiolitic, cholangitic,
cholostatic (primary) K74.3
congestive K76.1
Cruveilhier-Baumgarten K74.69
cryptogenic (liver) K74.69
due to
hepatolenticular degeneration
E83.01
Wilson's disease E83.01
xanthomatosis E78.2
fatty K76.0
alcoholic K70.0
Hanot's (hypertrophic) K74.3
hepatic —*see* Cirrhosis, liver
hypertrophic K74.3
Indian childhood K74.69
kidney —*see* Sclerosis, renal
Laennec's K70.30
with ascites K70.31
alcoholic K70.30
with ascites K70.31
nonalcoholic K74.69
liver K74.60
alcoholic K70.30
with ascites K70.31
fatty K70.0
congenital P78.81
syphilitic A52.74
lung (chronic) J84.10
macronodular K74.69
alcoholic K70.30
with ascites K70.31
micronodular K74.69
alcoholic K70.30
with ascites K70.31
mixed type K74.69
monolobular K74.3
nephritis —*see* Sclerosis, renal
nutritional K74.69
alcoholic K70.30
with ascites K70.31

Cirrhosis, cirrhotic (*continued*)
obstructive —*see* Cirrhosis, biliary
ovarian N83.8
pancreas (duct) K86.89
pigmentary E83.110
portal K74.69
alcoholic K70.30
with ascites K70.31
postnecrotic K74.69
alcoholic K70.30
with ascites K70.31
pulmonary J84.10
renal —*see* Sclerosis, renal
spleen D73.2
stasis K76.1
Todd's K74.3
unilobar K74.3
xanthomatous (biliary) K74.5
due to xanthomatosis (familial)
(metabolic) (primary) E78.2

Cistern, subarachnoid R93.0

Citrullinemia E72.23

Citrullinuria E72.23

Civatte's disease or poikiloderma
L57.3

Clam digger's itch B65.3

Clammy skin R23.1

Clap —*see* Gonorrhea

Clarke-Hadfield syndrome
(pancreatic infantilism) K86.89

Clark's paralysis G80.9

Clastothrix L67.8

Claude Bernard-Horner syndrome
G90.2
traumatic —*see* Injury, nerve,
cervical sympathetic

Claude's disease or syndrome
G46.3

Claudication (intermittent) I73.9
cerebral (artery) G45.9
spinal cord (arteriosclerotic) G95.19
syphilitic A52.09
venous (axillary) I87.8

Claudicatio venosa intermittens
I87.8

Claustrophobia F40.240

Clavus (infected) L84

Clawfoot (congenital) Q66.89
acquired —*see* Deformity, limb,
clawfoot

Clawhand (acquired) —*see also*
Deformity, limb, clawhand
congenital Q68.1

Clawtoe (congenital) Q66.89
acquired —*see* Deformity, toe,
specified NEC

Clay eating —*see* Pica

Cleansing of artificial opening —*see*
Attention to, artificial, opening

Cleft (congenital) —*see also*
Imperfect, closure
alveolar process M26.79
branchial (persistent) Q18.2
cyst Q18.0
fistula Q18.0
sinus Q18.0
cricoid cartilage, posterior
Q31.8
foot Q72.7
hand Q71.6
lip (unilateral) Q36.9
with cleft palate Q37.9
hard Q37.1
with soft Q37.5
soft Q37.3
with hard Q37.5

Cleft (continued)
lip (continued)
bilateral Q36.0
with cleft palate Q37.8
hard Q37.0
with soft Q37.4
soft Q37.2
with hard Q37.4
median Q36.1
nose Q30.2
palate Q35.9
with cleft lip (unilateral)
Q37.9
bilateral Q37.8
hard Q35.1
with
cleft lip (unilateral) Q37.1
bilateral Q37.0
soft Q35.5
with cleft lip (unilateral)
Q37.5
bilateral Q37.4
medial Q35.5
soft Q35.3
with
cleft lip (unilateral) Q37.3
bilateral Q37.2
hard Q35.5
with cleft lip (unilateral)
Q37.5
bilateral Q37.4
penis Q55.69
scrotum Q55.29
thyroid cartilage Q31.8
uvula Q35.7

Cleidocranial dysostosis Q74.0

Cleptomania F63.2

Clicking hip (newborn) R29.4

Climacteric (female) —see also
Menopause
arthritis (any site) NEC —see
Arthritis, specified form NEC
depression (single episode) F32.89
recurrent episode F33.8
melancholia (single episodie)
F32.89
recurrent episode F33.8
male (symptoms) (syndrome) NEC
N50.89
paranoid state F22
polyarthritis NEC —see Arthritis,
specified form NEC
symptoms (female) N95.1

Clinical research investigation
(clinical trial) (control subject)
(normal comparison) (participant)
Z00.6

Clitoris —see condition

Cloaca (persistent) Q43.7

Clonorchiasis, clonorchis infection
(liver) B66.1

Clonus R25.8

Closed bite M26.29

Clostridium (C.) **perfringens,
as cause of disease classified
elsewhere** B96.7

Closure
congenital, nose Q30.0
cranial sutures, premature Q75.0
defective or imperfect NEC —see
Imperfect, closure
fistula, delayed —see Fistula
foramen ovale, imperfect Q21.1
hymen N89.6
interauricular septum, defective
Q21.1
interventricular septum, defective
Q21.0

Closure (continued)
lacrimal duct —see also Stenosis,
lacrimal, duct
congenital Q10.5
nose (congenital) Q30.0
acquired M95.0
of artificial opening —see Attention
to, artificial, opening
primary angle, without glaucoma
damage H40.06-
vagina N89.5
valve —see Endocarditis
vulva N90.5

Clot (blood) —see also Embolism
artery (obstruction) (occlusion)
—see Embolism
bladder N32.89
brain (intradural or extradural) —
see Occlusion, artery, cerebral
circulation I74.9
heart —see also Infarct,
myocardium
not resulting in infarction I51.3
vein —see Thrombosis

Clouded state R40.1
epileptic —see Epilepsy, specified
NEC
paroxysmal —see Epilepsy,
specified NEC

Cloudy antrum, antra J32.0

Clouston's (hidrotic) **ectodermal
dysplasia** Q82.4

Clubbed nail pachydermoperiostosis
M89.40 [L62]

Clubbing of finger(s) (nails)
R68.3

Clubfinger R68.3
congenital Q68.1

Clubfoot (congenital) Q66.89
acquired —see Deformity, limb,
clubfoot
equinovarus Q66.0-
paralytic —see Deformity, limb,
clubfoot

Clubhand (congenital) (radial)
Q71.4-
acquired —see Deformity, limb,
clubhand

Clubnail R68.3
congenital Q84.6

Clump, kidney Q63.1

Clumsiness, clumsy child syndrome
F82

Cluttering F80.81

Clutton's joints A50.51 [M12.80]

Coagulation, intravascular
(diffuse) (disseminated) —see also
Defibrination syndrome
complicating abortion —see
Abortion, by type, complicated
by, intravascular coagulation
following ectopic or molar
pregnancy O08.1

Coagulopathy —see also Defect,
coagulation
consumption D65
intravascular D65
newborn P60

Coalition
calcaneo-scaphoid Q66.89
tarsal Q66.89

Coalminer's
elbow —see Bursitis, elbow,
olecranon
lung or pneumoconiosis J60

Coalworker's lung or
pneumoconiosis J60

Coarctation
aorta (preductal) (postductal) Q25.1
pulmonary artery Q25.71

Coated tongue K14.3

Coats' disease (exudative
retinopathy) —see Retinopathy,
exudative

Cocaine-induced
anxiety disorder F14.980
bipolar and related disorder
F14.94
depressive disorder F14.94
obsessive-compulsive and related
disorder F14.988
psychotic disorder F14.959
sleep disorder F14.982
sexual dysfunction F14.981

Cocainism —see Disorder, cocaine use

Coccidioidomycosis B38.9
cutaneous B38.3
disseminated B38.7
generalized B38.7
meninges B38.4
prostate B38.81
pulmonary B38.2
acute B38.0
chronic B38.1
skin B38.3
specified NEC B38.89

Coccidioidosis —see
Coccidioidomycosis

Coccidiosis (intestinal) A07.3

Coccydynia, coccygodynia M53.3

Coccyx —see condition

Cochin-China diarrhea K90.1

Cockayne's syndrome Q87.19

Cocked up toe —see Deformity, toe,
specified NEC

Cock's peculiar tumor L72.3

Codman's tumor —see Neoplasm,
bone, benign

Coenurosis B71.8

Coffee-worker's lung J67.8

Cogan's syndrome H16.32-
oculomotor apraxia H51.8

Coitus, painful (female) N94.10
male N53.12
psychogenic F52.6

Cold J00
with influenza, flu, or grippe —see
Influenza, with, respiratory
manifestations NEC
agglutinin disease or
hemoglobinuria (chronic) D59.12
bronchial —see Bronchitis
chest —see Bronchitis
common (head) J00
effects of T69.9
specified effect NEC T69.8
excessive, effects of T69.9
specified effect NEC T69.8
exhaustion from T69.8
exposure to T69.9
specified effect NEC T69.8
head J00
injury syndrome (newborn) P80.0
on lung —see Bronchitis
rose J30.1
sensitivity, auto-immune D59.12
symptoms J00
virus J00

Coldsore B00.1

Colibacillosis A49.8
as the cause of other disease (see
also Escherichia coli) B96.20
generalized A41.50

Colic (bilious) (infantile) (intestinal)
(recurrent) (spasmodic) R10.83
abdomen R10.83
psychogenic F45.8
appendix, appendicular K38.8
bile duct —see Calculus, bile duct
biliary —see Calculus, bile duct
common duct —see Calculus, bile
duct
cystic duct —see Calculus,
gallbladder
Devonshire NEC —see Poisoning,
lead
gallbladder —see Calculus,
gallbladder
gallstone —see Calculus,
gallbladder
gallbladder or cystic duct —see
Calculus, gallbladder
hepatic (duct) —see Calculus, bile
duct
hysterical F45.8
kidney N23
lead NEC —see Poisoning, lead
mucous K58.9
with diarrhea K58.0
psychogenic F54
nephritic N23
painter's NEC —see Poisoning,
lead
pancreas K86.89
psychogenic F45.8
renal N23
saturnine NEC —see Poisoning,
lead
ureter N23
urethral N36.8
due to calculus N21.1
uterus NEC N94.89
menstrual —see Dysmenorrhea
worm NOS B83.9

Colicystitis —see Cystitis

Colitis (acute) (catarrhal) (chronic)
(noninfective) (hemorrhagic) (see
also Enteritis) K52.9
allergic K52.29
with
food protein-induced
enterocolitis syndrome K52.21
proctocolitis K52.82
amebic (acute) (see also
Amebiasis) A06.0
nondysenteric A06.2
anthrax A22.2
bacillary —see Infection, Shigella
balantidial A07.0
Clostridium difficile
not specified as recurrent A04.72
recurrent A04.71
coccidial A07.3
collagenous K52.831
cystica superficialis K52.89
dietary counseling and surveillance
(for) Z71.3
dietetic (see also Colitis, allergic)
K52.29
drug-induced K52.1
due to radiation K52.0
eosinophilic K52.82
food hypersensitivity (see also
Colitis, allergic) K52.29
giardial A07.1
granulomatous —see Enteritis,
regional, large intestine

Colitis (continued)
indeterminate, so stated K52.3
infectious —see Enteritis, infectious
ischemic K55.9
acute (subacute) (see also Ischemia, intestine, acute) K55.039
chronic K55.1
due to mesenteric artery insufficiency K55.1
fulminant (acute) (see also Ischemia, intestine, acute) K55.039
left sided K51.50
with
abscess K51.514
complication K51.519
specified NEC K51.518
fistula K51.513
obstruction K51.512
rectal bleeding K51.511
lymphocytic K52.832
membranous
psychogenic F54
microscopic K52.839
specified NEC K52.838
mucous —see Syndrome, irritable, bowel
psychogenic F54
noninfective K52.9
specified NEC K52.89
polyposa —see Polyp, colon, inflammatory
protozoal A07.9
pseudomembranous
not specified as recurrent A04.72
recurrent A04.71
pseudomucinous —see Syndrome, irritable, bowel
regional —see Enteritis, regional, large intestine
infectious A09
segmental —see Enteritis, regional, large intestine
septic —see Enteritis, infectious
spastic K58.9
with diarrhea K58.0
psychogenic F54
staphylococcal A04.8
foodborne A05.0
subacute ischemic (see also Ischemia, intestine, acute) K55.039
thromboulcerative (see also Ischemia, intestine, acute) K55.039
toxic NEC K52.1
due to Clostridium difficile
not specified as recurrent A04.72
recurrent A04.71
transmural —see Enteritis, regional, large intestine
trichomonal A07.8
tuberculous (ulcerative) A18.32
ulcerative (chronic) K51.90
with
complication K51.919
abscess K51.914
fistula K51.913
obstruction K51.912
rectal bleeding K51.911
specified complication NEC K51.918
enterocolitis —see Enterocolitis, ulcerative
ileocolitis —see Ileocolitis, ulcerative
mucosal proctocolitis —see Proctocolitis, mucosal

Colitis (continued)
ulcerative (continued)
proctitis —see Proctitis, ulcerative
pseudopolyposis —see Polyp, colon, inflammatory
psychogenic F54
rectosigmoiditis —see Rectosigmoiditis, ulcerative
specified type NEC K51.80
with
complication K51.819
abscess K51.814
fistula K51.813
obstruction K51.812
rectal bleeding K51.811
specified complication NEC K51.818

Collagenosis, collagen disease
(nonvascular) (vascular) M35.9
cardiovascular I42.8
reactive perforating L87.1
specified NEC M35.8

Collapse R55
adrenal E27.2
cardiorespiratory R57.0
cardiovascular R57.0
newborn P29.89
circulatory (peripheral) R57.9
during or after labor and delivery O75.1
following ectopic or molar pregnancy O08.3
newborn P29.89
during or
after labor and delivery O75.1
resulting from a procedure, not elsewhere classified T81.10
external ear canal —see Stenosis, external ear canal
general R55
heart —see Disease, heart
heat T67.1
hysterical F44.89
labyrinth, membranous (congenital) Q16.5
lung (massive) (see also Atelectasis) J98.19
pressure due to anesthesia (general) (local) or other sedation T88.2
during labor and delivery O74.1
in pregnancy O29.02-
postpartum, puerperal O89.09
myocardial —see Disease, heart
nervous F48.8
neurocirculatory F45.8
nose M95.0
postoperative T81.10
pulmonary (see also Atelectasis) J98.19
newborn —see Atelectasis
trachea J39.8
tracheobronchial J98.09
valvular —see Endocarditis
vascular (peripheral) R57.9
during or after labor and delivery O75.1
following ectopic or molar pregnancy O08.3
newborn P29.89
vertebra M48.50-
cervical region M48.52-
cervicothoracic region M48.53-
in (due to)
metastasis —see Collapse, vertebra, in, specified disease NEC

Collapse (continued)
vertebra (continued)
in (continued)
osteoporosis (see also Osteoporosis) M80.88
cervical region M80.88
cervicothoracic region M80.88
lumbar region M80.88
lumbosacral region M80.88
multiple sites M80.88
occipito-atlanto-axial region M80.88
sacrococcygeal region M80.88
thoracic region M80.88
thoracolumbar region M80.88
specified disease NEC M48.50-
cervical region M48.52-
cervicothoracic region M48.53-
lumbar region M48.56-
lumbosacral region M48.57-
occipito-atlanto-axial region M48.51-
sacrococcygeal region M48.58-
thoracic region M48.54-
thoracolumbar region M48.55-
lumbar region M48.56-
lumbosacral region M48.57-
occipito-atlanto-axial region M48.51-
sacrococcygeal region M48.58-
thoracic region M48.54-
thoracolumbar region M48.55-

Collateral —see also condition
circulation (venous) I87.8
dilation, veins I87.8

Colles' fracture S52.53-

Collet (-Sicard) **syndrome** G52.7

Collier's asthma or lung J60

Collodion baby Q80.2

Colloid nodule (of thyroid) (cystic) E04.1

Coloboma (iris) Q13.0
eyelid Q10.3
fundus Q14.8
lens Q12.2
optic disc (congenital) Q14.2
acquired H47.31-

Coloenteritis —see Enteritis

Colon —see condition

Colonization
MRSA (Methicillin resistant Staphylococcus aureus) Z22.322
MSSA (Methicillin susceptible Staphylococcus aureus) Z22.321
status —see Carrier (suspected) of

Coloptosis K63.4

Color blindness —see Deficiency, color vision

Colostomy
attention to Z43.3
fitting or adjustment Z46.89
malfunctioning K94.03
status Z93.3

Colpitis (acute) —see Vaginitis

Colpocele N81.5

Colpocystitis —see Vaginitis

Colpospasm N94.2

Column, spinal, vertebral —see condition

Coma R40.20
with
motor response (none) R40.231
abnormal R40.233
abnormal extensor posturing to pain or noxious stimuli (<2 years of age) R40.232
abnormal flexure posturing to pain or noxious stimuli (0-5 years of age) R40.233
extension R40.232
extensor posturing to pain or noxious stimuli (2-5 years of age) R40.232
flexion/decorticate posturing (<2 years of age) R40.233
flexion withdrawal R40.234
localizes pain (2-5 years of age) R40.235
normal or spontaneous movement (<2 years of age) R40.236
obeys commands (2-5 years of age) R40.236
score of
1 R40.231
2 R40.232
3 R40.233
4 R40.234
5 R40.235
6 R40.236
withdraws from pain or noxious stimuli (0-5 years of age) R40.234
withdraws to touch (<2 years of age) R40.235
opening of eyes (never) R40.211
in response to pain R40.212
sound R40.213
score of
1 R40.211
2 R40.212
3 R40.213
4 R40.214
spontaneous R40.214
verbal response (none) R40.221
confused conversation R40.224
cooing or babbling or crying appropriately (<2 years of age) R40.225
inappropriate crying or screaming (<2 years of age) R40.223
inappropriate words (2-5 years of age) R40.224
incomprehensible sounds (2-5 years of age) R40.222
incomprehensible words R40.222
irritable cries (<2 years of age) R40.224
moans/grunts to pain; restless (<2 years of age) R40.222
oriented R40.225
score of
1 R40.221
2 R40.222
3 R40.223
4 R40.224
5 R40.225
screaming (2-5 years of age) R40.223
uses appropriate words (2-5 years of age) R40.225
eclamptic —see Eclampsia
epileptic —see Epilepsy
Glasgow, scale score —see Glasgow coma scale
hepatic —see Failure, hepatic, by type, with coma

Coma *(continued)*
hyperglycemic (diabetic)
—*see* Diabetes, by type, with
hyperosmolarity, with coma
hyperosmolar (diabetic) —*see*
Diabetes, by type, with
hyperosmolarity, with coma
hypoglycemic (diabetic) —*see*
Diabetes, by type, with
hypoglycemia, with coma
nondiabetic E15
in diabetes —*see* Diabetes, coma
insulin-induced —*see* Coma,
hypoglycemic
ketoacidotic (diabetic) —*see*
Diabetes, by type, with
ketoacidosis, with coma
myxedematous E03.5
newborn P91.5
persistent vegetative state R40.3
specified NEC, without documented
Glasgow coma scale score, or
with partial Glasgow coma scale
score reported R40.244

Comatose —*see* Coma

Combat fatigue F43.0

Combined —*see* condition

Comedo, comedones (giant) L70.0

Comedocarcinoma —*see also*
Neoplasm, breast, malignant
noninfiltrating
breast D05.8-
specified site —*see* Neoplasm, in
situ, by site
unspecified site D05.8-

Comedomastitis —*see* Ectasia,
mammary duct

**Comminuted fracture - code as
Fracture, closed**

Common
arterial trunk Q20.0
atrioventricular canal Q21.2
atrium Q21.1
cold (head) J00
truncus (arteriosus) Q20.0
variable immunodeficiency —*see*
Immunodeficiency, common
variable
ventricle Q20.4

Commotio, commotion (current)
brain —*see* Injury, intracranial,
concussion
cerebri —*see* Injury, intracranial,
concussion
retinae S05.8X-
spinal cord —*see* Injury, spinal
cord, by region
spinalis —*see* Injury, spinal cord,
by region

Communication
between
base of aorta and pulmonary
artery Q21.4
left ventricle and right atrium
Q20.5
pericardial sac and pleural sac
Q34.8
pulmonary artery and pulmonary
vein, congenital Q25.72
congenital between uterus and
digestive or urinary tract Q51.7

Compartment syndrome (deep)
(posterior) (traumatic) T79.A0
abdomen T79.A3
lower extremity (hip, buttock,
thigh, leg, foot, toes) T79.A2
nontraumatic
abdomen M79.A3

Compartment syndrome *(continued)*
nontraumatic *(continued)*
lower extremity (hip, buttock,
thigh, leg, foot, toes) M79.A2-
specified site NEC M79.A9
upper extremity (shoulder, arm,
forearm, wrist, hand, fingers)
M79.A1-
specified site NEC T79.A9
upper extremity (shoulder, arm,
forearm, wrist, hand, fingers)
T79.A1

Compensation
failure —*see* Disease, heart
neurosis, psychoneurosis —*see*
Disorder, factitious

Complaint —*see also* Disease
bowel, functional K59.9
psychogenic F45.8
intestine, functional K59.9
psychogenic F45.8
kidney —*see* Disease, renal
miners' J60

Complete —*see* condition

Complex
Addison-Schilder E71.528
cardiorenal —*see* Hypertension,
cardiorenal
Costen's M26.69
disseminated mycobacterium avium-
intracellulare (DMAC) A31.2
Eisenmenger's (ventricular septal
defect) I27.83
hypersexual F52.8
jumped process, spine —*see*
Dislocation, vertebra
primary, tuberculous A15.7
Schilder-Addison E71.528
subluxation (vertebral) M99.19
abdomen M99.19
acromioclavicular M99.17
cervical region M99.11
cervicothoracic M99.11
costochondral M99.18
costovertebral M99.18
head region M99.10
hip M99.15
lower extremity M99.16
lumbar region M99.13
lumbosacral M99.13
occipitocervical M99.10
pelvic region M99.15
pubic M99.15
rib cage M99.18
sacral region M99.14
sacrococcygeal M99.14
sacroiliac M99.14
specified NEC M99.19
sternochondral M99.18
sternoclavicular M99.17
thoracic region M99.12
thoracolumbar M99.12
upper extremity M99.17
Taussig-Bing (transposition, aorta
and overriding pulmonary artery)
Q20.1

Complication(s) (from) (of)
accidental puncture or laceration
during a procedure (of) —*see*
Complications, intraoperative
(intraprocedural), puncture or
laceration
amputation stump (surgical) (late)
NEC T87.9
dehiscence T87.81
infection or inflammation T87.40
lower limb T87.4-
upper limb T87.4-
necrosis T87.50

Complication *(continued)*
amputation stump *(continued)*
necrosis *(continued)*
amputation stump (surgical)
lower limb T87.5-
upper limb T87.5-
neuroma T87.30
lower limb T87.3-
upper limb T87.3-
specified type NEC T87.89
anastomosis (and bypass) —*see
also* Complications, prosthetic
device or implant
intestinal (internal) NEC K91.89
involving urinary tract N99.89
urinary tract (involving intestinal
tract) N99.89
vascular —*see* Complications,
cardiovascular device or
implant
anesthesia, anesthetic (*see also*
Anesthesia, complication) T88.59
general, unintended awareness
during procedure T88.53
unintended awareness under
general anesthesia during
procedure T88.53
brain, postpartum, puerperal O89.2
cardiac
in
labor and delivery O74.2
pregnancy O29.19-
postpartum, puerperal O89.1
central nervous system
in
labor and delivery O74.3
pregnancy O29.29-
postpartum, puerperal O89.2
difficult or failed intubation T88.4
in pregnancy O29.6-
failed sedation (conscious)
(moderate) during procedure
T88.52
hyperthermia, malignant T88.3
hypothermia T88.51
intubation failure T88.4
malignant hyperthermia T88.3
pulmonary
in
labor and delivery O74.1
pregnancy NEC O29.09-
postpartum, puerperal O89.09
shock T88.2
spinal and epidural
in
labor and delivery NEC O74.6
headache O74.5
pregnancy NEC O29.5X-
postpartum, puerperal NEC
O89.5
headache O89.4
anti-reflux device —*see*
Complications, esophageal anti-
reflux device
aortic (bifurcation) graft —*see*
Complications, graft, vascular
aortocoronary (bypass) graft —*see*
Complications, coronary artery
(bypass) graft
aortofemoral (bypass) graft —*see*
Complications, extremity artery
(bypass) graft
arteriovenous
fistula, surgically created T82.9
embolism T82.818
fibrosis T82.828
hemorrhage T82.838
infection or inflammation T82.7
mechanical
breakdown T82.510

Complication *(continued)*
arteriovenous *(continued)*
fistula, surgically created
(continued)
mechanical *(continued)*
displacement T82.520
leakage T82.530
malposition T82.520
obstruction T82.590
perforation T82.590
protrusion T82.590
pain T82.848
specified type NEC T82.898
stenosis T82.858
thrombosis T82.868
shunt, surgically created T82.9
embolism T82.818
fibrosis T82.828
hemorrhage T82.838
infection or inflammation T82.7
mechanical
breakdown T82.511
displacement T82.521
leakage T82.531
malposition T82.521
obstruction T82.591
perforation T82.591
protrusion T82.591
pain T82.848
specified type NEC T82.898
stenosis T82.858
thrombosis T82.868
arthroplasty —*see* Complications,
joint prosthesis
artificial
fertilization or insemination N98.9
attempted introduction (of)
embryo in embryo transfer
N98.3
ovum following in vitro
fertilization N98.2
hyperstimulation of ovaries
N98.1
infection N98.0
specified NEC N98.8
heart T82.9
embolism T82.817
fibrosis T82.827
hemorrhage T82.837
infection or inflammation
T82.7
mechanical
breakdown T82.512
displacement T82.522
leakage T82.532
malposition T82.522
obstruction T82.592
perforation T82.592
protrusion T82.592
pain T82.847
specified type NEC T82.897
stenosis T82.857
thrombosis T82.867
opening
cecostomy —*see*
Complications, colostomy
colostomy —*see*
Complications, colostomy
cystostomy —*see*
Complications, cystostomy
enterostomy —*see*
Complications, enterostomy
gastrostomy —*see*
Complications, gastrostomy
ileostomy —*see*
Complications, enterostomy
jejunostomy —*see*
Complications, enterostomy
nephrostomy —*see*
Complications, stoma,
urinary tract

Complication *(continued)*
  artificial *(continued)*
    opening *(continued)*
      tracheostomy —*see*
        Complications,
        tracheostomy
      ureterostomy —*see*
        Complications, stoma,
        urinary tract
      urethrostomy —*see*
        Complications, stoma,
        urinary tract
  balloon implant or device
    gastrointestinal T85.9
      embolism T85.818
      fibrosis T85.828
      hemorrhage T85.838
      infection and inflammation
        T85.79
      pain T85.848
      specified type NEC T85.898
      stenosis T85.858
      thrombosis T85.868
    vascular (counterpulsation)
      T82.9
      embolism T82.818
      fibrosis T82.828
      hemorrhage T82.838
      infection or inflammation
        T82.7
      mechanical
        breakdown T82.513
        displacement T82.523
        leakage T82.533
        malposition T82.523
        obstruction T82.593
        perforation T82.593
        protrusion T82.593
      pain T82.848
      specified type NEC T82.898
      stenosis T82.858
      thrombosis T82.868
  bariatric procedure
    gastric band procedure K95.09
      infection K95.01
    specified procedure NEC K95.89
      infection K95.81
  bile duct implant (prosthetic) T85.9
    embolism T85.818
    fibrosis T85.828
    hemorrhage T85.838
    infection and inflammation
      T85.79
    mechanical
      breakdown T85.510
      displacement T85.520
      malfunction T85.510
      malposition T85.520
      obstruction T85.590
      perforation T85.590
      protrusion T85.590
      specified NEC T85.590
    pain T85.848
    specified type NEC T85.898
    stenosis T85.858
    thrombosis T85.868
  bladder device (auxiliary) —*see*
    Complications, genitourinary,
    device or implant, urinary system
  bleeding (postoperative) —*see*
    Complication, postoperative,
    hemorrhage
    intraoperative —*see*
      Complication, intraoperative,
      hemorrhage
  blood vessel graft —*see*
    Complications, graft, vascular
  bone
    device NEC T84.9
      embolism T84.81
      fibrosis T84.82

Complication *(continued)*
  bone *(continued)*
    device NEC *(continued)*
      hemorrhage T84.83
      infection or inflammation T84.7
      mechanical
        breakdown T84.318
        displacement T84.328
        malposition T84.328
        obstruction T84.398
        perforation T84.398
        protrusion T84.398
      pain T84.84
      specified type NEC T84.89
      stenosis T84.85
      thrombosis T84.86
    graft —*see* Complications, graft,
      bone
    growth stimulator (electrode)
      —*see* Complications, electronic
      stimulator device, bone
    marrow transplant —*see*
      Complications, transplant,
      bone, marrow
  brain neurostimulator (electrode)
    —*see* Complications, electronic
    stimulator device, brain
  breast implant (prosthetic) T85.9
    capsular contracture T85.44
    embolism T85.818
    fibrosis T85.828
    hemorrhage T85.838
    infection and inflammation T85.79
    mechanical
      breakdown T85.41
      displacement T85.42
      leakage T85.43
      malposition T85.42
      obstruction T85.49
      perforation T85.49
      protrusion T85.49
      specified NEC T85.49
    pain T85.848
    specified type NEC T85.898
    stenosis T85.858
    thrombosis T85.868
  bypass —*see also* Complications,
    prosthetic device or implant
    aortocoronary —*see* Complications,
      coronary artery (bypass) graft
    arterial —*see also*
      Complications, graft, vascular
      extremity —*see*
        Complications, extremity
        artery (bypass) graft
  cardiac —*see also* Disease, heart
    device, implant or graft T82.9
      embolism T82.817
      fibrosis T82.827
      hemorrhage T82.837
      infection or inflammation T82.7
        valve prosthesis T82.6
      mechanical
        breakdown T82.519
          specified device NEC
            T82.518
        displacement T82.529
          specified device NEC
            T82.528
        leakage T82.539
          specified device NEC
            T82.538
        malposition T82.529
          specified device NEC
            T82.528
        obstruction T82.599
          specified device NEC
            T82.598
        perforation T82.599
          specified device NEC
            T82.598

Complication *(continued)*
  cardiac —*see also* Disease, heart
    (continued)
    device, implant or graft *(continued)*
      mechanical *(continued)*
        protrusion T82.599
          specified device NEC
            T82.598
        pain T82.847
        specified type NEC T82.897
        stenosis T82.857
        thrombosis T82.867
  cardiovascular device, graft or
    implant T82.9
    aortic graft —*see* Complications,
      graft, vascular
    arteriovenous
      fistula, artificial —*see*
        Complication, arteriovenous,
        fistula, surgically created
      shunt —*see* Complication,
        arteriovenous, shunt,
        surgically created
    artificial heart —*see*
      Complication, artificial, heart
    balloon (counterpulsation)
      device —*see* Complication,
        balloon implant, vascular
    carotid artery graft —*see*
      Complications, graft, vascular
    coronary bypass graft —*see*
      Complication, coronary artery
      (bypass) graft
    dialysis catheter (vascular) —*see*
      Complication, catheter, dialysis
    electronic T82.9
      electrode T82.9
        embolism T82.817
        fibrosis T82.827
        hemorrhage T82.837
        infection T82.7
        mechanical
          breakdown T82.110
          displacement T82.120
          leakage T82.190
          obstruction T82.190
          perforation T82.190
          protrusion T82.190
          specified type NEC
            T82.190
        pain T82.847
        specified NEC T82.897
        stenosis T82.857
        thrombosis T82.867
      embolism T82.817
      fibrosis T82.827
      hemorrhage T82.837
      infection T82.7
      mechanical
        breakdown T82.119
        displacement T82.129
        leakage T82.199
        obstruction T82.199
        perforation T82.199
        protrusion T82.199
        specified type NEC T82.199
      pain T82.847
      pulse generator T82.9
        embolism T82.817
        fibrosis T82.827
        hemorrhage T82.837
        infection T82.7
        mechanical
          breakdown T82.111
          displacement T82.121
          leakage T82.191
          obstruction T82.191
          perforation T82.191
          protrusion T82.191
          specified type NEC
            T82.191

Complication *(continued)*
  cardiovascular device, graft or
    implant *(continued)*
    electronic *(continued)*
      pulse generator *(continued)*
        pain T82.847
        specified NEC T82.897
        stenosis T82.857
        thrombosis T82.867
      specified condition NEC
        T82.897
    specified device NEC T82.9
      embolism T82.817
      fibrosis T82.827
      hemorrhage T82.837
      infection T82.7
      mechanical
        breakdown T82.118
        displacement T82.128
        leakage T82.198
        obstruction T82.198
        perforation T82.198
        protrusion T82.198
        specified type NEC
          T82.198
      pain T82.847
      specified NEC T82.897
      stenosis T82.857
      thrombosis T82.867
    stenosis T82.857
    thrombosis T82.867
    extremity artery graft —*see*
      Complication, extremity artery
      (bypass) graft
    femoral artery graft —*see*
      Complication, extremity artery
      (bypass) graft
    heart-lung transplant —*see*
      Complication, transplant,
      heart, with lung
    heart
      transplant —*see* Complication,
        transplant, heart
      valve —*see* Complication,
        prosthetic device, heart valve
        graft —*see* Complication,
          heart, valve, graft
    infection or inflammation T82.7
    umbrella device —*see*
      Complication, umbrella
      device, vascular
    vascular graft (or anastomosis)
      —*see* Complication, graft,
      vascular
  carotid artery (bypass) graft —*see*
    Complications, graft, vascular
  catheter (device) NEC —*see also*
    Complications, prosthetic device
    or implant
    cranial infusion
      infection and inflammation
        T85.735
      mechanical
        breakdown T85.610
        displacement T85.620
        leakage T85.630
        malfunction T85.690
        malposition T85.620
        obstruction T85.690
        perforation T85.690
        protrusion T85.690
        specified NEC T85.690
    cystostomy T83.9
      embolism T83.81
      fibrosis T83.82
      hemorrhage T83.83
      infection and inflammation
        T83.510
      mechanical
        breakdown T83.010
        displacement T83.020

Complication *(continued)*
catheter (device) NEC *(continued)*
  cystostomy *(continued)*
    mechanical *(continued)*
      leakage T83.030
      malposition T83.020
      obstruction T83.090
      perforation T83.090
      protrusion T83.090
      specified NEC T83.090
    pain T83.84
    specified type NEC T83.89
    stenosis T83.85
    thrombosis T83.86
  dialysis (vascular) T82.9
    embolism T82.818
    fibrosis T82.828
    hemorrhage T82.838
    infection and inflammation T82.7
    intraperitoneal —*see*
      Complications, catheter,
      intraperitoneal
    mechanical
      breakdown T82.41
      displacement T82.42
      leakage T82.43
      malposition T82.42
      obstruction T82.49
      perforation T82.49
      protrusion T82.49
    pain T82.848
    specified type NEC T82.898
    stenosis T82.858
    thrombosis T82.868
  epidural infusion T85.9
    embolism T85.810
    fibrosis T85.820
    hemorrhage T85.830
    infection and inflammation T85.735
    mechanical
      breakdown T85.610
      displacement T85.620
      leakage T85.630
      malfunction T85.610
      malposition T85.620
      obstruction T85.690
      perforation T85.690
      protrusion T85.690
      specified NEC T85.690
    pain T85.840
    specified type NEC T85.890
    stenosis T85.850
    thrombosis T85.860
  intraperitoneal dialysis T85.9
    embolism T85.818
    fibrosis T85.828
    hemorrhage T85.838
    infection and inflammation T85.735
    mechanical
      breakdown T85.611
      displacement T85.621
      leakage T85.631
      malfunction T85.611
      malposition T85.621
      obstruction T85.691
      perforation T85.691
      protrusion T85.691
      specified NEC T85.691
    pain T85.848
    specified type NEC T85.898
    stenosis T85.858
    thrombosis T85.868
  intrathecal infusion
    infection and inflammation T85.735
    mechanical
      breakdown T85.610
      displacement T85.620
      leakage T85.630

Complication *(continued)*
catheter (device) NEC *(continued)*
  intrathecal infusion *(continued)*
    mechanical *(continued)*
      malfunction T85.690
      malposition T85.620
      obstruction T85.690
      perforation T85.690
      protrusion T85.690
      specified NEC T85.690
  intravenous infusion T82.9
    embolism T82.818
    fibrosis T82.828
    hemorrhage T82.838
    infection or inflammation T82.7
    mechanical
      breakdown T82.514
      displacement T82.524
      leakage T82.534
      malposition T82.524
      obstruction T82.594
      perforation T82.594
      protrusion T82.594
    pain T82.848
    specified type NEC T82.898
    stenosis T82.858
    thrombosis T82.868
  spinal infusion
    infection and inflammation T85.735
    mechanical
      breakdown T85.610
      displacement T85.620
      leakage T85.630
      malfunction T85.690
      malposition T85.620
      obstruction T85.690
      perforation T85.690
      protrusion T85.690
      specified NEC T85.690
  subarachnoid infusion
    infection and inflammation T85.735
    mechanical
      breakdown T85.610
      displacement T85.620
      leakage T85.630
      malfunction T85.690
      malposition T85.620
      obstruction T85.690
      perforation T85.690
      protrusion T85.690
      specified NEC T85.690
  subdural infusion T85.9
    embolism T85.810
    fibrosis T85.820
    hemorrhage T85.830
    infection and inflammation T85.735
    mechanical
      breakdown T85.610
      displacement T85.620
      leakage T85.630
      malfunction T85.610
      malposition T85.620
      obstruction T85.690
      perforation T85.690
      protrusion T85.690
      specified NEC T85.690
    pain T85.840
    specified type NEC T85.890
    stenosis T85.850
    thrombosis T85.860
  urethral T83.9
    displacement T83.028
    embolism T83.81
    fibrosis T83.82
    hemorrhage T83.83
    indwelling
      breakdown T83.011
      displacement T83.021

Complication *(continued)*
catheter (device) NEC *(continued)*
  urethral *(continued)*
    indwelling *(continued)*
      infection and inflammation T83.511
      leakage T83.031
      specified complication NEC T83.091
    infection and inflammation T83.511
    leakage T83.038
    malposition T83.028
    mechanical
      breakdown T83.011
    obstruction (mechanical) T83.091
    pain T83.84
    perforation T83.091
    protrusion T83.091
    specified type NEC T83.091
    stenosis T83.85
    thrombosis T83.86
  urinary NEC
    breakdown T83.018
    displacement T83.028
    infection and inflammation T83.518
    leakage T83.038
    specified complication NEC T83.098
cecostomy (stoma) —*see* Complications, colostomy
cesarean delivery wound NEC O90.89
  disruption O90.0
  hematoma O90.2
  infection (following delivery) O86.00
chemotherapy (antineoplastic) NEC T88.7
chin implant (prosthetic) —*see* Complication, prosthetic device or implant, specified NEC
circulatory system I99.8
  intraoperative I97.88
  postprocedural I97.89
    following cardiac surgery (*see also* Infarct, myocardium, associated with revascularization procedure) I97.19-
      postcardiotomy syndrome I97.0
    hypertension I97.3
    lymphedema after mastectomy I97.2
    postcardiotomy syndrome I97.0
    seroma —*see* Complications, postprocedural, seroma (of), mastoid process
    specified NEC I97.89
colostomy (stoma) K94.00
  hemorrhage K94.01
  infection K94.02
  malfunction K94.03
  mechanical K94.03
  specified complication NEC K94.09
contraceptive device, intrauterine —*see* Complications, intrauterine, contraceptive device
cord (umbilical) —*see* Complications, umbilical cord
corneal graft —*see* Complications, graft, cornea
coronary artery (bypass) graft T82.9
  atherosclerosis —*see* Arteriosclerosis, coronary (artery)

Complication *(continued)*
coronary artery (bypass) graft *(continued)*
  embolism T82.818
  fibrosis T82.828
  hemorrhage T82.838
  infection and inflammation T82.7
  mechanical
    breakdown T82.211
    displacement T82.212
    leakage T82.213
    malposition T82.212
    obstruction T82.218
    perforation T82.218
    protrusion T82.218
    specified NEC T82.218
  pain T82.848
  specified type NEC T82.898
  stenosis T82.858
  thrombosis T82.868
counterpulsation device (balloon), intra- aortic —*see* Complications, balloon implant, vascular
cystostomy (stoma) N99.518
  catheter —*see* Complications, catheter, cystostomy
  hemorrhage N99.510
  infection N99.511
  malfunction N99.512
  specified type NEC N99.518
delivery (*see also* Complications, obstetric) O75.9
  procedure (instrumental) (manual) (surgical) O75.4
  specified NEC O75.89
dialysis (peritoneal) (renal) —*see also* Complications, infusion
  catheter (vascular) —*see* Complication, catheter, dialysis
  peritoneal, intraperitoneal —*see* Complications, catheter, intraperitoneal
dorsal column (spinal) neurostimulator —*see* Complications, electronic stimulator device, spinal cord
drug NEC T88.7
ear procedure —*see also* Disorder, ear
  intraoperative H95.88
    hematoma —*see* Complications, intraoperative, hemorrhage (hematoma) (of), ear
    hemorrhage —*see* Complications, intraoperative, hemorrhage (hematoma) (of), ear
    laceration —*see* Complications, intraoperative, puncture or laceration..., ear
    specified NEC H95.88
  postoperative H95.89
    external ear canal stenosis H95.81-
    hematoma —*see* Complications, postprocedural, hematoma (of), ear
    hemorrhage —*see* Complications, postprocedural, hemorrhage (of), ear
    postmastoidectomy —*see* Complications, postmastoidectomy
    specified NEC H95.89
    seroma — *see* Complications, postprocedural, seroma (of), mastoid process

Complication *(continued)*
ectopic pregnancy O08.9
  damage to pelvic organs O08.6
  embolism O08.2
  genital infection O08.0
  hemorrhage (delayed)
    (excessive) O08.1
  metabolic disorder O08.5
  renal failure O08.4
  shock O08.3
  specified type NEC O08.0
  venous complication NEC O08.7
electronic stimulator device
  bladder (urinary) —*see*
    Complications, electronic
    stimulator device, urinary
  bone T84.9
    breakdown T84.310
    displacement T84.320
    embolism T84.81
    fibrosis T84.82
    hemorrhage T84.83
    infection or inflammation
      T84.7
    malfunction T84.310
    malposition T84.320
    mechanical NEC T84.390
    obstruction T84.390
    pain T84.84
    perforation T84.390
    protrusion T84.390
    specified type NEC T84.89
    stenosis T84.85
    thrombosis T84.86
  brain T85.9
    embolism T85.810
    fibrosis T85.820
    hemorrhage T85.830
    infection and inflammation
      T85.731
    mechanical
      breakdown T85.110
      displacement T85.120
      leakage T85.190
      malposition T85.120
      obstruction T85.190
      perforation T85.190
      protrusion T85.190
      specified NEC T85.190
    pain T85.840
    specified type NEC T85.890
    stenosis T85.850
    thrombosis T85.860
  cardiac (defibrillator)
    (pacemaker) —*see*
    Complications,
    cardiovascular device or
    implant, electronic
  generator (brain) (gastric)
    (peripheral) (sacral) (spinal)
    breakdown T85.113
    displacement T85.123
    leakage T85.193
    malposition T85.123
    obstruction T85.193
    perforation T85.193
    protrusion T85.193
    specified NEC T85.193
  muscle T84.9
    breakdown T84.418
    displacement T84.428
    embolism T84.81
    fibrosis T84.82
    hemorrhage T84.83
    infection or inflammation
      T84.7
    mechanical NEC T84.498
    pain T84.84
    specified type NEC T84.89
    stenosis T84.85
    thrombosis T84.86

Complication *(continued)*
electronic stimulator device
(continued)
  nervous system T85.9
    brain —*see* Complications,
      electronic stimulator device,
      brain
    cranial nerve —*see*
      Complications, electronic
      stimulator device,
      peripheral nerve
    embolism T85.810
    fibrosis T85.820
    gastric nerve —*see*
      Complications, electronic
      stimulator device,
      peripheral nerve
    hemorrhage T85.830
    infection and inflammation
      T85.738
    mechanical
      breakdown T85.118
      displacement T85.128
      leakage T85.199
      malposition T85.128
      obstruction T85.199
      perforation T85.199
      protrusion T85.199
      specified NEC T85.199
    pain T85.840
    peripheral nerve —*see*
      Complications, electronic
      stimulator device,
      peripheral nerve
    sacral nerve —*see*
      Complications, electronic
      stimulator device,
      peripheral nerve
    specified type NEC T85.890
    spinal cord —*see*
      Complications, electronic
      stimulator device, spinal cord
    stenosis T85.850
    thrombosis T85.860
    vagal nerve —*see* Complications,
      electronic stimulator device,
      peripheral nerve
  peripheral nerve T85.9
    embolism T85.810
    fibrosis T85.820
    hemorrhage T85.830
    infection and inflammation
      T85.732
    mechanical
      breakdown T85.111
      displacement T85.121
      leakage T85.191
      malposition T85.121
      obstruction T85.191
      perforation T85.191
      protrusion T85.191
      specified NEC T85.191
    pain T85.840
    specified type NEC T85.890
    stenosis T85.850
    thrombosis T85.860
  spinal cord T85.9
    embolism T85.810
    fibrosis T85.820
    hemorrhage T85.830
    infection and inflammation
      T85.733
    mechanical
      breakdown T85.112
      displacement T85.122
      leakage T85.192
      malposition T85.122
      obstruction T85.192
      perforation T85.192
      protrusion T85.192
      specified NEC T85.192

Complication *(continued)*
electronic stimulator device
(continued)
  spinal cord *(continued)*
    pain T85.840
    specified type NEC T85.890
    stenosis T85.850
    thrombosis T85.860
  urinary T83.9
    embolism T83.81
    fibrosis T83.82
    hemorrhage T83.83
    infection and inflammation
      T83.598
    mechanical
      breakdown T83.110
      displacement T83.120
      malposition T83.120
      perforation T83.190
      protrusion T83.190
      specified NEC T83.190
    pain T83.84
    specified type NEC T83.89
    stenosis T83.85
    thrombosis T83.86
electroshock therapy T88.9
  specified NEC T88.8
endocrine E34.9
  postprocedural
    adrenal hypofunction E89.6
    hypoinsulinemia E89.1
    hypoparathyroidism E89.2
    hypopituitarism E89.3
    hypothyroidism E89.0
    ovarian failure E89.40
      asymptomatic E89.40
      symptomatic E89.41
    specified NEC E89.89
    testicular hypofunction E89.5
endodontic treatment NEC
  M27.59
enterostomy (stoma) K94.10
  hemorrhage K94.11
  infection K94.12
  malfunction K94.13
  mechanical K94.13
  specified complication NEC
    K94.19
episiotomy, disruption O90.1
esophageal anti-reflux device T85.9
  embolism T85.818
  fibrosis T85.828
  hemorrhage T85.838
  infection and inflammation
    T85.79
  mechanical
    breakdown T85.511
    displacement T85.521
    malfunction T85.511
    malposition T85.521
    obstruction T85.591
    perforation T85.591
    protrusion T85.591
    specified NEC T85.591
  pain T85.848
  specified type NEC T85.898
  stenosis T85.858
  thrombosis T85.868
esophagostomy K94.30
  hemorrhage K94.31
  infection K94.32
  malfunction K94.33
  mechanical K94.33
  specified complication NEC
    K94.39
extracorporeal circulation T80.90
extremity artery (bypass) graft
  T82.9
  arteriosclerosis —*see*
    Arteriosclerosis, extremities,
    bypass graft

Complication *(continued)*
extremity artery (bypass) graft
(continued)
  embolism T82.818
  fibrosis T82.828
  hemorrhage T82.838
  infection and inflammation
    T82.7
  mechanical
    breakdown T82.318
      femoral artery T82.312
    displacement T82.328
      femoral artery T82.322
    leakage T82.338
      femoral artery T82.332
    malposition T82.328
      femoral artery T82.322
    obstruction T82.398
      femoral artery T82.392
    perforation T82.398
      femoral artery T82.392
    protrusion T82.398
      femoral artery T82.392
  pain T82.848
  specified type NEC T82.898
  stenosis T82.858
  thrombosis T82.868
eye H57.9
  corneal graft —*see*
    Complications, graft, cornea
  implant (prosthetic) T85.9
    embolism T85.818
    fibrosis T85.828
    hemorrhage T85.838
    infection and inflammation
      T85.79
    mechanical
      breakdown T85.318
      displacement T85.328
      leakage T85.398
      malposition T85.328
      obstruction T85.398
      perforation T85.398
      protrusion T85.398
      specified NEC T85.398
    pain T85.848
    specified type NEC T85.898
    stenosis T85.858
    thrombosis T85.868
  intraocular lens —*see*
    Complications, intraocular lens
  orbital prosthesis —*see*
    Complications, orbital
    prosthesis
female genital N94.9
  device, implant or graft
    NEC —*see* Complications,
    genitourinary, device or
    implant, genital tract
femoral artery (bypass) graft —*see*
  Complication, extremity artery
  (bypass) graft
fixation device, internal
  (orthopedic) T84.9
  infection and inflammation T84.60
    arm T84.61-
      humerus T84.61-
      radius T84.61-
      ulna T84.61-
    leg T84.629
      femur T84.62-
      fibula T84.62-
      tibia T84.62-
    specified site NEC T84.69
    spine T84.63
  mechanical
    breakdown
      limb T84.119
        carpal T84.210
        femur T84.11-
        fibula T84.11-

Complication (*continued*)
  graft (*continued*)
    muscle (*continued*)
      embolism T84.81
      fibrosis T84.82
      hemorrhage T84.83
      infection and inflammation
        T84.7
      mechanical NEC T84.490
      pain T84.84
      specified type NEC T84.89
      stenosis T84.85
      thrombosis T84.86
    nerve —*see* Complication,
      prosthetic device or implant,
      specified NEC
    skin —*see* Complications,
      prosthetic device or implant,
      skin graft
    tendon T84.9
      breakdown T84.410
      displacement T84.420
      embolism T84.81
      fibrosis T84.82
      hemorrhage T84.83
      infection and inflammation
        T84.7
      mechanical NEC T84.490
      pain T84.84
      specified type NEC T84.89
      stenosis T84.85
      thrombosis T84.86
    urinary organ T83.9
      embolism T83.81
      fibrosis T83.82
      hemorrhage T83.83
      infection and inflammation
        T83.598
        indwelling urethral catheter
          T83.511
      mechanical
        breakdown T83.21
        displacement T83.22
        erosion T83.24
        exposure T83.25
        leakage T83.23
        malposition T83.22
        obstruction T83.29
        perforation T83.29
        protrusion T83.29
        specified NEC T83.29
      pain T83.84
      specified type NEC T83.89
      stenosis T83.85
      thrombosis T83.86
    vascular T82.9
      embolism T82.818
      femoral artery —*see*
        Complication, extremity
        artery (bypass) graft
        T82.828
      fibrosis T82.828
      hemorrhage T82.838
      mechanical
        breakdown T82.319
        aorta (bifurcation)
          T82.310
        carotid artery T82.311
        specified vessel NEC
          T82.318
        displacement T82.329
        aorta (bifurcation)
          T82.320
        carotid artery T82.321
        specified vessel NEC
          T82.328
        leakage T82.339
        aorta (bifurcation)
          T82.330
        carotid artery T82.331
        specified vessel NEC
          T82.338

Complication (*continued*)
  graft (*continued*)
    vascular (*continued*)
      mechanical (*continued*)
        malposition T82.329
        aorta (bifurcation) T82.320
        carotid artery T82.321
        specified vessel NEC
          T82.328
        obstruction T82.399
        aorta (bifurcation)
          T82.390
        carotid artery T82.391
        specified vessel NEC
          T82.398
        perforation T82.399
        aorta (bifurcation)
          T82.390
        carotid artery T82.391
        specified vessel NEC
          T82.398
        protrusion T82.399
        aorta (bifurcation)
          T82.390
        carotid artery T82.391
        specified vessel NEC
          T82.398
      pain T82.848
      specified complication NEC
        T82.898
      stenosis T82.858
      thrombosis T82.868
  heart I51.9
    assist device
      infection and inflammation
        T82.7
    following acute myocardial
      infarction —*see*
      Complications, following,
      acute myocardial infarction
    postoperative —*see*
      Complications, circulatory
      system
    transplant —*see* Complication,
      transplant, heart
      and lung(s) —*see*
        Complications, transplant,
        heart, with lung
    valve
      graft (biological) T82.9
        embolism T82.817
        fibrosis T82.827
        hemorrhage T82.837
        infection and inflammation
          T82.7
        mechanical T82.228
          breakdown T82.221
          displacement T82.222
          leakage T82.223
          malposition T82.222
          obstruction T82.228
          perforation T82.228
          protrusion T82.228
        pain T82.847
        specified type NEC T82.897
        stenosis T82.857
        thrombosis T82.867
      prosthesis T82.9
        embolism T82.817
        fibrosis T82.827
        hemorrhage T82.837
        infection or inflammation
          T82.6
        mechanical T82.09
          breakdown T82.01
          displacement T82.02
          leakage T82.03
          malposition T82.02
          obstruction T82.09
          perforation T82.09
          protrusion T82.09

Complication (*continued*)
  heart (*continued*)
    valve (*continued*)
      prosthesis (*continued*)
        pain T82.847
        specified type NEC T82.897
          mechanical T82.09
        stenosis T82.857
        thrombosis T82.867
  hematoma
    intraoperative —*see*
      Complication, intraoperative,
      hemorrhage
    postprocedural —*see*
      Complication, postprocedural,
      hematoma
  hemodialysis —*see* Complications,
    dialysis
  hemorrhage
    intraoperative —*see*
      Complication, intraoperative,
      hemorrhage
    postprocedural —*see*
      Complication, postprocedural,
      hemorrhage
  ileostomy (stoma) —*see*
    Complications, enterostomy
  immunization (procedure) —*see*
    Complications, vaccination
  implant —*see also* Complications,
    by site and type
    urinary sphincter T83.9
      embolism T83.81
      fibrosis T83.82
      hemorrhage T83.83
      infection and inflammation
        T83.591
      mechanical
        breakdown T83.111
        displacement T83.121
        leakage T83.191
        malposition T83.121
        obstruction T83.191
        perforation T83.191
        protrusion T83.191
        specified NEC T83.191
      pain T83.84
      specified type NEC T83.89
      stenosis T83.85
      thrombosis T83.86
  infusion (procedure) T80.90
    air embolism T80.0
    blood —*see* Complications,
      transfusion
    catheter —*see* Complications,
      catheter
    infection T80.29
    pump —*see* Complications,
      cardiovascular, device or
      implant
    sepsis T80.29
    serum reaction (*see also*
      Reaction, serum) T80.69
      anaphylactic shock (*see*
        also Shock, anaphylactic)
        T80.59
    specified type NEC T80.89
  inhalation therapy NEC
    T81.81
  injection (procedure) T80.90
    drug reaction —*see* Reaction, drug
    infection T80.29
    sepsis T80.29
    serum (prophylactic) (therapeutic)
      —*see* Complications,
      vaccination
    specified type NEC T80.89
    vaccine (any) —*see*
      Complications, vaccination
  inoculation (any) —*see*
    Complications, vaccination

Complication (*continued*)
  insulin pump
    infection and inflammation T85.72
    mechanical
      breakdown T85.614
      displacement T85.624
      leakage T85.633
      malposition T85.624
      obstruction T85.694
      perforation T85.694
      protrusion T85.694
      specified NEC T85.694
  intestinal pouch NEC K91.858
  intraocular lens (prosthetic) T85.9
    embolism T85.818
    fibrosis T85.828
    hemorrhage T85.838
    infection and inflammation T85.79
    mechanical
      breakdown T85.21
      displacement T85.22
      malposition T85.22
      obstruction T85.29
      perforation T85.29
      protrusion T85.29
      specified NEC T85.29
    pain T85.848
    specified type NEC T85.898
    stenosis T85.858
    thrombosis T85.868
  intraoperative (intraprocedural)
    cardiac arrest —*see also* Infarct,
      myocardium, associated with
      revascularization procedure
      during cardiac surgery I97.710
      during other surgery I97.711
    cardiac functional disturbance
      NEC —*see also* Infarct,
      myocardium, associated with
      revascularization procedure
      during cardiac surgery I97.790
      during other surgery I97.791
    hemorrhage (hematoma) (of)
      circulatory system organ or
        structure
        during cardiac bypass I97.411
        during cardiac
          catheterization I97.410
        during other circulatory
          system procedure I97.418
        during other procedure
          I97.42
      digestive system organ
        during procedure on
          digestive system K91.61
        during procedure on other
          organ K91.62
      ear
        during procedure on ear and
          mastoid process H95.21
        during procedure on other
          organ H95.22
      endocrine system organ or
        structure
        during procedure on
          endocrine system organ
          or structure E36.01
        during procedure on other
          organ E36.02
      eye and adnexa
        during ophthalmic
          procedure H59.11-
        during other procedure
          H59.12-
      genitourinary organ or
        structure
        during procedure on
          genitourinary organ or
          structure N99.61
        during procedure on other
          organ N99.62

musculoskeletal system —see also
Complication, intraoperative
(intraprocedural), by site
(continued)
joint prosthesis —see
Complications, joint prosthesis
postoperative (postprocedural)
M96.89
with osteoporosis —see
Osteoporosis
fracture following insertion
of device —see Fracture,
following insertion of
orthopedic implant, joint
prosthesis or bone plate
joint instability after
prosthesis removal M96.89
lordosis M96.4
postlaminectomy syndrome
NEC M96.1
kyphosis M96.3
pseudarthrosis M96.0
specified complication NEC
M96.89
post radiation M96.89
kyphosis M96.2
scoliosis M96.5
specified complication NEC
M96.89
nephrostomy (stoma) —see
Complications, stoma, urinary
tract, external NEC
nervous system G98.8
central G96.9
device, implant or graft —see
also Complication, prosthetic
device or implant, specified
NEC
electronic stimulator
(electrode(s)) —see
Complications, electronic
stimulator device
specified NEC
infection and inflammation
T85.738
mechanical T85.695
breakdown T85.615
displacement T85.625
leakage T85.635
malfunction T85.695
malposition T85.625
obstruction T85.695
perforation T85.695
protrusion T85.695
specified NEC T85.695
ventricular shunt —see
Complications, ventricular
shunt
electronic stimulator
(electrode(s)) —see
Complications, electronic
stimulator device
postprocedural G97.82
intracranial hypotension
G97.2
specified NEC G97.82
spinal fluid leak G97.0
newborn, due to intrauterine (fetal)
procedure P96.5
nonabsorbable (permanent) sutures
—see Complication, sutures,
permanent
obstetric O75.9
procedure (instrumental)
(manual) (surgical) specified
NEC O75.4
specified NEC O75.89
surgical wound NEC O90.89
hematoma O90.2
infection O86.00

ocular lens implant —see
Complications, intraocular lens
ophthalmologic
postprocedural bleb —see
Blebitis
orbital prosthesis T85.9
embolism T85.818
fibrosis T85.828
hemorrhage T85.838
infection and inflammation
T85.79
mechanical
breakdown T85.31-
displacement T85.32-
malposition T85.32-
obstruction T85.39-
perforation T85.39-
protrusion T85.39-
specified NEC T85.39-
pain T85.848
specified type NEC T85.898
stenosis T85.858
thrombosis T85.868
organ or tissue transplant (partial)
(total) —see Complications,
transplant
orthopedic —see also Disorder,
soft tissue
device or implant T84.9
bone
device or implant —see
Complication, bone,
device NEC
graft —see Complication,
graft, bone
breakdown T84.418
displacement T84.428
electronic bone stimulator
—see Complications,
electronic stimulator device,
bone
embolism T84.81
fibrosis T84.82
fixation device —see
Complication, fixation
device, internal
hemorrhage T84.83
infection or inflammation
T84.7
joint prosthesis —see
Complication, joint
prosthesis, internal
malfunction T84.418
malposition T84.428
mechanical NEC T84.498
muscle graft —see
Complications, graft, muscle
obstruction T84.498
pain T84.84
perforation T84.498
protrusion T84.498
specified complication NEC
T84.89
stenosis T84.85
tendon graft —see
Complications, graft,
tendon
thrombosis T84.86
fracture (following insertion
of device) —see Fracture,
following insertion of
orthopedic implant, joint
prosthesis or bone plate
postprocedural M96.89
fracture —see Fracture,
following insertion of
orthopedic implant, joint
prosthesis or bone plate
postlaminectomy syndrome
NEC M96.1

orthopedic (continued)
postprocedural (continued)
postlaminectomy syndrome
(continued)
kyphosis M96.3
lordosis M96.4
postradiation
kyphosis M96.2
scoliosis M96.5
pseudarthrosis post-fusion
M96.0
specified type NEC M96.89
pacemaker (cardiac) —see
Complications, cardiovascular
device or implant, electronic
pancreas transplant —see
Complications, transplant,
pancreas
penile prosthesis (implant) —see
Complications, prosthetic device,
penile
perfusion NEC T80.90
perineal repair (obstetrical) NEC
O90.89
disruption O90.1
hematoma O90.2
infection (following delivery)
O86.09
phototherapy T88.9
specified NEC T88.8
postmastoidectomy NEC H95.19-
cyst, mucosal H95.13-
granulation H95.12-
inflammation, chronic H95.11-
recurrent cholesteatoma H95.0-
postoperative —see Complications,
postprocedural
circulatory —see Complications,
circulatory system
ear —see Complications, ear
endocrine —see Complications,
endocrine
eye —see Complications, eye
lumbar puncture G97.1
cerebrospinal fluid leak
G97.0
nervous system (central)
(peripheral) —see
Complications, nervous
system
respiratory system —see
Complications, respiratory
system
postprocedural —see also
Complications, surgical procedure
cardiac arrest —see also Infarct,
myocardium, associated with
revascularization procedure
following cardiac surgery
I97.120
following other surgery
I97.121
cardiac functional disturbance
NEC —see also Infarct,
myocardium, associated with
revascularization procedure
following cardiac surgery
I97.190
following other surgery
I97.191
cardiac insufficiency
following cardiac surgery
I97.110
following other surgery
I97.111
chorioretinal scars following
retinal surgery H59.81-
following cataract surgery
cataract (lens) fragments
H59.02-

postprocedural (continued)
following cataract surgery
(continued)
cystoid macular edema H59.03-
specified NEC H59.09-
vitreous (touch) syndrome
H59.01-
heart failure
following cardiac surgery
I97.130
following other surgery
I97.131
hematoma (of)
circulatory system organ or
structure
following cardiac bypass
I97.631
following cardiac
catheterization I97.630
following other circulatory
system procedure I97.638
following other procedure
I97.621
digestive system
following procedure on
digestive system K91.870
following procedure on
other organ K91.871
ear
following other procedure
H95.52
following procedure on
ear and mastoid process
H95.51
endocrine system
following endocrine system
procedure E89.820
following other procedure
E89.821
eye and adnexa
following ophthalmic
procedure H59.33-
following other procedure
H59.34-
genitourinary organ or
structure
following procedure on
genitourinary organ or
structure N99.840
following procedure on
other organ N99.841
mastoid process
following other procedure
H95.52
following procedure on
ear and mastoid process
H95.51
musculoskeletal structure
following musculoskeletal
surgery M96.840
following non-orthopedic
surgery M96.841
following orthopedic
surgery M96.840
nervous system
following nervous system
procedure G97.61
following other procedure
G97.62
respiratory system
following other procedure
J95.861
following procedure on
respiratory system organ
or structure J95.860
skin and subcutaneous tissue
following dematologic
procedure L76.31
following procedure on
other organ L76.32

Complication (*continued*)
  postprocedural (*continued*)
    hematoma (*continued*)
      spleen
        following procedure on
          other organ D78.32
        following procedure on the
          spleen D78.31
    hemorrhage (of)
      circulatory system organ or
        structure
        following cardiac bypass
          I97.611
        following cardiac
          catheterization I97.610
        following other circulatory
          system procedure I97.618
        following other procedure
          I97.620
      digestive system
        following procedure on
          digestive system K91.840
        following procedure on
          other organ K91.841
      ear
        following other procedure
          H95.42
        following procedure on
          ear and mastoid process
          H95.41
      endocrine system
        following endocrine system
          procedure E89.810
        following other procedure
          E89.811
      eye and adnexa
        following ophthalmic
          procedure H59.31-
        following other procedure
          H59.32-
      genitourinary organ or
        structure
        following procedure on
          genitourinary organ or
          structure N99.820
        following procedure on
          other organ N99.821
      mastoid process
        following other procedure
          H95.42
        following procedure on
          ear and mastoid process
          H95.41
      musculoskeletal structure
        following musculoskeletal
          surgery M96.830
        following non-orthopedic
          surgery M96.831
        following orthopedic
          surgery M96.830
      nervous system
        following nervous system
          procedure G97.51
        following other procedure
          G97.52
      respiratory system
        following other procedure
          J95.831
        following procedure on
          respiratory system organ
          or structure J95.830
      skin and subcutaneous tissue
        following dermatologic
          procedure L76.21
        following a procedure on
          other organ L76.22
      spleen
        following procedure on
          other organ D78.22
        following procedure on the
          spleen D78.21

  postprocedural (*continued*)
    seroma (of)
      circulatory system organ or
        structure
        following cardiac bypass
          I97.641
        following cardiac
          catheterization I97.640
        following other circulatory
          system procedure
          I97.648
        following other procedure
          I97.622
      digestive system
        following procedure on
          digestive system K91.872
        following procedure on
          other organ K91.873
      ear
        following other procedure
          H95.54
        following procedure on
          ear and mastoid process
          H95.53
      endocrine system
        following endocrine system
          procedure E89.822
        following other procedure
          E89.823
      eye and adnexa
        following ophthalmic
          procedure H59.35-
        following other procedure
          H59.36-
      genitourinary organ or
        structure
        following procedure on
          genitourinary organ or
          structure N99.842
        following procedure on
          other organ N99.843
      mastoid process
        following other procedure
          H95.54
        following procedure on
          ear and mastoid process
          H95.53
      musculoskeletal structure
        following musculoskeletal
          surgery M96.842
        following non-orthopedic
          surgery M96.843
        following orthopedic
          surgery M96.842
      nervous system
        following nervous system
          procedure G97.63
        following other procedure
          G97.64
      respiratory system
        following other procedure
          J95.863
        following procedure on
          respiratory system organ
          or structure J95.862
      skin and subcutaneous tissue
        following dematologic
          procedure L76.33
        following procedure on
          other organ L76.34
      spleen
        following procedure on
          other organ D78.34
        following procedure on the
          spleen D78.33
    specified NEC
      circulatory system I97.89
      digestive K91.89
      ear H95.89
      endocrine E89.89

  postprocedural (*continued*)
    specified NEC (*continued*)
      eye and adnexa H59.89
      genitourinary N99.89
      mastoid process H95.89
      metabolic E89.89
      musculoskeletal structure
        M96.89
      nervous system G97.82
      respiratory system J95.89
      skin and subcutaneous tissue
        L76.82
      spleen D78.89
  pregnancy NEC —*see* Pregnancy,
    complicated by
  prosthetic device or implant T85.9
    bile duct —*see* Complications,
      bile duct implant
    breast —*see* Complications,
      breast implant
    bulking agent
      ureteral
        erosion T83.714
        exposure T83.724
      urethral
        erosion T83.713
        exposure T83.723
    cardiac and vascular NEC —*see*
      Complications, cardiovascular
      device or implant
    corneal transplant —*see*
      Complications, graft, cornea
    electronic nervous system
      stimulator —*see*
      Complications, electronic
      stimulator device
    epidural infusion catheter —*see*
      Complications, catheter, epidural
    esophageal anti-reflux device —
      see Complications, esophageal
      anti-reflux device
    genital organ or tract —*see*
      Complications, genitourinary,
      device or implant, genital
      tract
      specified NEC T83.79
    heart valve —*see* Complications,
      heart, valve, prosthesis
    infection or inflammation T85.79
      intestine transplant T86.892
      liver transplant T86.43
      lung transplant T86.812
      pancreas transplant T86.892
      skin graft T86.822
    intraocular lens —*see*
      Complications, intraocular
      lens
    intraperitoneal (dialysis) catheter
      —*see* Complications, catheter,
      intraperitoneal
    joint —*see* Complications, joint
      prosthesis, internal
    mechanical NEC T85.698
      dialysis catheter (vascular)
        —*see also* Complication,
        catheter, dialysis,
        mechanical
        peritoneal —*see*
          Complication, catheter,
          intraperitoneal,
          mechanical
      gastrointestinal device T85.598
      ocular device T85.398
      subdural (infusion) catheter
        T85.690
      suture, permanent T85.692
        that for bone repair —
          see Complications,
          fixation device, internal
          (orthopedic), mechanical

  prosthetic device or implant
    (*continued*)
    mechanical NEC (*continued*)
      ventricular shunt
        breakdown T85.01
        displacement T85.02
        leakage T85.03
        malposition T85.02
        obstruction T85.09
        perforation T85.09
        protrusion T85.09
        specified NEC T85.09
    mesh
      erosion (to surrounding organ
        or tissue) T83.718
        vaginal (into pelvic floor
          muscles) T83.711
        urethral (into pelvic floor
          muscles) T83.712
      exposure (into surrounding
        organ or tissue) T83.728
        vaginal (into vagina) (through
          vaginal wall) T83.721
        urethral (through urethral
          wall) T83.722
    orbital —*see* Complications,
      orbital prosthesis
    penile T83.9
      embolism T83.81
      fibrosis T83.82
      hemorrhage T83.83
      infection and inflammation
        T83.61
      mechanical
        breakdown T83.410
        displacement T83.420
        leakage T83.490
        malposition T83.420
        obstruction T83.490
        perforation T83.490
        protrusion T83.490
        specified NEC T83.490
      pain T83.848
      specified type NEC T83.89
      stenosis T83.85
      thrombosis T83.86
    prosthetic materials NEC
      erosion (to surrounding organ
        or tissue) T83.718
      exposure (into surrounding
        organ or tissue) T83.728
    skin graft T86.829
      artificial skin or decellularized
        allodermis
        embolism T85.818
        fibrosis T85.828
        hemorrhage T85.838
        infection and inflammation
          T85.79
        mechanical
          breakdown T85.613
          displacement T85.623
          malfunction T85.613
          malposition T85.623
          obstruction T85.693
          perforation T85.693
          protrusion T85.693
          specified NEC T85.693
        pain T85.848
        specified type NEC T85.898
        stenosis T85.858
        thrombosis T85.868
      failure T86.821
      infection T86.822
      rejection T86.820
      specified NEC T86.828
    sling
      urethral (female) (male)
        erosion T83.712
        exposure T83.722

Complication *(continued)*

prosthetic device or implant
(continued)
specified NEC T85.9
embolism T85.818
fibrosis T85.828
hemorrhage T85.838
infection and inflammation
T85.79
mechanical
breakdown T85.618
displacement T85.628
leakage T85.638
malfunction T85.618
malposition T85.628
obstruction T85.698
perforation T85.698
protrusion T85.698
specified NEC T85.698
pain T85.848
specified type NEC T85.898
stenosis T85.858
thrombosis T85.868
subdural infusion catheter —*see*
Complications, catheter,
subdural
sutures —*see* Complications,
sutures
urinary organ or tract NEC —*see*
Complications, genitourinary,
device or implant, urinary
system
vascular —*see* Complications,
cardiovascular device or
implant
ventricular shunt —*see*
Complications, ventricular
shunt (device)
puerperium —*see* Puerperal
puncture, spinal G97.1
cerebrospinal fluid leak G97.0
headache or reaction G97.1
pyelogram N99.89
radiation
kyphosis M96.2
scoliosis M96.5
reattached
extremity (infection) (rejection)
lower T87.1X-
upper T87.0X-
specified body part NEC T87.2
reconstructed breast
asymmetry between native and
reconstructed breast N65.1
deformity N65.0
disproportion between native and
reconstructed breast N65.1
excess tissue N65.0
misshappen N65.0
reimplant NEC —*see also*
Complications, prosthetic device
or implant
limb (infection) (rejection) —*see*
Complications, reattached,
extremity
organ (partial) (total) —*see*
Complications, transplant
prosthetic device NEC —*see*
Complications, prosthetic device
renal N28.9
allograft —*see* Complications,
transplant, kidney
dialysis —*see* Complications,
dialysis
respirator
mechanical J95.850
specified NEC J95.859
respiratory system J98.9
device, implant or graft —*see*
Complication, prosthetic device
or implant, specified NEC

Complication *(continued)*

respiratory system *(continued)*
lung transplant —*see*
Complications, prosthetic
device or implant, lung
transplant
postoperative J95.89
air leak J95.812
Mendelson's syndrome
(chemical pneumonitis) J95.4
pneumothorax J95.811
pulmonary insufficiency
(acute) (after nonthoracic
surgery) J95.2
chronic J95.3
following thoracic surgery
J95.1
respiratory failure (acute)
J95.821
acute and chronic J95.822
specified NEC J95.89
subglottic stenosis J95.5
tracheostomy complication
—*see* Complications,
tracheostomy
therapy T81.89
sedation during labor and delivery
O74.9
cardiac O74.2
central nervous system O74.3
pulmonary NEC O74.1
shunt —*see also* Complications,
prosthetic device or implant
arteriovenous —*see*
Complications, arteriovenous,
shunt
ventricular (communicating)
—*see* Complications,
ventricular shunt
skin
graft T86.829
failure T86.821
infection T86.822
rejection T86.820
specified type NEC T86.828
spinal
anesthesia —*see* Complications,
anesthesia, spinal
catheter (epidural) (subdural)
—*see* Complications, catheter
puncture or tap G97.1
cerebrospinal fluid leak G97.0
headache or reaction G97.1
stent
bile duct —*see* Complications,
bile duct prosthesis
ureteral indwelling
breakdown T83.112
displacement T83.122
leakage T83.192
malposition T83.122
obstruction T83.192
perforation T83.192
protrusion T83.192
specified NEC T83.192
urinary NEC (ileal conduit)
(nephroureteral) T83.193
embolism T83.81
fibrosis T83.82
hemorrhage T83.83
infection and inflammation
T83.593
mechanical
breakdown T83.113
displacement T83.123
leakage T83.193
malposition T83.123
obstruction T83.193
perforation T83.193
protrusion T83.193
specified NEC T83.193

Complication *(continued)*

stent *(continued)*
urinary NEC *(continued)*
pain T83.84
specified type NEC T83.89
stenosis T83.85
thrombosis T83.86
vascular
end stent stenosis —*see*
Restenosis, stent
in stent stenosis —*see*
Restenosis, stent
stoma
digestive tract
colostomy —*see*
Complications, colostomy
enterostomy —*see*
Complications, enterostomy
esophagostomy —*see*
Complications,
esophagostomy
gastrostomy —*see*
Complications, gastrostomy
urinary tract N99.528
continent N99.538
hemorrhage N99.530
herniation N99.533
infection N99.531
malfunction N99.532
specified type NEC
N99.538
stenosis N99.534
cystostomy —*see*
Complications, cystostomy
external NOS N99.528
hemorrhage N99.520
herniation N99.523
incontinent N99.528
hemorrhage N99.520
herniation N99.523
infection N99.521
malfunction N99.522
specified type NEC
N99.528
stenosis N99.524
infection N99.521
malfunction N99.522
specified type NEC N99.528
stenosis N99.524
stomach banding —*see*
Complication(s), bariatric
procedure
stomach stapling —*see*
Complication(s), bariatric
procedure
surgical material, nonabsorbable
—*see* Complication, suture,
permanent
surgical procedure (on) T81.9
amputation stump (late) —*see*
Complications, amputation
stump
cardiac —*see* Complications,
circulatory system
cholesteatoma, recurrent
—*see* Complications,
postmastoidectomy, recurrent
cholesteatoma
circulatory (early) —*see*
Complications, circulatory
system
digestive system —*see*
Complications,
gastrointestinal
dumping syndrome
(postgastrectomy) K91.1
ear —*see* Complications, ear
elephantiasis or lymphedema
I97.89
postmastectomy I97.2
emphysema (surgical) T81.82

Complication *(continued)*

surgical procedure *(continued)*
endocrine —*see* Complications,
endocrine
eye —*see* Complications, eye
fistula (persistent postoperative)
T81.83
foreign body inadvertently left
in wound (sponge) (suture)
(swab) —*see* Foreign body,
accidentally left during a
procedure
gastrointestinal —*see*
Complications,
gastrointestinal
genitourinary NEC N99.89
hematoma
intraoperative —*see*
Complication,
intraoperative, hemorrhage
postprocedural —
see Complication,
postprocedural, hematoma
hemorrhage
intraoperative —*see*
Complication,
intraoperative, hemorrhage
postprocedural —
see Complication,
postprocedural, hemorrhage
hepatic failure K91.82
hyperglycemia
(postpancreatectomy) E89.1
hypoinsulinemia
(postpancreatectomy) E89.1
hypoparathyroidism
(postparathyroidectomy)
E89.2
hypopituitarism
(posthypophysectomy) E89.3
hypothyroidism (post-
thyroidectomy) E89.0
intestinal obstruction (*see*
also Obstruction, intestine,
postoperative) K91.30
intracranial hypotension
following ventricular shunting
(ventriculostomy) G97.2
lymphedema I97.89
postmastectomy I97.2
malabsorption (postsurgical)
NEC K91.2
osteoporosis —*see*
Osteoporosis, postsurgical
malabsorption
mastoidectomy cavity NEC
—*see* Complications,
postmastoidectomy
metabolic E89.89
specified NEC E89.89
musculoskeletal —*see*
Complications,
musculoskeletal system
nervous system (central)
(peripheral) —*see*
Complications, nervous
system
ovarian failure E89.40
asymptomatic E89.40
symptomatic E89.41
peripheral vascular —*see*
Complications, surgical
procedure, vascular
postcardiotomy syndrome
I97.0
postcholecystectomy syndrome
K91.5
postcommissurotomy syndrome
I97.0
postgastrectomy dumping
syndrome K91.1

Complication (continued)

surgical procedure (continued)
postlaminectomy syndrome NEC
M96.1
kyphosis M96.3
postmastectomy lymphedema
syndrome I97.2
postmastoidectomy
cholesteatoma —see
Complications,
postmastoidectomy, recurrent
cholesteatoma
postvagotomy syndrome K91.1
postvalvulotomy syndrome I97.0
pulmonary insufficiency (acute)
J95.2
chronic J95.3
following thoracic surgery J95.1
reattached body part —see
Complications, reattached
respiratory —see Complications,
respiratory system
shock (hypovolemic) T81.19
spleen (postoperative) D78.89
intraoperative D78.81
stitch abscess T81.41
subglottic stenosis (postsurgical)
J95.5
testicular hypofunction E89.5
transplant —see Complications,
organ or tissue transplant
urinary NEC N99.89
vaginal vault prolapse
(posthysterectomy) N99.3
vascular (peripheral)
artery T81.719
mesenteric T81.710
renal T81.711
specified NEC T81.718
vein T81.72
wound infection T81.49
suture, permanent (wire) NEC T85.9
with repair of bone —see
Complications, fixation
device, internal
embolism T85.818
fibrosis T85.828
hemorrhage T85.838
infection and inflammation T85.79
mechanical
breakdown T85.612
displacement T85.622
malfunction T85.612
malposition T85.622
obstruction T85.692
perforation T85.692
protrusion T85.692
specified NEC T85.692
pain T85.848
specified type NEC T85.898
stenosis T85.858
thrombosis T85.868
tracheostomy J95.00
granuloma J95.09
hemorrhage J95.01
infection J95.02
malfunction J95.03
mechanical J95.03
obstruction J95.03
specified type NEC J95.09
tracheo-esophageal fistula J95.04
transfusion (blood) (lymphocytes)
(plasma) T80.92
air embolism T80.0
circulatory overload E87.71
febrile nonhemolytic transfusion
reaction R50.84
hemolysis T80.89
hemochromatosis E83.111
hemolytic reaction (antigen
unspecified) T80.919

Complication (continued)

transfusion (continued)
incompatibility reaction (antigen
unspecified) T80.919
ABO T80.30
delayed serologic (DSTR)
T80.39
hemolytic transfusion
reaction (HTR)
(unspecified time after
transfusion) T80.319
acute (AHTR) (less
than 24 hours after
transfusion) T80.310
delayed (DHTR) (24
hours or more after
transfusion) T80.311
specified NEC T80.39
acute (antigen unspecified)
T80.910
delayed (antigen unspecified)
T80.911
delayed serologic (DSTR)
T80.89
Non-ABO (minor antigens
(Duffy) (K) (Kell) (Kidd)
(Lewis) (M) (N) (P) (S))
T80.A0
delayed serologic (DSTR)
T80.A9
hemolytic transfusion
reaction (HTR)
(unspecified time after
transfusion) T80.A19
acute (AHTR) (less
than 24 hours after
transfusion) T80.A10
delayed (DHTR) (24
hours or more after
transfusion) T80.A11
specified NEC T80.A9
Rh (antigens (C) (c) (D) (E)
(e)) (factor) T80.40
delayed serologic (DSTR)
T80.49
hemolytic transfusion
reaction (HTR)
(unspecified time after
transfusion) T80.419
hemolytic transfusion acute
(AHTR) (less than 24
hours after transfusion)
T80.410
delayed (DHTR) (24
hours or more after
transfusion) T80.411
specified NEC T80.49
infection T80.29
acute T80.22
reaction NEC T80.89
sepsis T80.29
shock T80.89
transplant T86.90
bone T86.839
failure T86.831
infection T86.832
rejection T86.830
specified type NEC T86.838
bone marrow T86.00
failure T86.02
infection T86.03
rejection T86.01
specified type NEC T86.09
cornea T86.849-
failure T86.841-
infection T86.842-
rejection T86.840-
specified type NEC T86.848-
failure T86.92
heart T86.20
with lung T86.30

Complication (continued)

transplant (continued)
heart (continued)
cardiac allograft vasculopathy
T86.290
failure T86.32
infection T86.33
rejection T86.31
specified type NEC
T86.39
failure T86.22
infection T86.23
rejection T86.21
specified type NEC T86.298
infection T86.93
intestine T86.859
failure T86.851
infection T86.852
rejection T86.850
specified type NEC T86.858
kidney T86.10
failure T86.12
infection T86.13
rejection T86.11
specified type NEC T86.19
liver T86.40
failure T86.42
infection T86.43
rejection T86.41
specified type NEC T86.49
lung T86.819
with heart T86.30
failure T86.32
infection T86.33
rejection T86.31
specified type NEC T86.39
failure T86.811
infection T86.812
rejection T86.810
specified type NEC T86.818
malignant neoplasm C80.2
pancreas T86.899
failure T86.891
infection T86.892
rejection T86.890
specified type NEC T86.898
peripheral blood stem cells
T86.5
post-transplant
lymphoproliferative disorder
(PTLD) D47.Z1
rejection T86.91
skin T86.829
failure T86.821
infection T86.822
rejection T86.820
specified type NEC T86.828
specified
tissue T86.899
failure T86.891
infection T86.892
rejection T86.890
specified type NEC
T86.898
type NEC T86.99
stem cell (from peripheral blood)
(from umbilical cord) T86.5
umbilical cord stem cells
T86.5
trauma (early) T79.9
specified NEC T79.8
ultrasound therapy NEC T88.9
umbilical cord NEC
complicating delivery O69.9
specified NEC O69.89
umbrella device, vascular T82.9
embolism T82.818
fibrosis T82.828
hemorrhage T82.838
infection or inflammation
T82.7

Complication (continued)

umbrella device, vascular
(continued)
mechanical
breakdown T82.515
displacement T82.525
leakage T82.535
malposition T82.525
obstruction T82.595
perforation T82.595
protrusion T82.595
pain T82.848
specified type NEC T82.898
stenosis T82.858
thrombosis T82.868
urethral catheter —see
Complications, catheter, urethral,
indwelling
vaccination T88.1
anaphylaxis NEC T80.52
arthropathy —see Arthropathy,
postimmunization
cellulitis T88.0
encephalitis or encephalomyelitis
G04.02
infection (general) (local) NEC
T88.0
meningitis G03.8
myelitis G04.02
protein sickness T80.62
rash T88.1
reaction (allergic) T88.1
serum T80.62
sepsis T88.0
serum intoxication, sickness,
rash, or other serum reaction
NEC T80.62
anaphylactic shock T80.52
shock (allergic) (anaphylactic)
T80.52
vaccinia (generalized) (localized)
T88.1
vas deferens device or implant
—see Complications,
genitourinary, device or implant,
genital tract
vascular I99.9
device or implant T82.9
embolism T82.818
fibrosis T82.828
hemorrhage T82.838
infection or inflammation T82.7
mechanical
breakdown T82.519
specified device NEC
T82.518
displacement T82.529
specified device NEC
T82.528
leakage T82.539
specified device NEC
T82.538
malposition T82.529
specified device NEC
T82.528
obstruction T82.599
specified device NEC
T82.598
perforation T82.599
specified device NEC
T82.598
protrusion T82.599
specified device NEC
T82.598
pain T82.848
specified type NEC T82.898
stenosis T82.858
thrombosis T82.868
dialysis catheter —see
Complication, catheter,
dialysis

Complication *(continued)*
  vascular *(continued)*
    following infusion, therapeutic injection or transfusion T80.1
    graft T82.9
      embolism T82.818
      fibrosis T82.828
      hemorrhage T82.838
      mechanical
        breakdown T82.319
          aorta (bifurcation) T82.310
          carotid artery T82.311
          specified vessel NEC T82.318
        displacement T82.329
          aorta (bifurcation) T82.320
          carotid artery T82.321
          specified vessel NEC T82.328
        leakage T82.339
          aorta (bifurcation) T82.330
          carotid artery T82.331
          specified vessel NEC T82.338
        malposition T82.329
          aorta (bifurcation) T82.320
          carotid artery T82.321
          specified vessel NEC T82.328
        obstruction T82.399
          aorta (bifurcation) T82.390
          carotid artery T82.391
          specified vessel NEC T82.398
        perforation T82.399
          aorta (bifurcation) T82.390
          carotid artery T82.391
          specified vessel NEC T82.398
        protrusion T82.399
          aorta (bifurcation) T82.390
          carotid artery T82.391
          specified vessel NEC T82.398
      pain T82.848
      specified complication NEC T82.898
      stenosis T82.858
      thrombosis T82.868
    postoperative —*see* Complications, postoperative, circulatory
    vena cava device (filter) (sieve) (umbrella) —*see* Complications, umbrella device, vascular
    ventilation therapy NEC T81.81
    ventilator
      mechanical J95.850
        specified NEC J95.859
    ventricular (communicating) shunt (device) T85.9
      embolism T85.810
      fibrosis T85.820
      hemorrhage T85.830
      infection and inflammation T85.730
      mechanical
        breakdown T85.01
        displacement T85.02
        leakage T85.03
        malposition T85.02
        obstruction T85.09
        perforation T85.09
        protrusion T85.09
        specified NEC T85.09

Complication *(continued)*
  ventricular (communicating) shunt (device) *(continued)*
    pain T85.840
    specified type NEC T85.890
    stenosis T85.850
    thrombosis T85.860
  wire suture, permanent (implanted) —*see* Complications, suture, permanent

Compressed air disease T70.3

Compression
  with injury - code by Nature of injury
  artery I77.1
    celiac, syndrome I77.4
  brachial plexus G54.0
  brain (stem) G93.5
    due to
      contusion (diffuse) —*see* Injury, intracranial, diffuse
      focal —*see* Injury, intracranial, focal
      injury NEC —*see* Injury, intracranial, diffuse
      traumatic —*see* Injury, intracranial, diffuse
  bronchus J98.09
  cauda equina G83.4
  celiac (artery) (axis) I77.4
  cerebral —*see* Compression, brain
  cervical plexus G54.2
  cord
    spinal —*see* Compression, spinal
    umbilical —*see* Compression, umbilical cord
  cranial nerve G52.9
    eighth H93.3
    eleventh G52.8
    fifth G50.8
    first G52.0
    fourth —*see* Strabismus, paralytic, fourth nerve
    ninth G52.1
    second —*see* Disorder, nerve, optic
    seventh G51.8
    sixth —*see* Strabismus, paralytic, sixth nerve
    tenth G52.2
    third —*see* Strabismus, paralytic, third nerve
    twelfth G52.3
  diver's squeeze T70.3
  during birth (newborn) P15.9
  esophagus K22.2
  eustachian tube —*see* Obstruction, eustachian tube, cartilaginous
  facies Q67.1
  fracture
    nontraumatic NOS —*see* Collapse, vertebra
    pathological —*see* Fracture, pathological
    traumatic —*see* Fracture, traumatic
  heart —*see* Disease, heart
  intestine —*see* Obstruction, intestine
  laryngeal nerve, recurrent G52.2
    with paralysis of vocal cords and larynx J38.00
      bilateral J38.02
      unilateral J38.01
  lumbosacral plexus G54.1
  lung J98.4
  lymphatic vessel I89.0
  medulla —*see* Compression, brain
  nerve (see also Disorder, nerve) G58.9
    arm NEC —*see* Mononeuropathy, upper limb

Compression *(continued)*
  nerve *(continued)*
    axillary G54.0
    cranial —*see* Compression, cranial nerve
    leg NEC —*see* Mononeuropathy, lower limb
    median (in carpal tunnel) —*see* Syndrome, carpal tunnel
    optic —*see* Disorder, nerve, optic
    plantar —*see* Lesion, nerve, plantar
    posterior tibial (in tarsal tunnel) —*see* Syndrome, tarsal tunnel
    root or plexus NOS (in) G54.9
      intervertebral disc disorder NEC —*see* Disorder, disc, with, radiculopathy
        with myelopathy —*see* Disorder, disc, with, myelopathy
      neoplastic disease —*see also* Neoplasm D49.9 *[G55]*
      spondylosis —*see* Spondylosis, with radiculopathy
    sciatic (acute) —*see* Lesion, nerve, sciatic
    sympathetic G90.8
    traumatic —*see* Injury, nerve
    ulnar —*see* Lesion, nerve, ulnar
    upper extremity NEC —*see* Mononeuropathy, upper limb
  spinal (cord) G95.20
    by displacement of intervertebral disc NEC —*see also* Disorder, disc, with, myelopathy
    nerve root NOS G54.9
      due to displacement of intervertebral disc NEC —*see* Disorder, disc, with, radiculopathy
        with myelopathy —*see* Disorder, disc, with, myelopathy
    specified NEC G95.29
    spondylogenic (cervical) (lumbar, lumbosacral) (thoracic) —*see* Spondylosis, with myelopathy NEC
    anterior —*see* Syndrome, anterior, spinal artery, compression
    traumatic —*see* Injury, spinal cord, by region
  subcostal nerve (syndrome) —*see* Mononeuropathy, upper limb, specified NEC
  sympathetic nerve NEC G90.8
  syndrome T79.5
  trachea J39.8
  ulnar nerve (by scar tissue) —*see* Lesion, nerve, ulnar
  umbilical cord
    complicating delivery O69.2
      cord around neck O69.1
      prolapse O69.0
      specified NEC O69.2
  ureter N13.5
  vein I87.1
  vena cava (inferior) (superior) I87.1

Compulsion, compulsive
  gambling F63.0
  neurosis F42.8
  personality F60.5
  states F42.8

Compulsion, compulsive *(continued)*
  swearing F42.8
    in Gilles de la Tourette's syndrome F95.2
  tics and spasms F95.9

Concato's disease (pericardial polyserositis) A19.9
  nontubercular I31.1
  pleural —*see* Pleurisy, with effusion

Concavity chest wall M95.4

Concealed penis Q55.64

Concern (normal) about sick person in family Z63.6

Concrescence (teeth) K00.2

Concretio cordis I31.1
  rheumatic I09.2

Concretion —*see also* Calculus
  appendicular K38.1
  canaliculus —*see* Dacryolith
  clitoris N90.89
  conjunctiva H11.12-
  eyelid —*see* Disorder, eyelid, specified type NEC
  lacrimal passages —*see* Dacryolith
  prepuce (male) N47.8
  salivary gland (any) K11.5
  seminal vesicle N50.89
  tonsil J35.8

Concussion (brain) (cerebral) (current) S06.0X9
  with
    loss of consciousness of 30 minutes or less S06.0X1
    loss of consciousness of unspecified duration S06.0X9
  blast (air) (hydraulic) (immersion) (underwater)
    abdomen or thorax —*see* Injury, blast, by site
    ear with acoustic nerve injury —*see* Injury, nerve, acoustic, specified type NEC
  cauda equina S34.3
  conus medullaris S34.02
  ocular S05.8X-
  spinal (cord)
    cervical S14.0
    lumbar S34.01
    sacral S34.02
    thoracic S24.0
  syndrome F07.81
  without loss of consciousness S06.0X0

Condition —*see* Disease

Conditions arising in the perinatal period —*see* Newborn, affected by

Conduct disorder —*see* Disorder, conduct

Condyloma A63.0
  acuminatum A63.0
  gonorrheal A54.09
  latum A51.31
  syphilitic A51.31
    congenital A50.07
  venereal, syphilitic A51.31

Conflagration —*see also* Burn
  asphyxia (by inhalation of gases, fumes or vapors) (*see also* Table of Drugs and Chemicals) T59.9-

Conflict (with) —*see also* Discord
  family Z73.9
  marital Z63.0
    involving divorce or estrangement Z63.5
  parent-child Z62.820

Conflict (continued)

parent-child (continued)
- parent-adopted child Z62.821
- parent-biological child Z62.820
- parent-foster child Z62.822
- social role NEC Z73.5

Confluent —see condition

Confusion, confused R41.0
- epileptic F05
- mental state (psychogenic) F44.89
- psychogenic F44.89
- reactive (from emotional stress, psychological trauma) F44.89

Confusional arousals G47.51

Congelation T69.9

Congenital —see also condition
- aortic septum Q25.49
- intrinsic factor deficiency D51.0
- malformation —see Anomaly

Congestion, congestive
- bladder N32.89
- bowel K63.89
- brain G93.89
- breast N64.59
- bronchial J98.09
- catarrhal J31.0
- chest R09.89
- chill, malarial —see Malaria
- circulatory NEC I99.8
- duodenum K31.89
- eye —see Hyperemia, conjunctiva
- facial, due to birth injury P15.4
- general R68.89
- glottis J37.0
- heart —see Failure, heart, congestive
- hepatic K76.1
- hypostatic (lung) —see Edema, lung
- intestine K63.89
- kidney N28.89
- labyrinth —see subcategory H83.8
- larynx J37.0
- liver K76.1
- lung R09.89
  - active or acute —see Pneumonia
- malaria, malarial —see Malaria
- nasal R09.81
- nose R09.81
- orbit, orbital —see also Exophthalmos
  - inflammatory (chronic) —see Inflammation, orbit
- ovary N83.8
- pancreas K86.89
- pelvic, female N94.89
- pleural J94.8
- prostate (active) N42.1
- pulmonary —see Congestion, lung
- renal N28.89
- retina H35.81
- seminal vesicle N50.1
- spinal cord G95.19
- spleen (chronic) D73.2
- stomach K31.89
- trachea —see Tracheitis
- urethra N36.8
- uterus N85.8
  - with subinvolution N85.3
- venous (passive) I87.8
- viscera R68.89

Congestive —see Congestion

Conical
- cervix (hypertrophic elongation) N88.4
- cornea —see Keratoconus
- teeth K00.2

Conjoined twins Q89.4

Conjugal maladjustment Z63.0

involving divorce or estrangement Z63.5

Conjunctiva —see condition

Conjunctivitis (staphylococcal) (streptococcal) **NOS** H10.9
- Acanthamoeba B60.12
- acute H10.3-
  - atopic H10.1-
    - mucopurulent H10.02-
      - follicular H10.01-
  - chemical (see also Corrosion, cornea) H10.21-
  - pseudomembranous H10.22-
  - serous except viral H10.23-
    - viral —see Conjunctivitis, viral
  - toxic H10.21-
- adenoviral (acute) (follicular) B30.1
- allergic (acute) —see Conjunctivitis, acute, atopic
  - chronic H10.45
    - vernal H10.44
- anaphylactic —see Conjunctivitis, acute, atopic
- Apollo B30.3
- atopic (acute) —see Conjunctivitis, acute, atopic
- Béal's B30.2
- blennorrhagic (gonococcal) (neonatorum) A54.31
- chemical (acute) (see also Corrosion, cornea) H10.21-
- chlamydial A74.0
  - due to trachoma A71.1
  - neonatal P39.1
- chronic (nodosa) (petrificans) (phlyctenular) H10.40-
  - allergic H10.45
    - vernal H10.44
  - follicular H10.43-
  - giant papillary H10.41-
  - simple H10.42-
  - vernal H10.44
- coxsackievirus 24 B30.3
- diphtheritic A36.86
- due to
  - dust —see Conjunctivitis, acute, atopic
  - filariasis B74.9
  - mucocutaneous leishmaniasis B55.2
- enterovirus type 70 (hemorrhagic) B30.3
- epidemic (viral) B30.9
  - hemorrhagic B30.3
- gonococcal (neonatorum) A54.31
- granular (trachomatous) A71.1
  - sequelae (late effect) B94.0
- hemorrhagic (acute) (epidemic) B30.3
- herpes zoster B02.31
- in (due to)
  - Acanthamoeba B60.12
  - adenovirus (acute) (follicular) B30.1
  - Chlamydia A74.0
  - coxsackievirus 24 B30.3
  - diphtheria A36.86
  - enterovirus type 70 (hemorrhagic) B30.3
  - filariasis B74.9
  - gonococci A54.31
  - herpes (simplex) virus B00.53
    - zoster B02.31
  - infectious disease NEC B99
  - meningococci A39.89
  - mucocutaneous leishmaniasis B55.2
  - rosacea H10.82-
  - syphilis (late) A52.71
  - zoster B02.31

Conjunctivitis (continued)

- inclusion A74.0
- infantile P39.1
  - gonococcal A54.31
- Koch-Weeks' —see Conjunctivitis, acute, mucopurulent
- light —see Conjunctivitis, acute, atopic
- ligneous —see Blepharoconjunctivitis, ligneous
- meningococcal A39.89
- mucopurulent —see Conjunctivitis, acute, mucopurulent
- neonatal P39.1
  - gonococcal A54.31
- Newcastle B30.8
- of Béal B30.2
- parasitic
  - filariasis B74.9
  - mucocutaneous leishmaniasis B55.2
- Parinaud's H10.89
- petrificans H10.89
- rosacea H10.82-
- specified NEC H10.89
- swimming-pool B30.1
- trachomatous A71.1
  - acute A71.0
  - sequelae (late effect) B94.0
- traumatic NEC H10.89
- tuberculous A18.59
- tularemic A21.1
- tularensis A21.1
- viral B30.9
  - due to
    - adenovirus B30.1
    - enterovirus B30.3
  - specified NEC B30.8

Conjunctivochalasis H11.82-

Connective tissue —see condition

Conn's syndrome E26.01

Conradi (-Hünermann) **disease** Q77.3

Consanguinity Z84.3
- counseling Z71.89

Conscious simulation (of illness) Z76.5

Consecutive —see condition

Consolidation lung (base) —see Pneumonia, lobar

Constipation (atonic) (neurogenic) (simple) (spastic) K59.00
- chronic K59.09
  - idiopathic K59.04
- drug-induced K59.03
- functional K59.04
- outlet dysfunction K59.02
- psychogenic F45.8
- slow transit K59.01
- specified NEC K59.09

Constitutional —see also condition
- substandard F60.7

Constitutionally substandard F60.7

Constriction —see also Stricture
- auditory canal —see Stenosis, external ear canal
- bronchial J98.09
- duodenum K31.5
- esophagus K22.2
- external
  - abdomen, abdominal (wall) S30.841
  - alveolar process S00.542
  - ankle S90.54-
  - antecubital space —see Constriction, external, forearm

Constriction (continued)

external (continued)
- arm (upper) S40.84-
- auricle —see Constriction, external, ear
- axilla —see Constriction, external, arm
- back, lower S30.840
- breast S20.14-
- brow S00.84
- buttock S30.840
- calf —see Constriction, external, leg
- canthus —see Constriction, external, eyelid
- cheek S00.84
  - internal S00.542
- chest wall —see Constriction, external, thorax
- chin S00.84
- clitoris S30.844
- costal region —see Constriction, external, thorax
- digit(s)
  - foot —see Constriction, external, toe
  - hand —see Constriction, external, finger
- ear S00.44-
- elbow S50.34-
- epididymis S30.843
- epigastric region S30.841
- esophagus, cervical S10.14
- eyebrow —see Constriction, external, eyelid
- eyelid S00.24-
- face S00.84
- finger(s) S60.44-
  - index S60.44-
  - little S60.44-
  - middle S60.44-
  - ring S60.44-
- flank S30.841
- foot (except toe(s) alone) S90.84-
  - toe —see Constriction, external, toe
- forearm S50.84-
  - elbow only —see Constriction, external, elbow
- forehead S00.84
- genital organs, external
  - female S30.846
  - male S30.845
- groin S30.841
- gum S00.542
- hand S60.54-
- head S00.94
  - ear —see Constriction, external, ear
  - eyelid —see Constriction, external, eyelid
  - lip S00.541
  - nose S00.34
  - oral cavity S00.542
  - scalp S00.04
  - specified site NEC S00.84
- heel —see Constriction, external, foot
- hip S70.24-
- inguinal region S30.841
- interscapular region S20.449
- jaw S00.84
- knee S80.24-
- labium (majus) (minus) S30.844
- larynx S10.14
- leg (lower) S80.84-
  - knee —see Constriction, external, knee
  - upper —see Constriction, external, thigh

Contraction(s), contracture, contracted (continued)

joint (continued)
  elbow M24.52-
  foot joint M24.57-
  hand joint M24.54-
  hip M24.55-
    congenital Q65.89
  hysterical F44.4
  knee M24.56-
  shoulder M24.51-
  specified site NEC M24.59
  wrist M24.53-
kidney (granular) (secondary) N26.9
  congenital Q63.8
  hydronephritic —see Hydronephrosis Page N26.2
  pyelonephritic —see Pyelitis, chronic
  tuberculous A18.11
ligament —see also Disorder, ligament
  congenital Q79.8
muscle (postinfective) (postural) NEC M62.40
  with contracture of joint —see Contraction, joint
  ankle M62.47-
  congenital Q79.8
    sternocleidomastoid Q68.0
  extraocular —see Strabismus
  eye (extrinsic) —see Strabismus
  foot M62.47-
  forearm M62.43-
  hand M62.44-
  hysterical F44.4
  ischemic (Volkmann's) T79.6
  lower leg M62.46-
  multiple sites M62.49
  pelvic region M62.45-
  posttraumatic —see Strabismus, paralytic
  psychogenic F45.8
    conversion reaction F44.4
  shoulder region M62.41-
  specified site NEC M62.48
  thigh M62.45-
  upper arm M62.42-
neck —see Torticollis
ocular muscle —see Strabismus
organ or site, congenital NEC — see Atresia, by site
outlet (pelvis) —see Contraction, pelvis
palmar fascia M72.0
paralytic
  joint —see Contraction, joint
  muscle —see also Contraction, muscle NEC
    ocular —see Strabismus, paralytic
pelvis (acquired) (general) M95.5
  with disproportion (fetopelvic) O33.1
    causing obstructed labor O65.1
    inlet O33.2
    mid-cavity O33.3
    outlet O33.3
plantar fascia M72.2
premature
  atrium I49.1
  auriculoventricular I49.49
  heart I49.49
  junctional I49.2
  supraventricular I49.1
  ventricular I49.3
prostate N42.89

Contraction(s), contracture, contracted (continued)

pylorus NEC —see also Pylorospasm
  psychogenic F45.8
rectum, rectal (sphincter) K59.89
ring (Bandl's) (complicating delivery) O62.4
scar —see Cicatrix
spine —see Dorsopathy, deforming
sternocleidomastoid (muscle), congenital Q68.0
stomach K31.89
  hourglass K31.89
    congenital Q40.2
    psychogenic F45.8
  psychogenic F45.8
tendon (sheath) M62.40
  with contracture of joint —see Contraction, joint
  Achilles —see Short, tendon, Achilles
  ankle M62.47-
    Achilles —see Short, tendon, Achilles
  foot M62.47-
  forearm M62.43-
  hand M62.44-
  lower leg M62.46-
  multiple sites M62.49
  neck M62.48
  pelvic region M62.45-
  shoulder region M62.41-
  specified site NEC M62.48
  thigh M62.45-
  thorax M62.48
  trunk M62.48
  upper arm M62.42-
toe —see Deformity, toe, specified NEC

Contraction(s), contracture,

ureterovesical orifice (postinfectional) N13.5
  with infection N13.6
urethra —see also Stricture, urethra
  orifice N32.0
uterus N85.8
  abnormal NEC O62.9
  clonic (complicating delivery) O62.4
  dyscoordinate (complicating delivery) O62.4
  hourglass (complicating delivery) O62.4
  hypertonic O62.4
  hypotonic NEC O62.2
  inadequate
    primary O62.0
    secondary O62.1
  incoordinate (complicating delivery) O62.4
  poor O62.2
  tetanic (complicating delivery) O62.4
vagina (outlet) N89.5
vesical N32.89
  neck or urethral orifice N32.0
visual field —see Defect, visual field, generalized
Volkmann's (ischemic) T79.6

Contusion (skin surface intact) T14.8

abdomen, abdominal (muscle) (wall) S30.1
adnexa, eye NEC S05.8X-
adrenal gland S37.812
alveolar process S00.532
ankle S90.0-
antecubital space —see Contusion, forearm
anus S30.3

Contusion (continued)

arm (upper) S40.02-
  lower (with elbow) —see Contusion, forearm
auditory canal —see Contusion, ear
auricle —see Contusion, ear
axilla —see Contusion, arm, upper
back —see also Contusion, thorax, back
  lower S30.0
bile duct S36.13
bladder S37.22
bone NEC T14.8
brain (diffuse) —see Injury, intracranial, diffuse
  focal —see Injury, intracranial, focal
brainstem S06.38-
breast S20.0-
broad ligament S37.892
brow S00.83
buttock S30.0
canthus, eye S00.1-
cauda equina S34.3
cerebellar, traumatic S06.37-
cerebral S06.33-
  left side S06.32-
  right side S06.31-
cheek S00.83
  internal S00.532
chest (wall) —see Contusion, thorax
chin S00.83
clitoris S30.23
colon —see Injury, intestine, large, contusion
common bile duct S36.13
conjunctiva S05.1-
  with foreign body (in conjunctival sac) —see Foreign body, conjunctival sac
conus medullaris (spine) S34.139
cornea —see Contusion, eyeball
  with foreign body —see Foreign body, cornea
corpus cavernosum S30.21
cortex (brain) (cerebral) —see Injury, intracranial, diffuse
  focal —see Injury, intracranial, focal
costal region —see Contusion, thorax
cystic duct S36.13
diaphragm S27.802
duodenum S36.420
ear S00.43-
elbow S50.0-
  with forearm —see Contusion, forearm
epididymis S30.22
epigastric region S30.1
epiglottis S10.0
esophagus (thoracic) S27.812
  cervical S10.0
eyeball S05.1-
eyebrow S00.1-
eyelid (and periocular area) S00.1-
face NEC S00.83
fallopian tube S37.529
  bilateral S37.522
  unilateral S37.521
femoral triangle S30.1
finger(s) S60.00
  with damage to nail (matrix) S60.10
  index S60.02-
    with damage to nail S60.12-
  little S60.05-
    with damage to nail S60.15-
  middle S60.03-
    with damage to nail S60.13-
  ring S60.04-
    with damage to nail S60.14-
  thumb —see Contusion, thumb

Contusion (continued)

flank S30.1
foot (except toe(s) alone) S90.3-
  toe —see Contusion, toe
forearm S50.1-
  elbow only —see Contusion, elbow
forehead S00.83
gallbladder S36.122
genital organs, external
  female S30.202
  male S30.201
globe (eye) —see Contusion, eyeball
groin S30.1
gum S00.532
hand S60.22-
  finger(s) —see Contusion, finger
  wrist —see Contusion, wrist
head S00.93
  ear —see Contusion, ear
  eyelid —see Contusion, eyelid
  lip S00.531
  nose S00.33
  oral cavity S00.532
  scalp S00.03
  specified part NEC S00.83
heart (see also Injury, heart) S26.91
heel —see Contusion, foot
hepatic duct S36.13
hip S70.0-
ileum S36.428
iliac region S30.1
inguinal region S30.1
interscapular region S20.229
intra-abdominal organ S36.92
  colon —see Injury, intestine, large, contusion
  liver S36.112
  pancreas —see Contusion, pancreas
  rectum S36.62
  small intestine —see Injury, intestine, small, contusion
  specified organ NEC S36.892
  spleen —see Contusion, spleen
  stomach S36.32
iris (eye) —see Contusion, eyeball
jaw S00.83
jejunum S36.428
kidney S37.01-
  major (greater than 2 cm) S37.02-
  minor (less than 2 cm) S37.01-
knee S80.0-
labium (majus) (minus) S30.23
lacrimal apparatus, gland or sac S05.8X-
larynx S10.0
leg (lower) S80.1-
  knee —see Contusion, knee
lens —see Contusion, eyeball
lip S00.531
liver S36.112
lower back S30.0
lumbar region S30.0
lung S27.329
  bilateral S27.322
  unilateral S27.321
malar region S00.83
mastoid region S00.83
membrane, brain —see Injury, intracranial, diffuse
  focal —see Injury, intracranial, focal
mesentery S36.892
mesosalpinx S37.892
mouth S00.532
muscle —see Contusion, by site
nail
  finger —see Contusion, finger, with damage to nail
  toe —see Contusion, toe, with damage to nail

Contusion (*continued*)
nasal S00.33
neck S10.93
specified site NEC S10.83
throat S10.0
nerve —*see* Injury, nerve
newborn P54.5
nose S00.33
occipital
lobe (brain) —*see* Injury,
intracranial, diffuse
focal —*see* Injury,
intracranial, focal
region (scalp) S00.03
orbit (region) (tissues) S05.1-
ovary S37.429
bilateral S37.422
unilateral S37.421
palate S00.532
pancreas S36.229
body S36.221
head S36.220
tail S36.222
parietal
lobe (brain) —*see* Injury,
intracranial, diffuse
focal —*see* Injury,
intracranial, focal
region (scalp) S00.03
pelvic organ S37.92
adrenal gland S37.812
bladder S37.22
fallopian tube —*see* Contusion,
fallopian tube
kidney —*see* Contusion, kidney
ovary —*see* Contusion, ovary
prostate S37.822
specified organ NEC S37.892
ureter S37.12
urethra S37.32
uterus S37.62
pelvis S30.0
penis S30.21
perineum
female S30.23
male S30.0
periocular area S00.1-
peritoneum S36.81
periurethral tissue —*see* Contusion,
urethra
pharynx S10.0
pinna —*see* Contusion, ear
popliteal space —*see* Contusion, knee
prepuce S30.21
prostate S37.822
pubic region S30.1
pudendum
female S30.202
male S30.201
quadriceps femoris —*see*
Contusion, thigh
rectum S36.62
retroperitoneum S36.892
round ligament S37.892
sacral region S30.0
scalp S00.03
due to birth injury P12.3
scapular region —*see* Contusion,
shoulder
sclera —*see* Contusion, eyeball
scrotum S30.22
seminal vesicle S37.892
shoulder S40.01-
skin NEC T14.8
small intestine —*see* Injury,
intestine, small, contusion
spermatic cord S30.22
spinal cord —*see* Injury, spinal
cord, by region
cauda equina S34.3
conus medullaris S34.139

Contusion (*continued*)
spleen S36.029
major S36.021
minor S36.020
sternal region S20.219
stomach S36.32
subconjunctival S05.1-
subcutaneous NEC T14.8
submaxillary region S00.83
submental region S00.83
subperiosteal NEC T14.8
subungual
finger —*see* Contusion, finger,
with damage to nail
toe —*see* Contusion, toe, with
damage to nail
supraclavicular fossa S10.83
supraorbital S00.83
suprarenal gland S37.812
temple (region) S00.83
temporal
lobe (brain) —*see* Injury,
intracranial, diffuse
focal —*see* Injury,
intracranial, focal
region S00.83
testis S30.22
thigh S70.1-
thorax (wall) S20.20
back S20.22-
front S20.21-
throat S10.0
thumb S60.01-
with damage to nail S60.11-
toe(s) (lesser) S90.12-
with damage to nail S90.22-
great S90.11-
with damage to nail S90.21-
tongue S00.532
trachea (cervical) S10.0
thoracic S27.52
tunica vaginalis S30.22
tympanum, tympanic membrane
—*see* Contusion, ear
ureter S37.12
urethra S37.32
urinary organ NEC S37.892
uterus S37.62
uvula S00.532
vagina S30.23
vas deferens S37.892
vesical S37.22
vocal cord(s) S10.0
vulva S30.23
wrist S60.21-

Conus (congenital) (any type) Q14.8
cornea —*see* Keratoconus
medullaris syndrome G95.81

**Conversion hysteria, neurosis or
reaction** F44.9

Converter, tuberculosis (test
reaction) R76.11

Conviction (legal), **anxiety
concerning** Z65.0
with imprisonment Z65.1

Convulsions (idiopathic) (*see also*
Seizure(s)) R56.9
apoplectiform (cerebral ischemia)
I67.82
dissociative F44.5
epileptic —*see* Epilepsy
epileptiform, epileptoid —*see*
Seizure, epileptiform
ether (anesthetic) —*see* Table of
Drugs and Chemicals, by drug
febrile R56.00
with status epilepticus G40.901
complex R56.01
with status epilepticus G40.901
simple R56.00

Convulsions (*continued*)
hysterical F44.5
infantile P90
epilepsy —*see* Epilepsy
jacksonian —*see* Epilepsy,
localization-related,
symptomatic, with simple partial
seizures
myoclonic G25.3
newborn P90
obstetrical (nephritic) (uremic)
—*see* Eclampsia
paretic A52.17
post traumatic R56.1
psychomotor —*see* Epilepsy,
localization-related,
symptomatic, with complex
partial seizures
recurrent R56.9
reflex R25.8
scarlatinal A38.8
tetanus, tetanic —*see* Tetanus
thymic E32.8

Convulsive —*see also* Convulsions

Cooley's anemia D56.1

Coolie itch B76.9

Cooper's
disease —*see* Mastopathy, cystic
hernia —*see* Hernia, abdomen,
specified site NEC

Copra itch B88.0

Coprophagy F50.89

Coprophobia F40.298

Coproporphyria, hereditary
E80.29

Cor
biloculare Q20.8
bovis, bovinum —*see* Hypertrophy,
cardiac
pulmonale (chronic) I27.81
acute I26.09
triatriatum, triatrium Q24.2
triloculare Q20.8
biatrium Q20.4
biventriculare Q21.1

Corbus' disease (gangrenous
balanitis) N48.1

Cord —*see also* condition
around neck
complicating delivery O69.81
with compression O69.1
bladder G95.89
tabetic A52.19

Cordis ectopia Q24.8

Corditis (spermatic) N49.1

Corectopia Q13.2

Cori's disease (glycogen storage)
E74.03

Corkhandler's disease or lung J67.3

Corkscrew esophagus K22.4

Corkworker's disease or lung J67.3

Corn (infected) L84

Cornea —*see also* condition
donor Z52.5
plana Q13.4

Cornelia de Lange syndrome Q87.19

Cornu cutaneum L85.8

Cornual gestation or pregnancy
O00.80
with intrauterine pregnancy O00.81

Coronary (artery) —*see* condition

Coronavirus (infection)
as cause of disease classified
elsewhere B97.29

Coronavirus (*continued*)
coronavirus-19 U07.1
COVID-19 U07.1
SARS-associated B97.21

Corpora —*see also* condition
amylacea, prostate N42.89
cavernosa —*see* condition

Corpulence —*see* Obesity

Corpus —*see* condition

Corrected transposition Q20.5

Corrosion (injury) (acid) (caustic)
(chemical) (lime) (external)
(internal) T30.4
abdomen, abdominal (muscle)
(wall) T21.42
first degree T21.52
second degree T21.62
third degree T21.72
above elbow T22.439
first degree T22.539
left T22.432
first degree T22.532
second degree T22.632
third degree T22.732
right T22.431
first degree T22.531
second degree T22.631
third degree T22.731
second degree T22.639
third degree T22.739
alimentary tract NEC T28.7
ankle T25.419
first degree T25.519
left T25.412
first degree T25.512
second degree T25.612
third degree T25.712
multiple with foot —*see*
Corrosion, lower, limb,
multiple, ankle and foot
right T25.411
first degree T25.511
second degree T25.611
third degree T25.711
second degree T25.619
third degree T25.719
anus —*see* Corrosion, buttock
arm(s) (meaning upper
limb(s)) —*see* Corrosion, upper
limb
axilla T22.449
first degree T22.549
left T22.442
first degree T22.542
second degree T22.642
third degree T22.742
right T22.441
first degree T22.541
second degree T22.641
third degree T22.741
second degree T22.649
third degree T22.749
back (lower) T21.44
first degree T21.54
second degree T21.64
third degree T21.74
upper T21.43
first degree T21.53
second degree T21.63
third degree T21.73
blisters - code as Corrosion, second
degree, by site
breast(s) —*see* Corrosion,
chest wall
buttock(s) T21.45
first degree T21.55
second degree T21.65
third degree T21.75
calf T24.439
first degree T24.539

calf (continued)
left T24.432
first degree T24.532 sickle-cell D57.00
second degree T24.632
third degree T24.732
right T24.431
first degree T24.531
second degree T24.631
third degree T24.731
second degree T24.639
third degree T24.739
canthus (eye) —*see* Corrosion, eyelid
cervix T28.8
cheek T20.46
first degree T20.56
second degree T20.66
third degree T20.76
chest wall T21.41
first degree T21.51
second degree T21.61
third degree T21.71
chin T20.43
first degree T20.53
second degree T20.63
third degree T20.73
colon T28.7
conjunctiva (and cornea) —*see* Corrosion, cornea
cornea (and conjunctiva) T26.6-
deep necrosis of underlying tissue - code as Corrosion, third degree, by site
dorsum of hand T23.469
first degree T23.569
left T23.462
first degree T23.562
second degree T23.662
third degree T23.762
right T23.461
first degree T23.561
second degree T23.661
third degree T23.761
second degree T23.669
third degree T23.769
ear (auricle) (external) (canal) T20.41
drum T28.91
first degree T20.51
second degree T20.61
third degree T20.71
elbow T22.429
first degree T22.529
left T22.422
first degree T22.522
second degree T22.622
third degree T22.722
right T22.421
first degree T22.521
second degree T22.621
third degree T22.721
second degree T22.629
third degree T22.729
entire body —*see* Corrosion, multiple body regions
epidermal loss - code as Corrosion, second degree, by site
epiglottis T27.4
erythema, erythematous - code as Corrosion, first degree, by site
esophagus T28.6
extent (percentage of body surface)
less than 10 percent T32.0
10-19 percent (0-9 percent third degree) T32.10
with 10-19 percent third degree T32.11

extent (continued)
20-29 percent (0-9 percent third degree) T32.20
with
10-19 percent third degree T32.21
20-29 percent third degree T32.22
30-39 percent (0-9 percent third degree) T32.30
with
10-19 percent third degree T32.31
20-29 percent third degree T32.32
30-39 percent third degree T32.33
40-49 percent (0-9 percent third degree) T32.40
with
10-19 percent third degree T32.41
20-29 percent third degree T32.42
30-39 percent third degree T32.43
40-49 percent third degree T32.44
50-59 percent (0-9 percent third degree) T32.50
with
10-19 percent third degree T32.51
20-29 percent third degree T32.52
30-39 percent third degree T32.53
40-49 percent third degree T32.54
50-59 percent third degree T32.55
60-69 percent (0-9 percent third degree) T32.60
with
10-19 percent third degree T32.61
20-29 percent third degree T32.62
30-39 percent third degree T32.63
40-49 percent third degree T32.64
50-59 percent third degree T32.65
60-69 percent third degree T32.66
70-79 percent (0-9 percent third degree) T32.70
with
10-19 percent third degree T32.71
20-29 percent third degree T32.72
30-39 percent third degree T32.73
40-49 percent third degree T32.74
50-59 percent third degree T32.75
60-69 percent third degree T32.76
70-79 percent third degree T32.77
80-89 percent (0-9 percent third degree) T32.80
with
10-19 percent third degree T32.81
20-29 percent third degree T32.82

extent (continued)
80-89 percent (continued)
with (continued)
30-39 percent third degree T32.83
40-49 percent third degree T32.84
50-59 percent third degree T32.85
60-69 percent third degree T32.86
70-79 percent third degree T32.87
80-89 percent third degree T32.88
90 percent or more (0-9 percent third degree) T32.90
with
10-19 percent third degree T32.91
20-29 percent third degree T32.92
30-39 percent third degree T32.93
40-49 percent third degree T32.94
50-59 percent third degree T32.95
60-69 percent third degree T32.96
70-79 percent third degree T32.97
80-89 percent third degree T32.98
90-99 percent third degree T32.99
extremity —*see* Corrosion, limb
eye(s) and adnexa T26.9-
with resulting rupture and destruction of eyeball T26.7-
conjunctival sac —*see* Corrosion, cornea
cornea —*see* Corrosion, cornea
lid —*see* Corrosion, eyelid
periocular area —*see* Corrosion eyelid
specified site NEC T26.8-
eyeball —*see* Corrosion, eye
eyelid(s) T26.5-
face —*see* Corrosion, head
finger T23.429
first degree T23.529
left T23.422
first degree T23.522
second degree T23.622
third degree T23.722
multiple sites (without thumb) T23.439
with thumb T23.449
first degree T23.549
left T23.442
first degree T23.542
second degree T23.642
third degree T23.742
right T23.441
first degree T23.541
second degree T23.641
third degree T23.741
second degree T23.649
third degree T23.749
first degree T23.539
left T23.432
first degree T23.532
second degree T23.632
third degree T23.732
right T23.431
first degree T23.531
second degree T23.631
third degree T23.731

finger (continued)
multiple sites (continued)
second degree T23.639
third degree T23.739
right T23.421
first degree T23.521
second degree T23.621
third degree T23.721
second degree T23.629
third degree T23.729
flank —*see* Corrosion, abdomen
foot T25.429
first degree T25.529
left T25.422
first degree T25.522
second degree T25.622
third degree T25.722
multiple with ankle —*see* Corrosion, lower, limb, multiple, ankle and foot
right T25.421
first degree T25.521
second degree T25.621
third degree T25.721
second degree T25.629
third degree T25.729
forearm T22.419
first degree T22.519
left T22.412
first degree T22.512
second degree T22.612
third degree T22.712
right T22.411
first degree T22.511
second degree T22.611
third degree T22.711
second degree T22.619
third degree T22.719
forehead T20.46
first degree T20.56
second degree T20.66
third degree T20.76
fourth degree - code as Corrosion, third degree, by site
full thickness skin loss - code as Corrosion, third degree, by site
gastrointestinal tract NEC T28.7
genital organs
external
female T21.47
first degree T21.57
second degree T21.67
third degree T21.77
male T21.46
first degree T21.56
second degree T21.66
third degree T21.76
internal T28.8
groin —*see* Corrosion, abdominal wall
hand(s) T23.409
back —*see* Corrosion, dorsum of hand
finger —*see* Corrosion, finger
first degree T23.509
left T23.402
first degree T23.502
second degree T23.602
third degree T23.702
multiple sites with wrist T23.499
first degree T23.599
left T23.492
first degree T23.592
second degree T23.692
third degree T23.792
right T23.491
first degree T23.591
second degree T23.691
third degree T23.791
second degree T23.699
third degree T23.799

hand(s) *(continued)*
  palm —*see* Corrosion, palm
  right T23.401
    first degree T23.501
    second degree T23.601
    third degree T23.701
  second degree T23.609
  third degree T23.709
  thumb —*see* Corrosion, thumb
head (and face) (and neck) T20.40
  cheek —*see* Corrosion, cheek
  chin —*see* Corrosion, chin
  ear —*see* Corrosion, ear
  eye(s) only —*see* Corrosion, eye
  first degree T20.50
  forehead —*see* Corrosion,
    forehead
  lip —*see* Corrosion, lip
  multiple sites T20.49
    first degree T20.59
    second degree T20.69
    third degree T20.79
  neck —*see* Corrosion, neck
  nose —*see* Corrosion, nose
  scalp —*see* Corrosion, scalp
  second degree T20.60
  third degree T20.70
hip(s) —*see* Corrosion, lower, limb
inhalation —*see* Corrosion,
  respiratory tract
internal organ(s) *(see also*
  Corrosion, by site) T28.90
  alimentary tract T28.7
    esophagus T28.6
  esophagus T28.6
  genitourinary T28.8
  mouth T28.5
  pharynx T28.5
  specified organ NEC T28.99
interscapular region —*see*
  Corrosion, back, upper
intestine (large) (small) T28.7
knee T24.429
  first degree T24.529
  left T24.422
    first degree T24.522
    second degree T24.622
    third degree T24.722
  right T24.421
    first degree T24.521
    second degree T24.621
    third degree T24.721
  second degree T24.629
  third degree T24.729
labium (majus) (minus) —*see*
  Corrosion, genital organs,
  external, female
lacrimal apparatus, duct, gland
  or sac —*see* Corrosion, eye,
  specified site NEC
larynx T27.4
  with lung T27.5
leg(s) (meaning lower limb(s))
  —*see* Corrosion, lower limb
limb(s)
  lower —*see* Corrosion, lower,
    limb
  upper —*see* Corrosion, upper
    limb
lip(s) T20.42
  first degree T20.52
  second degree T20.62
  third degree T20.72
lower
  back —*see* Corrosion, back
  limb T24.409
    ankle —*see* Corrosion, ankle
    calf —*see* Corrosion, calf
    first degree T24.509
    foot —*see* Corrosion, foot

lower *(continued)*
  limb *(continued)*
    knee —*see* Corrosion, knee
    left T24.402
      first degree T24.502
      second degree T24.602
      third degree T24.702
    multiple sites, except ankle
      and foot T24.499
      ankle and foot T25.499
        first degree T25.599
        left T25.492
          first degree T25.592
          second degree T25.692
          third degree T25.792
        right T25.491
          first degree T25.591
          second degree T25.691
          third degree T25.791
        second degree T25.699
        third degree T25.799
      first degree T24.599
      left T24.492
        first degree T24.592
        second degree T24.692
        third degree T24.792
      right T24.491
        first degree T24.591
        second degree T24.691
        third degree T24.791
      second degree T24.699
      third degree T24.799
    right T24.401
      first degree T24.501
      second degree T24.601
      third degree T24.701
    second degree T24.609
    hip —*see* Corrosion, thigh
    thigh —*see* Corrosion, thigh
    third degree T24.709
lung (with larynx and trachea)
  T27.5
mouth T28.5
neck T20.47
  first degree T20.57
  second degree T20.67
  third degree T20.77
nose (septum) T20.44
  first degree T20.54
  second degree T20.64
  third degree T20.74
ocular adnexa —*see* Corrosion, eye
orbit region —*see* Corrosion, eyelid
palm T23.459
  first degree T23.559
  left T23.452
    first degree T23.552
    second degree T23.652
    third degree T23.752
  right T23.451
    first degree T23.551
    second degree T23.651
    third degree T23.751
  second degree T23.659
  third degree T23.759
partial thickness - code as
  Corrosion, unspecified degree,
  by site
pelvis —*see* Corrosion, trunk
penis —*see* Corrosion, genital
  organs, external, male
perineum
  female —*see* Corrosion, genital
    organs, external, female
  male —*see* Corrosion, genital
    organs, external, male
periocular area —*see* Corrosion,
  eyelid
pharynx T28.5
rectum T28.7

respiratory tract T27.7
  larynx —*see* Corrosion, larynx
  specified part NEC T27.6
  trachea —*see* Corrosion, larynx
sac, lacrimal —*see* Corrosion, eye,
  specified site NEC
scalp T20.45
  first degree T20.55
  second degree T20.65
  third degree T20.75
scapular region T22.469
  first degree T22.569
  left T22.462
    first degree T22.562
    second degree T22.662
    third degree T22.762
  right T22.461
    first degree T22.561
    second degree T22.661
    third degree T22.761
  second degree T22.669
  third degree T22.769
sclera —*see* Corrosion, eye,
  specified site NEC
scrotum —*see* Corrosion, genital
  organs, external, male
shoulder T22.459
  first degree T22.559
  left T22.452
    first degree T22.552
    second degree T22.652
    third degree T22.752
  right T22.451
    first degree T22.551
    second degree T22.651
    third degree T22.751
  second degree T22.659
  third degree T22.759
stomach T28.7
temple —*see* Corrosion, head
testis —*see* Corrosion, genital
  organs, external, male
thigh T24.419
  first degree T24.519
  left T24.412
    first degree T24.512
    second degree T24.612
    third degree T24.712
  right T24.411
    first degree T24.511
    second degree T24.611
    third degree T24.711
  second degree T24.619
  third degree T24.719
thorax (external) —*see* Corrosion,
  trunk
throat (meaning pharynx) T28.5
thumb(s) T23.419
  first degree T23.519
  left T23.412
    first degree T23.512
    second degree T23.612
    third degree T23.712
  multiple sites with fingers T23.449
    first degree T23.549
    left T23.442
      first degree T23.542
      second degree T23.642
      third degree T23.742
    right T23.441
      first degree T23.541
      second degree T23.641
      third degree T23.741
    second degree T23.649
    third degree T23.749
  right T23.411
    first degree T23.511
    second degree T23.611
    third degree T23.711
  second degree T23.619

thumb(s) *(continued)*
  third degree T23.719
toe T25.439
  first degree T25.539
  left T25.432
    first degree T25.532
    second degree T25.632
    third degree T25.732
  right T25.431
    first degree T25.531
    second degree T25.631
    third degree T25.731
  second degree T25.639
  third degree T25.739
tongue T28.5
tonsil(s) T28.5
total body —*see* Corrosion,
  multiple body regions
trachea T27.4
  with lung T27.5
trunk T21.40
  abdominal wall —*see* Corrosion,
    abdominal wall
  anus —*see* Corrosion, buttock
  axilla —*see* Corrosion, upper
    limb
  back —*see* Corrosion, back
  breast —*see* Corrosion, chest
    wall
  buttock —*see* Corrosion, buttock
  chest wall —*see* Corrosion, chest
    wall
  first degree T21.50
  flank —*see* Corrosion,
    abdominal wall
  genital
    female —*see* Corrosion, genital
      organs, external, female
    male —*see* Corrosion, genital
      organs, external, male
  groin —*see* Corrosion,
    abdominal wall
  interscapular region —*see*
    Corrosion, back, upper
  labia —*see* Corrosion, genital
    organs, external, female
  lower back —*see* Corrosion, back
  penis —*see* Corrosion, genital
    organs, external, male
  perineum
    female —*see* Corrosion, genital
      organs, external, female
    male —*see* Corrosion, genital
      organs, external, male
  scapular region —*see* Corrosion,
    upper limb
  scrotum —*see* Corrosion, genital
    organs, external, male
  second degree T21.60
  shoulder —*see* Corrosion, upper
    limb
  specified site NEC T21.49
    first degree T21.59
    second degree T21.69
    third degree T21.79
  testes —*see* Corrosion, genital
    organs, external, male
  third degree T21.70
  upper back —*see* Corrosion,
    back, upper
  vagina T28.8
  vulva —*see* Corrosion, genital
    organs, external, female
unspecified site with extent of
  body surface involved specified
  less than 10 percent T32.0
  10-19 percent (0-9 percent third
    degree) T32.10
    with 10-19 percent third
      degree T32.11

Corrosion (continued)
unspecified site with extent of
body surface involved specified
(continued)
20-29 percent (0-9 percent third
degree) T32.20
with
10-19 percent third degree
T32.21
20-29 percent third degree
T32.22
30-39 percent (0-9 percent third
degree) T32.30
with
10-19 percent third degree
T32.31
20-29 percent third degree
T32.32
30-39 percent third degree
T32.33
40-49 percent (0-9 percent third
degree) T32.40
with
10-19 percent third degree
T32.41
20-29 percent third degree
T32.42
30-39 percent third degree
T32.43
40-49 percent third degree
T32.44
50-59 percent (0-9 percent third
degree) T32.50
with
10-19 percent third degree
T32.51
20-29 percent third degree
T32.52
30-39 percent third degree
T32.53
40-49 percent third degree
T32.54
50-59 percent third degree
T32.55
60-69 percent (0-9 percent third
degree) T32.60
with
10-19 percent third degree
T32.61
20-29 percent third degree
T32.62
30-39 percent third degree
T32.63
40-49 percent third degree
T32.64
50-59 percent third degree
T32.65
60-69 percent third degree
T32.66
70-79 percent (0-9 percent third
degree) T32.70
with
10-19 percent third degree
T32.71
20-29 percent third degree
T32.72
30-39 percent third degree
T32.73
40-49 percent third degree
T32.74
50-59 percent third degree
T32.75
60-69 percent third degree
T32.76
70-79 percent third degree
T32.77
80-89 percent (0-9 percent third
degree) T32.80
with
10-19 percent third degree
T32.81

Corrosion (continued)
unspecified site with extent of
body surface involved specified
(continued)
80-89 percent (continued)
with (continued)
20-29 percent third degree
T32.82
30-39 percent third degree
T32.83
40-49 percent third degree
T32.84
50-59 percent third degree
T32.85
60-69 percent third degree
T32.86
70-79 percent third degree
T32.87
80-89 percent third degree
T32.88
90 percent or more (0-9 percent
third degree) T32.90
with
10-19 percent third degree
T32.91
20-29 percent third degree
T32.92
30-39 percent third degree
T32.93
40-49 percent third degree
T32.94
50-59 percent third degree
T32.95
60-69 percent third degree
T32.96
70-79 percent third degree
T32.97
80-89 percent third degree
T32.98
90-99 percent third degree
T32.99
upper limb (axilla) (scapular
region) T22.40
above elbow —see Corrosion,
above elbow
axilla —see Corrosion, axilla
elbow —see Corrosion, elbow
first degree T22.50
forearm —see Corrosion, forearm
hand —see Corrosion, hand
interscapular region —see
Corrosion, back, upper
multiple sites T22.499
first degree T22.599
left T22.492
first degree T22.592
second degree T22.692
third degree T22.792
right T22.491
first degree T22.591
second degree T22.691
third degree T22.791
second degree T22.699
third degree T22.799
scapular region —see Corrosion,
scapular region
second degree T22.60
shoulder —see Corrosion,
shoulder
third degree T22.70
wrist —see Corrosion, hand
uterus T28.8
vagina T28.8
vulva —see Corrosion, genital
organs, external, female
wrist T23.479
first degree T23.579
left T23.472
first degree T23.572
second degree T23.672
third degree T23.772

Corrosion (continued)
wrist (continued)
multiple sites with hand T23.499
first degree T23.599
left T23.492
first degree T23.592
second degree T23.692
third degree T23.792
right T23.491
first degree T23.591
second degree T23.691
third degree T23.791
second degree T23.699
third degree T23.799
right T23.471
first degree T23.571
second degree T23.671
third degree T23.771
second degree T23.679
third degree T23.779

Corrosive burn —see Corrosion

Corsican fever —see Malaria

Cortical —see condition

Cortico-adrenal —see condition

Coryza (acute) J00
with grippe or influenza —see
Influenza, with, respiratory
manifestations NEC
syphilitic
congenital (chronic) A50.05

Costen's syndrome or complex
M26.69

Costiveness —see Constipation

Costochondritis M94.0

Cotard's syndrome F22

Cot death R99

Cotia virus B08.8

Cotton wool spots (retinal) H35.81

Cotungo's disease —see Sciatica

Cough (affected) (chronic)
(epidemic) (nervous) R05
with hemorrhage —see
Hemoptysis
bronchial R05
with grippe or influenza —see
Influenza, with, respiratory
manifestations NEC
functional F45.8
hysterical F45.8
laryngeal, spasmodic R05
psychogenic F45.8
smokers' J41.0
tea taster's B49

Counseling (for) Z71.9
abuse NEC
perpetrator Z69.82
victim Z69.81
alcohol abuser Z71.41
family Z71.42
child abuse
nonparental
perpetrator Z69.021
victim Z69.020
parental
perpetrator Z69.011
victim Z69.010
consanguinity Z71.89
contraceptive Z30.09
dietary Z71.3
drug abuser Z71.51
family member Z71.52
exercise Z71.82
family Z71.89
fertility preservation (prior to
cancer therapy) (prior to removal
of gonads) Z31.62

Counseling (continued)
for non-attending third party Z71.0
related to sexual behavior or
orientation Z70.2
genetic
nonprocreative Z71.83
procreative NEC Z31.5
gestational carrier Z31.7
health (advice) (education)
(instruction) —see Counseling,
medical
risk for travel (international)
Z71.84
human immunodeficiency virus
(HIV) Z71.7
impotence Z70.1
insulin pump use Z46.81
medical (for) Z71.9
boarding school resident Z59.3
consanguinity Z71.89
feared complaint and no disease
found Z71.1
human immunodeficiency virus
(HIV) Z71.7
institutional resident Z59.3
on behalf of another Z71.0
related to sexual behavior or
orientation Z70.2
person living alone Z60.2
specified reason NEC Z71.89
natural family planning
procreative Z31.61
to avoid pregnancy Z30.02
perpetrator (of)
abuse NEC Z69.82
child abuse
non-parental Z69.021
parental Z69.011
rape NEC Z69.82
spousal abuse Z69.12
procreative NEC Z31.69
fertility preservation (prior to
cancer therapy) (prior to
removal of gonads) Z31.62
using natural family planning
Z31.61
promiscuity Z70.1
rape victim Z69.81
religious Z71.81
safety for travel (international) Z71.84
sex, sexual (related to) Z70.9
attitude(s) Z70.0
behavior or orientation Z70.1
combined concerns Z70.3
non-responsiveness Z70.1
on behalf of third party Z70.2
specified reason NEC Z70.8
specified reason NEC Z71.89
spiritual Z71.81
spousal abuse (perpetrator) Z69.12
victim Z69.11
substance abuse Z71.89
alcohol Z71.41
drug Z71.51
tobacco Z71.6
tobacco use Z71.6
travel (international) Z71.84
use (of)
insulin pump Z46.81
victim (of)
abuse Z69.81
child abuse
by parent Z69.010
non-parental Z69.020
rape NEC Z69.81

Coupled rhythm R00.8

Couvelaire syndrome or uterus
(complicating delivery) O45.8X-

Cowperitis —see Urethritis

Cowper's gland —see condition

Cowpox B08.010
    due to vaccination T88.1
Coxa
    magna M91.4-
    plana M91.2-
    valga (acquired) —see also
        Deformity, limb, specified type
        NEC, thigh
        congenital Q65.81
        sequelae (late effect) of rickets
            E64.3
    vara (acquired) —see also Deformity,
        limb, specified type NEC, thigh
        congenital Q65.82
        sequelae (late effect) of rickets
            E64.3
Coxalgia, coxalgic (nontuberculous)
    —see also Pain, joint, hip
    tuberculous A18.02
Coxitis —see Monoarthritis, hip
Coxsackie (virus) (infection) B34.1
    as cause of disease classified
        elsewhere B97.11
    carditis B33.20
    central nervous system NEC A88.8
    endocarditis B33.21
    enteritis A08.39
    meningitis (aseptic) A87.0
    myocarditis B33.22
    pericarditis B33.23
    pharyngitis B08.5
    pleurodynia B33.0
    specific disease NEC B33.8
Crabs, meaning pubic lice B85.3
Crack baby P04.41
Cracked nipple N64.0
    associated with
        lactation O92.13
        pregnancy O92.11-
        puerperium O92.12
Cracked tooth K03.81
Cradle cap L21.0
Craft neurosis F48.8
Cramp(s) R25.2
    abdominal —see Pain, abdominal
    bathing T75.1
    colic R10.83
        psychogenic F45.8
    due to immersion T75.1
    fireman T67.2
    heat T67.2
    immersion T75.1
    intestinal —see Pain, abdominal
        psychogenic F45.8
    leg, sleep related G47.62
    limb (lower) (upper) NEC R25.2
        sleep related G47.62
    linotypist's F48.8
        organic G25.89
    muscle (limb) (general) R25.2
        due to immersion T75.1
        psychogenic F45.8
    occupational (hand) F48.8
        organic G25.89
    salt-depletion E87.1
    sleep related, leg G47.62
    stoker's T67.2
    swimmer's T75.1
    telegrapher's F48.8
        organic G25.89
    typist's F48.8
        organic G25.89
    uterus N94.89
        menstrual —see Dysmenorrhea
    writer's F48.8
        organic G25.89
Cranial —see condition
Craniocleidodysostosis Q74.0

Craniofenestria (skull) Q75.8
Craniolacunia (skull) Q75.8
Craniopagus Q89.4
Craniopathy, metabolic M85.2
Craniopharyngeal —see condition
Craniopharyngioma D44.4
Craniorachischisis (totalis) Q00.1
Cranioschisis Q75.8
Craniostenosis Q75.0
Craniosynostosis Q75.0
Craniotabes (cause unknown) M83.8
    neonatal P96.3
    rachitic E64.3
    syphilitic A50.56
Cranium —see condition
Craw-craw —see Onchocerciasis
Creaking joint —see Derangement,
    joint, specified type NEC
Creeping
    eruption B76.9
    palsy or paralysis G12.22
Crenated tongue K14.8
Creotoxism A05.9
Crepitus
    caput Q75.8
    joint —see Derangement, joint,
        specified type NEC
Crescent or conus choroid,
    congenital Q14.3
CREST syndrome M34.1
Cretin, cretinism (congenital)
    (endemic) (nongoitrous) (sporadic)
    E00.9
    pelvis
        with disproportion (fetopelvic)
            O33.0
            causing obstructed labor
                O65.0
    type
        hypothyroid E00.1
        mixed E00.2
        myxedematous E00.1
        neurological E00.0
Creutzfeldt-Jakob disease or
    syndrome (with dementia) A81.00
    familial A81.09
    iatrogenic A81.09
    specified NEC A81.09
    sporadic A81.09
    variant (vCJD) A81.01
Crib death R99
Cribriform hymen Q52.3
Cri-du-chat syndrome Q93.4
Crigler-Najjar disease or syndrome
    E80.5
Crime, victim of Z65.4
Crimean hemorrhagic fever A98.0
Criminalism F60.2
Crisis
    abdomen R10.0
    acute reaction F43.0
    addisonian E27.2
    adrenal (cortical) E27.2
    celiac K90.0
    Dietl's N13.8
    emotional —see also Disorder,
        adjustment
        acute reaction to stress F43.0
        specific to childhood and
            adolescence F93.8
    glaucomatocyclitic —see Glaucoma,
        secondary, inflammation

Crisis (continued)
    heart —see Failure, heart
    nitritoid I95.2
        correct substance properly
            administered —see Table
            of Drugs and Chemicals, by
            drug, adverse effect
        overdose or wrong substance
            given or taken —see Table
            of Drugs and Chemicals, by
            drug, poisoning
    oculogyric H51.8
        psychogenic F45.8
    Pel's (tabetic) A52.11
    psychosexual identity F64.2
    renal N28.0
    sickle-cell D57.00
        with
            acute chest syndrome D57.01
            cerebral vascular involvement
                D57.03
            crisis (painful) D57.00
                with complication specified
                    NEC D57.09
            splenic sequestration D57.02
            vasoocclusive pain D57.00
    state (acute reaction) F43.0
    tabetic A52.11
    thyroid —see Thyrotoxicosis with
        thyroid storm
    thyrotoxic —see Thyrotoxicosis
        with thyroid storm
Crocq's disease (acrocyanosis) I73.89
Crohn's disease —see Enteritis,
    regional
Crooked septum, nasal J34.2
Cross syndrome E70.328
Crossbite (anterior) (posterior) M26.24
Cross-eye —see Strabismus,
    convergent concomitant
Croup, croupous (catarrhal)
    (infectious) (inflammatory)
    (nondiphtheritic) J05.0
    bronchial J20.9
    diphtheritic A36.2
    false J38.5
    spasmodic J38.5
        diphtheritic A36.2
    stridulous J38.5
        diphtheritic A36.2
Crouzon's disease Q75.1
Crowding, tooth, teeth, fully
    erupted M26.31
CRST syndrome M34.1
Cruchet's disease A85.8
Cruelty in children —see also
    Disorder, conduct
Crural ulcer —see Ulcer, lower limb
Crush, crushed, crushing T14.8
    abdomen S38.1
    ankle S97.0-
    arm (upper) (and shoulder) S47.-
    axilla —see Crush, arm
    back, lower S38.1
    buttock S38.1
    cheek S07.0
    chest S28.0
    cranium S07.1
    ear S07.0
    elbow S57.0-
    extremity
        lower
            ankle —see Crush, ankle
            below knee —see Crush, leg
            foot —see Crush, foot
            hip —see Crush, hip

Crush, crushed, crushing
(continued)
    extremity (continued)
        lower (continued)
            knee —see Crush, knee
            thigh —see Crush, thigh
            toe —see Crush, toe
        upper
            below elbow S67.9-
            elbow —see Crush, elbow
            finger —see Crush, finger
            forearm —see Crush, forearm
            hand —see Crush, hand
            thumb —see Crush, thumb
            upper arm —see Crush, arm
            wrist —see Crush, wrist
    face S07.0
    finger(s) S67.1-
        with hand (and wrist) —see
            Crush, hand, specified site
            NEC
        index S67.19-
        little S67.19-
        middle S67.19-
        ring S67.19-
        thumb —see Crush, thumb
    foot S97.8-
        toe —see Crush, toe
    forearm S57.8-
    genitalia, external
        female S38.002
            vagina S38.03
            vulva S38.03
        male S38.001
            penis S38.01
            scrotum S38.02
            testis S38.02
    hand (except fingers alone) S67.2-
        with wrist S67.4-
    head S07.9
        specified NEC S07.8
    heel —see Crush, foot
    hip S77.0-
        with thigh S77.2-
    internal organ (abdomen, chest, or
        pelvis) NEC T14.8
    knee S87.0-
    labium (majus) (minus) S38.03
    larynx S17.0
    leg (lower) S87.8-
        knee —see Crush, knee
    lip S07.0
    lower
        back S38.1
        leg —see Crush, leg
    neck S17.9
    nerve —see Injury, nerve
    nose S07.0
    pelvis S38.1
    penis S38.01
    scalp S07.8
    scapular region —see
        rush, arm
    scrotum S38.02
    severe, unspecified site T14.8
    shoulder (and upper arm) —see
        Crush, arm
    skull S07.1
    syndrome (complication of trauma)
        T79.5
    testis S38.02
    thigh S77.1-
        with hip S77.2-
    throat S17.8
    thumb S67.0-
        with hand (and wrist) —see
            Crush, hand, specified site
            NEC
    toe(s) S97.10-
        great S97.11-
        lesser S97.12-

Cyst *(continued)*

carcinomatous —*see* Neoplasm, malignant, by site
cauda equina G95.89
cavum septi pellucidi —*see* Cyst, brain
celomic (pericardium) Q24.8
cerebellopontine (angle) —*see* Cyst, brain
cerebellum —*see* Cyst, brain
cerebral —*see* Cyst, brain
cervical lateral Q18.0
cervix NEC N88.8
  embryonic Q51.6
  nabothian N88.8
chiasmal optic NEC —*see* Disorder, optic, chiasm
chocolate (ovary) N80.1
choledochus, congenital Q44.4
chorion O41.8X-
choroid plexus G93.0
  congenital Q04.6
ciliary body —*see* Cyst, iris
clitoris N90.7
colon K63.89
common (bile) duct K83.5
congenital NEC Q89.8
  adrenal gland Q89.1
  epiglottis Q31.8
  esophagus Q39.8
  fallopian tube Q50.4
  kidney Q61.00
    more than one (multiple) Q61.02
      specified as polycystic Q61.3
        adult type Q61.2
        infantile type NEC Q61.19
          collecting duct dilation Q61.11
    solitary Q61.01
  larynx Q31.8
  liver Q44.6
  lung Q33.0
  mediastinum Q34.1
  ovary Q50.1
  oviduct Q50.4
  periurethral (tissue) Q64.79
  prepuce Q55.69
  salivary gland (any) Q38.4
  sublingual Q38.6
  submaxillary gland Q38.6
  thymus (gland) Q89.2
  tongue Q38.3
  ureterovesical orifice Q62.8
  vulva Q52.79
conjunctiva H11.44-
cornea H18.89-
corpora quadrigemina G93.0
corpus
  albicans N83.29-
  luteum (hemorrhagic) (ruptured) N83.1-
Cowper's gland (benign) (infected) N36.8
cranial meninges G93.0
craniobuccal pouch E23.6
craniopharyngeal pouch E23.6
cystic duct K82.8
Cysticercus —*see* Cysticercosis
Dandy-Walker Q03.1
  with spina bifida —*see* Spina bifida
dental (root) K04.8
  developmental K09.0
  eruption K09.0
  primordial K09.0
dentigerous (mandible) (maxilla) K09.0

Cyst *(continued)*

dermoid —*see* Neoplasm, benign, by site
  with malignant transformation C56.-
  implantation
    external area or site (skin) NEC L72.0
    iris —*see* Cyst, iris, implantation
    vagina N89.8
    vulva N90.7
  mouth K09.8
  oral soft tissue K09.8
  sacrococcygeal —*see* Cyst, pilonidal
developmental K09.1
  odontogenic K09.0
  oral region (nonodontogenic) K09.1
  ovary, ovarian Q50.1
dura (cerebral) G93.0
  spinal G96.198
ear (external) Q18.1
echinococcal —*see* Echinococcus
embryonic
  cervix uteri Q51.6
  fallopian tube Q50.4
  vagina Q52.4
endometrium, endometrial (uterus) N85.8
  ectopic —*see* Endometriosis
enterogenous Q43.8
epidermal, epidermoid (inclusion) (*see also* Cyst, skin) L72.0
  mouth K09.8
  oral soft tissue K09.8
epididymis N50.3
epiglottis J38.7
epiphysis cerebri E34.8
epithelial (inclusion) L72.0
epoophoron Q50.5
eruption K09.0
esophagus K22.8
ethmoid sinus J34.1
external female genital organs NEC N90.7
eye NEC H57.89
  congenital Q15.8
eyelid (sebaceous) H02.829
  infected —*see* Hordeolum
  left H02.826
    lower H02.825
    upper H02.824
  right H02.823
    lower H02.822
    upper H02.821
fallopian tube N83.8
  congenital Q50.4
fimbrial (twisted) Q50.4
fissural (oral region) K09.1
follicle (graafian) (hemorrhagic) N83.0-
  nabothian N88.8
follicular (atretic) (hemorrhagic) (ovarian) N83.0-
  dentigerous K09.0
  odontogenic K09.0
  skin L72.9
    specified NEC L72.8
frontal sinus J34.1
gallbladder K82.8
ganglion —*see* Ganglion
Gartner's duct Q52.4
gingiva K09.0
gland of Moll —*see* Cyst, eyelid
globulomaxillary K09.1
graafian follicle (hemorrhagic) N83.0-
granulosal lutein (hemorrhagic) N83.1-

Cyst *(continued)*

hemangiomatous D18.00
  intra-abdominal D18.03
  intracranial D18.02
  skin D18.01
  specified site NEC D18.09
hemorrhagic M27.49
hydatid (*see also* Echinococcus) B67.90
  brain B67.99 *[G94]*
  liver (*see also* Cyst, liver, hydatid) B67.8
  lung NEC B67.99 *[J99]*
  Morgagni
    female Q50.5
    male (epididymal) Q55.4
      testicular Q55.29
  specified site NEC B67.99
hymen N89.8
  embryonic Q52.4
hypopharynx J39.2
hypophysis, hypophyseal (duct) (recurrent) E23.6
  cerebri E23.6
implantation (dermoid)
  external area or site (skin) NEC L72.0
  iris —*see* Cyst, iris, implantation
  vagina N89.8
  vulva N90.7
incisive canal K09.1
inclusion (epidermal) (epithelial) (epidermoid) (squamous) L72.0
  not of skin - code under Cyst, by site
intestine (large) (small) K63.89
intracranial —*see* Cyst, brain
intraligamentous —*see also* Disorder, ligament
  knee —*see* Derangement, knee
intrasellar E23.6
iris H21.309
  exudative H21.31-
  idiopathic H21.30-
  implantation H21.32-
  parasitic H21.33-
  pars plana (primary) H21.34-
    exudative H21.35-
jaw (bone) M27.40
  aneurysmal M27.49
  developmental (odontogenic) K09.0
  fissural K09.1
  hemorrhagic M27.49
  traumatic M27.49
joint NEC —*see* Disorder, joint, specified type NEC
kidney (acquired) N28.1
  calyceal —*see* Hydronephrosis
  congenital Q61.00
    more than one (multiple) Q61.02
      specified as polycystic Q61.3
        adult type (autosomal dominant) Q61.2
        infantile type (autosomal recessive) NEC Q61.19
          collecting duct dilation Q61.11
  pyelogenic —*see* Hydronephrosis
  simple N28.1
  solitary (single) Q61.01
    acquired N28.1
labium (majus) (minus) N90.7
  sebaceous N90.7
lacrimal —*see also* Disorder, lacrimal system, specified NEC
  gland H04.13-
  passages or sac —*see* Disorder, lacrimal system, specified NEC

Cyst *(continued)*

larynx J38.7
lateral periodontal K09.0
lens H27.8
  congenital Q12.8
lip (gland) K13.0
liver (idiopathic) (simple) K76.89
  congenital Q44.6
  hydatid B67.8
    granulosus B67.0
    multilocularis B67.5
lung J98.4
  congenital Q33.0
  giant bullous J43.9
lutein N83.1-
lymphangiomatous D18.1
lymphoepithelial, oral soft tissue K09.8
macula —*see* Degeneration, macula, hole
malignant —*see* Neoplasm, malignant, by site
mammary gland —*see* Cyst, breast
mandible M27.40
  dentigerous K09.0
  radicular K04.8
maxilla M27.40
  dentigerous K09.0
  radicular K04.8
medial, face and neck Q18.8
median
  anterior maxillary K09.1
  palatal K09.1
mediastinum, congenital Q34.1
meibomian (gland) —*see* Chalazion
  infected —*see* Hordeolum
membrane, brain G93.0
meninges (cerebral) G93.0
  spinal G96.198
meniscus, knee —*see* Derangement, knee, meniscus, cystic
mesentery, mesenteric K66.8
  chyle I89.8
mesonephric duct
  female Q50.5
  male Q55.4
milk N64.89
Morgagni (hydatid)
  female Q50.5
  male (epididymal) Q55.4
    testicular Q55.29
mouth K09.8
Müllerian duct Q50.4
  appendix testis Q55.29
  cervix Q51.6
  fallopian tube Q50.4
  female Q50.4
  male Q55.29
  prostatic utricle Q55.4
  vagina (embryonal) Q52.4
multilocular (ovary) D39.10
  benign —*see* Neoplasm, benign, by site
myometrium N85.8
nabothian (follicle) (ruptured) N88.8
nasoalveolar K09.1
nasolabial K09.1
nasopalatine (anterior) (duct) K09.1
nasopharynx J39.2
neoplastic —*see* Neoplasm, uncertain behavior, by site
  benign —*see* Neoplasm, benign, by site
nerve root
  cervical G96.191
  lumbar G96.191
  sacral G96.191
  thoracic G96.191

Cyst (*continued*)

nervous system NEC G96.89
neuroenteric (congenital) Q06.8
nipple —*see* Cyst, breast
nose (turbinates) J34.1
sinus J34.1
odontogenic, developmental K09.0
omentum (lesser) K66.8
congenital Q45.8
ora serrata —*see* Cyst, retina, ora serrata
oral
region K09.9
developmental (nonodontogenic) K09.1
specified NEC K09.8
soft tissue K09.9
specified NEC K09.8
orbit H05.81-
ovary, ovarian (twisted) N83.20-
adherent N83.20-
chocolate N80.1
corpus
albicans N83.29-
luteum (hemorrhagic) N83.1-
dermoid D27.9
developmental Q50.1
due to failure of involution NEC N83.20-
endometrial N80.1
follicular (graafian) (hemorrhagic) N83.0-
hemorrhagic N83.20-
in pregnancy or childbirth O34.8-
with obstructed labor O65.5
multilocular D39.10
pseudomucinous D27.9
retention N83.29-
serous N83.20-
specified NEC N83.29-
theca lutein (hemorrhagic) N83.1-
tuberculous A18.18
oviduct N83.8
palate (median) (fissural) K09.1
palatine papilla (jaw) K09.1
pancreas, pancreatic (hemorrhagic) (true) K86.2
congenital Q45.2
false K86.3
paralabral
hip M24.85-
shoulder S43.43-
paramesonephric duct Q50.4
female Q50.4
male Q55.29
paranephric N28.1
paraphysis, cerebri, congenital Q04.6
parasitic B89
parathyroid (gland) E21.4
paratubal N83.8
paraurethral duct N36.8
paroophoron Q50.5
parotid gland K11.6
parovarian Q50.5
pelvis, female N94.89
in pregnancy or childbirth O34.8-
causing obstructed labor O65.5
penis (sebaceous) N48.89
periapical K04.8
pericardial (congenital) Q24.8
acquired (secondary) I31.8
pericoronal K09.0
perineural G96.191
periodontal K04.8
lateral K09.0
peripelvic (lymphatic) N28.1
peritoneum K66.8
chylous I89.8

Cyst (*continued*)

periventricular, acquired, newborn P91.1
pharynx (wall) J39.2
pilar L72.11
pilonidal (infected) (rectum) L05.91
with abscess L05.01
malignant C44.59-
pituitary (duct) (gland) E23.6
placenta O43.19-
pleura J94.8
popliteal —*see* Cyst, Baker's
porencephalic Q04.6
acquired G93.0
postanal (infected) —*see* Cyst, pilonidal
postmastoidectomy cavity (mucosal) —*see* Complications, postmastoidectomy, cyst
preauricular Q18.1
prepuce N47.4
congenital Q55.69
primordial (jaw) K09.0
prostate N42.83
pseudomucinous (ovary) D27.9
pupillary, miotic H21.27-
radicular (residual) K04.8
radiculodental K04.8
ranular K11.8
Rathke's pouch E23.6
rectum (epithelium) (mucous) K62.89
renal —*see* Cyst, kidney
residual (radicular) K04.8
retention (ovary) N83.29-
salivary gland K11.6
retina H33.19-
ora serrata H33.11-
parasitic H33.12-
retroperitoneal K68.9
sacrococcygeal (dermoid) —*see* Cyst, pilonidal
salivary gland or duct (mucous extravasation or retention) K11.6
Sampson's N80.1
sclera H15.89
scrotum L72.9
sebaceous L72.3
sebaceous (duct) (gland) L72.3
breast —*see* Dysplasia, mammary, specified type NEC
eyelid —*see* Cyst, eyelid
genital organ NEC
female N94.89
male N50.89
scrotum L72.3
semilunar cartilage (knee) (multiple) —*see* Derangement, knee, meniscus, cystic
seminal vesicle N50.89
serous (ovary) N83.20-
sinus (accessory) (nasal) J34.1
Skene's gland N36.8
skin L72.9
breast —*see* Dysplasia, mammary, specified type NEC
epidermal, epidermoid L72.0
epithelial L72.0
eyelid —*see* Cyst, eyelid
genital organ NEC
female N90.7
male N50.89
inclusion L72.0
scrotum L72.9
sebaceous L72.3
sweat gland or duct L74.8
solitary
bone —*see* Cyst, bone, solitary
jaw M27.40
kidney N28.1

Cyst (*continued*)

spermatic cord N50.89
sphenoid sinus J34.1
spinal meninges G96.198
spleen NEC D73.4
congenital Q89.09
hydatid (*see also* Echinococcus) B67.99 *[D77]*
Stafne's M27.0
subarachnoid intrasellar R93.0
subcutaneous, pheomycotic (chromomycotic) B43.2
subdural (cerebral) G93.0
spinal cord G96.198
sublingual gland K11.6
submandibular gland K11.6
submaxillary gland K11.6
suburethral N36.8
suprarenal gland E27.8
suprasellar —*see* Cyst, brain
sweat gland or duct L74.8
synovial —*see also* Cyst, bursa
ruptured —*see* Rupture, synovium
Tarlov G96.191
tarsal —*see* Chalazion
tendon (sheath) —*see* Disorder, tendon, specified type NEC
testis N44.2
tunica albuginea N44.1
theca lutein (ovary) N83.1-
Thornwaldt's J39.2
thymus (gland) E32.8
thyroglossal duct (infected) (persistent) Q89.2
thyrolingual duct (infected) (persistent) Q89.2
thyroid (gland) E04.1
tongue K14.8
tonsil J35.8
tooth —*see* Cyst, dental
Tornwaldt's J39.2
trichilemmal (proliferating) L72.12
trichodermal L72.12
tubal (fallopian) N83.8
inflammatory —*see* Salpingitis, chronic
tubo-ovarian N83.8
inflammatory N70.13
tunica
albuginea testis N44.1
vaginalis N50.89
turbinate (nose) J34.1
Tyson's gland N48.89
urachus, congenital Q64.4
ureter N28.89
ureterovesical orifice N28.89
urethra, urethral (gland) N36.8
uterine ligament N83.8
uterus (body) (corpus) (recurrent) N85.8
embryonic Q51.818
cervix Q51.6
vagina, vaginal (implantation) (inclusion) (squamous cell) (wall) N89.8
embryonic Q52.4
vallecula, vallecular (epiglottis) J38.7
vesical (orifice) N32.89
vitreous body H43.89
vulva (implantation) (inclusion) N90.7
congenital Q52.79
sebaceous gland N90.7
vulvovaginal gland N90.7
wolffian
female Q50.5
male Q55.4

Cystadenocarcinoma —*see* Neoplasm, malignant, by site
bile duct C22.1

Cystadenocarcinoma (*continued*)

endometrioid —*see* Neoplasm, malignant, by site
specified site —*see* Neoplasm, malignant, by site
unspecified site
female C56.9
male C61
mucinous
papillary
specified site —*see* Neoplasm, malignant, by site
unspecified site C56.9
specified site —*see* Neoplasm, malignant, by site
unspecified site C56.9
papillary
mucinous
specified site —*see* Neoplasm, malignant, by site
unspecified site C56.9
pseudomucinous
specified site —*see* Neoplasm, malignant, by site
unspecified site C56.9
serous
specified site —*see* Neoplasm, malignant, by site
unspecified site C56.9
specified site —*see* Neoplasm, malignant, by site
unspecified site C56.9
pseudomucinous
papillary
specified site —*see* Neoplasm, malignant, by site
unspecified site C56.9
specified site —*see* Neoplasm, malignant, by site
unspecified site C56.9
serous
papillary
specified site —*see* Neoplasm, malignant, by site
unspecified site C56.9
specified site —*see* Neoplasm, malignant, by site
unspecified site C56.9

Cystadenofibroma

clear cell —*see* Neoplasm, benign, by site
endometrioid D27.9
borderline malignancy D39.1-
malignant C56.-
mucinous
specified site —*see* Neoplasm, benign, by site
unspecified site D27.9
serous
specified site —*see* Neoplasm, benign, by site
unspecified site D27.9
specified site —*see* Neoplasm, benign, by site
unspecified site D27.9

Cystadenoma —*see also* Neoplasm, benign, by site
bile duct D13.4
endometrioid —*see* Neoplasm, benign, by site
borderline malignancy —*see* Neoplasm, uncertain behavior, by site
malignant —*see* Neoplasm, malignant, by site
mucinous
borderline malignancy
ovary C56.-

Dacryocystoblenorrhea —*see* Inflammation, lacrimal, passages, chronic

Dacryocystocele —*see* Disorder, lacrimal system, changes

Dacryolith, dacryolithiasis H04.51-

Dacryoma —*see* Disorder, lacrimal system, changes

Dacryopericystitis —*see* Dacryocystitis

Dacryops H04.11-

Dacryostenosis —*see also* Stenosis, lacrimal
congenital Q10.5

Dactylitis
bone —*see* Osteomyelitis
sickle-cell D57.00
Hb C D57.219
Hb SS D57.00
specified NEC D57.819
skin L08.9
syphilitic A52.77
tuberculous A18.03

Dactylolysis spontanea (ainhum) L94.6

Dactylosymphysis Q70.9
fingers —*see* Syndactylism, complex, fingers
toes —*see* Syndactylism, complex, toes

Damage
arteriosclerotic —*see* Arteriosclerosis
brain (nontraumatic) G93.9
anoxic, hypoxic G93.1
resulting from a procedure G97.82
child NEC G80.9
due to birth injury P11.2
cardiorenal (vascular) —*see* Hypertension, cardiorenal
cerebral NEC —*see* Damage, brain
coccyx, complicating delivery O71.6
coronary —*see* Disease, heart, ischemic
deep tissue, pressure-induced —*see also* L89 with final character .6
eye, birth injury P15.3
liver (nontraumatic) K76.9
alcoholic K70.9
due to drugs —*see* Disease, liver, toxic
toxic —*see* Disease, liver, toxic
lung
dabbing (related) U07.0
electronic cigarette (related) U07.0
vaping (associated) (device) (product) (use) U07.0
medication T88.7
organ
dabbing (related) U07.0
electronic cigarette (related) U07.0
vaping (associated) (device) (product) (use) U07.0
pelvic
joint or ligament, during delivery O71.6
organ NEC
during delivery O71.5
following ectopic or molar pregnancy O08.6
renal —*see* Disease, renal
subendocardium, subendocardial —*see* Degeneration, myocardial
vascular I99.9

Dana-Putnam syndrome (subacute combined sclerosis with pernicious anemia) —*see* Degeneration, combined

Danbolt (-Cross) **syndrome** (acrodermatitis enteropathica) E83.2

Dandruff L21.0

Dandy-Walker syndrome Q03.1
with spina bifida —*see* Spina bifida

Danlos' syndrome (*see also* Syndrome, Ehlers-Danlos) Q79.60

Darier (-White) **disease** (congenital) Q82.8
meaning erythema annulare centrifugum L53.1

Darier-Roussy sarcoid D86.3

Darling's disease or histoplasmosis B39.4

Darwin's tubercle Q17.8

Dawson's (inclusion body) **encephalitis** A81.1

De Beurmann (-Gougerot) **disease** B42.1

De la Tourette's syndrome F95.2

De Lange's syndrome Q87.19

De Morgan's spots (senile angiomas) I78.1

De Quervain's
disease (tendon sheath) M65.4
syndrome E34.51
thyroiditis (subacute granulomatous thyroiditis) E06.1

De Toni-Fanconi (-Debré) **syndrome** E72.09
with cystinosis E72.04

Dead
fetus, retained (mother) O36.4
early pregnancy O02.1
labyrinth H83.2
ovum, retained O02.0

Deaf nonspeaking NEC H91.3

Deafmutism (acquired) (congenital) **NEC** H91.3
hysterical F44.6
syphilitic, congenital (*see also* subcategory H94.8) A50.09

Deafness (acquired) (complete) (hereditary) (partial) H91.9-
with blue sclera and fragility of bone Q78.0
auditory fatigue —*see* Deafness, specified type NEC
aviation T70.0
nerve injury —*see* Injury, nerve, acoustic, specified type NEC
boilermaker's —*see* subcategory H83.3
central —*see* Deafness, sensorineural
conductive H90.2
and sensorineural
mixed H90.8
bilateral H90.6
bilateral H90.0
unilateral H90.1-
with restricted hearing on the contralateral side H90.A-
congenital H90.5
with blue sclera and fragility of bone Q78.0
due to toxic agents —*see* Deafness, ototoxic
emotional (hysterical) F44.6

Deafness (continued)
functional (hysterical) F44.6
high frequency H91.9-
hysterical F44.6
low frequency H91.9-
mental R48.8
mixed conductive and sensorineural H90.8
bilateral H90.6
unilateral H90.7-
nerve —*see* Deafness, sensorineural
neural —*see* Deafness, sensorineural
noise-induced —*see also* subcategory H83.3
nerve injury —*see* Injury, nerve, acoustic, specified type NEC
nonspeaking H91.3
ototoxic H91.0
perceptive —*see* Deafness, sensorineural
psychogenic (hysterical) F44.6
sensorineural H90.5
and conductive
mixed H90.8
bilateral H90.6
bilateral H90.3
unilateral H90.4-
with restricted hearing on the contralateral side H90.A-
sensory —*see* Deafness, sensorineural
specified type NEC H91.8
sudden (idiopathic) H91.2-
syphilitic A52.15
transient ischemic H93.01-
traumatic —*see* Injury, nerve, acoustic, specified type NEC
word (developmental) H93.25

Death (cause unknown) (of) (unexplained) (unspecified cause) R99
brain G93.82
cardiac (sudden) (with successful resuscitation) - code to underlying disease
family history of Z82.41
personal history of Z86.74
family member (assumed) Z63.4

Debility (chronic) (general) (nervous) R53.81
congenital or neonatal NOS P96.9
nervous R53.81
old age R54
senile R54

Débove's disease (splenomegaly) R16.1

Decalcification
bone —*see* Osteoporosis
teeth K03.89

Decapsulation, kidney N28.89

Decay
dental —*see* Caries, dental
senile R54
tooth, teeth —*see* Caries, dental

Deciduitis (acute)
following ectopic or molar pregnancy O08.0

Decline (general) —*see* Debility
cognitive, age-associated R41.81

Decompensation
cardiac (acute) (chronic) —*see* Disease, heart
cardiovascular —*see* Disease, cardiovascular
heart —*see* Disease, heart

Decompensation (continued)
hepatic —*see* Failure, hepatic
myocardial (acute) (chronic) —*see* Disease, heart
respiratory J98.8

Decompression sickness T70.3

Decrease (d)
absolute neutrophile count —*see* Neutropenia
blood
platelets —*see* Thrombocytopenia
pressure R03.1
due to shock following injury T79.4
operation T81.19
estrogen E28.39
postablative E89.40
asymptomatic E89.40
symptomatic E89.41
fragility of erythrocytes D58.8
function
lipase (pancreatic) K90.3
ovary in hypopituitarism E23.0
parenchyma of pancreas K86.89
pituitary (gland) (anterior) (lobe) E23.0
posterior (lobe) E23.0
functional activity R68.89
glucose R73.09
hematocrit R71.0
hemoglobin R71.0
leukocytes D72.819
specified NEC D72.818
libido R68.82
lymphocytes D72.810
platelets D69.6
respiration, due to shock following injury T79.4
sexual desire R68.82
tear secretion NEC —*see* Syndrome, dry eye
tolerance
fat K90.49
glucose R73.09
pancreatic K90.3
salt and water E87.8
vision NEC H54.7
white blood cell count D72.819
specified NEC D72.818

Decubitus (ulcer) —*see* Ulcer, pressure, by site
cervix N86

Deepening acetabulum —*see* Derangement, joint, specified type NEC, hip

Defect, defective Q89.9
3-beta-hydroxysteroid dehydrogenase E25.0
11-hydroxylase E25.0
21-hydroxylase E25.0
abdominal wall, congenital Q79.59
antibody immunodeficiency D80.9
aorticopulmonary septum Q21.4
atrial septal (ostium secundum type) Q21.1
following acute myocardial infarction (current complication) I23.1
ostium primum type Q21.2
atrioventricular
canal Q21.2
septum Q21.2
auricular septal Q21.1
bilirubin excretion NEC E80.6
biosynthesis, androgen (testicular) E29.1
bulbar septum Q21.0

Defect, defective *(continued)*

catalase E80.3
cell membrane receptor complex (CR3) D71
circulation I99.9
  congenital Q28.9
  newborn Q28.9
coagulation (factor) *(see also Deficiency, factor)* D68.9
  with
    ectopic pregnancy O08.1
    molar pregnancy O08.1
  acquired D68.4
  antepartum with hemorrhage —*see* Hemorrhage, antepartum, with coagulation defect
  due to
    liver disease D68.4
    vitamin K deficiency D68.4
  hereditary NEC D68.2
  intrapartum O67.0
  newborn, transient P61.6
  postpartum O99.13
    with hemorrhage O72.3
  specified type NEC D68.8
complement system D84.1
conduction (heart) I45.9
  bone —*see* Deafness, conductive
congenital, organ or site not listed —*see* Anomaly, by site
coronary sinus Q21.1
cushion, endocardial Q21.2
degradation, glycoprotein E77.1
dental bridge, crown, fillings —*see* Defect, dental restoration
dental restoration K08.50
  specified NEC K08.59
dentin (hereditary) K00.5
Descemet's membrane, congenital Q13.89
developmental —*see also* Anomaly
  cauda equina Q06.3
diaphragm
  with elevation, eventration or hernia —*see* Hernia, diaphragm
  congenital Q79.1
    with hernia Q79.0
    gross (with hernia) Q79.0
ectodermal, congenital Q82.9
Eisenmenger's Q21.8
enzyme
  catalase E80.3
  peroxidase E80.3
esophagus, congenital Q39.9
extensor retinaculum M62.89
fibrin polymerization D68.2
filling
  bladder R93.41
  kidney R93.42-
  renal pelvis R93.41
  stomach R93.3
  ureter R93.41
  urinary organs, specified NEC R93.49
GABA (gamma aminobutyric acid) metabolic E72.81
Gerbode Q21.0
glucose transport, blood-brain barrier E74.810
glycoprotein degradation E77.1
Hageman (factor) D68.2
hearing —*see* Deafness
high grade F70
interatrial septal Q21.1
interauricular septal Q21.1
interventricular septal Q21.0
  with dextroposition of aorta, pulmonary stenosis and hypertrophy of right ventricle Q21.3
  in tetralogy of Fallot Q21.3

Defect, defective *(continued)*

learning (specific) —*see* Disorder, learning
lymphocyte function antigen-1(LFA-1) D84.0
lysosomal enzyme, post-translational modification E77.0
major osseous M89.70
  ankle M89.77-
  carpus M89.74-
  clavicle M89.71-
  femur M89.75-
  fibula M89.76-
  fingers M89.74-
  foot M89.77-
  forearm M89.73-
  hand M89.74-
  humerus M89.72-
  lower leg M89.76-
  metacarpus M89.74-
  metatarsus M89.77-
  multiple sites M89.79
  pelvic region M89.75-
  pelvis M89.75-
  radius M89.73-
  scapula M89.71-
  shoulder region M89.71-
  specified NEC M89.78
  tarsus M89.77-
  thigh M89.75-
  tibia M89.76-
  toes M89.77-
  ulna M89.73-
mental —*see* Disability, intellectual
modification, lysosomal enzymes, post-translational E77.0
obstructive, congenital
  renal pelvis Q62.39
  ureter Q62.39
    atresia —*see* Atresia, ureter
    cecoureterocele Q62.32
    megaureter Q62.2
    orthotopic ureterocele Q62.31
osseous, major M89.70
  ankle M89.77-
  carpus M89.74-
  clavicle M89.71-
  femur M89.75-
  fibula M89.76-
  fingers M89.74-
  foot M89.77-
  forearm M89.73-
  hand M89.74-
  humerus M89.72-
  lower leg M89.76-
  metacarpus M89.74-
  metatarsus M89.77-
  multiple sites M89.9
  pelvic region M89.75-
  pelvis M89.75-
  radius M89.73-
  scapula M89.71-
  shoulder region M89.71-
  specified NEC M89.78
  tarsus M89.77-
  thigh M89.75-
  tibia M89.76-
  toes M89.77-
  ulna M89.73-
osteochondral NEC *(see also Deformity)* M95.8
ostium
  primum Q21.2
  secundum Q21.1
peroxidase E80.3
placental blood supply —*see* Insufficiency, placental
platelets, qualitative D69.1
  constitutional D68.0
postural NEC, spine —*see* Dorsopathy, deforming

Defect, defective *(continued)*

reduction
  limb Q73.8
    lower Q72.9-
      absence —*see* Agenesis, leg
      foot —*see* Agenesis, foot
      longitudinal
        femur Q72.4-
        fibula Q72.6-
        tibia Q72.5-
      specified type NEC Q72.89-
      split foot Q72.7-
    specified type NEC Q73.8
    upper Q71.9-
      absence —*see* Agenesis, arm
        forearm —*see* Agenesis, forearm
        hand —*see* Agenesis, hand
      lobster-claw hand Q71.6-
      longitudinal
        radius Q71.4-
        ulna Q71.5-
      specified type NEC Q71.89-
  renal pelvis Q63.8
  obstructive Q62.39
respiratory system, congenital Q34.9
restoration, dental K08.50
  specified NEC K08.59
retinal nerve bundle fibers H35.89
septal (heart) NOS Q21.9
  acquired (atrial) (auricular) (ventricular) (old) I51.0
  atrial Q21.1
    concurrent with acute myocardial infarction —*see* Infarct, myocardium
    following acute myocardial infarction (current complication) I23.1
  ventricular *(see also Defect, ventricular septal)* Q21.0
sinus venosus Q21.1
speech —*see* disorder speech
  developmental F80.9
  specified NEC R47.89
Taussig-Bing (aortic transposition and overriding pulmonary artery) Q20.1
teeth, wedge K03.1
vascular (local) I99.9
  congenital Q27.9
ventricular septal Q21.0
  concurrent with acute myocardial infarction —*see* Infarct, myocardium
  following acute myocardial infarction (current complication) I23.2
  in tetralogy of Fallot Q21.3
vision NEC H54.7
visual field H53.40
  bilateral
    heteronymous H53.47
    homonymous H53.46-
  generalized contraction H53.48-
  localized
    arcuate H53.43-
    scotoma (central area) H53.41-
      blind spot area H53.42-
    sector H53.43-
    specified type NEC H53.45-
voice R49.9
  specified NEC R49.8
wedge, tooth, teeth (abrasion) K03.1

Deferentitis N49.1
  gonorrheal (acute) (chronic) A54.23

Defibrination (syndrome) D65
antepartum —*see* Hemorrhage, antepartum, with coagulation defect, disseminated intravascular coagulation
following ectopic or molar pregnancy O08.1
intrapartum O67.0
newborn P60
postpartum O72.3

Deficiency, deficient
3-beta hydroxysteroid dehydrogenase E25.0
5-alpha reductase (with male pseudohermaphroditism) E29.1
11-hydroxylase E25.0
21-hydroxylase E25.0
AADC (aromatic L-amino acid decarboxylase) E70.81
abdominal muscle syndrome Q79.4
accelerator globulin (Ac G) (blood) D68.2
AC globulin (congenital) (hereditary) D68.2
  acquired D68.4
acid phosphatase E83.39
activating factor (blood) D68.2
ADA2 (adenosine deaminase 2) D81.32
adenosine deaminase (ADA) D81.30
  with severe combined immuno-deficiency (SCID) D81.32
  partial (type 1) D81.39
  specified NEC D81.39
  type 1 (without SCID) (without severe combined immunodeficiency) D81.39
  type 2 D81.32
aldolase (hereditary) E74.19
alpha-1-antitrypsin E88.01
amino-acids E72.9
anemia —*see* Anemia
aneurin E51.9
antibody with
  hyperimmunoglobulinemia D80.6
  near-normal immunoglobins D80.6
antidiuretic hormone E23.2
anti-hemophilic
  factor (A) D66
    B D67
    C D68.1
  globulin (AHG) NEC D66
antithrombin (antithrombin III) D68.59
aromatic L-amino acid decarboxylase (AADC) E70.81
ascorbic acid E54
attention (disorder) (syndrome) F98.8
  with hyperactivity —*see* Disorder, attention-deficit hyperactivity
autoprothrombin
  I D68.2
  II D67
  C D68.2
beta-glucuronidase E76.29
biotin E53.8
biotin-dependent carboxylase D81.819
biotinidase D81.810
brancher enzyme (amylopectinosis) E74.03
calciferol E55.9
  with
    adult osteomalacia M83.8
    rickets —*see* Rickets
calcium (dietary) E58

Deficiency, deficient *(continued)*
  sodium (Na) E87.1
  SPCA(factor VII) D68.2
  sphincter, intrinsic N36.42
    with urethral hypermobility N36.43
  stable factor (congenital)
    (hereditary) D68.2
    acquired D68.4
  Stuart-Prower (factor X) D68.2
  succinic semialdehyde
    dehydrogenase E72.81
  sucrase E74.39
  sulfatase E75.26
  sulfite oxidase E72.19
  thiamin, thiaminic (chloride) E51.9
    beriberi (dry) E51.11
      wet E51.12
  thrombokinase D68.2
    newborn P53
  thyroid (gland) —*see*
    Hypothyroidism
  tocopherol E56.0
  tooth bud K00.0
  transcobalamine II (anemia) D51.2
  vanadium E61.6
  vascular I99.9
  vasopressin E23.2
  vertical ridge K06.8
  viosterol —*see* Deficiency, calciferol
  vitamin (multiple) NOS E56.9
    A E50.9
      with
        Bitot's spot (corneal) E50.1
        follicular keratosis E50.8
        keratomalacia E50.4
        manifestations NEC E50.8
        night blindness E50.5
        scar of cornea,
          xerophthalmic E50.6
        xeroderma E50.8
        xerophthalmia E50.7
        xerosis
          conjunctival E50.0
            and Bitot's spot E50.1
          cornea E50.2
            and ulceration E50.3
      sequelae E64.1
    B (complex) NOS E53.9
      with
        beriberi (dry) E51.11
          wet E51.12
        pellagra E52
    B1 NOS E51.9
      beriberi (dry) E51.11
        with circulatory system
          manifestations E51.11
        wet E51.12
    B12 E53.8
    B2 (riboflavin) E53.0
    B6 E53.1
    C E54
      sequelae E64.2
    D E55.9
      with
        adult osteomalacia M83.8
        rickets —*see* Rickets
      25-hydroxylase E83.32
    E E56.0
    folic acid E53.8
    G E53.0
    group B E53.9
      specified NEC E53.8
    H (biotin) E53.8
    K E56.1
      of newborn P53
    nicotinic E52
    P E56.8
    PP (pellagra-preventing) E52
    specified NEC E56.8
    thiamin E51.9
      beriberi —*see* Beriberi
  zinc, dietary E60

Deficit —*see also* Deficiency
  attention and concentration R41.840
    disorder —*see* Attention, deficit
    following
      cerebral infarction I69.310
      cerebrovascular disease I69.910
        specified disease NEC I69.810
      nontraumatic
        intracerebral hemorrhage
          I69.110
        specified intracranial
          hemorrhage NEC I69.210
        subarachnoid hemorrhage
          I69.010
  cognitive
    communication R41.841
    emotional
      following
        cerebral infarction I69.315
        cerebrovascular disease
          I69.915
          specified disease NEC
            I69.815
        nontraumantic
          intracerebral hemorrhage
            I69.115
          specified intracranial
            hemorrhage NEC
            I69.215
          subarachnoid hemorrhage
            I69.015
    following
      cerebral infarction I69.319
      cerebrovascular disease I69.919
        specified disease NEC
          I69.819
      nontraumatic
        intracerebral hemorrhage
          I69.119
        specified intracranial
          hemorrhage NEC I69.219
        subarachnoid hemorrhage
          I69.019
    social
      following
        cerebral infarction I69.315
        cerebrovascular disease
          I69.915
          specified disease NEC
            I69.815
        nontraumatic
          intracerebral hemorrhage
            I69.115
          specified intracranial
            hemorrhage NEC
            I69.215
          subarachnoid hemorrhage
            I69.015
  cognitive NEC R41.89
    following
      cerebral infarction I69.318
      cerebrovascular disease I69.918
        specified disease NEC
          I69.818
      nontraumatic
        intracerebral hemorrhage
          I69.118
        specified intracaranial
          hemorrhage NEC
          I69.218
        subarachnoid hemorrhage
          I69.018
  concentration R41.840
  executive function R41.844
    following
      cerebral infarction I69.314
      cerebrovascular disease
        I69.914
        specified disease NEC
          I69.814

Deficit *(continued)*
  executive function *(continued)*
    following *(continued)*
      nontraumatic
        intracerebral hemorrhage
          I69.114
        specified intracranial
          hemorrhage NEC I69.214
        subarachnoid hemorrhage
          I69.014
  frontal lobe R41.844
    following
      cerebral infarction I69.314
      cerebrovascular disease
        I69.914
        specified disease NEC
          I69.814
      nontraumatic
        intracerebral hemorrhage
          I69.114
        specified intracranial
          hemorrhage NEC I69.214
        subarachnoid hemorrhage
          I69.014
  memory
    following
      cerebral infarction I69.311
      cerebrovascular disease
        I69.911
        specified disease NEC
          I69.811
      nontraumatic
        intracerebral hemorrhage
          I69.111
        specified intracranial
          hemorrhage NEC I69.211
        subarachnoid hemorrhage
          I69.011
  neurologic NEC R29.818
    ischemic
      reversible (RIND) I63.9
        prolonged (PRIND) I63.9
  oxygen R09.02
  prolonged reversible ischemic
    neurologic (PRIND) I63.9
  psychomotor R41.843
    following
      cerebral infarction I69.313
      cerebrovascular disease
        I69.913
        specified disease NEC
          I69.813
      nontraumatic
        intracerebral hemorrhage
          I69.113
        specified intracranial
          hemorrhage NEC I69.213
        subarachnoid hemorrhage
          I69.013
  visuospatial R41.842
    following
      cerebral infarction I69.312
      cerebrovascular disease
        I69.912
        specified disease NEC
          I69.812
      nontraumatic
        intracerebral hemorrhage
          I69.112
        specified intracranial
          hemorrhage NEC I69.212
        subarachnoid hemorrhage
          I69.012

Deflection
  radius —*see* Deformity, limb,
    specified type NEC, forearm
  septum (acquired) (nasal) (nose)
    J34.2
  spine —*see* Curvature, spine
  turbinate (nose) J34.2

Defluvium
  capillorum —*see* Alopecia
  ciliorum —*see* Madarosis
  unguium L60.8

Deformity Q89.9
  abdomen, congenital Q89.9
  abdominal wall
    acquired M95.8
    congenital Q79.59
  acquired (unspecified site) M95.9
  adrenal gland Q89.1
  alimentary tract, congenital Q45.9
    upper Q40.9
  ankle (joint) (acquired) —*see also*
    Deformity, limb, lower leg
    abduction —*see* Contraction,
      joint, ankle
    congenital Q68.8
    contraction —*see* Contraction,
      joint, ankle
    specified type NEC —*see*
      Deformity, limb, foot, specified
      NEC
  anus (acquired) K62.89
    congenital Q43.9
  aorta (arch) (congenital) Q25.40
    acquired I77.89
  aortic
    arch, acquired I77.89
    cusp or valve (congenital) Q23.8
      acquired (*see also*
        Endocarditis, aortic) I35.8
  arm (acquired) (upper) —*see also*
    Deformity, limb, upper arm
    congenital Q68.8
    forearm —*see* Deformity, limb,
      forearm
  artery (congenital) (peripheral)
    NOS Q27.9
    acquired I77.89
    coronary (acquired) I25.9
      congenital Q24.5
    umbilical Q27.0
  atrial septal Q21.1
  auditory canal (external)
    (congenital) —*see also*
    Malformation, ear, external
    acquired —*see* Disorder, ear,
      external, specified type NEC
  auricle
    ear (congenital) —*see also*
      Malformation, ear, external
      acquired —*see* Disorder,
        pinna, deformity
  back —*see* Dorsopathy, deforming
  bile duct (common) (congenital)
    (hepatic) Q44.5
    acquired K83.8
  biliary duct or passage (congenital)
    Q44.5
    acquired K83.8
  bladder (neck) (trigone) (sphincter)
    (acquired) N32.89
    congenital Q64.79
  bone (acquired) NOS M95.9
    congenital Q79.9
    turbinate M95.0
  brain (congenital) Q04.9
    acquired G93.89
    reduction Q04.3
  breast (acquired) N64.89
    congenital Q83.9
    reconstructed N65.0
  bronchus (congenital) Q32.4
    acquired NEC J98.09
  bursa, congenital Q79.9
  canaliculi (lacrimalis) (acquired)
    —*see also* Disorder, lacrimal
    system, changes
    congenital Q10.6

canthus, acquired —*see* Disorder, eyelid, specified type NEC
capillary (acquired) I78.8
cardiovascular system, congenital Q28.9
caruncle, lacrimal (acquired) —*see also* Disorder, lacrimal system, changes
  congenital Q10.6
cascade, stomach K31.2
cecum (congenital) Q43.9
  acquired K63.89
cerebral, acquired G93.89
  congenital Q04.9
cervix (uterus) (acquired) NEC N88.8
  congenital Q51.9
cheek (acquired) M95.2
  congenital Q18.9
chest (acquired) (wall) M95.4
  congenital Q67.8
  sequelae (late effect) of rickets E64.3
chin (acquired) M95.2
  congenital Q18.9
choroid (congenital) Q14.3
  acquired H31.8
  plexus Q07.8
   acquired G96.198
cicatricial —*see* Cicatrix
cilia, acquired —*see* Disorder, eyelid, specified type NEC
clavicle (acquired) M95.8
  congenital Q68.8
clitoris (congenital) Q52.6
  acquired N90.89
clubfoot —*see* Clubfoot
coccyx (acquired) M43.8
colon (congenital) Q43.9
  acquired K63.89
concha (ear), congenital —*see also* Malformation, ear, external
  acquired —*see* Disorder, pinna, deformity
cornea (acquired) H18.70
  congenital Q13.4
  descemetocele —*see* Descemetocele
  ectasia —*see* Ectasia, cornea
  specified NEC H18.79-
  staphyloma —*see* Staphyloma, cornea
coronary artery (acquired) I25.9
  congenital Q24.5
cranium (acquired) —*see* Deformity, skull
cricoid cartilage (congenital) Q31.8
  acquired J38.7
cystic duct (congenital) Q44.5
  acquired K82.8
Dandy-Walker Q03.1
  with spina bifida —*see* Spina bifida
diaphragm (congenital) Q79.1
  acquired J98.6
digestive organ NOS Q45.9
ductus arteriosus Q25.0
duodenal bulb K31.89
duodenum (congenital) Q43.9
  acquired K31.89
dura —*see* Deformity, meninges
ear (acquired) —*see also* Disorder, pinna, deformity
  congenital (external) Q17.9
   internal Q16.5
   middle Q16.4
    ossicles Q16.3
   ossicles Q16.3
ectodermal (congenital) NEC Q84.9
ejaculatory duct (congenital) Q55.4
  acquired N50.89

elbow (joint) (acquired) —*see also* Deformity, limb, upper arm
  congenital Q68.8
  contraction —*see* Contraction, joint, elbow
endocrine gland NEC Q89.2
epididymis (congenital) Q55.4
  acquired N50.89
epiglottis (congenital) Q31.8
  acquired J38.7
esophagus (congenital) Q39.9
  acquired K22.8
eustachian tube (congenital) NEC Q17.8
eye, congenital Q15.9
eyebrow (congenital) Q18.8
eyelid (acquired) —*see also* Disorder, eyelid, specified type NEC
  congenital Q10.3
face (acquired) M95.2
  congenital Q18.9
fallopian tube, acquired N83.8
femur (acquired) —*see* Deformity, limb, specified type NEC, thigh
fetal
  with fetopelvic disproportion O33.7
  causing obstructed labor O66.3
finger (acquired) M20.00-
  boutonniere M20.02-
  congenital Q68.1
  flexion contracture —*see* Contraction, joint, hand
  mallet finger M20.01-
  specified NEC M20.09-
  swan-neck M20.03-
flexion (joint) (acquired) (*see also* Deformity, limb, flexion) M21.20
  congenital NOS Q74.9
  hip Q65.89
foot (acquired) —*see also* Deformity, limb, lower leg
  cavovarus (congenital) Q66.1-
  congenital NOS Q66.9-
   specified type NEC Q66.89
  specified type NEC —*see* Deformity, limb, foot, specified NEC
  valgus (congenital) Q66.6
   acquired —*see* Deformity, valgus, ankle
  varus (congenital) NEC Q66.3-
   acquired —*see* Deformity, varus, ankle
forearm (acquired) —*see also* Deformity, limb, forearm
  congenital Q68.8
forehead (acquired) M95.2
  congenital Q75.8
frontal bone (acquired) M95.2
  congenital Q75.8
gallbladder (congenital) Q44.1
  acquired K82.8
gastrointestinal tract (congenital) NOS Q45.9
  acquired K63.89
genitalia, genital organ(s) or system NEC
  female (congenital) Q52.9
   acquired N94.89
   external Q52.70
  male (congenital) Q55.9
   acquired N50.89
globe (eye) (congenital) Q15.8
  acquired H44.89
gum, acquired NEC K06.8
hand (acquired) —*see* Deformity, limb, hand

hand *(continued)*
  congenital Q68.1
head (acquired) M95.2
  congenital Q75.8
heart (congenital) Q24.9
  septum Q21.9
   auricular Q21.1
   ventricular Q21.0
  valve (congenital) NEC Q24.8
   acquired —*see* Endocarditis
heel (acquired) —*see* Deformity, foot
hepatic duct (congenital) Q44.5
  acquired K83.8
hip (joint) (acquired) —*see also* Deformity, limb, thigh
  congenital Q65.9
  due to (previous) juvenile osteochondrosis —*see* Coxa, plana
  flexion —*see* Contraction, joint, hip
hourglass —*see* Contraction, hourglass
humerus (acquired) M21.82-
  congenital Q74.0
hypophyseal (congenital) Q89.2
ileocecal (coil) (valve) (acquired) K63.89
  congenital Q43.9
ileum (congenital) Q43.9
  acquired K63.89
ilium (acquired) M95.5
  congenital Q74.2
integument (congenital) Q84.9
intervertebral cartilage or disc (acquired) —*see* Disorder, disc, specified NEC
intestine (large) (small) (congenital) NOS Q43.9
  acquired K63.89
intrinsic minus or plus (hand) —*see* Deformity, limb, specified type NEC, forearm
iris (acquired) H21.89
  congenital Q13.2
ischium (acquired) M95.5
  congenital Q74.2
jaw (acquired) (congenital) M26.9
joint (acquired) NEC M21.90
  congenital Q68.8
  elbow M21.92-
  hand M21.94-
  hip M21.95-
  knee M21.96-
  shoulder M21.92-
  wrist M21.93-
kidney(s) (calyx) (pelvis) (congenital) Q63.9
  acquired N28.89
  artery (congenital) Q27.2
   acquired I77.89
Klippel-Feil (brevicollis) Q76.1
knee (acquired) NEC —*see also* Deformity, limb, lower leg
  congenital Q68.2
labium (majus) (minus) (congenital) Q52.79
  acquired N90.89
lacrimal passages or duct (congenital) NEC Q10.6
  acquired —*see* Disorder, lacrimal system, changes
larynx (muscle) (congenital) Q31.8
  acquired J38.7
  web (glottic) Q31.0
leg (upper) (acquired) NEC —*see also* Deformity, limb, thigh
  congenital Q68.8

leg *(continued)*
  lower leg —*see* Deformity, limb, lower leg
lens (acquired) H27.8
  congenital Q12.9
lid (fold) (acquired) —*see also* Disorder, eyelid, specified type NEC
  congenital Q10.3
ligament (acquired) —*see* Disorder, ligament
  congenital Q79.9
limb (acquired) M21.90
  clawfoot M21.53-
  clawhand M21.51-
  clubfoot M21.54-
  clubhand M21.52-
  congenital, except reduction deformity Q74.9
  flat foot M21.4-
  flexion M21.20
   ankle M21.27-
   elbow M21.22-
   finger M21.24-
   hip M21.25-
   knee M21.26-
   shoulder M21.21-
   toe M21.27-
   wrist M21.23-
  foot
   claw —*see* Deformity, limb, clawfoot
   club —*see* Deformity, limb, clubfoot
   drop M21.37-
   flat —*see* Deformity, limb, flat foot
   specified NEC M21.6X-
  forearm M21.93-
  hand M21.94-
  lower leg M21.96-
  specified type NEC M21.80
   forearm M21.83-
   lower leg M21.86-
   thigh M21.85-
   upper arm M21.82-
  thigh M21.95-
  unequal length M21.70
   short site is
    femur M21.75-
    fibula M21.76-
    humerus M21.72-
    radius M21.73-
    tibia M21.76-
    ulna M21.73-
  upper arm M21.92-
  valgus —*see* Deformity, valgus
  varus —*see* Deformity, varus
  wrist drop M21.33-
lip (acquired) NEC K13.0
  congenital Q38.0
liver (congenital) Q44.7
  acquired K76.89
lumbosacral (congenital) (joint) (region) Q76.49
  acquired M43.8
  kyphosis —*see* Kyphosis, congenital
  lordosis —*see* Lordosis, congenital
lung (congenital) Q33.9
  acquired J98.4
lymphatic system, congenital Q89.9
Madelung's (radius) Q74.0
mandible (acquired) (congenital) M26.9
maxilla (acquired) (congenital) M26.9

Left side vertical text:
Degeneration, degenerative–Degeneration, degenerative

Degeneration, degenerative

(continued)

amyloid (*see also* Amyloidosis) E85.9
anterior cornua, spinal cord G12.29
anterior labral S43.49-
aorta, aortic I70.0
  fatty I77.89
aortic valve (heart) —*see* Endocarditis, aortic
arteriovascular —*see* Arteriosclerosis
artery, arterial (atheromatous) (calcareous) —*see also* Arteriosclerosis
  cerebral, amyloid E85.4 [I68.0]
  medial —*see* Arteriosclerosis, extremities
articular cartilage NEC —*see* Derangement, joint, articular cartilage, by site
atheromatous —*see* Arteriosclerosis
basal nuclei or ganglia G23.9
  specified NEC G23.8
bone NEC —*see* Disorder, bone, specified type NEC
brachial plexus G54.0
brain (cortical) (progressive) G31.9
  alcoholic G31.2
  arteriosclerotic I67.2
  childhood G31.9
    specified NEC G31.89
  cystic G31.89
    congenital Q04.6
  in
    alcoholism G31.2
    beriberi E51.2
    cerebrovascular disease I67.9
    congenital hydrocephalus Q03.9
      with spina bifida —*see also* Spina bifida
    Fabry-Anderson disease E75.21
    Gaucher's disease E75.22
    Hunter's syndrome E76.1
    lipidosis
      cerebral E75.4
      generalized E75.6
    mucopolysaccharidosis —*see* Mucopolysaccharidosis
    myxedema E03.9 [G32.89]
    neoplastic disease (*see also* Neoplasm) D49.6 [G32.89]
    Niemann-Pick disease E75.249 [G32.89]
    sphingolipidosis E75.3 [G32.89]
    vitamin B12 deficiency E53.8 [G32.89]
  senile NEC G31.1
breast N64.89
Bruch's membrane —*see* Degeneration, choroid
capillaries (fatty) I78.8
  amyloid E85.89 [I79.8]
cardiac —*see also* Degeneration, myocardial
  valve, valvular —*see* Endocarditis
cardiorenal —*see* Hypertension, cardiorenal
cardiovascular —*see also* Disease, cardiovascular
  renal —*see* Hypertension, cardiorenal
cerebellar NOS G31.9
  alcoholic G31.2
  primary (hereditary) (sporadic) G11.9

Degeneration, degenerative

(continued)

cerebral —*see* Degeneration, brain
cerebrovascular I67.9
  due to hypertension I67.4
cervical plexus G54.2
cervix N88.8
  due to radiation (intended effect) N88.8
    adverse effect or misadventure N99.89
chamber angle H21.21-
changes, spine or vertebra —*see* Spondylosis
chorioretinal —*see also* Degeneration, choroid
  hereditary H31.20
choroid (colloid) (drusen) H31.10-
  atrophy —*see* Atrophy, choroidal
  hereditary —*see* Dystrophy, choroidal, hereditary
ciliary body H21.22-
cochlear H83.8
combined (spinal cord) (subacute) E53.8 [G32.0]
  with anemia (pernicious) D51.0 [G32.0]
    due to dietary vitamin B12 deficiency D51.3 [G32.0]
  in (due to)
    vitamin B12 deficiency E53.8 [G32.0]
    anemia D51.9 [G32.0]
conjunctiva H11.10
  concretions —*see* Concretion, conjunctiva
  deposits —*see* Deposit, conjunctiva
  pigmentations —*see* Pigmentation, conjunctiva
  pinguecula —*see* Pinguecula
  xerosis —*see* Xerosis, conjunctiva
cornea H18.40
  calcerous H18.43
    band keratopathy H18.42-
  familial, hereditary —*see* Dystrophy, cornea
  hyaline (of old scars) H18.49
  keratomalacia —*see* Keratomalacia
  nodular H18.45-
  peripheral H18.46-
  senile H18.41-
  specified type NEC H18.49
cortical (cerebellar) (parenchymatous) G31.89
  alcoholic G31.2
  diffuse, due to arteriopathy I67.2
corticobasal G31.85
cutis L98.8
  amyloid E85.4 [L99]
dental pulp K04.2
disc disease —*see* Degeneration, intervertebral disc NEC
dorsolateral (spinal cord) —*see* Degeneration, combined
extrapyramidal G25.9
eye, macular —*see also* Degeneration, macula
  congenital or hereditary —*see* Dystrophy, retina
facet joints —*see* Spondylosis
fatty
  liver NEC K76.0
    alcoholic K70.0
grey matter (brain) (Alpers') G31.81
heart —*see also* Degeneration, myocardial
  amyloid E85.4 [I43]

Degeneration, degenerative

(continued)

heart *(continued)*
  atheromatous —*see* Disease, heart, ischemic, atherosclerotic
  ischemic —*see* Disease, heart, ischemic
hepatolenticular (Wilson's) E83.01
hepatorenal K76.7
hyaline (diffuse) (generalized)
  localized —*see* Degeneration, by site
infrapatellar fat pad M79.4
intervertebral disc NOS
  with
    myelopathy —*see* Disorder, disc, with, myelopathy
    radiculitis or radiculopathy —*see* Disorder, disc, with, radiculopathy
  cervical, cervicothoracic —*see* Disorder, disc, cervical, degeneration
    with
      myelopathy —*see* Disorder, disc, cervical, with myelopathy
      neuritis, radiculitis or radiculopathy —*see* Disorder, disc, cervical, with neuritis
  lumbar region M51.36
    with
      myelopathy M51.06
      neuritis, radiculitis, radiculopathy or sciatica M51.16
  lumbosacral region M51.37
    with
      neuritis, radiculitis, radiculopathy or sciatica M51.17
  sacrococcygeal region M53.3
  thoracic region M51.34
    with
      myelopathy M51.04
      neuritis, radiculitis, radiculopathy M51.14
  thoracolumbar region M51.35
    with
      myelopathy M51.05
      neuritis, radiculitis, radiculopathy M51.15
intestine, amyloid E85.4
iris (pigmentary) H21.23-
ischemic —*see* Ischemia
joint disease —*see* Osteoarthritis
kidney N28.89
  amyloid E85.4 [N29]
  cystic, congenital Q61.9
  fatty N28.89
  polycystic Q61.3
    adult type (autosomal dominant) Q61.2
    infantile type (autosomal recessive) NEC Q61.19
    collecting duct dilatation Q61.11
Kuhnt-Junius (*see also* Degeneration, macula) H35.32-
lens —*see* Cataract
lenticular (familial) (progressive) (Wilson's) (with cirrhosis of liver) E83.01
liver (diffuse) NEC K76.89
  amyloid E85.4 [K77]
  cystic K76.89
    congenital Q44.6
  fatty NEC K76.0
    alcoholic K70.0

Degeneration, degenerative

(continued)

liver *(continued)*
  hypertrophic K76.89
  parenchymatous, acute or subacute K72.00
    with coma K72.01
  pigmentary K76.89
  toxic (acute) K71.9
lung J98.4
lymph gland I89.8
  hyaline I89.8
macula, macular (acquired) (age-related) (senile) H35.30
  angioid streaks H35.33
  atrophic age-related H35.31-
  congenital or hereditary —*see* Dystrophy, retina
  cystoid H35.35-
  dry age-related H35.31-
  drusen H35.36-
  exudative H35.32-
  hole H35.34-
  nonexudative H35.31-
  puckering H35.37-
  toxic H35.38-
  wet age-related H35.32-
membranous labyrinth, congenital (causing impairment of hearing) Q16.5
meniscus —*see* Derangement, meniscus
mitral —*see* Insufficiency, mitral
Mönckeberg's —*see* Arteriosclerosis, extremities
motor centers, senile G31.1
multi-system G90.3
mural —*see* Degeneration, myocardial
muscle (fatty) (fibrous) (hyaline) (progressive) M62.89
  heart —*see* Degeneration, myocardial
myelin, central nervous system G37.9
myocardial, myocardium (fatty) (hyaline) (senile) I51.5
  with rheumatic fever (conditions in I00) I09.0
    active, acute or subacute I01.2
      with chorea I02.0
    inactive or quiescent (with chorea) I09.0
  hypertensive —*see* Hypertension, heart
  rheumatic —*see* Degeneration, myocardial, with rheumatic fever
  syphilitic A52.06
nasal sinus (mucosa) J32.9
  frontal J32.1
  maxillary J32.0
nerve —*see* Disorder, nerve
nervous system G31.9
  alcoholic G31.2
  amyloid E85.4 [G99.8]
  autonomic G90.9
  fatty G31.89
  specified NEC G31.89
nipple N64.89
olivopontocerebellar (hereditary) (familial) G23.8
osseous labyrinth —*see* subcategory H83.8
ovary N83.8
  cystic N83.20-
  microcystic N83.20-
pallidal pigmentary (progressive) G23.0
pancreas K86.89
  tuberculous A18.83

90

Degeneration, degenerative
(continued)
penis N48.89
pigmentary (diffuse) (general)
  localized —*see* Degeneration,
    by site
  pallidal (progressive) G23.0
pineal gland E34.8
pituitary (gland) E23.6
popliteal fat pad M79.4
posterolateral (spinal cord) —*see*
  Degeneration, combined
pulmonary valve (heart) I37.8
pulp (tooth) K04.2
pupillary margin H21.24-
renal —*see* Degeneration, kidney
retina H35.9
  hereditary (cerebroretinal)
    (congenital) (juvenile)
    (macula) (peripheral)
    (pigmentary) —*see* Dystrophy,
    retina
  Kuhnt-Junius (*see also*
    Degeneration, macula) H35.32-
  macula (cystic) (exudative)
    (hole) (nonexudative)
    (pseudohole) (senile) (toxic)
    —*see* Degeneration, macula
  peripheral H35.40
    lattice H35.41-
    microcystoid H35.42-
    paving stone H35.43-
    secondary
      pigmentary H35.45-
      vitreoretinal H35.46-
    senile reticular H35.44-
  pigmentary (primary) —*see also*
    Dystrophy, retina
  secondary —*see*
    Degeneration, retina,
    peripheral, secondary
  posterior pole —*see*
    Degeneration, macula
saccule, congenital (causing
  impairment of hearing) Q16.5
senile R54
  brain G31.1
  cardiac, heart or myocardium
    —*see* Degeneration,
    myocardial
  motor centers G31.1
  vascular —*see* Arteriosclerosis
sinus (cystic) —*see also* Sinusitis
  polypoid J33.1
skin L98.8
  amyloid E85.4 *[L99]*
  colloid L98.8
spinal (cord) G31.89
  amyloid E85.4 *[G32.89]*
  combined (subacute) —*see*
    Degeneration, combined
  dorsolateral —*see* Degeneration,
    combined
  familial NEC G31.89
  fatty G31.89
  funicular —*see* Degeneration,
    combined
  posterolateral —*see*
    Degeneration, combined
  subacute combined —*see*
    Degeneration, combined
  tuberculous A17.81
spleen D73.0
  amyloid E85.4 *[D77]*
stomach K31.89
striatonigral G23.2
suprarenal (capsule) (gland) E27.8
synovial membrane (pulpy) —*see*
  Disorder, synovium, specified
  type NEC
tapetoretinal —*see* Dystrophy, retina

Degeneration, degenerative
(continued)
thymus (gland) E32.8
  fatty E32.8
thyroid (gland) E07.89
tricuspid (heart) (valve) I07.9
tuberculous NEC —*see*
  Tuberculosis
turbinate J34.89
uterus (cystic) N85.8
vascular (senile) —*see*
  Arteriosclerosis
  hypertensive —*see* Hypertension
vitreoretinal, secondary —*see*
  Degeneration, retina, peripheral,
  secondary, vitreoretinal
vitreous (body) H43.81-
Wallerian —*see* Disorder, nerve
Wilson's hepatolenticular E83.01

Deglutition
paralysis R13.0
  hysterical F44.4
pneumonia J69.0

Degos' disease I77.89

Dehiscence (of)
amputation stump T87.81
cesarean wound O90.0
closure of
  cornea T81.31
  craniotomy T81.32
  fascia (muscular) (superficial)
    T81.32
  internal organ or tissue T81.32
  laceration (external) (internal)
    T81.33
  ligament T81.32
  mucosa T81.31
  muscle or muscle flap T81.32
  ribs or rib cage T81.32
  skin and subcutaneous tissue
    (full-thickness) (superficial)
    T81.31
  skull T81.32
  sternum (sternotomy) T81.32
  tendon T81.32
  traumatic laceration (external)
    (internal) T81.33
episiotomy O90.1
operation wound NEC T81.31
  external operation wound
    (superficial) T81.31
  internal operation wound (deep)
    T81.32
perineal wound (postpartum) O90.1
traumatic injury wound repair T81.33
wound T81.30
  traumatic repair T81.33

Dehydration E86.0
newborn P74.1

Déjérine-Roussy syndrome G89.0

**Déjérine-Sottas disease or
neuropathy** (hypertrophic) G60.0

Déjérine-Thomas atrophy G23.8

Delay, delayed
any plane in pelvis
  complicating delivery O66.9
birth or delivery NOS O63.9
closure, ductus arteriosus (Botalli)
  P29.38
coagulation —*see* Defect,
  coagulation
conduction (cardiac) (ventricular)
  I45.9
delivery, second twin, triplet, etc
  O63.2
development R62.50
  global F88
  intellectual (specific) F81.9

Delay, delayed *(continued)*
development *(continued)*
  language F80.9
    due to hearing loss F80.4
  learning F81.9
  pervasive F84.9
  physiological R62.50
    specified stage NEC R62.0
  reading F81.0
  sexual E30.0
  speech F80.9
    due to hearing loss F80.4
  spelling F81.81
ejaculation F52.32
gastric emptying K30
menarche E30.0
menstruation (cause unknown) N91.0
milestone R62.0
passage of meconium (newborn) P76.0
primary respiration P28.9
puberty (constitutional) E30.0
separation of umbilical cord P96.82
sexual maturation, female E30.0
sleep phase syndrome G47.21
union, fracture —*see* Fracture, by site
vaccination Z28.9

Deletion(s)
autosome Q93.9
  identified by fluorescence in situ
    hybridization (FISH) Q93.89
  identified by in situ hybridization
    (ISH) Q93.89
chromosome
  with complex rearrangements
    NEC Q93.7
  part of NEC Q93.59
  seen only at prometaphase Q93.89
  short arm
    4 Q93.3
    5p Q93.4
    22q11.2 Q93.81
  specified NEC Q93.89
long arm chromosome 18 or 21
  Q93.89
  with complex rearrangements
    NEC Q93.7
microdeletions NEC Q93.88

Delhi boil or button B55.1

Delinquency (juvenile) (neurotic)
F91.8
group Z72.810

Delinquent immunization status
Z28.3

Delirium, delirious (acute or
subacute) (not alcohol- or drug-
induced) (with dementia) R41.0
alcoholic (acute) (tremens)
  (withdrawal) F10.921
  with intoxication F10.921
    in
      abuse F10.121
      dependence F10.221
due to (secondary to)
  alcohol
    intoxication F10.921
      in
        abuse F10.121
        dependence F10.221
    withdrawal F10.231
  amphetamine intoxication F15.921
    in
      abuse F15.121
      dependence F15.221
  anxiolytic
    intoxication F13.921
      in
        abuse F13.121
        dependence F13.221
        withdrawal F13.231

Delirium, delirious *(continued)*
due to *(continued)*
  cannabis intoxication (acute)
    F12.921
    in
      abuse F12.121
      dependence F12.221
  cocaine intoxication (acute)
    F14.921
    in
      abuse F14.121
      dependence F14.221
  general medical condition F05
  hallucinogen intoxication
    F16.921
    in
      abuse F16.121
      dependence F16.221
  hypnotic
    intoxication F13.921
      in
        abuse F13.121
        dependence F13.221
    withdrawal F13.231
  inhalant intoxication (acute)
    F18.921
    in
      abuse F18.121
      dependence F18.221
  multiple etiologies F05
  opioid intoxication (acute)
    F11.921
    in
      abuse F11.121
      dependence F11.221
  other (or unknown) substance
    F19.921
  phencyclidine intoxication
    (acute) F16.921
    in
      abuse F16.121
      dependence F16.221
  psychoactive substance NEC
    intoxication (acute) F19.921
    in
      abuse F19.121
      dependence F19.221
  sedative
    intoxication F13.921
      in
        abuse F13.121
        dependence F13.221
    withdrawal F13.231
  unknown etiology R41.0
exhaustion F43.0
hysterical F44.89
postprocedural (postoperative) F05
puerperal F05
thyroid —*see* Thyrotoxicosis with
  thyroid storm
traumatic —*see* Injury, intracranial
tremens (alcohol-induced) F10.231
sedative-induced F13.231

Delivery (childbirth) (labor)
arrested active phase O62.1
cesarean (for)
  abnormal
    pelvis (bony) (deformity)
      (major) NEC with
      disproportion (fetopelvic)
      O33.0
      with obstructed labor O65.0
      presentation or position O32.9
  abruptio placentae (*see also*
    Abruptio placentae) O45.9-
  acromion presentation O32.2
  atony, uterus O62.2
  breech presentation O32.1
    incomplete O32.8
  brow presentation O32.3

Delivery (continued)

cesarean (continued)

cephalopelvic disproportion
O33.9

cerclage O34.3-

chin presentation O32.3

cicatrix of cervix O34.4-

contracted pelvis (general)

inlet O33.2

outlet O33.3

cord presentation or prolapse
O69.0

cystocele O34.8-

deformity (acquired) (congenital)

pelvic organs or tissues NEC
O34.8-

pelvis (bony) NEC O33.0

disproportion NOS O33.9

eclampsia —see Eclampsia

face presentation O32.3

failed

forceps O66.5

induction of labor O61.9

instrumental O61.1

mechanical O61.1

medical O61.0

specified NEC O61.8

surgical O61.1

trial of labor NOS O66.40

following previous cesarean
delivery O66.41

vacuum extraction O66.5

ventouse O66.5

fetal-maternal hemorrhage
O43.01-

hemorrhage (intrapartum)
O67.9

with coagulation defect O67.0

specified cause NEC O67.8

high head at term O32.4

hydrocephalic fetus O33.6

incarceration of uterus O34.51-

incoordinate uterine action O62.4

increased size, fetus O33.5

inertia, uterus O62.2

primary O62.0

secondary O62.1

isthmocele O34.22

lateroversion, uterus O34.59-

mal lie O32.9

malposition

fetus O32.9

pelvic organs or tissues NEC
O34.8-

uterus NEC O34.59-

malpresentation NOS O32.9

oblique presentation O32.2

occurring after 37 completed
weeks of gestation but before
39 completed weeks gestation
due to (spontaneous) onset of
labor O75.82

oversize fetus O33.5

pelvic tumor NEC O34.8-

placenta previa O44.0-

complete O44.0-

with hemorrhage O44.1-

placental insufficiency O36.51-

planned, occurring after 37
completed weeks of gestation
but before 39 completed
weeks gestation due to
(spontaneous) onset of labor
O75.82

polyp, cervix O34.4-

causing obstructed labor
O65.5

poor dilatation, cervix O62.0

pre-eclampsia O14.94

mild O14.04

moderate O14.04

Delivery (continued)

cesarean (continued)

pre-eclampsia (continued)

severe O14.14

with hemolysis, elevated
liver enzymes and low
platelet count (HELLP)
O14.24

previous

cesarean delivery O34.219

classical (vertical)
O34.212

isthmocele O34.22

low transverse scar O34.211

mid-transverse T incision
O34.218

scar

defect (isthmocele)
O34.22

specified type NEC
O34.218

surgery (to)

cervix O34.4-

gynecological NEC O34.8-

rectum O34.7-

uterus O34.29

vagina O34.6-

prolapse

arm or hand O32.2

uterus O34.52-

prolonged labor NOS O63.9

rectocele O34.8-

retroversion

uterus O34.53-

rigid

cervix O34.4-

pelvic floor O34.8-

perineum O34.7-

vagina O34.6-

vulva O34.7-

sacculation, pregnant uterus
O34.59-

scar(s)

cervix O34.4-

cesarean delivery O34.219

classical (vertical) O34.212

isthmocele O34.22

low transverse O34.211

mid-transverse T incision
O34.218

scar

defect (isthmocele)
O34.22

specified type NEC
O34.218

defect (isthmocele) O34.22

transmural uterine O34.29

uterus O34.29

Shirodkar suture in situ O34.3-

shoulder presentation O32.2

stenosis or stricture, cervix
O34.4-

streptococcus group B (GBS)
carrier state O99.824

transmural uterine scar O34.29

transverse presentation or lie
O32.2

tumor, pelvic organs or tissues
NEC O34.8-

cervix O34.4-

umbilical cord presentation or
prolapse O69.0

without indication O82

completely normal case O80

complicated O75.9

by

abnormal, abnormality (of)

forces of labor O62.9

specified type NEC
O62.8

glucose O99.814

Delivery (continued)

complicated (continued)

by (continued)

abnormal, abnormality
(continued)

uterine contractions NOS
O62.9

abruptio placentae (see also
Abruptio placentae) O45.9-

abuse

physical O9A.32

psychological O9A.52

sexual O9A.42

adherent placenta O72.0

without hemorrhage O73.0

alcohol use O99.314

anemia (pre-existing) O99.02

anesthetic death O74.8

annular detachment of cervix
O71.3

atony, uterus O62.2

attempted vacuum extraction
and forceps O66.5

Bandl's ring O62.4

bariatric surgery status O99.844

biliary tract disorder O26.62

bleeding —see Delivery,
complicated by, hemorrhage

blood disorder NEC O99.12

cervical dystocia (hypotonic)
O62.2

primary O62.0

secondary O62.1

circulatory system disorder
O99.42

compression of cord
(umbilical) NEC O69.2

condition NEC O99.892

contraction, contracted ring
O62.4

cord (umbilical)

around neck

with compression O69.1

without compression
O69.81

bruising O69.5

complication O69.9

specified NEC O69.89

compression NEC O69.2

entanglement O69.2

without compression
O69.82

hematoma O69.5

presentation O69.0

prolapse O69.0

short O69.3

thrombosis (vessels) O69.5

vascular lesion O69.5

Couvelaire uterus O45.8X-

damage to (injury to) NEC

perineum O71.82

periurethral tissue O71.82

vulva O71.82

delay following rupture of
membranes (spontaneous)
—see Pregnancy,
complicated by, premature
rupture of membranes

depressed fetal heart tones
O76

diabetes O24.92

gestational

diabetes O24.429

diet controlled
O24.420

insulin (and diet)
controlled O24.424

oral drug controlled
(antidiabetic)
(hypoglycemic)
O24.425

Delivery (continued)

complicated (continued)

by (continued)

diabetes (continued)

gestational (continued)

edema O12.04

with proteinuria O12.24

proteinuria O12.14

pre-existing O24.32

specified NEC O24.82

type 1 O24.02

type 2 O24.12

diastasis recti (abdominis)
O71.89

dilatation

bladder O66.8

cervix incomplete, poor or
slow O62.0

disease NEC O99.892

disruptio uteri —see Delivery,
complicated by, rupture,
uterus

drug use O99.324

dysfunction, uterus NOS O62.9

hypertonic O62.4

hypotonic O62.2

primary O62.0

secondary O62.1

incoordinate O62.4

eclampsia O15.1

embolism (pulmonary) —see
Embolism, obstetric

endocrine, nutritional or
metabolic disease NEC
O99.284

failed

attempted vaginal birth
after previous cesarean
delivery O66.41

induction of labor O61.9

instrumental O61.1

mechanical O61.1

medical O61.0

specified NEC O61.8

surgical O61.1

trial of labor O66.40

female genital mutilation O65.5

fetal

abnormal acid-base balance
O68

acidemia O68

acidosis O68

alkalosis O68

death, early O02.1

deformity O66.3

heart rate or rhythm
(abnormal) (non-
reassuring) O76

hypoxia O77.8

stress O77.9

due to drug
administration O77.1

electrocardiographic
evidence of O77.8

specified NEC O77.8

ultrasound evidence of
O77.8

fever during labor O75.2

gastric banding status O99.844

gastric bypass status O99.844

gastrointestinal disease NEC
O99.62

gestational

diabetes O24.429

diet controlled O24.420

insulin (and diet)
controlled O24.424

oral drug controlled
(antidiabetic)
(hypoglycemic)
O24.425

Delivery (*continued*)
  complicated (*continued*)
    by (*continued*)
      gestational (*continued*)
        edema O12.04
          with proteinuria O12.14
          proteinuria O12.14
        gonorrhea O98.22
      hematoma O71.7
        ischial spine O71.7
        pelvic O71.7
        vagina O71.7
        vulva or perineum O71.7
      hemorrhage (uterine) O67.9
        associated with
          afibrinogenemia O67.0
          coagulation defect O67.0
          hyperfibrinolysis O67.0
          hypofibrinogenemia
            O67.0
        due to
          low implantation of
            placenta O44.5-
          low-lying placenta
            O44.5-
          placenta previa O44.1-
            marginal O44.3-
            partial O44.3-
          premature separation of
            placenta (normally
            implanted) (*see also*
            Abruptio placentae)
            O45.9-
          retained placenta O72.0
          uterine leiomyoma O67.8
        placenta NEC O67.8
        postpartum NEC (atonic)
          (immediate) O72.1
          with retained or trapped
            placenta O72.0
          delayed O72.2
          secondary O72.2
          third stage O72.0
      hourglass contraction, uterus
        O62.4
      hypertension, hypertensive
        (pre-existing) —*see*
        Hypertension, complicated
        by, childbirth (labor)
      hypotension O26.5-
      incomplete dilatation (cervix)
        O62.0
      incoordinate uterus
        contractions O62.4
      inertia, uterus O62.2
        during latent phase of labor
          O62.0
        primary O62.0
        secondary O62.1
      infection (maternal) O98.92
        carrier state NEC O99.834
        gonorrhea O98.22
        human immunodeficiency
          virus (HIV) O98.72
        sexually transmitted NEC
          O98.32
        specified NEC O98.82
        syphilis O98.12
        tuberculosis O98.02
        viral hepatitis O98.42
        viral NEC O98.52
      injury (to mother) (*see also*
        Delivery, complicated by,
        damage to) O71.9
        nonobstetric O9A.22
          caused by abuse —*see*
            Delivery, complicated
            by, abuse
      intrauterine fetal death, early
        O02.1
      inversion, uterus O71.2

Delivery (*continued*)
  complicated (*continued*)
    by (*continued*)
      laceration (perineal) O70.9
        anus (sphincter) O70.4
          with third degree
            laceration (*see also*
            Delivery, complicated,
            by, laceration,
            perineum, third
            degree) O70.20
            with mucosa O70.3
          without third degree
            laceration O70.4
        bladder (urinary) O71.5
        bowel O71.5
        cervix (uteri) O71.3
        fourchette O70.0
        hymen O70.0
        labia O70.0
        pelvic
          floor O70.1
          organ NEC O71.5
        perineum, perineal O70.9
          first degree O70.0
          fourth degree O70.3
          muscles O70.1
          second degree O70.1
          skin O70.0
          slight O70.0
          third degree O70.20
           with
            both external anal
              sphincter (EAS)
              and internal anal
              sphincter (IAS)
              torm (IIIc) O70.23
            less than 50% of
              external anal
              sphincter (EAS)
              thickness torn
              (IIIa) O70.21
            more than 50% of
              external anal
              sphincter (EAS)
              thickness torn
              (IIIb) O70.22
            IIIa O70.21
            IIIb O70.22
            IIIc O70.23
        peritoneum (pelvic) O71.5
        rectovaginal (septum)
          (without perineal
          laceration) O71.4
          with perineum (*see also*
            Delivery, complicated,
            by, laceration, perineum,
            third degree) O70.20
            with anal or rectal
              mucosa O70.3
        specified NEC O71.89
        sphincter ani —*see*
          Delivery, complicated,
          by, laceration, anus
          (sphincter)
        urethra O71.5
        uterus O71.81
          before labor O71.81
        vagina, vaginal (deep)
          (high) (without perineal
          laceration) O71.4
          with perineum O70.0
          muscles, with perineum
           O70.1
        vulva O70.0
      liver disorder O26.62
      malignancy O9A.12
      malnutrition O25.2
      malposition, malpresentation
        placenta O44.0-
          with hemorrhage O44.1-

Delivery (*continued*)
  complicated (*continued*)
    by (*continued*)
      malposition, malpresentation
        (*continued*)
        uterus or cervix O65.5
        without obstruction
          (*see also* Delivery,
          complicated by,
          obstruction) O32.9
          breech O32.1
          compound O32.6
          face (brow) (chin) O32.3
          footling O32.8
          high head O32.4
          oblique O32.2
          specified NEC O32.8
          transverse O32.2
          unstable lie O32.0
      meconium in amniotic fluid
        O77.0
      mental disorder NEC O99.344
      metrorrhexis —*see* Delivery,
        complicated by, rupture,
        uterus
      nervous system disorder
        O99.354
      obesity (pre-existing) O99.214
      obesity surgery status O99.844
      obstetric trauma O71.9
        specified NEC O71.89
      obstructed labor
        due to
          breech (complete) (frank)
            presentation O64.1
            incomplete O64.8
          brow presentation O64.3
          buttock presentation O64.1
          chin presentation O64.2
          compound presentation
           O64.5
          contracted pelvis O65.1
          deep transverse arrest
           O64.0
          deformed pelvis O65.0
          dystocia (fetal) O66.9
           due to
            conjoined twins O66.3
            fetal
              abnormality NEC
               O66.3
              ascites O66.3
              hydrops O66.3
              meningomyelocele
               O66.3
              sacral teratoma
               O66.3
              tumor O66.3
            hydrocephalic fetus
              O66.3
            shoulder O66.0
          face presentation O64.2
          fetopelvic disproportion
           O65.4
          footling presentation O64.8
          impacted shoulders O66.0
          incomplete rotation of
           fetal head O64.0
          large fetus O66.2
          locked twins O66.1
          malposition O64.9
           specified NEC O64.8
          malpresentation O64.9
           specified NEC O64.8
          multiple fetuses NEC
           O66.6
          pelvic
           abnormality (maternal)
            O65.9
            organ O65.5
            specified NEC O65.8

Delivery (*continued*)
  complicated (*continued*)
    by (*continued*)
      obstructed labor (*continued*)
        due to (*continued*)
          pelvic (*continued*)
           abnormality (*continued*)
            contraction
             inlet O65.2
             mid-cavity O65.3
             outlet O65.3
           persistent (position)
            occipitoiliac O64.0
            occipitoposterior O64.0
            occipitosacral O64.0
            occipitotransverse
             O64.0
           prolapsed arm O64.4
           shoulder presentation
            O64.4
          specified NEC O66.8
        pathological retraction ring,
          uterus O62.4
      penetration, pregnant uterus
        by instrument O71.1
      perforation —*see* Delivery,
        complicated by, laceration
      placenta, placental
        ablatio (*see also* Abruptio
          placentae) O45.9-
        abnormality O43.9-
          specified NEC O43.89-
        abruptio (*see also* Abruptio
          placentae) O45.9-
        accreta O43.21-
        adherent (with hemorrhage)
          O72.0
          without hemorrhage O73.0
        detachment (premature)
          (*see also* Abruptio
          placentae) O45.9-
        disorder O43.9-
          specified NEC O43.89-
        hemorrhage NEC O67.8
        increta O43.22-
        low (implantation) (lying)
          O44.4-
          with hemorrhage O44.5-
        malformation O43.10-
        malposition O44.0-
          with hemorrhage O44.1-
        percreta O43.23-
        previa (central) (complete)
          (lateral) (total) O44.0-
          with hemorrhage O44.1-
          marginal O44.2-
           with hemorrhage
            O44.3-
          partial O44.2-
           with hemorrhage
            O44.3-
          with hemorrhage O44.1-
        retained (with hemorrhage)
          O72.0
          without hemorrhage
           O73.0
        separation (premature)
          O45.9-
          specified NEC O45.8X-
        vicious insertion O44.1-
      precipitate labor O62.3
      premature rupture, membranes
        (*see also* Pregnancy,
        complicated by, premature
        rupture of membranes)
        O42.90
      prolapse
        arm or hand O32.2
        cord (umbilical) O69.0
        foot or leg O32.8
        uterus O34.52-

Delivery *(continued)*
  complicated *(continued)*
    by *(continued)*
      prolonged labor O63.9
        first stage O63.0
        second stage O63.1
      protozoal disease (maternal) O98.62
      respiratory disease NEC O99.52
      retained membranes or portions of placenta O72.2
        without hemorrhage O73.1
      retarded birth O63.9
      retention of secundines (with hemorrhage) O72.0
        without hemorrhage O73.0
        partial O72.2
          without hemorrhage O73.1
      rupture
        bladder (urinary) O71.5
        cervix O71.3
        pelvic organ NEC O71.5
        urethra O71.5
        uterus (during or after labor) O71.1
          before labor O71.0-
      separation, pubic bone (symphysis pubis) O71.6
      shock O75.1
      shoulder presentation O64.4
      skin disorder NEC O99.72
      spasm, cervix O62.4
      stenosis or stricture, cervix O65.5
      streptococcus group B (GBS) carrier state O99.824
      subluxation of symphysis (pubis) O26.72
      syphilis (maternal) O98.12
      tear —*see* Delivery, complicated by, laceration
      tetanic uterus O62.4
      trauma (obstetrical) *(see also* Delivery, complicated by, damage to) O71.9
        non-obstetric O9A.22
        periurethral O71.82
        specified NEC O71.89
      tuberculosis (maternal) O98.02
      tumor, pelvic organs or tissues NEC O65.5
      umbilical cord around neck
        with compression O69.1
        without compression O69.81
      uterine inertia O62.2
        during latent phase of labor O62.0
        primary O62.0
        secondary O62.1
      vasa previa O69.4
      velamentous insertion of cord O43.12-
    specified complication NEC O75.89
  delayed NOS O63.9
    following rupture of membranes artificial O75.5
  second twin, triplet, etc. O63.2
  forceps, low following failed vacuum extraction O66.5
  missed (at or near term) O36.4
  normal O80
  obstructed —*see* Delivery, complicated by, obstructed labor
  precipitate O62.3
  preterm *(see also* Pregnancy, complicated by, preterm labor) O60.10

Dementia *(continued)*
  spontaneous O80
  term pregnancy NOS O80
  uncomplicated O80
  vaginal, following previous
    cesarean delivery O34.219
    classical (vertical) scar O34.212
    low transverse scar O34.211
    mid-transverse T incision O34.218
    scar
      defect (isthmocele)O34.22
      specified type NEC O34.218

Delusions (paranoid) —*see* Disorder, delusional

Dementia (degenerative (primary)) (old age) (persisting) F03.90
  with
    aggressive behavior F03.91
    behavioral disturbance F03.91
    combative behavior F03.91
    Lewy bodies G31.83 *[F02.80]*
      with behavioral disturbance G31.83 *[F02.81]*
    Parkinsonism G31.83 *[F02.80]*
      with behavioral disturbance G31.83 *[F02.81]*
    Parkinson's disease G20 *[F02.80]*
      with behavioral disturbance G20 *[F02.81]*
    violent behavior F03.91
  alcoholic F10.97
    with dependence F10.27
  Alzheimer's type —*see* Disease, Alzheimer's
  arteriosclerotic —*see* Dementia, vascular
  atypical, Alzheimer's type —*see* Disease, Alzheimer's, specified NEC
  congenital —*see* Disability, intellectual
  frontal (lobe) G31.09 *[F02.80]*
    with behavioral disturbance G31.09 *[F02.81]*
  frontotemporal G31.09 *[F02.80]*
    with behavioral disturbance G31.09 *[F02.81]*
    specified NEC G31.09 *[F02.80]*
      with behavioral disturbance G31.09 *[F02.81]*
  in (due to)
    alcohol F10.97
      with dependence F10.27
    Alzheimer's disease —*see* Disease, Alzheimer's
    arteriosclerotic brain disease —*see* Dementia, vascular
    cerebral lipidoses E75.- *[F02.80]*
      with behavioral disturbance E75.- *[F02.81]*
    Creutzfeldt-Jakob disease —*see also* Creutzfeldt-Jakob disease or syndrome (with dementia) A81.00
    epilepsy G40.- *[F02.80]*
      with behavioral disturbance G40.- *[F02.81]*
    hepatolenticular degeneration E83.01 *[F02.80]*
      with behavioral disturbance E83.01 *[F02.81]*
    human immunodeficiency virus (HIV) disease B20 *[F02.80]*
      with behavioral disturbance B20 *[F02.81]*
    Huntington's disease or chorea G10 *[F02.80]*
      with behavioral disturbance G10 *[F02.81]*

Dementia *(continued)*
  in *(continued)*
    hypercalcemia E83.52 *[F02.80]*
      with behavioral disturbance E83.52 *[F02.81]*
    hypothyroidism, acquired E03.9 *[F02.80]*
      with behavioral disturbance E03.9 *[F02.81]*
      due to iodine deficiency E01.8 *[F02.80]*
        with behavioral disturbance E01.8 *[F02.81]*
    inhalants F18.97
      with dependence F18.27
    multiple
      etiologies F03
      sclerosis G35 *[F02.80]*
        with behavioral disturbance G35 *[F02.81]*
    neurosyphilis A52.17 *[F02.80]*
      with behavioral disturbance A52.17 *[F02.81]*
      juvenile A50.49 *[F02.80]*
        with behavioral disturbance A50.49 *[F02.81]*
    niacin deficiency E52 *[F02.80]*
      with behavioral disturbance E52 *[F02.81]*
    paralysis agitans G20 *[F02.80]*
      with behavioral disturbance G20 *[F02.81]*
    Parkinson's disease G20 *[F02.80]*
    pellagra E52 *[F02.80]*
      with behavioral disturbance E52 *[F02.81]*
    Pick's G31.01 *[F02.80]*
      with behavioral disturbance G31.01 *[F02.81]*
    polyarteritis nodosa M30.0 *[F02.80]*
      with behavioral disturbance M30.0 *[F02.81]*
    psychoactive drug F19.97
      with dependence F19.27
      inhalants F18.97
        with dependence F18.27
      sedatives, hypnotics or anxiolytics F13.97
        with dependence F13.27
    sedatives, hypnotics or anxiolytics F13.97
      with dependence F13.27
    systemic lupus erythematosus M32.- *[F02.80]*
      with behavioral disturbance M32.- *[F02.81]*
    trypanosomiasis
      African B56.9 *[F02.80]*
        with behavioral disturbance B56.9 *[F02.81]*
    unknown etiology F03
    vitamin B12 deficiency E53.8 *[F02.80]*
      with behavioral disturbance E53.8 *[F02.81]*
    volatile solvents F18.97
      with dependence F18.27
    with behavioral disturbance G31.83 *[F02.81]*
  infantile, infantilis F84.3
  Lewy body G31.83 *[F02.80]*
    with behavioral disturbance G31.83 *[F02.81]*
  multi-infarct —*see* Dementia, vascular
  paralytica, paralytic (syphilitic) A52.17 *[F02.80]*

Dementia *(continued)*
  paralytica, paralytic *(continued)*
    with behavioral disturbance A52.17 *[F02.81]*
    juvenilis A50.45
  paretic A52.17
  praecox —*see* Schizophrenia
  presenile F03
    Alzheimer's type —*see* Disease, Alzheimer's, early onset
  primary degenerative F03
  progressive, syphilitic A52.17
  senile F03
    with acute confusional state F05
    Alzheimer's type —*see* Disease, Alzheimer's, late onset
    depressed or paranoid type F03
  vascular (acute onset) (mixed) (multi-infarct) (subcortical) F01.50
    with behavioral disturbance F01.51

Demineralization, bone —*see* Osteoporosis

Demodex folliculorum (infestation) B88.0

Demophobia F40.248

Demoralization R45.3

Demyelination, demyelinization
  central nervous system G37.9
    specified NEC G37.8
  corpus callosum (central) G37.1
  disseminated, acute G36.9
    specified NEC G36.8
  global G35
  in optic neuritis G36.0

Dengue (classical) (fever) A90
  hemorrhagic A91
  sandfly A93.1

Dennie-Marfan syphilitic syndrome A50.45

Dens evaginatus, in dente or invaginatus K00.2

Dense breasts R92.2

Density
  increased, bone (disseminated) (generalized) (spotted) —*see* Disorder, bone, density and structure, specified type NEC
  lung (nodular) J98.4

Dental —*see also* condition
  examination Z01.20
    with abnormal findings Z01.21
  restoration
    aesthetically inadequate or displeasing K08.56
    defective K08.50
      specified NEC K08.59
    failure of marginal integrity K08.51
    failure of periodontal anatomical integrity K08.54

Dentia praecox K00.6

Denticles (pulp) K04.2

Dentigerous cyst K09.0

Dentin
  irregular (in pulp) K04.3
  opalescent K00.5
  secondary (in pulp) K04.3
  sensitive K03.89

Dentinogenesis imperfecta K00.5

Dentinoma —*see* Cyst, calcifying odontogenic

Dentition (syndrome) K00.7
  delayed K00.6
  difficult K00.7

Dependence *(continued)*

heroin (salt) (any) —*see* Dependence, drug, opioid

hypnotic NEC —*see* Dependence, drug, sedative

Indian hemp —*see* Dependence, drug, cannabis

inhalants —*see* Dependence, drug, inhalant

khat —*see* Dependence, drug, stimulant NEC

laudanum —*see* Dependence, drug, opioid

LSD(-25) (derivatives) —*see* Dependence, drug, hallucinogen

luminal —*see* Dependence, drug, sedative

lysergic acid —*see* Dependence, drug, hallucinogen

maconha —*see* Dependence, drug, cannabis

marihuana —*see* Dependence, drug, cannabis

meprobamate —*see* Dependence, drug, sedative

mescaline —*see* Dependence, drug, hallucinogen

methadone —*see* Dependence, drug, opioid

methamphetamine(s) —*see* Dependence, drug, stimulant NEC

methaqualone —*see* Dependence, drug, sedative

methyl

  alcohol (without remission) F10.20

    with remission F10.21

  bromide —*see* Dependence, drug, sedative

  morphine —*see* Dependence, drug, opioid

  phenidate —*see* Dependence, drug, stimulant NEC

  sulfonal —*see* Dependence, drug, sedative

morphine (sulfate) (sulfite) (type) —*see* Dependence, drug, opioid

narcotic (drug) NEC —*see* Dependence, drug, opioid

nembutal —*see* Dependence, drug, sedative

neraval —*see* Dependence, drug, sedative

neravan —*see* Dependence, drug, sedative

neurobarb —*see* Dependence, drug, sedative

nicotine —*see* Dependence, drug, nicotine

nitrous oxide F19.20

nonbarbiturate sedatives and tranquilizers with similar effect —*see* Dependence, drug, sedative

on

  artificial heart (fully implantable) (mechanical) Z95.812

  aspirator Z99.0

  care provider (because of) Z74.9

    impaired mobility Z74.09

    need for

      assistance with personal care Z74.1

      continuous supervision Z74.3

      no other household member able to render care Z74.2

      specified reason NEC Z74.8

Dependence *(continued)*

on *(continued)*

  machine Z99.89

    enabling NEC Z99.89

    specified type NEC Z99.89

  renal dialysis (hemodialysis) (peritoneal) Z99.2

  respirator Z99.11

  ventilator Z99.11

  wheelchair Z99.3

opiate —*see* Dependence, drug, opioid

opioids —*see* Dependence, drug, opioid

opium (alkaloids) (derivatives) (tincture) —*see* Dependence, drug, opioid

oxygen (long-term) (supplemental) Z99.81

paraldehyde —*see* Dependence, drug, sedative

paregoric —*see* Dependence, drug, opioid

PCP (phencyclidine) (or related substance) —*see* Dependence, drug, hallucinogen

pentobarbital —*see* Dependence, drug, sedative

pentobarbitone (sodium) —*see* Dependence, drug, sedative

pentothal —*see* Dependence, drug, sedative

peyote —*see* Dependence, drug, hallucinogen

phencyclidine (PCP) (or related substance) —*see* Dependence, drug, hallucinogen

phenmetrazine —*see* Dependence, drug, stimulant NEC

phenobarbital —*see* Dependence, drug, sedative

polysubstance F19.20

psilocibin, psilocin, psilocyn, psilocyline —*see* Dependence, drug, hallucinogen

psychostimulant NEC —*see* Dependence, drug, stimulant NEC

secobarbital —*see* Dependence, drug, sedative

seconal —*see* Dependence, drug, sedative

sedative NEC —*see* Dependence, drug, sedative

specified drug NEC —*see* Dependence, drug

stimulant NEC —*see* Dependence, drug, stimulant NEC

substance NEC —*see* Dependence, drug

supplemental oxygen Z99.81

tobacco —*see* Dependence, drug, nicotine

  counseling and surveillance Z71.6

tranquilizer NEC —*see* Dependence, drug, sedative

vitamin B6 E53.1

volatile solvents —*see* Dependence, drug, inhalant

Dependency

care-provider Z74.9

passive F60.7

reactions (persistent) F60.7

Depersonalization (in neurotic state) (neurotic) (syndrome) F48.1

Depletion

extracellular fluid E86.9

plasma E86.1

potassium E87.6

  nephropathy N25.89

Depletion *(continued)*

salt or sodium E87.1

  causing heat exhaustion or prostration T67.4

  nephropathy N28.9

volume NOS E86.9

Deployment (current) (military)

status Z56.82

in theater or in support of military war, peacekeeping and humanitarian operations Z56.82

personal history of Z91.82

  military war, peacekeeping and humanitarian deployment (current or past conflict) Z91.82

returned from Z91.82

Depolarization, premature I49.40

atrial I49.1

junctional I49.2

specified NEC I49.49

ventricular I49.3

Deposit

bone in Boeck's sarcoid D86.89

calcareous, calcium —*see* Calcification

cholesterol

  retina H35.89

  vitreous (body) (humor) —*see* Deposit, crystalline

conjunctiva H11.11-

cornea H18.00-

  argentous H18.02-

  due to metabolic disorder H18.03-

  Kayser-Fleischer ring H18.04-

  pigmentation —*see* Pigmentation, cornea

crystalline, vitreous (body) (humor) H43.2-

hemosiderin in old scars of cornea —*see* Pigmentation, cornea, stromal

metallic in lens —*see* Cataract, specified NEC

skin R23.8

tooth, teeth (betel) (black) (green) (materia alba) (orange) (tobacco) K03.6

urate, kidney —*see* Calculus, kidney

Depraved appetite —*see* Pica

Depressed

HDL cholesterol E78.6

Depression (acute) (mental) F32.9

agitated (single episode) F32.2

anaclitic —*see* Disorder, adjustment

anxiety F41.8

  persistent F34.1

arches —*see also* Deformity, limb, flat foot

atypical (single episode) F32.89

  recurrent episode F33.8

basal metabolic rate R94.8

bone marrow D75.89

central nervous system R09.2

cerebral R29.818

  newborn P91.4

cerebrovascular I67.9

chest wall M95.4

climacteric (single episode) F32.89

  recurrent episode F33.8

endogenous (without psychotic symptoms) F33.2

  with psychotic symptoms F33.3

functional activity R68.89

hysterical F44.89

Depression *(continued)*

involutional (single episode) F32.89

  recurrent episode F33.8

major F32.9

  with psychotic symptoms F32.3

  recurrent —*see* Disorder, depressive, recurrent

manic-depressive —*see* Disorder, depressive, recurrent

masked (single episode) F32.89

medullary G93.89

menopausal (single episode) F32.89

  recurrent episode F33.8

metatarsus —*see* Depression, arches

monopolar F33.9

nervous F34.1

neurotic F34.1

nose M95.0

postnatal NOS F53.0

postpartum NOS F53.0

post-psychotic of schizophrenia F32.89

post-schizophrenic F32.89

psychogenic (reactive) (single episode) F32.9

psychoneurotic F34.1

psychotic (single episode) F32.3

  recurrent F33.3

reactive (psychogenic) (single episode) F32.9

  psychotic (single episode) F32.3

recurrent —*see* Disorder, depressive, recurrent

respiratory center G93.89

seasonal —*see* Disorder, depressive, recurrent

senile F03

severe, single episode F32.2

situational F43.21

skull Q67.4

specified NEC (single episode) F32.89

sternum M95.4

visual field —*see* Defect, visual field

vital (recurrent) (without psychotic symptoms) F33.2

  with psychotic symptoms F33.3

  single episode F32.2

Deprivation

cultural Z60.3

effects NOS T73.9

  specified NEC T73.8

emotional NEC Z65.8

  affecting infant or child —*see* Maltreatment, child, psychological

food T73.0

protein —*see* Malnutrition

sleep Z72.820

social Z60.4

  affecting infant or child —*see* Maltreatment, child, psychological

specified NEC T73.8

vitamins —*see* Deficiency, vitamin

water T73.1

Derangement

ankle (internal) —*see* Derangement, joint, ankle

cartilage (articular) NEC —*see* Derangement, joint, articular cartilage, by site

  recurrent —*see* Dislocation, recurrent

Dependence–Derangement

Derangement (continued)
cruciate ligament, anterior, current
   injury —see Sprain, knee,
   cruciate, anterior
elbow (internal) —see
   Derangement, joint, elbow
hip (joint) (internal) (old) —see
   Derangement, joint, hip
joint (internal) M24.9
   ankylosis —see Ankylosis
   articular cartilage M24.10
      ankle M24.17-
      elbow M24.12-
      foot M24.17-
      hand M24.14-
      hip M24.15-
      knee NEC M23.9-
      loose body —see Loose, body
      shoulder M24.11-
      specified site NEC M24.19
      wrist M24.13-
   contracture —see Contraction,
      joint
   current injury —see also
      Dislocation
      knee, meniscus or cartilage
         —see Tear, meniscus
   dislocation
      pathological —see
         Dislocation, pathological
      recurrent —see Dislocation,
         recurrent
   knee —see Derangement, knee
   ligament —see Disorder,
      ligament
   loose body —see Loose, body
   recurrent —see Dislocation,
      recurrent
   specified type NEC M24.80
      ankle M24.87-
      elbow M24.82-
      foot joint M24.87-
      hand joint M24.84-
      hip M24.85-
      shoulder M24.81-
      specified site NEC M24.89
      wrist M24.83-
   temporomandibular M26.69
knee (recurrent) M23.9-
   ligament disruption, spontaneous
      M23.60-
      anterior cruciate M23.61-
      capsular M23.67-
      instability, chronic M23.5-
      lateral collateral M23.64-
      medial collateral M23.63-
      posterior cruciate M23.62-
   loose body M23.4-
   meniscus M23.30-
      cystic M23.00-
         lateral M23.002
            anterior horn M23.04-
            posterior horn M23.05-
            specified NEC M23.06-
         medial M23.005
            anterior horn M23.01-
            posterior horn M23.02-
            specified NEC M23.03-
      degenerate —see
         Derangement, knee,
         meniscus, specified NEC
      detached —see Derangement,
         knee, meniscus, specified
         NEC
      due to old tear or injury
         M23.20-
         lateral M23.20-
            anterior horn M23.24-
            posterior horn M23.25-
            specified NEC M23.26-
         medial M23.20-

Derangement (continued)
knee (continued)
   meniscus (continued)
      due to old tear or injury
         (continued)
         medial (continued)
            anterior horn M23.21-
            posterior horn M23.22-
            specified NEC M23.23-
      retained —see Derangement,
         knee, meniscus, specified
         NEC
      specified NEC M23.30-
         lateral M23.30-
            anterior horn M23.34-
            posterior horn M23.35-
            specified NEC M23.36-
         medial M23.30-
            anterior horn M23.31-
            posterior horn M23.32-
            specified NEC M23.33-
      old M23.8X-
      specified NEC —see subcategory
         M23.8
   low back NEC —see Dorsopathy,
      specified NEC
   meniscus —see Derangement,
      knee, meniscus
   mental —see Psychosis
   patella, specified NEC —see Disorder,
      patella, derangement NEC
   semilunar cartilage (knee) —see
      Derangement, knee, meniscus,
      specified NEC
   shoulder (internal) —see
      Derangement, joint, shoulder

Dercum's disease E88.2

Derealization (neurotic) F48.1

Dermal —see condition

Dermaphytid —see Dermatophytosis

Dermatitis (eczematous) L30.9
   ab igne L59.0
   acarine B88.0
   actinic (due to sun) L57.8
      other than from sun L59.8
   allergic —see Dermatitis, contact,
      allergic
   ambustionis, due to burn or scald
      —see Burn
   amebic A06.7
   ammonia L22
   arsenical (ingested) L27.8
   artefacta L98.1
      psychogenic F54
   atopic L20.9
      psychogenic F54
      specified NEC L20.89
   autoimmune progesterone L30.8
   berlock, berloque L56.2
   blastomycotic B40.3
   blister beetle L24.89
   bullous, bullosa L13.9
      mucosynechial, atrophic L12.1
      seasonal L30.8
      specified NEC L13.8
   calorica L59.0
      due to burn or scald —see Burn
   caterpillar L24.89
   cercarial B65.3
   combustionis L59.0
      due to burn or scald —see Burn
   congelationis T69.1
   contact (occupational) L25.9
      allergic L23.9
         due to
            adhesives L23.1
            cement L23.5
            chemical products NEC L23.5

Dermatitis (continued)
contact (continued)
   allergic (continued)
      due to (continued)
         chromium L23.0
         cosmetics L23.2
         dander (cat) (dog) L23.81
         drugs in contact with skin
            L23.3
         dyes L23.4
         food in contact with skin
            L23.6
         hair (cat) (dog) L23.81
         insecticide L23.5
         metals L23.0
         nickel L23.0
         plants, non-food L23.7
         plastic L23.5
         rubber L23.5
         specified agent NEC L23.89
   due to
      cement L25.3
      chemical products NEC L25.3
      cosmetics L25.0
      dander (cat) (dog) L23.81
      drugs in contact with skin
         L25.1
      dyes L25.2
      food in contact with skin L25.4
      hair (cat) (dog) L23.81
      plants, non-food L25.5
      specified agent NEC L25.8
   irritant L24.9
      due to
         cement L24.5
         chemical products NEC L24.5
         cosmetics L24.3
         detergents L24.0
         drugs in contact with skin
            L24.4
         food in contact with skin
            L24.6
         oils and greases L24.1
         plants, non-food L24.7
         solvents L24.2
         specified agent NEC L24.89
   contusiformis L52
desquamative L30.8
diabetic —see E08-E13 with .620
diaper L22
diphtheritica A36.3
dry skin L85.3
due to
   acetone (contact) (irritant) L24.2
   acids (contact) (irritant) L24.5
   adhesive(s) (allergic) (contact)
      (plaster) L23.1
      irritant L24.5
   alcohol (irritant) (skin contact)
      (substances in category T51)
      L24.2
      taken internally L27.8
   alkalis (contact) (irritant) L24.5
   arsenic (ingested) L27.8
   carbon disulfide (contact)
      (irritant) L24.2
   caustics (contact) (irritant) L24.5
   cement (contact) L25.3
   cereal (ingested) L27.2
   chemical(s) NEC L25.3
      taken internally L27.8
   chlorocompounds L24.2
   chromium (contact) (irritant)
      L24.81
   coffee (ingested) L27.2
   cold weather L30.8
   cosmetics (contact) L25.0
      allergic L23.2
      irritant L24.3
   cyclohexanes L24.2
   dander (cat) (dog) L23.81

Dermatitis (continued)
due to (continued)
   Demodex species B88.0
   Dermanyssus gallinae B88.0
   detergents (contact) (irritant) L24.0
   dichromate L24.81
   drugs and medicaments
      (generalized) (internal use) L27.0
      external —see Dermatitis, due
         to, drugs, in contact with skin
      in contact with skin L25.1
         allergic L23.3
         irritant L24.4
      localized skin eruption L27.1
      specified substance —see Table
         of Drugs and Chemicals
   dyes (contact) L25.2
      allergic L23.4
      irritant L24.89
   epidermophytosis —see
      Dermatophytosis
   esters L24.2
   external irritant NEC L24.9
   fish (ingested) L27.2
   flour (ingested) L27.2
   food (ingested) L27.2
      in contact with skin L25.4
   fruit (ingested) L27.2
   furs (allergic) (contact) L23.81
   glues —see Dermatitis, due to,
      adhesives
   glycols L24.2
   greases NEC (contact) (irritant)
      L24.1
   hair (cat) (dog) L23.81
   hot
      objects and materials —see Burn
      weather or places L59.0
   hydrocarbons L24.2
   infrared rays L59.8
   ingestion, ingested substance L27.9
      chemical NEC L27.8
      drugs and medicaments —see
         Dermatitis, due to, drugs
      food L27.2
      specified NEC L27.8
   insecticide in contact with skin
      L24.5
   internal agent L27.9
      drugs and medicaments
         (generalized) —see
         Dermatitis, due to, drugs
      food L27.2
   irradiation —see Dermatitis, due
      to, radioactive substance
   ketones L24.2
   lacquer tree (allergic) (contact)
      L23.7
   light (sun) NEC L57.8
      acute L56.8
      other L59.8
   Liponyssoides sanguineus B88.0
   low temperature L30.8
   meat (ingested) L27.2
   metals, metal salts (contact)
      (irritant) L24.81
   milk (ingested) L27.2
   nickel (contact) (irritant) L24.81
   nylon (contact) (irritant) L24.5
   oils NEC (contact) (irritant) L24.1
   paint solvent (contact) (irritant)
      L24.2
   petroleum products (contact)
      (irritant) (substances in T52.0)
      L24.2
   plants NEC (contact) L25.5
      allergic L23.7
      irritant L24.7
   plasters (adhesive) (any)
      (allergic) (contact) L23.1
      irritant L24.5

Descensus uteri —*see* Prolapse, uterus

Desert
  rheumatism B38.0
  sore —*see* Ulcer, skin

Desertion (newborn) —*see* Maltreatment

Desmoid (extra-abdominal) (tumor) —*see* Neoplasm, connective tissue, uncertain behavior
  abdominal D48.1

Despondency F32.9

Desquamation, skin R23.4

Destruction, destructive —*see also* Damage
  articular facet —*see also* Derangement, joint, specified type NEC
    knee M23.8X-
    vertebra —*see* Spondylosis
  bone —*see also* Disorder, bone, specified type NEC
    syphilitic A52.77
  joint —*see also* Derangement, joint, specified type NEC
    sacroiliac M53.3
  rectal sphincter K62.89
  septum (nasal) J34.89
  tuberculous NEC —*see* Tuberculosis
  tympanum, tympanic membrane (nontraumatic) —*see* Disorder, tympanic membrane, specified NEC
  vertebral disc —*see* Degeneration, intervertebral disc

Destructiveness —*see also* Disorder, conduct
  adjustment reaction —*see* Disorder, adjustment

Desultory labor O62.2

Detachment
  cartilage —*see* Sprain
  cervix, annular N88.8
    complicating delivery O71.3
  choroid (old) (postinfectional) (simple) (spontaneous) H31.40-
    hemorrhagic H31.41-
    serous H31.42-
  ligament —*see* Sprain
  meniscus (knee) —*see also* Derangement, knee, meniscus, specified NEC
    current injury —*see* Tear, meniscus
    due to old tear or injury —*see* Derangement, knee, meniscus, due to old tear
  retina (without retinal break) (serous) H33.2-
    with retinal:
      break H33.00-
        giant H33.03-
        multiple H33.02-
        single H33.01-
      dialysis H33.04-
    pigment epithelium —*see* Degeneration, retina, separation of layers, pigment epithelium detachment
    rhegmatogenous —*see* Detachment, retina, with retinal, break
    specified NEC H33.8
    total H33.05-
    traction H33.4-
  vitreous (body) H43.81

Detergent asthma J69.8

Deterioration
  epileptic F06.8
  general physical R53.81
  heart, cardiac —*see* Degeneration, myocardial
  mental —*see* Psychosis
  myocardial, myocardium —*see* Degeneration, myocardial
  senile (simple) R54

Deuteranomaly (anomalous trichromat) H53.53

Deuteranopia (complete) (incomplete) H53.53

Development
  abnormal, bone Q79.9
  arrested R62.50
    bone —*see* Arrest, development or growth, bone
    child R62.50
    due to malnutrition E45
  defective, congenital —*see also* Anomaly, by site
    cauda equina Q06.3
    left ventricle Q24.8
      in hypoplastic left heart syndrome Q23.4
    valve Q24.8
      pulmonary Q22.3
  delayed —*see also* Delay, development R62.50
    arithmetical skills F81.2
    language (skills) (expressive) F80.1
    learning skill F81.9
    mixed skills F88
    motor coordination F82
    reading F81.0
    specified learning skill NEC F81.89
    speech F80.9
    spelling F81.81
    written expression F81.81
  imperfect, congenital —*see also* Anomaly, by site
    heart Q24.9
    lungs Q33.6
  incomplete
    bronchial tree Q32.4
    organ or site not listed —*see* Hypoplasia, by site
    respiratory system Q34.9
  sexual, precocious NEC E30.1
  tardy, mental (*see also* Disability, intellectual) F79

Developmental —*see* condition
  testing, infant or child —*see* Examination, child

Devergie's disease (pityriasis rubra pilaris) L44.0

Deviation (in)
  conjugate palsy (eye) (spastic) H51.0
  esophagus (acquired) K22.8
  eye, skew H51.8
  midline (jaw) (teeth) (dental arch) M26.29
    specified site NEC —*see* Malposition
  nasal septum J34.2
    congenital Q67.4
  opening and closing of the mandible M26.53
  organ or site, congenital NEC —*see* Malposition, congenital
  septum (nasal) (acquired) J34.2
    congenital Q67.4
  sexual F65.9
    bestiality F65.89
    erotomania F52.8
    exhibitionism F65.2

Deviation (continued)
  sexual (continued)
    fetishism, fetishistic F65.0
      transvestism F65.1
    frotteurism F65.81
    masochism F65.51
    multiple F65.89
    necrophilia F65.89
    nymphomania F52.8
    pederosis F65.4
    pedophilia F65.4
    sadism, sadomasochism F65.52
    satyriasis F52.8
    specified type NEC F65.89
    transvestism F64.1
    voyeurism F65.3
  teeth, midline M26.29
  trachea J39.8
  ureter, congenital Q62.61

Device
  cerebral ventricle (communicating) in situ Z98.2
  contraceptive —*see* Contraceptive, device
  drainage, cerebrospinal fluid, in situ Z98.2

Devic's disease G36.0

Devil's
  grip B33.0
  pinches (purpura simplex) D69.2

Devitalized tooth K04.99

Devonshire colic —*see* Poisoning, lead

Dextraposition, aorta Q20.3
  in tetralogy of Fallot Q21.3

Dextrinosis, limit (debrancher enzyme deficiency) E74.03

Dextrocardia (true) Q24.0
  with
    complete transposition of viscera Q89.3
    situs inversus Q89.3

Dextrotransposition, aorta Q20.3

d-glycericacidemia E72.59

Dhat syndrome F48.8

Dhobi itch B35.6

Di George's syndrome D82.1

Di Guglielmo's disease C94.0-

Diabetes, diabetic (mellitus) (sugar) E11.9
  with
    amyotrophy E11.44
    arthropathy NEC E11.618
    autonomic (poly)neuropathy E11.43
    cataract E11.36
    Charcot's joints E11.610
    chronic kidney disease E11.22
    circulatory complication NEC E11.59
    complication E11.8
      specified NEC E11.69
    dermatitis E11.620
    foot ulcer E11.621
    gangrene E11.52
    gastroparalysis E11.43
    gastroparesis E11.43
    glomerulonephrosis, intracapillary E11.21
    glomerulosclerosis, intercapillary E11.21
    hyperglycemia E11.65
    hyperosmolarity E11.00
      with coma E11.01
    hypoglycemia E11.649
      with coma E11.641
    ketoacidosis E11.10
      with coma E11.11

Diabetes, diabetic (continued)
  with (continued)
    kidney complications NEC E11.29
    Kimmelstiel-Wilson disease E11.21
    loss of protective sensation (LOPS) —*see* Diabetes, by type, with neuropathy
    mononeuropathy E11.41
    myasthenia E11.44
    necrobiosis lipoidica E11.620
    nephropathy E11.21
    neuralgia E11.42
    neurologic complication NEC E11.49
    neuropathic arthropathy E11.610
    neuropathy E11.40
    ophthalmic complication NEC E11.39
    oral complication NEC E11.638
    osteomyelitis E11.69
    periodontal disease E11.630
    peripheral angiopathy E11.51
      with gangrene E11.52
    polyneuropathy E11.42
    renal complication NEC E11.29
    renal tubular degeneration E11.29
    retinopathy E11.319
      with macular edema E11.311
        resolved following treatment E11.37
      nonproliferative E11.329
        with macular edema E11.321
        mild E11.329
          with macular edema E11.321
        moderate E11.339
          with macular edema E11.331
        severe E11.349
          with macular edema E11.341
        with
          combined traction retinal detachment and rhegmatogenous retinal detachment E11.354
          macular edema E11.351
          stable proliferative diabetic retinopathy E11.355
          traction retinal detachment involving the macula E11.352
          traction retinal detachment no involving the macula E11.353
      proliferative E11.359
        with
          combined traction retinal detachment and rhegmatogenous retinal detachment E11.354
          macular edema E11.351
          stable proliferative diabetic retinopathy E11.355
          traction retinal detachment involving the macula E11.352
          traction retinal detachement not involving the macula E11.353
    skin complication NEC E11.628
    skin ulcer NEC E11.622
  brittle —*see* Diabetes, type 1

Diabetes, diabetic *(continued)*

bronzed E83.110
complicating pregnancy —*see*
　Pregnancy, complicated by,
　diabetes
dietary counseling and surveillance
　Z71.3
due to
　autoimmune process —*see*
　　Diabetes, type 1
　immune mediated pancreatic
　　islet beta-cell destruction
　　—*see* Diabetes, type 1
due to drug or chemical E09.9
　with
　　amyotrophy E09.44
　　arthropathy NEC E09.618
　　autonomic (poly)neuropathy
　　　E09.43
　　cataract E09.36
　　Charcot's joints E09.610
　　chronic kidney disease
　　　E09.22
　　circulatory complication NEC
　　　E09.59
　　complication E09.8
　　　specified NEC E09.69
　　dermatitis E09.620
　　foot ulcer E09.621
　　gangrene E09.52
　　gastroparalysis E09.43
　　gastroparesis E09.43
　　glomerulonephrosis,
　　　intracapillary E09.21
　　glomerulosclerosis,
　　　intercapillary E09.21
　　hyperglycemia E09.65
　　hyperosmolarity E09.00
　　　with coma E09.01
　　hypoglycemia E09.649
　　　with coma E09.641
　　ketoacidosis E09.10
　　　with coma E09.11
　　kidney complications NEC
　　　E09.29
　　Kimmelstiel-Wilson disease
　　　E09.21
　　mononeuropathy E09.41
　　myasthenia E09.44
　　necrobiosis lipoidica E09.620
　　nephropathy E09.21
　　neuralgia E09.42
　　neurologic complication NEC
　　　E09.49
　　neuropathic arthropathy
　　　E09.610
　　neuropathy E09.40
　　ophthalmic complication NEC
　　　E09.39
　　oral complication NEC
　　　E09.638
　　periodontal disease E09.630
　　peripheral angiopathy
　　　E09.51
　　　with gangrene E09.52
　　polyneuropathy E09.42
　　renal complication NEC
　　　E09.29
　　renal tubular degeneration
　　　E09.29
　　retinopathy E09.319
　　　with macular edema
　　　　E09.311
　　　resolved following
　　　　treatment E09.37
　　　nonproliferative E09.329
　　　　with macular edema
　　　　　E09.321
　　　　mild E09.329
　　　　　with macular edema
　　　　　　E09.321

Diabetes, diabetic *(continued)*

due to underlying condition
　(continued)
　with *(continued)*
　　retinopathy *(continued)*
　　　nonproliferative *(continued)*
　　　　moderate E09.339
　　　　　with macular edema
　　　　　　E09.331
　　　　severe E09.349
　　　　　with macular edema
　　　　　　E09.341
　　　proliferative E09.359
　　　　with
　　　　　combined traction
　　　　　　retinal detachment
　　　　　　and rhegmatogenous
　　　　　　retinal detachment
　　　　　　E09.354
　　　　　macular edema
　　　　　　E09.351
　　　　　stable proliferative
　　　　　　diabetic retinopathy
　　　　　　E09.355
　　　　　traction retinal
　　　　　　detachment
　　　　　　involving the macula
　　　　　　E09.352
　　　　　traction retinal
　　　　　　detachment not
　　　　　　involving the macula
　　　　　　E09.353
　　skin complication NEC
　　　E09.628
　　skin ulcer NEC E09.622
due to underlying condition
　E08.9
　with
　　amyotrophy E08.44
　　arthropathy NEC E08.618
　　autonomic (poly)neuropathy
　　　E08.43
　　cataract E08.36
　　Charcot's joints E08.610
　　chronic kidney disease
　　　E08.22
　　circulatory complication NEC
　　　E08.59
　　complication E08.8
　　　specified NEC E08.69
　　dermatitis E08.620
　　foot ulcer E08.621
　　gangrene E08.52
　　gastroparalysis E08.43
　　gastroparesis E08.43
　　glomerulonephrosis,
　　　intracapillary E08.21
　　glomerulosclerosis,
　　　intercapillary E08.21
　　hyperglycemia E08.65
　　hyperosmolarity E08.00
　　　with coma E08.01
　　hypoglycemia E08.649
　　　with coma E08.641
　　ketoacidosis E08.10
　　　with coma E08.11
　　kidney complications NEC
　　　E08.29
　　Kimmelstiel-WIlson disease
　　　E08.21
　　mononeuropathy E08.41
　　myasthenia E08.44
　　necrobiosis lipoidica E08.620
　　nephropathy E08.21
　　neuralgia E08.42
　　neurologic complication NEC
　　　E08.49
　　neuropathic arthropathy E08.610
　　neuropathy E08.40
　　ophthalmic complication NEC
　　　E08.39

Diabetes, diabetic *(continued)*

due to underlying condition
　(continued)
　　oral complication NEC E08.638
　　periodontal disease E08.630
　　peripheral angiopathy E08.51
　　　with gangrene E08.52
　　polyneuropathy E08.42
　　renal complication NEC
　　　E08.29
　　renal tubular degeneration
　　　E08.29
　　retinopathy E08.319
　　　with macular edema
　　　　E08.311
　　　resolved following
　　　　treatment E08.37
　　　nonproliferative E08.329
　　　　with macular edema
　　　　　E08.321
　　　　mild E08.329
　　　　　with macular edema
　　　　　　E08.321
　　　　moderate E08.339
　　　　　with macular edema
　　　　　　E08.331
　　　　severe E08.349
　　　　　with macular edema
　　　　　　E08.341
　　　proliferative E08.359
　　　　with
　　　　　combined traction
　　　　　　retinal detachment
　　　　　　and rhegmatogenous
　　　　　　retinal detachment
　　　　　　E08.354
　　　　　macular edema E08.351
　　　　　stable proliferative
　　　　　　diabetic retinopathy
　　　　　　E08.355
　　　　　traction retinal
　　　　　　detachment
　　　　　　involving the macula
　　　　　　E08.352
　　　　　traction retinal
　　　　　　detachment not
　　　　　　involving the macula
　　　　　　E08.353
　　skin complication NEC E08.628
　　skin ulcer NEC E08.622
gestational (in pregnancy) O24.419
　affecting newborn P70.0
　diet controlled O24.410
　in childbirth O24.429
　　diet controlled O24.420
　　insulin (and diet) controlled
　　　O24.424
　　oral drug controlled
　　　(antidiabetic)
　　　(hypoglycemic) O24.425
　oral drug controlled
　　(antidiabetic) (hypoglycemic)
　　O24.415
　insulin (and diet) controlled
　　O24.414
　puerperal O24.439
　　diet controlled O24.430
　　insulin (and diet) controlled
　　　O24.434
　　oral drug controlled
　　　(antidiabetic)
　　　(hypoglycemic) O24.435
hepatogenous E13.9
idiopathic —*see* Diabetes, type 1
inadequately controlled - code
　to Diabetes, by type, with
　hyperglycemia
insipidus E23.2
　nephrogenic N25.1
　pituitary E23.2
　vasopressin resistant N25.1

Diabetes, diabetic *(continued)*

insulin dependent - code to type of
　diabetes
juvenile-onset —*see* Diabetes, type 1
ketosis-prone —*see* Diabetes, type 1
latent R73.03
neonatal (transient) P70.2
non-insulin dependent - code to
　type of diabetes
out of control - code to Diabetes,
　by type, with hyperglycemia
phosphate E83.39
poorly controlled - code to
　Diabetes, by type, with
　hyperglycemia
postpancreatectomy —*see*
　Diabetes, specified type NEC
postprocedural —*see* Diabetes,
　specified type NEC
secondary diabetes mellitus NEC
　—*see* Diabetes, specified type
　NEC
specified type NEC E13.9
　with
　　amyotrophy E13.44
　　arthropathy NEC E13.618
　　autonomic (poly)neuropathy
　　　E13.43
　　cataract E13.36
　　Charcot's joints E13.610
　　chronic kidney disease
　　　E13.22
　　circulatory complication NEC
　　　E13.59
　　complication E13.8
　　　specified NEC E13.69
　　dermatitis E13.620
　　foot ulcer E13.621
　　gangrene E13.52
　　gastroparalysis E13.43
　　gastroparesis E13.43
　　glomerulonephrosis,
　　　intracapillary E13.21
　　glomerulosclerosis,
　　　intercapillary E13.21
　　hyperglycemia E13.65
　　hyperosmolarity E13.00
　　　with coma E13.01
　　hypoglycemia E13.649
　　　with coma E13.641
　　ketoacidosis E13.10
　　　with coma E13.11
　　kidney complications NEC
　　　E13.29
　　Kimmelstiel-Wilson disease
　　　E13.21
　　mononeuropathy E13.41
　　myasthenia E13.44
　　necrobiosis lipoidica E13.620
　　nephropathy E13.21
　　neuralgia E13.42
　　neurologic complication NEC
　　　E13.49
　　neuropathic arthropathy E13.610
　　neuropathy E13.40
　　ophthalmic complication NEC
　　　E13.39
　　oral complication NEC
　　　E13.638
　　periodontal disease E13.630
　　peripheral angiopathy E13.51
　　　with gangrene E13.52
　　polyneuropathy E13.42
　　renal complication NEC
　　　E13.29
　　renal tubular degeneration
　　　E13.29
　　retinopathy E13.319
　　　with macular edema E13.311
　　　resolved following
　　　　treatment E13.37

specified type NEC *(continued)*
  with *(continued)*
    retinopathy *(continued)*
      nonproliferative E13.329
        with macular edema
          E13.321
        mild E13.329
          with macular edema
            E13.321
        moderate E13.339
          with macular edema
            E13.331
        severe E13.349
          with macular edema
            E13.341
      proliferative E13.359
        with
          combined traction
            retinal detachment
            and rhegmatogenous
            retinal detachment
            E13.354
          macular edema
            E13.351
          stable proliferative
            diabetic retinopathy
            E13.355
          traction retinal
            detachment
            involving the macula
            E13.352
          traction retinal
            detachment not
            involving the macula
            E13.353
    skin complication NEC
      E13.628
    skin ulcer NEC E13.622
steroid-induced —*see* Diabetes,
  due to, drug or chemical
type 1 E10.9
  with
    amyotrophy E10.44
    arthropathy NEC E10.618
    autonomic (poly)neuropathy
      E10.43
    cataract E10.36
    Charcot's joints E10.610
    chronic kidney disease E10.22
    circulatory complication NEC
      E10.59
    complication E10.8
      specified NEC E10.69
    dermatitis E10.620
    foot ulcer E10.621
    gangrene E10.52
    gastroparalysis E10.43
    gastroparesis E10.43
    glomerulonephrosis,
      intracapillary E10.21
    glomerulosclerosis,
      intercapillary E10.21
    hyperglycemia E10.65
    hypoglycemia E10.649
      with coma E10.641
    ketoacidosis E10.10
      with coma E10.11
    kidney complications NEC
      E10.29
    Kimmelsteil-Wilson disease
      E10.21
    mononeuropathy E10.41
    myasthenia E10.44
    necrobiosis lipoidica E10.620
    nephropathy E10.21
    neuralgia E10.42
    neurologic complication NEC
      E10.49
    neuropathic arthropathy E10.610
    neuropathy E10.40

type 1 *(continued)*
  with *(continued)*
    ophthalmic complication NEC
      E10.39
    oral complication NEC
      E10.638
    osteomyelitis E10.69
    periodontal disease E10.630
    peripheral angiopathy E10.51
      with gangrene E10.52
    polyneuropathy E10.42
    renal complication NEC
      E10.29
    renal tubular degeneration
      E10.29
    retinopathy E10.319
      with macular edema
        E10.311
      resolved following
        treatment E10.37
      nonproliferative E10.329
        with macular edema
          E10.321
        mild E10.329
          with macular edema
            E10.321
        moderate E10.339
          with macular edema
            E10.331
        severe E10.349
          with macular edema
            E10.341
      proliferative E10.359
        with
          combined traction
            retinal detachment
            and rhegmatogenous
            retinal detachment
            E10.354
        with
          macular edema
            E10.351
          stable proliferative
            diabetic retinopathy
            E10.355
          traction retinal
            detachment
            involving the macula
            E10.352
          traction retinal
            detachment not
            involving the macula
            E10.353
    skin complication NEC E10.628
    skin ulcer NEC E10.622
type 2 E11.9
  with
    amyotrophy E11.44
    arthropathy NEC E11.618
    autonomic (poly)neuropathy
      E11.43
    cataract E11.36
    Charcot's joints E11.610
    chronic kidney disease E11.22
    circulatory complication NEC
      E11.59
    complication E11.8
      specified NEC E11.69
    dermatitis E11.620
    foot ulcer E11.621
    gangrene E11.52
    gastroparalysis E11.43
    gastroparesis E11.43
    glomerulonephrosis,
      intracapillary E11.21
    glomerulosclerosis,
      intercapillary E11.21
    hyperglycemia E11.65
    hyperosmolarity E11.00
      with coma E11.01

type 2 *(continued)*
  with *(continued)*
    hypoglycemia E11.649
      with coma E11.641
    ketoacidosis E11.10
      with coma E11.11
    kidney complications NEC
      E11.29
    Kimmelsteil-Wilson disease
      E11.21
    mononeuropathy E11.41
    myasthenia E11.44
    necrobiosis lipoidica E11.620
    nephropathy E11.21
    neuralgia E11.42
    neurologic complication NEC
      E11.49
    neuropathic arthropathy
      E11.610
    neuropathy E11.40
    ophthalmic complication NEC
      E11.39
    oral complication NEC
      E11.638
    osteomyelitis E11.69
    periodontal disease E11.630
    peripheral angiopathy E11.51
      with gangrene E11.52
    polyneuropathy E11.42
    renal complication NEC
      E11.29
    renal tubular degeneration
      E11.29
    retinopathy E11.319
      with macular edema
        E11.311
      resolved following
        treatment E11.37
      nonproliferative E11.329
        with macular edema
          E11.321
        mild E11.329
          with macular edema
            E11.321
        moderate E11.339
          with macular edema
            E11.331
        severe E11.349
          with macular edema
            E11.341
      proliferative E11.359
        with
          combined traction
            retinal detachment
            and rhegmatogenous
            retinal detachment
            E11.354
          macular edema
            E11.351
          stable proliferative
            diabetic retinopathy
            E11.355
          traction retinal
            detachment
            involving the macula
            E11.352
          traction retinal
            detachment not
            involving the macula
            E11.353
    skin complication NEC E11.628
    skin ulcer NEC E11.622
  uncontrolled
  meaning
  hyperglycemia —*see* Diabetes, by
    type, with, hyperglycemia
  hypoglycemia —*see* Diabetes, by
    type, with, hypoglycemia

Diacyclothrombopathia D69.1

Diagnosis deferred R69

Dialysis (intermittent) (treatment)
  noncompliance (with) Z91.15
  renal (hemodialysis) (peritoneal),
    status Z99.2
  retina, retinal —*see* Detachment,
    retina, with retinal, dialysis

Diamond-Blackfan anemia
  (congenital hypoplastic) D61.01

Diamond-Gardener syndrome
  (autoerythrocyte sensitization)
  D69.2

Diaper rash L22

Diaphoresis (excessive) R61

Diaphragm —*see* condition

Diaphragmalgia R07.1

Diaphragmatitis, diaphragmitis
  J98.6

Diaphysial aclasis Q78.6

Diaphysitis —*see* Osteomyelitis,
  specified type NEC

Diarrhea, diarrheal (disease)
  (infantile) (inflammatory) R19.7
  achlorhydric K31.83
  allergic K52.29
    due to
      colitis —*see* Colitis, allergic
      enteritis —*see* Enteritis, allergic
  amebic (*see also* Amebiasis) A06.0
    with abscess —*see* Abscess,
      amebic
    acute A06.0
    chronic A06.1
    nondysenteric A06.2
  bacillary —*see* Dysentery, bacillary
  balantidial A07.0
  cachectic NEC K52.89
  Chilomastix A07.8
  choleriformis A00.1
  chronic (noninfectious) K52.9
  coccidial A07.3
  Cochin-China K90.1
    strongyloidiasis B78.0
  Dientamoeba A07.8
  dietetic (*see also* Diarrhea, allergic)
    K52.29
  drug-induced K52.1
  due to
    bacteria A04.9
      specified NEC A04.8
    Campylobacter A04.5
    Capillaria philippinensis B81.1
    Clostridium difficile
      not specified as recurrent A04.72
      recurrent A04.71
    Clostridium perfringens (C) (F)
      A04.8
    Cryptosporidium A07.2
    drugs K52.1
    Escherichia coli A04.4
      enteroaggregative A04.4
      enterohemorrhagic A04.3
      enteroinvasive A04.2
      enteropathogenic A04.0
      enterotoxigenic A04.1
      specified NEC A04.4
    food hypersensitivity (*see also*
      Diarrhea, allergic) K52.29
    Necator americanus B76.1
    S. japonicum B65.2
    specified organism NEC A08.8
      bacterial A04.8
      viral A08.39
    Staphylococcus A04.8
    Trichuris trichiuria B79
    virus —*see* Enteritis, viral
    Yersinia enterocolitica A04.6
  dysenteric A09

Diarrhea, diarrheal (continued)
endemic A09
epidemic A09
flagellate A07.9
Flexner's (ulcerative) A03.1
functional K59.1
  following gastrointestinal
    surgery K91.89
  psychogenic F45.8
Giardia lamblia A07.1
giardial A07.1
hill K90.1
infectious A09
malarial —see Malaria
mite B88.0
mycotic NEC B49
neonatal (noninfectious) P78.3
nervous F45.8
neurogenic K59.1
noninfectious K52.9
postgastrectomy K91.1
postvagotomy K91.1
protozoal A07.9
  specified NEC A07.8
psychogenic F45.8
specified
  bacterium NEC A04.8
  virus NEC A08.39
strongyloidiasis B78.0
toxic K52.1
trichomonal A07.8
tropical K90.1
tuberculous A18.32
viral —see Enteritis, viral

Diastasis
cranial bones M84.88
  congenital NEC Q75.8
joint (traumatic) —see Dislocation
muscle M62.00
  ankle M62.07-
  congenital Q79.8
  foot M62.07-
  forearm M62.03-
  hand M62.04-
  lower leg M62.06-
  pelvic region M62.05-
  shoulder region M62.01-
  specified site NEC M62.08
  thigh M62.05-
  upper arm M62.02-
recti (abdomen)
  complicating delivery O71.89
  congenital Q79.59

Diastema, tooth, teeth, fully erupted M26.32

Diastematomyelia Q06.2

Diataxia, cerebral G80.4

Diathesis
allergic —see History, allergy
bleeding (familial) D69.9
cystine (familial) E72.00
gouty —see Gout
hemorrhagic (familial) D69.9
  newborn NEC P53
spasmophilic R29.0

Diaz's disease or osteochondrosis
(juvenile) (talus) —see
Osteochondrosis, juvenile, tarsus

**Dibothriocephalus,
dibothriocephaliasis** (latus)
(infection) (infestation) B70.0
larval B70.1

Dicephalus, dicephaly Q89.4

Dichotomy, teeth K00.2

Dichromat, dichromatopsia
(congenital) —see Deficiency,
color vision

Dichuchwa A65

Dicroceliasis B66.2

Didelphia, didelphys —see Double
uterus

Didymytis N45.1
with orchitis N45.3

Dietary
inadequacy or deficiency E63.9
surveillance and counseling Z71.3

Dietl's crisis N13.8

Dieulafoy lesion (hemorrhagic)
duodenum K31.82
esophagus K22.8
intestine (colon) K63.81
stomach K31.82

Difficult, difficulty (in)
acculturation Z60.3
feeding R63.3
  newborn P92.9
    breast P92.5
    specified NEC P92.8
  nonorganic (infant or child) F98.29
intubation, in anesthesia T88.4
mechanical, gastroduodenal stoma
  K91.89
  causing obstruction (see also
    Obstruction, intestine,
    postoperative) K91.30
micturition
  need to immediately re-void
    R39.191
  position dependent R39.192
  specified NEC R39.198
reading (developmental) F81.0
  secondary to emotional disorders
    F93.9
spelling (specific) F81.81
  with reading disorder F81.89
  due to inadequate teaching Z55.8
swallowing —see Dysphagia
walking R26.2
work
  conditions NEC Z56.5
  schedule Z56.3

Diffuse —see condition

DiGeorge's syndrome (thymic
hypoplasia) D82.1

Digestive —see condition

**Dihydropyrimidine dehydrogenase
disease** (DPD) E88.89

Diktyoma —see Neoplasm,
malignant, by site

Dilaceration, tooth K00.4

Dilatation
anus K59.89
  venule —see Hemorrhoids
aorta (focal) (general) —see
  Ectasia, aorta
  with aneuysm —see Aneurysm,
    aorta
  congenital Q25.44
artery —see Aneurysm
bladder (sphincter) N32.89
  congenital Q64.79
blood vessel I99.8
bronchial J47.9
  with
    exacerbation (acute) J47.1
    lower respiratory infection J47.0
calyx (due to obstruction) —see
  Hydronephrosis
capillaries I78.8
cardiac (acute) (chronic) —see also
  Hypertrophy, cardiac
  congenital Q24.8
    valve NEC Q24.8
      pulmonary Q22.3
  valve —see Endocarditis

Dilatation (continued)
cavum septi pellucidi Q06.8
cervix (uteri) —see also
  Incompetency, cervix
  incomplete, poor, slow
    complicating delivery O62.0
colon K59.39
  congenital Q43.1
  psychogenic F45.8
  toxic K59.31
common duct (acquired) K83.8
  congenital Q44.5
cystic duct (acquired) K82.8
  congenital Q44.5
duct, mammary —see Ectasia,
  mammary duct
duodenum K59.89
esophagus K22.8
  congenital Q39.5
  due to achalasia K22.0
eustachian tube, congenital
  Q17.8
gallbladder K82.8
gastric —see Dilatation, stomach
heart (acute) (chronic) —see also
  Hypertrophy, cardiac
  congenital Q24.8
  valve —see Endocarditis
ileum K59.89
  psychogenic F45.8
jejunum K59.89
  psychogenic F45.8
kidney (calyx) (collecting
  structures) (cystic)
  (parenchyma) (pelvis)
  (idiopathic) N28.89
lacrimal passages or duct —see
  Disorder, lacrimal system,
  changes
lymphatic vessel I89.0
mammary duct —see Ectasia,
  mammary duct
Meckel's diverticulum (congenital)
  Q43.0
  malignant —see Table of
    Neoplasms, small intestine,
    malignant
myocardium (acute) (chronic)
  —see Hypertrophy, cardiac
organ or site, congenital NEC
  —see Distortion
pancreatic duct K86.89
pericardium —see Pericarditis
pharynx J39.2
prostate N42.89
pulmonary
  artery (idiopathic) I28.8
  valve, congenital Q22.3
pupil H57.04
rectum K59.39
saccule, congenital Q16.5
salivary gland (duct) K11.8
sphincter ani K62.89
stomach K31.89
  acute K31.0
  psychogenic F45.8
submaxillary duct K11.8
trachea, congenital Q32.1
ureter (idiopathic) N28.82
  congenital Q62.2
  due to obstruction N13.4
urethra (acquired) N36.8
vasomotor I73.9
vein I86.8
ventricular, ventricle (acute)
  (chronic) —see also Hypertrophy,
  cardiac
  cerebral, congenital Q04.8
venule NEC I86.8
vesical orifice N32.89

Dilated, dilation —see Dilatation

Diminished, diminution
hearing (acuity) —see Deafness
sense or sensation (cold) (heat)
  (tactile) (vibratory) R20.8
vision NEC H54.7
vital capacity R94.2

Diminuta taenia B71.0

Dimitri-Sturge-Weber disease
Q85.8

Dimple
congenital sacral Q82.6
parasacral Q82.6
pilonidal or postanal —see Cyst,
  pilonidal

Dioctophyme renalis (infection)
(infestation) B83.8

Dipetalonemiasis B74.4

Diphallus Q55.69

Diphtheria, diphtheritic
(gangrenous) (hemorrhagic)
A36.9
carrier (suspected) Z22.2
cutaneous A36.3
faucial A36.0
infection of wound A36.3
laryngeal A36.2
myocarditis A36.81
nasal, anterior A36.89
nasopharyngeal A36.1
neurological complication A36.89
pharyngeal A36.0
specified site NEC A36.89
tonsillar A36.0

Diphyllobothriasis (intestine) B70.0
larval B70.1

Diplacusis H93.22-

Diplegia (upper limbs) G83.0
congenital (cerebral) G80.8
facial G51.0
lower limbs G82.20
spastic G80.1

Diplococcus, diplococcal —see
condition

Diplopia H53.2

Dipsomania F10.20
with
  psychosis —see Psychosis,
    alcoholic
  remission F10.21

Dipylidiasis B71.1

**DIRA (deficiency of interleukin 1
receptor antagonist)** M04.8

**Direction, teeth, abnormal, fully
erupted** M26.30

Dirofilariasis B74.8

Dirt-eating child F98.3

Disability, disabilities
heart —see Disease, heart
intellectual F79
  with
    autistic features F84.9
  mild (I.Q.50-69) F70
  moderate (I.Q.35-49) F71
  profound (I.Q. under 20) F73
  severe (I.Q.20-34) F72
  specified level NEC F78
knowledge acquisition F81.9
learning F81.9
limiting activities Z73.6
spelling, specific F81.81

Disappearance of family member
Z63.4

Disarticulation —see Amputation
meaning traumatic amputation
  —see Amputation, traumatic

Discharge (from)
abnormal finding in —see
  Abnormal, specimen
breast (female) (male) N64.52
diencephalic autonomic idiopathic
  —see Epilepsy, specified NEC
ear —see also Otorrhea
  blood —see Otorrhagia
excessive urine R35.8
nipple N64.52
penile R36.9
postnasal R09.82
prison, anxiety concerning Z65.2
urethral R36.9
  without blood R36.0
  hematospermia R36.1
vaginal N89.8

Discitis, diskitis M46.40
cervical region M46.42
cervicothoracic region M46.43
lumbar region M46.46
lumbosacral region M46.47
multiple sites M46.49
occipito-atlanto-axial region M46.41
pyogenic —see Infection,
  intervertebral disc, pyogenic
sacrococcygeal region M46.48
thoracic region M46.44
thoracolumbar region M46.45

Discoid
meniscus (congenital) Q68.6
semilunar cartilage (congenital)
  —see Derangement, knee,
  meniscus, specified NEC

Discoloration
nails L60.8
teeth (posteruptive) K03.7
  during formation K00.8

Discomfort
chest R07.89
visual H53.14-

Discontinuity, ossicles, ear H74.2-

Discord (with)
boss Z56.4
classmates Z55.4
counselor Z64.4
employer Z56.4
family Z63.8
fellow employees Z56.4
in-laws Z63.1
landlord Z59.2
lodgers Z59.2
neighbors Z59.2
probation officer Z64.4
social worker Z64.4
teachers Z55.4
workmates Z56.4

Discordant connection
atrioventricular (congenital) Q20.5
ventriculoarterial Q20.3

Discrepancy
centric occlusion maximum
  intercuspation M26.55
leg length (acquired) —see
  Deformity, limb, unequal length
  congenital —see Defect,
  reduction, lower limb
uterine size date O26.84-

Discrimination
ethnic Z60.5
political Z60.5
racial Z60.5
religious Z60.5
sex Z60.5

Disease, diseased —see also
Syndrome
absorbent system I87.8

Discitis, diskitis (continued)
acid-peptic K30
Acosta's T70.29
Adams-Stokes (-Morgagni)
  (syncope with heart block) I45.9
Addison's anemia (pernicious)
  D51.0
adenoids (and tonsils) J35.9
adrenal (capsule) (cortex) (gland)
  (medullary) E27.9
  hyperfunction E27.0
  specified NEC E27.8
ainhum L94.6
airway
  obstructive, chronic J44.9
    due to
      cotton dust J66.0
      specific organic dusts NEC
        J66.8
  reactive —see Asthma
akamushi (scrub typhus) A75.3
Albers-Schönberg (marble bones)
  Q78.2
Albert's —see Tendinitis, Achilles
alimentary canal K63.9
alligator-skin Q80.9
  acquired L85.0
alpha heavy chain C88.3
alpine T70.29
altitude T70.20
alveolar ridge
  edentulous K06.9
    specified NEC K06.8
alveoli, teeth K08.9
Alzheimer's G30.9 [F02.80]
  with behavioral disturbance
    G30.9 [F02.81]
  early onset G30.0 [F02.80]
    with behavioral disturbance
      G30.0 [F02.81]
  late onset G30.1 [F02.80]
    with behavioral disturbance
      G30.1 [F02.81]
  specified NEC G30.8 [F02.80]
    with behavioral disturbance
      G30.8 [F02.81]
amyloid —see Amyloidosis
Andersen's (glycogenosis IV)
  E74.09
Andes T70.29
Andrews'(bacterid) L08.89
angiospastic I73.9
  cerebral G45.9
  vein I87.8
anterior
  chamber H21.9
  horn cell G12.29
antiglomerular basement membrane
  (anti- GBM) antibody M31.0
  tubulo-interstitial nephritis N12
antral —see Sinusitis, maxillary
anus K62.9
  specified NEC K62.89
aorta (nonsyphilitic) I77.9
  syphilitic NEC A52.02
aortic (heart) (valve) I35.9
  rheumatic I06.9
Apollo B30.3
aponeuroses —see Enthesopathy
appendix K38.9
  specified NEC K38.8
aqueous (chamber) H21.9
Arnold-Chiari —see Arnold-Chiari
  disease
arterial I77.9
  occlusive —see Occlusion, by
    site
    due to stricture or stenosis
      I77.1
  peripheral I73.9

Disease, diseased (continued)
arteriocardiorenal —see
  Hypertension, cardiorenal
arteriolar (generalized)
  (obliterative) I77.9
arteriorenal —see Hypertension, kidney
arteriosclerotic —see also
  Arteriosclerosis
  cardiovascular —see
    Disease, heart, ischemic,
    atherosclerotic
  coronary (artery) —see
    Disease, heart, ischemic,
    atherosclerotic
  heart —see Disease, heart,
    ischemic, atherosclerotic
artery I77.9
  cerebral I67.9
  coronary I25.10
    with angina pectoris —see
      Arteriosclerosis, coronary
      (artery)
  peripheral I73.9
arthropod-borne NOS (viral) A94
  specified type NEC A93.8
atticoantral, chronic H66.20
  left H66.22
    with right H66.23
  right H66.21
    with left H66.23
auditory canal —see Disorder, ear,
  external
auricle, ear NEC —see Disorder,
  pinna
Australian X A83.4
autoimmune (systemic) NOS M35.9
  hemolytic D59.10
    cold type (primary)
      (secondary) (symptomatic)
      D59.12
    drug-induced D59.0
    mixed type (primary)
      (secondary) (symptomatic)
      D59.13
    warm type (primary)
      (secondary) (symptomatic)
      D59.11
  thyroid E06.3
autoinflammatory M04.9
  NOD2-associated M04.8
  specified type NEC M04.8
aviator's —see Effect, adverse,
  high altitude
Ayerza's (pulmonary artery sclerosis
  with pulmonary hypertension) I27.0
Babington's (familial hemorrhagic
  telangiectasia) I78.0
bacterial A49.9
  specified NEC A48.8
  zoonotic A28.9
    specified type NEC A28.8
Baelz's (cheilitis glandularis
  apostematosa) K13.0
bagasse J67.1
balloon —see Effect, adverse, high
  altitude
Bang's (brucella abortus) A23.1
Bannister's T78.3
barometer makers' —see
  Poisoning, mercury
Barraquer (-Simons') (progressive
  lipodystrophy) E88.1
Barrett's —see Barrett's, esophagus
Bartholin's gland N75.9
basal ganglia G25.9
  degenerative G23.9
    specified NEC G23.8
  specified NEC G25.89
Basedow's (exophthalmic goiter)
  —see Hyperthyroidism, with,
  goiter (diffuse)

Disease, diseased (continued)
Bateman's B08.1
Batten-Steinert G71.11
Battey A31.0
Beard's (neurasthenia) F48.8
Becker
  idiopathic mural endomyocardial
    I42.3
  myotonia congenita G71.12
Begbie's (exophthalmic goiter)
  —see Hyperthyroidism, with,
  goiter (diffuse)
behavioral, organic F07.9
Beigel's (white piedra) B36.2
Benson's —see Deposit,
  crystalline
Bernard-Soulier (thrombopathy)
  D69.1
Bernhardt (-Roth) —see
  Mononeuropathy, lower limb,
  meralgia paresthetica
Biermer's (pernicious anemia)
  D51.0
bile duct (common) (hepatic)
  K83.9
  with calculus, stones —see
    Calculus, bile duct
  specified NEC K83.8
biliary (tract) K83.9
  specified NEC K83.8
Billroth's —see Spina bifida
bird fancier's J67.2
black lung J60
bladder N32.9
  in (due to)
    schistosomiasis (bilharziasis)
      B65.0 [N33]
  specified NEC N32.89
bleeder's D66
blood D75.9
  forming organs D75.9
  vessel I99.9
Bloodgood's —see Mastopathy,
  cystic
Blount M92.51-
Bodechtel-Guttmann (subacute
  sclerosing panencephalitis)
  A81.1
bone —see also Disorder, bone
  aluminum M83.4
  fibrocystic NEC
    jaw M27.49
bone-marrow D75.9
Borna A83.9
Bornholm (epidemic pleurodynia)
  B33.0
Bouchard's
  (myopathic dilatation of the
  stomach) K31.0
Bouillaud's (rheumatic heart
  disease) I01.9
Bourneville (-Brissaud) (tuberous
  sclerosis) Q85.1
Bouveret (-Hoffmann)
  (paroxysmal tachycardia) I47.9
bowel K63.9
  functional K59.9
    psychogenic F45.8
brain G93.9
  arterial, artery I67.9
  arteriosclerotic I67.2
  congenital Q04.9
  degenerative —see
    Degeneration, brain
  inflammatory —see
    Encephalitis
  organic G93.9
    arteriosclerotic I67.2
  parasitic NEC B71.9 [G94]
  senile NEC G31.1
  specified NEC G93.89

breast —*see also* Disorder, breast
N64.9
   cystic (chronic) —*see*
      Mastopathy, cystic
   fibrocystic —*see* Mastopathy,
      cystic
   Paget's
      female, unspecified side
         C50.91-
      male, unspecified side
         C50.92-
   specified NEC N64.89
Breda's —*see* Yaws
Bretonneau's (diphtheritic
   malignant angina) A36.0
Bright's —*see* Nephritis
   arteriosclerotic —*see*
      Hypertension, kidney
Brill's (recrudescent typhus)
   A75.1
Brill-Zinsser (recrudescent typhus)
   A75.1
Brion-Kayser —*see* Fever,
   paratyphoid
broad
   beta E78.2
   ligament (noninflammatory)
      N83.9
      inflammatory —*see* Disease,
         pelvis, inflammatory
      specified NEC N83.8
Brocq-Duhring (dermatitis
   herpetiformis) L13.0
Brocq's
   meaning
      dermatitis herpetiformis L13.0
      prurigo L28.2
bronchopulmonary J98.4
bronchus NEC J98.09
bronze Addison's E27.1
   tuberculous A18.7
budgerigar fancier's J67.2
bullous L13.9
   chronic of childhood L12.2
   specified NEC L13.8
Buerger's (thromboangiitis
   obliterans) I73.1
Bürger-Grütz (essential familial
   hyperlipemia) E78.3
bursa —*see* Bursopathy
caisson T70.3
California —*see*
   Coccidioidomycosis
capillaries I78.9
   specified NEC I78.8
Carapata A68.0
cardiac —*see* Disease, heart
cardiopulmonary, chronic I27.9
cardiorenal (hepatic) (hypertensive)
   (vascular) —*see* Hypertension,
   cardiorenal
cardiovascular (atherosclerotic)
   I25.10
   with angina pectoris —*see*
      Arteriosclerosis, coronary
      (artery),
   congenital Q28.9
   newborn P29.9
      specified NEC P29.89
   hypertensive —*see*
      Hypertension, heart
   renal (hypertensive) —*see*
      Hypertension, cardiorenal
   syphilitic (asymptomatic) A52.00
cartilage —*see* Disorder, cartilage
Castellani's A69.8
Castleman (unicentric)
   (multicentric) D47.Z2
   HHV-8-associated (*see also*
      Herpesvirus, human, 8) D47.Z2

cat-scratch A28.1
Cavare's (familial periodic
   paralysis) G72.3
cecum K63.9
celiac (adult) (infantile) (with
   steatorrhea) K90.0
cellular tissue L98.9
central core G71.29
cerebellar, cerebellum —*see*
   Disease, brain
cerebral —*see also* Disease, brain
   degenerative —*see*
      Degeneration, brain
cerebrospinal G96.9
cerebrovascular I67.9
   acute I67.89
      embolic I63.4-
      thrombotic I63.3-
   arteriosclerotic I67.2
   hereditary NEC I67.858
   specified NEC I67.89
cervix (uteri) (noninflammatory)
   N88.9
   inflammatory —*see* Cervicitis
   specified NEC N88.8
Chabert's A22.9
Chandler's (osteochondritis
   dissecans, hip) —*see*
   Osteochondritis, dissecans, hip
Charlouis —*see* Yaws
Chédiak-Steinbrinck (-Higashi)
   (congenital gigantism of
   peroxidase granules) E70.330
chest J98.9
Chiari's (hepatic vein thrombosis)
   I82.0
Chicago B40.9
Chignon B36.8
chigo, chigoe B88.1
childhood granulomatous D71
Chinese liver fluke B66.1
chlamydial A74.9
   specified NEC A74.89
cholecystic K82.9
choroid H31.9
   specified NEC H31.8
Christmas D67
chronic bullous of childhood
   L12.2
chylomicron retention E78.3
ciliary body H21.9
   specified NEC H21.89
circulatory (system) NEC I99.8
   newborn P29.9
   syphilitic A52.00
      congenital A50.54
coagulation factor deficiency
   (congenital) —*see* Defect,
   coagulation
coccidioidal —*see*
   Coccidioidomycosis
cold
   agglutinin or hemoglobinuria
      D59.12
      paroxysmal D59.6
   hemagglutinin (chronic)
      D59.12
collagen NOS (nonvascular)
   (vascular) M35.9
   specified NEC M35.8
colon K63.9
   functional K59.9
      congenital Q43.2
   ischemic (*see also* Ischemia,
      intestine, acute) K55.039
colonic inflammatory bowel,
   unclassified (IBDU) K52.3
combined system —*see*
   Degeneration, combined
compressed air T70.3

Concato's (pericardial
   polyserositis) A19.9
   nontubercular I31.1
   pleural —*see* Pleurisy, with effusion
conjunctiva H11.9
   chlamydial A74.0
   specified NEC H11.89
   viral B30.9
      specified NEC B30.8
connective tissue, systemic
   (diffuse) M35.9
   in (due to)
      hypogammaglobulinemia
         D80.1 *[M36.8]*
      ochronosis E70.29 *[M36.8]*
   specified NEC M35.8
Conor and Bruch's (boutonneuse
   fever) A77.1
Cooper's —*see* Mastopathy, cystic
Cori's (glycogenosis III) E74.03
corkhandler's or corkworker's J67.3
cornea H18.9
   specified NEC H18.89-
coronary (artery) —*see* Disease,
   heart, ischemic, atherosclerotic
   congenital Q24.5
   ostial, syphilitic (aortic) (mitral)
      (pulmonary) A52.03
corpus cavernosum N48.9
   specified NEC N48.89
Cotugno's —*see* Sciatica
COVID-19 U07.1
coxsackie (virus) NEC B34.1
cranial nerve NOS G52.9
Creutzfeldt-Jakob —*see*
   Creutzfeldt-Jakob disease or
   syndrome
Crocq's (acrocyanosis) I73.89
Crohn's —*see* Enteritis, regional
Curschmann G71.11
cystic
   breast (chronic) —*see*
      Mastopathy, cystic
   kidney, congenital Q61.9
   liver, congenital Q44.6
   lung J98.4
      congenital Q33.0
cytomegalic inclusion (generalized)
   B25.9
   with pneumonia B25.0
   congenital P35.1
cytomegaloviral B25.9
   specified NEC B25.8
Czerny's (periodic hydrarthrosis of the
   knee) —*see* Effusion, joint, knee
Daae (-Finsen) (epidemic
   pleurodynia) B33.0
Darling's —*see* Histoplasmosis
   capsulati
Débove's (splenomegaly) R16.1
deer fly —*see* Tularemia
Degos' I77.89
demyelinating, demyelinizating
   (nervous system) G37.9
   multiple sclerosis G35
   specified NEC G37.8
dense deposit (*see also* N00-N07
   with fourth character .6) N05.6
deposition, hydroxyapatite —
   see Disease, hydroxyapatite
   deposition
de Quervain's (tendon sheath)
   M65.4
   thyroid (subacute granulomatous
      thyroiditis) E06.1
Devergie's (pityriasis rubra pilaris)
   L44.0
Devic's G36.0
diaphorase deficiency D74.0
diaphragm J98.6

diarrheal, infectious NEC A09
digestive system K92.9
   specified NEC K92.89
disc, degenerative —*see*
   Degeneration, intervertebral disc
discogenic —*see also*
   Displacement, intervertebral disc
   NEC
   with myelopathy —*see* Disorder,
      disc, with, myelopathy
diverticular —*see* Diverticula
Dubois (thymus) A50.59 *[E35]*
Duchenne-Griesinger G71.01
Duchenne's
   muscular dystrophy G71.01
   pseudohypertrophy, muscles
      G71.01
ductless glands E34.9
Duhring's (dermatitis
   herpetiformis) L13.0
duodenum K31.9
   specified NEC K31.89
Dupré's (meningism) R29.1
Dupuytren's (muscle contracture)
   M72.0
Durand-Nicholas-Favre (climatic
   bubo) A55
Duroziez's (congenital mitral
   stenosis) Q23.2
ear —*see* Disorder, ear
Eberth's —*see* Fever, typhoid
Ebola (virus) A98.4
Ebstein's heart Q22.5
Echinococcus —*see* Echinococcus
echovirus NEC B34.1
Eddowes' (brittle bones and blue
   sclera) Q78.0
edentulous (alveolar) ridge K06.9
   specified NEC K06.8
Edsall's T67.2
Eichstedt's (pityriasis versicolor)
   B36.0
Eisenmenger's (irreversible) I27.83
Ellis-van Creveld (chondroectodermal
   dysplasia) Q77.6
end stage renal (ESRD) N18.6
   due to hypertension I12.0
endocrine glands or system NEC
   E34.9
endomyocardial (eosinophilic) I42.3
English (rickets) E55.0
enteroviral, enterovirus NEC B34.1
   central nervous system NEC A88.8
epidemic B99.9
   specified NEC B99.8
epididymis N50.9
Erb (-Landouzy) G71.02
Erdheim-Chester (ECD) E88.89
esophagus K22.9
   functional K22.4
   psychogenic F45.8
   specified NEC K22.8
Eulenburg's (congenital
   paramyotonia) G71.19
eustachian tube —*see* Disorder,
   eustachian tube
external
   auditory canal —*see* Disorder,
      ear, external
   ear —*see* Disorder, ear, external
extrapyramidal G25.9
   specified NEC G25.89
eye H57.9
   anterior chamber H21.9
   inflammatory NEC H57.89
   muscle (external) —*see*
      Strabismus
   specified NEC H57.89
   syphilitic —*see* Oculopathy,
      syphilitic

eyeball H44.9
  specified NEC H44.89
eyelid —see Disorder, eyelid
  specified NEC —see Disorder,
    eyelid, specified type NEC
eyeworm of Africa B74.3
facial nerve (seventh) G51.9
  newborn (birth injury) P11.3
Fahr (of brain) G23.8
Fahr Volhard (of kidney) I12.-
fallopian tube (noninflammatory)
    N83.9
  inflammatory —see Salpingo-
    oophoritis
  specified NEC N83.8
familial periodic paralysis G72.3
Fanconi's (congenital
    pancytopenia) D61.09
fascia NEC —see also Disorder,
    muscle
  inflammatory —see Myositis
  specified NEC M62.89
Fauchard's (periodontitis) —see
    Periodontitis
Favre-Durand-Nicolas (climatic
    bubo) A55
Fede's K14.0
Feer's —see Poisoning, mercury
female pelvic inflammatory
    —see also Disease, pelvis,
    inflammatory N73.9
  syphilitic (secondary) A51.42
  tuberculous A18.17
Fernels' (aortic aneurysm) I71.9
fibrocaseous of lung —see
    Tuberculosis, pulmonary
fibrocystic —see Fibrocystic
    disease
Fiedler's (leptospiral jaundice) A27.0
fifth B08.3
file-cutter's —see Poisoning, lead
fish-skin Q80.9
  acquired L85.0
Flajani (-Basedow) (exophthalmic
    goiter) —see Hyperthyroidism,
    with, goiter (diffuse)
flax-dresser's J66.1
fluke —see Infestation, fluke
foot and mouth B08.8
foot process N04.9
Forbes' (glycogenosis III) E74.03
Fordyce-Fox (apocrine miliaria)
    L75.2
Fordyce's (ectopic sebaceous
    glands) (mouth) Q38.6
Forestier's (rhizomelic
    pseudopolyarthritis) M35.3
  meaning ankylosing hyperostosis
    —see Hyperostosis,
    ankylosing
Fothergill's
  neuralgia —see Neuralgia,
    trigeminal
  scarlatina anginosa A38.9
Fournier (gangrene) N49.3
  female N76.89
fourth B08.8
Fox (-Fordyce) (apocrine miliaria)
    L75.2
Francis' —see Tularemia
Franklin C88.2
Frei's (climatic bubo) A55
Friedreich's
  combined systemic or ataxia
    G11.11
  myoclonia G25.3
frontal sinus —see Sinusitis, frontal
fungus NEC B49
Gaisböck's (polycythemia
    hypertonica) D75.1

gallbladder K82.9
  calculus —see Calculus,
    gallbladder
  cholecystitis —see Cholecystitis
  cholesterolosis K82.4
  fistula —see Fistula, gallbladder
  hydrops K82.1
  obstruction —see Obstruction,
    gallbladder
  perforation K82.2
  specified NEC K82.8
gamma heavy chain C88.2
Gamna's (siderotic splenomegaly)
    D73.2
Gamstorp's (adynamia episodica
    hereditaria) G72.3
Gandy-Nanta (siderotic
    splenomegaly) D73.2
ganister J62.8
gastric —see Disease, stomach
gastroesophageal reflux (GERD)
    K21.9
  with esophagitis (without
    bleeding) K21.00
    with bleeding K21.01
gastrointestinal (tract) K92.9
  amyloid E85.4
  functional K59.9
    psychogenic F45.8
  specified NEC K92.89
Gee (-Herter) (-Heubner) (-Thaysen)
    (nontropical sprue) K90.0
genital organs
  female N94.9
  male N50.9
Gerhardt's (erythromelalgia) I73.81
Gibert's (pityriasis rosea) L42
Gierke's (glycogenosis I) E74.01
Gilles de la Tourette's (motor-
    verbal tic) F95.2
gingiva K06.9
  plaque induced K05.00
  specified NEC K06.8
gland (lymph) I89.9
Glanzmann's (hereditary hemorrhagic
    thrombasthenia) D69.1
glass-blower's (cataract) —see
    Cataract, specified NEC
  salivary gland hypertrophy K11.1
Glisson's —see Rickets
globe H44.9
  specified NEC H44.89
glomerular —see also
    Glomerulonephritis
  with edema —see Nephrosis
  acute —see Nephritis, acute
  chronic —see Nephritis, chronic
  minimal change N05.0
  rapidly progressive N01.9
glycogen storage E74.00
  Andersen's E74.09
  Cori's E74.03
  Forbes' E74.03
  generalized E74.00
  glucose-6-phosphatase
    deficiency E74.01
  heart E74.02 [143]
  hepatorenal E74.09
  Hers' E74.09
  liver and kidney E74.09
  McArdle's E74.04
  muscle phosphofructokinase
    E74.09
  myocardium E74.02 [143]
  Pompe's E74.02
  Tauri's E74.04
  type 0 E74.09
  type I E74.01
  type II E74.02
  type III E74.03

glycogen storage (continued)
  type IV E74.09
  type V E74.04
  type VI-XI E74.09
  Von Gierke's E74.01
Goldstein's (familial hemorrhagic
    telangiectasia) I78.0
gonococcal NOS A54.9
graft-versus-host (GVH) D89.813
  acute D89.810
  acute on chronic D89.812
  chronic D89.811
grainhandler's J67.8
granulomatous (childhood)
    (chronic) D71
Graves' (exophthalmic goiter) —see
    Hyperthyroidism, with, goiter
    (diffuse)
Griesinger's —see Ancylostomiasis
Grisel's M43.6
Gruby's (tinea tonsurans) B35.0
Guillain-Barré G61.0
Guinon's (motor-verbal tic) F95.2
gum K06.9
gynecological N94.9
H (Hartnup) E72.02
Haff —see Poisoning, mercury
Hageman (congenital factor XII
    deficiency) D68.2
hair (color) (shaft) L67.9
  follicles L73.9
    specified NEC L73.8
Hamman's (spontaneous
    mediastinal emphysema) J98.2
hand, foot and mouth B08.4
Hansen's —see Leprosy
Hantavirus, with pulmonary
    manifestations B33.4
  with renal manifestations A98.5
Harada's H30.81-
Hartnup (pellagra-cerebellar ataxia-
    renal aminoaciduria) E72.02
Hart's (pellagra-cerebellar ataxia-
    renal aminoaciduria) E72.02
Hashimoto's (struma
    lymphomatosa) E06.3
Hb —see Disease, hemoglobin
heart (organic) I51.9
  with
    pulmonary edema (acute)
      —see also Failure,
      ventricular, left I50.1
    rheumatic fever (conditions
      in I00)
      active I01.9
        with chorea I02.0
        specified NEC I01.8
      inactive or quiescent (with
        chorea) I09.9
        specified NEC I09.89
  amyloid E85.4 [143]
  aortic (valve) I35.9
  arteriosclerotic or sclerotic
    (senile) —see Disease, heart,
    ischemic, atherosclerotic
  artery, arterial —see
    Disease, heart, ischemic,
    atherosclerotic
  beer drinkers' I42.6
  beriberi (wet) E51.12
  black I27.0
  congenital Q24.9
    cyanotic Q24.9
    specified NEC Q24.8
  coronary —see Disease, heart,
    ischemic
  cryptogenic I51.9
  fibroid —see Myocarditis
  functional I51.89
    psychogenic F45.8

heart (continued)
  glycogen storage E74.02 [143]
  gonococcal A54.83
  hypertensive —see
    Hypertension, heart
  hyperthyroid —see also
    Hyperthyroidism E05.90 [143]
    with thyroid storm E05.91 [143]
  ischemic (chronic or with a
    stated duration of over 4
    weeks) I25.9
    atherosclerotic (of) I25.10
      with angina pectoris —see
        Arteriosclerosis, coronary
        (artery)
      coronary artery bypass graft
        —see Arteriosclerosis,
        coronary (artery),
        cardiomyopathy I25.5
      diagnosed on ECG or other
        special investigation, but
        currently presenting no
        symptoms I25.6
    silent I25.6
    specified form NEC I25.89
  kyphoscoliotic I27.1
  meningococcal A39.50
    endocarditis A39.51
    myocarditis A39.52
    pericarditis A39.53
  mitral I05.9
    specified NEC I05.8
  muscular —see Degeneration,
    myocardial
  psychogenic (functional) F45.8
  pulmonary (chronic) I27.9
    in schistosomiasis B65.9 [152]
    specified NEC I27.89
  rheumatic (chronic) (inactive) (old)
    (quiescent) (with chorea) I09.9
    active or acute I01.9
      with chorea (acute) (rheumatic)
        (Sydenham's) I02.0
    specified NEC I09.89
  senile —see Myocarditis
  syphilitic A52.06
    aortic A52.03
      aneurysm A52.01
    congenital A50.54 [152]
  thyrotoxic (see also
    Thyrotoxicosis) E05.90 [143]
    with thyroid storm E05.91 [143]
  valve, valvular (obstructive)
    (regurgitant) —see also
    Endocarditis
    congenital NEC Q24.8
      pulmonary Q22.3
  vascular —see Disease,
    cardiovascular
heavy chain NEC C88.2
  alpha C88.3
  gamma C88.2
  mu C88.2
Hebra's
  pityriasis
    maculata et circinata L42
    rubra pilaris L44.0
  prurigo L28.2
hematopoietic organs D75.9
hemoglobin or Hb
  abnormal (mixed) NEC D58.2
    with thalassemia D56.9
  AS genotype D57.3
  Bart's D56.0
  C (Hb-C) D58.2
    with other abnormal
      hemoglobin NEC D58.2
    elliptocytosis D58.1
    Hb-S D57.2-
    sickle-cell D57.2-

Disease, diseased, diseased

hemoglobin or Hb *(continued)*
  C (Hb-C) *(continued)*
    thalassemia D56.8
    Constant Spring D58.2
  D(Hb-D) D58.2
  E(Hb-E) D58.2
  E-beta thalassemia D56.5
  elliptocytosis D58.1
  H(Hb-H) (thalassemia) D56.0
    with other abnormal
      hemoglobin NEC D56.9
    Constant Spring D56.0
  I thalassemia D56.9
  M D74.0
  S or SS D57.1
    with
      acute chest syndrome D57.01
      cerebral vascular
        involvement D57.03
      crisis (painful) D57.00
        with complication
          specified NEC D57.09
      splenic sequestration D57.02
      vasoocclusive pain D57.00
    beta plus D57.44
      with
        acute chest syndrome
          D57.451
        cerebral vascular
          involvement D57.453
        crisis D57.459
          with specified
            complication NEC
            D57.458
        splenic sequestration
          D57.452
        vasoocclusive pain
          D57.459
      without crisis D57.44
    beta zero D57.42
      with
        acute chest syndrome
          D57.431
        cerebral vascular
          involvement D57.433
        crisis D57.439
          with specified
            complication NEC
            D57.438
        splenic sequestration
          D57.432
        vasoocclusive pain D57.439
      without crisis D57.42
  SC D57.2-
  SD D57.8-
  SE D57.8-
  spherocytosis D58.0
  unstable, hemolytic D58.2
hemolytic (newborn) P55.9
  autoimmune D59.10
    cold type (primary)
      (secondary) (symptomatic)
      D59.12
    mixed type (primary)
      (secondary) (symptomatic)
      D59.13
    warm type (primary)
      (secondary) (symptomatic)
      D59.11
  drug-induced D59.0
  due to or with
    incompatibility
      ABO (blood group) P55.1
      blood (group) (Duffy) (K)
        (Kell) (Kidd) (Lewis)
        (M) (S) NEC P55.8
      Rh (blood group) (factor) P55.0
      Rh negative mother P55.0
    specified type NEC P55.8
  unstable hemoglobin D58.2

hemorrhagic D69.9
  newborn P53
Henoch (-Schönlein) (purpura
  nervosa) D69.0
hepatic —*see* Disease, liver
hepatobiliary K83.9
  toxic K71.9
hepatolenticular E83.01
heredodegenerative NEC
  spinal cord G95.89
herpesviral, disseminated B00.7
Hers' (glycogenosis VI) E74.09
Herter (-Gee) (-Heubner)
  (nontropical sprue) K90.0
Heubner-Herter (nontropical sprue)
  K90.0
high fetal gene or hemoglobin
  thalassemia D56.9
Hildenbrand's —*see* Typhus
hip (joint) M25.9
  congenital Q65.89
  suppurative M00.9
  tuberculous A18.02
His (-Werner) (trench fever) A79.0
Hodgson's I71.2
  ruptured I71.1
Holla —*see* Spherocytosis
hookworm B76.9
  specified NEC B76.8
host-versus-graft D89.813
  acute D89.810
  acute on chronic D89.812
  chronic D89.811
human immunodeficiency virus
  (HIV) B20
Huntington's G10
  with dementia G10 *[F02.80]*
Hutchinson's (cheiropompholyx)
  —*see* Hutchinson's disease
hyaline (diffuse) (generalized)
  membrane (lung) (newborn) P22.0
  adult J80
hydatid —*see* Echinococcus
hydroxyapatite deposition M11.00
  ankle M11.07-
  elbow M11.02-
  foot joint M11.07-
  hand joint M11.04-
  hip M11.05-
  knee M11.06-
  multiple site M11.09
  shoulder M11.01-
  vertebra M11.08
  wrist M11.03-
hyperkinetic —*see* Hyperkinesia
hypertensive —*see* Hypertension
hypophysis E23.7
Iceland G93.3
I-cell E77.0
immune D89.9
immunoproliferative (malignant)
  C88.9
  small intestinal C88.3
  specified NEC C88.8
inclusion B25.9
  salivary gland B25.9
infectious, infective B99.9
  congenital P37.9
    specified NEC P37.8
    viral P35.9
      specified type NEC P35.8
  specified NEC B99.8
inflammatory
  penis N48.29
    abscess N48.21
    cellulitis N48.22
  prepuce N47.7
    balanoposthitis N47.6
  tubo-ovarian —*see* Salpingo-
    oophoritis

intervertebral disc —*see also*
  Disorder, disc
  with myelopathy —*see* Disorder,
    disc, with, myelopathy
  cervical, cervicothoracic —*see*
    Disorder, disc, cervical
    with
      myelopathy —*see* Disorder,
        disc, cervical, with
        myelopathy
      neuritis, radiculitis or
        radiculopathy —*see*
        Disorder, disc, cervical,
        with neuritis
    specified NEC —*see*
      Disorder, disc, cervical,
      specified type NEC
  lumbar (with)
    myelopathy M51.06
    neuritis, radiculitis,
      radiculopathy or sciatica
      M51.16
    specified NEC M51.86
  lumbosacral (with)
    neuritis, radiculitis,
      radiculopathy or sciatica
      M51.17
    specified NEC M51.87
  specified NEC —*see* Disorder,
    disc, specified NEC
  thoracic (with)
    myelopathy M51.04
    neuritis, radiculitis or
      radiculopathy M51.14
    specified NEC M51.84
  thoracolumbar (with)
    myelopathy M51.05
    neuritis, radiculitis or
      radiculopathy M51.15
    specified NEC M51.85
intestine K63.9
  functional K59.9
    psychogenic F45.8
    specified NEC K59.89
  organic K63.9
  protozoal A07.9
  specified NEC K63.89
iris H21.9
  specified NEC H21.89
iron metabolism or storage E83.10
island (scrub typhus) A75.3
itai-itai —*see* Poisoning, cadmium
Jakob-Creutzfeldt —*see*
  Creutzfeldt-Jakob disease or
  syndrome
jaw M27.9
  fibrocystic M27.49
  specified NEC M27.8
jigger B88.1
joint —*see also* Disorder, joint
  Charcot's —*see* Arthropathy,
    neuropathic (Charcot)
  degenerative —*see* Osteoarthritis
    multiple M15.9
    spine —*see* Spondylosis
  hypertrophic —*see* Osteoarthritis
  sacroiliac M53.3
  specified NEC —*see* Disorder,
    joint, specified type NEC
  spine NEC —*see* Dorsopathy
  suppurative —*see* Arthritis,
    pyogenic or pyemic
Jourdain's (acute gingivitis) K05.00
  nonplaque induced K05.01
  plaque induced K05.00
Kaschin-Beck (endemic
  polyarthritis) M12.10
  ankle M12.17-
  elbow M12.12-
  foot joint M12.17-

Kaschin-Beck *(continued)*
  hand joint M12.14-
  hip M12.15-
  knee M12.16-
  multiple site M12.19
  shoulder M12.11-
  vertebra M12.18
  wrist M12.13-
Katayama B65.2
Kedani (scrub typhus) A75.3
Keshan E59
kidney (functional) (pelvis) N28.9
  chronic N18.9
    hypertensive —*see*
      Hypertension, kidney
    stage 1 N18.1
    stage 2(mild) N18.2
    stage 3(moderate) N18.30
    stage 3a N18.31
    stage 3b N18.32
    stage 4(severe) N18.4
    stage 5 N18.5
  complicating pregnancy —*see*
    Pregnancy, complicated by,
    renal disease
  cystic (congenital) Q61.9
  diabetic —*see* E08-E13 with .22
  fibrocystic (congenital) Q61.8
  hypertensive —*see*
    Hypertension, kidney
  in (due to)
    schistosomiasis (bilharziasis)
      B65.9 *[N29]*
  multicystic Q61.4
  polycystic Q61.3
    adult type Q61.2
    childhood type NEC Q61.19
      collecting duct dilatation
      Q61.11
Kimmelstiel (-Wilson)
  (intercapillary polycystic
  (congenital) glomerulosclerosis)
  —*see* E08-E13 with .21
Kimura D21.9
  specified site (*see* Neoplasm,
    connective tissue benign)
Kinnier Wilson's (hepatolenticular
  degeneration) E83.01
kissing —*see* Mononucleosis,
  infectious
Klebs' (*see also*
  Glomerulonephritis) N05.-
Klippel-Feil (brevicollis) Q76.1
Köhler-Pellegrini-Stieda
  (calcification, knee joint) —*see*
  Bursitis, tibial collateral
Kok Q89.8
König's (osteochondritis dissecans)
  —*see* Osteochondritis, dissecans
Korsakoff's (nonalcoholic) F04
  alcoholic F10.96
    with dependence F10.26
Kostmann's (infantile genetic
  agranulocytosis) D70.0
kuru A81.81
Kyasanur Forest A98.2
labyrinth, ear —*see* Disorder, ear, inner
lacrimal system —*see* Disorder,
  lacrimal system
Lafora's —*see* Epilepsy,
  generalized, idiopathic
Lancereaux-Mathieu (leptospiral
  jaundice) A27.0
Landry's G61.0
Larrey-Weil (leptospiral jaundice)
  A27.0
larynx J38.7
legionnaires' A48.1
  nonpneumonic A48.2
Lenegre's I44.2

lens H27.9
specified NEC H27.8
Lev's (acquired complete heart block) I44.2
Lewy body (dementia) G31.83 *[F02.80]*
with behavioral disturbance G31.83 *[F02.81]*
Lichtheim's (subacute combined sclerosis with pernicious anemia) D51.0
Lightwood's (renal tubular acidosis) N25.89
Lignac's (cystinosis) E72.04
lip K13.0
lipid-storage E75.6
specified NEC E75.5
Lipschütz's N76.6
liver (chronic) (organic) K76.9
alcoholic (chronic) K70.9
acute —*see* Disease, liver, alcoholic, hepatitis
cirrhosis K70.30
with ascites K70.31
failure K70.40
with coma K70.41
fatty liver K70.0
fibrosis K70.2
hepatitis K70.10
with ascites K70.11
sclerosis K70.2
cystic, congenital Q44.6
drug-induced (idiosyncratic) (toxic) (predictable) (unpredictable) —*see* Disease, liver, toxic
end stage K72.90
due to hepatitis —*see* Hepatitis
fatty, nonalcoholic (NAFLD) K76.0
alcoholic K70.0
fibrocystic (congenital) Q44.6
fluke
Chinese B66.1
oriental B66.1
sheep B66.3
gestational alloimmune (GALD) P78.84
glycogen storage E74.09 *[K77]*
in (due to)
schistosomiasis (bilharziasis) B65.9 *[K77]*
inflammatory K75.9
alcoholic K70.1
specified NEC K75.89
polycystic (congenital) Q44.6
toxic K71.9
with
cholestasis K71.0
cirrhosis (liver) K71.7
fibrosis (liver) K71.7
focal nodular hyperplasia K71.8
hepatic granuloma K71.8
hepatic necrosis K71.10
with coma K71.11
hepatitis NEC K71.6
acute K71.2
chronic
active K71.50
with ascites K71.51
lobular K71.4
persistent K71.3
lupoid K71.50
with ascites K71.51
peliosis hepatis K71.8
veno-occlusive disease (VOD) of liver K71.8
veno-occlusive K76.5

Lobo's (keloid blastomycosis) B48.0
Lobstein's (brittle bones and blue sclera) Q78.0
Ludwig's (submaxillary cellulitis) K12.2
lumbosacral region M53.87
lung J98.4
black J60
congenital Q33.9
cystic J98.4
congenital Q33.0
dabbing (related) U07.0
electronic cigarette (related) U07.0
fibroid (chronic) —*see* Fibrosis, lung
fluke B66.4
oriental B66.4
in
amyloidosis E85.4 *[J99]*
sarcoidosis D86.0
Sjögren's syndrome M35.02
systemic
lupus erythematosus M32.13
sclerosis M34.81
interstitial J84.9
with progressive fibrotic phenotype, in diseases classified elsewhere J84.170
of childhood, specified NEC J84.848
respiratory bronchiolitis J84.115
specified NEC J84.89
obstructive (chronic) J44.9
with
acute
bronchitis J44.0
exacerbation NEC J44.1
lower respiratory infection J44.0
alveolitis, allergic J67.9
asthma J44.9
bronchiectasis J47.9
with
exacerbation (acute) J47.1
lower respiratory infection J47.0
bronchitis J44.9
with
exacerbation (acute) J44.1
lower respiratory infection J44.0
emphysema J43.9
hypersensitivity pneumonitis J67.9
decompensated J44.1
with
exacerbation (acute) J44.1
polycystic J98.4
congenital Q33.0
rheumatoid (diffuse) (interstitial) —*see* Rheumatoid, lung
vaping (associated) (device) (product) (use) U07.0
Lutembacher's (atrial septal defect with mitral stenosis) Q21.1
Lyme A69.20
lymphatic (gland) (system) (channel) (vessel) I89.9
lymphoproliferative D47.9
specified NEC D47.Z9
T-gamma D47.Z9
X-linked D82.3
Magitot's M27.2
malarial —*see* Malaria
malignant —*see also* Neoplasm, malignant, by site

Manson's B65.1
maple bark J67.6
maple-syrup-urine E71.0
Marburg (virus) A98.3
Marion's (bladder neck obstruction) N32.0
Marsh's (exophthalmic goiter) —*see* Hyperthyroidism, with, goiter (diffuse)
mastoid (process) —*see* Disorder, ear, middle
Mathieu's (leptospiral jaundice) A27.0
Maxcy's A75.2
McArdle (-Schmid-Pearson) (glycogenosis V) E74.04
mediastinum J98.59
medullary center (idiopathic) (respiratory) G93.89
Meige's (chronic hereditary edema) Q82.0
meningococcal —*see* Infection, meningococcal
mental F99
organic F09
mesenchymal M35.9
mesenteric embolic (*see also* Ischemia, intestine, acute) K55.039
metabolic, metabolism E88.9
bilirubin E80.7
metal-polisher's J62.8
metastatic (*see also* Neoplasm, secondary, by site) C794.9
microvascular - code to condition
microvillus
atrophy Q43.8
inclusion (MVD) Q43.8
middle ear —*see* Disorder, ear, middle
Mikulicz'(dryness of mouth, absent or decreased lacrimation) K11.8
Milroy's (chronic hereditary edema) Q82.0
Minamata —*see* Poisoning, mercury
minicore G71.29
Minor's G95.19
Minot's (hemorrhagic disease, newborn) P53
Minot-von Willebrand-Jürgens (angiohemophilia) D68.0
Mitchell's (erythromelalgia) I73.81
mitral (valve) I05.9
nonrheumatic I34.9
mixed connective tissue M35.1
moldy hay J67.0
Monge's T70.29
Morgagni-Adams-Stokes (syncope with heart block) I45.9
Morgagni's (syndrome) (hyperostosis frontalis interna) M85.2
Morton's (with metatarsalgia) —*see* Lesion, nerve, plantar
Morvan's G60.8
motor neuron (bulbar) (mixed type) (spinal) G12.20
amyotrophic lateral sclerosis G12.21
familial G12.24
progressive bulbar palsy G12.22
specified NEC G12.29
moyamoya I67.5
mu heavy chain disease C88.2
multicore G71.29
multiminicore G71.29
muscle —*see also* Disorder, muscle
inflammatory —*see* Myositis
ocular (external) —*see* Strabismus

musculoskeletal system, soft tissue —*see also* Disorder, soft tissue
specified NEC —*see* Disorder, soft tissue, specified type NEC
mushroom workers' J67.5
mycotic B49
myelodysplastic, not classified C94.6
myeloproliferative, not classified C94.6
chronic D47.1
myocardium, myocardial (*see also* Degeneration, myocardial) I51.5
primary (idiopathic) I42.9
myoneural G70.9
Naegeli's D69.1
nails L60.9
specified NEC L60.8
Nairobi (sheep virus) A93.8
nasal J34.9
nemaline body G71.21
nerve —*see* Disorder, nerve
nervous system G98.8
autonomic G90.9
central G96.9
specified NEC G96.89
congenital Q07.9
parasympathetic G90.9
specified NEC G98.8
sympathetic G90.9
vegetative G90.9
neuromuscular system G70.9
Newcastle B30.8
Nicolas (-Durand)-Favre (climatic bubo) A55
nipple N64.9
Paget's C50.01-
female C50.01-
male C50.02-
Nishimoto (-Takeuchi) I67.5
nonarthropod-borne NOS (viral) B34.9
enterovirus NEC B34.1
nonautoimmune hemolytic D59.4
drug-induced D59.2
Nonne-Milroy-Meige (chronic hereditary edema) Q82.0
nose J34.9
nucleus pulposus —*see* Disorder, disc
nutritional E63.9
oast-house-urine E72.19
ocular
herpesviral B00.50
zoster B02.30
obliterative vascular I77.1
Ohara's —*see* Tularemia
Opitz's (congestive splenomegaly) D73.2
Oppenheim-Urbach (necrobiosis lipoidica diabeticorum) —*see* E08-E13 with .620
optic nerve NEC —*see* Disorder, nerve, optic
orbit —*see* Disorder, orbit
organ
dabbing (related) U07.0
electronic cigarette (related) U07.0
vaping (associated) (device) (product) (use) U07.0
Oriental liver fluke B66.1
Oriental lung fluke B66.4
Ormond's N13.5
Oropouche virus A93.0
Osler-Rendu (familial hemorrhagic telangiectasia) I78.0
osteofibrocystic E21.0
Otto's M24.7
outer ear —*see* Disorder, ear, external
ovary (noninflammatory) N83.9
cystic N83.20-

Disease, diseased (*continued*)

ovary (*continued*)
  inflammatory —*see* Salpingo-
    oophoritis
  polycystic E28.2
  specified NEC N83.8
Owren's (congenital) —*see* Defect,
  coagulation
pancreas K86.9
  cystic K86.2
  fibrocystic E84.9
  specified NEC K86.89
panvalvular I08.9
  specified NEC I08.8
parametrium (noninflammatory)
  N83.9
parasitic B89
  cerebral NEC B71.9 [*G94*]
  intestinal NOS B82.9
  mouth B37.0
  skin NOS B88.9
  specified type —*see* Infestation
  tongue B37.0
parathyroid (gland) E21.5
  specified NEC E21.4
Parkinson's G20
parodontal K05.6
Parrot's (syphilitic osteochondritis)
  A50.02
Parry's (exophthalmic goiter) —*see*
  Hyperthyroidism, with, goiter
  (diffuse)
Parson's (exophthalmic goiter)
  —*see* Hyperthyroidism, with,
  goiter (diffuse)
Paxton's (white piedra) B36.2
pearl-worker's —*see* Osteomyelitis,
  specified type NEC
Pellegrini-Stieda (calcification, knee
  joint) —*see* Bursitis, tibial collateral
pelvis, pelvic
  female NOS N94.9
    specified NEC N94.89
  gonococcal (acute) (chronic)
    A54.24
  inflammatory (female) N73.9
    acute N73.0
    chlamydial A56.11
    chronic N73.1
    specified NEC N73.8
    syphilitic (secondary) A51.42
      late A52.76
    tuberculous A18.17
  organ, female N94.9
  peritoneum, female NEC N94.89
penis N48.9
  inflammatory N48.29
    abscess N48.21
    cellulitis N48.22
    specified NEC N48.89
periapical tissues NOS K04.90
periodontal K05.6
  specified NEC K05.5
periosteum —*see* Disorder, bone,
  specified type NEC
peripheral
  arterial I73.9
  autonomic nervous system G90.9
  nerves —*see* Polyneuropathy
  vascular NOS I73.9
peritoneum K66.9
  pelvic, female NEC N94.89
  specified NEC K66.8
persistent mucosal (middle ear)
  H66.20
  left H66.22
    with right H66.23
  right H66.21
    with left H66.23
Petit's —*see* Hernia, abdomen,
  specified site NEC

pharynx J39.2
  specified NEC J39.2
Phocas' —*see* Mastopathy, cystic
photochromogenic (acid-fast
  bacilli) (pulmonary) A31.0
  nonpulmonary A31.9
Pick's G31.01 [*F02.80*]
  with behavioral disturbance
    G31.01 [*F02.81*]
  brain G31.01 [*F02.80*]
    with behavioral disturbance
      G31.01 [*F02.81*]
  of pericardium (pericardial
    pseudocirrhosis of liver) I31.1
pigeon fancier's J67.2
pineal gland E34.8
pink —*see* Poisoning, mercury
Pinkus' (lichen nitidus) L44.1
pinworm B80
Piry virus A93.8
pituitary (gland) E23.7
pituitary-snuff-taker's J67.8
pleura (cavity) J94.9
  specified NEC J94.8
pneumatic drill (hammer) T75.21
Pollitzer's (hidradenitis
  suppurativa) L73.2
polycystic
  kidney or renal Q61.3
    adult type Q61.2
    childhood type NEC Q61.19
      collecting duct dilatation
        Q61.11
  liver or hepatic Q44.6
  lung or pulmonary J98.4
    congenital Q33.0
  ovary, ovaries E28.2
  spleen Q89.09
polyethylene T84.05-
Pompe's (glycogenosis II) E74.02
Posadas-Wernicke B38.9
Potain's (pulmonary edema) —*see*
  Edema, lung
prepuce N47.8
  inflammatory N47.7
    balanoposthitis N47.6
Pringle's (tuberous sclerosis) Q85.1
prion, central nervous system A81.9
  specified NEC A81.89
prostate N42.9
  specified NEC N42.89
protozoal B64
  acanthamebiasis —*see*
    Acanthamebiasis
  African trypanosomiasis —*see*
    African trypanosomiasis
  babesiosis (*see also* Babesiosis)
    B60.00
  Chagas disease —*see* Chagas
    disease
  intestine, intestinal A07.9
  leishmaniasis —*see*
    Leishmaniasis
  malaria —*see* Malaria
  naegleriasis B60.2
  pneumocystosis B59
  specified organism NEC B60.8
  toxoplasmosis —*see*
    Toxoplasmosis
pseudo-Hurler's E77.0
psychiatric F99
psychotic —*see* Psychosis
Puente's (simple glandular
  cheilitis) K13.0
puerperal (*see also* Puerperal)
  O90.89
pulmonary —*see also* Disease, lung
  artery I28.9
  chronic obstructive J44.9
    with

pulmonary (*continued*)
  chronic obstructive (*continued*)
    with (*continued*)
      acute bronchitis J44.0
      exacerbation (acute) J44.1
      lower respiratory infection
        (acute) J44.0
    decompensated J44.1
      with
        exacerbation (acute) J44.1
  heart I27.9
    specified NEC I27.89
  hypertensive (vascular) (*see also*
    Hypertension, pulmonary)
    I27.20
    primary (idiopathic) I27.0
  valve I37.9
    rheumatic I09.89
  pulp (dental) NOS K04.90
pulseless M31.4
Putnam's (subacute combined
  sclerosis with pernicious anemia)
  D51.0
Pyle (-Cohn) (metaphyseal
  dysplasia) Q78.5
ragpicker's or ragsorter's A22.1
Raynaud's —*see* Raynaud's disease
reactive airway —*see* Asthma
Reclus'(cystic) —*see* Mastopathy,
  cystic
rectum K62.9
  specified NEC K62.89
Refsum's (heredopathia atactica
  polyneuritiformis) G60.1
renal (functional) (pelvis) (*see also*
  Disease, kidney) N28.9
  with
    edema —*see* Nephrosis
    glomerular lesion —*see*
      Glomerulonephritis
      with edema —*see* Nephrosis
    interstitial nephritis N12
  acute N28.9
  chronic (*see also* Disease,
    kidney, chronic) N18.9
  cystic, congenital Q61.9
  diabetic —*see* E08-E13 with .22
  end-stage (failure) N18.6
    due to hypertension I12.0
  fibrocystic (congenital) Q61.8
  hypertensive —*see*
    Hypertension, kidney
  lupus M32.14
  phosphate-losing (tubular) N25.0
  polycystic (congenital) Q61.3
    adult type Q61.2
    childhood type NEC Q61.19
      collecting duct dilatation
        Q61.11
  rapidly progressive N01.9
  subacute N01.9
Rendu-Osler-Weber (familial
  hemorrhagic telangiectasia) I78.0
renovascular (arteriosclerotic)
  —*see* Hypertension, kidney
respiratory (tract) J98.9
  acute or subacute NOS J06.9
    due to
      chemicals, gases, fumes or
        vapors (inhalation)
        J68.3
      external agent J70.9
        specified NEC J70.8
      radiation J70.0
      smoke inhalation J70.5
    noninfectious J39.8
  chronic NOS J98.9
    due to
      chemicals, gases, fumes or
        vapors J68.4

respiratory (*continued*)
  chronic (*continued*)
    due to (*continued*)
      external agent J70.9
        specified NEC J70.8
      radiation J70.1
    newborn P27.9
      specified NEC P27.8
  due to
    chemicals, gases, fumes or
      vapors J68.9
      acute or subacute NEC J68.3
      chronic J68.4
    external agent J70.9
      specified NEC J70.8
  newborn P28.9
    specified type NEC P28.89
  upper J39.9
    acute or subacute J06.9
    noninfectious NEC J39.8
    specified NEC J39.8
    streptococcal J06.9
retina, retinal H35.9
  Batten's or Batten-Mayou E75.4
    [*H36*]
  specified NEC H35.89
rheumatoid —*see* Arthritis,
  rheumatoid
rickettsial NOS A79.9
  specified type NEC A79.89
Riga (-Fede) (cachectic aphthae)
  K14.0
Riggs'(compound periodontitis)
  —*see* Periodontitis
Ritter's L00
Rivalta's (cervicofacial
  actinomycosis) A42.2
Robles'(onchocerciasis) B73.01
rod body G71.21
Roger's (congenital interventricular
  septal defect) Q21.0
Rosenthal's (factor XI deficiency)
  D68.1
Rossbach's (hyperchlorhydria) K31.89
  psychogenic F45.8
Ross River B33.1
Rotes Quérol —*see* Hyperostosis,
  ankylosing
Roth (-Bernhardt) —*see*
  Mononeuropathy, lower limb,
  meralgia paresthetica
Runeberg's (progressive pernicious
  anemia) D51.0
sacroiliac NEC M53.3
salivary gland or duct K11.9
  inclusion B25.9
  specified NEC K11.8
  virus B25.9
sandworm B76.9
Schimmelbusch's —*see*
  Mastopathy, cystic
Schmorl's —*see* Schmorl's disease
  or nodes
Schönlein (-Henoch) (purpura
  rheumatica) D69.0
Schottmüller's —*see* Fever,
  paratyphoid
Schultz's (agranulocytosis) —*see*
  Agranulocytosis
Schwalbe-Ziehen-Oppenheim G24.1
Schwartz-Jampel G71.13
sclera H15.9
  specified NEC H15.89
scrofulous (tuberculous) A18.2
scrotum N50.9
sebaceous glands L73.9
semilunar cartilage, cystic —*see*
  also Derangement, knee,
  meniscus, cystic
seminal vesicle N50.9

serum NEC (see also Reaction,
   serum) T80.69
sexually transmitted A64
   anogenital
      herpesviral infection —see
         Herpes, anogenital
      warts A63.0
   chancroid A57
   chlamydial infection —see
      Chlamydia
   gonorrhea —see Gonorrhea
   granuloma inguinale A58
   specified organism NEC A63.8
   syphilis —see Syphilis
   trichomoniasis —see
      Trichomoniasis
Sézary C84.1-
shimamushi (scrub typhus) A75.3
shipyard B30.0
sickle-cell D57.1
   with
      acute chest syndrome D57.01
      cerebral vascular involvement
         D57.03
      crisis (painful) D57.00
         with complication specified
            NEC D57.09
      splenic sequestration D57.02
      vasoocclusive pain D57.00
   elliptocytosis D57.8-
   Hb-C D57.20
      with
         acute chest syndrome
            D57.211
         cerebral vascular
            involvement D57.213
         crisis D57.219
            with specified
               complication NEC
               D57.218
         splenic sequestration D57.212
         vasoocclusive pain D57.219
      without crisis D57.20
   Hb-SD D57.80
      with
         acute chest syndrome
            D57.811
         cerebral vascular
            involvement D57.813
         crisis D57.819
            with complication
               specified NEC
               D57.818
         splenic sequestration D57.812
         vasoocclusive pain D57.819
      without crisis D57.80
   Hb-SE D57.80
      with
         acute chest syndrome
            D57.811
         cerebral vascular
            involvement D57.813
         crisis D57.819
            with complication
               specified NEC D57.818
         splenic sequestration D57.812
         vasoocclusive pain D57.819
      without crisis D57.80
   specified NEC D57.80
      with
         acute chest syndrome
            D57.811
         cerebral vascular
            involvement D57.813
         crisis D57.819
            with complication
               specified NEC
               D57.818
         splenic sequestration D57.812
         vasoocclusive pain D57.819

sickle-cell (continued)
   specified NEC (continued)
      without crisis D57.80
   spherocytosis D57.80
      with
         acute chest syndrome
            D57.811
         cerebral vascular
            involvement D57.813
         crisis D57.819
            with complication
               specified NEC D57.818
         splenic sequestration D57.812
         vasoocclusive pain D57.819
      without crisis D57.80
   thalassemia D57.40
      with
         acute chest syndrome D57.411
         cerebral vascular
            involvement D57.413
         crisis D57.419
            with specified complication
               NEC D57.418
         splenic sequestration D57.412
         vasoocclusive pain D57.419
      beta plus D57.44
         with
            acute chest syndrome
               D57.451
            cerebral vascular
               involvement D57.453
            crisis D57.459
               with specified
                  complication NEC
                  D57.458
            splenic sequestration
               D57.452
            vasoocclusive pain
               D57.459
         without crisis D57.44
      beta zero D57.42
         with
            acute chest syndrome
               D57.431
            cerebral vascular
               involvement D57.433
            crisis D57.439
               with specified
                  complication NEC
                  D57.438
            splenic sequestration
               D57.432
            vasoocclusive pain
               D57.439
         without crisis D57.42
silo-filler's J68.8
   bronchitis J68.0
   pneumonitis J68.0
   pulmonary edema J68.1
simian B B00.4
Simons'(progressive lipodystrophy)
   E88.1
sin nombre virus B33.4
sinus —see Sinusitis
Sirkari's B55.0
sixth B08.20
   due to human herpesvirus 6 B08.21
   due to human herpesvirus 7 B08.22
skin L98.9
   due to metabolic disorder NEC
      E88.9 [L99]
   specified NEC L98.8
slim (HIV) B20
small vessel I73.9
Sneddon-Wilkinson (subcorneal
   pustular dermatosis) L13.1
South African creeping B88.0
spinal (cord) G95.9
   congenital Q06.9
   specified NEC G95.89

spine —see also Spondylopathy
   joint —see Dorsopathy
   tuberculous A18.01
spinocerebellar (hereditary) G11.9
   specified NEC G11.8
spleen D73.9
   amyloid E85.4 [D77]
   organic D73.9
   polycystic Q89.09
   postinfectional D73.89
sponge-diver's —see Toxicity,
   venom, marine animal, sea
   anemone
Startle Q89.8
Steinert's G71.11
Sticker's (erythema infectiosum)
   B08.3
Stieda's (calcification, knee joint)
   —see Bursitis, tibial collateral
Stokes'(exophthalmic goiter) —see
   Hyperthyroidism, with, goiter
   (diffuse)
Stokes-Adams (syncope with heart
   block) I45.9
stomach K31.9
   functional, psychogenic F45.8
   specified NEC K31.89
stonemason's J62.8
storage
   glycogen —see Disease,
      glycogen storage
   mucopolysaccharide —see
      Mucopolysaccharidosis
striatopallidal system NEC G25.89
Stuart-Prower (congenital factor X
   deficiency) D68.2
Stuart's (congenital factor X
   deficiency) D68.2
subcutaneous tissue —see Disease,
   skin
supporting structures of teeth K08.9
   specified NEC K08.89
suprarenal (capsule) (gland) E27.9
   hyperfunction E27.0
   specified NEC E27.8
sweat glands L74.9
   specified NEC L74.8
Sweeley-Klionsky E75.21
Swift (-Feer) —see Poisoning,
   mercury
swimming-pool granuloma A31.1
Sylvest's (epidemic pleurodynia)
   B33.0
sympathetic nervous system
   G90.9
synovium —see Disorder, synovium
syphilitic —see Syphilis
systemic tissue mast cell D47.02
tanapox (virus) B08.71
Tangier E78.6
Tarral-Besnier (pityriasis rubra
   pilaris) L44.0
Tauri's E74.09
tear duct —see Disorder, lacrimal
   system
tendon, tendinous —see also
   Disorder, tendon
   nodular —see Trigger finger
terminal vessel I73.9
testis N50.9
thalassemia Hb-S —see Disease,
   sickle-cell, thalassemia
Thaysen-Gee (nontropical sprue)
   K90.0
Thomsen G71.12
throat J39.2
   septic J02.0
thromboembolic —see Embolism
thymus (gland) E32.9
   specified NEC E32.8

thyroid (gland) E07.9
   heart (see also Hyperthyroidism)
      E05.90 [I43]
      with thyroid storm E05.91 [I43]
   specified NEC E07.89
Tietze's M94.0
tongue K14.9
   specified NEC K14.8
tonsils, tonsillar (and adenoids) J35.9
tooth, teeth K08.9
   hard tissues K03.9
      specified NEC K03.89
   pulp NEC K04.99
   specified NEC K08.89
Tourette's F95.2
trachea NEC J39.8
tricuspid I07.9
   nonrheumatic I36.9
triglyceride-storage E75.5
trophoblastic —see Mole,
   hydatidiform
tsutsugamushi A75.3
tube (fallopian) (noninflammatory)
   N83.9
   inflammatory —see Salpingitis
   specified NEC N83.8
tuberculous NEC —see Tuberculosis
tubo-ovarian (noninflammatory)
   N83.9
   inflammatory —see Salpingo-
      oophoritis
   specified NEC N83.8
tubotympanic, chronic —see Otitis,
   media, suppurative, chronic,
   tubotympanic
tubulo-interstitial N15.9
   specified NEC N15.8
tympanum —see Disorder,
   tympanic membrane
Uhl's Q24.8
Underwood's (sclerema
   neonatorum) P83.0
Unverricht (-Lundborg) —see
   Epilepsy, generalized,
   idiopathic
Urbach-Oppenheim (necrobiosis
   lipoidica diabeticorum) —see
   E08-E13 with .620
ureter N28.9
   in (due to)
      schistosomiasis (bilharziasis)
         B65.0 [N29]
urethra N36.9
   specified NEC N36.8
urinary (tract) N39.9
   bladder N32.9
      specified NEC N32.89
   specified NEC N39.8
uterus (noninflammatory) N85.9
   infective —see Endometritis
   inflammatory —see Endometritis
   specified NEC N85.8
uveal tract (anterior) H21.9
   posterior H31.9
vagabond's B85.1
vagina, vaginal (noninflammatory)
   N89.9
   inflammatory NEC N76.89
   specified NEC N89.8
valve, valvular I38
   multiple I08.9
      specified NEC I08.8
van Creveld-von Gierke
   (glycogenosis I) E74.01
vas deferens N50.9
vascular I99.9
   arteriosclerotic —see
      Arteriosclerosis
   ciliary body NEC —see
      Disorder, iris, vascular

Disorder *(continued)*

alcohol use
  mild F10.10
    with
      alcohol-induced
        anxiety disorder F10.180
        bipolar and related
          disorder F10.14
        depressive disorder F10.14
        psychotic disorder
          F10.159
        sexual dysfunction F10.181
        sleep disorder F10.182
      alcohol intoxication
        F10.129
        delirium F10.121
    in remission (early)
      (sustained) F10.11
  moderate or severe F10.20
    with
      alcohol-induced
        anxiety disorder F10.280
        bipolar and related
          disorder F10.24
        depressive disorder
          F10.24
        major neurocognitive
          disorder, amnestic-
          confabulatory type
          F10.26
        major neurocognitive
          disorder, nonamnestic-
          confabulatory type
          F10.27
        mild neurocognitive
          disorder F10.288
        psychotic disorder
          F10.259
        sexual dysfunction
          F10.281
        sleep disorder F10.282
      alcohol intoxication F10.229
        delirium F10.221
    in remission (early)
      (sustained) F10.21
allergic —*see* Allergy
alveolar NEC J84.09
amino-acid
  cystathioninuria E72.19
  cystinosis E72.04
  cystinuria E72.01
  glycinuria E72.09
  homocystinuria E72.11
  metabolism —*see* Disturbance,
    metabolism, amino-acid
    specified NEC E72.89
  neonatal, transitory P74.8
  renal transport NEC E72.09
  transport NEC E72.09
amnesic, amnestic
  alcohol-induced F10.96
    with dependence F10.26
  due to (secondary to) general
    medical condition F04
  psychoactive NEC-induced F19.96
    with
      abuse F19.16
      dependence F19.26
  sedative, hypnotic or anxiolytic-
    induced F13.96
    with dependence F13.26
amphetamine-type substance use
  mild F15.10
    in remission (early)
      (sustained) F15.11
  moderate F15.20
    in remission (early)
      (sustained) F15.21
  severe 15.20
    in remission (early)
      (sustained) F15.21

Disorder *(continued)*

amphetamine (or other stimulant)
  use
  mild F15.10
    with
      amphetamine (or other
        stimulant) -induced
        anxiety disorder F15.180
        bipolar and related
          disorder F15.14
        depressive disorder
          F15.14
        obsessive-compulsive
          and related disorder
          F15.188
        psychotic disorder F15.159
        sexual dysfunction F15.181
      amphetamine, cocaine,
        or other stimulant
        intoxication
        with perceptual
          disturbances F15.122
        without perceptual
          disturbances F15.129
      intoxication delirium F15.121
    in remission (early)
      (sustained) F15.11
  moderate or severe
    with
      amphetamine (or other
        stimulant) -induced
        anxiety disorder F15.280
        bipolar and related
          disorder F15.14
        depressive disorder
          F15.24
        obsessive-compulsive
          and related disorder
          F15.288
        psychotic disorder
          F15.259
        sexual dysfunction
          F15.281
      amphetamine, cocaine,
        or other stimulant
        intoxication
        with perceptual
          disturbances F15.222
        without perceptual
          disturbances F15.229
      intoxication delirium
        F15.221
anaerobic glycolysis with anemia
  D55.2
anxiety F41.9
  due to (secondary to)
    alcohol F10.980
      in
        abuse F10.980
        dependence F10.280
    amphetamine F15.980
      in
        abuse F15.180
        dependence F15.280
    anxiolytic F13.980
      in
        abuse F13.180
        dependence F13.280
    caffeine F15.980
      in
        abuse F15.180
        dependence F15.280
    cannabis F12.980
      in
        abuse F12.180
        dependence F12.280
    cocaine F14.980
      in
        abuse F14.180
        dependence F14.180
    general medical condition F06.4

Disorder *(continued)*

anxiety *(continued)*
  due to *(continued)*
    hallucinogen F16.980
      in
        abuse F16.180
        dependence F16.280
    hypnotic F13.980
      in
        abuse F13.180
        dependence F13.280
    inhalant F18.980
      in
        abuse F18.180
        dependence F18.280
    phencyclidine F16.980
      in
        abuse F16.180
        dependence F16.280
    psychoactive substance NEC
      F19.980
      in
        abuse F19.180
        dependence F19.280
    sedative F13.980
      in
        abuse F13.180
        dependence F13.280
    volatile solvents F18.980
      in
        abuse F18.180
        dependence F18.280
  generalized F41.1
  illness F45.21
  mixed
    with depression (mild) F41.8
    specified NEC F41.3
  organic F06.4
  phobic F40.9
    of childhood F40.8
  specified NEC F41.8
aortic valve —*see* Endocarditis,
  aortic
aromatic amino-acid metabolism
  E70.9
  specified NEC E70.89
arteriole NEC I77.89
artery NEC I77.89
articulation —*see* Disorder, joint
attachment (childhood)
  disinhibited F94.2
  reactive F94.1
attention-deficit hyperactivity
  (adolescent) (adult) (child) F90.0
  combined
    presentation F90.2
    type F90.2
  hyperactive
    impulsive presentation F90.1
    type F90.1
  inattentive
    presentation F90.0
    type F90.0
  specified type NEC F90.8
attention-deficit without
  hyperactivity (adolescent) (adult)
  (child) F98.8
auditory processing (central) H93.25
autistic F84.0
autoimmune D89.89
autonomic nervous system G90.9
  specified NEC G90.8
autism spectrum F84.0
avoidant
  child or adolescent F40.10
  restrictive food intake F50.82
balance
  acid-base E87.8
    mixed E87.4
  electrolyte E87.8
  fluid NEC E87.8

Disorder *(continued)*

behavioral (disruptive) —*see*
  Disorder, conduct
beta-amino-acid metabolism
  E72.89
bile acid and cholesterol
  metabolism E78.70
  Barth syndrome E78.71
  other specified E78.79
  Smith-Lemli-Opitz syndrome
    E78.72
bilirubin excretion E80.6
binge eating F50.81
binocular
  movement H51.9
    convergence
      excess H51.12
      insufficiency H51.11
    internuclear ophthalmoplegia
      —*see* Ophthalmoplegia,
      internuclear
    palsy of conjugate gaze H51.0
    specified type NEC H51.8
  vision NEC —*see* Disorder,
    vision, binocular
bipolar (I) (type 1) F31.9
  and related due to a known
    physiological condition
    with
      manic features F06.33
      manic- or hypomanic-like
        episodes F06.33
      mixed features F06.34
  current (or most recent) episode
    depressed F31.9
      with psychotic features
        F31.5
      without psychotic features
        F31.30
        mild F31.31
        moderate F31.32
        severe (without psychotic
          features) F31.4
          with psychotic features
            F31.5
    hypomanic F31.0
    manic F31.9
      with psychotic features
        F31.2
      without psychotic features
        F31.10
        mild F31.11
        moderate F31.12
        severe (without psychotic
          features) F31.13
          with psychotic features
            F31.2
    mixed F31.60
      mild F31.61
      moderate F31.62
      severe (without psychotic
        features) F31.63
        with psychotic features
          F31.64
    severe depression (without
      psychotic features) F31.4
      with psychotic features
        F31.5
  in remission (currently) F31.70
    in full remission
      most recent episode
        depressed F31.76
        hypomanic F31.72
        manic F31.74
        mixed F31.78
    in partial remission
      most recent episode
        depressed F31.75
        hypomanic F31.71
        manic F31.73
        mixed F31.77

Disorder (continued)

bipolar (continued)
 specified NEC F31.89
 II (type 2) F31.81
 organic F06.30
 single manic episode F30.9
  mild F30.11
  moderate F30.12
  severe (without psychotic
   symptoms) F30.13
   with psychotic symptoms
    F30.2
bladder N32.9
 functional NEC N31.9
 in schistosomiasis B65.0 [N33]
 specified NEC N32.89
bleeding D68.9
blood D75.9
 in congenital early syphilis
  A50.09 [D77]
body dysmorphic F45.22
bone M89.9
 continuity M84.9
  specified type NEC M84.80
   ankle M84.87-
   fibula M84.86-
   foot M84.87-
   hand M84.84-
   humerus M84.82-
   neck M84.88
   pelvis M84.859
   radius M84.83-
   rib M84.88
   shoulder M84.81-
   skull M84.88
   thigh M84.85-
   tibia M84.86-
   ulna M84.83-
   vertebra M84.88
 density and structure M85.9
  cyst —see also Cyst, bone,
   specified type NEC
   aneurysmal —see Cyst,
    bone, aneurysmal
   solitary —see Cyst, bone,
    solitary
  diffuse idiopathic skeletal
   hyperostosis —see
   Hyperostosis, ankylosing
  fibrous dysplasia (monostotic)
   —see Dysplasia, fibrous,
   bone
  fluorosis —see Fluorosis,
   skeletal
  hyperostosis of skull M85.2
  osteitis condensans —see
   Osteitis, condensans
  specified type NEC M85.8-
   ankle M85.87-
   foot M85.87-
   forearm M85.83-
   hand M85.84-
   lower leg M85.86-
   multiple sites M85.89
   neck M85.88
   rib M85.88
   shoulder M85.81-
   skull M85.88
   thigh M85.85-
   upper arm M85.82-
   vertebra M85.88
 development and growth NEC
  M89.20
  carpus M89.24-
  clavicle M89.21-
  femur M89.25-
  fibula M89.26-
  finger M89.24-
  humerus M89.22-
  ilium M89.259
  ischium M89.259

Disorder (continued)

bone (continued)
 development and growth NEC
  (continued)
  metacarpus M89.24-
  metatarsus M89.27-
  multiple sites M89.29
  neck M89.28
  radius M89.23-
  rib M89.28
  scapula M89.21-
  skull M89.28
  tarsus M89.27-
  tibia M89.26-
  toe M89.27-
  ulna M89.23-
  vertebra M89.28
 specified type NEC M89.8X-
brachial plexus G54.0
branched-chain amino-acid
 metabolism E71.2
 specified NEC E71.19
breast N64.9
 agalactia —see Agalactia
 associated with
  lactation O92.70
   specified NEC O92.79
  pregnancy O92.20
   specified NEC O92.29
  puerperium O92.20
   specified NEC O92.29
 cracked nipple —see Cracked nipple
 galactorrhea —see Galactorrhea
 hypogalactia O92.4
 lactation disorder NEC O92.79
 mastitis —see Mastitis
 nipple infection —see Infection,
  nipple
 retracted nipple —see
  Retraction, nipple
 specified type NEC N64.89
Briquet's F45.0
bullous, in diseases classified
 elsewhere L14
caffeine use
 mild
  with
   caffeine-induced
    anxiety disorder F15.180
    sleep disorder F15.182
 moderate or severe
  with
   caffeine-induced
    anxiety disorder F15.280
    sleep disorder F15.282
cannabis use
 mild F12.10
  with
   cannabis-induced
    anxiety disorder F12.180
    psychotic disorder F12.159
    sleep disorder F12.188
   cannabis intoxication
    delirium F12.121
    with perceptual
     disturbances F12.122
    without perceptual
     disturbances F12.129
  in remission (early)
   (sustained) F12.11
 moderate or severe F12.20
  with
   cannabis-induced
    anxiety disorder F12.280
    psychotic disorder F12.259
    sleep disorder F12.288
   cannabis intoxication
    with perceptual
     disturbances F12.222
    without perceptual
     disturbances F12.229

Disorder (continued)

cannabis use (continued)
 moderate or severe (continued)
  with (continued)
   delirium F12.221
  in remission (early)
   (sustained) F12.21
carbohydrate
 absorption, intestinal NEC
  E74.39
 metabolism (congenital) E74.9
  specified NEC E74.89
cardiac, functional I51.89
carnitine metabolism E71.40
cartilage M94.9
 articular NEC —see
  Derangement, joint, articular
  cartilage
 chondrocalcinosis —see
  Chondrocalcinosis
 specified type NEC M94.8X-
  articular —see Derangement,
   joint, articular cartilage
  multiple sites M94.8X0
catatonia (due to known
 physiological condition) (with
 another mental disorder) F06.1
catatonic
 due to (secondary to) known
  physiological condition F06.1
 organic F06.1
central auditory processing H93.25
cervical
 region NEC M53.82
 root (nerve) NEC G54.2
character NOS F60.9
childhood disintegrative NEC
 F84.3
cholesterol and bile acid
 metabolism E78.70
 Barth syndrome E78.71
 other specified E78.79
 Smith-Lemli-Opitz syndrome
  E78.72
choroid H31.9
 atrophy —see Atrophy, choroid
 degeneration —see
  Degeneration, choroid
 detachment —see Detachment,
  choroid
 dystrophy —see Dystrophy,
  choroid
 hemorrhage —see Hemorrhage,
  choroid
 rupture —see Rupture, choroid
 scar —see Scar, chorioretinal
 solar retinopathy —see
  Retinopathy, solar
 specified type NEC H31.8
ciliary body —see Disorder, iris
 degeneration —see
  Degeneration, ciliary body
coagulation (factor) (see also
 Defect, coagulation) D68.9
 newborn, transient P61.6
cocaine use
 mild F14.10
  with
   amphetamine, cocaine,
    or other stimulant
    intoxication
    with perceptual
     disturbances F14.122
    without perceptual
     disturbances F14.129
   cocaine-induced
    anxiety disorder F14.180
    bipolar and related
     disorder F14.14
    depressive disorder
     F14.14

Disorder (continued)

cannabis use (continued)
 mild (continued)
  with (continued)
   cocaine-induced
    (continued)
    obsessive-compulsive
     and related disorder
     F14.188
    psychotic disorder F14.159
    sexual dysfunction F14.181
    sleep disorder F14.182
   cocaine intoxication
    delirium F14.121
  in remission (early)
   (sustained) F14.11
 moderate or severe
  with
   amphetamine, cocaine,
    or other stimulant
    intoxication
    with perceptual
     disturbances F14.222
    without perceptual
     disturbances F14.229
   cocaine-induced
    anxiety disorder F14.280
    bipolar and related
     disorder F14.24
    depressive disorder
     F14.24
    obsessive-compulsive
     and related disorder
     F14.288
    psychotic disorder F14.259
    sexual dysfunction
     F14.281
    sleep disorder F14.282
   cocaine intoxication
    delirium F14.221
  in remission (early)
   (sustained) F14.21
coccyx NEC M53.3
cognitive F09
 due to (secondary to) general
  medical condition F09
 persisting R41.89
  due to
   alcohol F10.97
    with dependence F10.27
   anxiolytics F13.97
    with dependence F13.27
   hypnotics F13.97
    with dependence F13.27
   sedatives F13.97
    with dependence F13.27
   specified substance NEC
    F19.97
    with
     abuse F19.17
     dependence F19.27
communication F80.9
 social pragmatic F80.82
conduct (childhood) F91.9
 adjustment reaction —see
  Disorder, adjustment
 adolescent onset type F91.2
 childhood onset type F91.1
 compulsive F63.9
 confined to family context
  F91.0
 depressive F91.8
 group type F91.2
 hyperkinetic —see Disorder,
  attention-deficit hyperactivity
 oppositional defiance F91.3
 socialized F91.2
 solitary aggressive type F91.1
 specified NEC F91.8
 unsocialized (aggressive) F91.1
conduction, heart I45.9

electrolyte (balance) NEC E87.8
  with
    abortion —see Abortion
      by type complicated by
        specified condition NEC
    ectopic pregnancy O08.5
    molar pregnancy O08.5
  acidosis (metabolic) (respiratory)
    E87.2
  alkalosis (metabolic)
    (respiratory) E87.3
elimination, transepidermal L87.9
  specified NEC L87.8
emotional (persistent) F34.9
  of childhood F93.9
    specified NEC F93.8
endocrine E34.9
  postprocedural E89.89
    specified NEC E89.89
erectile (male) (organic) (see also
  Dysfunction, sexual, male,
  erectile) N52.9
  nonorganic F52.21
erythematous —see Erythema
esophagus K22.9
  functional K22.4
  psychogenic F45.8
eustachian tube H69.9-
  infection —see Salpingitis,
    eustachian
  obstruction —see Obstruction,
    eustachian tube
  patulous —see Patulous,
    eustachian tube
  specified NEC H69.8-
exhibitionistic F65.2
extrapyramidal G25.9
  in diseases classified elsewhere
    —see category G26
  specified type NEC G25.89
eye H57.9
  postprocedural —see
    Complication, postprocedural,
    eye
eyelid H02.9
  cyst —see Cyst, eyelid
  degenerative H02.70
    chloasma —see Chloasma,
      eyelid
    madarosis —see Madarosis
    specified type NEC H02.79
    vitiligo —see Vitiligo, eyelid
    xanthelasma —see
      Xanthelasma
  dermatochalasis —see
    Dermatochalasis
  edema —see Edema, eyelid
  elephantiasis —see
    Elephantiasis, eyelid
  foreign body, retained —see
    Foreign body, retained, eyelid
  function H02.59
    abnormal innervation
      syndrome —see Syndrome,
      abnormal innervation
    blepharochalasis —see
      Blepharochalasis
    blepharoclonus —see
      Blepharoclonus
    blepharophimosis —see
      Blepharophimosis
    blepharoptosis —see
      Blepharoptosis
    lagophthalmos —see
      Lagophthalmos
    lid retraction —see
      Retraction, lid
  hypertrichosis —see
    Hypertrichosis, eyelid
  specified type NEC H02.89

eyelid (continued)
  vascular H02.879
    left H02.876
      lower H02.875
      upper H02.874
    right H02.873
      lower H02.872
      upper H02.871
factitious
  by proxy F68.A
  imposed on another F68.A
  imposed on self F68.10
    with predominantly
      psychological symptoms
      F68.11
      with physical symptoms
        F68.13
    physical symptoms F68.12
      with psychological
        symptoms F68.13
factor, coagulation —see Defect,
  coagulation
fatty acid
  metabolism E71.30
    specified NEC E71.39
  oxidation
    LCAD E71.310
    MCAD E71.311
    SCAD E71.312
    specified deficiency NEC
      E71.318
feeding (infant or child) (see also
  Disorder, eating) R63.3
  or eating disorder F50.9
  specified NEC F50.9
feigned (with obvious motivation)
  Z76.5
  without obvious motivation
    —see Disorder, factitious
female
  hypoactive sexual desire F52.0
  orgasmic F52.31
  sexual interest/arousal F52.22
fetishistic F65.0
fibroblastic M72.9
  specified NEC M72.8
fluency
  adult onset F98.5
  childhood onset F80.81
  following
    cerebral infarction I69.323
    cerebrovascular disease
      I69.923
      specified disease NEC
        I69.823
    intracerebral hemorrhage
      I69.123
    nontraumatic intracranial
      hemorrhage NEC I69.223
    subarachnoid hemorrhage
      I69.023
  in conditions classified elsewhere
    R47.82
fluid balance E87.8
follicular (skin) L73.9
  specified NEC L73.8
frotteuristic F65.81
fructose metabolism E74.10
  essential fructosuria E74.11
  fructokinase deficiency E74.11
  fructose-1, 6-diphosphatase
    deficiency E74.19
  hereditary fructose intolerance
    E74.12
  other specified E74.19
functional polymorphonuclear
  neutrophils D71
gallbladder, biliary tract and
  pancreas in diseases classified
  elsewhere K87

gambling F63.0
gamma aminobutyric acid (GABA)
  metabolism E72.81
gamma-glutamyl cycle E72.89
gastric (functional) K31.9
  motility K30
  psychogenic F45.8
  secretion K30
gastrointestinal (functional) NOS
  K92.9
  newborn P78.9
  psychogenic F45.8
gender-identity or -role F64.9
  childhood F64.2
  effect on relationship F66
  of adolescence or adulthood
    F64.0
    nontranssexual F64.8
  specified NEC F64.8
  uncertainty F66
genito-pelvic pain penetration
  F52.6
genitourinary system
  female N94.9
  male N50.9
  psychogenic F45.8
globe H44.9
  degenerated condition H44.50
    absolute glaucoma H44.51-
    atrophy H44.52-
    leucocoria H44.53-
  degenerative H44.30
    chalcosis H44.31-
    myopia (see also Myopia,
      degenerative) H44.2-
    siderosis H44.32-
    specified type NEC H44.39-
  endophthalmitis —see
    Endophthalmitis
  foreign body, retained —see
    Foreign body, intraocular, old,
    retained
  hemophthalmos —see
    Hemophthalmos
  hypotony H44.40
    due to
      ocular fistula H44.42-
      specified disorder NEC
        H44.43-
    flat anterior chamber
      H44.41-
    primary H44.44-
  luxation —see Luxation, globe
  specified type NEC H44.89
glomerular (in) N05.9
  amyloidosis E85.4 [N08]
  cryoglobulinemia D89.1 [N08]
  disseminated intravascular
    coagulation D65 [N08]
  Fabry's disease E75.21 [N08]
  familial lecithin cholesterol
    acyltransferase deficiency
    E78.6 [N08]
  Goodpasture's syndrome M31.0
  hemolytic-uremic syndrome
    D59.3
  Henoch (-Schönlein) purpura
    D69.0 [N08]
  malariae malaria B52.0
  microscopic polyangiitis M31.7
    [N08]
  multiple myeloma C90.0- [N08]
  mumps B26.83
  schistosomiasis B65.9 [N08]
  sepsis NEC A41.- [N08]
    streptococcal A40.- [N08]
  sickle-cell disorders D57.- [N08]
  strongyloidiasis B78.9 [N08]
  subacute bacterial endocarditis
    I33.0 [N08]

glomerular (continued)
  syphilis A52.75
  systemic lupus erythematosus
    M32.14
  thrombotic thrombocytopenic
    purpura M31.1 [N08]
  Waldenström macroglobulinemia
    C88.0 [N08]
  Wegener's granulomatosis M31.31
gluconeogenesis E74.4
glucosaminoglycan metabolism
  —see Disorder, metabolism,
  glucosaminoglycan
glucose transport E74.819
  specified NEC E74.818
glycine metabolism E72.50
  d-glycericacidemia E72.59
  hyperhydroxyprolinemia E72.59
  hyperoxaluria R82.992
    primary E72.53
  hyperprolinemia E72.59
  non-ketotic hyperglycinemia
    E72.51
  oxalosis E72.53
  oxaluria E72.53
  sarcosinemia E72.59
  trimethylaminuria E72.52
glycoprotein metabolism E77.9
  specified NEC E77.8
habit (and impulse) F63.9
  involving sexual behavior NEC
    F65.9
  specified NEC F63.89
hallucinogen use
  mild F16.10
    with
      hallucinogen-induced
        anxiety disorder
        F16.180
      bipolar and related
        disorder F16.14
      depressive disorder
        F16.14
      psychotic disorder
        F16.159
      hallucinogen intoxication
        delirium F16.121
      other hallucinogen
        intoxication F16.129
    in remission (early)
      (sustained) F16.11
  moderate or severe F16.20
    with
      hallucinogen-induced
        anxiety disorder F16.280
      bipolar and related
        disorder F16.24
      depressive disorder
        F16.24
      psychotic disorder
        F16.259
      hallucinogen intoxication
        delirium F16.221
      other hallucinogen
        intoxication F16.229
    in remission (early)
      (sustained) F16.21
heart action I49.9
hematological D75.9
  newborn (transient) P61.9
    specified NEC P61.8
hematopoietic organs D75.9
hemorrhagic NEC D69.9
  drug-induced D68.32
  due to
    extrinsic circulating
      anticoagulants D68.32
    increase in
      anti-IIa D68.32
      anti-Xa D68.32

Disorder *(continued)*

hemorrhagic NEC *(continued)*
  due to *(continued)*
    intrinsic
      circulating anticoagulants
        D68.318
      increase in
        antithrombin D68.318
        anti-VIIIa D68.318
        anti-IXa D68.318
        anti-XIa D68.318
    following childbirth O72.3
hemostasis —*see* Defect,
  coagulation
histidine metabolism E70.40
  histidinemia E70.41
  other specified E70.49
hoarding F42.3
hyperkinetic —*see* Disorder,
  attention-deficit hyperactivity
hyperleucine-isoleucinemia
  E71.19
hypervalinemia E71.19
hypoactive sexual desire F52.0
hypochondriacal F45.20
  body dysmorphic F45.22
  neurosis F45.21
  other specified F45.29
identity
  dissociative F44.81
  illness anxiety F45.21
  of childhood F93.8
immune mechanism (immunity)
  D89.9
  specified type NEC D89.89
impaired renal tubular function
  N25.9
  specified NEC N25.89
impulse (control) F63.9
inflammatory
  pelvic, in diseases classified
    elsewhere —*see* category
    N74
  penis N48.29
    abscess N48.21
    cellulitis N48.22
inhalant use
  mild F18.10
    with
      inhalant-induced
        anxiety disorder
          F18.180
        depressive disorder
          F18.14
        major neurocognitive
          disorder F18.17
        mild neurocognitive
          disorder F18.188
        psychotic disorder
          F18.159
      inhalant intoxication
        F18.129
      inhalant intoxication
        delirium F18.121
      in remission (early)
        (sustained) F18.11
  moderate or severe F18.20
    with
      inhalant-induced
        anxiety disorder
          F18.280
        depressive disorder
          F18.24
        major neurocognitive
          disorder F18.27
        mild neurocognitive
          disorder F18.288
        psychotic disorder
          F18.259
      inhalant intoxication
        F18.229

inhalant use *(continued)*
  moderate or severe *(continued)*
    with *(continued)*
      inhalant intoxication
        delirium F18.221
    in remission (early)
      (sustained) F18.21
integument, newborn P83.9
  specified NEC P83.88
intermittent explosive F63.81
internal secretion pancreas —*see*
  Increased, secretion, pancreas,
  endocrine
intestine, intestinal
  carbohydrate absorption NEC
    E74.39
    postoperative K91.2
  functional NEC K59.9
    postoperative K91.89
  psychogenic F45.8
  vascular K55.9
    chronic K55.1
    specified NEC K55.8
intraoperative (intraprocedural)
  —*see* Complications,
  intraoperative
involuntary emotional expression
  (IEED) F48.2
iris H21.9
  adhesions —*see* Adhesions, iris
  atrophy —*see* Atrophy, iris
  chamber angle recession —*see*
    Recession, chamber angle
  cyst —*see* Cyst, iris
  degeneration —*see*
    Degeneration, iris
  in diseases classified elsewhere
    H22
  iridodialysis —*see* Iridodialysis
  iridoschisis —*see* Iridoschisis
  miotic pupillary cyst —*see* Cyst,
    pupillary
  pupillary
    abnormality —*see*
      Abnormality, pupillary
    membrane —*see* Membrane,
      pupillary
  specified type NEC H21.89
  vascular NEC H21.1X-
iron metabolism E83.10
  specified NEC E83.19
isovaleric acidemia E71.110
jaw, developmental M27.0
  temporomandibular
    (*see* Anomaly, dentofacial,
    temporomandibular joint)
    M26.60-
joint M25.9
  derangement —*see*
    Derangement, joint
  effusion —*see* Effusion, joint
  fistula —*see* Fistula, joint
  hemarthrosis —*see*
    Hemarthrosis
  instability —*see* Instability,
    joint
  osteophyte —*see* Osteophyte
  pain —*see* Pain, joint
  psychogenic F45.8
  specified type NEC M25.80
    ankle M25.87-
    elbow M25.82-
    foot joint M25.87-
    hand joint M25.84-
    hip M25.85-
    knee M25.86-
    shoulder M25.81-
    wrist M25.83-
  stiffness —*see* Stiffness, joint
ketone metabolism E71.32

kidney N28.9
  functional (tubular) N25.9
  in
    schistosomiasis B65.9 *[N29]*
  tubular function N25.9
    specified NEC N25.89
lacrimal system H04.9
  changes H04.69
    fistula —*see* Fistula, lacrimal
  gland H04.19
    atrophy —*see* Atrophy,
      lacrimal gland
    cyst —*see* Cyst, lacrimal, gland
    dacryops —*see* Dacryops
    dislocation —*see* Dislocation,
      lacrimal gland
    dry eye syndrome —*see*
      Syndrome, dry eye
    infection —*see*
      Dacryoadenitis
    granuloma —*see* Granuloma,
      lacrimal
    inflammation —*see*
      Inflammation, lacrimal
    obstruction —*see* Obstruction,
      lacrimal
  specified NEC H04.89
lactation NEC O92.79
language (developmental) F80.9
  expressive F80.1
  mixed receptive and expressive
    F80.2
  receptive F80.2
late luteal phase dysphoric N94.89
learning (specific) F81.9
  acalculia R48.8
  alexia R48.0
  mathematics F81.2
  reading F81.0
  specified
    with impairment in
      mathematics F81.2
      reading F81.0
      written expression F81.81
  specified NEC F81.89
  spelling F81.81
  written expression F81.81
lens H27.9
  aphakia —*see* Aphakia
  cataract —*see* Cataract
  dislocation —*see* Dislocation,
    lens
  specified type NEC H27.8
ligament M24.20
  ankle M24.27-
  attachment, spine —*see*
    Enthesopathy, spinal
  elbow M24.22-
  foot joint M24.27-
  hand joint M24.24-
  hip M24.25-
  knee —*see* Derangement, knee,
    specified NEC
  shoulder M24.21-
  specified site NEC M24.29
  vertebra M24.28
  wrist M24.23-
ligamentous attachments —*see also*
  Enthesopathy
  spine —*see* Enthesopathy, spinal
lipid
  metabolism, congenital E78.9
  storage E75.6
    specified NEC E75.5
lipoprotein
  deficiency (familial) E78.6
  metabolism E78.9
    specified NEC E78.89
liver K76.9
  malarial B54 *[K77]*

low back —*see also* Dorsopathy,
  specified NEC
lumbosacral
  plexus G54.1
  root (nerve) NEC G54.4
lung, interstitial, drug-induced
  J70.4
  acute J70.2
  chronic J70.3
  dabbing (related) U07.0
  e-cigarette (related) U07.0
  electronic cigarette (related)
    U07.0
  vaping (associated) (device)
    (product) (related) (use)
    U07.0
lymphoproliferative, post-
  transplant (PTLD) D47.Z1
lysine and hydroxylysine
  metabolism E72.3
male
  erectile (organic) (*see also*
    Dysfunction, sexual, male,
    erectile) N52.9
    nonorganic F52.21
  hypoactive sexual desire F52.0
  orgasmic F52.32
major neurocognitive —*see*
  Dementia, in (due to)
manic F30.9
  organic F06.33
mast cell activation —*see*
  Activation, mast cell
mastoid —*see also* Disorder, ear,
  middle
  postprocedural —*see*
    Complications, ear,
    procedure
meninges, specified type NEC
  G96.198
meniscus —*see* Derangement,
  knee, meniscus
menopausal N95.9
  specified NEC N95.8
menstrual N92.6
  psychogenic F45.8
  specified NEC N92.5
mental (or behavioral)
  (nonpsychotic) F99
  due to (secondary to)
    amphetamine
      due to drug abuse —*see*
        Abuse, drug, stimulant
      due to drug dependence
        —*see* Dependence, drug,
        stimulant
    brain disease, damage and
      dysfunction F09
    caffeine use
      due to drug abuse —*see*
        Abuse, drug, stimulant
      due to drug dependence
        —*see* Dependence, drug,
        stimulant
    cannabis use
      due to drug abuse —*see*
        Abuse, drug, cannabis
      due to drug dependence
        —*see* Dependence, drug,
        cannabis
    general medical condition
      F09
    sedative or hypnotic use
      due to drug abuse —*see*
        Abuse, drug, sedative
      due to drug dependence
        —*see* Dependence, drug,
        sedative
    tobacco (nicotine) use —*see*
      Dependence, drug, nicotine

Disorder *(continued)*
  mental *(continued)*
    following organic brain damage
      F07.9
      frontal lobe syndrome F07.0
      personality change F07.0
      postconcussional syndrome
        F07.81
      specified NEC F07.89
    infancy, childhood or
      adolescence F98.9
    neurotic —*see* Neurosis
    organic or symptomatic F09
    presenile, psychotic F03
    problem NEC
    psychoneurotic —*see* Neurosis
    psychotic —*see* Psychosis
    puerperal F53.0
    senile, psychotic NEC F03
  metabolic, amino acid, transitory,
    newborn P74.8
  metabolism NOS E88.9
    amino-acid E72.9
      aromatic E70.9
        albinism —*see* Albinism
        histidine E70.40
          histidinemia E70.41
          other specified E70.49
        hyperphenylalaninemia
          E70.1
          classical phenylketonuria
            E70.0
          other specified E70.89
        tryptophan E70.5
        tyrosine E70.20
          hypertyrosinemia E70.21
          other specified E70.29
      branched chain E71.2
        3-methylglutaconic aciduria
          E71.111
        hyperleucine-isoleucinemia
          E71.19
        hypervalinemia E71.19
        isovaleric acidemia
          E71.110
        maple syrup urine disease
          E71.0
        methylmalonic acidemia
          E71.120
        organic aciduria NEC
          E71.118
        other specified E71.19
        proprionate NEC E71.128
        proprionic acidemia
          E71.121
      glycine E72.50
        d-glycericacidemia E72.59
        hyperhydroxyprolinemia
          E72.59
        hyperoxaluria R82.992
          primary E72.53
        hyperprolinemia E72.59
        non-ketotic
          hyperglycinemia E72.51
        other specified E72.59
        sarcosinemia E72.59
        trimethylaminuria E72.52
      hydroxylysine E72.3
      lysine E72.3
      ornithine E72.4
      other specified E72.89
        beta-amino acid E72.89
        gamma-glutamyl cycle
          E72.89
        straight-chain E72.89
        sulfur-bearing E72.10
          homocystinuria E72.11
          methylenetetrahydrofolate
            reductase deficiency
            E72.12
        other specified E72.19

Disorder *(continued)*
  metabolism NOS *(continued)*
    bile acid and cholesterol
      metabolism E78.70
    bilirubin E80.7
      specified NEC E80.6
    calcium E83.50
      hypercalcemia E83.52
      hypocalcemia E83.51
      other specified E83.59
    carbohydrate E74.9
      specified NEC E74.89
    cholesterol and bile acid
      metabolism E78.70
    congenital E88.9
    copper E83.00
      Wilson's disease E83.01
      specified type NEC E83.09
    cystinuria E72.01
    fructose E74.10
    galactose E74.20
    glucosaminoglycan E76.9
      mucopolysaccharidosis
        —*see*
        Mucopolysaccharidosis
      specified NEC E76.8
    glutamine E72.89
    glycine E72.50
    glycogen storage (hepatorenal)
      E74.09
    glycoprotein E77.9
      specified NEC E77.8
    glycosaminoglycan E76.9
      specified NEC E76.8
    in labor and delivery O75.89
    iron E83.10
    isoleucine E71.19
    leucine E71.19
    lipoid E78.9
    lipoprotein E78.9
      specified NEC E78.89
    magnesium E83.40
      hypermagnesemia E83.41
      hypomagnesemia E83.42
      other specified E83.49
    mineral E83.9
      specified NEC E83.89
    mitochondrial E88.40
      MELAS syndrome E88.41
      MERRF syndrome (myoclonic
        epilepsy associated with
        ragged-red fibers) E88.42
      other specified E88.49
    ornithine E72.4
    phosphatases E83.30
    phosphorus E83.30
      acid phosphatase deficiency
        E83.39
      hypophosphatasia E83.39
      hypophosphatemia E83.39
        familial E83.31
      other specified E83.39
      pseudovitamin D deficiency
        E83.32
    plasma protein NEC E88.09
    porphyrin —*see* Porphyria
    postprocedural E89.89
      specified NEC E89.89
    purine E79.9
      specified NEC E79.8
    pyrimidine E79.9
      specified NEC E79.8
    pyruvate E74.4
    serine E72.89
    sodium E87.8
    specified NEC E88.89
    threonine E72.89
    valine E71.19
    zinc E83.2
  methylmalonic acidemia
    E71.120

Disorder *(continued)*
  micturition NEC *(see also*
    Difficulty, micturition)
    R39.198
    feeling of incomplete emptying
      R39.14
    hesitancy R39.11
    poor stream R39.12
    psychogenic F45.8
    split stream R39.13
    straining R39.16
    urgency R39.15
  mild neurocognitive G31.84
  mitochondrial metabolism E88.40
  mitral (valve) —*see* Endocarditis,
    mitral
  mixed
    anxiety and depressive F41.8
    of scholastic skills
      (developmental) F81.89
    receptive expressive language
      F80.2
  mood F39
    bipolar —*see* Disorder, bipolar
    depressive —*see* Disorder,
      depressive
    due to (secondary to)
      alcohol F10.94
      amphetamine F15.94
        in
          abuse F15.14
          dependence F15.24
      anxiolytic F13.94
        in
          abuse F13.14
          dependence F13.24
      cocaine F14.94
        in
          abuse F14.14
          dependence F14.24
      general medical condition
        F06.30
      hallucinogen F16.94
        in
          abuse F16.14
          dependence F16.24
      hypnotic F13.94
        in
          abuse F13.14
          dependence F13.24
      inhalant F18.94
        in
          abuse F18.14
          dependence F18.24
      opioid F11.94
        in
          abuse F11.14
          dependence F11.24
      phencyclidine (PCP) F16.94
        in
          abuse F16.14
          dependence F16.24
      physiological condition
        F06.30
        with
          depressive features
            F06.31
          major depressive-like
            episode F06.32
          manic features F06.33
          mixed features F06.34
      psychoactive substance NEC
        F19.94
        in
          abuse F19.14
          dependence F19.24
      sedative F13.94
        in
          abuse F13.14
          dependence F13.24
      volatile solvents F18.94

Disorder *(continued)*
  mood *(continued)*
    due to *(continued)*
      volatile solvents *(continued)*
        in
          abuse F18.14
          dependence F18.24
    manic episode F30.9
      with psychotic symptoms
        F30.2
      in remission (full) F30.4
        partial F30.3
      specified type NEC F30.8
      without psychotic symptoms
        F30.10
        mild F30.11
        moderate F30.12
        severe F30.13
    organic F06.30
      right hemisphere F07.89
    persistent F34.9
      cyclothymia F34.0
      dysthymia F34.1
      specified type NEC F34.89
    recurrent F39
    right hemisphere organic F07.89
  movement G25.9
    drug-induced G25.70
      akathisia G25.71
      specified NEC G25.79
    hysterical F44.4
    in diseases classified elsewhere
      —*see* category G26
    periodic limb G47.61
      sleep related G47.61
    specified NEC G25.89
    sleep related NEC G47.69
    stereotyped F98.4
    treatment-induced G25.9
  multiple personality F44.81
  muscle M62.9
    attachment, spine —*see*
      Enthesopathy, spinal
    in trichinellosis —*see*
      Trichinellosis, with muscle
      disorder
    psychogenic F45.8
    specified type NEC M62.89
    tone, newborn P94.9
      specified NEC P94.8
  muscular
    attachments —*see also*
      Enthesopathy
      spine —*see* Enthesopathy,
      spinal
    urethra N36.44
  musculoskeletal system, soft tissue
    —*see* Disorder, soft tissue
    postprocedural M96.89
    psychogenic F45.8
  myoneural G70.9
    due to lead G70.1
    specified NEC G70.89
    toxic G70.1
  myotonic NEC G71.19
  nail, in diseases classified
    elsewhere L62
  neck region NEC —*see*
    Dorsopathy, specified NEC
  neonatal onset multisystemic
    inflammatory (NOMID) M04.2
  nerve G58.9
    abducent NEC —*see* Strabismus,
      paralytic, sixth nerve
    accessory G52.8
    acoustic —*see* subcategory
      H93.3
    auditory —*see* subcategory
      H93.3
    auriculotemporal G50.8
    axillary G54.0

nerve (continued)
cerebral —see Disorder, nerve, cranial
cranial G52.9
eighth —see subcategory H93.3
eleventh G52.8
fifth G50.9
first G52.0
fourth NEC —see Strabismus, paralytic, fourth nerve
multiple G52.7
ninth G52.1
second NEC —see Disorder, nerve, optic
seventh NEC G51.8
sixth NEC —see Strabismus, paralytic, sixth nerve
specified NEC G52.8
tenth G52.2
third NEC —see Strabismus, paralytic, third nerve
twelfth G52.3
entrapment —see Neuropathy, entrapment
facial G51.9
specified NEC G51.8
femoral —see Lesion, nerve, femoral
glossopharyngeal NEC G52.1
hypoglossal G52.3
intercostal G58.0
lateral
cutaneous of thigh —see Mononeuropathy, lower limb, meralgia paresthetica
popliteal —see Lesion, nerve, popliteal
lower limb —see Mononeuropathy, lower limb
medial popliteal —see Lesion, nerve, popliteal, medial
median NEC —see Lesion, nerve, median
multiple G58.7
oculomotor NEC —see Strabismus, paralytic, third nerve
olfactory G52.0
optic NEC H47.09-
hemorrhage into sheath —see Hemorrhage, optic nerve
ischemic H47.01-
peroneal —see Lesion, nerve, popliteal
phrenic G58.8
plantar —see Lesion, nerve, plantar
pneumogastric G52.2
posterior tibial —see Syndrome, tarsal tunnel
radial —see Lesion, nerve, radial
recurrent laryngeal G52.2
root G54.9
cervical G54.2
lumbosacral G54.1
specified NEC G54.8
thoracic G54.3
sciatic NEC —see Lesion, nerve, sciatic
specified NEC G58.8
lower limb —see Mononeuropathy, lower limb, specified NEC
upper limb —see Mononeuropathy, upper limb, specified NEC
sympathetic G90.9

nerve (continued)
tibial —see Lesion, nerve, popliteal, medial
trigeminal G50.9
specified NEC G50.8
trochlear NEC —see Strabismus, paralytic, fourth nerve
ulnar —see Lesion, nerve, ulnar
upper limb —see Mononeuropathy, upper limb
vagus G52.2
nervous system G98.8
autonomic (peripheral) G90.9
specified NEC G90.8
central G96.9
specified NEC G96.89
parasympathetic G90.9
specified NEC G98.8
sympathetic G90.9
vegetative G90.9
neurocognitive R41.9
major
with
aggressive behavior F01.51
combative behavior F01.51
violent behavior F01.51
due to vascular disease, with behavioral disturbance F01.51
in (due to) (other diseases classified elsewhere) (see also Dementia, in (due to)) F02.80
with
aggressive behavior F02.81
combative behavior F02.81
violent behavior F02.81
without behavioral disturbance F01.50
mild G31.84
neurodevelopment F89
specified NEC F88
neurohypophysis NEC E23.3
neurological NEC R29.818
neuromuscular G70.9
hereditary NEC G71.9
specified NEC G70.89
toxic G70.1
neurotic F48.9
specified NEC F48.8
neutrophil, polymorphonuclear D71
nicotine use —see Dependence, drug, nicotine
nightmare F51.5
non-rapid eye movement sleep arousal
sleep terror type F51.4
sleepwalking type F51.3
nose J34.9
specified NEC J34.89
obsessive-compulsive F42.9
and related disorder due to a known physiological condition F06.8
odontogenesis NOS K00.9
opioid use
with
opioid-induced psychotic disorder F11.959
with
delusions F11.950
hallucinations F11.951
due to drug abuse —see Abuse, drug, opioid
due to drug dependence —see Dependence, drug, opioid

opioid use (continued)
mild F11.10
with
opioid-induced
anxiety disorder F11.188
depressive disorder F11.14
sexual dysfunction F11.181
opioid intoxication
with perceptual disturbances F11.122
delirium F11.121
without perceptual disturbances F11.129
in remission (early) (sustained) F11.11
moderate or severe F11.20
with
opioid-induced
anxiety disorder F11.288
anxiety disorder F11.988
depressive disorder F11.24
depressive disorder F11.94
sexual dysfunction F11.281
sexual dysfunction F11.981
opioid intoxication
with perceptual disturbances F11.222
delirium F11.221
without perceptual disturbances F11.229
in remission (early) (sustained) F11.21
oppositional defiant F91.3
optic
chiasm H47.49
due to
inflammatory disorder H47.41
neoplasm H47.42
vascular disorder H47.43
disc H47.39-
coloboma —see Coloboma, optic disc
drusen —see Drusen, optic disc
pseudopapilledema —see Pseudopapilledema
radiations —see Disorder, visual, pathway
tracts —see Disorder, visual, pathway
orbit H05.9
cyst —see Cyst, orbit
deformity —see Deformity, orbit
edema —see Edema, orbit
enophthalmos —see Enophthalmos
exophthalmos —see Exophthalmos
hemorrhage —see Hemorrhage, orbit
inflammation —see Inflammation, orbit
myopathy —see Myopathy, extraocular muscles
retained foreign body —see Foreign body, orbit, old
specified type NEC H05.89
organic
anxiety F06.4
catatonic F06.1
delusional F06.2
dissociative F06.8

organic (continued)
emotionally labile (asthenic) F06.8
mood (affective) F06.30
schizophrenia-like F06.2
orgasmic (female) F52.31
male F52.32
ornithine metabolism E72.4
overanxious F41.1
of childhood F93.8
pain
with related psychological factors F45.42
exclusively related to psychological factors F45.41
genito-pelvic penetration disorder F52.6
pancreatic internal secretion E16.9
specified NEC E16.8
panic F41.0
with agoraphobia F40.01
papulosquamous L44.9
in diseases classified elsewhere L45
specified NEC L44.8
paranoid F22
induced F24
shared F24
paraphilic F65.9
specified NEC F65.89
parathyroid (gland) E21.5
specified NEC E21.4
parietoalveolar NEC J84.09
paroxysmal, mixed R56.9
patella M22.9-
chondromalacia —see Chondromalacia, patella
derangement NEC M22.3X-
recurrent
dislocation —see Dislocation, patella, recurrent
subluxation —see Dislocation, patella, recurrent, incomplete
specified NEC M22.8X-
patellofemoral M22.2X-
pedophilic F65.4
pentose phosphate pathway with anemia D55.1
perception, due to hallucinogens F16.983
in
abuse F16.183
dependence F16.283
peripheral nervous system NEC G64
peroxisomal E71.50
biogenesis
neonatal adrenoleukodystrophy E71.511
specified disorder NEC E71.518
Zellweger syndrome E71.510
rhizomelic chondrodysplasia punctata E71.540
specified form NEC E71.548
group 1 E71.518
group 2 E71.53
group 3 E71.542
X-linked adrenoleukodystrophy E71.529
adolescent E71.521
adrenomyeloneuropathy E71.522
childhood E71.520
specified form NEC E71.528
Zellweger-like syndrome E71.541

Disorder (*continued*)
substance use (*continued*)
  mild (*continued*)
    with substance-induced
      (*continued*)
        major neurocognitive
          disorder F19.17
        mild neurocognitive
          disorder F19.188
        obsessive-compulsive and
          related disorder F19.188
        sexual dysfunction F19.181
      substance intoxication
        F19.129
      substance intoxication
        delirium F19.121
  moderate or severe F19.20
    with substance-induced
      anxiety disorder F19.280
      bipolar and related disorder
        F19.24
      depressive disorder F19.24
      major neurocognitive
        disorder F19.27
      mild neurocognitive
        disorder F19.288
      obsessive-compulsive and
        related disorder F19.288
      sexual dysfunction F19.281
    in remission (early)
      (sustained) F19.21
    substance intoxication
      F19.229
    substance intoxication
      delirium F19.221
sulfur-bearing amino-acid
  metabolism E72.10
sweat gland (eccrine) L74.9
  apocrine L75.9
    specified NEC L75.8
  specified NEC L74.8
synovium M67.90
  acromioclavicular M67.91-
  ankle M67.97-
  elbow M67.92-
  foot M67.97-
  forearm M67.93-
  hand M67.94-
  hip M67.95-
  knee M67.96-
  multiple sites M67.99
  rupture —*see* Rupture, synovium
  shoulder M67.91-
  specified type NEC M67.80
    acromioclavicular M67.81-
    ankle M67.87-
    elbow M67.82-
    foot M67.87-
    hand M67.84-
    hip M67.85-
    knee M67.86-
    multiple sites M67.89
    wrist M67.83-
  synovitis —*see* Synovitis
  upper arm M67.92-
  wrist M67.93-
temperature regulation, newborn
  P81.9
  specified NEC P81.8
temporomandibular joint M26.60-
tendon M67.90
  acromioclavicular M67.91-
  ankle M67.97-
  contracture —*see* Contracture,
    tendon
  elbow M67.92-
  foot M67.97-
  forearm M67.93-
  hand M67.94-
  hip M67.95-
  knee M67.96-

Disorder (*continued*)
tendon (*continued*)
  multiple sites M67.99
  rupture —*see* Rupture, tendon
  shoulder M67.91-
  specified type NEC M67.80
    acromioclavicular M67.81-
    ankle M67.87-
    elbow M67.82-
    foot M67.87-
    hand M67.84-
    hip M67.85-
    knee M67.86-
    multiple sites M67.89
    trunk M67.88
    wrist M67.83-
  synovitis —*see* Synovitis
  tendinitis —*see* Tendinitis
  tenosynovitis —*see* Tenosynovitis
  trunk M67.98
  upper arm M67.92-
  wrist M67.93-
thoracic root (nerve) NEC G54.3
thyrocalcitonin hypersecretion
  E07.0
thyroid (gland) E07.9
  function NEC, neonatal,
    transitory P72.2
  iodine-deficiency related E01.8
  specified NEC E07.89
tic —*see* Tic
tobacco use
  chewing tobacco (mild)
    (moderate) (severe)
    in remission (early)
      (sustained) F17.221
  cigarettes (mild) (moderate)
    (severe)
    in remission (early)
      (sustained) F17.211
    mild F17.200
      in remission (early)
        (sustained) F17.201
    moderate F17.200
      in remission (early)
        (sustained) F17.201
    severe F17.200
      in remission (early)
        (sustained) F17.201
  specified product NEC (mild)
    (moderate) (severe)
    in remission (early)
      (sustained) F17.291
tooth K08.9
  development K00.9
    specified NEC K00.8
  eruption K00.6
Tourette's F95.2
trance and possession F44.89
transvestic F65.1
trauma and stressor-related F43.9
  other specified F43.8
tricuspid (valve) —*see*
  Endocarditis, tricuspid
tryptophan metabolism E70.5
tubular, phosphate-losing N25.0
tubulo-interstitial (in)
  brucellosis A23.9 *[N16]*
  cystinosis E72.04
  diphtheria A36.84
  glycogen storage disease E74.00
    [N16]
  leukemia NEC C95.9- *[N16]*
  lymphoma NEC C85.9- *[N16]*
  mixed cryoglobulinemia D89.1
    [N16]
  multiple myeloma C90.0- *[N16]*
  Salmonella infection A02.25
  sarcoidosis D86.84
  sepsis A41.9 *[N16]*
    streptococcal A40.9 *[N16]*

Disorder (*continued*)
tubulo-interstitial (*continued*)
  systemic lupus erythematosus
    M32.15
  toxoplasmosis B58.83
  transplant rejection T86.91
    [N16]
  Wilson's disease E83.01 *[N16]*
tubulo-renal function, impaired
  N25.9
  specified NEC N25.89
tympanic membrane H73.9-
  atrophy —*see* Atrophy, tympanic
    membrane
  infection —*see* Myringitis
  perforation —*see* Perforation,
    tympanum
  specified NEC H73.89-
unsocialized aggressive F91.1
urea cycle metabolism E72.20
  argininemia E72.21
  arginosuccinic aciduria E72.22
  citrullinemia E72.23
  ornithine transcarbamylase
    deficiency E72.4
  other specified E72.29
ureter (in) N28.9
  schistosomiasis B65.0 *[N29]*
  tuberculosis A18.11
urethra N36.9
  specified NEC N36.8
urinary system N39.9
  specified NEC N39.8
valve, heart
  aortic —*see* Endocarditis, aortic
  mitral —*see* Endocarditis, mitral
  pulmonary —*see* Endocarditis,
    pulmonary
  rheumatic
    aortic —*see* Endocarditis,
      aortic, rheumatic
    mitral —*see* Endocarditis,
      mitral
    pulmonary —*see* Endocarditis,
      pulmonary, rheumatic
    tricuspid —*see* Endocarditis,
      tricuspid
  tricuspid —*see* Endocarditis,
    tricuspid
vestibular function H81.9-
  specified NEC —*see* subcategory
    H81.8
  in diseases classified
    elsewhere H82.-
  vertigo —*see* Vertigo
vision, binocular H53.30
  abnormal retinal correspondence
    H53.31
  diplopia H53.2
  fusion with defective stereopsis
    H53.32
  simultaneous perception
    H53.33
  suppression H53.34
visual
  cortex
    blindness H47.619
      left brain H47.612
      right brain H47.611
    due to
      inflammatory disorder
        H47.629
        left brain H47.622
        right brain H47.621
      neoplasm H47.639
        left brain H47.632
        right brain H47.631
      vascular disorder H47.649
        left brain H47.642
        right brain H47.641
  pathway H47.9

Disorder (*continued*)
visual (*continued*)
  pathway (*continued*)
    due to
      inflammatory disorder
        H47.51-
      neoplasm H47.52-
      vascular disorder H47.53-
    optic chiasm —*see* Disorder,
      optic, chiasm
vitreous body H43.9
  crystalline deposits —*see*
    Deposit, crystalline
  degeneration —*see*
    Degeneration, vitreous
  hemorrhage —*see* Hemorrhage,
    vitreous
  opacities —*see* Opacity, vitreous
  prolapse —*see* Prolapse,
    vitreous
  specified type NEC H43.89
voice R49.9
  specified type NEC R49.8
volatile solvent use
  due to drug abuse —*see* Abuse,
    drug, inhalant
  due to drug dependence —*see*
    Dependence, drug, inhalant
voyeuristic F65.3
white blood cells D72.9
  specified NEC D72.89
withdrawing, child or adolescent
  F40.10

Disorientation R41.0

Displacement, displaced
  acquired traumatic of bone,
    cartilage, joint, tendon NEC
    —*see* Dislocation
  adrenal gland (congenital) Q89.1
  appendix, retrocecal (congenital)
    Q43.8
  auricle (congenital) Q17.4
  bladder (acquired) N32.89
    congenital Q64.19
  brachial plexus (congenital) Q07.8
  brain stem, caudal (congenital)
    Q04.8
  canaliculus (lacrimalis), congenital
    Q10.6
  cardia through esophageal hiatus
    (congenital) Q40.1
  cerebellum, caudal (congenital)
    Q04.8
  cervix —*see* Malposition, uterus
  colon (congenital) Q43.3
  device, implant or graft (*see also*
    Complications, by site and type,
    mechanical) T85.628
    arterial graft NEC —*see*
      Complication, cardiovascular
      device, mechanical, vascular
    breast (implant) T85.42
    catheter NEC T85.628
      dialysis (renal) T82.42
        intraperitoneal T85.621
      infusion NEC T82.524
        spinal (epidural) (subdural)
          T85.620
      urinary
        cystostomy T83.020
        Hopkins T83.028
        ileostomy T83.028
        indwelling T83.021
        nephrostomy T83.022
        specified NEC T83.028
        urostomy T83.028
  electronic (electrode) (pulse
    generator) (stimulator) —*see*
    Complication, electronic
    stimulator

Distortion (continued)

chest (wall) Q67.8
  bones Q76.8
clavicle Q74.0
clitoris Q52.6
coccyx Q76.49
common duct Q44.5
coronary Q24.5
cystic duct Q44.5
ear (auricle) (external) Q17.3
  inner Q16.5
  middle Q16.4
    ossicles Q16.3
endocrine NEC Q89.2
eustachian tube Q17.8
eye (adnexa) Q15.8
face bone(s) NEC Q75.8
fallopian tube Q50.6
femur NEC Q68.8
fibula NEC Q68.8
finger(s) Q68.1
foot Q66.9-
genitalia, genital organ(s)
  female Q52.8
    external Q52.79
    internal NEC Q52.8
gyri Q04.8
hand bone(s) Q68.1
heart (auricle) (ventricle) Q24.8
  valve (cusp) Q24.8
hepatic duct Q44.5
humerus NEC Q68.8
hymen Q52.4
intrafamilial communications
  Z63.8
jaw NEC M26.89
labium (majus) (minus) Q52.79
leg NEC Q68.8
lens Q12.8
liver Q44.7
lumbar spine Q76.49
  with disproportion O33.8
    causing obstructed labor
      O65.0
lumbosacral (joint) (region) Q76.49
  kyphosis —see Kyphosis,
    congenital
  lordosis —see Lordosis,
    congenital
nerve Q07.8
nose Q30.8
organ
  of Corti Q16.5
  or site not listed —see Anomaly,
    by site
ossicles, ear Q16.3
oviduct Q50.6
pancreas Q45.3
parathyroid (gland) Q89.2
pituitary (gland) Q89.2
radius NEC Q68.8
sacroiliac joint Q74.2
sacrum Q76.49
scapula Q74.0
shoulder girdle Q74.0
skull bone(s) NEC Q75.8
  with
    anencephalus Q00.0
    encephalocele —see
      Encephalocele
    hydrocephalus Q03.9
      with spina bifida —see
        Spina bifida, with
        hydrocephalus
    microcephaly Q02
spinal cord Q06.8
spine Q76.49
  kyphosis —see Kyphosis,
    congenital
  lordosis —see Lordosis,
    congenital

Distortion (continued)

spleen Q89.09
sternum NEC Q76.7
thorax (wall) Q67.8
  bony Q76.8
thymus (gland) Q89.2
thyroid (gland) Q89.2
tibia NEC Q68.8
toe(s) Q66.9-
tongue Q38.3
trachea (cartilage) Q32.1
ulna NEC Q68.8
ureter Q62.8
urethra Q64.79
  causing obstruction Q64.39
uterus Q51.9
vagina Q52.4
vertebra Q76.49
  kyphosis —see Kyphosis,
    congenital
  lordosis —see Lordosis,
    congenital
visual —see also Disturbance,
  vision
  shape and size H53.15
vulva Q52.79
wrist (bones) (joint) Q68.8

Distress

abdomen —see Pain, abdominal
acute respiratory R06.03
  syndrome (adult) (child) J80
epigastric R10.13
fetal P84
  complicating pregnancy —see
    Stress, fetal
gastrointestinal (functional) K30
  psychogenic F45.8
intestinal (functional) NOS K59.9
  psychogenic F45.8
maternal, during labor and delivery
  O75.0
relationship, with spouse or
  intimate partner Z63.0
respiratory (adult) (child) R06.03
  newborn P22.9
    specified NEC P22.8
  orthopnea R06.01
  psychogenic F45.8
  shortness of breath R06.02
  specified type NEC R06.09

Distribution vessel, atypical Q27.9
coronary artery Q24.5
precerebral Q28.1

Districhiasis L68.8

Disturbance(s) —see also Disease
absorption K90.9
  calcium E58
  carbohydrate K90.49
  fat K90.49
    pancreatic K90.3
  protein K90.49
  starch K90.49
  vitamin —see Deficiency, vitamin
acid-base equilibrium E87.8
  mixed E87.4
activity and attention (with
  hyperkinesis) —see Disorder,
  attention-deficit hyperactivity
amino acid transport E72.00
assimilation, food K90.9
auditory nerve, except deafness
  —see subcategory H93.3
behavior —see Disorder, conduct
blood clotting (mechanism) (see
  also Defect, coagulation) D68.9
cerebral
  nerve —see Disorder, nerve,
    cranial
  status, newborn P91.9
    specified NEC P91.88

Disturbance (continued)

circulatory I99.9
conduct (see also Disorder,
  conduct) F91.9
  adjustment reaction —see
    Disorder, adjustment
  compulsive F63.9
  disruptive F91.9
  hyperkinetic —see Disorder,
    attention-deficit hyperactivity
  socialized F91.2
  specified NEC F91.8
  unsocialized F91.1
coordination R27.8
cranial nerve —see Disorder, nerve,
  cranial
deep sensibility —see Disturbance,
  sensation
digestive K30
  psychogenic F45.8
electrolyte —see also Imbalance,
  electrolyte
  newborn, transitory P74.49
    hyperammonemia P74.6
    hyperchloremia P74.421
    hyperchloremic metabolic
      acidosis P74.421
    hypochloremia P74.422
    potassium balance
      hyperkalemia P74.31
      hypokalemia P74.32
    sodium balance
      hypernatremia P74.21
      hyponatremia P74.22
    specified type NEC P74.49
emotions specific to childhood and
  adolescence F93.9
  with
    anxiety and fearfulness NEC
      F93.8
    elective mutism F94.0
    oppositional disorder F91.3
    sensitivity (withdrawal)
      F40.10
    shyness F40.10
    social withdrawal F40.10
  involving relationship problems
    F93.8
  mixed F93.8
  specified NEC F93.8
endocrine (gland) E34.9
  neonatal, transitory P72.9
    specified NEC P72.8
equilibrium R42
fructose metabolism E74.10
gait —see Gait
  hysterical F44.4
  psychogenic F44.4
gastrointestinal (functional) K30
  psychogenic F45.8
habit, child F98.9
hearing, except deafness and
  tinnitus —see Abnormal,
  auditory perception
heart, functional (conditions in
  I44-I50)
  due to presence of (cardiac)
    prosthesis I97.19-
  postoperative I97.89
    cardiac surgery (see also
      Infarct, myocardium,
      associated with
      revascularization procedure)
      I97.19-
hormones E34.9
innervation uterus (parasympathetic)
  (sympathetic) N85.8
keratinization NEC
  gingiva K05.10
    nonplaque induced K05.11
    plaque induced K05.10

Disturbance (continued)

keratinization NEC (continued)
  lip K13.0
  oral (mucosa) (soft tissue)
    K13.29
  tongue K13.29
learning (specific) —see Disorder,
  learning
memory —see Amnesia
  mild, following organic brain
    damage F06.8
mental F99
  associated with diseases
    classified elsewhere F54
metabolism E88.9
  with
    abortion —see Abortion, by
      type with other specified
      complication
    ectopic pregnancy O08.5
    molar pregnancy O08.5
  amino-acid E72.9
    aromatic E70.9
    branched-chain E71.2
      straight-chain E72.89
    sulfur-bearing E72.10
  ammonia E72.20
  arginine E72.21
  arginosuccinic acid E72.22
  carbohydrate E74.9
  cholesterol E78.9
  citrulline E72.23
  cystathionine E72.19
  general E88.9
  glutamine E72.89
  histidine E70.40
  homocystine E72.19
  hydroxylysine E72.3
  in labor or delivery O75.89
  iron E83.10
  lipoid E78.9
  lysine E72.3
  methionine E72.19
  neonatal, transitory P74.9
    calcium and magnesium P71.9
      specified type NEC P71.8
    carbohydrate metabolism
      P70.9
      specified type NEC P70.8
    specified NEC P74.8
  ornithine E72.4
  phosphate E83.39
  sodium NEC E87.8
  threonine E72.89
  tryptophan E70.5
  tyrosine E70.20
  urea cycle E72.20
motor R29.2
nervous, functional R45.0
neuromuscular mechanism (eye),
  due to syphilis A52.15
nutritional E63.9
  nail L60.3
ocular motion H51.9
  psychogenic F45.8
oculogyric H51.8
  psychogenic F45.8
oculomotor H51.9
  psychogenic F45.8
olfactory nerve R43.1
optic nerve NEC —see Disorder,
  nerve, optic
oral epithelium, including tongue
  NEC K13.29
perceptual due to
  alcohol withdrawal F10.232
  amphetamine intoxication
    F15.922
    in
      abuse F15.122
      dependence F15.222

Disturbance *(continued)*

perceptual due to *(continued)*
anxiolytic withdrawal F13.232
cannabis intoxication (acute)
F12.922
in
abuse F12.122
dependence F12.222
cocaine intoxication (acute)
F14.922
in
abuse F14.122
dependence F14.222
hypnotic withdrawal F13.232
opioid intoxication (acute)
F19.122
phencyclidine intoxication
(acute) F16.122
sedative withdrawal F13.232
personality (pattern) (trait) —*see*
also Disorder, personality F60.9
following organic brain damage
F07.9
polyglandular E31.9
specified NEC E31.8
potassium balance, newborn
hyperkalemia P74.31
hypokalemia P74.32
psychogenic F45.9
psychomotor F44.4
psychophysical visual H53.16
pupillary —*see* Anomaly, pupil,
function
reflex R29.2
rhythm, heart I49.9
salivary secretion K11.7
sensation (cold) (heat)
(localization) (tactile
discrimination) (texture)
(vibratory) NEC R20.9
hysterical F44.6
skin R20.9
anesthesia R20.0
hyperesthesia R20.3
hypoesthesia R20.1
paresthesia R20.2
specified type NEC R20.8
smell R43.9
and taste (mixed) R43.8
anosmia R43.0
parosmia R43.1
specified NEC R43.8
taste R43.9
and smell (mixed) R43.8
parageusia R43.2
specified NEC R43.8
sensory —*see* Disturbance,
sensation
situational (transient) —*see also*
Disorder, adjustment
acute F43.0
sleep G47.9
nonorganic origin F51.9
smell —*see* Disturbance, sensation,
smell
sociopathic F60.2
sodium balance, newborn
hypernatremia P74.21
hyponatremia P74.22
speech R47.9
developmental F80.9
specified NEC R47.89
stomach (functional) K31.9
sympathetic (nerve) G90.9
taste —*see* Disturbance, sensation,
taste
temperature
regulation, newborn P81.9
specified NEC P81.8
sense R20.8
hysterical F44.6

Disturbance *(continued)*

tooth
eruption K00.6
formation K00.4
structure, hereditary NEC K00.5
touch —*see* Disturbance, sensation
vascular I99.9
arteriosclerotic —*see*
Arteriosclerosis
vasomotor I73.9
vasospastic I73.9
vision, visual H53.9
following
cerebral infarction I69.398
cerebrovascular disease
I69.998
specified NEC I69.898
intracerebral hemorrhage
I69.198
nontraumatic intracranial
hemorrhage NEC I69.298
specified disease NEC
I69.898
subarachnoid hemorrhage
I69.098
psychophysical H53.16
specified NEC H53.8
subjective H53.10
day blindness H53.11
discomfort H53.14-
distortions of shape and size
H53.15
loss
sudden H53.13-
transient H53.12-
specified type NEC H53.19
voice R49.9
psychogenic F44.4
specified NEC R49.8

Diuresis R35.8

Diver's palsy, paralysis or squeeze
T70.3

Diverticulitis (acute) K57.92
bladder —*see* Cystitis
ileum —*see* Diverticulitis,
intestine, small
intestine K57.92
with
abscess, perforation K57.80
with bleeding K57.81
bleeding K57.93
congenital Q43.8
large K57.32
with
abscess, perforation K57.20
with bleeding K57.21
bleeding K57.33
small intestine K57.52
with
abscess, perforation
K57.40
with bleeding
K57.41
bleeding K57.53
small K57.12
with
abscess, perforation
K57.00
with bleeding K57.01
bleeding K57.13
large intestine K57.52
with
abscess, perforation
K57.40
with bleeding
K57.41
bleeding K57.53

Diverticulosis K57.90
with bleeding K57.91

Diverticulosis *(continued)*
large intestine K57.30
with
bleeding K57.31
small intestine K57.50
with bleeding K57.51
small intestine K57.10
with
bleeding K57.11
large intestine K57.50
with bleeding K57.51

Diverticulum, diverticula (multiple)
K57.90
appendix (noninflammatory)
K38.2
bladder (sphincter) N32.3
congenital Q64.6
bronchus (congenital) Q32.4
acquired J98.09
calyx, calyceal (kidney) N28.89
cardia (stomach) K31.4
cecum —*see* Diverticulosis,
intestine, large
congenital Q43.8
colon —*see* Diverticulosis,
intestine, large
congenital Q43.8
duodenum —*see* Diverticulosis,
intestine, small
congenital Q43.8
epiphrenic (esophagus) K22.5
esophagus (congenital) Q39.6
acquired (epiphrenic) (pulsion)
(traction) K22.5
eustachian tube —*see* Disorder,
eustachian tube, specified NEC
fallopian tube N83.8
gastric K31.4
heart (congenital) Q24.8
ileum —*see* Diverticulosis,
intestine, small
jejunum —*see* Diverticulosis,
intestine, small
kidney (pelvis) (calyces) N28.89
with calculus —*see* Calculus,
kidney
Meckel's (displaced) (hypertrophic)
Q43.0
malignant —*see* Table of
Neoplasms, small intestine,
malignant
midthoracic K22.5
organ or site, congenital NEC
—*see* Distortion
pericardium (congenital) (cyst)
Q24.8
acquired I31.8
pharyngoesophageal (congenital)
Q39.6
acquired K22.5
pharynx (congenital) Q38.7
rectosigmoid —*see* Diverticulosis,
intestine, large
congenital Q43.8
rectum —*see* Diverticulosis,
intestine, large
Rokitansky's K22.5
seminal vesicle N50.89
sigmoid —*see* Diverticulosis,
intestine, large
congenital Q43.8
stomach (acquired) K31.4
congenital Q40.2
trachea (acquired) J39.8
ureter (acquired) N28.89
congenital Q62.8
ureterovesical orifice N28.89
urethra (acquired) N36.1
congenital Q64.79
ventricle, left (congenital) Q24.8

Diverticulum, diverticula
(continued)
vesical N32.3
congenital Q64.6
Zenker's (esophagus) K22.5

Division
cervix uteri (acquired) N88.8
glans penis Q55.69
labia minora (congenital) Q52.79
ligament (partial or complete)
(current) —*see also* Sprain
with open wound —*see* Wound,
open
muscle (partial or complete)
(current) —*see also* Injury,
muscle
with open wound —*see* Wound,
open
nerve (traumatic) —*see* Injury,
nerve
spinal cord —*see* Injury, spinal
cord, by region
vein I87.8

Divorce, causing family disruption
Z63.5

Dix-Hallpike neurolabyrinthitis
—*see* Neuronitis, vestibular

Dizziness R42
hysterical F44.89
psychogenic F45.8

DMAC (disseminated mycobacterium
avium- intracellulare complex)
A31.2

DNR (do not resuscitate) Z66

Doan-Wiseman syndrome (primary
splenic neutropenia) —*see*
Agranulocytosis

Doehle-Heller aortitis A52.02

Dog bite —*see* Bite

Dohle body panmyelopathic
syndrome D72.0

Dolichocephaly Q67.2

Dolichocolon Q43.8

Dolichostenomelia —*see* Syndrome,
Marfan's

Donohue's syndrome E34.8

Donor (organ or tissue) Z52.9
blood (whole) Z52.000
autologous Z52.010
specified component
(lymphocytes) (platelets) NEC
Z52.008
autologous Z52.018
specified donor NEC Z52.098
specified donor NEC Z52.090
stem cells Z52.001
autologous Z52.011
specified donor NEC Z52.091
bone Z52.20
autologous Z52.21
marrow Z52.3
specified type NEC Z52.29
cornea Z52.5
egg (Oocyte) Z52.819
age 35 and over Z52.812
anonymous recipient Z52.812
designated recipient Z52.813
under age 35 Z52.810
anonymous recipient Z52.810
designated recipient Z52.811
kidney Z52.4
liver Z52.6
lung Z52.89
lymphocyte —*see* Donor, blood,
specified components NEC

Donor *(continued)*
Oocyte —*see* Donor, egg
platelets Z52.008
potential, examination of Z00.5
semen Z52.89
skin Z52.10
autologous Z52.11
specified type NEC Z52.19
specified organ or tissue NEC
Z52.89
sperm Z52.89

Donovanosis A58

Dorsalgia M54.9
psychogenic F45.41
specified NEC M54.89

Dorsopathy M53.9
deforming M43.9
specified NEC —*see* subcategory
M43.8
specified NEC M53.80
cervical region M53.82
cervicothoracic region M53.83
lumbar region M53.86
lumbosacral region M53.87
occipito-atlanto-axial region
M53.81
sacrococcygeal region M53.88
thoracic region M53.84
thoracolumbar region M53.85

Double
albumin E88.09
aortic arch Q25.45
auditory canal Q17.8
auricle (heart) Q20.8
bladder Q64.79
cervix Q51.820
with doubling of uterus (and
vagina) Q51.10
with obstruction Q51.11
inlet ventricle Q20.4
kidney with double pelvis (renal)
Q63.0
meatus urinarius Q64.75
monster Q89.4
outlet
left ventricle Q20.2
right ventricle Q20.1
pelvis (renal) with double ureter
Q62.5
tongue Q38.3
ureter (one or both sides) Q62.5
with double pelvis (renal) Q62.5
urethra Q64.74
urinary meatus Q64.75
uterus Q51.28
with
doubling of cervix (and
vagina) Q51.10
with obstruction Q51.11
complete Q51.21
in pregnancy or childbirth
O34.0-
causing obstructed labor O65.5
partial Q51.22
specified NEC Q51.28
vagina Q52.10
with doubling of uterus (and
cervix) Q51.10
with obstruction Q51.11
vision H53.2
vulva Q52.79

Douglas' pouch, cul-de-sac —*see*
condition

Down syndrome Q90.9
meiotic nondisjunction Q90.0
mitotic nondisjunction Q90.1
mosaicism Q90.1
translocation Q90.2

DPD (dihydropyrimidine
dehydrogenase deficiency) E88.89

Dracontiasis B72

Dracunculiasis, dracunculosis
B72

Dream state, hysterical F44.89

Dreschlera (hawaiiensis) (infection)
B43.8

Drepanocytic anemia —*see* Disease,
sickle-cell

Dresbach's syndrome (elliptocytosis)
D58.1

Dressler's syndrome I24.1

Drift, ulnar —*see* Deformity, limb,
specified type NEC, forearm

Drinking (alcohol)
excessive, to excess NEC (without
dependence) F10.10
habitual (continual) (without
remission) F10.20
with remission F10.21

Drip, postnasal (chronic) R09.82
due to
allergic rhinitis —*see* Rhinitis,
allergic
common cold J00
gastroesophageal reflux —*see*
Reflux, gastroesophageal
nasopharyngitis —*see*
Nasopharyngitis
other know condition - code to
condition
sinusitis —*see* Sinusitis

Droop
facial R29.810
cerebrovascular disease I69.992
cerebral infarction I69.392
intracerebral hemorrhage
I69.192
nontraumatic intracranial
hemorrhage NEC I69.292
specified disease NEC I69.892
subarachnoid hemorrhage
I69.092

Drop (in)
attack NEC R55
finger —*see* Deformity, finger
foot —*see* Deformity, limb, foot,
drop
hematocrit (precipitous) R71.0
hemoglobin R71.0
toe —*see* Deformity, toe, specified
NEC
wrist —*see* Deformity, limb, wrist
drop

Dropped heart beats I45.9

Dropsy, dropsical —*see also*
Hydrops
abdomen R18.8
brain —*see* Hydrocephalus
cardiac, heart —*see* Failure, heart,
congestive
gangrenous —*see* Gangrene
heart —*see* Failure, heart,
congestive
kidney —*see* Nephrosis
lung —*see* Edema, lung
newborn due to isoimmunization
P56.0
pericardium —*see* Pericarditis

Drowned, drowning (near) T75.1

Drowsiness R40.0

Drug
abuse counseling and surveillance
Z71.51

Drug *(continued)*
addiction —*see* Dependence
dependence —*see* Dependence
habit —*see* Dependence
harmful use —*see* Abuse, drug
induced fever R50.2
overdose —*see* Table of Drugs and
Chemicals, by drug, poisoning
poisoning —*see* Table of Drugs and
Chemicals, by drug, poisoning
resistant organism infection (*see
also* Resistant, organism, to,
drug) Z16.30
therapy
long term (current)
(prophylactic) —*see* Therapy,
drug long-term (current)
(prophylactic)
short term - omit code
wrong substance given or taken in
error —*see* Table of Drugs and
Chemicals, by drug, poisoning

Drunkenness (without dependence)
F10.129
acute in alcoholism F10.229
chronic (without remission) F10.20
with remission F10.21
pathological (without dependence)
F10.129
with dependence F10.229
sleep F51.9

Drusen
macula (degenerative) (retina)
—*see* Degeneration, macula,
drusen
optic disc H47.32-

Dry, dryness —*see also* condition
larynx J38.7
mouth R68.2
due to dehydration E86.0
nose J34.89
socket (teeth) M27.3
throat J39.2

DSAP L56.5

Duane's syndrome H50.81-

**Dubin-Johnson disease or
syndrome** E80.6

Dubois' disease (thymus gland)
A50.59 *[E35]*

Dubowitz' syndrome Q87.19

Duchenne-Aran muscular atrophy
G12.21

Duchenne-Griesinger disease
G71.01

Duchenne's
disease or syndrome
motor neuron disease G12.22
muscular dystrophy G71.01
locomotor ataxia (syphilitic)
A52.11
paralysis
birth injury P14.0
due to or associated with
motor neuron disease G12.22
muscular dystrophy G71.01

Ducrey's chancre A57

Duct, ductus —*see* condition

Duhring's disease (dermatitis
herpetiformis) L13.0

Dullness, cardiac (decreased)
(increased) R01.2

Dumb ague —*see* Malaria

Dumbness —*see* Aphasia

Dumdum fever B55.0

Dumping syndrome
(postgastrectomy) K91.1

Duodenitis (nonspecific) (peptic)
K29.80
with bleeding K29.81

Duodenocholangitis —*see*
Cholangitis

Duodenum, duodenal —*see*
condition

Duplay's bursitis or periarthritis
—*see* Tendinitis, calcific, shoulder

Duplication, duplex —*see also*
Accessory
alimentary tract Q45.8
anus Q43.4
appendix (and cecum) Q43.4
biliary duct (any) Q44.5
bladder Q64.79
cecum (and appendix) Q43.4
cervix Q51.820
chromosome NEC
with complex rearrangements
NEC Q92.5
seen only at prometaphase Q92.8
cystic duct Q44.5
digestive organs Q45.8
esophagus Q39.8
frontonasal process Q75.8
intestine (large) (small) Q43.4
kidney Q63.0
liver Q44.7
pancreas Q45.3
penis Q55.69
respiratory organs NEC Q34.8
salivary duct Q38.4
spinal cord (incomplete) Q06.2
stomach Q40.2

Dupré's disease (meningism) R29.1

Dupuytren's contraction or disease
M72.0

Durand-Nicolas-Favre disease A55

Durotomy (inadvertent) (incidental)
G97.41

Duroziez's disease (congenital mitral
stenosis) Q23.2

Dutton's relapsing fever (West
African) A68.1

Dwarfism E34.3
achondroplastic Q77.4
congenital E34.3
constitutional E34.3
hypochondroplastic Q77.4
hypophyseal E23.0
infantile E34.3
Laron-type E34.3
Lorain (-Levi) type E23.0
metatropic Q77.8
nephrotic-glycosuric (with
hypophosphatemic rickets)
E72.09
nutritional E45
pancreatic K86.89
pituitary E23.0
renal N25.0
thanatophoric Q77.1

Dyke-Young anemia (secondary)
(symptomatic) D59.19

Dysacusis —*see* Abnormal, auditory
perception

Dysadrenocortism E27.9
hyperfunction E27.0

Dysarthria R47.1
following
cerebral infarction I69.322

Dysarthria *(continued)*
　following *(continued)*
　　cerebrovascular disease I69.922
　　　specified disease NEC I69.822
　　intracerebral hemorrhage
　　　I69.122
　　nontraumatic intracranial
　　　hemorrhage NEC I69.222
　　subarachnoid hemorrhage
　　　I69.022

Dysautonomia (familial) G90.1

Dysbarism T70.3

Dysbasia R26.2
　angiosclerotica intermittens I73.9
　hysterical F44.4
　lordotica (progressiva) G24.1
　nonorganic origin F44.4
　psychogenic F44.4

Dysbetalipoproteinemia (familial)
　E78.2

Dyscalculia R48.8
　developmental F81.2

Dyschezia K59.00

Dyschondroplasia (with
　hemangiomata) Q78.4

Dyschromia (skin) L81.9

Dyscollagenosis M35.9

Dyscranio-pygo-phalangy Q87.0

Dyscrasia
　blood (with) D75.9
　　antepartum hemorrhage —*see*
　　　Hemorrhage, antepartum, with
　　　coagulation defect
　　newborn P61.9
　　　specified type NEC P61.8
　　intrapartum hemorrhage O67.0
　　puerperal, postpartum O72.3
　polyglandular, pluriglandular E31.9

Dysendocrinism E34.9

Dysentery, dysenteric (catarrhal)
　(diarrhea) (epidemic)
　(hemorrhagic) (infectious)
　(sporadic) (tropical) A09
　abscess, liver A06.4
　amebic (*see also* Amebiasis) A06.0
　　with abscess —*see* Abscess,
　　　amebic
　　acute A06.0
　　chronic A06.1
　arthritis (*see also* category M01)
　　A09
　bacillary (*see also* category
　　M01) A03.9
　bacillary A03.9
　　arthritis (*see also* category M01)
　　　A03.9
　　Boyd A03.2
　　Flexner A03.1
　　Schmitz (-Stutzer) A03.0
　　Shiga (-Kruse) A03.0
　　Shigella A03.9
　　　boydii A03.2
　　　dysenteriae A03.0
　　　flexneri A03.1
　　　group A A03.0
　　　group B A03.1
　　　group C A03.2
　　　group D A03.3
　　　sonnei A03.3
　　　specified type NEC A03.8
　　Sonne A03.3
　　specified type NEC A03.8
　balantidial A07.0
　Balantidium coli A07.0
　Boyd's A03.2
　candidal B37.82
　Chilomastix A07.8

Dysentery, dysenteric *(continued)*
　Chinese A03.9
　coccidial A07.3
　Dientamoeba (fragilis) A07.8
　Embadomonas A07.8
　Entamoeba, entamebic —*see*
　　Dysentery, amebic
　Flexner-Boyd A03.2
　Flexner's A03.1
　Giardia lamblia A07.1
　Hiss-Russell A03.1
　Lamblia A07.1
　leishmanial B55.0
　malarial —*see* Malaria
　metazoal B82.0
　monilial B37.82
　protozoal A07.9
　Salmonella A02.0
　schistosomal B65.1
　Schmitz (-Stutzer) A03.0
　Shiga (-Kruse) A03.0
　Shigella NOS —*see* Dysentery,
　　bacillary
　Sonne A03.3
　strongyloidiasis B78.0
　trichomonal A07.8
　viral —*see also* Enteritis, viral
　　A08.4

Dysequilibrium R42

Dysesthesia R20.8
　hysterical F44.6

Dysfibrinogenemia (congenital)
　D68.2

Dysfunction
　adrenal E27.9
　　hyperfunction E27.0
　autonomic
　　due to alcohol G31.2
　　somatoform F45.8
　bladder N31.9
　　neurogenic NOS —*see*
　　　Dysfunction, bladder,
　　　neuromuscular
　　neuromuscular NOS N31.9
　　　atonic (motor) (sensory)
　　　　N31.2
　　　autonomous N31.2
　　　flaccid N31.2
　　　nonreflex N31.2
　　　reflex N31.1
　　　specified NEC N31.8
　　　uninhibited N31.0
　bleeding, uterus N93.8
　cerebral G93.89
　colon K59.9
　　psychogenic F45.8
　colostomy K94.03
　cystic duct K82.8
　cystostomy (stoma) —*see*
　　Complications, cystostomy
　ejaculatory N53.19
　　anejaculatory orgasm N53.13
　　painful N53.12
　　premature F52.4
　　retarded N53.11
　endocrine NOS E34.9
　endometrium N85.8
　enterostomy K94.13
　erectile —*see* Dysfunction, sexual,
　　male, erectile
　gallbladder K82.8
　gastrostomy (stoma) K94.23
　gland, glandular NOS E34.9
　　meibomian, of eyelid —*see*
　　　Dysfunction, meibomian
　　　gland
　heart I51.89
　hemoglobin D75.89
　hepatic K76.89

Dysfunction *(continued)*
　hypophysis E23.7
　hypothalamic NEC E23.3
　ileostomy (stoma) K94.13
　jejunostomy (stoma) K94.13
　kidney —*see* Disease, renal
　labyrinthine —*see* subcategory
　　H83.2
　left ventricular, following sudden
　　emotional stress I51.81
　liver K76.89
　male —*see* Dysfunction, sexual,
　　male
　meibomian gland, of eyelid
　　H02.889
　　left H02.886
　　　lower H02.885
　　　upper H02.884
　　　upper and lower eyelids
　　　　H02.88B
　　right H02.883
　　　lower H02.882
　　　upper H02.881
　　　upper and lower eyelids
　　　　H02.88A
　orgasmic (female) F52.31
　　male F52.32
　ovary E28.9
　　specified NEC E28.8
　papillary muscle I51.89
　parathyroid E21.4
　physiological NEC R68.89
　　psychogenic F59
　pineal gland E34.8
　pituitary (gland) E23.3
　platelets D69.1
　polyglandular E31.9
　　specified NEC E31.8
　psychophysiologic F59
　psychosexual F52.9
　　with
　　　dyspareunia F52.6
　　　premature ejaculation F52.4
　　　vaginismus F52.5
　pylorus K31.9
　rectum K59.9
　　psychogenic F45.8
　reflex (sympathetic) —*see*
　　Syndrome, pain, complex
　　regional I
　segmental —*see* Dysfunction,
　　somatic
　senile R54
　sexual (due to) R37
　　alcohol F10.981
　　amphetamine F15.981
　　　in
　　　　abuse F15.181
　　　　dependence F15.281
　　anxiolytic F13.981
　　　in
　　　　abuse F13.181
　　　　dependence F13.281
　　cocaine F14.981
　　　in
　　　　abuse F14.181
　　　　dependence F14.281
　　excessive sexual drive F52.8
　　failure of genital response (male)
　　　F52.21
　　　female F52.22
　　female N94.9
　　　aversion F52.1
　　　dyspareunia N94.10
　　　　psychogenic F52.6
　　　frigidity F52.22
　　　nymphomania F52.8
　　　orgasmic F52.31
　　　psychogenic F52.9
　　　　aversion F52.1
　　　　dyspareunia F52.6

Dysfunction *(continued)*
　sexual *(continued)*
　　female *(continued)*
　　　psychogenic *(continued)*
　　　　frigidity F52.22
　　　　nymphomania F52.8
　　　　orgasmic F52.31
　　　　vaginismus F52.5
　　　vaginismus N94.2
　　　　psychogenic F52.5
　　hypnotic F13.981
　　　in
　　　　abuse F13.181
　　　　dependence F13.281
　　inhibited orgasm (female)
　　　F52.31
　　　male F52.32
　　lack
　　　of sexual enjoyment F52.1
　　　or loss of sexual desire F52.0
　　male N53.9
　　　anejaculatory orgasm N53.13
　　　ejaculatory N53.19
　　　　painful N53.12
　　　　premature F52.4
　　　　retarded N53.11
　　　erectile N52.9
　　　　drug induced N52.2
　　　　due to
　　　　　disease classified
　　　　　　elsewhere N52.1
　　　　　drug N52.2
　　　　postoperative
　　　　　(postprocedural) N52.39
　　　　following
　　　　　cryotherapy N52.37
　　　　　interstitial *seed* therapy
　　　　　　N52.36
　　　　　prostate ablative
　　　　　　therapy N52.37
　　　　　prostatectomy N52.34
　　　　　　radical N52.31
　　　　　radical cystectomy
　　　　　　N52.32
　　　　　radiation therapy
　　　　　　N52.35
　　　　　ultrasound ablative
　　　　　　therapy N52.37
　　　　　urethral surgery
　　　　　　N52.33
　　　　psychogenic F52.21
　　　　specified cause NEC N52.8
　　　　vasculogenic
　　　　　arterial insufficiency
　　　　　　N52.01
　　　　　　with corporo-venous
　　　　　　　occlusive N52.03
　　　　　corporo-venous occlusive
　　　　　　N52.02
　　　　　　with arterial
　　　　　　　insufficiency N52.03
　　　impotence —*see* Dysfunction,
　　　　sexual, male, erectile
　　　psychogenic F52.9
　　　　aversion F52.1
　　　　erectile F52.21
　　　　orgasmic F52.32
　　　　premature ejaculation F52.4
　　　　satyriasis F52.8
　　　　specified type NEC F52.8
　　　specified type NEC N53.8
　　nonorganic F52.9
　　　specified NEC F52.8
　　opioid F11.981
　　　in
　　　　abuse F11.181
　　　　dependence F11.281
　　orgasmic dysfunction (female)
　　　F52.31
　　　male F52.32
　　premature ejaculation F52.4

Dysfunction *(continued)*
sexual *(continued)*
psychoactive substances NEC
F19.981
in
abuse F19.181
dependence F19.281
psychogenic F52.9
sedative F13.981
in
abuse F13.181
dependence F13.281
sexual aversion F52.1
vaginismus (nonorganic)
(psychogenic) F52.5
sinoatrial node I49.5
somatic M99.09
abdomen M99.09
acromioclavicular M99.07
cervical region M99.01
cervicothoracic M99.01
costochondral M99.08
costovertebral M99.08
head region M99.00
hip M99.05
lower extremity M99.06
lumbar region M99.03
lumbosacral M99.03
occipitocervical M99.00
pelvic region M99.05
pubic M99.05
rib cage M99.08
sacral region M99.04
sacrococcygeal M99.04
sacroiliac M99.04
specified NEC M99.09
sternochondral M99.08
sternoclavicular M99.07
thoracic region M99.02
thoracolumbar M99.02
upper extremity M99.07
somatoform autonomic F45.8
stomach K31.89
psychogenic F45.8
suprarenal E27.9
hyperfunction E27.0
symbolic R48.9
specified type NEC R48.8
temporomandibular (joint)
M26.69
joint-pain syndrome M26.62-
testicular (endocrine) E29.9
specified NEC E29.8
thymus E32.9
thyroid E07.9
ureterostomy (stoma) —*see*
Complications, stoma, urinary
tract
urethrostomy (stoma) —*see*
Complications, stoma, urinary
tract
uterus, complicating delivery O62.9
hypertonic O62.4
hypotonic O62.2
primary O62.0
secondary O62.1
ventricular I51.9
with congestive heart failure
(*see also* Failure, heart)
I50.9
left, reversible, following sudden
emotional stress I51.81

Dysgenesis
gonadal (due to chromosomal
anomaly) Q96.9
pure Q99.1
renal Q60.5
bilateral Q60.4
unilateral Q60.3
reticular D72.0
tidal platelet D69.3

Dysgerminoma
specified site —*see* Neoplasm,
malignant, by site
unspecified site
female C56.9
male C62.90

Dysgeusia R43.2

Dysgraphia R27.8

Dyshidrosis, dysidrosis L30.1

Dyskaryotic cervical smear R87.619

Dyskeratosis L85.8
cervix —*see* Dysplasia, cervix
congenital Q82.8
uterus NEC N85.8

Dyskinesia G24.9
biliary (cystic duct or gallbladder)
K82.8
drug induced
orofacial G24.01
esophagus K22.4
hysterical F44.4
intestinal K59.89
nonorganic origin F44.4
orofacial (idiopathic) G24.4
drug induced G24.01
psychogenic F44.4
subacute, drug induced G24.01
tardive G24.01
neuroleptic induced G24.01
trachea J39.8
tracheobronchial J98.09

Dyslalia (developmental) F80.0

Dyslexia R48.0
developmental F81.0

Dyslipidemia E78.5
depressed HDL cholesterol E78.6
elevated fasting triglycerides
E78.1

Dysmaturity —*see also* Light for
dates
pulmonary (newborn) (Wilson-
Mikity) P27.0

Dysmenorrhea (essential)
(exfoliative) N94.6
congestive (syndrome) N94.6
primary N94.4
psychogenic F45.8
secondary N94.5

Dysmetabolic syndrome X E88.81

Dysmetria R27.8

Dysmorphism (due to)
alcohol Q86.0
exogenous cause NEC Q86.8
hydantoin Q86.1
warfarin Q86.2

Dysmorphophobia (nondelusional)
F45.22
delusional F22

Dysnomia R47.01

Dysorexia R63.0
psychogenic F50.89

Dysostosis
cleidocranial, cleidocranialis Q74.0
craniofacial Q75.1
Fairbank's (idiopathic familial
generalized osteophytosis) Q78.9
mandibulofacial (incomplete)
Q75.4
multiplex E76.01
oculomandibular Q75.5

Dyspareunia (female) N94.10
deep N94.12
male N53.12
nonorganic F52.6
psychogenic F52.6

Dyspareunia *(continued)*
secondary N94.19
specified NEC N94.19
superficial (introital) N94.11

Dyspepsia R10.13
atonic K30
functional (allergic) (congenital)
(gastrointestinal) (occupational)
(reflex) K30
intestinal K59.89
nervous F45.8
neurotic F45.8
psychogenic F45.8

Dysphagia R13.10
cervical R13.19
following
cerebral infarction I69.391
cerebrovascular disease I69.991
specified NEC I69.891
intracerebral hemorrhage
I69.191
nontraumatic intracranial
hemorrhage NEC I69.291
specified disease NEC I69.891
subarachnoid hemorrhage
I69.091
functional (hysterical) F45.8
hysterical F45.8
nervous (hysterical) F45.8
neurogenic R13.19
oral phase R13.11
oropharyngeal phase R13.12
pharyngeal phase R13.13
pharyngoesophageal phase R13.14
psychogenic F45.8
sideropenic D50.1
spastica K22.4
specified NEC R13.19

Dysphagocytosis, congenital D71

Dysphasia R47.02
developmental
expressive type F80.1
receptive type F80.2
following
cerebrovascular disease I69.921
cerebral infarction I69.321
intracerebral hemorrhage
I69.121
nontraumatic intracranial
hemorrhage NEC I69.221
specified disease NEC I69.821
subarachnoid hemorrhage
I69.021

Dysphonia R49.0
functional F44.4
hysterical F44.4
psychogenic F44.4
spastica J38.3

Dysphoria
gender F64.9
in
adolescence and adulthood
F64.0
children F64.2
postpartal O90.6
specified NEC F64.8

Dyspituitarism E23.3

Dysplasia —*see also* Anomaly
acetabular, congenital Q65.89
alveolar capillary, with vein
misalignment J84.843
anus (histologically confirmed)
(mild) (moderate) K62.82
severe D01.3
arrhythmogenic right ventricular
I42.8
arterial, fibromuscular I77.3
asphyxiating thoracic (congenital)
Q77.2

Dysplasia *(continued)*
brain Q07.9
bronchopulmonary, perinatal P27.1
cervix (uteri) N87.9
mild N87.0
moderate N87.1
severe D06.9
chondroectodermal Q77.6
colon D12.6
craniometaphyseal Q78.8
dentinal K00.5
diaphyseal, progressive Q78.3
dystrophic Q77.5
ectodermal (anhidrotic)
(congenital) (hereditary) Q82.4
hydrotic Q82.8
epithelial, uterine cervix —*see*
Dysplasia, cervix
eye (congenital) Q11.2
fibrous
bone NEC (monostotic) M85.00
ankle M85.07-
foot M85.07-
forearm M85.03-
hand M85.04-
lower leg M85.06-
multiple site M85.09
neck M85.08
rib M85.08
shoulder M85.01-
skull M85.08
specified site NEC M85.08
thigh M85.05-
toe M85.07-
upper arm M85.02-
vertebra M85.08
diaphyseal, progressive Q78.3
jaw M27.8
polyostotic Q78.1
florid osseous —*see also* Cyst,
calcifying odontogenic
high grade, focal D12.6
hip, congenital Q65.89
joint, congenital Q74.8
kidney Q61.4
multicystic Q61.4
leg Q74.2
lung, congenital (not associated
with short gestation) Q33.6
mammary (gland) (benign) N60.9-
cyst (solitary) —*see* Cyst, breast
cystic —*see* Mastopathy, cystic
duct ectasia —*see* Ectasia,
mammary duct
fibroadenosis —*see*
Fibroadenosis, breast
fibrosclerosis —*see*
Fibrosclerosis, breast
specified type NEC N60.8-
metaphyseal Q78.5
specified NEC N42.39
muscle Q79.8
oculodentodigital Q87.0
periapical (cemental) (cemento-
osseous) —*see* Cyst, calcifying
odontogenic
periosteum —*see* Disorder, bone,
specified type NEC
polyostotic fibrous Q78.1
prostate (*see also* Neoplasia,
intraepithelial, prostate) N42.30
severe D07.5
specified NEC N42.39
renal Q61.4
multicystic Q61.4
retinal, congenital Q14.1
right ventricular, arrhythmogenic
I42.8
septo-optic Q04.4
skin L98.8
spinal cord Q06.1

Dysplasia (*continued*)
spondyloepiphyseal Q77.7
thymic, with immunodeficiency D82.1
vagina N89.3
mild N89.0
moderate N89.1
severe NEC D07.2
vulva N90.3
mild N90.0
moderate N90.1
severe NEC D07.1

Dysplasminogenemia E88.02

Dyspnea (nocturnal) (paroxysmal) R06.00
asthmatic (bronchial) J45.909
with
exacerbation (acute) J45.901
bronchitis J45.909
with
exacerbation (acute) J45.901
status asthmaticus J45.902
chronic J44.9
status asthmaticus J45.902
cardiac —*see* Failure, ventricular, left
cardiac —*see* Failure, ventricular, left
functional F45.8
hyperventilation R06.4
hysterical F45.8
newborn P28.89
orthopnea R06.01
psychogenic F45.8
shortness of breath R06.02
specified type NEC R06.09

Dyspraxia R27.8
developmental (syndrome) F82

Dysproteinemia E88.09

Dysreflexia, autonomic G90.4

Dysrhythmia
cardiac I49.9
newborn
bradycardia P29.12
occurring before birth P03.819
before onset of labor P03.810
during labor P03.811
tachycardia P29.11
postoperative I97.89
cerebral or cortical —*see* Epilepsy

Dyssomnia —*see* Disorder, sleep

Dyssynergia
biliary K83.8
bladder sphincter N36.44
cerebellaris myoclonica (Hunt's ataxia) G11.19

Dysthymia F34.1

Dysthyroidism E07.9

Dystocia O66.9
affecting newborn P03.1
cervical (hypotonic) O62.2
affecting newborn P03.6
primary O62.0
secondary O62.1
contraction ring O62.4
fetal O66.9
abnormality NEC O66.3
conjoined twins O66.3
oversize O66.2
maternal O66.9
positional O64.9
shoulder (girdle) O66.0
causing obstructed labor O66.0
uterine NEC O62.4

Dystonia G24.9
cervical G24.3
deformans progressiva G24.1
drug induced NEC G24.09
acute G24.02
specified NEC G24.09
familial G24.1
idiopathic G24.1
familial G24.1
nonfamilial G24.2
orofacial G24.4
lenticularis G24.8
musculorum deformans G24.1
neuroleptic induced (acute) G24.02
orofacial (idiopathic) G24.4
oromandibular G24.4
due to drug G24.01
specified NEC G24.8
torsion (familial) (idiopathic) G24.1
acquired G24.8
genetic G24.1
symptomatic (nonfamilial) G24.2

Dystonic movements R25.8

Dystrophy, dystrophia
adiposogenital E23.6
autosomal recessive, childhood type, muscular dystrophy resembling Duchenne or Becker G71.01
Becker's type G71.01
cervical sympathetic G90.2
choroid (hereditary) H31.20
central areolar H31.22
choroideremia H31.21
gyrate atrophy H31.23
specified type NEC H31.29
cornea (hereditary) H18.50-
endothelial H18.51-
epithelial H18.52-
granular H18.53-
lattice H18.54-
macular H18.55-
specified type NEC H18.59-
Duchenne's type G71.01
due to malnutrition E45
Erb's G71.02
Fuchs' H18.51-
Gower's muscular G71.01
hair L67.8
infantile neuraxonal G31.89
Landouzy-Déjérine G71.02
Leyden-Möbius G71.09
muscular G71.00
autosomal recessive, childhood type, muscular dystrophy resembling Duchenne or Becker G71.01
benign (Becker type) G71.01
scapuloperoneal with early contractures [Emery-Dreifuss] G71.09
congenital (hereditary) (progressive) (with specific morphological abnormalities of the muscle fiber) G71.09
myotonic G71.11
distal G71.09
Duchenne type G71.01
Emery-Dreifuss G71.09
Erb type G71.02
facioscapulohumeral G71.02
Gower's G71.01
hereditary (progressive) G71.09
Landouzy-Déjérine type G71.02
limb-girdle G71.09
myotonic G71.11
progressive (hereditary) G71.09
Charcot-Marie (-Tooth) type G60.0

Dystrophy, dystrophia (*continued*)
muscular (*continued*)
pseudohypertrophic (infantile) G71.01
scapulohumeral G71.02
scapuloperoneal G71.09
severe (Duchenne type) G71.01
specified type NEC G71.09
myocardium, myocardial —*see* Degeneration, myocardial
nail L60.3
congenital Q84.6
nutritional E45
ocular G71.09
oculocerebrorenal E72.03
oculopharyngeal G71.09
ovarian N83.8
polyglandular E31.8
reflex (neuromuscular) (sympathetic) —*see* Syndrome, pain, complex regional I
retinal (hereditary) H35.50
in
lipid storage disorders E75.6 [H36]
systemic lipidoses E75.6 [H36]
involving
pigment epithelium H35.54
sensory area H35.53
pigmentary H35.52
vitreoretinal H35.51
Salzmann's nodular —*see* Degeneration, cornea, nodular
scapuloperoneal G71.09
skin NEC L98.8
sympathetic (reflex) —*see* Syndrome, pain, complex regional I
cervical G90.2
tapetoretinal H35.54
thoracic, asphyxiating Q77.2
unguium L60.3
congenital Q84.6
vitreoretinal H35.51
vulva N90.4
yellow (liver) —*see* Failure, hepatic

Dysuria R30.0
psychogenic F45.8

E

Eales' disease H35.06-

Ear —*see also* condition
piercing Z41.3
tropical NEC B36.9 [H62.40]
in
aspergillosis B44.89
candidiasis B37.84
moniliasis B37.84
wax (impacted) H61.20
left H61.22
with right H61.23
right H61.21
with left H61.23

Earache —*see* subcategory H92.0

Early satiety R68.81

Eaton-Lambert syndrome —*see* Syndrome, Lambert-Eaton

Eberth's disease (typhoid fever) A01.00

Ebola virus disease A98.4

Ebstein's anomaly or syndrome (heart) Q22.5

Eccentro-osteochondrodysplasia E76.29

Ecchondroma —*see* Neoplasm, bone, benign

Ecchondrosis D48.0

Ecchymosis R58
conjunctiva —*see* Hemorrhage, conjunctiva
eye (traumatic) —*see* Contusion, eyeball
eyelid (traumatic) —*see* Contusion, eyelid
newborn P54.5
spontaneous R23.3
traumatic —*see* Contusion

Echinococciasis —*see* Echinococcus

Echinococcosis —*see* Echinococcus

Echinococcus (infection) B67.90
granulosus B67.4
bone D67.2
liver B67.0
lung B67.1
multiple sites B67.32
specified site NEC B67.39
thyroid B67.31
liver NOS B67.8
granulosus B67.0
multilocularis B67.5
lung NEC B67.99
granulosus B67.1
multilocularis B67.69
multilocularis B67.7
liver B67.5
multiple sites B67.61
specified site NEC B67.69
specified site NEC B67.99
granulosus B67.39
multilocularis B67.69
thyroid NEC B67.99
granulosus B67.31
multilocularis B67.69 [E35]

Echinorhynchiasis B83.8

Echinostomiasis B66.8

Echolalia R48.8

Echovirus, as cause of disease classified elsewhere B97.12

Eclampsia, eclamptic (coma) (convulsions) (delirium) (with hypertension) **NEC** O15.9
complicating
labor and delivery O15.1
postpartum O15.2
pregnancy O15.0-
puerperal O15.2

Economic circumstances affecting care Z59.9

Economo's disease A85.8

Ectasia, ectasis
annuloaortic I35.8
aorta I77.819
with aneurysm —*see* Aneurysm, aorta
abdominal I77.811
thoracic I77.810
thoracoabdominal I77.812
breast —*see* Ectasia, mammary duct
capillary I78.8
cornea H18.71-
gastric antral vascular (GAVE) K31.819
with hemorrhage K31.811
without hemorrhage K31.819
mammary duct N60.4-
salivary gland (duct) K11.8
sclera —*see* Sclerectasia

Ecthyma L08.0
contagiosum B08.02
gangrenosum L08.0
infectiosum B08.02

Ectocardia Q24.8

Ectodermal dysplasia (anhidrotic) Q82.4

Ectodermosis erosiva pluriorificialis L51.1

Ectopic, ectopia (congenital)
abdominal viscera Q45.8
    due to defect in anterior abdominal wall Q79.59
ACTH syndrome E24.3
adrenal gland Q89.1
anus Q43.5
atrial beats I49.1
beats I49.49
    atrial I49.1
    ventricular I49.3
bladder Q64.10
bone and cartilage in lung Q33.5
brain Q04.8
breast tissue Q83.8
cardiac Q24.8
cerebral Q04.8
cordis Q24.8
endometrium —see Endometriosis
gastric mucosa Q40.2
gestation —see Pregnancy, by site
heart Q24.8
hormone secretion NEC E34.2
kidney (crossed) (pelvis) Q63.2
lens, lentis Q12.1
mole —see Pregnancy, by site
organ or site NEC —see Malposition, congenital
pancreas Q45.3
pregnancy —see Pregnancy, ectopic
pupil —see Abnormality, pupillary
renal Q63.2
sebaceous glands of mouth Q38.6
spleen Q89.09
testis Q53.00
    bilateral Q53.02
    unilateral Q53.01
thyroid Q89.2
tissue in lung Q33.5
ureter Q62.63
ventricular beats I49.3
vesicae Q64.10

Ectromelia Q73.8
lower limb —see Defect, reduction, limb, lower, specified type NEC
upper limb —see Defect, reduction, limb, upper, specified type NEC

Ectropion H02.109
cervix N86
    with cervicitis N72
congenital Q10.1
eyelid H02.109
    cicatricial H02.119
        left H02.116
            lower H02.115
            upper H02.114
        right H02.113
            lower H02.112
            upper H02.111
    congenital Q10.1
    left H02.106
        lower H02.105
        upper H02.104
    mechanical H02.129
        left H02.126
            lower H02.125
            upper H02.124
        right H02.123
            lower H02.122
            upper H02.121
    paralytic H02.159
        left H02.156
            lower H02.155
            upper H02.154

Ectropion (continued)
eyelid (continued)
    paralytic (continued)
        right H02.153
            lower H02.152
            upper H02.151
        right H02.103
            lower H02.102
            upper H02.101
    senile H02.139
        left H02.136
            lower H02.135
            upper H02.134
        right H02.133
            lower H02.132
            upper H02.131
    spastic H02.149
        left H02.146
            lower H02.145
            upper H02.144
        right H02.143
            lower H02.142
            upper H02.141
iris H21.89
lip (acquired) K13.0
    congenital Q38.0
urethra N36.8
uvea H21.89

Eczema (acute) (chronic) (erythematous) (fissum) (rubrum) (squamous) —see also Dermatitis L30.9
contact —see Dermatitis, contact
dyshydrotic L30.1
external ear —see Otitis, externa, acute, eczematoid
flexural L20.82
herpeticum B00.0
hypertrophicum L28.0
hypostatic —see Varix, leg, with, inflammation
impetiginous L01.1
infantile (due to any substance) L20.83
    intertriginous L21.1
    seborrheic L21.1
intertriginous NEC L30.4
    infantile L21.1
intrinsic (allergic) L20.84
lichenified NEC L28.0
marginatum (hebrae) B35.6
pustular L30.3
stasis I87.2
    with varicose veins —see Varix, leg, with, inflammation
vaccination, vaccinatum T88.1
varicose —see Varix, leg, with, inflammation

Eczematid L30.2

Eddowes (-Spurway) syndrome Q78.0

Edema, edematous (infectious) (pitting) (toxic) R60.9
with nephritis —see Nephrosis
allergic T78.3
amputation stump (surgical) (sequelae (late effect)) T87.89
angioneurotic (allergic) (any site) (with urticaria) T78.3
    hereditary D84.1
angiospastic I73.9
Berlin's (traumatic) S05.8X-
brain (cytotoxic) (vasogenic) G93.6
    due to birth injury P11.0
    newborn (anoxia or hypoxia) P52.4
        birth injury P11.0
        traumatic —see Injury, intracranial, cerebral edema

Edema, edematous (continued)
cardiac —see Failure, heart, congestive
cardiovascular —see Failure, heart, congestive
cerebral —see Edema, brain
cerebrospinal —see Edema, brain
cervix (uteri) (acute) N88.8
    puerperal, postpartum O90.89
chronic hereditary Q82.0
circumscribed, acute T78.3
    hereditary D84.1
conjunctiva H11.42-
cornea H18.2-
    idiopathic H18.22-
    secondary H18.23-
        due to contact lens H18.21-
due to
    lymphatic obstruction I89.0
    salt retention E87.0
epiglottis —see Edema, glottis
essential, acute T78.3
    hereditary D84.1
extremities, lower —see Edema, legs
eyelid NEC H02.849
    left H02.846
        lower H02.845
        upper H02.844
    right H02.843
        lower H02.842
        upper H02.841
familial, hereditary Q82.0
famine —see Malnutrition, severe
generalized R60.1
glottis, glottic, glottidis (obstructive) (passive) J38.4
    allergic T78.3
        hereditary D84.1
heart —see Failure, heart, congestive
heat T67.7
hereditary Q82.0
inanition —see Malnutrition, severe
intracranial G93.6
iris H21.89
joint —see Effusion, joint
larynx —see Edema, glottis
legs R60.0
    due to venous obstruction I87.1
    hereditary Q82.0
localized R60.0
    due to venous obstruction I87.1
lower limbs —see Edema, legs
lung J81.1
    with heart condition or failure —see Failure, ventricular, left
    acute J81.0
        chemical (acute) J68.1
            chronic J68.1
    chronic J81.1
        due to
            chemicals, gases, fumes or vapors (inhalation) J68.1
            external agent J70.9
                specified NEC J70.8
            radiation J70.1
    due to
        chemicals, fumes or vapors (inhalation) J68.1
        external agent J70.9
            specified NEC J70.8
        high altitude T70.29
        near drowning T75.1
        radiation J70.0
    meaning failure, left ventricle I50.1
lymphatic I89.0
    due to mastectomy I97.2
macula H35.81

Edema, edematous (continued)
macula (continued)
    cystoid, following cataract surgery —see Complications, postprocedural, following cataract surgery
    diabetic —see Diabetes, by type, with, retinopathy, with macular edema
malignant —see Gangrene, gas
Milroy's Q82.0
nasopharynx J39.2
newborn P83.30
    hydrops fetalis —see Hydrops, fetalis
    specified NEC P83.39
nutritional —see also Malnutrition, severe
    with dyspigmentation, skin and hair E40
optic disc or nerve —see Papilledema
orbit H05.22-
pancreas K86.89
papilla, optic —see Papilledema
penis N48.89
periodic T78.3
    hereditary D84.1
pharynx J39.2
pulmonary —see Edema, lung
Quincke's T78.3
    hereditary D84.1
renal —see Nephrosis
retina H35.81
    diabetic —see Diabetes, by type, with, retinopathy, with macular edema
salt E87.0
scrotum N50.89
seminal vesicle N50.89
spermatic cord N50.89
spinal (cord) (vascular) (nontraumatic) G95.19
starvation —see Malnutrition, severe
stasis —see Hypertension, venous, (chronic)
subglottic —see Edema, glottis
supraglottic —see Edema, glottis
testis N44.8
tunica vaginalis N50.89
vas deferens N50.89
vulva (acute) N90.89

Edentulism —see Absence, teeth, acquired

Edsall's disease T67.2

Educational handicap Z55.9
specified NEC Z55.8

Edward's syndrome —see Trisomy, 18

Effect, adverse
abnormal gravitational (G) forces or states T75.81
abuse —see Maltreatment
air pressure T70.9
    specified NEC T70.8
altitude (high) —see Effect, adverse, high altitude
anesthesia (see also Anesthesia) T88.59
    in labor and delivery O74.9
    local, toxic
        in labor and delivery O74.4
        in pregnancy NEC O29.3-
        postpartum, puerperal O89.3
    postpartum, puerperal O89.9
    specified NEC T88.59
        in labor and delivery O74.8
        postpartum, puerperal O89.8

Effect, adverse (continued)

anesthesia (continued)
spinal and epidural T88.59
headache T88.59
in labor and delivery O74.5
postpartum, puerperal O89.4
specified NEC
in labor and delivery O74.6
postpartum, puerperal O89.5
antitoxin —see Complications, vaccination
atmospheric pressure T70.9
due to explosion T70.8
high T70.3
low —see Effect, adverse, high altitude
specified effect NEC T70.8
biological, correct substance
properly administered —see Effect, adverse, drug
blood (derivatives) (serum) (transfusion) —see Complications, transfusion
chemical substance —see Table of Drugs and Chemicals
cold (temperature) (weather) T69.9
chilblains T69.1
frostbite —see Frostbite
specified effect NEC T69.8
drugs and medicaments T88.7
specified drug —see Table of Drugs and Chemicals, by drug, adverse effect
specified effect - code to condition
electric current, electricity (shock) T75.4
burn —see Burn
exertion (excessive) T73.3
exposure —see Exposure
external cause NEC T75.89
foodstuffs T78.1
allergic reaction —see Allergy, food
causing anaphylaxis —see Shock, anaphylactic, due to food
noxious —see Poisoning, food, noxious
gases, fumes, or vapors T59.9-
specified agent —see Table of Drugs and Chemicals
glue (airplane) sniffing
due to drug abuse —see Abuse, drug, inhalant
due to drug dependence —see Dependence, drug, inhalant
heat —see Heat
high altitude NEC T70.29
anoxia T70.29
on
ears T70.0
sinuses T70.1
polycythemia D75.1
high pressure fluids T70.4
hot weather —see Heat
hunger T73.0
immersion, foot —see Immersion
immunization —see Complications, vaccination
immunological agents —see Complications, vaccination
infrared (radiation) (rays) NOS T66
dermatitis or eczema L59.8
infusion —see Complications, infusion
lack of care of infants —see Maltreatment, child
lightning —see Lightning
medical care T88.9
specified NEC T88.8

Effect, adverse (continued)

medicinal substance, correct, properly administered —see Effect, adverse, drug
motion T75.3
noise, on inner ear —see subcategory H83.3
overheated places —see Heat
psychosocial, of work environment Z56.5
radiation (diagnostic) (infrared) (natural source) (therapeutic) (ultraviolet) (X-ray) NOS T66
dermatitis or eczema —see Dermatitis, due to, radiation
fibrosis of lung J70.1
pneumonitis J70.0
pulmonary manifestations
acute J70.0
chronic J70.1
skin L59.9
radioactive substance NOS
dermatitis or eczema —see Radiodermatitis
reduced temperature T69.9
immersion foot or hand —see Immersion
specified effect NEC T69.8
serum NEC (see also Reaction, serum) T80.69
specified NEC T78.8
external cause NEC T75.89
strangulation —see Asphyxia, traumatic
submersion T75.1
thirst T73.1
toxic —see Toxicity
transfusion —see Complications, transfusion
ultraviolet (radiation) (rays) NOS T66
burn —see Burn
dermatitis or eczema —see Dermatitis, due to, ultraviolet rays
acute L56.8
vaccine (any) —see Complications, vaccination
vibration —see Vibration, adverse effects
water pressure NEC T70.9
specified NEC T70.8
weightlessness T75.82
whole blood —see Complications, transfusion
work environment Z56.5

Effect(s) (of) (from) —see Effect, adverse NEC

Effects, late —see Sequelae

Effluvium
anagen L65.1
telogen L65.0

Effort syndrome (psychogenic) F45.8

Effusion
amniotic fluid —see Pregnancy, complicated by, premature rupture of membranes
brain (serous) G93.6
bronchial —see Bronchitis
cerebral G93.6
cerebrospinal —see also Meningitis
vessel G93.6
chest —see Effusion, pleura
chylous, chyliform (pleura) J94.0
intracranial G93.6
joint M25.40
ankle M25.47-
elbow M25.42-
foot joint M25.47-
hand joint M25.44-

Effusion (continued)

joint (continued)
hip M25.45-
knee M25.46-
shoulder M25.41-
specified joint NEC M25.48
wrist M25.43-
malignant pleural J91.0
meninges —see Meningitis
pericardium, pericardial (noninflammatory) I31.3
acute —see Pericarditis, acute
peritoneal (chronic) R18.8
pleura, pleurisy, pleuritic, pleuropericardial J90
chylous, chyliform J94.0
due to systemic lupus erythematosis M32.13
in conditions classified elsewhere J91.8
influenzal —see Influenza, with, respiratory manifestations NEC
malignant J91.0
newborn P28.89
tuberculous NEC A15.6
primary (progressive) A15.7
spinal —see Meningitis
thorax, thoracic —see Effusion, pleura

Egg shell nails L60.3
congenital Q84.6

EGPA (eosinophilic granulomatosis with polyangitis) M30.1

Egyptian splenomegaly B65.1

Ehrlichiosis A77.40
due to
E. chafeensis A77.41
E. ewingii A77.49
E. muris euclairensis A77.49
E. sennetsu A79.81
specified organism NEC A77.49

Ehlers-Danlos syndrome (see also Syndrome, Ehlers-Danlos) Q79.60

Eichstedt's disease B36.0

Eisenmenger's
complex or syndrome I27.83
defect Q21.8

Ejaculation
delayed F52.32
painful N53.12
premature F52.4
retarded N53.11
retrograde N53.14
semen, painful N53.12
psychogenic F52.6

Ekbom's syndrome (restless legs) G25.81

Ekman's syndrome (brittle bones and blue sclera) Q78.0

Elastic skin Q82.8
acquired L57.4

Elastofibroma —see Neoplasm, connective tissue, benign

Elastoma (juvenile) Q82.8
Miescher's L87.2

Elastomyofibrosis I42.4

Elastosis
actinic, solar L57.8
atrophicans (senile) L57.4
perforans serpiginosa L87.2
senilis L57.4

Elbow —see condition

Electric current, electricity, effects (concussion) (fatal) (nonfatal) (shock) T75.4
burn —see Burn

Electric feet syndrome E53.8

Electrocution T75.4
from electroshock gun (taser) T75.4

Electrolyte imbalance E87.8
with
abortion —see Abortion by type, complicated by, electrolyte imbalance
ectopic pregnancy O08.5
molar pregnancy O08.5

Elephantiasis (nonfilarial) I89.0
arabicum —see Infestation, filarial
bancroftian B74.0
congenital (any site) (hereditary) Q82.0
due to
Brugia (malayi) B74.1
timori B74.2
mastectomy I97.2
Wuchereria (bancrofti) B74.0
eyelid H02.859
left H02.856
lower H02.855
upper H02.854
right H02.853
lower H02.852
upper H02.851
filarial, filariensis —see Infestation, filarial
glandular I89.0
graecorum A30.9
lymphangiectatic I89.0
lymphatic vessel I89.0
due to mastectomy I97.2
scrotum (nonfilarial) I89.0
streptococcal I89.0
surgical I97.89
postmastectomy I97.2
telangiectodes I89.0
vulva (nonfilarial) N90.89

Elevated, elevation
alanine transaminase (ALT) R74.01
ALT (alanine transaminase) R74.01
antibody titer R76.0
aspartate transaminase (AST) R74.01
AST (aspartate transaminase) R74.01
basal metabolic rate R94.8
blood pressure —see also Hypertension
reading (incidental) (isolated) (nonspecific), no diagnosis of hypertension R03.0
blood sugar R73.9
body temperature (of unknown origin) R50.9
C-reactive protein (CRP) R79.82
cancer antigen 125 [CA 125] R97.1
carcinoembryonic antigen [CEA] R97.0
cholesterol E78.00
with high triglycerides E78.2
conjugate, eye H51.0
diaphragm, congenital Q79.1
erythrocyte sedimentation rate R70.0
fasting glucose R73.01
fasting triglycerides E78.1
finding on laboratory examination —see Findings, abnormal, inconclusive, without diagnosis, by type of exam
GFR (glomerular filtration rate) —see Findings, abnormal, inconclusive, without diagnosis, by type of exam
glucose tolerance (oral) R73.02
immunoglobulin level R76.8
indoleacetic acid R82.5
lactic acid dehydrogenase (LDH) level R74.02

Elevated, elevation *(continued)*
  leukocytes D72.829
  lipoprotein a (Lp(a)) level E78.41
  liver function
    study R94.5
    test R79.89
      alkaline phosphatase R74.8
      aminotransferase R74.01
      bilirubin R17
      hepatic enzyme R74.8
      lactate dehydrogenase R74.02
  Lp(a) (lipoprotein(a)) E78.41
  lymphocytes D72.820
  prostate specific antigen [PSA]
    R97.20
  Rh titer —*see* Complication(s),
    transfusion, incompatibility
    reaction, Rh (factor)
  scapula, congenital Q74.0
  sedimentation rate R70.0
  SGOT R74.01
  SGPT R74.01
  transaminase level R74.01
  triglycerides E78.1
    with high cholesterol E78.2
  troponin R77.8
  tumor associated antigens [TAA]
    NEC R97.8
  tumor specific antigens [TSA] NEC
    R97.8
  urine level of
    catecholamine R82.5
    indoleacetic acid R82.5
    17-ketosteroids R82.5
    steroids R82.5
    vanillylmandelic acid (VMA)
      R82.5
  venous pressure I87.8
  white blood cell count D72.829
    specified NEC D72.828

Elliptocytosis (congenital)
  (hereditary) D58.1
  Hb C (disease) D58.1
  hemoglobin disease D58.1
  sickle-cell (disease) D57.8-
    trait D57.3

Ellison-Zollinger syndrome E16.4

Ellis-van Creveld syndrome
  (chondroectodermal dysplasia) Q77.6

Elongated, elongation (congenital)
  —*see also* Distortion
  bone Q79.9
  cervix (uteri) Q51.828
    acquired N88.4
    hypertrophic N88.4
  colon Q43.8
  common bile duct Q44.5
  cystic duct Q44.5
  frenulum, penis Q55.69
  labia minora (acquired) N90.69
  ligamentum patellae Q74.1
  petiolus (epiglottidis) Q31.8
  tooth, teeth K00.2
  uvula Q38.6

Eltor cholera A00.1

Emaciation (due to malnutrition) E43

Embadomoniasis A07.8

Embedded tooth, teeth K01.0
  root only K08.3

Embolic —*see* condition

Embolism (multiple) (paradoxical)
  I74.9
  air (any site) (traumatic) T79.0
    following
      abortion —*see* Abortion
        by type complicated by
        embolism

Embolism *(continued)*
  air *(continued)*
    following *(continued)*
      ectopic pregnancy O08.2
      infusion, therapeutic injection
        or transfusion T80.0
      molar pregnancy O08.2
      procedure NEC
        artery T81.719
          mesenteric T81.710
          renal T81.711
          specified NEC T81.718
        vein T81.72
    in pregnancy, childbirth or
      puerperium —*see* Embolism,
      obstetric
  amniotic fluid (pulmonary) —*see
    also* Embolism, obstetric
    following
      abortion —*see* Abortion
        by type complicated by
        embolism
      ectopic pregnancy O08.2
      molar pregnancy O08.2
  aorta, aortic I74.10
    abdominal I74.09
      saddle I74.01
    bifurcation I74.09
    saddle I74.01
    thoracic I74.11
  artery I74.9
    auditory, internal I65.8
    basilar —*see* Occlusion, artery,
      basilar
    carotid (common) (internal) —
      see Occlusion, artery, carotid
    cerebellar (anterior inferior)
      (posterior inferior) (superior)
      I66.3
    cerebral —*see* Occlusion, artery,
      cerebral
    choroidal (anterior) I65.8
    communicating posterior I65.8
    coronary —*see* Infarct,
      myocardium
      not resulting in infarction
      I24.0
    extremity I74.4
      lower I74.3
      upper I74.2
    hypophyseal I65.8
    iliac I74.5
    limb I74.4
      lower I74.3
      upper I74.2
    mesenteric (with gangrene) (*see
      also* Ischemia, intestine, acute)
      K55.059
    ophthalmic —*see* Occlusion,
      artery, retina
    peripheral I74.4
    pontine I65.8
    precerebral —*see* Occlusion,
      artery, precerebral
    pulmonary —*see* Embolism,
      pulmonary
    renal N28.0
    retinal —*see* Occlusion, artery,
      retina
    septic I76
    specified NEC I74.8
    vertebral —*see* Occlusion,
      artery, vertebral
  basilar (artery) I65.1
  blood clot
    following
      abortion —*see* Abortion
        by type complicated by
        embolism
      ectopic or molar pregnancy
        O08.2

Embolism *(continued)*
  blood clot *(continued)*
    in pregnancy, childbirth or
      puerperium —*see* Embolism,
      obstetric
  brain —*see also* Occlusion, artery,
    cerebral
    following
      abortion —*see* Abortion
        by type complicated by
        embolism
      ectopic or molar pregnancy
        O08.2
      puerperal, postpartum, childbirth
        —*see* Embolism, obstetric
  capillary I78.8
  cardiac —*see also* Infarct,
    myocardium
    not resulting in infarction I51.3
  carotid (artery) (common)
    (internal) —*see* Occlusion,
    artery, carotid
  cavernous sinus (venous) —*see*
    Embolism, intracranial venous
    sinus
  cerebral —*see* Occlusion, artery,
    cerebral
  cholesterol —*see* Atheroembolism
  coronary (artery or vein) (systemic)
    —*see* Occlusion, coronary
  due to device, implant or graft
    —*see also* Complications, by
    site and type, specified NEC
    arterial graft NEC T82.818
    breast (implant) T85.818
    catheter NEC T85.818
      dialysis (renal) T82.818
        intraperitoneal T85.818
      infusion NEC T82.818
        spinal (epidural) (subdural)
          T85.810
      urinary (indwelling) T83.81
    electronic (electrode) (pulse
      generator) (stimulator)
      bone T84.81
      cardiac T82.817
      nervous system (brain)
        (peripheral nerve) (spinal)
        T85.810
      urinary T83.81
    fixation, internal (orthopedic)
      NEC T84.81
    gastrointestinal (bile duct)
      (esophagus) T85.818
    genital NEC T83.81
    heart (graft) (valve) T82.817
    joint prosthesis T84.81
    ocular (corneal graft) (orbital
      implant) T85.818
    orthopedic (bone graft) NEC
      T86.838
    specified NEC T85.818
    urinary (graft) NEC T83.81
    vascular NEC T82.818
    ventricular intracranial shunt
      T85.810
  extremities
    lower —*see* Embolism, vein,
      lower extremity
      arterial I74.3
    upper I74.2
  eye H34.9
  fat (cerebral) (pulmonary)
    (systemic) T79.1
    following
      abortion —*see* Abortion by type
        complicated by embolism
      ectopic or molar pregnancy
        O08.2
    complicating delivery —*see*
      Embolism, obstetric

Embolism *(continued)*
  following
    abortion —*see* Abortion by
      type complicated by
      embolism
    ectopic or molar pregnancy
      O08.2
    infusion, therapeutic injection or
      transfusion
      air T80.0
  heart (fatty) —*see also* Infarct,
    myocardium
    not resulting in infarction I51.3
  hepatic (vein) I82.0
  in pregnancy, childbirth or
    puerperium —*see* Embolism,
    obstetric
  intestine (artery) (vein) (with
    gangrene) (*see also* Ischemia,
    intestine, acute) K55.039
  intracranial —*see also* Occlusion,
    artery, cerebral
    venous sinus (any) G08
      nonpyogenic I67.6
  intraspinal venous sinuses or veins
    G08
    nonpyogenic G95.19
  kidney (artery) N28.0
  lateral sinus (venous) —*see*
    Embolism, intracranial, venous
    sinus
  leg —*see* Embolism, vein, lower
    extremity
    arterial I74.3
  longitudinal sinus (venous) —*see*
    Embolism, intracranial, venous
    sinus
  lung (massive) —*see* Embolism,
    pulmonary
  meninges I66.8
  mesenteric (artery) (vein) (with
    gangrene) (*see also* Ischemia,
    intestine, acute) K55.059
  obstetric (in) (pulmonary)
    childbirth O88.22
      air O88.02
      amniotic fluid O88.12
      blood clot O88.22
      fat O88.82
      pyemic O88.32
      septic O88.32
      specified type NEC O88.82
    pregnancy O88.21-
      air O88.01-
      amniotic fluid O88.11-
      blood clot O88.21-
      fat O88.81-
      pyemic O88.31-
      septic O88.31-
      specified type NEC O88.81-
    puerperal O88.23
      air O88.03
      amniotic fluid O88.13
      blood clot O88.23
      fat O88.83
      pyemic O88.33
      septic O88.33
      specified type NEC O88.83
  ophthalmic —*see* Occlusion, artery,
    retina
  penis N48.81
  peripheral artery NOS I74.4
  pituitary E23.6
  popliteal (artery) I74.3
  portal (vein) I81
  postoperative, postprocedural
    artery T81.719
      mesenteric T81.710
      renal T81.711
      specified NEC T81.718
    vein T81.72

131

Embolism (*continued*)
precerebral artery —*see* Occlusion, artery, precerebral
puerperal —*see* Embolism, obstetric
pulmonary (acute) (artery) (vein) I26.99
  with acute cor pulmonale I26.09
  chronic I27.82
  following
    abortion —*see* Abortion
      by type complicated by embolism
    ectopic or molar pregnancy O08.2
  healed or old Z86.711
  in pregnancy, childbirth or puerperium —*see* Embolism, obstetric
  multiple subsegmental without acute cor pulmonale I26.94
  personal history of Z86.711
  saddle I26.92
    with acute cor pulmonale I26.02
  septic I26.90
    with acute cor pulmonale I26.01
  single subsegmental without acute cor pulmonale I26.93
  subsegmental NOS I26.93
pyemic (multiple) I76
  following
    abortion —*see* Abortion
      by type complicated by embolism
    ectopic or molar pregnancy O08.2
  Hemophilus influenzae A41.3
  pneumococcal A40.3
    with pneumonia J13
  puerperal, postpartum, childbirth (any organism) —*see* Embolism, obstetric
  specified organism NEC A41.89
  staphylococcal A41.2
  streptococcal A40.9
renal (artery) N28.0
  vein I82.3
retina, retinal —*see* Occlusion, artery, retina
saddle
  abdominal aorta I74.01
  pulmonary artery I26.92
    with acute cor pulmonale I26.02
septic (arterial) I76
  complicating abortion —*see* Abortion, by type, complicated by, embolism
sinus —*see* Embolism, intracranial, venous sinus
soap complicating abortion —*see* Abortion, by type, complicated by, embolism
spinal cord G95.19
  pyogenic origin G06.1
spleen, splenic (artery) I74.8
upper extremity I74.2
vein (acute) I82.90
  antecubital I82.61-
    chronic I82.71-
  axillary I82.A1-
    chronic I82.A2-
  basilic I82.61-
    chronic I82.71-
  brachial I82.62-
    chronic I82.72-
  brachiocephalic (innominate) I82.290
    chronic I82.291

Embolism (*continued*)
vein (*continued*)
  cephalic I82.61-
    chronic I82.71-
  chronic I82.91
  deep (DVT) I82.40-
    calf I82.4Z-
      chronic I82.5Z-
    lower leg I82.4Z-
      chronic I82.5Z-
    thigh I82.4Y-
      chronic I82.5Y-
    upper leg I82.4Y
      chronic I82.5y-
  femoral I82.41-
    chronic I82.51-
  iliac (iliofemoral) I82.42-
    chronic I82.52-
  innominate I82.290
    chronic I82.291
  internal jugular I82.C1-
    chronic I82.C2-
  lower extremity
    deep I82.40-
      chronic I82.50-
      specified NEC I82.49-
        chronic NEC I82.59-
    distal
      deep I82.4Z-
    proximal
      deep I82.4Y-
        chronic I82.5Y-
    superficial I82.81-
  popliteal I82.43-
    chronic I82.53-
  radial I82.62-
    chronic I82.72-
  renal I82.3
  saphenous (greater) (lesser) I82.81-
  specified NEC I82.890
    chronic NEC I82.891
  subclavian I82.B1-
    chronic I82.B2-
  thoracic NEC I82.290
    chronic I82.291
  tibial I82.44-
    chronic I82.54-
  ulnar I82.62-
    chronic I82.72-
  upper extremity I82.60-
    chronic I82.70-
    deep I82.62-
      chronic I82.72-
    superficial I82.61-
      chronic I82.71-
vena cava
  inferior (acute) I82.220
    chronic I82.221
  superior (acute) I82.210
    chronic I82.211
venous sinus G08
vessels of brain —*see* Occlusion, artery, cerebral

Embolus —*see* Embolism

Embryoma —*see also* Neoplasm, uncertain behavior, by site
benign —*see* Neoplasm, benign, by site
kidney C64.-
liver C22.0
malignant —*see also* Neoplasm, malignant, by site
kidney C64.-
liver C22.0
testis C62.9-
  descended (scrotal) C62.1-
  undescended C62.0-
testis C62.9-
  descended (scrotal) C62.1-
  undescended C62.0-

Embryonic
circulation Q28.9
heart Q28.9
vas deferens Q55.4

Embryopathia NOS Q89.9

Embryotoxon Q13.4

Emesis —*see* Vomiting

Emotional lability R45.86

Emotionality, pathological F60.3

Emotogenic disease —*see* Disorder, psychogenic

Emphysema (atrophic) (bullous) (chronic) (interlobular) (lung) (obstructive) (pulmonary) (senile) (vesicular) J43.9
cellular tissue (traumatic) T79.7
  surgical T81.82
centrilobular J43.2
compensatory J98.3
congenital (interstitial) P25.0
conjunctiva H11.89
connective tissue (traumatic) T79.7
  surgical T81.82
due to chemicals, gases, fumes or vapors J68.4
eyelid(s) —*see* Disorder, eyelid, specified type NEC
  surgical T81.82
  traumatic T79.7
interstitial J98.2
  congenital P25.0
  perinatal period P25.0
laminated tissue T79.7
  surgical T81.82
mediastinal J98.2
  newborn P25.2
orbit, orbital —*see* Disorder, orbit, specified type NEC
panacinar J43.1
panlobular J43.1
specified NEC J43.8
subcutaneous (traumatic) T79.7
  nontraumatic J98.2
  postprocedural T81.82
  surgical T81.82
surgical T81.82
thymus (gland) (congenital) E32.8
traumatic (subcutaneous) T79.7
unilateral J43.0

Empty nest syndrome Z60.0

Empyema (acute) (chest) (double) (pleura) (supradiaphragmatic) (thorax) J86.9
with fistula J86.0
accessory sinus (chronic) —*see* Sinusitis
antrum (chronic) —*see* Sinusitis, maxillary
brain (any part) —*see* Abscess, brain
ethmoidal (chronic) (sinus) —*see* Sinusitis, ethmoidal
extradural —*see* Abscess, extradural
frontal (chronic) (sinus) —*see* Sinusitis, frontal
gallbladder K81.0
mastoid (process) (acute) —*see* Mastoiditis, acute
maxilla, maxillary M27.2
  sinus (chronic) —*see* Sinusitis, maxillary
nasal sinus (chronic) —*see* Sinusitis
sinus (accessory) (chronic) (nasal) —*see* Sinusitis
sphenoidal (sinus) (chronic) —*see* Sinusitis, sphenoidal

Empyema (*continued*)
subarachnoid —*see* Abscess, extradural
subdural —*see* Abscess, subdural
tuberculous A15.6
ureter —*see* Ureteritis
ventricular —*see* Abscess, brain

En coup de sabre lesion L94.1

Enamel pearls K00.2

Enameloma K00.2

Enanthema, viral B09

Encephalitis (chronic) (hemorrhagic) (idiopathic) (nonepidemic) (spurious) (subacute) G04.90
acute (*see also* Encephalitis, viral) A86
  disseminated G04.00
    infectious G04.01
    noninfectious G04.81
    postimmunization (postvaccination) G04.02
    postinfectious G04.01
  inclusion body A85.8
  necrotizing hemorrhagic G04.30
    postimmunization G04.32
    postinfectious G04.31
    specified NEC G04.39
arboviral, arbovirus NEC A85.2
arthropod-borne NEC (viral) A85.2
Australian A83.4
California (virus) A83.5
Central European (tick-borne) A84.1
Czechoslovakian A84.1
Dawson's (inclusion body) A81.1
diffuse sclerosing A81.1
disseminated, acute G04.00
due to
  cat scratch disease A28.1
  human immunodeficiency virus (HIV) disease B20 [G05.3]
  malaria —*see* Malaria
  rickettsiosis —*see* Rickettsiosis
  smallpox inoculation G04.02
  typhus —*see* Typhus
Eastern equine A83.2
endemic (viral) A86
epidemic NEC (viral) A86
equine (acute) (infectious) (viral) A83.9
  Eastern A83.2
  Venezuelan A92.2
  Western A83.1
Far Eastern (tick-borne) A84.0
following vaccination or other immunization procedure G04.02
herpes zoster B02.0
herpesviral B00.4
  due to herpesvirus 6 B10.01
  due to herpesvirus 7 B10.09
  specified NEC B10.09
Ilheus (virus) A83.8
inclusion body A81.1
in (due to)
  actinomycosis A42.82
  adenovirus A85.1
  African trypanosomiasis B56.9 [G05.3]
  Chagas' disease (chronic) B57.42
  cytomegalovirus B25.8
  enterovirus A85.0
  herpes (simplex) virus B00.4
    due to herpesvirus 6 B10.01
    due to herpesvirus 7 B10.09
    specified NEC B10.09
  infectious disease NEC B99 [G05.3]

Encephalitis *(continued)*
  in *(continued)*
    influenza —*see* Influenza, with,
      encephalopathy
    listeriosis A32.12
    measles B05.0
    mumps B26.2
    naegleriasis B60.2
    parasitic disease NEC B89
      [G05.3]
    poliovirus A80.9 *[G05.3]*
    rubella B06.01
    syphilis
      congenital A50.42
      late A52.14
    systemic lupus erythematosus
      M32.19
    toxoplasmosis (acquired) B58.2
      congenital P37.1
    tuberculosis A17.82
    zoster B02.0
  infectious (acute) (virus) NEC A86
  Japanese (B type) A83.0
  La Crosse A83.5
  lead —*see* Poisoning, lead
  lethargica (acute) (infectious) A85.8
  louping ill A84.89
  lupus erythematosus, systemic
    M32.19
  lymphatica A87.2
  Mengo A85.8
  meningococcal A39.81
  Murray Valley A83.4
  otitic NEC H66.40 *[G05.3]*
  parasitic NOS B71.9
  periaxial G37.0
  periaxialis (concentrica) (diffuse)
    G37.5
  postchickenpox B01.11
  postexanthematous NEC B09
  postimmunization G04.02
  postinfectious NEC G04.01
  postmeasles B05.0
  postvaccinal G04.02
  postvaricella B01.11
  postviral NEC A86
  Powassan A84.81
  Rasmussen G04.81
  Rio Bravo A85.8
  Russian
    autumnal A83.0
    spring-summer (taiga) A84.0
  saturnine —*see* Poisoning, lead
  specified NEC G04.81
  St. Louis A83.3
  subacute sclerosing A81.1
  summer A83.0
  suppurative G04.81
  tick-borne A84.9
  Torula, torular (cryptococcal) B45.1
  toxic NEC G92
  trichinosis B75 *[G05.3]*
  type
    B A83.0
    C A83.3
  van Bogaert's A81.1
  Venezuelan equine A92.2
  Vienna A85.8
  viral, virus A86
    arthropod-borne NEC A85.2
      mosquito-borne A83.9
        Australian X disease A83.4
        California virus A83.5
        Eastern equine A83.2
        Japanese (B type) A83.0
        Murray Valley A83.4
        specified NEC A83.8
        St. Louis A83.3
        type B A83.0
        type C A83.3
        Western equine A83.1

Encephalitis *(continued)*
  viral, virus *(continued)*
    arthropod-borne NEC
      (continued)
      tick-borne A84.9
        biundulant A84.1
        central European A84.1
        Czechoslovakian A84.1
        diphasic
          meningoencephalitis
          A84.1
        Far Eastern A84.0
        Russian spring-summer
          (taiga) A84.0
        specified NEC A84.89
      specified type NEC A85.8
      tick-borne, specified NEC A84.89
    Western equine A83.1

Encephalocele Q01.9
  frontal Q01.0
  nasofrontal Q01.1
  occipital Q01.2
  specified NEC Q01.8

Encephalocystocele —*see*
  Encephalocele

**Encephaloduroarterio-
  myosynangiosis** (EDAMS) I67.5

Encephalomalacia (brain)
  (cerebellar) (cerebral) —*see*
  Softening, brain

Encephalomeningitis —*see*
  Meningoencephalitis

Encephalomeningocele —*see*
  Encephalocele

Encephalomeningomyelitis —*see*
  Meningoencephalitis

Encephalomyelitis —*see also*
  Encephalitis G04.90
  acute disseminated G04.00
    infectious G04.01
    noninfectious G04.81
    postimmunization G04.02
    postinfectious G04.01
  acute necrotizing hemorrhagic
    G04.30
    postimmunization G04.32
    postinfectious G04.31
    specified NEC G04.39
  benign myalgic G93.3
  equine A83.9
    Eastern A83.2
    Venezuelan A92.2
    Western A83.1
  in diseases classified elsewhere G05.3
  myalgic, benign G93.3
  postchickenpox B01.11
  postinfectious NEC G04.01
  postmeasles B05.0
  postvaccinal G04.02
  postvaricella B01.11
  rubella B06.01
  specified NEC G04.81
  Venezuelan equine A92.2

Encephalomyelocele —*see*
  Encephalocele

Encephalomyelomeningitis —*see*
  Meningoencephalitis

Encephalomyelopathy G96.9

Encephalomyeloradiculitis (acute)
  G61.0

Encephalomyeloradiculoneuritis
  (acute) (Guillain-Barré) G61.0

Encephalomyeloradiculopathy
  G96.9

**Encephalopathia
hyperbilirubinemica, newborn**
P57.9
  due to isoimmunization (conditions
    in P55) P57.0

Encephalopathy (acute) G93.40
  acute necrotizing hemorrhagic
    G04.30
    postimmunization G04.32
    postinfectious G04.31
    specified NEC G04.39
  alcoholic G31.2
  anoxic —*see* Damage, brain,
    anoxic
  arteriosclerotic I67.2
  centrolobar progressive (Schilder)
    G37.0
  congenital Q07.9
  degenerative, in specified disease
    NEC G32.89
  demyelinating callosal G37.1
  due to
    drugs (*see also* Table of Drugs
      and Chemicals) G92
  hepatic —*see* Failure, hepatic
  hyperbilirubinemic, newborn
    P57.9
    due to isoimmunization
      (conditions in P55) P57.0
  hypertensive I67.4
  hypoglycemic E16.2
  hypoxic —*see* Damage, brain,
    anoxic
  hypoxic ischemic P91.60
    mild P91.61
    moderate P91.62
    severe P91.63
  in (due to) (with)
    birth injury P11.1
    hyperinsulinism E16.1 *[G94]*
    influenza —*see* Influenza, with,
      encephalopathy
    lack of vitamin (*see also*
      Deficiency, vitamin) E56.9
      [G32.89]
    neoplastic disease (*see also*
      Neoplasm) D49.9 *[G13.1]*
    serum (*see also* Reaction, serum)
      T80.69
    syphilis A52.17
    trauma (postconcussional)
      F07.81
      current injury —*see* Injury,
        intracranial
    vaccination G04.02
  lead —*see* Poisoning, lead
  metabolic G93.41
    drug induced G92
    toxic G92
  myoclonic, early, symptomatic
    —*see* Epilepsy, generalized,
    specified NEC
  necrotizing, subacute (Leigh)
    G31.82
  neonatal P91.819
    in diseases classified elsewhere
      P91.811
  pellagrous E52 *[G32.89]*
  portosystemic —*see* Failure,
    hepatic
  postcontusional F07.81
    current injury —*see* Injury,
      intracranial, diffuse
  posthypoglycemic (coma) E16.1
    [G94]
  postradiation G93.89
  saturnine —*see* Poisoning, lead
  septic G93.41
  specified NEC G93.49
  spongiform, subacute (viral)
    A81.09

Encephalopathy *(continued)*
  toxic G92
    metabolic G92
  traumatic (postconcussional)
    F07.81
    current injury —*see* Injury,
      intracranial
  vitamin B deficiency NEC E53.9
    [G32.89]
    vitamin B1 E51.2
  Wernicke's E51.2

Encephalorrhagia —*see*
  Hemorrhage, intracranial,
  intracerebral

Encephalosis, posttraumatic F07.81

Enchondroma —*see also* Neoplasm,
  bone, benign

Enchondromatosis (cartilaginous)
  (multiple) Q78.4

Encopresis R15.9
  functional F98.1
  nonorganic origin F98.1
  psychogenic F98.1

Encounter (with health service) (for)
  Z76.89
  adjustment and management (of)
    breast implant Z45.81
    implanted device NEC Z45.89
    myringotomy device (stent)
      (tube) Z45.82
    neurostimulator (brain) (gastric)
      (peripheral nerve) (sacral
      nerve) (spinal cord) (vagus
      nerve) Z45.42
  administrative purpose only Z02.9
    examination for
      adoption Z02.82
      armed forces Z02.3
      disability determination
        Z02.71
      driving license Z02.4
      employment Z02.1
      insurance Z02.6
      medical certificate NEC
        Z02.79
      paternity testing Z02.81
      residential institution
        admission Z02.2
      school admission Z02.0
      sports Z02.5
    specified reason NEC Z02.89
  aftercare —*see* Aftercare
  antenatal screening Z36.9
    cervical length Z36.86
    chromosomal anomalies Z36.0
    congenital cardiac abnormalities
      Z36.83
    elevated maternal serum
      alphafetoprotein level Z36.1
    fetal growth retardation Z36.4
    fetal lung maturity Z36.84
    fetal macrosomia Z36.88
    hydrops fetalis Z36.81
    intrauterine growth restriction
      (IUGR)/small-for-dates Z36.4
    isoimmunization Z36.5
    large-for-dates Z36.88
    malformations Z36.3
    non-visualized anatomy on a
      previous scan Z36.2
    nuchal translucency Z36.82
    raised alphafetoprotein level
      Z36.1
    risk of pre-term labor Z36.86
    specified type NEC Z36.89
    specified follow-up NEC Z36.2
    specified genetic defects NEC
      Z36.8A
    Streptococcus B Z36.85

Encounter *(continued)*
- antenatal screening *(continued)*
  - suspected anomaly Z36.3
  - uncertain dates Z36.87
- assisted reproductive fertility procedure cycle Z31.83
- blood typing Z01.83
  - Rh typing Z01.83
- breast augmentation or reduction Z41.1
- breast implant exchange (different material) (different size) Z45.81
- breast reconstruction following mastectomy Z42.1
- check-up —*see* Examination
- chemotherapy for neoplasm Z51.11
- colonoscopy, screening Z12.11
- counseling —*see* Counseling
- delivery, full-term, uncomplicated O80
  - cesarean, without indication O82
- desensitization to allergens Z51.6
- ear piercing Z41.3
- examination —*see* Examination
- expectant parent(s) (adoptive)
  - pre-birth pediatrician visit Z76.81
- fertility preservation procedure (prior to cancer therapy) (prior to removal of gonads) Z31.84
- fitting (of) —*see* Fitting (and adjustment) (of)
- genetic
  - counseling
    - nonprocreative Z71.83
    - procreative Z31.5
  - testing —*see* Test, genetic
- hearing conservation and treatment Z01.12
- immunotherapy for neoplasm Z51.12
- in vitro fertilization cycle Z31.83
- instruction (in)
  - childbirth Z32.2
  - child care (postpartal) (prenatal) Z32.3
  - natural family planning
    - procreative Z31.61
    - to avoid pregnancy Z30.02
- insulin pump titration Z46.81
- joint prosthesis insertion following prior explantation of joint prosthesis (staged procedure)
  - hip Z47.32
  - knee Z47.33
  - shoulder Z47.31
- laboratory (as part of a general medical examination) Z00.00
  - with abnormal findings Z00.01
- mental health services (for)
  - abuse NEC
    - perpetrator Z69.82
    - victim Z69.81
  - child abuse
    - nonparental
      - perpetrator Z69.021
      - victim Z69.020
    - parental
      - perpetrator Z69.011
      - victim Z69.010
  - child neglect
    - nonparental
      - perpetrator Z69.021
      - victim Z69.020
    - parental
      - perpetrator Z69.011
      - victim Z69.010
  - child psychological abuse
    - nonparental
      - perpetrator Z69.021
      - victim Z69.020

Encounter *(continued)*
- mental health services *(continued)*
  - child psychological abuse *(continued)*
    - parental
      - perpetrator Z69.011
      - victim Z69.010
  - child sexual abuse
    - nonparental
      - perpetrator Z69.021
      - victim Z69.020
    - parental
      - perpetrator Z69.011
      - victim Z69.010
  - non-spousal adult abuse
    - perpetrator Z69.82
    - victim Z69.81
  - spousal or partner
    - abuse
      - perpetrator Z69.12
      - victim Z69.11
    - neglect
      - perpetrator Z69.12
      - victim Z69.11
    - psychological abuse
      - perpetrator Z69.12
      - victim Z69.11
    - violence
      - perpetrator (physical) (sexual) Z69.12
      - victim (physical) Z69.11
      - sexual Z69.81
- observation (for) (ruled out)
  - exposure to (suspected)
    - anthrax Z03.810
    - biological agent NEC Z03.818
- pediatrician visit, by expectant parent(s) (adoptive) Z76.81
- placental sample (taken vaginally) (*see also* Encounter, antenatal screening) Z36.9
- plastic and reconstructive surgery following medical procedure or healed injury NEC Z42.8
- pregnancy
  - supervision of —*see* Pregnancy, supervision of
  - test Z32.00
    - result negative Z32.02
    - result positive Z32.01
- procreative management and counseling for gestational carrier Z31.7
- prophylactic measures Z29.9
  - antivenin Z29.12
  - fluoride administration Z29.3
  - immunotherapy for respiratory syncytial virus (RSV) Z29.11
  - rabies immune globulin Z29.14
  - Rho (D) immune globulin Z29.13
  - specified NEC Z29.8
- radiation therapy (antineoplastic) Z51.0
- radiological (as part of a general medical examination) Z00.00
  - with abnormal findings Z00.01
- reconstructive surgery following medical procedure or healed injury NEC Z42.8
- removal (of) —*see also* Removal
  - artificial
    - arm Z44.00-
      - complete Z44.01-
      - partial Z44.02-
    - eye Z44.2-
    - leg Z44.10-
      - complete Z44.11-
      - partial Z44.12-
  - breast implant Z45.81

Encounter *(continued)*
- removal *(continued)*
  - breast implant *(continued)*
    - tissue expander (with or without synchronous insertion of permanent implant) Z45.81
  - device Z46.9
    - specified NEC Z46.89
  - external
    - fixation device - code to fracture with seventh character D
    - prosthesis, prosthetic device Z44.9
      - breast Z44.3-
        - specified NEC Z44.8
  - implanted device NEC Z45.89
  - insulin pump Z46.81
  - internal fixation device Z47.2
  - myringotomy device (stent) (tube) Z45.82
  - nervous system device NEC Z46.2
    - brain neuropacemaker Z46.2
    - visual substitution device Z46.2
      - implanted Z45.31
  - non-vascular catheter Z46.82
  - orthodontic device Z46.4
  - stent
    - ureteral Z46.6
  - urinary device Z46.6
- repeat cervical smear to confirm findings of recent normal smear following initial abnormal smear Z01.42
- respirator [ventilator] use during power failure Z99.12
- Rh typing Z01.83
- screening —*see* Screening
- specified NEC Z76.89
- sterilization Z30.2
- suspected condition, ruled out
  - amniotic cavity and membrane Z03.71
  - cervical shortening Z03.75
  - fetal anomaly Z03.73
  - fetal growth Z03.74
  - maternal and fetal conditions NEC Z03.79
  - oligohydramnios Z03.71
  - placental problem Z03.72
  - polyhydramnios Z03.71
- suspected exposure (to), ruled out
  - anthrax Z03.810
  - biological agents NEC Z03.818
- termination of pregnancy, elective Z33.2
- testing —*see* Test
- therapeutic drug level monitoring Z51.81
- titration, insulin pump Z46.81
- to determine fetal viability of pregnancy O36.80
- training
  - insulin pump Z46.81
- X-ray of chest (as part of a general medical examination) Z00.00
  - with abnormal findings Z00.01

Encystment —*see* Cyst

Endarteritis (bacterial, subacute) (infective) I77.6
- brain I67.7
- cerebral or cerebrospinal I67.7
- deformans —*see* Arteriosclerosis
- embolic —*see* Embolism
- obliterans —*see also* Arteriosclerosis
  - pulmonary I28.8

Endarteritis *(continued)*
- pulmonary I28.8
- retina —*see* Vasculitis, retina
- senile —*see* Arteriosclerosis
- syphilitic A52.09
  - brain or cerebral A52.04
  - congenital A50.54 *[I79.8]*
- tuberculous A18.89

Endemic —*see* condition

Endocarditis (chronic) (marantic) (nonbacterial) (thrombotic) (valvular) I38
- with rheumatic fever (conditions in I00)
  - active —*see* Endocarditis, acute, rheumatic
  - inactive or quiescent (with chorea) I09.1
- acute or subacute I33.9
  - infective I33.0
  - rheumatic (aortic) (mitral) (pulmonary) (tricuspid) I01.1
    - with chorea (acute) (rheumatic) (Sydenham's) I02.0
- aortic (heart) (nonrheumatic) (valve) I35.8
  - with
    - mitral disease I08.0
      - with tricuspid (valve) disease I08.3
      - active or acute I01.1
        - with chorea (acute) (rheumatic) (Sydenham's) I02.0
    - rheumatic fever (conditions in I00)
      - active —*see* Endocarditis, acute, rheumatic
      - inactive or quiescent (with chorea) I06.9
    - tricuspid (valve) disease I08.2
      - with mitral (valve) disease I08.3
  - acute or subacute I33.9
  - arteriosclerotic I35.8
  - rheumatic I06.9
    - with mitral disease I08.0
      - with tricuspid (valve) disease I08.3
      - active or acute I01.1
        - with chorea (acute) (rheumatic) (Sydenham's) I02.0
    - active or acute I01.1
      - with chorea (acute) (rheumatic) (Sydenham's) I02.0
    - specified NEC I06.8
  - specified cause NEC I35.8
  - syphilitic A52.03
- arteriosclerotic I38
- atypical verrucous (Libman-Sacks) M32.11
- bacterial (acute) (any valve) (subacute) I33.0
- candidal B37.6
- congenital Q24.8
- constrictive I33.0
- Coxiella burnetii A78 *[I39]*
- Coxsackie B33.21
- due to
  - prosthetic cardiac valve T82.6
  - Q fever A78 *[I39]*
  - Serratia marcescens I33.0
  - typhoid (fever) A01.02
- gonococcal A54.83
- infectious or infective (acute) (any valve) (subacute) I33.0

Endocarditis *(continued)*
  lenta (acute) (any valve) (subacute)
    I33.0
  Libman-Sacks M32.11
  listerial A32.82
  Löffler's I42.3
  malignant (acute) (any valve)
    (subacute) I33.0
  meningococcal A39.51
  mitral (chronic) (double) (fibroid)
    (heart) (inactive) (valve) (with
    chorea) I05.9
    with
      aortic (valve) disease I08.0
        with tricuspid (valve)
          disease I08.3
        active or acute I01.1
          with chorea (acute)
            (rheumatic)
            (Sydenham's) I02.0
        rheumatic fever (conditions
          in I00)
          active —*see* Endocarditis,
            acute, rheumatic
          inactive or quiescent (with
            chorea) I05.9
        tricuspid (valve) disease I08.1
          with aortic (valve) disease
            I08.3
      active or acute I01.1
        with chorea (acute)
          (rheumatic) (Sydenham's)
          I02.0
      bacterial I33.0
      arteriosclerotic I34.8
      nonrheumatic I34.8
        acute or subacute I33.9
      specified NEC I05.8
  monilial B37.6
  multiple valves I08.9
    specified disorders I08.8
  mycotic (acute) (any valve)
    (subacute) I33.0
  pneumococcal (acute) (any valve)
    (subacute) I33.0
  pulmonary (chronic) (heart) (valve)
    I37.8
    with rheumatic fever (conditions
      in I00)
      active —*see* Endocarditis,
        acute, rheumatic
      inactive or quiescent (with
        chorea) I09.89
        with aortic, mitral or
          tricuspid disease I08.8
    acute or subacute I33.9
      rheumatic I01.1
        with chorea (acute)
          (rheumatic) (Sydenham's)
          I02.0
    arteriosclerotic I37.8
    congenital Q22.2
    rheumatic (chronic) (inactive)
      (with chorea) I09.89
      active or acute I01.1
        with chorea (acute)
          (rheumatic) (Sydenham's)
          I02.0
    syphilitic A52.03
  purulent (acute) (any valve)
    (subacute) I33.0
  Q fever A78 *[I39]*
  rheumatic (chronic) (inactive) (with
    chorea) I09.1
    active or acute (aortic) (mitral)
      (pulmonary) (tricuspid) I01.1
      with chorea (acute)
        (rheumatic) (Sydenham's)
        I02.0
  rheumatoid —*see* Rheumatoid,
    carditis

Endocarditis *(continued)*
  septic (acute) (any valve)
    (subacute) I33.0
  streptococcal (acute) (any valve)
    (subacute) I33.0
  subacute —*see* Endocarditis, acute
  suppurative (acute) (any valve)
    (subacute) I33.0
  syphilitic A52.03
  toxic I33.9
  tricuspid (chronic) (heart) (inactive)
    (rheumatic) (valve) (with chorea)
    I07.9
    with
      aortic (valve) disease I08.2
        mitral (valve) disease I08.3
      mitral (valve) disease I08.1
        aortic (valve) disease I08.3
      rheumatic fever (conditions
        in I00)
        active —*see* Endocarditis,
          acute, rheumatic
        inactive or quiescent (with
          chorea) I07.8
    active or acute I01.1
      with chorea (acute)
        (rheumatic) (Sydenham's)
        I02.0
  arteriosclerotic I36.8
  nonrheumatic I36.8
    acute or subacute I33.9
    specified cause, except rheumatic
      I36.8
  tuberculous —*see* Tuberculosis,
    endocarditis
  typhoid A01.02
  ulcerative (acute) (any valve)
    (subacute) I33.0
  vegetative (acute) (any valve)
    (subacute) I33.0
  verrucous (atypical) (nonbacterial)
    (nonrheumatic) M32.11

Endocardium, endocardial —*see
  also* condition
  cushion defect Q21.2

Endocervicitis —*see also* Cervicitis
  due to intrauterine (contraceptive)
    device T83.69
  hyperplastic N72

Endocrine —*see* condition

Endocrinopathy, pluriglandular
  E31.9

Endodontic
  overfill M27.52
  underfill M27.53

Endodontitis K04.01
  irreversible K04.02
  reversible K04.01

Endomastoiditis —*see* Mastoiditis

Endometrioma N80.9

Endometriosis N80.9
  appendix N80.5
  bladder N80.8
  bowel N80.5
  broad ligament N80.3
  cervix N80.0
  colon N80.5
  cul-de-sac (Douglas') N80.3
  exocervix N80.0
  fallopian tube N80.2
  female genital organ NEC N80.8
  gallbladder N80.8
  in scar of skin N80.6
  internal N80.0
  intestine N80.5
  lung N80.8
  myometrium N80.0
  ovary N80.1

Endometriosis *(continued)*
  parametrium N80.3
  pelvic peritoneum N80.3
  peritoneal (pelvic) N80.3
  rectovaginal septum N80.4
  rectum N80.5
  round ligament N80.3
  skin (scar) N80.6
  specified site NEC N80.8
  stromal D39.0
  thorax N80.8
  umbilicus N80.8
  uterus (internal) N80.0
  vagina N80.4
  vulva N80.8

Endometritis (decidual) (nonspecific)
  (purulent) (senile) (atrophic)
  (suppurative) N71.9
  with ectopic pregnancy O08.0
  acute N71.0
  blenorrhagic (gonococcal) (acute)
    (chronic) A54.24
  cervix, cervical (with erosion or
    ectropion) —*see also* Cervicitis
    hyperplastic N72
  chlamydial A56.11
  chronic N71.1
  following
    abortion —*see* Abortion by
      type complicated by genital
      infection
    ectopic or molar pregnancy
      O08.0
  gonococcal, gonorrheal (acute)
    (chronic) A54.24
  hyperplastic (*see also* Hyperplasia,
    endometrial) N85.00-
    cervix N72
  puerperal, postpartum, childbirth
    O86.12
  subacute N71.0
  tuberculous A18.17

Endometrium —*see* condition

**Endomyocardiopathy, South
  African** I42.3

Endomyocarditis —*see* Endocarditis

Endomyofibrosis I42.3

Endomyometritis —*see* Endometritis

Endopericarditis —*see* Endocarditis

Endoperineuritis —*see* Disorder,
  nerve

Endophlebitis —*see* Phlebitis

Endophthalmia —*see*
  Endophthalmitis, purulent

Endophthalmitis (acute) (infective)
  (metastatic) (subacute) H44.009
  bleb associated H59.4 —*see also*
    Bleb, inflamed (infected),
    postprocedural
  gonorrheal A54.39
  in (due to)
    cysticercosis B69.1
    onchocerciasis B73.01
    toxocariasis B83.0
  panuveitis —*see* Panuveitis
  parasitic H44.12-
  purulent H44.00-
    panophthalmitis —*see*
      Panophthalmitis
    vitreous abscess H44.02-
  specified NEC H44.19
  sympathetic —*see* Uveitis,
    sympathetic

Endosalpingioma D28.2

Endosalpingiosis N94.89

Endosteitis —*see* Osteomyelitis

Endothelioma, bone —*see*
  Neoplasm, bone, malignant

Endotheliosis (hemorrhagic
  infectional) D69.8

Endotoxemia - code to condition

Endotrachelitis —*see* Cervicitis

Engelmann (-Camurati) **syndrome**
  Q78.3

English disease —*see* Rickets

Engman's disease L30.3

Engorgement
  breast N64.59
    newborn P83.4
    puerperal, postpartum O92.79
  lung (passive) —*see* Edema, lung
  pulmonary (passive) —*see* Edema,
    lung
  stomach K31.89
  venous, retina —*see* Occlusion,
    retina, vein, engorgement

Enlargement, enlarged —*see also*
  Hypertrophy
  adenoids J35.2
    with tonsils J35.3
  alveolar ridge K08.89
    congenital —*see* Anomaly,
      alveolar
  apertures of diaphragm (congenital)
    Q79.1
  gingival K06.1
  heart, cardiac —*see* Hypertrophy,
    cardiac
  labium majus, childhood
    asymmetric (CALME) N90.61
  lacrimal gland, chronic H04.03-
  liver —*see* Hypertrophy, liver
  lymph gland or node R59.9
    generalized R59.1
    localized R59.0
  orbit H05.34-
  organ or site, congenital NEC
    —*see* Anomaly, by site
  parathyroid (gland) E21.0
  pituitary fossa R93.0
  prostate N40.0
    with lower urinary tract
      symptoms (LUTS) N40.1
    without lower urinary tract
      symtpoms (LUTS) N40.0
  sella turcica R93.0
  spleen —*see* Splenomegaly
  thymus (gland) (congenital)
    E32.0
  thyroid (gland) —*see* Goiter
  tongue K14.8
  tonsils J35.1
    with adenoids J35.3
  uterus N85.2
  vestibular aqueduct A16.5

Enophthalmos H05.40-
  due to
    orbital tissue atrophy H05.41-
    trauma or surgery H05.42-

Enostosis M27.8

Entamebic, entamebiasis —*see*
  Amebiasis

Entanglement
  umbilical cord(s) O69.82
    with compression O69.2
    around neck (with compression)
      O69.81
      with compression O69.1
      without compression O69.81
    of twins in monoamniotic sac
      O69.2
    without compression O69.82

Enteralgia —*see* Pain, abdominal

Enteric —*see* condition

Enteritis (acute) (diarrheal)
(hemorrhagic) (noninfective) K52.9
adenovirus A08.2
aertrycke infection A02.0
allergic K52.29
with
eosinophilic gastritis or
gastroenteritis K52.81
food protein-induced
entercolitis syndrome
K52.21
food protein-induced
enteropathy K52.22
FPIES K52.21
amebic (acute) A06.0
with abscess —*see* Abscess,
amebic
chronic A06.1
with abscess —*see* Abscess,
amebic
nondysenteric A06.2
nondysenteric A06.2
astrovirus A08.32
bacillary NOS A03.9
bacterial A04.9
specified NEC A04.8
calicivirus A08.31
candidal B37.82
Chilomastix A07.8
choleriformis A00.1
chronic (noninfectious) K52.9
ulcerative —*see* Colitis,
ulcerative
cicatrizing (chronic) —*see*
Enteritis, regional, small
intestine
Clostridium
botulinum (food poisoning)
A05.1
difficile
not specified as recurrent
A04.72
recurrent A04.71
coccidial A07.3
coxsackie virus A08.39
dietetic (*see also* Enteritis, allergic)
K52.29
drug-induced K52.1
due to
astrovirus A08.32
calicivirus A08.31
coxsackie virus A08.39
drugs K52.1
echovirus A08.39
enterovirus NEC A08.39
food hypersensitivity (*see also*
Enteritis, allergic) K52.29
infectious organism (bacterial)
(viral) —*see* Enteritis,
infectious
torovirus A08.39
Yersinia enterocolitica A04.6
echovirus A08.39
eltor A00.1
enterovirus NEC A08.39
eosinophilic K52.81
epidemic (infectious) A09
fulminant (*see also* Ischemia,
intestine acute) K55.019
gangrenous —*see* Enteritis,
infectious
giardial A07.1
infectious NOS A09
due to
adenovirus A08.2
Aerobacter aerogenes A04.8
Arizona (bacillus) A02.0
bacteria NOS A04.9
specified NEC A04.8

Enteritis (continued)
infectious NOS (continued)
due to (continued)
Campylobacter A04.5
Clostridium difficile
not specified as recurrent
A04.72
recurrent A04.71
Clostridium perfringens A04.8
Enterobacter aerogenes A04.8
enterovirus A08.39
Escherichia coli A04.4
enteroaggregative A04.4
enterohemorrhagic A04.3
enteroinvasive A04.2
enteropathogenic A04.0
enterotoxigenic A04.1
specified NEC A04.4
specified
bacteria NEC A04.8
virus NEC A08.39
Staphylococcus A04.8
virus NEC A08.4
specified type NEC A08.39
Yersinia enterocolitica A04.6
specified organism NEC A08.8
influenzal —*see* Influenza, with,
digestive manifestations
ischemic K55.9
acute (*see also* Ischemia,
intestine acute) K55.019
chronic K55.1
microsporidial A07.8
mucomembranous,
myxomembranous —*see*
Syndrome, irritable bowel
mucous —*see* Syndrome, irritable
bowel
necroticans A05.2
necrotizing of newborn —*see*
Enterocolitis, necrotizing, in
newborn
neurogenic —*see* Syndrome,
irritable bowel
newborn necrotizing —*see*
Enterocolitis, necrotizing, in
newborn
noninfectious K52.9
norovirus A08.11
parasitic NEC B82.9
paratyphoid (fever) —*see* Fever,
paratyphoid
protozoal A07.9
specified NEC A07.8
radiation K52.0
regional (of) K50.90
with
complication K50.919
abscess K50.914
fistula K50.913
intestinal obstruction
K50.912
rectal bleeding K50.911
specified complication NEC
K50.918
colon —*see* Enteritis, regional,
large intestine
duodenum —*see* Enteritis,
regional, small intestine
ileum —*see* Enteritis, regional,
small intestine
jejunum —*see* Enteritis,
regional, small intestine
large bowel —*see* Enteritis,
regional, large intestine
large intestine (colon) (rectum)
K50.10
with
complication K50.119
abscess K50.114
fistula K50.113

Enteritis (continued)
regional (continued)
large intestine (continued)
with (continued)
complication (continued)
intestinal obstruction
K50.112
rectal bleeding K50.111
small intestine
(duodenum) (ileum)
(jejunum) involvement
K50.80
with
complication
K50.819
abscess K50.814
fistula K50.813
intestinal
obstruction
K50.812
rectal bleeding
K50.811
specified
complication
NEC K50.818
specified complication
NEC K50.118
rectum —*see* Enteritis, regional,
large intestine
small intestine (duodenum)
(ileum) (jejunum) K50.00
with
complication K50.019
abscess K50.014
fistula K50.013
intestinal obstruction
K50.012
large intestine (colon)
(rectum) involvement
K50.80
with
complication
K50.819
abscess K50.814
fistula K50.813
intestinal
obstruction
K50.812
rectal bleeding
K50.811
specified
complication
NEC K50.818
rectal bleeding K50.011
specified complication
NEC K50.018
rotaviral A08.0
Salmonella, salmonellosis
(arizonae) (cholerae-suis)
(enteritidis) (typhimurium)
A02.0
segmental —*see* Enteritis, regional
septic A09
Shigella —*see* Infection, Shigella
small round structured NEC
A08.19
spasmodic, spastic —*see*
Syndrome, irritable bowel
staphylococcal A04.8
due to food A05.0
torovirus A08.39
toxic NEC K52.1
due to Clostridium difficile
not specified as recurrent
A04.72
recurrent A04.71
trichomonal A07.8
tuberculous A18.32
typhosa A01.00
ulcerative (chronic) —*see* Colitis,
ulcerative

Enteritis (continued)
viral A08.4
adenovirus A08.2
enterovirus A08.39
Rotavirus A08.0
small round structured NEC
A08.19
specified NEC A08.39
virus specified NEC A08.39

Enterobiasis B80

Enterobius vermicularis (infection)
(infestation) B80

Enterocele —*see also* Hernia,
abdomen
pelvic, pelvis (acquired)
(congenital) N81.5
vagina, vaginal (acquired)
(congenital) NEC N81.5

Enterocolitis (*see also* Enteritis)
K52.9
due to Clostridium difficile
not specified as recurrent A04.72
recurrent A04.71
fulminant ischemic (*see also*
Ischemia, intestine acute)
K55.059
granulomatous —*see* Enteritis,
regional
hemorrhagic (acute) (*see also*
Ischemia, intestine acute)
K55.059
chronic K55.1
infectious NEC A09
ischemic K55.9
necrotizing K55.30
with
perforation K55.33
pneumatosis K55.32
and perforation K55.33
due to Clostridium difficile
not specified as recurrent
A04.72
recurrent A04.71
in newborn P77.9
stage 1 (without pneumatosis,
without perforation) P77.1
stage 2 (with pneumatosis,
without perforation) P77.2
stage 3 (with pneumatosis,
with perforation) P77.3
in non-newborn K55.30
stage 1 (without pneumatosis,
without perforation) K55.31
stage 2 (with pneumatosis,
without perforation) K55.32
stage 3 (with pneumatosis,
with perforation) K55.33
without pneumatosis or
perforation K55.31
noninfectious K52.9
newborn —*see* Enterocolitis,
necrotizing, in newborn
pseudomembranous (newborn)
not specified as recurrent A04.72
recurrent A04.71
radiation K52.0
newborn —*see* Enterocolitis,
necrotizing, in newborn
ulcerative (chronic) —*see*
Pancolitis, ulcerative (chronic)

Enterogastritis —*see* Enteritis

Enteropathy K63.9
celiac-gluten-sensitive K90.0
non-celiac K90.41
food protein-induced K52.22
hemorrhagic, terminal (*see also*
Ischemia, intestine, acute)
K55.059
protein-losing K90.49

Enteroperitonitis —*see* Peritonitis

Enteroptosis K63.4

Enterorrhagia K92.2

Enterospasm —*see also* Syndrome, irritable, bowel
psychogenic F45.8

Enterostenosis (*see also* Obstruction, intestine specified NEC) K56.699

Enterostomy
complication —*see* Complication, enterostomy
status Z93.4

Enterovirus, as cause of disease classified elsewhere B97.10
coxsackievirus B97.11
echovirus B97.12
other specified B97.19

Enthesopathy (peripheral) M77.9
Achilles tendinitis —*see* Tendinitis, Achilles
ankle and tarsus M77.5-
specified type NEC —*see* Enthesopathy, foot, specified type NEC
anterior tibial syndrome M76.81-
calcaneal spur —*see* Spur, bone, calcaneal
elbow region M77.8
lateral epicondylitis —*see* Epicondylitis, lateral
medial epicondylitis —*see* Epicondylitis, medial
foot NEC M77.8
metatarsalgia —*see* Metatarsalgia
specified type NEC M77.5-
forearm M77.8
gluteal tendinitis —*see* Tendinitis, gluteal
hand M77.8
hip —*see* Enthesopathy, lower limb, specified type NEC
iliac crest spur —*see* Spur, bone, iliac crest
iliotibial band syndrome —*see* Syndrome, iliotibial band
knee —*see* Enthesopathy, lower limb, lower leg, specified type NEC
lateral epicondylitis —*see* Epicondylitis, lateral
lower limb (excluding foot) M76.9
Achilles tendinitis —*see* Tendinitis, Achilles
ankle and tarsus M77.5-
specified type NEC —*see* Enthesopathy, foot, specified type NEC
anterior tibial syndrome M76.81-
gluteal tendinitis —*see* Tendinitis, gluteal
iliac crest spur —*see* Spur, bone, iliac crest
iliotibial band syndrome —*see* Syndrome, iliotibial band
patellar tendinitis —*see* Tendinitis, patellar
pelvic region —*see* Enthesopathy, lower limb, specified type NEC
peroneal tendinitis —*see* Tendinitis, peroneal
posterior tibial syndrome M76.82-
psoas tendinitis —*see* Tendinitis, psoas
specified type NEC M76.89-

Enthesopathy (continued)
lower limb (continued)
tibial collateral bursitis —*see* Bursitis, tibial collateral
medial epicondylitis —*see* Epicondylitis, medial
metatarsalgia —*see* Metatarsalgia
multiple sites M77.8
patellar tendinitis —*see* Tendinitis, patellar
pelvis M77.8
periarthritis of wrist —*see* Periarthritis, wrist
peroneal tendinitis —*see* Tendinitis, peroneal
posterior tibial syndrome M76.82-
psoas tendinitis —*see* Tendinitis, psoas
shoulder M77.8
shoulder region —*see* Lesion, shoulder
specified type NEC M77.8
spinal M46.00
cervical region M46.02
cervicothoracic region M46.03
lumbar region M46.06
lumbosacral region M46.07
multiple sites M46.09
occipito-atlanto-axial region M46.01
sacrococcygeal region M46.08
thoracic region M46.04
thoracolumbar region M46.05
tibial collateral bursitis —*see* Bursitis, tibial collateral
upper arm M77.8
wrist and carpus NEC M77.8
calcaneal spur —*see* Spur, bone, calcaneal
periarthritis of wrist —*see* Periarthritis, wrist

Entomophobia F40.218

Entomophthoromycosis B46.8

Entrance, air into vein —*see* Embolism, air

Entrapment, nerve —*see* Neuropathy, entrapment

Entropion (eyelid) (paralytic) H02.009
cicatricial H02.019
left H02.016
lower H02.015
upper H02.014
right H02.013
lower H02.012
upper H02.011
congenital Q10.2
left H02.006
lower H02.005
upper H02.004
mechanical H02.029
left H02.026
lower H02.025
upper H02.024
right H02.023
lower H02.022
upper H02.021
right H02.003
lower H02.002
upper H02.001
senile H02.039
left H02.036
lower H02.035
upper H02.034
right H02.033
lower H02.032
upper H02.031
spastic H02.049
left H02.046
lower H02.045
upper H02.044

Entropion (continued)
spastic (continued)
right H02.043
lower H02.042
upper H02.041

Enucleated eye (traumatic, current) S05.7-

Enuresis R32
functional F98.0
habit disturbance F98.0
nocturnal N39.44
psychogenic F98.0
nonorganic origin F98.0
psychogenic F98.0

Eosinopenia —*see* Agranulocytosis

Eosinophilia (allergic) (idiopathic) (secondary) D72.10
with
angiolymphoid hyperplasia (ALHE) D18.01
familial D71.19
hereditary D72.19
in diseases classified elsewhere D72.18
infiltrative —*see* Eosinophilia, pulmonary
Löffler's J82.89
peritoneal —*see* Peritonitis, eosinophilic
pulmonary NEC J82.89
acute J82.82
asthmatic J82.83
chronic J82.81
specified NEC D72.19
tropical (pulmonary) J82.89

Eosinophilia-myalgia syndrome M35.8

Ependymitis (acute) (cerebral) (chronic) (granular) —*see* Encephalomyelitis

Ependymoblastoma
specified site —*see* Neoplasm, malignant, by site
unspecified site C71.9

Ependymoma (epithelial) (malignant)
anaplastic
specified site —*see* Neoplasm, malignant, by site
unspecified site C71.9
benign
specified site —*see* Neoplasm, benign, by site
unspecified site D33.2
myxopapillary D43.2
specified site —*see* Neoplasm, uncertain behavior, by site
unspecified site D43.2
papillary D43.2
specified site —*see* Neoplasm, uncertain behavior, by site
unspecified site D43.2
specified site —*see* Neoplasm, malignant, by site
unspecified site C71.9

Ependymopathy G93.89

Ephelis, ephelides L81.2

Epiblepharon (congenital) Q10.3

Epicanthus, epicanthic fold (eyelid) (congenital) Q10.3

Epicondylitis (elbow)
lateral M77.1-
medial M77.0-

Epicystitis —*see* Cystitis

Epidemic —*see* condition

Epidermidalization, cervix —*see* Dysplasia, cervix

Epidermis, epidermal —*see* condition

Epidermodysplasia verruciformis B07.8

Epidermolysis
bullosa (congenital) Q81.9
acquired L12.30
drug-induced L12.31
specified cause NEC L12.35
dystrophica Q81.2
letalis Q81.1
simplex Q81.0
specified NEC Q81.8
necroticans combustiformis L51.2
due to drug —*see* Table of Drugs and Chemicals, by drug

Epidermophytid —*see* Dermatophytosis

Epidermophytosis (infected) —*see* Dermatophytosis

Epididymis —*see* condition

Epididymitis (acute) (nonvenereal) (recurrent) (residual) N45.1
with orchitis N45.3
blennorrhagic (gonococcal) A54.23
caseous (tuberculous) A18.15
chlamydial A56.19
filarial (*see also* Infestation, filarial) B74.9 *[N51]*
gonococcal A54.23
syphilitic A52.76
tuberculous A18.15

Epididymo-orchitis (*see also* Epididymitis) N45.3

Epidural —*see* condition

Epigastrium, epigastric —*see* condition

Epigastrocele —*see* Hernia, ventral

Epiglottis —*see* condition

Epiglottitis, epiglottiditis (acute) J05.10
with obstruction J05.11
chronic J37.0

Epignathus Q89.4

Epilepsia partialis continua (*see also* Kozhevnikof's epilepsy) G40.1-

Epilepsy, epileptic, epilepsia (attack) (cerebral) (convulsion) (fit) (seizure) G40.909

Note: the following terms are to be considered equivalent to intractable: pharmacoresistant (pharmacologically resistant), treatment resistant, refractory (medically) and poorly controlled

with
complex partial seizures —*see* Epilepsy, localization-related, symptomatic, with complex partial seizures
grand mal seizures on awakening —*see* Epilepsy, generalized, specified NEC
myoclonic absences —*see* Epilepsy, generalized, specified NEC
myoclonic-astatic seizures —*see* Epilepsy, generalized, specified NEC
simple partial seizures —*see* Epilepsy, localization-related, symptomatic, with simple partial seizures
akinetic —*see* Epilepsy, generalized, specified NEC

Epilepsy, epileptic, epilepsia
(continued)

benign childhood with
  centrotemporal EEG spikes
  —*see* Epilepsy, localization-
  related, idiopathic
benign myoclonic in infancy G
  40.80-
Bravais-jacksonian —*see*
  Epilepsy, localization-related,
  symptomatic, with simple partial
  seizures
childhood
  with occipital EEG paroxysms
  —*see* Epilepsy, localization-
  related, idiopathic
  absence G40.A09
    intractable G40.A19
      with status epilepticus G40.
      A11
      without status epilepticus
      G40.A19
    not intractable G40.A09
      with status epilepticus G40.
      A01
      without status epilepticus
      G40.A09
climacteric —*see* Epilepsy,
  specified NEC
cysticercosis B69.0
deterioration (mental) F06.8
due to syphilis A52.19
focal —*see* Epilepsy, localization-
  related, symptomatic, with
  simple partial seizures
generalized
  idiopathic G40.309
    intractable G40.319
      with status epilepticus
      G40.311
      without status epilepticus
      G40.319
    not intractable G40.309
      with status epilepticus
      G40.301
      without status epilepticus
      G40.309
  specified NEC G40.409
    intractable G40.419
      with status epilepticus
      G40.411
      without status epilepticus
      G40.419
    not intractable G40.409
      with status epilepticus
      G40.401
      without status epilepticus
      G40.409
impulsive petit mal —*see* Epilepsy,
  juvenile myoclonic
intractable G40.919
  with status epilepticus G40.911
  without status epilepticus
  G40.919
juvenile absence G40.A09
  intractable G40.A19
    with status epilepticus G40.A11
    without status epilepticus
    G40.A19
  not intractable G40.A09
    with status epilepticus G40.
    A01
    without status epilepticus
    G40.A09
juvenile myoclonic G40.B09
  intractable G40.B19
    with status epilepticus G40.B11
    without status epilepticus
    G40.B19
  not intractable G40.B09
    with status epilepticus G40.B01

Epilepsy, epileptic, epilepsia
(continued)

juvenile myoclonic *(continued)*
  not intractable *(continued)*
    without status epilepticus
    G40.B09
localization-related (focal) (partial)
  idiopathic G40.009
    with seizures of localized
    onset G40.009
    intractable G40.019
      with status epilepticus
      G40.011
      without status epilepticus
      G40.019
    not intractable G40.009
      with status epilepticus
      G40.001
      without status epilepticus
      G40.009
  symptomatic
    with complex partial seizures
    G40.209
    intractable G40.219
      with status epilepticus
      G40.211
      without status epilepticus
      G40.219
    not intractable G40.209
      with status epilepticus
      G40.201
      without status epilepticus
      G40.209
    with simple partial seizures
    G40.109
    intractable G40.119
      with status epilepticus
      G40.111
      without status epilepticus
      G40.119
    not intractable G40.109
      with status epilepticus
      G40.101
      without status epilepticus
      G40.109
myoclonus, myoclonic —*see also*
  Epilepsy, generalized, specified
  NEC
  progressive —*see* Epilepsy,
    generalized, idiopathic
  severe, in infancy (SMEI)
    G40.83-
not intractable G40.909
  with status epilepticus G40.901
  without status epilepticus
  G40.909
on awakening —*see* Epilepsy,
  generalized, specified NEC
parasitic NOS B71.9 *[G94]*
partialis continua (*see also*
  Kozhevnikof's epilepsy) G40.1-
peripheral —*see* Epilepsy, specified
  NEC
polymorphic, in infancy (PMEI)
  G40.83-
procursiva —*see* Epilepsy,
  localization-related,
  symptomatic, with simple partial
  seizures
progressive (familial) myoclonic
  —*see* Epilepsy, generalized,
  idiopathic
reflex —*see* Epilepsy, specified
  NEC
related to
  alcohol G40.509
    not intractable G40.509
      with status epilepticus
      G40.501
      without status epliepticus
      G40.509

Epilepsy, epileptic, epilepsia
(continued)

related to *(continued)*
  drugs G40.509
    not intractable G40.509
      with status epilepticus
      G40.501
      without status epliepticus
      G40.509
  external causes G40.509
    not intractable G40.509
      with status epilepticus
      G40.501
      without status epilepticus
      G40.509
  hormonal changes G40.509
    not intractable G40.509
      with status epilepticus
      G40.501
      without status epilepticus
      G40.509
  sleep deprivation G40.509
    not intractable G40.509
      with status epilepticus
      G40.501
      without status epliepticus
      G40.509
  stress G40.509
    not intractable G40.509
      with status epilepticus
      G40.501
      without status epilepticus
      G40.509
  somatomotor —*see* Epilepsy,
    localization-related,
    symptomatic, with simple partial
    seizures
  somatosensory —*see* Epilepsy,
    localization-related,
    symptomatic, with simple partial
    seizures
spasms G40.822
  intractable G40.824
    with status epilepticus G40.823
    without status epilepticus
    G40.824
  not intractable G40.822
    with status epilepticus
    G40.821
    without status epilepticus
    G40.822
specified NEC G40.802
  intractable G40.804
    with status epilepticus
    G40.803
    without status epilepticus
    G40.804
  not intractable G40.802
    with status epilepticus
    G40.801
    without status epilepticus
    G40.802
syndromes
  generalized
    idiopathic G40.309
      intractable G40.319
        with status epilepticus
        G40.311
        without status epilepticus
        G40.319
      not intractable G40.309
        with status epilepticus
        G40.301
        without status epilepticus
        G40.309
    specified NEC G40.409
      intractable G40.419
        with status epilepticus
        G40.411
        without status epilepticus
        G40.419

Epilepsy, epileptic, epilepsia
(continued)

syndromes *(continued)*
  generalized *(continued)*
    specified NEC *(continued)*
      not intractable G40.409
        with status epilepticus
        G40.401
        without status epilepticus
        G40.409
  localization-related (focal)
    (partial)
    idiopathic G40.009
      with seizures of localized
      onset G40.009
      intractable G40.019
        with status epilepticus
        G40.011
        without status
        epilepticus G40.019
      not intractable G40.009
        with status epilepticus
        G40.001
        without status
        epilepticus G40.009
    symptomatic
      with complex partial
      seizures G40.209
      intractable G40.219
        with status epilepticus
        G40.211
        without status
        epilepticus G40.219
      not intractable G40.209
        with status epilepticus
        G40.201
        without status
        epilepticus G40.209
      with simple partial seizures
      G40.109
      intractable G40.119
        with status epilepticus
        G40.111
        without status
        epilepticus
        G40.119
      not intractable G40.109
        with status epilepticus
        G40.101
        without status
        epilepticus G40.109
  specified NEC G40.802
    intractable G40.804
      with status epilepticus
      G40.803
      without status epilepticus
      G40.804
    not intractable G40.802
      with status epilepticus
      G40.801
      without status epilepticus
      G40.802
tonic (-clonic) —*see* Epilepsy,
  generalized, specified NEC
twilight F05
uncinate (gyrus) —*see*
  Epilepsy, localization-related,
  symptomatic, with complex
  partial seizures
Unverricht (-Lundborg) (familial
  myoclonic) —*see* Epilepsy,
  generalized, idiopathic
visceral —*see* Epilepsy, specified
  NEC
visual —*see* Epilepsy, specified
  NEC

Epiloia Q85.1

Epimenorrhea N92.0

Epipharyngitis —*see*
  Nasopharyngitis

Epiphora H04.20-
- due to
  - excess lacrimation H04.21-
  - insufficient drainage H04.22-

Epiphyseal arrest —*see* Arrest, epiphyseal

Epiphyseolysis, epiphysiolysis —*see* Osteochondropathy

Epiphysitis —*see also* Osteochondropathy
- juvenile M92.9
- syphilitic (congenital) A50.02

Epiplocele —*see* Hernia, abdomen

Epiploitis —*see* Peritonitis

Epiplosarcomphalocele —*see* Hernia, umbilicus

Episcleritis (suppurative) H15.10-
- in (due to)
  - syphilis A52.71
  - tuberculosis A18.51
- nodular H15.12-
- periodica fugax H15.11-
  - angioneurotic —*see* Edema, angioneurotic
- syphilitic (late) A52.71
- tuberculous A18.51

Episode
- affective, mixed F39
- depersonalization (in neurotic state) F48.1
- depressive F32.9
  - major F32.9
    - mild F32.0
    - moderate F32.1
    - severe (without psychotic symptoms) F32.2
      - with psychotic symptoms F32.3
  - recurrent F33.9
    - brief F33.8
  - specified NEC F32.89
- hypomanic F30.8
- manic F30.9
  - with
    - psychotic symptoms F30.2
    - remission (full) F30.4
      - partial F30.3
  - other specified F30.8
  - recurrent F31.89
  - without psychotic symptoms F30.10
    - mild F30.11
    - moderate F30.12
    - severe (without psychotic symptoms) F30.13
      - with psychotic symptoms F30.2
- psychotic F23
  - organic F06.8
- schizophrenic (acute) NEC, brief F23

Epispadias (female) (male) Q64.0

Episplenitis D73.89

Epistaxis (multiple) R04.0
- hereditary I78.0
- vicarious menstruation N94.89

Epithelioma (malignant) —*see also* Neoplasm, malignant, by site
- adenoides cysticum —*see* Neoplasm, skin, benign
- basal cell —*see* Neoplasm, skin, malignant
- benign —*see* Neoplasm, benign, by site
- Bowen's —*see* Neoplasm, skin, in situ

Epithelioma (continued)
- calcifying, of Malherbe —*see* Neoplasm, skin, benign
- external site —*see* Neoplasm, skin, malignant
- intraepidermal, Jadassohn —*see* Neoplasm, skin, benign
- squamous cell —*see* Neoplasm, malignant, by site

Epitheliomatosis pigmented Q82.1

Epitheliopathy, multifocal placoid pigment H30.14-

Epithelium, epithelial —*see* condition

Epituberculosis (with atelectasis) (allergic) A15.7

Eponychia Q84.6

Epstein's
- nephrosis or syndrome —*see* Nephrosis
- pearl K09.8

Epulis (gingiva) (fibrous) (giant cell) K06.8

Equinia A24.0

Equinovarus (congenital) (talipes) Q66.0-
- acquired —*see* Deformity, limb, clubfoot

Equivalent
- convulsive (abdominal) —*see* Epilepsy, specified NEC
- epileptic (psychic) —*see* Epilepsy, localization-related, symptomatic, with complex partial seizures

Erb (-Duchenne) **paralysis** (birth injury) (newborn) P14.0

Erb-Goldflam disease or syndrome G70.00
- with exacerbation (acute) G70.01
- in crisis G70.01

Erb's
- disease G71.02
- palsy, paralysis (brachial) (birth) (newborn) P14.0
  - spinal (spastic) syphilitic A52.17
- pseudohypertrophic muscular dystrophy G71.02

Erdheim's syndrome (acromegalic macrospondylitis) E22.0

Erection, painful (persistent) —*see* Priapism

Ergosterol deficiency (vitamin D) E55.9
- with
  - adult osteomalacia M83.8
  - rickets —*see* Rickets

Ergotism —*see also* Poisoning, food, noxious, plant
- from ergot used as drug (migraine therapy) —*see* Table of Drugs and Chemicals

Erosio interdigitalis blastomycetica B37.2

Erosion
- artery I77.2
  - without rupture I77.89
- bone —*see* Disorder, bone, density and structure, specified NEC
- bronchus J98.09
- cartilage (joint) —*see* Disorder, cartilage, specified type NEC
- cervix (uteri) (acquired) (chronic) (congenital) N86
  - with cervicitis N72

Erosion (continued)
- cornea (nontraumatic) —*see* Ulcer, cornea
  - recurrent H18.83-
  - traumatic —*see* Abrasion, cornea
- dental (idiopathic) (occupational) (due to diet, drugs or vomiting) K03.2
- duodenum, postpyloric —*see* Ulcer, duodenum
- esophagus K22.10
  - with bleeding K22.11
- gastric —*see* Ulcer, stomach
- gastrojejunal —*see* Ulcer, gastrojejunal
- implanted mesh —*see* Complications, prosthetic device or implant, mesh
- intestine K63.3
- lymphatic vessel I89.8
- pylorus, pyloric (ulcer) —*see* Ulcer, stomach
- spine, aneurysmal A52.09
- stomach —*see* Ulcer, stomach
- subcutaneous device pocket
  - nervous system prosthetic device, implant, or graft T85.890
  - other internal prosthetic device, implant, or graft T85.898
- teeth (idiopathic) (occupational) (due to diet, drugs or vomiting) K03.2
- urethra N36.8
- uterus N85.8

Erotomania F52.8

Error
- metabolism, inborn -- se Disorder, metabolism
- refractive —*see* Disorder, refraction

Eructation R14.2
- nervous or psychogenic F45.8

Eruption
- creeping B76.9
- drug (generalized) (taken internally) L27.0
  - fixed L27.1
  - in contact with skin —*see* Dermatitis, due to drugs
  - localized L27.1
- Hutchinson, summer L56.4
- Kaposi's varicelliform B00.0
- napkin L22
- polymorphous light (sun) L56.4
- recalcitrant pustular L13.8
- ringed R23.8
- skin (nonspecific) R21
  - creeping (meaning hookworm) B76.9
  - due to inoculation/vaccination (generalized) (*see also* Dermatitis, due to, vaccine) L27.0
    - localized L27.1
  - erysipeloid A26.0
  - feigned L98.1
  - Kaposi's varicelliform B00.0
  - lichenoid L28.0
  - meaning dermatitis —*see* Dermatitis
  - toxic NEC L53.0
- tooth, teeth, abnormal (incomplete) (late) (premature) (sequence) K00.6
- vesicular R23.8

Erysipelas (gangrenous) (infantile) (newborn) (phlegmonous) (suppurative) A46
- external ear A46 [H62.40]
- puerperal, postpartum O86.89

Erysipeloid A26.9
- cutaneous (Rosenbach's) A26.0
- disseminated A26.8
- sepsis A26.7
- specified NEC A26.8

Erythema, erythematous
(infectional) (inflammation) L53.9
- ab igne L59.0
- annulare (centrifugum) (rheumaticum) L53.1
- arthriticum epidemicum A25.1
- brucellum —*see* Brucellosis
- chronic figurate NEC L53.3
- chronicum migrans (Borrelia burgdorferi) A69.20
- diaper L22
- due to
  - chemical NEC L53.0
    - in contact with skin L24.5
  - drug (internal use) —*see* Dermatitis, due to, drugs
- elevatum diutinum L95.1
- endemic E52
- epidemic, arthritic A25.1
- figuratum perstans L53.3
- gluteal L22
- heat - code by site under Burn, first degree
- ichthyosiforme congenitum bullous Q80.3
- in diseases classified elsewhere L54
- induratum (nontuberculous) L52
  - tuberculous A18.4
- infectiosum B08.3
- intertrigo L30.4
- iris L51.9
- marginatum L53.2
  - in (due to) acute rheumatic fever I00
- medicamentosum —*see* Dermatitis, due to, drugs
- migrans A26.0
  - chronicum A69.20
  - tongue K14.1
- multiforme (major) (minor) L51.9
  - bullous, bullosum L51.1
  - conjunctiva L51.1
  - nonbullous L51.0
  - pemphigoides L12.0
  - specified NEC L51.8
- napkin L22
- neonatorum P83.88
  - toxic P83.1
- nodosum L52
  - tuberculous A18.4
- palmar L53.8
- pernio T69.1
- rash, newborn P83.88
- scarlatiniform (recurrent) (exfoliative) L53.8
- solare L55.0
- specified NEC L53.8
- toxic, toxicum NEC L53.0
  - newborn P83.1
- tuberculous (primary) A18.4

Erythematous, erythematosus —*see* condition

Erythermalgia (primary) I73.81

Erythralgia I73.81

Erythrasma L08.1

Erythredema (polyneuropathy) —*see* Poisoning, mercury

Erythremia (acute) C94.0-
- chronic D45
- secondary D75.1

Erythroblastopenia —*see also* Aplasia, red cell D60.9
- congenital D61.01

Erythroblastophthisis D61.09

Erythroblastosis (fetalis) (newborn) P55.9
- due to
  - ABO (antibodies) (incompatibility) (isoimmunization) P55.1
  - Rh (antibodies) (incompatibility) (isoimmunization) P55.0

Erythrocyanosis (crurum) I73.89

Erythrocythemia —see Erythremia

Erythrocytosis (megalosplenic) (secondary) D75.1
- familial D75.0
- oval, hereditary —see Elliptocytosis
- secondary D75.1
- stress D75.1

Erythroderma (secondary) (see also Erythema) L53.9
- bullous ichthyosiform, congenital Q80.3
- desquamativum L21.1
- ichthyosiform, congenital (bullous) Q80.3
- neonatorum P83.88
- psoriaticum L40.8

Erythrodysesthesia, palmar plantar (PPE) L27.1

Erythrogenesis imperfecta D61.09

Erythroleukemia C94.0-

Erythromelalgia I73.81

Erythrophagocytosis D75.89

Erythrophobia F40.298

Erythroplakia, oral epithelium, and tongue K13.29

Erythroplasia (Queyrat) D07.4
- specified site —see Neoplasm, skin, in situ
- unspecified site D07.4

Escherichia coli (E. coli), as cause of disease classified elsewhere B96.20
- non-O157 Shiga toxin-producing (with known O group) B96.22
- non-Shiga toxin-producing B96.29
- O157 B96.21
- O157 with confirmation of Shiga toxin when H antigen is unknown, or is not H7 B96.21
- O157:H-(nonmotile) with confirmation of Shiga toxin B96.21
- O157:H7 with or without confirmation of Shiga toxin-production B96.21
- Shiga toxin-producing (with unspecified O group) (STEC) B96.23
- specified NEC B96.29

Esophagismus K22.4

Esophagitis (acute) (alkaline) (chemical) (chronic) (infectional) (necrotic) (peptic) (postoperative) (without bleeding) K20.90
- with bleeding K20.91
- candidal B37.81
- due to gastrointestinal reflux disease (without bleeding) K21.00
  - with bleeding K21.01
- eosinophilic K20.0
- reflux K21.00
- specified NEC (without bleeding) K20.80
  - with bleeding K21.81

Esophagitis (continued)
- tuberculous A18.83
- ulcerative K22.10
  - with bleeding K22.11

Esophagocele K22.5

Esophagomalacia K22.8

Esophagospasm K22.4

Esophagostenosis K22.2

Esophagostomiasis B81.8

Esophagotracheal —see condition

Esophagus —see condition

Esophoria H50.51
- convergence, excess H51.12
- divergence, insufficiency H51.8

Esotropia —see Strabismus, convergent concomitant

Espundia B55.2

Essential —see condition

Esthesioneuroblastoma C30.0

Esthesioneurocytoma C30.0

Esthesioneuroepithelioma C30.0

Esthiomene A55

Estivo-autumnal malaria (fever) B50.9

Estrangement (marital) Z63.5
- parent-child NEC Z62.890

Estriasis —see Myiasis

Ethanolism —see Alcoholism

Etherism —see Dependence, drug, inhalant

Ethmoid, ethmoidal —see condition

Ethmoiditis (chronic) (nonpurulent) (purulent) —see also Sinusitis, ethmoidal
- influenzal —see Influenza, with, respiratory manifestations NEC Woakes' J33.1

Ethylism —see Alcoholism

Eulenburg's disease (congenital paramyotonia) G71.19

Eumycetoma B47.0

Eunuchoidism E29.1
- hypogonadotropic E23.0

European blastomycosis —see Cryptococcosis

Eustachian —see condition

Evaluation (for) (of)
- development state
  - adolescent Z00.3
  - period of
    - delayed growth in childhood Z00.70
      - with abnormal findings Z00.71
    - rapid growth in childhood Z00.2
  - puberty Z00.3
- growth and developmental state (period of rapid growth) Z00.2
  - delayed growth Z00.70
    - with abnormal findings Z00.71
- mental health (status) Z00.8
  - requested by authority Z04.6
- period of
  - delayed growth in childhood Z00.70
    - with abnormal findings Z00.71
  - rapid growth in childhood Z00.2
- suspected condition —see Observation

Evans syndrome D69.41

Event
- apparent life threatening in newborn and infact (ALTE) R68.13
- brief resolved unexplained event (BRUE) R68.13

Eventration —see also Hernia, ventral
- colon into chest —see Hernia, diaphragm
- diaphragm (congenital) Q79.1

Eversion
- bladder N32.89
- cervix (uteri) N86
  - with cervicitis N72
- foot NEC —see also Deformity, valgus, ankle
  - congenital Q66.6
- punctum lacrimale (postinfectional) (senile) H04.52-
- ureter (meatus) N28.89
- urethra (meatus) N36.8
- uterus N81.4

Evidence
- cytologic
  - of malignancy on anal smear R85.614
  - of malignancy on cervical smear R87.614
  - of malignancy on vaginal smear R87.624

Evisceration
- birth injury P15.8
- traumatic NEC
  - eye —see Enucleated eye

Evulsion —see Avulsion

Ewing's sarcoma or tumor —see Neoplasm, bone, malignant

Examination (for) (following) (general) (of) (routine) Z00.00
- with abnormal findings Z00.01
- abuse, physical (alleged), ruled out
  - adult Z04.71
  - child Z04.72
- adolescent (development state) Z00.3
- alleged rape or sexual assault (victim), ruled out
  - adult Z04.41
  - child Z04.42
- allergy Z01.82
- annual (adult) (periodic) (physical) Z00.00
  - with abnormal findings Z00.01
  - gynecological Z01.419
    - with abnormal findings Z01.411
- antibody response Z01.84
- blood —see Examination, laboratory
- blood pressure Z01.30
  - with abnormal findings Z01.31
- cancer staging —see Neoplasm, malignant, by site
- cervical Papanicolaou smear Z12.4
  - as part of routine gynecological examination Z01.419
    - with abnormal findings Z01.411
- child (over 28 days old) Z00.129
  - with abnormal findings Z00.121
  - under 28 days old —see Newborn, examination
- clinical research control or normal comparison (control) (participant) Z00.6
- contraceptive (drug) maintenance (routine) Z30.8
  - device (intrauterine) Z30.431
- dental Z01.20
  - with abnormal findings Z01.21
- developmental —see Examination, child
- donor (potential) Z00.5

Examination (continued)
- ear Z01.10
  - with abnormal findings NEC Z01.118
- eye Z01.00
  - with abnormal findings Z01.01
  - following failed vision screening Z01.020
    - with abnormal findings Z01.021
- following
  - accident NEC Z04.3
    - transport Z04.1
    - work Z04.2
  - assault, alleged, ruled out
    - adult Z04.71
    - child Z04.72
  - motor vehicle accident Z04.1
  - treatment (for) Z09
    - combined NEC Z09
      - fracture Z09
      - malignant neoplasm Z08
    - malignant neoplasm Z08
    - mental disorder Z09
    - specified condition NEC Z09
- follow-up (routine) (following) Z09
  - chemotherapy NEC Z09
    - malignant neoplasm Z08
  - fracture Z09
  - malignant neoplasm Z08
  - postpartum Z39.2
  - psychotherapy Z09
  - radiotherapy NEC Z09
    - malignant neoplasm Z08
  - surgery NEC Z09
    - malignant neoplasm Z08
- forced sexual exploitation Z04.81
- forced labor exploitation Z04.82
- gynecological Z01.419
  - with abnormal findings Z01.411
  - for contraceptive maintenance Z30.8
- health —see Examination, medical
- hearing Z01.10
  - with abnormal findings NEC Z01.118
  - following failed hearing screening Z01.110
  - infant or child (over 28 days old) Z00.129
    - with abnormal findings Z00.121
- immunity status testing Z01.84
- laboratory (as part of a general medical examination) Z00.00
  - with abnormal findings Z00.01
  - preprocedural Z01.812
- lactating mother Z39.1
- medical (adult) (for) (of) Z00.00
  - with abnormal findings Z00.01
  - administrative purpose only Z02.9
    - specified NEC Z02.89
  - admission to
    - armed forces Z02.3
    - old age home Z02.2
    - prison Z02.89
    - residential institution Z02.2
    - school Z02.0
      - following illness or medical treatment Z02.0
    - summer camp Z02.89
  - adoption Z02.82
  - blood alcohol or drug level Z02.83
  - camp (summer) Z02.89
  - clinical research, normal subject (control) (participant) Z00.6
  - control subject in clinical research (normal comparison) (participant) Z00.6
  - donor (potential) Z00.5

Examination (continued)
medical (continued)
driving license Z02.4
general (adult) Z00.00
with abnormal findings Z00.01
immigration Z02.89
insurance purposes Z02.6
marriage Z02.89
medicolegal reasons NEC Z04.89
naturalization Z02.89
participation in sport Z02.5
paternity testing Z02.81
population survey Z00.8
pre-employment Z02.1
pre-operative —see
Examination, pre-procedural
pre-procedural
cardiovascular Z01.810
respiratory Z01.811
specified NEC Z01.818
preschool children
for admission to school Z02.0
prisoners
for entrance into prison Z02.89
recruitment for armed forces
Z02.3
specified NEC Z00.8
sport competition Z02.5
medicolegal reason NEC Z04.89
following
forced sexual exploitation
Z04.81
forced labor exploitation
Z04.82
newborn —see Newborn,
examination
pelvic (annual) (periodic)
Z01.419
with abnormal findings
Z01.411
period of rapid growth in childhood
Z00.2
periodic (adult) (annual) (routine)
Z00.00
with abnormal findings Z00.01
physical (adult) (see also
Examination, medical) Z00.00
sports Z02.5
postpartum
immediately after delivery Z39.0
routine follow-up Z39.2
prenatal (normal pregnancy) (see
also Pregnancy, normal) Z34.9-
pre-chemotherapy (antineoplastic)
Z01.818
pre-procedural (pre-operative)
cardiovascular Z01.810
laboratory Z01.812
respiratory Z01.811
specified NEC Z01.818
prior to chemotherapy
(antineoplastic) Z01.818
psychiatric NEC Z00.8
follow-up not needing further
care Z09
requested by authority Z04.6
radiological (as part of a general
medical examination) Z00.00
with abnormal findings Z00.01
repeat cervical smear to confirm
findings of recent normal smear
following initial abnormal smear
Z01.42
skin (hypersensitivity) Z01.82
special (see also Examination, by
type) Z01.89
specified type NEC Z01.89
specified type or reason NEC
Z04.89
teeth Z01.20
with abnormal findings Z01.21

Examination (continued)
urine —see Examination, laboratory
vision Z01.00
with abnormal findings Z01.01
following failed vision screening
Z01.020
with abnormal findings
Z01.021
infant or child (over 28 days old)
Z00.129
with abnormal findings Z00.121

Exanthem, exanthema —see also
Rash
with enteroviral vesicular stomatitis
B08.4
Boston A88.0
epidemic with meningitis A88.0
[G02]
subitum B08.20
due to human herpesvirus 6
B08.21
due to human herpesvirus 7
B08.22
viral, virus B09
specified type NEC B08.8

Excess, excessive, excessively
alcohol level in blood R78.0
androgen (ovarian) E28.1
attrition, tooth, teeth K03.0
carotene, carotin (dietary) E67.1
cold, effects of T69.9
specified effect NEC T69.8
convergence H51.12
crying
in child, adolescent, or adult
R45.83
in infant R68.11
development, breast N62
divergence H51.8
drinking (alcohol) NEC (without
dependence) F10.10
habitual (continual) (without
remission) F10.20
eating R63.2
estrogen E28.0
fat —see also Obesity
in heart —see Degeneration,
myocardial
localized E65
foreskin N47.8
gas R14.0
glucagon E16.3
heat —see Heat
intermaxillary vertical dimension
of fully erupted teeth M26.37
interocclusal distance of fully
erupted teeth M26.37
kalium E87.5
large
colon K59.39
congenital Q43.8
infant P08.0
organ or site, congenital NEC
—see Anomaly, by site
long
organ or site, congenital NEC
—see Anomaly, by site
menstruation (with regular cycle)
N92.0
with irregular cycle N92.1
napping Z72.821
natrium E87.0
number of teeth K00.1
nutrient (dietary) NEC R63.2
potassium (K) E87.5
salivation K11.7
secretion —see also Hypersecretion
milk O92.6
sputum R09.3
sweat R61

Excess, excessive, excessively
(continued)
sexual drive F52.8
short
organ or site, congenital NEC
—see Anomaly, by site
umbilical cord in labor or
delivery O69.3
skin L98.7
and subcutaneous tissue L98.7
eyelid (acquired) —see
Blepharochalasis
congenital Q10.3
sodium (Na) E87.0
spacing of fully erupted teeth
M26.32
sputum R09.3
sweating R61
thirst R63.1
due to deprivation of water
T73.1
tuberosity of jaw M26.07
vitamin
A (dietary) E67.0
administered as drug
(prolonged intake) —see
Table of Drugs and
Chemicals, vitamins,
adverse effect
overdose or wrong substance
given or taken —see Table
of Drugs and Chemicals,
vitamins, poisoning
D (dietary) E67.3
administered as drug
(prolonged intake) —see
Table of Drugs and
Chemicals, vitamins,
adverse effect
overdose or wrong substance
given or taken —see Table
of Drugs and Chemicals,
vitamins, poisoning
weight
gain R63.5
loss R63.4

**Excitability, abnormal, under
minor stress** (personality disorder)
F60.3

Excitation
anomalous atrioventricular I45.6
psychogenic F30.8
reactive (from emotional stress,
psychological trauma) F30.8

Excitement
hypomanic F30.8
manic F30.9
mental, reactive (from emotional
stress, psychological trauma)
F30.8
state, reactive (from emotional
stress, psychological trauma)
F30.8

Excoriation (traumatic) —see also
Abrasion
neurotic L98.1
skin picking disorder F42.4

Exfoliation
due to erythematous conditions
according to extent of body
surface involved L49.0
10-19 percent of body surface
L49.1
20-29 percent of body surface
L49.2
30-39 percent of body surface
L49.3
40-49 percent of body surface
L49.4

Exfoliation (continued)
due to erythematous conditions
according to extent of body
surface involved L49.0
(continued)
50-59 percent of body surface
L49.5
60-69 percent of body surface
L49.6
70-79 percent of body surface
L49.7
80-89 percent of body surface
L49.8
90-99 percent of body surface
L49.9
less than 10 percent of body
surface L49.0
teeth, due to systemic causes K08.0

Exfoliative —see condition

Exhaustion, exhaustive (physical
NEC) R53.83
battle F43.0
cardiac —see Failure, heart
delirium F43.0
due to
cold T69.8
excessive exertion T73.3
exposure T73.2
neurasthenia F48.8
heart —see Failure, heart
heat (see also Heat, exhaustion)
T67.5
due to
salt depletion T67.4
water depletion T67.3
maternal, complicating delivery
O75.81
mental F48.8
myocardium, myocardial —see
Failure, heart
nervous F48.8
old age R54
psychogenic F48.8
psychosis F43.0
senile R54
vital NEC Z73.0

Exhibitionism F65.2

Exocervicitis —see Cervicitis

Exomphalos Q79.2
meaning hernia —see Hernia,
umbilicus

Exophoria H50.52
convergence, insufficiency
H51.11
divergence, excess H51.8

Exophthalmos H05.2-
congenital Q15.8
constant NEC H05.24-
displacement, globe —see
Displacement, globe
due to thyrotoxicosis
(hyperthyroidism) —see
Hyperthyroidism, with, goiter
(diffuse)
dysthyroid —see Hyperthyroidism,
with, goiter (diffuse)
goiter —see Hyperthyroidism,
with, goiter (diffuse)
intermittent NEC H05.25-
malignant —see Hyperthyroidism,
with, goiter (diffuse)
orbital
edema —see Edema, orbit
hemorrhage —see Hemorrhage,
orbit
pulsating NEC H05.26-
thyrotoxic, thyrotropic —see
Hyperthyroidism, with, goiter
(diffuse)

Exostosis —*see also* Disorder, bone
  cartilaginous —*see* Neoplasm, bone, benign
  congenital (multiple) Q78.6
  external ear canal H61.81-
  gonococcal A54.49
  jaw (bone) M27.8
  multiple, congenital Q78.6
  orbit H05.35-
  osteocartilaginous —*see* Neoplasm, bone, benign
  syphilitic A52.77

Exotropia —*see* Strabismus, divergent concomitant

Explanation of
  investigation finding Z71.2
  medication Z71.89

Exposure (to) (*see also* Contact, with) T75.89
  acariasis Z20.7
  AIDS virus Z20.6
  air pollution Z77.110
  algae and algae toxins Z77.121
  algae bloom Z77.121
  anthrax Z20.810
  aromatic amines Z77.020
  aromatic (hazardous) compounds NEC Z77.028
  aromatic dyes NOS Z77.028
  arsenic Z77.010
  asbestos Z77.090
  bacterial disease NEC Z20.818
  benzene Z77.021
  blue-green algae bloom Z77.121
  body fluids (potentially hazardous) Z77.21
  brown tide Z77.121
  chemicals (chiefly nonmedicinal) (hazardous) NEC Z77.098
  cholera Z20.09
  chromium compounds Z77.018
  cold, effects of T69.9
    specified effect NEC T69.8
  communicable disease Z20.9
    bacterial NEC Z20.818
    specified NEC Z20.89
    viral NEC Z20.828
    Zika virus Z20.821
  cyanobacteria bloom Z77.121
  disaster Z65.5
  discrimination Z60.5
  dyes Z77.098
  effects of T73.9
  environmental tobacco smoke (acute) (chronic) Z77.22
  Escherichia coli (E. coli) Z20.01
  exhaustion due to T73.2
  fiberglass —*see* Table of Drugs and Chemicals, fiberglass
  German measles Z20.4
  gonorrhea Z20.2
  hazardous metals NEC Z77.018
  hazardous substances NEC Z77.29
  hazards in the physical environment NEC Z77.128
  hazards to health NEC Z77.9
  human immunodeficiency virus (HIV) Z20.6
  human T-lymphotropic virus type-1 (HTLV-1) Z20.89
  implanted
    mesh —*see* Complications, prosthetic device or implant, mesh
    prosthetic materials NEC —*see* Complications, prosthetic materials NEC
  infestation (parasitic) NEC Z20.7
  intestinal infectious disease NEC Z20.09
    Escherichia coli (E. coli) Z20.01

Exposure (continued)
  lead Z77.011
  meningococcus Z20.811
  mold (toxic) Z77.120
  nickel dust Z77.018
  noise Z77.122
  occupational
    air contaminants NEC Z57.39
    dust Z57.2
    environmental tobacco smoke Z57.31
    extreme temperature Z57.6
    noise Z57.0
    radiation Z57.1
    risk factors Z57.9
      specified NEC Z57.8
    toxic agents (gases) (liquids) (solids) (vapors) in agriculture Z57.4
    toxic agents (gases) (liquids) (solids) (vapors) in industry NEC Z57.5
    vibration Z57.7
  parasitic disease NEC Z20.7
  pediculosis Z20.7
  persecution Z60.5
  pfiesteria piscicida Z77.121
  poliomyelitis Z20.89
  polycyclic aromatic hydrocarbons Z77.028
  pollution
    air Z77.110
    environmental NEC Z77.118
    soil Z77.112
    water Z77.111
  prenatal (drugs) (toxic chemicals) —*see* Newborn, affected by, noxious substances transmitted via placenta or breast milk
  rabies Z20.3
  radiation, naturally occurring NEC Z77.123
  radon Z77.123
  red tide (Florida) Z77.121
  rubella Z20.4
  second hand tobacco smoke (acute) (chronic) Z77.22
    in the perinatal period P96.81
  sexually-transmitted disease Z20.2
  smallpox (laboratory) Z20.89
  syphilis Z20.2
  terrorism Z65.4
  torture Z65.4
  tuberculosis Z20.1
  uranium Z77.012
  varicella Z20.820
  venereal disease Z20.2
  viral disease NEC Z20.828
  war Z65.5
  water pollution Z77.111
  Zika virus Z20.821

Exsanguination —*see* Hemorrhage

Exstrophy
  abdominal contents Q45.8
  bladder Q64.10
    cloacal Q64.12
    specified type NEC Q64.19
    supravesical fissure Q64.11

Extensive —*see* condition

Extra (*see also* Accessory marker chromosomes) (normal individual) Q92.61
  in abnormal individual Q92.62
  rib Q76.6
    cervical Q76.5

Extrasystoles (supraventricular) I49.49
  atrial I49.1
  auricular I49.1

Extrasystoles (continued)
  junctional I49.2
  ventricular I49.3

Extrauterine gestation or pregnancy —*see* Pregnancy, by site

Extravasation
  blood R58
  chyle into mesentery I89.8
  pelvicalyceal N13.8
  pyelosinus N13.8
  urine (from ureter) R39.0
  vesicant agent
    antineoplastic chemotherapy T80.810
    other agent NEC T80.818

Extremity —*see* condition, limb

Extrophy —*see* Exstrophy

Extroversion
  bladder Q64.19
  uterus N81.4
    complicating delivery O71.2
    postpartal (old) N81.4

Extruded tooth (teeth) M26.34

Extrusion
  breast implant (prosthetic) T85.42
  eye implant (globe) (ball) T85.328
  intervertebral disc —*see* Displacement, intervertebral disc
  ocular lens implant (prosthetic) —*see* Complications, intraocular lens
  vitreous —*see* Prolapse, vitreous

Exudate
  pleural —*see* Effusion, pleura
  retina H35.89

Exudative —*see* condition

Eye, eyeball, eyelid —*see* condition

Eyestrain —*see* Disturbance, vision, subjective

Eyeworm disease of Africa B74.3

F

Faber's syndrome (achlorhydric anemia) D50.9

Fabry (-Anderson) **disease** E75.21

Facet syndrome M47.89-

Faciocephalalgia, autonomic (*see also* Neuropathy, peripheral, autonomic) G90.09

Factor(s)
  psychic, associated with diseases classified elsewhere F54
  psychological
    affecting physical conditions F54
    or behavioral
      affecting general medical condition F54
      associated with disorders or diseases classified elsewhere F54

Fahr disease (of brain) G23.8

Fahr Volhard disease (of kidney) I12.-

Failure, failed
  abortion —*see* Abortion, attempted
  aortic (valve) I35.8
    rheumatic I06.8
  attempted abortion —*see* Abortion, attempted
  biventricular I50.82
    due to left heart failure I50.814
  bone marrow —*see* Anemia, aplastic

Failure, failed (continued)
  cardiac —*see* Failure, heart
  cardiorenal (chronic) (*see also* Failure, renal, and Failure, heart) I50.9
    hypertensive I13.2
  cardiorespiratory (*see also* Failure, heart) R09.2
  cardiovascular (chronic) —*see* Failure, heart
  cerebrovascular I67.9
  cervical dilatation in labor O62.0
  circulation, circulatory (peripheral) R57.9
    newborn P29.89
  compensation —*see* Disease, heart
  compliance with medical treatment or regimen —*see* Noncompliance
  congestive —*see* Failure, heart, congestive
  dental implant (endosseous) M27.69
    due to
      failure of dental prosthesis M27.63
      lack of attached gingiva M27.62
      occlusal trauma (poor prosthetic design) M27.62
      parafunctional habits M27.62
      periodontal infection (peri-implantitis) M27.62
      poor oral hygiene M27.62
      osseointegration M27.61
        due to
          complications of systemic disease M27.61
          poor bone quality M27.61
        iatrogenic M27.61
      post-osseointegration
        biological M27.62
          due to complications of systemic disease M27.62
          iatrogenic M27.62
        mechanical M27.63
      pre-integration M27.61
      pre-osseointegration M27.61
    specified NEC M27.69
  descent of head (at term) of pregnancy (mother) O32.4
  endosseous dental implant —*see* Failure, dental implant
  engagement of head (term of pregnancy) (mother) O32.4
  erection (penile) (*see also* Dysfunction, sexual, male, erectile) N52.9
    nonorganic F52.21
  examination(s), anxiety concerning Z55.2
  expansion terminal respiratory units (newborn) (primary) P28.0
  forceps NOS (with subsequent cesarean delivery) O66.5
  gain weight (child over 28 days old) R62.51
    adult R62.7
    newborn P92.6
  genital response (male) F52.21
    female F52.22
  heart (acute) (senile) (sudden) I50.9
    with
      acute pulmonary edema —*see* Failure, ventricular, left
      decompensation —*see also* Failure, heart, by type as diastolic or systolic, acute and chronic I50.9

Failure, failed (continued)
trial of labor (with
subsequent cesarean delivery)
O66.40
following previous cesarean
delivery O66.41
tubal ligation N99.89
urinary —see Disease, kidney,
chronic
vacuum extraction NOS (with
subsequent cesarean delivery)
O66.5
vasectomy N99.89
ventouse NOS (with subsequent
cesarean delivery) O66.5
ventricular (see also Failure, heart)
I50.9
left (see also Failure, heart)
I50.1
with rheumatic fever
(conditions in I00)
active I01.8
with chorea I02.0
inactive or quiescent (with
chorea) I09.81
rheumatic (chronic) (inactive)
(with chorea) I09.81
active or acute I01.8
with chorea I02.0
right —see Failure, heart, right
vital centers, newborn P91.88

Fainting (fit) R55

Fallen arches —see Deformity, limb,
flat foot

Falling, falls (repeated) R29.6
any organ or part —see Prolapse

Fallopian
insufflation Z31.41
tube —see condition

Fallot's
pentalogy Q21.8
tetrad or tetralogy Q21.3
triad or trilogy Q22.3

False —see also condition
croup J38.5
joint —see Nonunion, fracture
labor (pains) O47.9
at or after 37 completed weeks
of gestation O47.1
before 37 completed weeks of
gestation O47.0-
passage, urethra (prostatic) N36.5
pregnancy F45.8

Family, familial —see also condition
disruption Z63.8
involving divorce or separation
Z63.5
Li-Fraumeni (syndrome) Z15.01
planning advice Z30.09
problem Z63.9
specified NEC Z63.8
retinoblastoma C69.2-

Famine (effects of) T73.0
edema —see Malnutrition, severe

Fanconi (-de Toni) (-Debré)
syndrome E72.09
with cystinosis E72.04

Fanconi's anemia (congenital
pancytopenia) D61.09

Farber's disease or syndrome
E75.29

Farcy A24.0

Farmer's
lung J67.0
skin L57.8

Farsightedness —see Hypermetropia

Fascia —see condition

Fasciculation R25.3

Fasciitis M72.9
diffuse (eosinophilic) M35.4
infective M72.8
necrotizing M72.6
necrotizing M72.6
nodular M72.4
perirenal (with ureteral obstruction)
N13.5
with infection N13.6
plantar M72.2
specified NEC M72.8
traumatic (old) M72.8
current - code by site under
Sprain

Fascioliasis B66.3

Fasciolopsis, fasciolopsiasis
(intestinal) B66.5

Fascioscapulohumeral myopathy
G71.02

Fast pulse R00.0

Fat
embolism —see Embolism, fat
excessive —see also Obesity
in heart —see Degeneration,
myocardial
in stool R19.5
localized (pad) E65
heart —see Degeneration,
myocardial
knee M79.4
retropatellar M79.4
necrosis
breast N64.1
mesentery K65.4
omentum K65.4
pad E65
knee M79.4

Fatigue R53.83
auditory deafness —see Deafness
chronic R53.82
combat F43.0
general R53.83
psychogenic F48.8
heat (transient) T67.6
muscle M62.89
myocardium —see Failure, heart
neoplasm-related R53.0
nervous, neurosis F48.8
operational F48.8
psychogenic (general) F48.8
senile R54
voice R49.8

Fatness —see Obesity

Fatty —see also condition
apron E65
degeneration —see Degeneration,
fatty
heart (enlarged) —see
Degeneration, myocardial
liver NEC K76.0
alcoholic K70.0
nonalcoholic K76.0
necrosis —see Degeneration, fatty

Fauces —see condition

Fauchard's disease (periodontitis)
—see Periodontitis

Faucitis J02.9

Favism (anemia) D55.0

Favus —see Dermatophytosis

Fazio-Londe disease or syndrome
G12.1

Fear complex or reaction F40.9

Fear of —see Phobia

Feared complaint unfounded Z71.1

Febris, febrile —see also Fever
flava (see also Fever, yellow) A95.9
melitensis A23.0
pestis —see Plague
recurrens —see Fever, relapsing
rubra A38.9

Fecal
incontinence R15.9
smearing R15.1
soiling R15.1
urgency R15.2

Fecalith (impaction) K56.41
appendix K38.1
congenital P76.8

Fede's disease K14.0

**Feeble rapid pulse due to shock
following injury** T79.4

Feeble-minded F70

Feeding
difficulties R63.3
problem R63.3
newborn P92.9
specified NEC P92.8
nonorganic (adult) —see
Disorder, eating

Feeling (of)
foreign body in throat R09.89

Feer's disease —see Poisoning,
mercury

Feet —see condition

Feigned illness Z76.5

Feil-Klippel syndrome (brevicollis)
Q76.1

Feinmesser's (hidrotic) **ectodermal
dysplasia** Q82.4

Felinophobia F40.218

Felon —see also Cellulitis, digit
with lymphangitis —see
Lymphangitis, acute, digit

Felty's syndrome M05.00
ankle M05.07-
elbow M05.02-
foot joint M05.07-
hand joint M05.04-
hip M05.05-
knee M05.06-
multiple site M05.09
shoulder M05.01-
vertebra —see Spondylitis,
ankylosing
wrist M05.03-

Female genital cutting status —see
Female genital mutilation status
(FGM)

Female genital mutilation status
(FGM) N90.810
specified NEC N90.818
type I (clitorectomy status)
N90.811
type II (clitorectomy with excision
of labia minora status) N90.812
type III (infibulation status)
N90.813
type IV N90.818

Femur, femoral —see condition

Fenestration, fenestrated —see also
Imperfect, closure
aortico-pulmonary Q21.4
cusps, heart valve NEC Q24.8
pulmonary Q22.3
pulmonic cusps Q22.3

Fernell's disease (aortic aneurysm)
I71.9

Fertile eunuch syndrome E23.0

Fetid
breath R19.6
sweat L75.0

Fetishism F65.0
transvestic F65.1

Fetus, fetal —see also condition
alcohol syndrome (dysmorphic)
Q86.0
compressus O31.0-
hydantoin syndrome Q86.1
lung tissue P28.0
papyraceous O31.0-

Fever (inanition) (of unknown origin)
(persistent) (with chills) (with
rigor) R50.9
abortus A23.1
Aden (dengue) A90
African tick bite A77.8
African tick-borne A68.1
American
mountain (tick) A93.2
spotted A77.0
aphthous B08.8
arbovirus, arboviral A94
hemorrhagic A94
specified NEC A93.8
Argentinian hemorrhagic A96.0
Assam B55.0
Australian Q A78
Bangkok hemorrhagic A91
Barmah forest A92.8
Bartonella A44.0
bilious, hemoglobinuric B50.8
blackwater B50.8
blister B00.1
Bolivian hemorrhagic A96.1
Bonvale dam T73.3
boutonneuse A77.1
brain —see Encephalitis
Brazilian purpuric A48.4
breakbone A90
Bullis A77.0
Bunyamwera A92.8
Burdwan B55.0
Bwamba A92.8
Cameroon —see Malaria
Canton A75.9
catarrhal (acute) J00
chronic J31.0
cat-scratch A28.1
Central Asian hemorrhagic A98.0
cerebral —see Encephalitis
cerebrospinal meningococcal
A39.0
Chagres B50.9
Chandipura A92.8
Changuinola A93.1
Charcot's (biliary) (hepatic)
(intermittent) —see Calculus,
bile duct
Chikungunya (viral) (hemorrhagic)
A92.0
Chitral A93.1
Colombo —see Fever, paratyphoid
Colorado tick (virus) A93.2
congestive (remittent) —see
Malaria
Congo virus A98.0
continued malarial B50.9
Corsican —see Malaria
Crimean-Congo hemorrhagic A98.0
Cyprus —see Brucellosis
dandy A90
deer fly —see Tularemia
dengue (virus) A90
hemorrhagic A91
sandfly A93.1
desert B38.0
drug induced R50.2

Fever *(continued)*
  due to
    conditions classified elsewhere
      R50.81
    heat T67.01
  enteric A01.00
  enteroviral exanthematous (Boston
    exanthem) A88.0
  ephemeral (of unknown origin)
    R50.9
  epidemic hemorrhagic A98.5
  erysipelatous —*see* Erysipelas
  estivo-autumnal (malarial) B50.9
  famine A75.0
  five day A79.0
  following delivery O86.4
  Fort Bragg A27.89
  gastroenteric A01.00
  gastromalarial —*see* Malaria
  Gibraltar —*see* Brucellosis
  glandular —*see* Mononucleosis,
    infectious
  Guama (viral) A92.8
  Haverhill A25.1
  hay (allergic) J30.1
    with asthma (bronchial)
      J45.909
      with
        exacerbation (acute)
          J45.901
        status asthmaticus J45.902
    due to
      allergen other than pollen
        J30.89
      pollen, any plant or tree J30.1
  heat (effects) T67.01
  hematuric, bilious B50.8
  hemoglobinuric (malarial) (bilious)
    B50.8
  hemorrhagic (arthropod-borne)
    NOS A94
    with renal syndrome A98.5
    arenaviral A96.9
      specified NEC A96.8
    Argentinian A96.0
    Bangkok A91
    Bolivian A96.1
    Central Asian A98.0
    Chikungunya A92.0
    Crimean-Congo A98.0
    dengue (virus) A91
    epidemic A98.5
    Junin (virus) A96.0
    Korean A98.5
    Kyasanur forest A98.2
    Machupo (virus) A96.1
    mite-borne A93.8
    mosquito-borne A92.8
    Omsk A98.1
    Philippine A91
    Russian A98.5
    Singapore A91
    Southeast Asia A91
    Thailand A91
    tick-borne NEC A93.8
    viral A99
      specified NEC A98.8
  hepatic —*see* Cholecystitis
  herpetic —*see* Herpes
  icterohemorrhagic A27.0
  Indiana A93.8
  infective B99.9
    specified NEC B99.8
  intermittent (bilious) —*see also*
    Malaria
    of unknown origin R50.9
    pernicious B50.9
  iodide R50.2
  Japanese river A75.3
  jungle —*see also* Malaria
    yellow A95.0

Fever *(continued)*
  Junin (virus) hemorrhagic A96.0
  Katayama B65.2
  kedani A75.3
  Kenya (tick) A77.1
  Kew Garden A79.1
  Korean hemorrhagic A98.5
  Lassa A96.2
  Lone Star A77.0
  Machupo (virus) hemorrhagic
    A96.1
  malaria, malarial —*see* Malaria
  Malta A23.9
  Marseilles A77.1
  marsh —*see* Malaria
  Mayaro (viral) A92.8
  Mediterranean (*see also*
    Brucellosis) A23.9
    familial M04.1
    tick A77.1
  meningeal —*see* Meningitis
  Meuse A79.0
  Mexican A75.2
  mianeh A68.1
  miasmatic —*see* Malaria
  mosquito-borne (viral) A92.9
    hemorrhagic A92.8
  mountain (*see also* Brucellosis)
    meaning Rocky Mountain
      spotted fever A77.0
    tick (American) (Colorado)
      (viral) A93.2
  Mucambo (viral) A92.8
  mud A27.9
  Neapolitan —*see* Brucellosis
  neutropenic D70.9
  newborn P81.9
    environmental P81.0
  Nine-Mile A78
  non-exanthematous tick A93.2
  North Asian tick-borne A77.2
  Omsk hemorrhagic A98.1
  O'nyong-nyong (viral) A92.1
  Oropouche (viral) A93.0
  Oroya A44.0
  pacific coast tick A77.8
  paludal —*see* Malaria
  Panama (malarial) B50.9
  Pappataci A93.1
  paratyphoid A01.4
    A A01.1
    B A01.2
    C A01.3
  parrot A70
  periodic (Mediterranean) M04.1
  persistent (of unknown origin)
    R50.9
  petechial A39.0
  pharyngoconjunctival B30.2
  Philippine hemorrhagic A91
  phlebotomus A93.1
  Piry (virus) A93.8
  Pixuna (viral) A92.8
  Plasmodium ovale B53.0
  polioviral (nonparalytic) A80.4
  Pontiac A48.2
  postimmunization R50.83
  postoperative R50.82
    due to infection T81.40
  posttransfusion R50.84
  postvaccination R50.83
  presenting with conditions
    classified elsewhere R50.81
  pretibial A27.89
  puerperal O86.4
  Q A78
  quadrilateral A78
  quartan (malaria) B52.9
  Queensland (coastal) (tick) A77.3
  quintan A79.0
  rabbit —*see* Tularemia

Fever *(continued)*
  rat-bite A25.9
    due to
      Spirillum A25.0
      Streptobacillus moniliformis
        A25.1
  recurrent —*see* Fever, relapsing
  relapsing (Borrelia) A68.9
    Carter's (Asiatic) A68.1
    Dutton's (West African) A68.1
    Koch's A68.9
    louse-borne A68.0
    Novy's
      louse-borne A68.0
      tick-borne A68.1
    Obermeyer's (European) A68.0
    tick-borne A68.1
  remittent (bilious) (congestive)
    (gastric) —*see* Malaria
  rheumatic (active) (acute) (chronic)
    (subacute) I00
    with central nervous system
      involvement I02.9
    active with heart involvement
      —*see* category I01
    inactive or quiescent with
      cardiac hypertrophy I09.89
      carditis I09.9
      endocarditis I09.1
        aortic (valve) I06.9
          with mitral (valve)
            disease I08.0
        mitral (valve) I05.9
          with aortic (valve)
            disease I08.0
        pulmonary (valve) I09.89
        tricuspid (valve) I07.8
      heart disease NEC I09.89
      heart failure (congestive)
        (conditions in category I50.)
        I09.81
      left ventricular failure (conditions
        in I50.1-I50.4-) I09.81
      myocarditis, myocardial
        degeneration (conditions in
        I51.4) I09.0
      pancarditis I09.9
      pericarditis I09.2
  Rift Valley (viral) A92.4
  Rocky Mountain spotted A77.0
  rose J30.1
  Ross River B33.1
  Russian hemorrhagic A98.5
  San Joaquin (Valley) B38.0
  sandfly A93.1
  Sao Paulo A77.0
  scarlet A38.9
  seven day (leptospirosis) (autumnal)
    (Japanese) A27.89
    dengue A90
  shin-bone A79.0
  Singapore hemorrhagic A91
  solar A90
  Songo A98.5
  sore B00.1
  South African tick-bite A68.1
  Southeast Asia hemorrhagic A91
  spinal —*see* Meningitis
  spirillary A25.0
  splenic —*see* Anthrax
  spotted A77.9
    American A77.0
    Brazilian A77.0
    cerebrospinal meningitis A39.0
    Colombian A77.0
    due to Rickettsia
      africae (African tick bite
        fever) A77.8
      australis A77.3
      conorii A77.1
      parkeri A77.8

Fever *(continued)*
  spotted *(continued)*
    due to Rickettsia *(continued)*
      rickettsii A77.0
      sibirica A77.2
      specified type NEC A77.8
    Ehrlichiosis A77.40
      due to
        E. chafeensis A77.41
        specified organism NEC
          A77.49
    Rocky Mountain A77.0
  steroid R50.2
  streptobacillary A25.1
  subtertian B50.9
  Sumatran mite A75.3
  sun A90
  swamp A27.9
  swine A02.8
  sylvatic, yellow A95.0
  Tahyna B33.8
  tertian —*see* Malaria, tertian
  Thailand hemorrhagic A91
  thermic T67.01
  three-day A93.1
  tick
    American mountain A93.2
    Colorado A93.2
    Kemerovo A93.8
    Mediterranean A77.1
    mountain A93.2
    nonexanthematous A93.2
    Quaranfil A93.8
  tick-bite NEC A93.8
  tick-borne (hemorrhagic) NEC A93.8
  trench A79.0
  tsutsugamushi A75.3
  typhogastric A01.00
  typhoid (abortive) (hemorrhagic)
    (intermittent) (malignant)
    A01.00
    complicated by
      arthritis A01.04
      heart involvement A01.02
      meningitis A01.01
      osteomyelitis A01.05
      pneumonia A01.03
      specified NEC A01.09
  typhomalarial —*see* Malaria
  typhus —*see* Typhus (fever)
  undulant —*see* Brucellosis
  unknown origin R50.9
  uveoparotid D86.89
  valley B38.0
  Venezuelan equine A92.2
  vesicular stomatitis A93.8
  viral hemorrhagic —*see* Fever,
    hemorrhagic, by type of virus
  Volhynian A79.0
  Wesselsbron (viral) A92.8
  West
    African B50.8
    Nile (viral) A92.30
      with
        complications NEC A92.39
        cranial nerve disorders
          A92.32
        encephalitis A92.31
        encephalomyelitis A92.31
        neurologic manifestation
          NEC A92.32
        optic neuritis A92.32
        polyradiculitis A92.32
  Whitmore's —*see* Melioidosis
  Wolhynian A79.0
  worm B83.9
  yellow A95.9
    jungle A95.0
    sylvatic A95.0
    urban A95.1
  Zika virus A92.5

Fibrillation
atrial or auricular (established) I48.91
chronic I48.20
persistent I48.19
paroxysmal I48.0
permanent I48.21
persistent (chronic) (NOS)
(other) I48.19
longstanding I48.11
cardiac I49.8
heart I49.8
muscular M62.89
ventricular I49.01

Fibrin
ball or bodies, pleural (sac) J94.1
chamber, anterior (eye) (gelatinous
exudate) —see Iridocyclitis,
acute

Fibrinogenolysis —see Fibrinolysis

Fibrinogenopenia D68.8
acquired D65
congenital D68.2

Fibrinolysis (hemorrhagic) (acquired)
D65
antepartum hemorrhage —see
Hemorrhage, antepartum, with
coagulation defect
following
abortion —see Abortion by type
complicated by hemorrhage
ectopic or molar pregnancy
O08.1
intrapartum O67.0
newborn, transient P60
postpartum O72.3

Fibrinopenia (hereditary) D68.2
acquired D68.4

Fibrinopurulent —see condition

Fibrinous —see condition

Fibroadenoma
cellular intracanalicular D24-
giant D24-
intracanalicular
cellular D24-
giant D24-
specified site —see Neoplasm,
benign, by site
unspecified site D24-
juvenile D24-
pericanalicular
specified site —see Neoplasm,
benign, by site
unspecified site D24-
phyllodes D24-
prostate D29.1
specified site NEC —see
Neoplasm, benign, by site
unspecified site D24-

Fibroadenosis, breast (chronic)
(cystic) (diffuse) (periodic)
(segmental) N60.2-

Fibroangioma —see also Neoplasm,
benign, by site
juvenile
specified site —see Neoplasm,
benign, by site
unspecified site D10.6

Fibrochondrosarcoma —see
Neoplasm, cartilage, malignant

Fibrocystic
disease —see also Fibrosis, cystic
breast —see Mastopathy, cystic
jaw M27.49
kidney (congenital) Q61.8
liver Q44.6
pancreas E84.9
kidney (congenital) Q61.8

**Fibrodysplasia ossificans
progressiva** —see Myositis,
ossificans, progressiva

Fibroelastosis (cordis) (endocardial)
(endomyocardial) I42.4

Fibroid (tumor) —see also
Neoplasm, connective tissue,
benign
disease, lung (chronic) —see
Fibrosis, lung
heart (disease) —see Myocarditis
in pregnancy or childbirth O34.1-
causing obstructed labor O65.5
induration, lung (chronic) —see
Fibrosis, lung
lung —see Fibrosis, lung
pneumonia (chronic) —see
Fibrosis, lung
uterus (see also Leiomyoma,
uterus) D25.9

Fibrolipoma —see Lipoma

Fibroliposarcoma —see Neoplasm,
connective tissue, malignant

Fibroma —see also Neoplasm,
connective tissue, benign
ameloblastic —see Cyst, calcifying
odontogenic
bone (nonossifying) —see
Disorder, bone, specified type
NEC
ossifying —see Neoplasm, bone,
benign
cementifying —see Neoplasm,
bone, benign
chondromyxoid —see Neoplasm,
bone, benign
desmoplastic —see Neoplasm,
connective tissue, uncertain
behavior
durum —see Neoplasm, connective
tissue, benign
fascial —see Neoplasm, connective
tissue, benign
invasive —see Neoplasm,
connective tissue, uncertain
behavior
molle —see Lipoma
myxoid —see Neoplasm,
connective tissue, benign
nasopharynx, nasopharyngeal
(juvenile) D10.6
nonosteogenic (nonossifying)
—see Dysplasia, fibrous
odontogenic (central) —see Cyst,
calcifying odontogenic
ossifying —see Neoplasm, bone,
benign
periosteal —see Neoplasm, bone,
benign
soft —see Lipoma

Fibromatosis M72.9
abdominal —see Neoplasm,
connective tissue, uncertain
behavior
aggressive —see Neoplasm,
connective tissue, uncertain
behavior
congenital generalized —see
Neoplasm, connective tissue,
uncertain behavior
Dupuytren's M72.0
gingival K06.1
palmar (fascial) M72.0
plantar (fascial) M72.2
pseudosarcomatous (proliferative)
(subcutaneous) M72.4
retroperitoneal D48.3
specified NEC M72.8

Fibromyalgia M79.7

Fibromyoma —see also Neoplasm,
connective tissue, benign
uterus (corpus) —see also
Leiomyoma, uterus
in pregnancy or childbirth —see
Fibroid, in pregnancy or
childbirth
causing obstructed labor O65.5

Fibromyositis M79.7

Fibromyxolipoma D17.9

Fibromyxoma —see Neoplasm,
connective tissue, benign

Fibromyxosarcoma —see Neoplasm,
connective tissue, malignant

Fibro-odontoma, ameloblastic —see
Cyst, calcifying odontogenic

Fibro-osteoma —see Neoplasm,
bone, benign

Fibroplasia, retrolental H35.17-

Fibropurulent —see condition

Fibrosarcoma —see also Neoplasm,
connective tissue, malignant
ameloblastic C41.1
upper jaw (bone) C41.0
congenital —see Neoplasm,
connective tissue, malignant
fascial —see Neoplasm, connective
tissue, malignant
infantile —see Neoplasm,
connective tissue, malignant
odontogenic C41.1
upper jaw (bone) C41.0
periosteal —see Neoplasm, bone,
malignant

Fibrosclerosis
breast N60.3-
multifocal M35.5
penis (corpora cavernosa) N48.6

Fibrosis, fibrotic
adrenal (gland) E27.8
amnion O41.8X-
anal papillae K62.89
arteriocapillary —see
Arteriosclerosis
bladder N32.89
interstitial —see Cystitis,
chronic, interstitial
localized submucosal —see
Cystitis, chronic, interstitial
panmural —see Cystitis, chronic,
interstitial
breast —see Fibrosclerosis, breast
capillary (see also Arteriosclerosis)
I70.90
lung (chronic) —see Fibrosis,
lung
cardiac —see Myocarditis
cervix N88.8
chorion O41.8X-
corpus cavernosum (sclerosing)
N48.6
cystic (of pancreas) E84.9
with
distal intestinal obstruction
syndrome E84.19
fecal impaction E84.19
intestinal manifestations NEC
E84.19
pulmonary manifestations
E84.0
specified manifestations NEC
E84.8
due to device, implant or graft (see
also Complications, by site and
type, specified) NEC T85.828
arterial graft NEC T82.828
breast (implant) T85.828

Fibrosis, fibrotic (continued)
due to device, implant or graft
(continued)
catheter NEC T85.828
dialysis (renal) T82.828
intraperitoneal T85.828
infusion NEC T82.828
spinal (epidural) (subdural)
T85.820
urinary (indwelling) T83.82
electronic (electrode) (pulse
generator) (stimulator)
bone T84.82
cardiac T82.827
nervous system (brain)
(peripheral nerve) (spinal)
T85.820
urinary T83.82
fixation, internal (orthopedic)
NEC T84.82
gastrointestinal (bile duct)
(esophagus) T85.828
genital NEC T83.82
heart NEC T82.827
joint prosthesis T84.82
ocular (corneal graft) (orbital
implant) NEC T85.828
orthopedic NEC T84.82
specified NEC T85.828
urinary NEC T83.82
vascular NEC T82.828
ventricular intracranial shunt
T85.820
ejaculatory duct N50.89
endocardium —see Endocarditis
endomyocardial (tropical) I42.3
epididymis N50.89
eye muscle —see Strabismus,
mechanical
heart —see Myocarditis
hepatic —see Fibrosis, liver
hepatolienal (portal hypertension)
K76.6
hepatosplenic (portal hypertension)
K76.6
infrapatellar fat pad M79.4
intrascrotal N50.89
kidney N26.9
liver K74.00
with sclerosis K74.2
advanced K74.02
alcoholic K70.2
early K74.01
stage
F1 or F2 K74.01
F3 K74.02
lung (atrophic) (chronic) (confluent)
(massive) (perialveolar)
(peribronchial) J84.10
with
anthracosilicosis J60
anthracosis J60
asbestosis J61
bagassosis J67.1
bauxite J63.1
berylliosis J63.2
byssinosis J66.0
calcicosis J62.8
chalicosis J62.8
dust reticulation J64
farmer's lung J67.0
ganister disease J62.8
graphite J63.3
pneumoconiosis NOS J64
siderosis J63.4
silicosis J62.8
capillary J84.10
congenital P27.8
diffuse (idiopathic) J84.10
chemicals, gases, fumes or
vapors (inhalation) J68.4

Fissure, fissured (*continued*)
lip K13.0
   congenital —*see* Cleft, lip
nipple N64.0
   associated with
      lactation O92.13
      pregnancy O92.11-
      puerperium O92.12
nose Q30.2
palate (congenital) —*see* Cleft,
   palate
skin R23.4
spine (congenital) —*see also* Spina
   bifida
   with hydrocephalus —*see*
      Spina bifida, by site, with
      hydrocephalus
tongue (acquired) K14.5
   congenital Q38.3

Fistula (cutaneous) L98.8
abdomen (wall) K63.2
   bladder N32.2
   intestine NEC K63.2
   ureter N28.89
   uterus N82.5
abdominorectal K63.2
abdominosigmoidal K63.2
abdominothoracic J86.0
abdominouterine N82.5
   congenital Q51.7
abdominovesical N32.2
accessory sinuses —*see* Sinusitis
actinomycotic —*see* Actinomycosis
alveolar antrum —*see* Sinusitis,
   maxillary
alveolar process K04.6
anorectal K60.5
antrobuccal —*see* Sinusitis,
   maxillary
antrum —*see* Sinusitis, maxillary
anus, anal (recurrent) (infectional)
   K60.3
   congenital Q43.6
      with absence, atresia and
         stenosis Q42.2
   tuberculous A18.32
aorta-duodenal I77.2
appendix, appendicular K38.3
arteriovenous (acquired)
   (nonruptured) I77.0
   brain I67.1
      congenital Q28.2
         ruptured —*see* Fistula,
            arteriovenous, brain,
            ruptured
      ruptured I60.8
         intracerebral I61.8
         intraparenchymal I61.8
         Intraventricular I61.5
         subarachnoid I60.8
   cerebral —*see* Fistula,
      arteriovenous, brain
   congenital (peripheral) —*see
      also* Malformation,
      arteriovenous
      brain Q28.2
         ruptured —*see* Fistula,
            arteriovenous, brain,
            ruptured
      coronary Q24.5
      pulmonary Q25.72
   coronary I25.41
      congenital Q24.5
   pulmonary I28.0
      congenital Q25.72
   surgically created (for dialysis)
      Z99.2
      complication —*see*
         Complication,
         arteriovenous, fistula,
         surgically created

Fistula (*continued*)
arteriovenous (*continued*)
   traumatic —*see* Injury, blood
      vessel
artery I77.2
aural (mastoid) —*see* Mastoiditis,
   chronic
auricle —*see also* Disorder, pinna,
   specified type NEC
   congenital Q18.1
Bartholin's gland N82.8
bile duct (common) (hepatic) K83.3
   with calculus, stones (*see also*
      Calculus, bile duct) K83.3
biliary (tract) —*see* Fistula, bile
   duct
bladder (sphincter) NEC (*see also*
   Fistula, vesico-) N32.2
   into seminal vesicle N32.2
bone —*see also* Disorder, bone,
   specified type NEC
   with osteomyelitis, chronic —
      see Osteomyelitis, chronic,
      with draining sinus
brain G93.89
   arteriovenous (acquired) (*see
      also* Fistula, arteriovenous,
      brain) I67.1
   congenital Q28.2
branchial (cleft) Q18.0
branchiogenous Q18.0
breast N61.0
   puerperal, postpartum or
      gestational, due to mastitis
      (purulent) —*see* Mastitis,
      obstetric, purulent
bronchial J86.0
bronchocutaneous,
   bronchomediastinal,
   bronchopleural,
   bronchopleuromediastinal
   (infective) J86.0
   tuberculous NEC A15.5
bronchoesophageal J86.0
   congenital Q39.2
      with atresia of esophagus
         Q39.1
bronchovisceral J86.0
buccal cavity (infective) K12.2
cecosigmoidal K63.2
cecum K63.2
cerebrospinal (fluid) G96.08
cervical, lateral Q18.1
cervicoaural Q18.1
cervicosigmoidal N82.4
cervicovesical N82.1
cervix N82.8
chest (wall) J86.0
cholecystenteric —*see* Fistula,
   gallbladder
cholecystocolic —*see* Fistula,
   gallbladder
cholecystocolonic —*see* Fistula,
   gallbladder
cholecystoduodenal —*see* Fistula,
   gallbladder
cholecystogastric —*see* Fistula,
   gallbladder
cholecystointestinal —*see* Fistula,
   gallbladder
choledochoduodenal —*see* Fistula,
   bile duct
cholocolic K82.3
coccyx —*see* Sinus, pilonidal
colon K63.2
colostomy K94.09
colovesical N32.1
common duct —*see* Fistula, bile
   duct
congenital, site not listed —*see*
   Anomaly, by site

Fistula (*continued*)
coronary, arteriovenous I25.41
   congenital Q24.5
costal region J86.0
cul-de-sac, Douglas' N82.8
cystic duct —*see also* Fistula,
   gallbladder
   congenital Q44.5
dental K04.6
diaphragm J86.0
duodenum K31.6
ear (external) (canal) —*see*
   Disorder, ear, external, specified
   type NEC
enterocolic K63.2
enterocutaneous K63.2
enterouterine N82.4
   congenital Q51.7
enterovaginal N82.4
   congenital Q52.2
   large intestine N82.3
   small intestine N82.2
enterovesical N32.1
epididymis N50.89
   tuberculous A18.15
esophagobronchial J86.0
   congenital Q39.2
      with atresia of esophagus
         Q39.1
esophagocutaneous K22.8
esophagopleural-cutaneous J86.0
esophagotracheal J86.0
   congenital Q39.2
      with atresia of esophagus
         Q39.1
esophagus K22.8
   congenital Q39.2
      with atresia of esophagus
         Q39.1
ethmoid —*see* Sinusitis, ethmoidal
eyeball (cornea) (sclera) —*see*
   Disorder, globe, hypotony
eyelid H01.8
fallopian tube, external N82.5
fecal K63.2
   congenital Q43.6
   from periapical abscess K04.6
frontal sinus —*see* Sinusitis,
   frontal
gallbladder K82.3
   with calculus, cholelithiasis,
      stones —*see* Calculus,
      gallbladder
gastric K31.6
gastrocolic K31.6
   congenital Q40.2
   tuberculous A18.32
gastroenterocolic K31.6
gastroesophageal K31.6
gastrojejunal K31.6
gastrojejunocolic K31.6
genital tract (female) N82.9
   specified NEC N82.8
   to intestine NEC N82.4
   to skin N82.5
hepatic artery-portal vein,
   congenital Q26.6
hepatopleural J86.0
hepatopulmonary J86.0
ileorectal or ileosigmoidal K63.2
ileovaginal N82.2
ileovesical N32.1
ileum K63.2
in ano K60.3
   tuberculous A18.32
inner ear (labyrinth) H83.1
intestine NEC K63.2
intestinocolonic (abdominal)
   K63.2
intestinoureteral N28.89
intestinouterine N82.4

Fistula (*continued*)
intestinovaginal N82.4
   large intestine N82.3
   small intestine N82.2
intestinovesical N32.1
ischiorectal (fossa) K61.39
jejunum K63.2
joint M25.10
   ankle M25.17-
   elbow M25.12-
   foot joint M25.17-
   hand joint M25.14-
   hip M25.15-
   knee M25.16-
   shoulder M25.11-
   specified joint NEC M25.18
   tuberculous —*see* Tuberculosis,
      joint
   vertebrae M25.18
   wrist M25.13-
kidney N28.89
labium (majus) (minus) N82.8
labyrinth H83.1
lacrimal (gland) (sac) H04.61-
lacrimonasal duct —*see* Fistula,
   lacrimal
laryngotracheal, congenital Q34.8
larynx J38.7
lip K13.0
   congenital Q38.0
lumbar, tuberculous A18.01
lung J86.0
lymphatic I89.8
mammary (gland) N61.0
mastoid (process) (region) —*see*
   Mastoiditis, chronic
maxillary J32.0
medial, face and neck Q18.8
mediastinal J86.0
mediastinobronchial J86.0
mediastinocutaneous J86.0
middle ear H74.8
mouth K12.2
nasal J34.89
   sinus —*see* Sinusitis
nasopharynx J39.2
nipple N64.0
nose J34.89
oral (cutaneous) K12.2
   maxillary J32.0
   nasal (with cleft palate) —*see*
      Cleft, palate
orbit, orbital —*see* Disorder, orbit,
   specified type NEC
oroantral J32.0
oviduct, external N82.5
palate (hard) M27.8
pancreatic K86.89
pancreaticoduodenal K86.89
parotid (gland) K11.4
   region K12.2
penis N48.89
perianal K60.3
pericardium (pleura) (sac) —*see*
   Pericarditis
pericecal K63.2
perineorectal K60.4
perineosigmoidal K63.2
perineum, perineal (with urethral
   involvement) NEC N36.0
   tuberculous A18.13
   ureter N28.89
perirectal K60.4
   tuberculous A18.32
peritoneum K65.9
pharyngoesophageal J39.2
pharynx J39.2
   branchial cleft (congenital)
      Q18.0
pilonidal (infected) (rectum) —*see*
   Sinus, pilonidal

Fistula *(continued)*
pleura, pleural, pleurocutaneous,
    pleuroperitoneal J86.0
        tuberculous NEC A15.6
pleuropericardial I31.8
portal vein-hepatic artery,
    congenital Q26.6
postauricular H70.81-
postoperative, persistent T81.83
    specified site —*see* Fistula, by
        site
preauricular (congenital) Q18.1
prostate N42.89
pulmonary J86.0
    arteriovenous I28.0
        congenital Q25.72
    tuberculous —*see* Tuberculosis,
        pulmonary
pulmonoperitoneal J86.0
rectolabial N82.4
rectosigmoid (intercommunicating)
    K63.2
rectoureteral N28.89
rectourethral N36.0
    congenital Q64.73
rectouterine N82.4
    congenital Q51.7
rectovaginal N82.3
    congenital Q52.2
    tuberculous A18.18
rectovesical N32.1
    congenital Q64.79
rectovesicovaginal N82.3
rectovulval N82.4
    congenital Q52.79
rectum (to skin) K60.4
    congenital Q43.6
        with absence, atresia and
            stenosis Q42.0
    tuberculous A18.32
renal N28.89
retroauricular —*see* Fistula,
    postauricular
salivary duct or gland (any) K11.4
    congenital Q38.4
scrotum (urinary) N50.89
    tuberculous A18.15
semicircular canals H83.1
sigmoid K63.2
    to bladder N32.1
sinus —*see* Sinusitis
skin L98.8
    to genital tract (female) N82.5
splenocolic D73.89
stercoral K63.2
stomach K31.6
sublingual gland K11.4
submandibular gland K11.4
submaxillary (gland) K11.4
    region K12.2
thoracic J86.0
    duct I89.8
thoracoabdominal J86.0
thoracogastric J86.0
thoracointestinal J86.0
thorax J86.0
thyroglossal duct Q89.2
thyroid E07.89
trachea, congenital (external)
    (internal) Q32.1
tracheoesophageal J86.0
    congenital Q39.2
        with atresia of esophagus
            Q39.1
    following tracheostomy J95.04
traumatic arteriovenous —*see*
    Injury, blood vessel, by site
tuberculous - code by site under
    Tuberculosis
typhoid A01.09
umbilicourinary Q64.8

Fistula *(continued)*
urachus, congenital Q64.4
ureter (persistent) N28.89
ureteroabdominal N28.89
ureterorectal N28.89
ureterosigmoido-abdominal
    N28.89
ureterovaginal N82.1
ureterovesical N32.2
urethra N36.0
    congenital Q64.79
    tuberculous A18.13
urethroperineal N36.0
urethroperineovesical N32.2
urethrorectal N36.0
    congenital Q64.73
urethroscrotal N50.89
urethrovaginal N82.1
urethrovesical N32.2
urinary (tract) (persistent)
    (recurrent) N36.0
uteroabdominal N82.5
    congenital Q51.7
uteroenteric, uterointestinal N82.4
    congenital Q51.7
uterorectal N82.4
    congenital Q51.7
uteroureteric N82.1
uterourethral Q51.7
uterovaginal N82.8
uterovesical N82.1
    congenital Q51.7
uterus N82.8
vagina (postpartal) (wall) N82.8
vaginocutaneous (postpartal) N82.5
vaginointestinal NEC N82.4
    large intestine N82.3
    small intestine N82.2
vaginoperineal N82.5
vasocutaneous, congenital Q55.7
vesical NEC N32.2
vesicoabdominal N32.2
vesicocervicovaginal N82.1
vesicocolic N32.1
vesicocutaneous N32.2
vesicoenteric N32.1
vesicointestinal N32.1
vesicometrorectal N82.4
vesicoperineal N32.2
vesicorectal N32.1
    congenital Q64.79
vesicosigmoidal N32.1
vesicosigmoidovaginal N82.3
vesicoureteral N32.2
vesicoureterovaginal N82.1
vesicourethral N32.2
vesicourethrorectal N32.1
vesicouterine N82.1
    congenital Q51.7
vesicovaginal N82.0
vulvorectal N82.4
    congenital Q52.79

Fit R56.9
epileptic —*see* Epilepsy
fainting R55
hysterical F44.5
newborn P90

Fitting (and adjustment) (of)
artificial
    arm —*see* Admission,
        adjustment, artificial, arm
    breast Z44.3
    eye Z44.2
    leg —*see* Admission, adjustment,
        artificial, leg
automatic implantable cardiac
    defibrillator (with synchronous
    cardiac pacemaker) Z45.02
brain neuropacemaker Z46.2
    implanted Z45.42

Fitting *(continued)*
cardiac defibrillator —*see* Fitting
    (and adjustment) (of), automatic
    implantable cardiac defibrillator
catheter, non-vascular Z46.82
colostomy belt Z46.89
contact lenses Z46.0
CRT-D (resynchronization therapy
    defibrillator) Z45.02
CRT-P (cardiac resynchronization
    therapy pacemaker) Z45.018
    pulse generator Z45.010
cystostomy device Z46.6
defibrillator, cardiac —*see* Fitting
    (and adjustment) (of), automatic
    implantable cardiac defibrillator
dentures Z46.3
device NOS Z46.9
    abdominal Z46.89
    gastrointestinal NEC Z46.59
    implanted NEC Z45.89
    nervous system Z46.2
        implanted —*see* Admission,
            adjustment, device,
            implanted, nervous system
    orthodontic Z46.4
    orthoptic Z46.0
    orthotic Z46.89
    prosthetic (external) Z44.9
        breast Z44.3
        dental Z46.3
        eye Z44.2
        specified NEC Z44.8
    specified NEC Z46.89
    substitution
        auditory Z46.2
            implanted —*see* Admission,
                adjustment, device,
                implanted, hearing device
        nervous system Z46.2
            implanted —*see* Admission,
                adjustment, device,
                implanted, nervous
                system
        visual Z46.2
            implanted Z45.31
    urinary Z46.6
gastric lap band Z46.51
gastrointestinal appliance NEC
    Z46.59
glasses (reading) Z46.0
hearing aid Z46.1
ileostomy device Z46.89
insulin pump Z46.81
intestinal appliance NEC Z46.89
myringotomy device (stent) (tube)
    Z45.82
neuropacemaker Z46.2
    implanted Z45.42
non-vascular catheter Z46.82
orthodontic device Z46.4
orthopedic device (brace) (cast)
    (corset) (shoes) Z46.89
pacemaker (cardiac) (cardiac
    resynchronization therapy
    (CRT-P)) Z45.018
    nervous system (brain)
        (peripheral nerve) (spinal
        cord) Z46.2
        implanted Z45.42
    pulse generator Z45.010
portacath (port-a-cath) Z45.2
prosthesis (external) Z44.9
    arm —*see* Admission,
        adjustment, artificial, arm
    breast Z44.3
    dental Z46.3
    eye Z44.2
    leg —*see* Admission, adjustment,
        artificial, leg
    specified NEC Z44.8

Fitting *(continued)*
spectacles Z46.0
wheelchair Z46.89

Fitzhugh-Curtis syndrome
due to
    Chlamydia trachomatis
        A74.81
    Neisseria gonorrhorea
        (gonococcal peritonitis)
        A54.85

Fitz's syndrome (acute hemorrhagic
    pancreatitis) *(see also* Pancreatitis,
    acute) K85.80

Fixation
joint —*see* Ankylosis
larynx J38.7
stapes —*see* Ankylosis, ear
    ossicles
    deafness —*see* Deafness,
        conductive
uterus (acquired) —*see*
    Malposition, uterus
vocal cord J38.3

Flabby ridge K06.8

Flaccid —*see also* condition
palate, congenital Q38.5

Flail
chest S22.5
    newborn (birth injury) P13.8
joint (paralytic) M25.20
    ankle M25.27-
    elbow M25.22-
    foot joint M25.27-
    hand joint M25.24-
    hip M25.25-
    knee M25.26-
    shoulder M25.21-
    specified joint NEC M25.28
    wrist M25.23-

Flajani's disease —*see*
    Hyperthyroidism, with, goiter
    (diffuse)

Flap, liver K71.3

Flashbacks (residual to hallucinogen
    use) F16.283

Flat
chamber (eye) —*see* Disorder,
    globe, hypotony, flat anterior
    chamber
chest, congenital Q67.8
foot (acquired) (fixed type)
    (painful) (postural) —*see also*
    Deformity, limb, flat foot
    congenital (rigid) (spastic
        (everted)) Q66.5-
    rachitic sequelae (late effect)
        E64.3
organ or site, congenital NEC
    —*see* Anomaly, by site
pelvis M95.5
    with disproportion (fetopelvic)
        O33.0
        causing obstructed labor
            O65.0
    congenital Q74.2

Flatau-Schilder disease G37.0

Flatback syndrome M40.30
lumbar region M40.36
lumbosacral region M40.37
thoracolumbar region M40.35

Flattening
head, femur M89.8X5
hip —*see* Coxa, plana
lip (congenital) Q18.8
nose (congenital) Q67.4
    acquired M95.0

Flatulence R14.3
  psychogenic F45.8

Flatus R14.3
  vaginalis N89.8

Flax-dresser's disease J66.1

Flea bite —see Injury, bite, by site, superficial, insect

Flecks, glaucomatous (subcapsular) —see Cataract, complicated

Fleischer (-Kayser) **ring** (cornea) H18.04-

Fleshy mole O02.0

Flexibilitas cerea —see Catalepsy

Flexion
  amputation stump (surgical) T87.89
  cervix —see Malposition, uterus
  contracture, joint —see Contraction, joint
  deformity, joint (see also Deformity, limb, flexion) M21.20
    hip, congenital Q65.89
  uterus —see also Malposition, uterus
    lateral —see Lateroversion, uterus

Flexner-Boyd dysentery A03.2

Flexner's dysentery A03.1

Flexure —see Flexion

Flint murmur (aortic insufficiency) I35.1

Floater, vitreous —see Opacity, vitreous

Floating
  cartilage (joint) —see also Loose, body, joint
    knee —see Derangement, knee, loose body
  gallbladder, congenital Q44.1
  kidney N28.89
    congenital Q63.8
  spleen D73.89

Flooding N92.0

Floor —see condition

Floppy
  baby syndrome (nonspecific) P94.2
  iris syndrome (intraoperative) (IFIS) H21.81
  nonrheumatic mitral valve syndrome I34.1

Flu —see also Influenza
  avian (see also Influenza, due to, identified novel influenza A virus) J09.X2
  bird (see also Influenza, due to, identified novel influenza A virus) J09.X2
  intestinal NEC A08.4
  swine (viruses that normally cause infections in pigs) (see also Influenza, due to, identified novel influenza A virus) J09.X2

Fluctuating blood pressure I99.8

Fluid
  abdomen R18.8
  chest J94.8
  heart —see Failure, heart, congestive
  joint —see Effusion, joint
  loss (acute) E86.9
  lung —see Edema, lung
  overload E87.70
    specified NEC E87.79

Fluid (continued)
  peritoneal cavity R18.8
  pleural cavity J94.8
  retention R60.9

Flukes NEC —see also Infestation, fluke
  blood NEC —see Schistosomiasis
  liver B66.3

Fluor (vaginalis) N89.8
  trichomonal or due to Trichomonas (vaginalis) A59.00

Fluorosis
  dental K00.3
  skeletal M85.10
    ankle M85.17-
    foot M85.17-
    forearm M85.13-
    hand M85.14-
    lower leg M85.16-
    multiple site M85.19
    neck M85.18
    rib M85.18
    shoulder M85.11-
    skull M85.18
    specified site NEC M85.18
    thigh M85.15-
    toe M85.17-
    upper arm M85.12-
    vertebra M85.18

Flush syndrome E34.0

Flushing R23.2
  menopausal N95.1

Flutter
  atrial or auricular I48.92
    atypical I48.4
    type I I48.3
    type II I48.4
    typical I48.3
  heart I49.8
    atrial or auricular I48.92
      atypical I48.4
      type I I48.3
      type II I48.4
      typical I48.3
    ventricular I49.02
  ventricular I49.02

FNHTR (febrile nonhemolytic transfusion reaction) R50.84

Fochier's abscess - code by site under Abscess

Focus, Assmann's —see Tuberculosis, pulmonary

Fogo selvagem L10.3

Foix-Alajouanine syndrome G95.19

Fold, folds (anomalous) —see also Anomaly, by site
  Descemet's membrane —see Change, corneal membrane, Descemet's, fold
  epicanthic Q10.3
  heart Q24.8

Folie à deux F24

Follicle
  cervix (nabothian) (ruptured) N88.8
  graafian, ruptured, with hemorrhage N83.0-
  nabothian N88.8

Follicular —see condition

Folliculitis (superficial) L73.9
  abscedens et suffodiens L66.3
  cyst N83.0-
  decalvans L66.2
  deep —see Furuncle, by site

Folliculitis (continued)
  gonococcal (acute) (chronic) A54.01
  keloid, keloidalis L73.0
  pustular L01.02
  ulerythematosa reticulata L66.4

Folliculome lipidique
  specified site —see Neoplasm, benign, by site
  unspecified site
    female D27.9
    male D29.20

Følling's disease E70.0

Follow-up —see Examination, follow-up

Fong's syndrome (hereditary osteo-onychodysplasia) Q87.2

Food
  allergy L27.2
  asphyxia (from aspiration or inhalation) —see Foreign body, by site
  choked on —see Foreign body, by site
  deprivation T73.0
    specified kind of food NEC E63.8
  intoxication —see Poisoning, food
  lack of T73.0
  poisoning —see Poisoning, food
  rejection NEC —see Disorder, eating
  strangulation or suffocation —see Foreign body, by site
  toxemia —see Poisoning, food

Foot —see condition

Foramen ovale (nonclosure) (patent) (persistent) Q21.1

Forbes' glycogen storage disease E74.03

Fordyce-Fox disease L75.2

Fordyce's disease (mouth) Q38.6

Forearm —see condition

Foreign body
  with
    laceration —see Laceration, by site, with foreign body
    puncture wound —see Puncture, by site, with foreign body
  accidentally left following a procedure T81.509
    aspiration T81.506
      resulting in
        adhesions T81.516
        obstruction T81.526
        perforation T81.536
        specified complication NEC T81.596
    cardiac catheterization T81.505
      resulting in
        acute reaction T81.60
          aseptic peritonitis T81.61
          specified NEC T81.69
    accidentally left following a
    adhesions T81.515
      obstruction T81.525
      perforation T81.535
      specified complication NEC T81.595
    causing
      acute reaction T81.60
        aseptic peritonitis T81.61
        specified complication NEC T81.69
      adhesions T81.519
        aseptic peritonitis T81.61

Foreign body (continued)
  accidentally left following a
  adhesions (continued)
    causing (continued)
      obstruction T81.529
      perforation T81.539
      specified complication NEC T81.599
    endoscopy T81.504
      resulting in
        adhesions T81.514
        obstruction T81.524
        perforation T81.534
        specified complication NEC T81.594
    immunization T81.503
      resulting in
        adhesions T81.513
        obstruction T81.523
        perforation T81.533
        specified complication NEC T81.593
    infusion T81.501
      resulting in
        adhesions T81.511
        obstruction T81.521
        perforation T81.531
        specified complication NEC T81.591
    injection T81.503
      resulting in
        adhesions T81.513
        obstruction T81.523
        perforation T81.533
        specified complication NEC T81.593
    kidney dialysis T81.502
      resulting in
        adhesions T81.512
        obstruction T81.522
        perforation T81.532
        specified complication NEC T81.592
    packing removal T81.507
      resulting in
        acute reaction T81.60
          aseptic peritonitis T81.61
          specified NEC T81.69
        adhesions T81.517
        obstruction T81.527
        perforation T81.537
        specified complication NEC T81.597
    puncture T81.506
      resulting in
        adhesions T81.516
        obstruction T81.526
        perforation T81.536
        specified complication NEC T81.596
    specified procedure NEC T81.508
      resulting in
        acute reaction T81.60
          aseptic peritonitis T81.61
          specified NEC T81.69
        adhesions T81.518
        obstruction T81.528
        perforation T81.538
        specified complication NEC T81.598
    surgical operation T81.500
      resulting in
        acute reaction T81.60
          aseptic peritonitis T81.61
          specified NEC T81.69
        adhesions T81.510
        obstruction T81.520
        perforation T81.530
        specified complication NEC T81.590

accidentally left following a
  adhesions *(continued)*
    transfusion T81.501
      resulting in
        adhesions T81.511
        obstruction T81.521
        perforation T81.531
        specified complication NEC
          T81.591
alimentary tract T18.9
  anus T18.5
  colon T18.4
  esophagus —*see* Foreign body,
    esophagus
  mouth T18.0
  multiple sites T18.8
  rectosigmoid (junction) T18.5
  rectum T18.5
  small intestine T18.3
  specified site NEC T18.8
  stomach T18.2
anterior chamber (eye) S05.5-
auditory canal —*see* Foreign body,
  entering through orifice, ear
bronchus T17.508
  causing
    asphyxiation T17.500
      food (bone) (seed) T17.520
      gastric contents (vomitus)
        T17.510
      specified type NEC T17.590
    injury NEC T17.508
      food (bone) (*seed*) T17.528
      gastric contents (vomitus)
        T17.518
      specified type NEC
        T17.598
canthus —*see* Foreign body,
  conjunctival sac
ciliary body (eye) S05.5-
conjunctival sac T15.1-
cornea T15.0-
entering through orifice
  accessory sinus T17.0
  alimentary canal T18.9
    multiple parts T18.8
    specified part NEC T18.8
  alveolar process T18.0
  antrum (Highmore's) T17.0
  anus T18.5
  appendix T18.4
  auditory canal —*see* Foreign
    body, entering through orifice,
    ear
  auricle —*see* Foreign body,
    entering through orifice, ear
  bladder T19.1
  bronchioles —*see* Foreign body,
    respiratory tract, specified site
    NEC
  bronchus (main) —*see* Foreign
    body, bronchus
  buccal cavity T18.0
  canthus (inner) —*see* Foreign
    body, conjunctival sac
  cecum T18.4
  cervix (canal) (uteri) T19.3
  colon T18.4
  conjunctival sac —*see* Foreign
    body, conjunctival sac
  cornea —*see* Foreign body,
    cornea
  digestive organ or tract NOS
    T18.9
    multiple parts T18.8
    specified part NEC T18.8
  duodenum T18.3
  ear (external) T16.-
  esophagus —*see* Foreign body,
    esophagus

entering through orifice *(continued)*
  eye (external) NOS T15.9-
    conjunctival sac —*see* Foreign
      body, conjunctival sac
    cornea —*see* Foreign body,
      cornea
    specified part NEC T15.8-
  eyeball —*see also* Foreign body,
    entering through orifice, eye,
    specified part NEC
    with penetrating wound —*see*
      Puncture, eyeball
  eyelid —*see also* Foreign body,
    conjunctival sac
    with
      laceration —*see* Laceration,
        eyelid, with foreign body
      puncture —*see* Puncture,
        eyelid, with foreign body
      superficial injury —*see*
        Foreign body, superficial,
        eyelid
  gastrointestinal tract T18.9
    multiple parts T18.8
    specified part NEC T18.8
  genitourinary tract T19.9
    multiple parts T19.8
    specified part NEC T19.8
  globe —*see* Foreign body,
    entering through orifice,
    eyeball
  gum T18.0
  Highmore's antrum T17.0
  hypopharynx —*see* Foreign
    body, pharynx
  ileum T18.3
  intestine (small) T18.3
    large T18.4
  lacrimal apparatus (punctum)
    —*see* Foreign body, entering
    through orifice, eye, specified
    part NEC
  large intestine T18.4
  larynx —*see* Foreign body,
    larynx
  lung —*see* Foreign body,
    respiratory tract, specified site
    NEC
  maxillary sinus T17.0
  mouth T18.0
  nasal sinus T17.0
  nasopharynx —*see* Foreign
    body, pharynx
  nose (passage) T17.1
  nostril T17.1
  oral cavity T18.0
  palate T18.0
  penis T19.4
  pharynx —*see* Foreign body,
    pharynx
  piriform sinus —*see* Foreign
    body, pharynx
  rectosigmoid (junction) T18.5
  rectum T18.5
  respiratory tract —*see* Foreign
    body, respiratory tract
  sinus (accessory) (frontal)
    (maxillary) (nasal) T17.0
    piriform —*see* Foreign body,
      pharynx
  small intestine T18.3
  stomach T18.2
  suffocation by —*see* Foreign
    body, by site
  tear ducts or glands —*see*
    Foreign body, entering
    through orifice, eye, specified
    part NEC
  throat —*see* Foreign body,
    pharynx

entering through orifice *(continued)*
  tongue T18.0
  tonsil, tonsillar (fossa) —*see*
    Foreign body, pharynx
  trachea —*see* Foreign body,
    trachea
  ureter T19.8
  urethra T19.0
  uterus (any part) T19.3
  vagina T19.2
  vulva T19.2
esophagus T18.108
  causing
    injury NEC T18.108
      food (bone) (seed) T18.128
      gastric contents (vomitus)
        T18.118
      specified type NEC T18.198
    tracheal compression T18.100
      food (bone) (seed) T18.120
      gastric contents (vomitus)
        T18.110
      specified type NEC T18.190
feeling of, in throat R09.89
fragment —*see* Retained, foreign
  body fragments (type of)
genitourinary tract T19.9
  bladder T19.1
  multiple parts T19.8
  penis T19.4
  specified site NEC T19.8
  urethra T19.0
  uterus T19.3
    IUD Z97.5
  vagina T19.2
    contraceptive device Z97.5
  vulva T19.2
granuloma (old) (soft tissue) —*see*
  also Granuloma, foreign body
  skin L92.3
in
  laceration —*see* Laceration, by
    site, with foreign body
  puncture wound —*see* Puncture,
    by site, with foreign body
  soft tissue (residual) M79.5
inadvertently left in operation
  wound —*see* Foreign body,
    accidentally left during a
    procedure
ingestion, ingested NOS T18.9
inhalation or inspiration —*see*
  Foreign body, by site
internal organ, not entering through
  a natural orifice - code as specific
  injury with foreign body
intraocular S05.5-
  old, retained (nonmagnetic)
    H44.70-
    anterior chamber H44.71-
    ciliary body H44.72-
    iris H44.72-
    lens H44.73-
    magnetic H44.60-
      anterior chamber H44.61-
      ciliary body H44.62-
      iris H44.62-
      lens H44.63-
      posterior wall H44.64-
      specified site NEC
        H44.69-
      vitreous body H44.65-
    posterior wall H44.74-
    specified site NEC H44.79-
    vitreous body H44.75-
iris —*see* Foreign body,
  intraocular
lacrimal punctum —*see* Foreign
  body, entering through orifice,
  eye, specified part NEC

larynx T17.308
  causing
    asphyxiation T17.300
      food (bone) (seed) T17.320
      gastric contents (vomitus)
        T17.310
      specified type NEC T17.390
    injury NEC T17.308
      food (bone) (seed) T17.328
      gastric contents (vomitus)
        T17.318
      specified type NEC T17.398
lens —*see* Foreign body,
  intraocular
ocular muscle S05.4-
  old, retained —*see* Foreign body,
    orbit, old
old or residual
  soft tissue (residual) M79.5
operation wound, left accidentally
  —*see* Foreign body, accidentally
  left during a procedure
orbit S05.4-
  old, retained H05.5-
pharynx T17.208
  causing
    asphyxiation T17.200
      food (bone) (seed) T17.220
      gastric contents (vomitus)
        T17.210
      specified type NEC T17.290
    injury NEC T17.208
      food (bone) (seed) T17.228
      gastric contents (vomitus)
        T17.218
      specified type NEC T17.298
respiratory tract T17.908
  bronchioles —*see* Foreign body,
    respiratory tract, specified site
    NEC
  bronchus —*see* Foreign body,
    bronchus
  causing
    asphyxiation T17.900
      food (bone) (seed) T17.920
      gastric contents (vomitus)
        T17.910
      specified type NEC T17.990
    injury NEC T17.908
      food (bone) (seed) T17.928
      gastric contents (vomitus)
        T17.918
      specified type NEC T17.998
  larynx —*see* Foreign body,
    larynx
  lung —*see* Foreign body,
    respiratory tract, specified site
    NEC
  multiple parts —*see* Foreign
    body, respiratory tract,
    specified site NEC
  nasal sinus T17.0
  nasopharynx —*see* Foreign
    body, pharynx
  nose T17.1
  nostril T17.1
  pharynx —*see* Foreign body,
    pharynx
  specified site NEC T17.808
    causing
      asphyxiation T17.800
        food (bone) (seed)
          T17.820
        gastric contents (vomitus)
          T17.810
        specified type NEC
          T17.890
      injury NEC T17.808
        food (bone) (seed)
          T17.828

Foreign body (continued)
respiratory tract (continued)
specified site NEC (continued)
causing (continued)
injury NEC (continued)
gastric contents (vomitus) T17.818
specified type NEC T17.898
throat —see Foreign body, pharynx
trachea —see Foreign body, trachea
retained (old) (nonmagnetic) (in)
anterior chamber (eye) —see Foreign body, intraocular, old, retained, anterior chamber
magnetic —see Foreign body, intraocular, old, retained, magnetic, anterior chamber
ciliary body —see Foreign body, intraocular, old, retained, ciliary body
magnetic —see Foreign body, intraocular, old, retained, magnetic, ciliary body
eyelid H02.819
left H02.816
lower H02.815
upper H02.814
right H02.813
lower H02.812
upper H02.811
fragments —see Retained, foreign body fragments (type of)
globe —see Foreign body, intraocular, old, retained
magnetic —see Foreign body, intraocular, old, retained, magnetic
intraocular —see Foreign body, intraocular, old, retained
magnetic —see Foreign body, intraocular, old, retained, magnetic
iris —see Foreign body, intraocular, old, retained, iris
magnetic —see Foreign body, intraocular, old, retained, magnetic, iris
lens —see Foreign body, intraocular, old, retained, lens
magnetic —see Foreign body, intraocular, old, retained, magnetic, lens
muscle —see Foreign body, retained, soft tissue
orbit —see Foreign body, orbit, old
posterior wall of globe —see Foreign body, intraocular, old, retained, posterior wall
magnetic —see Foreign body, intraocular, old, retained, magnetic, posterior wall
retrobulbar —see Foreign body, orbit, old, retrobulbar
soft tissue M79.5
vitreous —see Foreign body, intraocular, old, retained, vitreous body
magnetic —see Foreign body, intraocular, old, retained, magnetic, vitreous body
retina S05.5-
superficial, without open wound
abdomen, abdominal (wall) S30.851
alveolar process S00.552
ankle S90.55-

Foreign body (continued)
superficial, without open wound (continued)
antecubital space —see Foreign body, superficial, forearm
anus S30.857
arm (upper) S40.85-
auditory canal —see Foreign body, superficial, ear
auricle —see Foreign body, superficial, ear
axilla —see Foreign body, superficial, arm
back, lower S30.850
breast S20.15-
brow S00.85
buttock S30.850
calf —see Foreign body, superficial, leg
canthus —see Foreign body, superficial, eyelid
cheek S00.85
internal S00.552
chest wall —see Foreign body, superficial, thorax
chin S00.85
clitoris S30.854
costal region —see Foreign body, superficial, thorax
digit(s)
hand —see Foreign body, superficial, finger
foot —see Foreign body, superficial, toe
ear S00.45-
elbow S50.35-
epididymis S30.853
epigastric region S30.851
epiglottis S10.15
esophagus, cervical S10.15
eyebrow —see Foreign body, superficial, eyelid
eyelid S00.25-
face S00.85
finger(s) S60.459
index S60.45-
little S60.45-
middle S60.45-
ring S60.45-
flank S30.851
foot (except toe(s) alone) S90.85-
toe —see Foreign body, superficial, toe
forearm S50.85-
elbow only —see Foreign body, superficial, elbow
forehead S00.85
genital organs, external
female S30.856
male S30.855
groin S30.851
gum S00.552
hand S60.55-
head S00.95
ear —see Foreign body, superficial, ear
eyelid —see Foreign body, superficial, eyelid
lip S00.551
nose S00.35
oral cavity S00.552
scalp S00.05
specified site NEC S00.85
heel —see Foreign body, superficial, foot
hip S70.25-
inguinal region S30.851
interscapular region S20.459
jaw S00.85
knee S80.25-

Foreign body (continued)
superficial, without open wound (continued)
labium (majus) (minus) S30.854
larynx S10.15
leg (lower) S80.85-
knee —see Foreign body, superficial, knee
upper —see Foreign body, superficial, thigh
lip S00.551
lower back S30.850
lumbar region S30.850
malar region S00.85
mammary —see Foreign body, superficial, breast
mastoid region S00.85
mouth S00.552
nail
finger —see Foreign body, superficial, finger
toe —see Foreign body, superficial, toe
nape S10.85
nasal S00.35
neck S10.95
specified site NEC S10.85
throat S10.15
nose S00.35
occipital region S00.05
oral cavity S00.552
orbital region —see Foreign body, superficial, eyelid
palate S00.552
palm —see Foreign body, superficial, hand
parietal region S00.05
pelvis S30.850
penis S30.852
perineum
female S30.854
male S30.850
periocular area —see Foreign body, superficial, eyelid
phalanges
finger —see Foreign body, superficial, finger
toe —see Foreign body, superficial, toe
pharynx S10.15
pinna —see Foreign body, superficial, ear
popliteal space —see Foreign body, superficial, knee
prepuce S30.852
pubic region S30.850
pudendum
female S30.856
male S30.855
sacral region S30.850
scalp S00.05
scapular region —see Foreign body, superficial, shoulder
scrotum S30.853
shin —see Foreign body, superficial, leg
shoulder S40.25-
sternal region S20.359
submaxillary region S00.85
submental region S00.85
subungual
finger(s) —see Foreign body, superficial, finger
toe(s) —see Foreign body, superficial, toe
supraclavicular fossa S10.85
supraorbital S00.85
temple S00.85
temporal region S00.85
testis S30.853
thigh S70.35-

Foreign body (continued)
superficial, without open wound (continued)
thorax, thoracic (wall) S20.95
back S20.45-
front S20.35-
throat S10.15
thumb S60.35-
toe(s) (lesser) S90.456
great S90.45-
tongue S00.552
trachea S10.15
tunica vaginalis S30.853
tympanum, tympanic membrane —see Foreign body, superficial, ear
uvula S00.552
vagina S30.854
vocal cords S10.15
vulva S30.854
wrist S60.85-
swallowed T18.9
trachea T17.408
causing
asphyxiation T17.400
food (bone) (seed) T17.420
gastric contents (vomitus) T17.410
specified type NEC T17.490
injury NEC T17.408
food (bone) (seed) T17.428
gastric contents (vomitus) T17.418
specified type NEC T17.498
type of fragment —see Retained, foreign body fragments (type of)
vitreous (humor) S05.5-

Forestier's disease (rhizomelic pseudopolyarthritis) M35.3
meaning ankylosing hyperostosis —see Hyperostosis, ankylosing

Formation
hyalin in cornea —see Degeneration, cornea
sequestrum in bone (due to infection) —see Osteomyelitis, chronic
valve
colon, congenital Q43.8
ureter (congenital) Q62.39

Formication R20.2

Fort Bragg fever A27.89

Fossa —see also condition
pyriform —see condition

Foster-Kennedy syndrome H47.14-

Fothergill's
disease (trigeminal neuralgia) —see also Neuralgia, trigeminal
scarlatina anginosa A38.9

Foul breath R19.6

Foundling Z76.1

Fournier disease or gangrene N49.3
female N76.89

Fourth
cranial nerve —see condition
molar K00.1

Foville's (peduncular) **disease or syndrome** G46.3

Fox (Fordyce) disease (apocrine miliaria) L75.2

FPIES (food protein-induced enterocolitis syndrome) K52.21

Fracture, burst —see Fracture, traumatic, by site

Fracture, chronic —see Fracture, pathological, by site

Fracture, insufficiency —see Fracture, pathologic, by site

Fracture, nontraumatic, NEC
  atypical
    femur M84.750-
      complete
        oblique M84.759
          left side M84.758
          right side M84.757
        transverse M84.756
          left side M84.755
          right side M84.754
      incomplete M84.753
        left side M84.752
        right side M84.751

Fracture, pathological (pathologic)
  —see also Fracture, traumatic
  M84.40
  ankle M84.47-
  carpus M84.44-
  clavicle M84.41-
  compression (not due to trauma)
    (see also Collapse, vertebra)
    M48.50-
  dental implant M27.63
  dental restorative material K08.539
    with loss of material K08.531
    without loss of material K08.530
  due to
    neoplastic disease NEC (see also
      Neoplasm) M84.50
      ankle M84.57-
      carpus M84.54-
      clavicle M84.51-
      femur M84.55-
      fibula M84.56-
      finger M84.54-
      hip M84.559
      humerus M84.52-
      ilium M84.550
      ischium M84.550
      metacarpus M84.54-
      metatarsus M84.57-
      neck M84.58
      pelvis M84.550
      radius M84.53-
      rib M84.58
      scapula M84.51-
      skull M84.58
      specified site NEC M84.58
      tarsus M84.57-
      tibia M84.56-
      toe M84.57-
      ulna M84.53-
      vertebra M84.58
    osteoporosis M80.00
      disuse —see Osteoporosis,
        specified type NEC, with
        pathological fracture
      drug-induced —see
        Osteoporosis, drug induced,
        with pathological fracture
      idiopathic —see Osteoporosis,
        specified type NEC, with
        pathological fracture
      postmenopausal —see
        Osteoporosis,
        postmenopausal, with
        pathological fracture
      postoophorectomy —see
        Osteoporosis,
        postoophorectomy, with
        pathological fracture

Fracture, pathological (continued)
  due to (continued)
    osteoporosis (continued)
      postsurgical malabsorption
        —see Osteoporosis,
        specified type NEC, with
        pathological fracture
      specified cause NEC —see
        Osteoporosis, specified type
        NEC, with pathological
        fracture
    specified disease NEC M84.60
      ankle M84.67-
      carpus M84.64-
      clavicle M84.61-
      femur M84.65-
      fibula M84.66-
      finger M84.64-
      hip M84.65-
      humerus M84.62-
      ilium M84.650
      ischium M84.650
      metacarpus M84.64-
      metatarsus M84.67-
      neck M84.68
      radius M84.63-
      rib M84.68
      scapula M84.61-
      skull M84.68
      tarsus M84.67-
      tibia M84.66-
      toe M84.67-
      ulna M84.63-
      vertebra M84.68
  femur M84.45-
  fibula M84.46-
  finger M84.44-
  hip M84.459
  humerus M84.42-
  ilium M84.454
  ischium M84.454
  joint prosthesis —see
    Complications, joint
    prosthesis, mechanical,
    breakdown, by site
    periprosthetic —see Fracture,
      pathological, periprosthetic
  metacarpus M84.44-
  metatarsus M84.47-
  neck M84.48
  pelvis M84.454
  periprosthetic M97.9
    ankle M97.2-
    elbow M97.4-
    finger M97.8
    hip M97.0-
    knee M97.1-
    other specified joint M97.8
    shoulder M97.3-
    spinal joint M97.8
    toe joint M97.8
    wrist joint M97.8
  radius M84.43-
  restorative material (dental)
    K08.539
    with loss of material K08.531
    without loss of material
      K08.530
  rib M84.48
  scapula M84.41-
  skull M84.48
  tarsus M84.47-
  tibia M84.46-
  toe M84.47-
  ulna M84.43-
  vertebra M84.48

Fracture, traumatic (abduction)
  (adduction) (separation) (see
  also Fracture, pathological)
  T14.8
  acetabulum S32.40-

Fracture, traumatic (continued)
  acetabulum (continued)
    column
      anterior (displaced) (iliopubic)
        S32.43-
        nondisplaced S32.436
      posterior (displaced)
        (ilioischial) S32.443
        nondisplaced S32.44-
    dome (displaced) S32.48-
      nondisplaced S32.48
    specified NEC S32.49-
    transverse (displaced) S32.45-
      with associated posterior wall
        fracture (displaced) S32.46-
        nondisplaced S32.46-
      nondisplaced S32.45-
    wall
      anterior (displaced) S32.41-
        nondisplaced S32.41-
      medial (displaced) S32.47-
        nondisplaced S32.47-
      posterior (displaced) S32.42-
        with associated transverse
          fracture (displaced)
          S32.46-
          nondisplaced S32.46-
        nondisplaced S32.42-
  acromion —see Fracture, scapula,
    acromial process
  ankle S82.899
    bimalleolar (displaced) S82.84-
      nondisplaced S82.84-
    lateral malleolus only (displaced)
      S82.6-
      nondisplaced S82.6-
    medial malleolus (displaced)
      S82.5-
      associated with Maisonneuve's
        fracture —see Fracture,
        Maisonneuve's
      nondisplaced S82.5-
    talus —see Fracture, tarsal, talus
    trimalleolar (displaced) S82.85-
      nondisplaced S82.85-
  arm (upper) —see also Fracture,
    humerus, shaft
    humerus —see Fracture,
      humerus
    radius —see Fracture, radius
    ulna —see Fracture, ulna
  astragalus —see Fracture, tarsal,
    talus
  atlas —see Fracture, neck, cervical
    vertebra, first
  axis —see Fracture, neck, cervical
    vertebra, second
  back —see Fracture, vertebra
  Barton's —see Barton's fracture
  base of skull —see Fracture, skull,
    base
  basicervical (basal) (femoral) S72.0
  Bennett's —see Bennett's fracture
  bimalleolar —see Fracture, ankle,
    bimalleolar
  blow-out S02.3-
  bone NEC T14.8
    birth injury P13.9
    following insertion of
      orthopedic implant, joint
      prosthesis or bone plate
      —see Fracture, following
      insertion of orthopedic
      implant, joint prosthesis or
      bone plate
    in (due to) neoplastic disease
      NEC —see Fracture,
      pathological, due to,
      neoplastic disease
    pathological (cause unknown)
      —see Fracture, pathological

Fracture, traumatic (continued)
  breast bone —see Fracture,
    sternum
  bucket handle (semilunar cartilage)
    —see Tear, meniscus
  buckle —see Fracture, by site,
    torus
  burst —see Fracture, traumatic,
    by site
  calcaneus —see Fracture, tarsal,
    calcaneus
  carpal bone(s) S62.10-
    capitate (displaced) S62.13-
      nondisplaced S62.13-
    cuneiform —see Fracture, carpal
      bone, triquetrum
    hamate (body) (displaced)
      S62.143
      hook process (displaced)
        S62.15-
        nondisplaced S62.15-
      nondisplaced S62.14-
    larger multangular —see
      Fracture, carpal bones,
      trapezium
    lunate (displaced) S62.12-
      nondisplaced S62.12-
    navicular S62.00-
      distal pole (displaced) S62.01-
        nondisplaced S62.01-
      middle third (displaced)
        S62.02-
        nondisplaced S62.02-
      proximal third (displaced)
        S62.03-
        nondisplaced S62.03-
      volar tuberosity —see
        Fracture, carpal bones,
        navicular, distal pole
    os magnum —see Fracture,
      carpal bones, capitate
    pisiform (displaced) S62.16-
      nondisplaced S62.16-
    semilunar —see Fracture, carpal
      bones, lunate
    smaller multangular —see
      Fracture, carpal bones,
      trapezoid
    trapezium (displaced) S62.17-
      nondisplaced S62.17-
    trapezoid (displaced) S62.18-
      nondisplaced S62.18-
    triquetrum (displaced) S62.11-
      nondisplaced S62.11-
    unciform —see Fracture, carpal
      bones, hamate
  cervical —see Fracture, vertebra,
    cervical
  clavicle S42.00-
    acromial end (displaced) S42.03-
      nondisplaced S42.03-
    birth injury P13.4
    lateral end —see Fracture,
      clavicle, acromial end
    shaft (displaced) S42.02-
      nondisplaced S42.02-
    sternal end (anterior) (displaced)
      S42.01-
      nondisplaced S42.01-
      posterior S42.01-
  coccyx S32.2
  collapsed —see Collapse, vertebra
  collar bone —see Fracture,
    clavicle
  Colles' —see Colles' fracture
  coronoid process —see Fracture,
    ulna, upper end, coronoid
    process
  corpus cavernosum penis
    S39.840
  costochondral cartilage S23.41

Fracture, traumatic *(continued)*
neck *(continued)*
  cervical vertebra *(continued)*
    first *(continued)*
      posterior arch (displaced)
        S12.030
        nondisplaced S12.031
      specified type NEC
        (displaced) S12.090
        nondisplaced S12.091
    fourth (displaced) S12.300
      nondisplaced S12.301
      specified type NEC
        (displaced) S12.390
        nondisplaced S12.391
    second (displaced) S12.100
      nondisplaced S12.101
      dens (anterior) (displaced)
        (type II) S12.110
        nondisplaced S12.112
        posterior S12.111
      specified type NEC
        (displaced) S12.120
        nondisplaced S12.121
      specified type NEC
        (displaced) S12.190
        nondisplaced S12.191
    seventh (displaced) S12.600
      nondisplaced S12.601
      specified type NEC
        (displaced) S12.690
        non displaced S12.691
    sixth (displaced) S12.500
      nondisplaced S12.501
      specified type NEC
        (displaced) S12.590
        non displaced S12.591
    third (displaced) S12.200
      nondisplaced S12.201
      specified type NEC
        (displaced) S12.290
        non displaced S12.291
  hyoid bone S12.8
  larynx S12.8
  specified site NEC S12.8
  thyroid cartilage S12.8
  trachea S12.8
neoplastic NEC —*see* Fracture,
  pathological, due to, neoplastic
  disease
neural arch —*see* Fracture, vertebra
newborn —*see* Birth, injury,
  fracture
nontraumatic —*see* Fracture,
  pathological
nonunion —*see* Nonunion, fracture
nose, nasal (bone) (septum) S02.2
occiput —*see* Fracture, skull, base,
  occiput
odontoid process —*see* Fracture,
  neck, cervical vertebra, second
olecranon (process) (ulna) —*see*
  Fracture, ulna, upper end,
  olecranon process
orbit, orbital (bone) (region) S02.85
  floor (blow-out) S02.3-
  roof S02.12-
    wall S02.85
      lateral S02.84-
      medial S02.83-
os
  calcis —*see* Fracture, tarsal,
    calcaneus
  magnum —*see* Fracture, carpal,
    capitate
  pubis —*see* Fracture, pubis
palate S02.8-
parietal bone (skull) S02.0
patella S82.00-
  comminuted (displaced) S82.04-
    nondisplaced S82.04-

Fracture, traumatic *(continued)*
patella *(continued)*
  longitudinal (displaced) S82.02-
    nondisplaced S82.02-
  osteochondral (displaced)
    S82.01-
    nondisplaced S82.01-
  specified NEC S82.09-
  transverse (displaced) S82.03-
    nondisplaced S82.03-
pedicle (of vertebral arch) —*see*
  Fracture, vertebra
pelvis, pelvic (bone) S32.9
  acetabulum —*see* Fracture,
    acetabulum
  circle —*see* Disruption, pelvic
    ring
  following insertion of implant,
    prosthesis or plate M96.65
  ilium —*see* Fracture, ilium
  ischium —*see* Fracture, ischium
  multiple
    with disruption of pelvic ring
      (circle) —*see* Disruption,
      pelvic ring
    without disruption of pelvic
      ring (circle) S32.82
  pubis —*see* Fracture, pubis
  specified site NEC S32.89
  sacrum —*see* Fracture, sacrum
periprosthetic, around internal
  prosthetic joint M97.9
  ankle M97.2-
  elbow M97.4-
  finger M97.8
  hip M97.0-
  knee M97.1-
  shoulder M97.3-
  specified joint NEC M97.8
  spine M97.8
  toe M97.8
  wrist M97.8
phalanx
  foot —*see* Fracture, toe
  hand —*see* Fracture, finger
pisiform —*see* Fracture, carpal,
  pisiform
pond —*see* Fracture, skull
prosthetic device, internal —*see*
  Complications, prosthetic device,
  by site, mechanical
pubis S32.50-
  with disruption of pelvic ring
    —*see* Disruption, pelvic ring
  specified site NEC S32.59-
  superior rim S32.51-
radius S52.9-
  distal end —*see* Fracture, radius,
    lower end
  following insertion of implant,
    prosthesis or plate M96.63-
  head —*see* Fracture, radius,
    upper end, head
  lower end S52.50-
    Barton's —*see* Barton's fracture
    Colles' —*see* Colles' fracture
    extraarticular NEC S52.55-
    intraarticular NEC S52.57-
    physeal S59.20-
      Salter-Harris
        Type I S59.21-
        Type II S59.22-
        Type III S59.23-
        Type IV S59.24-
      specified NEC S59.29-
    Smith's —*see* Smith's fracture
    specified NEC S52.59-
    styloid process (displaced)
      S52.51-
      nondisplaced S52.51-
      torus S52.52-

Fracture, traumatic *(continued)*
radius *(continued)*
  neck —*see* Fracture, radius,
    upper end
  proximal end —*see* Fracture,
    radius, upper end
  shaft S52.30-
    bent bone S52.38-
    comminuted (displaced)
      S52.35-
      nondisplaced S52.35-
    Galeazzi's —*see* Galeazzi's
      fracture
    greenstick S52.31-
    oblique (displaced) S52.33-
      nondisplaced S52.33-
    segmental (displaced) S52.36-
      nondisplaced S52.36-
    specified NEC S52.39-
    spiral (displaced) S52.34-
      nondisplaced S52.34-
    transverse (displaced) S52.32-
      nondisplaced S52.32-
  upper end S52.10-
    head (displaced) S52.12-
      nondisplaced S52.12-
    neck (displaced) S52.13-
      nondisplaced S52.13-
    specified NEC S52.18-
    physeal S59.10-
      Salter-Harris
        Type I S59.11-
        Type II S59.12-
        Type III S59.13-
        Type IV S59.14-
      specified NEC S59.19-
    torus S52.11-
ramus
  inferior or superior, pubis —*see*
    Fracture, pubis
  mandible —*see* Fracture,
    mandible
restorative material (dental)
  K08.539
  with loss of material K08.531
  without loss of material
    K08.530
rib S22.3-
  with flail chest —*see* Flail,
    chest
  multiple S22.4-
    with flail chest —*see* Flail,
      chest
root, tooth —*see* Fracture, tooth
sacrum S32.10
  specified NEC S32.19
  Type
    1 S32.14
    2 S32.15
    3 S32.16
    4 S32.17
  Zone
    I S32.119
      displaced (minimally)
        S32.111
        severely S32.112
      nondisplaced S32.110
    II S32.129
      displaced (minimally)
        S32.121
        severely S32.122
      nondisplaced S32.120
    III S32.139
      displaced (minimally)
        S32.131
        severely S32.132
      nondisplaced S32.130
scaphoid (hand) —*see also*
  Fracture, carpal, navicular
  foot —*see* Fracture, tarsal,
    navicular

Fracture, traumatic *(continued)*
scapula S42.10-
  acromial process (displaced)
    S42.12-
    nondisplaced S42.12-
  body (displaced) S42.11-
    nondisplaced S42.11-
  coracoid process (displaced)
    S42.13-
    nondisplaced S42.13-
  glenoid cavity (displaced)
    S42.14-
    nondisplaced S42.14-
  neck (displaced) S42.15-
    nondisplaced S42.15-
  specified NEC S42.19-
semilunar bone, wrist —*see*
  Fracture, carpal, lunate
sequelae —*see* Sequelae, fracture
sesamoid bone
  hand —*see* Fracture, carpal
  foot S92.81-
  other —*see* Fracture, traumatic,
    by site
shepherd's —*see* Fracture, tarsal,
  talus
shoulder (girdle) S42.9-
  blade —*see* Fracture, scapula
sinus (ethmoid) (frontal) S02.19
skull S02.91
  base S02.10-
    occiput S02.119
      condyle S02.113
        type I S02.110
          left side S02.11B
          right side S02.11A
        type II S02.111
          left side S02.11D
          right side S02.11C
        type III S02.112
          left side S02.11F
          right side S02.11E
        specified NEC S02.118
          left side S02.11H
          right side S02.11G
      specified NEC S02.19
  birth injury P13.0
  frontal bone S02.0
  parietal bone S02.0
  specified site NEC S02.8-
  temporal bone S02.19
  vault S02.0
Smith's —*see* Smith's fracture
sphenoid (bone) (sinus) S02.19
spine —*see* Fracture, vertebra
spinous process —*see* Fracture,
  vertebra
spontaneous (cause unknown)
  —*see* Fracture, pathological
stave (of thumb) —*see* Fracture,
  metacarpal, first
sternum S22.20
  with flail chest —*see* Flail,
    chest
  body S22.22
  manubrium S22.21
  xiphoid (process) S22.24
stress M84.30
  ankle M84.37-
  carpus M84.34-
  clavicle M84.31-
  femoral neck M84.359
  femur M84.35-
  fibula M84.36-
  finger M84.34-
  hip M84.359
  humerus M84.32-
  ilium M84.350
  ischium M84.350
  metacarpus M84.34-
  metatarsus M84.37-

Fracture, traumatic *(continued)*
  ulna *(continued)*
    lower end *(continued)*
      physeal *(continued)*
        Salter-Harris *(continued)*
          Type III S59.03-
          Type IV S59.04-
          specified NEC S59.09-
        specified NEC S52.69-
        styloid process (displaced)
          S52.61-
          nondisplaced S52.61-
        torus S52.62-
    proximal end *—see* Fracture,
      ulna, upper end
    shaft S52.20-
      comminuted (displaced)
        S52.25-
        nondisplaced S52.25-
      greenstick S52.21-
      Monteggia's *—see*
        Monteggia's fracture
      oblique (displaced) S52.23-
        nondisplaced S52.23-
      segmental (displaced) S52.26-
        nondisplaced S52.26-
      specified NEC S52.29-
      spiral (displaced) S52.24-
        nondisplaced S52.24-
      transverse (displaced) S52.22-
        nondisplaced S52.22-
    upper end S52.00-
      coronoid process (displaced)
        S52.04-
        nondisplaced S52.04-
      olecranon process (displaced)
        S52.02-
        with intraarticular extension
          S52.03-
        nondisplaced S52.02-
          with intraarticular
            extension S52.03-
      specified NEC S52.09-
      torus S52.01-
  unciform *—see* Fracture, carpal,
    hamate
  vault of skull S02.0
  vertebra, vertebral (arch) (body)
    (column) (neural arch) (pedicle)
    (spinous process) (transverse
    process)
    atlas *—see* Fracture, neck,
      cervical vertebra, first
    axis *—see* Fracture, neck,
      cervical vertebra, second
    cervical (teardrop) S12.9
      axis *—see* Fracture, neck,
        cervical vertebra, second
      first (atlas) *—see* Fracture,
        neck, cervical vertebra, first
      second (axis) *—see* Fracture,
        neck, cervical vertebra,
        second
    chronic M84.48
    coccyx S32.2
    dorsal *—see* Fracture, thorax,
      vertebra
    lumbar S32.009
      burst (stable) S32.001
        unstable S32.002
      fifth S32.059
        burst (stable) S32.051
          unstable S32.052
        specified type NEC S32.058
        wedge compression
          S32.050
      first S32.019
        burst (stable) S32.011
          unstable S32.012
        specified type NEC S32.018
        wedge compression S32.010

Fracture, traumatic *(continued)*
  vertebra, vertebral *(continued)*
    lumbar *(continued)*
      fourth S32.049
        burst (stable) S32.041
          unstable S32.042
        specified type NEC S32.048
        wedge compression
          S32.040
      second S32.029
        burst (stable) S32.021
          unstable S32.022
        specified type NEC S32.028
        wedge compression
          S32.020
      specified type NEC S32.008
      third S32.039
        burst (stable) S32.031
          unstable S32.032
        specified type NEC
          S32.038
        wedge compression
          S32.030
      wedge compression S32.000
    metastatic *—see* Collapse,
      vertebra, in, specified disease
      NEC *—see also* Neoplasm
    newborn (birth injury) P11.5
    sacrum S32.10
      specified NEC S32.19
      Type
        1 S32.14
        2 S32.15
        3 S32.16
        4 S32.17
      Zone
        I S32.119
          displaced (minimally)
            S32.111
            severely S32.112
          nondisplaced S32.110
        II S32.129
          displaced (minimally)
            S32.121
            severely S32.122
          nondisplaced S32.120
        III S32.139
          displaced (minimally)
            S32.131
            severely S32.132
          nondisplaced S32.130
    thoracic *—see* Fracture, thorax,
      vertebra
  vertex S02.0
  vomer (bone) S02.2
  wrist S62.10-
    carpal *—see* Fracture, carpal
      bone
    navicular (scaphoid) (hand) —
      see Fracture, carpal, navicular
  xiphisternum, xiphoid (process)
    S22.24
  zygoma S02.402
    left side S02.40F
    right side S02.40E

Fragile, fragility
  autosomal site Q95.5
  bone, congenital (with blue sclera)
    Q78.0
  capillary (hereditary) D69.8
  hair L67.8
  nails L60.3
  non-sex chromosome site Q95.5
  X chromosome Q99.2

Fragilitas
  crinium L67.8
  ossium (with blue sclerae)
    (hereditary) Q78.0
  unguium L60.3
    congenital Q84.6

Fragments, cataract (lens),
  following cataract surgery
  H59.02-
    retained foreign body *—see*
      Retained, foreign body
      fragments (type of)

Frailty (frail) R54
  mental R41.81

Frambesia, frambesial (tropica)
  —see also Yaws
  initial lesion or ulcer A66.0
  primary A66.0

Frambeside
  gummatous A66.4
  of early yaws A66.2

Frambesioma A66.1

Franceschetti-Klein (-Wildervanck)
  disease or syndrome Q75.4

Francis' disease *—see* Tularemia

Franklin disease C88.2

Frank's essential thrombocytopenia
  D69.3

Fraser's syndrome Q87.0

Freckle(s) L81.2
  malignant melanoma in *—see*
    Melanoma
  melanotic (Hutchinson's) *—see*
    Melanoma, in situ
  retinal D49.81

Frederickson's
  hyperlipoproteinemia, type
  I and V E78.3
  IIA E78.00
  IIB and III E78.2
  IV E78.1

Freeman Sheldon syndrome Q87.0

Freezing (*see also* Effect, adverse,
  cold) T69.9

Freiberg's disease (infraction of
  metatarsal head or osteochondrosis)
  see Osteochondrosis, juvenile,
  metatarsus

Frei's disease A55

Fremitus, friction, cardiac R01.2

Frenum, frenulum
  external os Q51.828
  tongue (shortening) (congenital)
    Q38.1

Frequency micturition (nocturnal)
  R35.0
  psychogenic F45.8

Frey's syndrome
  auriculotemporal G50.8
  hyperhidrosis L74.52

Friction
  burn *—see* Burn, by site
  fremitus, cardiac R01.2
  precordial R01.2
  sounds, chest R09.89

Friderichsen-Waterhouse syndrome
  or disease A39.1

Friedländer's B (bacillus) **NEC** (*see*
  also condition) A49.8

Friedreich's
  ataxia G11.11
  combined systemic disease G11.11
  facial hemihypertrophy Q67.4
  sclerosis (cerebellum) (spinal cord)
    G11.11

Frigidity F52.22

Fröhlich's syndrome E23.6

Frontal *—see also* condition
  lobe syndrome F07.0

Frostbite (superficial) T33.90
  with
    partial thickness skin loss
      —see Frostbite (superficial),
      by site
    tissue necrosis T34.90
  abdominal wall T33.3
    with tissue necrosis T34.3
  ankle T33.81-
    with tissue necrosis T34.81-
  arm T33.4-
    with tissue necrosis T34.4-
    finger(s) *—see* Frostbite,
      finger
    hand *—see* Frostbite, hand
    wrist *—see* Frostbite, wrist
  ear T33.01-
    with tissue necrosis T34.01-
  face T33.09
    with tissue necrosis T34.09
  finger T33.53-
    with tissue necrosis T34.53-
  foot T33.82-
    with tissue necrosis T34.82-
  hand T33.52-
    with tissue necrosis T34.52-
  head T33.09
    with tissue necrosis T34.09
    ear *—see* Frostbite, ear
    nose *—see* Frostbite, nose
  hip (and thigh) T33.6-
    with tissue necrosis T34.6-
  knee T33.7-
    with tissue necrosis T34.7-
  leg T33.9-
    with tissue necrosis T34.9-
    ankle *—see* Frostbite, ankle
    foot *—see* Frostbite, foot
    knee *—see* Frostbite, knee
    lower T33.7-
      with tissue necrosis T34.7-
    thigh *—see* Frostbite, hip
    toe *—see* Frostbite, toe
  limb
    lower T33.99
      with tissue necrosis T34.99
    upper *—see* Frostbite, arm
  neck T33.1
    with tissue necrosis T34.1
  nose T33.02
    with tissue necrosis T34.02
  pelvis T33.3
    with tissue necrosis T34.3
  specified site NEC T33.99
    with tissue necrosis T34.99
  thigh *—see* Frostbite, hip
  thorax T33.2
    with tissue necrosis T34.2
  toes T33.83-
    with tissue necrosis T34.83-
  trunk T33.99
    with tissue necrosis T34.99
  wrist T33.51-
    with tissue necrosis T34.51-

Frotteurism F65.81

Frozen *—see also* Effect, adverse,
  cold T69.9
  pelvis (female) N94.89
    male K66.8
  shoulder *—see* Capsulitis,
    adhesive

Fructokinase deficiency E74.11

Fructose 1,6 diphosphatase
  deficiency E74.19

Fructosemia (benign) (essential)
  E74.12

Fructosuria (benign) (essential)
  E74.11

Fuchs'
black spot (myopic) (*see also*
Myopia, degenerative) H44.2-
dystrophy (corneal endothelium)
H18.51-
heterochromic cyclitis —*see*
Cyclitis, Fuchs' heterochromic

Fucosidosis E77.1

Fugue R68.89
dissociative F44.1
hysterical (dissociative) F44.1
postictal in epilepsy —*see* Epilepsy
reaction to exceptional stress
(transient) F43.0

Fulminant, fulminating —*see*
condition

Functional —*see also* condition
bleeding (uterus) N93.8

Functioning, intellectual, borderline
R41.83

Fundus —*see* condition

Fungemia NOS B49

Fungus, fungous
cerebral G93.89
disease NOS B49
infection —*see* Infection, fungus

Funiculitis (acute) (chronic)
(endemic) N49.1
gonococcal (acute) (chronic)
A54.23
tuberculous A18.15

Funnel
breast (acquired) M95.4
congenital Q67.6
sequelae (late effect) of rickets
E64.3
chest (acquired) M95.4
congenital Q67.6
sequelae (late effect) of rickets
E64.3
pelvis (acquired) M95.5
with disproportion (fetopelvic)
O33.3
causing obstructed labor
O65.3
congenital Q74.2

FUO (fever of unknown origin) R50.9

Furfur L21.0
microsporon B36.0

Furrier's lung J67.8

Furrowed K14.5
nail(s) (transverse) L60.4
congenital Q84.6
tongue K14.5
congenital Q38.3

Furuncle L02.92
abdominal wall L02.221
ankle —*see* Furuncle, lower limb
anus K61.0
antecubital space —*see* Furuncle,
upper limb
arm —*see* Furuncle, upper limb
auditory canal, external —*see*
Abscess, ear, external
auricle (ear) —*see* Abscess, ear,
external
axilla (region) L02.42-
back (any part) L02.222
breast N61.1
buttock L02.32
cheek (external) L02.02
chest wall L02.223
chin L02.02
corpus cavernosum N48.21
ear, external —*see* Abscess, ear,
external

Furuncle (*continued*)
external auditory canal —*see*
Abscess, ear, external
eyelid —*see* Abscess, eyelid
face L02.02
femoral (region) —*see* Furuncle,
lower limb
finger —*see* Furuncle, hand
flank L02.221
foot L02.62-
forehead L02.02
gluteal (region) L02.32
groin L02.224
hand L02.52-
head L02.821
face L02.02
hip —*see* Furuncle, lower limb
kidney —*see* Abscess, kidney
knee —*see* Furuncle, lower limb
labium (majus) (minus) N76.4
lacrimal
gland —*see* Dacryoadenitis
passages (duct) (sac) —*see*
Inflammation, lacrimal,
passages, acute
leg (any part) —*see* Furuncle,
lower limb
lower limb L02.42-
malignant A22.0
mouth K12.2
navel L02.226
neck L02.12
nose J34.0
orbit, orbital —*see* Abscess, orbit
palmar (space) —*see* Furuncle, hand
partes posteriores L02.32
pectoral region L02.223
penis N48.21
perineum L02.225
pinna —*see* Abscess, ear, external
popliteal —*see* Furuncle, lower
limb
prepatellar —*see* Furuncle, lower
limb
scalp L02.821
seminal vesicle N49.0
shoulder —*see* Furuncle, upper
limb
specified site NEC L02.828
submandibular K12.2
temple (region) L02.02
thumb —*see* Furuncle, hand
toe —*see* Furuncle, foot
trunk L02.229
abdominal wall L02.221
back L02.222
chest wall L02.223
groin L02.224
perineum L02.225
umbilicus L02.226
umbilicus L02.226
upper limb L02.42-
vulva N76.4

Furunculosis —*see* Furuncle

Fused —*see* Fusion, fused

Fusion, fused (congenital)
astragaloscaphoid Q74.2
atria Q21.1
auditory canal Q16.1
auricles, heart Q21.1
binocular with defective stereopsis
H53.32
bone Q79.8
cervical spine M43.22
choanal Q30.0
commissure, mitral valve Q23.2
cusps, heart valve NEC Q24.8
mitral Q23.2
pulmonary Q22.1
tricuspid Q22.4

Fusion, fused (*continued*)
ear ossicles Q16.3
fingers Q70.0-
hymen Q52.3
joint (acquired) —*see also*
Ankylosis
congenital Q74.8
kidneys (incomplete) Q63.1
labium (majus) (minus) Q52.5
larynx and trachea Q34.8
limb, congenital Q74.8
lower Q74.2
upper Q74.0
lobes, lung Q33.8
lumbosacral (acquired) M43.27
arthrodesis status Z98.1
congenital Q76.49
postprocedural status Z98.1
nares, nose, nasal, nostril(s) Q30.0
organ or site not listed —*see*
Anomaly, by site
ossicles Q79.9
auditory Q16.3
pulmonic cusps Q22.1
ribs Q76.6
sacroiliac (joint) (acquired) M43.28
arthrodesis status Z98.1
congenital Q74.2
postprocedural status Z98.1
spine (acquired) NEC M43.20
arthrodesis status Z98.1
cervical region M43.22
cervicothoracic region M43.23
congenital Q76.49
lumbar M43.26
lumbosacral region M43.27
occipito-atlanto-axial region
M43.21
postoperative status Z98.1
sacrococcygeal region M43.28
thoracic region M43.24
thoracolumbar region M43.25
sublingual duct with submaxillary
duct at opening in mouth Q38.4
testes Q55.1
toes Q70.2-
tooth, teeth K00.2
trachea and esophagus Q39.8
twins Q89.4
vagina Q52.4
ventricles, heart Q21.0
vertebra (arch) —*see* Fusion, spine
vulva Q52.5

Fusospirillosis (mouth) (tongue)
(tonsil) A69.1

Fussy baby R68.12

G

Gain in weight (abnormal)
(excessive) —*see also* Weight, gain

Gaisböck's disease (polycythemia
hypertonica) D75.1

Gait abnormality R26.9
ataxic R26.0
falling R29.6
hysterical (ataxic) (staggering) F44.4
paralytic R26.1
spastic R26.1
specified type NEC R26.89
staggering R26.0
unsteadiness R26.81
walking difficulty NEC R26.2

Galactocele (breast) N64.89
puerperal, postpartum O92.79

Galactokinase deficiency E74.29

Galactophoritis N61.0
gestational, puerperal, postpartum
O91.2-

Galactorrhea O92.6
not associated with childbirth
N64.3

Galactosemia (classic) (congenital)
E74.21

Galactosuria E74.29

Galacturia R82.0
schistosomiasis (bilharziasis)
B65.0

GALD (gestational alloimmune liver
disease) P78.84

Galeazzi's fracture S52.37-

Galen's vein —*see* condition

Galeophobia F40.218

Gall duct —*see* condition

Gallbladder —*see also* condition
acute K81.0

Gallop rhythm R00.8

Gallstone (colic) (cystic duct)
(gallbladder) (impacted) (multiple)
—*see also* Calculus, gallbladder
with
cholecystitis —*see* Calculus,
gallbladder, with cholecystitis
bile duct (common) (hepatic) —*see*
Calculus, bile duct
causing intestinal obstruction
K56.3
specified NEC K80.80
with obstruction K80.81

Gambling Z72.6
pathological (compulsive) F63.0

Gammopathy (of undetermined
significance [MGUS]) D47.2
associated with lymphoplasmacytic
dyscrasia D47.2
monoclonal D47.2
polyclonal D89.0

Gamna's disease (siderotic
splenomegaly) D73.1

Gamophobia F40.298

Gampsodactylia (congenital) Q66.7-

Gamstorp's disease (adynamia
episodica hereditaria) G72.3

Gandy-Nanta disease (siderotic
splenomegaly) D73.1

Gang
membership offenses Z72.810

Gangliocytoma D36.10

Ganglioglioma —*see* Neoplasm,
uncertain behavior, by site

Ganglion (compound) (diffuse)
(joint) (tendon (sheath)) M67.40
ankle M67.47-
foot M67.47-
forearm M67.43-
hand M67.44-
lower leg M67.46-
multiple sites M67.49
of yaws (early) (late) A66.6
pelvic region M67.45-
periosteal —*see* Periostitis
shoulder region M67.41-
specified site NEC M67.48
thigh region M67.45-
tuberculous A18.09
upper arm M67.42-
wrist M67.43-

Ganglioneuroblastoma —*see*
Neoplasm, nerve, malignant

Ganglioneuroma D36.10
malignant —*see* Neoplasm, nerve,
malignant

Ganglioneuromatosis D36.10

Ganglionitis
- fifth nerve —*see* Neuralgia, trigeminal
- gasserian (postherpetic) (postzoster) B02.21
- geniculate G51.1
  - newborn (birth injury) P11.3
  - postherpetic, postzoster B02.21
  - herpes zoster B02.21
- postherpetic geniculate B02.21

Gangliosidosis E75.10
- GM1 E75.19
- GM2 E75.00
  - other specified E75.09
  - Sandhoff disease E75.01
  - Tay-Sachs disease E75.02
- GM3 E75.19
- mucolipidosis IV E75.11

Gangosa A66.5

Gangrene, gangrenous (connective tissue) (dropsical) (dry) (moist) (skin) (ulcer) —*see also* Necrosis I96
- with diabetes (mellitus) —*see* Diabetes, gangrene
- abdomen (wall) I96
- alveolar M27.3
- appendix K35.80
  - with
    - peritonitis, localized —*see also* Appendicitis K35.31
- arteriosclerotic (general) (senile) —*see* Arteriosclerosis, extremities, with, gangrene
- auricle I96
- Bacillus welchii A48.0
- bladder (infectious) —*see* Cystitis, specified type NEC
- bowel, cecum, or colon —*see* Gangrene, intestine
- Clostridium perfringens or welchii A48.0
- cornea H18.89-
- corpora cavernosa N48.29
  - noninfective N48.89
- cutaneous, spreading I96
- decubital —*see* Ulcer, pressure, by site
- diabetic (any site) —*see* Diabetes, gangrene
- epidemic —*see* Poisoning, food, noxious, plant
- epididymis (infectional) N45.1
- erysipelas —*see* Erysipelas
- emphysematous —*see* Gangrene, gas
- extremity (lower) (upper) I96
- Fournier N49.3
  - female N76.89
- fusospirochetal A69.0
- gallbladder —*see* Cholecystitis, acute
- gas (bacillus) A48.0
  - following
    - abortion —*see* Abortion by type complicated by infection
    - ectopic or molar pregnancy O08.0
- glossitis K14.0
- hernia —*see* Hernia, by site, with gangrene
- intestine, intestinal (hemorrhagic) (massive) (see also Infarct, intestine) K55.069
  - with
    - mesenteric embolism (see also Infarct, intestine) K55.069
    - obstruction —*see* Obstruction, intestine

Gangrene, gangrenous (continued)
- laryngitis J04.0
- limb (lower) (upper) I96
- lung J85.0
  - spirochetal A69.8
- lymphangitis I89.1
- Meleney's (synergistic) —*see* Ulcer, skin
- mesentery (see also Infarct, intestine) K55.069
  - with
    - embolism (see also Infarct, intestine) K55.069
    - intestinal obstruction —*see* Obstruction, intestine
- mouth A69.0
- ovary —*see* Oophoritis
- pancreas —*see* Pancreatitis, acute
- penis N48.29
  - noninfective N48.89
- perineum I96
- pharynx —*see also* Pharyngitis
  - Vincent's A69.1
- presenile I73.1
- progressive synergistic —*see* Ulcer, skin
- pulmonary J85.0
- pulpal (dental) K04.1
- quinsy J36
- Raynaud's (symmetric gangrene) I73.01
- retropharyngeal J39.2
- scrotum N49.3
  - noninfective N50.89
- senile (atherosclerotic) —*see* Arteriosclerosis, extremities, with, gangrene
- spermatic cord N49.1
  - noninfective N50.89
- spine I96
- spirochetal NEC A69.8
- spreading cutaneous I96
- stomatitis A69.0
- symmetrical I73.01
- testis (infectional) N45.2
  - noninfective N44.8
- throat —*see also* Pharyngitis
  - diphtheritic A36.0
  - Vincent's A69.1
- thyroid (gland) E07.89
- tooth (pulp) K04.1
- tuberculous NEC —*see* Tuberculosis
- tunica vaginalis N49.1
  - noninfective N50.89
- umbilicus I96
- uterus —*see* Endometritis
- uvulitis K12.2
- vas deferens N49.1
  - noninfective N50.89
- vulva N76.89

Ganister disease J62.8

Ganser's syndrome (hysterical) F44.89

Gardner-Diamond syndrome (autoerythrocyte sensitization) D69.2

Gargoylism E76.01

Garré's disease, osteitis (sclerosing), **osteomyelitis** —*see* Osteomyelitis, specified type NEC

Garrod's pad, knuckle M72.1

Gartner's duct
- cyst Q52.4
- persistent Q50.6

Gas R14.3
- asphyxiation, inhalation, poisoning, suffocation NEC —*see* Table of Drugs and Chemicals

Gas (continued)
- excessive R14.0
- gangrene A48.0
  - following
    - abortion —*see* Abortion by type complicated by infection
    - ectopic or molar pregnancy O08.0
- on stomach R14.0
- pains R14.1

Gastralgia —*see also* Pain, abdominal

Gastrectasis K31.0
- psychogenic F45.8

Gastric —*see* condition

Gastrinoma
- malignant
  - pancreas C25.4
  - specified site NEC —*see* Neoplasm, malignant, by site
  - unspecified site C25.4
- specified site —*see* Neoplasm, uncertain behavior
- unspecified site D37.9

Gastritis (simple) K29.70
- with bleeding K29.71
- acute (erosive) K29.00
  - with bleeding K29.01
- alcoholic K29.20
  - with bleeding K29.21
- allergic K29.60
  - with bleeding K29.61
- atrophic (chronic) K29.40
  - with bleeding K29.41
- chronic (antral) (fundal) K29.50
  - with bleeding K29.51
  - atrophic K29.40
    - with bleeding K29.41
  - superficial K29.30
    - with bleeding K29.31
- dietary counseling and surveillance Z71.3
- due to diet deficiency E63.9
- eosinophilic K52.81
- giant hypertrophic K29.60
  - with bleeding K29.61
- granulomatous K29.60
  - with bleeding K29.61
- hypertrophic (mucosa) K29.60
  - with bleeding K29.61
- nervous F54
- spastic K29.60
  - with bleeding K29.61
- specified NEC K29.60
  - with bleeding K29.61
- superficial chronic K29.30
  - with bleeding K29.31
- tuberculous A18.83
- viral NEC A08.4

Gastrocarcinoma —*see* Neoplasm, malignant, stomach

Gastrocolic —*see* condition

Gastrodisciasis, gastrodiscoidiasis B66.8

Gastroduodenitis K29.90
- with bleeding K29.91
- virus, viral A08.4
  - specified type NEC A08.39

Gastrodynia —*see* Pain, abdominal

Gastroenteritis (acute) (chronic) (noninfectious) (see also Enteritis) K52.9
- allergic K52.29
  - with
    - eosinophilic gastritis or gastroenteritis K52.81

Gastroenteritis (continued)
- allergic (continued)
  - with (continued)
    - food protein-induced enterocolitis syndrome K52.21
    - food protein-induced enteropathy K52.22
- dietetic (see also Gastroenteritis, allergic) K52.29
- drug-induced K52.1
- due to
  - Cryptosporidium A07.2
  - drugs K52.1
  - food poisoning —*see* Intoxication, foodborne
  - radiation K52.0
- eosinophilic K52.81
- epidemic (infectious) A09
- food hypersensitivity (see also Gastroenteritis, allergic) K52.29
- infectious —*see* Enteritis, infectious
- influenzal —*see* Influenza, with gastroenteritis
- noninfectious K52.9
  - specified NEC K52.89
- rotaviral A08.0
- Salmonella A02.0
- toxic K52.1
- viral NEC A08.4
  - acute infectious A08.39
    - type Norwalk A08.11
  - infantile (acute) A08.39
  - Norwalk agent A08.11
  - rotaviral A08.0
  - severe of infants A08.39
  - specified type NEC A08.39

Gastroenteropathy (see also Gastroenteritis) K52.9
- acute, due to Norwalk agent A08.11
- acute, due to Norovirus A08.11
- infectious A09

Gastroenteroptosis K63.4

Gastroesophageal laceration-hemorrhage syndrome K22.6

Gastrointestinal —*see* condition

Gastrojejunal —*see* condition

Gastrojejunitis (see also Enteritis) K52.9

Gastrojejunocolic —*see* condition

Gastroliths K31.89

Gastromalacia K31.89

Gastroparalysis K31.84
- diabetic —*see* Diabetes, gastroparalysis

Gastroparesis K31.84
- diabetic —*see* Diabetes, by type, with gastroparesis

Gastropathy K31.9
- congestive portal K31.89
- erythematous K29.70
- exudative K90.89
- portal hypertensive K31.89

Gastroptosis K31.89

Gastrorrhagia K92.2
- psychogenic F45.8

Gastroschisis (congenital) Q79.3

Gastrospasm (neurogenic) (reflex) K31.89
- neurotic F45.8
- psychogenic F45.8

Gastrostaxis —*see* Gastritis, with bleeding

Gastrostenosis K31.89

Gastrostomy
attention to Z43.1
status Z93.1

Gastrosuccorrhea (continuous) (intermittent) K31.89
neurotic F45.8
psychogenic F45.8

Gatophobia F40.218

Gaucher's disease or splenomegaly (adult) (infantile) E75.22

Gee (-Herter) (-Thaysen) **disease** (nontropical sprue) K90.0

Gélineau's syndrome G47.419
with cataplexy G47.411

Gemination, tooth, teeth K00.2

Gemistocytoma
specified site —*see* Neoplasm, malignant, by site
unspecified site C71.9

General, generalized —*see* condition

Genetic
carrier (status)
cystic fibrosis Z14.1
hemophilia A (asymptomatic) Z14.01
symptomatic Z14.02
specified NEC Z14.8
susceptibility to disease NEC Z15.89
malignant neoplasm Z15.09
breast Z15.01
endometrium Z15.04
ovary Z15.02
prostate Z15.03
specified NEC Z15.09
multiple endocrine neoplasia Z15.81

Genital —*see* condition

Genito-anorectal syndrome A55

Genitourinary system —*see* condition

Genu
congenital Q74.1
extrorsum (acquired) —*see also* Deformity, varus, knee
congenital Q74.1
sequelae (late effect) of rickets E64.3
introrsum (acquired) —*see also* Deformity, valgus, knee
congenital Q74.1
sequelae (late effect) of rickets E64.3
rachitic (old) E64.3
recurvatum (acquired) —*see also* Deformity, limb, specified type NEC, lower leg
congenital Q68.2
sequelae (late effect) of rickets E64.3
valgum (acquired) (knock-knee) M21.06-
congenital Q74.1
sequelae (late effect) of rickets E64.3
varum (acquired) (bowleg) M21.16-
congenital Q74.1
sequelae (late effect) of rickets E64.3

Geographic tongue K14.1

Geophagia —*see* Pica

Geotrichosis B48.3
stomatitis B48.3

Gephyrophobia F40.242

Gerbode defect Q21.0

GERD (gastroesophageal reflux disease) K21.9

Gerhardt's
disease (erythromelalgia) I73.81
syndrome (vocal cord paralysis) J38.00
bilateral J38.02
unilateral J38.01

German measles —*see also* Rubella
exposure to Z20.4

Germinoblastoma (diffuse) C85.9-
follicular C82.9-

Germinoma —*see* Neoplasm, malignant, by site

Gerontoxon —*see* Degeneration, cornea, senile

Gerstmann-Sträussler-Scheinker syndrome (GSS) A81.82

Gerstmann's syndrome R48.8
developmental F81.2

Gestation (period) —*see also* Pregnancy
ectopic —*see* Pregnancy, by site
multiple O30.9-
greater than quadruplets —*see* Pregnancy, multiple (gestation), specified NEC
specified NEC —*see* Pregnancy, multiple (gestation), specified NEC

Gestational
mammary abscess O91.11-
purulent mastitis O91.11-
subarcolar abscess O91.11-

Ghon tubercle, primary infection A15.7

Ghost
teeth K00.4
vessels (cornea) H16.41-

Ghoul hand A66.3

Gianotti-Crosti disease L44.4

Giant
cell
epulis K06.8
peripheral granuloma K06.8
esophagus, congenital Q39.5
kidney, congenital Q63.3
urticaria T78.3
hereditary D84.1

Giardiasis A07.1

Gibert's disease or pityriasis L42

Giddiness R42
hysterical F44.89
psychogenic F45.8

Gierke's disease (glycogenosis I) E74.01

Gigantism (cerebral) (hypophyseal) (pituitary) E22.0
constitutional E34.4

Gilbert's disease or syndrome E80.4

Gilchrist's disease B40.9

Gilford-Hutchinson disease E34.8

Gilles de la Tourette's disease or syndrome (motor-verbal tic) F95.2

Gingivitis K05.10
acute (catarrhal) K05.00
necrotizing A69.1
nonplaque induced K05.01
plaque induced K05.00
chronic (desquamative) (hyperplastic) (simple marginal) (pregnancy associated) (ulcerative) K05.10
nonplaque induced K05.11
plaque induced K05.10
expulsiva —*see* Periodontitis
necrotizing ulcerative (acute) A69.1
pellagrous E52
acute necrotizing A69.1
Vincent's A69.1

Gingivoglossitis K14.0

Gingivopericementitis —*see* Periodontitis

Gingivosis —*see* Gingivitis, chronic

Gingivostomatitis K05.10
herpesviral B00.2
necrotizing ulcerative (acute) A69.1

Gland, glandular —*see* condition

Glanders A24.0

Glanzmann (-Naegeli) **disease or thrombasthenia** D69.1

Glasgow coma scale
total score
3-8 R40.243
9-12 R40.242
13-15 R40.241

Glass-blower's disease (cataract) —*see* Cataract, specified NEC

Glaucoma H40.9
with
increased episcleral venous pressure H40.81-
pseudoexfoliation of lens —*see* Glaucoma, open angle, primary, capsular
absolute H44.51-
angle-closure (primary) H40.20-
acute (attack) (crisis) H40.21-
chronic H40.22-
intermittent H40.23-
residual stage H40.24-
borderline H40.00-
capsular (with pseudoexfoliation of lens) —*see* Glaucoma, open angle, primary, capsular
childhood Q15.0
closed angle —*see* Glaucoma, angle-closure
congenital Q15.0
corticosteroid-induced —*see* Glaucoma, secondary, drugs
hypersecretion H40.82-
in (due to)
amyloidosis E85.4 *[H42]*
aniridia Q13.1 *[H42]*
concussion of globe —*see* Glaucoma, secondary, trauma
dislocation of lens —*see* Glaucoma, secondary
disorder of lens NEC —*see* Glaucoma, secondary
drugs —*see* Glaucoma, secondary, drugs
endocrine disease NOS E34.9 *[H42]*
eye
inflammation —*see* Glaucoma, secondary, inflammation
trauma —*see* Glaucoma, secondary, trauma

Glaucoma (continued)
in (continued)
hypermature cataract —*see* Glaucoma, secondary
iridocyclitis —*see* Glaucoma, secondary, inflammation
lens disorder —*see* Glaucoma, secondary,
Lowe's syndrome E72.03 *[H42]*
metabolic disease NOS E88.9 *[H42]*
ocular disorders NEC —*see* Glaucoma, secondary
onchocerciasis B73.02
pupillary block —*see* Glaucoma, secondary
retinal vein occlusion —*see* Glaucoma, secondary
Rieger's anomaly Q13.81 *[H42]*
rubeosis of iris —*see* Glaucoma, secondary
tumor of globe —*see* Glaucoma, secondary
infantile Q15.0
low tension —*see* Glaucoma, open angle, primary, low-tension
malignant H40.83-
narrow angle —*see* Glaucoma, angle-closure
newborn Q15.0
noncongestive (chronic) —*see* Glaucoma, open angle
nonobstructive —*see* Glaucoma, open angle
obstructive —*see also* Glaucoma, angle-closure
due to lens changes —*see* Glaucoma, secondary
open angle H40.10-
primary H40.11-
capsular (with pseudoexfoliation of lens) H40.14-
low-tension H40.12-
pigmentary H40.13-
residual stage H40.15-
phacolytic —*see* Glaucoma, secondary
pigmentary —*see* Glaucoma, open angle, primary, pigmentary
postinfectious —*see* Glaucoma, secondary, inflammation
secondary (to) H40.5-
drugs H40.6-
inflammation H40.4-
trauma H40.3-
simple (chronic) H40.11-
simplex H40.11-
specified type NEC H40.89
suspect H40.00-
syphilitic A52.71
traumatic —*see also* Glaucoma, secondary, trauma
newborn (birth injury) P15.3
tuberculous A18.59

Glaucomatous flecks (subcapsular) —*see* Cataract, complicated

Glazed tongue K14.4

Gleet (gonococcal) A54.01

Glénard's disease K63.4

Glioblastoma (multiforme)
with sarcomatous component
specified site —*see* Neoplasm, malignant, by site
unspecified site C71.9
giant cell
specified site —*see* Neoplasm, malignant, by site

Glioblastoma (continued)
  giant cell (continued)
    unspecified site C71.9
    specified site —see Neoplasm,
      malignant, by site
    unspecified site C71.9

Glioma (malignant)
  astrocytic
    specified site —see Neoplasm,
      malignant, by site
    unspecified site C71.9
  mixed
    specified site —see Neoplasm,
      malignant, by site
    unspecified site C71.9
  nose Q30.8
  specified site NEC —see
    Neoplasm, malignant, by site
  subependymal D43.2
    specified site —see Neoplasm,
      uncertain behavior, by site
    unspecified site D43.2
  unspecified site C71.9

Gliomatosis cerebri C71.0

Glioneuroma —see Neoplasm,
  uncertain behavior, by site

Gliosarcoma
  specified site —see Neoplasm,
    malignant, by site
  unspecified site C71.9

Gliosis (cerebral) G93.89
  spinal G95.89

Glisson's disease —see Rickets

Globinuria R82.3

Globus (hystericus) F45.8

Glomangioma D18.00
  intra-abdominal D18.03
  intracranial D18.02
  skin D18.01
  specified site NEC D18.09

Glomangiomyoma D18.00
  intra-abdominal D18.03
  intracranial D18.02
  skin D18.01
  specified site NEC D18.09

Glomangiosarcoma —see Neoplasm,
  connective tissue, malignant

Glomerular
  disease in syphilis A52.75
  nephritis —see Glomerulonephritis

Glomerulitis —see
  Glomerulonephritis

Glomerulonephritis (see also
  Nephritis) N05.9
  with
    C3
      glomerulonephritis N05.A
      glomerulopathy N05.A
        with dense deposit disease
          N05.6
    edema —see Nephrosis
    minimal change N05.0
    minor glomerular abnormality
      N05.0
  acute N00.9
  chronic N03.9
  crescentic (diffuse) NEC (see
    also N00-N07 with fourth
    character .7) N05.7
  dense deposit (see also N00-N07
    with fourth character .6) N05.6
  diffuse
    crescentic (see also N00-N07
      with fourth character .7) N05.7
    endocapillary proliferative (see
      also N00-N07 with fourth
      character .4) N05.4

Glomerulonephritis (continued)
  diffuse (continued)
    membranous (see also N00-N07
      with fourth character .2) N05.2
    mesangial proliferative (see
      also N00-N07 with fourth
      character .3) N05.3
    mesangiocapillary (see also
      N00-N07 with fourth
      character .5) N05.5
    sclerosing N18.9
  endocapillary proliferative (diffuse)
    NEC (see also N00-N07 with
    fourth character .4) N05.4
  extracapillary NEC (see also
    N00-N07 with fourth
    character .7) N05.7
  focal (and segmental) (see also
    N00-N07 with fourth
    character .1) N05.1
  hypocomplementemic —see
    Glomerulonephritis,
    membranoproliferative
  IgA —see Nephropathy, IgA
  immune complex (circulating)
    NEC N05.8
  in (due to)
    amyloidosis E85.4 [N08]
    bilharziasis B65.9 [N08]
    cryoglobulinemia D89.1 [N08]
    defibrination syndrome D65
      [N08]
    diabetes mellitus —see Diabetes,
      glomerulosclerosis
    disseminated intravascular
      coagulation D65 [N08]
    Fabry (-Anderson) disease
      E75.21 [N08]
    Goodpasture's syndrome M31.0
    hemolytic-uremic syndrome
      D59.3
    Henoch (-Schönlein) purpura
      D69.0 [N08]
    lecithin cholesterol
      acyltransferase deficiency
      E78.6 [N08]
    microscopic polyangiitis M31.7
      [N08]
    multiple myeloma C90.0- [N08]
    Plasmodium malariae B52.0
    schistosomiasis B65.9 [N08]
    sepsis A41.9 [N08]
      streptococcal A40- [N08]
    sickle-cell disorders D57.-
      [N08]
    strongyloidiasis B78.9 [N08]
    subacute bacterial endocarditis
      I33.0 [N08]
    syphilis (late) congenital A50.59
      [N08]
    systemic lupus erythematosus
      M32.14
    thrombotic thrombocytopenic
      purpura M31.1 [N08]
    typhoid fever A01.09
    Waldenström macroglobulinemia
      C88.0 [N08]
    Wegener's granulomatosis M31.31
  latent or quiescent N03.9
  lobular, lobulonodular —see
    Glomerulonephritis,
    membranoproliferative
  membranoproliferative (diffuse) (type
    1 or 3) (see also N00-N07 with
    fourth character .5) N05.5
    dense deposit (type 2) NEC (see
      also N00-N07 with fourth
      character .6) N05.6
  membranous (diffuse) NEC (see
    also N00-N07 with fourth
    character .2) N05.2

Glomerulonephritis (continued)
  mesangial
    IgA/IgG —see Nephropathy, IgA
    proliferative (diffuse) NEC (see
      also N00-N07 with fourth
      character .3) N05.3
  mesangiocapillary (diffuse) NEC
    (see also N00-N07 with fourth
    character .5) N05.5
  necrotic, necrotizing NEC (see
    also N00-N07 with fourth
    character .8) N05.8
  nodular —see Glomerulonephritis,
    membranoproliferative
  poststreptococcal NEC N05.9
    acute N00.9
    chronic N03.9
    rapidly progressive N01.9
  proliferative NEC (see also
    N00-N07 with fourth character
    .8) N05.8
    diffuse (lupus) M32.14
  rapidly progressive N01.9
  sclerosing, diffuse N18.9
  specified pathology NEC (see
    also N00-N07 with fourth
    character .8) N05.8
  subacute N01.9

Glomerulopathy —see
  Glomerulonephritis

Glomerulosclerosis —see also
  Sclerosis, renal
  intercapillary (nodular) (with
    diabetes) —see Diabetes,
    glomerulosclerosis
  intracapillary —see Diabetes,
    glomerulosclerosis

Glossagra K14.6

Glossalgia K14.6

Glossitis (chronic superficial)
  (gangrenous) (Moeller's) K14.0
  areata exfoliativa K14.1
  atrophic K14.4
  benign migratory K14.1
  cortical superficial, sclerotic K14.0
  Hunter's D51.0
  interstitial, sclerous K14.0
  median rhomboid K14.2
  pellagrous E52
  superficial, chronic K14.0

Glossocele K14.8

Glossodynia K14.6
  exfoliativa K14.4

Glossoncus K14.8

Glossopathy K14.9

Glossophytia K14.3

Glossoplegia K14.8

Glossoptosis K14.8

Glossopyrosis K14.6

Glossotrichia K14.3

Glossy skin L90.8

Glottis —see condition

Glottitis —see also Laryngitis J04.0

Glucagonoma
  pancreas
    benign D13.7
    malignant C25.4
    uncertain behavior D37.8
  specified site NEC
    benign —see Neoplasm, benign,
      by site
    malignant —see Neoplasm,
      malignant, by site
    uncertain behavior —see
      Neoplasm, uncertain behavior,
      by site

Glucagonoma (continued)
  specified site NEC (continued)
    unspecified site
      benign D13.7
      malignant C25.4
      uncertain behavior D37.8

Glucoglycinuria E72.51

Glucose-galactose malabsorption
  E74.39

Glue
  ear —see Otitis, media,
    nonsuppurative, chronic, mucoid
  sniffing (airplane) —see Abuse,
    drug, inhalant
    dependence —see Dependence,
      drug, inhalant

GLUT1 deficiency syndrome 1,
  infantile onset E74.810

GLUT1 deficiency syndrome 2,
  childhood onset E74.810

Glutaric aciduria E72.3

Glycinemia E72.51

Glycinuria (renal) (with ketosis)
  E72.09

Glycogen
  infiltration —see Disease, glycogen
    storage
  storage disease —see Disease,
    glycogen storage

Glycogenosis (diffuse) (generalized)
  —see also Disease, glycogen
  storage
  cardiac E74.02 [I43]
  diabetic, secondary —see Diabetes,
    glycogenosis, secondary
  pulmonary interstitial J84.842

Glycopenia E16.2

Glycosuria R81
  renal (familial) E74.818

Gnathostoma spinigerum (infection)
  (infestation), gnathostomiasis
  (wandering swelling) B83.1

Goiter (plunging) (substernal) E04.9
  with
    hyperthyroidism (recurrent)
      —see Hyperthyroidism, with,
      goiter
    thyrotoxicosis —see
      Hyperthyroidism, with, goiter
  adenomatous —see Goiter, nodular
  cancerous C73
  congenital (nontoxic) E03.0
    diffuse E03.0
    parenchymatous E03.0
    transitory, with normal
      functioning P72.0
  cystic E04.2
    due to iodine-deficiency E01.1
  due to
    enzyme defect in synthesis of
      thyroid hormone E07.1
    iodine-deficiency (endemic)
      E01.2
  dyshormonogenetic (familial)
    E07.1
  endemic (iodine-deficiency) E01.2
    diffuse E01.0
    multinodular E01.1
  exophthalmic —see
    Hyperthyroidism, with, goiter
  iodine-deficiency (endemic) E01.2
    diffuse E01.0
    multinodular E01.1
    nodular E01.1
  lingual Q89.2
  lymphadenoid E06.3
  malignant C73

Goiter (continued)
multinodular (cystic) (nontoxic)
E04.2
toxic or with hyperthyroidism
E05.20
with thyroid storm E05.21
neonatal NEC P72.0
nodular (nontoxic) (due to) E04.9
with
hyperthyroidism E05.20
with thyroid storm E05.21
thyrotoxicosis E05.20
with thyroid storm E05.21
endemic E01.1
iodine-deficiency E01.1
sporadic E04.9
toxic E05.20
with thyroid storm E05.21
nontoxic E04.9
diffuse (colloid) E04.0
multinodular E04.2
simple E04.0
specified NEC E04.8
uninodular E04.1
simple E04.0
toxic —see Hyperthyroidism, with,
goiter
uninodular (nontoxic) E04.1
toxic or with hyperthyroidism
E05.10
with thyroid storm E05.11

Goiter-deafness syndrome E07.1

Goldberg syndrome Q89.8

Goldberg-Maxwell syndrome
E34.51

Goldblatt's hypertension or kidney
I70.1

Goldenhar (-Gorlin) **syndrome**
Q87.0

Goldflam-Erb disease or syndrome
G70.00
with exacerbation (acute) G70.01
in crisis G70.01

Goldscheider's disease Q81.8

Goldstein's disease (familial
hemorrhagic telangiectasia) I78.0

Golfer's elbow —see Epicondylitis,
medial

Gonadoblastoma
specified site —see Neoplasm,
uncertain behavior, by site
unspecified site
female D39.10
male D40.10

Gonecystitis —see Vesiculitis

Gongylonemiasis B83.8

Goniosynechiae —see Adhesions,
iris, goniosynechiae

Gonococcemia A54.86

Gonococcus, gonococcal (disease)
(infection) (see also condition)
A54.9
anus A54.6
bursa, bursitis A54.49
conjunctiva, conjunctivitis
(neonatorum) A54.31
endocardium A54.83
eye A54.30
conjunctivitis A54.31
iridocyclitis A54.32
keratitis A54.33
newborn A54.31
other specified A54.39
fallopian tubes (acute) (chronic)
A54.24

Gonococcus, gonococcal
(continued)
genitourinary (organ) (system)
(tract) (acute)
lower A54.00
with abscess (accessory gland)
(periurethral) A54.1
upper (see also condition)
A54.29
heart A54.83
iridocyclitis A54.32
joint A54.42
lymphatic (gland) (node) A54.89
meninges, meningitis A54.81
musculoskeletal A54.40
arthritis A54.42
osteomyelitis A54.43
other specified A54.49
spondylopathy A54.41
pelviperitonitis A54.24
pelvis (acute) (chronic) A54.24
pharynx A54.5
proctitis A54.6
pyosalpinx (acute) (chronic)
A54.24
rectum A54.6
skin A54.89
specified site NEC A54.89
tendon sheath A54.49
throat A54.5
urethra (acute) (chronic) A54.01
with abscess (accessory gland)
(periurethral) A54.1
vulva (acute) (chronic) A54.02

Gonocytoma
specified site —see Neoplasm,
uncertain behavior, by site
unspecified site
female D39.10
male D40.10

Gonorrhea (acute) (chronic) A54.9
Bartholin's gland (acute) (chronic)
(purulent) A54.02
with abscess (accessory gland)
(periurethral) A54.1
bladder A54.01
cervix A54.03
conjunctiva, conjunctivitis
(neonatorum) A54.31
contact Z20.2
Cowper's gland (with abscess)
A54.1
exposure to Z20.2
fallopian tube (acute) (chronic)
A54.24
kidney (acute) (chronic) A54.21
lower genitourinary tract
A54.00
with abscess (accessory gland)
(periurethral) A54.1
ovary (acute) (chronic) A54.24
pelvis (acute) (chronic) A54.24
female pelvic inflammatory
disease A54.24
penis A54.09
prostate (acute) (chronic) A54.22
seminal vesicle (acute) (chronic)
A54.23
specified site not listed (see also
Gonococcus) A54.89
spermatic cord (acute) (chronic)
A54.23
urethra A54.01
with abscess (accessory gland)
(periurethral) A54.1
vagina A54.02
vas deferens (acute) (chronic)
A54.23
vulva A54.02

Goodall's disease A08.19

Goodpasture's syndrome M31.0

Gopalan's syndrome (burning feet)
E53.0

Gorlin-Chaudry-Moss syndrome
Q87.0

Gottron's papules L94.4

Gougerot's syndrome
(trisymptomatic) L81.7

Gougerot-Blum syndrome
(pigmented purpuric lichenoid
dermatitis) L81.7

Gougerot-Carteaud disease or
syndrome (confluent reticulate
papillomatosis) L83

Gouley's syndrome (constrictive
pericarditis) I31.1

Goundou A66.6

Gout, gouty (acute) (attack) (flare)
(see also Gout, chronic) M10.9
drug-induced M10.20
ankle M10.27-
elbow M10.22-
foot joint M10.27-
hand joint M10.24-
hip M10.25-
knee M10.26-
multiple site M10.29
shoulder M10.21-
vertebrae M10.28
wrist M10.23-
idiopathic M10.00
ankle M10.07-
elbow M10.02-
foot joint M10.07-
hand joint M10.04-
hip M10.05-
knee M10.06-
multiple site M10.09
shoulder M10.01-
vertebrae M10.08
wrist M10.03-
in (due to) renal impairment
M10.30
ankle M10.37-
elbow M10.32-
foot joint M10.37-
hand joint M10.34-
hip M10.35-
knee M10.36-
multiple site M10.39
shoulder M10.31-
vertebrae M10.38
wrist M10.33-
lead-induced M10.10
ankle M10.17-
elbow M10.12-
foot joint M10.17-
hand joint M10.14-
hip M10.15-
knee M10.16-
multiple site M10.19
shoulder M10.11-
vertebrae M10.18
wrist M10.13-
primary —see Gout, idiopathic
saturnine —see Gout, lead-induced
secondary NEC M10.40
ankle M10.47-
elbow M10.42-
foot joint M10.47-
hand joint M10.44-
hip M10.45-
knee M10.46-
multiple site M10.49
shoulder M10.41-
vertebrae M10.48
wrist M10.43-

Gout, gouty (continued)
syphilitic (see also subcategory
M14.8-) A52.77
tophi —see Gout, chronic

Gout, chronic (see also Gout, gouty)
M1A.9
drug-induced M1A.20
ankle M1A.27-
elbow M1A.22-
foot joint M1A.27-
hand joint M1A.24-
hip M1A.25-
knee M1A.26-
multiple site M1A.29
shoulder M1A.21-
vertebrae M1A.28
wrist M1A.23-
idiopathic M1A.00
ankle M1A.07-
elbow M1A.02-
foot joint M1A.07-
hand joint M1A.04-
hip M1A.05-
knee M1A.06-
multiple site M1A.09
shoulder M1A.01-
vertebrae M1A.08
wrist M1A.03-
in (due to) renal impairment
M1A.30
ankle M1A.37-
elbow M1A.32-
foot joint M1A.37-
hand joint M1A.34-
hip M1A.35-
knee M1A.36-
multiple site M1A.39
shoulder M1A.31-
vertebrae M1A.38
wrist M1A.33-
lead-induced M1A.10
ankle M1A.17-
elbow M1A.12-
foot joint M1A.17-
hand joint M1A.14-
hip M1A.15-
knee M1A.16-
multiple site M1A.19
shoulder M1A.11-
vertebrae M1A.18
wrist M1A.13-
primary —see Gout, chronic,
idiopathic
saturnine —see Gout, chronic,
lead-induced
secondary NEC M1A.40
ankle M1A.47-
elbow M1A.42-
foot joint M1A.47-
hand joint M1A.44-
hip M1A.45-
knee M1A.46-
multiple site M1A.49
shoulder M1A.41-
vertebrae M1A.48
wrist M1A.43-
syphilitic (see also subcategory
M14.8-) A52.77
tophi M1A.9

Gower's
muscular dystrophy G71.01
syndrome (vasovagal attack)
R55

Gradenigo's syndrome —see Otitis,
media, suppurative, acute

Graefe's disease —see Strabismus,
paralytic, ophthalmoplegia,
progressive

Graft-versus-host disease
D89.813
acute D89.810
acute on chronic D89.812
chronic D89.811

Grainhandler's disease or lung J67.8

Grain mite (itch) B88.0

Grand mal —see Epilepsy,
generalized, specified NEC

Grand multipara status only (not
pregnant) Z64.1
pregnant —see Pregnancy,
complicated by, grand
multiparity

Granite worker's lung J62.8

Granular —see also condition
inflammation, pharynx J31.2
kidney (contracting) —see
Sclerosis, renal
liver K74.69

Granulation tissue (abnormal)
(excessive) L92.9
postmastoidectomy cavity
—see Complications,
postmastoidectomy, granulation

Granulocytopenia (primary)
(malignant) —see Agranulocytosis

Granuloma L92.9
abdomen K66.8
from residual foreign body L92.3
pyogenicum L98.0
actinic L57.5
annulare (perforating) L92.0
apical K04.5
aural —see Otitis, externa,
specified NEC
beryllium (skin) L92.3
bone
eosinophilic C96.6
from residual foreign body —see
Osteomyelitis, specified type
NEC
lung C96.6
brain (any site) G06.0
schistosomiasis B65.9 [G07]
canaliculus lacrimalis —see
Granuloma, lacrimal
candidal (cutaneous) B37.2
cerebral (any site) G06.0
coccidioidal (primary)
(progressive) B38.7
lung B38.1
meninges B38.4
colon K63.89
conjunctiva H11.22-
dental K04.5
ear, middle —see Cholesteatoma
eosinophilic C96.6
bone C96.6
lung C96.6
oral mucosa K13.4
skin L92.2
eyelid H01.8
facial (e) L92.2
foreign body (in soft tissue) NEC
M60.20
ankle M60.27-
foot M60.27-
forearm M60.23-
hand M60.24-
in operation wound —see
Foreign body, accidentally left
during a procedure
lower leg M60.26-
pelvic region M60.25-
shoulder region M60.21-
skin L92.3

Granuloma (continued)
foreign body NEC (continued)
specified site NEC M60.28
subcutaneous tissue L92.3
thigh M60.25-
upper arm M60.22-
gangraenescens M31.2
genito-inguinale A58
giant cell (central) (reparative)
(jaw) M27.1
gingiva (peripheral) K06.8
gland (lymph) I88.8
hepatic NEC K75.3
in (due to)
berylliosis J63.2 [K77]
sarcoidosis D86.89
Hodgkin C81.9
ileum K63.89
infectious B99.9
specified NEC B99.8
inguinale (Donovan) (venereal)
A58
intestine NEC K63.89
intracranial (any site) G06.0
intraspinal (any part) G06.1
iridocyclitis —see Iridocyclitis,
chronic
jaw (bone) (central) M27.1
reparative giant cell M27.1
kidney (see also Infection, kidney)
N15.8
lacrimal H04.81-
larynx J38.7
lethal midline (faciale(e)) M31.2
liver NEC —see Granuloma,
hepatic
lung (infectious) —see also
Fibrosis, lung
coccidioidal B38.1
eosinophilic C96.6
Majocchi's B35.8
malignant (facial(e)) M31.2
mandible (central) M27.1
midline (lethal) M31.2
monilial (cutaneous) B37.2
nasal sinus —see Sinusitis
operation wound T81.89
foreign body —see Foreign
body, accidentally left during
a procedure
stitch T81.89
talc —see Foreign body,
accidentally left during a
procedure
oral mucosa K13.4
orbit, orbital H05.11-
paracoccidioidal B41.8
penis, venereal A58
periapical K04.5
peritoneum K66.8
due to ova of helminths NOS
(see also Helminthiasis) B83.9
[K67]
postmastoidectomy cavity
—see Complications,
postmastoidectomy, recurrent
cholesteatoma
prostate N42.89
pudendi (ulcerating) A58
pulp, internal (tooth) K03.3
pyogenic, pyogenicum (of) (skin)
L98.0
gingiva K06.8
maxillary alveolar ridge K04.5
oral mucosa K13.4
rectum K62.89
reticulohistiocytic D76.3
rubrum nasi L74.8
Schistosoma —see
Schistosomiasis
septic (skin) L98.0

Granuloma (continued)
silica (skin) L92.3
sinus (accessory) (infective) (nasal)
—see Sinusitis
skin L92.9
from residual foreign body L92.3
pyogenicum L98.0
spine
syphilitic (epidural) A52.19
tuberculous A18.01
stitch (postoperative) T81.89
suppurative (skin) L98.0
swimming pool A31.1
talc —see also Granuloma, foreign
body
in operation wound —see
Foreign body, accidentally left
during a procedure
telangiectaticum (skin) L98.0
tracheostomy J95.09
trichophyticum B35.8
tropicum A66.4
umbilical P83.81
umbilicus P83.81
urethra N36.8
uveitis —see Iridocyclitis, chronic
vagina A58
venereum A58
vocal cord J38.3

Granulomatosis L92.9
with polyangiitis M31.3
eosinophilic, with polyangiitis
[EGPA] M30.1
lymphoid C83.8-
miliary (listerial) A32.89
necrotizing, respiratory M31.30
progressive septic D71
specified NEC L92.8
Wegener's M31.30
with renal involvement M31.31

Granulomatous tissue (abnormal)
(excessive) L92.9

Granulosis rubra nasi L74.8

Graphite fibrosis (of lung) J63.3

Graphospasm F48.8
organic G25.89

Grating scapula M89.8X1

Gravel (urinary) —see Calculus,
urinary

Graves' disease —see
Hyperthyroidism, with, goiter

Gravis —see condition

Grawitz tumor C64.-

Gray syndrome (newborn) P93.0

Grayness, hair (premature) L67.1
congenital Q84.2

Green sickness D50.8

Greenfield's disease
meaning
concentric sclerosis
(encephalitis periaxialis
concentrica) G37.5
metachromatic leukodystrophy
E75.25

Greenstick fracture - code as
Fracture, by site

Grey syndrome (newborn) P93.0

Grief F43.21
prolonged F43.29
reaction (see also Disorder,
adjustment) F43.20

Griesinger's disease B76.0

Grinder's lung or pneumoconiosis
J62.8

Grinding, teeth
psychogenic F45.8
sleep related G47.63

Grip
Dabney's B33.0
devil's B33.0

Grippe, grippal —see also Influenza
Balkan A78
summer, of Italy A93.1

Grisel's disease M43.6

Groin —see condition

Grooved tongue K14.5

Ground itch B76.9

Grover's disease or syndrome L11.1

Growing pains, children R29.898

Growth (fungoid) (neoplastic) (new)
—see also Neoplasm
adenoid (vegetative) J35.8
benign —see Neoplasm, benign,
by site
malignant —see Neoplasm,
malignant, by site
rapid, childhood Z00.2
secondary —see Neoplasm,
secondary, by site

Gruby's disease B35.0

Gubler-Millard paralysis or
syndrome G46.3

Guerin-Stern syndrome Q74.3

Guidance, insufficient anterior
(occlusal) M26.54

Guillain-Barré disease or syndrome
G61.0
sequelae G65.0

Guinea worms (infection)
(infestation) B72

Guinon's disease (motor-verbal tic)
F95.2

Gull's disease E03.4

Gum —see condition

Gumboil K04.7
with sinus K04.6

Gumma (syphilitic) A52.79
artery A52.09
cerebral A52.04
bone A52.77
of yaws (late) A66.6
brain A52.19
cauda equina A52.19
central nervous system A52.3
ciliary body A52.71
congenital A50.59
eyelid A52.71
heart A52.06
intracranial A52.19
iris A52.71
kidney A52.75
larynx A52.73
leptomeninges A52.19
liver A52.74
meninges A52.19
myocardium A52.06
nasopharynx A52.73
neurosyphilitic A52.3
nose A52.73
orbit A52.71
palate (soft) A52.79
penis A52.76
pericardium A52.06
pharynx A52.73
pituitary A52.79
scrofulous (tuberculous) A18.4
skin A52.79
specified site NEC A52.79

Gumma *(continued)*
  spinal cord A52.19
  tongue A52.79
  tonsil A52.73
  trachea A52.73
  tuberculous A18.4
  ulcerative due to yaws A66.4
  ureter A52.75
  yaws A66.4
    bone A66.6

Gunn's syndrome Q07.8

Gunshot wound —*see also* Puncture, open
  fracture - code as Fracture, by site
  internal organs —*see* Injury, by site

Gynandrism Q56.0

Gynandroblastoma
  specified site —*see* Neoplasm, uncertain behavior, by site
  unspecified site
    female D39.10
    male D40.10

Gynecological examination (periodic) (routine) Z01.419
  with abnormal findings Z01.411

Gynecomastia N62

Gynephobia F40.291

Gyrate scalp Q82.8

H

H (Hartnup's) **disease** E72.02

Haas' disease or osteochondrosis (juvenile) (head of humerus) —*see* Osteochondrosis, juvenile, humerus

Habit, habituation
  bad sleep Z72.821
  chorea F95.8
  disturbance, child F98.9
  drug —*see* Dependence, drug
  irregular sleep Z72.821
  laxative F55.2
  spasm —*see* Tic
  tic —*see* Tic

Haemophilus (H.) **influenzae, as cause of disease classified elsewhere** B96.3

Haff disease —*see* Poisoning, mercury

Hageman's factor defect, deficiency or disease D68.2

Haglund's disease or osteochondrosis (juvenile) (os tibiale externum) —*see* Osteochondrosis, juvenile, tarsus

Hailey-Hailey disease Q82.8

Hair —*see also* condition
  plucking F63.3
    in stereotyped movement disorder F98.4
  tourniquet syndrome —*see also* Constriction, external, by site
    finger S60.44-
    penis S30.842
    thumb S60.34-
    toe S90.44-

Hairball in stomach T18.2

Hair-pulling, pathological (compulsive) F63.3

Hairy black tongue K14.3

Half vertebra Q76.49

Halitosis R19.6

Hallerman-Streiff syndrome Q87.0

Hallervorden-Spatz disease G23.0

Hallopeau's acrodermatitis or disease L40.2

Hallucination R44.3
  auditory R44.0
  gustatory R44.2
  olfactory R44.2
  specified NEC R44.2
  tactile R44.2
  visual R44.1

Hallucinosis (chronic) F28
  alcoholic (acute) F10.951
    in
      abuse F10.151
      dependence F10.251
  drug-induced F19.951
    cannabis F12.951
    cocaine F14.951
    hallucinogen F16.151
    in
      abuse F19.151
        cannabis F12.151
        cocaine F14.151
        hallucinogen F16.151
        inhalant F18.151
        opioid F11.151
        sedative, anxiolytic or hypnotic F13.151
        stimulant NEC F15.151
      dependence F19.251
        cannabis F12.251
        cocaine F14.251
        hallucinogen F16.251
        inhalant F18.251
        opioid F11.251
        sedative, anxiolytic or hypnotic F13.251
        stimulant NEC F15.251
    inhalant F18.951
    opioid F11.951
    sedative, anxiolytic or hypnotic F13.951
    stimulant NEC F15.951
  organic F06.0

Hallux
  deformity (acquired) NEC M20.5X-
  limitus M20.5X-
  malleus (acquired) NEC M20.3-
  rigidus (acquired) M20.2-
    congenital Q74.2
    sequelae (late effect) of rickets E64.3
  valgus (acquired) M20.1-
    congenital Q66.6
  varus (acquired) M20.3-
    congenital Q66.3-

Halo, visual H53.19

Hamartoma, hamartoblastoma Q85.9
  epithelial (gingival), odontogenic, central or peripheral —*see* Cyst, calcifying odontogenic

Hamartosis Q85.9

Hamman-Rich syndrome J84.114

Hammer toe (acquired) **NEC** —*see also* Deformity, toe, hammer toe
  congenital Q66.89
  sequelae (late effect) of rickets E64.3

Hand —*see* condition

Hand-foot syndrome L27.1

Handicap, handicapped
  educational Z55.9
  specified NEC Z55.8

Hand-Schüller-Christian disease or syndrome C96.5

Hanging (asphyxia) (strangulation) (suffocation) —*see* Asphyxia, traumatic, due to mechanical threat

Hangnail —*see also* Cellulitis, digit
  with lymphangitis —*see* Lymphangitis, acute, digit

Hangover (alcohol) F10.129

Hanhart's syndrome Q87.0

Hanot-Chauffard (-Troisier) **syndrome** E83.19

Hanot's cirrhosis or disease K74.3

Hansen's disease —*see* Leprosy

Hantaan virus disease (Korean hemorrhagic fever) A98.5

Hantavirus disease (with renal manifestations) (Dobrava) (Puumala) (Seoul) A98.5
  with pulmonary manifestations (Andes) (Bayou) (Bermejo) (Black Creek Canal) (Choclo) (Juquitiba) (Laguna negra) (Lechiguanas) (New York) (Oran) (Sin nombre) B33.4

Happy puppet syndrome Q93.51

Harada's disease or syndrome H30.81-

Hardening
  artery —*see* Arteriosclerosis
  brain G93.89

Harelip (complete) (incomplete) —*see* Cleft, lip

Harlequin (newborn) Q80.4

Harley's disease D59.6

Harmful use (of)
  alcohol F10.10
  anxiolytics —*see* Abuse, drug, sedative
  cannabinoids —*see* Abuse, drug, cannabis
  cocaine —*see* Abuse, drug, cocaine
  drug —*see* Abuse, drug
  hallucinogens —*see* Abuse, drug, hallucinogen
  hypnotics —*see* Abuse, drug, sedative
  opioids —*see* Abuse, drug, opioid
  PCP (phencyclidine) —*see* Abuse, drug, hallucinogen
  sedatives —*see* Abuse, drug, sedative
  stimulants NEC —*see* Abuse, drug, stimulant

Harris' lines —*see* Arrest, epiphyseal

Hartnup's disease E72.02

Harvester's lung J67.0

Harvesting ovum for in vitro fertilization Z31.83

Hashimoto's disease or thyroiditis E06.3

Hashitoxicosis (transient) E06.3

Hassal-Henle bodies or warts (cornea) H18.49

Haut mal —*see* Epilepsy, generalized, specified NEC

Haverhill fever A25.1

Hay fever (*see also* Fever, hay) J30.1

Hayem-Widal syndrome D59.8

Haygarth's nodes M15.8

Haymaker's lung J67.0

Hb (abnormal)
  Bart's disease D56.0
  disease —*see* Disease, hemoglobin
  trait —*see* Trait

Head —*see* condition

Headache R51.9
  with
    orthostatic component NEC R51.0
    positional component NEC R51.0
  allergic NEC G44.89
  associated with sexual activity G44.82
  chronic daily R51.9
  cluster G44.009
    chronic G44.029
      intractable G44.021
      not intractable G44.029
    episodic G44.019
      intractable G44.011
      not intractable G44.019
    intractable G44.001
    not intractable G44.009
  cough (primary) G44.83
  daily chronic R51.9
  drug-induced NEC G44.40
    intractable G44.41
    not intractable G44.40
  exertional (primary) G44.84
  histamine G44.009
    intractable G44.001
    not intractable G44.009
  hypnic G44.81
  lumbar puncture G97.1
  medication overuse G44.40
    intractable G44.41
    not intractable G44.40
  menstrual —*see* Migraine, menstrual
  migraine (type) (*see also* Migraine) G43.909
  nasal septum R51.9
  neuralgiform, short lasting unilateral, with conjunctival injection and tearing (SUNCT) G44.059
    intractable G44.051
    not intractable G44.059
  new daily persistent (NDPH) G44.52
  orgasmic G44.82
  periodic syndromes in adults and children G43.C0
    with refractory migraine G43.C1
    intractable G43.C1
    not intractable G43.C0
    without refractory migraine G43.C0
  postspinal puncture G97.1
  post-traumatic G44.309
    acute G44.319
      intractable G44.311
      not intractable G44.319
    chronic G44.329
      intractable G44.321
      not intractable G44.329
    intractable G44.301
    not intractable G44.309
  pre-menstrual —*see* Migraine, menstrual
  preorgasmic G44.82
  primary
    cough G44.83
    exertional G44.84
    stabbing G44.85
    thunderclap G44.53
  rebound G44.40
    intractable G44.41
    not intractable G44.40
  short lasting unilateral
    neuralgiform, with conjunctival injection and tearing (SUNCT) G44.059
    intractable G44.051
    not intractable G44.059
  specified syndrome NEC G44.89

Headache *(continued)*
spinal and epidural anesthesia -
induced T88.59
in labor and delivery O74.5
in pregnancy O29.4-
postpartum, puerperal O89.4
spinal fluid loss (from puncture)
G97.1
stabbing (primary) G44.85
tension (-type) G44.209
chronic G44.229
intractable G44.221
not intractable G44.229
episodic G44.219
intractable G44.211
not intractable G44.219
intractable G44.201
not intractable G44.209
thunderclap (primary) G44.53
vascular NEC G44.1

Healthy
infant
accompanying sick mother Z76.3
receiving care Z76.2
person accompanying sick person
Z76.3

Hearing examination Z01.10
with abnormal findings NEC
Z01.118
following failed hearing screening
Z01.110
for hearing conservation and
treatment Z01.12
infant or child (over 28 days old)
Z00.129
with abnormal finding Z00.121

Heart —*see* condition

Heart beat
abnormality R00.9
specified NEC R00.8
awareness R00.2
rapid R00.0
slow R00.1

Heartburn R12
psychogenic F45.8

Heartland virus disease A93.8

Heat (effects) T67.9
apoplexy T67.01
burn (*see also* Burn) L55.9
collapse T67.1
cramps T67.2
dermatitis or eczema L59.0
edema T67.7
erythema - code by site under Burn,
first degree
excessive T67.9
specified effect NEC T67.8
exhaustion T67.5
anhydrotic T67.3
due to
salt (and water) depletion
T67.4
water depletion T67.3
with salt depletion T67.4
fatigue (transient) T67.6
fever T67.01
hyperpyrexia T67.01
prickly L74.0
prostration —*see* Heat,
exhaustion
pyrexia T67.01
rash L74.0
specified effect NEC T67.8
stroke T67.01
exertional T67.02
specified NEC T67.09
sunburn —*see* Sunburn
syncope T67.1

Heavy-for-dates NEC (infant)
(4000g to 4499g) P08.1
exceptionally (4500g or more)
P08.0

Hebephrenia, hebephrenic
(schizophrenia) F20.1

Heberden's disease or nodes (with
arthropathy) M15.1

Hebra's
pityriasis L26
prurigo L28.2

Heel —*see* condition

Heerfordt's disease D86.89

Hegglin's anomaly or syndrome
D72.0

Heilmeyer-Schoner disease D45

Heine-Medin disease A80.9

Heinz body anemia, congenital
D58.2

Heliophobia F40.228

Heller's disease or syndrome F84.3

HELLP syndrome (hemolysis,
elevated liver enzymes and low
platelet count) O14.2-
complicating
childbirth O14.24
puerperium O14.25

Helminthiasis —*see also* Infestation,
helminth
Ancylostoma B76.0
intestinal B82.0
mixed types (types classifiable
to more than one of the titles
B65.0-B81.3 and B81.8)
B81.4
specified type NEC B81.8
mixed types (intestinal) (types
classifiable to more than one
of the titles B65.0-B81.3 and
B81.8) B81.4
Necator (americanus) B76.1
specified type NEC B83.8

Heloma L84

Hemangioblastoma —*see* Neoplasm,
connective tissue, uncertain
behavior
malignant —*see* Neoplasm,
connective tissue, malignant

Hemangioendothelioma —*see also*
Neoplasm, uncertain behavior,
by site
benign D18.00
intra-abdominal D18.03
intracranial D18.02
skin D18.01
specified site NEC D18.09
bone (diffuse) —*see* Neoplasm,
bone, malignant
epithelioid —*see also* Neoplasm,
uncertain behavior, by site
malignant —*see* Neoplasm,
malignant, by site
malignant —*see* Neoplasm,
connective tissue,
malignant

Hemangiofibroma —*see* Neoplasm,
benign, by site

Hemangiolipoma —*see* Lipoma

Hemangioma D18.00
arteriovenous D18.00
intra-abdominal D18.03
intracranial D18.02
skin D18.01
specified site NEC D18.09

Hemangioma *(continued)*
capillary I78.1
intra-abdominal D18.03
intracranial D18.02
skin D18.01
specified site NEC D18.09
cavernous D18.00
intra-abdominal D18.03
intracranial D18.02
skin D18.01
specified site NEC D18.09
epithelioid D18.00
intra-abdominal D18.03
intracranial D18.02
skin D18.01
specified site NEC D18.09
histiocytoid D18.00
intra-abdominal D18.03
intracranial D18.02
skin D18.01
specified site NEC D18.09
infantile D18.00
intra-abdominal D18.03
intracranial D18.02
skin D18.01
specified site NEC D18.09
intra-abdominal D18.03
intracranial D18.02
intramuscular D18.00
intra-abdominal D18.03
intracranial D18.02
skin D18.01
specified site NEC D18.09
intrathoracic structures D18.09
juvenile D18.00
malignant —*see*
Neoplasm, connective tissue,
malignant
plexiform D18.00
intra-abdominal D18.03
intracranial D18.02
skin D18.01
specified site NEC D18.09
racemose D18.00
intra-abdominal D18.03
intracranial D18.02
skin D18.01
specified site NEC D18.09
sclerosing —*see* Neoplasm, skin,
benign
simplex D18.00
intra-abdominal D18.03
intracranial D18.02
skin D18.01
specified site NEC D18.09
skin D18.01
specified site NEC D18.09
venous D18.00
intra-abdominal D18.03
intracranial D18.02
skin D18.01
specified site NEC D18.09
verrucous keratotic D18.00
intra-abdominal D18.03
intracranial D18.02
skin D18.01
specified site NEC D18.09

Hemangiomatosis (systemic) I78.8
involving single site —*see*
Hemangioma

Hemangiopericytoma —*see also*
Neoplasm, connective tissue,
uncertain behavior
benign —*see* Neoplasm, connective
tissue, benign
malignant —*see* Neoplasm,
connective tissue, malignant

Hemangiosarcoma —*see* Neoplasm,
connective tissue, malignant

Hemarthrosis (nontraumatic)
M25.00
ankle M25.07-
elbow M25.02-
foot joint M25.07-
hand joint M25.04-
hip M25.05-
in hemophilic arthropathy —*see*
Arthropathy, hemophilic
knee M25.06-
shoulder M25.01-
specified joint NEC M25.08
traumatic —*see* Sprain, by site
vertebrae M25.08
wrist M25.03-

Hematemesis K92.0
with ulcer - code by site under
Ulcer, with hemorrhage K27.4
newborn, neonatal P54.0
due to swallowed maternal blood
P78.2

Hematidrosis L74.8

Hematinuria —*see also*
Hemoglobinuria
malarial B50.8

Hematobilia K83.8

Hematocele
female NEC N94.89
with ectopic pregnancy
O00.90
with intrauterine pregnancy
O00.91
ovary N83.8
male N50.1

Hematochezia (*see also* Melena)
K92.1

Hematochyluria —*see also*
Infestation, filarial
schistosomiasis (bilharziasis) B65.0

Hematocolpos (with hematometra or
hematosalpinx) N89.7

Hematocornea —*see* Pigmentation,
cornea, stromal

Hematogenous —*see* condition

Hematoma (traumatic) (skin surface
intact) —*see also* Contusion
with
injury of internal organs —*see*
Injury, by site
open wound —*see* Wound, open
amputation stump (surgical) (late)
T87.89
aorta, dissecting I71.00
abdominal I71.02
thoracic I71.01
thoracoabdominal I71.03
aortic intramural —*see* Dissection,
aorta
arterial (complicating trauma) —
see Injury, blood vessel, by site
auricle —*see* Contusion, ear
nontraumatic —*see* Disorder,
pinna, hematoma
birth injury NEC P15.8
brain (traumatic)
with
cerebral laceration or
contusion (diffuse) —*see*
Injury, intracranial, diffuse
focal —*see* Injury,
intracranial, focal
cerebellar, traumatic S06.37-
newborn NEC P52.4
birth injury P10.1
intracerebral, traumatic —
see Injury, intracranial,
intracerebral hemorrhage

Hematoma (*continued*)
brain (*continued*)
nontraumatic —*see* Hemorrhage,
intracranial
subarachnoid, arachnoid,
traumatic —*see* Injury,
intracranial, subarachnoid
hemorrhage
subdural, traumatic —*see*
Injury, intracranial, subdural
hemorrhage
breast (nontraumatic) N64.89
broad ligament (nontraumatic)
N83.7
traumatic S37.892
cerebellar, traumatic S06.37-
cerebral —*see* Hematoma, brain
cerebrum S06.36-
left S06.35-
right S06.34-
cesarean delivery wound O90.2
complicating delivery (perineal)
(pelvic) (vagina) (vulva) O71.7
corpus cavernosum (nontraumatic)
N48.89
epididymis (nontraumatic) N50.1
epidural (traumatic) —*see* Injury,
intracranial, epidural hemorrhage
spinal —*see* Injury, spinal cord,
by region
episiotomy O90.2
face, birth injury P15.4
genital organ NEC (nontraumatic)
female (nonobstetric) N94.89
traumatic S30.202
male N50.1
traumatic S30.201
internal organs —*see* Injury, by site
intracerebral, traumatic —*see*
Injury, intracranial, intracerebral
hemorrhage
intraoperative —*see* Complications,
intraoperative, hemorrhage
labia (nontraumatic) (nonobstetric)
N90.89
liver (subcapsular) (nontraumatic)
K76.89
birth injury P15.0
mediastinum —*see* Injury,
intrathoracic
mesosalpinx (nontraumatic) N83.7
traumatic S37.898
muscle - code by site under
Contusion
nontraumatic
muscle M79.81
soft tissue M79.81
obstetrical surgical wound O90.2
orbit, orbital (nontraumatic) —*see*
also Hemorrhage, orbit
traumatic —*see* Contusion, orbit
pelvis (female) (nontraumatic)
(nonobstetric) N94.89
obstetric O71.7
traumatic —*see* Injury, by site
penis (nontraumatic) N48.89
birth injury P15.5
perianal (nontraumatic) K64.5
perineal S30.23
complicating delivery O71.7
perirenal —*see* Injury, kidney
pinna —*see* Contusion, ear
nontraumatic —*see* Disorder,
pinna, hematoma
placenta O43.89-
postoperative (postprocedural)
—*see* Complication,
postprocedural, hematoma
retroperitoneal (nontraumatic)
K66.1
traumatic S36.892

Hematoma (*continued*)
scrotum, superficial S30.22
birth injury P15.5
seminal vesicle (nontraumatic) N50.1
traumatic S37.892
spermatic cord (traumatic) S37.892
nontraumatic N50.1
spinal (cord) (meninges) —*see also*
Injury, spinal cord, by region
newborn (birth injury) P11.5
spleen D73.5
intraoperative —*see*
Complications, intraoperative,
hemorrhage, spleen
postprocedural (postoperative)
—*see* Complications,
postprocedural, hemorrhage,
spleen
sternocleidomastoid, birth injury
P15.2
sternomastoid, birth injury P15.2
subarachnoid (traumatic) —*see*
Injury, intracranial, subarachnoid
hemorrhage
newborn (nontraumatic) P52.5
due to birth injury P10.3
nontraumatic —*see* Hemorrhage,
intracranial, subarachnoid
subdural (traumatic) —*see*
Injury, intracranial, subdural
hemorrhage
newborn (localized) P52.8
birth injury P10.0
nontraumatic —*see* Hemorrhage,
intracranial, subdural
superficial, newborn P54.5
testis (nontraumatic) N50.1
birth injury P15.5
tunica vaginalis (nontraumatic) N50.1
umbilical cord, complicating
delivery O69.5
uterine ligament (broad)
(nontraumatic) N83.7
traumatic S37.892
vagina (ruptured) (nontraumatic)
N89.8
complicating delivery O71.7
vas deferens (nontraumatic) N50.1
traumatic S37.892
vitreous —*see* Hemorrhage, vitreous
vulva (nontraumatic) (nonobstetric)
N90.89
complicating delivery O71.7
newborn (birth injury) P15.5

Hematometra N85.7
with hematocolpos N89.7

Hematomyelia (central) G95.19
newborn (birth injury) P11.5
traumatic T14.8

Hematomyelitis G04.90

Hematoperitoneum —*see*
Hemoperitoneum

Hematophobia F40.230

Hematopneumothorax (*see*
Hemothorax)

Hematopoiesis, cyclic D70.4

Hematoporphyria —*see* Porphyria

Hematorachis, hematorrhachis
G95.19
newborn (birth injury) P11.5

Hematosalpinx N83.6
with
hematocolpos N89.7
hematometra N85.7
with hematocolpos N89.7
infectional —*see* Salpingitis

Hematospermia R36.1

Hematothorax (see Hemothorax)

Hematuria R31.9
due to sulphonamide, sulfonamide
—*see* Table of Drugs and
Chemicals, by drug
benign (familial) (of childhood) —
see also Hematuria, idiopathic
essential microscopic R31.1
endemic (*see also* Schistosomiasis)
B65.0
gross R31.0
idiopathic N02.9
with glomerular lesion
C3
glomerulonepritis N02.A
glomerulopathy N02.A
with dense deposit
disease N02.6
crescentic (diffuse)
glomerulonephritis N02.7
dense deposit disease N02.6
endocapillary proliferative
glomerulonephritis N02.4
focal and segmental hyalinosis
or sclerosis N02.1
membranoproliferative
(diffuse) N02.5
membranous (diffuse) N02.2
mesangial proliferative
(diffuse) N02.3
mesangiocapillary (diffuse)
N02.5
minor abnormality N02.0
proliferative NEC N02.8
specified pathology NEC N02.8
intermittent —*see* Hematuria,
idiopathic
malarial B50.8
microscopic NEC (with symptoms)
R31.29
asymptomatic R31.21
benign essential R31.1
paroxysmal —*see also* Hematuria,
idiopathic
nocturnal D59.5
persistent —*see* Hematuria,
idiopathic
recurrent —*see* Hematuria,
idiopathic
tropical (*see also* Schistosomiasis)
B65.0
tuberculous A18.13

Hemeralopia (day blindness) H53.11
vitamin A deficiency E50.5

Hemi-akinesia R41.4

Hemianalgesia R20.0

Hemianencephaly Q00.0

Hemianesthesia R20.0

Hemianopia, hemianopsia
(heteronymous) H53.47
homonymous H53.46-
syphilitic A52.71

Hemiathetosis R25.8

Hemiatrophy R68.89
cerebellar G31.9
face, facial, progressive (Romberg)
G51.8
tongue K14.8

Hemiballism (us) G25.5

Hemicardia Q24.8

Hemicephalus, hemicephaly Q00.0

Hemichorea G25.5

Hemicolitis, left —*see* Colitis, left sided

Hemicrania
congenital malformation Q00.0
continua G44.51

Hemicrania (*continued*)
meaning migraine (*see also*
Migraine) G43.909
paroxysmal G44.039
chronic G44.049
intractable G44.041
not intractable G44.049
episodic G44.039
intractable G44.031
not intractable G44.039
intractable G44.031
not intractable G44.039

Hemidystrophy —*see* Hemiatrophy

Hemiectromelia Q73.8

Hemihypalgesia R20.8

Hemihypesthesia R20.1

Hemi-inattention R41.4

Hemimelia Q73.8
lower limb —*see* Defect, reduction,
lower limb, specified type NEC
upper limb —*see* Defect, reduction,
upper limb, specified type NEC

Hemiparalysis —*see* Hemiplegia

Hemiparesis —*see* Hemiplegia

Hemiparesthesia R20.2

Hemiparkinsonism G20

Hemiplegia G81.9-
alternans facialis G83.89
ascending NEC G81.90
spinal G95.89
congenital (cerebral) G80.8
spastic G80.2
embolic (current episode) I63.4-
flaccid G81.0-
following
cerebrovascular disease I69.959
cerebral infarction I69.35-
intracerebral hemorrhage
I69.15-
nontraumatic intracranial
hemorrhage NEC I69.25-
specified disease NEC I69.85-
stroke NOS I69.35-
subarachnoid hemorrhage
I69.05-
hysterical F44.4
newborn NEC P91.88
birth injury P11.9
spastic G81.1-
congenital G80.2
thrombotic (current episode)
I63.3-

Hemisection, spinal cord —*see*
Injury, spinal cord, by region

Hemispasm (facial) R25.2

Hemisporosis B48.8

Hemitremor R25.1

Hemivertebra Q76.49
failure of segmentation with
scoliosis Q76.3
fusion with scoliosis Q76.3

Hemochromatosis E83.119
with refractory anemia D46.1
due to repeated red blood cell
transfusion E83.111
hereditary (primary) E83.110
neonatal P78.84
primary E83.110
specified NEC E83.118

Hemoglobin —*see also* condition
abnormal (disease) —*see* Disease,
hemoglobin
AS genotype D57.3
Constant Spring D58.2

Hemoglobin (continued)
  E-beta thalassemia D56.5
  fetal, hereditary persistence
    (HPFH) D56.4
  H Constant Spring D56.0
  low NOS D64.9
  S (Hb S), heterozygous D57.3
Hemoglobinemia D59.9
  due to blood transfusion T80.89
  paroxysmal D59.6
    nocturnal D59.5
Hemoglobinopathy (mixed) D58.2
  with thalassemia D56.8
  sickle-cell D57.1
    with thalassemia D57.40
      with
        acute chest syndrome
          D57.411
        cerebral vascular
          involvement D57.413
        crisis (painful) D57.419
          with specified
            complication NEC
            D57.418
        splenic sequestration
          D57.412
        vasooclusive pain D57.419
      without crisis D57.40
Hemoglobinuria R82.3
  with anemia, hemolytic, acquired
    (chronic) NEC D59.6
  cold (paroxysmal) (with Raynaud's
    syndrome) D59.6
    agglutinin D59.12
  due to exertion or hemolysis NEC
    D59.6
  intermittent D59.6
  malarial B50.8
  march D59.6
  nocturnal (paroxysmal) D59.5
  paroxysmal (cold) D59.6
    nocturnal D59.5
Hemolymphangioma D18.1
Hemolysis
  intravascular
    with
      abortion —see Abortion,
        by type, complicated by,
        hemorrhage
      ectopic or molar pregnancy
        O08.1
      hemorrhage
        antepartum —see
          Hemorrhage, antepartum,
          with coagulation defect
        intrapartum (see also
          Hemorrhage, complicating,
          delivery) O67.0
      postpartum O72.3
  neonatal (excessive) P58.9
    specified NEC P58.8
Hemolytic —see condition
Hemopericardium I31.2
  following acute myocardial infarction
    (current complication) I23.0
  newborn P54.8
  traumatic —see Injury, heart, with
    hemopericardium
Hemoperitoneum K66.1
  infectional K65.9
  traumatic S36.899
    with open wound —see Wound,
      open, with penetration into
      peritoneal cavity
Hemophilia (classical) (familial)
  (hereditary) D66
  A D66
  B D67
  C D68.1

Hemophilia (continued)
  acquired D68.311
  autoimmune D68.311
Hemophilia
  calcipriva (see also Defect,
    coagulation) D68.4
  nonfamilial (see also Defect,
    coagulation) D68.4
  secondary D68.311
  vascular D68.0
Hemophthalmos H44.81-
Hemopneumothorax —see also
  Hemothorax
  traumatic S27.2
Hemoptysis R04.2
  newborn P26.9
  tuberculous —see Tuberculosis,
    pulmonary
Hemorrhage, hemorrhagic
  (concealed) R58
  abdomen R58
  accidental antepartum —see
    Hemorrhage, antepartum
  acute idiopathic pulmonary, in
    infants R04.81
  adenoid J35.8
  adrenal (capsule) (gland) E27.49
    medulla E27.8
    newborn P54.4
  after delivery —see Hemorrhage,
    postpartum
  alveolar
    lung, newborn P26.8
    process K08.89
  alveolus K08.89
  amputation stump (surgical) T87.89
  anemia (chronic) D50.0
    acute D62
  antepartum (with) O46.90
    with coagulation defect O46.00-
      afibrinogenemia O46.01-
      disseminated intravascular
        coagulation O46.02-
      hypofibrinogenemia O46.01-
      specified defect NEC O46.09-
    before 20 weeks gestation O20.9
      specified type NEC O20.8
      threatened abortion O20.0
    due to
      abruptio placenta (see also
        Abuptio placentae) O45.9-
      leiomyoma, uterus —see
        Hemorrhage, antepartum,
        specified cause NEC
      placenta previa O44.1-
    specified cause NEC O46.8X-
  anus (sphincter) K62.5
  apoplexy (stroke) —see
    Hemorrhage, intracranial,
    intracerebral
  arachnoid —see Hemorrhage,
    intracranial, subarachnoid
  artery R58
    brain —see Hemorrhage,
      intracranial, intracerebral
  basilar (ganglion) I61.0
  bladder N32.89
  bowel K92.2
    newborn P54.3
  brain (miliary) (nontraumatic) —
    see Hemorrhage, intracranial,
    intracerebral
    due to
      birth injury P10.1
      syphilis A52.05
    epidural or extradural (traumatic)
      —see Injury, intracranial,
      epidural hemorrhage
    newborn P52.4
      birth injury P10.1

Hemorrhage, hemorrhagic
(continued)
  brain (continued)
    subarachnoid —see Hemorrhage,
      intracranial, subarachnoid
    subdural —see Hemorrhage,
      intracranial, subdural
  brainstem (nontraumatic) I61.3
    traumatic S06.38-
  breast N64.59
  bronchial tube —see Hemorrhage,
    lung
  bronchopulmonary —see
    Hemorrhage, lung
  bronchus —see Hemorrhage, lung
  bulbar I61.5
  capillary I78.8
    primary D69.8
  cecum K92.2
  cerebellar, cerebellum
    (nontraumatic) I61.4
    newborn P52.6
    traumatic S06.37-
  cerebral, cerebrum —see also
    Hemorrhage, intracranial,
    intracerebral
    newborn (anoxic) P52.4
      birth injury P10.1
    lobe I61.1
  cerebromeningeal I61.8
  cerebrospinal —see Hemorrhage,
    intracranial, intracerebral
  cervix (uteri) (stump) NEC N88.8
  chamber, anterior (eye) —see
    Hyphema
  childbirth —see Hemorrhage,
    complicating, delivery
  choroid H31.30-
    expulsive H31.31-
  ciliary body —see Hyphema
  cochlea —see subcategory H83.8
  colon K92.2
  complicating
    abortion —see Abortion, by type,
      complicated by, hemorrhage
    delivery O67.9
      associated with coagulation
        defect (afibrinogenemia)
        (DIC) (hyperfibrinolysis)
        O67.0
      specified cause NEC O67.8
    surgical procedure —see
      Hemorrhage, intraoperative
  conjunctiva H11.3-
    newborn P54.8
  cord, newborn (stump) P51.9
  corpus luteum (ruptured) cyst N83.1-
  cortical (brain) I61.1
  cranial —see Hemorrhage,
    intracranial
  cutaneous R23.3
    due to autosensitivity,
      erythrocyte D69.2
    newborn P54.5
  delayed
    following ectopic or molar
      pregnancy O08.1
    postpartum O72.2
  diathesis (familial) D69.9
  disease D69.9
    newborn P53
    specified type NEC D69.8
  due to or associated with
    afibrinogenemia or other
      coagulation defect (conditions
      in categories D65-D69)
      antepartum —see
        Hemorrhage, antepartum,
        with coagulation defect
      intrapartum O67.0
    dental implant M27.61

Hemorrhage, hemorrhagic
(continued)
  due to or associated with
    (continued)
    device, implant or graft (see also
      Complications, by site and
      type, specified NEC) T85.838
      arterial graft NEC T82.838
      breast T85.838
      catheter NEC T85.838
        dialysis (renal) T82.838
          intraperitoneal T85.838
        infusion NEC T82.838
          spinal (epidural)
            (subdural) T85.830
        urinary (indwelling) T83.83
      electronic (electrode) (pulse
        generator) (stimulator)
        bone T84.83
        cardiac T82.837
        nervous system (brain)
          (peripheral nerve)
          (spinal) T85.830
        urinary T83.83
      fixation, internal (orthopedic)
        NEC T84.83
      gastrointestinal (bile duct)
        (esophagus) T85.838
      genital NEC T83.83
      heart NEC T82.837
      joint prosthesis T84.83
      ocular (corneal graft) (orbital
        implant) NEC T85.838
      orthopedic NEC T84.83
        bone graft T86.838
      specified NEC T85.838
      urinary NEC T83.83
      vascular NEC T82.838
      ventricular intracranial shunt
        T85.830
  duodenum, duodenal K92.2
    ulcer —see Ulcer, duodenum,
      with hemorrhage
  dura mater —see Hemorrhage,
    intracranial, subdural
  endotracheal —see Hemorrhage,
    lung
  epicranial subaponeurotic
    (massive), birth injury P12.2
  epidural (traumatic) —see also
    Injury, intracranial, epidural
    hemorrhage
    nontraumatic I62.1
  esophagus K22.8
    varix I85.01
      secondary I85.11
  excessive, following ectopic
    gestation (subsequent episode)
    O08.1
  extradural (traumatic) —see Injury,
    intracranial, epidural hemorrhage
    birth injury P10.8
    newborn (anoxic) (nontraumatic)
      P52.8
    nontraumatic I62.1
  eye NEC H57.89
    fundus —see Hemorrhage, retina
    lid —see Disorder, eyelid,
      specified type NEC
  fallopian tube N83.6
  fibrinogenolysis —see Fibrinolysis
  fibrinolytic (acquired) —see
    Fibrinolysis
  from
    ear (nontraumatic) —see
      Otorrhagia
    tracheostomy stoma J95.01
  fundus, eye —see Hemorrhage,
    retina
  funis —see Hemorrhage,
    umbilicus, cord

(continued)

gastric —*see* Hemorrhage, stomach
gastroenteric K92.2
  newborn P54.3
gastrointestinal (tract) K92.2
  newborn P54.3
genital organ, male N50.1
genitourinary (tract) NOS R31.9
gingiva K06.8
globe (eye) —*see* Hemophthalmos
graafian follicle cyst (ruptured) N83.0-
gum K06.8
heart I51.89
hypopharyngeal (throat) R04.1
intermenstrual (regular) N92.3
  irregular N92.1
internal (organs) NEC R58
  capsule I61.0
  ear H83.8
  newborn P54.8
intestine K92.2
  newborn P54.3
intra-abdominal R58
intra-alveolar (lung), newborn P26.8
intracerebral (nontraumatic) —*see* Hemorrhage, intracranial, intracerebral
intracranial (nontraumatic) I62.9
  birth injury P10.9
  epidural, nontraumatic I62.1
  extradural, nontraumatic I62.1
  newborn P52.9
   specified NEC P52.8
  intracerebral (nontraumatic) (in) I61.9
   brain stem I61.3
   cerebellum I61.4
   newborn P52.4
    birth injury P10.1
   hemisphere I61.2
    cortical (superficial) I61.1
    subcortical (deep) I61.0
   intraoperative
    during a nervous system procedure G97.31
    during other procedure G97.32
   intraventricular I61.5
   multiple localized I61.6
   postprocedural
    following a nervous system procedure G97.51
    following other procedure G97.52
   specified NEC I61.8
   superficial I61.1
   traumatic (diffuse) —*see* Injury, intracranial, diffuse
    focal —*see* Injury, intracranial, focal
  subarachnoid (nontraumatic) (from) I60.9
   newborn P52.5
    birth injury P10.3
   intracranial (cerebral) artery I60.7
    anterior communicating I60.2
    basilar I60.4
    carotid siphon and bifurcation I60.0-
    communicating I60.7
     anterior I60.2
     posterior I60.3-
    middle cerebral I60.1-
    posterior communicating I60.3-

(continued)

intracranial *(continued)*
  subarachnoid *(continued)*
   intracranial artery *(continued)*
    specified artery NEC I60.6
    vertebral I60.5-
   specified NEC I60.8
   traumatic S06.6X-
  subdural (nontraumatic) I62.00
   acute I62.01
   birth injury P10.0
   chronic I62.03
   newborn (anoxic) (hypoxic) P52.8
    birth injury P10.0
   spinal G95.19
   subacute I62.02
   traumatic —*see* Injury, intracranial, subdural hemorrhage
  traumatic —*see* Injury, intracranial, focal brain injury
intramedullary NEC G95.19
intraocular —*see* Hemophthalmos
intraoperative, intraprocedural —*see* Complication, hemorrhage (hematoma), intraoperative (intraprocedural), by site
intrapartum —*see* Hemorrhage, complicating, delivery
intrapelvic
  female N94.89
  male K66.1
intraperitoneal K66.1
intrapontine I61.3
intraprocedural —*see* Complication, hemorrhage (hematoma), intraoperative (intraprocedural), by site
intrauterine N85.7
  complicating delivery (*see also* Hemorrhage, complicating, delivery) O67.9
  postpartum —*see* Hemorrhage, postpartum
intraventricular I61.5
  newborn (nontraumatic) (*see also* Newborn, affected by, hemorrhage) P52.3
   due to birth injury P10.2
   grade
    1 P52.0
    2 P52.1
    3 P52.21
    4 P52.22
intravesical N32.89
iris (postinfectional) (postinflammatory) (toxic) —*see* Hyphema
joint (nontraumatic) —*see* Hemarthrosis
kidney N28.89
knee (joint) (nontraumatic) —*see* Hemarthrosis, knee
labyrinth —*see* subcategory H83.8
lenticular striate artery I61.0
ligature, vessel —*see* Hemorrhage, postoperative
liver K76.89
lung R04.89
  newborn P26.9
   massive P26.1
   specified NEC P26.8
  tuberculous —*see* Tuberculosis, pulmonary
massive umbilical, newborn P51.0
mediastinum —*see* Hemorrhage, lung
medulla I61.3

(continued)

membrane (brain) I60.8
  spinal cord —*see* Hemorrhage, spinal cord
meninges, meningeal (brain) (middle) I60.8
  spinal cord —*see* Hemorrhage, spinal cord
mesentery K66.1
metritis —*see* Endometritis
mouth K13.79
mucous membrane NEC R58
  newborn P54.8
muscle M62.89
nail (subungual) L60.8
nasal turbinate R04.0
  newborn P54.8
navel, newborn P51.9
newborn P54.9
  specified NEC P54.8
nipple N64.59
nose R04.0
  newborn P54.8
omentum K66.1
optic nerve (sheath) H47.02-
orbit, orbital H05.23-
ovary NEC N83.8
oviduct N83.6
pancreas K86.89
parathyroid (gland) (spontaneous) E21.4
parturition —*see* Hemorrhage, complicating, delivery
penis N48.89
pericardium, pericarditis I31.2
peritoneum, peritoneal K66.1
peritonsillar tissue J35.8
  due to infection J36
petechial R23.3
  due to autosensitivity, erythrocyte D69.2
pituitary (gland) E23.6
pleura —*see* Hemorrhage, lung
polioencephalitis, superior E51.2
polymyositis —*see* Polymyositis
pons, pontine I61.3
posterior fossa (nontraumatic) I61.8
  newborn P52.6
postmenopausal N95.0
postnasal R04.0
postoperative —*see* Complications, postprocedural, hemorrhage, by site
postpartum NEC (following delivery of placenta) O72.1
  delayed or secondary O72.2
  retained placenta O72.0
  third stage O72.0
pregnancy —*see* Hemorrhage, antepartum
preretinal —*see* Hemorrhage, retina
prostate N42.1
puerperal —*see* Hemorrhage, postpartum
  delayed or secondary O72.2
pulmonary R04.89
  newborn P26.9
   massive P26.1
   specified NEC P26.8
  tuberculous —*see* Tuberculosis, pulmonary
purpura (primary) D69.3
rectum (sphincter) K62.5
  newborn P54.2
recurring, following initial hemorrhage at time of injury T79.2
renal N28.89
respiratory passage or tract R04.9
  specified NEC R04.89

(continued)

retina, retinal (vessels) H35.6-
  diabetic —*see* Diabetes, retinal, hemorrhage
retroperitoneal R58
scalp R58
scrotum N50.1
secondary (nontraumatic) R58
  following initial hemorrhage at time of injury T79.2
seminal vesicle N50.1
skin R23.3
  newborn P54.5
slipped umbilical ligature P51.8
spermatic cord N50.1
spinal (cord) G95.19
  newborn (birth injury) P11.5
spleen D73.5
  intraoperative —*see* Complications, intraoperative, hemorrhage, spleen
  postprocedural —*see* Complications, postprocedural, hemorrhage, spleen
stomach K92.2
  newborn P54.3
  ulcer —*see* Ulcer, stomach, with hemorrhage
subarachnoid (nontraumatic) —*see* Hemorrhage, intracranial, subarachnoid
subconjunctival —*see also* Hemorrhage, conjunctiva
  birth injury P15.3
subcortical (brain) I61.0
subcutaneous R23.3
subdiaphragmatic R58
subdural (acute) (nontraumatic) —*see* Hemorrhage, intracranial, subdural
subependymal
  newborn P52.0
   with intraventricular extension P52.1
    and intracerebral extension P52.22
subgaleal P12.2
subhyaloid —*see* Hemorrhage, retina
subperiosteal —*see* Disorder, bone, specified type NEC
subretinal —*see* Hemorrhage, retina
subtentorial —*see* Hemorrhage, intracranial, subdural
subungual L60.8
suprarenal (capsule) (gland) E27.49
  newborn P54.4
tentorium (traumatic) NEC —*see* Hemorrhage, brain
  newborn (birth injury) P10.4
testis N50.1
third stage (postpartum) O72.0
thorax —*see* Hemorrhage, lung
throat R04.1
thymus (gland) E32.8
thyroid (cyst) (gland) E07.89
tongue K14.8
tonsil J35.8
trachea —*see* Hemorrhage, lung
tracheobronchial R04.89
  newborn P26.0
traumatic - code to specific injury
  cerebellar —*see* Hemorrhage, brain
  intracranial —*see* Hemorrhage, brain
  recurring or secondary (following initial hemorrhage at time of injury) T79.2

Hernia, hernial (continued)
bladder (mucosa) (sphincter)
congenital (female) (male)
Q79.51
female —see Cystocele
male N32.89
brain, congenital —see
Encephalocele
cartilage, vertebra —see
Displacement, intervertebral disc
cerebral, congenital —see also
Encephalocele
endaural Q01.8
ciliary body (traumatic) S05.2-
colon —see Hernia, abdomen
Cooper's —see Hernia, abdomen,
specified site NEC
crural —see Hernia, femoral
diaphragm, diaphragmatic K44.9
with
gangrene (and obstruction)
K44.1
obstruction K44.0
congenital Q79.0
direct (inguinal) —see Hernia,
inguinal
diverticulum, intestine —see
Hernia, abdomen
double (inguinal) —see Hernia,
inguinal, bilateral
due to adhesions (with obstruction)
K56.50
epigastric (see also Hernia, ventral)
K43.9
esophageal hiatus —see Hernia,
hiatal
external (inguinal) —see Hernia,
inguinal
fallopian tube N83.4-
fascia M62.89
femoral K41.90
with
gangrene (and obstruction)
K41.40
not specified as recurrent
K41.40
recurrent K41.41
obstruction K41.30
not specified as recurrent
K41.30
recurrent K41.31
bilateral K41.20
with
gangrene (and obstruction)
K41.10
not specified as recurrent
K41.10
recurrent K41.11
obstruction K41.00
not specified as recurrent
K41.00
recurrent K41.01
not specified as recurrent
K41.20
recurrent K41.21
unilateral K41.90
with
gangrene (and obstruction)
K41.40
not specified as recurrent
K41.40
recurrent K41.41
obstruction K41.30
not specified as recurrent
K41.30
recurrent K41.31
not specified as recurrent
K41.90
recurrent K41.91
not specified as recurrent K41.90
recurrent K41.91

Hernia, hernial (continued)
foramen magnum G93.5
congenital Q01.8
funicular (umbilical) —see also
Hernia, umbilicus
spermatic (cord) —see Hernia,
inguinal
gastrointestinal tract —see Hernia,
abdomen
Hesselbach's —see Hernia,
femoral, specified site NEC
hiatal (esophageal) (sliding) K44.9
with
gangrene (and obstruction)
K44.1
obstruction K44.0
congenital Q40.1
hypogastric —see Hernia, ventral
incarcerated —see also Hernia, by
site, with obstruction
with gangrene —see Hernia, by
site, with gangrene
incisional K43.2
with
gangrene (and obstruction)
K43.1
obstruction K43.0
indirect (inguinal) —see Hernia,
inguinal
inguinal (direct) (external)
(funicular) (indirect) (internal)
(oblique) (scrotal) (sliding)
K40.90
with
gangrene (and obstruction)
K40.40
not specified as recurrent
K40.40
recurrent K40.41
obstruction K40.30
not specified as recurrent
K40.30
recurrent K40.31
not specified as recurrent
K40.90
recurrent K40.91
bilateral K40.20
with
gangrene (and obstruction)
K40.10
not specified as recurrent
K40.10
recurrent K40.11
obstruction K40.00
not specified as recurrent
K40.00
recurrent K40.01
not specified as recurrent
K40.20
recurrent K40.21
unilateral K40.90
with
gangrene (and obstruction)
K40.40
not specified as recurrent
K40.40
recurrent K40.41
obstruction K40.30
not specified as recurrent
K40.30
recurrent K40.31
not specified as recurrent
K40.90
recurrent K40.91
internal —see also Hernia,
abdomen
inguinal —see Hernia, inguinal
interstitial —see Hernia, abdomen
intervertebral cartilage or disc —
see Displacement, intervertebral
disc

Hernia, hernial (continued)
intestine, intestinal —see Hernia,
by site
intra-abdominal —see Hernia,
abdomen
iris (traumatic) S05.2-
irreducible —see also Hernia, by
site, with obstruction
with gangrene —see Hernia, by
site, with gangrene
ischiatic —see Hernia, abdomen,
specified site NEC
ischiorectal —see Hernia,
abdomen, specified site NEC
lens (traumatic) S05.2-
linea (alba) (semilunaris) —see
Hernia, ventral
Littre's —see Hernia, abdomen
lumbar —see Hernia, abdomen,
specified site NEC
lung (subcutaneous) J98.4
mediastinum J98.59
mesenteric (internal) —see Hernia,
abdomen
midline —see Hernia, ventral
muscle (sheath) M62.89
nucleus pulposus —see
Displacement, intervertebral disc
oblique (inguinal) —see Hernia,
inguinal
obstructive —see also Hernia, by
site, with obstruction
with gangrene —see Hernia, by
site, with gangrene
obturator —see Hernia, abdomen,
specified site NEC
omental —see Hernia, abdomen
ovary N83.4-
oviduct N83.4-
paraesophageal —see also Hernia,
diaphragm
congenital Q40.1
parastomal K43.5
with
gangrene (and obstruction)
K43.4
obstruction K43.3
paraumbilical —see Hernia,
umbilicus
perineal —see Hernia, abdomen,
specified site NEC
Petit's —see Hernia, abdomen,
specified site NEC
postoperative —see Hernia,
incisional
pregnant uterus —see Abnormal,
uterus in pregnancy or
childbirth
prevesical N32.89
properitoneal —see Hernia,
abdomen, specified site NEC
pudendal —see Hernia, abdomen,
specified site NEC
rectovaginal N81.6
retroperitoneal —see Hernia,
abdomen, specified site NEC
Richter's —see Hernia, abdomen,
with obstruction
Rieux's, Riex's —see Hernia,
abdomen, specified site NEC
sac condition (adhesion) (dropsy)
(inflammation) (laceration)
(suppuration) - code by site
under Hernia
sciatic —see Hernia, abdomen,
specified site NEC
scrotum, scrotal —see Hernia,
inguinal
sliding (inguinal) —see also
Hernia, inguinal
hiatus —see Hernia, hiatal

Hernia, hernial (continued)
spigelian —see Hernia, ventral
spinal —see Spina bifida
strangulated —see also Hernia, by
site, with obstruction
with gangrene —see Hernia, by
site, with gangrene
subxiphoid —see Hernia, ventral
supra-umbilicus —see Hernia,
ventral
tendon —see Disorder, tendon,
specified type NEC
Treitz's (fossa) —see Hernia,
abdomen, specified site NEC
tunica vaginalis Q55.29
umbilicus, umbilical K42.9
with
gangrene (and obstruction)
K42.1
obstruction K42.0
ureter N28.89
urethra, congenital Q64.79
urinary meatus, congenital Q64.79
uterus N81.4
pregnant —see Abnormal, uterus
in pregnancy or childbirth
vaginal (anterior) (wall) —see
Cystocele
Velpeau's —see Hernia, femoral
ventral K43.9
with
gangrene (and obstruction)
K43.7
obstruction K43.6
recurrent —see Hernia,
incisional
incisional K43.2
with
gangrene (and obstruction)
K43.1
obstruction K43.0
specified NEC K43.9
with
gangrene (and obstruction)
K43.7
obstruction K43.6
vesical
congenital (female) (male)
Q79.51
female —see Cystocele
male N32.89
vitreous (into wound) S05.2-
into anterior chamber —see
Prolapse, vitreous

Herniation —see also Hernia
brain (stem) G93.5
cerebral G93.5
mediastinum J98.59
nucleus pulposus —see
Displacement, intervertebral disc

Herpangina B08.5

Herpes, herpesvirus, herpetic B00.9
anogenital A60.9
perianal skin A60.1
rectum A60.1
urogenital tract A60.00
cervix A60.03
male genital organ NEC
A60.02
penis A60.01
specified site NEC A60.09
vagina A60.04
vulva A60.04
blepharitis (zoster) B02.39
simplex B00.59
circinatus B35.4
bullosus L12.0
conjunctivitis (simplex) B00.53
zoster B02.31
cornea B02.33

Herpes, herpesvirus, herpetic
(continued)
encephalitis B00.4
  due to herpesvirus 6 B10.01
  due to herpesvirus 7 B10.09
  specified NEC B10.09
eye (zoster) B02.30
  simplex B00.50
eyelid (zoster) B02.39
  simplex B00.59
facialis B00.1
febrilis B00.1
geniculate ganglionitis B02.21
genital, genitalis A60.00
  female A60.09
  male A60.02
gestational, gestationis O26.4-
gingivostomatitis B00.2
human B00.9
  1 —*see* Herpes, simplex
  2 —*see* Herpes, simplex
  3 —*see* Varicella
  4 —*see* Mononucleosis, Epstein-
    Barr (virus)
  5 —*see* Disease, cytomegalic
    inclusion (generalized)
  6
    encephalitis B10.01
    specified NEC B10.81
  7
    encephalitis B10.09
    specified NEC B10.82
  8 B10.89
infection NEC B10.89
  Kaposi's sarcoma associated
    B10.89
iridocyclitis (simplex) B00.51
  zoster B02.32
iris (vesicular erythema
  multiforme) L51.9
iritis (simplex) B00.51
  Kaposi's sarcoma associated
    B10.89
keratitis (simplex) (dendritic)
  (disciform) (interstitial) B00.52
  zoster (interstitial) B02.33
keratoconjunctivitis (simplex)
  B00.52
  zoster B02.33
labialis B00.1
lip B00.1
meningitis (simplex) B00.3
  zoster B02.1
ophthalmicus (zoster) NEC B02.30
  simplex B00.50
penis A60.01
perianal skin A60.1
pharyngitis, pharyngotonsillitis
  B00.2
rectum A60.1
scrotum A60.02
sepsis B00.7
simplex B00.9
  complicated NEC B00.89
  congenital P35.2
  conjunctivitis B00.53
  external ear B00.1
  eyelid B00.59
  hepatitis B00.81
  keratitis (interstitial) B00.52
  myeletis B00.82
  specified complication NEC
    B00.89
  visceral B00.89
stomatitis B00.2
tonsurans B35.0
visceral B00.89
vulva A60.04
whitlow B00.89
zoster (*see also* condition) B02.9
  auricularis B02.21

Herpes, herpesvirus, herpetic
(continued)
zoster *(continued)*
  complicated NEC B02.8
  conjunctivitis B02.31
  disseminated B02.7
  encephalitis B02.0
  eye (lid) B02.39
  geniculate ganglionitis B02.21
  keratitis (interstitial) B02.33
  meningitis B02.1
  myelitis B02.24
  neuritis, neuralgia B02.29
  ophthalmicus NEC B02.30
  oticus B02.21
  polyneuropathy B02.23
  specified complication NEC
    B02.8
  trigeminal neuralgia B02.22

Herpesvirus (human) —*see* Herpes

Herpetophobia F40.218

Herrick's anemia —*see* Disease,
sickle-cell

Hers' disease E74.09

Herter-Gee syndrome K90.0

Herxheimer's reaction R68.89

Hesitancy
of micturition R39.11
urinary R39.11

Hesselbach's hernia —*see* Hernia,
femoral, specified site NEC

Heterochromia (congenital) Q13.2
cataract —*see* Cataract,
  complicated
cyclitis (Fuchs) —*see* Cyclitis,
  Fuchs' heterochromic
hair L67.1
iritis —*see* Cyclitis, Fuchs'
  heterochromic
retained metallic foreign body
  (nonmagnetic) —*see* Foreign
  body, intraocular, old, retained
  magnetic —*see* Foreign body,
  intraocular, old, retained,
  magnetic
uveitis —*see* Cyclitis, Fuchs'
  heterochromic

Heterophoria —*see* Strabismus,
heterophoria

Heterophyes, heterophyiasis (small
intestine) B66.8

Heterotopia, heterotopic —*see also*
Malposition, congenital
cerebralis Q04.8

Heterotropia —*see* Strabismus

Heubner-Herter disease K90.0

Hexadactylism Q69.9

HGSIL (cytology finding) (high
grade squamous intraepithelial
lesion on cytologic smear) (Pap
smear finding)
anus R85.613
cervix R87.613
  biopsy (histology) finding —*see*
    Neoplasia, intraepithelial,
    cervix, grade II or grade III
vagina R87.623
  biopsy (histology) finding —*see*
    Neoplasia, intraepithelial,
    vagina, grade II or grade III

Hibernoma —*see* Lipoma

Hiccup, hiccough R06.6
epidemic B33.0
psychogenic F45.8

Hidden penis (congenital) Q55.64
acquired N48.83

Hidradenitis (axillaris) (suppurative)
L73.2

Hidradenoma (nodular) —*see also*
Neoplasm, skin, benign
clear cell —*see* Neoplasm, skin,
  benign
papillary —*see* Neoplasm, skin,
  benign

Hidrocystoma —*see* Neoplasm, skin,
benign

High
altitude effects T70.20
  anoxia T70.29
  on
    ears T70.0
    sinuses T70.1
  polycythemia D75.1
arch
  foot Q66.7-
  palate, congenital Q38.5
arterial tension —*see* Hypertension
basal metabolic rate R94.8
blood pressure —*see also*
  Hypertension
  borderline R03.0
  reading (incidental) (isolated)
    (nonspecific), without
    diagnosis of hypertension
    R03.0
cholesterol E78.00
  with high triglycerides E78.2
diaphragm (congenital) Q79.1
expressed emotional level within
  family Z63.8
head at term O32.4
palate, congenital Q38.5
risk
  infant NEC Z76.2
  sexual behavior (heterosexual)
    Z72.51
    bisexual Z72.53
    homosexual Z72.52
scrotal testis, testes
  bilateral Q53.23
  unilateral Q53.13
temperature (of unknown origin)
  R50.9
thoracic rib Q76.6
triglycerides E78.1
  with high cholesterol E78.2

Hildenbrand's disease A75.0

Hilum —*see* condition

Hip —*see* condition

Hippel's disease Q85.8

Hippophobia F40.218

Hippus H57.09

**Hirschsprung's disease or
megacolon** Q43.1

Hirsutism, hirsuties L68.0

Hirudiniasis
external B88.3
internal B83.4

Hiss-Russell dysentery A03.1

Histidinemia, histidinuria E70.41

Histiocytoma —*see also* Neoplasm,
skin, benign
fibrous —*see also* Neoplasm, skin,
  benign
  atypical —*see* Neoplasm,
    connective tissue, uncertain
    behavior
  malignant —*see* Neoplasm,
    connective tissue, malignant

Histiocytosis D76.3
acute differentiated progressive
  C96.0
Langerhans' cell NEC C96.6
multifocal X
  multisystemic (disseminated)
    C96.0
  unisystemic C96.5
pulmonary, adult (adult PLCH)
  J84.82
unifocal (X) C96.6
lipid, lipoid D76.3
  essential E75.29
malignant C96.A
mononuclear phagocytes NEC
  D76.1
  Langerhans' cells C96.6
non-Langerhans cell D76.3
polyostotic sclerosing D76.3
sinus, with massive
  lymphadenopathy D76.3
syndrome NEC D76.3
X NEC C96.6
  acute (progressive) C96.0
  chronic C96.6
  multifocal C96.5
  multisystemic C96.0
  unifocal C96.6

Histoplasmosis B39.9
with pneumonia NEC B39.2
African B39.5
American —*see* Histoplasmosis,
  capsulati
capsulati B39.4
  disseminated B39.3
  generalized B39.3
  pulmonary B39.2
    acute B39.0
    chronic B39.1
Darling's B39.4
duboisii B39.5
lung NEC B39.2

History
family (of) —*see also* History,
  personal (of)
  alcohol abuse Z81.1
  allergy NEC Z84.89
  anemia Z83.2
  arthritis Z82.61
  asthma Z82.5
  blindness Z82.1
  cardiac death (sudden) Z82.41
  carrier of genetic disease Z84.81
  chromosomal anomaly Z82.79
  chronic
    disabling disease NEC Z82.8
    lower respiratory disease
      Z82.5
  colonic polyps Z83.71
  congenital malformations and
    deformations Z82.79
    polycystic kidney Z82.71
  consanguinity Z84.3
  deafness Z82.2
  diabetes mellitus Z83.3
  disability NEC Z82.8
  disease or disorder (of)
    allergic NEC Z84.89
    behavioral NEC Z81.8
    blood and blood-forming
      organs Z83.2
    cardiovascular NEC Z82.49
    chronic disabling NEC Z82.8
    digestive Z83.79
    ear NEC Z83.52
    elevated lipoprotein (a)
      (Lp(a)) Z83.430
    endocrine NEC Z83.49
    eye NEC Z83.518
      glaucoma Z83.511

Hordeolum (eyelid) (externum)
(recurrent) H00.019
internum H00.029
left H00.026
lower H00.025
upper H00.024
right H00.023
lower H00.022
upper H00.021
left H00.016
lower H00.015
upper H00.014
right H00.013
lower H00.012
upper H00.011

Horn
cutaneous L85.8
nail L60.2
congenital Q84.6

Horner (-Claude Bernard) **syndrome**
G90.2
traumatic —see Injury, nerve,
cervical sympathetic

Horseshoe kidney (congenital) Q63.1

Horton's headache or neuralgia
G44.099
intractable G44.091
not intractable G44.099

Hospital hopper syndrome —see
Disorder, factitious

Hospitalism in children —see
Disorder, adjustment

Hostility R45.5
towards child Z62.3

Hot flashes
menopausal N95.1

Hourglass (contracture) —see also
Contraction, hourglass
stomach K31.89
congenital Q40.2
stricture K31.2

Household, housing circumstance
affecting care Z59.9
specified NEC Z59.8

Housemaid's knee —see Bursitis,
prepatellar

Hudson (-Stähli) **line** (cornea) —see
Pigmentation, cornea, anterior

Human
bite (open wound) —see also Bite
intact skin surface —see Bite,
superficial
herpesvirus —see Herpes
immunodeficiency virus (HIV)
disease (infection) B20
asymptomatic status Z21
contact Z20.6
counseling Z71.7
dementia B20 [F02.80]
with behavioral disturbance
B20 [F02.81]
exposure to Z20.6
laboratory evidence R75
type-2(HIV 2) as cause of disease
classified elsewhere B97.35
papillomavirus (HPV)
DNA test positive
high risk
cervix R87.810
vagina R87.811
low risk
cervix R87.820
vagina R87.821
screening for Z11.51
T-cell lymphotropic virus
type-1(HTLV-I) infection B33.3
as cause of disease classified
elsewhere B97.33
carrier Z22.6

Human (continued)
T-cell lymphotropic virus (continued)
type-2(HTLV-II) as cause of
disease classified elsewhere
B97.34

Humidifier lung or pneumonitis
J67.7

Humiliation (experience) **in**
childhood Z62.898

Humpback (acquired) —see Kyphosis

Hunchback (acquired) —see Kyphosis

Hunger T73.0
air, psychogenic F45.8

Hungry bone syndrome E83.81

Hunner's ulcer —see Cystitis,
chronic, interstitial

Hunter's
glossitis D51.0
syndrome E76.1

Huntington's disease or chorea G10
with dementia G10 [F02.80]
with behavioral disturbance G10
[F02.81]

Hunt's
disease or syndrome (herpetic
geniculate ganglionitis) B02.21
dyssynergia cerebellaris
myoclonica G11.19
neuralgia B02.21

Hurler (-Scheie) **disease or**
syndrome E76.02

Hurst's disease G36.1

Hurthle cell
adenocarcinoma C73
adenoma D34
carcinoma C73
tumor D34

Hutchinson-Boeck disease or
syndrome —see Sarcoidosis

Hutchinson-Gilford disease or
syndrome E34.8

Hutchinson's
disease, meaning
angioma serpiginosum L81.7
pompholyx (cheiropompholyx)
L30.1
prurigo estivalis L56.4
summer eruption or summer
prurigo L56.4
melanotic freckle —see Melanoma,
in situ
malignant melanoma in —see
Melanoma
teeth or incisors (congenital
syphilis) A50.52
triad (congenital syphilis) A50.53

Hyalin plaque, sclera, senile H15.89

Hyaline membrane (disease) (lung)
(pulmonary) (newborn) P22.0

Hyalinosis
cutis (et mucosae) E78.89
focal and segmental (glomerular)
(see also N00-N07 with fourth
character .1) N05.1

Hyalitis, hyalosis, asteroid —see
also Deposit, crystalline
syphilitic (late) A52.71

Hydatid
cyst or tumor —see Echinococcus
mole —see Hydatidiform mole
Morgagni
female Q50.5
male (epididymal) Q55.4
testicular Q55.29

Hydatidiform mole (benign)
(complicating pregnancy)
(delivered) (undelivered) O01.9
classical O01.0
complete O01.0
incomplete O01.1
invasive D39.2
malignant D39.2
partial O01.1

Hydatidosis —see Echinococcus

Hydradenitis (axillaris) (suppurative)
L73.2

Hydradenoma —see Hidradenoma

Hydramnios O40.-

Hydrancephaly, hydranencephaly
Q04.3
with spina bifida —see Spina
bifida, with hydrocephalus

Hydrargyrism NEC —see
Poisoning, mercury

Hydrarthrosis —see also Effusion,
joint
gonococcal A54.42
intermittent M12.40
ankle M12.47-
elbow M12.42-
foot joint M12.47-
hand joint M12.44-
hip M12.45-
knee M12.46-
multiple site M12.49
shoulder M12.41-
specified joint NEC M12.48
wrist M12.43-
of yaws (early) (late) (see also
subcategory M14.8-) A66.6
syphilitic (late) A52.77
congenital A50.55 [M12.80]

Hydremia D64.89

Hydrencephalocele (congenital)
—see Encephalocele

Hydrencephalomeningocele
(congenital) —see Encephalocele

Hydroa R23.8
aestivale L56.4
vacciniforme L56.4

Hydroadenitis (axillaris)
(suppurative) L73.2

Hydrocalycosis —see
Hydronephrosis

Hydrocele (spermatic cord) (testis)
(tunica vaginalis) N43.3
canal of Nuck N94.89
communicating N43.2
congenital P83.5
congenital P83.5
encysted N43.0
female NEC N94.89
infected N43.1
newborn P83.5
round ligament N94.89
specified NEC N43.2
spinalis —see Spina bifida
vulva N90.89

Hydrocephalus (acquired) (external)
(internal) (malignant) (recurrent)
G91.9
aqueduct Sylvius stricture Q03.0
causing disproportion O33.6
with obstructed labor O66.3
communicating G91.0
congenital (external) (internal)
Q03.9
with spina bifida Q05.4
cervical Q05.0
dorsal Q05.1

Hydrocephalus (continued)
congenital (continued)
with spina bifida (continued)
lumbar Q05.2
lumbosacral Q05.2
sacral Q05.3
thoracic Q05.1
thoracolumbar Q05.1
specified NEC Q03.8
due to toxoplasmosis (congenital)
P37.1
foramen Magendie block
(acquired) G91.1
congenital (see also
Hydrocephalus, congenital)
Q03.1
in (due to)
infectious disease NEC B89
[G91.4]
neoplastic disease NEC (see also
Neoplasm) G91.4
parasitic disease B89 [G91.4]
newborn Q03.9
with spina bifida —see Spina
bifida, with hydrocephalus
noncommunicating G91.1
normal pressure G91.2
secondary G91.0
obstructive G91.1
otitic G93.2
post-traumatic NEC G91.3
secondary G91.4
post-traumatic G91.3
specified NEC G91.8
syphilitic, congenital A50.49

Hydrocolpos (congenital) N89.8

Hydrocystoma —see Neoplasm,
skin, benign

Hydroencephalocele (congenital)
—see Encephalocele

Hydroencephalomeningocele
(congenital) —see Encephalocele

Hydrohematopneumothorax —see
Hemothorax

Hydromeningitis —see Meningitis

Hydromeningocele (spinal) —see
also Spina bifida
cranial —see Encephalocele

Hydrometra N85.8

Hydrometrocolpos N89.8

Hydromicrocephaly Q02

Hydromphalos (since birth) Q45.8

Hydromyelia Q06.4

Hydromyelocele —see Spina bifida

Hydronephrosis (atrophic) (early)
(functionless) (intermittent)
(primary) (secondary) **NEC** N13.30
with
infection N13.6
obstruction (by) (of)
renal calculus N13.2
with infection N13.6
ureteral NEC N13.1
with infection N13.6
calculus N13.2
with infection N13.6
ureteropelvic junction
(congenital) Q62.11
acquired N13.0
with infection N13.6
ureteral stricture NEC N13.1
with infection N13.6
congenital Q62.0
due to acquired occlusion of
ureteropelvic junction N13.0
specified type NEC N13.39
tuberculous A18.11

Hydropericarditis —*see* Pericarditis

Hydropericardium —*see* Pericarditis

Hydroperitoneum R18.8

Hydrophobia —*see* Rabies

Hydrophthalmos Q15.0

Hydropneumohemothorax —*see* Hemothorax

Hydropneumopericarditis —*see* Pericarditis

Hydropneumopericardium —*see* Pericarditis

Hydropneumothorax J94.8
traumatic —*see* Injury, intrathoracic, lung
tuberculous NEC A15.6

Hydrops R60.9
abdominis R18.8
articulorum intermittens —*see* Hydrarthrosis, intermittent
cardiac —*see* Failure, heart, congestive
causing obstructed labor (mother) O66.3
endolymphatic H81.0-
fetal —*see* Pregnancy, complicated by, hydrops, fetalis
fetalis P83.2
due to
ABO isoimmunization P56.0
alpha thalassemia D56.0
hemolytic disease P56.90
specified NEC P56.99
isoimmunization (ABO) (Rh) P56.0
other specified nonhemolytic disease NEC P83.2
Rh incompatibility P56.0
during pregnancy —*see* Pregnancy, complicated by, hydrops, fetalis
gallbladder K82.1
joint —*see* Effusion, joint
labyrinth H81.0-
newborn (idiopathic) P83.2
due to
ABO isoimmunization P56.0
alpha thalassemia D56.0
hemolytic disease P56.90
specified NEC P56.99
isoimmunization (ABO) (Rh) P56.0
Rh incompatibility P56.0
nutritional —*see* Malnutrition, severe
pericardium —*see* Pericarditis
pleura —*see* Hydrothorax
spermatic cord —*see* Hydrocele

Hydropyonephrosis N13.6

Hydrorachis Q06.4

Hydrorrhea (nasal) J34.89
pregnancy —*see* Rupture, membranes, premature

Hydrosadenitis (axillaris) (suppurative) L73.2

Hydrosalpinx (fallopian tube) (follicularis) N70.11

Hydrothorax (double) (pleura) J94.8
chylous (nonfilarial) I89.8
filarial (*see also* Infestation, filarial) B74.9 *[J91.8]*
traumatic —*see* Injury, intrathoracic
tuberculous NEC (non primary) A15.6

Hydroureter (*see also* Hydronephrosis) N13.4
with infection N13.6
congenital Q62.39

Hydroureteronephrosis —*see* Hydronephrosis

Hydrourethra N36.8

Hydroxykynureninuria E70.89

Hydroxylysinemia E72.3

Hydroxyprolinemia E72.59

Hygiene, sleep
abuse Z72.821
inadequate Z72.821
poor Z72.821

Hygroma (congenital) (cystic) D18.1
praepatellare, prepatellar —*see* Bursitis, prepatellar

Hymen —*see* condition

Hymenolepis, hymenolepiasis (diminuta) (infection) (infestation) (nana) B71.0

Hypalgesia R20.8

Hyperacidity (gastric) K31.89
psychogenic F45.8

Hyperactive, hyperactivity F90.9
basal cell, uterine cervix —*see* Dysplasia, cervix
bowel sounds R19.12
cervix epithelial (basal) —*see* Dysplasia, cervix
child F90.9
attention deficit —*see* Disorder, attention-deficit hyperactivity
detrusor muscle N32.81
gastrointestinal K31.89
psychogenic F45.8
nasal mucous membrane J34.3
stomach K31.89
thyroid (gland) —*see* Hyperthyroidism

Hyperacusis H93.23-

Hyperadrenalism E27.5

Hyperadrenocorticism E24.9
congenital E25.0
iatrogenic E24.2
correct substance properly administered —*see* Table of Drugs and Chemicals, by drug, adverse effect
overdose or wrong substance given or taken —*see* Table of Drugs and Chemicals, by drug, poisoning
not associated with Cushing's syndrome E27.0
pituitary-dependent E24.0

Hyperaldosteronism E26.9
familial (type I) E26.02
glucocorticoid-remediable E26.02
primary (due to (bilateral) adrenal hyperplasia) E26.09
primary NEC E26.09
secondary E26.1
specified NEC E26.89

Hyperalgesia R20.8

Hyperalimentation R63.2
carotene, carotin E67.1
specified NEC E67.8
vitamin
A E67.0
D E67.3

Hyperaminoaciduria
arginine E72.21

Hyperaminoaciduria (continued)
cystine E72.01
lysine E72.3
ornithine E72.4

Hyperammonemia (congenital) E72.20

Hyperazotemia —*see* Uremia

Hyperbetalipoproteinemia (familial) E78.00
with prebetalipoproteinemia E78.2

Hyperbicarbonatemia P74.41

Hyperbilirubinemia
constitutional E80.6
familial conjugated E80.6
neonatal (transient) —*see* Jaundice, newborn

Hypercalcemia, hypocalciuric, familial E83.52

Hypercalciuria, idiopathic R82.994

Hypercapnia R06.89
newborn P84

Hypercarotenemia (dietary) E67.1

Hypercementosis K03.4

Hyperchloremia E87.8

Hyperchlorhydria K31.89
neurotic F45.8
psychogenic F45.8

Hypercholesterinemia —*see* Hypercholesterolemia

Hypercholesterolemia (essential) (primary) (pure) E78.00
with hyperglyceridemia, endogenous E78.2
dietary counseling and surveillance Z71.3
familial E78.01
hereditary E78.01

Hyperchylia gastrica, psychogenic F45.8

Hyperchylomicronemia (familial) (primary) E78.3
with hyperbetalipoproteinemia E78.3

Hypercoagulable (state) D68.59
activated protein C resistance D68.51
antithrombin (III) deficiency D68.59
factor V Leiden mutation D68.51
primary NEC D68.59
protein C deficiency D68.59
protein S deficiency D68.59
prothrombin gene mutation D68.52
secondary D68.69
specified NEC D68.69

Hypercoagulation (state) D68.59

Hypercorticalism, pituitary-dependent E24.0

Hypercorticosolism —*see* Cushing's, syndrome

Hypercorticosteronism E24.2
correct substance properly administered —*see* Table of Drugs and Chemicals, by drug, adverse effect
overdose or wrong substance given or taken —*see* Table of Drugs and Chemicals, by drug, poisoning

Hypercortisonism E24.2
correct substance properly administered —*see* Table of Drugs and Chemicals, by drug, adverse effect
overdose or wrong substance given or taken —*see* Table of Drugs and Chemicals, by drug, poisoning

Hyperekplexia Q89.8

Hyperelectrolytemia E87.8

Hyperemesis R11.10
with nausea R11.2
gravidarum (mild) O21.0
with
carbohydrate depletion O21.1
dehydration O21.1
electrolyte imbalance O21.1
metabolic disturbance O21.1
severe (with metabolic disturbance) O21.1
projectile R11.12
psychogenic F45.8

Hyperemia (acute) (passive) R68.89
anal mucosa K62.89
bladder N32.89
cerebral I67.89
conjunctiva H11.43-
ear internal, acute H83.0
enteric K59.89
eye —*see* Hyperemia, conjunctiva
eyelid (active) (passive) —*see* Disorder, eyelid, specified type NEC
intestine K59.89
iris —*see* Disorder, iris, vascular
kidney N28.89
labyrinth H83.0
liver (active) K76.89
lung (passive) —*see* Edema, lung
pulmonary (passive) —*see* Edema, lung
renal N28.89
retina H35.89
stomach K31.89

Hyperesthesia (body surface) R20.3
larynx (reflex) J38.7
hysterical F44.89
pharynx (reflex) J39.2
hysterical F44.89

Hyperestrogenism (drug-induced) (iatrogenic) E28.0

Hyperexplexia Q89.8

Hyperfibrinolysis —*see* Fibrinolysis

Hyperfructosemia E74.19

Hyperfunction
adrenal cortex, not associated with Cushing's syndrome E27.0
medulla E27.5
adrenomedullary E27.5
virilism E25.9
congenital E25.0
ovarian E28.8
pancreas K86.89
parathyroid (gland) E21.3
pituitary (gland) (anterior) E22.9
specified NEC E22.8
polyglandular E31.1
testicular E29.0

Hypergammaglobulinemia D89.2
polyclonal D89.0
Waldenström D89.0

Hypergastrinemia E16.4

Hyperglobulinemia R77.1

Hyperglycemia, hyperglycemic (transient) R73.9

Hyperglycemia, hyperglycemic
(continued)
coma —*see* Diabetes, by type, with coma
postpancreatectomy E89.1

Hyperglyceridemia (endogenous) (essential) (familial) (hereditary) (pure) E78.1
mixed E78.3

Hyperglycinemia (non-ketotic) E72.51

Hypergonadism
ovarian E28.8
testicular (primary) (infantile) E29.0

Hyperheparinemia D68.32

Hyperhidrosis, hyperidrosis R61
focal
primary L74.519
axilla L74.510
face L74.511
palms L74.512
soles L74.513
secondary L74.52
generalized R61
localized
primary L74.519
axilla L74.510
face L74.511
palms L74.512
soles L74.513
secondary L74.52
psychogenic F45.8
secondary R61
focal L74.52

Hyperhistidinemia E70.41

Hyperhomocysteinemia E72.11

Hyperhydroxyprolinemia E72.59

Hyperinsulinism (functional) E16.1
with
coma (hypoglycemic) E15
encephalopathy E16.1 *[G94]*
ectopic E16.1
therapeutic misadventure (from administration of insulin) T38.3

Hyperkalemia E87.5

Hyperkeratosis (*see also* Keratosis) L85.9
cervix N88.0
due to yaws (early) (late) (palmar or plantar) A66.3
follicularis Q82.8
penetrans (in cutem) L87.0
palmoplantaris climacterica L85.1
pinta A67.1
senile (with pruritus) L57.0
universalis congenita Q80.8
vocal cord J38.3
vulva N90.4

Hyperkinesia, hyperkinetic (disease) (reaction) (syndrome) (childhood) (adolescence) —*see also* Disorder, attention-deficit hyperactivity
heart I51.89

Hyperleucine-isoleucinemia E71.19

Hyperlipemia, hyperlipidemia E78.5
combined E78.2
familial E78.49
group
A E78.00
B E78.1
C E78.2
D E78.3
mixed E78.2
specified NEC E78.49

Hyperlipidosis E75.6
hereditary NEC E75.5

Hyperlipoproteinemia E78.5
Fredrickson's type
I E78.3
IIa E78.00
IIb E78.2
III E78.2
IV E78.1
V E78.3
low-density-lipoprotein-type (LDL) E78.00
very-low-density-lipoprotein-type (VLDL) E78.1

Hyperlucent lung, unilateral J43.0

Hyperlysinemia E72.3

Hypermagnesemia E83.41
neonatal P71.8

Hypermenorrhea N92.0

Hypermethioninemia E72.19

Hypermetropia (congenital) H52.0-

Hypermobility, hypermotility
cecum —*see* Syndrome, irritable bowel
coccyx —*see* subcategory M53.2
colon —*see* Syndrome, irritable bowel
psychogenic F45.8
ileum K58.9
intestine (*see also* Syndrome, irritable bowel) K58.9
psychogenic F45.8
meniscus (knee) —*see* Derangement, knee, meniscus
scapula —*see* Instability, joint, shoulder
stomach K31.89
psychogenic F45.8
syndrome M35.7
urethra N36.41
with intrinsic sphincter deficiency N36.43

Hypernasality R49.21

Hypernatremia E87.0

Hypernephroma C64.-

Hyperopia —*see* Hypermetropia

Hyperorexia nervosa F50.2

Hyperornithinemia E72.4

Hyperosmia R43.1

Hyperosmolality E87.0

Hyperostosis (monomelic) —*see also* Disorder, bone, density and structure, specified NEC
ankylosing (spine) M48.10
cervical region M48.12
cervicothoracic region M48.13
lumbar region M48.16
lumbosacral region M48.17
multiple sites M48.19
occipito-atlanto-axial region M48.11
sacrococcygeal region M48.18
thoracic region M48.14
thoracolumbar region M48.15
cortical (skull) M85.2
infantile M89.8X-
frontal, internal of skull M85.2
interna frontalis M85.2
skeletal, diffuse idiopathic —*see* Hyperostosis, ankylosing
skull M85.2
congenital Q75.8
vertebral, ankylosing —*see* Hyperostosis, ankylosing

Hyperovarism E28.8

Hyperoxaluria R82.992
primary E72.53

Hyperparathyroidism E21.3
primary E21.0
secondary (renal) N25.81
non-renal E21.1
specified NEC E21.2
tertiary E21.2

Hyperpathia R20.8

Hyperperistalsis R19.2
psychogenic F45.8

Hyperpermeability, capillary I78.8

Hyperphagia R63.2

Hyperphenylalaninemia NEC E70.1

Hyperphoria (alternating) H50.53

Hyperphosphatemia E83.39

Hyperpiesis, hyperpiesia —*see* Hypertension

Hyperpigmentation —*see also* Pigmentation
melanin NEC L81.4
postinflammatory L81.0

Hyperpinealism E34.8

Hyperpituitarism E22.9

Hyperplasia, hyperplastic
adenoids J35.2
adrenal (capsule) (cortex) (gland) E27.8
with
sexual precocity (male) E25.9
congenital E25.0
virilism, adrenal E25.9
congenital E25.0
virilization (female) E25.9
congenital E25.0
congenital E25.0
salt-losing E25.0
adrenomedullary E27.5
angiolymphoid, eosinophilia (ALHE) D18.01
appendix (lymphoid) K38.0
artery, fibromuscular I77.3
bone —*see also* Hypertrophy, bone
marrow D75.89
breast —*see also* Hypertrophy, breast
atypical, atypia N60.9-
ductal N60.9-
lobular N60.9-
C-cell, thyroid E07.0
cementation (tooth) (teeth) K03.4
cervical gland R59.0
cervix (uteri) (basal cell) (endometrium) (polypoid) —*see also* Dysplasia, cervix
congenital Q51.828
clitoris, congenital Q52.6
denture K06.2
endocervicitis N72
endometrium, endometrial (adenomatous) (cystic) (glandular) (glandular-cystic) (polypoid) N85.00
with atypia N85.02
benign N85.01
cervix —*see* Dysplasia, cervix
complex (without atypia) N85.01
simple (without atypia) N85.01
epithelial L85.9
focal, oral, including tongue K13.29
nipple N62
skin L85.9
tongue K13.29
vaginal wall N89.3
erythroid D75.89
fibromuscular of artery (carotid) (renal) I77.3

Hyperplasia, hyperplastic *(continued)*
genital
female NEC N94.89
male N50.89
gingiva K06.1
glandularis cystica uteri (interstitialis) (*see also* Hyperplasia, endometrial) N85.00-
gum K06.1
hymen, congenital Q52.4
irritative, edentulous (alveolar) K06.2
jaw M26.09
alveolar M26.79
lower M26.03
alveolar M26.72
upper M26.01
alveolar M26.71
kidney (congenital) Q63.3
labia N90.69
epithelial N90.3
liver (congenital) Q44.7
nodular, focal K76.89
lymph gland or node R59.9
mandible, mandibular M26.03
alveolar M26.72
unilateral condylar M27.8
maxilla, maxillary M26.01
alveolar M26.71
myometrium, myometrial N85.2
neuroendocrine cell, of infancy J84.841
nose
lymphoid J34.89
polypoid J33.9
oral mucosa (irritative) K13.6
organ or site, congenital NEC —*see* Anomaly, by site
ovary N83.8
palate, papillary (irritative) K13.6
pancreatic islet cells E16.9
alpha E16.8
with excess
gastrin E16.4
glucagon E16.3
beta E16.1
parathyroid (gland) E21.0
pharynx (lymphoid) J39.2
prostate (adenofibromatous) (nodular) N40.0
with lower urinary tract symptoms (LUTS) N40.1
without lower urinary tract symptoms (LUTS) N40.0
renal artery I77.89
reticulo-endothelial (cell) D75.89
salivary gland (any) K11.1
Schimmelbusch's —*see* Mastopathy, cystic
suprarenal capsule (gland) E27.8
thymus (gland) (persistent) E32.0
thyroid (gland) —*see* Goiter
tonsils (faucial) (infective) (lingual) (lymphoid) J35.1
with adenoids J35.3
unilateral condylar M27.8
uterus, uterine N85.2
endometrium (glandular) (*see also* Hyperplasia, endometrial) N85.00-
vulva N90.69
epithelial N90.3

Hyperpnea —*see* Hyperventilation

Hyperpotassemia E87.5

Hyperprebetalipoproteinemia (familial) E78.1

Hyperprolactinemia E22.1

Hypertension, hypertensive
(continued)
renal —see Hypertension, kidney
renovascular I15.0
secondary NEC I15.9
  due to
    endocrine disorders I15.2
    pheochromocytoma I15.2
    renal disorders NEC I15.1
      arterial I15.0
    renovascular disorders I15.0
    specified NEC I15.8
transient R03.0
  of pregnancy O13.-
urgency I16.0
venous (chronic)
  due to
    deep vein thrombosis —see
      Syndrome, postthrombotic
    idiopathic I87.309
      with
        inflammation I87.32-
          with ulcer I87.33-
          specified complication NEC
            I87.39-
        ulcer I87.31-
          with inflammation
            I87.33-
      asymptomatic I87.30-

Hypertensive urgency —see
Hypertension

Hyperthecosis ovary E28.8

Hyperthermia (of unknown origin)
—see also Hyperpyrexia
malignant, due to anesthesia T88.3
newborn P81.9
  environmental P81.0

Hyperthyroid (recurrent) —see
Hyperthyroidism

Hyperthyroidism (latent) (pre-adult)
(recurrent) E05.90
with
  goiter (diffuse) E05.00
    with thyroid storm E05.01
    nodular (multinodular) E05.20
      with thyroid storm E05.21
      uninodular E05.10
        with thyroid storm
          E05.11
  storm E05.91
due to ectopic thyroid tissue E05.30
  with thyroid storm E05.31
neonatal, transitory P72.1
specified NEC E05.80
  with thyroid storm E05.81

Hypertony, hypertonia,
hypertonicity
bladder N31.8
congenital P94.1
stomach K31.89
  psychogenic F45.8
uterus, uterine (contractions)
  (complicating delivery) O62.4

Hypertrichosis L68.9
congenital Q84.2
eyelid H02.869
  left H02.866
    lower H02.865
    upper H02.864
  right H02.863
    lower H02.862
    upper H02.861
lanuginosa Q84.2
  acquired L68.1
localized L68.2
specified NEC L68.8

Hypertriglyceridemia, essential
E78.1

Hypertrophy, hypertrophic
adenofibromatous, prostate —see
  Enlargement, enlarged, prostate
adenoids (infective) J35.2
  with tonsils J35.3
adrenal cortex E27.8
alveolar process or ridge —see
  Anomaly, alveolar
anal papillae K62.89
artery I77.89
  congenital NEC Q27.8
    digestive system Q27.8
    lower limb Q27.8
    specified site NEC Q27.8
    upper limb Q27.8
auricular —see Hypertrophy,
  cardiac
Bartholin's gland N75.8
bile duct (common) (hepatic)
  K83.8
bladder (sphincter) (trigone)
  N32.89
bone M89.30
  carpus M89.34-
  clavicle M89.31-
  femur M89.35-
  fibula M89.36-
  finger M89.34-
  humerus M89.32-
  ilium M89.359
  ischium M89.359
  metacarpus M89.34-
  metatarsus M89.37-
  multiple sites M89.39
  neck M89.38
  radius M89.33-
  rib M89.38
  scapula M89.31-
  skull M89.38
  tarsus M89.37-
  tibia M89.36-
  toe M89.37-
  ulna M89.33-
  vertebra M89.38
brain G93.89
breast N62
  cystic —see Mastopathy, cystic
  newborn P83.4
  pubertal, massive N62
  puerperal, postpartum —see
    Disorder, breast, specified
    type NEC
  senile (parenchymatous) N62
cardiac (chronic) (idiopathic) I51.7
  with rheumatic fever (conditions
    in I00)
    active I01.8
    inactive or quiescent (with
      chorea) I09.89
  congenital NEC Q24.8
  fatty —see Degeneration,
    myocardial
  hypertensive —see
    Hypertension, heart
  rheumatic (with chorea) I09.89
    active or acute I01.8
      with chorea I02.0
  valve —see Endocarditis
cartilage —see Disorder, cartilage,
  specified type NEC
cecum —see Megacolon
cervix (uteri) N88.8
  congenital Q51.828
  elongation N88.4
clitoris (cirrhotic) N90.89
  congenital Q52.6
colon —see also Megacolon
  congenital Q43.2
conjunctiva, lymphoid H11.89
corpora cavernosa N48.89
cystic duct K82.8

Hypertrophy, hypertrophic
(continued)
duodenum K31.89
endometrium (glandular) (see
  also Hyperplasia, endometrial)
  N85.00-
  cervix N88.8
epididymis N50.89
esophageal hiatus (congenital)
  Q79.1
  with hernia —see Hernia, hiatal
eyelid —see Disorder, eyelid,
  specified type NEC
fat pad E65
  knee (infrapatellar) (popliteal)
    (prepatellar) (retropatellar)
    M79.4
foot (congenital) Q74.2
frenulum, frenum (tongue) K14.8
  lip K13.0
gallbladder K82.8
gastric mucosa K29.60
  with bleeding K29.61
gland, glandular R59.9
  generalized R59.1
  localized R59.0
gum (mucous membrane) K06.1
heart (idiopathic) —see also
  Hypertrophy, cardiac
  valve (see also Endocarditis) I38
hemifacial Q67.4
hepatic —see Hypertrophy, liver
hiatus (esophageal) Q79.1
hilus gland R59.0
hymen, congenital Q52.4
ileum K63.89
intestine NEC K63.89
jejunum K63.89
kidney (compensatory) N28.81
  congenital Q63.3
labium (majus) (minus) N90.60
ligament —see Disorder, ligament
lingual tonsil (infective) J35.1
  with adenoids J35.3
lip K13.0
  congenital Q18.6
liver R16.0
  acute K76.89
  congenital Q44.7
  cirrhotic —see Cirrhosis, liver
  fatty —see Fatty, liver
lymph, lymphatic gland R59.9
  generalized R59.1
  localized R59.0
  tuberculous —see Tuberculosis,
    lymph gland
mammary gland —see
  Hypertrophy, breast
Meckel's diverticulum (congenital)
  Q43.0
  malignant —see Table of
    Neoplasms, small intestine,
    malignant
median bar —see Hyperplasia,
  prostate
meibomian gland —see Chalazion
meniscus, knee, congenital Q74.1
metatarsal head —see Hypertrophy,
  bone, metatarsus
metatarsus —see Hypertrophy,
  bone, metatarsus
mucous membrane
  alveolar ridge K06.2
  gum K06.1
  nose (turbinate) J34.3
muscle M62.89
muscular coat, artery I77.89
myocardium —see also
  Hypertrophy, cardiac
  idiopathic I42.2
myometrium N85.2

Hypertrophy, hypertrophic
(continued)
nail L60.2
  congenital Q84.5
nasal J34.89
  alae J34.89
  bone J34.89
  cartilage J34.89
  mucous membrane (septum) J34.3
  sinus J34.89
  turbinate J34.3
nasopharynx, lymphoid
  (infectional) (tissue) (wall) J35.2
nipple N62
organ or site, congenital NEC
  —see Anomaly, by site
ovary N83.8
palate (hard) M27.8
  soft K13.79
pancreas, congenital Q45.3
parathyroid (gland) E21.0
parotid gland K11.1
penis N48.89
pharyngeal tonsil J35.2
pharynx J39.2
  lymphoid (infectional) (tissue)
    (wall) J35.2
pituitary (anterior) (fossa) (gland)
  E23.6
prepuce (congenital) N47.8
  female N90.89
prostate —see Enlargement,
  enlarged, prostate
  congenital Q55.4
pseudomuscular G71.09
pylorus (adult) (muscle) (sphincter)
  K31.1
  congenital or infantile Q40.0
rectal, rectum (sphincter) K62.89
rhinitis (turbinate) J31.0
salivary gland (any) K11.1
  congenital Q38.4
scaphoid (tarsal) —see
  Hypertrophy, bone, tarsus
scar L91.0
scrotum N50.89
seminal vesicle N50.89
sigmoid —see Megacolon
skin L91.9
  specified NEC L91.8
spermatic cord N50.89
spleen —see Splenomegaly
spondylitis —see Spondylosis
stomach K31.89
sublingual gland K11.1
submandibular gland K11.1
suprarenal cortex (gland) E27.8
synovial NEC M67.20
  acromioclavicular M67.21-
  ankle M67.27-
  elbow M67.22-
  foot M67.27-
  hand M67.24-
  hip M67.25-
  knee M67.26-
  multiple sites M67.29
  specified site NEC M67.28
  wrist M67.23-
tendon —see Disorder, tendon,
  specified type NEC
testis N44.8
  congenital Q55.29
thymic, thymus (gland)
  (congenital) E32.0
thyroid (gland) —see Goiter
toe (congenital) Q74.2
  acquired —see also Deformity,
    toe, specified NEC
tongue K14.8
  congenital Q38.2
  papillae (foliate) K14.3

Hypertrophy, hypertrophic
(continued)
tonsils (faucial) (infective) (lingual) (lymphoid) J35.1
with adenoids J35.3
tunica vaginalis N50.89
ureter N28.89
urethra N36.8
uterus N85.2
neck (with elongation) N88.4
puerperal O90.89
uvula K13.79
vagina N89.8
vas deferens N50.89
vein I87.8
ventricle, ventricular (heart) —see also Hypertrophy, cardiac
congenital Q24.8
in tetralogy of Fallot Q21.3
verumontanum N36.8
vocal cord J38.3
vulva N90.60
stasis (nonfilarial) N90.69

Hypertropia H50.2-

Hypertyrosinemia E70.21

Hyperuricemia (asymptomatic) E79.0

Hyperuricosuria R82.993

Hypervalinemia E71.19

Hyperventilation (tetany) R06.4
hysterical F45.8
psychogenic F45.8
syndrome F45.8

Hypervitaminosis (dietary) **NEC** E67.8
A E67.0
administered as drug (prolonged intake) —see Table of Drugs and Chemicals, vitamins, adverse effect
overdose or wrong substance given or taken —see Table of Drugs and Chemicals, vitamins, poisoning
B6 E67.2
D E67.3
administered as drug (prolonged intake) —see Table of Drugs and Chemicals, vitamins, adverse effect
overdose or wrong substance given or taken —see Table of Drugs and Chemicals, vitamins, poisoning
K E67.8
administered as drug (prolonged intake) —see Table of Drugs and Chemicals, vitamins, adverse effect
overdose or wrong substance given or taken —see Table of Drugs and Chemicals, vitamins, poisoning

Hypervolemia E87.70
specified NEC E87.79

Hypesthesia R20.1
cornea —see Anesthesia, cornea

Hyphema H21.0-
traumatic S05.1-

Hypoacidity, gastric K31.89
psychogenic F45.8

Hypoadrenalism, hypoadrenia E27.40
primary E27.1
tuberculous A18.7

Hypoadrenocorticism E27.40
pituitary E23.0
primary E27.1

Hypoalbuminemia E88.09

Hypoaldosteronism E27.40

Hypoalphalipoproteinemia E78.6

Hypobarism T70.29

Hypobaropathy T70.29

Hypobetalipoproteinemia (familial) E78.6

Hypocalcemia E83.51
dietary E58
neonatal P71.1
due to cow's milk P71.0
phosphate-loading (newborn) P71.1

Hypochloremia E87.8

Hypochlorhydria K31.89
neurotic F45.8
psychogenic F45.8

Hypochondria, hypochondriac, hypochondriasis (reaction) F45.21
sleep F51.03

Hypochondrogenesis Q77.0

Hypochondroplasia Q77.4

Hypochromasia, blood cells D50.8

Hypocitraturia R82.991

Hypodontia —see Anodontia

Hypoeosinophilia D72.89

Hypoesthesia R20.1

Hypofibrinogenemia D68.8
acquired D65
congenital (hereditary) D68.2

Hypofunction
adrenocortical E27.40
drug-induced E27.3
postprocedural E89.6
primary E27.1
adrenomedullary, postprocedural E89.6
cerebral R29.818
corticoadrenal NEC E27.40
intestinal K59.89
labyrinth H83.2
ovary E28.39
pituitary (gland) (anterior) E23.0
testicular E29.1
postprocedural (postsurgical) (postirradiation) (iatrogenic) E89.5

Hypogalactia O92.4

Hypogammaglobulinemia (see also Agammaglobulinemia) D80.1
hereditary D80.0
nonfamilial D80.1
transient, of infancy D80.7

Hypogenitalism (congenital) —see Hypogonadism

Hypoglossia Q38.3

Hypoglycemia (spontaneous) E16.2
coma E15
diabetic —see Diabetes, by type, with hypoglycemia, with coma
diabetic —see Diabetes, hypoglycemia
dietary counseling and surveillance Z71.3
drug-induced E16.0
with coma (nondiabetic) E15
due to insulin E16.0
with coma (nondiabetic) E15
therapeutic misadventure —see subcategory T38.3
functional, nonhyperinsulinemic E16.1
iatrogenic E16.0
with coma (nondiabetic) E15

Hypoglycemia (continued)
in infant of diabetic mother P70.1
gestational diabetes P70.0
infantile E16.1
leucine-induced E71.19
neonatal (transitory) P70.4
iatrogenic P70.3
reactive (not drug-induced) E16.1
transitory neonatal P70.4

Hypogonadism
female E28.39
hypogonadotropic E23.0
male E29.1
ovarian (primary) E28.39
pituitary E23.0
testicular (primary) E29.1

Hypohidrosis, hypoidrosis L74.4

Hypoinsulinemia, postprocedural E89.1

Hypokalemia E87.6

Hypoleukocytosis —see Agranulocytosis

Hypolipoproteinemia (alpha) (beta) E78.6

Hypomagnesemia E83.42
neonatal P71.2

Hypomania, hypomanic reaction F30.8

Hypomenorrhea —see Oligomenorrhea

Hypometabolism R63.8

Hypomotility
gastrointestinal (tract) K31.89
psychogenic F45.8
intestine K59.89
psychogenic F45.8
stomach K31.89
psychogenic F45.8

Hyponasality R49.22

Hyponatremia E87.1

Hypo-osmolality E87.1

Hypo-ovarianism, hypo-ovarism E28.39

Hypoparathyroidism E20.9
familial E20.8
idiopathic E20.0
neonatal, transitory P71.4
postprocedural E89.2
specified NEC E20.8

Hypoperfusion (in)
newborn P96.89

Hypopharyngitis —see Laryngopharyngitis

Hypophoria H50.53

Hypophosphatemia, hypophosphatasia (acquired) (congenital) (renal) E83.39
familial E83.31

Hypophyseal, hypophysis —see also condition
dwarfism E23.0
gigantism E22.0

Hypopiesis —see Hypotension

Hypopinealism E34.8

Hypopituitarism (juvenile) E23.0
drug-induced E23.1
due to
hypophysectomy E89.3
radiotherapy E89.3
iatrogenic NEC E23.1
postirradiation E89.3
postpartum O99.285
postprocedural E89.3

Hypoplasia, hypoplastic
adrenal (gland), congenital Q89.1
alimentary tract, congenital Q45.8
upper Q40.8
anus, anal (canal) Q42.3
with fistula Q42.2
aorta, aortic Q25.42
ascending, in hypoplastic left heart syndrome Q23.4
valve Q23.1
in hypoplastic left heart syndrome Q23.4
areola, congenital Q83.8
arm (congenital) —see Defect, reduction, upper limb
artery (peripheral) Q27.8
brain (congenital) Q28.3
coronary Q24.5
digestive system Q27.8
lower limb Q27.8
pulmonary Q25.79
functional, unilateral J43.0
retinal (congenital) Q14.1
specified site NEC Q27.8
umbilical Q27.0
upper limb Q27.8
auditory canal Q17.8
causing impairment of hearing Q16.9
biliary duct or passage Q44.5
bone NOS Q79.9
face Q75.8
marrow D61.9
megakaryocytic D69.49
skull —see Hypoplasia, skull
brain Q02
gyri Q04.3
part of Q04.3
breast (areola) N64.82
bronchus Q32.4
cardiac Q24.8
carpus —see Defect, reduction, upper limb, specified type NEC
cartilage hair Q78.8
cecum Q42.8
cementum K00.4
cephalic Q02
cerebellum Q04.3
cervix (uteri), congenital Q51.821
clavicle (congenital) Q74.0
coccyx Q76.49
colon Q42.9
specified NEC Q42.8
corpus callosum Q04.0
cricoid cartilage Q31.2
digestive organ(s) or tract NEC Q45.8
upper (congenital) Q40.8
ear (auricle) (lobe) Q17.2
middle Q16.4
enamel of teeth (neonatal) (postnatal) (prenatal) K00.4
endocrine (gland) NEC Q89.2
endometrium N85.8
epididymis (congenital) Q55.4
epiglottis Q31.2
erythroid, congenital D61.01
esophagus (congenital) Q39.8
eustachian tube Q17.8
eye Q11.2
eyelid (congenital) Q10.3
face Q18.8
bone(s) Q75.8
femur (congenital) —see Defect, reduction, lower limb, specified type NEC
fibula (congenital) —see Defect, reduction, lower limb, specified type NEC

Hypoplasia, hypoplastic *(continued)*
finger (congenital) —*see* Defect, reduction, upper limb, specified type NEC
focal dermal Q82.8
foot —*see* Defect, reduction, lower limb, specified type NEC
gallbladder Q44.0
genitalia, genital organ(s)
  female, congenital Q52.8
    external Q52.79
    internal NEC Q52.8
  in adiposogenital dystrophy E23.6
glottis Q31.2
hair Q84.2
hand (congenital) —*see* Defect, reduction, upper limb, specified type NEC
heart Q24.8
humerus (congenital) —*see* Defect, reduction, upper limb, specified type NEC
intestine (small) Q41.9
  large Q42.9
    specified NEC Q42.8
jaw M26.09
  alveolar M26.79
  lower M26.04
    alveolar M26.74
  upper M26.02
    alveolar M26.73
kidney(s) Q60.5
  bilateral Q60.4
  unilateral Q60.3
labium (majus) (minus), congenital Q52.79
larynx Q31.2
left heart syndrome Q23.4
leg (congenital) —*see* Defect, reduction, lower limb
limb Q73.8
  lower (congenital) —*see* Defect, reduction, lower limb
  upper (congenital) —*see* Defect, reduction, upper limb
liver Q44.7
lung (lobe) (not associated with short gestation) Q33.6
  associated with immaturity, low birth weight, prematurity, or short gestation P28.0
mammary (areola), congenital Q83.8
mandible, mandibular M26.04
  alveolar M26.74
  unilateral condylar M27.8
maxillary M26.02
  alveolar M26.73
medullary D61.9
megakaryocytic D69.49
metacarpus —*see* Defect, reduction, upper limb, specified type NEC
metatarsus —*see* Defect, reduction, lower limb, specified type NEC
muscle Q79.8
nail(s) Q84.6
nose, nasal Q30.1
optic nerve H47.03-
osseous meatus (ear) Q17.8
ovary, congenital Q50.39
pancreas Q45.0
parathyroid (gland) Q89.2
parotid gland Q38.4
patella Q74.1
pelvis, pelvic girdle Q74.2
penis (congenital) Q55.62
peripheral vascular system Q27.8
  digestive system Q27.8
  lower limb Q27.8

Hypoplasia, hypoplastic *(continued)*
peripheral vascular system *(continued)*
  specified site NEC Q27.8
  upper limb Q27.8
pituitary (gland) (congenital) Q89.2
pulmonary (not associated with short gestation) Q33.6
  artery, functional J43.0
  associated with short gestation P28.0
radioulnar —*see* Defect, reduction, upper limb, specified type NEC
radius —*see* Defect, reduction, upper limb
rectum Q42.1
  with fistula Q42.0
respiratory system NEC Q34.8
rib Q76.6
right heart syndrome Q22.6
sacrum Q76.49
scapula Q74.0
scrotum Q55.1
shoulder girdle Q74.0
skin Q82.8
skull (bone) Q75.8
  with
    anencephaly Q00.0
    encephalocele —*see* Encephalocele
    hydrocephalus Q03.9
      with spina bifida —*see* Spina bifida, by site, with hydrocephalus
    microcephaly Q02
spinal (cord) (ventral horn cell) Q06.1
spine Q76.49
sternum Q76.7
tarsus —*see* Defect, reduction, lower limb, specified type NEC
testis Q55.1
thymic, with immunodeficiency D82.1
thymus (gland) Q89.2
  with immunodeficiency D82.1
thyroid (gland) E03.1
  cartilage Q31.2
tibiofibular (congenital) —*see* Defect, reduction, lower limb, specified type NEC
toe —*see* Defect, reduction, lower limb, specified type NEC
tongue Q38.3
Turner's K00.4
ulna (congenital) —*see* Defect, reduction, upper limb
umbilical artery Q27.0
unilateral condylar M27.8
ureter Q62.8
uterus, congenital Q51.811
vagina Q52.4
vascular NEC peripheral Q27.8
  brain Q28.3
  digestive system Q27.8
  lower limb Q27.8
  specified site NEC Q27.8
  upper limb Q27.8
  vein(s) (peripheral) Q27.8
    brain Q28.3
    digestive system Q27.8
    great Q26.8
    lower limb Q27.8
    specified site NEC Q27.8
    upper limb Q27.8
  vena cava (inferior) (superior) Q26.8
vertebra Q76.49
vulva, congenital Q52.79
zonule (ciliary) Q12.8

Hypoplasminogenemia E88.02

Hypopnea, obstructive sleep apnea G47.33
Hypopotassemia E87.6
Hypoproconvertinemia, congenital (hereditary) D68.2
Hypoproteinemia E77.8
Hypoprothrombinemia (congenital) (hereditary) (idiopathic) D68.2
  acquired D68.4
  newborn, transient P61.6
Hypoptyalism K11.7
Hypopyon (eye) (anterior chamber) —*see* Iridocyclitis, acute, hypopyon
Hypopyrexia R68.0
Hyporeflexia R29.2
Hyposecretion
  ACTH E23.0
  antidiuretic hormone E23.2
  ovary E28.39
  salivary gland (any) K11.7
  vasopressin E23.2
Hyposegmentation, leukocytic, hereditary D72.0
Hyposiderinemia D50.9
Hypospadias Q54.9
  balanic Q54.0
  coronal Q54.0
  glandular Q54.0
  penile Q54.1
  penoscrotal Q54.2
  perineal Q54.3
  specified NEC Q54.8
Hypospermatogenesis —*see* Oligospermia
Hyposplenism D73.0
Hypostasis pulmonary, passive —*see* Edema, lung
Hypostatic —*see* condition
Hyposthenuria N28.89
Hypotension (arterial) (constitutional) I95.9
  chronic I95.89
  due to (of) hemodialysis I95.3
  drug-induced I95.2
  iatrogenic I95.89
  idiopathic (permanent) I95.0
  intracranial G96.810
    following
      lumbar cerebrospinal fluid shunting G97.83
      specified procedure NEC G97.84
      ventricular shunting (ventriculostomy) G97.2
    specified NEC G96.819
    spontaneous G96.811
  intra-dialytic I95.3
  maternal, syndrome (following labor and delivery) O26.5-
  neurogenic, orthostatic G90.3
  orthostatic (chronic) I95.1
    due to drugs I95.2
    neurogenic G90.3
  postoperative I95.81
  postural I95.1
  specified NEC I95.89
Hypothermia (accidental) T68
  due to anesthesia, anesthetic T88.51
  low environmental temperature T68
  neonatal P80.9
    environmental (mild) NEC P80.8
    mild P80.8
    severe (chronic) (cold injury syndrome) P80.0
    specified NEC P80.8

Hypothermia *(continued)*
not associated with low environmental temperature R68.0
Hypothyroidism (acquired) E03.9
  autoimmune —*see* Thyroiditis, autoimmune
  congenital (without goiter) E03.1
    with goiter (diffuse) E03.0
  due to
    exogenous substance NEC E03.2
    iodine-deficiency, acquired E01.8
      subclinical E02
    irradiation therapy E89.0
    medicament NEC E03.2
    P-aminosalicylic acid (PAS) E03.2
    phenylbutazone E03.2
    resorcinol E03.2
    sulfonamide E03.2
    surgery E89.0
    thiourea group drugs E03.2
  iatrogenic NEC E03.2
  iodine-deficiency (acquired) E01.8
    congenital —*see* Syndrome, iodine- deficiency, congenital
    subclinical E02
  neonatal, transitory P72.2
  postinfectious E03.3
  postirradiation E89.0
  postprocedural E89.0
  postsurgical E89.0
  specified NEC E03.8
  subclinical, iodine-deficiency related E02
Hypotonia, hypotonicity, hypotony
  bladder N31.2
  congenital (benign) P94.2
  eye —*see* Disorder, globe, hypotony
Hypotrichosis —*see* Alopecia
Hypotropia H50.2-
Hypoventilation R06.89
  congenital central alveolar G47.35
  sleep related
    idiopathic nonobstructive alveolar G47.34
    in conditions classified elsewhere G47.36
Hypovitaminosis —*see* Deficiency, vitamin
Hypovolemia E86.1
  surgical shock T81.19
  traumatic (shock) T79.4
Hypoxemia R09.02
  newborn P84
  sleep related, in conditions classified elsewhere G47.36
Hypoxia (see also Anoxia) R09.02
  cerebral, during a procedure NEC G97.81
    postprocedural NEC G97.82
  intrauterine P84
  myocardial —*see* Insufficiency, coronary
  newborn P84
  sleep-related G47.34
Hypsarhythmia —*see* Epilepsy, generalized, specified NEC
Hysteralgia, pregnant uterus O26.89-
Hysteria, hysterical (conversion) (dissociative state) F44.9
  anxiety F41.8
  convulsions F44.5
  psychosis, acute F44.9
Hysteroepilepsy F44.5

IBDU (colonic inflammatory bowel disease unclassified) K52.3

Ichthyoparasitism due to Vandellia cirrhosa B88.8

Ichthyosis (congenital) Q80.9
  acquired L85.0
  fetalis Q80.4
  hystrix Q80.8
  lamellar Q80.2
  lingual K13.29
  palmaris and plantaris Q82.8
  simplex Q80.0
  vera Q80.8
  vulgaris Q80.0
  X-linked Q80.1

Ichthyotoxism —*see* Poisoning, fish
  bacterial —*see* Intoxication, foodborne

Icteroanemia, hemolytic (acquired) D59.9
  congenital —*see* Spherocytosis

Icterus —*see also* Jaundice
  conjunctiva R17
  newborn P59.9
  gravis, newborn P55.0
  hematogenous (acquired) D59.9
  hemolytic (acquired) D59.9
    congenital —*see* Spherocytosis
  hemorrhagic (acute) (leptospiral) (spirochetal) A27.0
    newborn P53
  infectious B15.9
    with hepatic coma B15.0
    leptospiral A27.0
    spirochetal A27.0
  neonatorum —*see* Jaundice, newborn
  spirochetal A27.0

Ictus solaris, solis T67.01

Ideation
  homicidal R45.850
  suicidal R45.851

Identity disorder (child) F64.9
  gender role F64.2
  psychosexual F64.2

Id reaction (due to bacteria) L30.2

Idioglossia F80.0

Idiopathic —*see* condition

Idiot, idiocy (congenital) F73
  amaurotic (Bielschowsky (-Jansky)) (family) (infantile (late)) (juvenile (late)) (Vogt-Spielmeyer) E75.4
  microcephalic Q02

IgE asthma J45.909

IIAC (idiopathic infantile arterial calcification) Q28.8

Ileitis (chronic) (noninfectious) —*see also* Enteritis K52.9
  backwash —*see* Pancolitis, ulcerative (chronic)
  infectious A09
  regional (ulcerative) —*see* Enteritis, regional, small intestine
  segmental —*see* Enteritis, regional
  terminal (ulcerative) —*see* Enteritis, regional, small intestine

Ileocolitis (*see also* Enteritis) K52.9
  regional —*see* Enteritis, regional
  infectious A09
  ulcerative K51.0-

Ileostomy
  attention to Z43.2
  malfunctioning K94.13
  status Z93.2
    with complication —*see* Complications, enterostomy

Ileotyphus —*see* Typhoid

Ileum —*see* condition

Ileus (bowel) (colon) (inhibitory) (intestine) K56.7
  adynamic K56.0
  due to gallstone (in intestine) K56.3
  duodenal (chronic) K31.5
  gallstone K56.3
  mechanical NEC (*see also* Obstruction, intestine, specified NEC) K56.699
  meconium P76.0
    in cystic fibrosis E84.11
    meaning meconium plug (without cystic fibrosis) P76.0
  myxedema K59.89
  neurogenic K56.0
    Hirschsprung's disease or megacolon Q43.1
  newborn
    due to meconium P76.0
      in cystic fibrosis E84.11
      meaning meconium plug (without cystic fibrosis) P76.0
    transitory P76.1
  obstructive (*see also* Obstruction, intestine, specified NEC) K56.699
  paralytic K56.0
  postoperative K91.89

Iliac —*see* condition

Iliotibial band syndrome M76.3-

Illiteracy Z55.0

Illness (*see also* Disease) R69
  manic-depressive —*see* Disorder, bipolar

Imbalance R26.89
  autonomic G90.8
  constituents of food intake E63.1
  electrolyte E87.8
    with
      abortion —*see* Abortion by type, complicated by, electrolyte imbalance
      molar pregnancy O08.5
    due to hyperemesis gravidarum O21.1
    following ectopic or molar pregnancy O08.5
    neonatal, transitory NEC P74.49
      potassium
        hyperkalemia P74.31
        hypokalemia P74.32
      sodium
        hypernatremia P74.21
        hyponatremia P74.22
  endocrine E34.9
  eye muscle NOS H50.9
  hormone E34.9
  hysterical F44.4
  labyrinth H83.2
  posture R29.3
  protein-energy —*see* Malnutrition
  sympathetic G90.8

Imbecile, imbecility (I.Q.35-49) F71

Imbedding, intrauterine device T83.39

Imbibition, cholesterol (gallbladder) K82.4

Imbrication, teeth,, fully erupted M26.30

Imerslund (-Gräsbeck) syndrome D51.1

Immature —*see also* Immaturity
  birth (less than 37 completed weeks) —*see* Preterm, newborn
  extremely (less than 28 completed weeks) —*see* Immaturity, extreme
  personality F60.89

Immaturity (less than 37 completed weeks) —*see also* Preterm, newborn
  extreme of newborn (less than 28 completed weeks of gestation) (less than 196 completed days of gestation) (unspecified weeks of gestation) P07.20
    gestational age
      23 completed weeks (23 weeks, 0 days through 23 weeks, 6 days) P07.22
      24 completed weeks (24 weeks, 0 days through 24 weeks, 6 days) P07.23
      25 completed weeks (25 weeks, 0 days through 25 weeks, 6 days) P07.24
      26 completed weeks (26 weeks, 0 days through 26 weeks, 6 days) P07.25
      27 completed weeks (27 weeks, 0 days through 27 weeks, 6 days) P07.26
      less than 23 completed weeks P07.21
  fetus or infant light-for-dates —*see* Light-for-dates
  lung, newborn P28.0
  organ or site NEC —*see* Hypoplasia
  pulmonary, newborn P28.0
  reaction F60.89
  sexual (female) (male), after puberty E30.0

Immersion T75.1
  hand T69.01-
  foot T69.02-

Immobile, immobility
  complete, due to severe physical disability or frailty R53.2
  intestine K59.89
  syndrome (paraplegic) M62.3

Immune reconstitution (inflammatory) **syndrome [IRIS]** D89.3

Immunization —*see also* Vaccination
  ABO —*see* Incompatibility, ABO
    in newborn P55.1
  appropriate for age
    child (over 28 days old) Z00.129
      with abnormal findings Z00.121
  complication —*see* Complications, vaccination
  encounter for Z23
  not done (not carried out) Z28.9
    because (of)
      acute illness of patient Z28.01
      allergy to vaccine (or component) Z28.04
      caregiver refusal Z28.82
      chronic illness of patient Z28.02
      contraindication NEC Z28.09
      delay in delivery of vaccine Z28.83
      group pressure Z28.1
      guardian refusal Z28.82
      immune compromised state of patient Z28.03

Immunization (*continued*)
      lack of availability of vaccine Z28.83
      manufacturer delay of vaccine Z28.83
      parent refusal Z28.82
      patient's belief Z28.1
      patient had disease being vaccinated against Z28.81
      patient refusal Z28.21
      religious beliefs of patient Z28.1
      specified reason NEC Z28.89
        of patient Z28.29
      unavailability of vaccine Z28.83
      unspecified patient reason Z28.20
  Rh factor
    affecting management of pregnancy NEC O36.09-
      anti-D antibody O36.01-
    from transfusion —*see* Complication(s), transfusion, incompatibility reaction, Rh (factor)

Immunocompromised NOS D84.9

Immunocytoma C83.0-

Immunodeficiency D84.9
  with
    adenosine-deaminase deficiency (*see also* Deficiency, adenosine deaminase) D81.30
    antibody defects D80.9
      specified type NEC D80.8
    hyperimmunoglobulinemia D80.6
    increased immunoglobulin M (IgM) D80.5
    major defect D82.9
      specified type NEC D82.8
    partial albinism D82.8
    short-limbed stature D82.2
    thrombocytopenia and eczema D82.0
  antibody with
    hyperimmunoglobulinemia D80.6
    near-normal immunoglobulins D80.6
  autosomal recessive, Swiss type D80.0
  combined D81.9
    biotin-dependent carboxylase D81.819
      biotinidase D81.810
      holocarboxylase synthetase D81.818
      specified type NEC D81.818
    severe (SCID) D81.9
      with
        low or normal B-cell numbers D81.2
        low T- and B-cell numbers D81.1
        reticular dysgenesis D81.0
    specified type NEC D81.89
  common variable D83.9
    with
      abnormalities of B-cell numbers and function D83.0
      autoantibodies to B- or T-cells D83.2
      immunoregulatory T-cell disorders D83.1
    specified type NEC D83.8
  due to
    conditions classified elsewhere D84.81
    drugs D84.821
    external causes D84.822
    medication (current or past) D84.821

Immunodeficiency (continued)
following hereditary defective
response to Epstein-Barr virus
(EBV) D82.3
selective, immunoglobulin
A (IgA) D80.2
G (IgG) (subclasses) D80.3
M (IgM) D80.4
severe combined (SCID) D81.9
due to adenosine deaminase
deficiency D81.31
specified type NEC D84.89
X-linked, with increased IgM D80.5

Immunodeficient NOS D84.9

Immunosuppressed NOS D84.9

Immunotherapy (encounter for)
antineoplastic Z51.12

Impaction, impacted
bowel, colon, rectum (see also
Impaction, fecal) K56.49
by gallstone K56.3
calculus —see Calculus
cerumen (ear) (external) H61.2-
cuspid —see Impaction, tooth
dental (same or adjacent tooth) K01.1
fecal, feces K56.41
fracture —see Fracture, by site
gallbladder —see Calculus,
gallbladder
gallstone(s) —see Calculus,
gallbladder
bile duct (common) (hepatic)
—see Calculus, bile duct
cystic duct —see Calculus,
gallbladder
in intestine, with obstruction
(any part) K56.3
intestine (calculous) NEC —see
also Impaction, fecal K56.49
gallstone, with ileus K56.3
intrauterine device (IUD) T83.39
molar —see Impaction, tooth
shoulder, causing obstructed labor
O66.0
tooth, teeth K01.1
turbinate J34.89

Impaired, impairment (function)
auditory discrimination —see
Abnormal, auditory perception
cognitive, mild, so stated G31.84
dual sensory Z73.82
fasting glucose R73.01
glucose tolerance (oral) R73.02
hearing —see Deafness
heart —see Disease, heart
kidney N28.9
disorder resulting from N25.9
specified NEC N25.89
liver K72.90
with coma K72.91
mastication K08.89
mild cognitive, so stated G31.84
mobility
ear ossicles —see Ankylosis, ear
ossicles
requiring care provider Z74.09
myocardium, myocardial —see
Insufficiency, myocardial
rectal sphincter R19.8
renal (acute) (chronic) N28.9
disorder resulting from N25.9
specified NEC N25.89
vision NEC H54.7
both eyes H54.3

Impediment, speech (see also
Disorder, speech) R47.9
psychogenic (childhood) F98.8
slurring R47.81
specified NEC R47.89

Impending
coronary syndrome I20.0
delirium tremens F10.239
myocardial infarction I20.0

Imperception auditory (acquired)
—see also Deafness
congenital H93.25

Imperfect
aeration, lung (newborn) NEC
—see Atelectasis
closure (congenital)
alimentary tract NEC Q45.8
lower Q43.8
upper Q40.8
atrioventricular ostium Q21.2
atrium (secundum) Q21.1
branchial cleft NOS Q18.2
cyst Q18.0
fistula Q18.0
sinus Q18.0
choroid Q14.3
cricoid cartilage Q31.8
cusps, heart valve NEC Q24.8
pulmonary Q22.3
ductus
arteriosus Q25.0
Botalli Q25.0
ear drum (causing impairment of
hearing) Q16.4
esophagus with communication
to bronchus or trachea Q39.1
eyelid Q10.3
foramen
botalli Q21.1
ovale Q21.1
genitalia, genital organ(s) or
system
female Q52.8
external Q52.79
internal NEC Q52.8
male Q55.8
glottis Q31.0
interatrial ostium or septum Q21.1
interauricular ostium or septum
Q21.1
interventricular ostium or septum
Q21.0
larynx Q31.8
lip —see Cleft, lip
nasal septum Q30.3
nose Q30.2
omphalomesenteric duct Q43.0
optic nerve entry Q14.2
organ or site not listed —see
Anomaly, by site
ostium
interatrial Q21.1
interauricular Q21.1
interventricular Q21.0
palate —see Cleft, palate
preauricular sinus Q18.1
retina Q14.1
roof of orbit Q75.8
sclera Q13.5
septum
aorticopulmonary Q21.4
atrial (secundum) Q21.1
between aorta and pulmonary
artery Q21.4
heart Q21.9
interatrial (secundum) Q21.1
interauricular (secundum) Q21.1
interventricular Q21.0
in tetralogy of Fallot Q21.3
nasal Q30.3
ventricular Q21.0
with pulmonary stenosis or
atresia, dextraposition of
aorta, and hypertrophy of
right ventricle Q21.3
in tetralogy of Fallot Q21.3

Imperfect (continued)
closure (continued)
skull Q75.0
with
anencephaly Q00.0
encephalocele —see
Encephalocele
hydrocephalus Q03.9
with spina bifida —see
Spina bifida, by site,
with hydrocephalus
microcephaly Q02
spine (with meningocele) —see
Spina bifida
trachea Q32.1
tympanic membrane (causing
impairment of hearing) Q16.4
uterus Q51.818
vitelline duct Q43.0
erection —see Dysfunction, sexual,
male, erectile
fusion —see Imperfect, closure
inflation, lung (newborn) —see
Atelectasis
posture R29.3
rotation, intestine Q43.3
septum, ventricular Q21.0

Imperfectly descended testis —see
Cryptorchid

Imperforate (congenital) —see also
Atresia
anus Q42.3
with fistula Q42.2
cervix (uteri) Q51.828
esophagus Q39.0
with tracheoesophageal fistula
Q39.1
hymen Q52.3
jejunum Q41.1
pharynx Q38.8
rectum Q42.1
with fistula Q42.0
urethra Q64.39
vagina Q52.4

Impervious (congenital) —see also
Atresia
anus Q42.3
with fistula Q42.2
bile duct Q44.2
esophagus Q39.0
with tracheoesophageal fistula
Q39.1
intestine (small) Q41.9
large Q42.9
specified NEC Q42.8
rectum Q42.1
with fistula Q42.0
ureter —see Atresia, ureter
urethra Q64.39

Impetiginization of dermatoses L01.1

Impetigo (any organism) (any site)
(circinate) (contagiosa) (simplex)
(vulgaris) L01.00
Bockhart's L01.02
bullous, bullosa L01.03
external ear L01.00 [H62.40]
follicularis L01.02
furfuracea L30.5
herpetiformis L40.1
nonobstetrical L40.1
neonatorum L01.03
nonbullous L01.01
specified type NEC L01.09
ulcerative L01.09

Impingement (on teeth)
joint —see Disorder, joint,
specified type NEC
soft tissue
anterior M26.81
posterior M26.82

Implant, endometrial N80.9

Implantation
anomalous —see Anomaly, by site
ureter Q62.63
cyst
external area or site (skin) NEC
L72.0
iris —see Cyst, iris,
implantation
vagina N89.8
vulva N90.7
dermoid (cyst) —see Implantation,
cyst

Impotence (sexual) N52.9
counseling Z70.1
organic origin (see also
Dysfunction, sexual, male,
erectile) N52.9
psychogenic F52.21

Impression, basilar Q75.8

Imprisonment, anxiety concerning
Z65.1

Improper care (child) (newborn)
—see Maltreatment

Improperly tied umbilical cord
(causing hemorrhage) P51.8

Impulsiveness (impulsive) R45.87

Inability to swallow —see Aphagia

Inaccessible, inaccessibility
health care NEC Z75.3
due to
waiting period Z75.2
for admission to facility
elsewhere Z75.1
other helping agencies Z75.4

Inactive —see condition

Inadequate, inadequacy
aesthetics of dental restoration
K08.56
biologic, constitutional, functional,
or social F60.7
development
child R62.50
genitalia
after puberty NEC E30.0
congenital
female Q52.8
external Q52.79
internal Q52.8
male Q55.8
lungs Q33.6
associated with short gestation
P28.0
organ or site not listed —see
Anomaly, by site
diet (causing nutritional deficiency)
E63.9
eating habits Z72.4
environment, household Z59.1
family support Z63.8
food (supply) NEC Z59.4
hunger effects T73.0
functional F60.7
household care, due to
family member
handicapped or ill Z74.2
on vacation Z75.5
temporarily away from home
Z74.2
technical defects in home Z59.1
temporary absence from home
of person rendering care
Z74.2
housing (heating) (space) Z59.1
income (financial) Z59.6
intrafamilial communication Z63.8
material resources Z59.9

Inadequate, inadequacy (continued)
mental —see Disability,
intellectual
parental supervision or control of
child Z62.0
personality F60.7
pulmonary
function R06.89
newborn P28.5
ventilation, newborn P28.5
sample of cytologic smear
anus R85.615
cervix R87.615
vagina R87.625
social F60.7
insurance Z59.7
skills NEC Z73.4
supervision of child by parent
Z62.0
teaching affecting education Z55.8
welfare support Z59.7

Inanition R64
with edema —see Malnutrition,
severe
due to
deprivation of food T73.0
malnutrition —see Malnutrition
fever R50.9

Inappropriate
change in quantitative human
chorionic gonadotropin (hCG) in
early pregnancy O02.81
diet or eating habits Z72.4
level of quantitative human
chorionic gonadotropin (hCG)
for gestational age in early
pregnancy O02.81
secretion
antidiuretic hormone (ADH)
(excessive) E22.2
deficiency E23.2
pituitary (posterior) E22.2

Inattention at or after birth —see
Neglect

Incarceration, incarcerated
enterocele K46.0
gangrenous K46.1
epiplocele K46.0
gangrenous K46.1
exomphalos K42.0
gangrenous K42.1
hernia —see also Hernia, by site,
with obstruction
with gangrene —see Hernia, by
site, with gangrene
iris, in wound —see Injury, eye,
laceration, with prolapse
lens, in wound —see Injury, eye,
laceration, with prolapse
omphalocele K42.0
prison, anxiety concerning Z65.1
rupture —see Hernia, by site
sarcoepiplocele K46.0
gangrenous K46.1
sarcoepiplomphalocele K42.0
with gangrene K42.1
uterus N85.8
gravid O34.51-
causing obstructed labor
O65.5

Incised wound
external —see Laceration
internal organs —see Injury, by site

Incision, incisional
hernia K43.2
with
gangrene (and obstruction)
K43.1
obstruction K43.0

Incision, incisional (continued)
surgical, complication —see
Complications, surgical
procedure
traumatic
external —see Laceration
internal organs —see Injury,
by site

Inclusion
azurophilic leukocytic D72.0
blennorrhea (neonatal) (newborn)
P39.1
gallbladder in liver (congenital)
Q44.1

Incompatibility
ABO
affecting management of
pregnancy O36.11-
anti-A sensitization O36.11-
anti-B sensitization O36.19-
specified NEC O36.19-
infusion or transfusion reaction
—see Complication(s),
transfusion, incompatibility
reaction, ABO
newborn P55.1
blood (group) (Duffy) (K) (Kell)
(Kidd) (Lewis) (M) (S) NEC
affecting management of
pregnancy O36.11-
anti-A sensitization O36.11-
anti-B sensitization O36.19-
infusion or transfusion reaction
T80.89
newborn P55.8
divorce or estrangement Z63.5
Rh (blood group) (factor) Z31.82
affecting management of
pregnancy NEC O36.09-
anti-D antibody O36.01-
infusion or transfusion reaction
—see Complication(s),
transfusion, incompatibility
reaction, Rh (factor)
newborn P55.0
rhesus —see Incompatibility, Rh

Incompetency, incompetent,
incompetence
annular
aortic (valve) —see
Insufficiency, aortic
mitral (valve) I34.0
pulmonary valve (heart) I37.1
aortic (valve) —see Insufficiency,
aortic
cardiac valve —see Endocarditis
cervix, cervical (os) N88.3
in pregnancy O34.3-
chronotropic I45.89
with
autonomic dysfunction G90.8
ischemic heart disease I25.89
left ventricular dysfunction
I51.89
sinus node dysfunction I49.8
esophagogastric (junction)
(sphincter) K22.0
mitral (valve) —see Insufficiency,
mitral
pelvic fundus N81.89
pubocervical tissue N81.82
pulmonary valve (heart) I37.1
congenital Q22.3
rectovaginal tissue N81.83
tricuspid (annular) (valve) —see
Insufficiency, tricuspid
valvular —see Endocarditis
congenital Q24.8
vein, venous (saphenous) (varicose)
—see Varix, leg

Incomplete —see also condition
bladder, emptying R33.9
defecation R15.0
expansion lungs (newborn) NEC
—see Atelectasis
rotation, intestine Q43.3

Inconclusive
diagnostic imaging due to excess
body fat of patient R93.9
findings on diagnostic imaging of
breast NEC R92.8
mammogram (due to dense breasts)
R92.2

Incontinence R32
anal sphincter R15.9
coital N39.491
feces R15.9
nonorganic origin F98.1
insensible (urinary) N39.42
overflow N39.490
postural (urinary) N39.492
psychogenic F45.8
rectal R15.9
reflex N39.498
stress (female) (male) N39.3
and urge N39.46
urethral sphincter R32
urge N39.41
and stress (female) (male)
N39.46
urine (urinary) R32
continuous N39.45
due to cognitive impairment, or
severe physical disability or
immobility R39.81
functional R39.81
insensible N39.42
mixed (stress and urge) N39.46
nocturnal N39.44
nonorganic origin F98.0
overflow N39.490
post dribbling N39.43
postural N39.492
reflex N39.498
specified NEC N39.498
stress (female) (male) N39.3
and urge N39.46
total N39.498
unaware N39.42
urge N39.41
and stress (female) (male)
N39.46

Incontinentia pigmenti Q82.3

Incoordinate, incoordination
esophageal-pharyngeal (newborn)
—see Dysphagia
muscular R27.8
uterus (action) (contractions)
(complicating delivery) O62.4

Increase, increased
abnormal, in development R63.8
androgens (ovarian) E28.1
anticoagulants (antithrombin)
(anti-VIIIa) (anti-IXa) (anti-Xa)
(anti-XIa) —see Circulating
anticoagulants
cold sense R20.8
estrogen E28.0
function
adrenal
cortex —see Cushing's,
syndrome
medulla E27.5
pituitary (gland) (anterior) (lobe)
E22.9
posterior E22.2
heat sense R20.8
intracranial pressure (benign)
G93.2

Increase, increased (continued)
permeability, capillaries I78.8
pressure, intracranial G93.2
secretion
gastrin E16.4
glucagon E16.3
pancreas, endocrine E16.9
growth hormone-releasing
hormone E16.8
pancreatic polypeptide E16.8
somatostatin E16.8
vasoactive-intestinal
polypeptide E16.8
sphericity, lens Q12.4
splenic activity D73.1
venous pressure I87.8
portal K76.6

Increta placenta O43.22-

Incrustation, cornea, foreign body
(lead) (zinc) —see Foreign body,
cornea

Incyclophoria H50.54

Incyclotropia —see Cyclotropia

Indeterminate sex Q56.4

India rubber skin Q82.8

Indigestion (acid) (bilious)
(functional) K30
catarrhal K31.89
due to decomposed food NOS
A05.9
nervous F45.8
psychogenic F45.8

Indirect —see condition

Induratio penis plastica N48.6

Induration, indurated
brain G93.89
breast (fibrous) N64.51
puerperal, postpartum O92.29
broad ligament N83.8
chancre
anus A51.1
congenital A50.07
extragenital NEC A51.2
corpora cavernosa (penis) (plastic)
N48.6
liver (chronic) K76.89
lung (black) (chronic) (fibroid)
—see also Fibrosis, lung J84.10
essential brown J84.03
penile (plastic) N48.6
phlebitic —see Phlebitis
skin R23.4

Inebriety (without dependence)
—see Alcohol, intoxication

Inefficiency, kidney N28.9

Inelasticity, skin R23.4

Inequality, leg (length) (acquired)
—see also Deformity, limb,
unequal length
congenital —see Defect, reduction,
lower limb
lower leg —see Deformity, limb,
unequal length

Inertia
bladder (neurogenic) N31.2
stomach K31.89
psychogenic F45.8
uterus, uterine during labor O62.2
during latent phase of labor
O62.2
primary O62.0
secondary O62.1
vesical (neurogenic) N31.2

Infancy, infantile, infantilism —see
also condition
celiac K90.0

Infancy, infantile, infantilism
(continued)
  genitalia, genitals (after puberty)
    E30.0
  Herter's (nontropical sprue) K90.0
  intestinal K90.0
  Lorain E23.0
  pancreatic K86.89
  pelvis M95.5
    with disproportion (fetopelvic)
      O33.1
      causing obstructed labor O65.1
  pituitary E23.0
  renal N25.0
  uterus —*see* Infantile, genitalia

Infant(s) —*see also* Infancy
  excessive crying R68.11
  irritable child R68.12
  lack of care —*see* Neglect
  liveborn (singleton) Z38.2
    born in hospital Z38.00
      by cesarean Z38.01
    born outside hospital Z38.1
    multiple NEC Z38.8
      born in hospital Z38.68
        by cesarean Z38.69
      born outside hospital Z38.7
    quadruplet Z38.8
      born in hospital Z38.63
        by cesarean Z38.64
      born outside hospital Z38.7
    quintuplet Z38.8
      born in hospital Z38.65
        by cesarean Z38.66
      born outside hospital Z38.7
    triplet Z38.8
      born in hospital Z38.61
        by cesarean Z38.62
      born outside hospital Z38.7
    twin Z38.5
      born in hospital Z38.30
        by cesarean Z38.31
      born outside hospital Z38.4
  of diabetic mother (syndrome of)
    P70.1
    gestational diabetes P70.0

Infantile —*see also* condition
  genitalia, genitals E30.0
  os, uterine E30.0
  penis E30.0
  testis E29.1
  uterus E30.0

Infantilism —*see* Infancy

Infarct, infarction
  adrenal (capsule) (gland) E27.49
  appendices epiploicae (*see also*
    Infarct, intestine) K55.069
  bowel (*see also* Infarct, intestine)
    K55.0 069
  brain (stem) —*see* Infarct, cerebral
  breast N64.89
  brewer's (kidney) N28.0
  cardiac —*see* Infarct, myocardium
  cerebellar —*see* Infarct, cerebral
  cerebral (acute) (chronic) —*see*
    also Occlusion, artery cerebral
    or precerebral, with infarction
    I63.9-
    aborted I63.9
    cortical I63.9
    due to
      cerebral venous thrombosis,
        nonpyogenic I63.6
      embolism
        cerebral arteries I63.4-
        precerebral arteries I63.1-
      occlusion NEC
        cerebral arteries I63.5-
        precerebral arteries I63.2-
        small artery I63.81

Infarct, infarction *(continued)*
  cerebral *(continued)*
    due to *(continued)*
      stenosis NEC
        cerebral arteries I63.5-
        precerebral arteries I63.2-
        small artery I63.81
      thrombosis
        cerebral artery I63.3-
        precerebral artery I63.0-
    intraoperative
      during cardiac surgery I97.810
      during other surgery I97.811
    neonatal P91.82-
    perinatal (arterial ischemic)
      P91.82-
    postprocedural
      following cardiac surgery
        I97.820
      following other surgery
        I97.821
    specified NEC I63.89
  colon (acute) (agnogenic) (embolic)
    (hemorrhagic) (nonocclusive)
    (nonthrombotic) (occlusive)
    (segmental) (thrombotic) (with
    gangrene) (*see also* Infarct,
    intestine) K55.049
  coronary artery —*see* Infarct,
    myocardium
  embolic —*see* Embolism
  fallopian tube N83.8
  gallbladder K82.8
  heart —*see* Infarct, myocardium
  hepatic K76.3
  hypophysis (anterior lobe) E23.6
  impending (myocardium) I20.0
  intestine (acute) (agnogenic)
    (embolic) (hemorrhagic)
    (nonocclusive) (nonthrombotic)
    (occlusive) (thrombotic) (with
    gangrene) K55.069
    diffuse K55.062
    focal K55.061
    large K55.049
      diffuse K55.042
      focal K55.041
    small K55.029
      diffuse K55.029
      focal K55.021
  kidney N28.0
  lacunar I63.81
  liver K76.3
  lung (embolic) (thrombotic) —*see*
    Embolism, pulmonary
  lymph node I89.8
  mesentery, mesenteric (embolic)
    (thrombotic) (with gangrene)
    (*see also* Infarct, intestine)
    K55.069
  muscle (ischemic) M62.20
    ankle M62.27-
    foot M62.27-
    forearm M62.23-
    hand M62.24-
    lower leg M62.26-
    pelvic region M62.25-
    shoulder region M62.21-
    specified site NEC M62.28
    thigh M62.25-
    upper arm M62.22-
  myocardium, myocardial (acute)
    (with stated duration of 4 weeks
    or less) I21.9
    associated with revascularization
      procedure I21.A9
    diagnosed on ECG, but
      presenting no symptoms I25.2
    due to
      demand ischemia I21.A1
      ischemic imbalance I21.A1
    healed or old I25.2

Infarct, infarction *(continued)*
  myocardium, myocardial
    (continued)
    intraoperative —*see also* Infarct,
      myocardium, associated with
      revascularization procedure
      during cardiac surgery
        I97.790
      during other surgery I97.791
    non-Q wave I21.4
    non-ST elevation (NSTEMI) I21.4
      subsequent I22.2
    nontransmural I21.4
    past (diagnosed on ECG or other
      investigation, but currently
      presenting no symptoms) I25.2
    postprocedural —*see also*
      Infarct, myocardium,
      associated with
      revascularization procedure
      following cardiac surgery (*see*
        also Infarct, myocardium,
        type 4 or type 5) I97.190
      following other surgery I97.191
    Q wave (*see also*, Infarct,
      myocardium, by site) I21.3
    secondary to
      demand ischemia I21.A1
      ischemic imbalance I21.A1
    ST elevation (STEMI) I21.3
      anterior (anteroapical)
        (anterolateral) (anteroseptal)
        (Q wave) (wall) I21.09
        subsequent I22.0
      inferior (diaphragmatic)
        (inferolateral)
        (inferoposterior) (wall)
        NEC I21.19
        subsequent I22.1
      inferoposterior transmural (Q
        wave) I21.11
      involving
        coronary artery of anterior
          wall NEC I21.09
        coronary artery of inferior
          wall NEC I21.19
        diagonal coronary artery
          I21.02
        left anterior descending
          coronary artery I21.02
        left circumflex coronary
          artery I21.21
        left main coronary artery
          I21.01
        oblique marginal coronary
          artery I21.21
        right coronary artery I21.11
      lateral (apical-lateral) (basal-
        lateral) (high) I21.29
        subsequent I22.8
      posterior (posterobasal)
        (posterolateral)
        (posteroseptal) (true) I21.29
        subsequent I22.8
      septal I21.29
        subsequent I22.8
      specified NEC I21.29
        subsequent I22.8
      subsequent I22.9
    subsequent (recurrent)
      (reinfarction) I22.9
      anterior (anteroapical)
        (anterolateral) (anteroseptal)
        (wall) I22.0
      diaphragmatic (wall) I22.1
      inferior (diaphragmatic)
        (inferolateral)
        (inferoposterior) (wall)
        I22.1
      lateral (apical-lateral) (basal-
        lateral) (high) I22.8

Infarct, infarction *(continued)*
  myocardium, myocardial
    (continued)
    subsequent *(continued)*
      non-ST elevation (NSTEMI)
        I22.2
      posterior (posterobasal)
        (posterolateral)
        (posteroseptal) (true) I22.8
      septal I22.8
      specified NEC I22.8
      ST elevation I22.9
        anterior (anteroapical)
          (anterolateral)
          (anteroseptal) (wall)
          I22.0
        inferior (diaphragmatic)
          (inferolateral)
          (inferoposterior) (wall)
          I22.1
        specified NEC I22.8
      subendocardial I22.2
      transmural I21.3
        anterior (anteroapical)
          (anterolateral)
          (anteroseptal) (wall)
          I22.0
      transmural
        diaphragmatic (wall) I22.1
        inferior (diaphragmatic)
          (inferolateral)
          (inferoposterior) (wall)
          I22.1
        lateral (apical-lateral)
          (basal-lateral) (high)
          I22.8
        posterior (posterobasal)
          (posterolateral)
          (posteroseptal) (true)
          I22.8
        specified NEC I22.8
      type 1 (*see also* Infarction,
        myocardial, subsequent, by
        site, or by ST elevation or
        non-ST elevation) I22.9
      type 2 I21.A1
      type 3 I21.A9
      type 4 I21.A9
      type 5 I21.A9
    syphilitic A52.06
    transmural I21.9
      anterior (anteroapical)
        (anterolateral)
        (anteroseptal) (Q wave)
        (wall) NEC I21.09
      inferior (diaphragmatic)
        (inferolateral)
        (inferoposterior) (Q wave)
        (wall) NEC I21.19
      inferoposterior (Q wave)
        I21.11
      lateral (apical-lateral) (basal-
        lateral) (high) NEC I21.29
      posterior (posterobasal)
        (posterolateral)
        (posteroseptal) (true) NEC
        I21.29
      septal NEC I21.29
      specified NEC I21.29
    type 1 (*see also* Infarction,
      myocardial, by site, or by ST
      elevation or non-ST elevation)
      I21.9
    type 2 I21.A1
    type 3 I21.A9
    type 4 (a) (b) (c) I21.A9
    type 5 I21.A9
  nontransmural I21.4
  omentum (*see also* Infarct,
    intestine) K55.069
  ovary N83.8

Infarct, infarction *(continued)*
pancreas K86.89
papillary muscle —*see* Infarct,
myocardium
parathyroid gland E21.4
pituitary (gland) E23.6
placenta O43.81-
prostate N42.89
pulmonary (artery) (vein)
(hemorrhagic) —*see* Embolism,
pulmonary
renal (embolic) (thrombotic) N28.0
retina, retinal (artery) —*see*
Occlusion, artery, retina
spinal (cord) (acute) (embolic)
(nonembolic) G95.11
spleen D73.5
embolic or thrombotic I74.8
subendocardial (acute)
(nontransmural) I21.4
suprarenal (capsule) (gland) E27.49
testis N50.1
thrombotic —*see also* Thrombosis
artery, arterial —*see* Embolism
thyroid (gland) E07.89
ventricle (heart) —*see* Infarct,
myocardium

Infecting —*see* condition

Infection, infected, infective
(opportunistic) B99.9
with
drug resistant organism —*see*
Resistance (to), drug —*see*
also specific organism
lymphangitis —*see*
Lymphangitis
organ dysfunction (acute)
R65.20
with septic shock R65.21
abscess (skin)- code by site under
Abscess
Absidia —*see* Mucormycosis
Acanthamoeba —*see*
Acanthamebiasis
Acanthocheilonema (perstans)
(streptocerca) B74.4
accessory sinus (chronic) —*see*
Sinusitis
achorion —*see* Dermatophytosis
Acremonium falciforme B47.0
acromioclavicular M00.9
Actinobacillus (actinomycetem-
comitans) A28.8
mallei A24.0
muris A25.1
Actinomadura B47.1
Actinomyces (israelii) (*see also*
Actinomycosis) A42.9
Actinomycetales —*see*
Actinomycosis
actinomycotic NOS —*see*
Actinomycosis
adenoid (and tonsil) J03.90
chronic J35.02
adenovirus NEC
as cause of disease classified
elsewhere B97.0
unspecified nature or site B34.0
aerogenes capsulatus A48.0
aertrycke —*see* Infection,
salmonella
alimentary canal NOS —*see*
Enteritis, infectious
Allescheria boydii B48.2
Alternaria B48.8
alveolus, alveolar (process) K04.7
Ameba, amebic (histolytica) —*see*
Amebiasis
amniotic fluid, sac or cavity
O41.10-

Infection, infected, infective
(continued)
amniotic fluid, sac or cavity
(continued)
chorioamnionitis O41.12-
placentitis O41.14-
amputation stump (surgical)
—*see* Complication, amputation
stump, infection
Ancylostoma (duodenalis) B76.0
Anisakiasis, Anisakis larvae
B81.0
anthrax —*see* Anthrax
antrum (chronic) —*see* Sinusitis,
maxillary
anus, anal (papillae) (sphincter)
K62.89
arbovirus (arbor virus) A94
specified type NEC A93.8
artificial insemination N98.0
Ascaris lumbricoides —*see*
Ascariasis
Ascomycetes B47.0
Aspergillus (flavus) (fumigatus)
(terreus) —*see* Aspergillosis
atypical
acid-fast (bacilli) —*see*
Mycobacterium, atypical
mycobacteria —*see*
Mycobacterium, atypical
virus A81.9
specified type NEC A81.89
auditory meatus (external) —*see*
Otitis, externa, infective
auricle (ear) —*see* Otitis, externa,
infective
axillary gland (lymph) L04.2
Bacillus A49.9
abortus A23.1
anthracis —*see* Anthrax
Ducrey's (any location) A57
Flexner's A03.1
Friedländer's NEC A49.8
gas (gangrene) A48.0
mallei A24.0
melitensis A23.0
paratyphoid, paratyphosus A01.4
A A01.1
B A01.2
C A01.3
Shiga (-Kruse) A03.0
suipestifer —*see* Infection,
salmonella
swimming pool A31.1
typhosa A01.00
welchii —*see* Gangrene, gas
bacterial NOS A49.9
as cause of disease classified
elsewhere B96.89
Clostridium perfringens
[C. perfringens] B96.7
Bacteroides fragilis
[B. fragilis] B96.6
Enterobacter sakazakii B96.89
Enterococcus B95.2
Escherichia coli [E. coli]
—*see also* Escherichia coli
B96.20
Helicobacter pylori [H.pylori]
B96.81
Hemophilus influenzae [H.
influenzae] B96.3
Klebsiella pneumoniae [K.
pneumoniae] B96.1
Mycoplasma pneumoniae [M.
pneumoniae] B96.0
Proteus (mirabilis) (morganii)
B96.4
Pseudomonas (aeruginosa)
(mallei) (pseudomallei)
B96.5

Infection, infected, infective
(continued)
bacterial NOS *(continued)*
as cause of disease classified
elsewhere *(continued)*
Staphylococcus B95.8
aureus (methicillin
susceptible) (MSSA)
B95.61
methicillin resistant
(MRSA) B95.62
specified NEC B95.7
Streptococcus B95.5
group A B95.0
group B B95.1
pneumoniae B95.3
specified NEC B95.4
Vibrio vulnificus B96.82
specified NEC A48.8
Bacterium
paratyphosum A01.4
A A01.1
B A01.2
C A01.3
typhosum A01.00
Bacteroides NEC A49.8
fragilis, as cause of disease
classified elsewhere B96.6
Balantidium coli A07.0
Bartholin's gland N75.8
Basidiobolus B46.8
bile duct (common) (hepatic) —*see*
Cholangitis
bladder —*see* Cystitis
Blastomyces, blastomycotic —*see*
also Blastomycosis
brasiliensis —*see*
Paracoccidioidomycosis
dermatitidis —*see* Blastomycosis
European —*see* Cryptococcosis
Loboi B48.0
North American B40.9
South American —*see*
Paracoccidioidomycosis
bleb, postprocedure   *see* Blebitis
bone —*see* Osteomyelitis
Bordetella —*see* Whooping cough
Borrelia bergdorfi A69.20
brain (*see also* Encephalitis)
G04.90
membranes —*see* Meningitis
septic G06.0
meninges —*see* Meningitis,
bacterial
branchial cyst Q18.0
breast —*see* Mastitis
bronchus —*see* Bronchitis
Brucella A23.9
abortus A23.1
canis A23.3
melitensis A23.0
mixed A23.8
specified NEC A23.8
suis A23.2
Brugia (malayi) B74.1
timori B74.2
bursa —*see* Bursitis, infective
buttocks (skin) L08.9
Campylobacter, intestinal A04.5
as cause of disease classified
elsewhere B96.81
Candida (albicans) (tropicalis)
—*see* Candidiasis
candiru B88.8
Capillaria (intestinal) B81.1
hepatica B83.8
philippinensis B81.1
cartilage —*see* Disorder, cartilage,
specified type NEC
catheter-related bloodstream
(CRBSI) T80.211

Infection, infected, infective
(continued)
cat liver fluke B66.0
cellulitis - code by site under
Cellulitis
central line-associated T80.219
bloodstream (CLABSI) T80.211
specified NEC T80.218
Cephalosporium falciforme B47.0
cerebrospinal —*see* Meningitis
cervical gland (lymph) L04.0
cervix —*see* Cervicitis
cesarean delivery wound
(puerperal) O86.00
cestodes —*see* Infestation, cestodes
chest J22
Chilomastix (intestinal) A07.8
Chlamydia, chlamydial A74.9
anus A56.3
genitourinary tract A56.2
lower A56.00
specified NEC A56.19
lymphogranuloma A55
pharynx A56.4
psittaci A70
rectum A56.3
sexually transmitted NEC
A56.8
cholera —*see* Cholera
Cladosporium
bantianum (brain abscess) B43.1
carrionii B43.0
castellanii B36.1
trichoides (brain abscess) B43.1
werneckii B36.1
Clonorchis (sinensis) (liver) B66.1
Clostridium NEC
bifermentans A48.0
botulinum (food poisoning)
A05.1
infant A48.51
wound A48.52
difficile
as cause of disease classified
elsewhere B96.89
foodborne (disease)
not specified as recurrent
A04.72
recurrent A04.71
gas gangrene A48.0
necrotizing enterocolitis
not specified as recurrent
A04.72
recurrent A04.71
sepsis A41.4
gas-forming NEC A48.0
histolyticum A48.0
novyi, causing gas gangrene
A48.0
oedematiens A48.0
perfringens
as cause of disease classified
elsewhere B96.7
due to food A05.2
foodborne (disease) A05.2
gas gangrene A48.0
sepsis A41.4
septicum, causing gas gangrene
A48.0
sordellii, causing gas gangrene
A48.0
welchii
as cause of disease classified
elsewhere B96.7
foodborne (disease) A05.2
gas gangrene A48.0
necrotizing enteritis A05.2
sepsis A41.4
Coccidioides (immitis) —*see*
Coccidioidomycosis
colon —*see* Enteritis, infectious

colostomy K94.02
common duct —*see* Cholangitis
congenital P39.9
  Candida (albicans) P37.5
  cytomegalovirus P35.1
  hepatitis, viral P35.3
  herpes simplex P35.2
  infectious or parasitic disease P37.9
    specified NEC P37.8
  listeriosis (disseminated) P37.2
  malaria NEC P37.4
    falciparum P37.3
  Plasmodium falciparum P37.3
  poliomyelitis P35.8
  rubella P35.0
  skin P39.4
  toxoplasmosis (acute) (subacute)
    (chronic) P37.1
  tuberculosis P37.0
  urinary (tract) P39.3
  vaccinia P35.8
  virus P35.9
    specified type NEC P35.8
Conidiobolus B46.8
coronavirus-2019 U07.1
coronavirus NEC B34.2
  as cause of disease classified
    elsewhere B97.29
  severe acute respiratory syndrome
    (SARS associated) B97.21
corpus luteum —*see* Salpingo-
  oophoritis
Corynebacterium diphtheriae
  —*see* Diphtheria
cotia virus B08.8
COVID-19 U07.1
Coxiella burnetii A78
coxsackie —*see* Coxsackie
Cryptococcus neoformans —*see*
  Cryptococcosis
Cryptosporidium A07.2
Cunninghamella —*see*
  Mucormycosis
cyst —*see* Cyst
cystic duct (*see also* Cholecystitis)
  K81.9
Cysticercus cellulosae —*see*
  Cysticercosis
cytomegalovirus, cytomegaloviral
  B25.9
  congenital P35.1
  maternal, maternal care for
    (suspected) damage to fetus
    O35.3
  mononucleosis B27.10
    with
      complication NEC B27.19
      meningitis B27.12
      polyneuropathy B27.11
delta-agent (acute), in hepatitis B
  carrier B17.0
dental (pulpal origin) K04.7
Deuteromycetes B47.0
Dicrocoelium dendriticum B66.2
Dipetalonema (perstans)
  (streptocerca) B74.4
diphtherial —*see* Diphtheria
Diphyllobothrium (adult) (latum)
  (pacificum) B70.0
  larval B70.1
Diplogonoporus (grandis) B71.8
Dipylidium caninum B67.4
Dirofilaria B74.8
Dracunculus medinensis B72
Drechslera (hawaiiensis) B43.8
Ducrey Haemophilus (any location)
  A57
due to or resulting from
  artificial insemination N98.0

due to or resulting from *(continued)*
  Babesia
    divergens (-like) strain B60.03
    duncani (-type) species B60.02
    microti B60.01
    species
      specified NEC B60.09
  central venous catheter T80.219
    bloodstream T80.211
    exit or insertion site T80.212
    localized T80.212
    port or reservoir T80.212
    specified NEC T80.218
    tunnel T80.212
  device, implant or graft (*see*
    also Complications, by
    site and type, infection or
    inflammation) T85.79
    arterial graft NEC T82.7
    breast (implant) T85.79
    catheter NEC T85.79
      dialysis (renal) T82.7
        central line T80.211
        intraperitoneal T85.71
      infusion NEC T82.7
        cranial T85.735
        intrathecal T85.735
        spinal (epidural)
          (subdural) T85.735
        subarachnoid T85.735
      urinary T83.518
        cystostomy T83.510
        Hopkins T83.518
        ileostomy T83.518
        nephrostomy T83.512
        specified NEC T83.518
        urethral indwelling
          T83.511
        urostomy T83.518
    electronic (electrode) (pulse
    generator) (stimulator)
      bone T84.7
      cardiac T82.7
      nervous system T85.738
        brain T85.731
        cranial nerve T85.732
        gastric nerve T85.732
        generator pocket T85.734
        neurostimulator generator
          T85.734
        peripheral nerve
          T85.732
        sacral nerve T85.732
        spinal cord T85.733
        vagal nerve T85.732
      urinary T83.590
    fixation, internal (orthopedic)
    NEC —*see* Complication,
    fixation device, infection
    gastrointestinal (bile duct)
    (esophagus) T85.79
      neurostimulator electrode
        (lead) T85.732
    genital NEC T83.69
    heart NEC T82.7
      valve (prosthesis) T82.6
        graft T82.7
    joint prosthesis —*see*
      Complication, joint
      prosthesis, infection
    ocular (corneal graft) (orbital
    implant) NEC T85.79
    orthopedic NEC T84.7
    penile (cylinder) (pump)
    (resevoir) T83.61
    specified NEC T85.79
    testicular T83.62
    urinary NEC T83.598
      ileal conduit stent T83.593

due to or resulting from *(continued)*
  device, implant or graft
  (continued)
    urinary NEC *(continued)*
      implanted neurostimulation
        T83.590
      implanted sphincter T83.591
      indwelling ureteral stent
        T83.592
      nephroureteral stent T83.593
      specified stent NEC T83.593
    vascular NEC T82.7
    ventricular intracranial
    (communicating) shunt
    T85.730
  Hickman catheter T80.219
    bloodstream T80.211
    localized T80.212
    specified NEC T80.218
  immunization or vaccination T88.0
  infusion, injection or transfusion
    NEC T80.29
    acute T80.22
  injury NEC - code by site under
    Wound, open
  peripherally inserted central
    catheter (PICC) T80.219
    bloodstream T80.211
    localized T80.212
    specified NEC T80.218
  portacath (port-a-cath) T80.219
    bloodstream T80.211
    localized T80.212
    specified NEC T80.218
  protozoa of the order
    Piroplasmida NEC B60.09
  pulmonary artery catheter —*see*
    Infection, due to or resulting
    from, central venous catheter
  surgery T81.40
  Swan Ganz catheter —*see*
    Infection, due to or resulting
    from, central venous catheter
  triple lumen catheter T80.219
    bloodstream T80.211
    localized T80.212
    specified NEC T80.218
  umbilical venous catheter T80.219
    bloodstream T80.211
    localized T80.212
    specified NEC T80.218
during labor NEC O75.3
ear (middle) —*see also* Otitis media
  external —*see* Otitis, externa,
    infective
  inner —*see* subcategory H83.0
Eberthella typhosa A01.00
Echinococcus —*see* Echinococcus
echovirus
  as cause of disease classified
    elsewhere B97.12
  unspecified nature or site B34.1
endocardium I33.0
endocervix —*see* Cervicitis
Entamoeba —*see* Amebiasis
enteric —*see* Enteritis, infectious
Enterobacter sakazakii B96.89
Enterobius vermicularis B80
enterostomy K94.12
enterovirus B34.1
  as cause of disease classified
    elsewhere B97.10
    coxsackievirus B97.11
    echovirus B97.12
    specified NEC B97.19
Entomophthora B46.8
Epidermophyton —*see*
  Dermatophytosis
epididymis —*see* Epididymitis

episiotomy (puerperal) O86.09
Erysipelothrix (insidiosa)
  (rhusiopathiae) —*see* Erysipeloid
erythema infectiosum B08.3
Escherichia (E.) coli NEC A49.8
  as cause of disease classified
    elsewhere (*see also*
    Escherichia coli) B96.20
  congenital P39.8
    sepsis P36.4
  generalized A41.51
  intestinal —*see* Enteritis,
    infectious, due to, Escherichia
    coli
ethmoidal (chronic) (sinus) —*see*
  Sinusitis, ethmoidal
eustachian tube (ear) —*see*
  Salpingitis, eustachian
external auditory canal (meatus) NEC
  —*see* Otitis, externa, infective
eye (purulent) —*see*
  Endophthalmitis, purulent
eyelid —*see* Inflammation, eyelid
fallopian tube —*see* Salpingo-
  oophoritis
Fasciola (gigantica) (hepatica)
  (indica) B66.3
Fasciolopsis (buski) B66.5
filarial —*see* Infestation, filarial
finger (skin) L08.9
  nail L03.01-
    fungus B35.1
fish tapeworm B70.0
  larval B70.1
flagellate, intestinal A07.9
fluke —*see* Infestation, fluke
focal
  teeth (pulpal origin) K04.7
  tonsils J35.01
Fonsecaea (compactum) (pedrosoi)
  B43.0
food —*see* Intoxication, foodborne
foot (skin) L08.9
  dermatophytic fungus B35.3
Francisella tularensis —*see*
  Tularemia
frontal (sinus) (chronic) —*see*
  Sinusitis, frontal
fungus NOS B49
  beard B35.0
  dermatophytic —*see*
    Dermatophytosis
  foot B35.3
  groin B35.6
  hand B35.2
  nail B35.1
  pathogenic to compromised host
    only B48.8
  perianal (area) B35.6
  scalp B35.0
  skin B36.9
    foot B35.3
    hand B35.2
    toenails B35.1
Fusarium B48.8
gallbladder —*see* Cholecystitis
gas bacillus —*see* Gangrene, gas
gastrointestinal —*see* Enteritis,
  infectious
generalized NEC —*see* Sepsis
generator pocket, implanted
  electronic neurostimulator
  T85.734
genital organ or tract
  female —*see* Disease, pelvis,
    inflammatory
  male N49.9
    multiple sites N49.8
    specified NEC N49.8

Infection, infected, infective
(continued)
Ghon tubercle, primary A15.7
Giardia lamblia A07.1
gingiva (chronic) K05.10
  acute K05.00
    nonplaque induced K05.01
    plaque induced K05.00
    nonplaque induced K05.11
    plaque induced K05.10
glanders A24.0
glenosporopsis B48.0
Gnathostoma (spinigerum) B83.1
Gongylonema B83.8
gonococcal —*see* Gonococcus
gram-negative bacilli NOS A49.9
guinea worm B72
gum (chronic) K05.10
  acute K05.00
    nonplaque induced K05.01
    plaque induced K05.00
    nonplaque induced K05.11
    plaque induced K05.10
Haemophilus —*see* Infection,
  Hemophilus
heart —*see* Carditis
Helicobacter pylori A04.8
  as cause of disease classified
    elsewhere B96.81
helminths B83.9
  intestinal B82.0
    mixed (types classifiable to
      more than one of the titles
      B65.0-B81.3 and B81.8)
      B81.4
    specified type NEC B81.8
  specified type NEC B83.8
Hemophilus
  aegyptius, systemic A48.4
  ducrey (any location) A57
  influenzae NEC A49.2
    as cause of disease classified
      elsewhere B96.3
    generalized A41.3
herpes (simplex) —*see also* Herpes
  congenital P35.2
  disseminated B00.7
  zoster B02.9
herpesvirus, herpesviral —*see*
  Herpes
hip (joint) NEC M00.9
  due to internal joint prosthesis
    left T84.52
    right T84.51
  skin NEC L08.9
Heterophyes (heterophyes) B66.8
Histoplasma —*see* Histoplasmosis
  American B39.4
  capsulatum B39.4
hookworm B76.9
human
  papilloma virus A63.0
  T-cell lymphotropic virus
    type-1(HTLV-1) B33.3
hydrocele N43.0
Hymenolepis B71.0
hypopharynx —*see* Pharyngitis
inguinal (lymph) glands L04.1
  due to soft chancre A57
intervertebral disc, pyogenic
  M46.30
  cervical region M46.32
  cervicothoracic region M46.33
  lumbar region M46.36
  lumbosacral region M46.37
  multiple sites M46.39
  occipito-atlanto-axial region
    M46.31
  sacrococcygeal region M46.38
  thoracic region M46.34
  thoracolumbar region M46.35

Infection, infected, infective
(continued)
intestine, intestinal —*see* Enteritis,
  infectious
  specified NEC A08.8
intra-amniotic affecting newborn
  NEC P39.2
intrauterine inflammation O41.12-
Isospora belli or hominis A07.3
Japanese B encephalitis A83.0
jaw (bone) (lower) (upper) M27.2
joint NEC M00.9
  due to internal joint prosthesis
    T84.50
kidney (cortex) (hematogenous)
  N15.9
  with calculus N20.0
    with hydronephrosis N13.6
  following ectopic gestation O08.83
  pelvis and ureter (cystic) N28.85
  puerperal (postpartum) O86.21
  specified NEC N15.8
Klebsiella (K.) pneumoniae NEC
  A49.8
  as cause of disease classified
    elsewhere B96.1
knee (joint) NEC M00.9
  joint M00.9
  due to internal joint prosthesis
    left T84.54
    right T84.53
  skin L08.9
Koch's —*see* Tuberculosis
labia (majora) (minora) (acute)
  —*see* Vulvitis
lacrimal
  gland —*see* Dacryoadenitis
  passages (duct) (sac) —*see*
    Inflammation, lacrimal,
    passages
lancet fluke B66.2
larynx NEC J38.7
leg (skin) NOS L08.9
Legionella pneumophila A48.1
  nonpneumonic A48.2
Leishmania —*see also*
  Leishmaniasis
  aethiopica B55.1
  braziliensis B55.2
  chagasi B55.0
  donovani B55.0
  infantum B55.0
  major B55.1
  mexicana B55.1
  tropica B55.1
lentivirus, as cause of disease
  classified elsewhere B97.31
Leptosphaeria senegalensis B47.0
Leptospira interrogans A27.9
  autumnalis A27.89
  canicola A27.89
  hebdomadis A27.89
  icterohaemorrhagiae A27.0
  pomona A27.89
  specified type NEC A27.89
leptospirochetal NEC —*see*
  Leptospirosis
Listeria monocytogenes —*see also*
  Listeriosis
  congenital P37.2
Loa loa B74.3
  with conjunctival infestation
    B74.3
  eyelid B74.3
Loboa loboi B48.0
local, skin (staphylococcal)
  (streptococcal) L08.9
  abscess - code by site under
    Abscess
  cellulitis - code by site under
    Cellulitis

Infection, infected, infective
(continued)
local, skin *(continued)*
  specified NEC L08.89
  ulcer —*see* Ulcer, skin
Loefflerella mallei A24.0
lung (*see also* Pneumonia) J18.9
  atypical Mycobacterium A31.0
  spirochetal A69.8
  tuberculous —*see* Tuberculosis,
    pulmonary
  virus —*see* Pneumonia, viral
lymph gland —*see also*
  Lymphadenitis, acute
  mesenteric I88.0
lymphoid tissue, base of tongue
  or posterior pharynx, NEC
  (chronic) J35.03
Madurella (grisea) (mycetomii)
  B47.0
major
  following ectopic or molar
    pregnancy O08.0
  puerperal, postpartum, childbirth
    O85
Malassezia furfur B36.0
Malleomyces
  mallei A24.0
  pseudomallei (whitmori) —*see*
    Melioidosis
mammary gland N61.0
Mansonella (ozzardi) (perstans)
  (streptocerca) B74.4
mastoid —*see* Mastoiditis
maxilla, maxillary M27.2
  sinus (chronic) —*see* Sinusitis,
    maxillary
mediastinum J98.51
Medina (worm) B72
meibomian cyst or gland —*see*
  Hordeolum
meninges —*see* Meningitis,
  bacterial
meningococcal (*see also* condition)
  A39.9
  adrenals A39.1
  brain A39.81
  cerebrospinal A39.0
  conjunctiva A39.89
  endocardium A39.51
  heart A39.50
    endocardium A39.51
    myocardium A39.52
    pericardium A39.53
  joint A39.83
  meninges A39.0
  meningococcemia A39.4
    acute A39.2
    chronic A39.3
  myocardium A39.52
  pericardium A39.53
  retrobulbar neuritis A39.82
  specified site NEC A39.89
mesenteric lymph nodes or glands
  NEC I88.0
Metagonimus B66.8
metatarsophalangeal M00.9
methicillin
  resistant Staphylococcus aureus
    (MRSA) A49.02
  susceptible Staphylococcus
    aureus (MSSA) A49.01
Microsporum, microsporic —*see*
  Dermatophytosis
mixed flora (bacterial) NEC A49.8
Monilia —*see* Candidiasis
Monosporium apiospermum B48.2
mouth, parasitic B37.0
Mucor —*see* Mucormycosis
muscle NEC —*see* Myositis,
  infective

Infection, infected, infective
(continued)
mycelium NOS B49
mycetoma B47.9
  actinomycotic NEC B47.1
  mycotic NEC B47.0
Mycobacterium, mycobacterial
  —*see* Mycobacterium
Mycoplasma NEC A49.3
  pneumoniae, as cause of disease
    classified elsewhere B96.0
mycotic NOS B49
  pathogenic to compromised host
    only B48.8
  skin NOS B36.9
myocardium NEC I40.0
nail (chronic)
  with lymphangitis —*see*
    Lymphangitis, acute, digit
  finger L03.01-
    fungus B35.1
  ingrowing L60.0
  toe L03.03-
    fungus B35.1
nasal sinus (chronic) —*see*
  Sinusitis
nasopharynx —*see*
  Nasopharyngitis
navel L08.82
Necator americanus B76.1
Neisseria —*see* Gonococcus
Neotestudina rosatii B47.0
newborn P39.9
  vintra-amniotic NEC P39.2
  skin P39.4
  specified type NEC P39.8
nipple N61.0
  associated with
    lactation O91.03
    pregnancy O91.01-
    puerperium O91.02
Nocardia —*see* Nocardiosis
obstetrical surgical wound
  (puerperal) O86.00
  incisional site
    deep O86.02
    superficial O86.01
  organ and space site O86.03
  surgical site specified NEC
    O86.09
Oesophagostomum (apiostomum)
  B81.8
Oestrus ovis —*see* Myiasis
Oidium albicans B37.9
Onchocerca (volvulus) —*see*
  Onchocerciasis
oncovirus, as cause of disease
  classified elsewhere B97.32
operation wound T81.49
Opisthorchis (felineus) (viverrini)
  B66.0
orbit, orbital —*see* Inflammation,
  orbit
orthopoxvirus NEC B08.09
ovary —*see* Salpingo-oophoritis
Oxyuris vermicularis B80
pancreas (acute) —*see* Pancreatitis,
  acute
  abscess —*see* Pancreatitis, acute
  specified NEC (*see also*
    Pancreatitis, acute) K85.80
papillomavirus, as cause of disease
  classified elsewhere B97.7
papovavirus NEC B34.4
Paracoccidioides brasiliensis —*see*
  Paracoccidioidomycosis
Paragonimus (westermani) B66.4
parainfluenza virus B34.8
parameningococcus NOS A39.9
parapoxvirus B08.60
  specified NEC B08.69

parasitic B89
Parastrongylus
  cantonensis B83.2
  costaricensis B81.3
  paratyphoid A01.4
    Type A A01.1
    Type B A01.2
    Type C A01.3
paraurethral ducts N34.2
parotid gland —*see* Sialoadenitis
parvovirus NEC B34.3
  as cause of disease classified
    elsewhere B97.6
Pasteurella NEC A28.0
  multocida A28.0
  pestis —*see* Plague
  pseudotuberculosis A28.0
  septica (cat bite) (dog bite)
    A28.0
  tularensis —*see* Tularemia
pelvic, female —*see* Disease,
  pelvis, inflammatory
Penicillium (marneffei) B48.4
penis (glans) (retention) NEC
  N48.29
periapical K04.5
peridental, periodontal K05.20
  generalized —*see* Periodontitis,
    aggressive, generalized
  localized —*see* Periodontitis,
    aggressive, localized
perinatal period P39.9
  specified type NEC P39.8
perineal repair (puerperal) O86.09
periorbital —*see* Inflammation,
  orbit
perirectal K62.89
perirenal —*see* Infection, kidney
peritoneal —*see* Peritonitis
periureteral N28.89
Petriellidium boydii B48.2
pharynx —*see also* Pharyngitis
  coxsackievirus B08.5
  posterior, lymphoid (chronic)
    J35.03
Phialophora
  gougerotii (subcutaneous abscess
    or cyst) B43.2
  jeanselmei (subcutaneous
    abscess or cyst) B43.2
  verrucosa (skin) B43.0
Piedraia hortae B36.3
pinta A67.9
  intermediate A67.1
  late A67.2
  mixed A67.3
  primary A67.0
pinworm B80
pityrosporum furfur B36.0
pleuro-pneumonia-like organism
  (PPLO) NEC A49.3
  as cause of disease classified
    elsewhere B96.0
pneumococcus, pneumococcal
  NEC A49.1
  as cause of disease classified
    elsewhere B95.3
  generalized (purulent) A40.3
    with pneumonia J13
Pneumocystis carinii (pneumonia)
  B59
Pneumocystis jiroveci (pneumonia)
  B59
port or reservoir T80.212
postoperative T81.40
postoperative wound T81.49
  surgical site
    deep incisional T81.42
    organ and space T81.43

postoperative wound *(continued)*
  surgical site *(continued)*
    specified NEC T81.49
    superficial incisional T81.41
postprocedural T81.40
postvaccinal T88.0
prepuce NEC N47.7
  with penile inflammation N47.6
prion —*see* Disease, prion, central
  nervous system
prostate (capsule) —*see* Prostatitis
Proteus (mirabilis) (morganii)
  (vulgaris) NEC A49.8
  as cause of disease classified
    elsewhere B96.4
protozoal NEC B64
  intestinal A07.9
    specified NEC A07.8
  specified NEC B60.8
Pseudoallescheria boydii B48.2
Pseudomonas NEC A49.8
  as cause of disease classified
    elsewhere B96.5
  mallei A24.0
  pneumonia J15.1
  pseudomallei —*see* Melioidosis
puerperal O86.4
  genitourinary tract NEC O86.89
  major or generalized O85
  minor O86.4
  specified NEC O86.89
pulmonary —*see* Infection, lung
purulent —*see* Abscess
Pyrenochaeta romeroi B47.0
Q fever A78
rectum (sphincter) K62.89
renal —*see also* Infection, kidney
  pelvis and ureter (cystic) N28.85
reovirus, as cause of disease
  classified elsewhere B97.5
respiratory (tract) NEC J98.8
  acute J22
  chronic J98.8
  influenzal (upper) (acute) —*see*
    Influenza, with, respiratory
    manifestations NEC
  lower (acute) J22
    chronic —*see* Bronchitis,
      chronic
    rhinovirus J00
  syncytial virus (RSV) —*see*
    Infection, virus, respiratory
    syncytial (RSV)
  upper (acute) NOS J06.9
    chronic J39.8
    streptococcal J06.9
    viral NOS J06.9
      due to respiratory syncytial
        virus (RSV) J06.9
        [B97.4]
resulting from
  presence of internal prosthesis,
    implant, graft —*see*
    Complications, by site and
    type, infection
retortamoniasis A07.8
retroperitoneal NEC K68.9
retrovirus B33.3
  as cause of disease classified
    elsewhere B97.30
  human
    immunodeficiency, type
      2(HIV 2) B97.35
    T-cell lymphotropic
      type I (HTLV-I) B97.33
      type II (HTLV-II) B97.34
  lentivirus B97.31
  oncovirus B97.32
  specified NEC B97.39

Rhinosporidium (*see*beri) B48.1
rhinovirus
  as cause of disease classified
    elsewhere B97.89
  unspecified nature or site B34.8
Rhizopus —*see* Mucormycosis
rickettsial NOS A79.9
roundworm (large) NEC B82.0
  Ascariasis (*see also* Ascariasis)
    B77.9
rubella —*see* Rubella
Saccharomyces —*see* Candidiasis
salivary duct or gland (any) —*see*
  Sialoadenitis
Salmonella (aertrycke) (arizonae)
  (callinarum) (cholerae-suis)
  (enteritidis) (suipestifer)
  (typhimurium) A02.9
  with
    (gastro)enteritis A02.0
    sepsis A02.1
    specified manifestation NEC
      A02.8
  due to food (poisoning) A02.9
  hirschfeldii A01.3
  localized A02.20
    arthritis A02.23
    meningitis A02.21
    osteomyelitis A02.24
    pneumonia A02.22
    pyelonephritis A02.25
    specified NEC A02.29
  paratyphi A01.4
    A A01.1
    B A01.2
    C A01.3
  schottmuelleri A01.2
  typhi, typhosa —*see* Typhoid
Sarcocystis A07.8
scabies B86
Schistosoma —*see* Infestation,
  Schistosoma
scrotum (acute) NEC N49.2
seminal vesicle —*see* Vesiculitis
septic
  localized, skin —*see* Abscess
sheep liver fluke B66.3
Shigella A03.9
  boydii A03.2
  dysenteriae A03.0
  flexneri A03.1
  group
    A A03.0
    B A03.1
    C A03.2
    D A03.3
  Schmitz (-Stutzer) A03.0
  schmitzii A03.0
  shigae A03.0
  sonnei A03.3
  specified NEC A03.8
shoulder (joint) NEC M00.9
  due to internal joint prosthesis
    T84.59
  skin NEC L08.9
sinus (accessory) (chronic) (nasal)
  —*see also* Sinusitis
  pilonidal —*see* Sinus, pilonidal
  skin NEC L08.89
Skene's duct or gland —*see*
  Urethritis
skin (local) (staphylococcal)
  (streptococcal) L08.9
  abscess - code by site under
    Abscess
  cellulitis - code by site under
    Cellulitis
  due to fungus B36.9
    specified type NEC B36.8

skin *(continued)*
  mycotic B36.9
    specified type NEC B36.8
  newborn P39.4
  ulcer —*see* Ulcer, skin
slow virus A81.9
  specified NEC A81.89
Sparganum (mansoni) (proliferum)
  (baxteri) B70.1
specific —*see also* Syphilis
  to perinatal period —*see*
    Infection, congenital
specified NEC B99.8
spermatic cord NEC N49.1
sphenoidal (sinus) —*see* Sinusitis,
  sphenoidal
spinal cord NOS —*see also*
  Myelitis G04.91
  abscess G06.1
  meninges —*see* Meningitis
  streptococcal G04.89
Spirillum A25.0
spirochetal NOS A69.9
  lung A69.8
  specified NEC A69.8
Spirometra larvae B70.1
spleen D73.89
Sporotrichum, Sporothrix
  (schenckii) —*see* Sporotrichosis
staphylococcal, unspecified site
  aureus (methicillin susceptible)
    (MSSA) A49.01
    methicillin resistant (MRSA)
      A49.02
  as cause of disease classified
    elsewhere B95.8
    aureus (methicillin
      susceptible) (MSSA)
      B95.61
      methicillin resistant
        (MRSA) B95.62
    specified NEC B95.7
  food poisoning A05.0
  generalized (purulent) A41.2
  pneumonia —*see* Pneumonia,
    staphylococcal
Stellantchasmus falcatus B66.8
streptobacillus moniliformis A25.1
streptococcal NEC A49.1
  as cause of disease classified
    elsewhere B95.5
  B genitourinary complicating
    childbirth O98.82
    pregnancy O98.81-
    puerperium O98.83
  congenital
    sepsis P36.10
      group B P36.0
      specified NEC P36.19
  generalized (purulent) A40.9
Streptomyces B47.1
Strongyloides (stercoralis) —*see*
  Strongyloidiasis
stump (amputation) (surgical)
  —*see* Complication, amputation
  stump, infection
subcutaneous tissue, local
  L08.9
suipestifer —*see* Infection,
  salmonella
swimming pool bacillus A31.1
Taenia —*see* Infestation, Taenia
Taeniarhynchus saginatus B68.1
tapeworm —*see* Infestation,
  tapeworm
tendon (sheath) —*see*
  Tenosynovitis, infective NEC
Ternidens diminutus B81.8
testis —*see* Orchitis

Infection, infected, infective
(continued)
threadworm B80
throat —*see* Pharyngitis
thyroglossal duct K14.8
toe (skin) L08.9
  cellulitis L03.03-
    fungus B35.1
  nail L03.03-
    fungus B35.1
tongue NEC K14.0
  parasitic B37.0
tonsil (and adenoid) (faucial)
  (lingual) (pharyngeal) —*see*
  Tonsillitis
tooth, teeth K04.7
  periapical K04.7
  peridental, periodontal K05.20
    generalized —*see*
      Periodontitis, aggressive,
      generalized
    localized —*see* Periodontitis,
      aggressive, localized
  pulp K04.01
    irreversible K04.02
    reversible K04.01
  socket M27.3
TORCH —*see* Infection, congenital
  without active infection P00.2
Torula histolytica —*see*
  Cryptococcosis
Toxocara (canis) (cati) (felis) B83.0
Toxoplasma gondii —*see*
  Toxoplasma
trachea, chronic J42
trematode NEC —*see* Infestation,
  fluke
trench fever A79.0
Treponema pallidum —*see* Syphilis
Trichinella (spiralis) B75
Trichomonas A59.9
  cervix A59.09
  intestine A07.8
  prostate A59.02
  specified site NEC A59.8
  urethra A59.03
  urogenitalis A59.00
  vagina A59.01
  vulva A59.01
Trichophyton, trichophytic —*see*
  Dermatophytosis
Trichosporon (beigelii) cutaneum
  B36.2
Trichostrongylus B81.2
Trichuris (trichiura) B79
Trombicula (irritans) B88.0
Trypanosoma
  brucei
    gambiense B56.0
    rhodesiense B56.1
  cruzi —*see* Chagas' disease
tubal —*see* Salpingo-oophoritis
tuberculous
  latent (LTBI) Z22.7
  NEC —*see* Tuberculosis
tubo-ovarian —*see* Salpingo-
  oophoritis
tunnel T80.212
tunica vaginalis N49.1
tympanic membrane NEC —*see*
  Myringitis
typhoid (abortive) (ambulant)
  (bacillus) —*see* Typhoid
typhus A75.9
  flea-borne A75.2
  mite-borne A75.3
  recrudescent A75.1
  tick-borne A77.9
    African A77.1
    North Asian A77.2
umbilicus L08.82

Infection, infected, infective
(continued)
ureter —*see* Ureteritis
urethra —*see* Urethritis
urinary (tract) N39.0
  bladder —*see* Cystitis
  complicating
    pregnancy O23.4-
      specified type NEC
      O23.3-
  kidney —*see* Infection, kidney
  newborn P39.3
  puerperal (postpartum) O86.20
  tuberculous A18.13
  urethra —*see* Urethritis
uterus, uterine —*see* Endometritis
vaccination T88.0
vaccinia not from vaccination
  B08.011
vagina (acute) —*see* Vaginitis
varicella B01.9
varicose veins —*see* Varix
vas deferens NEC N49.1
vesical —*see* Cystitis
Vibrio
  cholerae A00.0
    El Tor A00.1
  parahaemolyticus (food
    poisoning) A05.3
  vulnificus
    as cause of disease classified
      elsewhere B96.82
    foodborne intoxication A05.5
Vincent's (gum) (mouth) (tonsil)
  A69.1
virus, viral NOS B34.9
  adenovirus
    as cause of disease classified
      elsewhere B97.0
    unspecified nature or site
      B34.0
  arborvirus, arbovirus arthropod-
    borne A94
  as cause of disease classified
    elsewhere B97.89
    adenovirus B97.0
    coronavirus B97.29
      SARS-associated B97.21
    coxsackievirus B97.11
    echovirus B97.12
    enterovirus B97.10
      coxsackievirus B97.11
      echovirus B97.12
      specified NEC B97.19
    human
      immunodeficiency, type 2
      (HIV 2) B97.35
      T-cell lymphotropic,
        type I (HTLV-I) B97.33
        type II (HTLV-II)
        B97.34
    metapneumovirus B97.81
    papillomavirus B97.7
    parvovirus B97.6
    reovirus B97.5
    respiratory syncytial (RSV)
      —*see* Infection, virus,
      respiratory syncytial (RSV)
    retrovirus B97.30
      human
        immunodeficiency, type
        2(HIV 2) B97.35
        T-cell lymphotropic,
          type I (HTLV-I)
          B97.33
          type II (HTLV-II)
          B97.34
      lentivirus B97.31
      oncovirus B97.32
      specified NEC B97.39
    specified NEC B97.89

Infection, infected, infective
(continued)
virus, viral NOS *(continued)*
  central nervous system A89
    atypical A81.9
      specified NEC A81.89
    enterovirus NEC A88.8
      meningitis A87.0
    slow virus A81.9
      specified NEC A81.89
    specified NEC A88.8
  chest J98.8
  cotia B08.8
  COVID-19 U07.1
  coxsackie (*see also* Infection,
    coxsackie) B34.1
    as cause of disease classified
      elsewhere B97.11
  ECHO
    as cause of disease classified
      elsewhere B97.12
    unspecified nature or site B34.1
  encephalitis, tick-borne A84.9
  enterovirus, as cause of disease
    classified elsewhere B97.10
    coxsackievirus B97.11
    echovirus B97.12
    specified NEC B97.19
  exanthem NOS B09
  human papilloma as cause of
    disease classified elsewhere
    B97.7
  human metapneumovirus as
    cause of disease classified
    elsewhere B97.81
  intestine —*see* Enteritis, viral
  respiratory syncytial (RSV)
    as cause of disease classified
      elsewhere B97.4
    bronchiolitis J21.0
    bronchitis J20.5
    bronchopneumonia J12.1
    otitis media H65.- *[B97.4]*
    pneumonia J12.1
    upper respiratory infection
      J06.9 *[B97.4]*
  rhinovirus
    as cause of disease classified
      elsewhere B97.89
    unspecified nature or site
      B34.8
  slow A81.9
    specified NEC A81.89
  specified type NEC B33.8
    as cause of disease classified
      elsewhere B97.89
    unspecified nature or site
      B34.8
  unspecified nature or site B34.9
  West Nile —*see* Virus, West Nile
  vulva (acute) —*see* Vulvitis
West Nile —*see* Virus, West Nile
whipworm B79
worms B83.9
  specified type NEC B83.8
Wuchereria (bancrofti) B74.0
  malayi B74.1
yatapoxvirus B08.70
  specified NEC B08.79
yeast (*see also* Candidiasis)
  B37.9
yellow fever —*see* Fever, yellow
Yersinia
  enterocolitica (intestinal) A04.6
  pestis —*see* Plague
  pseudotuberculosis A28.2
Zeis' gland —*see* Hordeolum
Zika virus A92.5
  congenital P35.4
zoonotic bacterial NOS A28.9
Zopfia senegalensis B47.0

Infective, infectious —*see* condition

Infertility
female N97.9
  age-related N97.8
  associated with
    anovulation N97.0
    cervical (mucus) disease or
      anomaly N88.3
    congenital anomaly
      cervix N88.3
      fallopian tube N97.1
      uterus N97.2
      vagina N97.8
    dysmucorrhea N88.3
    fallopian tube disease or
      anomaly N97.1
    pituitary-hypothalamic origin
      E23.0
    specified origin NEC N97.8
    Stein-Leventhal syndrome
      E28.2
    uterine disease or anomaly
      N97.2
    vaginal disease or anomaly
      N97.8
  due to
    cervical anomaly N88.3
    fallopian tube anomaly N97.1
    ovarian failure E28.39
    Stein-Leventhal syndrome
      E28.2
    uterine anomaly N97.2
    vaginal anomaly N97.8
  nonimplantation N97.2
  origin
    cervical N88.3
    tubal (block) (occlusion)
      (stenosis) N97.1
    uterine N97.2
    vaginal N97.8
male N46.9
  azoospermia N46.01
    extratesticular cause N46.029
      drug therapy N46.021
      efferent duct obstruction
        N46.023
      infection N46.022
      radiation N46.024
      specified cause NEC
        N46.029
      systemic disease N46.025
  oligospermia N46.11
    extratesticular cause N46.129
      drug therapy N46.121
      efferent duct obstruction
        N46.123
      infection N46.122
      radiation N46.124
      specified cause NEC
        N46.129
      systemic disease N46.125
  specified type NEC N46.8

Infestation B88.9
Acanthocheilonema (perstans)
  (streptocerca) B74.4
Acariasis B88.0
  demodex folliculorum B88.0
  sarcoptes scabiei B86
  trombiculae B88.0
Agamofilaria streptocerca B74.4
Ancylostoma, ankylostoma
  (braziliense) (caninum)
  (ceylanicum) (duodenale) B76.0
  americanum B76.1
  new world B76.1
Anisakis larvae, anisakiasis B81.0
arthropod NEC B88.2
Ascaris lumbricoides —*see*
  Ascariasis
Balantidium coli A07.0

Infestation *(continued)*

beef tapeworm B68.1
Bothriocephalus (latus) B70.0
  larval B70.1
broad tapeworm B70.0
  larval B70.1
Brugia (malayi) B74.1
  timori B74.2
candiru B88.8
Capillaria
  hepatica B83.8
  philippinensis B81.1
cat liver fluke B66.0
cestodes B71.9
  diphyllobothrium —*see*
    Infestation, diphyllobothrium
  dipylidiasis B71.1
  hymenolepiasis B71.0
  specified type NEC B71.8
chigger B88.0
chigo, chigoe B88.1
Clonorchis (sinensis) (liver)
    B66.1
coccidial A07.3
crab-lice B85.3
Cysticercus cellulosae —*see*
    Cysticercosis
Demodex (folliculorum) B88.0
Dermanyssus gallinae B88.0
Dermatobia (hominis) —*see*
    Myiasis
Dibothriocephalus (latus) B70.0
  larval B70.1
Dicrocoelium dendriticum B66.2
Diphyllobothrium (adult)
    (latum) (intestinal) (pacificum)
    B70.0
  larval B70.1
Diplogonoporus (grandis) B71.8
Dipylidium caninum B67.4
Distoma hepaticum B66.3
dog tapeworm B67.4
dragon worm B72
dwarf tapeworm B71.0
Echinococcus —*see*
    Echinococcus
Echinostomum ilocanum B66.8
Entamoeba (histolytica) —*see*
    Infection, Ameba
Enterobius vermicularis B80
eyelid
  in (due to)
    leishmaniasis B55.1
    loiasis B74.3
    onchocerciasis B73.09
    phthiriasis B85.3
    parasitic NOS B89
eyeworm B74.3
Fasciola (gigantica) (hepatica)
    (indica) B66.3
Fasciolopsis (buski) (intestine)
    B66.5
filarial B74.9
  bancroftian B74.0
  conjunctiva B74.9
  due to
    Acanthocheilonema (perstans)
      (streptocerca) B74.4
    Brugia (malayi) B74.1
      timori B74.2
    Dracunculus medinensis B72
    guinea worm B72
    loa loa B74.3
    Mansonella (ozzardi)
      (perstans) (streptocerca)
      B74.4
    Onchocerca volvulus B73.00
      eye B73.00
      eyelid B73.09
    Wuchereria (bancrofti) B74.0

Infestation *(continued)*

filarial *(continued)*
  Malayan B74.1
  ozzardi B74.4
  specified type NEC B74.8
fish tapeworm B70.0
  larval B70.1
fluke B66.9
  blood NOS —*see*
    Schistosomiasis
  cat liver B66.0
  intestinal B66.5
  liver (sheep) B66.3
    cat B66.0
    Chinese B66.1
    due to clonorchiasis B66.1
    oriental B66.1
  lancet B66.2
  lung (oriental) B66.4
  sheep liver B66.3
  specified type NEC B66.8
fly larvae —*see* Myiasis
Gasterophilus (intestinalis) —*see*
    Myiasis
Gastrodiscoides hominis B66.8
Giardia lamblia A07.1
Gnathostoma (spinigerum) B83.1
Gongylonema B83.8
guinea worm B72
helminth B83.9
  angiostrongyliasis B83.2
    intestinal B81.3
  gnathostomiasis B83.1
  hirudiniasis, internal B83.4
  intestinal B82.0
    angiostrongyliasis B81.3
    anisakiasis B81.0
    ascariasis —*see* Ascariasis
    capillariasis B81.1
    cysticercosis —*see*
      Cysticercosis
    diphyllobothriasis —*see*
      Infestation,
      diphyllobothriasis
    dracunculiasis B72
    echinococcus —*see*
      Echinococcosis
    enterobiasis B80
    filariasis —*see* Infestation,
      filarial
    fluke —*see* Infestation, fluke
    hookworm —*see* Infestation,
      hookworm
    mixed (types classifiable to
      more than one of the titles
      B65.0-B81.3 and B81.8)
      B81.4
    onchocerciasis —*see*
      Onchocerciasis
    schistosomiasis —*see*
      Infestation, schistosoma
    specified
      cestode NEC —*see*
        Infestation, cestode
        type NEC B81.8
      strongyloidiasis —*see*
        Strongyloidiasis
      taenia —*see* Infestation, taenia
    trichinellosis B75
    trichostrongyliasis B81.2
    trichuriasis B79
  specified type NEC B83.8
  syngamiasis B83.3
  visceral larva migrans B83.0
Heterophyes (heterophyes) B66.8
hookworm B76.9
  ancylostomiasis B76.0
  necatoriasis B76.1
  specified type NEC B76.8
Hymenolepis (diminuta) (nana)
    B71.0

Infestation *(continued)*

intestinal NEC B82.9
leeches (aquatic) (land) —*see*
    Hirudiniasis
Leishmania —*see* Leishmaniasis
lice, louse —*see* Infestation,
    Pediculus
Linguatula B88.8
Liponyssoides sanguineus B88.0
Loa loa B74.3
  conjunctival B74.3
  eyelid B74.3
louse —*see* Infestation, Pediculus
maggots —*see* Myiasis
Mansonella (ozzardi) (perstans)
    (streptocerca) B74.4
Medina (worm) B72
Metagonimus (yokogawai) B66.8
microfilaria streptocerca —*see*
    Onchocerciasis
  eye B73.00
  eyelid B73.09
mites B88.9
  scabic B86
Monilia (albicans) —*see*
    Candidiasis
mouth B37.0
Necator americanus B76.1
nematode NEC (intestinal) B82.0
  Ancylostoma B76.0
  conjunctiva NEC B83.9
  Enterobius vermicularis B80
  Gnathostoma spinigerum B83.1
  physaloptera B80
  specified NEC B81.8
  trichostrongylus B81.2
  trichuris (trichuria) B79
Oesophagostomum (apiostomum)
    B81.8
Oestrus ovis (*see also* Myiasis)
    B87.9
Onchocerca (volvulus) —*see*
    Onchocerciasis
Opisthorchis (felineus) (viverrini)
    B66.0
orbit, parasitic NOS B89
Oxyuris vermicularis B80
Paragonimus (westermani) B66.4
parasite, parasitic B89
  eyelid B89
  intestinal NOS B82.9
  mouth B37.0
  skin B88.9
  tongue B37.0
Parastrongylus
  cantonensis B83.2
  costaricensis B81.3
Pediculus B85.2
  body B85.1
  capitis (humanus) (any site)
    B85.0
  corporis (humanus) (any site)
    B85.1
  head B85.0
  mixed (classifiable to more than
    one of the titles B85.0-B85.3)
    B85.4
  pubis (any site) B85.3
Pentastoma B88.8
Phthirus (pubis) (any site)
    B85.3
  with any infestation classifiable
    to B85.0-B85.2 B85.4
pinworm B80
pork tapeworm (adult) B68.0
protozoal NEC B64
  intestinal A07.9
    specified NEC A07.8
  specified NEC B60.8
pubic, louse B85.3
rat tapeworm B71.0

Infestation *(continued)*

red bug B88.0
roundworm (large) NEC B82.0
  Ascariasis (*see also* Ascariasis)
    B77.9
sandflea B88.1
Sarcoptes scabiei B86
scabies B86
Schistosoma B65.9
  bovis B65.8
  cercariae B65.3
  haematobium B65.0
  intercalatum B65.8
  japonicum B65.2
  mansoni B65.1
  mattheei B65.8
  mekongi B65.8
  specified type NEC B65.8
  spindale B65.8
screw worms —*see* Myiasis
skin NOS B88.9
Sparganum (mansoni) (proliferum)
    (baxteri) B70.1
  larval B70.1
specified type NEC B88.8
Spirometra larvae B70.1
Stellantchasmus falcatus B66.8
Strongyloides stercoralis —*see*
    Strongyloidiasis
Taenia B68.9
  diminuta B71.0
  echinococcus —*see*
    Echinococcus
  mediocanellata B68.1
  nana B71.0
  saginata B68.1
  solium (intestinal form) B68.0
    larval form —*see*
      Cysticercosis
Taeniarhynchus saginatus B68.1
tapeworm B71.9
  beef B68.1
  broad B70.0
    larval B70.1
  dog B67.4
  dwarf B71.0
  fish B70.0
    larval B70.1
  pork B68.0
  rat B71.0
Ternidens diminutus B81.8
Tetranychus molestissimus B88.0
threadworm B80
tongue B37.0
Toxocara (canis) (cati) (felis) B83.0
trematode(s) NEC —*see*
    Infestation, fluke
Trichinella (spiralis) B75
Trichocephalus B79
Trichomonas —*see* Trichomoniasis
Trichostrongylus B81.2
Trichuris (trichiura) B79
Trombicula (irritans) B88.0
Tunga penetrans B88.1
Uncinaria americana B76.1
Vandellia cirrhosa B88.8
whipworm B79
worms B83.9
  intestinal B82.0
Wuchereria (bancrofti) B74.0

Infiltrate, infiltration
amyloid (generalized) (localized)
    —*see* Amyloidosis
calcareous NEC R89.7
  localized —*see* Degeneration,
    by site
calcium salt R89.7
cardiac
  fatty —*see* Degeneration,
    myocardial
  glycogenic E74.02 *[143]*

Infiltrate, infiltration *(continued)*
corneal —*see* Edema, cornea
eyelid —*see* Inflammation, eyelid
glycogen, glycogenic —*see*
    Disease, glycogen storage
heart, cardiac
    fatty —*see* Degeneration,
        myocardial
    glycogenic E74.02 *[143]*
inflammatory in vitreous H43.89
kidney N28.89
leukemic —*see* Leukemia
liver K76.89
    fatty —*see* Fatty, liver NEC
    glycogen (*see also* Disease,
        glycogen storage) E74.03 *[K77]*
lung R91.8
    eosinophilic —*see* Eosinophilia,
        pulmonary
lymphatic (*see also* Leukemia,
    lymphatic) C91.9-
    gland I88.9
muscle, fatty M62.89
myocardium, myocardial
    fatty —*see* Degeneration,
        myocardial
    glycogenic E74.02 *[143]*
on chest x-ray R91.8
pulmonary R91.8
    with eosinophilia —*see*
        Eosinophilia, pulmonary
skin (lymphocytic) L98.6
thymus (gland) (fatty) E32.8
urine R39.0
vesicant agent
    antineoplastic chemotherapy
        T80.810
    other agent NEC T80.818
vitreous body H43.89

Infirmity R68.89
senile R54

Inflammation, inflamed,
inflammatory (with exudation)
abducent (nerve) —*see* Strabismus,
    paralytic, sixth nerve
accessory sinus (chronic) —*see*
    Sinusitis
adrenal (gland) E27.8
alveoli, teeth M27.3
    scorbutic E54
anal canal, anus K62.89
antrum (chronic) —*see* Sinusitis,
    maxillary
appendix —*see* Appendicitis
arachnoid —*see* Meningitis
areola N61.0
    puerperal, postpartum or
        gestational —*see* Infection,
        nipple
areolar tissue NOS L08.9
artery —*see* Arteritis
auditory meatus (external) —*see*
    Otitis, externa
Bartholin's gland N75.8
bile duct (common) (hepatic) or
    passage —*see* Cholangitis
bladder —*see* Cystitis
bone —*see* Osteomyelitis
brain —*see also* Encephalitis
    membrane —*see* Meningitis
breast N61.0
    puerperal, postpartum, gestational
        —*see* Mastitis, obstetric
broad ligament —*see* Disease,
    pelvis, inflammatory
bronchi —*see* Bronchitis
catarrhal J00
cecum —*see* Appendicitis
cerebral —*see also* Encephalitis
    membrane —*see* Meningitis

Inflammation, inflamed,
inflammatory *(continued)*
cerebrospinal
    meningococcal A39.0
cervix (uteri) —*see* Cervicitis
chest J98.8
chorioretinal H30.9-
    cyclitis —*see* Cyclitis
    disseminated H30.10-
        generalized H30.13-
        peripheral H30.12-
        posterior pole H30.11-
    epitheliopathy —*see*
        Epitheliopathy
    focal H30.00-
        juxtapapillary H30.01-
        macular H30.04-
        paramacular —*see*
            Inflammation, chorioretinal,
            focal, macular
        peripheral H30.03-
        posterior pole H30.02-
    specified type NEC H30.89-
choroid —*see* Inflammation,
    chorioretinal
chronic, postmastoidectomy
    cavity —*see* Complications,
        postmastoidectomy,
        inflammation
colon —*see* Enteritis
connective tissue (diffuse) NEC
    —*see* Disorder, soft tissue,
    specified type NEC
cornea —*see* Keratitis
corpora cavernosa N48.29
cranial nerve —*see* Disorder, nerve,
    cranial
Douglas' cul-de-sac or pouch
    (chronic) N73.0
due to device, implant or graft
    —*see also* Complications,
    by site and type, infection or
    inflammation
    arterial graft T82.7
    breast (implant) T85.79
    catheter T85.79
        dialysis (renal) T82.7
            intraperitoneal T85.71
        infusion T82.7
            cranial T85.735
            intrathecal T85.735
            spinal (epidural) (subdural)
                T85.735
            subarachnoid T85.735
        urinary T83.51
            cystostomy T83.510
            Hopkins T83.518
            ileostomy T83.518
            nephrostomy T83.512
            specified NEC T83.518
            urethral indwelling T83.511
            urostomy T83.518
    electronic (electrode) (pulse
        generator) (stimulator)
        bone T84.7
        cardiac T82.7
        nervous system T85.738
            brain T85.731
            cranial nerve T85.732
            gastric nerve T85.732
            neurostimulator generator
                T85.734
            peripheral nerve T85.732
            sacral nerve T85.732
            spinal cord T85.733
            vagal nerve T85.732
        urinary T83.590
    fixation, internal (orthopedic)
        NEC —*see* Complication,
        fixation device, infection

Inflammation, inflamed,
inflammatory *(continued)*
due to device, implant or graft
    (continued)
    gastrointestinal (bile duct)
        (esophagus) T85.79
    neurostimulator electrode
        (lead) T85.732
    genital NEC T83.69
    heart NEC T82.7
        valve (prosthesis) T82.6
            graft T82.7
    joint prosthesis —*see*
        Complication, joint prosthesis,
        infection
    ocular (corneal graft) (orbital
        implant) NEC T85.79
    orthopedic NEC T84.7
    penile (cylinder) (pump)
        (resevoir) T83.61
    specified NEC T85.79
    testicular T83.62
    urinary NEC T83.598
        ileal conduit stent T83.593
        implanted neurostimulation
            T83.590
        implanted sphincter T83.591
        indwelling ureteral stent
            T83.592
        nephroureteral stent T83.593
        specified stent NEC T83.593
    vascular NEC T82.7
    ventricular intracranial
        (communicating) shunt
        T85.730
duodenum K29.80
    with bleeding K29.81
dura mater —*see* Meningitis
ear (middle) —*see also* Otitis,
    media
    external —*see* Otitis, externa
    inner —*see* subcategory H83.0
epididymis —*see* Epididymitis
esophagus —*see* Esophagitis
ethmoidal (sinus) (chronic)
    —*see* Sinusitis, ethmoidal
eustachian tube (catarrhal)
    —*see* Salpingitis, eustachian
eyelid H01.9
    abscess —*see* Abscess, eyelid
    blepharitis —*see* Blepharitis
    chalazion —*see* Chalazion
    dermatosis (noninfectious)
        —*see* Dermatosis, eyelid
    hordeolum —*see* Hordeolum
    specified NEC H01.8
fallopian tube —*see* Salpingo-
    oophoritis
fascia —*see* Myositis
follicular, pharynx J31.2
frontal (sinus) (chronic)
    —*see* Sinusitis, frontal
gallbladder —*see* Cholecystitis
gastric —*see* Gastritis
gastrointestinal —*see* Enteritis
genital organ (internal) (diffuse)
    female —*see* Disease, pelvis,
        inflammatory
    male N49.9
        multiple sites N49.8
        specified NEC N49.8
gland (lymph) —*see* Lymphadenitis
glottis —*see* Laryngitis
granular, pharynx J31.2
gum K05.10
    nonplaque induced K05.11
    plaque induced K05.10
heart —*see* Carditis
hepatic duct —*see* Cholangitis
ileoanal (internal) pouch K91.850
ileum —*see also* Enteritis

Inflammation, inflamed,
inflammatory *(continued)*
ileum *(continued)*
    regional or terminal —*see*
        Enteritis, regional
intestine (any part) —*see* Enteritis
intestinal pouch K91.850
jaw (acute) (bone) (chronic) (lower)
    (suppurative) (upper) M27.2
joint NEC —*see* Arthritis
    sacroiliac M46.1
kidney —*see* Nephritis
knee (joint) M13.169
    tuberculous A18.02
labium (majus) (minus) —*see*
    Vulvitis
lacrimal
    gland —*see* Dacryoadenitis
    passages (duct) (sac) —*see also*
        Dacryocystitis
    canaliculitis —*see*
        Canaliculitis, lacrimal
larynx —*see* Laryngitis
leg NOS L08.9
lip K13.0
liver (capsule) —*see also* Hepatitis
    chronic K73.9
    suppurative K75.0
lung (acute) —*see also* Pneumonia
    chronic J98.4
lymph gland or node —*see*
    Lymphadenitis
lymphatic vessel —*see*
    Lymphangitis
maxilla, maxillary M27.2
    sinus (chronic) —*see* Sinusitis,
        maxillary
membranes of brain or spinal cord
    —*see* Meningitis
meninges —*see* Meningitis
mouth K12.1
muscle —*see* Myositis
myocardium —*see* Myocarditis
nasal sinus (chronic) —*see*
    Sinusitis
nasopharynx —*see*
    Nasopharyngitis
navel L08.82
nerve NEC —*see* Neuralgia
nipple N61.0
    puerperal, postpartum or
        gestational —*see* Infection,
        nipple
nose —*see* Rhinitis
oculomotor (nerve) —*see*
    Strabismus, paralytic, third nerve
optic nerve —*see* Neuritis, optic
orbit (chronic) H05.10
    acute H05.00
        abscess —*see* Abscess, orbit
        cellulitis —*see* Cellulitis, orbit
        osteomyelitis —*see*
            Osteomyelitis, orbit
        periostitis —*see* Periostitis,
            orbital
        tenonitis —*see* Tenonitis, eye
        granuloma —*see* Granuloma,
            orbit
        myositis —*see* Myositis, orbital
ovary —*see* Salpingo-oophoritis
oviduct —*see* Salpingo-oophoritis
pancreas (acute) —*see* Pancreatitis
parametrium N73.0
parotid region L08.9
pelvis, female —*see* Disease,
    pelvis, inflammatory
penis (corpora cavernosa) N48.29
perianal K62.89
pericardium —*see* Pericarditis
perineum (female) (male) L08.9
perirectal K62.89

Injury–Injury

adrenal *(continued)*
  laceration S37.813
  specified type NEC S37.818
alveolar (process) S09.93
ankle S99.91-
  contusion —*see* Contusion, ankle
  dislocation —*see* Dislocation, ankle
  fracture —*see* Fracture, ankle
  nerve —*see* Injury, nerve, ankle
  open —*see* Wound, open, ankle
  specified type NEC S99.81-
  sprain —*see* Sprain, ankle
  superficial —*see* Injury, superficial, ankle
anterior chamber, eye —*see* Injury, eye, specified site NEC
anus —*see* Injury, abdomen
aorta (thoracic) S25.00
  abdominal S35.00
    laceration (minor) (superficial) S35.01
      major S35.02
    specified type NEC S35.09
  laceration (minor) (superficial) S25.01
    major S25.02
  specified type NEC S25.09
arm (upper) S49.9-
  blood vessel —*see* Injury, blood vessel, arm
  contusion —*see* Contusion, arm, upper
  fracture —*see* Fracture, humerus
  lower —*see* Injury, forearm
  muscle —*see* Injury, muscle, shoulder
  nerve —*see* Injury, nerve, arm
  open —*see* Wound, open, arm
  specified type NEC S49.8-
  superficial —*see* Injury, superficial, arm
artery (complicating trauma) —*see also* Injury, blood vessel, by site
  cerebral or meningeal —*see* Injury, intracranial
auditory canal (external) (meatus) S09.91
auricle, auris, ear S09.91
axilla —*see* Injury, shoulder
back —*see* Injury, back, lower
bile duct S36.13
birth —*see also* Birth, injury P15.9
bladder (sphincter) S37.20
  at delivery O71.5
  contusion S37.22
  laceration S37.23
  obstetrical trauma O71.5
  specified type NEC S37.29
blast (air) (hydraulic) (immersion) (underwater) NEC T14.8
  acoustic nerve trauma —*see* Injury, nerve, acoustic
  bladder —*see* Injury, bladder
  brain —*see* Concussion
  colon —*see* Injury, intestine, large, blast injury
  ear (primary) S09.31-
    secondary S09.39-
  generalized T70.8
  lung —*see* Injury, intrathoracic, lung, blast injury
  multiple body organs T70.8
  peritoneum S36.81
  rectum S36.61
  retroperitoneum S36.898
  small intestine S36.419
    duodenum S36.410
    specified site NEC S36.418

blast *(continued)*
  specified
    intra-abdominal organ NEC S36.898
    pelvic organ NEC S37.899
blood vessel NEC T14.8
  abdomen S35.9-
    aorta —*see* Injury, aorta, abdominal
    celiac artery —*see* Injury, blood vessel, celiac artery
    iliac vessel —*see* Injury, blood vessel, iliac
    laceration S35.91
    mesenteric vessel —*see* Injury, mesenteric
    portal vein —*see* Injury, blood vessel, portal vein
    renal vessel —*see* Injury, blood vessel, renal
    specified vessel NEC S35.8X-
    splenic vessel —*see* Injury, blood vessel, splenic
    vena cava —*see* Injury, vena cava, inferior
  ankle —*see* Injury, blood vessel, foot
  aorta (abdominal) (thoracic) —*see* Injury, aorta
  arm (upper) NEC S45.90-
    forearm —*see* Injury, blood vessel, forearm
    laceration S45.91-
    specified
      site NEC S45.80-
        laceration S45.81-
          specified type NEC S45.89-
      type NEC S45.99-
    superficial vein S45.30-
      laceration S45.31-
        specified type NEC S45.39-
  axillary
    artery S45.00-
      laceration S45.01-
      specified type NEC S45.09-
    vein S45.20-
      laceration S45.21-
      specified type NEC S45.29-
  azygos vein —*see* Injury, blood vessel, thoracic, specified site NEC
  brachial
    artery S45.10-
      laceration S45.11-
      specified type NEC S45.19-
    vein S45.20-
      laceration S45.219
      specified type NEC S45.29-
  carotid artery (common) (external) (internal, extracranial) S15.00-
    internal, intracranial S06.8-
    laceration (minor) (superficial) S15.01-
      major S15.02-
    specified type NEC S15.09-
  celiac artery S35.219
    branch S35.299
      laceration (minor) (superficial) S35.291
        major S35.292
      specified NEC S35.298
    laceration (minor) (superficial) S35.211
      major S35.212
    specified type NEC S35.218
  cerebral —*see* Injury, intracranial

blood vessel NEC *(continued)*
  deep plantar —*see* Injury, blood vessel, plantar artery
  digital (hand) —*see* Injury, blood vessel, finger
  dorsal
    artery (foot) S95.00-
      laceration S95.01-
      specified type NEC S95.09-
    vein (foot) S95.20-
      laceration S95.21-
      specified type NEC S95.29-
  due to accidental laceration during procedure —*see* Laceration, accidental complicating surgery
  extremity —*see* Injury, blood vessel, limb
  femoral
    artery (common) (superficial) S75.00-
      laceration (minor) (superficial) S75.01-
        major S75.02-
      specified type NEC S75.09-
    vein (hip level) (thigh level) S75.10-
      laceration (minor) (superficial) S75.11-
        major S75.12-
      specified type NEC S75.19-
  finger S65.50-
    index S65.50-
      laceration S65.51-
      specified type NEC S65.59-
    laceration S65.51-
    little S65.50-
      laceration S65.51-
      specified type NEC S65.59-
    middle S65.50-
      laceration S65.51-
      specified type NEC S65.59-
    specified type NEC S65.59-
    thumb —*see* Injury, blood vessel, thumb
  foot S95.90-
    dorsal
      artery —*see* Injury, blood vessel, dorsal, artery
      vein —*see* Injury, blood vessel, dorsal, vein
    laceration S95.91-
    plantar artery —*see* Injury, blood vessel, plantar artery
    specified
      site NEC S95.80-
        laceration S95.81-
          specified type NEC S95.89-
      specified type NEC S95.99-
  forearm S55.90-
    laceration S55.91-
    radial artery —*see* Injury, blood vessel, radial artery
    specified
      site NEC S55.80-
        laceration S55.81-
          specified type NEC S55.89-
      type NEC S55.99-
    ulnar artery —*see* Injury, blood vessel, ulnar artery
    vein S55.20-
      laceration S55.21-
      specified type NEC S55.29-
  gastric
    artery —*see* Injury, mesenteric, artery, branch
    vein —*see* Injury, blood vessel, abdomen

blood vessel NEC *(continued)*
  gastroduodenal artery —*see* Injury, mesenteric, artery, branch
  greater saphenous vein (lower leg level) S85.30-
    hip (and thigh) level S75.20-
      laceration (minor) (superficial) S75.21-
        major S75.22-
      specified type NEC S75.29-
    laceration S85.31-
    specified type NEC S85.39-
  hand (level) S65.90-
    finger —*see* Injury, blood vessel, finger
    laceration S65.91-
    palmar arch —*see* Injury, blood vessel, palmar arch
    radial artery —*see* Injury, blood vessel, radial artery, hand
    specified
      site NEC S65.80-
        laceration S65.81-
          specified type NEC S65.89-
      type NEC S65.99-
    thumb —*see* Injury, blood vessel, thumb
    ulnar artery —*see* Injury, blood vessel, ulnar artery, hand
  head S09.0
    intracranial —*see* Injury, intracranial
    multiple S09.0
  hepatic
    artery —*see* Injury, mesenteric, artery
    vein —*see* Injury, vena cava, inferior
  hip S75.90-
    femoral artery —*see* Injury, blood vessel, femoral, artery
    femoral vein —*see* Injury, blood vessel, femoral, vein
    greater saphenous vein —*see* Injury, blood vessel, greater saphenous, hip level
    laceration S75.91-
    specified
      site NEC S75.80-
        laceration S75.81-
          specified type NEC S75.89-
      type NEC S75.99-
  hypogastric (artery) (vein) —*see* Injury, blood vessel, iliac
  iliac S35.5-
    artery S35.51-
    specified vessel NEC S35.5-
    uterine vessel —*see* Injury, blood vessel, uterine
    vein S35.51-
  innominate —*see* Injury, blood vessel, thoracic, innominate
  intercostal (artery) (vein) —*see* Injury, blood vessel, thoracic, intercostal
  jugular vein (external) S15.20-
    internal S15.30-
      laceration (minor) (superficial) S15.31-
        major S15.32-
      specified type NEC S15.39-
    laceration (minor) (superficial) S15.21-
      major S15.22-

Injury *(continued)*

eighth cranial nerve (acoustic or
    auditory) —*see* Injury, nerve,
    acoustic
elbow S59.90-
    contusion —*see* Contusion, elbow
    dislocation —*see* Dislocation,
        elbow
    fracture —*see* Fracture, ulna,
        upper end
    open —*see* Wound, open, elbow
    specified NEC S59.80-
    sprain —*see* Sprain, elbow
    superficial —*see* Injury,
        superficial, elbow
eleventh cranial nerve (accessory)
    —*see* Injury, nerve, accessory
epididymis S39.94
epigastric region S39.91
epiglottis NEC S19.89
esophageal plexus —*see* Injury,
    nerve, thorax, sympathetic
esophagus (thoracic part) —*see
    also* Injury, intrathoracic,
    esophagus
    cervical NEC S19.85
eustachian tube S09.30-
eye S05.9-
    avulsion S05.7-
    ball —*see* Injury, eyeball
    conjunctiva S05.0-
    cornea
        abrasion S05.0-
        laceration S05.3-
            with prolapse S05.2-
    lacrimal apparatus S05.8X-
    orbit penetration S05.4-
    specified site NEC S05.8X-
eyeball S05.8X-
    contusion S05.1-
    penetrating S05.6-
        with
            foreign body S05.5-
            prolapse or loss of
                intraocular tissue S05.2-
        without prolapse or loss of
            intraocular tissue S05.3-
    specified type NEC S05.8-
eyebrow S09.93
eyelid S09.93
    abrasion —*see* Abrasion, eyelid
    contusion —*see* Contusion,
        eyelid
    open —*see* Wound, open, eyelid
face S09.93
fallopian tube S37.509
    bilateral S37.502
        blast injury S37.512
        contusion S37.522
        laceration S37.532
        specified type NEC S37.592
    blast injury (primary) S37.519
        bilateral S37.512
        secondary —*see* Injury,
            fallopian tube, specified
            type NEC
        unilateral S37.511
    contusion S37.529
        bilateral S37.522
        unilateral S37.521
    laceration S37.539
        bilateral S37.532
        unilateral S37.531
    specified type NEC S37.599
        bilateral S37.592
        unilateral S37.591
    unilateral S37.501
        blast injury S37.511
        contusion S37.521
        laceration S37.531
        specified type NEC S37.591

Injury *(continued)*

fascia —*see* Injury, muscle
fifth cranial nerve (trigeminal) —
    see Injury, nerve, trigeminal
finger (nail) S69.9-
    blood vessel —*see* Injury, blood
        vessel, finger
    contusion —*see* Contusion,
        finger
    dislocation —*see* Dislocation,
        finger
    fracture —*see* Fracture, finger
    muscle —*see* Injury, muscle,
        finger
    nerve —*see* Injury, nerve, digital,
        finger
    open —*see* Wound, open, finger
    specified NEC S69.8-
    sprain —*see* Sprain, finger
    superficial —*see* Injury,
        superficial, finger
first cranial nerve (olfactory) —*see*
    Injury, nerve, olfactory
flank —*see* Injury, abdomen
foot S99.92-
    blood vessel —*see* Injury, blood
        vessel, foot
    contusion —*see* Contusion, foot
    dislocation —*see* Dislocation,
        foot
    fracture —*see* Fracture, foot
    muscle —*see* Injury, muscle,
        foot
    open —*see* Wound, open, foot
    specified type NEC S99.82-
    sprain —*see* Sprain, foot
    superficial —*see* Injury,
        superficial, foot
forceps NOS P15.9
forearm S59.91-
    blood vessel —*see* Injury, blood
        vessel, forearm
    contusion —*see* Contusion,
        forearm
    fracture —*see* Fracture, forearm
    muscle —*see* Injury, muscle,
        forearm
    nerve —*see* Injury, nerve,
        forearm
    open —*see* Wound, open,
        forearm
    specified NEC S59.81-
    superficial —*see* Injury,
        superficial, forearm
forehead S09.90
fourth cranial nerve (trochlear)
    —*see* Injury, nerve, trochlear
gallbladder S36.129
    contusion S36.122
    laceration S36.123
    specified NEC S36.128
ganglion
    celiac, coeliac —*see* Injury,
        nerve, lumbosacral,
        sympathetic
    gasserian —*see* Injury, nerve,
        trigeminal
    stellate —*see* Injury, nerve,
        thorax, sympathetic
    thoracic sympathetic —*see*
        Injury, nerve, thorax,
        sympathetic
gasserian ganglion —*see* Injury,
    nerve, trigeminal
gastric artery —*see* Injury, blood
    vessel, celiac artery, branch
gastroduodenal artery —*see* Injury,
    blood vessel, celiac artery,
    branch
gastrointestinal tract —*see* Injury,
    intra-abdominal

Injury *(continued)*

gastrointestinal tract *(continued)*
    with open wound into abdominal
        cavity —*see* Wound, open,
        with penetration into
        peritoneal cavity
    colon —*see* Injury, intestine,
        large
    rectum —*see* Injury, intestine,
        large, rectum
        with open wound into
            abdominal cavity S36.61
    specified site NEC —*see* Injury,
        intra-abdominal, specified,
        site NEC
    stomach —*see* Injury, stomach
    small intestine —*see* Injury,
        intestine, small
genital organ(s)
    external S39.94
        specified NEC S39.848
    internal S37.90
        fallopian tube —*see* Injury,
            fallopian tube
        ovary —*see* Injury, ovary
        prostate —*see* Injury,
            prostate
        seminal vesicle —*see* Injury,
            pelvis, organ, specified site
            NEC
        uterus —*see* Injury, uterus
        vas deferens —*see* Injury,
            pelvis, organ, specified site
            NEC
    obstetrical trauma O71.9
gland
    lacrimal laceration —*see* Injury,
        eye, specified site NEC
    salivary S09.93
    thyroid NEC S19.84
globe (eye) S05.90
    specified NEC S05.8X-
groin —*see* Injury, abdomen
gum S09.90
hand S69.9-
    blood vessel —*see* Injury, blood
        vessel, hand
    contusion —*see* Contusion, hand
    fracture —*see* Fracture, hand
    muscle —*see* Injury, muscle,
        hand
    nerve —*see* Injury, nerve, hand
    open —*see* Wound, open, hand
    specified NEC S69.8-
    sprain —*see* Sprain, hand
    superficial —*see* Injury,
        superficial, hand
head S09.90
    with loss of consciousness
        S06.9-
    specified NEC S09.8
heart S26.90
    with hemopericardium S26.00
        contusion S26.01
        laceration (mild) S26.020
            moderate S26.021
            major S26.022
        specified type NEC S26.09
    contusion S26.91
    laceration S26.92
    specified type NEC S26.99
    without hemopericardium
        S26.10
        contusion S26.11
        laceration S26.12
        specified type NEC S26.19
heel —*see* Injury, foot
hepatic
    artery —*see* Injury, blood vessel,
        celiac artery, branch
    duct —*see* Injury, liver

Injury *(continued)*

hepatic *(continued)*
    vein —*see* Injury, vena cava,
        inferior
hip S79.91-
    blood vessel —*see* Injury, blood
        vessel, hip
    contusion —*see* Contusion, hip
    dislocation —*see* Dislocation,
        hip
    fracture —*see* Fracture, femur,
        neck
    muscle —*see* Injury, muscle, hip
    nerve —*see* Injury, nerve, hip
    open —*see* Wound, open, hip
    sprain —*see* Sprain, hip
    superficial —*see* Injury,
        superficial, hip
    specified NEC S79.81-
hymen S39.94
hypogastric
    blood vessel —*see* Injury, blood
        vessel, iliac
    plexus —*see* Injury, nerve,
        lumbosacral, sympathetic
ileum —*see* Injury, intestine, small
iliac region S39.91
instrumental (during surgery)
    —*see* Laceration, accidental
    complicating surgery
    birth injury —*see* Birth, injury
    nonsurgical —*see* Injury, by site
    obstetrical O71.9
        bladder O71.5
        cervix O71.3
        high vaginal O71.4
        perineal NOS O70.9
        urethra O71.5
        uterus O71.5
            with rupture or perforation
                O71.1
internal T14.8
    aorta —*see* Injury, aorta
    bladder (sphincter) —*see* Injury,
        bladder
        with
            ectopic or molar pregnancy
                O08.6
            following ectopic or molar
                pregnancy O08.6
        obstetrical trauma O71.5
    bronchus, bronchi —*see* Injury,
        intrathoracic, bronchus
    cecum —*see* Injury, intestine,
        large
    cervix (uteri) —*see also* Injury,
        uterus
        with ectopic or molar
            pregnancy O08.6
        following ectopic or molar
            pregnancy O08.6
        obstetrical trauma O71.3
    chest —*see* Injury, intrathoracic
    gastrointestinal tract —*see*
        Injury, intra-abdominal
    heart —*see* Injury, heart
    intestine NEC —*see* Injury,
        intestine
    intrauterine —*see* Injury, uterus
    mesentery —*see* Injury,
        intra-abdominal, specified,
        site NEC
    pelvis, pelvic (organ) S37.90
        following ectopic or molar
            pregnancy (subsequent
            episode) O08.6
        obstetrical trauma NEC O71.5
            rupture or perforation O71.1
        specified NEC S39.83
    rectum —*see* Injury, intestine,
        large, rectum

Injury (continued)

nerve NEC (continued)

hip (continued)

sciatic —see Injury, nerve, sciatic

specified site NEC S74.8

hypoglossal S04.89-

specified type NEC S04.89-

lateral plantar S94.0-

leg (lower) S84.9-

cutaneous sensory —see Injury, nerve, cutaneous sensory, leg

peroneal —see Injury, nerve, peroneal

specified site NEC —see subcategory S84.8

tibial —see Injury, nerve, tibial

upper —see Injury, nerve, thigh

lower

back —see Injury, nerve, abdomen, specified site NEC

peripheral —see Injury, nerve, abdomen, peripheral

limb —see Injury, nerve, leg

lumbar spinal —see Injury, nerve, spinal, lumbar

lumbar plexus —see Injury, nerve, lumbosacral, sympathetic

lumbosacral

plexus —see Injury, nerve, lumbosacral, sympathetic

sympathetic S34.5

medial plantar S94.1-

median (forearm level) S54.1-

hand (level) S64.1-

upper arm (level) S44.1-

wrist (level) —see Injury, nerve, median, hand

musculocutaneous S44.4-

musculospiral (upper arm level) —see Injury, nerve, radial, upper arm

neck S14.9

peripheral S14.4

specified site NEC S14.8

sympathetic S14.5

ninth cranial (glossopharyngeal) —see Injury, nerve, glossopharyngeal

oculomotor S04.1-

contusion S04.1-

laceration S04.1-

specified type NEC S04.1-

olfactory S04.81-

specified type NEC S04.81-

optic S04.01-

contusion S04.01-

laceration S04.01-

specified type NEC S04.01-

pelvic girdle —see Injury, nerve, hip

pelvis —see Injury, nerve, abdomen, specified site NEC

peripheral —see Injury, nerve, abdomen, peripheral

peripheral NEC T14.8

abdomen —see Injury, nerve, abdomen, peripheral

lower back —see Injury, nerve, abdomen, peripheral

neck —see Injury, nerve, neck, peripheral

pelvis —see Injury, nerve, abdomen, peripheral

specified NEC T14.8

peroneal (lower leg level) S84.1-

foot S94.2-

Injury (continued)

nerve NEC (continued)

plexus

brachial —see Injury, brachial plexus

celiac, coeliac —see Injury, nerve, lumbosacral, sympathetic

mesenteric, inferior —see Injury, nerve, lumbosacral, sympathetic

sacral —see Injury, lumbosacral plexus

spinal

brachial —see Injury, brachial plexus

lumbosacral —see Injury, lumbosacral plexus

pneumogastric —see Injury, nerve, vagus

radial (forearm level) S54.2-

hand (level) S64.2-

upper arm (level) S44.2-

wrist (level) —see Injury, nerve, radial, hand

root —see Injury, nerve, spinal, root

sacral plexus —see Injury, lumbosacral plexus

sacral spinal —see Injury, nerve, spinal, sacral

sciatic (hip level) (thigh level) S74.0-

second cranial (optic) —see Injury, nerve, optic

seventh cranial (facial) —see Injury, nerve, facial

shoulder —see Injury, nerve, arm

sixth cranial (abducent) —see Injury, nerve, abducens

spinal

plexus —see Injury, nerve, plexus, spinal

root

cervical S14.2

dorsal S24.2

lumbar S34.21

sacral S34.22

thoracic —see Injury, nerve, spinal, root, dorsal

splanchnic —see Injury, nerve, lumbosacral, sympathetic

sympathetic NEC —see Injury, nerve, lumbosacral, sympathetic

cervical —see Injury, nerve, cervical sympathetic

tenth cranial (pneumogastric or vagus) —see Injury, nerve, vagus

thigh (level) —see Injury, nerve, hip

cutaneous sensory —see Injury, nerve, cutaneous sensory, hip

femoral —see Injury, nerve, femoral

sciatic —see Injury, nerve, sciatic

specified NEC —see Injury, nerve, hip

third cranial (oculomotor) —see Injury, nerve, oculomotor

thorax S24.9

peripheral S24.3

specified site NEC S24.8

sympathetic S24.4

thumb, digital —see Injury, nerve, digital, thumb

tibial (lower leg level) (posterior) S84.0-

Injury (continued)

nerve NEC (continued)

toe —see Injury, nerve, ankle

trigeminal S04.3-

contusion S04.3-

laceration S04.3-

specified type NEC S04.3-

trochlear S04.2-

contusion S04.2-

laceration S04.2-

specified type NEC S04.2-

twelfth cranial (hypoglossal) —see Injury, nerve, hypoglossal

ulnar (forearm level) S54.0-

arm (upper) (level) S44.0-

hand (level) S64.0-

wrist (level) —see Injury, nerve, ulnar, hand

vagus S04.89-

specified type NEC S04.89-

wrist (level) —see Injury, nerve, hand

ninth cranial nerve (glossopharyngeal) —see Injury, nerve, glossopharyngeal

nose (septum) S09.92

obstetrical O71.9

specified NEC O71.89

occipital (region) (scalp) S09.90

lobe —see Injury, intracranial

optic chiasm S04.02

optic radiation S04.03-

optic tract and pathways S04.03-

orbit, orbital (region) —see Injury, eye

penetrating (with foreign body) —see Injury, eye, orbit, penetrating

specified NEC —see Injury, eye, specified site NEC

ovary, ovarian S37.409

bilateral S37.402

contusion S37.422

laceration S37.432

specified type NEC S37.492

blood vessel —see Injury, blood vessel, ovarian

contusion S37.429

bilateral S37.422

unilateral S37.421

laceration S37.439

bilateral S37.432

unilateral S37.431

specified type NEC S37.499

bilateral S37.492

unilateral S37.491

unilateral S37.401

contusion S37.421

laceration S37.431

specified type NEC S37.491

palate (hard) (soft) S09.93

pancreas S36.209

body S36.201

contusion S36.221

laceration S36.231

major S36.261

minor S36.241

moderate S36.251

specified type NEC S36.291

contusion S36.229

head S36.200

contusion S36.220

laceration S36.230

major S36.260

minor S36.240

moderate S36.250

specified type NEC S36.290

laceration S36.239

major S36.269

minor S36.249

moderate S36.259

Injury (continued)

pancreas (continued)

specified type NEC S36.299

tail S36.202

contusion S36.222

laceration S36.232

major S36.262

minor S36.242

moderate S36.252

specified type NEC S36.292

parietal (region) (scalp) S09.90

lobe —see Injury, intracranial

patellar ligament (tendon) S76.10-

laceration S76.12-

specified NEC S76.19-

strain S76.11-

pelvis, pelvic (floor) S39.93

complicating delivery O70.1

joint or ligament, complicating delivery O71.6

organ S37.90

with ectopic or molar pregnancy O08.6

complication of abortion —see Abortion

contusion S37.92

following ectopic or molar pregnancy O08.6

laceration S37.93

obstetrical trauma NEC O71.5

specified

site NEC S37.899

contusion S37.892

laceration S37.893

specified type NEC S37.898

type NEC S37.99

specified NEC S39.83

penis S39.94

perineum S39.94

peritoneum S36.81

laceration S36.893

periurethral tissue —see Injury, urethra

complicating delivery O71.82

phalanges

foot —see Injury, foot

hand —see Injury, hand

pharynx NEC S19.85

pleura —see Injury, intrathoracic, pleura

plexus

brachial —see Injury, brachial plexus

cardiac —see Injury, nerve, thorax, sympathetic

celiac, coeliac —see Injury, nerve, lumbosacral, sympathetic

esophageal —see Injury, nerve, thorax, sympathetic

hypogastric —see Injury, nerve, lumbosacral, sympathetic

lumbar, lumbosacral —see Injury, lumbosacral plexus

mesenteric —see Injury, nerve, lumbosacral, sympathetic

pulmonary —see Injury, nerve, thorax, sympathetic

postcardiac surgery (syndrome) I97.0

prepuce S39.94

pressure

injury —see Ulcer, pressure, by site

prostate S37.829

contusion S37.822

laceration S37.823

specified type NEC S37.828

pubic region S39.94

pudendum S39.94

Injury *(continued)*

pulmonary plexus —*see* Injury, nerve, thorax, sympathetic

rectovaginal septum NEC S39.83

rectum —*see* Injury, intestine, large, rectum

retina —*see* Injury, eye, specified site NEC

  penetrating —*see* Injury, eyeball, penetrating

retroperitoneal —*see* Injury, intra-abdominal, specified site NEC

rotator cuff (muscle(s)) (tendon(s)) S46.00-

  laceration S46.02-

  specified type NEC S46.09-

  strain S46.01-

round ligament —*see* Injury, pelvic organ, specified site NEC

sacral plexus —*see* Injury, lumbosacral plexus

salivary duct or gland S09.93

scalp S09.90

  newborn (birth injury) P12.9

    due to monitoring (electrode) (sampling incision) P12.4

    specified NEC P12.89

      caput succedaneum P12.81

scapular region —*see* Injury, shoulder

sclera —*see* Injury, eye, specified site NEC

  penetrating —*see* Injury, eyeball, penetrating

scrotum S39.94

second cranial nerve (optic) —*see* Injury, nerve, optic

seminal vesicle —*see* Injury, pelvic organ, specified site NEC

seventh cranial nerve (facial) —*see* Injury, nerve, facial

shoulder S49.9-

  blood vessel —*see* Injury, blood vessel, arm

  contusion —*see* Contusion, shoulder

  dislocation —*see* Dislocation, shoulder

  fracture —*see* Fracture, shoulder

shoulder S49.9-

  muscle —*see* Injury, muscle, shoulder

  nerve —*see* Injury, nerve, shoulder

  open —*see* Wound, open, shoulder

  specified type NEC S49.8-

  sprain —*see* Sprain, shoulder girdle

  superficial —*see* Injury, superficial, shoulder

sinus

  cavernous —*see* Injury, intracranial

  nasal S09.92

sixth cranial nerve (abducent) —*see* Injury, nerve, abducens

skeleton, birth injury P13.9

  specified part NEC P13.8

skin NEC T14.8

  surface intact —*see* Injury, superficial

skull NEC S09.90

specified NEC T14.8

spermatic cord (pelvic region) S37.898

  scrotal region S39.848

spinal (cord)

  cervical (neck) S14.109

    anterior cord syndrome S14.139

Injury *(continued)*

spinal *(continued)*

cervical *(continued)*

  anterior cord syndrome *(continued)*

    C1 level S14.131

    C2 level S14.132

    C3 level S14.133

    C4 level S14.134

    C5 level S14.135

    C6 level S14.136

    C7 level S14.137

    C8 level S14.138

  Brown-Séquard syndrome S14.149

    C1 level S14.141

    C2 level S14.142

    C3 level S14.143

    C4 level S14.144

    C5 level S14.145

    C6 level S14.146

    C7 level S14.147

    C8 level S14.148

  C1 level S14.101

  C2 level S14.102

  C3 level S14.103

  C4 level S14.104

  C5 level S14.105

  C6 level S14.106

  C7 level S14.107

  C8 level S14.108

  central cord syndrome S14.129

    C1 level S14.121

    C2 level S14.122

    C3 level S14.123

    C4 level S14.124

    C5 level S14.125

    C6 level S14.126

    C7 level S14.127

    C8 level S14.128

  complete lesion S14.119

    C1 level S14.111

    C2 level S14.112

    C3 level S14.113

    C4 level S14.114

    C5 level S14.115

    C6 level S14.116

    C7 level S14.117

    C8 level S14.118

  concussion S14.0

  edema S14.0

  incomplete lesion specified NEC S14.159

    C1 level S14.151

    C2 level S14.152

    C3 level S14.153

    C4 level S14.154

    C5 level S14.155

    C6 level S14.156

    C7 level S14.157

    C8 level S14.158

  posterior cord syndrome S14.159

    C1 level S14.151

    C2 level S14.152

    C3 level S14.153

    C4 level S14.154

    C5 level S14.155

    C6 level S14.156

    C7 level S14.157

    C8 level S14.158

  dorsal —*see* Injury, spinal, thoracic

  lumbar S34.109

    complete lesion S34.119

      L1 level S34.111

      L2 level S34.112

      L3 level S34.113

      L4 level S34.114

      L5 level S34.115

    concussion S34.01

Injury *(continued)*

spinal *(continued)*

lumbar *(continued)*

  edema S34.01

  incomplete lesion S34.129

    L1 level S34.121

    L2 level S34.122

    L3 level S34.123

    L4 level S34.124

    L5 level S34.125

    L1 level S34.101

    L2 level S34.102

    L3 level S34.103

    L4 level S34.104

    L5 level S34.105

  nerve root NEC

    cervical —*see* Injury, nerve, spinal, root, cervical

    dorsal —*see* Injury, nerve, spinal, root, dorsal

    lumbar S34.21

    sacral S34.22

    thoracic —*see* Injury, nerve, spinal, root, dorsal

  plexus

    brachial —*see* Injury, brachial plexus

    lumbosacral —*see* Injury, lumbosacral plexus

  sacral S34.139

    complete lesion S34.131

    incomplete lesion S34.132

  thoracic S24.109

    anterior cord syndrome S24.139

      T1 level S24.131

      T2-T6 level S24.132

      T7-T10 level S24.133

      T11-T12 level S24.134

    Brown-Séquard syndrome S24.149

      T1 level S24.141

      T2-T6 level S24.142

      T7-T10 level S24.143

      T11-T12 level S24.144

    complete lesion S24.119

      T1 level S24.111

      T2-T6 level S24.112

      T7-T10 level S24.113

      T11-T12 level S24.114

    concussion S24.0

    edema S24.0

    incomplete lesion specified NEC S24.159

      T1 level S24.151

      T2-T6 level S24.152

      T7-T10 level S24.153

      T11-T12 level S24.154

    posterior cord syndrome S24.159

      T1 level S24.151

      T2-T6 level S24.152

      T7-T10 level S24.153

      T11-T12 level S24.154

    T1 level S24.101

    T2-T6 level S24.102

    T7-T10 level S24.103

    T11-T12 level S24.104

  splanchnic nerve —*see* Injury, nerve, lumbosacral, sympathetic

spleen S36.00

  contusion S36.029

    major S36.021

    minor S36.020

  laceration S36.039

    major (massive) (stellate) S36.032

    moderate S36.031

    superficial (capsular) (minor) S36.030

Injury *(continued)*

spleen *(continued)*

  specified type NEC S36.09

  splenic artery —*see* Injury, blood vessel, celiac artery, branch

  stellate ganglion —*see* Injury, nerve, thorax, sympathetic

sternal region S29.9

stomach S36.30

  contusion S36.32

  laceration S36.33

  specified type NEC S36.39

subconjunctival —*see* Injury, eye, conjunctiva

subcutaneous NEC T14.8

submaxillary region S09.93

submental region S09.93

subungual

  fingers —*see* Injury, hand

  toes —*see* Injury, foot

superficial NEC T14.8

  abdomen, abdominal (wall) S30.92

    abrasion S30.811

    bite S30.871

      insect S30.861

    contusion S30.1

    external constriction S30.841

    foreign body S30.851

  abrasion —*see* Abrasion, by site

  adnexa, eye NEC —*see* Injury, eye, specified site NEC

  alveolar process —*see* Injury, superficial, oral cavity

  ankle S90.91-

    abrasion —*see* Abrasion, ankle

    blister —*see* Blister, ankle

    bite —*see* Bite, ankle

    contusion —*see* Contusion, ankle

    external constriction —*see* Constriction, external, ankle

    foreign body —*see* Foreign body, superficial, ankle

  anus S30.98

  arm (upper) S40.92-

    abrasion —*see* Abrasion, arm

    bite —*see* Bite, superficial, arm

    blister —*see* Blister, arm (upper)

    contusion —*see* Contusion, arm

    external constriction —*see* Constriction, external, arm

    foreign body —*see* Foreign body, superficial, arm

  auditory canal (external) (meatus) —*see* Injury, superficial, ear

  auricle —*see* Injury, superficial, ear

  axilla —*see* Injury, superficial, arm

  back —*see also* Injury, superficial, thorax, back

    lower S30.91

      abrasion S30.810

      contusion S30.0

      external constriction S30.840

      superficial

        bite NEC S30.870

          insect S30.860

        foreign body S30.850

  bite NEC —*see* Bite, superficial NEC, by site

  blister —*see* Blister, by site

  breast S20.10-

Injury (*continued*)

superficial NEC (*continued*)

sternal region —*see* Injury, superficial, thorax, front

subconjunctival —*see* Injury, eye, specified site NEC

subcutaneous NEC T14.8

submaxillary region —*see* Injury, superficial, head, specified NEC

submental region —*see* Injury, superficial, head, specified NEC

subungual

finger(s) —*see* Injury, superficial, finger

toe(s) —*see* Injury, superficial, toe

supraclavicular fossa —*see* Injury, superficial, neck

supraorbital —*see* Injury, superficial, head, specified NEC

temple —*see* Injury, superficial, head, specified NEC

temporal region —*see* Injury, superficial, head, specified NEC

testis S30.94

thigh S70.92-

abrasion —*see* Abrasion, thigh

bite —*see* Bite, superficial, thigh

blister —*see* Blister, thigh

contusion —*see* Contusion, thigh

external constriction —*see* Constriction, external, thigh

foreign body —*see* Foreign body, superficial, thigh

thorax, thoracic (wall) S20.90

abrasion —*see* Abrasion, thorax

back S20.40-

bite —*see* Bite, thorax, superficial

blister —*see* Blister, thorax

contusion —*see* Contusion, thorax

external constriction —*see* Constriction, external, thorax

foreign body —*see* Foreign body, superficial, thorax

front S20.30-

throat S10.10

abrasion S10.11

bite S10.17

insect S10.16

blister S10.12

contusion S10.0

external constriction S10.14

foreign body S10.15

thumb S60.93-

abrasion —*see* Abrasion, thumb

bite —*see* Bite, superficial, thumb

blister —*see* Blister, thumb

contusion —*see* Contusion, thumb

external constriction —*see* Constriction, external, thumb

foreign body —*see* Foreign body, superficial, thumb

insect bite —*see* Bite, by site, superficial, insect

specified type NEC S60.39-

Injury (*continued*)

superficial NEC (*continued*)

toe(s) S90.93-

abrasion —*see* Abrasion, toe

bite —*see* Bite, toe

blister —*see* Blister, toe

contusion —*see* Contusion, toe

external constriction —*see* Constriction, external, toe

foreign body —*see* Foreign body, superficial, toe

great S90.93-

tongue —*see* Injury, superficial, oral cavity

tooth, teeth —*see* Injury, superficial, oral cavity

trachea S10.10

tunica vaginalis S30.94

tympanum, tympanic membrane —*see* Injury, superficial, ear

uvula —*see* Injury, superficial, oral cavity

vagina S30.95

vocal cords —*see* Injury, superficial, throat

vulva S30.95

wrist S60.91-

supraclavicular region —*see* Injury, neck

supraorbital S09.93

suprarenal gland (multiple) —*see* Injury, adrenal

surgical complication (external or internal site) —*see* Laceration, accidental complicating surgery

temple S09.90

temporal region S09.90

tendon —*see also* Injury, muscle, by site

abdomen —*see* Injury, muscle, abdomen

Achilles —*see* Injury, Achilles tendon

lower back —*see* Injury, muscle, lower back

pelvic organs —*see* Injury, muscle, pelvis

tenth cranial nerve (pneumogastric or vagus) —*see* Injury, nerve, vagus

testis S39.94

thigh S79.92-

blood vessel —*see* Injury, blood vessel, hip

contusion —*see* Contusion, thigh

fracture —*see* Fracture, femur

muscle —*see* Injury, muscle, thigh

nerve —*see* Injury, nerve, thigh

open —*see* Wound, open, thigh

specified NEC S79.82-

superficial —*see* Injury, superficial, thigh

third cranial nerve (oculomotor) —*see* Injury, nerve, oculomotor

thorax, thoracic S29.9

blood vessel —*see* Injury, blood vessel, thorax

cavity —*see* Injury, intrathoracic

dislocation —*see* Dislocation, thorax

external (wall) S29.9

contusion —*see* Contusion, thorax

nerve —*see* Injury, nerve, thorax

open —*see* Wound, open, thorax

specified NEC S29.8

sprain —*see* Sprain, thorax

Injury (*continued*)

thorax, thoracic (*continued*)

external (*continued*)

superficial —*see* Injury, superficial, thorax

fracture —*see* Fracture, thorax

internal —*see* Injury, intrathoracic

intrathoracic organ —*see* Injury, intrathoracic

sympathetic ganglion —*see* Injury, nerve, thorax, sympathetic

throat (*see also* Injury, neck) S19.9

thumb S69.9-

blood vessel —*see* Injury, blood vessel, thumb

contusion —*see* Contusion, thumb

dislocation —*see* Dislocation, thumb

fracture —*see* Fracture, thumb

muscle —*see* Injury, muscle, thumb

nerve —*see* Injury, nerve, digital, thumb

open —*see* Wound, open, thumb

specified NEC S69.8-

sprain —*see* Sprain, thumb

superficial —*see* Injury, superficial, thumb

thymus (gland) —*see* Injury, intrathoracic, specified organ NEC

thyroid (gland) NEC S19.84

toe S99.92-

contusion —*see* Contusion, toe

dislocation —*see* Dislocation, toe

fracture —*see* Fracture, toe

muscle —*see* Injury, muscle, toe

open —*see* Wound, open, toe

specified type NEC S99.82-

sprain —*see* Sprain, toe

superficial —*see* Injury, superficial, toe

tongue S09.93

tonsil S09.93

tooth S09.93

trachea (cervical) NEC S19.82

thoracic —*see* Injury, intrathoracic, trachea, thoracic

transfusion-related acute lung (TRALI) J95.84

tunica vaginalis S39.94

twelfth cranial nerve (hypoglossal) —*see* Injury, nerve, hypoglossal

ureter S37.10

contusion S37.12

laceration S37.13

specified type NEC S37.19

urethra (sphincter) S37.30

at delivery O71.5

contusion S37.32

laceration S37.33

specified type NEC S37.39

urinary organ S37.90

contusion S37.92

laceration S37.93

specified

site NEC S37.899

contusion S37.892

laceration S37.893

specified type NEC S37.898

type NEC S37.99

uterus, uterine S37.60

with ectopic or molar pregnancy O08.6

blood vessel —*see* Injury, blood vessel, iliac

contusion S37.62

Injury (*continued*)

uterus, uterine (*continued*)

laceration S37.63

cervix at delivery O71.3

rupture associated with obstetrics —*see* Rupture, uterus

specified type NEC S37.69

uvula S09.93

vagina S39.93

abrasion S30.814

bite S31.45

insect S30.864

superficial NEC S30.874

contusion S30.23

crush S38.03

during delivery —*see* Laceration, vagina, during delivery

external constriction S30.844

insect bite S30.864

laceration S31.41

with foreign body S31.42

open wound S31.40

puncture S31.43

with foreign body S31.44

superficial S30.95

foreign body S30.854

vas deferens —*see* Injury, pelvic organ, specified site NEC

vascular NEC T14.8

vein —*see* Injury, blood vessel

vena cava (superior) S25.20

inferior S35.10

laceration (minor) (superficial) S35.11

major S35.12

specified type NEC S35.19

laceration (minor) (superficial) S25.21

major S25.22

specified type NEC S25.29

vesical (sphincter) —*see* Injury, bladder

visual cortex S04.04-

vitreous (humor) S05.90

specified NEC S05.8X-

vocal cord NEC S19.83

vulva S39.94

abrasion S30.814

bite S31.45

insect S30.864

superficial NEC S30.874

contusion S30.23

crush S38.03

during delivery —*see* Laceration, perineum, female, during delivery

external constriction S30.844

insect bite S30.864

laceration S31.41

with foreign body S31.42

open wound S31.40

puncture S31.43

with foreign body S31.44

superficial S30.95

foreign body S30.854

whiplash (cervical spine) S13.4

wrist S69.9-

blood vessel —*see* Injury, blood vessel, hand

contusion —*see* Contusion, wrist

dislocation —*see* Dislocation, wrist

fracture —*see* Fracture, wrist

muscle —*see* Injury, muscle, hand

nerve —*see* Injury, nerve, hand

open —*see* Wound, open, wrist

specified NEC S69.8-

sprain —*see* Sprain, wrist

Injury *(continued)*
  wrist *(continued)*
    superficial —*see* Injury,
      superficial, wrist

Inoculation —*see also* Vaccination
  complication or reaction —*see*
    Complications, vaccination

Insanity, insane —*see also*
  Psychosis
  adolescent —*see* Schizophrenia
  confusional F28
    acute or subacute F05
  delusional F22
  senile F03

Insect
  bite —*see* Bite, by site, superficial,
    insect
  venomous, poisoning NEC (by)
    —*see* Venom, arthropod

Insensitivity
  adrenocorticotropin hormone
    (ACTH) E27.49
  androgen E34.50
    complete E34.51
    partial E34.52

Insertion
  cord (umbilical) lateral or
    velamentous O43.12-
  intrauterine contraceptive
    device (encounter for) —*see*
    Intrauterine contraceptive
    device

Insolation (sunstroke) T67.01

Insomnia (organic) G47.00
  adjustment F51.02
  adjustment disorder F51.02
  behavioral, of childhood Z73.819
    combined type Z73.812
    limit setting type Z73.811
    sleep-onset association type
      Z73.810
  childhood Z73.819
  chronic F51.04
    somatized tension F51.04
  conditioned F51.04
  due to
    alcohol
      abuse F10.182
      dependence F10.282
      use F10.982
    amphetamines
      abuse F15.182
      dependence F15.282
      use F15.982
    anxiety disorder F51.05
    caffeine
      abuse F15.182
      dependence F15.282
      use F15.982
    cocaine
      abuse F14.182
      dependence F14.282
      use F14.982
    depression F51.05
    drug NEC
      abuse F19.182
      dependence F19.282
      use F19.982
    medical condition G47.01
    mental disorder NEC F51.05
    opioid
      abuse F11.182
      dependence F11.282
      use F11.982
    psychoactive substance NEC
      abuse F19.182
      dependence F19.282
      use F19.982

Insomnia *(continued)*
  due to *(continued)*
    sedative, hypnotic, or anxiolytic
      abuse F13.182
      dependence F13.282
      use F13.982
    stimulant NEC
      abuse F15.182
      dependence F15.282
      use F15.982
  fatal familial (FFI) A81.83
  idiopathic F51.01
  learned F51.3
  nonorganic origin F51.01
  not due to a substance or known
    physiological condition F51.01
    specified NEC F51.09
  paradoxical F51.03
  primary F51.01
  psychiatric F51.05
  psychophysiologic F51.04
  related to psychopathology F51.05
  short-term F51.02
  specified NEC G47.09
  stress-related F51.02
  transient F51.02
  without objective findings F51.02

Inspiration
  food or foreign body —*see* Foreign
    body, by site
  mucus —*see* Asphyxia, mucus

Inspissated bile syndrome
  (newborn) P59.1

Instability
  emotional (excessive) F60.3
  joint (post-traumatic) M25.30
    ankle M25.37-
    due to old ligament injury —*see*
      Disorder, ligament
    elbow M25.32-
    flail —*see* Flail, joint
    foot M25.37-
    hand M25.34-
    hip M25.35-
    knee M25.36-
    lumbosacral M53.2
    prosthesis —*see* Complications,
      joint prosthesis, mechanical,
      displacement, by site
    sacroiliac M53.2
    secondary to
      old ligament injury —*see*
        Disorder, ligament
      removal of joint prosthesis
        M96.89
    shoulder (region) M25.31-
    specified site NEC M25.39
    spine M53.2
    wrist M25.33-
  knee (chronic) M23.5-
  lumbosacral M53.2
  nervous F48.8
  personality (emotional) F60.3
  spine —*see* Instability, joint, spine
  vasomotor R55

Institutional syndrome (childhood)
  F94.2

Institutionalization, affecting child
  Z62.22
  disinhibited attachment F94.2

Insufficiency, insufficient
  accommodation, old age H52.4
  adrenal (gland) E27.40
    primary E27.1
  adrenocortical E27.40
    drug-induced E27.3
    iatrogenic E27.3
    primary E27.1
  anatomic crown height K08.89

Insufficiency, insufficient *(continued)*
  anterior (occlusal) guidance M26.54
  anus K62.89
  aortic (valve) I35.1
    with
      mitral (valve) disease I08.0
        with tricuspid (valve)
          disease I08.3
      stenosis I35.2
      tricuspid (valve) disease I08.2
        with mitral (valve) disease
          I08.3
    congenital Q23.1
    rheumatic I06.1
      with
        mitral (valve) disease I08.0
          with tricuspid (valve)
            disease I08.3
        stenosis I06.2
          with mitral (valve)
            disease I08.0
            with tricuspid (valve)
              disease I08.3
        tricuspid (valve) disease
          I08.2
          with mitral (valve)
            disease I08.3
    specified cause NEC I35.1
    syphilitic A52.03
  arterial I77.1
    basilar G45.0
    carotid (hemispheric) G45.1
    cerebral I67.81
    coronary (acute or subacute) I24.8
    mesenteric K55.1
    peripheral I73.9
    precerebral (multiple) (bilateral)
      G45.2
    vertebral G45.0
  arteriovenous I99.8
  biliary K83.8
  cardiac —*see also* Insufficiency,
    myocardial
    due to presence of (cardiac)
      prosthesis I97.11-
    postprocedural I97.11-
  cardiorenal, hypertensive I13.2
  cardiovascular —*see* Disease,
    cardiovascular
  cerebrovascular (acute) I67.81
    with transient focal neurological
      signs and symptoms G45.8
  circulatory NEC I99.8
    newborn P29.89
  clinical crown height K08.89
  convergence H51.11
  coronary (acute or subacute) I24.8
    chronic or with a stated duration
      of over 4 weeks I25.89
  corticoadrenal E27.40
    primary E27.1
  dietary E63.9
  divergence H51.8
  food T73.0
  gastroesophageal K22.8
  gonadal
    ovary E28.39
    testis E29.1
  heart —*see also* Insufficiency,
    myocardial
    newborn P29.0
    valve —*see* Endocarditis
  hepatic —*see* Failure, hepatic
  idiopathic autonomic G90.09
  interocclusal distance of fully
    erupted teeth (ridge) M26.36
  kidney N28.9
    acute N28.9
    chronic N18.9
  lacrimal (secretion) H04.12-
    passages —*see* Stenosis, lacrimal

Insufficiency, insufficient *(continued)*
  liver —*see* Failure, hepatic
  lung —*see* Insufficiency,
    pulmonary
  mental (congenital) —*see*
    Disability, intellectual
  mesenteric K55.1
  mitral (valve) I34.0
    with
      aortic valve disease I08.0
        with tricuspid (valve)
          disease I08.3
      obstruction or stenosis I05.2
        with aortic valve disease
          I08.0
      tricuspid (valve) disease I08.1
        with aortic (valve) disease
          I08.3
    congenital Q23.3
    rheumatic I05.1
      with
        aortic valve disease I08.0
          with tricuspid (valve)
            disease I08.3
        obstruction or stenosis I05.2
          with aortic valve disease
            I08.0
            with tricuspid (valve)
              disease I08.3
        tricuspid (valve) disease
          I08.1
          with aortic (valve)
            disease I08.3
    active or acute I01.1
      with chorea, rheumatic
        (Sydenham's) I02.0
    specified cause, except rheumatic
      I34.0
  muscle —*see also* Disease, muscle
    heart —*see* Insufficiency,
      myocardial
  ocular NEC H50.9
  myocardial, myocardium (with
    arteriosclerosis) (*see also*
    Failure, heart) I50.9
    with
      rheumatic fever (conditions in
        I00) I09.0
        active, acute or subacute
          I01.2
          with chorea I02.0
        inactive or quiescent (with
          chorea) I09.0
    congenital Q24.8
    hypertensive —*see*
      Hypertension, heart
    newborn P29.0
    rheumatic I09.0
      active, acute, or subacute I01.2
    syphilitic A52.06
  nourishment T73.0
  pancreatic K86.89
    exocrine K86.81
  parathyroid (gland) E20.9
  peripheral vascular (arterial) I73.9
  pituitary E23.0
  placental (mother) O36.51-
  platelets D69.6
  prenatal care affecting management
    of pregnancy O09.3-
  progressive pluriglandular E31.0
  pulmonary J98.4
    acute, following surgery
      (nonthoracic) J95.2
      thoracic J95.1
    chronic, following surgery J95.3
    following
      shock J98.4
      trauma J98.4
    newborn P28.89
    valve I37.1

Insufficiency, insufficient *(continued)*
  pulmonary *(continued)*
    valve *(continued)*
      with stenosis I37.2
      congenital Q22.2
      rheumatic I09.89
        with aortic, mitral or tricuspid (valve) disease I08.8
  pyloric K31.89
  renal (acute) N28.9
    chronic N18.9
  respiratory R06.89
    newborn P28.5
  rotation —*see* Malrotation
  sleep syndrome F51.12
  social insurance Z59.7
  suprarenal E27.40
    primary E27.1
  tarso-orbital fascia, congenital Q10.3
  testis E29.1
  thyroid (gland) (acquired) E03.9
    congenital E03.1
  tricuspid (valve) (rheumatic) I07.1
    with
      aortic (valve) disease I08.2
        with mitral (valve) disease I08.3
      mitral (valve) disease I08.1
        with aortic (valve) disease I08.3
      obstruction or stenosis I07.2
        with aortic (valve) disease I08.2
          with mitral (valve) disease I08.3
    congenital Q22.8
    nonrheumatic I36.1
      with stenosis I36.2
  urethral sphincter R32
  valve, valvular (heart) I38
    aortic —*see* Insufficiency, aortic (valve)
    congenital Q24.8
    mitral —*see* Insufficiency, mitral (valve)
    pulmonary —*see* Insufficiency, pulmonary valve
    tricuspid —*see* Insufficiency, tricuspid (valve)
  vascular I99.8
    intestine K55.9
      acute (*see also* Ischemia, intestine, acute) K55.059
    mesenteric K55.1
    peripheral I73.9
    renal —*see* Hypertension, kidney
  velopharyngeal
    acquired K13.79
    congenital Q38.8
  venous (chronic) (peripheral) I87.2
  ventricular —*see* Insufficiency, myocardial
  welfare support Z59.7

Insufflation, fallopian Z31.41

Insular —*see* condition

Insulinoma
  pancreas
    benign D13.7
    malignant C25.4
    uncertain behavior D37.8
  specified site
    benign —*see* Neoplasm, by site, benign
    malignant —*see* Neoplasm, by site, malignant
    uncertain behavior —*see* Neoplasm, by site, uncertain behavior

Insulinoma *(continued)*
  unspecified site
    benign D13.7
    malignant C25.4
    uncertain behavior D37.8

Insuloma —*see* Insulinoma

Interference
  balancing side M26.56
  non-working side M26.56

Intermenstrual —*see* condition

Intermittent —*see* condition

Internal —*see* condition

Interrogation
  cardiac defibrillator (automatic) (implantable) Z45.02
  cardiac pacemaker Z45.018
  cardiac (event) (loop) recorder Z45.09
  infusion pump (implanted) (intrathecal) Z45.1
  neurostimulator Z46.2

Interruption
  aortic arch Q25.21
  bundle of His I44.30
  phase-shift, sleep cycle —*see* Disorder, sleep, circadian rhythm
  sleep phase-shift, or 24 hour sleep-wake cycle —*see* Disorder, sleep, circadian rhythm

Interstitial —*see* condition

Intertrigo L30.4
  labialis K13.0

Intervertebral disc —*see* condition

Intestine, intestinal —*see* condition

Intolerance
  carbohydrate K90.49
  disaccharide, hereditary E73.0
  fat NEC K90.49
    pancreatic K90.3
  food K90.49
    dietary counseling and surveillance Z71.3
  fructose E74.10
    hereditary E74.12
  glucose (-galactose) E74.39
  gluten K90.41
  lactose E73.9
    specified NEC E73.8
  lysine E72.3
  milk NEC K90.49
    lactose E73.9
  protein K90.49
  starch NEC K90.49
  sucrose (-isomaltose) E74.31

Intoxicated NEC (without dependence) —*see* Alcohol, intoxication

Intoxication
  acid E87.2
  alcoholic (acute) (without dependence) —*see* Alcohol, intoxication
  alimentary canal K52.1
  amphetamine (without dependence) —*see also* Abuse, drug, stimulant, with intoxication
    with dependence —*see* Dependence, drug, stimulant, with intoxication
  stimulant NEC F15.10
    with
      anxiety disorder F15.180
      intoxication F15.129
        with
          delirium F15.121
          perceptual disturbance F15.122

Intoxication *(continued)*
  anxiolytic (acute) (without dependence) —*see* Abuse, drug, sedative, with intoxication
    with dependence —*see* Dependence, drug, sedative, with intoxication
  caffeine F15.929
    with
      abuse —*see* Abuse, drug, cannabis, with intoxication
      dependence —*see* Dependence, drug, cannabis, with intoxication
  cannabinoids (acute) (without dependence) —*see* Use, cannabis, with intoxication
    with
      abuse —*see* Abuse, drug, cannabis, with intoxication
      dependence —*see* Dependence, drug, cannabis, with intoxication
  chemical —*see* Table of Drugs and Chemicals
    via placenta or breast milk —*see* - Absorption, chemical, through placenta
  cocaine (acute) (without dependence) —*see* Abuse, drug, cocaine, with intoxication
    with dependence —*see* Dependence, drug, cocaine, with intoxication
  drug
    acute (without dependence) —*see* Abuse, drug, by type with intoxication
      with dependence —*see* Dependence, drug, by type with intoxication
    addictive
      via placenta or breast milk —*see* Absorption, drug, addictive, through placenta
      newborn P93.8
        gray baby syndrome P93.0
    overdose or wrong substance given or taken —*see* Table of Drugs and Chemicals, by drug, poisoning
  enteric K52.1
  foodborne A05.9
    bacterial A05.9
    classical (Clostridium botulinum) A05.1
    due to
      Bacillus cereus A05.4
      bacterium A05.9
        specified NEC A05.8
      Clostridium
        botulinum A05.1
        perfringens A05.2
        welchii A05.2
      Salmonella A02.9
        with
          (gastro)enteritis A02.0
          localized infection(s) A02.20
            arthritis A02.23
            meningitis A02.21
            osteomyelitis A02.24
            pneumonia A02.22
            pyelonephritis A02.25
            specified NEC A02.29
          sepsis A02.1
          specified manifestation NEC A02.8
      Staphylococcus A05.0

Intoxication *(continued)*
  foodborne *(continued)*
    due to *(continued)*
      Vibrio
        parahaemolyticus A05.3
        vulnificus A05.5
      enterotoxin, staphylococcal A05.0
    noxious —*see* Poisoning, food, noxious
  gastrointestinal K52.1
  hallucinogenic (without dependence) —*see* Abuse, drug, hallucinogen, with intoxication
    with dependence —*see* Dependence, drug, hallucinogen, with intoxication
  hypnotic (acute) (without dependence) —*see* Abuse, drug, sedative, with intoxication
    with dependence —*see* Dependence, drug, sedative, with intoxication
  inhalant (acute) (without dependence) —*see* Abuse, drug, inhalant, with intoxication
    with dependence —*see* Dependence, drug, inhalant, with intoxication
  meaning
    inebriation F10
    poisoning —*see* Table of Drugs and Chemicals
  methyl alcohol (acute) (without dependence) —*see* Alcohol, intoxication
  opioid (acute) (without dependence) —*see* Abuse, drug, opioid, with intoxication
    with dependence —*see* Dependence, drug, opioid, with intoxication
  pathologic NEC (without dependence) —*see* Alcohol, intoxication
  phencyclidine (without dependence) —*see* Abuse, drug, hallucinogen, with intoxication
    with dependence —*see* Dependence, drug, hallucinogen, with intoxication
  potassium (K) E87.5
  psychoactive substance NEC (without dependence) —*see* Abuse, drug, psychoactive NEC, with intoxication
    with dependence —*see* Dependence, drug, psychoactive NEC, with intoxication
  sedative (acute) (without dependence) —*see* Abuse, drug, sedative, with intoxication
    with dependence —*see* Dependence, drug, sedative, with intoxication
  serum (*see also* Reaction, serum) T80.69
  uremic —*see* Uremia
  volatile solvents (acute) (without dependence) —*see* Abuse, drug, inhalant, with intoxication
    with dependence —*see* Dependence, drug, inhalant, with intoxication
  water E87.79

Intraabdominal testis, testes
  bilateral Q53.211
  unilateral Q53.111

Intracranial —see condition

Intrahepatic gallbladder Q44.1

Intraligamentous —see condition

Intrathoracic —see also condition
kidney Q63.2

Intrauterine contraceptive device
checking Z30.431
insertion Z30.430
immediately following removal
Z30.433
in situ Z97.5
management Z30.431
reinsertion Z30.433
removal Z30.432
replacement Z30.433
retention in pregnancy O26.3-

Intraventricular —see condition

Intrinsic deformity —see Deformity

Intubation, difficult or failed T88.4

Intumescence, lens (eye) (cataract)
—see Cataract

Intussusception (bowel) (colon)
(enteric) (ileocecal) (ileocolic)
(intestine) (rectum) K56.1
appendix K38.8
congenital Q43.8
ureter (with obstruction) N13.5

Invagination (bowel, colon, intestine
or rectum) K56.1

Inversion
albumin-globulin (A-G) ratio
E88.09
bladder N32.89
cecum —see Intussusception
cervix N88.8
chromosome in normal individual
Q95.1
circadian rhythm —see Disorder,
sleep, circadian rhythm
nipple N64.59
congenital Q83.8
gestational —see Retraction,
nipple
puerperal, postpartum
—see Retraction, nipple
nyctohemeral rhythm —see
Disorder, sleep, circadian rhythm
optic papilla Q14.2
organ or site, congenital NEC
—see Anomaly, by site
sleep rhythm —see Disorder, sleep,
circadian rhythm
testis (congenital) Q55.29
uterus (chronic) (postinfectional)
(postpartal, old) N85.5
postpartum O71.2
vagina (posthysterectomy) N99.3
ventricular Q20.5

Investigation (see also Examination)
Z04.9
clinical research subject
(control) (normal comparison)
(participant) Z00.6

Involuntary movement, abnormal
R25.9

Involution, involutional —see also
condition
breast, cystic —see Dysplasia,
mammary, specified type NEC
depression (single episode) F32.89
recurrent episode F33.9
melancholia (single episode)
F32.89
recurrent episode F33.8
ovary, senile —see Atrophy, ovary
thymus failure E32.8

I.Q.
under 20 F73
20-34 F72
35-49 F71
50-69 F70

IRDS (type I) P22.0
type II P22.1

Irideremia Q13.1

Iridis rubeosis —see Disorder, iris,
vascular

Iridochoroiditis (panuveitis)
—see Panuveitis

Iridocyclitis H20.9
acute H20.0-
hypopyon H20.05-
primary H20.01-
recurrent H20.02-
secondary (noninfectious)
H20.04-
infectious H20.03-
chronic H20.1-
due to allergy —see Iridocyclitis,
acute, secondary
endogenous —see Iridocyclitis,
acute, primary
Fuchs' —see Cyclitis, Fuchs'
heterochromic
gonococcal A54.32
granulomatous —see Iridocyclitis,
chronic
herpes, herpetic (simplex) B00.51
zoster B02.32
hypopyon —see Iridocyclitis,
acute, hypopyon
in (due to)
ankylosing spondylitis M45.9
gonococcal infection A54.32
herpes (simplex) virus B00.51
zoster B02.32
infectious disease NOS B99
parasitic disease NOS B89 [H22]
sarcoidosis D86.83
syphilis A51.43
tuberculosis A18.54
zoster B02.32
lens-induced H20.2-
nongranulomatous —see
Iridocyclitis, acute
recurrent —see Iridocyclitis, acute,
recurrent
rheumatic —see Iridocyclitis,
chronic
subacute —see Iridocyclitis, acute
sympathetic —see Uveitis,
sympathetic
syphilitic (secondary) A51.43
tuberculous (chronic) A18.54
Vogt-Koyanagi H20.82-

Iridocyclochoroiditis (panuveitis) —
see Panuveitis

Iridodialysis H21.53-

Iridodonesis H21.89

Iridoplegia (complete) (partial)
(reflex) H57.09

Iridoschisis H21.25-

Iris —see also condition
bombé —see Membrane, pupillary

Iritis —see also Iridocyclitis
chronic —see Iridocyclitis, chronic
diabetic —see E08-E13 with .39
due to
herpes simplex B00.51
leprosy A30.9 [H22]
gonococcal A54.32
gouty (see also Gout, by type)
M10.9 [H22]

Iritis (continued)
granulomatous —see Iridocyclitis,
chronic
lens induced —see Iridocyclitis,
lens-induced
papulosa (syphilitic) A52.71
rheumatic —see Iridocyclitis,
chronic
syphilitic (secondary) A51.43
congenital (early) A50.01
late A52.71
tuberculous A18.54

Iron —see condition

Iron-miner's lung J63.4

Irradiated enamel (tooth, teeth)
K03.89

Irradiation effects, adverse T66

Irreducible, irreducibility —see
condition

Irregular, irregularity
action, heart I49.9
alveolar process K08.89
bleeding N92.6
breathing R06.89
contour of cornea (acquired) —see
Deformity, cornea
congenital Q13.4
contour, reconstructed breast N65.0
dentin (in pulp) K04.3
eye movements H55.89
nystagmus —see Nystagmus
deficient
saccadic H55.81
smooth H55.82
labor O62.2
menstruation (cause unknown) N92.6
periods N92.6
prostate N42.9
pupil —see Abnormality, pupillary
reconstructed breast N65.0
respiratory R06.89
septum (nasal) J34.2
shape, organ or site, congenital
NEC —see Distortion
sleep-wake pattern (rhythm) G47.23

Irritable, irritability R45.4
bladder N32.89
bowel (syndrome) K58.9
with
constipation K58.1
diarrhea K58.0
mixed K58.2
psychogenic F45.8
specified NEC K58.8
bronchial —see Bronchitis
cerebral, in newborn P91.3
colon (see also Irritable, bowel)
K58.9
with diarrhea K58.0
psychogenic F45.8
duodenum K59.89
heart (psychogenic) F45.8
hip —see Derangement, joint,
specified type NEC, hip
ileum K59.89
infant R68.12
jejunum K59.89
rectum K59.89
stomach K31.89
psychogenic F45.8
sympathetic G90.8
urethra N36.8

Irritation
anus K62.89
axillary nerve G54.0
bladder N32.89
brachial plexus G54.0
bronchial —see Bronchitis

Irritation (continued)
cervical plexus G54.2
cervix —see Cervicitis
choroid, sympathetic —see
Endophthalmitis
cranial nerve —see Disorder, nerve,
cranial
gastric K31.89
psychogenic F45.8
globe, sympathetic —see Uveitis,
sympathetic
labyrinth —see subcategory H83.2
lumbosacral plexus G54.1
meninges (traumatic) —see Injury,
intracranial
nontraumatic —see
Meningismus
nerve —see Disorder, nerve
nervous R45.0
penis N48.89
perineum NEC L29.3
peripheral autonomic nervous
system G90.8
peritoneum —see Peritonitis
pharynx J39.2
plantar nerve —see Lesion, nerve,
plantar
spinal (cord) (traumatic) —see also
Injury, spinal cord, by region
nerve G58.9
root NEC —see Radiculopathy
nontraumatic —see Myelopathy
stomach K31.89
psychogenic F45.8
sympathetic nerve NEC G90.8
ulnar nerve —see Lesion, nerve,
ulnar
vagina N89.8

Ischemia, ischemic I99.8
brain —see Ischemia, cerebral
bowel (transient)
acute (see also Ischemia,
intestine, acute) K55.019
diffuse K55.012
focal K55.011
chronic K55.1
due to mesenteric artery
insufficiency K55.1
cardiac (see Disease, heart,
ischemic)
cardiomyopathy I25.5
cerebral (chronic) (generalized)
I67.82
arteriosclerotic I67.2
intermittent G45.9
newborn P91.0
recurrent focal G45.8
transient G45.9
colon chronic (due to mesenteric
artery insufficiency) K55.1
coronary —see Disease, heart,
ischemic
demand (coronary) (see also
Angina) I24.8
with myocardial infarction
I21.A1
resulting in myocardial
infarction I21.A1
heart (chronic or with a stated
duration of over 4 weeks)
I25.9
acute or with a stated duration of
4 weeks or less I24.9
subacute I24.9
infarction, muscle —see Infarct,
muscle
intestine (large) (small) (transient)
K55.9
acute K55.059
diffuse K55.052
focal K55.051

Ischemia, ischemic *(continued)*
intestine *(continued)*
large K55.039
diffuse K55.032
focal K55.031
small K55.019
diffuse K55.012
focal K55.011
chronic K55.1
due to mesenteric artery
insufficiency K55.1
kidney N28.0
limb, critical —*see* Arteriosclerosis,
with critical limb ischemia
limb-threatening, chronic —*see*
Arteriosclerosis, with critical
limb ischemia
mesenteric, acute *(see also* Ischemia,
intestine, acute) K55.059
muscle, traumatic T79.6
myocardium, myocardial (chronic
or with a stated duration of over
4 weeks) I25.9
acute, without myocardial
infarction I51.3
silent (asymptomatic) I25.6
transient of newborn P29.4
renal N28.0
retina, retinal —*see* Occlusion,
artery, retina
small bowel
acute K55.019
diffuse K55.012
focal K55.011
chronic K55.1
due to mesenteric artery
insufficiency K55.1
spinal cord G95.11
subendocardial —*see* Insufficiency,
coronary
supply (coronary) *(see also* Angina)
I25.9
due to vasospasm I20.1

Ischial spine —*see* condition

Ischialgia —*see* Sciatica

Ischiopagus Q89.4

Ischium, ischial —*see* condition

Ischuria R34

Iselin's disease or osteochondrosis
—*see* Osteochondrosis, juvenile,
metatarsus

Islands of
parotid tissue in
lymph nodes Q38.6
neck structures Q38.6
submaxillary glands in
fascia Q38.6
lymph nodes Q38.6
neck muscles Q38.6

Islet cell tumor, pancreas D13.7

Isoimmunization NEC —*see also*
Incompatibility
affecting management of pregnancy
(ABO) (with hydrops fetalis)
O36.11-
anti-A sensitization O36.11-
anti-B sensitization O36.19-
anti-c sensitization O36.09-
anti-C sensitization O36.09-
anti-e sensitization O36.09-
anti-E sensitization O36.09-
Rh NEC O36.09-
anti-D antibody O36.01-
specified NEC O36.19-
newborn P55.9
with
hydrops fetalis P56.0
kernicterus P57.0

Isoimmunization NEC *(continued)*
newborn *(continued)*
ABO (blood groups) P55.1
Rhesus (Rh) factor P55.0
specified type NEC P55.8

Isolation, isolated
dwelling Z59.8
family Z63.79
social Z60.4

Isoleucinosis E71.19

Isomerism atrial appendages (with
asplenia or polysplenia) Q20.6

Isosporiasis, isosporosis A07.3

Isovaleric acidemia E71.110

Issue of
medical certificate Z02.79
for disability determination
Z02.71
repeat prescription (appliance)
(glasses) (medicinal substance,
medicament, medicine) Z76.0
contraception —*see*
Contraception

Itch, itching —*see also* Pruritus
baker's L23.6
barber's B35.0
bricklayer's L24.5
cheese B88.0
clam digger's B65.3
coolie B76.9
copra B88.0
dew B76.9
dhobi B35.6
filarial —*see* Infestation, filarial
grain B88.0
grocer's B88.0
ground B76.9
harvest B88.0
jock B35.6
Malabar B35.5
beard B35.0
foot B35.3
scalp B35.0
meaning scabies B86
Norwegian B86
perianal L29.0
poultrymen's B88.0
sarcoptic B86
scabies B86
scrub B88.0
straw B88.0
swimmer's B65.3
water B76.9
winter L29.8

Ivemark's syndrome (asplenia
with congenital heart disease)
Q89.01

Ivory bones Q78.2

Ixodiasis NEC B88.8

J

Jaccoud's syndrome —*see*
Arthropathy, postrheumatic,
chronic

Jackson's
membrane Q43.3
paralysis or syndrome G83.89
veil Q43.3

Jacquet's dermatitis (diaper
dermatitis) L22

**Jadassohn-Pellizari's disease or
anetoderma** L90.2

Jadassohn's
blue nevus —*see* Nevus
intraepidermal epithelioma —*see*
Neoplasm, skin, benign

Jaffe-Lichtenstein (-Uehlinger)
syndrome —*see* Dysplasia,
fibrous, bone NEC

**Jakob-Creutzfeldt disease or
syndrome** —*see* Creutzfeldt-Jakob
disease or syndrome

Jaksch-Luzet disease D64.89

Jamaican
neuropathy G92
paraplegic tropical ataxic-spastic
syndrome G92

Janet's disease F48.8

Janiceps Q89.4

**Jansky-Bielschowsky amaurotic
idiocy** E75.4

Japanese
B-type encephalitis A83.0
river fever A75.3

Jaundice (yellow) R17
acholuric (familial) (splenomegalic)
—*see also* Spherocytosis
acquired D59.8
breast-milk (inhibitor) P59.3
catarrhal (acute) B15.9
with hepatic coma B15.0
cholestatic (benign) R17
due to or associated with
delayed conjugation P59.8
associated with (due to)
preterm delivery P59.0
preterm delivery P59.0
epidemic (catarrhal) B15.9
with hepatic coma B15.0
leptospiral A27.0
spirochetal A27.0
familial nonhemolytic (congenital)
(Gilbert) E80.4
Crigler-Najjar E80.5
febrile (acute) B15.9
with hepatic coma B15.0
leptospiral A27.0
spirochetal A27.0
hematogenous D59.9
hemolytic (acquired) D59.9
congenital —*see* Spherocytosis
hemorrhagic (acute) (leptospiral)
(spirochetal) A27.0
infectious (acute) (subacute) B15.9
with hepatic coma B15.0
leptospiral A27.0
spirochetal A27.0
leptospiral (hemorrhagic) A27.0
malignant (without coma) K72.90
with coma K72.91
newborn P59.9
due to or associated with
ABO
antibodies P55.1
incompatibility, maternal/
fetal P55.1
isoimmunization P55.1
absence or deficiency
of enzyme system for
bilirubin conjugation
(congenital) P59.8
bleeding P58.1
breast milk inhibitors to
conjugation P59.3
associated with preterm
delivery P59.0
bruising P58.0
Crigler-Najjar syndrome E80.5
delayed conjugation P59.8
associated with preterm
delivery P59.0
drugs or toxins
given to newborn P58.42
transmitted from mother
P58.41

Jaundice *(continued)*
newborn *(continued)*
due to or associated with
(continued)
excessive hemolysis P58.9
due to
bleeding P58.1
bruising P58.0
drugs or toxins
given to newborn
P58.42
transmitted from
mother P58.41
infection P58.2
polycythemia P58.3
swallowed maternal
blood P58.5
specified type NEC P58.8
galactosemia E74.21
Gilbert syndrome E80.4
hemolytic disease P55.9
ABO isoimmunization
P55.1
Rh isoimmunization P55.0
specified NEC P55.8
hepatocellular damage
P59.20
specified NEC P59.29
hereditary hemolytic anemia
P58.8
hypothyroidism, congenital
E03.1
incompatibility, maternal/fetal
NOS P55.9
infection P58.2
inspissated bile syndrome
P59.1
isoimmunization NOS P55.9
mucoviscidosis E84.9
polycythemia P58.3
preterm delivery P59.0
Rh
antibodies P55.0
incompatibility, maternal/
fetal P55.0
isoimmunization P55.0
specified cause NEC P59.8
swallowed maternal blood
P58.5
spherocytosis (congenital)
D58.0
neonatal —*see* Jaundice, newborn
nonhemolytic congenital familial
(Gilbert) E80.4
nuclear, newborn *(see also*
Kernicterus of newborn) P57.9
obstructive *(see also* Obstruction,
bile duct) K83.1
post-immunization —*see* Hepatitis,
viral, type, B
post-transfusion —*see* Hepatitis,
viral, type, B
regurgitation *(see also* Obstruction,
bile duct) K83.1
serum (homologous) (prophylactic)
(therapeutic) —*see* Hepatitis,
viral, type, B
spirochetal (hemorrhagic) A27.0
symptomatic R17
newborn P59.9

Jaw —*see* condition

**Jaw-winking phenomenon or
syndrome** Q07.8

Jealousy
alcoholic F10.988
childhood F93.8
sibling F93.8

Jejunitis —*see* Enteritis

Jejunostomy status Z93.4

Jejunum, jejunal —*see* condition

Jensen's disease —*see* Inflammation, chorioretinal, focal, juxtapapillary

Jerks, myoclonic G25.3

Jervell-Lange-Nielsen syndrome I45.81

Jeune's disease Q77.2

Jigger disease B88.1

Job's syndrome (chronic granulomatous disease) D71

Joint —*see also* condition
　mice —*see* Loose, body, joint
　　knee M23.4-

Jordan's anomaly or syndrome D72.0

Joseph-Diamond-Blackfan anemia (congenital hypoplastic) D61.01

Jungle yellow fever A95.0

Jüngling's disease —*see* Sarcoidosis

Juvenile —*see* condition

K

Kahler's disease C90.0-

Kakke E51.11

Kala-azar B55.0

Kallmann's syndrome E23.0

Kanner's syndrome (autism) —*see* Psychosis, childhood

Kaposi's
　dermatosis (xeroderma pigmentosum) Q82.1
　lichen ruber L44.0
　　acuminatus L44.0
　sarcoma
　　colon C46.4
　　connective tissue C46.1
　　gastrointestinal organ C46.4
　　lung C46.5-
　　lymph node (multiple) C46.3
　　palate (hard) (soft) C46.2
　　rectum C46.4
　　skin (multiple sites) C46.0
　　specified site NEC C46.7
　　stomach C46.4
　　unspecified site C46.9
　varicelliform eruption B00.0
　　vaccinia T88.1

Kartagener's syndrome or triad (sinusitis, bronchiectasis, situs inversus) Q89.3

Karyotype
　with abnormality except iso (Xq) Q96.2
　45,X Q96.0
　46,X
　　iso (Xq) Q96.1
　46,XX Q98.3
　　with streak gonads Q50.32
　　hermaphrodite (true) Q99.1
　　male Q98.3
　46,XY
　　with streak gonads Q56.1
　　female Q97.3
　　hermaphrodite (true) Q99.1
　47,XXX Q97.0
　47,XXY Q98.0
　47,XYY Q98.5

Kaschin-Beck disease —*see* Disease, Kaschin-Beck

Katayama's disease or fever B65.2

Kawasaki's syndrome M30.3

Kayser-Fleischer ring (cornea) (pseudosclerosis) H18.04-

Kaznelson's syndrome (congenital hypoplastic anemia) D61.01

Kearns-Sayre syndrome H49.81-

Kedani fever A75.3

Kelis L91.0

Kelly (-Patterson) syndrome (sideropenic dysphagia) D50.1

Keloid, cheloid L91.0
　acne L73.0
　Addison's L94.0
　cornea —*see* Opacity, cornea
　Hawkin's L91.0
　scar L91.0

Keloma L91.0

Kenya fever A77.1

Keratectasia —*see also* Ectasia, cornea
　congenital Q13.4

Keratinization of alveolar ridge mucosa
　excessive K13.23
　minimal K13.22

Keratinized residual ridge mucosa
　excessive K13.23
　minimal K13.22

Keratitis (nodular) (nonulcerative) (simple) (zonular) H16.9
　with ulceration (central) (marginal) (perforated) (ring) —*see* Ulcer, cornea
　actinic —*see* Photokeratitis
　arborescens (herpes simplex) B00.52
　areolar H16.11-
　bullosa H16.8
　deep H16.309
　　specified type NEC H16.399
　dendritic (a) (herpes simplex) B00.52
　disciform (is) (herpes simplex) B00.52
　　varicella B01.81
　filamentary H16.12-
　gonococcal (congenital or prenatal) A54.33
　herpes, herpetic (simplex) B00.52
　　zoster B02.33
　in (due to)
　　acanthamebiasis B60.13
　　adenovirus B30.0
　　exanthema (*see also* Exanthem) B09
　　herpes (simplex) virus B00.52
　　measles B05.81
　　syphilis A50.31
　　tuberculosis A18.52
　　zoster B02.33
　interstitial (nonsyphilitic) H16.30-
　　diffuse H16.32-
　　herpes, herpetic (simplex) B00.52
　　　zoster B02.33
　　sclerosing H16.33-
　　specified type NEC H16.39-
　　syphilitic (congenital) (late) A50.31
　　tuberculous A18.52
　macular H16.11-
　nummular H16.11-
　oyster shuckers' H16.8
　parenchymatous —*see* Keratitis, interstitial
　petrificans H16.8
　postmeasles B05.81

Keratitis (continued)
　punctata
　　leprosa A30.9 [H16.14-]
　　syphilitic (profunda) A50.31
　punctate H16.14-
　purulent H16.8
　rosacea L71.8
　sclerosing H16.33-
　specified type NEC H16.8
　stellate H16.11-
　striate H16.11-
　superficial H16.10-
　　with conjunctivitis —*see* Keratoconjunctivitis
　　due to light —*see* Photokeratitis
　suppurative H16.8
　syphilitic (congenital) (prenatal) A50.31
　trachomatous A71.1
　　sequelae B94.0
　tuberculous A18.52
　vesicular H16.8
　xerotic (*see also* Keratomlacia) H16.8
　　vitamin A deficiency E50.4

Keratoacanthoma L85.8

Keratocele —*see* Descemetocele

Keratoconjunctivitis H16.20-
　Acanthamoeba B60.13
　adenoviral B30.0
　epidemic B30.0
　exposure H16.21-
　herpes, herpetic (simplex) B00.52
　　zoster B02.33
　in exanthema (*see also* Exanthem) B09
　infectious B30.0
　lagophthalmic —*see* Keratoconjunctivitis, specified type NEC
　neurotrophic H16.23-
　phlyctenular H16.25-
　postmeasles B05.81
　shipyard B30.0
　sicca (Sjogren's) M35.0-
　　not Sjogren's H16.22-
　specified type NEC H16.29-
　tuberculous (phlyctenular) A18.52
　vernal H16.26-

Keratoconus H18.60-
　congenital Q13.4
　stable H18.61-
　unstable H18.62-

Keratocyst (dental) (odontogenic) —*see* Cyst, calcifying odontogenic

Keratoderma, keratodermia (congenital) (palmaris et plantaris) (symmetrical) Q82.8
　acquired L85.1
　　in diseases classified elsewhere L86
　climactericum L85.1
　gonococcal A54.89
　gonorrheal A54.89
　punctata L85.2
　Reiter's —*see* Reiter's disease

Keratodermatocele —*see* Descemetocele

Keratoglobus H18.79
　congenital Q15.8
　　with glaucoma Q15.0

Keratohemia —*see* Pigmentation, cornea, stromal

Keratoiritis —*see also* Iridocyclitis
　syphilitic A50.39
　tuberculous A18.54

Keratoma L57.0
　palmaris and plantaris hereditarium Q82.8
　senile L57.0

Keratomalacia H18.44-
　vitamin A deficiency E50.4

Keratomegaly Q13.4

Keratomycosis B49
　nigrans, nigricans (palmaris) B36.1

Keratopathy H18.9
　band H18.42-
　bullous H18.1-
　bullous (aphakic), following cataract surgery H59.01-

Keratoscleritis, tuberculous A18.52

Keratosis L57.0
　actinic L57.0
　arsenical L85.8
　congenital, specified NEC Q80.8
　female genital NEC N94.89
　follicularis Q82.8
　　acquired L11.0
　　congenita Q82.8
　　et parafollicularis in cutem penetrans L87.0
　　spinulosa (decalvans) Q82.8
　　vitamin A deficiency E50.8
　gonococcal A54.89
　male genital (external) N50.89
　nigricans L83
　obturans, external ear (canal) —*see* Cholesteatoma, external ear
　palmaris et plantaris (inherited) (symmetrical) Q82.8
　　acquired L85.1
　penile N48.89
　pharynx J39.2
　pilaris, acquired L85.8
　punctata (palmaris et plantaris) L85.2
　scrotal N50.89
　seborrheic L82.1
　　inflamed L82.0
　senile L57.0
　solar L57.0
　tonsillaris J35.8
　vagina N89.4
　vegetans Q82.8
　vitamin A deficiency E50.8
　vocal cord J38.3

Kerato-uveitis —*see* Iridocyclitis

Kerunoparalysis T75.09

Kerion (celsi) B35.0

Kernicterus of newborn (not due to isoimmunization) P57.9
　due to isoimmunization (conditions in P55.0-P55.9) P57.0
　specified type NEC P57.8

Keshan disease E59

Ketoacidosis E87.2
　diabetic —*see* Diabetes, by type, with ketoacidosis

Ketonuria R82.4

Ketosis NEC E88.89
　diabetic —*see* Diabetes, by type, with ketoacidosis

Kew Garden fever A79.1

Kidney —*see* condition

Kienböck's disease —*see also* Osteochondrosis, juvenile, hand, carpal lunate
　adult M93.1

Kimmelstiel (-Wilson) disease —*see* Diabetes, Kimmelstiel (-Wilson) disease

Kimura disease D21.9
specified site —*see* Neoplasm, connective tissue benign

Kink, kinking
artery I77.1
hair (acquired) L67.8
ileum or intestine —*see* Obstruction, intestine
Lane's —*see* Obstruction, intestine
organ or site, congenital NEC —*see* Anomaly, by site
ureter (pelvic junction) N13.5
with
hydronephrosis N13.1
with infection N13.6
pyelonephritis (chronic) N11.1
congenital Q62.39
vein(s) I87.8
caval I87.1
peripheral I87.1

Kinnier Wilson's disease
(hepatolenticular degeneration) E83.01

Kissing spine M48.20
cervical region M48.22
cervicothoracic region M48.23
lumbar region M48.26
lumbosacral region M48.27
occipito-atlanto-axial region M48.21
thoracic region M48.24
thoracolumbar region M48.25

Klatskin's tumor C24.0

Klauder's disease A26.8

Klebs' disease (*see also* Glomerulonephritis) N05.-

Klebsiella (K.) pneumoniae, as cause of disease classified elsewhere B96.1

Klein (e)-Levin syndrome G47.13

Kleptomania F63.2

Klinefelter's syndrome Q98.4
karyotype 47,XXY Q98.0
male with more than two X chromosomes Q98.1

Klippel-Feil deficiency, disease, or syndrome (brevicollis) Q76.1

Klippel's disease I67.2

Klippel-Trenaunay (-Weber) syndrome Q87.2

Klumpke (-Déjerine) palsy, paralysis (birth) (newborn) P14.1

Knee —*see* condition

Knock knee (acquired) M21.06-
congenital Q74.1

Knot(s)
intestinal, syndrome (volvulus) K56.2
surfer S89.8-
umbilical cord (true) O69.2

Knotting (of)
hair L67.8
intestine K56.2

Knuckle pad (Garrod's) M72.1

Koch's
infection —*see* Tuberculosis
relapsing fever A68.9

Koch-Weeks' conjunctivitis —*see* Conjunctivitis, acute, mucopurulent

Köebner's syndrome Q81.8

Köenig's disease (osteochondritis dissecans) —*see* Osteochondritis, dissecans

Köhler-Pellegrini-Steida disease or syndrome (calcification, knee joint) —*see* Bursitis, tibial collateral

Köhler's disease
patellar —*see* Osteochondrosis, juvenile, patella
tarsal navicular —*see* Osteochondrosis, juvenile, tarsus

Koilonychia L60.3
congenital Q84.6

Kojevnikov's, epilepsy —*see* Kozhevnikof's epilepsy

Koplik's spots B05.9

Kopp's asthma E32.8

Korsakoff's (Wernicke) disease, psychosis or syndrome (alcoholic) F10.96
with dependence F10.26
drug-induced
due to drug abuse —*see* Abuse, drug, by type, with amnestic disorder
due to drug dependence —*see* Dependence, drug, by type, with amnestic disorder
nonalcoholic F04

Korsakov's disease, psychosis or syndrome —*see* Korsakoff's disease

Korsakow's disease, psychosis or syndrome —*see* Korsakoff's disease

Kostmann's disease or syndrome (infantile genetic agranulocytosis) —*see* Agranulocytosis

Kozhevnikof's epilepsy G40.109
intractable G40.119
with status epilepticus G40.111
without status epilepticus G40.119
not intractable G40.109
with status epilepticus G40.101
without status epilepticus G40.109

Krabbe's
disease E75.23
syndrome, congenital muscle hypoplasia Q79.8

Kraepelin-Morel disease —*see* Schizophrenia

Kraft-Weber-Dimitri disease Q85.8

Kraurosis
ani K62.89
penis N48.0
vagina N89.8
vulva N90.4

Kreotoxism A05.9

Krukenberg's
spindle —*see* Pigmentation, cornea, posterior
tumor C79.6-

Kufs' disease E75.4

Kugelberg-Welander disease G12.1

Kuhnt-Junius degeneration (*see also* Degeneration, macula) H35.32 -

Kümmell's disease or spondylitis —*see* Spondylopathy, traumatic

Kupffer cell sarcoma C22.3

Kuru A81.81

Kussmaul's
disease M30.0
respiration E87.2
in diabetic acidosis —*see* Diabetes, by type, with ketoacidosis

Kwashiorkor E40
marasmic, marasmus type E42

Kyasanur Forest disease A98.2

Kyphoscoliosis, kyphoscoliotic (acquired) (*see also* Scoliosis) M41.9
congenital Q67.5
heart (disease) I27.1
sequelae of rickets E64.3
tuberculous A18.01

Kyphosis, kyphotic (acquired) M40.209
cervical region M40.202
cervicothoracic region M40.203
congenital Q76.419
cervical region Q76.412
cervicothoracic region Q76.413
occipito-atlanto-axial region Q76.411
thoracic region Q76.414
thoracolumbar region Q76.415
Morquio-Brailsford type (spinal) (*see also* subcategory M49.8) E76.219
postlaminectomy M96.3
postradiation therapy M96.2
postural (adolescent) M40.00
cervicothoracic region M40.03
thoracic region M40.04
thoracolumbar region M40.05
secondary NEC M40.10
cervical region M40.12
cervicothoracic region M40.13
thoracic region M40.14
thoracolumbar region M40.15
sequelae of rickets E64.3
specified type NEC M40.299
cervical region M40.292
cervicothoracic region M40.293
thoracic region M40.294
thoracolumbar region M40.295
syphilitic, congenital A50.56
thoracic region M40.204
thoracolumbar region M40.205
tuberculous A18.01

Kyrle disease L87.0

L

Labia, labium —*see* condition

Labile
blood pressure R09.89
vasomotor system I73.9

Labioglossal paralysis G12.29

Labium leporinum —*see* Cleft, lip

Labor —*see* Delivery

Labored breathing —*see* Hyperventilation

Labyrinthitis (circumscribed) (destructive) (diffuse) (inner ear) (latent) (purulent) (suppurative) —*see also* subcategory H83.0
syphilitic A52.79

Laceration
with abortion —*see* Abortion, by type, complicated by laceration of pelvic organs
abdomen, abdominal wall S31.119

Laceration (*continued*)
abdomen, abdominal (*continued*)
wall (*continued*)
with
foreign body S31.129
penetration into peritoneal cavity S31.619
with foreign body S31.629
epigastric region S31.112
with
foreign body S31.122
penetration into peritoneal cavity S31.612
with foreign body S31.622
left
lower quadrant S31.114
with
foreign body S31.124
penetration into peritoneal cavity S31.614
with foreign body S31.624
upper quadrant S31.111
with
foreign body S31.121
penetration into peritoneal cavity S31.611
with foreign body S31.621
periumbilic region S31.115
with
foreign body S31.125
penetration into peritoneal cavity S31.615
with foreign body S31.625
right
lower quadrant S31.113
with
foreign body S31.123
penetration into peritoneal cavity S31.613
with foreign body S31.623
upper quadrant S31.110
with
foreign body S31.120
penetration into peritoneal cavity S31.610
with foreign body S31.620
accidental, complicating surgery —*see* Complications, surgical, accidental puncture or laceration
Achilles tendon S86.02-
adrenal gland S37.813
alveolar (process) —*see* Laceration, oral cavity
ankle S91.01-
with
foreign body S91.02-
antecubital space —*see* Laceration, elbow
anus (sphincter) S31.831
with
ectopic or molar pregnancy O08.6
foreign body S31.832
complicating delivery —*see* Delivery, complicated by, laceration, anus (sphincter)

Laceration (*continued*)

anus (*continued*)
  following ectopic or molar
    pregnancy O08.6
  nontraumatic, nonpuerperal
    —*see* Fissure, anus
arm (upper) S41.11-
  with foreign body S41.12-
  lower —*see* Laceration,
  forearm
auditory canal (external) (meatus)
  —*see* Laceration, ear
auricle, ear —*see* Laceration,
  ear
axilla —*see* Laceration, arm
back —*see also* Laceration, thorax,
  back
  lower S31.010
    with
      foreign body S31.020
        with penetration into
          retroperitoneal space
          S31.021
        penetration into
          retroperitoneal space
          S31.011
bile duct S36.13
bladder S37.23
  with ectopic or molar pregnancy
    O08.6
  following ectopic or molar
    pregnancy O08.6
  obstetrical trauma O71.5
blood vessel —*see* Injury, blood
  vessel
bowel —*see also* Laceration,
  intestine
  with ectopic or molar pregnancy
    O08.6
  complicating abortion
    —*see* Abortion, by type,
    complicated by, specified
    condition NEC
  following ectopic or molar
    pregnancy O08.6
  obstetrical trauma O71.5
brain (any part) (cortex) (diffuse)
  (membrane) —*see also* Injury,
  intracranial, diffuse
  during birth P10.8
    with hemorrhage P10.1
  focal —*see* Injury, intracranial,
    focal brain injury
brainstem S06.38-
breast S21.01-
  with foreign body S21.02-
broad ligament S37.893
  with ectopic or molar pregnancy
    O08.6
  following ectopic or molar
    pregnancy O08.6
  laceration syndrome N83.8
  obstetrical trauma O71.6
  syndrome (laceration) N83.8
buttock S31.801
  with foreign body S31.802
  left S31.821
    with foreign body S31.822
  right S31.811
    with foreign body S31.812
calf —*see* Laceration, leg
canaliculus lacrimalis —*see*
  Laceration, eyelid
canthus, eye —*see* Laceration,
  eyelid
capsule, joint —*see* Sprain
causing eversion of cervix uteri
  (old) N86
central (perineal), complicating
  delivery O70.9
cerebellum, traumatic S06.37-

cerebral S06.33-
  left side S06.32-
  during birth P10.8
    with hemorrhage P10.1
  right side S06.31-
cervix (uteri)
  with ectopic or molar pregnancy
    O08.6
  following ectopic or molar
    pregnancy O08.6
  nonpuerperal, nontraumatic N88.1
  obstetrical trauma (current) O71.3
  old (postpartal) N88.1
  traumatic S37.63
cheek (external) S01.41-
  with foreign body S01.42-
  internal —*see* Laceration, oral
    cavity
chest wall —*see* Laceration, thorax
chin —*see* Laceration, head,
  specified site NEC
chordae tendinae NEC I51.1
  concurrent with acute
    myocardial infarction —*see*
    Infarct, myocardium
  following acute myocardial
    infarction (current
    complication) I23.4
clitoris —*see* Laceration, vulva
colon —*see* Laceration, intestine,
  large, colon
common bile duct S36.13
cortex (cerebral) —*see* Injury,
  intracranial, diffuse
costal region —*see* Laceration,
  thorax
cystic duct S36.13
diaphragm S27.803
digit(s)
  hand —*see* Laceration, finger
  foot —*see* Laceration, toe
duodenum S36.430
ear (canal) (external) S01.31-
  with foreign body S01.32-
  drum S09.2-
elbow S51.01-
  with
    foreign body S51.02-
epididymis —*see* Laceration, testis
epigastric region —*see* Laceration,
  abdomen, wall, epigastric region
esophagus K22.8
  traumatic
    cervical S11.21
      with foreign body S11.22
    thoracic S27.813
eye (ball) S05.3-
  with prolapse or loss of
    intraocular tissue S05.2-
  penetrating S05.6-
eyebrow —*see* Laceration, eyelid
eyelid S01.11-
  with foreign body S01.12-
face NEC —*see* Laceration, head,
  specified site NEC
fallopian tube S37.539
  bilateral S37.532
  unilateral S37.531
finger(s) S61.219
  with
    damage to nail S61.319
      with
        foreign body S61.329
    foreign body S61.229
  index S61.218
    with
      damage to nail S61.318
        with
          foreign body S61.328
      foreign body S61.228

finger(s) (*continued*)
  index (*continued*)
    left S61.211
      with
        damage to nail S61.311
          with
            foreign body
            S61.321
        foreign body S61.221
    right S61.210
      with
        damage to nail S61.310
          with
            foreign body
            S61.320
        foreign body S61.220
  little S61.218
    with
      damage to nail S61.318
        with
          foreign body S61.328
      foreign body S61.228
    left S61.217
      with
        damage to nail S61.317
          with
            foreign body
            S61.327
        foreign body S61.227
    right S61.216
      with
        damage to nail S61.316
          with
            foreign body
            S61.326
        foreign body S61.226
  middle S61.218
    with
      damage to nail S61.318
        with
          foreign body S61.328
      foreign body S61.228
    left S61.213
      with
        damage to nail S61.313
          with
            foreign body
            S61.323
        foreign body S61.223
    right S61.212
      with
        damage to nail S61.312
          with
            foreign body
            S61.322
        foreign body S61.222
  ring S61.218
    with
      damage to nail S61.318
        with
          foreign body S61.328
      foreign body S61.228
    left S61.215
      with
        damage to nail S61.315
          with
            foreign body
            S61.325
        foreign body S61.225
    right S61.214
      with
        damage to nail S61.314
          with
            foreign body
            S61.324
        foreign body S61.224
flank S31.119
  with foreign body S31.129
foot (except toe(s) alone) S91.319
  with foreign body S91.329

foot (*continued*)
  left S91.312
    with foreign body S91.322
  right S91.311
    with foreign body S91.321
  toe —*see* Laceration, toe
forearm S51.819
  with
    foreign body S51.829
  elbow only —*see* Laceration,
    elbow
  left S51.812
    with
      foreign body S51.822
  right S51.811
    with
      foreign body S51.821
forehead S01.81
  with foreign body S01.82
fourchette O70.0
  with ectopic or molar pregnancy
    O08.6
  complicating delivery O70.0
  following ectopic or molar
    pregnancy O08.6
gallbladder S36.123
genital organs, external
  female S31.512
    with foreign body S31.522
    vagina —*see* Laceration,
      vagina
    vulva —*see* Laceration,
      vulva
  male S31.511
    with foreign body S31.521
    penis —*see* Laceration, penis
    scrotum —*see* Laceration,
      scrotum
    testis —*see* Laceration,
      testis
groin —*see* Laceration, abdomen,
  wall
gum —*see* Laceration, oral cavity
hand S61.419
  with
    foreign body S61.429
  finger —*see* Laceration, finger
  left S61.412
    with
      foreign body S61.422
  right S61.411
    with
      foreign body S61.421
  thumb —*see* Laceration, thumb
head S01.91
  with foreign body S01.92
  cheek —*see* Laceration, cheek
  ear —*see* Laceration, ear
  eyelid —*see* Laceration, eyelid
  lip —*see* Laceration, lip
  nose —*see* Laceration, nose
  oral cavity —*see* Laceration, oral
    cavity
  scalp S01.01
    with foreign body S01.02
  specified site NEC S01.81
    with foreign body S01.82
  temporomandibular area —*see*
    Laceration, cheek
heart —*see* Injury, heart, laceration
heel —*see* Laceration, foot
hepatic duct S36.13
hip S71.019
  with foreign body S71.029
  left S71.012
    with foreign body S71.022
  right S71.011
    with foreign body S71.021
hymen —*see* Laceration,
  vagina

Laceration (*continued*)

hypochondrium —*see* Laceration,
abdomen, wall
hypogastric region —*see*
Laceration, abdomen, wall
ileum S36.438
inguinal region —*see* Laceration,
abdomen, wall
instep —*see* Laceration, foot
internal organ —*see* Injury,
by site
interscapular region —*see*
Laceration, thorax, back
intestine
large
colon S36.539
ascending S36.530
descending S36.532
sigmoid S36.533
specified site NEC S36.538
rectum S36.63
transverse S36.531
small S36.439
duodenum S36.430
specified site NEC S36.438
intra-abdominal organ S36.93
intestine —*see* Laceration,
intestine
liver —*see* Laceration, liver
pancreas —*see* Laceration,
pancreas
peritoneum S36.81
specified site NEC S36.893
spleen —*see* Laceration, spleen
stomach —*see* Laceration,
stomach
intracranial NEC —*see also* Injury,
intracranial, diffuse
birth injury P10.9
jaw —*see* Laceration, head,
specified site NEC
jejunum S36.438
joint capsule —*see* Sprain, by site
kidney S37.03-
major (greater than 3 cm)
(massive) (stellate) S37.06-
minor (less than 1 cm) S37.04-
moderate (1 to 3 cm) S37.05-
multiple S37.06-
knee S81.01-
with foreign body S81.02-
labium (majus) (minus) —*see*
Laceration, vulva
lacrimal duct —*see* Laceration,
eyelid
large intestine —*see* Laceration,
intestine, large
larynx S11.011
with foreign body S11.012
leg (lower) S81.819
with foreign body S81.829
foot —*see* Laceration, foot
knee —*see* Laceration, knee
left S81.812
with foreign body S81.822
right S81.811
with foreign body S81.821
upper —*see* Laceration, thigh
ligament —*see* Sprain
lip S01.511
with foreign body S01.521
liver S36.113
major (stellate) S36.116
minor S36.114
moderate S36.115
loin —*see* Laceration, abdomen,
wall
lower back —*see* Laceration, back,
lower
lumbar region —*see* Laceration,
back, lower

Laceration (*continued*)

lung S27.339
bilateral S27.332
unilateral S27.331
malar region —*see* Laceration,
head, specified site NEC
mammary —*see* Laceration, breast
mastoid region —*see* Laceration,
head, specified site NEC
meninges —*see* Injury, intracranial,
diffuse
meniscus —*see* Tear, meniscus
mesentery S36.893
mesosalpinx S37.893
mouth —*see* Laceration, oral cavity
muscle —*see* Injury, muscle, by
site, laceration
nail
finger —*see* Laceration, finger,
with damage to nail
toe —*see* Laceration, toe, with
damage to nail
nasal (septum) (sinus) —*see*
Laceration, nose
nasopharynx —*see* Laceration,
head, specified site NEC
neck S11.91
with foreign body S11.92
involving
cervical esophagus S11.21
with foreign body S11.22
larynx —*see* Laceration,
larynx
pharynx —*see* Laceration,
pharynx
thyroid gland —*see*
Laceration, thyroid gland
trachea —*see* Laceration,
trachea
specified site NEC S11.81
with foreign body S11.82
nerve —*see* Injury, nerve
nose (septum) (sinus) S01.21
with foreign body S01.22
ocular NOS S05.3-
adnexa NOS S01.11-
oral cavity S01.512
with foreign body S01.522
orbit (eye) —*see* Wound, open,
ocular, orbit
ovary S37.439
bilateral S37.432
unilateral S37.431
palate —*see* Laceration, oral cavity
palm —*see* Laceration, hand
pancreas S36.239
body S36.231
major S36.261
minor S36.241
moderate S36.251
head S36.230
major S36.260
minor S36.240
moderate S36.250
major S36.269
minor S36.249
moderate S36.259
tail S36.232
major S36.262
minor S36.242
moderate S36.252
pelvic S31.010
with
foreign body S31.020
penetration into
retroperitoneal cavity
S31.021
penetration into retroperitoneal
cavity S31.011
floor —*see also* Laceration,
back, lower

Laceration (*continued*)

pelvic (*continued*)
floor (*continued*)
with ectopic or molar
pregnancy O08.6
complicating delivery O70.1
following ectopic or molar
pregnancy O08.6
old (postpartal) N81.89
organ S37.93
with ectopic or molar
pregnancy O08.6
adrenal gland S37.813
bladder S37.23
fallopian tube —*see*
Laceration, fallopian tube
following ectopic or molar
pregnancy O08.6
kidney —*see* Laceration,
kidney
obstetrical trauma O71.5
ovary —*see* Laceration,
ovary
prostate S37.823
specified site NEC S37.893
ureter S37.13
urethra S37.33
uterus S37.63
penis S31.21
with foreign body S31.22
perineum
female S31.41
with
ectopic or molar pregnancy
O08.6
foreign body S31.42
during delivery O70.9
first degree O70.0
fourth degree O70.3
second degree O70.1
third degree (*see also*
Delivery, complicated,
by, laceraton, perineum,
third degree) O70.20
old (postpartal) N81.89
postpartal N81.89
secondary (postpartal) O90.1
male S31.119
with foreign body S31.129
periocular area (with or without
lacrimal passages) —*see*
Laceration, eyelid
peritoneum S36.893
periumbilic region —*see*
Laceration, abdomen, wall,
periumbilic
periurethral tissue —*see*
Laceration, urethra
phalanges
finger —*see* Laceration, finger
toe —*see* Laceration, toe
pharynx S11.21
with foreign body S11.22
pinna —*see* Laceration, ear
popliteal space —*see* Laceration,
knee
prepuce —*see* Laceration, penis
prostate S37.823
pubic region S31.119
with foreign body S31.129
pudendum —*see* Laceration,
genital organs, external
rectovaginal septum —*see*
Laceration, vagina
rectum S36.63
retroperitoneum S36.893
round ligament S37.893
sacral region —*see* Laceration,
back, lower
sacroiliac region —*see* Laceration,
back, lower

Laceration (*continued*)

salivary gland —*see* Laceration,
oral cavity
scalp S01.01
with foreign body S01.02
scapular region —*see* Laceration,
shoulder
scrotum S31.31
with foreign body S31.32
seminal vesicle S37.893
shin —*see* Laceration, leg
shoulder S41.019
with foreign body S41.029
left S41.012
with foreign body S41.022
right S41.011
with foreign body S41.021
small intestine —*see* Laceration,
intestine, small
spermatic cord —*see* Laceration,
testis
spinal cord (meninges) —*see also*
Injury, spinal cord, by region
due to injury at birth P11.5
newborn (birth injury) P11.5
spleen S36.039
major (massive) (stellate) S36.032
moderate S36.031
superficial (minor) S36.030
sternal region —*see* Laceration,
thorax, front
stomach S36.33
submaxillary region —*see*
Laceration, head, specified site
NEC
submental region —*see* Laceration,
head, specified site NEC
subungual
finger(s) —*see* Laceration,
finger, with damage to nail
toe(s) —*see* Laceration, toe, with
damage to nail
suprarenal gland —*see* Laceration,
adrenal gland
temple, temporal region —*see*
Laceration, head, specified site
NEC
temporomandibular area —*see*
Laceration, cheek
tendon —*see* Injury, muscle, by
site, laceration
Achilles S86.02-
tentorium cerebelli —*see* Injury,
intracranial, diffuse
testis S31.31
with foreign body S31.32
thigh S71.11-
with foreign body S71.12-
thorax, thoracic (wall) S21.91
with foreign body S21.92
back S21.22-
with penetration into
thoracic cavity S21.42-
front S21.12-
with penetration into
thoracic cavity S21.32-
back S21.21-
with
foreign body S21.22-
with penetration into
thoracic cavity S21.42-
penetration into thoracic
cavity S21.41-
breast —*see* Laceration, breast
front S21.11-
with
foreign body S21.12-
with penetration into
thoracic cavity S21.32-
penetration into thoracic
cavity S21.31-

Laceration (*continued*)
thumb S61.019
  with
    damage to nail S61.119
      with
        foreign body S61.129
    foreign body S61.029
  left S61.012
    with
      damage to nail S61.112
        with
          foreign body S61.122
      foreign body S61.022
  right S61.011
    with
      damage to nail S61.111
        with
          foreign body S61.121
      foreign body S61.021
thyroid gland S11.11
  with foreign body S11.12
toe(s) S91.119
  with
    damage to nail S91.219
      with
        foreign body S91.229
    foreign body S91.129
  great S91.113
    with
      damage to nail S91.213
        with
          foreign body S91.223
      foreign body S91.123
    left S91.112
      with
        damage to nail S91.212
          with
            foreign body S91.222
        foreign body S91.122
    right S91.111
      with
        damage to nail S91.211
          with
            foreign body S91.221
        foreign body S91.121
  lesser S91.116
    with
      damage to nail S91.216
        with
          foreign body S91.226
      foreign body S91.126
    left S91.115
      with
        damage to nail S91.215
          with
            foreign body S91.225
        foreign body S91.125
    right S91.114
      with
        damage to nail S91.214
          with
            foreign body S91.224
        foreign body S91.124
tongue —*see* Laceration, oral cavity
trachea S11.021
  with foreign body S11.022
tunica vaginalis —*see* Laceration, testis
tympanum, tympanic membrane —*see* Laceration, ear, drum
umbilical region S31.115
  with foreign body S31.125
ureter S37.13
urethra S37.33
  with or following ectopic or molar pregnancy O08.6
  obstetrical trauma O71.5
urinary organ NEC S37.893
uterus S37.63
  with ectopic or molar pregnancy O08.6

Laceration (*continued*)
uterus (*continued*)
    following ectopic or molar pregnancy O08.6
  nonpuerperal, nontraumatic N85.8
  obstetrical trauma NEC O71.81
  old (postpartal) N85.8
uvula —*see* Laceration, oral cavity
vagina S31.41
  with
    ectopic or molar pregnancy O08.6
    foreign body S31.42
  during delivery O71.4
    with perineal laceration —*see* Laceration, perineum, female, during delivery
  following ectopic or molar pregnancy O08.6
  nonpuerperal, nontraumatic N89.8
  old (postpartal) N89.8
vas deferens S37.893
vesical —*see* Laceration, bladder
vocal cords S11.031
  with foreign body S11.032
vulva S31.41
  with
    ectopic or molar pregnancy O08.6
    foreign body S31.42
  complicating delivery O70.0
  following ectopic or molar pregnancy O08.6
  nonpuerperal, nontraumatic N90.89
  old (postpartal) N90.89
wrist S61.519
  with
    foreign body S61.529
  left S61.512
    with
      foreign body S61.522
  right S61.511
    with
      foreign body S61.521

Lack of
achievement in school Z55.3
adequate
  food Z59.4
  intermaxillary vertical dimension of fully erupted teeth M26.36
  sleep Z72.820
appetite (*see* Anorexia) R63.0
awareness R41.9
care
  in home Z74.2
  of infant (at or after birth) T76.02
    confirmed T74.02
cognitive functions R41.9
coordination R27.9
  ataxia R27.0
  specified type NEC R27.8
development (physiological) R62.50
  failure to thrive (child over 28 days old) R62.51
    adult R62.7
    newborn P92.6
  short stature R62.52
  specified type NEC R62.59
energy R53.83
financial resources Z59.6
food T73.0
growth R62.52
heating Z59.1

Lack of (*continued*)
housing (permanent) (temporary) Z59.0
  adequate Z59.1
learning experiences in childhood Z62.898
leisure time (affecting life-style) Z73.2
material resources Z59.9
memory —*see also* Amnesia
  mild, following organic brain damage F06.8
ovulation N97.0
parental supervision or control of child Z62.0
person able to render necessary care Z74.2
physical exercise Z72.3
play experience in childhood Z62.898
posterior occlusal support M26.57
relaxation (affecting life-style) Z73.2
sexual
  desire F52.0
  enjoyment F52.1
shelter Z59.0
sleep (adequate) Z72.820
supervision of child by parent Z62.0
support, posterior occlusal M26.57
water T73.1

Lacrimal —*see* condition

Lacrimation, abnormal —*see* Epiphora

Lacrimonasal duct —*see* condition

Lactation, lactating (breast) (puerperal, postpartum)
associated
  cracked nipple O92.13
  retracted nipple O92.03
defective O92.4
disorder NEC O92.79
excessive O92.6
failed (complete) O92.3
  partial O92.4
mastitis NEC —*see* Mastitis, obstetric
mother (care and/or examination) Z39.1
nonpuerperal N64.3

Lacticemia, excessive E87.2

Lacunar skull Q75.8

Laennec's cirrhosis K70.30
  with ascites K70.31
  nonalcoholic K74.69

Lafora's disease —*see* Epilepsy, generalized, idiopathic

Lag, lid (nervous) — *see* Retraction, lid

Lagophthalmos (eyelid) (nervous) H02.209
  bilateral, upper and lower eyelids H02.20C
  cicatricial H02.219
    bilateral, upper and lower eyelids H02.21C
    left H02.216
      lower H02.215
      upper H02.214
      upper and lower eyelids H02.21B
    right H02.213
      lower H02.212
      upper H02.211
      upper and lower eyelids H02.21A
  keratoconjunctivitis —*see* Keratoconjunctivitis

Lagophthalmos (*continued*)
  left H02.206
    lower H02.205
    upper H02.204
    upper and lower eyelids H02.20B
  mechanical H02.229
    bilateral, upper and lower eyelids H02.22C
    left H02.226
      lower H02.225
      upper H02.224
      upper and lower eyelids H02.22B
    right H02.223
      lower H02.222
      upper H02.221
      upper and lower eyelids H02.22A
  paralytic H02.239
    bilateral, upper and lower eyelids H02.23C
    left H02.236
      lower H02.235
      upper H02.234
      upper and lower eyelids H02.23B
    right H02.233
      lower H02.232
      upper H02.231
      upper and lower eyelids H02.23A
  right H02.203
    lower H02.202
    upper H02.201
    upper and lower eyelids H02.20A

Laki-Lorand factor deficiency —*see* Defect, coagulation, specified type NEC

Lalling F80.0

Lambert-Eaton syndrome —*see* Syndrome, Lambert-Eaton

Lambliasis, lambliosis A07.1

Landau-Kleffner syndrome —*see* Epilepsy, specified NEC

Landouzy-Déjérine dystrophy or facioscapulohumeral atrophy G71.02

Landouzy's disease (icterohemorrhagic leptospirosis) A27.0

Landry-Guillain-Barré, syndrome or paralysis G61.0

Landry's disease or paralysis G61.0

Lane's
  band Q43.3
  kink —*see* Obstruction, intestine
  syndrome K90.2

Langdon Down syndrome —*see* Trisomy, 21

Lapsed immunization schedule status Z28.3

Large
  baby (regardless of gestational age) (4000g to 4499g) P08.1
  ear, congenital Q17.1
  physiological cup Q14.2
  stature R68.89

Large-for-dates NEC (infant) (4000g to 4499g) P08.1
  affecting management of pregnancy O36.6-
  exceptionally (4500g or more) P08.0

Larsen-Johansson disease orosteochondrosis —*see* Osteochondrosis, juvenile, patella

Larsen's syndrome (flattened facies and multiple congenital dislocations) Q74.8

Larva migrans
cutaneous B76.9
Ancylostoma B76.0
visceral B83.0

Laryngeal —*see* condition

Laryngismus (stridulus) J38.5
congenital P28.89
diphtheritic A36.2

Laryngitis (acute) (edematous) (fibrinous) (infective) (infiltrative) (malignant) (membranous) (phlegmonous) (pneumococcal) (pseudomembranous) (septic) (subglottic) (suppurative) (ulcerative) J04.0
with
influenza, flu, or grippe —*see* Influenza, with, laryngitis
tracheitis (acute) —*see* Laryngotracheitis
atrophic J37.0
catarrhal J37.0
chronic J37.0
with tracheitis (chronic) J37.1
diphtheritic A36.2
due to external agent —*see* Inflammation, respiratory, upper, due to
Hemophilus influenzae J04.0
H. influenzae J04.0
hypertrophic J37.0
influenzal —*see* Influenza, with, respiratory manifestations NEC
obstructive J05.0
sicca J37.0
spasmodic J05.0
acute J04.0
streptococcal J04.0
stridulous J05.0
syphilitic (late) A52.73
congenital A50.59 [*J99*]
early A50.03 [*J99*]
tuberculous A15.5
Vincent's A69.1

Laryngocele (congenital) (ventricular) Q31.3

Laryngofissure J38.7
congenital Q31.8

Laryngomalacia (congenital) Q31.5

Laryngopharyngitis (acute) J06.0
chronic J37.0
due to external agent —*see* Inflammation, respiratory, upper, due to

Laryngoplegia J38.00
bilateral J38.02
unilateral J38.01

Laryngoptosis J38.7

Laryngospasm J38.5

Laryngostenosis J38.6

Laryngotracheitis (acute) (Infectional) (infective) (viral) J04.2
atrophic J37.1
catarrhal J37.1
chronic J37.1
diphtheritic A36.2
due to external agent —*see* Inflammation, respiratory, upper, due to

Laryngotracheitis (*continued*)
Hemophilus influenzae J04.2
hypertrophic J37.1
influenzal —*see* Influenza, with, respiratory manifestations NEC
pachydermic J38.7
sicca J37.1
spasmodic J38.5
acute J05.0
streptococcal J04.2
stridulous J38.5
syphilitic (late) A52.73
congenital A50.59 [*J99*]
early A50.03 [*J99*]
tuberculous A15.5
Vincent's A69.1

Laryngotracheobronchitis —*see* Bronchitis

Larynx, laryngeal —*see* condition

Lassa fever A96.2

Lassitude —*see* Weakness

Late
talker R62.0
walker R62.0

Late effect(s) —*see* Sequelae

Latent —*see* condition

LTBI (latent tuberculosis infection) Z22.7

Laterocession —*see* Lateroversion

Lateroflexion —*see* Lateroversion

Lateroversion
cervix —*see* Lateroversion, uterus
uterus, uterine (cervix) (postinfectional) (postpartal, old) N85.4
congenital Q51.818
in pregnancy or childbirth O34.59-

Lathyrism —*see* Poisoning, food, noxious, plant

Launois' syndrome (pituitary gigantism) E22.0

Launois-Bensaude adenolipomatosis E88.89

Laurence-Moon (-Bardet)-**Biedl syndrome** Q87.89

Lax, laxity —*see also* Relaxation
ligament (ous) —*see also* Disorder, ligament
familial M35.7
knee —*see* Derangement, knee
skin (acquired) L57.4
congenital Q82.8

Laxative habit F55.2

Lazy leukocyte syndrome D70.8

Lead miner's lung J63.6

Leak, leakage
air NEC J93.82
postprocedural J95.812
amniotic fluid —*see* Rupture, membranes, premature
blood (microscopic), fetal, into maternal circulation affecting management of pregnancy —*see* Pregnancy, complicated by
cerebrospinal fluid G96.00
cranial
postoperative G96.08
specified NEC G96.08
spontaneous G96.01
traumatic G96.08
from spinal (lumbar) puncture G97.0

Leak, leakage (*continued*)
cerebrospinal fluid (*continued*)
spinal
postoperative G96.09
post-traumatic G96.09
specified NEC G96.09
spontaneous G96.02
spontaneous
from
skull base G96.01
spine G96.02
CSF —*see* Leak, cerebrospinal fluid
device, implant or graft —*see also* Complications, by site and type, mechanical
arterial graft NEC —*see* Complication, cardiovascular device, mechanical, vascular
breast (implant) T85.43
catheter NEC T85.638
urinary T83.038
cystostomy T83.030
Hopkins T83.038
ileostomy T83.038
indwelling T83.031
nephrostomy T83.032
specified NEC T83.038
urostomy T83.038
dialysis (renal) T82.43
intraperitoneal T85.631
infusion NEC T82.534
spinal (epidural) (subdural) T85.630
gastrointestinal —*see* Complications, prosthetic device, mechanical, gastrointestinal device
genital NEC T83.498
penile prosthesis (cylinder) (implanted) (pump) (resevoir) T83.490
testicular prosthesis T83.491
heart NEC —*see* Complication, cardiovascular device, mechanical
joint prosthesis —*see* Complications, joint prosthesis, mechanical, specified NEC, by site
ocular NEC —*see* Complications, prosthetic device, mechanical, ocular device
orthopedic NEC —*see* Complication, orthopedic, device, mechanical
persistent air J93.82
specified NEC T85.638
urinary NEC —*see also* Complication, genitourinary, device, urinary, mechanical graft T83.23
vascular NEC —*see* Complication, cardiovascular device, mechanical
ventricular intracranial shunt T85.03
urine —*see* Incontinence

Leaky heart —*see* Endocarditis

Learning defect (specific) F81.9

Leather bottle stomach C16.9

Leber's
congenital amaurosis H35.50
optic atrophy (hereditary) H47.22

Lederer's anemia D59.19

Leeches (external) —*see* Hirudiniasis

Leg —*see* condition

Legg (-Calvé)-**Perthes disease, syndrome or osteochondrosis** M91.1-

Legionellosis A48.1
nonpneumonic A48.2

Legionnaires'
disease A48.1
nonpneumonic A48.2
pneumonia A48.1

Leigh's disease G31.82

Leiner's disease L21.1

Leiofibromyoma —*see* Leiomyoma

Leiomyoblastoma —*see* Neoplasm, connective tissue, benign

Leiomyofibroma —*see also* Neoplasm, connective tissue, benign
uterus (cervix) (corpus) D25.9

Leiomyoma —*see also* Neoplasm, connective tissue, benign
bizarre —*see* Neoplasm, connective tissue, benign
cellular —*see* Neoplasm, connective tissue, benign
epithelioid —*see* Neoplasm, connective tissue, benign
uterus (cervix) (corpus) D25.9
intramural D25.1
submucous D25.0
subserosal D25.2
vascular —*see* Neoplasm, connective tissue, benign

Leiomyoma, leiomyomatosis (intravascular) —*see* Neoplasm, connective tissue, uncertain behavior

Leiomyosarcoma —*see also* Neoplasm, connective tissue, malignant
epithelioid —*see* Neoplasm, connective tissue, malignant
myxoid —*see* Neoplasm, connective tissue, malignant

Leishmaniasis B55.9
American (mucocutaneous) B55.2
cutaneous B55.1
Asian Desert B55.1
Brazilian B55.2
cutaneous (any type) B55.1
dermal —*see also* Leishmaniasis, cutaneous
post-kala-azar B55.0
eyelid B55.1
infantile B55.0
Mediterranean B55.0
mucocutaneous (American) (New World) B55.2
naso-oral B55.2
nasopharyngeal B55.2
old world B55.1
tegumentaria diffusa B55.1
visceral B55.0

Leishmanoid, dermal —*see also* Leishmaniasis, cutaneous
post-kala-azar B55.0

Lenegre's disease I44.2

Lengthening, leg —*see* Deformity, limb, unequal length

Lennert's lymphoma —*see* Lymphoma, Lennert's

Lennox-Gastaut syndrome G40.812
intractable G40.814
with status epilepticus G40.813
without status epilepticus G40.814

Lennox-Gastaut syndrome
(continued)
  not intractable G40.812
    with status epilepticus G40.811
    without status epilepticus
      G40.812

Lens —*see* condition

Lenticonus (anterior) (posterior)
  (congenital) Q12.8

**Lenticular degeneration,
  progressive** E83.01

Lentiglobus (posterior) (congenital)
  Q12.8

Lentigo (congenital) L81.4
  maligna —*see also* Melanoma, in
    situ
    melanoma —*see* Melanoma

**Lentivirus, as cause of disease
  classified elsewhere** B97.31

Leontiasis
  ossium M85.2
  syphilitic (late) A52.78
    congenital A50.59

Lepothrix A48.8

Lepra —*see* Leprosy

Leprechaunism E34.8

Leprosy A30.-
  with muscle disorder A30.9
    [M63.80]
    ankle A30.9 *[M63.87-]*
    foot A30.9 *[M63.87-]*
    forearm A30.9 *[M63.83-]*
    hand A30.9 *[M63.84-]*
    lower leg A30.9 *[M63.86-]*
    multiple sites A30.9 *[M63.89]*
    pelvic region A30.9 *[M63.85-]*
    shoulder region A30.9 *[M63.81-]*
    specified site NEC A30.9
      [M63.88]
    thigh A30.9 *[M63.85-]*
    upper arm A30.9 *[M63.82-]*
  anesthetic A30.9
  BB A30.3
  BL A30.4
  borderline (infiltrated) (neuritic)
    A30.3
    lepromatous A30.4
    tuberculoid A30.2
  BT A30.2
  dimorphous (infiltrated) (neuritic)
    A30.3
  I A30.0
  indeterminate (macular) (neuritic)
    A30.0
  lepromatous (diffuse) (infiltrated)
    (macular) (neuritic) (nodular)
    A30.5
  LL A30.5
  macular (early) (neuritic) (simple)
    A30.9
  maculoanesthetic A30.9
  mixed A30.3
  neural A30.9
  nodular A30.5
  primary neuritic A30.3
  specified type NEC A30.8
  TT A30.1
  tuberculoid (major) (minor) A30.1

Leptocytosis, hereditary D56.9

Leptomeningitis (chronic)
  (circumscribed) (hemorrhagic)
  (nonsuppurative) —*see* Meningitis

Leptomeningopathy G96.198

Leptospiral —*see* condition

Leptospirochetal —*see* condition

Leptospirosis A27.9
  canicola A27.89
  due to Leptospira interrogans
    serovar icterohaemorrhagiae
    A27.0
  icterohemorrhagica A27.0
  pomona A27.89
  Weil's disease A27.0

Leptus dermatitis B88.0

Leriche's syndrome (aortic
  bifurcation occlusion) I74.09

Leri's pleonosteosis Q78.8

Leri-Weill syndrome Q77.8

Lermoyez' syndrome —*see* Vertigo,
  peripheral NEC

Lesch-Nyhan syndrome E79.1

Leser-Trélat disease L82.1
  inflamed L82.0

Lesion(s) (nontraumatic)
  abducens nerve —*see* Strabismus,
    paralytic, sixth nerve
  alveolar process K08.9
  angiocentric immunoproliferative
    D47.Z9
  anorectal K62.9
  aortic (valve) I35.9
  auditory nerve —*see* subcategory
    H93.3
  basal ganglion G25.9
  bile duct —*see* Disease, bile duct
  biomechanical M99.9
    specified type NEC M99.89
      abdomen M99.89
      acromioclavicular M99.87
      cervical region M99.81
      cervicothoracic M99.81
      costochondral M99.88
      costovertebral M99.88
      head region M99.80
      hip M99.85
      lower extremity M99.86
      lumbar region M99.83
      lumbosacral M99.83
      occipitocervical M99.80
      pelvic region M99.85
      pubic M99.85
      rib cage M99.88
      sacral region M99.84
      sacrococcygeal M99.84
      sacroiliac M99.84
      specified NEC M99.89
      sternochondral M99.88
      sternoclavicular M99.87
      thoracic region M99.82
      thoracolumbar M99.82
      upper extremity M99.87
  bladder N32.9
  bone —*see* Disorder, bone
  brachial plexus G54.0
  brain G93.9
    congenital Q04.9
    vascular I67.9
      degenerative I67.9
      hypertensive I67.4
  buccal cavity K13.79
  calcified —*see* Calcification
  canthus —*see* Disorder, eyelid
  carate —*see* Pinta, lesions
  cardia K31.9
  cardiac (*see also* Disease, heart) I51.9
    congenital Q24.9
    valvular —*see* Endocarditis
  cauda equina G83.4
  cecum K63.9
  cerebral —*see* Lesion, brain
  cerebrovascular I67.9
    degenerative I67.9
    hypertensive I67.4

Lesion *(continued)*
  cervical (nerve) root NEC G54.2
  chiasmal —*see* Disorder, optic,
    chiasm
  chorda tympani G51.8
  coin, lung R91.1
  colon K63.9
  combined periodontic - endodontic
    K05.5
  congenital —*see* Anomaly, by site
  conjunctiva H11.9
  conus medullaris —*see* Injury,
    conus medullaris
  coronary artery —*see* Ischemia,
    heart
  cranial nerve G52.9
    eighth —*see* Disorder, ear
    eleventh G52.9
    fifth G50.9
    first G52.0
    fourth —*see* Strabismus,
      paralytic, fourth nerve
    seventh G51.9
    sixth —*see* Strabismus,
      paralytic, sixth nerve
    tenth G52.2
    twelfth G52.3
  cystic —*see* Cyst
  degenerative —*see* Degeneration
  duodenum K31.9
  edentulous (alveolar) ridge,
    associated with trauma, due to
    traumatic occlusion K06.2
  en coup de sabre L94.1
  eyelid —*see* Disorder, eyelid
  gasserian ganglion G50.8
  gastric K31.9
  gastroduodenal K31.9
  gastrointestinal K63.9
  gingiva, associated with trauma
    K06.2
  glomerular
    focal and segmental (*see also*
      N00-N07 with fourth
      character .1) N05.1
    minimal change (*see also*
      N00-N07 with fourth
      character .0) N05.0
  heart (organic) —*see* Disease, heart
  hyperchromic, due to pinta (carate)
    A67.1
  hyperkeratotic —*see*
    Hyperkeratosis
  hypothalamic E23.7
  ileocecal K63.9
  ileum K63.9
  iliohypogastric nerve G57.8-
  inflammatory —*see* Inflammation
  intestine K63.9
  intracerebral —*see* Lesion, brain
  intrachiasmal (optic) —*see*
    Disorder, optic, chiasm
  intracranial, space-occupying
    R90.0
  joint —*see* Disorder, joint
    sacroiliac (old) M53.3
  keratotic —*see* Keratosis
  kidney —*see* Disease, renal
  laryngeal nerve (recurrent) G52.2
  lip K13.0
  liver K76.9
  lumbosacral
    plexus G54.1
    root (nerve) NEC G54.4
  lung (coin) R91.1
  maxillary sinus J32.0
  mitral I05.9
  Morel-Lavallée —*see* Hematoma,
    by site
  motor cortex NEC G93.89
  mouth K13.79

Lesion *(continued)*
  nerve G58.9
    femoral G57.2-
    median G56.1-
      carpal tunnel syndrome —*see*
        Syndrome, carpal tunnel
    plantar G57.6-
    popliteal (lateral) G57.3-
      medial G57.4-
    radial G56.3-
    sciatic G57.0-
    spinal —*see* Injury, nerve,
      spinal
    ulnar G56.2-
  nervous system, congenital
    Q07.9
  nonallopathic —*see* Lesion,
    biomechanical
  nose (internal) J34.89
  obstructive —*see* Obstruction
  obturator nerve G57.8-
  oral mucosa K13.70
  organ or site NEC —*see* Disease,
    by site
  osteolytic —*see* Osteolysis
  peptic K27.9
  periodontal, due to traumatic
    occlusion K05.5
  pharynx J39.2
  pigment, pigmented (skin) L81.9
  pinta —*see* Pinta, lesions
  polypoid —*see* Polyp
  prechiasmal (optic) —*see* Disorder,
    optic, chiasm
  primary (*see also* Syphilis,
    primary) A51.0
    carate A67.0
    pinta A67.0
    yaws A66.0
  pulmonary J98.4
    valve I37.9
  pylorus K31.9
  rectosigmoid K63.9
  retina, retinal H35.9
  sacroiliac (joint) (old) M53.3
  salivary gland K11.9
    benign lymphoepithelial K11.8
  saphenous nerve G57.8-
  sciatic nerve G57.0-
  secondary —*see* Syphilis, secondary
  shoulder (region) M75.9-
    specified NEC M75.8-
  sigmoid K63.9
  sinus (accessory) (nasal) J34.89
  skin L98.9
    suppurative L08.0
  SLAP S43.43-
  spinal cord G95.9
    congenital Q06.9
  spleen D73.89
  stomach K31.9
  superior glenoid labrum S43.43-
  syphilitic —*see* Syphilis
  tertiary —*see* Syphilis, tertiary
  thoracic root (nerve) NEC G54.3
  tonsillar fossa J35.9
  tooth, teeth K08.9
    white spot
      chewing surface K02.51
      pit and fissure surface
        K02.51
      smooth surface K02.61
  traumatic —*see* specific type of
    injury by site
  tricuspid (valve) I07.9
    nonrheumatic I36.9
  trigeminal nerve G50.9
  ulcerated or ulcerative —*see* Ulcer,
    skin
  uterus N85.9

Lesion (*continued*)
  vagina N89.8
  vagus nerve G52.2
  valvular —*see* Endocarditis
  vascular I99.9
    affecting central nervous
      system I67.9
    following trauma NEC T14.8
    umbilical cord, complicating
      delivery O69.5
  vulva N90.89
  warty —*see* Verruca
  white spot (tooth)
    chewing surface K02.51
    pit and fissure surface K02.51
    smooth surface K02.61

Lethargic —*see* condition

Lethargy R53.83

Letterer-Siwe's disease C96.0

Leukemia, leukemic C95.9-
  acute basophilic C94.8-
  acute bilineal C95.0-
  acute erythroid C94.0-
  acute lymphoblastic C91.0-
  acute megakaryoblastic C94.2-
  acute megakaryocytic C94.2-
  acute mixed lineage C95.0-
  acute monoblastic (monoblastic/
    monocytic) C93.0-
  acute monocytic (monoblastic/
    monocytic) C93.0-
  acute myeloblastic (minimal
    differentiation) (with
    maturation) C92.0-
  acute myeloid, NOS C92.0-
    with
      11q23-abnormality C92.6-
      dysplasia of remaining
        hematopoesis and/or
        myelodysplastic disease in
        its history C92.A-
      multilineage dysplasia C92.A-
      variation of MLL-gene C92.6-
    M6 (a)(b) C94.0-
    M7 C94.2-
  acute myelomonocytic C92.5-
  acute promyelocytic C92.4-
  adult T-cell (HTLV-1-associated)
    (acute variant) (chronic variant)
    (lymphomatoid variant)
    (smouldering variant) C91.5-
  aggressive NK-cell C94.8-
  AML (1/ETO) (M0) (M1) (M2)
    (without a FAB classification)
    C92.0-
  AML M3 C92.4-
  AML M4 (Eo with inv (16) or
    t (16;16)) C92.5-
  AML M5 C93.0-
  AML M5a C93.0-
  AML M5b C93.0-
  AML Me with t (15;17) and
    variants C92.4-
  atypical chronic myeloid, BCR/
    ABL-negative C92.2-
  biphenotypic acute C95.0-
  blast cell C95.0-
  Burkitt-type, mature B-cell C91.A-
  chronic eosinophilic (*see also*
    Syndrome, hypereosinophilic,
    myeloid) C94.8-
  chronic lymphocytic, of B-cell
    type C91.1-
  chronic monocytic C93.1-
  chronic myelogenous
    (Philadelphia chromosome
    (Ph1) positive) (t (9;22))
    (q34;q11) (with crisis of blast
    cells) C92.1-

Leukemia, leukemic (*continued*)
  chronic myeloid, BCR/ABL-
    positive C92.1-
    atypical, BCR/ABL-negative C92.2-
  chronic myelomonocytic C93.1-
  chronic neutrophilic D47.1
  CMML (-1) (-2) (with
    eosinophilia) C93.1-
  granulocytic (*see also* Category
    C92) C92.9-
  hairy cell C91.4-
  juvenile myelomonocytic C93.3-
  lymphoid C91.9-
    specified NEC C91.Z-
  mast cell C94.3-
  mature B-cell, Burkitt-type C91.A-
  monocytic (subacute) C93.9-
    specified NEC C93.Z-
  myelogenous (*see also* Category
    C92) C92.9-
  myeloid C92.9-
    specified NEC C92.Z-
  plasma cell C90.1-
  plasmacytic C90.1-
  prolymphocytic
    of B-cell type C91.3-
    of T-cell type C91.6-
  specified NEC C94.8-
  stem cell, of unclear lineage C95.0-
  subacute lymphocytic C91.9-
  T-cell large granular lymphocytic
    C91.Z-
  unspecified cell type C95.9-
    acute C95.0-
    chronic C95.1-

Leukemoid reaction (*see also*
  Reaction, leukemoid) D72.823-

Leukoaraiosis (hypertensive) I67.81

Leukoariosis —*see* Leukoaraiosis

Leukocoria —*see* Disorder, globe,
  degenerated condition, leucocoria

Leukocytopenia D72.819

Leukocytosis D72.829
  eosinophilic D72.19

Leukoderma, leukodermia NEC L81.5
  syphilitic A51.39
    late A52.79

Leukodystrophy E75.29

Leukoedema, oral epithelium
  K13.29

Leukoencephalitis G04.81
  acute (subacute) hemorrhagic G36.1
    postimmunization or
      postvaccinal G04.02
  postinfectious G04.01
  subacute sclerosing A81.1
  van Bogaert's (sclerosing) A81.1

Leukoencephalopathy (*see also*
  Encephalopathy) G93.49
  Binswanger's I67.3
  heroin vapor G92
  metachromatic E75.25
  multifocal (progressive) A81.2
  postimmunization and postvaccinal
    G04.02
  progressive multifocal A81.2
  reversible, posterior G93.6
  van Bogaert's (sclerosing) A81.1
  vascular, progressive I67.3

Leukoerythroblastosis D75.9

Leukokeratosis —*see also*
  Leukoplakia
  mouth K13.21
  nicotina palati K13.24
  oral mucosa K13.21
  tongue K13.21
  vocal cord J38.3

Leukokraurosis vulva (e) N90.4

Leukoma (cornea) —*see also*
  Opacity, cornea
  adherent H17.0-
  interfering with central vision
    —*see* Opacity, cornea, central

Leukomalacia, cerebral, newborn
  P91.2
  periventricular P91.2

Leukomelanopathy, hereditary D72.0

Leukonychia (punctata) (striata)
  L60.8
  congenital Q84.4

Leukopathia unguium L60.8
  congenital Q84.4

Leukopenia D72.819
  basophilic D72.818
  chemotherapy (cancer) induced
    D70.1
  congenital D70.0
  cyclic D70.0
  drug induced NEC D70.2
    due to cytoreductive cancer
      chemotherapy D70.1
  eosinophilic D72.818
  familial D70.0
  infantile genetic D70.0
  malignant D70.9
  periodic D70.0
  transitory neonatal P61.5

Leukopenic —*see* condition

Leukoplakia
  anus K62.89
  bladder (postinfectional) N32.89
  buccal K13.21
  cervix (uteri) N88.0
  esophagus K22.8
  gingiva K13.21
  hairy (oral mucosa) (tongue)
    K13.3
  kidney (pelvis) N28.89
  larynx J38.7
  lip K13.21
  mouth K13.21
  oral epithelium, including tongue
    (mucosa) K13.21
  palate K13.21
  pelvis (kidney) N28.89
  penis (infectional) N48.0
  rectum K62.89
  syphilitic (late) A52.79
  tongue K13.21
  ureter (postinfectional) N28.89
  urethra (postinfectional) N36.8
  uterus N85.8
  vagina N89.4
  vocal cord J38.3
  vulva N90.4

Leukorrhea N89.8
  due to Trichomonas (vaginalis)
    A59.00
  trichomonal A59.00

Leukosarcoma C85.9-

Levocardia (isolated) Q24.1
  with situs inversus Q89.3

Levotransposition Q20.5

Lev's disease or syndrome (acquired
  complete heart block) I44.2

Levulosuria —*see* Fructosuria

Levurid L30.2

Lewy body (ies) (dementia) (disease)
  G31.83

Leyden-Moebius dystrophy
  G71.09

Leydig cell
  carcinoma
    specified site —*see* Neoplasm,
      malignant, by site
    unspecified site
      female C56.9
      male C62.9-
  tumor
    benign
      specified site —*see* Neoplasm,
        benign, by site
      unspecified site
        female D27.-
        male D29.2-
    malignant
      specified site —*see* Neoplasm,
        malignant, by site
      unspecified site
        female C56.-
        male C62.9-
    specified site —*see* Neoplasm,
      uncertain behavior, by site
    unspecified site
      female D39.1-
      male D40.1-

Leydig-Sertoli cell tumor
  specified site —*see* Neoplasm,
    benign, by site
  unspecified site
    female D27.-
    male D29.2-

LGSIL (Low grade squamous
  intraepithelial lesion on cytologic
  smear of)
  anus R85.612
  cervix R87.612
  vagina R87.622

Liar, pathologic F60.2

Libido
  decreased R68.82

Libman-Sacks disease M32.11

Lice (infestation) B85.2
  body (Pediculus corporis) B85.1
  crab B85.3
  head (Pediculus capitis) B85.0
  mixed (classifiable to more than
    one of the titles B85.0-B85.3)
    B85.4
  pubic (Phthirus pubis)
    B85.3

Lichen L28.0
  albus L90.0
    penis N48.0
    vulva N90.4
  amyloidosis E85.4 *[L99]*
  atrophicus L90.0
    penis N48.0
    vulva N90.4
  congenital Q82.8
  myxedematosus L98.5
  nitidus L44.1
  pilaris Q82.8
    acquired L85.8
  planopilaris L66.1
  planus (chronicus) L43.9
    annularis L43.8
    bullous L43.1
    follicular L66.1
    hypertrophic L43.0
    moniliformis L44.3
    of Wilson L43.9
    specified NEC L43.8
    subacute (active) L43.3
    tropicus L43.3
  ruber
    acuminatus L44.0
    moniliformis L44.3
    planus L43.9

Lichen (continued)
  sclerosus (et atrophicus) L90.0
    penis N48.0
    vulva N90.4
  scrofulosus (primary) (tuberculous) A18.4
  simplex (chronicus) (circumscriptus) L28.0
  striatus L44.2
  urticatus L28.2

Lichenification L28.0

Lichenoides tuberculosis (primary) A18.4

Lichtheim's disease or syndrome D51.0

Lien migrans D73.89

Ligament —see condition

Light
  for gestational age —see Light for dates
  headedness R42

Light-for-dates (infant) P05.00
  with weight of
    499 grams or less P05.01
    500-749 grams P05.02
    750-999 grams P05.03
    1000-1249 grams P05.04
    1250-1499 grams P05.05
    1500-1749 grams P05.06
    1750-1999 grams P05.07
    2000-2499 grams P05.08
    2500 grams and over P05.09
  and small-for-dates —see Small for dates
  affecting management of pregnancy O36.59-
  specified NEC P05.09

Lightning (effects) (stroke) (struck by) T75.00
  burn —see Burn
  foot E53.8
  shock T75.01
  specified effect NEC T75.09

Lightwood-Albright syndrome N25.89

Lightwood's disease or syndrome (renal tubular acidosis) N25.89

Lignac (-de Toni) (-Fanconi) (-Debré) **disease or syndrome** E72.09
  with cystinosis E72.04

Ligneous thyroiditis E06.5

Likoff's syndrome I20.8

Limb —see condition

Limbic epilepsy personality syndrome F07.0

Limitation, limited
  activities due to disability Z73.6
  cardiac reserve —see Disease, heart
  eye muscle duction, traumatic —see Strabismus, mechanical
  mandibular range of motion M26.52

Lindau (-von Hippel) **disease** Q85.8

Line(s)
  Beau's L60.4
  Harris' —see Arrest, epiphyseal
  Hudson's (cornea) —see Pigmentation, cornea, anterior
  Stähli's (cornea) —see Pigmentation, cornea, anterior

Linea corneae senilis —see Change, cornea, senile

Lingua
  geographica K14.1
  nigra (villosa) K14.3
  plicata K14.5
  tylosis K13.29

Lingual —see condition

Linguatulosis B88.8

Linitis (gastric) **plastica** C16.9

Lip —see condition

Lipedema —see Edema

Lipemia —see also Hyperlipidemia
  retina, retinalis E78.3

Lipidosis E75.6
  cerebral (infantile) (juvenile) (late) E75.4
  cerebroretinal E75.4
  cerebroside E75.22
  cholesterol (cerebral) E75.5
  glycolipid E75.21
  hepatosplenomegalic E78.3
  sphingomyelin —see Niemann-Pick disease or syndrome
  sulfatide E75.29

Lipoadenoma —see Neoplasm, benign, by site

Lipoblastoma —see Lipoma

Lipoblastomatosis —see Lipoma

Lipochondrodystrophy E76.01

Lipodermatosclerosis —see Varix, leg, with, inflammation
  ulcerated —see Varix, leg, with, ulcer, with inflammation by site

Lipochrome histiocytosis (familial) D71

Lipodystrophia progressiva E88.1

Lipodystrophy (progressive) E88.1
  insulin E88.1
  intestinal K90.81
  mesenteric K65.4

Lipofibroma —see Lipoma

Lipofuscinosis, neuronal (with ceroidosis) E75.4

Lipogranuloma, sclerosing L92.8

Lipogranulomatosis E78.89

Lipoid —see also condition
  histiocytosis D76.3
    essential E75.29
  nephrosis N04.9
  proteinosis of Urbach E78.89

Lipoidemia —see Hyperlipidemia

Lipoidosis —see Lipidosis

Lipoma D17.9
  fetal D17.9
    fat cell D17.9
  infiltrating D17.9
  intramuscular D17.9
  pleomorphic D17.9
  site classification
    arms (skin) (subcutaneous) D17.2-
    connective tissue D17.30
      intra-abdominal D17.5
      intrathoracic D17.4
      peritoneum D17.79
      retroperitoneum D17.79
      specified site NEC D17.39
      spermatic cord D17.6
    face (skin) (subcutaneous) D17.0
    genitourinary organ NEC D17.72
    head (skin) (subcutaneous) D17.0
      intra-abdominal D17.5
      intrathoracic D17.4

Lipoma (continued)
  site classification (continued)
    kidney D17.71
    legs (skin) (subcutaneous) D17.2-
    neck (skin) (subcutaneous) D17.0
    peritoneum D17.79
    retroperitoneum D17.79
    skin D17.30
      specified site NEC D17.39
    specified site NEC D17.79
    spermatic cord D17.6
    subcutaneous D17.30
      specified site NEC D17.39
    trunk (skin) (subcutaneous) D17.1
    unspecified D17.9
  spindle cell D17.9

Lipomatosis E88.2
  dolorosa (Dercum) E88.2
  fetal —see Lipoma
  Launois-Bensaude E88.89

Lipomyoma —see Lipoma

Lipomyxoma —see Lipoma

Lipomyxosarcoma —see Neoplasm, connective tissue, malignant

Lipoprotein metabolism disorder E78.9

Lipoproteinemia E78.5
  broad-beta E78.2
  floating-beta E78.2
  hyper-pre-beta E78.1

Liposarcoma —see also Neoplasm, connective tissue, malignant
  dedifferentiated —see Neoplasm, connective tissue, malignant
  differentiated type —see Neoplasm, connective tissue, malignant
  embryonal —see Neoplasm, connective tissue, malignant
  mixed type —see Neoplasm, connective tissue, malignant
  myxoid —see Neoplasm, connective tissue, malignant
  pleomorphic —see Neoplasm, connective tissue, malignant
  round cell —see Neoplasm, connective tissue, malignant
  well differentiated type —see Neoplasm, connective tissue, malignant

Liposynovitis prepatellaris E88.89

Lipping, cervix N86

Lipschütz disease or ulcer N76.6

Lipuria R82.0
  schistosomiasis (bilharziasis) B65.0

Lisping F80.0

Lissauer's paralysis A52.17

Lissencephalia, lissencephaly Q04.3

Listeriosis, listerellosis A32.9
  congenital (disseminated) P37.2
  cutaneous A32.0
  neonatal, newborn (disseminated) P37.2
  oculoglandular A32.81
  specified NEC A32.89

Lithemia E79.0

Lithiasis —see Calculus

Lithosis J62.8

Lithuria R82.998

Litigation, anxiety concerning Z65.3

Little leaguer's elbow —see Epicondylitis, medial

Little's disease G80.9

Littre's
  gland —see condition
  hernia —see Hernia, abdomen

Littritis —see Urethritis

Livedo (annularis) (racemosa) (reticularis) R23.1

Liver —see condition

Living alone (problems with) Z60.2
  with handicapped person Z74.2

Lloyd's syndrome —see Adenomatosis, endocrine

Loa loa, loaiasis, loasis B74.3

Lobar —see condition

Lobomycosis B48.0

Lobo's disease B48.0

Lobotomy syndrome F07.0

Lobstein (-Ekman) **disease or syndrome** Q78.0

Lobster-claw hand Q71.6-

Lobulation (congenital) —see also Anomaly, by site
  kidney, Q63.1
  liver, abnormal Q44.7
  spleen Q89.09

Lobule, lobular —see condition

Local, localized —see condition

Locked-in state G83.5

Locked twins causing obstructed labor O66.1

Locking
  joint —see Derangement, joint, specified type NEC
    knee —see Derangement, knee

Lockjaw —see Tetanus

Löffler's
  endocarditis I42.3
  eosinophilia J82.89
  pneumonia J82.89
  syndrome (eosinophilic pneumonitis) J82.89

Loiasis (with conjunctival infestation) (eyelid) B74.3

Lone Star fever A77.0

Long
  labor O63.9
    first stage O63.0
    second stage O63.1
  QT syndrome I45.81

Long-term (current) (prophylactic)
  drug therapy (use of)
    agents affecting estrogen receptors and estrogen levels NEC Z79.818
    anastrozole (Arimidex) Z79.811
    antibiotics Z79.2
      short-term use - omit code
    anticoagulants Z79.01
    anti-inflammatory, non-steroidal (NSAID) Z79.1
    antiplatelet Z79.02
    antithrombotics Z79.02
    aromatase inhibitors Z79.811
    aspirin Z79.82
    birth control pill or patch Z79.3
    bisphosphonates Z79.83
    contraceptive, oral Z79.3
    drug, specified NEC Z79.899

Lump *(continued)*
  breast *(continued)*
    left *(continued)*
      upper inner quadrant N63.22
      upper outer quadrant N63.21
    right
      lower inner quadrant N63.14
      lower outer quadrant N63.13
      overlapping quadrants N63.15
      unspecified quadrant N63.10
      upper inner quadrant N63.12
      upper outer quadrant N63.11
    subareolar
      left N63.42
      right N63.41

Lunacy —*see* Psychosis

Lung —*see* condition

Lupoid (miliary) **of Boeck** D86.3

Lupus
  anticoagulant D68.62
    with
      hemorrhagic disorder D68.312
      hypercoagulable state D68.62
      finding without diagnosis R76.0
  discoid (local) L93.0
  erythematosus (discoid) (local) L93.0
    disseminated —*see* Lupus,
      erythematosus, systemic
    eyelid H01.129
      left H01.126
        lower H01.125
        upper H01.124
      right H01.123
        lower H01.122
        upper H01.121
    profundus L93.2
    specified NEC L93.2
    subacute cutaneous L93.1
    systemic M32.9
      with organ or system
        involvement M32.10
        endocarditis M32.11
        lung M32.13
        pericarditis M32.12
        renal (glomerular) M32.14
          tubulo-interstitial M32.15
        specified organ or system
          NEC M32.19
      drug-induced M32.0
      inhibitor (presence of) D68.62
        with
          hemorrhagic disorder
            D68.312
          hypercoagulable state
            D68.62
        finding without diagnosis
          R76.0
      specified NEC M32.8
  exedens A18.4
  hydralazine M32.0
    correct substance properly
      administered —*see* Table
      of Drugs and Chemicals, by
      drug, adverse effect
    overdose or wrong substance
      given or taken —*see* Table
      of Drugs and Chemicals, by
      drug, poisoning
  nephritis (chronic) M32.14
  nontuberculous, not disseminated
    L93.0
  panniculitis L93.2
  pernio (Besnier) D86.3
  systemic —*see* Lupus,
    erythematosus, systemic
  tuberculous A18.4
    eyelid A18.4
  vulgaris A18.4
    eyelid A18.4

Luteinoma D27.-

Lutembacher's disease or syndrome
  (atrial septal defect with mitral
  stenosis) Q21.1

Luteoma D27.-

Lutz (-Splendore-de
  Almeida) **disease** —*see*
  Paracoccidioidomycosis

Luxation —*see also* Dislocation
  eyeball (nontraumatic) —*see*
    Luxation, globe
    birth injury P15.3
  globe, nontraumatic H44.82-
  lacrimal gland —*see* Dislocation,
    lacrimal gland
  lens (old) (partial)
    (spontaneous)
    congenital Q12.1
    syphilitic A50.39

Lycanthropy F22

Lyell's syndrome L51.2
  due to drug L51.2
    correct substance properly
      administered —*see* Table
      of Drugs and Chemicals, by
      drug, adverse effect
    overdose or wrong substance
      given or taken —*see* Table
      of Drugs and Chemicals, by
      drug, poisoning

Lyme disease A69.20

Lymph
  gland or node —*see* condition
  scrotum —*see* Infestation, filarial

Lymphadenitis I88.9
  with ectopic or molar pregnancy
    O08.0
  acute L04.9
    axilla L04.2
    face L04.0
    head L04.0
    hip L04.3
    limb
      lower L04.3
      upper L04.2
    neck L04.0
    shoulder L04.2
    specified site NEC L04.8
    trunk L04.1
  anthracosis (occupational) J60
  any site, except mesenteric I88.9
    chronic I88.1
    subacute I88.1
  breast
    gestational —*see* Mastitis,
      obstetric
    puerperal, postpartum
      (nonpurulent) O91.22
  chancroidal (congenital) A57
  chronic I88.1
    mesenteric I88.0
  due to
    Brugia (malayi) B74.1
      timori B74.2
    chlamydial lymphogranuloma
      A55
    diphtheria (toxin) A36.89
    lymphogranuloma venereum
      A55
    Wuchereria bancrofti B74.0
  following ectopic or molar
    pregnancy O08.0
  gonorrheal A54.89
  infective —*see* Lymphadenitis,
    acute
  mesenteric (acute) (chronic)
    (nonspecific) (subacute) I88.0

Lymphadenitis *(continued)*
  mesenteric *(continued)*
    due to Salmonella typhi A01.09
    tuberculous A18.39
  mycobacterial A31.8
  purulent —*see* Lymphadenitis, acute
  pyogenic —*see* Lymphadenitis, acute
  regional, nonbacterial I88.8
  septic —*see* Lymphadenitis, acute
  subacute, unspecified site I88.1
  suppurative —*see* Lymphadenitis,
    acute
  syphilitic (early) (secondary) A51.49
    late A52.79
  tuberculous —*see* Tuberculosis,
    lymph gland
  venereal (chlamydial) A55

Lymphadenoid goiter E06.3

Lymphadenopathy (generalized)
  R59.1
  angioimmunoblastic, with
    dysproteinemia (AILD) C86.5
  due to toxoplasmosis (acquired)
    B58.89
    congenital (acute) (subacute)
      (chronic) P37.1
  localized R59.0
  syphilitic (early) (secondary) A51.49

Lymphadenosis R59.1

Lymphangiectasis I89.0
  conjunctiva H11.89
  postinfectional I89.0
  scrotum I89.0

Lymphangiectatic elephantiasis,
  nonfilarial I89.0

Lymphangioendothelioma D18.1
  malignant —*see* Neoplasm,
    connective tissue, malignant

Lymphangioleiomyomatosis J84.81

Lymphangioma D18.1
  capillary D18.1
  cavernous D18.1
  cystic D18.1
  malignant —*see* Neoplasm,
    connective tissue, malignant

Lymphangiomyoma D18.1

Lymphangiomyomatosis J84.81

Lymphangiosarcoma —*see*
  Neoplasm, connective tissue,
  malignant

Lymphangitis I89.1
  with
    abscess - code by site under
      Abscess
    cellulitis - code by site under
      Cellulitis
    ectopic or molar pregnancy
      O08.0
  acute L03.91
    abdominal wall L03.321
    ankle —*see* Lymphangitis, acute,
      lower limb
    arm —*see* Lymphangitis, acute,
      upper limb
    auricle (ear) —*see* Lymphangitis,
      acute, ear
    axilla L03.12-
    back (any part) L03.322
    buttock L03.327
    cervical (meaning neck) L03.222
    cheek (external) L03.212
    chest wall L03.323
    digit
      finger —*see* Lymphangitis,
        acute, finger
      toe —*see* Lymphangitis, acute,
        toe

Lymphangitis *(continued)*
  acute *(continued)*
    ear (external) H60.1-
    external auditory canal —*see*
      Lymphangitis, acute, ear
    eyelid —*see* Abscess, eyelid
    face NEC L03.212
    finger (intrathecal) (periosteal)
      (subcutaneous) (subcuticular)
      L03.02-
    foot —*see* Lymphangitis, acute,
      lower limb
    gluteal (region) L03.327
    groin L03.324
    hand —*see* Lymphangitis, acute,
      upper limb
    head NEC L03.891
      face (any part, except ear, eye
        and nose) L03.212
    heel —*see* Lymphangitis, acute,
      lower limb
    hip —*see* Lymphangitis, acute,
      lower limb
    jaw (region) L03.212
    knee —*see* Lymphangitis, acute,
      lower limb
    leg —*see* Lymphangitis, acute,
      lower limb
    lower limb L03.12-
      toe —*see* Lymphangitis, acute,
        toe
    navel L03.326
    neck (region) L03.222
    orbit, orbital —*see* Cellulitis, orbit
    pectoral (region) L03.323
    perineal, perineum L03.325
    scalp (any part) L03.891
    shoulder —*see* Lymphangitis,
      acute, upper limb
    specified site NEC L03.898
    thigh —*see* Lymphangitis, acute,
      lower limb
    thumb (intrathecal) (periosteal)
      (subcutaneous) (subcuticular) —
      see Lymphangitis, acute, finger
    toe (intrathecal) (periosteal)
      (subcutaneous) (subcuticular)
      L03.04-
    trunk L03.329
      abdominal wall L03.321
      back (any part) L03.322
      buttock L03.327
      chest wall L03.323
      groin L03.324
      perineal, perineum L03.325
      umbilicus L03.326
    umbilicus L03.326
    upper limb L03.12-
      axilla —*see* Lymphangitis,
        acute, axilla
      finger —*see* Lymphangitis,
        acute, finger
      thumb —*see* Lymphangitis,
        acute, finger
    wrist —*see* Lymphangitis, acute,
      upper limb
  breast
    gestational —*see* Mastitis,
      obstetric
  chancroidal A57
  chronic (any site) I89.1
  due to
    Brugia (malayi) B74.1
      timori B74.2
    Wuchereria bancrofti B74.0
  following ectopic or molar
    pregnancy O08.89
  penis
    acute N48.29
    gonococcal (acute) (chronic)
      A54.09

Lymphangitis (continued)
puerperal, postpartum, childbirth O86.89
strumous, tuberculous A18.2
subacute (any site) I89.1
tuberculous —see Tuberculosis, lymph gland

Lymphatic (vessel) —see condition

Lymphatism E32.8

Lymphectasia I89.0

Lymphedema (acquired) —see also Elephantiasis
congenital Q82.0
hereditary (chronic) (idiopathic) Q82.0
postmastectomy I97.2
praecox I89.0
secondary I89.0
surgical NEC I97.89
postmastectomy (syndrome) I97.2

Lymphoblastic —see condition

Lymphoblastoma (diffuse) —see Lymphoma, lymphoblastic (diffuse)
giant follicular —see Lymphoma, lymphoblastic (diffuse)
macrofollicular —see Lymphoma, lymphoblastic (diffuse)

Lymphocele I89.8

Lymphocytic
chorioencephalitis (acute) (serous) A87.2
choriomeningitis (acute) (serous) A87.2
meningoencephalitis A87.2

Lymphocytoma, benign cutis L98.8

Lymphocytopenia D72.810

Lymphocytosis (symptomatic) D72.820
infectious (acute) B33.8

Lymphoepithelioma —see Neoplasm, malignant, by site

Lymphogranuloma (malignant) —see also Lymphoma, Hodgkin
chlamydial A55
inguinale A55
venereum (any site) (chlamydial) (with stricture of rectum) A55

Lymphogranulomatosis (malignant) —see also Lymphoma, Hodgkin
benign (Boeck's sarcoid) (Schaumann's) D86.1

Lymphohistiocytosis, hemophagocytic (familial) D76.1

Lymphoid —see condition

Lymphoma (of) (malignant) C85.90
adult T-cell (HTLV-1-associated) (acute variant) (chronic variant) (lymphomatoid variant) (smouldering variant) C91.5-
anaplastic large cell
ALK-negative C84.7-
ALK-positive C84.6-
CD30-positive C84.6-
primary cutaneous C86.6
angioimmunoblastic T-cell C86.5
BALT C88.4
B-cell C85.1-
B-precursor C83.5-
blastic NK-cell C86.4
blastic plasmacytoid dendritic cell neoplasm (BPDCN) C86.4
blastic plasmacytoid dendritic cell neoplasm (BPDCN) C86.4

Lymphoma (continued)
bronchial-associated lymphoid tissue [BALT-lymphoma] C88.4
Burkitt (atypical) C83.7-
Burkitt-like C83.7-
centrocytic C83.1-
cutaneous follicle center C82.6-
cutaneous T-cell C84.A-
diffuse follicle center C82.5-
diffuse large cell C83.3-
anaplastic C83.3-
B-cell C83.3-
diffuse large cell C83.3-
CD30-positive C83.3-
centroblastic C83.3-
immunoblastic C83.3-
plasmablastic C83.3-
subtype not specified C83.3-
T-cell rich C83.3-
enteropathy-type (associated) (intestinal) T-cell C86.2
extranodal NK/T-cell, nasal type C86.0
extranodal marginal zone B-cell lymphoma of mucosa-associated lymphoid tissue [MALT-lymphoma] C88.4
follicular C82.9-
grade
I C82.0-
II C82.1-
III C82.2-
IIIa C82.3-
IIIb C82.4-
specified NEC C82.8-
hepatosplenic T-cell (alpha-beta) (gamma-delta) C86.1
histiocytic C85.9-
true C96.A
Hodgkin C81.9
lymphocyte-rich (classical) C81.4-
lymphocyte depleted (classical) C81.3-
mixed cellularity (classical) C81.2-
nodular sclerosis (classical) C81.1
specified NEC (classical) C81.7-
nodular
lymphocyte predominant C81.0-
sclerosis (classical) C81.1-
intravascular large B-cell C83.8-
Lennert's C84.4-
lymphoblastic B-cell C83.5-
lymphoblastic (diffuse) C83.5-
lymphoblastic T-cell C83.5-
lymphoepithelioid C84.4-
lymphoplasmacytic C83.0-
with IgM-production C88.0
MALT C88.4
mantle cell C83.1-
mature T-cell NEC C84.4-
mature T/NK-cell C84.9-
specified NEC C84.Z-
mediastinal (thymic) large B-cell C85.2-
Mediterranean C88.3
mucosa-associated lymphoid tissue [MALT-lymphoma] C88.4
NK/T cell C84.9-
nodal marginal zone C83.0-
non-follicular (diffuse) C83.9-
specified NEC C83.8-
non-Hodgkin (see also Lymphoma, by type) C85.9-
specified NEC C85.8-
non-leukemic variant of B-CLL C83.0-

Lymphoma (continued)
peripheral T-cell, not classified C84.4-
primary cutaneous
anaplastic large cell C86.6
CD30-positive large T-cell C86.6
primary effusion B-cell C83.8-
SALT C88.4
skin-associated lymphoid tissue [SALT-lymphoma] C88.4
small cell B-cell C83.0-
splenic marginal zone C83.0-
subcutaneous panniculitis-like T-cell C86.3
T-precursor C83.5-
true histiocytic C96.A

Lymphomatosis —see Lymphoma

Lymphopathia venereum, veneris A55

Lymphopenia D72.810

Lymphoplasmacytic leukemia —see Leukemia, chronic lymphocytic, B-cell type

Lymphoproliferation, X-linked disease D82.3

Lymphoreticulosis, benign (of inoculation) A28.1

Lymphorrhea I89.8

Lymphosarcoma (diffuse) (see also Lymphoma) C85.9-

Lymphostasis I89.8

Lypemania —see Melancholia

Lysine and hydroxylysine metabolism disorder E72.3

Lyssa —see Rabies

M

Macacus ear Q17.3

Maceration, wet feet, tropical (syndrome) T69.02-

MacLeod's syndrome J43.0

Macrocephalia, macrocephaly Q75.3

Macrocheilia, macrochilia (congenital) Q18.6

Macrocolon (see also Megacolon) Q43.1

Macrocornea Q15.8
with glaucoma Q15.0

Macrocytic —see condition

Macrocytosis D75.89

Macrodactylia, macrodactylism (fingers) (thumbs) Q74.0
toes Q74.2

Macrodontia K00.2

Macrogenia M26.05

Macrogenitosomia (adrenal) (male) (praecox) E25.9
congenital E25.0

Macroglobulinemia (idiopathic) (primary) C88.0
monoclonal (essential) D47.2
Waldenström C88.0

Macroglossia (congenital) Q38.2
acquired K14.8

Macrognathia, macrognathism (congenital) (mandibular) (maxillary) M26.09

Macrogyria (congenital) Q04.8

Macrohydrocephalus —see Hydrocephalus

Macromastia —see Hypertrophy, breast

Macrophthalmos Q11.3
in congenital glaucoma Q15.0

Macropsia H53.15

Macrosigmoid K59.39
congenital Q43.2

Macrospondylitis, acromegalic E22.0

Macrostomia (congenital) Q18.4

Macrotia (external ear) (congenital) Q17.1

Macula
cornea, corneal —see Opacity, cornea
degeneration (atrophic) (exudative) (senile) —see also Degeneration, macula
hereditary —see Dystrophy, retina

Maculae ceruleae B85.1

Maculopathy, toxic —see Degeneration, macula, toxic

Madarosis (eyelid) H02.729
left H02.726
lower H02.725
upper H02.724
right H02.723
lower H02.722
upper H02.721

Madelung's
deformity (radius) Q74.0
disease
radial deformity Q74.0
symmetrical lipomas, neck E88.89

Madness —see Psychosis

Madura
foot B47.9
actinomycotic B47.1
mycotic B47.0

Maduromycosis B47.0

Maffucci's syndrome Q78.4

Magnesium metabolism disorder —see Disorder, metabolism, magnesium

Main en griffe (acquired) —see also Deformity, limb, clawhand
congenital Q74.0

Maintenance (encounter for)
antineoplastic chemotherapy Z51.11
antineoplastic radiation therapy Z51.0
methadone F11.20

Majocchi's
disease L81.7
granuloma B35.8

Major —see condition

Malabar itch (any site) B35.5

Malabsorption K90.9
calcium K90.89
carbohydrate K90.49
disaccharide E73.9
fat K90.49
galactose E74.20
glucose (-galactose) E74.39
intestinal K90.9
specified NEC K90.89

Malabsorption *(continued)*
  isomaltose E74.31
  lactose E73.9
  methionine E72.19
  monosaccharide E74.39
  postgastrectomy K91.2
  postsurgical K91.2
  protein K90.49
  starch K90.49
  sucrose E74.39
  syndrome K90.9
    postsurgical K91.2

Malacia, bone (adult) M83.9
  juvenile —*see* Rickets

Malacoplakia
  bladder N32.89
  pelvis (kidney) N28.89
  ureter N28.89
  urethra N36.8

Malacosteon, juvenile —*see* Rickets

Maladaptation —*see* Maladjustment

Maladie de Roger Q21.0

Maladjustment
  conjugal Z63.0
    involving divorce or
      estrangement Z63.5
  educational Z55.4
  family Z63.9
  marital Z63.0
    involving divorce or
      estrangement Z63.5
  occupational NEC Z56.89
  simple, adult —*see* Disorder,
    adjustment
  situational —*see* Disorder,
    adjustment
  social Z60.9
    due to
      acculturation difficulty Z60.3
      discrimination and persecution
        (perceived) Z60.5
      exclusion and isolation Z60.4
      life-cycle (phase of life)
        transition Z60.0
      rejection Z60.4
      specified reason NEC Z60.8

Malaise R53.81

Malakoplakia —*see* Malacoplakia

Malaria, malarial (fever) B54
  with
    blackwater fever B50.8
      hemoglobinuric (bilious)
        B50.8
      hemoglobinuria B50.8
  accidentally induced
    (therapeutically) -
    code by type under Malaria
  algid B50.9
  cerebral B50.0 *[G94]*
  clinically diagnosed (without
    parasitological confirmation)
    B54
  congenital NEC P37.4
    falciparum P37.3
  congestion, congestive B54
  continued (fever) B50.9
  estivo-autumnal B50.9
  falciparum B50.9
    with complications NEC
      B50.8
      cerebral B50.0 *[G94]*
    severe B50.8
  hemorrhagic B54
  malariae B52.9
    with
      complications NEC B52.8
      glomerular disorder B52.0

Malaria, malarial *(continued)*
  malignant (tertian) —*see* Malaria,
    falciparum
  mixed infections - code to first
    listed type in B50-B53
  ovale B53.0
  parasitologically confirmed NEC
    B53.8
  pernicious, acute —*see* Malaria,
    falciparum
  Plasmodium (P.)
    falciparum NEC —*see* Malaria,
      falciparum
    malariae NEC B52.9
      with Plasmodium
        falciparum (and or
          vivax) —*see* Malaria,
          falciparum
        vivax —*see also* Malaria,
          vivax
          and falciparum —*see*
            Malaria, falciparum
    ovale B53.0
      with Plasmodium malariae
        —*see also* Malaria, malariae
      and vivax —*see also*
        Malaria, vivax
      and falciparum —*see*
        Malaria, falciparum
    simian B53.1
      with Plasmodium malariae
        —*see also* Malaria, malariae
      and vivax —*see also*
        Malaria, vivax
      and falciparum —*see*
        Malaria, falciparum
    vivax NEC B51.9
      with Plasmodium falciparum
        —*see* Malaria, falciparum
  quartan —*see* Malaria, malariae
  quotidian —*see* Malaria,
    falciparum
  recurrent B54
  remittent B54
  specified type NEC
    (parasitologically confirmed)
    B53.8
  spleen B54
  subtertian (fever) —*see* Malaria,
    falciparum
  tertian (benign) —*see also* Malaria,
    vivax
    malignant B50.9
  tropical B50.9
  typhoid B54
  vivax B51.9
    with
      complications NEC B51.8
      ruptured spleen B51.0

Malassimilation K90.9

Malassez's disease (cystic) N50.89

Mal de los pintos —*see* Pinta

Mal de mer T75.3

Maldescent, testis Q53.9
  bilateral Q53.20
    abdominal Q53.211
    perineal Q53.22
  unilateral Q53.10
    abdominal Q53.111
    perineal Q53.12

Maldevelopment —*see also*
  Anomaly
  brain Q07.9
  colon Q43.9
  hip Q74.2
    congenital dislocation Q65.2
      bilateral Q65.1
      unilateral Q65.0-
  mastoid process Q75.8

Maldevelopment *(continued)*
  middle ear Q16.4
    except ossicles Q16.4
    ossicles Q16.3
  ossicles Q16.3
  spine Q76.49
  toe Q74.2

Male type pelvis Q74.2
  with disproportion (fetopelvic)
    O33.3
    causing obstructed labor
      O65.3

Malformation (congenital) —*see
  also* Anomaly
  adrenal gland Q89.1
  affecting multiple systems with
    skeletal changes NEC Q87.5
  alimentary tract Q45.9
    specified type NEC Q45.8
    upper Q40.9
      specified type NEC Q40.8
  aorta Q25.40
    absence Q25.41
    aneurysm, congenital Q25.43
    aplasia Q25.41
    atresia Q25.29
      aortic arch Q25.21
    coarctation (preductal)
      (postductal) Q25.1
    dilatation, congenital Q25.44
    hypoplasia Q25.42
    patent ductus arteriosus Q25.0
    specified type NEC Q25.49
    stenosis Q25.1
      supravalvular Q25.3
  aortic valve Q23.9
    specified NEC Q23.8
  arteriovenous, aneurysmatic
    (congenital) Q27.30
    brain Q28.2
      ruptured I60.8
        intracerebral I61.8
        intraparenchymal I61.8
        intraventricular I61.5
        subarachnoid I60.8
    cerebral (*see also* Malformation,
      arteriovenous, brain) Q28.2
    peripheral Q27.30
      digestive system —*see*
        Angiodysplasia
        congenital Q27.33
      lower limb Q27.32
      other specified site Q27.39
      renal vessel Q27.34
      upper limb Q27.31
    precerebral vessels (nonruptured)
      Q28.0
  auricle
    ear (congenital) Q17.3
      acquired H61.119
        left H61.112
          with right H61.113
        right H61.111
          with left H61.113
  bile duct Q44.5
  bladder Q64.79
    aplasia Q64.5
    diverticulum Q64.6
    exstrophy —*see* Exstrophy,
      bladder
    neck obstruction Q64.31
  bone Q79.9
    face Q75.9
      specified type NEC Q75.8
    skull Q75.9
      specified type NEC Q75.8
  brain (multiple) Q04.9
    arteriovenous Q28.2
    specified type NEC Q04.8
  branchial cleft Q18.2

Malformation *(continued)*
  breast Q83.9
    specified type NEC Q83.8
  broad ligament Q50.6
  bronchus Q32.4
  bursa Q79.9
  cardiac
    chambers Q20.9
      specified type NEC Q20.8
    septum Q21.9
      specified type NEC Q21.8
  cerebral Q04.9
    vessels Q28.3
  cervix uteri Q51.9
    specified type NEC Q51.828
  Chiari
    Type I G93.5
    Type II Q07.01
  choroid (congenital) Q14.3
    plexus Q07.8
  circulatory system Q28.9
  cochlea Q16.5
  cornea Q13.4
  coronary vessels Q24.5
  corpus callosum (congenital) Q04.0
  diaphragm Q79.1
  digestive system NEC, specified
    type NEC Q45.8
  dura Q07.9
    brain Q04.9
    spinal Q06.9
  ear Q17.9
    causing impairment of hearing
      Q16.9
    external Q17.9
      accessory auricle Q17.0
      causing impairment of hearing
        Q16.9
      absence of
        auditory canal Q16.1
        auricle Q16.0
      macrotia Q17.1
      microtia Q17.2
      misplacement Q17.4
      misshapen NEC Q17.3
      prominence Q17.5
      specified type NEC Q17.8
    inner Q16.5
    middle Q16.4
      absence of eustachian tube
        Q16.2
      ossicles (fusion) Q16.3
    ossicles Q16.3
    specified type NEC Q17.8
  epididymis Q55.4
  esophagus Q39.9
    specified type NEC Q39.8
  eye Q15.9
    lid Q10.3
    specified NEC Q15.8
  fallopian tube Q50.6
  genital organ —*see* Anomaly,
    genitalia
  great
    artery Q25.9
      aorta —*see* Malformation,
        aorta
      pulmonary artery —*see*
        Malformation, pulmonary,
        artery
      specified type NEC Q25.8
    vein Q26.9
      anomalous
        portal venous connection
          Q26.5
        pulmonary venous
          connection Q26.4
          partial Q26.3
          total Q26.2
      persistent left superior vena
        cava Q26.1

Malformation (*continued*)
  great (*continued*)
    vein (*continued*)
      portal vein-hepatic artery
        fistula Q26.6
      specified type NEC Q26.8
      vena cava stenosis, congenital
        Q26.0
  gum Q38.6
  hair Q84.2
  heart Q24.9
    specified type NEC Q24.8
  integument Q84.9
    specified type NEC Q84.8
  internal ear Q16.5
  intestine Q43.9
    specified type NEC Q43.8
  iris Q13.2
  joint Q74.9
    ankle Q74.2
    lumbosacral Q76.49
    sacroiliac Q74.2
    specified type NEC Q74.8
  kidney Q63.9
    accessory Q63.0
    giant Q63.3
    horseshoe Q63.1
    hydronephrosis Q62.0
    malposition Q63.2
    specified type NEC Q63.8
  lacrimal apparatus Q10.6
  lip Q38.0
  lingual Q38.3
  liver Q44.7
  lung Q33.9
  meninges or membrane
    (congenital) Q07.9
    cerebral Q04.8
    spinal (cord) Q06.9
  middle ear Q16.4
    ossicles Q16.3
  mitral valve Q23.9
    specified NEC Q23.8
  Mondini's (congenital)
    (malformation, cochlea) Q16.5
  mouth (congenital) Q38.6
  multiple types NEC Q89.7
  musculoskeletal system Q79.9
  myocardium Q24.8
  nail Q84.6
  nervous system (central) Q07.9
  nose Q30.9
    specified type NEC Q30.8
  optic disc Q14.2
  orbit Q10.7
  ovary Q50.39
  palate Q38.5
  parathyroid gland Q89.2
  pelvic organs or tissues NEC
    in pregnancy or childbirth
      O34.8-
      causing obstructed labor
        O65.5
  penis Q55.69
    aplasia Q55.5
    curvature (lateral) Q55.61
    hypoplasia Q55.62
  pericardium Q24.8
  peripheral vascular system Q27.9
    specified type NEC Q27.8
  pharynx Q38.8
  precerebral vessels Q28.1
  prostate Q55.4
  pulmonary
    arteriovenous Q25.72
    artery Q25.9
      atresia Q25.5
      specified type NEC Q25.79
      stenosis Q25.6
    valve Q22.3
  renal artery Q27.2

Malformation (*continued*)
  respiratory system Q34.9
  retina Q14.1
  scrotum —*see* Malformation,
    testis and scrotum
  seminal vesicles Q55.4
  sense organs NEC Q07.9
  skin Q82.9
    specified NEC Q89.8
  spinal
    cord Q06.9
    nerve root Q07.8
  spine Q76.49
    kyphosis —*see* Kyphosis,
      congenital
    lordosis —*see* Lordosis,
      congenital
  spleen Q89.09
  stomach Q40.3
    specified type NEC Q40.2
  teeth, tooth K00.9
  tendon Q79.9
  testis and scrotum Q55.20
    aplasia Q55.0
    hypoplasia Q55.1
    polyorchism Q55.21
    retractile testis Q55.22
    scrotal transposition Q55.23
    specified NEC Q55.29
  throat Q38.8
  thorax, bony Q76.9
  thyroid gland Q89.2
  tongue (congenital) Q38.3
    hypertrophy Q38.2
    tie Q38.1
  trachea Q32.1
  tricuspid valve Q22.9
    specified type NEC Q22.8
  umbilical cord NEC (complicating
    delivery) O69.89
  umbilicus Q89.9
  ureter Q62.8
    agenesis Q62.4
    duplication Q62.5
    malposition —*see* Malposition,
      congenital, ureter
    obstructive defect —*see* Defect,
      obstructive, ureter
    vesico-uretero-renal reflux Q62.7
  urethra Q64.79
    aplasia Q64.5
    duplication Q64.74
    posterior valves Q64.2
    prolapse Q64.71
    stricture Q64.32
  urinary system Q64.9
  uterus Q51.9
    specified type NEC Q51.818
  vagina Q52.4
  vascular system, peripheral Q27.9
  vas deferens Q55.4
    atresia Q55.3
  venous —*see* Anomaly, vein(s)
  vulva Q52.70

Malfunction —*see also* Dysfunction
  cardiac electronic device T82.119
    electrode T82.110
    pulse generator T82.111
    specified type NEC T82.118
  catheter device NEC T85.618
    cystostomy T83.010
    dialysis (renal) (vascular)
      T82.41
      intraperitoneal T85.611
    infusion NEC T82.514
      cranial T85.610
      epidural T85.610
      intrathecal T85.610
      spinal T85.610
      subarachnoid T85.610
      subdural T85.610

Malfunction (*continued*)
  catheter device NEC (*continued*)
    urinary (*see also* Breakdown,
      device, catheter), T83.018
  colostomy K94.03
    valve K94.03
  cystostomy (stoma) N99.512
    catheter T83.010
  enteric stoma K94.13
  enterostomy K94.13
  esophagostomy K94.33
  gastroenteric K31.89
  gastrostomy K94.23
  ileostomy K94.13
    valve K94.13
  intrathecal infusion pump T85.615
  jejunostomy K94.13
  nervous system device, implant
    or graft, specified NEC
    T85.615
  pacemaker —*see* Malfunction,
    cardiac electronic device
  prosthetic device, internal —*see*
    Complications, prosthetic device,
    by site, mechanical
  tracheostomy J95.03
  urinary device NEC —*see*
    Complication, genitourinary,
    device, urinary, mechanical
  valve
    colostomy K94.03
    heart T82.09
    ileostomy K94.13
  vascular graft or shunt NEC —*see*
    Complication, cardiovascular
    device, mechanical, vascular
  ventricular (communicating shunt)
    T85.01

Malherbe's tumor —*see* Neoplasm,
  skin, benign

Malibu disease L98.8

Malignancy —*see also* Neoplasm,
  malignant, by site
  unspecified site (primary) C80.1

Malignant —*see* condition

Malingerer, malingering Z76.5

Mallet finger (acquired) —*see*
  Deformity, finger, mallet finger
  congenital Q74.0
  sequelae of rickets E64.3

Malleus A24.0

Mallory's bodies R89.7

Mallory-Weiss syndrome K22.6

Malnutrition E46
  degree
    first E44.1
    mild (protein) E44.1
    moderate (protein) E44.0
    second E44.0
    severe (protein-energy) E43
      intermediate form E42
        with
          kwashiorkor (and
            marasmus) E42
          marasmus E41
    third E43
  following gastrointestinal surgery
    K91.2
  intrauterine
    light-for-dates —*see* Light for
      dates
    small-for-dates —*see* Small for
      dates
  lack of care, or neglect (child)
    (infant) T76.02
    confirmed T74.02
  malignant E40
  protein E46

Malnutrition (*continued*)
  protein (*continued*)
    calorie E46
      mild E44.1
      moderate E44.0
      severe E43
        intermediate form E42
          with
            kwashiorkor (and
              marasmus) E42
            marasmus E41
    energy E46
      mild E44.1
      moderate E44.0
      severe E43
        intermediate form E42
          with
            kwashiorkor (and
              marasmus) E42
            marasmus E41
  severe (protein-energy) E43
    with
      kwashiorkor (and marasmus)
        E42
      marasmus E41

Malocclusion (teeth) M26.4
  Angle's M26.219
    class I M26.211
    class II M26.212
    class III M26.213
  due to
    abnormal swallowing M26.59
    mouth breathing M26.59
    tongue, lip or finger habits
      M26.59
  temporomandibular (joint) M26.69

Malposition
  cervix —*see* Malposition, uterus
  congenital
    adrenal (gland) Q89.1
    alimentary tract Q45.8
      lower Q43.8
      upper Q40.8
    aorta Q25.49
    appendix Q43.8
    arterial trunk Q20.0
    artery (peripheral) Q27.8
      coronary Q24.5
      digestive system Q27.8
      lower limb Q27.8
      pulmonary Q25.79
      specified site NEC Q27.8
      upper limb Q27.8
    auditory canal Q17.8
      causing impairment of hearing
        Q16.9
    auricle (ear) Q17.4
      causing impairment of hearing
        Q16.9
    cervical Q18.2
    biliary duct or passage Q44.5
    bladder (mucosa) —*see*
      Exstrophy, bladder
    brachial plexus Q07.8
    brain tissue Q04.8
    breast Q83.8
    bronchus Q32.4
    cecum Q43.8
    clavicle Q74.0
    colon Q43.8
    digestive organ or tract NEC
      Q45.8
      lower Q43.8
      upper Q40.8
    ear (auricle) (external) Q17.4
      ossicles Q16.3
    endocrine (gland) NEC Q89.2
    epiglottis Q31.8
    eustachian tube Q17.8
    eye Q15.8

221

Malposition *(continued)*
  congenital *(continued)*
    facial features Q18.8
    fallopian tube Q50.6
    finger(s) Q68.1
      supernumerary Q69.0
    foot Q66.9-
    gallbladder Q44.1
    gastrointestinal tract Q45.8
    genitalia, genital organ(s) or
      tract
      female Q52.8
        external Q52.79
        internal NEC Q52.8
      male Q55.8
    glottis Q31.8
    hand Q68.1
    heart Q24.8
      dextrocardia Q24.0
        with complete transposition
          of viscera Q89.3
    hepatic duct Q44.5
    hip (joint) Q65.89
    intestine (large) (small) Q43.8
      with anomalous adhesions,
        fixation or malrotation
        Q43.3
    joint NEC Q68.8
    kidney Q63.2
    larynx Q31.8
    limb Q68.8
      lower Q68.8
      upper Q68.8
    liver Q44.7
    lung (lobe) Q33.8
    nail(s) Q84.6
    nerve Q07.8
    nervous system NEC Q07.8
    nose, nasal (septum) Q30.8
    organ or site not listed —*see*
      Anomaly, by site
    ovary Q50.39
    pancreas Q45.3
    parathyroid (gland) Q89.2
    patella Q74.1
    peripheral vascular system
      Q27.8
    pituitary (gland) Q89.2
    respiratory organ or system NEC
      Q34.8
    rib (cage) Q76.6
      supernumerary in cervical
        region Q76.5
    scapula Q74.0
    shoulder Q74.0
    spinal cord Q06.8
    spleen Q89.09
    sternum NEC Q76.7
    stomach Q40.2
    symphysis pubis Q74.2
    thymus (gland) Q89.2
    thyroid (gland) (tissue) Q89.2
      cartilage Q31.8
    toe(s) Q66.9-
      supernumerary Q69.2
    tongue Q38.3
    trachea Q32.1
    ureter Q62.60
      deviation Q62.61
      displacement Q62.62
      ectopia Q62.63
      specified type NEC
        Q62.69
    uterus Q51.818
    vein(s) (peripheral) Q27.8
      great Q26.8
    vena cava (inferior) (superior)
      Q26.8
  device, implant or graft *(see also*
    Complications, by site and type,
    mechanical) T85.628

Malposition *(continued)*
  device, implant or graft *(continued)*
    arterial graft NEC —*see*
      Complication, cardiovascular
      device, mechanical, vascular
    breast (implant) T85.42
    catheter NEC T85.628
      cystostomy T83.020
      dialysis (renal) T82.42
        intraperitoneal T85.621
      infusion NEC T82.524
        spinal (epidural) (subdural)
          T85.620
      urinary *(see also*
        Displacement, device,
        catheter, urinary), T83.028
    electronic (electrode) (pulse
      generator) (stimulator)
      bone T84.320
      cardiac T82.129
        electrode T82.120
        pulse generator T82.121
        specified type NEC T82.128
      nervous system —*see*
        Complication, prosthetic
        device, mechanical,
        electronic nervous system
        stimulator
      urinary —*see* Complication,
        genitourinary, device,
        urinary, mechanical
    fixation, internal (orthopedic)
      NEC —*see* Complication,
      fixation device, mechanical
    gastrointestinal —*see*
      Complications, prosthetic
      device, mechanical,
      gastrointestinal device
    genital NEC T83.428
      intrauterine contraceptive
        device (string) T83.32
      penile prosthesis (cylinder)
        (implanted) (pump)
        (resevoir) T83.420
      testicular prosthesis T83.421
    heart NEC —*see* Complication,
      cardiovascular device,
      mechanical
    joint prosthesis —*see*
      Complication, joint prosthesis,
      mechanical
    ocular NEC —*see*
      Complications, prosthetic
      device, mechanical, ocular
      device
    orthopedic NEC —*see*
      Complication, orthopedic,
      device, mechanical
    specified NEC T85.628
    urinary NEC —*see also*
      Complication, genitourinary,
      device, urinary, mechanical
      graft T83.22
    vascular NEC —*see*
      Complication, cardiovascular
      device, mechanical
    ventricular intracranial shunt
      T85.02
  fetus —*see* Pregnancy, complicated
    by (management affected by),
    presentation, fetal
  gallbladder K82.8
  gastrointestinal tract, congenital
    Q45.8
  heart, congenital NEC Q24.8
  joint prosthesis —*see*
    Complications, joint prosthesis,
    mechanical, displacement, by
    site
  stomach K31.89
    congenital Q40.2

Malposition *(continued)*
  tooth, teeth, fully erupted M26.30
  uterus (acute) (acquired) (adherent)
    (asymptomatic) (postinfectional)
    (postpartal) (old) N85.4
    anteflexion or anteversion N85.4
      congenital Q51.818
    flexion N85.4
      lateral —*see* Lateroversion,
        uterus
    inversion N85.5
    lateral (flexion) (version) —*see*
      Lateroversion, uterus
    in pregnancy or childbirth —
      see subcategory O34.5
    retroflexion or retroversion —*see*
      Retroversion, uterus

Malposture R29.3

Malrotation
  cecum Q43.3
  colon Q43.3
  intestine Q43.3
  kidney Q63.2

Maltreatment
  adult
    abandonment
      confirmed T74.01
      suspected T76.01
    bullying
      confirmed T74.31
      suspected T76.31
    confirmed T74.91
    history of Z91.419
    intimidation (through social media)
      confirmed T74.31
      suspected T76.31
    neglect
      confirmed T74.01
      suspected T76.01
    physical abuse
      confirmed T74.11
      suspected T76.11
    psychological abuse
      confirmed T74.31
      suspected of T76.31
      history of Z91.411
    sexual abuse
      confirmed T74.21
      suspected T76.21
    suspected T76.91
  child
    abandonment
      confirmed T74.02
      suspected T76.02
    bullying
      confirmed T74.32
      suspected T76.32
    confirmed T74.92
    history of —*see* History,
      personal (of), abuse
    intimidation (through social media)
      confirmed T74.32
      suspected T76.32
    neglect
      confirmed T74.02
      history of —*see* History,
        personal (of), abuse
      suspected T76.02
    physical abuse
      confirmed T74.12
      history of —*see* History,
        personal (of), abuse
      suspected T76.12
    psychological abuse
      confirmed T74.32
      history of —*see* History,
        personal (of), abuse
      suspected T76.32
    sexual abuse
      confirmed T74.22

Maltreatment *(continued)*
  child *(continued)*
    sexual abuse *(continued)*
      history of —*see* History,
        personal (of), abuse
      suspected T76.22
      suspected T76.92
    personal history of Z91.89

Malta fever —*see* Brucellosis

Maltworker's lung J67.4

Malunion, fracture —*see* Fracture,
  by site

Mammillitis N61.0
  puerperal, postpartum O91.02

Mammitis —*see* Mastitis

Mammogram (examination) Z12.39
  routine Z12.31

Mammoplasia N62

Management (of)
  bone conduction hearing device
    (implanted) Z45.320
  cardiac pacemaker NEC Z45.018
  cerebrospinal fluid drainage device
    Z45.41
  cochlear device (implanted)
    Z45.321
  contraceptive Z30.9
    specified NEC Z30.8
  implanted device Z45.9
    specified NEC Z45.89
  infusion pump Z45.1
  procreative Z31.9
    male factor infertility in female
      Z31.81
    specified NEC Z31.89
  prosthesis (external) *(see also*
    Fitting) Z44.9
    implanted Z45.9
      specified NEC Z45.89
  renal dialysis catheter Z49.01
  vascular access device Z45.2

Mangled —*see* specified injury by
  site

Mania (monopolar) —*see also*
  Disorder, mood, manic episode
  with psychotic symptoms F30.2
  without psychotic symptoms
    F30.10
    mild F30.11
    moderate F30.12
    severe F30.13
  Bell's F30.8
  chronic (recurrent) F31.89
  hysterical F44.89
  puerperal F30.8
  recurrent F31.89

Manic depression F31.9

**Manic-depressive insanity,
  psychosis, or syndrome** —*see*
  Disorder, bipolar

Mannosidosis E77.1

Mansonelliasis, mansonellosis
  B74.4

Manson's
  disease B65.1
  schistosomiasis B65.1

Manual —*see* condition

Maple-bark-stripper's lung
  (disease) J67.6

Maple-syrup-urine disease E71.0

Marable's syndrome (celiac artery
  compression) I77.4

Marasmus E41
  due to malnutrition E41
  intestinal E41
  nutritional E41
  senile R54
  tuberculous NEC —*see*
    Tuberculosis

Marble
  bones Q78.2
  skin R23.8

Marburg virus disease A98.3

March
  fracture —*see* Fracture, traumatic,
    stress, by site
  hemoglobinuria D59.6

Marchesani (-Weill) **syndrome**
  Q87.0

Marchiafava (-Bignami) **syndrome
  or disease** G37.1

Marchiafava-Micheli syndrome
  D59.5

Marcus Gunn's syndrome Q07.8

Marfan's syndrome —*see*
  Syndrome, Marfan's

Marie-Bamberger disease —*see*
  Osteoarthropathy, hypertrophic,
  specified NEC

**Marie-Charcot-Tooth neuropathic
  muscular atrophy** G60.0

Marie's
  cerebellar ataxia (late-onset) G11.2
  disease or syndrome (acromegaly)
    E22.0

**Marie-Strümpell arthritis, disease
  or spondylitis** —*see* Spondylitis,
  ankylosing

Marion's disease (bladder neck
  obstruction) N32.0

Marital conflict Z63.0

Mark
  port wine Q82.5
  raspberry Q82.5
  strawberry Q82.5
  stretch L90.6
  tattoo L81.8

Marker heterochromatin —*see*
  Extra, marker chromosomes

Maroteaux-Lamy syndrome (mild)
  (severe) E76.29

Marrow (bone)
  arrest D61.9
  poor function D75.89

Marseilles fever A77.1

Marsh fever —*see* Malaria

Marshall's (hidrotic) **ectodermal
  dysplasia** Q82.4

Marsh's disease (exophthalmic
  goiter) E05.00
  with storm E05.01

Masculinization (female) **with
  adrenal hyperplasia** E25.9
  congenital E25.0

Masculinovoblastoma D27.-

Masochism (sexual) F65.51

Mason's lung J62.8

Mass
  abdominal R19.00
    epigastric R19.06
    generalized R19.07
    left lower quadrant R19.04
    left upper quadrant R19.02
    periumbilic R19.05

Mass (*continued*)
  abdominal (*continued*)
    right lower quadrant R19.03
    right upper quadrant R19.01
    specified site NEC R19.09
  breast (*see also* Lump, breast)
    N63.0
  chest R22.2
  cystic —*see* Cyst
  ear H93.8-
  head R22.0
  intra-abdominal (diffuse)
    (generalized) —*see* Mass,
    abdominal
  kidney N28.89
  liver R16.0
  localized (skin) R22.9
    chest R22.2
    head R22.0
    limb
      lower R22.4-
      upper R22.3-
    neck R22.1
    trunk R22.2
  lung R91.8
  malignant —*see* Neoplasm,
    malignant, by site
  neck R22.1
  pelvic (diffuse) (generalized) —*see*
    Mass, abdominal
  specified organ NEC —*see*
    Disease, by site
  splenic R16.1
  substernal thyroid —*see* Goiter
  superficial (localized) R22.9
  umbilical (diffuse) (generalized)
    R19.09

Massive —*see* condition

Mast cell
  disease, systemic tissue D47.02
  neoplasm
    malignant C96.20
      specified type NEC C96.29
    of uncertain behavior NEC
      D47.09
  leukemia C94.3-
  sarcoma C96.22
  tumor D47.09

Mastalgia N64.4

Masters-Allen syndrome N83.8

Mastitis (acute) (diffuse)
  (nonpuerperal) (subacute) N61.0
  with abscess N61.1
  chronic (cystic) —*see* Mastopathy,
    cystic
  cystic (Schimmelbusch's type)
    —*see* Mastopathy, cystic
  fibrocystic —*see* Mastopathy, cystic
  granulomatous N61.2-
  infective N61.0
    newborn P39.0
  interstitial, gestational or puerperal
    —*see* Mastitis, obstetric
  neonatal (noninfective) P83.4
    infective P39.0
  obstetric (interstitial) (nonpurulent)
    associated with
      lactation O91.23
      pregnancy O91.21-
      puerperium O91.22
    purulent
      associated with
        lactation O91.13
        pregnancy O91.11-
        puerperium O91.12
  periductal —*see* Ectasia, mammary
    duct
  phlegmonous —*see* Mastopathy,
    cystic

Mastitis (*continued*)
  plasma cell —*see* Ectasia,
    mammary duct
  without abscess N61.0

Mastocytoma (extracutaneous)
  D47.09
  malignant C96.29
  solitary D47.01

Mastocytosis D47.09
  aggressive systemic C96.21
  cutaneous (diffuse)
    (maculopapular) D47.01
    congenital Q82.2
    of neonatal onset Q82.2
    of newborn onset Q82.2
  indolent systemic D47.02
  isolated bone marrow D47.02
  malignant C96.29
  systemic (indolent) (smoldering)
    with an associated hematological
      non-mast cell lineage disease
      (SM-AHNMD) D47.02

Mastodynia N64.4

Mastoid —*see* condition

Mastoidalgia —*see* subcategory
  H92.0

Mastoiditis (coalescent)
  (hemorrhagic) (suppurative) H70.9-
  acute, subacute H70.00-
    complicated NEC H70.09-
    subperiosteal H70.01-
  chronic (necrotic) (recurrent)
    H70.1-
  in (due to)
    infectious disease NEC B99
      [H75.0-]
    parasitic disease NEC B89
      [H75.0-]
    tuberculosis A18.03
  petrositis —*see* Petrositis
  postauricular fistula —*see* Fistula,
    postauricular
  specified NEC H70.89-
  tuberculous A18.03

Mastopathy, mastopathia N64.9
  chronica cystica —*see* Mastopathy,
    cystic
  cystic (chronic) (diffuse) N60.1-
    with epithelial proliferation
      N60.3-
  diffuse cystic —*see* Mastopathy,
    cystic
  estrogenic, oestrogenica N64.89
  ovarian origin N64.89

Mastoplasia, mastoplastia N62

Masturbation (excessive) F98.8

Maternal care (for) —*see* Pregnancy
  (complicated by) (management
  affected by)

Matheiu's disease (leptospiral
  jaundice) A27.0

**Mauclaire's disease or
  osteochondrosis** —*see*
  Osteochondrosis, juvenile, hand,
  metacarpal

Maxcy's disease A75.2

Maxilla, maxillary —*see* condition

May (-Hegglin) **anomaly or
  syndrome** D72.0

McArdle (-Schmid) (-Pearson)
  disease (glycogen storage) E74.04

McCune-Albright syndrome
  Q78.1

McQuarrie's syndrome (idiopathic
  familial hypoglycemia) E16.2

Meadow's syndrome Q86.1

Measles (black) (hemorrhagic)
  (suppressed) B05.9
  with
    complications NEC B05.89
    encephalitis B05.0
    intestinal complications B05.4
    keratitis (keratoconjunctivitis)
      B05.81
    meningitis B05.1
    otitis media B05.3
    pneumonia B05.2
  French —*see* Rubella
  German —*see* Rubella
  Liberty —*see* Rubella

Meatitis, urethral —*see* Urethritis

Meatus, meatal —*see* condition

Meat-wrappers' asthma J68.9

Meckel-Gruber syndrome Q61.9

Meckel's diverticulitis, diverticulum
  (displaced) (hypertrophic)
  Q43.0
  malignant —*see* Table of
    Neoplasms, small intestine,
    malignant

Meconium
  ileus, newborn P76.0
    in cystic fibrosis E84.11
    meaning meconium plug
      (without cystic fibrosis)
      P76.0
  obstruction, newborn P76.0
    due to fecaliths P76.0
    in mucoviscidosis E84.11
  peritonitis P78.0
  plug syndrome (newborn) NEC
    P76.0

Median —*see also* condition
  arcuate ligament syndrome I77.4
  bar (prostate) (vesical orifice) —*see*
    Hyperplasia, prostate
  rhomboid glossitis K14.2

Mediastinal shift R93.89

Mediastinitis (acute) (chronic)
  J98.51
  syphilitic A52.73
  tuberculous A15.8

Mediastinopericarditis —*see also*
  Pericarditis
  acute I30.9
  adhesive I31.0
  chronic I31.8
    rheumatic I09.2

Mediastinum, mediastinal —*see*
  condition

Medicine poisoning —*see* Table of
  Drugs and Chemicals, by drug,
  poisoning

Mediterranean
  fever —*see* Brucellosis
    familial M04.1
    tick A77.1
  kala-azar B55.0
  leishmaniasis B55.0
  tick fever A77.1

Medulla —*see* condition

Medullary cystic kidney Q61.5

Medullated fibers
  optic (nerve) Q14.8
  retina Q14.1

Medulloblastoma
  desmoplastic C71.6
  specified site —*see* Neoplasm,
    malignant, by site
  unspecified site C71.6

Medulloepithelioma —see also
  Neoplasm, malignant, by site
  teratoid —see Neoplasm,
    malignant, by site

Medullomyoblastoma
  specified site —see Neoplasm,
    malignant, by site
  unspecified site C71.6

Meekeren-Ehlers-Danlos syndrome
  (see also Syndrome, Ehlers-
  Danlos) Q79.69

Megacolon (acquired) (functional)
  (not Hirschsprung's disease) (in)
  K59.39
  Chagas' disease B57.32
  congenital, congenitum
    (aganglionic) Q43.1
  Hirschsprung's (disease) Q43.1
  toxic NEC K59.31
    due to Clostridium difficile
      not specified as recurrent A04.72
      recurrent A04.71

Megaesophagus (functional) K22.0
  congenital Q39.5
  in (due to) Chagas' disease B57.31

Megalencephaly Q04.5

Megalerythema (epidemic) B08.3

Megaloappendix Q43.8

Megalocephalus, megalocephaly
  NEC Q75.3

Megalocornea Q15.8
  with glaucoma Q15.0

Megalocytic anemia D53.1

Megalodactylia (fingers) (thumbs)
  (congenital) Q74.0
  toes Q74.2

Megaloduodenum Q43.8

Megaloesophagus (functional) K22.0
  congenital Q39.5

Megalogastria (acquired) K31.89
  congenital Q40.2

Megalophthalmos Q11.3

Megalopsia H53.15

Megalosplenia —see Splenomegaly

Megaloureter N28.82
  congenital Q62.2

Megarectum K62.89

Megasigmoid K59.39
  congenital Q43.2

Megaureter N28.82
  congenital Q62.2

Megavitamin-B6 syndrome E67.2

Megrim —see Migraine

Meibomian
  cyst, infected —see Hordeolum
  gland —see condition
  sty, stye —see Hordeolum

Meibomitis —see Hordeolum

Meige-Milroy disease (chronic
  hereditary edema) Q82.0

Meige's syndrome Q82.0

Melalgia, nutritional E53.8

Melancholia F32.9
  climacteric (single episode) F32.89
    recurrent episode F33.8
  hypochondriac F45.29
  intermittent (single episode) F32.89
    recurrent episode F33.8
  involutional (single episode)
    F32.89
    recurrent episode F33.8

Melancholia (continued)
  menopausal (single episode)
    F32.89
    recurrent episode F33.8
  puerperal F32.89
  reactive (emotional stress or
    trauma) F32.3
  recurrent F33.9
  senile F03
  stuporous (single episode) F32.89
    recurrent episode F33.8

Melanemia R79.89

Melanoameloblastoma —see
  Neoplasm, bone, benign

Melanoblastoma —see Melanoma

Melanocarcinoma —see Melanoma

Melanocytoma, eyeball D31.9-

Melanocytosis, neurocutaneous
  Q82.8

Melanoderma, melanodermia
  L81.4

Melanodontia, infantile K03.89

Melanodontoclasia K03.89

Melanoepithelioma —see Melanoma

Melanoma (malignant) C43.9
  acral lentiginous, malignant —see
    Melanoma, skin, by site
  amelanotic —see Melanoma, skin,
    by site
  balloon cell —see Melanoma, skin,
    by site
  benign —see Nevus
  desmoplastic, malignant —see
    Melanoma, skin, by site
  epithelioid cell —see Melanoma,
    skin, by site
    with spindle cell, mixed —see
      Melanoma, skin, by site
  in
    giant pigmented nevus —see
      Melanoma, skin, by site
    Hutchinson's melanotic freckle
      —see Melanoma, skin, by site
    junctional nevus —see
      Melanoma, skin, by site
    precancerous melanosis —see
      Melanoma, skin, by site
  in situ D03.9
    abdominal wall D03.59
    ala nasi D03.39
    ankle D03.7-
    anus, anal (margin) (skin)
      D03.51
    arm D03.6-
    auditory canal D03.2-
    auricle (ear) D03.2-
    auricular canal (external)
      D03.2-
    axilla, axillary fold D03.59
    back D03.59
    breast D03.52
    brow D03.39
    buttock D03.59
    canthus (eye) D03.1-
    cheek (external) D03.39
    chest wall D03.59
    chin D03.39
    choroid D03.8
    conjunctiva D03.8
    ear (external) D03.2-
    external meatus (ear) D03.2-
    eye D03.8
    eyebrow D03.39
    eyelid (lower) (upper) D03.1-
    face D03.30
      specified NEC D03.39

Melanoma (continued)
  in situ (continued)
    female genital organ (external)
      NEC D03.8
    finger D03.6-
    flank D03.59
    foot D03.7-
    forearm D03.6-
    forehead D03.39
    foreskin D03.8
    gluteal region D03.59
    groin D03.59
    hand D03.6-
    heel D03.7-
    helix D03.2-
    hip D03.7-
    interscapular region D03.59
    iris D03.8
    jaw D03.39
    knee D03.7-
    labium (majus) (minus) D03.8
    lacrimal gland D03.8
    leg D03.7-
    lip (lower) (upper) D03.0
    lower limb NEC D03.7-
    male genital organ (external)
      NEC D03.8
    nail D03.9
      finger D03.6-
      toe D03.7-
    neck D03.4
    nose (external) D03.39
    orbit D03.8
    penis D03.8
    perianal skin D03.51
    perineum D03.51
    pinna D03.2-
    popliteal fossa or space D03.7-
    prepuce D03.8
    pudendum D03.8
    retina D03.8
    retrobulbar D03.8
    scalp D03.4
    scrotum D03.8
    shoulder D03.6-
    specified site NEC D03.8
    submammary fold D03.52
    temple D03.39
    thigh D03.7-
    toe D03.7-
    trunk NEC D03.59
    umbilicus D03.59
    upper limb NEC D03.6-
    vulva D03.8
  juvenile —see Nevus
  malignant, of soft parts except
    skin —see Neoplasm, connective
    tissue, malignant
  metastatic
    breast C79.81
    genital organ C79.82
    specified site NEC C79.89
  neurotropic, malignant —see
    Melanoma, skin, by site
  nodular —see Melanoma, skin, by
    site
  regressing, malignant —see
    Melanoma, skin, by site
  skin C43.9
    abdominal wall C43.59
    ala nasi C43.31
    ankle C43.7-
    anus, anal (skin) C43.51
    arm C43.6-
    auditory canal (external) C43.2-
    auricle (ear) C43.2-
    auricular canal (external) C43.2-
    axilla, axillary fold C43.59
    back C43.59
    breast (female) (male) C43.52

Melanoma (continued)
  skin (continued)
    brow C43.39
    buttock C43.59
    canthus (eye) C43.1-
    cheek (external) C43.39
    chest wall C43.59
    chin C43.39
    ear (external) C43.2-
    elbow C43.6-
    external meatus (ear) C43.2-
    eyebrow C43.39
    eyelid (lower) (upper) C43.1-
    face C43.30
      specified NEC C43.39
    female genital organ (external)
      NEC C51.9
    finger C43.6-
    flank C43.59
    foot C43.7-
    forearm C43.6-
    forehead C43.39
    foreskin C60.0
    glabella C43.39
    gluteal region C43.59
    groin C43.59
    hand C43.6-
    heel C43.7-
    helix C43.2-
    hip C43.7-
    interscapular region C43.59
    jaw (external) C43.39
    knee C43.7-
    labium C51.9
      majus C51.0
      minus C51.1
    leg C43.7-
    lip (lower) (upper) C43.0
    lower limb NEC C43.7-
    male genital organ (external)
      NEC C63.9
    nail
      finger C43.6-
      toe C43.7-
    nasolabial groove C43.39
    nates C43.59
    neck C43.4
    nose (external) C43.31
    overlapping site C43.8
    palpebra C43.1-
    penis C60.9
    perianal skin C43.51
    perineum C43.51
    pinna C43.2-
    popliteal fossa or space C43.7-
    prepuce C60.0
    pudendum C51.9
    scalp C43.4
    scrotum C63.2
    shoulder C43.6-
    skin NEC C43.9
    submammary fold C43.52
    temple C43.39
    thigh C43.7-
    toe C43.7-
    trunk NEC C43.59
    umbilicus C43.59
    upper limb NEC C43.6-
    vulva C51.9
      overlapping sites C51.8
  spindle cell
    with epithelioid, mixed —see
      Melanoma, skin, by site
    type A C69.4-
    type B C69.4-
  superficial spreading —see
    Melanoma, skin, by site

Melanosarcoma —see also
  Melanoma
  epithelioid cell —see Melanoma

Melanosis L81.4
- addisonian E27.1
  - tuberculous A18.7
- adrenal E27.1
- colon K63.89
- conjunctiva —*see* Pigmentation, conjunctiva
  - congenital Q13.89
- cornea (presenile) (senile) —*see also* Pigmentation, cornea
  - congenital Q13.4
- eye NEC H57.89
  - congenital Q15.8
- lenticularis progressiva Q82.1
- liver K76.89
- precancerous —*see also* Melanoma, in situ
  - malignant melanoma in —*see* Melanoma
- Riehl's L81.4
- sclera H15.89
  - congenital Q13.89
- suprarenal E27.1
- tar L81.4
- toxic L81.4

Melanuria R82.998

MELAS syndrome E88.41

Melasma L81.1
- adrenal (gland) E27.1
- suprarenal (gland) E27.1

Melena K92.1
- with ulcer - code by site under Ulcer, with hemorrhage K27.4
- due to swallowed maternal blood P78.2
- newborn, neonatal P54.1
  - due to swallowed maternal blood P78.2

Meleney's
- gangrene (cutaneous) —*see* Ulcer, skin
- ulcer (chronic undermining) —*see* Ulcer, skin

Melioidosis A24.9
- acute A24.1
- chronic A24.2
- fulminating A24.1
- pneumonia A24.1
- pulmonary (chronic) A24.2
  - acute A24.1
  - subacute A24.2
- sepsis A24.1
- specified NEC A24.3
- subacute A24.2

Melitensis, febris A23.0

Melkersson (-Rosenthal) **syndrome** G51.2

Mellitus, diabetes —*see* Diabetes

Melorheostosis (bone) —*see* Disorder, bone, density and structure, specified NEC

Meloschisis Q18.4

Melotia Q17.4

Membrana
- capsularis lentis posterior Q13.89
- epipapillaris Q14.2

Membranacea placenta O43.19-

Membranaceous uterus N85.8

Membrane(s), membranous —*see also* condition
- cyclitic —*see* Membrane, pupillary
- folds, congenital —*see* Web
- Jackson's Q43.3

Membrane(s), membranous (continued)
- over face of newborn P28.9
- premature rupture —*see* Rupture, membranes, premature
- pupillary H21.4-
  - persistent Q13.89
- retained (with hemorrhage) (complicating delivery) O72.2
  - without hemorrhage O73.1
- secondary cataract —*see* Cataract, secondary
- unruptured (causing asphyxia) —*see* Asphyxia, newborn
- vitreous —*see* Opacity, vitreous, membranes and strands

Membranitis —*see* Chorioamnionitis

Memory disturbance, lack or loss —*see also* Amnesia
- mild, following organic brain damage F06.8

Menadione deficiency E56.1

Menarche
- delayed E30.0
- precocious E30.1

Mendacity, pathologic F60.2

Mendelson's syndrome (due to anesthesia) J95.4
- in labor and delivery O74.0
- in pregnancy O29.01-
- obstetric O74.0
- postpartum, puerperal O89.01

Ménétrier's disease or syndrome K29.60
- with bleeding K29.61

Ménière's disease, syndrome or vertigo H81.0-

Meninges, meningeal —*see* condition

Meningioma —*see also* Neoplasm, meninges, benign
- angioblastic —*see* Neoplasm, meninges, benign
- angiomatous —*see* Neoplasm, meninges, benign
- atypical —*see* Neoplasm, meninges, uncertain behavior
- endotheliomatous —*see* Neoplasm, meninges, benign
- fibroblastic —*see* Neoplasm, meninges, benign
- fibrous —*see* Neoplasm, meninges, benign
- hemangioblastic —*see* Neoplasm, meninges, benign
- hemangiopericytic —*see* Neoplasm, meninges, benign
- malignant —*see* Neoplasm, meninges, malignant
- meningiothelial —*see* Neoplasm, meninges, benign
- meningotheliomatous —*see* Neoplasm, meninges, benign
- mixed —*see* Neoplasm, meninges, benign
- multiple —*see* Neoplasm, meninges, uncertain behavior
- papillary —*see* Neoplasm, meninges, uncertain behavior
- psammomatous —*see* Neoplasm, meninges, benign
- syncytial —*see* Neoplasm, meninges, benign
- transitional —*see* Neoplasm, meninges, benign

Meningiomatosis (diffuse) —*see* Neoplasm, meninges, uncertain behavior

Meningism —*see* Meningismus

Meningismus (infectional) (pneumococcal) R29.1
- due to serum or vaccine R29.1
- influenzal —*see* Influenza, with, manifestations NEC

Meningitis (basal) (basic) (brain) (cerebral) (cervical) (congestive) (diffuse) (hemorrhagic) (infantile) (membranous) (metastatic) (nonspecific) (pontine) (progressive) (simple) (spinal) (subacute) (sympathetic) (toxic) G03.9
- abacterial G03.0
- actinomycotic A42.81
- adenoviral A87.1
- arbovirus A87.8
- aseptic (acute) G03.0
- bacterial G00.9
  - Escherichia coli (E. coli) G00.8
  - Friedländer (bacillus) G00.8
  - gram-negative G00.9
  - H. influenzae G00.0
  - Klebsiella G00.8
  - pneumococcal G00.1
  - specified organism NEC G00.8
  - staphylococcal G00.3
  - streptococcal (acute) G00.2
- benign recurrent (Mollaret) G03.2
- candidal B37.5
- caseous (tuberculous) A17.0
- cerebrospinal A39.0
- chronic NEC G03.1
- clear cerebrospinal fluid NEC G03.0
- coxsackievirus A87.0
- cryptococcal B45.1
- diplococcal (gram positive) A39.0
- echovirus A87.0
- enteroviral A87.0
- eosinophilic B83.2
- epidemic NEC A39.0
- Escherichia coli (E. coli) G00.8
- fibrinopurulent G00.9
  - specified organism NEC G00.8
- Friedländer (bacillus) G00.8
- gonococcal A54.81
- gram-negative cocci G00.9
- gram-positive cocci G00.9
- Haemophilus (influenzae) G00.0
- H. influenzae G00.0
- in (due to)
  - adenovirus A87.1
  - African trypanosomiasis B56.9 [G02]
  - anthrax A22.8
  - bacterial disease NEC A48.8 [G01]
  - Chagas' disease (chronic) B57.41
  - chickenpox B01.0
  - coccidioidomycosis B38.4
  - Diplococcus pneumoniae G00.1
  - enterovirus A87.0
  - herpes (simplex) virus B00.3
    - zoster B02.1
  - infectious mononucleosis B27.92
  - leptospirosis A27.81
  - Listeria monocytogenes A32.11
  - Lyme disease A69.21
  - measles B05.1
  - mumps (virus) B26.1
  - neurosyphilis (late) A52.13
  - parasitic disease NEC B89 [G02]
  - poliovirus A80.9 [G02]
  - preventive immunization, inoculation or vaccination G03.8

Meningitis (continued)
- in (continued)
  - rubella B06.02
  - Salmonella infection A02.21
  - specified cause NEC G03.8
  - Streptococcal pneumoniae G00.1
  - typhoid fever A01.01
  - varicella B01.0
  - viral disease NEC A87.8
  - whooping cough A37.90
  - zoster B02.1
- infectious G00.9
- influenzal (H. influenzae) G00.0
- Klebsiella G00.8
- leptospiral (aseptic) A27.81
- lymphocytic (acute) (benign) (serous) A87.2
- meningococcal A39.0
- Mima polymorpha G00.8
- Mollaret (benign recurrent) G03.2
- monilial B37.5
- mycotic NEC B49 [G02]
- Neisseria A39.0
- nonbacterial G03.0
- nonpyogenic NEC G03.0
- ossificans G96.198
- pneumococcal streptococcus pneumoniae G00.1
- poliovirus A80.9 [G02]
- postmeasles B05.1
- purulent G00.9
  - specified organism NEC G00.8
- pyogenic G00.9
  - specified organism NEC G00.8
- Salmonella (arizonae) (Cholerae-Suis) (enteritidis) (typhimurium) A02.21
- septic G00.9
  - specified organism NEC G00.8
- serosa circumscripta NEC G03.0
- serous NEC G93.2
- specified organism NEC G00.8
- sporotrichosis B42.81
- staphylococcal G00.3
- sterile G03.0
- Streptococcal (acute) G00.2
  - pneumoniae G00.1
- suppurative G00.9
  - specified organism NEC G00.8
- syphilitic (late) (tertiary) A52.13
  - acute A51.41
  - congenital A50.41
  - secondary A51.41
- Torula histolytica (cryptococcal) B45.1
- traumatic (complication of injury) T79.8
- tuberculous A17.0
- typhoid A01.01
- viral NEC A87.9
- Yersinia pestis A20.3

Meningocele (spinal) —*see also* Spina bifida
- with hydrocephalus —*see* Spina bifida, by site, with hydrocephalus
- acquired (traumatic) G96.198
- cerebral —*see* Encephalocele

Meningocerebritis —*see* Meningoencephalitis

Meningococcemia A39.4
- acute A39.2
- chronic A39.3

Meningococcus, meningococcal —*see also* condition A39.9
- adrenalitis, hemorrhagic A39.1
- carrier (suspected) of Z22.31
- meningitis (cerebrospinal) A39.0

Meningoencephalitis (*see also* Encephalitis) G04.90
  acute NEC (*see also* Encephalitis, viral) A86
  bacterial NEC G04.2
  California A83.5
  diphasic A84.1
  eosinophilic B83.2
  epidemic A39.81
  herpesviral, herpetic B00.4
    due to herpesvirus 6 B10.01
    due to herpesvirus 7 B10.09
    specified NEC B10.09
  in (due to)
    blastomycosis NEC B40.81
    diseases classified elsewhere G05.3
    free-living amebae B60.2
    Hemophilus influenzae (H .influenzae) G00.0
    herpes B00.4
      due to herpesvirus 6 B10.01
      due to herpesvirus 7 B10.09
      specified NEC B10.09
    H. influenzae G00.0
    Lyme disease A69.22
    mercury —*see* subcategory T56.1
    mumps B26.2
    Naegleria (amebae) (organisms) (fowleri) B60.2
    Parastrongylus cantonensis B83.2
    toxoplasmosis (acquired) B58.2
      congenital P37.1
  infectious (acute) (viral) A86
  influenzal (H. influenzae) G00.0
  Listeria monocytogenes A32.12
  lymphocytic (serous) A87.2
  mumps B26.2
  parasitic NEC B89 *[G05.3]*
  pneumococcal G04.2
  primary amebic B60.2
  specific (syphilitic) A52.14
  specified organism NEC G04.81
  staphylococcal G04.2
  streptococcal G04.2
  syphilitic A52.14
  toxic NEC G92
    due to mercury —*see* subcategory T56.1
  tuberculous A17.82
  virus NEC A86

Meningoencephalocele —*see also* Encephalocele
  syphilitic A52.19
    congenital A50.49

Meningoencephalomyelitis —*see also* Meningoencephalitis
  acute NEC (viral) A86
    disseminated G04.00
      postimmunization or postvaccination G04.02
      postinfectious G04.01
  due to
    actinomycosis A42.82
    Torula B45.1
    Toxoplasma or toxoplasmosis (acquired) B58.2
      congenital P37.1
  postimmunization or postvaccination G04.02

Meningoencephalomyelopathy G96.9

Meningoencephalopathy G96.9

Meningomyelitis —*see also* Meningoencephalitis
  bacterial NEC G04.2
  blastomycotic NEC B40.81

Meningomyelitis (*continued*)
  cryptococcal B45.1
  in diseases classified elsewhere G05.4
  meningococcal A39.81
  syphilitic A52.14
  tuberculous A17.82

Meningomyelocele —*see also* Spina bifida
  syphilitic A52.19

Meningomyeloneuritis —*see* Meningoencephalitis

Meningoradiculitis —*see* Meningitis

Meningovascular —*see* condition

Menkes' disease or syndrome E83.09
  meaning maple-syrup-urine disease E71.0

Menometrorrhagia N92.1

Menopause, menopausal
  (asymptomatic) (state) Z78.0
  arthritis (any site) NEC —*see* Arthritis, specified form NEC
  bleeding N92.4
  depression (single episode) F32.89
    agitated (single episode) F32.2
      recurrent episode F33.9
    psychotic (single episode) F32.89
      recurrent episode F33.8
    recurrent episode F33.9
    melancholia (single episode) F32.89
      recurrent episode F33.8
  paranoid state F22
  premature E28.319
    asymptomatic E28.319
      postirradiation E89.40
      postsurgical E89.40
    symptomatic E28.310
      postirradiation E89.41
      postsurgical E89.41
  psychosis NEC F28
  symptomatic N95.1
  toxic polyarthritis NEC —*see* Arthritis, specified form NEC

Menorrhagia (primary) N92.0
  climacteric N92.4
    menopausal N92.4
  menopausal N92.4
  perimenopausal N92.4
  postclimacteric N95.0
  postmenopausal N95.0
  preclimacteric or premenopausal N92.4
  pubertal (menses retained) N92.2

Menostaxis N92.0

Menses, retention N94.89

Menstrual —*see* Menstruation

Menstruation
  absent —*see* Amenorrhea
  anovulatory N97.0
  cycle, irregular N92.6
  delayed N91.0
  disorder N93.9
    psychogenic F45.8
  during pregnancy O20.8
  excessive (with regular cycle) N92.0
    with irregular cycle N92.1
    at puberty N92.2
  frequent N92.0
  infrequent —*see* Oligomenorrhea
  irregular N92.6
    specified NEC N92.5

Menstruation (*continued*)
  latent N92.5
  membranous N92.5
  painful (*see also* Dysmenorrhea) N94.6
    primary N94.4
    psychogenic F45.8
    secondary N94.5
  passage of clots N92.0
  precocious E30.1
  protracted N92.5
  rare —*see* Oligomenorrhea
  retained N94.89
  retrograde N92.5
  scanty —*see* Oligomenorrhea
  suppression N94.89
  vicarious (nasal) N94.89

Mental —*see also* condition
  deficiency —*see* Disability, intellectual
  deterioration —*see* Psychosis
  disorder —*see* Disorder, mental
  exhaustion F48.8
  insufficiency (congenital) —*see* Disability, intellectual
  observation without need for further medical care Z03.89
  retardation —*see* Disability, intellectual
  subnormality —*see* Disability, intellectuall
  upset —*see* Disorder, mental

Meralgia paresthetica G57.1-

Mercurial —*see* condition

Mercurialism —*see* subcategory T56.1

MERRF syndrome (myoclonic epilepsy associated with ragged-red fiber) E88.42

Merkel cell tumor —*see* Carcinoma, Merkel cell

Merocele —*see* Hernia, femoral

Meromelia
  lower limb —*see* Defect, reduction, lower limb
    intercalary
      femur —*see* Defect, reduction, lower limb, specified type NEC
      tibiofibular (complete) (incomplete) —*see* Defect, reduction, lower limb
  upper limb —*see* Defect, reduction, upper limb
    intercalary, humeral, radioulnar —*see* Agenesis, arm, with hand present

Merzbacher-Pelizaeus disease E75.29

Mesaortitis —*see* Aortitis

Mesarteritis —*see* Arteritis

Mesencephalitis —*see* Encephalitis

Mesenchymoma —*see also* Neoplasm, connective tissue, uncertain behavior
  benign —*see* Neoplasm, connective tissue, benign
  malignant —*see* Neoplasm, connective tissue, malignant

Mesenteritis
  retractile K65.4
  sclerosing K65.4

Mesentery, mesenteric —*see* condition

Mesiodens, mesiodentes K00.1

Mesio-occlusion M26.213

Mesocolon —*see* condition

Mesonephroma (malignant) —*see* Neoplasm, malignant, by site
  benign —*see* Neoplasm, benign, by site

Mesophlebitis —*see* Phlebitis

Mesostromal dysgenesia Q13.89

Mesothelioma (malignant) C45.9
  benign
    mesentery D19.1
    mesocolon D19.1
    omentum D19.1
    peritoneum D19.1
    pleura D19.0
    specified site NEC D19.7
    unspecified site D19.9
  biphasic C45.9
    benign
      mesentery D19.1
      mesocolon D19.1
      omentum D19.1
      peritoneum D19.1
      pleura D19.0
      specified site NEC D19.7
      unspecified site D19.9
  cystic D48.4
  epithelioid C45.9
    benign
      mesentery D19.1
      mesocolon D19.1
      omentum D19.1
      peritoneum D19.1
      pleura D19.0
      specified site NEC D19.7
      unspecified site D19.9
  fibrous C45.9
    benign
      mesentery D19.1
      mesocolon D19.1
      omentum D19.1
      peritoneum D19.1
      pleura D19.0
      specified site NEC D19.7
      unspecified site D19.9
  site classification
    liver C45.7
    lung C45.7
    mediastinum C45.7
    mesentery C45.1
    mesocolon C45.1
    omentum C45.1
    pericardium C45.2
    peritoneum C45.1
    pleura C45.0
      parietal C45.0
    retroperitoneum C45.7
    specified site NEC C45.7
    unspecified C45.9

Metabolic syndrome E88.81

Metagonimiasis B66.8

Metagonimus infestation (intestine) B66.8

Metal
  pigmentation L81.8
  polisher's disease J62.8

Metamorphopsia H53.15

Metaplasia
  apocrine (breast) —*see* Dysplasia, mammary, specified type NEC
  cervix (squamous) —*see* Dysplasia, cervix
  endometrium (squamous) (uterus) N85.8

Metaplasia (continued)
esophagus K22.7-
kidney (pelvis) (squamous) N28.89
myelogenous D73.1
myeloid (agnogenic)
(megakaryocytic) D73.1
spleen D73.1
squamous cell, bladder N32.89

Metastasis, metastatic
abscess —see Abscess
calcification E83.59
cancer
from specified site —see
Neoplasm, malignant, by site
to specified site —see Neoplasm,
secondary, by site
deposits (in) —see Neoplasm,
secondary, by site
disease (see also Neoplasm,
secondary, by site) C79.9
spread (to) —see Neoplasm,
secondary, by site

Metastrongyliasis B83.8

Metatarsalgia M77.4-
anterior G57.6-
Morton's G57.6-

Metatarsus, metatarsal —see also
condition
adductus, congenital Q66.22-
valgus (abductus), congenital Q66.6
varus (congenital) Q66.22-
primus Q66.21-

Methadone use —see Use, opioid

Methemoglobinemia D74.9
acquired (with
sulfhemoglobinemia) D74.8
congenital D74.0
enzymatic (congenital) D74.0
Hb M disease D74.0
hereditary D74.0
toxic D74.8

Methemoglobinuria —see
Hemoglobinuria

Methioninemia E72.19

Methylmalonic acidemia E71.120

Metritis (catarrhal) (hemorrhagic)
(septic) (suppurative) —see also
Endometritis
cervical —see Cervicitis

Metropathia hemorrhagica N93.8

Metroperitonitis —see Peritonitis,
pelvic, female

Metrorrhagia N92.1
climacteric N92.4
menopausal N92.4
perimenopausal N92.4
postpartum NEC (atonic)
(following delivery of placenta)
O72.1
delayed or secondary O72.2
preclimacteric or premenopausal
N92.4
psychogenic F45.8

Metrorrhexis —see Rupture, uterus

Metrosalpingitis N70.91

Metrostaxis N93.8

Metrovaginitis —see Endometritis

**Meyer-Schwickerath and Weyers
syndrome** Q87.0

Meynert's amentia (nonalcoholic) F04
alcoholic F10.96
with dependence F10.26

Mibelli's disease (porokeratosis)
Q82.8

Mice, joint —see Loose, body, joint
knee M23.4-

Micrencephalon, micrencephaly Q02

Microalbuminuria R80.9

Microaneurysm, retinal —
see also Disorder, retina,
microaneurysms
diabetic —see E08-E13 with .31

Microangiopathy (peripheral) I73.9
thrombotic M31.1

Microcalcifications, breast R92.0

**Microcephalus, microcephalic,
microcephaly** Q02
due to toxoplasmosis (congenital)
P37.1

Microcheilia Q18.7

Microcolon (congenital) Q43.8

Microcornea (congenital) Q13.4

Microcytic —see condition

Microdeletions NEC Q93.88

Microdontia K00.2

Microdrepanocytosis D57.40
with
acute chest syndrome D57.411
cerebral vascular involvement
D57.413
crisis (painful) D57.419
with specified complication
NEC D57.418
splenic sequestration D57.412
vasoocclusive pain D57.419

Microembolism
atherothrombotic —see
Atheroembolism
retinal —see Occlusion, artery, retina

Microencephalon Q02

Microfilaria streptocerca infestation
—see Onchocerciasis

Microgastria (congenital) Q40.2

Microgenia M26.06

Microgenitalia, congenital
female Q52.8
male Q55.8

Microglioma —see Lymphoma,
non-Hodgkin, specified NEC

Microglossia (congenital) Q38.3

Micrognathia, micrognathism
(congenital) (mandibular)
(maxillary) M26.09

Microgyria (congenital) Q04.3

Microinfarct of heart —see
Insufficiency, coronary

Microlentia (congenital) Q12.8

Microlithiasis, alveolar, pulmonary
J84.02

Micromastia N64.82

Micromyelia (congenital) Q06.8

Micropenis Q55.62

Microphakia (congenital) Q12.8

Microphthalmos, microphthalmia
(congenital) Q11.2
due to toxoplasmosis P37.1

Micropsia H53.15

Microscopic polyangiitis
(polyarteritis) M31.7

Microsporidiosis B60.8
intestinal A07.8

Microsporon furfur infestation
B36.0

Microsporosis —see also
Dermatophytosis
nigra B36.1

Microstomia (congenital) Q18.5

Microtia (congenital) (external ear)
Q17.2

Microtropia H50.40

Microvillus inclusion disease
(MVD) (MVID) Q43.8

Micturition
disorder NEC (see also Difficulty,
micturition) R39.198
psychogenic F45.8
frequency R35.0
psychogenic F45.8
hesitancy R39.11
incomplete emptying R39.14
nocturnal R35.1
painful R30.9
dysuria R30.0
psychogenic F45.8
tenesmus R30.1
poor stream R39.12
position dependent R39.192
split stream R39.13
straining R39.16
urgency R39.15

Mid plane —see condition

Middle
ear —see condition
lobe (right) syndrome J98.19

Miescher's elastoma L87.2

Mietens' syndrome Q87.2

Migraine (idiopathic) G43.909
with refractory migraine G43.919
with status migrainosus G43.911
without status migrainosus
G43.919
with aura (acute-onset) (prolonged)
(typical) (without headache)
G43.109
with refractory migraine
G43.119
with status migrainosus
G43.111
without status migrainosus
G43.119
intractable G43.119
with status migrainosus
G43.111
without status migrainosus
G43.119
not intractable G43.109
with status migrainosus
G43.101
without status migrainosus
G43.109
persistent G43.509
with cerebral infarction
G43.609
with refractory migraine
G43.619
with status migrainosus
G43.611
without status
migrainosus G43.619
intractable G43.619
with status migrainosus
G43.611
without status
migrainosus G43.619
not intractable G43.609
with status migrainosus
G43.601
without status
migrainosus G43.609
without refractory migraine
G43.609

Migraine (continued)
with aura (continued)
persistsent (continued)
with cerebral infarction
(continued)
without refractory migraine
(continued)
with status migrainosus
G43.601
without status
migrainosus G43.609
without cerebral infarction
G43.509
with refractory migraine
G43.519
with status migrainosus
G43.511
without status
migrainosus G43.519
intractable G43.519
with status migrainosus
G43.511
without status
migrainosus G43.519
not intractable G43.509
with status migrainosus
G43.501
without status
migrainosus G43.509
without refractory migraine
G43.509
with status migrainosus
G43.501
without status
migrainosus G43.509
without mention of refractory
migraine G43.109
with status migrainosus
G43.101
without status migrainosus
G43.109
abdominal G43.D0
with refractory migraine G43.D1
intractable G43.D1
not intractable G43.D0
without refractory migraine
G43.D0
basilar see Migraine, with aura
classical —see Migraine, with aura
common —see Migraine, without
aura
complicated G43.109
equivalents —see Migraine, with
aura
familiar —see Migraine,
hemiplegic
hemiplegic G43.409
with refractory migraine G43.419
with status migrainosus
G43.411
without status migrainosus
G43.419
intractable G43.419
with status migrainosus
G43.411
without status migrainosus
G43.419
not intractable G43.409
with status migrainosus
G43.401
without status migrainosus
G43.409
without refractory migraine
G43.409
with status migrainosus
G43.401
without status migrainosus
G43.409
intractable G43.919
with status migrainosus
G43.911

Migraine (continued)
  intractable (continued)
    without status migrainosus G43.919
  menstrual G43.829
    with refractory migraine G43.839
      with status migrainosus G43.831
      without status migrainosus G43.839
    intractable G43.839
      with status migrainosus G43.831
      without status migrainosus G43.839
    not intractable 4G43.829
      with status migrainosus G43.821
      without status migrainosus G43.829
    without refractory migraine G43.829
      with status migrainosus G43.821
      without status migrainosus G43.829
  menstrually related —see Migraine, menstrual
  not intractable G43.909
    with status migrainosus G43.901
    without status migrainosus G43.919
  ophthalmoplegic G43.B0
    with refractory migraine G43.B1
    intractable G43.B1
    not intractable G43.B0
    without refractory migraine G43.B0
  persistent aura (with, without) cerebral infarction —see Migraine, with aura, persistent
  preceded or accompanied by transient focal neurological phenomena —see Migraine, with aura
  pre-menstrual —see Migraine, menstrual
  pure menstrual —see Migraine, menstrual
  retinal —see Migraine, with aura
  specified NEC G43.809
    intractable G43.819
      with status migrainosus G43.811
      without status migrainosus G43.819
    not intractable G43.809
      with status migrainosus G43.801
      without status migrainosus G43.809
  sporadic —see Migraine, hemiplegic
  transformed —see Migraine, without aura, chronic
  triggered seizures —see Migraine, with aura
  without aura G43.009
    with refractory migraine G43.019
      with status migrainosus G43.011
      without status migrainosus G43.019
    chronic G43.709
      with refractory migraine G43.719
        with status migrainosus G43.711

Migraine (continued)
  without aura (continued)
    chronic (continued)
      with refractory migraine (continued)
        without status migrainosus G43.719
      intractable
        with status migrainosus G43.711
        without status migrainosus G43.719
      not intractable
        with status migrainosus G43.701
        without status migrainosus G43.709
      without refractory migraine G43.709
        with status migrainosus G43.701
        without status migrainosus G43.709
    intractable
      with status migrainosus G43.011
      without status migrainosus G43.019
    not intractable
      with status migrainosus G43.001
      without status migrainosus G43.009
    without mention of refractory migraine G43.009
      with status migrainosus G43.001
      without status migrainosus G43.009
    without refractory migraine G43.909
      with status migrainosus G43.901
      without status migrainosus G43.919

Migrant, social Z59.0

Migration, anxiety concerning Z60.3

Migratory, migrating —see also condition
  person Z59.0
  testis Q55.29

Mikity-Wilson disease or syndrome P27.0

Mikulicz' disease or syndrome K11.8

Miliaria L74.3
  alba L74.1
  apocrine L75.2
  crystallina L74.1
  profunda L74.2
  rubra L74.0
  tropicalis L74.2

Miliary —see condition

Milium L72.0
  colloid L57.8

Milk
  crust L21.0
  excessive secretion O92.6
  poisoning —see Poisoning, food, noxious
  retention O92.79
  sickness —see Poisoning, food, noxious
  spots I31.0

Milk-alkali disease or syndrome E83.52

Milk-leg (deep vessels) (nonpuerperal) —see Embolism, vein, lower extremity
  complicating pregnancy O22.3-
  puerperal, postpartum, childbirth O87.1

Milkman's disease or syndrome M83.8

Milky urine —see Chyluria

Millard-Gubler (-Foville) **paralysis or syndrome** G46.3

Millar's asthma J38.5

Miller Fisher syndrome G61.0

Mills' disease —see Hemiplegia

Millstone maker's pneumoconiosis J62.8

Milroy's disease (chronic hereditary edema) Q82.0

Minamata disease T56.1

Miners' asthma or lung J60

Minkowski-Chauffard syndrome —see Spherocytosis

Minor —see condition

Minor's disease (hematomyelia) G95.19

Minot's disease (hemorrhagic disease), **newborn** P53

Minot-von Willebrand-Jurgens disease or syndrome (angiohemophilia) D68.0

Minus (and plus) hand (intrinsic) —see Deformity, limb, specified type NEC, forearm

Miosis (pupil) H57.03

Mirizzi's syndrome (hepatic duct stenosis) K83.1

Mirror writing F81.0

Misadventure (of) (prophylactic) (therapeutic) (see also Complications) T88.9
  administration of insulin (by accident) T38.3
  infusion —see Complications, infusion
  local applications (of fomentations, plasters, etc.) T88.9
    burn or scald —see Burn
    specified NEC T88.8
  medical care (early) (late) T88.9
    adverse effect of drugs or chemicals —see Table of Drugs and Chemicals
    burn or scald —see Burn
    specified NEC T88.8
  specified NEC T88.8
  surgical procedure (early) (late) —see Complications, surgical procedure
  transfusion —see Complications, transfusion
  vaccination or other immunological procedure —see Complications, vaccination

Miscarriage O03.9

Misdirection, aqueous H40.83-

Misperception, sleep state F51.02

Misplaced, misplacement
  ear Q17.4
  kidney (acquired) N28.89
    congenital Q63.2
  organ or site, congenital NEC —see Malposition, congenital

Missed
  abortion O02.1
  delivery O36.4

Missing —see also Absence
  string of intrauterine contraceptive device T83.32

Misuse of drugs F19.99

Mitchell's disease (erythromelalgia) I73.81

Mite(s) (infestation) B88.9
  diarrhea B88.0
  grain (itch) B88.0
  hair follicle (itch) B88.0
  in sputum B88.0

Mitral —see condition

Mittelschmerz N94.0

Mixed —see condition

MMN (multifocal motor neuropathy) G61.82

MNGIE (Mitochondrial Neurogastrointestinal Encephalopathy) syndrome E88.49

Mobile, mobility
  cecum Q43.3
  excessive —see Hypermobility
  gallbladder, congenital Q44.1
  kidney N28.89
  organ or site, congenital NEC —see Malposition, congenital

Mobitz heart block (atrioventricular) I44.1

Moebius, Möbius
  disease (ophthalmoplegic migraine) —see Migraine, ophthalmoplegic
  syndrome Q87.0
    congenital oculofacial paralysis (with other anomalies) Q87.0
  ophthalmoplegic migraine —see Migraine, ophthalmoplegic

Moeller's glossitis K14.0

Mohr's syndrome (Types I and II) Q87.0

Mola destruens D39.2

Molar pregnancy O02.0

Molarization of premolars K00.2

Molding, head (during birth) - omit code

Mole (pigmented) —see also Nevus
  blood O02.0
  Breus' O02.0
  cancerous —see Melanoma
  carneous O02.0
  destructive D39.2
  fleshy O02.0
  hydatid, hydatidiform (benign) (complicating pregnancy) (delivered) (undelivered) O01.9
    classical O01.0
    complete O01.0
    incomplete O01.1
    invasive D39.2
    malignant D39.2
    partial O01.1
  intrauterine O02.0
  invasive (hydatidiform) D39.2
  malignant
    meaning
      malignant hydatidiform mole D39.2
      melanoma —see Melanoma
  nonhydatidiform O02.0
  nonpigmented —see Nevus

Mole (continued)
pregnancy NEC O02.0
skin —see Nevus
tubal O00.10-
with intrauterine pregnancy
O00.11-
vesicular —see Mole,
hydatidiform

Molimen, molimina (menstrual)
N94.3

Molluscum contagiosum
(epitheliale) B08.1

Mönckeberg's arteriosclerosis,
disease, or sclerosis —see
Arteriosclerosis, extremities

Mondini's malformation (cochlea)
Q16.5

Mondor's disease I80.8

Monge's disease T70.29

Monilethrix (congenital) Q84.1

Moniliasis (see also Candidiasis)
B37.9
neonatal P37.5

Monitoring (encounter for)
therapeutic drug level Z51.81

Monkey malaria B53.1

Monkeypox B04

Monoarthritis M13.10
ankle M13.17-
elbow M13.12-
foot joint M13.17-
hand joint M13.14-
hip M13.15-
knee M13.16-
shoulder M13.11-
wrist M13.13-

Monoblastic —see condition

Monochromat (ism),
monochromatopsia (acquired)
(congenital) H53.51

Monocytic —see condition

Monocytopenia D72.818

Monocytosis (symptomatic)
D72.821

Monomania —see Psychosis

Mononeuritis G58.9
cranial nerve —see Disorder, nerve,
cranial
femoral nerve G57.2-
lateral
cutaneous nerve of thigh
G57.1-
popliteal nerve G57.3-
lower limb G57.9-
specified nerve NEC G57.8-
medial popliteal nerve G57.4-
median nerve G56.1-
multiplex G58.7
plantar nerve G57.6-
posterior tibial nerve G57.5-
radial nerve G56.3-
sciatic nerve G57.0-
specified NEC G58.8
tibial nerve G57.4-
ulnar nerve G56.2-
upper limb G56.9-
specified nerve NEC G56.8-
vestibular —see subcategory
H93.3

Mononeuropathy G58.9
carpal tunnel syndrome —see
Syndrome, carpal tunnel
diabetic NEC —see E08-E13
with .41

Mononeuropathy (continued)
femoral nerve —see Lesion, nerve,
femoral
ilioinguinal nerve G57.8-
in diseases classified elsewhere
—see category G59
intercostal G58.0
lower limb G57.9-
causalgia —see Causalgia, lower
limb
femoral nerve —see Lesion,
nerve, femoral
meralgia paresthetica
G57.1-
plantar nerve —see Lesion,
nerve, plantar
popliteal nerve —see Lesion,
nerve, popliteal
sciatic nerve —see Lesion,
nerve, sciatic
specified NEC G57.8-
tarsal tunnel syndrome —see
Syndrome, tarsal tunnel
median nerve —see Lesion, nerve,
median
multiplex G58.7
obturator nerve G57.8-
popliteal nerve —see Lesion,
nerve, popliteal
radial nerve —see Lesion, nerve,
radial
saphenous nerve G57.8-
specified NEC G58.8
tarsal tunnel syndrome —see
Syndrome, tarsal tunnel
tuberculous A17.83
ulnar nerve —see Lesion, nerve,
ulnar
upper limb G56.9-
carpal tunnel syndrome —see
Syndrome, carpal tunnel
causalgia —see Causalgia
median nerve —see Lesion,
nerve, median
radial nerve —see Lesion, nerve,
radial
specified site NEC G56.8-
ulnar nerve —see Lesion, nerve,
ulnar

Mononucleosis, infectious
B27.90
with
complication NEC B27.99
meningitis B27.92
polyneuropathy B27.91
cytomegaloviral B27.10
with
complication NEC B27.19
meningitis B27.12
polyneuropathy B27.11
Epstein-Barr (virus) B27.00
with
complication NEC B27.09
meningitis B27.02
polyneuropathy B27.01
gammaherpesviral B27.00
with
complication NEC B27.09
meningitis B27.02
polyneuropathy B27.01
specified NEC B27.80
with
complication NEC B27.89
meningitis B27.82
polyneuropathy B27.81

Monoplegia G83.3-
congenital (cerebral) G80.8
spastic G80.1
embolic (current episode) I63.4-
following

Monoplegia (continued)
following (continued)
cerebrovascular disease
cerebral infarction
lower limb I69.34-
upper limb I69.33-
intracerebral hemorrhage
lower limb I69.14-
upper limb I69.13-
lower limb I69.94-
nontraumatic intracranial
hemorrhage NEC
lower limb I69.24-
upper limb I69.23-
specified disease NEC
lower limb I69.84-
upper limb I69.83-
stroke NOS
lower limb I69.34-
upper limb I69.33-
subarachnoid hemorrhage
lower limb I69.04-
upper limb I69.03-
upper limb I69.93-
hysterical (transient) F44.4
lower limb G83.1-
psychogenic (conversion reaction)
F44.4
thrombotic (current episode)
I63.3-
transient R29.818
upper limb G83.2-

Monorchism, monorchidism
Q55.0

Monosomy (see also Deletion,
chromosome) Q93.9
specified NEC Q93.89
whole chromosome
meiotic nondisjunction Q93.0
mitotic nondisjunction Q93.1
mosaicism Q93.1
X Q96.9

Monster, monstrosity (single)
Q89.7
acephalic Q00.0
twin Q89.4

Monteggia's fracture (-dislocation)
S52.27-

Mooren's ulcer (cornea) —see Ulcer,
cornea, Mooren's

Moore's syndrome —see Epilepsy,
specified NEC

Mooser-Neill reaction A75.2

Mooser's bodies A75.2

Morbidity not stated or unknown
R69

Morbilli —see Measles

Morbus —see also Disease
angelicus, anglorum E55.0
Beigel B36.2
caducus —see Epilepsy
celiacus K90.0
comitialis —see Epilepsy
cordis (see also Disease, heart)
I51.9
valvulorum —see Endocarditis
coxae senilis M16.9
tuberculous A18.02
hemorrhagicus neonatorum P53
maculosus neonatorum P54.5

Morel (-Stewart) (-Morgagni)
syndrome M85.2

Morel-Kraepelin disease —see
Schizophrenia

Morel-Moore syndrome M85.2

Morgagni's
cyst, organ, hydatid, or appendage
female Q50.5
male (epididymal) Q55.4
testicular Q55.29
syndrome M85.2

Morgagni-Stokes-Adams syndrome
I45.9

Morgagni-Stewart-Morel syndrome
M85.2

Morgagni-Turner (-Albright)
syndrome Q96.9

Moria F07.0

Moron (I.Q.50-69) F70

Morphea L94.0

Morphinism (without remission)
F11.20
with remission F11.21

Morphinomania (without remission)
F11.20
with remission F11.21

Morquio (-Ullrich) (-Brailsford)
disease or syndrome —see
Mucopolysaccharidosis

Mortification (dry) (moist) —see
Gangrene

Morton's metatarsalgia (neuralgia)
(neuroma) (syndrome) G57.6-

Morvan's disease or syndrome
G60.8

Mosaicism, mosaic (autosomal)
(chromosomal)
45,X/other cell lines NEC with
abnormal sex chromosome
Q96.4
45,X/46,XX Q96.3
sex chromosome
female Q97.8
lines with various numbers of X
chromosomes Q97.2
male Q98.7
XY Q96.3

Moschowitz' disease M31.1

Mother yaw A66.0

Motion sickness (from travel, any
vehicle) (from roundabouts or
swings) T75.3

Mottled, mottling, teeth (enamel)
(endemic) (nonendemic) K00.3

Mounier-Kuhn syndrome Q32.4
with bronchiectasis J47.9
exacerbation (acute) J47.1
lower respiratory infection
J47.0
acquired J98.09
with bronchiectasis J47.9
with
exacerbation (acute) J47.1
lower respiratory infection
J47.0

Mountain
sickness T70.29
with polycythemia, acquired
(acute) D75.1
tick fever A93.2

Mouse, joint —see Loose, body,
joint
knee M23.4-

Mouth —see condition

Movable
coccyx —see subcategory M53.2
kidney N28.89
congenital Q63.8
spleen D73.89

Movements, dystonic R25.8

Moyamoya disease I67.5

MRSA (Methicillin resistant Staphylococcus aureus) infection A49.02
  as the cause of diseases classified elsewhere B95.62
  sepsis A41.02

MSD (multiple sulfatase deficiency) E75.26

MSSA (Methicillin susceptible Staphylococcus aureus) infection A49.01
  as the cause of diseases classified elsewhere B95.61
  sepsis A41.01

Mucha-Habermann disease L41.0

Mucinosis (cutaneous) (focal) (papular) (reticular erythematous) (skin) L98.5
  oral K13.79

Mucocele
  appendix K38.8
  buccal cavity K13.79
  gallbladder K82.1
  lacrimal sac, chronic H04.43-
  nasal sinus J34.1
  nose J34.1
  salivary gland (any) K11.6
  sinus (accessory) (nasal) J34.1
  turbinate (bone) (middle) (nasal) J34.1
  uterus N85.8

Mucolipidosis
  I E77.1
  II, III E77.0
  IV E75.11

Mucopolysaccharidosis E76.3
  beta-gluduronidase deficiency E76.29
  cardiopathy E76.3 [I52]
  Hunter's syndrome E76.1
  Hurler's syndrome E76.01
  Hurler-Scheie syndrome E76.02
  Maroteaux-Lamy syndrome E76.29
  Morquio syndrome E76.219
    A E76.210
    B E76.211
    classic E76.210
  Sanfilippo syndrome E76.22
  Scheie's syndrome E76.03
  specified NEC E76.29
  type
    I
      Hurler's syndrome E76.01
      Hurler-Scheie syndrome E76.02
      Scheie's syndrome E76.03
    II E76.1
    III E76.22
    IV E76.219
    IVA E76.210
    IVB E76.211
    VI E76.29
    VII E76.29

Mucormycosis B46.5
  cutaneous B46.3
  disseminated B46.4
  gastrointestinal B46.2
  generalized B46.4
  pulmonary B46.0
  rhinocerebral B46.1
  skin B46.3
  subcutaneous B46.3

Mucositis (ulcerative) K12.30
  due to drugs NEC K12.32
  gastrointestinal K92.81

Mucositis (continued)
  mouth (oral) (oropharyngeal) K12.30
    due to antineoplastic therapy K12.31
    due to drugs NEC K12.32
    due to radiation K12.33
    specified NEC K12.39
    viral K12.39
  nasal J34.81
  oral cavity —see Mucositis, mouth
  oral soft tissues —see Mucositis, mouth
  vagina and vulva N76.81

Mucositis necroticans agranulocytica —see Agranulocytosis

Mucous —see also condition
  patches (syphilitic) A51.39
    congenital A50.07

Mucoviscidosis E84.9
  with meconium obstruction E84.11

Mucus
  asphyxia or suffocation —see Asphyxia, mucus
  in stool R19.5
  plug —see Asphyxia, mucus

Muguet B37.0

Mulberry molars (congenital syphilis) A50.52

Müllerian mixed tumor
  specified site —see Neoplasm, malignant, by site
  unspecified site C54.9

Multicystic kidney (development) Q61.4

Multiparity (grand) Z64.1
  affecting management of pregnancy, labor and delivery (supervision only) O09.4-
  requiring contraceptive management —see Contraception

Multipartita placenta O43.19-

Multiple, multiplex —see also condition
  digits (congenital) Q69.9
  endocrine neoplasia —see Neoplasia, endocrine, multiple (MEN)
  personality F44.81

Mumps B26.9
  arthritis B26.85
  complication NEC B26.89
  encephalitis B26.2
  hepatitis B26.81
  meningitis (aseptic) B26.1
  meningoencephalitis B26.2
  myocarditis B26.82
  oophoritis B26.89
  orchitis B26.0
  pancreatitis B26.3
  polyneuropathy B26.84

Mumu —see also Infestation, filarial B74.9 [N51]

Münchhausen's syndrome —see Disorder, factitious

Münchmeyer's syndrome —see Myositis, ossificans, progressiva

Mural —see condition

Murmur (cardiac) (heart) (organic) R01.1
  abdominal R19.15
  aortic (valve) —see Endocarditis, aortic

Murmur (continued)
  benign R01.0
  diastolic —see Endocarditis
  Flint I35.1
  functional R01.0
  Graham Steell I37.1
  innocent R01.0
  mitral (valve) —see Insufficiency, mitral
  nonorganic R01.0
  presystolic, mitral —see Insufficiency, mitral
  pulmonic (valve) I37.8
  systolic R01.1
  tricuspid (valve) I07.9
  valvular —see Endocarditis

Murri's disease (intermittent hemoglobinuria) D59.6

Muscle, muscular —see also condition
  carnitine (palmityltransferase) deficiency E71.314

Musculoneuralgia —see Neuralgia

Mushroom-workers'(pickers') **disease or lung** J67.5

Mushrooming hip —see Derangement, joint, specified NEC, hip

Mutation(s)
  factor V Leiden D68.51
  surfactant, of lung J84.83
  prothrombin gene D68.52

Mutism —see also Aphasia
  deaf (acquired) (congenital) NEC H91.3
  elective (adjustment reaction) (childhood) F94.0
  hysterical F44.4
  selective (childhood) F94.0

MVD (microvillus inclusion disease) Q43.8

MVID (microvillus inclusion disease) Q43.8

Myalgia M79.10
  auxiliary muscles, head and neck M79.12
  epidemic (cervical) B33.0
  mastication muscle M79.11
  site specified NEC M79.18
  traumatic NEC T14.8

Myasthenia G70.9
  congenital G70.2
  cordis —see Failure, heart
  developmental G70.2
  gravis G70.00
    with exacerbation (acute) G70.01
    in crisis G70.01
    neonatal, transient P94.0
    pseudoparalytica G70.00
      with exacerbation (acute) G70.01
      in crisis G70.01
  stomach, psychogenic F45.8
  syndrome
    in
      diabetes mellitus —see E08-E13 with .44
      neoplastic disease (see also Neoplasm) D49.9 [G73.3]
      pernicious anemia D51.0 [G73.3]
      thyrotoxicosis E05.90 [G73.3]
        with thyroid storm E05.91 [G73.3]

Myasthenic M62.81

Mycelium infection B49

Mycetismus —see Poisoning, food, noxious, mushroom

Mycetoma B47.9
  actinomycotic B47.1
  bone (mycotic) B47.9 [M90.80]
  eumycotic B47.0
  foot B47.9
    actinomycotic B47.1
    mycotic B47.0
  madurae NEC B47.9
    mycotic B47.0
  maduromycotic B47.0
  mycotic B47.0
  nocardial B47.1

Mycobacteriosis —see Mycobacterium

Mycobacterium, mycobacterial (infection) A31.9
  anonymous A31.9
  atypical A31.9
    cutaneous A31.1
    pulmonary A31.0
      tuberculous —see Tuberculosis, pulmonary
    specified site NEC A31.8
  avium (intracellulare complex) A31.0
  balnei A31.1
  Battey A31.0
  chelonei A31.8
  cutaneous A31.1
  extrapulmonary systemic A31.8
  fortuitum A31.8
  intracellulare (Battey bacillus) A31.0
  kansasii (yellow bacillus) A31.0
  kakaferifu A31.8
  kasongo A31.8
  leprae (see also Leprosy) A30.9
  luciflavum A31.1
  marinum (M. balnei) A31.1
  nonspecific —see Mycobacterium, atypical
  pulmonary (atypical) A31.0
    tuberculous —see Tuberculosis, pulmonary
  scrofulaceum A31.8
  simiae A31.8
  systemic, extrapulmonary A31.8
  szulgai A31.8
  terrae A31.8
  triviale A31.8
  tuberculosis (human, bovine) —see Tuberculosis
  ulcerans A31.1
  xenopi A31.8

Mycoplasma (M.) **pneumoniae, as cause of disease classified elsewhere** B96.0

Mycosis, mycotic B49
  cutaneous NEC B36.9
  ear B36.9
    in
      aspergillosis B44.89
      candidiasis B37.84
      moniliasis B37.84
  fungoides (extranodal) (solid organ) C84.0-
  mouth B37.0
  nails B35.1
  opportunistic B48.8
  skin NEC B36.9
  specified NEC B48.8
  stomatitis B37.0
  vagina, vaginitis (candidal) B37.3

Mydriasis (pupil) H57.04

Myelatelia Q06.1

Myelinolysis, pontine, central
G37.2

Myelitis (acute) (ascending)
(childhood) (chronic) (descending)
(diffuse) (disseminated)
(idiopathic) (pressure) (progressive)
(spinal cord) (subacute) (*see also*
Encephalitis) G04.91
flaccid G04.89
herpes simplex B00.82
herpes zoster B02.24
in diseases classified elsewhere
G05.4
necrotizing, subacute G37.4
optic neuritis in G36.0
postchickenpox B01.12
postherpetic B02.24
postimmunization G04.02
postinfectious NEC G04.89
postvaccinal G04.02
specified NEC G04.89
syphilitic (transverse) A52.14
toxic G92
transverse (in demyelinating
diseases of central nervous
system)
G37.3
tuberculous A17.82
varicella B01.12

Myeloblastic —*see* condition

Myeloblastoma
granular cell —*see also* Neoplasm,
connective tissue
malignant —*see* Neoplasm,
connective tissue, malignant
tongue D10.1

Myelocele —*see* Spina bifida

Myelocystocele —*see* Spina bifida

Myelocytic —*see* condition

Myelodysplasia D46.9
specified NEC D46.Z
spinal cord (congenital) Q06.1

Myelodysplastic syndrome (*see also*,
Syndrome, myelodysplastic)
D46.9
with
5q deletion D46.C
isolated del (5q) chromosomal
abnormality D46.C
specified NEC D46.Z

Myeloencephalitis —*see*
Encephalitis

Myelofibrosis D75.81
with myeloid metaplasia D47.4
acute C94.4-
idiopathic (chronic) D47.4
primary D47.1
secondary D75.81
in myeloproliferative disease
D47.4

Myelogenous —*see* condition

Myeloid —*see* condition

Myelokathexis D70.9

Myeloleukodystrophy E75.29

Myelolipoma —*see* Lipoma

Myeloma (multiple) C90.0-
monostotic C90.3
plasma cell C90.0-
plasma cell C90.0-
solitary (*see also* Plasmacytoma,
solitary) C90.3-

Myelomalacia G95.89

Myelomatosis C90.0-

Myelomeningitis —*see*
Meningoencephalitis

Myelomeningocele (spinal cord)
—*see* Spina bifida

**Myelo-osteo-musculodysplasia
hereditaria** Q79.8

Myelopathic
anemia D64.89
muscle atrophy —*see* Atrophy,
muscle, spinal
pain syndrome G89.0

Myelopathy (spinal cord) G95.9
drug-induced G95.89
in (due to)
degeneration or displacement,
intervertebral disc NEC
—*see* Disorder, disc, with,
myelopathy
infection —*see* Encephalitis
intervertebral disc disorder
—*see also* Disorder, disc,
with, myelopathy
mercury —*see* subcategory T56.1
neoplastic disease (*see also*
Neoplasm) D49.9 *[G99.2]*
pernicious anemia D51.0 *[G99.2]*
spondylosis —*see* Spondylosis,
with myelopathy NEC
necrotic (subacute) (vascular)
G95.19
radiation-induced G95.89
spondylogenic NEC —*see*
Spondylosis, with myelopathy
NEC
toxic G95.89
transverse, acute G37.3
vascular G95.19
vitamin B12 E53.8 *[G32.0]*

Myelophthisis D61.82

Myeloradiculitis G04.91

Myeloradiculodysplasia (spinal)
Q06.1

Myelosarcoma C92.3-

Myelosclerosis D75.89
with myeloid metaplasia D47.4
disseminated, of nervous system
G35
megakaryocytic D47.4
with myeloid metaplasia D47.4

Myelosis
acute C92.0-
aleukemic C92.9-
chronic D47.1
erythremic (acute) C94.0-
megakaryocytic C94.2-
nonleukemic D72.828
subacute C92.9-

Myiasis (cavernous) B87.9
aural B87.4
creeping B87.0
cutaneous B87.0
dermal B87.0
ear (external) (middle) B87.4
eye B87.2
genitourinary B87.81
intestinal B87.82
laryngeal B87.3
nasopharyngeal B87.3
ocular B87.2
orbit B87.2
skin B87.0
specified site NEC B87.89
traumatic B87.1
wound B87.1

Myoadenoma, prostate —*see*
Hyperplasia, prostate

Myoblastoma
granular cell —*see also* Neoplasm,
connective tissue, benign
malignant —*see* Neoplasm,
connective tissue, malignant
tongue D10.1

Myocardial —*see* condition

Myocardiopathy (congestive)
(constrictive) (familial)
(hypertrophic nonobstructive)
(idiopathic) (infiltrative)
(obstructive) (primary)
(restrictive) (sporadic) (*see also*
Cardiomyopathy) I42.9
alcoholic I42.6
cobalt-beer I42.6
glycogen storage E74.02 *[I43]*
hypertrophic obstructive I42.1
in (due to)
beriberi E51.12
cardiac glycogenosis E74.02
[I43]
Friedreich's ataxia G11.11 *[I43]*
myotonia atrophica G71.11 *[I43]*
progressive muscular dystrophy
G71.09 *[I43]*
obscure (African) I42.8
secondary I42.9
thyrotoxic E05.90 *[I43]*
with storm E05.91 *[I43]*
toxic NEC I42.7

Myocarditis (with arteriosclerosis)
(chronic) (fibroid) (interstitial)
(old) (progressive) (senile) I51.4
with
rheumatic fever (conditions in
I00) I09.0
active —*see* Myocarditis,
acute, rheumatic
inactive or quiescent (with
chorea) I09.0
active I40.9
rheumatic I01.2
with chorea (acute) (rheumatic)
(Sydenham's) I02.0
acute or subacute (interstitial) I40.9
due to
streptococcus (beta-hemolytic)
I01.2
idiopathic I40.1
rheumatic I01.2
with chorea (acute)
(rheumatic) (Sydenham's)
I02.0
specified NEC I40.8
aseptic of newborn B33.22
bacterial (acute) I40.0
Coxsackie (virus) B33.22
diphtheritic A36.81
eosinophilic I40.1
epidemic of newborn (Coxsackie)
B33.22
Fiedler's (acute) (isolated) I40.1
giant cell (acute) (subacute) I40.1
gonococcal A54.83
granulomatous (idiopathic)
(isolated) (nonspecific) I40.1
hypertensive —*see* Hypertension,
heart
idiopathic (granulomatous) I40.1
in (due to)
diphtheria A36.81
epidemic louse-borne typhus
A75.0 *[I41]*
Lyme disease A69.29
sarcoidosis D86.85
scarlet fever A38.1
toxoplasmosis (acquired) B58.81
typhoid A01.02
typhus NEC A75.9 *[I41]*

Myocarditis (continued)
infective I40.0
influenzal —*see* Influenza, with,
myocarditis
isolated (acute) I40.1
meningococcal A39.52
mumps B26.82
nonrheumatic, active I40.9
parenchymatous I40.9
pneumococcal I40.0
rheumatic (chronic) (inactive) (with
chorea) I09.0
active or acute I01.2
with chorea (acute)
(rheumatic) (Sydenham's)
I02.0
rheumatoid —*see* Rheumatoid,
carditis
septic I40.0
staphylococcal I40.0
suppurative I40.0
syphilitic (chronic) A52.06
toxic I40.8
rheumatic —*see* Myocarditis,
acute, rheumatic
tuberculous A18.84
typhoid A01.02
valvular —*see* Endocarditis
virus, viral I40.0
of newborn (Coxsackie) B33.22

Myocardium, myocardial —*see*
condition

Myocardosis —*see*
Cardiomyopathy

Myoclonus, myoclonic, myoclonia
(familial) (essential) (multifocal)
(simplex) G25.3
drug-induced G25.3
epilepsy (*see also* Epilepsy,
generalized, specified NEC)
G40.4-
familial (progressive) G25.3
epileptica G40.409
with status epilepticus G40.401
facial G51.3-
familial progressive G25.3
Friedreich's G25.3
jerks G25.3
massive G25.3
palatal G25.3
pharyngeal G25.3

Myocytolysis I51.5

Myodiastasis —*see* Diastasis,
muscle

Myoendocarditis —*see*
Endocarditis

Myoepithelioma —*see* Neoplasm,
benign, by site

Myofasciitis (acute) —*see* Myositis

Myofibroma —*see also* Neoplasm,
connective tissue, benign
uterus (cervix) (corpus) —*see*
Leiomyoma

Myofibromatosis D48.1
infantile Q89.8

Myofibrosis M62.89
heart —*see* Myocarditis
scapulohumeral —*see* Lesion,
shoulder, specified NEC

Myofibrositis M79.7
scapulohumeral —*see* Lesion,
shoulder, specified NEC

Myoglobulinuria, myoglobinuria
(primary) R82.1

Myokymia, facial G51.4

Myolipoma —*see* Lipoma

Myoma —see also Neoplasm, connective tissue, benign
  malignant —see Neoplasm, connective tissue, malignant
  prostate D29.1
  uterus (cervix) (corpus) —see Leiomyoma

Myomalacia M62.89

Myometritis —see Endometritis

Myometrium —see condition

Myonecrosis, clostridial A48.0

Myopathy G72.9
  acute
    necrotizing G72.81
    quadriplegic G72.81
  alcoholic G72.1
  benign congenital G71.20
  central core G71.29
  centronuclear G71.228
    autosomal (dominant) (recessive) G71.228
    other specified NEC G71.228
  congenital (benign) G71.20
  critical illness G72.81
  distal G71.09
  drug-induced G72.0
  endocrine NEC E34.9 [G73.7]
  extraocular muscles H05.82-
  facioscapulohumeral G71.02
  hereditary G71.9
    specified NEC G71.8
  hyaline body G71.29
  immune NEC G72.49
  in (due to)
    Addison's disease E27.1 [G73.7]
    alcohol G72.1
    amyloidosis E85.0 [G73.7]
    cretinism E00.9 [G73.7]
    Cushing's syndrome E24.9 [G73.7]
    drugs G72.0
    endocrine disease NEC E34.9 [G73.7]
    giant cell arteritis M31.6 [G73.7]
    glycogen storage disease E74.00 [G73.7]
    hyperadrenocorticism E24.9 [G73.7]
    hyperparathyroidism NEC E21.3 [G73.7]
    hypoparathyroidism E20.9 [G73.7]
    hypopituitarism E23.0 [G73.7]
    hypothyroidism E03.9 [G73.7]
    infectious disease NEC B99 [G73.7]
    lipid storage disease E75.6 [G73.7]
    metabolic disease NEC E88.9 [G73.7]
    myxedema E03.9 [G73.7]
    parasitic disease NEC B89 [G73.7]
    polyarteritis nodosa M30.0 [G73.7]
    rheumatoid arthritis —see Rheumatoid, myopathy
    sarcoidosis D86.87
    scleroderma M34.82
    sicca syndrome M35.03
    Sjögren's syndrome M35.03
    systemic lupus erythematosus M32.19
    thyrotoxicosis (hyperthyroidism) E05.90 [G73.7]
      with thyroid storm E05.91 [G73.7]
    toxic agent NEC G72.2
  inflammatory NEC G72.49
  intensive care (ICU) G72.81
  limb-girdle G71.09
  mitochondrial NEC G71.3

Myopathy (continued)
  myosin storage G71.29
  myotubular (centronuclear) G71.220
    X-linked G71.220
  mytonic, proximal (PROMM) G71.11
  nemaline G71.21
  ocular G71.09
  oculopharyngeal G71.09
  of critical illness G72.81
  primary G71.9
    specified NEC G71.8
  progressive NEC G72.89
  proximal myotonic (PROMM) G71.11
  rod (body) G71.21
  scapulohumeral G71.02
  specified NEC G72.89
  toxic G72.2

Myopericarditis —see also Pericarditis
  chronic rheumatic I09.2

Myopia (axial) (congenital) H52.1-
  degenerative (malignant) H44.20
    with
      choroidal neovascularization H44.2A-
      foveoschisis H44.2D-
      macular hole H44.2B-
      retinal detachment H44.2C-
      specified maculopathy NEC H44.2E-
    bilateral H44.23
    left eye H44.22
    right eye H44.21
  malignant (see also Myopia, degenerative) H44.2-
  pernicious (see also Myopia, degenerative) H44.2-
  progressive high (degenerative) (see also Myopia, degenerative) H44.2-

Myosarcoma —see Neoplasm, connective tissue, malignant

Myosis (pupil) H57.03
  stromal (endolymphatic) D39.0

Myositis M60.9
  clostridial A48.0
  due to posture —see Myositis, specified type NEC
  epidemic B33.0
  fibrosa or fibrous (chronic), Volkmann's T79.6
  foreign body granuloma —see Granuloma, foreign body
  in (due to)
    bilharziasis B65.9 [M63.8-]
    cysticercosis B69.81
    leprosy A30.9 [M63.8-]
    mycosis B49 [M63.8-]
    sarcoidosis D86.87
    schistosomiasis B65.9 [M63.8-]
    syphilis
      late A52.78
      secondary A51.49
    toxoplasmosis (acquired) B58.82
    trichinellosis B75 [M63.8-]
    tuberculosis A18.09
  inclusion body [IBM] G72.41
  infective M60.009
    arm M60.002
      left M60.001
      right M60.000
    leg M60.005
      left M60.004
      right M60.003
    lower limb M60.005
      ankle M60.07-
      foot M60.07-

Myositis (continued)
  infective (continued)
    lower limb (continued)
      lower leg M60.06-
      thigh M60.05-
      toe M60.07-
    multiple sites M60.09
    specified site NEC M60.08
    upper limb M60.002
      finger M60.04-
      forearm M60.03-
      hand M60.04-
      shoulder region M60.01-
      upper arm M60.02-
  interstitial M60.10
    ankle M60.17-
    foot M60.17-
    forearm M60.13-
    hand M60.14-
    lower leg M60.16-
    multiple sites M60.19
    shoulder region M60.11-
    specified site NEC M60.18
    thigh M60.15-
    upper arm M60.12-
  mycotic B49 [M63.8-]
  orbital, chronic H05.12-
  ossificans or ossifying (circumscripta) —see also Ossification, muscle, specified NEC
    in (due to)
      burns M61.30
        ankle M61.37-
        foot M61.37-
        forearm M61.33-
        hand M61.34-
        lower leg M61.36-
        multiple sites M61.39
        pelvic region M61.35-
        shoulder region M61.31-
        specified site NEC M61.38
        thigh M61.35-
        upper arm M61.32-
    quadriplegia or paraplegia M61.20
      ankle M61.27-
      foot M61.27-
      forearm M61.23-
      hand M61.24-
      lower leg M61.26-
      multiple sites M61.29
      pelvic region M61.25-
      shoulder region M61.21-
      specified site NEC M61.28
      thigh M61.25-
      upper arm M61.22-
  progressiva M61.10
    ankle M61.17-
    finger M61.14-
    foot M61.17-
    forearm M61.13-
    hand M61.14-
    lower leg M61.16-
    multiple sites M61.19
    pelvic region M61.15-
    shoulder region M61.11-
    specified site NEC M61.18
    thigh M61.15-
    toe M61.17-
    upper arm M61.12-
  traumatica M61.00
    ankle M61.07-
    foot M61.07-
    forearm M61.03-
    hand M61.04-
    lower leg M61.06-
    multiple sites M61.09
    pelvic region M61.05-

Myositis (continued)
  ossificans or ossifying (continued)
    traumatica (continued)
      shoulder region M61.01-
      specified site NEC M61.08
      thigh M61.05-
      upper arm M61.02-
  purulent —see Myositis, infective
  specified type NEC M60.80
    ankle M60.87-
    foot M60.87-
    forearm M60.83-
    hand M60.84-
    lower leg M60.86-
    multiple sites M60.89
    pelvic region M60.85-
    shoulder region M60.81-
    specified site NEC M60.88
    thigh M60.85-
    upper arm M60.82-
  suppurative —see Myositis, infective
  traumatic (old) —see Myositis, specified type NEC

Myospasia impulsiva F95.2

Myotonia (acquisita) (intermittens) M62.89
  atrophica G71.11
  chondrodystrophic G71.13
  congenita (acetazolamide responsive) (dominant) (recessive) G71.12
  drug-induced G71.14
  dystrophica G71.11
  fluctuans G71.19
  levior G71.12
  permanens G71.19
  symptomatic G71.19

Myotonic pupil —see Anomaly, pupil, function, tonic pupil

Myriapodiasis B88.2

Myringitis H73.2-
  with otitis media —see Otitis, media
  acute H73.00-
    bullous H73.01-
    specified NEC H73.09-
  bullous —see Myringitis, acute, bullous
  chronic H73.1-

Mysophobia F40.228

Mytilotoxism —see Poisoning, fish

Myxadenitis labialis K13.0

Myxedema (adult) (idiocy) (infantile) (juvenile) (see also Hypothyroidism) E03.9
  circumscribed E05.90
    with storm E05.91
  coma E03.5
  congenital E00.1
  cutis L98.5
  localized (pretibial) E05.90
    with storm E05.91
  papular L98.5

Myxochondrosarcoma —see Neoplasm, cartilage, malignant

Myxofibroma —see Neoplasm, connective tissue, benign
  odontogenic —see Cyst, calcifying odontogenic

Myxofibrosarcoma —see Neoplasm, connective tissue, malignant

Myxolipoma D17.9

Myxoliposarcoma —see Neoplasm, connective tissue, malignant

Myxoma —see also Neoplasm, connective tissue, benign
  nerve sheath —see Neoplasm, nerve, benign
  odontogenic —see Cyst, calcifying odontogenic

Myxosarcoma —see Neoplasm, connective tissue, malignant

N

Naegeli's
  disease Q82.8
  leukemia, monocytic C93.1-

Naegleriasis (with meningoencephalitis) B60.2

Naffziger's syndrome G54.0

Naga sore —see Ulcer, skin

Nägele's pelvis M95.5
  with disproportion (fetopelvic) O33.0
    causing obstructed labor O65.0

Nail —see also condition
  biting F98.8
  patella syndrome Q87.2

Nanism, nanosomia —see Dwarfism

Nanophyetiasis B66.8

Nanukayami A27.89

Napkin rash L22

Narcolepsy G47.419
  with cataplexy G47.411
  in conditions classified elsewhere G47.429
    with cataplexy G47.421

Narcosis R06.89

Narcotism —see Dependence

NARP (Neuropathy, Ataxia and Retinitis pigmentosa) **syndrome** E88.49

Narrow
  anterior chamber angle H40.03-
  gingival width (of periodontal soft tissue) K05.5
  pelvis —see Contraction, pelvis

Narrowing —see also Stenosis
  artery I77.1
    auditory, internal I65.8
    basilar —see Occlusion, artery, basilar
    carotid —see Occlusion, artery, carotid
    cerebellar —see Occlusion, artery, cerebellar
    cerebral —see Occlusion artery, cerebral
    choroidal —see Occlusion, artery, precerebral, specified NEC
    communicating posterior —see Occlusion, artery, precerebral, specified NEC
    coronary —see also Disease, heart, ischemic, atherosclerotic
      congenital Q24.5
        syphilitic A50.54 [152]
      due to syphilis NEC A52.06
    hypophyseal —see Occlusion, artery, precerebral, specified NEC
    pontine —see Occlusion, artery, precerebral, specified NEC
    precerebral —see Occlusion, artery, precerebral

Narrowing (continued)
  artery (continued)
    vertebral —see Occlusion, artery, vertebral
  auditory canal (external) —see Stenosis, external ear canal
  eustachian tube —see Obstruction, eustachian tube
  eyelid —see Disorder, eyelid function
  larynx J38.6
  mesenteric artery (see also Ischemia, intestine, acute) K55.059
  palate M26.89
  palpebral fissure —see Disorder, eyelid function
  ureter N13.5
    with infection N13.6
  urethra —see Stricture, urethra

Narrowness, abnormal, eyelid Q10.3

Nasal —see condition

Nasolachrymal, nasolacrimal —see condition

Nasopharyngeal —see also condition
  pituitary gland Q89.2
  torticollis M43.6

Nasopharyngitis (acute) (infective) (streptococcal) (subacute) J00
  chronic (suppurative) (ulcerative) J31.1

Nasopharynx, nasopharyngeal —see condition

Natal tooth, teeth K00.6

Nausea (without vomiting) R11.0
  with vomiting R11.2
  gravidarum —see Hyperemesis, gravidarum
  marina T75.3
  navalis T75.3

Navel —see condition

Neapolitan fever —see Brucellosis

Near drowning T75.1

Nearsightedness —see Myopia

Near-syncope R55

Nebula, cornea —see Opacity, cornea

Necator americanus infestation B76.1

Necatoriasis B76.1

Neck —see condition

Necrobiosis R68.89
  lipoidica NEC L92.1
    with diabetes —see E08-E13 with .620

Necrolysis, toxic epidermal L51.2
  due to drug
    correct substance properly administered —see Table of Drugs and Chemicals, by drug, adverse effect
    overdose or wrong substance given or taken —see Table of Drugs and Chemicals, by drug, poisoning

Necrophilia F65.89

Necrosis, necrotic (ischemic) —see also Gangrene
  adrenal (capsule) (gland) E27.49
  amputation stump (surgical) (late) T87.50

Necrosis, necrotic (continued)
  amputation stump (continued)
    arm T87.5-
    leg T87.5-
  antrum J32.0
  aorta (hyaline) —see also Aneurysm, aorta
    cystic medial —see Dissection, aorta
  artery I77.5
  bladder (aseptic) (sphincter) N32.89
  bone —see also Osteonecrosis M87.9
    aseptic or avascular —see Osteonecrosis
      idiopathic M87.00
    ethmoid J32.2
    jaw M27.2
    tuberculous —see Tuberculosis, bone
  brain I67.89
  breast (aseptic) (fat) (segmental) N64.1
  bronchus J98.09
  central nervous system NEC I67.89
  cerebellar I67.89
  cerebral I67.89
  colon (see also Infarct, intestine) K55.049
  cornea H18.89-
  cortical (acute) (renal) N17.1
  cystic medial (aorta) —see Dissection, aorta
  dental pulp K04.1
  esophagus K22.8
  ethmoid (bone) J32.2
  eyelid —see Disorder, eyelid, degenerative
  fat, fatty (generalized) —see also Disorder, soft tissue, specified type NEC
    abdominal wall K65.4
    breast (aseptic) (segmental) N64.1
    localized —see Degeneration, by site, fatty
    mesentery K65.4
    omentum K65.4
    pancreas K86.89
    peritoneum K65.4
    skin (subcutaneous), newborn P83.0
    subcutaneous, due to birth injury P15.6
  gallbladder —see Cholecystitis, acute
  heart —see Infarct, myocardium
  hip, aseptic or avascular —see Osteonecrosis, by type, femur
  intestine (acute) (hemorrhagic) (massive) (see also Infarct, intestine) K55.069
  jaw M27.2
  kidney (bilateral) N28.0
    acute N17.9
    cortical (acute) (bilateral) N17.1
      with ectopic or molar pregnancy O08.4
    medullary (bilateral) (in acute renal failure) (papillary) N17.2
    papillary (bilateral) (in acute renal failure) N17.2
    tubular N17.0
      with ectopic or molar pregnancy O08.4
      complicating
        abortion —see Abortion, by type, complicated by, tubular necrosis

Necrosis, necrotic (continued)
  kidney (continued)
    tubular (continued)
      complicating (continued)
        ectopic or molar pregnancy O08.4
        pregnancy —see Pregnancy, complicated by, diseases of, specified type or system NEC
      following ectopic or molar pregnancy O08.4
      traumatic T79.5
  larynx J38.7
  liver (with hepatic failure) (cell) —see Failure, hepatic
    hemorrhagic, central K76.2
  lung J85.0
  lymphatic gland —see Lymphadenitis, acute
  mammary gland (fat) (segmental) N64.1
  mastoid (chronic) —see Mastoiditis, chronic
  medullary (acute) (renal) N17.2
  mesentery (see also Infarct, intestine) K55.069
    fat K65.4
  mitral valve —see Insufficiency, mitral
  myocardium, myocardial —see Infarct, myocardium
  nose J34.0
  omentum (with mesenteric infarction) (see also Infarct, intestine) K55.069
    fat K65.4
  orbit, orbital —see Osteomyelitis, orbit
  ossicles, ear —see Abnormal, ear ossicles
  ovary N70.92
  pancreas (aseptic) (duct) (fat) K86.89
    acute (infective) —see Pancreatitis, acute
    infective —see Pancreatitis, acute
  papillary (acute) (renal) N17.2
  perineum N90.89
  peritoneum (with mesenteric infarction) (see also Infarct, intestine) K55.069
    fat K65.4
  pharynx J02.9
    in granulocytopenia —see Neutropenia
    Vincent's A69.1
  phosphorus —see subcategory T54.2
  pituitary (gland) E23.0
    postpartum O99.285
    Sheehan O99.285
  pressure —see Ulcer, pressure, by site
  pulmonary J85.0
  pulp (dental) K04.1
  radiation —see Necrosis, by site
  radium —see Necrosis, by site
  renal —see Necrosis, kidney
  sclera H15.89
  scrotum N50.89
  skin or subcutaneous tissue NEC I96
  spine, spinal (column) —see also Osteonecrosis, by type, vertebra
    cord G95.19
  spleen D73.5
  stomach K31.89
  stomatitis (ulcerative) A69.0
  subcutaneous fat, newborn P83.88

Neuritis *(continued)*
cranial nerve *(continued)*
tenth or vagus G52.2
third or oculomotor —*see*
Strabismus, paralytic, third nerve
twelfth or hypoglossal G52.3
Déjérine-Sottas G60.0
diabetic (mononeuropathy) —*see*
E08-E13 with .41
polyneuropathy —*see* E08-E13
with .42
due to
beriberi E51.11
displacement, prolapse or
rupture, intervertebral disc
—*see* Disorder, disc, with,
radiculopathy
herniation, nucleus pulposus
M51.9 *[G55]*
endemic E51.11
facial G51.8
newborn (birth injury) P11.3
general —*see* Polyneuropathy
geniculate ganglion G51.1
due to herpes (zoster) B02.21
gouty (*see also* Gout, by type)
M10.9 *[G63]*
hypoglossal (nerve) G52.3
ilioinguinal (nerve) G57.9-
infectious (multiple) NEC G61.0
interstitial hypertrophic progressive
G60.0
lumbar M54.16
lumbosacral M54.17
multiple —*see also* Polyneuropathy
endemic E51.11
infective, acute G61.0
multiplex endemica E51.11
nerve root —*see* Radiculopathy
oculomotor (nerve) —*see*
Strabismus, paralytic, third nerve
olfactory nerve G52.0
optic (nerve) (hereditary)
(sympathetic) H46.9
with demyelination G36.0
in myelitis G36.0
nutritional H46.2
papillitis —*see* Papillitis, optic
retrobulbar H46.1-
specified type NEC H46.8
toxic H46.3
peripheral (nerve) G62.9
multiple —*see* Polyneuropathy
single —*see* Mononeuritis
pneumogastric (nerve) G52.2
postherpetic, postzoster B02.29
progressive hypertrophic interstitial
G60.0
retrobulbar —*see also* Neuritis,
optic, retrobulbar
in (due to)
late syphilis A52.15
meningococcal infection
A39.82
meningococcal A39.82
syphilitic A52.15
sciatic (nerve) —*see also* Sciatica
due to displacement of
intervertebral disc —*see*
Disorder, disc, with,
radiculopathy
serum (*see also* Reaction, serum)
T80.69
shoulder-girdle G54.5
specified nerve NEC G58.8
spinal (nerve) root —*see*
Radiculopathy
syphilitic A52.15
thenar (median) G56.1-
thoracic M54.14
toxic NEC G62.2

Neuritis *(continued)*
trochlear (nerve) —*see* Strabismus,
paralytic, fourth nerve
vagus (nerve) G52.2

Neuroastrocytoma —*see* Neoplasm,
uncertain behavior, by site

Neuroavitaminosis E56.9 *[G99.8]*

Neuroblastoma
olfactory C30.0
specified site —*see* Neoplasm,
malignant, by site
unspecified site C74.90

Neurochorioretinitis —*see*
Chorioretinitis

Neurocirculatory asthenia F45.8

Neurocysticercosis B69.0

Neurocytoma —*see* Neoplasm,
benign, by site

Neurodermatitis (circumscribed)
(circumscripta) (local) L28.0
atopic L20.81
diffuse (Brocq) L20.81
disseminated L20.81

Neuroencephalomyelopathy, optic
G36.0

Neuroepithelioma —*see also*
Neoplasm, malignant, by site
olfactory C30.0

Neurofibroma —*see also* Neoplasm,
nerve, benign
melanotic —*see* Neoplasm, nerve,
benign
multiple —*see* Neurofibromatosis
plexiform —*see* Neoplasm, nerve,
benign

Neurofibromatosis (multiple)
(nonmalignant) Q85.00
acoustic Q85.02
malignant —*see* Neoplasm, nerve,
malignant
specified NEC Q85.09
type 1 (von Recklinghausen)
Q85.01
type 2 Q85.02

Neurofibrosarcoma —*see* Neoplasm,
nerve, malignant

Neurogenic —*see also* condition
bladder (*see also* Dysfunction
bladder, neuromuscular) N31.9
cauda equina syndrome G83.4
bowel NEC K59.2
heart F45.8

Neuroglioma —*see* Neoplasm,
uncertain behavior, by site

Neurolabyrinthitis (of Dix and
Hallpike) —*see* Neuronitis,
vestibular

Neurolathyrism —*see* Poisoning,
food, noxious, plant

Neuroleprosy A30.9

Neuroma —*see also* Neoplasm,
nerve, benign
acoustic (nerve) D33.3
amputation (stump) (traumatic)
(surgical complication) (late)
T87.3-
arm T87.3-
leg T87.3-
digital (toe) G57.6-
interdigital G58.8
lower limb (toe) G57.8-
upper limb G56.8-
intermetatarsal G57.8-
Morton's G57.6-

Neuroma *(continued)*
nonneoplastic
arm G56.9-
leg G57.9-
lower extremity G57.9-
upper extremity G56.9-
optic (nerve) D33.3
plantar G57.6-
plexiform —*see* Neoplasm, nerve,
benign
surgical (nonneoplastic)
arm G56.9-
leg G57.9-
lower extremity G57.9-
upper extremity G56.9-

Neuromyalgia —*see* Neuralgia

Neuromyasthenia (epidemic)
(postinfectious) G93.3

Neuromyelitis G36.9
ascending G61.0
optica G36.0

Neuromyopathy G70.9
paraneoplastic D49.9 *[G13.0]*

Neuromyotonia (Isaacs) G71.19

Neuronevus —*see* Nevus

Neuronitis G58.9
ascending (acute) G57.2-
vestibular H81.2-

Neuroparalytic —*see* condition

Neuropathy, neuropathic G62.9
acute motor G62.81
alcoholic G62.1
with psychosis —*see* Psychosis,
alcoholic
arm G56.9-
autonomic, peripheral —*see*
Neuropathy, peripheral,
autonomic
axillary G56.9-
bladder N31.9
atonic (motor) (sensory) N31.2
autonomous N31.2
flaccid N31.2
nonreflex N31.2
reflex N31.1
uninhibited N31.0
brachial plexus G54.0
cervical plexus G54.2
chronic
progressive segmentally
demyelinating G62.89
relapsing demyelinating G62.89
Déjérine-Sottas G60.0
diabetic —*see* E08-E13 with .40
mononeuropathy —*see* E08-E13
with .41
polyneuropathy —*see* E08-E13
with .42
entrapment G58.9
iliohypogastric nerve G57.8-
ilioinguinal nerve G57.8-
lateral cutaneous nerve of thigh
G57.1-
median nerve G56.0-
obturator nerve G57.8-
peroneal nerve G57.3-
posterior tibial nerve G57.5-
saphenous nerve G57.8-
ulnar nerve G56.2-
facial nerve G51.9
hereditary G60.9
motor and sensory (types I-IV)
G60.0
sensory G60.8
specified NEC G60.8
hypertrophic G60.0
Charcot-Marie-Tooth G60.0

Neuropathy, neuropathic
(continued)
hypertrophic *(continued)*
-Sottas G60.0
interstitial progressive G60.0
of infancy G60.0
Refsum G60.1
idiopathic G60.9
progressive G60.3
specified NEC G60.8
in association with hereditary
ataxia G60.2
intercostal G58.0
ischemic —*see* Disorder, nerve
Jamaica (ginger) G62.2
leg NEC G57.9-
lower extremity G57.9-
lumbar plexus G54.1
median nerve G56.1-
motor and sensory —*see also*
Polyneuropathy
hereditary (types I-IV) G60.0
multifocal motor (MMN) G61.82
multiple (acute) (chronic) —*see*
Polyneuropathy
optic (nerve) —*see also* Neuritis, optic
ischemic H47.01-
paraneoplastic (sensorial) (Denny
Brown) D49.9 *[G13.0]*
peripheral (nerve) (*see also*
Polyneuropathy) G62.9
autonomic G90.9
idiopathic G90.09
in (due to)
amyloidosis E85.4
[G99.0]
diabetes mellitus —*see*
E08-E13 with .43
endocrine disease NEC
E34.9 *[G99.0]*
gout M10.00 *[G99.0]*
hyperthyroidism E05.90
[G99.0]
with thyroid storm
E05.91 *[G99.0]*
metabolic disease NEC
E88.9 *[G99.0]*
idiopathic G60.9
progressive G60.3
in (due to)
antitetanus serum G62.0
arsenic G62.2
drugs NEC G62.0
lead G62.2
organophosphate compounds
G62.2
toxic agent NEC G62.2
plantar nerves G57.6-
progressive
hypertrophic interstitial G60.0
inflammatory G62.81
radicular NEC —*see*
Radiculopathy
sacral plexus G54.1
sciatic G57.0-
serum G61.1
toxic NEC G62.2
trigeminal sensory G50.8
ulnar nerve G56.2-
uremic N18.9 *[G63]*
vitamin B12 E53.8 *[G63]*
with anemia (pernicious) D51.0
[G63]
due to dietary deficiency
D51.3 *[G63]*

Neurophthisis —*see also* Disorder,
nerve
peripheral, diabetic —*see* E08-E13
with .42

Neuroretinitis —*see* Chorioretinitis

Neuroretinopathy, hereditary optic H47.22

Neurosarcoma —*see* Neoplasm, nerve, malignant

Neurosclerosis —*see* Disorder, nerve

Neurosis, neurotic F48.9
anankastic F42.8
anxiety (state) F41.1
panic type F41.0
asthenic F48.8
bladder F45.8
cardiac (reflex) F45.8
cardiovascular F45.8
character F60.9
colon F45.8
compensation F68.10
compulsive, compulsion F42.8
conversion F44.9
craft F48.8
cutaneous F45.8
depersonalization F48.1
depressive (reaction) (type) F34.1
environmental F48.8
excoriation L98.1
fatigue F48.8
functional —*see* Disorder, somatoform
gastric F45.8
gastrointestinal F45.8
heart F45.8
hypochondriacal F45.21
hysterical F44.9
incoordination F45.8
larynx F45.8
vocal cord F45.8
intestine F45.8
larynx (sensory) F45.8
hysterical F44.4
mixed NEC F48.8
musculoskeletal F45.8
obsessional F42.8
obsessive-compulsive F42.8
occupational F48.8
ocular NEC F45.8
organ —*see* Disorder, somatoform
pharynx F45.8
phobic F40.9
posttraumatic (situational) F43.10
acute F43.11
chronic F43.12
psychasthenic (type) F48.8
railroad F48.8
rectum F45.8
respiratory F45.8
rumination F45.8
sexual F65.9
situational F48.8
social F40.10
generalized F40.11
specified type NEC F48.8
state F48.9
with depersonalization episode F48.1
stomach F45.8
traumatic F43.10
acute F43.11
chronic F43.12
vasomotor F45.8
visceral F45.8
war F48.8

Neurospongioblastosis diffusa Q85.1

Neurosyphilis (arrested) (early) (gumma) (late) (latent) (recurrent) (relapse) A52.3
with ataxia (cerebellar) (locomotor) (spastic) (spinal) A52.19
aneurysm (cerebral) A52.05
arachnoid (adhesive) A52.13

Neurosyphilis (*continued*)
arteritis (any artery) (cerebral) A52.04
asymptomatic A52.2
congenital A50.40
dura (mater) A52.13
general paresis A52.17
hemorrhagic A52.05
juvenile (asymptomatic) (meningeal) A50.40
leptomeninges (aseptic) A52.13
meningeal, meninges (adhesive) A52.13
meningitis A52.13
meningovascular (diffuse) A52.13
optic atrophy A52.15
parenchymatous (degenerative) A52.19
paresis, paretic A52.17
juvenile A50.45
remission in (sustained) A52.3
serological (without symptoms) A52.2
specified nature or site NEC A52.19
tabes, tabetic (dorsalis) A52.11
juvenile A50.45
taboparesis A52.17
juvenile A50.45
thrombosis (cerebral) A52.05
vascular (cerebral) NEC A52.05

Neurothekeoma —*see* Neoplasm, nerve, benign

Neurotic —*see* Neurosis

Neurotoxemia —*see* Toxemia

Neutroclusion M26.211

Neutropenia, neutropenic (chronic) (genetic) (idiopathic) (immune) (infantile) (malignant) (pernicious) (splenic) D70.9
congenital (primary) D70.0
cyclic D70.4
cytoreductive cancer chemotherapy sequela D70.1
drug-induced D70.2
due to cytoreductive cancer chemotherapy D70.1
due to infection D70.3
fever D70.9
neonatal, transitory (isoimmune) (maternal transfer) P61.5
periodic D70.4
secondary (cyclic) (periodic) (splenic) D70.4
drug-induced D70.2
due to cytoreductive cancer chemotherapy D70.1
toxic D70.8

Neutrophilia, hereditary giant D72.0

Nevocarcinoma —*see* Melanoma

Nevus D22.9
achromic —*see* Neoplasm, skin, benign
amelanotic —*see* Neoplasm, skin, benign
angiomatous D18.00
intra-abdominal D18.03
intracranial D18.02
skin D18.01
specified site NEC D18.09
araneus I78.1
balloon cell —*see* Neoplasm, skin, benign
bathing trunk D48.5
blue —*see* Neoplasm, skin, benign
cellular —*see* Neoplasm, skin, benign
giant —*see* Neoplasm, skin, benign

Nevus (*continued*)
blue (*continued*)
Jadassohn's —*see* Neoplasm, skin, benign
malignant —*see* Melanoma
capillary D18.00
intra-abdominal D18.03
intracranial D18.02
skin D18.01
specified site NEC D18.09
cavernous D18.00
intra-abdominal D18.03
intracranial D18.02
skin D18.01
specified site NEC D18.09
cellular —*see* Neoplasm, skin, benign
blue —*see* Neoplasm, skin, benign
choroid D31.3-
comedonicus Q82.5
conjunctiva D31.0-
dermal —*see* Neoplasm, skin, benign
with epidermal nevus —*see* Neoplasm, skin, benign
dysplastic —*see* Neoplasm, skin, benign
eye D31.9-
flammeus Q82.5
hemangiomatous D18.00
intra-abdominal D18.03
intracranial D18.02
skin D18.01
specified site NEC D18.09
iris D31.4-
lacrimal gland D31.5-
lymphatic D18.1
magnocellular
specified site —*see* Neoplasm, benign, by site
unspecified site D31.40
malignant —*see* Melanoma
meaning hemangioma D18.00
intra-abdominal D18.03
intracranial D18.02
skin D18.01
specified site NEC D18.09
mouth (mucosa) D10.30
specified site NEC D10.39
white sponge Q38.6
multiplex Q85.1
non-neoplastic I78.1
oral mucosa D10.30
specified site NEC D10.39
white sponge Q38.6
orbit D31.6-
pigmented
giant (*see also* Neoplasm, skin, uncertain behavior) D48.5
malignant melanoma in —*see* Melanoma
portwine Q82.5
retina D31.2-
retrobulbar D31.6-
sanguineous Q82.5
senile I78.1
skin D22.9
abdominal wall D22.5
ala nasi D22.39
ankle D22.7-
anus, anal D22.5
arm D22.6-
auditory canal (external) D22.2-
auricle (ear) D22.2-
auricular canal (external) D22.2-
axilla, axillary fold D22.5
back D22.5
breast D22.5
brow D22.39
buttock D22.5
canthus (eye) D22.1-

Nevus (*continued*)
skin (*continued*)
cheek (external) D22.39
chest wall D22.5
chin D22.39
ear (external) D22.2-
external meatus (ear) D22.2-
eyebrow D22.39
eyelid (lower) (upper) D22.1-
face D22.30
specified NEC D22.39
female genital organ (external) NEC D28.0
finger D22.6-
flank D22.5
foot D22.7-
forearm D22.6-
forehead D22.39
foreskin D29.0
genital organ (external) NEC
female D28.0
male D29.9
gluteal region D22.5
groin D22.5
hand D22.6-
heel D22.7-
helix D22.2-
hip D22.7-
interscapular region D22.5
jaw D22.39
knee D22.7-
labium (majus) (minus) D28.0
leg D22.7-
lip (lower) (upper) D22.0
lower limb D22.7-
male genital organ (external) D29.9
nail D22.9
finger D22.6-
toe D22.7-
nasolabial groove D22.39
nates D22.5
neck D22.4
nose (external) D22.39
palpebra D22.1-
penis D29.0
perianal skin D22.5
perineum D22.5
pinna D22.2-
popliteal fossa or space D22.7-
prepuce D29.0
pudendum D28.0
scalp D22.4
scrotum D29.4
shoulder D22.6-
submammary fold D22.5
temple D22.39
thigh D22.7-
toe D22.7-
trunk NEC D22.5
umbilicus D22.5
upper limb D22.6-
vulva D28.0
specified site NEC —*see* Neoplasm, by site, benign
spider I78.1
stellar I78.1
strawberry Q82.5
Sutton's benign D22.9
unius lateris Q82.5
Unna's Q82.5
vascular Q82.5
verrucous Q82.5

Newborn (infant) (liveborn) (singleton) Z38.2
acne L70.4
abstinence syndrome P96.1
affected by
abnormalities of membranes P02.9
specified NEC P02.8
abruptio placenta P02.1

237

Newborn (*continued*)
  affected by (*continued*)
    amino-acid metabolic disorder, transitory P74.8
    amniocentesis (while in utero) P00.6
    amnionitis P02.78
    apparent life threatening event (ALTE) R68.13
    bleeding (into)
      cerebral cortex P52.22
      germinal matrix P52.0
      ventricles P52.1
    breech delivery P03.0
    cardiac arrest P29.81
    cardiomyopathy I42.8
      congenital I42.4
    cerebral ischemia P91.0
    Cesarean delivery P03.4
    chemotherapy agents P04.11
    chorioamnionitis P02.78
    cocaine (crack) P04.41
    complications of labor and delivery P03.9
      specified NEC P03.89
    compression of umbilical cord NEC P02.5
    contracted pelvis P03.1
    cyanosis P28.2
    delivery P03.9
      Cesarean P03.4
      forceps P03.2
      vacuum extractor P03.3
    drugs of addiction P04.40
      cocaine P04.41
      hallucinogens P04.42
      specified drug NEC P04.49
    environmental chemicals P04.6
    entanglement (knot) in umbilical cord P02.5
    fetal (intrauterine)
      growth retardation P05.9
      inflammatory response syndrome (FIRS) P02.70
      malnutrition not light or small for gestational age P05.2
    FIRS (fetal inflammatory response syndrome) P02.70
    forceps delivery P03.2
    heart rate abnormalities
      bradycardia P29.12
      intrauterine P03.819
        before onset of labor P03.810
        during labor P03.811
      tachycardia P29.11
    hemorrhage (antepartum) P02.1
      cerebellar (nontraumatic) P52.6
      intracerebral (nontraumatic) P52.4
      intracranial (nontraumatic) P52.9
        specified NEC P52.8
      intraventricular (nontraumatic) P52.3
        grade 1 P52.0
        grade 2 P52.1
        grade 3 P52.21
        grade 4 P52.22
      posterior fossa (nontraumatic) P52.6
      subarachnoid (nontraumatic) P52.5
      subependymal P52.0
        with intracerebral extension P52.22
        with intraventricular extension P52.1
          with enlargment of ventricles P52.21
        without intraventricular extension P52.0

Newborn (*continued*)
  affected by (*continued*)
    hypoxic ischemic encephalopathy [HIE] P91.60
      mild P91.61
      moderate P91.62
      severe P91.63
    induction of labor P03.89
    intestinal perforation P78.0
    intrauterine (fetal) blood loss P50.9
      due to (from)
        cut end of co-twin cord P50.5
        hemorrhage into
          co-twin P50.3
          maternal circulation P50.4
        placenta P50.2
        ruptured cord blood P50.1
        vasa previa P50.0
      specified NEC P50.8
    intrauterine (fetal) hemorrhage P50.9
    intrauterine (in utero) procedure P96.5
    malpresentation (malposition) NEC P03.1
    maternal (complication of) (use of)
      alcohol P04.3
      amphetamines P04.16
      analgesia (maternal) P04.0
      anesthesia (maternal) P04.0
      anticonvulsants P04.13
      antidepressants P04.15
      antineoplastic chemotherapy P04.11
      anxiolytics P04.1A
      blood loss P02.1
      cannabis P04.81
      circulatory disease P00.3
      condition P00.9
        specified NEC P00.89
      cytotoxic drugs P04.12
      delivery P03.9
        Cesarean P03.4
        forceps P03.2
        vacuum extractor P03.3
      diabetes mellitus (pre-existing) P70.1
      disorder P00.9
        specified NEC P00.89
      drugs (addictive) (illegal) NEC P04.49
      ectopic pregnancy P01.4
      gestational diabetes P70.0
      hemorrhage P02.1
      hypertensive disorder P00.0
      incompetent cervix P01.0
      infectious disease P00.2
      injury P00.5
      labor and delivery P03.9
      malpresentation before labor P01.7
      maternal death P01.6
      medical procedure P00.7
      medication P04.19
        specified type NEC P04.18
      multiple pregnancy P01.5
      nutritional disorder P00.4
      oligohydramnios P01.2
      opiates P04.14
        administered for procedures during pregnancy or labor and delivery P04.0
      parasitic disease P00.2
      periodontal disease P00.81
      placenta previa P02.0
      polyhydramnios P01.3
      precipitate delivery P03.5

Newborn (*continued*)
  affected by (*continued*)
    maternal (*continued*)
      pregnancy P01.9
        specified P01.8
      premature rupture of membranes P01.1
      renal disease P00.1
      respiratory disease P00.3
      sedative-hypnotics P04.17
      surgical procedure P00.6
      tranquilizers administered for procedures during pregnancy or labor and delivery P04.0
      urinary tract disease P00.1
      uterine contraction (abnormal) P03.6
    meconium peritonitis P78.0
    medication (legal) (maternal use) (prescribed) P04.19
    membrane abnormalities P02.9
      specified NEC P02.8
    membranitis P02.78
    methamphetamine(s) P04.49
    mixed metabolic and respiratory acidosis P84
    neonatal abstinence syndrome P96.1
    noxious substances transmitted via placenta or breast milk P04.9
      cannabis P04.81
      specified NEC P04.89
    nutritional supplements P04.5
    placenta previa P02.0
    placental
      abnormality (functional) (morphological) P02.20
        specified NEC P02.29
      dysfunction P02.29
      infarction P02.29
      insufficiency P02.29
      separation NEC P02.1
      transfusion syndromes P02.3
    placentitis P02.78
    precipitate delivery P03.5
    prolapsed cord P02.4
    respiratory arrest P28.81
    slow intrauterine growth P05.9
    tobacco P04.2
    twin to twin transplacental transfusion P02.3
    umbilical cord (tightly) around neck P02.5
    umbilical cord condition P02.60
      short cord P02.69
      specified NEC P02.69
    uterine contractions (abnormal) P03.6
    vasa previa P02.69
      from intrauterine blood loss P50.0
  apnea P28.4
    primary P28.3
    obstructive P28.4
    sleep (central) (obstructive) (primary) P28.3
  born in hospital Z38.00
    by cesarean Z38.01
  born outside hospital Z38.1
  breast buds P96.89
  breast engorgement P83.4
  check-up —*see* Newborn, examination
  convulsion P90
  dehydration P74.1
  examination
    8 to 28 days old Z00.111
    under 8 days old Z00.110
  fever P81.9
    environmentally-induced P81.0

Newborn (*continued*)
  hyperbilirubinemia P59.9
    of prematurity P59.0
  hypernatremia P74.21
  hyponatremia P74.22
  infection P39.9
    candidal P37.5
    specified NEC P39.8
    urinary tract P39.3
  jaundice P59.9
    due to
      breast milk inhibitor P59.3
      hepatocellular damage P59.20
        specified NEC P59.29
      preterm delivery P59.0
    of prematurity P59.0
    specified NEC P59.8
  late metabolic acidosis P74.0
  mastitis P39.0
    infective P39.0
    noninfective P83.4
  multiple born NEC Z38.8
    born in hospital Z38.68
      by cesarean Z38.69
    born outside hospital Z38.7
  omphalitis P38.9
    with mild hemorrhage P38.1
    without hemorrhage P38.9
  post-term P08.21
  prolonged gestation (over 42 completed weeks) P08.22
  quadruplet Z38.8
    born in hospital Z38.63
      by cesarean Z38.64
    born outside hospital Z38.7
  quintuplet Z38.8
    born in hospital Z38.65
      by cesarean Z38.66
    born outside hospital Z38.7
  seizure P90
  sepsis (congenital) P36.9
    due to
      anaerobes NEC P36.5
      Escherichia coli P36.4
      Staphylococcus P36.30
        aureus P36.2
        specified NEC P36.39
      Streptococcus P36.10
        group B P36.0
        specified NEC P36.19
    specified NEC P36.8
  triplet Z38.8
    born in hospital Z38.61
      by cesarean Z38.62
    born outside hospital Z38.7
  twin Z38.5
    born in hospital Z38.30
      by cesarean Z38.31
    born outside hospital Z38.4
  vomiting P92.09
    bilious P92.01
  weight check Z00.111

Newcastle conjunctivitis or disease B30.8

Nezelof's syndrome (pure alymphocytosis) D81.4

Niacin (amide) **deficiency** E52

Nicolas (-Durand)-**Favre disease** A55

Nicotine —*see* Tobacco

Nicotinic acid deficiency E52

Niemann-Pick disease or syndrome E75.249
  specified NEC E75.248
  type
    A E75.240
    B E75.241
    C E75.242
    D E75.243

Night
blindness —*see* Blindness, night
sweats R61
terrors (child) F51.4

Nightmares (REM sleep type) F51.5

NIHSS (National Institutes of Health Stroke Scale) score R29.7-

Nipple —*see* condition

Nisbet's chancre A57

Nishimoto (-Takeuchi) **disease** I67.5

Nitritoid crisis or reaction —*see* Crisis, nitritoid

Nitrosohemoglobinemia D74.8

Njovera A65

Nocardiosis, nocardiasis A43.9
cutaneous A43.1
lung A43.0
pneumonia A43.0
pulmonary A43.0
specified site NEC A43.8

Nocturia R35.1
psychogenic F45.8

Nocturnal —*see* condition

Nodal rhythm I49.8

Node(s) —*see also* Nodule
Bouchard's (with arthropathy) M15.2
Haygarth's M15.8
Heberden's (with arthropathy) M15.1
larynx J38.7
lymph —*see* condition
milker's B08.03
Osler's I33.0
Schmorl's —*see* Schmorl's disease
singer's J38.2
teacher's J38.2
tuberculous —*see* Tuberculosis, lymph gland
vocal cord J38.2

Nodule(s), **nodular**
actinomycotic —*see* Actinomycosis
breast NEC (*see also* Lump, breast) N63.0
colloid (cystic), thyroid E04.1
cutaneous —*see* Swelling, localized
endometrial (stromal) D26.1
Haygarth's M15.8
inflammatory —*see* Inflammation
juxta-articular
syphilitic A52.77
yaws A66.7
larynx J38.7
lung, solitary (subsegmental branch of the bronchial tree) R91.1
multiple R91.8
milker's B08.03
prostate N40.2
with lower urinary tract symptoms (LUTS) N40.3
without lower urinary tract symtpoms (LUTS) N40.2
pulmonary, solitary (subsegmental branch of the bronchial tree) R91.1
retrocardiac R09.89
rheumatoid M06.30
ankle M06.37-
elbow M06.32-
foot joint M06.37-
hand joint M06.34-
hip M06.35-
knee M06.36-
multiple site M06.39
shoulder M06.31-

Nodule(s), **nodular** (*continued*)
rheumatoid (*continued*)
vertebra M06.38
wrist M06.33-
scrotum (inflammatory) N49.2
singer's J38.2
solitary, lung (subsegmental branch of the bronchial tree) R91.1
multiple R91.8
subcutaneous —*see* Swelling, localized
teacher's J38.2
thyroid (cold) (gland) (nontoxic) E04.1
with thyrotoxicosis E05.20
with thyroid storm E05.21
toxic or with hyperthyroidism E05.20
with thyroid storm E05.21
vocal cord J38.2

Noma (gangrenous) (hospital) (infective) A69.0
auricle I96
mouth A69.0
pudendi N76.89
vulvae N76.89

Nomad, nomadism Z59.0

NOMID (neonatal onset multisystemic inflammatory disorder) M04.2

Nonadherence to medical treatment Z91.19

Nonautoimmune hemolytic anemia D59.4
drug-induced D59.2

Nonclosure —*see also* Imperfect, closure
ductus arteriosus (Botallo's) Q25.0
foramen
botalli Q21.1
ovale Q21.1

Noncompliance Z91.19
with
dietary regimen Z91.11
dialysis Z91.15
medical treatment Z91.19
medication regimen NEC Z91.14
underdosing (*see also* Table of Drugs and Chemicals, categories T36-T50, with final character 6) Z91.14
intentional NEC Z91.128
due to financial hardship of patient Z91.120
unintentional NEC Z91.138
due to patient's age related debility Z91.130
renal dialysis Z91.15

Nondescent (congenital) —*see also* Malposition, congenital
cecum Q43.3
colon Q43.3
testicle Q53.9
bilateral Q53.20
abdominal Q53.211
perineal Q53.22
unilateral Q53.10
abdominal Q53.111
perineal Q53.12

Nondevelopment
brain Q02
part of Q04.3
heart Q24.8
organ or site, congenital NEC —*see* Hypoplasia

Nonengagement
head NEC O32.4
in labor, causing obstructed labor O64.8

Nonexanthematous tick fever A93.2

Nonexpansion, lung (newborn) P28.0

Nonfunctioning
cystic duct (*see also* Disease, gallbladder) K82.8
gallbladder (*see also* Disease, gallbladder) K82.8
kidney N28.9
labyrinth H83.2

Non-Hodgkin lymphoma NEC —*see* Lymphoma, non-Hodgkin

Non-working side interference M26.56

Nonimplantation, ovum N97.2

Noninsufflation, fallopian tube N97.1

Non-ketotic hyperglycinemia E72.51

Nonne-Milroy syndrome Q82.0

Nonovulation N97.0

Nonpatent fallopian tube N97.1

Non-palpable testicle(s)
bilateral R39.84
unilateral R39.83

Nonpneumatization, lung NEC P28.0

Nonrotation —*see* Malrotation

Nonsecretion, urine —*see* Anuria

Nonunion
fracture —*see* Fracture, by site
joint, following fusion or arthrodesis M96.0
organ or site, congenital NEC —*see* Imperfect, closure
symphysis pubis, congenital Q74.2

Nonvisualization, gallbladder R93.2

Nonvital, nonvitalized tooth K04.99

Noonan's syndrome Q87.19

Normocytic anemia (infectional) **due to blood loss** (chronic) D50.0
acute D62

Norrie's disease (congenital) Q15.8

North American blastomycosis B40.9

Norwegian itch B86

Nose, nasal —*see* condition

Nosebleed R04.0

Nose-picking F98.8

Nosomania F45.21

Nosophobia F45.22

Nostalgia F43.20

Notch of iris Q13.2

Notching nose, congenital (tip) Q30.2

Nothnagel's
syndrome —*see* Strabismus, paralytic, third nerve
vasomotor acroparesthesia I73.89

Novy's relapsing fever A68.9
louse-borne A68.0
tick-borne A68.1

Noxious
foodstuffs, poisoning by —*see* Poisoning, food, noxious, plant
substances transmitted through placenta or breast milk P04.9

Nucleus pulposus —*see* condition

Numbness R20.0

Nuns' knee —*see* Bursitis, prepatellar

Nursemaid's elbow S53.03-

Nutcracker esophagus K22.4

Nutmeg liver K76.1

Nutrient element deficiency E61.9
specified NEC E61.8

Nutrition deficient or insufficient (*see also* Malnutrition) E46
due to
insufficient food T73.0
lack of
care (child) T76.02
adult T76.01
food T73.0

Nutritional stunting E45

Nyctalopia (night blindness) —*see* Blindness, night

Nycturia R35.1
psychogenic F45.8

Nymphomania F52.8

Nystagmus H55.00
benign paroxysmal —*see* Vertigo, benign paroxysmal
central positional H81.4
congenital H55.01
dissociated H55.04
latent H55.02
miners' H55.09
positional
benign paroxysmal H81.4
central H81.4
specified form NEC H55.09
visual deprivation H55.03

O

Obermeyer's relapsing fever (European) A68.0

Obesity E66.9
with alveolar hypoventilation E66.2
adrenal E27.8
complicating
childbirth O99.214
pregnancy O99.21-
puerperium O99.215
constitutional E66.8
dietary counseling and surveillance Z71.3
drug-induced E66.1
due to
drug E66.1
excess calories E66.09
morbid E66.01
severe E66.01
endocrine E66.8
endogenous E66.8
exogenous E66.09
familial E66.8
glandular E66.8
hypothyroid —*see* Hypothyroidism
hypoventilation syndrome (OHS) E66.2
morbid E66.01
with
alveolar hypoventilation E66.2
obesity hypoventilation syndrome (OHS) E66.2
due to excess calories E66.01
nutritional E66.09
pituitary E23.6
severe E66.01
specified type NEC E66.8

Oblique —*see* condition

Obliteration
appendix (lumen) K38.8
artery I77.1
bile duct (noncalculous) K83.1
common duct (noncalculous) K83.1
cystic duct —*see* Obstruction,
   gallbladder
disease, arteriolar I77.1
endometrium N85.8
eye, anterior chamber —*see*
   Disorder, globe, hypotony
fallopian tube N97.1
lymphatic vessel I89.0
   due to mastectomy I97.2
organ or site, congenital NEC
   —*see* Atresia, by site
ureter N13.5
   with infection N13.6
urethra —*see* Stricture, urethra
vein I87.8
vestibule (oral) K08.89

Observation (following) (for)
(without need for further medical
care) Z04.9
accident NEC Z04.3
   at work Z04.2
   transport Z04.1
adverse effect of drug Z03.6
alleged rape or sexual assault
   (victim), ruled out
   adult Z04.41
   child Z04.42
criminal assault Z04.89
development state
   adolescent Z00.3
   period of rapid growth in
      childhood Z00.2
   puberty Z00.3
disease, specified NEC Z03.89
following work accident Z04.2
forced sexual exploitation Z04.81
forced labor exploitation Z04.82
growth and development state
   —*see* Observation, development
   state
injuries (accidental) NEC —*see*
   also Observation, accident
newborn (for)
   suspected condition, related to
      exposure from the mother or
      birth process —*see* Newborn,
      affected by, maternal
      ruled out Z05.9
         cardiac Z05.0
         connective tissue Z05.73
         gastrointestinal Z05.5
         genetic Z05.41
         genitourinary Z05.6
         immunologic Z05.43
         infectious Z05.1
         metabolic Z05.42
         mesculoskeletal Z05.72
         neurological Z05.2
         respiratory Z05.3
         skin and subcutaneous
            tissue Z05.71
         specified condition NEC
            Z05.8
postpartum
   immediately after delivery Z39.0
   routine follow-up Z39.2
pregnancy (normal) (without
   complication) Z34.9-
   high risk O09.9-
suicide attempt, alleged NEC
   Z03.89
   self-poisoning Z03.6
suspected, ruled out —*see also*
   Suspected condition, ruled out

Observation (continued)
suspected, ruled out (continued)
abuse, physical
   adult Z04.71
   child Z04.72
accident at work Z04.2
adult battering victim Z04.71
child battering victim Z04.72
condition NEC Z03.89
   newborn (see also
      Observation, newborn (for),
      suspected condition, ruled
      out) Z05.9
drug poisoning or adverse effect
   Z03.6
exposure (to)
   anthrax Z03.810
   biological agent NEC Z03.818
   foreign body
      aspirated (inhaled) Z03.822
      ingested Z03.821
      inserted (injected), in (eye)
         (orifice) (skin) Z03.823
inflicted injury NEC Z04.89
suicide attempt, alleged Z03.89
   self-poisoning Z03.6
toxic effects from ingested
   substance (drug) (poison) Z03.6
toxic effects from ingested
   substance (drug) (poison) Z03.6

Obsession, obsessional state F42.8
mixed thoughts and acts F42.2

**Obsessive-compulsive neurosis or
reaction** F42.8

Obstetric embolism, septic —*see*
Embolism, obstetric, septic

Obstetrical trauma (complicating
delivery) O71.9
with or following ectopic or molar
   pregnancy O08.6
specified type NEC O71.89

Obstipation —*see* Constipation

**Obstruction, obstructed,
obstructive**
airway J98.8
   with
      allergic alveolitis J67.9
      asthma J45.909
         with
            exacerbation (acute)
               J45.901
            status asthmaticus
               J45.902
      bronchiectasis J47.9
         with
            exacerbation (acute)
               J47.1
            lower respiratory
               infection J47.0
      bronchitis (chronic) J44.9
      emphysema J43.9
   chronic J44.9
      with
         allergic alveolitis —*see*
            Pneumonitis,
            hypersensitivity
         bronchiectasis J47.9
            with
               exacerbation (acute)
                  J47.1
               lower respiratory
                  infection J47.0
   due to
      foreign body —*see* Foreign
         body, by site, causing
         asphyxia
      inhalation of fumes or vapors
         J68.9
      laryngospasm J38.5

**Obstruction, obstructed,
obstructive** (continued)
ampulla of Vater K83.1
aortic (heart) (valve) —*see*
   Stenosis, aortic
aortoiliac I74.09
aqueduct of Sylvius G91.1
   congenital Q03.0
      with spina bifida —*see*
         Spina bifida, by site, with
         hydrocephalus
Arnold-Chiari —*see* Arnold-Chiari
   disease
artery (see also Atherosclerosis,
   artery) I70.9
   basilar (complete) (partial) —*see*
      Occlusion, artery, basilar
   carotid (complete) (partial) —*see*
      Occlusion, artery, carotid
   cerebellar —*see* Occlusion,
      artery, cerebellar
   cerebral (anterior) (middle)
      (posterior) —*see* Occlusion,
      artery, cerebral
   precerebral —*see* Occlusion,
      artery, precerebral
   renal N28.0
   retinal NEC —*see* Occlusion,
      artery, retina
   stent —*see* Restenosis, stent
   vertebral (complete) (partial) —
      see Occlusion, artery, vertebral
band (intestinal) (see also
   Obstruction, intestine, specified
   NEC) K56.699
bile duct or passage (common)
   (hepatic) (noncalculous) K83.1
   with calculus K80.51
   congenital (causing jaundice)
      Q44.3
biliary (duct) (tract) K83.1
   gallbladder K82.0
bladder-neck (acquired) N32.0
   congenital Q64.31
   due to hyperplasia (hypertrophy)
      of prostate —*see* Hyperplasia,
      prostate
bowel —*see* Obstruction, intestine
bronchus J98.09
canal, ear —*see* Stenosis, external
   ear canal
cardia K22.2
caval veins (inferior) (superior) I87.1
cecum —*see* Obstruction, intestine
circulatory I99.8
colon —*see* Obstruction, intestine
common duct (noncalculous) K83.1
coronary (artery) —*see* Occlusion,
   coronary
cystic duct —*see also* Obstruction,
   gallbladder
   with calculus K80.21
device, implant or graft (see also
   Complications, by site and type,
   mechanical) T85.698
   arterial graft NEC —*see*
      Complication, cardiovascular
      device, mechanical, vascular
   catheter NEC T85.628
      cystostomy T83.090
      dialysis (renal) T82.49
         intraperitoneal T85.691
      Hopkins T83.098
      ileostomy T83.098
      infusion NEC T82.594
         spinal (epidural) (subdural)
            T85.690
      nephrostomy T83.092
      urethral indwelling T83.091
      urinary T83.098
      urostomy T83.098

**Obstruction, obstructed,
obstructive** (continued)
device, implant or graft (continued)
   due to infection T85.79
   gastrointestinal —*see*
      Complications, prosthetic
      device, mechanical,
      gastrointestinal device
   genital NEC T83.498
      intrauterine contraceptive
         device T83.39
      penile prosthesis (cylinder)
         (implanted) (pump)
         (resevoir) T83.490
      testicular prosthesis T83.491
   heart NEC —*see* Complication,
      cardiovascular device,
      mechanical
   joint prosthesis —*see*
      Complications, joint
      prosthesis, mechanical,
      specified NEC, by site
   orthopedic NEC —*see*
      Complication, orthopedic,
      device, mechanical
   specified NEC T85.628
   urinary NEC —*see also*
      Complication, genitourinary,
      device, urinary, mechanical
      graft T83.29
   vascular NEC —*see*
      Complication, cardiovascular
      device, mechanical
   ventricular intracranial shunt
      T85.09
due to foreign body accidentally
   left in operative wound T81.529
duodenum K31.5
ejaculatory duct N50.89
esophagus K22.2
eustachian tube (complete) (partial)
   H68.10-
   cartilagenous (extrinsic) H68.13-
   intrinsic H68.12-
   osseous H68.11-
fallopian tube (bilateral) N97.1
fecal K56.41
   with hernia —*see* Hernia, by
      site, with obstruction
foramen of Monro (congenital)
   Q03.8
   with spina bifida —*see*
      Spina bifida, by site, with
      hydrocephalus
foreign body —*see* Foreign body
gallbladder K82.0
   with calculus, stones K80.21
   congenital Q44.1
gastric outlet K31.1
gastrointestinal —*see* Obstruction,
   intestine
hepatic K76.89
   duct (noncalculous) K83.1
hepatobiliary K83.1
ileum —*see* Obstruction, intestine
iliofemoral (artery) I74.5
intestine K56.609
   complete K56.601
   incomplete K56.600
   partial K56.600
   with
      adhesions (intestinal)
         (peritoneal) K56.50
      complete K56.52
      incomplete K56.51
      partial K56.51
   adynamic K56.0
   by gallstone K56.3
   congenital (small) Q41.9
      large Q42.9
         specified part NEC Q42.8

Obstruction, obstructed, obstructive *(continued)*
intestine *(continued)*
  neurogenic K56.0
    Hirschsprung's disease or megacolon Q43.1
  newborn P76.9
    due to
      fecaliths P76.8
      inspissated milk P76.2
      meconium (plug) P76.0
        in mucoviscidosis E84.11
      specified NEC P76.8
  postoperative K91.30
    complete K91.32
    incomplete K91.31
    partial K91.31
  reflex K56.0
  specified NEC K56.699
    complete K56.691
    incomplete K56.690
    partial K56.690
  volvulus K56.2
intracardiac ball valve prosthesis T82.09
jejunum —*see* Obstruction, intestine
joint prosthesis —*see* Complications, joint prosthesis, mechanical, specified NEC, by site
kidney (calices) N28.89
labor —*see* Delivery
lacrimal (passages) (duct)
  by
    dacryolith —*see* Dacryolith
    stenosis —*see* Stenosis, lacrimal
  congenital Q10.5
  neonatal H04.53-
lacrimonasal duct —*see* Obstruction, lacrimal
lacteal, with steatorrhea K90.2
laryngitis —*see* Laryngitis
larynx NEC J38.6
  congenital Q31.8
lung J98.4
  disease, chronic J44.9
lymphatic I89.0
meconium (plug)
  newborn P76.0
    due to fecaliths P76.0
    in mucoviscidosis E84.11
mitral —*see* Stenosis, mitral
nasal J34.89
nasolacrimal duct —*see also* Obstruction, lacrimal
  congenital Q10.5
nasopharynx J39.2
nose J34.89
organ or site, congenital NEC —*see* Atresia, by site
pancreatic duct K86.89
parotid duct or gland K11.8
pelviureteral junction N13.5
  with hydronephrosis N13.0
  congenital Q62.39
pharynx J39.2
portal (circulation) (vein) I81
prostate —*see also* Hyperplasia, prostate
  valve (urinary) N32.0
pulmonary valve (heart) I37.0
pyelonephritis (chronic) N11.1
pylorus
  adult K31.1
  congenital or infantile Q40.0
rectosigmoid —*see* Obstruction, intestine
rectum K62.4

Obstruction, obstructed, obstructive *(continued)*
renal N28.89
  outflow N13.8
  pelvis, congenital Q62.39
respiratory J98.8
  chronic J44.9
retinal (vessels) H34.9
salivary duct (any) K11.8
  with calculus K11.5
sigmoid —*see* Obstruction, intestine
sinus (accessory) (nasal) J34.89
Stensen's duct K11.8
stomach NEC K31.89
  acute K31.0
  congenital Q40.2
  due to pylorospasm K31.3
submandibular duct K11.8
submaxillary gland K11.8
  with calculus K11.5
thoracic duct I89.0
thrombotic —*see* Thrombosis
trachea J39.8
tracheostomy airway J95.03
tricuspid (valve) —*see* Stenosis, tricuspid
upper respiratory, congenital Q34.8
ureter (functional) (pelvic junction) NEC N13.5
  with
    hydronephrosis N13.1
      with infection N13.6
    pyelonephritis (chronic) N11.1
  congenital Q62.39
  due to calculus —*see* Calculus, ureter
urethra NEC N36.8
  congenital Q64.39
urinary (moderate) N13.9
  due to hyperplasia (hypertrophy) of prostate —*see* Hyperplasia, prostate
  organ or tract (lower) N13.9
  prostatic valve N32.0
  specified NEC N13.8
uropathy N13.9
uterus N85.8
vagina N89.5
valvular —*see* Endocarditis
vein, venous I87.1
  caval (inferior) (superior) I87.1
  thrombotic —*see* Thrombosis
vena cava (inferior) (superior) I87.1
vesical NEC N32.0
vesicourethral orifice N32.0
  congenital Q64.31
vessel NEC I99.8
  stent —*see* Restenosis, stent

Obturator —*see* condition

Occlusal wear, teeth K03.0

Occlusio pupillae —*see* Membrane, pupillary

Occlusion, occluded
anus K62.4
  congenital Q42.3
    with fistula Q42.2
aortoiliac (chronic) I74.09
aqueduct of Sylvius G91.1
  congenital Q03.0
    with spina bifida —*see* Spina bifida, by site, with hydrocephalus
artery (*see also* Atherosclerosis, artery) I70.9
  auditory, internal I65.8
  basilar I65.1
    with
      infarction I63.22

Occlusion, occluded *(continued)*
artery *(continued)*
  basilar *(continued)*
    with *(continued)*
      infarction *(continued)*
        due to
          embolism I63.12
          thrombosis I63.02
  brain or cerebral I66.9
    with infarction (due to) I63.5-
      embolism I63.4-
      thrombosis I63.3-
  carotid I65.2-
    with
      infarction I63.23-
        due to
          embolism I63.13-
          thrombosis I63.03-
  cerebellar (anterior inferior) (posterior inferior) (superior) I66.3
    with infarction I63.54-
      due to
        embolism I63.44-
        thrombosis I63.34-
  cerebral I66.9
    with infarction I63.50
      due to
        embolism I63.40
          specified NEC I63.49
        thrombosis I63.30
          specified NEC I63.39
    anterior I66.1-
      with infarction I63.52-
        due to
          embolism I63.42-
          thrombosis I63.32-
    middle I66.0-
      with infarction I63.51-
        due to
          embolism I63.41-
          thrombosis I63.31-
    posterior I66.2-
      with infarction I63.53-
        due to
          embolism I63.43-
          thrombosis I63.33-
    specified NEC I66.8
      with infarction I63.59
        due to
          embolism I63.4-
          thrombosis I63.3-
  choroidal (anterior) —*see* Occlusion, artery, precerebral, specified NEC
  communicating posterior —*see* Occlusion, artery, precerebral, specified NEC
  complete
    coronary I25.82
    extremities I70.92
  coronary (acute) (thrombotic) (without myocardial infarction) I24.0
    with myocardial infarction —*see* Infarction, myocardium
    chronic total I25.82
    complete I25.82
    healed or old I25.2
    total (chronic) I25.82
  hypophyseal —*see* Occlusion, artery, precerebral, specified NEC
  iliac I74.5
  lower extremities due to stenosis or stricture I77.1
  mesenteric (embolic) (thrombotic) (*see also* Infarct, intestine) K55.069
  perforating —*see* Occlusion, artery, cerebral, specified NEC

Occlusion, occluded *(continued)*
artery *(continued)*
  peripheral I77.9
    thrombotic or embolic I74.4
  pontine —*see* Occlusion, artery, precerebral, specified NEC
  precerebral I65.9
    with infarction I63.20
      specified NEC I63.29
      due to
        embolism I63.10
          specified NEC I63.19
        thrombosis I63.09
          specified NEC I63.09
    basilar —*see* Occlusion, artery, basilar
    carotid —*see* Occlusion, artery, carotid
    puerperal O88.23
    specified NEC I65.8
      with infarction I63.29
        due to
          embolism I63.19
          thrombosis I63.09
    vertebral —*see* Occlusion, artery, vertebral
  renal N28.0
  retinal
    central H34.1-
    partial H34.21-
    branch H34.23-
    transient H34.0-
  spinal —*see* Occlusion, artery, precerebral, vertebral
  total (chronic)
    coronary I25.82
    extremities I70.92
  vertebral I65.0-
    with
      infarction I63.21-
        due to
          embolism I63.11-
          thrombosis I63.01-
basilar artery —*see* Occlusion, artery, basilar
bile duct (common) (hepatic) (noncalculous) K83.1
bowel —*see* Obstruction, intestine
carotid (artery) (common) (internal) —*see* Occlusion, artery, carotid
centric (of teeth) M26.59
  maximum intercuspation discrepancy M26.55
cerebellar (artery) —*see* Occlusion, artery, cerebellar
cerebral (artery) —*see* Occlusion, artery, cerebral
cerebrovascular —*see also* Occlusion, artery, cerebral
  with infarction I63.5-
cervical canal —*see* Stricture, cervix
cervix (uteri) —*see* Stricture, cervix
choanal Q30.0
choroidal (artery) —*see* Occlusion, artery, precerebral, specified NEC
colon —*see* Obstruction, intestine
communicating posterior artery —*see* Occlusion, artery, precerebral, specified NEC
coronary (artery) (vein) (thrombotic) —*see also* Infarct, myocardium
  chronic total I25.82
  healed or old I25.2
  not resulting in infarction I24.0
  total (chronic) I25.82
cystic duct —*see* Obstruction, gallbladder

Occlusion, occluded (continued)

embolic —see Embolism
fallopian tube N97.1
  congenital Q50.6
gallbladder —see also Obstruction, gallbladder
  congenital (causing jaundice) Q44.1
gingiva, traumatic K06.2
hymen N89.6
  congenital Q52.3
hypophyseal (artery) —see Occlusion, artery, precerebral, specified NEC
iliac artery I74.5
intestine —see Obstruction, intestine
lacrimal passages —see Obstruction, lacrimal
lung J98.4
lymph or lymphatic channel I89.0
mammary duct N64.89
mesenteric artery (embolic) (thrombotic) (see also Infarct, intestine) K55.069
nose J34.89
  congenital Q30.0
organ or site, congenital NEC —see Atresia, by site
oviduct N97.1
  congenital Q50.6
peripheral arteries
  due to stricture or stenosis I77.1
  upper extremity I74.2
pontine (artery) —see Occlusion, artery, precerebral, specified NEC
posterior lingual, of mandibular teeth M26.29
precerebral artery —see Occlusion, artery, precerebral
punctum lacrimale —see Obstruction, lacrimal
pupil —see Membrane, pupillary
pylorus, adult (see also Stricture, pylorus) K31.1
renal artery N28.0
retina, retinal
  artery —see Occlusion, artery, retinal
  vein (central) H34.81-
    engorgement H34.82-
    tributary H34.83-
    vessels H34.9
spinal artery —see Occlusion, artery, precerebral, vertebral
teeth (mandibular) (posterior lingual) M26.29
thoracic duct I89.0
thrombotic —see Thrombosis, artery
traumatic
  edentulous (alveolar) ridge K06.2
  gingiva K06.2
  periodontal K05.5
tubal N97.1
ureter (complete) (partial) N13.5
  congenital Q62.10
ureteropelvic junction N13.5
  congenital Q62.11
ureterovesical orifice N13.5
  congenital Q62.12
urethra —see Stricture, urethra
uterus N85.8
vagina N89.5
vascular NEC I99.8
vein —see Thrombosis
  retinal —see Occlusion, retinal, vein
vena cava (inferior) (superior) —see Embolism, vena cava

Occlusion, occluded (continued)

ventricle (brain) NEC G91.1
vertebral (artery) —see Occlusion, artery, vertebral
vessel (blood) I99.8
vulva N90.5

Occult
blood in feces (stools) R19.5

Occupational
problems NEC Z56.89

Ochlophobia —see Agoraphobia

Ochronosis (endogenous) E70.29

Ocular muscle —see condition

Oculogyric crisis or disturbance H51.8
psychogenic F45.8

Oculomotor syndrome H51.9

Oculopathy
syphilitic NEC A52.71
  congenital
    early A50.01
    late A50.30
  early (secondary) A51.43
  late A52.71

Oddi's sphincter spasm K83.4

Odontalgia K08.89

Odontoameloblastoma —see Cyst, calcifying odontogenic

Odontoclasia K03.89

Odontodysplasia, regional K00.4

Odontogenesis imperfecta K00.5

Odontoma (ameloblastic) (complex) (compound) (fibroameloblastic) —see Cyst, calcifying odontogenic

Odontomyelitis (closed) (open) K04.01
irreversible K04.02
reversible K04.01

Odontorrhagia K08.89

Odontosarcoma, ameloblastic C41.1
upper jaw (bone) C41.0

Oestriasis —see Myiasis

Oguchi's disease H53.63

Ohara's disease —see Tularemia

OHS (obesity hypoventilation syndrome) E66.2

Oidiomycosis —see Candidiasis

Oidium albicans infection —see Candidiasis

Old age (without mention of debility) R54
dementia F03

Old (previous) **myocardial infarction** I25.2

Olfactory —see condition

Oligemia —see Anemia

Oligoastrocytoma
specified site —see Neoplasm, malignant, by site
unspecified site C71.9

Oligocythemia D64.9

Oligodendroblastoma
specified site —see Neoplasm, malignant
unspecified site C71.9

Oligodendroglioma
anaplastic type
  specified site —see Neoplasm, malignant, by site
  unspecified site C71.9

Oligodendroglioma (continued)

specified site —see Neoplasm, malignant, by site
unspecified site C71.9

Oligodontia —see Anodontia

Oligoencephalon Q02

Oligohidrosis L74.4

Oligohydramnios O41.0-

Oligohydrosis L74.4

Oligomenorrhea N91.5
primary N91.3
secondary N91.4

Oligophrenia —see also Disability, intellectual
phenylpyruvic E70.0

Oligospermia N46.11
due to
  drug therapy N46.121
  efferent duct obstruction N46.123
  infection N46.122
  radiation N46.124
  specified cause NEC N46.129
  systemic disease N46.125

Oligotrichia —see Alopecia

Oliguria R34
with, complicating or following
  ectopic or molar pregnancy O08.4
postprocedural N99.0

Ollier's disease Q78.4

Omentitis —see Peritonitis

Omenotocele —see Hernia, abdomen, specified site NEC

Omentum, omental —see condition

Omphalitis (congenital) (newborn) P38.9
with mild hemorrhage P38.1
without hemorrhage P38.9
not of newborn L08.82
tetanus A33

Omphalocele Q79.2

Omphalomesenteric duct, persistent Q43.0

Omphalorrhagia, newborn P51.9

Omsk hemorrhagic fever A98.1

Onanism (excessive) F98.8

Onchocerciasis, onchocercosis B73.1
with
  eye disease B73.00
    endophthalmitis B73.01
    eyelid B73.09
    glaucoma B73.02
    specified NEC B73.09
  eye NEC B73.00
  eyelid B73.09

Oncocytoma —see Neoplasm, benign, by site

Oncovirus, as cause of disease classified elsewhere B97.32

Ondine's curse —see Apnea, sleep

Oneirophrenia F23

Onychauxis L60.2
congenital Q84.5

Onychia —see also Cellulitis, digit
with lymphangitis —see Lymphangitis, acute, digit
candidal B37.2
dermatophytic B35.1

Onychitis —see also Cellulitis, digit
with lymphangitis —see Lymphangitis, acute, digit

Onychocryptosis L60.0

Onychodystrophy L60.3
congenital Q84.6

Onychogryphosis, onychogryposis L60.2

Onycholysis L60.1

Onychomadesis L60.8

Onychomalacia L60.3

Onychomycosis (finger) (toe) B35.1

Onycho-osteodysplasia Q87.2

Onychophagia F98.8

Onychophosis L60.8

Onychoptosis L60.8

Onychorrhexis L60.3
congenital Q84.6

Onychoschizia L60.3

Onyxis (finger) (toe) L60.0

Onyxitis —see also Cellulitis, digit
with lymphangitis —see Lymphangitis, acute, digit

Oophoritis (cystic) (infectional) (interstitial) N70.92
with salpingitis N70.93
acute N70.02
  with salpingitis N70.03
chronic N70.12
  with salpingitis N70.13
complicating abortion —see Abortion, by type, complicated by, oophoritis

Oophorocele N83.4-

Opacity, opacities
cornea H17.-
  central H17.1-
  congenital Q13.3
  degenerative —see Degeneration, cornea
  hereditary —see Dystrophy, cornea
  inflammatory —see Keratitis
  minor H17.81-
  peripheral H17.82-
cornea
  sequelae of trachoma (healed) B94.0
  specified NEC H17.89
enamel (teeth) (fluoride) (nonfluoride) K00.3
lens —see Cataract
snowball —see Deposit, crystalline
vitreous (humor) NEC H43.39-
  congenital Q14.0
  membranes and strands H43.31-

Opalescent dentin (hereditary) K00.5

Open, opening
abnormal, organ or site, congenital —see Imperfect, closure
angle with
  borderline
    findings
      high risk H40.02-
      low risk H40.01-
    intraocular pressure H40.00-
  cupping of discs H40.01-
  glaucoma (primary) —see Glaucoma, open angle
bite
  anterior M26.220
  posterior M26.221

Open, opening *(continued)*
 false —*see* Imperfect, closure
 margin on tooth restoration K08.51
 restoration margins of tooth K08.51
 wound —*see* Wound, open

Operational fatigue F48.8

Operative —*see* condition

Operculitis —*see* Periodontitis

Operculum —*see* Break, retina

Ophiasis L63.2

Ophthalmia *(see also* Conjunctivitis)
 H10.9
 actinic rays —*see* Photokeratitis
 allergic (acute) —*see*
  Conjunctivitis, acute, atopic
 blennorrhagic (gonococcal)
  (neonatorum) A54.31
 diphtheritic A36.86
 Egyptian A71.1
 electrica —*see* Photokeratitis
 gonococcal (neonatorum) A54.31
 metastatic —*see* Endophthalmitis,
  purulent
 migraine —*see* Migraine,
  ophthalmoplegic
 neonatorum, newborn P39.1
  gonococcal A54.31
 nodosa H16.24-
 purulent —*see* Conjunctivitis,
  acute, mucopurulent
 spring —*see* Conjunctivitis, acute,
  atopic
 sympathetic —*see* Uveitis,
  sympathetic

Ophthalmitis —*see* Ophthalmia

Ophthalmocele (congenital) Q15.8

Ophthalmoneuromyelitis G36.0

Ophthalmoplegia —*see also*
 Strabismus, paralytic
 anterior internuclear —*see*
  Ophthalmoplegia, internuclear
 ataxia-areflexia G61.0
 diabetic —*see* E08-E13 with .39
 exophthalmic E05.00
  with thyroid storm E05.01
 external H49.88-
  progressive H49.4-
   with pigmentary retinopathy
    —*see* Kearns-Sayre
    syndrome
   total H49.3-
 internal (complete) (total) H52.51-
 internuclear H51.2-
 migraine —*see* Migraine,
  ophthalmoplegic
 Parinaud's H49.88-
 progressive external —*see*
  Ophthalmoplegia, external,
  progressive
 supranuclear, progressive G23.1
 total (external) —*see*
  Ophthalmoplegia, external, total

Opioid(s)
 abuse —*see* Abuse, drug, opioids
 dependence —*see* Dependence,
  drug, opioids
 induced, without use disorder
  anxiety disorder F11.988
  delirium F11.921
  depressive disorder F11.94
  sexual dysfunction F11.981
  sleep disorder F11.982

Opisthognathism M26.09

Opisthorchiasis (felineus) (viverrini)
 B66.0

Opitz' disease D73.2

Opiumism —*see* Dependence, drug,
 opioid

Oppenheim's disease G70.2

Oppenheim-Urbach disease
 (necrobiosis lipoidica
 diabeticorum) —*see* E08-E13 with
 .620

Optic nerve —*see* condition

Orbit —*see* condition

Orchioblastoma C62.9-

Orchitis (gangrenous) (nonspecific)
 (septic) (suppurative) N45.2
 blennorrhagic (gonococcal) (acute)
  (chronic) A54.23
 chlamydial A56.19
 filarial —*see also* Infestation,
  filarial B74.9 *[N51]*
 gonococcal (acute) (chronic)
  A54.23
 mumps B26.0
 syphilitic A52.76
 tuberculous A18.15

Orf (virus disease) B08.02

Organic —*see also* condition
 brain syndrome F09
 heart —*see* Disease, heart
 mental disorder F09
 psychosis F09

Orgasm
 anejaculatory N53.13

Oriental
 bilharziasis B65.2
 schistosomiasis B65.2

Orifice —*see* condition

**Origin of both great vessels from
 right ventricle** Q20.1

Ormond's disease (with ureteral
 obstruction) N13.5
 with infection N13.6

Ornithine metabolism disorder
 E72.4

Ornithinemia (Type I) (Type II)
 E72.4

Ornithosis A70

Orotaciduria, oroticaciduria
 (congenital) (hereditary)
 (pyrimidine deficiency) E79.8
 anemia D53.0

Orthodontics
 adjustment Z46.4
 fitting Z46.4

Orthopnea R06.01

Orthopoxvirus B08.09

Os, uterus —*see* condition

**Osgood-Schlatter disease or
 osteochondrosis** M92.52-

Osler (-Weber)-**Rendu disease**
 I78.0

Osler's nodes I33.0

Osmidrosis L75.0

Osseous —*see* condition

Ossification
 artery —*see* Arteriosclerosis
 auricle (ear) —*see* Disorder, pinna,
  specified type NEC
 bronchial J98.09
 cardiac —*see* Degeneration,
  myocardial
 cartilage (senile) —*see* Disorder,
  cartilage, specified type NEC
 coronary (artery) —*see* Disease,
  heart, ischemic, atherosclerotic

Ossification *(continued)*
 diaphragm J98.6
 ear, middle —*see* Otosclerosis
 falx cerebri G96.198
 fontanel, premature Q75.0
 heart —*see also* Degeneration,
  myocardial
  valve —*see* Endocarditis
 larynx J38.7
 ligament —*see* Disorder, tendon,
  specified type NEC
  posterior longitudinal —*see*
   Spondylopathy, specified
   NEC
 meninges (cerebral) (spinal)
  G96.198
 multiple, eccentric centers —*see*
  Disorder, bone, development or
  growth
 muscle —*see also* Calcification,
  muscle
  due to burns —*see* Myositis,
   ossificans, in, burns
  paralytic —*see* Myositis,
   ossificans, in, quadriplegia
  progressive —*see* Myositis,
   ossificans, progressiva
  specified NEC M61.50
   ankle M61.57-
   foot M61.57-
   forearm M61.53-
   hand M61.54-
   lower leg M61.56-
   multiple sites M61.59
   pelvic region M61.55-
   shoulder region M61.51-
   specified site NEC M61.58
   thigh M61.55-
   upper arm M61.52-
  traumatic —*see* Myositis,
   ossificans, traumatica
 myocardium, myocardial —*see*
  Degeneration, myocardial
 penis N48.89
 periarticular —*see* Disorder, joint,
  specified type NEC
 pinna —*see* Disorder, pinna,
  specified type NEC
 rider's bone —*see* Ossification,
  muscle, specified NEC
 sclera H15.89
 subperiosteal, post-traumatic
  M89.8X-
 tendon —*see* Disorder, tendon,
  specified type NEC
 trachea J39.8
 tympanic membrane —*see*
  Disorder, tympanic membrane,
  specified NEC
 vitreous (humor) —*see* Deposit,
  crystalline

Osteitis —*see also* Osteomyelitis
 alveolar M27.3
 condensans M85.30
  ankle M85.37-
  foot M85.37-
  forearm M85.33-
  hand M85.34-
  lower leg M85.36-
  multiple site M85.39
  neck M85.38
  rib M85.38
  shoulder M85.31-
  skull M85.38
  specified site NEC M85.38
  thigh M85.35-
  toe M85.37-
  upper arm M85.32-
  vertebra M85.38
 deformans M88.9

Osteitis *(continued)*
 deformans *(continued)*
  in (due to)
   malignant neoplasm of bone
    C41.9 *[M90.60]*
   neoplastic disease *(see also*
    Neoplasm) D49.9 *[M90.60]*
    carpus D49.9 *[M90.64-]*
    clavicle D49.9 *[M90.61-]*
    femur D49.9 *[M90.65-]*
    fibula D49.9 *[M90.66-]*
    finger D49.9 *[M90.64-]*
    humerus D49.9 *[M90.62-]*
    ilium D49.9 *[M90.65-]*
    ischium D49.9 *[M90.65-]*
    metacarpus D49.9 *[M90.64-]*
    metatarsus D49.9 *[M90.67-]*
    multiple sites D49.9
     [M90.69]
    neck D49.9 *[M90.68]*
    radius D49.9 *[M90.63-]*
    rib D49.9 *[M90.68]*
    scapula D49.9 *[M90.61-]*
    skull D49.9 *[M90.68]*
    tarsus D49.9 *[M90.67-]*
    tibia D49.9 *[M90.66-]*
    toe D49.9 *[M90.67-]*
    ulna D49.9 *[M90.63-]*
    vertebra D49.9 *[M90.68]*
  skull M88.0
  specified NEC —*see* Paget's
   disease, bone, by site
  vertebra M88.1
 due to yaws A66.6
 fibrosa NEC —*see* Cyst, bone,
  by site
  circumscripta —*see* Dysplasia,
   fibrous, bone NEC
  cystica (generalisata) E21.0
  disseminata Q78.1
  osteoplastica E21.0
 fragilitans Q78.0
 Garr's (sclerosing) —*see*
  Osteomyelitis, specified type NEC
 jaw (acute) (chronic) (lower)
  (suppurative) (upper) M27.2
 parathyroid E21.0
 petrous bone (acute) (chronic)
  —*see* Petrositis
 sclerotic, nonsuppurative —*see*
  Osteomyelitis, specified type
  NEC
 tuberculosa A18.09
  cystica D86.89
  multiplex cystoides D86.89

Osteoarthritis M19.90
 ankle M19.07-
 elbow M19.02-
 foot joint M19.07-
 generalized M15.9
  erosive M15.4
  primary M15.0
  specified NEC M15.8
 hand joint M19.04-
  first carpometacarpal joint
   M18.9
 hip M16.1-
  bilateral M16.0
  due to hip dysplasia (unilateral)
   M16.3-
   bilateral M16.2
 interphalangeal
  distal (Heberden) M15.1
  proximal (Bouchard) M15.2
 knee M17.1-
  bilateral M17.0
 post-traumatic NEC M19.92
  ankle M19.17-
  elbow M19.12-
  foot joint M19.17-

Osteochondrosis *(continued)*
  juvenile, juvenilis *(continued)*
    upper limb NEC M92.3-
    vertebra (body) (epiphyseal plates)
      (Calvé's) (Scheuermann's)
      —see Osteochondrosis,
      juvenile, spine
  Kienböck's *—see* Osteochondrosis,
    juvenile, hand, carpal lunate
    adult M93.1
  Köhler's
    patellar *—see* Osteochondrosis,
      juvenile, patella
    tarsal navicular *—see*
      Osteochondrosis, juvenile,
      tarsus
  Legg-Perthes (-Calvé)
    (-Waldenström) *—see* Legg-
    Calvé-Perthes disease
  limb
    lower NEC (juvenile) M92.8
      tibia and fibula M92.59-
    upper NEC (juvenile) *—see*
      Osteochondrosis, juvenile,
      upper limb NEC
  lunate bone (carpal) (juvenile)
    —see also Osteochondrosis,
    juvenile, hand, carpal lunate
    adult M93.1
  Mauclaire's *—see* Osteochondrosis,
    juvenile, hand, metacarpal
  metacarpal (head) (juvenile) *—see*
    Osteochondrosis, juvenile, hand,
    metacarpal
  metatarsus (fifth) (head) (juvenile)
    (second) *—see* Osteochondrosis,
    juvenile, metatarsus
  navicular (juvenile) *—see*
    Osteochondrosis, juvenile, tarsus
  os
    calcis (juvenile) *—see*
      Osteochondrosis, juvenile,
      tarsus
    tibiale externum (juvenile) *—see*
      Osteochondrosis, juvenile, tarsus
  Osgood-Schlatter M92.52-
  Panner's *—see* Osteochondrosis,
    juvenile, humerus
  patellar center (juvenile)
    (primary) (secondary) *—see*
    Osteochondrosis, juvenile, patella
  pelvis (juvenile) M91.0
  Pierson's M91.0
  radius (head) (juvenile) *—see*
    Osteochondrosis, juvenile, radius
  Scheuermann's *—see*
    Osteochondrosis, juvenile, spine
  Sever's *—see* Osteochondrosis,
    juvenile, tarsus
  Sinding-Larsen *—see*
    Osteochondrosis, juvenile, patella
  spine M42.9
    adult M42.10
      cervical region M42.12
      cervicothoracic region M42.13
      lumbar region M42.16
      lumbosacral region M42.17
      multiple sites M42.19
      occipito-atlanto-axial region
        M42.11
      sacrococcygeal region M42.18
      thoracic region M42.14
      thoracolumbar region M42.15
    juvenile *—see* Osteochondrosis,
      juvenile, spine
  symphysis pubis (juvenile) M91.0
  syphilitic (congenital) A50.02
  talus (juvenile) *—see*
    Osteochondrosis, juvenile, tarsus
  tarsus (navicular) (juvenile) *—see*
    Osteochondrosis, juvenile, tarsus

Osteochondrosis *(continued)*
  tibia (proximal) (tubercle)
    (juvenile) *—see*
    Osteochondrosis, juvenile, tibia
  tuberculous *—see* Tuberculosis, bone
  ulna (lower) (juvenile) *—see*
    Osteochondrosis, juvenile, ulna
  van Neck's M91.0
  vertebral *—see* Osteochondrosis,
    spine

Osteoclastoma D48.0
  malignant *—see* Neoplasm, bone,
    malignant

Osteodynia *—see* Disorder, bone,
  specified type NEC

Osteodystrophy Q78.9
  azotemic N25.0
  congenital Q78.9
  parathyroid, secondary E21.1
  renal N25.0

Osteofibroma *—see* Neoplasm, bone,
  benign

Osteofibrosarcoma *—see* Neoplasm,
  bone, malignant

Osteogenesis imperfecta Q78.0

Osteogenic *—see* condition

Osteolysis M89.50
  carpus M89.54-
  clavicle M89.51-
  femur M89.55-
  fibula M89.56-
  finger M89.54-
  humerus M89.52-
  ilium M89.559
  ischium M89.559
  joint prosthesis (periprosthetic)
    —see Complications, joint
    prosthesis, mechanical,
    periprosthetic, osteolysis, by site
  metacarpus M89.54-
  metatarsus M89.57-
  multiple sites M89.59
  neck M89.58
  periprosthetic *—see* Complications,
    joint prosthesis, mechanical,
    periprosthetic, osteolysis, by site
  radius M89.53-
  rib M89.58
  scapula M89.51-
  skull M89.58
  tarsus M89.57-
  tibia M89.56-
  toe M89.57-
  ulna M89.53-
  vertebra M89.58

Osteoma *—see also* Neoplasm, bone,
  benign
  osteoid *—see also* Neoplasm, bone,
    benign
    giant *—see* Neoplasm, bone,
      benign

Osteomalacia M83.9
  adult M83.9
    drug-induced NEC M83.5
    due to
      malabsorption (postsurgical)
        M83.2
      malnutrition M83.3
    specified NEC M83.8
  aluminium-induced M83.4
  infantile *—see* Rickets
  juvenile *—see* Rickets
  oncogenic E83.89
  pelvis M83.8
  puerperal M83.0
  senile M83.1
  vitamin-D-resistant in adults
    E83.31 *[M90.8-]*

Osteomalacia *(continued)*
  vitamin-D-resistant in adults
    (continued)
    carpus E83.31 *[M90.84-]*
    clavicle E83.31 *[M90.81-]*
    femur E83.31 *[M90.85-]*
    fibula E83.31 *[M90.86-]*
    finger E83.31 *[M90.84-]*
    humerus E83.31 *[M90.82-]*
    ilium E83.31 *[M90.859]*
    ischium E83.31 *[M90.859]*
    metacarpus E83.31 *[M90.84-]*
    metatarsus E83.31 *[M90.87-]*
    multiple sites E83.31 *[M90.89]*
    neck E83.31 *[M90.88]*
    radius E83.31 *[M90.83-]*
    rib E83.31 *[M90.88]*
    scapula E83.31 *[M90.819]*
    skull E83.31 *[M90.88]*
    tarsus E83.31 *[M90.879]*
    tibia E83.31 *[M90.869]*
    toe E83.31 *[M90.879]*
    ulna E83.31 *[M90.839]*
    vertebra E83.31 *[M90.88]*

Osteomyelitis (general) (infective)
  (localized) (neonatal) (purulent)
  (septic) (staphylococcal)
  (streptococcal) (suppurative) (with
  periostitis) M86.9
  acute M86.10
    carpus M86.14-
    clavicle M86.11-
    femur M86.15-
    fibula M86.16-
    finger M86.14-
    hematogenous M86.00
      carpus M86.04-
      clavicle M86.01-
      femur M86.05-
      fibula M86.06-
      finger M86.04-
      humerus M86.02-
      ilium M86.059
      ischium M86.059
      mandible M27.2
      metacarpus M86.04-
      metatarsus M86.07-
      multiple sites M86.09
      neck M86.08
      orbit H05.02-
      petrous bone *—see* Petrositis
      radius M86.03-
      rib M86.08
      scapula M86.01-
      skull M86.08
      tarsus M86.07-
      tibia M86.06-
      toe M86.07-
      ulna M86.03-
      vertebra *—see* Osteomyelitis,
        vertebra
    humerus M86.12-
    ilium M86.18
    ischium M86.18
    mandible M27.2
    metacarpus M86.14-
    metatarsus M86.17-
    multiple sites M86.19
    neck M86.18
    orbit H05.02-
    petrous bone *—see* Petrositis
    radius M86.13-
    rib M86.18
    scapula M86.11-
    skull M86.18
    tarsus M86.17-
    tibia M86.16-
    toe M86.17-
    ulna M86.13-
    vertebra *—see* Osteomyelitis,
      vertebra

Osteomyelitis *(continued)*
  chronic (or old) M86.60
    with draining sinus M86.40
      carpus M86.44-
      clavicle M86.41-
      femur M86.45-
      fibula M86.46-
      finger M86.44-
      humerus M86.42-
      ilium M86.459
      ischium M86.459
      mandible M27.2
      metacarpus M86.44-
      metatarsus M86.47-
      multiple sites M86.49
      neck M86.48
      orbit H05.02-
      petrous bone *—see*
        Petrositis
      radius M86.43-
      rib M86.48
      scapula M86.41-
      skull M86.48
      tarsus M86.47-
      tibia M86.46-
      toe M86.47-
      ulna M86.43-
      vertebra *—see* Osteomyelitis,
        vertebra
    carpus M86.64-
    clavicle M86.61-
    femur M86.65-
    fibula M86.66-
    finger M86.64-
    hematogenous NEC M86.50
      carpus M86.54-
      clavicle M86.51-
      femur M86.55-
      fibula M86.56-
      finger M86.54-
      humerus M86.52-
      ilium M86.559
      ischium M86.559
      mandible M27.2
      metacarpus M86.54-
      metatarsus M86.57-
      multifocal M86.30
        carpus M86.34
        clavicle M86.31-
        femur M86.35-
        fibula M86.36-
        finger M86.34-
        humerus M86.32-
        ilium M86.359
        ischium M86.359
        metacarpus M86.34-
        metatarsus M86.37-
        multiple sites M86.39
        neck M86.38
        radius M86.33-
        rib M86.38
        scapula M86.31-
        skull M86.38
        tarsus M86.37-
        tibia M86.36-
        toe M86.37-
        ulna M86.33-
        vertebra *—see*
          Osteomyelitis, vertebra
      multiple sites M86.59
      neck M86.58
      orbit H05.02-
      petrous bone *—see* Petrositis
      radius M86.53-
      rib M86.58
      scapula M86.51-
      skull M86.58
      tarsus M86.57-
      tibia M86.56-
      toe M86.57-
      ulna M86.53-

Osteomyelitis *(continued)*
  chronic *(continued)*
    hematogenous NEC *(continued)*
      vertebra —*see* Osteomyelitis, vertebra
    humerus M86.62-
    ilium M86.659
    ischium M86.659
    mandible M27.2
    metacarpus M86.64-
    metatarsus M86.67-
    multifocal —*see* Osteomyelitis, chronic, hematogenous, multifocal
    multiple sites M86.69
    neck M86.68
    orbit H05.02-
    petrous bone —*see* Petrositis
    radius M86.63-
    rib M86.68
    scapula M86.61-
    skull M86.68
    tarsus M86.67-
    tibia M86.66-
    toe M86.67-
    ulna M86.63-
    vertebra —*see* Osteomyelitis, vertebra
  echinococcal B67.2
  Garr's —*see* Osteomyelitis, specified type NEC
  in diabetes mellitus —*see* E08-E13 with .69
  jaw (acute) (chronic) (lower) (neonatal) (suppurative) (upper) M27.2
  nonsuppurating —*see* Osteomyelitis, specified type NEC
  orbit H05.02-
  petrous bone —*see* Petrositis
  Salmonella (arizonae) (cholerae-suis) (enteritidis) (typhimurium) A02.24
  sclerosing, nonsuppurative —*see* Osteomyelitis, specified type NEC
  specified type NEC *(see also subcategory)* M86.8X-
    mandible M27.2
    orbit H05.02-
    petrous bone —*see* Petrositis
    vertebra —*see* Osteomyelitis, vertebra
  subacute M86.20
    carpus M86.24-
    clavicle M86.21-
    femur M86.25-
    fibula M86.26-
    finger M86.24-
    humerus M86.22-
    mandible M27.2
    metacarpus M86.24-
    metatarsus M86.27-
    multiple sites M86.29
    neck M86.28
    orbit H05.02-
    petrous bone —*see* Petrositis
    radius M86.23-
    rib M86.28
    scapula M86.21-
    skull M86.28
    tarsus M86.27-
    tibia M86.26-
    toe M86.27-
    ulna M86.23-
    vertebra —*see* Osteomyelitis, vertebra
  syphilitic A52.77
    congenital (early) A50.02 *[M90.80]*

Osteomyelitis *(continued)*
  tuberculous —*see* Tuberculosis, bone
  typhoid A01.05
  vertebra M46.20
    cervical region M46.22
    cervicothoracic region M46.23
    lumbar region M46.26
    lumbosacral region M46.27
    occipito-atlanto-axial region M46.21
    sacrococcygeal region M46.28
    thoracic region M46.24
    thoracolumbar region M46.25

Osteomyelofibrosis D47.4

Osteomyelosclerosis D75.89

Osteonecrosis M87.9
  due to
    drugs —*see* Osteonecrosis, secondary, due to, drugs
    trauma —*see* Osteonecrosis, secondary, due to, trauma
  idiopathic aseptic M87.00
    ankle M87.07-
    carpus M87.03-
    clavicle M87.01-
    femur M87.05-
    fibula M87.06-
    finger M87.04-
    humerus M87.02-
    ilium M87.050
    ischium M87.050
    metacarpus M87.04-
    metatarsus M87.07-
    multiple sites M87.09
    neck M87.08
    pelvis M87.050
    radius M87.03-
    rib M87.08
    scapula M87.01-
    skull M87.08
    tarsus M87.07-
    tibia M87.06-
    toe M87.07-
    ulna M87.03-
    vertebra M87.08
  secondary NEC M87.30
    carpus M87.33-
    clavicle M87.31-
    due to
      drugs M87.10
        carpus M87.13-
        clavicle M87.11-
        femur M87.15-
        fibula M87.16-
        finger M87.14-
        humerus M87.12-
        ilium M87.159
        ischium M87.159
        jaw M87.180
        metacarpus M87.14-
        metatarsus M87.17-
        multiple sites M87.19
        neck M87.18
        radius M87.13-
        rib M87.18
        scapula M87.11-
        skull M87.18
        tarsus M87.17-
        tibia M87.16-
        toe M87.17-
        ulna M87.13-
        vertebra M87.18
      hemoglobinopathy NEC D58.2 *[M90.50]*
        carpus D58.2 *[M90.54-]*
        clavicle D58.2 *[M90.51-]*
        femur D58.2 *[M90.55-]*
        fibula D58.2 *[M90.56-]*
        finger D58.2 *[M90.54-]*

Osteonecrosis *(continued)*
  secondary NEC *(continued)*
    due to *(continued)*
      hemoglobinopathy NEC *(continued)*
        humerus D58.2 *[M90.52-]*
        ilium D58.2 *[M90.55-]*
        ischium D58.2 *[M90.55-]*
        metacarpus D58.2 *[M90.54-]*
        metatarsus D58.2 *[M90.57-]*
        multiple sites D58.2 *[M90.58]*
        neck D58.2 *[M90.58]*
        radius D58.2 *[M90.53-]*
        rib D58.2 *[M90.58]*
        scapula D58.2 *[M90.51-]*
        skull D58.2 *[M90.58]*
        tarsus D58.2 *[M90.57-]*
        tibia D58.2 *[M90.56-]*
        toe D58.2 *[M90.57-]*
        ulna D58.2 *[M90.53-]*
        vertebra D58.2 *[M90.58]*
      trauma (previous) M87.20
        carpus M87.23-
        clavicle M87.21-
        femur M87.25-
        fibula M87.26-
        finger M87.24-
        humerus M87.22-
        ilium M87.25-
        ischium M87.25-
        metacarpus M87.24-
        metatarsus M87.27-
        multiple sites M87.29
        neck M87.28
        radius M87.23-
        rib M87.28
        scapula M87.21-
        skull M87.28
        tarsus M87.27-
        tibia M87.26-
        toe M87.27-
        ulna M87.23-
        vertebra M87.28
    femur M87.35-
    fibula M87.36-
    finger M87.34-
    humerus M87.32-
    ilium M87.350
    in
      caisson disease T70.3 *[M90.50]*
        carpus T70.3 *[M90.54-]*
        clavicle T70.3 *[M90.51-]*
        femur T70.3 *[M90.55-]*
        fibula T70.3 *[M90.56-]*
        finger T70.3 *[M90.54-]*
        humerus T70.3 *[M90.52-]*
        ilium T70.3 *[M90.55-]*
        ischium T70.3 *[M90.55-]*
        metacarpus T70.3 *[M90.54-]*
        metatarsus T70.3 *[M90.57-]*
        multiple sites T70.3 *[M90.59]*
        neck T70.3 *[M90.58]*
        radius T70.3 *[M90.53-]*
        rib T70.3 *[M90.58]*
        scapula T70.3 *[M90.51-]*
        skull T70.3 *[M90.58]*
        tarsus T70.3 *[M90.57-]*
        tibia T70.3 *[M90.56-]*
        toe T70.3 *[M90.57-]*
        ulna T70.3 *[M90.53-]*
        vertebra T70.3 *[M90.58]*
    ischium M87.350
    metacarpus M87.34-
    metatarsus M87.37-
    multiple site M87.39
    neck M87.38
    radius M87.33-
    rib M87.38

Osteonecrosis *(continued)*
  secondary NEC *(continued)*
    scapula M87.319
    skull M87.38
    tarsus M87.379
    tibia M87.366
    toe M87.379
    ulna M87.33-
    vertebra M87.38
  specified type NEC M87.80
    carpus M87.83-
    clavicle M87.81-
    femur M87.85-
    fibula M87.86-
    finger M87.84-
    humerus M87.82-
    ilium M87.85-
    ischium M87.85-
    metacarpus M87.84-
    metatarsus M87.87-
    multiple sites M87.89
    neck M87.88
    radius M87.83-
    rib M87.88
    scapula M87.81-
    skull M87.88
    tarsus M87.87-
    tibia M87.86-
    toe M87.87-
    ulna M87.83-
    vertebra M87.88

Osteo-onycho-arthro-dysplasia Q87.2

Osteo-onychodysplasia, hereditary Q87.2

Osteopathia condensans disseminata Q78.8

Osteopathy —*see also* Osteomyelitis, Osteonecrosis, Osteoporosis
  after poliomyelitis M89.60
    carpus M89.64-
    clavicle M89.61-
    femur M89.65-
    fibula M89.66-
    finger M89.64-
    humerus M89.62-
    ilium M89.659
    ischium M89.659
    metacarpus M89.64-
    metatarsus M89.67-
    multiple sites M89.69
    neck M89.68
    radius M89.63-
    rib M89.68
    scapula M89.61-
    skull M89.68
    tarsus M89.67-
    tibia M89.66-
    toe M89.67-
    ulna M89.63-
    vertebra M89.68
  in (due to)
    renal osteodystrophy N25.0
    specified diseases classified elsewhere M90.8

Osteopenia M85.8-
  borderline M85.8-

Osteoperiostitis —*see* Osteomyelitis, specified type NEC

Osteopetrosis (familial) Q78.2

Osteophyte M25.70
  ankle M25.77-
  elbow M25.72-
  foot joint M25.77-
  hand joint M25.74-
  hip M25.75-
  knee M25.76-
  shoulder M25.71-

Osteophyte (continued)
  spine M25.78
  vertebrae M25.78
  wrist M25.73-

Osteopoikilosis Q78.8

Osteoporosis (female) (male) M81.0
  with current pathological fracture M80.00
  age-related M81.0
    with current pathologic fracture M80.00
      carpus M80.04-
      clavicle M80.01-
      fibula M80.06-
      finger M80.04-
      humerus M80.02-
      ilium M80.05-
      ischium M80.05-
      metacarpus M80.04-
      metatarsus M80.07-
      pelvis M80.05-
      radius M80.03-
      scapula M80.01-
      specified site NEC M80.0A
      tarsus M80.07-
      tibia M80.06-
      toe M80.07-
      ulna M80.03-
      vertebra M80.08
  disuse M81.8
    with current pathological fracture M80.80
      carpus M80.84-
      clavicle M80.81-
      fibula M80.86-
      finger M80.84-
      humerus M80.82-
      ilium M80.85-
      ischium M80.85-
      metacarpus M80.84-
      metatarsus M80.87-
      pelvis M80.85-
      radius M80.83-
      scapula M80.81-
      specified site NEC M80.8A
      tarsus M80.87-
      tibia M80.86-
      toe M80.87-
      ulna M80.83-
      vertebra M80.88
  drug-induced —*see* Osteoporosis, specified type NEC
  idiopathic —*see* Osteoporosis, specified type NEC
  involutional —*see* Osteoporosis, age-related
  Lequesne M81.6
  localized M81.6
  postmenopausal M81.0
    with pathological fracture M80.00
      carpus M80.04-
      clavicle M80.01-
      fibula M80.06-
      finger M80.04-
      humerus M80.02-
      ilium M80.05-
      ischium M80.05-
      metacarpus M80.04-
      metatarsus M80.07-
      pelvis M80.05-
      radius M80.03-
      scapula M80.01-
      specified site NEC M80.0A
      tarsus M80.07-
      tibia M80.06-
      toe M80.07-
      ulna M80.03-
      vertebra M80.08
  postoophorectomy —*see* Osteoporosis, specified type NEC

Osteoporosis (continued)
  postsurgical malabsorption —*see* Osteoporosis, specified type NEC
  post-traumatic —*see* Osteoporosis, specified type NEC
  senile —*see* Osteoporosis, age-related
  specified type NEC M81.8
    with pathological fracture M80.80
      carpus M80.84-
      clavicle M80.81-
      fibula M80.86-
      finger M80.84-
      humerus M80.82-
      ilium M80.85-
      ischium M80.85-
      metacarpus M80.84-
      metatarsus M80.87-
      pelvis M80.85-
      radius M80.83-
      scapula M80.81-
      specified site NEC M80.8A
      tarsus M80.87-
      tibia M80.86-
      toe M80.87-
      ulna M80.83-
      vertebra M80.88

Osteopsathyrosis (idiopathica) Q78.0

Osteoradionecrosis, jaw (acute) (chronic) (lower) (suppurative) (upper) M27.2

Osteosarcoma (any form) —*see* Neoplasm, bone, malignant

Osteosclerosis Q78.2
  acquired M85.8-
  congenita Q77.4
  fragilitas (generalisata) Q78.2
  myelofibrosis D75.81

Osteosclerotic anemia D64.89

Osteosis
  cutis L94.2
  renal fibrocystic N25.0

Österreicher-Turner syndrome Q87.2

Ostium
  atrioventriculare commune Q21.2
  primum (arteriosum) (defect) (persistent) Q21.2
  secundum (arteriosum) (defect) (patent) (persistent) Q21.1

Ostrum-Furst syndrome Q75.8

Otalgia —*see* subcategory H92.0

Otitis (acute) H66.90
  with effusion —*see also* Otitis, media, nonsuppurative
    purulent —*see* Otitis, media, suppurative
  adhesive H74.1
  chronic —*see also* Otitis, media, chronic
    with effusion —*see also* Otitis, media, nonsuppurative, chronic
  externa H60.9-
    abscess —*see* Abscess, ear, external
    acute (noninfective) H60.50-
      actinic H60.51-
      chemical H60.52-
      contact H60.53-
      eczematoid H60.54-
      infective —*see* Otitis, externa, infective
      reactive H60.55-
      specified NEC H60.59-
    cellulitis —*see* Cellulitis, ear
    chronic H60.6-
    diffuse —*see* Otitis, externa, infective, diffuse
    hemorrhagic —*see* Otitis, externa, infective, hemorrhagic

Otitis (continued)
  externa (continued)
    in (due to)
      aspergillosis B44.89
      candidiasis B37.84
      erysipelas A46 *[H62.40]*
      herpes (simplex) virus
        infection B00.1
        zoster B02.8
      impetigo L01.00 *[H62.40]*
      infectious disease NEC B99 *[H62.4-]*
      mycosis NEC B36.9 *[H62.40]*
      parasitic disease NEC B89 *[H62.40]*
      viral disease NEC B34.9 *[H62.40]*
      zoster B02.8
    infective NEC H60.39-
      abscess —*see* Abscess, ear, external
      cellulitis —*see* Cellulitis, ear
      diffuse H60.31-
      hemorrhagic H60.32-
      swimmer's ear —*see* Swimmer's, ear
    malignant H60.2-
    mycotic NEC B36.9 *[H62.40]*
      in
        aspergillosis B44.89
        candidiasis B37.84
        moniliasis B37.84
    necrotizing —*see* Otitis, externa, malignant
    Pseudomonas aeruginosa —*see* Otitis, externa, malignant
    reactive —*see* Otitis, externa, acute, reactive
    specified NEC —*see* subcategory H60.8
    tropical NEC B36.9 *[H62.40]*
      in
        aspergillosis B44.89
        candidiasis B37.84
        moniliasis B37.84
  insidiosa —*see* Otosclerosis
  interna —*see* subcategory H83.0
  media (hemorrhagic) (staphylococcal) (streptococcal) H66.9-
    with effusion (nonpurulent) —*see* Otitis, media, nonsuppurative
    acute, subacute H66.90
      allergic —*see* Otitis, media, nonsuppurative, acute, allergic
      exudative —*see* Otitis, media, suppurative, acute
      mucoid —*see* Otitis, media, nonsuppurative, acute
      necrotizing —*see also* Otitis, media, suppurative, acute
        in
          measles B05.3
          scarlet fever A38.0
      nonsuppurative NEC —*see* Otitis, media, nonsuppurative, acute
      purulent —*see* Otitis, media, suppurative, acute
      sanguinous —*see* Otitis, media, nonsuppurative, acute
      secretory —*see* Otitis, media, nonsuppurative, acute, serous
      seromucinous —*see* Otitis, media, nonsuppurative, acute

Otitis (continued)
  media (continued)
    acute, subacute (continued)
      serous —*see* Otitis, media, nonsuppurative, acute, serous
      suppurative —*see* Otitis, media, suppurative, acute
    allergic —*see* Otitis, media, nonsuppurative
    catarrhal —*see* Otitis, media, nonsuppurative
    chronic H66.90
      with effusion (nonpurulent) —*see* Otitis, media, nonsuppurative, chronic
      allergic —*see* Otitis, media, nonsuppurative, chronic, allergic
      benign suppurative —*see* Otitis, media, suppurative, chronic, tubotympanic
      catarrhal —*see* Otitis, media, nonsuppurative, chronic, serous
      exudative —*see* Otitis, media, nonsuppurative, chronic
      mucinous —*see* Otitis, media, nonsuppurative, chronic, mucoid
      mucoid —*see* Otitis, media, nonsuppurative, chronic, mucoid
      nonsuppurative NEC —*see* Otitis, media, nonsuppurative, chronic
      purulent —*see* Otitis, media, suppurative, chronic
      secretory —*see* Otitis, media, nonsuppurative, chronic, mucoid
      seromucinous —*see* Otitis, media, nonsuppurative, chronic
      serous —*see* Otitis, media, nonsuppurative, chronic, serous
      suppurative —*see* Otitis, media, suppurative, chronic
      transudative —*see* Otitis, media, nonsuppurative, chronic, mucoid
    exudative —*see* Otitis, media, suppurative
    in (due to) (with)
      influenza —*see* Influenza, with, otitis media
      measles B05.3
      scarlet fever A38.0
      tuberculosis A18.6
      viral disease NEC B34.- *[H67.-]*
    mucoid —*see* Otitis, media, nonsuppurative
    nonsuppurative H65.9-
      acute or subacute NEC H65.19-
        allergic H65.11-
          recurrent H65.11-
        recurrent H65.19-
        secretory —*see* Otitis, media, nonsuppurative, serous
        serous H65.0-
          recurrent H65.0-
      chronic H65.49-
        allergic H65.41-
        mucoid H65.3-
        serous H65.2-
    postmeasles B05.3

Otitis (continued)
media (continued)
purulent —see Otitis, media, suppurative
secretory —see Otitis, media, nonsuppurative
seromucinous —see Otitis, media, nonsuppurative
serous —see Otitis, media, nonsuppurative
suppurative H66.4-
acute H66.00-
with rupture of ear drum H66.01-
recurrent H66.00-
with rupture of ear drum H66.01-
chronic (see also subcategory) H66.3
atticoantral H66.2-
benign —see Otitis, media, suppurative, chronic, tubotympanic
tubotympanic H66.1-
transudative —see Otitis, media, nonsuppurative
tuberculous A18.6

Otocephaly Q18.2

Otolith syndrome —see subcategory H81.8

Otomycosis (diffuse) **NEC** B36.9 *[H62.40]*
in
aspergillosis B44.89
candidiasis B37.84
moniliasis B37.84

Otoporosis —see Otosclerosis

Otorrhagia (nontraumatic) H92.2-
traumatic - code by Type of injury

Otorrhea H92.1-
cerebrospinal (fluid) G96.01
postoperative G96.08
specified NEC G96.08
spontaneous G96.01
traumatic G96.08

Otosclerosis (general) H80.9-
cochlear (endosteal) H80.2-
involving
otic capsule —see Otosclerosis, cochlear
oval window
nonobliterative H80.0-
obliterative H80.1-
round window —see Otosclerosis, cochlear
nonobliterative —see Otosclerosis, involving, oval window, nonobliterative
obliterative —see Otosclerosis, involving, oval window, obliterative
specified NEC H80.8-

Otospongiosis —see Otosclerosis

Otto's disease or pelvis M24.7

Outcome of delivery Z37.9
multiple births Z37.9
all liveborn Z37.50
quadruplets Z37.52
quintuplets Z37.53
sextuplets Z37.54
specified number NEC Z37.59
triplets Z37.51
all stillborn Z37.7
some liveborn Z37.60
quadruplets Z37.62
quintuplets Z37.63
sextuplets Z37.64
specified number NEC Z37.69
triplets Z37.61
single NEC Z37.9

Outcome of delivery (continued)
single NEC (continued)
liveborn Z37.0
stillborn Z37.1
twins NEC Z37.9
both liveborn Z37.2
both stillborn Z37.4
one liveborn, one stillborn Z37.3

Outlet —see condition

Ovalocytosis (congenital) (hereditary) —see Elliptocytosis

Ovarian —see Condition

Ovariocele N83.4-

Ovaritis (cystic) —see Oophoritis

Ovary, ovarian —see also condition
resistant syndrome E28.39
vein syndrome N13.8

Overactive —see also Hyperfunction
adrenal cortex NEC E27.0
bladder N32.81
hypothalamus E23.3
thyroid —see Hyperthyroidism

Overactivity R46.3
child —see Disorder, attention-deficit hyperactivity

Overbite (deep) (excessive) (horizontal) (vertical) M26.29

Overbreathing —see Hyperventilation

Overconscientious personality vF60.5

Overdevelopment —see Hypertrophy

Overdistension —see Distension

Overdose, overdosage (drug) —see Table of Drugs and Chemicals, by drug, poisoning

Overeating R63.2
nonorganic origin F50.89
psychogenic F50.89

Overexertion (effects) (exhaustion) T73.3

Overexposure (effects) T73.9
exhaustion T73.2

Overfeeding —see Overeating
newborn P92.4

Overfill, endodontic M27.52

Overgrowth, bone —see Hypertrophy, bone

Overhanging of dental restorative material (unrepairable) K08.52

Overheated (places) (effects) —see Heat

Overjet (excessive horizontal) M26.23

Overlaid, overlying (suffocation) —see Asphyxia, traumatic, due to mechanical threat

Overlap, excessive horizontal (teeth) M26.23

Overlapping toe (acquired) — see also Deformity, toe, specified NEC
congenital (fifth toe) Q66.89

Overload
circulatory, due to transfusion (blood) (blood components) (TACO) E87.71
fluid E87.70
due to transfusion (blood) (blood components) E87.71
specified NEC E87.79
iron, due to repeated red blood cell transfusions E83.111

Overload (continued)
potassium (K) E87.5
sodium (Na) E87.0

Overnutrition —see Hyperalimentation

Overproduction —see also Hypersecretion
ACTH E27.0
catecholamine E27.5
growth hormone E22.0

Overprotection, child by parent Z62.1

Overriding
aorta Q25.49
finger (acquired) —see Deformity, finger
congenital Q68.1
toe (acquired) —see also Deformity, toe, specified NEC
congenital Q66.89

Overstrained R53.83
heart —see Hypertrophy, cardiac

Overuse, muscle NEC M70.8-

Overweight E66.3

Overworked R53.83

Oviduct —see condition

Ovotestis Q56.0

Ovulation (cycle)
failure or lack of N97.0
pain N94.0

Ovum —see condition

Owren's disease or syndrome (parahemophilia) D68.2

Ox heart —see Hypertrophy, cardiac

Oxalosis E72.53

Oxaluria E72.53

Oxycephaly, oxycephalic Q75.0
syphilitic, congenital A50.02

Oxyuriasis D80

Oxyuris vermicularis (infestation) B80

Ozena J31.0

P

Pachyderma, pachydermia L85.9
larynx (verrucosa) J38.7

Pachydermatocele (congenital) Q82.8

Pachydermoperiostosis —see also Osteoarthropathy, hypertrophic, specified type NEC
clubbed nail M89.40 *[L62]*

Pachygyria Q04.3

Pachymeningitis (adhesive) (basal) (brain) (cervical) (chronic) (circumscribed) (external) (fibrous) (hemorrhagic) (hypertrophic) (internal) (purulent) (spinal) (suppurative) —see Meningitis

Pachyonychia (congenital) Q84.5

Pacinian tumor —see Neoplasm, skin, benign

Pad, knuckle or Garrod's M72.1

Paget-Schroetter syndrome I82.890

Paget's disease
with infiltrating duct carcinoma — see Neoplasm, breast, malignant
bone M88.9

Paget's disease (continued)
bone (continued)
carpus M88.84-
clavicle M88.81-
femur M88.85-
fibula M88.86-
finger M88.84-
humerus M88.82-
ilium M88.85-
in neoplastic disease —see Osteitis, deformans, in neoplastic disease
ischium M88.85-
metacarpus M88.84-
metatarsus M88.87-
multiple sites M88.89
neck M88.88
radius M88.83-
rib M88.88
scapula M88.81-
skull M88.0
specified NEC M88.88
tarsus M88.87-
tibia M88.86-
toe M88.87-
ulna M88.83-
vertebra M88.1
breast (female) C50.01-
male C50.02-
extramammary —see also Neoplasm, skin, malignant
anus C21.0
margin C44.590
skin C44.590
intraductal carcinoma —see Neoplasm, breast, malignant
malignant —see Neoplasm, skin, malignant
breast (female) C50.01-
male C50.02-
unspecified site (female) C50.01-
male C50.02-
mammary —see Paget's disease, breast
nipple —see Paget's disease, breast
osteitis deformans —see Paget's disease, bone

Pain(s) (see also Painful) R52
abdominal R10.9
colic R10.83
generalized R10.84
with acute abdomen R10.0
lower R10.30
left quadrant R10.32
pelvic or perineal R10.2
periumbilical R10.33
right quadrant R10.31
rebound —see Tenderness, abdominal, rebound
severe with abdominal rigidity R10.0
tenderness —see Tenderness, abdominal
upper R10.10
epigastric R10.13
left quadrant R10.12
right quadrant R10.11
acute R52
due to trauma G89.11
neoplasm related G89.3
postprocedural NEC G89.18
post-thoracotomy G89.12
specified by site - code to Pain, by site
adnexa (uteri) R10.2
anginoid —see Pain, precordial
anus K62.89
arm —see Pain, limb, upper
axillary (axilla) M79.62-
back (postural) M54.9

248

Pain (continued)

bladder R39.89
  associated with micturition —see
    Micturition, painful
  chronic R39.82
bone —see Disorder, bone,
  specified type NEC
breast N64.4
broad ligament R10.2
cancer associated (acute) (chronic)
  G89.3
cecum —see Pain, abdominal
cervicobrachial M53.1
chest (central) R07.9
  anterior wall R07.89
  atypical R07.89
  ischemic I20.9
  musculoskeletal R07.89
  non-cardiac R07.89
  on breathing R07.1
  pleurodynia R07.81
  precordial R07.2
  wall (anterior) R07.89
chronic G89.29
  associated with significant
    psychosocial dysfunction
    G89.4
  due to trauma G89.21
  neoplasm related G89.3
  postoperative NEC G89.28
  postprocedural NEC G89.28
  post-thoracotomy G89.22
  specified NEC G89.29
coccyx M53.3
colon —see Pain, abdominal
coronary —see Angina
costochondral R07.1
diaphragm R07.1
due to cancer G89.3
due to device, implant or graft
  (see also Complications, by
  site and type, specified NEC)
  T85.848
  arterial graft NEC T82.848
  breast (implant) T85.848
  catheter NEC T85.848
    dialysis (renal) T82.848
      intraperitoneal T85.848
    infusion NEC T82.848
      spinal (epidural) (subdural)
      T85.840
    urinary (indwelling) T83.84
  electronic (electrode) (pulse
    generator) (stimulator)
    bone T84.84
    cardiac T82.847
    nervous system (brain)
      (peripheral nerve) (spinal)
      T85.840
    urinary T83.84
  fixation, internal (orthopedic)
    NEC T84.84
  gastrointestinal (bile duct)
    (esophagus) T85.848
  genital NEC T83.84
  heart NEC T82.847
  infusion NEC T85.848
  joint prosthesis T84.84
  ocular (corneal graft) (orbital
    implant) NEC T85.848
  orthopedic NEC T84.84
  specified NEC T85.848
  urinary NEC T83.84
  vascular NEC T82.848
  ventricular intracranial shunt
    T85.840
due to malignancy (primary)
  (secondary) G89.3
ear —see subcategory H92.0
epigastric, epigastrium R10.13
eye —see Pain, ocular

Pain (continued)

face, facial R51.9
  atypical G50.1
female genital organs NEC N94.89
finger —see Pain, limb, upper
flank —see Pain, abdominal
foot —see Pain, limb, lower
gallbladder K82.9
gas (intestinal) R14.1
gastric —see Pain, abdominal
generalized NOS R52
genital organ
  female N94.89
  male N50.89
groin —see Pain, abdominal, lower
hand —see Pain, limb, upper
head —see Headache
heart —see Pain, precordial
infra-orbital —see Neuralgia,
  trigeminal
intercostal R07.82
intermenstrual N94.0
jaw R68.84
joint M25.50
  ankle M25.57-
  elbow M25.52-
  finger M25.54-
  foot M25.57-
  hand M25.54-
  hip M25.55-
  knee M25.56-
  shoulder M25.51-
  specified site NEC M25.59
  toe M25.57-
  wrist M25.53-
kidney N23
laryngeal R07.0
leg —see Pain, limb, lower
limb M79.609
  lower M79.60-
    foot M79.67-
    lower leg M79.66-
    thigh M79.65-
    toe M79.67-
  upper M79.60-
    axilla M79.62-
    finger M79.64-
    forearm M79.63-
    hand M79.64-
    upper arm M79.62-
loin M54.5
low back M54.5
lumbar region M54.5
mandibular R68.84
mastoid —see subcategory H92.0
maxilla R68.84
menstrual (see also Dysmenorrhea)
  N94.6
metacarpophalangeal (joint) —see
  Pain, joint, hand
metatarsophalangeal (joint) —see
  Pain, joint, foot
mouth K13.79
muscle —see Myalgia
musculoskeletal (see also Pain, by
  site) M79.18
myofascial M79.18
nasal J34.89
nasopharynx J39.2
neck NEC M54.2
nerve NEC —see Neuralgia
neuromuscular —see Neuralgia
nose J34.89
ocular H57.1-
ophthalmic —see Pain, ocular
orbital region —see Pain, ocular
ovary N94.89
ovulation N94.0
pelvic (female) R10.2
penis N48.89

Pain (continued)

pericardial —see Pain, precordial
perineal, perineum R10.2
pharynx J39.2
pleura, pleural, pleuritic R07.81
postoperative NOS G89.18
postprocedural NOS G89.18
post-thoracotomy G89.12
precordial (region) R07.2
premenstrual N94.3
psychogenic (persistent) (any site)
  F45.41
radicular (spinal) —see
  Radiculopathy
rectum K62.89
respiration R07.1
retrosternal R07.2
rheumatoid, muscular —see
  Myalgia
rib R07.81
root (spinal) —see Radiculopathy
round ligament (stretch) R10.2
sacroiliac M53.3
sciatic —see Sciatica
scrotum N50.82
seminal vesicle N50.89
shoulder M25.51-
spermatic cord N50.89
spinal root —see Radiculopathy
spine M54.9
  cervical M54.2
  low back M54.5
    with sciatica M54.4-
  thoracic M54.6
stomach —see Pain, abdominal
substernal R07.2
temporomandibular (joint) M26.62-
testis N50.81-
thoracic spine M54.6
  with radicular and visceral pain
    M54.14
throat R07.0
tibia —see Pain, limb, lower
toe —see Pain, limb, lower
tongue K14.6
tooth K08.89
trigeminal —see Neuralgia,
  trigeminal
tumor associated G89.3
ureter N23
urinary (organ) (system) N23
uterus NEC N94.89
vagina R10.2
vertebrogenic (syndrome) M54.89
vesical R39.89
  associated with micturition —see
    Micturition, painful
vulva R10.2

Painful —see also Pain
coitus
  female N94.10
  male N53.12
  psychogenic F52.6
ejaculation (semen) N53.12
  psychogenic F52.6
erection —see Priapism
feet syndrome E53.8
joint replacement (hip) (knee)
  T84.84
menstruation —see Dysmenorrhea
  psychogenic F45.8
micturition —see Micturition, painful
respiration R07.1
scar NEC L90.5
wire sutures T81.89

Painter's colic —see subcategory
  T56.0

Palate —see condition

Palatoplegia K13.79

Palatoschisis —see Cleft, palate

Palilalia R48.8

Palliative care Z51.5

Pallor R23.1
optic disc, temporal —see Atrophy,
  optic

Palmar —see also condition
fascia —see condition

Palpable
cecum K63.89
kidney N28.89
ovary N83.8
prostate N42.9
spleen —see Splenomegaly

Palpitations (heart) R00.2
psychogenic F45.8

Palsy (see also Paralysis) G83.9
atrophic diffuse (progressive)
  G12.22
Bell's —see also Palsy, facial
  newborn P11.3
brachial plexus NEC G54.0
  newborn (birth injury)
    P14.3
brain —see Palsy, cerebral
bulbar (progressive) (chronic)
  G12.22
  of childhood (Fazio-Londe)
    G12.1
  pseudo NEC G12.29
  supranuclear (progressive)
    G23.1
cerebral (congenital) G80.9
  ataxic G80.4
  athetoid G80.3
  choreathetoid G80.3
  diplegic G80.8
    spastic G80.1
  dyskinetic G80.3
    athetoid G80.3
    choreathetoid G80.3
    distonic G80.3
  dystonic G80.3
  hemiplegic G80.8
    spastic G80.2
  mixed G80.8
  monoplegic G80.8
    spastic G80.1
  paraplegic G80.8
    spastic G80.1
  quadriplegic G80.8
    spastic G80.0
  spastic G80.1
    diplegic G80.1
    hemiplegic G80.2
    monoplegic G80.1
    quadriplegic G80.0
    specified NEC G80.1
    tetrapelgic G80.0
  specified NEC G80.8
  syphilitic A52.12
    congenital A50.49
  tetraplegic G80.8
    spastic G80.0
cranial nerve —see also Disorder,
  nerve, cranial
  multiple G52.7
    in
      infectious disease B99
        [G53]
      neoplastic disease (see also
        Neoplasm) D49.9 [G53]
      parasitic disease B89 [G53]
      sarcoidosis D86.82
creeping G12.22
diver's T70.3
Erb's P14.0
facial G51.0
  newborn (birth injury) P11.3
glossopharyngeal G52.1

Palsy *(continued)*
  Klumpke (-Déjérine) P14.1
  lead —*see* subcategory T56.0
  median nerve (tardy) G56.1-
  nerve G58.9
    specified NEC G58.8
  peroneal nerve (acute) (tardy)
    G57.3-
  progressive supranuclear G23.1
  pseudobulbar NEC G12.29
  radial nerve (acute) G56.3-
  seventh nerve —*see also* Palsy,
    facial
    newborn P11.3
  shaking —*see* Parkinsonism
  spastic (cerebral) (spinal) G80.1
  ulnar nerve (tardy) G56.2-
  wasting G12.29

Paludism —*see* Malaria

Panangiitis M30.0

Panaris, panaritium —*see also*
  Cellulitis, digit
  with lymphangitis —*see*
    Lymphangitis, acute, digit

Panarteritis nodosa M30.0
  brain or cerebral I67.7

Pancake heart R93.1
  with cor pulmonale (chronic)
    I27.81

Pancarditis (acute) (chronic) I51.89
  rheumatic I09.89
    active or acute I01.8

Pancoast's syndrome or tumor
  C34.1-

Pancolitis, ulcerative (chronic)
  K51.00
  with
    complication K51.019
      abscess K51.014
      fistula K51.013
      obstruction K51.012
      rectal bleeding K51.011
      specified complication NEC
        K51.018

Pancreas, pancreatic —*see* condition

Pancreatitis (annular) (apoplectic)
  (calcareous) (edematous)
  (hemorrhagic) (malignant)
  (subacute) (suppurative) K85.90
  with necrosis (uninfected)
    K85.91
    infected K85.92
  acute (without necrosis or
    infection) K85.90
    with necrosis (uninfected)
      K85.91
      infected K85.92
    alcohol induced (without
      necrosis or infection) K85.20
      with necrosis (uninfected)
        K85.21
        infected K85.22
    biliary (without necrosis or
      infection) K85.10
      with necrosis (uninfected)
        K85.11
        infected K85.12
    drug induced (without necrosis
      or infection) K85.30
      with necrosis (uninfected)
        K85.31
        infected K85.32
    gallstone (without necrosis or
      infection) K85.10
      with necrosis (uninfected)
        K85.11
        infected K85.12

Pancreatitis *(continued)*
  acute *(continued)*
    idiopathic (without necrosis or
      infection) K85.00
      with necrosis (uninfected)
        K85.01
        infected K85.02
    specified NEC (without necrosis
      or infection) K85.80
      with necrosis (uninfected)
        K85.81
        infected K85.82
  chronic (infectious) K86.1
    alcohol-induced K86.0
    recurrent K86.1
    relapsing K86.1
  cystic (chronic) K86.1
  cytomegaloviral B25.2
  fibrous (chronic) K86.1
  gangrenous —*see* Pancreatitis,
    acute
  gallstone (without necrosis or
    infection) K85.10
    with necrosis (uninfected)
      K85.11
      infected K85.12
  interstitial (chronic) K86.1
    acute (*see also* Pancreatitis,
      acute) K85.80
  mumps B26.3
  recurrent
    acute K85.50
    chronic K86.1
  relapsing, chronic K86.1
  syphilitic A52.74

Pancreatoblastoma —*see* Neoplasm,
  pancreas, malignant

Pancreolithiasis K86.89

Pancytolysis D75.89

Pancytopenia (acquired) D61.818
  with
    malformations D61.09
    myelodysplastic syndrome
      —*see* Syndrome,
      myelodysplastic
  antineoplastic chemotherapy
    induced D61.810
  congenital D61.09
  drug-induced NEC D61.811

PANDAS (pediatric autoimmune
  neuropsychiatric disorders
  associated with streptococcal
  infections syndrome) D89.89

**Panencephalitis, subacute,
  sclerosing** A81.1

Panhematopenia D61.9
  congenital D61.09
  constitutional D61.09
  splenic, primary D73.1

Panhemocytopenia D61.9
  congenital D61.09
  constitutional D61.09

Panhypogonadism E29.1

Panhypopituitarism E23.0
  prepubertal E23.0

Panic (attack) (state) F41.0
  reaction to exceptional stress
    (transient) F43.0

**Panmyelopathy, familial,
  constitutional** D61.09

Panmyelophthisis D61.82
  congenital D61.09

Panmyelosis (acute) (with
  myelofibrosis) C94.4-

Panner's disease —*see*
  Osteochondrosis, juvenile, humerus

Panneuritis endemica E51.11

Panniculitis (nodular)
  (nonsuppurative) M79.3
  back M54.00
    cervical region M54.02
    cervicothoracic region M54.03
    lumbar region M54.06
    lumbosacral region M54.07
    multiple sites M54.09
    occipito-atlanto-axial region
      M54.01
    sacrococcygeal region M54.08
    thoracic region M54.04
    thoracolumbar region M54.05
  lupus L93.2
  mesenteric K65.4
  neck M54.02
    cervicothoracic region M54.03
    occipito-atlanto-axial region
      M54.01
  relapsing M35.6

Panniculus adiposus (abdominal) E65

Pannus (allergic) (cornea)
  (degenerativus) (keratic) H16.42-
  abdominal (symptomatic) E65
  trachomatosus, trachomatous
    (active) A71.1

Panophthalmitis H44.01-

Pansinusitis (chronic) (hyperplastic)
  (nonpurulent) (purulent) J32.4
  acute J01.40
    recurrent J01.41
  tuberculous A15.8

Panuveitis (sympathetic) H44.11-

Panvalvular disease I08.9
  specified NEC I08.8

**PAPA (pyogenic arthritis,
  pyoderma gangrenosum, and
  acne syndrome)** M04.8

Papanicolaou smear, cervix Z12.4
  as part of routine gynecological
    examination Z01.419
    with abnormal findings Z01.411
  for suspected neoplasm Z12.4
  nonspecific abnormal finding
    R87.619
  routine Z01.419
    with abnormal findings Z01.411

Papilledema (choked disc) H47.10
  associated with
    decreased ocular pressure
      H47.12
    increased intracranial pressure
      H47.11
    retinal disorder H47.13
  Foster-Kennedy syndrome H47.14-

Papillitis H46.00
  anus K62.89
  chronic lingual K14.4
  necrotizing, kidney N17.2
  optic H46.0-
  rectum K62.89
  renal, necrotizing N17.2
  tongue K14.0

Papilloma —*see also* Neoplasm,
  benign, by site
  basal cell L82.1
    inflamed L82.0
  acuminatum (female) (male)
    (anogenital) A63.0
  benign pinta (primary) A67.0
  bladder (urinary) (transitional cell)
    D41.4
  choroid plexus (lateral ventricle)
    (third ventricle) D33.0
    anaplastic C71.5
    fourth ventricle D33.1
    malignant C71.5

Papilloma *(continued)*
  renal pelvis (transitional cell)
    D41.1-
    benign D30.1-
  Schneiderian
    specified site —*see* Neoplasm,
      benign, by site
    unspecified site D14.0
  serous surface
    borderline malignancy
      specified site —*see* Neoplasm,
        uncertain behavior, by site
      unspecified site D39.10
    specified site —*see* Neoplasm,
      benign, by site
    unspecified site D27.9
  transitional (cell)
    bladder (urinary) D41.4
    inverted type —*see* Neoplasm,
      uncertain behavior, by site
    renal pelvis D41.1-
    ureter D41.2-
  ureter (transitional cell) D41.2-
    benign D30.2-
  urothelial —*see* Neoplasm,
    uncertain behavior, by site
  villous —*see* Neoplasm, uncertain
    behavior, by site
    adenocarcinoma in —*see*
      Neoplasm, malignant, by site
    in situ —*see* Neoplasm, in situ
  yaws, plantar or palmar A66.1

Papillomata, multiple, of yaws
  A66.1

Papillomatosis —*see also* Neoplasm,
  benign, by site
  confluent and reticulated L83
  cystic, breast —*see* Mastopathy,
    cystic
  ductal, breast —*see* Mastopathy,
    cystic
  intraductal (diffuse) —*see*
    Neoplasm, benign, by site
  subareolar duct D24-

**Papillomavirus, as cause of disease
  classified elsewhere** B97.7

**Papillon-Léage and Psaume
  syndrome** Q87.0

Papule(s) R23.8
  carate (primary) A67.0
  fibrous, of nose D22.39
  Gottron's L94.4
  pinta (primary) A67.0

Papulosis
  lymphomatoid C86.6
  malignant I77.89

Papyraceous fetus O31.0-

Para-albuminemia E88.09

Paracephalus Q89.7

Parachute mitral valve Q23.2

Paracoccidioidomycosis B41.9
  disseminated B41.7
  generalized B41.7
  mucocutaneous-lymphangitic
    B41.8
  pulmonary B41.0
  specified NEC B41.8
  visceral B41.8

Paradentosis K05.4

Paraffinoma T88.8

Paraganglioma D44.7
  adrenal D35.0-
    malignant C74.1-
  aortic body D44.7
    malignant C75.5
  carotid body D44.6
    malignant C75.4

Paraganglioma (continued)
  chromaffin —see also Neoplasm,
    benign, by site
    malignant —see Neoplasm,
      malignant, by site
  extra-adrenal D44.7
    malignant C75.5
      specified site —see Neoplasm,
        malignant, by site
      unspecified site C75.5
    specified site —see Neoplasm,
      uncertain behavior, by site
    unspecified site D44.7
  gangliocytic D13.2
    specified site —see Neoplasm,
      benign, by site
    unspecified site D13.2
  glomus jugulare D44.7
    malignant C75.5
  jugular D44.7
  malignant C75.5
    specified site —see Neoplasm,
      malignant, by site
    unspecified site C75.5
  nonchromaffin D44.7
    malignant C75.5
      specified site —see Neoplasm,
        malignant, by site
      unspecified site C75.5
    specified site —see Neoplasm,
      uncertain behavior, by site
    unspecified site D44.7
  parasympathetic D44.7
    specified site —see Neoplasm,
      uncertain behavior, by site
    unspecified site D44.7
  specified site —see Neoplasm,
    uncertain behavior, by site
  sympathetic D44.7
    specified site —see Neoplasm,
      uncertain behavior, by site
    unspecified site D44.7
  unspecified site D44.7

Parageusia R43.2
  psychogenic F45.8

Paragonimiasis B66.4

Paragranuloma, Hodgkin —see
  Lymphoma, Hodgkin, specified
  NEC

Parahemophilia (see also Defect,
  coagulation) D68.2

Parakeratosis R23.4
  variegata L41.0

Paralysis, paralytic (complete)
  (incomplete) G83.9
  with
    syphilis A52.17
  abducens, abducent (nerve) —see
    Strabismus, paralytic, sixth nerve
  abductor, lower extremity G57.9-
  accessory nerve G52.8
  accommodation —see also Paresis,
    of accommodation
    hysterical F44.89
  acoustic nerve (except Deafness)
    —see subcategory H93.3
  agitans (see also Parkinsonism)
    G20
    arteriosclerotic G21.4
  alternating (oculomotor) G83.89
  amyotrophic G12.21
  ankle G57.9-
  anus (sphincter) K62.89
  arm —see Monoplegia, upper limb
  ascending (spinal), acute G61.0
  association G12.29
  asthenic bulbar G70.00
    with exacerbation (acute) G70.01
    in crisis G70.01

Paralysis, paralytic (continued)
  ataxic (hereditary) G11.9
    general (syphilitic) A52.17
  atrophic G58.9
    infantile, acute —see
      Poliomyelitis, paralytic
    progressive G12.22
    spinal (acute) —see
      Poliomyelitis, paralytic
  axillary G54.0
  Babinski-Nageotte's G83.89
  Bell's G51.0
    newborn P11.3
  Benedikt's G46.3
  birth injury P14.9
    spinal cord P11.5
  bladder (neurogenic) (sphincter)
    N31.2
  bowel, colon or intestine K56.0
  brachial plexus G54.0
    birth injury P14.3
    newborn (birth injury) P14.3
  brain G83.9
    diplegia G83.0
    triplegia G83.89
  bronchial J98.09
  Brown-Séquard G83.81
  bulbar (chronic) (progressive) G12.22
    infantile —see Poliomyelitis,
      paralytic
    poliomyelitic —see
      Poliomyelitis, paralytic
    pseudo G12.29
  bulbospinal G70.00
    with exacerbation (acute) G70.01
    in crisis G70.01
  cardiac (see also Failure, heart) I50.9
  cerebrocerebellar, diplegic G80.1
  cervical
    plexus G54.2
    sympathetic G90.09
  Céstan-Chenais G46.3
  Charcot-Marie-Tooth type G60.0
  Clark's G80.9
  colon K56.0
  compressed air T70.3
  compression
    arm G56.9-
    leg G57.9-
    lower extremity G57.9-
    upper extremity G56.9-
  congenital (cerebral) —see Palsy,
    cerebral
  conjugate movement (gaze) (of
    eye) H51.0
    cortical (nuclear) (supranuclear)
      H51.0
  cordis —see Failure, heart
  cranial or cerebral nerve G52.9
  creeping G12.22
  crossed leg G83.89
  crutch —see Injury, brachial plexus
  deglutition R13.0
    hysterical F44.4
  dementia A52.17
  descending (spinal) NEC G12.29
  diaphragm (flaccid) J98.6
    due to accidental dissection
      of phrenic nerve during
      procedure —see Puncture,
      accidental complicating
      surgery
  digestive organs NEC K59.89
  diplegic —see Diplegia
  divergence (nuclear) H51.8
  diver's T70.3
  Duchenne's
    birth injury P14.0
    due to or associated with
      motor neuron disease G12.22
      muscular dystrophy G71.01

Paralysis, paralytic (continued)
  due to intracranial or spinal birth
    injury —see Palsy, cerebral
  embolic (current episode) I63.4-
  Erb (-Duchenne) (birth) (newborn)
    P14.0
  Erb's syphilitic spastic spinal
    A52.17
  esophagus K22.8
  eye muscle (extrinsic) H49.9
    intrinsic —see also Paresis, of
      accommodation
  facial (nerve) G51.0
    birth injury P11.3
    congenital P11.3
    following operation NEC
      —see Puncture, accidental
      complicating surgery
    newborn (birth injury) P11.3
  familial (recurrent) (periodic)
    G72.3
    spastic G11.4
  fauces J39.2
  finger G56.9-
  gait R26.1
  gastric nerve (nondiabetic) G52.2
  gaze, conjugate H51.0
  general (progressive) (syphilitic)
    A52.17
    juvenile A50.45
  glottis J38.00
    bilateral J38.02
    unilateral J38.01
  gluteal G54.1
  Gubler (-Millard) G46.3
  hand —see Monoplegia, upper
    limb
  heart —see Arrest, cardiac
  hemiplegic —see Hemiplegia
  hyperkalemic periodic (familial)
    G72.3
  hypoglossal (nerve) G52.3
  hypokalemic periodic G72.3
  hysterical F44.4
  ileus K56.0
  infantile (see also Poliomyelitis,
    paralytic) A80.30
    bulbar —see Poliomyelitis,
      paralytic
    cerebral —see Palsy, cerebral
    spastic —see Palsy, cerebral,
      spastic
  infective —see Poliomyelitis,
    paralytic
  inferior nuclear G83.9
  internuclear —see
    Ophthalmoplegia, internuclear
  intestine K56.0
  iris H57.09
    due to diphtheria (toxin) A36.89
  ischemic, Volkmann's
    (complicating trauma) T79.6
  Jackson's G83.89
  jake —see Poisoning, food,
    noxious, plant
  Jamaica ginger (jake) G62.2
  juvenile general A50.45
  Klumpke (-Déjérine) (birth)
    (newborn) P14.1
  labioglossal (laryngeal)
    (pharyngeal) G12.29
  Landry's G61.0
  laryngeal nerve (recurrent)
    (superior) (unilateral) J38.00
    bilateral J38.02
    unilateral J38.01
  larynx J38.00
    bilateral J38.02
    due to diphtheria (toxin) A36.2
    unilateral J38.01
  lateral G12.23

Paralysis, paralytic (continued)
  lead —see subcategory T56.0
  left side —see Hemiplegia
  leg G83.1-
    both —see Paraplegia
    crossed G83.89
    hysterical F44.4
    psychogenic F44.4
    transient or transitory R29.818
      traumatic NEC —see Injury,
      nerve, leg
  levator palpebrae superioris —see
    Blepharoptosis, paralytic
  limb —see Monoplegia
  lip K13.0
  Lissauer's A52.17
  lower limb —see Monoplegia,
    lower limb
    both —see Paraplegia
  lung J98.4
  median nerve G56.1-
  medullary (tegmental) G83.89
  mesencephalic NEC G83.89
    tegmental G83.89
  middle alternating G83.89
  Millard-Gubler-Foville G46.3
  monoplegic —see Monoplegia
  motor G83.9
  muscle, muscular NEC G72.89
    due to nerve lesion G58.9
    eye (extrinsic) H49.9
      intrinsic —see Paresis, of
      accommodation
      oblique —see Strabismus,
      paralytic, fourth nerve
    iris sphincter H21.9
    ischemic (Volkmann's)
      (complicating trauma)
      T79.6
    progressive G12.21
    progressive, spinal G12.25
    pseudohypertrophic G71.02
    spinal progressive G12.25
  musculocutaneous nerve G56.9-
  musculospiral G56.9-
  nerve —see also Disorder, nerve
    abducent —see Strabismus,
      paralytic, sixth nerve
    accessory G52.8
    auditory (except Deafness)
      —see subcategory H93.3
    birth injury P14.9
    cranial or cerebral G52.9
    facial G51.0
      birth injury P11.3
      congenital P11.3
      newborn (birth injury) P11.3
    fourth or trochlear —see
      Strabismus, paralytic, fourth
      nerve
    newborn (birth injury) P14.9
    oculomotor —see Strabismus,
      paralytic, third nerve
    phrenic (birth injury) P14.2
    radial G56.3-
    seventh or facial G51.0
      newborn (birth injury) P11.3
    sixth or abducent —see
      Strabismus, paralytic, sixth
      nerve
    syphilitic A52.15
    third or oculomotor —see
      Strabismus, paralytic, third
      nerve
    trigeminal G50.9
    trochlear —see Strabismus,
      paralytic, fourth nerve
    ulnar G56.2-
  normokalemic periodic G72.3
  ocular H49.9
    alternating G83.89

Paralysis, paralytic *(continued)*

oculofacial, congenital (Moebius)
Q87.0
oculomotor (external bilateral)
(nerve) —*see* Strabismus,
paralytic, third nerve
palate (soft) K13.79
paratrigeminal G50.9
periodic (familial) (hyperkalemic)
(hypokalemic) (myotonic)
(normokalemic) (potassium
sensitive) (secondary) G72.3
peripheral autonomic nervous
system —*see* Neuropathy,
peripheral, autonomic
peroneal (nerve) G57.3-
pharynx J39.2
phrenic nerve G56.8-
plantar nerve(s) G57.6-
pneumogastric nerve G52.2
poliomyelitis (current) —*see*
Poliomyelitis, paralytic
popliteal nerve G57.3-
postepileptic transitory G83.84
progressive (atrophic) (bulbar)
(spinal) G12.22
general A52.17
infantile acute —*see*
Poliomyelitis, paralytic
supranuclear G23.1
pseudobulbar G12.29
pseudohypertrophic (muscle)
G71.09
psychogenic F44.4
quadriceps G57.9-
quadriplegic —*see* Tetraplegia
radial nerve G56.3-
rectus muscle (eye) H49.9
recurrent isolated sleep G47.53
respiratory (muscle) (system)
(tract) R06.81
center NEC G93.89
congenital P28.89
newborn P28.89
right side —*see* Hemiplegia
saturnine —*see* subcategory
T56.0
sciatic nerve G57.0-
senile G83.9
shaking —*see* Parkinsonism
shoulder G56.9-
sleep, recurrent isolated G47.53
spastic G83.9
cerebral —*see* Palsy, cerebral,
spastic
congenital (cerebral) —*see*
Palsy, cerebral, spastic
familial G11.4
hereditary G11.4
quadriplegic G80.0
syphilitic (spinal) A52.17
sphincter, bladder —*see* Paralysis,
bladder
spinal (cord) G83.9
accessory nerve G52.8
acute —*see* Poliomyelitis,
paralytic
ascending acute G61.0
atrophic (acute) —*see also*
Poliomyelitis, paralytic
spastic, syphilitic A52.17
congenital NEC —*see* Palsy,
cerebral
infantile —*see* Poliomyelitis,
paralytic
hereditary G95.89
progressive G12.21
muscle G12.25
sequelae NEC G83.89
sternomastoid G52.8
stomach K31.84

Paralysis, paralytic *(continued)*

stomach *(continued)*
diabetic —*see* Diabetes, by type,
with gastroparesis
nerve G52.2
diabetic —*see* Diabetes, by
type, with gastroparesis
stroke —*see* Infarct, brain
subcapsularis G56.8-
supranuclear (progressive) G23.1
sympathetic G90.8
cervical G90.09
nervous system —*see*
Neuropathy, peripheral,
autonomic
syndrome G83.9
specified NEC G83.89
syphilitic spastic spinal (Erb's)
A52.17
thigh G57.9-
throat J39.2
diphtheritic A36.0
muscle J39.2
thrombotic (current episode) I63.3-
thumb G56.9-
tick —*see* Toxicity, venom,
arthropod, specified NEC
Todd's (postepileptic transitory
paralysis) G83.84
toe G57.6-
tongue K14.8
transient R29.5
arm or leg NEC R29.818
traumatic NEC —*see* Injury,
nerve
trapezius G52.8
traumatic, transient NEC —*see*
Injury, nerve
trembling —*see* Parkinsonism
triceps brachii G56.9-
trigeminal nerve G50.9
trochlear (nerve) —*see* Strabismus,
paralytic, fourth nerve
ulnar nerve G56.2-
upper limb —*see* Monoplegia,
upper limb
uremic N18.9 *[G99.8]*
uveoparotitic D86.89
uvula K13.79
postdiphtheritic A36.0
vagus nerve G52.2
vasomotor NEC G90.8
velum palati K13.79
vesical —*see* Paralysis, bladder
vestibular nerve (except Vertigo)
—*see* subcategory H93.3
vocal cords J38.00
bilateral J38.02
unilateral J38.01
Volkmann's (complicating trauma)
T79.6
wasting G12.29
Weber's G46.3
wrist G56.9-

Paramedial urethrovesical orifice
Q64.79

Paramenia N92.6

Parametritis (*see also* Disease,
pelvis, inflammatory) N73.2
acute N73.0
complicating abortion —*see*
Abortion, by type, complicated
by, parametritis

Parametrium, parametric —*see*
condition

Paramnesia —*see* Amnesia

Paramolar K00.1

Paramyloidosis E85.89

Paramyoclonus multiplex G25.3

Paramyotonia (congenita) G71.19

Parangi —*see* Yaws

Paranoia (querulans) F22
senile F03

Paranoid
dementia (senile) F03
praecox —*see* Schizophrenia
personality F60.0
psychosis (climacteric)
(involutional) (menopausal) F22
psychogenic (acute) F23
senile F03
reaction (acute) F23
chronic F22
schizophrenia F20.0
state (climacteric) (involutional)
(menopausal) (simple) F22
senile F03
tendencies F60.0
traits F60.0
trends F60.0
type, psychopathic personality
F60.0

Paraparesis —*see* Paraplegia

Paraphasia R47.02

Paraphilia F65.9

Paraphimosis (congenital) N47.2
chancroidal A57

Paraphrenia, paraphrenic (late) F22
schizophrenia F20.0

Paraplegia (lower) G82.20
ataxic —*see* Degeneration,
combined, spinal cord
complete G82.21
congenital (cerebral) G80.8
spastic G80.1
familial spastic G11.4
functional (hysterical) F44.4
hereditary, spastic G11.4
hysterical F44.4
incomplete G82.22
Pott's A18.01
psychogenic F44.4
spastic
Erb's spinal, syphilitic A52.17
hereditary G11.4
tropical G04.1
syphilitic (spastic) A52.17
traumatic
current injury - code to injury
with seventh character A
sequela of previous injury -
code to injury with seventh
character S
tropical spastic G04.1

Parapoxvirus B08.60
specified NEC B08.69

Paraproteinemia D89.2
benign (familial) D89.2
monoclonal D47.2
secondary to malignant disease
D47.2

Parapsoriasis L41.9
en plaques L41.4
guttata L41.1
large plaque L41.4
retiform, retiformis L41.5
small plaque L41.3
specified NEC L41.8
varioliformis (acuta) L41.0

Parasitic —*see also* condition
disease NEC B89
stomatitis B37.0
sycosis (beard) (scalp) B35.0
twin Q89.4

Parasitism B89
intestinal B82.9
skin B88.9
specified —*see* Infestation

Parasitophobia F40.218

Parasomnia G47.50
due to
alcohol
abuse F10.182
dependence F10.282
use F10.982
amphetamines
abuse F15.182
dependence F15.282
use F15.982
caffeine
abuse F15.182
dependence F15.282
use F15.982
cocaine
abuse F14.182
dependence F14.282
use F14.982
drug NEC
abuse F19.182
dependence F19.282
use F19.982
opioid
abuse F11.182
dependence F11.282
use F11.982
psychoactive substance NEC
abuse F19.182
dependence F19.282
use F19.982
sedative, hypnotic, or anxiolytic
abuse F13.182
dependence F13.282
use F13.982
stimulant NEC
abuse F15.182
dependence F15.282
use F15.982
in conditions classified elsewhere
G47.54
nonorganic origin F51.8
organic G47.50
specified NEC G47.59

Paraspadias Q54.9

Paraspasmus facialis G51.8

Parasuicide (attempt)
history of (personal) Z91.5
in family Z81.8

Parathyroid gland —*see* condition

Parathyroid tetany E20.9

Paratrachoma A74.0

Paratyphilitis —*see* Appendicitis

Paratyphoid (fever) —*see* Fever,
paratyphoid

Paratyphus —*see* Fever, paratyphoid

Paraurethral duct Q64.79

Paraurethritis —*see also*
Urethritis
gonococcal (acute) (chronic) (with
abscess) A54.1

Paravaccinia NEC B08.04

Paravaginitis —*see* Vaginitis

Parencephalitis —*see also*
Encephalitis
sequelae G09

Parent-child conflict —*see* Conflict,
parent-child
estrangement NEC Z62.890

Paresis —*see also* Paralysis
accommodation —*see* Paresis, of
accommodation

Paralysis, paralytic–Paresis

Paresis (continued)
  Bernhardt's G57.1-
  bladder (sphincter) —see also
    Paralysis, bladder
    tabetic A52.17
  bowel, colon or intestine K56.0
  extrinsic muscle, eye H49.9
  general (progressive) (syphilitic)
    A52.17
    juvenile A50.45
  heart —see Failure, heart
  insane (syphilitic) A52.17
  juvenile (general) A50.45
  of accommodation H52.52-
  peripheral progressive (idiopathic)
    G60.3
  pseudohypertrophic G71.09
  senile G83.9
  syphilitic (general) A52.17
    congenital A50.45
  vesical NEC N31.2

Paresthesia (see also Disturbance, sensation, skin) R20.2
  Bernhardt G57.1-

Paretic —see condition

Parinaud's
  conjunctivitis H10.89
  oculoglandular syndrome H10.89
  ophthalmoplegia H49.88-

Parkinsonism (idiopathic) (primary) G20
  with neurogenic orthostatic
    hypotension (symptomatic)
    G90.3
  arteriosclerotic G21.4
  dementia G31.83 [F02.80]
    with behavioral disturbance
      G31.83 [F02.81]
  due to
    drugs NEC G21.19
      neuroleptic G21.11
    medication-induced NEC G21.19
  neuroleptic induced G21.11
  postencephalitic G21.3
  secondary G21.9
    due to
      arteriosclerosis G21.4
      drugs NEC G21.19
        neuroleptic G21.11
      encephalitis G21.3
      external agents NEC G21.2
      syphilis A52.19
    specified NEC G21.8
  syphilitic A52.19
  treatment-induced NEC G21.19
  vascular G21.4

Parkinson's disease, syndrome or tremor —see Parkinsonism

Parodontitis —see Periodontitis

Parodontosis K05.4

Paronychia —see also Cellulitis, digit
  with lymphangitis —see
    Lymphangitis, acute, digit
  candidal (chronic) B37.2
  tuberculous (primary) A18.4

Parorexia (psychogenic) F50.89

Parosmia R43.1
  psychogenic F45.8

Parotid gland —see condition

Parotitis, parotiditis (allergic) (nonspecific toxic) (purulent) (septic) (suppurative) —see also Sialoadenitis
  epidemic —see Mumps
  infectious —see Mumps

Parotitis, parotiditis (continued)
  postoperative K91.89
  surgical K91.89

Parrot fever A70

Parrot's disease (early congenital syphilitic pseudoparalysis) A50.02

Parry-Romberg syndrome G51.8

Parry's disease or syndrome E05.00
  with thyroid storm E05.01

Pars planitis —see Cyclitis

Parsonage (-Aldren)-**Turner syndrome** G54.5

Parson's disease (exophthalmic goiter) E05.00
  with thyroid storm E05.01

Particolored infant Q82.8

Parturition —see Delivery

Parulis K04.7
  with sinus K04.6

Parvovirus, as cause of disease classified elsewhere B97.6

Pasini and Pierini's atrophoderma L90.3

Passage
  false, urethra N36.5
  meconium (newborn) during
    delivery P03.82
  of sounds or bougies —see
    Attention to, artificial, opening

Passive —see condition
  smoking Z77.22

Pasteurella septica A28.0

Pasteurellosis —see Infection, Pasteurella

PAT (paroxysmal atrial tachycardia) I47.1

Patau's syndrome —see Trisomy, 13

Patches
  mucous (syphilitic) A51.39
    congenital A50.07
  smokers' (mouth) K13.24

Patellar —see condition

Patent —see also Imperfect, closure
  canal of Nuck Q52.4
  cervix N88.3
  ductus arteriosus or Botallo's
    Q25.0
  foramen
    botalli Q21.1
    ovale Q21.1
  interauricular septum Q21.1
  interventricular septum Q21.0
  omphalomesenteric duct Q43.0
  os (uteri) —see Patent, cervix
  ostium secundum Q21.1
  urachus Q64.4
  vitelline duct Q43.0

Paterson (-Brown) (-Kelly) **syndrome or web** D50.1

Pathologic, pathological —see also condition
  asphyxia R09.01
  fire-setting F63.1
  gambling F63.0
  ovum O02.0
  resorption, tooth K03.3
  stealing F63.2

Pathology (of) —see Disease
  periradicular, associated with
    previous endodontic treatment
    NEC M27.59

Pattern, sleep-wake, irregular G47.23

Patulous —see also Imperfect, closure (congenital)
  alimentary tract Q45.8
    lower Q43.8
    upper Q40.8
  eustachian tube H69.0-

Pause, sinoatrial I49.5

Paxton's disease B36.2

Pearl(s)
  enamel K00.2
  Epstein's K09.8

Pearl-worker's disease —see Osteomyelitis, specified type NEC

Pectenosis K62.4

Pectoral —see condition

Pectus
  carinatum (congenital) Q67.7
    acquired M95.4
      rachitic sequelae (late effect)
        E64.3
  excavatum (congenital) Q67.6
    acquired M95.4
      rachitic sequelae (late effect)
        E64.3
  recurvatum (congenital) Q67.6

Pedatrophia E41

Pederosis F65.4

Pediculosis (infestation) B85.2
  capitis (head-louse) (any site)
    B85.0
  corporis (body-louse) (any site)
    B85.1
  eyelid B85.0
  mixed (classifiable to more than
    one of the titles B85.0-B85.3)
    B85.4
  pubis (pubic louse) (any site)
    B85.3
  vestimenti B85.1
  vulvae B85.3

Pediculus (infestation) —see Pediculosis

Pedophilia F65.4

Peg-shaped teeth K00.2

Pelade —see Alopecia, areata

Pelger-Huët anomaly or syndrome D72.0

Peliosis (rheumatica) D69.0
  hepatis K76.4
    with toxic liver disease K71.8

Pelizaeus-Merzbacher disease E75.29

Pellagra (alcoholic) (with polyneuropathy) E52

Pellagra-cerebellar-ataxia-renal aminoaciduria syndrome E72.02

Pellegrini (-Stieda) **disease or syndrome** —see Bursitis, tibial collateral

Pellizzi's syndrome E34.8

Pel's crisis A52.11

Pelvic —see also condition
  examination (periodic) (routine)
    Z01.419
    with abnormal findings Z01.411
  kidney, congenital Q63.2

Pelviolithiasis —see Calculus, kidney

Pelviperitonitis —see also
  Peritonitis, pelvic
  gonococcal A54.24
  puerperal O85

Pelvis —see condition or type

Pemphigoid L12.9
  benign, mucous membrane L12.1
  bullous L12.0
  cicatricial L12.1
  juvenile L12.2
  ocular L12.1
  specified NEC L12.8

Pemphigus L10.9
  benign familial (chronic) Q82.8
  Brazilian L10.3
  circinatus L13.0
  conjunctiva L12.1
  drug-induced L10.5
  erythematosus L10.4
  foliaceous L10.2
  gangrenous —see Gangrene
  neonatorum L01.03
  ocular L12.1
  paraneoplastic L10.81
  specified NEC L10.89
  syphilitic (congenital) A50.06
  vegetans L10.1
  vulgaris L10.0
  wildfire L10.3

Pendred's syndrome E07.1

Pendulous
  abdomen, in pregnancy —see
    Pregnancy, complicated by,
    abnormal, pelvic organs or
    tissues NEC
  breast N64.89

Penetrating wound —see also
  Puncture
  with internal injury —see Injury,
    by site
  eyeball —see Puncture,
    eyeball
  orbit (with or without foreign body)
    —see Puncture, orbit
  uterus by instrument with or
    following ectopic or molar
    pregnancy O08.6

Penicillosis B48.4

Penis —see condition

Penitis N48.29

Pentalogy of Fallot Q21.8

Pentasomy X syndrome Q97.1

Pentosuria (essential) E74.89

Percreta placenta O43.23-

Peregrinating patient —see
  Disorder, factitious

Perforation, perforated
  (nontraumatic) (of)
  accidental during procedure
    (blood vessel) (nerve) (organ)
    —see Complication, accidental
    puncture or laceration
  antrum —see Sinusitis, maxillary
  appendix K35.32
    with localized peritonitis
      K35.32
  atrial septum, multiple Q21.1
  attic, ear —see Perforation,
    tympanum, attic
  bile duct (common) (hepatic)
    K83.2
    cystic K82.2
  bladder (urinary)
    with or following ectopic or
      molar pregnancy O08.6
    obstetrical trauma O71.5
    traumatic S37.29
      at delivery O71.5
  bowel K63.1
    with or following ectopic or
      molar pregnancy O08.6
    newborn P78.0

Perforation, perforated *(continued)*
bowel *(continued)*
obstetrical trauma O71.5
traumatic —*see* Laceration,
intestine
broad ligament N83.8
with or following ectopic or
molar pregnancy O08.6
obstetrical trauma O71.6
by
device, implant or graft *(see also*
Complications, by site and
type, mechanical) T85.628
arterial graft NEC —*see*
Complication,
cardiovascular device,
mechanical, vascular
breast (implant) T85.49
catheter NEC T85.698
cystostomy T83.090
dialysis (renal) T82.49
intraperitoneal T85.691
infusion NEC T82.594
spinal (epidural)
(subdural) T85.690
urinary *(see also*
Complications, catheter,
urinary) T83.098
electronic (electrode) (pulse
generator) (stimulator)
bone T84.390
cardiac T82.199
electrode T82.190
pulse generator T82.191
specified type NEC
T82.198
nervous system —*see*
Complication, prosthetic
device, mechanical,
electronic nervous system
stimulator
urinary —*see* Complication,
genitourinary, device,
urinary, mechanical
fixation, internal (orthopedic)
NEC —*see* Complication,
fixation device, mechanical
gastrointestinal —*see*
Complications, prosthetic
device, mechanical,
gastrointestinal device
genital NEC T83.498
intrauterine contraceptive
device T83.39
penile prosthesis T83.490
heart NEC —*see*
Complication,
cardiovascular device,
mechanical
joint prosthesis —*see*
Complications, joint
prosthesis, mechanical,
specified NEC, by site
ocular NEC —*see*
Complications, prosthetic
device, mechanical, ocular
device
orthopedic NEC —*see*
Complication, orthopedic,
device, mechanical
specified NEC T85.628
urinary NEC —*see also*
Complication, genitourinary,
device, urinary, mechanical
graft T83.29
vascular NEC —*see*
Complication,
cardiovascular device,
mechanical
ventricular intracranial shunt
T85.09

Perforation, perforated *(continued)*
by *(continued)*
foreign body left accidentally in
operative wound T81.539
instrument (any) during a
procedure, accidental —
see Puncture, accidental
complicating surgery
cecum K35.32
with localized peritonitis K35.32
cervix (uteri) N88.8
with or following ectopic or
molar pregnancy O08.6
obstetrical trauma O71.3
colon K63.1
newborn P78.0
obstetrical trauma O71.5
traumatic —*see* Laceration,
intestine, large
common duct (bile) K83.2
cornea (due to ulceration) —*see*
Ulcer, cornea, perforated
cystic duct K82.2
diverticulum (intestine) K57.80
with bleeding K57.81
large intestine K57.20
with
bleeding K57.21
small intestine K57.40
with bleeding K57.41
small intestine K57.00
with
bleeding K57.01
large intestine K57.40
with bleeding K57.41
ear drum —*see* Perforation,
tympanum
esophagus K22.3
ethmoidal sinus —*see* Sinusitis,
ethmoidal
frontal sinus —*see* Sinusitis, frontal
gallbladder K82.2
heart valve —*see* Endocarditis
ileum K63.1
newborn P78.0
obstetrical trauma O71.5
traumatic —*see* Laceration,
intestine, small
instrumental, surgical (accidental)
(blood vessel) (nerve) (organ)
—*see* Puncture, accidental
complicating surgery
intestine NEC K63.1
with ectopic or molar pregnancy
O08.6
newborn P78.0
obstetrical trauma O71.5
traumatic —*see* Laceration,
intestine
ulcerative NEC K63.1
newborn P78.0
jejunum, jejunal K63.1
obstetrical trauma O71.5
traumatic —*see* Laceration,
intestine, small
ulcer —*see* Ulcer, gastrojejunal,
with perforation
joint prosthesis —*see*
Complications, joint prosthesis,
mechanical, specified NEC, by
site
mastoid (antrum) (cell) —*see*
Disorder, mastoid, specified NEC
maxillary sinus —*see* Sinusitis,
maxillary
membrana tympani —*see*
Perforation, tympanum
nasal
septum J34.89
congenital Q30.3
syphilitic A52.73

Perforation, perforated *(continued)*
nasal *(continued)*
sinus J34.89
congenital Q30.8
due to sinusitis —*see* Sinusitis
palate *(see also* Cleft, palate) Q35.9
syphilitic A52.79
palatine vault *(see also* Cleft,
palate, hard) Q35.1
syphilitic A52.79
congenital A50.59
pars flaccida (ear drum) —*see*
Perforation, tympanum, attic
pelvic
floor S31.030
with
ectopic or molar pregnancy
O08.6
penetration into
retroperitoneal space
S31.031
retained foreign body
S31.040
with penetration into
retroperitoneal space
S31.041
following ectopic or molar
pregnancy O08.6
obstetrical trauma O70.1
organ S37.99
adrenal gland S37.818
bladder —*see* Perforation,
bladder
fallopian tube S37.599
bilateral S37.592
unilateral S37.591
kidney S37.09-
obstetrical trauma O71.5
ovary S37.499
bilateral S37.492
unilateral S37.491
prostate S37.828
specified organ NEC S37.898
ureter —*see* Perforation,
ureter
urethra —*see* Perforation,
urethra
uterus —*see* Perforation,
uterus
perineum —*see* Laceration,
perineum
pharynx J39.2
rectum K63.1
newborn P78.0
obstetrical trauma O71.5
traumatic S36.63
root canal space due to endodontic
treatment M27.51
sigmoid K63.1
newborn P78.0
obstetrical trauma O71.5
traumatic S36.533
sinus (accessory) (chronic) (nasal)
J34.89
sphenoidal sinus —*see* Sinusitis,
sphenoidal
surgical (accidental) (by
instrument) (blood vessel)
(nerve) (organ) —*see* Puncture,
accidental complicating surgery
traumatic
external —*see* Puncture
eye —*see* Puncture, eyeball
internal organ —*see* Injury, by
site
tympanum, tympanic (membrane)
(persistent post-traumatic)
(postinflammatory) H72.9-
attic H72.1-
multiple —*see* Perforation,
tympanum, multiple

Perforation, perforated *(continued)*
tympanum, tympanic *(continued)*
attic *(continued)*
total —*see* Perforation,
tympanum, total
central H72.0-
multiple —*see* Perforation,
tympanum, multiple
total —*see* Perforation,
tympanum, total
marginal NEC —*see* subcategory
H72.2
multiple H72.81-
pars flaccida —*see* Perforation,
tympanum, attic
total H72.82-
traumatic, current episode
S09.2-
typhoid, gastrointestinal —*see*
Typhoid
ulcer —*see* Ulcer, by site, with
perforation
ureter N28.89
traumatic S37.19
urethra N36.8
with ectopic or molar pregnancy
O08.6
following ectopic or molar
pregnancy O08.6
obstetrical trauma O71.5
traumatic S37.39
at delivery O71.5
uterus
with ectopic or molar pregnancy
O08.6
by intrauterine contraceptive
device T83.39
following ectopic or molar
pregnancy O08.6
obstetrical trauma O71.1
traumatic S37.69
obstetric O71.1
uvula K13.79
syphilitic A52.79
vagina
obstetrical trauma O71.4
other trauma —*see* Puncture,
vagina

**Periadenitis mucosa necrotica
recurrens** K12.0

Periappendicitis (acute) —*see*
Appendicitis

Periarteritis nodosa (disseminated)
(infectious) (necrotizing) M30.0

Periarthritis (joint) —*see also*
Enthesopathy
Duplay's M75.0-
gonococcal A54.42
humeroscapularis —*see* Capsulitis,
adhesive
scapulohumeral —*see* Capsulitis,
adhesive
shoulder —*see* Capsulitis,
adhesive
wrist M77.2-

Periarthrosis (angioneural) —*see*
Enthesopathy

Pericapsulitis, adhesive (shoulder)
—*see* Capsulitis, adhesive

Pericarditis (with decompensation)
(with effusion) I31.9
with rheumatic fever (conditions
in I00)
active —*see* Pericarditis,
rheumatic
inactive or quiescent I09.2
acute (hemorrhagic)
(nonrheumatic) (Sicca) I30.9

Pericarditis (continued)

acute *(continued)*
  with chorea (acute) (rheumatic)
    (Sydenham's) I02.0
  benign I30.8
  nonspecific I30.0
  rheumatic I01.0
    with chorea (acute)
      (Sydenham's) I02.0
adhesive or adherent (chronic)
  (external) (internal) I31.0
  acute —*see* Pericarditis, acute
  rheumatic I09.2
bacterial (acute) (subacute) (with
  serous or seropurulent effusion)
  I30.1
calcareous I31.1
cholesterol (chronic) I31.8
  acute I30.9
chronic (nonrheumatic) I31.9
  rheumatic I09.2
constrictive (chronic) I31.1
coxsackie B33.23
fibrinocaseous (tuberculous)
  A18.84
fibrinopurulent I30.1
fibrinous I30.8
fibrous I31.0
gonococcal A54.83
idiopathic I30.0
in systemic lupus erythematosus
  M32.12
infective I30.1
meningococcal A39.53
neoplastic (chronic) I31.8
  acute I30.9
obliterans, obliterating I31.0
plastic I31.0
pneumococcal I30.1
postinfarction I24.1
purulent I30.1
rheumatic (active) (acute) (with
  effusion) (with pneumonia)
  I01.0
  with chorea (acute) (rheumatic)
    (Sydenham's) I02.0
  chronic or inactive (with chorea)
    I09.2
rheumatoid —*see* Rheumatoid,
  carditis
septic I30.1
serofibrinous I30.8
staphylococcal I30.1
streptococcal I30.1
suppurative I30.1
syphilitic A52.06
tuberculous A18.84
uremic N18.9 *[I32]*
viral I30.1

Pericardium, pericardial —*see*
condition

Pericellulitis —*see* Cellulitis

Pericementitis (chronic)
(suppurative) —*see also*
Periodontitis
acute K05.20
  generalized —*see* Periodontitis,
    aggressive, generalized
  localized —*see* Periodontitis,
    aggressive, localized

Perichondritis

auricle —*see* Perichondritis, ear
bronchus J98.09
ear (external) H61.00-
  acute H61.01-
  chronic H61.02-
  external auditory canal —*see*
    Perichondritis, ear

Perichondritis (continued)

larynx J38.7
  syphilitic A52.73
  typhoid A01.09
nose J34.89
pinna —*see* Perichondritis, ear
trachea J39.8

Periclasia K05.4

Pericoronitis —*see* Periodontitis

Pericystitis N30.90
with hematuria N30.91

Peridiverticulitis (intestine) K57.92
cecum —*see* Diverticulitis,
  intestine, large
colon —*see* Diverticulitis, intestine,
  large
duodenum —*see* Diverticulitis,
  intestine, small
intestine —*see* Diverticulitis,
  intestine
jejunum —*see* Diverticulitis,
  intestine, small
rectosigmoid —*see* Diverticulitis,
  intestine, large
rectum —*see* Diverticulitis,
  intestine, large
sigmoid —*see* Diverticulitis,
  intestine, large

Periendocarditis —*see* Endocarditis

Periepididymitis N45.1

Perifolliculitis L01.02
abscedens, caput, scalp L66.3
capitis, abscedens (et suffodiens)
  L66.3
superficial pustular L01.02

Perihepatitis K65.8

Perilabyrinthitis (acute) —*see*
subcategory H83.0

Perimeningitis —*see* Meningitis

Perimetritis —*see* Endometritis

Perimetrosalpingitis —*see* Salpingo-
oophoritis

Perineocele N81.81

Perinephric, perinephritic —*see*
condition

Perinephritis —*see also* Infection,
kidney
purulent —*see* Abscess, kidney

Perineum, perineal —*see* condition

Perineuritis NEC —*see* Neuralgia

Periodic —*see* condition

Periodontitis (chronic) (complex)
(compound) (local) (simplex)
K05.30
acute K05.20
  generalized K05.229
    moderate K05.222
    severe K05.223
    slight K05.221
  localized K05.219
    moderate K05.212
    severe K05.213
    slight K05.211
apical K04.5
  acute (pulpal origin) K04.4
generalized K05.329
  moderate K05.322
  severe K05.323
  slight K05.321
localized K05.319
  moderate K05.312
  severe K05.313
  slight K05.311

Periodontoclasia K05.4

Periodontosis (juvenile) K05.4

Periods —*see also* Menstruation
heavy N92.0
irregular N92.6
shortened intervals (irregular)
  N92.1

Perionychia —*see also* Cellulitis,
digit
with lymphangitis —*see*
  Lymphangitis, acute, digit

Perioophoritis —*see* Salpingo-
oophoritis

Periorchitis N45.2

Periosteum, periosteal —*see*
condition

Periostitis (albuminosa)
(circumscribed) (diffuse)
(infective) (monomelic) —*see also*
Osteomyelitis
alveolar M27.3
alveolodental M27.3
dental M27.3
gonorrheal A54.43
jaw (lower) (upper) M27.2
orbit H05.03-
syphilitic A52.77
  congenital (early) A50.02
    [M90.80]
  secondary A51.46
tuberculous —*see* Tuberculosis,
  bone
yaws (hypertrophic) (early) (late)
  A66.6 *[M90.80]*

Periostosis (hyperplastic) —*see also*
Disorder, bone, specified type NEC
with osteomyelitis —*see*
  Osteomyelitis, specified type
  NEC

Peripartum
cardiomyopathy O90.3

Periphlebitis —*see* Phlebitis

Periproctitis K62.89

Periprostatitis —*see* Prostatitis

Perirectal —*see* condition

Perirenal —*see* condition

Perisalpingitis —*see* Salpingo-
oophoritis

Perisplenitis (infectional) D73.89

Peristalsis, visible or reversed
R19.2

Peritendinitis —*see* Enthesopathy

Peritoneum, peritoneal —*see*
condition

Peritonitis (adhesive) (bacterial)
(fibrinous) (hemorrhagic)
(idiopathic) (localized) (perforative)
(primary) (with adhesions) (with
effusion) K65.9
with or following
  abscess K65.1
  appendicitis
    with perforation or rupture
      K35.32
    generalized (*see also*
      Appendicitis) K35.20
    localized (*see also*
      Appendicitis) K35.30
  diverticular disease (intestine)
    K57.80
    with bleeding K57.81
    large intestine K57.20
      with
        bleeding K57.21
        small intestine K57.40
          with bleeding K57.41

Peritonitis (continued)

with or following *(continued)*
  diverticular disease *(continued)*
    small intestine K57.00
      with
        bleeding K57.01
        large intestine K57.40
          with bleeding K57.41
  ectopic or molar pregnancy
    O08.0
acute (generalized) K65.0
aseptic T81.61
bile, biliary K65.3
chemical T81.61
chlamydial A74.81
complicating abortion —*see*
  Abortion, by type, complicated
  by, pelvic peritonitis
congenital P78.1
chronic proliferative K65.8
diaphragmatic K65.0
diffuse K65.0
diphtheritic A36.89
disseminated K65.0
due to
  bile K65.3
  foreign
    body or object accidentally
      left during a procedure
      (instrument) (sponge)
      (swab) T81.599
    substance accidentally
      left during a procedure
      (chemical) (powder) (talc)
      T81.61
  talc T81.61
  urine K65.8
eosinophilic K65.8
  acute K65.0
fibrocaseous (tuberculous) A18.31
fibropurulent K65.0
following ectopic or molar
  pregnancy O08.0
general (ized) K65.0
gonococcal A54.85
meconium (newborn) P78.0
neonatal P78.1
  meconium P78.0
pancreatic K65.0
paroxysmal, familial E85.0
  benign E85.0
pelvic
  female N73.5
    acute N73.3
    chronic N73.4
      with adhesions N73.6
  male K65.0
periodic, familial E85.0
proliferative, chronic K65.8
puerperal, postpartum, childbirth
  O85
purulent K65.0
septic K65.0
specified NEC K65.8
spontaneous bacterial K65.2
subdiaphragmatic K65.0
subphrenic K65.0
suppurative K65.0
syphilitic A52.74
  congenital (early) A50.08
    [K67]
talc T81.61
tuberculous A18.31
urine K65.8

Peritonsillar —*see* condition

Peritonsillitis J36

Perityphlitis K37

Periureteritis N28.89

Periurethral —*see* condition

Periurethritis (gangrenous) —*see*
Urethritis

Periuterine —*see* condition

Perivaginitis —*see* Vaginitis

Perivasculitis, retinal H35.06-

Perivasitis (chronic) N49.1

Perivesiculitis (seminal) —*see*
Vesiculitis

Perlèche NEC K13.0
due to
candidiasis B37.83
moniliasis B37.83
riboflavin deficiency E53.0
vitamin B2 (riboflavin)
deficiency E53.0

Pernicious —*see* condition

Pernio, perniosis T69.1

Perpetrator (of abuse) —*see* Index
to External Causes of Injury,
Perpetrator

Persecution
delusion F22
social Z60.5

Perseveration (tonic) R48.8

Persistence, persistent (congenital)
anal membrane Q42.3
with fistula Q42.2
arteria stapedia Q16.3
atrioventricular canal Q21.2
branchial cleft NOS Q18.2
cyst Q18.0
fistula Q18.0
sinus Q18.0
bulbus cordis in left ventricle Q21.8
canal of Cloquet Q14.0
capsule (opaque) Q12.8
cilioretinal artery or vein Q14.8
cloaca Q43.7
communication —*see* Fistula,
congenital
convolutions
aortic arch Q25.46
fallopian tube Q50.6
oviduct Q50.6
uterine tube Q50.6
double aortic arch Q25.45
ductus arteriosus (Botalli) Q25.0
fetal
circulation P29.38
form of cervix (uteri) Q51.828
hemoglobin, hereditary (HPFH)
D56.4
foramen
Botalli Q21.1
ovale Q21.1
Gartner's duct Q52.4
hemoglobin, fetal (hereditary)
(HPFH) D56.4
hyaloid
artery (generally incomplete)
Q14.0
system Q14.8
hymen, in pregnancy or childbirth
—*see* Pregnancy, complicated
by, abnormal, vulva
lanugo Q84.2
left
posterior cardinal vein Q26.8
root with right arch of aorta
Q25.49
superior vena cava Q26.1
Meckel's diverticulum Q43.0
malignant —*see* Table of
Neoplasms, small intestine,
malignant
mucosal disease (middle ear)
—*see* Otitis, media, suppurative,
chronic, tubotympanic

Persistence, persistent *(continued)*
nail(s), anomalous Q84.6
omphalomesenteric duct Q43.0
organ or site not listed —*see*
Anomaly, by site
ostium
atrioventriculare commune
Q21.2
primum Q21.2
secundum Q21.1
ovarian rests in fallopian tube
Q50.6
pancreatic tissue in intestinal tract
Q43.8
primary (deciduous)
teeth K00.6
vitreous hyperplasia Q14.0
pupillary membrane Q13.89
right aortic arch Q25.47
rhesus (Rh) titer —*see*
Complication(s), transfusion,
incompatibility reaction, Rh
(factor)
sinus
urogenitalis
female Q52.8
male Q55.8
venosus with imperfect
incorporation in right auricle
Q26.8
thymus (gland) (hyperplasia) E32.0
thyroglossal duct Q89.2
thyrolingual duct Q89.2
truncus arteriosus or communis
Q20.0
tunica vasculosa lentis Q12.2
umbilical sinus Q64.4
urachus Q64.4
vitelline duct Q43.0

Person (with)
admitted for clinical research,
as a control subject (normal
comparison) (participant) Z00.6
awaiting admission to adequate
facility elsewhere Z75.1
concern (normal) about sick person
in family Z63.6
consulting on behalf of another
Z71.0
feigning illness Z76.5
living (in)
alone Z60.2
boarding school Z59.3
residential institution Z59.3
without
adequate housing (heating)
(space) Z59.1
housing (permanent)
(temporary) Z59.0
person able to render
necessary care Z74.2
shelter Z59.0
on waiting list Z75.1
sick or handicapped in family
Z63.6

Personality (disorder) F60.9
accentuation of traits (type A
pattern) Z73.1
affective F34.0
aggressive F60.3
amoral F60.2
anacastic, anankastic F60.5
antisocial F60.2
anxious F60.6
asocial F60.2
asthenic F60.7
avoidant F60.6
borderline F60.3
change due to organic condition
(enduring) F07.0

Personality *(continued)*
compulsive F60.5
cycloid F34.0
cyclothymic F34.0
dependent F60.7
depressive F34.1
dissocial F60.2
dual F44.81
eccentric F60.89
emotionally unstable F60.3
expansive paranoid F60.0
explosive F60.3
fanatic F60.0
haltlose type F60.89
histrionic F60.4
hyperthymic F34.0
hypothymic F34.1
hysterical F60.4
immature F60.89
inadequate F60.7
labile (emotional) F60.3
mixed (nonspecific) F60.89
morally defective F60.2
multiple F44.81
narcissistic F60.81
obsessional F60.5
obsessive (-compulsive) F60.5
organic F07.0
overconscientious F60.5
paranoid F60.0
passive (-dependent) F60.7
passive-aggressive F60.89
pathologic F60.9
pattern defect or disturbance F60.9
pseudopsychopathic (organic)
F07.0
pseudoretarded (organic) F07.0
psychoinfantile F60.4
psychoneurotic NEC F60.89
psychopathic F60.2
querulant F60.0
sadistic F60.89
schizoid F60.1
self-defeating F60.89
sensitive paranoid F60.0
sociopathic (amoral) (antisocial)
(asocial) (dissocial) F60.2
specified NEC F60.89
type A Z73.1
unstable (emotional) F60.3

Perthes' disease —*see* Legg-Calvé-
Perthes disease

Pertussis (*see also* Whooping cough)
A37.90

Perversion, perverted
appetite F50.89
psychogenic F50.89
function
pituitary gland E23.2
posterior lobe E22.2
sense of smell and taste R43.8
psychogenic F45.8
sexual —*see* Deviation, sexual

Pervious, congenital —*see also*
Imperfect, closure
ductus arteriosus Q25.0

Pes (congenital) —*see also* Talipes
acquired —*see also* Deformity,
limb, foot, specified NEC
planus —*see* Deformity, limb,
flat foot
adductus Q66.89
cavus Q66.7-
deformity NEC, acquired —*see*
Deformity, limb, foot, specified
NEC
planus (acquired) (any degree)
—*see also* Deformity, limb, flat
foot

Pes *(continued)*
planus *(continued)*
rachitic sequelae (late effect)
E64.3
valgus Q66.6

Pest, pestis —*see* Plague

Petechia, petechiae R23.3
newborn P54.5

Petechial typhus A75.9

Peter's anomaly Q13.4

Petit mal seizure —*see* Epilepsy,
childhood, absence

Petit's hernia —*see* Hernia,
abdomen, specified site NEC

Petrellidosis B48.2

Petrositis H70.20-
acute H70.21-
chronic H70.22-

Peutz-Jeghers disease or syndrome
Q85.8

Peyronie's disease N48.6

**PFAPA (periodic fever, aphthous
stomatitis, pharyngitis, and
adenopathy syndrome)** M04.8

Pfeiffer's disease —*see*
Mononucleosis, infectious

Phagedena (dry) (moist) (sloughing)
—*see also* Gangrene
geometric L88
penis N48.29
tropical —*see* Ulcer, skin
vulva N76.6

Phagedenic —*see* condition

Phakoma H35.89

Phakomatosis (*see also* specific
eponymous syndromes) Q85.9
Bourneville's Q85.1
specified NEC Q85.8

Phantom limb syndrome (without
pain) G54.7
with pain G54.6

Pharyngeal pouch syndrome
D82.1

Pharyngitis (acute)
(catarrhal) (gangrenous)
(infective) (malignant)
(membranous) (phlegmonous)
(pseudomembranous) (simple)
(subacute) (suppurative)
(ulcerative) (viral) J02.9
with influenza, flu, or grippe —*see*
Influenza, with, pharyngitis
aphthous B08.5
atrophic J31.2
chlamydial A56.4
chronic (atrophic) (granular)
(hypertrophic) J31.2
coxsackievirus B08.5
diphtheritic A36.0
enteroviral vesicular B08.5
follicular (chronic) J31.2
fusospirochetal A69.1
gonococcal A54.5
granular (chronic) J31.2
herpesviral B00.2
hypertrophic J31.2
infectional, chronic J31.2
influenzal —*see* Influenza,
with, respiratory manifestations
NEC
lymphonodular, acute (enteroviral)
B08.8
pneumococcal J02.8
purulent J02.9
putrid J02.9

Pharyngitis *(continued)*
  septic J02.0
  sicca J31.2
  specified organism NEC J02.8
  staphylococcal J02.8
  streptococcal J02.0
  syphilitic, congenital (early)
    A50.03
  tuberculous A15.8
  vesicular, enteroviral B08.5
  viral NEC J02.8

Pharyngoconjunctivitis, viral B30.2

Pharyngolaryngitis (acute) J06.0
  chronic J37.0

Pharyngoplegia J39.2

Pharyngotonsillitis, herpesviral B00.2

Pharyngotracheitis, chronic J42

Pharynx, pharyngeal —*see*
  condition

Phencyclidine-induced
  anxiety disorder F16.980
  bipolar and related disorder F16.94
  depressive disorder F16.94
  psychotic disorder F16.959

Phenomenon
  Arthus' —*see* Arthus' phenomenon
  jaw-winking Q07.8
  lupus erythematosus (LE) cell
    M32.9
  Raynaud's (secondary) I73.00
    with gangrene I73.01
  vasomotor R55
  vasospastic I73.9
  vasovagal R55
  Wenckebach's I44.1

Phenylketonuria E70.1
  classical E70.0
  maternal E70.1

Pheochromoblastoma
  specified site —*see* Neoplasm,
    malignant, by site
  unspecified site C74.10

Pheochromocytoma
  malignant
    specified site —*see* Neoplasm,
      malignant, by site
    unspecified site C74.10
  specified site —*see* Neoplasm,
    benign, by site
  unspecified site D35.00

Pheohyphomycosis —*see*
  Chromomycosis

Pheomycosis —*see* Chromomycosis

Phimosis (congenital) (due to
  infection) N47.1
  chancroidal A57

Phlebectasia —*see also* Varix
  congenital Q27.4

Phlebitis (infective) (pyemic) (septic)
  (suppurative) I80.9
  antepartum —*see*
    Thrombophlebitis, antepartum
  blue —*see* Phlebitis, leg, deep
  breast, superficial I80.8
  calf muscular vein (NOS) I80.25-
  cavernous (venous) sinus —*see*
    Phlebitis, intracranial (venous)
    sinus
  cerebral (venous) sinus —*see*
    Phlebitis, intracranial (venous)
    sinus
  chest wall, superficial I80.8
  cranial (venous) sinus —*see*
    Phlebitis, intracranial (venous)
    sinus

Phlebitis *(continued)*
  deep (vessels) —*see* Phlebitis, leg,
    deep
  due to implanted device —*see*
    Complications, by site and type,
    specified NEC
  during or resulting from a
    procedure T81.72
  femoral vein (superficial) I80.1-
  femoropopliteal vein I80.0-
  gastrocnemial vein I80.25-
  gestational —*see* Phlebopathy,
    gestational
  hepatic veins I80.8
  iliac vein (common) (external)
    (internal) I80.21-
  iliofemoral —*see* Phlebitis, femoral
    vein
  intracranial (venous) sinus (any)
    G08
    nonpyogenic I67.6
  intraspinal venous sinuses and
    veins G08
    nonpyogenic G95.19
  lateral (venous) sinus —*see*
    Phlebitis, intracranial (venous)
    sinus
  leg I80.3
    antepartum —*see*
      Thrombophlebitis, antepartum
    deep (vessels) NEC I80.20-
      iliac I80.21-
      popliteal vein I80.22-
      specified vessel NEC I80.29-
      tibial vein (anterior)
        (posterior) I80.23-
    femoral vein (superficial) I80.1-
    superficial (vessels) I80.0-
  longitudinal sinus —*see* Phlebitis,
    intracranial (venous) sinus
  lower limb —*see* Phlebitis, leg
  migrans, migrating (superficial)
    I82.1
  pelvic
    with ectopic or molar pregnancy
      O08.0
    following ectopic or molar
      pregnancy O08.0
    puerperal, postpartum O87.1
  peroneal vein I80.24-
  popliteal vein —*see* Phlebitis, leg,
    deep, popliteal
  portal (vein) K75.1
  postoperative T81.72
  pregnancy —*see* Thrombophlebitis,
    antepartum
  puerperal, postpartum, childbirth
    O87.0
    deep O87.1
    pelvic O87.1
    superficial O87.0
  retina —*see* Vasculitis, retina
  saphenous (accessory) (great)
    (long) (small) —*see* Phlebitis,
    leg, superficial
  sinus (meninges) —*see* Phlebitis,
    intracranial (venous) sinus
  soleal vein I80.25-
  specified site NEC I80.8
  syphilitic A52.09
  tibial vein —*see* Phlebitis, leg,
    deep, tibial
  ulcerative I80.9
    leg —*see* Phlebitis, leg
  umbilicus I80.8
  uterus (septic) —*see* Endometritis
  varicose (leg) (lower limb) —*see*
    Varix, leg, with, inflammation

Phlebofibrosis I87.8

Phleboliths I87.8

Phlebopathy,
  gestational O22.9-
  puerperal O87.9

Phlebosclerosis I87.8

Phlebothrombosis —*see also*
  Thrombosis
  antepartum —*see*
    Thrombophlebitis, antepartum
  pregnancy —*see* Thrombophlebitis,
    antepartum
  puerperal —*see* Thrombophlebitis,
    puerperal

Phlebotomus fever A93.1

Phlegmasia
  alba dolens O87.1
    nonpuerperal —*see* Phlebitis,
      femoral vein
  cerulea dolens —*see* Phlebitis, leg,
    deep

Phlegmon —*see* Abscess

Phlegmonous —*see* condition

Phlyctenulosis (allergic)
  (keratoconjunctivitis)
  (nontuberculous) —*see also*
  Keratoconjunctivitis
  cornea —*see* Keratoconjunctivitis
  tuberculous A18.52

Phobia, phobic F40.9
  animal F40.218
    spiders F40.210
  examination F40.298
  reaction F40.9
  simple F40.298
  social F40.10
    generalized F40.11
  specific (isolated) F40.298
    animal F40.218
      spiders F40.210
    blood F40.230
    injection F40.231
    injury F40.233
    men F40.290
    natural environment F40.228
      thunderstorms F40.220
    situational F40.248
      bridges F40.242
      closed in spaces F40.240
      flying F40.243
      heights F40.241
    specified focus NEC F40.298
    transfusion F40.231
    women F40.291
  specified NEC F40.8
    medical care NEC F40.232
  state F40.9

Phocas' disease —*see* Mastopathy,
  cystic

Phocomelia Q73.1
  lower limb —*see* Agenesis, leg,
    with foot present
  upper limb —*see* Agenesis, arm,
    with hand present

Phoria H50.50

Phosphate-losing tubular disorder
  N25.0

Phosphatemia E83.39

Phosphaturia E83.39

Photodermatitis (sun) L56.8
  chronic L57.8
  due to drug L56.8
  light other than sun L59.8

Photokeratitis H16.13-

Photophobia H53.14-

Photophthalmia —*see* Photokeratitis

Photopsia H53.19

Photoretinitis —*see* Retinopathy,
  solar

Photosensitivity, photosensitization
  (sun) **skin** L56.8
  light other than sun L59.8

Phrenitis —*see* Encephalitis

Phrynoderma (vitamin A deficiency)
  E50.8

Phthiriasis (pubis) B85.3
  with any infestation classifiable to
    B85.0-B85.2 *[B85.4]*

Phthirus infestation —*see*
  Phthiriasis

Phthisis —*see also* Tuberculosis
  bulbi (infectional) —*see* Disorder,
    globe, degenerated condition,
    atrophy
  eyeball (due to infection) —*see*
    Disorder, globe, degenerated
    condition, atrophy

Phycomycosis —*see* Zygomycosis

Physalopteriasis B81.8

Physical restraint status Z78.1

Phytobezoar T18.9
  intestine T18.3
  stomach T18.2

Pian —*see* Yaws

Pianoma A66.1

Pica F50.89
  in adults F50.89
  infant or child F98.3

Picking, nose F98.8

Pick-Niemann disease —*see*
  Niemann-Pick disease or syndrome

Pick's
  cerebral atrophy G31.01 *[F02.80]*
    with behavioral disturbance
      G31.01 *[F02.81]*
  disease or syndrome (brain) G31.01
    [F02.80]
    with behavioral disturbance
      G31.01 *[F02.81]*
    brain G31.01 *[F02.80]*
      with behavioral disturbance
        G31.01 *[F02.81]*
    pericardium (pericardial
      pseudocirrhosis of liver) I31.1
  syndrome
    brain G31.01 *[F02.80]*
      with behavioral disturbance
        G31.01 *[F02.81]*
    of heart (pericardial
      pseudocirrhosis of liver)
      I31.1

Pickwickian syndrome E66.2

Piebaldism E70.39

Piedra (beard) (scalp) B36.8
  black B36.3
  white B36.2

**Pierre Robin deformity or
syndrome** Q87.0

Pierson's disease or osteochondrosis
  M91.0

Pig-bel A05.2

Pigeon
  breast or chest (acquired) M95.4
    congenital Q67.7
      rachitic sequelae (late effect)
        E64.3
  breeder's disease or lung J67.2
  fancier's disease or lung J67.2
  toe —*see* Deformity, toe, specified
    NEC

Pigmentation (abnormal) (anomaly) L81.9
conjunctiva H11.13-
cornea (anterior) H18.01-
posterior H18.05-
stromal H18.06-
diminished melanin formation NEC L81.6
iron L81.8
lids, congenital Q82.8
limbus corneae —see Pigmentation, cornea
metals L81.8
optic papilla, congenital Q14.2
retina, congenital (grouped) (nevoid) Q14.1
scrotum, congenital Q82.8
tattoo L81.8

Piles (see also Hemorrhoids) K64.9

Pili
annulati or torti (congenital) Q84.1
incarnati L73.1

Pill roller hand (intrinsic) —see Parkinsonism

Pilomatrixoma —see Neoplasm, skin, benign
malignant —see Neoplasm, skin, malignant

Pilonidal —see condition

Pimple R23.8

PIN —see Neoplasia, intraepithelial, prostate

Pinched nerve —see Neuropathy, entrapment

Pindborg tumor —see Cyst, calcifying odontogenic

Pineal body or gland —see condition

Pinealoblastoma C75.3

Pinealoma D44.5
malignant C75.3

Pineoblastoma C75.3

Pineocytoma D44.5

Pinguecula H11.15-

Pingueculitis H10.81-

Pinhole meatus (see also Stricture, urethra) N35.919

Pink
disease —see subcategory T56.1
eye —see Conjunctivitis, acute, mucopurulent

Pinkus' disease (lichen nitidus) L44.1

Pinpoint
meatus —see Stricture, urethra
os (uteri) —see Stricture, cervix

Pins and needles R20.2

Pinta A67.9
cardiovascular lesions A67.2
chancre (primary) A67.0
erythematous plaques A67.1
hyperchromic lesions A67.1
hyperkeratosis A67.1
lesions A67.9
cardiovascular A67.2
hyperchromic A67.1
intermediate A67.1
late A67.2
mixed A67.3
primary A67.0
skin (achromic) (cicatricial) (dyschromic) A67.2
hyperchromic A67.1

Pinta (continued)
lesions (continued)
skin (continued)
mixed (achromic and hyperchromic) A67.3
papule (primary) A67.0
skin lesions (achromic) (cicatricial) (dyschromic) A67.2
hyperchromic A67.1
mixed (achromic and hyperchromic) A67.3
vitiligo A67.2

Pintids A67.1

Pinworm (disease) (infection) (infestation) B80

Piroplasmosis (see also Babesiosis) B60.00
specified NEC B60.09

Pistol wound —see Gunshot wound

Pitchers' elbow —see Derangement, joint, specified type NEC, elbow

Pithecoid pelvis Q74.2
with disproportion (fetopelvic) O33.0
causing obstructed labor O65.0

Pithiatism F48.8

Pitted —see Pitting

Pitting (see also Edema) R60.9
lip R60.0
nail L60.8
teeth K00.4

Pituitary gland —see condition

Pituitary-snuff-taker's disease J67.8

Pityriasis (capitis) L21.0
alba L30.5
circinata (et maculata) L42
furfuracea L21.0
Hebra's L26
lichenoides L41.0
chronica L41.1
et varioliformis (acuta) L41.0
maculata (et circinata) L30.5
nigra B36.1
pilaris, Hebra's L44.0
rosea L42
rotunda L44.8
rubra (Hebra) pilaris L44.0
simplex L30.5
specified type NEC L30.5
streptogenes L30.5
versicolor (scrotal) B36.0

Placenta, placental —see Pregnancy, complicated by (care of) (management affected by), specified condition

Placentitis O41.14-

Plagiocephaly Q67.3

Plague A20.9
abortive A20.8
ambulatory A20.8
asymptomatic A20.8
bubonic A20.0
cellulocutaneous A20.1
cutaneobubonic A20.1
lymphatic gland A20.0
meningitis A20.3
pharyngeal A20.8
pneumonic (primary) (secondary) A20.2
pulmonary, pulmonic A20.2
septicemic A20.7
tonsillar A20.8
septicemic A20.7

Planning, family
contraception Z30.9
procreation Z31.69

Plaque(s)
artery, arterial —see Arteriosclerosis
calcareous —see Calcification
coronary, lipid rich I25.83
epicardial I31.8
erythematous, of pinta A67.1
Hollenhorst's —see Occlusion, artery, retina
lipid rich, coronary I25.83
pleural (without asbestos) J92.9
with asbestos J92.0
tongue K13.29

Plasmacytoma C90.3-
extramedullary C90.2-
medullary C90.0-
solitary C90.3-

Plasmacytopenia D72.818

Plasmacytosis D72.822

Plaster ulcer —see Ulcer, pressure, by site

Plateau iris syndrome (post-iridectomy) (postprocedural) (without glaucoma) H21.82
with glaucoma H40.22-

Platybasia Q75.8

Platyonychia (congenital) Q84.6
acquired L60.8

Platypelloid pelvis M95.5
with disproportion (fetopelvic) O33.0
causing obstructed labor O65.0
congenital Q74.2

Platyspondylisis Q76.49

Plaut (-Vincent) **disease** (see also Vincent's) A69.1

Plethora R23.2
newborn P61.1

Pleura, pleural —see condition

Pleuralgia R07.81

Pleurisy (acute) (adhesive) (chronic) (costal) (diaphragmatic) (double) (dry) (fibrinous) (fibrous) (interlobar) (latent) (plastic) (primary) (residual) (sicca) (sterile) (subacute) (unresolved) R09.1
with
adherent pleura J86.0
effusion J90
chylous, chyliform J94.0
tuberculous (non primary) A15.6
primary (progressive) A15.7
tuberculosis —see Pleurisy, tuberculous (non primary)
encysted —see Pleurisy, with effusion
exudative —see Pleurisy, with effusion
fibrinopurulent, fibropurulent —see Pyothorax
hemorrhagic —see Hemothorax
pneumococcal J90
purulent —see Pyothorax
septic —see Pyothorax
serofibrinous —see Pleurisy, with effusion
seropurulent —see Pyothorax
serous —see Pleurisy, with effusion
staphylococcal J86.9
streptococcal J90
suppurative —see Pyothorax
traumatic (post) (current) —see Injury, intrathoracic, pleura
tuberculous (with effusion) (non primary) A15.6
primary (progressive) A15.7

Pleuritis sicca —see Pleurisy

Pleurobronchopneumonia —see Pneumonia, broncho-

Pleurodynia R07.81
epidemic B33.0
viral B33.0

Pleuropericarditis —see also Pericarditis
acute I30.9

Pleuropneumonia (acute) (bilateral) (double) (septic) (see also Pneumonia) J18.8
chronic —see Fibrosis, lung

Pleuro-pneumonia-like-organism (PPLO), as cause of disease classified elsewhere B96.0

Pleurorrhea —see Pleurisy, with effusion

Plexitis, brachial G54.0

Plica
polonica B85.0
syndrome, knee M67.5-
tonsil J35.8

Plicated tongue K14.5

Plug
bronchus NEC J98.09
meconium (newborn) NEC syndrome P76.0
mucus —see Asphyxia, mucus

Plumbism —see subcategory T56.0

Plummer's disease E05.20
with thyroid storm E05.21

Plummer-Vinson syndrome D50.1

Pluricarential syndrome of infancy E40

Plus (and minus) hand (intrinsic) —see Deformity, limb, specified type NEC, forearm

PMEI (polymorphic epilepsy in infancy) G40.83-

Pneumathemia —see Air, embolism

Pneumatic hammer (drill) **syndrome** T75.21

Pneumatocele (lung) J98.4
intracranial G93.89
tension J44.9

Pneumatosis
cystoides intestinalis K63.89
intestinalis K63.89
peritonei K66.8

Pneumaturia R39.89

Pneumoblastoma —see Neoplasm, lung, malignant

Pneumocephalus G93.89

Pneumococcemia A40.3

Pneumococcus, pneumococcal —see condition

Pneumoconiosis (due to) (inhalation of) J64
with tuberculosis (any type in A15) J65
aluminum J63.0
asbestos J61
bagasse, bagassosis J67.1
bauxite J63.1
beryllium J63.2
coal miners' (simple) J60
coalworkers' (simple) J60
collier's J60
cotton dust J66.0
diatomite (diatomaceous earth) J62.8
dust
inorganic NEC J63.6
lime J62.8
marble J62.8
organic NEC J66.8

Pneumoconiosis *(continued)*
- fumes or vapors (from silo) J68.9
- graphite J63.3
- grinder's J62.8
- kaolin J62.8
- mica J62.8
- millstone maker's J62.8
- mineral fibers NEC J61
- miner's J60
- moldy hay J67.0
- potter's J62.8
- rheumatoid —*see* Rheumatoid, lung
- sandblaster's J62.8
- silica, silicate NEC J62.8
  - with carbon J60
- stonemason's J62.8
- talc (dust) J62.0

Pneumocystis carinii pneumonia B59

Pneumocystis jiroveci (pneumonia) B59

Pneumocystosis (with pneumonia) B59

Pneumohemopericardium I31.2

Pneumohemothorax J94.2
- traumatic S27.2

Pneumohydropericardium —*see* Pericarditis

Pneumohydrothorax —*see* Hydrothorax

Pneumomediastinum J98.2
- congenital or perinatal P25.2

Pneumomycosis B49 *[J99]*

Pneumonia (acute) (double) (migratory) (purulent) (septic) (unresolved) J18.9
- with
  - lung abscess J85.1
    - due to specified organism —*see* Pneumonia, in (due to)
  - influenza —*see* Influenza, with, pneumonia
- adenoviral J12.0
- adynamic J18.2
- alba A50.04
- allergic (*see also* Pneumonitis, hypersensitivity) J82.89
- alveolar —*see* Pneumonia, lobar
- anaerobes J15.8
- anthrax A22.1
- apex, apical —*see* Pneumonia, lobar
- Ascaris B77.81
- aspiration J69.0
  - due to
    - aspiration of microorganisms
      - bacterial J15.9
      - viral J12.9
    - food (regurgitated) J69.0
    - gastric secretions J69.0
    - milk (regurgitated) J69.0
    - oils, essences J69.1
    - solids, liquids NEC J69.8
    - vomitus J69.0
  - newborn P24.81
    - amniotic fluid (clear) P24.11
    - blood P24.21
    - liquor (amnii) P24.11
    - meconium P24.01
    - milk P24.31
    - mucus P24.11
    - food (regurgitated) P24.31
    - specified NEC P24.81
    - stomach contents P24.31
  - postprocedural J95.4
- atypical NEC J18.9

Pneumonia *(continued)*
- bacillus J15.9
  - specified NEC J15.8
- bacterial J15.9
  - specified NEC J15.8
- Bacteroides (fragilis) (oralis) (melaninogenicus) J15.8
- basal, basic, basilar —*see* Pneumonia, by type
- bronchiolitis obliterans organized (BOOP) J84.89
- broncho-, bronchial (confluent) (croupous) (diffuse) (disseminated) (hemorrhagic) (involving lobes) (lobar) (terminal) J18.0
  - allergic (*see also* Pneumonitis, hypersensitivity) J82.89
  - aspiration —*see* Pneumonia, aspiration
  - bacterial J15.9
    - specified NEC J15.8
  - chronic —*see* Fibrosis, lung
  - diplococcal J13
  - Eaton's agent J15.7
  - Escherichia coli (E. coli) J15.5
  - Friedländer's bacillus J15.0
  - Hemophilus influenzae J14
  - hypostatic J18.2
  - inhalation —*see also* Pneumonia, aspiration
    - due to fumes or vapors (chemical) J68.0
    - of oils or essences J69.1
  - Klebsiella (pneumoniae) J15.0
  - lipid, lipoid J69.1
    - endogenous J84.89
  - Mycoplasma (pneumoniae) J15.7
  - pleuro-pneumonia-like-organisms (PPLO) J15.7
  - pneumococcal J13
  - Proteus J15.6
  - Pseudomonas J15.1
  - Serratia marcescens J15.6
  - specified organism NEC J16.8
  - staphylococcal —*see* Pneumonia, staphylococcal
  - streptococcal NEC J15.4
    - group B J15.3
    - pneumoniae J13
  - viral, virus —*see* Pneumonia, viral
- Butyrivibrio (fibriosolvens) J15.8
- Candida B37.1
- caseous —*see* Tuberculosis, pulmonary
- catarrhal —*see* Pneumonia, broncho
- chlamydial J16.0
  - congenital P23.1
- cholesterol J84.89
- cirrhotic (chronic) —*see* Fibrosis, lung
- Clostridium (haemolyticum) (novyi) J15.8
- confluent —*see* Pneumonia, broncho
- congenital (infective) P23.9
  - due to
    - bacterium NEC P23.6
    - Chlamydia P23.1
    - Escherichia coli P23.4
    - Haemophilus influenzae P23.6
    - infective organism NEC P23.8
    - Klebsiella pneumoniae P23.6
    - Mycoplasma P23.6
    - Pseudomonas P23.5
    - Staphylococcus P23.2
    - Streptococcus (except group B) P23.6

Pneumonia *(continued)*
- congenital *(continued)*
  - due to *(continued)*
    - Streptococcus *(continued)*
      - group B P23.3
    - viral agent P23.0
  - specified NEC P23.8
- croupous —*see* Pneumonia, lobar
- cryptogenic organizing J84.116
- cytomegalic inclusion B25.0
- cytomegaloviral B25.0
- deglutition —*see* Pneumonia, aspiration
- desquamative interstitial J84.117
- diffuse —*see* Pneumonia, broncho
- diplococcal, diplococcus (broncho-) (lobar) J13
- disseminated (focal) —*see* Pneumonia, broncho
- Eaton's agent J15.7
- embolic, embolism —*see* Embolism, pulmonary
- Enterobacter J15.6
- eosinophilic J82.81
  - acute J82.82
  - chronic J82.81
- Escherichia coli (E. coli) J15.5
- Eubacterium J15.8
- fibrinous —*see* Pneumonia, lobar
- fibroid, fibrous (chronic) —*see* Fibrosis, lung
- Friedländer's bacillus J15.0
- Fusobacterium (nucleatum) J15.8
- gangrenous J85.0
- giant cell (measles) B05.2
- gonococcal A54.84
- gram-negative bacteria NEC J15.6
  - anaerobic J15.8
- Hemophilus influenzae (broncho) (lobar) J14
- human metapneumovirus J12.3
- hypostatic (broncho) (lobar) J18.2
- in (due to)
  - actinomycosis A42.0
  - adenovirus J12.0
  - anthrax A22.1
  - ascariasis B77.81
  - aspergillosis B44.9
  - Bacillus anthracis A22.1
  - Bacterium anitratum J15.6
  - candidiasis B37.1
  - chickenpox B01.2
  - Chlamydia J16.0
    - neonatal P23.1
  - coccidioidomycosis B38.2
    - acute B38.0
    - chronic B38.1
  - cytomegalovirus disease B25.0
  - Diplococcus (pneumoniae) J13
  - Eaton's agent J15.7
  - Enterobacter J15.6
  - Escherichia coli (E. coli) J15.5
  - Friedländer's bacillus J15.0
  - fumes and vapors (chemical) (inhalation) J68.0
  - gonorrhea A54.84
  - Hemophilus influenzae (H. influenzae) J14
  - Herellea J15.6
  - histoplasmosis B39.2
    - acute B39.0
    - chronic B39.1
  - human metapneumovirus J12.3
  - Klebsiella (pneumoniae) J15.0
  - measles B05.2
  - Mycoplasma (pneumoniae) J15.7
  - nocardiosis, nocardiasis A43.0
  - ornithosis A70
  - parainfluenza virus J12.2
  - pleuro-pneumonia-like-organism (PPLO) J15.7

Pneumonia *(continued)*
- in *(continued)*
  - pneumococcus J13
  - pneumocystosis (Pneumocystis carinii) (Pneumocystis jiroveci) B59
  - Proteus J15.6
  - Pseudomonas NEC J15.1
    - pseudomallei A24.1
  - psittacosis A70
  - Q fever A78
  - respiratory syncytial virus (RSV) J12.1
  - rheumatic fever I00 *[J17]*
  - rubella B06.81
  - Salmonella (infection) A02.22
    - typhi A01.03
  - schistosomiasis B65.9 *[J17]*
  - Serratia marcescens J15.6
  - specified
    - bacterium NEC J15.8
    - organism NEC J16.8
    - spirochetal NEC A69.8
  - Staphylococcus J15.20
    - aureus (methicillin susceptible) (MSSA) J15.211
    - methicillin resistant (MRSA) J15.212
    - specified NEC J15.29
  - Streptococcus J15.4
    - group B J15.3
    - pneumoniae J13
    - specified NEC J15.4
  - toxoplasmosis B58.3
  - tularemia A21.2
  - typhoid (fever) A01.03
  - varicella B01.2
  - virus —*see* Pneumonia, viral
  - whooping cough A37.91
    - due to
      - Bordetella parapertussis A37.11
      - Bordetella pertussis A37.01
      - specified NEC A37.81
  - Yersinia pestis A20.2
- inhalation of food or vomit —*see* Pneumonia, aspiration
- interstitial J84.9
  - chronic J84.111
  - desquamative J84.117
  - due to
    - collagen vascular disease J84.178
    - known underlying cause J84.178
  - idiopathic NOS J84.111
  - in disease classified elsewhere J84.178
  - lymphocytic (due to collagen vascular disease) (in diseases classified elsewhere) J84.178
  - lymphoid J84.2
  - non-specific J84.89
    - due to
      - collagen vascular disease J84.178
      - known underlying cause J84.178
    - idiopathic J84.113
    - in diseases classified elsewhere J84.178
  - plasma cell B59
  - pseudomonas J15.1
  - usual J84.112
    - due to collagen vascular disease J84.178
    - idiopathic J84.112
    - in diseases classified elsewhere J84.178
- Klebsiella (pneumoniae) J15.0

Pneumonia *(continued)*
lipid, lipoid (exogenous) J69.1
    endogenous J84.89
lobar (disseminated) (double)
    (interstitial) J18.1
    bacterial J15.9
        specified NEC J15.8
    chronic —*see* Fibrosis, lung
    Escherichia coli (E. coli) J15.5
    Friedländer's bacillus J15.0
    Hemophilus influenzae J14
    hypostatic J18.2
    Klebsiella (pneumoniae) J15.0
    pneumococcal J13
    Proteus J15.6
    Pseudomonas J15.1
    specified organism NEC J16.8
    staphylococcal —*see*
        Pneumonia, staphylococcal
    streptococcal NEC J15.4
    Streptococcus pneumoniae J13
    viral, virus —*see* Pneumonia, viral
lobular —*see* Pneumonia, broncho
Löffler's J82.89
lymphoid interstitial J84.2
massive —*see* Pneumonia, lobar
meconium P24.01
MRSA (Methicillin resistant
    Staphylococcus aureus)
    J15.212
MSSA (methicillin susceptible
    Staphylococcus aureus) J15.211
multilobar —*see* Pneumonia, by
    type
Mycoplasma (pneumoniae) J15.7
necrotic J85.0
neonatal P23.9
    aspiration —*see* Aspiration, by
        substance, with pneumonia
nitrogen dioxide J68.0
organizing J84.89
    due to
        collagen vascular disease
            J84.178
        known underlying cause
            J84.178
        in diseases classified elsewhere
            J84.178
orthostatic J18.2
parainfluenza virus J12.2
parenchymatous —*see* Fibrosis,
    lung
passive J18.2
patchy —*see* Pneumonia, broncho
Peptococcus J15.8
Peptostreptococcus J15.8
plasma cell (of infants) B59
pleurolobar —*see* Pneumonia,
    lobar
pleuro-pneumonia-like organism
    (PPLO) J15.7
pneumococcal (broncho) (lobar) J13
Pneumocystis (carinii) (jiroveci)
    B59
postinfectional NEC B99 *[J17]*
postmeasles B05.2
Proteus J15.6
Pseudomonas J15.1
psittacosis A70
radiation J70.0
respiratory syncytial virus (RSV)
    J12.1
resulting from a procedure J95.89
rheumatic I00 *[J17]*
Salmonella (arizonae) (cholerae-
    suis) (enteritidis) (typhimurium)
    A02.22
    typhi A01.03
    typhoid fever A01.03
SARS-associated coronavirus
    J12.81

Pneumonia *(continued)*
segmented, segmental —*see*
    Pneumonia, broncho-
Serratia marcescens J15.6
specified NEC J18.8
    bacterium NEC J15.8
    organism NEC J16.8
    virus NEC J12.89
spirochetal NEC A69.8
staphylococcal (broncho) (lobar)
    J15.20
    aureus (methicillin susceptible)
        (MSSA) J15.211
        methicillin resistant (MRSA)
            J15.212
    specified NEC J15.29
static, stasis J18.2
streptococcal NEC (broncho)
    (lobar) J15.4
    group
        A J15.4
        B J15.3
        specified NEC J15.4
Streptococcus pneumoniae J13
syphilitic, congenital (early)
    A50.04
traumatic (complication) (early)
    (secondary) T79.8
tuberculous (any) —*see*
    Tuberculosis, pulmonary
tularemic A21.2
varicella B01.2
Veillonella J15.8
ventilator associated J95.851
viral, virus (broncho) (interstitial)
    (lobar) J12.9
    adenoviral J12.0
    congenital P23.0
    human metapneumovirus J12.3
    parainfluenza J12.2
    respiratory syncytial (RSV)
        J12.1
    SARS-associated coronavirus
        J12.81
    specified NEC J12.89
white (congenital) A50.04

Pneumonic —*see* condition

Pneumonitis (acute) (primary) —*see*
    also Pneumonia
air-conditioner J67.7
allergic (due to) J67.9
    organic dust NEC J67.8
    red cedar dust J67.8
    sequoiosis J67.8
    wood dust J67.8
aspiration J69.0
    due to
        anesthesia J95.4
            during
                labor and delivery
                    O74.0
                pregnancy O29.01-
                puerperium O89.01
        fumes or gases J68.0
    obstetric O74.0
chemical (due to gases, fumes or
    vapors) (inhalation) J68.0
    due to anesthesia J95.4
cholesterol J84.89
crack (cocaine) J68.0
chronic —*see* Fibrosis, lung
congenital rubella P35.0
due to
    beryllium J68.0
    cadmium J68.0
    crack (cocaine) J68.0
    detergent J69.8
    fluorocarbon-polymer J68.0
    food, vomit (aspiration) J69.0
    fumes or vapors J68.0

Pneumonitis *(continued)*
due to *(continued)*
    gases, fumes or vapors
        (inhalation) J68.0
    inhalation
        blood J69.8
        essences J69.1
        food (regurgitated), milk,
            vomit J69.0
        oils, essences J69.1
        saliva J69.0
        solids, liquids NEC J69.8
    manganese J68.0
    nitrogen dioxide J68.0
    oils, essences J69.1
    solids, liquids NEC J69.8
    toxoplasmosis (acquired) B58.3
        congenital P37.1
    vanadium J68.0
    ventilator J95.851
eosinophilic J82.81
    acute J82.82
    chronic J82.81
hypersensitivity J67.9
    air conditioner lung J67.7
    bagassosis J67.1
    bird fancier's lung J67.2
    farmer's lung J67.0
    maltworker's lung J67.4
    maple bark-stripper's lung J67.6
    mushroom worker's lung J67.5
    specified organic dust NEC J67.8
    suberosis J67.3
interstitial (chronic) J84.89
    acute J84.114
    lymphoid J84.2
    non-specific J84.89
        idiopathic J84.113
lymphoid, interstitial J84.2
meconium P24.01
postanesthetic J95.4
    correct substance properly
        administered —*see* Table
        of Drugs and Chemicals, by
        drug, adverse effect
    in labor and delivery O74.0
    in pregnancy O29.01-
        obstetric O74.0
    overdose or wrong substance
        given or taken (by accident)
        —*see* Table of Drugs and
        Chemicals, by drug, poisoning
    postpartum, puerperal O89.01
postoperative J95.4
    obstetric O74.0
radiation J70.0
rubella, congenital P35.0
ventilation (air-conditioning) J67.7
ventilator associated J95.851
wood-dust J67.8

Pneumonoconiosis —*see*
    Pneumoconiosis

Pneumoparotid K11.8

Pneumopathy NEC J98.4
alveolar J84.09
due to organic dust NEC J66.8
parietoalveolar J84.09

Pneumopericarditis —*see also*
    Pericarditis
acute I30.9

Pneumopericardium —*see also*
    Pericarditis
congenital P25.3
newborn P25.3
traumatic (post) —*see* Injury, heart

Pneumophagia (psychogenic) F45.8

Pneumopleurisy, pneumopleuritis
    (see also Pneumonia) J18.8

Pneumopyopericardium I30.1

Pneumopyothorax —*see*
    Pyopneumothorax
    with fistula J86.0

Pneumorrhagia —*see also*
    Hemorrhage, lung
    tuberculous —*see* Tuberculosis,
        pulmonary

Pneumothorax NOS J93.9
acute J93.83
chronic J93.81
congenital P25.1
    perinatal period P25.1
postprocedural J95.811
specified NEC J93.83
spontaneous NOS J93.83
    newborn P25.1
    primary J93.11
    secondary J93.12
    tension J93.0
tense valvular, infectional J93.0
tension (spontaneous) J93.0
traumatic S27.0
    with hemothorax S27.2
tuberculous —*see* Tuberculosis,
    pulmonary

Podagra (*see also* Gout) M10.9

Podencephalus Q01.9

Poikilocytosis R71.8

Poikiloderma L81.6
Civatte's L57.3
congenital Q82.8
vasculare atrophicans L94.5

Poikilodermatomyositis M33.10
with
    myopathy M33.12
    respiratory involvement M33.11
    specified organ involvement
        NEC M33.19

Pointed ear (congenital) Q17.3

**Poison ivy, oak, sumac or other
plant dermatitis** (allergic)
    (contact) L23.7

Poisoning (acute) —*see also* Table of
    Drugs and Chemicals
algae and toxins T65.82-
Bacillus B (aertrycke) (cholerae
    (suis)) (paratyphosus)
    (suipestifer) A02.9
    botulinus A05.1
bacterial toxins A05.9
berries, noxious —*see* Poisoning,
    food, noxious, berries
botulism A05.1
ciguatera fish T61.0-
Clostridium botulinum A05.1
death-cap (Amanita phalloides)
    (Amanita verna) —*see* Poisoning,
    food, noxious, mushrooms
drug —*see* Table of Drugs
    and Chemicals, by drug,
    poisoning
epidemic, fish (noxious) —*see*
    Poisoning, seafood
    bacterial A05.9
fava bean D55.0
fish (noxious) T61.9-
    bacterial —*see* Intoxication,
        foodborne, by agent
    ciguatera fish —*see* Poisoning,
        ciguatera fish
    scombroid fish —*see* Poisoning,
        scombroid fish
    specified type NEC T61.77-
food NEC A05.9
    bacterial —*see* Intoxication,
        foodborne, by agent

Polyneuropathy (continued)

in (continued)

infectious

disease NEC B99 [G63]

mononucleosis B27.91

lack of vitamin NEC E56.9 [G63]

lead G62.2

sequelae G65.2

leprosy A30.9 [G63]

Lyme disease A69.22

metabolic disease NEC E88.9 [G63]

microscopic polyangiitis M31.7 [G63]

mumps B26.84

neoplastic disease (see also Neoplasm) D49.9 [G63]

nutritional deficiency NEC E63.9 [G63]

organophosphate compounds G62.2

sequelae G65.2

parasitic disease NEC B89 [G63]

pellagra E52 [G63]

polyarteritis nodosa M30.0

porphyria E80.20 [G63]

radiation G62.82

rheumatoid arthritis —see Rheumatoid, polyneuropathy

sarcoidosis D86.89

serum G61.1

syphilis (late) A52.15

congenital A50.43

systemic

connective tissue disorder M35.9 [G63]

lupus erythematosus M32.19

toxic agent NEC G62.2

sequelae G65.2

inflammatory G61.9

chronic demyelinating (CIDP) G61.81

sequelae G65.1

specified NEC G61.89

lead G62.2

sequelae G65.2

nutritional NEC E63.9 [G63]

postherpetic (zoster) B02.23

progressive G60.3

radiation-induced G62.82

sensory (hereditary) (idiopathic) G60.8

specified NEC G62.89

syphilitic (late) A52.15

congenital A50.43

transthyretin-related (ATTR)

familial amyloid E85.1

triorthocresyl phosphate G62.2

sequelae G65.2

tuberculosis A17.89

uremia N18.9 [G63]

vitamin B12 deficiency E53.8 [G63]

with anemia (pernicious) D51.0 [G63]

due to dietary deficiency D51.3 [G63]

zoster B02.23

Polyopia H53.8

Polyorchism, polyorchidism Q55.21

Polyosteoarthritis (see also Osteoarthritis, generalized) M15.9-

post-traumatic M15.3

specified NEC M15.8

Polyostotic fibrous dysplasia Q78.1

Polyotia Q17.0

Polyp, polypus

accessory sinus J33.8

adenocarcinoma in —see Neoplasm, malignant, by site

adenocarcinoma in situ in —see Neoplasm, in situ, by site

adenoid tissue J33.0

adenomatous —see also Neoplasm, benign, by site

adenocarcinoma in —see Neoplasm, malignant, by site

adenocarcinoma in situ in —see Neoplasm, in situ, by site

carcinoma in —see Neoplasm, malignant, by site

carcinoma in situ in —see Neoplasm, in situ, by site

multiple —see Neoplasm, benign

adenocarcinoma in —see Neoplasm, malignant, by site

adenocarcinoma in situ in —see Neoplasm, in situ, by site

antrum J33.8

anus, anal (canal) K62.0

Bartholin's gland N84.3

bladder D41.4

carcinoma in —see Neoplasm, malignant, by site

carcinoma in situ in —see Neoplasm, in situ, by site

cecum D12.0

cervix (uteri) N84.1

in pregnancy or childbirth —see Pregnancy, complicated by, abnormal, cervix

mucous N84.1

nonneoplastic N84.1

choanal J33.0

cholesterol K82.4

clitoris N84.3

colon K63.5

adenomatous D12.6

ascending D12.2

cecum D12.0

descending D12.4

hyperplastic, (any site) K63.5

inflammatory K51.40

with

abscess K51.414

complication K51.419

specified NEC K51.418

fistula K51.413

intestinal obstruction K51.412

rectal bleeding K51.411

sigmoid D12.5

transverse D12.3

corpus uteri N84.0

dental K04.01

irreversible K04.02

reversible K04.01

duodenum K31.7

ear (middle) H74.4-

endometrium N84.0

ethmoidal (sinus) J33.8

fallopian tube N84.8

female genital tract N84.9

specified NEC N84.8

frontal (sinus) J33.8

gallbladder K82.4

gingiva, gum K06.8

labia, labium (majus) (minus) N84.3

larynx (mucous) J38.1

adenomatous D14.1

malignant —see Neoplasm, malignant, by site

maxillary (sinus) J33.8

middle ear —see Polyp, ear (middle)

Polyp, polypus (continued)

myometrium N84.0

nares

anterior J33.9

posterior J33.0

nasal (mucous) J33.9

cavity J33.0

septum J33.0

nasopharyngeal J33.0

nose (mucous) J33.9

oviduct N84.8

pharynx J39.2

placenta O90.89

prostate —see Enlargement, enlarged, prostate

pudenda, pudendum N84.3

pulpal (dental) K04.01

irreversible K04.02

reversible K04.01

rectum (nonadenomatous) K62.1

adenomatous —see Polyp, adenomatous

septum (nasal) J33.0

sinus (accessory) (ethmoidal) (frontal) (maxillary) (sphenoidal) J33.8

sphenoidal (sinus) J33.8

stomach K31.7

adenomatous D13.1

tube, fallopian N84.8

turbinate, mucous membrane J33.8

umbilical, newborn P83.6

ureter N28.89

urethra N36.2

uterus (body) (corpus) (mucous) N84.0

cervix N84.1

in pregnancy or childbirth —see Pregnancy, complicated by, tumor, uterus

vagina N84.2

vocal cord (mucous) J38.1

vulva N84.3

Polyphagia R63.2

Polyploidy Q92.7

Polypoid —see condition

Polyposis —see also Polyp

coli (adenomatous) D12.6

adenocarcinoma in C18.9

adenocarcinoma in situ in —see Neoplasm, in situ, by site

carcinoma in C18.9

colon (adenomatous) D12.6

familial D12.6

adenocarcinoma in situ in —see Neoplasm, in situ, by site

intestinal (adenomatous) D12.6

malignant lymphomatous C83.1-

multiple, adenomatous (see also Neoplasm, benign) D36.9

Polyradiculitis —see Polyneuropathy

Polyradiculoneuropathy (acute) (postinfective) (segmentally demyelinating) G61.0

Polyserositis

due to pericarditis I31.1

pericardial I31.1

periodic, familial E85.0

tuberculous A19.9

acute A19.1

chronic A19.8

Polysplenia syndrome Q89.09

Polysyndactyly (see also Syndactylism, syndactyly) Q70.4

Polytrichia L68.3

Polyunguia Q84.6

Polyuria R35.8

nocturnal R35.1

psychogenic F45.8

Pompe's disease (glycogen storage) E74.02

Pompholyx L30.1

Poncet's disease (tuberculous rheumatism) A18.09

Pond fracture —see Fracture, skull

Ponos B55.0

Pons, pontine —see condition

Poor

aesthetic of existing restoration of tooth K08.56

contractions, labor O62.2

gingival margin to tooth restoration K08.51

personal hygiene R46.0

prenatal care, affecting management of pregnancy —see Pregnancy, complicated by, insufficient, prenatal care

sucking reflex (newborn) R29.2

urinary stream R39.12

vision NEC H54.7

Poradenitis, nostras inguinalis or venerea A55

Porencephaly (congenital) (developmental) (true) Q04.6

acquired G93.0

nondevelopmental G93.0

traumatic (post) F07.89

Porocephaliasis B88.8

Porokeratosis Q82.8

Poroma, eccrine —see Neoplasm, skin, benign

Porphyria (South African) E80.20

acquired E80.20

acute intermittent (hepatic) (Swedish) E80.21

cutanea tarda (hereditary) (symptomatic) E80.1

due to drugs E80.20

correct substance properly administered —see Table of Drugs and Chemicals, by drug, adverse effect

overdose or wrong substance given or taken —see Table of Drugs and Chemicals, by drug, poisoning

erythropoietic (congenital) (hereditary) E80.0

hepatocutaneous type E80.1

secondary E80.20

toxic NEC E80.20

variegata E80.20

Porphyrinuria —see Porphyria

Porphyruria —see Porphyria

Portal —see condition

Port wine nevus, mark, or stain Q82.5

Posadas-Wernicke disease B38.9

Positive

culture (nonspecific)

blood R78.81

bronchial washings R84.5

cerebrospinal fluid R83.5

cervix uteri R87.5

nasal secretions R84.5

nipple discharge R89.5

nose R84.5

staphylococcus (Methicillin susceptible) Z22.321

Methicillin resistant Z22.322

Positive (continued)
culture (continued)
peritoneal fluid R85.5
pleural fluid R84.5
prostatic secretions R86.5
saliva R85.5
seminal fluid R86.5
sputum R84.5
synovial fluid R89.5
throat scrapings R84.5
urine R82.79
vagina R87.5
vulva R87.5
wound secretions R89.5
PPD (skin test) R76.11
serology for syphilis A53.0
false R76.8
with signs or symptoms - code as
Syphilis, by site and stage
skin test, tuberculin (without active
tuberculosis) R76.11
test, human immunodeficiency
virus (HIV) R75
VDRL A53.0
with signs or symptoms - code
by site and stage under
Syphilis A53.9
Wassermann reaction A53.0

Postcardiotomy syndrome I97.0

Postcaval ureter Q62.62

Postcholecystectomy syndrome
K91.5

Postclimacteric bleeding N95.0

Postcommissurotomy syndrome
I97.0

Postconcussional syndrome F07.81

Postcontusional syndrome F07.81

Postcricoid region —see condition

Post-dates (40-42 weeks)
(pregnancy) (mother) O48.0
more than 42 weeks gestation
O48.1

Postencephalitic syndrome F07.89

Posterior —see condition

Posterolateral sclerosis (spinal
cord) —see Degeneration,
combined

Postexanthematous —see
condition

Postfebrile —see condition

**Postgastrectomy dumping
syndrome** K91.1

Posthemiplegic chorea —see
Monoplegia

Posthemorrhagic anemia (chronic)
D50.0
acute D62
newborn P61.3

Postherpetic neuralgia (zoster)
B02.29
trigeminal B02.22

Posthitis N47.7

**Postimmunization complication
or reaction** —see Complications,
vaccination

Postinfectious —see condition

Postlaminectomy syndrome NEC
M96.1

Postleukotomy syndrome F07.0

Postmastectomy lymphedema
(syndrome) I97.2

Postmaturity, postmature (over 42
weeks)
maternal (over 42 weeks gestation)
O48.1
newborn P08.22

Postmeasles complication NEC —
see also condition B05.89

Postmenopausal
endometrium (atrophic) N95.8
suppurative (see also
Endometritis) N71.9
osteoporosis —see Osteoporosis,
postmenopausal

Postnasal drip R09.82
due to
allergic rhinitis —see Rhinitis,
allergic
common cold J00
gastroesophageal reflux —see
Reflux, gastroesophageal
nasopharyngitis —see
Nasopharyngitis
other know condition - code to
condition
sinusitis —see Sinusitis

Postnatal —see condition

Postoperative (postprocedural) —see
Complication, postoperative
pneumothorax, therapeutic Z98.3
state NEC Z98.890

Postpancreatectomy hyperglycemia
E89.1

Postpartum —see Puerperal

Postphlebitic syndrome —see
Syndrome, postthrombotic

Postpoliomyelitic —see also
condition
osteopathy —see Osteopathy, after
poliomyelitis

Postpolio (myelitic) **syndrome** G14

Postprocedural —see also
Postoperative
hypolnsullnemla E89.1

Postschizophrenic depression
F32.89

Postsurgery status —see also Status
(post)
pneumothorax, therapeutic Z98.3

Post-term (40-42 weeks) (pregnancy)
(mother) O48.0
infant P08.21
more than 42 weeks gestation
(mother) O48.1

**Post-traumatic brain syndrome,
nonpsychotic** F07.81

Post-typhoid abscess A01.09

Postures, hysterical F44.2

**Postvaccinal reaction or
complication** —see Complications,
vaccination

Postvalvulotomy syndrome I97.0

Potain's
disease (pulmonary edema) —see
Edema, lung
syndrome (gastrectasis with
dyspepsia) K31.0

Potter's
asthma J62.8
facies Q60.6
lung J62.8
syndrome (with renal agenesis) Q60.6

Pott's
curvature (spinal) A18.01

Pott's (continued)
disease or paraplegia A18.01
spinal curvature A18.01
tumor, puffy —see Osteomyelitis,
specified type NEC

Pouch
bronchus Q32.4
Douglas' —see condition
esophagus, esophageal, congenital
Q39.6
acquired K22.5
gastric K31.4
Hartmann's K82.8
pharynx, pharyngeal (congenital)
Q38.7

Pouchitis K91.850

Poultrymen's itch B88.0

Poverty NEC Z59.6
extreme Z59.5

Poxvirus NEC B08.8

Prader-Willi syndrome Q87.11

Prader-Willi-like syndrome Q87.19

Preauricular appendage or tag
Q17.0

Prebetalipoproteinemia (acquired)
(essential) (familial) (hereditary)
(primary) (secondary) E78.1
with chylomicronemia E78.3

Precipitate labor or delivery
O62.3

Preclimacteric bleeding
(menorrhagia) N92.4

Precocious
adrenarche E30.1
menarche E30.1
menstruation E30.1
pubarche E30.1
puberty E30.1
central E22.8
sexual development NEC
E30.1
thelarche E30,8

Precocity, sexual (constitutional)
(cryptogenic) (female) (idiopathic)
(male) E30.1
with adrenal hyperplasia E25.9
congenital E25.0

Precordial pain R07.2

Predeciduous teeth K00.2

Prediabetes, prediabetic R73.03
complicating
pregnancy —see Pregnancy,
complicated by, diseases of,
specified type or system
NEC
puerperium O99.893

Predislocation status of hip at birth
Q65.6

Pre-eclampsia O14.9-
with pre-existing hypertension
—see Hypertension,
complicating pregnancy,
pre-existing, with, pre-eclampsia
complicating
childbirth O14.94
puerperium O14.95
mild O14.0-
complicating
childbirth O14.04
puerperium O14.05
moderate O14.0-
complicating
childbirth O14.04
puerperium O14.05

Pre-eclampsia (continued)
severe O14.1-
with hemolysis, elevated liver
enzymes and low platelet
count (HELLP) O14.2-
complicating
childbirth O14.24
puerperium O14.25
complicating
childbirth O14.14
puerperium O14.15

**Pre-eruptive color change, teeth,
tooth** K00.8

**Pre-excitation atrioventricular
conduction** I45.6

Preglaucoma H40.00-

Pregnancy (single) (uterine) —see
also Delivery and Puerperal Z33.1

> Note: The Tabular must be
> reviewed for assignment of
> the appropriate character
> indicating the trimester of the
> pregnancy
> Note: The Tabular must be
> reviewed for assignment of
> appropriate seventh character
> for multiple gestation codes in
> Chapter 15

abdominal (ectopic) O00.00
with intrauterine pregnancy
O00.01
with viable fetus O36.7-
ampullar O00.10-
with intrauterine pregnancy
O00.11-
biochemical O02.81
broad ligament O00.80
with intrauterine pregnancy
O00.81
cervical O00.80
with intrauterine pregnancy
O00.81
chemical O02.81
complicated NOS O26.9-
complicated by (care of)
(management affected by)
abnormal, abnormality
cervix O34.4-
causing obstructed labor
O65.5
cord (umbilical) O69.9
fetal heart rate or rhythm
O36.83-
findings on antenatal
screening of mother O28.9
biochemical O28.1
cytological O28.2
chromosomal O28.5
genetic O28.5
hematological O28.0
radiological O28.4
specified NEC O28.8
ultrasonic O28.3
glucose (tolerance) NEC
O99.810
pelvic organs O34.9-
specified NEC O34.8-
causing obstructed labor
O65.5
pelvis (bony) (major) NEC
O33.0
perineum O34.7-
position
placenta O44.0
with hemorrhage
O44.1-
uterus O34.59-
uterus O34.59-

Pregnancy (*continued*)
complicated by (*continued*)
abnormal, abnormality
(*continued*)
uterus (*continued*)
causing obstructed labor
O65.5
congenital O34.0-
vagina O34.6-
causing obstructed labor
O65.5
vulva O34.7-
causing obstructed labor
O65.5
abruptio placentae —*see*
Abruptio placentae
abscess or cellulitis
bladder O23.1-
breast O91.11-
genital organ or tract O23.9-
abuse
physical O9A.31-
psychological O9A.51-
sexual O9A.41-
adverse effect anesthesia
O29.9-
aspiration pneumonitis O29.01-
cardiac arrest O29.11-
cardiac complication NEC
O29.19-
cardiac failure O29.12-
central nervous system
complication NEC O29.29-
cerebral anoxia O29.21-
failed or difficult intubation
O29.6-
inhalation of stomach
contents or secretions NOS
O29.01-
local, toxic reaction O29.3X
Mendelson's syndrome
O29.01-
pressure collapse of lung
O29.02-
pulmonary complications
NEC O29.09-
specified NEC O29.8X-
spinal and epidural type NEC
O29.5X
induced headache O29.4-
albuminuria (*see also*
Proteinuria, gestational)
O12.1-
alcohol use O99.31-
amnionitis O41.12-
anaphylactoid syndrome of
pregnancy O88.01-
anemia (conditions in D50-D64)
(pre-existing) O99.01-
complicating the puerperium
O99.03
antepartum hemorrhage O46.9-
with coagulation defect —*see*
Hemorrhage, antepartum,
with coagulation defect
specified NEC O46.8X-
appendicitis O99.61-
atrophy (yellow) (acute) liver
(subacute) O26.61-
bariatric surgery status O99.84-
bicornis or bicornuate uterus
O34.0-
biliary tract problems O26.61-
breech presentation O32.1
cardiovascular diseases
(conditions in I00-I09,
I20-I52, I70-I99) O99.41-
cerebrovascular disorders
(conditions in I60-I69)
O99.41-
cervical shortening O26.87-

complicated by (*continued*)
cervicitis O23.51-
cesarean scar defect (isthmocele)
O34.22
chloasma (gravidarum) O26.89-
cholestasis (intrahepatic)
O26.61-
cholecystitis O99.61-
chorioamnionitis O41.12-
circulatory system disorder
(conditions in I00-I09,
I20-I99, O99.41-)
compound presentation O32.6
conjoined twins O30.02-
connective system disorders
(conditions in M00-M99)
O99.891
contracted pelvis (general)
O33.1
inlet O33.2
outlet O33.3
convulsions (eclamptic) (uremic)
(*see also* Eclampsia) O15.9-
cracked nipple O92.11-
cystitis O23.1-
cystocele O34.8-
death of fetus (near term) O36.4
early pregnancy O02.1
of one fetus or more in
multiple gestation O31.2-
deciduitis O41.14-
decreased fetal movement
O36.81-
dental problems O99.61-
diabetes (mellitus) O24.91-
gestational (pregnancy
induced) —*see* Diabetes,
gestational
pre-existing O24.31-
specified NEC O24.81-
type 1 O24.01-
type 2 O24.11-
digestive system disorders
(conditions in K00-K93)
O99.61-
diseases of —*see* Pregnancy,
complicated by, specified body
system disease
biliary tract O26.61-
blood NEC (conditions in
D65-D77) O99.11-
liver O26.61-
specified NEC O99.891
disorders of —*see* Pregnancy,
complicated by, specified body
system disorder
amniotic fluid and membranes
O41.9-
specified NEC O41.8X-
biliary tract O26.61-
ear and mastoid process
(conditions in H60-H95)
O99.891
eye and adnexa (conditions in
H00-H59) O99.891
liver O26.61-
skin (conditions in L00-L99)
O99.71-
specified NEC O99.891
displacement, uterus NEC
O34.59-
causing obstructed labor O65.5
disproportion (due to) O33.9
fetal (ascites) (hydrops)
(meningomyelocele)
(sacral teratoma) (tumor)
deformities NEC O33.7
generally contracted pelvis
O33.1
hydrocephalic fetus O33.6

complicated by (*continued*)
disproportion (*continued*)
inlet contraction of pelvis
O33.2
mixed maternal and fetal
origin O33.4
specified NEC O33.8
double uterus O34.0-
causing obstructed labor
O65.5
drug use (conditions in F11-F19)
O99.32-
eclampsia, eclamptic (coma)
(convulsions) (delirium)
(nephritis) (uremia) (*see also*
Eclampsia) O15.-
ectopic pregnancy —*see*
Pregnancy, ectopic
edema O12.0-
with
gestational hypertension,
mild (*see also* Pre-
eclampsia) O14.0-
proteinuria O12.2-
effusion, amniotic fluid —*see*
Pregnancy, complicated
by, premature rupture of
membranes
elderly
multigravida O09.52-
primigravida O09.51-
embolism (*see also* Embolism,
obstetric, pregnancy) O88.-
endocrine diseases NEC O99.28-
endometritis O86.12
excessive weight gain O26.0-
exhaustion O26.81-
during labor and delivery
O75.81
face presentation O32.3
failed induction of labor O61.9
instrumental O61.1
mechanical O61.1
medical O61.0
specified NEC O61.8
surgical O61.1
failed or difficult intubation for
anesthesia O29.6-
false labor (pains) O47.9
at or after 37 completed weeks
of pregnancy O47.1
before 37 completed weeks of
pregnancy O47.0-
fatigue O26.81-
during labor and delivery
O75.81
fatty metamorphosis of liver
O26.61-
female genital mutilation O34.8-
[N90.81-]
fetal (maternal care for)
abnormality or damage
O35.9
acid-base balance O68
specified type NEC O35.8
acidemia O68
acidosis O68
alkalosis O68
anemia and thrombocytopenia
O36.82-
anencephaly O35.0
bradycardia O36.83-
chromosomal abnormality
(conditions in Q90-Q99)
O35.1
conjoined twins O30.02-
damage from
amniocentesis O35.7
biopsy procedures O35.7
drug addiction O35.5

complicated by (*continued*)
fetal (*continued*)
damage from (*continued*)
hematological investigation
O35.7
intrauterine contraceptive
device O35.7
maternal
alcohol addiction O35.4
cytomegalovirus
infection O35.3
disease NEC O35.8
drug addiction O35.5
listeriosis O35.8
rubella O35.3
toxoplasmosis O35.8
viral infection O35.3
medical procedure NEC
O35.7
radiation O35.6
death (near term) O36.4
early pregnancy O02.1
decreased movement O36.81-
depressed heart rate tones
O36.83-
disproportion due to deformity
(fetal) O33.7
excessive growth (large for
dates) O36.6-
growth retardation O36.59-
light for dates O36.59-
small for dates O36.59-
heart rate irregularity
(abnormal variability)
(bradycardia)
(decelerations)
(tachycardia) O36.83-
hereditary disease O35.2
hydrocephalus O35.0
intrauterine death O36.4
non-reassuring heart rate or
rhythm O36.83-
poor growth O36.59-
light for dates O36.59-
small for dates O36.59-
problem O36.9-
specified NEC O36.89-
reduction (elective) O31.3-
selective termination O31.3-
spina bifida O35.0
thrombocytopenia O36.82-
fibroid (tumor) (uterus) O34.1-
fissure of nipple O92.11-
gallstones O99.61-
gastric banding status O99.84-
gastric bypass status O99.84-
genital herpes (asymptomatic)
(history of) (inactive) O98.3-
genital tract infection O23.9-
glomerular diseases (conditions
in N00-N07) O26.83-
with hypertension,
pre-existing —*see*
Hypertension, complicating,
pregnancy, pre-existing,
with, renal disease
gonorrhea O98.21-
grand multiparity O09.4
habitual aborter —*see*
Pregnancy, complicated by,
recurrent pregnancy loss
HELLP syndrome (hemolysis,
elevated liver enzymes and
low platelet count) O14.2-
hemorrhage
antepartum —*see*
Hemorrhage, antepartum
before 20 completed weeks
gestation O20.9
specified NEC O20.8

Pregnancy *(continued)*
  complicated by *(continued)*
    PUPPP (pruritic urticarial papules and plaques of pregnancy) O26.86
    pyelitis O23.0-
    recurrent pregnancy loss O26.2-
    renal disease or failure NEC O26.83-
      with secondary hypertension, pre-existing —*see* Hypertension, complicating, pregnancy, pre-existing, secondary
      hypertensive, pre-existing —*see* Hypertension, complicating, pregnancy, pre-existing, with, renal disease
    respiratory condition (conditions in J00-J99) O99.51-
    retained, retention
      dead ovum O02.0
      intrauterine contraceptive device O26.3-
    retroversion, uterus O34.53-
    Rh immunization, incompatibility or sensitization NEC O36.09-
      anti-D antibody O36.01-
    rupture
      amnion (premature) (*see also* Pregnancy, complicated by, premature rupture of membranes) O42-
      membranes (premature) (*see also* Pregnancy, complicated by, premature rupture of membranes) O42-
      uterus (during labor) O71.1
        before onset of labor O71.0-
    salivation (excessive) O26.89-
    salpingitis O23.52-
    salpingo-oophoritis O23.52-
    sepsis (conditions in A40, A41) O98.81-
    size date discrepancy (uterine) O26.84-
    skin condition (conditions in L00-L99) O99.71-
    smoking (tobacco) O99.33-
    social problem O09.7-
    specified condition NEC O26.89-
    spotting O26.85-
    streptococcus group B (GBS) carrier state O99.820
    subluxation of symphysis (pubis) O26.71-
    syphilis (conditions in A50-A53) O98.11-
    threatened
      abortion O20.0
      labor O47.9
        at or after 37 completed weeks of gestation O47.1
        before 37 completed weeks of gestation O47.0-
    thrombophlebitis (superficial) O22.2-
    thrombosis O22.9-
      cerebral venous O22.5-
      cerebrovenous sinus O22.5-
      deep O22.3-
    tobacco use disorder (smoking) O99.33-
    torsion of uterus O34.59-
    toxemia O14.9-
    transverse lie or presentation O32.2
    tuberculosis (conditions in A15-A19) O98.01-

Pregnancy *(continued)*
  complicated by *(continued)*
    tumor (benign)
      cervix O34.4-
        malignant O9A.11-
      uterus O34.1-
    unstable lie O32.0
    upper respiratory infection O99.51-
    urethritis O23.2-
    uterine size date discrepancy O26.84-
    vaginitis or vulvitis O23.59-
    varicose veins (lower extremities) O22.0-
      genitals O22.1-
      legs O22.0-
      perineal O22.1-
      vaginal or vulval O22.1-
    venereal disease NEC (conditions in A63.8) O98.31-
    venous disorders O22.9-
      specified NEC O22.8X-
    viral diseases (conditions in A80-B09, B25-B34) O98.51-
    very young mother —*see* Pregnancy, complicated by, young mother
    vomiting O21.9
      due to diseases classified elsewhere O21.8
      hyperemesis gravidarum (mild) (*see also* Hyperemesis, gravidarum) O21.0-
      late (occurring after 20 weeks of gestation) O21.2
    young mother
      multigravida O09.62-
      primigravida O09.61-
  concealed O09.3-
  continuing following
    elective fetal reduction of one or more fetus O31.3-
    intrauterine death of one or more fetus O31.2-
    spontaneous abortion of one or more fetus O31.1-
  cornual O00.80
    with intrauterine pregnancy O00.81
  ectopic (ruptured) O00.90
    with intrauterine pregnancy O00.91
    abdominal O00.00
      with
        intrauterine pregnancy O00.01
        viable fetus O36.7-
    cervical O00.80
      with intrauterine pregnancy O00.81
    complicated (by) O08.9
      afibrinogenemia O08.1
      cardiac arrest O08.81
      chemical damage of pelvic organ(s) O08.6
      circulatory collapse O08.3
      defibrination syndrome O08.1
      electrolyte imbalance O08.5
      embolism (amniotic fluid) (blood clot) (pulmonary) (septic) O08.2
      endometritis O08.0
      genital tract and pelvic infection O08.0
      hemorrhage (delayed) (excessive) O08.1
      infection
        genital tract or pelvic O08.0
        kidney 008.83
        urinary tract O08.83

Pregnancy *(continued)*
  ectopic *(continued)*
    complicated *(continued)*
      intravascular coagulation O08.1
      laceration of pelvic organ(s) O08.6
      metabolic disorder O08.5
      oliguria O08.4
      oophoritis O08.0
      parametritis O08.0
      pelvic peritonitis O08.0
      perforation of pelvic organ(s) O08.6
      renal failure or shutdown O08.4
      salpingitis or salpingo-oophoritis O08.0
      sepsis O08.82
      shock O08.83
        septic O08.82
      specified condition NEC O08.89
      tubular necrosis (renal) O08.4
      uremia O08.4
      urinary infection O08.83
      venous complication NEC O08.7
        embolism O08.2
    cornual O00.80
      with intrauterine pregnancy O00.81
    intraligamentous O00.80
      with intrauterine pregnancy O00.81
    mural O00.80
      with intrauterine pregnancy O00.81
    ovarian O00.20-
      with intrauterine pregnancy O00.21-
    specified site NEC O00.80
      with intrauterine pregnancy O00.81
    tubal (ruptured) O00.10-
      with intrauterine pregnancy O00.11-
  examination (normal) Z34.9-
    high-risk —*see* Pregnancy, supervision of, high-risk
    first Z34.0-
    specified Z34.8-
  extrauterine —*see* Pregnancy, ectopic
  fallopian O00.10-
    with intrauterine pregnancy O00.11-
  false F45.8
  gestational carrier Z33.3
  heptachorionic, hepta-amniotic (septuplets) O30.83-
  hexachorionic, hexa-amniotic (septuplets) O30.83-
  hidden O09.3-
  high-risk —*see* Pregnancy, supervision of, high-risk
  incidental finding Z33.1
  interstitial O00.80
    with intrauterine pregnancy O00.81
  intraligamentous O00.80
    with intrauterine pregnancy O00.81
  intramural O00.80
    with intrauterine pregnancy O00.81
  intraperitoneal O00.00
    with intrauterine pregnancy O00.01
  isthmian O00.10-
    with intrauterine pregnancy O00.11-

Pregnancy *(continued)*
  mesometric (mural) O00.80
    with intrauterine pregnancy O00.81
  molar NEC O02.0
    complicated (by) O08.9
      afibrinogenemia O08.1
      cardiac arrest O08.81
      chemical damage of pelvic organ(s) O08.6
      circulatory collapse O08.3
      defibrination syndrome O08.1
      electrolyte imbalance O08.5
      embolism (amniotic fluid) (blood clot) (pulmonary) (septic) O08.2
      endometritis O08.0
      genital tract and pelvic infection O08.0
      hemorrhage (delayed) (excessive) O08.1
      infection
        genital tract or pelvic O08.0
        kidney O08.83
        urinary tract O08.83
      intravascular coagulation O08.1
      laceration of pelvic organ(s) O08.6
      metabolic disorder O08.5
      oliguria O08.4
      oophoritis O08.0
      parametritis O08.0
      pelvic peritonitis O08.0
      perforation of pelvic organ(s) O08.6
      renal failure or shutdown O08.4
      salpingitis or salpingo-oophoritis O08.0
      sepsis O08.82
      shock O08.3
        septic O08.82
      specified condition NEC O08.89
      tubular necrosis (renal) O08.4
      uremia O08.4
      urinary infection O08.83
      venous complication NEC O08.7
        embolism O08.2
    hydatidiform (*see also* Mole, hydatidiform) O01.9-
  multiple (gestation) O30.9-
    greater than quadruplets —*see* Pregnancy, multiple (gestation), specified NEC
    specified NEC O30.80-
      with
        two or more monoamniotic fetuses O30.82-
        two or more monochorionic fetuses O30.81-
      number of chorions and amnions are both equal to the number of fetuses O30.83-
      two or more monoamniotic fetuses O30.82-
      two or more monochorionic fetuses O30.81-
      unable to determine number of placenta and number of amniotic sacs O30.89-
      unspecified number of placenta and unspecified number of amniotic sacs O30.80-

Presence *(continued)*
cardiac *(continued)*
  implant or graft Z95.9
    specified type NEC Z95.818
  pacemaker Z95.0
  resynchronization therapy
    defibrillator Z95.810
    pacemaker Z95.0
cardioverter-defibrillator (ICD)
  Z95.810
cerebrospinal fluid drainage device
  Z98.2
cochlear implant (functional)
  Z96.21
contact lens (es) Z97.3
coronary artery graft or prosthesis
  Z95.5
CRT-D (cardiac resynchronization
  therapy defibrillator) Z95.810
CRT-P (cardiac resynchronization
  therapy pacemaker) Z95.0
CSF shunt Z98.2
dental prosthesis device Z97.2
dentures Z97.2
device (external) NEC Z97.8
  cardiac NEC Z95.818
  heart assist Z95.811
  implanted (functional) Z96.9
    specified NEC Z96.89
  prosthetic Z97.8
ear implant Z96.20
  cochlear implant Z96.21
  myringotomy tube Z96.22
  specified type NEC Z96.29
elbow-joint implant (functional)
  (prosthesis) Z96.62-
endocrine implant (functional)
  NEC Z96.49
eustachian tube stent or device
  (functional) Z96.29
external hearing-aid or device
  Z97.4
finger-joint implant (functional)
  (prosthetic) Z96.69-
functional implant Z96.9
  specified NEC Z96.89
graft
  cardiac NEC Z95.818
  vascular NEC Z95.828
hearing-aid or device (external)
  Z97.4
  implant (bone) (cochlear)
    (functional) Z96.21
heart assist device Z95.811
heart valve implant (functional)
  Z95.2
  prosthetic Z95.2
  specified type NEC Z95.4
  xenogenic Z95.3
hip-joint implant (functional)
  (prosthesis) Z96.64-
ICD (cardioverter-defibrillator)
  Z95.810
implanted device (artificial)
  (functional) (prosthetic) Z96.9
  automatic cardiac defibrillator
    (with synchronous cardiac
    pacemaker) Z95.810
  cardiac pacemaker Z95.0
  cochlear Z96.21
  dental Z96.5
  heart Z95.812
  heart valve Z95.2
    prosthetic Z95.2
    specified NEC Z95.4
    xenogenic Z95.3
  insulin pump Z96.41
  intraocular lens Z96.1
  joint Z96.60
    ankle Z96.66-
    elbow Z96.62-

Presence *(continued)*
implanted device *(continued)*
  joint *(continued)*
    finger Z96.69-
    hip Z96.64-
    knee Z96.65-
    shoulder Z96.61-
    specified NEC Z96.698
    wrist Z96.63-
  larynx Z96.3
  myringotomy tube Z96.22
  otological Z96.20
    cochlear Z96.21
    eustachian stent Z96.29
    myringotomy Z96.22
    specified NEC Z96.29
    stapes Z96.29
  skin Z96.81
  skull plate Z96.7
  specified NEC Z96.89
  urogenital Z96.0
insulin pump (functional) Z96.41
intestinal bypass or anastomosis
  Z98.0
intraocular lens (functional)
  Z96.1
intrauterine contraceptive device
  (IUD) Z97.5
intravascular implant (functional)
  (prosthetic) NEC Z95.9
  coronary artery Z95.5
  defibrillator (with synchronous
    cardiac pacemaker) Z95.810
  peripheral vessel (with
    angioplasty) Z95.820
joint implant (prosthetic) (any)
  Z96.60
  ankle —see Presence, ankle joint
    implant
  elbow —see Presence, elbow
    joint implant
  finger —see Presence, finger
    joint implant
  hip —see Presence, hip joint
    implant
  knee —see Presence, knee joint
    implant
  shoulder —see Presence,
    shoulder joint implant
  specified joint NEC Z96.698
  wrist —see Presence, wrist joint
    implant
knee-joint implant (functional)
  (prosthesis) Z96.65-
laryngeal implant (functional)
  Z96.3
mandibular implant (dental)
  Z96.5
myringotomy tube(s) Z96.22
neurostimulator (brain) (gastric)
  (peripheral nerve) (sacral nerve)
  (spinal cord) (vagus nerve)
  Z96.82
orthopedic-joint implant
  (prosthetic) (any) —see
  Presence, joint implant
otological implant (functional)
  Z96.29
shoulder-joint implant (functional)
  (prosthesis) Z96.61-
skull-plate implant Z96.7
spectacles Z97.3
stapes implant (functional)
  Z96.29
systemic lupus erythematosus
  [SLE] inhibitor D68.62
tendon implant (functional) (graft)
  Z96.7
tooth root(s) implant Z96.5
ureteral stent Z96.0
urethral stent Z96.0

Presence *(continued)*
urogenital implant (functional) Z96.0
vascular implant or device Z95.9
  access port device Z95.828
  specified type NEC Z95.828
wrist-joint implant (functional)
  (prosthesis) Z96.63-

Presenile —see also condition
dementia F03
premature aging E34.8

Presentation, fetal —see Delivery,
complicated by, malposition

Prespondylolisthesis (congenital)
Q76.2

Pressure
area, skin —see Ulcer, pressure,
  by site
brachial plexus G54.0
brain G93.5
  injury at birth NEC P11.1
cerebral —see Pressure, brain
chest R07.89
cone, tentorial G93.5
hyposystolic —see also
  Hypotension
  incidental reading, without
    diagnosis of hypotension
    R03.1
increased
  intracranial benign, G93.2
    injury at birth P11.0
  intraocular H40.05-
injury —see Ulcer, pressure,
  by site
lumbosacral plexus G54.1
mediastinum J98.59
necrosis (chronic) —see Ulcer,
  pressure, by site
parental, inappropriate (excessive)
  Z62.6
sore (chronic) —see Ulcer,
  pressure, by site
spinal cord G95.20
ulcer (chronic) —see Ulcer,
  pressure, by site
venous, increased I87.8

Pre-syncope R55

Preterm
delivery (see also Pregnancy,
  complicated by, preterm labor)
  O60.10
labor —see Pregnancy, complicated
  by, preterm labor
newborn (infant) P07.30
  gestational age
    28 completed weeks (28
      weeks, 0 days through 28
      weeks, 6 days) P07.31
    29 completed weeks (29
      weeks, 0 days through 29
      weeks, 6 days) P07.32
    30 completed weeks (30
      weeks, 0 days through 30
      weeks, 6 days) P07.33
    31 completed weeks (31
      weeks, 0 days through 31
      weeks, 6 days) P07.34
    32 completed weeks (32
      weeks, 0 days through 32
      weeks, 6 days) P07.35
    33 completed weeks (33
      weeks, 0 days through 33
      weeks, 6 days) P07.36
    34 completed weeks (34
      weeks, 0 days through 34
      weeks, 6 days) P07.37
    35 completed weeks (35
      weeks, 0 days through 35
      weeks, 6 days) P07.38

Preterm *(continued)*
newborn *(continued)*
  gestational age *(continued)*
    36 completed weeks (36
      weeks, 0 days through 36
      weeks, 6 days) P07.39

Previa
placenta (total) (without
  hemorrhage) O44.0-
  with hemorrhage O44.1-
  complete O44.0-
    with hemorrhage O44.1-
  low (see also Delivery,
    complicated, by, placenta,
    low) O44.4-
    with hemorrhage O44.5-
  marginal O44.2-
    with hemorrhage O44.3-
  partial O44.2-
    with hemorrhage O44.3-
vasa O69.4

Priapism N48.30
due to
  disease classified elsewhere
    N48.32
  drug N48.33
  specified cause NEC N48.39
  trauma N48.31

Prickling sensation (skin) R20.2

Prickly heat L74.0

Primary —see condition

Primigravida
elderly, affecting management of
  pregnancy, labor and delivery
  (supervision only) —see
  Pregnancy, complicated by,
  elderly, primigravida
older, affecting management of
  pregnancy, labor and delivery
  (supervision only) —see
  Pregnancy, complicated by,
  elderly, primigravida
very young, affecting management
  of pregnancy, labor and delivery
  (supervision only) —see
  Pregnancy, complicated by,
  young mother, primigravida

Primipara
elderly, affecting management of
  pregnancy, labor and delivery
  (supervision only) —see
  Pregnancy, complicated by,
  elderly, primigravida
older, affecting management of
  pregnancy, labor and delivery
  (supervision only) —see
  Pregnancy, complicated by,
  elderly, primigravida
very young, affecting management
  of pregnancy, labor and delivery
  (supervision only) —see
  Pregnancy, complicated by,
  young mother, primigravida

Primus varus Q66.21-

PRIND (Prolonged reversible
ischemic neurologic deficit) I63.9

Pringle's disease (tuberous sclerosis)
Q85.1

Prinzmetal angina I20.1

Prizefighter ear —see Cauliflower
ear

Problem (with) (related to)
academic Z55.8
acculturation Z60.3
adjustment (to)
  change of job Z56.1
  life-cycle transition Z60.0

Prolapse, prolapsed (*continued*)
bladder (mucosa) (sphincter)
(acquired)
congenital Q79.4
female —*see* Cystocele
male N32.89
breast implant (prosthetic) T85.49
cecostomy K94.09
cecum K63.4
cervix, cervical (hypertrophied)
N81.2
anterior lip, obstructing labor
O65.5
congenital Q51.828
postpartal, old N81.2
stump N81.85
ciliary body (traumatic) —*see*
Laceration, eye (ball), with
prolapse or loss of interocular
tissue
colon (pedunculated) K63.4
colostomy K94.09
disc (intervertebral) —*see*
Displacement, intervertebral
disc
eye implant (orbital) T85.398
lens (ocular) —*see*
Complications, intraocular
lens
fallopian tube N83.4-
gastric (mucosa) K31.89
genital, female N81.9
specified NEC N81.89
globe, nontraumatic —*see*
Luxation, globe
ileostomy bud K94.19
intervertebral disc —*see*
Displacement, intervertebral disc
intestine (small) K63.4
iris (traumatic) —*see* Laceration,
eye (ball), with prolapse or loss
of interocular tissue
nontraumatic H21.89
kidney N28.83
congenital Q63.2
laryngeal muscles or ventricle
J38.7
liver K76.89
meatus urinarius N36.8
mitral (valve) I34.1
ocular lens implant —*see*
Complications, intraocular lens
organ or site, congenital NEC
—*see* Malposition, congenital
ovary N83.4-
pelvic floor, female N81.89
perineum, female N81.89
rectum (mucosa) (sphincter) K62.3
due to trichuris trichuria B79
spleen D73.89
stomach K31.89
umbilical cord
complicating delivery O69.0
urachus, congenital Q64.4
ureter N28.89
with obstruction N13.5
with infection N13.6
ureterovesical orifice N28.89
urethra (acquired) (infected)
(mucosa) N36.8
congenital Q64.71
urinary meatus N36.8
congenital Q64.72
uterovaginal N81.4
complete N81.3
incomplete N81.2
uterus (with prolapse of vagina)
N81.4
complete N81.3
congenital Q51.818
first degree N81.2

Prolapse, prolapsed (*continued*)
uterus (*continued*)
in pregnancy or childbirth —*see*
Pregnancy, complicated by,
abnormal, uterus
incomplete N81.2
postpartal (old) N81.4
second degree N81.2
third degree N81.3
uveal (traumatic) —*see* Laceration,
eye (ball), with prolapse or loss
of interocular tissue
vagina (anterior) (wall) —*see*
Cystocele
with prolapse of uterus N81.4
complete N81.3
incomplete N81.2
posterior wall N81.6
posthysterectomy N99.3
vitreous (humor) H43.0-
in wound —*see* Laceration, eye
(ball), with prolapse or loss of
interocular tissue
womb —*see* Prolapse, uterus

Prolapsus, female N81.9
specified NEC N81.89

Proliferation(s)
primary cutaneous CD30-positive
large T-cell C86.6
prostate, atypical small acinar
N42.32

Proliferative —*see* condition

Prolonged, prolongation (of)
bleeding (time) (idiopathic) R79.1
coagulation (time) R79.1
gestation (over 42 completed
weeks)
mother O48.1
newborn P08.22
interval I44.0
labor O63.9
first stage O63.0
second stage O63.1
partial thromboplastin time (PTT)
R79.1
pregnancy (more than 42 weeks
gestation) O48.1
prothrombin time R79.1
QT interval R94.31
uterine contractions in labor
O62.4

Prominence, prominent
auricle (congenital) (ear) Q17.5
ischial spine or sacral promontory
with disproportion (fetopelvic)
O33.0
causing obstructed labor O65.0
nose (congenital) acquired M95.0

Promiscuity —*see* High, risk, sexual
behavior

Pronation
ankle —*see* Deformity, limb, foot,
specified NEC
foot —*see also* Deformity, limb,
foot, specified NEC
congenital Q74.2

Prophylactic
administration of
antibiotics, long-term Z79.2
short-term use - omit code
drug (*see also* Long-term
(current) drug therapy (use
of)) Z79.899-
medication Z79.899
organ removal (for neoplasia
management) Z40.00
breast Z40.01
fallopian tube(s) Z40.03
with ovary(s) Z40.02

Prophylactic (*continued*)
organ removal (*continued*)
ovary(s) Z40.02
specified site NEC Z40.09
surgery Z40.9
for risk factors related to
malignant neoplasm —*see*
Prophylactic, organ removal
specified NEC Z40.8
vaccination Z23

Propionic acidemia E71.121

Proptosis (ocular) —*see also*
Exophthalmos
thyroid —*see* Hyperthyroidism,
with goiter

Prosecution, anxiety concerning
Z65.3

Prosopagnosia R48.3

Prostadynia N42.81

Prostate, prostatic —*see* condition

Prostatism —*see* Hyperplasia,
prostate

Prostatitis (congestive) (suppurative)
(with cystitis) N41.9
acute N41.0
cavitary N41.8
chronic N41.1
diverticular N41.8
due to Trichomonas (vaginalis)
A59.02
fibrous N41.1
gonococcal (acute) (chronic)
A54.22
granulomatous N41.4
hypertrophic N41.1
subacute N41.1
trichomonal A59.02
tuberculous A18.14

Prostatocystitis N41.3

Prostatorrhea N42.89

Prostatosis N42.82

Prostration R53.83
heat —*see also* Heat, exhaustion
anhydrotic T67.3
due to
salt (and water) depletion
T67.4
water depletion T67.3
nervous F48.8
senile R54

Protanomaly (anomalous trichromat)
H53.54

Protanopia (complete) (incomplete)
H53.54

Protection (against) (from) —*see*
Prophylactic

Protein
deficiency NEC —*see* Malnutrition
malnutrition —*see* Malnutrition
sickness (*see also* Reaction, serum)
T80.69

Proteinemia R77.9

Proteinosis
alveolar (pulmonary) J84.01
lipid or lipoid (of Urbach) E78.89

Proteinuria R80.9
Bence Jones R80.3
complicating pregnancy —*see*
Proteinuria, gestational
gestational
complicating
childbirth O12.14
pregnancy O12.1-
with edema O12.2-
puerperium O12.15

Proteinuria (*continued*)
idiopathic R80.0
isolated R80.0
with glomerular lesion N06.9
C3
glomerulonephritis N06.A
glomerulopathy N06.A
with dense deposit
disease N06.6
dense deposit disease N06.6
diffuse
crescentic
glomerulonephritis N06.7
endocapillary proliferative
glomerulonephritis N06.4
mesangiocapillary
glomerulonephritis N06.5
focal and segmental hyalinosis
or sclerosis N06.1
membranous (diffuse) N06.2
mesangial proliferative
(diffuse) N06.3
minimal change N06.0
specified pathology NEC N06.8
orthostatic R80.2
with glomerular lesion —*see*
Proteinuria, isolated, with
glomerular lesion
persistent R80.1
with glomerular lesion —*see*
Proteinuria, isolated, with
glomerular lesion
postural R80.2
with glomerular lesion —*see*
Proteinuria, isolated, with
glomerular lesion
pre-eclamptic —*see* Pre-eclampsia
puerperal O12.15
specified type NEC R80.8

Proteolysis, pathologic D65

Proteus (mirabilis) (morganii), **as
cause of disease classified
elsewhere** B96.4

Prothrombin gene mutation D68.52

Protoporphyria, erythropoietic E80.0

Protozoal —*see also* condition
disease B64
specified NEC B60.8

Protrusion, protrusio
acetabuli M24.7
acetabulum (into pelvis) M24.7
device, implant or graft (*see also*
Complications, by site and type,
mechanical) T85.698
arterial graft NEC —*see*
Complication, cardiovascular
device, mechanical, vascular
breast (implant) T85.49
catheter NEC T85.698
cystostomy T83.090
dialysis (renal) T82.49
intraperitoneal T85.691
infusion NEC T82.594
spinal (epidural) (subdural)
T85.690
urinary (*see also*
Complications, catheter,
urinary), T83.098
electronic (electrode) (pulse
generator) (stimulator)
bone T84.390
nervous system —*see*
Complication, prosthetic
device, mechanical,
electronic nervous system
stimulator
fixation, internal (orthopedic)
NEC —*see* Complication,
fixation device, mechanical

Protrusion, protrusio (continued)
device, implant or graft (continued)
gastrointestinal —see
Complications, prosthetic
device, mechanical,
gastrointestinal device
genital NEC T83.498
intrauterine contraceptive
device T83.39
penile prosthesis (cylinder)
(implanted) (pump)
(resevoir) T83.490
testicular prosthesis T83.491
heart NEC —see Complication,
cardiovascular device,
mechanical
joint prosthesis —see
Complications, joint
prosthesis, mechanical,
specified NEC, by site
ocular NEC —see Complications,
prosthetic device, mechanical,
ocular device
orthopedic NEC —see
Complication, orthopedic,
device, mechanical
specified NEC T85.628
urinary NEC —see also
Complication, genitourinary,
device, urinary, mechanical
graft T83.29
vascular NEC —see
Complication, cardiovascular
device, mechanical
ventricular intracranial shunt
T85.09
intervertebral disc —see
Displacement, intervertebral disc
joint prosthesis —see
Complications, joint prosthesis,
mechanical, specified NEC, by
site
nucleus pulposus —see
Displacement, intervertebral disc

Prune belly (syndrome) Q79.4

Prurigo (ferox) (gravis) (Hebrae)
(Hebra's) (mitis) (simplex) L28.2
Besnier's L20.0
estivalis L56.4
nodularis L28.1
psychogenic F45.8

Pruritus, pruritic (essential) L29.9
ani, anus L29.0
psychogenic F45.8
anogenital L29.3
psychogenic F45.8
due to onchocerca volvulus B73.1
gravidarum —see Pregnancy,
complicated by, specified
pregnancy-related condition
NEC
hiemalis L29.8
neurogenic (any site) F45.8
perianal L29.0
psychogenic (any site) F45.8
scroti, scrotum L29.1
psychogenic F45.8
senile, senilis L29.8
specified NEC L29.8
psychogenic F45.8
Trichomonas A59.9
vulva, vulvae L29.2
psychogenic F45.8

Pseudarthrosis, pseudoarthrosis
(bone) —see Nonunion,
fracture
clavicle, congenital Q74.0
joint, following fusion or
arthrodesis M96.0

Pseudoaneurysm —see Aneurysm

Pseudoangioma I81

Pseudoangina (pectoris) —see Angina

Pseudoarteriosus Q28.8

Pseudoarthrosis —see Pseudarthrosis

Pseudobulbar affect (PBA) F48.2

Pseudochromhidrosis L67.8

Pseudocirrhosis, liver, pericardial
I31.1

Pseudocowpox B08.03

Pseudocoxalgia M91.3-

Pseudocroup J38.5

**Pseudo-Cushing's syndrome,
alcohol-induced** E24.4

Pseudocyesis F45.8

Pseudocyst
lung J98.4
pancreas K86.3
retina —see Cyst, retina

Pseudoelephantiasis neuroarthritica
Q82.0

Pseudoexfoliation, capsule (lens)
—see Cataract, specified NEC

Pseudofolliculitis barbae L73.1

Pseudoglioma H44.89

Pseudohemophilia (Bernuth's)
(hereditary) (type B) D68.0
Type A D69.8
vascular D69.8

Pseudohermaphroditism Q56.3
adrenal E25.8
female Q56.2
with adrenocortical disorder E25.8
without adrenocortical disorder
Q56.2
adrenal (congenital) E25.0
unspecified E25.9
male Q56.1
with
adrenocortical disorder E25.8
androgen resistance E34.51
cleft scrotum Q56.1
feminizing testis E34.51
5-alpha-reductase deficiency
E29.1
without gonadal disorder Q56.1
adrenal E25.8
unspecified E25.9

Pseudo-Hurler's polydystrophy E77.0

Pseudohydrocephalus G93.2

**Pseudohypertrophic muscular
dystrophy** (Erb's) G71.02

Pseudohypertrophy, muscle G71.09

Pseudohypoparathyroidism E20.1

Pseudoinsomnia F51.03

Pseudoleukemia, infantile D64.89

Pseudomembranous —see condition

Pseudomenses (newborn) P54.6

Pseudomenstruation (newborn) P54.6

Pseudomeningocele (cerebral)
(infective) (post-traumatic) G96.198
postprocedural (spinal) G97.82

Pseudomonas
aeruginosa, as cause of disease
classified elsewhere B96.5
mallei infection A24.0
as cause of disease classified
elsewhere B96.5
pseudomallei, as cause of disease
classified elsewhere B96.5

Pseudomyotonia G71.19

Pseudomyxoma peritonei C78.6

Pseudoneuritis, optic (nerve) (disc)
(papilla), congenital Q14.2

Pseudo-obstruction intestine (acute)
(chronic) (idiopathic) (intermittent
secondary) (primary) K59.89
colonic K59.81

Pseudopapilledema H47.33-
congenital Q14.2

Pseudoparalysis
arm or leg R29.818
atonic, congenital P94.2

Pseudopelade L66.0

Pseudophakia Z96.1

Pseudopolyarthritis, rhizomelic
M35.3

Pseudopolycythemia D75.1

Pseudopseudohypoparathyroidism
E20.1

Pseudopterygium H11.81-

Pseudoptosis (eyelid) —see
Blepharochalasis

Pseudopuberty, precocious
female heterosexual E25.8
male isosexual E25.8

Pseudorickets (renal) N25.0

Pseudorubella B08.20

Pseudosclerema, newborn P83.88

Pseudosclerosis (brain)
of Westphal (Strümpell) E83.01
Jakob's —see Creutzfeldt-Jakob
disease or syndrome
spastic —see Creutzfeldt-Jakob
disease or syndrome

Pseudotetanus —see Convulsions

Pseudotetany R29.0
hysterical F44.5

Pseudotruncus arteriosus Q25.49

Pseudotuberculosis A28.2
enterocolitis A04.8
pasteurella (infection) A28.0

Pseudotumor G93.2
cerebri G93.2
orbital H05.11-

Pseudoxanthoma elasticum Q82.8

Psilosis (sprue) (tropical) K90.1
nontropical K90.0

Psittacosis A70

Psoitis M60.88

Psoriasis L40.9
arthropathic L40.50
arthritis mutilans L40.52
distal interphalangeal L40.51
juvenile L40.54
other specified L40.59
spondylitis L40.53
buccal K13.29
flexural L40.8
guttate L40.4
mouth K13.29
nummular L40.0
plaque L40.0
psychogenic F54
pustular (generalized) L40.1
palmaris et plantaris L40.3
specified NEC L40.8
vulgaris L40.0

Psychasthenia F48.8

Psychiatric disorder or problem F99

Psychogenic —see also condition

Psychogenic (continued)
factors associated with physical
conditions F54

**Psychological and behavioral
factors affecting medical
condition** F59

Psychoneurosis, psychoneurotic
—see also Neurosis
anxiety (state) F41.1
depersonalization F48.1
hypochondriacal F45.21
hysteria F44.9
neurasthenic F48.8
personality NEC F60.89

Psychopathy, psychopathic
affectionless F94.2
autistic F84.5
constitution, post-traumatic F07.81
personality —see Disorder,
personality
sexual —see Deviation, sexual
state F60.2

**Psychosexual identity disorder of
childhood** F64.2

Psychosis, psychotic F29
acute (transient) F23
hysterical F44.9
affective —see Disorder, mood
alcoholic F10.959
with
abuse F10.159
anxiety disorder F10.980
with
abuse F10.180
dependence F10.280
delirium tremens F10.231
delusions F10.950
with
abuse F10.150
dependence F10.250
dementia F10.97
with dependence F10.27
dependence F10.259
hallucinosis F10.951
with
abuse F10.151
dependence F10.251
mood disorder F10.94
with
abuse F10.14
dependence F10.24
paranoia F10.950
with
abuse F10.150
dependence F10.250
persisting amnesia F10.96
with dependence F10.26
amnestic confabulatory F10.96
with dependence F10.26
delirium tremens F10.231
Korsakoff's, Korsakov's,
Korsakow's F10.26
paranoid type F10.950
with
abuse F10.150
dependence F10.250
anergastic —see Psychosis, organic
arteriosclerotic (simple type)
(uncomplicated) F01.50
with behavioral disturbance
F01.51
childhood F84.0
atypical F84.8
climacteric —see Psychosis,
involutional
confusional F29
acute or subacute F05
reactive F23
cycloid F23

Psychosis, psychotic *(continued)*
depressive —*see* Disorder,
depressive
disintegrative (childhood) F84.3
drug-induced —*see* F11-F19 with
.x59
paranoid and hallucinatory states
—*see* F11-F19 with .x50 or
.x51
due to or associated with
addiction, drug —*see* F11-F19
with .x59
dependence
alcohol F10.259
drug —*see* F11-F19 with .x59
epilepsy F06.8
Huntington's chorea F06.8
ischemia, cerebrovascular
(generalized) F06.8
multiple sclerosis F06.8
physical disease F06.8
presenile dementia F03
senile dementia F03
vascular disease (arteriosclerotic)
(cerebral) F01.50
with behavioral disturbance
F01.51
epileptic F06.8
episode F23
due to or associated with
physical condition F06.8
exhaustive F43.0
hallucinatory, chronic F28
hypomanic F30.8
hysterical (acute) F44.9
induced F24
infantile F84.0
atypical F84.8
infective (acute) (subacute) F05
involutional F28
depressive —*see* Disorder,
depressive
melancholic —*see* Disorder,
depressive
paranoid (state) F22
Korsakoff's, Korsakov's,
Korsakow's (nonalcoholic) F04
alcoholic F10.96
in dependence F10.26
induced by other psychoactive
substance —*see* categories
F11-F19 with .x5x
mania, manic (single episode)
F30.2
recurrent type F31.89
manic-depressive —*see* Disorder,
bipolar
menopausal —*see* Psychosis,
involutional
mixed schizophrenic and affective
F25.8
multi-infarct (cerebrovascular)
F01.50
with behavioral disturbance
F01.51
nonorganic F29
specified NEC F28
organic F09
due to or associated with
arteriosclerosis (cerebral)
—*see* Psychosis,
arteriosclerotic
cerebrovascular disease,
arteriosclerotic —*see*
Psychosis, arteriosclerotic
childbirth —*see* Psychosis,
puerperal
Creutzfeldt-Jakob disease
or syndrome —*see*
Creutzfeldt-Jakob disease
or syndrome

Psychosis, psychotic *(continued)*
organic *(continued)*
due to or associated with
(continued)
dependence, alcohol F10.259
disease
alcoholic liver F10.259
brain, arteriosclerotic
—*see* Psychosis,
arteriosclerotic
cerebrovascular F01.50
with behavioral
disturbance F01.51
Creutzfeldt-Jakob —*see*
Creutzfeldt-Jakob disease
or syndrome
endocrine or metabolic F06.8
acute or subacute F05
liver, alcoholic F10.259
epilepsy transient (acute) F05
infection
brain (intracranial) F06.8
acute or subacute F05
intoxication
alcoholic (acute) F10.259
drug F11-F19 with .x59
ischemia, cerebrovascular
(generalized) —*see*
Psychosis, arteriosclerotic
puerperium —*see* Psychosis,
puerperal
trauma, brain (birth) (from
electric current) (surgical)
F06.8
acute or subacute F05
infective F06.8
acute or subacute F05
post-traumatic F06.8
acute or subacute F05
paranoiac F22
paranoid (climacteric)
(involutional) (menopausal) F22
psychogenic (acute) F23
schizophrenic F20.0
senile F03
postpartum (NOS) F53.1
presbyophrenic (type) F03
presenile F03
psychogenic (paranoid) F23
depressive (NOS) F32.3
puerperal F53
specified type —*see* Psychosis,
by type
reactive (brief) (transient)
(emotional stress) (psychological
trauma) F23
depressive F32.3
recurrent F33.3
excitative type F30.8
schizoaffective F25.9
depressive type F25.1
manic type F25.0
schizophrenia, schizophrenic —*see*
Schizophrenia
schizophrenia-like, in epilepsy
F06.2
schizophreniform F20.81
affective type F25.9
brief F23
confusional type F23
mixed type F25.0
senile NEC F03
depressed or paranoid type F03
simple deterioration F03
specified type - code to condition
shared F24
situational (reactive) F23
symbiotic (childhood) F84.3
symptomatic F09

Psychosomatic —*see* Disorder,
psychosomatic

Psychosyndrome, organic F07.9

**Psychotic episode due to or
associated with physical
condition** F06.8

Pterygium (eye) H11.00-
amyloid H11.01-
central H11.02-
colli Q18.3
double H11.03-
peripheral
progressive H11.05-
stationary H11.04-
recurrent H11.06-

Ptilosis (eyelid) —*see* Madarosis

Ptomaine (poisoning) —*see*
Poisoning, food

Ptosis —*see also* Blepharoptosis
adiposa (false) —*see*
Blepharoptosis
breast N64.81
brow H57.81-
cecum K63.4
colon K63.4
congenital (eyelid) Q10.0
specified site NEC —*see*
Anomaly, by site
eyebrow H57.81-
eyelid —*see* Blepharoptosis
congenital Q10.0
gastric K31.89
intestine K63.4
kidney N28.83
liver K76.89
renal N28.83
splanchnic K63.4
spleen D73.89
stomach K31.89
viscera K63.4

PTP D69.51

Ptyalism (periodic) K11.7
hysterical F45.8
pregnancy —*see* Pregnancy,
complicated by, specified
pregnancy-related condition
NEC
psychogenic F45.8

Ptyalolithiasis K11.5

Pubarche, precocious E30.1

Pubertas praecox E30.1

Puberty (development state) Z00.3
bleeding (excessive) N92.2
delayed E30.0
precocious (constitutional)
(cryptogenic) (idiopathic) E30.1
central E22.8
due to
ovarian hyperfunction E28.1
estrogen E28.0
testicular hyperfunction E29.0
premature E30.1
due to
adrenal cortical hyperfunction
E25.8
pineal tumor E34.8
pituitary (anterior)
hyperfunction E22.8

Puckering, macula —*see*
Degeneration, macula, puckering

Pudenda, pudendum —*see*
condition

Puente's disease (simple glandular
cheilitis) K13.0

Puerperal, puerperium (complicated
by, complications)
abnormal glucose (tolerance test)
O99.815

Puerperal, puerperium *(continued)*
abscess
areola O91.02
associated with lactation
O91.03
Bartholin's gland O86.19
breast O91.12
associated with lactation
O91.13
cervix (uteri) O86.11
genital organ NEC O86.19
kidney O86.21
mammary O91.12
associated with lactation
O91.13
nipple O91.02
associated with lactation
O91.03
peritoneum O85
subareolar O91.12
associated with lactation
O91.13
urinary tract —*see* Puerperal,
infection, urinary
uterus O86.12
vagina (wall) O86.13
vaginorectal O86.13
vulvovaginal gland O86.13
adnexitis O86.19
afibrinogenemia, or other
coagulation defect O72.3
albuminuria (acute) (subacute)
—*see* Proteinuria, gestational
alcohol use O99.315
anemia O90.81
pre-existing (pre-pregnancy)
O99.03
anesthetic death O89.8
apoplexy O99.43
bariatric surgery status O99.845
blood disorder NEC O99.13
blood dyscrasia O72.3
cardiomyopathy O90.3
cerebrovascular disorder
(conditions in I60-I69) O99.43
cervicitis O86.11
circulatory system disorder O99.43
coagulopathy (any) O99.13
with hemorrhage O72.3
complications O90.9
specified NEC O90.89
convulsions —*see* Eclampsia
cystitis O86.22
cystopyelitis O86.29
delirium NEC F05
diabetes O24.93
gestational —*see* Puerperal,
gestational diabetes
pre-existing O24.33
specified NEC O24.83
type 1 O24.03
type 2 O24.13
digestive system disorder O99.63
disease O90.9
breast NEC O92.29
cerebrovascular (acute) O99.43
nonobstetric NEC O99.893
tubo-ovarian O86.19
Valsuani's O99.03
disorder O90.9
biliary tract O26.63
lactation O92.70
liver O26.63
nonobstetric NEC O99.893
disruption
cesarean wound O90.0
episiotomy wound O90.1
perineal laceration wound O90.1
drug use O99.325
eclampsia (with pre-existing
hypertension) O15.2

Puerperal, puerperium *(continued)*
embolism (pulmonary) (blood
  clot) —*see* Embolism, obstetric,
  puerperal
endocrine, nutritional or metabolic
  disease NEC O99.285
endophlebitis —*see* Puerperal,
  phlebitis
endotrachelitis O86.11
failure
  lactation (complete) O92.3
    partial O92.4
  renal, acute O90.4
fever (of unknown origin) O86.4
  septic O85
fissure, nipple O92.12
  associated with lactation O92.13
fistula
  breast (due to mastitis) O91.12
    associated with lactation
      O91.13
  nipple O91.02
    associated with lactation
      O91.03
galactophoritis O91.22
  associated with lactation O91.23
galactorrhea O92.6
gastric banding status O99.845
gastric bypass status O99.845
gastrointestinal disease NEC
  O99.63
gestational
  diabetes O24.439
    diet controlled O24.430
    insulin (and diet) controlled
      O24.434
    oral drug controlled
      (antidiabetic)
      (hypoglycemic) O24.435
  edema O12.05
    with proteinuria O12.25
  proteinuria O12.15
gonorrhea O98.23
hematoma, subdural O99.43
hemiplegia, cerebral O99.355
  due to cerbrovascular disorder
    O99.43
hemorrhage O72.1
  brain O99.43
  bulbar O99.43
  cerebellar O99.43
  cerebral O99.43
  cortical O99.43
  delayed or secondary O72.2
  extradural O99.43
  internal capsule O99.43
  intracranial O99.43
  intrapontine O99.43
  meningeal O99.43
  pontine O99.43
  retained placenta O72.0
  subarachnoid O99.43
  subcortical O99.43
  subdural O99.43
  third stage O72.0
  uterine, delayed O72.2
  ventricular O99.43
hemorrhoids O87.2
hepatorenal syndrome O90.4
hypertension —*see* Hypertension,
  complicating, puerperium
hypertrophy, breast O92.29
induration breast (fibrous) O92.29
infection O86.4
  cervix O86.11
  generalized O85
  genital tract NEC O86.19
    obstetric surgical wound
      O86.09
  kidney (bacillus coli) O86.21
  maternal O98.93

Puerperal, puerperium *(continued)*
infection *(continued)*
  maternal *(continued)*
    carrier state NEC O99.835
    gonorrhea O98.23
    human immunodeficiency
      virus (HIV) O98.73
    protozoal O98.63
    sexually transmitted NEC
      O98.33
    specified NEC O98.83
    streptococcus group B (GBS)
      carrier state O99.825
    syphilis O98.13
    tuberculosis O98.03
    viral hepatitis O98.43
    viral NEC O98.53
  nipple O91.02
    associated with lactation
      O91.03
  peritoneum O85
  renal O86.21
  specified NEC O86.89
  urinary (asymptomatic) (tract)
    NEC O86.20
    bladder O86.22
    kidney O86.21
    specified site NEC O86.29
    urethra O86.22
  vagina O86.13
  vein —*see* Puerperal, phlebitis
ischemia, cerebral O99.43
lymphangitis O86.89
  breast O91.22
    associated with lactation
      O91.23
malignancy O9A.13
malnutrition O25.3
mammillitis O91.02
  associated with lactation O91.03
mammitis O91.22
  associated with lactation O91.23
mania F30.8
mastitis O91.22
  associated with lactation O91.23
  purulent O91.12
    associated with lactation
      O91.13
melancholia —*see* Disorder,
  depressive
mental disorder NEC O99.345
metroperitonitis O85
metrorrhagia —*see* Hemorrhage,
  postpartum
metrosalpingitis O86.19
metrovaginitis O86.13
milk leg O87.1
monoplegia, cerebral O99.43
mood disturbance O90.6
necrosis, liver (acute) (subacute)
  (conditions in subcategory
  K72.0) O26.63
  with renal failure O90.4
nervous system disorder O99.355
neuritis O90.89
obesity (pre-existing prior to
  pregnancy) O99.215
obesity surgery status O99.845
occlusion, precerebral artery O99.43
paralysis
  bladder (sphincter) O90.89
  cerebral O99.43
paralytic stroke O99.43
parametritis O85
paravaginitis O86.13
pelviperitonitis O85
perimetritis O86.12
perimetrosalpingitis O86.19
perinephritis O86.21
periphlebitis —*see* Puerperal
  phlebitis

Puerperal, puerperium *(continued)*
peritoneal infection O85
peritonitis (pelvic) O85
perivaginitis O86.13
phlebitis O87.0
  deep O87.1
  pelvic O87.1
  superficial O87.0
phlebothrombosis, deep O87.1
phlegmasia alba dolens O87.1
placental polyp O90.89
pneumonia, embolic —*see*
  Embolism, obstetric, puerperal
pre-eclampsia (NOS) —*see*
  Pre-eclampsia
psychosis F53.1
pyelitis O86.21
pyelocystitis O86.29
pyelonephritis O86.21
pyelonephrosis O86.21
pyemia O85
pyocystitis O86.29
pyohemia O85
pyometra O86.12
pyonephritis O86.21
pyosalpingitis O86.19
pyrexia (of unknown origin) O86.4
renal
  disease NEC O90.89
  failure O90.4
respiratory disease NEC O99.53
retention
  decidua —*see* Retention, decidua
  placenta O72.0
  secundines —*see* Retention,
    secundines
retrated nipple O92.02
salpingo-ovaritis O86.19
salpingoperitonitis O85
secondary perineal tear O90.1
sepsis (pelvic) O85
sepsis O85
septic thrombophlebitis O86.81
skin disorder NEC O99.73
specified condition NEC O99.893
stroke O99.43
subinvolution (uterus) O90.89
subluxation of symphysis (pubis)
  O26.73
suppuration —*see* Puerperal,
  abscess
tetanus A34
thelitis O91.02
  associated with lactation O91.03
thrombocytopenia O72.3
thrombophlebitis (superficial)
  O87.0
  deep O87.1
  pelvic O87.1
  septic O86.81
thrombosis (venous) —*see*
  Thrombosis, puerperal
thyroiditis O90.5
toxemia (eclamptic) (pre-
  eclamptic) (with convulsions)
  O15.2
trauma, non-obstetric O9A.23
  caused by abuse (physical)
    (suspected) O9A.33
    confirmed O9A.33
  psychological (suspected)
    O9A.53
    confirmed O9A.53
  sexual (suspected) O9A.43
    confirmed O9A.43
uremia (due to renal failure) O90.4
urethritis O86.22
vaginitis O86.13
varicose veins (legs) O87.4
  vulva or perineum O87.8
venous O87.9

Puerperal, puerperium *(continued)*
vulvitis O86.19
vulvovaginitis O86.13
white leg O87.1

Puerperium —*see* Puerperal

Pulmolithiasis J98.4

Pulmonary —*see* condition

Pulpitis (acute) (anachoretic)
  (chronic) (hyperplastic)
  (putrescent) (suppurative)
  (ulcerative) K04.01
  irreversible K04.02
  reversible K04.01

Pulpless tooth K04.99

Pulse
  alternating R00.8
  bigeminal R00.8
  fast R00.0
  feeble, rapid due to shock
    following injury T79.4
  rapid R00.0
  weak R09.89

Pulsus alternans or trigeminus R00.8

Punch drunk F07.81

Punctum lacrimale occlusion —*see*
  Obstruction, lacrimal

Puncture
abdomen, abdominal
  wall S31.139
    with
      foreign body S31.149
      penetration into peritoneal
        cavity S31.639
        with foreign body S31.649
  wall S31.139
    epigastric region S31.132
      with
        foreign body S31.142
        penetration into
          peritoneal cavity
          S31.632
          with foreign body
            S31.642
    left
      lower quadrant S31.134
        with
          foreign body S31.144
          penetration into
            peritoneal cavity
            S31.634
            with foreign body
              S31.644
      upper quadrant S31.131
        with
          foreign body S31.141
          penetration into
            peritoneal cavity
            S31.631
            with foreign body
              S31.641
    periumbilic region S31.135
      with
        foreign body S31.145
        penetration into
          peritoneal cavity
          S31.635
          with foreign body
            S31.645
    right
      lower quadrant S31.133
        with
          foreign body S31.143
          penetration into
            peritoneal cavity
            S31.633
            with foreign body
              S31.643

Puncture *(continued)*
abdomen, abdominal *(continued)*
  wall *(continued)*
    right *(continued)*
      upper quadrant S31.130
        with
          foreign body S31.140
          penetration into
            peritoneal cavity
            S31.630
              with foreign body
              S31.640
accidental, complicating surgery
  —*see* Complication, accidental
  puncture or laceration
alveolar (process) —*see* Puncture,
  oral cavity
ankle S91.039
  with
    foreign body S91.049
  left S91.032
    with
      foreign body S91.042
  right S91.031
    with
      foreign body S91.041
anus S31.833
  with foreign body S31.834
arm (upper) S41.139
  with foreign body S41.149
  left S41.132
    with foreign body S41.142
  lower —*see* Puncture, forearm
  right S41.131
    with foreign body S41.141
auditory canal (external) (meatus)
  —*see* Puncture, ear
auricle, ear —*see* Puncture, ear
axilla —*see* Puncture, arm
back —*see also* Puncture, thorax,
  back
  lower S31.030
    with
      foreign body S31.040
        with penetration into
          retroperitoneal space
          S31.041
        penetration into
          retroperitoneal space
          S31.031
bladder (traumatic) S37.29
  nontraumatic N32.89
breast S21.039
  with foreign body S21.049
  left S21.032
    with foreign body S21.042
  right S21.031
    with foreign body S21.041
buttock S31.803
  with foreign body S31.804
  left S31.823
    with foreign body S31.824
  right S31.813
    with foreign body S31.814
by
  device, implant or graft —*see*
    Complications, by site and
    type, mechanical
  foreign body left accidentally in
    operative wound T81.539
  instrument (any) during a
    procedure, accidental
    —*see* Puncture, accidental
    complicating surgery
calf —*see* Puncture, leg
canaliculus lacrimalis —*see*
  Puncture, eyelid
canthus, eye —*see* Puncture, eyelid
cervical esophagus S11.23
  with foreign body S11.24
cheek (external) S01.439

Puncture *(continued)*
cheek *(continued)*
  with foreign body S01.449
  left S01.432
    with foreign body S01.442
  right S01.431
    with foreign body S01.441
  internal —*see* Puncture, oral
    cavity
chest wall —*see* Puncture, thorax
chin —*see* Puncture, head,
  specified site NEC
clitoris —*see* Puncture, vulva
costal region —*see* Puncture,
  thorax
digit(s)
  hand —*see* Puncture, finger
  foot —*see* Puncture, toe
ear (canal) (external) S01.339
  with foreign body S01.349
  left S01.332
    with foreign body S01.342
  right S01.331
    with foreign body S01.341
  drum S09.2-
elbow S51.039
  with
    foreign body S51.049
  left S51.032
    with
      foreign body S51.042
  right S51.031
    with
      foreign body S51.041
epididymis —*see* Puncture,
  testis
epigastric region —*see* Puncture,
  abdomen, wall, epigastric
epiglottis S11.83
  with foreign body S11.84
esophagus
  cervical S11.23
    with foreign body S11.24
  thoracic S27.818
eyeball S05.6-
  with foreign body S05.5-
eyebrow —*see* Puncture, eyelid
eyelid S01.13-
  with foreign body S01.14-
  left S01.132
    with foreign body S01.142
  right S01.131
    with foreign body S01.141
face NEC —*see* Puncture, head,
  specified site NEC
finger(s) S61.239
  with
    damage to nail S61.339
      with
        foreign body S61.349
    foreign body S61.249
  index S61.238
    with
      damage to nail S61.338
        with
          foreign body S61.348
      foreign body S61.248
    left S61.231
      with
        damage to nail S61.331
          with
            foreign body
            S61.341
        foreign body S61.241
    right S61.230
      with
        damage to nail S61.330
          with
            foreign body
            S61.340
        foreign body S61.240

Puncture *(continued)*
finger *(continued)*
  little S61.238
    with
      damage to nail S61.338
        with
          foreign body S61.348
      foreign body S61.248
    left S61.237
      with
        damage to nail S61.337
          with
            foreign body
            S61.347
        foreign body S61.247
    right S61.236
      with
        damage to nail S61.336
          with
            foreign body
            S61.346
        foreign body S61.246
  middle S61.238
    with
      damage to nail S61.338
        with
          foreign body S61.348
      foreign body S61.248
    left S61.233
      with
        damage to nail S61.333
          with
            foreign body
            S61.343
        foreign body S61.243
    right S61.232
      with
        damage to nail S61.332
          with
            foreign body
            S61.342
        foreign body S61.242
  ring S61.238
    with
      damage to nail S61.338
        with
          foreign body S61.348
      foreign body S61.248
    left S61.235
      with
        damage to nail S61.335
          with
            foreign body
            S61.345
        foreign body S61.245
    right S61.234
      with
        damage to nail S61.334
          with
            foreign body
            S61.344
        foreign body S61.244
flank S31.139
  with foreign body S31.149
foot (except toe(s) alone) S91.339
  with foreign body S91.349
  left S91.332
    with foreign body S91.342
  right S91.331
    with foreign body S91.341
  toe —*see* Puncture, toe
forearm S51.839
  with
    foreign body S51.849
  elbow only —*see* Puncture, elbow
  left S51.832
    with
      foreign body S51.842
  right S51.831
    with
      foreign body S51.841

Puncture *(continued)*
forehead —*see* Puncture, head,
  specified site NEC
genital organs, external
  female S31.532
    with foreign body S31.542
    vagina —*see* Puncture, vagina
    vulva —*see* Puncture, vulva
  male S31.531
    with foreign body S31.541
    penis —*see* Puncture, penis
    scrotum —*see* Puncture,
      scrotum
    testis —*see* Puncture, testis
groin —*see* Puncture, abdomen,
  wall
gum —*see* Puncture, oral cavity
hand S61.439
  with
    foreign body S61.449
  finger —*see* Puncture, finger
  left S61.432
    with
      foreign body S61.442
  right S61.431
    with
      foreign body S61.441
  thumb —*see* Puncture, thumb
head S01.93
  with foreign body S01.94
  cheek —*see* Puncture, cheek
  ear —*see* Puncture, ear
  eyelid —*see* Puncture, eyelid
  lip —*see* Puncture, oral cavity
  nose —*see* Puncture, nose
  oral cavity —*see* Puncture, oral
    cavity
  scalp S01.03
    with foreign body S01.04
  specified site NEC S01.83
    with foreign body S01.84
  temporomandibular area —*see*
    Puncture, cheek
heart S26.99
  with hemopericardium S26.09
  without hemopericardium
    S26.19
heel —*see* Puncture, foot
hip S71.039
  with foreign body S71.049
  left S71.032
    with foreign body S71.042
  right S71.031
    with foreign body S71.041
hymen —*see* Puncture, vagina
hypochondrium —*see* Puncture,
  abdomen, wall
hypogastric region —*see* Puncture,
  abdomen, wall
inguinal region —*see* Puncture,
  abdomen, wall
instep —*see* Puncture, foot
internal organs —*see* Injury, by site
interscapular region —*see*
  Puncture, thorax, back
intestine
  large
    colon S36.599
      ascending S36.590
      descending S36.592
      sigmoid S36.593
      specified site NEC S36.598
      transverse S36.591
    rectum S36.69
  small S36.499
    duodenum S36.490
    specified site NEC S36.498
intra-abdominal organ S36.99
  gallbladder S36.128
  intestine —*see* Puncture,
    intestine

Purpura *(continued)*
  thrombocytopenic D69.49
    congenital D69.42
    hemorrhagic D69.3
    hereditary D69.42
    idiopathic D69.3
    immune D69.3
    neonatal, transitory P61.0
    thrombotic M31.1
  thrombohemolytic —*see*
    Fibrinolysis
  thrombolytic —*see* Fibrinolysis
  thrombopenic D69.49
  thrombotic, thrombocytopenic
    M31.1
  toxic D69.0
  vascular D69.0
  visceral symptoms D69.0

Purpuric spots R23.3

Purulent —*see* condition

Pus
  in
    stool R19.5
    urine N39.0
  tube (rupture) —*see* Salpingo-
    oophoritis

Pustular rash L08.0

Pustule (nonmalignant) L08.9
  malignant A22.0

Pustulosis palmaris et plantaris
  L40.3

Putnam (-Dana) **disease or**
  syndrome —*see* Degeneration,
  combined

Putrescent pulp (dental) K04.1

Pyarthritis, pyarthrosis —*see*
  Arthritis, pyogenic or pyemic
  tuberculous —*see* Tuberculosis,
    joint

Pyelectasis —*see* Hydronephrosis

Pyelitis (congenital) (uremic) —*see*
  also Pyelonephritis
  with
    calculus —*see* category N20
      with hydronephrosis N13.6
    contracted kidney N11.9
  acute N10
  chronic N11.9
    with calculus —*see* category
      N20
      with hydronephrosis N13.6
  cystica N28.84
  puerperal (postpartum) O86.21
  tuberculous A18.11

Pyelocystitis —*see* Pyelonephritis

Pyelonephritis —*see also* Nephritis,
  tubulo-interstitial
  with
    calculus —*see* category N20
      with hydronephrosis N13.6
    contracted kidney N11.9
  acute N10
  calculous —*see* category N20
    with hydronephrosis N13.6
  chronic N11.9
    with calculus —*see* category
      N20
      with hydronephrosis N13.6
    associated with ureteral
      obstruction or stricture
      N11.1
    nonobstructive N11.8
      with reflux (vesicoureteral)
        N11.0
    obstructive N11.1
    specified NEC N11.8

Pyelonephritis *(continued)*
  in (due to)
    brucellosis A23.9 *[N16]*
    cryoglobulinemia (mixed) D89.1
      [N16]
    cystinosis E72.04
    diphtheria A36.84
    glycogen storage disease E74.09
      [N16]
    leukemia NEC C95.9- *[N16]*
    lymphoma NEC C85.90 *[N16]*
    multiple myeloma C90.0- *[N16]*
    obstruction N11.1
    Salmonella infection A02.25
    sarcoidosis D86.84
    sepsis A41.9 *[N16]*
    Sjögren's disease M35.04
    toxoplasmosis B58.83
    transplant rejection T86.91
      [N16]
    Wilson's disease E83.01 *[N16]*
  nonobstructive N12
    with reflux (vesicoureteral)
      N11.0
    chronic N11.8
  syphilitic A52.75

Pyelonephrosis (obstructive) N11.1
  chronic N11.9

Pyelophlebitis I80.8

Pyeloureteritis cystica N28.85

Pyemia, pyemic (fever) (infection)
  (purulent) —*see also* Sepsis
  joint —*see* Arthritis, pyogenic or
    pyemic
  liver K75.1
  pneumococcal A40.3
  portal K75.1
  postvaccinal T88.0
  puerperal, postpartum, childbirth
    O85
  specified organism NEC A41.89
  tuberculous —*see* Tuberculosis,
    miliary

Pygopagus Q89.4

Pyknoepilepsy (idiopathic) —*see*
  Pyknolepsy

Pyknolepsy G40.A09
  intractable G40.A19
    with status epilepticus G40.A11
    without status epilepticus G40.
      A19
  not intractable G40.A09
    with status epilepticus G40.A01
    without status epilepticus G40.
      A09

Pylephlebitis K75.1

Pyle's syndrome Q78.5

Pylethrombophlebitis K75.1

Pylethrombosis K75.1

Pyloritis K29.90
  with bleeding K29.91

Pylorospasm (reflex) NEC K31.3
  congenital or infantile Q40.0
  newborn Q40.0
  neurotic F45.8
  psychogenic F45.8

Pylorus, pyloric —*see* condition

Pyoarthrosis —*see* Arthritis,
  pyogenic or pyemic

Pyocele
  mastoid —*see* Mastoiditis, acute
  sinus (accessory) —*see* Sinusitis
  turbinate (bone) J32.9
  urethra (*see also* Urethritis)
    N34.0

Pyocolpos —*see* Vaginitis

Pyocystitis N30.80
  with hematuria N30.81

Pyoderma, pyodermia L08.0
  gangrenosum L88
  newborn P39.4
  phagedenic L88
  vegetans L08.81

Pyodermatitis L08.0
  vegetans L08.81

Pyogenic —*see* condition

Pyohydronephrosis N13.6

Pyometra, pyometrium, pyometritis
  —*see* Endometritis

Pyomyositis (tropical) —*see*
  Myositis, infective

Pyonephritis N12

Pyonephrosis N13.6
  tuberculous A18.11

Pyo-oophoritis —*see* Salpingo-
  oophoritis

Pyo-ovarium —*see* Salpingo-
  oophoritis

Pyopericarditis, pyopericardium
  I30.1

Pyophlebitis —*see* Phlebitis

Pyopneumopericardium I30.1

Pyopneumothorax (infective) J86.9
  with fistula J86.0
  tuberculous NEC A15.6

Pyosalpinx, pyosalpingitis —*see*
  also Salpingo-oophoritis

Pyothorax J86.9
  with fistula J86.0
  tuberculous NEC A15.6

Pyoureter N28.89
  tuberculous A18.11

Pyramidopallidonigral syndrome
  G20

Pyrexia (of unknown origin) R50.9
  atmospheric T67.01
  during labor NEC O75.2
  heat T67.01
  newborn P81.9
    environmentally-induced P81.0
  persistent R50.9
  puerperal O86.4

Pyroglobulinemia NEC E88.09

Pyromania F63.1

Pyrosis R12

Pyuria (bacterial) (sterile) R82.81

Q

Q fever A78
  with pneumonia A78

Quadricuspid aortic valve Q23.8

Quadrilateral fever A78

Quadriparesis —*see* Quadriplegia
  meaning muscle weakness M62.81

Quadriplegia G82.50
  complete
    C1-C4 level G82.51
    C5-C7 level G82.53
  congenital (cerebral) (spinal) G80.8
    spastic G80.0
  embolic (current episode) I63.4-
  functional R53.2
  incomplete
    C1-C4 level G82.52
    C5-C7 level G82.54

Quadriplegia *(continued)*
  thrombotic (current episode) I63.3-
  traumatic -- code to injury with
    seventh character S
    current episode —*see* Injury,
      spinal (cord), cervical

Quadruplet, pregnancy —*see*
  Pregnancy, quadruplet

Quarrelsomeness F60.3

Queensland fever A77.3

Quervain's disease M65.4
  thyroid E06.1

Queyrat's erythroplasia D07.4
  penis D07.4
  specified site —*see* Neoplasm,
    skin, in situ
  unspecified site D07.4

Quincke's disease or edema T78.3
  hereditary D84.1

Quinsy (gangrenous) J36

Quintan fever A79.0

Quintuplet, pregnancy —*see*
  Pregnancy, quintuplet

R

Rabbit fever —*see* Tularemia

Rabies A82.9
  contact Z20.3
  exposure to Z20.3
  inoculation reaction —*see*
    Complications, vaccination
  sylvatic A82.0
  urban A82.1

Rachischisis —*see* Spina bifida

Rachitic —*see also* condition
  deformities of spine (late effect)
    (sequelae) E64.3
  pelvis (late effect) (sequelae) E64.3
    with disproportion (fetopelvic)
      O33.0
      causing obstructed labor
        O65.0

Rachitis, rachitism (acute) (tarda)
  —*see also* Rickets
  renalis N25.0
  sequelae E64.3

Radial nerve —*see* condition

Radiation
  burn —*see* Burn
  effects NOS T66
  sickness NOS T66
  therapy, encounter for Z51.0

Radiculitis (pressure) (vertebrogenic)
  —*see* Radiculopathy

Radiculomyelitis —*see also*
  Encephalitis
  toxic, due to
    Clostridium tetani A35
    Corynebacterium diphtheriae
      A36.82

Radiculopathy M54.10
  cervical region M54.12
  cervicothoracic region M54.13
  due to
    disc disorder
      C3 M50.11
      C4 M50.11
      C5 M50.121
      C6 M50.122
      C7 M50.123
      C8 M50.13
    displacement of intervertebral
      disc —*see* Disorder, disc,
      with, radiculopathy

Radiculopathy *(continued)*
 leg M54.1-
 lumbar region M54.16
 lumbosacral region M54.17
 occipito-atlanto-axial region
  M54.11
 postherpetic B02.29
 sacrococcygeal region M54.18
 syphilitic A52.11
 thoracic region (with visceral pain)
  M54.14
 thoracolumbar region M54.15

Radiodermal burns (acute, chronic,
 or occupational) —*see* Burn

Radiodermatitis L58.9
 acute L58.0
 chronic L58.1

Radiotherapy session Z51.0

**RAEB (refractory anemia with
 excess blasts)** D46.2-

Rage, meaning rabies —*see* Rabies

Ragpicker's disease A22.1

Ragsorter's disease A22.1

Raillietiniasis B71.8

Railroad neurosis F48.8

Railway spine F48.8

Raised —*see also* Elevated
 antibody titer R76.0

Rake teeth, tooth M26.39

Rales R09.89

Ramifying renal pelvis Q63.8

Ramsay-Hunt disease or syndrome
 (*see also* Hunt's disease) B02.21
 meaning dyssynergia cerebellaris
  myoclonica G11.19

Ranula K11.6
 congenital Q38.4

Rape
 adult
  confirmed T74.21
  suspected T76.21
 alleged, observation or
  examination, ruled out
  adult Z04.41
  child Z04.42
 child
  confirmed T74.22
  suspected T76.22

Rapid
 feeble pulse, due to shock,
  following injury T79.4
 heart (beat) R00.0
  psychogenic F45.8
 second stage (delivery) O62.3
 time-zone change syndrome
  G47.25

Rarefaction, bone —*see* Disorder,
 bone, density and structure,
 specified NEC

Rash (toxic) R21
 canker A38.9
 diaper L22
 drug (internal use) L27.0
  contact (*see also* Dermatitis, due
   to, drugs, external) L25.1
 following immunization T88.1
 food —*see* Dermatitis, due to, food
 heat L74.0
 napkin (psoriasiform) L22
 nettle —*see* Urticaria
 pustular L08.0
 rose R21
  epidemic B06.9
 scarlet A38.9

Rash *(continued)*
 serum (*see also* Reaction, serum)
  T80.69
 wandering tongue K14.1

Rasmussen aneurysm —*see*
 Tuberculosis, pulmonary

Rasmussen encephalitis G04.81

Rat-bite fever A25.9
 due to Streptobacillus moniliformis
  A25.1
 spirochetal (morsus muris) A25.0

Rathke's pouch tumor D44.3

Raymond (-Céstan) **syndrome** I65.8

**Raynaud's disease, phenomenon or
 syndrome** (secondary) I73.00
 with gangrene (symmetric) I73.01

RDS (newborn) (type I) P22.0
 type II P22.1

Reaction —*see also* Disorder
 adaptation —*see* Disorder,
  adjustment
 adjustment (anxiety) (conduct
  disorder) (depressiveness)
  (distress) —*see* Disorder,
  adjustment
  with
   mutism, elective (child)
    (adolescent) F94.0
 adverse
  food (any) (ingested) NEC T78.1
   anaphylactic —*see* Shock,
    anaphylactic, due to food
 affective —*see* Disorder, mood
 allergic —*see* Allergy
 anaphylactic —*see* Shock,
  anaphylactic
 anaphylactoid —*see* Shock,
  anaphylactic
 anesthesia —*see* Anesthesia,
  complication
 antitoxin (prophylactic)
  (therapeutic) —*see*
  Complications, vaccination
 anxiety F41.1
 Arthus —*see* Arthus' phenomenon
 asthenic F48.8
 combat and operational stress F43.0
 compulsive F42.8
 conversion F44.9
 crisis, acute F43.0
 deoxyribonuclease (DNA) (DNase)
  hypersensitivity D69.2
 depressive (single episode) F32.9
  affective (single episode) F31.4
   recurrent episode F33.9
  neurotic F34.1
  psychoneurotic F34.1
  psychotic F32.3
  recurrent —*see* Disorder,
   depressive, recurrent
 dissociative F44.9
 drug NEC T88.7
  addictive —*see* Dependence,
   drug
   transmitted via placenta
    or breast milk —*see*
    Absorption, drug, addictive,
    through placenta
  allergic —*see* Allergy, drug
  lichenoid L43.2
  newborn P93.8
   gray baby syndrome P93.0
  overdose or poisoning (by
   accident) —*see* Table of
   Drugs and Chemicals, by
   drug, poisoning
  photoallergic L56.1
  phototoxic L56.0

Reaction *(continued)*
 drug NEC *(continued)*
  withdrawal —*see* Dependence,
   by drug, with, withdrawal
   infant of dependent mother
    P96.1
   newborn P96.1
  wrong substance given or taken
   (by accident) —*see* Table
   of Drugs and Chemicals, by
   drug, poisoning
 fear F40.9
  child (abnormal) F93.8
 febrile nonhemolytic transfusion
  (FNHTR) R50.84
 fluid loss, cerebrospinal G97.1
 foreign
  body NEC —*see* Granuloma,
   foreign body
   in operative wound
    (inadvertently left) —*see*
    Foreign body, accidentally
    left during a procedure
  substance accidentally left
   during a procedure (chemical)
   (powder) (talc) T81.60
   aseptic peritonitis T81.61
   body or object (instrument)
    (sponge) (swab) —*see*
    Foreign body, accidentally
    left during a procedure
   specified reaction NEC T81.69
 grief —*see* Disorder, adjustment
 Herxheimer's R68.89
 hyperkinetic —*see* Hyperkinesia
 hypochondriacal F45.20
 hypoglycemic, due to insulin E16.0
  with coma (diabetic) —*see*
   Diabetes, coma
   nondiabetic E15
  therapeutic misadventure —*see*
   subcategory T38.3
 hypomanic F30.8
 hysterical F44.9
 immunization —*see* Complications,
  vaccination
 incompatibility
  ABO blood group (infusion)
   (transfusion) —*see*
   Complication(s), transfusion,
   incompatibility reaction, ABO
   delayed serologic T80.39
  minor blood group (Duffy) (E)
   (K) (Kell) (Kidd) (Lewis) (M)
   (N) (P) (S) T80.89
  Rh (factor) (infusion)
   (transfusion) —*see*
   Complication(s), transfusion,
   incompatibility reaction, Rh
   (factor)
 inflammatory —*see* Infection
 infusion —*see* Complications,
  infusion
 inoculation (immune serum) —*see*
  Complications, vaccination
 insulin T38.3-
 involutional psychotic —*see*
  Disorder, depressive
 leukemoid D72.823
  basophilic D72.823
  lymphocytic D72.823
  monocytic D72.823
  myelocytic D72.823
  neutrophilic D72.823
 LSD (acute)
  due to drug abuse —*see* Abuse,
   drug, hallucinogen
  due to drug dependence —*see*
   Dependence, drug,
   hallucinogen
 lumbar puncture G97.1

Reaction *(continued)*
 manic-depressive —*see* Disorder,
  bipolar
 neurasthenic F48.8
 neurogenic —*see* Neurosis
 neurotic F48.9
 neurotic-depressive F34.1
 nitritoid —*see* Crisis, nitritoid
 nonspecific
  to
   cell mediated immunity
    measurement of gamma
    interferon antigen response
    without active tuberculosis
    R76.12
   QuantiFERON-TB test (QFT)
    without active tuberculosis
    R76.12
   tuberculin test (*see also*
    Reaction, tuberculin skin
    test) R76.11
 obsessive-compulsive F42.8
 organic, acute or subacute —*see*
  Delirium
 paranoid (acute) F23
  chronic F22
  senile F03
 passive dependency F60.7
 phobic F40.9
 post-traumatic stress,
  uncomplicated Z73.3
 psychogenic F99
 psychoneurotic —*see also* Neurosis
  compulsive F42.8
  depersonalization F48.1
  depressive F34.1
  hypochondriacal F45.20
  neurasthenic F48.8
  obsessive F42.8
 psychophysiologic —*see* Disorder,
  somatoform
 psychosomatic —*see* Disorder,
  somatoform
 psychotic —*see* Psychosis
 scarlet fever toxin —*see*
  Complications, vaccination
 schizophrenic F23
  acute (brief) (undifferentiated)
   F23
  latent F21
  undifferentiated (acute) (brief) F23
 serological for syphilis —*see*
  Serology for syphilis
 serum T80.69
  anaphylactic (immediate) —*see
   also* Shock, anaphylactic T80.59
  specified reaction NEC
   due to
    administration of blood and
     blood products T80.61
    immunization T80.62
    serum specified NEC
     T80.69
    vaccination T80.62
 situational —*see* Disorder,
  adjustment
 somatization —*see* Disorder,
  somatoform
 spinal puncture G97.1
  dural G97.1
 stress (severe) F43.9
  acute (agitation) ("daze")
   (disorientation) (disturbance
   of consciousness) (flight
   reaction) (fugue) F43.0
  specified NEC F43.8
 surgical procedure —*see*
  Complications, surgical
  procedure
 tetanus antitoxin —*see*
  Complications, vaccination

Reaction *(continued)*
toxic, to local anesthesia T88.59
in labor and delivery O74.4
in pregnancy O29.3X-
postpartum, puerperal O89.3
toxin-antitoxin —*see*
Complications, vaccination
transfusion (blood) (bone marrow)
(lymphocytes) (allergic) —*see*
Complications, transfusion
tuberculin skin test, abnormal R76.11
vaccination (any) —*see*
Complications, vaccination
withdrawing, child or adolescent
F93.8

Reactive airway disease —*see*
Asthma

Reactive depression —*see* Reaction,
depressive

Rearrangement
chromosomal
balanced (in) Q95.9
abnormal individual
(autosomal) Q95.2
non-sex (autosomal)
chromosomes Q95.2
sex/non-sex chromosomes
Q95.3
specified NEC Q95.8

Recalcitrant patient —*see*
Noncompliance

Recanalization, thrombus —*see*
Thrombosis

Recession, receding
chamber angle (eye) H21.55-
chin M26.09
gingival (postinfective)
(postoperative)
generalized K06.020
minimal K06.021
moderate K06.022
severe K06.023
localized K06.010
minimal K06.011
moderate K06.012
severe K06.013

Recklinghausen disease Q85.01
bones E21.0

Reclus' disease (cystic) —*see*
Mastopathy, cystic

Recrudescent typhus (fever) A75.1

Recruitment, auditory H93.21-

Rectalgia K62.89

Rectitis K62.89

Rectocele
female (without uterine prolapse)
N81.6
with uterine prolapse N81.4
incomplete N81.2
in pregnancy —*see* Pregnancy,
complicated by, abnormal, pelvic
organs or tissues NEC
male K62.3

Rectosigmoid junction —*see*
condition

Rectosigmoiditis K63.89
ulcerative (chronic) K51.30
with
complication K51.319
abscess K51.314
fistula K51.313
obstruction K51.312
rectal bleeding K51.311
specified NEC K51.318

Rectourethral —*see* condition

Rectovaginal —*see* condition

Rectovesical —*see* condition

Rectum, rectal —*see* condition

Recurrent —*see* condition
pregnancy loss —*see* Loss (of),
pregnancy, recurrent

Red bugs B88.0

Red-cedar lung or pneumonitis
J67.8

Red tide (*see also* Table of Drugs and
Chemicals) T65.82-

Reduced
mobility Z74.09
ventilatory or vital capacity R94.2

Redundant, redundancy
anus (congenital) Q43.8
clitoris N90.89
colon (congenital) Q43.8
foreskin (congenital) N47.8
intestine (congenital) Q43.8
labia N90.69
organ or site, congenital NEC
—*see* Accessory
panniculus (abdominal) E65
prepuce (congenital) N47.8
pylorus K31.89
rectum (congenital) Q43.8
scrotum N50.89
sigmoid (congenital) Q43.8
skin L98.7
and subcutaneous tissue L98.7
of face L57.4
eyelids —*see* Blepharochalasis
stomach K31.89

Reduplication —*see* Duplication

Reflex R29.2
hyperactive gag J39.2
pupillary, abnormal —*see*
Anomaly, pupil, function
vasoconstriction I73.9
vasovagal R55

Reflux K21.9
acid K21.9
esophageal K21.9
with esophagitis (without
bleeding) K21.00
with bleeding K21.01
newborn P78.83
gastroesophageal K21.9
with esophagitis (without
bleeding) K21.00
with bleeding K21.01
mitral —*see* Insufficiency, mitral
ureteral —*see* Reflux,
vesicoureteral
vesicoureteral (with scarring) N13.70
with
nephropathy N13.729
with hydroureter N13.739
bilateral N13.732
unilateral N13.731
bilateral N13.722
unilateral N13.721
without hydroureter
N13.729
bilateral N13.722
unilateral N13.721
pyelonephritis (chronic) N11.0
congenital Q62.7
without nephropathy N13.71

Reforming, artificial openings —*see*
Attention to, artificial, opening

Refractive error —*see* Disorder,
refraction

Refsum's disease or syndrome G60.1

Refusal of
food, psychogenic F50.89

Refusal of *(continued)*
treatment (because of) Z53.20
left against medical advice
(AMA) Z53.21
patient's decision NEC Z53.29
reasons of belief or group
pressure Z53.1

Regional —*see* condition

Regurgitation R11.10
aortic (valve) —*see* Insufficiency,
aortic
food —*see also* Vomiting
with reswallowing —*see*
Rumination
newborn P92.1
gastric contents —*see* Vomiting
heart —*see* Endocarditis
mitral (valve) —*see* Insufficiency,
mitral
congenital Q23.3
myocardial —*see* Endocarditis
pulmonary (valve) (heart) I37.1
congenital Q22.2
syphilitic A52.03
tricuspid —*see* Insufficiency,
tricuspid
valve, valvular —*see* Endocarditis
congenital Q24.8
vesicoureteral —*see* Reflux,
vesicoureteral

Reifenstein syndrome
E34.52

Reinsertion
implantable subdermal
contraceptive Z30.46
intrauterine contraceptive device
Z30.433

**Reiter's disease, syndrome, or
urethritis** M02.30
ankle M02.37-
elbow M02.32-
foot joint M02.37-
hand joint M02.34-
hip M02.35-
knee M02.36-
multiple site M02.39
shoulder M02.31-
vertebra M02.38
wrist M02.33-

Reichmann's disease or syndrome
K31.89

Rejection
food, psychogenic F50.89
transplant T86.91
bone T86.830
marrow T86.01
cornea T86.840-
heart T86.21
with lung(s) T86.31
intestine T86.850
kidney T86.11
liver T86.41
lung(s) T86.810
with heart T86.31
organ (immune or nonimmune
cause) T86.91
pancreas T86.890
skin (allograft) (autograft) T86.820
specified NEC T86.890
stem cell (peripheral blood)
(umbilical cord) T86.5

Relapsing fever A68.9
Carter's (Asiatic) A68.1
Dutton's (West African) A68.1
Koch's A68.9
louse-borne (epidemic) A68.0

Relapsing fever *(continued)*
Novy's (American) A68.1
Obermeyers's (European) A68.0
Spirillum A68.9
tick-borne (endemic) A68.1

Relationship
occlusal
open anterior M26.220
open posterior M26.221

Relaxation
anus (sphincter) K62.89
psychogenic F45.8
arch (foot) —*see also* Deformity,
limb, flat foot
back ligaments —*see* Instability,
joint, spine
bladder (sphincter) N31.2
cardioesophageal K21.9
cervix —*see* Incompetency, cervix
diaphragm J98.6
joint (capsule) (ligament)
(paralytic) —*see* Flail, joint
congenital NEC Q74.8
lumbosacral (joint) —*see*
subcategory M53.2
pelvic floor N81.89
perineum N81.89
posture R29.3
rectum (sphincter) K62.89
sacroiliac (joint) —*see* subcategory
M53.2
scrotum N50.89
urethra (sphincter) N36.44
vesical N31.2

**Release from prison, anxiety
concerning** Z65.2

Remains
canal of Cloquet Q14.0
capsule (opaque) Q14.8

Remittent fever (malarial) B54

Remnant
canal of Cloquet Q14.0
capsule (opaque) Q14.8
cervix, cervical stump (acquired)
(postoperative) N88.8
cystic duct, postcholecystectomy
K91.5
fingernail L60.8
congenital Q84.6
meniscus, knee —*see*
Derangement, knee, meniscus,
specified NEC
thyroglossal duct Q89.2
tonsil J35.8
infected (chronic) J35.01
urachus Q64.4

Removal (from) (of)
artificial
arm Z44.00-
complete Z44.01-
partial Z44.02-
eye Z44.2-
leg Z44.10-
complete Z44.11-
partial Z44.12-
breast implant Z45.81
cardiac pulse generator (battery)
(end-of-life) Z45.010
catheter (urinary) (indwelling) Z46.6
from artificial opening —*see*
Attention to, artificial, opening
non-vascular Z46.82
vascular NEC Z45.2
drains Z48.03
device Z46.9
contraceptive Z30.432
implantable subdermal Z30.46
implanted NEC Z45.89
specified NEC Z46.89

Removal *(continued)*
  dressing (nonsurgical) Z48.00
    surgical Z48.01
  external
    fixation device - code to fracture
      with seventh character D
    prosthesis, prosthetic device
      Z44.9
      breast Z44.3-
      specified NEC Z44.8
  home in childhood (to foster home
    or institution) Z62.29
  ileostomy Z43.2
  insulin pump Z46.81
  myringotomy device (stent) (tube)
    Z45.82
  nervous system device NEC Z46.2
    brain neuropacemaker Z46.2
    visual substitution device Z46.2
      implanted Z45.31
  non-vascular catheter Z46.82
  orthodontic device Z46.4
  organ, prophylactic (for
    neoplasia management) —*see*
    Prophylactic, organ removal
  staples Z48.02
  stent
    ureteral Z46.6
  suture Z48.02
  urinary device Z46.6
  vascular access device or catheter
    Z45.2

Ren
  arcuatus Q63.1
  mobile, mobilis N28.89
    congenital Q63.8
  unguliformis Q63.1

Renal —*see* condition

**Rendu-Osler-Weber disease or
  syndrome** I78.0

Reninoma D41.0-

Renon-Delille syndrome E23.3

**Reovirus, as cause of disease
  classified elsewhere** B97.5

Repeated falls NEC R29.6

**Replaced chromosome by dicentric
  ring** Q93.2

**Replacement by artificial or
  mechanical device or prosthesis
  of**
  bladder Z96.0
  blood vessel NEC Z95.828
  bone NEC Z96.7
  cochlea Z96.21
  coronary artery Z95.5
  eustachian tube Z96.29
  eye globe Z97.0
  heart Z95.812
    valve Z95.2
      prosthetic Z95.2
      specified NEC Z95.4
      xenogenic Z95.3
  intestine Z96.89
  joint Z96.60
    hip —*see* Presence, hip joint
      implant
    knee —*see* Presence, knee joint
      implant
    specified site NEC Z96.698
  larynx Z96.3
  lens Z96.1
  limb(s) —*see* Presence, artificial,
    limb
  mandible NEC (for tooth root
    implant(s)) Z96.5
  organ NEC Z96.89
  peripheral vessel NEC Z95.828
  stapes Z96.29

**Replacement by artificial or
  mechanical device or prosthesis
  of** *(continued)*
  teeth Z97.2
  tendon Z96.7
  tissue NEC Z96.89
  tooth root(s) Z96.5
  vessel NEC Z95.828
    coronary (artery) Z95.5

Request for expert evidence Z04.89

Reserve, decreased or low
  cardiac —*see* Disease, heart
  kidney N28.89

Residual —*see also* condition
  ovary syndrome N99.83
  state, schizophrenic F20.5
  urine R39.198

Resistance, resistant (to)
  activated protein C D68.51
  complicating pregnancy O26.89
  insulin E88.81
  organism(s)
    to
      drug Z16.30
        aminoglycosides Z16.29
        amoxicillin Z16.11
        ampicillin Z16.11
        antibiotic(s) Z16.20
          multiple Z16.24
          specified NEC Z16.29
        antifungal Z16.32
        antimicrobial (single)
          Z16.30
          multiple Z16.35
          specified NEC Z16.39
        antimycobacterial (single)
          Z16.341
          multiple Z16.342
        antiparasitic Z16.31
        antiviral Z16.33
        beta lactam antibiotics
          Z16.10
          specified NEC Z16.19
        cephalosporins Z16.19
        extended beta lactamase
          (ESBL) Z16.12
        fluoroquinolones Z16.23
        macrolides Z16.29
        methicillin —*see* MRSA
        multiple drugs (MDRO)
          antibiotics Z16.24
          antimicrobial Z16.35
          antimycobacterials
            Z16.342
        penicillins Z16.11
        quinine (and related
          compounds) Z16.31
        quinolones Z16.23
        sulfonamides Z16.29
        tetracyclines Z16.29
        tuberculostatics (single)
          Z16.341
          multiple Z16.342
        vancomycin Z16.21
          related antibiotics
            Z16.22
  thyroid hormone E07.89

Resorption
  dental (roots) K03.3
    alveoli M26.79
  teeth (external) (internal)
    (pathological) (roots) K03.3

Respiration
  Cheyne-Stokes R06.3
  decreased due to shock, following
    injury T79.4
  disorder of, psychogenic F45.8
  insufficient, or poor R06.89
    newborn P28.5

Respiration *(continued)*
  painful R07.1
  sighing, psychogenic F45.8

Respiratory —*see also* condition
  distress syndrome (newborn) (type
    I) P22.0
    type II P22.1
  syncytial virus, as cause of disease
    classified elsewhere (*see also*
    Virus, respiratory syncytial
    (RSV)) B97.4

Respite care Z75.5

Response (drug)
  photoallergic L56.1
  phototoxic L56.0

Restenosis
  stent
    vascular
      end stent
        adjacent to stent —*see*
          Arteriosclerosis
        within the stent
          coronary T82.855
          peripheral T82.856
      in stent
        coronary vessel T82.855
        peripheral vessel T82.856

Restless legs (syndrome) G25.81

Restlessness R45.1

Restriction of housing space Z59.1

Restoration (of)
  dental
    aesthetically inadequate or
      displeasing K08.56
    defective K08.50
      specified NEC K08.59
    failure of marginal integrity
      K08.51
    failure of periodontal anatomical
      intergrity K08.54
  organ continuity from previous
    sterilization (tuboplasty)
    (vasoplasty) Z31.0
    aftercare Z31.42
  tooth (existing)
    contours biologically incompatible
      with oral health K08.54
    open margins K08.51
    overhanging K08.52
    poor aesthetic K08.56
    poor gingival margins K08.51
  unsatisfactory, of tooth K08.50
    specified NEC K08.59

Restorative material (dental)
  allergy to K08.55
  fractured K08.539
    with loss of material K08.531
    without loss of material K08.530
  unrepairable overhanging of
    K08.52

Rests, ovarian, in fallopian tube
  Q50.6

Restzustand (schizophrenic) F20.5

Retained —*see also* Retention
  cholelithiasis following
    cholecystectomy K91.86
  foreign body fragments (type of)
    Z18.9
    acrylics Z18.2
    animal quill(s) or spines Z18.31
    cement Z18.83
    concrete Z18.83
    crystalline Z18.83
    depleted isotope Z18.09
    depleted uranium Z18.01
    diethylhexyl phthalates Z18.2
    glass Z18.81

Retained *(continued)*
  foreign body fragments *(continued)*
    isocyanate Z18.2
    magnetic metal Z18.11
    metal Z18.10
    nonmagnetic metal Z18.12
    nontherapeutic radioactive
      Z18.09
    organic NEC Z18.39
    plastic Z18.2
    quill(s) (animal) Z18.31
    radioactive (nontherapeutic)
      NEC Z18.09
    specified NEC Z18.89
    spine(s) (animal) Z18.31
    stone Z18.83
    tooth (teeth) Z18.32
    wood Z18.33
  fragments (type of) Z18.9
    acrylics Z18.2
    animal quill(s) or spines Z18.31
    cement Z18.83
    concrete Z18.83
    crystalline Z18.83
    depleted isotope Z18.09
    depleted uranium Z18.01
    diethylhexyl phthalates Z18.2
    glass Z18.81
    isocyanate Z18.2
    magnetic metal Z18.11
    metal Z18.10
    nonmagnectic metal Z18.12
    nontherapeutic radioactive Z18.09
    organic NEC Z18.39
    plastic Z18.2
    quill(s) (animal) Z18.31
    radioactive (nontherapeutic)
      NEC Z18.09
    specified NEC Z18.89
    spine(s) (animal) Z18.31
    stone Z18.83
    tooth (teeth) Z18.32
    wood Z18.33
  gallstones, following
    cholecystectomy K91.86

Retardation
  development, developmental,
    specific —*see* Disorder,
    developmental
  endochondral bone growth —*see*
    Disorder, bone, development or
    growth
  growth R62.50
    due to malnutrition E45
  mental —*see* Disability, intellectual
  motor function, specific F82
  physical (child) R62.52
    due to malnutrition E45
  reading (specific) F81.0
  spelling (specific) (without reading
    disorder) F81.81

Retching —*see* Vomiting

Retention —*see also* Retained
  bladder —*see* Retention, urine
  carbon dioxide E87.2
  cholelithiasis following
    cholecystectomy K91.86
  cyst —*see* Cyst
  dead
    fetus (at or near term) (mother)
      O36.4
      early fetal death O02.1
    ovum O02.0
  decidua (fragments) (following
    delivery) (with hemorrhage)
    O72.2
    without hemorrhage O73.1
  deciduous tooth K00.6
  dental root K08.3
  fecal —*see* Constipation

Retention (continued)
  fetus
    dead O36.4
      early O02.1
  fluid R60.9
  foreign body —see also Foreign
      body, retained
    current trauma - code as Foreign
        body, by site or type
  gallstones, following
      cholecystectomy K91.86
  gastric K31.89
  intrauterine contraceptive device,
      in pregnancy —see Pregnancy,
      complicated by, retention,
      intrauterine device
  membranes (complicating delivery)
      (with hemorrhage) O72.2
    with abortion —see Abortion,
        by type
    without hemorrhage O73.1
  meniscus —see Derangement,
      meniscus
  menses N94.89
  milk (puerperal, postpartum) O92.79
  nitrogen, extrarenal R39.2
  ovary syndrome N99.83
  placenta (total) (with hemorrhage)
      O72.0
    without hemorrhage O73.0
    portions or fragments (with
        hemorrhage) O72.2
      without hemorrhage O73.1
  products of conception
    early pregnancy (dead fetus)
        O02.1
    following
        delivery (with hemorrhage)
            O72.2
          without hemorrhage O73.1
  secundines (following delivery)
      (with hemorrhage) O72.0
    without hemorrhage O73.0
    complicating puerperium
        (delayed hemorrhage) O72.2
    partial O72.2
      without hemorrhage O73.1
  smegma, clitoris N90.89
  urine R33.9
    due to hyperplasia (hypertrophy)
        of prostate —see Hyperplasia,
        prostate
    drug-induced R33.0
    organic R33.8
      drug-induced R33.0
    psychogenic F45.8
    specified NEC R33.8
  water (in tissues) —see Edema

Reticular erythematous mucinosis
    L98.5

Reticulation, dust —see
    Pneumoconiosis

Reticulocytosis R70.1

Reticuloendotheliosis
  acute infantile C96.0
  leukemic C91.4-
  nonlipid C96.0

Reticulohistiocytoma (giant-cell)
    D76.3

Reticuloid, actinic L57.1

Reticulosis (skin)
  acute of infancy C96.0
  hemophagocytic, familial D76.1
  histiocytic medullary C96.A
  lipomelanotic I89.8
  malignant (midline) C86.0
  polymorphic C86.0
  Sézary —see Sézary disease

Retina, retinal —see also condition
  dark area D49.81

Retinitis —see also Inflammation,
    chorioretinal
  albuminurica N18.9 [H32]
  diabetic —see Diabetes, retinitis
  disciformis —see Degeneration,
      macula
  focal —see Inflammation,
      chorioretinal, focal
  gravidarum —see Pregnancy,
      complicated by, specified
      pregnancy-related condition
      NEC
  juxtapapillaris —see Inflammation,
      chorioretinal, focal,
      juxtapapillary
  luetic —see Retinitis, syphilitic
  pigmentosa H35.52
  proliferans —see Disorder, globe,
      degenerative, specified type
      NEC
  proliferating —see Disorder,
      globe, degenerative, specified
      type NEC
  renal N18.9 [H32]
  syphilitic (early) (secondary)
      A51.43
    central, recurrent A52.71
    congenital (early) A50.01 [H32]
    late A52.71
  tuberculous A18.53

Retinoblastoma C69.2-
  differentiated C69.2-
  undifferentiated C69.2-

Retinochoroiditis —see also
    Inflammation, chorioretinal
  disseminated —see Inflammation,
      chorioretinal, disseminated
    syphilitic A52.71
  focal —see Inflammation,
      chorioretinal
  juxtapapillaris see Inflammation,
      chorioretinal, focal,
      juxtapapillary

Retinopathy (background) H35.00
  arteriosclerotic I70.8 [H35.0-]
  atherosclerotic I70.8 [H35.0-]
  central serous —see
      Chorioretinopathy, central serous
  Coats H35.02-
  diabetic —see Diabetes,
      retinopathy
  exudative H35.02-
  hypertensive H35.03-
  in (due to)
    diabetes —see Diabetes,
        retinopathy
    sickle-cell disorders D57.- H36
  of prematurity H35.10-
    stage 0 H35.11-
    stage 1 H35.12-
    stage 2 H35.13-
    stage 3 H35.14-
    stage 4 H35.15-
    stage 5 H35.16-
  pigmentary, congenital —see
      Dystrophy, retina
  proliferative NEC H35.2-
    diabetic —see Diabetes,
        retinopathy, proliferative
    sickle-cell D57.- [H36]
  solar H31.02-

Retinoschisis H33.10-
  congenital Q14.1
  specified type NEC H33.19-

Retortamoniasis A07.8

Retractile testis Q55.22

Retraction
  cervix —see Retroversion, uterus
  drum (membrane) —see Disorder,
      tympanic membrane, specified
      NEC
  finger —see Deformity, finger
  lid H02.539
    left H02.536
      lower H02.535
      upper H02.534
    right H02.533
      lower H02.532
      upper H02.531
  lung J98.4
  mediastinum J98.59
  nipple N64.53
    associated with
        lactation O92.03
        pregnancy O92.01-
        puerperium O92.02
    congenital Q83.8
  palmar fascia M72.0
  pleura —see Pleurisy
  ring, uterus (Bandl's) (pathological)
      O62.4
  sternum (congenital) Q76.7
    acquired M95.4
  uterus —see Retroversion, uterus
  valve (heart) —see Endocarditis

Retrobulbar —see condition

Retrocecal —see condition

Retrocession —see Retroversion

Retrodisplacement —see
    Retroversion

Retroflection, retroflexion —see
    Retroversion

Retrognathia, retrognathism
    (mandibular) (maxillary) M26.19

Retrograde menstruation N92.5

Retroperineal —see condition

Retroperitoneal —see condition

Retroperitonitis K68.9

Retropharyngeal —see condition

Retroplacental —see condition

Retroposition —see Retroversion

Retroprosthetic membrane T85.398

Retrosternal thyroid (congenital)
    Q89.2

Retroversion, retroverted
  cervix —see Retroversion, uterus
  female NEC —see Retroversion,
      uterus
  iris H21.89
  testis (congenital) Q55.29
  uterus (acquired) (acute) (any
      degree) (asymptomatic) (cervix)
      (postinfectional) (postpartal, old)
      N85.4
    congenital Q51.818
    in pregnancy O34.53-

**Retrovirus, as cause of disease
    classified elsewhere** B97.30
  human
      immunodeficiency, type 2 (HIV
          2) B97.35
      T-cell lymphotropic
          type I (HTLV-I) B97.33
          type II (HTLV-II) B97.34
  lentivirus B97.31
  oncovirus B97.32
  specified NEC B97.39

Retrusion, premaxilla
    (developmental) M26.09

Rett's disease or syndrome F84.2

Reverse peristalsis R19.2

Reye's syndrome G93.7

Rh (factor)
  hemolytic disease (newborn) P55.0
  incompatibility, immunization or
      sensitization
    affecting management of
        pregnancy NEC O36.09-
        anti-D antibody O36.01-
    newborn P55.0
    transfusion reaction —see
        Complication(s), transfusion,
        incompatibility reaction, Rh
        (factor)
  negative mother affecting newborn
      P55.0
  titer elevated —see
      Complication(s), transfusion,
      incompatibility reaction, Rh
      (factor)
  transfusion reaction —see
      Complication(s), transfusion,
      incompatibility reaction, Rh
      (factor)

Rhabdomyolysis (idiopathic) **NEC**
    M62.82
  traumatic T79.6

Rhabdomyoma —see also
    Neoplasm, connective tissue,
    benign
  adult —see Neoplasm, connective
      tissue, benign
  fetal —see Neoplasm, connective
      tissue, benign
  glycogenic —see Neoplasm,
      connective tissue, benign

Rhabdomyosarcoma (any type)
    —see Neoplasm, connective tissue,
    malignant

Rhabdosarcoma —see
    Rhabdomyosarcoma

Rhesus (factor) **incompatibility**
    —see Rh, incompatibility

Rheumatic (acute) (subacute)
  adherent pericardium I09.2
  chronic I09.89
  coronary arteritis I01.8
  degeneration, myocardium I09.0
  fever (acute) —see Fever,
      rheumatic
  heart —see Disease, heart,
      rheumatic
  myocardial degeneration —see
      Degeneration, myocardium
  myocarditis (chronic) (inactive)
      (with chorea) I09.0
    active or acute I01.2
      with chorea (acute) (rheumatic)
          (Sydenham's) I02.0
  pancarditis, acute I01.8
    with chorea (acute (rheumatic)
        Sydenham's) I02.0
  pericarditis (active) (acute) (with
      effusion) (with pneumonia) I01.0
    with chorea (acute) (rheumatic)
        (Sydenham's) I02.0
    chronic or inactive I09.2
  pneumonia I00 [J17]
  torticollis M43.6
  typhoid fever A01.09

Rheumatism (articular) (neuralgic)
    (nonarticular) M79.0
  gout —see Arthritis, rheumatoid
  intercostal, meaning Tietze's
      disease M94.0
  palindromic (any site) M12.30
    ankle M12.37-

Rheumatism *(continued)*
  palindromic *(continued)*
    elbow M12.32-
    foot joint M12.37-
    hand joint M12.34-
    hip M12.35-
    knee M12.36-
    multiple site M12.39
    shoulder M12.31-
    specified joint NEC M12.38
    vertebrae M12.38
    wrist M12.33-
  sciatic M54.4-
Rheumatoid —*see also* condition
  arthritis —*see also* Arthritis,
    rheumatoid
    with involvement of organs NEC
      M05.60
      ankle M05.67-
      elbow M05.62-
      foot joint M05.67-
      hand joint M05.64-
      hip M05.65-
      knee M05.66-
      multiple site M05.69
      shoulder M05.61-
      vertebra —*see* Spondylitis,
        ankylosing
      wrist M05.63-
    seronegative —*see* Arthritis,
      rheumatoid, seronegative
    seropositive —*see* Arthritis,
      rheumatoid, seropositive
  carditis M05.30
    ankle M05.37-
    elbow M05.32-
    foot joint M05.37-
    hand joint M05.34-
    hip M05.35-
    knee M05.36-
    multiple site M05.39
    shoulder M05.31-
    vertebra —*see* Spondylitis,
      ankylosing
    wrist M05.33-
  endocarditis —*see* Rheumatoid,
    carditis
  lung (disease) M05.10
    ankle M05.17-
    elbow M05.12-
    foot joint M05.17-
    hand joint M05.14-
    hip M05.15-
    knee M05.16-
    multiple site M05.19
    shoulder M05.11-
    vertebra —*see* Spondylitis,
      ankylosing
    wrist M05.13-
  myocarditis —*see* Rheumatoid,
    carditis
  myopathy M05.40
    ankle M05.47-
    elbow M05.42-
    foot joint M05.47-
    hand joint M05.44-
    hip M05.45-
    knee M05.46-
    multiple site M05.49
    shoulder M05.41-
    vertebra —*see* Spondylitis,
      ankylosing
    wrist M05.43-
  pericarditis —*see* Rheumatoid,
    carditis
  polyarthritis —*see* Arthritis,
    rheumatoid
  polyneuropathy M05.50
    ankle M05.57-
    elbow M05.52-
    foot joint M05.57-

Rheumatoid *(continued)*
  polyneuropathy *(continued)*
    hand joint M05.54-
    hip M05.55-
    knee M05.56-
    multiple site M05.59
    shoulder M05.51-
    vertebra —*see* Spondylitis,
      ankylosing
    wrist M05.53-
  vasculitis M05.20
    ankle M05.27-
    elbow M05.22-
    foot joint M05.27-
    hand joint M05.24-
    hip M05.25-
    knee M05.26-
    multiple site M05.29
    shoulder M05.21-
    vertebra —*see* Spondylitis,
      ankylosing
    wrist M05.23-

Rhinitis (atrophic) (catarrhal)
  (chronic) (croupous) (fibrinous)
  (granulomatous) (hyperplastic)
  (hypertrophic) (membranous)
  (obstructive) (purulent)
  (suppurative) (ulcerative) J31.0
  with
    sore throat —*see*
      Nasopharyngitis
  acute J00
  allergic J30.9
    with asthma J45.909
      with
        exacerbation (acute)
          J45.901
        status asthmaticus J45.902
    due to
      food J30.5
      pollen J30.1
    nonseasonal J30.89
    perennial J30.89
    seasonal NEC J30.2
    specified NEC J30.89
  infective J00
  pneumococcal J00
  syphilitic A52.73
    congenital A50.05 *[J99]*
  tuberculous A15.8
  vasomotor J30.0
Rhinoantritis (chronic) —*see*
  Sinusitis, maxillary
Rhinodacryolith —*see* Dacryolith
Rhinolith (nasal sinus) J34.89
Rhinomegaly J34.89
Rhinopharyngitis (acute) (subacute)
  —*see also* Nasopharyngitis
  chronic J31.1
  destructive ulcerating A66.5
  mutilans A66.5
Rhinophyma L71.1
Rhinorrhea J34.89
  cerebrospinal (fluid) G96.01
    postoperative G96.08
    specified NEC G96.08
    spontaneous G96.01
    traumatic G96.08
  paroxysmal —*see* Rhinitis,
    allergic
  spasmodic —*see* Rhinitis, allergic
Rhinosalpingitis —*see* Salpingitis,
  eustachian
Rhinoscleroma A48.8
Rhinosporidiosis B48.1
Rhinovirus infection NEC B34.8
Rhizomelic chondrodysplasia
  punctata E71.540

Rhythm
  atrioventricular nodal I49.8
  disorder I49.9
    coronary sinus I49.8
    ectopic I49.8
    nodal I49.8
  escape I49.9
  heart, abnormal I49.9
  idioventricular I44.2
  nodal I49.8
  sleep, inversion G47.2-
    nonorganic origin —*see*
      Disorder, sleep, circadian
      rhythm, psychogenic
Rhytidosis facialis L98.8
Rib —*see also* condition
  cervical Q76.5
Riboflavin deficiency E53.0
Rice bodies —*see also* Loose, body,
  joint
  knee M23.4-
Richter syndrome —*see* Leukemia,
  chronic lymphocytic, B-cell type
Richter's hernia —*see* Hernia,
  abdomen, with obstruction
Ricinism —*see* Poisoning, food,
  noxious, plant
Rickets (active) (acute) (adolescent)
  (chest wall) (congenital) (current)
  (infantile) (intestinal) E55.0
  adult —*see* Osteomalacia
  celiac K90.0
  hypophosphatemic with nephrotic-
    glycosuric dwarfism E72.09
  inactive E64.3
  kidney N25.0
  renal N25.0
  sequelae, any E64.3
  vitamin-D-resistant E83.31
    [M90.80]
Rickettsia 364D/R. philipii (Pacific
  Coast tick fever) A77.8
Rickettsial disease A79.9
  specified type NEC A79.89
Rickettsialpox (Rickettsia akari)
  A79.1
Rickettsiosis A79.9
  due to
    Ehrlichia sennetsu A79.81
    Neorickettsia sennetsu
      A79.81
    Rickettsia akari (rickettsialpox)
      A79.1
  specified type NEC A79.89
  tick-borne A77.9
  vesicular A79.1
Rider's bone —*see* Ossification,
  muscle, specified NEC
Ridge, alveolus —*see also* condition
  flabby K06.8
Ridged ear, congenital Q17.3
Riedel's
  lobe, liver Q44.7
  struma, thyroiditis or disease
    E06.5
Rieger's anomaly or syndrome
  Q13.81
Riehl's melanosis L81.4
Rietti-Greppi-Micheli anemia
  D56.9
Rieux's hernia —*see* Hernia,
  abdomen, specified site NEC
Riga (-Fede) **disease** K14.0

Riggs' disease —*see* Periodontitis
Right aortic arch Q25.47
Right middle lobe syndrome J98.11
Rigid, rigidity —*see also* condition
  abdominal R19.30
    with severe abdominal pain
      R10.0
    epigastric R19.36
    generalized R19.37
    left lower quadrant R19.34
    left upper quadrant R19.32
    periumbilic R19.35
    right lower quadrant R19.33
    right upper quadrant R19.31
  articular, multiple, congenital Q68.8
  cervix (uteri) in pregnancy —*see*
    Pregnancy, complicated by,
    abnormal, cervix
  hymen (acquired) (congenital) N89.6
  nuchal R29.1
  pelvic floor in pregnancy —*see*
    Pregnancy, complicated by,
    abnormal, pelvic organs or
    tissues NEC
  perineum or vulva in pregnancy
    —*see* Pregnancy, complicated
    by, abnormal, vulva
  spine —*see* Dorsopathy, specified
    NEC
  vagina in pregnancy —*see*
    Pregnancy, complicated by,
    abnormal, vagina
Rigors R68.89
  with fever R50.9
Riley-Day syndrome G90.1
RIND (reversible ischemic neurologic
  deficit) I63.9
Ring(s)
  aorta (vascular) Q25.45
  Bandl's O62.4
  contraction, complicating delivery
    O62.4
  esophageal, lower (muscular) K22.2
  Fleischer's (cornea) H18.04-
  hymenal, tight (acquired)
    (congenital) N89.6
  Kayser-Fleischer (cornea)
    H18.04-
  retraction, uterus, pathological
    O62.4
  Schatzki's (esophagus) (lower) K22.2
    congenital Q39.3
  Soemmerring's —*see* Cataract,
    secondary
  vascular (congenital) Q25.8
    aorta Q25.45
Ringed hair (congenital) Q84.1
Ringworm B35.9
  beard B35.0
  black dot B35.0
  body B35.4
  Burmese B35.5
  corporeal B35.4
  foot B35.3
  groin B35.6
  hand B35.2
  honeycomb B35.0
  nails B35.1
  perianal (area) B35.6
  scalp B35.0
  specified NEC B35.8
  Tokelau B35.5
Rise, venous pressure I87.8
Rising, PSA following treatment for
  malignant neoplasm of prostate
  R97.21

Risk
for
dental caries Z91.849
high Z91.843
low Z91.841
moderate Z91.842
suicidal
meaning personal history of
attempted suicide Z91.5
meaning suicidal ideation
—see Ideation, suicidal

Ritter's disease L00

Rivalry, sibling Z62.891

Rivalta's disease A42.2

River blindness B73.01

Robert's pelvis Q74.2
with disproportion (fetopelvic)
O33.0
causing obstructed labor O65.0

Robin (-Pierre) **syndrome** Q87.0

**Robinow-Silvermann-Smith
syndrome** Q87.19

Robinson's (hidrotic) **ectodermal
dysplasia or syndrome** Q82.4

Robles' disease B73.01

Rocky Mountain (spotted) **fever**
A77.0

Roetheln —see Rubella

Roger's disease Q21.0

Rokitansky-Aschoff sinuses
(gallbladder) K82.8

Rolando's fracture (displaced)
S62.22-
nondisplaced S62.22-

Romano-Ward (prolonged QT
interval) **syndrome** I45.81

Romberg's disease or syndrome
G51.8

Roof, mouth —see condition

Rosacea L71.9
acne L71.9
keratitis L71.8
specified NEC L71.8

Rosary, rachitic E55.0

Rose
cold J30.1
fever J30.1
rash R21
epidemic B06.9

Rosenbach's erysipeloid A26.0

Rosenthal's disease or syndrome
D68.1

Roseola B09
infantum B08.20
due to human herpesvirus 6
B08.21
due to human herpesvirus 7
B08.22

Rossbach's disease K31.89
psychogenic F45.8

Ross River disease or fever B33.1

Rostan's asthma (cardiac) —see
Failure, ventricular, left

Rotation
anomalous, incomplete or
insufficient, intestine Q43.3
cecum (congenital) Q43.3
colon (congenital) Q43.3
spine, incomplete or insufficient
—see Dorsopathy, deforming,
specified NEC

Rotation (continued)
tooth, teeth, fully erupted M26.35
vertebra, incomplete or insufficient
—see Dorsopathy, deforming,
specified NEC

Rotes Quérol disease or syndrome
—see Hyperostosis, ankylosing

Roth (-Bernhardt) **disease or
syndrome** —see Meralgia
paraesthetica

Rothmund (-Thomson) **syndrome**
Q82.8

Rotor's disease or syndrome E80.6

Round
back (with wedging of vertebrae)
—see Kyphosis
sequelae (late effect) of rickets
E64.3
worms (large) (infestation) NEC
B82.0
Ascariasis (see also Ascariasis)
B77.9

Roussy-Lévy syndrome G60.0

Rubella (German measles) B06.9
complication NEC B06.09
neurological B06.00
congenital P35.0
contact Z20.4
exposure to Z20.4
maternal
manifest rubella in infant P35.0
care for (suspected) damage to
fetus O35.3
suspected damage to fetus
affecting management of
pregnancy O35.3
specified complications NEC
B06.89

Rubeola (meaning measles) —see
Measles
meaning rubella —see Rubella

Rubeosis, iris —see Disorder, iris,
vascular

Rubinstein-Taybi syndrome Q87.2

Rudimentary (congenital) —see also
Agenesis
arm —see Defect, reduction, upper
limb
bone Q79.9
cervix uteri Q51.828
eye Q11.2
lobule of ear Q17.3
patella Q74.1
respiratory organs in thoracopagus
Q89.4
tracheal bronchus Q32.4
uterus Q51.818
in male Q56.1
vagina Q52.0

Ruled out condition —see
Observation, suspected

Rumination R11.10
with nausea R11.2
disorder of infancy F98.21
neurotic F42.8
newborn P92.1
obsessional F42.8
psychogenic F42.8

Runeberg's disease D51.0

Runny nose R09.89

Rupia (syphilitic) A51.39
congenital A50.06
tertiary A52.79

Rupture, ruptured
abscess (spontaneous) - code by
site under Abscess

Rupture, ruptured (continued)
aneurysm —see Aneurysm
anus (sphincter) —see Laceration,
anus
aorta, aortic I71.8
abdominal I71.3
arch I71.1
ascending I71.1
descending I71.8
abdominal I71.3
thoracic I71.1
syphilitic A52.01
thoracoabdominal I71.5
thorax, thoracic I71.1
transverse I71.1
traumatic —see Injury, aorta,
laceration, major
valve or cusp (see also
Endocarditis, aortic) I35.8
appendix (with peritonitis) (see
also Appendicitis) K35.32
with localized peritonitis (see
also Appendicitis) K35.32
arteriovenous fistula, brain —see
Fistula, arteriovenous, brain,
ruptured
artery I77.2
brain —see Hemorrhage,
intracranial, intracerebral
coronary —see Infarct,
myocardium
heart —see Infarct, myocardium
pulmonary I28.8
traumatic (complication) —see
Injury, blood vessel
bile duct (common) (hepatic)
K83.2
cystic K82.2
bladder (sphincter) (nontraumatic)
(spontaneous) N32.89
following ectopic or molar
pregnancy O08.6
obstetrical trauma O71.5
traumatic S37.29
blood vessel —see also
Hemorrhage
brain —see Hemorrhage,
intracranial, intracerebral
heart —see Infarct, myocardium
traumatic (complication) —
see Injury, blood vessel,
laceration, major, by site
bone —see Fracture
bowel (nontraumatic) K63.1
brain
aneurysm (congenital) —see
also Hemorrhage, intracranial,
subarachnoid
syphilitic A52.05
hemorrhagic —see Hemorrhage,
intracranial, intracerebral
capillaries I78.8
cardiac (auricle) (ventricle) (wall)
I23.3
with hemopericardium I23.0
infectional I40.9
traumatic —see Injury, heart
cartilage (articular) (current) —see
also Sprain
knee S83.3-
semilunar —see Tear, meniscus
cecum (with peritonitis) K65.0
with peritoneal abscess
K35.33
traumatic S36.598
celiac artery, traumatic —see
Injury, blood vessel, celiac
artery, laceration, major
cerebral aneurysm (congenital)
(see Hemorrhage, intracranial,
subarachnoid)

Rupture, ruptured (continued)
cervix (uteri)
with ectopic or molar pregnancy
O08.6
following ectopic or molar
pregnancy O08.6
obstetrical trauma O71.3
traumatic S37.69
chordae tendineae NEC I51.1
concurrent with acute
myocardial infarction —see
Infarct, myocardium
following acute myocardial
infarction (current
complication) I23.4
choroid (direct) (indirect)
(traumatic) H31.32-
circle of Willis I60.6
colon (nontraumatic) K63.1
traumatic —see Injury, intestine,
large
cornea (traumatic) —see Injury,
eye, laceration
coronary (artery) (thrombotic)
—see Infarct, myocardium
corpus luteum (infected) (ovary)
N83.1-
cyst —see Cyst
cystic duct K82.2
Descemet's membrane —see
Change, corneal membrane,
Descemet's, rupture
traumatic —see Injury, eye,
laceration
diaphragm, traumatic —see Injury,
intrathoracic, diaphragm
disc —see Rupture, intervertebral
disc
diverticulum (intestine) K57.80
with bleeding K57.81
bladder N32.3
large intestine K57.20
with
bleeding K57.21
small intestine K57.40
with bleeding K57.41
small intestine K57.00
with
bleeding K57.01
large intestine K57.40
with bleeding K57.41
duodenal stump K31.89
ear drum (nontraumatic) —see also
Perforation, tympanum
traumatic S09.2-
due to blast injury —see
Injury, blast, ear
esophagus K22.3
eye (without prolapse or loss of
intraocular tissue) —see Injury,
eye, laceration
fallopian tube NEC (nonobstetric)
(nontraumatic) N83.8
due to pregnancy O00.10-
with intrauterine pregnancy
O00.11-
fontanel P13.1
gallbladder K82.2
traumatic S36.128
gastric —see also Rupture,
stomach
vessel K92.2
globe (eye) (traumatic) —see
Injury, eye, laceration
graafian follicle (hematoma)
N83.0-
heart —see Rupture, cardiac
hymen (nontraumatic)
(nonintentional) N89.8
internal organ, traumatic —see
Injury, by site

Rupture, ruptured *(continued)*

intervertebral disc —*see*
 Displacement, intervertebral disc
 traumatic —*see* Rupture,
  traumatic, intervertebral disc
intestine NEC (nontraumatic) K63.1
 traumatic —*see* Injury, intestine
iris —*see also* Abnormality,
 pupillary
 traumatic —*see* Injury, eye,
  laceration
joint capsule, traumatic —*see*
 Sprain
kidney (traumatic) S37.06-
 birth injury P15.8
 nontraumatic N28.89
lacrimal duct (traumatic) —*see*
 Injury, eye, specified site NEC
lens (cataract) (traumatic) —*see*
 Cataract, traumatic
ligament, traumatic —*see* Rupture,
 traumatic, ligament, by site
liver S36.116
 birth injury P15.0
lymphatic vessel I89.8
marginal sinus (placental) (with
 hemorrhage) —*see* Hemorrhage,
 antepartum, specified cause NEC
membrana tympani (nontraumatic)
 —*see* Perforation, tympanum
membranes (spontaneous)
 artificial
  delayed delivery following
   O75.5
 delayed delivery following
  —*see* Pregnancy, complicated
  by, premature rupture of
  membranes
meningeal artery I60.8
meniscus (knee) —*see also* Tear,
 meniscus
 old —*see* Derangement,
  meniscus
 site other than knee - code as
  Sprain
mesenteric artery, traumatic —*see*
 Injury, mesenteric, artery,
 laceration, major
mesentery (nontraumatic) K66.8
 traumatic —*see* Injury, intra-
  abdominal, specified, site
  NEC
mitral (valve) I34.8
muscle (traumatic) —*see also*
 Strain
 diastasis —*see* Diastasis, muscle
 nontraumatic M62.10
  ankle M62.17-
  foot M62.17-
  forearm M62.13-
  hand M62.14-
  lower leg M62.16-
  pelvic region M62.15-
  shoulder region M62.11-
  specified site NEC M62.18
  thigh M62.15-
  upper arm M62.12-
 traumatic —*see* Strain, by site
musculotendinous junction NEC,
 nontraumatic —*see* Rupture,
 tendon, spontaneous
mycotic aneurysm causing cerebral
 hemorrhage —*see* Hemorrhage,
 intracranial, subarachnoid
myocardium, myocardial —*see*
 Rupture, cardiac
 traumatic —*see* Injury, heart
nontraumatic, meaning hernia
 —*see* Hernia
obstructed —*see* Hernia, by site,
 obstructed

operation wound —*see* Disruption,
 wound, operation
ovary, ovarian N83.8
 corpus luteum cyst N83.1-
 follicle (graafian) N83.0-
oviduct (nonobstetric)
 (nontraumatic) N83.8
 due to pregnancy O00.10-
  with intrauterine pregnancy
   O00.11-
pancreas (nontraumatic) K86.89
 traumatic S36.299
papillary muscle NEC I51.2
 following acute myocardial
  infarction (current
  complication) I23.5
pelvic
 floor, complicating delivery
  O70.1
 organ NEC, obstetrical trauma
  O71.5
perineum (nonobstetric)
 (nontraumatic) N90.89
 complicating delivery —*see*
  Delivery, complicated, by,
  laceration, anus (sphincter)
postoperative wound —*see*
 Disruption, wound, operation
prostate (traumatic) S37.828
pulmonary
 artery I28.8
 valve (heart) I37.8
 vein I28.8
 vessel I28.8
pus tube —*see* Salpingitis
pyosalpinx —*see* Salpingitis
rectum (nontraumatic) K63.1
 traumatic S36.69
retina, retinal (traumatic) (without
 detachment) —*see also* Break,
 retina
 with detachment —*see*
  Detachment, retina, with
  retinal, break
rotator cuff (nontraumatic)
 M75.10-
 complete M75.12-
 incomplete M75.11-
sclera —*see* Injury, eye, laceration
sigmoid (nontraumatic) K63.1
 traumatic S36.593
spinal cord —*see also* Injury, spinal
 cord, by region
 due to injury at birth P11.5
 newborn (birth injury) P11.5
spleen (traumatic) S36.09
 birth injury P15.1
 congenital (birth injury) P15.1
 due to P. vivax malaria B51.0
 nontraumatic D73.5
 spontaneous D73.5
splenic vein R58
 traumatic —*see* Injury, blood
  vessel, splenic vein
stomach (nontraumatic)
 (spontaneous) K31.89
 traumatic S36.39
supraspinatus (complete)
 (incomplete) (nontraumatic)
 —*see* Tear, rotator cuff
symphysis pubis
 obstetric O71.6
 traumatic S33.4
synovium (cyst) M66.10
 ankle M66.17-
 elbow M66.12-
 finger M66.14-
 foot M66.17-
 forearm M66.13-
 hand M66.14-

synovium (cyst) *(continued)*
 pelvic region M66.15-
 shoulder region M66.11-
 specified site NEC M66.18
 thigh M66.15-
 toe M66.17-
 upper arm M66.12-
 wrist M66.13-
tendon (traumatic) —*see* Strain
 nontraumatic (spontaneous)
  M66.9
  ankle M66.87-
  extensor M66.20
   ankle M66.27-
   foot M66.27-
   forearm M66.23-
   hand M66.24-
   lower leg M66.26-
   multiple sites M66.29
   pelvic region M66.25-
   shoulder region M66.21-
   specified site NEC M66.28
   thigh M66.25-
   upper arm M66.22-
  flexor M66.30
   ankle M66.37-
   foot M66.37-
   forearm M66.33-
   hand M66.34-
   lower leg M66.36-
   multiple sites M66.39
   pelvic region M66.35-
   shoulder region M66.31-
   specified site NEC M66.38
   thigh M66.35-
   upper arm M66.32-
  foot M66.87-
  forearm M66.83-
  hand M66.84-
  lower leg M66.86-
  multiple sites M66.89
  pelvic region M66.85-
  shoulder region M66.81-
  specified
   site NEC M66.88
   tendon M66.80
  thigh M66.85-
  upper arm M66.82-
thoracic duct I89.8
tonsil J35.8
traumatic
 aorta —*see* Injury, aorta,
  laceration, major
 diaphragm —*see* Injury,
  intrathoracic, diaphragm
 external site —*see* Wound, open,
  by site
 eye —*see* Injury, eye, laceration
 internal organ —*see* Injury, by
  site
 intervertebral disc
  cervical S13.0
  lumbar S33.0
  thoracic S23.0
 kidney S37.06-
 ligament —*see also* Sprain
  ankle —*see* Sprain, ankle
  carpus —*see* Rupture,
   traumatic, ligament, wrist
  collateral (hand) —*see*
   Rupture, traumatic,
   ligament, finger, collateral
  finger (metacarpophalangeal)
   (interphalangeal) S63.40-
   collateral S63.41-
    index S63.41-
    little S63.41-
    middle S63.41-
    ring S63.41-
   index S63.40-

traumatic *(continued)*
 ligament *(continued)*
  finger *(continued)*
   little S63.40-
   middle S63.40-
   palmar S63.42-
    index S63.42-
    little S63.42-
    middle S63.42-
    ring S63.42-
   ring S63.40-
   specified site NEC S63.499
    index S63.49-
    little S63.49-
    middle S63.49-
    ring S63.49-
   volar plate S63.43-
    index S63.43-
    little S63.43-
    middle S63.43-
    ring S63.43-
  foot —*see* Sprain, foot
  radial collateral S53.2-
  radiocarpal —*see* Rupture,
   traumatic, ligament, wrist,
   radiocarpal
  ulnar collateral S53.3-
  ulnocarpal —*see* Rupture,
   traumatic, ligament, wrist,
   ulnocarpal
  wrist S63.30-
   collateral S63.31-
   radiocarpal S63.32-
   specified site NEC S63.39-
   ulnocarpal (palmar)
    S63.33-
 liver S36.116
 membrana tympani —*see*
  Rupture, ear drum,
  traumatic
 muscle or tendon —*see* Strain
 myocardium —*see* Injury, heart
 pancreas S36.299
 rectum S36.69
 sigmoid S36.593
 spleen S36.09
 stomach S36.39
 symphysis pubis S33.4
 tympanum, tympanic
  (membrane) —*see* Rupture,
  ear drum, traumatic
 ureter S37.19
 uterus S37.69
 vagina —*see* Injury, vagina
 vena cava —*see* Injury, vena
  cava, laceration, major
tricuspid (heart) (valve) I07.8
tube, tubal (nonobstetric)
 (nontraumatic) N83.8
 abscess —*see* Salpingitis
 due to pregnancy O00.10-
  with intrauterine pregnancy
   O00.11-
tympanum, tympanic (membrane)
 (nontraumatic) (*see also*
 Perforation, tympanic
 membrane) H72.9-
 traumatic —*see* Rupture, ear
  drum, traumatic
umbilical cord, complicating
 delivery O69.89
ureter (traumatic) S37.19
 nontraumatic N28.89
urethra (nontraumatic) N36.8
 with ectopic or molar pregnancy
  O08.6
 following ectopic or molar
  pregnancy O08.6
 obstetrical trauma O71.5
 traumatic S37.39

Rupture, ruptured *(continued)*
 uterosacral ligament (nonobstetric)
  (nontraumatic) N83.8
 uterus (traumatic) S37.69
  before labor O71.0-
  during or after labor O71.1
  nonpuerperal, nontraumatic
   N85.8
  pregnant (during labor) O71.1
   before labor O71.0-
 vagina —*see* Injury, vagina
 valve, valvular (heart) —*see*
  Endocarditis
 varicose vein —*see* Varix
 varix —*see* Varix
 vena cava R58
  traumatic —*see* Injury, vena
   cava, laceration, major
 vesical (urinary) N32.89
 vessel (blood) R58
  pulmonary I28.8
  traumatic —*see* Injury, blood
   vessel
 viscus R19.8
 vulva complicating delivery O70.0

Russell-Silver syndrome Q87.19

**Russian spring-summer type
 encephalitis** A84.0

Rust's disease (tuberculous cervical
 spondylitis) A18.01

Ruvalcaba-Myhre-Smith syndrome
 E71.440

Rytand-Lipsitch syndrome I44.2

S

Saber, sabre shin or tibia (syphilitic)
 A50.56 *[M90.8-]*

Sac lacrimal —*see* condition

Saccharomyces infection B37.9

Saccharopinuria E72.3

Saccular —*see* condition

Sacculation
 aorta (nonsyphilitic) —*see*
  Aneurysm, aorta
 bladder N32.3
 intralaryngeal (congenital)
  (ventricular) Q31.3
 larynx (congenital) (ventricular)
  Q31.3
 organ or site, congenital —*see*
  Distortion
 pregnant uterus —*see* Pregnancy,
  complicated by, abnormal, uterus
 ureter N28.89
 urethra N36.1
 vesical N32.3

**Sachs' amaurotic familial idiocy or
 disease** E75.02

Sachs-Tay disease E75.02

Sacks-Libman disease M32.11

Sacralgia M53.3

Sacralization Q76.49

Sacrodynia M53.3

Sacroiliac joint —*see* condition

Sacroiliitis NEC M46.1

Sacrum —*see* condition

Saddle
 back —*see* Lordosis
 embolus
  abdominal aorta I74.01
  pulmonary artery I26.92
   with acute cor pulmonale
    I26.02

Saddle *(continued)*
 injury - code to condition
 nose M95.0
  due to syphilis A50.57

Sadism (sexual) F65.52

Sadness, postpartal O90.6

Sadomasochism F65.50

Saemisch's ulcer (cornea) —*see*
 Ulcer, cornea, central

Sagging
 skin and subcutaneous tissue
  (following bariatric surgery
  weight loss) (following dietary
  weight loss) L98.7

Sahib disease B55.0

Sailors' skin L57.8

Saint
 Anthony's fire —*see* Erysipelas
 triad —*see* Hernia, diaphragm
 Vitus' dance —*see* Chorea,
  Sydenham's

Salaam
 attack(s) —*see* Epilepsy, spasms
 tic R25.8

Salicylism
 abuse F55.8
 overdose or wrong substance
  given —*see* Table of Drugs and
  Chemicals, by drug, poisoning

Salivary duct or gland —*see*
 condition

Salivation, excessive K11.7

Salmonella —*see* Infection,
 Salmonella

Salmonellosis A02.0

Salpingitis (catarrhal) (fallopian
 tube) (nodular) (pseudofollicular)
 (purulent) (septic) N70.91
 with oophoritis N70.93
 acute N70.01
  with oophoritis N70.03
 chlamydial A56.11
 chronic N70.11
  with oophoritis N70.13
 complicating abortion —*see*
  Abortion, by type, complicated
  by, salpingitis
 ear —*see* Salpingitis, eustachian
 eustachian (tube) H68.00-
  acute H68.01-
  chronic H68.02-
 follicularis N70.11
  with oophoritis N70.13
 gonococcal (acute) (chronic)
  A54.24
 interstitial, chronic N70.11
  with oophoritis N70.13
 isthmica nodosa N70.11
  with oophoritis N70.13
 specific (gonococcal) (acute)
  (chronic) A54.24
 tuberculous (acute) (chronic)
  A18.17
 venereal (gonococcal) (acute)
  (chronic) A54.24

Salpingocele N83.4-

Salpingo-oophoritis (catarrhal)
 (purulent) (ruptured) (septic)
 (suppurative) N70.93
 acute N70.03
  with ectopic or molar pregnancy
   O08.0
  following ectopic or molar
   pregnancy O08.0
  gonococcal A54.24

Salpingo-oophoritis *(continued)*
 chronic N70.13
 following ectopic or molar
  pregnancy O08.0
 gonococcal (acute) (chronic)
  A54.24
 puerperal O86.19
 specific (gonococcal) (acute)
  (chronic) A54.24
 subacute N70.03
 tuberculous (acute) (chronic) A18.17
 venereal (gonococcal) (acute)
  (chronic) A54.24

Salpingo-ovaritis —*see* Salpingo-
 oophoritis

Salpingoperitonitis —*see* Salpingo-
 oophoritis

Salzmann's nodular dystrophy
 —*see* Degeneration, cornea,
 nodular

Sampson's cyst or tumor N80.1

San Joaquin (Valley) **fever** B38.0

**Sandblaster's asthma, lung or
 pneumoconiosis** J62.8

Sander's disease (paranoia) F22

Sandfly fever A93.1

Sandhoff's disease E75.01

Sanfilippo (Type B) (Type C) (Type
 D) **syndrome** E76.22

Sanger-Brown ataxia G11.2

Sao Paulo fever or typhus A77.0

Saponification, mesenteric K65.8

Sarcocele (benign)
 syphilitic A52.76
  congenital A50.59

Sarcocystosis A07.8

Sarcoepiplocele —*see* Hernia

Sarcoeplplomphalocele Q79.2

Sarcoid —*see also* Sarcoidosis
 arthropathy D86.86
 Boeck's D86.9
 Darier-Roussy D86.3
 iridocyclitis D86.83
 meningitis D86.81
 myocarditis D86.85
 myositis D86.87
 pyelonephritis D86.84
 Spiegler-Fendt L08.89

Sarcoidosis D86.9
 with
  cranial nerve palsies D86.82
  hepatic granuloma D86.89
  polyarthritis D86.86
  tubulo-interstitial nephropathy
   D86.84
 combined sites NEC D86.89
 lung D86.0
  and lymph nodes D86.2
 lymph nodes D86.1
  and lung D86.2
 meninges D86.81
 skin D86.3
 specified type NEC D86.89

Sarcoma (of) —*see also* Neoplasm,
 connective tissue, malignant
 alveolar soft part —*see* Neoplasm,
  connective tissue, malignant
 ameloblastic C41.1
  upper jaw (bone) C41.0
 botryoid —*see* Neoplasm,
  connective tissue, malignant
 botryoides —*see* Neoplasm,
  connective tissue, malignant

Sarcoma *(continued)*
 cerebellar C71.6
  circumscribed (arachnoidal)
   C71.6
 circumscribed (arachnoidal)
  cerebellar C71.6
 clear cell —*see also* Neoplasm,
  connective tissue, malignant
  kidney C64.-
 dendritic cells (accessory cells)
  C96.4
 embryonal —*see* Neoplasm,
  connective tissue, malignant
 endometrial (stromal) C54.1
  isthmus C54.0
 epithelioid (cell) —*see* Neoplasm,
  connective tissue, malignant
 Ewing's —*see* Neoplasm, bone,
  malignant
 follicular dendritic cell C96.4
 germinoblastic (diffuse) —*see*
  Lymphoma, diffuse large
  cell
  follicular —*see* Lymphoma,
   follicular, specified NEC
 giant cell (except of bone) —*see
  also* Neoplasm, connective
  tissue, malignant
  bone —*see* Neoplasm, bone,
   malignant
 glomoid —*see* Neoplasm,
  connective tissue, malignant
 granulocytic C92.3-
 hemangioendothelial —*see*
  Neoplasm, connective tissue,
  malignant
 hemorrhagic, multiple —*see*
  Sarcoma, Kaposi's
 histiocytic C96.A
 Hodgkin —*see* Lymphoma,
  Hodgkin
 immunoblastic (diffuse) —*see*
  Lymphoma, diffuse large cell
 interdigitating dendritic cell C96.4
 Kaposi's
  colon C46.4
  connective tissue C46.1
  gastrointestinal organ C46.4
  lung C46.5-
  lymph node(s) C46.3
  palate (hard) (soft) C46.2
  rectum C46.4
  skin C46.0
  specified site NEC C46.7
  stomach C46.4
  unspecified site C46.9
 Kupffer cell C22.3
 Langerhans cell C96.4
 leptomeningeal —*see* Neoplasm,
  meninges, malignant
 liver NEC C22.4
 lymphangioendothelial —*see*
  Neoplasm, connective tissue,
  malignant
 lymphoblastic —*see* Lymphoma,
  lymphoblastic (diffuse)
 lymphocytic —*see* Lymphoma,
  small cell B-cell
 mast cell C96.22
 melanotic —*see* Melanoma
 meningeal —*see* Neoplasm,
  meninges, malignant
 meningothelial —*see* Neoplasm,
  meninges, malignant
 mesenchymal —*see also*
  Neoplasm, connective tissue,
  malignant
  mixed —*see* Neoplasm,
   connective tissue, malignant
 mesothelial —*see* Mesothelioma
 monstrocellular

Schwartz-Bartter syndrome E22.2

Schweniger-Buzzi anetoderma
L90.1

Sciatic —*see* condition

Sciatica (infective)
with lumbago M54.4-
due to intervertebral disc
disorder —*see* Disorder, disc,
with, radiculopathy
due to displacement of
intervertebral disc (with
lumbago) —*see* Disorder, disc,
with, radiculopathy
wallet M54.3-

Scimitar syndrome Q26.8

Sclera —*see* condition

Sclerectasia H15.84-

Scleredema
adultorum —*see* Sclerosis,
systemic
Buschke's —*see* Sclerosis,
systemic
newborn P83.0

Sclerema (adiposum) (edematosum)
(neonatorum) (newborn) P83.0
adultorum —*see* Sclerosis,
systemic

Scleriasis —*see* Scleroderma

Scleritis H15.00-
with corneal involvement H15.04-
anterior H15.01-
brawny H15.02-
in (due to) zoster B02.34
posterior H15.03-
specified type NEC H15.09-
syphilitic A52.71
tuberculous (nodular) A18.51

Sclerochoroiditis H31.8

Scleroconjunctivitis —*see* Scleritis

Sclerocystic ovary syndrome E28.2

Sclerodactyly, sclerodactylia L94.3

Scleroderma, sclerodermia
(acrosclerotic) (diffuse)
(generalized) (progressive)
(pulmonary) (*see also* Sclerosis,
systemic) M34.9-
circumscribed L94.0
linear L94.1
localized L94.0
newborn P83.88
systemic M34.9

Sclerokeratitis H16.8
tuberculous A18.52

Scleroma nasi A48.8

Scleromalacia (perforans) H15.05-

Scleromyxedema L98.5

Sclérose en plaques G35

Sclerosis, sclerotic
adrenal (gland) E27.8
Alzheimer's —*see* Disease,
Alzheimer's
amyotrophic (lateral) G12.21
aorta, aortic I70.0
valve —*see* Endocarditis, aortic
artery, arterial, arteriolar,
arteriovascular —*see*
Arteriosclerosis
ascending multiple G35
brain (generalized) (lobular) G37.9
artery, arterial I67.2
diffuse G37.0
disseminated G35
insular G35
Krabbe's E75.23

Sclerosis, sclerotic *(continued)*
brain *(continued)*
miliary G35
multiple G35
presenile (Alzheimer's) —*see*
Disease, Alzheimer's, early
onset
senile (arteriosclerotic) I67.2
stem, multiple G35
tuberous Q85.1
bulbar, multiple G35
bundle of His I44.39
cardiac —*see* Disease, heart,
ischemic, atherosclerotic
cardiorenal —*see* Hypertension,
cardiorenal
cardiovascular —*see also* Disease,
cardiovascular
renal —*see* Hypertension,
cardiorenal
cerebellar —*see* Sclerosis, brain
cerebral —*see* Sclerosis, brain
cerebrospinal (disseminated)
(multiple) G35
cerebrovascular I67.2
choroid —*see* Degeneration,
choroid
combined (spinal cord) —*see also*
Degeneration, combined
multiple G35
concentric (Balo) G37.5
cornea —*see* Opacity, cornea
coronary (artery) I25.10
with angina pectoris —*see*
Arteriosclerosis, coronary
(artery),
corpus cavernosum
female N90.89
male N48.6
diffuse (brain) (spinal cord)
G37.0
disseminated G35
dorsal G35
dorsolateral (spinal cord) —*see*
Degeneration, combined
endometrium N85.5
extrapyramidal G25.9
eye, nuclear (senile) —*see*
Cataract, senile, nuclear
focal and segmental (glomerular)
(*see also* N00-N07 with fourth
character .1) N05.1
Friedreich's (spinal cord) G11.11
funicular (spermatic cord)
N50.89
general (vascular) —*see*
Arteriosclerosis
gland (lymphatic) I89.8
hepatic K74.1
alcoholic K70.2
hereditary
cerebellar G11.9
spinal (Friedreich's ataxia)
G11.11
hippocampal G93.81
insular G35
kidney —*see* Sclerosis, renal
larynx J38.7
lateral (amyotrophic) (descending)
(spinal) G12.21
primary G12.23
lens, senile nuclear —*see* Cataract,
senile, nuclear
liver K74.1
with fibrosis K74.2
alcoholic K70.2
alcoholic K70.2
cardiac K76.1
lung —*see* Fibrosis, lung
mastoid —*see* Mastoiditis, chronic
mesial temporal G93.81

Sclerosis, sclerotic *(continued)*
mitral I05.8
Mönckeberg's (medial) —*see*
Arteriosclerosis, extremities
multiple (brain stem) (cerebral)
(generalized) (spinal cord) G35
myocardium, myocardial —*see*
Disease, heart, ischemic,
atherosclerotic
nuclear (senile), eye —*see*
Cataract, senile, nuclear
ovary N83.8
pancreas K86.89
penis N48.6
peripheral arteries —*see*
Arteriosclerosis, extremities
plaques G35
pluriglandular E31.8
polyglandular E31.8
posterolateral (spinal cord) —*see*
Degeneration, combined
presenile (Alzheimer's) —*see*
Disease, Alzheimer's, early onset
primary, lateral G12.23
progressive, systemic M34.0
pulmonary —*see* Fibrosis, lung
artery I27.0
valve (heart) —*see* Endocarditis,
pulmonary
renal N26.9
with
cystine storage disease E72.09
hypertensive heart disease
(conditions in I11) —*see*
Hypertension, cardiorenal
arteriolar (hyaline) (hyperplastic)
—*see* Hypertension, kidney
retina (senile) (vascular) H35.00
senile (vascular) —*see*
Arteriosclerosis
spinal (cord) (progressive) G95.89
ascending G61.0
combined —*see also*
Degeneration, combined
multiple G35
syphilitic A52.11
disseminated G35
dorsolateral —*see* Degeneration,
combined
hereditary (Friedreich's) (mixed
form) G11.11
lateral (amyotrophic) G12.21
progressive G12.23
multiple G35
posterior (syphilitic) A52.11
stomach K31.89
subendocardial, congenital I42.4
systemic M34.9
with
lung involvement M34.81
myopathy M34.82
polyneuropathy M34.83
drug-induced M34.2
due to chemicals NEC M34.2
progressive M34.0
specified NEC M34.89
temporal (mesial) G93.81
tricuspid (heart) (valve) I07.8
tuberous (brain) Q85.1
tympanic membrane —*see*
Disorder, tympanic membrane,
specified NEC
valve, valvular (heart) —*see*
Endocarditis
vascular —*see* Arteriosclerosis
vein I87.8

Scoliosis (acquired) (postural) M41.9
adolescent (idiopathic) —*see*
Scoliosis, idiopathic, adolescent
congenital Q67.5
due to bony malformation Q76.3

Scoliosis *(continued)*
congenital *(continued)*
failure of segmentation
(hemivertebra) Q76.3
hemivertebra fusion Q76.3
postural Q67.5
degenerative M41.8-
idiopathic M41.20
adolescent M41.129
cervical region M41.122
cervicothoracic region
M41.123
lumbar region M41.126
lumbosacral region M41.127
thoracic region M41.124
thoracolumbar region
M41.125
cervical region M41.22
cervicothoracic region M41.23
infantile M41.00
cervical region M41.02
cervicothoracic region M41.03
lumbar region M41.06
lumbosacral region M41.07
sacrococcygeal region M41.08
thoracic region M41.04
thoracolumbar region M41.05
juvenile M41.119
cervical region M41.112
cervicothoracic region M41.113
lumbar region M41.116
lumbosacral region M41.117
thoracic region M41.114
thoracolumbar region
M41.115
lumbar region M41.26
lumbosacral region M41.27
thoracic region M41.24
thoracolumbar region M41.25
infantile —*see* Scoliosis,
idiopathic, infantile
neuromuscular M41.40
cervical region M41.42
cervicothoracic region M41.43
lumbar region M41.46
lumbosacral region M41.47
occipito-atlanto-axial region
M41.41
thoracic region M41.44
thoracolumbar region M41.45
paralytic —*see* Scoliosis,
neuromuscular
postradiation therapy M96.5
rachitic (late effect or sequelae)
E64.3 *[M49.80]*
cervical region E64.3 *[M49.82]*
cervicothoracic region E64.3
[M49.83]
lumbar region E64.3 *[M49.86]*
lumbosacral region E64.3
[M49.87]
multiple sites E64.3 *[M49.89]*
occipito-atlanto-axial region
E64.3 *[M49.81]*
sacrococcygeal region E64.3
[M49.88]
thoracic region E64.3 *[M49.84]*
thoracolumbar region E64.3
[M49.85]
sciatic M54.4-
secondary (to) NEC M41.50
cerebral palsy, Friedreich's
ataxia, poliomyelitis,
neuromuscular disorders —*see*
Scoliosis, neuromuscular
cervical region M41.52
cervicothoracic region M41.53
lumbar region M41.56
lumbosacral region M41.57
thoracic region M41.54
thoracolumbar region M41.55

Scoliosis (continued)
specified form NEC M41.80
cervical region M41.82
cervicothoracic region M41.83
lumbar region M41.86
lumbosacral region M41.87
thoracic region M41.84
thoracolumbar region M41.85
thoracogenic M41.30
thoracic region M41.34
thoracolumbar region M41.35
tuberculous A18.01

Scoliotic pelvis
with disproportion (fetopelvic)
O33.0
causing obstructed labor O65.0

Scorbutus, scorbutic —see also
Scurvy
anemia D53.2

**Score, NIHSS (National Institutes
of Health Stoke Scale)** R29.7-

Scotoma (arcuate) (Bjerrum) (central)
(ring) —see also Defect, visual
field, localized, scotoma
scintillating H53.19

Scratch —see Abrasion

Scratchy throat R09.89

Screening (for) Z13.9
alcoholism Z13.39
anemia Z13.0
anomaly, congenital Z13.89
antenatal, of mother (see also
Encounter, antenatal screening)
Z36.9
arterial hypertension Z13.6
arthropod-borne viral disease NEC
Z11.59
autism Z13.41
bacteriuria, asymptomatic Z13.89
behavioral disorder Z13.30
specified NEC Z13.39
brain injury, traumatic Z13.850
bronchitis, chronic Z13.83
brucellosis Z11.2
cardiovascular disorder Z13.6
cataract Z13.5
chlamydial diseases Z11.8
cholera Z11.0
chromosomal abnormalities
(nonprocreative) NEC Z13.79
colonoscopy Z12.11
congenital
dislocation of hip Z13.89
eye disorder Z13.5
malformation or deformation
Z13.89
contamination NEC Z13.88
cystic fibrosis Z13.228
dengue fever Z11.59
dental disorder Z13.84
depression (adult) (adolescent)
(child) Z13.31
maternal Z13.32
perinatal Z13.32
developmental
delays Z13.40
global (milestones) Z13.42
specified NEC Z13.49
handicap Z13.42
in early childhood Z13.42
diabetes mellitus Z13.1
diphtheria Z11.2
disability, intellectual Z13.39
disease or disorder Z13.9
bacterial NEC Z11.2
intestinal infectious Z11.0
respiratory tuberculosis Z11.1
behavioral Z13.30
specified NEC Z13.39

Screening (continued)
disease or disorder (continued)
blood or blood-forming organ
Z13.0
cardiovascular Z13.6
Chagas' Z11.6
chlamydial Z11.8
dental Z13.89
developmental delays Z13.40
global (milestones) Z13.42
specified NEC Z13.49
digestive tract NEC Z13.818
lower GI Z13.811
upper GI Z13.810
ear Z13.5
endocrine Z13.29
eye Z13.5
genitourinary Z13.89
heart Z13.6
human immunodeficiency virus
(HIV) infection Z11.4
immunity Z13.0
infection
intestinal Z11.0
specified NEC Z11.6
infectious Z11.9
mental health and behavioral
Z13.30
specified NEC Z13.39
metabolic Z13.228
neurological Z13.89
nutritional Z13.21
metabolic Z13.228
lipoid disorders Z13.220
protozoal Z11.6
intestinal Z11.0
respiratory Z13.83
rheumatic Z13.828
rickettsial Z11.8
sexually-transmitted NEC Z11.3
human immunodeficiency
virus (HIV) Z11.4
sickle-cell (trait) Z13.0
skin Z13.89
specified NEC Z13.89
spirochetal Z11.8
thyroid Z13.29
vascular Z13.6
venereal Z11.3
viral NEC Z11.59
human immunodeficiency
virus (HIV) Z11.4
intestinal Z11.0
elevated titer Z13.89
emphysema Z13.83
encephalitis, viral (mosquito- or
tick-borne) Z11.59
exposure to contaminants (toxic)
Z13.88
fever
dengue Z11.59
hemorrhagic Z11.59
yellow Z11.59
filariasis Z11.6
galactosemia Z13.228
gastrointestinal condition Z13.818
genetic (nonprocreative) - for
procreative management —see
Testing, genetic, for procreative
management
disease carrier status
(nonprocreative) Z13.71
specified NEC (nonprocreative)
Z13.79
genitourinary condition Z13.89
glaucoma Z13.5
gonorrhea Z11.3
gout Z13.89
helminthiasis (intestinal) Z11.6
hematopoietic malignancy Z12.89
hemoglobinopathies NEC Z13.0

Screening (continued)
hemorrhagic fever Z11.59
Hodgkin disease Z12.89
human immunodeficiency virus
(HIV) Z11.4
human papillomavirus Z11.51
hypertension Z13.6
immunity disorders Z13.0
infant or child (over 28 days old)
Z00.129
with abnormal findings Z00.121
infection
mycotic Z11.8
parasitic Z11.8
ingestion of radioactive substance
Z13.88
intellectual disability Z13.39
intestinal
helminthiasis Z11.6
infectious disease Z11.0
leishmaniasis Z11.6
leprosy Z11.2
leptospirosis Z11.8
leukemia Z12.89
lymphoma Z12.89
malaria Z11.6
malnutrition Z13.29
metabolic Z13.228
nutritional Z13.21
measles Z11.59
mental health disorder Z13.30
specified NEC Z13.39
metabolic errors, inborn Z13.228
multiphasic Z13.89
musculoskeletal disorder Z13.828
osteoporosis Z13.820
mycoses Z11.8
myocardial infarction (acute) Z13.6
neoplasm (malignant) (of) Z12.9
bladder Z12.6
blood Z12.89
breast Z12.39
routine mammogram Z12.31
cervix Z12.4
colon Z12.11
genitourinary organs NEC
Z12.79
bladder Z12.6
cervix Z12.4
ovary Z12.73
prostate Z12.5
testis Z12.71
vagina Z12.72
hematopoietic system Z12.89
intestinal tract Z12.10
colon Z12.11
rectum Z12.12
small intestine Z12.13
lung Z12.2
lymph (glands) Z12.89
nervous system Z12.82
oral cavity Z12.81
prostate Z12.5
rectum Z12.12
respiratory organs Z12.2
skin Z12.83
small intestine Z12.13
specified site NEC Z12.89
stomach Z12.0
nephropathy Z13.89
nervous system disorders NEC
Z13.858
neurological condition Z13.89
osteoporosis Z13.820
parasitic infestation Z11.9
specified NEC Z11.8
phenylketonuria Z13.228
plague Z11.2
poisoning (chemical) (heavy metal)
Z13.88
poliomyelitis Z11.59

Screening (continued)
postnatal, chromosomal
abnormalities Z13.89
prenatal, of mother (see also
Encounter, antenatal screening)
Z36.9
protozoal disease Z11.6
intestinal Z11.0
pulmonary tuberculosis Z11.1
radiation exposure Z13.88
respiratory condition Z13.83
respiratory tuberculosis Z11.1
rheumatoid arthritis Z13.828
rubella Z11.59
schistosomiasis Z11.6
sexually-transmitted disease NEC
Z11.3
human immunodeficiency virus
(HIV) Z11.4
sickle-cell disease or trait Z13.0
skin condition Z13.89
sleeping sickness Z11.6
special Z13.9
specified NEC Z13.89
syphilis Z11.3
tetanus Z11.2
trachoma Z11.8
traumatic brain injury Z13.850
trypanosomiasis Z11.6
tuberculosis, respiratory Z11.1
active Z11.1
latent Z11.7
venereal disease Z11.3
viral encephalitis (mosquito- or
tick-borne) Z11.59
whooping cough Z11.2
worms, intestinal Z11.6
yaws Z11.8
yellow fever Z11.59

Scrofula, scrofulosis (tuberculosis of
cervical lymph glands) A18.2

Scrofulide (primary) (tuberculous)
A18.4

Scrofuloderma, scrofulodermia
(any site) (primary) A18.4

Scrofulosus lichen (primary)
(tuberculous) A18.4

Scrofulous —see condition

Scrotal tongue K14.5

Scrotum —see condition

Scurvy, scorbutic E54
anemia D53.2
gum E54
infantile E54
rickets E55.0 [M90.80]

Sealpox B08.62

Seasickness T75.3

Seatworm (infection) (infestation)
B80

Sebaceous —see also condition
cyst —see Cyst, sebaceous

Seborrhea, seborrheic L21.9
capillitii R23.8
capitis L21.0
dermatitis L21.9
infantile L21.1
eczema L21.9
infantile L21.1
sicca L21.0

Seckel's syndrome Q87.19

Seclusion, pupil —see Membrane,
pupillary

**Second hand tobacco smoke
exposure** (acute) (chronic)
Z77.22
in the perinatal period P96.81

Sepsis *(continued)*
- following *(continued)*
  - infusion, therapeutic injection or transfusion NEC T80.29
  - obstetrical procedure O86.04
- gangrenous A41.9
- gonococcal A54.86
- Gram-negative (organism) A41.5
  - anaerobic A41.4
- Haemophilus influenzae A41.3
- herpesviral B00.7
- intra-abdominal K65.1
- intraocular —*see* Endophthalmitis, purulent
- Listeria monocytogenes A32.7
- localized - code to specific localized infection
  - in operation wound T81.49
  - skin —*see* Abscess
- malleus A24.0
- melioidosis A24.1
- meningeal —*see* Meningitis
- meningococcal A39.4
  - acute A39.2
  - chronic A39.3
- MSSA (Methicillin susceptible Staphylococcus aureus) A41.01
- newborn P36.9
  - due to
    - anaerobes NEC P36.5
    - Escherichia coli P36.4
    - Staphylococcus P36.30
      - aureus P36.2
      - specified NEC P36.39
    - Streptococcus P36.10
      - group B P36.0
      - specified NEC P36.19
    - specified NEC P36.8
- Pasteurella multocida A28.0
- pelvic, puerperal, postpartum, childbirth O85
- postprocedural T81.44
- pneumococcal A40.3
- puerperal, postpartum, childbirth (pelvic) O85
- Salmonella (arizonae) (choleraesuis) (enteritidis) (typhimurium) A02.1
- severe R65.20
  - with septic shock R65.21
- skin, localized —*see* Abscess
- Shigella (*see also* Dysentery, bacillary) A03.9
- specified organism NEC A41.89
- Staphylococcus, staphylococcal A41.2
  - aureus (methicillin susceptible) (MSSA) A41.01
    - methicillin resistant (MRSA) A41.02
  - coagulase-negative A41.1
  - specified NEC A41.1
- Streptococcus, streptococcal A40.9
  - agalactiae A40.1
  - group
    - A A40.0
    - B A40.1
    - D A41.81
  - neonatal P36.10
    - group B P36.0
    - specified NEC P36.19
  - pneumoniae A40.3
  - pyogenes A40.0
  - specified NEC A40.8
- tracheostomy stoma J95.02
- tularemic A21.7
- umbilical, umbilical cord (newborn) —*see* Sepsis, newborn
- Yersinia pestis A20.7

Septate —*see* Septum

Septic —*see* condition
- arm —*see* Cellulitis, upper limb
  - with lymphangitis —*see* Lymphangitis, acute, upper limb
- embolus —*see* Embolism
- finger —*see* Cellulitis, digit
  - with lymphangitis —*see* Lymphangitis, acute, digit
- foot —*see* Cellulitis, lower limb
  - with lymphangitis —*see* Lymphangitis, acute, lower limb
- gallbladder (acute) K81.0
- hand —*see* Cellulitis, upper limb
  - with lymphangitis —*see* Lymphangitis, acute, upper limb
- joint —*see* Arthritis, pyogenic or pyemic
- leg —*see* Cellulitis, lower limb
  - with lymphangitis —*see* Lymphangitis, acute, lower limb
- nail —*see also* Cellulitis, digit
  - with lymphangitis —*see* Lymphangitis, acute, digit
- sore —*see also* Abscess
  - throat J02.0
    - streptococcal J02.0
- spleen (acute) D73.89
- teeth, tooth (pulpal origin) K04.4
- throat —*see* Pharyngitis
- thrombus —*see* Thrombosis
- toe —*see* Cellulitis, digit
  - with lymphangitis —*see* Lymphangitis, acute, digit
- tonsils, chronic J35.01
  - with adenoiditis J35.03
- uterus —*see* Endometritis

Septicemia A41.9
- meaning sepsis —*see* Sepsis

Septum, septate (congenital) —*see also* Anomaly, by site
- anal Q42.3
  - with fistula Q42.2
- aqueduct of Sylvius Q03.0
  - with spina bifida —*see* Spina bifida, by site, with hydrocephalus
- uterus Q51.28
  - complete Q51.21
  - partial Q51.22
  - specified NEC Q51.28
- vagina Q52.10
  - in pregnancy —*see* Pregnancy, complicated by, abnormal vagina
    - causing obstructed labor O65.5
  - longitudinal Q52.129
    - microperforate
      - left side Q52.124
      - right side Q52.123
    - nonobstruction Q52.120
    - obstructing Q52.129
      - left side Q52.122
      - right side Q52.1221
  - transverse Q52.11

Sequelae (of) —*see also* condition
- abscess, intracranial or intraspinal (conditions in G06) G09
- amputation -- code to injury with seventh character S
- burn and corrosion -- code to injury with seventh character S
- calcium deficiency E64.8
- cerebrovascular disease — *see* Sequelae, disease, cerebrovascular

Sequelae *(continued)*
- childbirth O94
- contusion -- code to injury with seventh character S
- corrosion —*see* Sequelae, burn and corrosion
- crushing injury -- code to injury with seventh character S
- disease
  - cerebrovascular I69.90
    - alteration of sensation I69.998
    - aphasia I69.920
    - apraxia I69.990
    - ataxia I69.993
    - cognitive deficits I69.91
    - disturbance of vision I69.998
    - dysarthria I69.922
    - dysphagia I69.991
    - dysphasia I69.921
    - facial droop I69.992
    - facial weakness I69.992
    - fluency disorder I69.923
    - hemiplegia I69.95-
    - hemorrhage
      - intracerebral —*see* Sequelae, hemorrhage, intracerebral
      - intracranial, nontraumatic NEC —*see* Sequelae, hemorrhage, intracranial, nontraumatic
      - subarachnoid —*see* Sequelae, hemorrhage, subarachnoid
    - language deficit I69.928
    - monoplegia
      - lower limb I69.94-
      - upper limb I69.93-
    - paralytic syndrome I69.96-
    - specified effect NEC I69.998
    - specified type NEC I69.80
      - alteration of sensation I69.898
      - aphasia I69.820
      - apraxia I69.890
      - ataxia I69.893
      - cognitive deficits I69.81
      - disturbance of vision I69.898
      - dysarthria I69.822
      - dysphagia I69.891
      - dysphasia I69.821
      - facial droop I69.892
      - facial weakness I69.892
      - fluency disorder I69.823
      - hemiplegia I69.85-
      - language deficit I69.828
      - monoplegia
        - lower limb I69.84-
        - upper limb I69.83-
      - paralytic syndrome I69.86-
      - specified effect NEC I69.898
    - speech deficit I69.928
      - speech deficit I69.828
    - stroke NOS —*see* Sequelae, stroke NOS
- dislocation -- code to injury with seventh character S
- encephalitis or encephalomyelitis (conditions in G04) G09
  - in infectious disease NEC B94.8
  - viral B94.1
- external cause -- code to injury with seventh character S
- foreign body entering natural orifice -- code to injury with seventh character S
- fracture -- code to injury with seventh character S
- frostbite -- code to injury with seventh character S

Sequelae *(continued)*
- Hansen's disease B92
- hemorrhage
  - intracerebral I69.10
    - alteration of sensation I69.198
    - aphasia I69.120
    - apraxia I69.190
    - ataxia I69.193
    - cognitive deficits I69.11
    - disturbance of vision I69.198
    - dysarthria I69.122
    - dysphagia I69.191
    - dysphasia I69.121
    - facial droop I69.192
    - facial weakness I69.192
    - fluency disorder I69.123
    - hemiplegia I69.15-
    - language deficit NEC I69.128
    - monoplegia
      - lower limb I69.14-
      - upper limb I69.13-
    - paralytic syndrome I69.16-
    - specified effect NEC I69.198
    - speech deficit NEC I69.128
  - intracranial, nontraumatic NEC I69.20
    - alteration of sensation I69.298
    - aphasia I69.220
    - apraxia I69.290
    - ataxia I69.293
    - cognitive deficits I69.21
    - disturbance of vision I69.298
    - dysarthria I69.222
    - dysphagia I69.291
    - dysphasia I69.221
    - facial droop I69.292
    - facial weakness I69.292
    - fluency disorder I69.223
    - hemiplegia I69.25-
    - language deficit NEC I69.228
    - monoplegia
      - lower limb I69.24-
      - upper limb I69.23-
    - paralytic syndrome I69.26-
    - specified effect NEC I69.298
    - speech deficit NEC I69.228
  - subarachnoid I69.00
    - alteration of sensation I69.098
    - aphasia I69.020
    - apraxia I69.090
    - ataxia I69.093
    - cognitive deficits —*see* subcategory I69.01-
    - disturbance of vision I69.098
    - dysarthria I69.022
    - dysphagia I69.091
    - dysphasia I69.021
    - facial droop I69.092
    - facial weakness I69.092
    - fluency disorder I69.023
    - hemiplegia I69.05-
    - language deficit NEC I69.028
    - monoplegia
      - lower limb I69.04-
      - upper limb I69.03-
    - paralytic syndrome I69.06-
    - specified effect NEC I69.098
    - speech deficit NEC I69.028
- hepatitis, viral B94.2
- hyperalimentation E68
- infarction
  - cerebral I69.30
    - alteration of sensation I69.398
    - aphasia I69.320
    - apraxia I69.390
    - ataxia I69.393
    - cognitive deficits I69.31
    - disturbance of vision I69.398
    - dysarthria I69.322
    - dysphagia I69.391
    - dysphasia I69.321

Sequelae (*continued*)
infarction (*continued*)
cerebral (*continued*)
facial droop I69.392
facial weakness I69.392
fluency disorder I69.323
hemiplegia I69.35-
language deficit NEC I69.328
monoplegia
lower limb I69.34-
upper limb I69.33-
paralytic syndrome I69.36-
specified effect NEC I69.398
speech deficit NEC I69.328
infection, pyogenic, intracranial or intraspinal G09
infectious disease B94.9
specified NEC B94.8
injury -- code to injury with seventh character S
leprosy B92
meningitis
bacterial (conditions in G00) G09
other or unspecified cause (conditions in G03) G09
muscle (and tendon) injury - code to injury with seventh character S
myelitis —*see* Sequelae, encephalitis
niacin deficiency E64.8
nutritional deficiency E64.9
specified NEC E64.8
obstetrical condition O94
parasitic disease B94.9
phlebitis or thrombophlebitis of intracranial or intraspinal venous sinuses and veins (conditions in G08) G09
poisoning -- code to poisoning with seventh character S
nonmedicinal substance — *see* Sequelae, toxic effect, nonmedicinal substance
poliomyelitis (acute) B91
pregnancy O94
protein-energy malnutrition E64.0
puerperium O94
rickets E64.3
selenium deficiency E64.8
sprain and strain - code to injury with seventh character S
stroke NOS I69.30
alteration in sensation I69.398
aphasia I69.320
apraxia I69.390
ataxia I69.393
cognitive deficits I69.31
disturbance of vision I69.398
dysarthria I69.322
dysphagia I69.391
dysphasia I69.321
facial droop I69.392
facial weakness I69.392
hemiplegia I69.35-
language deficit NEC I69.328
monoplegia
lower limb I69.34-
upper limb I69.33-
paralytic syndrome I69.36-
specified effect NEC I69.398
speech deficit NEC I69.328
tendon and muscle injury - code to injury with seventh character S
thiamine deficiency E64.8
trachoma B94.0
tuberculosis B90.9
bones and joints B90.2
central nervous system B90.0
genitourinary B90.1
pulmonary (respiratory) B90.9
specified organs NEC B90.8

Sequelae (*continued*)
viral
encephalitis B94.1
hepatitis B94.2
vitamin deficiency NEC E64.8
A E64.1
B E64.8
C E64.2
wound, open - code to injury with seventh character S

Sequestration —*see also* Sequestrum
disc —*see* Displacement, intervertebral disc
lung, congenital Q33.2

Sequestrum
bone —*see* Osteomyelitis, chronic
dental M27.2
jaw bone M27.2
orbit —*see* Osteomyelitis, orbit
sinus (accessory) (nasal) —*see* Sinusitis

Sequoiosis lung or pneumonitis J67.8

Serology for syphilis
doubtful
with signs or symptoms - code by site and stage under Syphilis
follow-up of latent syphilis —*see* Syphilis, latent
negative, with signs or symptoms - code by site and stage under Syphilis
positive A53.0
with signs or symptoms - code by site and stage under Syphilis
reactivated A53.0

Seroma —*see also* Hematoma
postprocedural —*see* Complication, postprocedural, seroma
traumatic, secondary and recurrent T79.2

Seropurulent —*see* condition

Serositis, multiple K65.8
pericardial I31.1
peritoneal K65.8

Serous —*see* condition

Sertoli cell
adenoma
specified site —*see* Neoplasm, benign, by site
unspecified site
female D27.9
male D29.20
carcinoma
specified site —*see* Neoplasm, malignant, by site
unspecified site (male) C62.9-
female C56.9
tumor
with lipid storage
specified site —*see* Neoplasm, benign, by site
unspecified site
female D27.9
male D29.20
specified site —*see* Neoplasm, benign, by site
unspecified site
female D27.9
male D29.20

Sertoli-Leydig cell tumor —*see* Neoplasm, benign, by site
specified site —*see* Neoplasm, benign, by site
unspecified site
female D27.9
male D29.20

Serum
allergy, allergic reaction (*see also* Reaction, serum) T80.69
shock (*see also* Shock, anaphylactic) T80.59
arthritis (*see also* Reaction, serum) T80.69
complication or reaction NEC (*see also* Reaction, serum) T80.69
disease NEC (*see also* Reaction, serum) T80.69
hepatitis —*see also* Hepatitis, viral, type B
carrier (suspected) of B18.1
intoxication (*see also* Reaction, serum) T80.69
neuritis (*see also* Reaction, serum) T80.69
neuropathy G61.1
poisoning NEC (*see also* Reaction, serum) T80.69
rash NEC (*see also* Reaction, serum) T80.69
reaction NEC (*see also* Reaction, serum) T80.69
sickness NEC (*see also* Reaction, serum) T80.69
urticaria (*see also* Reaction, serum) T80.69

Sesamoiditis M25.8-

Sever's disease or osteochondrosis —*see* Osteochondrosis, juvenile, tarsus

Severe sepsis R65.20
with septic shock R65.21

Sex
chromosome mosaics Q97.8
lines with various numbers of X chromosomes Q97.2
education Z70.8
reassignment surgery status Z87.890

Sextuplet pregnancy —*see* Pregnancy, sextuplet

Sexual
function, disorder of (psychogenic) F52.9
immaturity (female) (male) E30.0
impotence (psychogenic) organic origin NEC —*see* Dysfunction, sexual, male
precocity (constitutional) (cryptogenic) (female) (idiopathic) (male) E30.1

Sexuality, pathologic —*see* Deviation, sexual

Sézary disease C84.1-

Shadow, lung R91.8

Shaking palsy or paralysis —*see* Parkinsonism

Shallowness, acetabulum —*see* Derangement, joint, specified type NEC, hip

Shaver's disease J63.1

Sheath (tendon) —*see* condition

Sheathing, retinal vessels H35.01-

Shedding
nail L60.8
premature, primary (deciduous) teeth K00.6

Sheehan's disease or syndrome E23.0

Shelf, rectal K62.89

Shell teeth K00.5

Shellshock (current) F43.0
lasting state —*see* Disorder, post-traumatic stress

Shield kidney Q63.1

Shift
auditory threshold (temporary) H93.24-
mediastinal R93.89

Shifting sleep-work schedule (affecting sleep) G47.26

Shiga (-Kruse) **dysentery** A03.0

Shiga's bacillus A03.0

Shigella (dysentery) —*see* Dysentery, bacillary

Shigellosis A03.9
Group A A03.0
Group B A03.1
Group C A03.2
Group D A03.3

Shin splints S86.89

Shingles —*see* Herpes, zoster

Shipyard disease or eye B30.0

Shirodkar suture, in pregnancy —*see* Pregnancy, complicated by, incompetent cervix

Shock R57.9
with ectopic or molar pregnancy O08.3
adrenal (cortical) (Addisonian) E27.2
adverse food reaction (anaphylactic) —*see* Shock, anaphylactic, due to food
allergic —*see* Shock, anaphylactic
anaphylactic T78.2
chemical —*see* Table of Drugs and Chemicals
due to drug or medicinal substance
correct substance properly administered T88.6
overdose or wrong substance given or taken (by accident) —*see* Table of Drugs and Chemicals, by drug, poisoning
due to food (nonpoisonous) T78.00
additives T78.06
dairy products T78.07
eggs T78.08
fish T78.03
shellfish T78.02
fruit T78.04
milk T78.07
nuts T78.05
multiple types T78.05
peanuts T78.01
peanuts T78.01
seeds T78.05
specified type NEC T78.09
vegetable T78.04
following sting(s) —*see* Venom
immunization T80.52
serum T80.59
blood and blood products T80.51
immunization T80.52
specified NEC T80.59
vaccination T80.52
anaphylactoid —*see* Shock, anaphylactic
anesthetic
correct substance properly administered T88.2

Shock *(continued)*
  anesthetic *(continued)*
    overdose or wrong substance
      given or taken —*see* Table
        of Drugs and Chemicals, by
        drug, poisoning
      specified anesthetic —*see*
        Table of Drugs and
        Chemicals, by drug,
        poisoning
  cardiogenic R57.0
  chemical substance —*see* Table of
    Drugs and Chemicals
  complicating ectopic or molar
    pregnancy O08.3
  culture —*see* Disorder, adjustment
  drug
    due to correct substance properly
      administered T88.6
    overdose or wrong substance
      given or taken (by accident)
      —*see* Table of Drugs and
      Chemicals, by drug, poisoning
  during or after labor and delivery
    O75.1
  electric T75.4
    (taser) T75.4
  endotoxic R65.21
    postprocedural (resulting from
      a procedure, not elsewhere
      classified) T81.12
  following
    ectopic or molar pregnancy
      O08.3
    injury (immediate) (delayed)
      T79.4
    labor and delivery O75.1
  food (anaphylactic) —*see* Shock,
    anaphylactic, due to food
  from electroshock gun (taser)
    T75.4
  gram-negative R65.21
    postprocedural (resulting from
      a procedure, not elsewhere
      classified) T81.12
  hematologic R57.8
  hemorrhagic R57.8
    surgery (intraoperative)
      (postoperative) T81.19
    trauma T79.4
  hypovolemic R57.1
    surgical T81.19
    traumatic T79.4
  insulin E15
    therapeutic misadventure —*see*
      subcategory T38.3
  kidney N17.0
    traumatic (following crushing)
      T79.5
  lightning T75.01
  liver K72.00
  lung J80
  obstetric O75.1
    with ectopic or molar pregnancy
      O08.3
    following ectopic or molar
      pregnancy O08.3
  pleural (surgical) T81.19
    due to trauma T79.4
  postprocedural (postoperative)
    T81.10
    with ectopic or molar pregnancy
      O08.3
    cardiogenic T81.11
    endotoxic T81.12
    following ectopic or molar
      pregnancy O08.3
    gram-negative T81.12
    hypovolemic T81.19
    septic T81.12
    specified type NEC T81.19

Shock *(continued)*
  psychic F43.0
  septic (due to severe sepsis) R65.21
  specified NEC R57.8
  surgical T81.10
  taser gun (taser) T75.4
  therapeutic misadventure NEC
    T81.10
  thyroxin
    overdose or wrong substance
      given or taken —*see* Table
      of Drugs and Chemicals, by
      drug, poisoning
  toxic, syndrome A48.3
  transfusion —*see* Complications,
    transfusion
  traumatic (immediate) (delayed)
    T79.4

Shoemaker's chest M95.4

Short, shortening, shortness
  arm (acquired) —*see also*
    Deformity, limb, unequal length
    congenital Q71.81-
      forearm —*see* Deformity, limb,
        unequal length
  bowel syndrome K91.2
  breath R06.02
  cervical (complicating pregnancy)
    O26.87-
    non-gravid uterus N88.3
  common bile duct, congenital Q44.5
  cord (umbilical), complicating
    delivery O69.3
  cystic duct, congenital Q44.5
  esophagus (congenital) Q39.8
  femur (acquired) —*see* Deformity,
    limb, unequal length, femur
    congenital —*see* Defect,
      reduction, lower limb,
      longitudinal, femur
  frenum, frenulum, linguae
    (congenital) Q38.1
  hip (acquired) —*see also*
    Deformity, limb, unequal length
    congenital Q65.89
  leg (acquired) —*see also*
    Deformity, limb, unequal length
    congenital Q72.81-
    lower leg —*see also* Deformity,
      limb, unequal length
  limbed stature, with
    immunodeficiency D82.2
  lower limb (acquired) —*see also*
    Deformity, limb, unequal length
    congenital Q72.81-
  organ or site, congenital NEC
    —*see* Distortion
  palate, congenital Q38.5
  radius (acquired) —*see also*
    Deformity, limb, unequal length
    congenital —*see* Defect,
      reduction, upper limb,
      longitudinal, radius
  rib syndrome Q77.2
  stature (child) (hereditary)
    (idiopathic) NEC R62.52
    constitutional E34.3
    due to endocrine disorder
      E34.3
    Laron-type E34.3
  tendon —*see also* Contraction,
    tendon
    with contracture of joint —*see*
      Contraction, joint
    Achilles (acquired) M67.0-
      congenital Q66.89
    congenital Q79.8
  thigh (acquired) —*see also*
    Deformity, limb, unequal length,
    femur

Short, shortening, shortness
(continued)
  thigh *(continued)*
    congenital —*sese* Defect,
      reduction, lower limb,
      longitudinal, femur
  tibialis anterior (tendon) —*see*
    Contraction, tendon
  umbilical cord
    complicating delivery O69.3
  upper limb, congenital —*see*
    Defect, reduction, upper limb,
    specified type NEC
  urethra N36.8
  uvula, congenital Q38.5
  vagina (congenital) Q52.4

Shortsightedness —*see* Myopia

Shoshin (acute fulminating beriberi)
  E51.11

Shoulder —*see* condition

Shovel-shaped incisors K00.2

Shower, thromboembolic —*see*
  Embolism

Shunt
  arterial-venous (dialysis) Z99.2
  arteriovenous, pulmonary
    (acquired) I28.0
    congenital Q25.72
  cerebral ventricle (communicating)
    in situ Z98.2
  surgical, prosthetic, with
    complications —*see*
    Complications, cardiovascular,
    device or implant

Shutdown, renal N28.9

Shy-Drager syndrome G90.3

Sialadenitis, sialadenosis (any gland)
  (chronic) (periodic) (suppurative)
  —*see* Sialoadenitis

Sialectasia K11.8

Sialidosis E77.1

Sialitis, silitis (any gland) (chronic)
  (suppurative) —*see* Sialoadenitis

Sialoadenitis (any gland) (periodic)
  (suppurative) K11.20
  acute K11.21
    recurrent K11.22
  chronic K11.23

Sialoadenopathy K11.9

Sialoangitis —*see* Sialoadenitis

Sialodochitis (fibrinosa) —*see*
  Sialoadenitis

Sialodocholithiasis K11.5

Sialolithiasis K11.5

Sialometaplasia, necrotizing
  K11.8

Sialorrhea —*see also* Ptyalism
  periodic —*see* Sialoadenitis

Sialosis K11.7

Siamese twin Q89.4

Sibling rivalry Z62.891

Sicard's syndrome G52.7

Sicca syndrome M35.00
  with
    keratoconjunctivitis M35.01
    lung involvement M35.02
    myopathy M35.03
    renal tubulo-interstitial disorders
      M35.04
  specified organ involvement NEC
    M35.09

Sick R69

Sick *(continued)*
  or handicapped person in family
    Z63.79
    needing care at home Z63.6
  sinus (syndrome) I49.5

Sick-euthyroid syndrome E07.81

Sickle-cell
  anemia —*see* Disease, sickle-cell
  beta plus —*see* Disease, sickle-cell,
    thalassemia, beta plus
  beta zero —*see* Disease, sickle-cell,
    thalassemia, beta zero
  trait D57.3

Sicklemia —*see also* Disease, sickle-
  cell
  trait D57.3

Sickness
  air (travel) T75.3
  airplane T75.3
  alpine T70.29
  altitude T70.20
  Andes T70.29
  aviator's T70.29
  balloon T70.29
  car T75.3
  compressed air T70.3
  decompression T70.3
  green D50.8
  milk —*see* Poisoning, food, noxious
  motion T75.3
  mountain T70.29
    acute D75.1
  protein (*see also* Reaction, serum)
    T80.69
  radiation T66
  roundabout (motion) T75.3
  sea T75.3
  serum NEC (*see also* Reaction,
    serum) T80.69
  sleeping (African) B56.9
    by Trypanosoma B56.9
      brucei
        gambiense B56.0
        rhodesiense B56.1
    East African B56.1
    Gambian B56.0
    Rhodesian B56.1
    West African B56.0
  swing (motion) T75.3
  train (railway) (travel) T75.3
  travel (any vehicle) T75.3

Sideropenia —*see* Anemia, iron
  deficiency

Siderosilicosis J62.8

Siderosis (lung) J63.4
  brain G93.89
  eye (globe) —*see* Disorder, globe,
    degenerative, siderosis

Siemens' syndrome (ectodermal
  dysplasia) Q82.8

Sighing R06.89
  psychogenic F45.8

Sigmoid —*see also* condition
  flexure —*see* condition
  kidney Q63.1

Sigmoiditis (*see also* Enteritis) K52.9
  infectious A09
  noninfectious K52.9

Silfversköld's syndrome Q78.9

Silicosiderosis J62.8

Silicosis, silicotic (simple)
  (complicated) J62.8
  with tuberculosis J65

Silicotuberculosis J65

Silo-fillers' disease J68.8

Silo-fillers' disease *(continued)*
  bronchitis J68.0
  pneumonitis J68.0
  pulmonary edema J68.1

Silver's syndrome Q87.19

Simian malaria B53.1

Simmonds' cachexia or disease E23.0

Simons' disease or syndrome
  (progressive lipodystrophy) E88.1

Simple, simplex —*see* condition

Simulation, conscious (of illness) Z76.5

Simultanagnosia (asimultagnosia)
  R48.3

Sin Nombre virus disease
  (Hantavirus) (cardio)-**pulmonary syndrome**) B33.4

Sinding-Larsen disease or osteochondrosis —*see*
  Osteochondrosis, juvenile, patella

Singapore hemorrhagic fever A91

Singer's node or nodule J38.2

Single
  atrium Q21.2
  coronary artery Q24.5
  umbilical artery Q27.0
  ventricle Q20.4

Singultus R06.6
  epidemicus B33.0

Sinus —*see also* Fistula
  abdominal K63.89
  arrest I45.5
  arrhythmia I49.8
  bradycardia R00.1
  branchial cleft (internal) (external)
    Q18.0
  coccygeal —*see* Sinus, pilonidal
  dental K04.6
  dermal (congenital) Q06.8
    with abscess Q06.8
    coccygeal, pilonidal —*see* Sinus,
      coccygeal
  infected, skin NEC L08.89
  marginal, ruptured or bleeding —
    see Hemorrhage, antepartum,
    specified cause NEC
  medial, face and neck Q18.8
  pause I45.5
  pericranii Q01.9
  pilonidal (infected) (rectum) L05.92
    with abscess L05.02
  preauricular Q18.1
  rectovaginal N82.3
  Rokitansky-Aschoff (gallbladder)
    K82.8
  sacrococcygeal (dermoid)
    (infected) —*see* Sinus, pilonidal
  tachycardia R00.0
    paroxysmal I47.1
  tarsi syndrome M25.57-
  testis N50.89
  tract (postinfective) —*see* Fistula
  urachus Q64.4

Sinusitis (accessory) (chronic)
  (hyperplastic) (nasal) (nonpurulent)
  (purulent) J32.9
  acute J01.90
    ethmoidal J01.20
      recurrent J01.21
    frontal J01.10
      recurrent J01.11
    involving more than one sinus,
      other than pansinusitis J01.80
      recurrent J01.81
    maxillary J01.00
      recurrent J01.01

Sinusitis *(continued)*
  acute *(continued)*
    pansinusitis J01.40
      recurrent J01.41
    recurrent J01.91
    specified NEC J01.80
      recurrent J01.81
    sphenoidal J01.30
      recurrent J01.31
  allergic —*see* Rhinitis, allergic
  due to high altitude T70.1
  ethmoidal J32.2
    acute J01.20
      recurrent J01.21
  frontal J32.1
    acute J01.10
      recurrent J01.11
  influenzal —*see* Influenza, with,
    respiratory manifestations NEC
  involving more than one sinus but
    not pansinusitis J32.8
    acute J01.80
      recurrent J01.81
  maxillary J32.0
    acute J01.00
      recurrent J01.01
  sphenoidal J32.3
    acute J01.30
      recurrent J01.31
  tuberculous, any sinus A15.8

Sinusitis-bronchiectasis-situs inversus (syndrome) (triad) Q89.3

Sipple's syndrome E31.22

Sirenomelia (syndrome) Q87.2

Siriasis T67.01

Sirkari's disease B55.0

Siti A65

Situation, psychiatric F99

Situational
  disturbance (transient) —*see*
    Disorder, adjustment
    acute F43.0
  maladjustment —*see* Disorder,
    adjustment
  reaction —*see* Disorder, adjustment
    acute F43.0

Situs inversus or transversus
  (abdominalis) (thoracis) Q89.3

Sixth disease B08.20
  due to human herpesvirus 6 B08.21
  due to human herpesvirus 7 B08.22

Sjögren-Larsson syndrome Q87.19

Sjögren's syndrome or disease —
  see Sicca syndrome

Skeletal —*see* condition

Skene's gland —*see* condition

Skenitis —*see* Urethritis

Skerljevo A65

Skevas-Zerfus disease —*see*
  Toxicity, venom, marine animal,
  sea anemone

Skin —*see also* condition
  clammy R23.1
  donor —*see* Donor, skin
  hidebound M35.9

Slate-dressers' or slate-miners' lung J62.8

Sleep
  apnea —*see* Apnea, sleep
  deprivation Z72.820
  disorder or disturbance G47.9
    child F51.9
    nonorganic origin F51.9
    specified NEC G47.8

Sleep *(continued)*
  disturbance G47.9
    nonorganic origin F51.9
  drunkenness F51.9
  rhythm inversion G47.2-
  terrors F51.4
  walking F51.3
    hysterical F44.89

Sleep hygiene
  abuse Z72.821
  inadequate Z72.821
  poor Z72.821

Sleeping sickness —*see* Sickness,
  sleeping

Sleeplessness —*see* Insomnia
  menopausal N95.1

Sleep-wake schedule disorder G47.20

Slim disease (in HIV infection) B20

Slipped, slipping
  epiphysis (traumatic) —*see also*
    Osteochondropathy, specified
    type NEC
    capital femoral (traumatic)
      acute (on chronic) S79.01-
    current traumatic - code as
      Fracture, by site
    upper femoral (nontraumatic)
      M93.00-
      acute M93.01-
        on chronic M93.03-
      chronic M93.02-
  intervertebral disc —*see*
    Displacement, intervertebral disc
  ligature, umbilical P51.8
  patella —*see* Disorder, patella,
    derangement NEC
  rib M89.8X8
  sacroiliac joint —*see* subcategory
    M53.2
  tendon —*see* Disorder, tendon
  ulnar nerve, nontraumatic —*see*
    Lesion, nerve, ulnar
  vertebra NEC —*see*
    Spondylolisthesis

Slocumb's syndrome E27.0

Sloughing (multiple) (phagedena)
  (skin) —*see also* Gangrene
  abscess —*see* Abscess
  appendix K38.8
  sfascia —*see* Disorder, soft tissue,
    specified type NEC
  scrotum N50.89
  tendon —*see* Disorder, tendon
  transplanted organ —*see* Rejection,
    transplant
  ulcer —*see* Ulcer, skin

Slow
  feeding, newborn P92.2
  flow syndrome, coronary I20.8
  heart (beat) R00.1

Slowing, urinary stream R39.198

Sluder's neuralgia (syndrome) G44.89

Slurred, slurring speech R47.81

Small (ness)
  for gestational age —*see* Small for
    dates
  introitus, vagina N89.6
  kidney (unknown cause) N27.9
    bilateral N27.1
    unilateral N27.0
  ovary (congenital) Q50.39
  pelvis
    with disproportion (fetopelvic)
      O33.1
      causing obstructed labor O65.1
  uterus N85.8
  white kidney N03.9

Small-and-light-for-dates —*see*
  Small for dates

Small-for-dates (infant) P05.10
  with weight of
    499 grams or less P05.11
    500-749 grams P05.12
    750-999 grams P05.13
    1000-1249 grams P05.14
    1250-1499 grams P05.15
    1500-1749 grams P05.16
    1750-1999 grams P05.17
    2000-2499 grams P05.18
    2500 grams and over P05.19
  specified NEC P05.19

Smallpox B03

Smearing, fecal R15.1

SMEI (severe myoclonic epilepsy in
  infancy) G40.83-

Smith-Lemli-Opitz syndrome
  E78.72

Smith's fracture S52.54-

Smoker —*see* Dependence, drug,
  nicotine

Smoker's
  bronchitis J41.0
  cough J41.0
  palate K13.24
  throat J31.2
  tongue K13.24

Smoking
  passive Z77.22

Smothering spells R06.81

Snaggle teeth, tooth M26.39

Snapping
  finger —*see* Trigger finger
  hip —*see* Derangement, joint,
    specified type NEC, hip
    involving the iliotibial band
    M76.3-
  knee —*see* Derangement, knee
    involving the iliotibial band
    M76.3-

Sneddon-Wilkinson disease or syndrome (sub-corneal pustular
  dermatosis) L13.1

Sneezing (intractable) R06.7

Sniffing
  cocaine
    abuse —*see* Abuse, drug, cocaine
    dependence —*see* Dependence,
      drug, cocaine
  gasoline
    abuse —*see* Abuse, drug,
      inhalant
    dependence —*see* Dependence,
      drug, inhalant
  glue (airplane)
    abuse —*see* Abuse, drug,
      inhalant
    drug dependence —*see*
      Dependence, drug, inhalant

Sniffles
  newborn P28.89

Snoring R06.83

Snow blindness —*see* Photokeratitis

Snuffles (non-syphilitic) R06.5
  newborn P28.89
  syphilitic (infant) A50.05 *[J99]*

Social
  exclusion Z60.4
    due to discrimination or
      persecution (perceived) Z60.5
  migrant Z59.0
  acculturation difficulty Z60.3

Silo-fillers' disease–Social

Social *(continued)*
  rejection Z60.4
    due to discrimination or
      persecution Z60.5
    role conflict NEC Z73.5
    skills inadequacy NEC Z73.4
    transplantation Z60.3

Sodoku A25.0

Soemmerring's ring *—see* Cataract, secondary

Soft *—see also* condition
  nails L60.3

Softening
  bone *—see* Osteomalacia
  brain (necrotic) (progressive)
    G93.89
    congenital Q04.8
    embolic I63.4-
    hemorrhagic *—see* Hemorrhage,
      intracranial, intracerebral
    occlusive I63.5-
    thrombotic I63.3-
  cartilage M94.2-
    patella M22.4-
  cerebellar *—see* Softening, brain
  cerebral *—see* Softening, brain
  cerebrospinal *—see* Softening,
    brain
  myocardial, heart *—see*
    Degeneration, myocardial
  spinal cord G95.89
  stomach K31.89

Soldier's
  heart F45.8
  patches I31.0

Solitary
  cyst, kidney N28.1
  kidney, congenital Q60.0

Solvent abuse *—see* Abuse, drug,
  inhalant
  dependence *—see* Dependence,
    drug, inhalant

**Somatization reaction, somatic
reaction** *see* Disorder,
  somatoform

Somnambulism F51.3
  hysterical F44.89

Somnolence R40.0
  nonorganic origin F51.11

Sonne dysentery A03.3

Soor B37.0

Sore
  bed *—see* Ulcer, pressure, by site
  chiclero B55.1
  Delhi B55.1
  desert *—see* Ulcer, skin
  eye H57.1-
  Lahore B55.1
  mouth K13.79
    canker K12.0
  muscle M79.10
  Naga *—see* Ulcer, skin
  of skin *—see* Ulcer, skin
  oriental B55.1
  pressure *—see* Ulcer, pressure,
    by site
  skin L98.9
  soft A57
  throat (acute) *—see also*
    Pharyngitis
    with influenza, flu, or grippe
      —see Influenza, with,
      respiratory manifestations
      NEC
    chronic J31.2
    coxsackie (virus) B08.5

Sore *(continued)*
  throat *(continued)*
    diphtheritic A36.0
    herpesviral B00.2
    influenzal *—see* Influenza, with,
      respiratory manifestations NEC
    septic J02.0
    streptococcal (ulcerative) J02.0
    viral NEC J02.8
      coxsackie B08.5
    tropical *—see* Ulcer, skin
    veldt *—see* Ulcer, skin

Soto's syndrome (cerebral gigantism)
  Q87.3

**South African cardiomyopathy
syndrome** I42.8

Southeast Asian hemorrhagic fever
  A91

Spacing
  abnormal, tooth, teeth, fully
    erupted M26.30
  excessive, tooth, fully erupted
    M26.32

Spade-like hand (congenital) Q68.1

Spading nail L60.8
  congenital Q84.6

Spanish collar N47.1

Sparganosis B70.1

Spasm(s), spastic, spasticity *(see
also* condition) R25.2
  accommodation *—see* Spasm, of
    accommodation
  ampulla of Vater K83.4
  anus, ani (sphincter) (reflex) K59.4
    psychogenic F45.8
  artery I73.9
    cerebral G45.9
  Bell's G51.3-
  bladder (sphincter, external or
    internal) N32.89
    psychogenic F45.8
  bronchus, bronchiole J98.01
  cardia K22.0
  cardiac I20.1
  carpopedal *—see* Tetany
  cerebral (arteries) (vascular) G45.9
  cervix, complicating delivery
    O62.4
  ciliary body (of accommodation)
    —see Spasm, of accommodation
  colon (*see also* Irritable, bowel)
    K58.9
    with diarrhea K58.0
    psychogenic F45.8
  common duct K83.8
  compulsive *—see* Tic
  conjugate H51.8
  coronary (artery) I20.1
  diaphragm (reflex) R06.6
    epidemic B33.0
    psychogenic F45.8
  duodenum K59.89
  epidemic diaphragmatic (transient)
    B33.0
  esophagus (diffuse) K22.4
    psychogenic F45.8
  facial G51.3-
  fallopian tube N83.8
  gastrointestinal (tract) K31.89
    psychogenic F45.8
  glottis J38.5
    hysterical F44.4
    psychogenic F45.8
      conversion reaction F44.4
    reflex through recurrent
      laryngeal nerve J38.5
  habit *—see* Tic
  heart I20.1

Spasm(s), spastic, spasticity
(continued)
  hemifacial (clonic) G51.3-
  hourglass *—see* Contraction,
    hourglass
  hysterical F44.4
  infantile *—see* Epilepsy, spasms
  inferior oblique, eye H51.8
  intestinal (*see also* Syndrome,
    irritable bowel) K58.9
    psychogenic F45.8
  larynx, laryngeal J38.5
    hysterical F44.4
    psychogenic F45.8
      conversion reaction F44.4
  levator palpebrae superioris *—see*
    Disorder, eyelid function
  muscle NEC M62.838
    back M62.830
  nerve, trigeminal G51.0
  nervous F45.8
  nodding F98.4
  occupational F48.8
  oculogyric H51.8
    psychogenic F45.8
  of accommodation H52.53-
  ophthalmic artery *—see* Occlusion,
    artery, retina
  perineal, female N94.89
  peroneo-extensor *—see also*
    Deformity, limb, flat foot
  pharynx (reflex) J39.2
    hysterical F45.8
    psychogenic F45.8
  psychogenic F45.8
  pylorus NEC K31.3
    adult hypertrophic K31.89
    congenital or infantile Q40.0
    psychogenic F45.8
  rectum (sphincter) K59.4
    psychogenic F45.8
  retinal (artery) *—see* Occlusion,
    artery, retina
  sigmoid (*see also* Syndrome,
    irritable bowel) K58.9
    psychogenic F45.8
  sphincter of Oddi K83.4
  stomach K31.89
    neurotic F45.8
  throat J39.2
    hysterical F45.8
    psychogenic F45.8
  tic F95.9
    chronic F95.1
    transient of childhood F95.0
  tongue K14.8
  torsion (progressive) G24.1
  trigeminal nerve *—see* Neuralgia,
    trigeminal
  ureter N13.5
  urethra (sphincter) N35.919
  uterus N85.8
    complicating labor O62.4
  vagina N94.2
    psychogenic F52.5
  vascular I73.9
  vasomotor I73.9
  vein NEC I87.8
  viscera *—see* Pain, abdominal

Spasmodic *—see* condition

Spasmophilia *—see* Tetany

Spasmus nutans F98.4

Spastic, spasticity *—see also*
  Spasm
  child (cerebral) (congenital)
    (paralysis) G80.1

Speaker's throat R49.8

Specific, specified *—see* condition

Speech
  defect, disorder, disturbance,
    impediment *—see* Disorder,
    speech R47.9
    psychogenic, in childhood and
      adolescence F98.8
    slurring R47.81
    specified NEC R47.89

Spencer's disease A08.19

Spens' syndrome (syncope with
  heart block) I45.9

Sperm counts (fertility testing) Z31.41
  postvasectomy Z30.8
  reversal Z31.42

Spermatic cord *—see* condition

Spermatocele N43.40
  congenital Q55.4
  multiple N43.42
  single N43.41

Spermatocystitis N49.0

Spermatocytoma C62.9-
  specified site *—see* Neoplasm,
    malignant, by site

Spermatorrhea N50.89

Sphacelus *—see* Gangrene

Sphenoidal *—see* condition

Sphenoiditis (chronic) *—see*
  Sinusitis, sphenoidal

Sphenopalatine ganglion neuralgia
  G90.09

Sphericity, increased, lens
  (congenital) Q12.4

Spherocytosis (congenital) (familial)
  (hereditary) D58.0
  hemoglobin disease D58.0
  sickle-cell (disease) D57.8-

Spherophakia Q12.4

Sphincter *—see* condition

Sphincteritis, sphincter of Oddi *—
  see* Cholangitis

Sphingolipidosis E75.3
  specified NEC E75.29

Sphingomyelinosis E75.3

Spicule tooth K00.2

Spider
  bite *—see* Toxicity, venom, spider
    nonvenomous *—see* Bite, by
      site, superficial, insect
  fingers *—see* Syndrome, Marfan's
  nevus I78.1
  toes *—see* Syndrome, Marfan's
  vascular I78.1

Spiegler-Fendt
  benign lymphocytoma L98.8
  sarcoid L08.89

Spielmeyer-Vogt disease E75.4

Spina bifida (aperta) Q05.9
  with hydrocephalus NEC Q05.4
  cervical Q05.5
    with hydrocephalus Q05.0
  dorsal Q05.6
    with hydrocephalus Q05.1
  lumbar Q05.7
    with hydrocephalus Q05.2
  lumbosacral Q05.7
    with hydrocephalus Q05.2
  occulta Q76.0
  sacral Q05.8
    with hydrocephalus Q05.3
  thoracic Q05.6
    with hydrocephalus Q05.1
  thoracolumbar Q05.6
    with hydrocephalus Q05.1

Spindle, Krukenberg's —*see*
    Pigmentation, cornea, posterior

Spine, spinal —*see* condition

Spiradenoma (eccrine) —*see*
    Neoplasm, skin, benign

Spirillosis A25.0

Spirillum
    minus A25.0
    obermeieri infection A68.0

Spirochetal —*see* condition

Spirochetosis A69.9
    arthritic, arthritica A69.9
    bronchopulmonary A69.8
    icterohemorrhagic A27.0
    lung A69.8

Spirometrosis B70.1

Spitting blood —*see* Hemoptysis

Splanchnoptosis K63.4

Spleen, splenic —*see* condition

Splenectasis —*see* Splenomegaly

Splenitis (interstitial) (malignant)
    (nonspecific) D73.89
    malarial (*see also* Malaria) B54 *[D77]*
    tuberculous A18.85

Splenocele D73.89

Splenomegaly, splenomegalia
    (Bengal) (cryptogenic) (idiopathic)
    (tropical) R16.1
    with hepatomegaly R16.2
    cirrhotic D73.2
    congenital Q89.09
    congestive, chronic D73.2
    Egyptian B65.1
    Gaucher's E75.22
    malarial (*see also* Malaria) B54
      [D77]
    neutropenic D73.81
    Niemann-Pick —*see* Niemann-Pick
      disease or syndrome
    siderotic D73.2
    syphilitic A52.79
      congenital (early) A50.08 *[D77]*

Splenopathy D73.9

Splenoptosis D73.89

Splenosis D73.89

Splinter —*see* Foreign body,
    superficial, by site

Split, splitting
    foot Q72.7-
    hand Q71.6
    heart sounds R01.2
    lip, congenital —*see* Cleft, lip
    nails L60.3
    urinary stream R39.13

Spondylarthrosis —*see* Spondylosis

Spondylitis (chronic) —*see also*
    Spondylopathy, inflammatory
    ankylopoietica —*see* Spondylitis,
      ankylosing
    ankylosing (chronic) M45.9
      with lung involvement M45.9 *[J99]*
      cervical region M45.2
      cervicothoracic region M45.3
      juvenile M08.1
      lumbar region M45.6
      lumbosacral region M45.7
      multiple sites M45.0
      occipito-atlanto-axial region M45.1
      sacrococcygeal region M45.8
      thoracic region M45.4
      thoracolumbar region M45.5
    atrophic (ligamentous) —*see*
      Spondylitis, ankylosing

Spondylitis (continued)
    deformans (chronic) —*see*
      Spondylosis
    gonococcal A54.41
    gouty (*see also* Gout, by type,
      vertebrae) M10.08
    in (due to)
      brucellosis A23.9 *[M49.80]*
        cervical region A23.9
        [M49.82]
        cervicothoracic region A23.9
        [M49.83]
        lumbar region A23.9
        [M49.86]
        lumbosacral region A23.9
        [M49.87]
        multiple sites A23.9 *[M49.89]*
        occipito-atlanto-axial region
        A23.9 *[M49.81]*
        sacrococcygeal region A23.9
        [M49.88]
        thoracic region A23.9
        [M49.84]
        thoracolumbar region A23.9
        [M49.85]
      enterobacteria (*see also*
        subcategory M49.8) A04.9
      tuberculosis A18.01
    infectious NEC —*see*
      Spondylopathy, infective
    juvenile ankylosing (chronic) M08.1
    Kümmell's —*see* Spondylopathy,
      traumatic
    Marie-Strümpell —*see* Spondylitis,
      ankylosing
    muscularis —*see* Spondylopathy,
      specified NEC
    psoriatic L40.53
    rheumatoid —*see* Spondylitis,
      ankylosing
    rhizomelica —*see* Spondylitis,
      ankylosing
    sacroiliac NEC M46.1
    senescent, senile —*see* Spondylosis
    traumatic (chronic) or post-
      traumatic —*see* Spondylopathy,
      traumatic
    tuberculous A18.01
    typhosa A01.05

Spondyloarthritis
    axial —*see also* Spondlyitis,
      ankylosing
      non-radiographic M46.80
        cervical M46.82
        cervicothoracic M46.83
        lumbar M46.84
        lumbosacral M46.87
        multiple sites M46.89
        occipito-atlanto-axial region
        M46.81
        sacral and sacrococcygeal
        M46.88
        thoracic M46.84
        thoracolumbar M46.85

Spondylolisthesis (acquired)
    (degenerative) M43.10
    with disproportion (fetopelvic)
      O33.0
      causing obstructed labor O65.0
    cervical region M43.12
    cervicothoracic region M43.13
    congenital Q76.2
    lumbar region M43.16
    lumbosacral region M43.17
    multiple sites M43.19
    occipito-atlanto-axial region
      M43.11
    sacrococcygeal region M43.18
    thoracic region M43.14
    thoracolumbar region M43.15

Spondylolisthesis (continued)
    traumatic (old) M43.10
      acute
        fifth cervical (displaced)
        S12.430
          nondisplaced S12.431
          specified type NEC
            (displaced) S12.450
            nondisplaced S12.451
          type III S12.44
        fourth cervical (displaced)
        S12.330
          nondisplaced S12.331
          specified type NEC
            (displaced) S12.350
            nondisplaced S12.351
          type III S12.34
        second cervical (displaced)
        S12.130
          nondisplaced S12.131
          specified type NEC
            (displaced) S12.150
            nondisplaced S12.151
          type III S12.14
        seventh cervical (displaced)
        S12.630
          nondisplaced S12.631
          specified type NEC
            (displaced) S12.650
            nondisplaced S12.651
          type III S12.64
        sixth cervical (displaced)
        S12.530
          nondisplaced S12.531
          specified type NEC
            (displaced) S12.550
            nondisplaced S12.551
          type III S12.54
        third cervical (displaced)
        S12.230
          nondisplaced S12.231
          specified type NEC
            (displaced) S12.250
            nondisplaced S12.251
          type III S12.24

Spondylolysis (acquired) M43.00
    cervical region M43.02
    cervicothoracic region M43.03
    congenital Q76.2
    lumbar region M43.06
    lumbosacral region M43.07
      with disproportion (fetopelvic)
      O33.0
      causing obstructed labor
      O65.8
    multiple sites M43.09
    occipito-atlanto-axial region M43.01
    sacrococcygeal region M43.08
    thoracic region M43.04
    thoracolumbar region M43.05

Spondylopathy M48.9
    infective NEC M46.50
      cervical region M46.52
      cervicothoracic region M46.53
      lumbar region M46.56
      lumbosacral region M46.57
      multiple sites M46.59
      occipito-atlanto-axial region
        M46.51
      sacrococcygeal region M46.58
      thoracic region M46.54
      thoracolumbar region M46.55
    inflammatory M46.90
      cervical region M46.92
      cervicothoracic region M46.93
      lumbar region M46.96
      lumbosacral region M46.97
      multiple sites M46.99
      occipito-atlanto-axial region
        M46.91
      sacrococcygeal region M46.98

Spondylopathy (continued)
    inflammatory (continued)
      specified type NEC M46.80
        cervical region M46.82
        cervicothoracic region M46.83
        lumbar region M46.86
        lumbosacral region M46.87
        multiple sites M46.89
        occipito-atlanto-axial region
        M46.81
        sacrococcygeal region M46.88
        thoracic region M46.84
        thoracolumbar region M46.85
      thoracic region M46.94
      thoracolumbar region M46.95
    neuropathic, in
      syringomyelia and syringobulbia
      G95.0
      tabes dorsalis A52.11
    specified NEC M48.8
    traumatic M48.30
      cervical region M48.32
      cervicothoracic region M48.33
      lumbar region M48.36
      lumbosacral region M48.37
      occipito-atlanto-axial region
        M48.31
      sacrococcygeal region M48.38
      thoracic region M48.34
      thoracolumbar region M48.35

Spondylosis M47.9
    with
      disproportion (fetopelvic) O33.0
        causing obstructed labor O65.0
      myelopathy NEC M47.10
        cervical region M47.12
        cervicothoracic region M47.13
        lumbar region M47.16
        occipito-atlanto-axial region
        M47.11
        thoracic region M47.14
        thoracolumbar region M47.15
      radiculopathy M47.20
        cervical region M47.22
        cervicothoracic region M47.23
        lumbar region M47.26
        lumbosacral region M47.27
        occipito-atlanto-axial region
        M47.21
        sacrococcygeal region M47.28
        thoracic region M47.24
        thoracolumbar region M47.25
    specified NEC M47.899
      cervical region M47.892
      cervicothoracic region M47.893
      lumbar region M47.896
      lumbosacral region M47.897
      occipito-atlanto-axial region
        M47.891
      sacrococcygeal region M47.898
      thoracic region M47.894
      thoracolumbar region M47.895
    traumatic —*see* Spondylopathy,
      traumatic
    without myelopathy or
      radiculopathy M47.819
      cervical region M47.812
      cervicothoracic region M47.813
      lumbar region M47.816
      lumbosacral region M47.817
      occipito-atlanto-axial region
        M47.811
      sacrococcygeal region M47.818
      thoracic region M47.814
      thoracolumbar region M47.815

Sponge
    inadvertently left in operation
      wound —*see* Foreign body,
      accidentally left during a procedure
    kidney (medullary) Q61.5

Sprain *(continued)*
  ulna, collateral —*see* Rupture, traumatic, ligament, ulnar collateral
  ulnohumeral —*see* Sprain, elbow
  wrist S63.50-
    carpal S63.51-
    radiocarpal S63.52-
    specified site NEC S63.59-
  xiphoid cartilage —*see* Sprain, sternum

Sprengel's deformity (congenital) Q74.0

Sprue (tropical) K90.1
  celiac K90.0
  idiopathic K90.49
  meaning thrush B37.0
  nontropical K90.0

Spur, bone —*see also* Enthesopathy
  calcaneal M77.3-
  iliac crest M76.2-
  nose (septum) J34.89

Spurway's syndrome Q78.0

Sputum
  abnormal (amount) (color) (odor) (purulent) R09.3
  blood-stained R04.2
  excessive (cause unknown) R09.3

Squamous —*see also* condition
  epithelium in
    cervical canal (congenital) Q51.828
    uterine mucosa (congenital) Q51.818

Squashed nose M95.0
  congenital Q67.4

Squeeze, diver's T70.3

Squint —*see also* Strabismus
  accommodative —*see* Strabismus, convergent concomitant

SSADHD (succinic semialdehyde dehydrogenase deficiency) E72.81

St. Hubert's disease A82.9

Stab —*see also* Laceration
  internal organs —*see* Injury, by site

Stafne's cyst or cavity M27.0

Staggering gait R26.0
  hysterical F44.4

Staghorn calculus —*see* Calculus, kidney

Stähli's line (cornea) (pigment) —*see* Pigmentation, cornea, anterior

Stain, staining
  meconium (newborn) P96.83
  port wine Q82.5
  tooth, teeth (hard tissues) (extrinsic) K03.6
    due to
      accretions K03.6
      deposits (betel) (black) (green) (materia alba) (orange) (soft) (tobacco) K03.6
      metals (copper) (silver) K03.7
      nicotine K03.6
      pulpal bleeding K03.7
      tobacco K03.6
    intrinsic K00.8

Stammering *(see also* Disorder, fluency) F80.81

Standstill
  auricular I45.5
  cardiac —*see* Arrest, cardiac
  sinoatrial I45.5
  ventricular —*see* Arrest, cardiac

Stannosis J63.5

Stanton's disease —*see* Melioidosis

Staphylitis (acute) (catarrhal) (chronic) (gangrenous) (membranous) (suppurative) (ulcerative) K12.2

Staphylococcal scalded skin syndrome L00

Staphylococcemia A41.2

Staphylococcus, staphylococcal
  —*see also* condition
  as cause of disease classified elsewhere B95.8
    aureus (methicillin susceptible) (MSSA) B95.61
      methicillin resistant (MRSA) B95.62
    specified NEC, as cause of disease classified elsewhere B95.7

Staphyloma (sclera)
  cornea H18.72-
  equatorial H15.81-
  localized (anterior) H15.82-
  posticum H15.83-
  ring H15.85-

Stargardt's disease —*see* Dystrophy, retina

Starvation (inanition) (due to lack of food) T73.0
  edema —*see* Malnutrition, severe

Stasis
  bile (noncalculous) K83.1
  bronchus J98.09
    with infection —*see* Bronchitis
  cardiac —*see* Failure, heart, congestive
  cecum K59.89
  colon K59.89
  dermatitis I87.2
    with
      varicose ulcer —*see* Varix, leg, with ulcer, with inflammation
      varicose veins —*see* Varix, leg, with inflammation
    due to postthrombotic syndrome —*see* Syndrome, postthombotic
  duodenal K31.5
  eczema —*see* Varix, leg, with, inflammation
  edema —*see* Hypertension, venous (chronic), idiopathic
  foot T69.0-
  ileocecal coil K59.89
  ileum K59.89
  intestinal K59.89
  jejunum K59.89
  kidney N19
  liver (cirrhotic) K76.1
  lymphatic I89.8
  pneumonia J18.2
  pulmonary —*see* Edema, lung
  rectal K59.89
  renal N19
    tubular N17.0
  ulcer —*see* Varix, leg, with, ulcer
    without varicose veins I87.2
  urine —*see* Retention, urine
  venous I87.8

State (of)
  affective and paranoid, mixed, organic psychotic F06.8
  agitated R45.1
    acute reaction to stress F43.0
  anxiety (neurotic) F41.1
  apprehension F41.1
  burn-out Z73.0
  climacteric, female Z78.0
    symptomatic N95.1

State *(continued)*
  compulsive F42.8
    mixed with obsessional thoughts F42.2
  confusional (psychogenic) F44.89
    acute —*see also* Delirium
      with
        arteriosclerotic dementia F01.50
          with behavioral disturbance F01.51
        senility or dementia F05
      alcoholic F10.231
    epileptic F05
    reactive (from emotional stress, psychological trauma) F44.89
    subacute —*see* Delirium
  convulsive —*see* Convulsions
  crisis F43.0
  depressive F32.9
    neurotic F34.1
  dissociative F44.9
  emotional shock (stress) R45.7
  hypercoagulation —*see* Hypercoagulable
  locked-in G83.5
  menopausal Z78.0
    symptomatic N95.1
  neurotic F48.9
    with depersonalization F48.1
  obsessional F42.8
  oneiroid (schizophrenia-like) F23
  organic
    hallucinatory (nonalcoholic) F06.0
    paranoid (-hallucinatory) F06.2
  panic F41.0
  paranoid F22
    climacteric F22
    involutional F22
    menopausal F22
    organic F06.2
    senile F03
    simple F22
  persistent vegetative R40.3
  phobic F40.9
  postleukotomy F07.0
  pregnant
    gestational carrier Z33.3
    incidental Z33.1
  psychogenic, twilight F44.89
  psychopathic (constitutional) F60.2
  psychotic, organic —*see also* Psychosis, organic
    mixed paranoid and affective F06.8
    senile or presenile F03
    transient NEC F06.8
      with
        hallucinations F06.0
        depression F06.31
  residual schizophrenic F20.5
  restlessness R45.1
  stress (emotional) R45.7
  tension (mental) F48.9
    specified NEC F48.8
  transient organic psychotic NEC F06.8
    depressive type F06.31
    hallucinatory type F06.0
  twilight
    epileptic F05
    psychogenic F44.89
  vegetative, persistent R40.3
  vital exhaustion Z73.0
  withdrawal, —*see* Withdrawal, state

Status (post) —*see also* Presence (of)
  absence, epileptic —*see* Epilepsy, by type, with status epilepticus

Status *(continued)*
  administration of tPA (rtPA) in a different facility within the last 24 hours prior to admission to current facility Z92.82
  adrenalectomy (unilateral) (bilateral) E89.6
  anastomosis Z98.0
  angioplasty (peripheral) Z98.62
    with implant Z95.820
    coronary artery Z98.61
      with implant Z95.5
  anginosus I20.9
  aortocoronary bypass Z95.1
  arthrodesis Z98.1
  artificial opening (of) Z93.9
    gastrointestinal tract Z93.4
    specified NEC Z93.8
    urinary tract Z93.6
    vagina Z93.8
  asthmaticus —*see* Asthma, by type, with status asthmaticus
  awaiting organ transplant Z76.82
  bariatric surgery Z98.84
  bed confinement Z74.01
  bleb, filtering (vitreous), after glaucoma surgery Z98.83
  breast implant Z98.82
    removal Z98.86
  cataract extraction Z98.4-
  cholecystectomy Z90.49
  clitorectomy N90.811
    with excision of labia minora N90.812
  colectomy (complete) (partial) Z90.49
  colonization —*see* Carrier (suspected) of
  colostomy Z93.3
  convulsivus idiopathicus —*see* Epilepsy, by type, with status epilepticus
  coronary artery angioplasty —*see* Status, angioplasty, coronary artery
  coronary artery bypass graft Z95.1
  cystectomy (urinary bladder) Z90.6
  cystostomy Z93.50
    appendico-vesicostomy Z93.52
    cutaneous Z93.51
    specified NEC Z93.59
  delinquent immunization Z28.3
  dental Z98.818
    crown Z98.811
    fillings Z98.811
    restoration Z98.811
    sealant Z98.810
    specified NEC Z98.818
  deployment (current) (military) Z56.82
  dialysis (hemodialysis) (peritoneal) Z99.2
  do not resuscitate (DNR) Z66
  donor —*see* Donor
  embedded fragments —*see* Retained, foreign body fragments (type of)
  embedded splinter —*see* Retained, foreign body fragments (type of)
  enterostomy Z93.4
  epileptic, epilepticus *(see also* Epilepsy, by type, with status epilepticus) G40.901
  estrogen receptor
    negative Z17.1
    positive Z17.0
  female genital cutting —*see* Female genital mutilation status
  female genital mutilation —*see* Female genital mutilation status

filtering (vitreous) bleb after glaucoma surgery Z98.83
gastrectomy (complete) (partial) Z90.3
gastric banding Z98.84
gastric bypass for obesity Z98.84
gastrostomy Z93.1
human immunodeficiency virus (HIV) infection, asymptomatic Z21
hysterectomy (complete) (total) Z90.710
  partial (with remaining cervial stump) Z90.711
ileostomy Z93.2
implant
  breast Z98.82
infibulation N90.813
intestinal bypass Z98.0
jejunostomy Z93.4
laryngectomy Z90.02
lapsed immunization schedule Z28.3
lymphaticus E32.8
malignancy
  castrate resistant prostate Z19.2
  hormone resistant Z19.2
  hormone sensitive Z19.1
marmoratus G80.3
mastectomy (unilateral) (bilateral) Z90.1-
military deployment status (current) Z56.82
  in theater or in support of military war, peacekeeping and humanitarian operations Z56.82
nephrectomy (unilateral) (bilateral) Z90.5
nephrostomy Z93.6
obesity surgery Z98.84
oophorectomy
  bilateral Z90.722
  unilateral Z90.721
organ replacement
  by artificial or mechanical device or prosthesis of
    artery Z95.828
    bladder Z96.0
    blood vessel Z95.828
    breast Z97.8
    eye globe Z97.0
    heart Z95.812
      valve Z95.2
    intestine Z97.8
    joint Z96.60
      hip —*see* Presence, hip joint implant
      knee —*see* Presence, knee joint implant
      specified site NEC Z96.698
    kidney Z97.8
    larynx Z96.3
    lens Z96.1
    limbs —*see* Presence, artificial, limb
    liver Z97.8
    lung Z97.8
    pancreas Z97.8
  by organ transplant (heterologous)(homologous) —*see* Transplant
pacemaker
  brain Z96.89
  cardiac Z95.0
  specified NEC Z96.89
pancreatectomy Z90.410
  complete Z90.410
  partial Z90.411
  total Z90.410

physical restraint Z78.1
pneumonectomy (complete) (partial) Z90.2
pneumothorax, therapeutic Z98.3
postcommotio cerebri F07.81
postoperative (postprocedural) NEC Z98.890
  breast implant Z98.82
  dental Z98.818
    crown Z98.811
    fillings Z98.811
    restoration Z98.811
    sealant Z98.810
    specified NEC Z98.818
  pneumothorax, therapeutic Z98.3
  uterine scar Z98.891
postpartum (routine follow-up) Z39.2
  care immediately after delivery Z39.0
postsurgical (postprocedural) NEC Z98.890
  pneumothorax, therapeutic Z98.3
pregnancy, incidental Z33.1
prosthesis coronary angioplasty Z95.5
pseudophakia Z96.1
renal dialysis (hemodialysis) (peritoneal) Z99.2
retained foreign body —*see* Retained, foreign body fragments (type of)
reversed jejunal transposition (for bypass) Z98.0
salpingo-oophorectomy
  bilateral Z90.722
  unilateral Z90.721
sex reassignment surgery status Z87.890
shunt
  arteriovenous (for dialysis) Z99.2
  cerebrospinal fluid Z98.2
  ventricular (communicating) (for drainage) Z98.2
splenectomy Z90.81
thymicolymphaticus E32.8
thymicus E32.8
thymolymphaticus E32.8
thyroidectomy (hypothyroidism) E89.0
tooth (teeth) extraction (*see also* Absence, teeth, acquired) K08.409
tPA (rtPA) administration in a different facility within the last 24 hours prior to admission to current facility Z92.82
tracheostomy Z93.0
transplant —*see* Transplant
  organ removed Z98.85
tubal ligation Z98.51
underimmunization Z28.3
ureterostomy Z93.6
urethrostomy Z93.6
vagina, artificial Z93.8
vasectomy Z98.52
wheelchair confinement Z99.3

Stealing
child problem F91.8
  in company with others Z72.810
pathological (compulsive) F63.2

Steam burn —*see* Burn

Steatocystoma multiplex L72.2

Steatohepatitis (nonalcoholic) (NASH) K75.81

Steatoma L72.3
eyelid (cystic) —*see* Dermatosis, eyelid
  infected —*see* Hordeolum

Steatorrhea (chronic) K90.4
with lacteal obstruction K90.2
idiopathic (adult) (infantile) K90.9
pancreatic K90.3
primary K90.0
tropical K90.1

Steatosis E88.89
heart —*see* Degeneration, myocardial
kidney N28.89
liver NEC K76.0

Steele-Richardson-Olszewski disease or syndrome G23.1

Steinbrocker's syndrome G90.8

Steinert's disease G71.11

Stein-Leventhal syndrome E28.2

Stein's syndrome E28.2

STEMI (*see also* Infarct, myocardium ST elevation) I21.3

Stenocardia I20.8

Stenocephaly Q75.8

Stenosis, stenotic (cicatricial) —*see also* Stricture
ampulla of Vater K83.1
anus, anal (canal) (sphincter) K62.4
  and rectum K62.4
  congenital Q42.3
    with fistula Q42.2
aorta (ascending) (supraventricular) (congenital) Q25.1
  arteriosclerotic I70.0
  calcified I70.0
  supravalvular Q25.3
aortic (valve) I35.0
  with insufficiency I35.2
  congenital Q23.0
  rheumatic I06.0
    with
      incompetency, insufficiency or regurgitation I06.2
      with mitral (valve) disease I08.0
        with tricuspid (valve) disease I08.3
      mitral (valve) disease I08.0
        with tricuspid (valve) disease I08.3
      tricuspid (valve) disease I08.2
        with mitral (valve) disease I08.3
  specified cause NEC I35.0
  syphilitic A52.03
aqueduct of Sylvius (congenital) Q03.0
  with spina bifida —*see* Spina bifida, by site, with hydrocephalus
  acquired G91.1
artery NEC (*see also* Arteriosclerosis) I77.1
  celiac I77.4
  cerebral —*see* Occlusion, artery, cerebral
  extremities —*see* Arteriosclerosis, extremities
  precerebral —*see* Occlusion, artery, precerebral
  pulmonary (congenital) Q25.6
    acquired I28.8
  renal I70.1
  stent
    coronary T82.855
    peripheral T82.856

bile duct (common) (hepatic) K83.1
  congenital Q44.3
bladder-neck (acquired) N32.0
  congenital Q64.31
brain G93.89
bronchus J98.09
  congenital Q32.3
  syphilitic A52.72
cardia (stomach) K22.2
  congenital Q39.3
cardiovascular —*see* Disease, cardiovascular
caudal M48.08
cervix, cervical (canal) N88.2
  congenital Q51.828
  in pregnancy or childbirth —*see* Pregnancy, complicated by, abnormal cervix
colon —*see also* Obstruction, intestine
  congenital Q42.9
  specified NEC Q42.8
colostomy K94.03
common (bile) duct K83.1
  congenital Q44.3
coronary (artery) —*see* Disease, heart, ischemic, atherosclerotic
cystic duct —*see* Obstruction, gallbladder
due to presence of device, implant or graft (*see also* Complications, by site and type, specified NEC) T85.858
  arterial graft NEC T82.858
  breast (implant) T85.858
  catheter T85.858
    dialysis (renal) T82.858
      intraperitoneal T85.858
    infusion NEC T82.858
      spinal (epidural) (subdural) T85.850
    urinary (indwelling) T83.85
  fixation, internal (orthopedic) NEC T84.85
  gastrointestinal (bile duct) (esophagus) T85.858
  genital NEC T83.85
  heart NEC T82.857
  joint prosthesis T84.85
  ocular (corneal graft) (orbital implant) NEC T85.858
  orthopedic NEC T84.85
  specified NEC T85.858
  urinary NEC T83.85
  vascular NEC T82.858
  ventricular intracranial shunt T85.850
duodenum K31.5
  congenital Q41.0
ejaculatory duct NEC N50.89
endocervical os —*see* Stenosis, cervix
enterostomy K94.13
esophagus K22.2
  congenital Q39.3
  syphilitic A52.79
    congenital A50.59 *[K23]*
eustachian tube —*see* Obstruction, eustachian tube
external ear canal (acquired) H61.30-
  congenital Q16.1
  due to
    inflammation H61.32-
    trauma H61.31-
  postprocedural H95.81-
  specified cause NEC H61.39-
gallbladder —*see* Obstruction, gallbladder

Stenosis, stenotic (continued)

glottis J38.6
heart valve (congenital) Q24.8
  aortic Q23.0
  mitral Q23.2
  pulmonary Q22.1
  tricuspid Q22.4
hepatic duct K83.1
hymen N89.6
hypertrophic subaortic (idiopathic) I42.1
ileum (see also Obstruction, intestine, specified NEC) K56.699
  congenital Q41.2
infundibulum cardia Q24.3
intervertebral foramina —see also Lesion, biomechanical, specified NEC
  connective tissue M99.79
    abdomen M99.79
    cervical region M99.71
    cervicothoracic M99.71
    head region M99.70
    lumbar region M99.73
    lumbosacral M99.73
    occipitocervical M99.70
    sacral region M99.74
    sacrococcygeal M99.74
    sacroiliac M99.74
    specified NEC M99.79
    thoracic region M99.72
    thoracolumbar M99.72
  disc M99.79
    abdomen M99.79
    cervical region M99.71
    cervicothoracic M99.71
    head region M99.70
    lower extremity M99.76
    lumbar region M99.73
    lumbosacral M99.73
    occipitocervical M99.70
    pelvic M99.75
    rib cage M99.78
    sacral region M99.74
    sacrococcygeal M99.74
    sacroiliac M99.74
    specified NEC M99.79
    thoracic region M99.72
    thoracolumbar M99.72
    upper extremity M99.77
  osseous M99.69
    abdomen M99.69
    cervical region M99.61
    cervicothoracic M99.61
    head region M99.60
    lower extremity M99.66
    lumbar region M99.63
    lumbosacral M99.63
    occipitocervical M99.60
    pelvic M99.65
    rib cage M99.68
    sacral region M99.64
    sacrococcygeal M99.64
    sacroiliac M99.64
    specified NEC M99.69
    thoracic region M99.62
    thoracolumbar M99.62
    upper extremity M99.67
  subluxation —see Stenosis, intervertebral foramina, Vosseous
intestine —see also Obstruction, intestine
  congenital (small) Q41.9
    large Q42.9
      specified NEC Q42.8
    specified NEC Q41.8
jejunum (see also Obstruction, intestine, specified NEC) K56.699
  congenital Q41.1

Stenosis, stenotic (continued)

lacrimal (passage)
  canaliculi H04.54-
  congenital Q10.5
  duct H04.55-
  punctum H04.56-
  sac H04.57-
lacrimonasal duct —see Stenosis, lacrimal, duct
  congenital Q10.5
larynx J38.6
  congenital NEC Q31.8
    subglottic Q31.1
  syphilitic A52.73
    congenital A50.59 [J99]
mitral (chronic) (inactive) (valve) I05.0
  with
    aortic valve disease I08.0
    incompetency, insufficiency or regurgitation I05.2
  active or acute I01.1
    with rheumatic or Sydenham's chorea I02.0
  congenital Q23.2
  specified cause, except rheumatic I34.2
  syphilitic A52.03
myocardium, myocardial —see also Degeneration, myocardial
  hypertrophic subaortic (idiopathic) I42.1
nares (anterior) (posterior) J34.89
  congenital Q30.0
nasal duct —see also Stenosis, lacrimal, duct
  congenital Q10.5
nasolacrimal duct —see also Stenosis, lacrimal, duct
  congenital Q10.5
neural canal —see also Lesion, biomechanical, specified NEC
  connective tissue M99.49
    abdomen M99.49
    cervical region M99.41
    cervicothoracic M99.41
    head region M99.40
    lower extremity M99.46
    lumbar region M99.43
    lumbosacral M99.43
    occipitocervical M99.40
    pelvic M99.45
    rib cage M99.48
    sacral region M99.44
    sacrococcygeal M99.44
    sacroiliac M99.44
    specified NEC M99.49
    thoracic region M99.42
    thoracolumbar M99.42
    upper extremity M99.47
  intervertebral disc M99.59
    abdomen M99.59
    cervical region M99.51
    cervicothoracic M99.51
    head region M99.50
    lower extremity M99.56
    lumbar region M99.53
    lumbosacral M99.53
    occipitocervical M99.50
    pelvic M99.55
    rib cage M99.58
    sacral region M99.54
    sacrococcygeal M99.54
    sacroiliac M99.54
    specified NEC M99.59
    thoracic region M99.52
    thoracolumbar M99.52
    upper extremity M99.57
  osseous M99.39
    abdomen M99.39
    cervical region M99.31

Stenosis, stenotic (continued)

neural canal (continued)
  osseous (continued)
    cervicothoracic M99.31
    head region M99.30
    lower extremity M99.36
    lumbar region M99.33
    lumbosacral M99.33
    pelvic M99.35
    rib cage M99.38
    occipitocervical M99.30
    sacral region M99.34
    sacrococcygeal M99.34
    sacroiliac M99.34
    specified NEC M99.39
    thoracic region M99.32
    thoracolumbar M99.32
    upper extremity M99.37
  subluxation M99.29
    cervical region M99.21
    cervicothoracic M99.21
    head region M99.20
    lower extremity M99.26
    lumbar region M99.23
    lumbosacral M99.23
    occipitocervical M99.20
    pelvic M99.25
    rib cage M99.28
    sacral region M99.24
    sacrococcygeal M99.24
    sacroiliac M99.24
    specified NEC M99.29
    thoracic region M99.22
    thoracolumbar M99.22
    upper extremity M99.27
organ or site, congenital NEC —see Atresia, by site
papilla of Vater K83.1
pulmonary (artery) (congenital) Q25.6
  with ventricular septal defect, transposition of aorta, and hypertrophy of right ventricle Q21.3
  acquired I28.8
  in tetralogy of Fallot Q21.3
  infundibular Q24.3
  subvalvular Q24.3
  supravalvular Q25.6
  valve I37.0
    with insufficiency I37.2
    congenital Q22.1
    rheumatic I09.89
      with aortic, mitral or tricuspid (valve) disease I08.8
  vein, acquired I28.8
  vessel NEC I28.8
pulmonic (congenital) Q22.1
  infundibular Q24.3
  subvalvular Q24.3
pylorus (hypertrophic) (acquired) K31.1
  adult K31.1
  congenital Q40.0
  infantile Q40.0
rectum (sphincter) —see Stricture, rectum
renal artery I70.1
  congenital Q27.1
salivary duct (any) K11.8
sphincter of Oddi K83.1
spinal M48.00
  cervical region M48.02
  cervicothoracic region M48.03
  lumbar region (NOS) (without neurogenic claudication) M48.061
    with neurogenic claudication M48.062
  lumbosacral region M48.07

Stenosis, stenotic (continued)

spinal (continued)
  occipito-atlanto-axial region M48.01
  sacrococcygeal region M48.08
  thoracic region M48.04
  thoracolumbar region M48.05
stent
  vascular
    end stent
      adjacent to stent —see Arteriosclerosis
    within the stent
      coronary T82.855
      peripheral T82.856
    in stent
      coronary vessel T82.855
      peripheral vessel T82.856
stomach, hourglass K31.2
subaortic (congenital) Q24.4
  hypertrophic (idiopathic) I42.1
subglottic J38.6
  congenital Q31.1
  postprocedural J95.5
trachea J39.8
  congenital Q32.1
  syphilitic A52.73
  tuberculous NEC A15.5
tracheostomy J95.03
tricuspid (valve) I07.0
  with
    aortic (valve) disease I08.2
    incompetency, insufficiency or regurgitation I07.2
      with aortic (valve) disease I08.2
        with mitral (valve) disease I08.3
    mitral (valve) disease I08.1
      with aortic (valve) disease I08.3
  congenital Q22.4
  nonrheumatic I36.0
    with insufficiency I36.2
tubal N97.1
ureter —see Atresia, ureter
ureteropelvic junction, congenital Q62.11
ureterovesical orifice, congenital Q62.12
urethra (valve) —see also Stricture, urethra
  congenital Q64.32
urinary meatus, congenital Q64.33
vagina N89.5
  congenital Q52.4
  in pregnancy —see Pregnancy, complicated by, abnormal vagina
    causing obstructed labor O65.5
valve (cardiac) (heart) (see also Endocarditis) I38
  congenital Q24.8
    aortic Q23.0
    mitral Q23.2
    pulmonary Q22.1
    tricuspid Q22.4
vena cava (inferior) (superior) I87.1
  congenital Q26.0
vesicourethral orifice Q64.31
vulva N90.5

Stent jail T82.897

Stercolith (impaction) K56.41
  appendix K38.1

Stercoraceous, stercoral ulcer K63.3
  anus or rectum K62.6

Stereotypies NEC F98.4

Sterility —see Infertility

Sterilization —see Encounter (for), sterilization

Sternalgia —see Angina

Sternopagus Q89.4

Sternum bifidum Q76.7

Steroid
  effects (adverse) (adrenocortical)
    (iatrogenic)
    cushingoid E24.2
      correct substance properly
        administered —see Table
        of Drugs and Chemicals, by
        drug, adverse effect
      overdose or wrong substance
        given or taken —see Table
        of Drugs and Chemicals, by
        drug, poisoning
    diabetes —see category E09
      correct substance properly
        administered —see Table
        of Drugs and Chemicals, by
        drug, adverse effect
      overdose or wrong substance
        given or taken —see Table
        of Drugs and Chemicals, by
        drug, poisoning
    fever R50.2
    insufficiency E27.3
      correct substance properly
        administered —see Table
        of Drugs and Chemicals, by
        drug, adverse effect
      overdose or wrong substance
        given or taken —see Table
        of Drugs and Chemicals, by
        drug, poisoning
  responder H40.04-

Stevens-Johnson disease or
  syndrome L51.1
  toxic epidermal necrolysis overlap
    L51.3

Stewart-Morel syndrome M85.2

Sticker's disease B08.3

Sticky eye —see Conjunctivitis,
  acute, mucopurulent

Stieda's disease —see Bursitis, tibial
  collateral

Stiff neck —see Torticollis

Stiff-man syndrome G25.82

Stiffness, joint NEC M25.60-
  ankle M25.67-
  ankylosis —see Ankylosis, joint
  contracture —see Contraction, joint
  elbow M25.62-
  foot M25.67-
  hand M25.64-
  hip M25.65-
  knee M25.66-
  shoulder M25.61-
  specified site NEC M25.69
  wrist M25.63-

Stigmata congenital syphilis A50.59

Stillbirth P95

Still-Felty syndrome —see Felty's
  syndrome

Still's disease or syndrome
  (juvenile) M08.20
  adult-onset M06.1
  ankle M08.27-
  elbow M08.22-
  foot joint M08.27-
  hand joint M08.24-
  hip M08.25-
  knee M08.26-
  multiple site M08.29
  shoulder M08.21-
  specified site NEC M08.2A

Still's disease or syndrome
  (continued)
  vertebra M08.28
  wrist M08.23-

Stimulation, ovary E28.1

Sting (venomous) (with allergic or
  anaphylactic shock) —see Table of
  Drugs and Chemicals, by animal or
  substance, poisoning

Stippled epiphyses Q78.8

Stitch
  abscess T81.41
  burst (in operation wound) —see
    Disruption, wound, operation

Stokes-Adams disease or syndrome
  I45.9

Stokes' disease E05.00
  with thyroid storm E05.01

Stokvis (-Talma) disease D74.8

Stoma malfunction
  colostomy K94.03
  enterostomy K94.13
  gastrostomy K94.23
  ileostomy K94.13
  tracheostomy J95.03

Stomach —see condition

Stomatitis (denture) (ulcerative) K12.1
  angular K13.0
    due to dietary or vitamin
      deficiency E53.0
  aphthous K12.0
  bovine B08.61
  candidal B37.0
  catarrhal K12.1
  diphtheritic A36.89
  due to
    dietary deficiency E53.0
    thrush B37.0
    vitamin deficiency
      B group NEC E53.9
      B2(riboflavin) E53.0
  epidemic B08.8
  epizootic B08.8
  follicular K12.1
  gangrenous A69.0
  Geotrichum B48.3
  herpesviral, herpetic B00.2
  herpetiformis K12.0
  malignant K12.1
  membranous acute K12.1
  monilial B37.0
  mycotic B37.0
  necrotizing ulcerative A69.0
  parasitic B37.0
  septic K12.1
  spirochetal A69.1
  suppurative (acute) K12.2
  ulceromembranous A69.1
  vesicular K12.1
    with exanthem (enteroviral)
      B08.4
    virus disease A93.8
  Vincent's A69.1

Stomatocytosis D58.8

Stomatomycosis B37.0

Stomatorrhagia K13.79

Stone(s) —see also Calculus
  bladder (diverticulum) N21.0
  cystine E72.09
  heart syndrome I50.1
  kidney N20.0
  prostate N42.0
  pulpal (dental) K04.2
  renal N20.0
  salivary gland or duct (any) K11.5
  urethra (impacted) N21.1

Stone *(continued)*
  urinary (duct) (impacted) (passage)
    N20.9
    bladder (diverticulum) N21.0
    lower tract N21.9
    specified NEC N21.8
  xanthine E79.8 *[N22]*

Stonecutter's lung J62.8

Stonemason's asthma, disease, lung
  or pneumoconiosis J62.8

Stoppage
  heart —see Arrest, cardiac
  urine —see Retention, urine

Storm, thyroid —see Thyrotoxicosis

Strabismus (congenital)
  (nonparalytic) H50.9
  concomitant H50.40
    convergent —see Strabismus,
      convergent concomitant
    divergent —see Strabismus,
      divergent concomitant
  convergent concomitant H50.00
    accommodative component
      H50.43
    alternating H50.05
      with
        A pattern H50.06
        specified nonconcomitances
          NEC H50.08
        V pattern H50.07
    monocular H50.01-
      with
        A pattern H50.02-
        specified nonconcomitances
          NEC H50.04-
        V pattern H50.03-
      intermittent H50.31-
        alternating H50.32
  cyclotropia H50.41
  divergent concomitant H50.10
    alternating H50.15
      with
        A pattern H50.16
        specified noncomitances
          NEC H50.18
        V pattern H50.17
    monocular H50.11-
      with
        A pattern H50.12-
        specified noncomitances
          NEC H50.14-
        V pattern H50.13-
      intermittent H50.33
        alternating H50.34
  Duane's syndrome H50.81-
  due to adhesions, scars H50.69
  heterophoria H50.50
    alternating H50.55
    cyclophoria H50.54
    esophoria H50.51
    exophoria H50.52
    vertical H50.53
  heterotropia H50.40
    intermittent H50.30
  hypertropia H50.2-
  hypotropia —see Hypertropia
  latent H50.50
  mechanical H50.60
    Brown's sheath syndrome H50.61-
    specified type NEC H50.69
  monofixation syndrome H50.42
  paralytic H49.9
    abducens nerve H49.2-
    fourth nerve H49.1-
    Kearns-Sayre syndrome H49.81-
    ophthalmoplegia (external)
      progressive H49.4-
        with pigmentary retinopathy
          H49.81-
      total H49.3-

Strabismus *(continued)*
  paralytic *(continued)*
    sixth nerve H49.2-
    specified type NEC H49.88-
    third nerve H49.0-
    trochlear nerve H49.1-
  specified type NEC H50.89
  vertical H50.2-

Strain
  back S39.012
  cervical S16.1
  eye NEC —see Disturbance,
    vision, subjective
  heart —see Disease, heart
  low back S39.012
  mental NOS Z73.3
    work-related Z56.6
  muscle (tendon) —see Injury,
    muscle, by site, strain
  neck S16.1
  postural —see also Disorder, soft
    tissue, due to use
  physical NOS Z73.3
    work-related Z56.6
  psychological NEC Z73.3
  tendon —see Injury, muscle, by
    site, strain

Straining, on urination R39.16

Strand, vitreous —see Opacity,
  vitreous, membranes and strands

Strangulation, strangulated
  —see also Asphyxia, traumatic
  appendix K38.8
  bladder-neck N32.0
  bowel or colon K56.2
  food or foreign body —see Foreign
    body, by site
  hemorrhoids —see Hemorrhoids,
    with complication
  hernia —see also Hernia, by site,
    with obstruction
    with gangrene —see Hernia, by
      site, with gangrene
  intestine (large) (small) K56.2
    with hernia —see also Hernia,
      by site, with obstruction
      with gangrene —see Hernia,
        by site, with gangrene
  mesentery K56.2
  mucus —see Asphyxia, mucus
  omentum K56.2
  organ or site, congenital NEC
    —see Atresia, by site
  ovary —see Torsion, ovary
  penis N48.89
    foreign body T19.4
  rupture —see Hernia, by site, with
    obstruction
  stomach due to hernia —see also
    Hernia, by site, with obstruction
    with gangrene —see Hernia, by
      site, with gangrene
  vesicourethral orifice N32.0

Strangury R30.0

Straw itch B88.0

Strawberry
  gallbladder K82.4
  mark Q82.5
  tongue (red) (white) K14.3

Streak(s)
  macula, angioid H35.33
  ovarian Q50.32

Strephosymbolia F81.0
  secondary to organic lesion R48.8

Streptobacillary fever A25.1

Streptobacillosis A25.1

Streptobacillus moniliformis A25.1

Streptococcus, streptococcal —*see also* condition
as cause of disease classified elsewhere B95.5
group
A, as cause of disease classified elsewhere B95.0
B, as cause of disease classified elsewhere B95.1
D, as cause of disease classified elsewhere B95.2
pneumoniae, as cause of disease classified elsewhere B95.3
specified NEC, as cause of disease classified elsewhere B95.4

Streptomycosis B47.1

Streptotrichosis A48.8

Stress F43.9
family —*see* Disruption, family
fetal P84
complicating pregnancy O77.9
due to drug administration O77.1
mental NEC Z73.3
work-related Z56.6
physical NEC Z73.3
work-related Z56.6
polycythemia D75.1
reaction (*see also* Reaction, stress) F43.9
work schedule Z56.3

Stretching, nerve —*see* Injury, nerve

Striae albicantes, atrophicae or distensae (cutis) L90.6

Stricture —*see also* Stenosis
ampulla of Vater K83.1
anus (sphincter) K62.4
congenital Q42.3
with fistula Q42.2
infantile Q42.3
with fistula Q42.2
aorta (ascending) (congenital) Q25.1
arteriosclerotic I70.0
calcified I70.0
supravalvular, congenital Q25.3
aortic (valve) —*see* Stenosis, aortic
aqueduct of Sylvius (congenital) Q03.0
with spina bifida —*see* Spina bifida, by site, with hydrocephalus
acquired G91.1
artery I77.1
basilar —*see* Occlusion, artery, basilar
carotid —*see* Occlusion, artery, carotid
celiac I77.4
congenital (peripheral) Q27.8
cerebral Q28.3
coronary Q24.5
digestive system Q27.8
lower limb Q27.8
retinal Q14.1
specified site NEC Q27.8
umbilical Q27.0
upper limb Q27.8
coronary —*see* Disease, heart, ischemic, atherosclerotic
congenital Q24.5
precerebral —*see* Occlusion, artery, precerebral
pulmonary (congenital) Q25.6
acquired I28.8
renal I70.1
vertebral —*see* Occlusion, artery, vertebral

Stricture (*continued*)
auditory canal (external) (congenital)
acquired —*see* Stenosis, external ear canal
bile duct (common) (hepatic) K83.1
congenital Q44.3
postoperative K91.89
bladder N32.89
neck N32.0
bowel —*see* Obstruction, intestine
brain G93.89
bronchus J98.09
congenital Q32.3
syphilitic A52.72
cardia (stomach) K22.2
congenital Q39.3
cardiac —*see also* Disease, heart
orifice (stomach) K22.2
cecum —*see* Obstruction, intestine
cervix, cervical (canal) N88.2
congenital Q51.828
in pregnancy —*see* Pregnancy, complicated by, abnormal cervix
causing obstructed labor O65.5
colon —*see also* Obstruction, intestine
congenital Q42.9
specified NEC Q42.8
colostomy K94.03
common (bile) duct K83.1
coronary (artery) —*see* Disease, heart, ischemic, atherosclerotic
cystic duct —*see* Obstruction, gallbladder
digestive organs NEC, congenital Q45.8
duodenum K31.5
congenital Q41.0
ear canal (external) (congenital) Q16.1
acquired —*see* Stricture, auditory canal, acquired
ejaculatory duct N50.89
enterostomy K94.13
esophagus K22.2
congenital Q39.3
syphilitic A52.79
congenital A50.59 [K23]
eustachian tube —*see also* Obstruction, eustachian tube
congenital Q17.8
fallopian tube N97.1
gonococcal A54.24
tuberculous A18.17
gallbladder —*see* Obstruction, gallbladder
glottis J38.6
heart —*see also* Disease, heart
valve (*see also* Endocarditis) I38
aortic Q23.0
mitral Q23.2
pulmonary Q22.1
tricuspid Q22.4
hepatic duct K83.1
hourglass, of stomach K31.2
hymen N89.6
hypopharynx J39.2
ileum (*see also* Obstruction, intestine, specified NEC) K56.699
congenital Q41.2
intestine —*see also* Obstruction, intestine
congenital (small) Q41.9
large Q42.9
specified NEC Q42.8
specified NEC Q41.8
ischemic K55.1

Stricture (*continued*)
jejunum (*see also* Obstruction, intestine, specified NEC) K56.699
congenital Q41.1
lacrimal passages —*see also* Stenosis, lacrimal
congenital Q10.5
larynx J38.6
congenital NEC Q31.8
subglottic Q31.1
syphilitic A52.73
congenital A50.59 [J99]
meatus
ear (congenital) Q16.1
acquired —*see* Stricture, auditory canal, acquired
osseous (ear) (congenital) Q16.1
acquired —*see* Stricture, auditory canal, acquired
urinarius —*see also* Stricture, urethra
congenital Q64.33
mitral (valve) —*see* Stenosis, mitral
myocardium, myocardial I51.5
hypertrophic subaortic (idiopathic) I42.1
nares (anterior) (posterior) J34.89
congenital Q30.0
nasal duct —*see also* Stenosis, lacrimal, duct
congenital Q10.5
nasolacrimal duct —*see also* Stenosis, lacrimal, duct
congenital Q10.5
nasopharynx J39.2
syphilitic A52.73
nose J34.89
congenital Q30.0
nostril (anterior) (posterior) J34.89
congenital Q30.0
syphilitic A52.73
congenital A50.59 [J99]
organ or site, congenital NEC —*see* Atresia, by site
os uteri —*see* Stricture, cervix
osseous meatus (ear) (congenital) Q16.1
acquired —*see* Stricture, auditory canal, acquired
oviduct —*see* Stricture, fallopian tube
pelviureteric junction (congenital) Q62.11
acquired, with hydronephrosis N13.0
penis, by foreign body T19.4
pharynx J39.2
prostate N42.89
pulmonary, pulmonic
artery (congenital) Q25.6
acquired I28.8
noncongenital I28.8
infundibulum (congenital) Q24.3
valve I37.0
congenital Q22.1
vein, acquired I28.8
vessel NEC I28.8
punctum lacrimale —*see also* Stenosis, lacrimal, punctum
congenital Q10.5
pylorus (hypertrophic) K31.1
adult K31.1
congenital Q40.0
infantile Q40.0
rectosigmoid (*see also* Obstruction, intestine, specified NEC) K56.699

Stricture (*continued*)
rectum (sphincter) K62.4
congenital Q42.1
with fistula Q42.0
due to
chlamydial lymphogranuloma A55
irradiation K91.89
lymphogranuloma venereum A55
gonococcal A54.6
inflammatory (chlamydial) A55
syphilitic A52.74
tuberculous A18.32
renal artery I70.1
congenital Q27.1
salivary duct or gland (any) K11.8
sigmoid (flexure) —*see* Obstruction, intestine
spermatic cord N50.89
stoma (following) (of)
colostomy K94.03
enterostomy K94.13
gastrostomy K94.23
ileostomy K94.13
tracheostomy J95.03
stomach K31.89
congenital Q40.2
hourglass K31.2
subaortic Q24.4
hypertrophic (acquired) (idiopathic) I42.1
subglottic J38.6
syphilitic NEC A52.79
trachea J39.8
congenital Q32.1
syphilitic A52.73
tuberculous NEC A15.5
tracheostomy J95.03
tricuspid (valve) —*see* Stenosis, tricuspid
tunica vaginalis N50.89
ureter (postoperative) N13.5
with
hydronephrosis N13.1
with infection N13.6
pyelonephritis (chronic) N11.1
congenital —*see* Atresia, ureter
tuberculous A18.11
ureteropelvic junction (congenital) Q62.11
acquired, with hydronephrosis N13.0
ureterovesical orifice N13.5
with infection N13.6
urethra (organic) (spasmodic) (*see also* Stricture, urethra, male) N35.919
associated with schistosomiasis B65.0 [N37]
congenital Q64.39
valvular (posterior) Q64.2
due to
infection —*see* Stricture, urethra, postinfective
trauma —*see* Stricture, urethra, post-traumatic
female N35.92
gonococcal, gonorrheal A54.01
infective NEC —*see* Stricture, urethra, postinfective
late effect (sequelae) of injury —*see* Stricture, urethra, post-traumatic
male N35.919
anterior urethra N35.914
bulbous urethra N35.912
meatal N35.911
membranous urethra N35.913
overlapping site N35.916

Subluxation (continued)
  metacarpophalangeal (joint)
    finger S63.21-
      index S63.21-
      little S63.21-
      middle S63.21-
      ring S63.21-
      thumb S63.11-
  metatarsophalangeal joint S93.14-
    great toe S93.14-
    lesser toe S93.14-
  midcarpal (joint) S63.03-
  patella S83.00-
    lateral S83.01-
    recurrent (nontraumatic) —see
      Dislocation, patella, recurrent,
      incomplete
    specified type NEC S83.09-
  pathological —see Dislocation,
    pathological
  radial head S53.00-
    anterior S53.01-
    nursemaid's elbow S53.03-
    posterior S53.02-
    specified type NEC S53.09-
  radiocarpal (joint) S63.02-
  radioulnar (joint)
    distal S63.01-
    proximal —see Subluxation,
      elbow
  shoulder
    congenital Q68.8
    girdle S43.30-
      scapula S43.31-
      specified site NEC S43.39-
    traumatic S43.00-
      anterior S43.01-
      inferior S43.03-
      posterior S43.02-
      specified type NEC S43.08-
  sternoclavicular (joint) S43.20-
    anterior S43.21-
    posterior S43.22-
  symphysis (pubis)
  thumb S63.103
    interphalangeal joint —see
      Subluxation, interphalangeal
      (joint), thumb
    metacarpophalangeal
      joint —see Subluxation,
      metacarpophalangeal (joint),
      thumb
  toe(s) S93.10-
    great S93.10-
      interphalangeal joint
        S93.13-
      metatarsophalangeal joint
        S93.14-
    interphalangeal joint S93.13-
    lesser S93.10-
      interphalangeal joint S93.13-
      metatarsophalangeal joint
        S93.14-
    metatarsophalangeal joint
      S93.149
  ulna
    distal end S63.07-
    proximal end —see Subluxation,
      elbow
  ulnohumeral joint —see
    Subluxation, elbow
  vertebral
    recurrent NEC —see
      subcategory M43.5
    traumatic
      cervical S13.100
        atlantoaxial joint S13.120
        atlantooccipital joint
          S13.110
        atloidooccipital joint
          S13.110

Subluxation (continued)
  vertebral (continued)
    traumatic (continued)
      cervical (continued)
        joint between
          C0 and C1 S13.110
          C1 and C2 S13.120
          C2 and C3 S13.130
          C3 and C4 S13.140
          C4 and C5 S13.150
          C5 and C6 S13.160
          C6 and C7 S13.170
          C7 and T1 S13.180
        occipitoatloid joint S13.110
      lumbar S33.100
        joint between
          L1 and L2 S33.110
          L2 and L3 S33.120
          L3 and L4 S33.130
          L4 and L5 S33.140
      thoracic S23.100
        joint between
          T1 and T2 S23.110
          T2 and T3 S23.120
          T3 and T4 S23.122
          T4 and T5 S23.130
          T5 and T6 S23.132
          T6 and T7 S23.140
          T7 and T8 S23.142
          T8 and T9 S23.150
          T9 and T10 S23.152
          T10 and T11 S23.160
          T11 and T12 S23.162
          T12 and L1 S23.170
    wrist (carpal bone) S63.00-
      carpometacarpal joint —see
        Subluxation, carpometacarpal
        (joint)
      distal radioulnar joint —see
        Subluxation, radioulnar
        (joint), distal
      metacarpal bone, proximal
        —see Subluxation, metacarpal
        (bone), proximal end
      midcarpal —see Subluxation,
        midcarpal (joint)
      radiocarpal joint —see
        Subluxation, radiocarpal
        (joint)
      recurrent —see Dislocation,
        recurrent, wrist
      specified site NEC S63.09-
      ulna —see Subluxation, ulna,
        distal end

Submaxillary —see condition

Submersion (fatal) (nonfatal) T75.1

Submucous —see condition

Subnormal, subnormality
  accommodation (old age) H52.4
  mental —see Disability, intellectual
  temperature (accidental) T68

Subphrenic —see condition

Subscapular nerve —see condition

Subseptus uterus Q51.28

Subsiding appendicitis K36

**Substance (other psychoactive)
-induced**
  anxiety disorder F19.980
  bipolar and related disorder F19.94
  delirium F19.921
  depressive disorder F19.94
  major neurocognitive disorder
    F19.97
  mild neurocognitive disorder
    F19.988
  obsessive-compulsive and related
    disorder F19.988
  psychotic disorder F19.959

Substance (continued)
  sexual dysfunction F19.981
  sleep disorder F19.982

Substernal thyroid E04.9
  congenital Q89.2

Substitution disorder F44.9

Subtentorial —see condition

Subthyroidism (acquired) —see also
  Hypothyroidism
  congenital E03.1

Succenturiate placenta O43.19-

Sucking thumb, child (excessive)
  F98.8

Sudamen, sudamina L74.1

Sudanese kala-azar B55.0

Sudden
  heart failure —see Failure, heart
  hearing loss —see Deafness,
    sudden

**Sudeck's atrophy, disease,
or syndrome** —see
  Algoneurodystrophy

Suffocation —see Asphyxia,
  traumatic

Sugar
  blood
    high (transient) R73.9
    low (transient) E16.2
  in urine R81

Suicide, suicidal (attempted) T14.91
  by poisoning —see Table of Drugs
    and Chemicals
  history of (personal) Z91.5
    in family Z81.8
  ideation —see Ideation, suicidal
  risk
    meaning personal history of
      attempted suicide Z91.5
    meaning suicidal ideation —see
      Ideation, suicidal
  tendencies
    meaning personal history of
      attempted suicide Z91.5
    meaning suicidal ideation —see
      Ideation, suicidal
  trauma —see nature of injury by
    site

Suipestifer infection —see Infection,
  salmonella

**Sulfhemoglobinemia,
sulphemoglobinemia** (acquired)
  (with methemoglobinemia) D74.8

Sumatran mite fever A75.3

Summer —see condition

Sunburn L55.9
  due to
    tanning bed (acute) L56.8
      chronic L57.8
    ultraviolet radiation (acute)
      L56.8
      chronic L57.8
  first degree L55.0
  second degree L55.1
  third degree L55.2

SUNCT (short lasting unilateral
  neuralgiform headache with
  conjunctival injection and tearing)
  G44.059
  intractable G44.051
  not intractable G44.059

Sundowning F05

Sunken acetabulum —see
  Derangement, joint, specified type
  NEC, hip

Sunstroke T67.01
  specified NEC T67.09

Superfecundation —see Pregnancy,
  multiple

Superfetation —see Pregnancy,
  multiple

Superinvolution (uterus) N85.8

Supernumerary (congenital)
  aortic cusps Q23.8
  auditory ossicles Q16.3
  bone Q79.8
  breast Q83.1
  carpal bones Q74.0
  cusps, heart valve NEC Q24.8
    aortic Q23.8
    mitral Q23.2
    pulmonary Q22.3
  digit(s) Q69.9
  ear (lobule) Q17.0
  fallopian tube Q50.6
  finger Q69.0
  hymen Q52.4
  kidney Q63.0
  lacrimonasal duct Q10.6
  lobule (ear) Q17.0
  mitral cusps Q23.2
  muscle Q79.8
  nipple(s) Q83.3
  organ or site not listed —see
    Accessory
  ossicles, auditory Q16.3
  ovary Q50.31
  oviduct Q50.6
  pulmonary, pulmonic cusps Q22.3
  rib Q76.6
    cervical or first (syndrome)
      Q76.5
  roots (of teeth) K00.2
  spleen Q89.09
  tarsal bones Q74.2
  teeth K00.1
  testis Q55.29
  thumb Q69.1
  toe Q69.2
  uterus Q51.28
  vagina Q52.1
  vertebra Q76.49

Supervision (of)
  contraceptive —see Prescription,
    contraceptives
  dietary (for) Z71.3
    allergy (food) Z71.3
    colitis Z71.3
    diabetes mellitus Z71.3
    food allergy or intolerance
      Z71.3
    gastritis Z71.3
    hypercholesterolemia Z71.3
    hypoglycemia Z71.3
    intolerance (food) Z71.3
    obesity Z71.3
    specified NEC Z71.3
  healthy infant or child Z76.2
    foundling Z76.1
  high-risk pregnancy —see
    Pregnancy, complicated by, high,
    risk
  lactation Z39.1
  pregnancy —see Pregnancy,
    supervision of

Supplemental teeth K00.1

Suppression
  binocular vision H53.34
  lactation O92.5
  menstruation N94.89
  ovarian secretion E28.39
  renal N28.9
  urine, urinary secretion R34

Suppuration, suppurative —*see also* condition
  accessory sinus (chronic) —*see* Sinusitis
  adrenal gland
  antrum (chronic) —*see* Sinusitis, maxillary
  bladder —*see* Cystitis
  brain G06.0
    sequelae G09
  breast N61.1
    puerperal, postpartum or gestational —*see* Mastitis, obstetric, purulent
  dental periosteum M27.3
  ear (middle) —*see also* Otitis, media
    external NEC —*see* Otitis, externa, infective
    internal —*see* subcategory H83.0
  ethmoidal (chronic) (sinus) —*see* Sinusitis, ethmoidal
  fallopian tube —*see* Salpingo-oophoritis
  frontal (chronic) (sinus) —*see* Sinusitis, frontal
  gallbladder (acute) K81.0
  gum K05.20
    generalized —*see* Periodontitis, aggressive, generalized
    localized —*see* Periodontitis, aggressive, localized
  intracranial G06.0
  joint —*see* Arthritis, pyogenic or pyemic
  labyrinthine —*see* subcategory H83.0
  lung —*see* Abscess, lung
  mammary gland N61.1
    puerperal, postpartum O91.12
    associated with lactation O91.13
  maxilla, maxillary M27.2
    sinus (chronic) —*see* Sinusitis, maxillary
  muscle —*see* Myositis, infective
  nasal sinus (chronic) —*see* Sinusitis
  pancreas, acute (*see also* Pancreatitis, acute) K85.80
  parotid gland —*see* Sialoadenitis
  pelvis, pelvic
    female —*see* Disease, pelvis, inflammatory
    male K65.0
  pericranial —*see* Osteomyelitis
  salivary duct or gland (any) —*see* Sialoadenitis
  sinus (accessory) (chronic) (nasal) —*see* Sinusitis
  sphenoidal sinus (chronic) —*see* Sinusitis, sphenoidal
  thymus (gland) E32.1
  thyroid (gland) E06.0
  tonsil —*see* Tonsillitis
  uterus —*see* Endometritis

Supraeruption of tooth (teeth) M26.34

Supraglottitis J04.30
  with obstruction J04.31

Suprarenal (gland) —*see* condition

Suprascapular nerve —*see* condition

Suprasellar —*see* condition

Surfer's knots or nodules S89.8-

Surgical
  emphysema T81.82

Surgical (*continued*)
  procedures, complication or misadventure —*see* Complications, surgical procedures
  shock T81.10

Surveillance (of) (for) —*see also* Observation
  alcohol abuse Z71.41
  contraceptive —*see* Prescription, contraceptives
  dietary Z71.3
  drug abuse Z71.51

Susceptibility to disease, genetic Z15.89
  malignant neoplasm Z15.09
    breast Z15.01
    endometrium Z15.04
    ovary Z15.02
    prostate Z15.03
    specified NEC Z15.09
  multiple endocrine neoplasia Z15.81

Suspected condition, ruled out — *see also* Observation, suspected
  amniotic cavity and membrane Z03.71
  cervical shortening Z03.75
  fetal anomaly Z03.73
  fetal growth Z03.74
  maternal and fetal conditions NEC Z03.79
  newborn (*see also* Observation, newborn, suspected condition ruled out) Z05.9
  oligohydramnios Z03.71
  placental problem Z03.72
  polyhydramnios Z03.71

Suspended uterus
  in pregnancy or childbirth —*see* Pregnancy, complicated by, abnormal uterus

Sutton's nevus D22.9

Suture
  burst (in operation wound) T81.31
    external operation wound T81.31
    internal operation wound T81.32
  inadvertently left in operation wound —*see* Foreign body, accidentally left during a procedure
  removal Z48.02

Swab inadvertently left in operation wound —*see* Foreign body, accidentally left during a procedure

Swallowed, swallowing
  difficulty —*see* Dysphagia
  foreign body —*see* Foreign body, alimentary tract

Swan-neck deformity (finger) —*see* Deformity, finger, swan-neck

Swearing, compulsive F42.8
  in Gilles de la Tourette's syndrome F95.2

Sweat, sweats
  fetid L75.0
  night R61

Sweating, excessive R61

Sweeley-Klionsky disease E75.21

Sweet's disease or dermatosis L98.2

Swelling (of) R60.9
  abdomen, abdominal (not referable to any particular organ) —*see* Mass, abdominal
  ankle —*see* Effusion, joint, ankle
  arm M79.89
    forearm M79.89

Swelling (*continued*)
  breast (*see also* Lump, breast) N63.0
  Calabar B74.3
  cervical gland R59.0
  chest, localized R22.2
  ear H93.8-
  extremity (lower) (upper) —*see* Disorder, soft tissue, specified type NEC
  finger M79.89
  foot M79.89
  glands R59.9
    generalized R59.1
    localized R59.0
  hand M79.89
  head (localized) R22.0
  inflammatory —*see* Inflammation
  intra-abdominal —*see* Mass, abdominal
  joint —*see* Effusion, joint
  leg M79.89
    lower M79.89
  limb —*see* Disorder, soft tissue, specified type NEC
  localized (skin) R22.9
    chest R22.2
    head R22.0
    limb
      lower —*see* Mass, localized, limb, lower
      upper —*see* Mass, localized, limb, upper
    neck R22.1
    trunk R22.2
  neck (localized) R22.1
  pelvic —*see* Mass, abdominal
  scrotum N50.89
  splenic —*see* Splenomegaly
  testis N50.89
  toe M79.89
  umbilical R19.09
  wandering, due to Gnathostoma (spinigerum) B83.1
  white —*see* Tuberculosis, arthritis

Swift (-Feer) **disease**
  overdose or wrong substance given or taken —*see* Table of Drugs and Chemicals, by drug, poisoning

Swimmer's
  cramp T75.1
  ear H60.33-
  itch B65.3

Swimming in the head R42

Swollen —*see* Swelling

Swyer syndrome Q99.1

Sycosis L73.8
  barbae (not parasitic) L73.8
  contagiosa (mycotic) B35.0
  lupoides L73.8
  mycotic B35.0
  parasitic B35.0
  vulgaris L73.8

Sydenham's chorea —*see* Chorea, Sydenham's

Sylvatic yellow fever A95.0

Sylvest's disease B33.0

Symblepharon H11.23-
  congenital Q10.3

Symond's syndrome G93.2

Sympathetic —*see* condition

Sympatheticotonia G90.8

Sympathicoblastoma
  specified site —*see* Neoplasm, malignant, by site
  unspecified site C74.90

Sympathogonioma —*see* Sympathicoblastoma

Symphalangy (fingers) (toes) Q70.9

Symptoms NEC R68.89
  breast NEC N64.59
  cold J00
  development NEC R63.8
  factitious, self-induced —*see* Disorder, factitious
  genital organs, female R10.2
  involving
    abdomen NEC R19.8
    appearance NEC R46.89
    awareness R41.9
      altered mental status R41.82
      amnesia —*see* Amnesia
      borderline intellectual functioning R41.83
      coma —*see* Coma
      disorientation R41.0
      neurologic neglect syndrome R41.4
      senile cognitive decline R41.81
      specified symptom NEC R41.89
    behavior NEC R46.89
    cardiovascular system NEC R09.89
    chest NEC R09.89
    circulatory system NEC R09.89
    cognitive functions R41.9
      altered mental status R41.82
      amnesia —*see* Amnesia
      borderline intellectual functioning R41.83
      coma —*see* Coma
      disorientation R41.0
      neurologic neglect syndrome R41.4
      senile cognitive decline R41.81
      specified symptom NEC R41.89
    development NEC R62.50
    digestive system NEC R19.8
    emotional state NEC R45.89
      emotional lability R45.86
    food and fluid intake R63.8
    general perceptions and sensations R44.9
      specified NEC R44.8
    musculoskeletal system R29.91
      specified NEC R29.898
    nervous system R29.90
      specified NEC R29.818
    pelvis NEC R19.8
    respiratory system NEC R09.89
    skin and integument R23.9
    urinary system R39.9
  menopausal N95.1
  metabolism NEC R63.8
  neurotic F48.8
  of infancy R68.19
  pelvis NEC, female R10.2
  skin and integument NEC R23.9
  subcutaneous tissue NEC R23.9
  viral cold J00

Sympus Q74.2

Syncephalus Q89.4

Synchondrosis
  abnormal (congenital) Q78.8
  ischiopubic M91.0

Synchysis (scintillans) (senile) (vitreous body) H43.89

Syncope (near) (pre-) R55
  anginosa I20.8
  bradycardia R00.1
  cardiac R55

Syncope *(continued)*
 carotid sinus G90.01
 due to spinal (lumbar) puncture
  G97.1
 heart R55
 heat T67.1
 laryngeal R05
 psychogenic F48.8
 tussive R05
 vasoconstriction R55
 vasodepressor R55
 vasomotor R55
 vasovagal R55

Syndactylism, syndactyly Q70.9
 complex (with synostosis)
  fingers Q70.0-
  toes Q70.2-
 simple (without synostosis)
  fingers Q70.1-
  toes Q70.3-

Syndrome *—see also* Disease
 5q minus NOS D46.C
 48, XXXX Q97.1
 49, XXXXX Q97.1
 abdominal
  acute R10.0
  muscle deficiency Q79.4
 abnormal innervation H02.519
  left H02.516
   lower H02.515
   upper H02.514
  right H02.513
   lower H02.512
   upper H02.511
 abstinence, neonatal P96.1
 acid pulmonary aspiration, obstetric
  O74.0
 acquired immunodeficiency *—see*
  Human, immunodeficiency virus
  (HIV) disease
 acute abdominal R10.0
 acute respiratory distress (adult)
  (child) J80
  idiopathic J84.114
 Adair-Dighton Q78.0
 Adams-Stokes (-Morgagni) I45.9
 adiposogenital E23.6
 adrenal
  hemorrhage (meningococcal)
   A39.1
  meningococcic A39.1
 adrenocortical *—see* Cushing's,
  syndrome
 adrenogenital E25.9
  congenital, associated with
   enzyme deficiency E25.0
 afferent loop NEC K91.89
 Alagille's Q44.7
 alcohol withdrawal (without
  convulsions) *—see* Dependence,
  alcohol, with, withdrawal
 Alder's D72.0
 Aldrich (-Wiskott) D82.0
 alien hand R41.4
 Alport Q87.81
 alveolar hypoventilation E66.2
 alveolocapillary block J84.10
 amnesic, amnestic (confabulatory)
  (due to) *—see* Disorder, amnesic
 amyostatic (Wilson's disease)
  E83.01
 androgen insensitivity E34.50
  complete E34.51
  partial E34.52
 androgen resistance (*see*
  also Syndrome, androgen
  insensitivity) E34.50
 Angelman Q93.51
 anginal *—see* Angina
 ankyloglossia superior Q38.1

Syndrome *(continued)*
 anterior
  chest wall R07.89
  cord G83.82
  spinal artery G95.19
   compression M47.019
    cervical region M47.012
    cervicothoracic region
     M47.013
    lumbar region M47.016
    occipito-atlanto-axial region
     M47.011
    thoracic region M47.014
    thoracolumbar region
     M47.015
  tibial M76.81-
 antibody deficiency D80.9
  agammaglobulinemic D80.1
   hereditary D80.0
  congenital D80.0
  hypogammaglobulinemic D80.1
   hereditary D80.0
 anticardiolipin (-antibody) D68.61
 antidepressant discontinuation
  T43.205
 antiphospholipid (-antibody) D68.61
 aortic
  arch M31.4
  bifurcation I74.09
 aortomesenteric duodenum
  occlusion K31.5
 apical ballooning (transient left
  ventricular) I51.81
 arcuate ligament I77.4
 argentaffin, argintaffinoma E34.0
 Arnold-Chiari *—see* Arnold-Chiari
  disease
 Arrillaga-Ayerza I27.0
 arterial tortuosity Q87.82
 arteriovenous steal T82.898-
 Asherman's N85.6
 aspiration, of newborn *—see*
  Aspiration, by substance, with
  pneumonia
  meconium P24.01
 ataxia-telangiectasia G11.3
 auriculotemporal G50.8
 autoerythrocyte sensitization
  (Gardner-Diamond) D69.2
 autoimmune polyglandular E31.0
 autoimmune lymphoproliferative
  [ALPS] D89.82
 autoinflammatory M04.9
  specified type NEC M04.8
 autosomal *—see* Abnormal,
  autosomes
 Avellis' G46.8
 Ayerza (-Arrillaga) I27.0
 Babinski-Nageotte G83.89
 Bakwin-Krida Q78.5
 bare lymphocyte D81.6
 Barré-Guillain G61.0
 Barré-Liéou M53.0
 Barrett's *—see* Barrett's, esophagus
 Barsony-Polgar K22.4
 Barsony-Teschendorf K22.4
 Barth E78.71
 Bartter's E26.81
 basal cell nevus Q87.89
 Basedow's E05.00
  with thyroid storm E05.01
 basilar artery G45.0
 Batten-Steinert G71.11
 battered
  baby or child *—see*
   Maltreatment, child, physical
   abuse
  spouse *—see* Maltreatment,
   adult, physical abuse
 Beals Q87.40
 Beau's I51.5

Syndrome *(continued)*
 Beck's I65.8
 Benedikt's G46.3
 Béquez César (-Steinbrinck-
  Chédiak-Higashi) E70.330
 Bernhardt-Roth *—see* Meralgia
  paresthetica
 Bernheim's *—see* Failure, heart,
  right
 big spleen D73.1
 bilateral polycystic ovarian E28.2
 Bing-Horton's *—see* Horton's
  headache
 Birt-Hogg-Dube syndrome
  Q87.89
 Björck (-Thorsen) E34.0
 black
  lung J60
  widow spider bite *—see* Toxicity,
   venom, spider, black widow
 Blackfan-Diamond D61.01
 Blau M04.8
 blind loop K90.2
  congenital Q43.8
  postsurgical K91.2
 blue sclera Q78.0
 blue toe I75.02-
 Boder-Sedgewick G11.3
 Boerhaave's K22.3
 Borjeson Forssman Lehmann
  Q89.8
 Bouillaud's I01.9
 Bourneville (-Pringle) Q85.1
 Bouveret (-Hoffman) I47.9
 brachial plexus G54.0
 bradycardia-tachycardia I49.5
 brain (nonpsychotic) F09
  with psychosis, psychotic
   reaction F09
  acute or subacute *—see* Delirium
  congenital *—see* Disability,
   intellectual
  organic F09
   post-traumatic (nonpsychotic)
    F07.81
   psychotic F09
  personality change F07.0
  postcontusional F07.81
  post-traumatic, nonpsychotic
   F07.81
  psycho-organic F09
  psychotic F06.8
 brain stem stroke G46.3
 Brandt's (acrodermatitis
  enteropathica) E83.2
 broad ligament laceration N83.8
 Brock's J98.11
 bronze baby P83.88
 Brown-Sequard G83.81
 Brugada I49.8
 bubbly lung P27.0
 Buchem's M85.2
 Budd-Chiari I82.0
 bulbar (progressive) G12.22
 Bürger-Grütz E78.3
 Burke's K86.89
 Burnett's (milk-alkali) E83.52
 burning feet E53.9
 Bywaters' T79.5
 Call-Fleming I67.841
 carbohydrate-deficient glycoprotein
  (CDGS) E77.8
 carcinogenic thrombophlebitis
  I82.1
 carcinoid E34.0
 cardiac asthma I50.1
 cardiacos negros I27.0
 cardiofaciocutaneous Q87.89
 cardiopulmonary-obesity E66.2
 cardiorenal *—see* Hypertension,
  cardiorenal

Syndrome *(continued)*
 cardiorespiratory distress
  (idiopathic), newborn P22.0
 cardiovascular renal *—see*
  Hypertension, cardiorenal
 carotid
  artery (hemispheric) (internal)
   G45.1
  body G90.01
  sinus G90.01
 carpal tunnel G56.0-
 Cassidy (-Scholte) E34.0
 cat cry Q93.4
 cat eye Q92.8
 cauda equina G83.4
 causalgia *—see* Causalgia
 celiac K90.0
  artery compression I77.4
  axis I77.4
 central pain G89.0
 cerebellar
  hereditary G11.9
  stroke G46.4
 cerebellomedullary malformation
  —see Spina bifida
 cerebral
  artery
   anterior G46.1
   middle G46.0
   posterior G46.2
  gigantism E22.0
 cervical (root) M53.1
  disc *—see* Disorder, disc,
   cervical, with neuritis
  fusion Q76.1
  posterior, sympathicus M53.0
  rib Q76.5
  sympathetic paralysis G90.2
 cervicobrachial (diffuse) M53.1
 cervicocranial G90.09
 cervicodorsal outlet G54.2
 cervicothoracic outlet G54.0
 Céstan (-Raymond) I65.8
 Charcot's (angina cruris)
  (intermittent claudication)
  I73.9
 Charcot-Weiss-Baker G90.09
 CHARGE Q89.8
 Chédiak-Higashi (-Steinbrinck)
  E70.330
 chest wall R07.1
 Chiari's (hepatic vein thrombosis)
  I82.0
 Chilaiditi's Q43.3
 child maltreatment *—see*
  Maltreatment, child
 chondrocostal junction M94.0
 chondroectodermal dysplasia
  Q77.6
 chromosome 4 short arm deletion
  Q93.3
 chromosome 5 short arm deletion
  Q93.4
 chronic
  infantile neurological, cutaneous
   and articular (CINCA) M04.2
  pain G89.4
  personality F68.8
 Churg-Strauss M30.1
 Clarke-Hadfield K86.89
 Clerambault's automatism G93.89
 Clouston's (hidrotic ectodermal
  dysplasia) Q82.4
 clumsiness, clumsy child F82
 cluster headache G44.009
  intractable G44.001
  not intractable G44.009
 Coffin-Lowry Q89.8
 cold injury (newborn) P80.0
 combined immunity deficiency
  D81.9

Syndrome *(continued)*
- compartment (deep) (posterior) (traumatic) T79.A0
  - abdomen T79.A3
  - lower extremity (hip, buttock, thigh, leg, foot, toes) T79.A2
  - nontraumatic
    - abdomen M79.A3
    - lower extremity (hip, buttock, thigh, leg, foot, toes) M79.A2-
    - specified site NEC M79.A9
    - upper extremity (shoulder, arm, forearm, wrist, hand, fingers) M79.A1-
  - postprocedural —*see* Syndrome, compartment, nontraumatic
  - specified site NEC T79.A9
  - upper extremity (shoulder, arm, forearm, wrist, hand, fingers) T79.A1
- complex regional pain —*see* Syndrome, pain, complex regional
- compression T79.5
  - anterior spinal —*see* Syndrome, anterior, spinal artery, compression
  - cauda equina G83.4
  - celiac artery I77.4
  - vertebral artery M47.029
    - occipito-atlanto-axial region M47.021
    - cervical region M47.022
- concussion F07.81
- congenital
  - affecting multiple systems NEC Q87.89
  - central alveolar hypoventilation G47.35
  - facial diplegia Q87.0
  - muscular hypertrophy-cerebral Q87.89
  - oculo-auriculovertebral Q87.0
  - oculofacial diplegia (Moebius) Q87.0
  - rubella (manifest) P35.0
- congestion-fibrosis (pelvic), female N94.89
- congestive dysmenorrhea N94.6
- Conn's E26.01
- connective tissue M35.9
  - overlap NEC M35.1
- conus medullaris G95.81
- cord
  - anterior G83.82
  - posterior G83.83
- coronary
  - acute NEC I24.9
  - insufficiency or intermediate I20.0
  - slow flow I20.8
- Costen's (complex) M26.69
- costochondral junction M94.0
- costoclavicular G54.0
- costovertebral E22.0
- Cowden Q85.8
- craniovertebral M53.0
- Creutzfeldt-Jakob —*see* Creutzfeldt-Jakob disease or syndrome
- cri-du-chat Q93.4
- crib death R99
- cricopharyngeal —*see* Dysphagia
- croup J05.0
- CRPS I —*see* Syndrome, pain, complex regional I
- crush T79.5
- cryopyrin-associated periodic M04.2
- cryptophthalmos Q87.0
- cubital tunnel —*see* Lesion, nerve, ulnar

Syndrome *(continued)*
- Curschmann (-Batten) (-Steinert) G71.11
- Cushing's E24.9
  - alcohol-induced E24.4
  - due to
    - alcohol
    - drugs E24.2
    - ectopic ACTH E24.3
    - overproduction of pituitary ACTH E24.0
  - drug-induced E24.2
  - overdose or wrong substance given or taken —*see* Table of Drugs and Chemicals, by drug, poisoning
  - pituitary-dependent E24.0
  - specified type NEC E24.8
- cystic duct stump K91.5
- cytokine release D89.839
  - grade 1 D89.831
  - grade 2 D89.832
  - grade 3 D89.833
  - grade 4 D89.834
  - grade 5 D89.835
- Dana-Putnam D51.0
- Danbolt (-Cross) (acrodermatitis enteropathica) E83.2
- Dandy-Walker Q03.1
  - with spina bifida Q07.01
- Danlos' (*see also* Syndrome, Ehlers-Danlos) Q79.60
- defibrination —*see also* Fibrinolysis
  - with
    - antepartum hemorrhage —*see* Hemorrhage, antepartum, with coagulation defect
    - intrapartum hemorrhage —*see* Hemorrhage, complicating, delivery
  - newborn P60
  - postpartum O72.3
- Degos' I77.89
- Déjérine-Roussy G89.0
- delayed sleep phase G47.21
- demyelinating G37.9
- dependence —*see* F10-F19 with fourth character .2
- depersonalization (-derealization) F48.1
- De Quervain E34.51
- de Toni-Fanconi (-Debré) E72.09
  - with cystinosis E72.04
- diabetes mellitus-hypertension-nephrosis —*see* Diabetes, nephrosis
- de Vivo syndrome E74.810
- diabetes mellitus in newborn infant P70.2
- diabetes-nephrosis —*see* Diabetes, nephrosis
- diabetic amyotrophy —*see* Diabetes, amyotrophy
- dialysis associated steal T82.898-
- Diamond-Blackfan D61.01
- Diamond-Gardener D69.2
- DIC (diffuse or disseminated intravascular coagulopathy) D65
- di George's D82.1
- Dighton's Q78.0
- disequilibrium E87.8
- Döhle body-panmyelopathic D72.0
- dorsolateral medullary G46.4
- double athetosis G80.3
- Down (*see also* Down syndrome) Q90.9
- Dravet (intractable) G40.834
  - with status epilepticus G40.833
  - without status epilepticus G40.834

Syndrome *(continued)*
- DRESS (drug rash with eosinophilia and systemic symptoms) D72.12
- Dresbach's (elliptocytosis) D58.1
- Dressler's (postmyocardial infarction) I24.1
  - postcardiotomy I97.0
- drug rash with eosinophilia and systemic symptoms (DRESS) D72.12
- drug withdrawal, infant of dependent mother P96.1
- dry eye H04.12-
- due to abnormality
  - chromosomal Q99.9
    - sex
      - female phenotype Q97.9
      - male phenotype Q98.9
    - specified NEC Q99.8
- dumping (postgastrectomy) K91.1
  - nonsurgical K31.89
- Dupré's (meningism) R29.1
- dysmetabolic X E88.81
- dyspraxia, developmental F82
- Eagle-Barrett Q79.4
- Eaton-Lambert —*see* Syndrome, Lambert-Eaton
- Ebstein's Q22.5
- ectopic ACTH E24.3
- eczema-thrombocytopenia D82.0
- Eddowes' Q78.0
- effort (psychogenic) F45.8
- Eisenmenger's I27.83
- Ehlers-Danlos Q79.60
  - classical (cEDS) (classical EDS) Q79.61
  - hypermobile (hEDS) (hypermobile EDS) Q79.62
  - specified NEC Q79.69
  - vascular (vascular EDS) (vEDS) Q79.63
- Ekman's Q78.0
- electric feet E53.8
- Ellis-van Creveld Q77.6
- empty nest Z60.0
- endocrine hypertensive E27.0
- entrapment —*see* Neuropathy, entrapment
- eosinophilia-myalgia M35.8
- epileptic —*see also* Epilepsy, by type
  - absence G40.A09
    - intractable G40.A19
      - with status epilepticus G40.A11
      - without status epilepticus G40.A19
    - not intractable G40.A09
      - with status epilepticus G40.A01
      - without status epilepticus G40.A09
- Erdheim-Chester (ECD) E88.89
- Erdheim's E22.0
- erythrocyte fragmentation D59.4
- Evans D69.41
- exhaustion F48.8
- extrapyramidal G25.9
  - specified NEC G25.89
- eye retraction —*see* Strabismus
- eyelid-malar-mandible Q87.0
- Faber's D50.9
- facet M47.89-
- facial pain, paroxysmal G50.0
- Fallot Q21.3
- familial cold autoinflammatory M04.2
- familial eczema-thrombocytopenia (Wiskott-Aldrich) D82.0
- Fanconi (-de Toni) (-Debré) E72.09
  - with cystinosis E72.04

Syndrome *(continued)*
- Fanconi's (anemia) (congenital pancytopenia) D61.09
- fatigue
  - chronic R53.82
  - psychogenic F48.8
- faulty bowel habit K59.39
- Feil-Klippel (brevicollis) Q76.1
- Felty's —*see* Felty's syndrome
- fertile eunuch E23.0
- fetal
  - alcohol (dysmorphic) Q86.0
  - hydantoin Q86.1
- Fiedler's I40.1
- first arch Q87.0
- fish odor E72.89
- Fisher's G61.0
- Fitzhugh-Curtis
  - due to
    - Chlamydia trachomatis A74.81
    - Neisseria gonorrhorea (gonococcal peritonitis) A54.85
- Fitz's (*see also* Pancreatitis, acute) K85.80
- Flajani (-Basedow) E05.00
  - with thyroid storm E05.01
- flatback —*see* Flatback syndrome
- floppy
  - baby P94.2
  - iris (intraoeprative) (IFIS) H21.81
  - mitral valve I34.1
- flush E34.0
- Foix-Alajouanine G95.19
- Fong's Q87.2
- food protein-induced enterocolitis (FPIES) K52.21
- foramen magnum G93.5
- Foster-Kennedy H47.14-
- Foville's (peduncular) G46.3
- fragile X Q99.2
- Franceschetti Q75.4
- Frey's
  - auriculotemporal G50.8
  - hyperhidrosis L74.52
- Friderichsen-Waterhouse A39.1
- Froin's G95.89
- frontal lobe F07.0
- Fukuhara E88.49
- functional
  - bowel K59.9
  - prepubertal castrate E29.1
- Gaisböck's D75.1
- ganglion (basal ganglia brain) G25.9
  - geniculi G51.1
- Gardner-Diamond D69.2
- gastroesophageal
  - junction K22.0
  - laceration-hemorrhage K22.6
- gastrojejunal loop obstruction K91.89
- Gee-Herter-Heubner K90.0
- Gelineau's G47.419
  - with cataplexy G47.411
- genito-anorectal A55
- Gerstmann-Sträussler-Scheinker (GSS) A81.82
- Gianotti-Crosti L44.4
- giant platelet (Bernard-Soulier) D69.1
- Gilles de la Tourette's F95.2
- Glass Q87.89
- Gleich's D72.118
- goiter-deafness E07.1
- Goldberg Q89.8
- Goldberg-Maxwell E34.51
- Good's D83.8
- Gopalan' (burning feet) E53.8
- Gorlin's Q87.89
- Gougerot-Blum L81.7

Syndrome *(continued)*
Gouley's I31.1
Gower's R55
gray or grey (newborn) P93.0
platelet D69.1
Gubler-Millard G46.3
Guillain-Barré (-Strohl) G61.0
gustatory sweating G50.8
Hadfield-Clarke K86.89
hair tourniquet —*see* Constriction,
external, by site
Hamman's J98.19
hand-foot L27.1
hand-shoulder G90.8
hantavirus (cardio)-pulmonary
(HPS) (HCPS) B33.4
happy puppet Q93.51
Harada's H30.81-
Hayem-Faber D50.9
headache NEC G44.89
complicated NEC G44.59
Heberden's I20.8
Hedinger's E34.0
Hegglin's D72.0
HELLP (hemolysis, elevated liver
enzymes and low platelet count)
O14.2-
complicating
childbirth O14.24
puerperium O14.25
hemolytic-uremic D59.3
hemophagocytic, infection-
associated D76.2
Henoch-Schönlein D69.0
hepatic flexure K59.89
hepatopulmonary K76.81
hepatorenal K76.7
following delivery O90.4
postoperative or postprocedural
K91.83
postpartum, puerperal O90.4
hepatourologic K76.7
Herter (-Gee) (nontropical sprue)
K90.0
Heubner-Herter K90.0
Heyd's K76.7
Hilger's G90.09
histamine-like (fish poisoning)
—*see* Poisoning, fish
histiocytic D76.3
histiocytosis NEC D76.3
HIV infection, acute B20
Hoffmann-Werdnig G12.0
Hollander-Simons E88.1
Hoppe-Goldflam G70.00
with exacerbation (acute) G70.01
in crisis G70.01
Horner's G90.2
hungry bone E83.81
hunterian glossitis D51.0
Hutchinson's triad A50.53
hyperabduction G54.0
hyperammonemia-
hyperornithinemia-
homocitrullinemia E72.4
hypereosinophilic (HES) D72.119
idiopathic (IHES) D72.110
lymphocytic variant (LHES)
D72.111
specified NEC D72.118
hyperimmunoglobulin D M04.1
hyperimmunoglobulin E (IgE) D82.4
hyperkalemic E87.5
hyperkinetic —*see* Hyperkinesia
hypermobility M35.7
hypernatremia E87.0
hyperosmolarity E87.0
hyperperfusion G97.82
hypersplenic D73.1
hypertransfusion, newborn P61.1
hyperventilation F45.8

Syndrome *(continued)*
hyperviscosity (of serum)
polycythemic D75.1
sclerothymic D58.8
hypoglycemic (familial) (neonatal)
E16.2
hypokalemic E87.6
hyponatremic E87.1
hypopituitarism E23.0
hypoplastic left-heart Q23.4
hypopotassemia E87.6
hyposmolality E87.1
hypotension, maternal O26.5-
hypothenar hammer I73.89
hypoventilation, obesity (OHS) E66.2
ICF (intravascular coagulation-
fibrinolysis) D65
idiopathic
cardiorespiratory distress,
newborn P22.0
nephrotic (infantile) N04.9
iliotibial band M76.3-
immobility, immobilization
(paraplegic) M62.3
immune reconstitution D89.3
immune reconstitution
inflammatory [IRIS] D89.3
immunity deficiency, combined D81.9
immunodeficiency
acquired —*see* Human,
immunodeficiency virus (HIV)
disease
combined D81.9
impending coronary I20.0
impingement, shoulder M75.4-
inappropriate secretion of
antidiuretic hormone E22.2
infant
of diabetic mother P70.1
gestational diabetes P70.0
infantilism (pituitary) E23.0
inferior vena cava I87.1
inspissated bile (newborn) P59.1
institutional (childhood) F94.2
insufficient sleep F51.12
intermediate coronary (artery) I20.0
interspinous ligament —*see*
Spondylopathy, specified NEC
intestinal
carcinoid E34.0
knot K56.2
intravascular coagulation-
fibrinolysis (ICF) D65
iodine-deficiency, congenital E00.9
type
mixed E00.2
myxedematous E00.1
neurological E00.0
IRDS (idiopathic respiratory
distress, newborn) P22.0
irritable
bowel K58.9
with
constipation K58.1
diarrhea K58.0
mixed K58.2
psychogenic F45.8
specified NEC K58.8
heart (psychogenic) F45.8
weakness F48.8
ischemic
bowel (transient) K55.9
chronic K55.1
due to mesenteric artery
insufficiency K55.1
steal T82.898
IVC (intravascular coagulopathy)
D65
Ivemark's Q89.01
Jaccoud's —*see* Arthropathy,
postrheumatic, chronic

Syndrome *(continued)*
Jackson's G83.89
Jakob-Creutzfeldt —*see*
Creutzfeldt-Jakob disease or
syndrome
jaw-winking Q07.8
Jervell-Lange-Nielsen I45.81
jet lag G47.25
Job's D71
Joseph-Diamond-Blackfan D61.01
jugular foramen G52.7
Kabuki Q89.8
Kanner's (autism) F84.0
Kartagener's Q89.3
Kelly's D50.1
Kimmelstiel-Wilson —*see*
Diabetes, specified type, with
Kimmelstiel-Wilson disease
Klein (e)-Levine G47.13
Klippel-Feil (brevicollis) Q76.1
Köhler-Pellegrini-Steida —*see*
Bursitis, tibial collateral
König's K59.89
Korsakoff (-Wernicke)
(nonalcoholic) F04
alcoholic F10.26
Kostmann's D70.0
Krabbe's congenital muscle
hypoplasia Q79.8
labyrinthine H83.2
lacunar NEC G46.7
Lambert-Eaton G70.80
in
neoplastic disease G73.1
specified disease NEC G70.81
Landau-Kleffner —*see* Epilepsy,
specified NEC
Larsen's Q74.8
lateral
cutaneous nerve of thigh G57.1-
medullary G46.4
Launois' E22.0
lazy
leukocyte D70.8
posture M62.3
Lemiere I80.8
Lennox-Gastaut G40.812
intractable G40.814
with status epilepticus G40.813
without status epilepticus
G40.814
not intractable G40.812
with status epilepticus G40.811
without status epilepticus
G40.812
lenticular, progressive E83.01
Leopold-Levi's E05.90
Lev's I44.2
Li-Fraumeni Z15.01
Lichtheim's D51.0
Lightwood's N25.89
Lignac (de Toni) (-Fanconi)
(-Debré) E72.09
with cystinosis E72.04
Likoff's I20.8
limbic epilepsy personality F07.0
liver-kidney K76.7
lobotomy F07.0
Loffler's J82.89
long arm 18 or 21 deletion Q93.89
long QT I45.81
Louis-Barré G11.3
low
atmospheric pressure T70.29
back M54.5
output (cardiac) I50.9
lower radicular, newborn (birth
injury) P14.8
Luetscher's (dehydration) E86.0
Lupus anticoagulant D68.62
Lutembacher's Q21.1

Syndrome *(continued)*
macrophage activation D76.1
due to infection D76.2
magnesium-deficiency R29.0
Majeed M04.8
Mal de Debarquement R42
malabsorption K90.9
postsurgical K91.2
malformation, congenital, due to
alcohol Q86.0
exogenous cause NEC Q86.8
hydantoin Q86.1
warfarin Q86.2
malignant
carcinoid E34.0
neuroleptic G21.0
Mallory-Weiss K22.6
mandibulofacial dysostosis Q75.4
manic-depressive —*see* Disorder,
bipolar
maple-syrup-urine E71.0
Marable's I77.4
Marfan's Q87.40
with
cardiovascular manifestations
Q87.418
aortic dilation Q87.410
ocular manifestations Q87.42
skeletal manifestations Q87.43
Marie's (acromegaly) E22.0
mast cell activation —*see*
Activation, mast cell
maternal hypotension —*see*
Syndrome, hypotension, maternal
May (-Hegglin) D72.0
McArdle (-Schmidt) (-Pearson)
E74.04
McQuarrie's E16.2
meconium plug (newborn) P76.0
median arcuate ligament I77.4
Meekeren-Ehlers-Danlos Q79.6
megavitamin-B6 E67.2
Meige G24.4
MELAS E88.41
Mendelson's O74.0
MERRF (myoclonic epilepsy
associated with ragged-red
fibers) E88.42
mesenteric
artery (superior) K55.1
vascular insufficiency K55.1
metabolic E88.81
metastatic carcinoid E34.0
micrognathia-glossoptosis Q87.0
midbrain NEC G93.89
middle lobe (lung) J98.19
middle radicular G54.0
migraine (*see also* Migraine)
G43.909-
Mikulicz' K11.8
milk-alkali E83.52
Millard-Gubler G46.3
Miller-Dieker Q93.88
Miller-Fisher G61.0
Minkowski-Chauffard D58.0
Mirizzi's K83.1
MNGIE (Mitochondrial
Neurogastrointestinal
Encephalopathy) E88.49
Möbius, ophthalmoplegic migraine
—*see* Migraine, ophthalmoplegic
monofixation H50.42
Morel-Moore M85.2
Morel-Morgagni M85.2
Morgagni (-Morel) (-Stewart) M85.2
Morgagni-Adams-Stokes I45.9
mucocutaneous lymph node (acute
febrile) (MCLS) M30.3
multiple endocrine neoplasia
(MEN) —*see* Neoplasia,
endocrine, multiple (MEN)

Syndrome (*continued*)

right
  heart, hypoplastic Q22.6
    ventricular obstruction —*see*
      Failure, heart, right
Romano-Ward (prolonged QT
  interval) I45.81
rotator cuff, shoulder (*see also*
  Tear, rotator cuff) M75.10-
Rotes Quérol —*see* Hyperostosis,
  ankylosing
Roth —*see* Meralgia paresthetica
rubella (congenital) P35.0
Ruvalcaba-Myhre-Smith E71.440
Rytand-Lipsitch I44.2
salt
  depletion E87.1
    due to heat NEC T67.8
      causing heat exhaustion or
        prostration T67.4
  low E87.1
salt-losing N28.89
SATB2-associated Q87.89
Scaglietti-Dagnini E22.0
scalenus anticus (anterior) G54.0
scapulocostal —*see*
  Mononeuropathy, upper limb,
  specified site NEC
scapuloperoneal G71.09
schizophrenic, of childhood NEC
  F84.5
Schnitzler D47.2
Scholte's E34.0
Schroeder's E27.0
Schüller-Christian C96.5
Schwachman's —*see* Syndrome,
  Shwachman's
Schwartz (-Jampel) G71.13
Schwartz-Bartter E22.2
scimitar Q26.8
sclerocystic ovary E28.2
Seitelberger's G31.89
septicemic adrenal hemorrhage A39.1
seroconversion, retroviral (acute) Z21
serous meningitis G93.2
severe acute respiratory (SARS)
  J12.81
shaken infant T74.4
shock (traumatic) T79.4
  kidney N17.0
    following crush injury T79.5
  toxic A48.3
shock-lung J80
Shone's - code to specific
  anomalies
short
  bowel K91.2
  rib Q77.2
shoulder-hand —*see*
  Algoneurodystrophy
Shwachman's D70.4
sicca —*see* Sicca syndrome
sick
  cell E87.1
  sinus I49.5
sick-euthyroid E07.81
sideropenic D50.1
Siemens' ectodermal dysplasia Q82.4
Silfversköld's Q78.9
Simons' E88.1
sinus tarsi M25.57-
sinusitis-bronchiectasis-situs
  inversus Q89.3
Sipple's E31.22
sirenomelia Q87.2
Slocumb's E27.0
slow flow, coronary I20.8
Sluder's G44.89
Smith-Magenis Q93.88
Sneddon-Wilkinson L13.1
Sotos' Q87.3

Syndrome (*continued*)

South African cardiomyopathy I42.8
spasmodic
  upward movement, eyes H51.8
  winking F95.8
Spen's I45.9
splenic
  agenesis Q89.01
  flexure K59.89
  neutropenia D73.81
Spurway's Q78.0
staphylococcal scalded skin L00
steal
  arteriovenous T82.898-
  ischemic T82.898-
  subclavian G45.8
Stein-Leventhal E28.2
Stein's E28.2
Stevens-Johnson syndrome L51.1
  toxic epidermal necrolysis
    overlap L51.3
Stewart-Morel M85.2
Stickler Q89.8
stiff baby Q89.8
stiff man G25.82
Still-Felty —*see* Felty's syndrome
Stokes (-Adams) I45.9
stone heart I50.1
straight back, congenital Q76.49
subclavian steal G45.8
subcoracoid-pectoralis minor G54.0
subcostal nerve compression I77.89
subphrenic interposition Q43.3
superior
  cerebellar artery I63.89
  mesenteric artery K55.1
  semi-circular canal dehiscence
    H83.8X-
  vena cava I87.1
supine hypotensive (maternal) —*see*
  Syndrome, hypotension, maternal
suprarenal cortical E27.0
supraspinatus (*see also* Tear, rotator
  cuff) M75.10-
Susac G93.49
swallowed blood P78.2
sweat retention L74.0
Swyer Q99.1
Symond's G93.2
sympathetic
  cervical paralysis G90.2
  pelvic, female N94.89
systemic inflammatory response
  (SIRS), of non-infectious origin
  (without organ dysfunction)
  R65.10
  with acute organ dysfunction
    R65.11
tachycardia-bradycardia I49.5
takotsubo I51.81
TAR (thrombocytopenia with
  absent radius) Q87.2
tarsal tunnel G57.5-
teething K00.7
tegmental G93.89
telangiectasic-pigmentation-
  cataract Q82.8
temporal pyramidal apex —*see*
  Otitis, media, suppurative, acute
temporomandibular joint-pain-
  dysfunction M26.62-
Terry's (*see also* Myopia,
  degenerative) H44.2-
testicular feminization (*see
  also* Syndrome, androgen
  insensitivity) E34.51
thalamic pain (hyperesthetic) G89.0
thoracic outlet (compression) G54.0
Thorson-Björck E34.0
thrombocytopenia with absent
  radius (TAR) Q87.2

Syndrome (*continued*)

thyroid-adrenocortical insufficiency
  E31.0
tibial
  anterior M76.81-
  posterior M76.82-
Tietze's M94.0
time-zone (rapid) G47.25
Toni-Fanconi E72.09
  with cystinosis E72.04
Touraine's Q79.8
tourniquet —*see* Constriction,
  external, by site
toxic shock A48.3
transient left ventricular apical
  ballooning I51.81
traumatic vasospastic T75.22
Treacher Collins Q75.4
triple X, female Q97.0
trisomy Q92.9
  13 Q91.7
    meiotic nondisjunction Q91.4
    mitotic nondisjunction Q91.5
    mosaicism Q91.5
    translocation Q91.6
  18 Q91.3
    meiotic nondisjunction Q91.0
    mitotic nondisjunction Q91.1
    mosaicism Q91.1
    translocation Q91.2
  20 (q)(p) Q92.8
  21 Q90.9
    meiotic nondisjunction Q90.0
    mitotic nondisjunction Q90.1
    mosaicism Q90.1
    translocation Q90.2
  22 Q92.8
tropical wet feet T69.0-
Trousseau's I82.1
tumor lysis (following
  antineoplastic chemotherapy)
  (spontaneous) NEC E88.3
tumor necrosis factor receptor
  associated periodic (TRAPS)
  M04.1
Twiddler's (due to)
  automatic implantable
    defibrillator T82.198
  cardiac pacemaker T82.198
Unverricht (-Lundborg) —
  see Epilepsy, generalized,
  idiopathic
upward gaze H51.8
uremia, chronic (*see also* Disease,
  kidney, chronic) N18.9
urethral N34.3
urethro-oculo-articular —*see*
  Reiter's disease
urohepatic K76.7
vago-hypoglossal G52.7
vascular NEC in cerebrovascular
  disease G46.8
vasoconstriction, reversible
  cerebrovascular I67.841
vasomotor I73.9
vasospastic (traumatic) T75.22
vasovagal R55
van Buchem's M85.2
van der Hoeve's Q78.0
VATER Q87.2
velo-cardio-facial Q93.81
vena cava (inferior) (superior)
  (obstruction) I87.1
vertebral
  artery G45.0
    compression —*see* Syndrome,
      anterior, spinal artery,
      compression
  steal G45.0
vertebro-basilar artery G45.0
vertebrogenic (pain) M54.89

Syndrome (*continued*)

vertiginous —*see* Disorder,
  vestibular function
Vinson-Plummer D50.1
virus B34.9
visceral larva migrans B83.0
visual disorientation H53.8
vitamin B6 deficiency E53.1
vitreal corneal H59.01-
vitreous (touch) H59.01-
Vogt-Koyanagi H20.82-
Volkmann's T79.6
von Schroetter's I82.890
von Willebrand (-Jürgen) D68.0
Waldenström-Kjellberg D50.1
Wallenberg's G46.3
water retention E87.79
Waterhouse (-Friderichsen) A39.1
Weber-Gubler G46.3
Weber-Leyden G46.3
Weber's G46.3
Wegener's M31.30
  with
    kidney involvement M31.31
    lung involvement M31.30
      with kidney involvement
        M31.31
Weingarten's (tropical eosinophilia)
  J82.89
Weiss-Baker G90.09
Werdnig-Hoffman G12.0
Wermer's E31.21
Werner's E34.8
Wernicke-Korsakoff (nonalcoholic)
  F04
  alcoholic F10.26
West's —*see* Epilepsy, spasms
Westphal-Strümpell E83.01
wet
  feet (maceration) (tropical)
    T69.0-
  lung, newborn P22.1
whiplash S13.4
whistling face Q87.0
Wilkie's K55.1
Wilkinson-Sneddon L13.1
Willebrand (-Jürgens) D68.0
Williams Q93.82
Wilson's (hepatolenticular
  degeneration) E83.01
Wiskott-Aldrich D82.0
withdrawal —*see* Withdrawal, state
  drug
    infant of dependent mother
      P96.1
    therapeutic use, newborn
      P96.2
Woakes' (ethmoiditis) J33.1
Wright's (hyperabduction) G54.0
X I20.9
XXXX Q97.1
XXXXX Q97.1
XXXXY Q98.1
XXY Q98.0
Yao M04.8
yellow nail L60.5
Zahorsky's B08.5
Zellweger syndrome E71.510
Zellweger-like syndrome E71.541

Synechia (anterior) (iris) (posterior)
  (pupil) —*see also* Adhesions, iris
  intra-uterine (traumatic) N85.6

Synesthesia R20.8

Syngamiasis, syngamosis B83.3

Synodontia K00.2

Synorchidism, synorchism Q55.1

Synostosis (congenital) Q78.8
  astragalo-scaphoid Q74.2
  radioulnar Q74.0

Synovial sarcoma —see Neoplasm, connective tissue, malignant

Synovioma (malignant) —see also Neoplasm, connective tissue, malignant
  benign —see Neoplasm, connective tissue, benign

Synoviosarcoma —see Neoplasm, connective tissue, malignant

Synovitis (see also Tenosynovitis) M65.9
  crepitant
    hand M70.0-
    wrist M70.03-
  gonococcal A54.49
  gouty —see Gout,
  in (due to)
    crystals M65.8-
    gonorrhea A54.49
    syphilis (late) A52.78
    use, overuse, pressure —see Disorder, soft tissue, due to use
  infective NEC —see Tenosynovitis, infective NEC
  specified NEC —see Tenosynovitis, specified type NEC
  syphilitic A52.78
    congenital (early) A50.02
  toxic —see Synovitis, transient
  transient M67.3-
    ankle M67.37-
    elbow M67.32-
    foot joint M67.37-
    hand joint M67.34-
    hip M67.35-
    knee M67.36-
    multiple site M67.39
    pelvic region M67.35-
    shoulder M67.31-
    specified joint NEC M67.38
    wrist M67.33-
  traumatic, current —see Sprain
  tuberculous —see Tuberculosis, synovitis
  villonodular (pigmented) M12.2-
    ankle M12.27-
    elbow M12.22-
    foot joint M12.27-
    hand joint M12.24-
    hip M12.25-
    knee M12.26-
    multiple site M12.29
    pelvic region M12.25-
    shoulder M12.21-
    specified joint NEC M12.28
    vertebrae M12.28
    wrist M12.23-

Syphilid A51.39
  congenital A50.06
  newborn A50.06
  tubercular (late) A52.79

Syphilis, syphilitic (acquired) A53.9
  abdomen (late) A52.79
  acoustic nerve A52.15
  adenopathy (secondary) A51.49
  adrenal (gland) (with cortical hypofunction) A52.79
  age under 2 years NOS —see also Syphilis, congenital, early
    acquired A51.9
  alopecia (secondary) A51.32
  anemia (late) A52.79 [D63.8]
  aneurysm (aorta) (ruptured) A52.01
    central nervous system A52.05
    congenital A50.54 [I79.0]
  anus (late) A52.74
    primary A51.1
    secondary A51.39

Syphilis, syphilitic (continued)
  aorta (arch) (abdominal) (thoracic) A52.02
    aneurysm A52.01
  aortic (insufficiency) (regurgitation) (stenosis) A52.03
    aneurysm A52.01
  arachnoid (adhesive) (cerebral) (spinal) A52.13
  asymptomatic —see Syphilis, latent
  ataxia (locomotor) A52.11
  atrophoderma maculatum A51.39
  auricular fibrillation A52.06
  bladder (late) A52.76
  bone A52.77
    secondary A51.46
  brain A52.17
  breast (late) A52.79
  bronchus (late) A52.72
  bubo (primary) A51.0
  bulbar palsy A52.19
  bursa (late) A52.78
  cardiac decompensation A52.06
  cardiovascular A52.00
  central nervous system (late) (recurrent) (relapse) (tertiary) A52.3
    with
      ataxia A52.11
      general paralysis A52.17
        juvenile A50.45
      paresis (general) A52.17
        juvenile A50.45
      tabes (dorsalis) A52.11
        juvenile A50.45
      taboparesis A52.17
        juvenile A50.45
    aneurysm A52.05
    congenital A50.40
    juvenile A50.40
    remission in (sustained) A52.3
    serology doubtful, negative, or positive A52.3
    specified nature or site NEC A52.19
    vascular A52.05
  cerebral A52.17
    meningovascular A52.13
    nerves (multiple palsies) A52.15
    sclerosis A52.17
    thrombosis A52.05
  cerebrospinal (tabetic type) A52.12
  cerebrovascular A52.05
  cervix (late) A52.76
  chancre (multiple) A51.0
    extragenital A51.2
    Rollet's A51.0
  Charcot's joint A52.16
  chorioretinitis A51.43
    congenital A50.01
    late A52.71
    prenatal A50.01
  choroiditis —see Syphilitic chorioretinitis
  choroidoretinitis —see Syphilitic chorioretinitis
  ciliary body (secondary) A51.43
    late A52.71
  colon (late) A52.74
  combined spinal sclerosis A52.11
  condyloma (latum) A51.31
  congenital A50.9
    with
      paresis (general) A50.45
      tabes (dorsalis) A50.45
      taboparesis A50.45
    chorioretinitis, choroiditis A50.01 [H32]
    early, or less than 2 years after birth NEC A50.2

Syphilis, syphilitic (continued)
  congenital (continued)
    early, or less than 2 years after birth NEC (continued)
      with manifestations —see Syphilis, congenital, early, symptomatic
      latent (without manifestations) A50.1
        negative spinal fluid test A50.1
        serology positive A50.1
      symptomatic A50.09
        cutaneous A50.06
        mucocutaneous A50.07
        oculopathy A50.01
        osteochondropathy A50.02
        pharyngitis A50.03
        pneumonia A50.04
        rhinitis A50.05
        visceral A50.08
    interstitial keratitis A50.31
    juvenile neurosyphilis A50.45
    late, or 2 years or more after birth NEC A50.7
      chorioretinitis, choroiditis A50.32
      interstitial keratitis A50.31
      juvenile neurosyphilis A50.45
      latent (without manifestations) A50.6
        negative spinal fluid test A50.6
        serology positive A50.6
      symptomatic or with manifestations NEC A50.59
        arthropathy A50.55
        cardiovascular A50.54
        Clutton's joints A50.51
        Hutchinson's teeth A50.52
        Hutchinson's triad A50.53
        osteochondropathy A50.56
        saddle nose A50.57
  conjugal A53.9
    tabes A52.11
  conjunctiva (late) A52.71
  contact Z20.2
  cord bladder A52.19
  cornea, late A52.71
  coronary (artery) (sclerosis) A52.06
  coryza, congenital A50.05
  cranial nerve A52.15
    multiple palsies A52.15
  cutaneous —see Syphilis, skin
  dacryocystitis (late) A52.71
  degeneration, spinal cord A52.12
  dementia paralytica A52.17
    juvenilis A50.45
  destruction of bone A52.77
  dilatation, aorta A52.01
  due to blood transfusion A53.9
  dura mater A52.13
  ear A52.79
    inner A52.79
      nerve (eighth) A52.15
      neurorecurrence A52.15
  early A51.9
    cardiovascular A52.00
    central nervous system A52.3
    latent (without manifestations) (less than 2 years after infection) A51.5
      negative spinal fluid test A51.5
      serological relapse after treatment A51.5
      serology positive A51.5
    relapse (treated, untreated) A51.9
    skin A51.39
    symptomatic A51.9
      extragenital chancre A51.2

Syphilis, syphilitic (continued)
  early (continued)
    symptomatic (continued)
      primary, except extragenital chancre A51.0
      secondary (see also Syphilis, secondary) A51.39
        relapse (treated, untreated) A51.49
      ulcer A51.39
  eighth nerve (neuritis) A52.15
  endemic A65
  endocarditis A52.03
    aortic A52.03
    pulmonary A52.03
  epididymis (late) A52.76
  epiglottis (late) A52.73
  epiphysitis (congenital) (early) A50.02
  episcleritis (late) A52.71
  esophagus A52.79
  eustachian tube A52.73
  exposure to Z20.2
  eye A52.71
  eyelid (late) (with gumma) A52.71
  fallopian tube (late) A52.76
  fracture A52.77
  gallbladder (late) A52.74
  gastric (polyposis) (late) A52.74
  general A53.9
    paralysis A52.17
      juvenile A50.45
  genital (primary) A51.0
  glaucoma A52.71
  gumma NEC A52.79
    cardiovascular system A52.00
    central nervous system A52.3
    congenital A50.59
  heart (block) (decompensation) (disease) (failure) A52.06 [I52]
    valve NEC A52.03
  hemianesthesia A52.19
  hemianopsia A52.71
  hemiparesis A52.17
  hemiplegia A52.17
  hepatic artery A52.09
  hepatic A52.74
  hepatomegaly, congenital A50.08
  hereditaria tarda —see Syphilis, congenital, late
  hereditary —see Syphilis, congenital
  Hutchinson's teeth A50.52
  hyalitis A52.71
  inactive —see Syphilis, latent
  infantum —see Syphilis, congenital
  inherited —see Syphilis, congenital
  internal ear A52.79
  intestine (late) A52.74
  iris, iritis (secondary) A51.43
    late A52.71
  joint (late) A52.77
  keratitis (congenital) (interstitial) (late) A50.31
  kidney (late) A52.75
  lacrimal passages (late) A52.71
  larynx (late) A52.73
  late A52.9
    cardiovascular A52.00
    central nervous system A52.3
    kidney A52.75
    latent or 2 years or more after infection (without manifestations) A52.8
      negative spinal fluid test A52.8
      serology positive A52.8
    paresis A52.17
    specified site NEC A52.79
    symptomatic or with manifestations A52.79
    tabes A52.11

Syphilis, syphilitic *(continued)*
 latent A53.0
  with signs or symptoms - code
   by site and stage under
   Syphilis
  central nervous system A52.2
  date of infection unspecified
   A53.0
  early, or less than 2 years after
   infection A51.5
  follow-up of latent syphilis
   A53.0
   date of infection unspecified
    A53.0
   late, or 2 years or more after
    infection A52.8
  late, or 2 years or more after
   infection A52.8
  positive serology (only finding)
   A53.0
   date of infection unspecified
    A53.0
   early, or less than 2 years after
    infection A51.5
   late, or 2 years or more after
    infection A52.8
 lens (late) A52.71
 leukoderma A51.39
  late A52.79
 lienitis A52.79
 lip A51.39
  chancre (primary) A51.2
  late A52.79
 Lissauer's paralysis A52.17
 liver A52.74
 locomotor ataxia A52.11
 lung A52.72
 lymph gland (early) (secondary)
  A51.49
  late A52.79
 lymphadenitis (secondary) A51.49
 macular atrophy of skin A51.39
  striated A52.79
 mediastinum (late) A52.73
 meninges (adhesive) (brain) (spinal
  cord) A52.13
 meningitis A52.13
  acute (secondary) A51.41
  congenital A50.41
 meningoencephalitis A52.14
 meningovascular A52.13
  congenital A50.41
 mesarteritis A52.09
  brain A52.04
 middle ear A52.77
 mitral stenosis A52.03
 monoplegia A52.17
 mouth (secondary) A51.39
  late A52.79
 mucocutaneous (secondary) A51.39
  late A52.79
 mucous
  membrane (secondary) A51.39
   late A52.79
  patches A51.39
   congenital A50.07
 mulberry molars A50.52
 muscle A52.78
 myocardium A52.06
 nasal sinus (late) A52.73
 neonatorum —*see* Syphilis,
  congenital
 nephrotic syndrome (secondary)
  A51.44
 nerve palsy (any cranial nerve)
  A52.15
  multiple A52.15
 nervous system, central A52.3
 neuritis A52.15
  acoustic A52.15
 neurorecidive of retina A52.19

Syphilis, syphilitic *(continued)*
 neuroretinitis A52.19
 newborn —*see* Syphilis, congenital
 nodular superficial (late) A52.79
 nonvenereal A65
 nose (late) A52.73
  saddle back deformity A50.57
 occlusive arterial disease A52.09
 oculopathy A52.71
 ophthalmic (late) A52.71
 optic nerve (atrophy) (neuritis)
  (papilla) A52.15
 orbit (late) A52.71
 organic A53.9
 osseous (late) A52.77
 osteochondritis (congenital) (early)
  A50.02 *[M90.80]*
 osteoporosis A52.77
 ovary (late) A52.76
 oviduct (late) A52.76
 palate (late) A52.79
 pancreas (late) A52.74
 paralysis A52.17
  general A52.17
   juvenile A50.45
 paresis (general) A52.17
  juvenile A50.45
 paresthesia A52.19
 Parkinson's disease or syndrome
  A52.19
 paroxysmal tachycardia A52.06
 pemphigus (congenital) A50.06
 penis (chancre) A51.0
  late A52.76
 pericardium A52.06
 perichondritis, larynx (late) A52.73
 periosteum (late) A52.77
  congenital (early) A50.02
   [M90.80]
  early (secondary) A51.46
 peripheral nerve A52.79
 petrous bone (late) A52.77
 pharynx (late) A52.73
  secondary A51.39
 pituitary (gland) A52.79
 pleura (late) A52.73
 pneumonia, white A50.04
 pontine lesion A52.17
 portal vein A52.09
 primary A51.0
  anal A51.1
  and secondary —*see* Syphilis,
   secondary
  central nervous system A52.3
  extragenital chancre NEC A51.2
  fingers A51.2
  genital A51.0
  lip A51.2
  specified site NEC A51.2
  tonsils A51.2
 prostate (late) A52.76
 ptosis (eyelid) A52.71
 pulmonary (late) A52.72
  artery A52.09
 pyelonephritis (late) A52.75
 recently acquired, symptomatic
  A51.9
 rectum (late) A52.74
 respiratory tract (late) A52.73
 retina, late A52.71
 retrobulbar neuritis A52.15
 salpingitis A52.76
 sclera (late) A52.71
 sclerosis
  cerebral A52.17
  coronary A52.06
  multiple A52.11
 scotoma (central) A52.71
 scrotum (late) A52.76
 secondary (and primary) A51.49
  adenopathy A51.49

Syphilis, syphilitic *(continued)*
 secondary *(continued)*
  anus A51.39
  bone A51.46
  chorioretinitis, choroiditis A51.43
  hepatitis A51.45
  liver A51.45
  lymphadenitis A51.49
  meningitis (acute) A51.41
  mouth A51.39
  mucous membranes A51.39
  periosteum, periostitis A51.46
  pharynx A51.39
  relapse (treated, untreated) A51.49
  skin A51.39
  specified form NEC A51.49
  tonsil A51.39
  ulcer A51.39
  viscera NEC A51.49
  vulva A51.39
 seminal vesicle (late) A52.76
 seronegative with signs or
  symptoms - code by site and
  stage under Syphilis
 seropositive
  with signs or symptoms - code
   by site and stage under
   Syphilis
  follow-up of latent syphilis —*see*
   Syphilis, latent
  only finding —*see* Syphilis,
   latent
 seventh nerve (paralysis) A52.15
 sinus, sinusitis (late) A52.73
 skeletal system A52.77
 skin (with ulceration) (early)
  (secondary) A51.39
  late or tertiary A52.79
 small intestine A52.74
 spastic spinal paralysis A52.17
 spermatic cord (late) A52.76
 spinal (cord) A52.12
 spleen A52.79
 splenomegaly A52.79
 spondylitis A52.77
 staphyloma A52.71
 stigmata (congenital) A50.59
 stomach A52.74
 synovium A52.78
 tabes dorsalis (late) A52.11
  juvenile A50.45
 tabetic type A52.11
  juvenile A50.45
 taboparesis A52.17
  juvenile A50.45
 tachycardia A52.06
 tendon (late) A52.78
 tertiary A52.9
  with symptoms NEC A52.79
  cardiovascular A52.00
  central nervous system A52.3
  multiple NEC A52.79
  specified site NEC A52.79
 testis A52.76
 thorax A52.73
 throat A52.73
 thymus (gland) (late) A52.79
 thyroid (late) A52.79
 tongue (late) A52.79
 tonsil (lingual) (late) A52.73
  primary A51.2
  secondary A51.39
 trachea (late) A52.73
 tunica vaginalis (late) A52.76
 ulcer (any site) (early) (secondary)
  A51.39
  late A52.79
  perforating A52.79
   foot A52.11
 urethra (late) A52.76
 urogenital (late) A52.76

Syphilis, syphilitic *(continued)*
 uterus (late) A52.76
 uveal tract (secondary) A51.43
  late A52.71
 uveitis (secondary) A51.43
  late A52.71
 uvula (late) (perforated) A52.79
 vagina A51.0
  late A52.76
 valvulitis NEC A52.03
 vascular A52.00
  brain (cerebral) A52.05
 ventriculi A52.74
 vesicae urinariae (late) A52.76
 viscera (abdominal) (late) A52.74
  secondary A51.49
 vitreous (opacities) (late) A52.71
  hemorrhage A52.71
 vulva A51.0
  late A52.76
  secondary A51.39

Syphiloma A52.79
 cardiovascular system A52.00
 central nervous system A52.3
 circulatory system A52.00
 congenital A50.59

Syphilophobia F45.29

Syringadenoma —*see also*
  Neoplasm, skin, benign
 papillary —*see* Neoplasm, skin,
  benign

Syringobulbia G95.0

Syringocystadenoma —*see*
  Neoplasm, skin, benign
 papillary —*see* Neoplasm, skin,
  benign

Syringoma —*see also* Neoplasm,
  skin, benign
 chondroid —*see* Neoplasm, skin,
  benign

Syringomyelia G95.0

Syringomyelitis —*see* Encephalitis

Syringomyelocele —*see* Spina bifida

Syringopontia G95.0

System, systemic —*see also*
  condition
 disease, combined —*see*
  Degeneration, combined
 inflammatory response syndrome
  (SIRS) of non-infectious origin
  (without organ dysfunction)
  R65.10
  with acute organ dysfunction
   R65.11
 lupus erythematosus M32.9
  inhibitor present D68.62

T

Tabacism, tabacosis, tabagism
  —*see also* Poisoning, tobacco
 meaning dependence (without
  remission) F17.200
  with
   disorder F17.299
    in remission F17.211
    specified disorder NEC
     F17.298
   withdrawal F17.203

Tabardillo A75.9
 flea-borne A75.2
 louse-borne A75.0

Tabes, tabetic A52.10
 with
  central nervous system syphilis
   A52.10

Tabes, tabetic *(continued)*
- with *(continued)*
  - Charcot's joint A52.16
  - cord bladder A52.19
  - crisis, viscera (any) A52.19
  - paralysis, general A52.17
  - paresis (general) A52.17
  - perforating ulcer (foot) A52.19
  - arthropathy (Charcot) A52.16
  - bladder A52.19
  - bone A52.11
  - cerebrospinal A52.12
  - congenital A50.45
  - conjugal A52.10
  - dorsalis A52.11
    - juvenile A50.49
  - juvenile A50.49
  - latent A52.19
  - mesenterica A18.39
  - paralysis, insane, general A52.17
  - spasmodic A52.17
  - syphilis (cerebrospinal) A52.12

Taboparalysis A52.17

Taboparesis (remission) A52.17
- juvenile A50.45

TAC (trigeminal autonomic cephalgia) **NEC** G44.099
- intractable G44.091
- not intractable G44.099

Tache noir S60.22-

Tachyalimentation K91.2

Tachyarrhythmia, tachyrhythmia —*see* Tachycardia

Tachycardia R00.0
- atrial (paroxysmal) I47.1
- auricular I47.1
- AV nodal re-entry (re-entrant) I47.1
- junctional (paroxysmal) I47.1
- newborn P29.11
- nodal (paroxysmal) I47.1
- non-paroxysmal AV nodal I45.89
- paroxysmal (sustained)
  - (nonsustained) I47.9
    - with sinus bradycardia I49.5
    - atrial (PAT) I47.1
    - atrioventricular (AV) (re-entrant) I47.1
      - psychogenic F54
    - junctional I47.1
      - ectopic I47.1
    - nodal I47.1
    - psychogenic (atrial) (supraventricular) (ventricular) F54
    - supraventricular (sustained) I47.1
      - psychogenic F54
    - ventricular I47.2
      - psychogenic F54
- psychogenic F45.8
- sick sinus I49.5
- sinoauricular NOS R00.0
  - paroxysmal I47.1
- sinus [sinusal] NOS R00.0
  - paroxysmal I47.1
- supraventricular I47.1
- ventricular (paroxysmal) (sustained) I47.2
  - psychogenic F54

Tachygastria K31.89

Tachypnea R06.82
- hysterical F45.8
- newborn (idiopathic) (transitory) P22.1
- psychogenic F45.8
- transitory, of newborn P22.1

Taenia (infection) (infestation) B68.9
- diminuta B71.0

Taenia *(continued)*
- echinococcal infestation B67.90
- mediocanellata B68.1
- nana B71.0
- saginata B68.1
- solium (intestinal form) B68.0
  - larval form —*see* Cysticercosis

Taeniasis (intestine) —*see* Taenia

TACO (transfusion associated circulatory overload) E87.71

Tag (hypertrophied skin) (infected) L91.8
- adenoid J35.8
- anus K64.4
- hemorrhoidal K64.4
- hymen N89.8
- perineal N90.89
- preauricular Q17.0
- sentinel K64.4
- skin L91.8
  - accessory (congenital) Q82.8
  - anus K64.4
  - congenital Q82.8
  - preauricular Q17.0
- tonsil J35.8
- urethra, urethral N36.8
- vulva N90.89

Tahyna fever B33.8

Takahara's disease E80.3

Takayasu's disease or syndrome M31.4

Talaromycosis B48.4

Talcosis (pulmonary) J62.0

Talipes (congenital) Q66.89
- acquired, planus —*see* Deformity, limb, flat foot
- asymmetric Q66.89
- calcaneovalgus Q66.4-
- calcaneovarus Q66.1-
- calcaneus Q66.89
- cavus Q66.7-
- equinovalgus Q66.6
- equinovarus Q66.0-
- equinus Q66.89
- percavus Q66.7-
- planovalgus Q66.6
- planus (acquired) (any degree) —*see also* Deformity, limb, flat foot
  - congenital Q66.5-
  - due to rickets (sequelae) E64.3
- valgus Q66.6
- varus Q66.3-

Tall stature, constitutional E34.4

Talma's disease M62.89

Talon noir S90.3-
- hand S60.22-
- heel S90.3-
- toe S90.1-

Tamponade, heart I31.4

Tanapox (virus disease) B08.71

Tangier disease E78.6

Tantrum, child problem F91.8

Tapeworm (infection) (infestation) —*see* Infestation, tapeworm

Tapia's syndrome G52.7

TAR (thrombocytopenia with absent radius) **syndrome** Q87.2

Tarral-Besnier disease L44.0

Tarsal tunnel syndrome —*see* Syndrome, tarsal tunnel

Tarsalgia —*see* Pain, limb, lower

Tarsitis (eyelid) H01.8
- syphilitic A52.71
- tuberculous A18.4

Tartar (teeth) (dental calculus) K03.6

Tattoo (mark) L81.8

Tauri's disease E74.09

Taurodontism K00.2

Taussig-Bing syndrome Q20.1

Taybi's syndrome Q87.2

Tay-Sachs amaurotic familial idiocy or disease E75.02

TBI (traumatic brain injury) S06.9

Teacher's node or nodule J38.2

Tear, torn (traumatic) —*see also* Laceration
- with abortion —*see* Abortion
- annular fibrosis M51.35
- anus, anal (sphincter) S31.831
  - complicating delivery
    - with third degree perineal laceration (*see also* Delivery, complicated, by, laceration, perineum, third degree) O70.20
      - with mucosa O70.3
    - without third degree perineal laceration O70.4
  - nontraumatic (healed) (old) K62.81
- articular cartilage, old —*see* Derangement, joint, articular cartilage, by site
- bladder
  - with ectopic or molar pregnancy O08.6
  - following ectopic or molar pregnancy O08.6
  - obstetrical O71.5
  - traumatic —*see* Injury, bladder
- bowel
  - with ectopic or molar pregnancy O08.6
  - following ectopic or molar pregnancy O08.6
  - obstetrical trauma O71.5
- broad ligament
  - with ectopic or molar pregnancy O08.6
- broad ligament
  - following ectopic or molar pregnancy O08.6
  - obstetrical trauma O71.6
- bucket handle (knee) (meniscus) —*see* Tear, meniscus
- capsule, joint —*see* Sprain
- cartilage —*see also* Sprain
  - articular, old —*see* Derangement, joint, articular cartilage, by site
- cervix
  - with ectopic or molar pregnancy O08.6
  - following ectopic or molar pregnancy O08.6
  - obstetrical trauma (current) O71.3
  - old N88.1
  - traumatic —*see* Injury, uterus
- dural G97.41
  - nontraumatic G96.11
- internal organ —*see* Injury, by site
- knee cartilage
  - articular (current) S83.3-
  - old —*see* Derangement, knee, meniscus, due to old tear
- ligament —*see* Sprain
- meniscus (knee) (current injury) S83.209
  - bucket-handle S83.20-
  - lateral
    - bucket-handle S83.25-
    - complex S83.27-

Tear, torn *(continued)*
- meniscus *(continued)*
  - lateral *(continued)*
    - peripheral S83.26-
    - specified type NEC S83.28-
  - medial
    - bucket-handle S83.21-
    - complex S83.23-
    - peripheral S83.22-
    - specified type NEC S83.24-
  - old —*see* Derangement, knee, meniscus, due to old tear
  - site other than knee - code as Sprain
  - specified type NEC S83.20-
- muscle —*see* Strain
- pelvic
  - floor, complicating delivery O70.1
  - organ NEC, obstetrical trauma O71.5
    - with ectopic or molar pregnancy O08.6
    - following ectopic or molar pregnancy O08.6
- perineal, secondary O90.1
- periurethral tissue, obstetrical trauma O71.82
  - with ectopic or molar pregnancy O08.6
  - following ectopic or molar pregnancy O08.6
- rectovaginal septum —*see* Laceration, vagina
- retina, retinal (without detachment) (horseshoe) —*see also* Break, retina, horseshoe
  - with detachment —*see* Detachment, retina, with retinal, break
- rotator cuff (nontraumatic) M75.10-
  - complete M75.12-
  - incomplete M75.11-
  - traumatic S46.01-
    - capsule S43.42-
- semilunar cartilage, knee *see* Tear, meniscus
- supraspinatus (complete) (incomplete) (nontraumatic) (*see also* Tear, rotator cuff) M75.10-
- tendon —*see* Strain
- tentorial, at birth P10.4
- umbilical cord
  - complicating delivery O69.89
- urethra
  - with ectopic or molar pregnancy O08.6
  - following ectopic or molar pregnancy O08.6
  - obstetrical trauma O71.5
- uterus —*see* Injury, uterus
- vagina —*see* Laceration, vagina
- vessel, from catheter —*see* Puncture, accidental complicating surgery
- vulva, complicating delivery O70.0

Tear-stone —*see* Dacryolith

Teeth —*see also* condition
- grinding
  - psychogenic F45.8
  - sleep related G47.63

Teething (syndrome) K00.7

Telangiectasia, telangiectasis (verrucous) I78.1
- ataxic (cerebellar) (Louis-Bar) G11.3
- familial I78.0

Telangiectasia, telangiectasis
  (continued)
  hemorrhagic, hereditary
    (congenital) (senile) I78.0
  hereditary, hemorrhagic
    (congenital) (senile) I78.0
  juxtafoveal H35.07-
  macular H35.07-
  macularis eruptiva perstans
    D47.01
  parafoveal H35.07-
  retinal (idiopathic) (juxtafoveal)
    (macular) (parafoveal)
    H35.07-
  spider I78.1

Telephone scatologia F65.89

Telescoped bowel or intestine
  K56.1
  congenital Q43.8

Temperature
  body, high (of unknown origin)
    R50.9
  cold, trauma from T69.9
    newborn P80.0
    specified effect NEC T69.8

Temple —*see* condition

Temporal —*see* condition

Temporomandibular joint pain-dysfunction syndrome M26.62-

Temporosphenoidal —*see* condition

Tendency
  bleeding —*see* Defect, coagulation
  suicide
    meaning personal history of
      attempted suicide Z91.5
    meaning suicidal ideation —*see*
      Ideation, suicidal
  to fall R29.6

Tenderness, abdominal R10.819
  epigastric R10.816
  generalized R10.817
  left lower quadrant R10.814
  left upper quadrant R10.812
  periumbilic R10.815
  right lower quadrant R10.813
  right upper quadrant R10.811
  rebound R10.829
    epigastric R10.826
    generalized R10.827
    left lower quadrant R10.824
    left upper quadrant R10.822
    periumbilic R10.825
    right lower quadrant R10.823
    right upper quadrant R10.821

Tendinitis, tendonitis —*see also*
  Enthesopathy
  Achilles M76.6-
  adhesive —*see* Tenosynovitis,
    specified type NEC
    shoulder —*see* Capsulitis,
      adhesive
  bicipital M75.2-
  calcific M65.2-
    ankle M65.27-
    foot M65.27-
    forearm M65.23-
    hand M65.24-
    lower leg M65.26-
    multiple sites M65.29
    pelvic region M65.25-
    shoulder M75.3-
    specified site NEC M65.28
    thigh M65.25-
    upper arm M65.22-
  due to use, overuse, pressure —*see
    also* Disorder, soft tissue, due
    to use

Tendinitis, tendonitis *(continued)*
  due to use, overuse, pressure
    (continued)
    specified NEC —*see* Disorder,
      soft tissue, due to use,
      specified NEC
  gluteal M76.0-
  patellar M76.5-
  peroneal M76.7-
  psoas M76.1-
  tibial (posterior) M76.82-
    anterior M76.81-
  trochanteric —*see* Bursitis, hip,
    trochanteric

Tendon —*see* condition

Tendosynovitis —*see* Tenosynovitis

Tenesmus (rectal) R19.8
  vesical R30.1

Tennis elbow —*see* Epicondylitis,
  lateral

Tenonitis —*see also* Tenosynovitis
  eye (capsule) H05.04-

Tenontosynovitis —*see*
  Tenosynovitis

Tenontothecitis —*see*
  Tenosynovitis

Tenophyte —*see* Disorder, synovium,
  specified type NEC

Tenosynovitis (*see also* Synovitis)
  M65.9
  adhesive —*see* Tenosynovitis,
    specified type NEC
    shoulder —*see* Capsulitis,
      adhesive
  bicipital (calcifying) —*see*
    Tendinitis, bicipital
  gonococcal A54.49
  in (due to)
    crystals M65.8-
    gonorrhea A54.49
    syphilis (late) A52.78
    use, overuse, pressure —*see
      also* Disorder, soft tissue, due
      to use
      specified NEC —*see* Disorder,
        soft tissue, due to use,
        specified NEC
  infective NEC M65.1-
    ankle M65.17-
    foot M65.17-
    forearm M65.13-
    hand M65.14-
    lower leg M65.16-
    multiple sites M65.19
    pelvic region M65.15-
    shoulder region M65.11-
    specified site NEC M65.18
    thigh M65.15-
    upper arm M65.12-
  radial styloid M65.4
  shoulder region M65.81-
    adhesive —*see* Capsulitis,
      adhesive
  specified type NEC M65.88
    ankle M65.87-
    foot M65.87-
    forearm M65.83-
    hand M65.84-
    lower leg M65.86-
    multiple sites M65.89
    pelvic region M65.85-
    shoulder region M65.81-
    specified site NEC M65.88
    thigh M65.85-
    upper arm M65.82-
  tuberculous —*see* Tuberculosis,
    tenosynovitis

Tenovaginitis —*see* Tenosynovitis

Tension
  arterial, high —*see also*
    Hypertension
    without diagnosis of
      hypertension R03.0
  headache G44.209
    intractable G44.201
    not intractable G44.209
  nervous R45.0
  pneumothorax J93.0
  premenstrual N94.3
  state (mental) F48.9

Tentorium —*see* condition

Teratencephalus Q89.8

Teratism Q89.7

Teratoblastoma (malignant) —*see*
  Neoplasm, malignant, by site

Teratocarcinoma —*see also*
  Neoplasm, malignant, by site
  liver C22.7

Teratoma (solid) —*see also*
  Neoplasm, uncertain behavior, by
  site
  with embryonal carcinoma, mixed
    —*see* Neoplasm, malignant,
    by site
  with malignant transformation —
    see Neoplasm, malignant, by
    site
  adult (cystic) —*see* Neoplasm,
    benign, by site
  benign —*see* Neoplasm, benign,
    by site
  combined with choriocarcinoma
    —*see* Neoplasm, malignant,
    by site
  cystic (adult) —*see* Neoplasm,
    benign, by site
  differentiated —*see* Neoplasm,
    benign, by site
  embryonal —*see also* Neoplasm,
    malignant, by site
    liver C22.7
  immature —*see* Neoplasm,
    malignant, by site
  liver C22.7
    adult, benign, cystic,
      differentiated type or mature
      D13.4
  malignant —*see also* Neoplasm,
    malignant, by site
    anaplastic —*see* Neoplasm,
      malignant, by site
    intermediate —*see* Neoplasm,
      malignant, by site
      specified site —*see* Neoplasm,
        malignant, by site
      unspecified site C62.90
    undifferentiated —*see*
      Neoplasm, malignant, by
      site
  mature —*see* Neoplasm, uncertain
    behavior, by site
    malignant —*see* Neoplasm, by
      site, malignant, by site
  ovary D27.-
    embryonal, immature or
      malignant C56-
  solid —*see* Neoplasm, uncertain
    behavior, by site
  testis C62.9-
    adult, benign, cystic, differentiated
      type or mature D29.2-
    scrotal C62.1-
    undescended C62.0-

Termination
  anomalous —*see also* Malposition,
    congenital
    right pulmonary vein Q26.3
  pregnancy, elective Z33.2

Ternidens diminutus infestation
  B81.8

Ternidensiasis B81.8

Terror(s) night (child) F51.4

Terrorism, victim of Z65.4

Terry's syndrome (*see also* Myopia,
  degenerative) H44.2-

Tertiary —*see* condition

Test, tests, testing (for)
  adequacy (for dialysis)
    hemodialysis Z49.31
    peritoneal Z49.32
  blood pressure Z01.30
    abnormal reading —*see* Blood,
      pressure
  blood-alcohol Z04.89
    positive —*see* Findings,
      abnormal, in blood
  blood-drug Z04.89
    positive —*see* Findings,
      abnormal, in blood
  blood typing Z01.83
    Rh typing Z01.83
  cardiac pulse generator (battery)
    Z45.010
  fertility Z31.41
  genetic
    disease carrier status for
      procreative management
      female Z31.430
      male Z31.440
    male partner of patient with
      recurrent pregnancy loss
      Z31.441
    procreative management NEC
      female Z31.438
      male Z31.448
  hearing Z01.10
    with abnormal findings NEC
      Z01.118
    infant or child (over 28 days old)
      Z00.129
      with abnormal findings
        Z00.121
  HIV (human immunodeficiency
    virus)
    nonconclusive (in infants) R75
    positive Z21
    seropositive Z21
  immunity status Z01.84
  intelligence NEC Z01.89
  laboratory (as part of a general
    medical examination) Z00.00
    with abnormal finding Z00.01
    for medicolegal reason NEC
      Z04.89
  male partner of patient with
    recurrent pregnancy loss
    Z31.441
  Mantoux (for tuberculosis)
    Z11.1
    abnormal result R76.11
  pregnancy, positive first pregnancy
    —*see* Pregnancy, normal, first
  procreative Z31.49
    fertility Z31.41
  skin, diagnostic
    allergy Z01.82
      special screening examination
        —*see* Screening, by name
        of disease
    Mantoux Z11.1
    tuberculin Z11.1
  specified NEC Z01.89

Test, tests, testing *(continued)*
tuberculin Z11.1
abnormal result R76.11
vision Z01.00
with abnormal findings Z01.01
following failed vision screening Z01.020
with abnormal findings Z01.021
infant or child (over 28 days old) Z00.129
with abnormal findings Z00.121
Wassermann Z11.3
positive —*see* Serology for syphilis, positive

Testicle, testicular, testis —*see also* condition
feminization syndrome (*see also* Syndrome, androgen insensitivity) E34.51
migrans Q55.29

Tetanus, tetanic (cephalic) (convulsions) A35
with
abortion A34
ectopic or molar pregnancy O08.0
following ectopic or molar pregnancy O08.0
inoculation reaction (due to serum) —*see* Complications, vaccination
neonatorum A33
obstetrical A34
puerperal, postpartum, childbirth A34

Tetany (due to) R29.0
alkalosis E87.3
associated with rickets E55.0
convulsions R29.0
hysterical F44.5
functional (hysterical) F44.5
hyperkinetic R29.0
hysterical F44.5
hyperpnea R06.4
hysterical F44.5
psychogenic F45.8
hyperventilation (*see also* Hyperventilation) R06.4
hysterical F44.5
neonatal (without calcium or magnesium deficiency) P71.3
parathyroid (gland) E20.9
parathyroprival E89.2
post- (para)thyroidectomy E89.2
postoperative E89.2
pseudotetany R29.0
psychogenic (conversion reaction) F44.5

Tetralogy of Fallot Q21.3

Tetraplegia (chronic) (*see also* Quadriplegia) G82.50

Thailand hemorrhagic fever A91

Thalassanemia —*see* Thalassemia

Thalassemia (anemia) (disease) D56.9
with other hemoglobinopathy D56.8
alpha (major) (severe) (triple gene defect) D56.0
minor D56.3
silent carrier D56.3
trait D56.3
beta (severe) D56.1
homozygous D56.1
major D56.1

Thalassemia *(continued)*
beta *(continued)*
minor D56.3
trait D56.3
delta-beta (homozygous) D56.2
minor D56.3
trait D56.3
dominant D56.8
hemoglobin
C D56.8
E-beta D56.5
intermedia D56.1
major D56.1
minor D56.3
mixed D56.8
sickle-cell —*see* Disease, sickle-cell, thalassemia
specified type NEC D56.8
trait D56.3
variants D56.8

Thanatophoric dwarfism or short stature Q77.1

Thaysen-Gee disease (nontropical sprue) K90.0

Thaysen's disease K90.0

Thecoma D27-
luteinized D27-
malignant C56-

Thelarche, premature E30.8

Thelaziasis B83.8

Thelitis N61.0
puerperal, postpartum or gestational —*see* Infection, nipple

Therapeutic —*see* condition

Therapy
drug, long-term (current) (prophylactic)
agents affecting estrogen receptors and estrogen levels NEC Z79.818
anastrozole (Arimidex) Z79.811
antibiotics Z79.2
short-term use - omit code
anticoagulants Z79.01
anti-inflammatory Z79.1
antiplatelet Z79.02
antithrombotics Z79.02
aromatase inhibitors Z79.811
aspirin Z79.82
birth control pill or patch Z79.3
bisphosphonates Z79.83
contraceptive, oral Z79.3
drug, specified NEC Z79.899
estrogen receptor downregulators Z79.818
Evista Z79.810
exemestane (Aromasin) Z79.811
Fareston Z79.810
fulvestrant (Faslodex) Z79.818
gonadotropin-releasing hormone (GnRH) agonist Z79.818
goserelin acetate (Zoladex) Z79.818
hormone replacement Z79.890
insulin Z79.4
letrozole (Femara) Z79.811
leuprolide acetate (leuprorelin) (Lupron) Z79.818
megestrol acetate (Megace) Z79.818
methadone
for pain management Z79.891
maintenance therapy F11.20
Nolvadex Z79.810
opiate analgesic Z79.891

Therapy *(continued)*
drug, long-term *(continued)*
oral contraceptive Z79.3
raloxifene (Evista) Z79.810
selective estrogen receptor modulators (SERMs) Z79.810
short term - omit code
steroids
inhaled Z79.51
systemic Z79.52
tamoxifen (Nolvadex) Z79.810
toremifene (Fareston) Z79.810

Thermic —*see* condition

Thermography (abnormal) (*see also* Abnormal, diagnostic imaging) R93.89
breast R92.8

Thermoplegia T67.01

Thesaurismosis, glycogen —*see* Disease, glycogen storage

Thiamin deficiency E51.9
specified NEC E51.8

Thiaminic deficiency with beriberi E51.11

Thibierge-Weissenbach syndrome —*see* Sclerosis, systemic

Thickening
bone —*see* Hypertrophy, bone
breast N64.59
endometrium R93.89
epidermal L85.9
specified NEC L85.8
hymen N89.6
larynx J38.7
nail L60.2
congenital Q84.5
periosteal —*see* Hypertrophy, bone
pleura J92.9
with asbestos J92.0
skin R23.4
subepiglottic J38.7
tongue K14.8
valve, heart —*see* Endocarditis

Thigh —*see* condition

Thinning vertebra —*see* Spondylopathy, specified NEC

Thirst, excessive R63.1
due to deprivation of water T73.1

Thomsen disease G71.12

Thoracic —*see also* condition
kidney Q63.2
outlet syndrome G54.0

Thoracogastroschisis (congenital) Q79.8

Thoracopagus Q89.4

Thorax —*see* condition

Thorn's syndrome N28.89

Thorson-Björck syndrome E34.0

Threadworm (infection) (infestation) B80

Threatened
abortion O20.0
with subsequent abortion O03.9
job loss, anxiety concerning Z56.2
labor (without delivery) O47.9
at or after 37 completed weeks of gestation O47.1
before 37 completed weeks of gestation O47.0-
loss of job, anxiety concerning Z56.2

Threatened *(continued)*
miscarriage O20.0
unemployment, anxiety concerning Z56.2

Three-day fever A93.1

Threshers' lung J67.0

Thrix annulata (congenital) Q84.1

Throat —*see* condition

Thrombasthenia (Glanzmann) (hemorrhagic) (hereditary) D69.1

Thromboangiitis I73.1
obliterans (general) I73.1
cerebral I67.89
vessels
brain I67.89
spinal cord I67.89

Thromboarteritis —*see* Arteritis

Thromboasthenia (Glanzmann) (hemorrhagic) (hereditary) D69.1

Thrombocytasthenia (Glanzmann) D69.1

Thrombocythemia (essential) (hemorrhagic) (idiopathic) (primary) D47.3

Thrombocytopathy (dystrophic) (granulopenic) D69.1

Thrombocytopenia, thrombocytopenic D69.6
with absent radius (TAR) Q87.2
congenital D69.42
dilutional D69.59
due to
drugs D69.59
extracorporeal circulation of blood D69.59
(massive) blood transfusion D69.59
platelet alloimmunization D69.59
essential D69.3
heparin induced (HIT) D75.82
hereditary D69.42
idiopathic D69.3
neonatal, transitory P61.0
due to
exchange transfusion P61.0
idiopathic maternal thrombocytopenia P61.0
isoimmunization P61.0
primary NEC D69.49
idiopathic D69.3
puerperal, postpartum O72.3
secondary D69.59
transient neonatal P61.0

Thrombocytosis, essential D47.3
primary D47.3

Thromboembolism —*see* Embolism

Thrombopathy (Bernard-Soulier) D69.1
constitutional D68.0
Willebrand-Jurgens D68.0

Thrombopenia —*see* Thrombocytopenia

Thrombophilia D68.59
primary NEC D68.59
secondary NEC D68.69
specified NEC D68.69

Thrombophlebitis I80.9
antepartum O22.2-
deep O22.3-
superficial O22.2-
calf muscular vein (NOS) I80.25-

Thrombophlebitis *(continued)*
  cavernous (venous) sinus G08
    complicating pregnancy O22.5-
    nonpyogenic I67.6
  cerebral (sinus) (vein) G08
    nonpyogenic I67.6
    sequelae G09
  due to implanted device —*see*
    Complications, by site and type,
    specified NEC
  during or resulting from a
    procedure NEC T81.72
  femoral vein (superficial) I80.1-
  femoropopliteal vein I80.0-
  gastrocnemial vein I80.25
  hepatic (vein) I80.8
  idiopathic, recurrent I82.1
  iliac vein (common) (external)
    (internal) I80.21-
  iliofemoral I80.1-
  intracranial venous sinus (any)
    G08
    nonpyogenic I67.6
    sequelae G09
  intraspinal venous sinuses and
    veins G08
    nonpyogenic G95.19
  lateral (venous) sinus G08
    nonpyogenic I67.6
  leg I80.3
    superficial I80.0-
  longitudinal (venous) sinus G08
    nonpyogenic I67.6
  lower extremity I80.299
  migrans, migrating I82.1
  pelvic
    with ectopic or molar pregnancy
      O08.0
    following ectopic or molar
      pregnancy O08.0
    puerperal O87.1
  peroneal vein I80.24-
  popliteal vein —*see* Phlebitis, leg,
    deep, popliteal
  portal (vein) K75.1
  postoperative T81.72
  pregnancy —*see* Thrombophlebitis,
    antepartum
  puerperal, postpartum, childbirth
    O87.0
    deep O87.1
    pelvic O87.1
    septic O86.81
    superficial O87.0
  saphenous (greater) (lesser) I80.0-
  sinus (intracranial) G08
    nonpyogenic I67.6
  soleal vein I80.25-
  specified site NEC I80.8
  tibial vein (anterior) (posterior)
    I80.23-

Thrombosis, thrombotic (bland)
  (multiple) (progressive) (silent)
  (vessel) I82.90
  anal K64.5
  antepartum —*see*
    Thrombophlebitis, antepartum
  aorta, aortic I74.10
    abdominal I74.09
      saddle I74.01
    bifurcation I74.09
    saddle I74.01
    specified site NEC I74.19
    terminal I74.09
    thoracic I74.11
    valve —*see* Endocarditis, aortic
  apoplexy I63.3-
  artery, arteries (postinfectional) I74.9
    auditory, internal —*see*
      Occlusion, artery, precerebral,
      specified NEC

artery, arteries *(continued)*
  basilar —*see* Occlusion, artery,
    basilar
  carotid (common) (internal)
    —*see* Occlusion, artery,
    carotid
  cerebellar (anterior inferior)
    (posterior inferior) (superior)
    —*see* Occlusion, artery,
    cerebellar
  cerebral —*see* Occlusion, artery,
    cerebral
  choroidal (anterior) —*see*
    Occlusion, artery, precerebral,
    specified NEC
  communicating, posterior —*see*
    Occlusion, artery, precerebral,
    specified NEC
  coronary —*see also* Infarct,
    myocardium
    not resulting in infarction
      I24.0
  hepatic I74.8
  hypophyseal —*see* Occlusion,
    artery, precerebral, specified
    NEC
  iliac I74.5
  limb I74.4
    lower I74.3
    upper I74.2
  meningeal, anterior or posterior
    —*see* Occlusion, artery,
    cerebral, specified NEC
  mesenteric (with gangrene) (*see*
    also Infarct, intestine)
    K55.069
  ophthalmic —*see* Occlusion,
    artery, retina
  pontine —*see* Occlusion,
    artery, precerebral, specified
    NEC
  precerebral —*see* Occlusion,
    artery, precerebral
  pulmonary (iatrogenic) —*see*
    Embolism, pulmonary
  renal N28.0
  retinal —*see* Occlusion, artery,
    retina
  spinal, anterior or posterior
    G95.11
  traumatic NEC T14.8
  vertebral —*see* Occlusion,
    artery, vertebral
  atrium, auricular —*see also* Infarct,
    myocardium
    following acute myocardial
      infarction (current
      complication) I23.6
    not resulting in infarction I51.3
    old I51.3
  basilar (artery) —*see* Occlusion,
    artery, basilar
  brain (artery) (stem) —*see also*
    Occlusion, artery, cerebral
    due to syphilis A52.05
    puerperal O99.43
    sinus —*see* Thrombosis,
      intracranial venous sinus
  capillary I78.8
  cardiac —*see also* Infarct,
    myocardium
    not resulting in infarction I51.3
    old I51.3
    valve —*see* Endocarditis
  carotid (artery) (common)
    (internal) —*see* Occlusion,
    artery, carotid
  cavernous (venous) sinus —*see*
    Thrombosis, intracranial venous
    sinus

cerebellar artery (anterior inferior)
  (posterior inferior) (superior)
  I66.3
cerebral (artery) —*see* Occlusion,
  artery, cerebral
cerebrovenous sinus —*see also*
  Thrombosis, intracranial venous
  sinus
  puerperium O87.3
chronic I82.91
coronary (artery) (vein) —*see also*
  Infarct, myocardium
  not resulting in infarction I24.0
corpus cavernosum N48.89
cortical I66.9
deep —*see* Embolism, vein, lower
  extremity
due to device, implant or graft
  (*see also* Complications, by
  site and type, specified NEC)
  T85.868
  arterial graft NEC T82.868
  breast (implant) T85.868
  catheter NEC T85.868
    dialysis (renal) T82.868
      intraperitoneal T85.868
    infusion NEC T82.868
      spinal (epidural) (subdural)
        T85.860
    urinary (indwelling) T83.86
  electronic (electrode) (pulse
    generator) (stimulator)
    bone T84.86
    cardiac T82.867
    nervous system (brain)
      (peripheral nerve) (spinal)
      T85.860
    urinary T83.86
  fixation, internal (orthopedic)
    NEC T84.86
  gastrointestinal (bile duct)
    (esophagus) T85.868
  genital NEC T83.86
  heart T82.867
  joint prosthesis T84.86
  ocular (corneal graft) (orbital
    implant) NEC T85.868
  orthopedic NEC T84.86
  specified NEC T85.868
  urinary NEC T83.86
  vascular NEC T82.868
  ventricular intracranial shunt
    T85.860
during the puerperium —*see*
  Thrombosis, puerperal
endocardial —*see also* Infarct,
  myocardium
  not resulting in infarction I51.3
eye —*see* Occlusion, retina
genital organ
  female NEC N94.89
    pregnancy —*see*
      Thrombophlebitis,
      antepartum
  male N50.1
gestational —*see* Phlebopathy,
  gestational
heart (chamber) —*see also* Infarct,
  myocardium
  not resulting in infarction I51.3
  old I51.3
hepatic (vein) I82.0
  artery I74.8
history (of) Z86.718
intestine (with gangrene (*see also*
  Infarct, intestine)) K55.069
intracardiac NEC (apical) (atrial)
  (auricular) (ventricular)
  (old) I51.3
intracranial (arterial) I66.9

intracranial *(continued)*
  venous sinus (any) G08
    nonpyogenic origin I67.6
    puerperium O87.3
intramural —*see also* Infarct,
  myocardium
  not resulting in infarction I51.3
  old I51.3
intraspinal venous sinuses and
  veins G08
  nonpyogenic G95.19
kidney (artery) N28.0
lateral (venous) sinus —*see*
  Thrombosis, intracranial venous
  sinus
leg —*see* Thrombosis, vein, lower
  extremity
  arterial I74.3
liver (venous) I82.0
  artery I74.8
  portal vein I81
longitudinal (venous) sinus —*see*
  Thrombosis, intracranial venous
  sinus
lower limb —*see* Thrombosis, vein,
  lower extremity
lung (iatrogenic) (postoperative)
  —*see* Embolism, pulmonary
meninges (brain) (arterial) I66.8
mesenteric (artery) (with gangrene)
  (*see also* Infarct, intestine)
  K55.069
  vein (inferior) (superior) K55.0-
mitral I34.8
mural —*see also* Infarct,
  myocardium
  due to syphilis A52.06
  not resulting in infarction I51.3
  old I51.3
omentum (with gangrene) (*see*
  also Infarct, intestine)
  K55.069
ophthalmic —*see* Occlusion,
  retina
pampiniform plexus (male) N50.1
parietal —*see also* Infarct,
  myocardium
  not resulting in infarction I24.0
penis, superficial vein N48.81
perianal venous K64.5
peripheral arteries I74.4
  upper I74.2
personal history (of) Z86.718
portal I81
  due to syphilis A52.09
precerebral artery —*see* Occlusion,
  artery, precerebral
puerperal, postpartum O87.0
  brain (artery) O99.43
    venous (sinus) O87.3
  cardiac O99.43
  cerebral (artery) O99.43
    venous (sinus) O87.3
  superficial O87.0
pulmonary (artery) (iatrogenic)
  (postoperative) (vein) —*see*
  Embolism, pulmonary
renal (artery) N28.0
  vein I82.3
resulting from presence of
  device, implant or graft —*see*
  Complications, by site and type,
  specified NEC
retina, retinal —*see* Occlusion,
  retina
scrotum N50.1
seminal vesicle N50.1
sigmoid (venous) sinus —*see*
  Thrombosis, intracranial venous
  sinus

Thrombosis, thrombotic *(continued)*
  sinus, intracranial (any) —*see*
    Thrombosis, intracranial venous
    sinus
  specified site NEC I82.890
    chronic I82.891
  spermatic cord N50.1
  spinal cord (arterial) G95.11
    due to syphilis A52.09
    pyogenic origin G06.1
  spleen, splenic D73.5
    artery I74.8
  testis N50.1
  tumor —*see* Neoplasm, unspecified
    behavior, by site
  traumatic NEC T14.8
  tricuspid I07.8
  tunica vaginalis N50.1
  umbilical cord (vessels),
    complicating delivery O69.5
  vas deferens N50.1
  vein (acute) I82.90
    antecubital I82.61-
      chronic I82.71-
    axillary I82.A1-
      chronic I82.A2-
    basilic I82.61-
      chronic I82.71-
    brachial I82.62-
      chronic I82.72-
    brachiocephalic (innominate)
      I82.290
      chronic I82.291
    cerebral, nonpyogenic I67.6
    cephalic I82.61-
      chronic I82.71-
    chronic I82.91
    deep (DVT) I82.40-
      calf I82.4Z-
        chronic I82.5Z-
      lower leg I82.4Z-
        chronic I82.5Z-
      thigh I82.4Y-
        chronic I82.5Y-
      upper leg I82.4Y
        chronic I82.5y--
    femoral I82.41-
      chronic I82.51-
    iliac (iliofemoral) I82.42-
      chronic I82.52-
    innominate I82.290
      chronic I82.291
    internal jugular I82.C1-
      chronic I82.C2-
    lower extremity
      deep I82.40-
        chronic I82.50-
        specified NEC I82.49-
          chronic NEC I82.59-
      distal
        deep I82.4Z-
      proximal
        deep I82.4Y-
          chronic I82.5Y-
      superficial I82.81-
    perianal K64.5
    popliteal I82.43-
      chronic I82.53-
    radial I82.62-
      chronic I82.72-
    renal I82.3
    saphenous (greater) (lesser)
      I82.81-
    specified NEC I82.890
      chronic NEC I82.891
    subclavian I82.B1-
      chronic I82.B2-
    thoracic NEC I82.290
      chronic I82.291
    tibial I82.44-
      chronic I82.54-

Thrombosis, thrombotic *(continued)*
  vein *(continued)*
    ulnar I82.62-
      chronic I82.72-
    upper extremity I82.60-
      chronic I82.70-
      deep I82.62-
        chronic I82.72-
      superficial I82.61-
        chronic I82.71-
    vena cava
      inferior I82.220
        chronic I82.221
      superior I82.210
        chronic I82.211
    venous, perianal K64.5
    ventricle —*see also* Infarct,
      myocardium
      following acute myocardial
        infarction (current
        complication) I23.6
      not resulting in infarction I24.0
      old I51.3

Thrombus —*see* Thrombosis

Thrush —*see also* Candidiasis
  oral B37.0
  newborn P37.5
  vaginal B37.3

Thumb —*see also* condition
  sucking (child problem) F98.8

Thymitis E32.8

Thymoma —*see also* Neoplasm,
  thymus, by type
  malignant C37
  metaplastic C37
  microscopic D15.0
  sclerosing C37
  type A C37
  type AB C37
  type B1 C37
  type B2 C37
  type B3 C37

Thymus, thymic (gland) —*see*
  condition

Thyrocele —*see* Goiter

Thyroglossal —*see also* condition
  cyst Q89.2
  duct, persistent Q89.2

Thyroid (gland) (body) —*see also*
  condition
  hormone resistance E07.89
  lingual Q89.2
  nodule (cystic) (nontoxic) (single)
    E04.1

Thyroiditis E06.9
  acute (nonsuppurative) (pyogenic)
    (suppurative) E06.0
  autoimmune E06.3
  chronic (nonspecific) (sclerosing)
    E06.5
    with thyrotoxicosis, transient E06.2
    fibrous E06.5
    lymphadenoid E06.3
    lymphocytic E06.3
    lymphoid E06.3
  de Quervain's E06.1
  drug-induced E06.4
  fibrous (chronic) E06.5
  giant-cell (follicular) E06.1
  granulomatous (de Quervain)
    (subacute) E06.1
  Hashimoto's (struma
    lymphomatosa) E06.3
  iatrogenic E06.4
  ligneous E06.5
  lymphocytic (chronic) E06.3
  lymphoid E06.3

Thyroiditis *(continued)*
  lymphomatous E06.3
  nonsuppurative E06.1
  postpartum, puerperal O90.5
  pseudotuberculous E06.1
  pyogenic E06.0
  radiation E06.4
  Riedel's E06.5
  subacute (granulomatous) E06.1
  suppurative E06.0
  tuberculous A18.81
  viral E06.1
  woody E06.5

Thyrolingual duct, persistent Q89.2

Thyromegaly E01.0

Thyrotoxic
  crisis —*see* Thyrotoxicosis
  heart disease or failure (*see also*
    Thyrotoxicosis) E05.90 *[I43]*
    with thyroid storm E05.91 *[I43]*
  storm —*see* Thyrotoxicosis

Thyrotoxicosis (recurrent) E05.90
  with
    goiter (diffuse) E05.00
      with thyroid storm E05.01
      adenomatous uninodular E05.10
        with thyroid storm E05.11
      multinodular E05.20
        with thyroid storm E05.21
      nodular E05.20
        with thyroid storm E05.21
      uninodular E05.10
        with thyroid storm E05.11
    infiltrative
      dermopathy E05.00
        with thyroid storm E05.01
      ophthalmopathy E05.00
        with thyroid storm E05.01
    single thyroid nodule E05.10
      with thyroid storm E05.11
    thyroid storm E05.91
  due to
    ectopic thyroid nodule or tissue
      E05.30
      with thyroid storm E05.31
    ingestion of (excessive) thyroid
      material E05.40
      with thyroid storm E05.41
    overproduction of thyroid-
      stimulating hormone E05.80
      with thyroid storm E05.81
    specified cause NEC E05.80
      with thyroid storm E05.81
  factitia E05.40
    with thyroid storm E05.41
  heart (*see also* Failure, heart, high-
    output) E05.90 *[I43]*
    with thyroid storm (*see also*
      Failure, heart, high-output)
      E05.91 *[I43]*
    failure (*see also* Failure, heart,
      high-output) E05.90 *[I43]*
  neonatal (transient) P72.1
  transient with chronic thyroiditis
    E06.2

Tibia vara M92.51-

Tic (disorder) F95.9
  breathing F95.8
  child problem F95.0
  compulsive F95.1
  de la Tourette F95.2
  degenerative (generalized)
    (localized) G25.69
    facial G25.69
  disorder
    chronic
      motor F95.1
      vocal F95.1

Tic *(continued)*
  disorder *(continued)*
    combined vocal and multiple
      motor F95.2
    transient F95.0
  douloureux G50.0
    atypical G50.1
    postherpetic, postzoster B02.22
  drug-induced G25.61
  eyelid F95.8
  habit F95.9
    chronic F95.1
    transient of childhood F95.0
  lid, transient of childhood F95.0
  motor-verbal F95.2
  occupational F48.8
  orbicularis F95.8
    transient of childhood F95.0
  organic origin G25.69
  postchoreic G25.69
  provisional F95.0
  psychogenic, compulsive F95.1
  salaam R25.8
  spasm (motor or vocal) F95.9
    chronic F95.1
    transient of childhood F95.0
  specified NEC F95.8

Tick-borne —*see* condition

Tietze's disease or syndrome M94.0

Tight, tightness
  anus K62.89
  chest R07.89
  fascia (lata) M62.89
  foreskin (congenital) N47.1
  hymen, hymenal ring N89.6
  introitus (acquired) (congenital) N89.6
  rectal sphincter K62.89
  tendon —*see* Short, tendon
  urethral sphincter N35.919

Tilting vertebra —*see* Dorsopathy,
  deforming, specified NEC

Timidity, child F93.8

Tin-miner's lung J63.5

Tinea (intersecta) (tarsi) B35.9
  amiantacea L44.8
  asbestina B35.0
  barbae B35.0
  beard B35.0
  black dot B35.0
  blanca B36.2
  capitis B35.0
  corporis B35.4
  cruris B35.6
  flava B36.0
  foot B35.3
  furfuracea B36.0
  imbricata (Tokelau) B35.5
  kerion B35.0
  manuum B35.2
  microsporic —*see* Dermatophytosis
  nigra B36.1
  nodosa —*see* Piedra
  pedis B35.3
  scalp B35.0
  specified NEC B35.8
  sycosis B35.0
  tonsurans B35.0
  trichophytic —*see*
    Dermatophytosis
  unguium B35.1
  versicolor B36.0

Tingling sensation (skin) R20.2

Tinnitus NOS H93.1-
  audible H93.1-
  aurium H93.1-
  pulsatile H93.A-
  subjective H93.1-

Tipped tooth (teeth) M26.33

Tipping
pelvis M95.5
with disproportion (fetopelvic)
O33.0
causing obstructed labor
O65.0
tooth (teeth), fully erupted M26.33

Tiredness R53.83

Tissue —*see* condition

Tobacco (nicotine)
abuse —*see* Tobacco, use
dependence —*see* Dependence,
drug, nicotine
harmful use Z72.0
heart —*see* Tobacco, toxic effect
maternal use, affecting newborn
P04.2
toxic effect —*see* Table of Drugs
and Chemicals, by substance,
poisoning
chewing tobacco —*see* Table
of Drugs and Chemicals, by
substance, poisoning
cigarettes —*see* Table of Drugs
and Chemicals, by substance,
poisoning
use Z72.0
complicating
childbirth O99.334
pregnancy O99.33-
puerperium O99.335
counseling and surveillance
Z71.6
history Z87.891
withdrawal state (*see also*
Dependence, drug, nicotine)
F17.203

Tocopherol deficiency E56.0

Todd's
cirrhosis K74.3
paralysis (postepileptic) (transitory)
G83.84

Toe —*see* condition

Toilet, artificial opening —*see*
Attention to, artificial, opening

Tokelau (ringworm) B35.5

Tollwut —*see* Rabies

Tommaselli's disease R31.9
correct substance properly
administered —*see* Table of
Drugs and Chemicals, by drug,
adverse effect
overdose or wrong substance given
or taken —*see* Table of Drugs and
Chemicals, by drug, poisoning

Tongue —*see also* condition
tie Q38.1

Tonic pupil —*see* Anomaly, pupil,
function, tonic pupil

Toni-Fanconi syndrome (cystinosis)
E72.09
with cystinosis E72.04

Tonsil —*see* condition

Tonsillitis (acute) (catarrhal)
(croupous) (follicular) (gangrenous)
(infective) (lacunar) (lingual)
(malignant) (membranous)
(parenchymatous) (phlegmonous)
(pseudomembranous) (purulent)
(septic) (subacute) (suppurative)
(toxic) (ulcerative) (vesicular)
(viral) J03.90
chronic J35.01
with adenoiditis J35.03

Tonsillitis (*continued*)
diphtheritic A36.0
hypertrophic J35.01
with adenoiditis J35.03
recurrent J03.91
specified organism NEC J03.80
recurrent J03.81
staphylococcal J03.80
recurrent J03.81
streptococcal J03.00
recurrent J03.01
tuberculous A15.8
Vincent's A69.1

Tooth, teeth —*see* condition

Toothache K08.89

Topagnosis R20.8

Tophi —*see* Gout, chronic

TORCH infection —*see* Infection,
congenital
without active infection P00.2

Torn —*see* Tear

Tornwaldt's cyst or disease J39.2

Torsion
accessory tube —*see* Torsion,
fallopian tube
adnexa (female) —*see* Torsion,
fallopian tube
aorta, acquired I77.1
appendix epididymis N44.04
appendix testis N44.03
bile duct (common) (hepatic)
K83.8
congenital Q44.5
bowel, colon or intestine K56.2
cervix —*see* Malposition, uterus
cystic duct K82.8
dystonia —*see* Dystonia, torsion
epididymis (appendix) N44.04
fallopian tube N83.52-
with ovary N83.53
gallbladder K82.8
congenital Q44.1
hydatid of Morgagni
female N83.52-
male N44.03
kidney (pedicle) (leading to
infarction) N28.0
Meckel's diverticulum (congenital)
Q43.0
malignant —*see* Table of
Neoplasms, small intestine,
malignant
mesentery K56.2
omentum K56.2
organ or site, congenital NEC
—*see* Anomaly, by site
ovary (pedicle) N83.51-
with fallopian tube N83.53
congenital Q50.2
oviduct —*see* Torsion, fallopian
tube
penis (acquired) N48.82
congenital Q55.63
spasm —*see* Dystonia, torsion
spermatic cord N44.02
extravaginal N44.01
intravaginal N44.02
spleen D73.5
testis, testicle N44.00
appendix N44.03
tibia —*see* Deformity, limb,
specified type NEC, lower leg
uterus —*see* Malposition, uterus

Torticollis (intermittent) (spastic)
M43.6
congenital (sternomastoid) Q68.0
due to birth injury P15.8
hysterical F44.4

Torticollis (*continued*)
ocular R29.891
psychogenic F45.8
conversion reaction F44.4
rheumatic M43.6
rheumatoid M06.88
spasmodic G24.3
traumatic, current S13.4

Tortipelvis G24.1

Tortuous
aortic arch Q25.46
artery I77.1
organ or site, congenital NEC
—*see* Distortion
retinal vessel, congenital Q14.1
ureter N13.8
urethra N36.8
vein —*see* Varix

Torture, victim of Z65.4

Torula, torular (histolytica)
(infection) —*see* Cryptococcosis

Torulosis —*see* Cryptococcosis

Torus (mandibularis) (palatinus)
M27.0
fracture —*see* Fracture, by site,
torus

Touraine's syndrome Q79.8

Tourette's syndrome F95.2

Tourniquet syndrome —*see*
Constriction, external, by site

Tower skull Q75.0
with exophthalmos Q87.0

Toxemia R68.89
bacterial —*see* Sepsis
burn —*see* Burn
eclamptic (with pre-existing
hypertension) —*see* Eclampsia
erysipelatous —*see* Erysipelas
fatigue R68.89
food —*see* Poisoning, food
gastrointestinal K52.1
intestinal K52.1
kidney —*see* Uremia
malarial —*see* Malaria
myocardial —*see* Myocarditis,
toxic
of pregnancy —*see* Pre-eclampsia
pre-eclamptic —*see* Pre-eclampsia
small intestine K52.1
staphylococcal, due to food A05.0
stasis R68.89
uremic —*see* Uremia
urinary —*see* Uremia

Toxemica cerebropathia psychica
(nonalcoholic) F04
alcoholic —*see* Alcohol, amnestic
disorder

Toxic (poisoning) (*see also* condition)
T65.91
effect —*see* Table of Drugs and
Chemicals, by substance,
poisoning
shock syndrome A48.3
thyroid (gland) —*see*
Thyrotoxicosis

Toxicemia —*see* Toxemia

Toxicity —*see* Table of Drugs and
Chemicals, by substance, poisoning
fava bean D55.0
food, noxious —*see* Poisoning,
food
from drug or nonmedicinal
substance —*see* Table of Drugs
and Chemicals, by drug

Toxicosis —*see also* Toxemia
capillary, hemorrhagic D69.0

Toxinfection, gastrointestinal K52.1

Toxocariasis B83.0

Toxoplasma, toxoplasmosis
(acquired) B58.9
with
hepatitis B58.1
meningoencephalitis B58.2
ocular involvement B58.00
other organ involvement B58.89
pneumonia, pneumonitis B58.3
congenital (acute) (subacute)
(chronic) P37.1
maternal, manifest toxoplasmosis
in infant (acute) (subacute)
(chronic) P37.1

tPA (rtPA) **administation in a
different facility within the last
24 hours prior to admission to
current facility** Z92.82

Trabeculation, bladder N32.89

Trachea —*see* condition

Tracheitis (catarrhal) (infantile)
(membranous) (plastic) (septal)
(suppurative) (viral) J04.10
with
bronchitis (15 years of age and
above) J40
acute or subacute —*see*
Bronchitis, acute
chronic J42
tuberculous NEC A15.5
under 15 years of age J20.9
laryngitis (acute) J04.2
chronic J37.1
tuberculous NEC A15.5
acute J04.10
with obstruction J04.11
chronic J42
with
bronchitis (chronic) J42
laryngitis (chronic) J37.1
diphtheritic (membranous) A36.89
due to external agent —*see*
Inflammation, respiratory, upper,
due to
syphilitic A52.73
tuberculous A15.5

Trachelitis (nonvenereal) —*see*
Cervicitis

Tracheobronchial —*see* condition

Tracheobronchitis (15 years of age
and above) —*see also* Bronchitis
due to
Bordetella bronchiseptica
A37.80
with pneumonia A37.81
Francisella tularensis A21.8

Tracheobronchomegaly Q32.4
with bronchiectasis J47.9
with
exacerbation (acute) J47.1
lower respiratory infection
J47.0
acquired J98.09
with bronchiectasis J47.9
with
exacerbation (acute) J47.1
lower respiratory infection
J47.0

Tracheobronchopneumonitis —*see*
Pneumonia, broncho-

Tracheocele (external) (internal)
J39.8
congenital Q32.1

Tracheomalacia J39.8
  congenital Q32.0

Tracheopharyngitis (acute) J06.9
  chronic J42
  due to external agent —*see*
    Inflammation, respiratory, upper,
    due to

Tracheostenosis J39.8

Tracheostomy
  complication —*see* Complication,
    tracheostomy
  status Z93.0
    attention to Z43.0
    malfunctioning J95.03

Trachoma, trachomatous A71.9
  active (stage) A71.1
  contraction of conjunctiva
    A71.1
  dubium A71.0
  initial (stage) A71.0
  healed or sequelae B94.0
  pannus A71.1
  Türck's J37.0

Traction, vitreomacular H43.82-

Train sickness T75.3

Trait(s)
  Hb-S D57.3
  hemoglobin
    abnormal NEC D58.2
      with thalassemia D56.3
    C —*see* Disease, hemoglobin C
    S (Hb-S) D57.3
  Lepore D56.3
  personality, accentuated Z73.1
  sickle-cell D57.3
    with elliptocytosis or
      spherocytosis D57.3
  type A personality Z73.1

Tramp Z59.0

Trance R41.89
  hysterical F44.89

Transaminasemia R74.01

Transection
  abdomen (partial) S38.3
  aorta (incomplete) —*see also*
    Injury, aorta
    complete —*see* Injury, aorta,
      laceration, major
  carotid artery (incomplete) —*see*
    also Injury, blood vessel, carotid,
    laceration
    complete —*see* Injury, blood
      vessel, carotid, laceration,
      major
  celiac artery (incomplete) S35.211
    branch (incomplete) S35.291
      complete S35.292
    complete S35.212
  innominate
    artery (incomplete) —*see also*
      Injury, blood vessel, thoracic,
      innominate, artery, laceration
      complete —*see* Injury, blood
        vessel, thoracic, innominate,
        artery, laceration, major
    vein (incomplete) —*see also*
      Injury, blood vessel, thoracic,
      innominate, vein, laceration
      complete —*see* Injury, blood
        vessel, thoracic, innominate,
        vein, laceration, major
  jugular vein (external) (incomplete)
    —*see also* Injury, blood vessel,
    jugular vein, laceration
    complete —*see* Injury,
      blood vessel, jugular vein,
      laceration, major

Transection (*continued*)
  jugular vein (*continued*)
    internal (incomplete) —*see*
      also Injury, blood vessel,
      jugular vein, internal,
      laceration
      complete —*see* Injury,
        blood vessel, jugular
        vein, internal, laceration,
        major
  mesenteric artery (incomplete)
    —*see also* Injury, mesenteric,
    artery, laceration
    complete —*see* Injury,
      mesenteric artery, laceration,
      major
  pulmonary vessel (incomplete)
    —*see also* Injury, blood
    vessel, thoracic, pulmonary,
    laceration
    complete —*see* Injury, blood
      vessel, thoracic, pulmonary,
      laceration, major
  subclavian —*see* Transection,
    innominate
  vena cava (incomplete) —*see also*
    Injury, vena cava
    complete —*see* Injury, vena
      cava, laceration, major
  vertebral artery (incomplete)
    —*see also* Injury, blood vessel,
    vertebral, laceration
    complete —*see* Injury, blood
      vessel, vertebral, laceration,
      major

Transfusion
  associated (red blood cell)
    hemochromatosis E83.111
  blood
    ABO incompatible —*see*
      Complication(s), transfusion,
      incompatibility reaction,
      ABO
    minor blood group (Duffy)
      (E) (K) (Kell) (Kidd) (Lewis)
      (M) (N) (P) (S) T80.89
    reaction or complication —*see*
      Complications, transfusion
  fetomaternal (mother) —*see*
    Pregnancy, complicated
    by, placenta, transfusion
    syndrome
  maternofetal (mother) —*see*
    Pregnancy, complicated by,
    placenta, transfusion syndrome
  placental (syndrome) (mother)
    —*see* Pregnancy, complicated
    by, placenta, transfusion
    syndrome
  reaction (adverse) —*see*
    Complications, transfusion
  related acute lung injury (TRALI)
    J95.84
  twin-to-twin —*see* Pregnancy,
    complicated by, placenta,
    transfusion syndrome, fetus to
    fetus

Transient (meaning homeless) —*see*
  also condition Z59.0

Translocation
  balanced autosomal Q95.9
    in normal individual Q95.0
  chromosomes NEC Q99.8
    balanced and insertion in normal
      individual Q95.0
  Down syndrome Q90.2
  trisomy
    13 Q91.6
    18 Q91.2
    21 Q90.2

Translucency, iris —*see*
  Degeneration, iris

Transmission of chemical
  substances through the placenta
  —*see* Absorption, chemical,
  through placenta

Transparency, lung, unilateral
  J43.0

Transplant (ed) (status) Z94.9
  awaiting organ Z76.82
  bone Z94.6
    marrow Z94.81
  candidate Z76.82
  complication —*see* Complication,
    transplant
  cornea Z94.7
  heart Z94.1
    and lung(s) Z94.3
    valve Z95.2
      prosthetic Z95.2
      specified NEC Z95.4
      xenogenic Z95.3
  intestine Z94.82
  kidney Z94.0
  liver Z94.4
  lung(s) Z94.2
    and heart Z94.3
  organ (failure) (infection)
    (rejection) Z94.9
    removal status Z98.85
  pancreas Z94.83
  skin Z94.5
  social Z60.3
  specified organ or tissue NEC
    Z94.89
  stem cells Z94.84
  tissue Z94.9

Transplants, ovarian, endometrial
  N80.1

Transposed —*see* Transposition

Transposition (congenital) —*see*
  also Malposition, congenital
  abdominal viscera Q89.3
  aorta (dextra) Q20.3
  appendix Q43.8
  colon Q43.8
  corrected Q20.5
  great vessels (complete) (partial)
    Q20.3
  heart Q24.0
    with complete transposition of
      viscera Q89.3
  intestine (large) (small) Q43.8
  reversed jejunal (for bypass)
    (status) Z98.0
  scrotum Q55.23
  stomach Q40.2
    with general transposition of
      viscera Q89.3
  tooth, teeth, fully erupted M26.30
  vessels, great (complete) (partial)
    Q20.3
  viscera (abdominal) (thoracic) Q89.3

Transsexualism F64.0

Transverse —*see also* condition
  arrest (deep), in labor O64.0
  lie (mother) O32.2
    causing obstructed labor O64.8

Transvestism, transvestitism (dual-
  role) F64.1
  fetishistic F65.1

Trapped placenta (with hemorrhage)
  O72.0
  without hemorrhage O73.0

TRAPS (tumor necrosis factor
  receptor associated periodic
  syndrome) M04.1

Trauma, traumatism —*see also*
  Injury
  acoustic —*see* subcategory
    H83.3
  birth —*see* Birth, injury
  complicating ectopic or molar
    pregnancy O08.6
  during delivery O71.9
  following ectopic or molar
    pregnancy O08.6
  obstetric O71.9
    specified NEC O71.89
  occlusal
    primary K08.81
    secondary K08.82

Traumatic —*see also* condition
  brain injury S06.9

Treacher Collins syndrome Q75.4

Treitz's hernia —*see* Hernia,
  abdomen, specified site NEC

Trematode infestation —*see*
  Infestation, fluke

Trematodiasis —*see* Infestation,
  fluke

Trembling paralysis —*see*
  Parkinsonism

Tremor(s) R25.1
  drug induced G25.1
  essential (benign) G25.0
  familial G25.0
  hereditary G25.0
  hysterical F44.4
  intention G25.2
  medication induced postural
    G25.1
  mercurial —*see* subcategory
    T56.1
  Parkinson's —*see* Parkinsonism
  psychogenic (conversion reaction)
    F44.4
  senilis R54
  specified type NEC G25.2

Trench
  fever A79.0
  foot —*see* Immersion, foot
  mouth A69.1

Treponema pallidum infection
  —*see* Syphilis

Treponematosis
  due to
    T. pallidum —*see* Syphilis
    T. pertenue —*see* Yaws

Triad
  Hutchinson's (congenital syphilis)
    A50.53
  Kartagener's Q89.3
  Saint's —*see* Hernia, diaphragm

Trichiasis (eyelid) H02.059
  with entropion —*see* Entropion
  left H02.056
    lower H02.055
    upper H02.054
  right H02.053
    lower H02.052
    upper H02.051

Trichinella spiralis (infection)
  (infestation) B75

Trichinellosis, trichiniasis,
  trichinelliasis, trichinosis B75
  with muscle disorder B75
    [M63.80]
    ankle B75 *[M63.87-]*
    foot B75 *[M63.87-]*
    forearm B75 *[M63.83-]*
    hand B75 *[M63.84-]*

Trichinellosis, trichiniasis, trichinelliasis, trichinosis *(continued)*
- with muscle disorder *(continued)*
  - lower leg B75 *[M63.86-]*
  - multiple sites B75 *[M63.89]*
  - pelvic region B75 *[M63.85-]*
  - shoulder region B75 *[M63.81-]*
  - specified site NEC B75 *[M63.88]*
  - thigh B75 *[M63.85-]*
  - upper arm B75 *[M63.82-]*

Trichobezoar T18.9
- intestine T18.3
- stomach T18.2

Trichocephaliasis, trichocephalosis B79

Trichocephalus infestation B79

Trichoclasis L67.8

Trichoepithelioma —*see also* Neoplasm, skin, benign
- malignant —*see* Neoplasm, skin, malignant

Trichofolliculoma —*see* Neoplasm, skin, benign

Tricholemmoma —*see* Neoplasm, skin, benign

Trichomoniasis A59.9
- bladder A59.03
- cervix A59.09
- intestinal A07.8
- prostate A59.02
- seminal vesicles A59.09
- specified site NEC A59.8
- urethra A59.03
- urogenitalis A59.00
- vagina A59.01
- vulva A59.01

Trichomycosis
- axillaris A48.8
- nodosa, nodularis B36.8

Trichonodosis L67.8

Trichophytid, trichophyton infection —*see* Dermatophytosis

Trichophytobezoar T18.9
- intestine T18.3
- stomach T18.2

Trichophytosis —*see* Dermatophytosis

Trichoptilosis L67.8

Trichorrhexis (nodosa) (invaginata) L67.0

Trichosis axillaris A48.8

Trichosporosis nodosa B36.2

Trichostasis spinulosa (congenital) Q84.1

Trichostrongyliasis, trichostrongylosis (small intestine) B81.2

Trichostrongylus infection B81.2

Trichotillomania F63.3

Trichromat, trichromatopsia, anomalous (congenital) H53.55

Trichuriasis B79

Trichuris trichiura (infection) (infestation) (any site) B79

Tricuspid (valve) —*see* condition

Trifid —*see also* Accessory
- kidney (pelvis) Q63.8
- tongue Q38.3

Trigeminal neuralgia —*see* Neuralgia, trigeminal

Trigeminy R00.8

Trigger finger (acquired) M65.30
- congenital Q74.0
- index finger M65.32-
- little finger M65.35-
- middle finger M65.33-
- ring finger M65.34-
- thumb M65.31-

Trigonitis (bladder) (chronic) (pseudomembranous) N30.30
- with hematuria N30.31

Trigonocephaly Q75.0

Trilocular heart —*see* Cor triloculare

Trimethylaminuria E72.52

Tripartite placenta O43.19-

Triphalangeal thumb Q74.0

Triple —*see also* Accessory
- kidneys Q63.0
- uteri Q51.818
- X, female Q97.0

Triple I O41.12-

Triplegia G83.89
- congenital G80.8

Triplet (newborn) —*see also* Newborn, triplet
- complicating pregnancy —*see* Pregnancy, triplet

Triplication —*see* Accessory

Triploidy Q92.7

Trismus R25.2
- neonatorum A33
- newborn A33

Trisomy (syndrome) Q92.9
- autosomes Q92.9
- chromosome specified NEC Q92.8
  - partial Q92.2
    - due to unbalanced translocation Q92.5
  - whole (nonsex chromosome)
    - meiotic nondisjunction Q92.0
    - mitotic nondisjunction Q92.1
    - mosaicism Q92.1
  - specified NEC Q92.8
- due to
  - dicentrics —*see* Extra, marker chromosomes
  - extra rings —*see* Extra, marker chromosomes
  - isochromosomes —*see* Extra, marker chromosomes
- specified NEC Q92.8
- whole chromosome Q92.9
  - meiotic nondisjunction Q92.0
  - mitotic nondisjunction Q92.1
  - mosaicism Q92.1
  - partial Q92.9
  - specified NEC Q92.8
- 13 (partial) Q91.7
  - meiotic nondisjunction Q91.4
  - mitotic nondisjunction Q91.5
  - mosaicism Q91.5
  - translocation Q91.6
- 18 (partial) Q91.3
  - meiotic nondisjunction Q91.0
  - mitotic nondisjunction Q91.1
  - mosaicism Q91.1
  - translocation Q91.2
- 20 Q92.8
- 21 (partial) Q90.9
  - meiotic nondisjunction Q90.0
  - mitotic nondisjunction Q90.1
  - mosaicism Q90.1
  - translocation Q90.2
- 22 Q92.8

Tritanomaly, tritanopia H53.55

Trombiculosis, trombiculiasis, trombidiosis B88.0

Trophedema (congenital) (hereditary) Q82.0

Trophoblastic disease (see also Mole, hydatidiform) O01.9

Tropholymphedema Q82.0

Trophoneurosis NEC G96.89
- disseminated M34.9

Tropical —*see* condition

Trouble —*see also* Disease
- heart —*see* Disease, heart
- kidney —*see* Disease, renal
- nervous R45.0
- sinus —*see* Sinusitis

Trousseau's syndrome (thrombophlebitis migrans) I82.1

Truancy, childhood
- from school Z72.810

Truncus
- arteriosus (persistent) Q20.0
- communis Q20.0

Trunk —*see* condition

Trypanosomiasis
- African B56.9
  - by Trypanosoma brucei
    - gambiense B56.0
    - rhodesiense B56.1
- American —*see* Chagas' disease
- Brazilian —*see* Chagas' disease
- by Trypanosoma
  - brucei gambiense B56.0
  - brucei rhodesiense B56.1
  - cruzi —*see* Chagas' disease
- gambiensis, Gambian B56.0
- rhodesiensis, Rhodesian B56.1
- South American —*see* Chagas' disease
- where
  - African trypanosomiasis is prevalent B56.9
  - Chagas' disease is prevalent B57.2

T-shaped incisors K00.2

Tsutsugamushi (disease) (fever) A75.3

Tube, tubal, tubular —*see* condition

Tubercle —*see also* Tuberculosis
- brain, solitary A17.81
- Darwin's Q17.8
- Ghon, primary infection A15.7

Tuberculid, tuberculide (indurating, subcutaneous) (lichenoid) (miliary) (papulonecrotic) (primary) (skin) A18.4

Tuberculoma —*see also* Tuberculosis
- brain A17.81
- meninges (cerebral) (spinal) A17.1
- spinal cord A17.81

Tuberculosis, tubercular, tuberculous (calcification) (calcified) (caseous) (chromogenic acid-fast bacilli) (degeneration) (fibrocaseous) (fistula) (interstitial) (isolated circumscribed lesions) (necrosis) (parenchymatous) (ulcerative) A15.9
- with pneumoconiosis (any condition in J60-J64) J65

Tuberculosis, tubercular, tuberculous *(continued)*
- abdomen (lymph gland) A18.39
- abscess (respiratory) A15.9
  - bone A18.03
    - hip A18.02
    - knee A18.02
    - sacrum A18.01
    - specified site NEC A18.03
    - spinal A18.01
    - vertebra A18.01
  - brain A17.81
  - breast A18.89
  - Cowper's gland A18.15
  - dura (mater) (cerebral) (spinal) A17.81
  - epidural (cerebral) (spinal) A17.81
  - female pelvis A18.17
  - frontal sinus A15.8
  - genital organs NEC A18.10
  - genitourinary A18.10
  - gland (lymphatic) —*see* Tuberculosis, lymph gland
  - hip A18.02
  - intestine A18.32
  - ischiorectal A18.32
  - joint NEC A18.02
    - hip A18.02
    - knee A18.02
    - specified NEC A18.02
    - vertebral A18.01
  - kidney A18.11
  - knee A18.02
  - latent Z22.7
  - lumbar (spine) A18.01
  - lung —*see* Tuberculosis, pulmonary
  - meninges (cerebral) (spinal) A17.0
  - muscle A18.09
  - perianal (fistula) A18.32
  - perinephritic A18.11
  - perirectal A18.32
  - rectum A18.32
  - retropharyngeal A15.8
  - sacrum A18.01
  - scrofulous A18.2
  - scrotum A18.15
  - skin (primary) A18.4
  - spinal cord A17.81
  - spine or vertebra (column) A18.01
  - subdiaphragmatic A18.31
  - testis A18.15
  - urinary A18.13
  - uterus A18.17
- accessory sinus —*see* Tuberculosis, sinus
- Addison's disease A18.7
- adenitis —*see* Tuberculosis, lymph gland
- adenoids A15.8
- adenopathy —*see* Tuberculosis, lymph gland
- adherent pericardium A18.84
- adnexa (uteri) A18.17
- adrenal (capsule) (gland) A18.7
- alimentary canal A18.32
- anemia A18.89
- ankle (joint) (bone) A18.02
- anus A18.32
- apex, apical —*see* Tuberculosis, pulmonary
- appendicitis, appendix A18.32
- arachnoid A17.0
- artery, arteritis A18.89
  - cerebral A18.89
- arthritis (chronic) (synovial) A18.02
  - spine or vertebra (column) A18.01

Tuberculosis, tubercular, tuberculous *(continued)*
articular —*see* Tuberculosis, joint
ascites A18.31
asthma —*see* Tuberculosis, pulmonary
axilla, axillary (gland) A18.2
bladder A18.12
bone A18.03
  hip A18.02
  knee A18.02
  limb NEC A18.03
  sacrum A18.01
  spine or vertebral column A18.01
bowel (miliary) A18.32
brain A17.81
breast A18.89
broad ligament A18.17
bronchi, bronchial, bronchus A15.5
  ectasia, ectasis (bronchiectasis) —*see* Tuberculosis, pulmonary
  fistula A15.5
    primary (progressive) A15.7
  gland or node A15.4
    primary (progressive) A15.7
  lymph gland or node A15.4
    primary (progressive) A15.7
bronchiectasis —*see* Tuberculosis, pulmonary
bronchitis A15.5
bronchopleural A15.6
bronchopneumonia, bronchopneumonic —*see* Tuberculosis, pulmonary
bronchorrhagia A15.5
bronchotracheal A15.5
bronze disease A18.7
buccal cavity A18.83
bulbourethral gland A18.15
bursa A18.09
cachexia A15.9
cardiomyopathy A18.84
caries —*see* Tuberculosis, bone
cartilage A18.02
  intervertebral A18.01
catarrhal —*see* Tuberculosis, respiratory
cecum A18.32
cellulitis (primary) A18.4
cerebellum A17.81
cerebral, cerebrum A17.81
cerebrospinal A17.81
  meninges A17.0
cervical (lymph gland or node) A18.2
cervicitis, cervix (uteri) A18.16
chest —*see* Tuberculosis, respiratory
chorioretinitis A18.53
choroid, choroiditis A18.53
ciliary body A18.54
colitis A18.32
collier's J65
colliquativa (primary) A18.4
colon A18.32
complex, primary A15.7
congenital P37.0
conjunctiva A18.59
connective tissue (systemic) A18.89
contact Z20.1
cornea (ulcer) A18.52
Cowper's gland A18.15
coxae A18.02
coxalgia A18.02
cul-de-sac of Douglas A18.17
curvature, spine A18.01
cutis (colliquativa) (primary) A18.4

Tuberculosis, tubercular, tuberculous *(continued)*
cyst, ovary A18.18
cystitis A18.12
dactylitis A18.03
diarrhea A18.32
diffuse —*see* Tuberculosis, miliary
digestive tract A18.32
disseminated —*see* Tuberculosis, miliary
duodenum A18.32
dura (mater) (cerebral) (spinal) A17.0
  abscess (cerebral) (spinal) A17.81
dysentery A18.32
ear (inner) (middle) A18.6
  bone A18.03
  external (primary) A18.4
  skin (primary) A18.4
elbow A18.02
emphysema —*see* Tuberculosis, pulmonary
empyema A15.6
encephalitis A17.82
endarteritis A18.89
endocarditis A18.84
  aortic A18.84
  mitral A18.84
  pulmonary A18.84
  tricuspid A18.84
endocrine glands NEC A18.82
endometrium A18.17
enteric, enterica, enteritis A18.32
enterocolitis A18.32
epididymis, epididymitis A18.15
epidural abscess (cerebral) (spinal) A17.81
epiglottis A15.5
episcleritis A18.51
erythema (induratum) (nodosum) (primary) A18.4
esophagus A18.83
eustachian tube A18.6
exposure (to) Z20.1
exudative —*see* Tuberculosis, pulmonary
eye A18.50
eyelid (primary) (lupus) A18.4
fallopian tube (acute) (chronic) A18.17
fascia A18.09
fauces A15.8
female pelvic inflammatory disease A18.17
finger A18.03
first infection A15.7
gallbladder A18.83
ganglion A18.09
gastritis A18.83
gastrocolic fistula A18.32
gastroenteritis A18.32
gastrointestinal tract A18.32
general, generalized —*see* Tuberculosis, miliary
genital organs A18.10
genitourinary A18.10
genu A18.02
glandula suprarenalis A18.7
glandular, general A18.2
glottis A15.5
grinder's J65
gum A18.83
hand A18.03
heart A18.84
hematogenous —*see* Tuberculosis, miliary
hemoptysis —*see* Tuberculosis, pulmonary
hemorrhage NEC —*see* Tuberculosis, pulmonary

Tuberculosis, tubercular, tuberculous *(continued)*
hemothorax A15.6
hepatitis A18.83
hilar lymph nodes A15.4
  primary (progressive) A15.7
hip (joint) (disease) (bone) A18.02
hydropneumothorax A15.6
hydrothorax A15.6
hypoadrenalism A18.7
hypopharynx A15.8
ileocecal (hyperplastic) A18.32
ileocolitis A18.32
ileum A18.32
iliac spine (superior) A18.03
immunological findings only A15.7
indurativa (primary) A18.4
infantile A15.7
infection A15.9
  without clinical manifestations A15.7
infraclavicular gland A18.2
inguinal gland A18.2
inguinalis A18.2
intestine (any part) A18.32
iridocyclitis A18.54
iris, iritis A18.54
ischiorectal A18.32
jaw A18.03
jejunum A18.32
joint A18.02
  vertebral A18.01
keratitis (interstitial) A18.52
keratoconjunctivitis A18.52
kidney A18.11
knee (joint) A18.02
kyphosis, kyphoscoliosis A18.01
laryngitis A15.5
larynx A15.5
latent Z22.7
leptomeninges, leptomeningitis (cerebral) (spinal) A17.0
lichenoides (primary) A18.4
linguae A18.83
lip A18.83
liver A18.83
lordosis A18.01
lung —*see* Tuberculosis, pulmonary
lupus vulgaris A18.4
lymph gland or node (peripheral) A18.2
  abdomen A18.39
  bronchial A15.4
    primary (progressive) A15.7
  cervical A18.2
  hilar A15.4
    primary (progressive) A15.7
  intrathoracic A15.4
    primary (progressive) A15.7
  mediastinal A15.4
    primary (progressive) A15.7
  mesenteric A18.39
  retroperitoneal A18.39
  tracheobronchial A15.4
    primary (progressive) A15.7
lymphadenitis —*see* Tuberculosis, lymph gland
lymphangitis —*see* Tuberculosis, lymph gland
lymphatic (gland) (vessel) —*see* Tuberculosis, lymph gland
mammary gland A18.89
marasmus A15.9
mastoiditis A18.03
mediastinal lymph gland or node A15.4
  primary (progressive) A15.7
mediastinitis A15.8

Tuberculosis, tubercular, tuberculous *(continued)*
mediastinitis *(continued)*
  primary (progressive) A15.7
mediastinum A15.8
  primary (progressive) A15.7
medulla A17.81
melanosis, Addisonian A18.7
meninges, meningitis (basilar) (cerebral) (cerebrospinal) (spinal) A17.0
meningoencephalitis A17.82
mesentery, mesenteric (gland or node) A18.39
miliary A19.9
  acute A19.2
    multiple sites A19.1
    single specified site A19.0
  chronic A19.8
  specified NEC A19.8
millstone makers' J65
miner's J65
molder's J65
mouth A18.83
multiple A19.9
  acute A19.1
  chronic A19.8
muscle A18.09
myelitis A17.82
myocardium, myocarditis A18.84
nasal (passage) (sinus) A15.8
nasopharynx A15.8
neck gland A18.2
nephritis A18.11
nerve (mononeuropathy) A17.83
nervous system A17.9
nose (septum) A15.8
ocular A18.50
omentum A18.31
oophoritis (acute) (chronic) A18.17
optic (nerve trunk) (papilla) A18.59
orbit A18.59
orchitis A18.15
organ, specified NEC A18.89
osseous —*see* Tuberculosis, bone
osteitis —*see* Tuberculosis, bone
osteomyelitis —*see* Tuberculosis, bone
otitis media A18.6
ovary, ovaritis (acute) (chronic) A18.17
oviduct (acute) (chronic) A18.17
pachymeningitis A17.0
palate (soft) A18.83
pancreas A18.83
papulonecrotic (a) (primary) A18.4
parathyroid glands A18.82
paronychia (primary) A18.4
parotid gland or region A18.83
pelvis (bony) A18.03
penis A18.15
peribronchitis A15.5
pericardium, pericarditis A18.84
perichondritis, larynx A15.5
periostitis —*see* Tuberculosis, bone
perirectal fistula A18.32
peritoneum NEC A18.31
peritonitis A18.31
pharynx, pharyngitis A15.8
phlyctenulosis (keratoconjunctivitis) A18.52
phthisis NEC —*see* Tuberculosis, pulmonary
pituitary gland A18.82
pleura, pleural, pleurisy, pleuritis (fibrinous) (obliterative) (purulent) (simple plastic) (with effusion) A15.6

Codman's —*see* Neoplasm, bone, benign

dentigerous, mixed —*see* Cyst, calcifying odontogenic

dermoid —*see* Neoplasm, benign, by site
  with malignant transformation C56-

desmoid (extra-abdominal) —*see also* Neoplasm, connective tissue, uncertain behavior
  abdominal —*see* Neoplasm, connective tissue, uncertain behavior

embolus —*see* Neoplasm, secondary, by site

embryonal (mixed) —*see also* Neoplasm, uncertain behavior, by site
  liver C22.7

endodermal sinus
  specified site —*see* Neoplasm, malignant, by site
  unspecified site
    female C56.-
    male C62.90

epithelial
  benign —*see* Neoplasm, benign, by site
  malignant —*see* Neoplasm, malignant, by site

Ewing's —*see* Neoplasm, bone, malignant, by site

fatty —*see* Lipoma

fibroid —*see* Leiomyoma

G cell
  malignant
    pancreas C25.4
    specified site NEC —*see* Neoplasm, malignant, by site
    unspecified site C25.4
  specified site —*see* Neoplasm, uncertain behavior, by site
  unspecified site D37.8

germ cell —*see also* Neoplasm, malignant, by site
  mixed —*see* Neoplasm, malignant, by site

ghost cell, odontogenic —*see* Cyst, calcifying odontogenic

giant cell —*see also* Neoplasm, uncertain behavior, by site
  bone D48.0
    malignant —*see* Neoplasm, bone, malignant
  chondromatous —*see* Neoplasm, bone, benign
  malignant —*see* Neoplasm, malignant, by site
  soft parts —*see* Neoplasm, connective tissue, uncertain behavior
    malignant —*see* Neoplasm, connective tissue, malignant

glomus D18.00
  intra-abdominal D18.03
  intracranial D18.02
  jugulare D44.7
    malignant C75.5
  skin D18.01
  specified site NEC D18.09

gonadal stromal —*see* Neoplasm, uncertain behavior, by site

granular cell —*see also* Neoplasm, connective tissue, benign
  malignant —*see* Neoplasm, connective tissue, malignant

granulosa cell D39.1-
  juvenile D39.1-
  malignant C56-

granulosa cell-theca cell D39.1-
  malignant C56-

Grawitz's C64-

hemorrhoidal —*see* Hemorrhoids

hilar cell D27-

hilus cell D27-

Hurthle cell (benign) D34
  malignant C73

hydatid —*see* Echinococcus

hypernephroid —*see also* Neoplasm, uncertain behavior, by site

interstitial cell —*see also* Neoplasm, uncertain behavior, by site
  benign —*see* Neoplasm, benign, by site
  malignant —*see* Neoplasm, malignant, by site

intravascular bronchial alveolar D38.1

islet cell —*see* Neoplasm, benign, by site
  malignant —*see* Neoplasm, malignant, by site
    pancreas C25.4
    specified site NEC —*see* Neoplasm, malignant, by site
    unspecified site C25.4
  pancreas D13.7
  specified site NEC —*see* Neoplasm, benign, by site
  unspecified site D13.7

juxtaglomerular D41.0-

Klatskin's C24.0

Krukenberg's C79.6-

Leydig cell —*see* Neoplasm, uncertain behavior, by site
  benign —*see* Neoplasm, benign, by site
    specified site —*see* Neoplasm, benign, by site
    unspecified site
      female D27.9
      male D29.20
  malignant —*see* Neoplasm, malignant, by site
    specified site —*see* Neoplasm, malignant, by site
    unspecified site
      female C56.9
      male C62.90
  specified site —*see* Neoplasm, uncertain behavior, by site
  unspecified site
    female D39.10
    male D40.10

lipid cell, ovary D27-

lipoid cell, ovary D27-

malignant (*see also* Neoplasm, malignant, by site) C80.1
  fusiform cell (type) C80.1
  giant cell (type) C80.1
  localized, plasma cell —*see* Plasmacytoma, solitary
  mixed NEC C80.1
  small cell (type) C80.1
  spindle cell (type) C80.1
  unclassified C80.1

mast cell D47.09

melanotic, neuroectodermal —*see* Neoplasm, benign, by site

Merkel cell —*see* Carcinoma, Merkel cell

mesenchymal
  malignant —*see* Neoplasm, connective tissue, malignant

mesenchymal *(continued)*
  mixed —*see* Neoplasm, connective tissue, uncertain behavior

mesodermal, mixed —*see also* Neoplasm, malignant, by site
  liver C22.4

mesonephric —*see also* Neoplasm, uncertain behavior, by site
  malignant —*see* Neoplasm, malignant, by site

metastatic
  from specified site —*see* Neoplasm, malignant, by site
  of specified site —*see* Neoplasm, malignant, by site
  to specified site —*see* Neoplasm, secondary, by site

mixed NEC —*see also* Neoplasm, benign, by site
  malignant —*see* Neoplasm, malignant, by site

mucinous of low malignant potential
  specified site —*see* Neoplasm, malignant, by site
  unspecified site C56.9

mucocarcinoid
  specified site —*see* Neoplasm, malignant, by site
  unspecified site C18.1

mucoepidermoid —*see* Neoplasm, uncertain behavior, by site

Müllerian, mixed
  specified site —*see* Neoplasm, malignant, by site
  unspecified site C54.9

myoepithelial —*see* Neoplasm, benign, by site

neuroectodermal (peripheral) —*see* Neoplasm, malignant, by site
  primitive
    specified site —*see* Neoplasm, malignant, by site
    unspecified C71.9

neuroendocrine D3A.8
  malignant poorly differentiated C7A.1
  secondary NEC C7B.8
  specified NEC C7A.8

neurogenic olfactory C30.0

nonencapsulated sclerosing C73

odontogenic (adenomatoid) (benign) (calcifying epithelial) (keratocystic) (squamous) —*see* Cyst, calcifying odontogenic
  malignant C41.1
    upper jaw (bone) C41.0

ovarian stromal D39.1-

ovary, in pregnancy —*see* Pregnancy, complicated by

pacinian —*see* Neoplasm, skin, benign

Pancoast's —*see* Pancoast's syndrome

papillary —*see also* Papilloma
  cystic D37.9
    mucinous of low malignant potential C56-
      specified site —*see* Neoplasm, malignant, by site
      unspecified site C56.9
    serous of low malignant potential
      specified site —*see* Neoplasm, malignant, by site
      unspecified site C56.9

pelvic, in pregnancy or childbirth —*see* Pregnancy, complicated by

phantom F45.8

phyllodes D48.6-
  benign D24-
  malignant —*see* Neoplasm, breast, malignant

Pindborg —*see* Cyst, calcifying odontogenic

placental site trophoblastic D39.2

plasma cell (malignant) (localized) —*see* Plasmacytoma, solitary

polyvesicular vitelline
  specified site —*see* Neoplasm, malignant, by site
  unspecified site
    female C56.9
    male C62.90

Pott's puffy —*see* Osteomyelitis, specified NEC

Rathke's pouch D44.3

retinal anlage —*see* Neoplasm, benign, by site

salivary gland type, mixed —*see* Neoplasm, salivary gland, benign
  malignant —*see* Neoplasm, salivary gland, malignant

Sampson's N80.1

Schmincke's —*see* Neoplasm, nasopharynx, malignant

sclerosing stromal D27-

sebaceous —*see* Cyst, sebaceous

secondary —*see* Neoplasm, secondary, by site
  carcinoid C7B.00
    bone C7B.03
    distant lymph nodes C7B.01
    liver C7B.02
    peritoneum C7B.04
    specified NEC C7B.09
  neuroendocrine NEC C7B.8

serous of low malignant potential
  specified site —*see* Neoplasm, malignant, by site
  unspecified site C56.9

Sertoli cell —*see* Neoplasm, benign, by site
  with lipid storage
    specified site —*see* Neoplasm, benign, by site
    unspecified site
      female D27.9
      male D29.20
  specified site —*see* Neoplasm, benign, by site
  unspecified site
    female D27.9
    male D29.20

Sertoli-Leydig cell —*see* Neoplasm, benign, by site
  specified site —*see* Neoplasm, benign, by site
  unspecified site
    female D27.9
    male D29.20

sex cord (-stromal) —*see* Neoplasm, uncertain behavior, by site
  with annular tubules D39.1-

skin appendage —*see* Neoplasm, skin, benign

smooth muscle —*see* Neoplasm, connective tissue, uncertain behavior

soft tissue
  benign —*see* Neoplasm, connective tissue, benign
  malignant —*see* Neoplasm, connective tissue, malignant

sternomastoid (congenital) Q68.0

Ulcer, ulcerated, ulcerating, ulceration, ulcerative
(continued)
cornea *(continued)*
  with hypopyon H16.03-
    central H16.01-
    dendritic (herpes simplex)
      B00.52
    marginal H16.04-
    Mooren's H16.05-
    mycotic H16.06-
    perforated H16.07-
    ring H16.02-
    tuberculous (phlyctenular)
      A18.52
corpus cavernosum (chronic)
  N48.5
crural —*see* Ulcer, lower limb
Curling's —*see* Ulcer, peptic, acute
Cushing's —*see* Ulcer, peptic,
  acute
cystic duct K82.8
cystitis (interstitial) —*see* Cystitis,
  interstitial
decubitus —*see* Ulcer, pressure,
  by site
dendritic, cornea (herpes simplex)
  B00.52
diabetes, diabetic —*see* Diabetes,
  ulcer
Dieulafoy's K25.0
due to
  infection NEC —*see* Ulcer,
    skin
  radiation NEC L59.8
  trophic disturbance (any region)
    —*see* Ulcer, skin
  X-ray L58.1
duodenum, duodenal (eroded)
  (peptic) K26.9
  with
    hemorrhage K26.4
      and perforation K26.6
    perforation K26.5
  acute K26.3
    with
      hemorrhage K26.0
        and perforation K26.2
      perforation K26.1
  chronic K26.7
    with
      hemorrhage K26.4
        and perforation K26.6
      perforation K26.5
dysenteric A09
elusive —*see* Cystitis, interstitial
endocarditis (acute) (chronic)
  (subacute) I28.8
epiglottis J38.7
esophagus (peptic) K22.10
  with bleeding K22.11
  due to
    aspirin K22.10
      with bleeding K22.11
    gastrointestinal reflux disease
      (without bleeding) K21.00
      with bleeding K21.01
    ingestion of chemical or
      medicament K22.10
      with bleeding K22.11
  fungal K22.10
    with bleeding K22.11
  infective K22.10
    with bleeding K22.11
  varicose —*see* Varix,
    esophagus
eyelid (region) H01.8
fauces J39.2
Fenwick (-Hunner) (solitary)
  —*see* Cystitis, interstitial

Ulcer, ulcerated, ulcerating, ulceration, ulcerative
(continued)
fistulous —*see* Ulcer, skin
foot (indolent) (trophic) —*see*
  Ulcer, lower limb
frambesial, initial A66.0
frenum (tongue) K14.0
gallbladder or duct K82.8
gangrenous —*see* Gangrene
gastric —*see* Ulcer, stomach
gastrocolic —*see* Ulcer,
  gastrojejunal
gastroduodenal —*see* Ulcer,
  peptic
gastroesophageal —*see* Ulcer,
  stomach
gastrointestinal —*see* Ulcer,
  gastrojejunal
gastrojejunal (peptic) K28.9
  with
    hemorrhage K28.4
      and perforation K28.6
    perforation K28.5
  acute K28.3
    with
      hemorrhage K28.0
        and perforation K28.2
      perforation K28.1
  chronic K28.7
    with
      hemorrhage K28.4
        and perforation K28.6
      perforation K28.5
gastrojejunocolic —*see* Ulcer,
  gastrojejunal
gingiva K06.8
gingivitis K05.10
  nonplaque induced K05.11
  plaque induced K05.10
glottis J38.7
granuloma of pudenda A58
gum K06.8
gumma, due to yaws A66.4
heel —*see* Ulcer, lower limb
hemorrhoid (*see also* Hemorrhoids,
  by degree) K64.8
Hunner's —*see* Cystitis, interstitial
hypopharynx J39.2
hypopyon (chronic) (subacute)
  —*see* Ulcer, cornea, with
  hypopyon
hypostaticum —*see* Ulcer,
  varicose
ileum —*see* Ulcer, intestine
intestine, intestinal K63.3
  with perforation K63.1
  amebic A06.1
  duodenal —*see* Ulcer, duodenum
  granulocytopenic (with
    hemorrhage) —*see*
    Neutropenia
  marginal —*see* Ulcer,
    gastrojejunal
  perforating K63.1
    newborn P78.0
  primary, small intestine K63.3
  rectum K62.6
  stercoraceous, stercoral K63.3
  tuberculous A18.32
  typhoid (fever) —*see* Typhoid
  varicose I86.8
jejunum, jejunal —*see* Ulcer,
  gastrojejunal
keratitis —*see* Ulcer, cornea
knee —*see* Ulcer, lower limb
labium (majus) (minus) N76.6
laryngitis —*see* Laryngitis
larynx (aphthous) (contact) J38.7
  diphtheritic A36.2
leg —*see* Ulcer, lower limb

Ulcer, ulcerated, ulcerating, ulceration, ulcerative
(continued)
lip K13.0
Lipschütz's N76.6
lower limb (atrophic) (chronic)
  (neurogenic) (perforating)
  (pyogenic) (trophic) (tropical)
  L97.909
  with
    bone involvement without
      evidence of necrosis
      L97.906
    bone necrosis L97.904
    exposed fat layer L97.902
    muscle involvement without
      evidence of necrosis
      L97.905
    muscle necrosis L97.903
    skin breakdown only
      L97.901
    specified severity NEC
      L97.908
  ankle L97.309
    with
      bone involvement without
        evidence of necrosis
        L97.306
      bone necrosis L97.304
      exposed fat layer L97.302
      muscle involvement without
        evidence of necrosis
        L97.305
      muscle necrosis L97.303
      skin breakdown only
        L97.301
      specified severity NEC
        L97.308
    left L97.329
      with
        bone involvement
          without evidence of
          necrosis L97.326
        bone necrosis L97.324
        exposed fat layer
          L97.322
        muscle involvement
          without evidence of
          necrosis L97.325
        muscle necrosis L97.323
        skin breakdown only
          L97.321
        specified severity NEC
          L97.328
    right L97.319
      with
        bone involvement
          without evidence of
          necrosis L97.316
        bone necrosis L97.314
        exposed fat layer
          L97.312
        muscle involvement
          without evidence of
          necrosis L97.315
        muscle necrosis L97.313
        skin breakdown only
          L97.311
        specified severity NEC
          L97.318
  calf L97.209
    with
      bone involvement without
        evidence of necrosis
        L97.206
      bone necrosis L97.204
      exposed fat layer L97.202
      muscle involvement without
        evidence of necrosis
        L97.205
      muscle necrosis L97.203

Ulcer, ulcerated, ulcerating, ulceration, ulcerative
(continued)
lower limb *(continued)*
  calf *(continued)*
    with *(continued)*
      skin breakdown only
        L97.201
      specified severity NEC
        L97.208
    left L97.229
      with
        bone involvement
          without evidence of
          necrosis L97.226
        bone necrosis L97.224
        exposed fat layer
          L97.222
        muscle involvement
          without evidence of
          necrosis L97.225
        muscle necrosis
          L97.223
        skin breakdown only
          L97.221
        specified severity NEC
          L97.228
    right L97.219
      with
        bone involvement
          without evidence of
          necrosis L97.216
        bone necrosis L97.214
        exposed fat layer
          L97.212
        muscle involvement
          without evidence of
          necrosis L97.215
        muscle necrosis L97.213
        skin breakdown only
          L97.211
        specified severity NEC
          L97.218
  decubitus —*see* Ulcer, pressure,
    by site
  foot specified NEC L97.509
    with
      bone involvement without
        evidence of necrosis
        L97.506
      bone necrosis L97.504
      exposed fat layer L97.502
      muscle involvement without
        evidence of necrosis
        L97.505
      muscle necrosis L97.503
      skin breakdown only
        L97.501
      specified severity NEC
        L97.508
    left L97.529
      with
        bone involvement
          without evidence of
          necrosis L97.526
        bone necrosis L97.524
        exposed fat layer
          L97.522
        muscle involvement
          without evidence of
          necrosis L97.525
        muscle necrosis L97.523
        skin breakdown only
          L97.521
        specified severity NEC
          L97.528
    right L97.519
      with
        bone involvement
          without evidence of
          necrosis L97.516

Ulcer, ulcerated, ulcerating, ulceration, ulcerative *(continued)*
lower limb *(continued)*
foot specified NEC *(continued)*
right *(continued)*
with *(continued)*
bone necrosis L97.514
exposed fat layer L97.512
muscle involvement without evidence of necrosis L97.515
muscle necrosis L97.513
skin breakdown only L97.511
specified severity NEC L97.518
heel L97.409
with
bone involvement without evidence of necrosis L97.406
bone necrosis L97.404
exposed fat layer L97.402
muscle involvement without evidence of necrosis L97.405
muscle necrosis L97.403
skin breakdown only L97.401
specified severity NEC L97.408
left L97.429
with
bone involvement without evidence of necrosis L97.426
bone necrosis L97.424
exposed fat layer L97.422
muscle involvement without evidence of necrosis L97.425
muscle necrosis L97.423
skin breakdown only L97.421
specified severity NEC L97.428
right L97.419
with
bone involvement without evidence of necrosis L97.416
bone necrosis L97.414
exposed fat layer L97.412
muscle involvement without evidence of necrosis L97.415
muscle necrosis L97.413
skin breakdown only L97.411
specified severity NEC L97.418
left L97.929
with
bone involvement without evidence of necrosis L97.926
bone necrosis L97.924
exposed fat layer L97.922
muscle involvement without evidence of necrosis L97.925
muscle necrosis L97.923
skin breakdown only L97.921
specified severity NEC L97.928

Ulcer, ulcerated, ulcerating, ulceration, ulcerative *(continued)*
lower limb *(continued)*
lower leg NOS L97.909
with
bone involvement without evidence of necrosis L97.906
bone necrosis L97.904
exposed fat layer L97.902
muscle involvement without evidence of necrosis L97.905
muscle necrosis L97.903
skin breakdown only L97.901
specified severity NEC L97.908
left L97.929
with
bone involvement without evidence of necrosis L97.926
bone necrosis L97.924
exposed fat layer L97.922
muscle involvement without evidence of necrosis L97.925
muscle necrosis L97.923
skin breakdown only L97.921
specified severity NEC L97.928
right L97.919
with
bone involvement without evidence of necrosis L97.916
bone necrosis L97.914
exposed fat layer L97.912
muscle involvement without evidence of necrosis L97.915
muscle necrosis L97.913
skin breakdown only L97.911
specified severity NEC L97.918
specified site NEC L97.809
with
bone involvement without evidence of necrosis L97.806
bone necrosis L97.804
exposed fat layer L97.802
muscle involvement without evidence of necrosis L97.805
muscle necrosis L97.803
skin breakdown only L97.801
specified severity NEC L97.808
left L97.829
with
bone involvement without evidence of necrosis L97.826
bone necrosis L97.824
exposed fat layer L97.822
muscle involvement without evidence of necrosis L97.825

Ulcer, ulcerated, ulcerating, ulceration, ulcerative *(continued)*
lower limb *(continued)*
lower leg NOS *(continued)*
specified site NEC *(continued)*
left *(continued)*
with *(continued)*
muscle necrosis L97.823
skin breakdown only L97.821
specified severity NEC L97.828
right L97.819
with
bone involvement without evidence of necrosis L97.816
bone necrosis L97.814
exposed fat layer L97.812
muscle involvement without evidence of necrosis L97.815
muscle necrosis L97.813
skin breakdown only L97.811
specified severity NEC L97.818
midfoot L97.409
with
bone involvement without evidence of necrosis L97.406
bone necrosis L97.404
exposed fat layer L97.402
muscle involvement without evidence of necrosis L97.405
muscle necrosis L97.403
skin breakdown only L97.401
specified severity NEC L97.408
left L97.429
with
bone involvement without evidence of necrosis L97.426
bone necrosis L97.424
exposed fat layer L97.422
muscle involvement without evidence of necrosis L97.425
muscle necrosis L97.423
skin breakdown only L97.421
specified severity NEC L97.428
right L97.419
with
bone involvement without evidence of necrosis L97.416
bone necrosis L97.414
exposed fat layer L97.412
muscle involvement without evidence of necrosis L97.415
muscle necrosis L97.413
skin breakdown only L97.411

Ulcer, ulcerated, ulcerating, ulceration, ulcerative *(continued)*
lower limb *(continued)*
midfoot *(continued)*
right *(continued)*
with *(continued)*
specified severity NEC L97.418
right L97.919
with
bone involvement without evidence of necrosis L97.916
bone necrosis L97.914
exposed fat layer L97.912
muscle involvement without evidence of necrosis L97.915
muscle necrosis L97.913
skin breakdown only L97.911
specified severity NEC L97.918
thigh L97.109
with
bone involvement without evidence of necrosis L97.106
bone necrosis L97.104
exposed fat layer L97.102
muscle involvement without evidence of necrosis L97.105
muscle necrosis L97.103
skin breakdown only L97.101
specified severity NEC L97.108
left L97.129
with
bone involvement without evidence of necrosis L97.126
bone necrosis L97.124
exposed fat layer L97.122
muscle involvement without evidence of necrosis L97.125
muscle necrosis L97.123
skin breakdown only L97.121
specified severity NEC L97.128
right L97.119
with
bone involvement without evidence of necrosis L97.116
bone necrosis L97.114
exposed fat layer L97.112
muscle involvement without evidence of necrosis L97.115
muscle necrosis L97.113
skin breakdown only L97.111
specified severity NEC L97.118
toe L97.509
with
bone involvement without evidence of necrosis L97.506
bone necrosis L97.504
exposed fat layer L97.502

lower limb *(continued)*
  toe *(continued)*
    with *(continued)*
      muscle involvement without evidence of necrosis L97.505
      muscle necrosis L97.503
      skin breakdown only L97.501
      specified severity NEC L97.508
    left L97.529
      with
        bone involvement without evidence of necrosis L97.526
        bone necrosis L97.524
        exposed fat layer L97.522
        muscle involvement without evidence of necrosis L97.525
        muscle necrosis L97.523
        skin breakdown only L97.521
        specified severity NEC L97.528
    right L97.519
      with
        bone involvement without evidence of necrosis L97.516
        bone necrosis L97.514
        exposed fat layer L97.512
        muscle involvement without evidence of necrosis L97.515
        muscle necrosis L97.513
        skin breakdown only L97.511
        specified severity NEC L97.518
leprous A30.1
syphilitic A52.19
varicose —*see* Varix, leg, with, ulcer
luetic —*see* Ulcer, syphilitic
lung J98.4
  tuberculous —*see* Tuberculosis, pulmonary
malignant —*see* Neoplasm, malignant, by site
marginal NEC —*see* Ulcer, gastrojejunal
meatus (urinarius) N34.2
Meckel's diverticulum Q43.0
  malignant —*see* Table of Neoplasms, small intestine, malignant
Meleney's (chronic undermining) —*see* Ulcer, skin
Mooren's (cornea) —*see* Ulcer, cornea, Mooren's
mycobacterial (skin) A31.1
nasopharynx J39.2
neck, uterus N86
neurogenic NEC —*see* Ulcer, skin
nose, nasal (passage) (infective) (septum) J34.0
  skin —*see* Ulcer, skin
spirochetal A69.8
varicose (bleeding) I86.8
oral mucosa (traumatic) K12.1

palate (soft) K12.1
penis (chronic) N48.5
peptic (site unspecified) K27.9
  with
    hemorrhage K27.4
      and perforation K27.6
    perforation K27.5
  acute K27.3
    with
      hemorrhage K27.0
        and perforation K27.2
      perforation K27.1
  chronic K27.7
    with
      hemorrhage K27.4
        and perforation K27.6
      perforation K27.5
  esophagus K22.10
    with bleeding K22.11
  newborn P78.82
perforating K27.5
  skin —*see* Ulcer, skin
peritonsillar J35.8
phagedenic (tropical) —*see* Ulcer, skin
pharynx J39.2
phlebitis —*see* Phlebitis
plaster —*see* Ulcer, pressure, by site
popliteal space —*see* Ulcer, lower limb
postpyloric —*see* Ulcer, duodenum
prepuce N47.7
prepyloric —*see* Ulcer, stomach
pressure (pressure area) L89.9-
  ankle L89.5-
  back L89.1-
  buttock L89.3-
  coccyx L89.15-
  contiguous site of back, buttock, hip L89.4-
  elbow L89.0-
  face L89.81-
  head L89.81-
  heel L89.6-
  hip L89.2-
  sacral region (tailbone) L89.15-
  specified site NEC L89.89-
  stage 1 (healing) (pre-ulcer skin changes limited to persistent focal edema)
    ankle L89.5-
    back L89.1-
    buttock L89.3-
    coccyx L89.15-
    contiguous site of back, buttock, hip L89.4-
    elbow L89.0-
    face L89.81-
    head L89.81-
    heel L89.6-
    hip L89.2-
    sacral region (tailbone) L89.15-
    specified site NEC L89.89-
  stage 2 (healing) (abrasion, blister, partial thickness skin loss involving epidermis and/or dermis)
    ankle L89.5-
    back L89.1-
    buttock L89.3-
    coccyx L89.15-
    contiguous site of back, buttock, hip L89.4-
    elbow L89.0-
    face L89.81-

pressure *(continued)*
  stage 2 *(continued)*
    head L89.81-
    heel L89.6-
    hip L89.2-
    sacral region (tailbone) L89.15-
    specified site NEC L89.89-
  stage 3 (healing) (full thickness skin loss involving damage or necrosis of subcutaneous tissue)
    ankle L89.5-
    back L89.1-
    buttock L89.3-
    coccyx L89.15-
    contiguous site of back, buttock, hip L89.4-
    elbow L89.0-
    face L89.81-
    head L89.81-
    heel L89.6-
    hip L89.2-
    sacral region (tailbone) L89.15-
    specified site NEC L89.89-
  stage 4 (healing) (necrosis of soft tissues through to underlying muscle, tendon, or bone)
    ankle L89.5-
    back L89.1-
    buttock L89.3-
    coccyx L89.15-
    contiguous site of back, buttock, hip L89.4-
    elbow L89.0-
    face L89.81-
    head L89.81-
    heel L89.6-
    hip L89.2-
    sacral region (tailbone) L89.15-
    specified site NEC L89.89-
  unspecified stage
    ankle L89.5-
    back L89.1-
    buttock L89.3-
    coccyx L89.15-
    contiguous site of back, buttock, hip L89.4-
    elbow L89.0-
    face L89.81-
    head L89.81-
    heel L89.6-
    hip L89.2-
    sacral region (tailbone) L89.15-
    specified site NEC L89.89-
  unstageable
    ankle L89.5-
    back L89.1-
    buttock L89.3-
    coccyx L89.15-
    contiguous site of back, buttock, hip L89.4-
    elbow L89.0-
    face L89.81-
    head L89.81-
    heel L89.6-
    hip L89.2-
    sacral region (tailbone) L89.15-
    specified site NEC L89.89-
primary of intestine K63.3
  with perforation K63.1
prostate N41.9

pyloric —*see* Ulcer, stomach
rectosigmoid K63.3
  with perforation K63.1
rectum (sphincter) (solitary) K62.6
  stercoraceous, stercoral K62.6
retina —*see* Inflammation, chorioretinal
rodent —*see also* Neoplasm, skin, malignant
sclera —*see* Scleritis
scrofulous (tuberculous) A18.2
scrotum N50.89
  tuberculous A18.15
  varicose I86.1
seminal vesicle N50.89
sigmoid —*see* Ulcer, intestine
skin (atrophic) (chronic) (neurogenic) (non-healing) (perforating) (pyogenic) (trophic) (tropical) L98.499
  with gangrene —*see* Gangrene
  amebic A06.7
  back —*see* Ulcer, back
  buttock —*see* Ulcer, buttock
  decubitus —*see* Ulcer, pressure
  lower limb —*see* Ulcer, lower limb
  mycobacterial A31.1
  specified site NEC L98.499
    with
      bone involvement without evidence of necrosis L98.496
      bone necrosis L98.494
      exposed fat layer L98.492
      muscle involvement without evidence of necrosis L98.495
      muscle necrosis L98.493
      skin breakdown only L98.491
      specified severity NEC L98.498
  tuberculous (primary) A18.4
  varicose —*see* Ulcer, varicose
sloughing —*see* Ulcer, skin
solitary, anus or rectum (sphincter) K62.6
sore throat J02.9
  streptococcal J02.0
spermatic cord N50.89
spine (tuberculous) A18.01
stasis (venous) —*see* Varix, leg, with, ulcer
  without varicose veins I87.2
stercoraceous, stercoral K63.3
  with perforation K63.1
  anus or rectum K62.6
stoma, stomal —*see* Ulcer, gastrojejunal
stomach (eroded) (peptic) (round) K25.9
  with
    hemorrhage K25.4
      and perforation K25.6
    perforation K25.5
  acute K25.3
    with
      hemorrhage K25.0
        and perforation K25.2
      perforation K25.1
  chronic K25.7
    with
      hemorrhage K25.4
        and perforation K25.6
      perforation K25.5
stomal —*see* Ulcer, gastrojejunal

Ulcer, ulcerated, ulcerating, ulceration, ulcerative
(continued)
stomatitis K12.1
stress —*see* Ulcer, peptic
strumous (tuberculous) A18.2
submucosal, bladder —*see* Cystitis, interstitial
syphilitic (any site) (early) (secondary) A51.39
late A52.79
perforating A52.79
foot A52.11
testis N50.89
thigh —*see* Ulcer, lower limb
throat J39.2
diphtheritic A36.0
toe —*see* Ulcer, lower limb
tongue (traumatic) K14.0
tonsil J35.8
diphtheritic A36.0
trachea J39.8
trophic —*see* Ulcer, skin
tropical —*see* Ulcer, skin
tuberculous —*see* Tuberculosis, ulcer
tunica vaginalis N50.89
turbinate J34.89
typhoid (perforating) —*see* Typhoid
unspecified site —*see* Ulcer, skin
urethra (meatus) —*see* Urethritis
uterus N85.8
cervix N86
with cervicitis N72
neck N86
with cervicitis N72
vagina N76.5
in Behçet's disease M35.2 *[N77.0]*
pessary N89.8
valve, heart I33.0
varicose (lower limb, any part) —*see also* Varix, leg, with, ulcer
broad ligament I86.2
esophagus —*see* Varix, esophagus
inflamed or infected —*see* Varix, leg, with ulcer, with inflammation
nasal septum I86.8
perineum I86.3
scrotum I86.1
specified site NEC I86.8
sublingual I86.0
vulva I86.3
vas deferens N50.89
vulva (acute) (infectional) N76.6
in (due to)
Behçet's disease M35.2 *[N77.0]*
herpesviral (herpes simplex) infection A60.04
tuberculosis A18.18
vulvobuccal, recurring N76.6
X-ray L58.1
yaws A66.4

Ulcerosa scarlatina A38.8

Ulcus —*see also* Ulcer
cutis tuberculosum A18.4
duodeni —*see* Ulcer, duodenum
durum (syphilitic) A51.0
extragenital A51.2
gastrojejunale —*see* Ulcer, gastrojejunal
hypostaticum —*see* Ulcer, varicose
molle (cutis) (skin) A57
serpens corneae —*see* Ulcer, cornea, central
ventriculi —*see* Ulcer, stomach

Ulegyria Q04.8

Ulerythema
ophryogenes, congenital Q84.2
sycosiforme L73.8

Ullrich (-Bonnevie) (-Turner) **syndrome** (*see also* Turner's syndrome) Q87.19

Ullrich-Feichtiger syndrome Q87.0

Ulnar —*see* condition

Ulorrhagia, ulorrhea K06.8

Umbilicus, umbilical —*see* condition

Unacceptable
contours of tooth K08.54
morphology of tooth K08.54

Unavailability (of)
bed at medical facility Z75.1
health service-related agencies Z75.4
medical facilities (at) Z75.3
due to
investigation by social service agency Z75.2
lack of services at home Z75.0
remoteness from facility Z75.3
waiting list Z75.1
home Z75.0
outpatient clinic Z75.3
schooling Z55.1
social service agencies Z75.4

Uncinaria americana infestation B76.1

Uncinariasis B76.9

Uncongenial work Z56.5

Unconscious (ness) —*see* Coma

Under observation —*see* Observation

Underachievement in school Z55.3

Underdevelopment —*see also* Undeveloped
nose Q30.1
sexual E30.0

Underdosing (*see also* Tables of Drugs and Chemicals, categories T36-T50, with final character 6) Z91.14
intentional NEC Z91.128
due to financial hardship of patient Z91.120
unintentional NEC Z91.138
due to patient's age related debility Z91.130

Underfeeding, newborn P92.3

Underfill, endodontic M27.53

Underimmunization status Z28.3

Undernourishment —*see* Malnutrition

Undernutrition —*see* Malnutrition

Underweight R63.6
for gestational age —*see* Light for dates

Underwood's disease P83.0

Undescended —*see also* Malposition, congenital
cecum Q43.3
colon Q43.3
testicle —*see* Cryptorchid

Undeveloped, undevelopment —*see also* Hypoplasia
brain (congenital) Q02

Undeveloped, undevelopment
(continued)
cerebral (congenital) Q02
heart Q24.8
lung Q33.6
testis E29.1
uterus E30.0

Undiagnosed (disease) R69

Undulant fever —*see* Brucellosis

Unemployment, anxiety concerning Z56.0
threatened Z56.2

Unequal length (acquired) (limb) —*see also* Deformity, limb, unequal length
leg —*see also* Deformity, limb, unequal length
congenital Q72.9-

Unextracted dental root K08.3

Unguis incarnatus L60.0

Unhappiness R45.2

Unicornate uterus Q51.4
in pregnancy or childbirth O34.00

Unilateral —*see also* condition
development, breast N64.89
organ or site, congenital NEC —*see* Agenesis, by site

Unilocular heart Q20.8

Union, abnormal —*see also* Fusion
larynx and trachea Q34.8

Universal mesentery Q43.3

Unrepairable overhanging of dental restorative materials K08.52

Unsatisfactory
restoration of tooth K08.50
specified NEC K08.59
sample of cytologic smear
anus R85.615
cervix R87.615
vagina R87.625
surroundings Z59.1
work Z56.5

Unsoundness of mind —*see* Psychosis

Unstable
back NEC —*see* Instability, joint, spine
hip (congenital) Q65.6
acquired —*see* Derangement, joint, specified type NEC, hip
joint —*see* Instability, joint
secondary to removal of joint prosthesis M96.89
lie (mother) O32.0
lumbosacral joint (congenital) —*see* subcategory M53.2
sacroiliac —*see* subcategory M53.2
spine NEC —*see* Instability, joint, spine

Unsteadiness on feet R26.81

Untruthfulness, child problem F91.8

Unverricht (-Lundborg) **disease or epilepsy** —*see* Epilepsy, generalized, idiopathic

Unwanted pregnancy Z64.0

Upbringing, institutional Z62.22
away from parents NEC Z62.29
in care of non-parental family member Z62.21
in foster care Z62.21

Upbringing, institutional
(continued)
in orphanage or group home Z62.22
in welfare custody Z62.21

Upper respiratory —*see* condition

Upset
gastric K30
gastrointestinal K30
psychogenic F45.8
intestinal (large) (small) K59.9
psychogenic F45.8
menstruation N93.9
mental F48.9
stomach K30
psychogenic F45.8

Urachus —*see also* condition
patent or persistent Q64.4

Urbach-Oppenheim disease (necrobiosis lipoidica diabeticorum) —*see* E08-E13 with .620

Urbach's lipoid proteinosis E78.89

Urbach-Wiethe disease E78.89

Urban yellow fever A95.1

Urea
blood, high —*see* Uremia
cycle metabolism disorder —*see* Disorder, urea cycle metabolism

Uremia, uremic N19
with
ectopic or molar pregnancy O08.4
polyneuropathy N18.9 *[G63]*
chronic NOS (*see also* Disease, kidney, chronic) N18.9
due to hypertension —*see* Hypertensive, kidney
complicating
ectopic or molar pregnancy O08.4
congenital P96.0
extrarenal R39.2
following ectopic or molar pregnancy O08.4
newborn P96.0
prerenal R39.2

Ureter, ureteral —*see* condition

Ureteralgia N23

Ureterectasis —*see* Hydroureter

Ureteritis N28.89
cystica N28.86
due to calculus N20.1
with calculus, kidney N20.2
with hydronephrosis N13.2
gonococcal (acute) (chronic) A54.21
nonspecific N28.89

Ureterocele N28.89
congenital (orthotopic) Q62.31
ectopic Q62.32

Ureterolith, ureterolithiasis —*see* Calculus, ureter

Ureterostomy
attention to Z43.6
status Z93.6

Urethra, urethral —*see* condition

Urethralgia R39.89

Urethritis (anterior) (posterior) N34.2
calculous N21.1
candidal B37.41
chlamydial A56.01
diplococcal (gonococcal) A54.01

Urethritis *(continued)*
diplococcal *(continued)*
with abscess (accessory gland)
(periurethral) A54.1
gonococcal A54.01
with abscess (accessory gland)
(periurethral) A54.1
nongonococcal N34.1
Reiter's —*see* Reiter's disease
nonspecific N34.1
nonvenereal N34.1
postmenopausal N34.2
puerperal O86.22
Reiter's —*see* Reiter's disease
specified NEC N34.2
trichomonal or due to Trichomonas
(vaginalis) A59.03

Urethrocele N81.0
with
cystocele —*see* Cystocele
prolapse of uterus —*see*
Prolapse, uterus

Urethrolithiasis (with colic or
infection) N21.1

Urethrorectal —*see* condition

Urethrorrhagia N36.8

Urethrorrhea R36.9

Urethrostomy
attention to Z43.6
status Z93.6

Urethrotrigonitis —*see* Trigonitis

Urethrovaginal —*see* condition

Urgency
fecal R15.2
hypertensive —*see* Hypertension
urinary R39.15

Urhidrosis, uridrosis L74.8

Uric acid in blood (increased) E79.0

Uricacidemia (asymptomatic) E79.0

Uricemia (asymptomatic) E79.0

Uricosuria R82.998

Urinary —*see* condition

Urination
frequent R35.0
painful R30.9

Urine
blood in —*see* Hematuria
discharge, excessive R35.8
enuresis, nonorganic origin F98.0
extravasation R39.0
frequency R35.0
incontinence R32
nonorganic origin F98.0
intermittent stream R39.198
pus in N39.0
retention or stasis R33.9
organic R33.8
drug-induced R33.0
psychogenic F45.8
secretion
deficient R34
excessive R35.8
frequency R35.0
stream
intermittent R39.198
slowing R39.198
splitting R39.13
weak R39.12

Urinemia —*see* Uremia

Urinoma, urethra N36.8

Uroarthritis, infectious (Reiter's)
—*see* Reiter's disease

Urodialysis R34

Urolithiasis —*see* Calculus, urinary

Uronephrosis —*see* Hydronephrosis

Uropathy N39.9
obstructive N13.9
specified NEC N13.8
reflux N13.9
specified NEC N13.8
vesicoureteral reflux-associated
—*see* Reflux, vesicoureteral

Urosepsis - code to condition

Urticaria L50.9
with angioneurotic edema T78.3
hereditary D84.1
allergic L50.0
cholinergic L50.5
chronic L50.8
cold, familial L50.2
contact L50.6
dermatographic L50.3
due to
cold or heat L50.2
drugs L50.0
food L50.0
inhalants L50.0
plants L50.6
serum (*see also* Reaction, serum)
T80.69
factitial L50.3
familial cold M04.2
giant T78.3
hereditary D84.1
gigantea T78.3
idiopathic L50.1
larynx T78.3
hereditary D84.1
neonatorum P83.88
nonallergic L50.1
papulosa (Hebra) L28.2
pigmentosa D47.01
congenital Q82.2
of neonatal onset Q82.2
of newborn onset Q82.2
recurrent periodic L50.8
serum (*see also* Reaction, serum)
T80.69
solar L56.3
specified type NEC L50.8
thermal (cold) (heat) L50.2
vibratory L50.4
xanthelasmoidea —*see* Urticaria
pigmentosa

Use (of)
alcohol Z72.89
with
intoxication F10.929
sleep disorder F10.982
withdrawal F10.939
with
perceptual disturbance
F10.932
delirium F10.931
uncomplicated F10.930
harmful —*see* Abuse, alcohol
amphetamines —*see* Use, stimulant
NEC
caffeine —*see* Use, stimulant NEC
cannabis F12.90
with
anxiety disorder F12.980
intoxication F12.929
with
delirium F12.921
perceptual disturbance
F12.922
uncomplicated F12.920
other specified disorder
F12.988
psychosis F12.959
delusions F12.950
hallucinations F12.951
unspecified disorder F12.99
withdrawal F12.93

Use *(continued)*
cocaine F14.90
with
anxiety disorder F14.980
intoxication F14.929
with
delirium F14.921
perceptual disturbance
F14.922
uncomplicated F14.920
other specified disorder
F14.988
psychosis F14.959
delusions F14.950
hallucinations F14.951
sexual dysfunction F14.981
sleep disorder F14.982
unspecified disorder F14.99
withdrawal F14.93
harmful —*see* Abuse, drug,
cocaine
drug(s) NEC F19.90
with sleep disorder F19.982
harmful —*see* Abuse, drug, by
type
hallucinogen NEC F16.90
with
anxiety disorder F16.980
intoxication F16.929
with
delirium F16.921
uncomplicated F16.920
mood disorder F16.94
other specified disorder
F16.988
perception disorder
(flashbacks) F16.983
psychosis F16.959
delusions F16.950
hallucinations F16.951
unspecified disorder F16.99
harmful —*see* Abuse, drug,
hallucinogen NEC
inhalants F18.90
with
anxiety disorder F18.980
intoxication F18.929
with delirium F18.921
uncomplicated F18.920
mood disorder F18.94
other specified disorder
F18.988
persisting dementia F18.97
psychosis F18.959
delusions F18.950
hallucinations F18.951
unspecified disorder F18.99
harmful —*see* Abuse, drug,
inhalant
methadone —*see* Use, opioid
nonprescribed drugs F19.90
harmful —*see* Abuse, non-
psychoactive substance
opioid F11.90
with
disorder F11.99
mood F11.94
sleep F11.982
specified type NEC F11.988
intoxication F11.929
with
delirium F11.921
perceptual disturbance
F11.922
uncomplicated F11.920
withdrawal F11.93
harmful —*see* Abuse, drug,
opioid
patent medicines F19.90
harmful —*see* Abuse, non-
psychoactive substance

Use *(continued)*
psychoactive drug NEC F19.90
with
anxiety disorder F19.980
intoxication F19.929
with
delirium F19.921
perceptual disturbance
F19.922
uncomplicated F19.920
mood disorder F19.94
other specified disorder F19.988
persisting
amnestic disorder F19.96
dementia F19.97
psychosis F19.959
delusions F19.950
hallucinations F19.951
sexual dysfunction F19.981
sleep disorder F19.982
unspecified disorder F19.99
withdrawal F19.939
with
delirium F19.931
perceptual disturbance
F19.932
uncomplicated F19.930
harmful —*see* Abuse, drug NEC,
psychoactive NEC
sedative, hypnotic, or anxiolytic
F13.90
with
anxiety disorder F13.980
intoxication F13.929
with
delirium F13.921
uncomplicated F13.920
other specified disorder
F13.988
persisting
amnestic disorder F13.96
dementia F13.97
psychosis F13.959
delusions F13.950
hallucinations F13.951
sexual dysfunction F13.981
sleep disorder F13.982
unspecified disorder F13.99
harmful —*see* Abuse, drug,
sedative, hypnotic, or
anxiolytic
stimulant NEC F15.90
with
anxiety disorder F15.980
intoxication F15.929
with
delirium F15.921
perceptual disturbance
F15.922
uncomplicated F15.920
mood disorder F15.94
other specified disorder
F15.988
psychosis F15.959
delusions F15.950
hallucinations F15.951
sexual dysfunction F15.981
sleep disorder F15.982
unspecified disorder F15.99
withdrawal F15.93
harmful —*see* Abuse, drug,
stimulant NEC
volatile solvents (*see also* Use,
inhalant) F18.90
harmful —*see* Abuse, drug,
inhalant
tobacco Z72.0
with dependence —*see*
Dependence, drug, nicotine

Usher-Senear disease or syndrome
L10.4

Uta B55.1

Uteromegaly N85.2

Uterovaginal —see condition

Uterovesical —see condition

Uveal —see condition

Uveitis (anterior) —see also
    Iridocyclitis
    acute —see Iridocyclitis, acute
    chronic —see Iridocyclitis,
        chronic
    due to toxoplasmosis (acquired)
        B58.09
        congenital P37.1
    granulomatous —see Iridocyclitis,
        chronic
    heterochromic —see Cyclitis,
        Fuchs' heterochromic
    lens-induced —see Iridocyclitis,
        lens-induced
    posterior —see Chorioretinitis
    sympathetic H44.13-
    syphilitic (secondary) A51.43
        congenital (early) A50.01
        late A52.71
    tuberculous A18.54

Uveoencephalitis —see
    Inflammation, chorioretinal

Uveokeratitis —see Iridocyclitis

Uveoparotitis D86.89

Uvula —see condition

Uvulitis (acute) (catarrhal) (chronic)
    (membranous) (suppurative)
    (ulcerative) K12.2

V

Vaccination (prophylactic)
    complication or reaction —see
        Complications, vaccination
    delayed Z28.9
    encounter for Z23
    not done —see Immunization, not
        done, because (of)

Vaccinia (generalized) (localized)
    T88.1
    congenital P35.8
    without vaccination B08.011

Vacuum, in sinus (accessory) (nasal)
    J34.89

Vagabond, vagabondage Z59.0

Vagabond's disease B85.1

Vagina, vaginal —see condition

Vaginalitis (tunica) (testis) N49.1

Vaginismus (reflex) N94.2
    functional F52.5
    nonorganic F52.5
    psychogenic F52.5
    secondary N94.2

Vaginitis (acute) (circumscribed)
    (diffuse) (emphysematous)
    (nonvenereal) (ulcerative)
    N76.0
    with ectopic or molar pregnancy
        O08.0
    amebic A06.82
    atrophic, postmenopausal N95.2
    bacterial N76.0
    blennorrhagic (gonococcal)
        A54.02
    candidal B37.3
    chlamydial A56.02
    chronic N76.1
    due to Trichomonas (vaginalis)
        A59.01

Vaginitis (continued)
    following ectopic or molar
        pregnancy O08.0
    gonococcal A54.02
        with abscess (accessory gland)
            (periurethral) A54.1
    granuloma A58
    in (due to)
        candidiasis B37.3
        herpesviral (herpes simplex)
            infection A60.04
        pinworm infection B80
            [N77.1]
    monilial B37.3
    mycotic (candidal) B37.3
    postmenopausal atrophic N95.2
    puerperal (postpartum) O86.13
    senile (atrophic) N95.2
    subacute or chronic N76.1
    syphilitic (early) A51.0
        late A52.76
    trichomonal A59.01
    tuberculous A18.18

Vaginosis —see Vaginitis

Vagotonia G52.2

Vagrancy Z59.0

VAIN —see Neoplasia,
    intraepithelial, vagina

Vallecula —see condition

Valley fever B38.0

Valsuani's disease —see Anemia,
    obstetric

Valve, valvular (formation) —see
    also condition
    cerebral ventricle (communicating)
        in situ Z98.2
    cervix, internal os Q51.828
    congenital NEC —see Atresia, by
        site
    ureter (pelvic junction) (vesical
        orifice) Q62.39
    urethra (congenital) (posterior)
        Q64.2

Valvulitis (chronic) —see
    Endocarditis

Valvulopathy —see Endocarditis

Van Bogaert's leukoencephalopathy
    (sclerosing) (subacute) A81.1

Van Bogaert-Scherer-Epstein
    disease or syndrome E75.5

Van Buchem's syndrome M85.2

Van Creveld-von Gierke disease
    E74.01

Van der Hoeve (-de Kleyn)
    syndrome Q78.0

Van der Woude's syndrome Q38.0

Van Neck's disease or
    osteochondrosis M91.0

Vanishing lung J44.9

Vapor asphyxia or suffocation
    T59.9
    specified agent —see Table of
        Drugs and Chemicals

Variance, lethal ball, prosthetic
    heart valve T82.09

Variants, thalassemic D56.8

Variations in hair color L67.1

Varicella B01.9
    with
        complications NEC B01.89
        encephalitis B01.11
        encephalomyelitis B01.11
        meningitis B01.0

Varicella (continued)
    with (continued)
        myelitis B01.12
        pneumonia B01.2
    congenital P35.8

Varices —see Varix

Varicocele (scrotum) (thrombosed)
    I86.1
    ovary I86.2
    perineum I86.3
    spermatic cord (ulcerated) I86.1

Varicose
    aneurysm (ruptured) I77.0
    dermatitis —see Varix, leg, with,
        inflammation
    eczema —see Varix, leg, with,
        inflammation
    phlebitis —see Varix, with,
        inflammation
    tumor —see Varix
    ulcer (lower limb, any part) —see
        also Varix, leg, with, ulcer
        anus (see also Hemorrhoids)
            K64.8
        esophagus —see Varix,
            esophagus
        inflamed or infected —see
            Varix, leg, with ulcer, with
            inflammation
        nasal septum I86.8
        perineum I86.3
        scrotum I86.1
        specified site NEC I86.8
    vein —see Varix
    vessel —see Varix, leg

Varicosis, varicosities, varicosity
    —see Varix

Variola (major) (minor) B03

Varioloid B03

Varix (lower limb) (ruptured) I83.90
    with
        bleeding I83.899
        edema I83.899
        inflammation I83.10
            with ulcer (venous) I83.209
        pain I83.819
        rupture I83.899
        specified complication NEC
            I83.899
        stasis dermatitis I83.10
            with ulcer (venous) I83.209
        swelling I83.899
        ulcer I83.009
            with inflammation I83.209
    aneurysmal I77.0
    asymptomatic I83.9-
    bladder I86.2
    broad ligament I86.2
    complicating
        childbirth (lower extremity)
            O87.4
            anus or rectum O87.2
            genital (vagina, vulva or
                perineum) O87.8
        pregnancy (lower extremity)
            O22.0-
            anus or rectum O22.4-
            genital (vagina, vulva or
                perineum) O22.1-
        puerperium (lower extremity)
            O87.4
            anus or rectum O87.2
            genital (vagina, vulva,
                perineum) O87.8
    congenital (any site) Q27.8
    esophagus (idiopathic) (primary)
        (ulcerated) I85.00
        bleeding I85.01

Varix (continued)
    esophagus (continued)
        congenital Q27.8
        in (due to)
            alcoholic liver disease I85.10
                bleeding I85.11
            cirrhosis of liver I85.10
                bleeding I85.11
            portal hypertension I85.10
                bleeding I85.11
            schistosomiasis I85.10
                bleeding I85.11
            toxic liver disease I85.10
                bleeding I85.11
        secondary I85.10
            bleeding I85.11
    gastric I86.4
    inflamed or infected I83.10
        ulcerated I83.209
    labia (majora) I86.3
    leg (asymptomatic) I83.90
        with
            edema I83.899
            inflammation I83.10
                with ulcer —see Varix,
                    leg, with, ulcer, with
                    inflammation by site
            pain I83.819
            specified complication NEC
                I83.899
            swelling I83.899
            ulcer I83.009
                with inflammation I83.209
                ankle I83.003
                    with inflammation
                        I83.203
                calf I83.002
                    with inflammation
                        I83.202
                foot NEC I83.005
                    with inflammation
                        I83.205
                heel I83.004
                    with inflammation
                        I83.204
                lower leg NEC I83.008
                    with inflammation
                        I83.208
                midfoot I83.004
                    with inflammation
                        I83.204
                thigh I83.001
                    with inflammation
                        I83.201
        bilateral (asymptomatic) I83.93
            with
                edema I83.893
                pain I83.813
                specified complication NEC
                    I83.893
                swelling I83.893
                ulcer I83.0-
                    with inflammation
                        I83.209
        left (asymptomatic) I83.92
            with
                edema I83.892
                pain I83.812
                specified complication NEC
                    I83.892
                swelling I83.892
                inflammation I83.12
                    with ulcer —see
                        Varix, leg, with, ulcer,
                        with inflammation
                        by site
                ulcer I83.029
                    with inflammation
                        I83.229
                    ankle I83.023

Watsoniasis B66.8

Wax in ear —see Impaction, cerumen

Weak, weakening, weakness
(generalized) R53.1
arches (acquired) —see also
Deformity, limb, flat foot
bladder (sphincter) R32
facial R29.810
following
cerebrovascular disease
I69.992
cerebral infarction
I69.392
intracerebral hemorrhage
I69.192
nontraumatic intracranial
hemorrhage NEC
I69.292
specified disease NEC
I69.892
stroke I69.392
subarachnoid hemorrhage
I69.092
foot (double) —see also Weak,
arches
heart, cardiac —see Failure, heart
mind F70
muscle M62.81
myocardium —see Failure, heart
newborn P96.89
pelvic fundus N81.89
pubocervical tissue N81.82
senile R54
rectovaginal tissue N81.83
urinary stream R39.12
valvular —see Endocarditis

Wear, worn (with normal or routine
use)
articular bearing surface of
internal joint prosthesis —see
Complications, joint prosthesis,
mechanical, wear of articular
bearing surfaces, by site
device, implant or graft —see
Complications, by site,
mechanical complication
tooth, teeth (approximal) (hard
tissues) (interproximal)
(occlusal) K03.0

Weather, weathered
effects of
cold T69.9
specified effect NEC T69.8
hot —see Heat
skin L57.8

Weaver's syndrome Q87.3

Web, webbed (congenital)
duodenal Q43.8
esophagus Q39.4
fingers Q70.1-
larynx (glottic) (subglottic)
Q31.0
neck (pterygium colli) Q18.3
Paterson-Kelly D50.1
popliteal syndrome Q87.89
toes Q70.3-

Weber-Christian disease M35.6

Weber-Cockayne syndrome
(epidermolysis bullosa) Q81.8

Weber-Gubler syndrome G46.3

Weber-Leyden syndrome G46.3

Weber-Osler syndrome I78.0

Weber's paralysis or syndrome
G46.3

Wedge-shaped or wedging vertebra
—see Collapse, vertebra NEC

Wegener's granulomatosis or
syndrome M31.30
with
kidney involvement M31.31
lung involvement M31.30
with kidney involvement
M31.31

Wegner's disease A50.02

Weight
1000-2499 grams at birth (low)
—see Low, birthweight
999 grams or less at birth
(extremely low) —see Low,
birthweight, extreme
and length below 10th percentile
for gestational age P05.1-
below but length above 10th
percentile for gestational age
P05.0-
gain (abnormal) (excessive)
R63.5
in pregnancy —see Pregnancy,
complicated by, excessive
weight gain
low —see Pregnancy,
complicated by, insufficient,
weight gain
loss (abnormal) (cause unknown)
R63.4

Weightlessness (effect of) T75.82

Weil (l)-Marchesani syndrome
Q87.19

Weil's disease A27.0

Weingarten's syndrome J82.89

Weir Mitchell's disease I73.81

Weiss-Baker syndrome G90.09

Wells' disease L98.3

Wen —see Cyst, sebaceous

Wenckebach's block or
phenomenon I44.1

Werdnig-Hoffmann syndrome
(muscular atrophy) G12.0

Werlhof's disease D69.3

Wermer's disease or syndrome
E31.21

Werner-His disease A79.0

Werner's disease or syndrome
E34.8

Wernicke-Korsakoff's syndrome or
psychosis (alcoholic) F10.96
with dependence F10.26
drug-induced
due to drug abuse —see Abuse,
drug, by type, with amnestic
disorder
due to drug dependence —see
Dependence, drug, by type,
with amnestic disorder
nonalcoholic F04

Wernicke-Posadas disease B38.9

Wernicke's
developmental aphasia F80.2
disease or syndrome E51.2
encephalopathy E51.2
polioencephalitis, superior E51.2

West African fever B50.8

Westphal-Strümpell syndrome
E83.01

West's syndrome —see Epilepsy,
spasms

Wet
feet, tropical (maceration)
(syndrome) —see Immersion,
foot
lung (syndrome), newborn P22.1

Wharton's duct —see condition

Wheal —see Urticaria

Wheezing R06.2

Whiplash injury S13.4

Whipple's disease (see also
subcategory M14.8-) K90.81

Whipworm (disease) (infection)
(infestation) B79

Whistling face Q87.0

White —see also condition
kidney, small N03.9
leg, puerperal, postpartum,
childbirth O87.1
mouth B37.0
patches of mouth K13.29
spot lesions, teeth
chewing surface K02.51
pit and fissure surface K02.51
smooth surface K02.61

Whitehead L70.0

Whitlow —see also Cellulitis, digit
with lymphangitis —see
Lymphangitis, acute, digit
herpesviral B00.89

Whitmore's disease or fever —see
Melioidosis

Whooping cough A37.90
with pneumonia A37.91
due to Bordetella
bronchiseptica A37.81
parapertussis A37.11
pertussis A37.01
specified organism NEC
A37.81
due to
Bordetella
bronchiseptica A37.80
with pneumonia A37.81
parapertussis A37.10
with pneumonia A37.11
pertussis A37.00
with pneumonia A37.01
specified NEC A37.80
with pneumonia A37.81

Wichman's asthma J38.5

Wide cranial sutures, newborn
P96.3

Widening aorta —see Ectasia, aorta
with aneurysm —see Aneurysm,
aorta

Wilkie's disease or syndrome K55.1

Wilkinson-Sneddon disease or
syndrome L13.1

Willebrand (-Jürgens)
thrombopathy D68.0

Willige-Hunt disease or syndrome
G23.1

Williams syndrome Q93.82

Wilms' tumor C64-

Wilson-Mikity syndrome P27.0

Wilson's
disease or syndrome E83.01
hepatolenticular degeneration
E83.01
lichen ruber L43.9

Window —see also Imperfect,
closure
aorticopulmonary Q21.4

Winter —see condition

Wiskott-Aldrich syndrome D82.0

Withdrawal state —see also
Dependence, drug by type, with
withdrawal
alcohol
with perceptual disturbances
F10.232
without perceptual disturbances
F10.239
caffeine F15.93
cannabis F12.23
newborn
correct therapeutic substance
properly administered
P96.2
infant of dependent mother
P96.1
therapeutic substance, neonatal
P96.2

Witts' anemia D50.8

Witzelsucht F07.0

Woakes' ethmoiditis or syndrome
J33.1

Wolff-Hirschorn syndrome Q93.3

Wolff-Parkinson-White syndrome
I45.6

Wolhynian fever A79.0

Wolman's disease E75.5

Wood lung or pneumonitis J67.8

Woolly, wooly hair (congenital)
(nevus) Q84.1

Woolsorter's disease A22.1

Word
blindness (congenital)
(developmental) F81.0
deafness (congenital)
(developmental) H93.25

Worm(s) (infection) (infestation)
—see also Infestation, helminth
guinea B72
in intestine NEC B82.0

Worm-eaten soles A66.3

Worn out —see Exhaustion
cardiac
defibrillator (with synchronous
cardiac pacemaker) Z45.02
pacemaker
battery Z45.010
lead Z45.018
device, implant or graft —see
Complications, by site,
mechanical

Worried well Z71.1

Worries R45.82

Wound check Z48.0-
due to injury - code to Injury, by
site, using appropriate seventh
character for subsequent
encounter

Wound, open T14.8-
abdomen, abdominal
wall S31.109
with penetration into
peritoneal cavity S31.609
bite —see Bite, abdomen,
wall
epigastric region S31.102
with penetration into
peritoneal cavity S31.602

Wound, open *(continued)*

abdomen, abdominal *(continued)*
wall *(continued)*
epigastric region *(continued)*
bite —*see* Bite, abdomen, wall, epigastric region
laceration —*see* Laceration, abdomen, wall, epigastric region
puncture —*see* Puncture, abdomen, wall, epigastric region
laceration —*see* Laceration, abdomen, wall
left
lower quadrant S31.104
with penetration into peritoneal cavity S31.604
bite —*see* Bite, abdomen, wall, left, lower quadrant
laceration —*see* Laceration, abdomen, wall, left, lower quadrant
puncture —*see* Puncture, abdomen, wall, left, lower quadrant
upper quadrant S31.101
with penetration into peritoneal cavity S31.601
bite —*see* Bite, abdomen, wall, left, upper quadrant
laceration —*see* Laceration, abdomen, wall, left, upper quadrant
puncture —*see* Puncture, abdomen, wall, left, upper quadrant
periumbilic region S31.105
with penetration into peritoneal cavity S31.605
bite —*see* Bite, abdomen, wall, periumbilic region
laceration —*see* Laceration, abdomen, wall, periumbilic region
puncture —*see* Puncture, abdomen, wall, periumbilic region
puncture —*see* Puncture, abdomen, wall
right
lower quadrant S31.103
with penetration into peritoneal cavity S31.603
bite —*see* Bite, abdomen, wall, right, lower quadrant
laceration —*see* Laceration, abdomen, wall, right, lower quadrant
puncture —*see* Puncture, abdomen, wall, right, lower quadrant
upper quadrant S31.100
with penetration into peritoneal cavity S31.600
bite —*see* Bite, abdomen, wall, right, upper quadrant

Wound, open *(continued)*

abdomen, abdominal *(continued)*
wall *(continued)*
right *(continued)*
upper quadrant *(continued)*
laceration —*see* Laceration, abdomen, wall, right, upper quadrant
puncture —*see* Puncture, abdomen, wall, right, upper quadrant
alveolar (process) —*see* Wound, open, oral cavity
ankle S91.00-
bite —*see* Bite, ankle
laceration —*see* Laceration, ankle
puncture —*see* Puncture, ankle
antecubital space —*see* Wound, open, elbow
anterior chamber, eye —*see* Wound, open, ocular
anus S31.839
bite S31.835
laceration —*see* Laceration, anus
puncture —*see* Puncture, anus
arm (upper) S41.10-
with amputation —*see* Amputation, traumatic, arm
bite —*see* Bite, arm
forearm —*see* Wound, open, forearm
laceration —*see* Laceration, arm
puncture —*see* Puncture, arm
auditory canal (external) (meatus) —*see* Wound, open, ear
auricle, ear —*see* Wound, open, ear
axilla —*see* Wound, open, arm
back —*see also* Wound, open, thorax, back
lower S31.000
with penetration into retroperitoneal space S31.001
bite —*see* Bite, back, lower
laceration —*see* Laceration, back, lower
puncture —*see* Puncture, back, lower
bite —*see* Bite
blood vessel —*see* Injury, blood vessel
breast S21.00-
with amputation —*see* Amputation, traumatic, breast
bite —*see* Bite, breast
laceration —*see* Laceration, breast
puncture —*see* Puncture, breast
buttock S31.809
bite —*see* Bite, buttock
laceration —*see* Laceration, buttock
left S31.829
puncture —*see* Puncture, buttock
right S31.819
calf —*see* Wound, open, leg
canaliculus lacrimalis —*see* Wound, open, eyelid
canthus, eye —*see* Wound, open, eyelid
cervical esophagus S11.20
bite S11.25
laceration —*see* Laceration, esophagus, traumatic, cervical
puncture —*see* Puncture, cervical esophagus

Wound, open *(continued)*

cheek (external) S01.40-
bite —*see* Bite, cheek
laceration —*see* Laceration, cheek
puncture —*see* Puncture, cheek
internal —*see* Wound, open, oral cavity
chest wall —*see* Wound, open, thorax
chin —*see* Wound, open, head, specified site NEC
choroid —*see* Wound, open, ocular
ciliary body (eye) —*see* Wound, open, ocular
clitoris S31.40
with amputation —*see* Amputation, traumatic, clitoris
bite S31.45
laceration —*see* Laceration, vulva
puncture —*see* Puncture, vulva
conjunctiva —*see* Wound, open, ocular
cornea —*see* Wound, open, ocular
costal region —*see* Wound, open, thorax
Descemet's membrane —*see* Wound, open, ocular
digit(s)
foot —*see* Wound, open, toe
hand —*see* Wound, open, finger
ear (canal) (external) S01.30-
with amputation —*see* Amputation, traumatic, ear
bite —*see* Bite, ear
laceration —*see* Laceration, ear
puncture —*see* Puncture, ear
drum S09.2-
elbow S51.00-
bite —*see* Bite, elbow
laceration —*see* Laceration, elbow
puncture —*see* Puncture, elbow
epididymis —*see* Wound, open, testis
epigastric region S31.102
with penetration into peritoneal cavity S31.602
bite —*see* Bite, abdomen, wall, epigastric region
laceration —*see* Laceration, abdomen, wall, epigastric region
puncture —*see* Puncture, abdomen, wall, epigastric region
epiglottis —*see* Wound, open, neck, specified site NEC
esophagus (thoracic) S27.819
cervical —*see* Wound, open, cervical esophagus
laceration S27.813
specified type NEC S27.818
eye —*see* Wound, open, ocular
eyeball —*see* Wound, open, ocular
eyebrow —*see* Wound, open, eyelid
eyelid S01.10-
bite —*see* Bite, eyelid
laceration —*see* Laceration, eyelid
puncture —*see* Puncture, eyelid
face NEC —*see* Wound, open, head, specified site NEC
finger(s) S61.209

Wound, open *(continued)*

finger *(continued)*
with
amputation —*see* Amputation, traumatic, finger
damage to nail S61.309
bite —*see* Bite, finger
index S61.208
with
damage to nail S61.308
left S61.201
with
damage to nail S61.301
right S61.200
with
damage to nail S61.300
laceration —*see* Laceration, finger
little S61.208
with
damage to nail S61.308
left S61.207
with damage to nail S61.307
right S61.206
with damage to nail S61.306
middle S61.208
with
damage to nail S61.308
left S61.203
with damage to nail S61.303
right S61.202
with damage to nail S61.302
puncture —*see* Puncture, finger
ring S61.208
with
damage to nail S61.308
left S61.205
with damage to nail S61.305
right S61.204
with damage to nail S61.304
flank —*see* Wound, open, abdomen, wall
foot (except toe(s) alone) S91.30-
with amputation —*see* Amputation, traumatic, foot
bite —*see* Bite, foot
laceration —*see* Laceration, foot
puncture —*see* Puncture, foot
toe —*see* Wound, open, toe
forearm S51.80-
with
amputation —*see* Amputation, traumatic, forearm
bite —*see* Bite, forearm
elbow only —*see* Wound, open, elbow
laceration —*see* Laceration, forearm
puncture —*see* Puncture, forearm
forehead —*see* Wound, open, head, specified site NEC
genital organs, external
with amputation —*see* Amputation, traumatic, genital organs
bite —*see* Bite, genital organ
female S31.502
vagina S31.40
vulva S31.40
laceration —*see* Laceration, genital organ
male S31.501

Wound, open (continued)
  scrotum (continued)
    with amputation —see
      Amputation, traumatic,
      scrotum
    bite S31.35
    laceration —see Laceration,
      scrotum
    puncture —see Puncture,
      scrotum
  shin —see Wound, open, leg
  shoulder S41.00-
    with amputation —see
      Amputation, traumatic, arm
    bite —see Bite, shoulder
    laceration —see Laceration,
      shoulder
    puncture —see Puncture,
      shoulder
  skin NOS T14.8
  spermatic cord —see Wound, open,
    testis
  sternal region —see Wound, open,
    thorax, front wall
  submaxillary region —see
    Wound, open, head, specified
    site NEC
  submental region —see
    Wound, open, head, specified
    site NEC
  subungual
    finger(s) —see Wound, open,
      finger
    toe(s) —see Wound, open, toe
  supraclavicular region —see
    Wound, open, neck, specified
    site NEC
  temple, temporal region —see
    Wound, open, head, specified
    site NEC
  temporomandibular area —see
    Wound, open, cheek
  testis S31.30
    with amputation —see
      Amputation, traumatic, testes
    bite S31.35
    laceration —see Laceration,
      testis
    puncture —see Puncture, testis
  thigh S71.10-
    with amputation —see
      Amputation, traumatic, hip
    bite —see Bite, thigh
    laceration —see Laceration,
      thigh
    puncture —see Puncture, thigh
  thorax, thoracic (wall) S21.90
    back S21.20-
      with penetration S21.40
    bite —see Bite, thorax
    breast —see Wound, open, breast
    front S21.10-
      with penetration S21.30
    laceration —see Laceration,
      thorax
    puncture —see Puncture, thorax
  throat —see Wound, open, neck
  thumb S61.009
    with
      amputation —see Amputation,
        traumatic, thumb
      damage to nail S61.109
    bite —see Bite, thumb
    laceration —see Laceration,
      thumb
    left S61.002
      with
        damage to nail S61.102
    puncture —see Puncture, thumb
    right S61.001

Wound, open (continued)
  thumb (continued)
    right (continued)
      with
        damage to nail S61.101
  thyroid (gland) —see Wound, open,
    neck, thyroid
  toe(s) S91.109
    with
      amputation —see Amputation,
        traumatic, toe
      damage to nail S91.209
    bite —see Bite, toe
    great S91.103
      with
        damage to nail S91.203
      left S91.102
        with
          damage to nail S91.202
      right S91.101
        with
          damage to nail S91.201
      laceration —see Laceration, toe
    lesser S91.106
      with
        damage to nail S91.206
      left S91.105
        with
          damage to nail S91.205
      right S91.104
        with
          damage to nail S91.204
    puncture —see Puncture, toe
  tongue —see Wound, open, oral
    cavity
  trachea (cervical region) —see
    Wound, open, neck, trachea
  tunica vaginalis —see Wound,
    open, testis
  tympanum, tympanic membrane
    S09.2-
    laceration —see Laceration, ear,
      drum
    puncture —see Puncture,
      tympanum
  umbilical region —see Wound,
    open, abdomen, wall,
    periumbilic region
  uvula —see Wound, open, oral
    cavity
  vagina S31.40
    bite S31.45
    laceration —see Laceration,
      vagina
    puncture —see Puncture, vagina
  vocal cord S11.039
    bite —see Bite, vocal cord
    laceration S11.031
      with foreign body S11.032
    puncture S11.033
      with foreign body S11.034
  vitreous (humor) —see Wound,
    open, ocular
  vulva S31.40
    with amputation —see
      Amputation, traumatic, vulva
    bite S31.45
    laceration —see Laceration,
      vulva
    puncture —see Puncture, vulva
  wrist S61.50-
    bite —see Bite, wrist
    laceration —see Laceration,
      wrist
    puncture —see Puncture, wrist

Wound, superficial —see Injury —
  see also specified injury type

Wright's syndrome G54.0

Wrist —see condition

Wrong drug (by accident) (given in
  error) —see Table of Drugs and
  Chemicals, by drug, poisoning

Wry neck —see Torticollis

Wuchereria (bancrofti) **infestation**
  B74.0

Wuchereriasis B74.0

Wuchernde Struma Langhans C73

X

Xanthelasma (eyelid) (palpebrarum)
  H02.60
  left H02.66
    lower H02.65
    upper H02.64
  right H02.63
    lower H02.62
    upper H02.61

Xanthelasmatosis (essential) E78.2

Xanthinuria, hereditary E79.8

Xanthoastrocytoma
  specified site —see Neoplasm,
    malignant, by site
  unspecified site C71.9

Xanthofibroma —see Neoplasm,
  connective tissue, benign

Xanthogranuloma D76.3

Xanthoma(s), xanthomatosis (primary)
  (familial) (hereditary) E75.5
  with
    hyperlipoproteinemia
      Type I E78.3
      Type III E78.2
      Type IV E78.1
      Type V E78.3
  bone (generalisata) C96.5
  cerebrotendinous E75.5
  cutaneotendinous E75.5
  disseminatum (skin) E78.2
  eruptive E78.2
  hypercholesterinemic E78.00
  hypercholesterolemic E78.00
  hyperlipidemic E78.5
  joint E75.5
  multiple (skin) E78.2
  tendon (sheath) E75.5
  tubo-eruptive E78.2
  tuberosum E78.2
  tuberous E78.2
  verrucous, oral mucosa K13.4

Xanthosis R23.8

Xenophobia F40.10

Xeroderma —see also Ichthyosis
  acquired L85.0
    eyelid H01.149
      left H01.146
        lower H01.145
        upper H01.144
      right H01.143
        lower H01.142
        upper H01.141
  pigmentosum Q82.1
  vitamin A deficiency E50.8

Xerophthalmia (vitamin A
  deficiency) E50.7
  unrelated to vitamin A deficiency
    —see Keratoconjunctivitis

Xerosis
  conjunctiva H11.14-
    with Bitot's spots —see also
      Pigmentation, conjunctiva
      vitamin A deficiency E50.1
    vitamin A deficiency E50.0

Xerosis (continued)
  cornea H18.89-
    with ulceration —see Ulcer,
      cornea
      vitamin A deficiency E50.3
    vitamin A deficiency E50.2
  cutis L85.3
  skin L85.3

Xerostomia K11.7

Xiphopagus Q89.4

XO syndrome Q96.9

X-ray (of)
  abnormal findings —see Abnormal,
    diagnostic imaging
  breast (mammogram) (routine)
    Z12.31
  chest
    routine (as part of a general
      medical examination) Z00.00
      with abnormal findings
        Z00.01
  routine (as part of a general
    medical examination) Z00.00
    with abnormal findings Z00.01

XXXXY syndrome Q98.1

XXY syndrome Q98.0

Y

Yaba pox (virus disease) B08.72

Yatapoxvirus B08.70
  specified NEC B08.79

Yawning R06.89
  psychogenic F45.8

Yaws A66.9
  bone lesions A66.6
  butter A66.1
  chancre A66.0
  cutaneous, less than five years after
    infection A66.2
  early (cutaneous) (macular)
    (maculopapular) (micropapular)
    (papular) A66.2
    frambeside A66.2
    skin lesions NEC A66.2
  eyelid A66.2
  ganglion A66.6
  gangosis, gangosa A66.5
  gumma, gummata A66.4
    bone A66.6
  gummatous
    frambeside A66.4
    osteitis A66.6
    periostitis A66.6
  hydrarthrosis (see also subcategory
    M14.8-) A66.6
  hyperkeratosis (early) (late)
    A66.3
  initial lesions A66.0
  joint lesions (see also subcategory
    M14.8-) A66.6
  juxta-articular nodules A66.7
  late nodular (ulcerated) A66.4
  latent (without clinical
    manifestations) (with positive
    serology) A66.8
  mother A66.0
  mucosal A66.7
  multiple papillomata A66.1
  nodular, late (ulcerated) A66.4
  osteitis A66.6
  papilloma, plantar or palmar
    A66.1
  periostitis (hypertrophic) A66.6
  specified NEC A66.7
  ulcers A66.4
  wet crab A66.1

Yeast infection (*see also* Candidiasis)
B37.9

Yellow
atrophy (liver) —*see* Failure,
hepatic
fever —*see* Fever, yellow
jack —*see* Fever, yellow
jaundice —*see* Jaundice
nail syndrome L60.5

Yersiniosis —*see also* Infection,
Yersinia

Yersiniosis *(continued)*
extraintestinal A28.2
intestinal A04.6

Z

Zahorsky's syndrome (herpangina)
B08.5

Zellweger's syndrome E71.510

Zenker's diverticulum (esophagus)
K22.5

Ziehen-Oppenheim disease G24.1

Zieve's syndrome K70.0

Zika NOS A92.5
congenital P35.4

Zinc
deficiency, dietary E60
metabolism disorder E83.2

Zollinger-Ellison syndrome
E16.4

Zona —*see* Herpes, zoster

Zoophobia F40.218

Zoster (herpes) —*see* Herpes,
zoster

Zygomycosis B46.9
specified NEC B46.8

Zymotic —*see* condition

The Neoplasm Table gives the code numbers for neoplasms by anatomical site. For each site there are six possible code numbers according to whether the neoplasm in question is malignant, benign, in situ, of uncertain behavior, or of unspecified nature. The description of the neoplasm will often indicate which of the six columns is appropriate; e.g., malignant melanoma of skin, benign fibroadenoma of breast, carcinoma in situ of cervix uteri.

Where such descriptors are not present, the remainder of the Index should be consulted where guidance is given to the appropriate column for each morphological (histological) variety listed; e.g., Mesonephroma—see Neoplasm, malignant; Embryoma—see also Neoplasm, uncertain behavior; Disease, Bowen's—see Neoplasm, skin, in situ. However, the guidance in the Index can be overridden if one of the descriptors mentioned above is present; e.g., malignant adenoma of colon is coded to C18.9 and not to D12.6 as the adjective "malignant" overrides the Index entry "Adenoma—see also Neoplasm, benign."

Codes listed with a dash -, following the code have a required additional character for laterality. The tabular must be reviewed for the complete code.

Table of Neoplasms

	Malignant Primary	Malignant Secondary	Ca in situ	Benign	Uncertain Behavior	Unspecified Behavior
Neoplasm, neoplastic	C80.1	C79.9	D09.9	D36.9	D48.9	D49.9
A						
abdomen, abdominal	C76.2	C79.8-	D09.8	D36.7	D48.7	D49.89
cavity	C76.2	C79.8-	D09.8	D36.7	D48.7	D49.89
organ	C76.2	C79.8-	D09.8	D36.7	D48.7	D49.89
viscera	C76.2	C79.8-	D09.8	D36.7	D48.7	D49.89
wall—see also Neoplasm, abdomen, wall, skin	C44.509	C79.2	D04.5	D23.5	D48.5	D49.2
connective tissue	C49.4	C79.8-	-	D21.4	D48.1	D49.2
skin	C44.509					
basal cell carcinoma	C44.519	-	-	-	-	-
specified type NEC	C44.599	-	-	-	-	-
squamous cell carcinoma	C44.529	-	-	-	-	-
abdominopelvic	C76.8	C79.8-		D36.7	D48.7	D49.89
accessory sinus—see Neoplasm, sinus						
acoustic nerve	C72.4-	C79.49	-	D33.3	D43.3	D49.7
adenoid (pharynx) (tissue)	C11.1	C79.89	D00.08	D10.6	D37.05	D49.0
adipose tissue —see also Neoplasm, connective tissue	C49.4	C79.89	-	D21.9	D48.1	D49.2
adnexa (uterine)	C57.4	C79.89	D07.39	D28.7	D39.8	D49.59
adrenal	C74.9-	C79.7-	D09.3	D35.0-	D44.1-	D49.7
capsule	C74.9-	C79.7-	D09.3	D35.0-	D44.1-	D49.7
cortex	C74.0-	C79.7-	D09.3	D35.0-	D44.1-	D49.7
gland	C74.9-	C79.7-	D09.3	D35.0-	D44.1-	D49.7
medulla	C74.1-	C79.7-	D09.3	D35.0-	D44.1-	D49.7
ala nasi (external)—see also Neoplasm, skin, nose	C44.301	C79.2	D04.39	D23.39	D48.5	D49.2
alimentary canal or tract NEC	C26.9	C78.80	D01.9	D13.9	D37.9	D49.0
alveolar	C03.9	C79.89	D00.03	D10.39	D37.09	D49.0
mucosa	C03.9	C79.89	D00.03	D10.39	D37.09	D49.0
lower	C03.1	C79.89	D00.03	D10.39	D37.09	D49.0
upper	C03.0	C79.89	D00.03	D10.39	D37.09	D49.0
ridge or process	C41.1	C79.51	-	D16.5	D48.0	D49.2
carcinoma	C03.9	C79.8-	-	-	-	-
lower	C03.1	C79.8-	-	-	-	-
upper	C03.0	C79.8-	-	-	-	-
lower	C41.1	C79.51	-	D16.5-	D48.0	D49.2
mucosa	C03.9	C79.89	D00.03	D10.39	D37.09	D49.0
lower	C03.1	C79.89	D00.03	D10.39	D37.09	D49.0
upper	C03.0	C79.89	D00.03	D10.39	D37.09	D49.0
upper	C41.0	C79.51	-	D16.4-	D48.0	D49.2
sulcus	C06.1	C79.89	D00.02	D10.39	D37.09	D49.0
alveolus	C03.9	C79.89	D00.03	D10.39	D37.09	D49.0
lower	C03.1	C79.89	D00.03	D10.39	D37.09	D49.0
upper	C03.0	C79.89	D00.03	D10.39	D37.09	D49.0
ampulla of Vater	C24.1	C78.89	D01.5	D13.5	D37.6	D49.0
ankle NEC	C76.5-	C79.89	D04.7-	D36.7	D48.7	D49.89
anorectum, anorectal (junction)	C21.8	C78.5	D01.3	D12.9	D37.8	D49.0
antecubital fossa or space	C76.4-	C79.89	D04.6-	D36.7	D48.7	D49.89
antrum (Highmore) (maxillary)	C31.0	C78.39	D02.3	D14.0	D38.5	D49.1
pyloric	C16.3	C78.89	D00.2	D13.1	D37.1	D49.0
tympanicum	C30.1	C78.39	D02.3	D14.0	D38.5	D49.1
anus, anal	C21.0	C78.5	D01.3	D12.9	D37.8	D49.0
canal	C21.1	C78.5	D01.3	D12.9	D37.8	D49.0
cloacogenic zone	C21.2	C78.5	D01.3	D12.9	D37.8	D49.0
margin—see also Neoplasm, anus, skin	C44.500	C79.2	D04.5	D23.5	D48.5	D49.2
overlapping lesion with rectosigmoid junction or rectum	C21.8	-	-	-	-	-
skin	C44.500	C79.2	D04.5	D23.5	D48.5	D49.2
basal cell carcinoma	C44.510	-	-	-	-	-
specified type NEC	C44.590	-	-	-	-	-
squamous cell carcinoma	C44.520	-	-	-	-	-
sphincter	C21.1	C78.5	D01.3	D12.9	D37.8	D49.0
aorta (thoracic)	C49.3	C79.89	-	D21.3	D48.1	D49.2
abdominal	C49.4	C79.89	-	D21.4	D48.1	D49.2
aortic body	C75.5	C79.89	-	D35.6	D44.7	D49.7
aponeurosis	C49.9	C79.89	-	D21.9	D48.1	D49.2
palmar	C49.1-	C79.89	-	D21.1-	D48.1	D49.2
plantar	C49.2-	C79.89	-	D21.2-	D48.1	D49.2
appendix	C18.1	C78.5	D01.0	D12.1	D37.3	D49.0
arachnoid	C70.9	C79.49	-	D32.9	D42.9	D49.7
cerebral	C70.0	C79.32	-	D32.0	D42.0	D49.7
spinal	C70.1	C79.49	-	D32.1	D42.1	D49.7
areola	C50.0-	C79.81	D05.-	D24.-	D48.6-	D49.3
arm NEC	C76.4-	C79.89	D04.6-	D36.7	D48.7	D49.89
artery—see Neoplasm, connective tissue						
aryepiglottic fold	C13.1	C79.89	D00.08	D10.7	D37.05	D49.0
hypopharyngeal aspect	C13.1	C79.89	D00.08	D10.7	D37.05	D49.0
laryngeal aspect	C32.1	C78.39	D02.0	D14.1	D38.0	D49.1
marginal zone	C13.1	C79.89	D00.08	D10.7	D37.05	D49.0
arytenoid (cartilage)	C32.3	C78.39	D02.0	D14.1	D38.0	D49.1
fold—see Neoplasm, aryepiglottic						
associated with transplanted organ	C80.2	-	-	-	-	-
atlas	C41.2	C79.51	-	D16.6	D48.0	D49.2
atrium, cardiac	C38.0	C79.89	-	D15.1	D48.7	D49.89
auditory						
canal (external) (skin)	C44.20-	C79.2	D04.2-	D23.2-	D48.5	D49.2
internal	C30.1	C78.39	D02.3	D14.0	D38.5	D49.1
nerve	C72.4-	C79.49	-	D33.3	D43.3	D49.7
tube	C30.1	C78.39	D02.3	D14.0	D38.5	D49.1
opening	C11.2	C79.89	D00.08	D10.6	D37.05	D49.0

	Malignant Primary	Malignant Secondary	Ca in situ	Benign	Uncertain Behavior	Unspecified Behavior
auricle, ear—see also Neoplasm, skin, ear	C44.20-	C79.2	D04.2-	D23.2-	D48.5	D49.2
auricular canal (external)—see also Neoplasm, skin, ear	C44.20-	C79.2	D04.2-	D23.2-	D48.5	D49.2
internal	C30.1	C78.39	D02.3	D14.0	D38.5	D49.2
autonomic nerve or nervous system NEC (see Neoplasm, nerve, peripheral)						
axilla, axillary	C76.1	C79.89	D09.8	D36.7	D48.7	D49.89
fold—see also Neoplasm, skin, trunk	C44.509	C79.2	D04.5	D23.5	D48.5	D49.2
B						
back NEC	C76.8	C79.89	D04.5	D36.7	D48.7	D49.89
Bartholin's gland	C51.0	C79.82	D07.1	D28.0	D39.8	D49.59
basal ganglia	C71.0	C79.31	-	D33.0	D43.0	D49.6
basis pedunculi	C71.7	C79.31	-	D33.1	D43.1	D49.6
bile or biliary (tract)	C24.9	C78.89	D01.5	D13.5	D37.6	D49.0
canaliculi (biliferi) (intrahepatic)	C22.1	C78.7	D01.5	D13.4	D37.6	D49.0
canals, interlobular	C22.1	C78.89	D01.5	D13.4	D37.6	D49.0
duct or passage (common) (cystic) (extrahepatic)	C24.0	C78.89	D01.5	D13.5	D37.6	D49.0
interlobular	C22.1	C78.89	D01.5	D13.4	D37.6	D49.0
intrahepatic	C22.1	C78.7	D01.5	D13.4	D37.6	D49.0
and extrahepatic	C24.8	C78.89	D01.5	D13.5	D37.6	D49.0
bladder (urinary)	C67.9	C79.11	D09.0	D30.3	D41.4	D49.4
dome	C67.1	C79.11	D09.0	D30.3	D41.4	D49.4
neck	C67.5	C79.11	D09.0	D30.3	D41.4	D49.4
orifice	C67.9	C79.11	D09.0	D30.3	D41.4	D49.4
ureteric	C67.6	C79.11	D09.0	D30.3	D41.4	D49.4
urethral	C67.5	C79.11	D09.0	D30.3	D41.4	D49.4
overlapping lesion	C67.8	-	-	-	-	-
sphincter	C67.8	C79.11	D09.0	D30.3	D41.4	D49.4
trigone	C67.0	C79.11	D09.0	D30.3	D41.4	D49.4
urachus	C67.7	C79.11	D09.0	D30.3	D41.4	D49.4
wall	C67.9	C79.11	D09.0	D30.3	D41.4	D49.4
anterior	C67.3	C79.11	D09.0	D30.3	D41.4	D49.4
lateral	C67.2	C79.11	D09.0	D30.3	D41.4	D49.4
posterior	C67.4	C79.11	D09.0	D30.3	D41.4	D49.4
blood vessel—see Neoplasm, connective tissue						
bone (periosteum)	C41.9	C79.51	-	D16.9	D48.0	D49.2
acetabulum	C41.4	C79.51	-	D16.8	D48.0	D49.2
ankle	C40.3-	C79.51	-	D16.3-	-	-
arm NEC	C40.0-	C79.51	-	D16.0-	-	-
astragalus	C40.3-	C79.51	-	D16.3-	-	-
atlas	C41.2	C79.51	-	D16.6	D48.0	D49.2
axis	C41.2	C79.51	-	D16.6	D48.0	D49.2
back NEC	C41.2	C79.51	-	D16.6	D48.0	D49.2
calcaneus	C40.3-	C79.51	-	D16.3-	-	-
calvarium	C41.0	C79.51	-	D16.4	D48.0	D49.2
carpus (any)	C40.1-	C79.51	-	D16.1-	-	-
cartilage NEC	C41.9	C79.51	-	D16.9	D48.0	D49.2

	Malignant Primary	Malignant Secondary	Ca in situ	Benign	Uncertain Behavior	Unspecified Behavior
bone — *continued*						
clavicle	C41.3	C79.51	-	D16.7	D48.0	D49.2
clivus	C41.0	C79.51	-	D16.4	D48.0	D49.2
coccygeal vertebra	C41.4	C79.51	-	D16.8	D48.0	D49.2
coccyx	C41.4	C79.51	-	D16.8	D48.0	D49.2
costal cartilage	C41.3	C79.51	-	D16.7	D48.0	D49.2
costovertebral joint	C41.3	C79.51	-	D16.7	D48.0	D49.2
cranial	C41.0	C79.51	-	D16.4	D48.0	D49.2
cuboid	C40.3-	C79.51	-	D16.3-	-	-
cuneiform	C41.9	C79.51	-	D16.9	D48.0	D49.2
elbow	C40.0-	C79.51	-	D16.0-	-	-
ethmoid (labyrinth)	C41.0	C79.51	-	D16.4	D48.0	D49.2
face	C41.0	C79.51	-	D16.4	D48.0	D49.2
femur (any part)	C40.2-	C79.51	-	D16.2-	-	-
fibula (any part)	C40.2-	C79.51	-	D16.2-	-	-
finger (any)	C40.1-	C79.51	-	D16.1-	-	-
foot	C40.3-	C79.51	-	D16.3-	-	-
forearm	C40.0-	C79.51	-	D16.0-	-	-
frontal	C41.0	C79.51	-	D16.4	D48.0	D49.2
hand	C40.1-	C79.51	-	D16.1-	-	-
heel	C40.3-	C79.51	-	D16.3-	-	-
hip	C41.4	C79.51	-	D16.8	D48.0	D49.2
humerus (any part)	C40.0-	C79.51	-	D16.0-	-	-
hyoid	C41.0	C79.51	-	D16.4	D48.0	D49.2
ilium	C41.4	C79.51	-	D16.8	D48.0	D49.2
innominate	C41.4	C79.51	-	D16.8	D48.0	D49.2
intervertebral cartilage or disc	C41.2	C79.51	-	D16.6	D48.0	D49.2
ischium	C41.4	C79.51	-	D16.8	D48.0	D49.2
jaw (lower)	C41.1	C79.51	-	D16.5	D48.0	D49.2
knee	C40.2-	C79.51	-	D16.2-	-	-
leg NEC	C40.2-	C79.51	-	D16.2-	-	-
limb NEC	C40.9-	C79.51	-	D16.9	-	-
lower (long bones)	C40.2-	C79.51	-	D16.2-	-	-
short bones	C40.3-	C79.51	-	D16.3-	-	-
upper (long bones)	C40.0-	C79.51	-	D16.0-	-	-
short bones	C40.1-	C79.51	-	D16.1-	-	-
malar	C41.0	C79.51	-	D16.4	D48.0	D49.2
mandible	C41.1	C79.51	-	D16.5	D48.0	D49.2
marrow NEC (any bone)	C96.9	C79.52	-	-	D47.9	D49.89
mastoid	C41.0	C79.51	-	D16.4	D48.0	D49.2
maxilla, maxillary (superior)	C41.0	C79.51	-	D16.4	D48.0	D49.2
inferior	C41.1	C79.51	-	D16.4	D48.0	D49.2
metacarpus (any)	C40.1-	C79.51	-	D16.1-	-	-
metatarsus (any)	C40.3-	C79.51	-	D16.3-	-	-
navicular						
ankle	C40.3-	C79.51	-	-	-	-
hand	C40.1-	C79.51	-	-	-	-
nose, nasal	C41.0	C79.51	-	D16.4	D48.0	D49.2
occipital	C41.0	C79.51	-	D16.4	D48.0	D49.2
orbit	C41.0	C79.51	-	D16.4	D48.0	D49.2

	Malignant Primary	Malignant Secondary	Ca in situ	Benign	Uncertain Behavior	Unspecified Behavior
bone — *continued*						
overlapping sites	C40.8-	-	-	-	-	-
parietal	C41.0	C79.51	-	D16.4	D48.0	D49.2
patella	C40.2-	C79.51	-	-	-	-
pelvic	C41.4	C79.51	-	D16.8	D48.0	D49.2
phalanges						
foot	C40.3-	C79.51	-	-	-	-
hand	C40.1-	C79.51	-	-	-	-
pubic	C41.4	C79.51	-	D16.8	D48.0	D49.2
radius (any part)	C40.0-	C79.51	-	D16.0-	-	-
rib	C41.3	C79.51	-	D16.7	D48.0	D49.2
sacral vertebra	C41.4	C79.51	-	D16.8	D48.0	D49.2
sacrum	C41.4	C79.51	-	D16.8	D48.0	D49.2
scaphoid	-	-	-	-	-	-
of ankle	C40.3-	C79.51	-	-	-	-
of hand	C40.1-	C79.51	-	-	-	-
scapula (any part)	C40.0-	C79.51	-	D16.0-	-	-
sella turcica	C41.0	C79.51	-	D16.4	D48.0	D49.2
shoulder	C40.0-	C79.51	-	D16.0-	-	-
skull	C41.0	C79.51	-	D16.4	D48.0	D49.2
sphenoid	C41.0	C79.51	-	D16.4	D48.0	D49.2
spine, spinal (column)	C41.2	C79.51	-	D16.6	D48.0	D49.2
coccyx	C41.4	C79.51	-	D16.8	D48.0	D49.2
sacrum	C41.4	C79.51	-	D16.8	D48.0	D49.2
sternum	C41.3	C79.51	-	D16.7	D48.0	D49.2
tarsus (any)	C40.3-	C79.51	-	-	-	-
temporal	C41.0	C79.51	-	D16.4	D48.0	D49.2
thumb	C40.1-	C79.51	-	-	-	-
tibia (any part)	C40.2-	C79.51	-	-	-	-
toe (any)	C40.3-	C79.51	-	-	-	-
trapezium	C40.1-	C79.51	-	-	-	-
trapezoid	C40.1-	C79.51	-	-	-	-
turbinate	C41.0	C79.51	-	D16.4	D48.0	D49.2
ulna (any part)	C40.0-	C79.51	-	D16.0-	-	-
unciform	C40.1-	C79.51	-	-	-	-
vertebra (column)	C41.2	C79.51	-	D16.6	D48.0	D49.2
coccyx	C41.4	C79.51	-	D16.8	D48.0	D49.2
sacrum	C41.4	C79.51	-	D16.8	D48.0	D49.2
vomer	C41.0	C79.51	-	D16.4	D48.0	D49.2
wrist	C40.1-	C79.51	-	-	-	-
xiphoid process	C41.3	C79.51	-	D16.7	D48.0	D49.2
zygomatic	C41.0	C79.51	-	D16.4	D48.0	D49.2
book-leaf (mouth)	C06.89	C79.89	D00.00	D10.39	D37.09	D49.0
bowel—see Neoplasm, intestine						
brachial plexus	C47.1-	C79.89	-	D36.12	D48.2	D49.2
brain NEC	C71.9	C79.31	-	D33.2	D43.2	D49.6
basal ganglia	C71.0	C79.31	-	D33.0	D43.0	D49.6
cerebellopontine angle	C71.6	C79.31	-	D33.1	D43.1	D49.6
cerebellum NOS	C71.6	C79.31	-	D33.1	D43.1	D49.6
cerebrum	C71.0	C79.31	-	D33.0	D43.0	D49.6
choroid plexus	C71.7	C79.31	-	D33.1	D43.1	D49.6
corpus callosum	C71.8	C79.31	-	D33.2	D43.2	D49.6

	Malignant Primary	Malignant Secondary	Ca in situ	Benign	Uncertain Behavior	Unspecified Behavior
brain NEC — *continued*						
corpus striatum	C71.0	C79.31	-	D33.0	D43.0	D49.6
cortex (cerebral)	C71.0	C79.31	-	D33.0	D43.0	D49.6
frontal lobe	C71.1	C79.31	-	D33.0	D43.0	D49.6
globus pallidus	C71.0	C79.31	-	D33.0	D43.0	D49.6
hippocampus	C71.2	C79.31	-	D33.0	D43.0	D49.6
hypothalamus	C71.0	C79.31	-	D33.0	D43.0	D49.6
internal capsule	C71.0	C79.31	-	D33.0	D43.0	D49.6
medulla oblongata	C71.7	C79.31	-	D33.1	D43.1	D49.6
meninges	C70.0	C79.32	-	D32.0	D42.0	D49.7
midbrain	C71.7	C79.31	-	D33.1	D43.1	D49.6
occipital lobe	C71.4	C79.31	-	D33.0	D43.0	D49.6
overlapping lesion	C71.8	C79.31	-	-	-	-
parietal lobe	C71.3	C79.31	-	D33.0	D43.0	D49.6
peduncle	C71.7	C79.31	-	D33.1	D43.1	D49.6
pons	C71.7	C79.31	-	D33.1	D43.1	D49.6
stem	C71.7	C79.31	-	D33.1	D43.1	D49.6
tapetum	C71.8	C79.31	-	D33.2	D43.2	D49.6
temporal lobe	C71.2	C79.31	-	D33.0	D43.0	D49.6
thalamus	C71.0	C79.31	-	D33.0	D43.0	D49.6
uncus	C71.2	C79.31	-	D33.0	D43.0	D49.6
ventricle (floor)	C71.5	C79.31	-	D33.0	D43.0	D49.6
fourth	C71.7	C79.31	-	D33.1	D43.1	D49.6
branchial (cleft) (cyst) (vestiges)	C10.4	C79.89	D00.08	D10.5	D37.05	D49.0
breast (connective tissue) (glandular tissue) (soft parts)	C50.9-	C79.81	D05.-	D24.-	D48.6-	D49.3
areola	C50.0-	C79.81	D05.-	D24.-	D48.6-	D49.3
axillary tail	C50.6-	C79.81	D05.-	D24.-	D48.6-	D49.3
central portion	C50.1-	C79.81	D05.-	D24.-	D48.6-	D49.3
inner	C50.8-	C79.81	D05.-	D24.-	D48.6-	D49.3
lower	C50.8-	C79.81	D05.-	D24.-	D48.6-	D49.3
lower-inner quadrant	C50.3-	C79.81	D05.-	D24.-	D48.6-	D49.3
lower-outer quadrant	C50.5-	C79.81	D05.-	D24.-	D48.6-	D49.3
mastectomy site (skin)— see also Neoplasm, breast, skin	C44.501	C79.2	-	-	-	-
specified as breast tissue	C50.8-	C79.81	-	-	-	-
midline	C50.8-	C79.81	D05.-	D24.-	D48.6-	D49.3
nipple	C50.0-	C79.81	D05.-	D24.-	D48.6-	D49.3
outer	C50.8-	C79.81	D05.-	D24.-	D48.6-	D49.3
overlapping lesion	C50.8-	-	-	-	-	-
skin	C44.501	C79.2	D04.5	D23.5	D48.5	D49.2
basal cell carcinoma	C44.511	-	-	-	-	-
specified type NEC	C44.591	-	-	-	-	-
squamous cell carcinoma	C44.521	-	-	-	-	-
tail (axillary)	C50.6-	C79.81	D05.-	D24.-	D48.6-	D49.3
upper	C50.8-	C79.81	D05.-	D24.-	D48.6-	D49.3
upper-inner quadrant	C50.2-	C79.81	D05.-	D24.-	D48.6-	D49.3
upper-outer quadrant	C50.4-	C79.81	D05.-	D24.-	D48.6-	D49.3
broad ligament	C57.1-	C79.82	D07.39	D28.2	D39.8	D49.59

	Malignant Primary	Malignant Secondary	Ca in situ	Benign	Uncertain Behavior	Unspecified Behavior
bronchiogenic, bronchogenic (lung)	C34.9-	C78.0-	D02.2-	D14.3-	D38.1	D49.1
bronchiole	C34.9-	C78.0-	D02.2-	D14.3-	D38.1	D49.1
bronchus	C34.9-	C78.0-	D02.2-	D14.3-	D38.1	D49.1
carina	C34.0-	C78.0-	D02.2-	D14.3-	D38.1	D49.1
lower lobe of lung	C34.3-	C78.0-	D02.2-	D14.3-	D38.1	D49.1
main	C34.0-	C78.0-	D02.2-	D14.3-	D38.1	D49.1
middle lobe of lung	C34.2	C78.0-	D02.21	D14.31	D38.1	D49.1
overlapping lesion	C34.8-	-	-	-	-	-
upper lobe of lung	C34.1-	C78.0-	D02.2-	D14.3-	D38.1	D49.1
brow	C44.309	C79.2	D04.39	D23.39	D48.5	D49.2
basal cell carcinoma	C44.319	-	-	-	-	-
specified type NEC	C44.399	-	-	-	-	-
squamous cell carcinoma	C44.329	-	-	-	-	-
buccal (cavity)	C06.9	C79.89	D00.00	D10.39	D37.09	D49.0
commissure	C06.0	C79.89	D00.02	D10.39	D37.09	D49.0
groove (lower) (upper)	C06.1	C79.89	D00.02	D10.39	D37.09	D49.0
mucosa	C06.0	C79.89	D00.02	D10.39	D37.09	D49.0
sulcus (lower) (upper)	C06.1	C79.89	D00.02	D10.39	D37.09	D49.0
bulbourethral gland	C68.0	C79.19	D09.19	D30.4	D41.3	D49.59
bursa—see Neoplasm, connective tissue						
buttock NEC	C76.3	C79.89	D04.5	D36.7	D48.7	D49.89
C						
calf	C76.5-	C79.89	D04.7-	D36.7	D48.7	D49.89
calvarium	C41.0	C79.51	-	D16.4	D48.0	D49.2
calyx, renal	C65.-	C79.0-	D09.19	D30.1-	D41.1-	D49.51-
canal						
anal	C21.1	C78.5	D01.3	D12.9	D37.8	D49.0
auditory (external)—see also Neoplasm, skin, ear	C44.20-	C79.2	D04.2-	D23.2-	D48.5	D49.2
auricular (external)—see also Neoplasm, skin, ear	C44.20-	C79.2	D04.2-	D23.2-	D48.5	D49.2
canaliculi, biliary (biliferi) (intrahepatic)	C22.1	C78.7	D01.5	D13.4	D37.6	D49.0
canthus (eye) (inner) (outer)	C44.10-	C79.2	D04.1-	D23.1-	D48.5	D49.2
basal cell carcinoma	C44.11-	-	-	-	-	-
sebaceous cell	C44.13-	-	-	-	-	-
specified type NEC	C44.19-	-	-	-	-	-
squamous cell carcinoma	C44.12-	-	-	-	-	-
capillary—see Neoplasm, connective tissue						
caput coli	C18.0	C78.5	D01.0	D12.0	D37.4	D49.0
carcinoid—see Tumor, carcinoid						
cardia (gastric)	C16.0	C78.89	D00.2	D13.1	D37.1	D49.0
cardiac orifice (stomach)	C16.0	C78.89	D00.2	D13.1	D37.1	D49.0
cardio-esophageal junction	C16.0	C78.89	D00.2	D13.1	D37.1	D49.0
cardio-esophagus	C16.0	C78.89	D00.2	D13.1	D37.1	D49.0
carina (bronchus)	C34.0-	C78.0-	D02.2-	D14.3-	D38.1	D49.1
carotid (artery)	C49.0	C79.89	-	D21.0	D48.1	D49.2
body	C75.4	C79.89	-	D35.5	D44.6	D49.7
carpus (any bone)	C40.1-	C79.51	-	D16.1-	-	-
cartilage (articular) (joint) NEC—see also Neoplasm, bone	C41.9	C79.51	-	D16.9	D48.0	D49.2
arytenoid	C32.3	C78.39	D02.0	D14.1	D38.0	D49.1

	Malignant Primary	Malignant Secondary	Ca in situ	Benign	Uncertain Behavior	Unspecified Behavior
cartilage NEC — *continued*						
auricular	C49.0	C79.89	-	D21.0	D48.1	D49.2
bronchi	C34.0-	C78.39	-	D14.3-	D38.1	D49.1
costal	C41.3	C79.51	-	D16.7	D48.0	D49.2
cricoid	C32.3	C78.39	D02.0	D14.1	D38.0	D49.1
cuneiform	C32.3	C78.39	D02.0	D14.1	D38.0	D49.1
ear (external)	C49.0	C79.89	-	D21.0	D48.1	D49.2
ensiform	C41.3	C79.51	-	D16.7	D48.0	D49.2
epiglottis	C32.1	C78.39	D02.0	D14.1	D38.0	D49.1
anterior surface	C10.1	C79.89	D00.08	D10.5	D37.05	D49.0
eyelid	C49.0	C79.89	-	D21.0	D48.1	D49.2
intervertebral	C41.2	C79.51	-	D16.6	D48.0	D49.2
larynx, laryngeal	C32.3	C78.39	D02.0	D14.1	D38.0	D49.1
nose, nasal	C30.0	C78.39	D02.3	D14.0	D38.5	D49.1
pinna	C49.0	C79.89	-	D21.0	D48.1	D49.2
rib	C41.3	C79.51	-	D16.7	D48.0	D49.2
semilunar (knee)	C40.2-	C79.51	-	D16.2-	D48.0	D49.2
thyroid	C32.3	C78.39	D02.0	D14.1	D38.0	D49.1
trachea	C33	C78.39	D02.1	D14.2	D38.1	D49.1
cauda equina	C72.1	C79.49	-	D33.4	D43.4	D49.7
cavity						
buccal	C06.9	C79.89	D00.00	D10.30	D37.09	D49.0
nasal	C30.0	C78.39	D02.3	D14.0	D38.5	D49.1
oral	C06.9	C79.89	D00.00	D10.30	D37.09	D49.0
peritoneal	C48.2	C78.6	-	D20.1	D48.4	D49.0
tympanic	C30.1	C78.39	D02.3	D14.0	D38.5	D49.1
cecum	C18.0	C78.5	D01.0	D12.0	D37.4	D49.0
central nervous system	C72.9	C79.40	-	-	-	-
cerebellopontine (angle)	C71.6	C79.31	-	D33.1	D43.1	D49.6
cerebellum, cerebellar	C71.6	C79.31	-	D33.1	D43.1	D49.6
cerebrum, cerebral (cortex) (hemisphere) (white matter)	C71.0	C79.31	-	D33.0	D43.0	D49.6
meninges	C70.0	C79.32	-	D32.0	D42.0	D49.7
peduncle	C71.7	C79.31	-	D33.1	D43.1	D49.6
ventricle	C71.5	C79.31	-	D33.0	D43.0	D49.6
fourth	C71.7	C79.31	-	D33.1	D43.1	D49.6
cervical region	C76.0	C79.89	D09.8	D36.7	D48.7	D49.89
cervix (cervical) (uteri) (uterus)	C53.9	C79.82	D06.9	D26.0	D39.0	D49.59
canal	C53.0	C79.82	D06.0	D26.0	D39.0	D49.59
endocervix (canal) (gland)	C53.0	C79.82	D06.0	D26.0	D39.0	D49.59
exocervix	C53.1	C79.82	D06.1	D26.0	D39.0	D49.59
external os	C53.1	C79.82	D06.1	D26.0	D39.0	D49.59
internal os	C53.0	C79.82	D06.0	D26.0	D39.0	D49.59
nabothian gland	C53.0	C79.82	D06.0	D26.0	D39.0	D49.59
overlapping lesion	C53.8	-	-	-	-	-
squamocolumnar junction	C53.8	C79.82	D06.7	D26.0	D39.0	D49.59
stump	C53.8	C79.82	D06.7	D26.0	D39.0	D49.59
cheek	C76.0	C79.89	D09.8	D36.7	D48.7	D49.89
external	C44.309	C79.2	D04.39	D23.39	D48.5	D49.2
basal cell carcinoma	C44.319	-	-	-	-	-
specified type NEC	C44.399	-	-	-	-	-
squamous cell carcinoma	C44.329	-	-	-	-	-

	Malignant Primary	Malignant Secondary	Ca in situ	Benign	Uncertain Behavior	Unspecified Behavior
cheek — *continued*						
inner aspect	C06.0	C79.89	D00.02	D10.39	D37.09	D49.0
internal	C06.0	C79.89	D00.02	D10.39	D37.09	D49.0
mucosa	C06.0	C79.89	D00.02	D10.39	D37.09	D49.0
chest (wall) NEC	C76.1	C79.89	D09.8	D36.7	D48.7	D49.89
chiasma opticum	C72.3-	C79.49	-	D33.3	D43.3	D49.7
chin	C44.309	C79.2	D04.39	D23.39	D48.5	D49.2
basal cell carcinoma	C44.319	-	-	-	-	-
specified type NEC	C44.399	-	-	-	-	-
squamous cell carcinoma	C44.329	-	-	-	-	-
choana	C11.3	C79.89	D00.08	D10.6	D37.05	D49.0
cholangiole	C22.1	C78.89	D01.5	D13.4	D37.6	D49.0
choledochal duct	C24.0	C78.89	D01.5	D13.5	D37.6	D49.0
choroid	C69.3-	C79.49	D09.2-	D31.3-	D48.7	D49.81
plexus	C71.5	C79.31	-	D33.0	D43.0	D49.6
ciliary body	C69.4-	C79.49	D09.2-	D31.4-	D48.7	D49.89
clavicle	C41.3	C79.51	-	D16.7	D48.0	D49.2
clitoris	C51.2	C79.82	D07.1	D28.0	D39.8	D49.59
clivus	C41.0	C79.51	-	D16.4-	D48.0	D49.2
cloacogenic zone	C21.2	C78.5	D01.3	D12.9	D37.8	D49.0
coccygeal						
body or glomus	C49.5	C79.89	-	D21.5	D48.1	D49.2
vertebra	C41.4	C79.51	-	D16.8	D48.0	D49.2
coccyx	C41.4	C79.51	-	D16.8	D48.0	D49.2
colon—see also Neoplasm, intestine, large	C18.9	C78.5	-	-	-	-
with rectum	C19	C78.5	D01.1	D12.7	D37.5	D49.0
column, spinal—see Neoplasm, spine						
columnella—see also Neoplasm, skin, face	C44.390	C79.2	D04.39	D23.39	D48.5	D49.2
commissure						
labial, lip	C00.6	C79.89	D00.01	D10.39	D37.01	D49.0
laryngeal	C32.0	C78.39	D02.0	D14.1	D38.0	D49.1
common (bile) duct	C24.0	C78.89	D01.5	D13.5	D37.6	D49.0
concha—see also Neoplasm, skin, ear	C44.20-	C79.2	D04.2-	D23.2-	D48.5	D49.2
nose	C30.0	C78.39	D02.3	D14.0	D38.5	D49.1
conjunctiva	C69.0-	C79.49	D09.2-	D31.0-	D48.7	D49.89
connective tissue NEC	C49.9	C79.89	-	D21.9	D48.1	D49.2

Note: For neoplasms of connective tissue (blood vessel, bursa, fascia, ligament, muscle, peripheral nerves, sympathetic and parasympathetic nerves and ganglia, synovia, tendon, etc.) or of morphological types that indicate connective tissue, code according to the list under "Neoplasm, connective tissue". For sites that do not appear in this list, code to neoplasm of that site; e.g., fibrosarcoma, pancreas (C25.9)

	Malignant Primary	Malignant Secondary	Ca in situ	Benign	Uncertain Behavior	Unspecified Behavior
connective tissue NEC — *continued*						
Note: Morphological types that indicate connective tissue appear in their proper place in the alphabetic index with the instruction "see Neoplasm, connective tissue …."						
abdomen	C49.4	C79.89	-	D21.4	D48.1	D49.2
abdominal wall	C49.4	C79.89	-	D21.4	D48.1	D49.2
ankle	C49.2-	C79.89	-	D21.2-	D48.1	D49.2
antecubital fossa or space	C49.1-	C79.89	-	D21.1-	D48.1	D49.2
arm	C49.1-	C79.89	-	D21.1-	D48.1	D49.2
auricle (ear)	C49.0	C79.89	-	D21.0	D48.1	D49.2
axilla	C49.3	C79.89	-	D21.3	D48.1	D49.2
back	C49.6	C79.89	-	D21.6	D48.1	D49.2
breast—see Neoplasm, breast						
buttock	C49.5	C79.89	-	D21.5	D48.1	D49.2
calf	C49.2-	C79.89	-	D21.2-	D48.1	D49.2
cervical region	C49.0	C79.89	-	D21.0	D48.1	D49.2
cheek	C49.0	C79.89	-	D21.0	D48.1	D49.2
chest (wall)	C49.3	C79.89	-	D21.3	D48.1	D49.2
chin	C49.0	C79.89	-	D21.0	D48.1	D49.2
diaphragm	C49.3	C79.89	-	D21.3	D48.1	D49.2
ear (external)	C49.0	C79.89	-	D21.0	D48.1	D49.2
elbow	C49.1-	C79.89	-	D21.1-	D48.1	D49.2
extrarectal	C49.5	C79.89	-	D21.5	D48.1	D49.2
extremity	C49.9	C79.89	-	D21.9	D48.1	D49.2
lower	C49.2-	C79.89	-	D21.2-	D48.1	D49.2
upper	C49.1-	C79.89	-	D21.1-	D48.1	D49.2
eyelid	C49.0	C79.89	-	D21.0	D48.1	D49.2
face	C49.0	C79.89	-	D21.0	D48.1	D49.2
finger	C49.1-	C79.89	-	D21.1-	D48.1	D49.2
flank	C49.6	C79.89	-	D21.6	D48.1	D49.2
foot	C49.2-	C79.89	-	D21.2-	D48.1	D49.2
forearm	C49.1-	C79.89	-	D21.1-	D48.1	D49.2
forehead	C49.0	C79.89	-	D21.0	D48.1	D49.2
gastric	C49.4	C79.89	-	D21.4	D48.1	D49.2
gastrointestinal	C49.4	C79.89	-	D21.4	D48.1	D49.2
gluteal region	C49.5	C79.89	-	D21.5	D48.1	D49.2
great vessels NEC	C49.3	C79.89	-	D21.3	D48.1	D49.2
groin	C49.5	C79.89	-	D21.5	D48.1	D49.2
hand	C49.1-	C79.89	-	D21.1-	D48.1	D49.2
head	C49.0	C79.89	-	D21.0	D48.1	D49.2
heel	C49.2-	C79.89	-	D21.2-	D48.1	D49.2
hip	C49.2-	C79.89	-	D21.2-	D48.1	D49.2
hypochondrium	C49.4	C79.89	-	D21.4	D48.1	D49.2
iliopsoas muscle	C49.5	C79.89	-	D21.5	D48.1	D49.2
infraclavicular region	C49.3	C79.89	-	D21.3	D48.1	D49.2
inguinal (canal) (region)	C49.5	C79.89	-	D21.5	D48.1	D49.2
intestinal	C49.4	C79.89	-	D21.4	D48.1	D49.2
intrathoracic	C49.3	C79.89	-	D21.3	D48.1	D49.2
ischiorectal fossa	C49.5	C79.89	-	D21.5	D48.1	D49.2

	Malignant Primary	Malignant Secondary	Ca in situ	Benign	Uncertain Behavior	Unspecified Behavior
connective tissue NEC — *continued*						
jaw	C03.9	C79.89	D00.03	D10.39	D48.1	D49.0
knee	C49.2-	C79.89	-	D21.2-	D48.1	D49.2
leg	C49.2-	C79.89	-	D21.2-	D48.1	D49.2
limb NEC	C49.9	C79.89	-	D21.9	D48.1	D49.2
lower	C49.2-	C79.89	-	D21.2-	D48.1	D49.2
upper	C49.1-	C79.89	-	D21.1-	D48.1	D49.2
nates	C49.5	C79.89	-	D21.5	D48.1	D49.2
neck	C49.0	C79.89	-	D21.0	D48.1	D49.2
orbit	C69.6-	C79.49	D09.2-	D31.6-	D48.1	D49.89
overlapping lesion	C49.8	-	-	-	-	-
pararectal	C49.5	C79.89	-	D21.5	D48.1	D49.2
para-urethral	C49.5	C79.89	-	D21.5	D48.1	D49.2
paravaginal	C49.5	C79.89	-	D21.5	D48.1	D49.2
pelvis (floor)	C49.5	C79.89	-	D21.5	D48.1	D49.2
pelvo-abdominal	C49.8	C79.89	-	D21.6	D48.1	D49.2
perineum	C49.5	C79.89	-	D21.5	D48.1	D49.2
perirectal (tissue)	C49.5	C79.89	-	D21.5	D48.1	D49.2
periurethral (tissue)	C49.5	C79.89	-	D21.5	D48.1	D49.2
popliteal fossa or space	C49.2-	C79.89	-	D21.2-	D48.1	D49.2
presacral	C49.5	C79.89	-	D21.5	D48.1	D49.2
psoas muscle	C49.4	C79.89	-	D21.4	D48.1	D49.2
pterygoid fossa	C49.0	C79.89	-	D21.0	D48.1	D49.2
rectovaginal septum or wall	C49.5	C79.89	-	D21.5	D48.1	D49.2
rectovesical	C49.5	C79.89	-	D21.5	D48.1	D49.2
retroperitoneum	C48.0	C78.6	-	D20.0	D48.3	D49.0
sacrococcygeal region	C49.5	C79.89	-	D21.5	D48.1	D49.2
scalp	C49.0	C79.89	-	D21.0	D48.1	D49.2
scapular region	C49.3	C79.89	-	D21.3	D48.1	D49.2
shoulder	C49.1-	C79.89	-	D21.1-	D48.1	D49.2
skin (dermis) NEC—see also Neoplasm, skin, by site	C44.90	C79.2	D04.9	D23.9	D48.5	D49.2
stomach	C49.4	C79.89	-	D21.4	D48.1	D49.2
submental	C49.0	C79.89	-	D21.0	D48.1	D49.2
supraclavicular region	C49.0	C79.89	-	D21.0	D48.1	D49.2
temple	C49.0	C79.89	-	D21.0	D48.1	D49.2
temporal region	C49.0	C79.89	-	D21.0	D48.1	D49.2
thigh	C49.2-	C79.89	-	D21.2-	D48.1	D49.2
thoracic (duct) (wall)	C49.3	C79.89	-	D21.3	D48.1	D49.2
thorax	C49.3	C79.89	-	D21.3	D48.1	D49.2
thumb	C49.1-	C79.89	-	D21.1-	D48.1	D49.2
toe	C49.2-	C79.89	-	D21.2-	D48.1	D49.2
trunk	C49.6	C79.89	-	D21.6	D48.1	D49.2
umbilicus	C49.4	C79.89	-	D21.4	D48.1	D49.2
vesicorectal	C49.5	C79.89	-	D21.5	D48.1	D49.2
wrist	C49.1-	C79.89	-	D21.1-	D48.1	D49.2
conus medullaris	C72.0	C79.49	-	D33.4	D43.4	D49.7
cord (true) (vocal)	C32.0	C78.39	D02.0	D14.1	D38.0	D49.1
false	C32.1	C78.39	D02.0	D14.1	D38.0	D49.1
spermatic	C63.1-	C79.82	D07.69	D29.8	D40.8	D49.59

	Malignant Primary	Malignant Secondary	Ca in situ	Benign	Uncertain Behavior	Unspecified Behavior
cord (true) (vocal) — *continued*						
spinal (cervical) (lumbar) (thoracic)	C72.0	C79.49	-	D33.4	D43.4	D49.7
cornea (limbus)	C69.1-	C79.49	D09.2-	D31.1-	D48.7	D49.89
corpus						
albicans	C56.-	C79.6-	D07.39	D27.-	D39.1-	D49.59
callosum, brain	C71.0	C79.31	-	D33.2	D43.2	D49.6
cavernosum	C60.2	C79.82	D07.4	D29.0	D40.8	D49.59
gastric	C16.2	C78.89	D00.2	D13.1	D37.1	D49.0
overlapping sites	C54.8	-	-	-	-	-
penis	C60.2	C79.82	D07.4	D29.0	D40.8	D49.59
striatum, cerebrum	C71.0	C79.31	-	D33.0	D43.0	D49.6
uteri	C54.9	C79.82	D07.0	D26.1	D39.0	D49.59
isthmus	C54.0	C79.82	D07.0	D26.1	D39.0	D49.59
cortex						
adrenal	C74.0-	C79.7-	D09.3	D35.0-	D44.1-	D49.7
cerebral	C71.0	C79.31	-	D33.0	D43.0	D49.6
costal cartilage	C41.3	C79.51	-	D16.7	D48.0	D49.2
costovertebral joint	C41.3	C79.51	-	D16.7	D48.0	D49.2
Cowper's gland	C68.0	C79.19	D09.19	D30.4	D41.3	D49.59
cranial (fossa, any)	C71.9	C79.31	-	D33.2	D43.2	D49.6
meninges	C70.0	C79.32	-	D32.0	D42.0	D49.7
nerve	C72.50	C79.49	-	D33.3	D43.3	D49.7
specified NEC	C72.59	C79.49	-	D33.3	D43.3	D49.7
craniobuccal pouch	C75.2	C79.89	D09.3	D35.2	D44.3	D49.7
craniopharyngeal (duct) (pouch)	C75.2	C79.89	D09.3	D35.3	D44.4	D49.7
cricoid	C13.0	C79.89	D00.08	D10.7	D37.05	D49.0
cartilage	C32.3	C78.39	D02.0	D14.1	D38.0	D49.1
cricopharynx	C13.0	C79.89	D00.08	D10.7	D37.05	D49.0
crypt of Morgagni	C21.8	C78.5	D01.3	D12.9	D37.8	D49.0
crystalline lens	C69.4-	C79.49	D09.2-	D31.4-	D48.7	D49.89
cul-de-sac (Douglas')	C48.1	C78.6	-	D20.1	D48.4	D49.0
cuneiform cartilage	C32.3	C78.39	D02.0	D14.1	D38.0	D49.1
cutaneous—see Neoplasm, skin						
cutis—see Neoplasm, skin						
cystic (bile) duct (common)	C24.0	C78.89	D01.5	D13.5	D37.6	D49.0
D						
dermis—see Neoplasm, skin						
diaphragm	C49.3	C79.89	-	D21.3	D48.1	D49.2
digestive organs, system, tube, or tract NEC	C26.9	C78.89	D01.9	D13.9	D37.9	D49.0
disc, intervertebral	C41.2	C79.51	-	D16.6	D48.0	D49.2
disease, generalized	C80.0	-	-	-	-	-
disseminated	C80.0	-	-	-	-	-
Douglas' cul-de-sac or pouch	C48.1	C78.6	-	D20.1	D48.4	D49.0
duodenojejunal junction	C17.8	C78.4	D01.49	D13.39	D37.2	D49.0
duodenum	C17.0	C78.4	D01.49	D13.2	D37.2	D49.0
dura (cranial) (mater)	C70.9	C79.49	-	D32.9	D42.9	D49.7
cerebral	C70.0	C79.32	-	D32.0	D42.0	D49.7
spinal	C70.1	C79.49	-	D32.1	D42.1	D49.7

	Malignant Primary	Malignant Secondary	Ca in situ	Benign	Uncertain Behavior	Unspecified Behavior
E						
ear (external)—see also Neoplasm, skin, ear	C44.20-	C79.2	D04.2-	D23.2-	D48.5	D49.2
auricle or auris—see also Neoplasm, skin, ear	C44.20-	C79.2	D04.2-	D23.2-	D48.5	D49.2
canal, external—see also Neoplasm, skin, ear	C44.20-	C79.2	D04.2-	D23.2-	D48.5	D49.2
cartilage	C49.0	C79.89	-	D21.0	D48.1	D49.2
external meatus—see also Neoplasm, skin, ear	C44.20-	C79.2	D04.2-	D23.2-	D48.5	D49.2
inner	C30.1	C78.39	D02.3	D14.0	D38.5	D49.1
lobule—see also Neoplasm, skin, ear	C44.20-	C79.2	D04.2-	D23.2-	D48.5	D49.2
middle	C30.1	C78.39	D02.3	D14.0	D38.5	D49.1
overlapping lesion with accessory sinuses	C31.8	-	-	-	-	-
skin	C44.20-	C79.2	D04.2-	D23.2-	D48.5	D49.2
basal cell carcinoma	C44.21-	-	-	-	-	-
specified type NEC	C44.29-	-	-	-	-	-
squamous cell carcinoma	C44.22-	-	-	-	-	-
earlobe	C44.20-	C79.2	D04.2-	D23.2-	D48.5	D49.2
basal cell carcinoma	C44.21-	-	-	-	-	-
specified type NEC	C44.29-	-	-	-	-	-
squamous cell carcinoma	C44.22-	-	-	-	-	-
ejaculatory duct	C63.7	C79.82	D07.69	D29.8	D40.8	D49.59
elbow NEC	C76.4-	C79.89	D04.6-	D36.7	D48.7	D49.89
endocardium	C38.0	C79.89	-	D15.1	D48.7	D49.89
endocervix (canal) (gland)	C53.0	C79.82	D06.0	D26.0	D39.0	D49.59
endocrine gland NEC	C75.9	C79.89	D09.3	D35.9	D44.9	D49.7
pluriglandular	C75.8	C79.89	D09.3	D35.7	D44.9	D49.7
endometrium (gland) (stroma)	C54.1	C79.82	D07.0	D26.1	D39.0	D49.59
ensiform cartilage	C41.3	C79.51	-	D16.7	D48.0	D49.2
enteric—see Neoplasm, intestine						
ependyma (brain)	C71.5	C79.31	-	D33.0	D43.0	D49.6
fourth ventricle	C71.7	C79.31	-	D33.1	D43.1	D49.6
epicardium	C38.0	C79.89	-	D15.1	D48.7	D49.89
epididymis	C63.0-	C79.82	D07.69	D29.3-	D40.8	D49.59
epidural	C72.9	C79.49	-	D33.9	D43.9	D49.7
epiglottis	C32.1	C78.39	D02.0	D14.1	D38.0	D49.1
anterior aspect or surface	C10.1	C79.89	D00.08	D10.5	D37.05	D49.0
cartilage	C32.3	C78.39	D02.0	D14.1	D38.0	D49.1
free border (margin)	C10.1	C79.89	D00.08	D10.5	D37.05	D49.0
junctional region	C10.8	C79.89	D00.08	D10.5	D37.05	D49.0
posterior (laryngeal) surface	C32.1	C78.39	D02.0	D14.1	D38.0	D49.1
suprahyoid portion	C32.1	C78.39	D02.0	D14.1	D38.0	D49.1
esophagogastric junction	C16.0	C78.89	D00.2	D13.1	D37.1	D49.0
esophagus	C15.9	C78.89	D00.1	D13.0	D37.8	D49.0
abdominal	C15.5	C78.89	D00.1	D13.0	D37.8	D49.0
cervical	C15.3	C78.89	D00.1	D13.0	D37.8	D49.0
distal (third)	C15.5	C78.89	D00.1	D13.0	D37.8	D49.0
lower (third)	C15.5	C78.89	D00.1	D13.0	D37.8	D49.0

	Malignant Primary	Malignant Secondary	Ca in situ	Benign	Uncertain Behavior	Unspecified Behavior
esophagus — *continued*						
middle (third)	C15.4	C78.89	D00.1	D13.0	D37.8	D49.0
overlapping lesion	C15.8	-	-	-	-	-
proximal (third)	C15.3	C78.89	D00.1	D13.0	D37.8	D49.0
thoracic	C15.4	C78.89	D00.1	D13.0	D37.8	D49.0
upper (third)	C15.3	C78.89	D00.1	D13.0	D37.8	D49.0
ethmoid (sinus)	C31.1	C78.39	D02.3	D14.0	D38.5	D49.1
bone or labyrinth	C41.0	C79.51	-	D16.4-	D48.0	D49.2
eustachian tube	C30.1	C78.39	D02.3	D14.0	D38.5	D49.1
exocervix	C53.1	C79.82	D06.1	D26.0	D39.0	D49.59
external						
meatus (ear)—see also Neoplasm, skin, ear	C44.20-	C79.2	D04.2-	D23.2-	D48.5	D49.2
os, cervix uteri	C53.1	C79.82	D06.1	D26.0	D39.0	D49.59
extradural	C72.9	C79.49	-	D33.9	D43.9	D49.7
extrahepatic (bile) duct	C24.0	C78.89	D01.5	D13.5	D37.6	D49.0
overlapping lesion with gallbladder	C24.8	-	-	-	-	-
extraocular muscle	C69.6-	C79.49	D09.2-	D31.6-	D48.7	D49.89
extrarectal	C76.3	C79.89	D09.8	D36.7	D48.7	D49.89
extremity	C76.8	C79.89	D04.8	D36.7	D48.7	D49.89
lower	C76.5-	C79.89	D04.7-	D36.7	D48.7	D49.89
upper	C76.4-	C79.89	D04.6-	D36.7	D48.7	D49.89
eye NEC	C69.9-	C79.49	D09.2-	D31.9	D48.7	D49.89
overlapping sites	C69.8-	-	-	-	-	-
eyeball	C69.9-	C79.49	D09.2-	D31.9-	D48.7	D49.89
eyebrow	C44.309	C79.2	D04.39	D23.39	D48.5	D49.2
basal cell carcinoma	C44.319	-	-	-	-	-
specified type NEC	C44.399	-	-	-	-	-
squamous cell carcinoma	C44.329	-	-	-	-	-
eyelid (lower) (skin) (upper)	C44.10-	-	-	-	-	-
basal cell carcinoma	C44.11-	-	-	-	-	-
sebaceous cell	C44.13-	-	-	-	-	-
specified type NEC	C44.19-	-	-	-	-	-
squamous cell carcinoma	C44.12-	-	-	-	-	-
cartilage	C49.0	C79.89	-	D21.0	D48.1	D49.2
F						
face NEC	C76.0	C79.89	D04.39	D36.7	D48.7	D49.89
fallopian tube (accessory)	C57.0-	C79.82	D07.39	D28.2	D39.8	D49.59
falx (cerebella) (cerebri)	C70.0	C79.32	-	D32.0	D42.0	D49.7
fascia—see also Neoplasm, connective tissue						
palmar	C49.1-	C79.89	-	D21.1-	D48.1	D49.2
plantar	C49.2-	C79.89	-	D21.2-	D48.1	D49.2
fatty tissue—see Neoplasm, connective tissue						
fauces, faucial NEC	C10.9	C79.89	D00.08	D10.5	D37.05	D49.0
pillars	C09.1	C79.89	D00.08	D10.5	D37.05	D49.0
tonsil	C09.9	C79.89	D00.08	D10.4	D37.05	D49.0
femur (any part)	C40.2-	-	-	D16.2-	-	-
fetal membrane	C58	C79.82	D07.0	D26.7	D39.2	D49.59
fibrous tissue—see Neoplasm, connective tissue						

343

	Malignant Primary	Malignant Secondary	Ca in situ	Benign	Uncertain Behavior	Unspecified Behavior
fibula (any part)	C40.2-	C79.51	-	D16.2-	-	-
filum terminale	C72.0	C79.49	-	D33.4	D43.4	D49.7
finger NEC	C76.4-	C79.89	D04.6-	D36.7	D48.7	D49.89
flank NEC	C76.8	C79.89	D04.5	D36.7	D48.7	D49.89
follicle, nabothian	C53.0	C79.82	D06.0	D26.0	D39.0	D49.59
foot NEC	C76.5-	C79.89	D04.7-	D36.7	D48.7	D49.89
forearm NEC	C76.4-	C79.89	D04.6-	D36.7	D48.7	D49.89
forehead (skin)	C44.309	C79.2	D04.39	D23.39	D48.5	D49.2
basal cell carcinoma	C44.319	-	-	-	-	-
specified type NEC	C44.399	-	-	-	-	-
squamous cell carcinoma	C44.329	-	-	-	-	-
foreskin	C60.0	C79.82	D07.4	D29.0	D40.8	D49.59
fornix						
pharyngeal	C11.3	C79.89	D00.08	D10.6	D37.05	D49.0
vagina	C52	C79.82	D07.2	D28.1	D39.8	D49.59
fossa (of)						
anterior (cranial)	C71.9	C79.31	-	D33.2	D43.2	D49.6
cranial	C71.9	C79.31	-	D33.2	D43.2	D49.6
ischiorectal	C76.3	C79.89	D09.8	D36.7	D48.7	D49.89
middle (cranial)	C71.9	C79.31	-	D33.2	D43.2	D49.6
piriform	C12	C79.89	D00.08	D10.7	D37.05	D49.0
pituitary	C75.1	C79.89	D09.3	D35.2	D44.3	D49.7
posterior (cranial)	C71.9	C79.31	-	D33.2	D43.2	D49.6
pterygoid	C49.0	C79.89	-	D21.0	D48.1	D49.2
pyriform	C12	C79.89	D00.08	D10.7	D37.05	D49.0
Rosenmuller	C11.2	C79.89	D00.08	D10.6	D37.05	D49.0
tonsillar	C09.0	C79.89	D00.08	D10.5	D37.05	D49.0
fourchette	C51.9	C79.82	D07.1	D28.0	D39.8	D49.59
frenulum						
labii—see Neoplasm, lip, internal						
linguae	C02.2	C79.89	D00.07	D10.1	D37.02	D49.0
frontal						
bone	C41.0	C79.51	-	D16.4	D48.0	D49.2
lobe, brain	C71.1	C79.31	-	D33.0	D43.0	D49.6
pole	C71.1	C79.31	-	D33.0	D43.0	D49.6
sinus	C31.2	C78.39	D02.3	D14.0	D38.5	D49.1
fundus						
stomach	C16.1	C78.89	D00.2	D13.1	D37.1	D49.0
uterus	C54.3	C79.82	D07.0	D26.1	D39.0	D49.59
G						
gall duct (extrahepatic)	C24.0	C78.89	D01.5	D13.5	D37.6	D49.0
intrahepatic	C22.1	C78.7	D01.5	D13.4	D37.6	D49.0
gallbladder	C23	C78.89	D01.5	D13.5	D37.6	D49.0
overlapping lesion with extrahepatic bile ducts	C24.8	-	-	-	-	-
ganglia—see also Neoplasm, nerve, peripheral	C47.9	C79.89	-	D36.10	D48.2	D49.2
basal	C71.0	C79.31	-	D33.0	D43.0	D49.6
cranial nerve	C72.50	C79.49	-	D33.3	D43.3	D49.7
Gartner's duct	C52	C79.82	D07.2	D28.1	D39.8	D49.59
gastric—see Neoplasm, stomach						
gastrocolic	C26.9	C78.89	D01.9	D13.9	D37.9	D49.0
gastroesophageal junction	C16.0	C78.89	D00.2	D13.1	D37.1	D49.0
gastrointestinal (tract) NEC	C26.9	C78.89	D01.9	D13.9	D37.9	D49.0
generalized	C80.0	-	-	-	-	-
genital organ or tract						
female NEC	C57.9	C79.82	D07.30	D28.9	D39.9	D49.59
overlapping lesion	C57.8	-	-	-	-	-
specified site NEC	C57.7	C79.82	D07.39	D28.7	D39.8	D49.59
male NEC	C63.9	C79.82	D07.60	D29.9	D40.9	D49.59
overlapping lesion	C63.8	-	-	-	-	-
specified site NEC	C63.7	C79.82	D07.69	D29.8	D40.8	D49.59
genitourinary tract						
female	C57.9	C79.82	D07.30	D28.9	D39.9	D49.59
male	C63.9	C79.82	D07.60	D29.9	D40.9	D49.59
gingiva (alveolar) (marginal)	C03.9	C79.89	D00.03	D10.39	D37.09	D49.0
lower	C03.1	C79.89	D00.03	D10.39	D37.09	D49.0
mandibular	C03.1	C79.89	D00.03	D10.39	D37.09	D49.0
maxillary	C03.0	C79.89	D00.03	D10.39	D37.09	D49.0
upper	C03.0	C79.89	D00.03	D10.39	D37.09	D49.0
gland, glandular (lymphatic) (system)—see also Neoplasm, lymph gland						
endocrine NEC	C75.9	C79.89	D09.3	D35.9	D44.9	D49.7
salivary—see Neoplasm, salivary gland						
glans penis	C60.1	C79.82	D07.4	D29.0	D40.8	D49.59
globus pallidus	C71.0	C79.31	-	D33.0	D43.0	D49.6
glomus						
coccygeal	C49.5	C79.89	-	D21.5	D48.1	D49.2
jugularis	C75.5	C79.89	-	D35.6	D44.7	D49.7
glosso-epiglottic fold(s)	C10.1	C79.89	D00.08	D10.5	D37.05	D49.0
glossopalatine fold	C09.1	C79.89	D00.08	D10.5	D37.05	D49.0
glossopharyngeal sulcus	C09.0	C79.89	D00.08	D10.5	D37.05	D49.0
glottis	C32.0	C78.39	D02.0	D14.1	D38.0	D49.1
gluteal region	C76.3	C79.89	D04.5	D36.7	D48.7	D49.89
great vessels NEC	C49.3	C79.89	-	D21.3	D48.1	D49.2
groin NEC	C76.3	C79.89	D04.5	D36.7	D48.7	D49.89
gum	C03.9	C79.89	D00.03	D10.39	D37.09	D49.0
lower	C03.1	C79.89	D00.03	D10.39	D37.09	D49.0
upper	C03.0	C79.89	D00.03	D10.39	D37.09	D49.0
H						
hand NEC	C76.4-	C79.89	D04.6-	D36.7	D48.7	D49.89
head NEC	C76.0	C79.89	D04.4	D36.7	D48.7	D49.89
heart	C38.0	C79.89	-	D15.1	D48.7	D49.89
heel NEC	C76.5-	C79.89	D04.7-	D36.7	D48.7	D49.89
helix—see also Neoplasm, skin, ear	C44.20-	C79.2	D04.2-	D23.2-	D48.5	D49.2
hematopoietic, hemopoietic tissue NEC	C96.9	-	-	-	-	-
specified NEC	C96.Z	-	-	-	-	-
hemisphere, cerebral	C71.0	C79.31	-	D33.0	D43.0	D49.6
hemorrhoidal zone	C21.1	C78.5	D01.3	D12.9	D37.8	D49.0
hepatic—see also Index to disease, by histology	C22.9	C78.7	D01.5	D13.4	D37.6	D49.0

	Malignant Primary	Malignant Secondary	Ca in situ	Benign	Uncertain Behavior	Unspecified Behavior
hepatic — *continued*						
duct (bile)	C24.0	C78.89	D01.5	D13.5	D37.6	D49.0
flexure (colon)	C18.3	C78.5	D01.0	D12.3	D37.4	D49.0
primary	C22.8	C78.7	D01.5	D13.4	D37.6	D49.0
hepatobiliary	C24.9	C78.89	D01.5	D13.5	D37.6	D49.0
hepatoblastoma	C22.2	C78.7	D01.5	D13.4	D37.6	D49.0
hepatoma	C22.0	C78.7	D01.5	D13.4	D37.6	D49.0
hilus of lung	C34.0-	C78.0-	D02.2-	D14.3-	D38.1	D49.1
hip NEC	C76.5-	C79.89	D04.7-	D36.7	D48.7	D49.89
hippocampus, brain	C71.2	C79.31	-	D33.0	D43.0	D49.6
humerus (any part)	C40.0-	C79.51	-	D16.0-	-	-
hymen	C52	C79.82	D07.2	D28.1	D39.8	D49.59
hypopharynx, hypopharyngeal NEC	C13.9	C79.89	D00.08	D10.7	D37.05	D49.0
overlapping lesion	C13.8	-	-	-	-	-
postcricoid region	C13.0	C79.89	D00.08	D10.7	D37.05	D49.0
posterior wall	C13.2	C79.89	D00.08	D10.7	D37.05	D49.0
pyriform fossa (sinus)	C12	C79.89	D00.08	D10.7	D37.05	D49.0
hypophysis	C75.1	C79.89	D09.3	D35.2	D44.3	D49.7
hypothalamus	C71.0	C79.31	-	D33.0	D43.0	D49.6
I						
ileocecum, ileocecal (coil) (junction) (valve)	C18.0	C78.5	D01.0	D12.0	D37.4	D49.0
ileum	C17.2	C78.4	D01.49	D13.39	D37.2	D49.0
ilium	C41.4	C79.51	-	D16.8	D48.0	D49.2
immunoproliferative NEC	C88.9	-	-	-	-	-
infraclavicular (region)	C76.1	C79.89	D04.5	D36.7	D48.7	D49.89
inguinal (region)	C76.3	C79.89	D04.5	D36.7	D48.7	D49.89
insula	C71.0	C79.31	-	D33.0	D43.0	D49.6
insular tissue (pancreas)	C25.4	C78.89	D01.7	D13.7	D37.8	D49.0
brain	C71.0	C79.31	-	D33.0	D43.0	D49.6
interarytenoid fold	C13.1	C79.89	D00.08	D10.7	D37.05	D49.0
hypopharyngeal aspect	C13.1	C79.89	D00.08	D10.7	D37.05	D49.0
laryngeal aspect	C32.1	C78.39	D02.0	D14.1	D38.0	D49.1
marginal zone	C13.1	C79.89	D00.08	D10.7	D37.05	D49.0
interdental papillae	C03.9	C79.89	D00.03	D10.39	D37.09	D49.0
lower	C03.1	C79.89	D00.03	D10.39	D37.09	D49.0
upper	C03.0	C79.89	D00.03	D10.39	D37.09	D49.0
internal						
capsule	C71.0	C79.31	-	D33.0	D43.0	D49.6
os (cervix)	C53.0	C79.82	D06.0	D26.0	D39.0	D49.59
intervertebral cartilage or disc	C41.2	C79.51	-	D16.6	D48.0	D49.2
intestine, intestinal	C26.0	C78.80	D01.40	D13.9	D37.8	D49.0
large	C18.9	C78.5	D01.0	D12.6	D37.4	D49.0
appendix	C18.1	C78.5	D01.0	D12.1	D37.3	D49.0
caput coli	C18.0	C78.5	D01.0	D12.0	D37.4	D49.0
cecum	C18.0	C78.5	D01.0	D12.0	D37.4	D49.0
colon	C18.9	C78.5	D01.0	D12.6	D37.4	D49.0
and rectum	C19	C78.5	D01.1	D12.7	D37.5	D49.0
ascending	C18.2	C78.5	D01.0	D12.2	D37.4	D49.0
caput	C18.0	C78.5	D01.0	D12.0	D37.4	D49.0

	Malignant Primary	Malignant Secondary	Ca in situ	Benign	Uncertain Behavior	Unspecified Behavior
intestine, intestinal, large, colon — *continued*						
descending	C18.6	C78.5	D01.0	D12.4	D37.4	D49.0
distal	C18.6	C78.5	D01.0	D12.4	D37.4	D49.0
left	C18.6	C78.5	D01.0	D12.4	D37.4	D49.0
overlapping lesion	C18.8	-	-	-	-	-
pelvic	C18.7	C78.5	D01.0	D12.5	D37.4	D49.0
right	C18.2	C78.5	D01.0	D12.2	D37.4	D49.0
sigmoid (flexure)	C18.7	C78.5	D01.0	D12.5	D37.4	D49.0
transverse	C18.4	C78.5	D01.0	D12.3	D37.4	D49.0
hepatic flexure	C18.3	C78.5	D01.0	D12.3	D37.4	D49.0
ileocecum, ileocecal (coil) (valve)	C18.0	C78.5	D01.0	D12.0	D37.4	D49.0
overlapping lesion	C18.8	-	-	-	-	-
sigmoid flexure (lower) (upper)	C18.7	C78.5	D01.0	D12.5	D37.4	D49.0
splenic flexure	C18.5	C78.5	D01.0	D12.3	D37.4	D49.0
small	C17.9	C78.4	D01.40	D13.30	D37.2	D49.0
duodenum	C17.0	C78.4	D01.49	D13.2	D37.2	D49.0
ileum	C17.2	C78.4	D01.49	D13.39	D37.2	D49.0
jejunum	C17.1	C78.4	D01.49	D13.39	D37.2	D49.0
overlapping lesion	C17.8	-	-	-	-	-
tract NEC	C26.0	C78.89	D01.40	D13.9	D37.8	D49.0
intra-abdominal	C76.2	C79.89	D09.8	D36.7	D48.7	D49.89
intracranial NEC	C71.9	C79.31	-	D33.2	D43.2	D49.6
intrahepatic (bile) duct	C22.1	C78.7	D01.5	D13.4	D37.6	D49.0
intraocular	C69.9-	C79.49	D09.2-	D31.9-	D48.7	D49.89
intraorbital	C69.6-	C79.49	D09.2-	D31.6-	D48.7	D49.89
intrasellar	C75.1	C79.89	D09.3	D35.2	D44.3	D49.7
intrathoracic (cavity) (organs)	C76.1	C79.89	D09.8	D15.9	D48.7	D49.89
specified NEC	C76.1	C79.89	D09.8	D15.7	-	-
iris	C69.4-	C79.49	D09.2-	D31.4-	D48.7	D49.89
ischiorectal (fossa)	C76.3	C79.89	D09.8	D36.7	D48.7	D49.89
ischium	C41.4	C79.51	-	D16.8	D48.0	D49.2
island of Reil	C71.0	C79.31	-	D33.0	D43.0	D49.6
islands or islets of Langerhans	C25.4	C78.89	D01.7	D13.7	D37.8	D49.0
isthmus uteri	C54.0	C79.82	D07.0	D26.1	D39.0	D49.59
J						
jaw	C76.0	C79.89	D09.8	D36.7	D48.7	D49.89
bone	C41.1	C79.51	-	D16.5	D48.0	D49.2
lower	C41.1	C79.51	-	D16.5	-	-
upper	C41.0	C79.51	-	D16.4	-	-
carcinoma (any type) (lower) (upper)	C76.0	C79.89	-	-	-	-
skin—see also Neoplasm, skin, face	C44.309	C79.2	D04.39	D23.39	D48.5	D49.2
soft tissues	C03.9	C79.89	D00.03	D10.39	D37.09	D49.0
lower	C03.1	C79.89	D00.03	D10.39	D37.09	D49.0
upper	C03.0	C79.89	D00.03	D10.39	D37.09	D49.0
jejunum	C17.1	C78.4	D01.49	D13.39	D37.2	D49.0
joint NEC—see also Neoplasm, bone	C41.9	C79.51	-	D16.9	D48.0	D49.2

	Malignant Primary	Malignant Secondary	Ca in situ	Benign	Uncertain Behavior	Unspecified Behavior
joint NEC — *continued*						
acromioclavicular	C40.0-	C79.51	-	D16.0-	-	-
bursa or synovial membrane—see Neoplasm, connective tissue						
costovertebral	C41.3	C79.51	-	D16.7	D48.0	D49.2
sternocostal	C41.3	C79.51	-	D16.7	D48.0	D49.2
temporomandibular	C41.1	C79.51	-	D16.5	D48.0	D49.2
junction						
anorectal	C21.8	C78.5	D01.3	D12.9	D37.8	D49.0
cardioesophageal	C16.0	C78.89	D00.2	D13.1	D37.1	D49.0
esophagogastric	C16.0	C78.89	D00.2	D13.1	D37.1	D49.0
gastroesophageal	C16.0	C78.89	D00.2	D13.1	D37.1	D49.0
hard and soft palate	C05.9	C79.89	D00.00	D10.39	D37.09	D49.0
ileocecal	C18.0	C78.5	D01.0	D12.0	D37.4	D49.0
pelvirectal	C19	C78.5	D01.1	D12.7	D37.5	D49.0
pelviureteric	C65.-	C79.0-	D09.19	D30.1-	D41.1-	D49.59
rectosigmoid	C19	C78.5	D01.1	D12.7	D37.5	D49.0
squamocolumnar, of cervix	C53.8	C79.82	D06.7	D26.0	D39.0	D49.59
K						
Kaposi's sarcoma—see Kaposi's, sarcoma						
kidney (parenchymal)	C64.-	C79.0-	D09.19	D30.0-	D41.0-	D49.51-
calyx	C65.-	C79.0-	D09.19	D30.1-	D41.1-	D49.51-
hilus	C65.-	C79.0-	D09.19	D30.1-	D41.1-	D49.51-
pelvis	C65.-	C79.0-	D09.19	D30.1-	D41.1-	D49.51-
knee NEC	C76.5-	C79.89	D04.7-	D36.7	D48.7	D49.89
L						
labia (skin)	C51.9	C79.82	D07.1	D28.0	D39.8	D49.59
majora	C51.0	C79.82	D07.1	D28.0	D39.8	D49.59
minora	C51.1	C79.82	D07.1	D28.0	D39.8	D49.59
labial—see also Neoplasm, lip	C00.9	C79.89	D00.01	D10.0	D37.01	D49.0
sulcus (lower) (upper)	C06.1	C79.89	D00.02	D10.39	D37.09	D49.0
labium (skin)	C51.9	C79.82	D07.1	D28.0	D39.8	D49.59
majus	C51.0	C79.82	D07.1	D28.0	D39.8	D49.59
minus	C51.1	C79.82	D07.1	D28.0	D39.8	D49.59
lacrimal						
canaliculi	C69.5-	C79.49	D09.2-	D31.5-	D48.7	D49.89
duct (nasal)	C69.5-	C79.49	D09.2-	D31.5-	D48.7	D49.89
gland	C69.5-	C79.49	D09.2-	D31.5-	D48.7	D49.89
punctum	C69.5-	C79.49	D09.2-	D31.5-	D48.7	D49.89
sac	C69.5-	C79.49	D09.2-	D31.5-	D48.7	D49.89
Langerhans, islands or islets	C25.4	C78.89	D01.7	D13.7	D37.8	D49.0
laryngopharynx	C13.9	C79.89	D00.08	D10.7	D37.05	D49.0
larynx, laryngeal NEC	C32.9	C78.39	D02.0	D14.1	D38.0	D49.1
aryepiglottic fold	C32.1	C78.39	D02.0	D14.1	D38.0	D49.1
cartilage (arytenoid) (cricoid) (cuneiform) (thyroid)	C32.3	C78.39	D02.0	D14.1	D38.0	D49.1
commissure (anterior) (posterior)	C32.0	C78.39	D02.0	D14.1	D38.0	D49.1

	Malignant Primary	Malignant Secondary	Ca in situ	Benign	Uncertain Behavior	Unspecified Behavior
larynx, laryngeal NEC — *continued*						
extrinsic NEC	C32.1	C78.39	D02.0	D14.1	D38.0	D49.1
meaning hypopharynx	C13.9	C79.89	D00.08	D10.7	D37.05	D49.0
interarytenoid fold	C32.1	C78.39	D02.0	D14.1	D38.0	D49.1
intrinsic	C32.0	C78.39	D02.0	D14.1	D38.0	D49.1
overlapping lesion	C32.8	-	-	-	-	-
ventricular band	C32.1	C78.39	D02.0	D14.1	D38.0	D49.1
leg NEC	C76.5-	C79.89	D04.7-	D36.7	D48.7	D49.89
lens, crystalline	C69.4-	C79.49	D09.2-	D31.4-	D48.7	D49.89
lid (lower) (upper)	C44.10-	C79.2	D04.1-	D23.1-	D48.5	D49.2
basal cell carcinoma	C44.11-	-	-	-	-	-
sebaceous cell	C44.13-	-	-	-	-	-
specified type NEC	C44.19-	-	-	-	-	-
squamous cell carcinoma	C44.12-	-	-	-	-	-
ligament—see also Neoplasm, connective tissue						
broad	C57.1-	C79.82	D07.39	D28.2	D39.8	D49.59
Mackenrodt's	C57.7	C79.82	D07.39	D28.7	D39.8	D49.59
non-uterine—see Neoplasm, connective tissue						
round	C57.2-	C79.82	-	D28.2	D39.8	D49.59
sacro-uterine	C57.3	C79.82	-	D28.2	D39.8	D49.59
uterine	C57.3	C79.82	-	D28.2	D39.8	D49.59
utero-ovarian	C57.7	C79.82	D07.39	D28.2	D39.8	D49.59
uterosacral	C57.3	C79.82	-	D28.2	D39.8	D49.59
limb	C76.8	C79.89	D04.8	D36.7	D48.7	D49.89
lower	C76.5-	C79.89	D04.7-	D36.7	D48.7	D49.89
upper	C76.4-	C79.89	D04.6-	D36.7	D48.7	D49.89
limbus of cornea	C69.1-	C79.49	D09.2-	D31.1-	D48.7	D49.89
lingual NEC—see also Neoplasm, tongue	C02.9	C79.89	D00.07	D10.1	D37.02	D49.0
lingula, lung	C34.1-	C78.0-	D02.2-	D14.3-	D38.1	D49.1
lip	C00.9	C79.89	D00.01	D10.0	D37.01	D49.0
buccal aspect—see Neoplasm, lip, internal						
commissure	C00.6	C79.89	D00.01	D10.0	D37.01	D49.0
external	C00.2	C79.89	D00.01	D10.0	D37.01	D49.0
lower	C00.1	C79.89	D00.01	D10.0	D37.01	D49.0
upper	C00.0	C79.89	D00.01	D10.0	D37.01	D49.0
frenulum—see Neoplasm, lip, internal						
inner aspect—see Neoplasm, lip, internal						
internal	C00.5	C79.89	D00.01	D10.0	D37.01	D49.0
lower	C00.4	C79.89	D00.01	D10.0	D37.01	D49.0
upper	C00.3	C79.89	D00.01	D10.0	D37.01	D49.0
lipstick area	C00.2	C79.89	D00.01	D10.0	D37.01	D49.0
lower	C00.1	C79.89	D00.01	D10.0	D37.01	D49.0
upper	C00.0	C79.89	D00.01	D10.0	D37.01	D49.0
lower	C00.1	C79.89	D00.01	D10.0	D37.01	D49.0
internal	C00.4	C79.89	D00.01	D10.0	D37.01	D49.0

lip — continued	Malignant Primary	Malignant Secondary	Ca in situ	Benign	Uncertain Behavior	Unspecified Behavior
mucosa—see Neoplasm, lip, intervnal						
oral aspect—see Neoplasm, lip, internal						
overlapping lesion	C00.8	-	-	-	-	-
with oral cavity or pharynx	C14.8	-	-	-	-	-
skin (commissure) (lower) (upper)	C44.00	C79.2	D04.0	D23.0	D48.5	D49.2
basal cell carcinoma	C44.01	-	-	-	-	-
specified type NEC	C44.09	-	-	-	-	-
squamous cell carcinoma	C44.02	-	-	-	-	-
upper	C00.0	C79.89	D00.01	D10.0	D37.01	D49.0
internal	C00.3	C79.89	D00.01	D10.0	D37.01	D49.0
vermilion border	C00.2	C79.89	D00.01	D10.0	D37.01	D49.0
lower	C00.1	C79.89	D00.01	D10.0	D37.01	D49.0
upper	C00.0	C79.89	D00.01	D10.0	D37.01	D49.0
lipomatous—see Lipoma, by site						
liver—see also Index to disease, by histology	C22.9	C78.7	D01.5	D13.4	D37.6	D49.0
primary	C22.8	C78.7	D01.5	D13.4	D37.6	D49.0
lumbosacral plexus	C47.5	C79.89	-	D36.16	D48.2	D49.2
lung	C34.9-	C78.0-	D02.2-	D14.3-	D38.1	D49.1
azygos lobe	C34.1-	C78.0-	D02.2-	D14.3-	D38.1	D49.1
carina	C34.0-	C78.0-	D02.2-	D14.3-	D38.1	D49.1
hilus	C34.0-	C78.0-	D02.2-	D14.3-	D38.1	D49.1
linqula	C34.1-	C78.0-	D02.2-	D14.3-	D38.1	D49.1
lobe NEC	C34.9-	C78.0-	D02.2-	D14.3-	D38.1	D49.1
lower lobe	C34.3-	C78.0-	D02.2-	D14.3-	D38.1	D49.1
main bronchus	C34.0-	C78.0-	D02.2-	D14.3-	D38.1	D49.1
mesothelioma—see Mesothelioma						
middle lobe	C34.2	C78.0-	D02.21	D14.31	D38.1	D49.1
overlapping lesion	C34.8-	-	-	-	-	-
upper lobe	C34.1-	C78.0-	D02.2-	D14.3-	D38.1	D49.1
lymph, lymphatic channel NEC	C49.9	C79.89	-	D21.9	D48.1	D49.2
gland (secondary)	-	C77.9	-	D36.0	D48.7	D49.89
abdominal	-	C77.2	-	D36.0	D48.7	D49.89
aortic	-	C77.2	-	D36.0	D48.7	D49.89
arm	-	C77.3	-	D36.0	D48.7	D49.89
auricular (anterior) (posterior)	-	C77.0	-	D36.0	D48.7	D49.89
axilla, axillary	-	C77.3	-	D36.0	D48.7	D49.89
brachial	-	C77.3	-	D36.0	D48.7	D49.89
bronchial	-	C77.1	-	D36.0	D48.7	D49.89
bronchopulmonary	-	C77.1	-	D36.0	D48.7	D49.89
celiac	-	C77.2	-	D36.0	D48.7	D49.89
cervical	-	C77.0	-	D36.0	D48.7	D49.89
cervicofacial	-	C77.0	-	D36.0	D48.7	D49.89
Cloquet	-	C77.4	-	D36.0	D48.7	D49.89
colic	-	C77.2	-	D36.0	D48.7	D49.89
common duct	-	C77.2	-	D36.0	D48.7	D49.89

lymph, lymphatic channel NEC, gland — continued	Malignant Primary	Malignant Secondary	Ca in situ	Benign	Uncertain Behavior	Unspecified Behavior
cubital	-	C77.3	-	D36.0	D48.7	D49.89
diaphragmatic	-	C77.1	-	D36.0	D48.7	D49.89
epigastric, inferior	-	C77.1	-	D36.0	D48.7	D49.89
epitrochlear	-	C77.3	-	D36.0	D48.7	D49.89
esophageal	-	C77.1	-	D36.0	D48.7	D49.89
face	-	C77.0	-	D36.0	D48.7	D49.89
femoral	-	C77.4	-	D36.0	D48.7	D49.89
gastric	-	C77.2	-	D36.0	D48.7	D49.89
groin	-	C77.4	-	D36.0	D48.7	D49.89
head	-	C77.0	-	D36.0	D48.7	D49.89
hepatic	-	C77.2	-	D36.0	D48.7	D49.89
hilar (pulmonary)	-	C77.1	-	D36.0	D48.7	D49.89
splenic	-	C77.2	-	D36.0	D48.7	D49.89
hypogastric	-	C77.5	-	D36.0	D48.7	D49.89
ileocolic	-	C77.2	-	D36.0	D48.7	D49.89
iliac	-	C77.5	-	D36.0	D48.7	D49.89
infraclavicular	-	C77.3	-	D36.0	D48.7	D49.89
inguina, inguinal	-	C77.4	-	D36.0	D48.7	D49.89
innominate	-	C77.1	-	D36.0	D48.7	D49.89
intercostal	-	C77.1	-	D36.0	D48.7	D49.89
intestinal	-	C77.2	-	D36.0	D48.7	D49.89
intrabdominal	-	C77.2	-	D36.0	D48.7	D49.89
intrapelvic	-	C77.5	-	D36.0	D48.7	D49.89
intrathoracic	-	C77.1	-	D36.0	D48.7	D49.89
jugular	-	C77.0	-	D36.0	D48.7	D49.89
leg	-	C77.4	-	D36.0	D48.7	D49.89
limb						
lower	-	C77.4	-	D36.0	D48.7	D49.89
upper	-	C77.3	-	D36.0	D48.7	D49.89
lower limb	-	C77.4	-	D36.0	D48.7	D49.89
lumbar	-	C77.2	-	D36.0	D48.7	D49.89
mandibular	-	C77.0	-	D36.0	D48.7	D49.89
mediastinal	-	C77.1	-	D36.0	D48.7	D49.89
mesenteric (inferior) (superior)	-	C77.2	-	D36.0	D48.7	D49.89
midcolic	-	C77.2	-	D36.0	D48.7	D49.89
multiple sites in categories C77.0 - C77.5	-	C77.8	-	D36.0	D48.7	D49.89
neck	-	C77.0	-	D36.0	D48.7	D49.89
obturator	-	C77.5	-	D36.0	D48.7	D49.89
occipital	-	C77.0	-	D36.0	D48.7	D49.89
pancreatic	-	C77.2	-	D36.0	D48.7	D49.89
para-aortic	-	C77.2	-	D36.0	D48.7	D49.89
paracervical	-	C77.5	-	D36.0	D48.7	D49.89
parametrial	-	C77.5	-	D36.0	D48.7	D49.89
parasternal	-	C77.1	-	D36.0	D48.7	D49.89
parotid	-	C77.0	-	D36.0	D48.7	D49.89
pectoral	-	C77.3	-	D36.0	D48.7	D49.89
pelvic	-	C77.5	-	D36.0	D48.7	D49.89
peri-aortic	-	C77.2	-	D36.0	D48.7	D49.89
peripancreatic	-	C77.2	-	D36.0	D48.7	D49.89

	Malignant Primary	Malignant Secondary	Ca in situ	Benign	Uncertain Behavior	Unspecified Behavior
lymph, lymphatic channel NEC, gland — *continued*						
popliteal	-	C77.4	-	D36.0	D48.7	D49.89
porta hepatis	-	C77.2	-	D36.0	D48.7	D49.89
portal	-	C77.2	-	D36.0	D48.7	D49.89
preauricular	-	C77.0	-	D36.0	D48.7	D49.89
prelaryngeal	-	C77.0	-	D36.0	D48.7	D49.89
presymphysial	-	C77.5	-	D36.0	D48.7	D49.89
pretracheal	-	C77.0	-	D36.0	D48.7	D49.89
primary (any site) NEC	C96.9	-	-	-	-	-
pulmonary (hiler)	-	C77.1	-	D36.0	D48.7	D49.89
pyloric	-	C77.2	-	D36.0	D48.7	D49.89
retroperitoneal	-	C77.2	-	D36.0	D48.7	D49.89
retropharyngeal	-	C77.0	-	D36.0	D48.7	D49.89
Rosenmuller's	-	C77.4	-	D36.0	D48.7	D49.89
sacral	-	C77.5	-	D36.0	D48.7	D49.89
scalene	-	C77.0	-	D36.0	D48.7	D49.89
site NEC	-	C77.9	-	D36.0	D48.7	D49.89
splenic (hilar)	-	C77.2	-	D36.0	D48.7	D49.89
subclavicular	-	C77.3	-	D36.0	D48.7	D49.89
subinguinal	-	C77.4	-	D36.0	D48.7	D49.89
sublingual	-	C77.0	-	D36.0	D48.7	D49.89
submandibular	-	C77.0	-	D36.0	D48.7	D49.89
submaxillary	-	C77.0	-	D36.0	D48.7	D49.89
submental	-	C77.0	-	D36.0	D48.7	D49.89
subscapular	-	C77.3	-	D36.0	D48.7	D49.89
supraclavicular	-	C77.0	-	D36.0	D48.7	D49.89
thoracic	-	C77.1	-	D36.0	D48.7	D49.89
tibial	-	C77.4	-	D36.0	D48.7	D49.89
tracheal	-	C77.1	-	D36.0	D48.7	D49.89
tracheobronchial	-	C77.1	-	D36.0	D48.7	D49.89
upper limb	-	C77.3	-	D36.0	D48.7	D49.89
Virchow's	-	C77.0	-	D36.0	D48.7	D49.89
node—see also Neoplasm, lymph gland						
primary NEC	C96.9	-	-	-	-	-
vessel—see also Neoplasm, connective tissue	C49.9	C79.89	-	D21.9	D48.1	D49.2
M						
Mackenrodt's ligament	C57.7	C79.82	D07.39	D28.7	D39.8	D49.59
malar	C41.0	C79.51	-	D16.4	D48.0	D49.2
region—see Neoplasm, cheek						
mammary gland—see Neoplasm, breast						
mandible	C41.1	C79.51	-	D16.5	D48.0	D49.2
alveolar						
mucosa (carcinoma)	C03.1	C79.89	D00.03	D10.39	D37.09	D49.0
ridge or process	C41.1	C79.51	-	D16.5	D48.0	D49.2
marrow (bone) NEC	C96.9	C79.52	-	-	D47.9	D49.89
mastectomy site (skin)—see also Neoplasm, breast, skin	C44.501	C79.2	-	-	-	-
specified as breast tissue	C50.8-	C79.81	-	-	-	-

	Malignant Primary	Malignant Secondary	Ca in situ	Benign	Uncertain Behavior	Unspecified Behavior
mastoid (air cells) (antrum) (cavity)	C30.1	C78.39	D02.3	D14.0	D38.5	D49.1
bone or process	C41.0	C79.51	-	D16.4	D48.0	D49.2
maxilla, maxillary (superior)	C41.0	C79.51	-	D16.4	D48.0	D49.2
alveolar						
mucosa	C03.0	C79.89	D00.03	D10.39	D37.09	D49.0
ridge or process (carcinoma)	C41.0	C79.51	-	D16.4	D48.0	D49.2
antrum	C31.0	C78.39	D02.3	D14.0	D38.5	D49.1
carcinoma	C03.0	C79.51	-	-	-	-
inferior—see Neoplasm, mandible						
sinus	C31.0	C78.39	D02.3	D14.0	D38.5	D49.1
meatus external (ear)—see also Neoplasm, skin, ear	C44.20-	C79.2	D04.2-	D23.2-	D48.5	D49.2
Meckel diverticulum, malignant	C17.3	C78.4	D01.49	D13.39	D37.2	D49.0
mediastinum, mediastinal	C38.3	C78.1	-	D15.2	D38.3	D49.89
anterior	C38.1	C78.1	-	D15.2	D38.3	D49.89
posterior	C38.2	C78.1	-	D15.2	D38.3	D49.89
medulla						
adrenal	C74.1-	C79.7-	D09.3	D35.0-	D44.1-	D49.7
oblongata	C71.7	C79.31	-	D33.1	D43.1	D49.6
meibomian gland	C44.10-	C79.2	D04.1-	D23.1-	D48.5	D49.2
basal cell carcinoma	C44.11-	-	-	-	-	-
sebaceous cell	C44.13-	-	-	-	-	-
specified type NEC	C44.19-	-	-	-	-	-
squamous cell carcinoma	C44.12-	-	-	-	-	-
melanoma—see Melanoma						
meninges	C70.9	C79.49	-	D32.9	D42.9	D49.7
brain	C70.0	C79.32	-	D32.0	D42.0	D49.7
cerebral	C70.0	C79.32	-	D32.0	D42.0	D49.7
crainial	C70.0	C79.32	-	D32.0	D42.0	D49.7
intracranial	C70.0	C79.32	-	D32.0	D42.0	D49.7
spinal (cord)	C70.1	C79.49	-	D32.1	D42.1	D49.7
meniscus, knee joint (lateral) (medial)	C40.2-	C79.51	-	D16.2-	D48.0	D49.2
Merkel cell—see Carcinoma, Merkel cell						
mesentery, mesenteric	C48.1	C78.6	-	D20.1	D48.4	D49.0
mesoappendix	C48.1	C78.6	-	D20.1	D48.4	D49.0
mesocolon	C48.1	C78.6	-	D20.1	D48.4	D49.0
mesopharynx—see Neoplasm, oropharynx						
mesosalpinx	C57.1-	C79.82	D07.39	D28.2	D39.8	D49.59
mesothelial tissue—see Mesothelioma						
mesothelioma—see Mesothelioma						
mesovarium	C57.1-	C79.82	D07.39	D28.2	D39.8	D49.59
metacarpus (any bone)	C40.1-	C79.51	-	D16.1-	-	-
metastatic NEC—see also Neoplasm, by site, secondary	-	C79.9	-	-	-	-
metatarsus (any bone)	C40.3-	C79.51	-	D16.3-	-	-
midbrain	C71.7	C79.31	-	D33.1	D43.1	D49.6

	Malignant Primary	Malignant Secondary	Ca in situ	Benign	Uncertain Behavior	Unspecified Behavior
milk duct—see Neoplasm, breast						
mons						
pubis	C51.9	C79.82	D07.1	D28.0	D39.8	D49.59
veneris	C51.9	C79.82	D07.1	D28.0	D39.8	D49.59
motor tract	C72.9	C79.49	-	D33.9	D43.9	D49.7
brain	C71.9	C79.31	-	D33.2	D43.2	D49.6
cauda equina	C72.1	C79.49	-	D33.4	D43.4	D49.7
spinal	C72.0	C79.49	-	D33.4	D43.4	D49.7
mouth	C06.9	C79.89	D00.00	D10.30	D37.09	D49.0
book-leaf	C06.89	C79.89	-	-	-	-
floor	C04.9	C79.89	D00.06	D10.2	D37.09	D49.0
anterior portion	C04.0	C79.89	D00.06	D10.2	D37.09	D49.0
lateral portion	C04.1	C79.89	D00.06	D10.2	D37.09	D49.0
overlapping lesion	C04.8	-	-	-	-	-
overlapping NEC	C06.80	-	-	-	-	-
roof	C05.9	C79.89	D00.00	D10.39	D37.09	D49.0
specified part NEC	C06.89	C79.89	D00.00	D10.39	D37.09	D49.0
vestibule	C06.1	C79.89	D00.00	D10.39	D37.09	D49.0
mucosa						
alveolar (ridge or process)	C03.9	C79.89	D00.03	D10.39	D37.09	D49.0
lower	C03.1	C79.89	D00.03	D10.39	D37.09	D49.0
upper	C03.0	C79.89	D00.03	D10.39	D37.09	D49.0
buccal	C06.0	C79.89	D00.02	D10.39	D37.09	D49.0
cheek	C06.0	C79.89	D00.02	D10.39	D37.09	D49.0
lip—see Neoplasm, lip, internal						
nasal	C30.0	C78.39	D02.3	D14.0	D38.5	D49.1
oral	C06.0	C79.89	D00.02	D10.39	D37.09	D49.0
Mullerian duct						
female	C57.7	C79.82	D07.39	D28.7	D39.8	D49.59
male	C63.7	C79.82	D07.69	D29.8	D40.8	D49.59
muscle—see also Neoplasm, connective tissue						
extraocular	C69.6-	C79.49	D09.2-	D31.6-	D48.7	D49.89
myocardium	C38.0	C79.89	-	D15.1	D48.7	D49.89
myometrium	C54.2	C79.82	D07.0	D26.1	D39.0	D49.59
myopericardium	C38.0	C79.89	-	D15.1	D48.7	D49.89
N						
nabothian gland (follicle)	C53.0	C79.82	D06.0	D26.0	D39.0	D49.59
nail—see also Neoplasm, skin, limb	C44.90	C79.2	D04.9	D23.9	D48.5	D49.2
finger—see also Neoplasm, skin, limb, upper	C44.60-	C79.2	D04.6-	D23.6-	D48.5	D49.2
toe—see also Neoplasm, skin, limb, lower	C44.70-	C79.2	D04.7-	D23.7-	D48.5	D49.2
nares, naris (anterior) (posterior)	C30.0	C78.39	D02.3	D14.0	D38.5	D49.1
nasal—see Neoplasm, nose						
nasolabial groove—see also Neoplasm, skin, face	C44.309	C79.2	D04.39	D23.39	D48.5	D49.2
nasolacrimal duct	C69.5-	C79.49	D09.2-	D31.5-	D48.7	D49.89

	Malignant Primary	Malignant Secondary	Ca in situ	Benign	Uncertain Behavior	Unspecified Behavior
nasopharynx, nasopharyngeal	C11.9	C79.89	D00.08	D10.6	D37.05	D49.0
floor	C11.3	C79.89	D00.08	D10.6	D37.05	D49.0
overlapping lesion	C11.8	-	-	-	-	-
roof	C11.0	C79.89	D00.08	D10.6	D37.05	D49.0
wall	C11.9	C79.89	D00.08	D10.6	D37.05	D49.0
anterior	C11.3	C79.89	D00.08	D10.6	D37.05	D49.0
lateral	C11.2	C79.89	D00.08	D10.6	D37.05	D49.0
posterior	C11.1	C79.89	D00.08	D10.6	D37.05	D49.0
superior	C11.0	C79.89	D00.08	D10.6	D37.05	D49.0
nates—see also Neoplasm, skin, trunk	C44.509	C79.2	D04.5	D23.5	D48.5	D49.2
neck NEC	C76.0	C79.89	D09.8	D36.7	D48.7	D49.89
skin	C44.40	-	-	-	-	-
basal cell carcinoma	C44.41	-	-	-	-	-
specified type NEC	C44.49	-	-	-	-	-
squamous cell carcinoma	C44.42	-	-	-	-	-
nerve (ganglion)	C47.9	C79.89	-	D36.10	D48.2	D49.2
abducens	C72.59	C79.49	-	D33.3	D43.3	D49.7
accessory (spinal)	C72.59	C79.49	-	D33.3	D43.3	D49.7
acoustic	C72.4-	C79.49	-	D33.3	D43.3	D49.7
auditory	C72.4-	C79.49	-	D33.3	D43.3	D49.7
autonomic NEC—see also Neoplasm, nerve, peripheral	C47.9	C79.89	-	D36.10	D48.2	D49.2
brachial	C47.1-	C79.89	-	D36.12	D48.2	D49.2
cranial	C72.50	C79.49	-	D33.3	D43.3	D49.7
specified NEC	C72.59	C79.49	-	D33.3	D43.3	D49.7
facial	C72.59	C79.49	-	D33.3	D43.3	D49.7
femoral	C47.2-	C79.89	-	D36.13	D48.2	D49.2
ganglion NEC—see also Neoplasm, nerve, peripheral	C47.9	C79.89	-	D36.10	D48.2	D49.2
glossopharyngeal	C72.59	C79.49	-	D33.3	D43.3	D49.7
hypoglossal	C72.59	C79.49	-	D33.3	D43.3	D49.7
intercostal	C47.3	C79.89	-	D36.14	D48.2	D49.2
lumbar	C47.6	C79.89	-	D36.17	D48.2	D49.2
median	C47.1-	C79.89	-	D36.12	D48.2	D49.2
obturator	C47.2-	C79.89	-	D36.13	D48.2	D49.2
oculomotor	C72.59	C79.49	-	D33.3	D43.3	D49.7
olfactory	C47.2-	C79.49	-	D33.3	D43.3	D49.7
optic	C72.3-	C79.49	-	D33.3	D43.3	D49.7
parasympathetic NEC	C47.9	C79.89	-	D36.10	D48.2	D49.2
peripheral NEC	C47.9	C79.89	-	D36.10	D48.2	D49.2
abdomen	C47.4	C79.89	-	D36.15	D48.2	D49.2
abdominal wall	C47.4	C79.89	-	D36.15	D48.2	D49.2
ankle	C47.2-	C79.89	-	D36.13	D48.2	D49.2
antecubital fossa or space	C47.1-	C79.89	-	D36.12	D48.2	D49.2
arm	C47.1-	C79.89	-	D36.12	D48.2	D49.2
auricle (ear)	C47.0	C79.89	-	D36.11	D48.2	D49.2
axilla	C47.3	C79.89	-	D36.12	D48.2	D49.2
back	C47.6	C79.89	-	D36.17	D48.2	D49.2
buttock	C47.5	C79.89	-	D36.16	D48.2	D49.2

	Malignant Primary	Malignant Secondary	Ca in situ	Benign	Uncertain Behavior	Unspecified Behavior
nerve (ganglion), peripheral NEC — *continued*						
calf	C47.2-	C79.89	-	D36.13	D48.2	D49.2
cervical region	C47.0	C79.89	-	D36.11	D48.2	D49.2
cheek	C47.0	C79.89	-	D36.11	D48.2	D49.2
chest (wall)	C47.3	C79.89	-	D36.14	D48.2	D49.2
chin	C47.0	C79.89	-	D36.11	D48.2	D49.2
ear (external)	C47.0	C79.89	-	D36.11	D48.2	D49.2
elbow	C47.1-	C79.89	-	D36.12	D48.2	D49.2
extrarectal	C47.5	C79.89	-	D36.16	D48.2	D49.2
extremity	C47.9	C79.89	-	D36.10	D48.2	D49.2
lower	C47.2-	C79.89	-	D36.13	D48.2	D49.2
upper	C47.1-	C79.89	-	D36.12	D48.2	D49.2
eyelid	C47.0	C79.89	-	D36.11	D48.2	D49.2
face	C47.0	C79.89	-	D36.11	D48.2	D49.2
finger	C47.1-	C79.89	-	D36.12	D48.2	D49.2
flank	C47.6	C79.89	-	D36.17	D48.2	D49.2
foot	C47.2-	C79.89	-	D36.13	D48.2	D49.2
forearm	C47.1-	C79.89	-	D36.12	D48.2	D49.2
forehead	C47.0	C79.89	-	D36.11	D48.2	D49.2
gluteal region	C47.5	C79.89	-	D36.16	D48.2	D49.2
groin	C47.5	C79.89	-	D36.16	D48.2	D49.2
hand	C47.1-	C79.89	-	D36.12	D48.2	D49.2
head	C47.0	C79.89	-	D36.11	D48.2	D49.2
heel	C47.2-	C79.89	-	D36.13	D48.2	D49.2
hip	C47.2-	C79.89	-	D36.13	D48.2	D49.2
infraclavicular region	C47.3	C79.89	-	D36.14	D48.2	D49.2
inguinal (canal) (region)	C47.5	C79.89	-	D36.16	D48.2	D49.2
intrathoracic	C47.3	C79.89	-	D36.14	D48.2	D49.2
ischiorectal fossa	C47.5	C79.89	-	D36.16	D48.2	D49.2
knee	C47.2-	C79.89	-	D36.13	D48.2	D49.2
leg	C47.2-	C79.89	-	D36.13	D48.2	D49.2
limb NEC	C47.9	C79.89	-	D36.10	D48.2	D49.2
lower	C47.2-	C79.89	-	D36.13	D48.2	D49.2
upper	C47.1-	C79.89	-	D36.12	D48.2	D49.2
nates	C47.5	C79.89	-	D36.16	D48.2	D49.2
neck	C47.0	C79.89	-	D36.11	D48.2	D49.2
orbit	C69.6-	C79.49	-	D31.6-	D48.7	D49.2
pararectal	C47.5	C79.89	-	D36.16	D48.2	D49.2
paraurethral	C47.5	C79.89	-	D36.16	D48.2	D49.2
paravaginal	C47.5	C79.89	-	D36.16	D48.2	D49.2
pelvis (floor)	C47.5	C79.89	-	D36.16	D48.2	D49.2
pelvoabdominal	C47.8	C79.89	-	D36.17	D48.2	D49.2
perineum	C47.5	C79.89	-	D36.16	D48.2	D49.2
perirectal (tissue)	C47.5	C79.89	-	D36.16	D48.2	D49.2
periurethral (tissue)	C47.5	C79.89	-	D36.16	D48.2	D49.2
popliteal fossa or space	C47.2-	C79.89	-	D36.13	D48.2	D49.2
presacral	C47.5	C79.89	-	D36.16	D48.2	D49.2
pterygoid fossa	C47.0	C79.89	-	D36.11	D48.2	D49.2
rectovaginal septum or wall	C47.5	C79.89	-	D36.16	D48.2	D49.2
rectovesical	C47.5	C79.89	-	D36.16	D48.2	D49.2
sacrococcygeal region	C47.5	C79.89	-	D36.16	D48.2	D49.2

	Malignant Primary	Malignant Secondary	Ca in situ	Benign	Uncertain Behavior	Unspecified Behavior
nerve (ganglion), peripheral NEC — *continued*						
scalp	C47.0	C79.89	-	D36.11	D48.2	D49.2
scapular region	C47.3	C79.89	-	D36.14	D48.2	D49.2
shoulder	C47.1-	C79.89	-	D36.12	D48.2	D49.2
submental	C47.0	C79.89	-	D36.11	D48.2	D49.2
supraclavicular region	C47.0	C79.89	-	D36.11	D48.2	D49.2
temple	C47.0	C79.89	-	D36.11	D48.2	D49.2
temporal region	C47.0	C79.89	-	D36.11	D48.2	D49.2
thigh	C47.2-	C79.89	-	D36.13	D48.2	D49.2
thoracic (duct) (wall)	C47.3	C79.89	-	D36.14	D48.2	D49.2
thorax	C47.3	C79.89	-	D36.14	D48.2	D49.2
thumb	C47.1-	C79.89	-	D36.12	D48.2	D49.2
toe	C47.2-	C79.89	-	D36.13	D48.2	D49.2
trunk	C47.6	C79.89	-	D36.17	D48.2	D49.2
umbilicus	C47.4	C79.89	-	D36.15	D48.2	D49.2
vesicorectal	C47.5	C79.89	-	D36.16	D48.2	D49.2
wrist	C47.1-	C79.89	-	D36.12	D48.2	D49.2
radial	C47.1-	C79.89	-	D36.12	D48.2	D49.2
sacral	C47.5	C79.89	-	D36.16	D48.2	D49.2
sciatic	C47.2-	C79.89	-	D36.13	D48.2	D49.2
spinal NEC	C47.9	C79.89	-	D36.10	D48.2	D49.2
accessory	C72.59	C79.49	-	D33.3	D43.3	D49.7
sympathetic NEC—see also Neoplasm, nerve, peripheral	C47.9	C79.89	-	D36.10	D48.2	D49.2
trigeminal	C72.59	C79.49	-	D33.3	D43.3	D49.7
trochlear	C72.59	C79.49	-	D33.3	D43.3	D49.7
ulnar	C47.1-	C79.89	-	D36.12	D48.2	D49.2
vagus	C72.59	C79.49	-	D33.3	D43.3	D49.7
nervous system (central)	C72.9	C79.40	-	D33.9	D43.9	D49.7
autonomic—see Neoplasm, nerve, peripheral						
parasympathetic—see Neoplasm, nerve, peripheral						
specified site NEC	-	C79.49	-	D33.7	D43.8	-
sympathetic—see Neoplasm, nerve, peripheral						
nevus—see Nevus						
nipple	C50.0-	C79.81	D05.-	D24.-	-	-
nose, nasal	C76.0	C79.89	D09.8	D36.7	D48.7	D49.89
ala (external) (nasi)—see also Neoplasm, nose, skin	C44.301	C79.2	D04.39	D23.39	D48.5	D49.2
bone	C41.0	C79.51	-	D16.4	D48.0	D49.2
cartilage	C30.0	C78.39	D02.3	D14.0	D38.5	D49.1
cavity	C30.0	C78.39	D02.3	D14.0	D38.5	D49.1
choana	C11.3	C79.89	D00.08	D10.6	D37.05	D49.0
external (skin)—see also Neoplasm, nose, skin	C44.301	C79.2	D04.39	D23.39	D48.5	D49.2
fossa	C30.0	C78.39	D02.3	D14.0	D38.5	D49.1
internal	C30.0	C78.39	D02.3	D14.0	D38.5	D49.1
mucosa	C30.0	C78.39	D02.3	D14.0	D38.5	D49.1
septum	C30.0	C78.39	D02.3	D14.0	D38.5	D49.1

	Malignant Primary	Malignant Secondary	Ca in situ	Benign	Uncertain Behavior	Unspecified Behavior
nose, nasal, septum — *continued*						
posterior margin	C11.3	C79.89	D00.08	D10.6	D37.05	D49.0
sinus—see Neoplasm, sinus						
skin	C44.301	C79.2	D04.39	D23.39	D48.5	D49.2
basal cell carcinoma	C44.311	-	-	-	-	-
specified type NEC	C44.391	-	-	-	-	-
squamous cell carcinoma	C44.321	-	-	-	-	-
turbinate (mucosa)	C30.0	C78.39	D02.3	D14.0	D38.5	D49.1
bone	C41.0	C79.51	-	D16.4	D48.0	D49.2
vestibule	C30.0	C78.39	D02.3	D14.0	D38.5	D49.1
nostril	C30.0	C78.39	D02.3	D14.0	D38.5	D49.1
nucleus pulposus	C41.2	C79.51	-	D16.6	D48.0	D49.2
O						
occipital						
bone	C41.0	C79.51	-	D16.4	D48.0	D49.2
lobe or pole, brain	C71.4	C79.31	-	D33.0	D43.0	D49.6
odontogenic—see Neoplasm, jaw bone						
olfactory nerve or bulb	C72.2-	C79.49	-	D33.3	D43.3	D49.7
olive (brain)	C71.7	C79.31	-	D33.1	D43.1	D49.6
omentum	C48.1	C78.6	-	D20.1	D48.4	D49.0
operculum (brain)	C71.0	C79.31	-	D33.0	D43.0	D49.6
optic nerve, chiasm, or tract	C72.3-	C79.49	-	D33.3	D43.3	D49.7
oral (cavity)	C06.9	C79.89	D00.00	D10.30	D37.09	D49.0
ill-defined	C14.8	C79.89	D00.00	D10.30	D37.09	D49.0
mucosa	C06.0	C79.89	D00.02	D10.39	D37.09	D49.0
orbit	C69.6-	C79.49	D09.2-	D31.6-	D48.7	D49.89
autonomic nerve	C69.6-	C79.49	-	D31.6-	D48.7	D49.2
bone	C41.0	C79.51	-	D16.4	D48.0	D49.2
eye	C69.6-	C79.49	D09.2-	D31.6-	D48.7	D49.89
peripheral nerves	C69.6-	C79.49	-	D31.6-	D48.7	D49.2
soft parts	C69.6-	C79.49	D09.2-	D31.6-	D48.7	D49.89
organ of Zuckerkandl	C75.5	C79.89	-	D35.6	D44.7	D49.7
oropharynx	C10.9	C79.89	D00.08	D10.5	D37.05	D49.0
branchial cleft (vestige)	C10.4	C79.89	D00.08	D10.5	D37.05	D49.0
junctional region	C10.8	C79.89	D00.08	D10.5	D37.05	D49.0
lateral wall	C10.2	C79.89	D00.08	D10.5	D37.05	D49.0
overlapping lesion	C10.8	-	-	-	-	-
pillars or fauces	C09.1	C79.89	D00.08	D10.5	D37.05	D49.0
posterior wall	C10.3	C79.89	D00.08	D10.5	D37.05	D49.0
vallecula	C10.0	C79.89	D00.08	D10.5	D37.05	D49.0
os						
external	C53.1	C79.82	D06.1	D26.0	D39.0	D49.59
internal	C53.0	C79.82	D06.0	D26.0	D39.0	D49.59
ovary	C56.-	C79.6-	D07.39	D27.-	D39.1-	D49.59
oviduct	C57.0-	C79.82	D07.39	D28.2	D39.8	D49.59
P						
palate	C05.9	C79.89	D00.00	D10.39	D37.09	D49.0
hard	C05.0	C79.89	D00.05	D10.39	D37.09	D49.0
junction of hard and soft palate	C05.9	C79.89	D00.00	D10.39	D37.09	D49.0

	Malignant Primary	Malignant Secondary	Ca in situ	Benign	Uncertain Behavior	Unspecified Behavior
palate — *continued*						
overlapping lesions	C05.8	-	-	-	-	-
soft	C05.1	C79.89	D00.04	D10.39	D37.09	D49.0
nasopharyngeal surface	C11.3	C79.89	D00.08	D10.6	D37.05	D49.0
posterior surface	C11.3	C79.89	D00.08	D10.6	D37.05	D49.0
superior surface	C11.3	C79.89	D00.08	D10.6	D37.05	D49.0
palatoglossal arch	C09.1	C79.89	D00.00	D10.5	D37.09	D49.0
palatopharyngeal arch	C09.1	C79.89	D00.00	D10.5	D37.09	D49.0
pallium	C71.0	C79.31	-	D33.0	D43.0	D49.6
palpebra	C44.10-	C79.2	D04.1-	D23.1-	D48.5	D49.2
basal cell carcinoma	C44.11-	-	-	-	-	-
sebaceous cell	C44.13-	-	-	-	-	-
specified type NEC	C44.19-	-	-	-	-	-
squamous cell carcinoma	C44.12-	-	-	-	-	-
pancreas	C25.9	C78.89	D01.7	D13.6	D37.8	D49.0
body	C25.1	C78.89	D01.7	D13.6	D37.8	D49.0
duct (of Santorini) (of Wirsung)	C25.3	C78.89	D01.7	D13.6	D37.8	D49.0
ectopic tissue	C25.7	C78.89	-	D13.6	D37.8	D49.0
head	C25.0	C78.89	D01.7	D13.6	D37.8	D49.0
islet cells	C25.4	C78.89	D01.7	D13.7	D37.8	D49.0
neck	C25.7	C78.89	D01.7	D13.6	D37.8	D49.0
overlapping lesion	C25.8	-	-	-	-	-
tail	C25.2	C78.89	D01.7	D13.6	D37.8	D49.0
para-aortic body	C75.5	C79.89	-	D35.6	D44.7	D49.7
paraganglion NEC	C75.5	C79.89	-	D35.6	D44.7	D49.7
parametrium	C57.3	C79.82	-	D28.2	D39.8	D49.59
paranephric	C48.0	C78.6	-	D20.0	D48.3	D49.0
pararectal	C76.3	C79.89	-	D36.7	D48.7	D49.89
parasagittal (region)	C76.0	C79.89	D09.8	D36.7	D48.7	D49.89
parasellar	C72.9	C79.49	-	D33.9	D43.8	D49.7
parathyroid (gland)	C75.0	C79.89	D09.3	D35.1	D44.2	D49.7
paraurethral	C76.3	C79.89	-	D36.7	D48.7	D49.89
gland	C68.1	C79.19	D09.19	D30.8	D41.8	D49.59
paravaginal	C76.3	C79.89	-	D36.7	D48.7	D49.89
parenchyma, kidney	C64.-	C79.0-	D09.19	D30.0-	D41.0-	D49.51-
parietal						
bone	C41.0	C79.51	-	D16.4	D48.0	D49.2
lobe, brain	C71.3	C79.31	-	D33.0	D43.0	D49.6
paroophoron	C57.1-	C79.82	D07.39	D28.2	D39.8	D49.59
parotid (duct) (gland)	C07	C79.89	D00.00	D11.0	D37.030	D49.0
parovarium	C57.1-	C79.82	D07.39	D28.2	D39.8	D49.59
patella	C40.20	C79.51	-	-	-	-
peduncle, cerebral	C71.7	C79.31	-	D33.1	D43.1	D49.6
pelvirectal junction	C19	C78.5	D01.1	D12.7	D37.5	D49.0
pelvis, pelvic	C76.3	C79.89	D09.8	D36.7	D48.7	D49.89
bone	C41.4	C79.51	-	D16.8	D48.0	D49.2
floor	C76.3	C79.89	D09.8	D36.7	D48.7	D49.89
renal	C65.-	C79.0-	D09.19	D30.1-	D41.1-	D49.51-
viscera	C76.3	C79.89	D09.8	D36.7	D48.7	D49.89
wall	C76.3	C79.89	D09.8	D36.7	D48.7	D49.89
pelvo-abdominal	C76.8	C79.89	D09.8	D36.7	D48.7	D49.89

	Malignant Primary	Malignant Secondary	Ca in situ	Benign	Uncertain Behavior	Unspecified Behavior
penis	C60.9	C79.82	D07.4	D29.0	D40.8	D49.59
body	C60.2	C79.82	D07.4	D29.0	D40.8	D49.59
corpus (cavernosum)	C60.2	C79.82	D07.4	D29.0	D40.8	D49.59
glans	C60.1	C79.82	D07.4	D29.0	D40.8	D49.59
overlapping sites	C60.8	-	-	-	-	-
skin NEC	C60.9	C79.82	D07.4	D29.0	D40.8	D49.59
periadrenal (tissue)	C48.0	C78.6	-	D20.0	D48.3	D49.0
perianal (skin)—see also Neoplasm, anus, skin	C44.500	C79.2	D04.5	D23.5	D48.5	D49.2
pericardium	C38.0	C79.89		D15.1	D48.7	D49.89
perinephric	C48.0	C78.6	-	D20.0	D48.3	D49.0
perineum	C76.3	C79.89	D09.8	D36.7	D48.7	D49.89
periodontal tissue NEC	C03.9	C79.89	D00.03	D10.39	D37.09	D49.0
periosteum—see Neoplasm, bone						
peripancreatic	C48.0	C78.6	-	D20.0	D48.3	D49.0
peripheral nerve NEC	C47.9	C79.89		D36.10	D48.2	D49.2
perirectal (tissue)	C76.3	C79.89		D36.7	D48.7	D49.89
perirenal (tissue)	C48.0	C78.6	-	D20.0	D48.3	D49.0
peritoneum, peritoneal (cavity)	C48.2	C78.6		D20.1	D48.4	D49.0
benign mesothelial tissue—see Mesothelioma, benign						
overlapping lesion	C48.8	-	-	-	-	-
with digestive organs	C26.9	-	-	-	-	-
parietal	C48.1	C78.6		D20.1	D48.4	D49.0
pelvic	C48.1	C78.6		D20.1	D48.4	D49.0
specified part NEC	C48.1	C78.6		D20.1	D48.4	D49.0
peritonsillar (tissue)	C76.0	C79.89	D09.8	D36.7	D48.7	D49.89
periurethral tissue	C76.3	C79.89		D36.7	D48.7	D49.89
phalanges						
foot	C40.3-	C79.51	-	D16.3-	-	-
hand	C40.1-	C79.51	-	D16.1-	-	-
pharynx, pharyngeal	C14.0	C79.89	D00.08	D10.9	D37.05	D49.0
bursa	C11.1	C79.89	D00.08	D10.6	D37.05	D49.0
fornix	C11.3	C79.89	D00.08	D10.6	D37.05	D49.0
recess	C11.2	C79.89	D00.08	D10.6	D37.05	D49.0
region	C14.0	C79.89	D00.08	D10.9	D37.05	D49.0
tonsil	C11.1	C79.89	D00.08	D10.6	D37.05	D49.0
wall (lateral) (posterior)	C14.0	C79.89	D00.08	D10.9	D37.05	D49.0
pia mater	C70.9	C79.40	-	D32.9	D42.9	D49.7
cerebral	C70.0	C79.32	-	D32.0	D42.0	D49.7
cranial	C70.0	C79.32	-	D32.0	D42.0	D49.7
spinal	C70.1	C79.49	-	D32.1	D42.1	D49.7
pillars of fauces	C09.1	C79.89	D00.08	D10.5	D37.05	D49.0
pineal (body) (gland)	C75.3	C79.89	D09.3	D35.4	D44.5	D49.7
pinna (ear) NEC—see also Neoplasm, skin, ear	C44.20-	C79.2	D04.2-	D23.2-	D48.5	D49.2
piriform fossa or sinus	C12	C79.89	D00.08	D10.7	D37.05	D49.0
pituitary (body) (fossa) (gland) (lobe)	C75.1	C79.89	D09.3	D35.2	D44.3	D49.7
placenta	C58	C79.82	D07.0	D26.7	D39.2	D49.59
pleura, pleural (cavity)	C38.4	C78.2	-	D19.0	D38.2	D49.1
overlapping lesion with heart or mediastinum	C38.8	-	-	-	-	-
parietal	C38.4	C78.2	-	D19.0	D38.2	D49.1
visceral	C38.4	C78.2	-	D19.0	D38.2	D49.1
plexus						
brachial	C47.1-	C79.89	-	D36.12	D48.2	D49.2
cervical	C47.0	C79.89	-	D36.11	D48.2	D49.2
choroid	C71.5	C79.31		D33.0	D43.0	D49.6
lumbosacral	C47.5	C79.89		D36.16	D48.2	D49.2
sacral	C47.5	C79.89		D36.16	D48.2	D49.2
pluriendocrine	C75.8	C79.89	D09.3	D35.7	D44.9	D49.7
pole						
frontal	C71.1	C79.31		D33.0	D43.0	D49.6
occipital	C71.4	C79.31		D33.0	D43.0	D49.6
pons (varolii)	C71.7	C79.31		D33.1	D43.1	D49.6
popliteal fossa or space	C76.5-	C79.89	D04.7-	D36.7	D48.7	D49.89
postcricoid (region)	C13.0	C79.89	D00.08	D10.7	D37.05	D49.0
posterior fossa (cranial)	C71.9	C79.31		D33.2	D43.2	D49.6
postnasal space	C11.9	C79.89	D00.08	D10.6	D37.05	D49.0
prepuce	C60.0	C79.82	D07.4	D29.0	D40.8	D49.59
prepylorus	C16.4	C78.89	D00.2	D13.1	D37.1	D49.0
presacral (region)	C76.3	C79.89	-	D36.7	D48.7	D49.89
prostate (gland)	C61	C79.82	D07.5	D29.1	D40.0	D49.59
utricle	C68.0	C79.19	D09.19	D30.4	D41.3	D49.59
pterygoid fossa	C49.0	C79.89	-	D21.0	D48.1	D49.2
pubic bone	C41.4	C79.51		D16.8	D48.0	D49.2
pudenda, pudendum (female)	C51.9	C79.82	D07.1	D28.0	D39.8	D49.59
pulmonary—see also Neoplasm, lung	C34.9-	C78.0-	D02.2-	D14.3-	D38.1	D49.1
putamen	C71.0	C79.31		D33.0	D43.0	D49.6
pyloric						
antrum	C16.3	C78.89	D00.2	D13.1	D37.1	D49.0
canal	C16.4	C78.89	D00.2	D13.1	D37.1	D49.0
pylorus	C16.4	C78.89	D00.2	D13.1	D37.1	D49.0
pyramid (brain)	C71.7	C79.31		D33.1	D43.1	D49.6
pyriform fossa or sinus	C12	C79.89	D00.08	D10.7	D37.05	D49.0
R						
radius (any part)	C40.0-	C79.51	-	D16.0-	-	-
Rathke's pouch	C75.1	C79.89	D09.3	D35.2	D44.3	D49.7
rectosigmoid (junction)	C19	C78.5	D01.1	D12.7	D37.5	D49.0
overlapping lesion with anus or rectum	C21.8	-	-	-	-	-
rectouterine pouch	C48.1	C78.6	-	D20.1	D48.4	D49.0
rectovaginal septum or wall	C76.3	C79.89	D09.8	D36.7	D48.7	D49.89
rectovesical septum	C76.3	C79.89	D09.8	D36.7	D48.7	D49.89
rectum (ampulla)	C20	C78.5	D01.2	D12.8	D37.5	D49.0
and colon	C19	C78.5	D01.1	D12.7	D37.5	D49.0
overlapping lesion with anus or rectosigmoid junction	C21.8	-	-	-	-	-

	Malignant Primary	Malignant Secondary	Ca in situ	Benign	Uncertain Behavior	Unspecified Behavior
renal	C64.-	C79.0-	D09.19	D30.0-	D41.0-	D49.51-
calyx	C65.-	C79.0-	D09.19	D30.1-	D41.1-	D49.51-
hilus	C65.-	C79.0-	D09.19	D30.1-	D41.1-	D49.51-
parenchyma	C64.-	C79.0-	D09.19	D30.0-	D41.0-	D49.51-
pelvis	C65.-	C79.0-	D09.19	D30.1-	D41.1-	D49.51-
respiratory						
organs or system NEC	C39.9	C78.30	D02.4	D14.4	D38.6	D49.1
tract NEC	C39.9	C78.30	D02.4	D14.4	D38.5	D49.1
upper	C39.0	C78.30	D02.4	D14.4	D38.5	D49.1
retina	C69.2-	C79.49	D09.2-	D31.2-	D48.7	D49.81
retrobulbar	C69.6-	C79.49	-	D31.6-	D48.7	D49.89
retrocecal	C48.0	C78.6	-	D20.0	D48.3	D49.0
retromolar (area) (triangle) (trigone)	C06.2	C79.89	D00.00	D10.39	D37.09	D49.0
retro-orbital	C76.0	C79.89	D09.8	D36.7	D48.7	D49.89
retroperitoneal (space) (tissue)	C48.0	C78.6	-	D20.0	D48.3	D49.0
retroperitoneum	C48.0	C78.6	-	D20.0	D48.3	D49.0
retropharyngeal	C14.0	C79.89	D00.08	D10.9	D37.05	D49.0
retrovesical (septum)	C76.3	C79.89	D09.8	D36.7	D48.7	D49.89
rhinencephalon	C71.0	C79.31		D33.0	D43.0	D49.6
rib	C41.3	C79.51		D16.7	D48.0	D49.2
Rosenmuller's fossa	C11.2	C79.89	D00.08	D10.6	D37.05	D49.0
round ligament	C57.2-	C79.82	-	D28.2	D39.8	D49.59
S						
sacrococcyx, sacrococcygeal	C41.4	C79.51		D16.8	D48.0	D49.2
region	C76.3	C79.89	D09.8	D36.7	D48.7	D49.89
sacrouterine ligament	C57.3	C79.82	-	D28.2	D39.8	D49.59
sacrum, sacral (vertebra)	C41.4	C79.51	-	D16.8	D48.0	D49.2
salivary gland or duct (major)	C08.9	C79.89	D00.00	D11.9	D37.039	D49.0
minor NEC	C06.9	C79.89	D00.00	D10.39	D37.04	D49.0
overlapping lesion	C08.9	-	-	-	-	-
parotid	C07	C79.89	D00.00	D11.0	D37.030	D49.0
pluriglandular	C08.9	C79.89	D00.00	D11.9	D37.039	D49.0
sublingual	C08.1	C79.89	D00.00	D11.7	D37.031	D49.0
submandibular	C08.0	C79.89	D00.00	D11.7	D37.032	D49.0
submaxillary	C08.0	C79.89	D00.00	D11.7	D37.032	D49.0
salpinx (uterine)	C57.0-	C79.82	D07.39	D28.2	D39.8	D49.59
Santorini's duct	C25.3	C78.89	D01.7	D13.6	D37.8	D49.0
scalp	C44.40	C79.2	D04.4	D23.4	D48.5	D49.2
basal cell carcinoma	C44.41	-	-	-	-	-
specified type NEC	C44.49	-	-	-	-	-
squamous cell carcinoma	C44.42	-	-	-	-	-
scapula (any part)	C40.0-	C79.51	-	D16.0-	-	-
scapular region	C76.1	C79.89	D09.8	D36.7	D48.7	D49.89
scar NEC—see also Neoplasm, skin, by site	C44.90	C79.2	D04.9	D23.9	D48.5	D49.2
sciatic nerve	C47.2-	C79.89	-	D36.13	D48.2	D49.2
sclera	C69.4-	C79.49	D09.2-	D31.4-	D48.7	D49.89
scrotum (skin)	C63.2	C79.82	D07.61	D29.4	D40.8	D49.59
sebaceous gland—see Neoplasm, skin						
sella turcica	C75.1	C79.89	D09.3	D35.2	D44.3	D49.7
bone	C41.0	C79.51	-	D16.4	D48.0	D49.2
semilunar cartilage (knee)	C40.2-	C79.51	-	D16.2-	D48.0	D49.2
seminal vesicle	C63.7	C79.82	D07.69	D29.8	D40.8	D49.59
septum						
nasal	C30.0	C78.39	D02.3	D14.0	D38.5	D49.1
posterior margin	C11.3	C79.89	D00.08	D10.6	D37.05	D49.0
rectovaginal	C76.3	C79.89	D09.8	D36.7	D48.7	D49.89
rectovesical	C76.3	C79.89	D09.8	D36.7	D48.7	D49.89
urethrovaginal	C57.9	C79.82	D07.30	D28.9	D39.9	D49.59
vesicovaginal	C57.9	C79.82	D07.30	D28.9	D39.9	D49.59
shoulder NEC	C76.4-	C79.89	D04.6-	D36.7	D48.7	D49.89
sigmoid flexure (lower) (upper)	C18.7	C78.5	D01.0	D12.5	D37.4	D49.0
sinus (accessory)	C31.9	C78.39	D02.3	D14.0	D38.5	D49.1
bone (any)	C41.0	C79.51	-	D16.4	D48.0	D49.2
ethmoidal	C31.1	C78.39	D02.3	D14.0	D38.5	D49.1
frontal	C31.2	C78.39	D02.3	D14.0	D38.5	D49.1
maxillary	C31.0	C78.39	D02.3	D14.0	D38.5	D49.1
nasal, paranasal NEC	C31.9	C78.39	D02.3	D14.0	D38.5	D49.1
overlapping lesion	C31.8	-	-	-	-	-
pyriform	C12	C79.89	D00.08	D10.7	D37.05	D49.0
sphenoid	C31.3	C78.39	D02.3	D14.0	D38.5	D49.1
skeleton, skeletal NEC	C41.9	C79.51	-	D16.9	D48.0	D49.2
Skene's gland	C68.1	C79.19	D09.19	D30.8	D41.8	D49.59
skin NOS	C44.90	C79.2	D04.9	D23.9	D48.5	D49.2
abdominal wall	C44.509	C79.2	D04.5	D23.5	D48.5	D49.2
basal cell carcinoma	C44.519	-	-	-	-	-
specified type NEC	C44.599	-	-	-	-	-
squamous cell carcinoma	C44.529	-	-	-	-	-
ala nasi—see also Neoplasm, nose, skin	C44.301	C79.2	D04.39	D23.39	D48.5	D49.2
ankle—see also Neoplasm, skin, limb, lower	C44.70-	C79.2	D04.7-	D23.7-	D48.5	D49.2
antecubital space—see also Neoplasm, skin, limb, upper	C44.60-	C79.2	D04.6-	D23.6-	D48.5	D49.2
anus	C44.500	C79.2	D04.5	D23.5	D48.5	D49.2
basal cell carcinoma	C44.510	-	-	-	-	-
specified type NEC	C44.590	-	-	-	-	-
squamous cell carcinoma	C44.520	-	-	-	-	-
arm—see also Neoplasm, skin, limb, upper	C44.60-	C79.2	D04.6-	D23.6-	D48.5	D49.2
auditory canal (external)—see also Neoplasm, skin, ear	C44.20-	C79.2	D04.2-	D23.2-	D48.5	D49.2
auricle (ear)—see also Neoplasm, skin, ear	C44.20-	C79.2	D04.2-	D23.2-	D48.5	D49.2
auricular canal (external)—see also Neoplasm, skin, ear	C44.20-	C79.2	D04.2-	D23.2-	D48.5	D49.2
axilla, axillary fold—see also Neoplasm, skin, trunk	C44.509	C79.2	D04.5	D23.5	D48.5	D49.2

skin NOS — *continued*	Malignant Primary	Malignant Secondary	Ca in situ	Benign	Uncertain Behavior	Unspecified Behavior
back—see also Neoplasm, skin, trunk	C44.509	C79.2	D04.5	D23.5	D48.5	D49.2
basal cell carcinoma	C44.91					
breast	C44.501	C79.2	D04.5	D23.5	D48.5	D49.2
basal cell carcinoma	C44.511	-	-	-	-	-
specified type NEC	C44.591	-	-	-	-	-
squamous cell carcinoma	C44.521	-	-	-	-	-
brow—see also Neoplasm, skin, face	C44.309	C79.2	D04.39	D23.39	D48.5	D49.2
buttock—see also Neoplasm, skin, trunk	C44.509	C79.2	D04.5	D23.5	D48.5	D49.2
calf—see also Neoplasm, skin, limb, lower	C44.70-	C79.2	D04.7-	D23.7-	D48.5	D49.2
canthus (eye) (inner) (outer)	C44.10-	C79.2	D04.1-	D23.1-	D48.5	D49.2
basal cell carcinoma	C44.11-	-	-	-	-	-
sebaceous cell	C44.13-	-	-	-	-	-
specified type NEC	C44.19-	-	-	-	-	-
squamous cell carcinoma	C44.12-	-	-	-	-	-
cervical region—see also Neoplasm, skin, neck	C44.40	C79.2	D04.4	D23.4	D48.5	D49.2
cheek (external) —see also Neoplasm, skin, face	C44.309	C79.2	D04.39	D23.39	D48.5	D49.2
chest (wall)—see also Neoplasm, skin, trunk	C44.509	C79.2	D04.5	D23.5	D48.5	D49.2
chin—see also Neoplasm, skin, face	C44.309	C79.2	D04.39	D23.39	D48.5	D49.2
clavicular area—see also Neoplasm, skin, trunk	C44.509	C79.2	D04.5	D23.5	D48.5	D49.2
clitoris	C51.2	C79.82	D07.1	D28.0	D39.8	D49.59
columnella—see also Neoplasm, skin, face	C44.309	C79.2	D04.39	D23.39	D48.5	D49.2
concha—see also Neoplasm, skin, ear	C44.20-	C79.2	D04.2-	D23.2-	D48.5	D49.2
ear (external)	C44.20-	C79.2	D04.2-	D23.2-	D48.5	D49.2
basal cell carcinoma	C44.21-	-	-	-	-	-
specified type NEC	C44.29-	-	-	-	-	-
squamous cell carcinoma	C44.22-	-	-	-	-	-
elbow—see also Neoplasm, skin, limb, upper	C44.60-	C79.2	D04.6-	D23.6-	D48.5	D49.2
eyebrow—see also Neoplasm, skin, face	C44.309	C79.2	D04.39	D23.39	D48.5	D49.2
eyelid	C44.10-	C79.2	D04.1-	D23.1-	D48.5	D49.2
basal cell carcinoma	C44.11-	-	-	-	-	-
sebaceous cell	C44.13-	-	-	-	-	-
specified type NEC	C44.19-	-	-	-	-	-
squamous cell carcinoma	C44.12-	-	-	-	-	-
face NOS	C44.300	C79.2	D04.30	D23.30	D48.5	D49.2
basal cell carcinoma	C44.310	-	-	-	-	-
specified type NEC	C44.390	-	-	-	-	-

skin NOS, face NOS — *continued*	Malignant Primary	Malignant Secondary	Ca in situ	Benign	Uncertain Behavior	Unspecified Behavior
squamous cell carcinoma	C44.320	-	-	-	-	-
female genital organs (external)	C51.9	C79.82	D07.1	D28.0	D39.8	D49.59
clitoris	C51.2	C79.82	D07.1	D28.0	D39.8	D49.59
labium NEC	C51.9	C79.82	D07.1	D28.0	D39.8	D49.59
majus	C51.0	C79.82	D07.1	D28.0	D39.8	D49.59
minus	C51.1	C79.82	D07.1	D28.0	D39.8	D49.59
pudendum	C51.9	C79.82	D07.1	D28.0	D39.8	D49.59
vulva	C51.9	C79.82	D07.1	D28.0	D39.8	D49.59
finger—see also Neoplasm, skin, limb, upper	C44.60-	C79.2	D04.6-	D23.6-	D48.5	D49.2
flank—see also Neoplasm, skin, trunk	C44.509	C79.2	D04.5	D23.5	D48.5	D49.2
foot—see also Neoplasm, skin, limb, lower	C44.70-	C79.2	D04.7-	D23.7-	D48.5	D49.2
forearm—see also Neoplasm, skin, limb, upper	C44.60-	C79.2	D04.6-	D23.6-	D48.5	D49.2
forehead—see also *Neoplasm, skin, face*	C44.309	C79.2	D04.39	D23.39	D48.5	D49.2
glabella—see also Neoplasm, skin, face	C44.309	C79.2	D04.39	D23.39	D48.5	D49.2
gluteal region—see also Neoplasm, skin, trunk	C44.509	C79.2	D04.5	D23.5	D48.5	D49.2
groin—see also Neoplasm, skin, trunk	C44.509	C79.2	D04.5	D23.5	D48.5	D49.2
hand—see also Neoplasm, skin, limb, upper	C44.60-	C79.2	D04.6-	D23.6-	D48.5	D49.2
head NEC—see also Neoplasm, skin, scalp	C44.40	C79.2	D04.4	D23.4	D48.5	D49.2
heel—see also Neoplasm, skin, limb, lower	C44.70-	C79.2	D04.7-	D23.7-	D48.5	D49.2
helix—see also Neoplasm, skin, ear	C44.20-	C79.2	D04.2-	D23.2-	D48.5	D49.2
hip—see also Neoplasm, skin, limb, lower	C44.70-	C79.2	D04.7-	D23.7-	D48.5	D49.2
infraclavicular region— see also Neoplasm, skin, trunk	C44.509	C79.2	D04.5	D23.5	D48.5	D49.2
inguinal region—see also Neoplasm, skin, trunk	C44.509	C79.2	D04.5	D23.5	D48.5	D49.2
jaw—see also Neoplasm, skin, face	C44.309	C79.2	D04.39	D23.39	D48.5	D49.2
Kaposi's sarcoma —see Kaposi's, sarcoma, skin						
knee—see also Neoplasm, skin, limb, lower	C44.70-	C79.2	D04.7-	D23.7-	D48.5	D49.2
labia						
majora	C51.0	C79.82	D07.1	D28.0	D39.8	D49.59
minora	C51.1	C79.82	D07.1	D28.0	D39.8	D49.59
leg—see also Neoplasm, skin, limb, lower	C44.70-	C79.2	D04.7-	D23.7-	D48.5	D49.2
lid (lower) (upper)	C44.10-	C79.2	D04.1-	D23.1-	D48.5	D49.2
basal cell carcinoma	C44.11-	-	-	-	-	-

skin NOS, lid (lower) (upper) — continued	Malignant Primary	Malignant Secondary	Ca in situ	Benign	Uncertain Behavior	Unspecified Behavior
sebaceous cell	C44.13-	-	-	-	-	-
specified type NEC	C44.19-	-	-	-	-	-
squamous cell carcinoma	C44.12-	-	-	-	-	-
limb NEC	C44.90	C79.2	D04.9	D23.9	D48.5	D49.2
basal cell carcinoma	C44.91					
lower	C44.70-	C79.2	D04.7-	D23.7-	D48.5	D49.2
basal cell carcinoma	C44.71-	-	-	-	-	-
specified type NEC	C44.79-	-	-	-	-	-
squamous cell carcinoma	C44.72-	-	-	-	-	-
upper	C44.60-	C79.2	D04.6-	D23.6-	D48.5	D49.2
basal cell carcinoma	C44.61-	-	-	-	-	-
specified type NEC	C44.69-	-	-	-	-	-
squamous cell carcinoma	C44.62-	-	-	-	-	-
lip (lower) (upper)	C44.00	C79.2	D04.0	D23.0	D48.5	D49.2
basal cell carcinoma	C44.01	-	-	-	-	-
specified type NEC	C44.09	-	-	-	-	-
squamous cell carcinoma	C44.02	-	-	-	-	-
male genital organs	C63.9	C79.82	D07.60	D29.9	D40.8	D49.59
penis	C60.9	C79.82	D07.4	D29.0	D40.8	D49.59
prepuce	C60.0	C79.82	D07.4	D29.0	D40.8	D49.59
scrotum	C63.2	C79.82	D07.61	D29.4	D40.8	D49.59
mastectomy site (skin)—see also Neoplasm, skin, breast	C44.501	C79.2	-	-	-	-
specified as breast tissue	C50.8-	C79.81	-	-	-	-
meatus, acoustic (external)—see also Neoplasm, skin, ear	C44.20-	C79.2	D04.2-	D23.2-	D48.5	D49.2
melanotic—see Melanoma						
Merkel cell—see Carcinoma, Merkel cell						
nates—see also Neoplasm, skin, trunk	C44.509	C79.2	D04.5	D23.5	D48.5	D49.2
neck	C44.40	C79.2	D04.4	D23.4	D48.5	D49.2
basal cell carcinoma	C44.41	-	-	-	-	-
specified type NEC	C44.49	-	-	-	-	-
squamous cell carcinoma	C44.42	-	-	-	-	-
nevus—see Nevus, skin						
nose (external)—see also Neoplasm, nose, skin	C44.301	C79.2	D04.39	D23.39	D48.5	D49.2
overlapping lesion	C44.80					
basal cell carcinoma	C44.81	-	-	-	-	-
specified type NEC	C44.89	-	-	-	-	-
squamous cell carcinoma	C44.82	-	-	-	-	-
palm—see also Neoplasm, skin, limb, upper	C44.60-	C79.2	D04.6-	D23.6-	D48.5	D49.2
palpebra	C44.10-	C79.2	D04.1-	D23.1-	D48.5	D49.2
basal cell carcinoma	C44.11-	-	-	-	-	-
sebaceous cell	C44.13-	-	-	-	-	-

skin NOS, palpebra — continued	Malignant Primary	Malignant Secondary	Ca in situ	Benign	Uncertain Behavior	Unspecified Behavior
specified type NEC	C44.19-	-	-	-	-	-
squamous cell carcinoma	C44.12-	-	-	-	-	-
penis NEC	C60.9	C79.82	D07.4	D29.0	D40.8	D49.59
perianal—see also Neoplasm, skin, anus	C44.500	C79.2	D04.5	D23.5	D48.5	D49.2
perineum—see also Neoplasm, skin, anus	C44.500	C79.2	D04.5	D23.5	D48.5	D49.2
pinna—see also Neoplasm, skin, ear	C44.20-	C79.2	D04.2-	D23.2-	D48.5	D49.2
plantar—see also Neoplasm, skin, limb, lower	C44.70-	C79.2	D04.7-	D23.7-	D48.5	D49.2
popliteal fossa or space—see also Neoplasm, skin, limb, lower	C44.70-	C79.2	D04.7-	D23.7-	D48.5	D49.2
prepuce	C60.0	C79.82	D07.4	D29.0	D40.8	D49.59
pubes—see also Neoplasm, skin, trunk	C44.509	C79.2	D04.5	D23.5	D48.5	D49.2
sacrococcygeal region—see also Neoplasm, skin, trunk	C44.509	C79.2	D04.5	D23.5	D48.5	D49.2
scalp	C44.40	C79.2	D04.4	D23.4	D48.5	D49.2
basal cell carcinoma	C44.41	-	-	-	-	-
specified type NEC	C44.49	-	-	-	-	-
squamous cell carcinoma	C44.42	-	-	-	-	-
scapular region—see also Neoplasm, skin, trunk	C44.509	C79.2	D04.5	D23.5	D48.5	D49.2
scrotum	C63.2	C79.82	D07.61	D29.4	D40.8	D49.59
shoulder—see also Neoplasm, skin, limb, upper	C44.60-	C79.2	D04.6-	D23.6-	D48.5	D49.2
sole (foot)—see also Neoplasm, skin, limb, lower	C44.70-	C79.2	D04.7-	D23.7-	D48.5	D49.2
specified sites NEC	C44.80	C79.2	D04.8	D23.9	D48.5	D49.2
basal cell carcinoma	C44.81	-	-	-	-	-
specified type NEC	C44.89	-	-	-	-	-
squamous cell carcinoma	C44.82	-	-	-	-	-
specified type NEC	C44.99	-	-	-	-	-
squamous cell carcinoma	C44.92	-	-	-	-	-
submammary fold—see also Neoplasm, skin, trunk	C44.509	C79.2	D04.5	D23.5	D48.5	D49.2
supraclavicular region—see also Neoplasm, skin, neck	C44.40	C79.2	D04.4	D23.4	D48.5	D49.2
temple—see also Neoplasm, skin, face	C44.309	C79.2	D04.39	D23.39	D48.5	D49.2
thigh—see also Neoplasm, skin, limb, lower	C44.70-	C79.2	D04.7-	D23.7-	D48.5	D49.2
thoracic wall—see also Neoplasm, skin, trunk	C44.509	C79.2	D04.5	D23.5	D48.5	D49.2
thumb—see also Neoplasm, skin, limb, upper	C44.60-	C79.2	D04.6-	D23.6-	D48.5	D49.2

skin NOS — continued	Malignant Primary	Malignant Secondary	Ca in situ	Benign	Uncertain Behavior	Unspecified Behavior
toe—see also Neoplasm, skin, limb, lower	C44.70-	C79.2	D04.7-	D23.7-	D48.5	D49.2
tragus—see also Neoplasm, skin, ear	C44.20-	C79.2	D04.2-	D23.2-	D48.5	D49.2
trunk	C44.509	C79.2	D04.5	D23.5	D48.5	D49.2
basal cell carcinoma	C44.519	-	-	-	-	-
specified type NEC	C44.599	-	-	-	-	-
squamous cell carcinoma	C44.529	-	-	-	-	-
umbilicus—see also Neoplasm, skin, trunk	C44.509	C79.2	D04.5	D23.5	D48.5	D49.2
vulva	C51.9	C79.82	D07.1	D28.0	D39.8	D49.59
overlapping lesion	C51.8	-	-	-	-	-
wrist—see also Neoplasm, skin, limb, upper	C44.60-	C79.2	D04.6-	D23.6-	D48.5	D49.2
skull	C41.0	C79.51	-	D16.4	D48.0	D49.2
soft parts or tissues—see Neoplasm, connective tissue						
specified site NEC	C76.8	C79.89	D09.8	D36.7	D48.7	D49.89
spermatic cord	C63.1-	C79.82	D07.69	D29.8	D40.8	D49.59
sphenoid	C31.3	C78.39	D02.3	D14.0	D38.5	D49.1
bone	C41.0	C79.51	-	D16.4	D48.0	D49.2
sinus	C31.3	C78.39	D02.3	D14.0	D38.5	D49.1
sphincter						
anal	C21.1	C78.5	D01.3	D12.9	D37.8	D49.0
of Oddi	C24.0	C78.89	D01.5	D13.5	D37.6	D49.0
spine, spinal (column)	C41.2	C79.51	-	D16.6	D48.0	D49.2
bulb	C71.7	C79.31	-	D33.1	D43.1	D49.6
coccyx	C41.4	C79.51	-	D16.8	D48.0	D49.2
cord (cervical) (lumbar) (sacral) (thoracic)	C72.0	C79.49	-	D33.4	D43.4	D49.7
dura mater	C70.1	C79.49	-	D32.1	D42.1	D49.7
lumbosacral	C41.2	C79.51	-	D16.6	D48.0	D49.2
marrow NEC	C96.9	C79.52	-	-	D47.9	D49.89
membrane	C70.1	C79.49	-	D32.1	D42.1	D49.7
meninges	C70.1	C79.49	-	D32.1	D42.1	D49.7
nerve (root)	C47.9	C79.89	-	D36.10	D48.2	D49.2
pia mater	C70.1	C79.49	-	D32.1	D42.1	D49.7
root	C47.9	C79.89	-	D36.10	D48.2	D49.2
sacrum	C41.4	C79.51	-	D16.8	D48.0	D49.2
spleen, splenic NEC	C26.1	C78.89	D01.7	D13.9	D37.8	D49.0
flexure (colon)	C18.5	C78.5	D01.0	D12.3	D37.4	D49.0
stem, brain	C71.7	C79.31	-	D33.1	D43.1	D49.6
Stensen's duct	C07	C79.89	D00.00	D11.0	D37.030	D49.0
sternum	C41.3	C79.51	-	D16.7	D48.0	D49.2
stomach	C16.9	C78.89	D00.2	D13.1	D37.1	D49.0
antrum (pyloric)	C16.3	C78.89	D00.2	D13.1	D37.1	D49.0
body	C16.2	C78.89	D00.2	D13.1	D37.1	D49.0
cardia	C16.0	C78.89	D00.2	D13.1	D37.1	D49.0
cardiac orifice	C16.0	C78.89	D00.2	D13.1	D37.1	D49.0
corpus	C16.2	C78.89	D00.2	D13.1	D37.1	D49.0
fundus	C16.1	C78.89	D00.2	D13.1	D37.1	D49.0

stomach — continued	Malignant Primary	Malignant Secondary	Ca in situ	Benign	Uncertain Behavior	Unspecified Behavior
greater curvature NEC	C16.6	C78.89	D00.2	D13.1	D37.1	D49.0
lesser curvature NEC	C16.5	C78.89	D00.2	D13.1	D37.1	D49.0
overlapping lesion	C16.8	-	-	-	-	-
prepylorus	C16.4	C78.89	D00.2	D13.1	D37.1	D49.0
pylorus	C16.4	C78.89	D00.2	D13.1	D37.1	D49.0
wall NEC	C16.9	C78.89	D00.2	D13.1	D37.1	D49.0
anterior NEC	C16.8	C78.89	D00.2	D13.1	D37.1	D49.0
posterior NEC	C16.8	C78.89	D00.2	D13.1	D37.1	D49.0
stroma, endometrial	C54.1	C79.82	D07.0	D26.1	D39.0	D49.59
stump, cervical	C53.8	C79.82	D06.7	D26.0	D39.0	D49.59
subcutaneous (nodule) (tissue) NEC—see Neoplasm, connective tissue						
subdural	C70.9	C79.32	-	D32.9	D42.9	D49.7
subglottis, subglottic	C32.2	C78.39	D02.0	D14.1	D38.0	D49.1
sublingual	C04.9	C79.89	D00.06	D10.2	D37.09	D49.0
gland or duct	C08.1	C79.89	D00.00	D11.7	D37.031	D49.0
submandibular gland	C08.0	C79.89	D00.00	D11.7	D37.032	D49.0
submaxillary gland or duct	C08.0	C79.89	D00.00	D11.7	D37.032	D49.0
submental	C76.0	C79.89	D09.8	D36.7	D48.7	D49.89
subpleural	C34.9-	C78.0-	D02.2-	D14.3-	D38.1	D49.1
substernal	C38.1	C78.1	-	D15.2	D38.3	D49.89
sudoriferous, sudoriparous gland, site unspecified	C44.90	C79.2	D04.9	D23.9	D48.5	D49.2
specified site—see Neoplasm, skin						
supraclavicular region	C76.0	C79.89	D09.8	D36.7	D48.7	D49.89
supraglottis	C32.1	C78.39	D02.0	D14.1	D38.0	D49.1
suprarenal	C74.9-	C79.7-	D09.3	D35.0-	D44.1-	D49.7
capsule	C74.9-	C79.7-	D09.3	D35.0-	D44.1-	D49.7
cortex	C74.0-	C79.7-	D09.3	D35.0-	D44.1-	D49.7
gland	C74.9-	C79.7-	D09.3	D35.0-	D44.1-	D49.7
medulla	C74.1-	C79.7-	D09.3	D35.0-	D44.1-	D49.7
suprasellar (region)	C71.9	C79.31	-	D33.2	D43.2	D49.6
supratentorial (brain) NEC	C71.0	C79.31	-	D33.0	D43.0	D49.6
sweat gland (apocrine) (eccrine), site unspecified	C44.90	C79.2	D04.9	D23.9	D48.5	D49.2
specified site— see Neoplasm, skin						
sympathetic nerve or nervous system NEC	C47.9	C79.89	-	D36.10	D48.2	D49.2
symphysis pubis	C41.4	C79.51	-	D16.8	D48.0	D49.2
synovial membrane—see Neoplasm, connective tissue						
T						
tapetum, brain	C71.8	C79.31	-	D33.2	D43.2	D49.6
tarsus (any bone)	C40.3-	C79.51	-	D16.3-	-	-
temple (skin)—see also Neoplasm, skin, face	C44.309	C79.2	D04.39	D23.39	D48.5	D49.2
temporal						
bone	C41.0	C79.51	-	D16.4	D48.0	D49.2

	Malignant Primary	Malignant Secondary	Ca in situ	Benign	Uncertain Behavior	Unspecified Behavior
temporal — *continued*						
lobe or pole	C71.2	C79.31	-	D33.0	D43.0	D49.6
region	C76.0	C79.89	D09.8	D36.7	D48.7	D49.89
skin—see also Neoplasm, skin, face	C44.309	C79.2	D04.39	D23.39	D48.5	D49.2
tendon (sheath)—see Neoplasm, connective tissue						
tentorium (cerebelli)	C70.0	C79.32	-	D32.0	D42.0	D49.7
testis, testes	C62.9-	C79.82	D07.69	D29.2-	D40.1-	D49.59
descended	C62.1-	C79.82	D07.69	D29.2-	D40.1-	D49.59
ectopic	C62.0-	C79.82	D07.69	D29.2-	D40.1-	D49.59
retained	C62.0-	C79.82	D07.69	D29.2-	D40.1-	D49.59
scrotal	C62.1-	C79.82	D07.69	D29.2-	D40.1-	D49.59
undescended	C62.0-	C79.82	D07.69	D29.2-	D40.1-	D49.59
unspecified whether descended or undescended	C62.9-	C79.82	D07.69	D29.2-	D40.1-	D49.59
thalamus	C71.0	C79.31	-	D33.0	D43.0	D49.6
thigh NEC	C76.5-	C79.89	D04.7-	D36.7	D48.7	D49.89
thorax, thoracic (cavity) (organs NEC)	C76.1	C79.89	D09.8	D36.7	D48.7	D49.89
duct	C49.3	C79.89	-	D21.3	D48.1	D49.2
wall NEC	C76.1	C79.89	D09.8	D36.7	D48.7	D49.89
throat	C14.0	C79.89	D00.08	D10.9	D37.05	D49.0
thumb NEC	C76.4-	C79.89	D04.6-	D36.7	D48.7	D49.89
thymus (gland)	C37	C79.89	D09.3	D15.0	D38.4	D49.89
thyroglossal duct	C73	C79.89	D09.3	D34	D44.0	D49.7
thyroid (gland)	C73	C79.89	D09.3	D34	D44.0	D49.7
cartilage	C32.3	C78.39	D02.0	D14.1	D38.0	D49.1
tibia (any part)	C40.2-	C79.51	-	D16.2-	-	-
toe NEC	C76.5-	C79.89	D04.7-	D36.7	D48.7	D49.89
tongue	C02.9	C79.89	D00.07	D10.1	D37.02	D49.0
anterior (two-thirds) NEC	C02.3	C79.89	D00.07	D10.1	D37.02	D49.0
dorsal surface	C02.0	C79.89	D00.07	D10.1	D37.02	D49.0
ventral surface	C02.2	C79.89	D00.07	D10.1	D37.02	D49.0
base (dorsal surface)	C01	C79.89	D00.07	D10.1	D37.02	D49.0
border (lateral)	C02.1	C79.89	D00.07	D10.1	D37.02	D49.0
dorsal surface NEC	C02.0	C79.89	D00.07	D10.1	D37.02	D49.0
fixed part NEC	C01	C79.89	D00.07	D10.1	D37.02	D49.0
foreamen cecum	C02.0	C79.89	D00.07	D10.1	D37.02	D49.0
frenulum linguae	C02.2	C79.89	D00.07	D10.1	D37.02	D49.0
junctional zone	C02.8	C79.89	D00.07	D10.1	D37.02	D49.0
margin (lateral)	C02.1	C79.89	D00.07	D10.1	D37.02	D49.0
midline NEC	C02.0	C79.89	D00.07	D10.1	D37.02	D49.0
mobile part NEC	C02.3	C79.89	D00.07	D10.1	D37.02	D49.0
overlapping lesion	C02.8	-	-	-	-	-
posterior (third)	C01	C79.89	D00.07	D10.1	D37.02	D49.0
root	C01	C79.89	D00.07	D10.1	D37.02	D49.0
surface (dorsal)	C02.0	C79.89	D00.07	D10.1	D37.02	D49.0
base	C01	C79.89	D00.07	D10.1	D37.02	D49.0
ventral	C02.2	C79.89	D00.07	D10.1	D37.02	D49.0
tip	C02.1	C79.89	D00.07	D10.1	D37.02	D49.0
tonsil	C02.4	C79.89	D00.07	D10.1	D37.02	D49.0

	Malignant Primary	Malignant Secondary	Ca in situ	Benign	Uncertain Behavior	Unspecified Behavior
tonsil	C09.9	C79.89	D00.08	D10.4	D37.05	D49.0
fauces, faucial	C09.9	C79.89	D00.08	D10.4	D37.05	D49.0
lingual	C02.4	C79.89	D00.07	D10.1	D37.02	D49.0
overlapping sites	C09.8	-	-	-	-	-
palatine	C09.9	C79.89	D00.08	D10.4	D37.05	D49.0
pharyngeal	C11.1	C79.89	D00.08	D10.6	D37.05	D49.0
pillar (anterior) (posterior)	C09.1	C79.89	D00.08	D10.5	D37.05	D49.0
tonsillar fossa	C09.0	C79.89	D00.08	D10.5	D37.05	D49.0
tooth socket NEC	C03.9	C79.89	D00.03	D10.39	D37.09	D49.0
trachea (cartilage) (mucosa)	C33	C78.39	D02.1	D14.2	D38.1	D49.1
overlapping lesion with bronchus or lung	C34.8-	-	-	-	-	-
tracheobronchial	C34.8-	C78.39	D02.1	D14.2	D38.1	D49.1
overlapping lesion with lung	C34.8-	-	-	-	-	-
tragus—see also Neoplasm, skin, ear	C44.20-	C79.2	D04.2-	D23.2-	D48.5	D49.2
trunk NEC	C76.8	C79.89	D04.5	D36.7	D48.7	D49.89
tubo-ovarian	C57.8	C79.82	D07.39	D28.7	D39.8	D49.59
tunica vaginalis	C63.7	C79.82	D07.69	D29.8	D40.8	D49.59
turbinate (bone)	C41.0	C79.51	-	D16.4	D48.0	D49.2
nasal	C30.0	C78.39	D02.3	D14.0	D38.5	D49.1
tympanic cavity	C30.1	C78.39	D02.3	D14.0	D38.5	D49.1
U						
ulna (any part)	C40.0-	C79.51	-	D16.0-	-	-
umbilicus, umbilical—see also Neoplasm, skin, trunk	C44.509	C79.2	D04.5	D23.5	D48.5	D49.2
uncus, brain	C71.2	C79.31	-	D33.0	D43.0	D49.6
unknown site or unspecified	C80.1	C79.9	D09.9	D36.9	D48.9	D49.9
urachus	C67.7	C79.11	D09.0	D30.3	D41.4	D49.4
ureter, ureteral	C66.-	C79.19	D09.19	D30.2-	D41.2-	D49.59
orifice (bladder)	C67.6	C79.11	D09.0	D30.3	D41.4	D49.4
ureter-bladder (junction)	C67.6	C79.11	D09.0	D30.3	D41.4	D49.4
urethra, urethral (gland)	C68.0	C79.19	D09.19	D30.4	D41.3	D49.59
orifice, internal	C67.5	C79.11	D09.0	D30.3	D41.4	D49.4
urethrovaginal (septum)	C57.9	C79.82	D07.30	D28.9	D39.8	D49.59
urinary organ or system	C68.9	C79.10	D09.10	D30.9	D41.9	D49.59
bladder—see Neoplasm, bladder						
overlapping lesion	C68.8	-	-	-	-	-
specified sites NEC	C68.8	C79.19	D09.19	D30.8	D41.8	D49.59
utero-ovarian	C57.8	C79.82	D07.39	D28.7	D39.8	D49.59
ligament	C57.1	C79.82	D07.39	D28.2	D39.8	D49.59
uterosacral ligament	C57.3	C79.82	-	D28.2	D39.8	D49.59
uterus, uteri, uterine	C55	C79.82	D07.0	D26.9	D39.0	D49.59
adnexa NEC	C57.4	C79.82	D07.39	D28.7	D39.8	D49.59
body	C54.9	C79.82	D07.0	D26.1	D39.0	D49.59
cervix	C53.9	C79.82	D06.9	D26.0	D39.0	D49.59
cornu	C54.9	C79.82	D07.0	D26.1	D39.0	D49.59
corpus	C54.9	C79.82	D07.0	D26.1	D39.0	D49.59
endocervix (canal) (gland)	C53.0	C79.82	D06.0	D26.0	D39.0	D49.59
endometrium	C54.1	C79.82	D07.0	D26.1	D39.0	D49.59
exocervix	C53.1	C79.82	D06.1	D26.0	D39.0	D49.59

uterus, uteri, uterine — *continued*	Malignant Primary	Malignant Secondary	Ca in situ	Benign	Uncertain Behavior	Unspecified Behavior
external os	C53.1	C79.82	D06.1	D26.0	D39.0	D49.59
fundus	C54.3	C79.82	D07.0	D26.1	D39.0	D49.59
internal os	C53.0	C79.82	D06.0	D26.0	D39.0	D49.59
isthmus	C54.0	C79.82	D07.0	D26.1	D39.0	D49.59
ligament	C57.3	C79.82	-	D28.2	D39.8	D49.59
broad	C57.1	C79.82	D07.39	D28.2	D39.8	D49.59
round	C57.2	C79.82	-	D28.2	D39.8	D49.59
lower segment	C54.0	C79.82	D07.0	D26.1	D39.0	D49.59
myometrium	C54.2	C79.82	D07.0	D26.1	D39.0	D49.59
overlapping sites	C54.8	-	-	-	-	-
squamocolumnar junction	C53.8	C79.82	D06.7	D26.0	D39.0	D49.59
tube	C57.0-	C79.82	D07.39	D28.2	D39.8	D49.59
utricle, prostatic	C68.0	C79.19	D09.19	D30.4	D41.3	D49.59
uveal tract	C69.4-	C79.49	D09.2-	D31.4-	D48.7	D49.89
uvula	C05.2	C79.89	D00.04	D10.39	D37.09	D49.0
V						
vagina, vaginal (fornix) (vault) (wall)	C52	C79.82	D07.2	D28.1	D39.8	D49.59
vaginovesical	C57.9	C79.82	D07.30	D28.9	D39.9	D49.59
septum	C57.9	C79.82	D07.30	D28.9	D39.9	D49.59
vallecula (epigiottis)	C10.0	C79.89	D00.08	D10.5	D37.05	D49.0
vas deferens	C63.1-	C79.82	D07.69	D29.8	D40.8	D49.59
vascular—see Neoplasm, connective tissue						
Vater's ampulla	C24.1	C78.89	D01.5	D13.5	D37.6	D49.0
vein, venous—see Neoplasm, connective tissue						
vena cava (abdominal) (inferior)	C49.4	C79.89	-	D21.4	D48.1	D49.2
superior	C49.3	C79.89	-	D21.3	D48.1	D49.2
ventricle (cerebral) (floor) (lateral) (third)	C71.5	C79.31	-	D33.0	D43.0	D49.6
cardiac (left) (right)	C38.0	C79.89	-	D15.1	D48.7	D49.89
fourth	C71.7	C79.31	-	D33.1	D43.1	D49.6
ventricular band of larynx	C32.1	C78.39	D02.0	D14.1	D38.0	D49.1
ventriculus—see Neoplasm, stomach						
vermillion border—see Neoplasm, lip						
vermis, cerebellum	C71.6	C79.31	-	D33.1	D43.1	D49.6

	Malignant Primary	Malignant Secondary	Ca in situ	Benign	Uncertain Behavior	Unspecified Behavior
vertebra (column)	C41.2	C79.51	-	D16.6	D48.0	D49.2
coccyx	C41.4	C79.51	-	D16.8	D48.0	D49.2
marrow NEC	C96.9	C79.52	-	-	D47.9	D49.89
sacrum	C41.4	C79.51	-	D16.8	D48.0	D49.2
vesical—see Neoplasm, bladder						
vesicle, seminal	C63.7	C79.82	D07.69	D29.8	D40.8	D49.59
vesicocervical tissue	C57.9	C79.82	D07.30	D28.9	D39.9	D49.59
vesicorectal	C76.3	C79.82	D09.8	D36.7	D48.7	D49.89
vesicovaginal	C57.9	C79.82	D07.30	D28.9	D39.9	D49.59
septum	C57.9	C79.82	D07.30	D28.9	D39.8	D49.59
vessel (blood)—see Neoplasm, connective tissue						
vestibular gland, greater	C51.0	C79.82	D07.1	D28.0	D39.8	D49.59
vestibule						
mouth	C06.1	C79.89	D00.00	D10.39	D37.09	D49.0
nose	C30.0	C78.39	D02.3	D14.0	D38.5	D49.1
Virchow's gland	C77.0	C77.0	-	D36.0	D48.7	D49.89
viscera NEC	C76.8	C79.89	D09.8	D36.7	D48.7	D49.89
vocal cords (true)	C32.0	C78.39	D02.0	D14.1	D38.0	D49.1
false	C32.1	C78.39	D02.0	D14.1	D38.0	D49.1
vomer	C41.0	C79.51	-	D16.4	D48.0	D49.2
vulva	C51.9	C79.82	D07.1	D28.0	D39.8	D49.59
vulvovaginal gland	C51.0	C79.82	D07.1	D28.0	D39.8	D49.59
W						
Waldeyer's ring	C14.2	C79.89	D00.08	D10.9	D37.05	D49.0
Wharton's duct	C08.0	C79.89	D00.00	D11.7	D37.032	D49.0
white matter (central) (cerebral)	C71.0	C79.31	-	D33.0	D43.0	D49.6
windpipe	C33	C78.39	D02.1	D14.2	D38.1	D49.1
Wirsung's duct	C25.3	C78.89	D01.7	D13.6	D37.8	D49.0
wolffian (body) (duct)						
female	C57.7	C79.82	D07.39	D28.7	D39.8	D49.59
male	C63.7	C79.82	D07.69	D29.8	D40.8	D49.59
womb—see Neoplasm, uterus						
wrist NEC	C76.4-	C79.89	D04.6-	D36.7	D48.7	D49.89
X						
xiphoid process	C41.3	C79.51	-	D16.7	D48.0	D49.2
Z						
Zuckerkandl organ	C75.5	C79.89	-	D35.6	D44.7	D49.7

Substance	Poisoning, Accidental (unintentional)	Poisoning, Intentional self-harm	Poisoning, Assault	Poisoning, Undetermined	Adverse effect	Underdosing
1-propanol	T51.3X1	T51.3X2	T51.3X3	T51.3X4	—	—
2-propanol	T51.2X1	T51.2X2	T51.2X3	T51.2X4	—	—
2,4-D (dichlorophen-oxyacetic acid)	T60.3X1	T60.3X2	T60.3X3	T60.3X4	—	—
2,4-toluene diisocyanate	T65.0X1	T65.0X2	T65.0X3	T65.0X4	—	—
2,4,5-T (trichloro-phenoxyacetic acid)	T60.1X1	T60.1X2	T60.1X3	T60.1X4	—	—
3,4-methylenedioxy-methamphetamine	T43.641	T43.642	T43.643	T43.644	—	—
14-hydroxydihydro-morphinone	T40.2X1	T40.2X2	T40.2X3	T40.2X4	T40.2X5	T40.2X6
A						
ABOB	T37.5X1	T37.5X2	T37.5X3	T37.5X4	T37.5X5	T37.5X6
Abrine	T62.2X1	T62.2X2	T62.2X3	T62.2X4	—	—
Abrus (seed)	T62.2X1	T62.2X2	T62.2X3	T62.2X4	—	—
Absinthe	T51.0X1	T51.0X2	T51.0X3	T51.0X4	—	—
beverage	T51.0X1	T51.0X2	T51.0X3	T51.0X4	—	—
Acaricide	T60.8X1	T60.8X2	T60.8X3	T60.8X4	—	—
Acebutolol	T44.7X1	T44.7X2	T44.7X3	T44.7X4	T44.7X5	T44.7X6
Acecarbromal	T42.6X1	T42.6X2	T42.6X3	T42.6X4	T42.6X5	T42.6X6
Aceclidine	T44.1X1	T44.1X2	T44.1X3	T44.1X4	T44.1X5	T44.1X6
Acedapsone	T37.0X1	T37.0X2	T37.0X3	T37.0X4	T37.0X5	T37.0X6
Acefylline piperazine	T48.6X1	T48.6X2	T48.6X3	T48.6X4	T48.6X5	T48.6X6
Acemorphan	T40.2X1	T40.2X2	T40.2X3	T40.2X4	T40.2X5	T40.2X6
Acenocoumarin	T45.511	T45.512	T45.513	T45.514	T45.515	T45.516
Acenocoumarol	T45.511	T45.512	T45.513	T45.514	T45.515	T45.516
Acepifylline	T48.6X1	T48.6X2	T48.6X3	T48.6X4	T48.6X5	T48.6X6
Acepromazine	T43.3X1	T43.3X2	T43.3X3	T43.3X4	T43.3X5	T43.3X6
Acesulfamethoxy-pyridazine	T37.0X1	T37.0X2	T37.0X3	T37.0X4	T37.0X5	T37.0X6
Acetal	T52.8X1	T52.8X2	T52.8X3	T52.8X4	—	—
Acetaldehyde (vapor)	T52.8X1	T52.8X2	T52.8X3	T52.8X4	—	—
liquid	T65.891	T65.892	T65.893	T65.894	—	—
P-Acetamidophenol	T39.1X1	T39.1X2	T39.1X3	T39.1X4	T39.1X5	T39.1X6
Acetaminophen	T39.1X1	T39.1X2	T39.1X3	T39.1X4	T39.1X5	T39.1X6
Acetaminosalol	T39.1X1	T39.1X2	T39.1X3	T39.1X4	T39.1X5	T39.1X6
Acetanilide	T39.1X1	T39.1X2	T39.1X3	T39.1X4	T39.1X5	T39.1X6
Acetarsol	T37.3X1	T37.3X2	T37.3X3	T37.3X4	T37.3X5	T37.3X6
Acetazolamide	T50.2X1	T50.2X2	T50.2X3	T50.2X4	T50.2X5	T50.2X6
Acetiamine	T45.2X1	T45.2X2	T45.2X3	T45.2X4	T45.2X5	T45.2X6
Acetic						
acid	T54.2X1	T54.2X2	T54.2X3	T54.2X4	—	—
with sodium acetate (ointment)	T49.3X1	T49.3X2	T49.3X3	T49.3X4	T49.3X5	T49.3X6
ester (solvent) (vapor)	T52.8X1	T52.8X2	T52.8X3	T52.8X4	—	—
irrigating solution	T50.3X1	T50.3X2	T50.3X3	T50.3X4	T50.3X5	T50.3X6
medicinal (lotion)	T49.2X1	T49.2X2	T49.2X3	T49.2X4	T49.2X5	T49.2X6
anhydride	T65.891	T65.892	T65.893	T65.894	—	—
ether (vapor)	T52.8X1	T52.8X2	T52.8X3	T52.8X4	—	—
Acetohexamide	T38.3X1	T38.3X2	T38.3X3	T38.3X4	T38.3X5	T38.3X6
Acetohydroxamic acid	T50.991	T50.992	T50.993	T50.994	T50.995	T50.996
Acetomenaphthone	T45.7X1	T45.7X2	T45.7X3	T45.7X4	T45.7X5	T45.7X6
Acetomorphine	T40.1X1	T40.1X2	T40.1X3	T40.1X4	—	—
Acetone (oils)	T52.4X1	T52.4X2	T52.4X3	T52.4X4	—	—
chlorinated	T52.4X1	T52.4X2	T52.4X3	T52.4X4	—	—
vapor	T52.4X1	T52.4X2	T52.4X3	T52.4X4	—	—
Acetonitrile	T52.8X1	T52.8X2	T52.8X3	T52.8X4	—	—
Acetophenazine	T43.3X1	T43.3X2	T43.3X3	T43.3X4	T43.3X5	T43.3X6
Acetophenetedin	T39.1X1	T39.1X2	T39.1X3	T39.1X4	T39.1X5	T39.1X6
Acetophenone	T52.4X1	T52.4X2	T52.4X3	T52.4X4	—	—
Acetorphine	T40.2X1	T40.2X2	T40.2X3	T40.2X4	—	—
Acetosulfone (sodium)	T37.1X1	T37.1X2	T37.1X3	T37.1X4	T37.1X5	T37.1X6
Acetrizoate (sodium)	T50.8X1	T50.8X2	T50.8X3	T50.8X4	T50.8X5	T50.8X6
Acetrizoic acid	T50.8X1	T50.8X2	T50.8X3	T50.8X4	T50.8X5	T50.8X6
Acetyl						
bromide	T53.6X1	T53.6X2	T53.6X3	T53.6X4	—	—
chloride	T53.6X1	T53.6X2	T53.6X3	T53.6X4	—	—
Acetylcarbromal	T42.6X1	T42.6X2	T42.6X3	T42.6X4	T42.6X5	T42.6X6
Acetylcholine						
chloride	T44.1X1	T44.1X2	T44.1X3	T44.1X4	T44.1X5	T44.1X6
derivative	T44.1X1	T44.1X2	T44.1X3	T44.1X4	T44.1X5	T44.1X6
Acetylcysteine	T48.4X1	T48.4X2	T48.4X3	T48.4X4	T48.4X5	T48.4X6
Acetyldigitoxin	T46.0X1	T46.0X2	T46.0X3	T46.0X4	T46.0X5	T46.0X6
Acetyldigoxin	T46.0X1	T46.0X2	T46.0X3	T46.0X4	T46.0X5	T46.0X6
Acetyldihydrocodeine	T40.2X1	T40.2X2	T40.2X3	T40.2X4	—	—
Acetyldihydroco-deinone	T40.2X1	T40.2X2	T40.2X3	T40.2X4	—	—
Acetylene (gas)	T59.891	T59.892	T59.893	T59.894	—	—
dichloride	T53.6X1	T53.6X2	T53.6X3	T53.6X4	—	—
incomplete combustion of	T58.11	T58.12	T58.13	T58.14	—	—
industrial	T59.891	T59.892	T59.893	T59.894	—	—
tetrachloride	T53.6X1	T53.6X2	T53.6X3	T53.6X4	—	—
vapor	T53.6X1	T53.6X2	T53.6X3	T53.6X4	—	—
Acetylpheneturide	T42.6X1	T42.6X2	T42.6X3	T42.6X4	T42.6X5	T42.6X6
Acetylphenylhydra-zine	T39.8X1	T39.8X2	T39.8X3	T39.8X4	T39.8X5	T39.8X6
Acetylsalicylic acid (salts)	T39.011	T39.012	T39.013	T39.014	T39.015	T39.016
enteric coated	T39.011	T39.012	T39.013	T39.014	T39.015	T39.016
Acetylsulfamethoxy-pyridazine	T37.0X1	T37.0X2	T37.0X3	T37.0X4	T37.0X5	T37.0X6
Achromycin	T36.4X1	T36.4X2	T36.4X3	T36.4X4	T36.4X5	T36.4X6
ophthalmic preparation	T49.5X1	T49.5X2	T49.5X3	T49.5X4	T49.5X5	T49.5X6
topical NEC	T49.0X1	T49.0X2	T49.0X3	T49.0X4	T49.0X5	T49.0X6
Aciclovir	T37.5X1	T37.5X2	T37.5X3	T37.5X4	T37.5X5	T37.5X6
Acid (corrosive) NEC	T54.2X1	T54.2X2	T54.2X3	T54.2X4	—	—
Acidifying agent NEC	T50.901	T50.902	T50.903	T50.904	T50.905	T50.906

Substance	Poisoning, Accidental (unintentional)	Poisoning, Intentional self-harm	Poisoning, Assault	Poisoning, Undetermined	Adverse effect	Underdosing
Acipimox	T46.6X1	T46.6X2	T46.6X3	T46.6X4	T46.6X5	T46.6X6
Acitretin	T50.991	T50.992	T50.993	T50.994	T50.995	T50.996
Aclarubicin	T45.1X1	T45.1X2	T45.1X3	T45.1X4	T45.1X5	T45.1X6
Aclatonium napadisilate	T48.1X1	T48.1X2	T48.1X3	T48.1X4	T48.1X5	T48.1X6
Aconite (wild)	T46.991	T46.992	T46.993	T46.994	T46.995	T46.996
Aconitine	T46.991	T46.992	T46.993	T46.994	T46.995	T46.996
Aconitum ferox	T46.991	T46.992	T46.993	T46.994	T46.995	T46.996
Acridine	T65.6X1	T65.6X2	T65.6X3	T65.6X4	—	—
vapor	T59.891	T59.892	T59.893	T59.894	—	—
Acriflavine	T37.91	T37.92	T37.93	T37.94	T37.95	T37.96
Acriflavinium chloride	T49.0X1	T49.0X2	T49.0X3	T49.0X4	T49.0X5	T49.0X6
Acrinol	T49.0X1	T49.0X2	T49.0X3	T49.0X4	T49.0X5	T49.0X6
Acrisorcin	T49.0X1	T49.0X2	T49.0X3	T49.0X4	T49.0X5	T49.0X6
Acrivastine	T45.0X1	T45.0X2	T45.0X3	T45.0X4	T45.0X5	T45.0X6
Acrolein (gas)	T59.891	T59.892	T59.893	T59.894	—	—
liquid	T54.1X1	T54.1X2	T54.1X3	T54.1X4		
Acrylamide	T65.891	T65.892	T65.893	T65.894	—	—
Acrylic resin	T49.3X1	T49.3X2	T49.3X3	T49.3X4	T49.3X5	T49.3X6
Acrylonitrile	T65.891	T65.892	T65.893	T65.894	—	—
Actaea spicata	T62.2X1	T62.2X2	T62.2X3	T62.2X4		
berry	T62.1X1	T62.1X2	T62.1X3	T62.1X4		
Acterol	T37.3X1	T37.3X2	T37.3X3	T37.3X4	T37.3X5	T37.3X6
ACTH	T38.811	T38.812	T38.813	T38.814	T38.815	T38.816
Actinomycin C	T45.1X1	T45.1X2	T45.1X3	T45.1X4	T45.1X5	T45.1X6
Actinomycin D	T45.1X1	T45.1X2	T45.1X3	T45.1X4	T45.1X5	T45,1X6
Activated charcoal—see also Charcoal, medicinal	T47.6X1	T47.6X2	T47.6X3	T47.6X4	T47.6X5	T47.6X6
Acyclovir	T37.5X1	T37.5X2	T37.5X3	T37.5X4	T37.5X5	T37.5X6
Adenine	T45.2X1	T45.2X2	T45.2X3	T45.2X4	T45.2X5	T45.2X6
arabinoside	T37.5X1	T37.5X2	T37.5X3	T37.5X4	T37.5X5	T37.5X6
Adenosine (phosphate)	T46.2X1	T46.2X2	T46.2X3	T46.2X4	T46.2X5	T46.2X6
ADH	T38.891	T38.892	T38.893	T38.894	T38.895	T38.896
Adhesive NEC	T65.891	T65.892	T65.893	T65.894	—	—
Adicillin	T36.0X1	T36.0X2	T36.0X3	T36.0X4	T36.0X5	T36.0X6
Adiphenine	T44.3X1	T44.3X2	T44.3X3	T44.3X4	T44.3X5	T44.3X6
Adipiodone	T50.8X1	T50.8X2	T50.8X3	T50.8X4	T50.8X5	T50.8X6
Adjunct, pharmaceutical	T50.901	T50.902	T50.903	T50.904	T50.905	T50.906
Adrenal (extract, cortex or medulla) (glucocorticoids) (hormones) (mineralocorticoids)	T38.0X1	T38.0X2	T38.0X3	T38.0X4	T38.0X5	T38.0X6
ENT agent	T49.6X1	T49.6X2	T49.6X3	T49.6X4	T49.6X5	T49.6X6
ophthalmic preparation	T49.5X1	T49.5X2	T49.5X3	T49.5X4	T49.5X5	T49.5X6
topical NEC	T49.0X1	T49.0X2	T49.0X3	T49.0X4	T49.0X5	T49.0X6
Adrenaline	T44.5X1	T44.5X2	T44.5X3	T44.5X4	T44.5X5	T44.5X6
Adrenalin—see Adrenaline						
Adrenergic NEC	T44.901	T44.902	T44.903	T44.904	T44.905	T44.906
blocking agent NEC	T44.8X1	T44.8X2	T44.8X3	T44.8X4	T44.8X5	T44.8X6
beta, heart	T44.7X1	T44.7X2	T44.7X3	T44.7X4	T44.7X5	T44.7X6
specified NEC	T44.991	T44.992	T44.993	T44.994	T44.995	T44.996
Adrenochrome						
(mono) semicarbazone	T46.991	T46.992	T46.993	T46.994	T46.995	T46.996
derivative	T46.991	T46.992	T46.993	T46.994	T46.995	T46.996
Adrenocorticotrophic hormone	T38.811	T38.812	T38.813	T38.814	T38.815	T38.816
Adrenocorticotro-phin	T38.811	T38.812	T38.813	T38.814	T38.815	T38.816
Adriamycin	T45.1X1	T45.1X2	T45.1X3	T45.1X4	T45.1X5	T45.1X6
Aerosol spray NEC	T65.91	T65.92	T65.93	T65.94	—	—
Aerosporin	T36.8X1	T36.8X2	T36.8X3	T36.8X4	T36.8X5	T36.8X6
ENT agent	T49.6X1	T49.6X2	T49.6X3	T49.6X4	T49.6X5	T49.6X6
ophthalmic preparation	T49.5X1	T49.5X2	T49.5X3	T49.5X4	T49.5X5	T49.5X6
topical NEC	T49.0X1	T49.0X2	T49.0X3	T49.0X4	T49.0X5	T49.0X6
Aethusa cynapium	T62.2X1	T62.2X2	T62.2X3	T62.2X4	—	—
Afghanistan black	T40.7X1	T40.7X2	T40.7X3	T40.7X4	T40.7X5	T40.7X6
Aflatoxin	T64.01	T64.02	T64.03	T64.04	—	—
Afloqualone	T42.8X1	T42.8X2	T42.8X3	T42.8X4	T42.8X5	T42.8X6
African boxwood	T62.2X1	T62.2X2	T62.2X3	T62.2X4	—	—
Agar	T47.4X1	T47.4X2	T47.4X3	T47.4X4	T47.4X5	T47.4X6
Agonist						
predominantly						
alpha-adrenoreceptor	T44.4X1	T44.4X2	T44.4X3	T44.4X4	T44.4X5	T44.4X6
beta-adrenoreceptor	T44.5X1	T44.5X2	T44.5X3	T44.5X4	T44.5X5	T44.5X6
Agricultural agent NEC	T65.91	T65.92	T65.93	T65.94	—	—
Agrypnal	T42.3X1	T42.3X2	T42.3X3	T42.3X4	T42.3X5	T42.3X6
AHLG	T50.Z11	T50.Z12	T50.Z13	T50.Z14	T50.Z15	T50.Z16
Air contaminant (s), source/type NOS	T65.91	T65.92	T65.93	T65.94		
Ajmaline	T46.2X1	T46.2X2	T46.2X3	T46.2X4	T46.2X5	T46.2X6
Akee	T62.1X1	T62.1X2	T62.1X3	T62.1X4	—	—
Akrinol	T49.0X1	T49.0X2	T49.0X3	T49.0X4	T49.0X5	T49.0X6
Akritoin	T37.8X1	T37.8X2	T37.8X3	T37.8X4	T37.8X5	T37.8X6
Alacepril	T46.4X1	T46.4X2	T46.4X3	T46.4X4	T46.4X5	T46.4X6
Alantolactone	T37.4X1	T37.4X2	T37.4X3	T37.4X4	T37.4X5	T37.4X6
Albamycin	T36.8X1	T36.8X2	T36.8X3	T36.8X4	T36.8X5	T36.8X6
Albendazole	T37.4X1	T37.4X2	T37.4X3	T37.4X4	T37.4X5	T37.4X6
Albumin						
bovine	T45.8X1	T45.8X2	T45.8X3	T45.8X4	T45.8X5	T45.8X6
human serum	T45.8X1	T45.8X2	T45.8X3	T45.8X4	T45.8X5	T45.8X6
salt-poor	T45.8X1	T45.8X2	T45.8X3	T45.8X4	T45.8X5	T45.8X6
normal human serum	T45.8X1	T45.8X2	T45.8X3	T45.8X4	T45.8X5	T45.8X6
Albuterol	T48.6X1	T48.6X2	T48.6X3	T48.6X4	T48.6X5	T48.6X6
Albutoin	T42.0X1	T42.0X2	T42.0X3	T42.0X4	T42.0X5	T42.0X6
Alclometasone	T49.0X1	T49.0X2	T49.0X3	T49.0X4	T49.0X5	T49.0X6
Alcohol	T51.91	T51.92	T51.93	T51.94	—	—
absolute	T51.0X1	T51.0X2	T51.0X3	T51.0X4		
beverage	T51.0X1	T51.0X2	T51.0X3	T51.0X4		
allyl	T51.8X1	T51.8X2	T51.8X3	T51.8X4		
amyl	T51.3X1	T51.3X2	T51.3X3	T51.3X4		
antifreeze	T51.1X1	T51.1X2	T51.1X3	T51.1X4		
beverage	T51.0X1	T51.0X2	T51.0X3	T51.0X4		
butyl	T51.3X1	T51.3X2	T51.3X3	T51.3X4		

Substance	Poisoning, Accidental (unintentional)	Poisoning, Intentional self-harm	Poisoning, Assault	Poisoning, Undetermined	Adverse effect	Underdosing
Alcohol — *Continued*						
dehydrated	T51.0X1	T51.0X2	T51.0X3	T51.0X4	—	—
beverage	T51.0X1	T51.0X2	T51.0X3	T51.0X4	—	—
denatured	T51.0X1	T51.0X2	T51.0X3	T51.0X4	—	—
deterrent NEC	T50.6X1	T50.6X2	T50.6X3	T50.6X4	T50.6X5	T50.6X6
diagnostic (gastric function)	T50.8X1	T50.8X2	T50.8X3	T50.8X4	T50.8X5	T50.8X6
ethyl	T51.0X1	T51.0X2	T51.0X3	T51.0X4	—	—
beverage	T51.0X1	T51.0X2	T51.0X3	T51.0X4	—	—
grain	T51.0X1	T51.0X2	T51.0X3	T51.0X4	—	—
beverage	T51.0X1	T51.0X2	T51.0X3	T51.0X4	—	—
industrial	T51.0X1	T51.0X2	T51.0X3	T51.0X4	—	—
isopropyl	T51.2X1	T51.2X2	T51.2X3	T51.2X4	—	—
methyl	T51.1X1	T51.1X2	T51.1X3	T51.1X4	—	—
preparation for consumption	T51.0X1	T51.0X2	T51.0X3	T51.0X4	—	—
propyl	T51.3X1	T51.3X2	T51.3X3	T51.3X4	—	—
secondary	T51.2X1	T51.2X2	T51.2X3	T51.2X4	—	—
radiator	T51.1X1	T51.1X2	T51.1X3	T51.1X4	—	—
rubbing	T51.2X1	T51.2X2	T51.2X3	T51.2X4	—	—
specified type NEC	T51.8X1	T51.8X2	T51.8X3	T51.8X4	—	—
surgical	T51.0X1	T51.0X2	T51.0X3	T51.0X4	—	—
vapor (from any type of Alcohol)	T59.891	T59.892	T59.893	T59.894	—	—
wood	T51.1X1	T51.1X2	T51.1X3	T51.1X4	—	—
Alcuronium (chloride)	T48.1X1	T48.1X2	T48.1X3	T48.1X4	T48.1X5	T48.1X6
Aldactone	T50.0X1	T50.0X2	T50.0X3	T50.0X4	T50.0X5	T50.0X6
Aldesulfone sodium	T37.1X1	T37.1X2	T37.1X3	T37.1X4	T37.1X5	T37.1X6
Aldicarb	T60.0X1	T60.0X2	T60.0X3	T60.0X4	—	—
Aldomet	T46.5X1	T46.5X2	T46.5X3	T46.5X4	T46.5X5	T46.5X6
Aldosterone	T50.0X1	T50.0X2	T50.0X3	T50.0X4	T50.0X5	T50.0X6
Aldrin (dust)	T60.1X1	T60.1X2	T60.1X3	T60.1X4	—	—
Aleve—see Naproxen						
Alexitol sodium	T47.1X1	T47.1X2	T47.1X3	T47.1X4	T47.1X5	T47.1X6
Alfacalcidol	T45.2X1	T45.2X2	T45.2X3	T45.2X4	T45.2X5	T45.2X6
Alfadolone	T41.1X1	T41.1X2	T41.1X3	T41.1X4	T41.1X5	T41.1X6
Alfaxalone	T41.1X1	T41.1X2	T41.1X3	T41.1X4	T41.1X5	T41.1X6
Alfentanil	T40.411	T40.412	T40.413	T40.414	T40.415	T40.416
Alfuzosin (hydrochloride)	T44.8X1	T44.8X2	T44.8X3	T44.8X4	T44.8X5	T44.8X6
Algae (harmful) (toxin)	T65.821	T65.822	T65.823	T65.824	—	—
Algeldrate	T47.1X1	T47.1X2	T47.1X3	T47.1X4	T47.1X5	T47.1X6
Algin	T47.8X1	T47.8X2	T47.8X3	T47.8X4	T47.8X5	T47.8X6
Alglucerase	T45.3X1	T45.3X2	T45.3X3	T45.3X4	T45.3X5	T45.3X6
Alidase	T45.3X1	T45.3X2	T45.3X3	T45.3X4	T45.3X5	T45.3X6
Alimemazine	T43.3X1	T43.3X2	T43.3X3	T43.3X4	T43.3X5	T43.3X6
Aliphatic thiocyanates	T65.0X1	T65.0X2	T65.0X3	T65.0X4	—	—
Alizapride	T45.0X1	T45.0X2	T45.0X3	T45.0X4	T45.0X5	T45.0X6
Alkali (caustic)	T54.3X1	T54.3X2	T54.3X3	T54.3X4	—	—
Alkaline antiseptic solution (aromatic)	T49.6X1	T49.6X2	T49.6X3	T49.6X4	T49.6X5	T49.6X6
Alkalinizing agents (medicinal)	T50.901	T50.902	T50.903	T50.904	T50.905	T50.906
Alkalizing agent NEC	T50.901	T50.902	T50.903	T50.904	T50.905	T50.906
Alka-seltzer	T39.011	T39.012	T39.013	T39.014	T39.015	T39.016
Alkavervir	T46.5X1	T46.5X2	T46.5X3	T46.5X4	T46.5X5	T46.5X6
Alkonium (bromide)	T49.0X1	T49.0X2	T49.0X3	T49.0X4	T49.0X5	T49.0X6
Alkylating drug NEC	T45.1X1	T45.1X2	T45.1X3	T45.1X4	T45.1X5	T45.1X6
antimyeloprolifera-tive	T45.1X1	T45.1X2	T45.1X3	T45.1X4	T45.1X5	T45.1X6
lymphatic	T45.1X1	T45.1X2	T45.1X3	T45.1X4	T45.1X5	T45.1X6
Alkylisocyanate	T65.0X1	T65.0X2	T65.0X3	T65.0X4	—	—
Allantoin	T49.4X1	T49.4X2	T49.4X3	T49.4X4	T49.4X5	T49.4X6
Allegron	T43.011	T43.012	T43.013	T43.014	T43.015	T43.016
Allethrin	T49.0X1	T49.0X2	T49.0X3	T49.0X4	T49.0X5	T49.0X6
Allobarbital	T42.3X1	T42.3X2	T42.3X3	T42.3X4	T42.3X5	T42.3X6
Allopurinol	T50.4X1	T50.4X2	T50.4X3	T50.4X4	T50.4X5	T50.4X6
Allyl						
Alcohol	T51.8X1	T51.8X2	T51.8X3	T51.8X4	—	—
disulfide	T46.6X1	T46.6X2	T46.6X3	T46.6X4	T46.6X5	T46.6X6
Allylestrenol	T38.5X1	T38.5X2	T38.5X3	T38.5X4	T38.5X5	T38.5X6
Allylisopropyl-acetylurea	T42.6X1	T42.6X2	T42.6X3	T42.6X4	T42.6X5	T42.6X6
Allylisopropyl-malonylurea	T42.3X1	T42.3X2	T42.3X3	T42.3X4	T42.3X5	T42.3X6
Allylthiourea	T49.3X1	T49.3X2	T49.3X3	T49.3X4	T49.3X5	T49.3X6
Allyltribromide	T42.6X1	T42.6X2	T42.6X3	T42.6X4	T42.6X5	T42.6X6
Allypropymal	T42.3X1	T42.3X2	T42.3X3	T42.3X4	T42.3X5	T42.3X6
Almagate	T47.1X1	T47.1X2	T47.1X3	T47.1X4	T47.1X5	T47.1X6
Almasilate	T47.1X1	T47.1X2	T47.1X3	T47.1X4	T47.1X5	T47.1X6
Almitrine	T50.7X1	T50.7X2	T50.7X3	T50.7X4	T50.7X5	T50.7X6
Aloes	T47.2X1	T47.2X2	T47.2X3	T47.2X4	T47.2X5	T47.2X6
Aloglutamol	T47.1X1	T47.1X2	T47.1X3	T47.1X4	T47.1X5	T47.1X6
Aloin	T47.2X1	T47.2X2	T47.2X3	T47.2X4	T47.2X5	T47.2X6
Aloxidone	T42.2X1	T42.2X2	T42.2X3	T42.2X4	T42.2X5	T42.2X6
Alpha						
acetyldigoxin	T46.0X1	T46.0X2	T46.0X3	T46.0X4	T46.0X5	T46.0X6
adrenergic blocking drug	T44.6X1	T44.6X2	T44.6X3	T44.6X4	T44.6X5	T44.6X6
amylase	T45.3X1	T45.3X2	T45.3X3	T45.3X4	T45.3X5	T45.3X6
tocoferol (acetate)	T45.2X1	T45.2X2	T45.2X3	T45.2X4	T45.2X5	T45.2X6
tocopherol	T45.2X1	T45.2X2	T45.2X3	T45.2X4	T45.2X5	T45.2X6
Alphadolone	T41.1X1	T41.1X2	T41.1X3	T41.1X4	T41.1X5	T41.1X6
Alphaprodine	T40.491	T40.492	T40.493	T40.494	T40.495	T40.496
Alphaxalone	T41.1X1	T41.1X2	T41.1X3	T41.1X4	T41.1X5	T41.1X6
Alprazolam	T42.4X1	T42.4X2	T42.4X3	T42.4X4	T42.4X5	T42.4X6
Alprenolol	T44.7X1	T44.7X2	T44.7X3	T44.7X4	T44.7X5	T44.7X6
Alprostadil	T46.7X1	T46.7X2	T46.7X3	T46.7X4	T46.7X5	T46.7X6
Alsactide	T38.811	T38.812	T38.813	T38.814	T38.815	T38.816
Alseroxylon	T46.5X1	T46.5X2	T46.5X3	T46.5X4	T46.5X5	T46.5X6
Alteplase	T45.611	T45.612	T45.613	T45.614	T45.615	T45.616
Altizide	T50.2X1	T50.2X2	T50.2X3	T50.2X4	T50.2X5	T50.2X6

Substance	Poisoning, Accidental (unintentional)	Poisoning, Intentional self-harm	Poisoning, Assault	Poisoning, Undetermined	Adverse effect	Underdosing
Altretamine	T45.1X1	T45.1X2	T45.1X3	T45.1X4	T45.1X5	T45.1X6
Alum (medicinal)	T49.4X1	T49.4X2	T49.4X3	T49.4X4	T49.4X5	T49.4X6
nonmedicinal (ammonium) (potassium)	T56.891	T56.892	T56.893	T56.894	—	—
Aluminium, aluminum						
acetate	T49.2X1	T49.2X2	T49.2X3	T49.2X4	T49.2X5	T49.2X6
solution	T49.0X1	T49.0X2	T49.0X3	T49.0X4	T49.0X5	T49.0X6
aspirin	T39.011	T39.012	T39.013	T39.014	T39.015	T39.016
bis (acetylsalicylate)	T39.011	T39.012	T39.013	T39.014	T39.015	T39.016
carbonate (gel, basic)	T47.1X1	T47.1X2	T47.1X3	T47.1X4	T47.1X5	T47.1X6
chlorhydroxide-complex	T47.1X1	T47.1X2	T47.1X3	T47.1X4	T47.1X5	T47.1X6
chloride	T49.2X1	T49.2X2	T49.2X3	T49.2X4	T49.2X5	T49.2X6
clofibrate	T46.6X1	T46.6X2	T46.6X3	T46.6X4	T46.6X5	T46.6X6
diacetate	T49.2X1	T49.2X2	T49.2X3	T49.2X4	T49.2X5	T49.2X6
glycinate	T47.1X1	T47.1X2	T47.1X3	T47.1X4	T47.1X5	T47.1X6
hydroxide (gel)	T47.1X1	T47.1X2	T47.1X3	T47.1X4	T47.1X5	T47.1X6
hydroxide-magnesium carb. gel	T47.1X1	T47.1X2	T47.1X3	T47.1X4	T47.1X5	T47.1X6
magnesium silicate	T47.1X1	T47.1X2	T47.1X3	T47.1X4	T47.1X5	T47.1X6
nicotinate	T46.7X1	T46.7X2	T46.7X3	T46.7X4	T46.7X5	T46.7X6
ointment (surgical) (topical)	T49.3X1	T49.3X2	T49.3X3	T49.3X4	T49.3X5	T49.3X6
phosphate	T47.1X1	T47.1X2	T47.1X3	T47.1X4	T47.1X5	T47.1X6
salicylate	T39.091	T39.092	T39.093	T39.094	T39.095	T39.096
silicate	T47.1X1	T47.1X2	T47.1X3	T47.1X4	T47.1X5	T47.1X6
sodium silicate	T47.1X1	T47.1X2	T47.1X3	T47.1X4	T47.1X5	T47.1X6
subacetate	T49.2X1	T49.2X2	T49.2X3	T49.2X4	T49.2X5	T49.2X6
sulfate	T49.0X1	T49.0X2	T49.0X3	T49.0X4	T49.0X5	T49.0X6
tannate	T47.6X1	T47.6X2	T47.6X3	T47.6X4	T47.6X5	T47.6X6
topical NEC	T49.3X1	T49.3X2	T49.3X3	T49.3X4	T49.3X5	T49.3X6
Alurate	T42.3X1	T42.3X2	T42.3X3	T42.3X4	T42.3X5	T42.3X6
Alverine	T44.3X1	T44.3X2	T44.3X3	T44.3X4	T44.3X5	T44.3X6
Alvodine	T40.2X1	T40.2X2	T40.2X3	T40.2X4	T40.2X5	T40.2X6
Amanita phalloides	T62.0X1	T62.0X2	T62.0X3	T62.0X4	—	—
Amanitine	T62.0X1	T62.0X2	T62.0X3	T62.0X4	—	—
Amantadine	T42.8X1	T42.8X2	T42.8X3	T42.8X4	T42.8X5	T42.8X6
Ambazone	T49.6X1	T49.6X2	T49.6X3	T49.6X4	T49.6X5	T49.6X6
Ambenonium (chloride)	T44.0X1	T44.0X2	T44.0X3	T44.0X4	T44.0X5	T44.0X6
Ambroxol	T48.4X1	T48.4X2	T48.4X3	T48.4X4	T48.4X5	T48.4X6
Ambuphylline	T48.6X1	T48.6X2	T48.6X3	T48.6X4	T48.6X5	T48.6X6
Ambutonium bromide	T44.3X1	T44.3X2	T44.3X3	T44.3X4	T44.3X5	T44.3X6
Amcinonide	T49.0X1	T49.0X2	T49.0X3	T49.0X4	T49.0X5	T49.0X6
Amdinocilline	T36.0X1	T36.0X2	T36.0X3	T36.0X4	T36.0X5	T36.0X6
Ametazole	T50.8X1	T50.8X2	T50.8X3	T50.8X4	T50.8X5	T50.8X6
Amethocaine	T41.3X1	T41.3X2	T41.3X3	T41.3X4	T41.3X5	T41.3X6
regional	T41.3X1	T41.3X2	T41.3X3	T41.3X4	T41.3X5	T41.3X6
spinal	T41.3X1	T41.3X2	T41.3X3	T41.3X4	T41.3X5	T41.3X6
Amethopterin	T45.1X1	T45.1X2	T45.1X3	T45.1X4	T45.1X5	T45.1X6
Amezinium metilsulfate	T44.991	T44.992	T44.993	T44.994	T44.995	T44.996

Substance	Poisoning, Accidental (unintentional)	Poisoning, Intentional self-harm	Poisoning, Assault	Poisoning, Undetermined	Adverse effect	Underdosing
Amfebutamone	T43.291	T43.292	T43.293	T43.294	T43.295	T43.296
Amfepramone	T50.5X1	T50.5X2	T50.5X3	T50.5X4	T50.5X5	T50.5X6
Amfetamine	T43.621	T43.622	T43.623	T43.624	T43.625	T43.626
Amfetaminil	T43.621	T43.622	T43.623	T43.624	T43.625	T43.626
Amfomycin	T36.8X1	T36.8X2	T36.8X3	T36.8X4	T36.8X5	T36.8X6
Amidefrine mesilate	T48.5X1	T48.5X2	T48.5X3	T48.5X4	T48.5X5	T48.5X6
Amidone	T40.3X1	T40.3X2	T40.3X3	T40.3X4	T40.3X5	T40.3X6
Amidopyrine	T39.2X1	T39.2X2	T39.2X3	T39.2X4	T39.2X5	T39.2X6
Amidotrizoate	T50.8X1	T50.8X2	T50.8X3	T50.8X4	T50.8X5	T50.8X6
Amiflamine	T43.1X1	T43.1X2	T43.1X3	T43.1X4	T43.1X5	T43.1X6
Amikacin	T36.5X1	T36.5X2	T36.5X3	T36.5X4	T36.5X5	T36.5X6
Amikhelline	T46.3X1	T46.3X2	T46.3X3	T46.3X4	T46.3X5	T46.3X6
Amiloride	T50.2X1	T50.2X2	T50.2X3	T50.2X4	T50.2X5	T50.2X6
Aminacrine	T49.0X1	T49.0X2	T49.0X3	T49.0X4	T49.0X5	T49.0X6
Amineptine	T43.011	T43.012	T43.013	T43.014	T43.015	T43.016
Aminitrozole	T37.3X1	T37.3X2	T37.3X3	T37.3X4	T37.3X5	T37.3X6
Amino acids	T50.3X1	T50.3X2	T50.3X3	T50.3X4	T50.3X5	T50.3X6
Aminoacetic acid (derivatives)	T50.3X1	T50.3X2	T50.3X3	T50.3X4	T50.3X5	T50.3X6
Aminoacridine	T49.0X1	T49.0X2	T49.0X3	T49.0X4	T49.0X5	T49.0X6
Aminobenzoic acid(-p)	T49.3X1	T49.3X2	T49.3X3	T49.3X4	T49.3X5	T49.3X6
4-Aminobutyric acid	T43.8X1	T43.8X2	T43.8X3	T43.8X4	T43.8X5	T43.8X6
Aminocaproic acid	T45.621	T45.622	T45.623	T45.624	T45.625	T45.626
Aminoethyl-isothiourium	T45.8X1	T45.8X2	T45.8X3	T45.8X4	T45.8X5	T45.8X6
Aminofenazone	T39.2X1	T39.2X2	T39.2X3	T39.2X4	T39.2X5	T39.2X6
Aminoglutethimide	T45.1X1	T45.1X2	T45.1X3	T45.1X4	T45.1X5	T45.1X6
Aminohippuric acid	T50.8X1	T50.8X2	T50.8X3	T50.8X4	T50.8X5	T50.8X6
Aminomethylbenzoic acid	T45.691	T45.692	T45.693	T45.694	T45.695	T45.696
Aminometradine	T50.2X1	T50.2X2	T50.2X3	T50.2X4	T50.2X5	T50.2X6
Aminopentamide	T44.3X1	T44.3X2	T44.3X3	T44.3X4	T44.3X5	T44.3X6
Aminophenazone	T39.2X1	T39.2X2	T39.2X3	T39.2X4	T39.2X5	T39.2X6
Aminophenol	T54.0X1	T54.0X2	T54.0X3	T54.0X4	—	—
4-Aminophenol derivatives	T39.1X1	T39.1X2	T39.1X3	T39.1X4	T39.1X5	T39.1X6
Aminophenylpyri-done	T43.591	T43.592	T43.593	T43.594	T43.595	T43.596
Aminophylline	T48.6X1	T48.6X2	T48.6X3	T48.6X4	T48.6X5	T48.6X6
Aminopterin sodium	T45.1X1	T45.1X2	T45.1X3	T45.1X4	T45.1X5	T45.1X6
Aminopyrine	T39.2X1	T39.2X2	T39.2X3	T39.2X4	T39.2X5	T39.2X6
8-Aminoquinoline drugs	T37.2X1	T37.2X2	T37.2X3	T37.2X4	T37.2X5	T37.2X6
Aminorex	T50.5X1	T50.5X2	T50.5X3	T50.5X4	T50.5X5	T50.5X6
Aminosalicylic acid	T37.1X1	T37.1X2	T37.1X3	T37.1X4	T37.1X5	T37.1X6
Aminosalylum	T37.1X1	T37.1X2	T37.1X3	T37.1X4	T37.1X5	T37.1X6
Amiodarone	T46.2X1	T46.2X2	T46.2X3	T46.2X4	T46.2X5	T46.2X6
Amiphenazole	T50.7X1	T50.7X2	T50.7X3	T50.7X4	T50.7X5	T50.7X6
Amiquinsin	T46.5X1	T46.5X2	T46.5X3	T46.5X4	T46.5X5	T46.5X6
Amisometradine	T50.2X1	T50.2X2	T50.2X3	T50.2X4	T50.2X5	T50.2X6
Amisulpride	T43.591	T43.592	T43.593	T43.594	T43.595	T43.596
Amitriptyline	T43.011	T43.012	T43.013	T43.014	T43.015	T43.016
Amitriptylinoxide	T43.011	T43.012	T43.013	T43.014	T43.015	T43.016

Substance	Poisoning, Accidental (unintentional)	Poisoning, Intentional self-harm	Poisoning, Assault	Poisoning, Undetermined	Adverse effect	Underdosing
Amlexanox	T48.6X1	T48.6X2	T48.6X3	T48.6X4	T48.6X5	T48.6X6
Ammonia (fumes) (gas) (vapor)	T59.891	T59.892	T59.893	T59.894	—	—
aromatic spirit	T48.991	T48.992	T48.993	T48.994	T48.995	T48.996
liquid (household)	T54.3X1	T54.3X2	T54.3X3	T54.3X4	—	—
Ammoniated mercury	T49.0X1	T49.0X2	T49.0X3	T49.0X4	T49.0X5	T49.0X6
Ammonium						
acid tartrate	T49.5X1	T49.5X2	T49.5X3	T49.5X4	T49.5X5	T49.5X6
bromide	T42.6X1	T42.6X2	T42.6X3	T42.6X4	T42.6X5	T42.6X6
carbonate	T54.3X1	T54.3X2	T54.3X3	T54.3X4	—	—
chloride	T50.991	T50.992	T50.993	T50.994	T50.995	T50.996
expectorant	T48.4X1	T48.4X2	T48.4X3	T48.4X4	T48.4X5	T48.4X6
compounds (household) NEC	T54.3X1	T54.3X2	T54.3X3	T54.3X4	—	—
fumes (any usage)	T59.891	T59.892	T59.893	T59.894	—	—
industrial	T54.3X1	T54.3X2	T54.3X3	T54.3X4	—	—
ichthyosulronate	T49.4X1	T49.4X2	T49.4X3	T49.4X4	T49.4X5	T49.4X6
mandelate	T37.91	T37.92	T37.93	T37.94	T37.95	T37.96
sulfamate	T60.3X1	T60.3X2	T60.3X3	T60.3X4	—	—
sulfonate resin	T47.8X1	T47.8X2	T47.8X3	T47.8X4	T47.8X5	T47.8X6
Amobarbital (sodium)	T42.3X1	T42.3X2	T42.3X3	T42.3X4	T42.3X5	T42.3X6
Amodiaquine	T37.2X1	T37.2X2	T37.2X3	T37.2X4	T37.2X5	T37.2X6
Amopyroquin(e)	T37.2X1	T37.2X2	T37.2X3	T37.2X4	T37.2X5	T37.2X6
Amoxapine	T43.011	T43.012	T43.013	T43.014	T43.015	T43.016
Amoxicillin	T36.0X1	T36.0X2	T36.0X3	T36.0X4	T36.0X5	T36.0X6
Amperozide	T43.591	T43.592	T43.593	T43.594	T43.595	T43.596
Amphenidone	T43.591	T43.592	T43.593	T43.594	T43.595	T43.596
Amphetamine NEC	T43.621	T43.622	T43.623	T43.624	T43.625	T43.626
Amphomycin	T36.8X1	T36.8X2	T36.8X3	T36.8X4	T36.8X5	T36.8X6
Amphotalide	T37.4X1	T37.4X2	T37.4X3	T37.4X4	T37.4X5	T37.4X6
Amphotericin B	T36.7X1	T36.7X2	T36.7X3	T36.7X4	T36.7X5	T36.7X6
topical	T49.0X1	T49.0X2	T49.0X3	T49.0X4	T49.0X5	T49.0X6
Ampicillin	T36.0X1	T36.0X2	T36.0X3	T36.0X4	T36.0X5	T36.0X6
Amprotropine	T44.3X1	T44.3X2	T44.3X3	T44.3X4	T44.3X5	T44.3X6
Amsacrine	T45.1X1	T45.1X2	T45.1X3	T45.1X4	T45.1X5	T45.1X6
Amygdaline	T62.2X1	T62.2X2	T62.2X3	T62.2X4	—	—
Amyl						
acetate	T52.8X1	T52.8X2	T52.8X3	T52.8X4	—	—
vapor	T59.891	T59.892	T59.893	T59.894	—	—
alcohol	T51.3X1	T51.3X2	T51.3X3	T51.3X4	—	—
chloride	T53.6X1	T53.6X2	T53.6X3	T53.6X4	—	—
formate	T52.8X1	T52.8X2	T52.8X3	T52.8X4	—	—
nitrite	T46.3X1	T46.3X2	T46.3X3	T46.3X4	T46.3X5	T46.3X6
propionate	T65.891	T65.892	T65.893	T65.894	—	—
Amylase	T47.5X1	T47.5X2	T47.5X3	T47.5X4	T47.5X5	T47.5X6
Amyleine, regional	T41.3X1	T41.3X2	T41.3X3	T41.3X4	T41.3X5	T41.3X6
Amylene						
dichloride	T53.6X1	T53.6X2	T53.6X3	T53.6X4	—	—
hydrate	T51.3X1	T51.3X2	T51.3X3	T51.3X4	—	—
Amylmetacresol	T49.6X1	T49.6X2	T49.6X3	T49.6X4	T49.6X5	T49.6X6
Amylobarbitone	T42.3X1	T42.3X2	T42.3X3	T42.3X4	T42.3X5	T42.3X6

Substance	Poisoning, Accidental (unintentional)	Poisoning, Intentional self-harm	Poisoning, Assault	Poisoning, Undetermined	Adverse effect	Underdosing
Amylocaine, regional	T41.3X1	T41.3X2	T41.3X3	T41.3X4	T41.3X5	T41.3X6
infiltration (subcutaneous)	T41.3X1	T41.3X2	T41.3X3	T41.3X4	T41.3X5	T41.3X6
nerve block (peripheral) (plexus)	T41.3X1	T41.3X2	T41.3X3	T41.3X4	T41.3X5	T41.3X6
spinal	T41.3X1	T41.3X2	T41.3X3	T41.3X4	T41.3X5	T41.3X6
topical (surface)	T41.3X1	T41.3X2	T41.3X3	T41.3X4	T41.3X5	T41.3X6
Amylopectin	T47.6X1	T47.6X2	T47.6X3	T47.6X4	T47.6X5	T47.6X6
Amytal (sodium)	T42.3X1	T42.3X2	T42.3X3	T42.3X4	T42.3X5	T42.3X6
Anabolic steroid	T38.7X1	T38.7X2	T38.7X3	T38.7X4	T38.7X5	T38.7X6
Analeptic NEC	T50.7X1	T50.7X2	T50.7X3	T50.7X4	T50.7X5	T50.7X6
Analgesic	T39.91	T39.92	T39.93	T39.94	T39.95	T39.96
anti-inflammatory NEC	T39.91	T39.92	T39.93	T39.94	T39.95	T39.96
propionic acid derivative	T39.311	T39.312	T39.313	T39.314	T39.315	T39.316
antirheumatic NEC	T39.4X1	T39.4X2	T39.4X3	T39.4X4	T39.4X5	T39.4X6
aromatic NEC	T39.1X1	T39.1X2	T39.1X3	T39.1X4	T39.1X5	T39.1X6
narcotic NEC	T40.601	T40.602	T40.603	T40.604	T40.605	T40.606
combination	T40.601	T40.602	T40.603	T40.604	T40.605	T40.606
obstetric	T40.601	T40.602	T40.603	T40.604	T40.605	T40.606
non-narcotic NEC	T39.91	T39.92	T39.93	T39.94	T39.95	T39.96
combination	T39.91	T39.92	T39.93	T39.94	T39.95	T39.96
pyrazole	T39.2X1	T39.2X2	T39.2X3	T39.2X4	T39.2X5	T39.2X6
specified NEC	T39.8X1	T39.8X2	T39.8X3	T39.8X4	T39.8X5	T39.8X6
Analgin	T39.2X1	T39.2X2	T39.2X3	T39.2X4	T39.2X5	T39.2X6
Anamirta cocculus	T62.1X1	T62.1X2	T62.1X3	T62.1X4	—	—
Ancillin	T36.0X1	T36.0X2	T36.0X3	T36.0X4	T36.0X5	T36.0X6
Ancrod	T45.691	T45.692	T45.693	T45.694	T45.695	T45.696
Androgen	T38.7X1	T38.7X2	T38.7X3	T38.7X4	T38.7X5	T38.7X6
Androgen-estrogen mixture	T38.7X1	T38.7X2	T38.7X3	T38.7X4	T38.7X5	T38.7X6
Androstalone	T38.7X1	T38.7X2	T38.7X3	T38.7X4	T38.7X5	T38.7X6
Androstanolone	T38.7X1	T38.7X2	T38.7X3	T38.7X4	T38.7X5	T38.7X6
Androsterone	T38.7X1	T38.7X2	T38.7X3	T38.7X4	T38.7X5	T38.7X6
Anemone pulsatilla	T62.2X1	T62.2X2	T62.2X3	T62.2X4	—	—
Anesthesia						
caudal	T41.3X1	T41.3X2	T41.3X3	T41.3X4	T41.3X5	T41.3X6
endotracheal	T41.0X1	T41.0X2	T41.0X3	T41.0X4	T41.0X5	T41.0X6
epidural	T41.3X1	T41.3X2	T41.3X3	T41.3X4	T41.3X5	T41.3X6
inhalation	T41.0X1	T41.0X2	T41.0X3	T41.0X4	T41.0X5	T41.0X6
local	T41.3X1	T41.3X2	T41.3X3	T41.3X4	T41.3X5	T41.3X6
mucosal	T41.3X1	T41.3X2	T41.3X3	T41.3X4	T41.3X5	T41.3X6
muscle relaxation	T48.1X1	T48.1X2	T48.1X3	T48.1X4	T48.1X5	T48.1X6
nerve blocking	T41.3X1	T41.3X2	T41.3X3	T41.3X4	T41.3X5	T41.3X6
plexus blocking	T41.3X1	T41.3X2	T41.3X3	T41.3X4	T41.3X5	T41.3X6
potentiated	T41.201	T41.202	T41.203	T41.204	T41.205	T41.206
rectal	T41.201	T41.202	T41.203	T41.204	T41.205	T41.206
general	T41.201	T41.202	T41.203	T41.204	T41.205	T41.206
local	T41.3X1	T41.3X2	T41.3X3	T41.3X4	T41.3X5	T41.3X6
regional	T41.3X1	T41.3X2	T41.3X3	T41.3X4	T41.3X5	T41.3X6
surface	T41.3X1	T41.3X2	T41.3X3	T41.3X4	T41.3X5	T41.3X6

Substance	Poisoning, Accidental (unintentional)	Poisoning, Intentional self-harm	Poisoning, Assault	Poisoning, Undetermined	Adverse effect	Underdosing
Anesthetic NEC —see also Anesthesia	T41.41	T41.42	T41.43	T41.44	T41.45	T41.46
with muscle relaxant	T41.201	T41.202	T41.203	T41.204	T41.205	T41.206
general	T41.201	T41.202	T41.203	T41.204	T41.205	T41.206
local	T41.3X1	T41.3X2	T41.3X3	T41.3X4	T41.3X5	T41.3X6
gaseous NEC	T41.0X1	T41.0X2	T41.0X3	T41.0X4	T41.0X5	T41.0X6
general NEC	T41.201	T41.202	T41.203	T41.204	T41.205	T41.206
halogenated hydrocarbon derivatives NEC	T41.0X1	T41.0X2	T41.0X3	T41.0X4	T41.0X5	T41.0X6
infiltration NEC	T41.3X1	T41.3X2	T41.3X3	T41.3X4	T41.3X5	T41.3X6
intravenous NEC	T41.1X1	T41.1X2	T41.1X3	T41.1X4	T41.1X5	T41.1X6
local NEC	T41.3X1	T41.3X2	T41.3X3	T41.3X4	T41.3X5	T41.3X6
rectal	T41.201	T41.202	T41.203	T41.204	T41.205	T41.206
general	T41.201	T41.202	T41.203	T41.204	T41.205	T41.206
local	T41.3X1	T41.3X2	T41.3X3	T41.3X4	T41.3X5	T41.3X6
regional NEC	T41.3X1	T41.3X2	T41.3X3	T41.3X4	T41.3X5	T41.3X6
spinal NEC	T41.3X1	T41.3X2	T41.3X3	T41.3X4	T41.3X5	T41.3X6
thiobarbiturate	T41.1X1	T41.1X2	T41.1X3	T41.1X4	T41.1X5	T41.1X6
topical	T41.3X1	T41.3X2	T41.3X3	T41.3X4	T41.3X5	T41.3X6
Aneurine	T45.2X1	T45.2X2	T45.2X3	T45.2X4	T45.2X5	T45.2X6
Angio-Conray	T50.8X1	T50.8X2	T50.8X3	T50.8X4	T50.8X5	T50.8X6
Angiotensin	T44.5X1	T44.5X2	T44.5X3	T44.5X4	T44.5X5	T44.5X6
Angiotensinamide	T44.991	T44.992	T44.993	T44.994	T44.995	T44.996
Anhydrohydroxy-progesterone	T38.5X1	T38.5X2	T38.5X3	T38.5X4	T38.5X5	T38.5X6
Anhydron	T50.2X1	T50.2X2	T50.2X3	T50.2X4	T50.2X5	T50.2X6
Anileridine	T40.491	T40.492	T40.493	T40.494	T40.495	T40.496
Aniline (dye) (liquid)	T65.3X1	T65.3X2	T65.3X3	T65.3X4	—	—
analgesic	T39.1X1	T39.1X2	T39.1X3	T39.1X4	T39.1X5	T39.1X6
derivatives, therapeutic NEC	T39.1X1	T39.1X2	T39.1X3	T39.1X4	T39.1X5	T39.1X6
vapor	T65.3X1	T65.3X2	T65.3X3	T65.3X4	—	—
Aniscoropine	T44.3X1	T44.3X2	T44.3X3	T44.3X4	T44.3X5	T44.3X6
Anise oil	T47.5X1	T47.5X2	T47.5X3	T47.5X4	T47.5X5	T47.5X6
Anisidine	T65.3X1	T65.3X2	T65.3X3	T65.3X4	—	—
Anisindione	T45.511	T45.512	T45.513	T45.514	T45.515	T45.516
Anisotropine methyl-bromide	T44.3X1	T44.3X2	T44.3X3	T44.3X4	T44.3X5	T44.3X6
Anistreplase	T45.611	T45.612	T45.613	T45.614	T45.615	T45.616
Anorexiant (central)	T50.5X1	T50.5X2	T50.5X3	T50.5X4	T50.5X5	T50.5X6
Anorexic agents	T50.5X1	T50.5X2	T50.5X3	T50.5X4	T50.5X5	T50.5X6
Ansamycin	T36.6X1	T36.6X2	T36.6X3	T36.6X4	T36.6X5	T36.6X6
Ant (bite) (sting)	T63.421	T63.422	T63.423	T63.424	—	—
Ant poison—see Insecticide						
Antabuse	T50.6X1	T50.6X2	T50.6X3	T50.6X4	T50.6X5	T50.6X6
Antacid NEC	T47.1X1	T47.1X2	T47.1X3	T47.1X4	T47.1X5	T47.1X6
Antagonist						
Aldosterone	T50.0X1	T50.0X2	T50.0X3	T50.0X4	T50.0X5	T50.0X6
alpha-adrenoreceptor	T44.6X1	T44.6X2	T44.6X3	T44.6X4	T44.6X5	T44.6X6
anticoagulant	T45.7X1	T45.7X2	T45.7X3	T45.7X4	T45.7X5	T45.7X6

Substance	Poisoning, Accidental (unintentional)	Poisoning, Intentional self-harm	Poisoning, Assault	Poisoning, Undetermined	Adverse effect	Underdosing
Antagonist — *Continued*						
beta-adrenoreceptor	T44.7X1	T44.7X2	T44.7X3	T44.7X4	T44.7X5	T44.7X6
extrapyramidal NEC	T44.3X1	T44.3X2	T44.3X3	T44.3X4	T44.3X5	T44.3X6
folic acid	T45.1X1	T45.1X2	T45.1X3	T45.1X4	T45.1X5	T45.1X6
H2 receptor	T47.0X1	T47.0X2	T47.0X3	T47.0X4	T47.0X5	T47.0X6
heavy metal	T45.8X1	T45.8X2	T45.8X3	T45.8X4	T45.8X5	T45.8X6
narcotic analgesic	T50.7X1	T50.7X2	T50.7X3	T50.7X4	T50.7X5	T50.7X6
opiate	T50.7X1	T50.7X2	T50.7X3	T50.7X4	T50.7X5	T50.7X6
pyrimidine	T45.1X1	T45.1X2	T45.1X3	T45.1X4	T45.1X5	T45.1X6
serotonin	T46.5X1	T46.5X2	T46.5X3	T46.5X4	T46.5X5	T46.5X6
Antazolin(e)	T45.0X1	T45.0X2	T45.0X3	T45.0X4	T45.0X5	T45.0X6
Anterior pituitary hormone NEC	T38.811	T38.812	T38.813	T38.814	T38.815	T38.816
Anthelmintic NEC	T37.4X1	T37.4X2	T37.4X3	T37.4X4	T37.4X5	T37.4X6
Anthiolimine	T37.4X1	T37.4X2	T37.4X3	T37.4X4	T37.4X5	T37.4X6
Anthralin	T49.4X1	T49.4X2	T49.4X3	T49.4X4	T49.4X5	T49.4X6
Anthramycin	T45.1X1	T45.1X2	T45.1X3	T45.1X4	T45.1X5	T45.1X6
Antiadrenergic NEC	T44.8X1	T44.8X2	T44.8X3	T44.8X4	T44.8X5	T44.8X6
Antiallergic NEC	T45.0X1	T45.0X2	T45.0X3	T45.0X4	T45.0X5	T45.0X6
Anti-anemic (drug) (preparation)	T45.8X1	T45.8X2	T45.8X3	T45.8X4	T45.8X5	T45.8X6
Antiandrogen NEC	T38.6X1	T38.6X2	T38.6X3	T38.6X4	T38.6X5	T38.6X6
Antianxiety drug NEC	T43.501	T43.502	T43.503	T43.504	T43.505	T43.506
Antiaris toxicaria	T65.891	T65.892	T65.893	T65.894	—	—
Antiarteriosclerotic drug	T46.6X1	T46.6X2	T46.6X3	T46.6X4	T46.6X5	T46.6X6
Antiasthmatic drug NEC	T48.6X1	T48.6X2	T48.6X3	T48.6X4	T48.6X5	T48.6X6
Antibiotic NEC	T36.91	T36.92	T36.93	T36.94	T36.95	T36.96
aminoglycoside	T36.5X1	T36.5X2	T36.5X3	T36.5X4	T36.5X5	T36.5X6
anticancer	T45.1X1	T45.1X2	T45.1X3	T45.1X4	T45.1X5	T45.1X6
antifungal	T36.7X1	T36.7X2	T36.7X3	T36.7X4	T36.7X5	T36.7X6
antimycobacterial	T36.5X1	T36.5X2	T36.5X3	T36.5X4	T36.5X5	T36.5X6
antineoplastic	T45.1X1	T45.1X2	T45.1X3	T45.1X4	T45.1X5	T45.1X6
cephalosporin (group)	T36.1X1	T36.1X2	T36.1X3	T36.1X4	T36.1X5	T36.1X6
chloramphenicol (group)	T36.2X1	T36.2X2	T36.2X3	T36.2X4	T36.2X5	T36.2X6
ENT	T49.6X1	T49.6X2	T49.6X3	T49.6X4	T49.6X5	T49.6X6
eye	T49.5X1	T49.5X2	T49.5X3	T49.5X4	T49.5X5	T49.5X6
fungicidal (local)	T49.0X1	T49.0X2	T49.0X3	T49.0X4	T49.0X5	T49.0X6
intestinal	T36.8X1	T36.8X2	T36.8X3	T36.8X4	T36.8X5	T36.8X6
b-lactam NEC	T36.1X1	T36.1X2	T36.1X3	T36.1X4	T36.1X5	T36.1X6
local	T49.0X1	T49.0X2	T49.0X3	T49.0X4	T49.0X5	T49.0X6
macrolides	T36.3X1	T36.3X2	T36.3X3	T36.3X4	T36.3X5	T36.3X6
polypeptide	T36.8X1	T36.8X2	T36.8X3	T36.8X4	T36.8X5	T36.8X6
specified NEC	T36.8X1	T36.8X2	T36.8X3	T36.8X4	T36.8X5	T36.8X6
tetracycline (group)	T36.4X1	T36.4X2	T36.4X3	T36.4X4	T36.4X5	T36.4X6
throat	T49.6X1	T49.6X2	T49.6X3	T49.6X4	T49.6X5	T49.6X6
Anticancer agents NEC	T45.1X1	T45.1X2	T45.1X3	T45.1X4	T45.1X5	T45.1X6
Anticholesterolemic drug NEC	T46.6X1	T46.6X2	T46.6X3	T46.6X4	T46.6X5	T46.6X6
Anticholinergic NEC	T44.3X1	T44.3X2	T44.3X3	T44.3X4	T44.3X5	T44.3X6

Substance	Poisoning, Accidental (unintentional)	Poisoning, Intentional self-harm	Poisoning, Assault	Poisoning, Undetermined	Adverse effect	Underdosing
Anticholinesterase	T44.0X1	T44.0X2	T44.0X3	T44.0X4	T44.0X5	T44.0X6
organophosphorus	T44.0X1	T44.0X2	T44.0X3	T44.0X4	T44.0X5	T44.0X6
insecticide	T60.0X1	T60.0X2	T60.0X3	T60.0X4	—	—
nerve gas	T59.891	T59.892	T59.893	T59.894	—	—
reversible	T44.0X1	T44.0X2	T44.0X3	T44.0X4	T44.0X5	T44.0X6
ophthalmological	T49.5X1	T49.5X2	T49.5X3	T49.5X4	T49.5X5	T49.5X6
Anticoagulant NEC	T45.511	T45.512	T45.513	T45.514	T45.515	T45.516
Antagonist	T45.7X1	T45.7X2	T45.7X3	T45.7X4	T45.7X5	T45.7X6
Anti-common-cold drug NEC	T48.5X1	T48.5X2	T48.5X3	T48.5X4	T48.5X5	T48.5X6
Anticonvulsant	T42.71	T42.72	T42.73	T42.74	T42.75	T42.76
barbiturate	T42.3X1	T42.3X2	T42.3X3	T42.3X4	T42.3X5	T42.3X6
combination (with barbiturate)	T42.3X1	T42.3X2	T42.3X3	T42.3X4	T42.3X5	T42.3X6
hydantoin	T42.0X1	T42.0X2	T42.0X3	T42.0X4	T42.0X5	T42.0X6
hypnotic NEC	T42.6X1	T42.6X2	T42.6X3	T42.6X4	T42.6X5	T42.6X6
oxazolidinedione	T42.2X1	T42.2X2	T42.2X3	T42.2X4	T42.2X5	T42.2X6
pyrimidinedione	T42.6X1	T42.6X2	T42.6X3	T42.6X4	T42.6X5	T42.6X6
specified NEC	T42.6X1	T42.6X2	T42.6X3	T42.6X4	T42.6X5	T42.6X6
succinimide	T42.2X1	T42.2X2	T42.2X3	T42.2X4	T42.2X5	T42.2X6
Anti-D immuno-globulin (human)	T50.Z11	T50.Z12	T50.Z13	T50.Z14	T50.Z15	T50.Z16
Antidepressant	T43.201	T43.202	T43.203	T43.204	T43.205	T43.206
monoamine oxidase inhibitor	T43.1X1	T43.1X2	T43.1X3	T43.1X4	T43.1X5	T43.1X6
selective serotonin norepinephrine reuptake inhibitor	T43.211	T43.212	T43.213	T43.214	T43.215	T43.216
selective serotonin reuptake inhibitor	T43.221	T43.222	T43.223	T43.224	T43.225	T43.226
specified NEC	T43.291	T43.292	T43.293	T43.294	T43.295	T43.296
tetracyclic	T43.021	T43.022	T43.023	T43.024	T43.025	T43.026
triazolopyridine	T43.211	T43.212	T43.213	T43.214	T43.215	T43.216
tricyclic	T43.011	T43.012	T43.013	T43.014	T43.015	T43.016
Antidiabetic NEC	T38.3X1	T38.3X2	T38.3X3	T38.3X4	T38.3X5	T38.3X6
biguanide	T38.3X1	T38.3X2	T38.3X3	T38.3X4	T38.3X5	T38.3X6
and sulfonyl combined	T38.3X1	T38.3X2	T38.3X3	T38.3X4	T38.3X5	T38.3X6
combined	T38.3X1	T38.3X2	T38.3X3	T38.3X4	T38.3X5	T38.3X6
sulfonylurea	T38.3X1	T38.3X2	T38.3X3	T38.3X4	T38.3X5	T38.3X6
Antidiarrheal drug NEC	T47.6X1	T47.6X2	T47.6X3	T47.6X4	T47.6X5	T47.6X6
absorbent	T47.6X1	T47.6X2	T47.6X3	T47.6X4	T47.6X5	T47.6X6
Antidiphtheria serum	T50.Z11	T50.Z12	T50.Z13	T50.Z14	T50.Z15	T50.Z16
Antidiuretic hormone	T38.891	T38.892	T38.893	T38.894	T38.895	T38.896
Antidote NEC	T50.6X1	T50.6X2	T50.6X3	T50.6X4	T50.6X5	T50.6X6
heavy metal	T45.8X1	T45.8X2	T45.8X3	T45.8X4	T45.8X5	T45.8X6
Antidysrhythmic NEC	T46.2X1	T46.2X2	T46.2X3	T46.2X4	T46.2X5	T46.2X6
Antiemetic drug	T45.0X1	T45.0X2	T45.0X3	T45.0X4	T45.0X5	T45.0X6
Antiepilepsy agent	T42.71	T42.72	T42.73	T42.74	T42.75	T42.76
combination	T42.5X1	T42.5X2	T42.5X3	T42.5X4	T42.5X5	T42.5X6
mixed	T42.5X1	T42.5X2	T42.5X3	T42.5X4	T42.5X5	T42.5X6
specified, NEC	T42.6X1	T42.6X2	T42.6X3	T42.6X4	T42.6X5	T42.6X6
Antiestrogen NEC	T38.6X1	T38.6X2	T38.6X3	T38.6X4	T38.6X5	T38.6X6
Antifertility pill	T38.4X1	T38.4X2	T38.4X3	T38.4X4	T38.4X5	T38.4X6
Antifibrinolytic drug	T45.621	T45.622	T45.623	T45.624	T45.625	T45.626
Antifilarial drug	T37.4X1	T37.4X2	T37.4X3	T37.4X4	T37.4X5	T37.4X6
Antiflatulent	T47.5X1	T47.5X2	T47.5X3	T47.5X4	T47.5X5	T47.5X6
Antifreeze	T65.91	T65.92	T65.93	T65.94	—	—
alcohol	T51.1X1	T51.1X2	T51.1X3	T51.1X4	—	—
ethylene glycol	T51.8X1	T51.8X2	T51.8X3	T51.8X4	—	—
Antifungal						
antibiotic (systemic)	T36.7X1	T36.7X2	T36.7X3	T36.7X4	T36.7X5	T36.7X6
anti-infective NEC	T37.91	T37.92	T37.93	T37.94	T37.95	T37.96
disinfectant, local	T49.0X1	T49.0X2	T49.0X3	T49.0X4	T49.0X5	T49.0X6
nonmedicinal (spray)	T60.3X1	T60.3X2	T60.3X3	T60.3X4	—	—
topical	T49.0X1	T49.0X2	T49.0X3	T49.0X4	T49.0X5	T49.0X6
Anti-gastric-secretion drug NEC	T47.1X1	T47.1X2	T47.1X3	T47.1X4	T47.1X5	T47.1X6
Antigonadotrophin NEC	T38.6X1	T38.6X2	T38.6X3	T38.6X4	T38.6X5	T38.6X6
Antihallucinogen	T43.501	T43.502	T43.503	T43.504	T43.505	T43.506
Antihelmintics	T37.4X1	T37.4X2	T37.4X3	T37.4X4	T37.4X5	T37.4X6
Antihemophilic						
factor	T45.8X1	T45.8X2	T45.8X3	T45.8X4	T45.8X5	T45.8X6
fraction	T45.8X1	T45.8X2	T45.8X3	T45.8X4	T45.8X5	T45.8X6
globulin concentrate	T45.7X1	T45.7X2	T45.7X3	T45.7X4	T45.7X5	T45.7X6
human plasma	T45.8X1	T45.8X2	T45.8X3	T45.8X4	T45.8X5	T45.8X6
plasma, dried	T45.7X1	T45.7X2	T45.7X3	T45.7X4	T45.7X5	T45.7X6
Antihemorrhoidal preparation	T49.2X1	T49.2X2	T49.2X3	T49.2X4	T49.2X5	T49.2X6
Antiheparin drug	T45.7X1	T45.7X2	T45.7X3	T45.7X4	T45.7X5	T45.7X6
Antihistamine	T45.0X1	T45.0X2	T45.0X3	T45.0X4	T45.0X5	T45.0X6
Antihookworm drug	T37.4X1	T37.4X2	T37.4X3	T37.4X4	T37.4X5	T37.4X6
Anti-human lymphocytic globulin	T50.Z11	T50.Z12	T50.Z13	T50.Z14	T50.Z15	T50.Z16
Antihyperlipidemic drug	T46.6X1	T46.6X2	T46.6X3	T46.6X4	T46.6X5	T46.6X6
Antihypertensive drug NEC	T46.5X1	T46.5X2	T46.5X3	T46.5X4	T46.5X5	T46.5X6
Anti-infective NEC	T37.91	T37.92	T37.93	T37.94	T37.95	T37.96
anthelmintic	T37.4X1	T37.4X2	T37.4X3	T37.4X4	T37.4X5	T37.4X6
antibiotics	T36.91	T36.92	T36.93	T36.94	T36.95	T36.96
specified NEC	T36.8X1	T36.8X2	T36.8X3	T36.8X4	T36.8X5	T36.8X6
antimalarial	T37.2X1	T37.2X2	T37.2X3	T37.2X4	T37.2X5	T37.2X6
antimycobacterial NEC	T37.1X1	T37.1X2	T37.1X3	T37.1X4	T37.1X5	T37.1X6
antibiotics	T36.5X1	T36.5X2	T36.5X3	T36.5X4	T36.5X5	T36.5X6
antiprotozoal NEC	T37.3X1	T37.3X2	T37.3X3	T37.3X4	T37.3X5	T37.3X6
blood	T37.2X1	T37.2X2	T37.2X3	T37.2X4	T37.2X5	T37.2X6
antiviral	T37.5X1	T37.5X2	T37.5X3	T37.5X4	T37.5X5	T37.5X6
arsenical	T37.8X1	T37.8X2	T37.8X3	T37.8X4	T37.8X5	T37.8X6
bismuth, local	T49.0X1	T49.0X2	T49.0X3	T49.0X4	T49.0X5	T49.0X6
ENT	T49.6X1	T49.6X2	T49.6X3	T49.6X4	T49.6X5	T49.6X6
eye NEC	T49.5X1	T49.5X2	T49.5X3	T49.5X4	T49.5X5	T49.5X6
heavy metals NEC	T37.8X1	T37.8X2	T37.8X3	T37.8X4	T37.8X5	T37.8X6

Substance	Poisoning, Accidental (unintentional)	Poisoning, Intentional self-harm	Poisoning, Assault	Poisoning, Undetermined	Adverse effect	Underdosing
Anti-infective NEC — *Continued*						
local NEC	T49.0X1	T49.0X2	T49.0X3	T49.0X4	T49.0X5	T49.0X6
specified NEC	T49.0X1	T49.0X2	T49.0X3	T49.0X4	T49.0X5	T49.0X6
mixed	T37.91	T37.92	T37.93	T37.94	T37.95	T37.96
ophthalmic preparation	T49.5X1	T49.5X2	T49.5X3	T49.5X4	T49.5X5	T49.5X6
topical NEC	T49.0X1	T49.0X2	T49.0X3	T49.0X4	T49.0X5	T49.0X6
Anti-inflammatory drug NEC	T39.391	T39.392	T39.393	T39.394	T39.395	T39.396
local	T49.0X1	T49.0X2	T49.0X3	T49.0X4	T49.0X5	T49.0X6
nonsteroidal NEC	T39.391	T39.392	T39.393	T39.394	T39.395	T39.396
propionic acid derivative	T39.311	T39.312	T39.313	T39.314	T39.315	T39.316
specified NEC	T39.391	T39.392	T39.393	T39.394	T39.395	T39.396
Antikaluretic	T50.3X1	T50.3X2	T50.3X3	T50.3X4	T50.3X5	T50.3X6
Antiknock (tetraethyl lead)	T56.0X1	T56.0X2	T56.0X3	T56.0X4	—	—
Antilipemic drug NEC	T46.6X1	T46.6X2	T46.6X3	T46.6X4	T46.6X5	T46.6X6
Antimalarial	T37.2X1	T37.2X2	T37.2X3	T37.2X4	T37.2X5	T37.2X6
prophylactic NEC	T37.2X1	T37.2X2	T37.2X3	T37.2X4	T37.2X5	T37.2X6
pyrimidine derivative	T37.2X1	T37.2X2	T37.2X3	T37.2X4	T37.2X5	T37.2X6
Antimetabolite	T45.1X1	T45.1X2	T45.1X3	T45.1X4	T45.1X5	T45.1X6
Antimitotic agent	T45.1X1	T45.1X2	T45.1X3	T45.1X4	T45.1X5	T45.1X6
Antimony (compounds) (vapor)NEC	T56.891	T56.892	T56.893	T56.894	—	—
anti-infectives	T37.8X1	T37.8X2	T37.8X3	T37.8X4	T37.8X5	T37.8X6
dimercaptosuccinate	T37.3X1	T37.3X2	T37.3X3	T37.3X4	T37.3X5	T37.3X6
hydride	T56.891	T56.892	T56.893	T56.894	—	—
pesticide (vapor)	T60.8X1	T60.8X2	T60.8X3	T60.8X4	—	—
potassium (sodium) tartrate	T37.8X1	T37.8X2	T37.8X3	T37.8X4	T37.8X5	T37.8X6
sodium dimercaptosuccinate	T37.3X1	T37.3X2	T37.3X3	T37.3X4	T37.3X5	T37.3X6
tartrated	T37.8X1	T37.8X2	T37.8X3	T37.8X4	T37.8X5	T37.8X6
Antimuscarinic NEC	T44.3X1	T44.3X2	T44.3X3	T44.3X4	T44.3X5	T44.3X6
Antimycobacterial drug NEC	T37.1X1	T37.1X2	T37.1X3	T37.1X4	T37.1X5	T37.1X6
antibiotics	T36.5X1	T36.5X2	T36.5X3	T36.5X4	T36.5X5	T36.5X6
combination	T37.1X1	T37.1X2	T37.1X3	T37.1X4	T37.1X5	T37.1X6
Antinausea drug	T45.0X1	T45.0X2	T45.0X3	T45.0X4	T45.0X5	T45.0X6
Antinematode drug	T37.4X1	T37.4X2	T37.4X3	T37.4X4	T37.4X5	T37.4X6
Antineoplastic NEC	T45.1X1	T45.1X2	T45.1X3	T45.1X4	T45.1X5	T45.1X6
alkaloidal	T45.1X1	T45.1X2	T45.1X3	T45.1X4	T45.1X5	T45.1X6
antibiotics	T45.1X1	T45.1X2	T45.1X3	T45.1X4	T45.1X5	T45.1X6
combination	T45.1X1	T45.1X2	T45.1X3	T45.1X4	T45.1X5	T45.1X6
estrogen	T38.5X1	T38.5X2	T38.5X3	T38.5X4	T38.5X5	T38.5X6
steroid	T38.7X1	T38.7X2	T38.7X3	T38.7X4	T38.7X5	T38.7X6
Antiparasitic drug (systemic)	T37.91	T37.92	T37.93	T37.94	T37.95	T37.96
local	T49.0X1	T49.0X2	T49.0X3	T49.0X4	T49.0X5	T49.0X6
specified NEC	T37.8X1	T37.8X2	T37.8X3	T37.8X4	T37.8X5	T37.8X6
Antiparkinsonism drug NEC	T42.8X1	T42.8X2	T42.8X3	T42.8X4	T42.8X5	T42.8X6
Antiperspirant NEC	T49.2X1	T49.2X2	T49.2X3	T49.2X4	T49.2X5	T49.2X6
Antiphlogistic NEC	T39.4X1	T39.4X2	T39.4X3	T39.4X4	T39.4X5	T39.4X6
Antiplatyhelmintic drug	T37.4X1	T37.4X2	T37.4X3	T37.4X4	T37.4X5	T37.4X6
Antiprotozoal drug NEC	T37.3X1	T37.3X2	T37.3X3	T37.3X4	T37.3X5	T37.3X6
blood	T37.2X1	T37.2X2	T37.2X3	T37.2X4	T37.2X5	T37.2X6
local	T49.0X1	T49.0X2	T49.0X3	T49.0X4	T49.0X5	T49.0X6
Antipruritic drug NEC	T49.1X1	T49.1X2	T49.1X3	T49.1X4	T49.1X5	T49.1X6
Antipsychotic drug	T43.501	T43.502	T43.503	T43.504	T43.505	T43.506
specified NEC	T43.591	T43.592	T43.593	T43.594	T43.595	T43.596
Antipyretic	T39.91	T39.92	T39.93	T39.94	T39.95	T39.96
specified NEC	T39.8X1	T39.8X2	T39.8X3	T39.8X4	T39.8X5	T39.8X6
Antipyrine	T39.2X1	T39.2X2	T39.2X3	T39.2X4	T39.2X5	T39.2X6
Antirabies hyperimmune serum	T50.Z11	T50.Z12	T50.Z13	T50.Z14	T50.Z15	T50.Z16
Antirheumatic NEC	T39.4X1	T39.4X2	T39.4X3	T39.4X4	T39.4X5	T39.4X6
Antirigidity drug NEC	T42.8X1	T42.8X2	T42.8X3	T42.8X4	T42.8X5	T42.8X6
Antischistosomal drug	T37.4X1	T37.4X2	T37.4X3	T37.4X4	T37.4X5	T37.4X6
Antiscorpion sera	T50.Z11	T50.Z12	T50.Z13	T50.Z14	T50.Z15	T50.Z16
Antiseborrheics	T49.4X1	T49.4X2	T49.4X3	T49.4X4	T49.4X5	T49.4X6
Antiseptics (external) (medicinal)	T49.0X1	T49.0X2	T49.0X3	T49.0X4	T49.0X5	T49.0X6
Antistine	T45.0X1	T45.0X2	T45.0X3	T45.0X4	T45.0X5	T45.0X6
Antitapeworm drug	T37.4X1	T37.4X2	T37.4X3	T37.4X4	T37.4X5	T37.4X6
Antitetanus immunoglobulin	T50.Z11	T50.Z12	T50.Z13	T50.Z14	T50.Z15	T50.Z16
Antithrombotic	T45.521	T45.522	T45.523	T45.524	T45.525	T45.526
Antithyroid drug NEC	T38.2X1	T38.2X2	T38.2X3	T38.2X4	T38.2X5	T38.2X6
Antitoxin	T50.Z11	T50.Z12	T50.Z13	T50.Z14	T50.Z15	T50.Z16
diphtheria	T50.Z11	T50.Z12	T50.Z13	T50.Z14	T50.Z15	T50.Z16
gas gangrene	T50.Z11	T50.Z12	T50.Z13	T50.Z14	T50.Z15	T50.Z16
tetanus	T50.Z11	T50.Z12	T50.Z13	T50.Z14	T50.Z15	T50.Z16
Antitrichomonal drug	T37.3X1	T37.3X2	T37.3X3	T37.3X4	T37.3X5	T37.3X6
Antituberculars	T37.1X1	T37.1X2	T37.1X3	T37.1X4	T37.1X5	T37.1X6
antibiotics	T36.5X1	T36.5X2	T36.5X3	T36.5X4	T36.5X5	T36.5X6
Antitussive NEC	T48.3X1	T48.3X2	T48.3X3	T48.3X4	T48.3X5	T48.3X6
codeine mixture	T40.2X1	T40.2X2	T40.2X3	T40.2X4	T40.2X5	T40.2X6
opiate	T40.2X1	T40.2X2	T40.2X3	T40.2X4	T40.2X5	T40.2X6
Antivaricose drug	T46.8X1	T46.8X2	T46.8X3	T46.8X4	T46.8X5	T46.8X6
Antivenin, antivenom (sera)	T50.Z11	T50.Z12	T50.Z13	T50.Z14	T50.Z15	T50.Z16
crotaline	T50.Z11	T50.Z12	T50.Z13	T50.Z14	T50.Z15	T50.Z16
spider bite	T50.Z11	T50.Z12	T50.Z13	T50.Z14	T50.Z15	T50.Z16
Antivertigo drug	T45.0X1	T45.0X2	T45.0X3	T45.0X4	T45.0X5	T45.0X6
Antiviral drug NEC	T37.5X1	T37.5X2	T37.5X3	T37.5X4	T37.5X5	T37.5X6
eye	T49.5X1	T49.5X2	T49.5X3	T49.5X4	T49.5X5	T49.5X6
Antiwhipworm drug	T37.4X1	T37.4X2	T37.4X3	T37.4X4	T37.4X5	T37.4X6
Antrol—see also by specific chemical substance	T60.91	T60.92	T60.93	T60.94	—	—
fungicide	T60.91	T60.92	T60.93	T60.94	—	—
ANTU (alpha naphthylthiourea)	T60.4X1	T60.4X2	T60.4X3	T60.4X4	—	—
Apalcillin	T36.0X1	T36.0X2	T36.0X3	T36.0X4	T36.0X5	T36.0X6

Substance	Poisoning, Accidental (unintentional)	Poisoning, Intentional self-harm	Poisoning, Assault	Poisoning, Undetermined	Adverse effect	Underdosing
APC	T48.5X1	T48.5X2	T48.5X3	T48.5X4	T48.5X5	T48.5X6
Aplonidine	T44.4X1	T44.4X2	T44.4X3	T44.4X4	T44.4X5	T44.4X6
Apomorphine	T47.7X1	T47.7X2	T47.7X3	T47.7X4	T47.7X5	T47.7X6
Appetite depressants, central	T50.5X1	T50.5X2	T50.5X3	T50.5X4	T50.5X5	T50.5X6
Apraclonidine (hydrochloride)	T44.4X1	T44.4X2	T44.4X3	T44.4X4	T44.4X5	T44.4X6
Apresoline	T46.5X1	T46.5X2	T46.5X3	T46.5X4	T46.5X5	T46.5X6
Aprindine	T46.2X1	T46.2X2	T46.2X3	T46.2X4	T46.2X5	T46.2X6
Aprobarbital	T42.3X1	T42.3X2	T42.3X3	T42.3X4	T42.3X5	T42.3X6
Apronalide	T42.6X1	T42.6X2	T42.6X3	T42.6X4	T42.6X5	T42.6X6
Aprotinin	T45.621	T45.622	T45.623	T45.624	T45.625	T45.626
Aptocaine	T41.3X1	T41.3X2	T41.3X3	T41.3X4	T41.3X5	T41.3X6
Aqua fortis	T54.2X1	T54.2X2	T54.2X3	T54.2X4	—	—
Ara-A	T37.5X1	T37.5X2	T37.5X3	T37.5X4	T37.5X5	T37.5X6
Ara-C	T45.1X1	T45.1X2	T45.1X3	T45.1X4	T45.1X5	T45.1X6
Arachis oil	T49.3X1	T49.3X2	T49.3X3	T49.3X4	T49.3X5	T49.3X6
cathartic	T47.4X1	T47.4X2	T47.4X3	T47.4X4	T47.4X5	T47.4X6
Aralen	T37.2X1	T37.2X2	T37.2X3	T37.2X4	T37.2X5	T37.2X6
Arecoline	T44.1X1	T44.1X2	T44.1X3	T44.1X4	T44.1X5	T44.1X6
Arginine	T50.991	T50.992	T50.993	T50.994	T50.995	T50.996
glutamate	T50.991	T50.992	T50.993	T50.994	T50.995	T50.996
Argyrol	T49.0X1	T49.0X2	T49.0X3	T49.0X4	T49.0X5	T49.0X6
ENT agent	T49.6X1	T49.6X2	T49.6X3	T49.6X4	T49.6X5	T49.6X6
ophthalmic preparation	T49.5X1	T49.5X2	T49.5X3	T49.5X4	T49.5X5	T49.5X6
Aristocort	T38.0X1	T38.0X2	T38.0X3	T38.0X4	T38.0X5	T38.0X6
ENT agent	T49.6X1	T49.6X2	T49.6X3	T49.6X4	T49.6X5	T49.6X6
ophthalmic preparation	T49.5X1	T49.5X2	T49.5X3	T49.5X4	T49.5X5	T49.5X6
topical NEC	T49.0X1	T49.0X2	T49.0X3	T49.0X4	T49.0X5	T49.0X6
Aromatics, corrosive	T54.1X1	T54.1X2	T54.1X3	T54.1X4	—	—
disinfectants	T54.1X1	T54.1X2	T54.1X3	T54.1X4	—	—
Arsenate of lead	T57.0X1	T57.0X2	T57.0X3	T57.0X4	—	—
herbicide	T57.0X1	T57.0X2	T57.0X3	T57.0X4	—	—
Arsenic, arsenicals (compounds) (dust) (vapor) NEC	T57.0X1	T57.0X2	T57.0X3	T57.0X4	—	—
anti-infectives	T37.8X1	T37.8X2	T37.8X3	T37.8X4	T37.8X5	T37.8X6
pesticide (dust) (fumes)	T57.0X1	T57.0X2	T57.0X3	T57.0X4	—	—
Arsine (gas)	T57.0X1	T57.0X2	T57.0X3	T57.0X4	—	—
Arsphenamine (silver)	T37.8X1	T37.8X2	T37.8X3	T37.8X4	T37.8X5	T37.8X6
Arsthinol	T37.3X1	T37.3X2	T37.3X3	T37.3X4	T37.3X5	T37.3X6
Artane	T44.3X1	T44.3X2	T44.3X3	T44.3X4	T44.3X5	T44.3X6
Arthropod (venomous) NEC	T63.481	T63.482	T63.483	T63.484	—	—
Articaine	T41.3X1	T41.3X2	T41.3X3	T41.3X4	T41.3X5	T41.3X6
Asbestos	T57.8X1	T57.8X2	T57.8X3	T57.8X4	—	—
Ascaridole	T37.4X1	T37.4X2	T37.4X3	T37.4X4	T37.4X5	T37.4X6
Ascorbic acid	T45.2X1	T45.2X2	T45.2X3	T45.2X4	T45.2X5	T45.2X6
Asiaticoside	T49.0X1	T49.0X2	T49.0X3	T49.0X4	T49.0X5	T49.0X6
Asparaginase	T45.1X1	T45.1X2	T45.1X3	T45.1X4	T45.1X5	T45.1X6
Aspidium (oleoresin)	T37.4X1	T37.4X2	T37.4X3	T37.4X4	T37.4X5	T37.4X6

Substance	Poisoning, Accidental (unintentional)	Poisoning, Intentional self-harm	Poisoning, Assault	Poisoning, Undetermined	Adverse effect	Underdosing
Aspirin (aluminum) (soluble)	T39.011	T39.012	T39.013	T39.014	T39.015	T39.016
Aspoxicillin	T36.0X1	T36.0X2	T36.0X3	T36.0X4	T36.0X5	T36.0X6
Astemizole	T45.0X1	T45.0X2	T45.0X3	T45.0X4	T45.0X5	T45.0X6
Astringent (local)	T49.2X1	T49.2X2	T49.2X3	T49.2X4	T49.2X5	T49.2X6
specified NEC	T49.2X1	T49.2X2	T49.2X3	T49.2X4	T49.2X5	T49.2X6
Astromicin	T36.5X1	T36.5X2	T36.5X3	T36.5X4	T36.5X5	T36.5X6
Ataractic drug NEC	T43.501	T43.502	T43.503	T43.504	T43.505	T43.506
Atenolol	T44.7X1	T44.7X2	T44.7X3	T44.7X4	T44.7X5	T44.7X6
Atonia drug, intestinal	T47.4X1	T47.4X2	T47.4X3	T47.4X4	T47.4X5	T47.4X6
Atophan	T50.4X1	T50.4X2	T50.4X3	T50.4X4	T50.4X5	T50.4X6
Atracurium besilate	T48.1X1	T48.1X2	T48.1X3	T48.1X4	T48.1X5	T48.1X6
Atropine	T44.3X1	T44.3X2	T44.3X3	T44.3X4	T44.3X5	T44.3X6
derivative	T44.3X1	T44.3X2	T44.3X3	T44.3X4	T44.3X5	T44.3X6
methonitrate	T44.3X1	T44.3X2	T44.3X3	T44.3X4	T44.3X5	T44.3X6
Attapulgite	T47.6X1	T47.6X2	T47.6X3	T47.6X4	T47.6X5	T47.6X6
Auramine	T65.891	T65.892	T65.893	T65.894	—	—
dye	T65.6X1	T65.6X2	T65.6X3	T65.6X4	—	—
fungicide	T60.3X1	T60.3X2	T60.3X3	T60.3X4	—	—
Auranofin	T39.4X1	T39.4X2	T39.4X3	T39.4X4	T39.4X5	T39.4X6
Aurantiin	T46.991	T46.992	T46.993	T46.994	T46.995	T46.996
Aureomycin	T36.4X1	T36.4X2	T36.4X3	T36.4X4	T36.4X5	T36.4X6
ophthalmic preparation	T49.5X1	T49.5X2	T49.5X3	T49.5X4	T49.5X5	T49.5X6
topical NEC	T49.0X1	T49.0X2	T49.0X3	T49.0X4	T49.0X5	T49.0X6
Aurothioglucose	T39.4X1	T39.4X2	T39.4X3	T39.4X4	T39.4X5	T39.4X6
Aurothioglycanide	T39.4X1	T39.4X2	T39.4X3	T39.4X4	T39.4X5	T39.4X6
Aurothiomalate sodium	T39.4X1	T39.4X2	T39.4X3	T39.4X4	T39.4X5	T39.4X6
Aurotioprol	T39.4X1	T39.4X2	T39.4X3	T39.4X4	T39.4X5	T39.4X6
Automobile fuel	T52.0X1	T52.0X2	T52.0X3	T52.0X4	—	—
Autonomic nervous system agent NEC	T44.901	T44.902	T44.903	T44.904	T44.905	T44.906
Avlosulfon	T37.1X1	T37.1X2	T37.1X3	T37.1X4	T37.1X5	T37.1X6
Avomine	T42.6X1	T42.6X2	T42.6X3	T42.6X4	T42.6X5	T42.6X6
Axerophthol	T45.2X1	T45.2X2	T45.2X3	T45.2X4	T45.2X5	T45.2X6
Azacitidine	T45.1X1	T45.1X2	T45.1X3	T45.1X4	T45.1X5	T45.1X6
Azacyclonol	T43.591	T43.592	T43.593	T43.594	T43.595	T43.596
Azadirachta	T60.2X1	T60.2X2	T60.2X3	T60.2X4	—	—
Azanidazole	T37.3X1	T37.3X2	T37.3X3	T37.3X4	T37.3X5	T37.3X6
Azapetine	T46.7X1	T46.7X2	T46.7X3	T46.7X4	T46.7X5	T46.7X6
Azapropazone	T39.2X1	T39.2X2	T39.2X3	T39.2X4	T39.2X5	T39.2X6
Azaribine	T45.1X1	T45.1X2	T45.1X3	T45.1X4	T45.1X5	T45.1X6
Azaserine	T45.1X1	T45.1X2	T45.1X3	T45.1X4	T45.1X5	T45.1X6
Azatadine	T45.0X1	T45.0X2	T45.0X3	T45.0X4	T45.0X5	T45.0X6
Azatepa	T45.1X1	T45.1X2	T45.1X3	T45.1X4	T45.1X5	T45.1X6
Azathioprine	T45.1X1	T45.1X2	T45.1X3	T45.1X4	T45.1X5	T45.1X6
Azelaic acid	T49.0X1	T49.0X2	T49.0X3	T49.0X4	T49.0X5	T49.0X6
Azelastine	T45.0X1	T45.0X2	T45.0X3	T45.0X4	T45.0X5	T45.0X6
Azidocillin	T36.0X1	T36.0X2	T36.0X3	T36.0X4	T36.0X5	T36.0X6
Azidothymidine	T37.5X1	T37.5X2	T37.5X3	T37.5X4	T37.5X5	T37.5X6

Substance	Poisoning, Accidental (unintentional)	Poisoning, Intentional self-harm	Poisoning, Assault	Poisoning, Undetermined	Adverse effect	Underdosing
Azinphos (ethyl) (methyl)	T60.0X1	T60.0X2	T60.0X3	T60.0X4	—	—
Aziridine (chelating)	T54.1X1	T54.1X2	T54.1X3	T54.1X4	—	—
Azithromycin	T36.3X1	T36.3X2	T36.3X3	T36.3X4	T36.3X5	T36.3X6
Azlocillin	T36.0X1	T36.0X2	T36.0X3	T36.0X4	T36.0X5	T36.0X6
Azobenzene smoke	T65.3X1	T65.3X2	T65.3X3	T65.3X4	—	—
acaricide	T60.8X1	T60.8X2	T60.8X3	T60.8X4	—	—
Azosulfamide	T37.0X1	T37.0X2	T37.0X3	T37.0X4	T37.0X5	T37.0X6
AZT	T37.5X1	T37.5X2	T37.5X3	T37.5X4	T37.5X5	T37.5X6
Aztreonam	T36.1X1	T36.1X2	T36.1X3	T36.1X4	T36.1X5	T36.1X6
Azulfidine	T37.0X1	T37.0X2	T37.0X3	T37.0X4	T37.0X5	T37.0X6
Azuresin	T50.8X1	T50.8X2	T50.8X3	T50.8X4	T50.8X5	T50.8X6
B						
Bacampicillin	T36.0X1	T36.0X2	T36.0X3	T36.0X4	T36.0X5	T36.0X6
Bacillus						
lactobacillus	T47.8X1	T47.8X2	T47.8X3	T47.8X4	T47.8X5	T47.8X6
subtilis	T47.6X1	T47.6X2	T47.6X3	T47.6X4	T47.6X5	T47.6X6
Bacimycin	T49.0X1	T49.0X2	T49.0X3	T49.0X4	T49.0X5	T49.0X6
ophthalmic preparation	T49.5X1	T49.5X2	T49.5X3	T49.5X4	T49.5X5	T49.5X6
Bacitracin zinc	T49.0X1	T49.0X2	T49.0X3	T49.0X4	T49.0X5	T49.0X6
with neomycin	T49.0X1	T49.0X2	T49.0X3	T49.0X4	T49.0X5	T49.0X6
ENT agent	T49.6X1	T49.6X2	T49.6X3	T49.6X4	T49.6X5	T49.6X6
ophthalmic preparation	T49.5X1	T49.5X2	T49.5X3	T49.5X4	T49.5X5	T49.5X6
topical NEC	T49.0X1	T49.0X2	T49.0X3	T49.0X4	T49.0X5	T49.0X6
Baclofen	T42.8X1	T42.8X2	T42.8X3	T42.8X4	T42.8X5	T42.8X6
Baking soda	T50.991	T50.992	T50.993	T50.994	T50.995	T50.996
BAL	T45.8X1	T45.8X2	T45.8X3	T45.8X4	T45.8X5	T45.8X6
Bambuterol	T48.6X1	T48.6X2	T48.6X3	T48.6X4	T48.6X5	T48.6X6
Bamethan (sulfate)	T46.7X1	T46.7X2	T46.7X3	T46.7X4	T46.7X5	T46.7X6
Bamifylline	T48.6X1	T48.6X2	T48.6X3	T48.6X4	T48.6X5	T48.6X6
Bamipine	T45.0X1	T45.0X2	T45.0X3	T45.0X4	T45.0X5	T45.0X6
Baneberry—see Actausea spicata						
Banewort—see Belladonna						
Barbenyl	T42.3X1	T42.3X2	T42.3X3	T42.3X4	T42.3X5	T42.3X6
Barbexaclone	T42.6X1	T42.6X2	T42.6X3	T42.6X4	T42.6X5	T42.6X6
Barbital	T42.3X1	T42.3X2	T42.3X3	T42.3X4	T42.3X5	T42.3X6
sodium	T42.3X1	T42.3X2	T42.3X3	T42.3X4	T42.3X5	T42.3X6
Barbitone	T42.3X1	T42.3X2	T42.3X3	T42.3X4	T42.3X5	T42.3X6
Barbiturate NEC	T42.3X1	T42.3X2	T42.3X3	T42.3X4	T42.3X5	T42.3X6
with tranquilizer	T42.3X1	T42.3X2	T42.3X3	T42.3X4	T42.3X5	T42.3X6
anesthetic (intravenous)	T41.1X1	T41.1X2	T41.1X3	T41.1X4	T41.1X5	T41.1X6
Barium (carbonate) (chloride) (sulfite)	T57.8X1	T57.8X2	T57.8X3	T57.8X4	—	—
diagnostic agent	T50.8X1	T50.8X2	T50.8X3	T50.8X4	T50.8X5	T50.8X6
pesticide	T60.4X1	T60.4X2	T60.4X3	T60.4X4	—	—
rodenticide	T60.4X1	T60.4X2	T60.4X3	T60.4X4	—	—
sulfate (medicinal)	T50.8X1	T50.8X2	T50.8X3	T50.8X4	T50.8X5	T50.8X6
Barrier cream	T49.3X1	T49.3X2	T49.3X3	T49.3X4	T49.3X5	T49.3X6
Basic fuchsin	T49.0X1	T49.0X2	T49.0X3	T49.0X4	T49.0X5	T49.0X6

Substance	Poisoning, Accidental (unintentional)	Poisoning, Intentional self-harm	Poisoning, Assault	Poisoning, Undetermined	Adverse effect	Underdosing
Battery acid or fluid	T54.2X1	T54.2X2	T54.2X3	T54.2X4	—	—
Bay rum	T51.8X1	T51.8X2	T51.8X3	T51.8X4	—	—
BCG (vaccine)	T50.A91	T50.A92	T50.A93	T50.A94	T50.A95	T50.A96
BCNU	T45.1X1	T45.1X2	T45.1X3	T45.1X4	T45.1X5	T45.1X6
Bearsfoot	T62.2X1	T62.2X2	T62.2X3	T62.2X4	—	—
Beclamide	T42.6X1	T42.6X2	T42.6X3	T42.6X4	T42.6X5	T42.6X6
Beclomethasone	T44.5X1	T44.5X2	T44.5X3	T44.5X4	T44.5X5	T44.5X6
Bee (sting) (venom)	T63.441	T63.442	T63.443	T63.444	—	—
Befunolol	T49.5X1	T49.5X2	T49.5X3	T49.5X4	T49.5X5	T49.5X6
Bekanamycin	T36.5X1	T36.5X2	T36.5X3	T36.5X4	T36.5X5	T36.5X6
Belladonna—see also Nightshade						
alkaloids	T44.3X1	T44.3X2	T44.3X3	T44.3X4	T44.3X5	T44.3X6
extract	T44.3X1	T44.3X2	T44.3X3	T44.3X4	T44.3X5	T44.3X6
herb	T44.3X1	T44.3X2	T44.3X3	T44.3X4	T44.3X5	T44.3X6
Bemegride	T50.7X1	T50.7X2	T50.7X3	T50.7X4	T50.7X5	T50.7X6
Benactyzine	T44.3X1	T44.3X2	T44.3X3	T44.3X4	T44.3X5	T44.3X6
Benadryl	T45.0X1	T45.0X2	T45.0X3	T45.0X4	T45.0X5	T45.0X6
Benaprizine	T44.3X1	T44.3X2	T44.3X3	T44.3X4	T44.3X5	T44.3X6
Benazepril	T46.4X1	T46.4X2	T46.4X3	T46.4X4	T46.4X5	T46.4X6
Bencyclane	T46.7X1	T46.7X2	T46.7X3	T46.7X4	T46.7X5	T46.7X6
Bendazol	T46.3X1	T46.3X2	T46.3X3	T46.3X4	T46.3X5	T46.3X6
Bendrofluazide	T50.2X1	T50.2X2	T50.2X3	T50.2X4	T50.2X5	T50.2X6
Bendroflumethiazide	T50.2X1	T50.2X2	T50.2X3	T50.2X4	T50.2X5	T50.2X6
Benemid	T50.4X1	T50.4X2	T50.4X3	T50.4X4	T50.4X5	T50.4X6
Benethamine penicillin	T36.0X1	T36.0X2	T36.0X3	T36.0X4	T36.0X5	T36.0X6
Benexate	T47.1X1	T47.1X2	T47.1X3	T47.1X4	T47.1X5	T47.1X6
Benfluorex	T46.6X1	T46.6X2	T46.6X3	T46.6X4	T46.6X5	T46.6X6
Benfotiamine	T45.2X1	T45.2X2	T45.2X3	T45.2X4	T45.2X5	T45.2X6
Benisone	T49.0X1	T49.0X2	T49.0X3	T49.0X4	T49.0X5	T49.0X6
Benomyl	T60.0X1	T60.0X2	T60.0X3	T60.0X4	—	—
Benoquin	T49.8X1	T49.8X2	T49.8X3	T49.8X4	T49.8X5	T49.8X6
Benoxinate	T41.3X1	T41.3X2	T41.3X3	T41.3X4	T41.3X5	T41.3X6
Benperidol	T43.4X1	T43.4X2	T43.4X3	T43.4X4	T43.4X5	T43.4X6
Benproperine	T48.3X1	T48.3X2	T48.3X3	T48.3X4	T48.3X5	T48.3X6
Benserazide	T42.8X1	T42.8X2	T42.8X3	T42.8X4	T42.8X5	T42.8X6
Bentazepam	T42.4X1	T42.4X2	T42.4X3	T42.4X4	T42.4X5	T42.4X6
Bentiromide	T50.8X1	T50.8X2	T50.8X3	T50.8X4	T50.8X5	T50.8X6
Bentonite	T49.3X1	T49.3X2	T49.3X3	T49.3X4	T49.3X5	T49.3X6
Benzalbutyramide	T46.6X1	T46.6X2	T46.6X3	T46.6X4	T46.6X5	T46.6X6
Benzalkonium (chloride)	T49.0X1	T49.0X2	T49.0X3	T49.0X4	T49.0X5	T49.0X6
ophthalmic preparation	T49.5X1	T49.5X2	T49.5X3	T49.5X4	T49.5X5	T49.5X6
Benzamidosali cylate (calcium)	T37.1X1	T37.1X2	T37.1X3	T37.1X4	T37.1X5	T37.1X6
Benzamine	T41.3X1	T41.3X2	T41.3X3	T41.3X4	T41.3X5	T41.3X6
lactate	T49.1X1	T49.1X2	T49.1X3	T49.1X4	T49.1X5	T49.1X6
Benzamphetamine	T50.5X1	T50.5X2	T50.5X3	T50.5X4	T50.5X5	T50.5X6
Benzapril hydrochloride	T46.5X1	T46.5X2	T46.5X3	T46.5X4	T46.5X5	T46.5X6
Benzathine benzylpenicillin	T36.0X1	T36.0X2	T36.0X3	T36.0X4	T36.0X5	T36.0X6
Benzathine penicillin	T36.0X1	T36.0X2	T36.0X3	T36.0X4	T36.0X5	T36.0X6

Substance	Poisoning, Accidental (unintentional)	Poisoning, Intentional self-harm	Poisoning, Assault	Poisoning, Undetermined	Adverse effect	Underdosing
Benzatropine	T42.8X1	T42.8X2	T42.8X3	T42.8X4	T42.8X5	T42.8X6
Benzbromarone	T50.4X1	T50.4X2	T50.4X3	T50.4X4	T50.4X5	T50.4X6
Benzcarbimine	T45.1X1	T45.1X2	T45.1X3	T45.1X4	T45.1X5	T45.1X6
Benzedrex	T44.991	T44.992	T44.993	T44.994	T44.995	T44.996
Benzedrine (amphetamine)	T43.621	T43.622	T43.623	T43.624	T43.625	T43.626
Benzenamine	T65.3X1	T65.3X2	T65.3X3	T65.3X4	—	—
Benzene	T52.1X1	T52.1X2	T52.1X3	T52.1X4	—	—
homologues (acetyl) (dimethyl) (methyl) (solvent)	T52.2X1	T52.2X2	T52.2X3	T52.2X4	—	—
Benzethonium (chloride)	T49.0X1	T49.0X2	T49.0X3	T49.0X4	T49.0X5	T49.0X6
Benzfetamine	T50.5X1	T50.5X2	T50.5X3	T50.5X4	T50.5X5	T50.5X6
Benzhexol	T44.3X1	T44.3X2	T44.3X3	T44.3X4	T44.3X5	T44.3X6
Benzhydramine (chloride)	T45.0X1	T45.0X2	T45.0X3	T45.0X4	T45.0X5	T45.0X6
Benzidine	T65.891	T65.892	T65.893	T65.894	—	—
Benzilonium bromide	T44.3X1	T44.3X2	T44.3X3	T44.3X4	T44.3X5	T44.3X6
Benzimidazole	T60.3X1	T60.3X2	T60.3X3	T60.3X4		
Benzin(e)—see Ligroin						
Benziodarone	T46.3X1	T46.3X2	T46.3X3	T46.3X4	T46.3X5	T46.3X6
Benznidazole	T37.3X1	T37.3X2	T37.3X3	T37.3X4	T37.3X5	T37.3X6
Benzocaine	T41.3X1	T41.3X2	T41.3X3	T41.3X4	T41.3X5	T41.3X6
Benzodiapin	T42.4X1	T42.4X2	T42.4X3	T42.4X4	T42.4X5	T42.4X6
Benzodiazepine NEC	T42.4X1	T42.4X2	T42.4X3	T42.4X4	T42.4X5	T42.4X6
Benzoic acid	T49.0X1	T49.0X2	T49.0X3	T49.0X4	T49.0X5	T49.0X6
with salicylic acid	T49.0X1	T49.0X2	T49.0X3	T49.0X4	T49.0X5	T49.0X6
Benzoin (tincture)	T48.5X1	T48.5X2	T48.5X3	T48.5X4	T48.5X5	T48.5X6
Benzol (benzene)	T52.1X1	T52.1X2	T52.1X3	T52.1X4	—	—
vapor	T52.0X1	T52.0X2	T52.0X3	T52.0X4	—	—
Benzomorphan	T40.2X1	T40.2X2	T40.2X3	T40.2X4	T40.2X5	T40.2X6
Benzonatate	T48.3X1	T48.3X2	T48.3X3	T48.3X4	T48.3X5	T48.3X6
Benzophenones	T49.3X1	T49.3X2	T49.3X3	T49.3X4	T49.3X5	T49.3X6
Benzopyrone	T46.991	T46.992	T46.993	T46.994	T46.995	T46.996
Benzothiadiazides	T50.2X1	T50.2X2	T50.2X3	T50.2X4	T50.2X5	T50.2X6
Benzoxonium chloride	T49.0X1	T49.0X2	T49.0X3	T49.0X4	T49.0X5	T49.0X6
Benzoyl peroxide	T49.0X1	T49.0X2	T49.0X3	T49.0X4	T49.0X5	T49.0X6
Benzoylpas calcium	T37.1X1	T37.1X2	T37.1X3	T37.1X4	T37.1X5	T37.1X6
Benzperidin	T43.591	T43.592	T43.593	T43.594	T43.595	T43.596
Benzperidol	T43.591	T43.592	T43.593	T43.594	T43.595	T43.596
Benzphetamine	T50.5X1	T50.5X2	T50.5X3	T50.5X4	T50.5X5	T50.5X6
Benzpyrinium bromide	T44.1X1	T44.1X2	T44.1X3	T44.1X4	T44.1X5	T44.1X6
Benzquinamide	T45.0X1	T45.0X2	T45.0X3	T45.0X4	T45.0X5	T45.0X6
Benzthiazide	T50.2X1	T50.2X2	T50.2X3	T50.2X4	T50.2X5	T50.2X6
Benztropine						
anticholinergic	T44.3X1	T44.3X2	T44.3X3	T44.3X4	T44.3X5	T44.3X6
antiparkinson	T42.8X1	T42.8X2	T42.8X3	T42.8X4	T42.8X5	T42.8X6
Benzydamine	T49.0X1	T49.0X2	T49.0X3	T49.0X4	T49.0X5	T49.0X6
Benzyl						
acetate	T52.8X1	T52.8X2	T52.8X3	T52.8X4	—	—
alcohol	T49.0X1	T49.0X2	T49.0X3	T49.0X4	T49.0X5	T49.0X6

Substance	Poisoning, Accidental (unintentional)	Poisoning, Intentional self-harm	Poisoning, Assault	Poisoning, Undetermined	Adverse effect	Underdosing
Benzyl — *Continued*						
benzoate	T49.0X1	T49.0X2	T49.0X3	T49.0X4	T49.0X5	T49.0X6
Benzoic acid	T49.0X1	T49.0X2	T49.0X3	T49.0X4	T49.0X5	T49.0X6
morphine	T40.2X1	T40.2X2	T40.2X3	T40.2X4	—	—
nicotinate	T46.6X1	T46.6X2	T46.6X3	T46.6X4	T46.6X5	T46.6X6
penicillin	T36.0X1	T36.0X2	T36.0X3	T36.0X4	T36.0X5	T36.0X6
Benzylhydrochl-orthia-zide	T50.2X1	T50.2X2	T50.2X3	T50.2X4	T50.2X5	T50.2X6
Benzylpenicillin	T36.0X1	T36.0X2	T36.0X3	T36.0X4	T36.0X5	T36.0X6
Benzylthiouracil	T38.2X1	T38.2X2	T38.2X3	T38.2X4	T38.2X5	T38.2X6
Bephenium hydroxy-naphthoate	T37.4X1	T37.4X2	T37.4X3	T37.4X4	T37.4X5	T37.4X6
Bepridil	T46.1X1	T46.1X2	T46.1X3	T46.1X4	T46.1X5	T46.1X6
Bergamot oil	T65.891	T65.892	T65.893	T65.894	—	—
Bergapten	T50.991	T50.992	T50.993	T50.994	T50.995	T50.996
Berries, poisonous	T62.1X1	T62.1X2	T62.1X3	T62.1X4	—	—
Beryllium (compounds)	T56.7X1	T56.7X2	T56.7X3	T56.7X4	—	—
b-acetyldigoxin	T46.0X1	T46.0X2	T46.0X3	T46.0X4	T46.0X5	T46.0X6
beta adrenergic blocking agent, heart	T44.7X1	T44.7X2	T44.7X3	T44.7X4	T44.7X5	T44.7X6
b-benzalbutyramide	T46.6X1	T46.6X2	T46.6X3	T46.6X4	T46.6X5	T46.6X6
Betacarotene	T45.2X1	T45.2X2	T45.2X3	T45.2X4	T45.2X5	T45.2X6
b-eucaine	T49.1X1	T49.1X2	T49.1X3	T49.1X4	T49.1X5	T49.1X6
Beta-Chlor	T42.6X1	T42.6X2	T42.6X3	T42.6X4	T42.6X5	T42.6X6
b-galactosidase	T47.5X1	T47.5X2	T47.5X3	T47.5X4	T47.5X5	T47.5X6
Betahistine	T46.7X1	T46.7X2	T46.7X3	T46.7X4	T46.7X5	T46.7X6
Betaine	T47.5X1	T47.5X2	T47.5X3	T47.5X4	T47.5X5	T47.5X6
Betamethasone	T49.0X1	T49.0X2	T49.0X3	T49.0X4	T49.0X5	T49.0X6
topical	T49.0X1	T49.0X2	T49.0X3	T49.0X4	T49.0X5	T49.0X6
Betamicin	T36.8X1	T36.8X2	T36.8X3	T36.8X4	T36.8X5	T36.8X6
Betanidine	T46.5X1	T46.5X2	T46.5X3	T46.5X4	T46.5X5	T46.5X6
b-sitosterol(s)	T46.6X1	T46.6X2	T46.6X3	T46.6X4	T46.6X5	T46.6X6
Betaxolol	T44.7X1	T44.7X2	T44.7X3	T44.7X4	T44.7X5	T44.7X6
Betazole	T50.8X1	T50.8X2	T50.8X3	T50.8X4	T50.8X5	T50.8X6
Bethanechol	T44.1X1	T44.1X2	T44.1X3	T44.1X4	T44.1X5	T44.1X6
chloride	T44.1X1	T44.1X2	T44.1X3	T44.1X4	T44.1X5	T44.1X6
Bethanidine	T46.5X1	T46.5X2	T46.5X3	T46.5X4	T46.5X5	T46.5X6
Betoxycaine	T41.3X1	T41.3X2	T41.3X3	T41.3X4	T41.3X5	T41.3X6
Betula oil	T49.3X1	T49.3X2	T49.3X3	T49.3X4	T49.3X5	T49.3X6
Bevantolol	T44.7X1	T44.7X2	T44.7X3	T44.7X4	T44.7X5	T44.7X6
Bevonium metilsulfate	T44.3X1	T44.3X2	T44.3X3	T44.3X4	T44.3X5	T44.3X6
Bezafibrate	T46.6X1	T46.6X2	T46.6X3	T46.6X4	T46.6X5	T46.6X6
Bezitramide	T40.491	T40.492	T40.493	T40.494	T40.495	T40.496
BHA	T50.991	T50.992	T50.993	T50.994	T50.995	T50.996
Bhang	T40.7X1	T40.7X2	T40.7X3	T40.7X4	T40.7X5	T40.7X6
BHC (medicinal)	T49.0X1	T49.0X2	T49.0X3	T49.0X4	T49.0X5	T49.0X6
nonmedicinal (vapor)	T53.6X1	T53.6X2	T53.6X3	T53.6X4	—	—
Bialamicol	T37.3X1	T37.3X2	T37.3X3	T37.3X4	T37.3X5	T37.3X6
Bibenzonium bromide	T48.3X1	T48.3X2	T48.3X3	T48.3X4	T48.3X5	T48.3X6
Bibrocathol	T49.5X1	T49.5X2	T49.5X3	T49.5X4	T49.5X5	T49.5X6
Bichloride of mercury— see Mercury, chloride						

Substance	Poisoning, Accidental (unintentional)	Poisoning, Intentional self-harm	Poisoning, Assault	Poisoning, Undetermined	Adverse effect	Underdosing
Bichromates (calcium) (potassium) (sodium) (crystals)	T57.8X1	T57.8X2	T57.8X3	T57.8X4	—	—
fumes	T56.2X1	T56.2X2	T56.2X3	T56.2X4	—	—
Biclotymol	T49.6X1	T49.6X2	T49.6X3	T49.6X4	T49.6X5	T49.6X6
Bicucculine	T50.7X1	T50.7X2	T50.7X3	T50.7X4	T50.7X5	T50.7X6
Bifemelane	T43.291	T43.292	T43.293	T43.294	T43.295	T43.296
Biguanide derivatives, oral	T38.3X1	T38.3X2	T38.3X3	T38.3X4	T38.3X5	T38.3X6
Bile salts	T47.5X1	T47.5X2	T47.5X3	T47.5X4	T47.5X5	T47.5X6
Biligrafin	T50.8X1	T50.8X2	T50.8X3	T50.8X4	T50.8X5	T50.8X6
Bilopaque	T50.8X1	T50.8X2	T50.8X3	T50.8X4	T50.8X5	T50.8X6
Binifibrate	T46.6X1	T46.6X2	T46.6X3	T46.6X4	T46.6X5	T46.6X6
Binitrobenzol	T65.3X1	T65.3X2	T65.3X3	T65.3X4	—	—
Bioflavonoid(s)	T46.991	T46.992	T46.993	T46.994	T46.995	T46.996
Biological substance NEC	T50.901	T50.902	T50.903	T50.904	T50.905	T50.906
Biotin	T45.2X1	T45.2X2	T45.2X3	T45.2X4	T45.2X5	T45.2X6
Biperiden	T44.3X1	T44.3X2	T44.3X3	T44.3X4	T44.3X5	T44.3X6
Bisacodyl	T47.2X1	T47.2X2	T47.2X3	T47.2X4	T47.2X5	T47.2X6
Bisbentiamine	T45.2X1	T45.2X2	T45.2X3	T45.2X4	T45.2X5	T45.2X6
Bisbutiamine	T45.2X1	T45.2X2	T45.2X3	T45.2X4	T45.2X5	T45.2X6
Bisdequalinium (salts) (diacetate)	T49.6X1	T49.6X2	T49.6X3	T49.6X4	T49.6X5	T49.6X6
Bishydroxycoumarin	T45.511	T45.512	T45.513	T45.514	T45.515	T45.516
Bismarsen	T37.8X1	T37.8X2	T37.8X3	T37.8X4	T37.8X5	T37.8X6
Bismuth salts	T47.6X1	T47.6X2	T47.6X3	T47.6X4	T47.6X5	T47.6X6
aluminate	T47.1X1	T47.1X2	T47.1X3	T47.1X4	T47.1X5	T47.1X6
anti-infectives	T37.8X1	T37.8X2	T37.8X3	T37.8X4	T37.8X5	T37.8X6
formic iodide	T49.0X1	T49.0X2	T49.0X3	T49.0X4	T49.0X5	T49.0X6
glycolylarsenate	T49.0X1	T49.0X12	T49.0X3	T49.0X4	T49.0X5	T49.0X6
nonmedicinal (compounds) NEC	T65.91	T65.92	T65.93	T65.94	—	—
subcarbonate	T47.6X1	T47.6X2	T47.6X3	T47.6X4	T47.6X5	T47.6X6
subsalicylate	T37.8X1	T37.8X2	T37.8X3	T37.8X4	T37.8X5	T37.8X6
sulfarsphenamine	T37.8X1	T37.8X2	T37.8X3	T37.8X4	T37.8X5	T37.8X6
Bisoprolol	T44.7X1	T44.7X2	T44.7X3	T44.7X4	T44.7X5	T44.7X6
Bisoxatin	T47.2X1	T47.2X2	T47.2X3	T47.2X4	T47.2X5	T47.2X6
Bisulepin (hydrochloride)	T45.0X1	T45.0X2	T45.0X3	T45.0X4	T45.0X5	T45.0X6
Bithionol	T37.8X1	T37.8X2	T37.8X3	T37.8X4	T37.8X5	T37.8X6
anthelminthic	T37.4X1	T37.4X2	T37.4X3	T37.4X4	T37.4X5	T37.4X6
Bitolterol	T48.6X1	T48.6X2	T48.6X3	T48.6X4	T48.6X5	T48.6X6
Bitoscanate	T37.4X1	T37.4X2	T37.4X3	T37.4X4	T37.4X5	T37.4X6
Bitter almond oil	T62.8X1	T62.8X2	T62.8X3	T62.8X4	—	—
Bittersweet	T62.2X1	T62.2X2	T62.2X3	T62.2X4	—	—
Black						
flag	T60.91	T60.92	T60.93	T60.94	—	—
henbane	T62.2X1	T62.2X2	T62.2X3	T62.2X4	—	—
leaf (40)	T60.91	T60.92	T60.93	T60.94	—	—
widow spider (bite)	T63.311	T63.312	T63.313	T63.314	—	—
antivenin	T50.Z11	T50.Z12	T50.Z13	T50.Z14	T50.Z15	T50.Z16

Substance	Poisoning, Accidental (unintentional)	Poisoning, Intentional self-harm	Poisoning, Assault	Poisoning, Undetermined	Adverse effect	Underdosing
Blast furnace gas (carbon monoxide from)	T58.8X1	T58.8X2	T58.8X3	T58.8X4	—	—
Bleach	T54.91	T54.92	T54.93	T54.94	—	—
Bleaching agent (medicinal)	T49.4X1	T49.4X2	T49.4X3	T49.4X4	T49.4X5	T49.4X6
Bleomycin	T45.1X1	T45.1X2	T45.1X3	T45.1X4	T45.1X5	T45.1X6
Blockain	T41.3X1	T41.3X2	T41.3X3	T41.3X4	T41.3X5	T41.3X6
infiltration (subcutaneous)	T41.3X1	T41.3X2	T41.3X3	T41.3X4	T41.3X5	T41.3X6
nerve block (peripheral) (plexus)	T41.3X1	T41.3X2	T41.3X3	T41.3X4	T41.3X5	T41.3X6
topical (surface)	T41.3X1	T41.3X2	T41.3X3	T41.3X4	T41.3X5	T41.3X6
Blockers, calcium channel	T46.1X1	T46.1X2	T46.1X3	T46.1X4	T46.1X5	T46.1X6
Blood (derivatives) (natural) (plasma) (whole)	T45.8X1	T45.8X2	T45.8X3	T45.8X4	T45.8X5	T45.8X6
dried	T45.8X1	T45.8X2	T45.8X3	T45.8X4	T45.8X5	T45.8X6
drug affecting NEC	T45.91	T45.92	T45.93	T45.94	T45.95	T45.96
expander NEC	T45.8X1	T45.8X2	T45.8X3	T45.8X4	T45.8X5	T45.8X6
fraction NEC	T45.8X1	T45.8X2	T45.8X3	T45.8X4	T45.8X5	T45.8X6
substitute (macromolecular)	T45.8X1	T45.8X2	T45.8X3	T45.8X4	T45.8X5	T45.8X6
Blue velvet	T40.2X1	T40.2X2	T40.2X3	T40.2X4	—	—
Bone meal	T62.8X1	T62.8X2	T62.8X3	T62.8X4	—	—
Bonine	T45.0X1	T45.0X2	T45.0X3	T45.0X4	T45.0X5	T45.0X6
Bopindolol	T44.7X1	T44.7X2	T44.7X3	T44.7X4	T44.7X5	T44.7X6
Boracic acid	T49.0X1	T49.0X2	T49.0X3	T49.0X4	T49.0X5	T49.0X6
ENT agent	T49.6X1	T49.6X2	T49.6X3	T49.6X4	T49.6X5	T49.6X6
ophthalmic preparation	T49.5X1	T49.5X2	T49.5X3	T49.5X4	T49.5X5	T49.5X6
Borane complex	T57.8X1	T57.8X2	T57.8X3	T57.8X4	—	—
Borate (s)	T57.8X1	T57.8X2	T57.8X3	T57.8X4	—	—
buffer	T50.991	T50.992	T50.993	T50.994	T50.995	T50.996
cleanser	T54.91	T54.92	T54.93	T54.94	—	—
sodium	T57.8X1	T57.8X2	T57.8X3	T57.8X4	—	—
Borax (cleanser)	T54.91	T54.92	T54.93	T54.94	—	—
Bordeaux mixture	T60.3X1	T60.3X2	T60.3X3	T60.3X4	—	—
Boric acid	T49.0X1	T49.0X2	T49.0X3	T49.0X4	T49.0X5	T49.0X6
ENT agent	T49.6X1	T49.6X2	T49.6X3	T49.6X4	T49.6X5	T49.6X6
ophthalmic preparation	T49.5X1	T49.5X2	T49.5X3	T49.5X4	T49.5X5	T49.5X6
Bornaprine	T44.3X1	T44.3X2	T44.3X3	T44.3X4	T44.3X5	T44.3X6
Boron	T57.8X1	T57.8X2	T57.8X3	T57.8X4	—	—
hydride NEC	T57.8X1	T57.8X2	T57.8X3	T57.8X4	—	—
fumes or gas	T57.8X1	T57.8X2	T57.8X3	T57.8X4	—	—
trifluoride	T59.891	T59.892	T59.893	T59.894		
Botox	T48.291	T48.292	T48.293	T48.294	T48.295	T48.296
Botulinus anti-toxin (type A, B)	T50.Z11	T50.Z12	T50.Z13	T50.Z14	T50.Z15	T50.Z16
Brake fluid vapor	T59.891	T59.892	T59.893	T59.894	—	—
Brallobarbital	T42.3X1	T42.3X2	T42.3X3	T42.3X4	T42.3X5	T42.3X6
Bran (wheat)	T47.4X1	T47.4X2	T47.4X3	T47.4X4	T47.4X5	T47.4X6
Brass (fumes)	T56.891	T56.892	T56.893	T56.894		

Substance	Poisoning, Accidental (unintentional)	Poisoning, Intentional self-harm	Poisoning, Assault	Poisoning, Undetermined	Adverse effect	Underdosing
Brasso	T52.0X1	T52.0X2	T52.0X3	T52.0X4	—	—
Bretylium tosilate	T46.2X1	T46.2X2	T46.2X3	T46.2X4	T46.2X5	T46.2X6
Brevital (sodium)	T41.1X1	T41.1X2	T41.1X3	T41.1X4	T41.1X5	T41.1X6
Brinase	T45.3X1	T45.3X2	T45.3X3	T45.3X4	T45.3X5	T45.3X6
British antilewisite	T45.8X1	T45.8X2	T45.8X3	T45.8X4	T45.8X5	T45.8X6
Brodifacoum	T60.4X1	T60.4X2	T60.4X3	T60.4X4	—	—
Bromal (hydrate)	T42.6X1	T42.6X2	T42.6X3	T42.6X4	T42.6X5	T42.6X6
Bromazepam	T42.4X1	T42.4X2	T42.4X3	T42.4X4	T42.4X5	T42.4X6
Bromazine	T45.0X1	T45.0X2	T45.0X3	T45.0X4	T45.0X5	T45.0X6
Brombenzylcyanide	T59.3X1	T59.3X2	T59.3X3	T59.3X4	—	—
Bromelains	T45.3X1	T45.3X2	T45.3X3	T45.3X4	T45.3X5	T45.3X6
Bromethalin	T60.4X1	T60.4X2	T60.4X3	T60.4X4	—	—
Bromhexine	T48.4X1	T48.4X2	T48.4X3	T48.4X4	T48.4X5	T48.4X6
Bromide salts	T42.6X1	T42.6X2	T42.6X3	T42.6X4	T42.6X5	T42.6X6
Bromindione	T45.511	T45.512	T45.513	T45.514	T45.515	T45.516
Bromine						
compounds (medicinal)	T42.6X1	T42.6X2	T42.6X3	T42.6X4	T42.6X5	T42.6X6
sedative	T42.6X1	T42.6X2	T42.6X3	T42.6X4	T42.6X5	T42.6X6
vapor	T59.891	T59.892	T59.893	T59.894	—	—
Bromisoval	T42.6X1	T42.6X2	T42.6X3	T42.6X4	T42.6X5	T42.6X6
Bromisovalum	T42.6X1	T42.6X2	T42.6X3	T42.6X4	T42.6X5	T42.6X6
Bromobenzylcyanide	T59.3X1	T59.3X2	T59.3X3	T59.3X4	—	—
Bromochloro-salicylanilide	T49.0X1	T49.0X2	T49.0X3	T49.0X4	T49.0X5	T49.0X6
Bromocriptine	T42.8X1	T42.8X2	T42.8X3	T42.8X4	T42.8X5	T42.8X6
Bromodiphenhydramine	T45.0X1	T45.0X2	T45.0X3	T45.0X4	T45.0X5	T45.0X6
Bromoform	T42.6X1	T42.6X2	T42.6X3	T42.6X4	T42.6X5	T42.6X6
Bromophenol blue reagent	T50.991	T50.992	T50.993	T50.994	T50.995	T50.996
Bromopride	T47.8X1	T47.8X2	T47.8X3	T47.8X4	T47.8X5	T47.8X6
Bromosalicyl chloranitide	T49.0X1	T49.0X2	T49.0X3	T49.0X4	T49.0X5	T49.0X6
Bromosalicyl hydroxamic acid	T37.1X1	T37.1X2	T37.1X3	T37.1X4	T37.1X5	T37.1X6
Bromo-seltzer	T39.1X1	T39.1X2	T39.1X3	T39.1X4	T39.1X5	T39.1X6
Bromoxynil	T60.3X1	T60.3X2	T60.3X3	T60.3X4	—	—
Bromperidol	T43.4X1	T43.4X2	T43.4X3	T43.4X4	T43.4X5	T43.4X6
Brompheniramine	T45.0X1	T45.0X2	T45.0X3	T45.0X4	T45.0X5	T45.0X6
Bromsulfophthalein	T50.8X1	T50.8X2	T50.8X3	T50.8X4	T50.8X5	T50.8X6
Bromural	T42.6X1	T42.6X2	T42.6X3	T42.6X4	T42.6X5	T42.6X6
Bromvaletone	T42.6X1	T42.6X2	T42.6X3	T42.6X4	T42.6X5	T42.6X6
Bronchodilator NEC	T48.6X1	T48.6X2	T48.6X3	T48.6X4	T48.6X5	T48.6X6
Brotizolam	T42.4X1	T42.4X2	T42.4X3	T42.4X4	T42.4X5	T42.4X6
Brovincamine	T46.7X1	T46.7X2	T46.7X3	T46.7X4	T46.7X5	T46.7X6
Brown recluse spider (bite) (venom)	T63.331	T63.332	T63.333	T63.334	—	—
Brown spider (bite) (venom)	T63.391	T63.392	T63.393	T63.394	—	—
Broxaterol	T48.6X1	T48.6X2	T48.6X3	T48.6X4	T48.6X5	T48.6X6
Broxuridine	T45.1X1	T45.1X2	T45.1X3	T45.1X4	T45.1X5	T45.1X6
Broxyquinoline	T37.8X1	T37.8X2	T37.8X3	T37.8X4	T37.8X5	T37.8X6
Bruceine	T48.291	T48.292	T48.293	T48.294	T48.295	T48.296
Brucia	T62.2X1	T62.2X2	T62.2X3	T62.2X4	—	—
Brucine	T65.1X1	T65.1X2	T65.1X3	T65.1X4	—	—
Brunswick green—see Copper						
Bruten—see Ibuprofen						
Bryonia	T47.2X1	T47.2X2	T47.2X3	T47.2X4	T47.2X5	T47.2X6
Buclizine	T45.0X1	T45.0X2	T45.0X3	T45.0X4	T45.0X5	T45.0X6
Buclosamide	T49.0X1	T49.0X2	T49.0X3	T49.0X4	T49.0X5	T49.0X6
Budesonide	T44.5X1	T44.5X2	T44.5X3	T44.5X4	T44.5X5	T44.5X6
Budralazine	T46.5X1	T46.5X2	T46.5X3	T46.5X4	T46.5X5	T46.5X6
Bufferin	T39.011	T39.012	T39.013	T39.014	T39.015	T39.016
Buflomedil	T46.7X1	T46.7X2	T46.7X3	T46.7X4	T46.7X5	T46.7X6
Buformin	T38.3X1	T38.3X2	T38.3X3	T38.3X4	T38.3X5	T38.3X6
Bufotenine	T40.991	T40.992	T40.993	T40.994	—	—
Bufrolin	T48.6X1	T48.6X2	T48.6X3	T48.6X4	T48.6X5	T48.6X6
Bufylline	T48.6X1	T48.6X2	T48.6X3	T48.6X4	T48.6X5	T48.6X6
Bulk filler	T50.5X1	T50.5X2	T50.5X3	T50.5X4	T50.5X5	T50.5X6
cathartic	T47.4X1	T47.4X2	T47.4X3	T47.4X4	T47.4X5	T47.4X6
Bumetanide	T50.1X1	T50.1X2	T50.1X3	T50.1X4	T50.1X5	T50.1X6
Bunaftine	T46.2X1	T46.2X2	T46.2X3	T46.2X4	T46.2X5	T46.2X6
Bunamiodyl	T50.8X1	T50.8X2	T50.8X3	T50.8X4	T50.8X5	T50.8X6
Bunazosin	T44.6X1	T44.6X2	T44.6X3	T44.6X4	T44.6X5	T44.6X6
Bunitrolol	T44.7X1	T44.7X2	T44.7X3	T44.7X4	T44.7X5	T44.7X6
Buphenine	T46.7X1	T46.7X2	T46.7X3	T46.7X4	T46.7X5	T46.7X6
Bupivacaine	T41.3X1	T41.3X2	T41.3X3	T41.3X4	T41.3X5	T41.3X6
infiltration (subcutaneous)	T41.3X1	T41.3X2	T41.3X3	T41.3X4	T41.3X5	T41.3X6
nerve block (peripheral) (plexus)	T41.3X1	T41.3X2	T41.3X3	T41.3X4	T41.3X5	T41.3X6
spinal	T41.3X1	T41.3X2	T41.3X3	T41.3X4	T41.3X5	T41.3X6
Bupranolol	T44.7X1	T44.7X2	T44.7X3	T44.7X4	T44.7X5	T44.7X6
Buprenorphine	T40.491	T40.492	T40.493	T40.494	T40.495	T40.496
Bupropion	T43.291	T43.292	T43.293	T43.294	T43.295	T43.296
Burimamide	T47.1X1	T47.1X2	T47.1X3	T47.1X4	T47.1X5	T47.1X6
Buserelin	T38.891	T38.892	T38.893	T38.894	T38.895	T38.896
Buspirone	T43.591	T43.592	T43.593	T43.594	T43.595	T43.596
Busulfan, busulphan	T45.1X1	T45.1X2	T45.1X3	T45.1X4	T45.1X5	T45.1X6
Butabarbital (sodium)	T42.3X1	T42.3X2	T42.3X3	T42.3X4	T42.3X5	T42.3X6
Butabarbitone	T42.3X1	T42.3X2	T42.3X3	T42.3X4	T42.3X5	T42.3X6
Butabarpal	T42.3X1	T42.3X2	T42.3X3	T42.3X4	T42.3X5	T42.3X6
Butacaine	T41.3X1	T41.3X2	T41.3X3	T41.3X4	T41.3X5	T41.3X6
Butalamine	T46.7X1	T46.7X2	T46.7X3	T46.7X4	T46.7X5	T46.7X6
Butalbital	T42.3X1	T42.3X2	T42.3X3	T42.3X4	T42.3X5	T42.3X6
Butallylonal	T42.3X1	T42.3X2	T42.3X3	T42.3X4	T42.3X5	T42.3X6
Butamben	T41.3X1	T41.3X2	T41.3X3	T41.3X4	T41.3X5	T41.3X6
Butamirate	T48.3X1	T48.3X2	T48.3X3	T48.3X4	T48.3X5	T48.3X6

Substance	Poisoning, Accidental (unintentional)	Poisoning, Intentional self-harm	Poisoning, Assault	Poisoning, Undetermined	Adverse effect	Underdosing
Butane (distributed in mobile container)	T59.891	T59.892	T59.893	T59.894	—	—
distributed through pipes	T59.891	T59.892	T59.893	T59.894	—	—
incomplete combustion	T58.11	T58.12	T58.13	T58.14	—	—
Butanilicaine	T41.3X1	T41.3X2	T41.3X3	T41.3X4	T41.3X5	T41.3X6
Butanol	T51.3X1	T51.3X2	T51.3X3	T51.3X4	—	—
Butanone, 2-butanone	T52.4X1	T52.4X2	T52.4X3	T52.4X4	—	—
Butantrone	T49.4X1	T49.4X2	T49.4X3	T49.4X4	T49.4X5	T49.4X6
Butaperazine	T43.3X1	T43.3X2	T43.3X3	T43.3X4	T43.3X5	T43.3X6
Butazolidin	T39.2X1	T39.2X2	T39.2X3	T39.2X4	T39.2X5	T39.2X6
Butetamate	T48.6X1	T48.6X2	T48.6X3	T48.6X4	T48.6X5	T48.6X6
Butethal	T42.3X1	T42.3X2	T42.3X3	T42.3X4	T42.3X5	T42.3X6
Butethamate	T44.3X1	T44.3X2	T44.3X3	T44.3X4	T44.3X5	T44.3X6
Buthalitone (sodium)	T41.1X1	T41.1X2	T41.1X3	T41.1X4	T41.1X5	T41.1X6
Butisol (sodium)	T42.3X1	T42.3X2	T42.3X3	T42.3X4	T42.3X5	T42.3X6
Butizide	T50.2X1	T50.2X2	T50.2X3	T50.2X4	T50.2X5	T50.2X6
Butobarbital	T42.3X1	T42.3X2	T42.3X3	T42.3X4	T42.3X5	T42.3X6
sodium	T42.3X1	T42.3X2	T42.3X3	T42.3X4	T42.3X5	T42.3X6
Butobarbitone	T42.3X1	T42.3X2	T42.3X3	T42.3X4	T42.3X5	T42.3X6
Butoconazole (nitrate)	T49.0X1	T49.0X2	T49.0X3	T49.0X4	T49.0X5	T49.0X6
Butorphanol	T40.491	T40.492	T40.493	T40.494	T40.495	T40.496
Butriptyline	T43.011	T43.012	T43.013	T43.014	T43.015	T43.016
Butropium bromide	T44.3X1	T44.3X2	T44.3X3	T44.3X4	T44.3X5	T44.3X6
Butter of antimony—see Antimony						
Buttercups	T62.2X1	T62.2X2	T62.2X3	T62.2X4	—	—
Butyl						
acetate (secondary)	T52.8X1	T52.8X2	T52.8X3	T52.8X4	—	—
alcohol	T51.3X1	T51.3X2	T51.3X3	T51.3X4	—	—
aminobenzoate	T41.3X1	T41.3X2	T41.3X3	T41.3X4	T41.3X5	T41.3X6
butyrate	T52.8X1	T52.8X2	T52.8X3	T52.8X4	—	—
carbinol	T51.3X1	T51.3X2	T51.3X3	T51.3X4	—	—
carbitol	T52.3X1	T52.3X2	T52.3X3	T52.3X4	—	—
cellosolve	T52.3X1	T52.3X2	T52.3X3	T52.3X4	—	—
chloral (hydrate)	T42.6X1	T42.6X2	T42.6X3	T42.6X4	T42.6X5	T42.6X6
formate	T52.8X1	T52.8X2	T52.8X3	T52.8X4	—	—
lactate	T52.8X1	T52.8X2	T52.8X3	T52.8X4	—	—
propionate	T52.8X1	T52.8X2	T52.8X3	T52.8X4	—	—
scopolamine bromide	T44.3X1	T44.3X2	T44.3X3	T44.3X4	T44.3X5	T44.3X6
thiobarbital sodium	T41.1X1	T41.1X2	T41.1X3	T41.1X4	T41.1X5	T41.1X6
Butylated hydroxy-anisole	T50.991	T50.992	T50.993	T50.994	T50.995	T50.996
Butylchloral hydrate	T42.6X1	T42.6X2	T42.6X3	T42.6X4	T42.6X5	T42.6X6
Butyltoluene	T52.2X1	T52.2X2	T52.2X3	T52.2X4	—	—
Butyn	T41.3X1	T41.3X2	T41.3X3	T41.3X4	T41.3X5	T41.3X6
Butyrophenone (-based tranquilizers)	T43.4X1	T43.4X2	T43.4X3	T43.4X4	T43.4X5	T43.4X6
C						
Cabergoline	T42.8X1	T42.8X2	T42.8X3	T42.8X4	T42.8X5	T42.8X6
Cacodyl, cacodylic acid	T57.0X1	T57.0X2	T57.0X3	T57.0X4	—	—
Cactinomycin	T45.1X1	T45.1X2	T45.1X3	T45.1X4	T45.1X5	T45.1X6
Cade oil	T49.4X1	T49.4X2	T49.4X3	T49.4X4	T49.4X5	T49.4X6
Cadexomer iodine	T49.0X1	T49.0X2	T49.0X3	T49.0X4	T49.0X5	T49.0X6
Cadmium (chloride) (fumes) (oxide)	T56.3X1	T56.3X2	T56.3X3	T56.3X4	—	—
sulfide (medicinal) NEC	T49.4X1	T49.4X2	T49.4X3	T49.4X4	T49.4X5	T49.4X6
Cadralazine	T46.5X1	T46.5X2	T46.5X3	T46.5X4	T46.5X5	T46.5X6
Caffeine	T43.611	T43.612	T43.613	T43.614	T43.615	T43.616
Calabar bean	T62.2X1	T62.2X2	T62.2X3	T62.2X4	—	—
Caladium seguinum	T62.2X1	T62.2X2	T62.2X3	T62.2X4	—	—
Calamine (lotion)	T49.3X1	T49.3X2	T49.3X3	T49.3X4	T49.3X5	T49.3X6
Calcifediol	T45.2X1	T45.2X2	T45.2X3	T45.2X4	T45.2X5	T45.2X6
Calciferol	T45.2X1	T45.2X2	T45.2X3	T45.2X4	T45.2X5	T45.2X6
Calcitonin	T50.991	T50.992	T50.993	T50.994	T50.995	T50.996
Calcitriol	T45.2X1	T45.2X2	T45.2X3	T45.2X4	T45.2X5	T45.2X6
Calcium	T50.3X1	T50.3X2	T50.3X3	T50.3X4	T50.3X5	T50.3X6
actylsalicylate	T39.011	T39.012	T39.013	T39.014	T39.015	T39.016
benzamidosalicylate	T37.1X1	T37.1X2	T37.1X3	T37.1X4	T37.1X5	T37.1X6
bromide	T42.6X1	T42.6X2	T42.6X3	T42.6X4	T42.6X5	T42.6X6
bromolactobionate	T42.6X1	T42.6X2	T42.6X3	T42.6X4	T42.6X5	T42.6X6
carbaspirin	T39.011	T39.012	T39.013	T39.014	T39.015	T39.016
carbimide	T50.6X1	T50.6X2	T50.6X3	T50.6X4	T50.6X5	T50.6X6
carbonate	T47.1X1	T47.1X2	T47.1X3	T47.1X4	T47.1X5	T47.1X6
chloride	T50.991	T50.992	T50.993	T50.994	T50.995	T50.996
anhydrous	T50.991	T50.992	T50.993	T50.994	T50.995	T50.996
cyanide	T57.8X1	T57.8X2	T57.8X3	T57.8X4	—	—
dioctyl sulfosuccinate	T47.4X1	T47.4X2	T47.4X3	T47.4X4	T47.4X5	T47.4X6
disodium edathamil	T45.8X1	T45.8X2	T45.8X3	T45.8X4	T45.8X5	T45.8X6
disodium edetate	T45.8X1	T45.8X2	T45.8X3	T45.8X4	T45.8X5	T45.8X6
dobesilate	T46.991	T46.992	T46.993	T46.994	T46.995	T46.996
EDTA	T45.8X1	T45.8X2	T45.8X3	T45.8X4	T45.8X5	T45.8X6
ferrous citrate	T45.4X1	T45.4X2	T45.4X3	T45.4X4	T45.4X5	T45.4X6
folinate	T45.8X1	T45.8X2	T45.8X3	T45.8X4	T45.8X5	T45.8X6
glubionate	T50.3X1	T50.3X2	T50.3X3	T50.3X4	T50.3X5	T50.3X6
gluconate	T50.3X1	T50.3X2	T50.3X3	T50.3X4	T50.3X5	T50.3X6
gluconoga-lactogluconate	T50.3X1	T50.3X2	T50.3X3	T50.3X4	T50.3X5	T50.3X6
hydrate, hydroxide	T54.3X1	T54.3X2	T54.3X3	T54.3X4	—	—
hypochlorite	T54.3X1	T54.3X2	T54.3X3	T54.3X4	—	—
iodide	T48.4X1	T48.4X2	T48.4X3	T48.4X4	T48.4X5	T48.4X6
ipodate	T50.8X1	T50.8X2	T50.8X3	T50.8X4	T50.8X5	T50.8X6
lactate	T50.3X1	T50.3X2	T50.3X3	T50.3X4	T50.3X5	T50.3X6
leucovorin	T45.8X1	T45.8X2	T45.8X3	T45.8X4	T45.8X5	T45.8X6
mandelate	T37.91	T37.92	T37.93	T37.94	T37.95	T37.96
oxide	T54.3X1	T54.3X2	T54.3X3	T54.3X4	—	—
pantothenate	T45.2X1	T45.2X2	T45.2X3	T45.2X4	T45.2X5	T45.2X6
phosphate	T50.3X1	T50.3X2	T50.3X3	T50.3X4	T50.3X5	T50.3X6
salicylate	T39.091	T39.092	T39.093	T39.094	T39.095	T39.096
salts	T50.3X1	T50.3X2	T50.3X3	T50.3X4	T50.3X5	T50.3X6
Calculus-dissolving drug	T50.991	T50.992	T50.993	T50.994	T50.995	T50.996
Calomel	T49.0X1	T49.0X2	T49.0X3	T49.0X4	T49.0X5	T49.0X6
Caloric agent	T50.3X1	T50.3X2	T50.3X3	T50.3X4	T50.3X5	T50.3X6

Substance	Poisoning, Accidental (unintentional)	Poisoning, Intentional self-harm	Poisoning, Assault	Poisoning, Undetermined	Adverse effect	Underdosing
Calusterone	T38.7X1	T38.7X2	T38.7X3	T38.7X4	T38.7X5	T38.7X6
Camazepam	T42.4X1	T42.4X2	T42.4X3	T42.4X4	T42.4X5	T42.4X6
Camomile	T49.0X1	T49.0X2	T49.0X3	T49.0X4	T49.0X5	T49.0X6
Camoquin	T37.2X1	T37.2X2	T37.2X3	T37.2X4	T37.2X5	T37.2X6
Camphor						
insecticide	T60.2X1	T60.2X2	T60.2X3	T60.2X4	—	—
medicinal	T49.8X1	T49.8X2	T49.8X3	T49.8X4	T49.8X5	T49.8X6
Camylofin	T44.3X1	T44.3X2	T44.3X3	T44.3X4	T44.3X5	T44.3X6
Cancer chemotherapy drug regimen	T45.1X1	T45.1X2	T45.1X3	T45.1X4	T45.1X5	T45.1X6
Candeptin	T49.0X1	T49.0X2	T49.0X3	T49.0X4	T49.0X5	T49.0X6
Candicidin	T49.0X1	T49.0X2	T49.0X3	T49.0X4	T49.0X5	T49.0X6
Cannabinol	T40.7X1	T40.7X2	T40.7X3	T40.7X4	T40.7X5	T40.7X6
Cannabis (derivatives)	T40.7X1	T40.7X2	T40.7X3	T40.7X4	T40.7X5	T40.7X6
Canned heat	T51.1X1	T51.1X2	T51.1X3	T51.1X4	—	—
Canrenoic acid	T50.0X1	T50.0X2	T50.0X3	T50.0X4	T50.0X5	T50.0X6
Canrenone	T50.0X1	T50.0X2	T50.0X3	T50.0X4	T50.0X5	T50.0X6
Cantharides, cantharidin, cantharis	T49.8X1	T49.8X2	T49.8X3	T49.8X4	T49.8X5	T49.8X6
Canthaxanthin	T50.991	T50.992	T50.993	T50.994	T50.995	T50.996
Capillary-active drug NEC	T46.901	T46.902	T46.903	T46.904	T46.905	T46.906
Capreomycin	T36.8X1	T36.8X2	T36.8X3	T36.8X4	T36.8X5	T36.8X6
Capsicum	T49.4X1	T49.4X2	T49.4X3	T49.4X4	T49.4X5	T49.4X6
Captafol	T60.3X1	T60.3X2	T60.3X3	T60.3X4	—	—
Captan	T60.3X1	T60.3X2	T60.3X3	T60.3X4	—	—
Captodiame, captodiamine	T43.591	T43.592	T43.593	T43.594	T43.595	T43.596
Captopril	T46.4X1	T46.4X2	T46.4X3	T46.4X4	T46.4X5	T46.4X6
Caramiphen	T44.3X1	T44.3X2	T44.3X3	T44.3X4	T44.3X5	T44.3X6
Carazolol	T44.7X1	T44.7X2	T44.7X3	T44.7X4	T44.7X5	T44.7X6
Carbachol	T44.1X1	T44.1X2	T44.1X3	T44.1X4	T44.1X5	T44.1X6
Carbacrylamine (resin)	T50.3X1	T50.3X2	T50.3X3	T50.3X4	T50.3X5	T50.3X6
Carbamate (insecticide)	T60.0X1	T60.0X2	T60.0X3	T60.0X4	—	—
Carbamate (sedative)	T42.6X1	T42.6X2	T42.6X3	T42.6X4	T42.6X5	T42.6X6
herbicide	T60.0X1	T60.0X2	T60.0X3	T60.0X4	—	—
insecticide	T60.0X1	T60.0X2	T60.0X3	T60.0X4	—	—
Carbamazepine	T42.1X1	T42.1X2	T42.1X3	T42.1X4	T42.1X5	T42.1X6
Carbamide	T47.3X1	T47.3X2	T47.3X3	T47.3X4	T47.3X5	T47.3X6
peroxide	T49.0X1	T49.0X2	T49.0X3	T49.0X4	T49.0X5	T49.0X6
topical	T49.8X1	T49.8X2	T49.8X3	T49.8X4	T49.8X5	T49.8X6
Carbamylcholine chloride	T44.1X1	T44.1X2	T44.1X3	T44.1X4	T44.1X5	T44.1X6
Carbaril	T60.0X1	T60.0X2	T60.0X3	T60.0X4	—	—
Carbarsone	T37.3X1	T37.3X2	T37.3X3	T37.3X4	T37.3X5	T37.3X6
Carbaryl	T60.0X1	T60.0X2	T60.0X3	T60.0X4	—	—
Carbaspirin	T39.011	T39.012	T39.013	T39.014	T39.015	T39.016
Carbazochrome (salicylate) (sodium sulfonate)	T49.4X1	T49.4X2	T49.4X3	T49.4X4	T49.4X5	T49.4X6
Carbenicillin	T36.0X1	T36.0X2	T36.0X3	T36.0X4	T36.0X5	T36.0X6
Carbenoxolone	T47.1X1	T47.1X2	T47.1X3	T47.1X4	T47.1X5	T47.1X6
Carbetapentane	T48.3X1	T48.3X2	T48.3X3	T48.3X4	T48.3X5	T48.3X6
Carbethyl salicylate	T39.091	T39.092	T39.093	T39.094	T39.095	T39.096
Carbidopa (with levodopa)	T42.8X1	T42.8X2	T42.8X3	T42.8X4	T42.8X5	T42.8X6
Carbimazole	T38.2X1	T38.2X2	T38.2X3	T38.2X4	T38.2X5	T38.2X6
Carbinol	T51.1X1	T51.1X2	T51.1X3	T51.1X4	—	—
Carbinoxamine	T45.0X1	T45.0X2	T45.0X3	T45.0X4	T45.0X5	T45.0X6
Carbiphene	T39.8X1	T39.8X2	T39.8X3	T39.8X4	T39.8X5	T39.8X6
Carbitol	T52.3X1	T52.3X2	T52.3X3	T52.3X4	—	—
Carbo medicinalis	T47.6X1	T47.6X2	T47.6X3	T47.6X4	T47.6X5	T47.6X6
Carbocaine	T41.3X1	T41.3X2	T41.3X3	T41.3X4	T41.3X5	T41.3X6
infiltration (subcutaneous)	T41.3X1	T41.3X2	T41.3X3	T41.3X4	T41.3X5	T41.3X6
nerve block (peripheral) (plexus)	T41.3X1	T41.3X2	T41.3X3	T41.3X4	T41.3X5	T41.3X6
topical (surface)	T41.3X1	T41.3X2	T41.3X3	T41.3X4	T41.3X5	T41.3X6
Carbocisteine	T48.4X1	T48.4X2	T48.4X3	T48.4X4	T48.4X5	T48.4X6
Carbocromen	T46.3X1	T46.3X2	T46.3X3	T46.3X4	T46.3X5	T46.3X6
Carbol fuchsin	T49.0X1	T49.0X2	T49.0X3	T49.0X4	T49.0X5	T49.0X6
Carbolic acid—see also Phenol	T54.0X1	T54.0X2	T54.0X3	T54.0X4	—	—
Carbolonium (bromide)	T48.1X1	T48.1X2	T48.1X3	T48.1X4	T48.1X5	T48.1X6
Carbomycin	T36.8X1	T36.8X2	T36.8X3	T36.8X4	T36.8X5	T36.8X6
Carbon						
bisulfide (liquid)	T65.4X1	T65.4X2	T65.4X3	T65.4X4	—	—
vapor	T65.4X1	T65.4X2	T65.4X3	T65.4X4	—	—
dioxide (gas)	T59.7X1	T59.7X2	T59.7X3	T59.7X4	—	—
medicinal	T41.5X1	T41.5X2	T41.5X3	T41.5X4	T41.5X5	T41.5X6
nonmedicinal	T59.7X1	T59.7X2	T59.7X3	T59.7X4	—	—
snow	T49.4X1	T49.4X2	T49.4X3	T49.4X4	T49.4X5	T49.4X6
disulfide (liquid)	T65.4X1	T65.4X2	T65.4X3	T65.4X4	—	—
vapor	T65.4X1	T65.4X2	T65.4X3	T65.4X4	—	—
monoxide (from incomplete combustion)	T58.91	T58.92	T58.93	T58.94	—	—
blast furnace gas	T58.8X1	T58.8X2	T58.8X3	T58.8X4	—	—
butane (distributed in mobile container)	T58.11	T58.12	T58.13	T58.14	—	—
distributed through pipes	T58.11	T58.12	T58.13	T58.14	—	—
charcoal fumes	T58.2X1	T58.2X2	T58.2X3	T58.2X4	—	—
coal	T58.2X1	T58.2X2	T58.2X3	T58.2X4	—	—
coke (in domestic stoves, fireplaces)	T58.2X1	T58.2X2	T58.2X3	T58.2X4	—	—
gas (piped)	T58.11	T58.12	T58.13	T58.14	—	—
solid (in domestic stoves, fireplaces)	T58.2X1	T58.2X2	T58.2X3	T58.2X4	—	—
exhaust gas (motor) not in transit	T58.01	T58.02	T58.03	T58.04	—	—
combustion engine, any not in watercraft	T58.01	T58.02	T58.03	T58.04	—	—
farm tractor, not in transit	T58.01	T58.02	T58.03	T58.04	—	—

Substance	Poisoning, Accidental (unintentional)	Poisoning, Intentional self-harm	Poisoning, Assault	Poisoning, Undetermined	Adverse effect	Underdosing
Carbon — *Continued*						
gas engine	T58.01	T58.02	T58.03	T58.04	—	—
motor pump	T58.01	T58.02	T58.03	T58.04	—	—
motor vehicle, not in transit	T58.01	T58.02	T58.03	T58.04	—	—
fuel (in domestic use)	T58.2X1	T58.2X2	T58.2X3	T58.2X4	—	—
gas (piped)	T58.11	T58.12	T58.13	T58.14	—	—
in mobile container	T58.11	T58.12	T58.13	T58.14	—	—
piped (natural)	T58.11	T58.12	T58.13	T58.14	—	—
utility	T58.11	T58.12	T58.13	T58.14	—	—
in mobile container	T58.11	T58.12	T58.13	T58.14	—	—
illuminating gas	T58.11	T58.12	T58.13	T58.14	—	—
industrial fuels or gases, any	T58.8X1	T58.8X2	T58.8X3	T58.8X4	—	—
kerosene (in domestic stoves, fireplaces)	T58.2X1	T58.2X2	T58.2X3	T58.2X4	—	—
kiln gas or vapor	T58.8X1	T58.8X2	T58.8X3	T58.8X4	—	—
motor exhaust gas, not in transit	T58.01	T58.02	T58.03	T58.04	—	—
piped gas (manufactured) (natural)	T58.11	T58.12	T58.13	T58.14	—	—
producer gas	T58.8X1	T58.8X2	T58.8X3	T58.8X4	—	—
propane (distributed in mobile container)	T58.11	T58.12	T58.13	T58.14	—	—
distributed through pipes	T58.11	T58.12	T58.13	T58.14	—	—
specified source NEC	T58.8X1	T58.8X2	T58.8X3	T58.8X4	—	—
stove gas	T58.11	T58.12	T58.13	T58.14	—	—
piped	T58.11	T58.12	T58.13	T58.14	—	—
utility gas	T58.11	T58.12	T58.13	T58.14	—	—
piped	T58.11	T58.12	T58.13	T58.14	—	—
water gas	T58.11	T58.12	T58.13	T58.14	—	—
wood (in domestic stoves, fireplaces)	T58.2X1	T58.2X2	T58.2X3	T58.2X4	—	—
tetrachloride (vapor) NEC	T53.0X1	T53.0X2	T53.0X3	T53.0X4	—	—
liquid (cleansing agent) NEC	T53.0X1	T53.0X2	T53.0X3	T53.0X4	—	—
solvent	T53.0X1	T53.0X2	T53.0X3	T53.0X4	—	—
Carbonic acid gas	T59.7X1	T59.7X2	T59.7X3	T59.7X4	—	—
anhydrase inhibitor NEC	T50.2X1	T50.2X2	T50.2X3	T50.2X4	T50.2X5	T50.2X6
Carbophenothion	T60.0X1	T60.0X2	T60.0X3	T60.0X4	—	—
Carboplatin	T45.1X1	T45.1X2	T45.1X3	T45.1X4	T45.1X5	T45.1X6
Carboprost	T48.0X1	T48.0X2	T48.0X3	T48.0X4	T48.0X5	T48.0X6
Carboquone	T45.1X1	T45.1X2	T45.1X3	T45.1X4	T45.1X5	T45.1X6
Carbowax	T49.3X1	T49.3X2	T49.3X3	T49.3X4	T49.3X5	T49.3X6
Carboxymethyl-cellulose	T47.4X1	T47.4X2	T47.4X3	T47.4X4	T47.4X5	T47.4X6
S-Carboxymethyl-cysteine	T48.4X1	T48.4X2	T48.4X3	T48.4X4	T48.4X5	T48.4X6
Carbrital	T42.3X1	T42.3X2	T42.3X3	T42.3X4	T42.3X5	T42.3X6

Substance	Poisoning, Accidental (unintentional)	Poisoning, Intentional self-harm	Poisoning, Assault	Poisoning, Undetermined	Adverse effect	Underdosing
Carbromal	T42.6X1	T42.6X2	T42.6X3	T42.6X4	T42.6X5	T42.6X6
Carbutamide	T38.3X1	T38.3X2	T38.3X3	T38.3X4	T38.3X5	T38.3X6
Carbuterol	T48.6X1	T48.6X2	T48.6X3	T48.6X4	T48.6X5	T48.6X6
Cardiac						
depressants	T46.2X1	T46.2X2	T46.2X3	T46.2X4	T46.2X5	T46.2X6
rhythm regulator	T46.2X1	T46.2X2	T46.2X3	T46.2X4	T46.2X5	T46.2X6
specified NEC	T46.2X1	T46.2X2	T46.2X3	T46.2X4	T46.2X5	T46.2X6
Cardiografin	T50.8X1	T50.8X2	T50.8X3	T50.8X4	T50.8X5	T50.8X6
Cardio-green	T50.8X1	T50.8X2	T50.8X3	T50.8X4	T50.8X5	T50.8X6
Cardiotonic (glycoside)NEC	T46.0X1	T46.0X2	T46.0X3	T46.0X4	T46.0X5	T46.0X6
Cardiovascular drug NEC	T46.901	T46.902	T46.903	T46.904	T46.905	T46.906
Cardrase	T50.2X1	T50.2X2	T50.2X3	T50.2X4	T50.2X5	T50.2X6
Carfecillin	T36.0X1	T36.0X2	T36.0X3	T36.0X4	T36.0X5	T36.0X6
Carfenazine	T43.3X1	T43.3X2	T43.3X3	T43.3X4	T43.3X5	T43.3X6
Carfusin	T49.0X1	T49.0X2	T49.0X3	T49.0X4	T49.0X5	T49.0X6
Carindacillin	T36.0X1	T36.0X2	T36.0X3	T36.0X4	T36.0X5	T36.0X6
Carisoprodol	T42.8X1	T42.8X2	T42.8X3	T42.8X4	T42.8X5	T42.8X6
Carmellose	T47.4X1	T47.4X2	T47.4X3	T47.4X4	T47.4X5	T47.4X6
Carminative	T47.5X1	T47.5X2	T47.5X3	T47.5X4	T47.5X5	T47.5X6
Carmofur	T45.1X1	T45.1X2	T45.1X3	T45.1X4	T45.1X5	T45.1X6
Carmustine	T45.1X1	T45.1X2	T45.1X3	T45.1X4	T45.1X5	T45.1X6
Carotene	T45.2X1	T45.2X2	T45.2X3	T45.2X4	T45.2X5	T45.2X6
Carphenazine	T43.3X1	T43.3X2	T43.3X3	T43.3X4	T43.3X5	T43.3X6
Carpipramine	T42.4X1	T42.4X2	T42.4X3	T42.4X4	T42.4X5	T42.4X6
Carprofen	T39.311	T39.312	T39.313	T39.314	T39.315	T39.316
Carpronium chloride	T44.3X1	T44.3X2	T44.3X3	T44.3X4	T44.3X5	T44.3X6
Carrageenan	T47.8X1	T47.8X2	T47.8X3	T47.8X4	T47.8X5	T47.8X6
Carteolol	T44.7X1	T44.7X2	T44.7X3	T44.7X4	T44.7X5	T44.7X6
Carter's Little Pills	T47.2X1	T47.2X2	T47.2X3	T47.2X4	T47.2X5	T47.2X6
Cascara (sagrada)	T47.2X1	T47.2X2	T47.2X3	T47.2X4	T47.2X5	T47.2X6
Cassava	T62.2X1	T62.2X2	T62.2X3	T62.2X4	—	—
Castellani's paint	T49.0X1	T49.0X2	T49.0X3	T49.0X4	T49.0X5	T49.0X6
Castor						
bean	T62.2X1	T62.2X2	T62.2X3	T62.2X4	—	—
oil	T47.2X1	T47.2X2	T47.2X3	T47.2X4	T47.2X5	T47.2X6
Catalase	T45.3X1	T45.3X2	T45.3X3	T45.3X4	T45.3X5	T45.3X6
Caterpillar (sting)	T63.431	T63.432	T63.433	T63.434	—	—
Catha (edulis) (tea)	T43.691	T43.692	T43.693	T43.694	—	—
Cathartic NEC	T47.4X1	T47.4X2	T47.4X3	T47.4X4	T47.4X5	T47.4X6
anthacene derivative	T47.2X1	T47.2X2	T47.2X3	T47.2X4	T47.2X5	T47.2X6
bulk	T47.4X1	T47.4X2	T47.4X3	T47.4X4	T47.4X5	T47.4X6
contact	T47.2X1	T47.2X2	T47.2X3	T47.2X4	T47.2X5	T47.2X6
emollient NEC	T47.4X1	T47.4X2	T47.4X3	T47.4X4	T47.4X5	T47.4X6
irritant NEC	T47.2X1	T47.2X2	T47.2X3	T47.2X4	T47.2X5	T47.2X6
mucilage	T47.4X1	T47.4X2	T47.4X3	T47.4X4	T47.4X5	T47.4X6
saline	T47.3X1	T47.3X2	T47.3X3	T47.3X4	T47.3X5	T47.3X6
vegetable	T47.2X1	T47.2X2	T47.2X3	T47.2X4	T47.2X5	T47.2X6
Cathine	T50.5X1	T50.5X2	T50.5X3	T50.5X4	T50.5X5	T50.5X6
Cathomycin	T36.8X1	T36.8X2	T36.8X3	T36.8X4	T36.8X5	T36.8X6

Substance	Poisoning, Accidental (unintentional)	Poisoning, Intentional self-harm	Poisoning, Assault	Poisoning, Undetermined	Adverse effect	Underdosing
Cation exchange resin	T50.3X1	T50.3X2	T50.3X3	T50.3X4	T50.3X5	T50.3X6
Caustic(s) NEC	T54.91	T54.92	T54.93	T54.94	—	—
alkali	T54.3X1	T54.3X2	T54.3X3	T54.3X4	—	—
hydroxide	T54.3X1	T54.3X2	T54.3X3	T54.3X4	—	—
potash	T54.3X1	T54.3X2	T54.3X3	T54.3X4	—	—
soda	T54.3X1	T54.3X2	T54.3X3	T54.3X4	—	—
specified NEC	T54.91	T54.92	T54.93	T54.94	—	—
Ceepryn	T49.0X1	T49.0X2	T49.0X3	T49.0X4	T49.0X5	T49.0X6
ENT agent	T49.6X1	T49.6X2	T49.6X3	T49.6X4	T49.6X5	T49.6X6
lozenges	T49.6X1	T49.6X2	T49.6X3	T49.6X4	T49.6X5	T49.6X6
Cefacetrile	T36.1X1	T36.1X2	T36.1X3	T36.1X4	T36.1X5	T36.1X6
Cefaclor	T36.1X1	T36.1X2	T36.1X3	T36.1X4	T36.1X5	T36.1X6
Cefadroxil	T36.1X1	T36.1X2	T36.1X3	T36.1X4	T36.1X5	T36.1X6
Cefalexin	T36.1X1	T36.1X2	T36.1X3	T36.1X4	T36.1X5	T36.1X6
Cefaloglycin	T36.1X1	T36.1X2	T36.1X3	T36.1X4	T36.1X5	T36.1X6
Cefaloridine	T36.1X1	T36.1X2	T36.1X3	T36.1X4	T36.1X5	T36.1X6
Cefalosporins	T36.1X1	T36.1X2	T36.1X3	T36.1X4	T36.1X5	T36.1X6
Cefalotin	T36.1X1	T36.1X2	T36.1X3	T36.1X4	T36.1X5	T36.1X6
Cefamandole	T36.1X1	T36.1X2	T36.1X3	T36.1X4	T36.1X5	T36.1X6
Cefamycin antibiotic	T36.1X1	T36.1X2	T36.1X3	T36.1X4	T36.1X5	T36.1X6
Cefapirin	T36.1X1	T36.1X2	T36.1X3	T36.1X4	T36.1X5	T36.1X6
Cefatrizine	T36.1X1	T36.1X2	T36.1X3	T36.1X4	T36.1X5	T36.1X6
Cefazedone	T36.1X1	T36.1X2	T36.1X3	T36.1X4	T36.1X5	T36.1X6
Cefazolin	T36.1X1	T36.1X2	T36.1X3	T36.1X4	T36.1X5	T36.1X6
Cefbuperazone	T36.1X1	T36.1X2	T36.1X3	T36.1X4	T36.1X5	T36.1X6
Cefetamet	T36.1X1	T36.1X2	T36.1X3	T36.1X4	T36.1X5	T36.1X6
Cefixime	T36.1X1	T36.1X2	T36.1X3	T36.1X4	T36.1X5	T36.1X6
Cefmenoxime	T36.1X1	T36.1X2	T36.1X3	T36.1X4	T36.1X5	T36.1X6
Cefmetazole	T36.1X1	T36.1X2	T36.1X3	T36.1X4	T36.1X5	T36.1X6
Cefminox	T36.1X1	T36.1X2	T36.1X3	T36.1X4	T36.1X5	T36.1X6
Cefonicid	T36.1X1	T36.1X2	T36.1X3	T36.1X4	T36.1X5	T36.1X6
Cefoperazone	T36.1X1	T36.1X2	T36.1X3	T36.1X4	T36.1X5	T36.1X6
Ceforanide	T36.1X1	T36.1X2	T36.1X3	T36.1X4	T36.1X5	T36.1X6
Cefotaxime	T36.1X1	T36.1X2	T36.1X3	T36.1X4	T36.1X5	T36.1X6
Cefotetan	T36.1X1	T36.1X2	T36.1X3	T36.1X4	T36.1X5	T36.1X6
Cefotiam	T36.1X1	T36.1X2	T36.1X3	T36.1X4	T36.1X5	T36.1X6
Cefoxitin	T36.1X1	T36.1X2	T36.1X3	T36.1X4	T36.1X5	T36.1X6
Cefpimizole	T36.1X1	T36.1X2	T36.1X3	T36.1X4	T36.1X5	T36.1X6
Cefpiramide	T36.1X1	T36.1X2	T36.1X3	T36.1X4	T36.1X5	T36.1X6
Cefradine	T36.1X1	T36.1X2	T36.1X3	T36.1X4	T36.1X5	T36.1X6
Cefroxadine	T36.1X1	T36.1X2	T36.1X3	T36.1X4	T36.1X5	T36.1X6
Cefsulodin	T36.1X1	T36.1X2	T36.1X3	T36.1X4	T36.1X5	T36.1X6
Ceftazidime	T36.1X1	T36.1X2	T36.1X3	T36.1X4	T36.1X5	T36.1X6
Cefteram	T36.1X1	T36.1X2	T36.1X3	T36.1X4	T36.1X5	T36.1X6
Ceftezole	T36.1X1	T36.1X2	T36.1X3	T36.1X4	T36.1X5	T36.1X6
Ceftizoxime	T36.1X1	T36.1X2	T36.1X3	T36.1X4	T36.1X5	T36.1X6
Ceftriaxone	T36.1X1	T36.1X2	T36.1X3	T36.1X4	T36.1X5	T36.1X6
Cefuroxime	T36.1X1	T36.1X2	T36.1X3	T36.1X4	T36.1X5	T36.1X6
Cefuzonam	T36.1X1	T36.1X2	T36.1X3	T36.1X4	T36.1X5	T36.1X6
Celestone	T38.0X1	T38.0X2	T38.0X3	T38.0X4	T38.0X5	T38.0X6
topical	T49.0X1	T49.0X2	T49.0X3	T49.0X4	T49.0X5	T49.0X6

Substance	Poisoning, Accidental (unintentional)	Poisoning, Intentional self-harm	Poisoning, Assault	Poisoning, Undetermined	Adverse effect	Underdosing
Celiprolol	T44.7X1	T44.7X2	T44.7X3	T44.7X4	T44.7X5	T44.7X6
Cell stimulants and proliferants	T49.8X1	T49.8X2	T49.8X3	T49.8X4	T49.8X5	T49.8X6
Cellosolve	T52.91	T52.92	T52.93	T52.94	—	—
Cellulose						
cathartic	T47.4X1	T47.4X2	T47.4X3	T47.4X4	T47.4X5	T47.4X6
hydroxyethyl	T47.4X1	T47.4X2	T47.4X3	T47.4X4	T47.4X5	T47.4X6
nitrates (topical)	T49.3X1	T49.3X2	T49.3X3	T49.3X4	T49.3X5	T49.3X6
oxidized	T49.4X1	T49.4X2	T49.4X3	T49.4X4	T49.4X5	T49.4X6
Centipede (bite)	T63.411	T63.412	T63.413	T63.414	—	—
Central nervous system						
depressants	T42.71	T42.72	T42.73	T42.74	T42.75	T42.76
anesthetic (general) NEC	T41.201	T41.202	T41.203	T41.204	T41.205	T41.206
gases NEC	T41.0X1	T41.0X2	T41.0X3	T41.0X4	T41.0X5	T41.0X6
intravenous	T41.1X1	T41.1X2	T41.1X3	T41.1X4	T41.1X5	T41.1X6
barbiturates	T42.3X1	T42.3X2	T42.3X3	T42.3X4	T42.3X5	T42.3X6
benzodiazepines	T42.4X1	T42.4X2	T42.4X3	T42.4X4	T42.4X5	T42.4X6
bromides	T42.6X1	T42.6X2	T42.6X3	T42.6X4	T42.6X5	T42.6X6
cannabis sativa	T40.7X1	T40.7X2	T40.7X3	T40.7X4	T40.7X5	T40.7X6
chloral hydrate	T42.6X1	T42.6X2	T42.6X3	T42.6X4	T42.6X5	T42.6X6
ethanol	T51.0X1	T51.0X2	T51.0X3	T51.0X4	—	—
hallucinogenics	T40.901	T40.902	T40.903	T40.904	T40.905	T40.906
hypnotics	T42.71	T42.72	T42.73	T42.74	T42.75	T42.76
specified NEC	T42.6X1	T42.6X2	T42.6X3	T42.6X4	T42.6X5	T42.6X6
muscle relaxants	T42.8X1	T42.8X2	T42.8X3	T42.8X4	T42.8X5	T42.8X6
paraldehyde	T42.6X1	T42.6X2	T42.6X3	T42.6X4	T42.6X5	T42.6X6
sedatives; sedative-hypnotics	T42.71	T42.72	T42.73	T42.74	T42.75	T42.76
mixed NEC	T42.6X1	T42.6X2	T42.6X3	T42.6X4	T42.6X5	T42.6X6
specified NEC	T42.6X1	T42.6X2	T42.6X3	T42.6X4	T42.6X5	T42.6X6
muscle-tone depressants	T42.8X1	T42.8X2	T42.8X3	T42.8X4	T42.8X5	T42.8X6
stimulants	T43.601	T43.602	T43.603	T43.604	T43.605	T43.606
amphetamines	T43.621	T43.622	T43.623	T43.624	T43.625	T43.626
analeptics	T50.7X1	T50.7X2	T50.7X3	T50.7X4	T50.7X5	T50.7X6
antidepressants	T43.201	T43.202	T43.203	T43.204	T43.205	T43.206
opiate antagonists	T50.7X1	T50.7X2	T50.7X3	T50.7X4	T50.7X5	T50.7X6
specified NEC	T43.691	T43.692	T43.693	T43.694	T43.695	T43.696
Cephalexin	T36.1X1	T36.1X2	T36.1X3	T36.1X4	T36.1X5	T36.1X6
Cephaloglycin	T36.1X1	T36.1X2	T36.1X3	T36.1X4	T36.1X5	T36.1X6
Cephaloridine	T36.1X1	T36.1X2	T36.1X3	T36.1X4	T36.1X5	T36.1X6
Cephalosporins	T36.1X1	T36.1X2	T36.1X3	T36.1X4	T36.1X5	T36.1X6
N(adicillin)	T36.0X1	T36.0X2	T36.0X3	T36.0X4	T36.0X5	T36.0X6
Cephalothin	T36.1X1	T36.1X2	T36.1X3	T36.1X4	T36.1X5	T36.1X6
Cephalotin	T36.1X1	T36.1X2	T36.1X3	T36.1X4	T36.1X5	T36.1X6
Cephradine	T36.1X1	T36.1X2	T36.1X3	T36.1X4	T36.1X5	T36.1X6
Cerbera (odallam)	T62.2X1	T62.2X2	T62.2X3	T62.2X4	—	—
Cerberin	T46.0X1	T46.0X2	T46.0X3	T46.0X4	T46.0X5	T46.0X6
Cerebral stimulants	T43.601	T43.602	T43.603	T43.604	T43.605	T43.606
psychotherapeutic	T43.601	T43.602	T43.603	T43.604	T43.605	T43.606
specified NEC	T43.691	T43.692	T43.693	T43.694	T43.695	T43.696

Substance	Poisoning, Accidental (unintentional)	Poisoning, Intentional self-harm	Poisoning, Assault	Poisoning, Undetermined	Adverse effect	Underdosing
Cerium oxalate	T45.0X1	T45.0X2	T45.0X3	T45.0X4	T45.0X5	T45.0X6
Cerous oxalate	T45.0X1	T45.0X2	T45.0X3	T45.0X4	T45.0X5	T45.0X6
Ceruletide	T50.8X1	T50.8X2	T50.8X3	T50.8X4	T50.8X5	T50.8X6
Cetalkonium (chloride)	T49.0X1	T49.0X2	T49.0X3	T49.0X4	T49.0X5	T49.0X6
Cethexonium chloride	T49.0X1	T49.0X2	T49.0X3	T49.0X4	T49.0X5	T49.0X6
Cetiedil	T46.7X1	T46.7X2	T46.7X3	T46.7X4	T46.7X5	T46.7X6
Cetirizine	T45.0X1	T45.0X2	T45.0X3	T45.0X4	T45.0X5	T45.0X6
Cetomacrogol	T50.991	T50.992	T50.993	T50.994	T50.995	T50.996
Cetotiamine	T45.2X1	T45.2X2	T45.2X3	T45.2X4	T45.2X5	T45.2X6
Cetoxime	T45.0X1	T45.0X2	T45.0X3	T45.0X4	T45.0X5	T45.0X6
Cetraxate	T47.1X1	T47.1X2	T47.1X3	T47.1X4	T47.1X5	T47.1X6
Cetrimide	T49.0X1	T49.0X2	T49.0X3	T49.0X4	T49.0X5	T49.0X6
Cetrimonium (bromide)	T49.0X1	T49.0X2	T49.0X3	T49.0X4	T49.0X5	T49.0X6
Cetylpyridinium chloride	T49.0X1	T49.0X2	T49.0X3	T49.0X4	T49.0X5	T49.0X6
ENT agent	T49.6X1	T49.6X2	T49.6X3	T49.6X4	T49.6X5	T49.6X6
lozenges	T49.6X1	T49.6X2	T49.6X3	T49.6X4	T49.6X5	T49.6X6
Cevadilla—see Sabadilla						
Cevitamic acid	T45.2X1	T45.2X2	T45.2X3	T45.2X4	T45.2X5	T45.2X6
Chalk, precipitated	T47.1X1	T47.1X2	T47.1X3	T47.1X4	T47.1X5	T47.1X6
Chamomile	T49.0X1	T49.0X2	T49.0X3	T49.0X4	T49.0X5	T49.0X6
Ch'an su	T46.0X1	T46.0X2	T46.0X3	T46.0X4	T46.0X5	T46.0X6
Charcoal	T47.6X1	T47.6X2	T47.6X3	T47.6X4	T47.6X5	T47.6X6
activated—see also Charcoal, medicinal	T47.6X1	T47.6X2	T47.6X3	T47.6X4	T47.6X5	T47.6X6
fumes (Carbon monoxide)	T58.2X1	T58.2X2	T58.2X3	T58.2X4	—	—
industrial	T58.8X1	T58.8X2	T58.8X3	T58.8X4	—	—
medicinal (activated)	T47.6X1	T47.6X2	T47.6X3	T47.6X4	T47.6X5	T47.6X6
antidiarrheal	T47.6X1	T47.6X2	T47.6X3	T47.6X4	T47.6X5	T47.6X6
poison control	T47.8X1	T47.8X2	T47.8X3	T47.8X4	T47.8X5	T47.8X6
specified use other than for diarrhea	T47.8X1	T47.8X2	T47.8X3	T47.8X4	T47.8X5	T47.8X6
topical	T49.8X1	T49.8X2	T49.8X3	T49.8X4	T49.8X5	T49.8X6
Chaulmosulfone	T37.1X1	T37.1X2	T37.1X3	T37.1X4	T37.1X5	T37.1X6
Chelating agent NEC	T50.6X1	T50.6X2	T50.6X3	T50.6X4	T50.6X5	T50.6X6
Chelidonium majus	T62.2X1	T62.2X2	T62.2X3	T62.2X4	—	—
Chemical substance NEC	T65.91	T65.92	T65.93	T65.94	—	—
Chenodeoxycholic acid	T47.5X1	T47.5X2	T47.5X3	T47.5X4	T47.5X5	T47.5X6
Chenodiol	T47.5X1	T47.5X2	T47.5X3	T47.5X4	T47.5X5	T47.5X6
Chenopodium	T37.4X1	T37.4X2	T37.4X3	T37.4X4	T37.4X5	T37.4X6
Cherry laurel	T62.2X1	T62.2X2	T62.2X3	T62.2X4	—	—
Chinidin(e)	T46.2X1	T46.2X2	T46.2X3	T46.2X4	T46.2X5	T46.2X6
Chiniofon	T37.8X1	T37.8X2	T37.8X3	T37.8X4	T37.8X5	T37.8X6
Chlophedianol	T48.3X1	T48.3X2	T48.3X3	T48.3X4	T48.3X5	T48.3X6
Chloral	T42.6X1	T42.6X2	T42.6X3	T42.6X4	T42.6X5	T42.6X6
derivative	T42.6X1	T42.6X2	T42.6X3	T42.6X4	T42.6X5	T42.6X6
hydrate	T42.6X1	T42.6X2	T42.6X3	T42.6X4	T42.6X5	T42.6X6
Chloralamide	T42.6X1	T42.6X2	T42.6X3	T42.6X4	T42.6X5	T42.6X6
Chloralodol	T42.6X1	T42.6X2	T42.6X3	T42.6X4	T42.6X5	T42.6X6
Chloralose	T60.4X1	T60.4X2	T60.4X3	T60.4X4	—	—
Chlorambucil	T45.1X1	T45.1X2	T45.1X3	T45.1X4	T45.1X5	T45.1X6
Chloramine	T57.8X1	T57.8X2	T57.8X3	T57.8X4	—	—
T	T49.0X1	T49.0X2	T49.0X3	T49.0X4	T49.0X5	T49.0X6
topical	T49.0X1	T49.0X2	T49.0X3	T49.0X4	T49.0X5	T49.0X6
Chloramphenicol	T36.2X1	T36.2X2	T36.2X3	T36.2X4	T36.2X5	T36.2X6
ENT agent	T49.6X1	T49.6X2	T49.6X3	T49.6X4	T49.6X5	T49.6X6
ophthalmic preparation	T49.5X1	T49.5X2	T49.5X3	T49.5X4	T49.5X5	T49.5X6
topical NEC	T49.0X1	T49.0X2	T49.0X3	T49.0X4	T49.0X5	T49.0X6
Chlorate (potassium) (sodium) NEC	T60.3X1	T60.3X2	T60.3X3	T60.3X4	—	—
herbicide	T60.3X1	T60.3X2	T60.3X3	T60.3X4	—	—
Chlorazanil	T50.2X1	T50.2X2	T50.2X3	T50.2X4	T50.2X5	T50.2X6
Chlorbenzene, chlorbenzol	T53.7X1	T53.7X2	T53.7X3	T53.7X4	—	—
Chlorbenzoxamine	T44.3X1	T44.3X2	T44.3X3	T44.3X4	T44.3X5	T44.3X6
Chlorbutol	T42.6X1	T42.6X2	T42.6X3	T42.6X4	T42.6X5	T42.6X6
Chlorcyclizine	T45.0X1	T45.0X2	T45.0X3	T45.0X4	T45.0X5	T45.0X6
Chlordan(e) (dust)	T60.1X1	T60.1X2	T60.1X3	T60.1X4	—	—
Chlordantoin	T49.0X1	T49.0X2	T49.0X3	T49.0X4	T49.0X5	T49.0X6
Chlordiazepoxide	T42.4X1	T42.4X2	T42.4X3	T42.4X4	T42.4X5	T42.4X6
Chlordiethyl benzamide	T49.3X1	T49.3X2	T49.3X3	T49.3X4	T49.3X5	T49.3X6
Chloresium	T49.8X1	T49.8X2	T49.8X3	T49.8X4	T49.8X5	T49.8X6
Chlorethiazol	T42.6X1	T42.6X2	T42.6X3	T42.6X4	T42.6X5	T42.6X6
Chlorethyl—see Ethyl chloride						
Chloretone	T42.6X1	T42.6X2	T42.6X3	T42.6X4	T42.6X5	T42.6X6
Chlorex	T53.6X1	T53.6X2	T53.6X3	T53.6X4	—	—
insecticide	T60.1X1	T60.1X2	T60.1X3	T60.1X4	—	—
Chlorfenvinphos	T60.0X1	T60.0X2	T60.0X3	T60.0X4	—	—
Chlorhexadol	T42.6X1	T42.6X2	T42.6X3	T42.6X4	T42.6X5	T42.6X6
Chlorhexamide	T45.1X1	T45.1X2	T45.1X3	T45.1X4	T45.1X5	T45.1X6
Chlorhexidine	T49.0X1	T49.0X2	T49.0X3	T49.0X4	T49.0X5	T49.0X6
Chlorhydro-xyquinolin	T49.0X1	T49.0X2	T49.0X3	T49.0X4	T49.0X5	T49.0X6
Chloride of lime (bleach)	T54.3X1	T54.3X2	T54.3X3	T54.3X4	—	—
Chlorimipramine	T43.011	T43.012	T43.013	T43.014	T43.015	T43.016
Chlorinated						
camphene	T53.6X1	T53.6X2	T53.6X3	T53.6X4	—	—
diphenyl	T53.7X1	T53.7X2	T53.7X3	T53.7X4	—	—
hydrocarbons NEC	T53.91	T53.92	T53.93	T53.94	—	—
solvents	T53.91	T53.92	T53.93	T53.94	—	—
lime (bleach)	T54.3X1	T54.3X2	T54.3X3	T54.3X4	—	—
and boric acid solution	T49.0X1	T49.0X2	T49.0X3	T49.0X4	T49.0X5	T49.0X6
naphthalene (insecticide)	T60.1X1	T60.1X2	T60.1X3	T60.1X4	—	—
industrial (non-pesticide)	T53.7X1	T53.7X2	T53.7X3	T53.7X4	—	—
pesticide NEC	T60.8X1	T60.8X2	T60.8X3	T60.8X4	—	—
soda—see also sodium hypochlorite						
solution	T49.0X1	T49.0X2	T49.0X3	T49.0X4	T49.0X5	T49.0X6

Substance	Poisoning, Accidental (unintentional)	Poisoning, Intentional self-harm	Poisoning, Assault	Poisoning, Undetermined	Adverse effect	Underdosing
Chlorine (fumes) (gas)	T59.4X1	T59.4X2	T59.4X3	T59.4X4	—	—
bleach	T54.3X1	T54.3X2	T54.3X3	T54.3X4	—	—
compound gas NEC	T59.4X1	T59.4X2	T59.4X3	T59.4X4	—	—
disinfectant	T59.4X1	T59.4X2	T59.4X3	T59.4X4	—	—
releasing agents NEC	T59.4X1	T59.4X2	T59.4X3	T59.4X4	—	—
Chlorisondamine chloride	T46.991	T46.992	T46.993	T46.994	T46.995	T46.996
Chlormadinone	T38.5X1	T38.5X2	T38.5X3	T38.5X4	T38.5X5	T38.5X6
Chlormephos	T60.0X1	T60.0X2	T60.0X3	T60.0X4		
Chlormerodrin	T50.2X1	T50.2X2	T50.2X3	T50.2X4	T50.2X5	T50.2X6
Chlormethiazole	T42.6X1	T42.6X2	T42.6X3	T42.6X4	T42.6X5	T42.6X6
Chlormethine	T45.1X1	T45.1X2	T45.1X3	T45.1X4	T45.1X5	T45.1X6
Chlormethyle-necycline	T36.4X1	T36.4X2	T36.4X3	T36.4X4	T36.4X5	T36.4X6
Chlormezanone	T42.6X1	T42.6X2	T42.6X3	T42.6X4	T42.6X5	T42.6X6
Chloroacetic acid	T60.3X1	T60.3X2	T60.3X3	T60.3X4	—	—
Chloroacetone	T59.3X1	T59.3X2	T59.3X3	T59.3X4	—	—
Chloroacetophenone	T59.3X1	T59.3X2	T59.3X3	T59.3X4	—	—
Chloroaniline	T53.7X1	T53.7X2	T53.7X3	T53.7X4	—	—
Chlorobenzene, chlorobenzol	T53.7X1	T53.7X2	T53.7X3	T53.7X4	—	—
Chlorobromo methane (fire extinguisher)	T53.6X1	T53.6X2	T53.6X3	T53.6X4	—	—
Chlorobutanol	T49.0X1	T49.0X2	T49.0X3	T49.0X4	T49.0X5	T49.0X6
Chlorocresol	T49.0X1	T49.0X2	T49.0X3	T49.0X4	T49.0X5	T49.0X6
Chlorodehydro-methyltestosterone	T38.7X1	T38.7X2	T38.7X3	T38.7X4	T38.7X5	T38.7X6
Chlorodinitro-benzene	T53.7X1	T53.7X2	T53.7X3	T53.7X4	—	—
dust or vapor	T53.7X1	T53.7X2	T53.7X3	T53.7X4	—	—
Chlorodiphenyl	T53.7X1	T53.7X2	T53.7X3	T53.7X4	—	—
Chloroethane—see Ethyl chloride						
Chloroethylene	T53.6X1	T53.6X2	T53.6X3	T53.6X4	—	—
Chlorofluorocarbons	T53.5X1	T53.5X2	T53.5X3	T53.5X4	—	—
Chloroform (fumes) (vapor)	T53.1X1	T53.1X2	T53.1X3	T53.1X4	—	—
anesthetic	T41.0X1	T41.0X2	T41.0X3	T41.0X4	T41.0X5	T41.0X6
solvent	T53.1X1	T53.1X2	T53.1X3	T53.1X4	—	—
water, concentrated	T41.0X1	T41.0X2	T41.0X3	T41.0X4	T41.0X5	T41.0X6
Chloroguanide	T37.2X1	T37.2X2	T37.2X3	T37.2X4	T37.2X5	T37.2X6
Chloromycetin	T36.2X1	T36.2X2	T36.2X3	T36.2X4	T36.2X5	T36.2X6
ENT agent	T49.6X1	T49.6X2	T49.6X3	T49.6X4	T49.6X5	T49.6X6
ophthalmic preparation	T49.5X1	T49.5X2	T49.5X3	T49.5X4	T49.5X5	T49.5X6
otic solution	T49.6X1	T49.6X2	T49.6X3	T49.6X4	T49.6X5	T49.6X6
topical NEC	T49.0X1	T49.0X2	T49.0X3	T49.0X4	T49.0X5	T49.0X6
Chloronitrobenzene	T53.7X1	T53.7X2	T53.7X3	T53.7X4	—	—
dust or vapor	T53.7X1	T53.7X2	T53.7X3	T53.7X4	—	—
Chlorophacinone	T60.4X1	T60.4X2	T60.4X3	T60.4X4	—	—
Chlorophenol	T53.7X1	T53.7X2	T53.7X3	T53.7X4	—	—
Chlorophenothane	T60.1X1	T60.1X2	T60.1X3	T60.1X4	—	—
Chlorophyll	T50.991	T50.992	T50.993	T50.994	T50.995	T50.996
Chloropicrin (fumes)	T53.6X1	T53.6X2	T53.6X3	T53.6X4	—	—
fumigant	T60.8X1	T60.8X2	T60.8X3	T60.8X4	—	—

Substance	Poisoning, Accidental (unintentional)	Poisoning, Intentional self-harm	Poisoning, Assault	Poisoning, Undetermined	Adverse effect	Underdosing
Chloropicrin — *Continued*						
fungicide	T60.3X1	T60.3X2	T60.3X3	T60.3X4	—	—
pesticide	T60.8X1	T60.8X2	T60.8X3	T60.8X4	—	—
Chloroprocaine	T41.3X1	T41.3X2	T41.3X3	T41.3X4	T41.3X5	T41.3X6
infiltration (subcutaneous)	T41.3X1	T41.3X2	T41.3X3	T41.3X4	T41.3X5	T41.3X6
nerve block (peripheral) (plexus)	T41.3X1	T41.3X2	T41.3X3	T41.3X4	T41.3X5	T41.3X6
spinal	T41.3X1	T41.3X2	T41.3X3	T41.3X4	T41.3X5	T41.3X6
Chloroptic	T49.5X1	T49.5X2	T49.5X3	T49.5X4	T49.5X5	T49.5X6
Chloropurine	T45.1X1	T45.1X2	T45.1X3	T45.1X4	T45.1X5	T45.1X6
Chloropyramine	T45.0X1	T45.0X2	T45.0X3	T45.0X4	T45.0X5	T45.0X6
Chloropyrifos	T60.0X1	T60.0X2	T60.0X3	T60.0X4	—	—
Chloropyrilene	T45.0X1	T45.0X2	T45.0X3	T45.0X4	T45.0X5	T45.0X6
Chloroquine	T37.2X1	T37.2X2	T37.2X3	T37.2X4	T37.2X5	T37.2X6
Chlorothalonil	T60.3X1	T60.3X2	T60.3X3	T60.3X4	—	—
Chlorothen	T45.0X1	T45.0X2	T45.0X3	T45.0X4	T45.0X5	T45.0X6
Chlorothiazide	T50.2X1	T50.2X2	T50.2X3	T50.2X4	T50.2X5	T50.2X6
Chlorothymol	T49.4X1	T49.4X2	T49.4X3	T49.4X4	T49.4X5	T49.4X6
Chlorotrianisene	T38.5X1	T38.5X2	T38.5X3	T38.5X4	T38.5X5	T38.5X6
Chlorovinyldichloro-arsine, not in war	T57.0X1	T57.0X2	T57.0X3	T57.0X4	—	—
Chloroxine	T49.4X1	T49.4X2	T49.4X3	T49.4X4	T49.4X5	T49.4X6
Chloroxylenol	T49.0X1	T49.0X2	T49.0X3	T49.0X4	T49.0X5	T49.0X6
Chlorphenamine	T45.0X1	T45.0X2	T45.0X3	T45.0X4	T45.0X5	T45.0X6
Chlorphenesin	T42.8X1	T42.8X2	T42.8X3	T42.8X4	T42.8X5	T42.8X6
topical (antifungal)	T49.0X1	T49.0X2	T49.0X3	T49.0X4	T49.0X5	T49.0X6
Chlorpheniramine	T45.0X1	T45.0X2	T45.0X3	T45.0X4	T45.0X5	T45.0X6
Chlorphenoxamine	T45.0X1	T45.0X2	T45.0X3	T45.0X4	T45.0X5	T45.0X6
Chlorphentermine	T50.5X1	T50.5X2	T50.5X3	T50.5X4	T50.5X5	T50.5X6
Chlorprocaine—see Chloroprocaine						
Chlorproguanil	T37.2X1	T37.2X2	T37.2X3	T37.2X4	T37.2X5	T37.2X6
Chlorpromazine	T43.3X1	T43.3X2	T43.3X3	T43.3X4	T43.3X5	T43.3X6
Chlorpropamide	T38.3X1	T38.3X2	T38.3X3	T38.3X4	T38.3X5	T38.3X6
Chlorprothixene	T43.4X1	T43.4X2	T43.4X3	T43.4X4	T43.4X5	T43.4X6
Chlorquinaldol	T49.0X1	T49.0X2	T49.0X3	T49.0X4	T49.0X5	T49.0X6
Chlorquinol	T49.0X1	T49.0X2	T49.0X3	T49.0X4	T49.0X5	T49.0X6
Chlortalidone	T50.2X1	T50.2X2	T50.2X3	T50.2X4	T50.2X5	T50.2X6
Chlortetracycline	T36.4X1	T36.4X2	T36.4X3	T36.4X4	T36.4X5	T36.4X6
Chlorthalidone	T50.2X1	T50.2X2	T50.2X3	T50.2X4	T50.2X5	T50.2X6
Chlorthiophos	T60.0X1	T60.0X2	T60.0X3	T60.0X4	—	—
Chlortrianisene	T38.5X1	T38.5X2	T38.5X3	T38.5X4	T38.5X5	T38.5X6
Chlor-Trimeton	T45.0X1	T45.0X2	T45.0X3	T45.0X4	T45.0X5	T45.0X6
Chlorthion	T60.0X1	T60.0X2	T60.0X3	T60.0X4	—	—
Chlorzoxazone	T42.8X1	T42.8X2	T42.8X3	T42.8X4	T42.8X5	T42.8X6
Choke damp	T59.7X1	T59.7X2	T59.7X3	T59.7X4	—	—
Cholagogues	T47.5X1	T47.5X2	T47.5X3	T47.5X4	T47.5X5	T47.5X6
Cholebrine	T50.8X1	T50.8X2	T50.8X3	T50.8X4	T50.8X5	T50.8X6
Cholecalciferol	T45.2X1	T45.2X2	T45.2X3	T45.2X4	T45.2X5	T45.2X6

Substance	Poisoning, Accidental (unintentional)	Poisoning, Intentional self-harm	Poisoning, Assault	Poisoning, Undetermined	Adverse effect	Underdosing
Cholecystokinin	T50.8X1	T50.8X2	T50.8X3	T50.8X4	T50.8X5	T50.8X6
Cholera vaccine	T50.A91	T50.A92	T50.A93	T50.A94	T50.A95	T50.A96
Choleretic	T47.5X1	T47.5X2	T47.5X3	T47.5X4	T47.5X5	T47.5X6
Cholesterol-lowering agents	T46.6X1	T46.6X2	T46.6X3	T46.6X4	T46.6X5	T46.6X6
Cholestyramine (resin)	T46.6X1	T46.6X2	T46.6X3	T46.6X4	T46.6X5	T46.6X6
Cholic acid	T47.5X1	T47.5X2	T47.5X3	T47.5X4	T47.5X5	T47.5X6
Choline	T48.6X1	T48.6X2	T48.6X3	T48.6X4	T48.6X5	T48.6X6
chloride	T50.991	T50.992	T50.993	T50.994	T50.995	T50.996
dihydrogen citrate	T50.991	T50.992	T50.993	T50.994	T50.995	T50.996
salicylate	T39.091	T39.092	T39.093	T39.094	T39.095	T39.096
theophyllinate	T48.6X1	T48.6X2	T48.6X3	T48.6X4	T48.6X5	T48.6X6
Cholinergic (drug) NEC	T44.1X1	T44.1X2	T44.1X3	T44.1X4	T44.1X5	T44.1X6
muscle tone enhancer	T44.1X1	T44.1X2	T44.1X3	T44.1X4	T44.1X5	T44.1X6
organophosphorus	T44.0X1	T44.0X2	T44.0X3	T44.0X4	T44.0X5	T44.0X6
insecticide	T60.0X1	T60.0X2	T60.0X3	T60.0X4	—	—
nerve gas	T59.891	T59.892	T59.893	T59.894	—	—
trimethyl ammonium propanediol	T44.1X1	T44.1X2	T44.1X3	T44.1X4	T44.1X5	T44.1X6
Cholinesterase reactivator	T50.6X1	T50.6X2	T50.6X3	T50.6X4	T50.6X5	T50.6X6
Chologafin	T50.8X1	T50.8X2	T50.8X3	T50.8X4	T50.8X5	T50.8X6
Chorionic gonadotropin	T38.891	T38.892	T38.893	T38.894	T38.895	T38.896
Chromate	T56.2X1	T56.2X2	T56.2X3	T56.2X4	—	—
dust or mist	T56.2X1	T56.2X2	T56.2X3	T56.2X4	—	—
lead—see also lead	T56.0X1	T56.0X2	T56.0X3	T56.0X4	—	—
paint	T56.0X1	T56.0X2	T56.0X3	T56.0X4	—	—
Chromic						
acid	T56.2X1	T56.2X2	T56.2X3	T56.2X4	—	—
dust or mist	T56.2X1	T56.2X2	T56.2X3	T56.2X4	—	—
phosphate 32P	T45.1X1	T45.1X2	T45.1X3	T45.1X4	T45.1X5	T45.1X6
Chromium	T56.2X1	T56.2X2	T56.2X3	T56.2X4	—	—
compounds—see Chromate						
sesquioxide	T50.8X1	T50.8X2	T50.8X3	T50.8X4	T50.8X5	T50.8X6
Chromomycin A3	T45.1X1	T45.1X2	T45.1X3	T45.1X4	T45.1X5	T45.1X6
Chromonar	T46.3X1	T46.3X2	T46.3X3	T46.3X4	T46.3X5	T46.3X6
Chromyl chloride	T56.2X1	T56.2X2	T56.2X3	T56.2X4	—	—
Chrysarobin	T49.4X1	T49.4X2	T49.4X3	T49.4X4	T49.4X5	T49.4X6
Chrysazin	T47.2X1	T47.2X2	T47.2X3	T47.2X4	T47.2X5	T47.2X6
Chymar	T45.3X1	T45.3X2	T45.3X3	T45.3X4	T45.3X5	T45.3X6
ophthalmic preparation	T49.5X1	T49.5X2	T49.5X3	T49.5X4	T49.5X5	T49.5X6
Chymopapain	T45.3X1	T45.3X2	T45.3X3	T45.3X4	T45.3X5	T45.3X6
Chymotrypsin	T45.3X1	T45.3X2	T45.3X3	T45.3X4	T45.3X5	T45.3X6
ophthalmic preparation	T49.5X1	T49.5X2	T49.5X3	T49.5X4	T49.5X5	T49.5X6
Cianidanol	T50.991	T50.992	T50.993	T50.994	T50.995	T50.996
Cianopramine	T43.011	T43.012	T43.013	T43.014	T43.015	T43.016
Cibenzoline	T46.2X1	T46.2X2	T46.2X3	T46.2X4	T46.2X5	T46.2X6
Ciclacillin	T36.0X1	T36.0X2	T36.0X3	T36.0X4	T36.0X5	T36.0X6
Ciclobarbital—see Hexobarbital						
Ciclonicate	T46.7X1	T46.7X2	T46.7X3	T46.7X4	T46.7X5	T46.7X6
Ciclopirox (olamine)	T49.0X1	T49.0X2	T49.0X3	T49.0X4	T49.0X5	T49.0X6
Ciclosporin	T45.1X1	T45.1X2	T45.1X3	T45.1X4	T45.1X5	T45.1X6
Cicuta maculata or virosa	T62.2X1	T62.2X2	T62.2X3	T62.2X4	—	—
Cicutoxin	T62.2X1	T62.2X2	T62.2X3	T62.2X4	—	—
Cigarette lighter fluid	T52.0X1	T52.0X2	T52.0X3	T52.0X4	—	—
Cigarettes (tobacco)	T65.221	T65.222	T65.223	T65.224	—	—
Ciguatoxin	T61.01	T61.02	T61.03	T61.04	—	—
Cilazapril	T46.4X1	T46.4X2	T46.4X3	T46.4X4	T46.4X5	T46.4X6
Cimetidine	T47.0X1	T47.0X2	T47.0X3	T47.0X4	T47.0X5	T47.0X6
Cimetropium bromide	T44.3X1	T44.3X2	T44.3X3	T44.3X4	T44.3X5	T44.3X6
Cinchocaine	T41.3X1	T41.3X2	T41.3X3	T41.3X4	T41.3X5	T41.3X6
topical (surface)	T41.3X1	T41.3X2	T41.3X3	T41.3X4	T41.3X5	T41.3X6
Cinchona	T37.2X1	T37.2X2	T37.2X3	T37.2X4	T37.2X5	T37.2X6
Cinchonine alkaloids	T37.2X1	T37.2X2	T37.2X3	T37.2X4	T37.2X5	T37.2X6
Cinchophen	T50.4X1	T50.4X2	T50.4X3	T50.4X4	T50.4X5	T50.4X6
Cinepazide	T46.7X1	T46.7X2	T46.7X3	T46.7X4	T46.7X5	T46.7X6
Cinnamedrine	T48.5X1	T48.5X2	T48.5X3	T48.5X4	T48.5X5	T48.5X6
Cinnarizine	T45.0X1	T45.0X2	T45.0X3	T45.0X4	T45.0X5	T45.0X6
Cinoxacin	T37.8X1	T37.8X2	T37.8X3	T37.8X4	T37.8X5	T37.8X6
Ciprofibrate	T46.6X1	T46.6X2	T46.6X3	T46.6X4	T46.6X5	T46.6X6
Ciprofloxacin	T36.8X1	T36.8X2	T36.8X3	T36.8X4	T36.8X5	T36.8X6
Cisapride	T47.8X1	T47.8X2	T47.8X3	T47.8X4	T47.8X5	T47.8X6
Cisplatin	T45.1X1	T45.1X2	T45.1X3	T45.1X4	T45.1X5	T45.1X6
Citalopram	T43.221	T43.222	T43.223	T43.224	T43.225	T43.226
Citanest	T41.3X1	T41.3X2	T41.3X3	T41.3X4	T41.3X5	T41.3X6
infiltration (subcutaneous)	T41.3X1	T41.3X2	T41.3X3	T41.3X4	T41.3X5	T41.3X6
nerve block (peripheral) (plexus)	T41.3X1	T41.3X2	T41.3X3	T41.3X4	T41.3X5	T41.3X6
Citric acid	T47.5X1	T47.5X2	T47.5X3	T47.5X4	T47.5X5	T47.5X6
Citrovorum (factor)	T45.8X1	T45.8X2	T45.8X3	T45.8X4	T45.8X5	T45.8X6
Claviceps purpurea	T62.2X1	T62.2X2	T62.2X3	T62.2X4	—	—
Clavulanic acid	T36.1X1	T36.1X2	T36.1X3	T36.1X4	T36.1X5	T36.1X6
Cleaner, cleansing agent, type not specified	T65.891	T65.892	T65.893	T65.894	—	—
of paint or varnish	T52.91	T52.92	T52.93	T52.94	—	—
specified type NEC	T65.891	T65.892	T65.893	T65.894	—	—
Clebopride	T47.8X1	T47.8X2	T47.8X3	T47.8X4	T47.8X5	T47.8X6
Clefamide	T37.3X1	T37.3X2	T37.3X3	T37.3X4	T37.3X5	T37.3X6
Clemastine	T45.0X1	T45.0X2	T45.0X3	T45.0X4	T45.0X5	T45.0X6
Clematis vitalba	T62.2X1	T62.2X2	T62.2X3	T62.2X4	—	—
Clemizole	T45.0X1	T45.0X2	T45.0X3	T45.0X4	T45.0X5	T45.0X6
penicillin	T36.0X1	T36.0X2	T36.0X3	T36.0X4	T36.0X5	T36.0X6
Clenbuterol	T48.6X1	T48.6X2	T48.6X3	T48.6X4	T48.6X5	T48.6X6
Clidinium bromide	T44.3X1	T44.3X2	T44.3X3	T44.3X4	T44.3X5	T44.3X6
Clindamycin	T36.8X1	T36.8X2	T36.8X3	T36.8X4	T36.8X5	T36.8X6
Clinofibrate	T46.6X1	T46.6X2	T46.6X3	T46.6X4	T46.6X5	T46.6X6
Clioquinol	T37.8X1	T37.8X2	T37.8X3	T37.8X4	T37.8X5	T37.8X6
Cliradon	T40.2X1	T40.2X2	T40.2X3	T40.2X4	—	—

Substance	Poisoning, Accidental (unintentional)	Poisoning, Intentional self-harm	Poisoning, Assault	Poisoning, Undetermined	Adverse effect	Underdosing
Clobazam	T42.4X1	T42.4X2	T42.4X3	T42.4X4	T42.4X5	T42.4X6
Clobenzorex	T50.5X1	T50.5X2	T50.5X3	T50.5X4	T50.5X5	T50.5X6
Clobetasol	T49.0X1	T49.0X2	T49.0X3	T49.0X4	T49.0X5	T49.0X6
Clobetasone	T49.0X1	T49.0X2	T49.0X3	T49.0X4	T49.0X5	T49.0X6
Clobutinol	T48.3X1	T48.3X2	T48.3X3	T48.3X4	T48.3X5	T48.3X6
Clocortolone	T38.0X1	T38.0X2	T38.0X3	T38.0X4	T38.0X5	T38.0X6
Clodantoin	T49.0X1	T49.0X2	T49.0X3	T49.0X4	T49.0X5	T49.0X6
Clodronic acid	T50.991	T50.992	T50.993	T50.994	T50.995	T50.996
Clofazimine	T37.1X1	T37.1X2	T37.1X3	T37.1X4	T37.1X5	T37.1X6
Clofedanol	T48.3X1	T48.3X2	T48.3X3	T48.3X4	T48.3X5	T48.3X6
Clofenamide	T50.2X1	T50.2X2	T50.2X3	T50.2X4	T50.2X5	T50.2X6
Clofenotane	T49.0X1	T49.0X2	T49.0X3	T49.0X4	T49.0X5	T49.0X6
Clofezone	T39.2X1	T39.2X2	T39.2X3	T39.2X4	T39.2X5	T39.2X6
Clofibrate	T46.6X1	T46.6X2	T46.6X3	T46.6X4	T46.6X5	T46.6X6
Clofibride	T46.6X1	T46.6X2	T46.6X3	T46.6X4	T46.6X5	T46.6X6
Cloforex	T50.5X1	T50.5X2	T50.5X3	T50.5X4	T50.5X5	T50.5X6
Clomethiazole	T42.6X1	T42.6X2	T42.6X3	T42.6X4	T42.6X5	T42.6X6
Clometocillin	T36.0X1	T36.0X2	T36.0X3	T36.0X4	T36.0X5	T36.0X6
Clomifene	T38.5X1	T38.5X2	T38.5X3	T38.5X4	T38.5X5	T38.5X6
Clomiphene	T38.5X1	T38.5X2	T38.5X3	T38.5X4	T38.5X5	T38.5X6
Clomipramine	T43.011	T43.012	T43.013	T43.014	T43.015	T43.016
Clomocycline	T36.4X1	T36.4X2	T36.4X3	T36.4X4	T36.4X5	T36.4X6
Clonazepam	T42.4X1	T42.4X2	T42.4X3	T42.4X4	T42.4X5	T42.4X6
Clonidine	T46.5X1	T46.5X2	T46.5X3	T46.5X4	T46.5X5	T46.5X6
Clonixin	T39.8X1	T39.8X2	T39.8X3	T39.8X4	T39.8X5	T39.8X6
Clopamide	T50.2X1	T50.2X2	T50.2X3	T50.2X4	T50.2X5	T50.2X6
Clopenthixol	T43.4X1	T43.4X2	T43.4X3	T43.4X4	T43.4X5	T43.4X6
Cloperastine	T48.3X1	T48.3X2	T48.3X3	T48.3X4	T48.3X5	T48.3X6
Clophedianol	T48.3X1	T48.3X2	T48.3X3	T48.3X4	T48.3X5	T48.3X6
Cloponone	T36.2X1	T36.2X2	T36.2X3	T36.2X4	T36.2X5	T36.2X6
Cloprednol	T38.0X1	T38.0X2	T38.0X3	T38.0X4	T38.0X5	T38.0X6
Cloral betaine	T42.6X1	T42.6X2	T42.6X3	T42.6X4	T42.6X5	T42.6X6
Cloramfenicol	T36.2X1	T36.2X2	T36.2X3	T36.2X4	T36.2X5	T36.2X6
Clorazepate (dipotassium)	T42.4X1	T42.4X2	T42.4X3	T42.4X4	T42.4X5	T42.4X6
Clorexolone	T50.2X1	T50.2X2	T50.2X3	T50.2X4	T50.2X5	T50.2X6
Clorfenamine	T45.0X1	T45.0X2	T45.0X3	T45.0X4	T45.0X5	T45.0X6
Clorgiline	T43.1X1	T43.1X2	T43.1X3	T43.1X4	T43.1X5	T43.1X6
Clorotepine	T44.3X1	T44.3X2	T44.3X3	T44.3X4	T44.3X5	T44.3X6
Clorox (bleach)	T54.91	T54.92	T54.93	T54.94	—	—
Clorprenaline	T48.6X1	T48.6X2	T48.6X3	T48.6X4	T48.6X5	T48.6X6
Clortermine	T50.5X1	T50.5X2	T50.5X3	T50.5X4	T50.5X5	T50.5X6
Clotiapine	T43.591	T43.592	T43.593	T43.594	T43.595	T43.596
Clotiazepam	T42.4X1	T42.4X2	T42.4X3	T42.4X4	T42.4X5	T42.4X6
Clotibric acid	T46.6X1	T46.6X2	T46.6X3	T46.6X4	T46.6X5	T46.6X6
Clotrimazole	T49.0X1	T49.0X2	T49.0X3	T49.0X4	T49.0X5	T49.0X6
Cloxacillin	T36.0X1	T36.0X2	T36.0X3	T36.0X4	T36.0X5	T36.0X6
Cloxazolam	T42.4X1	T42.4X2	T42.4X3	T42.4X4	T42.4X5	T42.4X6
Cloxiquine	T49.0X1	T49.0X2	T49.0X3	T49.0X4	T49.0X5	T49.0X6
Clozapine	T42.4X1	T42.4X2	T42.4X3	T42.4X4	T42.4X5	T42.4X6

Substance	Poisoning, Accidental (unintentional)	Poisoning, Intentional self-harm	Poisoning, Assault	Poisoning, Undetermined	Adverse effect	Underdosing
Coagulant NEC	T45.7X1	T45.7X2	T45.7X3	T45.7X4	T45.7X5	T45.7X6
Coal (carbon monoxide from)—see also Carbon, monoxide, coal	T58.2X1	T58.2X2	T58.2X3	T58.2X4	—	—
oil—see Kerosene						
tar	T49.1X1	T49.1X2	T49.1X3	T49.1X4	T49.1X5	T49.1X6
fumes	T59.891	T59.892	T59.893	T59.894	—	—
medicinal (ointment)	T49.4X1	T49.4X2	T49.4X3	T49.4X4	T49.4X5	T49.4X6
analgesics NEC	T39.2X1	T39.2X2	T39.2X3	T39.2X4	T39.2X5	T39.2X6
naphtha (solvent)	T52.0X1	T52.0X2	T52.0X3	T52.0X4	—	—
Cobalamine	T45.2X1	T45.2X2	T45.2X3	T45.2X4	T45.2X5	T45.2X6
Cobalt (nonmedicinal) (fumes) (industrial)	T56.891	T56.892	T56.893	T56.894	—	—
medicinal (trace) (chloride)	T45.8X1	T45.8X2	T45.8X3	T45.8X4	T45.8X5	T45.8X6
Cobra (venom)	T63.041	T63.042	T63.043	T63.044	—	—
Coca (leaf)	T40.5X1	T40.5X2	T40.5X3	T40.5X4	T40.5X5	T40.5X6
Cocaine	T40.5X1	T40.5X2	T40.5X3	T40.5X4	T40.5X5	T40.5X6
topical anesthetic	T41.3X1	T41.3X2	T41.3X3	T41.3X4	T41.3X5	T41.3X6
Cocarboxylase	T45.3X1	T45.3X2	T45.3X3	T45.3X4	T45.3X5	T45.3X6
Coccidioidin	T50.8X1	T50.8X2	T50.8X3	T50.8X4	T50.8X5	T50.8X6
Cocculus indicus	T62.1X1	T62.1X2	T62.1X3	T62.1X4	—	—
Cochineal	T65.6X1	T65.6X2	T65.6X3	T65.6X4	—	—
medicinal products	T50.991	T50.992	T50.993	T50.994	T50.995	T50.996
Codeine	T40.2X1	T40.2X2	T40.2X3	T40.2X4	T40.2X5	T40.2X6
Cod-liver oil	T45.2X1	T45.2X2	T45.2X3	T45.2X4	T45.2X5	T45.2X6
Coenzyme A	T50.991	T50.992	T50.993	T50.994	T50.995	T50.996
Coffee	T62.8X1	T62.8X2	T62.8X3	T62.8X4	—	—
Cogalactoiso-merase	T50.991	T50.992	T50.993	T50.994	T50.995	T50.996
Cogentin	T44.3X1	T44.3X2	T44.3X3	T44.3X4	T44.3X5	T44.3X6
Coke fumes or gas (carbon monoxide)	T58.2X1	T58.2X2	T58.2X3	T58.2X4	—	—
industrial use	T58.8X1	T58.8X2	T58.8X3	T58.8X4	—	—
Colace	T47.4X1	T47.4X2	T47.4X3	T47.4X4	T47.4X5	T47.4X6
Colaspase	T45.1X1	T45.1X2	T45.1X3	T45.1X4	T45.1X5	T45.1X6
Colchicine	T50.4X1	T50.4X2	T50.4X3	T50.4X4	T50.4X5	T50.4X6
Colchicum	T62.2X1	T62.2X2	T62.2X3	T62.2X4	—	—
Cold cream	T49.3X1	T49.3X2	T49.3X3	T49.3X4	T49.3X5	T49.3X6
Colecalciferol	T45.2X1	T45.2X2	T45.2X3	T45.2X4	T45.2X5	T45.2X6
Colestipol	T46.6X1	T46.6X2	T46.6X3	T46.6X4	T46.6X5	T46.6X6
Colestyramine	T46.6X1	T46.6X2	T46.6X3	T46.6X4	T46.6X5	T46.6X6
Colimycin	T36.8X1	T36.8X2	T36.8X3	T36.8X4	T36.8X5	T36.8X6
Colistimethate	T36.8X1	T36.8X2	T36.8X3	T36.8X4	T36.8X5	T36.8X6
Colistin	T36.8X1	T36.8X2	T36.8X3	T36.8X4	T36.8X5	T36.8X6
sulfate (eye preparation)	T49.5X1	T49.5X2	T49.5X3	T49.5X4	T49.5X5	T49.5X6
Collagen	T50.991	T50.992	T50.993	T50.994	T50.995	T50.996
Collagenase	T49.4X1	T49.4X2	T49.4X3	T49.4X4	T49.4X5	T49.4X6
Collodion	T49.3X1	T49.3X2	T49.3X3	T49.3X4	T49.3X5	T49.3X6
Colocynth	T47.2X1	T47.2X2	T47.2X3	T47.2X4	T47.2X5	T47.2X6
Colophony adhesive	T49.3X1	T49.3X2	T49.3X3	T49.3X4	T49.3X5	T49.3X6
Colorant—see also Dye	T50.991	T50.992	T50.993	T50.994	T50.995	T50.996

Substance	Poisoning, Accidental (unintentional)	Poisoning, Intentional self-harm	Poisoning, Assault	Poisoning, Undetermined	Adverse effect	Underdosing
Coloring matter—see Dye(s)						
Combustion gas (after combustion)—see Carbon, monoxide						
prior to combustion	T59.891	T59.892	T59.893	T59.894	—	—
Compazine	T43.3X1	T43.3X2	T43.3X3	T43.3X4	T43.3X5	T43.3X6
Compound						
42 (warfarin)	T60.4X1	T60.4X2	T60.4X3	T60.4X4	—	—
269 (endrin)	T60.1X1	T60.1X2	T60.1X3	T60.1X4	—	—
497 (dieldrin)	T60.1X1	T60.1X2	T60.1X3	T60.1X4	—	—
1080 (sodium fluoroacetate)	T60.4X1	T60.4X2	T60.4X3	T60.4X4	—	—
3422 (parathion)	T60.0X1	T60.0X2	T60.0X3	T60.0X4	—	—
3911 (phorate)	T60.0X1	T60.0X2	T60.0X3	T60.0X4	—	—
3956 (toxaphene)	T60.1X1	T60.1X2	T60.1X3	T60.1X4	—	—
4049 (malathion)	T60.0X1	T60.0X2	T60.0X3	T60.0X4	—	—
4069 (malathion)	T60.0X1	T60.0X2	T60.0X3	T60.0X4	—	—
4124 (dicapthon)	T60.0X1	T60.0X2	T60.0X3	T60.0X4	—	—
E (cortisone)	T38.0X1	T38.0X2	T38.0X3	T38.0X4	T38.0X5	T38.0X6
F (hydrocortisone)	T38.0X1	T38.0X2	T38.0X3	T38.0X4	T38.0X5	T38.0X6
Congener, avwnabolic	T38.7X1	T38.7X2	T38.7X3	T38.7X4	T38.7X5	T38.7X6
Congo red	T50.8X1	T50.8X2	T50.8X3	T50.8X4	T50.8X5	T50.8X6
Coniine, conine	T62.2X1	T62.2X2	T62.2X3	T62.2X4	—	—
Conium (maculatum)	T62.2X1	T62.2X2	T62.2X3	T62.2X4	—	—
Conjugated estrogenic substances	T38.5X1	T38.5X2	T38.5X3	T38.5X4	T38.5X5	T38.5X6
Contac	T48.5X1	T48.5X2	T48.5X3	T48.5X4	T48.5X5	T48.5X6
Contact lens solution	T49.5X1	T49.5X2	T49.5X3	T49.5X4	T49.5X5	T49.5X6
Contraceptive (oral)	T38.4X1	T38.4X2	T38.4X3	T38.4X4	T38.4X5	T38.4X6
vaginal	T49.8X1	T49.8X2	T49.8X3	T49.8X4	T49.8X5	T49.8X6
Contrast medium, radiography	T50.8X1	T50.8X2	T50.8X3	T50.8X4	T50.8X5	T50.8X6
Convallaria glycosides	T46.0X1	T46.0X2	T46.0X3	T46.0X4	T46.0X5	T46.0X6
Convallaria majalis	T62.2X1	T62.2X2	T62.2X3	T62.2X4	—	—
berry	T62.1X1	T62.1X2	T62.1X3	T62.1X4	—	—
Copper (dust) (fumes) (nonmedicinal) NEC	T56.4X1	T56.4X2	T56.4X3	T56.4X4	—	—
arsenate, arsenite	T57.0X1	T57.0X2	T57.0X3	T57.0X4	—	—
insecticide	T60.2X1	T60.2X2	T60.2X3	T60.2X4	—	—
emetic	T47.7X1	T47.7X2	T47.7X3	T47.7X4	T47.7X5	T47.7X6
fungicide	T60.3X1	T60.3X2	T60.3X3	T60.3X4	—	—
gluconate	T49.0X1	T49.0X2	T49.0X3	T49.0X4	T49.0X5	T49.0X6
insecticide	T60.2X1	T60.2X2	T60.2X3	T60.2X4	—	—
medicinal (trace)	T45.8X1	T45.8X2	T45.8X3	T45.8X4	T45.8X5	T45.8X6
oleate	T49.0X1	T49.0X2	T49.0X3	T49.0X4	T49.0X5	T49.0X6
sulfate	T56.4X1	T56.4X2	T56.4X3	T56.4X4	—	—
cupric	T56.4X1	T56.4X2	T56.4X3	T56.4X4	—	—
fungicide	T60.3X1	T60.3X2	T60.3X3	T60.3X4	—	—
medicinal						
ear	T49.6X1	T49.6X2	T49.6X3	T49.6X4	T49.6X5	T49.6X6
emetic	T47.7X1	T47.7X2	T47.7X3	T47.7X4	T47.7X5	T47.7X6

Substance	Poisoning, Accidental (unintentional)	Poisoning, Intentional self-harm	Poisoning, Assault	Poisoning, Undetermined	Adverse effect	Underdosing
Copper NEC — Continued						
eye	T49.5X1	T49.5X2	T49.5X3	T49.5X4	T49.5X5	T49.5X6
cuprous	T56.4X1	T56.4X2	T56.4X3	T56.4X4	—	—
fungicide	T60.3X1	T60.3X2	T60.3X3	T60.3X4	—	—
medicinal						
ear	T49.6X1	T49.6X2	T49.6X3	T49.6X4	T49.6X5	T49.6X6
emetic	T47.7X1	T47.7X2	T47.7X3	T47.7X4	T47.7X5	T47.7X6
eye	T49.5X1	T49.5X2	T49.5X3	T49.5X4	T49.5X5	T49.5X6
Copperhead snake (bite) (venom)	T63.061	T63.062	T63.063	T63.064	—	—
Coral (sting)	T63.691	T63.692	T63.693	T63.694	—	—
snake (bite) (venom)	T63.021	T63.022	T63.023	T63.024	—	—
Corbadrine	T49.6X1	T49.6X2	T49.6X3	T49.6X4	T49.6X5	T49.6X6
Cordite	T65.891	T65.892	T65.893	T65.894	—	—
vapor	T59.891	T59.892	T59.893	T59.894	—	—
Cordran	T49.0X1	T49.0X2	T49.0X3	T49.0X4	T49.0X5	T49.0X6
Corn cures	T49.4X1	T49.4X2	T49.4X3	T49.4X4	T49.4X5	T49.4X6
Corn starch	T49.3X1	T49.3X2	T49.3X3	T49.3X4	T49.3X5	T49.3X6
Cornhusker's lotion	T49.3X1	T49.3X2	T49.3X3	T49.3X4	T49.3X5	T49.3X6
Coronary vasodilator NEC	T46.3X1	T46.3X2	T46.3X3	T46.3X4	T46.3X5	T46.3X6
Corrosive NEC	T54.91	T54.92	T54.93	T54.94	—	—
acid NEC	T54.2X1	T54.2X2	T54.2X3	T54.2X4	—	—
aromatics	T54.1X1	T54.1X2	T54.1X3	T54.1X4	—	—
disinfectant	T54.1X1	T54.1X2	T54.1X3	T54.1X4	—	—
fumes NEC	T54.91	T54.92	T54.93	T54.94	—	—
specified NEC	T54.91	T54.92	T54.93	T54.94	—	—
sublimate	T56.1X1	T56.1X2	T56.1X3	T56.1X4	—	—
Cortate	T38.0X1	T38.0X2	T38.0X3	T38.0X4	T38.0X5	T38.0X6
Cort-Dome	T38.0X1	T38.0X2	T38.0X3	T38.0X4	T38.0X5	T38.0X6
ENT agent	T49.6X1	T49.6X2	T49.6X3	T49.6X4	T49.6X5	T49.6X6
ophthalmic preparation	T49.5X1	T49.5X2	T49.5X3	T49.5X4	T49.5X5	T49.5X6
topical NEC	T49.0X1	T49.0X2	T49.0X3	T49.0X4	T49.0X5	T49.0X6
Cortef	T38.0X1	T38.0X2	T38.0X3	T38.0X4	T38.0X5	T38.0X6
ENT agent	T49.6X1	T49.6X2	T49.6X3	T49.6X4	T49.6X5	T49.6X6
ophthalmic preparation	T49.5X1	T49.5X2	T49.5X3	T49.5X4	T49.5X5	T49.5X6
topical NEC	T49.0X1	T49.0X2	T49.0X3	T49.0X4	T49.0X5	T49.0X6
Corticosteroid	T38.0X1	T38.0X2	T38.0X3	T38.0X4	T38.0X5	T38.0X6
ENT agent	T49.6X1	T49.6X2	T49.6X3	T49.6X4	T49.6X5	T49.6X6
mineral	T50.0X1	T50.0X2	T50.0X3	T50.0X4	T50.0X5	T50.0X6
ophthalmic	T49.5X1	T49.5X2	T49.5X3	T49.5X4	T49.5X5	T49.5X6
topical NEC	T49.0X1	T49.0X2	T49.0X3	T49.0X4	T49.0X5	T49.0X6
Corticotropin	T38.811	T38.812	T38.813	T38.814	T38.815	T38.816
Cortisol	T49.0X1	T49.0X2	T49.0X3	T49.0X4	T49.0X5	T49.0X6
ENT agent	T49.6X1	T49.6X2	T49.6X3	T49.6X4	T49.6X5	T49.6X6
ophthalmic preparation	T49.5X1	T49.5X2	T49.5X3	T49.5X4	T49.5X5	T49.5X6
topical NEC	T49.0X1	T49.0X2	T49.0X3	T49.0X4	T49.0X5	T49.0X6
Cortisone (acetate)	T38.0X1	T38.0X2	T38.0X3	T38.0X4	T38.0X5	T38.0X6
ENT agent	T49.6X1	T49.6X2	T49.6X3	T49.6X4	T49.6X5	T49.6X6

Substance	Poisoning, Accidental (unintentional)	Poisoning, Intentional self-harm	Poisoning, Assault	Poisoning, Undetermined	Adverse effect	Underdosing
Cortisone — *Continued*						
ophthalmic preparation	T49.5X1	T49.5X2	T49.5X3	T49.5X4	T49.5X5	T49.5X6
topical NEC	T49.0X1	T49.0X2	T49.0X3	T49.0X4	T49.0X5	T49.0X6
Cortivazol	T38.0X1	T38.0X2	T38.0X3	T38.0X4	T38.0X5	T38.0X6
Cortogen	T38.0X1	T38.0X2	T38.0X3	T38.0X4	T38.0X5	T38.0X6
ENT agent	T49.6X1	T49.6X2	T49.6X3	T49.6X4	T49.6X5	T49.6X6
ophthalmic preparation	T49.5X1	T49.5X2	T49.5X3	T49.5X4	T49.5X5	T49.5X6
Cortone	T38.0X1	T38.0X2	T38.0X3	T38.0X4	T38.0X5	T38.0X6
ENT agent	T49.6X1	T49.6X2	T49.6X3	T49.6X4	T49.6X5	T49.6X6
ophthalmic preparation	T49.5X1	T49.5X2	T49.5X3	T49.5X4	T49.5X5	T49.5X6
Cortril	T38.0X1	T38.0X2	T38.0X3	T38.0X4	T38.0X5	T38.0X6
ENT agent	T49.6X1	T49.6X2	T49.6X3	T49.6X4	T49.6X5	T49.6X6
ophthalmic preparation	T49.5X1	T49.5X2	T49.5X3	T49.5X4	T49.5X5	T49.5X6
topical NEC	T49.0X1	T49.0X2	T49.0X3	T49.0X4	T49.0X5	T49.0X6
Corynebacterium parvum	T45.1X1	T45.1X2	T45.1X3	T45.1X4	T45.1X5	T45.1X6
Cosmetic preparation	T49.8X1	T49.8X2	T49.8X3	T49.8X4	T49.8X5	T49.8X6
Cosmetics	T49.8X1	T49.8X2	T49.8X3	T49.8X4	T49.8X5	T49.8X6
Cosyntropin	T38.811	T38.812	T38.813	T38.814	T38.815	T38.816
Cotarnine	T45.7X1	T45.7X2	T45.7X3	T45.7X4	T45.7X5	T45.7X6
Co-trimoxazole	T36.8X1	T36.8X2	T36.8X3	T36.8X4	T36.8X5	T36.8X6
Cottonseed oil	T49.3X1	T49.3X2	T49.3X3	T49.3X4	T49.3X5	T49.3X6
Cough mixture (syrup)	T48.4X1	T48.4X2	T48.4X3	T48.4X4	T48.4X5	T48.4X6
containing opiates	T40.2X1	T40.2X2	T40.2X3	T40.2X4	T40.2X5	T40.2X6
expectorants	T48.4X1	T48.4X2	T48.4X3	T48.4X4	T48.4X5	T48.4X6
Coumadin	T45.511	T45.512	T45.513	T45.514	T45.515	T45.516
rodenticide	T60.4X1	T60.4X2	T60.4X3	T60.4X4	—	—
Coumaphos	T60.0X1	T60.0X2	T60.0X3	T60.0X4	—	—
Coumarin	T45.511	T45.512	T45.513	T45.514	T45.515	T45.516
Coumetarol	T45.511	T45.512	T45.513	T45.514	T45.515	T45.516
Cowbane	T62.2X1	T62.2X2	T62.2X3	T62.2X4	—	—
Cozyme	T45.2X1	T45.2X2	T45.2X3	T45.2X4	T45.2X5	T45.2X6
Crack	T40.5X1	T40.5X2	T40.5X3	T40.5X4		
Crataegus extract	T46.0X1	T46.0X2	T46.0X3	T46.0X4	T46.0X5	T46.0X6
Creolin	T54.1X1	T54.1X2	T54.1X3	T54.1X4		
disinfectant	T54.1X1	T54.1X2	T54.1X3	T54.1X4		
Creosol (compound)	T49.0X1	T49.0X2	T49.0X3	T49.0X4	T49.0X5	T49.0X6
Creosote (coal tar) (beechwood)	T49.0X1	T49.0X2	T49.0X3	T49.0X4	T49.0X5	T49.0X6
medicinal (expectorant)	T48.4X1	T48.4X2	T48.4X3	T48.4X4	T48.4X5	T48.4X6
syrup	T48.4X1	T48.4X2	T48.4X3	T48.4X4	T48.4X5	T48.4X6
Cresol(s)	T49.0X1	T49.0X2	T49.0X3	T49.0X4	T49.0X5	T49.0X6
and soap solution	T49.0X1	T49.0X2	T49.0X3	T49.0X4	T49.0X5	T49.0X6
Cresyl acetate	T49.0X1	T49.0X2	T49.0X3	T49.0X4	T49.0X5	T49.0X6
Cresylic acid	T49.0X1	T49.0X2	T49.0X3	T49.0X4	T49.0X5	T49.0X6
Crimidine	T60.4X1	T60.4X2	T60.4X3	T60.4X4	—	—
Croconazole	T37.8X1	T37.8X2	T37.8X3	T37.8X4	T37.8X5	T37.8X6
Cromoglicic acid	T48.6X1	T48.6X2	T48.6X3	T48.6X4	T48.6X5	T48.6X6
Cromolyn	T48.6X1	T48.6X2	T48.6X3	T48.6X4	T48.6X5	T48.6X6
Cromonar	T46.3X1	T46.3X2	T46.3X3	T46.3X4	T46.3X5	T46.3X6
Cropropamide	T39.8X1	T39.8X2	T39.8X3	T39.8X4	T39.8X5	T39.8X6

Substance	Poisoning, Accidental (unintentional)	Poisoning, Intentional self-harm	Poisoning, Assault	Poisoning, Undetermined	Adverse effect	Underdosing
Cropropamide — *Continued*						
with crotethamide	T50.7X1	T50.7X2	T50.7X3	T50.7X4	T50.7X5	T50.7X6
Crotamiton	T49.0X1	T49.0X2	T49.0X3	T49.0X4	T49.0X5	T49.0X6
Crotethamide	T39.8X1	T39.8X2	T39.8X3	T39.8X4	T39.8X5	T39.8X6
with cropropamide	T50.7X1	T50.7X2	T50.7X3	T50.7X4	T50.7X5	T50.7X6
Croton (oil)	T47.2X1	T47.2X2	T47.2X3	T47.2X4	T47.2X5	T47.2X6
chloral	T42.6X1	T42.6X2	T42.6X3	T42.6X4	T42.6X5	T42.6X6
Crude oil	T52.0X1	T52.0X2	T52.0X3	T52.0X4	—	—
Cryogenine	T39.8X1	T39.8X2	T39.8X3	T39.8X4	T39.8X5	T39.8X6
Cryolite (vapor)	T60.1X1	T60.1X2	T60.1X3	T60.1X4	—	—
insecticide	T60.1X1	T60.1X2	T60.1X3	T60.1X4	—	—
Cryptenamine (tannates)	T46.5X1	T46.5X2	T46.5X3	T46.5X4	T46.5X5	T46.5X6
Crystal violet	T49.0X1	T49.0X2	T49.0X3	T49.0X4	T49.0X5	T49.0X6
Cuckoopint	T62.2X1	T62.2X2	T62.2X3	T62.2X4	—	—
Cumetharol	T45.511	T45.512	T45.513	T45.514	T45.515	T45.516
Cupric						
acetate	T60.3X1	T60.3X2	T60.3X3	T60.3X4	—	—
acetoarsenite	T57.0X1	T57.0X2	T57.0X3	T57.0X4	—	—
arsenate	T57.0X1	T57.0X2	T57.0X3	T57.0X4	—	—
gluconate	T49.0X1	T49.0X2	T49.0X3	T49.0X4	T49.0X5	T49.0X6
oleate	T49.0X1	T49.0X2	T49.0X3	T49.0X4	T49.0X5	T49.0X6
sulfate	T56.4X1	T56.4X2	T56.4X3	T56.4X4	—	—
Cuprous sulfate—see also Copper sulfate	T56.4X1	T56.4X2	T56.4X3	T56.4X4	—	—
Curare, curarine	T48.1X1	T48.1X2	T48.1X3	T48.1X4	T48.1X5	T48.1X6
Cyamemazine	T43.3X1	T43.3X2	T43.3X3	T43.3X4	T43.3X5	T43.3X6
Cyamopsis tetragono-loba	T46.6X1	T46.6X2	T46.6X3	T46.6X4	T46.6X5	T46.6X6
Cyanacetyl hydrazide	T37.1X1	T37.1X2	T37.1X3	T37.1X4	T37.1X5	T37.1X6
Cyanic acid (gas)	T59.891	T59.892	T59.893	T59.894	—	—
Cyanide(s) (compounds) (potassium) (sodium) NEC	T65.0X1	T65.0X2	T65.0X3	T65.0X4		
dust or gas (inhalation) NEC	T57.3X1	T57.3X2	T57.3X3	T57.3X4		
fumigant	T65.0X1	T65.0X2	T65.0X3	T65.0X4	—	—
hydrogen	T57.3X1	T57.3X2	T57.3X3	T57.3X4		
mercuric—see *Mercury*						
pesticide (dust) (fumes)	T65.0X1	T65.0X2	T65.0X3	T65.0X4		
Cyanoacrylate adhesive	T49.3X1	T49.3X2	T49.3X3	T49.3X4	T49.3X5	T49.3X6
Cyanocobalamin	T45.8X1	T45.8X2	T45.8X3	T45.8X4	T45.8X5	T45.8X6
Cyanogen (chloride) (gas) NEC	T59.891	T59.892	T59.893	T59.894	—	—
Cyclacillin	T36.0X1	T36.0X2	T36.0X3	T36.0X4	T36.0X5	T36.0X6
Cyclaine	T41.3X1	T41.3X2	T41.3X3	T41.3X4	T41.3X5	T41.3X6
Cyclamate	T50.991	T50.992	T50.993	T50.994	T50.995	T50.996
Cyclamen europaeum	T62.2X1	T62.2X2	T62.2X3	T62.2X4	—	—
Cyclandelate	T46.7X1	T46.7X2	T46.7X3	T46.7X4	T46.7X5	T46.7X6
Cyclazocine	T50.7X1	T50.7X2	T50.7X3	T50.7X4	T50.7X5	T50.7X6
Cyclizine	T45.0X1	T45.0X2	T45.0X3	T45.0X4	T45.0X5	T45.0X6
Cyclobarbital	T42.3X1	T42.3X2	T42.3X3	T42.3X4	T42.3X5	T42.3X6

Substance	Poisoning, Accidental (unintentional)	Poisoning, Intentional self-harm	Poisoning, Assault	Poisoning, Undetermined	Adverse effect	Underdosing
Cyclobarbitone	T42.3X1	T42.3X2	T42.3X3	T42.3X4	T42.3X5	T42.3X6
Cyclobenzaprine	T48.1X1	T48.1X2	T48.1X3	T48.1X4	T48.1X5	T48.1X6
Cyclodrine	T44.3X1	T44.3X2	T44.3X3	T44.3X4	T44.3X5	T44.3X6
Cycloguanil embonate	T37.2X1	T37.2X2	T37.2X3	T37.2X4	T37.2X5	T37.2X6
Cyclohexane	T52.8X1	T52.8X2	T52.8X3	T52.8X4	—	—
Cyclohexanol	T51.8X1	T51.8X2	T51.8X3	T51.8X4	—	—
Cyclohexanone	T52.4X1	T52.4X2	T52.4X3	T52.4X4	—	—
Cycloheximide	T60.3X1	T60.3X2	T60.3X3	T60.3X4	—	—
Cyclohexyl acetate	T52.8X1	T52.8X2	T52.8X3	T52.8X4	—	—
Cycloleucin	T45.1X1	T45.1X2	T45.1X3	T45.1X4	T45.1X5	T45.1X6
Cyclomethycaine	T41.3X1	T41.3X2	T41.3X3	T41.3X4	T41.3X5	T41.3X6
Cyclopentamine	T44.4X1	T44.4X2	T44.4X3	T44.4X4	T44.4X5	T44.4X6
Cyclopenthiazide	T50.2X1	T50.2X2	T50.2X3	T50.2X4	T50.2X5	T50.2X6
Cyclopentolate	T44.3X1	T44.3X2	T44.3X3	T44.3X4	T44.3X5	T44.3X6
Cyclophosphamide	T45.1X1	T45.1X2	T45.1X3	T45.1X4	T45.1X5	T45.1X6
Cycloplegic drug	T49.5X1	T49.5X2	T49.5X3	T49.5X4	T49.5X5	T49.5X6
Cyclopropane	T41.291	T41.292	T41.293	T41.294	T41.295	T41.296
Cyclopyrabital	T39.8X1	T39.8X2	T39.8X3	T39.8X4	T39.8X5	T39.8X6
Cycloserine	T37.1X1	T37.1X2	T37.1X3	T37.1X4	T37.1X5	T37.1X6
Cyclosporin	T45.1X1	T45.1X2	T45.1X3	T45.1X4	T45.1X5	T45.1X6
Cyclothiazide	T50.2X1	T50.2X2	T50.2X3	T50.2X4	T50.2X5	T50.2X6
Cycrimine	T44.3X1	T44.3X2	T44.3X3	T44.3X4	T44.3X5	T44.3X6
Cyhalothrin	T60.1X1	T60.1X2	T60.1X3	T60.1X4	—	—
Cymarin	T46.0X1	T46.0X2	T46.0X3	T46.0X4	T46.0X5	T46.0X6
Cypermethrin	T60.1X1	T60.1X2	T60.1X3	T60.1X4	—	—
Cyphenothrin	T60.2X1	T60.2X2	T60.2X3	T60.2X4	—	—
Cyproheptadine	T45.0X1	T45.0X2	T45.0X3	T45.0X4	T45.0X5	T45.0X6
Cyproterone	T38.6X1	T38.6X2	T38.6X3	T38.6X4	T38.6X5	T38.6X6
Cysteamine	T50.6X1	T50.6X2	T50.6X3	T50.6X4	T50.6X5	T50.6X6
Cytarabine	T45.1X1	T45.1X2	T45.1X3	T45.1X4	T45.1X5	T45.1X6
Cytisus						
laburnum	T62.2X1	T62.2X2	T62.2X3	T62.2X4	—	—
scoparius	T62.2X1	T62.2X2	T62.2X3	T62.2X4	—	—
Cytochrome C	T47.5X1	T47.5X2	T47.5X3	T47.5X4	T47.5X5	T47.5X6
Cytomel	T38.1X1	T38.1X2	T38.1X3	T38.1X4	T38.1X5	T38.1X6
Cytosine arabinoside	T45.1X1	T45.1X2	T45.1X3	T45.1X4	T45.1X5	T45.1X6
Cytoxan	T45.1X1	T45.1X2	T45.1X3	T45.1X4	T45.1X5	T45.1X6
Cytozyme	T45.7X1	T45.7X2	T45.7X3	T45.7X4	T45.7X5	T45.7X6
2,4-D	T60.3X1	T60.3X2	T60.3X3	T60.3X4	—	—
D						
Dacarbazine	T45.1X1	T45.1X2	T45.1X3	T45.1X4	T45.1X5	T45.1X6
Dactinomycin	T45.1X1	T45.1X2	T45.1X3	T45.1X4	T45.1X5	T45.1X6
DADPS	T37.1X1	T37.1X2	T37.1X3	T37.1X4	T37.1X5	T37.1X6
Dakin's solution	T49.0X1	T49.0X2	T49.0X3	T49.0X4	T49.0X5	T49.0X6
Dalapon (sodium)	T60.3X1	T60.3X2	T60.3X3	T60.3X4	—	—
Dalmane	T42.4X1	T42.4X2	T42.4X3	T42.4X4	T42.4X5	T42.4X6
Danazol	T38.6X1	T38.6X2	T38.6X3	T38.6X4	T38.6X5	T38.6X6
Danilone	T45.511	T45.512	T45.513	T45.514	T45.515	T45.516
Danthron	T47.2X1	T47.2X2	T47.2X3	T47.2X4	T47.2X5	T47.2X6
Dantrolene	T42.8X1	T42.8X2	T42.8X3	T42.8X4	T42.8X5	T42.8X6

Substance	Poisoning, Accidental (unintentional)	Poisoning, Intentional self-harm	Poisoning, Assault	Poisoning, Undetermined	Adverse effect	Underdosing
Dantron	T47.2X1	T47.2X2	T47.2X3	T47.2X4	T47.2X5	T47.2X6
Daphne (gnidium) (mezereum)	T62.2X1	T62.2X2	T62.2X3	T62.2X4	—	—
berry	T62.1X1	T62.1X2	T62.1X3	T62.1X4	—	—
Dapsone	T37.1X1	T37.1X2	T37.1X3	T37.1X4	T37.1X5	T37.1X6
Daraprim	T37.2X1	T37.2X2	T37.2X3	T37.2X4	T37.2X5	T37.2X6
Darnel	T62.2X1	T62.2X2	T62.2X3	T62.2X4	—	—
Darvon	T39.8X1	T39.8X2	T39.8X3	T39.8X4	T39.8X5	T39.8X6
Daunomycin	T45.1X1	T45.1X2	T45.1X3	T45.1X4	T45.1X5	T45.1X6
Daunorubicin	T45.1X1	T45.1X2	T45.1X3	T45.1X4	T45.1X5	T45.1X6
DBI	T38.3X1	T38.3X2	T38.3X3	T38.3X4	T38.3X5	T38.3X6
D-Con	T60.91	T60.92	T60.93	T60.94	—	—
insecticide	T60.2X1	T60.2X2	T60.2X3	T60.2X4	—	—
rodenticide	T60.4X1	T60.4X2	T60.4X3	T60.4X4	—	—
DDAVP	T38.891	T38.892	T38.893	T38.894	T38.895	T38.896
DDE (bis (chlorophenyl)-dichloroethylene)	T60.2X1	T60.2X2	T60.2X3	T60.2X4	—	—
DDS	T37.1X1	T37.1X2	T37.1X3	T37.1X4	T37.1X5	T37.1X6
DDT (dust)	T60.1X1	T60.1X2	T60.1X3	T60.1X4	—	—
Deadly nightshade—see also Belladonna	T62.2X1	T62.2X2	T62.2X3	T62.2X4	—	—
berry	T62.1X1	T62.1X2	T62.1X3	T62.1X4	—	—
Deamino-D-arginine vasopressin	T38.891	T38.892	T38.893	T38.894	T38.895	T38.896
Deanol (aceglumate)	T50.991	T50.992	T50.993	T50.994	T50.995	T50.996
Debrisoquine	T46.5X1	T46.5X2	T46.5X3	T46.5X4	T46.5X5	T46.5X6
Decaborane	T57.8X1	T57.8X2	T57.8X3	T57.8X4	—	—
fumes	T59.891	T59.892	T59.893	T59.894	—	—
Decadron	T38.0X1	T38.0X2	T38.0X3	T38.0X4	T38.0X5	T38.0X6
ENT agent	T49.6X1	T49.6X2	T49.6X3	T49.6X4	T49.6X5	T49.6X6
ophthalmic preparation	T49.5X1	T49.5X2	T49.5X3	T49.5X4	T49.5X5	T49.5X6
topical NEC	T49.0X1	T49.0X2	T49.0X3	T49.0X4	T49.0X5	T49.0X6
Decahydro-naphthalene	T52.8X1	T52.8X2	T52.8X3	T52.8X4	—	—
Decalin	T52.8X1	T52.8X2	T52.8X3	T52.8X4	—	—
Decametho-nium (bromide)	T48.1X1	T48.1X2	T48.1X3	T48.1X4	T48.1X5	T48.1X6
Decholin	T47.5X1	T47.5X2	T47.5X3	T47.5X4	T47.5X5	T47.5X6
Declomycin	T36.4X1	T36.4X2	T36.4X3	T36.4X4	T36.4X5	T36.4X6
Decongestant, nasal (mucosa)	T48.5X1	T48.5X2	T48.5X3	T48.5X4	T48.5X5	T48.5X6
combination	T48.5X1	T48.5X2	T48.5X3	T48.5X4	T48.5X5	T48.5X6
Deet	T60.8X1	T60.8X2	T60.8X3	T60.8X4	—	—
Deferoxamine	T45.8X1	T45.8X2	T45.8X3	T45.8X4	T45.8X5	T45.8X6
Deflazacort	T38.0X1	T38.0X2	T38.0X3	T38.0X4	T38.0X5	T38.0X6
Deglycyrrhizinized extract of licorice	T48.4X1	T48.4X2	T48.4X3	T48.4X4	T48.4X5	T48.4X6
Dehydrocholic acid	T47.5X1	T47.5X2	T47.5X3	T47.5X4	T47.5X5	T47.5X6
Dehydroemetine	T37.3X1	T37.3X2	T37.3X3	T37.3X4	T37.3X5	T37.3X6
Dekalin	T52.8X1	T52.8X2	T52.8X3	T52.8X4	—	—
Delalutin	T38.5X1	T38.5X2	T38.5X3	T38.5X4	T38.5X5	T38.5X6
Delorazepam	T42.4X1	T42.4X2	T42.4X3	T42.4X4	T42.4X5	T42.4X6
Delphinium	T62.2X1	T62.2X2	T62.2X3	T62.2X4	—	—

Substance	Poisoning, Accidental (unintentional)	Poisoning, Intentional self-harm	Poisoning, Assault	Poisoning, Undetermined	Adverse effect	Underdosing
Deltamethrin	T60.1X1	T60.1X2	T60.1X3	T60.1X4	—	—
Deltasone	T38.0X1	T38.0X2	T38.0X3	T38.0X4	T38.0X5	T38.0X6
Deltra	T38.0X1	T38.0X2	T38.0X3	T38.0X4	T38.0X5	T38.0X6
Delvinal	T42.3X1	T42.3X2	T42.3X3	T42.3X4	T42.3X5	T42.3X6
Demecarium (bromide)	T49.5X1	T49.5X2	T49.5X3	T49.5X4	T49.5X5	T49.5X6
Demeclocycline	T36.4X1	T36.4X2	T36.4X3	T36.4X4	T36.4X5	T36.4X6
Demecolcine	T45.1X1	T45.1X2	T45.1X3	T45.1X4	T45.1X5	T45.1X6
Demegestone	T38.5X1	T38.5X2	T38.5X3	T38.5X4	T38.5X5	T38.5X6
Demelanizing agents	T49.8X1	T49.8X2	T49.8X3	T49.8X4	T49.8X5	T49.8X6
Demephion -O and -S	T60.0X1	T60.0X2	T60.0X3	T60.0X4	—	—
Demerol	T40.2X1	T40.2X2	T40.2X3	T40.2X4	T40.2X5	T40.2X6
Demethylchlor-tetracycline	T36.4X1	T36.4X2	T36.4X3	T36.4X4	T36.4X5	T36.4X6
Demethyltetracycline	T36.4X1	T36.4X2	T36.4X3	T36.4X4	T36.4X5	T36.4X6
Demeton -O and -S	T60.0X1	T60.0X2	T60.0X3	T60.0X4		
Demulcent (external)	T49.3X1	T49.3X2	T49.3X3	T49.3X4	T49.3X5	T49.3X6
specified NEC	T49.3X1	T49.3X2	T49.3X3	T49.3X4	T49.3X5	T49.3X6
Demulen	T38.4X1	T38.4X2	T38.4X3	T38.4X4	T38.4X5	T38.4X6
Denatured alcohol	T51.0X1	T51.0X2	T51.0X3	T51.0X4	—	—
Dendrid	T49.5X1	T49.5X2	T49.5X3	T49.5X4	T49.5X5	T49.5X6
Dental drug, topical application NEC	T49.7X1	T49.7X2	T49.7X3	T49.7X4	T49.7X5	T49.7X6
Dentifrice	T49.7X1	T49.7X2	T49.7X3	T49.7X4	T49.7X5	T49.7X6
Deodorant spray (feminine hygiene)	T49.8X1	T49.8X2	T49.8X3	T49.8X4	T49.8X5	T49.8X6
Deoxycortone	T50.0X1	T50.0X2	T50.0X3	T50.0X4	T50.0X5	T50.0X6
2-Deoxy-5-fluorouridine	T45.1X1	T45.1X2	T45.1X3	T45.1X4	T45.1X5	T45.1X6
5-Deoxy-5-fluorouridine	T45.1X1	T45.1X2	T45.1X3	T45.1X4	T45.1X5	T45.1X6
Deoxyribonuclease (pancreatic)	T45.3X1	T45.3X2	T45.3X3	T45.3X4	T45.3X5	T45.3X6
Depilatory	T49.4X1	T49.4X2	T49.4X3	T49.4X4	T49.4X5	T49.4X6
Deprenalin	T42.8X1	T42.8X2	T42.8X3	T42.8X4	T42.8X5	T42.8X6
Deprenyl	T42.8X1	T42.8X2	T42.8X3	T42.8X4	T42.8X5	T42.8X6
Depressant, appetite	T50.5X1	T50.5X2	T50.5X3	T50.5X4	T50.5X5	T50.5X6
Depressant						
appetite (central)	T50.5X1	T50.5X2	T50.5X3	T50.5X4	T50.5X5	T50.5X6
cardiac	T46.2X1	T46.2X2	T46.2X3	T46.2X4	T46.2X5	T46.2X6
central nervous system (anesthetic)—see also Central nervous system, depressants	T42.71	T42.72	T42.73	T42.74	T42.75	T42.76
general anesthetic	T41.201	T41.202	T41.203	T41.204	T41.205	T41.206
muscle tone	T42.8X1	T42.8X2	T42.8X3	T42.8X4	T42.8X5	T42.8X6
muscle tone, central	T42.8X1	T42.8X2	T42.8X3	T42.8X4	T42.8X5	T42.8X6
psychotherapeutic	T43.501	T43.502	T43.503	T43.504	T43.505	T43.506
Deptropine	T45.0X1	T45.0X2	T45.0X3	T45.0X4	T45.0X5	T45.0X6
Dequalinium (chloride)	T49.0X1	T49.0X2	T49.0X3	T49.0X4	T49.0X5	T49.0X6
Derris root	T60.2X1	T60.2X2	T60.2X3	T60.2X4	—	—
Deserpidine	T46.5X1	T46.5X2	T46.5X3	T46.5X4	T46.5X5	T46.5X6
Desferrioxamine	T45.8X1	T45.8X2	T45.8X3	T45.8X4	T45.8X5	T45.8X6
Desipramine	T43.011	T43.012	T43.013	T43.014	T43.015	T43.016
Deslanoside	T46.0X1	T46.0X2	T46.0X3	T46.0X4	T46.0X5	T46.0X6

Substance	Poisoning, Accidental (unintentional)	Poisoning, Intentional self-harm	Poisoning, Assault	Poisoning, Undetermined	Adverse effect	Underdosing
Desloughing agent	T49.4X1	T49.4X2	T49.4X3	T49.4X4	T49.4X5	T49.4X6
Desmethy-limipramine	T43.011	T43.012	T43.013	T43.014	T43.015	T43.016
Desmopressin	T38.891	T38.892	T38.893	T38.894	T38.895	T38.896
Desocodeine	T40.2X1	T40.2X2	T40.2X3	T40.2X4	T40.2X5	T40.2X6
Desogestrel	T38.5X1	T38.5X2	T38.5X3	T38.5X4	T38.5X5	T38.5X6
Desomorphine	T40.2X1	T40.2X2	T40.2X3	T40.2X4	—	—
Desonide	T49.0X1	T49.0X2	T49.0X3	T49.0X4	T49.0X5	T49.0X6
Desoximetasone	T49.0X1	T49.0X2	T49.0X3	T49.0X4	T49.0X5	T49.0X6
Desoxycorticosteroid	T50.0X1	T50.0X2	T50.0X3	T50.0X4	T50.0X5	T50.0X6
Desoxycortone	T50.0X1	T50.0X2	T50.0X3	T50.0X4	T50.0X5	T50.0X6
Desoxyephedrine	T43.621	T43.622	T43.623	T43.624	T43.625	T43.626
Detaxtran	T46.6X1	T46.6X2	T46.6X3	T46.6X4	T46.6X5	T46.6X6
Detergent	T49.2X1	T49.2X2	T49.2X3	T49.2X4	T49.2X5	T49.2X6
external medication	T49.2X1	T49.2X2	T49.2X3	T49.2X4	T49.2X5	T49.2X6
local	T49.2X1	T49.2X2	T49.2X3	T49.2X4	T49.2X5	T49.2X6
medicinal	T49.2X1	T49.2X2	T49.2X3	T49.2X4	T49.2X5	T49.2X6
nonmedicinal	T55.1X1	T55.1X2	T55.1X3	T55.1X4	—	—
specified NEC	T55.1X1	T55.1X2	T55.1X3	T55.1X4	—	—
Deterrent, alcohol	T50.6X1	T50.6X2	T50.6X3	T50.6X4	T50.6X5	T50.6X6
Detoxifying agent	T50.6X1	T50.6X2	T50.6X3	T50.6X4	T50.6X5	T50.6X6
Detrothyronine	T38.1X1	T38.1X2	T38.1X3	T38.1X4	T38.1X5	T38.1X6
Dettol (external medication)	T49.0X1	T49.0X2	T49.0X3	T49.0X4	T49.0X5	T49.0X6
Dexamethasone	T38.0X1	T38.0X2	T38.0X3	T38.0X4	T38.0X5	T38.0X6
ENT agent	T49.6X1	T49.6X2	T49.6X3	T49.6X4	T49.6X5	T49.6X6
ophthalmic preparation	T49.5X1	T49.5X2	T49.5X3	T49.5X4	T49.5X5	T49.5X6
topical NEC	T49.0X1	T49.0X2	T49.0X3	T49.0X4	T49.0X5	T49.0X6
Dexamfetamine	T43.621	T43.622	T43.623	T43.624	T43.625	T43.626
Dexamphetamine	T43.621	T43.622	T43.623	T43.624	T43.625	T43.626
Dexbrom-pheniramine	T45.0X1	T45.0X2	T45.0X3	T45.0X4	T45.0X5	T45.0X6
Dexchlorpheniramine	T45.0X1	T45.0X2	T45.0X3	T45.0X4	T45.0X5	T45.0X6
Dexedrine	T43.621	T43.622	T43.623	T43.624	T43.625	T43.626
Dexetimide	T44.3X1	T44.3X2	T44.3X3	T44.3X4	T44.3X5	T44.3X6
Dexfenfluramine	T50.5X1	T50.5X2	T50.5X3	T50.5X4	T50.5X5	T50.5X6
Dexpanthenol	T45.2X1	T45.2X2	T45.2X3	T45.2X4	T45.2X5	T45.2X6
Dextran (40) (70) (150)	T45.8X1	T45.8X2	T45.8X3	T45.8X4	T45.8X5	T45.8X6
Dextriferron	T45.4X1	T45.4X2	T45.4X3	T45.4X4	T45.4X5	T45.4X6
Dextro calcium pantothenate	T45.2X1	T45.2X2	T45.2X3	T45.2X4	T45.2X5	T45.2X6
Dextro pantothenyl alcohol	T45.2X1	T45.2X2	T45.2X3	T45.2X4	T45.2X5	T45.2X6
Dextroamphetamine	T43.621	T43.622	T43.623	T43.624	T43.625	T43.626
Dextromethorphan	T48.3X1	T48.3X2	T48.3X3	T48.3X4	T48.3X5	T48.3X6
Dextromoramide	T40.491	T40.492	T40.493	T40.494	—	—
topical	T49.8X1	T49.8X2	T49.8X3	T49.8X4	T49.8X5	T49.8X6
Dextropropoxyphene	T40.491	T40.492	T40.493	T40.494	T40.495	T40.496
Dextrorphan	T40.2X1	T40.2X2	T40.2X3	T40.2X4	T40.2X5	T40.2X6
Dextrose	T50.3X1	T50.3X2	T50.3X3	T50.3X4	T50.3X5	T50.3X6
concentrated solution, intravenous	T46.8X1	T46.8X2	T46.8X3	T46.8X4	T46.8X5	T46.8X6
Dextrothyroxin	T38.1X1	T38.1X2	T38.1X3	T38.1X4	T38.1X5	T38.1X6

Substance	Poisoning, Accidental (unintentional)	Poisoning, Intentional self-harm	Poisoning, Assault	Poisoning, Undetermined	Adverse effect	Underdosing
Dextrothyroxine sodium	T38.1X1	T38.1X2	T38.1X3	T38.1X5	T38.1X5	T38.1X6
DFP	T44.0X1	T44.0X2	T44.0X3	T44.0X4	T44.0X5	T44.0X6
DHE	T37.3X1	T37.3X2	T37.3X3	T37.3X4	T37.3X5	T37.3X6
45	T46.5X1	T46.5X2	T46.5X3	T46.5X4	T46.5X5	T46.5X6
Diabinese	T38.3X1	T38.3X2	T38.3X3	T38.3X4	T38.3X5	T38.3X6
Diacetone alcohol	T52.4X1	T52.4X2	T52.4X3	T52.4X4	—	—
Diacetyl monoxime	T50.991	T50.992	T50.993	T50.994	—	—
Diacetylmorphine	T40.1X1	T40.1X2	T40.1X3	T40.1X4	—	—
Diachylon plaster	T49.4X1	T49.4X2	T49.4X3	T49.4X4	T49.4X5	T49.4X6
Diaethylst-ilboestrolum	T38.5X1	T38.5X2	T38.5X3	T38.5X4	T38.5X5	T38.5X6
Diagnostic agent NEC	T50.8X1	T50.8X2	T50.8X3	T50.8X4	T50.8X5	T50.8X6
Dial (soap)	T49.2X1	T49.2X2	T49.2X3	T49.2X4	T49.2X5	T49.2X6
sedative	T42.3X1	T42.3X2	T42.3X3	T42.3X4	T42.3X5	T42.3X6
Dialkyl carbonate	T52.91	T52.92	T52.93	T52.94	—	—
Diallylbarbituric acid	T42.3X1	T42.3X2	T42.3X3	T42.3X4	T42.3X5	T42.3X6
Diallymal	T42.3X1	T42.3X2	T42.3X3	T42.3X4	T42.3X5	T42.3X6
Dialysis solution (intraperitoneal)	T50.3X1	T50.3X2	T50.3X3	T50.3X4	T50.3X5	T50.3X6
Diaminodi-phenylsulfone	T37.1X1	T37.1X2	T37.1X3	T37.1X4	T37.1X5	T37.1X6
Diamorphine	T40.1X1	T40.1X2	T40.1X3	T40.1X4	—	—
Diamox	T50.2X1	T50.2X2	T50.2X3	T50.2X4	T50.2X5	T50.2X6
Diamthazole	T49.0X1	T49.0X2	T49.0X3	T49.0X4	T49.0X5	T49.0X6
Dianthone	T47.2X1	T47.2X2	T47.2X3	T47.2X4	T47.2X5	T47.2X6
Diaphenylsulfone	T37.0X1	T37.0X2	T37.0X3	T37.0X4	T37.0X5	T37.0X6
Diasone (sodium)	T37.1X1	T37.1X2	T37.1X3	T37.1X4	T37.1X5	T37.1X6
Diastase	T47.5X1	T47.5X2	T47.5X3	T47.5X4	T47.5X5	T47.5X6
Diatrizoate	T50.8X1	T50.8X2	T50.8X3	T50.8X4	T50.8X5	T50.8X6
Diazepam	T42.4X1	T42.4X2	T42.4X3	T42.4X4	T42.4X5	T42.4X6
Diazinon	T60.0X1	T60.0X2	T60.0X3	T60.0X4	—	—
Diazomethane (gas)	T59.891	T59.892	T59.893	T59.894	—	—
Diazoxide	T46.5X1	T46.5X2	T46.5X3	T46.5X4	T46.5X5	T46.5X6
Dibekacin	T36.5X1	T36.5X2	T36.5X3	T36.5X4	T36.5X5	T36.5X6
Dibenamine	T44.6X1	T44.6X2	T44.6X3	T44.6X4	T44.6X5	T44.6X6
Dibenzepin	T43.011	T43.012	T43.013	T43.014	T43.015	T43.016
Dibenzheptropine	T45.0X1	T45.0X2	T45.0X3	T45.0X4	T45.0X5	T45.0X6
Dibenzyline	T44.6X1	T44.6X2	T44.6X3	T44.6X4	T44.6X5	T44.6X6
Diborane (gas)	T59.891	T59.892	T59.893	T59.894	—	—
Dibromoch-loropropane	T60.8X1	T60.8X2	T60.8X3	T60.8X4	—	—
Dibromodulcitol	T45.1X1	T45.1X2	T45.1X3	T45.1X4	T45.1X5	T45.1X6
Dibromoethane	T53.6X1	T53.6X2	T53.6X3	T53.6X4	—	—
Dibromomannitol	T45.1X1	T45.1X2	T45.1X3	T45.1X4	T45.1X5	T45.1X6
Dibromopropamidine isethionate	T49.0X1	T49.0X2	T49.0X3	T49.0X4	T49.0X5	T49.0X6
Dibrompropamidine	T49.0X1	T49.0X2	T49.0X3	T49.0X4	T49.0X5	T49.0X6
Dibucaine	T41.3X1	T41.3X2	T41.3X3	T41.3X4	T41.3X5	T41.3X6
topical (surface)	T41.3X1	T41.3X2	T41.3X3	T41.3X4	T41.3X5	T41.3X6
Dibunate sodium	T48.3X1	T48.3X2	T48.3X3	T48.3X4	T48.3X5	T48.3X6
Dibutoline sulfate	T44.3X1	T44.3X2	T44.3X3	T44.3X4	T44.3X5	T44.3X6
Dicamba	T60.3X1	T60.3X2	T60.3X3	T60.3X4	—	—
Dicapthon	T60.0X1	T60.0X2	T60.0X3	T60.0X4	—	—

Substance	Poisoning, Accidental (unintentional)	Poisoning, Intentional self-harm	Poisoning, Assault	Poisoning, Undetermined	Adverse effect	Underdosing
Dichlobenil	T60.3X1	T60.3X2	T60.3X3	T60.3X4	—	—
Dichlone	T60.3X1	T60.3X2	T60.3X3	T60.3X4	—	—
Dichloralphenozone	T42.6X1	T42.6X2	T42.6X3	T42.6X4	T42.6X5	T42.6X6
Dichlorbenzidine	T65.3X1	T65.3X2	T65.3X3	T65.3X4	—	—
Dichlorhydrin	T52.8X1	T52.8X2	T52.8X3	T52.8X4	—	—
Dichlorhydroxy-quinoline	T37.8X1	T37.8X2	T37.8X3	T37.8X4	T37.8X5	T37.8X6
Dichlorobenzene	T53.7X1	T53.7X2	T53.7X3	T53.7X4	—	—
Dichlorobenzyl alcohol	T49.6X1	T49.6X2	T49.6X3	T49.6X4	T49.6X5	T49.6X6
Dichlorodifluoro-methane	T53.5X1	T53.5X2	T53.5X3	T53.5X4	—	—
Dichloroethane	T52.8X1	T52.8X2	T52.8X3	T52.8X4	—	—
Sym-Dichloroethyl ether	T53.6X1	T53.6X2	T53.6X3	T53.6X4	—	—
Dichloroethyl sulfide, not in war	T59.891	T59.892	T59.893	T59.894	—	—
Dichloroethylene	T53.6X1	T53.6X2	T53.6X3	T53.6X4	—	—
Dichloroformoxine, not in war	T59.891	T59.892	T59.893	T59.894	—	—
Dichlorohydrin, alpha-dichlorohydrin	T52.8X1	T52.8X2	T52.8X3	T52.8X4	—	—
Dichloromethane (solvent)	T53.4X1	T53.4X2	T53.4X3	T53.4X4	—	—
vapor	T53.4X1	T53.4X2	T53.4X3	T53.4X4	—	—
Dichloronaphtho-quinone	T60.3X1	T60.3X2	T60.3X3	T60.3X4	—	—
Dichlorophen	T37.4X1	T37.4X2	T37.4X3	T37.4X4	T37.4X5	T37.4X6
2,4-Dichlorophenoxy-acetic acid	T60.3X1	T60.3X2	T60.3X3	T60.3X4	—	—
Dichloropropene	T60.3X1	T60.3X2	T60.3X3	T60.3X4	—	—
Dichloropropionic acid	T60.3X1	T60.3X2	T60.3X3	T60.3X4	—	—
Dichlorphenamide	T50.2X1	T50.2X2	T50.2X3	T50.2X4	T50.2X5	T50.2X6
Dichlorvos	T60.0X1	T60.0X2	T60.0X3	T60.0X4	—	—
Diclofenac	T39.391	T39.392	T39.393	T39.394	T39.395	T39.396
Diclofenamide	T50.2X1	T50.2X2	T50.2X3	T50.2X4	T50.2X5	T50.2X6
Diclofensine	T43.291	T43.292	T43.293	T43.294	T43.295	T43.296
Diclonixine	T39.8X1	T39.8X2	T39.8X3	T39.8X4	T39.8X5	T39.8X6
Dicloxacillin	T36.0X1	T36.0X2	T36.0X3	T36.0X4	T36.0X5	T36.0X6
Dicophane	T49.0X1	T49.0X2	T49.0X3	T49.0X4	T49.0X5	T49.0X6
Dicoumarol, dicoumarin, dicumarol	T45.511	T45.512	T45.513	T45.514	T45.515	T45.516
Dicrotophos	T60.0X1	T60.0X2	T60.0X3	T60.0X4	—	—
Dicyanogen (gas)	T65.0X1	T65.0X2	T65.0X3	T65.0X4	—	—
Dicyclomine	T44.3X1	T44.3X2	T44.3X3	T44.3X4	T44.3X5	T44.3X6
Dicycloverine	T44.3X1	T44.3X2	T44.3X3	T44.3X4	T44.3X5	T44.3X6
Dideoxycytidine	T37.5X1	T37.5X2	T37.5X3	T37.5X4	T37.5X5	T37.5X6
Dideoxyinosine	T37.5X1	T37.5X2	T37.5X3	T37.5X4	T37.5X5	T37.5X6
Dieldrin (vapor)	T60.1X1	T60.1X2	T60.1X3	T60.1X4	—	—
Diemal	T42.3X1	T42.3X2	T42.3X3	T42.3X4	T42.3X5	T42.3X6
Dienestrol	T38.5X1	T38.5X2	T38.5X3	T38.5X4	T38.5X5	T38.5X6
Dienoestrol	T38.5X1	T38.5X2	T38.5X3	T38.5X4	T38.5X5	T38.5X6
Dietetic drug NEC	T50.901	T50.902	T50.903	T50.904	T50.905	T50.906
Diethazine	T42.8X1	T42.8X2	T42.8X3	T42.8X4	T42.8X5	T42.8X6

Substance	Poisoning, Accidental (unintentional)	Poisoning, Intentional self-harm	Poisoning, Assault	Poisoning, Undetermined	Adverse effect	Underdosing
Diethyl						
barbituric acid	T42.3X1	T42.3X2	T42.3X3	T42.3X4	T42.3X5	T42.3X6
carbamazine	T37.4X1	T37.4X2	T37.4X3	T37.4X4	T37.4X5	T37.4X6
carbinol	T51.3X1	T51.3X2	T51.3X3	T51.3X4	—	—
carbonate	T52.8X1	T52.8X2	T52.8X3	T52.8X4	—	—
ether (vapor)—see also ether	T41.0X1	T41.0X2	T41.0X3	T41.0X4	T41.0X5	T41.0X6
oxide	T52.8X1	T52.8X2	T52.8X3	T52.8X4	—	—
propion	T50.5X1	T50.5X2	T50.5X3	T50.5X4	T50.5X5	T50.5X6
stilbestrol	T38.5X1	T38.5X2	T38.5X3	T38.5X4	T38.5X5	T38.5X6
toluamide (nonmedicinal)	T60.8X1	T60.8X2	T60.8X3	T60.8X4		
medicinal	T49.3X1	T49.3X2	T49.3X3	T49.3X4	T49.3X5	T49.3X6
Diethylcarbamazine	T37.4X1	T37.4X2	T37.4X3	T37.4X4	T37.4X5	T37.4X6
Diethylene						
dioxide	T52.8X1	T52.8X2	T52.8X3	T52.8X4		
glycol (monoacetate) (monobutyl ether) (monoethyl ether)	T52.3X1	T52.3X2	T52.3X3	T52.3X4		
Diethylhexy-lphthalate	T65.891	T65.892	T65.893	T65.894	—	—
Diethylpropion	T50.5X1	T50.5X2	T50.5X3	T50.5X4	T50.5X5	T50.5X6
Diethylstilbestrol	T38.5X1	T38.5X2	T38.5X3	T38.5X4	T38.5X5	T38.5X6
Diethylstilboestrol	T38.5X1	T38.5X2	T38.5X3	T38.5X4	T38.5X5	T38.5X6
Diethylsulfone-diethylmethane	T42.6X1	T42.6X2	T42.6X3	T42.6X4	T42.6X5	T42.6X6
Diethyltoluamide	T49.0X1	T49.0X2	T49.0X3	T49.0X4	T49.0X5	T49.0X6
Diethyltryptamine (DET)	T40.991	T40.992	T40.993	T40.994	—	—
Difebarbamate	T42.3X1	T42.3X2	T42.3X3	T42.3X4	T42.3X5	T42.3X6
Difencloxazine	T40.2X1	T40.2X2	T40.2X3	T40.2X4	T40.2X5	T40.2X6
Difenidol	T45.0X1	T45.0X2	T45.0X3	T45.0X4	T45.0X5	T45.0X6
Difenoxin	T47.6X1	T47.6X2	T47.6X3	T47.6X4	T47.6X5	T47.6X6
Difetarsone	T37.3X1	T37.3X2	T37.3X3	T37.3X4	T37.3X5	T37.3X6
Diffusin	T45.3X1	T45.3X2	T45.3X3	T45.3X4	T45.3X5	T45.3X6
Diflorasone	T49.0X1	T49.0X2	T49.0X3	T49.0X4	T49.0X5	T49.0X6
Diflos	T44.0X1	T44.0X2	T44.0X3	T44.0X4	T44.0X5	T44.0X6
Diflubenzuron	T60.1X1	T60.1X2	T60.1X3	T60.1X4	—	—
Diflucortolone	T49.0X1	T49.0X2	T49.0X3	T49.0X4	T49.0X5	T49.0X6
Diflunisal	T39.091	T39.092	T39.093	T39.094	T39.095	T39.096
Difluoromethyldopa	T42.8X1	T42.8X2	T42.8X3	T42.8X4	T42.8X5	T42.8X6
Difluorophate	T44.0X1	T44.0X2	T44.0X3	T44.0X4	T44.0X5	T44.0X6
Digestant NEC	T47.5X1	T47.5X2	T47.5X3	T47.5X4	T47.5X5	T47.5X6
Digitalin(e)	T46.0X1	T46.0X2	T46.0X3	T46.0X4	T46.0X5	T46.0X6
Digitalis (leaf) (glycoside)	T46.0X1	T46.0X2	T46.0X3	T46.0X4	T46.0X5	T46.0X6
lanata	T46.0X1	T46.0X2	T46.0X3	T46.0X4	T46.0X5	T46.0X6
purpurea	T46.0X1	T46.0X2	T46.0X3	T46.0X4	T46.0X5	T46.0X6
Digitoxin	T46.0X1	T46.0X2	T46.0X3	T46.0X4	T46.0X5	T46.0X6
Digitoxose	T46.0X1	T46.0X2	T46.0X3	T46.0X4	T46.0X5	T46.0X6
Digoxin	T46.0X1	T46.0X2	T46.0X3	T46.0X4	T46.0X5	T46.0X6
Digoxine	T46.0X1	T46.0X2	T46.0X3	T46.0X4	T46.0X5	T46.0X6
Dihydralazine	T46.5X1	T46.5X2	T46.5X3	T46.5X4	T46.5X5	T46.5X6
Dihydrazine	T46.5X1	T46.5X2	T46.5X3	T46.5X4	T46.5X5	T46.5X6

Substance	Poisoning, Accidental (unintentional)	Poisoning, Intentional self-harm	Poisoning, Assault	Poisoning, Undetermined	Adverse effect	Underdosing
Dihydrocodeine	T40.2X1	T40.2X2	T40.2X3	T40.2X4	T40.2X5	T40.2X6
Dihydrocodeinone	T40.2X1	T40.2X2	T40.2X3	T40.2X4	T40.2X5	T40.2X6
Dihydroergocornine	T46.7X1	T46.7X2	T46.7X3	T46.7X4	T46.7X5	T46.7X6
Dihydroergocristine (mesilate)	T46.7X1	T46.7X2	T46.7X3	T46.7X4	T46.7X5	T46.7X6
Dihydroergokryptine	T46.7X1	T46.7X2	T46.7X3	T46.7X4	T46.7X5	T46.7X6
Dihydroergotamine	T46.5X1	T46.5X2	T46.5X3	T46.5X4	T46.5X5	T46.5X6
Dihydroergotoxine	T46.7X1	T46.7X2	T46.7X3	T46.7X4	T46.7X5	T46.7X6
mesilate	T46.7X1	T46.7X2	T46.7X3	T46.7X4	T46.7X5	T46.7X6
Dihydrohydroxy-codeinone	T40.2X1	T40.2X2	T40.2X3	T40.2X4	T40.2X5	T40.2X6
Dihydrohydroxy-morphinone	T40.2X1	T40.2X2	T40.2X3	T40.2X4	T40.2X5	T40.2X6
Dihydroisocodeine	T40.2X1	T40.2X2	T40.2X3	T40.2X4	T40.2X5	T40.2X6
Dihydromorphine	T40.2X1	T40.2X2	T40.2X3	T40.2X4	—	—
Dihydromorphinone	T40.2X1	T40.2X2	T40.2X3	T40.2X4	T40.2X5	T40.2X6
Dihydrostreptomycin	T36.5X1	T36.5X2	T36.5X3	T36.5X4	T36.5X5	T36.5X6
Dihydrotachysterol	T45.2X1	T45.2X2	T45.2X3	T45.2X4	T45.2X5	T45.2X6
Dihydroxyaluminum aminoacetate	T47.1X1	T47.1X2	T47.1X3	T47.1X4	T47.1X5	T47.1X6
Dihydroxyaluminum sodium carbonate	T47.1X1	T47.1X2	T47.1X3	T47.1X4	T47.1X5	T47.1X6
Dihydroxyanthra-quinone	T47.2X1	T47.2X2	T47.2X3	T47.2X4	T47.2X5	T47.2X6
Dihydroxycodeinone	T40.2X1	T40.2X2	T40.2X3	T40.2X4	T40.2X5	T40.2X6
Dihydroxypropyl theophylline	T50.2X1	T50.2X2	T50.2X3	T50.2X4	T50.2X5	T50.2X6
Diiodohydroxyquin	T37.8X1	T37.8X2	T37.8X3	T37.8X4	T37.8X5	T37.8X6
topical	T49.0X1	T49.0X2	T49.0X3	T49.0X4	T49.0X5	T49.0X6
Diiodo-hydroxyquinoline	T37.8X1	T37.8X2	T37.8X3	T37.8X4	T37.8X5	T37.8X6
Diiodotyrosine	T38.2X1	T38.2X2	T38.2X3	T38.2X4	T38.2X5	T38.2X6
Diisopromine	T44.3X1	T44.3X2	T44.3X3	T44.3X4	T44.3X5	T44.3X6
Diisopropylamine	T46.3X1	T46.3X2	T46.3X3	T46.3X4	T46.3X5	T46.3X6
Diisopropyl-fluorophos-phonate	T44.0X1	T44.0X2	T44.0X3	T44.0X4	T44.0X5	T44.0X6
Dilantin	T42.0X1	T42.0X2	T42.0X3	T42.0X4	T42.0X5	T42.0X6
Dilaudid	T40.2X1	T40.2X2	T40.2X3	T40.2X4	T40.2X5	T40.2X6
Dilazep	T46.3X1	T46.3X2	T46.3X3	T46.3X4	T46.3X5	T46.3X6
Dill	T47.5X1	T47.5X2	T47.5X3	T47.5X4	T47.5X5	T47.5X6
Diloxanide	T37.3X1	T37.3X2	T37.3X3	T37.3X4	T37.3X5	T37.3X6
Diltiazem	T46.1X1	T46.1X2	T46.1X3	T46.1X4	T46.1X5	T46.1X6
Dimazole	T49.0X1	T49.0X2	T49.0X3	T49.0X4	T49.0X5	T49.0X6
Dimefline	T50.7X1	T50.7X2	T50.7X3	T50.7X4	T50.7X5	T50.7X6
Dimefox	T60.0X1	T60.0X2	T60.0X3	T60.0X4	—	—
Dimemorfan	T48.3X1	T48.3X2	T48.3X3	T48.3X4	T48.3X5	T48.3X6
Dimenhydrinate	T45.0X1	T45.0X2	T45.0X3	T45.0X4	T45.0X5	T45.0X6
Dimercaprol (British anti-lewisite)	T45.8X1	T45.8X2	T45.8X3	T45.8X4	T45.8X5	T45.8X6
Dimercaptopropanol	T45.8X1	T45.8X2	T45.8X3	T45.8X4	T45.8X5	T45.8X6
Dimestrol	T38.5X1	T38.5X2	T38.5X3	T38.5X4	T38.5X5	T38.5X6
Dimetane	T45.0X1	T45.0X2	T45.0X3	T45.0X4	T45.0X5	T45.0X6
Dimethicone	T47.1X1	T47.1X2	T47.1X3	T47.1X4	T47.1X5	T47.1X6
Dimethindene	T45.0X1	T45.0X2	T45.0X3	T45.0X4	T45.0X5	T45.0X6

Substance	Poisoning, Accidental (unintentional)	Poisoning, Intentional self-harm	Poisoning, Assault	Poisoning, Undetermined	Adverse effect	Underdosing
Dimethisoquin	T49.1X1	T49.1X2	T49.1X3	T49.1X4	T49.1X5	T49.1X6
Dimethisterone	T38.5X1	T38.5X2	T38.5X3	T38.5X4	T38.5X5	T38.5X6
Dimethoate	T60.0X1	T60.0X2	T60.0X3	T60.0X4	—	—
Dimethocaine	T41.3X1	T41.3X2	T41.3X3	T41.3X4	T41.3X5	T41.3X6
Dimethoxanate	T48.3X1	T48.3X2	T48.3X3	T48.3X4	T48.3X5	T48.3X6
Dimethyl						
arsine, arsinic acid	T57.0X1	T57.0X2	T57.0X3	T57.0X4	—	—
carbinol	T51.2X1	T51.2X2	T51.2X3	T51.2X4	—	—
carbonate	T52.8X1	T52.8X2	T52.8X3	T52.8X4	—	—
diguanide	T38.3X1	T38.3X2	T38.3X3	T38.3X4	T38.3X5	T38.3X6
ketone	T52.4X1	T52.4X2	T52.4X3	T52.4X4	—	—
vapor	T52.4X1	T52.4X2	T52.4X3	T52.4X4	—	—
meperidine	T40.2X1	T40.2X2	T40.2X3	T40.2X4	T40.2X5	T40.2X6
parathion	T60.0X1	T60.0X2	T60.0X3	T60.0X4	—	—
phthlate	T49.3X1	T49.3X2	T49.3X3	T49.3X4	T49.3X5	T49.3X6
polysiloxane	T47.8X1	T47.8X2	T47.8X3	T47.8X4	T47.8X5	T47.8X6
sulfate (fumes)	T59.891	T59.892	T59.893	T59.894	—	—
liquid	T65.891	T65.892	T65.893	T65.894	—	—
sulfoxide (nonmedicinal)	T52.8X1	T52.8X2	T52.8X3	T52.8X4	—	—
medicinal	T49.4X1	T49.4X2	T49.4X3	T49.4X4	T49.4X5	T49.4X6
tryptamine	T40.991	T40.992	T40.993	T40.994	—	—
tubocurarine	T48.1X1	T48.1X2	T48.1X3	T48.1X4	T48.1X5	T48.1X6
Dimethylamine sulfate	T49.4X1	T49.4X2	T49.4X3	T49.4X4	T49.4X5	T49.4X6
Dimethylformamide	T52.8X1	T52.8X2	T52.8X3	T52.8X4	—	—
Dimethyltubocurari-nium chloride	T48.1X1	T48.1X2	T48.1X3	T48.1X4	T48.1X5	T48.1X6
Dimeticone	T47.1X1	T47.1X2	T47.1X3	T47.1X4	T47.1X5	T47.1X6
Dimetilan	T60.0X1	T60.0X2	T60.0X3	T60.0X4	—	—
Dimetindene	T45.0X1	T45.0X2	T45.0X3	T45.0X4	T45.0X5	T45.0X6
Dimetotiazine	T43.3X1	T43.3X2	T43.3X3	T43.3X4	T43.3X5	T43.3X6
Dimorpholamine	T50.7X1	T50.7X2	T50.7X3	T50.7X4	T50.7X5	T50.7X6
Dimoxyline	T46.3X1	T46.3X2	T46.3X3	T46.3X4	T46.3X5	T46.3X6
Dinitrobenzene	T65.3X1	T65.3X2	T65.3X3	T65.3X4	—	—
vapor	T59.891	T59.892	T59.893	T59.894	—	—
Dinitrobenzol	T65.3X1	T65.3X2	T65.3X3	T65.3X4	—	—
vapor	T59.891	T59.892	T59.893	T59.894	—	—
Dinitrobutylphenol	T65.3X1	T65.3X2	T65.3X3	T65.3X4	—	—
Dinitro (-ortho-)cresol (pesticide) (spray)	T65.3X1	T65.3X2	T65.3X3	T65.3X4	—	—
Dinitro-cyclohexylphenol	T65.3X1	T65.3X2	T65.3X3	T65.3X4	—	—
Dinitrophenol	T65.3X1	T65.3X2	T65.3X3	T65.3X4	—	—
Dinoprost	T48.0X1	T48.0X2	T48.0X3	T48.0X4	T48.0X5	T48.0X6
Dinoprostone	T48.0X1	T48.0X2	T48.0X3	T48.0X4	T48.0X5	T48.0X6
Dinoseb	T60.3X1	T60.3X2	T60.3X3	T60.3X4	—	—
Dioctyl sulfosuccinate (calcium) (sodium)	T47.4X1	T47.4X2	T47.4X3	T47.4X4	T47.4X5	T47.4X6
Diodone	T50.8X1	T50.8X2	T50.8X3	T50.8X4	T50.8X5	T50.8X6
Diodoquin	T37.8X1	T37.8X2	T37.8X3	T37.8X4	T37.8X5	T37.8X6
Dionin	T40.2X1	T40.2X2	T40.2X3	T40.2X4	T40.2X5	T40.2X6
Diosmin	T46.991	T46.992	T46.993	T46.994	T46.995	T46.996

Substance	Poisoning, Accidental (unintentional)	Poisoning, Intentional self-harm	Poisoning, Assault	Poisoning, Undetermined	Adverse effect	Underdosing
Dioxane	T52.8X1	T52.8X2	T52.8X3	T52.8X4	—	—
Dioxathion	T60.0X1	T60.0X2	T60.0X3	T60.0X4	—	—
Dioxin	T53.7X1	T53.7X2	T53.7X3	T53.7X4	—	—
Dioxopromethazine	T43.3X1	T43.3X2	T43.3X3	T43.3X4	T43.3X5	T43.3X6
Dioxyline	T46.3X1	T46.3X2	T46.3X3	T46.3X4	T46.3X5	T46.3X6
Dipentene	T52.8X1	T52.8X2	T52.8X3	T52.8X4	—	—
Diperodon	T41.3X1	T41.3X2	T41.3X3	T41.3X4	T41.3X5	T41.3X6
Diphacinone	T60.4X1	T60.4X2	T60.4X3	T60.4X4	—	—
Diphemanil	T44.3X1	T44.3X2	T44.3X3	T44.3X4	T44.3X5	T44.3X6
metilsulfate	T44.3X1	T44.3X2	T44.3X3	T44.3X4	T44.3X5	T44.3X6
Diphenadione	T45.511	T45.512	T45.513	T45.514	T45.515	T45.516
rodenticide	T60.4X1	T60.4X2	T60.4X3	T60.4X4	—	—
Diphenhydramine	T45.0X1	T45.0X2	T45.0X3	T45.0X4	T45.0X5	T45.0X6
Diphenidol	T45.0X1	T45.0X2	T45.0X3	T45.0X4	T45.0X5	T45.0X6
Diphenoxylate	T47.6X1	T47.6X2	T47.6X3	T47.6X4	T47.6X5	T47.6X6
Diphenylamine	T65.3X1	T65.3X2	T65.3X3	T65.3X4	—	—
Diphenylbutazone	T39.2X1	T39.2X2	T39.2X3	T39.2X4	T39.2X5	T39.2X6
Diphenyl-chloroarsine, not in war	T57.0X1	T57.0X2	T57.0X3	T57.0X4	—	—
Diphenylhydantoin	T42.0X1	T42.0X2	T42.0X3	T42.0X4	T42.0X5	T42.0X6
Diphenylmethane dye	T52.1X1	T52.1X2	T52.1X3	T52.1X4	—	—
Diphenylpyraline	T45.0X1	T45.0X2	T45.0X3	T45.0X4	T45.0X5	T45.0X6
Diphtheria						
antitoxin	T50.Z11	T50.Z12	T50.Z13	T50.Z14	T50.Z15	T50.Z16
toxoid	T50.A91	T50.A92	T50.A93	T50.A94	T50.A95	T50.A96
with tetanus toxoid	T50.A21	T50.A22	T50.A23	T50.A24	T50.A25	T50.A26
with pertussis component	T50.A11	T50.A12	T50.A13	T50.A14	T50.A15	T50.A16
vaccine	T50.A91	T50.A92	T50.A93	T50.A94	T50.A95	T50.A96
combination						
including pertussis	T50.A11	T50.A12	T50.A13	T50.A14	T50.A15	T50.A16
without pertussis	T50.A21	T50.A22	T50.A23	T50.A24	T50.A25	T50.A26
Diphylline	T50.2X1	T50.2X2	T50.2X3	T50.2X4	T50.2X5	T50.2X6
Dipipanone	T40.491	T40.492	T40.493	T40.494	—	—
Dipivefrine	T49.5X1	T49.5X2	T49.5X3	T49.5X4	T49.5X5	T49.5X6
Diplovax	T50.B91	T50.B92	T50.B93	T50.B94	T50.B95	T50.B96
Diprophylline	T50.2X1	T50.2X2	T50.2X3	T50.2X4	T50.2X5	T50.2X6
Dipropyline	T48.291	T48.292	T48.293	T48.294	T48.295	T48.296
Dipyridamole	T46.3X1	T46.3X2	T46.3X3	T46.3X4	T46.3X5	T46.3X6
Dipyrone	T39.2X1	T39.2X2	T39.2X3	T39.2X4	T39.2X5	T39.2X6
Diquat (dibromide)	T60.3X1	T60.3X2	T60.3X3	T60.3X4	—	—
Disinfectant	T65.891	T65.892	T65.893	T65.894	—	—
alkaline	T54.3X1	T54.3X2	T54.3X3	T54.3X4	—	—
aromatic	T54.1X1	T54.1X2	T54.1X3	T54.1X4	—	—
intestinal	T37.8X1	T37.8X2	T37.8X3	T37.8X4	T37.8X5	T37.8X6
Disipal	T42.8X1	T42.8X2	T42.8X3	T42.8X4	T42.8X5	T42.8X6
Disodium edetate	T50.6X1	T50.6X2	T50.6X3	T50.6X4	T50.6X5	T50.6X6
Disoprofol	T41.291	T41.292	T41.293	T41.294	T41.295	T41.296
Disopyramide	T46.2X1	T46.2X2	T46.2X3	T46.2X4	T46.2X5	T46.2X6
Distigmine (bromide)	T44.0X1	T44.0X2	T44.0X3	T44.0X4	T44.0X5	T44.0X6
Disulfamide	T50.2X1	T50.2X2	T50.2X3	T50.2X4	T50.2X5	T50.2X6

Substance	Poisoning, Accidental (unintentional)	Poisoning, Intentional self-harm	Poisoning, Assault	Poisoning, Undetermined	Adverse effect	Underdosing
Disulfanilamide	T37.0X1	T37.0X2	T37.0X3	T37.0X4	T37.0X5	T37.0X6
Disulfiram	T50.6X1	T50.6X2	T50.6X3	T50.6X4	T50.6X5	T50.6X6
Disulfoton	T60.0X1	T60.0X2	T60.0X3	T60.0X4	—	—
Dithiazanine iodide	T37.4X1	T37.4X2	T37.4X3	T37.4X4	T37.4X5	T37.4X6
Dithiocarbamate	T60.0X1	T60.0X2	T60.0X3	T60.0X4	—	—
Dithranol	T49.4X1	T49.4X2	T49.4X3	T49.4X4	T49.4X5	T49.4X6
Diucardin	T50.2X1	T50.2X2	T50.2X3	T50.2X4	T50.2X5	T50.2X6
Diupres	T50.2X1	T50.2X2	T50.2X3	T50.2X4	T50.2X5	T50.2X6
Diuretic NEC	T50.2X1	T50.2X2	T50.2X3	T50.2X4	T50.2X5	T50.2X6
benzothiadiazine	T50.2X1	T50.2X2	T50.2X3	T50.2X4	T50.2X5	T50.2X6
carbonic acid anhydrase inhibitors	T50.2X1	T50.2X2	T50.2X3	T50.2X4	T50.2X5	T50.2X6
furfuryl NEC	T50.2X1	T50.2X2	T50.2X3	T50.2X4	T50.2X5	T50.2X6
loop (high-ceiling)	T50.1X1	T50.1X2	T50.1X3	T50.1X4	T50.1X5	T50.1X6
mercurial NEC	T50.2X1	T50.2X2	T50.2X3	T50.2X4	T50.2X5	T50.2X6
osmotic	T50.2X1	T50.2X2	T50.2X3	T50.2X4	T50.2X5	T50.2X6
purine NEC	T50.2X1	T50.2X2	T50.2X3	T50.2X4	T50.2X5	T50.2X6
saluretic NEC	T50.2X1	T50.2X2	T50.2X3	T50.2X4	T50.2X5	T50.2X6
sulfonamide	T50.2X1	T50.2X2	T50.2X3	T50.2X4	T50.2X5	T50.2X6
thiazide NEC	T50.2X1	T50.2X2	T50.2X3	T50.2X4	T50.2X5	T50.2X6
xanthine	T50.2X1	T50.2X2	T50.2X3	T50.2X4	T50.2X5	T50.2X6
Diurgin	T50.2X1	T50.2X2	T50.2X3	T50.2X4	T50.2X5	T50.2X6
Diuril	T50.2X1	T50.2X2	T50.2X3	T50.2X4	T50.2X5	T50.2X6
Diuron	T60.3X1	T60.3X2	T60.3X3	T60.3X4	—	—
Divalproex	T42.6X1	T42.6X2	T42.6X3	T42.6X4	T42.6X5	T42.6X6
Divinyl ether	T41.0X1	T41.0X2	T41.0X3	T41.0X4	T41.0X5	T41.0X6
Dixanthogen	T49.0X1	T49.0X2	T49.0X3	T49.0X4	T49.0X5	T49.0X6
Dixyrazine	T43.3X1	T43.3X2	T43.3X3	T43.3X4	T43.3X5	T43.3X6
D-lysergic acid diethylamide	T40.8X1	T40.8X2	T40.8X3	T40.8X4	—	—
DMCT	T36.4X1	T36.4X2	T36.4X3	T36.4X4	T36.4X5	T36.4X6
DMSO—see Dimethyl sulfoxide						
DNBP	T60.3X1	T60.3X2	T60.3X3	T60.3X4	—	—
DNOC	T65.3X1	T65.3X2	T65.3X3	T65.3X4	—	—
Dobutamine	T44.5X1	T44.5X2	T44.5X3	T44.5X4	T44.5X5	T44.5X6
DOCA	T38.0X1	T38.0X2	T38.0X3	T38.0X4	T38.0X5	T38.0X6
Docusate sodium	T47.4X1	T47.4X2	T47.4X3	T47.4X4	T47.4X5	T47.4X6
Dodicin	T49.0X1	T49.0X2	T49.0X3	T49.0X4	T49.0X5	T49.0X6
Dofamium chloride	T49.0X1	T49.0X2	T49.0X3	T49.0X4	T49.0X5	T49.0X6
Dolophine	T40.3X1	T40.3X2	T40.3X3	T40.3X4	T40.3X5	T40.3X6
Doloxene	T39.8X1	T39.8X2	T39.8X3	T39.8X4	T39.8X5	T39.8X6
Domestic gas (after combustion)—see Gas, utility						
prior to combustion	T59.891	T59.892	T59.893	T59.894	—	—
Domiodol	T48.4X1	T48.4X2	T48.4X3	T48.4X4	T48.4X5	T48.4X6
Domiphen (bromide)	T49.0X1	T49.0X2	T49.0X3	T49.0X4	T49.0X5	T49.0X6
Domperidone	T45.0X1	T45.0X2	T45.0X3	T45.0X4	T45.0X5	T45.0X6
Dopa	T42.8X1	T42.8X2	T42.8X3	T42.8X4	T42.8X5	T42.8X6
Dopamine	T44.991	T44.992	T44.993	T44.994	T44.995	T44.996
Doriden	T42.6X1	T42.6X2	T42.6X3	T42.6X4	T42.6X5	T42.6X6

Substance	Poisoning, Accidental (unintentional)	Poisoning, Intentional self-harm	Poisoning, Assault	Poisoning, Undetermined	Adverse effect	Underdosing
Dormiral	T42.3X1	T42.3X2	T42.3X3	T42.3X4	T42.3X5	T42.3X6
Dormison	T42.6X1	T42.6X2	T42.6X3	T42.6X4	T42.6X5	T42.6X6
Dornase	T48.4X1	T48.4X2	T48.4X3	T48.4X4	T48.4X5	T48.4X6
Dorsacaine	T41.3X1	T41.3X2	T41.3X3	T41.3X4	T41.3X5	T41.3X6
Dosulepin	T43.011	T43.012	T43.013	T43.014	T43.015	T43.016
Dothiepin	T43.011	T43.012	T43.013	T43.014	T43.015	T43.016
Doxantrazole	T48.6X1	T48.6X2	T48.6X3	T48.6X4	T48.6X5	T48.6X6
Doxapram	T50.7X1	T50.7X2	T50.7X3	T50.7X4	T50.7X5	T50.7X6
Doxazosin	T44.6X1	T44.6X2	T44.6X3	T44.6X4	T44.6X5	T44.6X6
Doxepin	T43.011	T43.012	T43.013	T43.014	T43.015	T43.016
Doxifluridine	T45.1X1	T45.1X2	T45.1X3	T45.1X4	T45.1X5	T45.1X6
Doxorubicin	T45.1X1	T45.1X2	T45.1X3	T45.1X4	T45.1X5	T45.1X6
Doxycycline	T36.4X1	T36.4X2	T36.4X3	T36.4X4	T36.4X5	T36.4X6
Doxylamine	T45.0X1	T45.0X2	T45.0X3	T45.0X4	T45.0X5	T45.0X6
Dramamine	T45.0X1	T45.0X2	T45.0X3	T45.0X4	T45.0X5	T45.0X6
Drano (drain cleaner)	T54.3X1	T54.3X2	T54.3X3	T54.3X4	—	—
Dressing, live pulp	T49.7X1	T49.7X2	T49.7X3	T49.7X4	T49.7X5	T49.7X6
Drocode	T40.2X1	T40.2X2	T40.2X3	T40.2X4	T40.2X5	T40.2X6
Dromoran	T40.2X1	T40.2X2	T40.2X3	T40.2X4	T40.2X5	T40.2X6
Dromostanolone	T38.7X1	T38.7X2	T38.7X3	T38.7X4	T38.7X5	T38.7X6
Dronabinol	T40.7X1	T40.7X2	T40.7X3	T40.7X4	T40.7X5	T40.7X6
Droperidol	T43.591	T43.592	T43.593	T43.594	T43.595	T43.596
Dropropizine	T48.3X1	T48.3X2	T48.3X3	T48.3X4	T48.3X5	T48.3X6
Drostanolone	T38.7X1	T38.7X2	T38.7X3	T38.7X4	T38.7X5	T38.7X6
Drotaverine	T44.3X1	T44.3X2	T44.3X3	T44.3X4	T44.3X5	T44.3X6
Drotrecogin alfa	T45.511	T45.512	T45.513	T45.514	T45.515	T45.516
Drug NEC	T50.901	T50.902	T50.903	T50.904	T50.905	T50.906
specified NEC	T50.991	T50.992	T50.993	T50.994	T50.995	T50.996
DTIC	T45.1X1	T45.1X2	T45.1X3	T45.1X4	T45.1X5	T45.1X6
Duboisine	T44.3X1	T44.3X2	T44.3X3	T44.3X4	T44.3X5	T44.3X6
Dulcolax	T47.2X1	T47.2X2	T47.2X3	T47.2X4	T47.2X5	T47.2X6
Duponol (C) (EP)	T49.2X1	T49.2X2	T49.2X3	T49.2X4	T49.2X5	T49.2X6
Durabolin	T38.7X1	T38.7X2	T38.7X3	T38.7X4	T38.7X5	T38.7X6
Dyclone	T41.3X1	T41.3X2	T41.3X3	T41.3X4	T41.3X5	T41.3X6
Dyclonine	T41.3X1	T41.3X2	T41.3X3	T41.3X4	T41.3X5	T41.3X6
Dydrogesterone	T38.5X1	T38.5X2	T38.5X3	T38.5X4	T38.5X5	T38.5X6
Dye NEC	T65.6X1	T65.6X2	T65.6X3	T65.6X4	—	—
antiseptic	T49.0X1	T49.0X2	T49.0X3	T49.0X4	T49.0X5	T19.0X6
diagnostic agents	T50.8X1	T50.8X2	T50.8X3	T50.8X4	T50.8X5	T50.8X6
pharmaceutical NEC	T50.901	T50.902	T50.903	T50.904	T50.905	T50.906
Dyflos	T44.0X1	T44.0X2	T44.0X3	T44.0X4	T44.0X5	T44.0X6
Dymelor	T38.3X1	T38.3X2	T38.3X3	T38.3X4	T38.3X5	T38.3X6
Dynamite	T65.3X1	T65.3X2	T65.3X3	T65.3X4	—	—
fumes	T59.891	T59.892	T59.893	T59.894	—	—
Dyphylline	T44.3X1	T44.3X2	T44.3X3	T44.3X4	T44.3X5	T44.3X6
E						
Ear drug NEC	T49.6X1	T49.6X2	T49.6X3	T49.6X4	T49.6X5	T49.6X6
Ear preparations	T49.6X1	T49.6X2	T49.6X3	T49.6X4	T49.6X5	T49.6X6
Echothiophate, echothiopate, ecothiopate	T49.5X1	T49.5X2	T49.5X3	T49.5X4	T49.5X5	T49.5X6

Substance	Poisoning, Accidental (unintentional)	Poisoning, Intentional self-harm	Poisoning, Assault	Poisoning, Undetermined	Adverse effect	Underdosing
Econazole	T49.0X1	T49.0X2	T49.0X3	T49.0X4	T49.0X5	T49.0X6
Ecothiopate iodide	T49.5X1	T49.5X2	T49.5X3	T49.5X4	T49.5X5	T49.5X6
Ecstasy	T43.641	T43.642	T43.643	T43.644	—	—
Ectylurea	T42.6X1	T42.6X2	T42.6X3	T42.6X4	T42.6X5	T42.6X6
Edathamil disodium	T45.8X1	T45.8X2	T45.8X3	T45.8X4	T45.8X5	T45.8X6
Edecrin	T50.1X1	T50.1X2	T50.1X3	T50.1X4	T50.1X5	T50.1X6
Edetate, disodium (calcium)	T45.8X1	T45.8X2	T45.8X3	T45.8X4	T45.8X5	T45.8X6
Edoxudine	T49.5X1	T49.5X2	T49.5X3	T49.5X4	T49.5X5	T49.5X6
Edrophonium	T44.0X1	T44.0X2	T44.0X3	T44.0X4	T44.0X5	T44.0X6
chloride	T44.0X1	T44.0X2	T44.0X3	T44.0X4	T44.0X5	T44.0X6
EDTA	T50.6X1	T50.6X2	T50.6X3	T50.6X4	T50.6X5	T50.6X6
Eflornithine	T37.2X1	T37.2X2	T37.2X3	T37.2X4	T37.2X5	T37.2X6
Efloxate	T46.3X1	T46.3X2	T46.3X3	T46.3X4	T46.3X5	T46.3X6
Elase	T49.8X1	T49.8X2	T49.8X3	T49.8X4	T49.8X5	T49.8X6
Elastase	T47.5X1	T47.5X2	T47.5X3	T47.5X4	T47.5X5	T47.5X6
Elaterium	T47.2X1	T47.2X2	T47.2X3	T47.2X4	T47.2X5	T47.2X6
Elcatonin	T50.991	T50.992	T50.993	T50.994	T50.995	T50.996
Elder	T62.2X1	T62.2X2	T62.2X3	T62.2X4	—	—
berry,(unripe)	T62.1X1	T62.1X2	T62.1X3	T62.1X4	—	—
Electrolyte balance drug	T50.3X1	T50.3X2	T50.3X3	T50.3X4	T50.3X5	T50.3X6
Electrolytes NEC	T50.3X1	T50.3X2	T50.3X3	T50.3X4	T50.3X5	T50.3X6
Electrolytic agent NEC	T50.3X1	T50.3X2	T50.3X3	T50.3X4	T50.3X5	T50.3X6
Elemental diet	T50.901	T50.902	T50.903	T50.904	T50.905	T50.906
Elliptinium acetate	T45.1X1	T45.1X2	T45.1X3	T45.1X4	T45.1X5	T45.1X6
Embramine	T45.0X1	T45.0X2	T45.0X3	T45.0X4	T45.0X5	T45.0X6
Emepronium (salts)	T44.3X1	T44.3X2	T44.3X3	T44.3X4	T44.3X5	T44.3X6
bromide	T44.3X1	T44.3X2	T44.3X3	T44.3X4	T44.3X5	T44.3X6
Emetic NEC	T47.7X1	T47.7X2	T47.7X3	T47.7X4	T47.7X5	T47.7X6
Emetine	T37.3X1	T37.3X2	T37.3X3	T37.3X4	T37.3X5	T37.3X6
Emollient NEC	T49.3X1	T49.3X2	T49.3X3	T49.3X4	T49.3X5	T49.3X6
Emorfazone	T39.8X1	T39.8X2	T39.8X3	T39.8X4	T39.8X5	T39.8X6
Emylcamate	T43.591	T43.592	T43.593	T43.594	T43.595	T43.596
Enalapril	T46.4X1	T46.4X2	T46.4X3	T46.4X4	T46.4X5	T46.4X6
Enalaprilat	T46.4X1	T46.4X2	T46.4X3	T46.4X4	T46.4X5	T46.4X6
Encainide	T46.2X1	T46.2X2	T46.2X3	T46.2X4	T46.2X5	T46.2X6
Endocaine	T41.3X1	T41.3X2	T41.3X3	T41.3X4	T41.3X5	T41.3X6
Endosulfan	T60.2X1	T60.2X2	T60.2X3	T60.2X4	—	—
Endothall	T60.3X1	T60.3X2	T60.3X3	T60.3X4	—	—
Endralazine	T46.5X1	T46.5X2	T46.5X3	T46.5X4	T46.5X5	T46.5X6
Endrin	T60.1X1	T60.1X2	T60.1X3	T60.1X4	—	—
Enflurane	T41.0X1	T41.0X2	T41.0X3	T41.0X4	T41.0X5	T41.0X6
Enhexymal	T42.3X1	T42.3X2	T42.3X3	T42.3X4	T42.3X5	T42.3X6
Enocitabine	T45.1X1	T45.1X2	T45.1X3	T45.1X4	T45.1X5	T45.1X6
Enovid	T38.4X1	T38.4X2	T38.4X3	T38.4X4	T38.4X5	T38.4X6
Enoxacin	T36.8X1	T36.8X2	T36.8X3	T36.8X4	T36.8X5	T36.8X6
Enoxaparin (sodium)	T45.511	T45.512	T45.513	T45.514	T45.515	T45.516
Enpiprazole	T43.591	T43.592	T43.593	T43.594	T43.595	T43.596
Enprofylline	T48.6X1	T48.6X2	T48.6X3	T48.6X4	T48.6X5	T48.6X6
Enprostil	T47.1X1	T47.1X2	T47.1X3	T47.1X4	T47.1X5	T47.1X6
ENT preparations (anti-infectives)	T49.6X1	T49.6X2	T49.6X3	T49.6X4	T49.6X5	T49.6X6
Enterogastrone	T38.891	T38.892	T38.893	T38.894	T38.895	T38.896
Enviomycin	T36.8X1	T36.8X2	T36.8X3	T36.8X4	T36.8X5	T36.8X6
Enzodase	T45.3X1	T45.3X2	T45.3X3	T45.3X4	T45.3X5	T45.3X6
Enzyme NEC	T45.3X1	T45.3X2	T45.3X3	T45.3X4	T45.3X5	T45.3X6
depolymerizing	T49.8X1	T49.8X2	T49.8X3	T49.8X4	T49.8X5	T49.8X6
fibrolytic	T45.3X1	T45.3X2	T45.3X3	T45.3X4	T45.3X5	T45.3X6
gastric	T47.5X1	T47.5X2	T47.5X3	T47.5X4	T47.5X5	T47.5X6
intestinal	T47.5X1	T47.5X2	T47.5X3	T47.5X4	T47.5X5	T47.5X6
local action	T49.4X1	T49.4X2	T49.4X3	T49.4X4	T49.4X5	T49.4X6
proteolytic	T49.4X1	T49.4X2	T49.4X3	T49.4X4	T49.4X5	T49.4X6
thrombolytic	T45.3X1	T45.3X2	T45.3X3	T45.3X4	T45.3X5	T45.3X6
EPAB	T41.3X1	T41.3X2	T41.3X3	T41.3X4	T41.3X5	T41.3X6
Epanutin	T42.0X1	T42.0X2	T42.0X3	T42.0X4	T42.0X5	T42.0X6
Ephedra	T44.991	T44.992	T44.993	T44.994	T44.995	T44.996
Ephedrine	T44.991	T44.992	T44.993	T44.994	T44.995	T44.996
Epichlorhydrin, epichlorohydrin	T52.8X1	T52.8X2	T52.8X3	T52.8X4	—	—
Epicillin	T36.0X1	T36.0X2	T36.0X3	T36.0X4	T36.0X5	T36.0X6
Epiestriol	T38.5X1	T38.5X2	T38.5X3	T38.5X4	T38.5X5	T38.5X6
Epilim—see Sodium valproate						
Epimestrol	T38.5X1	T38.5X2	T38.5X3	T38.5X4	T38.5X5	T38.5X6
Epinephrine	T44.5X1	T44.5X2	T44.5X3	T44.5X4	T44.5X5	T44.5X6
Epirubicin	T45.1X1	T45.1X2	T45.1X3	T45.1X4	T45.1X5	T45.1X6
Epitiostanol	T38.7X1	T38.7X2	T38.7X3	T38.7X4	T38.7X5	T38.7X6
Epitizide	T50.2X1	T50.2X2	T50.2X3	T50.2X4	T50.2X5	T50.2X6
EPN	T60.0X1	T60.0X2	T60.0X3	T60.0X4	—	—
EPO	T45.8X1	T45.8X2	T45.8X3	T45.8X4	T45.8X5	T45.8X6
Epoetin alpha	T45.8X1	T45.8X2	T45.8X3	T45.8X4	T45.8X5	T45.8X6
Epomediol	T50.991	T50.992	T50.993	T50.994	T50.995	T50.996
Epoprostenol	T45.521	T45.522	T45.523	T45.524	T45.525	T45.526
Epoxy resin	T65.891	T65.892	T65.893	T65.894	—	—
Eprazinone	T48.4X1	T48.4X2	T48.4X3	T48.4X4	T48.4X5	T48.4X6
Epsilon amino-caproic acid	T45.621	T45.622	T45.623	T45.624	T45.625	T45.626
Epsom salt	T47.3X1	T47.3X2	T47.3X3	T47.3X4	T47.3X5	T47.3X6
Eptazocine	T40.491	T40.492	T40.493	T40.494	T40.495	T40.496
Equanil	T43.591	T43.592	T43.593	T43.594	T43.595	T43.596
Equisetum	T62.2X1	T62.2X2	T62.2X3	T62.2X4	—	—
diuretic	T50.2X1	T50.2X2	T50.2X3	T50.2X4	T50.2X5	T50.2X6
Ergobasine	T48.0X1	T48.0X2	T48.0X3	T48.0X4	T48.0X5	T48.0X6
Ergocalciferol	T45.2X1	T45.2X2	T45.2X3	T45.2X4	T45.2X5	T45.2X6
Ergoloid mesylates	T46.7X1	T46.7X2	T46.7X3	T46.7X4	T46.7X5	T46.7X6
Ergometrine	T48.0X1	T48.0X2	T48.0X3	T48.0X4	T48.0X5	T48.0X6
Ergonovine	T48.0X1	T48.0X2	T48.0X3	T48.0X4	T48.0X5	T48.0X6
Ergot NEC	T64.81	T64.82	T64.83	T64.84	—	—
derivative	T48.0X1	T48.0X2	T48.0X3	T48.0X4	T48.0X5	T48.0X6
medicinal (alkaloids)	T48.0X1	T48.0X2	T48.0X3	T48.0X4	T48.0X5	T48.0X6
prepared	T48.0X1	T48.0X2	T48.0X3	T48.0X4	T48.0X5	T48.0X6

Substance	Poisoning, Accidental (unintentional)	Poisoning, Intentional self-harm	Poisoning, Assault	Poisoning, Undetermined	Adverse effect	Underdosing
Ergotamine	T46.5X1	T46.5X2	T46.5X3	T46.5X4	T46.5X5	T46.5X6
Ergotocine	T48.0X1	T48.0X2	T48.0X3	T48.0X4	T48.0X5	T48.0X6
Ergotrate	T48.0X1	T48.0X2	T48.0X3	T48.0X4	T48.0X5	T48.0X6
Eritrityl tetranitrate	T46.3X1	T46.3X2	T46.3X3	T46.3X4	T46.3X5	T46.3X6
Erythrityl tetranitrate	T46.3X1	T46.3X2	T46.3X3	T46.3X4	T46.3X5	T46.3X6
Erythrol tetranitrate	T46.3X1	T46.3X2	T46.3X3	T46.3X4	T46.3X5	T46.3X6
Erythromycin (salts)	T36.3X1	T36.3X2	T36.3X3	T36.3X4	T36.3X5	T36.3X6
ophthalmic preparation	T49.5X1	T49.5X2	T49.5X3	T49.5X4	T49.5X5	T49.5X6
topical NEC	T49.0X1	T49.0X2	T49.0X3	T49.0X4	T49.0X5	T49.0X6
Erythropoietin	T45.8X1	T45.8X2	T45.8X3	T45.8X4	T45.8X5	T45.8X6
human	T45.8X1	T45.8X2	T45.8X3	T45.8X4	T45.8X5	T45.8X6
Escin	T46.991	T46.992	T46.993	T46.994	T46.995	T46.996
Esculin	T45.2X1	T45.2X2	T45.2X3	T45.2X4	T45.2X5	T45.2X6
Esculoside	T45.2X1	T45.2X2	T45.2X3	T45.2X4	T45.2X5	T45.2X6
ESDT (ether-soluble tar distillate)	T49.1X1	T49.1X2	T49.1X3	T49.1X4	T49.1X5	T49.1X6
Eserine	T49.5X1	T49.5X2	T49.5X3	T49.5X4	T49.5X5	T49.5X6
Esflurbiprofen	T39.311	T39.312	T39.313	T39.314	T39.315	T39.316
Eskabarb	T42.3X1	T42.3X2	T42.3X3	T42.3X4	T42.3X5	T42.3X6
Eskalith	T43.8X1	T43.8X2	T43.8X3	T43.8X4	T43.8X5	T43.8X6
Esmolol	T44.7X1	T44.7X2	T44.7X3	T44.7X4	T44.7X5	T44.7X6
Estanozolol	T38.7X1	T38.7X2	T38.7X3	T38.7X4	T38.7X5	T38.7X6
Estazolam	T42.4X1	T42.4X2	T42.4X3	T42.4X4	T42.4X5	T42.4X6
Estradiol	T38.5X1	T38.5X2	T38.5X3	T38.5X4	T38.5X5	T38.5X6
with testosterone	T38.7X1	T38.7X2	T38.7X3	T38.7X4	T38.7X5	T38.7X6
benzoate	T38.5X1	T38.5X2	T38.5X3	T38.5X4	T38.5X5	T38.5X6
Estramustine	T45.1X1	T45.1X2	T45.1X3	T45.1X4	T45.1X5	T45.1X6
Estriol	T38.5X1	T38.5X2	T38.5X3	T38.5X4	T38.5X5	T38.5X6
Estrogen	T38.5X1	T38.5X2	T38.5X3	T38.5X4	T38.5X5	T38.5X6
with progesterone	T38.5X1	T38.5X2	T38.5X3	T38.5X4	T38.5X5	T38.5X6
conjugated	T38.5X1	T38.5X2	T38.5X3	T38.5X4	T38.5X5	T38.5X6
Estrone	T38.5X1	T38.5X2	T38.5X3	T38.5X4	T38.5X5	T38.5X6
Estropipate	T38.5X1	T38.5X2	T38.5X3	T38.5X4	T38.5X5	T38.5X6
Etacrynate sodium	T50.1X1	T50.1X2	T50.1X3	T50.1X4	T50.1X5	T50.1X6
Etacrynic acid	T50.1X1	T50.1X2	T50.1X3	T50.1X4	T50.1X5	T50.1X6
Etafedrine	T48.6X1	T48.6X2	T48.6X3	T48.6X4	T48.6X5	T48.6X6
Etafenone	T46.3X1	T46.3X2	T46.3X3	T46.3X4	T46.3X5	T46.3X6
Etambutol	T37.1X1	T37.1X2	T37.1X3	T37.1X4	T37.1X5	T37.1X6
Etamiphyllin	T48.6X1	T48.6X2	T48.6X3	T48.6X4	T48.6X5	T48.6X6
Etamivan	T50.7X1	T50.7X2	T50.7X3	T50.7X4	T50.7X5	T50.7X6
Etamsylate	T45.7X1	T45.7X2	T45.7X3	T45.7X4	T45.7X5	T45.7X6
Etebenecid	T50.4X1	T50.4X2	T50.4X3	T50.4X4	T50.4X5	T50.4X6
Ethacridine	T49.0X1	T49.0X2	T49.0X3	T49.0X4	T49.0X5	T49.0X6
Ethacrynic acid	T50.1X1	T50.1X2	T50.1X3	T50.1X4	T50.1X5	T50.1X6
Ethadione	T42.2X1	T42.2X2	T42.2X3	T42.2X4	T42.2X5	T42.2X6
Ethambutol	T37.1X1	T37.1X2	T37.1X3	T37.1X4	T37.1X5	T37.1X6
Ethamide	T50.2X1	T50.2X2	T50.2X3	T50.2X4	T50.2X5	T50.2X6
Ethamivan	T50.7X1	T50.7X2	T50.7X3	T50.7X4	T50.7X5	T50.7X6
Ethamsylate	T45.7X1	T45.7X2	T45.7X3	T45.7X4	T45.7X5	T45.7X6

Substance	Poisoning, Accidental (unintentional)	Poisoning, Intentional self-harm	Poisoning, Assault	Poisoning, Undetermined	Adverse effect	Underdosing
Ethanol	T51.0X1	T51.0X2	T51.0X3	T51.0X4	—	—
beverage	T51.0X1	T51.0X2	T51.0X3	T51.0X4	—	—
Ethanolamine oleate	T46.8X1	T46.8X2	T46.8X3	T46.8X4	T46.8X5	T46.8X6
Ethaverine	T44.3X1	T44.3X2	T44.3X3	T44.3X4	T44.3X5	T44.3X6
Ethchlorvynol	T42.6X1	T42.6X2	T42.6X3	T42.6X4	T42.6X5	T42.6X6
Ethebenecid	T50.4X1	T50.4X2	T50.4X3	T50.4X4	T50.4X5	T50.4X6
Ether (vapor)	T41.0X1	T41.0X2	T41.0X3	T41.0X4	T41.0X5	T41.0X6
anesthetic	T41.0X1	T41.0X2	T41.0X3	T41.0X4	T41.0X5	T41.0X6
divinyl	T41.0X1	T41.0X2	T41.0X3	T41.0X4	T41.0X5	T41.0X6
ethyl (medicinal)	T41.0X1	T41.0X2	T41.0X3	T41.0X4	T41.0X5	T41.0X6
nonmedicinal	T52.8X1	T52.8X2	T52.8X3	T52.8X4	—	—
petroleum—see Ligroin						
solvent	T52.8X1	T52.8X2	T52.8X3	T52.8X4	—	—
Ethiazide	T50.2X1	T50.2X2	T50.2X3	T50.2X4	T50.2X5	T50.2X6
Ethidium chloride (vapor)	T59.891	T59.892	T59.893	T59.894	—	—
Ethinamate	T42.6X1	T42.6X2	T42.6X3	T42.6X4	T42.6X5	T42.6X6
Ethinylestradiol, ethinyloestradiol	T38.5X1	T38.5X2	T38.5X3	T38.5X4	T38.5X5	T38.5X6
with						
levonorgestrel	T38.4X1	T38.4X2	T38.4X3	T38.4X4	T38.4X5	T38.4X6
norethisterone	T38.4X1	T38.4X2	T38.4X3	T38.4X4	T38.4X5	T38.4X6
Ethiodized oil (131 I)	T50.8X1	T50.8X2	T50.8X3	T50.8X4	T50.8X5	T50.8X6
Ethion	T60.0X1	T60.0X2	T60.0X3	T60.0X4	—	—
Ethionamide	T37.1X1	T37.1X2	T37.1X3	T37.1X4	T37.1X5	T37.1X6
Ethioniamide	T37.1X1	T37.1X2	T37.1X3	T37.1X4	T37.1X5	T37.1X6
Ethisterone	T38.5X1	T38.5X2	T38.5X3	T38.5X4	T38.5X5	T38.5X6
Ethobral	T42.3X1	T42.3X2	T42.3X3	T42.3X4	T42.3X5	T42.3X6
Ethocaine (infiltration) (topical)	T41.3X1	T41.3X2	T41.3X3	T41.3X4	T41.3X5	T41.3X6
nerve block (peripheral) (plexus)	T41.3X1	T41.3X2	T41.3X3	T41.3X4	T41.3X5	T41.3X6
spinal	T41.3X1	T41.3X2	T41.3X3	T41.3X4	T41.3X5	T41.3X6
Ethoheptazine	T40.491	T40.492	T40.493	T40.494	T40.495	T40.496
Ethopropazine	T44.3X1	T44.3X2	T44.3X3	T44.3X4	T44.3X5	T44.3X6
Ethosuximide	T42.2X1	T42.2X2	T42.2X3	T42.2X4	T42.2X5	T42.2X6
Ethotoin	T42.0X1	T42.0X2	T42.0X3	T42.0X4	T42.0X5	T42.0X6
Ethoxazene	T37.91	T37.92	T37.93	T37.94	T37.95	T37.96
Ethoxazorutoside	T46.991	T46.992	T46.993	T46.994	T46.995	T46.996
2-Ethoxyethanol	T52.3X1	T52.3X2	T52.3X3	T52.3X4	—	—
Ethoxzolamide	T50.2X1	T50.2X2	T50.2X3	T50.2X4	T50.2X5	T50.2X6
Ethyl						
acetate	T52.8X1	T52.8X2	T52.8X3	T52.8X4	—	—
alcohol	T51.0X1	T51.0X2	T51.0X3	T51.0X4	—	—
beverage	T51.0X1	T51.0X2	T51.0X3	T51.0X4	—	—
aldehyde (vapor)	T59.891	T59.892	T59.893	T59.894	—	—
liquid	T52.8X1	T52.8X2	T52.8X3	T52.8X4	—	—
aminobenzoate	T41.3X1	T41.3X2	T41.3X3	T41.3X4	T41.3X5	T41.3X6
aminophenothiazine	T43.3X1	T43.3X2	T43.3X3	T43.3X4	T43.3X5	T43.3X6
benzoate	T52.8X1	T52.8X2	T52.8X3	T52.8X4	—	—

Substance	Poisoning, Accidental (unintentional)	Poisoning, Intentional self-harm	Poisoning, Assault	Poisoning, Undetermined	Adverse effect	Underdosing
Ethyl — *Continued*						
biscoumacetate	T45.511	T45.512	T45.513	T45.514	T45.515	T45.516
bromide (anesthetic)	T41.0X1	T41.0X2	T41.0X3	T41.0X4	T41.0X5	T41.0X6
carbamate	T45.1X1	T45.1X2	T45.1X3	T45.1X4	T45.1X5	T45.1X6
carbinol	T51.3X1	T51.3X2	T51.3X3	T51.3X4	—	—
carbonate	T52.8X1	T52.8X2	T52.8X3	T52.8X4	—	—
chaulmoograte	T37.1X1	T37.1X2	T37.1X3	T37.1X4	T37.1X5	T37.1X6
chloride (anesthetic)	T41.0X1	T41.0X2	T41.0X3	T41.0X4	T41.0X5	T41.0X6
anesthetic (local)	T41.3X1	T41.3X2	T41.3X3	T41.3X4	T41.3X5	T41.3X6
inhaled	T41.0X1	T41.0X2	T41.0X3	T41.0X4	T41.0X5	T41.0X6
local	T49.4X1	T49.4X2	T49.4X3	T49.4X4	T49.4X5	T49.4X6
solvent	T53.6X1	T53.6X2	T53.6X3	T53.6X4	—	—
dibunate	T48.3X1	T48.3X2	T48.3X3	T48.3X4	T48.3X5	T48.3X6
dichloroarsine (vapor)	T57.0X1	T57.0X2	T57.0X3	T57.0X4	—	—
estranol	T38.7X1	T38.7X2	T38.7X3	T38.7X4	T38.7X5	T38.7X6
ether—see also ether	T52.8X1	T52.8X2	T52.8X3	T52.8X4	—	—
formate NEC (solvent)	T52.0X1	T52.0X2	T52.0X3	T52.0X4	—	—
fumarate	T49.4X1	T49.4X2	T49.4X3	T49.4X4	T49.4X5	T49.4X6
hydroxyisobutyrate NEC (solvent)	T52.8X1	T52.8X2	T52.8X3	T52.8X4	—	—
iodoacetate	T59.3X1	T59.3X2	T59.3X3	T59.3X4	—	—
lactate NEC (solvent)	T52.8X1	T52.8X2	T52.8X3	T52.8X4	—	—
loflazepate	T42.4X1	T42.4X2	T42.4X3	T42.4X4	T42.4X5	T42.4X6
mercuric chloride	T56.1X1	T56.1X2	T56.1X3	T56.1X4	—	—
methylcarbinol	T51.8X1	T51.8X2	T51.8X3	T51.8X4	—	—
morphine	T40.2X1	T40.2X2	T40.2X3	T40.2X4	T40.2X5	T40.2X6
noradrenaline	T48.6X1	T48.6X2	T48.6X3	T48.6X4	T48.6X5	T48.6X6
oxybutyrate NEC (solvent)	T52.8X1	T52.8X2	T52.8X3	T52.8X4	—	—
Ethylene (gas)	T59.891	T59.892	T59.893	T59.894		
anesthetic (general)	T41.0X1	T41.0X2	T41.0X3	T41.0X4	T41.0X5	T41.0X6
chlorohydrin	T52.8X1	T52.8X2	T52.8X3	T52.8X4	—	—
vapor	T53.6X1	T53.6X2	T53.6X3	T53.6X4	—	—
dichloride	T52.8X1	T52.8X2	T52.8X3	T52.8X4	—	—
vapor	T53.6X1	T53.6X2	T53.6X3	T53.6X4	—	—
dinitrate	T52.3X1	T52.3X2	T52.3X3	T52.3X4	—	—
glycol(s)	T52.8X1	T52.8X2	T52.8X3	T52.8X4	—	—
dinitrate	T52.3X1	T52.3X2	T52.3X3	T52.3X4	—	—
monobutyl ether	T52.3X1	T52.3X2	T52.3X3	T52.3X4	—	—
imine	T54.1X1	T54.1X2	T54.1X3	T54.1X4	—	—
oxide (fumigant) (nonmedicinal)	T59.891	T59.892	T59.893	T59.894	—	—
medicinal	T49.0X1	T49.0X2	T49.0X3	T49.0X4	T49.0X5	T49.0X6
Ethylenediamine theophylline	T48.6X1	T48.6X2	T48.6X3	T48.6X4	T48.6X5	T48.6X6
Ethylenediaminetetra-acetic acid	T50.6X1	T50.6X2	T50.6X3	T50.6X4	T50.6X5	T50.6X6
Ethylen-edinitrilotetra-acetate	T50.6X1	T50.6X2	T50.6X3	T50.6X4	T50.6X5	T50.6X6
Ethylestrenol	T38.7X1	T38.7X2	T38.7X3	T38.7X4	T38.7X5	T38.7X6
Ethylhydro-xycellulose	T47.4X1	T47.4X2	T47.4X3	T47.4X4	T47.4X5	T47.4X6

Substance	Poisoning, Accidental (unintentional)	Poisoning, Intentional self-harm	Poisoning, Assault	Poisoning, Undetermined	Adverse effect	Underdosing
Ethylidene						
chloride NEC	T53.6X1	T53.6X2	T53.6X3	T53.6X4	—	—
diacetate	T60.3X1	T60.3X2	T60.3X3	T60.3X4	—	—
dicoumarin	T45.511	T45.512	T45.513	T45.514	T45.515	T45.516
dicoumarol	T45.511	T45.512	T45.513	T45.514	T45.515	T45.516
diethyl ether	T52.0X1	T52.0X2	T52.0X3	T52.0X4	—	—
Ethylmorphine	T40.2X1	T40.2X2	T40.2X3	T40.2X4	T40.2X5	T40.2X6
Ethylnorepinephrine	T48.6X1	T48.6X2	T48.6X3	T48.6X4	T48.6X5	T48.6X6
Ethylparachloro-phenoxyisobutyrate	T46.6X1	T46.6X2	T46.6X3	T46.6X4	T46.6X5	T46.6X6
Ethynodiol	T38.4X1	T38.4X2	T38.4X3	T38.4X4	T38.4X5	T38.4X6
with mestranol diacetate	T38.4X1	T38.4X2	T38.4X3	T38.4X4	T38.4X5	T38.4X6
Etidocaine	T41.3X1	T41.3X2	T41.3X3	T41.3X4	T41.3X5	T41.3X6
infiltration (subcutaneous)	T41.3X1	T41.3X2	T41.3X3	T41.3X4	T41.3X5	T41.3X6
nerve (peripheral) (plexus)	T41.3X1	T41.3X2	T41.3X3	T41.3X4	T41.3X5	T41.3X6
Etidronate	T50.991	T50.992	T50.993	T50.994	T50.995	T50.996
Etidronic acid (disodium salt)	T50.991	T50.992	T50.993	T50.994	T50.995	T50.996
Etifoxine	T42.6X1	T42.6X2	T42.6X3	T42.6X4	T42.6X5	T42.6X6
Etilefrine	T44.4X1	T44.4X2	T44.4X3	T44.4X4	T44.4X5	T44.4X6
Etilfen	T42.3X1	T42.3X2	T42.3X3	T42.3X4	T42.3X5	T42.3X6
Etinodiol	T38.4X1	T38.4X2	T38.4X3	T38.4X4	T38.4X5	T38.4X6
Etiroxate	T46.6X1	T46.6X2	T46.6X3	T46.6X4	T46.6X5	T46.6X6
Etizolam	T42.4X1	T42.4X2	T42.4X3	T42.4X4	T42.4X5	T42.4X6
Etodolac	T39.391	T39.392	T39.393	T39.394	T39.395	T39.396
Etofamide	T37.3X1	T37.3X2	T37.3X3	T37.3X4	T37.3X5	T37.3X6
Etofibrate	T46.6X1	T46.6X2	T46.6X3	T46.6X4	T46.6X5	T46.6X6
Etofylline	T46.7X1	T46.7X2	T46.7X3	T46.7X4	T46.7X5	T46.7X6
clofibrate	T46.6X1	T46.6X2	T46.6X3	T46.6X4	T46.6X5	T46.6X6
Etoglucid	T45.1X1	T45.1X2	T45.1X3	T45.1X4	T45.1X5	T45.1X6
Etomidate	T41.1X1	T41.1X2	T41.1X3	T41.1X4	T41.1X5	T41.1X6
Etomide	T39.8X1	T39.8X2	T39.8X3	T39.8X4	T39.8X5	T39.8X6
Etomidoline	T44.3X1	T44.3X2	T44.3X3	T44.3X4	T44.3X5	T44.3X6
Etoposide	T45.1X1	T45.1X2	T45.1X3	T45.1X4	T45.1X5	T45.1X6
Etorphine	T40.2X1	T40.2X2	T40.2X3	T40.2X4	T40.2X5	T40.2X6
Etoval	T42.3X1	T42.3X2	T42.3X3	T42.3X4	T42.3X5	T42.3X6
Etozolin	T50.1X1	T50.1X2	T50.1X3	T50.1X4	T50.1X5	T50.1X6
Etretinate	T50.991	T50.992	T50.993	T50.994	T50.995	T50.996
Etryptamine	T43.691	T43.692	T43.693	T43.694	T43.695	T43.696
Etybenzatropine	T44.3X1	T44.3X2	T44.3X3	T44.3X4	T44.3X5	T44.3X6
Etynodiol	T38.4X1	T38.4X2	T38.4X3	T38.4X4	T38.4X5	T38.4X6
Eucaine	T41.3X1	T41.3X2	T41.3X3	T41.3X4	T41.3X5	T41.3X6
Eucalyptus oil	T49.7X1	T49.7X2	T49.7X3	T49.7X4	T49.7X5	T49.7X6
Eucatropine	T49.5X1	T49.5X2	T49.5X3	T49.5X4	T49.5X5	T49.5X6
Eucodal	T40.2X1	T40.2X2	T40.2X3	T40.2X4	T40.2X5	T40.2X6
Euneryl	T42.3X1	T42.3X2	T42.3X3	T42.3X4	T42.3X5	T42.3X6
Euphthalmine	T44.3X1	T44.3X2	T44.3X3	T44.3X4	T44.3X5	T44.3X6

Substance	Poisoning, Accidental (unintentional)	Poisoning, Intentional self-harm	Poisoning, Assault	Poisoning, Undetermined	Adverse effect	Underdosing
Eurax	T49.0X1	T49.0X2	T49.0X3	T49.0X4	T49.0X5	T49.0X6
Euresol	T49.4X1	T49.4X2	T49.4X3	T49.4X4	T49.4X5	T49.4X6
Euthroid	T38.1X1	T38.1X2	T38.1X3	T38.1X4	T38.1X5	T38.1X6
Evans blue	T50.8X1	T50.8X2	T50.8X3	T50.8X4	T50.8X5	T50.8X6
Evipal	T42.3X1	T42.3X2	T42.3X3	T42.3X4	T42.3X5	T42.3X6
sodium	T41.1X1	T41.1X2	T41.1X3	T41.1X4	T41.1X5	T41.1X6
Evipan	T42.3X1	T42.3X2	T42.3X3	T42.3X4	T42.3X5	T42.3X6
sodium	T41.1X1	T41.1X2	T41.1X3	T41.1X4	T41.1X5	T41.1X6
Exalamide	T49.0X1	T49.0X2	T49.0X3	T49.0X4	T49.0X5	T49.0X6
Exalgin	T39.1X1	T39.1X2	T39.1X3	T39.1X4	T39.1X5	T39.1X6
Excipients, pharmaceutical	T50.901	T50.902	T50.903	T50.904	T50.905	T50.906
Exhaust gas (engine) (motor vehicle)	T58.01	T58.02	T58.03	T58.04	—	—
Ex-Lax (phenolphthalein)	T47.2X1	T47.2X2	T47.2X3	T47.2X4	T47.2X5	T47.2X6
Expectorant NEC	T48.4X1	T48.4X2	T48.4X3	T48.4X4	T48.4X5	T48.4X6
Extended insulin zinc suspension	T38.3X1	T38.3X2	T38.3X3	T38.3X4	T38.3X5	T38.3X6
External medications (skin) (mucous membrane)	T49.91	T49.92	T49.93	T49.94	T49.95	T49.96
dental agent	T49.7X1	T49.7X2	T49.7X3	T49.7X4	T49.7X5	T49.7X6
ENT agent	T49.6X1	T49.6X2	T49.6X3	T49.6X4	T49.6X5	T49.6X6
ophthalmic preparation	T49.5X1	T49.5X2	T49.5X3	T49.5X4	T49.5X5	T49.5X6
specified NEC	T49.8X1	T49.8X2	T49.8X3	T49.8X4	T49.8X5	T49.8X6
Extrapyramidal antagonist NEC	T44.3X1	T44.3X2	T44.3X3	T44.3X4	T44.3X5	T44.3X6
Eye agents (anti-infective)	T49.5X1	T49.5X2	T49.5X3	T49.5X4	T49.5X5	T49.5X6
Eye drug NEC	T49.5X1	T49.5X2	T49.5X3	T49.5X4	T49.5X5	T49.5X6
F						
FAC (fluorouracil + doxorubicin + cyclophosphamide)	T45.1X1	T45.1X2	T45.1X3	T45.1X4	T45.1X5	T45.1X6
Factor						
I (fibrinogen)	T45.8X1	T45.8X2	T45.8X3	T45.8X4	T45.8X5	T45.8X6
III (thromboplastin)	T45.8X1	T45.8X2	T45.8X3	T45.8X4	T45.8X5	T45.8X6
VIII (antihemophilic Factor) (concentrate)	T45.8X1	T45.8X2	T45.8X3	T45.8X4	T45.8X5	T45.8X6
IX complex	T45.7X1	T45.7X2	T45.7X3	T45.7X4	T45.7X5	T45.7X6
human	T45.8X1	T45.8X2	T45.8X3	T45.8X4	T45.8X5	T45.8X6
Famotidine	T47.0X1	T47.0X2	T47.0X3	T47.0X4	T47.0X5	T47.0X6
Fat suspension, intravenous	T50.991	T50.992	T50.993	T50.994	T50.995	T50.996
Fazadinium bromide	T48.1X1	T48.1X2	T48.1X3	T48.1X4	T48.1X5	T48.1X6
Febarbamate	T42.3X1	T42.3X2	T42.3X3	T42.3X4	T42.3X5	T42.3X6
Fecal softener	T47.4X1	T47.4X2	T47.4X3	T47.4X4	T47.4X5	T47.4X6
Fedrilate	T48.3X1	T48.3X2	T48.3X3	T48.3X4	T48.3X5	T48.3X6
Felodipine	T46.1X1	T46.1X2	T46.1X3	T46.1X4	T46.1X5	T46.1X6
Felypressin	T38.891	T38.892	T38.893	T38.894	T38.895	T38.896
Femoxetine	T43.221	T43.222	T43.223	T43.224	T43.225	T43.226
Fenalcomine	T46.3X1	T46.3X2	T46.3X3	T46.3X4	T46.3X5	T46.3X6
Fenamisal	T37.1X1	T37.1X2	T37.1X3	T37.1X4	T37.1X5	T37.1X6
Fenazone	T39.2X1	T39.2X2	T39.2X3	T39.2X4	T39.2X5	T39.2X6
Fenbendazole	T37.4X1	T37.4X2	T37.4X3	T37.4X4	T37.4X5	T37.4X6
Fenbutrazate	T50.5X1	T50.5X2	T50.5X3	T50.5X4	T50.5X5	T50.5X6
Fencamfamine	T43.691	T43.692	T43.693	T43.694	T43.695	T43.696
Fendiline	T46.1X1	T46.1X2	T46.1X3	T46.1X4	T46.1X5	T46.1X6
Fenetylline	T43.691	T43.692	T43.693	T43.694	T43.695	T43.696
Fenflumizole	T39.391	T39.392	T39.393	T39.394	T39.395	T39.396
Fenfluramine	T50.5X1	T50.5X2	T50.5X3	T50.5X4	T50.5X5	T50.5X6
Fenobarbital	T42.3X1	T42.3X2	T42.3X3	T42.3X4	T42.3X5	T42.3X6
Fenofibrate	T46.6X1	T46.6X2	T46.6X3	T46.6X4	T46.6X5	T46.6X6
Fenoprofen	T39.311	T39.312	T39.313	T39.314	T39.315	T39.316
Fenoterol	T48.6X1	T48.6X2	T48.6X3	T48.6X4	T48.6X5	T48.6X6
Fenoverine	T44.3X1	T44.3X2	T44.3X3	T44.3X4	T44.3X5	T44.3X6
Fenoxazoline	T48.5X1	T48.5X2	T48.5X3	T48.5X4	T48.5X5	T48.5X6
Fenproporex	T50.5X1	T50.5X2	T50.5X3	T50.5X4	T50.5X5	T50.5X6
Fenquizone	T50.2X1	T50.2X2	T50.2X3	T50.2X4	T50.2X5	T50.2X6
Fentanyl (analogs)	T40.411	T40.412	T40.413	T40.414	T40.415	T40.416
Fentazin	T43.3X1	T43.3X2	T43.3X3	T43.3X4	T43.3X5	T43.3X6
Fenthion	T60.0X1	T60.0X2	T60.0X3	T60.0X4	—	—
Fenticlor	T49.0X1	T49.0X2	T49.0X3	T49.0X4	T49.0X5	T49.0X6
Fenylbutazone	T39.2X1	T39.2X2	T39.2X3	T39.2X4	T39.2X5	T39.2X6
Feprazone	T39.2X1	T39.2X2	T39.2X3	T39.2X4	T39.2X5	T39.2X6
Fer de lance (bite) (venom)	T63.061	T63.062	T63.063	T63.064	—	—
Ferric—see also Iron						
chloride	T45.4X1	T45.4X2	T45.4X3	T45.4X4	T45.4X5	T45.4X6
citrate	T45.4X1	T45.4X2	T45.4X3	T45.4X4	T45.4X5	T45.4X6
hydroxide						
colloidal	T45.4X1	T45.4X2	T45.4X3	T45.4X4	T45.4X5	T45.4X6
polymaltose	T45.4X1	T45.4X2	T45.4X3	T45.4X4	T45.4X5	T45.4X6
pyrophosphate	T45.4X1	T45.4X2	T45.4X3	T45.4X4	T45.4X5	T45.4X6
Ferritin	T45.4X1	T45.4X2	T45.4X3	T45.4X4	T45.4X5	T45.4X6
Ferrocholinate	T45.4X1	T45.4X2	T45.4X3	T45.4X4	T45.4X5	T45.4X6
Ferrodextrane	T45.4X1	T45.4X2	T45.4X3	T45.4X4	T45.4X5	T45.4X6
Ferropolimaler	T45.4X1	T45.4X2	T45.4X3	T45.4X4	T45.4X5	T45.4X6
Ferrous—see also Iron						
phosphate	T45.4X1	T45.4X2	T45.4X3	T45.4X4	T45.4X5	T45.4X6
salt	T45.4X1	T45.4X2	T45.4X3	T45.4X4	T45.4X5	T45.4X6
with folic acid	T45.4X1	T45.4X2	T45.4X3	T45.4X4	T45.4X5	T45.4X6
Ferrous fumarate, gluconate, lactate, salt NEC, sulfate (medicinal)	T45.4X1	T45.4X2	T45.4X3	T45.4X4	T45.4X5	T45.4X6
Ferrovanadium (fumes)	T59.891	T59.892	T59.893	T59.894	—	—
Ferrum—see Iron						
Fertilizers NEC	T65.891	T65.892	T65.893	T65.894		
with herbicide mixture	T60.3X1	T60.3X2	T60.3X3	T60.3X4	—	—
Fetoxilate	T47.6X1	T47.6X2	T47.6X3	T47.6X4	T47.6X5	T47.6X6
Fiber, dietary	T47.4X1	T47.4X2	T47.4X3	T47.4X4	T47.4X5	T47.4X6
Fiberglass	T65.831	T65.832	T65.833	T65.834	—	—
Fibrinogen (human)	T45.8X1	T45.8X2	T45.8X3	T45.8X4	T45.8X5	T45.8X6
Fibrinolysin (human)	T45.691	T45.692	T45.693	T45.694	T45.695	T45.696

Substance	Poisoning, Accidental (unintentional)	Poisoning, Intentional self-harm	Poisoning, Assault	Poisoning, Undetermined	Adverse effect	Underdosing
Fibrinolysis						
affecting drug	T45.601	T45.602	T45.603	T45.604	T45.605	T45.606
inhibitor NEC	T45.621	T45.622	T45.623	T45.624	T45.625	T45.626
Fibrinolytic drug	T45.611	T45.612	T45.613	T45.614	T45.615	T45.616
Filix mas	T37.4X1	T37.4X2	T37.4X3	T37.4X4	T37.4X5	T37.4X6
Filtering cream	T49.3X1	T49.3X2	T49.3X3	T49.3X4	T49.3X5	T49.3X6
Fiorinal	T39.011	T39.012	T39.013	T39.014	T39.015	T39.016
Firedamp	T59.891	T59.892	T59.893	T59.894	—	—
Fish, noxious, nonbacterial	T61.91	T61.92	T61.93	T61.94	—	—
ciguatera	T61.01	T61.02	T61.03	T61.04	—	—
scombroid	T61.11	T61.12	T61.13	T61.14	—	—
shell	T61.781	T61.782	T61.783	T61.784	—	—
specified NEC	T61.771	T61.772	T61.773	T61.774	—	—
Flagyl	T37.3X1	T37.3X2	T37.3X3	T37.3X4	T37.3X5	T37.3X6
Flavine adenine dinucleotide	T45.2X1	T45.2X2	T45.2X3	T45.2X4	T45.2X5	T45.2X6
Flavodic acid	T46.991	T46.992	T46.993	T46.994	T46.995	T46.996
Flavoxate	T44.3X1	T44.3X2	T44.3X3	T44.3X4	T44.3X5	T44.3X6
Flaxedil	T48.1X1	T48.1X2	T48.1X3	T48.1X4	T48.1X5	T48.1X6
Flaxseed (medicinal)	T49.3X1	T49.3X2	T49.3X3	T49.3X4	T49.3X5	T49.3X6
Flecainide	T46.2X1	T46.2X2	T46.2X3	T46.2X4	T46.2X5	T46.2X6
Fleroxacin	T36.8X1	T36.8X2	T36.8X3	T36.8X4	T36.8X5	T36.8X6
Floctafenine	T39.8X1	T39.8X2	T39.8X3	T39.8X4	T39.8X5	T39.8X6
Flomax	T44.6X1	T44.6X2	T44.6X3	T44.6X4	T44.6X5	T44.6X6
Flomoxef	T36.1X1	T36.1X2	T36.1X3	T36.1X4	T36.1X5	T36.1X6
Flopropione	T44.3X1	T44.3X2	T44.3X3	T44.3X4	T44.3X5	T44.3X6
Florantyrone	T47.5X1	T47.5X2	T47.5X3	T47.5X4	T47.5X5	T47.5X6
Floraquin	T37.8X1	T37.8X2	T37.8X3	T37.8X4	T37.8X5	T37.8X6
Florinef	T38.0X1	T38.0X2	T38.0X3	T38.0X4	T38.0X5	T38.0X6
ENT agent	T49.6X1	T49.6X2	T49.6X3	T49.6X4	T49.6X5	T49.6X6
ophthalmic preparation	T49.5X1	T49.5X2	T49.5X3	T49.5X4	T49.5X5	T49.5X6
topical NEC	T49.0X1	T49.0X2	T49.0X3	T49.0X4	T49.0X5	T49.0X6
Flowers of sulfur	T49.4X1	T49.4X2	T49.4X3	T49.4X4	T49.4X5	T49.4X6
Floxuridine	T45.1X1	T45.1X2	T45.1X3	T45.1X4	T45.1X5	T45.1X6
Fluanisone	T43.4X1	T43.4X2	T43.4X3	T43.4X4	T43.4X5	T43.4X6
Flubendazole	T37.4X1	T37.4X2	T37.4X3	T37.4X4	T37.4X5	T37.4X6
Fluclorolone acetonide	T49.0X1	T49.0X2	T49.0X3	T49.0X4	T49.0X5	T49.0X6
Flucloxacillin	T36.0X1	T36.0X2	T36.0X3	T36.0X4	T36.0X5	T36.0X6
Fluconazole	T37.8X1	T37.8X2	T37.8X3	T37.8X4	T37.8X5	T37.8X6
Flucytosine	T37.8X1	T37.8X2	T37.8X3	T37.8X4	T37.8X5	T37.8X6
Fludeoxyglucose (18F)	T50.8X1	T50.8X2	T50.8X3	T50.8X4	T50.8X5	T50.8X6
Fludiazepam	T42.4X1	T42.4X2	T42.4X3	T42.4X4	T42.4X5	T42.4X6
Fludrocortisone	T50.0X1	T50.0X2	T50.0X3	T50.0X4	T50.0X5	T50.0X6
ENT agent	T49.6X1	T49.6X2	T49.6X3	T49.6X4	T49.6X5	T49.6X6
ophthalmic preparation	T49.5X1	T49.5X2	T49.5X3	T49.5X4	T49.5X5	T49.5X6
topical NEC	T49.0X1	T49.0X2	T49.0X3	T49.0X4	T49.0X5	T49.0X6
Fludroxycortide	T49.0X1	T49.0X2	T49.0X3	T49.0X4	T49.0X5	T49.0X6
Flufenamic acid	T39.391	T39.392	T39.393	T39.394	T39.395	T39.396
Fluindione	T45.511	T45.512	T45.513	T45.514	T45.515	T45.516
Flumequine	T37.8X1	T37.8X2	T37.8X3	T37.8X4	T37.8X5	T37.8X6

Substance	Poisoning, Accidental (unintentional)	Poisoning, Intentional self-harm	Poisoning, Assault	Poisoning, Undetermined	Adverse effect	Underdosing
Flumethasone	T49.0X1	T49.0X2	T49.0X3	T49.0X4	T49.0X5	T49.0X6
Flumethiazide	T50.2X1	T50.2X2	T50.2X3	T50.2X4	T50.2X5	T50.2X6
Flumidin	T37.5X1	T37.5X2	T37.5X3	T37.5X4	T37.5X5	T37.5X6
Flunarizine	T46.7X1	T46.7X2	T46.7X3	T46.7X4	T46.7X5	T46.7X6
Flunidazole	T37.8X1	T37.8X2	T37.8X3	T37.8X4	T37.8X5	T37.8X6
Flunisolide	T48.6X1	T48.6X2	T48.6X3	T48.6X4	T48.6X5	T48.6X6
Flunitrazepam	T42.4X1	T42.4X2	T42.4X3	T42.4X4	T42.4X5	T42.4X6
Fluocinolone (acetonide)	T49.0X1	T49.0X2	T49.0X3	T49.0X4	T49.0X5	T49.0X6
Fluocinonide	T49.0X1	T49.0X2	T49.0X3	T49.0X4	T49.0X5	T49.0X6
Fluocortin (butyl)	T49.0X1	T49.0X2	T49.0X3	T49.0X4	T49.0X5	T49.0X6
Fluocortolone	T49.0X1	T49.0X2	T49.0X3	T49.0X4	T49.0X5	T49.0X6
Fluohydrocortisone	T38.0X1	T38.0X2	T38.0X3	T38.0X4	T38.0X5	T38.0X6
ENT agent	T49.6X1	T49.6X2	T49.6X3	T49.6X4	T49.6X5	T49.6X6
ophthalmic preparation	T49.5X1	T49.5X2	T49.5X3	T49.5X4	T49.5X5	T49.5X6
topical NEC	T49.0X1	T49.0X2	T49.0X3	T49.0X4	T49.0X5	T49.0X6
Fluonid	T49.0X1	T49.0X2	T49.0X3	T49.0X4	T49.0X5	T49.0X6
Fluopromazine	T43.3X1	T43.3X2	T43.3X3	T43.3X4	T43.3X5	T43.3X6
Fluoracetate	T60.8X1	T60.8X2	T60.8X3	T60.8X4	—	—
Fluorescein	T50.8X1	T50.8X2	T50.8X3	T50.8X4	T50.8X5	T50.8X6
Fluorhydrocortisone	T50.0X1	T50.0X2	T50.0X3	T50.0X4	T50.0X5	T50.0X6
Fluoride (nonmedicinal)(pesticide) (sodium) NEC	T60.8X1	T60.8X2	T60.8X3	T60.8X4	—	—
hydrogen—see Hydrofluoric acid						
medicinal NEC	T50.991	T50.992	T50.993	T50.994	T50.995	T50.996
dental use	T49.7X1	T49.7X2	T49.7X3	T49.7X4	T49.7X5	T49.7X6
not pesticide NEC	T54.91	T54.92	T54.93	T54.94	—	—
stannous	T49.7X1	T49.7X2	T49.7X3	T49.7X4	T49.7X5	T49.7X6
Fluorinated corticosteroids	T38.0X1	T38.0X2	T38.0X3	T38.0X4	T38.0X5	T38.0X6
Fluorine (gas)	T59.5X1	T59.5X2	T59.5X3	T59.5X4	—	—
salt—see Fluoride(s)						
Fluoristan	T49.7X1	T49.7X2	T49.7X3	T49.7X4	T49.7X5	T49.7X6
Fluormetholone	T49.0X1	T49.0X2	T49.0X3	T49.0X4	T49.0X5	T49.0X6
Fluoroacetate	T60.8X1	T60.8X2	T60.8X3	T60.8X4	—	—
Fluorocarbon monomer	T53.6X1	T53.6X2	T53.6X3	T53.6X4	—	—
Fluorocytosine	T37.8X1	T37.8X2	T37.8X3	T37.8X4	T37.8X5	T37.8X6
Fluorodeoxyuridine	T45.1X1	T45.1X2	T45.1X3	T45.1X4	T45.1X5	T45.1X6
Fluorometholone	T49.0X1	T49.0X2	T49.0X3	T49.0X4	T49.0X5	T49.0X6
ophthalmic preparation	T49.5X1	T49.5X2	T49.5X3	T49.5X4	T49.5X5	T49.5X6
Fluorophosphate insecticide	T60.0X1	T60.0X2	T60.0X3	T60.0X4	—	—
Fluorosol	T46.3X1	T46.3X2	T46.3X3	T46.3X4	T46.3X5	T46.3X6
Fluorouracil	T45.1X1	T45.1X2	T45.1X3	T45.1X4	T45.1X5	T45.1X6
Fluorphenylalanine	T49.5X1	T49.5X2	T49.5X3	T49.5X4	T49.5X5	T49.5X6
Fluothane	T41.0X1	T41.0X2	T41.0X3	T41.0X4	T41.0X5	T41.0X6
Fluoxetine	T43.221	T43.222	T43.223	T43.224	T43.225	T43.226
Fluoxymesterone	T38.7X1	T38.7X2	T38.7X3	T38.7X4	T38.7X5	T38.7X6
Flupenthixol	T43.4X1	T43.4X2	T43.4X3	T43.4X4	T43.4X5	T43.4X6
Flupentixol	T43.4X1	T43.4X2	T43.4X3	T43.4X4	T43.4X5	T43.4X6

Substance	Poisoning, Accidental (unintentional)	Poisoning, Intentional self-harm	Poisoning, Assault	Poisoning, Undetermined	Adverse effect	Underdosing
Fluphenazine	T43.3X1	T43.3X2	T43.3X3	T43.3X4	T43.3X5	T43.3X6
Fluprednidene	T49.0X1	T49.0X2	T49.0X3	T49.0X4	T49.0X5	T49.0X6
Fluprednisolone	T38.0X1	T38.0X2	T38.0X3	T38.0X4	T38.0X5	T38.0X6
Fluradoline	T39.8X1	T39.8X2	T39.8X3	T39.8X4	T39.8X5	T39.8X6
Flurandrenolide	T49.0X1	T49.0X2	T49.0X3	T49.0X4	T49.0X5	T49.0X6
Flurandrenolone	T49.0X1	T49.0X2	T49.0X3	T49.0X4	T49.0X5	T49.0X6
Flurazepam	T42.4X1	T42.4X2	T42.4X3	T42.4X4	T42.4X5	T42.4X6
Flurbiprofen	T39.311	T39.312	T39.313	T39.314	T39.315	T39.316
Flurobate	T49.0X1	T49.0X2	T49.0X3	T49.0X4	T49.0X5	T49.0X6
Fluroxene	T41.0X1	T41.0X2	T41.0X3	T41.0X4	T41.0X5	T41.0X6
Fluspirilene	T43.591	T43.592	T43.593	T43.594	T43.595	T43.596
Flutamide	T38.6X1	T38.6X2	T38.6X3	T38.6X4	T38.6X5	T38.6X6
Flutazolam	T42.4X1	T42.4X2	T42.4X3	T42.4X4	T42.4X5	T42.4X6
Fluticasone propionate	T38.0X1	T38.0X2	T38.0X3	T38.0X4	T38.0X5	T38.0X6
Flutoprazepam	T42.4X1	T42.4X2	T42.4X3	T42.4X4	T42.4X5	T42.4X6
Flutropium bromide	T48.6X1	T48.6X2	T48.6X3	T48.6X4	T48.6X5	T48.6X6
Fluvoxamine	T43.221	T43.222	T43.223	T43.224	T43.225	T43.226
Folacin	T45.8X1	T45.8X2	T45.8X3	T45.8X4	T45.8X5	T45.8X6
Folic acid	T45.8X1	T45.8X2	T45.8X3	T45.8X4	T45.8X5	T45.8X6
with ferrous salt	T45.2X1	T45.2X2	T45.2X3	T45.2X4	T45.2X5	T45.2X6
antagonist	T45.1X1	T45.1X2	T45.1X3	T45.1X4	T45.1X5	T45.1X6
Folinic acid	T45.8X1	T45.8X2	T45.8X3	T45.8X4	T45.8X5	T45.8X6
Folium stramoniae	T48.6X1	T48.6X2	T48.6X3	T48.6X4	T48.6X5	T48.6X6
Follicle-stimulating hormone, human	T38.811	T38.812	T38.813	T38.814	T38.815	T38.816
Folpet	T60.3X1	T60.3X2	T60.3X3	T60.3X4	—	—
Fominoben	T48.3X1	T48.3X2	T48.3X3	T48.3X4	T48.3X5	T48.3X6
Food, foodstuffs, noxious, nonbacterial, NEC	T62.91	T62.92	T62.93	T62.94	—	—
berries	T62.1X1	T62.1X2	T62.1X3	T62.1X4	—	—
fish—see also Fish	T61.91	T61.92	T61.93	T61.94	—	—
mushrooms	T62.0X1	T62.0X2	T62.0X3	T62.0X4	—	—
plants	T62.2X1	T62.2X2	T62.2X3	T62.2X4	—	—
seafood	T61.91	T61.92	T61.93	T61.94	—	—
specified NEC	T61.8X1	T61.8X2	T61.8X3	T61.8X4	—	—
seeds	T62.2X1	T62.2X2	T62.2X3	T62.2X4	—	—
shellfish	T61.781	T61.782	T61.783	T61.784	—	—
specified NEC	T62.8X1	T62.8X2	T62.8X3	T62.8X4	—	—
Fool's parsley	T62.2X1	T62.2X2	T62.2X3	T62.2X4	—	—
Formaldehyde (solution), gas or vapor	T59.2X1	T59.2X2	T59.2X3	T59.2X4	—	—
fungicide	T60.3X1	T60.3X2	T60.3X3	T60.3X4	—	—
Formalin	T59.2X1	T59.2X2	T59.2X3	T59.2X4	—	—
fungicide	T60.3X1	T60.3X2	T60.3X3	T60.3X4	—	—
vapor	T59.2X1	T59.2X2	T59.2X3	T59.2X4	—	—
Formic acid	T54.2X1	T54.2X2	T54.2X3	T54.2X4	—	—
vapor	T59.891	T59.892	T59.893	T59.894	—	—
Foscarnet sodium	T37.5X1	T37.5X2	T37.5X3	T37.5X4	T37.5X5	T37.5X6
Fosfestrol	T38.5X1	T38.5X2	T38.5X3	T38.5X4	T38.5X5	T38.5X6
Fosfomycin	T36.8X1	T36.8X2	T36.8X3	T36.8X4	T36.8X5	T36.8X6
Fosfonet sodium	T37.5X1	T37.5X2	T37.5X3	T37.5X4	T37.5X5	T37.5X6

Substance	Poisoning, Accidental (unintentional)	Poisoning, Intentional self-harm	Poisoning, Assault	Poisoning, Undetermined	Adverse effect	Underdosing
Fosinopril	T46.4X1	T46.4X2	T46.4X3	T46.4X4	T46.4X5	T46.4X6
sodium	T46.4X1	T46.4X2	T46.4X3	T46.4X4	T46.4X5	T46.4X6
Fowler's solution	T57.0X1	T57.0X2	T57.0X3	T57.0X4	—	—
Foxglove	T62.2X1	T62.2X2	T62.2X3	T62.2X4	—	—
Framycetin	T36.5X1	T36.5X2	T36.5X3	T36.5X4	T36.5X5	T36.5X6
Frangula	T47.2X1	T47.2X2	T47.2X3	T47.2X4	T47.2X5	T47.2X6
extract	T47.2X1	T47.2X2	T47.2X3	T47.2X4	T47.2X5	T47.2X6
Frei antigen	T50.8X1	T50.8X2	T50.8X3	T50.8X4	T50.8X5	T50.8X6
Freon	T53.5X1	T53.5X2	T53.5X3	T53.5X4	—	—
Fructose	T50.3X1	T50.3X2	T50.3X3	T50.3X4	T50.3X5	T50.3X6
Frusemide	T50.1X1	T50.1X2	T50.1X3	T50.1X4	T50.1X5	T50.1X6
FSH	T38.811	T38.812	T38.813	T38.814	T38.815	T38.816
Ftorafur	T45.1X1	T45.1X2	T45.1X3	T45.1X4	T45.1X5	T45.1X6
Fuel						
automobile	T52.0X1	T52.0X2	T52.0X3	T52.0X4	—	—
exhaust gas, not in transit	T58.01	T58.02	T58.03	T58.04	—	—
vapor NEC	T52.0X1	T52.0X2	T52.0X3	T52.0X4	—	—
gas (domestic use)—see also Carbon, monoxide, fuel, utility	T59.891	T59.892	T59.893	T59.894	—	—
utility	T59.891	T59.892	T59.893	T59.894	—	—
in mobile container	T59.891	T59.892	T59.893	T59.894	—	—
incomplete combustion of—see Carbon, monoxide, fuel, utility						
piped (natural)	T59.891	T59.892	T59.893	T59.894	—	—
industrial, incomplete combustion	T58.8X1	T58.8X2	T58.8X3	T58.8X4	—	—
Fugillin	T36.8X1	T36.8X2	T36.8X3	T36.8X4	T36.8X5	T36.8X6
Fulminate of mercury	T56.1X1	T56.1X2	T56.1X3	T56.1X4	—	—
Fulvicin	T36.7X1	T36.7X2	T36.7X3	T36.7X4	T36.7X5	T36.7X6
Fumadil	T36.8X1	T36.8X2	T36.8X3	T36.8X4	T36.8X5	T36.8X6
Fumagillin	T36.8X1	T36.8X2	T36.8X3	T36.8X4	T36.8X5	T36.8X6
Fumaric acid	T49.4X1	T49.4X2	T49.4X3	T49.4X4	T49.4X5	T49.4X6
Fumes (from)	T59.91	T59.92	T59.93	T59.94	—	—
carbon monoxide—see Carbon, monoxide						
charcoal (domestic use)—see Charcoal, fumes						
chloroform—see Chloroform						
coke (in domestic stoves, fireplaces)—see Coke fumes						
corrosive NEC	T54.91	T54.92	T54.93	T54.94	—	—
ether—see ether						
freons	T53.5X1	T53.5X2	T53.5X3	T53.5X4	—	—
hydrocarbons	T59.891	T59.892	T59.893	T59.894	—	—
petroleum (liquefied)	T59.891	T59.892	T59.893	T59.894	—	—
distributed through pipes (pure or mixed with air)	T59.891	T59.892	T59.893	T59.894	—	—

Substance	Poisoning, Accidental (unintentional)	Poisoning, Intentional self-harm	Poisoning, Assault	Poisoning, Undetermined	Adverse effect	Underdosing
Fumes — *Continued*						
lead—see lead						
metal—see Metals, or the specified metal						
nitrogen dioxide	T59.0X1	T59.0X2	T59.0X3	T59.0X4	—	—
pesticides—see Pesticides						
petroleum (liquefied)	T59.891	T59.892	T59.893	T59.894		
distributed through pipes (pure or mixed with air)	T59.891	T59.892	T59.893	T59.894	—	—
polyester	T59.891	T59.892	T59.893	T59.894	—	—
specified source NEC— see also substance specified	T59.891	T59.892	T59.893	T59.894	—	—
sulfur dioxide	T59.1X1	T59.1X2	T59.1X3	T59.1X4	—	—
Fumigant NEC	T60.91	T60.92	T60.93	T60.94		
Fungi, noxious, used as food	T62.0X1	T62.0X2	T62.0X3	T62.0X4	—	—
Fungicide NEC (nonmedicinal)	T60.3X1	T60.3X2	T60.3X3	T60.3X4	—	—
Fungizone	T36.7X1	T36.7X2	T36.7X3	T36.7X4	T36.7X5	T36.7X6
topical	T49.0X1	T49.0X2	T49.0X3	T49.0X4	T49.0X5	T49.0X6
Furacin	T49.0X1	T49.0X2	T49.0X3	T49.0X4	T49.0X5	T49.0X6
Furadantin	T37.91	T37.92	T37.93	T37.94	T37.95	T37.96
Furazolidone	T37.8X1	T37.8X2	T37.8X3	T37.8X4	T37.8X5	T37.8X6
Furazolium chloride	T49.0X1	T49.0X2	T49.0X3	T49.0X4	T49.0X5	T49.0X6
Furfural	T52.8X1	T52.8X2	T52.8X3	T52.8X4	—	—
Furnace (coal burning) (domestic), gas from	T58.2X1	T58.2X2	T58.2X3	T58.2X4	—	—
industrial	T58.8X1	T58.8X2	T58.8X3	T58.8X4	—	—
Furniture polish	T65.891	T65.892	T65.893	T65.894	—	—
Furosemide	T50.1X1	T50.1X2	T50.1X3	T50.1X4	T50.1X5	T50.1X6
Furoxone	T37.91	T37.92	T37.93	T37.94	T37.95	T37.96
Fursultiamine	T45.2X1	T45.2X2	T45.2X3	T45.2X4	T45.2X5	T45.2X6
Fusafungine	T36.8X1	T36.8X2	T36.8X3	T36.8X4	T36.8X5	T36.8X6
Fusel oil (any) (amyl) (butyl) (propyl), vapor	T51.3X1	T51.3X2	T51.3X3	T51.3X4	—	—
Fusidate (ethanolamine) (sodium)	T36.8X1	T36.8X2	T36.8X3	T36.8X4	T36.8X5	T36.8X6
Fusidic acid	T36.8X1	T36.8X2	T36.8X3	T36.8X4	T36.8X5	T36.8X6
Fytic acid, nonasodium	T50.6X1	T50.6X2	T50.6X3	T50.6X4	T50.6X5	T50.6X6
G						
GABA	T43.8X1	T43.8X2	T43.8X3	T43.8X4	T43.8X5	T43.8X6
Gadopentetic acid	T50.8X1	T50.8X2	T50.8X3	T50.8X4	T50.8X5	T50.8X6
Galactose	T50.3X1	T50.3X2	T50.3X3	T50.3X4	T50.3X5	T50.3X6
b-Galactosidase	T47.5X1	T47.5X2	T47.5X3	T47.5X4	T47.5X5	T47.5X6
Galantamine	T44.0X1	T44.0X2	T44.0X3	T44.0X4	T44.0X5	T44.0X6
Gallamine (triethiodide)	T48.1X1	T48.1X2	T48.1X3	T48.1X4	T48.1X5	T48.1X6
Gallium citrate	T50.991	T50.992	T50.993	T50.994	T50.995	T50.996
Gallopamil	T46.1X1	T46.1X2	T46.1X3	T46.1X4	T46.1X5	T46.1X6
Gamboge	T47.2X1	T47.2X2	T47.2X3	T47.2X4	T47.2X5	T47.2X6

Substance	Poisoning, Accidental (unintentional)	Poisoning, Intentional self-harm	Poisoning, Assault	Poisoning, Undetermined	Adverse effect	Underdosing
Gamimune	T50.Z11	T50.Z12	T50.Z13	T50.Z14	T50.Z15	T50.Z16
Gamma globulin	T50.Z11	T50.Z12	T50.Z13	T50.Z14	T50.Z15	T50.Z16
Gamma-aminobutyric acid	T43.8X1	T43.8X2	T43.8X3	T43.8X4	T43.8X5	T43.8X6
Gamma-benzene hexachloride (medicinal)	T49.0X1	T49.0X2	T49.0X3	T49.0X4	T49.0X5	T49.0X6
nonmedicinal, vapor	T53.6X1	T53.6X2	T53.6X3	T53.6X4	—	—
Gamma-BHC (medicinal)—see also Gamma-benzene hexachloride	T49.0X1	T49.0X2	T49.0X3	T49.0X4	T49.0X5	T49.0X6
Gamulin	T50.Z11	T50.Z12	T50.Z13	T50.Z14	T50.Z15	T50.Z16
Ganciclovir (sodium)	T37.5X1	T37.5X2	T37.5X3	T37.5X4	T37.5X5	T37.5X6
Ganglionic blocking drug NEC	T44.2X1	T44.2X2	T44.2X3	T44.2X4	T44.2X5	T44.2X6
specified NEC	T44.2X1	T44.2X2	T44.2X3	T44.2X4	T44.2X5	T44.2X6
Ganja	T40.7X1	T40.7X2	T40.7X3	T40.7X4	T40.7X5	T40.7X6
Garamycin	T36.5X1	T36.5X2	T36.5X3	T36.5X4	T36.5X5	T36.5X6
ophthalmic preparation	T49.5X1	T49.5X2	T49.5X3	T49.5X4	T49.5X5	T49.5X6
topical NEC	T49.0X1	T49.0X2	T49.0X3	T49.0X4	T49.0X5	T49.0X6
Gardenal	T42.3X1	T42.3X2	T42.3X3	T42.3X4	T42.3X5	T42.3X6
Gardepanyl	T42.3X1	T42.3X2	T42.3X3	T42.3X4	T42.3X5	T42.3X6
Gas NEC	T59.91	T59.92	T59.93	T59.94	—	—
acetylene	T59.891	T59.892	T59.893	T59.894	—	—
incomplete combustion of	T58.11	T58.12	T58.13	T58.14	—	—
air contaminants, source or type not specified	T59.91	T59.92	T59.93	T59.94	—	—
anesthetic	T41.0X1	T41.0X2	T41.0X3	T41.0X4	T41.0X5	T41.0X6
blast furnace	T58.8X1	T58.8X2	T58.8X3	T58.8X4	—	—
butane—see butane						
carbon monoxide—see Carbon, monoxide						
chlorine	T59.4X1	T59.4X2	T59.4X3	T59.4X4	—	—
coal	T58.2X1	T58.2X2	T58.2X3	T58.2X4	—	—
cyanide	T57.3X1	T57.3X2	T57.3X3	T57.3X4	—	—
dicyanogen	T65.0X1	T65.0X2	T65.0X3	T65.0X4	—	—
domestic—see Domestic gas						
exhaust	T58.01	T58.02	T58.03	T58.04	—	—
from utility (for cooking, heating, or lighting) (after combustion)—see Carbon, monoxide, fuel, utility						
prior to combustion	T59.891	T59.892	T59.893	T59.894	—	—
from wood- or coal-burning stove or fireplace	T58.2X1	T58.2X2	T58.2X3	T58.2X4	—	—
fuel (domestic use) (after combustion)—see also Carbon, monoxide, fuel						

Substance	Poisoning, Accidental (unintentional)	Poisoning, Intentional self-harm	Poisoning, Assault	Poisoning, Undetermined	Adverse effect	Underdosing
Gas NEC — *Continued*						
industrial use	T58.8X1	T58.8X2	T58.8X3	T58.8X4	—	—
prior to combustion	T59.891	T59.892	T59.893	T59.894	—	—
utility	T59.891	T59.892	T59.893	T59.894	—	—
in mobile container	T59.891	T59.892	T59.893	T59.894	—	—
incomplete combustion of—see Carbon, monoxide, fuel, utility						
piped (natural)	T59.891	T59.892	T59.893	T59.894	—	—
garage	T58.01	T58.02	T58.03	T58.04	—	—
hydrocarbon NEC	T59.891	T59.892	T59.893	T59.894	—	—
incomplete combustion of—see Carbon, monoxide, fuel, utility						
liquefied—see butane						
piped	T59.891	T59.892	T59.893	T59.894	—	—
hydrocyanic acid	T65.0X1	T65.0X2	T65.0X3	T65.0X4	—	—
illuminating (after combustion)	T58.11	T58.12	T58.13	T58.14	—	—
prior to combustion	T59.891	T59.892	T59.893	T59.894	—	—
incomplete combustion, any—see Carbon, monoxide						
kiln	T58.8X1	T58.8X2	T58.8X3	T58.8X4	—	—
lacrimogenic	T59.3X1	T59.3X2	T59.3X3	T59.3X4	—	—
liquefied petroleum—see butane						
marsh	T59.891	T59.892	T59.893	T59.894	—	—
motor exhaust, not in transit	T58.01	T58.02	T58.03	T58.04	—	—
mustard, not in war	T59.891	T59.892	T59.893	T59.894	—	—
natural	T59.891	T59.892	T59.893	T59.894	—	—
nerve, not in war	T59.91	T59.92	T59.93	T59.94	—	—
oil	T52.0X1	T52.0X2	T52.0X3	T52.0X4	—	—
petroleum (liquefied) (distributed in mobile containers)	T59.891	T59.892	T59.893	T59.894	—	—
piped (pure or mixed with air)	T59.891	T59.892	T59.893	T59.894	—	—
pipcd (manufactured) (natural) NEC	T59.891	T59.892	T59.893	T59.894	—	—
producer	T58.8X1	T58.8X2	T58.8X3	T58.8X4	—	—
propane—see propane						
refrigerant (chlorofluoro-carbon)	T53.5X1	T53.5X2	T53.5X3	T53.5X4	—	—
not chlorofluoro-carbon	T59.891	T59.892	T59.893	T59.894	—	—
sewer	T59.91	T59.92	T59.93	T59.94	—	—
specified source NEC	T59.91	T59.92	T59.93	T59.94	—	—
stove (after combustion)	T58.11	T58.12	T58.13	T58.14	—	—
prior to combustion	T59.891	T59.892	T59.893	T59.894	—	—
tear	T59.3X1	T59.3X2	T59.3X3	T59.3X4	—	—
therapeutic	T41.5X1	T41.5X2	T41.5X3	T41.5X4	T41.5X5	T41.5X6

Substance	Poisoning, Accidental (unintentional)	Poisoning, Intentional self-harm	Poisoning, Assault	Poisoning, Undetermined	Adverse effect	Underdosing
Gas NEC — *Continued*						
utility (for cooking, heating, or lighting) (piped) NEC	T59.891	T59.892	T59.893	T59.894	—	—
in mobile container	T59.891	T59.892	T59.893	T59.894	—	—
incomplete combustion of—see Carbon, monoxide, fuel, utlity						
piped (natural)	T59.891	T59.892	T59.893	T59.894	—	—
water	T58.11	T58.12	T58.13	T58.14	—	—
incomplete combustion of—see Carbon, monoxide, fuel, utility						
Gaseous substance—see Gas						
Gasoline	T52.0X1	T52.0X2	T52.0X3	T52.0X4	—	—
vapor	T52.0X1	T52.0X2	T52.0X3	T52.0X4	—	—
Gastric enzymes	T47.5X1	T47.5X2	T47.5X3	T47.5X4	T47.5X5	T47.5X6
Gastrografin	T50.8X1	T50.8X2	T50.8X3	T50.8X4	T50.8X5	T50.8X6
Gastrointestinal drug	T47.91	T47.92	T47.93	T47.94	T47.95	T47.96
biological	T47.8X1	T47.8X2	T47.8X3	T47.8X4	T47.8X5	T47.8X6
specified NEC	T47.8X1	T47.8X2	T47.8X3	T47.8X4	T47.8X5	T47.8X6
Gaultheria procumbens	T62.2X1	T62.2X2	T62.2X3	T62.2X4	—	—
Gefarnate	T44.3X1	T44.3X2	T44.3X3	T44.3X4	T44.3X5	T44.3X6
Gelatin (intravenous)	T45.8X1	T45.8X2	T45.8X3	T45.8X4	T45.8X5	T45.8X6
absorbable (sponge)	T45.7X1	T45.7X2	T45.7X3	T45.7X4	T45.7X5	T45.7X6
Gelfilm	T49.8X1	T49.8X2	T49.8X3	T49.8X4	T49.8X5	T49.8X6
Gelfoam	T45.7X1	T45.7X2	T45.7X3	T45.7X4	T45.7X5	T45.7X6
Gelsemine	T50.991	T50.992	T50.993	T50.994	T50.995	T50.996
Gelsemium (sempervirens)	T62.2X1	T62.2X2	T62.2X3	T62.2X4	—	—
Gemeprost	T48.0X1	T48.0X2	T48.0X3	T48.0X4	T48.0X5	T48.0X6
Gemfibrozil	T46.6X1	T46.6X2	T46.6X3	T46.6X4	T46.6X5	T46.6X6
Gemonil	T42.3X1	T42.3X2	T42.3X3	T42.3X4	T42.3X5	T42.3X6
Gentamicin	T36.5X1	T36.5X2	T36.5X3	T36.5X4	T36.5X5	T36.5X6
ophthalmic preparation	T49.5X1	T49.5X2	T49.5X3	T49.5X4	T49.5X5	T49.5X6
topical NEC	T49.0X1	T49.0X2	T49.0X3	T49.0X4	T49.0X5	T49.0X6
Gentian	T47.5X1	T47.5X2	T47.5X3	T47.5X4	T47.5X5	T47.5X6
violet	T49.0X1	T49.0X2	T49.0X3	T49.0X4	T49.0X5	T49.0X6
Gepefrine	T44.4X1	T44.4X2	T44.4X3	T44.4X4	T44.4X5	T44.4X6
Gestonorone caproate	T38.5X1	T38.5X2	T38.5X3	T38.5X4	T38.5X5	T38.5X6
Gexane	T49.0X1	T49.0X2	T49.0X3	T49.0X4	T49.0X5	T49.0X6
Gila monster (venom)	T63.111	T63.112	T63.113	T63.114	—	—
Ginger	T47.5X1	T47.5X2	T47.5X3	T47.5X4	T47.5X5	T47.5X6
Jamaica—see Jamaica, ginger						
Gitalin	T46.0X1	T46.0X2	T46.0X3	T46.0X4	T46.0X5	T46.0X6
amorphous	T46.0X1	T46.0X2	T46.0X3	T46.0X4	T46.0X5	T46.0X6
Gitaloxin	T46.0X1	T46.0X2	T46.0X3	T46.0X4	T46.0X5	T46.0X6
Gitoxin	T46.0X1	T46.0X2	T46.0X3	T46.0X4	T46.0X5	T46.0X6
Glafenine	T39.8X1	T39.8X2	T39.8X3	T39.8X4	T39.8X5	T39.8X6

Substance	Poisoning, Accidental (unintentional)	Poisoning, Intentional self-harm	Poisoning, Assault	Poisoning, Undetermined	Adverse effect	Underdosing
Glandular extract (medicinal) NEC	T50.Z91	T50.Z92	T50.Z93	T50.Z94	T50.Z95	T50.Z96
Glaucarubin	T37.3X1	T37.3X2	T37.3X3	T37.3X4	T37.3X5	T37.3X6
Glibenclamide	T38.3X1	T38.3X2	T38.3X3	T38.3X4	T38.3X5	T38.3X6
Glibornuride	T38.3X1	T38.3X2	T38.3X3	T38.3X4	T38.3X5	T38.3X6
Gliclazide	T38.3X1	T38.3X2	T38.3X3	T38.3X4	T38.3X5	T38.3X6
Glimidine	T38.3X1	T38.3X2	T38.3X3	T38.3X4	T38.3X5	T38.3X6
Glipizide	T38.3X1	T38.3X2	T38.3X3	T38.3X4	T38.3X5	T38.3X6
Gliquidone	T38.3X1	T38.3X2	T38.3X3	T38.3X4	T38.3X5	T38.3X6
Glisolamide	T38.3X1	T38.3X2	T38.3X3	T38.3X4	T38.3X5	T38.3X6
Glisoxepide	T38.3X1	T38.3X2	T38.3X3	T38.3X4	T38.3X5	T38.3X6
Globin zinc insulin	T38.3X1	T38.3X2	T38.3X3	T38.3X4	T38.3X5	T38.3X6
Globulin						
antilymphocytic	T50.Z11	T50.Z12	T50.Z13	T50.Z14	T50.Z15	T50.Z16
antirhesus	T50.Z11	T50.Z12	T50.Z13	T50.Z14	T50.Z15	T50.Z16
antivenin	T50.Z11	T50.Z12	T50.Z13	T50.Z14	T50.Z15	T50.Z16
antiviral	T50.Z11	T50.Z12	T50.Z13	T50.Z14	T50.Z15	T50.Z16
Glucagon	T38.3X1	T38.3X2	T38.3X3	T38.3X4	T38.3X5	T38.3X6
Glucocorticoids	T38.0X1	T38.0X2	T38.0X3	T38.0X4	T38.0X5	T38.0X6
Glucocorticosteroid	T38.0X1	T38.0X2	T38.0X3	T38.0X4	T38.0X5	T38.0X6
Gluconic acid	T50.991	T50.992	T50.993	T50.994	T50.995	T50.996
Glucosamine sulfate	T39.4X1	T39.4X2	T39.4X3	T39.4X4	T39.4X5	T39.4X6
Glucose	T50.3X1	T50.3X2	T50.3X3	T50.3X4	T50.3X5	T50.3X6
with sodium chloride	T50.3X1	T50.3X2	T50.3X3	T50.3X4	T50.3X5	T50.3X6
Glucosulfone sodium	T37.1X1	T37.1X2	T37.1X3	T37.1X4	T37.1X5	T37.1X6
Glucurolactone	T47.8X1	T47.8X2	T47.8X3	T47.8X4	T47.8X5	T47.8X6
Glue NEC	T52.8X1	T52.8X2	T52.8X3	T52.8X4	—	—
Glutamic acid	T47.5X1	T47.5X2	T47.5X3	T47.5X4	T47.5X5	T47.5X6
Glutaral (medicinal)	T49.0X1	T49.0X2	T49.0X3	T49.0X4	T49.0X5	T49.0X6
nonmedicinal	T65.891	T65.892	T65.893	T65.894	—	—
Glutaraldehyde (nonmedicinal)	T65.891	T65.892	T65.893	T65.894	—	—
medicinal	T49.0X1	T49.0X2	T49.0X3	T49.0X4	T49.0X5	T49.0X6
Glutathione	T50.6X1	T50.6X2	T50.6X3	T50.6X4	T50.6X5	T50.6X6
Glutethimide	T42.6X1	T42.6X2	T42.6X3	T42.6X4	T42.6X5	T42.6X6
Glyburide	T38.3X1	T38.3X2	T38.3X3	T38.3X4	T38.3X5	T38.3X6
Glycerin	T47.4X1	T47.4X2	T47.4X3	T47.4X4	T47.4X5	T47.4X6
Glycerol	T47.4X1	T47.4X2	T47.4X3	T47.4X4	T47.4X5	T47.4X6
borax	T49.6X1	T49.6X2	T49.6X3	T49.6X4	T49.6X5	T49.6X6
intravenous	T50.3X1	T50.3X2	T50.3X3	T50.3X4	T50.3X5	T50.3X6
iodinated	T48.4X1	T48.4X2	T48.4X3	T48.4X4	T48.4X5	T48.4X6
Glycerophosphate	T50.991	T50.992	T50.993	T50.994	T50.995	T50.996
Glyceryl						
gualacolate	T48.4X1	T48.4X2	T48.4X3	T48.4X4	T48.4X5	T48.4X6
nitrate	T46.3X1	T46.3X2	T46.3X3	T46.3X4	T46.3X5	T46.3X6
triacetate (topical)	T49.0X1	T49.0X2	T49.0X3	T49.0X4	T49.0X5	T49.0X6
trinitrate	T46.3X1	T46.3X2	T46.3X3	T46.3X4	T46.3X5	T46.3X6
Glycine	T50.3X1	T50.3X2	T50.3X3	T50.3X4	T50.3X5	T50.3X6
Glyclopyramide	T38.3X1	T38.3X2	T38.3X3	T38.3X4	T38.3X5	T38.3X6
Glycobiarsol	T37.3X1	T37.3X2	T37.3X3	T37.3X4	T37.3X5	T37.3X6
Glycols (ether)	T52.3X1	T52.3X2	T52.3X3	T52.3X4	—	—

Substance	Poisoning, Accidental (unintentional)	Poisoning, Intentional self-harm	Poisoning, Assault	Poisoning, Undetermined	Adverse effect	Underdosing
Glyconiazide	T37.1X1	T37.1X2	T37.1X3	T37.1X4	T37.1X5	T37.1X6
Glycopyrrolate	T44.3X1	T44.3X2	T44.3X3	T44.3X4	T44.3X5	T44.3X6
Glycopyrronium	T44.3X1	T44.3X2	T44.3X3	T44.3X4	T44.3X5	T44.3X6
bromide	T44.3X1	T44.3X2	T44.3X3	T44.3X4	T44.3X5	T44.3X6
Glycoside, cardiac (stimulant)	T46.0X1	T46.0X2	T46.0X3	T46.0X4	T46.0X5	T46.0X6
Glycyclamide	T38.3X1	T38.3X2	T38.3X3	T38.3X4	T38.3X5	T38.3X6
Glycyrrhiza extract	T48.4X1	T48.4X2	T48.4X3	T48.4X4	T48.4X5	T48.4X6
Glycyrrhizic acid	T48.4X1	T48.4X2	T48.4X3	T48.4X4	T48.4X5	T48.4X6
Glycyrrhizinate potassium	T48.4X1	T48.4X2	T48.4X3	T48.4X4	T48.4X5	T48.4X6
Glymidine sodium	T38.3X1	T38.3X2	T38.3X3	T38.3X4	T38.3X5	T38.3X6
Glyphosate	T60.3X1	T60.3X2	T60.3X3	T60.3X4	—	—
Glyphylline	T48.6X1	T48.6X2	T48.6X3	T48.6X4	T48.6X5	T48.6X6
Gold						
colloidal (l98Au)	T45.1X1	T45.1X2	T45.1X3	T45.1X4	T45.1X5	T45.1X6
salts	T39.4X1	T39.4X2	T39.4X3	T39.4X4	T39.4X5	T39.4X6
Golden sulfide of antimony	T56.891	T56.892	T56.893	T56.894	—	—
Goldylocks	T62.2X1	T62.2X2	T62.2X3	T62.2X4		
Gonadal tissue extract	T38.901	T38.902	T38.903	T38.904	T38.905	T38.906
female	T38.5X1	T38.5X2	T38.5X3	T38.5X4	T38.5X5	T38.5X6
male	T38.7X1	T38.7X2	T38.7X3	T38.7X4	T38.7X5	T38.7X6
Gonadorelin	T38.891	T38.892	T38.893	T38.894	T38.895	T38.896
Gonadotropin	T38.891	T38.892	T38.893	T38.894	T38.895	T38.896
chorionic	T38.891	T38.892	T38.893	T38.894	T38.895	T38.896
pituitary	T38.811	T38.812	T38.813	T38.814	T38.815	T38.816
Goserelin	T45.1X1	T45.1X2	T45.1X3	T45.1X4	T45.1X5	T45.1X6
Grain alcohol	T51.0X1	T51.0X2	T51.0X3	T51.0X4	—	—
Gramicidin	T49.0X1	T49.0X2	T49.0X3	T49.0X4	T49.0X5	T49.0X6
Granisetron	T45.0X1	T45.0X2	T45.0X3	T45.0X4	T45.0X5	T45.0X6
Gratiola officinalis	T62.2X1	T62.2X2	T62.2X3	T62.2X4	—	—
Grease	T65.891	T65.892	T65.893	T65.894	—	—
Green hellebore	T62.2X1	T62.2X2	T62.2X3	T62.2X4	—	—
Green soap	T49.2X1	T49.2X2	T49.2X3	T49.2X4	T49.2X5	T49.2X6
Grifulvin	T36.7X1	T36.7X2	T36.7X3	T36.7X4	T36.7X5	T36.7X6
Griseofulvin	T36.7X1	T36.7X2	T36.7X3	T36.7X4	T36.7X5	T36.7X6
Growth hormone	T38.811	T38.812	T38.813	T38.814	T38.815	T38.816
Guaiac reagent	T50.991	T50.992	T50.993	T50.994	T50.995	T50.996
Guaiacol derivatives	T48.4X1	T48.4X2	T48.4X3	T48.4X4	T48.4X5	T48.4X6
Guaifenesin	T48.4X1	T48.4X2	T48.4X3	T48.4X4	T48.4X5	T48.4X6
Guaimesal	T48.4X1	T48.4X2	T48.4X3	T48.4X4	T48.4X5	T48.4X6
Guaiphenesin	T48.4X1	T48.4X2	T48.4X3	T48.4X4	T48.4X5	T48.4X6
Guamecycline	T36.4X1	T36.4X2	T36.4X3	T36.4X4	T36.4X5	T36.4X6
Guanabenz	T46.5X1	T46.5X2	T46.5X3	T46.5X4	T46.5X5	T46.5X6
Guanacline	T46.5X1	T46.5X2	T46.5X3	T46.5X4	T46.5X5	T46.5X6
Guanadrel	T46.5X1	T46.5X2	T46.5X3	T46.5X4	T46.5X5	T46.5X6
Guanatol	T37.2X1	T37.2X2	T37.2X3	T37.2X4	T37.2X5	T37.2X6
Guanethidine	T46.5X1	T46.5X2	T46.5X3	T46.5X4	T46.5X5	T46.5X6
Guanfacine	T46.5X1	T46.5X2	T46.5X3	T46.5X4	T46.5X5	T46.5X6
Guano	T65.891	T65.892	T65.893	T65.894	—	—

Substance	Poisoning, Accidental (unintentional)	Poisoning, Intentional self-harm	Poisoning, Assault	Poisoning, Undetermined	Adverse effect	Underdosing
Guanochlor	T46.5X1	T46.5X2	T46.5X3	T46.5X4	T46.5X5	T46.5X6
Guanoclor	T46.5X1	T46.5X2	T46.5X3	T46.5X4	T46.5X5	T46.5X6
Guanoctine	T46.5X1	T46.5X2	T46.5X3	T46.5X4	T46.5X5	T46.5X6
Guanoxabenz	T46.5X1	T46.5X2	T46.5X3	T46.5X4	T46.5X5	T46.5X6
Guanoxan	T46.5X1	T46.5X2	T46.5X3	T46.5X4	T46.5X5	T46.5X6
Guar gum (medicinal)	T46.6X1	T46.6X2	T46.6X3	T46.6X4	T46.6X5	T46.6X6
H						
Hachimycin	T36.7X1	T36.7X2	T36.7X3	T36.7X4	T36.7X5	T36.7X6
Hair						
dye	T49.4X1	T49.4X2	T49.4X3	T49.4X4	T49.4X5	T49.4X6
preparation NEC	T49.4X1	T49.4X2	T49.4X3	T49.4X4	T49.4X5	T49.4X6
Halazepam	T42.4X1	T42.4X2	T42.4X3	T42.4X4	T42.4X5	T42.4X6
Halcinolone	T49.0X1	T49.0X2	T49.0X3	T49.0X4	T49.0X5	T49.0X6
Halcinonide	T49.0X1	T49.0X2	T49.0X3	T49.0X4	T49.0X5	T49.0X6
Halethazole	T49.0X1	T49.0X2	T49.0X3	T49.0X4	T49.0X5	T49.0X6
Hallucinogen NOS	T40.901	T40.902	T40.903	T40.904	T40.905	T40.906
specified NEC	T40.991	T40.992	T40.993	T40.994	T40.995	T40.996
Halofantrine	T37.2X1	T37.2X2	T37.2X3	T37.2X4	T37.2X5	T37.2X6
Halofenate	T46.6X1	T46.6X2	T46.6X3	T46.6X4	T46.6X5	T46.6X6
Halometasone	T49.0X1	T49.0X2	T49.0X3	T49.0X4	T49.0X5	T49.0X6
Haloperidol	T43.4X1	T43.4X2	T43.4X3	T43.4X4	T43.4X5	T43.4X6
Haloprogin	T49.0X1	T49.0X2	T49.0X3	T49.0X4	T49.0X5	T49.0X6
Halotex	T49.0X1	T49.0X2	T49.0X3	T49.0X4	T49.0X5	T49.0X6
Halothane	T41.0X1	T41.0X2	T41.0X3	T41.0X4	T41.0X5	T41.0X6
Haloxazolam	T42.4X1	T42.4X2	T42.4X3	T42.4X4	T42.4X5	T42.4X6
Halquinols	T49.0X1	T49.0X2	T49.0X3	T49.0X4	T49.0X5	T49.0X6
Hamamelis	T49.2X1	T49.2X2	T49.2X3	T49.2X4	T49.2X5	T49.2X6
Haptendextran	T45.8X1	T45.8X2	T45.8X3	T45.8X4	T45.8X5	T45.8X6
Harmonyl	T46.5X1	T46.5X2	T46.5X3	T46.5X4	T46.5X5	T46.5X6
Hartmann's solution	T50.3X1	T50.3X2	T50.3X3	T50.3X4	T50.3X5	T50.3X6
Hashish	T40.7X1	T40.7X2	T40.7X3	T40.7X4	T40.7X5	T40.7X6
Hawaiian Woodrose seeds	T40.991	T40.992	T40.993	T40.994	—	—
HCB	T60.3X1	T60.3X2	T60.3X3	T60.3X4	—	—
HCH	T53.6X1	T53.6X2	T53.6X3	T53.6X4	—	—
medicinal	T49.0X1	T49.0X2	T49.0X3	T49.0X4	T49.0X5	T49.0X6
HCN	T57.3X1	T57.3X2	T57.3X3	T57.3X4	—	—
Headache cures, drugs, powders NEC	T50.901	T50.902	T50.903	T50.904	T50.905	T50.906
Heavenly Blue (morning glory)	T40.991	T40.992	T40.993	T40.994	—	—
Heavy metal antidote	T45.8X1	T45.8X2	T45.8X3	T45.8X4	T45.8X5	T45.8X6
Hedaquinium	T49.0X1	T49.0X2	T49.0X3	T49.0X4	T49.0X5	T49.0X6
Hedge hyssop	T62.2X1	T62.2X2	T62.2X3	T62.2X4	—	—
Heet	T49.8X1	T49.8X2	T49.8X3	T49.8X4	T49.8X5	T49.8X6
Helenin	T37.4X1	T37.4X2	T37.4X3	T37.4X4	T37.4X5	T37.4X6
Helium (nonmedicinal) NEC	T59.891	T59.892	T59.893	T59.894	—	—
medicinal	T48.991	T48.992	T48.993	T48.994	T48.995	T48.996
Hellebore (black) (green) (white)	T62.2X1	T62.2X2	T62.2X3	T62.2X4	—	—
Hematin	T45.8X1	T45.8X2	T45.8X3	T45.8X4	T45.8X5	T45.8X6

Substance	Poisoning, Accidental (unintentional)	Poisoning, Intentional self-harm	Poisoning, Assault	Poisoning, Undetermined	Adverse effect	Underdosing
Hematinic preparation	T45.8X1	T45.8X2	T45.8X3	T45.8X4	T45.8X5	T45.8X6
Hematological agent	T45.91	T45.92	T45.93	T45.94	T45.95	T45.96
specified NEC	T45.8X1	T45.8X2	T45.8X4	T45.8X4	T45.8X5	T45.8X6
Hemlock	T62.2X1	T62.2X2	T62.2X3	T62.2X4	—	—
Hemostatic	T45.621	T45.622	T45.623	T45.624	T45.625	T45.626
drug, systemic	T45.621	T45.622	T45.623	T45.624	T45.625	T45.626
Hemostyptic	T49.4X1	T49.4X2	T49.4X3	T49.4X4	T49.4X5	T49.4X6
Henbane	T62.2X1	T62.2X2	T62.2X3	T62.2X4	—	—
Heparin (sodium)	T45.511	T45.512	T45.513	T45.514	T45.515	T45.516
action reverser	T45.7X1	T45.7X2	T45.7X3	T45.7X4	T45.7X5	T45.7X6
Heparin-fraction	T45.511	T45.512	T45.513	T45.514	T45.515	T45.516
Heparinoid (systemic)	T45.511	T45.512	T45.513	T45.514	T45.515	T45.516
Hepatic secretion stimulant	T47.8X1	T47.8X2	T47.8X3	T47.8X4	T47.8X5	T47.8X6
Hepatitis B						
immune globulin	T50.Z11	T50.Z12	T50.Z13	T50.Z14	T50.Z15	T50.Z16
vaccine	T50.B91	T50.B92	T50.B93	T50.B94	T50.B95	T50.B96
Hepronicate	T46.7X1	T46.7X2	T46.7X3	T46.7X4	T46.7X5	T46.7X6
Heptabarb	T42.3X1	T42.3X2	T42.3X3	T42.3X4	T42.3X5	T42.3X6
Heptabarbital	T42.3X1	T42.3X2	T42.3X3	T42.3X4	T42.3X5	T42.3X6
Heptabarbitone	T42.3X1	T42.3X2	T42.3X3	T42.3X4	T42.3X5	T42.3X6
Heptachlor	T60.1X1	T60.1X2	T60.1X3	T60.1X4	—	—
Heptalgin	T40.2X1	T40.2X2	T40.2X3	T40.2X4	T40.2X5	T40.2X6
Heptaminol	T46.3X1	T46.3X2	T46.3X3	T46.3X4	T46.3X5	T46.3X6
Herbicide NEC	T60.3X1	T60.3X2	T60.3X3	T60.3X4	—	—
Heroin	T40.1X1	T40.1X2	T40.1X3	T40.1X4	—	—
Herplex	T49.5X1	T49.5X2	T49.5X3	T49.5X4	T49.5X5	T49.5X6
HES	T45.8X1	T45.8X2	T45.8X3	T45.8X4	T45.8X5	T45.8X6
Hesperidin	T46.991	T46.992	T46.993	T46.994	T46.995	T46.996
Hetacillin	T36.0X1	T36.0X2	T36.0X3	T36.0X4	T36.0X5	T36.0X6
Hetastarch	T45.8X1	T45.8X2	T45.8X3	T45.8X4	T45.8X5	T45.8X6
HETP	T60.0X1	T60.0X2	T60.0X3	T60.0X4	—	—
Hexachlorobenzene (vapor)	T60.3X1	T60.3X2	T60.3X3	T60.3X4	—	—
Hexachlorocyclohexane	T53.6X1	T53.6X2	T53.6X3	T53.6X4	—	—
Hexachlorophene	T49.0X1	T49.0X2	T49.0X3	T49.0X4	T49.0X5	T49.0X6
Hexadiline	T46.3X1	T46.3X2	T46.3X3	T46.3X4	T46.3X5	T46.3X6
Hexadimethrine (bromide)	T45.7X1	T45.7X2	T45.7X3	T45.7X4	T45.7X5	T45.7X6
Hexadylamine	T46.3X1	T46.3X2	T46.3X3	T46.3X4	T46.3X4	T46.3X6
Hexaethyl tetraphosphate	T60.0X1	T60.0X2	T60.0X3	T60.0X4	—	—
Hexafluorenium bromide	T48.1X1	T48.1X2	T48.1X3	T48.1X4	T48.1X5	T48.1X6
Hexafluronium (bromide)	T48.1X1	T48.1X2	T48.1X3	T48.1X4	T48.1X5	T48.1X6
Hexa-germ	T49.2X1	T49.2X2	T49.2X3	T49.2X4	T49.2X5	T49.2X6
Hexahydrobenzol	T52.8X1	T52.8X2	T52.8X3	T52.8X4	—	—
Hexahydrocresol(s)	T51.8X1	T51.8X2	T51.8X3	T51.8X4	—	—
arsenide	T57.0X1	T57.0X2	T57.0X3	T57.0X4	—	—
arseniurated	T57.0X1	T57.0X2	T57.0X3	T57.0X4	—	—
cyanide	T57.3X1	T57.3X2	T57.3X3	T57.3X4	—	—

Substance	Poisoning, Accidental (unintentional)	Poisoning, Intentional self-harm	Poisoning, Assault	Poisoning, Undetermined	Adverse effect	Underdosing
Hexahydrocresol(s) — *Continued*						
gas	T59.891	T59.892	T59.893	T59.894	—	—
Fluoride (liquid)	T57.8X1	T57.8X2	T57.8X3	T57.8X4	—	—
vapor	T59.891	T59.892	T59.893	T59.894		
phophorated	T60.0X1	T60.0X2	T60.0X3	T60.0X4	—	—
sulfate	T57.8X1	T57.8X2	T57.8X3	T57.8X4	—	—
sulfide (gas)	T59.6X1	T59.6X2	T59.6X3	T59.6X4	—	—
arseniurated	T57.0X1	T57.0X2	T57.0X3	T57.0X4	—	—
sulfurated	T57.8X1	T57.8X2	T57.8X3	T57.8X4	—	—
Hexahydrophenol	T51.8X1	T51.8X2	T51.8X3	T51.8X4	—	—
Hexalen	T51.8X1	T51.8X2	T51.8X3	T51.8X4	—	—
Hexamethonium bromide	T44.2X1	T44.2X2	T44.2X3	T44.2X4	T44.2X5	T44.2X6
Hexamethylene	T52.8X1	T52.8X2	T52.8X3	T52.8X4		
Hexamethylmelamine	T45.1X1	T45.1X2	T45.1X3	T45.1X4	T45.1X5	T45.1X6
Hexamidine	T49.0X1	T49.0X2	T49.0X3	T49.0X4	T49.0X5	T49.0X6
Hexamine (mandelate)	T37.8X1	T37.8X2	T37.8X3	T37.8X4	T37.8X5	T37.8X6
Hexanone, 2-hexanone	T52.4X1	T52.4X2	T52.4X3	T52.4X4	—	—
Hexanuorenium	T48.1X1	T48.1X2	T48.1X3	T48.1X4	T48.1X5	T48.1X6
Hexapropymate	T42.6X1	T42.6X2	T42.6X3	T42.6X4	T42.6X5	T42.6X6
Hexasonium iodide	T44.3X1	T44.3X2	T44.3X3	T44.3X4	T44.3X5	T44.3X6
Hexcarbacholine bromide	T48.1X1	T48.1X2	T48.1X3	T48.1X4	T48.1X5	T48.1X6
Hexemal	T42.3X1	T42.3X2	T42.3X3	T42.3X4	T42.3X5	T42.3X6
Hexestrol	T38.5X1	T38.5X2	T38.5X3	T38.5X4	T38.5X5	T38.5X6
Hexethal (sodium)	T42.3X1	T42.3X2	T42.3X3	T42.3X4	T42.3X5	T42.3X6
Hexetidine	T37.8X1	T37.8X2	T37.8X3	T37.8X4	T37.8X5	T37.8X6
Hexobarbital	T42.3X1	T42.3X2	T42.3X3	T42.3X4	T42.3X5	T42.3X6
rectal	T41.291	T41.292	T41.293	T41.294	T41.295	T41.296
sodium	T41.1X1	T41.1X2	T41.1X3	T41.1X4	T41.1X5	T41.1X6
Hexobendine	T46.3X1	T46.3X2	T46.3X3	T46.3X4	T46.3X5	T46.3X6
Hexocyclium	T44.3X1	T44.3X2	T44.3X3	T44.3X4	T44.3X5	T44.3X6
metilsulfate	T44.3X1	T44.3X2	T44.3X3	T44.3X4	T44.3X5	T44.3X6
Hexoestrol	T38.5X1	T38.5X2	T38.5X3	T38.5X4	T38.5X5	T38.5X6
Hexone	T52.4X1	T52.4X2	T52.4X3	T52.4X4	—	—
Hexoprenaline	T48.6X1	T48.6X2	T48.6X3	T48.6X4	T48.6X5	T48.6X6
Hexylcaine	T41.3X1	T41.3X2	T41.3X3	T41.3X4	T41.3X5	T41.3X6
Hexylresorcinol	T52.2X1	T52.2X2	T52.2X3	T52.2X4	—	—
HGH (human growth hormone)	T38.811	T38.812	T38.813	T38.814	T38.815	T38.816
Hinkle's pills	T47.2X1	T47.2X2	T47.2X3	T47.2X4	T47.2X5	T47.2X6
Histalog	T50.8X1	T50.8X2	T50.8X3	T50.8X4	T50.8X5	T50.8X6
Histamine (phosphate)	T50.8X1	T50.8X2	T50.8X3	T50.8X4	T50.8X5	T50.8X6
Histoplasmin	T50.8X1	T50.8X2	T50.8X3	T50.8X4	T50.8X5	T50.8X6
Holly berries	T62.2X1	T62.2X2	T62.2X3	T62.2X4	—	—
Homatropine	T44.3X1	T44.3X2	T44.3X3	T44.3X4	T44.3X5	T44.3X6
methylbromide	T44.3X1	T44.3X2	T44.3X3	T44.3X4	T44.3X5	T44.3X6
Homochlorcyclizine	T45.0X1	T45.0X2	T45.0X3	T45.0X4	T45.0X5	T45.0X6
Homosalate	T49.3X1	T49.3X2	T49.3X3	T49.3X4	T49.3X5	T49.3X6
Homo-tet	T50.Z11	T50.Z12	T50.Z13	T50.Z14	T50.Z15	T50.Z16

Substance	Poisoning, Accidental (unintentional)	Poisoning, Intentional self-harm	Poisoning, Assault	Poisoning, Undetermined	Adverse effect	Underdosing
Hormone	T38.801	T38.802	T38.803	T38.804	T38.805	T38.806
adrenal cortical steroids	T38.0X1	T38.0X2	T38.0X3	T38.0X4	T38.0X5	T38.0X6
androgenic	T38.7X1	T38.7X2	T38.7X3	T38.7X4	T38.7X5	T38.7X6
anterior pituitary NEC	T38.811	T38.812	T38.813	T38.814	T38.815	T38.816
antidiabetic agents	T38.3X1	T38.3X2	T38.3X3	T38.3X4	T38.3X5	T38.3X6
antidiuretic	T38.891	T38.892	T38.893	T38.894	T38.895	T38.896
cancer therapy	T45.1X1	T45.1X2	T45.1X3	T45.1X4	T45.1X5	T45.1X6
follicle stimulating	T38.811	T38.812	T38.813	T38.814	T38.815	T38.816
gonadotropic	T38.891	T38.892	T38.893	T38.894	T38.895	T38.896
pituitary	T38.811	T38.812	T38.813	T38.814	T38.815	T38.816
growth	T38.811	T38.812	T38.813	T38.814	T38.815	T38.816
luteinizing	T38.811	T38.812	T38.813	T38.814	T38.815	T38.816
ovarian	T38.5X1	T38.5X2	T38.5X3	T38.5X4	T38.5X5	T38.5X6
oxytocic	T48.0X1	T48.0X2	T48.0X3	T48.0X4	T48.0X5	T48.0X6
parathyroid (derivatives)	T50.991	T50.992	T50.993	T50.994	T50.995	T50.996
pituitary (posterior) NEC	T38.891	T38.892	T38.893	T38.894	T38.895	T38.896
anterior	T38.811	T38.812	T38.813	T38.814	T38.815	T38.816
specified, NEC	T38.891	T38.892	T38.893	T38.894	T38.895	T38.896
thyroid	T38.1X1	T38.1X2	T38.1X3	T38.1X4	T38.1X5	T38.1X6
Hornet (sting)	T63.451	T63.452	T63.453	T63.454	—	—
Horse anti-human lymphocytic serum	T50.Z11	T50.Z12	T50.Z13	T50.Z14	T50.Z15	T50.Z16
Horticulture agent NEC	T65.91	T65.92	T65.93	T65.94	—	—
with pesticide	T60.91	T60.92	T60.93	T60.94	—	—
Human						
albumin	T45.8X1	T45.8X2	T45.8X3	T45.8X4	T45.8X5	T45.8X6
growth hormone (HGH)	T38.811	T38.812	T38.813	T38.814	T38.815	T38.816
immune serum	T50.Z11	T50.Z12	T50.Z13	T50.Z14	T50.Z15	T50.Z16
Hyaluronidase	T45.3X1	T45.3X2	T45.3X3	T45.3X4	T45.3X5	T45.3X6
Hyazyme	T45.3X1	T45.3X2	T45.3X3	T45.3X4	T45.3X5	T45.3X6
Hycodan	T40.2X1	T40.2X2	T40.2X3	T40.2X4	T40.2X5	T40.2X6
Hydantoin derivative NEC	T42.0X1	T42.0X2	T42.0X3	T42.0X4	T42.0X5	T42.0X6
Hydeltra	T38.0X1	T38.0X2	T38.0X3	T38.0X4	T38.0X5	T38.0X6
Hydergine	T44.6X1	T44.6X2	T44.6X3	T44.6X4	T44.6X5	T44.6X6
Hydrabamine penicillin	T36.0X1	T36.0X2	T36.0X3	T36.0X4	T36.0X5	T36.0X6
Hydralazine	T46.5X1	T46.5X2	T46.5X3	T46.5X4	T46.5X5	T46.5X6
Hydrargaphen	T49.0X1	T49.0X2	T49.0X3	T49.0X4	T49.0X5	T49.0X6
Hydrargyri amino-chloridum	T49.0X1	T49.0X2	T49.0X3	T49.0X4	T49.0X5	T49.0X6
Hydrastine	T48.291	T48.292	T48.293	T48.294	T48.295	T48.296
Hydrazine	T54.1X1	T54.1X2	T54.1X3	T54.1X4	—	—
monoamine oxidase inhibitors	T43.1X1	T43.1X2	T43.1X3	T43.1X4	T43.1X5	T43.1X6
Hydrazoic acid, azides	T54.2X1	T54.2X2	T54.2X3	T54.2X4	—	—
Hydriodic acid	T48.4X1	T48.4X2	T48.4X3	T48.4X4	T48.4X5	T48.4X6
Hydrocarbon gas	T59.891	T59.892	T59.893	T59.894	—	—
incomplete combustion of—see Carbon, monoxide, fuel, utility						

Substance	Poisoning, Accidental (unintentional)	Poisoning, Intentional self-harm	Poisoning, Assault	Poisoning, Undetermined	Adverse effect	Underdosing
Hydrocarbon gas — *Continued*						
liquefied (mobile container)	T59.891	T59.892	T59.893	T59.894	—	—
piped (natural)	T59.891	T59.892	T59.893	T59.894	—	—
Hydrochloric acid (liquid)	T54.2X1	T54.2X2	T54.2X3	T54.2X4	—	—
medicinal (digestant)	T47.5X1	T47.5X2	T47.5X3	T47.5X4	T47.5X5	T47.5X6
vapor	T59.891	T59.892	T59.893	T59.894	—	—
Hydrochlorothiazide	T50.2X1	T50.2X2	T50.2X3	T50.2X4	T50.2X5	T50.2X6
Hydrocodone	T40.2X1	T40.2X2	T40.2X3	T40.2X4	T40.2X5	T40.2X6
Hydrocortisone (derivatives)	T38.0X1	T38.0X2	T38.0X3	T38.0X4	T38.0X5	T38.0X6
aceponate	T49.0X1	T49.0X2	T49.0X3	T49.0X4	T49.0X5	T49.0X6
ENT agent	T49.6X1	T49.6X2	T49.6X3	T49.6X4	T49.6X5	T49.6X6
ophthalmic preparation	T49.5X1	T49.5X2	T49.5X3	T49.5X4	T49.5X5	T49.5X5
topical NEC	T49.0X1	T49.0X2	T49.0X3	T49.0X4	T49.0X5	T49.0X6
Hydrocortone	T38.0X1	T38.0X2	T38.0X3	T38.0X4	T38.0X5	T38.0X6
ENT agent	T49.6X1	T49.6X2	T49.6X3	T49.6X4	T49.6X5	T49.6X6
ophthalmic preparation	T49.5X1	T49.5X2	T49.5X3	T49.5X4	T49.5X5	T49.5X5
topical NEC	T49.0X1	T49.0X2	T49.0X3	T49.0X4	T49.0X5	T49.0X6
Hydrocyanic acid (liquid)	T57.3X1	T57.3X2	T57.3X3	T57.3X4	—	—
gas	T65.0X1	T65.0X2	T65.0X3	T65.0X4	—	—
Hydroflumethiazide	T50.2X1	T50.2X2	T50.2X3	T50.2X4	T50.2X5	T50.2X6
Hydrofluoric acid (liquid)	T54.2X1	T54.2X2	T54.2X3	T54.2X4	—	—
vapor	T59.891	T59.892	T59.893	T59.894	—	—
Hydrogen	T59.891	T59.892	T59.893	T59.894	—	—
arsenide	T57.0X1	T57.0X2	T57.0X3	T57.0X4	—	—
arseniureted	T57.0X1	T57.0X2	T57.0X3	T57.0X4	—	—
chloride	T57.8X1	T57.8X2	T57.8X3	T57.8X4	—	—
cyanide (salts)	T57.3X1	T57.3X2	T57.3X3	T57.3X4	—	—
gas	T57.3X1	T57.3X2	T57.3X3	T57.3X4	—	—
Fluoride	T59.5X1	T59.5X2	T59.5X3	T59.5X4	—	—
vapor	T59.5X1	T59.5X2	T59.5X3	T59.5X4	—	—
peroxide	T49.0X1	T49.0X2	T49.0X3	T49.0X4	T49.0X5	T49.0X6
phosphureted	T57.1X1	T57.1X2	T57.1X3	T57.1X4	—	—
sulfide	T59.6X1	T59.6X2	T59.6X3	T59.6X4	—	—
arseniureted	T57.0X1	T57.0X2	T57.0X3	T57.0X4	—	—
sulfureted	T59.6X1	T59.6X2	T59.6X3	T59.6X4	—	—
Hydromethylpyridine	T46.7X1	T46.7X2	T46.7X3	T46.7X4	T46.7X5	T46.7X6
Hydromorphinol	T40.2X1	T40.2X2	T40.2X3	T40.2X4	—	—
Hydromorphinone	T40.2X1	T40.2X2	T40.2X3	T40.2X4	T40.2X5	T40.2X6
Hydromorphone	T40.2X1	T40.2X2	T40.2X3	T40.2X4	T40.2X5	T40.2X6
Hydromox	T50.2X1	T50.2X2	T50.2X3	T50.2X4	T50.2X5	T50.2X6
Hydrophilic lotion	T49.3X1	T49.3X2	T49.3X3	T49.3X4	T49.3X5	T49.3X6
Hydroquinidine	T46.2X1	T46.2X2	T46.2X3	T46.2X4	T46.2X5	T46.2X6
Hydroquinone	T52.2X1	T52.2X2	T52.2X3	T52.2X4	—	—
vapor	T59.891	T59.892	T59.893	T59.894	—	—
Hydrosulfuric acid (gas)	T59.6X1	T59.6X2	T59.6X3	T59.6X4	—	—

Substance	Poisoning, Accidental (unintentional)	Poisoning, Intentional self-harm	Poisoning, Assault	Poisoning, Undetermined	Adverse effect	Underdosing
Hydrotalcite	T47.1X1	T47.1X2	T47.1X3	T47.1X4	T47.1X5	T47.1X6
Hydrous wool fat	T49.3X1	T49.3X2	T49.3X3	T49.3X4	T49.3X5	T49.3X6
Hydroxide, caustic	T54.3X1	T54.3X2	T54.3X3	T54.3X4	—	—
Hydroxocobalamin	T45.8X1	T45.8X2	T45.8X3	T45.8X4	T45.8X5	T45.8X6
Hydroxyamp-hetamine	T49.5X1	T49.5X2	T49.5X3	T49.5X4	T49.5X5	T49.5X6
Hydroxycarbamide	T45.1X1	T45.1X2	T45.1X3	T45.1X4	T45.1X5	T45.1X6
Hydroxychloroquine	T37.8X1	T37.8X2	T37.8X3	T37.8X4	T37.8X5	T37.8X6
Hydroxydihydro-codeinone	T40.2X1	T40.2X2	T40.2X3	T40.2X4	T40.2X5	T40.2X6
Hydroxyestrone	T38.5X1	T38.5X2	T38.5X3	T38.5X4	T38.5X5	T38.5X6
Hydroxyethyl starch	T45.8X1	T45.8X2	T45.8X3	T45.8X4	T45.8X5	T45.8X6
Hydroxyme-thylpentanone	T52.4X1	T52.4X2	T52.4X3	T52.4X4	—	—
Hydroxyphenamate	T43.591	T43.592	T43.593	T43.594	T43.595	T43.596
Hydroxypheny-lbutazone	T39.2X1	T39.2X2	T39.2X3	T39.2X4	T39.2X5	T39.2X6
Hydroxyprogesterone	T38.5X1	T38.5X2	T38.5X3	T38.5X4	T38.5X5	T38.5X6
caproate	T38.5X1	T38.5X2	T38.5X3	T38.5X4	T38.5X5	T38.5X6
Hydroxyquinoline (derivatives) NEC	T37.8X1	T37.8X2	T37.8X3	T37.8X4	T37.8X5	T37.8X6
Hydroxystilbamidine	T37.3X1	T37.3X2	T37.3X3	T37.3X4	T37.3X5	T37.3X6
Hydroxytoluene (nonmedicinal)	T54.0X1	T54.0X2	T54.0X3	T54.0X4	—	—
medicinal	T49.0X1	T49.0X2	T49.0X3	T49.0X4	T49.0X5	T49.0X6
Hydroxyurea	T45.1X1	T45.1X2	T45.1X3	T45.1X4	T45.1X5	T45.1X6
Hydroxyzine	T43.591	T43.592	T43.593	T43.594	T43.595	T43.596
Hyoscine	T44.3X1	T44.3X2	T44.3X3	T44.3X4	T44.3X5	T44.3X6
Hyoscyamine	T44.3X1	T44.3X2	T44.3X3	T44.3X4	T44.3X5	T44.3X6
Hyoscyamus	T44.3X1	T44.3X2	T44.3X3	T44.3X4	T44.3X5	T44.3X6
dry extract	T44.3X1	T44.3X2	T44.3X3	T44.3X4	T44.3X5	T44.3X6
Hypaque	T50.8X1	T50.8X2	T50.8X3	T50.8X4	T50.8X5	T50.8X6
Hypertussis	T50.Z11	T50.Z12	T50.Z13	T50.Z14	T50.Z15	T50.Z16
Hypnotic	T42.71	T42.72	T42.73	T42.74	T42.75	T42.76
anticonvulsant	T42.71	T42.72	T42.73	T42.74	T42.75	T42.76
specified NEC	T42.6X1	T42.6X2	T42.6X3	T42.6X4	T42.6X5	T42.6X6
Hypochlorite	T49.0X1	T49.0X2	T49.0X3	T49.0X4	T49.0X5	T49.0X6
Hypophysis, posterior	T38.891	T38.892	T38.893	T38.894	T38.895	T38.896
Hypotensive NEC	T46.5X1	T46.5X2	T46.5X3	T46.5X4	T46.5X5	T46.5X6
Hypromellose	T49.5X1	T49.5X2	T49.5X3	T49.5X4	T49.5X5	T49.5X6
I						
Ibacitabine	T37.5X1	T37.5X2	T37.5X3	T37.5X4	T37.5X5	T37.5X6
Ibopamine	T44.991	T44.992	T44.993	T44.994	T44.995	T44.996
Ibufenac	T39.311	T39.312	T39.313	T39.314	T39.315	T39.316
Ibuprofen	T39.311	T39.312	T39.313	T39.314	T39.315	T39.316
Ibuproxam	T39.311	T39.312	T39.313	T39.314	T39.315	T39.316
Ibuterol	T48.6X1	T48.6X2	T48.6X3	T48.6X4	T48.6X5	T48.6X6
Ichthammol	T49.0X1	T49.0X2	T49.0X3	T49.0X4	T49.0X5	T49.0X6
Ichthyol	T49.4X1	T49.4X2	T49.4X3	T49.4X4	T49.4X5	T49.4X6
Idarubicin	T45.1X1	T45.1X2	T45.1X3	T45.1X4	T45.1X5	T45.1X6
Idrocilamide	T42.8X1	T42.8X2	T42.8X3	T42.8X4	T42.8X5	T42.8X6
Ifenprodil	T46.7X1	T46.7X2	T46.7X3	T46.7X4	T46.7X5	T46.7X6

Substance	Poisoning, Accidental (unintentional)	Poisoning, Intentional self-harm	Poisoning, Assault	Poisoning, Undetermined	Adverse effect	Underdosing
Ifosfamide	T45.1X1	T45.1X2	T45.1X3	T45.1X4	T45.1X5	T45.1X6
Iletin	T38.3X1	T38.3X2	T38.3X3	T38.3X4	T38.3X5	T38.3X6
Ilex	T62.2X1	T62.2X2	T62.2X3	T62.2X4	—	—
Illuminating gas (after combustion)	T58.11	T58.12	T58.13	T58.14	—	—
prior to combustion	T59.891	T59.892	T59.893	T59.894	—	—
Ilopan	T45.2X1	T45.2X2	T45.2X3	T45.2X4	T45.2X5	T45.2X6
Iloprost	T46.7X1	T46.7X2	T46.7X3	T46.7X4	T46.7X5	T46.7X6
Ilotycin	T36.3X1	T36.3X2	T36.3X3	T36.3X4	T36.3X5	T36.3X6
ophthalmic preparation	T49.5X1	T49.5X2	T49.5X3	T49.5X4	T49.5X5	T49.5X6
topical NEC	T49.0X1	T49.0X2	T49.0X3	T49.0X4	T49.0X5	T49.0X6
Imidazole-4-carboxamide	T45.1X1	T45.1X2	T45.1X3	T45.1X4	T45.1X5	T45.1X6
Imipenem	T36.0X1	T36.0X2	T36.0X3	T36.0X4	T36.0X5	T36.0X6
Imipramine	T43.011	T43.012	T43.013	T43.014	T43.015	T43.016
Iminostilbene	T42.1X1	T42.1X2	T42.1X3	T42.1X4	T42.1X5	T42.1X6
Immu-G	T50.Z11	T50.Z12	T50.Z13	T50.Z14	T50.Z15	T50.Z16
Immuglobin	T50.Z11	T50.Z12	T50.Z13	T50.Z14	T50.Z15	T50.Z16
Immune						
globulin	T50.Z11	T50.Z12	T50.Z13	T50.Z14	T50.Z15	T50.Z16
serum globulin	T50.Z11	T50.Z12	T50.Z13	T50.Z14	T50.Z15	T50.Z16
Immunoglobin human (intravenous) (normal)	T50.Z11	T50.Z12	T50.Z13	T50.Z14	T50.Z15	T50.Z16
unmodified	T50.Z11	T50.Z12	T50.Z13	T50.Z14	T50.Z15	T50.Z16
Immunosuppressive drug	T45.1X1	T45.1X2	T45.1X3	T45.1X4	T45.1X5	T45.1X6
Immu-tetanus	T50.Z11	T50.Z12	T50.Z13	T50.Z14	T50.Z15	T50.Z16
Indalpine	T43.221	T43.222	T43.223	T43.224	T43.225	T43.226
Indanazoline	T48.5X1	T48.5X2	T48.5X3	T48.5X4	T48.5X5	T48.5X6
Indandione (derivatives)	T45.511	T45.512	T45.513	T45.514	T45.515	T45.516
Indapamide	T46.5X1	T46.5X2	T46.5X3	T46.5X4	T46.5X5	T46.5X6
Indendione (derivatives)	T45.511	T45.512	T45.513	T45.514	T45.515	T45.516
Indenolol	T44.7X1	T44.7X2	T44.7X3	T44.7X4	T44.7X5	T44.7X6
Inderal	T44.7X1	T44.7X2	T44.7X3	T44.7X4	T44.7X5	T44.7X6
Indian						
hemp	T40.7X1	T40.7X2	T40.7X3	T40.7X4	T40.7X5	T40.7X6
tobacco	T62.2X1	T62.2X2	T62.2X3	T62.2X4	—	—
Indigo carmine	T50.8X1	T50.8X2	T50.8X3	T50.8X4	T50.8X5	T50.8X6
Indobufen	T45.521	T45.522	T45.523	T45.524	T45.525	T45.526
Indocin	T39.2X1	T39.2X2	T39.2X3	T39.2X4	T39.2X5	T39.2X6
Indocyanine green	T50.8X1	T50.8X2	T50.8X3	T50.8X4	T50.8X5	T50.8X6
Indometacin	T39.391	T39.392	T39.393	T39.394	T39.395	T39.396
Indomethacin	T39.391	T39.392	T39.393	T39.394	T39.395	T39.396
farnesil	T39.4X1	T39.4X2	T39.4X3	T39.4X4	T39.4X5	T39.4X6
Indoramin	T44.6X1	T44.6X2	T44.6X3	T44.6X4	T44.6X5	T44.6X6
Industrial						
alcohol	T51.0X1	T51.0X2	T51.0X3	T51.0X4	—	—
fumes	T59.891	T59.892	T59.893	T59.894	—	—
solvents (fumes) (vapors)	T52.91	T52.92	T52.93	T52.94	—	—
Influenza vaccine	T50.B91	T50.B92	T50.B93	T50.B94	T50.B95	T50.B96
Ingested substance NEC	T65.91	T65.92	T65.93	T65.94	—	—

Substance	Poisoning, Accidental (unintentional)	Poisoning, Intentional self-harm	Poisoning, Assault	Poisoning, Undetermined	Adverse effect	Underdosing
INH	T37.1X1	T37.1X2	T37.1X3	T37.1X4	T37.1X5	T37.1X6
Inhalation, gas (noxious)—see Gas						
Inhibitor						
angiotensin-converting enzyme	T46.4X1	T46.4X2	T46.4X3	T46.4X4	T46.4X5	T46.4X6
carbonic anhydrase	T50.2X1	T50.2X2	T50.2X3	T50.2X4	T50.2X5	T50.2X6
fibrinolysis	T45.621	T45.622	T45.623	T45.624	T45.625	T45.626
monoamine oxidase NEC	T43.1X1	T43.1X2	T43.1X3	T43.1X4	T43.1X5	T43.1X6
hydrazine	T43.1X1	T43.1X2	T43.1X3	T43.1X4	T43.1X5	T43.1X6
postsynaptic	T43.8X1	T43.8X2	T43.8X3	T43.8X4	T43.8X5	T43.8X6
prothrombin synthesis	T45.511	T45.512	T45.513	T45.514	T45.515	T45.516
Ink	T65.891	T65.892	T65.893	T65.894	—	—
Inorganic substance NEC	T57.91	T57.92	T57.93	T57.94	—	—
Inosine pranobex	T37.5X1	T37.5X2	T37.5X3	T37.5X4	T37.5X5	T37.5X6
Inositol	T50.991	T50.992	T50.993	T50.994	T50.995	T50.996
nicotinate	T46.7X1	T46.7X2	T46.7X3	T46.7X4	T46.7X5	T46.7X6
Inproquone	T45.1X1	T45.1X2	T45.1X3	T45.1X4	T45.1X5	T45.1X6
Insect (sting), venomous	T63.481	T63.482	T63.483	T63.484	—	—
ant	T63.421	T63.422	T63.423	T63.424	—	—
bee	T63.441	T63.442	T63.443	T63.444	—	—
caterpillar	T63.431	T63.432	T63.433	T63.434	—	—
hornet	T63.451	T63.452	T63.453	T63.454	—	—
wasp	T63.461	T63.462	T63.463	T63.464	—	—
Insecticide NEC	T60.91	T60.92	T60.93	T60.94	—	—
carbamate	T60.0X1	T60.0X2	T60.0X3	T60.0X4	—	—
chlorinated	T60.1X1	T60.1X2	T60.1X3	T60.1X4	—	—
mixed	T60.91	T60.92	T60.93	T60.94	—	—
organochlorine	T60.1X1	T60.1X2	T60.1X3	T60.1X4	—	—
organophosphorus	T60.0X1	T60.0X2	T60.0X3	T60.0X4	—	—
Insular tissue extract	T38.3X1	T38.3X2	T38.3X3	T38.3X4	T38.3X5	T38.3X6
Insulin (amorphous) (globin) (isophane) (Lente) (NPH) (Semilente) (Ultralente)	T38.3X1	T38.3X2	T38.3X3	T38.3X4	T38.3X5	T38.3X6
defalan	T38.3X1	T38.3X2	T38.3X3	T38.3X4	T38.3X5	T38.3X6
human	T38.3X1	T38.3X2	T38.3X3	T38.3X4	T38.3X5	T38.3X6
injection, soluble	T38.3X1	T38.3X2	T38.3X3	T38.3X4	T38.3X5	T38.3X6
biphasic	T38.3X1	T38.3X2	T38.3X3	T38.3X4	T38.3X5	T38.3X6
intermediate acting	T38.3X1	T38.3X2	T38.3X3	T38.3X4	T38.3X5	T38.3X6
protamine zinc	T38.3X1	T38.3X2	T38.3X3	T38.3X4	T38.3X5	T38.3X6
slow acting	T38.3X1	T38.3X2	T38.3X3	T38.3X4	T38.3X5	T38.3X6
zinc						
protamine injection	T38.3X1	T38.3X2	T38.3X3	T38.3X4	T38.3X5	T38.3X6
suspension (amorphous) (crystalline)	T38.3X1	T38.3X2	T38.3X3	T38.3X4	T38.3X5	T38.3X6
Interferon (alpha) (beta) (gamma)	T37.5X1	T37.5X2	T37.5X3	T37.5X4	T37.5X5	T37.5X6
Intestinal motility control drug	T47.6X1	T47.6X2	T47.6X3	T47.6X4	T47.6X5	T47.6X6
biological	T47.8X1	T47.8X2	T47.8X3	T47.8X4	T47.8X5	T47.8X6

Substance	Poisoning, Accidental (unintentional)	Poisoning, Intentional self-harm	Poisoning, Assault	Poisoning, Undetermined	Adverse effect	Underdosing
Intranarcon	T41.1X1	T41.1X2	T41.1X3	T41.1X4	T41.1X5	T41.1X6
Intravenous						
amino acids	T50.991	T50.992	T50.993	T50.994	T50.995	T50.996
fat suspension	T50.991	T50.992	T50.993	T50.994	T50.995	T50.996
Inulin	T50.8X1	T50.8X2	T50.8X3	T50.8X4	T50.8X5	T50.8X6
Invert sugar	T50.3X1	T50.3X2	T50.3X3	T50.3X4	T50.3X5	T50.3X6
Inza—see Naproxen						
Iobenzamic acid	T50.8X1	T50.8X2	T50.8X3	T50.8X4	T50.8X5	T50.8X6
Iocarmic acid	T50.8X1	T50.8X2	T50.8X3	T50.8X4	T50.8X5	T50.8X6
Iocetamic acid	T50.8X1	T50.8X2	T50.8X3	T50.8X4	T50.8X5	T50.8X6
Iodamide	T50.8X1	T50.8X2	T50.8X3	T50.8X4	T50.8X5	T50.8X6
Iodide NEC—see also Iodine	T49.0X1	T49.0X2	T49.0X3	T49.0X4	T49.0X5	T49.0X6
mercury (ointment)	T49.0X1	T49.0X2	T49.0X3	T49.0X4	T49.0X5	T49.0X6
methylate	T49.0X1	T49.0X2	T49.0X3	T49.0X4	T49.0X5	T49.0X6
potassium (expectorant) NEC	T48.4X1	T48.4X2	T48.4X3	T48.4X4	T48.4X5	T48.4X6
Iodinated						
contrast medium	T50.8X1	T50.8X2	T50.8X3	T50.8X4	T50.8X5	T50.8X6
glycerol	T48.4X1	T48.4X2	T48.4X3	T48.4X4	T48.4X5	T48.4X6
human serum albumin (131I)	T50.8X1	T50.8X2	T50.8X3	T50.8X4	T50.8X5	T50.8X6
Iodine (antiseptic, external) (tincture) NEC	T49.0X1	T49.0X2	T49.0X3	T49.0X4	T49.0X5	T49.0X6
125—see also Radiation sickness, and Exposure to radioactivce isotopes	T50.8X1	T50.8X2	T50.8X3	T50.8X4	T50.8X5	T50.8X6
therapeutic	T50.991	T50.992	T50.993	T50.994	T50.995	T50.996
131—see also Radiation sickness, and Exposure to radioactivce isotopes	T50.8X1	T50.8X2	T50.8X3	T50.8X4	T50.8X5	T50.8X6
therapeutic	T38.2X1	T38.2X2	T38.2X3	T38.2X4	T38.2X5	T38.2X6
diagnostic	T50.8X1	T50.8X2	T50.8X3	T50.8X4	T50.8X5	T50.8X6
for thyroid conditions (antithyroid)	T38.2X1	T38.2X2	T38.2X3	T38.2X4	T38.2X5	T38.2X6
solution	T49.0X1	T49.0X2	T49.0X3	T49.0X4	T49.0X5	T49.0X6
vapor	T59.891	T59.892	T59.893	T59.894	—	—
Iodipamide	T50.8X1	T50.8X2	T50.8X3	T50.8X4	T50.8X5	T50.8X6
Iodized (poppy seed) oil	T50.8X1	T50.8X2	T50.8X3	T50.8X4	T50.8X5	T50.8X6
Iodobismitol	T37.8X1	T37.8X2	T37.8X3	T37.8X4	T37.8X5	T37.8X6
Iodochlorhyd-roxyquin	T37.8X1	T37.8X2	T37.8X3	T37.8X4	T37.8X5	T37.8X6
topical	T49.0X1	T49.0X2	T49.0X3	T49.0X4	T49.0X5	T49.0X6
Iodochlorhydroxy-quinoline	T37.8X1	T37.8X2	T37.8X3	T37.8X4	T37.8X5	T37.8X6
Iodocholesterol (131I)	T50.8X1	T50.8X2	T50.8X3	T50.8X4	T50.8X5	T50.8X6
Iodoform	T49.0X1	T49.0X2	T49.0X3	T49.0X4	T49.0X5	T49.0X6
Iodohippuric acid	T50.8X1	T50.8X2	T50.8X3	T50.8X4	T50.8X5	T50.8X6
Iodopanoic acid	T50.8X1	T50.8X2	T50.8X3	T50.8X4	T50.8X5	T50.8X6
Iodophthalein (sodium)	T50.8X1	T50.8X2	T50.8X3	T50.8X4	T50.8X5	T50.8X6
Iodopyracet	T50.8X1	T50.8X2	T50.8X3	T50.8X4	T50.8X5	T50.8X6
Iodoquinol	T37.8X1	T37.8X2	T37.8X3	T37.8X4	T37.8X5	T37.8X6
Iodoxamic acid	T50.8X1	T50.8X2	T50.8X3	T50.8X4	T50.8X5	T50.8X6
Iofendylate	T50.8X1	T50.8X2	T50.8X3	T50.8X4	T50.8X5	T50.8X6
Ioglycamic acid	T50.8X1	T50.8X2	T50.8X3	T50.8X4	T50.8X5	T50.8X6
Iohexol	T50.8X1	T50.8X2	T50.8X3	T50.8X4	T50.8X5	T50.8X6
Ion exchange resin						
anion	T47.8X1	T47.8X2	T47.8X3	T47.8X4	T47.8X5	T47.8X6
cation	T50.3X1	T50.3X2	T50.3X3	T50.3X4	T50.3X5	T50.3X6
cholestyramine	T46.6X1	T46.6X2	T46.6X3	T46.6X4	T46.6X5	T46.6X6
intestinal	T47.8X1	T47.8X2	T47.8X3	T47.8X4	T47.8X5	T47.8X6
Iopamidol	T50.8X1	T50.8X2	T50.8X3	T50.8X4	T50.8X5	T50.8X6
Iopanoic acid	T50.8X1	T50.8X2	T50.8X3	T50.8X4	T50.8X5	T50.8X6
Iophenoic acid	T50.8X1	T50.8X2	T50.8X3	T50.8X4	T50.8X5	T50.8X6
Iopodate, sodium	T50.8X1	T50.8X2	T50.8X3	T50.8X4	T50.8X5	T50.8X6
Iopodic acid	T50.8X1	T50.8X2	T50.8X3	T50.8X4	T50.8X5	T50.8X6
Iopromide	T50.8X1	T50.8X2	T50.8X3	T50.8X4	T50.8X5	T50.8X6
Iopydol	T50.8X1	T50.8X2	T50.8X3	T50.8X4	T50.8X5	T50.8X6
Iotalamic acid	T50.8X1	T50.8X2	T50.8X3	T50.8X4	T50.8X5	T50.8X6
Iothalamate	T50.8X1	T50.8X2	T50.8X3	T50.8X4	T50.8X5	T50.8X6
Iothiouracil	T38.2X1	T38.2X2	T38.2X3	T38.2X4	T38.2X5	T38.2X6
Iotrol	T50.8X1	T50.8X2	T50.8X3	T50.8X4	T50.8X5	T50.8X6
Iotrolan	T50.8X1	T50.8X2	T50.8X3	T50.8X4	T50.8X5	T50.8X6
Iotroxate	T50.8X1	T50.8X2	T50.8X3	T50.8X4	T50.8X5	T50.8X6
Iotroxic acid	T50.8X1	T50.8X2	T50.8X3	T50.8X4	T50.8X5	T50.8X6
Ioversol	T50.8X1	T50.8X2	T50.8X3	T50.8X4	T50.8X5	T50.8X6
Ioxaglate	T50.8X1	T50.8X2	T50.8X3	T50.8X4	T50.8X5	T50.8X6
Ioxaglic acid	T50.8X1	T50.8X2	T50.8X3	T50.8X4	T50.8X5	T50.8X6
Ioxitalamic acid	T50.8X1	T50.8X2	T50.8X3	T50.8X4	T50.8X5	T50.8X6
Ipecac	T47.7X1	T47.7X2	T47.7X3	T47.7X4	T47.7X5	T47.7X6
Ipecacuanha	T48.4X1	T48.4X2	T48.4X3	T48.4X4	T48.4X5	T48.4X6
Ipodate, calcium	T50.8X1	T50.8X2	T50.8X3	T50.8X4	T50.8X5	T50.8X6
Ipral	T42.3X1	T42.3X2	T42.3X3	T42.3X4	T42.3X5	T42.3X6
Ipratropium (bromide)	T48.6X1	T48.6X2	T48.6X3	T48.6X4	T48.6X5	T48.6X6
Ipriflavone	T46.3X1	T46.3X2	T46.3X3	T46.3X4	T46.3X5	T46.3X6
Iprindole	T43.011	T43.012	T43.013	T43.014	T43.015	T43.016
Iproclozide	T43.1X1	T43.1X2	T43.1X3	T43.1X4	T43.1X5	T43.1X6
Iprofenin	T50.8X1	T50.8X2	T50.8X3	T50.8X4	T50.8X5	T50.8X6
Iproheptine	T49.2X1	T49.2X2	T49.2X3	T49.2X4	T49.2X5	T49.2X6
Iproniazid	T43.1X1	T43.1X2	T43.1X3	T43.1X4	T43.1X5	T43.1X6
Iproplatin	T45.1X1	T45.1X2	T45.1X3	T45.1X4	T45.1X5	T45.1X6
Iproveratril	T46.1X1	T46.1X2	T46.1X3	T46.1X4	T46.1X5	T46.1X6
Iron (compounds) (medicinal) NEC	T45.4X1	T45.4X2	T45.4X3	T45.4X4	T45.4X5	T45.4X6
ammonium	T45.4X1	T45.4X2	T45.4X3	T45.4X4	T45.4X5	T45.4X6
dextran injection	T45.4X1	T45.4X2	T45.4X3	T45.4X4	T45.4X5	T45.4X6
nonmedicinal	T56.891	T56.892	T56.893	T56.894	—	—
salts	T45.4X1	T45.4X2	T45.4X3	T45.4X4	T45.4X5	T45.4X6
sorbitex	T45.4X1	T45.4X2	T45.4X3	T45.4X4	T45.4X5	T45.4X6
sorbitol citric acid complex	T45.4X1	T45.4X2	T45.4X3	T45.4X4	T45.4X5	T45.4X6
Irrigating fluid (vaginal)	T49.8X1	T49.8X2	T49.8X3	T49.8X4	T49.8X5	T49.8X6
eye	T49.5X1	T49.5X2	T49.5X3	T49.5X4	T49.5X5	T49.5X6
Isepamicin	T36.5X1	T36.5X2	T36.5X3	T36.5X4	T36.5X5	T36.5X6
Isoaminile (citrate)	T48.3X1	T48.3X2	T48.3X3	T48.3X4	T48.3X5	T48.3X6
Isoamyl nitrite	T46.3X1	T46.3X2	T46.3X3	T46.3X4	T46.3X5	T46.3X6
Isobenzan	T60.1X1	T60.1X2	T60.1X3	T60.1X4	—	—

Substance	Poisoning, Accidental (unintentional)	Poisoning, Intentional self-harm	Poisoning, Assault	Poisoning, Undetermined	Adverse effect	Underdosing
Isobutyl acetate	T52.8X1	T52.8X2	T52.8X3	T52.8X4	—	—
Isocarboxazid	T43.1X1	T43.1X2	T43.1X3	T43.1X4	T43.1X5	T43.1X6
Isoconazole	T49.0X1	T49.0X2	T49.0X3	T49.0X4	T49.0X5	T49.0X6
Isocyanate	T65.0X1	T65.0X2	T65.0X3	T65.0X4	—	—
Isoephedrine	T44.991	T44.992	T44.993	T44.994	T44.995	T44.996
Isoetarine	T48.6X1	T48.6X2	T48.6X3	T48.6X4	T48.6X5	T48.6X6
Isoethadione	T42.2X1	T42.2X2	T42.2X3	T42.2X4	T42.2X5	T42.2X6
Isoetharine	T44.5X1	T44.5X2	T44.5X3	T44.5X4	T44.5X5	T44.5X6
Isoflurane	T41.0X1	T41.0X2	T41.0X3	T41.0X4	T41.0X5	T41.0X6
Isoflurophate	T44.0X1	T44.0X2	T44.0X3	T44.0X4	T44.0X5	T44.0X6
Isomaltose, ferric complex	T45.4X1	T45.4X2	T45.4X3	T45.4X4	T45.4X5	T45.4X6
Isometheptene	T44.3X1	T44.3X2	T44.3X3	T44.3X4	T44.3X5	T44.3X6
Isoniazid	T37.1X1	T37.1X2	T37.1X3	T37.1X4	T37.1X5	T37.1X6
with						
rifampicin	T36.6X1	T36.6X2	T36.6X3	T36.6X4	T36.6X5	T36.6X6
thioacetazone	T37.1X1	T37.1X2	T37.1X3	T37.1X4	T37.1X5	T37.1X6
Isonicotinic acid hydrazide	T37.1X1	T37.1X2	T37.1X3	T37.1X4	T37.1X5	T37.1X6
Isonipecaine	T40.491	T40.492	T40.493	T40.494	T40.495	T40.496
Isopentaquine	T37.2X1	T37.2X2	T37.2X3	T37.2X4	T37.2X5	T37.2X6
Isophane insulin	T38.3X1	T38.3X2	T38.3X3	T38.3X4	T38.3X5	T38.3X6
Isophorone	T65.891	T65.892	T65.893	T65.894	—	—
Isophosphamide	T45.1X1	T45.1X2	T45.1X3	T45.1X4	T45.1X5	T45.1X6
Isopregnenone	T38.5X1	T38.5X2	T38.5X3	T38.5X4	T38.5X5	T38.5X6
Isoprenaline	T48.6X1	T48.6X2	T48.6X3	T48.6X4	T48.6X5	T48.6X6
Isopromethazine	T43.3X1	T43.3X2	T43.3X3	T43.3X4	T43.3X5	T43.3X6
Isopropamide	T44.3X1	T44.3X2	T44.3X3	T44.3X4	T44.3X5	T44.3X6
iodide	T44.3X1	T44.3X2	T44.3X3	T44.3X4	T44.3X5	T44.3X6
Isopropanol	T51.2X1	T51.2X2	T51.2X3	T51.2X4	—	—
Isopropyl						
acetate	T52.8X1	T52.8X2	T52.8X3	T52.8X4	—	—
alcohol	T51.2X1	T51.2X2	T51.2X3	T51.2X4	—	—
medicinal	T49.4X1	T49.4X2	T49.4X3	T49.4X4	T49.4X5	T49.4X6
ether	T52.8X1	T52.8X2	T52.8X3	T52.8X4	—	—
Isopropylamino-phenazone	T39.2X1	T39.2X2	T39.2X3	T39.2X4	T39.2X5	T39.2X6
Isoproterenol	T48.6X1	T48.6X2	T48.6X3	T48.6X4	T48.6X5	T48.6X6
Isosorbide dinitrate	T46.3X1	T46.3X2	T46.3X3	T46.3X4	T46.3X5	T46.3X6
Isothipendyl	T45.0X1	T45.0X2	T45.0X3	T45.0X4	T45.0X5	T45.0X6
Isotretinoin	T50.991	T50.992	T50.993	T50.994	T50.995	T50.996
Isoxazolyl penicillin	T36.0X1	T36.0X2	T36.0X3	T36.0X4	T36.0X5	T36.0X6
Isoxicam	T39.391	T39.392	T39.393	T39.394	T39.395	T39.396
Isoxsuprine	T46.7X1	T46.7X2	T46.7X3	T46.7X4	T46.7X5	T46.7X6
Ispagula	T47.4X1	T47.4X2	T47.4X3	T47.4X4	T47.4X5	T47.4X6
husk	T47.4X1	T47.4X2	T47.4X3	T47.4X4	T47.4X5	T47.4X6
Isradipine	T46.1X1	T46.1X2	T46.1X3	T46.1X4	T46.1X5	T46.1X6
I-thyroxine sodium	T38.1X1	T38.1X2	T38.1X3	T38.1X4	T38.1X5	T38.1X6
Itraconazole	T37.8X1	T37.8X2	T37.8X3	T37.8X4	T37.8X5	T37.8X6
Itramin tosilate	T46.3X1	T46.3X2	T46.3X3	T46.3X4	T46.3X5	T46.3X6
Ivermectin	T37.4X1	T37.4X2	T37.4X3	T37.4X4	T37.4X5	T37.4X6
Izoniazid	T37.1X1	T37.1X2	T37.1X3	T37.1X4	T37.1X5	T37.1X6
with thioacetazone	T37.1X1	T37.1X2	T37.1X3	T37.1X4	T37.1X5	T37.1X6

Substance	Poisoning, Accidental (unintentional)	Poisoning, Intentional self-harm	Poisoning, Assault	Poisoning, Undetermined	Adverse effect	Underdosing
J						
Jalap	T47.2X1	T47.2X2	T47.2X3	T47.2X4	T47.2X5	T47.2X6
Jamaica						
dogwood (bark)	T39.8X1	T39.8X2	T39.8X3	T39.8X4	T39.8X5	T39.8X6
ginger	T65.891	T65.892	T65.893	T65.894	—	—
root	T62.2X1	T62.2X2	T62.2X3	T62.2X4	—	—
Jatropha	T62.2X1	T62.2X2	T62.2X3	T62.2X4	—	—
curcas	T62.2X1	T62.2X2	T62.2X3	T62.2X4	—	—
Jectofer	T45.4X1	T45.4X2	T45.4X3	T45.4X4	T45.4X5	T45.4X6
Jellyfish (sting)	T63.621	T63.622	T63.623	T63.624	—	—
Jequirity (bean)	T62.2X1	T62.2X2	T62.2X3	T62.2X4	—	—
Jimson weed (stramonium)	T62.2X1	T62.2X2	T62.2X3	T62.2X4	—	—
seeds	T62.2X1	T62.2X2	T62.2X3	T62.2X4	—	—
Josamycin	T36.3X1	T36.3X2	T36.3X3	T36.3X4	T36.3X5	T36.3X6
Juniper tar	T49.1X1	T49.1X2	T49.1X3	T49.1X4	T49.1X5	T49.1X6
K						
Kallidinogenase	T46.7X1	T46.7X2	T46.7X3	T46.7X4	T46.7X5	T46.7X6
Kallikrein	T46.7X1	T46.7X2	T46.7X3	T46.7X4	T46.7X5	T46.7X6
Kanamycin	T36.5X1	T36.5X2	T36.5X3	T36.5X4	T36.5X5	T36.5X6
Kantrex	T36.5X1	T36.5X2	T36.5X3	T36.5X4	T36.5X5	T36.5X6
Kaolin	T47.6X1	T47.6X2	T47.6X3	T47.6X4	T47.6X5	T47.6X6
light	T47.6X1	T47.6X2	T47.6X3	T47.6X4	T47.6X5	T47.6X6
Karaya (gum)	T47.4X1	T47.4X2	T47.4X3	T47.4X4	T47.4X5	T47.4X6
Kebuzone	T39.2X1	T39.2X2	T39.2X3	T39.2X4	T39.2X5	T39.2X6
Kelevan	T60.1X1	T60.1X2	T60.1X3	T60.1X4	—	—
Kemithal	T41.1X1	T41.1X2	T41.1X3	T41.1X4	T41.1X5	T41.1X6
Kenacort	T38.0X1	T38.0X2	T38.0X3	T38.0X4	T38.0X5	T38.0X6
Keratolytic drug NEC	T49.4X1	T49.4X2	T49.4X3	T49.4X4	T49.4X5	T49.4X6
anthracene	T49.4X1	T49.4X2	T49.4X3	T49.4X4	T49.4X5	T49.4X6
Keratoplastic NEC	T49.4X1	T49.4X2	T49.4X3	T49.4X4	T49.4X5	T49.4X6
Kerosene, kerosine (fuel) (solvent) NEC	T52.0X1	T52.0X2	T52.0X3	T52.0X4	—	—
insecticide	T52.0X1	T52.0X2	T52.0X3	T52.0X4	—	—
vapor	T52.0X1	T52.0X2	T52.0X3	T52.0X4	—	—
Ketamine	T41.291	T41.292	T41.293	T41.294	T41.295	T41.296
Ketazolam	T42.4X1	T42.4X2	T42.4X3	T42.4X4	T42.4X5	T42.4X6
Ketazon	T39.2X1	T39.2X2	T39.2X3	T39.2X4	T39.2X5	T39.2X6
Ketobemidone	T40.491	T40.492	T40.493	T40.494	—	—
Ketoconazole	T49.0X1	T49.0X2	T49.0X3	T49.0X4	T49.0X5	T49.0X6
Ketols	T52.4X1	T52.4X2	T52.4X3	T52.4X4	—	—
Ketone oils	T52.4X1	T52.4X2	T52.4X3	T52.4X4	—	—
Ketoprofen	T39.311	T39.312	T39.313	T39.314	T39.315	T39.316
Ketorolac	T39.8X1	T39.8X2	T39.8X3	T39.8X4	T39.8X5	T39.8X6
Ketotifen	T45.0X1	T45.0X2	T45.0X3	T45.0X4	T45.0X5	T45.0X6
Khat	T43.691	T43.692	T43.693	T43.694	—	—
Khellin	T46.3X1	T46.3X2	T46.3X3	T46.3X4	T46.3X5	T46.3X6
Khelloside	T46.3X1	T46.3X2	T46.3X3	T46.3X4	T46.3X5	T46.3X6
Kiln gas or vapor (carbon monoxide)	T58.8X1	T58.8X2	T58.8X3	T58.8X4	—	—
Kitasamycin	T36.3X1	T36.3X2	T36.3X3	T36.3X4	T36.3X5	T36.3X6
Konsyl	T47.4X1	T47.4X2	T47.4X3	T47.4X4	T47.4X5	T47.4X6

Substance	Poisoning, Accidental (unintentional)	Poisoning, Intentional self-harm	Poisoning, Assault	Poisoning, Undetermined	Adverse effect	Underdosing
Kosam seed	T62.2X1	T62.2X2	T62.2X3	T62.2X4	—	—
Krait (venom)	T63.091	T63.092	T63.093	T63.094	—	—
Kwell (insecticide)	T60.1X1	T60.1X2	T60.1X3	T60.1X4	—	—
anti-infective (topical)	T49.0X1	T49.0X2	T49.0X3	T49.0X4	T49.0X5	T49.0X6
L						
Labetalol	T44.8X1	T44.8X2	T44.8X3	T44.8X4	T44.8X5	T44.8X6
Laburnum (seeds)	T62.2X1	T62.2X2	T62.2X3	T62.2X4	—	—
leaves	T62.2X1	T62.2X2	T62.2X3	T62.2X4	—	—
Lachesine	T49.5X1	T49.5X2	T49.5X3	T49.5X4	T49.5X5	T49.5X6
Lacidipine	T46.5X1	T46.5X2	T46.5X3	T46.5X4	T46.5X5	T46.5X6
Lacquer	T65.6X1	T65.6X2	T65.6X3	T65.6X4	—	—
Lacrimogenic gas	T59.3X1	T59.3X2	T59.3X3	T59.3X4	—	—
Lactated potassic saline	T50.3X1	T50.3X2	T50.3X3	T50.3X4	T50.3X5	T50.3X6
Lactic acid	T49.8X1	T49.8X2	T49.8X3	T49.8X4	T49.8X5	T49.8X6
Lactobacillus						
acidophilus	T47.6X1	T47.6X2	T47.6X3	T47.6X4	T47.6X5	T47.6X6
compound	T47.6X1	T47.6X2	T47.6X3	T47.6X4	T47.6X5	T47.6X6
bifidus, lyophilized	T47.6X1	T47.6X2	T47.6X3	T47.6X4	T47.6X5	T47.6X6
bulgaricus	T47.6X1	T47.6X2	T47.6X3	T47.6X4	T47.6X5	T47.6X6
sporogenes	T47.6X1	T47.6X2	T47.6X3	T47.6X4	T47.6X5	T47.6X6
Lactoflavin	T45.2X1	T45.2X2	T45.2X3	T45.2X4	T45.2X5	T45.2X6
Lactose (as excipient)	T50.901	T50.902	T50.903	T50.904	T50.905	T50.906
Lactuca (virosa) (extract)	T42.6X1	T42.6X2	T42.6X3	T42.6X4	T42.6X5	T42.6X6
Lactucarium	T42.6X1	T42.6X2	T42.6X3	T42.6X4	T42.6X5	T42.6X6
Lactulose	T47.3X1	T47.3X2	T47.3X3	T47.3X4	T47.3X5	T47.3X6
Laevo—see Levo-						
Lanatosides	T46.0X1	T46.0X2	T46.0X3	T46.0X4	T46.0X5	T46.0X6
Lanolin	T49.3X1	T49.3X2	T49.3X3	T49.3X4	T49.3X5	T49.3X6
Largactil	T43.3X1	T43.3X2	T43.3X3	T43.3X4	T43.3X5	T43.3X6
Larkspur	T62.2X1	T62.2X2	T62.2X3	T62.2X4	—	—
Laroxyl	T43.011	T43.012	T43.013	T43.014	T43.015	T43.016
Lasix	T50.1X1	T50.1X2	T50.1X3	T50.1X4	T50.1X5	T50.1X6
Lassar's paste	T49.4X1	T49.4X2	T49.4X3	T49.4X4	T49.4X5	T49.4X6
Latamoxef	T36.1X1	T36.1X2	T36.1X3	T36.1X4	T36.1X5	T36.1X6
Latex	T65.811	T65.812	T65.813	T65.814	—	—
Lathyrus (seed)	T62.2X1	T62.2X2	T62.2X3	T62.2X4	—	—
Laudanum	T40.0X1	T40.0X2	T40.0X3	T40.0X4	T40.0X5	T40.0X6
Laudexium	T48.1X1	T48.1X2	T48.1X3	T48.1X4	T48.1X5	T48.1X6
Laughing gas	T41.0X1	T41.0X2	T41.0X3	T41.0X4	T41.0X5	T41.0X6
Laurel, black or cherry	T62.2X1	T62.2X2	T62.2X3	T62.2X4	—	—
Laurolinium	T49.0X1	T49.0X2	T49.0X3	T49.0X4	T49.0X5	T49.0X6
Lauryl sulfoacetate	T49.2X1	T49.2X2	T49.2X3	T49.2X4	T49.2X5	T49.2X6
Laxative NEC	T47.4X1	T47.4X2	T47.4X3	T47.4X4	T47.4X5	T47.4X6
osmotic	T47.3X1	T47.3X2	T47.3X3	T47.3X4	T47.3X5	T47.3X6
saline	T47.3X1	T47.3X2	T47.3X3	T47.3X4	T47.3X5	T47.3X6
stimulant	T47.2X1	T47.2X2	T47.2X3	T47.2X4	T47.2X5	T47.2X6
L-dopa	T42.8X1	T42.8X2	T42.8X3	T42.8X4	T42.8X5	T42.8X6
Lead (dust) (fumes) (vapor) NEC	T56.0X1	T56.0X2	T56.0X3	T56.0X4	—	—
acetate	T49.2X1	T49.2X2	T49.2X3	T49.2X4	T49.2X5	T49.2X6

Substance	Poisoning, Accidental (unintentional)	Poisoning, Intentional self-harm	Poisoning, Assault	Poisoning, Undetermined	Adverse effect	Underdosing
Lead NEC — *Continued*						
alkyl (fuel additive)	T56.0X1	T56.0X2	T56.0X3	T56.0X4	—	—
anti-infectives	T37.8X1	T37.8X2	T37.8X3	T37.8X4	T37.8X5	T37.8X6
antiknock compound (tetraethyl)	T56.0X1	T56.0X2	T56.0X3	T56.0X4	—	—
arsenate, arsenite (dust) (herbicide) (insecticide) (vapor)	T57.0X1	T57.0X2	T57.0X3	T57.0X4	—	—
carbonate	T56.0X1	T56.0X2	T56.0X3	T56.0X4	—	—
paint	T56.0X1	T56.0X2	T56.0X3	T56.0X4	—	—
chromate	T56.0X1	T56.0X2	T56.0X3	T56.0X4	—	—
paint	T56.0X1	T56.0X2	T56.0X3	T56.0X4	—	—
dioxide	T56.0X1	T56.0X2	T56.0X3	T56.0X4	—	—
inorganic	T56.0X1	T56.0X2	T56.0X3	T56.0X4	—	—
iodide	T56.0X1	T56.0X2	T56.0X3	T56.0X4	—	—
pigment (paint)	T56.0X1	T56.0X2	T56.0X3	T56.0X4	—	—
monoxide (dust)	T56.0X1	T56.0X2	T56.0X3	T56.0X4	—	—
paint	T56.0X1	T56.0X2	T56.0X3	T56.0X4	—	—
organic	T56.0X1	T56.0X2	T56.0X3	T56.0X4	—	—
oxide	T56.0X1	T56.0X2	T56.0X3	T56.0X4	—	—
paint	T56.0X1	T56.0X2	T56.0X3	T56.0X4	—	—
paint	T56.0X1	T56.0X2	T56.0X3	T56.0X4	—	—
salts	T56.0X1	T56.0X2	T56.0X3	T56.0X4	—	—
specified compound NEC	T56.0X1	T56.0X2	T56.0X3	T56.0X4	—	—
tetra-ethyl	T56.0X1	T56.0X2	T56.0X3	T56.0X4	—	—
Lebanese red	T40.7X1	T40.7X2	T40.7X3	T40.7X4	T40.7X5	T40.7X6
Lefetamine	T39.8X1	T39.8X2	T39.8X3	T39.8X4	T39.8X5	T39.8X6
Lenperone	T43.4X1	T43.4X2	T43.4X3	T43.4X4	T43.4X5	T43.4X6
Lente lietin (insulin)	T38.3X1	T38.3X2	T38.3X3	T38.3X4	T38.3X5	T38.3X6
Leptazol	T50.7X1	T50.7X2	T50.7X3	T50.7X4	T50.7X5	T50.7X6
Leptophos	T60.0X1	T60.0X2	T60.0X3	T60.0X4	—	—
Leritine	T40.2X1	T40.2X2	T40.2X3	T40.2X4	T40.2X5	T40.2X6
Letosteine	T48.4X1	T48.4X2	T48.4X3	T48.4X4	T48.4X5	T48.4X6
Letter	T38.1X1	T38.1X2	T38.1X3	T38.1X4	T38.1X5	T38.1X6
Lettuce opium	T42.6X1	T42.6X2	T42.6X3	T42.6X4	T42.6X5	T42.6X6
Leucinocaine	T41.3X1	T41.3X2	T41.3X3	T41.3X4	T41.3X5	T41.3X6
Leucocianidol	T46.991	T46.992	T46.993	T46.994	T46.995	T46.996
Leucovorin (factor)	T45.8X1	T45.8X2	T45.8X3	T45.8X4	T45.8X5	T45.8X6
Leukeran	T45.1X1	T45.1X2	T45.1X3	T45.1X4	T45.1X5	T45.1X6
Leuprolide	T38.891	T38.892	T38.893	T38.894	T38.895	T38.896
Levalbuterol	T48.6X1	T48.6X2	T48.6X3	T48.6X4	T48.6X5	T48.6X6
Levallorphan	T50.7X1	T50.7X2	T50.7X3	T50.7X4	T50.7X5	T50.7X6
Levamisole	T37.4X1	T37.4X2	T37.4X3	T37.4X4	T37.4X5	T37.4X6
Levanil	T42.6X1	T42.6X2	T42.6X3	T42.6X4	T42.6X5	T42.6X6
Levarterenol	T44.4X1	T44.4X2	T44.4X3	T44.4X4	T44.4X5	T44.4X6
Levdropropizine	T48.3X1	T48.3X2	T48.3X3	T48.3X4	T48.3X5	T48.3X6
Levobunolol	T49.5X1	T49.5X2	T49.5X3	T49.5X4	T49.5X5	T49.5X6
Levocabastine (hydrochloride)	T45.0X1	T45.0X2	T45.0X3	T45.0X4	T45.0X5	T45.0X6
Levocarnitine	T50.991	T50.992	T50.993	T50.994	T50.995	T50.996

Substance	Poisoning, Accidental (unintentional)	Poisoning, Intentional self-harm	Poisoning, Assault	Poisoning, Undetermined	Adverse effect	Underdosing
Levodopa	T42.8X1	T42.8X2	T42.8X3	T42.8X4	T42.8X5	T42.8X6
with carbidopa	T42.8X1	T42.8X2	T42.8X3	T42.8X4	T42.8X5	T42.8X6
Levo-dromoran	T40.2X1	T40.2X2	T40.2X3	T40.2X4	T40.2X5	T40.2X6
Levoglutamide	T50.991	T50.992	T50.993	T50.994	T50.995	T50.996
Levoid	T38.1X1	T38.1X2	T38.1X3	T38.1X4	T38.1X5	T38.1X6
Levo-iso-methadone	T40.3X1	T40.3X2	T40.3X3	T40.3X4	T40.3X5	T40.3X6
Levomepromazine	T43.3X1	T43.3X2	T43.3X3	T43.3X4	T43.3X5	T43.3X6
Levonordefrin	T49.6X1	T49.6X2	T49.6X3	T49.6X4	T49.6X5	T49.6X6
Levonorgestrel	T38.4X1	T38.4X2	T38.4X3	T38.4X4	T38.4X5	T38.4X6
with ethinylestradiol	T38.5X1	T38.5X2	T38.5X3	T38.5X4	T38.5X5	T38.5X6
Levopromazine	T43.3X1	T43.3X2	T43.3X3	T43.3X4	T43.3X5	T43.3X6
Levoprome	T42.6X1	T42.6X2	T42.6X3	T42.6X4	T42.6X5	T42.6X6
Levopropoxyphene	T40.491	T40.492	T40.493	T40.494	T40.495	T40.496
Levopropylhexedrine	T50.5X1	T50.5X2	T50.5X3	T50.5X4	T50.5X5	T50.5X6
Levoproxyphylline	T48.6X1	T48.6X2	T48.6X3	T48.6X4	T48.6X5	T48.6X6
Levorphanol	T40.491	T40.492	T40.493	T40.494	T40.495	T40.496
Levothyroxine	T38.1X1	T38.1X2	T38.1X3	T38.1X4	T38.1X5	T38.1X6
sodium	T38.1X1	T38.1X2	T38.1X3	T38.1X4	T38.1X5	T38.1X6
Levsin	T44.3X1	T44.3X2	T44.3X3	T44.3X4	T44.3X5	T44.3X6
Levulose	T50.3X1	T50.3X2	T50.3X3	T50.3X4	T50.3X5	T50.3X6
Lewisite (gas), not in war	T57.0X1	T57.0X2	T57.0X3	T57.0X4	—	—
Librium	T42.4X1	T42.4X2	T42.4X3	T42.4X4	T42.4X5	T42.4X6
Lidex	T49.0X1	T49.0X2	T49.0X3	T49.0X4	T49.0X5	T49.0X6
Lidocaine	T41.3X1	T41.3X2	T41.3X3	T41.3X4	T41.3X5	T41.3X6
regional	T41.3X1	T41.3X2	T41.3X3	T41.3X4	T41.3X5	T41.3X6
spinal	T41.3X1	T41.3X2	T41.3X3	T41.3X4	T41.3X5	T41.3X6
Lidofenin	T50.8X1	T50.8X2	T50.8X3	T50.8X4	T50.8X5	T50.8X6
Lidoflazine	T46.1X1	T46.1X2	T46.1X3	T46.1X4	T46.1X5	T46.1X6
Lighter fluid	T52.0X1	T52.0X2	T52.0X3	T52.0X4	—	—
Lignin hemicellulose	T47.6X1	T47.6X2	T47.6X3	T47.6X4	T47.6X5	T47.6X6
Lignocaine	T41.3X1	T41.3X2	T41.3X3	T41.3X4	T41.3X5	T41.3X6
regional	T41.3X1	T41.3X2	T41.3X3	T41.3X4	T41.3X5	T41.3X6
spinal	T41.3X1	T41.3X2	T41.3X3	T41.3X4	T41.3X5	T41.3X6
Ligroin(e) (solvent)	T52.0X1	T52.0X2	T52.0X3	T52.0X4	—	—
vapor	T59.891	T59.892	T59.893	T59.894	—	—
Ligustrum vulgare	T62.2X1	T62.2X2	T62.2X3	T62.2X4	—	—
Lily of the valley	T62.2X1	T62.2X2	T62.2X3	T62.2X4	—	—
Lime (chloride)	T54.3X1	T54.3X2	T54.3X3	T54.3X4	—	—
Limonene	T52.8X1	T52.8X2	T52.8X3	T52.8X4	—	—
Lincomycin	T36.8X1	T36.8X2	T36.8X3	T36.8X4	T36.8X5	T36.8X6
Lindane (insecticide) (nonmedicinal) (vapor)	T53.6X1	T53.6X2	T53.6X3	T53.6X4	—	—
medicinal	T49.0X1	T49.0X2	T49.0X3	T49.0X4	T49.0X5	T49.0X6
Liniments NEC	T49.91	T49.92	T49.93	T49.94	T49.95	T49.96
Linoleic acid	T46.6X1	T46.6X2	T46.6X3	T46.6X4	T46.6X5	T46.6X6
Linolenic acid	T46.6X1	T46.6X2	T46.6X3	T46.6X4	T46.6X5	T46.6X6
Linseed	T47.4X1	T47.4X2	T47.4X3	T47.4X4	T47.4X5	T47.4X6
Liothyronine	T38.1X1	T38.1X2	T38.1X3	T38.1X4	T38.1X5	T38.1X6
Liotrix	T38.1X1	T38.1X2	T38.1X3	T38.1X4	T38.1X5	T38.1X6
Lipancreatin	T47.5X1	T47.5X2	T47.5X3	T47.5X4	T47.5X5	T47.5X6

Substance	Poisoning, Accidental (unintentional)	Poisoning, Intentional self-harm	Poisoning, Assault	Poisoning, Undetermined	Adverse effect	Underdosing
Lipo-alprostadil	T46.7X1	T46.7X2	T46.7X3	T46.7X4	T46.7X5	T46.7X6
Lipo-Lutin	T38.5X1	T38.5X2	T38.5X3	T38.5X4	T38.5X5	T38.5X6
Lipotropic drug NEC	T50.901	T50.902	T50.903	T50.904	T50.905	T50.906
Liquefied petroleum gases	T59.891	T59.892	T59.893	T59.894	—	—
piped (pure or mixed with air)	T59.891	T59.892	T59.893	T59.894	—	—
Liquid						
paraffin	T47.4X1	T47.4X2	T47.4X3	T47.4X4	T47.4X5	T47.4X6
petrolatum	T47.4X1	T47.4X2	T47.4X3	T47.4X4	T47.4X5	T47.4X6
topical	T49.3X1	T49.3X2	T49.3X3	T49.3X4	T49.3X5	T49.3X6
specified NEC	T65.891	T65.892	T65.893	T65.894	—	—
substance	T65.91	T65.92	T65.93	T65.94	—	—
Liquor creosolis compositus	T65.891	T65.892	T65.893	T65.894	—	—
Liquorice	T48.4X1	T48.4X2	T48.4X3	T48.4X4	T48.4X5	T48.4X6
extract	T47.8X1	T47.8X2	T47.8X3	T47.8X4	T47.8X5	T47.8X6
Lisinopril	T46.4X1	T46.4X2	T46.4X3	T46.4X4	T46.4X5	T46.4X6
Lisuride	T42.8X1	T42.8X2	T42.8X3	T42.8X4	T42.8X5	T42.8X6
Lithane	T43.8X1	T43.8X2	T43.8X3	T43.8X4	T43.8X5	T43.8X6
Lithium	T56.891	T56.892	T56.893	T56.894	—	—
gluconate	T43.591	T43.592	T43.593	T43.594	T43.595	T43.596
salts (carbonate)	T43.591	T43.592	T43.593	T43.594	T43.595	T43.596
Lithonate	T43.8X1	T43.8X2	T43.8X3	T43.8X4	T43.8X5	T43.8X6
Liver						
extract	T45.8X1	T45.8X2	T45.8X3	T45.8X4	T45.8X5	T45.8X6
for parenteral use	T45.8X1	T45.8X2	T45.8X3	T45.8X4	T45.8X5	T45.8X6
fraction 1	T45.8X1	T45.8X2	T45.8X3	T45.8X4	T45.8X5	T45.8X6
hydrolysate	T45.8X1	T45.8X2	T45.8X3	T45.8X4	T45.8X5	T45.8X6
Lizard (bite) (venom)	T63.121	T63.122	T63.123	T63.124	—	—
LMD	T45.8X1	T45.8X2	T45.8X3	T45.8X4	T45.8X5	T45.8X6
Lobelia	T62.2X1	T62.2X2	T62.2X3	T62.2X4	—	—
Lobeline	T50.7X1	T50.7X2	T50.7X3	T50.7X4	T50.7X5	T50.7X6
Local action drug NEC	T49.8X1	T49.8X2	T49.8X3	T49.8X4	T49.8X5	T49.8X6
Locorten	T49.0X1	T49.0X2	T49.0X3	T49.0X4	T49.0X5	T49.0X6
Lofepramine	T43.011	T43.012	T43.013	T43.014	T43.015	T43.016
Lolium temulentum	T62.2X1	T62.2X2	T62.2X3	T62.2X4	—	—
Lomotil	T47.6X1	T47.6X2	T47.6X3	T47.6X4	T47.6X5	T47.6X6
Lomustine	T45.1X1	T45.1X2	T45.1X3	T45.1X4	T45.1X5	T45.1X6
Lonidamine	T45.1X1	T45.1X2	T45.1X3	T45.1X4	T45.1X5	T45.1X6
Loperamide	T47.6X1	T47.6X2	T47.6X3	T47.6X4	T47.6X5	T47.6X6
Loprazolam	T42.4X1	T42.4X2	T42.4X3	T42.4X4	T42.4X5	T42.4X6
Lorajmine	T46.2X1	T46.2X2	T46.2X3	T46.2X4	T46.2X5	T46.2X6
Loratidine	T45.0X1	T45.0X2	T45.0X3	T45.0X4	T45.0X5	T45.0X6
Lorazepam	T42.4X1	T42.4X2	T42.4X3	T42.4X4	T42.4X5	T42.4X6
Lorcainide	T46.2X1	T46.2X2	T46.2X3	T46.2X4	T46.2X5	T46.2X6
Lormetazepam	T42.4X1	T42.4X2	T42.4X3	T42.4X4	T42.4X5	T42.4X6
Lotions NEC	T49.91	T49.92	T49.93	T49.94	T49.95	T49.96
Lotusate	T42.3X1	T42.3X2	T42.3X3	T42.3X4	T42.3X5	T42.3X6
Lovastatin	T46.6X1	T46.6X2	T46.6X3	T46.6X4	T46.6X5	T46.6X6
Lowila	T49.2X1	T49.2X2	T49.2X3	T49.2X4	T49.2X5	T49.2X6

Substance	Poisoning, Accidental (unintentional)	Poisoning, Intentional self-harm	Poisoning, Assault	Poisoning, Undetermined	Adverse effect	Underdosing
Loxapine	T43.591	T43.592	T43.593	T43.594	T43.595	T43.596
Lozenges (throat)	T49.6X1	T49.6X2	T49.6X3	T49.6X4	T49.6X5	T49.6X6
LSD	T40.8X1	T40.8X2	T40.8X3	T40.8X4	—	—
L-Tryptophan—see amino acid						
Lubricant, eye	T49.5X1	T49.5X2	T49.5X3	T49.5X4	T49.5X5	T49.5X6
Lubricating oil NEC	T52.0X1	T52.0X2	T52.0X3	T52.0X4	—	—
Lucanthone	T37.4X1	T37.4X2	T37.4X3	T37.4X4	T37.4X5	T37.4X6
Luminal	T42.3X1	T42.3X2	T42.3X3	T42.3X4	T42.3X5	T42.3X6
Lung irritant (gas) NEC	T59.91	T59.92	T59.93	T59.94	—	—
Luteinizing hormone	T38.811	T38.812	T38.813	T38.814	T38.815	T38.816
Lutocylol	T38.5X1	T38.5X2	T38.5X3	T38.5X4	T38.5X5	T38.5X6
Lutromone	T38.5X1	T38.5X2	T38.5X3	T38.5X4	T38.5X5	T38.5X6
Lututrin	T48.291	T48.292	T48.293	T48.294	T48.295	T48.296
Lye (concentrated)	T54.3X1	T54.3X2	T54.3X3	T54.3X4	—	—
Lygranum (skin test)	T50.8X1	T50.8X2	T50.8X3	T50.8X4	T50.8X5	T50.8X6
Lymecycline	T36.4X1	T36.4X2	T36.4X3	T36.4X4	T36.4X5	T36.4X6
Lymphogranuloma venereum antigen	T50.8X1	T50.8X2	T50.8X3	T50.8X4	T50.8X5	T50.8X6
Lynestrenol	T38.4X1	T38.4X2	T38.4X3	T38.4X4	T38.4X5	T38.4X6
Lyovac Sodium Edecrin	T50.1X1	T50.1X2	T50.1X3	T50.1X4	T50.1X5	T50.1X6
Lypressin	T38.891	T38.892	T38.893	T38.894	T38.895	T38.896
Lysergic acid diethylamide	T40.8X1	T40.8X2	T40.8X3	T40.8X4	—	—
Lysergide	T40.8X1	T40.8X2	T40.8X3	T40.8X4	—	—
Lysine vasopressin	T38.891	T38.892	T38.893	T38.894	T38.895	T38.896
Lysol	T54.1X1	T54.1X2	T54.1X3	T54.1X4	—	—
Lysozyme	T49.0X1	T49.0X2	T49.0X3	T49.0X4	T49.0X5	T49.0X6
Lytta (vitatta)	T49.8X1	T49.8X2	T49.8X3	T49.8X4	T49.8X5	T49.8X6
M						
Mace	T59.3X1	T59.3X2	T59.3X3	T59.3X4	—	—
Macrogol	T50.991	T50.992	T50.993	T50.994	T50.995	T50.996
Macrolide						
anabolic drug	T38.7X1	T38.7X2	T38.7X3	T38.7X4	T38.7X5	T38.7X6
antibiotic	T36.3X1	T36.3X2	T36.3X3	T36.3X4	T36.3X5	T36.3X6
Mafenide	T49.0X1	T49.0X2	T49.0X3	T49.0X4	T49.0X5	T49.0X6
Magaldrate	T47.1X1	T47.1X2	T47.1X3	T47.1X4	T47.1X5	T47.1X6
Magic mushroom	T40.991	T40.992	T40.993	T40.994	—	—
Magnamycin	T36.8X1	T36.8X2	T36.8X3	T36.8X4	T36.8X5	T36.8X6
Magnesia magma	T47.1X1	T47.1X2	T47.1X3	T47.1X4	T47.1X5	T47.1X6
Magnesium NEC	T56.891	T56.892	T56.893	T56.894	—	—
carbonate	T47.1X1	T47.1X2	T47.1X3	T47.1X4	T47.1X5	T47.1X6
citrate	T47.4X1	T47.4X2	T47.4X3	T47.4X4	T47.4X5	T47.4X6
hydroxide	T47.1X1	T47.1X2	T47.1X3	T47.1X4	T47.1X5	T47.1X6
oxide	T47.1X1	T47.1X2	T47.1X3	T47.1X4	T47.1X5	T47.1X6
peroxide	T49.0X1	T49.0X2	T49.0X3	T49.0X4	T49.0X5	T49.0X6
salicylate	T39.091	T39.092	T39.093	T39.094	T39.095	T39.096
silicofluoride	T50.3X1	T50.3X2	T50.3X3	T50.3X4	T50.3X5	T50.3X6
sulfate	T47.4X1	T47.4X2	T47.4X3	T47.4X4	T47.4X5	T47.4X6
thiosulfate	T45.0X1	T45.0X2	T45.0X3	T45.0X4	T45.0X5	T45.0X6
trisilicate	T47.1X1	T47.1X2	T47.1X3	T47.1X4	T47.1X5	T47.1X6

Substance	Poisoning, Accidental (unintentional)	Poisoning, Intentional self-harm	Poisoning, Assault	Poisoning, Undetermined	Adverse effect	Underdosing
Malathion (medicinal)	T49.0X1	T49.0X2	T49.0X3	T49.0X4	T49.0X5	T49.0X6
insecticide	T60.0X1	T60.0X2	T60.0X3	T60.0X4	—	—
Male fern extract	T37.4X1	T37.4X2	T37.4X3	T37.4X4	T37.4X5	T37.4X6
M-AMSA	T45.1X1	T45.1X2	T45.1X3	T45.1X4	T45.1X5	T45.1X6
Mandelic acid	T37.8X1	T37.8X2	T37.8X3	T37.8X4	T37.8X5	T37.8X6
Manganese (dioxide) (salts)	T57.2X1	T57.2X2	T57.2X3	T57.2X4	—	—
medicinal	T50.991	T50.992	T50.993	T50.994	T50.995	T50.996
Mannitol	T47.3X1	T47.3X2	T47.3X3	T47.3X4	T47.3X5	T47.3X6
hexanitrate	T46.3X1	T46.3X2	T46.3X3	T46.3X4	T46.3X5	T46.3X6
Mannomustine	T45.1X1	T45.1X2	T45.1X3	T45.1X4	T45.1X5	T45.1X6
MAO inhibitors	T43.1X1	T43.1X2	T43.1X3	T43.1X4	T43.1X5	T43.1X6
Mapharsen	T37.8X1	T37.8X2	T37.8X3	T37.8X4	T37.8X5	T37.8X6
Maphenide	T49.0X1	T49.0X2	T49.0X3	T49.0X4	T49.0X5	T49.0X6
Maprotiline	T43.021	T43.022	T43.023	T43.024	T43.025	T43.026
Marcaine	T41.3X1	T41.3X2	T41.3X3	T41.3X4	T41.3X5	T41.3X6
infiltration (subcutaneous)	T41.3X1	T41.3X2	T41.3X3	T41.3X4	T41.3X5	T41.3X6
nerve block (peripheral) (plexus)	T41.3X1	T41.3X2	T41.3X3	T41.3X4	T41.3X5	T41.3X6
Marezine	T45.0X1	T45.0X2	T45.0X3	T45.0X4	T45.0X5	T45.0X6
Marihuana	T40.7X1	T40.7X2	T40.7X3	T40.7X4	T40.7X5	T40.7X6
Marijuana	T40.7X1	T40.7X2	T40.7X3	T40.7X4	T40.7X5	T40.7X6
Marine (sting)	T63.691	T63.692	T63.693	T63.694	—	—
animals (sting)	T63.691	T63.692	T63.693	T63.694	—	—
plants (sting)	T63.711	T63.712	T63.713	T63.714	—	—
Marplan	T43.1X1	T43.1X2	T43.1X3	T43.1X4	T43.1X5	T43.1X6
Marsh gas	T59.891	T59.892	T59.893	T59.894	—	—
Marsilid	T43.1X1	T43.1X2	T43.1X3	T43.1X4	T43.1X5	T43.1X6
Matulane	T45.1X1	T45.1X2	T45.1X3	T45.1X4	T45.1X5	T45.1X6
Mazindol	T50.5X1	T50.5X2	T50.5X3	T50.5X4	T50.5X5	T50.5X6
MCPA	T60.3X1	T60.3X2	T60.3X3	T60.3X4	—	—
MDMA	T43.641	T43.642	T43.643	T43.644		
Meadow saffron	T62.2X1	T62.2X2	T62.2X3	T62.2X4		
Measles virus vaccine (attenuated)	T50.B91	T50.B92	T50.B93	T50.B94	T50.B95	T50.B96
Meat, noxious	T62.8X1	T62.8X2	T62.8X3	T62.8X4	—	—
Meballymal	T42.3X1	T42.3X2	T42.3X3	T42.3X4	T42.3X5	T42.3X6
Mebanazine	T43.1X1	T43.1X2	T43.1X3	T43.1X4	T43.1X5	T43.1X6
Mebaral	T42.3X1	T42.3X2	T42.3X3	T42.3X4	T42.3X5	T42.3X6
Mebendazole	T37.4X1	T37.4X2	T37.4X3	T37.4X4	T37.4X5	T37.4X6
Mebeverine	T44.3X1	T44.3X2	T44.3X3	T44.3X4	T44.3X5	T44.3X6
Mebhydrolin	T45.0X1	T45.0X2	T45.0X3	T45.0X4	T45.0X5	T45.0X6
Mebumal	T42.3X1	T42.3X2	T42.3X3	T42.3X4	T42.3X5	T42.3X6
Mebutamate	T43.591	T43.592	T43.593	T43.594	T43.595	T43.596
Mecamylamine	T44.2X1	T44.2X2	T44.2X3	T44.2X4	T44.2X5	T44.2X6
Mechlorethamine	T45.1X1	T45.1X2	T45.1X3	T45.1X4	T45.1X5	T45.1X6
Mecillinam	T36.0X1	T36.0X2	T36.0X3	T36.0X4	T36.0X5	T36.0X6
Meclizine (hydrochloride)	T45.0X1	T45.0X2	T45.0X3	T45.0X4	T45.0X5	T45.0X6
Meclocycline	T36.4X1	T36.4X2	T36.4X3	T36.4X4	T36.4X5	T36.4X6

Substance	Poisoning, Accidental (unintentional)	Poisoning, Intentional self-harm	Poisoning, Assault	Poisoning, Undetermined	Adverse effect	Underdosing
Meclofenamate	T39.391	T39.392	T39.393	T39.394	T39.395	T39.396
Meclofenamic acid	T39.391	T39.392	T39.393	T39.394	T39.395	T39.396
Meclofenoxate	T43.691	T43.692	T43.693	T43.694	T43.695	T43.696
Meclozine	T45.0X1	T45.0X2	T45.0X3	T45.0X4	T45.0X5	T45.0X6
Mecobalamin	T45.8X1	T45.8X2	T45.8X3	T45.8X4	T45.8X5	T45.8X6
Mecoprop	T60.3X1	T60.3X2	T60.3X3	T60.3X4	—	—
Mecrilate	T49.3X1	T49.3X2	T49.3X3	T49.3X4	T49.3X5	T49.3X6
Mecysteine	T48.4X1	T48.4X2	T48.4X3	T48.4X4	T48.4X5	T48.4X6
Medazepam	T42.4X1	T42.4X2	T42.4X3	T42.4X4	T42.4X5	T42.4X6
Medicament NEC	T50.901	T50.902	T50.903	T50.904	T50.905	T50.906
Medinal	T42.3X1	T42.3X2	T42.3X3	T42.3X4	T42.3X5	T42.3X6
Medomin	T42.3X1	T42.3X2	T42.3X3	T42.3X4	T42.3X5	T42.3X6
Medrogestone	T38.5X1	T38.5X2	T38.5X3	T38.5X4	T38.5X5	T38.5X6
Medroxalol	T44.8X1	T44.8X2	T44.8X3	T44.8X4	T44.8X5	T44.8X6
Medroxyprogesteron eacetate (depot)	T38.5X1	T38.5X2	T38.5X3	T38.5X4	T38.5X5	T38.5X6
Medrysone	T49.0X1	T49.0X2	T49.0X3	T49.0X4	T49.0X5	T49.0X6
Mefenamic acid	T39.391	T39.392	T39.393	T39.394	T39.395	T39.396
Mefenorex	T50.5X1	T50.5X2	T50.5X3	T50.5X4	T50.5X5	T50.5X6
Mefloquine	T37.2X1	T37.2X2	T37.2X3	T37.2X4	T37.2X5	T37.2X6
Mefruside	T50.2X1	T50.2X2	T50.2X3	T50.2X4	T50.2X5	T50.2X6
Megahallucinogen	T40.901	T40.902	T40.903	T40.904	T40.905	T40.906
Megestrol	T38.5X1	T38.5X2	T38.5X3	T38.5X4	T38.5X5	T38.5X6
Meglumine						
antimoniate	T37.8X1	T37.8X2	T37.8X3	T37.8X4	T37.8X5	T37.8X6
diatrizoate	T50.8X1	T50.8X2	T50.8X3	T50.8X4	T50.8X5	T50.8X6
iodipamide	T50.8X1	T50.8X2	T50.8X3	T50.8X4	T50.8X5	T50.8X6
iotroxate	T50.8X1	T50.8X2	T50.8X3	T50.8X4	T50.8X5	T50.8X6
MEK (methyl ethyl ketone)	T52.4X1	T52.4X2	T52.4X3	T52.4X4	—	—
Meladinin	T49.3X1	T49.3X2	T49.3X3	T49.3X4	T49.3X5	T49.3X6
Meladrazine	T44.3X1	T44.3X2	T44.3X3	T44.3X4	T44.3X5	T44.3X6
Melaleuca alternifolia oil	T49.0X1	T49.0X2	T49.0X3	T49.0X4	T49.0X5	T49.0X6
Melanizing agents	T49.3X1	T49.3X2	T49.3X3	T49.3X4	T49.3X5	T49.3X6
Melanocyte-stimulating hormone	T38.891	T38.892	T38.893	T38.894	T38.895	T38.896
Melarsonyl potassium	T37.3X1	T37.3X2	T37.3X3	T37.3X4	T37.3X5	T37.3X6
Melarsoprol	T37.3X1	T37.3X2	T37.3X3	T37.3X4	T37.3X5	T37.3X6
Melia azedarach	T62.2X1	T62.2X2	T62.2X3	T62.2X4	—	—
Melitracen	T43.011	T43.012	T43.013	T43.014	T43.015	T43.016
Mellaril	T43.3X1	T43.3X2	T43.3X3	T43.3X4	T43.3X5	T43.3X6
Meloxine	T49.3X1	T49.3X2	T49.3X3	T49.3X4	T49.3X5	T49.3X6
Melperone	T43.4X1	T43.4X2	T43.4X3	T43.4X4	T43.4X5	T43.4X6
Melphalan	T45.1X1	T45.1X2	T45.1X3	T45.1X4	T45.1X5	T45.1X6
Memantine	T43.8X1	T43.8X2	T43.8X3	T43.8X4	T43.8X5	T43.8X6
Menadiol	T45.7X1	T45.7X2	T45.7X3	T45.7X4	T45.7X5	T45.7X6
sodium sulfate	T45.7X1	T45.7X2	T45.7X3	T45.7X4	T45.7X5	T45.7X6
Menadione	T45.7X1	T45.7X2	T45.7X3	T45.7X4	T45.7X5	T45.7X6
sodium bisulfite	T45.7X1	T45.7X2	T45.7X3	T45.7X4	T45.7X5	T45.7X6

Substance	Poisoning, Accidental (unintentional)	Poisoning, Intentional self-harm	Poisoning, Assault	Poisoning, Undetermined	Adverse effect	Underdosing
Menaphthone	T45.7X1	T45.7X2	T45.7X3	T45.7X4	T45.7X5	T45.7X6
Menaquinone	T45.7X1	T45.7X2	T45.7X3	T45.7X4	T45.7X5	T45.7X6
Menatetrenone	T45.7X1	T45.7X2	T45.7X3	T45.7X4	T45.7X5	T45.7X6
Meningococcal vaccine	T50.A91	T50.A92	T50.A93	T50.A94	T50.A95	T50.A96
Menningovax (-AC) (-C)	T50.A91	T50.A92	T50.A93	T50.A94	T50.A95	T50.A96
Menotropins	T38.811	T38.812	T38.813	T38.814	T38.815	T38.816
Menthol	T48.5X1	T48.5X2	T48.5X3	T48.5X4	T48.5X5	T48.5X6
Mepacrine	T37.2X1	T37.2X2	T37.2X3	T37.2X4	T37.2X5	T37.2X6
Meparfynol	T42.6X1	T42.6X2	T42.6X3	T42.6X4	T42.6X5	T42.6X6
Mepartricin	T36.7X1	T36.7X2	T36.7X3	T36.7X4	T36.7X5	T36.7X6
Mepazine	T43.3X1	T43.3X2	T43.3X3	T43.3X4	T43.3X5	T43.3X6
Mepenzolate	T44.3X1	T44.3X2	T44.3X3	T44.3X4	T44.3X5	T44.3X6
bromide	T44.3X1	T44.3X2	T44.3X3	T44.3X4	T44.3X5	T44.3X6
Meperidine	T40.491	T40.492	T40.493	T40.494	T40.495	T40.496
Mephebarbital	T42.3X1	T42.3X2	T42.3X3	T42.3X4	T42.3X5	T42.3X6
Mephenamin (e)	T42.8X1	T42.8X2	T42.8X3	T42.8X4	T42.8X5	T42.8X6
Mephenesin	T42.8X1	T42.8X2	T42.8X3	T42.8X4	T42.8X5	T42.8X6
Mephenhydramine	T45.0X1	T45.0X2	T45.0X3	T45.0X4	T45.0X5	T45.0X6
Mephenoxalone	T42.8X1	T42.8X2	T42.8X3	T42.8X4	T42.8X5	T42.8X6
Mephentermine	T44.991	T44.992	T44.993	T44.994	T44.995	T44.996
Mephenytoin	T42.0X1	T42.0X2	T42.0X3	T42.0X4	T42.0X5	T42.0X6
with phenobarbital	T42.3X1	T42.3X2	T42.3X3	T42.3X4	T42.3X5	T42.3X6
Mephobarbital	T42.3X1	T42.3X2	T42.3X3	T42.3X4	T42.3X5	T42.3X6
Mephosfolan	T60.0X1	T60.0X2	T60.0X3	T60.0X4	—	—
Mepindolol	T44.7X1	T44.7X2	T44.7X3	T44.7X4	T44.7X5	T44.7X6
Mepiperphenidol	T44.3X1	T44.3X2	T44.3X3	T44.3X4	T44.3X5	T44.3X6
Mepitiostane	T38.7X1	T38.7X2	T38.7X3	T38.7X4	T38.7X5	T38.7X6
Mepivacaine	T41.3X1	T41.3X2	T41.3X3	T41.3X4	T41.3X5	T41.3X6
epidural	T41.3X1	T41.3X2	T41.3X3	T41.3X4	T41.3X5	T41.3X6
Meprednisone	T38.0X1	T38.0X2	T38.0X3	T38.0X4	T38.0X5	T38.0X6
Meprobam	T43.591	T43.592	T43.593	T43.594	T43.595	T43.596
Meprobamate	T43.591	T43.592	T43.593	T43.594	T43.595	T43.596
Meproscillarin	T46.0X1	T46.0X2	T46.0X3	T46.0X4	T46.0X5	T46.0X6
Meprylcaine	T41.3X1	T41.3X2	T41.3X3	T41.3X4	T41.3X5	T41.3X6
Meptazinol	T39.8X1	T39.8X2	T39.8X3	T39.8X4	T39.8X5	T39.8X6
Mepyramine	T45.0X1	T45.0X2	T45.0X3	T45.0X4	T45.0X5	T45.0X6
Mequitazine	T43.3X1	T43.3X2	T43.3X3	T43.3X4	T43.3X5	T43.3X6
Meralluride	T50.2X1	T50.2X2	T50.2X3	T50.2X4	T50.2X5	T50.2X6
Merbaphen	T50.2X1	T50.2X2	T50.2X3	T50.2X4	T50.2X5	T50.2X6
Merbromin	T49.0X1	T49.0X2	T49.0X3	T49.0X4	T49.0X5	T49.0X6
Mercaptoben-zothiazole salts	T49.0X1	T49.0X2	T49.0X3	T49.0X4	T49.0X5	T49.0X6
Mercaptomerin	T50.2X1	T50.2X2	T50.2X3	T50.2X4	T50.2X5	T50.2X6
Mercaptopurine	T45.1X1	T45.1X2	T45.1X3	T45.1X4	T45.1X5	T45.1X6
Mercumatilin	T50.2X1	T50.2X2	T50.2X3	T50.2X4	T50.2X5	T50.2X6
Mercuramide	T50.2X1	T50.2X2	T50.2X3	T50.2X4	T50.2X5	T50.2X6
Mercurochrome	T49.0X1	T49.0X2	T49.0X3	T49.0X4	T49.0X5	T49.0X6
Mercurophylline	T50.2X1	T50.2X2	T50.2X3	T50.2X4	T50.2X5	T50.2X6

Substance	Poisoning, Accidental (unintentional)	Poisoning, Intentional self-harm	Poisoning, Assault	Poisoning, Undetermined	Adverse effect	Underdosing
Mercury, mercurial, mercuric, mercurous (compounds) (cyanide) (fumes) (nonmedicinal) (vapor) NEC	T56.1X1	T56.1X2	T56.1X3	T56.1X4	—	—
ammoniated	T49.0X1	T49.0X2	T49.0X3	T49.0X4	T49.0X5	T49.0X6
anti-infective						
local	T49.0X1	T49.0X2	T49.0X3	T49.0X4	T49.0X5	T49.0X6
systemic	T37.8X1	T37.8X2	T37.8X3	T37.8X4	T37.8X5	T37.8X6
topical	T49.0X1	T49.0X2	T49.0X3	T49.0X4	T49.0X5	T49.0X6
chloride (ammoniated)	T49.0X1	T49.0X2	T49.0X3	T49.0X4	T49.0X5	T49.0X6
fungicide	T56.1X1	T56.1X2	T56.1X3	T56.1X4	—	—
diuretic NEC	T50.2X1	T50.2X2	T50.2X3	T50.2X4	T50.2X5	T50.2X6
fungicide	T56.1X1	T56.1X2	T56.1X3	T56.1X4	—	—
organic (fungicide)	T56.1X1	T56.1X2	T56.1X3	T56.1X4	—	—
oxide, yellow	T49.0X1	T49.0X2	T49.0X3	T49.0X4	T49.0X5	T49.0X6
Mersalyl	T50.2X1	T50.2X2	T50.2X3	T50.2X4	T50.2X5	T50.2X6
Merthiolate	T49.0X1	T49.0X2	T49.0X3	T49.0X4	T49.0X5	T49.0X6
ophthalmic preparation	T49.5X1	T49.5X2	T49.5X3	T49.5X4	T49.5X5	T49.5X6
Meruvax	T50.B91	T50.B92	T50.B93	T50.B94	T50.B95	T50.B96
Mesalazine	T47.8X1	T47.8X2	T47.8X3	T47.8X4	T47.8X5	T47.8X6
Mescal buttons	T40.991	T40.992	T40.993	T40.994	—	—
Mescaline	T40.991	T40.992	T40.993	T40.994	—	—
Mesna	T48.4X1	T48.4X2	T48.4X3	T48.4X4	T48.4X5	T48.4X6
Mesoglycan	T46.6X1	T46.6X2	T46.6X3	T46.6X4	T46.6X5	T46.6X6
Mesoridazine	T43.3X1	T43.3X2	T43.3X3	T43.3X4	T43.3X5	T43.3X6
Mestanolone	T38.7X1	T38.7X2	T38.7X3	T38.7X4	T38.7X5	T38.7X6
Mesterolone	T38.7X1	T38.7X2	T38.7X3	T38.7X4	T38.7X5	T38.7X6
Mestranol	T38.5X1	T38.5X2	T38.5X3	T38.5X4	T38.5X5	T38.5X6
Mesulergine	T42.8X1	T42.8X2	T42.8X3	T42.8X4	T42.8X5	T42.8X6
Mesulfen	T49.0X1	T49.0X2	T49.0X3	T49.0X4	T49.0X5	T49.0X6
Mesuximide	T42.2X1	T42.2X2	T42.2X3	T42.2X4	T42.2X5	T42.2X6
Metabutethamine	T41.3X1	T41.3X2	T41.3X3	T41.3X4	T41.3X5	T41.3X6
Metactesylacetate	T49.0X1	T49.0X2	T49.0X3	T49.0X4	T49.0X5	T49.0X6
Metacycline	T36.4X1	T36.4X2	T36.4X3	T36.4X4	T36.4X5	T36.4X6
Metaldehyde (snail killer) NEC	T60.8X1	T60.8X2	T60.8X3	T60.8X4	—	—
Metals (heavy) (nonmedicinal)	T56.91	T56.92	T56.93	T56.94	—	—
dust, fumes, or vapor NEC	T56.91	T56.92	T56.93	T56.94	—	—
light NEC	T56.91	T56.92	T56.93	T56.94	—	—
dust, fumes, or vapor NEC	T56.91	T56.92	T56.93	T56.94	—	—
specified NEC	T56.891	T56.892	T56.893	T56.894	—	—
thallium	T56.811	T56.812	T56.813	T56.814	—	—
Metamfetamine	T43.621	T43.622	T43.623	T43.624	T43.625	T43.626
Metamizole sodium	T39.2X1	T39.2X2	T39.2X3	T39.2X4	T39.2X5	T39.2X6
Metampicillin	T36.0X1	T36.0X2	T36.0X3	T36.0X4	T36.0X5	T36.0X6
Metamucil	T47.4X1	T47.4X2	T47.4X3	T47.4X4	T47.4X5	T47.4X6
Metandienone	T38.7X1	T38.7X2	T38.7X3	T38.7X4	T38.7X5	T38.7X6
Metandrostenolone	T38.7X1	T38.7X2	T38.7X3	T38.7X4	T38.7X5	T38.7X6
Metaphen	T49.0X1	T49.0X2	T49.0X3	T49.0X4	T49.0X5	T49.0X6

Substance	Poisoning, Accidental (unintentional)	Poisoning, Intentional self-harm	Poisoning, Assault	Poisoning, Undetermined	Adverse effect	Underdosing
Metaphos	T60.0X1	T60.0X2	T60.0X3	T60.0X4	—	—
Metapramine	T43.011	T43.012	T43.013	T43.014	T43.015	T43.016
Metaproterenol	T48.291	T48.292	T48.293	T48.294	T48.295	T48.296
Metaraminol	T44.4X1	T44.4X2	T44.4X3	T44.4X4	T44.4X5	T44.4X6
Metaxalone	T42.8X1	T42.8X2	T42.8X3	T42.8X4	T42.8X5	T42.8X6
Metenolone	T38.7X1	T38.7X2	T38.7X3	T38.7X4	T38.7X5	T38.7X6
Metergoline	T42.8X1	T42.8X2	T42.8X3	T42.8X4	T42.8X5	T42.8X6
Metescufylline	T46.991	T46.992	T46.993	T46.994	T46.995	T46.996
Metetoin	T42.0X1	T42.0X2	T42.0X3	T42.0X4	T42.0X5	T42.0X6
Metformin	T38.3X1	T38.3X2	T38.3X3	T38.3X4	T38.3X5	T38.3X6
Methacholine	T44.1X1	T44.1X2	T44.1X3	T44.1X4	T44.1X5	T44.1X6
Methacycline	T36.4X1	T36.4X2	T36.4X3	T36.4X4	T36.4X5	T36.4X6
Methadone	T40.3X1	T40.3X2	T40.3X3	T40.3X4	T40.3X5	T40.3X6
Methallenestril	T38.5X1	T38.5X2	T38.5X3	T38.5X4	T38.5X5	T38.5X6
Methallenoestril	T38.5X1	T38.5X2	T38.5X3	T38.5X4	T38.5X5	T38.5X6
Methamphetamine	T43.621	T43.622	T43.623	T43.624	T43.625	T43.626
Methampyrone	T39.2X1	T39.2X2	T39.2X3	T39.2X4	T39.2X5	T39.2X6
Methandienone	T38.7X1	T38.7X2	T38.7X3	T38.7X4	T38.7X5	T38.7X6
Methandriol	T38.7X1	T38.7X2	T38.7X3	T38.7X4	T38.7X5	T38.7X6
Methandrostenolone	T38.7X1	T38.7X2	T38.7X3	T38.7X4	T38.7X5	T38.7X6
Methane	T59.891	T59.892	T59.893	T59.894	—	—
Methanethiol	T59.891	T59.892	T59.893	T59.894	—	—
Methaniazide	T37.1X1	T37.1X2	T37.1X3	T37.1X4	T37.1X5	T37.1X6
Methanol (vapor)	T51.1X1	T51.1X2	T51.1X3	T51.1X4	—	—
Methantheline	T44.3X1	T44.3X2	T44.3X3	T44.3X4	T44.3X5	T44.3X6
Methanthelinium bromide	T44.3X1	T44.3X2	T44.3X3	T44.3X4	T44.3X5	T44.3X6
Methaphenilene	T45.0X1	T45.0X2	T45.0X3	T45.0X4	T45.0X5	T45.0X6
Methapyrilene	T45.0X1	T45.0X2	T45.0X3	T45.0X4	T45.0X5	T45.0X6
Methaqualone (compound)	T42.6X1	T42.6X2	T42.6X3	T42.6X4	T42.6X5	T42.6X6
Metharbital	T42.3X1	T42.3X2	T42.3X3	T42.3X4	T42.3X5	T42.3X6
Methazolamide	T50.2X1	T50.2X2	T50.2X3	T50.2X4	T50.2X5	T50.2X6
Methdilazine	T43.3X1	T43.3X2	T43.3X3	T43.3X4	T43.3X5	T43.3X6
Methedrine	T43.621	T43.622	T43.623	T43.624	T43.625	T43.626
Methenamine (mandelate)	T37.8X1	T37.8X2	T37.8X3	T37.8X4	T37.8X5	T37.8X6
Methenolone	T38.7X1	T38.7X2	T38.7X3	T38.7X4	T38.7X5	T38.7X6
Methergine	T48.0X1	T48.0X2	T48.0X3	T48.0X4	T48.0X5	T48.0X6
Methetoin	T42.0X1	T42.0X2	T42.0X3	T42.0X4	T42.0X5	T42.0X6
Methiacil	T38.2X1	T38.2X2	T38.2X3	T38.2X4	T38.2X5	T38.2X6
Methicillin	T36.0X1	T36.0X2	T36.0X3	T36.0X4	T36.0X5	T36.0X6
Methimazole	T38.2X1	T38.2X2	T38.2X3	T38.2X4	T38.2X5	T38.2X6
Methiodal sodium	T50.8X1	T50.8X2	T50.8X3	T50.8X4	T50.8X5	T50.8X6
Methionine	T50.991	T50.992	T50.993	T50.994	T50.995	T50.996
Methisazone	T37.5X1	T37.5X2	T37.5X3	T37.5X4	T37.5X5	T37.5X6
Methisoprinol	T37.5X1	T37.5X2	T37.5X3	T37.5X4	T37.5X5	T37.5X6
Methitural	T42.3X1	T42.3X2	T42.3X3	T42.3X4	T42.3X5	T42.3X6
Methixene	T44.3X1	T44.3X2	T44.3X3	T44.3X4	T44.3X5	T44.3X6
Methobarbital, methobarbitone	T42.3X1	T42.3X2	T42.3X3	T42.3X4	T42.3X5	T42.3X6

Methocarbamol–Methyldopate

Substance	Poisoning, Accidental (unintentional)	Poisoning, Intentional self-harm	Poisoning, Assault	Poisoning, Undetermined	Adverse effect	Underdosing
Methocarbamol	T42.8X1	T42.8X2	T42.8X3	T42.8X4	T42.8X5	T42.8X6
skeletal muscle relaxant	T48.1X1	T48.1X2	T48.1X3	T48.1X4	T48.1X5	T48.1X6
Methohexital	T41.1X1	T41.1X2	T41.1X3	T41.1X4	T41.1X5	T41.1X6
Methohexitone	T41.1X1	T41.1X2	T41.1X3	T41.1X4	T41.1X5	T41.1X6
Methoin	T42.0X1	T42.0X2	T42.0X3	T42.0X4	T42.0X5	T42.0X6
Methopholine	T39.8X1	T39.8X2	T39.8X3	T39.8X4	T39.8X5	T39.8X6
Methopromazine	T43.3X1	T43.3X2	T43.3X3	T43.3X4	T43.3X5	T43.3X6
Methorate	T48.3X1	T48.3X2	T48.3X3	T48.3X4	T48.3X5	T48.3X6
Methoserpidine	T46.5X1	T46.5X2	T46.5X3	T46.5X4	T46.5X5	T46.5X6
Methotrexate	T45.1X1	T45.1X2	T45.1X3	T45.1X4	T45.1X5	T45.1X6
Methotrimeprazine	T43.3X1	T43.3X2	T43.3X3	T43.3X4	T43.3X5	T43.3X6
Methoxa-Dome	T49.3X1	T49.3X2	T49.3X3	T49.3X4	T49.3X5	T49.3X6
Methoxamine	T44.4X1	T44.4X2	T44.4X3	T44.4X4	T44.4X5	T44.4X6
Methoxsalen	T50.991	T50.992	T50.993	T50.994	T50.995	T50.996
Methoxyaniline	T65.3X1	T65.3X2	T65.3X3	T65.3X4	—	—
Methoxybenzyl penicillin	T36.0X1	T36.0X2	T36.0X3	T36.0X4	T36.0X5	T36.0X6
Methoxychlor	T53.7X1	T53.7X2	T53.7X3	T53.7X4	—	—
Methoxy-DDT	T53.7X1	T53.7X2	T53.7X3	T53.7X4	—	—
2-Methoxyethanol	T52.3X1	T52.3X2	T52.3X3	T52.3X4	—	—
Methoxyflurane	T41.0X1	T41.0X2	T41.0X3	T41.0X4	T41.0X5	T41.0X6
Methoxyphenamine	T48.6X1	T48.6X2	T48.6X3	T48.6X4	T48.6X5	T48.6X6
Methoxypromazine	T43.3X1	T43.3X2	T43.3X3	T43.3X4	T43.3X5	T43.3X6
5-Methoxypsoralen (5-MOP)	T50.991	T50.992	T50.993	T50.994	T50.995	T50.996
8-Methoxypsoralen (8-MOP)	T50.991	T50.992	T50.993	T50.994	T50.995	T50.996
Methscopolamine bromide	T44.3X1	T44.3X2	T44.3X3	T44.3X4	T44.3X5	T44.3X6
Methsuximide	T42.2X1	T42.2X2	T42.2X3	T42.2X4	T42.2X5	T42.2X6
Methyclothiazide	T50.2X1	T50.2X2	T50.2X3	T50.2X4	T50.2X5	T50.2X6
Methyl						
acetate	T52.4X1	T52.4X2	T52.4X3	T52.4X4	—	—
acetone	T52.4X1	T52.4X2	T52.4X3	T52.4X4	—	—
acrylate	T65.891	T65.892	T65.893	T65.894	—	—
alcohol	T51.1X1	T51.1X2	T51.1X3	T51.1X4	—	—
aminophenol	T65.3X1	T65.3X2	T65.3X3	T65.3X4	—	—
amphetamine	T43.621	T43.622	T43.623	T43.624	T43.625	T43.626
androstanolone	T38.7X1	T38.7X2	T38.7X3	T38.7X4	T38.7X5	T38.7X6
atropine	T44.3X1	T44.3X2	T44.3X3	T44.3X4	T44.3X5	T44.3X6
benzene	T52.2X1	T52.2X2	T52.2X3	T52.2X4	—	—
benzoate	T52.8X1	T52.8X2	T52.8X3	T52.8X4	—	—
benzol	T52.2X1	T52.2X2	T52.2X3	T52.2X4	—	—
bromide (gas)	T59.891	T59.892	T59.893	T59.894	—	—
fumigant	T60.8X1	T60.8X2	T60.8X3	T60.8X4	—	—
butanol	T51.3X1	T51.3X2	T51.3X3	T51.3X4	—	—
carbinol	T51.1X1	T51.1X2	T51.1X3	T51.1X4	—	—
carbonate	T52.8X1	T52.8X2	T52.8X3	T52.8X4	—	—
CCNU	T45.1X1	T45.1X2	T45.1X3	T45.1X4	T45.1X5	T45.1X6
cellosolve	T52.91	T52.92	T52.93	T52.94	—	—
cellulose	T47.4X1	T47.4X2	T47.4X3	T47.4X4	T47.4X5	T47.4X6

Substance	Poisoning, Accidental (unintentional)	Poisoning, Intentional self-harm	Poisoning, Assault	Poisoning, Undetermined	Adverse effect	Underdosing
Methyl — Continued						
chloride (gas)	T59.891	T59.892	T59.893	T59.894	—	—
chloroformate	T59.3X1	T59.3X2	T59.3X3	T59.3X4	—	—
cyclohexane	T52.8X1	T52.8X2	T52.8X3	T52.8X4	—	—
cyclohexanol	T51.8X1	T51.8X2	T51.8X3	T51.8X4	—	—
cyclohexanone	T52.8X1	T52.8X2	T52.8X3	T52.8X4	—	—
cyclohexyl acetate	T52.8X1	T52.8X2	T52.8X3	T52.8X4	—	—
demeton	T60.0X1	T60.0X2	T60.0X3	T60.0X4	—	—
dihydromorphinone	T40.2X1	T40.2X2	T40.2X3	T40.2X4	T40.2X5	T40.2X6
ergometrine	T48.0X1	T48.0X2	T48.0X3	T48.0X4	T48.0X5	T48.0X6
ergonovine	T48.0X1	T48.0X2	T48.0X3	T48.0X4	T48.0X5	T48.0X6
ethyl ketone	T52.4X1	T52.4X2	T52.4X3	T52.4X4	—	—
glucamine antimonate	T37.8X1	T37.8X2	T37.8X3	T37.8X4	T37.8X5	T37.8X6
hydrazine	T65.891	T65.892	T65.893	T65.894	—	—
iodide	T65.891	T65.892	T65.893	T65.894	—	—
isobutyl ketone	T52.4X1	T52.4X2	T52.4X3	T52.4X4	—	—
isothiocyanate	T60.3X1	T60.3X2	T60.3X3	T60.3X4	—	—
mercaptan	T59.891	T59.892	T59.893	T59.894	—	—
morphine NEC	T40.2X1	T40.2X2	T40.2X3	T40.2X4	T40.2X5	T40.2X6
nicotinate	T49.4X1	T49.4X2	T49.4X3	T49.4X4	T49.4X5	T49.4X6
paraben	T49.0X1	T49.0X2	T49.0X3	T49.0X4	T49.0X5	T49.0X6
parafynol	T42.6X1	T42.6X2	T42.6X3	T42.6X4	T42.6X5	T42.6X6
parathion	T60.0X1	T60.0X2	T60.0X3	T60.0X4	—	—
peridol	T43.4X1	T43.4X2	T43.4X3	T43.4X4	T43.4X5	T43.4X6
phenidate	T43.631	T43.632	T43.633	T43.634	T43.635	T43.636
prednisolone	T38.0X1	T38.0X2	T38.0X3	T38.0X4	T38.0X5	T38.0X6
ENT agent	T49.6X1	T49.6X2	T49.6X3	T49.6X4	T49.6X5	T49.6X6
ophthalmic preparation	T49.5X1	T49.5X2	T49.5X3	T49.5X4	T49.5X5	T49.5X6
topical NEC	T49.0X1	T49.0X2	T49.0X3	T49.0X4	T49.0X5	T49.0X6
propylcarbinol	T51.3X1	T51.3X2	T51.3X3	T51.3X4	—	—
rosaniline NEC	T49.0X1	T49.0X2	T49.0X3	T49.0X4	T49.0X5	T49.0X6
salicylate	T49.2X1	T49.2X2	T49.2X3	T49.2X4	T49.2X5	T49.2X6
sulfate (fumes)	T59.891	T59.892	T59.893	T59.894	—	—
liquid	T52.8X1	T52.8X2	T52.8X3	T52.8X4	—	—
sulfonal	T42.6X1	T42.6X2	T42.6X3	T42.6X4	T42.6X5	T42.6X6
testosterone	T38.7X1	T38.7X2	T38.7X3	T38.7X4	T38.7X5	T38.7X6
thiouracil	T38.2X1	T38.2X2	T38.2X3	T38.2X4	T38.2X5	T38.2X6
Methylamphetamine	T43.621	T43.622	T43.623	T43.624	T43.625	T43.626
Methylated spirit	T51.1X1	T51.1X2	T51.1X3	T51.1X4	—	—
Methylatropine nitrate	T44.3X1	T44.3X2	T44.3X3	T44.3X4	T44.3X5	T44.3X6
Methylbenactyzium bromide	T44.3X1	T44.3X2	T44.3X3	T44.3X4	T44.3X5	T44.3X6
Methylbenzethonium chloride	T49.0X1	T49.0X2	T49.0X3	T49.0X4	T49.0X5	T49.0X6
Methylcellulose	T47.4X1	T47.4X2	T47.4X3	T47.4X4	T47.4X5	T47.4X6
laxative	T47.4X1	T47.4X2	T47.4X3	T47.4X4	T47.4X5	T47.4X6
Methylchlorophenoxy-acetic acid	T60.3X1	T60.3X2	T60.3X3	T60.3X4	—	—
Methyldopa	T46.5X1	T46.5X2	T46.5X3	T46.5X4	T46.5X5	T46.5X6
Methyldopate	T46.5X1	T46.5X2	T46.5X3	T46.5X4	T46.5X5	T46.5X6

Substance	Poisoning, Accidental (unintentional)	Poisoning, Intentional self-harm	Poisoning, Assault	Poisoning, Undetermined	Adverse effect	Underdosing
Methylene						
blue	T50.6X1	T50.6X2	T50.6X3	T50.6X4	T50.6X5	T50.6X6
chloride or dichloride (solvent) NEC	T53.4X1	T53.4X2	T53.4X3	T53.4X4	—	—
Methylenedioxy-amphetamine	T43.621	T43.622	T43.623	T43.624	T43.625	T43.626
Methylenedioxy-methamphetamine	T43.641	T43.642	T43.643	T43.644	—	—
Methylergometrine	T48.0X1	T48.0X2	T48.0X3	T48.0X4	T48.0X5	T48.0X6
Methylergonovine	T48.0X1	T48.0X2	T48.0X3	T48.0X4	T48.0X5	T48.0X6
Methylestrenolone	T38.5X1	T38.5X2	T38.5X3	T38.5X4	T38.5X5	T38.5X6
Methylethyl cellulose	T50.991	T50.992	T50.993	T50.994	T50.995	T50.996
Methylhexabital	T42.3X1	T42.3X2	T42.3X3	T42.3X4	T42.3X5	T42.3X6
Methylmorphine	T40.2X1	T40.2X2	T40.2X3	T40.2X4	T40.2X5	T40.2X6
Methylparaben (ophthalmic)	T49.5X1	T49.5X2	T49.5X3	T49.5X4	T49.5X5	T49.5X6
Methylparafynol	T42.6X1	T42.6X2	T42.6X3	T42.6X4	T42.6X5	T42.6X6
Methylpentynol, methylpenthynol	T42.6X1	T42.6X2	T42.6X3	T42.6X4	T42.6X5	T42.6X6
Methylphenidate	T43.631	T43.632	T43.633	T43.634	T43.635	T43.636
Methylphenobarbital	T42.3X1	T42.3X2	T42.3X3	T42.3X4	T42.3X5	T42.3X6
Methylpolysiloxane	T47.1X1	T47.1X2	T47.1X3	T47.1X4	T47.1X5	T47.1X6
Methylprednisolone— see Methyl, prednisolone						
Methylrosaniline	T49.0X1	T49.0X2	T49.0X3	T49.0X4	T49.0X5	T49.0X6
Methylrosanilinium chloride	T49.0X1	T49.0X2	T49.0X3	T49.0X4	T49.0X5	T49.0X6
Methyltestosterone	T38.7X1	T38.7X2	T38.7X3	T38.7X4	T38.7X5	T38.7X6
Methylthionine chloride	T50.6X1	T50.6X2	T50.6X3	T50.6X4	T50.6X5	T50.6X6
Methylthioninium chloride	T50.6X1	T50.6X2	T50.6X3	T50.6X4	T50.6X5	T50.6X6
Methylthiouracil	T38.2X1	T38.2X2	T38.2X3	T38.2X4	T38.2X5	T38.2X6
Methyprylon	T42.6X1	T42.6X2	T42.6X3	T42.6X4	T42.6X5	T42.6X6
Methysergide	T46.5X1	T46.5X2	T46.5X3	T46.5X4	T46.5X5	T46.5X6
Metiamide	T47.1X1	T47.1X2	T47.1X3	T47.1X4	T47.1X5	T47.1X6
Meticillin	T36.0X1	T36.0X2	T36.0X3	T36.0X4	T36.0X5	T36.0X6
Meticrane	T50.2X1	T50.2X2	T50.2X3	T50.2X4	T50.2X5	T50.2X6
Metildigoxin	T46.0X1	T46.0X2	T46.0X3	T46.0X4	T46.0X5	T46.0X6
Metipranolol	T49.5X1	T49.5X2	T49.5X3	T49.5X4	T49.5X5	T49.5X6
Metirosine	T46.5X1	T46.5X2	T46.5X3	T46.5X4	T46.5X5	T46.5X6
Metisazone	T37.5X1	T37.5X2	T37.5X3	T37.5X4	T37.5X5	T37.5X6
Metixene	T44.3X1	T44.3X2	T44.3X3	T44.3X4	T44.3X5	T44.3X6
Metizoline	T48.5X1	T48.5X2	T48.5X3	T48.5X4	T48.5X5	T48.5X6
Metoclopramide	T45.0X1	T45.0X2	T45.0X3	T45.0X4	T45.0X5	T45.0X6
Metofenazate	T43.3X1	T43.3X2	T43.3X3	T43.3X4	T43.3X5	T43.3X6
Metofoline	T39.8X1	T39.8X2	T39.8X3	T39.8X4	T39.8X5	T39.8X6
Metolazone	T50.2X1	T50.2X2	T50.2X3	T50.2X4	T50.2X5	T50.2X6
Metopon	T40.2X1	T40.2X2	T40.2X3	T40.2X4	T40.2X5	T40.2X6
Metoprine	T45.1X1	T45.1X2	T45.1X3	T45.1X4	T45.1X5	T45.1X6
Metoprolol	T44.7X1	T44.7X2	T44.7X3	T44.7X4	T44.7X5	T44.7X6
Metrifonate	T60.0X1	T60.0X2	T60.0X3	T60.0X4	—	—
Metrizamide	T50.8X1	T50.8X2	T50.8X3	T50.8X4	T50.8X5	T50.8X6
Metrizoic acid	T50.8X1	T50.8X2	T50.8X3	T50.8X4	T50.8X5	T50.8X6

Substance	Poisoning, Accidental (unintentional)	Poisoning, Intentional self-harm	Poisoning, Assault	Poisoning, Undetermined	Adverse effect	Underdosing
Metronidazole	T37.8X1	T37.8X2	T37.8X3	T37.8X4	T37.8X5	T37.8X6
Metycaine	T41.3X1	T41.3X2	T41.3X3	T41.3X4	T41.3X5	T41.3X6
infiltration (subcutaneous)	T41.3X1	T41.3X2	T41.3X3	T41.3X4	T41.3X5	T41.3X6
nerve block (peripheral) (plexus)	T41.3X1	T41.3X2	T41.3X3	T41.3X4	T41.3X5	T41.3X6
topical (surface)	T41.3X1	T41.3X2	T41.3X3	T41.3X4	T41.3X5	T41.3X6
Metyrapone	T50.8X1	T50.8X2	T50.8X3	T50.8X4	T50.8X5	T50.8X6
Mevinphos	T60.0X1	T60.0X2	T60.0X3	T60.0X4	—	—
Mexazolam	T42.4X1	T42.4X2	T42.4X3	T42.4X4	T42.4X5	T42.4X6
Mexenone	T49.3X1	T49.3X2	T49.3X3	T49.3X4	T49.3X5	T49.3X6
Mexiletine	T46.2X1	T46.2X2	T46.2X3	T46.2X4	T46.2X5	T46.2X6
Mezereon	T62.2X1	T62.2X2	T62.2X3	T62.2X4	—	—
berries	T62.1X1	T62.1X2	T62.1X3	T62.1X4	—	—
Mezlocillin	T36.0X1	T36.0X2	T36.0X3	T36.0X4	T36.0X5	T36.0X6
Mianserin	T43.021	T43.022	T43.023	T43.024	T43.025	T43.026
Micatin	T49.0X1	T49.0X2	T49.0X3	T49.0X4	T49.0X5	T49.0X6
Miconazole	T49.0X1	T49.0X2	T49.0X3	T49.0X4	T49.0X5	T49.0X6
Micronomicin	T36.5X1	T36.5X2	T36.5X3	T36.5X4	T36.5X5	T36.5X6
Midazolam	T42.4X1	T42.4X2	T42.4X3	T42.4X4	T42.4X5	T42.4X6
Midecamycin	T36.3X1	T36.3X2	T36.3X3	T36.3X4	T36.3X5	T36.3X6
Mifepristone	T38.6X1	T38.6X2	T38.6X3	T38.6X4	T38.6X5	T38.6X6
Milk of magnesia	T47.1X1	T47.1X2	T47.1X3	T47.1X4	T47.1X5	T47.1X6
Millipede (tropical) (venomous)	T63.411	T63.412	T63.413	T63.414	—	—
Miltown	T43.591	T43.592	T43.593	T43.594	T43.595	T43.596
Milverine	T44.3X1	T44.3X2	T44.3X3	T44.3X4	T44.3X5	T44.3X6
Minaprine	T43.291	T43.292	T43.293	T43.294	T43.295	T43.296
Minaxolone	T41.291	T41.292	T41.293	T41.294	T41.295	T41.296
Mineral						
acids	T54.2X1	T54.2X2	T54.2X3	T54.2X4	—	—
oil (laxative) (medicinal)	T47.4X1	T47.4X2	T47.4X3	T47.4X4	T47.4X5	T47.4X6
emulsion	T47.2X1	T47.2X2	T47.2X3	T47.2X4	T47.2X5	T47.2X6
nonmedicinal	T52.0X1	T52.0X2	T52.0X3	T52.0X4	—	—
topical	T49.3X1	T49.3X2	T49.3X3	T49.3X4	T49.3X5	T49.3X6
salt NEC	T50.3X1	T50.3X2	T50.3X3	T50.3X4	T50.3X5	T50.3X6
spirits	T52.0X1	T52.0X2	T52.0X3	T52.0X4	—	—
Mineralocorticosteroid	T50.0X1	T50.0X2	T50.0X3	T50.0X4	T50.0X5	T50.0X6
Minocycline	T36.4X1	T36.4X2	T36.4X3	T36.4X4	T36.4X5	T36.4X6
Minoxidil	T46.7X1	T46.7X2	T46.7X3	T46.7X4	T46.7X5	T46.7X6
Miokamycin	T36.3X1	T36.3X2	T36.3X3	T36.3X4	T36.3X5	T36.3X6
Miotic drug	T49.5X1	T49.5X2	T49.5X3	T49.5X4	T49.5X5	T49.5X6
Mipafox	T60.0X1	T60.0X2	T60.0X3	T60.0X4	—	—
Mirex	T60.1X1	T60.1X2	T60.1X3	T60.1X4	—	—
Mirtazapine	T43.021	T43.022	T43.023	T43.024	T43.025	T43.026
Misonidazole	T37.3X1	T37.3X2	T37.3X3	T37.3X4	T37.3X5	T37.3X6
Misoprostol	T47.1X1	T47.1X2	T47.1X3	T47.1X4	T47.1X5	T47.1X6
Mithramycin	T45.1X1	T45.1X2	T45.1X3	T45.1X4	T45.1X5	T45.1X6
Mitobronitol	T45.1X1	T45.1X2	T45.1X3	T45.1X4	T45.1X5	T45.1X6
Mitoguazone	T45.1X1	T45.1X2	T45.1X3	T45.1X4	T45.1X5	T45.1X6

Substance	Poisoning, Accidental (unintentional)	Poisoning, Intentional self-harm	Poisoning, Assault	Poisoning, Undetermined	Adverse effect	Underdosing
Mitolactol	T45.1X1	T45.1X2	T45.1X3	T45.1X4	T45.1X5	T45.1X6
Mitomycin	T45.1X1	T45.1X2	T45.1X3	T45.1X4	T45.1X5	T45.1X6
Mitopodozide	T45.1X1	T45.1X2	T45.1X3	T45.1X4	T45.1X5	T45.1X6
Mitotane	T45.1X1	T45.1X2	T45.1X3	T45.1X4	T45.1X5	T45.1X6
Mitoxantrone	T45.1X1	T45.1X2	T45.1X3	T45.1X4	T45.1X5	T45.1X6
Mivacurium chloride	T48.1X1	T48.1X2	T48.1X3	T48.1X4	T48.1X5	T48.1X6
Miyari bacteria	T47.6X1	T47.6X2	T47.6X3	T47.6X4	T47.6X5	T47.6X6
Moclobemide	T43.1X1	T43.1X2	T43.1X3	T43.1X4	T43.1X5	T43.1X6
Moderil	T46.5X1	T46.5X2	T46.5X3	T46.5X4	T46.5X5	T46.5X6
Mofebutazone	T39.2X1	T39.2X2	T39.2X3	T39.2X4	T39.2X5	T39.2X6
Mogadon—see Nitrazepam						
Molindone	T43.591	T43.592	T43.593	T43.594	T43.595	T43.596
Molsidomine	T46.3X1	T46.3X2	T46.3X3	T46.3X4	T46.3X5	T46.3X6
Mometasone	T49.0X1	T49.0X2	T49.0X3	T49.0X4	T49.0X5	T49.0X6
Monistat	T49.0X1	T49.0X2	T49.0X3	T49.0X4	T49.0X5	T49.0X6
Monkshood	T62.2X1	T62.2X2	T62.2X3	T62.2X4	—	—
Monoamine oxidase inhibitor NEC	T43.1X1	T43.1X2	T43.1X3	T43.1X4	T43.1X5	T43.1X6
hydrazine	T43.1X1	T43.1X2	T43.1X3	T43.1X4	T43.1X5	T43.1X6
Monobenzone	T49.4X1	T49.4X2	T49.4X3	T49.4X4	T49.4X5	T49.4X6
Monochloroacetic acid	T60.3X1	T60.3X2	T60.3X3	T60.3X4	—	—
Monochlorobenzene	T53.7X1	T53.7X2	T53.7X3	T53.7X4	—	—
Monoethanolamine	T46.8X1	T46.8X2	T46.8X3	T46.8X4	T46.8X5	T46.8X6
oleate	T46.8X1	T46.8X2	T46.8X3	T46.8X4	T46.8X5	T46.8X6
Monooctanoin	T50.991	T50.992	T50.993	T50.994	T50.995	T50.996
Monophenylbutazone	T39.2X1	T39.2X2	T39.2X3	T39.2X4	T39.2X5	T39.2X6
Monosodium glutamate	T65.891	T65.892	T65.893	T65.894		
Monosulfiram	T49.0X1	T49.0X2	T49.0X3	T49.0X4	T49.0X5	T49.0X6
Monoxide, carbon—see Carbon, monoxide						
Monoxidine hydrochloride	T46.1X1	T46.1X2	T46.1X3	T46.1X4	T46.1X5	T46.1X6
Monuron	T60.3X1	T60.3X2	T60.3X3	T60.3X4	—	—
Moperone	T43.4X1	T43.4X2	T43.4X3	T43.4X4	T43.4X5	T43.4X6
Mopidamol	T45.1X1	T45.1X2	T45.1X3	T45.1X4	T45.1X5	T45.1X6
MOPP (mechloreth-amine + vincristine + prednisone + procarba-zine)	T45.1X1	T45.1X2	T45.1X3	T45.1X4	T45.1X5	T45.1X6
Morfin	T40.2X1	T40.2X2	T40.2X3	T40.2X4	T40.2X5	T40.2X6
Morinamide	T37.1X1	T37.1X2	T37.1X3	T37.1X4	T37.1X5	T37.1X6
Morning glory seeds	T40.991	T40.992	T40.993	T40.994	—	—
Moroxydine	T37.5X1	T37.5X2	T37.5X3	T37.5X4	T37.5X5	T37.5X6
Morphazinamide	T37.1X1	T37.1X2	T37.1X3	T37.1X4	T37.1X5	T37.1X6
Morphine	T40.2X1	T40.2X2	T40.2X3	T40.2X4	T40.2X5	T40.2X6
antagonist	T50.7X1	T50.7X2	T50.7X3	T50.7X4	T50.7X5	T50.7X6
Morpholinylethyl-morphine	T40.2X1	T40.2X2	T40.2X3	T40.2X4	—	—
Morsuximide	T42.2X1	T42.2X2	T42.2X3	T42.2X4	T42.2X5	T42.2X6
Mosapramine	T43.591	T43.592	T43.593	T43.594	T43.595	T43.596

Substance	Poisoning, Accidental (unintentional)	Poisoning, Intentional self-harm	Poisoning, Assault	Poisoning, Undetermined	Adverse effect	Underdosing
Moth balls—see also Pesticides	T60.2X1	T60.2X2	T60.2X3	T60.2X4	—	—
naphthalene	T60.2X1	T60.2X2	T60.2X3	T60.2X4	—	—
paradichlorobenzene	T60.1X1	T60.1X2	T60.1X3	T60.1X4	—	—
Motor exhaust gas	T58.01	T58.02	T58.03	T58.04	—	—
Mouthwash (antiseptic) (zincchloride)	T49.6X1	T49.6X2	T49.6X3	T49.6X4	T49.6X5	T49.6X6
Moxastine	T45.0X1	T45.0X2	T45.0X3	T45.0X4	T45.0X5	T45.0X6
Moxaverine	T44.3X1	T44.3X2	T44.3X3	T44.3X4	T44.3X5	T44.3X6
Moxisylyte	T46.7X1	T46.7X2	T46.7X3	T46.7X4	T46.7X5	T46.7X6
Mucilage, plant	T47.4X1	T47.4X2	T47.4X3	T47.4X4	T47.4X5	T47.4X6
Mucolytic drug	T48.4X1	T48.4X2	T48.4X3	T48.4X4	T48.4X5	T48.4X6
Mucomyst	T48.4X1	T48.4X2	T48.4X3	T48.4X4	T48.4X5	T48.4X6
Mucous membrane agents (external)	T49.91	T49.92	T49.93	T49.94	T49.95	T49.96
specified NEC	T49.8X1	T49.8X2	T49.8X3	T49.8X4	T49.8X5	T49.8X6
Multiple unspecified drugs, medicaments and biological substances	T50.911	T50.912	T50.913	T50.914	T50.915	T50.916
Mumps						
immune globulin (human)	T50.Z11	T50.Z12	T50.Z13	T50.Z14	T50.Z15	T50.Z16
skin test antigen	T50.8X1	T50.8X2	T50.8X3	T50.8X4	T50.8X5	T50.8X6
vaccine	T50.B91	T50.B92	T50.B93	T50.B94	T50.B95	T50.B96
Mumpsvax	T50.B91	T50.B92	T50.B93	T50.B94	T50.B95	T50.B96
Mupirocin	T49.0X1	T49.0X2	T49.0X3	T49.0X4	T49.0X5	T49.0X6
Muriatic acid—see Hydrochloric acid						
Muromonab-CD3	T45.1X1	T45.1X2	T45.1X3	T45.1X4	T45.1X5	T45.1X6
Muscle-action drug NEC	T48.201	T48.202	T48.203	T48.204	T48.205	T48.206
Muscle affecting agents NEC	T48.201	T48.202	T48.203	T48.204	T48.205	T48.206
oxytocic	T48.0X1	T48.0X2	T48.0X3	T48.0X4	T48.0X5	T48.0X6
relaxants	T48.201	T48.202	T48.203	T48.204	T48.205	T48.206
central nervous system	T42.8X1	T42.8X2	T42.8X3	T42.8X4	T42.8X5	T42.8X6
skeletal	T48.1X1	T48.1X2	T48.1X3	T48.1X4	T48.1X5	T48.1X6
smooth	T44.3X1	T44.3X2	T44.3X3	T44.3X4	T44.3X5	T44.3X6
Muscle relaxant—see Relaxant, muscle						
Muscle-tone depressant, central NEC	T42.8X1	T42.8X2	T42.8X3	T42.8X4	T42.8X5	T42.8X6
specified NEC	T42.8X1	T42.8X2	T42.8X3	T42.8X4	T42.8X5	T42.8X6
Mushroom, noxious	T62.0X1	T62.0X2	T62.0X3	T62.0X4	—	—
Mussel, noxious	T61.781	T61.782	T61.783	T61.784	—	—
Mustard (emetic)	T47.7X1	T47.7X2	T47.7X3	T47.7X4	T47.7X5	T47.7X6
black	T47.7X1	T47.7X2	T47.7X3	T47.7X4	T47.7X5	T47.7X6
gas, not in war	T59.91	T59.92	T59.93	T59.94	—	—
nitrogen	T45.1X1	T45.1X2	T45.1X3	T45.1X4	T45.1X5	T45.1X6
Mustine	T45.1X1	T45.1X2	T45.1X3	T45.1X4	T45.1X5	T45.1X6
M-vac	T45.1X1	T45.1X2	T45.1X3	T45.1X4	T45.1X5	T45.1X6
Mycifradin	T36.5X1	T36.5X2	T36.5X3	T36.5X4	T36.5X5	T36.5X6
topical	T49.0X1	T49.0X2	T49.0X3	T49.0X4	T49.0X5	T49.0X6

Substance	Poisoning, Accidental (unintentional)	Poisoning, Intentional self-harm	Poisoning, Assault	Poisoning, Undetermined	Adverse effect	Underdosing
Mycitracin	T36.8X1	T36.8X2	T36.8X3	T36.8X4	T36.8X5	T36.8X6
ophthalmic preparation	T49.5X1	T49.5X2	T49.5X3	T49.5X4	T49.5X5	T49.5X6
Mycostatin	T36.7X1	T36.7X2	T36.7X3	T36.7X4	T36.7X5	T36.7X6
topical	T49.0X1	T49.0X2	T49.0X3	T49.0X4	T49.0X5	T49.0X6
Mycotoxins	T64.81	T64.82	T64.83	T64.84	—	—
aflatoxin	T64.01	T64.02	T64.03	T64.04	—	—
specified NEC	T64.81	T64.82	T64.83	T64.84	—	—
Mydriacyl	T44.3X1	T44.3X2	T44.3X3	T44.3X4	T44.3X5	T44.3X6
Mydriatic drug	T49.5X1	T49.5X2	T49.5X3	T49.5X4	T49.5X5	T49.5X6
Myelobromal	T45.1X1	T45.1X2	T45.1X3	T45.1X4	T45.1X5	T45.1X6
Myleran	T45.1X1	T45.1X2	T45.1X3	T45.1X4	T45.1X5	T45.1X6
Myochrysin(e)	T39.2X1	T39.2X2	T39.2X3	T39.2X4	T39.2X5	T39.2X6
Myoneural blocking agents	T48.1X1	T48.1X2	T48.1X3	T48.1X4	T48.1X5	T48.1X6
Myralact	T49.0X1	T49.0X2	T49.0X3	T49.0X4	T49.0X5	T49.0X6
Myristica fragrans	T62.2X1	T62.2X2	T62.2X3	T62.2X4	—	—
Myristicin	T65.891	T65.892	T65.893	T65.894	—	—
Mysoline	T42.3X1	T42.3X2	T42.3X3	T42.3X4	T42.3X5	T42.3X6
N						
Nabilone	T40.7X1	T40.7X2	T40.7X3	T40.7X4	T40.7X5	T40.7X6
Nabumetone	T39.391	T39.392	T39.393	T39.394	T39.395	T39.396
Nadolol	T44.7X1	T44.7X2	T44.7X3	T44.7X4	T44.7X5	T44.7X6
Nafcillin	T36.0X1	T36.0X2	T36.0X3	T36.0X4	T36.0X5	T36.0X6
Nafoxidine	T38.6X1	T38.6X2	T38.6X3	T38.6X4	T38.6X5	T38.6X6
Naftazone	T46.991	T46.992	T46.993	T46.994	T46.995	T46.996
Naftidrofuryl (oxalate)	T46.7X1	T46.7X2	T46.7X3	T46.7X4	T46.7X5	T46.7X6
Naftifine	T49.0X1	T49.0X2	T49.0X3	T49.0X4	T49.0X5	T49.0X6
Nail polish remover	T52.91	T52.92	T52.93	T52.94	—	—
Nalbuphine	T40.491	T40.492	T40.493	T40.494	T40.495	T40.496
Naled	T60.0X1	T60.0X2	T60.0X3	T60.0X4	—	—
Nalidixic acid	T37.8X1	T37.8X2	T37.8X3	T37.8X4	T37.8X5	T37.8X6
Nalorphine	T50.7X1	T50.7X2	T50.7X3	T50.7X4	T50.7X5	T50.7X6
Naloxone	T50.7X1	T50.7X2	T50.7X3	T50.7X4	T50.7X5	T50.7X6
Naltrexone	T50.7X1	T50.7X2	T50.7X3	T50.7X4	T50.7X5	T50.7X6
Namenda	T43.8X1	T43.8X2	T43.8X3	T43.8X4	T43.8X5	T43.8X6
Nandrolone	T38.7X1	T38.7X2	T38.7X3	T38.7X4	T38.7X5	T38.7X6
Naphazoline	T48.5X1	T48.5X2	T48.5X3	T48.5X4	T48.5X5	T48.5X6
Naphtha (painters') (petroleum)	T52.0X1	T52.0X2	T52.0X3	T52.0X4	—	—
solvent	T52.0X1	T52.0X2	T52.0X3	T52.0X4	—	—
vapor	T52.0X1	T52.0X2	T52.0X3	T52.0X4	—	—
Naphthalene (non-chlorinated)	T60.2X1	T60.2X2	T60.2X3	T60.2X4	—	—
chlorinated	T60.1X1	T60.1X2	T60.1X3	T60.1X4	—	—
vapor	T60.1X1	T60.1X2	T60.1X3	T60.1X4	—	—
insecticide or moth repellent	T60.2X1	T60.2X2	T60.2X3	T60.2X4	—	—
chlorinated	T60.1X1	T60.1X2	T60.1X3	T60.1X4	—	—
vapor	T60.2X1	T60.2X2	T60.2X3	T60.2X4	—	—
chlorinated	T60.1X1	T60.1X2	T60.1X3	T60.1X4	—	—
Naphthol	T65.891	T65.892	T65.893	T65.894		

Substance	Poisoning, Accidental (unintentional)	Poisoning, Intentional self-harm	Poisoning, Assault	Poisoning, Undetermined	Adverse effect	Underdosing
Naphthylamine	T65.891	T65.892	T65.893	T65.894	—	—
Naphthylthiourea (ANTU)	T60.4X1	T60.4X2	T60.4X3	T60.4X4	—	—
Naprosyn—see Naproxen						
Naproxen	T39.311	T39.312	T39.313	T39.314	T39.315	T39.316
Narcotic (drug)	T40.601	T40.602	T40.603	T40.604	T40.605	T40.606
analgesic NEC	T40.601	T40.602	T40.603	T40.604	T40.605	T40.606
antagonist	T50.7X1	T50.7X2	T50.7X3	T50.7X4	T50.7X5	T50.7X6
specified NEC	T40.691	T40.692	T40.693	T40.694	T40.695	T40.696
synthetic	T40.491	T40.492	T40.493	T40.494	T40.495	T40.496
Narcotine	T48.3X1	T48.3X2	T48.3X3	T48.3X4	T48.3X5	T48.3X6
Nardil	T43.1X1	T43.1X2	T43.1X3	T43.1X4	T43.1X5	T43.1X6
Nasal drug NEC	T49.6X1	T49.6X2	T49.6X3	T49.6X4	T49.6X5	T49.6X6
Natamycin	T49.0X1	T49.0X2	T49.0X3	T49.0X4	T49.0X5	T49.0X6
Natrium cyanide—see Cyanide (s)						
Natural						
blood (product)	T45.8X1	T45.8X2	T45.8X3	T45.8X4	T45.8X5	T45.8X6
gas (piped)	T59.891	T59.892	T59.893	T59.894	—	—
incomplete combustion	T58.11	T58.12	T58.13	T58.14	—	—
Nealbarbital	T42.3X1	T42.3X2	T42.3X3	T42.3X4	T42.3X5	T42.3X6
Nectadon	T48.3X1	T48.3X2	T48.3X3	T48.3X4	T48.3X5	T48.3X6
Nedocromil	T48.6X1	T48.6X2	T48.6X3	T48.6X4	T48.6X5	T48.6X6
Nefopam	T39.8X1	T39.8X2	T39.8X3	T39.8X4	T39.8X5	T39.8X6
Nematocyst (sting)	T63.691	T63.692	T63.693	T63.694	—	—
Nembutal	T42.3X1	T42.3X2	T42.3X3	T42.3X4	T42.3X5	T42.3X6
Nemonapride	T43.591	T43.592	T43.593	T43.594	T43.595	T43.596
Neoarsphenamine	T37.8X1	T37.8X2	T37.8X3	T37.8X4	T37.8X5	T37.8X6
Neocinchophen	T50.4X1	T50.4X2	T50.4X3	T50.4X4	T50.4X5	T50.4X6
Neomycin (derivatives)	T36.5X1	T36.5X2	T36.5X3	T36.5X4	T36.5X5	T36.5X6
with						
bacitracin	T49.0X1	T49.0X2	T49.0X3	T49.0X4	T49.0X5	T49.0X6
neostigmine	T44.0X1	T44.0X2	T44.0X3	T44.0X4	T44.0X5	T44.0X6
ENT agent	T49.6X1	T49.6X2	T49.6X3	T49.6X4	T49.6X5	T49.6X6
ophthalmic preparation	T49.5X1	T49.5X2	T49.5X3	T49.5X4	T49.5X5	T49.5X6
topical NEC	T49.0X1	T49.0X2	T49.0X3	T49.0X4	T49.0X5	T49.0X6
Neonal	T42.3X1	T42.3X2	T42.3X3	T42.3X4	T42.3X5	T42.3X6
Neoprontosil	T37.0X1	T37.0X2	T37.0X3	T37.0X4	T37.0X5	T37.0X6
Neosalvarsan	T37.8X1	T37.8X2	T37.8X3	T37.8X4	T37.8X5	T37.8X6
Neosilversalvarsan	T37.8X1	T37.8X2	T37.8X3	T37.8X4	T37.8X5	T37.8X6
Neosporin	T36.8X1	T36.8X2	T36.8X3	T36.8X4	T36.8X5	T36.8X6
ENT agent	T49.6X1	T49.6X2	T49.6X3	T49.6X4	T49.6X5	T49.6X6
opthalmic preparation	T49.5X1	T49.5X2	T49.5X3	T49.5X4	T49.5X5	T49.5X6
topical NEC	T49.0X1	T49.0X2	T49.0X3	T49.0X4	T49.0X5	T49.0X6
Neostigmine bromide	T44.0X1	T44.0X2	T44.0X3	T44.0X4	T44.0X5	T44.0X6
Neraval	T42.3X1	T42.3X2	T42.3X3	T42.3X4	T42.3X5	T42.3X6
Neravan	T42.3X1	T42.3X2	T42.3X3	T42.3X4	T42.3X5	T42.3X6
Nerium oleander	T62.2X1	T62.2X2	T62.2X3	T62.2X4	—	—
Nerve gas, not in war	T59.91	T59.92	T59.93	T59.94	—	—

Substance	Poisoning, Accidental (unintentional)	Poisoning, Intentional self-harm	Poisoning, Assault	Poisoning, Undetermined	Adverse effect	Underdosing
Nesacaine	T41.3X1	T41.3X2	T41.3X3	T41.3X4	T41.3X5	T41.3X6
infiltration (subcutaneous)	T41.3X1	T41.3X2	T41.3X3	T41.3X4	T41.3X5	T41.3X6
nerve block (peripheral) (plexus)	T41.3X1	T41.3X2	T41.3X3	T41.3X4	T41.3X5	T41.3X6
Netilmicin	T36.5X1	T36.5X2	T36.5X3	T36.5X4	T36.5X5	T36.5X6
Neurobarb	T42.3X1	T42.3X2	T42.3X3	T42.3X4	T42.3X5	T42.3X6
Neuroleptic drug NEC	T43.501	T43.502	T43.503	T43.504	T43.505	T43.506
Neuromuscular blocking drug	T48.1X1	T48.1X2	T48.1X3	T48.1X4	T48.1X5	T48.1X6
Neutral insulin injection	T38.3X1	T38.3X2	T38.3X3	T38.3X4	T38.3X5	T38.3X6
Neutral spirits	T51.0X1	T51.0X2	T51.0X3	T51.0X4	—	—
beverage	T51.0X1	T51.0X2	T51.0X3	T51.0X4	—	—
Niacin	T46.7X1	T46.7X2	T46.7X3	T46.7X4	T46.7X5	T46.7X6
Niacinamide	T45.2X1	T45.2X2	T45.2X3	T45.2X4	T45.2X5	T45.2X6
Nialamide	T43.1X1	T43.1X2	T43.1X3	T43.1X4	T43.1X5	T43.1X6
Niaprazine	T42.6X1	T42.6X2	T42.6X3	T42.6X4	T42.6X5	T42.6X6
Nicametate	T46.7X1	T46.7X2	T46.7X3	T46.7X4	T46.7X5	T46.7X6
Nicardipine	T46.1X1	T46.1X2	T46.1X3	T46.1X4	T46.1X5	T46.1X6
Nicergoline	T46.7X1	T46.7X2	T46.7X3	T46.7X4	T46.7X5	T46.7X6
Nickel (carbonyl) (tetra-carbonyl) (fumes) (vapor)	T56.891	T56.892	T56.893	T56.894	—	—
Nickelocene	T56.891	T56.892	T56.893	T56.894	—	—
Niclosamide	T37.4X1	T37.4X2	T37.4X3	T37.4X4	T37.4X5	T37.4X6
Nicofuranose	T46.7X1	T46.7X2	T46.7X3	T46.7X4	T46.7X5	T46.7X6
Nicomorphine	T40.2X1	T40.2X2	T40.2X3	T40.2X4	—	—
Nicorandil	T46.3X1	T46.3X2	T46.3X3	T46.3X4	T46.3X5	T46.3X6
Nicotiana (plant)	T62.2X1	T62.2X2	T62.2X3	T62.2X4	—	—
Nicotinamide	T45.2X1	T45.2X2	T45.2X3	T45.2X4	T45.2X5	T45.2X6
Nicotine (insecticide) (spray) (sulfate) NEC	T60.2X1	T60.2X2	T60.2X3	T60.2X4		
from tobacco	T65.291	T65.292	T65.293	T65.294	—	—
cigarettes	T65.221	T65.222	T65.223	T65.224	—	—
not insecticide	T65.291	T65.292	T65.293	T65.294	—	—
Nicotinic acid	T46.7X1	T46.7X2	T46.7X3	T46.7X4	T46.7X5	T46.7X6
Nicotinyl alcohol	T46.7X1	T46.7X2	T46.7X3	T46.7X4	T46.7X5	T46.7X6
Nicoumalone	T45.511	T45.512	T45.513	T45.514	T45.515	T45.516
Nifedipine	T46.1X1	T46.1X2	T46.1X3	T46.1X4	T46.1X5	T46.1X6
Nifenazone	T39.2X1	T39.2X2	T39.2X3	T39.2X4	T39.2X5	T39.2X6
Nifuraldezone	T37.91	T37.92	T37.93	T37.94	T37.95	T37.96
Nifuratel	T37.8X1	T37.8X2	T37.8X3	T37.8X4	T37.8X5	T37.8X6
Nifurtimox	T37.3X1	T37.3X2	T37.3X3	T37.3X4	T37.3X5	T37.3X6
Nifurtoinol	T37.8X1	T37.8X2	T37.8X3	T37.8X4	T37.8X5	T37.8X6
Nightshade, deadly (solanum)—see also Belladonna	T62.2X1	T62.2X2	T62.2X3	T62.2X4	—	—
berry	T62.1X1	T62.1X2	T62.1X3	T62.1X4	—	—
Nikethamide	T50.7X1	T50.7X2	T50.7X3	T50.7X4	T50.7X5	T50.7X6
Nilstat	T36.7X1	T36.7X2	T36.7X3	T36.7X4	T36.7X5	T36.7X6
topical	T49.0X1	T49.0X2	T49.0X3	T49.0X4	T49.0X5	T49.0X6
Nilutamide	T38.6X1	T38.6X2	T38.6X3	T38.6X4	T38.6X5	T38.6X6

Substance	Poisoning, Accidental (unintentional)	Poisoning, Intentional self-harm	Poisoning, Assault	Poisoning, Undetermined	Adverse effect	Underdosing
Nimesulide	T39.391	T39.392	T39.393	T39.394	T39.395	T39.396
Nimetazepam	T42.4X1	T42.4X2	T42.4X3	T42.4X4	T42.4X5	T42.4X6
Nimodipine	T46.1X1	T46.1X2	T46.1X3	T46.1X4	T46.1X5	T46.1X6
Nimorazole	T37.3X1	T37.3X2	T37.3X3	T37.3X4	T37.3X5	T37.3X6
Nimustine	T45.1X1	T45.1X2	T45.1X3	T45.1X4	T45.1X5	T45.1X6
Niridazole	T37.4X1	T37.4X2	T37.4X3	T37.4X4	T37.4X5	T37.4X6
Nisentil	T40.2X1	T40.2X2	T40.2X3	T40.2X4	T40.2X5	T40.2X6
Nisoldipine	T46.1X1	T46.1X2	T46.1X3	T46.1X4	T46.1X5	T46.1X6
Nitramine	T65.3X1	T65.3X2	T65.3X3	T65.3X4	—	—
Nitrate, organic	T46.3X1	T46.3X2	T46.3X3	T46.3X4	T46.3X5	T46.3X6
Nitrazepam	T42.4X1	T42.4X2	T42.4X3	T42.4X4	T42.4X5	T42.4X6
Nitrefazole	T50.6X1	T50.6X2	T50.6X3	T50.6X4	T50.6X5	T50.6X6
Nitrendipine	T46.1X1	T46.1X2	T46.1X3	T46.1X4	T46.1X5	T46.1X6
Nitric						
acid (liquid)	T54.2X1	T54.2X2	T54.2X3	T54.2X4	—	—
vapor	T59.891	T59.892	T59.893	T59.894		
oxide (gas)	T59.0X1	T59.0X2	T59.0X3	T59.0X4		
Nitrimidazine	T37.3X1	T37.3X2	T37.3X3	T37.3X4	T37.3X5	T37.3X6
Nitrite, amyl (medicinal) (vapor)	T46.3X1	T46.3X2	T46.3X3	T46.3X4	T46.3X5	T46.3X6
Nitroaniline	T65.3X1	T65.3X2	T65.3X3	T65.3X4		
vapor	T59.891	T59.892	T59.893	T59.894		
Nitrobenzene, nitrobenzol	T65.3X1	T65.3X2	T65.3X3	T65.3X4	—	—
vapor	T65.3X1	T65.3X2	T65.3X3	T65.3X4		
Nitrocellulose	T65.891	T65.892	T65.893	T65.894		
lacquer	T65.891	T65.892	T65.893	T65.894		
Nitrodiphenyl	T65.3X1	T65.3X2	T65.3X3	T65.3X4		
Nitrofural	T49.0X1	T49.0X2	T49.0X3	T49.0X4	T49.0X5	T49.0X6
Nitrofurantoin	T37.8X1	T37.8X2	T37.8X3	T37.8X4	T37.8X5	T37.8X6
Nitrofurazone	T49.0X1	T49.0X2	T49.0X3	T49.0X4	T49.0X5	T49.0X6
Nitrogen	T59.0X1	T59.0X2	T59.0X3	T59.0X4	—	—
mustard	T45.1X1	T45.1X2	T45.1X3	T45.1X4	T45.1X5	T45.1X6
Nitroglycerin, nitro-glycerol (medicinal)	T46.3X1	T46.3X2	T46.3X3	T46.3X4	T46.3X5	T46.3X6
nonmedicinal	T65.5X1	T65.5X2	T65.5X3	T65.5X4	—	—
fumes	T65.5X1	T65.5X2	T65.5X3	T65.5X4	—	—
Nitroglycol	T52.3X1	T52.3X2	T52.3X3	T52.3X4		
Nitrohydrochloric acid	T54.2X1	T54.2X2	T54.2X3	T54.2X4		
Nitromersol	T49.0X1	T49.0X2	T49.0X3	T49.0X4	T49.0X5	T49.0X6
Nitronaphthalene	T65.891	T65.892	T65.893	T65.894	—	—
Nitrophenol	T54.0X1	T54.0X2	T54.0X3	T54.0X4	—	—
Nitropropane	T52.8X1	T52.8X2	T52.8X3	T52.8X4	—	—
Nitroprusside	T46.5X1	T46.5X2	T46.5X3	T46.5X4	T46.5X5	T46.5X6
Nitrosodimethylamine	T65.3X1	T65.3X2	T65.3X3	T65.3X4	—	—
Nitrothiazol	T37.4X1	T37.4X2	T37.4X3	T37.4X4	T37.4X5	T37.4X6
Nitrotoluene, nitrotoluol	T65.3X1	T65.3X2	T65.3X3	T65.3X4	—	—
vapor	T65.3X1	T65.3X2	T65.3X3	T65.3X4	—	—
Nitrous						
acid (liquid)	T54.2X1	T54.2X2	T54.2X3	T54.2X4	—	—
fumes	T59.891	T59.892	T59.893	T59.894	—	—

Substance	Poisoning, Accidental (unintentional)	Poisoning, Intentional self-harm	Poisoning, Assault	Poisoning, Undetermined	Adverse effect	Underdosing
Nitrous — *Continued*						
ether spirit	T46.3X1	T46.3X2	T46.3X3	T46.3X4	T46.3X5	T46.3X6
oxide	T41.0X1	T41.0X2	T41.0X3	T41.0X4	T41.0X5	T41.0X6
Nitroxoline	T37.8X1	T37.8X2	T37.8X3	T37.8X4	T37.8X5	T37.8X6
Nitrozone	T49.0X1	T49.0X2	T49.0X3	T49.0X4	T49.0X5	T49.0X6
Nizatidine	T47.0X1	T47.0X2	T47.0X3	T47.0X4	T47.0X5	T47.0X6
Nizofenone	T43.8X1	T43.8X2	T43.8X3	T43.8X4	T43.8X5	T43.8X6
Noctec	T42.6X1	T42.6X2	T42.6X3	T42.6X4	T42.6X5	T42.6X6
Noludar	T42.6X1	T42.6X2	T42.6X3	T42.6X4	T42.6X5	T42.6X6
Nomegestrol	T38.5X1	T38.5X2	T38.5X3	T38.5X4	T38.5X5	T38.5X6
Nomifensine	T43.291	T43.292	T43.293	T43.294	T43.295	T43.296
Nonoxinol	T49.8X1	T49.8X2	T49.8X3	T49.8X4	T49.8X5	T49.8X6
Nonylphenoxy (polyethoxy-ethanol)	T49.8X1	T49.8X2	T49.8X3	T49.8X4	T49.8X5	T49.8X6
Noptil	T42.3X1	T42.3X2	T42.3X3	T42.3X4	T42.3X5	T42.3X6
Noradrenaline	T44.4X1	T44.4X2	T44.4X3	T44.4X4	T44.4X5	T44.4X6
Noramidopyrine	T39.2X1	T39.2X2	T39.2X3	T39.2X4	T39.2X5	T39.2X6
methanesulfonate sodium	T39.2X1	T39.2X2	T39.2X3	T39.2X4	T39.2X5	T39.2X6
Norbormide	T60.4X1	T60.4X2	T60.4X3	T60.4X4	—	—
Nordazepam	T42.4X1	T42.4X2	T42.4X3	T42.4X4	T42.4X5	T42.4X6
Norepinephrine	T44.4X1	T44.4X2	T44.4X3	T44.4X4	T44.4X5	T44.4X6
Norethandrolone	T38.7X1	T38.7X2	T38.7X3	T38.7X4	T38.7X5	T38.7X6
Norethindrone	T38.4X1	T38.4X2	T38.4X3	T38.4X4	T38.4X5	T38.4X6
Norethisterone (acetate) (enantate)	T38.4X1	T38.4X2	T38.4X3	T38.4X4	T38.4X5	T38.4X6
with ethinylestradiol	T38.5X1	T38.5X2	T38.5X3	T38.5X4	T38.5X5	T38.5X6
Noretynodrel	T38.5X1	T38.5X2	T38.5X3	T38.5X4	T38.5X5	T38.5X6
Norfenefrine	T44.4X1	T44.4X2	T44.4X3	T44.4X4	T44.4X5	T44.4X6
Norfloxacin	T36.8X1	T36.8X2	T36.8X3	T36.8X4	T36.8X5	T36.8X6
Norgestrel	T38.4X1	T38.4X2	T38.4X3	T38.4X4	T38.4X5	T38.4X6
Norgestrienone	T38.4X1	T38.4X2	T38.4X3	T38.4X4	T38.4X5	T38.4X6
Norlestrin	T38.4X1	T38.4X2	T38.4X3	T38.4X4	T38.4X5	T38.4X6
Norlutin	T38.4X1	T38.4X2	T38.4X3	T38.4X4	T38.4X5	T38.4X6
Normal serum albumin (human), salt-poor	T45.8X1	T45.8X2	T45.8X3	T45.8X4	T45.8X5	T45.8X6
Normethandrone	T38.5X1	T38.5X2	T38.5X3	T38.5X4	T38.5X5	T38.5X6
Normison—see Benzodiazepines						
Normorphine	T40.2X1	T40.2X2	T40.2X3	T40.2X4	—	—
Norpseudoephedrine	T50.5X1	T50.5X2	T50.5X3	T50.5X4	T50.5X5	T50.5X6
Nortestosterone (furanpro pionate)	T38.7X1	T38.7X2	T38.7X3	T38.7X4	T38.7X5	T38.7X6
Nortriptyline	T43.011	T43.012	T43.013	T43.014	T43.015	T43.016
Noscapine	T48.3X1	T48.3X2	T48.3X3	T48.3X4	T48.3X5	T48.3X6
Nose preparations	T49.6X1	T49.6X2	T49.6X3	T49.6X4	T49.6X5	T49.6X6
Novobiocin	T36.5X1	T36.5X2	T36.5X3	T36.5X4	T36.5X5	T36.5X6
Novocain (infiltration) (topical)	T41.3X1	T41.3X2	T41.3X3	T41.3X4	T41.3X5	T41.3X6
nerve block (peripheral) (plexus)	T41.3X1	T41.3X2	T41.3X3	T41.3X4	T41.3X5	T41.3X6
spinal	T41.3X1	T41.3X2	T41.3X3	T41.3X4	T41.3X5	T41.3X6

Substance	Poisoning, Accidental (unintentional)	Poisoning, Intentional self-harm	Poisoning, Assault	Poisoning, Undetermined	Adverse effect	Underdosing
Noxious foodstuff	T62.91	T62.92	T62.93	T62.94	—	—
specified NEC	T62.8X1	T62.8X2	T62.8X3	T62.8X4	—	—
Noxiptiline	T43.011	T43.012	T43.013	T43.014	T43.015	T43.016
Noxytiolin	T49.0X1	T49.0X2	T49.0X3	T49.0X4	T49.0X5	T49.0X6
NPH Iletin (insulin)	T38.3X1	T38.3X2	T38.3X3	T38.3X4	T38.3X5	T38.3X6
Numorphan	T40.2X1	T40.2X2	T40.2X3	T40.2X4	T40.2X5	T40.2X6
Nunol	T42.3X1	T42.3X2	T42.3X3	T42.3X4	T42.3X5	T42.3X6
Nupercaine (spinal anesthetic)	T41.3X1	T41.3X2	T41.3X3	T41.3X4	T41.3X5	T41.3X6
topical (surface)	T41.3X1	T41.3X2	T41.3X3	T41.3X4	T41.3X5	T41.3X6
Nutmeg oil (liniment)	T49.3X1	T49.3X2	T49.3X3	T49.3X4	T49.3X5	T49.3X6
Nutritional supplement	T50.901	T50.902	T50.903	T50.904	T50.905	T50.906
Nux vomica	T65.1X1	T65.1X2	T65.1X3	T65.1X4	—	—
Nydrazid	T37.1X1	T37.1X2	T37.1X3	T37.1X4	T37.1X5	T37.1X6
Nylidrin	T46.7X1	T46.7X2	T46.7X3	T46.7X4	T46.7X5	T46.7X6
Nystatin	T36.7X1	T36.7X2	T36.7X3	T36.7X4	T36.7X5	T36.7X6
topical	T49.0X1	T49.0X2	T49.0X3	T49.0X4	T49.0X5	T49.0X6
Nytol	T45.0X1	T45.0X2	T45.0X3	T45.0X4	T45.0X5	T45.0X6
O						
Obidoxime chloride	T50.6X1	T50.6X2	T50.6X3	T50.6X4	T50.6X5	T50.6X6
Octafonium (chloride)	T49.3X1	T49.3X2	T49.3X3	T49.3X4	T49.3X5	T49.3X6
Octamethyl pyrophosphoramide	T60.0X1	T60.0X2	T60.0X3	T60.0X4	—	—
Octanoin	T50.991	T50.992	T50.993	T50.994	T50.995	T50.996
Octatropine methylbromide	T44.3X1	T44.3X2	T44.3X3	T44.3X4	T44.3X5	T44.3X6
Octotiamine	T45.2X1	T45.2X2	T45.2X3	T45.2X4	T45.2X5	T45.2X6
Octoxinol (9)	T49.8X1	T49.8X2	T49.8X3	T49.8X4	T49.8X5	T49.8X6
Octreotide	T38.991	T38.992	T38.993	T38.994	T38.995	T38.996
Octyl nitrite	T46.3X1	T46.3X2	T46.3X3	T46.3X4	T46.3X5	T46.3X6
Oestradiol	T38.5X1	T38.5X2	T38.5X3	T38.5X4	T38.5X5	T38.5X6
Oestriol	T38.5X1	T38.5X2	T38.5X3	T38.5X4	T38.5X5	T38.5X6
Oestrogen	T38.5X1	T38.5X2	T38.5X3	T38.5X4	T38.5X5	T38.5X6
Oestrone	T38.5X1	T38.5X2	T38.5X3	T38.5X4	T38.5X5	T38.5X6
Ofloxacin	T36.8X1	T36.8X2	T36.8X3	T36.8X4	T36.8X5	T36.8X6
Oil (of)	T65.891	T65.892	T65.893	T65.894	—	—
bitter almond	T62.8X1	T62.8X2	T62.8X3	T62.8X4	—	—
cloves	T49.7X1	T49.7X2	T49.7X3	T49.7X4	T49.7X5	T49.7X6
colors	T65.6X1	T65.6X2	T65.6X3	T65.6X4	—	—
fumes	T59.891	T59.892	T59.893	T59.894	—	—
lubricating	T52.0X1	T52.0X2	T52.0X3	T52.0X4	—	—
Niobe	T52.8X1	T52.8X2	T52.8X3	T52.8X4	—	—
vitriol (liquid)	T54.2X1	T54.2X2	T54.2X3	T54.2X4	—	—
fumes	T54.2X1	T54.2X2	T54.2X3	T54.2X4	—	—
wintergreen (bitter) NEC	T49.3X1	T49.3X2	T49.3X3	T49.3X4	T49.3X5	T49.3X6
Oily preparation (for skin)	T49.3X1	T49.3X2	T49.3X3	T49.3X4	T49.3X5	T49.3X6
Ointment NEC	T49.3X1	T49.3X2	T49.3X3	T49.3X4	T49.3X5	T49.3X6
Olanzapine	T43.591	T43.592	T43.593	T43.594	T43.595	T43.596
Oleander	T62.2X1	T62.2X2	T62.2X3	T62.2X4	—	—
Oleandomycin	T36.3X1	T36.3X2	T36.3X3	T36.3X4	T36.3X5	T36.3X6

Substance	Poisoning, Accidental (unintentional)	Poisoning, Intentional self-harm	Poisoning, Assault	Poisoning, Undetermined	Adverse effect	Underdosing
Oleandrin	T46.0X1	T46.0X2	T46.0X3	T46.0X4	T46.0X5	T46.0X6
Oleic acid	T46.6X1	T46.6X2	T46.6X3	T46.6X4	T46.6X5	T46.6X6
Oleovitamin A	T45.2X1	T45.2X2	T45.2X3	T45.2X4	T45.2X5	T45.2X6
Oleum ricini	T47.2X1	T47.2X2	T47.2X3	T47.2X4	T47.2X5	T47.2X6
Olive oil (medicinal) NEC	T47.4X1	T47.4X2	T47.4X3	T47.4X4	T47.4X5	T47.4X6
Olivomycin	T45.1X1	T45.1X2	T45.1X3	T45.1X4	T45.1X5	T45.1X6
Olsalazine	T47.8X1	T47.8X2	T47.8X3	T47.8X4	T47.8X5	T47.8X6
Omeprazole	T47.1X1	T47.1X2	T47.1X3	T47.1X4	T47.1X5	T47.1X6
OMPA	T60.0X1	T60.0X2	T60.0X3	T60.0X4	—	—
Oncovin	T45.1X1	T45.1X2	T45.1X3	T45.1X4	T45.1X5	T45.1X6
Ondansetron	T45.0X1	T45.0X2	T45.0X3	T45.0X4	T45.0X5	T45.0X6
Ophthaine	T41.3X1	T41.3X2	T41.3X3	T41.3X4	T41.3X5	T41.3X6
Ophthetic	T41.3X1	T41.3X2	T41.3X3	T41.3X4	T41.3X5	T41.3X6
Opiate NEC	T40.601	T40.602	T40.603	T40.604	T40.605	T40.606
antagonists	T50.7X1	T50.7X2	T50.7X3	T50.7X4	T50.7X5	T50.7X6
Opioid NEC	T40.2X1	T40.2X2	T40.2X3	T40.2X4	T40.2X5	T40.2X6
Opipramol	T43.011	T43.012	T43.013	T43.014	T43.015	T43.016
Opium alkaloids (total)	T40.0X1	T40.0X2	T40.0X3	T40.0X4	T40.0X5	T40.0X6
standardized powdered	T40.0X1	T40.0X2	T40.0X3	T40.0X4	T40.0X5	T40.0X6
tincture (camphorated)	T40.0X1	T40.0X2	T40.0X3	T40.0X4	T40.0X5	T40.0X6
Oracon	T38.4X1	T38.4X2	T38.4X3	T38.4X4	T38.4X5	T38.4X6
Oragrafin	T50.8X1	T50.8X2	T50.8X3	T50.8X4	T50.8X5	T50.8X6
Oral contraceptives	T38.4X1	T38.4X2	T38.4X3	T38.4X4	T38.4X5	T38.4X6
Oral rehydration salts	T50.3X1	T50.3X2	T50.3X3	T50.3X4	T50.3X5	T50.3X6
Orazamide	T50.991	T50.992	T50.993	T50.994	T50.995	T50.996
Orciprenaline	T48.291	T48.292	T48.293	T48.294	T48.295	T48.296
Organidin	T48.4X1	T48.4X2	T48.4X3	T48.4X4	T48.4X5	T48.4X6
Organonitrate NEC	T46.3X1	T46.3X2	T46.3X3	T46.3X4	T46.3X5	T46.3X6
Organophosphates	T60.0X1	T60.0X2	T60.0X3	T60.0X4	—	—
Orimune	T50.B91	T50.B92	T50.B93	T50.B94	T50.B95	T50.B96
Orinase	T38.3X1	T38.3X2	T38.3X3	T38.3X4	T38.3X5	T38.3X6
Ormeloxifene	T38.6X1	T38.6X2	T38.6X3	T38.6X4	T38.6X5	T38.6X6
Ornidazole	T37.3X1	T37.3X2	T37.3X3	T37.3X4	T37.3X5	T37.3X6
Ornithine aspartate	T50.991	T50.992	T50.993	T50.994	T50.995	T50.996
Ornoprostil	T47.1X1	T47.1X2	T47.1X3	T47.1X4	T47.1X5	T47.1X6
Orphenadrine (hydrochloride)	T42.8X1	T42.8X2	T42.8X3	T42.8X4	T42.8X5	T42.8X6
Ortal (sodium)	T42.3X1	T42.3X2	T42.3X3	T42.3X4	T42.3X5	T42.3X6
Orthoboric acid	T49.0X1	T49.0X2	T49.0X3	T49.0X4	T49.0X5	T49.0X6
ENT agent	T49.6X1	T49.6X2	T49.6X3	T49.6X4	T49.6X5	T49.6X6
ophthalmic preparation	T49.5X1	T49.5X2	T49.5X3	T49.5X4	T49.5X5	T49.5X6
Orthocaine	T41.3X1	T41.3X2	T41.3X3	T41.3X4	T41.3X5	T41.3X6
Orthodichlorobenzene	T53.7X1	T53.7X2	T53.7X3	T53.7X4	—	—
Ortho-Novum	T38.4X1	T38.4X2	T38.4X3	T38.4X4	T38.4X5	T38.4X6
Orthotolidine (reagent)	T54.2X1	T54.2X2	T54.2X3	T54.2X4	—	—
Osmic acid (liquid)	T54.2X1	T54.2X2	T54.2X3	T54.2X4	—	—
fumes	T54.2X1	T54.2X2	T54.2X3	T54.2X4	—	—
Osmotic diuretics	T50.2X1	T50.2X2	T50.2X3	T50.2X4	T50.2X5	T50.2X6
Otilonium bromide	T44.3X1	T44.3X2	T44.3X3	T44.3X4	T44.3X5	T44.3X6

Substance	Poisoning, Accidental (unintentional)	Poisoning, Intentional self-harm	Poisoning, Assault	Poisoning, Undetermined	Adverse effect	Underdosing
Otorhinolaryngological drug NEC	T49.6X1	T49.6X2	T49.6X3	T49.6X4	T49.6X5	T49.6X6
Ouabain(e)	T46.0X1	T46.0X2	T46.0X3	T46.0X4	T46.0X5	T46.0X6
Ovarian						
hormone	T38.5X1	T38.5X2	T38.5X3	T38.5X4	T38.5X5	T38.5X6
stimulant	T38.5X1	T38.5X2	T38.5X3	T38.5X4	T38.5X5	T38.5X6
Ovral	T38.4X1	T38.4X2	T38.4X3	T38.4X4	T38.4X5	T38.4X6
Ovulen	T38.4X1	T38.4X2	T38.4X3	T38.4X4	T38.4X5	T38.4X6
Oxacillin	T36.0X1	T36.0X2	T36.0X3	T36.0X4	T36.0X5	T36.0X6
Oxalic acid	T54.2X1	T54.2X2	T54.2X3	T54.2X4	—	—
ammonium salt	T50.991	T50.992	T50.993	T50.994	T50.995	T50.996
Oxamniquine	T37.4X1	T37.4X2	T37.4X3	T37.4X4	T37.4X5	T37.4X6
Oxanamide	T43.591	T43.592	T43.593	T43.594	T43.595	T43.596
Oxandrolone	T38.7X1	T38.7X2	T38.7X3	T38.7X4	T38.7X5	T38.7X6
Oxantel	T37.4X1	T37.4X2	T37.4X3	T37.4X4	T37.4X5	T37.4X6
Oxapium iodide	T44.3X1	T44.3X2	T44.3X3	T44.3X4	T44.3X5	T44.3X6
Oxaprotiline	T43.021	T43.022	T43.023	T43.024	T43.025	T43.026
Oxaprozin	T39.311	T39.312	T39.313	T39.314	T39.315	T39.316
Oxatomide	T45.0X1	T45.0X2	T45.0X3	T45.0X4	T45.0X5	T45.0X6
Oxazepam	T42.4X1	T42.4X2	T42.4X3	T42.4X4	T42.4X5	T42.4X6
Oxazimedrine	T50.5X1	T50.5X2	T50.5X3	T50.5X4	T50.5X5	T50.5X6
Oxazolam	T42.4X1	T42.4X2	T42.4X3	T42.4X4	T42.4X5	T42.4X6
Oxazolidine derivatives	T42.2X1	T42.2X2	T42.2X3	T42.2X4	T42.2X5	T42.2X6
Oxazolidinedione (derivative)	T42.2X1	T42.2X2	T42.2X3	T42.2X4	T42.2X5	T42.2X6
Ox bile extract	T47.5X1	T47.5X2	T47.5X3	T47.5X4	T47.5X5	T47.5X6
Oxcarbazepine	T42.1X1	T42.1X2	T42.1X3	T42.1X4	T42.1X5	T42.1X6
Oxedrine	T44.4X1	T44.4X2	T44.4X3	T44.4X4	T44.4X5	T44.4X6
Oxeladin (citrate)	T48.3X1	T48.3X2	T48.3X3	T48.3X4	T48.3X5	T48.3X6
Oxendolone	T38.5X1	T38.5X2	T38.5X3	T38.5X4	T38.5X5	T38.5X6
Oxetacaine	T41.3X1	T41.3X2	T41.3X3	T41.3X4	T41.3X5	T41.3X6
Oxethazine	T41.3X1	T41.3X2	T41.3X3	T41.3X4	T41.3X5	T41.3X6
Oxetorone	T39.8X1	T39.8X2	T39.8X3	T39.8X4	T39.8X5	T39.8X6
Oxiconazole	T49.0X1	T49.0X2	T49.0X3	T49.0X4	T49.0X5	T49.0X6
Oxidizing agent NEC	T54.91	T54.92	T54.93	T54.94	—	—
Oxipurinol	T50.4X1	T50.4X2	T50.4X3	T50.4X4	T50.4X5	T50.4X6
Oxitriptan	T43.291	T43.292	T43.293	T43.294	T43.295	T43.296
Oxitropium bromide	T48.6X1	T48.6X2	T48.6X3	T48.6X4	T48.6X5	T48.6X6
Oxodipine	T46.1X1	T46.1X2	T46.1X3	T46.1X4	T46.1X5	T46.1X6
Oxolamine	T48.3X1	T48.3X2	T48.3X3	T48.3X4	T48.3X5	T48.3X6
Oxolinic acid	T37.8X1	T37.8X2	T37.8X3	T37.8X4	T37.8X5	T37.8X6
Oxomemazine	T43.3X1	T43.3X2	T43.3X3	T43.3X4	T43.3X5	T43.3X6
Oxophenarsine	T37.3X1	T37.3X2	T37.3X3	T37.3X4	T37.3X5	T37.3X6
Oxprenolol	T44.7X1	T44.7X2	T44.7X3	T44.7X4	T44.7X5	T44.7X6
Oxsoralen	T49.3X1	T49.3X2	T49.3X3	T49.3X4	T49.3X5	T49.3X6
Oxtriphylline	T48.6X1	T48.6X2	T48.6X3	T48.6X4	T48.6X5	T48.6X6
Oxybate sodium	T41.291	T41.292	T41.293	T41.294	T41.295	T41.296
Oxybuprocaine	T41.3X1	T41.3X2	T41.3X3	T41.3X4	T41.3X5	T41.3X6
Oxybutynin	T44.3X1	T44.3X2	T44.3X3	T44.3X4	T44.3X5	T44.3X6
Oxychlorosene	T49.0X1	T49.0X2	T49.0X3	T49.0X4	T49.0X5	T49.0X6

Substance	Poisoning, Accidental (unintentional)	Poisoning, Intentional self-harm	Poisoning, Assault	Poisoning, Undetermined	Adverse effect	Underdosing
Oxycodone	T40.2X1	T40.2X2	T40.2X3	T40.2X4	T40.2X5	T40.2X6
Oxyfedrine	T46.3X1	T46.3X2	T46.3X3	T46.3X4	T46.3X5	T46.3X6
Oxygen	T41.5X1	T41.5X2	T41.5X3	T41.5X4	T41.5X5	T41.5X6
Oxylone	T49.0X1	T49.0X2	T49.0X3	T49.0X4	T49.0X5	T49.0X6
ophthalmic preparation	T49.5X1	T49.5X2	T49.5X3	T49.5X4	T49.5X5	T49.5X6
Oxymesterone	T38.7X1	T38.7X2	T38.7X3	T38.7X4	T38.7X5	T38.7X6
Oxymetazoline	T48.5X1	T48.5X2	T48.5X3	T48.5X4	T48.5X5	T48.5X6
Oxymetholone	T38.7X1	T38.7X2	T38.7X3	T38.7X4	T38.7X5	T38.7X6
Oxymorphone	T40.2X1	T40.2X2	T40.2X3	T40.2X4	T40.2X5	T40.2X6
Oxypertine	T43.591	T43.592	T43.593	T43.594	T43.595	T43.596
Oxyphenbutazone	T39.2X1	T39.2X2	T39.2X3	T39.2X4	T39.2X5	T39.2X6
Oxyphencyclimine	T44.3X1	T44.3X2	T44.3X3	T44.3X4	T44.3X5	T44.3X6
Oxyphenisatine	T47.2X1	T47.2X2	T47.2X3	T47.2X4	T47.2X5	T47.2X6
Oxyphenonium bromide	T44.3X1	T44.3X2	T44.3X3	T44.3X4	T44.3X5	T44.3X6
Oxypolygelatin	T45.8X1	T45.8X2	T45.8X3	T45.8X4	T45.8X5	T45.8X6
Oxyquinoline (derivatives)	T37.8X1	T37.8X2	T37.8X3	T37.8X4	T37.8X5	T37.8X6
Oxytetracycline	T36.4X1	T36.4X2	T36.4X3	T36.4X4	T36.4X5	T36.4X6
Oxytocic drug NEC	T48.0X1	T48.0X2	T48.0X3	T48.0X4	T48.0X5	T48.0X6
Oxytocin (synthetic)	T48.0X1	T48.0X2	T48.0X3	T48.0X4	T48.0X5	T48.0X6
Ozone	T59.891	T59.892	T59.893	T59.894	—	—
P						
PABA	T49.3X1	T49.3X2	T49.3X3	T49.3X4	T49.3X5	T49.3X6
Packed red cells	T45.8X1	T45.8X2	T45.8X3	T45.8X4	T45.8X5	T45.8X6
Padimate	T49.3X1	T49.3X2	T49.3X3	T49.3X4	T49.3X5	T49.3X6
Paint NEC	T65.6X1	T65.6X2	T65.6X3	T65.6X4	—	—
cleaner	T52.91	T52.92	T52.93	T52.94	—	—
fumes NEC	T59.891	T59.892	T59.893	T59.894	—	—
lead (fumes)	T56.0X1	T56.0X2	T56.0X3	T56.0X4	—	—
solvent NEC	T52.8X1	T52.8X2	T52.8X3	T52.8X4	—	—
stripper	T52.8X1	T52.8X2	T52.8X3	T52.8X4	—	—
Palfium	T40.2X1	T40.2X2	T40.2X3	T40.2X4	—	—
Palm kernel oil	T50.991	T50.992	T50.993	T50.994	T50.995	T50.996
Paludrine	T37.2X1	T37.2X2	T37.2X3	T37.2X4	T37.2X5	T37.2X6
PAM (pralidoxime)	T50.6X1	T50.6X2	T50.6X3	T50.6X4	T50.6X5	T50.6X6
Pamaquine (naphthoute)	T37.2X1	T37.2X2	T37.2X3	T37.2X4	T37.2X5	T37.2X6
Panadol	T39.1X1	T39.1X2	T39.1X3	T39.1X4	T39.1X5	T39.1X6
Pancreatic						
digestive secretion stimulant	T47.8X1	T47.8X2	T47.8X3	T47.8X4	T47.8X5	T47.8X6
dornase	T45.3X1	T45.3X2	T45.3X3	T45.3X4	T45.3X5	T45.3X6
Pancreatin	T47.5X1	T47.5X2	T47.5X3	T47.5X4	T47.5X5	T47.5X6
Pancrelipase	T47.5X1	T47.5X2	T47.5X3	T47.5X4	T47.5X5	T47.5X6
Pancuronium (bromide)	T48.1X1	T48.1X2	T48.1X3	T48.1X4	T48.1X5	T48.1X6
Pangamic acid	T45.2X1	T45.2X2	T45.2X3	T45.2X4	T45.2X5	T45.2X6
Panthenol	T45.2X1	T45.2X2	T45.2X3	T45.2X4	T45.2X5	T45.2X6
topical	T49.8X1	T49.8X2	T49.8X3	T49.8X4	T49.8X5	T49.8X6
Pantopon	T40.0X1	T40.0X2	T40.0X3	T40.0X4	T40.0X5	T40.0X6
Pantothenic acid	T45.2X1	T45.2X2	T45.2X3	T45.2X4	T45.2X5	T45.2X6
Panwarfin	T45.511	T45.512	T45.513	T45.514	T45.515	T45.516
Papain	T47.5X1	T47.5X2	T47.5X3	T47.5X4	T47.5X5	T47.5X6
digestant	T47.5X1	T47.5X2	T47.5X3	T47.5X4	T47.5X5	T47.5X6
Papaveretum	T40.0X1	T40.0X2	T40.0X3	T40.0X4	T40.0X5	T40.0X6
Papaverine	T44.3X1	T44.3X2	T44.3X3	T44.3X4	T44.3X5	T44.3X6
Para-acetamidophenol	T39.1X1	T39.1X2	T39.1X3	T39.1X4	T39.1X5	T39.1X6
Para-aminobenzoic acid	T49.3X1	T49.3X2	T49.3X3	T49.3X4	T49.3X5	T49.3X6
Para-aminophenol derivatives	T39.1X1	T39.1X2	T39.1X3	T39.1X4	T39.1X5	T39.1X6
Para-aminosalicylic acid	T37.1X1	T37.1X2	T37.1X3	T37.1X4	T37.1X5	T37.1X6
Paracetaldehyde	T42.6X1	T42.6X2	T42.6X3	T42.6X4	T42.6X5	T42.6X6
Paracetamol	T39.1X1	T39.1X2	T39.1X3	T39.1X4	T39.1X5	T39.1X6
Parachlorophenol (camphorated)	T49.0X1	T49.0X2	T49.0X3	T49.0X4	T49.0X5	T49.0X6
Paracodin	T40.2X1	T40.2X2	T40.2X3	T40.2X4	T40.2X5	T40.2X6
Paradione	T42.2X1	T42.2X2	T42.2X3	T42.2X4	T42.2X5	T42.2X6
Paraffin(s) (wax)	T52.0X1	T52.0X2	T52.0X3	T52.0X4	—	—
liquid (medicinal)	T47.4X1	T47.4X2	T47.4X3	T47.4X4	T47.4X5	T47.4X6
nonmedicinal	T52.0X1	T52.0X2	T52.0X3	T52.0X4	—	—
Paraformaldehyde	T60.3X1	T60.3X2	T60.3X3	T60.3X4	—	—
Paraldehyde	T42.6X1	T42.6X2	T42.6X3	T42.6X4	T42.6X5	T42.6X6
Paramethadione	T42.2X1	T42.2X2	T42.2X3	T42.2X4	T42.2X5	T42.2X6
Paramethasone	T38.0X1	T38.0X2	T38.0X3	T38.0X4	T38.0X5	T38.0X6
acetate	T49.0X1	T49.0X2	T49.0X3	T49.0X4	T49.0X5	T49.0X6
Paraoxon	T60.0X1	T60.0X2	T60.0X3	T60.0X4	—	—
Paraquat	T60.3X1	T60.3X2	T60.3X3	T60.3X4	—	—
Parasympatholytic NEC	T44.3X1	T44.3X2	T44.3X3	T44.3X4	T44.3X5	T44.3X6
Parasympathomimetic drug NEC	T44.1X1	T44.1X2	T44.1X3	T44.1X4	T44.1X5	T44.1X6
Parathion	T60.0X1	T60.0X2	T60.0X3	T60.0X4	—	—
Parathormone	T50.991	T50.992	T50.993	T50.994	T50.995	T50.996
Parathyroid extract	T50.991	T50.992	T50.993	T50.994	T50.995	T50.996
Paratyphoid vaccine	T50.A91	T50.A92	T50.A93	T50.A94	T50.A95	T50.A96
Paredrine	T44.4X1	T44.4X2	T44.4X3	T44.4X4	T44.4X5	T44.4X6
Paregoric	T40.0X1	T40.0X2	T40.0X3	T40.0X4	T40.0X5	T40.0X6
Pargyline	T46.5X1	T46.5X2	T46.5X3	T46.5X4	T46.5X5	T46.5X6
Paris green	T57.0X1	T57.0X2	T57.0X3	T57.0X4	—	—
insecticide	T57.0X1	T57.0X2	T57.0X3	T57.0X4	—	—
Parnate	T43.1X1	T43.1X2	T43.1X3	T43.1X4	T43.1X5	T43.1X6
Paromomycin	T36.5X1	T36.5X2	T36.5X3	T36.5X4	T36.5X5	T36.5X6
Paroxypropione	T45.1X1	T45.1X2	T45.1X3	T45.1X4	T45.1X5	T45.1X6
Parzone	T40.2X1	T40.2X2	T40.2X3	T40.2X4	T40.2X5	T40.2X6
PAS	T37.1X1	T37.1X2	T37.1X3	T37.1X4	T37.1X5	T37.1X6
Pasiniazid	T37.1X1	T37.1X2	T37.1X3	T37.1X4	T37.1X5	T37.1X6
PBB (polybrominated biphenyls)	T65.891	T65.892	T65.893	T65.894	—	—
PCB	T65.891	T65.892	T65.893	T65.894	—	—
PCP						
meaning pentachlorophenol	T60.1X1	T60.1X2	T60.1X3	T60.1X4	—	—
fungicide	T60.3X1	T60.3X2	T60.3X3	T60.3X4	—	—
herbicide	T60.3X1	T60.3X2	T60.3X3	T60.3X4	—	—
insecticide	T60.1X1	T60.1X2	T60.1X3	T60.1X4	—	—
meaning phencyclidine	T40.991	T40.992	T40.993	T40.994	—	—

Substance	Poisoning, Accidental (unintentional)	Poisoning, Intentional self-harm	Poisoning, Assault	Poisoning, Undetermined	Adverse effect	Underdosing
Peach kernel oil (emulsion)	T47.4X1	T47.4X2	T47.4X3	T47.4X4	T47.4X5	T47.4X6
Peanut oil (emulsion) NEC	T47.4X1	T47.4X2	T47.4X3	T47.4X4	T47.4X5	T47.4X6
topical	T49.3X1	T49.3X2	T49.3X3	T49.3X4	T49.3X5	T49.3X6
Pearly Gates (morning glory seeds)	T40.991	T40.992	T40.993	T40.994	—	—
Pecazine	T43.3X1	T43.3X2	T43.3X3	T43.3X4	T43.3X5	T43.3X6
Pectin	T47.6X1	T47.6X2	T47.6X3	T47.6X4	T47.6X5	T47.6X6
Pefloxacin	T37.8X1	T37.8X2	T37.8X3	T37.8X4	T37.8X5	T37.8X6
Pegademase, bovine	T50.Z91	T50.Z92	T50.Z93	T50.Z94	T50.Z95	T50.Z96
Pelletierine tannate	T37.4X1	T37.4X2	T37.4X3	T37.4X4	T37.4X5	T37.4X6
Pemirolast (potassium)	T48.6X1	T48.6X2	T48.6X3	T48.6X4	T48.6X5	T48.6X6
Pemoline	T50.7X1	T50.7X2	T50.7X3	T50.7X4	T50.7X5	T50.7X6
Pempidine	T44.2X1	T44.2X2	T44.2X3	T44.2X4	T44.2X5	T44.2X6
Penamecillin	T36.0X1	T36.0X2	T36.0X3	T36.0X4	T36.0X5	T36.0X6
Penbutolol	T44.7X1	T44.7X2	T44.7X3	T44.7X4	T44.7X5	T44.7X6
Penethamate	T36.0X1	T36.0X2	T36.0X3	T36.0X4	T36.0X5	T36.0X6
Penfluridol	T43.591	T43.592	T43.593	T43.594	T43.595	T43.596
Penflutizide	T50.2X1	T50.2X2	T50.2X3	T50.2X4	T50.2X5	T50.2X6
Pengitoxin	T46.0X1	T46.0X2	T46.0X3	T46.0X4	T46.0X5	T46.0X6
Penicillamine	T50.6X1	T50.6X2	T50.6X3	T50.6X4	T50.6X5	T50.6X6
Penicillin (any)	T36.0X1	T36.0X2	T36.0X3	T36.0X4	T36.0X5	T36.0X6
Penicillinase	T45.3X1	T45.3X2	T45.3X3	T45.3X4	T45.3X5	T45.3X6
Penicilloyl polylysine	T50.8X1	T50.8X2	T50.8X3	T50.8X4	T50.8X5	T50.8X6
Penimepicycline	T36.4X1	T36.4X2	T36.4X3	T36.4X4	T36.4X5	T36.4X6
Pentachloroethane	T53.6X1	T53.6X2	T53.6X3	T53.6X4	—	—
Pentachloronaphthalene	T53.7X1	T53.7X2	T53.7X3	T53.7X4	—	—
Pentachlorophenol (pesticide)	T60.1X1	T60.1X2	T60.1X3	T60.1X4		
fungicide	T60.3X1	T60.3X2	T60.3X3	T60.3X4		
herbicide	T60.3X1	T60.3X2	T60.3X3	T60.3X4		
insecticide	T60.1X1	T60.1X2	T60.1X3	T60.1X4		
Pentaerythritol	T46.3X1	T46.3X2	T46.3X3	T46.3X4	T46.3X5	T46.3X6
chloral	T42.6X1	T42.6X2	T42.6X3	T42.6X4	T42.6X5	T42.6X6
tetranitrate NEC	T46.3X1	T46.3X2	T46.3X3	T46.3X4	T46.3X5	T46.3X6
Pentaerythrityl tetranitrate	T46.3X1	T46.3X2	T46.3X3	T46.3X4	T46.3X5	T46.3X6
Pentagastrin	T50.8X1	T50.8X2	T50.8X3	T50.8X4	T50.8X5	T50.8X6
Pentalin	T53.6X1	T53.6X2	T53.6X3	T53.6X4	—	—
Pentamethonium bromide	T44.2X1	T44.2X2	T44.2X3	T44.2X4	T44.2X5	T44.2X6
Pentamidine	T37.3X1	T37.3X2	T37.3X3	T37.3X4	T37.3X5	T37.3X6
Pentanol	T51.3X1	T51.3X2	T51.3X3	T51.3X4	—	—
Pentapyrrolinium (bitartrate)	T44.2X1	T44.2X2	T44.2X3	T44.2X4	T44.2X5	T44.2X6
Pentaquine	T37.2X1	T37.2X2	T37.2X3	T37.2X4	T37.2X5	T37.2X6
Pentazocine	T40.491	T40.492	T40.493	T40.494	T40.495	T40.496
Pentetrazole	T50.7X1	T50.7X2	T50.7X3	T50.7X4	T50.7X5	T50.7X6
Penthienate bromide	T44.3X1	T44.3X2	T44.3X3	T44.3X4	T44.3X5	T44.3X6
Pentifylline	T46.7X1	T46.7X2	T46.7X3	T46.7X4	T46.7X5	T46.7X6

Substance	Poisoning, Accidental (unintentional)	Poisoning, Intentional self-harm	Poisoning, Assault	Poisoning, Undetermined	Adverse effect	Underdosing
Pentobarbital	T42.3X1	T42.3X2	T42.3X3	T42.3X4	T42.3X5	T42.3X6
sodium	T42.3X1	T42.3X2	T42.3X3	T42.3X4	T42.3X5	T42.3X6
Pentobarbitone	T42.3X1	T42.3X2	T42.3X3	T42.3X4	T42.3X5	T42.3X6
Pentolonium tartrate	T44.2X1	T44.2X2	T44.2X3	T44.2X4	T44.2X5	T44.2X6
Pentosan polysulfate (sodium)	T39.8X1	T39.8X2	T39.8X3	T39.8X4	T39.8X5	T39.8X6
Pentostatin	T45.1X1	T45.1X2	T45.1X3	T45.1X4	T45.1X5	T45.1X6
Pentothal	T41.1X1	T41.1X2	T41.1X3	T41.1X4	T41.1X5	T41.1X6
Pentoxifylline	T46.7X1	T46.7X2	T46.7X3	T46.7X4	T46.7X5	T46.7X6
Pentoxyverine	T48.3X1	T48.3X2	T48.3X3	T48.3X4	T48.3X5	T48.3X6
Pentrinat	T46.3X1	T46.3X2	T46.3X3	T46.3X4	T46.3X5	T46.3X6
Pentylenetetrazole	T50.7X1	T50.7X2	T50.7X3	T50.7X4	T50.7X5	T50.7X6
Pentylsalicylamide	T37.1X1	T37.1X2	T37.1X3	T37.1X4	T37.1X5	T37.1X6
Pentymal	T42.3X1	T42.3X2	T42.3X3	T42.3X4	T42.3X5	T42.3X6
Peplomycin	T45.1X1	T45.1X2	T45.1X3	T45.1X4	T45.1X5	T45.1X6
Peppermint (oil)	T47.5X1	T47.5X2	T47.5X3	T47.5X4	T47.5X5	T47.5X6
Pepsin	T47.5X1	T47.5X2	T47.5X3	T47.5X4	T47.5X5	T47.5X6
digestant	T47.5X1	T47.5X2	T47.5X3	T47.5X4	T47.5X5	T47.5X6
Pepstatin	T47.1X1	T47.1X2	T47.1X3	T47.1X4	T47.1X5	T47.1X6
Peptavlon	T50.8X1	T50.8X2	T50.8X3	T50.8X4	T50.8X5	T50.8X6
Perazine	T43.3X1	T43.3X2	T43.3X3	T43.3X4	T43.3X5	T43.3X6
Percaine (spinal)	T41.3X1	T41.3X2	T41.3X3	T41.3X4	T41.3X5	T41.3X6
topical (surface)	T41.3X1	T41.3X2	T41.3X3	T41.3X4	T41.3X5	T41.3X6
Perchloroethylene	T53.3X1	T53.3X2	T53.3X3	T53.3X4	—	—
medicinal	T37.4X1	T37.4X2	T37.4X3	T37.4X4	T37.4X5	T37.4X6
vapor	T53.3X1	T53.3X2	T53.3X3	T53.3X4	—	—
Percodan	T40.2X1	T40.2X2	T40.2X3	T40.2X4	T40.2X5	T40.2X6
Percogesic—see also acetaminophen	T45.0X1	T45.0X2	T45.0X3	T45.0X4	T45.0X5	T45.0X6
Percorten	T38.0X1	T38.0X2	T38.0X3	T38.0X4	T38.0X5	T38.0X6
Pergolide	T42.8X1	T42.8X2	T42.8X3	T42.8X4	T42.8X5	T42.8X6
Pergonal	T38.811	T38.812	T38.813	T38.814	T38.815	T38.816
Perhexilene	T46.3X1	T46.3X2	T46.3X3	T46.3X4	T46.3X5	T46.3X6
Perhexiline (maleate)	T46.3X1	T46.3X2	T46.3X3	T46.3X4	T46.3X5	T46.3X6
Periactin	T45.0X1	T45.0X2	T45.0X3	T45.0X4	T45.0X5	T45.0X6
Periciazine	T43.3X1	T43.3X2	T43.3X3	T43.3X4	T43.3X5	T43.3X6
Periclor	T42.6X1	T42.6X2	T42.6X3	T42.6X4	T42.6X5	T42.6X6
Perindopril	T46.4X1	T46.4X2	T46.4X3	T46.4X4	T46.4X5	T46.4X6
Perisoxal	T39.8X1	T39.8X2	T39.8X3	T39.8X4	T39.8X5	T39.8X6
Peritoneal dialysis solution	T50.3X1	T50.3X2	T50.3X3	T50.3X4	T50.3X5	T50.3X6
Peritrate	T46.3X1	T46.3X2	T46.3X3	T46.3X4	T46.3X5	T46.3X6
Perlapine	T42.4X1	T42.4X2	T42.4X3	T42.4X4	T42.4X5	T42.4X6
Permanganate	T65.891	T65.892	T65.893	T65.894	—	—
Permethrin	T60.1X1	T60.1X2	T60.1X3	T60.1X4	—	—
Pernocton	T42.3X1	T42.3X2	T42.3X3	T42.3X4	T42.3X5	T42.3X6
Pernoston	T42.3X1	T42.3X2	T42.3X3	T42.3X4	T42.3X5	T42.3X6
Peronine	T40.2X1	T40.2X2	T40.2X3	T40.2X4	—	—
Perphenazine	T43.3X1	T43.3X2	T43.3X3	T43.3X4	T43.3X5	T43.3X6
Pertofrane	T43.011	T43.012	T43.013	T43.014	T43.015	T43.016

Substance	Poisoning, Accidental (unintentional)	Poisoning, Intentional self-harm	Poisoning, Assault	Poisoning, Undetermined	Adverse effect	Underdosing
Pertussis						
immune serum (human)	T50.Z11	T50.Z12	T50.Z13	T50.Z14	T50.Z15	T50.Z16
vaccine (with diphtheria toxoid) (with tetanus toxoid)	T50.A11	T50.A12	T50.A13	T50.A14	T50.A15	T50.A16
Peruvian balsam	T49.0X1	T49.0X2	T49.0X3	T49.0X4	T49.0X5	T49.0X6
Peruvoside	T46.0X1	T46.0X2	T46.0X3	T46.0X4	T46.0X5	T46.0X6
Pesticide (dust) (fumes) (vapor) NEC	T60.91	T60.92	T60.93	T60.94	—	—
arsenic	T57.0X1	T57.0X2	T57.0X3	T57.0X4	—	—
chlorinated	T60.1X1	T60.1X2	T60.1X3	T60.1X4	—	—
cyanide	T65.0X1	T65.0X2	T65.0X3	T65.0X4	—	—
kerosene	T52.0X1	T52.0X2	T52.0X3	T52.0X4	—	—
mixture (of compounds)	T60.91	T60.92	T60.93	T60.94	—	—
naphthalene	T60.2X1	T60.2X2	T60.2X3	T60.2X4	—	—
organochlorine (compounds)	T60.1X1	T60.1X2	T60.1X3	T60.1X4	—	—
petroleum (distillate) (products) NEC	T60.8X1	T60.8X2	T60.8X3	T60.8X4	—	—
specified ingredient NEC	T60.8X1	T60.8X2	T60.8X3	T60.8X4	—	—
strychnine	T65.1X1	T65.1X2	T65.1X3	T65.1X4	—	—
thallium	T60.4X1	T60.4X2	T60.4X3	T60.4X4	—	—
Pethidine	T40.491	T40.492	T40.493	T40.494	T40.495	T40.496
Petrichloral	T42.6X1	T42.6X2	T42.6X3	T42.6X4	T42.6X5	T42.6X6
Petrol	T52.0X1	T52.0X2	T52.0X3	T52.0X4	—	—
vapor	T52.0X1	T52.0X2	T52.0X3	T52.0X4	—	—
Petrolatum	T49.3X1	T49.3X2	T49.3X3	T49.3X4	T49.3X5	T49.3X6
hydrophilic	T49.3X1	T49.3X2	T49.3X3	T49.3X4	T49.3X5	T49.3X6
liquid	T47.4X1	T47.4X2	T47.4X3	T47.4X4	T47.4X5	T47.4X6
topical	T49.3X1	T49.3X2	T49.3X3	T49.3X4	T49.3X5	T49.3X6
nonmedicinal	T52.0X1	T52.0X2	T52.0X3	T52.0X4	—	—
red veterinary	T49.3X1	T49.3X2	T49.3X3	T49.3X4	T49.3X5	T49.3X6
white	T49.3X1	T49.3X2	T49.3X3	T49.3X4	T49.3X5	T49.3X6
Petroleum (products) NEC	T52.0X1	T52.0X2	T52.0X3	T52.0X4	—	—
benzine(s)—see Ligroin						
ether—see Ligroin						
jelly—see Petrolatum						
naphtha—see Ligroin						
pesticide	T60.8X1	T60.8X2	T60.8X3	T60.8X4	—	—
solids	T52.0X1	T52.0X2	T52.0X3	T52.0X4	—	—
solvents	T52.0X1	T52.0X2	T52.0X3	T52.0X4	—	—
vapor	T52.0X1	T52.0X2	T52.0X3	T52.0X4	—	—
Peyote	T40.991	T40.992	T40.993	T40.994	—	—
Phanodorm, phanodorn	T42.3X1	T42.3X2	T42.3X3	T42.3X4	T42.3X5	T42.3X6
Phanquinone	T37.3X1	T37.3X2	T37.3X3	T37.3X4	T37.3X5	T37.3X6
Phanquone	T37.3X1	T37.3X2	T37.3X3	T37.3X4	T37.3X5	T37.3X6
Pharmaceutical						
adjunct NEC	T50.901	T50.902	T50.903	T50.904	T50.905	T50.906
excipient NEC	T50.901	T50.902	T50.903	T50.904	T50.905	T50.906
sweetener	T50.901	T50.902	T50.903	T50.904	T50.905	T50.906
viscous agent	T50.901	T50.902	T50.903	T50.904	T50.905	T50.906

Substance	Poisoning, Accidental (unintentional)	Poisoning, Intentional self-harm	Poisoning, Assault	Poisoning, Undetermined	Adverse effect	Underdosing
Phemitone	T42.3X1	T42.3X2	T42.3X3	T42.3X4	T42.3X5	T42.3X6
Phenacaine	T41.3X1	T41.3X2	T41.3X3	T41.3X4	T41.3X5	T41.3X6
Phenacemide	T42.6X1	T42.6X2	T42.6X3	T42.6X4	T42.6X5	T42.6X6
Phenacetin	T39.1X1	T39.1X2	T39.1X3	T39.1X4	T39.1X5	T39.1X6
Phenadoxone	T40.2X1	T40.2X2	T40.2X3	T40.2X4	—	—
Phenaglycodol	T43.591	T43.592	T43.593	T43.594	T43.595	T43.596
Phenantoin	T42.0X1	T42.0X2	T42.0X3	T42.0X4	T42.0X5	T42.0X6
Phenaphthazine reagent	T50.991	T50.992	T50.993	T50.994	T50.995	T50.996
Phenazocine	T40.491	T40.492	T40.493	T40.494	T40.495	T40.496
Phenazone	T39.2X1	T39.2X2	T39.2X3	T39.2X4	T39.2X5	T39.2X6
Phenazopyridine	T39.8X1	T39.8X2	T39.8X3	T39.8X4	T39.8X5	T39.8X6
Phenbenicillin	T36.0X1	T36.0X2	T36.0X3	T36.0X4	T36.0X5	T36.0X6
Phenbutrazate	T50.5X1	T50.5X2	T50.5X3	T50.5X4	T50.5X5	T50.5X6
Phencyclidine	T40.991	T40.992	T40.993	T40.994	T40.995	T40.996
Phendimetrazine	T50.5X1	T50.5X2	T50.5X3	T50.5X4	T50.5X5	T50.5X6
Phenelzine	T43.1X1	T43.1X2	T43.1X3	T43.1X4	T43.1X5	T43.1X6
Phenemal	T42.3X1	T42.3X2	T42.3X3	T42.3X4	T42.3X5	T42.3X6
Phenergan	T42.6X1	T42.6X2	T42.6X3	T42.6X4	T42.6X5	T42.6X6
Pheneticillin	T36.0X1	T36.0X2	T36.0X3	T36.0X4	T36.0X5	T36.0X6
Pheneturide	T42.6X1	T42.6X2	T42.6X3	T42.6X4	T42.6X5	T42.6X6
Phenformin	T38.3X1	T38.3X2	T38.3X3	T38.3X4	T38.3X5	T38.3X6
Phenglutarimide	T44.3X1	T44.3X2	T44.3X3	T44.3X4	T44.3X5	T44.3X6
Phenicarbazide	T39.8X1	T39.8X2	T39.8X3	T39.8X4	T39.8X5	T39.8X6
Phenindamine	T45.0X1	T45.0X2	T45.0X3	T45.0X4	T45.0X5	T45.0X6
Phenindione	T45.511	T45.512	T45.513	T45.514	T45.515	T45.516
Pheniprazine	T43.1X1	T43.1X2	T43.1X3	T43.1X4	T43.1X5	T43.1X6
Pheniramine	T45.0X1	T45.0X2	T45.0X3	T45.0X4	T45.0X5	T45.0X6
Phenisatin	T47.2X1	T47.2X2	T47.2X3	T47.2X4	T47.2X5	T47.2X6
Phenmetrazine	T50.5X1	T50.5X2	T50.5X3	T50.5X4	T50.5X5	T50.5X6
Phenobal	T42.3X1	T42.3X2	T42.3X3	T42.3X4	T42.3X5	T42.3X6
Phenobarbital	T42.3X1	T42.3X2	T42.3X3	T42.3X4	T42.3X5	T42.3X6
with						
mephenytoin	T42.3X1	T42.3X2	T42.3X3	T42.3X4	T42.3X5	T42.3X6
phenytoin	T42.3X1	T42.3X2	T42.3X3	T42.3X4	T42.3X5	T42.3X6
sodium	T42.3X1	T42.3X2	T42.3X3	T42.3X4	T42.3X5	T42.3X6
Phenobarbitone	T42.3X1	T42.3X2	T42.3X3	T42.3X4	T42.3X5	T42.3X6
Phenobutiodil	T50.8X1	T50.8X2	T50.8X3	T50.8X4	T50.8X5	T50.8X6
Phenoctide	T49.0X1	T49.0X2	T49.0X3	T49.0X4	T49.0X5	T49.0X6
Phenol	T49.0X1	T49.0X2	T49.0X3	T49.0X4	T49.0X5	T49.0X6
disinfectant	T54.0X1	T54.0X2	T54.0X3	T54.0X4	—	—
in oil injection	T46.8X1	T46.8X2	T46.8X3	T46.8X4	T46.8X5	T46.8X6
medicinal	T49.1X1	T49.1X2	T49.1X3	T49.1X4	T49.1X5	T49.1X6
nonmedicinal NEC	T54.0X1	T54.0X2	T54.0X3	T54.0X4	—	—
pesticide	T60.8X1	T60.8X2	T60.8X3	T60.8X4	—	—
red	T50.8X1	T50.8X2	T50.8X3	T50.8X4	T50.8X5	T50.8X6
Phenolic preparation	T49.1X1	T49.1X2	T49.1X3	T49.1X4	T49.1X5	T49.1X6
Phenolphthalein	T47.2X1	T47.2X2	T47.2X3	T47.2X4	T47.2X5	T47.2X6
Phenolsulfonphthalein	T50.8X1	T50.8X2	T50.8X3	T50.8X4	T50.8X5	T50.8X6
Phenomorphan	T40.2X1	T40.2X2	T40.2X3	T40.2X4	—	—
Phenonyl	T42.3X1	T42.3X2	T42.3X3	T42.3X4	T42.3X5	T42.3X6

Substance	Poisoning, Accidental (unintentional)	Poisoning, Intentional self-harm	Poisoning, Assault	Poisoning, Undetermined	Adverse effect	Underdosing
Phenoperidine	T40.491	T40.492	T40.493	T40.494	—	—
Phenopyrazone	T46.991	T46.992	T46.993	T46.994	T46.995	T46.996
Phenoquin	T50.4X1	T50.4X2	T50.4X3	T50.4X4	T50.4X5	T50.4X6
Phenothiazine (psychotropic) NEC	T43.3X1	T43.3X2	T43.3X3	T43.3X4	T43.3X5	T43.3X6
insecticide	T60.2X1	T60.2X2	T60.2X3	T60.2X4	—	—
Phenothrin	T49.0X1	T49.0X2	T49.0X3	T49.0X4	T49.0X5	T49.0X6
Phenoxybenzamine	T46.7X1	T46.7X2	T46.7X3	T46.7X4	T46.7X5	T46.7X6
Phenoxyethanol	T49.0X1	T49.0X2	T49.0X3	T49.0X4	T49.0X5	T49.0X6
Phenoxymethyl penicillin	T36.0X1	T36.0X2	T36.0X3	T36.0X4	T36.0X5	T36.0X6
Phenprobamate	T42.8X1	T42.8X2	T42.8X3	T42.8X4	T42.8X5	T42.8X6
Phenprocoumon	T45.511	T45.512	T45.513	T45.514	T45.515	T45.516
Phensuximide	T42.2X1	T42.2X2	T42.2X3	T42.2X4	T42.2X5	T42.2X6
Phentermine	T50.5X1	T50.5X2	T50.5X3	T50.5X4	T50.5X5	T50.5X6
Phenthicillin	T36.0X1	T36.0X2	T36.0X3	T36.0X4	T36.0X5	T36.0X6
Phentolamine	T46.7X1	T46.7X2	T46.7X3	T46.7X4	T46.7X5	T46.7X6
Phenyl						
butazone	T39.2X1	T39.2X2	T39.2X3	T39.2X4	T39.2X5	T39.2X6
enediamine	T65.3X1	T65.3X2	T65.3X3	T65.3X4	—	—
hydrazine	T65.3X1	T65.3X2	T65.3X3	T65.3X4	—	—
antineoplastic	T45.1X1	T45.1X2	T45.1X3	T45.1X4	T45.1X5	T45.1X6
mercuric compounds— see Mercury						
salicylate	T49.3X1	T49.3X2	T49.3X3	T49.3X4	T49.3X5	T49.3X6
Phenylalanine mustard	T45.1X1	T45.1X2	T45.1X3	T45.1X4	T45.1X5	T45.1X6
Phenylbutazone	T39.2X1	T39.2X2	T39.2X3	T39.2X4	T39.2X5	T39.2X6
Phenylenediamine	T65.3X1	T65.3X2	T65.3X3	T65.3X4	—	—
Phenylephrine	T44.4X1	T44.4X2	T44.4X3	T44.4X4	T44.4X5	T44.4X6
Phenylethylbiguanide	T38.3X1	T38.3X2	T38.3X3	T38.3X4	T38.3X5	T38.3X6
Phenylmercuric						
acetate	T49.0X1	T49.0X2	T49.0X3	T49.0X4	T49.0X5	T49.0X6
borate	T49.0X1	T49.0X2	T49.0X3	T49.0X4	T49.0X5	T49.0X6
nitrate	T49.0X1	T49.0X2	T49.0X3	T49.0X4	T49.0X5	T49.0X6
Phenylmethylbarbitone	T42.3X1	T42.3X2	T42.3X3	T42.3X4	T42.3X5	T42.3X6
Phenylpropanol	T47.5X1	T47.5X2	T47.5X3	T47.5X4	T47.5X5	T47.5X6
Phenylpropanolamine	T44.991	T44.992	T44.993	T44.994	T44.995	T44.996
Phenylsulfthion	T60.0X1	T60.0X2	T60.0X3	T60.0X4	—	—
Phenyltoloxamine	T45.0X1	T45.0X2	T45.0X3	T45.0X4	T45.0X5	T45.0X6
Phenyramidol, phenyramidon	T39.8X1	T39.8X2	T39.8X3	T39.8X4	T39.8X5	T39.8X6
Phenytoin	T42.0X1	T42.0X2	T42.0X3	T42.0X4	T42.0X5	T42.0X6
with Phenobarbital	T42.3X1	T42.3X2	T42.3X3	T42.3X4	T42.3X5	T42.3X6
pHisoHex	T49.2X1	T49.2X2	T49.2X3	T49.2X4	T49.2X5	T49.2X6
Pholcodine	T48.3X1	T48.3X2	T48.3X3	T48.3X4	T48.3X5	T48.3X6
Pholedrine	T46.991	T46.992	T46.993	T46.994	T46.995	T46.996
Phorate	T60.0X1	T60.0X2	T60.0X3	T60.0X4	—	—
Phosdrin	T60.0X1	T60.0X2	T60.0X3	T60.0X4	—	—
Phosfolan	T60.0X1	T60.0X2	T60.0X3	T60.0X4	—	—
Phosgene (gas)	T59.891	T59.892	T59.893	T59.894	—	—
Phosphamidon	T60.0X1	T60.0X2	T60.0X3	T60.0X4	—	—

Substance	Poisoning, Accidental (unintentional)	Poisoning, Intentional self-harm	Poisoning, Assault	Poisoning, Undetermined	Adverse effect	Underdosing
Phosphate	T65.891	T65.892	T65.893	T65.894	—	—
laxative	T47.4X1	T47.4X2	T47.4X3	T47.4X4	T47.4X5	T47.4X6
organic	T60.0X1	T60.0X2	T60.0X3	T60.0X4	—	—
solvent	T52.91	T52.92	T52.93	T52.94	—	—
tricresyl	T65.891	T65.892	T65.893	T65.894	—	—
Phosphine	T57.1X1	T57.1X2	T57.1X3	T57.1X4	—	—
fumigant	T57.1X1	T57.1X2	T57.1X3	T57.1X4	—	—
Phospholine	T49.5X1	T49.5X2	T49.5X3	T49.5X4	T49.5X5	T49.5X6
Phosphoric acid	T54.2X1	T54.2X2	T54.2X3	T54.2X4	—	—
Phosphorus (compound) NEC	T57.1X1	T57.1X2	T57.1X3	T57.1X4	—	—
pesticide	T60.0X1	T60.0X2	T60.0X3	T60.0X4	—	—
Phthalates	T65.891	T65.892	T65.893	T65.894	—	—
Phthalic anhydride	T65.891	T65.892	T65.893	T65.894	—	—
Phthalimidoglutarimide	T42.6X1	T42.6X2	T42.6X3	T42.6X4	T42.6X5	T42.6X6
Phthalylsulfathiazole	T37.0X1	T37.0X2	T37.0X3	T37.0X4	T37.0X5	T37.0X6
Phylloquinone	T45.7X1	T45.7X2	T45.7X3	T45.7X4	T45.7X5	T45.7X6
Physeptone	T40.3X1	T40.3X2	T40.3X3	T40.3X4	T40.3X5	T40.3X6
Physostigma venenosum	T62.2X1	T62.2X2	T62.2X3	T62.2X4	—	—
Physostigmine	T49.5X1	T49.5X2	T49.5X3	T49.5X4	T49.5X5	T49.5X6
Phytolacca decandra	T62.2X1	T62.2X2	T62.2X3	T62.2X4	—	—
berries	T62.1X1	T62.1X2	T62.1X3	T62.1X4	—	—
Phytomenadione	T45.7X1	T45.7X2	T45.7X3	T45.7X4	T45.7X5	T45.7X6
Phytonadione	T45.7X1	T45.7X2	T45.7X3	T45.7X4	T45.7X5	T45.7X6
Picoperine	T48.3X1	T48.3X2	T48.3X3	T48.3X4	T48.3X5	T48.3X6
Picosulfate (sodium)	T47.2X1	T47.2X2	T47.2X3	T47.2X4	T47.2X5	T47.2X6
Picric (acid)	T54.2X1	T54.2X2	T54.2X3	T54.2X4	—	—
Picrotoxin	T50.7X1	T50.7X2	T50.7X3	T50.7X4	T50.7X5	T50.7X6
Piketoprofen	T49.0X1	T49.0X2	T49.0X3	T49.0X4	T49.0X5	T49.0X6
Pilocarpine	T44.1X1	T44.1X2	T44.1X3	T44.1X4	T44.1X5	T44.1X6
Pilocarpus (jaborandi) extract	T44.1X1	T44.1X2	T44.1X3	T44.1X4	T44.1X5	T44.1X6
Pilsicainide (hydrochloride)	T46.2X1	T46.2X2	T46.2X3	T46.2X4	T46.2X5	T46.2X6
Pimaricin	T36.7X1	T36.7X2	T36.7X3	T36.7X4	T36.7X5	T36.7X6
Pimeclone	T50.7X1	T50.7X2	T50.7X3	T50.7X4	T50.7X5	T50.7X6
Pimelic ketone	T52.8X1	T52.8X2	T52.8X3	T52.8X4	—	—
Pimethixene	T45.0X1	T45.0X2	T45.0X3	T45.0X4	T45.0X5	T45.0X6
Piminodine	T40.2X1	T40.2X2	T40.2X3	T40.2X4	T40.2X5	T40.2X6
Pimozide	T43.591	T43.592	T43.593	T43.594	T43.595	T43.596
Pinacidil	T46.5X1	T46.5X2	T46.5X3	T46.5X4	T46.5X5	T46.5X6
Pinaverium bromide	T44.3X1	T44.3X2	T44.3X3	T44.3X4	T44.3X5	T44.3X6
Pinazepam	T42.4X1	T42.4X2	T42.4X3	T42.4X4	T42.4X5	T42.4X6
Pindolol	T44.7X1	T44.7X2	T44.7X3	T44.7X4	T44.7X5	T44.7X6
Pindone	T60.4X1	T60.4X2	T60.4X3	T60.4X4	—	—
Pine oil (disinfectant)	T65.891	T65.892	T65.893	T65.894	—	—
Pinkroot	T37.4X1	T37.4X2	T37.4X3	T37.4X4	T37.4X5	T37.4X6
Pipadone	T40.2X1	T40.2X2	T40.2X3	T40.2X4	—	—
Pipamazine	T45.0X1	T45.0X2	T45.0X3	T45.0X4	T45.0X5	T45.0X6
Pipamperone	T43.4X1	T43.4X2	T43.4X3	T43.4X4	T43.4X5	T43.4X6
Pipazetate	T48.3X1	T48.3X2	T48.3X3	T48.3X4	T48.3X5	T48.3X6

Substance	Poisoning, Accidental (unintentional)	Poisoning, Intentional self-harm	Poisoning, Assault	Poisoning, Undetermined	Adverse effect	Underdosing
Pipemidic acid	T37.8X1	T37.8X2	T37.8X3	T37.8X4	T37.8X5	T37.8X6
Pipenzolate bromide	T44.3X1	T44.3X2	T44.3X3	T44.3X4	T44.3X5	T44.3X6
Piperacetazine	T43.3X1	T43.3X2	T43.3X3	T43.3X4	T43.3X5	T43.3X6
Piperacillin	T36.0X1	T36.0X2	T36.0X3	T36.0X4	T36.0X5	T36.0X6
Piperazine	T37.4X1	T37.4X2	T37.4X3	T37.4X4	T37.4X5	T37.4X6
estrone sulfate	T38.5X1	T38.5X2	T38.5X3	T38.5X4	T38.5X5	T38.5X6
Piper cubeba	T62.2X1	T62.2X2	T62.2X3	T62.2X4	—	—
Piperidione	T48.3X1	T48.3X2	T48.3X3	T48.3X4	T48.3X5	T48.3X6
Piperidolate	T44.3X1	T44.3X2	T44.3X3	T44.3X4	T44.3X5	T44.3X6
Piperocaine	T41.3X1	T41.3X2	T41.3X3	T41.3X4	T41.3X5	T41.3X6
infiltration (subcutaneous)	T41.3X1	T41.3X2	T41.3X3	T41.3X4	T41.3X5	T41.3X6
nerve block (peripheral) (plexus)	T41.3X1	T41.3X2	T41.3X3	T41.3X4	T41.3X5	T41.3X6
topical (surface)	T41.3X1	T41.3X2	T41.3X3	T41.3X4	T41.3X5	T41.3X6
Piperonyl butoxide	T60.8X1	T60.8X2	T60.8X3	T60.8X4	—	—
Pipethanate	T44.3X1	T44.3X2	T44.3X3	T44.3X4	T44.3X5	T44.3X6
Pipobroman	T45.1X1	T45.1X2	T45.1X3	T45.1X4	T45.1X5	T45.1X6
Pipotiazine	T43.3X1	T43.3X2	T43.3X3	T43.3X4	T43.3X5	T43.3X6
Pipoxizine	T45.0X1	T45.0X2	T45.0X3	T45.0X4	T45.0X5	T45.0X6
Pipradrol	T43.691	T43.692	T43.693	T43.694	T43.695	T43.696
Piprinhydrinate	T45.0X1	T45.0X2	T45.0X3	T45.0X4	T45.0X5	T45.0X6
Pirarubicin	T45.1X1	T45.1X2	T45.1X3	T45.1X4	T45.1X5	T45.1X6
Pirazinamide	T37.1X1	T37.1X2	T37.1X3	T37.1X4	T37.1X5	T37.1X6
Pirbuterol	T48.6X1	T48.6X2	T48.6X3	T48.6X4	T48.6X5	T48.6X6
Pirenzepine	T47.1X1	T47.1X2	T47.1X3	T47.1X4	T47.1X5	T47.1X6
Piretanide	T50.1X1	T50.1X2	T50.1X3	T50.1X4	T50.1X5	T50.1X6
Piribedil	T42.8X1	T42.8X2	T42.8X3	T42.8X4	T42.8X5	T42.8X6
Piridoxilate	T46.3X1	T46.3X2	T46.3X3	T46.3X4	T46.3X5	T46.3X6
Piritramide	T40.491	T40.492	T40.493	T40.494	—	—
Piromidic acid	T37.8X1	T37.8X2	T37.8X3	T37.8X4	T37.8X5	T37.8X6
Piroxicam	T39.391	T39.392	T39.393	T39.394	T39.395	T39.396
beta-cyclodextrin complex	T39.8X1	T39.8X2	T39.8X3	T39.8X4	T39.8X5	T39.8X6
Pirozadil	T46.6X1	T46.6X2	T46.6X3	T46.6X4	T46.6X5	T46.6X6
Piscidia (bark) (erythrina)	T39.8X1	T39.8X2	T39.8X3	T39.8X4	T39.8X5	T39.8X6
Pitch	T65.891	T65.892	T65.893	T65.894	—	—
Pitkin's solution	T41.3X1	T41.3X2	T41.3X3	T41.3X4	T41.3X5	T41.3X6
Pitocin	T48.0X1	T48.0X2	T48.0X3	T48.0X4	T48.0X5	T48.0X6
Pitressin (tannate)	T38.891	T38.892	T38.893	T38.894	T38.895	T38.896
Pituitary extracts (posterior)	T38.891	T38.892	T38.893	T38.894	T38.895	T38.896
anterior	T38.811	T38.812	T38.813	T38.814	T38.815	T38.816
Pituitrin	T38.891	T38.892	T38.893	T38.894	T38.895	T38.896
Pivampicillin	T36.0X1	T36.0X2	T36.0X3	T36.0X4	T36.0X5	T36.0X6
Pivmecillinam	T36.0X1	T36.0X2	T36.0X3	T36.0X4	T36.0X5	T36.0X6
Placental hormone	T38.891	T38.892	T38.893	T38.894	T38.895	T38.896
Placidyl	T42.6X1	T42.6X2	T42.6X3	T42.6X4	T42.6X5	T42.6X6
Plague vaccine	T50.A91	T50.A92	T50.A93	T50.A94	T50.A95	T50.A96

Substance	Poisoning, Accidental (unintentional)	Poisoning, Intentional self-harm	Poisoning, Assault	Poisoning, Undetermined	Adverse effect	Underdosing
Plant						
food or fertilizer NEC	T65.891	T65.892	T65.893	T65.894	—	—
containing herbicide	T60.3X1	T60.3X2	T60.3X3	T60.3X4	—	—
noxious, used as food	T62.2X1	T62.2X2	T62.2X3	T62.2X4	—	—
berries	T62.1X1	T62.1X2	T62.1X3	T62.1X4	—	—
seeds	T62.2X1	T62.2X2	T62.2X3	T62.2X4	—	—
specified type NEC	T62.2X1	T62.2X2	T62.2X3	T62.2X4	—	—
Plasma	T45.8X1	T45.8X2	T45.8X3	T45.8X4	T45.8X5	T45.8X6
expander NEC	T45.8X1	T45.8X2	T45.8X3	T45.8X4	T45.8X5	T45.8X6
protein fraction (human)	T45.8X1	T45.8X2	T45.8X3	T45.8X4	T45.8X5	T45.8X6
Plasmanate	T45.8X1	T45.8X2	T45.8X3	T45.8X4	T45.8X5	T45.8X6
Plasminogen (tissue) activator	T45.611	T45.612	T45.613	T45.614	T45.615	T45.616
Plaster dressing	T49.3X1	T49.3X2	T49.3X3	T49.3X4	T49.3X5	T49.3X6
Plastic dressing	T49.3X1	T49.3X2	T49.3X3	T49.3X4	T49.3X5	T49.3X6
Plegicil	T43.3X1	T43.3X2	T43.3X3	T43.3X4	T43.3X5	T43.3X6
Plicamycin	T45.1X1	T45.1X2	T45.1X3	T45.1X4	T45.1X5	T45.1X6
Podophyllotoxin	T49.8X1	T49.8X2	T49.8X3	T49.8X4	T49.8X5	T49.8X6
Podophyllum (resin)	T49.4X1	T49.4X2	T49.4X3	T49.4X4	T49.4X5	T49.4X6
Poison NEC	T65.91	T65.92	T65.93	T65.94	—	—
Poisonous berries	T62.1X1	T62.1X2	T62.1X3	T62.1X4	—	—
Pokeweed (any part)	T62.2X1	T62.2X2	T62.2X3	T62.2X4	—	—
Poldine metilsulfate	T44.3X1	T44.3X2	T44.3X3	T44.3X4	T44.3X5	T44.3X6
Polidexide (sulfate)	T46.6X1	T46.6X2	T46.6X3	T46.6X4	T46.6X5	T46.6X6
Polidocanol	T46.8X1	T46.8X2	T46.8X3	T46.8X4	T46.8X5	T46.8X6
Poliomyelitis vaccine	T50.B91	T50.B92	T50.B93	T50.B94	T50.B95	T50.B96
Polish (car) (floor) (furniture) (metal) (porcelain) (silver)	T65.891	T65.892	T65.893	T65.894		
abrasive	T65.891	T65.892	T65.893	T65.894	—	—
porcelain	T65.891	T65.892	T65.893	T65.894	—	—
Poloxalkol	T47.4X1	T47.4X2	T47.4X3	T47.4X4	T47.4X5	T47.4X6
Poloxamer	T47.4X1	T47.4X2	T47.4X3	T47.4X4	T47.4X5	T47.4X6
Polyaminostyrene resins	T50.3X1	T50.3X2	T50.3X3	T50.3X4	T50.3X5	T50.3X6
Polycarbophil	T47.4X1	T47.4X2	T47.4X3	T47.4X4	T47.4X5	T47.4X6
Polychlorinated biphenyl	T65.891	T65.892	T65.893	T65.894	—	—
Polycycline	T36.4X1	T36.4X2	T36.4X3	T36.4X4	T36.4X5	T36.4X6
Polyester fumes	T59.891	T59.892	T59.893	T59.894	—	—
Polyester resin hardener	T52.91	T52.92	T52.93	T52.94	—	—
fumes	T59.891	T59.892	T59.893	T59.894	—	—
Polyestradiol phosphate	T38.5X1	T38.5X2	T38.5X3	T38.5X4	T38.5X5	T38.5X6
Polyethanolamine alkyl sulfate	T49.2X1	T49.2X2	T49.2X3	T49.2X4	T49.2X5	T49.2X6
Polyethylene adhesive	T49.3X1	T49.3X2	T49.3X3	T49.3X4	T49.3X5	T49.3X6
Polyferose	T45.4X1	T45.4X2	T45.4X3	T45.4X4	T45.4X5	T45.4X6
Polygeline	T45.8X1	T45.8X2	T45.8X3	T45.8X4	T45.8X5	T45.8X6
Polymyxin	T36.8X1	T36.8X2	T36.8X3	T36.8X4	T36.8X5	T36.8X6
B	T36.8X1	T36.8X2	T36.8X3	T36.8X4	T36.8X5	T36.8X6
ENT agent	T49.6X1	T49.6X2	T49.6X3	T49.6X4	T49.6X5	T49.6X6

Substance	Poisoning, Accidental (unintentional)	Poisoning, Intentional self-harm	Poisoning, Assault	Poisoning, Undetermined	Adverse effect	Underdosing
Polymyxin — *Continued*						
ophthalmic preparation	T49.5X1	T49.5X2	T49.5X3	T49.5X4	T49.5X5	T49.5X6
topical NEC	T49.0X1	T49.0X2	T49.0X3	T49.0X4	T49.0X5	T49.0X6
E sulfate (eye preparation)	T49.5X1	T49.5X2	T49.5X3	T49.5X4	T49.5X5	T49.5X6
Polynoxylin	T49.0X1	T49.0X2	T49.0X3	T49.0X4	T49.0X5	T49.0X6
Polyoestradiol phosphate	T38.5X1	T38.5X2	T38.5X3	T38.5X4	T38.5X5	T38.5X6
Polyoxymethyleneurea	T49.0X1	T49.0X2	T49.0X3	T49.0X4	T49.0X5	T49.0X6
Polysilane	T47.8X1	T47.8X2	T47.8X3	T47.8X4	T47.8X5	T47.8X6
Polytetrafluoroethylene (inhaled)	T59.891	T59.892	T59.893	T59.894	—	—
Polythiazide	T50.2X1	T50.2X2	T50.2X3	T50.2X4	T50.2X5	T50.2X6
Polyvidone	T45.8X1	T45.8X2	T45.8X3	T45.8X4	T45.8X5	T45.8X6
Polyvinylpyrrolidone	T45.8X1	T45.8X2	T45.8X3	T45.8X4	T45.8X5	T45.8X6
Pontocaine (hydrochloride) (infiltration) (topical)	T41.3X1	T41.3X2	T41.3X3	T41.3X4	T41.3X5	T41.3X6
nerve block (peripheral) (plexus)	T41.3X1	T41.3X2	T41.3X3	T41.3X4	T41.3X5	T41.3X6
spinal	T41.3X1	T41.3X2	T41.3X3	T41.3X4	T41.3X5	T41.3X6
Porfiromycin	T45.1X1	T45.1X2	T45.1X3	T45.1X4	T45.1X5	T45.1X6
Posterior pituitary hormone NEC	T38.891	T38.892	T38.893	T38.894	T38.895	T38.896
Pot	T40.7X1	T40.7X2	T40.7X3	T40.7X4	T40.7X5	T40.7X6
Potash (caustic)	T54.3X1	T54.3X2	T54.3X3	T54.3X4	—	—
Potassic saline injection (lactated)	T50.3X1	T50.3X2	T50.3X3	T50.3X4	T50.3X5	T50.3X6
Potassium (salts) NEC	T50.3X1	T50.3X2	T50.3X3	T50.3X4	T50.3X5	T50.3X6
aminobenzoate	T45.8X1	T45.8X2	T45.8X3	T45.8X4	T45.8X5	T45.8X6
aminosalicylate	T37.1X1	T37.1X2	T37.1X3	T37.1X4	T37.1X5	T37.1X6
antimony 'tartrate'	T37.8X1	T37.8X2	T37.8X3	T37.8X4	T37.8X5	T37.8X6
arsenite (solution)	T57.0X1	T57.0X2	T57.0X3	T57.0X4	—	—
bichromate	T56.2X1	T56.2X2	T56.2X3	T56.2X4	—	—
bisulfate	T47.3X1	T47.3X2	T47.3X3	T47.3X4	T47.3X5	T47.3X6
bromide	T42.6X1	T42.6X2	T42.6X3	T42.6X4	T42.6X5	T42.6X6
canrenoate	T50.0X1	T50.0X2	T50.0X3	T50.0X4	T50.0X5	T50.0X6
carbonate	T54.3X1	T54.3X2	T54.3X3	T54.3X4	—	—
chlorate NEC	T65.891	T65.892	T65.893	T65.894	—	—
chloride	T50.3X1	T50.3X2	T50.3X3	T50.3X4	T50.3X5	T50.3X6
citrate	T50.991	T50.992	T50.993	T50.994	T50.995	T50.996
cyanide	T65.0X1	T65.0X2	T65.0X3	T65.0X4	—	—
ferric hexacyano-ferrate (medicinal)	T50.6X1	T50.6X2	T50.6X3	T50.6X4	T50.6X5	T50.6X6
nonmedicinal	T65.891	T65.892	T65.893	T65.894	—	—
Fluoride	T57.8X1	T57.8X2	T57.8X3	T57.8X4	—	—
glucaldrate	T47.1X1	T47.1X2	T47.1X3	T47.1X4	T47.1X5	T47.1X6
hydroxide	T54.3X1	T54.3X2	T54.3X3	T54.3X4	—	—
iodate	T49.0X1	T49.0X2	T49.0X3	T49.0X4	T49.0X5	T49.0X6
iodide	T48.4X1	T48.4X2	T48.4X3	T48.4X4	T48.4X5	T48.4X6
nitrate	T57.8X1	T57.8X2	T57.8X3	T57.8X4	—	—
oxalate	T65.891	T65.892	T65.893	T65.894	—	—

Substance	Poisoning, Accidental (unintentional)	Poisoning, Intentional self-harm	Poisoning, Assault	Poisoning, Undetermined	Adverse effect	Underdosing
Potassium — *Continued*						
perchlorate (nonmedicinal) NEC	T65.891	T65.892	T65.893	T65.894	—	—
antithyroid	T38.2X1	T38.2X2	T38.2X3	T38.2X4	T38.2X5	T38.2X6
medicinal	T38.2X1	T38.2X2	T38.2X3	T38.2X4	T38.2X5	T38.2X6
Permanganate (nonmedicinal)	T65.891	T65.892	T65.893	T65.894		
medicinal	T49.0X1	T49.0X2	T49.0X3	T49.0X4	T49.0X5	T49.0X6
sulfate	T47.2X1	T47.2X2	T47.2X3	T47.2X4	T47.2X5	T47.2X6
Potassium-removing resin	T50.3X1	T50.3X2	T50.3X3	T50.3X4	T50.3X5	T50.3X6
Potassium-retaining drug	T50.3X1	T50.3X2	T50.3X3	T50.3X4	T50.3X5	T50.3X6
Povidone	T45.8X1	T45.8X2	T45.8X3	T45.8X4	T45.8X5	T45.8X6
iodine	T49.0X1	T49.0X2	T49.0X3	T49.0X4	T49.0X5	T49.0X6
Practolol	T44.7X1	T44.7X2	T44.7X3	T44.7X4	T44.7X5	T44.7X6
Prajmalium bitartrate	T46.2X1	T46.2X2	T46.2X3	T46.2X4	T46.2X5	T46.2X6
Pralidoxime (iodide)	T50.6X1	T50.6X2	T50.6X3	T50.6X4	T50.6X5	T50.6X6
chloride	T50.6X1	T50.6X2	T50.6X3	T50.6X4	T50.6X5	T50.6X6
Pramiverine	T44.3X1	T44.3X2	T44.3X3	T44.3X4	T44.3X5	T44.3X6
Pramocaine	T49.1X1	T49.1X2	T49.1X3	T49.1X4	T49.1X5	T49.1X6
Pramoxine	T49.1X1	T49.1X2	T49.1X3	T49.1X4	T49.1X5	T49.1X6
Prasterone	T38.7X1	T38.7X2	T38.7X3	T38.7X4	T38.7X5	T38.7X6
Pravastatin	T46.6X1	T46.6X2	T46.6X3	T46.6X4	T46.6X5	T46.6X6
Prazepam	T42.4X1	T42.4X2	T42.4X3	T42.4X4	T42.4X5	T42.4X6
Praziquantel	T37.4X1	T37.4X2	T37.4X3	T37.4X4	T37.4X5	T37.4X6
Prazitone	T43.291	T43.292	T43.293	T43.294	T43.295	T43.296
Prazosin	T44.6X1	T44.6X2	T44.6X3	T44.6X4	T44.6X5	T44.6X6
Prednicarbate	T49.0X1	T49.0X2	T49.0X3	T49.0X4	T49.0X5	T49.0X6
Prednimustine	T45.1X1	T45.1X2	T45.1X3	T45.1X4	T45.1X5	T45.1X6
Prednisolone	T38.0X1	T38.0X2	T38.0X3	T38.0X4	T38.0X5	T38.0X6
ENT agent	T49.6X1	T49.6X2	T49.6X3	T49.6X4	T49.6X5	T49.6X6
ophthalmic preparation	T49.5X1	T49.5X2	T49.5X3	T49.5X4	T49.5X5	T49.5X6
steaglate	T49.0X1	T49.0X2	T49.0X3	T49.0X4	T49.0X5	T49.0X6
topical NEC	T49.0X1	T49.0X2	T49.0X3	T49.0X4	T49.0X5	T49.0X6
Prednisone	T38.0X1	T38.0X2	T38.0X3	T38.0X4	T38.0X5	T38.0X6
Prednylidene	T38.0X1	T38.0X2	T38.0X3	T38.0X4	T38.0X5	T38.0X6
Pregnandiol	T38.5X1	T38.5X2	T38.5X3	T38.5X4	T38.5X5	T38.5X6
Pregneninolone	T38.5X1	T38.5X2	T38.5X3	T38.5X4	T38.5X5	T38.5X6
Preludin	T43.691	T43.692	T43.693	T43.694	T43.695	T43.696
Premarin	T38.5X1	T38.5X2	T38.5X3	T38.5X4	T38.5X5	T38.5X6
Premedication anesthetic	T41.201	T41.202	T41.203	T41.204	T41.205	T41.206
Prenalterol	T44.5X1	T44.5X2	T44.5X3	T44.5X4	T44.5X5	T44.5X6
Prenoxdiazine	T48.3X1	T48.3X2	T48.3X3	T48.3X4	T48.3X5	T48.3X6
Prenylamine	T46.3X1	T46.3X2	T46.3X3	T46.3X4	T46.3X5	T46.3X6
Preparation H	T49.8X1	T49.8X2	T49.8X3	T49.8X4	T49.8X5	T49.8X6
Preparation, local	T49.4X1	T49.4X2	T49.4X3	T49.4X4	T49.4X5	T49.4X6
Preservative (nonmedicinal)	T65.891	T65.892	T65.893	T65.894	—	—
medicinal	T50.901	T50.902	T50.903	T50.904	T50.905	T50.906
wood	T60.91	T60.92	T60.93	T60.94	—	—

Substance	Poisoning, Accidental (unintentional)	Poisoning, Intentional self-harm	Poisoning, Assault	Poisoning, Undetermined	Adverse effect	Underdosing
Prethcamide	T50.7X1	T50.7X2	T50.7X3	T50.7X4	T50.7X5	T50.7X6
Pride of China	T62.2X1	T62.2X2	T62.2X3	T62.2X4	—	—
Pridinol	T44.3X1	T44.3X2	T44.3X3	T44.3X4	T44.3X5	T44.3X6
Prifinium bromide	T44.3X1	T44.3X2	T44.3X3	T44.3X4	T44.3X5	T44.3X6
Prilocaine	T41.3X1	T41.3X2	T41.3X3	T41.3X4	T41.3X5	T41.3X6
infiltration (subcutaneous)	T41.3X1	T41.3X2	T41.3X3	T41.3X4	T41.3X5	T41.3X6
nerve block (peripheral) (plexus)	T41.3X1	T41.3X2	T41.3X3	T41.3X4	T41.3X5	T41.3X6
regional	T41.3X1	T41.3X2	T41.3X3	T41.3X4	T41.3X5	T41.3X6
Primaquine	T37.2X1	T37.2X2	T37.2X3	T37.2X4	T37.2X5	T37.2X6
Primidone	T42.6X1	T42.6X2	T42.6X3	T42.6X4	T42.6X5	T42.6X6
Primula (veris)	T62.2X1	T62.2X2	T62.2X3	T62.2X4	—	—
Prinadol	T40.2X1	T40.2X2	T40.2X3	T40.2X4	T40.2X5	T40.2X6
Priscol, Priscoline	T44.6X1	T44.6X2	T44.6X3	T44.6X4	T44.6X5	T44.6X6
Pristinamycin	T36.3X1	T36.3X2	T36.3X3	T36.3X4	T36.3X5	T36.3X6
Privet	T62.2X1	T62.2X2	T62.2X3	T62.2X4	—	—
berries	T62.1X1	T62.1X2	T62.1X3	T62.1X4	—	—
Privine	T44.4X1	T44.4X2	T44.4X3	T44.4X4	T44.4X5	T44.4X6
Pro-Banthine	T44.3X1	T44.3X2	T44.3X3	T44.3X4	T44.3X5	T44.3X6
Probarbital	T42.3X1	T42.3X2	T42.3X3	T42.3X4	T42.3X5	T42.3X6
Probenecid	T50.4X1	T50.4X2	T50.4X3	T50.4X4	T50.4X5	T50.4X6
Probucol	T46.6X1	T46.6X2	T46.6X3	T46.6X4	T46.6X5	T46.6X6
Procainamide	T46.2X1	T46.2X2	T46.2X3	T46.2X4	T46.2X5	T46.2X6
Procaine	T41.3X1	T41.3X2	T41.3X3	T41.3X4	T41.3X5	T41.3X6
benzylpenicillin	T36.0X1	T36.0X2	T36.0X3	T36.0X4	T36.0X5	T36.0X6
nerve block (periphreal) (plexus)	T41.3X1	T41.3X2	T41.3X3	T41.3X4	T41.3X5	T41.3X6
penicillin G	T36.0X1	T36.0X2	T36.0X3	T36.0X4	T36.0X5	T36.0X6
regional	T41.3X1	T41.3X2	T41.3X3	T41.3X4	T41.3X5	T41.3X6
spinal	T41.3X1	T41.3X2	T41.3X3	T41.3X4	T41.3X5	T41.3X6
Procalmidol	T43.591	T43.592	T43.593	T43.594	T43.595	T43.596
Procarbazine	T45.1X1	T45.1X2	T45.1X3	T45.1X4	T45.1X5	T45.1X6
Procaterol	T44.5X1	T44.5X2	T44.5X3	T44.5X4	T44.5X5	T44.5X6
Prochlorperazine	T43.3X1	T43.3X2	T43.3X3	T43.3X4	T43.3X5	T43.3X6
Procyclidine	T44.3X1	T44.3X2	T44.3X3	T44.3X4	T44.3X5	T44.3X6
Producer gas	T58.8X1	T58.8X2	T58.8X3	T58.8X4	—	—
Profadol	T40.491	T40.492	T40.493	T40.494	T40.495	T40.496
Profenamine	T44.3X1	T44.3X2	T44.3X3	T44.3X4	T44.3X5	T44.3X6
Profenil	T44.3X1	T44.3X2	T44.3X3	T44.3X4	T44.3X5	T44.3X6
Proflavine	T49.0X1	T49.0X2	T49.0X3	T49.0X4	T49.0X5	T49.0X6
Progabide	T42.6X1	T42.6X2	T42.6X3	T42.6X4	T42.6X5	T42.6X6
Progesterone	T38.5X1	T38.5X2	T38.5X3	T38.5X4	T38.5X5	T38.5X6
Progestin	T38.5X1	T38.5X2	T38.5X3	T38.5X4	T38.5X5	T38.5X6
oral contraceptive	T38.4X1	T38.4X2	T38.4X3	T38.4X4	T38.4X5	T38.4X6
Progestogen NEC	T38.5X1	T38.5X2	T38.5X3	T38.5X4	T38.5X5	T38.5X6
Progestone	T38.5X1	T38.5X2	T38.5X3	T38.5X4	T38.5X5	T38.5X6
Proglumide	T47.1X1	T47.1X2	T47.1X3	T47.1X4	T47.1X5	T47.1X6
Proguanil	T37.2X1	T37.2X2	T37.2X3	T37.2X4	T37.2X5	T37.2X6
Prolactin	T38.811	T38.812	T38.813	T38.814	T38.815	T38.816

Substance	Poisoning, Accidental (unintentional)	Poisoning, Intentional self-harm	Poisoning, Assault	Poisoning, Undetermined	Adverse effect	Underdosing
Prolintane	T43.691	T43.692	T43.693	T43.694	T43.695	T43.696
Proloid	T38.1X1	T38.1X2	T38.1X3	T38.1X4	T38.1X5	T38.1X6
Proluton	T38.5X1	T38.5X2	T38.5X3	T38.5X4	T38.5X5	T38.5X6
Promacetin	T37.1X1	T37.1X2	T37.1X3	T37.1X4	T37.1X5	T37.1X6
Promazine	T43.3X1	T43.3X2	T43.3X3	T43.3X4	T43.3X5	T43.3X6
Promedol	T40.2X1	T40.2X2	T40.2X3	T40.2X4	—	—
Promegestone	T38.5X1	T38.5X2	T38.5X3	T38.5X4	T38.5X5	T38.5X6
Promethazine (teoclate)	T43.3X1	T43.3X2	T43.3X3	T43.3X4	T43.3X5	T43.3X6
Promin	T37.1X1	T37.1X2	T37.1X3	T37.1X4	T37.1X5	T37.1X6
Pronase	T45.3X1	T45.3X2	T45.3X3	T45.3X4	T45.3X5	T45.3X6
Pronestyl (hydrochloride)	T46.2X1	T46.2X2	T46.2X3	T46.2X4	T46.2X5	T46.2X6
Pronetalol	T44.7X1	T44.7X2	T44.7X3	T44.7X4	T44.7X5	T44.7X6
Prontosil	T37.0X1	T37.0X2	T37.0X3	T37.0X4	T37.0X5	T37.0X6
Propachlor	T60.3X1	T60.3X2	T60.3X3	T60.3X4	—	—
Propafenone	T46.2X1	T46.2X2	T46.2X3	T46.2X4	T46.2X5	T46.2X6
Propallylonal	T42.3X1	T42.3X2	T42.3X3	T42.3X4	T42.3X5	T42.3X6
Propamidine	T49.0X1	T49.0X2	T49.0X3	T49.0X4	T49.0X5	T49.0X6
Propane (distributed in mobile container)	T59.891	T59.892	T59.893	T59.894	—	—
distributed through pipes	T59.891	T59.892	T59.893	T59.894	—	—
incomplete combustion	T58.11	T58.12	T58.13	T58.14	—	—
Propanidid	T41.291	T41.292	T41.293	T41.294	T41.295	T41.296
Propanil	T60.3X1	T60.3X2	T60.3X3	T60.3X4	—	—
1-Propanol	T51.3X1	T51.3X2	T51.3X3	T51.3X4		
2-Propanol	T51.2X1	T51.2X2	T51.2X3	T51.2X4		
Propantheline	T44.3X1	T44.3X2	T44.3X3	T44.3X4	T44.3X5	T44.3X6
bromide	T44.3X1	T44.3X2	T44.3X3	T44.3X4	T44.3X5	T44.3X6
Proparacaine	T41.3X1	T41.3X2	T41.3X3	T41.3X4	T41.3X5	T41.3X6
Propatylnitrate	T46.3X1	T46.3X2	T46.3X3	T46.3X4	T46.3X5	T46.3X6
Propicillin	T36.0X1	T36.0X2	T36.0X3	T36.0X4	T36.0X5	T36.0X6
Propiolactone	T49.0X1	T49.0X2	T49.0X3	T49.0X4	T49.0X5	T49.0X6
Propiomazine	T45.0X1	T45.0X2	T45.0X3	T45.0X4	T45.0X5	T45.0X6
Propionaldehyde (medicinal)	T42.6X1	T42.6X2	T42.6X3	T42.6X4	T42.6X5	T42.6X6
Propionate (calcium) (sodium)	T49.0X1	T49.0X2	T49.0X3	T49.0X4	T49.0X5	T49.0X6
Propion gel	T49.0X1	T49.0X2	T49.0X3	T49.0X4	T49.0X5	T49.0X6
Propitocaine	T41.3X1	T41.3X2	T41.3X3	T41.3X4	T41.3X5	T41.3X6
infiltration (subcutaneous)	T41.3X1	T41.3X2	T41.3X3	T41.3X4	T41.3X5	T41.3X6
nerve block (peripheral) (plexus)	T41.3X1	T41.3X2	T41.3X3	T41.3X4	T41.3X5	T41.3X6
Propofol	T41.291	T41.292	T41.293	T41.294	T41.295	T41.296
Propoxur	T60.0X1	T60.0X2	T60.0X3	T60.0X4	—	—
Propoxycaine	T41.3X1	T41.3X2	T41.3X3	T41.3X4	T41.3X5	T41.3X6
infiltration (subcutaneous)	T41.3X1	T41.3X2	T41.3X3	T41.3X4	T41.3X5	T41.3X6
nerve block (peripheral) (plexus)	T41.3X1	T41.3X2	T41.3X3	T41.3X4	T41.3X5	T41.3X6
topical (surface)	T41.3X1	T41.3X2	T41.3X3	T41.3X4	T41.3X5	T41.3X6

Substance	Poisoning, Accidental (unintentional)	Poisoning, Intentional self-harm	Poisoning, Assault	Poisoning, Undetermined	Adverse effect	Underdosing
Propoxyphene	T40.491	T40.492	T40.493	T40.494	T40.495	T40.496
Propranolol	T44.7X1	T44.7X2	T44.7X3	T44.7X4	T44.7X5	T44.7X6
Propyl						
alcohol	T51.3X1	T51.3X2	T51.3X3	T51.3X4	—	—
carbinol	T51.3X1	T51.3X2	T51.3X3	T51.3X4	—	—
hexadrine	T44.4X1	T44.4X2	T44.4X3	T44.4X4	T44.4X5	T44.4X6
iodone	T50.8X1	T50.8X2	T50.8X3	T50.8X4	T50.8X5	T50.8X6
thiouracil	T38.2X1	T38.2X2	T38.2X3	T38.2X4	T38.2X5	T38.2X6
Propylaminopheno-thiazine	T43.3X1	T43.3X2	T43.3X3	T43.3X4	T43.3X5	T43.3X6
Propylene	T59.891	T59.892	T59.893	T59.894	—	—
Propylhexedrine	T48.5X1	T48.5X2	T48.5X3	T48.5X4	T48.5X5	T48.5X6
Propyliodone	T50.8X1	T50.8X2	T50.8X3	T50.8X4	T50.8X5	T50.8X6
Propylparaben (ophthalmic)	T49.5X1	T49.5X2	T49.5X3	T49.5X4	T49.5X5	T49.5X6
Propylthiouracil	T38.2X1	T38.2X2	T38.2X3	T38.2X4	T38.2X5	T38.2X6
Propyphenazone	T39.2X1	T39.2X2	T39.2X3	T39.2X4	T39.2X5	T39.2X6
Proquazone	T39.391	T39.392	T39.393	T39.394	T39.395	T39.396
Proscillaridin	T46.0X1	T46.0X2	T46.0X3	T46.0X4	T46.0X5	T46.0X6
Prostacyclin	T45.521	T45.522	T45.523	T45.524	T45.525	T45.526
Prostaglandin (I2)	T45.521	T45.522	T45.523	T45.524	T45.525	T45.526
E1	T46.7X1	T46.7X2	T46.7X3	T46.7X4	T46.7X5	T46.7X6
E2	T48.0X1	T48.0X2	T48.0X3	T48.0X4	T48.0X5	T48.0X6
F2 alpha	T48.0X1	T48.0X2	T48.0X3	T48.0X4	T48.0X5	T48.0X6
Prostigmin	T44.0X1	T44.0X2	T44.0X3	T44.0X4	T44.0X5	T44.0X6
Prosultiamine	T45.2X1	T45.2X2	T45.2X3	T45.2X4	T45.2X5	T45.2X6
Protamine sulfate	T45.7X1	T45.7X2	T45.7X3	T45.7X4	T45.7X5	T45.7X6
zinc insulin	T38.3X1	T38.3X2	T38.3X3	T38.3X4	T38.3X5	T38.3X6
Protease	T47.5X1	T47.5X2	T47.5X3	T47.5X4	T47.5X5	T47.5X6
Protectant, skin NEC	T49.3X1	T49.3X2	T49.3X3	T49.3X4	T49.3X5	T49.3X6
Protein hydrolysate	T50.991	T50.992	T50.993	T50.994	T50.995	T50.996
Prothiaden—see Dothiepin hydrochloride						
Prothionamide	T37.1X1	T37.1X2	T37.1X3	T37.1X4	T37.1X5	T37.1X6
Prothipendyl	T43.591	T43.592	T43.593	T43.594	T43.595	T43.596
Prothoate	T60.0X1	T60.0X2	T60.0X3	T60.0X4	—	—
Prothrombin						
activator	T45.7X1	T45.7X2	T45.7X3	T45.7X4	T45.7X5	T45.7X6
synthesis inhibitor	T45.511	T45.512	T45.513	T45.514	T45.515	T45.516
Protionamide	T37.1X1	T37.1X2	T37.1X3	T37.1X4	T37.1X5	T37.1X6
Protirelin	T38.891	T38.892	T38.893	T38.894	T38.895	T38.896
Protokylol	T48.6X1	T48.6X2	T48.6X3	T48.6X4	T48.6X5	T48.6X6
Protopam	T50.6X1	T50.6X2	T50.6X3	T50.6X4	T50.6X5	T50.6X6
Protoveratrine (s) (A) (B)	T46.5X1	T46.5X2	T46.5X3	T46.5X4	T46.5X5	T46.5X6
Protriptyline	T43.011	T43.012	T43.013	T43.014	T43.015	T43.016
Provera	T38.5X1	T38.5X2	T38.5X3	T38.5X4	T38.5X5	T38.5X6
Provitamin A	T45.2X1	T45.2X2	T45.2X3	T45.2X4	T45.2X5	T45.2X6
Proxibarbal	T42.3X1	T42.3X2	T42.3X3	T42.3X4	T42.3X5	T42.3X6
Proxymetacaine	T41.3X1	T41.3X2	T41.3X3	T41.3X4	T41.3X5	T41.3X6
Proxyphylline	T48.6X1	T48.6X2	T48.6X3	T48.6X4	T48.6X5	T48.6X6

Substance	Poisoning, Accidental (unintentional)	Poisoning, Intentional self-harm	Poisoning, Assault	Poisoning, Undetermined	Adverse effect	Underdosing
Prozac—see Fluoxetine hydrochloride						
Prunus						
laurocerasus	T62.2X1	T62.2X2	T62.2X3	T62.2X4	—	—
virginiana	T62.2X1	T62.2X2	T62.2X3	T62.2X4	—	—
Prussian blue						
commercial	T65.891	T65.892	T65.893	T65.894	—	—
therapeutic	T50.6X1	T50.6X2	T50.6X3	T50.6X4	T50.6X5	T50.6X6
Prussic acid	T65.0X1	T65.0X2	T65.0X3	T65.0X4	—	—
vapor	T57.3X1	T57.3X2	T57.3X3	T57.3X4	—	—
Pseudoephedrine	T44.991	T44.992	T44.993	T44.994	T44.995	T44.996
Psilocin	T40.991	T40.992	T40.993	T40.994		
Psilocybin	T40.991	T40.992	T40.993	T40.994		
Psilocybine	T40.991	T40.992	T40.993	T40.994		
Psoralene (nonmedicinal)	T65.891	T65.892	T65.893	T65.894		
Psoralens (medicinal)	T50.991	T50.992	T50.993	T50.994	T50.995	T50.996
PSP (phenolsulfon-phthalein)	T50.8X1	T50.8X2	T50.8X3	T50.8X4	T50.8X5	T50.8X6
Psychodysleptic drug NOS	T40.901	T40.902	T40.903	T40.904	T40.905	T40.906
specified NEC	T40.991	T40.992	T40.993	T40.994	T40.995	T40.996
Psychostimulant	T43.601	T43.602	T43.603	T43.604	T43.605	T43.606
amphetamine	T43.621	T43.622	T43.623	T43.624	T43.625	T43.626
caffeine	T43.611	T43.612	T43.613	T43.614	T43.615	T43.616
methylphenidate	T43.631	T43.632	T43.633	T43.634	T43.635	T43.636
specified NEC	T43.691	T43.692	T43.693	T43.694	T43.695	T43.696
Psychotherapeutic drug NEC	T43.91	T43.92	T43.93	T43.94	T43.95	T43.96
antidepressants—see also Antidepressant	T43.201	T43.202	T43.203	T43.204	T43.205	T43.206
specified NEC	T43.8X1	T43.8X2	T43.8X3	T43.8X4	T43.8X5	T43.8X6
tranquilizers NEC	T43.501	T43.502	T43.503	T43.504	T43.505	T43.506
Psychotomimetic agents	T40.901	T40.902	T40.903	T40.904	T40.905	T40.906
Psychotropic drug NEC	T43.91	T43.92	T43.93	T43.94	T43.95	T43.96
specified NEC	T43.8X1	T43.8X2	T43.8X3	T43.8X4	T43.8X5	T43.8X6
Psyllium hydrophilic mucilloid	T47.4X1	T47.4X2	T47.4X3	T47.4X4	T47.4X5	T47.4X6
Pteroylglutamic acid	T45.8X1	T45.8X2	T45.8X3	T45.8X4	T45.8X5	T45.8X6
Pteroyltriglutamate	T45.1X1	T45.1X2	T45.1X3	T45.1X4	T45.1X5	T45.1X6
PTFE—see Polytetra-fluoroethylene						
Pulp						
devitalizing paste	T49.7X1	T49.7X2	T49.7X3	T49.7X4	T49.7X5	T49.7X6
dressing	T49.7X1	T49.7X2	T49.7X3	T49.7X4	T49.7X5	T49.7X6
Pulsatilla	T62.2X1	T62.2X2	T62.2X3	T62.2X4		
Pumpkin seed extract	T37.4X1	T37.4X2	T37.4X3	T37.4X4	T37.4X5	T37.4X6
Purex (bleach)	T54.91	T54.92	T54.93	T54.94	—	—
Purgative NEC—see also Cathartic	T47.4X1	T47.4X2	T47.4X3	T47.4X4	T47.4X5	T47.4X6
Purine analogue (antineoplastic)	T45.1X1	T45.1X2	T45.1X3	T45.1X4	T45.1X5	T45.1X6

Substance	Poisoning, Accidental (unintentional)	Poisoning, Intentional self-harm	Poisoning, Assault	Poisoning, Undetermined	Adverse effect	Underdosing
Purine diuretics	T50.2X1	T50.2X2	T50.2X3	T50.2X4	T50.2X5	T50.2X6
Purinethol	T45.1X1	T45.1X2	T45.1X3	T45.1X4	T45.1X5	T45.1X6
PVP	T45.8X1	T45.8X2	T45.8X3	T45.8X4	T45.8X5	T45.8X6
Pyrabital	T39.8X1	T39.8X2	T39.8X3	T39.8X4	T39.8X5	T39.8X6
Pyramidon	T39.2X1	T39.2X2	T39.2X3	T39.2X4	T39.2X5	T39.2X6
Pyrantel	T37.4X1	T37.4X2	T37.4X3	T37.4X4	T37.4X5	T37.4X6
Pyrathiazine	T45.0X1	T45.0X2	T45.0X3	T45.0X4	T45.0X5	T45.0X6
Pyrazinamide	T37.1X1	T37.1X2	T37.1X3	T37.1X4	T37.1X5	T37.1X6
Pyrazinoic acid (amide)	T37.1X1	T37.1X2	T37.1X3	T37.1X4	T37.1X5	T37.1X6
Pyrazole (derivatives)	T39.2X1	T39.2X2	T39.2X3	T39.2X4	T39.2X5	T39.2X6
Pyrazolone analgesic NEC	T39.2X1	T39.2X2	T39.2X3	T39.2X4	T39.2X5	T39.2X6
Pyrethrin, pyrethrum (nonmedicinal)	T60.2X1	T60.2X2	T60.2X3	T60.2X4	—	—
Pyrethrum extract	T49.0X1	T49.0X2	T49.0X3	T49.0X4	T49.0X5	T49.0X6
Pyribenzamine	T45.0X1	T45.0X2	T45.0X3	T45.0X4	T45.0X5	T45.0X6
Pyridine	T52.8X1	T52.8X2	T52.8X3	T52.8X4		
aldoxime methiodide	T50.6X1	T50.6X2	T50.6X3	T50.6X4	T50.6X5	T50.6X6
aldoxime methyl chloride	T50.6X1	T50.6X2	T50.6X3	T50.6X4	T50.6X5	T50.6X6
vapor	T59.891	T59.892	T59.893	T59.894	—	—
Pyridium	T39.8X1	T39.8X2	T39.8X3	T39.8X4	T39.8X5	T39.8X6
Pyridostigmine bromide	T44.0X1	T44.0X2	T44.0X3	T44.0X4	T44.0X5	T44.0X6
Pyridoxal phosphate	T45.2X1	T45.2X2	T45.2X3	T45.2X4	T45.2X5	T45.2X6
Pyridoxine	T45.2X1	T45.2X2	T45.2X3	T45.2X4	T45.2X5	T45.2X6
Pyrilamine	T45.0X1	T45.0X2	T45.0X3	T45.0X4	T45.0X5	T45.0X6
Pyrimethamine	T37.2X1	T37.2X2	T37.2X3	T37.2X4	T37.2X5	T37.2X6
with sulfadoxine	T37.2X1	T37.2X2	T37.2X3	T37.2X4	T37.2X5	T37.2X6
Pyrimidine antagonist	T45.1X1	T45.1X2	T45.1X3	T45.1X4	T45.1X5	T45.1X6
Pyriminil	T60.4X1	T60.4X2	T60.4X3	T60.4X4	—	—
Pyrithione zinc	T49.4X1	T49.4X2	T49.4X3	T49.4X4	T49.4X5	T49.4X6
Pyrithyldione	T42.6X1	T42.6X2	T42.6X3	T42.6X4	T42.6X5	T42.6X6
Pyrogallic acid	T49.0X1	T49.0X2	T49.0X3	T49.0X4	T49.0X5	T49.0X6
Pyrogallol	T49.0X1	T49.0X2	T49.0X3	T49.0X4	T49.0X5	T49.0X6
Pyroxylin	T49.3X1	T49.3X2	T49.3X3	T49.3X4	T49.3X5	T49.3X6
Pyrrobutamine	T45.0X1	T45.0X2	T45.0X3	T45.0X4	T45.0X5	T45.0X6
Pyrrolizidine alkaloids	T62.8X1	T62.8X2	T62.8X3	T62.8X4	—	—
Pyrvinium chloride	T37.4X1	T37.4X2	T37.4X3	T37.4X4	T37.4X5	T37.4X6
PZI	T38.3X1	T38.3X2	T38.3X3	T38.3X4	T38.3X5	T38.3X6
Q						
Quaalude	T42.6X1	T42.6X2	T42.6X3	T42.6X4	T42.6X5	T42.6X6
Quarternary ammonium						
anti-infective	T49.0X1	T49.0X2	T49.0X3	T49.0X4	T49.0X5	T49.0X6
ganglion blocking	T44.2X1	T44.2X2	T44.2X3	T44.2X4	T44.2X5	T44.2X6
parasympatholytic	T44.3X1	T44.3X2	T44.3X3	T44.3X4	T44.3X5	T44.3X6
Quazepam	T42.4X1	T42.4X2	T42.4X3	T42.4X4	T42.4X5	T42.4X6
Quicklime	T54.3X1	T54.3X2	T54.3X3	T54.3X4	—	—
Quillaja extract	T48.4X1	T48.4X2	T48.4X3	T48.4X4	T48.4X5	T48.4X6
Quinacrine	T37.2X1	T37.2X2	T37.2X3	T37.2X4	T37.2X5	T37.2X6
Quinaglute	T46.2X1	T46.2X2	T46.2X3	T46.2X4	T46.2X5	T46.2X6
Quinalbarbital	T42.3X1	T42.3X2	T42.3X3	T42.3X4	T42.3X5	T42.3X6

Substance	Poisoning, Accidental (unintentional)	Poisoning, Intentional self-harm	Poisoning, Assault	Poisoning, Undetermined	Adverse effect	Underdosing
Quinalbarbitone sodium	T42.3X1	T42.3X2	T42.3X3	T42.3X4	T42.3X5	T42.3X6
Quinalphos	T60.0X1	T60.0X2	T60.0X3	T60.0X4	—	—
Quinapril	T46.4X1	T46.4X2	T46.4X3	T46.4X4	T46.4X5	T46.4X6
Quinestradiol	T38.5X1	T38.5X2	T38.5X3	T38.5X4	T38.5X5	T38.5X6
Quinestradol	T38.5X1	T38.5X2	T38.5X3	T38.5X4	T38.5X5	T38.5X6
Quinestrol	T38.5X1	T38.5X2	T38.5X3	T38.5X4	T38.5X5	T38.5X6
Quinethazone	T50.2X1	T50.2X2	T50.2X3	T50.2X4	T50.2X5	T50.2X6
Quingestanol	T38.4X1	T38.4X2	T38.4X3	T38.4X4	T38.4X5	T38.4X6
Quinidine	T46.2X1	T46.2X2	T46.2X3	T46.2X4	T46.2X5	T46.2X6
Quinine	T37.2X1	T37.2X2	T37.2X3	T37.2X4	T37.2X5	T37.2X6
Quiniobine	T37.8X1	T37.8X2	T37.8X3	T37.8X4	T37.8X5	T37.8X6
Quinisocaine	T49.1X1	T49.1X2	T49.1X3	T49.1X4	T49.1X5	T49.1X6
Quinocide	T37.2X1	T37.2X2	T37.2X3	T37.2X4	T37.2X5	T37.2X6
Quinoline (derivatives) NEC	T37.8X1	T37.8X2	T37.8X3	T37.8X4	T37.8X5	T37.8X6
Quinupramine	T43.011	T43.012	T43.013	T43.014	T43.015	T43.016
Quotane	T41.3X1	T41.3X2	T41.3X3	T41.3X4	T41.3X5	T41.3X6
R						
Rabies						
immune globulin (human)	T50.Z11	T50.Z12	T50.Z13	T50.Z14	T50.Z15	T50.Z16
vaccine	T50.B91	T50.B92	T50.B93	T50.B94	T50.B95	T50.B96
Racemoramide	T40.2X1	T40.2X2	T40.2X3	T40.2X4	—	—
Racemorphan	T40.2X1	T40.2X2	T40.2X3	T40.2X4	T40.2X5	T40.2X6
Racepinefrin	T44.5X1	T44.5X2	T44.5X3	T44.5X4	T44.5X5	T44.5X6
Raclopride	T43.591	T43.592	T43.593	T43.594	T43.595	T43.596
Radiator alcohol	T51.1X1	T51.1X2	T51.1X3	T51.1X4	—	—
Radioactive drug NEC	T50.8X1	T50.8X2	T50.8X3	T50.8X4	T50.8X5	T50.8X6
Radio-opaque (drugs) (materials)	T50.8X1	T50.8X2	T50.8X3	T50.8X4	T50.8X5	T50.8X6
Ramifenazone	T39.2X1	T39.2X2	T39.2X3	T39.2X4	T39.2X5	T39.2X6
Ramipril	T46.4X1	T46.4X2	T46.4X3	T46.4X4	T46.4X5	T46.4X6
Ranitidine	T47.0X1	T47.0X2	T47.0X3	T47.0X4	T47.0X5	T47.0X6
Ranunculus	T62.2X1	T62.2X2	T62.2X3	T62.2X4	—	—
Rat poison NEC	T60.4X1	T60.4X2	T60.4X3	T60.4X4	—	—
Rattlesnake (venom)	T63.011	T63.012	T63.013	T63.014		
Raubasine	T46.7X1	T46.7X2	T46.7X3	T46.7X4	T46.7X5	T46.7X6
Raudixin	T46.5X1	T46.5X2	T46.5X3	T46.5X4	T46.5X5	T46.5X6
Rautensin	T46.5X1	T46.5X2	T46.5X3	T46.5X4	T46.5X5	T46.5X6
Rautina	T46.5X1	T46.5X2	T46.5X3	T46.5X4	T46.5X5	T46.5X6
Rautotal	T46.5X1	T46.5X2	T46.5X3	T46.5X4	T46.5X5	T46.5X6
Rauwiloid	T46.5X1	T46.5X2	T46.5X3	T46.5X4	T46.5X5	T46.5X6
Rauwoldin	T46.5X1	T46.5X2	T46.5X3	T46.5X4	T46.5X5	T46.5X6
Rauwolfia (alkaloids)	T46.5X1	T46.5X2	T46.5X3	T46.5X4	T46.5X5	T46.5X6
Razoxane	T45.1X1	T45.1X2	T45.1X3	T45.1X4	T45.1X5	T45.1X6
Realgar	T57.0X1	T57.0X2	T57.0X3	T57.0X4	—	—
Recombinant(R)—see specific protein						
Red blood cells, packed	T45.8X1	T45.8X2	T45.8X3	T45.8X4	T45.8X5	T45.8X6
Red squill (scilliroside)	T60.4X1	T60.4X2	T60.4X3	T60.4X4	—	—
Reducing agent, industrial NEC	T65.891	T65.892	T65.893	T65.894	—	—

Substance	Poisoning, Accidental (unintentional)	Poisoning, Intentional self-harm	Poisoning, Assault	Poisoning, Undetermined	Adverse effect	Underdosing
Refrigerant gas (chlorofluoro-carbon)	T53.5X1	T53.5X2	T53.5X3	T53.5X4	—	—
not chlorofluoro-carbon	T59.891	T59.892	T59.893	T59.894	—	—
Regroton	T50.2X1	T50.2X2	T50.2X3	T50.2X4	T50.2X5	T50.2X6
Rehydration salts (oral)	T50.3X1	T50.3X2	T50.3X3	T50.3X4	T50.3X5	T50.3X6
Rela	T42.8X1	T42.8X2	T42.8X3	T42.8X4	T42.8X5	T42.8X6
Relaxant, muscle						
anesthetic	T48.1X1	T48.1X2	T48.1X3	T48.1X4	T48.1X5	T48.1X6
central nervous system	T42.8X1	T42.8X2	T42.8X3	T42.8X4	T42.8X5	T42.8X6
skeletal NEC	T48.1X1	T48.1X2	T48.1X3	T48.1X4	T48.1X5	T48.1X6
smooth NEC	T44.3X1	T44.3X2	T44.3X3	T44.3X4	T44.3X5	T44.3X6
Remoxipride	T43.591	T43.592	T43.593	T43.594	T43.595	T43.596
Renese	T50.2X1	T50.2X2	T50.2X3	T50.2X4	T50.2X5	T50.2X6
Renografin	T50.8X1	T50.8X2	T50.8X3	T50.8X4	T50.8X5	T50.8X6
Replacement solution	T50.3X1	T50.3X2	T50.3X3	T50.3X4	T50.3X5	T50.3X6
Reproterol	T48.6X1	T48.6X2	T48.6X3	T48.6X4	T48.6X5	T48.6X6
Rescinnamine	T46.5X1	T46.5X2	T46.5X3	T46.5X4	T46.5X5	T46.5X6
Reserpin(e)	T46.5X1	T46.5X2	T46.5X3	T46.5X4	T46.5X5	T46.5X6
Resorcin, resorcinol (nonmedicinal)	T65.891	T65.892	T65.893	T65.894	—	—
medicinal	T49.4X1	T49.4X2	T49.4X3	T49.4X4	T49.4X5	T49.4X6
Respaire	T48.4X1	T48.4X2	T48.4X3	T48.4X4	T48.4X5	T48.4X6
Respiratory drug NEC	T48.901	T48.902	T48.903	T48.904	T48.905	T48.906
antiasthmatic NEC	T48.6X1	T48.6X2	T48.6X3	T48.6X4	T48.6X5	T48.6X6
anti-common-cold NEC	T48.5X1	T48.5X2	T48.5X3	T48.5X4	T48.5X5	T48.5X6
expectorant NEC	T48.4X1	T48.4X2	T48.4X3	T48.4X4	T48.4X5	T48.4X6
stimulant	T48.901	T48.902	T48.903	T48.904	T48.905	T48.906
Retinoic acid	T49.0X1	T49.0X2	T49.0X3	T49.0X4	T49.0X5	T49.0X6
Retinol	T45.2X1	T45.2X2	T45.2X3	T45.2X4	T45.2X5	T45.2X6
Rh(D) immune globulin (human)	T50.Z11	T50.Z12	T50.Z13	T50.Z14	T50.Z15	T50.Z16
Rhodine	T39.011	T39.012	T39.013	T39.014	T39.015	T39.016
RhoGAM	T50.Z11	T50.Z12	T50.Z13	T50.Z14	T50.Z15	T50.Z16
Rhubarb						
dry extract	T47.2X1	T47.2X2	T47.2X3	T47.2X4	T47.2X5	T47.2X6
tincture, compound	T47.2X1	T47.2X2	T47.2X3	T47.2X4	T47.2X5	T47.2X6
Ribavirin	T37.5X1	T37.5X2	T37.5X3	T37.5X4	T37.5X5	T37.5X6
Riboflavin	T45.2X1	T45.2X2	T45.2X3	T45.2X4	T45.2X5	T45.2X6
Ribostamycin	T36.5X1	T36.5X2	T36.5X3	T36.5X4	T36.5X5	T36.5X6
Ricin	T62.2X1	T62.2X2	T62.2X3	T62.2X4	—	—
Ricinus communis	T62.2X1	T62.2X2	T62.2X3	T62.2X4	—	—
Rickettsial vaccine NEC	T50.A91	T50.A92	T50.A93	T50.A94	T50.A95	T50.A96
Rifabutin	T36.6X1	T36.6X2	T36.6X3	T36.6X4	T36.6X5	T36.6X6
Rifamide	T36.6X1	T36.6X2	T36.6X3	T36.6X4	T36.6X5	T36.6X6
Rifampicin	T36.6X1	T36.6X2	T36.6X3	T36.6X4	T36.6X5	T36.6X6
with isoniazid	T37.1X1	T37.1X2	T37.1X3	T37.1X4	T37.1X5	T37.1X6
Rifampin	T36.6X1	T36.6X2	T36.6X3	T36.6X4	T36.6X5	T36.6X6
Rifamycin	T36.6X1	T36.6X2	T36.6X3	T36.6X4	T36.6X5	T36.6X6
Rifaximin	T36.6X1	T36.6X2	T36.6X3	T36.6X4	T36.6X5	T36.6X6

Substance	Poisoning, Accidental (unintentional)	Poisoning, Intentional self-harm	Poisoning, Assault	Poisoning, Undetermined	Adverse effect	Underdosing
Rimantadine	T37.5X1	T37.5X2	T37.5X3	T37.5X4	T37.5X5	T37.5X6
Rimazolium metilsulfate	T39.8X1	T39.8X2	T39.8X3	T39.8X4	T39.8X5	T39.8X6
Rimifon	T37.1X1	T37.1X2	T37.1X3	T37.1X4	T37.1X5	T37.1X6
Rimiterol	T48.6X1	T48.6X2	T48.6X3	T48.6X4	T48.6X5	T48.6X6
Ringer (lactate) solution	T50.3X1	T50.3X2	T50.3X3	T50.3X4	T50.3X5	T50.3X6
Ristocetin	T36.8X1	T36.8X2	T36.8X3	T36.8X4	T36.8X5	T36.8X6
Ritalin	T43.631	T43.632	T43.633	T43.634	T43.635	T43.636
Ritodrine	T44.5X1	T44.5X2	T44.5X3	T44.5X4	T44.5X5	T44.5X6
Roach killer—see Insecticide						
Rociverine	T44.3X1	T44.3X2	T44.3X3	T44.3X4	T44.3X5	T44.3X6
Rocky Mountain spotted fever vaccine	T50.A91	T50.A92	T50.A93	T50.A94	T50.A95	T50.A96
Rodenticide NEC	T60.4X1	T60.4X2	T60.4X3	T60.4X4	—	—
Rohypnol	T42.4X1	T42.4X2	T42.4X3	T42.4X4	T42.4X5	T42.4X6
Rokitamycin	T36.3X1	T36.3X2	T36.3X3	T36.3X4	T36.3X5	T36.3X6
Rolaids	T47.1X1	T47.1X2	T47.1X3	T47.1X4	T47.1X5	T47.1X6
Rolitetracycline	T36.4X1	T36.4X2	T36.4X3	T36.4X4	T36.4X5	T36.4X6
Romilar	T48.3X1	T48.3X2	T48.3X3	T48.3X4	T48.3X5	T48.3X6
Ronifibrate	T46.6X1	T46.6X2	T46.6X3	T46.6X4	T46.6X5	T46.6X6
Rosaprostol	T47.1X1	T47.1X2	T47.1X3	T47.1X4	T47.1X5	T47.1X6
Rose bengal sodium (131I)	T50.8X1	T50.8X2	T50.8X3	T50.8X4	T50.8X5	T50.8X6
Rose water ointment	T49.3X1	T49.3X2	T49.3X3	T49.3X4	T49.3X5	T49.3X6
Rosoxacin	T37.8X1	T37.8X2	T37.8X3	T37.8X4	T37.8X5	T37.8X6
Rotenone	T60.2X1	T60.2X2	T60.2X3	T60.2X4	—	—
Rotoxamine	T45.0X1	T45.0X2	T45.0X3	T45.0X4	T45.0X5	T45.0X6
Rough-on-rats	T60.4X1	T60.4X2	T60.4X3	T60.4X4	—	—
Roxatidine	T47.0X1	T47.0X2	T47.0X3	T47.0X4	T47.0X5	T47.0X6
Roxithromycin	T36.3X1	T36.3X2	T36.3X3	T36.3X4	T36.3X5	T36.3X6
Rt-PA	T45.611	T45.612	T45.613	T45.614	T45.615	T45.616
Rubbing alcohol	T51.2X1	T51.2X2	T51.2X3	T51.2X4	—	—
Rubefacient	T49.4X1	T49.4X2	T49.4X3	T49.4X4	T49.4X5	T49.4X6
Rubella vaccine	T50.B91	T50.B92	T50.B93	T50.B94	T50.B95	T50.B96
Rubeola vaccine	T50.B91	T50.B92	T50.B93	T50.B94	T50.B95	T50.B96
Rubidium chloride Rb82	T50.8X1	T50.8X2	T50.8X3	T50.8X4	T50.8X5	T50.8X6
Rubidomycin	T45.1X1	T45.1X2	T45.1X3	T45.1X4	T45.1X5	T45.1X6
Rue	T62.2X1	T62.2X2	T62.2X3	T62.2X4	—	—
Rufocromomycin	T45.1X1	T45.1X2	T45.1X3	T45.1X4	T45.1X5	T45.1X6
Russel's viper venin	T45.7X1	T45.7X2	T45.7X3	T45.7X4	T45.7X5	T45.7X6
Ruta (graveolens)	T62.2X1	T62.2X2	T62.2X3	T62.2X4	—	—
Rutinum	T46.991	T46.992	T46.993	T46.994	T46.995	T46.996
Rutoside	T46.991	T46.992	T46.993	T46.994	T46.995	T46.996
S						
Sabadilla (plant)	T62.2X1	T62.2X2	T62.2X3	T62.2X4		
pesticide	T60.2X1	T60.2X2	T60.2X3	T60.2X4	—	—
Saccharated iron oxide	T45.8X1	T45.8X2	T45.8X3	T45.8X4	T45.8X5	T45.8X6
Saccharin	T50.901	T50.902	T50.903	T50.904	T50.905	T50.906
Saccharomyces boulardii	T47.6X1	T47.6X2	T47.6X3	T47.6X4	T47.6X5	T47.6X6
Safflower oil	T46.6X1	T46.6X2	T46.6X3	T46.6X4	T46.6X5	T46.6X6
Safrazine	T43.1X1	T43.1X2	T43.1X3	T43.1X4	T43.1X5	T43.1X6

Substance	Poisoning, Accidental (unintentional)	Poisoning, Intentional self-harm	Poisoning, Assault	Poisoning, Undetermined	Adverse effect	Underdosing
Salazosulfapyridine	T37.0X1	T37.0X2	T37.0X3	T37.0X4	T37.0X5	T37.0X6
Salbutamol	T48.6X1	T48.6X2	T48.6X3	T48.6X4	T48.6X5	T48.6X6
Salicylamide	T39.091	T39.092	T39.093	T39.094	T39.095	T39.096
Salicylate NEC	T39.091	T39.092	T39.093	T39.094	T39.095	T39.096
methyl	T49.3X1	T49.3X2	T49.3X3	T49.3X4	T49.3X5	T49.3X6
theobromine calcium	T50.2X1	T50.2X2	T50.2X3	T50.2X4	T50.2X5	T50.2X6
Salicylazosulfapyridine	T37.0X1	T37.0X2	T37.0X3	T37.0X4	T37.0X5	T37.0X6
Salicylhydroxamic acid	T49.0X1	T49.0X2	T49.0X3	T49.0X4	T49.0X5	T49.0X6
Salicylic acid	T49.4X1	T49.4X2	T49.4X3	T49.4X4	T49.4X5	T49.4X6
with benzoic acid	T49.4X1	T49.4X2	T49.4X3	T49.4X4	T49.4X5	T49.4X6
congeners	T39.091	T39.092	T39.093	T39.094	T39.095	T39.096
derivative	T39.091	T39.092	T39.093	T39.094	T39.095	T39.096
salts	T39.091	T39.092	T39.093	T39.094	T39.095	T39.096
Salinazid	T37.1X1	T37.1X2	T37.1X3	T37.1X4	T37.1X5	T37.1X6
Salmeterol	T48.6X1	T48.6X2	T48.6X3	T48.6X4	T48.6X5	T48.6X6
Salol	T49.3X1	T49.3X2	T49.3X3	T49.3X4	T49.3X5	T49.3X6
Salsalate	T39.091	T39.092	T39.093	T39.094	T39.095	T39.096
Salt substitute	T50.901	T50.902	T50.903	T50.904	T50.905	T50.906
Salt-replacing drug	T50.901	T50.902	T50.903	T50.904	T50.905	T50.906
Salt-retaining mineralocorticoid	T50.0X1	T50.0X2	T50.0X3	T50.0X4	T50.0X5	T50.0X6
Saluretic NEC	T50.2X1	T50.2X2	T50.2X3	T50.2X4	T50.2X5	T50.2X6
Saluron	T50.2X1	T50.2X2	T50.2X3	T50.2X4	T50.2X5	T50.2X6
Salvarsan 606 (neosilver) (silver)	T37.8X1	T37.8X2	T37.8X3	T37.8X4	T37.8X5	T37.8X6
Sambucus canadensis	T62.2X1	T62.2X2	T62.2X3	T62.2X4	—	—
berry	T62.1X1	T62.1X2	T62.1X3	T62.1X4	—	—
Sandril	T46.5X1	T46.5X2	T46.5X3	T46.5X4	T46.5X5	T46.5X6
Sanguinaria canadensis	T62.2X1	T62.2X2	T62.2X3	T62.2X4	—	—
Saniflush (cleaner)	T54.2X1	T54.2X2	T54.2X3	T54.2X4	—	—
Santonin	T37.4X1	T37.4X2	T37.4X3	T37.4X4	T37.4X5	T37.4X6
Santyl	T49.8X1	T49.8X2	T49.8X3	T49.8X4	T49.8X5	T49.8X6
Saralasin	T46.5X1	T46.5X2	T46.5X3	T46.5X4	T46.5X5	T46.5X6
Sarcolysin	T45.1X1	T45.1X2	T45.1X3	T45.1X4	T45.1X5	T45.1X6
Sarkomycin	T45.1X1	T45.1X2	T45.1X3	T45.1X4	T45.1X5	T45.1X6
Saroten	T43.011	T43.012	T43.013	T43.014	T43.015	T43.016
Saturnine—see Lead						
Savin (oil)	T49.4X1	T49.4X2	T49.4X3	T49.4X4	T49.4X5	T49.4X6
Scammony	T47.2X1	T47.2X2	T47.2X3	T47.2X4	T47.2X5	T47.2X6
Scarlet red	T49.8X1	T49.8X2	T49.8X3	T49.8X4	T49.8X5	T49.8X6
Scheele's green	T57.0X1	T57.0X2	T57.0X3	T57.0X4	—	—
insecticide	T57.0X1	T57.0X2	T57.0X3	T57.0X4	—	—
Schizontozide (blood) (tissue)	T37.2X1	T37.2X2	T37.2X3	T37.2X4	T37.2X5	T37.2X6
Schradan	T60.0X1	T60.0X2	T60.0X3	T60.0X4	—	—
Schweinfurth green	T57.0X1	T57.0X2	T57.0X3	T57.0X4	—	—
insecticide	T57.0X1	T57.0X2	T57.0X3	T57.0X4	—	—
Scilla, rat poison	T60.4X1	T60.4X2	T60.4X3	T60.4X4	—	—
Scillaren	T60.4X1	T60.4X2	T60.4X3	T60.4X4	—	—
Sclerosing agent	T46.8X1	T46.8X2	T46.8X3	T46.8X4	T46.8X5	T46.8X6
Scombrotoxin	T61.11	T61.12	T61.13	T61.14	—	—

Substance	Poisoning, Accidental (unintentional)	Poisoning, Intentional self-harm	Poisoning, Assault	Poisoning, Undetermined	Adverse effect	Underdosing
Scopolamine	T44.3X1	T44.3X2	T44.3X3	T44.3X4	T44.3X5	T44.3X6
Scopolia extract	T44.3X1	T44.3X2	T44.3X3	T44.3X4	T44.3X5	T44.3X6
Scouring powder	T65.891	T65.892	T65.893	T65.894	—	—
Sea						
anemone (sting)	T63.631	T63.632	T63.633	T63.634	—	—
cucumber (sting)	T63.691	T63.692	T63.693	T63.694	—	—
snake (bite) (venom)	T63.091	T63.092	T63.093	T63.094	—	—
urchin spine (puncture)	T63.691	T63.692	T63.693	T63.694	—	—
Seafood	T61.91	T61.92	T61.93	T61.94	—	—
specified NEC	T61.8X1	T61.8X2	T61.8X3	T61.8X4	—	—
Secbutabarbital	T42.3X1	T42.3X2	T42.3X3	T42.3X4	T42.3X5	T42.3X6
Secbutabarbitone	T42.3X1	T42.3X2	T42.3X3	T42.3X4	T42.3X5	T42.3X6
Secnidazole	T37.3X1	T37.3X2	T37.3X3	T37.3X4	T37.3X5	T37.3X6
Secobarbital	T42.3X1	T42.3X2	T42.3X3	T42.3X4	T42.3X5	T42.3X6
Seconal	T42.3X1	T42.3X2	T42.3X3	T42.3X4	T42.3X5	T42.3X6
Secretin	T50.8X1	T50.8X2	T50.8X3	T50.8X4	T50.8X5	T50.8X6
Sedative NEC	T42.71	T42.72	T42.73	T42.74	T42.75	T42.76
mixed NEC	T42.6X1	T42.6X2	T42.6X3	T42.6X4	T42.6X5	T42.6X6
Sedormid	T42.6X1	T42.6X2	T42.6X3	T42.6X4	T42.6X5	T42.6X6
Seed disinfectant or dressing	T60.8X1	T60.8X2	T60.8X3	T60.8X4	—	—
Seeds (poisonous)	T62.2X1	T62.2X2	T62.2X3	T62.2X4	—	—
Selegiline	T42.8X1	T42.8X2	T42.8X3	T42.8X4	T42.8X5	T42.8X6
Selenium NEC	T56.891	T56.892	T56.893	T56.894	—	—
disulfide or sulfide	T49.4X1	T49.4X2	T49.4X3	T49.4X4	T49.4X5	T49.4X6
fumes	T59.891	T59.892	T59.893	T59.894	—	—
sulfide	T49.4X1	T49.4X2	T49.4X3	T49.4X4	T49.4X5	T49.4X6
Selenomethionine (75Se)	T50.8X1	T50.8X2	T50.8X3	T50.8X4	T50.8X5	T50.8X6
Selsun	T49.4X1	T49.4X2	T49.4X3	T49.4X4	T49.4X5	T49.4X6
Semustine	T45.1X1	T45.1X2	T45.1X3	T45.1X4	T45.1X5	T45.1X6
Senega syrup	T48.4X1	T48.4X2	T48.4X3	T48.4X4	T48.4X5	T48.4X6
Senna	T47.2X1	T47.2X2	T47.2X3	T47.2X4	T47.2X5	T47.2X6
Sennoside A+B	T47.2X1	T47.2X2	T47.2X3	T47.2X4	T47.2X5	T47.2X6
Septisol	T49.2X1	T49.2X2	T49.2X3	T49.2X4	T49.2X5	T49.2X6
Seractide	T38.811	T38.812	T38.813	T38.814	T38.815	T38.816
Serax	T42.4X1	T42.4X2	T42.4X3	T42.4X4	T42.4X5	T42.4X6
Serenesil	T42.6X1	T42.6X2	T42.6X3	T42.6X4	T42.6X5	T42.6X6
Serenium (hydrochloride)	T37.91	T37.92	T37.93	T37.94	T37.95	T37.96
Serepax—see Oxazepam						
Sermorelin	T38.891	T38.892	T38.893	T38.894	T38.895	T38.896
Sernyl	T41.1X1	T41.1X2	T41.1X3	T41.1X4	T41.1X5	T41.1X6
Serotonin	T50.991	T50.992	T50.993	T50.994	T50.995	T50.996
Serpasil	T46.5X1	T46.5X2	T46.5X3	T46.5X4	T46.5X5	T46.5X6
Serrapeptase	T45.3X1	T45.3X2	T45.3X3	T45.3X4	T45.3X5	T45.3X6
Serum						
antibotulinus	T50.Z11	T50.Z12	T50.Z13	T50.Z14	T50.Z15	T50.Z16
anticytotoxic	T50.Z11	T50.Z12	T50.Z13	T50.Z14	T50.Z15	T50.Z16
antidiphtheria	T50.Z11	T50.Z12	T50.Z13	T50.Z14	T50.Z15	T50.Z16
antimeningococcus	T50.Z11	T50.Z12	T50.Z13	T50.Z14	T50.Z15	T50.Z16
anti-Rh	T50.Z11	T50.Z12	T50.Z13	T50.Z14	T50.Z15	T50.Z16

Substance	Poisoning, Accidental (unintentional)	Poisoning, Intentional self-harm	Poisoning, Assault	Poisoning, Undetermined	Adverse effect	Underdosing
Serum — *Continued*						
anti-snake-bite	T50.Z11	T50.Z12	T50.Z13	T50.Z14	T50.Z15	T50.Z16
antitetanic	T50.Z11	T50.Z12	T50.Z13	T50.Z14	T50.Z15	T50.Z16
antitoxic	T50.Z11	T50.Z12	T50.Z13	T50.Z14	T50.Z15	T50.Z16
complement (inhibitor)	T45.8X1	T45.8X2	T45.8X3	T45.8X4	T45.8X5	T45.8X6
convalescent	T50.Z11	T50.Z12	T50.Z13	T50.Z14	T50.Z15	T50.Z16
hemolytic complement	T45.8X1	T45.8X2	T45.8X3	T45.8X4	T45.8X5	T45.8X6
immune (human)	T50.Z11	T50.Z12	T50.Z13	T50.Z14	T50.Z15	T50.Z16
protective NEC	T50.Z11	T50.Z12	T50.Z13	T50.Z14	T50.Z15	T50.Z16
Setastine	T45.0X1	T45.0X2	T45.0X3	T45.0X4	T45.0X5	T45.0X6
Setoperone	T43.591	T43.592	T43.593	T43.594	T43.595	T43.596
Sewer gas	T59.91	T59.92	T59.93	T59.94	—	—
Shampoo	T55.0X1	T55.0X2	T55.0X3	T55.0X4		
Shellfish, noxious, nonbacterial	T61.781	T61.782	T61.783	T61.784	—	—
Sildenafil	T46.7X1	T46.7X2	T46.7X3	T46.7X4	T46.7X5	T46.7X6
Silibinin	T50.991	T50.992	T50.993	T50.994	T50.995	T50.996
Silicone NEC	T65.891	T65.892	T65.893	T65.894	—	—
medicinal	T49.3X1	T49.3X2	T49.3X3	T49.3X4	T49.3X5	T49.3X6
Silvadene	T49.0X1	T49.0X2	T49.0X3	T49.0X4	T49.0X5	T49.0X6
Silver	T49.0X1	T49.0X2	T49.0X3	T49.0X4	T49.0X5	T49.0X6
anti-infectives	T49.0X1	T49.0X2	T49.0X3	T49.0X4	T49.0X5	T49.0X6
arsphenamine	T37.8X1	T37.8X2	T37.8X3	T37.8X4	T37.8X5	T37.8X6
colloidal	T49.0X1	T49.0X2	T49.0X3	T49.0X4	T49.0X5	T49.0X6
nitrate	T49.0X1	T49.0X2	T49.0X3	T49.0X4	T49.0X5	T49.0X6
ophthalmic preparation	T49.5X1	T49.5X2	T49.5X3	T49.5X4	T49.5X5	T49.5X6
toughened (keratolytic)	T49.4X1	T49.4X2	T49.4X3	T49.4X4	T49.4X5	T49.4X6
nonmedicinal (dust)	T56.891	T56.892	T56.893	T56.894	—	—
protein	T49.5X1	T49.5X2	T49.5X3	T49.5X4	T49.5X5	T49.5X6
salvarsan	T37.8X1	T37.8X2	T37.8X3	T37.8X4	T37.8X5	T37.8X6
sulfadiazine	T49.4X1	T49.4X2	T49.4X3	T49.4X4	T49.4X5	T49.4X6
Silymarin	T50.991	T50.992	T50.993	T50.994	T50.995	T50.996
Simaldrate	T47.1X1	T47.1X2	T47.1X3	T47.1X4	T47.1X5	T47.1X6
Simazine	T60.3X1	T60.3X2	T60.3X3	T60.3X4	—	—
Simethicone	T47.1X1	T47.1X2	T47.1X3	T47.1X4	T47.1X5	T47.1X6
Simfibrate	T46.6X1	T46.6X2	T46.6X3	T46.6X4	T46.6X5	T46.6X6
Simvastatin	T46.6X1	T46.6X2	T46.6X3	T46.6X4	T46.6X5	T46.6X6
Sincalide	T50.8X1	T50.8X2	T50.8X3	T50.8X4	T50.8X5	T50.8X6
Sinequan	T43.011	T43.012	T43.013	T43.014	T43.015	T43.016
Singoserp	T46.5X1	T46.5X2	T46.5X3	T46.5X4	T46.5X5	T46.5X6
Sintrom	T45.511	T45.512	T45.513	T45.514	T45.515	T45.516
Sisomicin	T36.5X1	T36.5X2	T36.5X3	T36.5X4	T36.5X5	T36.5X6
Sitosterols	T46.6X1	T46.6X2	T46.6X3	T46.6X4	T46.6X5	T46.6X6
Skeletal muscle relaxants	T48.1X1	T48.1X2	T48.1X3	T48.1X4	T48.1X5	T48.1X6
Skin						
agents (external)	T49.91	T49.92	T49.93	T49.94	T49.95	T49.96
specified NEC	T49.8X1	T49.8X2	T49.8X3	T49.8X4	T49.8X5	T49.8X6
test antigen	T50.8X1	T50.8X2	T50.8X3	T50.8X4	T50.8X5	T50.8X6

Substance	Poisoning, Accidental (unintentional)	Poisoning, Intentional self-harm	Poisoning, Assault	Poisoning, Undetermined	Adverse effect	Underdosing
Sleep-eze	T45.0X1	T45.0X2	T45.0X3	T45.0X4	T45.0X5	T45.0X6
Sleeping draught, pill	T42.71	T42.72	T42.73	T42.74	T42.75	T42.76
Smallpox vaccine	T50.B11	T50.B12	T50.B13	T50.B14	T50.B15	T50.B16
Smelter fumes NEC	T56.91	T56.92	T56.93	T56.94	—	—
Smog	T59.1X1	T59.1X2	T59.1X3	T59.1X4	—	—
Smoke NEC	T59.811	T59.812	T59.813	T59.814		
Smooth muscle relaxant	T44.3X1	T44.3X2	T44.3X3	T44.3X4	T44.3X5	T44.3X6
Snail killer NEC	T60.8X1	T60.8X2	T60.8X3	T60.8X4	—	—
Snake venom or bite	T63.001	T63.002	T63.003	T63.004	—	—
hemocoagulase	T45.7X1	T45.7X2	T45.7X3	T45.7X4	T45.7X5	T45.7X6
Snuff	T65.211	T65.212	T65.213	T65.214		
Soap (powder) (product)	T55.0X1	T55.0X2	T55.0X3	T55.0X4		
enema	T47.4X1	T47.4X2	T47.4X3	T47.4X4	T47.4X5	T47.4X6
medicinal, soft	T49.2X1	T49.2X2	T49.2X3	T49.2X4	T49.2X5	T49.2X6
superfatted	T49.2X1	T49.2X2	T49.2X3	T49.2X4	T49.2X5	T49.2X6
Sobrerol	T48.4X1	T48.4X2	T48.4X3	T48.4X4	T48.4X5	T48.4X6
Soda (caustic)	T54.3X1	T54.3X2	T54.3X3	T54.3X4	—	—
bicarb	T47.1X1	T47.1X2	T47.1X3	T47.1X4	T47.1X5	T47.1X6
chlorinated—see Sodium, hypochlorite						
Sodium						
acetosulfone	T37.1X1	T37.1X2	T37.1X3	T37.1X4	T37.1X5	T37.1X6
acetrizoate	T50.8X1	T50.8X2	T50.8X3	T50.8X4	T50.8X5	T50.8X6
acid phosphate	T50.3X1	T50.3X2	T50.3X3	T50.3X4	T50.3X5	T50.3X6
alginate	T47.8X1	T47.8X2	T47.8X3	T47.8X4	T47.8X5	T47.8X6
amidotrizoate	T50.8X1	T50.8X2	T50.8X3	T50.8X4	T50.8X5	T50.8X6
aminopterin	T45.1X1	T45.1X2	T45.1X3	T45.1X4	T45.1X5	T45.1X6
amylosulfate	T47.8X1	T47.8X2	T47.8X3	T47.8X4	T47.8X5	T47.8X6
amytal	T42.3X1	T42.3X2	T42.3X3	T42.3X4	T42.3X5	T42.3X6
antimony gluconate	T37.3X1	T37.3X2	T37.3X3	T37.3X4	T37.3X5	T37.3X6
arsenate	T57.0X1	T57.0X2	T57.0X3	T57.0X4	—	—
aurothiomalate	T39.4X1	T39.4X2	T39.4X3	T39.4X4	T39.4X5	T39.4X6
aurothiosulfate	T39.4X1	T39.4X2	T39.4X3	T39.4X4	T39.4X5	T39.4X6
barbiturate	T42.3X1	T42.3X2	T42.3X3	T42.3X4	T42.3X5	T42.3X6
basic phosphate	T47.4X1	T47.4X2	T47.4X3	T47.4X4	T47.4X5	T47.4X6
bicarbonate	T47.1X1	T47.1X2	T47.1X3	T47.1X4	T47.1X5	T47.1X6
bichromate	T57.8X1	T57.8X2	T57.8X3	T57.8X4	—	—
biphosphate	T50.3X1	T50.3X2	T50.3X3	T50.3X4	T50.3X5	T50.3X6
bisulfate	T65.891	T65.892	T65.893	T65.894		
borate						
cleanser	T57.8X1	T57.8X2	T57.8X3	T57.8X4	—	—
eye	T49.5X1	T49.5X2	T49.5X3	T49.5X4	T49.5X5	T49.5X6
therapeutic	T49.8X1	T49.8X2	T49.8X3	T49.8X4	T49.8X5	T49.8X6
bromide	T42.6X1	T42.6X2	T42.6X3	T42.6X4	T42.6X5	T42.6X6
cacodylate (nonmedicinal) NEC	T50.8X1	T50.8X2	T50.8X3	T50.8X4	T50.8X5	T50.8X6
anti-infective	T37.8X1	T37.8X2	T37.8X3	T37.8X4	T37.8X5	T37.8X6
herbicide	T60.3X1	T60.3X2	T60.3X3	T60.3X4	—	—
calcium edetate	T45.8X1	T45.8X2	T45.8X3	T45.8X4	T45.8X5	T45.8X6
carbonate NEC	T54.3X1	T54.3X2	T54.3X3	T54.3X4	—	—
chlorate NEC	T65.891	T65.892	T65.893	T65.894	—	—

Substance	Poisoning, Accidental (unintentional)	Poisoning, Intentional self-harm	Poisoning, Assault	Poisoning, Undetermined	Adverse effect	Underdosing
Sodium — *Continued*						
herbicide	T54.91	T54.92	T54.93	T54.94	—	—
chloride	T50.3X1	T50.3X2	T50.3X3	T50.3X4	T50.3X5	T50.3X6
with glucose	T50.3X1	T50.3X2	T50.3X3	T50.3X4	T50.3X5	T50.3X6
chromate	T65.891	T65.892	T65.893	T65.894	—	—
citrate	T50.991	T50.992	T50.993	T50.994	T50.995	T50.996
cromoglicate	T48.6X1	T48.6X2	T48.6X3	T48.6X4	T48.6X5	T48.6X6
cyanide	T65.0X1	T65.0X2	T65.0X3	T65.0X4	—	—
cyclamate	T50.3X1	T50.3X2	T50.3X3	T50.3X4	T50.3X5	T50.3X6
dehydrocholate	T45.8X1	T45.8X2	T45.8X3	T45.8X4	T45.8X5	T45.8X6
diatrizoate	T50.8X1	T50.8X2	T50.8X3	T50.8X4	T50.8X5	T50.8X6
dibunate	T48.4X1	T48.4X2	T48.4X3	T48.4X4	T48.4X5	T48.4X6
dioctyl sulfosuccinate	T47.4X1	T47.4X2	T47.4X3	T47.4X4	T47.4X5	T47.4X6
dipantoyl ferrate	T45.8X1	T45.8X2	T45.8X3	T45.8X4	T45.8X5	T45.8X6
edetate	T45.8X1	T45.8X2	T45.8X3	T45.8X4	T45.8X5	T45.8X6
ethacrynate	T50.1X1	T50.1X2	T50.1X3	T50.1X4	T50.1X5	T50.1X6
feredetate	T45.8X1	T45.8X2	T45.8X3	T45.8X4	T45.8X5	T45.8X6
Fluoride—see Fluoride						
fluoroacetate (dust) (pesticide)	T60.4X1	T60.4X2	T60.4X3	T60.4X4	—	—
free salt	T50.3X1	T50.3X2	T50.3X3	T50.3X4	T50.3X5	T50.3X6
fusidate	T36.8X1	T36.8X2	T36.8X3	T36.8X4	T36.8X5	T36.8X6
glucaldrate	T47.1X1	T47.1X2	T47.1X3	T47.1X4	T47.1X5	T47.1X6
glucosulfone	T37.1X1	T37.1X2	T37.1X3	T37.1X4	T37.1X5	T37.1X6
glutamate	T45.8X1	T45.8X2	T45.8X3	T45.8X4	T45.8X5	T45.8X6
hydrogen carbonate	T50.3X1	T50.3X2	T50.3X3	T50.3X4	T50.3X5	T50.3X6
hydroxide	T54.3X1	T54.3X2	T54.3X3	T54.3X4	—	—
hypochlorite (bleach) NEC	T54.3X1	T54.3X2	T54.3X3	T54.3X4	—	—
disinfectant	T54.3X1	T54.3X2	T54.3X3	T54.3X4	—	—
medicinal (anti-infective) (external)	T49.0X1	T49.0X2	T49.0X3	T49.0X4	T49.0X5	T49.0X6
vapor	T54.3X1	T54.3X2	T54.3X3	T54.3X4	—	—
hyposulfite	T49.0X1	T49.0X2	T49.0X3	T49.0X4	T49.0X5	T49.0X6
indigotin disulfonate	T50.8X1	T50.8X2	T50.8X3	T50.8X4	T50.8X5	T50.8X6
iodide	T50.991	T50.992	T50.993	T50.994	T50.995	T50.996
I-131	T50.8X1	T50.8X2	T50.8X3	T50.8X4	T50.8X5	T50.8X6
therapeutic	T38.2X1	T38.2X2	T38.2X3	T38.2X4	T38.2X5	T38.2X6
iodohippurate (131I)	T50.8X1	T50.8X2	T50.8X3	T50.8X4	T50.8X5	T50.8X6
iopodate	T50.8X1	T50.8X2	T50.8X3	T50.8X4	T50.8X5	T50.8X6
iothalamate	T50.8X1	T50.8X2	T50.8X3	T50.8X4	T50.8X5	T50.8X6
iron edetate	T45.4X1	T45.4X2	T45.4X3	T45.4X4	T45.4X5	T45.4X6
lactate (compound solution)	T45.8X1	T45.8X2	T45.8X3	T45.8X4	T45.8X5	T45.8X6
lauryl (sulfate)	T49.2X1	T49.2X2	T49.2X3	T49.2X4	T49.2X5	T49.2X6
L-triiodothyronine	T38.1X1	T38.1X2	T38.1X3	T38.1X4	T38.1X5	T38.1X6
magnesium citrate	T50.991	T50.992	T50.993	T50.994	T50.995	T50.996
mersalate	T50.2X1	T50.2X2	T50.2X3	T50.2X4	T50.2X5	T50.2X6
metasilicate	T65.891	T65.892	T65.893	T65.894	—	—
metrizoate	T50.8X1	T50.8X2	T50.8X3	T50.8X4	T50.8X5	T50.8X6
monofluoroacetate (pesticide)	T60.1X1	T60.1X2	T60.1X3	T60.1X4	—	—
Sodium — *Continued*						
morrhuate	T46.8X1	T46.8X2	T46.8X3	T46.8X4	T46.8X5	T46.8X6
nafcillin	T36.0X1	T36.0X2	T36.0X3	T36.0X4	T36.0X5	T36.0X6
nitrate (oxidizing agent)	T65.891	T65.892	T65.893	T65.894	—	—
nitrite	T50.6X1	T50.6X2	T50.6X3	T50.6X4	T50.6X5	T50.6X6
nitroferricyanide	T46.5X1	T46.5X2	T46.5X3	T46.5X4	T46.5X5	T46.5X6
nitroprusside	T46.5X1	T46.5X2	T46.5X3	T46.5X4	T46.5X5	T46.5X6
oxalate	T65.891	T65.892	T65.893	T65.894	—	—
oxide/peroxide	T65.891	T65.892	T65.893	T65.894	—	—
oxybate	T41.291	T41.292	T41.293	T41.294	T41.295	T41.296
para-aminohippurate	T50.8X1	T50.8X2	T50.8X3	T50.8X4	T50.8X5	T50.8X6
perborate (nonmedicinal) NEC	T65.891	T65.892	T65.893	T65.894	—	—
medicinal	T49.0X1	T49.0X2	T49.0X3	T49.0X4	T49.0X5	T49.0X6
soap	T55.0X1	T55.0X2	T55.0X3	T55.0X4	—	—
percarbonate—see Sodium, perborate						
pertechnetate Tc99m	T50.8X1	T50.8X2	T50.8X3	T50.8X4	T50.8X5	T50.8X6
phosphate						
cellulose	T45.8X1	T45.8X2	T45.8X3	T45.8X4	T45.8X5	T45.8X6
dibasic	T47.2X1	T47.2X2	T47.2X3	T47.2X4	T47.2X5	T47.2X6
monobasic	T47.2X1	T47.2X2	T47.2X3	T47.2X4	T47.2X5	T47.2X6
phytate	T50.6X1	T50.6X2	T50.6X3	T50.6X4	T50.6X5	T50.6X6
picosulfate	T47.2X1	T47.2X2	T47.2X3	T47.2X4	T47.2X5	T47.2X6
polyhydroxyaluminium monocarbonate	T47.1X1	T47.1X2	T47.1X3	T47.1X4	T47.1X5	T47.1X6
polystyrene sulfonate	T50.3X1	T50.3X2	T50.3X3	T50.3X4	T50.3X5	T50.3X6
propionate	T49.0X1	T49.0X2	T49.0X3	T49.0X4	T49.0X5	T49.0X6
propyl hydroxybenzoate	T50.991	T50.992	T50.993	T50.994	T50.995	T50.996
psylliate	T46.8X1	T46.8X2	T46.8X3	T46.8X4	T46.8X5	T46.8X6
removing resins	T50.3X1	T50.3X2	T50.3X3	T50.3X4	T50.3X5	T50.3X6
salicylate	T39.091	T39.092	T39.093	T39.094	T39.095	T39.096
salt NEC	T50.3X1	T50.3X2	T50.3X3	T50.3X4	T50.3X5	T50.3X6
selenate	T60.2X1	T60.2X2	T60.2X3	T60.2X4	—	—
stibogluconate	T37.3X1	T37.3X2	T37.3X3	T37.3X4	T37.3X5	T37.3X6
sulfate	T47.4X1	T47.4X2	T47.4X3	T47.4X4	T47.4X5	T47.4X6
sulfoxone	T37.1X1	T37.1X2	T37.1X3	T37.1X4	T37.1X5	T37.1X6
tetradecyl sulfate	T46.8X1	T46.8X2	T46.8X3	T46.8X4	T46.8X5	T46.8X6
thiopental	T41.1X1	T41.1X2	T41.1X3	T41.1X4	T41.1X5	T41.1X6
thiosalicylate	T39.091	T39.092	T39.093	T39.094	T39.095	T39.096
thiosulfate	T50.6X1	T50.6X2	T50.6X3	T50.6X4	T50.6X5	T50.6X6
tolbutamide	T38.3X1	T38.3X2	T38.3X3	T38.3X4	T38.3X5	T38.3X6
(L)-triiodothyronine	T38.1X1	T38.1X2	T38.1X3	T38.1X4	T38.1X5	T38.1X6
tyropanoate	T50.8X1	T50.8X2	T50.8X3	T50.8X4	T50.8X5	T50.8X6
valproate	T42.6X1	T42.6X2	T42.6X3	T42.6X4	T42.6X5	T42.6X6
versenate	T50.6X1	T50.6X2	T50.6X3	T50.6X4	T50.6X5	T50.6X6
Sodium-free salt	T50.901	T50.902	T50.903	T50.904	T50.905	T50.906
Sodium-removing resin	T50.3X1	T50.3X2	T50.3X3	T50.3X4	T50.3X5	T50.3X6
Soft soap	T55.0X1	T55.0X2	T55.0X3	T55.0X4	—	—
Solanine	T62.2X1	T62.2X2	T62.2X3	T62.2X4	—	—
berries	T62.1X1	T62.1X2	T62.1X3	T62.1X4	—	—

Substance	Poisoning, Accidental (unintentional)	Poisoning, Intentional self-harm	Poisoning, Assault	Poisoning, Undetermined	Adverse effect	Underdosing
Solanum dulcamara	T62.2X1	T62.2X2	T62.2X3	T62.2X4	—	—
berries	T62.1X1	T62.1X2	T62.1X3	T62.1X4	—	—
Solapsone	T37.1X1	T37.1X2	T37.1X3	T37.1X4	T37.1X5	T37.1X6
Solar lotion	T49.3X1	T49.3X2	T49.3X3	T49.3X4	T49.3X5	T49.3X6
Solasulfone	T37.1X1	T37.1X2	T37.1X3	T37.1X4	T37.1X5	T37.1X6
Soldering fluid	T65.891	T65.892	T65.893	T65.894	—	—
Solid substance	T65.91	T65.92	T65.93	T65.94	—	—
specified NEC	T65.891	T65.892	T65.893	T65.894	—	—
Solvent, industrial NEC	T52.91	T52.92	T52.93	T52.94	—	—
naphtha	T52.0X1	T52.0X2	T52.0X3	T52.0X4	—	—
petroleum	T52.0X1	T52.0X2	T52.0X3	T52.0X4	—	—
specified NEC	T52.8X1	T52.8X2	T52.8X3	T52.8X4	—	—
Soma	T42.8X1	T42.8X2	T42.8X3	T42.8X4	T42.8X5	T42.8X6
Somatorelin	T38.891	T38.892	T38.893	T38.894	T38.895	T38.896
Somatostatin	T38.991	T38.992	T38.993	T38.994	T38.995	T38.996
Somatotropin	T38.811	T38.812	T38.813	T38.814	T38.815	T38.816
Somatrem	T38.811	T38.812	T38.813	T38.814	T38.815	T38.816
Somatropin	T38.811	T38.812	T38.813	T38.814	T38.815	T38.816
Sominex	T45.0X1	T45.0X2	T45.0X3	T45.0X4	T45.0X5	T45.0X6
Somnos	T42.6X1	T42.6X2	T42.6X3	T42.6X4	T42.6X5	T42.6X6
Somonal	T42.3X1	T42.3X2	T42.3X3	T42.3X4	T42.3X5	T42.3X6
Soneryl	T42.3X1	T42.3X2	T42.3X3	T42.3X4	T42.3X5	T42.3X6
Soothing syrup	T50.901	T50.902	T50.903	T50.904	T50.905	T50.906
Sopor	T42.6X1	T42.6X2	T42.6X3	T42.6X4	T42.6X5	T42.6X6
Soporific	T42.71	T42.72	T42.73	T42.74	T42.75	T42.76
Soporific drug	T42.71	T42.72	T42.73	T42.74	T42.75	T42.76
specified type NEC	T42.6X1	T42.6X2	T42.6X3	T42.6X4	T42.6X5	T42.6X6
Sorbide nitrate	T46.3X1	T46.3X2	T46.3X3	T46.3X4	T46.3X5	T46.3X6
Sorbitol	T47.4X1	T47.4X2	T47.4X3	T47.4X4	T47.4X5	T47.4X6
Sotalol	T44.7X1	T44.7X2	T44.7X3	T44.7X4	T44.7X5	T44.7X6
Sotradecol	T46.8X1	T46.8X2	T46.8X3	T46.8X4	T46.8X5	T46.8X6
Soysterol	T46.6X1	T46.6X2	T46.6X3	T46.6X4	T46.6X5	T46.6X6
Spacoline	T44.3X1	T44.3X2	T44.3X3	T44.3X4	T44.3X5	T44.3X6
Spanish fly	T49.8X1	T49.8X2	T49.8X3	T49.8X4	T49.8X5	T49.8X6
Sparine	T43.3X1	T43.3X2	T43.3X3	T43.3X4	T43.3X5	T43.3X6
Sparteine	T48.0X1	T48.0X2	T48.0X3	T48.0X4	T48.0X5	T48.0X6
Spasmolytic						
anticholinergics	T44.3X1	T44.3X2	T44.3X3	T44.3X4	T44.3X5	T44.3X6
autonomic	T44.3X1	T44.3X2	T44.3X3	T44.3X4	T44.3X5	T44.3X6
bronchial NEC	T48.6X1	T48.6X2	T48.6X3	T48.6X4	T48.6X5	T48.6X6
quaternary ammonium	T44.3X1	T44.3X2	T44.3X3	T44.3X4	T44.3X5	T44.3X6
skeletal muscle NEC	T48.1X1	T48.1X2	T48.1X3	T48.1X4	T48.1X5	T48.1X6
Spectinomycin	T36.5X1	T36.5X2	T36.5X3	T36.5X4	T36.5X5	T36.5X6
Speed	T43.621	T43.622	T43.623	T43.624	T43.625	T43.626
Spermicide	T49.8X1	T49.8X2	T49.8X3	T49.8X4	T49.8X5	T49.8X6
Spider (bite) (venom)	T63.391	T63.392	T63.393	T63.394	—	—
antivenin	T50.Z11	T50.Z12	T50.Z13	T50.Z14	T50.Z15	T50.Z16
Spigelia (root)	T37.4X1	T37.4X2	T37.4X3	T37.4X4	T37.4X5	T37.4X6
Spindle inactivator	T50.4X1	T50.4X2	T50.4X3	T50.4X4	T50.4X5	T50.4X6
Spiperone	T43.4X1	T43.4X2	T43.4X3	T43.4X4	T43.4X5	T43.4X6

Substance	Poisoning, Accidental (unintentional)	Poisoning, Intentional self-harm	Poisoning, Assault	Poisoning, Undetermined	Adverse effect	Underdosing
Spiramycin	T36.3X1	T36.3X2	T36.3X3	T36.3X4	T36.3X5	T36.3X6
Spirapril	T46.4X1	T46.4X2	T46.4X3	T46.4X4	T46.4X5	T46.4X6
Spirilene	T43.591	T43.592	T43.593	T43.594	T43.595	T43.596
Spirit(s) (neutral) NEC	T51.0X1	T51.0X2	T51.0X3	T51.0X4	—	—
beverage	T51.0X1	T51.0X2	T51.0X3	T51.0X4	—	—
industrial	T51.0X1	T51.0X2	T51.0X3	T51.0X4	—	—
mineral	T52.0X1	T52.0X2	T52.0X3	T52.0X4	—	—
of salt—see Hydrochloric acid						
surgical	T51.0X1	T51.0X2	T51.0X3	T51.0X4	—	—
Spironolactone	T50.0X1	T50.0X2	T50.0X3	T50.0X4	T50.0X5	T50.0X6
Spiroperidol	T43.4X1	T43.4X2	T43.4X3	T43.4X4	T43.4X5	T43.4X6
Sponge, absorbable (gelatin)	T45.7X1	T45.7X2	T45.7X3	T45.7X4	T45.7X5	T45.7X6
Sporostacin	T49.0X1	T49.0X2	T49.0X3	T49.0X4	T49.0X5	T49.0X6
Spray (aerosol)	T65.91	T65.92	T65.93	T65.94	—	—
cosmetic	T65.891	T65.892	T65.893	T65.894	—	—
medicinal NEC	T50.901	T50.902	T50.903	T50.904	T50.905	T50.906
pesticides—see Pesticides						
specified content—see specific substance						
Spurge flax	T62.2X1	T62.2X2	T62.2X3	T62.2X4	—	—
Spurges	T62.2X1	T62.2X2	T62.2X3	T62.2X4	—	—
Sputum viscosity-lowering drug	T48.4X1	T48.4X2	T48.4X3	T48.4X4	T48.4X5	T48.4X6
Squill	T46.0X1	T46.0X2	T46.0X3	T46.0X4	T46.0X5	T46.0X6
rat poison	T60.4X1	T60.4X2	T60.4X3	T60.4X4	—	—
Squirting cucumber (cathartic)	T47.2X1	T47.2X2	T47.2X3	T47.2X4	T47.2X5	T47.2X6
Stains	T65.6X1	T65.6X2	T65.6X3	T65.6X4	—	—
Stannous fluoride	T49.7X1	T49.7X2	T49.7X3	T49.7X4	T49.7X5	T49.7X6
Stanolone	T38.7X1	T38.7X2	T38.7X3	T38.7X4	T38.7X5	T38.7X6
Stanozolol	T38.7X1	T38.7X2	T38.7X3	T38.7X4	T38.7X5	T38.7X6
Staphisagria or stavesacre (pediculicide)	T49.0X1	T49.0X2	T49.0X3	T49.0X4	T49.0X5	T49.0X6
Starch	T50.901	T50.902	T50.903	T50.904	T50.905	T50.906
Stelazine	T43.3X1	T43.3X2	T43.3X3	T43.3X4	T43.3X5	T43.3X6
Stemetil	T43.3X1	T43.3X2	T43.3X3	T43.3X4	T43.3X5	T43.3X6
Stepronin	T48.4X1	T48.4X2	T48.4X3	T48.4X4	T48.4X5	T48.4X6
Sterculia	T47.4X1	T47.4X2	T47.4X3	T47.4X4	T47.4X5	T47.4X6
Sternutator gas	T59.891	T59.892	T59.893	T59.894	—	—
Steroid	T38.0X1	T38.0X2	T38.0X3	T38.0X4	T38.0X5	T38.0X6
anabolic	T38.7X1	T38.7X2	T38.7X3	T38.7X4	T38.7X5	T38.7X6
androgenic	T38.7X1	T38.7X2	T38.7X3	T38.7X4	T38.7X5	T38.7X6
antineoplastic, hormone	T38.7X1	T38.7X2	T38.7X3	T38.7X4	T38.7X5	T38.7X6
estrogen	T38.5X1	T38.5X2	T38.5X3	T38.5X4	T38.5X5	T38.5X6
ENT agent	T49.6X1	T49.6X2	T49.6X3	T49.6X4	T49.6X5	T49.6X6
ophthalmic preparation	T49.5X1	T49.5X2	T49.5X3	T49.5X4	T49.5X5	T49.5X6
topical NEC	T49.0X1	T49.0X2	T49.0X3	T49.0X4	T49.0X5	T49.0X6
Stibine	T56.891	T56.892	T56.893	T56.894	—	—
Stibogluconate	T37.3X1	T37.3X2	T37.3X3	T37.3X4	T37.3X5	T37.3X6

Substance	Poisoning, Accidental (unintentional)	Poisoning, Intentional self-harm	Poisoning, Assault	Poisoning, Undetermined	Adverse effect	Underdosing
Stibophen	T37.4X1	T37.4X2	T37.4X3	T37.4X4	T37.4X5	T37.4X6
Stilbamidine (isetionate)	T37.3X1	T37.3X2	T37.3X3	T37.3X4	T37.3X5	T37.3X6
Stilbestrol	T38.5X1	T38.5X2	T38.5X3	T38.5X4	T38.5X5	T38.5X6
Stilboestrol	T38.5X1	T38.5X2	T38.5X3	T38.5X4	T38.5X5	T38.5X6
Stimulant						
central nervous system—see also Psychostimulant	T43.601	T43.602	T43.603	T43.604	T43.605	T43.606
analeptics	T50.7X1	T50.7X2	T50.7X3	T50.7X4	T50.7X5	T50.7X6
opiate antagonist	T50.7X1	T50.7X2	T50.7X3	T50.7X4	T50.7X5	T50.7X6
psychotherapeutic NEC—see also Psychotherapeutic drug	T43.601	T43.602	T43.603	T43.604	T43.605	T43.606
specified NEC	T43.691	T43.692	T43.693	T43.694	T43.695	T43.696
respiratory	T48.901	T48.902	T48.903	T48.904	T48.905	T48.906
Stone-dissolving drug	T50.901	T50.902	T50.903	T50.904	T50.905	T50.906
Storage battery (cells) (acid)	T54.2X1	T54.2X2	T54.2X3	T54.2X4	—	—
Stovaine	T41.3X1	T41.3X2	T41.3X3	T41.3X4	T41.3X5	T41.3X6
infiltration (subcutaneous)	T41.3X1	T41.3X2	T41.3X3	T41.3X4	T41.3X5	T41.3X6
nerve block (peripheral) (plexus)	T41.3X1	T41.3X2	T41.3X3	T41.3X4	T41.3X5	T41.3X6
spinal	T41.3X1	T41.3X2	T41.3X3	T41.3X4	T41.3X5	T41.3X6
topical (surface)	T41.3X1	T41.3X2	T41.3X3	T41.3X4	T41.3X5	T41.3X6
Stovarsal	T37.8X1	T37.8X2	T37.8X3	T37.8X4	T37.8X5	T37.8X6
Stove gas—see Gas, stove						
Stoxil	T49.5X1	T49.5X2	T49.5X3	T49.5X4	T49.5X5	T49.5X6
Stramonium	T48.6X1	T48.6X2	T48.6X3	T48.6X4	T48.6X5	T48.6X6
natural state	T62.2X1	T62.2X2	T62.2X3	T62.2X4	—	—
Streptodornase	T45.3X1	T45.3X2	T45.3X3	T45.3X4	T45.3X5	T45.3X6
Streptoduocin	T36.5X1	T36.5X2	T36.5X3	T36.5X4	T36.5X5	T36.5X6
Streptokinase	T45.611	T45.612	T45.613	T45.614	T45.615	T45.616
Streptomycin (derivative)	T36.5X1	T36.5X2	T36.5X3	T36.5X4	T36.5X5	T36.5X6
Streptonivicin	T36.5X1	T36.5X2	T36.5X3	T36.5X4	T36.5X5	T36.5X6
Streptovarycin	T36.5X1	T36.5X2	T36.5X3	T36.5X4	T36.5X5	T36.5X6
Streptozocin	T45.1X1	T45.1X2	T45.1X3	T45.1X4	T45.1X5	T45.1X6
Streptozotocin	T45.1X1	T45.1X2	T45.1X3	T45.1X4	T45.1X5	T45.1X6
Stripper (paint) (solvent)	T52.8X1	T52.8X2	T52.8X3	T52.8X4	—	—
Strobane	T60.1X1	T60.1X2	T60.1X3	T60.1X4	—	—
Strofantina	T46.0X1	T46.0X2	T46.0X3	T46.0X4	T46.0X5	T46.0X6
Strophanthin (g) (k)	T46.0X1	T46.0X2	T46.0X3	T46.0X4	T46.0X5	T46.0X6
Strophanthus	T46.0X1	T46.0X2	T46.0X3	T46.0X4	T46.0X5	T46.0X6
Strophantin	T46.0X1	T46.0X2	T46.0X3	T46.0X4	T46.0X5	T46.0X6
Strophantin-g	T46.0X1	T46.0X2	T46.0X3	T46.0X4	T46.0X5	T46.0X6
Strychnine (nonmedicinal) (pesticide) (salts)	T65.1X1	T65.1X2	T65.1X3	T65.1X4	—	—
medicinal	T48.291	T48.292	T48.293	T48.294	T48.295	T48.296
Strychnos (ignatii)—see Strychnine						

Substance	Poisoning, Accidental (unintentional)	Poisoning, Intentional self-harm	Poisoning, Assault	Poisoning, Undetermined	Adverse effect	Underdosing
Styramate	T42.8X1	T42.8X2	T42.8X3	T42.8X4	T42.8X5	T42.8X6
Styrene	T65.891	T65.892	T65.893	T65.894	—	—
Succinimide, antiepileptic or anticonvulsant	T42.2X1	T42.2X2	T42.2X3	T42.2X4	T42.2X5	T42.2X6
mercuric—see Mercury						
Succinylcholine	T48.1X1	T48.1X2	T48.1X3	T48.1X4	T48.1X5	T48.1X6
Succinylsulfathiazole	T37.0X1	T37.0X2	T37.0X3	T37.0X4	T37.0X5	T37.0X6
Sucralfate	T47.1X1	T47.1X2	T47.1X3	T47.1X4	T47.1X5	T47.1X6
Sucrose	T50.3X1	T50.3X2	T50.3X3	T50.3X4	T50.3X5	T50.3X6
Sufentanil	T40.411	T40.412	T40.413	T40.414	T40.415	T40.416
Sulbactam	T36.0X1	T36.0X2	T36.0X3	T36.0X4	T36.0X5	T36.0X6
Sulbenicillin	T36.0X1	T36.0X2	T36.0X3	T36.0X4	T36.0X5	T36.0X6
Sulbentine	T49.0X1	T49.0X2	T49.0X3	T49.0X4	T49.0X5	T49.0X6
Sulfacetamide	T49.0X1	T49.0X2	T49.0X3	T49.0X4	T49.0X5	T49.0X6
ophthalmic preparation	T49.5X1	T49.5X2	T49.5X3	T49.5X4	T49.5X5	T49.5X6
Sulfachlorpyridazine	T37.0X1	T37.0X2	T37.0X3	T37.0X4	T37.0X5	T37.0X6
Sulfacitine	T37.0X1	T37.0X2	T37.0X3	T37.0X4	T37.0X5	T37.0X6
Sulfadiasulfone sodium	T37.0X1	T37.0X2	T37.0X3	T37.0X4	T37.0X5	T37.0X6
Sulfadiazine	T37.0X1	T37.0X2	T37.0X3	T37.0X4	T37.0X5	T37.0X6
silver (topical)	T49.0X1	T49.0X2	T49.0X3	T49.0X4	T49.0X5	T49.0X6
Sulfadimethoxine	T37.0X1	T37.0X2	T37.0X3	T37.0X4	T37.0X5	T37.0X6
Sulfadimidine	T37.0X1	T37.0X2	T37.0X3	T37.0X4	T37.0X5	T37.0X6
Sulfadoxine	T37.0X1	T37.0X2	T37.0X3	T37.0X4	T37.0X5	T37.0X6
with pyrimethamine	T37.2X1	T37.2X2	T37.2X3	T37.2X4	T37.2X5	T37.2X6
Sulfaethidole	T37.0X1	T37.0X2	T37.0X3	T37.0X4	T37.0X5	T37.0X6
Sulfafurazole	T37.0X1	T37.0X2	T37.0X3	T37.0X4	T37.0X5	T37.0X6
Sulfaguanidine	T37.0X1	T37.0X2	T37.0X3	T37.0X4	T37.0X5	T37.0X6
Sulfalene	T37.0X1	T37.0X2	T37.0X3	T37.0X4	T37.0X5	T37.0X6
Sulfaloxate	T37.0X1	T37.0X2	T37.0X3	T37.0X4	T37.0X5	T37.0X6
Sulfaloxic acid	T37.0X1	T37.0X2	T37.0X3	T37.0X4	T37.0X5	T37.0X6
Sulfamazone	T39.2X1	T39.2X2	T39.2X3	T39.2X4	T39.2X5	T39.2X6
Sulfamerazine	T37.0X1	T37.0X2	T37.0X3	T37.0X4	T37.0X5	T37.0X6
Sulfameter	T37.0X1	T37.0X2	T37.0X3	T37.0X4	T37.0X5	T37.0X6
Sulfamethazine	T37.0X1	T37.0X2	T37.0X3	T37.0X4	T37.0X5	T37.0X6
Sulfamethizole	T37.0X1	T37.0X2	T37.0X3	T37.0X4	T37.0X5	T37.0X6
Sulfamethoxazole	T37.0X1	T37.0X2	T37.0X3	T37.0X4	T37.0X5	T37.0X6
with trimethoprim	T36.8X1	T36.8X2	T36.8X3	T36.8X4	T36.8X5	T36.8X6
Sulfamethoxydiazine	T37.0X1	T37.0X2	T37.0X3	T37.0X4	T37.0X5	T37.0X6
Sulfamethoxypyridazine	T37.0X1	T37.0X2	T37.0X3	T37.0X4	T37.0X5	T37.0X6
Sulfamethylthiazole	T37.0X1	T37.0X2	T37.0X3	T37.0X4	T37.0X5	T37.0X6
Sulfametoxydiazine	T37.0X1	T37.0X2	T37.0X3	T37.0X4	T37.0X5	T37.0X6
Sulfamidopyrine	T39.2X1	T39.2X2	T39.2X3	T39.2X4	T39.2X5	T39.2X6
Sulfamonomethoxine	T37.0X1	T37.0X2	T37.0X3	T37.0X4	T37.0X5	T37.0X6
Sulfamoxole	T37.0X1	T37.0X2	T37.0X3	T37.0X4	T37.0X5	T37.0X6
Sulfamylon	T49.0X1	T49.0X2	T49.0X3	T49.0X4	T49.0X5	T49.0X6
Sulfan blue (diagnostic dye)	T50.8X1	T50.8X2	T50.8X3	T50.8X4	T50.8X5	T50.8X6
Sulfanilamide	T37.0X1	T37.0X2	T37.0X3	T37.0X4	T37.0X5	T37.0X6
Sulfanilylguanidine	T37.0X1	T37.0X2	T37.0X3	T37.0X4	T37.0X5	T37.0X6
Sulfaperin	T37.0X1	T37.0X2	T37.0X3	T37.0X4	T37.0X5	T37.0X6

Substance	Poisoning, Accidental (unintentional)	Poisoning, Intentional self-harm	Poisoning, Assault	Poisoning, Undetermined	Adverse effect	Underdosing
Sulfaphenazole	T37.0X1	T37.0X2	T37.0X3	T37.0X4	T37.0X5	T37.0X6
Sulfaphenylthiazole	T37.0X1	T37.0X2	T37.0X3	T37.0X4	T37.0X5	T37.0X6
Sulfaproxyline	T37.0X1	T37.0X2	T37.0X3	T37.0X4	T37.0X5	T37.0X6
Sulfapyridine	T37.0X1	T37.0X2	T37.0X3	T37.0X4	T37.0X5	T37.0X6
Sulfapyrimidine	T37.0X1	T37.0X2	T37.0X3	T37.0X4	T37.0X5	T37.0X6
Sulfarsphenamine	T37.8X1	T37.8X2	T37.8X3	T37.8X4	T37.8X5	T37.8X6
Sulfasalazine	T37.0X1	T37.0X2	T37.0X3	T37.0X4	T37.0X5	T37.0X6
Sulfasuxidine	T37.0X1	T37.0X2	T37.0X3	T37.0X4	T37.0X5	T37.0X6
Sulfasymazine	T37.0X1	T37.0X2	T37.0X3	T37.0X4	T37.0X5	T37.0X6
Sulfated amylopectin	T47.8X1	T47.8X2	T47.8X3	T47.8X4	T47.8X5	T47.8X6
Sulfathiazole	T37.0X1	T37.0X2	T37.0X3	T37.0X4	T37.0X5	T37.0X6
Sulfatostearate	T49.2X1	T49.2X2	T49.2X3	T49.2X4	T49.2X5	T49.2X6
Sulfinpyrazone	T50.4X1	T50.4X2	T50.4X3	T50.4X4	T50.4X5	T50.4X6
Sulfiram	T49.0X1	T49.0X2	T49.0X3	T49.0X4	T49.0X5	T49.0X6
Sulfisomidine	T37.0X1	T37.0X2	T37.0X3	T37.0X4	T37.0X5	T37.0X6
Sulfisoxazole	T37.0X1	T37.0X2	T37.0X3	T37.0X4	T37.0X5	T37.0X6
ophthalmic preparation	T49.5X1	T49.5X2	T49.5X3	T49.5X4	T49.5X5	T49.5X6
Sulfobromophthalein (sodium)	T50.8X1	T50.8X2	T50.8X3	T50.8X4	T50.8X5	T50.8X6
Sulfobromphthalein	T50.8X1	T50.8X2	T50.8X3	T50.8X4	T50.8X5	T50.8X6
Sulfogaiacol	T48.4X1	T48.4X2	T48.4X3	T48.4X4	T48.4X5	T48.4X6
Sulfomyxin	T36.8X1	T36.8X2	T36.8X3	T36.8X4	T36.8X5	T36.8X6
Sulfonal	T42.6X1	T42.6X2	T42.6X3	T42.6X4	T42.6X5	T42.6X6
Sulfonamide NEC	T37.0X1	T37.0X2	T37.0X3	T37.0X4	T37.0X5	T37.0X6
eye	T49.5X1	T49.5X2	T49.5X3	T49.5X4	T49.5X5	T49.5X6
Sulfonazide	T37.1X1	T37.1X2	T37.1X3	T37.1X4	T37.1X5	T37.1X6
Sulfones	T37.1X1	T37.1X2	T37.1X3	T37.1X4	T37.1X5	T37.1X6
Sulfonethylmethane	T42.6X1	T42.6X2	T42.6X3	T42.6X4	T42.6X5	T42.6X6
Sulfonmethane	T42.6X1	T42.6X2	T42.6X3	T42.6X4	T42.6X5	T42.6X6
Sulfonphthal, sulfonphthol	T50.8X1	T50.8X2	T50.8X3	T50.8X4	T50.8X5	T50.8X6
Sulfonylurea derivatives, oral	T38.3X1	T38.3X2	T38.3X3	T38.3X4	T38.3X5	T38.3X6
Sulforidazine	T43.3X1	T43.3X2	T43.3X3	T43.3X4	T43.3X5	T43.3X6
Sulfoxone	T37.1X1	T37.1X2	T37.1X3	T37.1X4	T37.1X5	T37.1X6
Sulfur, sulfurated, sulfuric, sulfurous, sulfuryl (compounds NEC) (medicinal)	T49.4X1	T49.4X2	T49.4X3	T49.4X4	T49.4X5	T49.4X6
acid	T54.2X1	T54.2X2	T54.2X3	T54.2X4	—	—
dioxide (gas)	T59.1X1	T59.1X2	T59.1X3	T59.1X4	—	—
ether—see Ether(s)						
hydrogen	T59.6X1	T59.6X2	T59.6X3	T59.6X4	—	—
medicinal (keratolytic) (ointment) NEC	T49.4X1	T49.4X2	T49.4X3	T49.4X4	T49.4X5	T49.4X6
ointment	T49.0X1	T49.0X2	T49.0X3	T49.0X4	T49.0X5	T49.0X6
pesticide (vapor)	T60.91	T60.92	T60.93	T60.94	—	—
vapor NEC	T59.891	T59.892	T59.893	T59.894		
Sulfuric acid	T54.2X1	T54.2X2	T54.2X3	T54.2X4	—	—
Sulglicotide	T47.1X1	T47.1X2	T47.1X3	T47.1X4	T47.1X5	T47.1X6
Sulindac	T39.391	T39.392	T39.393	T39.394	T39.395	T39.396
Sulisatin	T47.2X1	T47.2X2	T47.2X3	T47.2X4	T47.2X5	T47.2X6

Substance	Poisoning, Accidental (unintentional)	Poisoning, Intentional self-harm	Poisoning, Assault	Poisoning, Undetermined	Adverse effect	Underdosing
Sulisobenzone	T49.3X1	T49.3X2	T49.3X3	T49.3X4	T49.3X5	T49.3X6
Sulkowitch's reagent	T50.8X1	T50.8X2	T50.8X3	T50.8X4	T50.8X5	T50.8X6
Sulmetozine	T44.3X1	T44.3X2	T44.3X3	T44.3X4	T44.3X5	T44.3X6
Suloctidil	T46.7X1	T46.7X2	T46.7X3	T46.7X4	T46.7X5	T46.7X6
Sulph——see also Sulf-						
Sulphadiazine	T37.0X1	T37.0X2	T37.0X3	T37.0X4	T37.0X5	T37.0X6
Sulphadimethoxine	T37.0X1	T37.0X2	T37.0X3	T37.0X4	T37.0X5	T37.0X6
Sulphadimidine	T37.0X1	T37.0X2	T37.0X3	T37.0X4	T37.0X5	T37.0X6
Sulphadione	T37.1X1	T37.1X2	T37.1X3	T37.1X4	T37.1X5	T37.1X6
Sulphafurazole	T37.0X1	T37.0X2	T37.0X3	T37.0X4	T37.0X5	T37.0X6
Sulphamethizole	T37.0X1	T37.0X2	T37.0X3	T37.0X4	T37.0X5	T37.0X6
Sulphamethoxazole	T37.0X1	T37.0X2	T37.0X3	T37.0X4	T37.0X5	T37.0X6
Sulphan blue	T50.8X1	T50.8X2	T50.8X3	T50.8X4	T50.8X5	T50.8X6
Sulphaphenazole	T37.0X1	T37.0X2	T37.0X3	T37.0X4	T37.0X5	T37.0X6
Sulphapyridine	T37.0X1	T37.0X2	T37.0X3	T37.0X4	T37.0X5	T37.0X6
Sulphasalazine	T37.0X1	T37.0X2	T37.0X3	T37.0X4	T37.0X5	T37.0X6
Sulphinpyrazone	T50.4X1	T50.4X2	T50.4X3	T50.4X4	T50.4X5	T50.4X6
Sulpiride	T43.591	T43.592	T43.593	T43.594	T43.595	T43.596
Sulprostone	T48.0X1	T48.0X2	T48.0X3	T48.0X4	T48.0X5	T48.0X6
Sulpyrine	T39.2X1	T39.2X2	T39.2X3	T39.2X4	T39.2X5	T39.2X6
Sultamicillin	T36.0X1	T36.0X2	T36.0X3	T36.0X4	T36.0X5	T36.0X6
Sulthiame	T42.6X1	T42.6X2	T42.6X3	T42.6X4	T42.6X5	T42.6X6
Sultiame	T42.6X1	T42.6X2	T42.6X3	T42.6X4	T42.6X5	T42.6X6
Sultopride	T43.591	T43.592	T43.593	T43.594	T43.595	T43.596
Sumatriptan	T39.8X1	T39.8X2	T39.8X3	T39.8X4	T39.8X5	T39.8X6
Sunflower seed oil	T46.6X1	T46.6X2	T46.6X3	T46.6X4	T46.6X5	T46.6X6
Superinone	T48.4X1	T48.4X2	T48.4X3	T48.4X4	T48.4X5	T48.4X6
Suprofen	T39.311	T39.312	T39.313	T39.314	T39.315	T39.316
Suramin (sodium)	T37.4X1	T37.4X2	T37.4X3	T37.4X4	T37.4X5	T37.4X6
Surfacaine	T41.3X1	T41.3X2	T41.3X3	T41.3X4	T41.3X5	T41.3X6
Surital	T41.1X1	T41.1X2	T41.1X3	T41.1X4	T41.1X5	T41.1X6
Sutilains	T45.3X1	T45.3X2	T45.3X3	T45.3X4	T45.3X5	T45.3X6
Suxamethonium (chloride)	T48.1X1	T48.1X2	T48.1X3	T48.1X4	T48.1X5	T48.1X6
Suxethonium (chloride)	T48.1X1	T48.1X2	T48.1X3	T48.1X4	T48.1X5	T48.1X6
Suxibuzone	T39.2X1	T39.2X2	T39.2X3	T39.2X4	T39.2X5	T39.2X6
Sweet niter spirit	T46.3X1	T46.3X2	T46.3X3	T46.3X4	T46.3X5	T46.3X6
Sweet oil (birch)	T49.3X1	T49.3X2	T49.3X3	T49.3X4	T49.3X5	T49.3X6
Sweetener	T50.901	T50.902	T50.903	T50.904	T50.905	T50.906
Sym-dichloroethyl ether	T53.6X1	T53.6X2	T53.6X3	T53.6X4	—	—
Sympatholytic NEC	T44.8X1	T44.8X2	T44.8X3	T44.8X4	T44.8X5	T44.8X6
haloalkylamine	T44.8X1	T44.8X2	T44.8X3	T44.8X4	T44.8X5	T44.8X6
Sympathomimetic NEC	T44.901	T44.902	T44.903	T44.904	T44.905	T44.906
anti-common-cold	T48.5X1	T48.5X2	T48.5X3	T48.5X4	T48.5X5	T48.5X6
bronchodilator	T48.6X1	T48.6X2	T48.6X3	T48.6X4	T48.6X5	T48.6X6
specified NEC	T44.991	T44.992	T44.993	T44.994	T44.995	T44.996
Synagis	T50.B91	T50.B92	T50.B93	T50.B94	T50.B95	T50.B96
Synalar	T49.0X1	T49.0X2	T49.0X3	T49.0X4	T49.0X5	T49.0X6
Synthroid	T38.1X1	T38.1X2	T38.1X3	T38.1X4	T38.1X5	T38.1X6
Syntocinon	T48.0X1	T48.0X2	T48.0X3	T48.0X4	T48.0X5	T48.0X6

Substance	Poisoning, Accidental (unintentional)	Poisoning, Intentional self-harm	Poisoning, Assault	Poisoning, Undetermined	Adverse effect	Underdosing
Syrosingopine	T46.5X1	T46.5X2	T46.5X3	T46.5X4	T46.5X5	T46.5X6
Systemic drug	T45.91	T45.92	T45.93	T45.94	T45.95	T45.96
specified NEC	T45.8X1	T45.8X2	T45.8X3	T45.8X4	T45.8X5	T45.8X6
2,4,5-T	T60.3X1	T60.3X2	T60.3X3	T60.3X4	—	—
T						
Tablets—see also specified substance	T50.901	T50.902	T50.903	T50.904	T50.905	T50.906
Tace	T38.5X1	T38.5X2	T38.5X3	T38.5X4	T38.5X5	T38.5X6
Tacrine	T44.0X1	T44.0X2	T44.0X3	T44.0X4	T44.0X5	T44.0X6
Tadalafil	T46.7X1	T46.7X2	T46.7X3	T46.7X4	T46.7X5	T46.7X6
Talampicillin	T36.0X1	T36.0X2	T36.0X3	T36.0X4	T36.0X5	T36.0X6
Talbutal	T42.3X1	T42.3X2	T42.3X3	T42.3X4	T42.3X5	T42.3X6
Talc powder	T49.3X1	T49.3X2	T49.3X3	T49.3X4	T49.3X5	T49.3X6
Talcum	T49.3X1	T49.3X2	T49.3X3	T49.3X4	T49.3X5	T49.3X6
Taleranol	T38.6X1	T38.6X2	T38.6X3	T38.6X4	T38.6X5	T38.6X6
Tamoxifen	T38.6X1	T38.6X2	T38.6X3	T38.6X4	T38.6X5	T38.6X6
Tamsulosin	T44.6X1	T44.6X2	T44.6X3	T44.6X4	T44.6X5	T44.6X6
Tandearil, tanderil	T39.2X1	T39.2X2	T39.2X3	T39.2X4	T39.2X5	T39.2X6
Tannic acid	T49.2X1	T49.2X2	T49.2X3	T49.2X4	T49.2X5	T49.2X6
medicinal (astringent)	T49.2X1	T49.2X2	T49.2X3	T49.2X4	T49.2X5	T49.2X6
Tannin—see Tannic acid						
Tansy	T62.2X1	T62.2X2	T62.2X3	T62.2X4	—	—
TAO	T36.3X1	T36.3X2	T36.3X3	T36.3X4	T36.3X5	T36.3X6
Tapazole	T38.2X1	T38.2X2	T38.2X3	T38.2X4	T38.2X5	T38.2X6
Tar NEC	T52.0X1	T52.0X2	T52.0X3	T52.0X4	—	—
camphor	T60.1X1	T60.1X2	T60.1X3	T60.1X4	—	—
distillate	T49.1X1	T49.1X2	T49.1X3	T49.1X4	T49.1X5	T49.1X6
fumes	T59.891	T59.892	T59.893	T59.894	—	—
medicinal	T49.1X1	T49.1X2	T49.1X3	T49.1X4	T49.1X5	T49.1X6
ointment	T49.1X1	T49.1X2	T49.1X3	T49.1X4	T49.1X5	T49.1X6
Taractan	T43.591	T43.592	T43.593	T43.594	T43.595	T43.596
Tarantula (venomous)	T63.321	T63.322	T63.323	T63.324		
Tartar emetic	T37.8X1	T37.8X2	T37.8X3	T37.8X4	T37.8X5	T37.8X6
Tartaric acid	T65.891	T65.892	T65.893	T65.894	—	—
Tartrate, laxative	T47.4X1	T47.4X2	T47.4X3	T47.4X4	T47.4X5	T47.4X6
Tartrated antimony (anti-infective)	T37.8X1	T37.8X2	T37.8X3	T37.8X4	T37.8X5	T37.8X6
Tauromustine	T45.1X1	T45.1X2	T45.1X3	T45.1X4	T45.1X5	T45.1X6
TCA—see Trichloroacetic acid						
TCDD	T53.7X1	T53.7X2	T53.7X3	T53.7X4	—	—
TDI (vapor)	T65.0X1	T65.0X2	T65.0X3	T65.0X4	—	—
Tear						
gas	T59.3X1	T59.3X2	T59.3X3	T59.3X4	—	—
solution	T49.5X1	T49.5X2	T49.5X3	T49.5X4	T49.5X5	T49.5X6
Teclothiazide	T50.2X1	T50.2X2	T50.2X3	T50.2X4	T50.2X5	T50.2X6
Teclozan	T37.3X1	T37.3X2	T37.3X3	T37.3X4	T37.3X5	T37.3X6
Tegafur	T45.1X1	T45.1X2	T45.1X3	T45.1X4	T45.1X5	T45.1X6
Tegretol	T42.1X1	T42.1X2	T42.1X3	T42.1X4	T42.1X5	T42.1X6
Teicoplanin	T36.8X1	T36.8X2	T36.8X3	T36.8X4	T36.8X5	T36.8X6
Telepaque	T50.8X1	T50.8X2	T50.8X3	T50.8X4	T50.8X5	T50.8X6

Substance	Poisoning, Accidental (unintentional)	Poisoning, Intentional self-harm	Poisoning, Assault	Poisoning, Undetermined	Adverse effect	Underdosing
Tellurium	T56.891	T56.892	T56.893	T56.894	—	—
fumes	T56.891	T56.892	T56.893	T56.894	—	—
TEM	T45.1X1	T45.1X2	T45.1X3	T45.1X4	T45.1X5	T45.1X6
Temazepam	T42.4X1	T42.4X2	T42.4X3	T42.4X4	T42.4X5	T42.4X6
Temocillin	T36.0X1	T36.0X2	T36.0X3	T36.0X4	T36.0X5	T36.0X6
Tenamfetamine	T43.621	T43.622	T43.623	T43.624	T43.625	T43.626
Teniposide	T45.1X1	T45.1X2	T45.1X3	T45.1X4	T45.1X5	T45.1X6
Tenitramine	T46.3X1	T46.3X2	T46.3X3	T46.3X4	T46.3X5	T46.3X6
Tenoglicin	T48.4X1	T48.4X2	T48.4X3	T48.4X4	T48.4X5	T48.4X6
Tenonitrozole	T37.3X1	T37.3X2	T37.3X3	T37.3X4	T37.3X5	T37.3X6
Tenoxicam	T39.391	T39.392	T39.393	T39.394	T39.395	T39.396
TEPA	T45.1X1	T45.1X2	T45.1X3	T45.1X4	T45.1X5	T45.1X6
TEPP	T60.0X1	T60.0X2	T60.0X3	T60.0X4	—	—
Teprotide	T46.5X1	T46.5X2	T46.5X3	T46.5X4	T46.5X5	T46.5X6
Terazosin	T44.6X1	T44.6X2	T44.6X3	T44.6X4	T44.6X5	T44.6X6
Terbufos	T60.0X1	T60.0X2	T60.0X3	T60.0X4		
Terbutaline	T48.6X1	T48.6X2	T48.6X3	T48.6X4	T48.6X5	T48.6X6
Terconazole	T49.0X1	T49.0X2	T49.0X3	T49.0X4	T49.0X5	T49.0X6
Terfenadine	T45.0X1	T45.0X2	T45.0X3	T45.0X4	T45.0X5	T45.0X6
Teriparatide (acetate)	T50.991	T50.992	T50.993	T50.994	T50.995	T50.996
Terizidone	T37.1X1	T37.1X2	T37.1X3	T37.1X4	T37.1X5	T37.1X6
Terlipressin	T38.891	T38.892	T38.893	T38.894	T38.895	T38.896
Terodiline	T46.3X1	T46.3X2	T46.3X3	T46.3X4	T46.3X5	T46.3X6
Teroxalene	T37.4X1	T37.4X2	T37.4X3	T37.4X4	T37.4X5	T37.4X6
Terpin(cis) hydrate	T48.4X1	T48.4X2	T48.4X3	T48.4X4	T48.4X5	T48.4X6
Terramycin	T36.4X1	T36.4X2	T36.4X3	T36.4X4	T36.4X5	T36.4X6
Tertatolol	T44.7X1	T44.7X2	T44.7X3	T44.7X4	T44.7X5	T44.7X6
Tessalon	T48.3X1	T48.3X2	T48.3X3	T48.3X4	T48.3X5	T48.3X6
Testolactone	T38.7X1	T38.7X2	T38.7X3	T38.7X4	T38.7X5	T38.7X6
Testosterone	T38.7X1	T38.7X2	T38.7X3	T38.7X4	T38.7X5	T38.7X6
Tetanus toxoid or vaccine	T50.A91	T50.A92	T50.A93	T50.A94	T50.A95	T50.A96
antitoxin	T50.Z11	T50.Z12	T50.Z13	T50.Z14	T50.Z15	T50.Z16
immune globulin (human)	T50.Z11	T50.Z12	T50.Z13	T50.Z14	T50.Z15	T50.Z16
toxoid	T50.A91	T50.A92	T50.A93	T50.A94	T50.A95	T50.A96
with diphtheria toxoid	T50.A21	T50.A22	T50.A23	T50.A24	T50.A25	T50.A26
with pertussis	T50.A11	T50.A12	T50.A13	T50.A14	T50.A15	T50.A16
Tetrabenazine	T43.591	T43.592	T43.593	T43.594	T43.595	T43.596
Tetracaine	T41.3X1	T41.3X2	T41.3X3	T41.3X4	T41.3X5	T41.3X6
nerve block (peripheral) (plexus)	T41.3X1	T41.3X2	T41.3X3	T41.3X4	T41.3X5	T41.3X6
regional	T41.3X1	T41.3X2	T41.3X3	T41.3X4	T41.3X5	T41.3X6
spinal	T41.3X1	T41.3X2	T41.3X3	T41.3X4	T41.3X5	T41.3X6
Tetrachlorethylene—see Tetrachloroethylene						
Tetrachlormethiazide	T50.2X1	T50.2X2	T50.2X3	T50.2X4	T50.2X5	T50.2X6
2,3,7,8-Tetrachlorodi-benzo-p-dioxin	T53.7X1	T53.7X2	T53.7X3	T53.7X4	—	—
Tetrachloroethane	T53.6X1	T53.6X2	T53.6X3	T53.6X4	—	—
vapor	T53.6X1	T53.6X2	T53.6X3	T53.6X4	—	—

Substance	Poisoning, Accidental (unintentional)	Poisoning, Intentional self-harm	Poisoning, Assault	Poisoning, Undetermined	Adverse effect	Underdosing
Tetrachloroethane — *Continued*						
paint or varnish	T53.6X1	T53.6X2	T53.6X3	T53.6X4	—	—
Tetrachloroethylene (liquid)	T53.3X1	T53.3X2	T53.3X3	T53.3X4		
medicinal	T37.4X1	T37.4X2	T37.4X3	T37.4X4	T37.4X5	T37.4X6
vapor	T53.3X1	T53.3X2	T53.3X3	T53.3X4		
Tetrachloromethane— see Carbon tetrachloride						
Tetracosactide	T38.811	T38.812	T38.813	T38.814	T38.815	T38.816
Tetracosactrin	T38.811	T38.812	T38.813	T38.814	T38.815	T38.816
Tetracycline	T36.4X1	T36.4X2	T36.4X3	T36.4X4	T36.4X5	T36.4X6
ophthalmic preparation	T49.5X1	T49.5X2	T49.5X3	T49.5X4	T49.5X5	T49.5X6
topical NEC	T49.0X1	T49.0X2	T49.0X3	T49.0X4	T49.0X5	T49.0X6
Tetradifon	T60.8X1	T60.8X2	T60.8X3	T60.8X4	—	—
Tetradotoxin	T61.771	T61.772	T61.773	T61.774	—	—
Tetraethyl						
lead	T56.0X1	T56.0X2	T56.0X3	T56.0X4		
pyrophosphate	T60.0X1	T60.0X2	T60.0X3	T60.0X4	—	—
Tetraethylammonium chloride	T44.2X1	T44.2X2	T44.2X3	T44.2X4	T44.2X5	T44.2X6
Tetraethylthiuram disulfide	T50.6X1	T50.6X2	T50.6X3	T50.6X4	T50.6X5	T50.6X6
Tetrahydroamino-acridine	T44.0X1	T44.0X2	T44.0X3	T44.0X4	T44.0X5	T44.0X6
Tetrahydrocannabinol	T40.7X1	T40.7X2	T40.7X3	T40.7X4	T40.7X5	T40.7X6
Tetrahydrofuran	T52.8X1	T52.8X2	T52.8X3	T52.8X4	—	—
Tetrahydronaphthalene	T52.8X1	T52.8X2	T52.8X3	T52.8X4	—	—
Tetrahydrozoline	T49.5X1	T49.5X2	T49.5X3	T49.5X4	T49.5X5	T49.5X6
Tetralin	T52.8X1	T52.8X2	T52.8X3	T52.8X4	—	—
Tetramethrin	T60.2X1	T60.2X2	T60.2X3	T60.2X4		
Tetramethylthiuram (disulfide) NEC	T60.3X1	T60.3X2	T60.3X3	T60.3X4		
medicinal	T49.0X1	T49.0X2	T49.0X3	T49.0X4	T49.0X5	T49.0X6
Tetramisole	T37.4X1	T37.4X2	T37.4X3	T37.4X4	T37.4X5	T37.4X6
Tetranicotinoyl fructose	T46.7X1	T46.7X2	T46.7X3	T46.7X4	T46.7X5	T46.7X6
Tetrazepam	T42.4X1	T42.4X2	T42.4X3	T42.4X4	T42.4X5	T42.4X6
Tetronal	T42.6X1	T42.6X2	T42.6X3	T42.6X4	T42.6X5	T42.6X6
Tetryl	T65.3X1	T65.3X2	T65.3X3	T65.3X4	—	—
Tetrylammonium chloride	T44.2X1	T44.2X2	T44.2X3	T44.2X4	T44.2X5	T44.2X6
Tetryzoline	T49.5X1	T49.5X2	T49.5X3	T49.5X4	T49.5X5	T49.5X6
Thalidomide	T45.1X1	T45.1X2	T45.1X3	T45.1X4	T45.1X5	T45.1X6
Thallium (compounds) (dust) NEC	T56.811	T56.812	T56.813	T56.814	—	—
pesticide	T60.4X1	T60.4X2	T60.4X3	T60.4X4	—	—
THC	T40.7X1	T40.7X2	T40.7X3	T40.7X4	T40.7X5	T40.7X6
Thebacon	T48.3X1	T48.3X2	T48.3X3	T48.3X4	T48.3X5	T48.3X6
Thebaine	T40.2X1	T40.2X2	T40.2X3	T40.2X4	T40.2X5	T40.2X6
Thenoic acid	T49.6X1	T49.6X2	T49.6X3	T49.6X4	T49.6X5	T49.6X6
Thenyldiamine	T45.0X1	T45.0X2	T45.0X3	T45.0X4	T45.0X5	T45.0X6

Substance	Poisoning, Accidental (unintentional)	Poisoning, Intentional self-harm	Poisoning, Assault	Poisoning, Undetermined	Adverse effect	Underdosing
Theobromine (calcium salicylate)	T48.6X1	T48.6X2	T48.6X3	T48.6X4	T48.6X5	T48.6X6
sodium salicylate	T48.6X1	T48.6X2	T48.6X3	T48.6X4	T48.6X5	T48.6X6
Theophyllamine	T48.6X1	T48.6X2	T48.6X3	T48.6X4	T48.6X5	T48.6X6
Theophylline	T48.6X1	T48.6X2	T48.6X3	T48.6X4	T48.6X5	T48.6X6
aminobenzoic acid	T48.6X1	T48.6X2	T48.6X3	T48.6X4	T48.6X5	T48.6X6
ethylenediamine	T48.6X1	T48.6X2	T48.6X3	T48.6X4	T48.6X5	T48.6X6
piperazine p-amino-benzoate	T48.6X1	T48.6X2	T48.6X3	T48.6X4	T48.6X5	T48.6X6
Thiabendazole	T37.4X1	T37.4X2	T37.4X3	T37.4X4	T37.4X5	T37.4X6
Thialbarbital	T41.1X1	T41.1X2	T41.1X3	T41.1X4	T41.1X5	T41.1X6
Thiamazole	T38.2X1	T38.2X2	T38.2X3	T38.2X4	T38.2X5	T38.2X6
Thiambutosine	T37.1X1	T37.1X2	T37.1X3	T37.1X4	T37.1X5	T37.1X6
Thiamine	T45.2X1	T45.2X2	T45.2X3	T45.2X4	T45.2X5	T45.2X6
Thiamphenicol	T36.2X1	T36.2X2	T36.2X3	T36.2X4	T36.2X5	T36.2X6
Thiamylal	T41.1X1	T41.1X2	T41.1X3	T41.1X4	T41.1X5	T41.1X6
sodium	T41.1X1	T41.1X2	T41.1X3	T41.1X4	T41.1X5	T41.1X6
Thiazesim	T43.291	T43.292	T43.293	T43.294	T43.295	T43.296
Thiazides (diuretics)	T50.2X1	T50.2X2	T50.2X3	T50.2X4	T50.2X5	T50.2X6
Thiazinamium metilsulfate	T43.3X1	T43.3X2	T43.3X3	T43.3X4	T43.3X5	T43.3X6
Thiethylperazine	T43.3X1	T43.3X2	T43.3X3	T43.3X4	T43.3X5	T43.3X6
Thimerosal	T49.0X1	T49.0X2	T49.0X3	T49.0X4	T49.0X5	T49.0X6
ophthalmic preparation	T49.5X1	T49.5X2	T49.5X3	T49.5X4	T49.5X5	T49.5X6
Thioacetazone	T37.1X1	T37.1X2	T37.1X3	T37.1X4	T37.1X5	T37.1X6
with isoniazid	T37.1X1	T37.1X2	T37.1X3	T37.1X4	T37.1X5	T37.1X6
Thiobarbital sodium	T41.1X1	T41.1X2	T41.1X3	T41.1X4	T41.1X5	T41.1X6
Thiobarbiturate anesthetic	T41.1X1	T41.1X2	T41.1X3	T41.1X4	T41.1X5	T41.1X6
Thiobismol	T37.8X1	T37.8X2	T37.8X3	T37.8X4	T37.8X5	T37.8X6
Thiobutabarbital sodium	T41.1X1	T41.1X2	T41.1X3	T41.1X4	T41.1X5	T41.1X6
Thiocarbamate (insecticide)	T60.0X1	T60.0X2	T60.0X3	T60.0X4	—	—
Thiocarbamide	T38.2X1	T38.2X2	T38.2X3	T38.2X4	T38.2X5	T38.2X6
Thiocarbarsone	T37.8X1	T37.8X2	T37.8X3	T37.8X4	T37.8X5	T37.8X6
Thiocarlide	T37.1X1	T37.1X2	T37.1X3	T37.1X4	T37.1X5	T37.1X6
Thioctamide	T50.991	T50.992	T50.993	T50.994	T50.995	T50.996
Thioctic acid	T50.991	T50.992	T50.993	T50.994	T50.995	T50.996
Thiofos	T60.0X1	T60.0X2	T60.0X3	T60.0X4	—	—
Thioglycolate	T49.4X1	T49.4X2	T49.4X3	T49.4X4	T49.4X5	T49.4X6
Thioglycolic acid	T65.891	T65.892	T65.893	T65.894	—	—
Thioguanine	T45.1X1	T45.1X2	T45.1X3	T45.1X4	T45.1X5	T45.1X6
Thiomercaptomerin	T50.2X1	T50.2X2	T50.2X3	T50.2X4	T50.2X5	T50.2X6
Thiomerin	T50.2X1	T50.2X2	T50.2X3	T50.2X4	T50.2X5	T50.2X6
Thiomersal	T49.0X1	T49.0X2	T49.0X3	T49.0X4	T49.0X5	T49.0X6
Thionazin	T60.0X1	T60.0X2	T60.0X3	T60.0X4	—	—
Thiopental (sodium)	T41.1X1	T41.1X2	T41.1X3	T41.1X4	T41.1X5	T41.1X6
Thiopentone (sodium)	T41.1X1	T41.1X2	T41.1X3	T41.1X4	T41.1X5	T41.1X6
Thiopropazate	T43.3X1	T43.3X2	T43.3X3	T43.3X4	T43.3X5	T43.3X6
Thioproperazine	T43.3X1	T43.3X2	T43.3X3	T43.3X4	T43.3X5	T43.3X6

Substance	Poisoning, Accidental (unintentional)	Poisoning, Intentional self-harm	Poisoning, Assault	Poisoning, Undetermined	Adverse effect	Underdosing
Thioridazine	T43.3X1	T43.3X2	T43.3X3	T43.3X4	T43.3X5	T43.3X6
Thiosinamine	T49.3X1	T49.3X2	T49.3X3	T49.3X4	T49.3X5	T49.3X6
Thiotepa	T45.1X1	T45.1X2	T45.1X3	T45.1X4	T45.1X5	T45.1X6
Thiothixene	T43.4X1	T43.4X2	T43.4X3	T43.4X4	T43.4X5	T43.4X6
Thiouracil (benzyl) (methyl) (propyl)	T38.2X1	T38.2X2	T38.2X3	T38.2X4	T38.2X5	T38.2X6
Thiourea	T38.2X1	T38.2X2	T38.2X3	T38.2X4	T38.2X5	T38.2X6
Thiphenamil	T44.3X1	T44.3X2	T44.3X3	T44.3X4	T44.3X5	T44.3X6
Thiram	T60.3X1	T60.3X2	T60.3X3	T60.3X4	—	—
medicinal	T49.2X1	T49.2X2	T49.2X3	T49.2X4	T49.2X5	T49.2X6
Thonzylamine (systemic)	T45.0X1	T45.0X2	T45.0X3	T45.0X4	T45.0X5	T45.0X6
mucosal decongestant	T48.5X1	T48.5X2	T48.5X3	T48.5X4	T48.5X5	T48.5X6
Thorazine	T43.3X1	T43.3X2	T43.3X3	T43.3X4	T43.3X5	T43.3X6
Thorium dioxide suspension	T50.8X1	T50.8X2	T50.8X3	T50.8X4	T50.8X5	T50.8X6
Thornapple	T62.2X1	T62.2X2	T62.2X3	T62.2X4	—	—
Throat drug NEC	T49.6X1	T49.6X2	T49.6X3	T49.6X4	T49.6X5	T49.6X6
Thrombin	T45.7X1	T45.7X2	T45.7X3	T45.7X4	T45.7X5	T45.7X6
Thrombolysin	T45.611	T45.612	T45.613	T45.614	T45.615	T45.616
Thromboplastin	T45.7X1	T45.7X2	T45.7X3	T45.7X4	T45.7X5	T45.7X6
Thurfyl nicotinate	T46.7X1	T46.7X2	T46.7X3	T46.7X4	T46.7X5	T46.7X6
Thymol	T49.0X1	T49.0X2	T49.0X3	T49.0X4	T49.0X5	T49.0X6
Thymopentin	T37.5X1	T37.5X2	T37.5X3	T37.5X4	T37.5X5	T37.5X6
Thymoxamine	T46.7X1	T46.7X2	T46.7X3	T46.7X4	T46.7X5	T46.7X6
Thymus extract	T38.891	T38.892	T38.893	T38.894	T38.895	T38.896
Thyreotrophic hormone	T38.811	T38.812	T38.813	T38.814	T38.815	T38.816
Thyroglobulin	T38.1X1	T38.1X2	T38.1X3	T38.1X4	T38.1X5	T38.1X6
Thyroid (hormone)	T38.1X1	T38.1X2	T38.1X3	T38.1X4	T38.1X5	T38.1X6
Thyrolar	T38.1X1	T38.1X2	T38.1X3	T38.1X4	T38.1X5	T38.1X6
Thyrotrophin	T38.811	T38.812	T38.813	T38.814	T38.815	T38.816
Thyrotropic hormone	T38.811	T38.812	T38.813	T38.814	T38.815	T38.816
Thyroxine	T38.1X1	T38.1X2	T38.1X3	T38.1X4	T38.1X5	T38.1X6
Tiabendazole	T37.4X1	T37.4X2	T37.4X3	T37.4X4	T37.4X5	T37.4X6
Tiamizide	T50.2X1	T50.2X2	T50.2X3	T50.2X4	T50.2X5	T50.2X6
Tianeptine	T43.291	T43.292	T43.293	T43.294	T43.295	T43.296
Tiapamil	T46.1X1	T46.1X2	T46.1X3	T46.1X4	T46.1X5	T46.1X6
Tiapride	T43.591	T43.592	T43.593	T43.594	T43.595	T43.596
Tiaprofenic acid	T39.311	T39.312	T39.313	T39.314	T39.315	T39.316
Tiaramide	T39.8X1	T39.8X2	T39.8X3	T39.8X4	T39.8X5	T39.8X6
Ticarcillin	T36.0X1	T36.0X2	T36.0X3	T36.0X4	T36.0X5	T36.0X6
Ticlatone	T49.0X1	T49.0X2	T49.0X3	T49.0X4	T49.0X5	T49.0X6
Ticlopidine	T45.521	T45.522	T45.523	T45.524	T45.525	T45.526
Ticrynafen	T50.1X1	T50.1X2	T50.1X3	T50.1X4	T50.1X5	T50.1X6
Tidiacic	T50.991	T50.992	T50.993	T50.994	T50.995	T50.996
Tiemonium	T44.3X1	T44.3X2	T44.3X3	T44.3X4	T44.3X5	T44.3X6
iodide	T44.3X1	T44.3X2	T44.3X3	T44.3X4	T44.3X5	T44.3X6
Tienilic acid	T50.1X1	T50.1X2	T50.1X3	T50.1X4	T50.1X5	T50.1X6
Tifenamil	T44.3X1	T44.3X2	T44.3X3	T44.3X4	T44.3X5	T44.3X6
Tigan	T45.0X1	T45.0X2	T45.0X3	T45.0X4	T45.0X5	T45.0X6
Tigloidine	T44.3X1	T44.3X2	T44.3X3	T44.3X4	T44.3X5	T44.3X6

Substance	Poisoning, Accidental (unintentional)	Poisoning, Intentional self-harm	Poisoning, Assault	Poisoning, Undetermined	Adverse effect	Underdosing
Tilactase	T47.5X1	T47.5X2	T47.5X3	T47.5X4	T47.5X5	T47.5X6
Tiletamine	T41.291	T41.292	T41.293	T41.294	T41.295	T41.296
Tilidine	T40.491	T40.492	T40.493	T40.494	—	—
Timepidium bromide	T44.3X1	T44.3X2	T44.3X3	T44.3X4	T44.3X5	T44.3X6
Timiperone	T43.4X1	T43.4X2	T43.4X3	T43.4X4	T43.4X5	T43.4X6
Timolol	T44.7X1	T44.7X2	T44.7X3	T44.7X4	T44.7X5	T44.7X6
Tin (chloride) (dust) (oxide) NEC	T56.6X1	T56.6X2	T56.6X3	T56.6X4		
anti-infectives	T37.8X1	T37.8X2	T37.8X3	T37.8X4	T37.8X5	T37.8X6
Tincture, iodine—see Iodine						
Tindal	T43.3X1	T43.3X2	T43.3X3	T43.3X4	T43.3X5	T43.3X6
Tinidazole	T37.3X1	T37.3X2	T37.3X3	T37.3X4	T37.3X5	T37.3X6
Tinoridine	T39.8X1	T39.8X2	T39.8X3	T39.8X4	T39.8X5	T39.8X6
Tiocarlide	T37.1X1	T37.1X2	T37.1X3	T37.1X4	T37.1X5	T37.1X6
Tioclomarol	T45.511	T45.512	T45.513	T45.514	T45.515	T45.516
Tioconazole	T49.0X1	T49.0X2	T49.0X3	T49.0X4	T49.0X5	T49.0X6
Tioguanine	T45.1X1	T45.1X2	T45.1X3	T45.1X4	T45.1X5	T45.1X6
Tiopronin	T50.991	T50.992	T50.993	T50.994	T50.995	T50.996
Tiotixene	T43.4X1	T43.4X2	T43.4X3	T43.4X4	T43.4X5	T43.4X6
Tioxolone	T49.4X1	T49.4X2	T49.4X3	T49.4X4	T49.4X5	T49.4X6
Tipepidine	T48.3X1	T48.3X2	T48.3X3	T48.3X4	T48.3X5	T48.3X6
Tiquizium bromide	T44.3X1	T44.3X2	T44.3X3	T44.3X4	T44.3X5	T44.3X6
Tiratricol	T38.1X1	T38.1X2	T38.1X3	T38.1X4	T38.1X5	T38.1X6
Tisopurine	T50.4X1	T50.4X2	T50.4X3	T50.4X4	T50.4X5	T50.4X6
Titanium (compounds) (vapor)	T56.891	T56.892	T56.893	T56.894	—	—
dioxide	T49.3X1	T49.3X2	T49.3X3	T49.3X4	T49.3X5	T49.3X6
ointment	T49.3X1	T49.3X2	T49.3X3	T49.3X4	T49.3X5	T49.3X6
oxide	T49.3X1	T49.3X2	T49.3X3	T49.3X4	T49.3X5	T49.3X6
tetrachloride	T56.891	T56.892	T56.893	T56.894	—	—
Titanocene	T56.891	T56.892	T56.893	T56.894	—	—
Titroid	T38.1X1	T38.1X2	T38.1X3	T38.1X4	T38.1X5	T38.1X6
Tizanidine	T42.8X1	T42.8X2	T42.8X3	T42.8X4	T42.8X5	T42.8X6
TMTD	T60.3X1	T60.3X2	T60.3X3	T60.3X4	—	—
TNT (fumes)	T65.3X1	T65.3X2	T65.3X3	T65.3X4	—	—
Toadstool	T62.0X1	T62.0X2	T62.0X3	T62.0X4	—	—
Tobacco NEC	T65.291	T65.292	T65.293	T65.294	—	—
cigarettes	T65.221	T65.222	T65.223	T65.224	—	—
Indian	T62.2X1	T62.2X2	T62.2X3	T62.2X4	—	—
smoke, second-hand	T65.221	T65.222	T65.223	T65.224	—	—
Tobramycin	T36.5X1	T36.5X2	T36.5X3	T36.5X4	T36.5X5	T36.5X6
Tocainide	T46.2X1	T46.2X2	T46.2X3	T46.2X4	T46.2X5	T46.2X6
Tocoferol	T45.2X1	T45.2X2	T45.2X3	T45.2X4	T45.2X5	T45.2X6
Tocopherol	T45.2X1	T45.2X2	T45.2X3	T45.2X4	T45.2X5	T45.2X6
acetate	T45.2X1	T45.2X2	T45.2X3	T45.2X4	T45.2X5	T45.2X6
Tocosamine	T48.0X1	T48.0X2	T48.0X3	T48.0X4	T48.0X5	T48.0X6
Todralazine	T46.5X1	T46.5X2	T46.5X3	T46.5X4	T46.5X5	T46.5X6
Tofisopam	T42.4X1	T42.4X2	T42.4X3	T42.4X4	T42.4X5	T42.4X6
Tofranil	T43.011	T43.012	T43.013	T43.014	T43.015	T43.016
Toilet deodorizer	T65.891	T65.892	T65.893	T65.894	—	—

Substance	Poisoning, Accidental (unintentional)	Poisoning, Intentional self-harm	Poisoning, Assault	Poisoning, Undetermined	Adverse effect	Underdosing
Tolamolol	T44.7X1	T44.7X2	T44.7X3	T44.7X4	T44.7X5	T44.7X6
Tolazamide	T38.3X1	T38.3X2	T38.3X3	T38.3X4	T38.3X5	T38.3X6
Tolazoline	T46.7X1	T46.7X2	T46.7X3	T46.7X4	T46.7X5	T46.7X6
Tolbutamide (sodium)	T38.3X1	T38.3X2	T38.3X3	T38.3X4	T38.3X5	T38.3X6
Tolciclate	T49.0X1	T49.0X2	T49.0X3	T49.0X4	T49.0X5	T49.0X6
Tolmetin	T39.391	T39.392	T39.393	T39.394	T39.395	T39.396
Tolnaftate	T49.0X1	T49.0X2	T49.0X3	T49.0X4	T49.0X5	T49.0X6
Tolonidine	T46.5X1	T46.5X2	T46.5X3	T46.5X4	T46.5X5	T46.5X6
Toloxatone	T42.6X1	T42.6X2	T42.6X3	T42.6X4	T42.6X5	T42.6X6
Tolperisone	T44.3X1	T44.3X2	T44.3X3	T44.3X4	T44.3X5	T44.3X6
Tolserol	T42.8X1	T42.8X2	T42.8X3	T42.8X4	T42.8X5	T42.8X6
Toluene (liquid)	T52.2X1	T52.2X2	T52.2X3	T52.2X4	—	—
diisocyanate	T65.0X1	T65.0X2	T65.0X3	T65.0X4	—	—
Toluidine	T65.891	T65.892	T65.893	T65.894	—	—
vapor	T59.891	T59.892	T59.893	T59.894	—	—
Toluol (liquid)	T52.2X1	T52.2X2	T52.2X3	T52.2X4	—	—
vapor	T52.2X1	T52.2X2	T52.2X3	T52.2X4	—	—
Toluylenediamine	T65.3X1	T65.3X2	T65.3X3	T65.3X4	—	—
Tolylene-2,4-diisocyanate	T65.0X1	T65.0X2	T65.0X3	T65.0X4	—	—
Tonic NEC	T50.901	T50.902	T50.903	T50.904	T50.905	T50.906
Topical action drug NEC	T49.91	T49.92	T49.93	T49.94	T49.95	T49.96
ear, nose or throat	T49.6X1	T49.6X2	T49.6X3	T49.6X4	T49.6X5	T49.6X6
eye	T49.5X1	T49.5X2	T49.5X3	T49.5X4	T49.5X5	T49.5X6
skin	T49.91	T49.92	T49.93	T49.94	T49.95	T49.96
specified NEC	T49.8X1	T49.8X2	T49.8X3	T49.8X4	T49.8X5	T49.8X6
Toquizine	T44.3X1	T44.3X2	T44.3X3	T44.3X4	T44.3X5	T44.3X6
Toremifene	T38.6X1	T38.6X2	T38.6X3	T38.6X4	T38.6X5	T38.6X6
Tosylchloramide sodium	T49.8X1	T49.8X2	T49.8X3	T49.8X4	T49.8X5	T49.8X6
Toxaphene (dust) (spray)	T60.1X1	T60.1X2	T60.1X3	T60.1X4	—	—
Toxin, diphtheria (Schick Test)	T50.8X1	T50.8X2	T50.8X3	T50.8X4	T50.8X5	T50.8X6
Toxoid						
combined	T50.A21	T50.A22	T50.A23	T50.A24	T50.A25	T50.A26
diphtheria	T50.A91	T50.A92	T50.A93	T50.A94	T50.A95	T50.A96
tetanus	T50.A91	T50.A92	T50.A93	T50.A94	T50.A95	T50.A96
Trace element NEC	T45.8X1	T45.8X2	T45.8X3	T45.8X4	T45.8X5	T45.8X6
Tractor fuel NEC	T52.0X1	T52.0X2	T52.0X3	T52.0X4	—	—
Tragacanth	T50.991	T50.992	T50.993	T50.994	T50.995	T50.996
Tramadol	T40.421	T40.422	T40.423	T40.424	T40.425	T40.426
Tramazoline	T48.5X1	T48.5X2	T48.5X3	T48.5X4	T48.5X5	T48.5X6
Tranexamic acid	T45.621	T45.622	T45.623	T45.624	T45.625	T45.626
Tranilast	T45.0X1	T45.0X2	T45.0X3	T45.0X4	T45.0X5	T45.0X6
Tranquilizer NEC	T43.501	T43.502	T43.503	T43.504	T43.505	T43.506
with hypnotic or sedative	T42.6X1	T42.6X2	T42.6X3	T42.6X4	T42.6X5	T42.6X6
benzodiazepine NEC	T42.4X1	T42.4X2	T42.4X3	T42.4X4	T42.4X5	T42.4X6
butyrophenone NEC	T43.4X1	T43.4X2	T43.4X3	T43.4X4	T43.4X5	T43.4X6
carbamate	T43.591	T43.592	T43.593	T43.594	T43.595	T43.596
dimethylamine	T43.3X1	T43.3X2	T43.3X3	T43.3X4	T43.3X5	T43.3X6
ethylamine	T43.3X1	T43.3X2	T43.3X3	T43.3X4	T43.3X5	T43.3X6

Substance	Poisoning, Accidental (unintentional)	Poisoning, Intentional self-harm	Poisoning, Assault	Poisoning, Undetermined	Adverse effect	Underdosing
Tranquilizer NEC — Continued						
hydroxyzine	T43.591	T43.592	T43.593	T43.594	T43.595	T43.596
major NEC	T43.501	T43.502	T43.503	T43.504	T43.505	T43.506
penothiazine NEC	T43.3X1	T43.3X2	T43.3X3	T43.3X4	T43.3X5	T43.3X6
phenothiazine-based	T43.3X1	T43.3X2	T43.3X3	T43.3X4	T43.3X5	T43.3X6
piperazine NEC	T43.3X1	T43.3X2	T43.3X3	T43.3X4	T43.3X5	T43.3X6
piperidine	T43.3X1	T43.3X2	T43.3X3	T43.3X4	T43.3X5	T43.3X6
propylamine	T43.3X1	T43.3X2	T43.3X3	T43.3X4	T43.3X5	T43.3X6
specified NEC	T43.591	T43.592	T43.593	T43.594	T43.595	T43.596
thioxanthene NEC	T43.591	T43.592	T43.593	T43.594	T43.595	T43.596
Tranxene	T42.4X1	T42.4X2	T42.4X3	T42.4X4	T42.4X5	T42.4X6
Tranylcypromine	T43.1X1	T43.1X2	T43.1X3	T43.1X4	T43.1X5	T43.1X6
Trapidil	T46.3X1	T46.3X2	T46.3X3	T46.3X4	T46.3X5	T46.3X6
Trasentine	T44.3X1	T44.3X2	T44.3X3	T44.3X4	T44.3X5	T44.3X6
Travert	T50.3X1	T50.3X2	T50.3X3	T50.3X4	T50.3X5	T50.3X6
Trazodone	T43.211	T43.212	T43.213	T43.214	T43.215	T43.216
Trecator	T37.1X1	T37.1X2	T37.1X3	T37.1X4	T37.1X5	T37.1X6
Treosulfan	T45.1X1	T45.1X2	T45.1X3	T45.1X4	T45.1X5	T45.1X6
Tretamine	T45.1X1	T45.1X2	T45.1X3	T45.1X4	T45.1X5	T45.1X6
Tretinoin	T49.0X1	T49.0X2	T49.0X3	T49.0X4	T49.0X5	T49.0X6
Tretoquinol	T48.6X1	T48.6X2	T48.6X3	T48.6X4	T48.6X5	T48.6X6
Triacetin	T49.0X1	T49.0X2	T49.0X3	T49.0X4	T49.0X5	T49.0X6
Triacetoxyanthracene	T49.4X1	T49.4X2	T49.4X3	T49.4X4	T49.4X5	T49.4X6
Triacetyloleandomycin	T36.3X1	T36.3X2	T36.3X3	T36.3X4	T36.3X5	T36.3X6
Triamcinolone	T38.0X1	T38.0X2	T38.0X3	T38.0X4	T38.0X5	T38.0X6
ENT agent	T49.6X1	T49.6X2	T49.6X3	T49.6X4	T49.6X5	T49.6X6
hexacetonide	T49.0X1	T49.0X2	T49.0X3	T49.0X4	T49.0X5	T49.0X6
ophthalmic preparation	T49.5X1	T49.5X2	T49.5X3	T49.5X4	T49.5X5	T49.5X6
topical NEC	T49.0X1	T49.0X2	T49.0X3	T49.0X4	T49.0X5	T49.0X6
Triampyzine	T44.3X1	T44.3X2	T44.3X3	T44.3X4	T44.3X5	T44.3X6
Triamterene	T50.2X1	T50.2X2	T50.2X3	T50.2X4	T50.2X5	T50.2X6
Triazine (herbicide)	T60.3X1	T60.3X2	T60.3X3	T60.3X4	—	—
Triaziquone	T45.1X1	T45.1X2	T45.1X3	T45.1X4	T45.1X5	T45.1X6
Triazolam	T42.4X1	T42.4X2	T42.4X3	T42.4X4	T42.4X5	T42.4X6
Triazole (herbicide)	T60.3X1	T60.3X2	T60.3X3	T60.3X4	—	—
Tribenoside	T46.991	T46.992	T46.993	T46.994	T46.995	T46.996
Tribromacetaldehyde	T42.6X1	T42.6X2	T42.6X3	T42.6X4	T42.6X5	T42.6X6
Tribromoethanol, rectal	T41.291	T41.292	T41.293	T41.294	T41.295	T41.296
Tribromomethane	T42.6X1	T42.6X2	T42.6X3	T42.6X4	T42.6X5	T42.6X6
Trichlorethane	T53.2X1	T53.2X2	T53.2X3	T53.2X4	—	—
Trichlorethylene	T53.2X1	T53.2X2	T53.2X3	T53.2X4	—	—
Trichlorfon	T60.0X1	T60.0X2	T60.0X3	T60.0X4	—	—
Trichlormethiazide	T50.2X1	T50.2X2	T50.2X3	T50.2X4	T50.2X5	T50.2X6
Trichlormethine	T45.1X1	T45.1X2	T45.1X3	T45.1X4	T45.1X5	T45.1X6
Trichloroacetic acid, Trichloracetic acid	T54.2X1	T54.2X2	T54.2X3	T54.2X4	—	—
medicinal	T49.4X1	T49.4X2	T49.4X3	T49.4X4	T49.4X5	T49.4X6
Trichloroethane	T53.2X1	T53.2X2	T53.2X3	T53.2X4	—	—
Trichloroethanol	T42.6X1	T42.6X2	T42.6X3	T42.6X4	T42.6X5	T42.6X6

Substance	Poisoning, Accidental (unintentional)	Poisoning, Intentional self-harm	Poisoning, Assault	Poisoning, Undetermined	Adverse effect	Underdosing
Trichloroethyl phosphate	T42.6X1	T42.6X2	T42.6X3	T42.6X4	T42.6X5	T42.6X6
Trichloroethylene (liquid) (vapor)	T53.2X1	T53.2X2	T53.2X3	T53.2X4	—	—
anesthetic (gas)	T41.0X1	T41.0X2	T41.0X3	T41.0X4	T41.0X5	T41.0X6
vapor NEC	T53.2X1	T53.2X2	T53.2X3	T53.2X4	—	—
Trichlorofluoromethane NEC	T53.5X1	T53.5X2	T53.5X3	T53.5X4	—	—
Trichloronate	T60.0X1	T60.0X2	T60.0X3	T60.0X4	—	—
2,4,5-Trichlorophen-oxyacetic acid	T60.3X1	T60.3X2	T60.3X3	T60.3X4	—	—
Trichloropropane	T53.6X1	T53.6X2	T53.6X3	T53.6X4	—	—
Trichlorotriethylamine	T45.1X1	T45.1X2	T45.1X3	T45.1X4	T45.1X5	T45.1X6
Trichomonacides NEC	T37.3X1	T37.3X2	T37.3X3	T37.3X4	T37.3X5	T37.3X6
Trichomycin	T36.7X1	T36.7X2	T36.7X3	T36.7X4	T36.7X5	T36.7X6
Triclobisonium chloride	T49.0X1	T49.0X2	T49.0X3	T49.0X4	T49.0X5	T49.0X6
Triclocarban	T49.0X1	T49.0X2	T49.0X3	T49.0X4	T49.0X5	T49.0X6
Triclofos	T42.6X1	T42.6X2	T42.6X3	T42.6X4	T42.6X5	T42.6X6
Triclosan	T49.0X1	T49.0X2	T49.0X3	T49.0X4	T49.0X5	T49.0X6
Tricresyl phosphate	T65.891	T65.892	T65.893	T65.894	—	—
solvent	T52.91	T52.92	T52.93	T52.94	—	—
Tricyclamol chloride	T44.3X1	T44.3X2	T44.3X3	T44.3X4	T44.3X5	T44.3X6
Tridesilon	T49.0X1	T49.0X2	T49.0X3	T49.0X4	T49.0X5	T49.0X6
Tridihexethyl iodide	T44.3X1	T44.3X2	T44.3X3	T44.3X4	T44.3X5	T44.3X6
Tridione	T42.2X1	T42.2X2	T42.2X3	T42.2X4	T42.2X5	T42.2X6
Trientine	T45.8X1	T45.8X2	T45.8X3	T45.8X4	T45.8X5	T45.8X6
Triethanolamine NEC	T54.3X1	T54.3X2	T54.3X3	T54.3X4	—	—
detergent	T54.3X1	T54.3X2	T54.3X3	T54.3X4	—	—
trinitrate (biphosphate)	T46.3X1	T46.3X2	T46.3X3	T46.3X4	T46.3X5	T46.3X6
Triethanomelamine	T45.1X1	T45.1X2	T45.1X3	T45.1X4	T45.1X5	T45.1X6
Triethylenemelamine	T45.1X1	T45.1X2	T45.1X3	T45.1X4	T45.1X5	T45.1X6
Triethylenephos-phoramide	T45.1X1	T45.1X2	T45.1X3	T45.1X4	T45.1X5	T45.1X6
Triethylenethiophos-phoramide	T45.1X1	T45.1X2	T45.1X3	T45.1X4	T45.1X5	T45.1X6
Trifluoperazine	T43.3X1	T43.3X2	T43.3X3	T43.3X4	T43.3X5	T43.3X6
Trifluoroethyl vinyl ether	T41.0X1	T41.0X2	T41.0X3	T41.0X4	T41.0X5	T41.0X6
Trifluperidol	T43.4X1	T43.4X2	T43.4X3	T43.4X4	T43.4X5	T43.4X6
Triflupromazine	T43.3X1	T43.3X2	T43.3X3	T43.3X4	T43.3X5	T43.3X6
Trifluridine	T37.5X1	T37.5X2	T37.5X3	T37.5X4	T37.5X5	T37.5X6
Triflusal	T45.521	T45.522	T45.523	T45.524	T45.525	T45.526
Trihexyphenidyl	T44.3X1	T44.3X2	T44.3X3	T44.3X4	T44.3X5	T44.3X6
Triiodothyronine	T38.1X1	T38.1X2	T38.1X3	T38.1X4	T38.1X5	T38.1X6
Trilene	T41.0X1	T41.0X2	T41.0X3	T41.0X4	T41.0X5	T41.0X6
Trilostane	T38.991	T38.992	T38.993	T38.994	T38.995	T38.996
Trimebutine	T44.3X1	T44.3X2	T44.3X3	T44.3X4	T44.3X5	T44.3X6
Trimecaine	T41.3X1	T41.3X2	T41.3X3	T41.3X4	T41.3X5	T41.3X6
Trimeprazine (tartrate)	T44.3X1	T44.3X2	T44.3X3	T44.3X4	T44.3X5	T44.3X6
Trimetaphan camsilate	T44.2X1	T44.2X2	T44.2X3	T44.2X4	T44.2X5	T44.2X6
Trimetazidine	T46.7X1	T46.7X2	T46.7X3	T46.7X4	T46.7X5	T46.7X6
Trimethadione	T42.2X1	T42.2X2	T42.2X3	T42.2X4	T42.2X5	T42.2X6

Substance	Poisoning, Accidental (unintentional)	Poisoning, Intentional self-harm	Poisoning, Assault	Poisoning, Undetermined	Adverse effect	Underdosing
Trimethaphan	T44.2X1	T44.2X2	T44.2X3	T44.2X4	T44.2X5	T44.2X6
Trimethidinium	T44.2X1	T44.2X2	T44.2X3	T44.2X4	T44.2X5	T44.2X6
Trimethobenzamide	T45.0X1	T45.0X2	T45.0X3	T45.0X4	T45.0X5	T45.0X6
Trimethoprim	T37.8X1	T37.8X2	T37.8X3	T37.8X4	T37.8X5	T37.8X6
with sulfamethoxazole	T36.8X1	T36.8X2	T36.8X3	T36.8X4	T36.8X5	T36.8X6
Trimethylcarbinol	T51.3X1	T51.3X2	T51.3X3	T51.3X4	—	—
Trimethylpsoralen	T49.3X1	T49.3X2	T49.3X3	T49.3X4	T49.3X5	T49.3X6
Trimeton	T45.0X1	T45.0X2	T45.0X3	T45.0X4	T45.0X5	T45.0X6
Trimetrexate	T45.1X1	T45.1X2	T45.1X3	T45.1X4	T45.1X5	T45.1X6
Trimipramine	T43.011	T43.012	T43.013	T43.014	T43.015	T43.016
Trimustine	T45.1X1	T45.1X2	T45.1X3	T45.1X4	T45.1X5	T45.1X6
Trinitrine	T46.3X1	T46.3X2	T46.3X3	T46.3X4	T46.3X5	T46.3X6
Trinitrobenzol	T65.3X1	T65.3X2	T65.3X3	T65.3X4	—	—
Trinitrophenol	T65.3X1	T65.3X2	T65.3X3	T65.3X4	—	—
Trinitrotoluene (fumes)	T65.3X1	T65.3X2	T65.3X3	T65.3X4	—	—
Trional	T42.6X1	T42.6X2	T42.6X3	T42.6X4	T42.6X5	T42.6X6
Triorthocresyl phosphate	T65.891	T65.892	T65.893	T65.894	—	—
Trioxide of arsenic	T57.0X1	T57.0X2	T57.0X3	T57.0X4	—	—
Trioxysalen	T49.4X1	T49.4X2	T49.4X3	T49.4X4	T49.4X5	T49.4X6
Tripamide	T50.2X1	T50.2X2	T50.2X3	T50.2X4	T50.2X5	T50.2X6
Triparanol	T46.6X1	T46.6X2	T46.6X3	T46.6X4	T46.6X5	T46.6X6
Tripelennamine	T45.0X1	T45.0X2	T45.0X3	T45.0X4	T45.0X5	T45.0X6
Triperiden	T44.3X1	T44.3X2	T44.3X3	T44.3X4	T44.3X5	T44.3X6
Triperidol	T43.4X1	T43.4X2	T43.4X3	T43.4X4	T43.4X5	T43.4X6
Triphenylphosphate	T65.891	T65.892	T65.893	T65.894		
Triple						
bromides	T42.6X1	T42.6X2	T42.6X3	T42.6X4	T42.6X5	T42.6X6
carbonate	T47.1X1	T47.1X2	T47.1X3	T47.1X4	T47.1X5	T47.1X6
vaccine						
DPT	T50.A11	T50.A12	T50.A13	T50.A14	T50.A15	T50.A16
including pertussis	T50.A11	T50.A12	T50.A13	T50.A14	T50.A15	T50.A16
MMR	T50.B91	T50.B92	T50.B93	T50.B94	T50.B95	T50.B96
Triprolidine	T45.0X1	T45.0X2		T45.0X4	T45.0X5	T45.0X6
Trisodium hydrogen edetate	T50.6X1	T50.6X2	T50.6X3	T50.6X4	T50.6X5	T50.6X6
Trisoralen	T49.3X1	T49.3X2	T49.3X3	T49.3X4	T49.3X5	T49.3X6
Trisulfapyrimidines	T37.0X1	T37.0X2	T37.0X3	T37.0X4	T37.0X5	T37.0X6
Trithiozine	T44.3X1	T44.3X2	T44.3X3	T44.3X4	T44.3X5	T44.3X6
Tritiozine	T44.3X1	T44.3X2	T44.3X3	T44.3X4	T44.3X5	T44.3X6
Tritoqualine	T45.0X1	T45.0X2	T45.0X3	T45.0X4	T45.0X5	T45.0X6
Trofosfamide	T45.1X1	T45.1X2	T45.1X3	T45.1X4	T45.1X5	T45.1X6
Troleandomycin	T36.3X1	T36.3X2	T36.3X3	T36.3X4	T36.3X5	T36.3X6
Trolnitrate (phosphate)	T46.3X1	T46.3X2	T46.3X3	T46.3X4	T46.3X5	T46.3X6
Tromantadine	T37.5X1	T37.5X2	T37.5X3	T37.5X4	T37.5X5	T37.5X6
Trometamol	T50.2X1	T50.2X2	T50.2X3	T50.2X4	T50.2X5	T50.2X6
Tromethamine	T50.2X1	T50.2X2	T50.2X3	T50.2X4	T50.2X5	T50.2X6
Tronothane	T41.3X1	T41.3X2	T41.3X3	T41.3X4	T41.3X5	T41.3X6
Tropacine	T44.3X1	T44.3X2	T44.3X3	T44.3X4	T44.3X5	T44.3X6
Tropatepine	T44.3X1	T44.3X2	T44.3X3	T44.3X4	T44.3X5	T44.3X6

Substance	Poisoning, Accidental (unintentional)	Poisoning, Intentional self-harm	Poisoning, Assault	Poisoning, Undetermined	Adverse effect	Underdosing
Tropicamide	T44.3X1	T44.3X2	T44.3X3	T44.3X4	T44.3X5	T44.3X6
Trospium chloride	T44.3X1	T44.3X2	T44.3X3	T44.3X4	T44.3X5	T44.3X6
Troxerutin	T46.991	T46.992	T46.993	T46.994	T46.995	T46.996
Troxidone	T42.2X1	T42.2X2	T42.2X3	T42.2X4	T42.2X5	T42.2X6
Tryparsamide	T37.3X1	T37.3X2	T37.3X3	T37.3X4	T37.3X5	T37.3X6
Trypsin	T45.3X1	T45.3X2	T45.3X3	T45.3X4	T45.3X5	T45.3X6
Tryptizol	T43.011	T43.012	T43.013	T43.014	T43.015	T43.016
TSH	T38.811	T38.812	T38.813	T38.814	T38.815	T38.816
Tuaminoheptane	T48.5X1	T48.5X2	T48.5X3	T48.5X4	T48.5X5	T48.5X6
Tuberculin, purified protein derivative (PPD)	T50.8X1	T50.8X2	T50.8X3	T50.8X4	T50.8X5	T50.8X6
Tubocurare	T48.1X1	T48.1X2	T48.1X3	T48.1X4	T48.1X5	T48.1X6
Tubocurarine (chloride)	T48.1X1	T48.1X2	T48.1X3	T48.1X4	T48.1X5	T48.1X6
Tulobuterol	T48.6X1	T48.6X2	T48.6X3	T48.6X4	T48.6X5	T48.6X6
Turpentine (spirits of)	T52.8X1	T52.8X2	T52.8X3	T52.8X4	—	—
vapor	T52.8X1	T52.8X2	T52.8X3	T52.8X4	—	—
Tybamate	T43.591	T43.592	T43.593	T43.594	T43.595	T43.596
Tyloxapol	T48.4X1	T48.4X2	T48.4X3	T48.4X4	T48.4X5	T48.4X6
Tymazoline	T48.5X1	T48.5X2	T48.5X3	T48.5X4	T48.5X5	T48.5X6
Typhoid-paratyphoid vaccine	T50.A91	T50.A92	T50.A93	T50.A94	T50.A95	T50.A96
Typhus vaccine	T50.A91	T50.A92	T50.A93	T50.A94	T50.A95	T50.A96
Tyropanoate	T50.8X1	T50.8X2	T50.8X3	T50.8X4	T50.8X5	T50.8X6
Tyrothricin	T49.6X1	T49.6X2	T49.6X3	T49.6X4	T49.6X5	T49.6X6
ENT agent	T49.6X1	T49.6X2	T49.6X3	T49.6X4	T49.6X5	T49.6X6
ophthalmic preparation	T49.5X1	T49.5X2	T49.5X3	T49.5X4	T49.5X5	T49.5X6
U						
Ufenamate	T39.391	T39.392	T39.393	T39.394	T39.395	T39.396
Ultraviolet light protectant	T49.3X1	T49.3X2	T49.3X3	T49.3X4	T49.3X5	T49.3X6
Undecenoic acid	T49.0X1	T49.0X2	T49.0X3	T49.0X4	T49.0X5	T49.0X6
Undecoylium	T49.0X1	T49.0X2	T49.0X3	T49.0X4	T49.0X5	T49.0X6
Undecylenic acid (derivatives)	T49.0X1	T49.0X2	T49.0X3	T49.0X4	T49.0X5	T49.0X6
Unna's boot	T49.3X1	T49.3X2	T49.3X3	T49.3X4	T49.3X5	T49.3X6
Unsaturated fatty acid	T46.6X1	T46.6X2	T46.6X3	T46.6X4	T46.6X5	T46.6X6
Uracil mustard	T45.1X1	T45.1X2	T45.1X3	T45.1X4	T45.1X5	T45.1X6
Uramustine	T45.1X1	T45.1X2	T45.1X3	T45.1X4	T45.1X5	T45.1X6
Urapidil	T46.5X1	T46.5X2	T46.5X3	T46.5X4	T46.5X5	T46.5X6
Urari	T48.1X1	T48.1X2	T48.1X3	T48.1X4	T48.1X5	T48.1X6
Urate oxidase	T50.4X1	T50.4X2	T50.4X3	T50.4X4	T50.4X5	T50.4X6
Urea	T47.3X1	T47.3X2	T47.3X3	T47.3X4	T47.3X5	T47.3X6
peroxide	T49.0X1	T49.0X2	T49.0X3	T49.0X4	T49.0X5	T49.0X6
stibamine	T37.4X1	T37.4X2	T37.4X3	T37.4X4	T37.4X5	T37.4X6
topical	T49.8X1	T49.8X2	T49.8X3	T49.8X4	T49.8X5	T49.8X6
Urethane	T45.1X1	T45.1X2	T45.1X3	T45.1X4	T45.1X5	T45.1X6
Urginea (maritima) (scilla)—see Squill						
Uric acid metabolism drug NEC	T50.4X1	T50.4X2	T50.4X3	T50.4X4	T50.4X5	T50.4X6
Uricosuric agent	T50.4X1	T50.4X2	T50.4X3	T50.4X4	T50.4X5	T50.4X6
Urinary anti-infective	T37.8X1	T37.8X2	T37.8X3	T37.8X4	T37.8X5	T37.8X6

Substance	Poisoning, Accidental (unintentional)	Poisoning, Intentional self-harm	Poisoning, Assault	Poisoning, Undetermined	Adverse effect	Underdosing
Urofollitropin	T38.811	T38.812	T38.813	T38.814	T38.815	T38.816
Urokinase	T45.611	T45.612	T45.613	T45.614	T45.615	T45.616
Urokon	T50.8X1	T50.8X2	T50.8X3	T50.8X4	T50.8X5	T50.8X6
Ursodeoxycholic acid	T50.991	T50.992	T50.993	T50.994	T50.995	T50.996
Ursodiol	T50.991	T50.992	T50.993	T50.994	T50.995	T50.996
Urtica	T62.2X1	T62.2X2	T62.2X3	T62.2X4	—	—
Utility gas—see Gas, utility						
V						
Vaccine NEC	T50.Z91	T50.Z92	T50.Z93	T50.Z94	T50.Z95	T50.Z96
antineoplastic	T50.Z91	T50.Z92	T50.Z93	T50.Z94	T50.Z95	T50.Z96
bacterial NEC	T50.A91	T50.A92	T50.A93	T50.A94	T50.A95	T50.A96
with						
other bacterial component	T50.A21	T50.A22	T50.A23	T50.A24	T50.A25	T50.A26
pertussis component	T50.A11	T50.A12	T50.A13	T50.A14	T50.A15	T50.A16
viral-rickettsial component	T50.A21	T50.A22	T50.A23	T50.A24	T50.A25	T50.A26
mixed NEC	T50.A21	T50.A22	T50.A23	T50.A24	T50.A25	T50.A26
BCG	T50.A91	T50.A92	T50.A93	T50.A94	T50.A95	T50.A96
cholera	T50.A91	T50.A92	T50.A93	T50.A94	T50.A95	T50.A96
diphtheria	T50.A91	T50.A92	T50.A93	T50.A94	T50.A95	T50.A96
with tetanus	T50.A21	T50.A22	T50.A23	T50.A24	T50.A25	T50.A26
and pertussis	T50.A11	T50.A12	T50.A13	T50.A14	T50.A15	T50.A16
influenza	T50.B91	T50.B92	T50.B93	T50.B94	T50.B95	T50.B96
measles	T50.B91	T50.B92	T50.B93	T50.B94	T50.B95	T50.B96
with mumps and rubella	T50.B91	T50.B92	T50.B93	T50.B94	T50.B95	T50.B96
meningococcal	T50.A91	T50.A92	T50.A93	T50.A94	T50.A95	T50.A96
mumps	T50.B91	T50.B92	T50.B93	T50.B94	T50.B95	T50.B96
paratyphoid	T50.A91	T50.A92	T50.A93	T50.A94	T50.A95	T50.A96
pertussis	T50.A11	T50.A12	T50.A13	T50.A14	T50.A15	T50.A16
with diphtheria	T50.A11	T50.A12	T50.A13	T50.A14	T50.A15	T50.A16
and tetanus	T50.A11	T50.A12	T50.A13	T50.A14	T50.A15	T50.A16
with other component	T50.A11	T50.A12	T50.A13	T50.A14	T50.A15	T50.A16
plague	T50.A91	T50.A92	T50.A93	T50.A94	T50.A95	T50.A96
poliomyelitis	T50.B91	T50.B92	T50.B93	T50.B94	T50.B95	T50.B96
poliovirus	T50.B91	T50.B92	T50.B93	T50.B94	T50.B95	T50.B96
rabies	T50.B91	T50.B92	T50.B93	T50.B94	T50.B95	T50.B96
respiratory syncytial virus	T50.B91	T50.B92	T50.B93	T50.B94	T50.B95	T50.B96
rickettsial NEC	T50.A91	T50.A92	T50.A93	T50.A94	T50.A95	T50.A96
with						
bacterial component	T50.A21	T50.A22	T50.A23	T50.A24	T50.A25	T50.A26
Rocky Mountain spotted fever	T50.A91	T50.A92	T50.A93	T50.A94	T50.A95	T50.A96
rubella	T50.B91	T50.B92	T50.B93	T50.B94	T50.B95	T50.B96
sabin oral	T50.B91	T50.B92	T50.B93	T50.B94	T50.B95	T50.B96
smallpox	T50.B11	T50.B12	T50.B13	T50.B14	T50.B15	T50.B16
TAB	T50.A91	T50.A92	T50.A93	T50.A94	T50.A95	T50.A96
tetanus	T50.A91	T50.A92	T50.A93	T50.A94	T50.A95	T50.A96

Substance	Poisoning, Accidental (unintentional)	Poisoning, Intentional self-harm	Poisoning, Assault	Poisoning, Undetermined	Adverse effect	Underdosing
Vaccine NEC — *Continued*						
typhoid	T50.A91	T50.A92	T50.A93	T50.A94	T50.A95	T50.A96
typhus	T50.A91	T50.A92	T50.A93	T50.A94	T50.A95	T50.A96
viral NEC	T50.B91	T50.B92	T50.B93	T50.B94	T50.B95	T50.B96
yellow fever	T50.B91	T50.B92	T50.B93	T50.B94	T50.B95	T50.B96
Vaccinia immune globulin	T50.Z11	T50.Z12	T50.Z13	T50.Z14	T50.Z15	T50.Z16
Vaginal contraceptives	T49.8X1	T49.8X2	T49.8X3	T49.8X4	T49.8X5	T49.8X6
Valerian						
root	T42.6X1	T42.6X2	T42.6X3	T42.6X4	T42.6X5	T42.6X6
tincture	T42.6X1	T42.6X2	T42.6X3	T42.6X4	T42.6X5	T42.6X6
Valethamate bromide	T44.3X1	T44.3X2	T44.3X3	T44.3X4	T44.3X5	T44.3X6
Valisone	T49.0X1	T49.0X2	T49.0X3	T49.0X4	T49.0X5	T49.0X6
Valium	T42.4X1	T42.4X2	T42.4X3	T42.4X4	T42.4X5	T42.4X6
Valmid	T42.6X1	T42.6X2	T42.6X3	T42.6X4	T42.6X5	T42.6X6
Valnoctamide	T42.6X1	T42.6X2	T42.6X3	T42.6X4	T42.6X5	T42.6X6
Valproate (sodium)	T42.6X1	T42.6X2	T42.6X3	T42.6X4	T42.6X5	T42.6X6
Valproic acid	T42.6X1	T42.6X2	T42.6X3	T42.6X4	T42.6X5	T42.6X6
Valpromide	T42.6X1	T42.6X2	T42.6X3	T42.6X4	T42.6X5	T42.6X6
Vanadium	T56.891	T56.892	T56.893	T56.894	—	—
Vancomycin	T36.8X1	T36.8X2	T36.8X3	T36.8X4	T36.8X5	T36.8X6
Vapor—see also Gas	T59.91	T59.92	T59.93	T59.94		
kiln (carbon monoxide)	T58.8X1	T58.8X2	T58.8X3	T58.8X4	—	—
lead—see lead						
specified source NEC	T59.891	T59.892	T59.893	T59.894	—	—
Vardenafil	T46.7X1	T46.7X2	T46.7X3	T46.7X4	T46.7X5	T46.7X6
Varicose reduction drug	T46.8X1	T46.8X2	T46.8X3	T46.8X4	T46.8X5	T46.8X6
Varnish	T65.4X1	T65.4X2	T65.4X3	T65.4X4	—	—
cleaner	T52.91	T52.92	T52.93	T52.94	—	—
Vaseline	T49.3X1	T49.3X2	T49.3X3	T49.3X4	T49.3X5	T49.3X6
Vasodilan	T46.7X1	T46.7X2	T46.7X3	T46.7X4	T46.7X5	T46.7X6
Vasodilator						
coronary NEC	T46.3X1	T46.3X2	T46.3X3	T46.3X4	T46.3X5	T46.3X6
peripheral NEC	T46.7X1	T46.7X2	T46.7X3	T46.7X4	T46.7X5	T46.7X6
Vasopressin	T38.891	T38.892	T38.893	T38.894	T38.895	T38.896
Vasopressor drugs	T38.891	T38.892	T38.893	T38.894	T38.895	T38.896
Vecuronium bromide	T48.1X1	T48.1X2	T48.1X3	T48.1X4	T48.1X5	T48.1X6
Vegetable extract, astringent	T49.2X1	T49.2X2	T49.2X3	T49.2X4	T49.2X5	T49.2X6
Venlafaxine	T43.211	T43.212	T43.213	T43.214	T43.215	T43.216
Venom, venomous (bite) (sting)	T63.91	T63.92	T63.93	T63.94	—	—
amphibian NEC	T63.831	T63.832	T63.833	T63.834		
animal NEC	T63.891	T63.892	T63.893	T63.894		
ant	T63.421	T63.422	T63.423	T63.424		
arthropod NEC	T63.481	T63.482	T63.483	T63.484		
bee	T63.441	T63.442	T63.443	T63.444		
centipede	T63.411	T63.412	T63.413	T63.414		
fish	T63.591	T63.592	T63.593	T63.594		
frog	T63.811	T63.812	T63.813	T63.814	—	—

Substance	Poisoning, Accidental (unintentional)	Poisoning, Intentional self-harm	Poisoning, Assault	Poisoning, Undetermined	Adverse effect	Underdosing
Venom, venomous — *Continued*						
hornet	T63.451	T63.452	T63.453	T63.454	—	—
insect NEC	T63.481	T63.482	T63.483	T63.484		
lizard	T63.121	T63.122	T63.123	T63.124		
marine						
animals	T63.691	T63.692	T63.693	T63.694	—	—
bluebottle	T63.611	T63.612	T63.613	T63.614		
jellyfish NEC	T63.621	T63.622	T63.623	T63.624		
Portegese Man-o-war	T63.611	T63.612	T63.613	T63.614		
sea anemone	T63.631	T63.632	T63.633	T63.634		
specified NEC	T63.691	T63.692	T63.693	T63.694		
fish	T63.591	T63.592	T63.593	T63.594		
plants	T63.711	T63.712	T63.713	T63.714		
sting ray	T63.511	T63.512	T63.513	T63.514		
millipede (tropical)	T63.411	T63.412	T63.413	T63.414		
plant NEC	T63.791	T63.792	T63.793	T63.794		
marine	T63.711	T63.712	T63.713	T63.714		
reptile	T63.191	T63.192	T63.193	T63.194		
gila monster	T63.111	T63.112	T63.113	T63.114		
lizard NEC	T63.121	T63.122	T63.123	T63.124		
scorpion	T63.2X1	T63.2X2	T63.2X3	T63.2X4		
snake	T63.001	T63.002	T63.003	T63.004		
African NEC	T63.081	T63.082	T63.083	T63.084		
American (North) (South) NEC	T63.061	T63.062	T63.063	T63.064		
Asian	T63.081	T63.082	T63.083	T63.084		
Australian	T63.071	T63.072	T63.073	T63.074		
cobra	T63.041	T63.042	T63.043	T63.044		
coral snake	T63.021	T63.022	T63.023	T63.024		
rattlesnake	T63.011	T63.012	T63.013	T63.014		
specified NEC	T63.091	T63.092	T63.093	T63.094		
taipan	T63.031	T63.032	T63.033	T63.034		
specified NEC	T63.891	T63.892	T63.893	T63.894		
spider	T63.301	T63.302	T63.303	T63.304		
black widow	T63.311	T63.312	T63.313	T63.314		
brown recluse	T63.331	T63.332	T63.333	T63.334		
specified NEC	T63.391	T63.392	T63.393	T63.394		
tarantula	T63.321	T63.322	T63.323	T63.324		
sting ray	T63.511	T63.512	T63.513	T63.514		
toad	T63.821	T63.822	T63.823	T63.824		
wasp	T63.461	T63.462	T63.463	T63.464		
Venous sclerosing drug NEC	T46.8X1	T46.8X2	T46.8X3	T46.8X4	T46.8X5	T46.8X6
Ventolin—see Albuterol						
Veramon	T42.3X1	T42.3X2	T42.3X3	T42.3X4	T42.3X5	T42.3X6
Verapamil	T46.1X1	T46.1X2	T46.1X3	T46.1X4	T46.1X5	T46.1X6
Veratrine	T46.5X1	T46.5X2	T46.5X3	T46.5X4	T46.5X5	T46.5X6
Veratrum						
album	T62.2X1	T62.2X2	T62.2X3	T62.2X4	—	—
alkaloids	T46.5X1	T46.5X2	T46.5X3	T46.5X4	T46.5X5	T46.5X6

Substance	Poisoning, Accidental (unintentional)	Poisoning, Intentional self-harm	Poisoning, Assault	Poisoning, Undetermined	Adverse effect	Underdosing
Veratrum — *Continued*						
viride	T62.2X1	T62.2X2	T62.2X3	T62.2X4	—	—
Verdigris	T60.3X1	T60.3X2	T60.3X3	T60.3X4	—	—
Veronal	T42.3X1	T42.3X2	T42.3X3	T42.3X4	T42.3X5	T42.3X6
Veroxil	T37.4X1	T37.4X2	T37.4X3	T37.4X4	T37.4X5	T37.4X6
Versenate	T50.6X1	T50.6X2	T50.6X3	T50.6X4	T50.6X5	T50.6X6
Versidyne	T39.8X1	T39.8X2	T39.8X3	T39.8X4	T39.8X5	T39.8X6
Vetrabutine	T48.0X1	T48.0X2	T48.0X3	T48.0X4	T48.0X5	T48.0X6
Vidarabine	T37.5X1	T37.5X2	T37.5X3	T37.5X4	T37.5X5	T37.5X6
Vienna						
green	T57.0X1	T57.0X2	T57.0X3	T57.0X4	—	—
insecticide	T60.2X1	T60.2X2	T60.2X3	T60.2X4	—	—
red	T57.0X1	T57.0X2	T57.0X3	T57.0X4	—	—
pharmaceutical dye	T50.991	T50.992	T50.993	T50.994	T50.995	T50.996
Vigabatrin	T42.6X1	T42.6X2	T42.6X3	T42.6X4	T42.6X5	T42.6X6
Viloxazine	T43.291	T43.292	T43.293	T43.294	T43.295	T43.296
Viminol	T39.8X1	T39.8X2	T39.8X3	T39.8X4	T39.8X5	T39.8X6
Vinbarbital, vinbarbitone	T42.3X1	T42.3X2	T42.3X3	T42.3X4	T42.3X5	T42.3X6
Vinblastine	T45.1X1	T45.1X2	T45.1X3	T45.1X4	T45.1X5	T45.1X6
Vinburnine	T46.7X1	T46.7X2	T46.7X3	T46.7X4	T46.7X5	T46.7X6
Vincamine	T45.1X1	T45.1X2	T45.1X3	T45.1X4	T45.1X5	T45.1X6
Vincristine	T45.1X1	T45.1X2	T45.1X3	T45.1X4	T45.1X5	T45.1X6
Vindesine	T45.1X1	T45.1X2	T45.1X3	T45.1X4	T45.1X5	T45.1X6
Vinesthene, vinethene	T41.0X1	T41.0X2	T41.0X3	T41.0X4	T41.0X5	T41.0X6
Vinorelbine tartrate	T45.1X1	T45.1X2	T45.1X3	T45.1X4	T45.1X5	T45.1X6
Vinpocetine	T46.7X1	T46.7X2	T46.7X3	T46.7X4	T46.7X5	T46.7X6
Vinyl						
acetate	T65.891	T65.892	T65.893	T65.894	—	—
bital	T42.3X1	T42.3X2	T42.3X3	T42.3X4	T42.3X5	T42.3X6
bromide	T65.891	T65.892	T65.893	T65.894	—	—
chloride	T59.891	T59.892	T59.893	T59.894	—	—
ether	T41.0X1	T41.0X2	T41.0X3	T41.0X4	T41.0X5	T41.0X6
Vinylbital	T42.3X1	T42.3X2	T42.3X3	T42.3X4	T42.3X5	T42.3X6
Vinylidene chloride	T65.891	T65.892	T65.893	T65.894	—	—
Vioform	T37.8X1	T37.8X2	T37.8X3	T37.8X4	T37.8X5	T37.8X6
topical	T49.0X1	T49.0X2	T49.0X3	T49.0X4	T49.0X5	T49.0X6
Viomycin	T36.8X1	T36.8X2	T36.8X3	T36.8X4	T36.8X5	T36.8X6
Viosterol	T45.2X1	T45.2X2	T45.2X3	T45.2X4	T45.2X5	T45.2X6
Viper (venom)	T63.091	T63.092	T63.093	T63.094	—	—
Viprynium	T37.4X1	T37.4X2	T37.4X3	T37.4X4	T37.4X5	T37.4X6
Viquidil	T46.7X1	T46.7X2	T46.7X3	T46.7X4	T46.7X5	T46.7X6
Viral vaccine NEC	T50.B91	T50.B92	T50.B93	T50.B94	T50.B95	T50.B96
Virginiamycin	T36.8X1	T36.8X2	T36.8X3	T36.8X4	T36.8X5	T36.8X6
Virugon	T37.5X1	T37.5X2	T37.5X3	T37.5X4	T37.5X5	T37.5X6
Viscous agent	T50.901	T50.902	T50.903	T50.904	T50.905	T50.906
Visine	T49.5X1	T49.5X2	T49.5X3	T49.5X4	T49.5X5	T49.5X6
Visnadine	T46.3X1	T46.3X2	T46.3X3	T46.3X4	T46.3X5	T46.3X6
Vitamin NEC	T45.2X1	T45.2X2	T45.2X3	T45.2X4	T45.2X5	T45.2X6
A	T45.2X1	T45.2X2	T45.2X3	T45.2X4	T45.2X5	T45.2X6
B NEC	T45.2X1	T45.2X2	T45.2X3	T45.2X4	T45.2X5	T45.2X6

Substance	Poisoning, Accidental (unintentional)	Poisoning, Intentional self-harm	Poisoning, Assault	Poisoning, Undetermined	Adverse effect	Underdosing
Vitamin NEC — *Continued*						
nicotinic acid	T46.7X1	T46.7X2	T46.7X3	T46.7X4	T46.7X5	T46.7X6
B1	T45.2X1	T45.2X2	T45.2X3	T45.2X4	T45.2X5	T45.2X6
B2	T45.2X1	T45.2X2	T45.2X3	T45.2X4	T45.2X5	T45.2X6
B6	T45.2X1	T45.2X2	T45.2X3	T45.2X4	T45.2X5	T45.2X6
B12	T45.2X1	T45.2X2	T45.2X3	T45.2X4	T45.2X5	T45.2X6
B15	T45.2X1	T45.2X2	T45.2X3	T45.2X4	T45.2X5	T45.2X6
C	T45.2X1	T45.2X2	T45.2X3	T45.2X4	T45.2X5	T45.2X6
D	T45.2X1	T45.2X2	T45.2X3	T45.2X4	T45.2X5	T45.2X6
D2	T45.2X1	T45.2X2	T45.2X3	T45.2X4	T45.2X5	T45.2X6
D3	T45.2X1	T45.2X2	T45.2X3	T45.2X4	T45.2X5	T45.2X6
E	T45.2X1	T45.2X2	T45.2X3	T45.2X4	T45.2X5	T45.2X6
E acetate	T45.2X1	T45.2X2	T45.2X3	T45.2X4	T45.2X5	T45.2X6
hematopoietic	T45.8X1	T45.8X2	T45.8X3	T45.8X4	T45.8X5	T45.8X6
K NEC	T45.7X1	T45.7X2	T45.7X3	T45.7X4	T45.7X5	T45.7X6
K1	T45.7X1	T45.7X2	T45.7X3	T45.7X4	T45.7X5	T45.7X6
K2	T45.7X1	T45.7X2	T45.7X3	T45.7X4	T45.7X5	T45.7X6
PP	T45.2X1	T45.2X2	T45.2X3	T45.2X4	T45.2X5	T45.2X6
ulceroprotectant	T47.1X1	T47.1X2	T47.1X3	T47.1X4	T47.1X5	T47.1X6
Vleminckx's solution	T49.4X1	T49.4X2	T49.4X3	T49.4X4	T49.4X5	T49.4X6
Voltaren—see Diclofenac sodium						
			W			
Warfarin	T45.511	T45.512	T45.513	T45.514	T45.515	T45.516
rodenticide	T60.4X1	T60.4X2	T60.4X3	T60.4X4	—	—
sodium	T45.511	T45.512	T45.513	T45.514	T45.515	T45.516
Wasp (sting)	T63.461	T63.462	T63.463	T63.464	—	—
Water						
balance drug	T50.3X1	T50.3X2	T50.3X3	T50.3X4	T50.3X5	T50.3X6
distilled	T50.3X1	T50.3X2	T50.3X3	T50.3X4	T50.3X5	T50.3X6
gas—see Gas, water						
incomplete combustion of—see Carbon, monoxide, fuel, utility						
hemlock	T62.2X1	T62.2X2	T62.2X3	T62.2X4	—	—
moccasin (venom)	T63.061	T63.062	T63.063	T63.064	—	—
purified	T50.3X1	T50.3X2	T50.3X3	T50.3X4	T50.3X5	T50.3X6
Wax (paraffin) (petroleum)	T52.0X1	T52.0X2	T52.0X3	T52.0X4		
automobile	T65.891	T65.892	T65.893	T65.894	—	—
floor	T52.0X1	T52.0X2	T52.0X3	T52.0X4		
Weed killers NEC	T60.3X1	T60.3X2	T60.3X3	T60.3X4	—	—
Welldorm	T42.6X1	T42.6X2	T42.6X3	T42.6X4	T42.6X5	T42.6X6
White						
arsenic	T57.0X1	T57.0X2	T57.0X3	T57.0X4	—	—
hellebore	T62.2X1	T62.2X2	T62.2X3	T62.2X4	—	—
lotion (keratolytic)	T49.4X1	T49.4X2	T49.4X3	T49.4X4	T49.4X5	T49.4X6
spirit	T52.0X1	T52.0X2	T52.0X3	T52.0X4	—	—
Whitewash	T65.891	T65.892	T65.893	T65.894	—	—
Whole blood (human)	T45.8X1	T45.8X2	T45.8X3	T45.8X4	T45.8X5	T45.8X6

Substance	Poisoning, Accidental (unintentional)	Poisoning, Intentional self-harm	Poisoning, Assault	Poisoning, Undetermined	Adverse effect	Underdosing
Wild						
black cherry	T62.2X1	T62.2X2	T62.2X3	T62.2X4	—	—
poisonous plants NEC	T62.2X1	T62.2X2	T62.2X3	T62.2X4	—	—
Window cleaning fluid	T65.891	T65.892	T65.893	T65.894	—	—
Wintergreen (oil)	T49.3X1	T49.3X2	T49.3X3	T49.3X4	T49.3X5	T49.3X6
Wisterine	T62.2X1	T62.2X2	T62.2X3	T62.2X4	—	—
Witch hazel	T49.2X1	T49.2X2	T49.2X3	T49.2X4	T49.2X5	T49.2X6
Wood alcohol or spirit	T51.1X1	T51.1X2	T51.1X3	T51.1X4	—	—
Wool fat (hydrous)	T49.3X1	T49.3X2	T49.3X3	T49.3X4	T49.3X5	T49.3X6
Woorali	T48.1X1	T48.1X2	T48.1X3	T48.1X4	T48.1X5	T48.1X6
Wormseed, American	T37.4X1	T37.4X2	T37.4X3	T37.4X4	T37.4X5	T37.4X6
X						
Xamoterol	T44.5X1	T44.5X2	T44.5X3	T44.5X4	T44.5X5	T44.5X6
Xanthine diuretics	T50.2X1	T50.2X2	T50.2X3	T50.2X4	T50.2X5	T50.2X6
Xanthinol nicotinate	T46.7X1	T46.7X2	T46.7X3	T46.7X4	T46.7X5	T46.7X6
Xanthotoxin	T49.3X1	T49.3X2	T49.3X3	T49.3X4	T49.3X5	T49.3X6
Xantinol nicotinate	T46.7X1	T46.7X2	T46.7X3	T46.7X4	T46.7X5	T46.7X6
Xantocillin	T36.0X1	T36.0X2	T36.0X3	T36.0X4	T36.0X5	T36.0X6
Xenon (127Xe) (133Xe)	T50.8X1	T50.8X2	T50.8X3	T50.8X4	T50.8X5	T50.8X6
Xenysalate	T49.4X1	T49.4X2	T49.4X3	T49.4X4	T49.4X5	T49.4X6
Xibornol	T37.8X1	T37.8X2	T37.8X3	T37.8X4	T37.8X5	T37.8X6
Xigris	T45.511	T45.512	T45.513	T45.514	T45.515	T45.516
Xipamide	T50.2X1	T50.2X2	T50.2X3	T50.2X4	T50.2X5	T50.2X6
Xylene (vapor)	T52.2X1	T52.2X2	T52.2X3	T52.2X4	—	—
Xylocaine (infiltration) (topical)	T41.3X1	T41.3X2	T41.3X3	T41.3X4	T41.3X5	T41.3X6
nerve block (peripheral) (plexus)	T41.3X1	T41.3X2	T41.3X3	T41.3X4	T41.3X5	T41.3X6
spinal	T41.3X1	T41.3X2	T41.3X3	T41.3X4	T41.3X5	T41.3X6
Xylol (vapor)	T52.2X1	T52.2X2	T52.2X3	T52.2X4	—	—
Xylometazoline	T48.5X1	T48.5X2	T48.5X3	T48.5X4	T48.5X5	T48.5X6
Y						
Yeast	T45.2X1	T45.2X2	T45.2X3	T45.2X4	T45.2X5	T45.2X6
dried	T45.2X1	T45.2X2	T45.2X3	T45.2X4	T45.2X5	T45.2X6
Yellow						
fever vaccine	T50.B91	T50.B92	T50.B93	T50.B94	T50.B95	T50.B96
jasmine	T62.2X1	T62.2X2	T62.2X3	T62.2X4	—	—
phenolphthalein	T47.2X1	T47.2X2	T47.2X3	T47.2X4	T47.2X5	T47.2X6
Yew	T62.2X1	T62.2X2	T62.2X3	T62.2X4	—	—
Yohimbic acid	T40.991	T40.992	T40.993	T40.994	T40.995	T40.996
Z						
Zactane	T39.8X1	T39.8X2	T39.8X3	T39.8X4	T39.8X5	T39.8X6

Substance	Poisoning, Accidental (unintentional)	Poisoning, Intentional self-harm	Poisoning, Assault	Poisoning, Undetermined	Adverse effect	Underdosing
Zalcitabine	T37.5X1	T37.5X2	T37.5X3	T37.5X4	T37.5X5	T37.5X6
Zaroxolyn	T50.2X1	T50.2X2	T50.2X3	T50.2X4	T50.2X5	T50.2X6
Zephiran (topical)	T49.0X1	T49.0X2	T49.0X3	T49.0X4	T49.0X5	T49.0X6
ophthalmic preparation	T49.5X1	T49.5X2	T49.5X3	T49.5X4	T49.5X5	T49.5X6
Zeranol	T38.7X1	T38.7X2	T38.7X3	T38.7X4	T38.7X5	T38.7X6
Zerone	T51.1X1	T51.1X2	T51.1X3	T51.1X4	—	—
Zidovudine	T37.5X1	T37.5X2	T37.5X3	T37.5X4	T37.5X5	T37.5X6
Zimeldine	T43.221	T43.222	T43.223	T43.224	T43.225	T43.226
Zinc (compounds) (fumes) (vapor) NEC	T56.5X1	T56.5X2	T56.5X3	T56.5X4	—	—
anti-infectives	T49.0X1	T49.0X2	T49.0X3	T49.0X4	T49.0X5	T49.0X6
antivaricose	T46.8X1	T46.8X2	T46.8X3	T46.8X4	T46.8X5	T46.8X6
bacitracin	T49.0X1	T49.0X2	T49.0X3	T49.0X4	T49.0X5	T49.0X6
chloride (mouthwash)	T49.6X1	T49.6X2	T49.6X3	T49.6X4	T49.6X5	T49.6X6
chromate	T56.5X1	T56.5X2	T56.5X3	T56.5X4	—	—
gelatin	T49.3X1	T49.3X2	T49.3X3	T49.3X4	T49.3X5	T49.3X6
oxide	T49.3X1	T49.3X2	T49.3X3	T49.3X4	T49.3X5	T49.3X6
plaster	T49.3X1	T49.3X2	T49.3X3	T49.3X4	T49.3X5	T49.3X6
peroxide	T49.0X1	T49.0X2	T49.0X3	T49.0X4	T49.0X5	T49.0X6
pesticides	T56.5X1	T56.5X2	T56.5X3	T56.5X4	—	—
phosphide	T60.4X1	T60.4X2	T60.4X3	T60.4X4	—	—
pyrithionate	T49.4X1	T49.4X2	T49.4X3	T49.4X4	T49.4X5	T49.4X6
stearate	T49.3X1	T49.3X2	T49.3X3	T49.3X4	T49.3X5	T49.3X6
sulfate	T49.5X1	T49.5X2	T49.5X3	T49.5X4	T49.5X5	T49.5X6
ENT agent	T49.6X1	T49.6X2	T49.6X3	T49.6X4	T49.6X5	T49.6X6
ophthalmic solution	T49.5X1	T49.5X2	T49.5X3	T49.5X4	T49.5X5	T49.5X6
topical NEC	T49.0X1	T49.0X2	T49.0X3	T49.0X4	T49.0X5	T49.0X6
undecylenate	T49.0X1	T49.0X2	T49.0X3	T49.0X4	T49.0X5	T49.0X6
Zineb	T60.0X1	T60.0X2	T60.0X3	T60.0X4	—	—
Zinostatin	T45.1X1	T45.1X2	T45.1X3	T45.1X4	T45.1X5	T45.1X6
Zipeprol	T48.3X1	T48.3X2	T48.3X3	T48.3X4	T48.3X5	T48.3X6
Zofenopril	T46.4X1	T46.4X2	T46.4X3	T46.4X4	T46.4X5	T46.4X6
Zolpidem	T42.6X1	T42.6X2	T42.6X3	T42.6X4	T42.6X5	T42.6X6
Zomepirac	T39.391	T39.392	T39.393	T39.394	T39.395	T39.396
Zopiclone	T42.6X1	T42.6X2	T42.6X3	T42.6X4	T42.6X5	T42.6X6
Zorubicin	T45.1X1	T45.1X2	T45.1X3	T45.1X4	T45.1X5	T45.1X6
Zotepine	T43.591	T43.592	T43.593	T43.594	T43.595	T43.596
Zovant	T45.511	T45.512	T45.513	T45.514	T45.515	T45.516
Zoxazolamine	T42.8X1	T42.8X2	T42.8X3	T42.8X4	T42.8X5	T42.8X6
Zuclopenthixol	T43.4X1	T43.4X2	T43.4X3	T43.4X4	T43.4X5	T43.4X6
Zygadenus (venenosus)	T62.2X1	T62.2X2	T62.2X3	T62.2X4	—	—
Zyprexa	T43.591	T43.592	T43.593	T43.594	T43.595	T43.596

A

Abandonment (causing exposure to weather conditions) (with intent to injure or kill) NEC X58

Abuse (adult) (child) (mental) (physical) (sexual) X58

Accident (to) X58
aircraft (in transit) (powered) —*see also* Accident, transport, aircraft
  due to, caused by cataclysm — *see* Forces of nature, by type
animal-rider —*see* Accident, transport, animal-rider
animal-drawn vehicle —*see* Accident, transport, animal-drawn vehicle occupant
automobile —*see* Accident, transport, car occupant
bare foot water skiier V94.4
boat, boating —*see also* Accident, watercraft
  striking swimmer
    powered V94.11
    unpowered V94.12
bus —*see* Accident, transport, bus occupant
cable car, not on rails V98.0
  on rails —*see* Accident, transport, streetcar occupant
car —*see* Accident, transport, car occupant
caused by, due to
  animal NEC W64
  chain hoist W24.0
  cold (excessive) —*see* Exposure, cold
  corrosive liquid, substance —*see* Table of Drugs and Chemicals
  cutting or piercing instrument —*see* Contact, with, by type of instrument
  drive belt W24.0
  electric
    current —*see* Exposure, electric current
    motor —*see also* Contact, with, by type of machine W31.3
    current (of) W86.8
  environmental factor NEC X58
  explosive material —*see* Explosion
  fire, flames —*see* Exposure, fire
  firearm missile —*see* Discharge, firearm by type
  heat (excessive) —*see* Heat
  hot —*see* Contact, with, hot
  ignition —*see* Ignition
  lifting device W24.0
  lightning —*see subcategory* T75.0
    causing fire —*see* Exposure, fire
  machine, machinery —*see* Contact, with, by type of machine
  natural factor NEC X58
  pulley (block) W24.0
  radiation —*see* Radiation
  steam X13.1
    inhalation X13.0
    pipe X16

Accident *(continued)*
caused by, due to *(continued)*
  thunderbolt —*see subcategory* T75.0
    causing fire —*see* Exposure, fire
  transmission device W24.1
coach —*see* Accident, transport, bus occupant
coal car —*see* Accident, transport, industrial vehicle occupant
diving —*see also* Fall, into, water with
  drowning or submersion —*see* Drowning
forklift —*see* Accident, transport, industrial vehicle occupant
heavy transport vehicle NOS — *see* Accident, transport, truck occupant
ice yacht V98.2
in
  medical, surgical procedure
    as, or due to misadventure —*see* Misadventure
    causing an abnormal reaction or later complication without mention of misadventure —*see also* Complication of or following, by type of procedure Y84.9
land yacht V98.1
late effect of —*see* W00-X58 with 7th character S
logging car —*see* Accident, transport, industrial vehicle occupant
machine, machinery —*see also* Contact, with, by type of machine
  on board watercraft V93.69
    explosion —*see* Explosion, in, watercraft
    fire —*see* Burn, on board watercraft
    powered craft V93.63
      ferry boat V93.61
      fishing boat V93.62
      jetskis V93.63
      liner V93.61
      merchant ship V93.60
      passenger ship V93.61
      sailboat V93.64
mine tram —*see* Accident, transport, industrial vehicle occupant
mobility scooter (motorized) —*see* Accident, transport, pedestrian, conveyance, specified type NEC
motor scooter —*see* Accident, transport, motorcyclist
motor vehicle NOS (traffic) —*see also* Accident, transport V89.2
  nontraffic V89.0
  three-wheeled NOS —*see* Accident, transport, three-wheeled motor vehicle occupant
motorcycle NOS —*see* Accident, transport, motorcyclist
nonmotor vehicle NOS (nontraffic) —*see also* Accident, transport V89.1
  traffic NOS V89.3
nontraffic (victim's mode of transport NOS) V88.9

Accident *(continued)*
nontraffic *(continued)*
  collision (between) V88.7
    bus and truck V88.5
    car and:
      bus V88.3
      pickup V88.2
      three-wheeled motor vehicle V88.0
      train V88.6
      truck V88.4
      two-wheeled motor vehicle V88.0
      van V88.2
    specified vehicle NEC and:
      three-wheeled motor vehicle V88.1
      two-wheeled motor vehicle V88.1
  known mode of transport —*see* Accident, transport, by type of vehicle
  noncollision V88.8
  on board watercraft V93.89
    powered craft V93.83
      ferry boat V93.81
      fishing boat V93.82
      jetskis V93.83
      liner V93.81
      merchant ship V93.80
      passenger ship V93.81
    unpowered craft V93.88
      canoe V93.85
      inflatable V93.86
        in tow
          recreational V94.31
          specified NEC V94.32
      kayak V93.85
      sailboat V93.84
      surf-board V93.88
      water skis V93.87
      windsurfer V93.88
parachutist V97.29
  entangled in object V97.21
  injured on landing V97.22
pedal cycle —*see* Accident, transport, pedal cyclist
pedestrian (on foot)
  with
    another pedestrian W51
      with fall W03
        due to ice or snow W00.0
      on pedestrian conveyance NEC V00.09
    rider of
      hoverboard V00.038
      Segway V00.038
      standing
        electric scooter V00.031
        micro-mobility pedestrian conveyance NEC V00.038
    roller skater (in-line) V00.01
    skate boarder V00.02
    transport vehicle —*see* Accident, transport
  on pedestrian conveyance —*see* Accident, transport, pedestrian, conveyance
pick-up truck or van —*see* Accident, transport, pickup truck occupant
quarry truck —*see* Accident, transport, industrial vehicle occupant

Accident *(continued)*
railway vehicle (any) (in motion) — *see* Accident, transport, railway vehicle occupant
  due to cataclysm —*see* Forces of nature, by type
scooter (non-motorized) —*see* Accident, transport, pedestrian, conveyance, scooter
sequelae of —*see* W00-X58 with 7th character S
skateboard —*see* Accident, transport, pedestrian, conveyance, skateboard
ski (ing) —*see* Accident, transport, pedestrian, conveyance
  lift V98.3
specified cause NEC X58
streetcar —*see* Accident, transport, streetcar occupant
traffic (victim's mode of transport NOS) V87.9
  collision (between) V87.7
    bus and truck V87.5
    car and:
      bus V87.3
      pickup V87.2
      three-wheeled motor vehicle V87.0
      train V87.6
      truck V87.4
      two-wheeled motor vehicle V87.0
      van V87.2
    specified vehicle NEC V86.39
      and
        three-wheeled motor vehicle V87.1
        two-wheeled motor vehicle V87.1
    driver V86.09
    person on outside V86.29
    passenger V86.19
    while boarding or alighting V86.49
  known mode of transport —*see* Accident, transport, by type of vehicle
  noncollision V87.8
transport (involving injury to) V99
  18 wheeler —*see* Accident, transport, truck occupant
  agricultural vehicle occupant (nontraffic) V84.9
    driver V84.5
    hanger-on V84.7
    passenger V84.6
    traffic V84.3
      driver V84.0
      hanger-on V84.2
      passenger V84.1
    while boarding or alighting V84.4
  aircraft NEC V97.89
    military NEC V97.818
      with civilian aircraft V97.810
      civilian injured by V97.811
    occupant injured (in)
      nonpowered craft accident V96.9
        balloon V96.00
          collision V96.03
          crash V96.01
          explosion V96.05

Accident (continued)
  transport (continued)
    pedestrian (continued)
      conveyance (continued)
        hoverboard (continued)
          collision with (continued)
            bus or heavy transport V04.938
              nontraffic V04.038
              traffic V04.138
            car V03.938
              nontraffic V03.038
              traffic V03.138
            pedal cycle V01.938
              nontraffic V01.038
              traffic V01.138
            pick-up or van V03.938
              nontraffic V03.038
              traffic V03.138
            railway (train) (vehicle) V05.938
              nontraffic V05.038
              traffic V05.138
            streetcar V06.938
              nontraffic V06.038
              traffic V06.138
            three-wheeled motor vehicle V02.938
              nontraffic V02.038
              traffic V02.138
            two-wheeled motor vehicle V02.938
              nontraffic V02.038
              traffic V02.138
            vehicle, nonmotor, specified NEC V06.938
              nontraffic V06.038
              traffic V06.138
          fall V00.838
        ice skates V00.218
          collision (with) V09.9
            animal being ridden or animal drawn vehicle V06.99
              nontraffic V06.09
              traffic V06.19
            bus or heavy transport V04.99
              nontraffic V04.09
              traffic V04.19
            car V03.99
              nontraffic V03.09
              traffic V03.19
            pedal cycle V01.99
              nontraffic V01.09
              traffic V01.19
            pick-up truck or van V03.99
              nontraffic V03.09
              traffic V03.19
            railway (train) (vehicle) V05.99
              nontraffic V05.09
              traffic V05.19
            streetcar V06.99
              nontraffic V06.09
              traffic V06.19
            stationary object V00.212
            two- or three-wheeled motor vehicle V02.99
              nontraffic V02.09
              traffic V02.19

Accident (continued)
  transport (continued)
    pedestrian (continued)
      conveyance (continued)
        ice skates (continued)
          collision (continued)
            vehicle V09.9
              animal-drawn V06.99
                nontraffic V06.09
                traffic V06.19
              motor
                nontraffic V09.00
                traffic V09.20
          fall V00.211
          nontraffic V09.1
            involving motor vehicle NEC V09.00
          traffic V09.3
            involving motor vehicle NEC V09.20
        motorized mobility scooter V00.838
          collision with stationary object V00.832
          fall from V00.831
          nontraffic V09.1
            involving motor vehicle V09.00
              military V09.01
              specified type NEC V09.09
        roller skates (non in-line) V00.128
          collision (with) V09.9
            animal being ridden or animal drawn vehicle V06.91
              nontraffic V06.01
              traffic V06.11
            bus or heavy transport V04.91
              nontraffic V04.01
              traffic V04.11
            car V03.91
              nontraffic V03.01
              traffic V03.11
            pedal cycle V01.91
              nontraffic V01.01
              traffic V01.11
            pick-up truck or van V03.91
              nontraffic V03.01
              traffic V03.11
            railway (train) (vehicle) V05.91
              nontraffic V05.01
              traffic V05.11
            streetcar V06.91
              nontraffic V06.01
              traffic V06.11
            stationary object V00.122
            two- or three-wheeled motor vehicle V02.91
              nontraffic V02.01
              traffic V02.11
            vehicle V09.9
              animal-drawn V06.91
                nontraffic V06.01
                traffic V06.11
              motor
                nontraffic V09.00
                traffic V09.20
          fall V00.121

Accident (continued)
  transport (continued)
    pedestrian (continued)
      conveyance (continued)
        roller skates (continued)
          in-line V00.118
            collision —see also Accident, transport, pedestrian, conveyance, occupant, roller skates, collision with stationary object V00.112
            fall V00.111
            nontraffic V09.1
              involving motor vehicle NEC V09.00
            traffic V09.3
              involving motor vehicle NEC V09.20
        rolling shoes V00.158
          colliding with stationary object V00.152
          fall V00.151
        rolling type NEC V00.188
          collision (with) V09.9
            animal being ridden or animal drawn vehicle V06.99
              nontraffic V06.09
              traffic V06.19
            bus or heavy transport V04.99
              nontraffic V04.09
              traffic V04.19
            car V03.99
              nontraffic V03.09
              traffic V03.19
            pedal cycle V01.99
              nontraffic V01.09
              traffic V01.19
            pick-up truck or van V03.99
              nontraffic V03.09
              traffic V03.19
            railway (train) (vehicle) V05.99
              nontraffic V05.09
              traffic V05.19
            stationary object V00.182
            streetcar V06.99
              nontraffic V06.09
              traffic V06.19
            two- or three-wheeled motor vehicle V02.99
              nontraffic V02.09
              traffic V02.19
            vehicle V09.9
              animal-drawn V06.99
                nontraffic V06.09
                traffic V06.19
              motor
                nontraffic V09.00
                traffic V09.20
          fall V00.181
          in-line roller skate —see Accident, transport, pedestrian, conveyance, roller skate, in-line
          nontraffic V09.1
            involving motor vehicle NEC V09.00
          roller skate —see Accident, transport, pedestrian, conveyance, roller skate

Accident (continued)
  transport (continued)
    pedestrian (continued)
      conveyance (continued)
        rolling type NEC (continued)
          scooter (non-motorized) —see Accident, transport, pedestrian, conveyance, scooter
          skateboard —see Accident, transport, pedestrian, conveyance, skateboard
          traffic V09.3
            involving motor vehicle NEC V09.20
        scooter (non-motorized) V00.148
          collision (with) V09.9
            animal being ridden or animal drawn vehicle V06.99
              nontraffic V06.09
              traffic V06.19
            bus or heavy transport V04.99
              nontraffic V04.09
              traffic V04.19
            car V03.99
              nontraffic V03.09
              traffic V03.19
            pedal cycle V01.99
              nontraffic V01.09
              traffic V01.19
            pick-up truck or van V03.99
              nontraffic V03.09
              traffic V03.19
            railway (train) (vehicle) V05.99
              nontraffic V05.09
              traffic V05.19
            streetcar V06.99
              nontraffic V06.09
              traffic V06.19
            stationary object V00.142
            two- or three-wheeled motor vehicle V02.99
              nontraffic V02.09
              traffic V02.19
            vehicle V09.9
              animal-drawn V06.99
                nontraffic V06.09
                traffic V06.19
              motor
                nontraffic V09.00
                traffic V09.20
          fall V00.141
          nontraffic V09.1
            involving motor vehicle NEC V09.00
          traffic V09.3
            involving motor vehicle NEC V09.20
        Segway
          collision with
            animal being ridden or animal drawn vehicle V06.938
              nontraffic V06.038
              traffic V06.138
            bus or heavy transport V04.938
              nontraffic V04.038
              traffic V04.138
            car V03.938
              nontraffic V03.038
              traffic V03.138

Accident (continued)
transport (continued)
three-wheeled motor vehicle
occupant (continued)
collision (continued)
stationary object (traffic)
V37.9
nontraffic V37.3
while boarding or
alighting V37.4
streetcar (traffic) V36.9
nontraffic V36.3
while boarding or
alighting V36.4
three wheeled motor vehicle
(traffic) V32.9
nontraffic V32.3
while boarding or
alighting V32.4
truck (traffic) V34.9
nontraffic V34.3
while boarding or
alighting V34.4
two wheeled motor vehicle
(traffic) V32.9
nontraffic V32.3
while boarding or
alighting V32.4
van (traffic) V33.9
nontraffic V33.3
while boarding or
alighting V33.4
driver
collision (with)
animal (traffic) V30.5
being ridden (traffic)
V36.5
nontraffic V36.0
nontraffic V30.0
animal-drawn vehicle
(traffic) V36.5
nontraffic V36.0
bus (traffic) V34.5
nontraffic V34.0
car (traffic) V33.5
nontraffic V33.0
motor vehicle NOS
(traffic) V39.40
nontraffic V39.00
specified type NEC
(traffic) V39.49
nontraffic V39.09
pedal cycle (traffic) V31.5
nontraffic V31.0
pickup truck (traffic) V33.5
nontraffic V33.0
railway vehicle (traffic)
V35.5
nontraffic V35.0
specified vehicle NEC
(traffic) V36.5
nontraffic V36.0
stationary object (traffic)
V37.5
nontraffic V37.0
streetcar (traffic) V36.5
nontraffic V36.0
three wheeled motor
vehicle (traffic) V32.5
nontraffic V32.0
truck (traffic) V34.5
nontraffic V34.0
two wheeled motor
vehicle (traffic)
V32.5
nontraffic V32.0
van (traffic) V33.5
nontraffic V33.0
noncollision accident
(traffic) V38.5
nontraffic V38.0

Accident (continued)
transport (continued)
three-wheeled motor vehicle
occupant (continued)
noncollision accident (traffic)
V38.9
nontraffic V38.3
while boarding or alighting
V38.4
nontraffic V39.3
hanger-on
collision (with)
animal (traffic) V30.7
being ridden (traffic)
V36.7
nontraffic V36.2
nontraffic V30.2
animal-drawn vehicle
(traffic) V36.7
nontraffic V36.2
bus (traffic) V34.7
nontraffic V34.2
car (traffic) V33.7
nontraffic V33.2
pedal cycle (traffic) V31.7
nontraffic V31.2
pickup truck (traffic) V33.7
nontraffic V33.2
railway vehicle (traffic)
V35.7
nontraffic V35.2
specified vehicle NEC
(traffic) V36.7
nontraffic V36.2
stationary object (traffic)
V37.7
nontraffic V37.2
streetcar (traffic) V36.7
nontraffic V36.2
three wheeled motor
vehicle (traffic)
V32.7
nontraffic V32.2
truck (traffic) V34.7
nontraffic V34.2
two wheeled motor
vehicle (traffic)
V32.7
nontraffic V32.2
van (traffic) V33.7
nontraffic V33.2
noncollision accident
(traffic) V38.7
nontraffic V38.2
passenger
collision (with)
animal (traffic) V30.6
being ridden (traffic)
V36.6
nontraffic V36.1
nontraffic V30.1
animal-drawn vehicle
(traffic) V36.6
nontraffic V36.1
bus (traffic) V34.6
nontraffic V34.1
car (traffic) V33.6
nontraffic V33.1
motor vehicle NOS
(traffic) V39.50
nontraffic V39.10
specified type NEC
(traffic) V39.59
nontraffic V39.19
pedal cycle (traffic) V31.6
nontraffic V31.1
pickup truck (traffic) V33.6
nontraffic V33.1
railway vehicle (traffic)
V35.6
nontraffic V35.1

Accident (continued)
transport (continued)
three-wheeled motor vehicle
occupant (continued)
passenger (continued)
collision (continued)
specified vehicle NEC
(traffic) V36.6
nontraffic V36.1
stationary object (traffic)
V37.6
nontraffic V37.1
streetcar (traffic) V36.6
nontraffic V36.1
three wheeled motor
vehicle (traffic) V32.6
nontraffic V32.1
truck (traffic) V34.6
nontraffic V34.1
two wheeled motor
vehicle (traffic) V32.6
nontraffic V32.1
van (traffic) V33.6
nontraffic V33.1
noncollision accident
(traffic) V38.6
nontraffic V38.1
specified type NEC V39.89
military vehicle V39.81
tractor (farm) (and trailer)
—see Accident, transport,
agricultural vehicle occupant
tram —see Accident, transport,
streetcar
in mine or quarry —see
Accident, transport,
industrial vehicle occupant
trolley —see Accident, transport,
streetcar
in mine or quarry
—see Accident, transport,
industrial vehicle occupant
truck occupant V69.9
collision (with)
animal (traffic) V60.9
being ridden (traffic)
V66.9
nontraffic V66.3
while boarding or
alighting V66.4
nontraffic V60.3
while boarding or
alighting V60.4
animal-drawn vehicle
(traffic) V66.9
nontraffic V66.3
while boarding or
alighting V66.4
bus (traffic) V64.9
nontraffic V64.3
while boarding or
alighting V64.4
car (traffic) V63.9
nontraffic V63.3
while boarding or
alighting V63.4
motor vehicle NOS (traffic)
V69.60
nontraffic V69.20
specified type NEC
(traffic) V69.69
nontraffic V69.29
pedal cycle (traffic) V61.9
nontraffic V61.3
while boarding or
alighting V61.4
pickup truck (traffic)
V63.9
nontraffic V63.3
while boarding or
alighting V63.4

Accident (continued)
transport (continued)
truck occupant (continued)
collision (continued)
railway vehicle (traffic) V65.9
nontraffic V65.3
while boarding or
alighting V65.4
specified vehicle NEC
(traffic) V66.9
nontraffic V66.3
while boarding or
alighting V66.4
stationary object (traffic)
V67.9
nontraffic V67.3
while boarding or
alighting V67.4
streetcar (traffic) V66.9
nontraffic V66.3
while boarding or
alighting V66.4
three wheeled motor vehicle
(traffic) V62.9
nontraffic V62.3
while boarding or
alighting V62.4
truck (traffic) V64.9
nontraffic V64.3
while boarding or
alighting V64.4
two wheeled motor vehicle
(traffic) V62.9
nontraffic V62.3
while boarding or
alighting V62.4
van (traffic) V63.9
nontraffic V63.3
while boarding or
alighting V63.4
driver
collision (with)
animal (traffic) V60.5
being ridden (traffic)
V66.5
nontraffic V66.0
nontraffic V60.0
animal-drawn vehicle
(traffic) V66.5
nontraffic V66.0
bus (traffic) V64.5
nontraffic V64.0
car (traffic) V63.5
nontraffic V63.0
motor vehicle NOS
(traffic) V69.40
nontraffic V69.00
specified type NEC
(traffic) V69.49
nontraffic V69.09
pedal cycle (traffic)
V61.5
nontraffic V61.0
pickup truck (traffic) V63.5
nontraffic V63.0
railway vehicle (traffic)
V65.5
nontraffic V65.0
specified vehicle NEC
(traffic) V66.5
nontraffic V66.0
stationary object (traffic)
V67.5
nontraffic V67.0
streetcar (traffic) V66.5
nontraffic V66.0
three wheeled motor
vehicle (traffic) V62.5
nontraffic V62.0
truck (traffic) V64.5
nontraffic V64.0

Activity *(continued)*
jumping rope Y93.56
karate Y93.75
kayaking (in calm and turbulent water) Y93.16
keyboarding (computer) Y93.C1
kickball Y93.6A
knitting Y93.D1
lacrosse Y93.65
land maintenance NEC Y93.H9
landscaping Y93.H2
laundry Y93.E2
machines (exercise)
primarily for cardiorespiratory conditioning Y93.A1
primarily for muscle strengthening Y93.B1
maintenance
exterior building NEC Y93.H9
household (interior) NEC Y93.E9
land Y93.H9
property Y93.H9
marching (on level or elevated terrain) Y93.01
martial arts Y93.75
microwave oven Y93.G3
milking an animal Y93.K2
mopping (floor) Y93.E5
mountain climbing Y93.31
muscle strengthening
exercises (non-machine) NEC Y93.B9
machines Y93.B1
musical keyboard (electronic) playing Y93.J1
nordic skiing Y93.24
obstacle course Y93.A5
oven (microwave) Y93.G3
packing up and unpacking in moving to a new residence Y93.E6
parasailing Y93.19
pass out game Y93.85
percussion instrument playing NEC Y93.J2
personal
bathing and showering Y93.E1
hygiene NEC Y93.E8
showering Y93.E1
physical games generally associated with school recess, summer camp and children Y93.6A
physical training NEC Y93.A9
piano playing Y93.J1
pilates Y93.B4
platform diving Y93.12
playing musical instrument
brass instrument Y93.J4
drum Y93.J2
musical keyboard (electronic) Y93.J1
percussion instrument NEC Y93.J2
piano Y93.J1
string instrument Y93.J3
winds instrument Y93.J4
property maintenance
exterior NEC Y93.H9
interior NEC Y93.E9
pruning (garden and lawn) Y93.H2
pull-ups Y93.B2
push-ups Y93.B2
racquetball Y93.73
rafting (in calm and turbulent water) Y93.16
raking (leaves) Y93.H1
rappelling Y93.32
refereeing a sports activity Y93.81
residential relocation Y93.E6
rhythmic gymnastics Y93.43
rhythmic movement NEC Y93.49
riding
horseback Y93.52
rollercoaster Y93.I1

Activity *(continued)*
rock climbing Y93.31
rollercoaster riding Y93.I1
roller skating (inline) Y93.51
rough housing and horseplay Y93.83
rowing (in calm and turbulent water) Y93.16
rugby Y93.63
running Y93.02
SCUBA diving Y93.15
sewing Y93.D2
shoveling Y93.H1
dirt Y93.H1
snow Y93.H1
showering (personal) Y93.E1
sit-ups Y93.B2
skateboarding Y93.51
skating (ice) Y93.21
roller Y93.51
skiing (alpine) (downhill) Y93.23
cross country Y93.24
nordic Y93.24
water Y93.17
sledding (snow) Y93.23
sleeping (sleep) Y93.84
smoking and grilling food Y93.G2
snorkeling Y93.15
snow NEC Y93.29
boarding Y93.23
shoveling Y93.H1
sledding Y93.23
tubing Y93.23
soccer Y93.66
softball Y93.64
specified NEC Y93.89
spectator at an event Y93.82
sports NEC Y93.79
sports played as a team or group NEC Y93.69
sports played individually NEC Y93.59
springboard diving Y93.12
squash Y93.73
stationary bike Y93.A1
step (stepping) exercise (class) Y93.A3
stepper machine Y93.A1
stove Y93.G3
string instrument playing Y93.J3
surfing Y93.18
wind Y93.18
swimming Y93.11
tackle football Y93.61
tap dancing Y93.41
tennis Y93.73
toboggoning Y93.23
touch football Y93.62
track and field events (non-running) Y93.57
running Y93.02
trampoline Y93.44
treadmill Y93.A1
trimming shrubs Y93.H2
tubing (in calm and turbulent water) Y93.16
snow Y93.23
ultimate frisbee Y93.74
underwater diving Y93.15
unpacking in moving to a new residence Y93.E6
use of stove, oven and microwave oven Y93.G3
vacuuming Y93.E3
volleyball (beach) (court) Y93.68
wake boarding Y93.17
walking an animal Y93.K1
walking (on level or elevated terrain) Y93.01
an animal Y93.K1
wall climbing Y93.31
warm up and cool down exercises Y93.A2

Activity *(continued)*
water NEC Y93.19
aerobics Y93.14
craft NEC Y93.19
exercise Y93.14
polo Y93.13
skiing Y93.17
sliding Y93.18
survival training and testing Y93.19
weeding (garden and lawn) Y93.H2
wind instrument playing Y93.J4
windsurfing Y93.18
wrestling Y93.72
yoga Y93.42

Adverse effect of drugs *—see* Table of Drugs and Chemicals

Aerosinusitis *—see* Air, pressure

After-effect, late *—see* Sequelae

Air
blast in war operations *—see* War operations, air blast
pressure
change, rapid
during
ascent W94.29
while (in) (surfacing from)
aircraft W94.23
deep water diving W94.21
underground W94.22
descent W94.39
in
aircraft W94.31
water W94.32
high, prolonged W94.0
low, prolonged W94.12
due to residence or long visit at high altitude W94.11

Alpine sickness W94.11

Altitude sickness W94.11

Anaphylactic shock, anaphylaxis *—see* Table of Drugs and Chemicals

Andes disease W94.11

Arachnidism, arachnoidism X58

Arson (with intent to injure or kill) X97

Asphyxia, asphyxiation
by
food (bone) (*seed*) *—see* categories T17 and T18
gas *—see also* Table of Drugs and Chemicals
legal
execution *—see* Legal, intervention, gas
intervention *—see* Legal, intervention, gas
from
fire *—see also* Exposure, fire
in war operations *—see* War operations, fire
ignition *—see* Ignition
vomitus T17.81
in war operations *—see* War operations, restriction of airway

Aspiration
food (any type) (into respiratory tract) (with asphyxia, obstruction respiratory tract, suffocation) *—see* categories T17 and T18
foreign body *—see* Foreign body, aspiration
vomitus (with asphyxia, obstruction respiratory tract, suffocation) T17.81

Assassination (attempt) *—see* Assault

Assault (homicidal) (by) (in) Y09
arson X97
bite (of human being) Y04.1
bodily force Y04.8
bite Y04.1
bumping into Y04.2
sexual *—see* subcategories T74.0, T76.0
unarmed fight Y04.0
bomb X96.9
antipersonnel X96.0
fertilizer X96.3
gasoline X96.1
letter X96.2
petrol X96.1
pipe X96.3
specified NEC X96.8
brawl (hand) (fists) (foot) (unarmed) Y04.0
burning, burns (by fire) NEC X97
acid Y08.89
caustic, corrosive substance Y08.89
chemical from swallowing caustic, corrosive substance *—see* Table of Drugs and Chemicals
cigarette(s) X97
hot object X98.9
fluid NEC X98.2
household appliance X98.3
specified NEC X98.8
steam X98.0
tap water X98.1
vapors X98.0
scalding *—see* Assault, burning
steam X98.0
vitriol Y08.89
caustic, corrosive substance (gas) Y08.89
crashing of
aircraft Y08.81
motor vehicle Y03.8
pushed in front of Y02.0
run over Y03.0
specified NEC Y03.8
cutting or piercing instrument X99.9
dagger X99.2
glass X99.0
knife X99.1
specified NEC X99.8
sword X99.2
dagger X99.2
drowning (in) X92.9
bathtub X92.0
natural water X92.3
specified NEC X92.8
swimming pool X92.1
following fall X92.2
dynamite X96.8
explosive(s) (material) X96.9
fight (hand) (fists) (foot) (unarmed) Y04.0
with weapon *—see* Assault, by type of weapon
fire X97
firearm X95.9
airgun X95.01
handgun X93
hunting rifle X94.1
larger X94.9
specified NEC X94.8
machine gun X94.2
shotgun X94.0
specified NEC X95.8

Assault (continued)
  gunshot (wound) NEC
    —see Assault, firearm, by type
  incendiary device X97
  injury Y09
    to child due to criminal abortion
      attempt NEC Y08.89
  knife X99.1
  late effect of —see X92-Y08 with
    7th character S
  placing before moving object NEC
    Y02.8
    motor vehicle Y02.0
  poisoning —see categories
    T36-T65 with 7th character S
  puncture, any part of body
    —see Assault, cutting or piercing
    instrument
  pushing
    before moving object NEC
      Y02.8
      motor vehicle Y02.0
      subway train Y02.1
      train Y02.1
    from high place Y01
  rape T74.2-
  scalding —see Assault, burning
  sequelae of —see X92-Y08 with
    7th character S
  sexual (by bodily force) T74.2-
  shooting —see Assault, firearm
  specified means NEC Y08.89
  stab, any part of body
    —see Assault, cutting or piercing
    instrument
  steam X98.0
  striking against
    other person Y04.2
    sports equipment Y08.09
      baseball bat Y08.02
      hockey stick Y08.01
  struck by
    sports equipment Y08.09
      baseball bat Y08.02
      hockey stick Y08.01
  submersion —see Assault,
    drowning
  violence Y09
  weapon Y09
    blunt Y00
    cutting or piercing —see
      Assault, cutting or piercing
      instrument
    firearm —see Assault, firearm
  wound Y09
    cutting —see Assault, cutting or
      piercing instrument
    gunshot —see Assault, firearm
    knife X99.1
    piercing —see Assault, cutting or
      piercing instrument
    puncture —see Assault, cutting
      or piercing instrument
    stab —see Assault, cutting or
      piercing instrument

Attack by mammals NEC W55.89

Avalanche —see Landslide

Aviator's disease —see Air,
pressure

B

Barotitis, barodontalgia,
barosinusitis, barotrauma (otitic)
(sinus) —see Air, pressure

Battered (baby) (child) (person)
(syndrome) X58

Bayonet wound W26.1
  in

Bayonet wound (continued)
  in (continued)
    legal intervention —see Legal,
      intervention, sharp object,
      bayonet
    war operations —see War
      operations, combat
  stated as undetermined whether
    accidental or intentional Y28.8
  suicide (attempt) X78.2

Bean in nose —see categories T17
and T18

Bed set on fire NEC
  —see Exposure, fire, uncontrolled,
  building, bed

Beheading (by guillotine)
  homicide X99.9
  legal execution —see Legal,
    intervention

Bending, injury in (prolonged)
(static) X50.1

Bends —see Air, pressure, change

Bite, bitten by
  alligator W58.01
  arthropod (nonvenomous)
    NEC W57
  bull W55.21
  cat W55.01
  cow W55.21
  crocodile W58.11
  dog W54.0
  goat W55.31
  hoof stock NEC W55.31
  horse W55.11
  human being (accidentally) W50.3
    with intent to injure or kill Y04.1
    as, or caused by, a crowd or
      human stampede (with fall)
      W52
    assault Y04.1
    homicide (attempt) Y04.1
    in
      fight Y04.1
  insect (nonvenomous) W57
  lizard (nonvenomous) W59.01
  mammal NEC W55.81
    marine W56.31
  marine animal (nonvenomous)
    W56.81
  millipede W57
  moray eel W56.51
  mouse W53.01
  person(s) (accidentally) W50.3
    with intent to injure or kill Y04.1
    as, or caused by, a crowd or
      human stampede (with fall)
      W52
    assault Y04.1
    homicide (attempt) Y04.1
    in
      fight Y04.1
  pig W55.41
  raccoon W55.51
  rat W53.11
  reptile W59.81
    lizard W59.01
    snake W59.11
    turtle W59.21
      terrestrial W59.81
  rodent W53.81
    mouse W53.01
    rat W53.11
    specified NEC W53.81
    squirrel W53.21
  shark W56.41
  sheep W55.31
  snake (nonvenomous) W59.11
  spider (nonvenomous) W57
  squirrel W53.21

Blast (air) **in war operations**
  —see War operations, blast

Blizzard X37.2

Blood alcohol level Y90.9
  less than 20mg/100ml Y90.0
  presence in blood, level not
    specified Y90.9
  20-39mg/100ml Y90.1
  40-59mg/100ml Y90.2
  60-79mg/100ml Y90.3
  80-99mg/100ml Y90.4
  100-119mg/100ml Y90.5
  120-199mg/100ml Y90.6
  200-239mg/100ml Y90.7

Blow X58
  by law-enforcing agent, police (on
    duty) —see Legal, intervention,
    manhandling
    blunt object —see Legal,
      intervention, blunt object

Blowing up —see Explosion

Brawl (hand) (fists) (foot) Y04.0

Breakage (accidental) (part of)
  ladder (causing fall) W11
  scaffolding (causing fall) W12

Broken
  glass, contact with —see Contact,
    with, glass
  power line (causing electric
    shock) W85

Bumping against, into
(accidentally)
  object NEC W22.8
    with fall —see Fall, due to,
      bumping against, object
    caused by crowd or human
      stampede (with fall) W52
    sports equipment W21.9
  person(s) W51
    with fall W03
      due to ice or snow W00.0
    assault Y04.2
    caused by, a crowd or human
      stampede (with fall) W52
    homicide (attempt) Y04.2
  sports equipment W21.9

Burn, burned, burning (accidental)
(by) (from) (on)
  acid NEC —see Table of Drugs and
    Chemicals
  bed linen —see Exposure, fire,
    uncontrolled, in building, bed
  blowtorch X08.8
    with ignition of clothing
      NEC X06.2
      nightwear X05
  bonfire, campfire (controlled) —see
    also Exposure, fire, controlled,
    not in building
    uncontrolled —see Exposure,
      fire, uncontrolled, not in
      building
  candle X08.8
    with ignition of clothing NEC
      X06.2
      nightwear X05
  caustic liquid, substance (external)
    (internal) NEC —see Table of
    Drugs and Chemicals
  chemical (external) (internal) —
    see also Table of Drugs and
    Chemicals
    in war operations —see War
      operations. fire
  cigar(s) or cigarette(s) X08.8
    with ignition of clothing NEC
      X06.2
      nightwear X05
  clothes, clothing NEC (from
    controlled fire) X06.2
    with conflagration —see
      Exposure, fire, uncontrolled,
      building

Burn, burned, burning (continued)
  clothes, clothing NEC (continued)
    with conflagration (continued)
      not in building or structure
        —see Exposure, fire,
        uncontrolled, not in
        building
  cooker (hot) X15.8
    stated as undetermined whether
      accidental or intentional
      Y27.3
    suicide (attempt) X77.3
  electric blanket X16
  engine (hot) X17
  fire, flames —see Exposure, fire
  flare, Very pistol —see Discharge,
    firearm NEC
  heat
    from appliance (electrical)
      (household) X15.8
      cooker X15.8
      hotplate X15.2
      kettle X15.8
      light bulb X15.8
      saucepan X15.3
      skillet X15.3
      stove X15.0
      stated as undetermined whether
        accidental or intentional
        Y27.3
      suicide (attempt) X77.3
      toaster X15.1
    in local application or packing
      during medical or surgical
      procedure Y63.5
  heating
    appliance, radiator or pipe X16
  homicide (attempt) —see Assault,
    burning
  hot
    air X14.1
    cooker X15.8
    drink X10.0
    engine X17
    fat X10.2
    fluid NEC X12
    food X10.1
    gases X14.1
    heating appliance X16
    household appliance NEC X15.8
    kettle X15.8
    liquid NEC X12
    machinery X17
    metal (molten) (liquid)
      NEC X18
    object (not producing fire or
      flames) NEC X19
    oil (cooking) X10.2
    pipe(s) X16
    radiator X16
    saucepan (glass) (metal) X15.3
    stove (kitchen) X15.0
    substance NEC X19
      caustic or corrosive NEC
        —see Table of Drugs and
        Chemicals
    toaster X15.1
    tool X17
    vapor X13.1
    water (tap) —see Contact, with,
      hot, tap water
  hotplate X15.2
    suicide (attempt) X77.3
  ignition —see Ignition
  in war operations —see War
    operations, fire
  inflicted by other person X97
    by hot objects, hot vapor,
      and steam —see
      Assault, burning, hot
      object

Burn, burned, burning (*continued*)
internal, from swallowed caustic,
   corrosive liquid, substance
   —*see* Table of Drugs and
   Chemicals
iron (hot) X15.8
   stated as undetermined whether
      accidental or intentional Y27.3
   suicide (attempt) X77.3
kettle (hot) X15.8
   stated as undetermined whether
      accidental or intentional Y27.3
   suicide (attempt) X77.3
lamp (flame) X08.8
   with ignition of clothing NEC
      X06.2
      nightwear X05
lighter (cigar) (cigarette) X08.8
   with ignition of clothing NEC
      X06.2
      nightwear X05
lightning —*see* subcategory T75.0
   causing fire —*see* Exposure, fire
liquid (boiling) (hot) NEC X12
   stated as undetermined whether
      accidental or intentional Y27.2
   suicide (attempt) X77.2
local application of externally
   applied substance in medical or
   surgical care Y63.5
machinery (hot) X17
matches X08.8
   with ignition of clothing
      NEC X06.2
      nightwear X05
mattress —*see* Exposure, fire,
   uncontrolled, building, bed
medicament, externally applied
   Y63.5
metal (hot) (liquid) (molten) NEC
   X18
nightwear (nightclothes, nightdress,
   gown, pajamas, robe) X05
object (hot) NEC X19
on board watercraft
   due to
      accident to watercraft V91.09
         powered craft V91.03
            ferry boat V91.01
            fishing boat V91.02
            jetskis V91.03
            liner V91.01
            merchant ship V91.00
            passenger ship V91.01
         unpowered craft V91.08
            canoe V91.05
            inflatable V91.06
            kayak V91.05
            sailboat V91.04
            surf-board V91.08
            water skis V91.07
            windsurfer V91.08
      fire on board V93.09
         ferry boat V93.01
         fishing boat V93.02
         jetskis V93.03
         liner V93.01
         merchant ship V93.00
         passenger ship V93.01
         powered craft NEC V93.03
         sailboat V93.04
         specified heat source NEC on
            board V93.19
            ferry boat V93.11
            fishing boat V93.12
            jetskis V93.13
            liner V93.11
            merchant ship V93.10
            passenger ship V93.11
            powered craft NEC V93.13
            sailboat V93.14

Burn, burned, burning (*continued*)
pipe (hot) X16
   smoking X08.8
      with ignition of clothing NEC
         X06.2
         nightwear X05
powder —*see* Powder burn
radiator (hot) X16
saucepan (hot) (glass) (metal) X15.3
   stated as undetermined whether
      accidental or intentional Y27.3
   suicide (attempt) X77.3
self-inflicted X76
   stated as undetermined
      whether accidental or
      intentional Y26
steam X13.1
   pipe X16
      stated as undetermined
         whether accidental or
         intentional Y27.8
   stated as undetermined whether
      accidental or intentional Y27.0
   suicide (attempt) X77.0
stove (hot) (kitchen) X15.0
   stated as undetermined whether
      accidental or intentional Y27.3
   suicide (attempt) X77.3
substance (hot) NEC X19
   boiling X12
      stated as undetermined whether
         accidental or intentional
         Y27.2
      suicide (attempt) X77.2
   molten (metal) X18
suicide (attempt) NEC X76
   hot
      household appliance X77.3
      object X77.9
therapeutic misadventure
   heat in local application or
      packing during medical or
      surgical procedure Y63.5
   overdose of radiation Y63.2
toaster (hot) X15.1
   stated as undetermined whether
      accidental or intentional
      Y27.3
   suicide (attempt) X77.3
tool (hot) X17
torch, welding X08.8
   with ignition of clothing NEC
      X06.2
      nightwear X05
trash fire (controlled)
   —*see* Exposure, fire, controlled,
   not in building
   uncontrolled —*see* Exposure, fire,
      uncontrolled, not in building
vapor (hot) X13.1
   stated as undetermined whether
      accidental or intentional Y27.0
   suicide (attempt) X77.0
Very pistol —*see* Discharge,
   firearm NEC

Butted by animal W55.82
bull W55.22
cow W55.22
goat W55.32
horse W55.12
pig W55.42
sheep W55.32

C

Caisson disease —*see* Air, pressure,
change
Campfire (exposure to) (controlled)
—*see also* Exposure, fire,
controlled, not in building

Camfire (*continued*)
uncontrolled —*see* Exposure, fire,
   uncontrolled, not in building
Capital punishment (any means)
—*see* Legal, intervention
Car sickness T75.3
Casualty (not due to war) NEC X58
war —*see* War operations
Cat
bite W55.01
scratch W55.03
Cataclysm, cataclysmic (any injury)
NEC —*see* Forces of nature
Catching fire —*see* Exposure, fire
Caught
between
   folding object W23.0
   objects (moving) (stationary and
      moving) W23.0
      and machinery —*see* Contact,
         with, by type of machine
      stationary W23.1
   sliding door and door frame
      W23.0
by, in
   machinery (moving parts of) —
      see Contact, with, by type of
      machine
   washing-machine wringer W23.0
under packing crate (due to losing
   grip) W23.1
**Cave-in caused by cataclysmic
earth surface movement or
eruption** —*see* Landslide
Change(s) in air pressure —*see* Air,
pressure, change
Choked, choking (on) (any object
except food or vomitus)
food (bone) (*seed*) —*see* categories
   T17 and T18
vomitus T17.81-
Civil insurrection —*see* War
operations
Cloudburst (any injury) X37.8
Cold, exposure to (accidental)
(excessive) (extreme) (natural)
(place) NEC —*see* Exposure, cold
Collapse
building W20.1
   burning (uncontrolled fire) X00.2
dam or man-made structure
   (causing earth movement)
   X36.0
machinery —*see* Contact, with, by
   type of machine
structure W20.1
   burning (uncontrolled fire)
      X00.2
Collision (accidental) NEC —*see
also* Accident, transport V89.9
pedestrian W51
   with fall W03
   due to ice or snow W00.0
      involving pedestrian
         conveyance —*see* Accident,
         transport, pedestrian,
         conveyance
      and
         crowd or human stampede
            (with fall) W52
         object W22.8
            with fall —*see* Fall, due to,
               bumping against, object
person(s) —*see* Collision,
   pedestrian
transport vehicle NEC V89.9

Collision (*continued*)
transport vehicle NEC (*continued*)
   and
      avalanche, fallen or not
         moving —*see* Accident,
         transport
         falling or moving
            —*see* Landslide
      landslide, fallen or not moving
         —*see* Accident, transport
         falling or moving
            —*see* Landslide
   due to cataclysm —*see* Forces of
      nature, by type
   intentional, purposeful suicide
      (attempt) —*see* Suicide,
      collision

Combustion, spontaneous
—*see* Ignition

Complication (delayed) of or
following (medical or surgical
procedure) Y84.9
with misadventure
   —*see* Misadventure
amputation of limb(s) Y83.5
anastomosis (arteriovenous) (blood
   vessel) (gastrojejunal) (tendon)
   (natural or artificial material) Y83.2
aspiration (of fluid) Y84.4
   tissue Y84.8
biopsy Y84.8
blood
   sampling Y84.7
   transfusion
      procedure Y84.8
bypass Y83.2
catheterization (urinary) Y84.6
   cardiac Y84.0
colostomy Y83.3
cystostomy Y83.3
dialysis (kidney) Y84.1
drug —*see* Table of Drugs and
   Chemicals
due to misadventure
   —*see* Misadventure
duodenostomy Y83.3
electroshock therapy Y84.3
external stoma, creation of
   Y83.3
formation of external stoma
   Y83.3
gastrostomy Y83.3
graft Y83.2
hypothermia (medically-induced)
   Y84.8
implant, implantation (of)
   artificial
      internal device (cardiac
         pacemaker) (electrodes
         in brain) (heart valve
         prosthesis) (orthopedic)
         Y83.1
      material or tissue (for
         anastomosis or bypass) Y83.2
         with creation of external stoma
            Y83.3
   natural tissues (for anastomosis
      or bypass) Y83.2
      with creation of external
         stoma Y83.3
infusion
   procedure Y84.8
injection —*see* Table of Drugs and
   Chemicals
   procedure Y84.8
insertion of gastric or duodenal
   sound Y84.5
insulin-shock therapy Y84.3
paracentesis (abdominal) (thoracic)
   (aspirative) Y84.4

Deprivation X58

Derailment (accidental)
railway (rolling stock) (train) (vehicle) (without antecedent collision) V81.7
  with antecedent collision —see Accident, transport, railway vehicle occupant
streetcar (without antecedent collision) V82.7
  with antecedent collision —see Accident, transport, streetcar occupant

Descent
parachute (voluntary) (without accident to aircraft) V97.29
  due to accident to aircraft —see Accident, transport, aircraft

Desertion X58

Destitution X58

Disability, late effect or sequela of injury —see Sequelae

Discharge (accidental)
airgun W34.010
  assault X95.01
  homicide (attempt) X95.01
  stated as undetermined whether accidental or intentional Y24.0
  suicide (attempt) X74.01
BB gun —see Discharge, airgun
firearm (accidental) W34.00
  assault X95.9
  handgun (pistol) (revolver) W32.0
    assault X93
    homicide (attempt) X93
    legal intervention —see Legal, intervention, firearm, handgun
    stated as undetermined whether accidental or intentional Y22
    suicide (attempt) X72
  homicide (attempt) X95.9
  hunting rifle W33.02
    assault X94.1
    homicide (attempt) X94.1
    legal intervention injuring
      bystander Y35.032
      law enforcement personnel Y35.031
      suspect Y35.033
      unspecified person Y35.039
    stated as undetermined whether accidental or intentional Y23.1
    suicide (attempt) X73.1
  larger W33.00
    assault X94.9
    homicide (attempt) X94.9
    hunting rifle —see Discharge, firearm, hunting rifle
    legal intervention —see Legal, intervention, firearm by type of firearm
    machine gun —see Discharge, firearm, machine gun
    shotgun —see Discharge, firearm, shotgun
    specified NEC W33.09
      assault X94.8
      homicide (attempt) X94.8
      legal intervention injuring
        bystander Y35.092
        law enforcement personnel Y35.091

Discharge (continued)
firearm (continued)
  larger (continued)
    specified NEC (continued)
      legal intervention (continued)
        injuring (continued)
          suspect Y35.093
          unspecified person Y35.099
      stated as undetermined whether accidental or intentional Y23.8
    specified NEC W33.09
      suicide (attempt) X73.8
    stated as undetermined whether accidental or intentional Y23.9
    suicide (attempt) X73.9
  legal intervention injuring
    bystander Y35.002
    law enforcement personnel Y35.001
    suspect Y35.03
    unspecified person Y35.049
  using rubber bullet injuring
    bystander Y35.042
    law enforcement personnel Y35.041
    suspect Y35.043
    unspecified person Y35.049
  machine gun W33.03
    assault X94.2
    homicide (attempt) X94.2
    legal intervention —see Legal, intervention, firearm, machine gun
    stated as undetermined whether accidental or intentional Y23.3
    suicide (attempt) X73.2
  pellet gun —see Discharge, airgun
  shotgun W33.01
    assault X94.0
    homicide (attempt) X94.0
    legal intervention —see Legal, intervention, firearm, specified NEC
    stated as undetermined whether accidental or intentional Y23.0
    suicide (attempt) X73.0
  specified NEC W34.09
    assault X95.8
    homicide (attempt) X95.8
    legal intervention —see Legal, intervention, firearm, specified NEC
    stated as undetermined whether accidental or intentional Y24.8
    suicide (attempt) X74.8
    stated as undetermined whether accidental or intentional Y24.9
    suicide (attempt) X74.9
  Very pistol W34.09
    assault X95.8
    homicide (attempt) X95.8
    stated as undetermined whether accidental or intentional Y24.8
    suicide (attempt) X74.8
firework(s) W39
  stated as undetermined whether accidental or intentional Y25
gas-operated gun NEC W34.018

Discharge (continued)
gas-operated gun NEC (continued)
  airgun —see Discharge, airgun
  assault X95.09
  homicide (attempt) X95.09
  paintball gun —see Discharge, paintball gun
  stated as undetermined whether accidental or intentional Y24.8
  suicide (attempt) X74.09
gun NEC —see also Discharge, firearm NEC
  air —see Discharge, airgun
  BB —see Discharge, airgun
  for single hand use —see Discharge, firearm, handgun
  hand —see Discharge, firearm, handgun
  machine —see Discharge, firearm, machine gun
  other specified —see Discharge, firearm NEC
  paintball —see Discharge, paintball gun
  pellet —see Discharge, airgun
handgun —see Discharge, firearm, handgun
machine gun —see Discharge, firearm, machine gun
paintball gun W34.011
  assault X95.02
  homicide (attempt) X95.02
  stated as undetermined whether accidental or intentional Y24.8
  suicide (attempt) X74.02
pistol —see Discharge, firearm, handgun
  flare —see Discharge, firearm, Very pistol
  pellet —see Discharge, airgun
  Very —see Discharge, firearm, Very pistol
revolver —see Discharge, firearm, handgun
rifle (hunting) —see Discharge, firearm, hunting rifle
shotgun —see Discharge, firearm, shotgun
spring-operated gun NEC W34.018
  assault X95.09
  homicide (attempt) X95.09
  stated as undetermined whether accidental or intentional Y24.8
  suicide (attempt) X74.09

Disease
Andes W94.11
aviator's —see Air, pressure
range W94.11

Diver's disease, palsy, paralysis, squeeze —see Air, pressure

Diving (into water) —see Accident, diving

Dog bite W54.0

Dragged by transport vehicle NEC —see also Accident, transport V09.9

Drinking poison (accidental) —see Table of Drugs and Chemicals

Dropped (accidentally) while being carried or supported by other person W04

Drowning (accidental) W74
assault X92.9
due to
  accident (to)
    machinery —see Contact, with, by type of machine
    watercraft V90.89

Drowning (continued)
due to (continued)
  accident (continued)
    watercraft (continued)
      burning V90.29
        powered V90.23
          fishing boat V90.22
          jetskis V90.23
          merchant ship V90.20
          passenger ship V90.21
        unpowered V90.28
          canoe V90.25
          inflatable V90.26
          kayak V90.25
          sailboat V90.24
          water skis V90.27
      crushed V90.39
        powered V90.33
          fishing boat V90.32
          jetskis V90.33
          merchant ship V90.30
          passenger ship V90.31
        unpowered V90.38
          canoe V90.35
          inflatable V90.36
          kayak V90.35
          sailboat V90.34
          water skis V90.37
      overturning V90.09
        powered V90.03
          fishing boat V90.02
          jetskis V90.03
          merchant ship V90.00
          passenger ship V90.01
        unpowered V90.08
          canoe V90.05
          inflatable V90.06
          kayak V90.05
          sailboat V90.04
      sinking V90.19
        powered V90.13
          fishing boat V90.12
          jetskis V90.13
          merchant ship V90.10
          passenger ship V90.11
        unpowered V90.18
          canoe V90.15
          inflatable V90.16
          kayak V90.15
          sailboat V90.14
      specified type NEC V90.89
        powered V90.83
          fishing boat V90.82
          jetskis V90.83
          merchant ship V90.80
          passenger ship V90.81
        unpowered V90.88
          canoe V90.85
          inflatable V90.86
          kayak V90.85
          sailboat V90.84
          water skis V90.87
  avalanche —see Landslide
  cataclysmic
    earth surface movement NEC —see Forces of nature, earth movement
    storm —see Forces of nature, cataclysmic storm
  cloudburst X37.8
  cyclone X37.1
  fall overboard (from) V92.09
    powered craft V92.03
      ferry boat V92.01
      fishing boat V92.02
      jetskis V92.03
      liner V92.01
      merchant ship V92.00
      passenger ship V92.01
    unpowered craft V92.08

Drowning (continued)
  due to (continued)
    fall overboard (continued)
      unpowered craft (continued)
        canoe V92.05
        inflatable V92.06
        kayak V92.05
        sailboat V92.04
        surf-board V92.08
        water skis V92.07
        windsurfer V92.08
      resulting from
        accident to watercraft —
          see Drowning, due to,
          accident to, watercraft
        being washed overboard
          (from) V92.29
          powered craft V92.23
            ferry boat V92.21
            fishing boat V92.22
            jetskis V92.23
            liner V92.21
            merchant ship V92.20
            passenger ship V92.21
          unpowered craft V92.28
            canoe V92.25
            inflatable V92.26
            kayak V92.25
            sailboat V92.24
            surf-board V92.28
            water skis V92.27
            windsurfer V92.28
        motion of watercraft V92.19
          powered craft V92.13
            ferry boat V92.11
            fishing boat V92.12
            jetskis V92.13
            liner V92.11
            merchant ship V92.10
            passenger ship V92.11
          unpowered craft
            canoe V92.15
            inflatable V92.16
            kayak V92.15
            sailboat V92.14
  hurricane X37.0
  jumping into water from
    watercraft (involved in
    accident) —see also Drowning,
    due to, accident to, watercraft
    without accident to or on
      watercraft W16.711
  tidal wave NEC —see Forces of
    nature, tidal wave
  torrential rain X37.8
  following
    fall
      into
        bathtub W16.211
        bucket W16.221
        fountain —see Drowning,
          following, fall, into,
          water, specified NEC
        quarry —see Drowning,
          following, fall, into,
          water, specified NEC
        reservoir —see Drowning,
          following, fall, into,
          water, specified NEC
        swimming-pool W16.011
          striking
            bottom W16.021
            wall W16.031
          stated as undetermined
            whether accidental or
            intentional Y21.3
          suicide (attempt) X71.2
        water NOS W16.41
          natural (lake) (open sea)
            (river) (stream) (pond)
            W16.111

Drowning (continued)
  following (continued)
    fall (continued)
      into (continued)
        water NOS (continued)
          natural (continued)
            striking
              bottom W16.121
              side W16.131
            specified NEC W16.311
              striking
                bottom W16.321
                wall W16.331
      overboard NEC
        —see Drowning, due to, fall
        overboard
    jump or dive
      from boat W16.711
        striking bottom W16.721
      into
        fountain —see Drowning,
          following, jump or dive,
          into, water, specified
          NEC
        quarry —see Drowning,
          following, jump or dive,
          into, water, specified
          NEC
        reservoir —see Drowning,
          following, jump or dive,
          into, water, specified
          NEC
        swimming-pool W16.511
          striking
            bottom W16.521
            wall W16.531
          suicide (attempt) X71.2
        water NOS W16.91
          natural (lake) (open sea)
            (river) (stream) (pond)
            W16.611
          specified NEC W16.811
            striking
              bottom W16.821
              wall W16.831
          striking bottom W16.621
  homicide (attempt) X92.9
  in
    bathtub (accidental) W65
      assault X92.0
      following fall W16.211
        stated as undetermined
          whether accidental or
          intentional Y21.1
      stated as undetermined
        whether accidental or
        intentional Y21.0
      suicide (attempt) X71.0
    lake —see Drowning, in, natural
      water
    natural water (lake) (open sea)
      (river) (stream) (pond) W69
      assault X92.3
      following
        dive or jump W16.611
          striking bottom
            W16.621
        fall W16.111
          striking
            bottom W16.121
            side W16.131
      stated as undetermined
        whether accidental or
        intentional Y21.4
      suicide (attempt) X71.3
    quarry —see Drowning, in,
      specified place NEC
    quenching tank —see Drowning,
      in, specified place NEC
    reservoir —see Drowning, in,
      specified place NEC

Drowning (continued)
  in (continued)
    river —see Drowning, in, natural
      water
    sea —see Drowning, in, natural
      water
    specified place NEC W73
      assault X92.8
      following
        dive or jump W16.811
          striking
            bottom W16.821
            wall W16.831
        fall W16.311
          striking
            bottom W16.321
            wall W16.331
      stated as undetermined
        whether accidental or
        intentional Y21.8
      suicide (attempt) X71.8
    stream —see Drowning, in,
      natural water
    swimming-pool W67
      assault X92.1
        following fall X92.2
      following
        dive or jump W16.511
          striking
            bottom W16.521
            wall W16.531
        fall W16.011
          striking
            bottom W16.021
            wall W16.031
      stated as undetermined
        whether accidental or
        intentional Y21.2
        following fall Y21.3
      suicide (attempt) X71.1
        following fall X71.2
    war operations —see War opera-
      tions, restriction of airway
  resulting from accident to
    watercraft see Drowning, due to,
    accident, watercraft
  self-inflicted X71.9
  stated as undetermined whether
    accidental or intentional Y21.9
  suicide (attempt) X71.9

E

Earth (surface) movement NEC
  —see
  Forces of nature, earth movement

Earth falling (on) W20.0
  caused by cataclysmic earth
    surface movement or eruption
    —see Landslide

Earthquake (any injury) X34

Effect(s) (adverse) of
  air pressure (any)- —see Air,
    pressure
  cold, excessive (exposure to)
    —see Exposure, cold
  heat (excessive) —see Heat
  hot place (weather) —see Heat
  insolation X30
  late —see Sequelae
  motion —see Motion
  nuclear explosion or weapon in war
    operations —see War operations,
    nuclear weapon
  radiation —see Radiation
  travel —see Travel

Electric shock (accidental) (by)
  (in) —see Exposure, electric
  current

Electrocution (accidental)
  —see Exposure, electric current

Endotracheal tube wrongly placed
  during anesthetic procedure

Entanglement
  in
    bed linen, causing suffocation
      —see categories T71
    wheel of pedal cycle V19.88

Entry of foreign body or material
  —see Foreign body

Environmental pollution related
  condition —see Z57

Execution, legal (any method)
  —see Legal, intervention

Exhaustion
  cold —see Exposure, cold
  due to excessive exertion (see also
    Overexertion) X50.9
  heat —see Heat

Explosion (accidental) (of) (with
  secondary fire) W40.9
  acetylene W40.1
  aerosol can W36.1
  air tank (compressed) (in
    machinery) W36.2
  aircraft (in transit) (powered) NEC
    V95.9
    balloon V96.05
    fixed wing NEC (private) V95.25
      commercial V95.35
    glider V96.25
      hang V96.15
      powered V95.15
    helicopter V95.05
    in war operations —see War
      operations, destruction of
      aircraft
    microlight V95.15
    nonpowered V96.9
      specified NEC V96.8
    powered NEC V95.8
    stated as
      homicide (attempt) Y03.8
      suicide (attempt) X83.0
    ultralight V95.15
  anesthetic gas in operating room
    W40.1
  antipersonnel bomb W40.8
    assault X96.0
    homicide (attempt) X96.0
    suicide (attempt) X75
  assault X96.9
  bicycle tire W37.0
  blasting (cap) (materials) W40.0
  boiler (machinery), not on transport
    vehicle W35
    on watercraft —see Explosion,
      in, watercraft
  butane W40.1
  caused by other person X96.9
  coal gas W40.1
  detonator W40.0
  dump (munitions) W40.8
  dynamite W40.0
    in
      assault X96.8
      homicide (attempt) X96.8
      legal intervention
        injuring
          bystander Y35.112
          law enforcement
            personnel Y35.111
          unspecified person
            Y35.119
            suspect Y35.113
            unspecified person Y35.119
      suicide (attempt) X75

Fall, falling (*continued*)

  from, off, out of (*continued*)
    playground equipment (*continued*)
      slide W09.0
      swing W09.1
    quarry W17.89
    railing W13.9
    ramp W10.2
    roof W13.2
    scaffolding W12
    scooter (nonmotorized) W05.1
      motorized mobility W05.2
    sky lift W17.89
    stairs, steps W10.9
      curb W10.1
      due to ice or snow W00.1
      escalator W10.0
      incline W10.2
      ramp W10.2
      sidewalk curb W10.1
      specified NEC W10.8
      standing
        electric scooter V00.841
        micro-mobility pedestrian
          conveyance V00.848
    stepladder W11
    storm drain W17.1
    streetcar NEC V82.6
      with antecedent collision
        —*see* Accident, transport,
        streetcar occupant
      while boarding or alighting
        V82.4
    structure NEC W13.8
      burning (uncontrolled fire)
        X00.3
    table W08
    toilet W18.11
      with subsequent striking
        against object W18.12
    train NEC V81.6
      during derailment (without
        antecedent collision) V81.7
      with antecedent collision
        —*see* Accident, transport,
        railway vehicle occupant
      while boarding or alighting
        V81.4
    transport vehicle after collision
      —*see* Accident, transport, by
      type of vehicle, collision
    tree W14
    vehicle (in motion) NEC —*see
      also* Accident, transport V89.9
      motor NEC —*see also*
        Accident, transport,
        occupant, by type of vehicle
        V87.8
      stationary W17.89
        while boarding or alighting
          —*see* Accident, transport,
          by type of vehicle, while
          boarding or alighting
    viaduct W13.8
    wall W13.8
    watercraft —*see also* Drowning,
      due to, fall overboard
      with hitting bottom or object
        V94.0
    well W17.0
    wheelchair, non-moving W05.0
      powered —*see* Accident,
        transport, pedestrian,
        conveyance occupant,
        specified type NEC
    window W13.4
  in, on
    aircraft NEC V97.0
      with accident to aircraft V97.0
      while boarding or alighting
        V97.1

Fall, falling (*continued*)

  in, on (*continued*)
    bathtub (empty) W18.2
      filled W16.212
        causing drowning W16.211
    escalator W10.0
    incline W10.2
    ladder W11
    machine, machinery
      —*see* Contact, with, by type of
      machine
    object, edged, pointed or sharp
      (with cut) —*see* Fall, by type
    playground equipment W09.8
      jungle gym W09.2
      slide W09.0
      swing W09.1
    ramp W10.2
    scaffolding W12
    shower W18.2
      causing drowning W16.211
    staircase, stairs, steps W10.9
      curb W10.1
      due to ice or snow W00.1
      escalator W10.0
      incline W10.2
      specified NEC W10.8
    streetcar (without antecedent
      collision) V82.5
      with antecedent collision
        —*see* Accident, transport,
        streetcar occupant
      while boarding or alighting
        V82.4
    train (without antecedent
      collision) V81.5
      with antecedent collision
        —*see* Accident, transport,
        railway vehicle occupant
      during derailment (without
        antecedent collision) V81.7
      with antecedent collision
        —*see* Accident, transport,
        railway vehicle occupant
      while boarding or alighting
        V81.4
    transport vehicle after collision
      —*see* Accident, transport, by
      type of vehicle, collision
    watercraft V93.39
      due to
        accident to craft V91.29
          powered craft V91.23
            ferry boat V91.21
            fishing boat V91.22
            jetskis V91.23
            liner V91.21
            merchant ship V91.20
            passenger ship V91.21
          unpowered craft
            canoe V91.25
            inflatable V91.26
            kayak V91.25
            sailboat V91.24
        powered craft V93.33
          ferry boat V93.31
          fishing boat V93.32
          jetskis V93.33
          liner V93.31
          merchant ship V93.30
          passenger ship V93.31
        unpowered craft V93.38
          canoe V93.35
          inflatable V93.36
          kayak V93.35
          sailboat V93.34
          surf-board V93.38
          windsurfer V93.38
  into
    cavity W17.2
    dock W17.4

Fall, falling (*continued*)

  into (*continued*)
    fire —*see* Exposure, fire, by type
    haystack W17.89
    hole W17.2
    manhole W17.1
    moving part of machinery —*see*
      Contact, with, by type of
      machine
    ocean —*see* Fall, into, water
    opening in surface NEC
      W17.89
    pit W17.2
    pond —*see* Fall, into, water
    quarry W17.89
    river —*see* Fall, into, water
    shaft W17.89
    storm drain W17.1
    stream —*see* Fall, into, water
    swimming pool —*see also* Fall,
      into, water, in, swimming pool
      empty W17.3
    tank W17.89
    water W16.42
      causing drowning W16.41
      from watercraft —*see*
        Drowning, due to, fall
        overboard
      hitting diving board W21.4
      in
        bathtub W16.212
          causing drowning
            W16.211
        bucket W16.222
          causing drowning
            W16.221
        natural body of water
          W16.112
          causing drowning
            W16.111
          striking
            bottom W16.122
              causing drowning
                W16.121
            side W16.132
              causing drowning
                W16.131
        specified water NEC
          W16.312
          causing drowning
            W16.311
          striking
            bottom W16.322
              causing drowning
                W16.321
            wall W16.332
              causing drowning
                W16.331
        swimming pool W16.012
          causing drowning
            W16.011
          striking
            bottom W16.022
              causing drowning
                W16.021
            wall W16.032
              causing drowning
                W16.031
        utility bucket W16.222
          causing drowning
            W16.221
    well W17.0
  involving
    bed W06
    chair W07
    furniture NEC W08
    glass —*see* Fall, by type
    playground equipment W09.8
      jungle gym W09.2
      slide W09.0
      swing W09.1

Fall, falling (*continued*)

  involvin (*continued*)
    roller blades —*see* Accident,
      transport, pedestrian,
      conveyance
    skateboard(s) —*see* Accident,
      transport, pedestrian,
      conveyance
    skates (ice) (in line) (roller)
      —*see* Accident, transport,
      pedestrian, conveyance
    skis —*see* Accident, transport,
      pedestrian, conveyance
    table W08
    wheelchair, non-moving W05.0
      powered —*see* Accident,
        transport, pedestrian,
        conveyance, specified type
        NEC
  object —*see* Struck by, object,
    falling
  off
    toilet W18.11
      with subsequent striking
        against object W18.12
  on same level W18.30
    due to
      specified NEC W18.39
      stepping on an object W18.31
  out of
    bed W06
    building NEC W13.8
    chair W07
    furniture NEC W08
    wheelchair, non-moving W05.0
      powered —*see* Accident,
        transport, pedestrian,
        conveyance, specified type
        NEC
    window W13.4
  over
    animal W01.0
    cliff W15
    embankment W17.81
    small object W01.0
  rock W20.8
  same level W18.30
    from
      being crushed, pushed, or
        stepped on by a crowd or
        human stampede W52
      collision, pushing, shoving, by
        or with other person W03
      slipping, stumbling, tripping
        W01.0
    involving ice or snow W00.0
      involving skates (ice)
        (roller), skateboard, skis
        —*see* Accident, transport,
        pedestrian, conveyance
  snowslide (avalanche)
    —*see* Landslide
  stone W20.8
  structure W20.1
    burning (uncontrolled fire)
      X00.3
  through
    bridge W13.1
    floor W13.3
    roof W13.2
    wall W13.8
    window W13.4
  timber W20.8
  tree (caused by lightning) W20.8
  while being carried or supported by
    other person(s) W04

Fallen on by

  animal (not being ridden) NEC
    W55.89

Felo-de-se —*see* Suicide

Incident, adverse *(continued)*
device *(continued)*
neurological Y75.8
accessory Y75.2
diagnostic Y75.0
miscellaneous Y75.8
monitoring Y75.0
prosthetic Y75.2
rehabilitative Y75.1
surgical Y75.3
therapeutic Y75.1
obstetrical Y76.8
accessory Y76.2
diagnostic Y76.0
miscellaneous Y76.8
monitoring Y76.0
prosthetic Y76.2
rehabilitative Y76.1
surgical Y76.3
therapeutic Y76.1
ophthalmic Y77.8
accessory Y77.2
contact lens (rigid gas
permeable) (soft
(hydrophilic)) Y77.11
diagnostic Y77.0
miscellaneous Y77.8
monitoring Y77.0
prosthetic Y77.2
rehabilitative Y77.19
surgical Y77.3
therapeutic Y77.19
orthopedic Y79.8
accessory Y79.2
diagnostic Y79.0
miscellaneous Y79.8
monitoring Y79.0
prosthetic Y79.2
rehabilitative Y79.1
surgical Y79.3
therapeutic Y79.1
otorhinolaryngological
Y72.8
accessory Y72.2
diagnostic Y72.0
miscellaneous Y72.8
monitoring Y72.0
prosthetic Y72.2
rehabilitative Y72.1
surgical Y72.3
therapeutic Y72.1
personal use Y74.8
accessory Y74.2
diagnostic Y74.0
miscellaneous Y74.8
monitoring Y74.0
prosthetic Y74.2
rehabilitative Y74.1
surgical Y74.3
therapeutic Y74.1
physical medicine Y80.8
accessory Y80.2
diagnostic Y80.0
miscellaneous Y80.8
monitoring Y80.0
prosthetic Y80.2
rehabilitative Y80.1
surgical Y80.3
therapeutic Y80.1
plastic surgical Y81.8
accessory Y81.2
diagnostic Y81.0
miscellaneous Y81.8
monitoring Y81.0
prosthetic Y81.2
rehabilitative Y81.1
surgical Y81.3
therapeutic Y81.1
radiological Y78.8
accessory Y78.2
diagnostic Y78.0

Incident, adverse *(continued)*
device *(continued)*
radiological *(continued)*
miscellaneous Y78.8
monitoring Y78.0
prosthetic Y78.2
rehabilitative Y78.1
surgical Y78.3
therapeutic Y78.1
urology Y73.8
accessory Y73.2
diagnostic Y73.0
miscellaneous Y73.8
monitoring Y73.0
prosthetic Y73.2
rehabilitative Y73.1
surgical Y73.3
therapeutic Y73.1

Incineration (accidental)
—*see* Exposure, fire

Infanticide —*see* Assault

Infrasound waves (causing injury)
W49.9

Ingestion
foreign body (causing injury)
(with obstruction) —*see* Foreign
body, alimentary canal
poisonous
plant(s) X58
substance NEC —*see* Table of
Drugs and Chemicals

Inhalation
excessively cold substance, man-made
—*see* Exposure, cold, man-made
food (any type) (into respiratory
tract) (with asphyxia, obstruction
respiratory tract, suffocation)
—*see* categories T17 and T18
foreign body —*see* Foreign body,
aspiration
gastric contents (with
asphyxia, obstruction
respiratory passage,
suffocation) T17.81-
hot air or gases X14.0
liquid air, hydrogen, nitrogen W93.12
suicide (attempt) X83.2
steam X13.0
assault X98.0
stated as undetermined whether
accidental or intentional Y27.0
suicide (attempt) X77.0
toxic gas —*see* Table of Drugs and
Chemicals
vomitus (with asphyxia, obstruction
respiratory passage, suffocation)
T17.81-

Injury, injured (accidental(ly))
NOS X58
by, caused by, from
assault —*see* Assault
law-enforcing agent, police, in
course of legal intervention
—*see* Legal intervention
suicide (attempt) X83.8
due to, in
civil insurrection —*see* War
operations
fight —*see also* Assault, fight Y04.0
war operations —*see* War
operations
homicide —*see also* Assault Y09
inflicted (by)
in course of arrest (attempted),
suppression of disturbance,
maintenance of order, by law-
enforcing agents —*see* Legal
intervention

Injury *(continued)*
inflicted *(continued)*
other person
stated as
accidental X58
intentional, homicide
(attempt) —*see* Assault
undetermined whether
accidental or intentional
Y33
purposely (inflicted) by other
person(s) —*see* Assault
self-inflicted X83.8
stated as accidental X58
specified cause NEC X58
undetermined whether accidental or
intentional Y33

Insolation, effects X30

Insufficient nourishment X58

Interruption of respiration (by)
food (lodged in esophagus) —*see*
categories T17 and T18
vomitus (lodged in esophagus)
T17.81-

Intervention, legal —*see* Legal
intervention

Intoxication
drug —*see* Table of Drugs and
Chemicals
poison —*see* Table of Drugs and
Chemicals

J

Jammed (accidentally)
between objects (moving)
(stationary and moving) W23.0
stationary W23.1

Jumped, jumping
before moving object NEC X81.8
motor vehicle X81.0
subway train X81.1
train X81.1
undetermined whether accidental
or intentional Y31
from
boat (into water) voluntarily,
without accident (to or on
boat) W16.712
with
accident to or on boat —*see*
Accident, watercraft
drowning or submersion
W16.711
suicide (attempt) X71.3
striking bottom W16.722
causing drowning W16.721
building —*see also* Jumped,
from, high place W13.9
burning (uncontrolled fire)
X00.5
high place NEC W17.89
suicide (attempt) X80
undetermined whether
accidental or intentional Y30
structure —*see also* Jumped,
from, high place W13.9
burning (uncontrolled fire)
X00.5
into water W16.92
causing drowning W16.91
from, off watercraft
—*see* Jumped, from, boat
in
natural body W16.612
causing drowning W16.611
striking bottom W16.622
causing drowning
W16.621

Jumped *(continued)*
into water *(continued)*
in *(continued)*
specified place NEC
W16.812
causing drowning
W16.811
striking
bottom W16.822
causing drowning
W16.821
wall W16.832
causing drowning
W16.831
swimming pool W16.512
causing drowning
W16.511
striking
bottom W16.522
causing drowning
W16.521
wall W16.532
causing drowning
W16.531
suicide (attempt) X71.3

K

Kicked by
animal NEC W55.82
person(s) (accidentally) W50.1
with intent to injure or kill Y04.0
as, or caused by, a crowd or human
stampede (with fall) W52
assault Y04.0
homicide (attempt) Y04.0
in
fight Y04.0
legal intervention
injuring
bystander Y35.812
law enforcement
personnel Y35.811
suspect Y35.813
unspecified person
Y35.819

Kicking
against
object W22.8
sports equipment W21.9
stationary W22.09
sports equipment W21.89
person —*see* Striking against,
person
sports equipment W21.9
carpet stretcher with knee X50.3

Killed, killing (accidentally)
NOS —*see also* Injury X58
in action —*see* War operations
brawl, fight (hand) (fists) (foot)
Y04.0
by weapon —*see also* Assault
cutting, piercing
—*see* Assault, cutting or
piercing instrument
firearm —*see* Discharge,
firearm, by type, homicide
self
stated as
accident NOS X58
suicide —*see* Suicide
undetermined whether
accidental or intentional
Y33

Kneeling (prolonged) (static) X50.1

Knocked down (accidentally) (by)
NOS X58
animal (not being ridden) NEC
—*see also* Struck by, by type of
animal

Misadventure(s) to patient(s) during surgical or medical care *(continued)*
  puncture —*see* Index to Diseases and Injuries, Complication(s)
  specified type NEC Y65.8
    failure
      suture or ligature during surgical operation Y65.2
      to introduce or to remove tube or instrument —*see* Failure, to
    infusion of wrong fluid Y65.1
    performance of inappropriate operation —*see* Inappropriate operation performed
    transfusion of mismatched blood Y65.0
    wrong
      drug given in error —*see* Table of Drugs and Chemicals
      fluid in infusion Y65.1
      placement of endotracheal tube during anesthetic procedure Y65.3
  transfusion —*see* Misadventure, by type, transfusion
    excessive amount of blood Y63.0
    mismatched blood Y65.0
  wrong
    drug given in error —*see* Table of Drugs and Chemicals
    fluid in infusion Y65.1
    placement of endotracheal tube during anesthetic procedure Y65.3

Mismatched blood in transfusion Y65.0

Motion sickness T75.3

Mountain sickness W94.11

Mudslide (of cataclysmic nature) —*see* Landslide

Murder (attempt) —*see* Assault

N

Nail
  contact with W45.0
    gun W29.4
  embedded in skin W45.0

Neglect (criminal) (homicidal intent) X58

Noise (causing injury) (pollution) W42.9
  supersonic W42.0

Nonadministration (of)
  drug or biological substance (necessary) Y63.6
  surgical and medical care Y66

Nosocomial condition Y95

O

Object
  falling
    from, in, on, hitting
      machinery —*see* Contact, with, by type of machine
  set in motion by
    accidental explosion or rupture of pressure vessel W38
    firearm —*see* Discharge, firearm, by type
    machine (ry) —*see* Contact, with, by type of machine

Overdose (drug) —*see* Table of Drugs and Chemicals
  radiation Y63.2

Overexertion X50.9
  from
    prolonged static or awkward postures X50.1
    repetitive movements X50.3
    specified strenuous movements or postures NEC X50.9
    strenuous movement or load X50.0

Overexposure (accidental) (to)
  cold —*see also* Exposure, cold X31
    due to man-made conditions —*see* Exposure, cold, man-made
  heat —*see also* Heat X30
  radiation —*see* Radiation
  radioactivity W88.0
  sun (sunburn) X32
  weather NEC —*see* Forces of nature
  wind NEC —*see* Forces of nature

Overheated —*see* Heat

Overturning (accidental)
  machinery —*see* Contact, with, by type of machine
  transport vehicle NEC —*see also* Accident, transport V89.9
  watercraft (causing drowning, submersion) —*see also* Drowning, due to, accident to, watercraft, overturning
    causing injury except drowning or submersion —*see* Accident, watercraft, causing, injury NEC

P

Parachute descent (voluntary) (without accident to aircraft) V97.29
  due to accident to aircraft —*see* Accident, transport, aircraft

Pecked by bird W61.99

Perforation during medical or surgical treatment as misadventure —*see* Index to Diseases and Injuries, Complication(s)

Perpetrator, perpetration, of assault, maltreatment and neglect (by) Y07.9
  boyfriend Y07.03
  brother Y07.410
    stepbrother Y07.435
  coach Y07.53
  cousin
    female Y07.491
    male Y07.490
  daycare provider Y07.519
    at-home
      adult care Y07.512
      childcare Y07.510
    care center
      adult care Y07.513
      childcare Y07.511
  family member NEC Y07.499
  father Y07.11
    adoptive Y07.13
    foster Y07.420
    stepfather Y07.430
  foster father Y07.420
  foster mother X07.421

Perpetrator, perpetration, of assault, maltreatment and neglect *(continued)*
  girl friend Y07.04
  healthcare provider Y07.529
    mental health Y07.521
    specified NEC Y07.528
  husband Y07.01
  instructor Y07.53
  mother Y07.12
    adoptive Y07.14
    foster Y07.421
    stepmother Y07.433
  multiple perpetrators Y07.6
  nonfamily member Y07.50
    specified NEC Y07.59
  nurse Y07.528
  occupational therapist Y07.528
  partner of parent
    female Y07.434
    male Y07.432
  physical therapist Y07.528
  sister Y07.411
  speech therapist Y07.528
  stepbrother Y07.435
  stepfather Y07.430
  stepmother Y07.433
  stepsister Y07.436
  teacher Y07.53
  wife Y07.02

Piercing —*see* Contact, with, by type of object or machine

Pinched
  between objects (moving) (stationary and moving) W23.0
    stationary W23.1

Pinned under machine (ry) —*see* Contact, with, by type of machine

Place of occurrence Y92.9
  abandoned house Y92.89
  airplane Y92.813
  airport Y92.520
  ambulatory health services establishment NEC Y92.538
  ambulatory surgery center Y92.530
  amusement park Y92.831
  apartment (co-op) —*see* Place of occurrence, residence, apartment
  assembly hall Y92.29
  bank Y92.510
  barn Y92.71
  baseball field Y92.320
  basketball court Y92.310
  beach Y92.832
  boarding house —*see* Place of occurrence, residence, boarding house
  boat Y92.814
  bowling alley Y92.39
  bridge Y92.89
  building under construction Y92.61
  bus Y92.811
    station Y92.521
  cafe Y92.511
  campsite Y92.833
  campus —*see* Place of occurrence, school
  canal Y92.89
  car Y92.810
  casino Y92.59
  children's home —*see* Place of occurrence, residence, institutional, orphanage
  church Y92.22
  cinema Y92.26
  clubhouse Y92.29
  coal pit Y92.64
  college (community) Y92.214

Place of occurrence *(continued)*
  condominium —*see* Place of occurrence, residence, apartment
  construction area —*see* Place of occurrence, industrial and construction area
  convalescent home —*see* Place of occurrence, residence, institutional, nursing home
  court-house Y92.240
  cricket ground Y92.328
  cultural building Y92.258
    art gallery Y92.250
    museum Y92.251
    music hall Y92.252
    opera house Y92.253
    specified NEC Y92.258
    theater Y92.254
  dancehall Y92.252
  day nursery Y92.210
  dentist office Y92.531
  derelict house Y92.89
  desert Y92.820
  dock NOS Y92.89
  dockyard Y92.62
  doctor's office Y92.531
  dormitory —*see* Place of occurrence, residence, institutional, school dormitory
  dry dock Y92.62
  factory (building) (premises) Y92.63
  farm (land under cultivation) (outbuildings) Y92.79
    barn Y92.71
    chicken coop Y92.72
    field Y92.73
    hen house Y92.72
    house —*see* Place of occurrence, residence, house
    orchard Y92.74
    specified NEC Y92.79
  football field Y92.321
  forest Y92.821
  freeway Y92.411
  gallery Y92.250
  garage (commercial) Y92.59
    boarding house Y92.044
    military base Y92.135
    mobile home Y92.025
    nursing home Y92.124
    orphanage Y92.114
    private house Y92.015
    reform school Y92.155
  gas station Y92.524
  gasworks Y92.69
  golf course Y92.39
  gravel pit Y92.64
  grocery Y92.512
  gymnasium Y92.39
  handball court Y92.318
  harbor Y92.89
  harness racing course Y92.39
  healthcare provider office Y92.531
  highway (interstate) Y92.411
  hill Y92.828
  hockey rink Y92.330
  home —*see* Place of occurrence, residence
  hospice —*see* Place of occurrence, residence, institutional, nursing home
  hospital Y92.239
    cafeteria Y92.233
    corridor Y92.232
    operating room Y92.234
    patient
      bathroom Y92.231
      room Y92.230
    specified NEC Y92.238

Place of occurrence (continued)
  swimming pool (continued)
    private (continued)
      single family residence
        Y92.016
  synagogue Y92.22
  television station Y92.59
  tennis court Y92.312
  theater Y92.254
  trade area Y92.59
    bank Y92.510
    cafe Y92.511
    casino Y92.59
    garage Y92.59
    hotel Y92.59
    market Y92.512
    office building Y92.59
    radio station Y92.59
    restaurant Y92.511
    shop Y92.513
    shopping mall Y92.59
    store Y92.512
    supermarket Y92.512
    television station Y92.59
    warehouse Y92.59
  trailer park, residential —see Place
    of occurrence, residence, mobile
    home
  trailer site NOS Y92.89
  train Y92.815
    station Y92.522
  truck Y92.812
  tunnel under construction Y92.69
  urgent (health) care center Y92.532
  university Y92.214
  vehicle (transport) Y92.818
    airplane Y92.813
    boat Y92.814
    bus Y92.811
    car Y92.810
    specified NEC Y92.818
    subway car Y92.816
    train Y92.815
    truck Y92.812
  warehouse Y92.59
  water reservoir Y92.89
  wilderness area Y92.828
    desert Y92.820
    forest Y92.821
    marsh Y92.828
    mountain Y92.828
    prairie Y92.828
    specified NEC Y92.828
    swamp Y92.828
  workshop Y92.69
  yard, private Y92.096
    boarding house Y92.046
    single family house Y92.017
    mobile home Y92.027
  youth center Y92.29
  zoo (zoological garden)
    Y92.834

Plumbism —see Table of Drugs and
  Chemicals, lead

Poisoning (accidental) (by)
  —see also Table of Drugs and
  Chemicals
  by plant, thorns, spines, sharp
    leaves or other mechanisms NEC
    X58
  carbon monoxide
    generated by
      motor vehicle —see Accident,
        transport
      watercraft (in transit) (not in
        transit) V93.89
        ferry boat V93.81
        fishing boat V93.82
        jet skis V93.83
        liner V93.81

Poisoning (continued)
  carbon monoxide (continued)
    generated by (continued)
      watercraft (continued)
        merchant ship V93.80
        passenger ship V93.81
        powered craft NEC
          V93.83
  caused by injection of poisons into
    skin by plant thorns, spines,
    sharp leaves X58
    marine or sea plants (venomous)
    X58
  exhaust gas
    generated by
      motor vehicle —see Accident,
        transport
      watercraft (in transit) (not in
        transit) V93.89
        ferry boat V93.81
        fishing boat V93.82
        jet skis V93.83
        liner V93.81
        merchant ship V93.80
        passenger ship V93.81
        powered craft NEC
          V93.83
  fumes or smoke due to
    explosion —see also Explosion
      W40.9
    fire —see Exposure, fire
    ignition —see Ignition gas
    in legal intervention —see Legal,
      intervention, gas
    legal execution —see Legal,
      intervention, gas
  in war operations —see War
    operations

Powder burn (by) (from)
  airgun W34.110
  BB gun W34.110
  firearm NEC W34.19
  gas, air or spring-operated gun
    NEC W34.118
  handgun W32.1
  hunting rifle W33.12
  larger firearm W33.10
    specified NEC W33.19
  machine gun W33.13
  paintball gun W34.111
  pellet gun W34.110
  shotgun W33.11
  Very pistol [flare] W34.19

**Premature cessation (of) surgical
and medical care** Y66

Privation (food) (water) X58

Procedure (operation)
  correct, on wrong side or body
    part (wrong side) (wrong site)
    Y65.53
  intended for another patient
    done on wrong patient Y65.52
  performed on patient not scheduled
    for surgery Y65.52
  performed on wrong patient
    Y65.52
  wrong, performed on correct
    patient Y65.51

Prolonged
  sitting in transport vehicle
    —see Travel, by type of
    vehicle
  stay in
    high altitude as cause of anoxia,
      barodontalgia, barotitis or
      hypoxia W94.11
    weightless environment X52

Pulling, excessive (see also
  Overexertion) X50.9

Puncture, puncturing —see also
  Contact, with, by type of object
  or machine
  by
    plant thorns, spines, sharp leaves
      or other mechanisms NEC
      W60
  during medical or surgical
    treatment as misadventure
    —see Index to Diseases and
    Injuries, Complication(s)

Pushed, pushing (accidental) (injury in)
  by other person(s) (accidental) W51
    with fall W03
      due to ice or snow W00.0
    as, or caused by, a crowd or
      human stampede (with fall)
      W52
    before moving object NEC
      Y02.8
      motor vehicle Y02.0
      subway train Y02.1
      train Y02.1
    from
      high place NEC
        in accidental circumstances
          W17.89
        stated as
          intentional, homicide
            (attempt) Y01
          undetermined whether
            accidental or
            intentional Y30
      transport vehicle NEC —see
        also Accident, transport
        V89.9
        stated as
          intentional, homicide
            (attempt) Y08.89
  overexertion X50.9

R

Radiation (exposure to)
  arc lamps W89.0
  atomic power plant (malfunction)
    NEC W88.1
  complication of or abnormal
    reaction to medical radiotherapy
    Y84.2
  electromagnetic, ionizing W88.0
  gamma rays W88.1
  in
    war operations (from or
      following nuclear explosion)
      —see War operations
  inadvertent exposure of patient
    (receiving test or therapy)
    Y63.3
  infrared (heaters and lamps) W90.1
    excessive heat from W92
  ionized, ionizing (particles,
    artificially accelerated)
    radioisotopes W88.1
    specified NEC W88.8
    x-rays W88.0
  isotopes, radioactive
    —see Radiation, radioactive
    isotopes
  laser(s) W90.2
    in war operations —see War
      operations
    misadventure in medical care
      Y63.2
  light sources (man-made visible
    and ultraviolet) W89.9
    natural X32
    specified NEC W89.8
    tanning bed W89.1
    welding light W89.0

Radiation (continued)
  man-made visible light W89.9
    specified NEC W89.8
    tanning bed W89.1
    welding light W89.0
  microwave W90.8
  misadventure in medical or surgical
    procedure Y63.2
  natural NEC X39.08
    radon X39.01
  overdose (in medical or surgical
    procedure) Y63.2
  radar W90.0
  radioactive isotopes (any) W88.1
    atomic power plant malfunction
      W88.1
    misadventure in medical or
      surgical treatment Y63.2
  radiofrequency W90.0
  radium NEC W88.1
  sun X32
  ultraviolet (light) (man-made) W89.9
    natural X32
    specified NEC W89.8
    tanning bed W89.1
    welding light W89.0
  welding arc, torch, or light W89.0
    excessive heat from W92
  x-rays (hard) (soft) W88.0

Range disease W94.11

Rape (attempted) T74.2-

Rat bite W53.11

Reaching (prolonged) (static) X50.1

**Reaction, abnormal to medical
  procedure** —see also
  Complication of or following, by
  type of procedure Y84.9
  with misadventure
    —see Misadventure
  biologicals —see Table of Drugs
    and Chemicals
  drugs —see Table of Drugs and
    Chemicals
  vaccine —see Table of Drugs and
    Chemicals

Recoil
  airgun W34.110
  BB gun W34.110
  firearm NEC W34.19
  gas, air or spring-operated gun
    NEC W34.118
  handgun W32.1
  hunting rifle W33.12
  larger firearm W33.10
    specified NEC W33.19
  machine gun W33.13
  paintball gun W34.111
  pellet W34.110
  shotgun W33.11
  Very pistol [flare] W34.19

Reduction in
  atmospheric pressure —see Air,
    pressure, change

**Rock falling on or hitting
  (accidentally) (person)** W20.8
  in cave-in W20.0

Run over (accidentally) (by)
  animal (not being ridden) NEC
    W55.89
  machinery —see Contact, with,
    by specified type of machine
  transport vehicle NEC —see also
    Accident, transport V09.9
    intentional homicide (attempt)
      Y03.0
    motor NEC V09.20
      intentional homicide (attempt)
        Y03.0

Running
before moving object X81.8
motor vehicle X81.0

Running off, away
animal (being ridden) —*see also*
Accident, transport V80.918
not being ridden W55.89
animal-drawn vehicle NEC —*see
also* Accident, transport V80.928
highway, road (way), street
transport vehicle NEC —*see also*
Accident, transport V89.9

**Rupture pressurized devices —*see*
Explosion, by type of device**

S

Saturnism —*see* Table of Drugs and
Chemicals, lead

Scald, scalding (accidental) (by)
(from) (in) X19
air (hot) X14.1
gases (hot) X14.1
homicide (attempt) —*see* Assault,
burning, hot object
inflicted by other person
stated as intentional, homicide
(attempt) —*see* Assault,
burning, hot object
liquid (boiling) (hot) NEC X12
stated as undetermined whether
accidental or intentional Y27.2
suicide (attempt) X77.2
local application of externally
applied substance in medical or
surgical care Y63.5
metal (molten) (liquid) (hot) NEC
X18
self-inflicted X77.9
stated as undetermined whether
accidental or intentional Y27.8
steam X13.1
assault X98.0
stated as undetermined whether
accidental or intentional Y27.0
suicide (attempt) X77.0
suicide (attempt) X77.9
vapor (hot) X13.1
assault X98.0
stated as undetermined whether
accidental or intentional
Y27.0
suicide (attempt) X77.0

Scratched by
cat W55.03
person(s) (accidentally) W50.4
with intent to injure or kill
Y04.0
as, or caused by, a crowd or
human stampede (with fall)
W52
assault Y04.0
homicide (attempt) Y04.0
in
fight Y04.0
legal intervention
injuring
bystander Y35.892
law enforcement
personnel Y35.891
suspect Y35.893

Seasickness T75.3

Self-harm NEC —*see also* External
cause by type, undetermined
whether
accidental or intentional
intentional —*see* Suicide
poisoning NEC —*see* Table of
drugs and biologicals, accident

Self-inflicted (injury) NEC
—*see also* External cause by
type, undetermined whether
accidental or intentional
intentional —*see* Suicide
poisoning NEC —*see* Table
of drugs and biologicals,
accident

Sequelae (of)
accident NEC —*see* W00-X58 with
7th character S
assault (homicidal) (any means) —*see*
X92-Y08 with 7th character S
homicide, attempt (any means) —*see*
X92-Y08 with 7th character S
injury undetermined whether
accidentally or purposely
inflicted —*see* Y21-Y33 with 7th
character S
intentional self-harm (classifiable
to X71-X83) —*see* X71-X83
with 7th character S
legal intervention —*see* with 7th
character S Y35
motor vehicle accident —*see*
V00-V99 with 7th character S
suicide, attempt (any means) —*see*
X71-X83 with 7th character S
transport accident —*see* V00-V99
with 7th character S
war operations —*see* War
operations

Shock
electric —*see* Exposure, electric
current
from electric appliance (any)
(faulty) W86.8
domestic W86.0
suicide (attempt) X83.1

Shooting, shot (accidental(ly)) —*see
also* Discharge, firearm, by type
herself or himself —*see* Discharge,
firearm by type, self-inflicted
homicide (attempt)
—*see* Discharge, firearm by type,
homicide
in war operations —*see* War
operations
inflicted by other person
—*see* Discharge, firearm by type,
homicide
accidental —*see* Discharge,
firearm, by type of firearm
legal
execution —*see* Legal,
intervention, firearm
intervention —*see* Legal,
intervention, firearm
self-inflicted —*see* Discharge,
firearm by type, suicide
accidental —*see* Discharge,
firearm, by type of firearm
suicide (attempt) —*see* Discharge,
firearm by type, suicide

Shoving (accidentally) by other person
—*see* Pushed, by other person

Sickness
alpine W94.11
motion —*see* Motion
mountain W94.11

Sinking (accidental)
watercraft (causing
drowning, submersion)
—*see also* Drowning, due to,
accident to, watercraft, sinking
causing injury except drowning
or submersion —*see* Accident,
watercraft, causing, injury
NEC

Siriasis X32

Sitting (prolonged) (static) X50.1

Slashed wrists —*see* Cut, self-inflicted

Slipping (accidental) (on same level)
(with fall) W01.0
on
ice W00.0
with skates —*see* Accident,
transport, pedestrian,
conveyance
mud W01.0
oil W01.0
snow W00.0
with skis —*see* Accident,
transport, pedestrian,
conveyance
surface (slippery) (wet) NEC
W01.0
without fall W18.40
due to
specified NEC W18.49
stepping from one level to
another W18.43
stepping into hole or opening
W18.42
stepping on object W18.41

Sliver, wood, contact with W45.8

Smoldering (due to fire)
—*see* Exposure, fire

Sodomy (attempted) by force
T74.2-

Sound waves (causing injury) W42.9
supersonic W42.0

Splinter, contact with W45.8

Stab, stabbing —*see* Cut

Standing (prolonged) (static) X50.1

Starvation X58

Status of external cause Y99.9
child assisting in compensated
work for family Y99.8
civilian activity done for financial
or other compensation Y99.0
civilian activity done for income or
pay Y99.0
family member assisting in
compensated work for other
family member Y99.8
hobby not done for income Y99.8
leisure activity Y99.8
military activity Y99.1
off-duty activity of military
personnel Y99.8
recreation or sport not for income
or while a student Y99.8
specified NEC Y99.8
student activity Y99.8
volunteer activity Y99.2

Stepped on
by
animal (not being ridden) NEC
W55.89
crowd or human stampede W52
person W50.0

Stepping on
object W22.8
with fall W18.31
sports equipment W21.9
stationary W22.09
sports equipment W21.89
person W51
by crowd or human stampede
W52
sports equipment W21.9

Sting
arthropod, nonvenomous W57
insect, nonvenomous W57

Storm (cataclysmic) —*see* Forces of
nature, cataclysmic storm

Straining, excessive —(*see also*
Overexertion) X50.9

Strangling —*see* Strangulation

Strangulation (accidental) —*see*
categories T71

Strenuous movements (*see also*
Overexertion) X50.9

Striking against
airbag (automobile) W22.10
driver side W22.11
front passenger side W22.12
specified NEC W22.19
bottom when
diving or jumping into water (in)
W16.822
causing drowning W16.821
from boat W16.722
causing drowning W16.721
natural body W16.622
causing drowning W16.821
swimming pool W16.522
causing drowning W16.521
falling into water (in) W16.322
causing drowning W16.321
fountain —*see* Striking
against, bottom when,
falling into water, specified
NEC
natural body W16.122
causing drowning W16.121
reservoir —*see* Striking
against, bottom when,
falling into water, specified
NEC
specified NEC W16.322
causing drowning W16.321
swimming pool W16.022
causing drowning W16.021
diving board (swimming-pool)
W21.4
object W22.8
with
drowning or submersion —*see*
Drowning
fall —*see* Fall, due to,
bumping against, object
caused by crowd or human
stampede (with fall) W52
furniture W22.03
lamppost W22.02
sports equipment W21.9
stationary W22.09
sports equipment W21.89
wall W22.01
person(s) W51
with fall W03
due to ice or snow W00.0
as, or caused by, a crowd or
human stampede (with fall)
W52
assault Y04.2
homicide (attempt) Y04.2
sports equipment W21.9
wall (when) W22.01
diving or jumping into water (in)
W16.832
causing drowning W16.831
swimming pool W16.532
causing drowning
W16.531
falling into water (in) W16.332
causing drowning W16.331
fountain —*see* Striking
against, wall when, falling
into water, specified NEC
natural body W16.132
causing drowning W16.131

Striking against (continued)

wall (continued)

  falling into water (continued)

    reservoir —see Striking

      against, wall when, falling

      into water, specified NEC

    specified NEC W16.332

      causing drowning W16.331

    swimming pool W16.032

      causing drowning W16.031

  swimming pool (when) W22.042

    causing drowning W22.041

    diving or jumping into water

      W16.532

      causing drowning W16.531

    falling into water W16.032

      causing drowning W16.031

Struck (accidentally) by

airbag (automobile) W22.10

  driver side W22.11

  front passenger side W22.12

  specified NEC W22.19

alligator W58.02

animal (not being ridden) NEC

  W55.89

avalanche —see Landslide

ball (hit) (thrown) W21.00

  assault Y08.09

  baseball W21.03

  basketball W21.05

  golf ball W21.04

  football W21.01

  soccer W21.02

  softball W21.07

  specified NEC W21.09

  volleyball W21.06

bat or racquet

  baseball bat W21.11

    assault Y08.02

  golf club W21.13

    assault Y08.09

  specified NEC W21.19

    assault Y08.09

  tennis racquet W21.12

    assault Y08.09

bullet —see also Discharge, firearm

  by type

  in war operations —see War

    operations

crocodile W58.12

dog W54.1

flare, Very pistol —see Discharge,

  firearm NEC

hailstones X39.8

hockey (ice)

  field

    puck W21.221

    stick W21.211

  puck W21.220

  stick W21.210

    assault Y08.01

landslide —see Landslide

law-enforcement agent (on duty)

  —see Legal, intervention,

  manhandling

  with blunt object —see Legal,

    intervention, blunt object

lightning —see subcategory T75.0

  causing fire —see Exposure, fire

machine —see Contact, with, by

  type of machine

mammal NEC W55.89

  marine W56.32

marine animal W56.82

missile

  firearm —see Discharge, firearm

    by type

  in war operations —see War

    operations, missile

object W22.8

  blunt W22.8

Struck (continued)

object (continued)

  blunt (continued)

    assault Y00

    suicide (attempt) X79

    undetermined whether

      accidental or intentional

      Y29

  falling W20.8

    from, in, on

      building W20.1

        burning (uncontrolled

          fire) X00.4

      cataclysmic

        earth surface movement

          NEC —see Landslide

        storm —see Forces of

          nature, cataclysmic

          storm

      cave-in W20.0

      earthquake X34

      machine (in operation)

        —see Contact, with, by

        type of machine

      structure W20.1

        burning X00.4

      transport vehicle (in motion)

        —see Accident, transport,

        by type of vehicle

      watercraft V93.49

        due to

          accident to craft

            V91.39

            powered craft

              V91.33

              ferry boat V91.31

              fishing boat

                V91.32

              jetskis V91.33

              liner V91.31

              merchant ship

                V91.30

              passenger ship

                V91.31

            unpowered craft

              V91.38

              canoe V91.35

              inflatable V91.36

              kayak V91.35

              sailboat V91.34

              surf-board

                V91.38

              windsurfer

                V91.38

        powered craft V93.43

          ferry boat V93.41

          fishing boat V93.42

          jetskis V93.43

          liner V93.41

          merchant ship V93.40

          passenger ship V93.41

        unpowered craft V93.48

          sailboat V93.44

          surf-board V93.48

          windsurfer V93.48

  moving NEC W20.8

  projected W20.8

    assault Y00

    in sports W21.9

      assault Y08.09

      ball W21.00

        baseball W21.03

        basketball W21.05

        football W21.01

        golf ball W21.04

        soccer W21.02

        softball W21.07

        specified NEC W21.09

        volleyball W21.06

      bat or racquet

        baseball bat W21.11

Struck (continued)

object (continued)

  projected (continued)

    in sports (continued)

      bat or racquet (continued)

        baseball bat (continued)

          assault Y08.02

        golf club W21.13

          assault Y08.09

        specified NEC W21.19

          assault Y08.09

        tennis racquet W21.12

          assault Y08.09

      hockey (ice)

        field

          puck W21.221

          stick W21.211

        puck W21.220

        stick W21.210

          assault Y08.01

      specified NEC W21.89

    set in motion by explosion —see

      Explosion

  thrown W20.8

    assault Y00

    in sports W21.9

      assault Y08.09

      ball W21.00

        baseball W21.03

        basketball W21.05

        football W21.01

        golf ball W21.04

        soccer W21.02

        soft ball W21.07

        specified NEC W21.09

        volleyball W21.06

      bat or racquet

        baseball bat W21.11

          assault Y08.02

        golf club W21.13

          assault Y08.09

        specified NEC W21.19

          assault Y08.09

        tennis racquet W21.12

          assault Y08.09

      hockey (ice)

        field

          puck W21.221

          stick W21.211

        puck W21.220

        stick W21.210

          assault Y08.01

      specified NEC W21.89

other person(s) W50.0

  with

    blunt object W22.8

      intentional, homicide

        (attempt) Y00

      sports equipment W21.9

      undetermined whether acci-

        dental or intentional Y29

    fall W03

      due to ice or snow W00.0

  as, or caused by, a crowd or

    human stampede (with fall)

    W52

  assault Y04.2

  homicide (attempt) Y04.2

  in legal intervention

    injuring

      bystander Y35.812

      law enforcement personnel

        Y35.811

      suspect Y35.813

      unspecified person Y35.819

  sports equipment W21.9

police (on duty) —see Legal,

  intervention, manhandling

  with blunt object —see Legal,

    intervention, blunt object

sports equipment W21.9

Struck (continued)

sports equipment (continued)

  assault Y08.09

  ball W21.00

    baseball W21.03

    basketball W21.05

    football W21.01

    golf ball W21.04

    soccer W21.02

    soft ball W21.07

    specified NEC W21.09

    volleyball W21.06

  bat or racquet

    baseball bat W21.11

      assault Y08.02

    golf club W21.13

      assault Y08.09

    specified NEC W21.19

      assault Y08.09

    tennis racquet W21.12

      assault Y08.09

  cleats (shoe) W21.31

  foot wear NEC W21.39

  football helmet W21.81

  hockey (ice)

    field

      puck W21.221

      stick W21.211

    puck W21.220

    stick W21.210

      assault Y08.01

  skate blades W21.32

  specified NEC W21.89

    assault Y08.09

thunderbolt —see subcategory T75.0

  causing fire —see Exposure, fire

transport vehicle NEC —see

  also Accident, transport V09.9

  intentional, homicide (attempt)

    Y03.0

  motor NEC —see also Accident,

    transport V09.20

    homicide Y03.0

vehicle (transport) NEC

  —see Accident, transport, by

  type of vehicle

  stationary (falling from jack,

    hydraulic lift, ramp) W20.8

Stumbling

over

  animal NEC W01.0

    with fall W18.09

  carpet, rug or (small) object

    W22.8

    with fall W18.09

  person W51

    with fall W03

      due to ice or snow W00.0

without fall W18.40

  due to

    specified NEC W18.49

    stepping from one level to

      another W18.43

    stepping into hole or opening

      W18.42

    stepping on object W18.41

Submersion (accidental)

  —see Drowning

Suffocation (accidental) (by external

  means) (by pressure) (mechanical)

  —see also category T71

due to, by

  avalanche —see Landslide

  explosion —see Explosion

  fire —see Exposure, fire

  food, any type (aspiration)

    (ingestion) (inhalation)

    —see categories T17 and T18

  ignition —see Ignition

  landslide —see Landslide

Suffocation (continued)
due to, by (continued)
machine (ry) —see Contact,
with, by type of machine
vomitus (aspiration) (inhalation)
T17.81-
in
burning building X00.8

Suicide, suicidal (attempted) (by)
X83.8
blunt object X79
burning, burns X76
hot object X77.9
fluid NEC X77.2
household appliance X77.3
specified NEC X77.8
steam X77.0
tap water X77.1
vapors X77.0
caustic substance —see Table of
Drugs and Chemicals
cold, extreme X83.2
collision of motor vehicle with
motor vehicle X82.0
specified NEC X82.8
train X82.1
tree X82.2
crashing of aircraft X83.0
cut (any part of body)
X78.9
cutting or piercing instrument
X78.9
dagger X78.2
glass X78.0
knife X78.1
specified NEC X78.8
sword X78.2
drowning (in) X71.9
bathtub X71.0
natural water X71.3
specified NEC X71.8
swimming pool X71.1
following fall X71.2
electrocution X83.1
explosive(s) (material) X75
fire, flames X76
firearm X74.9
airgun X74.01
handgun X72
hunting rifle X73.1
larger X73.9
specified NEC X73.8
machine gun X73.2
shotgun X73.0
specified NEC X74.8
hanging X83.8
hot object —see Suicide, burning,
hot object
jumping
before moving object X81.8
motor vehicle X81.0
subway train X81.1
train X81.1
from high place X80
late effect of attempt
—see X71-X83 with 7th
character S
lying before moving object, train,
vehicle X81.8
poisoning —see Table of Drugs and
Chemicals
puncture (any part of body)
—see Suicide, cutting or piercing
instrument
scald —see Suicide, burning, hot
object
sequelae of attempt —see X71-X83
with 7th character S
sharp object (any) —see Suicide,
cutting or piercing instrument

Suicide, suicidal (continued)
shooting —see Suicide, firearm
specified means NEC X83.8
stab (any part of body)
—see Suicide, cutting or piercing
instrument
steam, hot vapors X77.0
strangulation X83.8
submersion —see Suicide,
drowning
suffocation X83.8
wound NEC X83.8

Sunstroke X32

Supersonic waves (causing injury)
W42.0

**Surgical procedure, complication
of** (delayed or as an
abnormal reaction without
mention of misadventure)
—see also Complication of
or following, by type of procedure
due to or as a result of
misadventure —see
Misadventure

Swallowed, swallowing
foreign body —see Foreign body,
alimentary canal
poison —see Table of Drugs and
Chemicals
substance
caustic or corrosive —see Table
of Drugs and Chemicals
poisonous —see Table of Drugs
and Chemicals

T

Tackle in sport W03

Terrorism (involving) Y38.80
biological weapons Y38.6X-
chemical weapons Y37.7X-
conflagration Y38.3X-
drowning and submersion
Y38.89-
explosion Y38.2X-
destruction of aircraft
Y38.1X-
marine weapons Y38.0X-
fire Y38.3X-
firearms Y38.4X-
hot substances Y38.3X-
lasers Y38.89-
nuclear weapons Y38.3X-
piercing or stabbing instruments
Y38.89-
secondary effects Y38.9X-
specified method NEC Y38.89-
suicide bomber Y38.81-

Thirst X58

Threat to breathing
aspiration —see Aspiration
due to cave-in, falling earth
or substance NEC —see
categories T71

Thrown (accidentally)
against part (any) of or object in
transport vehicle (in motion)
NEC —see also Accident,
transport
from
high place, homicide (attempt)
Y01
machinery —see Contact, with,
by type of machine
transport vehicle NEC —see also
Accident, transport V89.9
off —see Thrown, from

Thunderbolt —see subcategory
T75.0
causing fire —see Exposure, fire

Tidal wave (any injury) NEC
—see Forces of nature, tidal wave

Took
overdose (drug) —see Table of
Drugs and Chemicals
poison —see Table of Drugs and
Chemicals

Tornado (any injury) X37.1

Torrential rain (any injury) X37.8

Torture X58

Trampled by animal NEC W55.89

Trapped (accidentally)
between objects (moving)
(stationary and moving)
—see Caught
by part (any) of
motorcycle V29.88
pedal cycle V19.88
transport vehicle NEC —see also
Accident, transport V89.9

Travel (effects) (sickness) T75.3

Tree falling on or hitting
(accidentally) (person) W20.8

Tripping
over
animal W01.0
with fall W01.0
carpet, rug or (small) object W22.8
with fall W18.09
person W51
with fall W03
due to ice or snow W00.0
without fall W18.40
due to
specified NEC W18.49
stepping from one level to
another W18.43
stepping into hole or opening
W18.42
stepping on object W18.41

Twisted by person(s) (accidentally)
W50.2
with intent to injure or kill Y04.0
as, or caused by, a crowd or human
stampede (with fall) W52
assault Y04.0
homicide (attempt) Y04.0
in
fight Y04.0
legal intervention —see Legal,
intervention, manhandling

Twisting (prolonged) (static) X50.1

U

**Underdosing of necessary drugs,
medicaments or biological
substances** Y63.6

Undetermined intent (contact)
(exposure)
automobile collision Y32
blunt object Y29
drowning (submersion) (in) Y21.9
bathtub Y21.0
after fall Y21.1
natural water (lake) (ocean)
(pond) (river) (stream) Y21.4
specified place NEC Y21.8
swimming pool Y21.2
after fall Y21.3
explosive material Y25
fall, jump or push from high place
Y30

Undetermined intent (continued)
falling, lying or running before
moving object Y31
fire Y26
firearm discharge Y24.9
airgun (BB) (pellet) Y24.0
handgun (pistol) (revolver) Y22
hunting rifle Y23.1
larger Y23.9
hunting rifle Y23.1
machine gun Y23.3
military Y23.2
shotgun Y23.0
specified type NEC Y23.8
machine gun Y23.3
military Y23.2
shotgun Y23.0
specified type NEC Y24.8
Very pistol Y24.8
hot object Y27.9
fluid NEC Y27.2
household appliance Y27.3
specified object NEC Y27.8
steam Y27.0
tap water Y27.1
vapor Y27.0
jump, fall or push from high place
Y30
lying, falling or running before
moving object Y31
motor vehicle crash Y32
push, fall or jump from high place
Y30
running, falling or lying before
moving object Y31
sharp object Y28.9
dagger Y28.2
glass Y28.0
knife Y28.1
specified object NEC Y28.8
sword Y28.2
smoke Y26
specified event NEC Y33

Use of hand as hammer X50.3

V

Vibration (causing injury) W49.9

Victim (of)
avalanche —see Landslide
earth movements NEC —see Forces
of nature, earth movement
earthquake X34
flood —see Flood
landslide —see Landslide
lightning —see subcategory T75.0
causing fire —see Exposure, fire
storm (cataclysmic) NEC
—see Forces of nature,
cataclysmic storm
volcanic eruption X35

Volcanic eruption (any injury) X35

**Vomitus, gastric contents in
air passages** (with asphyxia,
obstruction or suffocation) T17.81-

W

Walked into stationary object (any)
W22.09
furniture W22.03
lamppost W22.02
wall W22.01

War operations (injuries to
military personnel and civilians
during war, civil insurrection
and peacekeeping missions) (by)
(from) (involving) Y36.90
after cessation of hostilities Y36.89-
explosion (of)

War operations (continued)
after cessation of hostilities
(continued)
explosion (continued)
bomb placed during war
operations Y36.82-
mine placed during war
operations Y36.81-
specified NEC Y36.88-
air blast Y36.20-
aircraft
destruction —see War operations,
destruction of aircraft
airway restriction —see War
operations, restriction of airways
asphyxiation —see War operations,
restriction of airways
biological weapons Y36.6X-
blast Y36.20-
blast fragments Y36.20-
blast wave Y36.20-
blast wind Y36.20-
bomb Y36.20-
dirty Y36.50-
gasoline Y36.31-
incendiary Y36.31-
petrol Y36.31-
bullet Y36.43-
incendiary Y36.32-
rubber Y36.41-
chemical weapons Y36.7X-
combat
hand to hand (unarmed) combat
Y36.44-
using blunt or piercing object
Y36.45-
conflagration —see War operations,
fire
conventional warfare NEC Y36.49-
depth-charge Y36.01-
destruction of aircraft Y36.10-
due to
air to air missile Y36.11-
collision with other aircraft
Y36.12-
detonation (accidental) of
onboard munitions and
explosives Y36.14-
enemy fire or explosives
Y36.11-
explosive placed on aircraft
Y36.11-

War operations (continued)
destruction of aircraft (continued)
due to (continued)
onboard fire Y36.13-
rocket propelled grenade
[RPG] Y36.11-
small arms fire Y36.11-
surface to air missile Y36.11-
specified NEC Y36.19-
detonation (accidental) of
onboard marine weapons Y36.05-
own munitions or munitions
launch device Y36.24-
dirty bomb Y36.50-
explosion (of) Y36.20-
after cessation of hostilities
bomb placed during war
operations Y36.82-
mine placed during war
operations Y36.81-
aerial bomb Y36.21-
bomb NOS —see also War
operations, bomb(s) Y36.20-
own munitions or munitions
launch device (accidental)
Y36.24-
fragments Y36.20-
grenade Y36.29-
guided missile Y36.22-
improvised explosive device
[IED] (person-borne) (roadside)
(vehicle-borne) Y36.23-
land mine Y36.29-
marine mine (at sea) (in harbor)
Y36.02-
marine weapon Y36.00-
specified NEC Y36.09-
sea-based artillery shell
Y36.03-
specified NEC Y36.29-
torpedo Y36.04-
fire Y36.30-
specified NEC Y36.39-
firearms
discharge Y36.43-
pellets Y36.42-
flamethrower Y36.33-
fragments (from) (of)
improvised explosive device
[IED] (person-borne)
(roadside) (vehicle-borne)
Y36.26-

War operations (continued)
fragments (continued)
munitions Y36.25-
specified NEC Y36.29-
weapons Y36.27-
friendly fire Y36.92
hand to hand (unarmed) combat
Y36.44-
hot substances —see War
operations, fire
incendiary bullet Y36.32-
nuclear weapon (effects of) Y36.50-
acute radiation exposure Y36.54-
blast pressure Y36.51-
direct blast Y36.51-
direct heat Y36.53-
fallout exposure Y36.54-
fireball Y36.53-
indirect blast (struck or crushed
by blast debris) (being thrown
by blast) Y36.52-
ionizing radiation (immediate
exposure) Y36.54-
nuclear radiation Y36.54-
radiation
ionizing (immediate
exposure) Y36.54-
nuclear Y36.54-
thermal Y36.53-
specified NEC Y36.59-
secondary effects Y36.54-
thermal radiation Y36.53-
restriction of air (airway)
intentional Y36.46-
unintentional Y36.47-
rubber bullets Y36.41-
shrapnel NOS Y36.29-
suffocation —see War operations,
restriction of airways
unconventional warfare NEC
Y36.7X-
underwater blast NOS Y36.00-
warfare
conventional NEC Y36.49-
unconventional NEC Y36.7X-
weapons
biological weapons Y36.6X-
chemical Y36.7X-
nuclear (effects of) Y36.50-
acute radiation exposure
Y36.54-

War operations (continued)
weapons (continued)
nuclear (continued)
blast pressure Y36.51-
direct blast Y36.51-
direct heat Y36.53-
fallout exposure Y36.54-
fireball Y36.53-
radiation
ionizing (immediate
exposure) Y36.54-
nuclear Y36.54-
thermal Y36.53-
secondary effects Y36.54-
specified NEC Y36.59-
of mass destruction [WMD]
Y36.91
weapon of mass destruction
[WMD] Y36.91

Washed
away by flood —see Flood
off road by storm (transport
vehicle) —see Forces of nature,
cataclysmic storm

Weather exposure NEC
—see Forces of nature

Weightlessness (causing injury)
(effects of) (in spacecraft,
real or simulated) X52

Work related condition Y99.0

Wound (accidental) NEC
—see also Injury X58
battle —see also War operations
Y36.90
gunshot —see Discharge, firearm
by type

Wreck transport vehicle NEC
—see also Accident, transport
V89.9

Wrong
device implanted into correct
surgical site Y65.51
fluid in infusion Y65.1
procedure (operation) on correct
patient Y65.51
patient, procedure performed on
Y65.52

Tabular List of Diseases and Injuries

Table of Contents

Instructional Notations

Includes:

The word 'Includes' appears immediately under certain categories to further define, or give examples of, the content of the category.

Excludes Notes

The ICD-10-CM has two types of excludes notes. Each note has a different definition for use but they are both similar in that they indicate that codes excluded from each other are independent of each other.

Excludes1

A type 1 Excludes note is a pure excludes. It means 'NOT CODED HERE!' An Excludes1 note indicates that the code excluded should never be used at the same time as the code above the Excludes1 note. An Excludes1 is used when two conditions cannot occur together, such as a congenital form versus an acquired form of the same condition.

Excludes2

A type 2 excludes note represents 'Not included here'. An Excludes2 note indicates that the condition excluded is not part of the condition it is excluded from but a patient may have both conditions at the same time. When an Excludes2 note appears under a code it is acceptable to use both the code and the excluded code together.

Code First/Use Additional Code notes (etiology/manifestation paired codes)

Certain conditions have both an underlying etiology and multiple body system manifestations due to the underlying etiology. For such conditions the ICD-10-CM has a coding convention that requires the underlying condition be sequenced first followed by the manifestation. Wherever such a combination exists there is a 'use additional code' note at the etiology code, and a 'code first' note at the manifestation code. These instructional notes indicate the proper sequencing order of the codes, etiology followed by manifestation.

In most cases the manifestation codes will have in the code title, 'in diseases classified elsewhere.' Codes with this title are a component of the etiology/ manifestation convention. The code title indicates that it is a manifestation code. 'In diseases classified elsewhere' codes are never permitted to be used as first listed or principal diagnosis codes. They must be used in conjunction with an underlying condition code and they must be listed following the underlying condition.

Code Also

A "code also" note instructs that two codes may be required to fully describe a condition, but this note does not provide sequencing direction. **The sequencing depends on the circumstances of the encounter**.

7th characters and placeholder X

Certain ICD-10-CM categories have applicable 7th characters. The applicable 7th character is required for all codes within the category, or as the notes in the Tabular List instruct. The 7th character must always be the 7th character in the data field. If a code that requires a 7th character is not 6 characters, a placeholder X must be used to fill in the empty characters.

475

+, +7th, X + 7th • Newborn • Pediatric • Maternity • Adult ♀ Female ♂ Male Manifestation Unacceptable PDX HCC CC MCC HAC

Chapter 1: Certain Infectious and Parasitic Diseases (A00-B99)

Includes: diseases generally recognized as communicable or transmissible

Use additional code to identify resistance to antimicrobial drugs (Z16-)

Excludes1: *certain localized infections - see body system-related chapters*

Excludes2: *carrier or suspected carrier of infectious disease (Z22.-)*
infectious and parasitic diseases specific to the perinatal period (P35-P39)
infectious and parasitic diseases complicating pregnancy, childbirth and the puerperium (O98.-)
influenza and other acute respiratory infections (J00-J22)

This chapter contains the following category blocks:

A00-A09	Intestinal infectious diseases
A15-A19	Tuberculosis
A20-A28	Certain zoonotic bacterial diseases
A30-A49	Other bacterial diseases
A50-A64	Infections with a predominantly sexual mode of transmission
A65-A69	Other spirochetal diseases
A70-A74	Other diseases caused by chlamydiae
A75-A79	Rickettsioses
A80-A89	Viral and prion infections of the central nervous system
A90-A99	Arthropod-borne viral fevers and viral hemorrhagic fevers
B00-B09	Viral infections characterized by skin and mucous membrane lesions
B10	Other human herpesviruses
B15-B19	Viral hepatitis
B20	Human immunodeficiency virus [HIV] disease
B25-B34	Other viral diseases
B35-B49	Mycoses
B50-B64	Protozoal diseases
B65-B83	Helminthiases
B85-B89	Pediculosis, acariasis and other infestations
B90-B94	Sequelae of infectious and parasitic diseases
B95-B97	Bacterial and viral infectious agents
B99	Other infectious diseases

C. Chapter-Specific Coding Guidelines

In addition to general coding guidelines, there are guidelines for specific diagnoses and/or conditions in the classification. Unless otherwise indicated, these guidelines apply to all health care settings. Please refer to Section II for guidelines on the selection of principal diagnosis.

1. Chapter 1: Certain Infectious and Parasitic Diseases (A00-B99), *U07.1*

a. Human Immunodeficiency Virus (HIV) Infections

1) Code only confirmed cases

Code only confirmed cases of HIV infection/illness. This is an exception to the hospital inpatient guideline Section II, H.

In this context, "confirmation" does not require documentation of positive serology or culture for HIV; the provider's diagnostic statement that the patient is HIV positive, or has an HIV-related illness is sufficient.

2) Selection and sequencing of HIV codes

(a) Patient admitted for HIV-related condition

If a patient is admitted for an HIV-related condition, the principal diagnosis should be B20, Human immunodeficiency virus [HIV] disease followed by additional diagnosis codes for all reported HIV-related conditions.

(b) Patient with HIV disease admitted for unrelated condition

If a patient with HIV disease is admitted for an unrelated condition (such as a traumatic injury), the code for the unrelated condition (e.g., the nature of injury code) should be the principal diagnosis. Other diagnoses would be B20 followed by additional diagnosis codes for all reported HIV-related conditions.

(c) Whether the patient is newly diagnosed

Whether the patient is newly diagnosed or has had previous admissions/encounters for HIV conditions is irrelevant to the sequencing decision.

(d) Asymptomatic human immunodeficiency virus

Z21, Asymptomatic human immunodeficiency virus [HIV] infection status, is to be applied when the patient without any documentation of symptoms is listed as being "HIV positive," "known HIV," "HIV test positive," or similar terminology. Do not use this code if the term "AIDS" is used or if the patient is treated for any HIV-related illness or is described as having any condition(s) resulting from his/her HIV positive status; use B20 in these cases.

(e) Patients with inconclusive HIV serology

Patients with inconclusive HIV serology, but no definitive diagnosis or manifestations of the illness, may be assigned code R75, Inconclusive laboratory evidence of human immunodeficiency virus [HIV].

(f) Previously diagnosed HIV-related illness

Patients with any known prior diagnosis of an HIV-related illness should be coded to B20. Once a patient has developed an HIV-related illness, the patient should always be assigned code B20 on every subsequent admission/encounter. Patients previously diagnosed with any HIV illness (B20) should never be assigned to R75 or Z21, Asymptomatic human immunodeficiency virus [HIV] infection status.

(g) HIV Infection in Pregnancy, Childbirth and the Puerperium

During pregnancy, childbirth or the puerperium, a patient admitted (or presenting for a health care encounter) because of an HIV-related illness should receive a principal diagnosis code of O98.7-, Human immunodeficiency [HIV] disease complicating pregnancy, childbirth and the puerperium, followed by B20 and the code(s) for the HIV-related illness(es). Codes from Chapter 15 always take sequencing priority. Patients with asymptomatic HIV infection status admitted (or presenting for a health care encounter) during pregnancy, childbirth, or the puerperium should receive codes of O98.7- and Z21.

(h) Encounters for testing for HIV

If a patient is being seen to determine his/her HIV status, use code Z11.4, Encounter for screening for human immunodeficiency virus [HIV]. Use additional codes for any associated high risk behavior.

If a patient with signs or symptoms is being seen for HIV testing, code the signs and symptoms. An additional counseling code Z71.7, Human immunodeficiency virus [HIV] counseling, may be used if counseling is provided during the encounter for the test.

When a patient returns to be informed of his/her HIV test results and the test result is negative, use code Z71.7, Human immunodeficiency virus [HIV] counseling.

If the results are positive, see previous guidelines and assign codes as appropriate.

b. Infectious agents as the cause of diseases classified to other chapters

Certain infections are classified in chapters other than Chapter 1 and no organism is identified as part of the infection code. In these instances, it is necessary to use an additional code from Chapter 1 to identify the organism. A code from category B95, Streptococcus, Staphylococcus, and Enterococcus as the cause of diseases classified to other chapters, B96, Other bacterial agents as the cause of diseases classified to other chapters, or B97, Viral agents as the cause of diseases classified to other chapters, is to be used as an additional code to identify the organism. An instructional note will be found at the infection code advising that an additional organism code is required.

c. Infections resistant to antibiotics

Many bacterial infections are resistant to current antibiotics. It is necessary to identify all infections documented as antibiotic resistant. Assign a code from category Z16, Resistance to antimicrobial drugs, following the infection code only if the infection code does not identify drug resistance.

d. Sepsis, Severe Sepsis, and Septic Shock

1) Coding of Sepsis and Severe Sepsis

(a) Sepsis

For a diagnosis of sepsis, assign the appropriate code for the underlying systemic infection. If the type of infection or causal organism is not further specified, assign code A41.9, Sepsis, unspecified organism.

A code from subcategory R65.2, Severe sepsis, should not be assigned unless severe sepsis or an associated acute organ dysfunction is documented.

(i) Negative or inconclusive blood cultures and sepsis

Negative or inconclusive blood cultures do not preclude a diagnosis of sepsis in patients with clinical evidence of the condition, however, the provider should be queried.

(ii) Urosepsis

The term urosepsis is a nonspecific term. It is not to be considered synonymous with sepsis. It has no default code in the Alphabetic Index. Should a provider use this term, he/she must be queried for clarification.

+, +7th, X + 7th   ● Newborn   ● Pediatric   ● Maternity   ● Adult   ♀ Female   ♂ Male   Manifestation   Unacceptable PDX   HCC   CC   MCC   HAC

(iii) Sepsis with organ dysfunction

If a patient has sepsis and associated acute organ dysfunction or multiple organ dysfunction (MOD), follow the instructions for coding severe sepsis.

(iv) Acute organ dysfunction that is not clearly associated with the sepsis

If a patient has sepsis and an acute organ dysfunction, but the medical record documentation indicates that the acute organ dysfunction is related to a medical condition other than the sepsis, do not assign a code from subcategory R65.2, Severe sepsis. An acute organ dysfunction must be associated with the sepsis in order to assign the severe sepsis code. If the documentation is not clear as to whether an acute organ dysfunction is related to the sepsis or another medical condition, query the provider.

(b) Severe sepsis

The coding of severe sepsis requires a minimum of 2 codes: first a code for the underlying systemic infection, followed by a code from subcategory R65.2, Severe sepsis. If the causal organism is not documented, assign code A41.9, Sepsis, unspecified organism, for the infection. Additional code(s) for the associated acute organ dysfunction are also required.

Due to the complex nature of severe sepsis, some cases may require querying the provider prior to assignment of the codes.

2) Septic shock

(a) Septic shock generally refers to circulatory failure associated with severe sepsis, and therefore, it represents a type of acute organ dysfunction.

For cases of septic shock, the code for the systemic infection should be sequenced first, followed by code R65.21, Severe sepsis with septic shock or code T81.12, Postprocedural septic shock. Any additional codes for the other acute organ dysfunctions should also be assigned. As noted in the sequencing instructions in the Tabular List, the code for septic shock cannot be assigned as a principal diagnosis.

3) Sequencing of severe sepsis

If severe sepsis is present on admission, and meets the definition of principal diagnosis, the underlying systemic infection should be assigned as principal diagnosis followed by the appropriate code from subcategory R65.2 as required by the sequencing rules in the Tabular List. A code from subcategory R65.2 can never be assigned as a principal diagnosis.

When severe sepsis develops during an encounter (it was not present on admission) the underlying systemic infection and the appropriate code from subcategory R65.2 should be assigned as secondary diagnoses.

Severe sepsis may be present on admission but the diagnosis may not be confirmed until sometime after admission. If the documentation is not clear whether severe sepsis was present on admission, the provider should be queried.

4) Sepsis or severe sepsis with a localized infection

If the reason for admission is both sepsis or severe sepsis and a localized infection, such as pneumonia or cellulitis, a code(s) for the underlying systemic infection should be assigned first and the code for the localized infection should be assigned as a secondary diagnosis. If the patient has severe sepsis, a code from subcategory R65.2 should also be assigned as a secondary diagnosis. If the patient is admitted with a localized infection, such as pneumonia, and sepsis/severe sepsis doesn't develop until after admission, the localized infection should be assigned first, followed by the appropriate sepsis/severe sepsis codes.

5) Sepsis due to a postprocedural infection

(a) Documentation of causal relationship

As with all postprocedural complications, code assignment is based on the provider's documentation of the relationship between the infection and the procedure.

(b) Sepsis due to a postprocedural infection

For infections following a procedure, a code from T81.40, to T81.43, Infection following a procedure, or a code from O86.00 to O86.03, Infection of obstetric surgical wound, that identifies the site of the infection should be coded first, if known. Assign an additional code for sepsis following a procedure (T81.44) or sepsis following an obstetrical procedure (O86.04). Use an additional code to identify the infectious agent. If the patient has severe sepsis the appropriate code from subcategory R65.2 should also be assigned with the additional code(s) for any acute organ dysfunction.

For infections following infusion, transfusion, therapeutic injection, or immunization, a code from subcategory T80.2, Infections following infusion, transfusion, and therapeutic injection, or code

T88.0-, Infection following immunization, should be coded first, followed by the code for the specific infection. If the patient has severe sepsis, the appropriate code from subcategory R65.2 should also be assigned, with the additional code(s) for any acute organ dysfunction.

(c) Postprocedural infection and postprocedural septic shock

If a postprocedural infection has resulted in postprocedural septic shock, assign the codes indicated above for sepsis due to a postprocedural infection, followed by code T81.12-, Postprocedural septic shock. Do not assign code R65.21, Severe sepsis with septic shock. Additional code(s) should be assigned for any acute organ dysfunction.

6) Sepsis and severe sepsis associated with a noninfectious process (condition)

In some cases a noninfectious process (condition), such as trauma, may lead to an infection which can result in sepsis or severe sepsis. If sepsis or severe sepsis is documented as associated with a noninfectious condition, such as a burn or serious injury, and this condition meets the definition for principal diagnosis, the code for the noninfectious condition should be sequenced first, followed by the code for the resulting infection. If severe sepsis, is present a code from subcategory R65.2 should also be assigned with any associated organ dysfunction(s) codes. It is not necessary to assign a code from subcategory R65.1, Systemic inflammatory response syndrome (SIRS) of non-infectious origin, for these cases.

If the infection meets the definition of principal diagnosis it should be sequenced before the non-infectious condition. When both the associated non-infectious condition and the infection meet the definition of principal diagnosis either may be assigned as principal diagnosis.

Only one code from category R65, Symptoms and signs specifically associated with systemic inflammation and infection, should be assigned. Therefore, when a non-infectious condition leads to an infection resulting in severe sepsis, assign the appropriate code from subcategory R65.2, Severe sepsis. Do not additionally assign a code from subcategory R65.1, Systemic inflammatory response syndrome (SIRS) of non-infectious origin.

See Section I.C.18. SIRS due to non-infectious process

7) Sepsis and septic shock complicating abortion, pregnancy, childbirth, and the puerperium

See Section I.C.15. Sepsis and septic shock complicating abortion, pregnancy, childbirth and the puerperium

8) Newborn sepsis

See Section I.C.16. f. Bacterial sepsis of Newborn

e. Methicillin Resistant *Staphylococcus aureus* (MRSA) Conditions

1) Selection and sequencing of MRSA codes

(a) Combination codes for MRSA infection

When a patient is diagnosed with an infection that is due to methicillin resistant Staphylococcus aureus (MRSA), and that infection has a combination code that includes the causal organism (e.g., sepsis, pneumonia) assign the appropriate combination code for the condition (e.g., code A41.02, Sepsis due to Methicillin resistant Staphylococcus aureus or code J15.212, Pneumonia due to Methicillin resistant Staphylococcus aureus). Do not assign code B95.62, Methicillin resistant Staphylococcus aureus infection as the cause of diseases classified elsewhere, as an additional code because the combination code includes the type of infection and the MRSA organism. Do not assign a code from subcategory Z16.11, Resistance to penicillins, as an additional diagnosis.

See Section C.1. for instructions on coding and sequencing of sepsis and severe sepsis.

(b) Other codes for MRSA infection

When there is documentation of a current infection (e.g., wound infection, stitch abscess, urinary tract infection) due to MRSA, and that infection does not have a combination code that includes the causal organism, assign the appropriate code to identify the condition along with code B95.62, Methicillin resistant Staphylococcus aureus infection as the cause of diseases classified elsewhere for the MRSA infection. Do not assign a code from subcategory Z16.11, Resistance to penicillins.

(c) Methicillin susceptible *Staphylococcus aureus* (MSSA) and MRSA colonization

The condition or state of being colonized or carrying MSSA or MRSA is called colonization or carriage, while an individual person is described as being colonized or being a carrier. Colonization means that MSSA

+, +7th, X + 7th   ● Newborn   ● Pediatric   ● Maternity   ● Adult   ♀ Female   ♂ Male   Manifestation   Unacceptable PDX   HCC   CC   MCC   HAC

or MSRA is present on or in the body without necessarily causing illness. A positive MRSA colonization test might be documented by the provider as "MRSA screen positive" or "MRSA nasal swab positive".

Assign code Z22.322, Carrier or suspected carrier of Methicillin resistant Staphylococcus aureus, for patients documented as having MRSA colonization. Assign code Z22.321, Carrier or suspected carrier of Methicillin susceptible Staphylococcus aureus, for patient documented as having MSSA colonization. Colonization is not necessarily indicative of a disease process or as the cause of a specific condition the patient may have unless documented as such by the provider.

(d) MRSA colonization and infection

If a patient is documented as having both MRSA colonization and infection during a hospital admission, code Z22.322, Carrier or suspected carrier of Methicillin resistant Staphylococcus aureus, and a code for the MRSA infection may both be assigned.

f. Zika virus infections

1) Code only confirmed cases

Code only a confirmed diagnosis of Zika virus (A92.5, Zika virus disease) as documented by the provider. This is an exception to the hospital inpatient guideline Section II, H. In this context, "confirmation" does not require documentation of the type of test performed; the provider's diagnostic statement that the condition is confirmed is sufficient. This code should be assigned regardless of the stated mode of transmission.

If the provider documents "suspected", "possible" or "provable" Zika, do not assign code A92.5. Assign a code(s) explaining the reason for encounter (such as fever, rash, or joint pain) or Z20.821, Contact with and (suspected) exposure to Zika virus.

g. Coronavirus infections

1) COVID-19 infection (infection due to SARS-CoV-2)

(a) Code only confirmed cases

Code only a confirmed diagnosis of the 2019 novel coronavirus disease (COVID-19) as documented by the provider or documentation of a positive COVID-19 test result. For a confirmed diagnosis, assign code U07.1, COVID-19. This is an exception to the hospital inpatient guideline Section II, H. In this context, "confirmation" does not require documentation of a positive test result for COVID-19; the provider's documentation that the individual has COVID-19 is sufficient.

If the provider documents "suspected," "possible," "probable," or "inconclusive" COVID-19, do not assign code U07.1. Instead, code the signs and symptoms reported.

See guideline I.C.1.g.1.g.

(b) Sequencing of codes

When COVID-19 meets the definition of principle diagnosis, code U07.1, COVID-19, should be sequenced first, followed by the appropriate codes for associated manifestations, except when another guideline requires that certain codes be sequenced first, such as obstetrics, sepsis, or transplant complications.

For a COVID-19 infection that progresses to sepsis, see Section I.C.1.d Sepsis, Severe Sepsis, and Septic Shock

See Section I.C.15.s. for COVID-19 infection in pregnancy, childbirth, and the puerperium

See Section I.C.16.h. for COVID-19 infection in newborn

For a COVID-19 infection in a lung transplant patient, see Section I.C.19.g.3.a. Transplant complications other than kidney

(c) Acute respiratory manifestations of COVID-19

When the reason for the encounter/admission is a respiratory manifestation of COVID-19, assign code U07.1, COVID-19, as the principal/first-listed diagnosis and assign code(s) for the respiratory manifestation(s) as additional diagnoses.

The following conditions are examples of common respiratory manifestations of COVID-19.

(i) Pneumonia

For a patient with pneumonia confirmed as due to COVID-19, assign codes U07.1, COVID-19, and J12.89, Other viral pneumonia.

(ii) Acute bronchitis

For a patient with acute bronchitis confirmed as due to COVID-19, assign codes U07.1, and J20.8, Acute bronchitis due to other specified organisms.

Bronchitis not otherwise specified (NOS) due to COVID-19 should be coded using code U07.1 and J40, Bronchitis, not specified as acute or chronic.

(iii) Lower respiratory infection

If the COVID-19 is documented as being associated with lower respiratory infection, not otherwise specified (NOS), or an acute respiratory infection, NOS, codes U07.1 and J22, Unspecified acute lower respiratory infection, should be assigned.

If the COVID-19 is documented as being associated with a respiratory infection, NOS, codes U07.1 and J98.8, Other specified respiratory disorders, should be assigned.

(iv) Acute respiratory distress syndrome

For acute respiratory distress syndrome (ARDS) due to COVID-19, assign codes U07.1 and J80, Acute respiratory distress syndrome.

(v) Acute respiratory failure

For acute respiratory failure due to COVID-19, assign code U07.1 and code J96.0-, Acute respiratory failure.

(d) Non-respiratory manifestations of COVID-19

When the reason for the encounter/admission is a non-respiratory manifestation (e.g., viral enteritis) of COVID-19, assign code U07.1, COVID-19, as the principal/first-listed diagnosis and assign code(s) for the manifestation(s) as additional diagnoses.

(e) Exposure to COVID-19

For asymptomatic individuals with actual or suspected exposure to COVID-19, assign code Z20.828, Contact with and (suspected) exposure to other viral communicable diseases.

For symptomatic individuals with actual or suspected exposure to COVID-19 and the infection has been ruled out, or test results are inconclusive or unknown, assign code Z20.828, Contact with and (suspected) exposure to other viral communicable diseases.

See guidelines I.C.21.c.1, Contact/Exposure, for additional guidance regarding the use of category Z20 codes.

If COVID-19 is confirmed, see guidelines I.C.1.g.1.a.

(f) Screening for COVID-19

During the COVID-19 pandemic, a screening code is generally not appropriate. For encounters for COVID-19 testing, including preoperative testing, code as exposure to COVID-19 (guideline I.C.1.g.1.e).

Coding guidance will be updated as new information concerning any changes in the pandemic status becomes available.

(g) Signs and symptoms without definitive diagnosis of COVID-19

For patient presenting with any signs/symptoms associated with COVID-19 (such as fever, etc.) but a definitive diagnosis has not been established, assign the appropriate code(s) for each of the presenting signs and symptoms such as:

- R05 Cough
- R06.02 Shortness of breath
- R50.9 Fever, unspecified

If a patient with signs/symptoms associated with COVID-19 also has an actual or suspected contact with or exposure to COVID-19, assign Z20.828, Contact with and (suspected) exposure to other viral communicable diseases, as an additional code.

(h) Asymptomatic individuals who test positive for COVID-19

For asymptomatic individuals who test positive for COVID-19, *see guideline I.C.1.g.1.a.* Although the individual is asymptomatic, the individual has tested positive and is considered to have a COVID-19 infection.

(i) Personal history of COVID-19

For patients with a history of COVID-19, assign code Z86.19, Personal history of other infectious and parasitic diseases.

(j) Follow-up visits after COVID-19 infection has resolved

For individuals who previously had COVID-19 and are being seen for follow-up evaluation, and COVID-19 test results are negative, assign codes Z09, Encounter for follow-up examination after completed treatment for conditions other than malignant neoplasm, and Z86.19, Personal history of other infections and parasitic diseases.

(k) Encounter for antibody testing

For an encounter for antibody testing that is not being performed to confirm a current COVID-19 infection, nor is a follow-up test after resolution of COVID-19, assign Z01.84, Encounter for antibody response examination.

Follow the applicable guidelines above if the individual is being tested to confirm a current COVID-19 infection.

For follow-up testing after a COVID-19 infection, see guideline I.C.1.g.1.j

Intestinal infectious diseases (A00-A09)

A00 Cholera

  CC **A00.0** **Cholera due to Vibrio cholerae 01, biovar cholerae**
      Classical cholera

  CC **A00.1** **Cholera due to Vibrio cholerae 01, biovar eltor**
      Cholera eltor

  CC **A00.9** **Cholera, unspecified**

A01 Typhoid and paratyphoid fevers

  + **A01.0** **Typhoid fever**
      Infection due to Salmonella typhi

    CC **A01.00** **Typhoid fever, unspecified**

    CC **A01.01** **Typhoid meningitis**

    CC **A01.02** **Typhoid fever with heart involvement**
        Typhoid endocarditis
        Typhoid myocarditis

    CC **A01.03** **Typhoid pneumonia**

    CC **A01.04** **Typhoid arthritis**

    CC **A01.05** **Typhoid osteomyelitis**

    CC **A01.09** **Typhoid fever with other complications**

  CC **A01.1** **Paratyphoid fever A**

  CC **A01.2** **Paratyphoid fever B**

  CC **A01.3** **Paratyphoid fever C**

  CC **A01.4** **Paratyphoid fever, unspecified**
      Infection due to Salmonella paratyphi NOS

A02 Other salmonella infections

  Includes: infection or foodborne intoxication due to any Salmonella species other than S. typhi and S. paratyphi

  CC **A02.0** **Salmonella enteritis**
      Salmonellosis

  MCC **A02.1** **Salmonella sepsis**
      Review coding guideline C.1.d

  + **A02.2** **Localized salmonella infections**

      A02.20 **Localized salmonella infection, unspecified**

    MCC **A02.21** **Salmonella meningitis**

    MCC **A02.22** **Salmonella pneumonia**

    CC **A02.23** **Salmonella arthritis**

    CC **A02.24** **Salmonella osteomyelitis**

    CC **A02.25** **Salmonella pyelonephritis**
        Salmonella tubulo-interstitial nephropathy

    CC **A02.29** **Salmonella with other localized infection**

  CC **A02.8** **Other specified salmonella infections**

  CC **A02.9** **Salmonella infection, unspecified**

A03 Shigellosis

  CC **A03.0** **Shigellosis due to Shigella dysenteriae**
      Group A shigellosis [Shiga-Kruse dysentery]

    A03.1 **Shigellosis due to Shigella flexneri**
      Group B shigellosis

    A03.2 **Shigellosis due to Shigella boydii**
      Group C shigellosis

    A03.3 **Shigellosis due to Shigella sonnei**
      Group D shigellosis

    A03.8 **Other shigellosis**

    A03.9 **Shigellosis, unspecified**
      Bacillary dysentery NOS

A04 Other bacterial intestinal infections

  Excludes1: bacterial foodborne intoxications, NEC (A05.-)
         tuberculous enteritis (A18.32)

  CC **A04.0** **Enteropathogenic Escherichia coli infection**

  CC **A04.1** **Enterotoxigenic Escherichia coli infection**

  CC **A04.2** **Enteroinvasive Escherichia coli infection**

  CC **A04.3** **Enterohemorrhagic Escherichia coli infection**

  CC **A04.4** **Other intestinal Escherichia coli infections**
      Escherichia coli enteritis NOS

  CC **A04.5** **Campylobacter enteritis**

  CC **A04.6** **Enteritis due to Yersinia enterocolitica**
      Excludes1: extraintestinal yersiniosis (A28.2)

  + **A04.7** **Enterocolitis due to Clostridium difficile**
      Foodborne intoxication by Clostridium difficile
      Pseudomembranous colitis
      AHA CC: 4Q, 2017, 4

    CC **A04.71** **Enterocolitis due to clostridium difficile, recurrent**
        AHA CC: 1Q, 2020, 18

    CC **A04.72** **Enterocolitis due to clostridium difficile, not specified as recurrent**

  CC **A04.8** **Other specified bacterial intestinal infections**

  CC **A04.9** **Bacterial intestinal infection, unspecified**
      Bacterial enteritis NOS

A05 Other bacterial foodborne intoxications, not elsewhere classified

  Excludes1: Clostridium difficile foodborne intoxication and infection (A04.7-)
        Escherichia coli infection (A04.0-A04.4)
        listeriosis (A32.-)
        salmonella foodborne intoxication and infection (A02.-)
        toxic effect of noxious foodstuffs (T61-T62)

  CC **A05.0** **Foodborne staphylococcal intoxication**

  CC **A05.1** **Botulism food poisoning**
      Botulism NOS
      Classical foodborne intoxication due to Clostridium botulinum
      Excludes1: infant botulism (A48.51)
            wound botulism (A48.52)

  CC **A05.2** **Foodborne Clostridium perfringens [Clostridium welchii] intoxication**
      Enteritis necroticans
      Pig-bel

  CC **A05.3** **Foodborne Vibrio parahaemolyticus intoxication**

  CC **A05.4** **Foodborne Bacillus cereus intoxication**

  CC **A05.5** **Foodborne Vibrio vulnificus intoxication**

  CC **A05.8** **Other specified bacterial foodborne intoxications**

    A05.9 **Bacterial foodborne intoxication, unspecified**

A06 Amebiasis

  Includes: infection due to Entamoeba histolytica
  Excludes1: other protozoal intestinal diseases (A07.-)
  Excludes2: acanthamebiasis (B60.1-)
        Naegleriasis (B60.2)

  CC **A06.0** **Acute amebic dysentery**
      Acute amebiasis
      Intestinal amebiasis NOS

  CC **A06.1** **Chronic intestinal amebiasis**

  CC **A06.2** **Amebic nondysenteric colitis**

  CC **A06.3** **Ameboma of intestine**
      Ameboma NOS

  MCC **A06.4** **Amebic liver abscess**
      Hepatic amebiasis

  MCC **A06.5** **Amebic lung abscess**
      Amebic abscess of lung (and liver)

  MCC **A06.6** **Amebic brain abscess**
      Amebic abscess of brain (and liver) (and lung)

    A06.7 **Cutaneous amebiasis**

  + **A06.8** **Amebic infection of other sites**

    CC **A06.81** **Amebic cystitis**

    CC **A06.82** **Other amebic genitourinary infections**
        Amebic balanitis
        Amebic vesiculitis
        Amebic vulvovaginitis

    CC **A06.89** **Other amebic infections**
        Amebic appendicitis
        Amebic splenic abscess

    A06.9 **Amebiasis, unspecified**

A07 Other protozoal intestinal diseases

    A07.0 **Balantidiasis**
      Balantidial dysentery

  CC **A07.1** **Giardiasis [lambliasis]**

  CC **A07.2** **Cryptosporidiosis**

  CC **A07.3** **Isosporiasis**
      Infection due to Isospora belli and Isospora hominis
      Intestinal coccidiosis
      Isosporosis

  CC **A07.4** **Cyclosporiasis**

  CC **A07.8** **Other specified protozoal intestinal diseases**
      Intestinal microsporidiosis
      Intestinal trichomoniasis
      Sarcocystosis
      Sarcosporidiosis

  CC **A07.9** **Protozoal intestinal disease, unspecified**
      Flagellate diarrhea
      Protozoal colitis
      Protozoal diarrhea
      Protozoal dysentery

A08 Viral and other specified intestinal infections

> *Excludes1:* *influenza with involvement of gastrointestinal tract (J09.X3, J10.2, J11.2)*

> CC **A08.0 Rotaviral enteritis**

> + **A08.1 Acute gastroenteropathy due to Norwalk agent and other small round viruses**

>> CC **A08.11 Acute gastroenteropathy due to Norwalk agent**
>>> Acute gastroenteropathy due to Norovirus
>>> Acute gastroenteropathy due to Norwalk-like agent

>> CC **A08.19 Acute gastroenteropathy due to other small round viruses**
>>> Acute gastroenteropathy due to small round virus [SRV] NOS

> CC **A08.2 Adenoviral enteritis**

> + **A08.3 Other viral enteritis**

>> CC **A08.31 Calicivirus enteritis**

>> CC **A08.32 Astrovirus enteritis**

>> CC **A08.39 Other viral enteritis**
>>> Coxsackie virus enteritis
>>> Echovirus enteritis
>>> Enterovirus enteritis NEC
>>> Torovirus enteritis

> **A08.4 Viral intestinal infection, unspecified**
>> Viral enteritis NOS
>> Viral gastroenteritis NOS
>> Viral gastroenteropathy NOS
>> *AHA CC: 3Q, 2016, 12*

> **A08.8 Other specified intestinal infections**

CC **A09 Infectious gastroenteritis and colitis, unspecified**

> Infectious colitis NOS
> Infectious enteritis NOS
> Infectious gastroenteritis NOS
> *Excludes1:* *colitis NOS (K52.9)*
>> *diarrhea NOS (R19.7)*
>> *enteritis NOS (K52.9)*
>> *gastroenteritis NOS (K52.9)*
>> *noninfective gastroenteritis and colitis, unspecified (K52.9)*
> Valid 3-character code, no further characters required

Tuberculosis (A15-A19)

Includes: infections due to Mycobacterium tuberculosis and Mycobacterium bovis

Excludes1: *congenital tuberculosis (P37.0)*
> *nonspecific reaction to test for tuberculosis without active tuberculosis (R76.1-)*
> *pneumoconiosis associated with tuberculosis, any type in A15 (J65)*
> *positive PPD (R76.11)*
> *positive tuberculin skin test without active tuberculosis (R76.11)*
> *sequelae of tuberculosis (B90.-)*
> *silicotuberculosis (J65)*

A15 Respiratory tuberculosis

> CC **A15.0 Tuberculosis of lung**
>> Tuberculous bronchiectasis
>> Tuberculous fibrosis of lung
>> Tuberculous pneumonia
>> Tuberculous pneumothorax

> CC **A15.4 Tuberculosis of intrathoracic lymph nodes**
>> Tuberculosis of hilar lymph nodes
>> Tuberculosis of mediastinal lymph nodes
>> Tuberculosis of tracheobronchial lymph nodes
>> *Excludes1:* *tuberculosis specified as primary (A15.7)*

> CC **A15.5 Tuberculosis of larynx, trachea and bronchus**
>> Tuberculosis of bronchus
>> Tuberculosis of glottis
>> Tuberculosis of larynx
>> Tuberculosis of trachea

> CC **A15.6 Tuberculous pleurisy**
>> Tuberculosis of pleura Tuberculous empyema
>> *Excludes1:* *primary respiratory tuberculosis (A15.7)*

> CC **A15.7 Primary respiratory tuberculosis**

> CC **A15.8 Other respiratory tuberculosis**
>> Mediastinal tuberculosis
>> Nasopharyngeal tuberculosis
>> Tuberculosis of nose
>> Tuberculosis of sinus [any nasal]

> CC **A15.9 Respiratory tuberculosis unspecified**

A17 Tuberculosis of nervous system

> MCC **A17.0 Tuberculous meningitis**
>> Tuberculosis of meninges (cerebral)(spinal)
>> Tuberculous leptomeningitis
>> *Excludes1:* *tuberculous meningoencephalitis (A17.82)*

> MCC **A17.1 Meningeal tuberculoma**
>> Tuberculoma of meninges (cerebral) (spinal)
>> *Excludes2:* *tuberculoma of brain and spinal cord (A17.81)*

> + **A17.8 Other tuberculosis of nervous system**

>> MCC **A17.81 Tuberculoma of brain and spinal cord**
>>> Tuberculous abscess of brain and spinal cord

>> MCC **A17.82 Tuberculous meningoencephalitis**
>>> Tuberculous myelitis

>> MCC **A17.83 Tuberculous neuritis**
>>> Tuberculous mononeuropathy

>> MCC **A17.89 Other tuberculosis of nervous system**
>>> Tuberculous polyneuropathy

> CC **A17.9 Tuberculosis of nervous system, unspecified**

A18 Tuberculosis of other organs

> + **A18.0 Tuberculosis of bones and joints**

>> CC **A18.01 Tuberculosis of spine**
>>> Pott's disease or curvature of spine
>>> Tuberculous arthritis
>>> Tuberculous osteomyelitis of spine
>>> Tuberculous spondylitis

>> CC **A18.02 Tuberculous arthritis of other joints**
>>> Tuberculosis of hip (joint)
>>> Tuberculosis of knee (joint)

>> CC **A18.03 Tuberculosis of other bones**
>>> Tuberculous mastoiditis
>>> Tuberculous osteomyelitis

>> CC **A18.09 Other musculoskeletal tuberculosis**
>>> Tuberculous myositis
>>> Tuberculous synovitis
>>> Tuberculous tenosynovitis

> + **A18.1 Tuberculosis of genitourinary system**

>> CC **A18.10 Tuberculosis of genitourinary system, unspecified**

>> CC **A18.11 Tuberculosis of kidney and ureter**

>> CC **A18.12 Tuberculosis of bladder**

>> CC **A18.13 Tuberculosis of other urinary organs**
>>> Tuberculous urethritis

>> ● ♂ CC **A18.14 Tuberculosis of prostate**

>> ♂ CC **A18.15 Tuberculosis of other male genital organs**

>> ♀ CC **A18.16 Tuberculosis of cervix**

>> ♀ CC **A18.17 Tuberculous female pelvic inflammatory disease**
>>> Tuberculous endometritis
>>> Tuberculous oophoritis and salpingitis

>> ♀ CC **A18.18 Tuberculosis of other female genital organs**
>>> Tuberculous ulceration of vulva

> CC **A18.2 Tuberculous peripheral lymphadenopathy**
>> Tuberculous adenitis
>> *Excludes2:* *tuberculosis of bronchial and mediastinal lymph nodes (A15.4)*
>>> *tuberculosis of mesenteric and retroperitoneal lymph nodes (A18.39)*
>>> *tuberculous tracheobronchial adenopathy (A15.4)*

> + **A18.3 Tuberculosis of intestines, peritoneum and mesenteric glands**

>> MCC **A18.31 Tuberculous peritonitis**
>>> Tuberculous ascites

>> CC **A18.32 Tuberculous enteritis**
>>> Tuberculosis of anus and rectum
>>> Tuberculosis of intestine (large) (small)

>> CC **A18.39 Retroperitoneal tuberculosis**
>>> Tuberculosis of mesenteric glands
>>> Tuberculosis of retroperitoneal (lymph glands)

> CC **A18.4 Tuberculosis of skin and subcutaneous tissue**
>> Erythema induratum, tuberculous
>> Lupus excedens
>> Lupus vulgaris NOS
>> Lupus vulgaris of eyelid
>> Scrofuloderma
>> Tuberculosis of external ear
>> *Excludes2:* *lupus erythematosus (L93.-)*
>>> *systemic lupus erythematosus (M32.-)*

> + **A18.5 Tuberculosis of eye**
>> *Excludes2:* *lupus vulgaris of eyelid (A18.4)*

>> CC **A18.50 Tuberculosis of eye, unspecified**

>> CC **A18.51 Tuberculous episcleritis**

CC **A18.52 Tuberculous keratitis**
Tuberculous interstitial keratitis
Tuberculous keratoconjunctivitis (interstitial) (phlyctenular)
CC **A18.53 Tuberculous chorioretinitis**
CC **A18.54 Tuberculous iridocyclitis**
CC **A18.59 Other tuberculosis of eye**
Tuberculous conjunctivitis
CC **A18.6 Tuberculosis of (inner) (middle) ear**
Tuberculous otitis media
Excludes2: *tuberculosis of external ear (A18.4)*
tuberculous mastoiditis (A18.03)
CC **A18.7 Tuberculosis of adrenal glands**
Tuberculous Addison's disease
+ **A18.8 Tuberculosis of other specified organs**
CC **A18.81 Tuberculosis of thyroid gland**
CC **A18.82 Tuberculosis of other endocrine glands**
Tuberculosis of pituitary gland
Tuberculosis of thymus gland
CC **A18.83 Tuberculosis of digestive tract organs, not elsewhere classified**
Excludes1: *tuberculosis of intestine (A18.32)*
CC **A18.84 Tuberculosis of heart**
Tuberculous cardiomyopathy
Tuberculous endocarditis
Tuberculous myocarditis
Tuberculous pericarditis
CC **A18.85 Tuberculosis of spleen**
CC **A18.89 Tuberculosis of other sites**
Tuberculosis of muscle
Tuberculous cerebral arteritis

A19 Miliary tuberculosis

Includes: disseminated tuberculosis
generalized tuberculosis
tuberculous polyserositis
MCC **A19.0 Acute miliary tuberculosis of a single specified site**
MCC **A19.1 Acute miliary tuberculosis of multiple sites**
MCC **A19.2 Acute miliary tuberculosis, unspecified**
MCC **A19.8 Other miliary tuberculosis**
MCC **A19.9 Miliary tuberculosis, unspecified**

Certain zoonotic bacterial diseases (A20-A28)

A20 Plague

Includes: infection due to Yersinia pestis
MCC **A20.0 Bubonic plague**
MCC **A20.1 Cellulocutaneous plague**
MCC **A20.2 Pneumonic plague**
MCC **A20.3 Plague meningitis**
MCC **A20.7 Septicemic plague**
Review coding guideline C.1.d
MCC **A20.8 Other forms of plague**
Abortive plague
Asymptomatic plague
Pestis minor
MCC **A20.9 Plague, unspecified**

A21 Tularemia

Includes: deer-fly fever
infection due to Francisella tularensis
rabbit fever
CC **A21.0 Ulceroglandular tularemia**
CC **A21.1 Oculoglandular tularemia**
Ophthalmic tularemia
CC **A21.2 Pulmonary tularemia**
CC **A21.3 Gastrointestinal tularemia**
Abdominal tularemia
CC **A21.7 Generalized tularemia**
Review coding guideline C.1.d
CC **A21.8 Other forms of tularemia**
CC **A21.9 Tularemia, unspecified**

A22 Anthrax

Includes: infection due to Bacillus anthracis
CC **A22.0 Cutaneous anthrax**
Malignant carbuncle
Malignant pustule
MCC **A22.1 Pulmonary anthrax**
Inhalation anthrax
Ragpicker's disease
Woolsorter's disease

CC **A22.2 Gastrointestinal anthrax**
MCC **A22.7 Anthrax sepsis**
Review coding guideline C.1.d
CC **A22.8 Other forms of anthrax**
Anthrax meningitis
CC **A22.9 Anthrax, unspecified**

A23 Brucellosis

Includes: Malta fever
Mediterranean fever
undulant fever
A23.0 Brucellosis due to Brucella melitensis
A23.1 Brucellosis due to Brucella abortus
A23.2 Brucellosis due to Brucella suis
A23.3 Brucellosis due to Brucella canis
CC **A23.8 Other brucellosis**
CC **A23.9 Brucellosis, unspecified**
Review coding guideline C.1.d

A24 Glanders and melioidosis

CC **A24.0 Glanders**
Infection due to Pseudomonas mallei
Malleus
Review coding guideline C.1.d
CC **A24.1 Acute and fulminating melioidosis**
Melioidosis pneumonia
Melioidosis sepsis
Review coding guideline C.1.d
CC **A24.2 Subacute and chronic melioidosis**
CC **A24.3 Other melioidosis**
CC **A24.9 Melioidosis, unspecified**
Infection due to Pseudomonas pseudomallei NOS
Whitmore's disease

A25 Rat-bite fevers

CC **A25.0 Spirillosis**
Sodoku
CC **A25.1 Streptobacillosis**
Epidemic arthritic erythema
Haverhill fever
Streptobacillary rat-bite fever
CC **A25.9 Rat-bite fever, unspecified**

A26 Erysipeloid

A26.0 Cutaneous erysipeloid
Erythema migrans
MCC **A26.7 Erysipelothrix sepsis**
Review coding guideline C.1.d
A26.8 Other forms of erysipeloid
A26.9 Erysipeloid, unspecified

A27 Leptospirosis

CC **A27.0 Leptospirosis icterohemorrhagica**
Leptospiral or spirochetal jaundice (hemorrhagic)
Weil's disease
+ **A27.8 Other forms of leptospirosis**
MCC **A27.81 Aseptic meningitis in leptospirosis**
CC **A27.89 Other forms of leptospirosis**
CC **A27.9 Leptospirosis, unspecified**

A28 Other zoonotic bacterial diseases, not elsewhere classified

CC **A28.0 Pasteurellosis**
Review coding guideline C.1.d
CC **A28.1 Cat-scratch disease**
Cat-scratch fever
CC **A28.2 Extraintestinal yersiniosis**
Excludes1: *enteritis due to Yersinia enterocolitica (A04.6)*
plague (A20.-)
Review coding guideline C.1.d
CC **A28.8 Other specified zoonotic bacterial diseases, not elsewhere classified**
CC **A28.9 Zoonotic bacterial disease, unspecified**

Other bacterial diseases (A30-A49)

A30 Leprosy [Hansen's disease]

Includes: infection due to Mycobacterium leprae
Excludes1: *sequelae of leprosy (B92)*
CC **A30.0 Indeterminate leprosy**
I leprosy
CC **A30.1 Tuberculoid leprosy**
TT leprosy
CC **A30.2 Borderline tuberculoid leprosy**
BT leprosy

+, +7th, X + 7th ● Newborn ● Pediatric ● Maternity ● Adult ♀ Female ♂ Male | Manifestation | Unacceptable PDX | HCC | CC | MCC | HAC

CC **A30.3** **Borderline leprosy**
BB leprosy
CC **A30.4** **Borderline lepromatous leprosy**
BL leprosy
CC **A30.5** **Lepromatous leprosy**
LL leprosy
CC **A30.8** **Other forms of leprosy**
CC **A30.9** **Leprosy, unspecified**

A31 **Infection due to other mycobacteria**

Excludes2: *leprosy (A30.-)*
tuberculosis (A15-A19)

CC **A31.0** **Pulmonary mycobacterial infection**
Infection due to Mycobacterium avium
Infection due to Mycobacterium intracellulare
[Battey bacillus]
Infection due to Mycobacterium kansasii

CC **A31.1** **Cutaneous mycobacterial infection**
Buruli ulcer
Infection due to Mycobacterium marinum
Infection due to Mycobacterium ulcerans

CC **A31.2** **Disseminated mycobacterium avium-intracellulare complex (DMAC)**
MAC sepsis

CC **A31.8** **Other mycobacterial infections**

CC **A31.9** **Mycobacterial infection, unspecified**
Atypical mycobacterial infection NOS
Mycobacteriosis NOS

A32 **Listeriosis**

Includes: listerial foodborne infection
Excludes1: *neonatal (disseminated) listeriosis (P37.2)*

CC **A32.0** **Cutaneous listeriosis**
+ **A32.1** **Listerial meningitis and meningoencephalitis**
CC **A32.11** **Listerial meningitis**
CC **A32.12** **Listerial meningoencephalitis**
MCC **A32.7** **Listerial sepsis**
Review coding guideline C.1.d
+ **A32.8** **Other forms of listeriosis**
CC **A32.81** **Oculoglandular listeriosis**
CC **A32.82** **Listerial endocarditis**
CC **A32.89** **Other forms of listeriosis**
Listerial cerebral arteritis
CC **A32.9** **Listeriosis, unspecified**

A33 **Tetanus neonatorum**
MCC
● Valid 3-character code, no further characters required

A34 **Obstetrical tetanus**
♀ CC
● Valid 3-character code, no further characters required

A35 **Other tetanus**
MCC
Tetanus NOS
Excludes1: *obstetrical tetanus (A34)*
tetanus neonatorum (A33)
Valid 3-character code, no further characters required

A36 **Diphtheria**

CC **A36.0** **Pharyngeal diphtheria**
Diphtheritic membranous angina
Tonsillar diphtheria
CC **A36.1** **Nasopharyngeal diphtheria**
CC **A36.2** **Laryngeal diphtheria**
Diphtheritic laryngotracheitis
CC **A36.3** **Cutaneous diphtheria**
Excludes2: *erythrasma (L08.1)*
+ **A36.8** **Other diphtheria**
CC **A36.81** **Diphtheritic cardiomyopathy**
Diphtheritic myocarditis
CC **A36.82** **Diphtheritic radiculomyelitis**
CC **A36.83** **Diphtheritic polyneuritis**
CC **A36.84** **Diphtheritic tubulo-interstitial nephropathy**
CC **A36.85** **Diphtheritic cystitis**
CC **A36.86** **Diphtheritic conjunctivitis**
CC **A36.89** **Other diphtheritic complications**
Diphtheritic peritonitis
CC **A36.9** **Diphtheria, unspecified**

A37 **Whooping cough**

+ **A37.0** **Whooping cough due to Bordetella pertussis**
CC **A37.00** **Whooping cough due to Bordetella pertussis without pneumonia**
MCC **A37.01** **Whooping cough due to Bordetella pertussis with pneumonia**

+ **A37.1** **Whooping cough due to Bordetella parapertussis**
CC **A37.10** **Whooping cough due to Bordetella parapertussis without pneumonia**
MCC **A37.11** **Whooping cough due to Bordetella parapertussis with pneumonia**
+ **A37.8** **Whooping cough due to other Bordetella species**
CC **A37.80** **Whooping cough due to other Bordetella species without pneumonia**
MCC **A37.81** **Whooping cough due to other Bordetella species with pneumonia**
+ **A37.9** **Whooping cough, unspecified species**
CC **A37.90** **Whooping cough, unspecified species without pneumonia**
MCC **A37.91** **Whooping cough, unspecified species with pneumonia**

A38 **Scarlet fever**

Includes: scarlatina
Excludes2: *streptococcal sore throat (J02.0)*
CC **A38.0** **Scarlet fever with otitis media**
CC **A38.1** **Scarlet fever with myocarditis**
CC **A38.8** **Scarlet fever with other complications**
CC **A38.9** **Scarlet fever, uncomplicated**
Scarlet fever, NOS

A39 **Meningococcal infection**

MCC **A39.0** **Meningococcal meningitis**
MCC **A39.1** **Waterhouse-Friderichsen syndrome**
Meningococcal hemorrhagic adrenalitis
Meningococcic adrenal syndrome
Review coding guideline C.1.d
MCC **A39.2** **Acute meningococcemia**
Review coding guideline C.1.d
MCC **A39.3** **Chronic meningococcemia**
Review coding guideline C.1.d
MCC **A39.4** **Meningococcemia, unspecified**
Review coding guideline C.1.d
+ **A39.5** **Meningococcal heart disease**
MCC **A39.50** **Meningococcal carditis, unspecified**
MCC **A39.51** **Meningococcal endocarditis**
MCC **A39.52** **Meningococcal myocarditis**
MCC **A39.53** **Meningococcal pericarditis**
+ **A39.8** **Other meningococcal infections**
MCC **A39.81** **Meningococcal encephalitis**
CC **A39.82** **Meningococcal retrobulbar neuritis**
CC **A39.83** **Meningococcal arthritis**
CC **A39.84** **Postmeningococcal arthritis**
CC **A39.89** **Other meningococcal infections**
Meningococcal conjunctivitis
CC **A39.9** **Meningococcal infection, unspecified**
Meningococcal disease NOS

A40 **Streptococcal sepsis**

Code first:
postprocedural streptococcal sepsis (T81.4-)
streptococcal sepsis during labor (O75.3)
streptococcal sepsis following abortion or ectopic or molar pregnancy (O03-O07, O08.0)
streptococcal sepsis following immunization (T88.0)
streptococcal sepsis following infusion, transfusion or therapeutic injection (T80.2-)
Excludes1: *neonatal (P36.0-P36.1)*
puerperal sepsis (O85)
sepsis due to Streptococcus, group D (A41.81)
Review coding guideline C.1.d
MCC **A40.0** **Sepsis due to streptococcus, group A**
MCC **A40.1** **Sepsis due to streptococcus, group B**
AHA CC: 4Q, 2018, 89; 1Q, 2019, 14
MCC **A40.3** **Sepsis due to Streptococcus pneumoniae**
Pneumococcal sepsis
MCC **A40.8** **Other streptococcal sepsis**
MCC **A40.9** **Streptococcal sepsis, unspecified**

A41 **Other sepsis**

Code first:
postprocedural sepsis (T81.4-)
sepsis during labor (O75.3)
sepsis following abortion, ectopic or molar pregnancy (O03-O07, O08.0)
sepsis following immunization (T88.0)
sepsis following infusion, transfusion or therapeutic injection (T80.2-)
Excludes1: *bacteremia NOS (R78.81)*
neonatal (P36.-)
puerperal sepsis (O85)

+, +7th, X + 7th ● Newborn ● Pediatric ● Maternity ● Adult ♀ Female ♂ Male Manifestation Unacceptable PDX HCC CC MCC HAC

streptococcal sepsis (A40.-)

Excludes2: *sepsis (due to) (in) actinomycotic (A42.7)*
sepsis (due to) (in) anthrax (A22.7)
sepsis (due to) (in) candidal (B37.7)
sepsis (due to) (in) Erysipelothrix (A26.7)
sepsis (due to) (in) extraintestinal yersiniosis (A28.2)
sepsis (due to) (in) gonococcal (A54.86)
sepsis (due to) (in) herpesviral (B00.7)
sepsis (due to) (in) listerial (A32.7)
sepsis (due to) (in) melioidosis (A24.1)
sepsis (due to) (in) meningococcal (A39.2-A39.4)
sepsis (due to) (in) plague (A20.7)
sepsis (due to) (in) tularemia (A21.7)
toxic shock syndrome (A48.3)
Review coding guideline C.1.d

+ **A41.0 Sepsis due to Staphylococcus aureus**

MCC **A41.01 Sepsis due to Methicillin susceptible Staphylococcus aureus**
MSSA sepsis
Staphylococcus aureus sepsis NOS
AHA CC: 2Q, 2020, 17-18

MCC **A41.02 Sepsis due to Methicillin resistant Staphylococcus aureus**
Review coding guideline C.1.e.1.a

MCC **A41.1 Sepsis due to other specified staphylococcus**
Coagulase negative staphylococcus sepsis

MCC **A41.2 Sepsis due to unspecified staphylococcus**

MCC **A41.3 Sepsis due to Hemophilus influenzae**

MCC **A41.4 Sepsis due to anaerobes**
Excludes1: *gas gangrene (A48.0)*

+ **A41.5 Sepsis due to other Gram-negative organisms**

MCC **A41.50 Gram-negative sepsis, unspecified**
Gram-negative sepsis NOS
AHA CC: 2Q, 2020, 29

MCC **A41.51 Sepsis due to Escherichia coli [E. coli]**
AHA CC: 1Q, 2018, 16; 2Q, 2020, 17-18

MCC **A41.52 Sepsis due to Pseudomonas**
Pseudomonas aeroginosa

MCC **A41.53 Sepsis due to Serratia**

MCC **A41.59 Other Gram-negative sepsis**
AHA CC: 1Q, 2019, 13

+ **A41.8 Other specified sepsis**

MCC **A41.81 Sepsis due to Enterococcus**

MCC **A41.89 Other specified sepsis**
AHA CC: 3Q, 2016, 9-14; 2Q, 2020, 8

MCC **A41.9 Sepsis, unspecified organism**
Septicemia NOS
AHA CC: 4Q, 2018, 18; 2Q, 2020, 28

A42 Actinomycosis

Excludes1: *actinomycetoma (B47.1)*

CC **A42.0 Pulmonary actinomycosis**
CC **A42.1 Abdominal actinomycosis**
CC **A42.2 Cervicofacial actinomycosis**
MCC **A42.7 Actinomycotic sepsis**
Review coding guideline C.1.d

+ **A42.8 Other forms of actinomycosis**
CC **A42.81 Actinomycotic meningitis**
CC **A42.82 Actinomycotic encephalitis**
CC **A42.89 Other forms of actinomycosis**
CC **A42.9 Actinomycosis, unspecified**

A43 Nocardiosis

CC **A43.0 Pulmonary nocardiosis**
CC **A43.1 Cutaneous nocardiosis**
CC **A43.8 Other forms of nocardiosis**
CC **A43.9 Nocardiosis, unspecified**

A44 Bartonellosis

CC **A44.0 Systemic bartonellosis**
Oroya fever
CC **A44.1 Cutaneous and mucocutaneous bartonellosis**
Verruga peruana
CC **A44.8 Other forms of bartonellosis**
CC **A44.9 Bartonellosis, unspecified**

A46 Erysipelas

Excludes1: *postpartum or puerperal erysipelas (O86.89)*
Valid 3-character code, no further characters required

A48 Other bacterial diseases, not elsewhere classified

Excludes1: *actinomycetoma (B47.1)*

MCC **A48.0 Gas gangrene**
Clostridial cellulitis
Clostridial myonecrosis
AHA CC: 4Q, 2017, 102

MCC **A48.1 Legionnaires' disease**
A48.2 Nonpneumonic Legionnaires' disease [Pontiac fever]

MCC **A48.3 Toxic shock syndrome**
Use additional code to identify the organism (B95, B96)
Excludes1: *endotoxic shock NOS (R57.8)*
sepsis NOS (A41.9)

A48.4 Brazilian purpuric fever
Systemic Hemophilus aegyptius infection

+ **A48.5 Other specified botulism**
Non-foodborne intoxication due to toxins of Clostridium botulinum [C. botulinum]
Excludes1: *food poisoning due to toxins of Clostridium botulinum (A05.1)*

• CC **A48.51 Infant botulism**
CC **A48.52 Wound botulism**
Non-foodborne botulism NOS
Use additional code for associated wound

A48.8 Other specified bacterial diseases

A49 Bacterial infection of unspecified site

Excludes1: *bacterial agents as the cause of diseases classified elsewhere (B95-B96)*
chlamydial infection NOS (A74.9)
meningococcal infection NOS (A39.9)
rickettsial infection NOS (A79.9)
spirochetal infection NOS (A69.9)

+ **A49.0 Staphylococcal infection, unspecified site**
A49.01 Methicillin susceptible Staphylococcus aureus infection, unspecified site
Methicillin susceptible Staphylococcus aureus (MSSA) infection
Staphylococcus aureus infection NOS
A49.02 Methicillin resistant Staphylococcus aureus infection, unspecified site
Methicillin resistant Staphylococcus aureus (MRSA) infection

A49.1 Streptococcal infection, unspecified site
A49.2 Hemophilus influenzae infection, unspecified site
A49.3 Mycoplasma infection, unspecified site
A49.8 Other bacterial infections of unspecified site
A49.9 Bacterial infection, unspecified
Excludes1: *bacteremia NOS (R78.81)*

Infections with a predominantly sexual mode of transmission (A50-A64)

Excludes1: *human immunodeficiency virus [HIV] disease (B20)*
nonspecific and nongonococcal urethritis (N34.1)
Reiter's disease (M02.3-)

A50 Congenital syphilis

+ **A50.0 Early congenital syphilis, symptomatic**
Any congenital syphilitic condition specified as early or manifest less than two years after birth.
CC **A50.01 Early congenital syphilitic oculopathy**
CC **A50.02 Early congenital syphilitic osteochondropathy**
CC **A50.03 Early congenital syphilitic pharyngitis**
Early congenital syphilitic laryngitis
CC **A50.04 Early congenital syphilitic pneumonia**
CC **A50.05 Early congenital syphilitic rhinitis**
CC **A50.06 Early cutaneous congenital syphilis**
CC **A50.07 Early mucocutaneous congenital syphilis**
CC **A50.08 Early visceral congenital syphilis**
CC **A50.09 Other early congenital syphilis, symptomatic**

A50.1 Early congenital syphilis, latent
Congenital syphilis without clinical manifestations, with positive serological reaction and negative spinal fluid test, less than two years after birth.

CC **A50.2 Early congenital syphilis, unspecified**
Congenital syphilis NOS less than two years after birth.

+ **A50.3 Late congenital syphilitic oculopathy**
Excludes1: *Hutchinson's triad (A50.53)*
CC **A50.30 Late congenital syphilitic oculopathy, unspecified**
CC **A50.31 Late congenital syphilitic interstitial keratitis**
CC **A50.32 Late congenital syphilitic chorioretinitis**
CC **A50.39 Other late congenital syphilitic oculopathy**

+ **A50.4 Late congenital neurosyphilis [juvenile neurosyphilis]**
Use additional code to identify any associated mental disorder
Excludes1: *Hutchinson's triad (A50.53)*
CC **A50.40 Late congenital neurosyphilis, unspecified**
Juvenile neurosyphilis NOS

MCC **A50.41** **Late congenital syphilitic meningitis**
MCC **A50.42** **Late congenital syphilitic encephalitis**
CC **A50.43** **Late congenital syphilitic polyneuropathy**
CC **A50.44** **Late congenital syphilitic optic nerve atrophy**
CC **A50.45** **Juvenile general paresis**
 Dementia paralytica juvenilis
 Juvenile tabetoparetic neurosyphilis
CC **A50.49** **Other late congenital neurosyphilis**
 Juvenile tabes dorsalis
+ **A50.5** **Other late congenital syphilis, symptomatic**
 Any congenital syphilitic condition specified as late or manifest two years or more after birth.
CC **A50.51** **Clutton's joints**
CC **A50.52** **Hutchinson's teeth**
CC **A50.53** **Hutchinson's triad**
CC **A50.54** **Late congenital cardiovascular syphilis**
CC **A50.55** **Late congenital syphilitic arthropathy**
CC **A50.56** **Late congenital syphilitic osteochondropathy**
CC **A50.57** **Syphilitic saddle nose**
CC **A50.59** **Other late congenital syphilis, symptomatic**
A50.6 **Late congenital syphilis, latent**
 Congenital syphilis without clinical manifestations, with positive serological reaction and negative spinal fluid test, two years or more after birth.
A50.7 **Late congenital syphilis, unspecified**
 Congenital syphilis NOS two years or more after birth.
A50.9 **Congenital syphilis, unspecified**

A51 **Early syphilis**

A51.0 **Primary genital syphilis**
 Syphilitic chancre NOS
A51.1 **Primary anal syphilis**
A51.2 **Primary syphilis of other sites**
+ **A51.3** **Secondary syphilis of skin and mucous membranes**
CC **A51.31** **Condyloma latum**
CC **A51.32** **Syphilitic alopecia**
CC **A51.39** **Other secondary syphilis of skin**
 Syphilitic leukoderma
 Syphilitic mucous patch
 Excludes1: *late syphilitic leukoderma (A52.79)*
+ **A51.4** **Other secondary syphilis**
MCC **A51.41** **Secondary syphilitic meningitis**
♀ CC **A51.42** **Secondary syphilitic female pelvic disease**
CC **A51.43** **Secondary syphilitic oculopathy**
 Secondary syphilitic chorioretinitis
 Secondary syphilitic iridocyclitis, iritis
 Secondary syphilitic uveitis
CC **A51.44** **Secondary syphilitic nephritis**
CC **A51.45** **Secondary syphilitic hepatitis**
CC **A51.46** **Secondary syphilitic osteopathy**
CC **A51.49** **Other secondary syphilitic conditions**
 Secondary syphilitic lymphadenopathy
 Secondary syphilitic myositis
A51.5 **Early syphilis, latent**
 Syphilis (acquired) without clinical manifestations, with positive serological reaction and negative spinal fluid test, less than two years after infection.
A51.9 **Early syphilis, unspecified**

A52 **Late syphilis**

+ **A52.0** **Cardiovascular and cerebrovascular syphilis**
CC **A52.00** **Cardiovascular syphilis, unspecified**
CC **A52.01** **Syphilitic aneurysm of aorta**
CC **A52.02** **Syphilitic aortitis**
CC **A52.03** **Syphilitic endocarditis**
 Syphilitic aortic valve incompetence or stenosis
 Syphilitic mitral valve stenosis
 Syphilitic pulmonary valve regurgitation
CC **A52.04** **Syphilitic cerebral arteritis**
CC **A52.05** **Other cerebrovascular syphilis**
 Syphilitic cerebral aneurysm (ruptured) (non-ruptured)
 Syphilitic cerebral thrombosis
CC **A52.06** **Other syphilitic heart involvement**
 Syphilitic coronary artery disease
 Syphilitic myocarditis
 Syphilitic pericarditis
CC **A52.09** **Other cardiovascular syphilis**
+ **A52.1** **Symptomatic neurosyphilis**
CC **A52.10** **Symptomatic neurosyphilis, unspecified**
CC **A52.11** **Tabes dorsalis**
 Locomotor ataxia (progressive)
 Tabetic neurosyphilis
CC **A52.12** **Other cerebrospinal syphilis**
MCC **A52.13** **Late syphilitic meningitis**
MCC **A52.14** **Late syphilitic encephalitis**
CC **A52.15** **Late syphilitic neuropathy**
 Late syphilitic acoustic neuritis
 Late syphilitic optic (nerve) atrophy
 Late syphilitic polyneuropathy
 Late syphilitic retrobulbar neuritis
CC **A52.16** **Charcôt's arthropathy (tabetic)**
CC **A52.17** **General paresis**
 Dementia paralytica
CC **A52.19** **Other symptomatic neurosyphilis**
 Syphilitic parkinsonism
CC **A52.2** **Asymptomatic neurosyphilis**
CC **A52.3** **Neurosyphilis, unspecified**
 Gumma (syphilitic)
 Syphilis (late)
 Syphiloma
+ **A52.7** **Other symptomatic late syphilis**
CC **A52.71** **Late syphilitic oculopathy**
 Late syphilitic chorioretinitis
 Late syphilitic episcleritis
CC **A52.72** **Syphilis of lung and bronchus**
CC **A52.73** **Symptomatic late syphilis of other respiratory organs**
CC **A52.74** **Syphilis of liver and other viscera**
 Late syphilitic peritonitis
CC **A52.75** **Syphilis of kidney and ureter**
 Syphilitic glomerular disease
CC **A52.76** **Other genitourinary symptomatic late syphilis**
 Late syphilitic female pelvic inflammatory disease
CC **A52.77** **Syphilis of bone and joint**
CC **A52.78** **Syphilis of other musculoskeletal tissue**
 Late syphilitic bursitis
 Syphilis [stage unspecified] of bursa
 Syphilis [stage unspecified] of muscle
 Syphilis [stage unspecified] of synovium
 Syphilis [stage unspecified] of tendon
CC **A52.79** **Other symptomatic late syphilis**
 Late syphilitic leukoderma
 Syphilis of adrenal gland
 Syphilis of pituitary gland
 Syphilis of thyroid gland
 Syphilitic splenomegaly
 Excludes1: *syphilitic leukoderma (secondary) (A51.39)*
A52.8 **Late syphilis, latent**
 Syphilis (acquired) without clinical manifestations, with positive serological reaction and negative spinal fluid test, two years or more after infection
A52.9 **Late syphilis, unspecified**

A53 **Other and unspecified syphilis**

A53.0 **Latent syphilis, unspecified as early or late**
 Latent syphilis NOS
 Positive serological reaction for syphilis
A53.9 **Syphilis, unspecified**
 Infection due to Treponema pallidum NOS
 Syphilis (acquired) NOS
 Excludes1: *syphilis NOS under two years of age (A50.2)*

A54 **Gonococcal infection**

+ **A54.0** **Gonococcal infection of lower genitourinary tract without periurethral or accessory gland abscess**
 Excludes1: *gonococcal infection with genitourinary gland abscess (A54.1)*
  gonococcal infection with periurethral abscess (A54.1)
CC **A54.00** **Gonococcal infection of lower genitourinary tract, unspecified**
CC **A54.01** **Gonococcal cystitis and urethritis, unspecified**
♀ CC **A54.02** **Gonococcal vulvovaginitis, unspecified**
♀ CC **A54.03** **Gonococcal cervicitis, unspecified**
CC **A54.09** **Other gonococcal infection of lower genitourinary tract**
CC **A54.1** **Gonococcal infection of lower genitourinary tract with periurethral and accessory gland abscess**
 Gonococcal Bartholin's gland abscess
+ **A54.2** **Gonococcal pelviperitonitis and other gonococcal genitourinary infection**
CC **A54.21** **Gonococcal infection of kidney and ureter**

♂ CC **A54.22 Gonococcal prostatitis**
♂ CC **A54.23 Gonococcal infection of other male genital organs**
  Gonococcal epididymitis
  Gonococcal orchitis
♀ CC **A54.24 Gonococcal female pelvic inflammatory disease**
  Gonococcal pelviperitonitis
  Excludes1: *gonococcal peritonitis (A54.85)*
CC **A54.29 Other gonococcal genitourinary infections**
+ **A54.3 Gonococcal infection of eye**
CC **A54.30 Gonococcal infection of eye, unspecified**
CC **A54.31 Gonococcal conjunctivitis**
  Ophthalmia neonatorum due to gonococcus
CC **A54.32 Gonococcal iridocyclitis**
CC **A54.33 Gonococcal keratitis**
CC **A54.39 Other gonococcal eye infection**
  Gonococcal endophthalmia
+ **A54.4 Gonococcal infection of musculoskeletal system**
CC **A54.40 Gonococcal infection of musculoskeletal system, unspecified**
CC **A54.41 Gonococcal spondylopathy**
CC **A54.42 Gonococcal arthritis**
  Excludes2: *gonococcal infection of spine (A54.41)*
CC **A54.43 Gonococcal osteomyelitis**
  Excludes2: *gonococcal infection of spine (A54.41)*
CC **A54.49 Gonococcal infection of other musculoskeletal tissue**
  Gonococcal bursitis
  Gonococcal myositis
  Gonococcal synovitis
  Gonococcal tenosynovitis
A54.5 Gonococcal pharyngitis
A54.6 Gonococcal infection of anus and rectum
+ **A54.8 Other gonococcal infections**
MCC **A54.81 Gonococcal meningitis**
CC **A54.82 Gonococcal brain abscess**
CC **A54.83 Gonococcal heart infection**
  Gonococcal endocarditis
  Gonococcal myocarditis
  Gonococcal pericarditis
CC **A54.84 Gonococcal pneumonia**
CC **A54.85 Gonococcal peritonitis**
  Excludes1: *gonococcal pelviperitonitis (A54.24)*
MCC **A54.86 Gonococcal sepsis**
  Review coding guideline C.1.d
CC **A54.89 Other gonococcal infections**
  Gonococcal keratoderma
  Gonococcal lymphadenitis
CC **A54.9 Gonococcal infection, unspecified**
A55 Chlamydial lymphogranuloma (venereum)

  Climatic or tropical bubo
  Durand-Nicolas-Favre disease
  Esthiomene
  Lymphogranuloma inguinale
  Valid 3-character code, no further characters required
A56 Other sexually transmitted chlamydial diseases

  Includes: sexually transmitted diseases due to Chlamydia
    trachomatis
  Excludes1: *neonatal chlamydial conjunctivitis (P39.1)*
    neonatal chlamydial pneumonia (P23.1)
  Excludes2: *chlamydial lymphogranuloma (A55)*
    conditions classified to A74.-
+ **A56.0 Chlamydial infection of lower genitourinary tract**
  A56.00 Chlamydial infection of lower genitourinary tract, unspecified
  A56.01 Chlamydial cystitis and urethritis
  ♀ **A56.02 Chlamydial vulvovaginitis**
  A56.09 Other chlamydial infection of lower genitourinary tract
    Chlamydial cervicitis
+ **A56.1 Chlamydial infection of pelviperitoneum and other genitourinary organs**
  ♀ **A56.11 Chlamydial female pelvic inflammatory disease**
  A56.19 Other chlamydial genitourinary infection
    Chlamydial epididymitis
    Chlamydial orchitis
A56.2 Chlamydial infection of genitourinary tract, unspecified
A56.3 Chlamydial infection of anus and rectum
A56.4 Chlamydial infection of pharynx
A56.8 Sexually transmitted chlamydial infection of other sites
A57 Chancroid

  Ulcus molle

Valid 3-character code, no further characters required
A58 Granuloma inguinale

  Donovanosis
  Valid 3-character code, no further characters required
A59 Trichomoniasis

  Excludes2: *intestinal trichomoniasis (A07.8)*
+ **A59.0 Urogenital trichomoniasis**
  A59.00 Urogenital trichomoniasis, unspecified
    Fluor (vaginalis) due to Trichomonas
    Leukorrhea (vaginalis) due to Trichomonas
  ♀ **A59.01 Trichomonal vulvovaginitis**
  ♂ **A59.02 Trichomonal prostatitis**
  A59.03 Trichomonal cystitis and urethritis
  A59.09 Other urogenital trichomoniasis
    Trichomonas cervicitis
A59.8 Trichomoniasis of other sites
A59.9 Trichomoniasis, unspecified
A60 Anogenital herpesviral [herpes simplex] infections

+ **A60.0 Herpesviral infection of genitalia and urogenital tract**
  A60.00 Herpesviral infection of urogenital system, unspecified
  ♂ **A60.01 Herpesviral infection of penis**
  ♂ **A60.02 Herpesviral infection of other male genital organs**
  ♀ **A60.03 Herpesviral cervicitis**
  ♀ **A60.04 Herpesviral vulvovaginitis**
    Herpesviral [herpes simplex] ulceration
    Herpesviral [herpes simplex] vaginitis
    Herpesviral [herpes simplex] vulvitis
  A60.09 Herpesviral infection of other urogenital tract
A60.1 Herpesviral infection of perianal skin and rectum
A60.9 Anogenital herpesviral infection, unspecified
  AHA CC: 1Q, 2020, 20
A63 Other predominantly sexually transmitted diseases, not elsewhere classified

  Excludes2: *molluscum contagiosum (B08.1)*
    papilloma of cervix (D26.0)
A63.0 Anogenital (venereal) warts
    Anogenital warts due to (human) papillomavirus [HPV]
    Condyloma acuminatum
A63.8 Other specified predominantly sexually transmitted diseases
A64 Unspecified sexually transmitted disease

  Valid 3-character code, no further characters required

Other spirochetal diseases (A65-A69)

Excludes2: *leptospirosis (A27.-)*
    syphilis (A50-A53)
A65 Nonvenereal syphilis

  Bejel
  Endemic syphilis
  Njovera
  Valid 3-character code, no further characters required
A66 Yaws

  Includes: bouba
    frambesia (tropica)
    pian
A66.0 Initial lesions of yaws
    Chancre of yaws
    Frambesia, initial or primary
    Initial frambesial ulcer
    Mother yaw
A66.1 Multiple papillomata and wet crab yaws
    Frambesioma
    Pianoma
    Plantar or palmar papilloma of yaws
A66.2 Other early skin lesions of yaws
    Cutaneous yaws, less than five years after infection
    Early yaws (cutaneous)(macular)(maculopapular)
      (micropapular)(papular)
    Frambeside of early yaws
A66.3 Hyperkeratosis of yaws
    Ghoul hand
    Hyperkeratosis, palmar or plantar (early) (late) due to yaws
    Worm-eaten soles
A66.4 Gummata and ulcers of yaws
    Gummatous frambeside
    Nodular late yaws (ulcerated)

+, +7th, X + 7th   ● Newborn   ● Pediatric   ● Maternity   ● Adult   ♀ Female   ♂ Male   Manifestation   Unacceptable PDX   HCC   CC   MCC   HAC

A66.5 **Gangosa**
Rhinopharyngitis mutilans

A66.6 **Bone and joint lesions of yaws**
Yaws ganglion
Yaws goundou
Yaws gumma, bone
Yaws gummatous osteitis or periostitis
Yaws hydrarthrosis
Yaws osteitis
Yaws periostitis (hypertrophic)

A66.7 **Other manifestations of yaws**
Juxta-articular nodules of yaws
Mucosal yaws

A66.8 **Latent yaws**
Yaws without clinical manifestations, with positive serology

A66.9 **Yaws, unspecified**

A67 **Pinta [carate]**

A67.0 **Primary lesions of pinta**
Chancre (primary) of pinta
Papule (primary) of pinta

A67.1 **Intermediate lesions of pinta**
Erythematous plaques of pinta
Hyperchromic lesions of pinta
Hyperkeratosis of pinta
Pintids

A67.2 **Late lesions of pinta**
Achromic skin lesions of pinta
Cicatricial skin lesions of pinta
Dyschromic skin lesions of pinta

A67.3 **Mixed lesions of pinta**
Achromic with hyperchromic skin lesions of pinta
[carate]

A67.9 **Pinta, unspecified**

A68 **Relapsing fevers**

Includes: recurrent fever
Excludes2: *Lyme disease (A69.2-)*

CC A68.0 **Louse-borne relapsing fever**
Relapsing fever due to Borrelia recurrentis

CC A68.1 **Tick-borne relapsing fever**
Relapsing fever due to any Borrelia species other than Borrelia recurrentis

CC A68.9 **Relapsing fever, unspecified**

A69 **Other spirochetal infections**

A69.0 **Necrotizing ulcerative stomatitis**
Cancrum oris
Fusospirochetal gangrene
Noma
Stomatitis gangrenosa

CC A69.1 **Other Vincent's infections**
Fusospirochetal pharyngitis
Necrotizing ulcerative (acute) gingivitis
Necrotizing ulcerative (acute) gingivostomatitis
Spirochetal stomatitis
Trench mouth
Vincent's angina
Vincent's gingivitis

+ A69.2 **Lyme disease**
Erythema chronicum migrans due to Borrelia burgdorferi

CC A69.20 **Lyme disease, unspecified**
CC A69.21 **Meningitis due to Lyme disease**
CC A69.22 **Other neurologic disorders in Lyme disease**
Cranial neuritis
Meningoencephalitis
Polyneuropathy
CC A69.23 **Arthritis due to Lyme disease**
CC A69.29 **Other conditions associated with Lyme disease**
Myopericarditis due to Lyme disease
AHA CC: 3Q, 2016, 12

A69.8 **Other specified spirochetal infections**
A69.9 **Spirochetal infection, unspecified**

Other diseases caused by chlamydiae (A70-A74)

Excludes1: *sexually transmitted chlamydial diseases (A55-A56)*

CC A70 **Chlamydia psittaci infections**

Ornithosis
Parrot fever
Psittacosis

Valid 3-character code, no further characters required

A71 **Trachoma**

Excludes1: *sequelae of trachoma (B94.0)*

A71.0 **Initial stage of trachoma**
Trachoma dubium

A71.1 **Active stage of trachoma**
Granular conjunctivitis (trachomatous)
Trachomatous follicular conjunctivitis
Trachomatous pannus

A71.9 **Trachoma, unspecified**

A74 **Other diseases caused by chlamydiae**

Excludes1: *neonatal chlamydial conjunctivitis (P39.1)*
neonatal chlamydial pneumonia (P23.1)
Reiter's disease (M02.3-)
sexually transmitted chlamydial diseases (A55-A56)
Excludes2: *chlamydial pneumonia (J16.0)*

A74.0 **Chlamydial conjunctivitis**
Paratrachoma

+ A74.8 **Other chlamydial diseases**
A74.81 **Chlamydial peritonitis**
A74.89 **Other chlamydial diseases**

A74.9 **Chlamydial infection, unspecified**
Chlamydiosis NOS

Rickettsioses (A75-A79)

A75 **Typhus fever**

Excludes1: *rickettsiosis due to Ehrlichia sennetsu (A79.81)*

CC A75.0 **Epidemic louse-borne typhus fever due to Rickettsia prowazekii**
Classical typhus (fever)
Epidemic (louse-borne) typhus

CC A75.1 **Recrudescent typhus [Brill's disease]**
Brill-Zinsser disease

CC A75.2 **Typhus fever due to Rickettsia typhi**
Murine (flea-borne) typhus

CC A75.3 **Typhus fever due to Rickettsia tsutsugamushi**
Scrub (mite-borne) typhus
Typhus fever due to Orientia Tsutsugamushi (scrub typhus)
Tsutsugamushi fever

CC A75.9 **Typhus fever, unspecified**
Typhus (fever) NOS

A77 **Spotted fever [tick-borne rickettsioses]**

CC A77.0 **Spotted fever due to Rickettsia rickettsii**
Rocky Mountain spotted fever
Sao Paulo fever

CC A77.1 **Spotted fever due to Rickettsia conorii**
African tick typhus
Boutonneuse fever
India tick typhus
Kenya tick typhus
Marseilles fever
Mediterranean tick fever

CC A77.2 **Spotted fever due to Rickettsia siberica**
North Asian tick fever
Siberian tick typhus

CC A77.3 **Spotted fever due to Rickettsia australis**
Queensland tick typhus

+ A77.4 **Ehrlichiosis**
Excludes1: *Rickettsiosis due to Ehrlichia sennetsu (A79.81)*
CC A77.40 **Ehrlichiosis, unspecified**
CC A77.41 **Ehrlichiosis chafeensis [E. chafeensis]**
CC A77.49 **Other ehrlichiosis**
Ehrlichiosis due to E. ewingii
Ehrlichiosis due to E. muris euclairensis

CC A77.8 **Other spotted fevers**
Rickettsia 364D/R. philipii (Pacific Coast tick fever)
Spotted fever due to Rickettsia africae (African tick bite fever)
Spotted fever due to Rickettsia parkeri

CC A77.9 **Spotted fever, unspecified**
Tick-borne typhus NOS

CC A78 **Q fever**

Infection due to Coxiella burnetii
Nine Mile fever
Quadrilateral fever
Valid 3-character code, no further characters required

+, +7th, X + 7th • Newborn • Pediatric • Maternity • Adult ♀ Female ♂ Male Manifestation Unacceptable PDX HCC CC MCC HAC

A79 Other rickettsioses

CC **A79.0** **Trench fever**
Quintan fever
Wolhynian fever

CC **A79.1** **Rickettsialpox due to Rickettsia akari**
Kew Garden fever
Vesicular rickettsiosis

A79.8 **Other specified rickettsioses**

CC **A79.81** **Rickettsiosis due to Ehrlichia sennetsu**
Rickettsiosis due to Neorickettsia sennetsu
Excludes1: *rickettsiosis due to Ehrlichia sennetsu (A79.81)*

CC **A79.89** **Other specified rickettsioses**

CC **A79.9** **Rickettsiosis, unspecified**
Rickettsial infection NOS

Viral and prion infections of the central nervous system (A80-A89)

Excludes1: *postpolio syndrome (G14)*
sequelae of poliomyelitis (B91)
sequelae of viral encephalitis (B94.1)

A80 Acute poliomyelitis

MCC **A80.0** **Acute paralytic poliomyelitis, vaccine-associated**
MCC **A80.1** **Acute paralytic poliomyelitis, wild virus, imported**
MCC **A80.2** **Acute paralytic poliomyelitis, wild virus, indigenous**
+ **A80.3** **Acute paralytic poliomyelitis, other and unspecified**
MCC **A80.30** **Acute paralytic poliomyelitis, unspecified**
MCC **A80.39** **Other acute paralytic poliomyelitis**
A80.4 **Acute nonparalytic poliomyelitis**
A80.9 **Acute poliomyelitis, unspecified**

A81 Atypical virus infections of central nervous system

Includes: diseases of the central nervous system caused by prions
Use additional code to identify:
dementia with behavioral disturbance (F02.81)
dementia without behavioral disturbance (F02.80)

+ **A81.0** **Creutzfeldt-Jakob disease**
CC **A81.00** **Creutzfeldt-Jakob disease, unspecified**
Jakob-Creutzfeldt disease, unspecified
CC **A81.01** **Variant Creutzfeldt-Jakob disease**
CJD
CC **A81.09** **Other Creutzfeldt-Jakob disease**
CJD
Familial Creutzfeldt-Jakob disease
Iatrogenic Creutzfeldt-Jakob disease
Sporadic Creutzfeldt-Jakob disease
Subacute spongiform encephalopathy (with dementia)

CC **A81.1** **Subacute sclerosing panencephalitis**
Dawson's inclusion body encephalitis
Van Bogaert's sclerosing leukoencephalopathy

CC **A81.2** **Progressive multifocal leukoencephalopathy**
Multifocal leukoencephalopathy NOS

+ **A81.8** **Other atypical virus infections of central nervous system**
CC **A81.81** **Kuru**
CC **A81.82** **Gerstmann-Sträussler-Scheinker syndrome**
GSS syndrome
CC **A81.83** **Fatal familial insomnia**
FFI
CC **A81.89** **Other atypical virus infections of central nervous system**

CC **A81.9** **Atypical virus infection of central nervous system, unspecified**
Prion diseases of the central nervous system NOS

A82 Rabies

CC **A82.0** **Sylvatic rabies**
CC **A82.1** **Urban rabies**
CC **A82.9** **Rabies, unspecified**

A83 Mosquito-borne viral encephalitis

Includes: mosquito-borne viral meningoencephalitis
Excludes2: *Venezuelan equine encephalitis (A92.2)*
West Nile fever (A92.3-)
West Nile virus (A92.3-)

MCC **A83.0** **Japanese encephalitis**
MCC **A83.1** **Western equine encephalitis**
MCC **A83.2** **Eastern equine encephalitis**
MCC **A83.3** **St Louis encephalitis**
MCC **A83.4** **Australian encephalitis**

Kunjin virus disease
MCC **A83.5** **California encephalitis**
California meningoencephalitis
La Crosse encephalitis
MCC **A83.6** **Rocio virus disease**
MCC **A83.8** **Other mosquito-borne viral encephalitis**
MCC **A83.9** **Mosquito-borne viral encephalitis, unspecified**

A84 Tick-borne viral encephalitis

Includes: tick-borne viral meningoencephalitis
MCC **A84.0** **Far Eastern tick-borne encephalitis [Russian spring-summer encephalitis]**
MCC **A84.1** **Central European tick-borne encephalitis**
+ **A84.8** **Other tick-borne viral encephalitis**
MCC **A84.81** **Powassan virus disease**
MCC **A84.89** **Other tick-borne viral encephalitis**
Louping ill
Code first, if applicable, transfusion related infection (T80.22-)

MCC **A84.9** **Tick-borne viral encephalitis, unspecified**

A85 Other viral encephalitis, not elsewhere classified

Includes: specified viral encephalomyelitis NEC
specified viral meningoencephalitis NEC
Excludes1: *benign myalgic encephalomyelitis (G93.3)*
encephalitis due to cytomegalovirus (B25.8)
encephalitis due to herpesvirus NEC (B10.0-)
encephalitis due to herpesvirus [herpes simplex] (B00.4)
encephalitis due to measles virus (B05.0)
encephalitis due to mumps virus (B26.2)
encephalitis due to poliomyelitis virus (A80.-)
encephalitis due to zoster (B02.0)
lymphocytic choriomeningitis (A87.2)

CC **A85.0** **Enteroviral encephalitis**
Enteroviral encephalomyelitis
CC **A85.1** **Adenoviral encephalitis**
Adenoviral meningoencephalitis
MCC **A85.2** **Arthropod-borne viral encephalitis, unspecified**
Excludes1: *West nile virus with encephalitis (A92.31)*
CC **A85.8** **Other specified viral encephalitis**
Encephalitis lethargica
Von Economo-Cruchet disease

CC **A86** **Unspecified viral encephalitis**
Viral encephalomyelitis NOS
Viral meningoencephalitis NOS
Valid 3-character code, no further characters required

A87 Viral meningitis

Excludes1: *meningitis due to herpesvirus [herpes simplex] (B00.3)*
meningitis due to herpesvirus [herpes simplex] (B00.3)
meningitis due to measles virus (B05.1)
meningitis due to mumps virus (B26.1)
meningitis due to poliomyelitis virus (A80.-)
meningitis due to zoster (B02.1)

CC **A87.0** **Enteroviral meningitis**
Coxsackievirus meningitis
Echovirus meningitis
CC **A87.1** **Adenoviral meningitis**
CC **A87.2** **Lymphocytic choriomeningitis**
Lymphocytic meningoencephalitis
CC **A87.8** **Other viral meningitis**
CC **A87.9** **Viral meningitis, unspecified**

A88 Other viral infections of central nervous system, not elsewhere classified

Excludes1: *viral encephalitis NOS (A86)*
viral meningitis NOS (A87.9)

CC **A88.0** **Enteroviral exanthematous fever [Boston exanthem]**
A88.1 **Epidemic vertigo**
CC **A88.8** **Other specified viral infections of central nervous system**

CC **A89** **Unspecified viral infection of central nervous system**
Valid 3-character code, no further characters required

Arthropod-borne viral fevers and viral hemorrhagic fevers (A90-A99)

CC **A90** **Dengue fever [classical dengue]**
Excludes1: *dengue hemorrhagic fever (A91)*
AHA CC: 3Q, 2016, 13

+, +7th, X + 7th ● Newborn ● Pediatric ● Maternity ● Adult ♀ Female ♂ Male Manifestation Unacceptable PDX HCC CC MCC HAC

Valid 3-character code, no further characters required

CC **A91** **Dengue hemorrhagic fever**

Valid 3-character code, no further characters required

A92 **Other mosquito-borne viral fevers**

Excludes1: *Ross River disease (B33.1)*

CC **A92.0** **Chikungunya virus disease**
Chikungunya (hemorrhagic) fever

CC **A92.1** **O'nyong-nyong fever**

CC **A92.2** **Venezuelan equine fever**
Venezuelan equine encephalitis
Venezuelan equine encephalomyelitis virus disease

+ **A92.3** **West Nile virus infection**
West Nile fever

MCC **A92.30** **West Nile virus infection, unspecified**
West Nile fever NOS
West Nile fever without complications
West Nile virus NOS

MCC **A92.31** **West Nile virus infection with encephalitis**
West Nile encephalitis
West Nile encephalomyelitis
AHA CC: 3Q, 2016, 12-13

MCC **A92.32** **West Nile virus infection with other neurologic manifestation**
Use additional code to specify the neurologic manifestation

MCC **A92.39** **West Nile virus infection with other complications**
Use additional code to specify the other conditions

CC **A92.4** **Rift Valley fever**

CC **A92.5** **Zika virus disease**
Zika virus fever
Zika virus infection
Zika NOS
Excludes1: *congenital Zika virus disease (P35.4)*
Review coding guideline C.1.f
AHA CC: 4Q, 2016, 4-7

CC **A92.8** **Other specified mosquito-borne viral fevers**

CC **A92.9** **Mosquito-borne viral fever, unspecified**

A93 **Other arthropod-borne viral fevers, not elsewhere classified**

CC **A93.0** **Oropouche virus disease**
Oropouche fever

CC **A93.1** **Sandfly fever**
Pappataci fever
Phlebotomus fever

CC **A93.2** **Colorado tick fever**

CC **A93.8** **Other specified arthropod-borne viral fevers**
Piry virus disease
Vesicular stomatitis virus disease [Indiana fever]

CC **A94** **Unspecified arthropod-borne viral fever**
Arboviral fever NOS
Arbovirus infection NOS
Valid 3-character code, no further characters required

A95 **Yellow fever**

CC **A95.0** **Sylvatic yellow fever**
Jungle yellow fever

CC **A95.1** **Urban yellow fever**

CC **A95.9** **Yellow fever, unspecified**

A96 **Arenaviral hemorrhagic fever**

CC **A96.0** **Junin hemorrhagic fever**
Argentinian hemorrhagic fever

CC **A96.1** **Machupo hemorrhagic fever**
Bolivian hemorrhagic fever

A96.2 **Lassa fever**

CC **A96.8** **Other arenaviral hemorrhagic fevers**

CC **A96.9** **Arenaviral hemorrhagic fever, unspecified**

A98 **Other viral hemorrhagic fevers, not elsewhere classified**

Excludes1: *chikungunya hemorrhagic fever (A92.0)*
dengue hemorrhagic fever (A91)

CC **A98.0** **Crimean-Congo hemorrhagic fever**
Central Asian hemorrhagic fever

CC **A98.1** **Omsk hemorrhagic fever**

CC **A98.2** **Kyasanur Forest disease**

A98.3 **Marburg virus disease**

A98.4 **Ebola virus disease**

CC **A98.5** **Hemorrhagic fever with renal syndrome**
Epidemic hemorrhagic fever
Korean hemorrhagic fever
Russian hemorrhagic fever

Hantaan virus disease
Hantavirus disease with renal manifestations
Nephropathia epidemica
Songo fever
Excludes1: *hantavirus (cardio)-pulmonary syndrome (B33.4)*

CC **A98.8** **Other specified viral hemorrhagic fevers**

CC **A99** **Unspecified viral hemorrhagic fever**

Valid 3-character code, no further characters

Viral infections characterized by skin and mucous membrane lesions (B00-B09)

B00 **Herpesviral [herpes simplex] infections**

Excludes1: *congenital herpesviral infections (P35.2)*
Excludes2: *anogenital herpesviral infection (A60.-)*
gammaherpesviral mononucleosis (B27.0-)
herpangina (B08.5)

B00.0 **Eczema herpeticum**
Kaposi's varicelliform eruption

B00.1 **Herpesviral vesicular dermatitis**
Herpes simplex facialis
Herpes simplex labialis
Herpes simplex otitis externa
Vesicular dermatitis of ear
Vesicular dermatitis of lip

CC **B00.2** **Herpesviral gingivostomatitis and pharyngotonsillitis**
Herpesviral pharyngitis

MCC **B00.3** **Herpesviral meningitis**

MCC **B00.4** **Herpesviral encephalitis**
Herpesviral meningoencephalitis
Simian B disease
Excludes1: *herpesviral encephalitis due to herpesvirus 6 and 7 (B10.01, B10.09)*
non-simplex herpesviral encephalitis (B10.0-)

+ **B00.5** **Herpesviral ocular disease**

CC **B00.50** **Herpesviral ocular disease, unspecified**

CC **B00.51** **Herpesviral iridocyclitis**
Herpesviral iritis
Herpesviral uveitis, anterior

CC **B00.52** **Herpesviral keratitis**
Herpesviral keratoconjunctivitis

CC **B00.53** **Herpesviral conjunctivitis**

CC **B00.59** **Other herpesviral disease of eye**
Herpesviral dermatitis of eyelid

MCC **B00.7** **Disseminated herpesviral disease**
Herpesviral sepsis
Review coding guideline C.1.d

+ **B00.8** **Other forms of herpesviral infections**

CC **B00.81** **Herpesviral hepatitis**

MCC **B00.82** **Herpes simplex myelitis**

CC **B00.89** **Other herpesviral infection**
Herpesviral whitlow

B00.9 **Herpesviral infection, unspecified**
Herpes simplex infection NOS

B01 **Varicella [chickenpox]**

CC **B01.0** **Varicella meningitis**

+ **B01.1** **Varicella encephalitis, myelitis and encephalomyelitis**
Postchickenpox encephalitis, myelitis and encephalomyelitis

MCC **B01.11** **Varicella encephalitis and encephalomyelitis**
Postchickenpox encephalitis and encephalomyelitis

MCC **B01.12** **Varicella myelitis**
Postchickenpox myelitis

MCC **B01.2** **Varicella pneumonia**

+ **B01.8** **Varicella with other complications**

CC **B01.81** **Varicella keratitis**

CC **B01.89** **Other varicella complications**

CC **B01.9** **Varicella without complication**
Varicella NOS

B02 **Zoster [herpes zoster]**

Includes: shingles
zona

CC **B02.0** **Zoster encephalitis**
Zoster meningoencephalitis

MCC **B02.1** **Zoster meningitis**
AHA CC: 1Q, 2019, 18

+ **B02.2** **Zoster with other nervous system involvement**

CC **B02.21** **Postherpetic geniculate ganglionitis**

CC **B02.22** **Postherpetic trigeminal neuralgia**

CC B02.23 **Posptherpetic polyneuropathy**
MCC **B02.24** **Postherpetic myelitis**
Herpes zoster myelitis
CC B02.29 **Other postherpetic nervous system involvement**
Posptherpetic radiculopathy
+ B02.3 **Zoster ocular disease**
CC B02.30 **Zoster ocular disease, unspecified**
CC B02.31 **Zoster conjunctivitis**
CC B02.32 **Zoster iridocyclitis**
CC B02.33 **Zoster keratitis**
Herpes zoster keratoconjunctivitis
CC B02.34 **Zoster scleritis**
CC B02.39 **Other herpes zoster eye disease**
Zoster blepharitis
CC B02.7 **Disseminated zoster**
CC B02.8 **Zoster with other complications**
Herpes zoster otitis externa
B02.9 **Zoster without complications**
Zoster NOS

CC **B03** **Smallpox**

> **NOTE** In 1980 the 33rd World Health Assembly declared that smallpox
> had been eradicated.
> The classification is maintained for surveillance purposes.
> **Valid 3-character code, no further characters required**

CC **B04** **Monkeypox**

> **Valid 3-character code, no further characters required**

B05 **Measles**

> **Includes:** morbilli
> **Excludes1:** *subacute sclerosing panencephalitis (A81.1)*

MCC B05.0 **Measles complicated by encephalitis**
Postmeasles encephalitis
CC B05.1 **Measles complicated by meningitis**
Postmeasles meningitis
MCC B05.2 **Measles complicated by pneumonia**
Postmeasles pneumonia
B05.3 **Measles complicated by otitis media**
Postmeasles otitis media
CC B05.4 **Measles with intestinal complications**
+ B05.8 **Measles with other complications**
CC B05.81 **Measles keratitis and keratoconjunctivitis**
CC B05.89 **Other measles complications**
B05.9 **Measles without complication**
Measles NOS

B06 **Rubella [German measles]**

> **Excludes1:** *congenital rubella (P35.0)*

+ B06.0 **Rubella with neurological complications**
CC B06.00 **Rubella with neurological complication, unspecified**
MCC B06.01 **Rubella encephalitis**
Rubella meningoencephalitis
CC B06.02 **Rubella meningitis**
CC B06.09 **Other neurological complications of rubella**
+ B06.8 **Rubella with other complications**
CC B06.81 **Rubella pneumonia**
CC **B06.82** **Rubella arthritis**
CC B06.89 **Other rubella complications**
B06.9 **Rubella without complication**
Rubella NOS

B07 **Viral warts**

> **Includes:** verruca simplex
> verruca vulgaris
> viral warts due to human papillomavirus
> **Excludes2:** *anogenital (venereal) warts (A63.0)*
> *papilloma of bladder (D41.4)*
> *papilloma of cervix (D26.0)*
> *papilloma larynx (D14.1)*

B07.0 **Plantar wart**
Verruca plantaris
B07.8 **Other viral warts**
Common wart
Flat wart
Verruca plana
B07.9 **Viral wart, unspecified**

B08 **Other viral infections characterized by skin and mucous membrane lesions, not elsewhere classified**

> **Excludes1:** *vesicular stomatitis virus disease (A93.8)*

B08.0 **Other orthopoxvirus infections**

> **Excludes2:** *monkeypox (B04)*

+ B08.01 **Cowpox and vaccinia not from vaccine**
B08.010 **Cowpox**
B08.011 **Vaccinia not from vaccine**

> **Excludes1:** *vaccinia (from vaccination)*
> *(generalized) (T88.1)*

B08.02 **Orf virus disease**
Contagious pustular dermatitis
Ecthyma contagiosum
B08.03 **Pseudocowpox [milker's node]**
B08.04 **Paravaccinia, unspecified**
B08.09 **Other orthopoxvirus infections**
Orthopoxvirus infection NOS
B08.1 **Molluscum contagiosum**
+ B08.2 **Exanthema subitum [sixth disease]**
Roseola infantum
• B08.20 **Exanthema subitum [sixth disease], unspecified**
Roseola infantum, unspecified
• B08.21 **Exanthema subitum [sixth disease] due to human herpesvirus 6**
Roseola infantum due to human herpesvirus 6
• B08.22 **Exanthema subitum [sixth disease] due to human herpesvirus 7**
Roseola infantum due to human herpesvirus 7
CC B08.3 **Erythema infectiosum [fifth disease]**
B08.4 **Enteroviral vesicular stomatitis with exanthem**
Hand, foot and mouth disease
B08.5 **Enteroviral vesicular pharyngitis**
Herpangina
+ B08.6 **Parapoxvirus infections**
B08.60 **Parapoxvirus infection, unspecified**
B08.61 **Bovine stomatitis**
B08.62 **Sealpox**
B08.69 **Other parapoxvirus infections**
+ B08.7 **Yatapoxvirus infections**
B08.70 **Yatapoxvirus infection, unspecified**
CC B08.71 **Tanapox virus disease**
B08.72 **Yaba pox virus disease**
Yaba monkey tumor disease
B08.79 **Other yatapoxvirus infections**
B08.8 **Other specified viral infections characterized by skin and mucous membrane lesions**
Enteroviral lymphonodular pharyngitis
Foot-and-mouth disease
Poxvirus NEC

B09 **Unspecified viral infection characterized by skin and mucous membrane lesions**

Viral enanthema NOS
Viral exanthema NOS

> **Valid 3-character code, no further characters required**

Other human herpesviruses (B10)

B10 **Other human herpesviruses**

> **Excludes2:** *cytomegalovirus (B25.9)*
> *Epstein-Barr virus (B27.0-)*
> *herpes NOS (B00.9)*
> *herpes simplex (B00.-)*
> *herpes zoster (B02.-)*
> *human herpesvirus NOS (B00.-)*
> *human herpesvirus 1 and 2 (B00.-)*
> *human herpesvirus 3 (B01.-, B02.-)*
> *human herpesvirus 4 (B27.0-)*
> *human herpesvirus 5 (B25.-)*
> *varicella (B01.-)*
> *zoster (B02.-)*

+ B10.0 **Other human herpesvirus encephalitis**

> **Excludes2:** *herpes encephalitis NOS (B00.4)*
> *herpes simplex encephalitis (B00.4)*
> *human herpesvirus encephalitis (B00.4)*
> *simian B herpes virus encephalitis (B00.4)*

MCC B10.01 **Human herpesvirus 6 encephalitis**
MCC B10.09 **Other human herpesvirus encephalitis**
Human herpesvirus 7 encephalitis
+ B10.8 **Other human herpesvirus infection**
B10.81 **Human herpesvirus 6 infection**
B10.82 **Human herpesvirus 7 infection**
B10.89 **Other human herpesvirus infection**
Human herpesvirus 8 infection
Kaposi's sarcoma-associated herpesvirus infection

Viral hepatitis (B15-B19)

Excludes1: *sequelae of viral hepatitis (B94.2)*

Excludes2: *cytomegaloviral hepatitis (B25.1)*
herpesviral [herpes simplex] hepatitis (B00.81)

B15 Acute hepatitis A

MCC **B15.0 Hepatitis A with hepatic coma**
CC **B15.9 Hepatitis A without hepatic coma**
Hepatitis A (acute)(viral) NOS

B16 Acute hepatitis B

MCC **B16.0 Acute hepatitis B with delta-agent with hepatic coma**
CC **B16.1 Acute hepatitis B with delta-agent without hepatic coma**
MCC **B16.2 Acute hepatitis B without delta-agent with hepatic coma**
CC **B16.9 Acute hepatitis B without delta-agent and without hepatic coma**
Hepatitis B (acute) (viral) NOS
AHA CC: 3Q, 2016, 13

B17 Other acute viral hepatitis

CC **B17.0 Acute delta-(super) infection of hepatitis B carrier**
+ **B17.1 Acute hepatitis C**
CC **B17.10 Acute hepatitis C without hepatic coma**
Acute hepatitis C NOS
MCC **B17.11 Acute hepatitis C with hepatic coma**
CC **B17.2 Acute hepatitis E**
CC **B17.8 Other specified acute viral hepatitis**
Hepatitis non-A non-B (acute) (viral) NEC
CC **B17.9 Acute viral hepatitis, unspecified**
Acute hepatitis NOS
Acute infectious hepatitis NOS

B18 Chronic viral hepatitis

Includes: Carrier of viral hepatitis
CC **B18.0 Chronic viral hepatitis B with delta-agent**
CC **B18.1 Chronic viral hepatitis B without delta-agent**
Carrier of viral hepatitis B
Chronic (viral) hepatitis B
B18.2 Chronic viral hepatitis C
Carrier of viral hepatitis C
AHA CC: 1Q, 2017, 41; 1Q, 2018, 4-5
CC **B18.8 Other chronic viral hepatitis**
Carrier of other viral hepatitis
CC **B18.9 Chronic viral hepatitis, unspecified**
Carrier of unspecified viral hepatitis

B19 Unspecified viral hepatitis

MCC **B19.0 Unspecified viral hepatitis with hepatic coma**
+ **B19.1 Unspecified viral hepatitis B**
CC **B19.10 Unspecified viral hepatitis B without hepatic coma**
Unspecified viral hepatitis B NOS
MCC **B19.11 Unspecified viral hepatitis B with hepatic coma**
+ **B19.2 Unspecified viral hepatitis C**
B19.20 Unspecified viral hepatitis C without hepatic coma
Viral hepatitis C NOS
MCC **B19.21 Unspecified viral hepatitis C with hepatic coma**
CC **B19.9 Unspecified viral hepatitis without hepatic coma**
Viral hepatitis NOS

Human immunodeficiency virus [HIV] disease (B20)

CC **B20 Human immunodeficiency virus [HIV] disease**

Includes: acquired immune deficiency syndrome [AIDS]
AIDS-related complex [ARC]
HIV infection, symptomatic
Code first Human immunodeficiency virus [HIV] disease complicating pregnancy, childbirth and the puerperium, if applicable (O98.7-)

Use additional code(s) to identify all manifestations of HIV infection
Excludes1: *asymptomatic human immunodeficiency virus [HIV] infection status (Z21)*
exposure to HIV virus (Z20.6)
inconclusive serologic evidence of HIV (R75)
Review coding guideline C.1.a
AHA CC: 1Q, 2019, 8-11
Valid 3-character code, no further characters required

Other viral diseases (B25-B34)

B25 Cytomegaloviral disease

Excludes1: *congenital cytomegalovirus infection (P35.1)*
cytomegaloviral mononucleosis (B27.1-)

MCC **B25.0 Cytomegaloviral pneumonitis**
CC **B25.1 Cytomegaloviral hepatitis**
MCC **B25.2 Cytomegaloviral pancreatitis**
CC **B25.8 Other cytomegaloviral diseases**
Cytomegaloviral encephalitis
CC **B25.9 Cytomegaloviral disease, unspecified**

B26 Mumps

Includes: epidemic parotitis
infectious parotitis
♂ CC **B26.0 Mumps orchitis**
MCC **B26.1 Mumps meningitis**
MCC **B26.2 Mumps encephalitis**
CC **B26.3 Mumps pancreatitis**
+ **B26.8 Mumps with other complications**
CC **B26.81 Mumps hepatitis**
CC **B26.82 Mumps myocarditis**
CC **B26.83 Mumps nephritis**
CC **B26.84 Mumps polyneuropathy**
CC **B26.85 Mumps arthritis**
CC **B26.89 Other mumps complications**
B26.9 Mumps without complication
Mumps NOS
Mumps parotitis NOS

B27 Infectious mononucleosis

Includes: glandular fever
monocytic angina
Pfeiffer's disease
+ **B27.0 Gammaherpesviral mononucleosis**
Mononucleosis due to Epstein-Barr virus
B27.00 Gammaherpesviral mononucleosis without complication
B27.01 Gammaherpesviral mononucleosis with polyneuropathy
B27.02 Gammaherpesviral mononucleosis with meningitis
B27.09 Gammaherpesviral mononucleosis with other complications
Hepatomegaly in gammaherpesviral mononucleosis
+ **B27.1 Cytomegaloviral mononucleosis**
B27.10 Cytomegaloviral mononucleosis without complications
B27.11 Cytomegaloviral mononucleosis with polyneuropathy
B27.12 Cytomegaloviral mononucleosis with meningitis
B27.19 Cytomegaloviral mononucleosis with other complication
Hepatomegaly in cytomegaloviral mononucleosis
+ **B27.8 Other infectious mononucleosis**
B27.80 Other infectious mononucleosis without complication
B27.81 Other infectious mononucleosis with polyneuropathy
B27.82 Other infectious mononucleosis with meningitis
B27.89 Other infectious mononucleosis with other complication
Hepatomegaly in other infectious mononucleosis
+ **B27.9 Infectious mononucleosis, unspecified**
B27.90 Infectious mononucleosis, unspecified without complication
B27.91 Infectious mononucleosis, unspecified with polyneuropathy
B27.92 Infectious mononucleosis, unspecified with meningitis
B27.99 Infectious mononucleosis, unspecified with other complication
Hepatomegaly in unspecified infectious mononucleosis

B30 Viral conjunctivitis

Excludes1: *herpesviral [herpes simplex] ocular disease (B00.5)*
ocular zoster (B02.3)
B30.0 Keratoconjunctivitis due to adenovirus
Epidemic keratoconjunctivitis
Shipyard eye
B30.1 Conjunctivitis due to adenovirus
Acute adenoviral follicular conjunctivitis
Swimming-pool conjunctivitis
B30.2 Viral pharyngoconjunctivitis

B30.3 **Acute epidemic hemorrhagic conjunctivitis (enteroviral)**
    Conjunctivitis due to coxsackievirus 24
    Conjunctivitis due to enterovirus 70
    Hemorrhagic conjunctivitis (acute)(epidemic)

B30.8 **Other viral conjunctivitis**
    Newcastle conjunctivitis

B30.9 **Viral conjunctivitis, unspecified**

B33 **Other viral diseases, not elsewhere classified**

  B33.0 **Epidemic myalgia**
    Bornholm disease

CC B33.1 **Ross River disease**
    Epidemic polyarthritis and exanthema
    Ross River fever

+ B33.2 **Viral carditis**
    Coxsackie (virus) carditis

    CC B33.20 **Viral carditis, unspecified**
    CC B33.21 **Viral endocarditis**
    CC B33.22 **Viral myocarditis**
    CC B33.23 **Viral pericarditis**
    B33.24 **Viral cardiomyopathy**

B33.3 **Retrovirus infections, not elsewhere classified**
    Retrovirus infection NOS

CC B33.4 **Hantavirus (cardio)-pulmonary syndrome [HPS] [HCPS]**
    Hantavirus disease with pulmonary manifestations
    Sin nombre virus disease
    Use additional code to identify any associated acute kidney failure (N17.9)
    Excludes1: hantavirus disease with renal manifestations (A98.5)
        hemorrhagic fever with renal manifestations (A98.5)

B33.8 **Other specified viral diseases**
    Excludes1: anogenital human papillomavirus infection (A63.0)
        viral warts due to human papillomavirus infection (B07)

B34 **Viral infection of unspecified site**

  Excludes1: anogenital human papillomavirus infection (A63.0)
    cytomegaloviral disease NOS (B25.9)
    herpesvirus [herpes simplex] infection NOS (B00.9)
    retrovirus infection NOS (B33.3)
    viral agents as the cause of diseases classified elsewhere (B97.-)
    viral warts due to human papillomavirus infection (B07)

B34.0 **Adenovirus infection, unspecified**

B34.1 **Enterovirus infection, unspecified**
    Coxsackievirus infection NOS
    Echovirus infection NOS

B34.2 **Coronavirus infection, unspecified**
    Excludes1: COVID-19 (U07.1)
        pneumonia due to SARS associated coronavirus (J12.81)
    AHA CC: 1Q, 2020, 34-36

CC B34.3 **Parvovirus infection, unspecified**

B34.4 **Papovavirus infection, unspecified**

B34.8 **Other viral infections of unspecified site**

B34.9 **Viral infection, unspecified**
    Viremia NOS
    AHA CC: 3Q, 2016, 10

Mycoses (B35-B49)

Excludes2: hypersensitivity pneumonitis due to organic dust (J67.-)
    mycosis fungoides (C84.0-)

B35 **Dermatophytosis**

  Includes: favus
    infections due to species of Epidermophyton, Micro-sporum and Trichophyton
    tinea, any type except those in B36.-

B35.0 **Tinea barbae and tinea capitis**
    Beard ringworm
    Kerion
    Scalp ringworm
    Sycosis, mycotic

B35.1 **Tinea unguium**
    Dermatophytic onychia
    Dermatophytosis of nail
    Onychomycosis
    Ringworm of nails

B35.2 **Tinea manuum**
    Dermatophytosis of hand
    Hand ringworm

B35.3 **Tinea pedis**
    Athlete's foot
    Dermatophytosis of foot
    Foot ringworm

B35.4 **Tinea corporis**
    Ringworm of the body

B35.5 **Tinea imbricata**
    Tokelau

B35.6 **Tinea cruris**
    Dhobi itch
    Groin ringworm
    Jock itch

B35.8 **Other dermatophytoses**
    Disseminated dermatophytosis
    Granulomatous dermatophytosis

B35.9 **Dermatophytosis, unspecified**
    Ringworm NOS

B36 **Other superficial mycoses**

B36.0 **Pityriasis versicolor**
    Tinea flava
    Tinea versicolor

B36.1 **Tinea nigra**
    Keratomycosis nigricans palmaris
    Microsporosis nigra
    Pityriasis nigra

B36.2 **White piedra**
    Tinea blanca

B36.3 **Black piedra**

B36.8 **Other specified superficial mycoses**

B36.9 **Superficial mycosis, unspecified**

B37 **Candidiasis**

  Includes: candidosis
    moniliasis
  Excludes1: neonatal candidiasis (P37.5)

CC B37.0 **Candidal stomatitis**
    Oral thrush

MCC B37.1 **Pulmonary candidiasis**
    Candidal bronchitis
    Candidal pneumonia

B37.2 **Candidiasis of skin and nail**
    Candidal onychia
    Candidal paronychia
    Excludes2: diaper dermatitis (L22)

♀ B37.3 **Candidiasis of vulva and vagina**
    Candidal vulvovaginitis
    Monilial vulvovaginitis
    Vaginal thrush

+ B37.4 **Candidiasis of other urogenital sites**
    CC B37.41 **Candidal cystitis and urethritis**
        HAC see Appendix B for HAC conditional logic
    ♂ B37.42 **Candidal balanitis**
    CC B37.49 **Other urogenital candidiasis**
        Candidal pyelonephritis
        HAC see Appendix B for HAC conditional logic

MCC B37.5 **Candidal meningitis**

MCC B37.6 **Candidal endocarditis**

MCC B37.7 **Candidal sepsis**
    Disseminated candidiasis
    Systemic candidiasis
    Review coding guideline C.1.d
    AHA CC: 4Q, 2014, 46

+ B37.8 **Candidiasis of other sites**
    CC B37.81 **Candidal esophagitis**
    CC B37.82 **Candidal enteritis**
        Candidal proctitis
    CC B37.83 **Candidal cheilitis**
    CC B37.84 **Candidal otitis externa**
    CC B37.89 **Other sites of candidiasis**
        Candidal osteomyelitis

B37.9 **Candidiasis, unspecified**
    Thrush NOS

B38 **Coccidioidomycosis**

CC B38.0 **Acute pulmonary coccidioidomycosis**

CC B38.1 **Chronic pulmonary coccidioidomycosis**

CC B38.2 **Pulmonary coccidioidomycosis, unspecified**

+, +7th, X + 7th   ● Newborn   ● Pediatric   ● Maternity   ● Adult   ♀ Female   ♂ Male   Manifestation   Unacceptable PDX   HCC   CC   MCC   HAC

CC **B38.3 Cutaneous coccidioidomycosis**
MCC **B38.4 Coccidioidomycosis meningitis**
CC **B38.7 Disseminated coccidioidomycosis**
　　　　Generalized coccidioidomycosis
 + **B38.8 Other forms of coccidioidomycosis**
 ♂ CC **B38.81 Prostatic coccidioidomycosis**
　 CC **B38.89 Other forms of coccidioidomycosis**
CC **B38.9 Coccidioidomycosis, unspecified**

B39 Histoplasmosis

Code first associated AIDS (B20)

Use additional code for any associated manifestations, such as:
　endocarditis (I39)
　meningitis (G02)
　pericarditis (I32)
　retinitis (H32)

MCC **B39.0 Acute pulmonary histoplasmosis capsulati**
MCC **B39.1 Chronic pulmonary histoplasmosis capsulati**
MCC **B39.2 Pulmonary histoplasmosis capsulati, unspecified**
CC **B39.3 Disseminated histoplasmosis capsulati**
　　　　Generalized histoplasmosis capsulati
 B39.4 Histoplasmosis capsulati, unspecified
　　　American histoplasmosis
 B39.5 Histoplasmosis duboisii
　　　African histoplasmosis
 B39.9 Histoplasmosis, unspecified

B40 Blastomycosis

Excludes1: *Brazilian blastomycosis (B41.-)*
　　　　keloidal blastomycosis (B48.0)

CC **B40.0 Acute pulmonary blastomycosis**
CC **B40.1 Chronic pulmonary blastomycosis**
CC **B40.2 Pulmonary blastomycosis, unspecified**
CC **B40.3 Cutaneous blastomycosis**
CC **B40.7 Disseminated blastomycosis**
　　　　Generalized blastomycosis
 + **B40.8 Other forms of blastomycosis**
　 CC **B40.81 Blastomycotic meningoencephalitis**
　　　　　Meningomyelitis due to blastomycosis
　 CC **B40.89 Other forms of blastomycosis**
CC **B40.9 Blastomycosis, unspecified**

B41 Paracoccidioidomycosis

Includes: Brazilian blastomycosis
　　　　Lutz' disease
CC **B41.0 Pulmonary paracoccidioidomycosis**
CC **B41.7 Disseminated paracoccidioidomycosis**
　　　　Generalized paracoccidioidomycosis
CC **B41.8 Other forms of paracoccidioidomycosis**
CC **B41.9 Paracoccidioidomycosis, unspecified**

B42 Sporotrichosis

 B42.0 Pulmonary sporotrichosis
 B42.1 Lymphocutaneous sporotrichosis
 B42.7 Disseminated sporotrichosis
　　　　Generalized sporotrichosis
 + **B42.8 Other forms of sporotrichosis**
　 B42.81 Cerebral sporotrichosis
　　　　　Meningitis due to sporotrichosis
　 B42.82 Sporotrichosis arthritis
　 B42.89 Other forms of sporotrichosis
 B42.9 Sporotrichosis, unspecified

B43 Chromomycosis and pheomycotic abscess

 B43.0 Cutaneous chromomycosis
　　　　Dermatitis verrucosa
 B43.1 Pheomycotic brain abscess
　　　　Cerebral chromomycosis
 B43.2 Subcutaneous pheomycotic abscess and cyst
 B43.8 Other forms of chromomycosis
 B43.9 Chromomycosis, unspecified

B44 Aspergillosis

Includes: aspergilloma
MCC **B44.0 Invasive pulmonary aspergillosis**
CC **B44.1 Other pulmonary aspergillosis**
CC **B44.2 Tonsillar aspergillosis**
CC **B44.7 Disseminated aspergillosis**
　　　　Generalized aspergillosis
 + **B44.8 Other forms of aspergillosis**
　 CC **B44.81 Allergic bronchopulmonary aspergillosis**
　 CC **B44.89 Other forms of aspergillosis**

CC **B44.9 Aspergillosis, unspecified**

B45 Cryptococcosis

CC **B45.0 Pulmonary cryptococcosis**
MCC **B45.1 Cerebral cryptococcosis**
　　　　Cryptococcal meningitis
　　　　Cryptococcosis meningocerebralis
CC **B45.2 Cutaneous cryptococcosis**
CC **B45.3 Osseous cryptococcosis**
CC **B45.7 Disseminated cryptococcosis**
　　　　Generalized cryptococcosis
CC **B45.8 Other forms of cryptococcosis**
CC **B45.9 Cryptococcosis, unspecified**

B46 Zygomycosis

MCC **B46.0 Pulmonary mucormycosis**
MCC **B46.1 Rhinocerebral mucormycosis**
MCC **B46.2 Gastrointestinal mucormycosis**
MCC **B46.3 Cutaneous mucormycosis**
　　　　Subcutaneous mucormycosis
MCC **B46.4 Disseminated mucormycosis**
　　　　Generalized mucormycosis
MCC **B46.5 Mucormycosis, unspecified**
MCC **B46.8 Other zygomycoses**
　　　　Entomophthoromycosis
MCC **B46.9 Zygomycosis, unspecified**
　　　　Phycomycosis NOS

B47 Mycetoma

CC **B47.0 Eumycetoma**
　　　　Madura foot, mycotic
　　　　Maduromycosis
CC **B47.1 Actinomycetoma**
CC **B47.9 Mycetoma, unspecified**
　　　　Madura foot NOS

B48 Other mycoses, not elsewhere classified

 B48.0 Lobomycosis
　　　　Keloidal blastomycosis
　　　　Lobo's disease
 B48.1 Rhinosporidiosis
CC **B48.2 Allescheriasis**
　　　　Infection due to Pseudallescheria boydii
　　　　Excludes1: *eumycetoma (B47.0)*
CC **B48.3 Geotrichosis**
　　　　Geotrichum stomatitis
CC **B48.4 Penicillosis**
　　　　Talaromycosis
CC **B48.8 Other specified mycoses**
　　　　Adiaspiromycosis
　　　　Infection of tissue and organs by Alternaria
　　　　Infection of tissue and organs by Drechslera
　　　　Infection of tissue and organs by Fusarium
　　　　Infection of tissue and organs by saprophytic fungi NEC
　　　　AHA CC: 2Q, 2014, 13; 4Q, 2014, 46

CC **B49 Unspecified mycosis**

Fungemia NOS
Valid 3-character code, no further characters required

Protozoal diseases (B50-B64)

Excludes1: *amebiasis (A06.-)*
　　　　　other protozoal intestinal diseases (A07.-)

B50 Plasmodium falciparum malaria

Includes: mixed infections of Plasmodium falciparum with any
　　　　　other Plasmodium species
CC **B50.0 Plasmodium falciparum malaria with cerebral complications**
　　　　Cerebral malaria NOS
CC **B50.8 Other severe and complicated Plasmodium falciparum malaria**
　　　　Severe or complicated Plasmodium falciparum malaria NOS
MCC **B50.9 Plasmodium falciparum malaria, unspecified**

B51 Plasmodium vivax malaria

Includes: mixed infections of Plasmodium vivax with other
　　　　　Plasmodium species, except Plasmodium falciparum
　　　Excludes1: *plasmodium vivax with Plasmodium falciparum (B50.-)*
CC **B51.0 Plasmodium vivax malaria with rupture of spleen**
CC **B51.8 Plasmodium vivax malaria with other complications**
CC **B51.9 Plasmodium vivax malaria without complication**
　　　　Plasmodium vivax malaria NOS

B52 Plasmodium malariae malaria

Includes: mixed infections of Plasmodium malariae with other
Plasmodium species, except Plasmodium falciparum
and Plasmodium vivax

Excludes1: *Plasmodium falciparum (B50.-)*
Plasmodium vivax (B51.-)

CC B52.0 **Plasmodium malariae malaria with nephropathy**

CC B52.8 **Plasmodium malariae malaria with other complications**

CC B52.9 **Plasmodium malariae malaria without complication**
Plasmodium malariae malaria NOS

B53 **Other specified malaria**

CC B53.0 **Plasmodium ovale malaria**

Excludes1: *Plasmodium ovale with Plasmodium falciparum*
(B50.-)
Plasmodium ovale with Plasmodium malariae
(B52.-)
Plasmodium ovale with Plasmodium vivax (B51.-)

CC B53.1 **Malaria due to simian plasmodia**

Excludes1: *Malaria due to simian plasmodia with*
Plasmodium falciparum (B50.-)
Malaria due to simian plasmodia with
Plasmodium malariae (B52.-)
Malaria due to simian plasmodia with
Plasmodium ovale (B53.0)
Malaria due to simian plasmodia with
Plasmodium vivax (B51.-)

CC B53.8 **Other malaria, not elsewhere classified**

CC B54 **Unspecified malaria**

Valid 3-character code, no further characters required

B55 **Leishmaniasis**

CC B55.0 **Visceral leishmaniasis**
Kala-azar
Post-kala-azar dermal leishmaniasis

CC B55.1 **Cutaneous leishmaniasis**

CC B55.2 **Mucocutaneous leishmaniasis**

CC B55.9 **Leishmaniasis, unspecified**

B56 **African trypanosomiasis**

CC B56.0 **Gambiense trypanosomiasis**
Infection due to Trypanosoma brucei gambiense
West African sleeping sickness

CC B56.1 **Rhodesiense trypanosomiasis**
East African sleeping sickness
Infection due to Trypanosoma brucei rhodesiense

CC B56.9 **African trypanosomiasis, unspecified**
Sleeping sickness NOS

B57 **Chagas' disease**

Includes: American trypanosomiasis
infection due to Trypanosoma cruzi

CC B57.0 **Acute Chagas' disease with heart involvement**
Acute Chagas' disease with myocarditis

CC B57.1 **Acute Chagas' disease without heart involvement**
Acute Chagas' disease NOS

CC B57.2 **Chagas' disease (chronic) with heart involvement**
American trypanosomiasis NOS
Chagas' disease (chronic) NOS
Chagas' disease (chronic) with myocarditis
Trypanosomiasis NOS

+ B57.3 **Chagas' disease (chronic) with digestive system involvement**

CC B57.30 **Chagas' disease with digestive system
involvement, unspecified**

CC B57.31 **Megaesophagus in Chagas' disease**

CC B57.32 **Megacolon in Chagas' disease**

CC B57.39 **Other digestive system involvement in Chagas'
disease**

+ B57.4 **Chagas' disease (chronic) with nervous system involvement**

CC B57.40 **Chagas' disease with nervous system involvement,
unspecified**

CC B57.41 **Meningitis in Chagas' disease**

CC B57.42 **Meningoencephalitis in Chagas' disease**

CC B57.49 **Other nervous system involvement in Chagas'
disease**

CC B57.5 **Chagas' disease (chronic) with other organ involvement**

B58 **Toxoplasmosis**

Includes: infection due to Toxoplasma gondii

Excludes1: *congenital toxoplasmosis (P37.1)*

+ B58.0 **Toxoplasma oculopathy**

CC B58.00 **Toxoplasma oculopathy, unspecified**

CC B58.01 **Toxoplasma chorioretinitis**

CC B58.09 **Other toxoplasma oculopathy**
Toxoplasma uveitis

CC B58.1 **Toxoplasma hepatitis**

MCC B58.2 **Toxoplasma meningoencephalitis**

MCC B58.3 **Pulmonary toxoplasmosis**

+ B58.8 **Toxoplasmosis with other organ involvement**

MCC B58.81 **Toxoplasma myocarditis**

CC B58.82 **Toxoplasma myositis**

CC B58.83 **Toxoplasma tubulo-interstitial nephropathy**
Toxoplasma pyelonephritis

CC B58.89 **Toxoplasmosis with other organ involvement**

CC B58.9 **Toxoplasmosis, unspecified**

B59 **Pneumocystosis**

MCC Pneumonia due to Pneumocystis carinii
Pneumonia due to Pneumocystis jiroveci
Valid 3-character code, no further characters required

B60 **Other protozoal diseases, not elsewhere classified**

Excludes1: *cryptosporidiosis (A07.2)*
intestinal microsporidiosis (A07.8)
isosporiasis (A07.3)

+ B60.0 **Babesiosis**

CC B60.00 **Babesiosis, unspecified**
Babesiosis due to unspecified Babesia species
Piroplasmosis, unspecified

CC B60.01 **Babesiosis due to Babesia microti**
Infection due to B. microti

CC B60.02 **Babesiosis due to Babesia duncani**
Infection due to B. duncani and B. duncani-type
species

CC B60.03 **Babesiosis due to Babesia divergens**
Babesiosis due to Babesia MO-1
Infection due to B. divergens and B. divergens-like
strains

CC B60.09 **Other babesiosis**
Babesiosis due to Babesia KO-1
Babesiosis due to Babesia venatorum
Infection due to other Babesia species
Infection due to other protozoa of the order
Piroplasmida
Other piroplasmosis

+ B60.1 **Acanthamebiasis**

CC B60.10 **Acanthamebiasis, unspecified**

B60.11 **Meningoencephalitis due to Acanthamoeba
(culbertsoni)**

B60.12 **Conjunctivitis due to Acanthamoeba**

B60.13 **Keratoconjunctivitis due to Acanthamoeba**

CC B60.19 **Other acanthamebic disease**

CC B60.2 **Naegleriasis**
Primary amebic meningoencephalitis

B60.8 **Other specified protozoal diseases**
Microsporidiosis

B64 **Unspecified protozoal disease**

Valid 3-character code, no further characters required

Helminthiases (B65-B83)

B65 **Schistosomiasis [bilharziasis]**

Includes: snail fever

CC B65.0 **Schistosomiasis due to Schistosoma haematobium [urinary
schistosomiasis]**

CC B65.1 **Schistosomiasis due to Schistosoma mansoni [intestinal
schistosomiasis]**

CC B65.2 **Schistosomiasis due to Schistosoma japonicum**
Asiatic schistosomiasis

CC B65.3 **Cercarial dermatitis**
Swimmer's itch

CC B65.8 **Other schistosomiasis**
Infection due to Schistosoma intercalatum
Infection due to Schistosoma mattheei
Infection due to Schistosoma mekongi

CC B65.9 **Schistosomiasis, unspecified**

B66 **Other fluke infections**

CC B66.0 **Opisthorchiasis**
Infection due to cat liver fluke
Infection due to Opisthorchis (felineus)(viverrini)

CC B66.1 **Clonorchiasis**
Chinese liver fluke disease
Infection due to Clonorchis sinensis
Oriental liver fluke disease

+, +7th, X + 7th   ● Newborn   ● Pediatric   ● Maternity   ● Adult   ♀ Female   ♂ Male   Manifestation   Unacceptable PDX   HCC   CC   MCC   HAC

CC **B66.2 Dicroceliasis**
Infection due to Dicrocoelium dendriticum
Lancet fluke infection

CC **B66.3 Fascioliasis**
Infection due to Fasciola gigantica
Infection due to Fasciola hepatica
Infection due to Fasciola indica
Sheep liver fluke disease

CC **B66.4 Paragonimiasis**
Infection due to Paragonimus species
Lung fluke disease
Pulmonary distomiasis

CC **B66.5 Fasciolopsiasis**
Infection due to Fasciolopsis buski
Intestinal distomiasis

CC **B66.8 Other specified fluke infections**
Echinostomiasis
Heterophyiasis
Metagonimiasis
Nanophyetiasis
Watsoniasis

B66.9 Fluke infection, unspecified

B67 Echinococcosis

Includes: hydatidosis

CC **B67.0 Echinococcus granulosus infection of liver**
CC **B67.1 Echinococcus granulosus infection of lung**
CC **B67.2 Echinococcus granulosus infection of bone**
+ **B67.3 Echinococcus granulosus infection, other and multiple sites**
    CC **B67.31 Echinococcus granulosus infection, thyroid gland**
    CC **B67.32 Echinococcus granulosus infection, multiple sites**
    CC **B67.39 Echinococcus granulosus infection, other sites**
CC **B67.4 Echinococcus granulosus infection, unspecified**
Dog tapeworm (infection)
CC **B67.5 Echinococcus multilocularis infection of liver**
+ **B67.6 Echinococcus multilocularis infection, other and multiple sites**
    CC **B67.61 Echinococcus multilocularis infection, multiple sites**
    CC **B67.69 Echinococcus multilocularis infection, other sites**
CC **B67.7 Echinococcus multilocularis infection, unspecified**
CC **B67.8 Echinococcosis, unspecified, of liver**
+ **B67.9 Echinococcosis, other and unspecified**
    CC **B67.90 Echinococcosis, unspecified**
Echinococcosis NOS
    CC **B67.99 Other echinococcosis**

B68 Taeniasis

Excludes1: *cysticercosis (B69.-)*

CC **B68.0 Taenia solium taeniasis**
Pork tapeworm (infection)
CC **B68.1 Taenia saginata taeniasis**
Beef tapeworm (infection)
Infection due to adult tapeworm Taenia saginata
CC **B68.9 Taeniasis, unspecified**

B69 Cysticercosis

Includes: cysticerciasis infection due to larval form of Taenia solium

CC **B69.0 Cysticercosis of central nervous system**
CC **B69.1 Cysticercosis of eye**
+ **B69.8 Cysticercosis of other sites**
    CC **B69.81 Myositis in cysticercosis**
    CC **B69.89 Cysticercosis of other sites**
CC **B69.9 Cysticercosis, unspecified**

B70 Diphyllobothriasis and sparganosis

CC **B70.0 Diphyllobothriasis**
Diphyllobothrium (adult) (latum) (pacificum) infection
Fish tapeworm (infection)
Excludes2: *larval diphyllobothriasis (B70.1)*
CC **B70.1 Sparganosis**
Infection due to Sparganum (mansoni) (proliferum)
Infection due to Spirometra larva
Larval diphyllobothriasis
Spirometrosis

B71 Other cestode infections

CC **B71.0 Hymenolepiasis**
Dwarf tapeworm infection
Rat tapeworm (infection)
CC **B71.1 Dipylidiasis**
CC **B71.8 Other specified cestode infections**

Coenurosis

B71.9 Cestode infection, unspecified
Tapeworm (infection) NOS

CC **B72 Dracunculiasis**

Includes: guinea worm infection
infection due to Dracunculus medinensis
Valid 3-character code, no further characters required

B73 Onchocerciasis

Includes: onchocerca volvulus infection
onchocercosis
river blindness

+ **B73.0 Onchocerciasis with eye disease**
    CC **B73.00 Onchocerciasis with eye involvement, unspecified**
    CC **B73.01 Onchocerciasis with endophthalmitis**
    CC **B73.02 Onchocerciasis with glaucoma**
    CC **B73.09 Onchocerciasis with other eye involvement**
Infestation of eyelid due to onchocerciasis
CC **B73.1 Onchocerciasis without eye disease**

B74 Filariasis

Excludes2: *onchocerciasis (B73)*
tropical (pulmonary) eosinophilia NOS (J82)

CC **B74.0 Filariasis due to Wuchereria bancrofti**
Bancroftian elephantiasis
Bancroftian filariasis
CC **B74.1 Filariasis due to Brugia malayi**
CC **B74.2 Filariasis due to Brugia timori**
CC **B74.3 Loiasis**
Calabar swelling
Eyeworm disease of Africa
Loa loa infection
CC **B74.4 Mansonelliasis**
Infection due to Mansonella ozzardi
Infection due to Mansonella perstans
Infection due to Mansonella streptocerca
CC **B74.8 Other filariases**
Dirofilariasis
CC **B74.9 Filariasis, unspecified**

CC **B75 Trichinellosis**

Includes: infection due to Trichinella species
trichiniasis
Valid 3-character code, no further characters required

B76 Hookworm diseases

Includes: uncinariasis

CC **B76.0 Ancylostomiasis**
Infection due to Ancylostoma species
CC **B76.1 Necatoriasis**
Infection due to Necator americanus
CC **B76.8 Other hookworm diseases**
CC **B76.9 Hookworm disease, unspecified**
Cutaneous larva migrans NOS

B77 Ascariasis

Includes: ascaridiasis
roundworm infection

CC **B77.0 Ascariasis with intestinal complications**
+ **B77.8 Ascariasis with other complications**
    MCC **B77.81 Ascariasis pneumonia**
    CC **B77.89 Ascariasis with other complications**
CC **B77.9 Ascariasis, unspecified**

B78 Strongyloidiasis

Excludes1: *trichostrongyliasis (B81.2)*

CC **B78.0 Intestinal strongyloidiasis**
B78.1 Cutaneous strongyloidiasis
CC **B78.7 Disseminated strongyloidiasis**
CC **B78.9 Strongyloidiasis, unspecified**

CC **B79 Trichuriasis**

Includes: trichocephaliasis
whipworm (disease)(infection)
Valid 3-character code, no further characters required

CC **B80 Enterobiasis**

Includes: oxyuriasis
pinworm infection
threadworm infection
Valid 3-character code, no further characters required

B81   Other intestinal helminthiases, not elsewhere classified

> *Excludes1:* angiostrongyliasis due to:
> > Angiostrongylus cantonensis (B83.2)
> > Parastrongylus cantonensis (B83.2)

CC **B81.0   Anisakiasis**
> Infection due to Anisakis larva

CC **B81.1   Intestinal capillariasis**
> Capillariasis NOS
> Infection due to Capillaria philippinensis
> *Excludes2:* hepatic capillariasis (B83.8)

CC **B81.2   Trichostrongyliasis**

CC **B81.3   Intestinal angiostrongyliasis**
> Angiostrongyliasis due to:
> > Angiostrongylus costaricensis
> > Parastrongylus cantonensis

CC **B81.4   Mixed intestinal helminthiases**
> Infection due to intestinal helminths classified to more than
> > one of the categories B65.0-B81.3 and B81.8
> Mixed helminthiasis NOS

CC **B81.8   Other specified intestinal helminthiases**
> Infection due to Oesophagostomum species
> > [esophagostomiasis]
> Infection due to Ternidens diminutus [ternidensiasis]

B82   Unspecified intestinal parasitism

CC **B82.0   Intestinal helminthiasis, unspecified**

B82.9   Intestinal parasitism, unspecified

B83   Other helminthiases

> *Excludes1:* capillariasis NOS (B81.1)
> *Excludes2:* intestinal capillariasis (B81.1)

B83.0   Visceral larva migrans
> Toxocariasis

B83.1   Gnathostomiasis
> Wandering swelling

B83.2   Angiostrongyliasis due to Parastrongylus cantonensis
> Eosinophilic meningoencephalitis due to Parastrongylus
> > cantonensis
> *Excludes2:* intestinal angiostrongyliasis (B81.3)

B83.3   Syngamiasis
> Syngamosis

B83.4   Internal hirudiniasis
> *Excludes2:* external hirudiniasis (B88.3)

B83.8   Other specified helminthiases
> Acanthocephaliasis
> Gongylonemiasis
> Hepatic capillariasis
> Metastrongyliasis
> Thelaziasis

B83.9   Helminthiasis, unspecified
> Worms NOS
> *Excludes1:* intestinal helminthiasis NOS (B82.0)

Pediculosis, acariasis and other infestations (B85-B89)

B85   Pediculosis and phthiriasis

B85.0   Pediculosis due to Pediculus humanus capitis
> Head-louse infestation

B85.1   Pediculosis due to Pediculus humanus corporis
> Body-louse infestation

B85.2   Pediculosis, unspecified

B85.3   Phthiriasis
> Infestation by crab-louse
> Infestation by Phthirus pubis

B85.4   Mixed pediculosis and phthiriasis
> Infestation classifiable to more than one of the categories
> > B85.0-B85.3

B86   Scabies

> Sarcoptic itch
> **Valid 3-character code, no further characters required**

B87   Myiasis

> **Includes:** infestation by larva of flies

B87.0   Cutaneous myiasis
> Creeping myiasis

B87.1   Wound myiasis
> Traumatic myiasis

B87.2   Ocular myiasis

B87.3   Nasopharyngeal myiasis
> Laryngeal myiasis

B87.4   Aural myiasis

+ **B87.8   Myiasis of other sites**
> **B87.81   Genitourinary myiasis**
> **B87.82   Intestinal myiasis**
> **B87.89   Myiasis of other sites**

B87.9   Myiasis, unspecified

B88   Other infestations

B88.0   Other acariasis
> Acarine dermatitis
> Dermatitis due to Demodex species
> Dermatitis due to Dermanyssus gallinae
> Dermatitis due to Liponyssoides sanguineus
> Trombiculosis
> *Excludes2:* scabies (B86)

B88.1   Tungiasis [sandflea infestation]

B88.2   Other arthropod infestations
> Scarabiasis

B88.3   External hirudiniasis
> Leech infestation NOS
> *Excludes2:* internal hirudiniasis (B83.4)

B88.8   Other specified infestations
> Ichthyoparasitism due to Vandellia cirrhosa
> Linguatulosis
> Porocephaliasis

B88.9   Infestation, unspecified
> Infestation (skin) NOS
> Infestation by mites NOS
> Skin parasites NOS

B89   Unspecified parasitic disease

> **Valid 3-character code, no further characters required**

Sequelae of infectious and parasitic diseases (B90-B94)

NOTE   Categories B90-B94 are to be used to indicate conditions in categories A00-B89 as the cause of sequelae, which are themselves classified elsewhere. The 'sequelae' include conditions specified as such; they also include residuals of diseases classifiable to the above categories if there is evidence that the disease itself is no longer present. Codes from these categories are not to be used for chronic infections. Code chronic current infections to active infectious disease as appropriate.

Code first condition resulting from (sequela) the infectious or parasitic disease

B90   Sequelae of tuberculosis

B90.0   Sequelae of central nervous system tuberculosis
B90.1   Sequelae of genitourinary tuberculosis
B90.2   Sequelae of tuberculosis of bones and joints
B90.8   Sequelae of tuberculosis of other organs
> *Excludes2:* sequelae of respiratory tuberculosis (B90.9)
B90.9   Sequelae of respiratory and unspecified tuberculosis
> Sequelae of tuberculosis NOS

B91   Sequelae of poliomyelitis

> *Excludes1:* postpolio syndrome (G14)
> **Valid 3-character code, no further characters required**

B92   Sequelae of leprosy

> **Valid 3-character code, no further characters required**

B94   Sequelae of other and unspecified infectious and parasitic diseases

B94.0   Sequelae of trachoma
B94.1   Sequelae of viral encephalitis
B94.2   Sequelae of viral hepatitis
B94.8   Sequelae of other specified infectious and parasitic diseases
> AHA CC: 4Q, 2017, 109
B94.9   Sequelae of unspecified infectious and parasitic disease

Bacterial and viral infectious agents (B95-B97)

NOTE   These categories are provided for use as supplementary or additional codes to identify the infectious agent(s) in diseases classified elsewhere.

B95   Streptococcus, Staphylococcus, and Enterococcus as the cause of diseases classified elsewhere

> Review coding guideline C.1.b

B95.0   Streptococcus, group A, as the cause of diseases classified elsewhere

B95.1   Streptococcus, group B, as the cause of diseases classified elsewhere
> AHA CC: 4Q, 2018, 23; 2Q, 2019, 9-10; 1Q, 2020, 10

B95.2   Enterococcus as the cause of diseases classified elsewhere

B95.3   Streptococcus pneumoniae as the cause of diseases classified elsewhere

+, +7th, X + 7th   ● Newborn   ● Pediatric   ● Maternity   ● Adult   ♀ Female   ♂ Male   Manifestation   Unacceptable PDX   HCC   CC   MCC   HAC

B95.4 Other streptococcus as the cause of diseases classified elsewhere

B95.5 Unspecified streptococcus as the cause of diseases classified elsewhere

+ **B95.6** Staphylococcus aureus as the cause of diseases classified elsewhere

    B95.61 Methicillin susceptible Staphylococcus aureus infection as the cause of diseases classified elsewhere

        Methicillin susceptible Staphylococcus aureus (MSSA) infection as the cause of diseases classified elsewhere

        Staphylococcus aureus infection NOS as the cause of diseases classified elsewhere

    B95.62 Methicillin resistant Staphylococcus aureus infection as the cause of diseases classified elsewhere

        Methicillin resistant staphylococcus aureus (MRSA) infection as the cause of diseases classified elsewhere

        Review coding guidelines C.1.e.1.a and C.1.e.1.b

        AHA CC: 1Q, 2016, 12-13

B95.7 Other staphylococcus as the cause of diseases classified elsewhere

B95.8 Unspecified staphylococcus as the cause of diseases classified elsewhere

B96 Other bacterial agents as the cause of diseases classified elsewhere

    Review coding guideline C.1.b

B96.0 Mycoplasma pneumoniae [M. pneumoniae] as the cause of diseases classified elsewhere

    Pleuro-pneumonia-like-organism [PPLO]

B96.1 Klebsiella pneumoniae [K. pneumoniae] as the cause of diseases classified elsewhere

+ **B96.2** Escherichia coli [E. coli] as the cause of diseases classified elsewhere

    B96.20 Unspecified Escherichia coli [E. coli] as the cause of diseases classified elsewhere

        Escherichia coli [E. coli] NOS

        AHA CC: 1Q, 2018, 16; 4Q, 2018, 34

    B96.21 Shiga toxin-producing Escherichia coli [E. coli] [STEC] O157 as the cause of diseases classified elsewhere

        E. coli O157:H- (nonmotile) with confirmation of Shiga toxin

        E. coli O157 with confirmation of Shiga toxin when H antigen is unknown, or is not H7

        O157:H7 Escherichia coli [E.coli] with or without confirmation of Shiga toxin-production

        Shiga toxin-producing Escherichia coli [E.coli] O157:H7 with or without confirmation of Shiga toxin-production

        STEC O157:H7 with or without confirmation of Shiga toxin-production

    B96.22 Other specified Shiga toxin-producing Escherichia coli [E. coli] [STEC] as the cause of diseases classified elsewhere

        Non-O157 Shiga toxin-producing Escherichia coli [E.coli]

        Non-O157 Shiga toxin-producing Escherichia coli [E.coli] with known O group

    B96.23 Unspecified Shiga toxin-producing Escherichia coli [E. coli] [STEC] as the cause of diseases classified elsewhere

        Shiga toxin-producing Escherichia coli [E. coli] with unspecified O group

        STEC NOS

    B96.29 Other Escherichia coli [E. coli] as the cause of diseases classified elsewhere

        Non-Shiga toxin-producing E. coli

B96.3 Hemophilus influenzae [H. influenzae] as the cause of diseases classified elsewhere

B96.4 Proteus (mirabilis) (morganii) as the cause of diseases classified elsewhere

B96.5 Pseudomonas (aeruginosa) (mallei) (pseudomallei) as the cause of diseases classified elsewhere

    AHA CC: 1Q, 2015, 18-19

B96.6 Bacteroides fragilis [B. fragilis] as the cause of diseases classified elsewhere

B96.7 Clostridium perfringens [C. perfringens] as the cause of diseases classified elsewhere

+ **B96.8** Other specified bacterial agents as the cause of diseases classified elsewhere

    B96.81 Helicobacter pylori [H. pylori] as the cause of diseases classified elsewhere

    B96.82 Vibrio vulnificus as the cause of diseases classified elsewhere

    B96.89 Other specified bacterial agents as the cause of diseases classified elsewhere

B97 Viral agents as the cause of diseases classified elsewhere

    Review coding guideline C.1.b

B97.0 Adenovirus as the cause of diseases classified elsewhere

+ **B97.1** Enterovirus as the cause of diseases classified elsewhere

    B97.10 Unspecified enterovirus as the cause of diseases classified elsewhere

    B97.11 Coxsackievirus as the cause of diseases classified elsewhere

    B97.12 Echovirus as the cause of diseases classified elsewhere

    B97.19 Other enterovirus as the cause of diseases classified elsewhere

+ **B97.2** Coronavirus as the cause of diseases classified elsewhere

CC **B97.21** SARS-associated coronavirus as the cause of diseases classified elsewhere

    Excludes1: *pneumonia due to SARS-associated coronavirus (J12.81)*

    B97.29 Other coronavirus as the cause of diseases classified elsewhere

    AHA CC: 1Q, 2020, 34-36

+ **B97.3** Retrovirus as the cause of diseases classified elsewhere

    Excludes1: *Human immunodeficiency virus [HIV] disease (B20)*

    B97.30 Unspecified retrovirus as the cause of diseases classified elsewhere

    B97.31 Lentivirus as the cause of diseases classified elsewhere

    B97.32 Oncovirus as the cause of diseases classified elsewhere

CC **B97.33** Human T-cell lymphotrophic virus, type I [HTLV-I] as the cause of diseases classified elsewhere

CC **B97.34** Human T-cell lymphotrophic virus, type II [HTLV-II] as the cause of diseases classified elsewhere

CC **B97.35** Human immunodeficiency virus, type 2 [HIV 2] as the cause of diseases classified elsewhere

    B97.39 Other retrovirus as the cause of diseases classified elsewhere

B97.4 Respiratory syncytial virus as the cause of diseases classified elsewhere

    RSV as the cause of diseases classified elsewhere

    Code first related disorders, such as:

        otitis media (H65.-)

        upper respiratory infection (J06.9)

    Excludes2: *acute bronchiolitis due to respiratory syncytial virus (RSV) (J21.0)*

        acute bronchitis due to respiratory syncytial virus (RSV) (J20.5)

        respiratory syncytial virus (RSV) pneumonia (J12.1)

B97.5 Reovirus as the cause of diseases classified elsewhere

B97.6 Parvovirus as the cause of diseases classified elsewhere

B97.7 Papillomavirus as the cause of diseases classified elsewhere

+ **B97.8** Other viral agents as the cause of diseases classified elsewhere

    B97.81 Human metapneumovirus as the cause of diseases classified elsewhere

    B97.89 Other viral agents as the cause of diseases classified elsewhere

    AHA CC: 3Q, 2016, 9-14

Other infectious diseases (B99)

B99 Other and unspecified infectious diseases

    B99.8 Other infectious disease

    B99.9 Unspecified infectious disease

Chapter 2: Neoplasms (C00-D49)

NOTE **Functional activity**

All neoplasms are classified in this chapter, whether they are functionally active or not. An additional code from Chapter 4 may be used, to identify functional activity associated with any neoplasm.

Morphology [Histology]

Chapter 2 classifies neoplasms primarily by site (topography), with broad groupings for behavior, malignant, in situ, benign, etc. The Table of Neoplasms should be used to identify the correct topography code. In a few cases, such as for malignant melanoma and certain neuroendocrine tumors, the morphology (histologic type) is included in the category and codes.

Primary malignant neoplasms overlapping site boundaries

A primary malignant neoplasm that overlaps two or more contiguous (next to each other) sites should be classified to the subcategory/ code .8 ('overlapping lesion'), unless the combination is specifically indexed elsewhere. For multiple neoplasms of the same site that are not contiguous, such as tumors in different quadrants of the same breast, codes for each site should be assigned.

Malignant neoplasm of ectopic tissue

Malignant neoplasms of ectopic tissue are to be coded to the site mentioned, e.g., ectopic pancreatic malignant neoplasms are coded to pancreas, unspecified (C25.9).

This chapter contains the following category blocks:

C00-C14	Malignant neoplasms of lip, oral cavity and pharynx
C15-C26	Malignant neoplasms of digestive organs
C30-C39	Malignant neoplasms of respiratory and intrathoracic organs
C40-C41	Malignant neoplasms of bone and articular cartilage
C43-C44	Melanoma and other malignant neoplasms of skin
C45-C49	Malignant neoplasms of mesothelial and soft tissue
C50	Malignant neoplasms of breast
C51-C58	Malignant neoplasms of female genital organs
C60-C63	Malignant neoplasms of male genital organs
C64-C68	Malignant neoplasms of urinary tract
C69-C72	Malignant neoplasms of eye, brain and other parts of central nervous system
C73-C75	Malignant neoplasms of thyroid and other endocrine glands
C7A	Malignant neuroendocrine tumors
C7B	Secondary neuroendocrine tumors
C76-C80	Malignant neoplasms of ill-defined, other secondary and unspecified sites
C81-C96	Malignant neoplasms of lymphoid, hematopoietic and related tissue
D00-D09	In situ neoplasms
D10-D36	Benign neoplasms, except benign neuroendocrine tumors
D3A	Benign neuroendocrine tumors
D37-D48	Neoplasms of uncertain behavior, polycythemia vera and myelodysplastic syndromes
D49	Neoplasms of unspecified behavior

C. Chapter-Specific Coding Guidelines

In addition to general coding guidelines, there are guidelines for specific diagnoses and/or conditions in the classification. Unless otherwise indicated, these guidelines apply to all health care settings. Please refer to Section II for guidelines on the selection of principal diagnosis.

2. Chapter 2: Neoplasms (C00-D49)

General guidelines

Chapter 2 of the ICD-10-CM contains the codes for most benign and all malignant neoplasms. Certain benign neoplasms, such as prostatic adenomas, may be found in the specific body system chapters. To properly code a neoplasm it is necessary to determine from the record if the neoplasm is benign, in-situ, malignant, or of uncertain histologic behavior. If malignant, any secondary (metastatic) sites should also be determined.

Primary malignant neoplasms overlapping site boundaries

A primary malignant neoplasm that overlaps two or more contiguous (next to each other) sites should be classified to the subcategory/code .8 ('overlapping lesion'), unless the combination is specifically indexed elsewhere. For multiple neoplasms of the same site that are not contiguous such as tumors in different quadrants of the same breast, codes for each site should be assigned.

Malignant neoplasm of ectopic tissue

Malignant neoplasms of ectopic tissue are to be coded to the site of origin mentioned, e.g., ectopic pancreatic malignant neoplasms involving the stomach are coded to malignant neoplasm of pancreas, unspecified (C25.9).

The neoplasm table in the Alphabetic Index should be referenced first. However, if the histological term is documented, that term should be referenced first, rather than going immediately to the Neoplasm Table, in order to determine which column in the Neoplasm Table is appropriate. For example, if the documentation indicates "adenoma," refer to the term in the Alphabetic Index to review the entries under this term and the instructional note to "see also neoplasm, by site, benign." The table provides the proper code based on the type of neoplasm and the site. It is important to select the proper column in the table that corresponds to the type of neoplasm. The Tabular List should then be referenced to verify that the correct code has been selected from the table and that a more specific site code does not exist.

See Section I.C.21. Factors influencing health status and contact with health services, Status, for information regarding Z15.0, codes for genetic susceptibility to cancer.

a. Treatment directed at the malignancy

If the treatment is directed at the malignancy, designate the malignancy as the principal diagnosis.

The only exception to this guideline is if a patient admission/encounter is solely for the administration of chemotherapy, immunotherapy or **external beam** radiation therapy, assign the appropriate Z51.-- code as the first-listed or principal diagnosis, and the diagnosis or problem for which the service is being performed as a secondary diagnosis.

b. Treatment of secondary site

When a patient is admitted because of a primary neoplasm with metastasis and treatment is directed toward the secondary site only, the secondary neoplasm is designated as the principal diagnosis even though the primary malignancy is still present.

c. Coding and sequencing of complications

Coding and sequencing of complications associated with the malignancies or with the therapy thereof are subject to the following guidelines:

1) Anemia associated with malignancy

When admission/encounter is for management of an anemia associated with the malignancy, and the treatment is only for anemia, the appropriate code for the malignancy is sequenced as the principal or first-listed diagnosis followed by the appropriate code for the anemia (such as code D63.0, Anemia in neoplastic disease).

2) Anemia associated with chemotherapy, immunotherapy and radiation therapy

When the admission/encounter is for management of an anemia associated with an adverse effect of the administration of chemotherapy or immunotherapy and the only treatment is for the anemia, the anemia code is sequenced first followed by the appropriate codes for the neoplasm and the adverse effect (T45.1X5-, Adverse effect of antineoplastic and immunosuppressive drugs).

When the admission/encounter is for management of an anemia associated with an adverse effect of radiotherapy, the anemia code should be sequenced first, followed by the appropriate neoplasm code and code Y84.2, Radiological procedure and radiotherapy as the cause of abnormal reaction of the patient, or of later complication, without mention of misadventure at the time of the procedure.

3) Management of dehydration due to the malignancy

When the admission/encounter is for management of dehydration due to the malignancy and only the dehydration is being treated (intravenous rehydration), the dehydration is sequenced first, followed by the code(s) for the malignancy.

4) Treatment of a complication resulting from a surgical procedure

When the admission/encounter is for treatment of a complication resulting from a surgical procedure, designate the complication as the principal or first-listed diagnosis if treatment is directed at resolving the complication.

d. Primary malignancy previously excised

When a primary malignancy has been previously excised or eradicated from its site and there is no further treatment directed to that site and there is no evidence of any existing primary malignancy at that site, a code from category Z85, Personal history of malignant neoplasm, should be used to indicate the former site of the malignancy. Any mention of extension, invasion, or metastasis to another site is coded as a secondary malignant neoplasm to that site. The secondary site may be the principal or first-listed diagnosis with the Z85 code used as a secondary code.

e. Admissions/Encounters involving chemotherapy, immunotherapy and radiation therapy

1) Episode of care involves surgical removal of neoplasm

When an episode of care involves the surgical removal of a neoplasm, primary or secondary site, followed by adjunct chemotherapy or radiation treatment during the same episode of care, the code for the neoplasm should be assigned as principal or first-listed diagnosis.

+, +7th, X + 7th   ● Newborn   ● Pediatric   ● Maternity   ● Adult   ♀ Female   ♂ Male   Manifestation   Unacceptable PDX   HCC   CC   MCC   HAC

2) Patient admission/encounter solely for administration of chemotherapy, immunotherapy and radiation therapy

If a patient admission/encounter is solely for the administration of chemotherapy, immunotherapy or external beam radiation therapy assign code Z51.0, Encounter for antineoplastic radiation therapy, or Z51.11, Encounter for antineoplastic chemotherapy, or Z51.12, Encounter for antineoplastic immunotherapy as the first-listed or principal diagnosis. If a patient receives more than one of these therapies during the same admission more than one of these codes may be assigned, in any sequence.

The malignancy for which the therapy is being administered should be assigned as a secondary diagnosis.

If a patient admission/encounter is for the insertion or implantation of radioactive elements (e.g., brachytherapy) the appropriate code for the malignancy is sequenced as the principal or first-listed diagnosis. Code Z51.0 should not be assigned.

3) Patient admitted for radiation therapy, chemotherapy or immunotherapy and develops complications

When a patient is admitted for the purpose of external beam radiotherapy, immunotherapy or chemotherapy and develops complications such as uncontrolled nausea and vomiting or dehydration, the principal or first-listed diagnosis is Z51.0, Encounter for antineoplastic radiation therapy, or Z51.11, Encounter for antineoplastic chemotherapy, or Z51.12, Encounter for antineoplastic immunotherapy followed by any codes for the complications.

When a patient is admitted for the purpose of insertion or implantation of radioactive elements (e.g., brachytherapy) and develops complications such as uncontrolled nausea and vomiting or dehydration, the principal or first-listed diagnosis is the appropriate code for the malignancy followed by any codes for the complications.

f. Admission/encounter to determine extent of malignancy

When the reason for admission/encounter is to determine the extent of the malignancy, or for a procedure such as paracentesis or thoracentesis, the primary malignancy or appropriate metastatic site is designated as the principal or first-listed diagnosis, even though chemotherapy or radiotherapy is administered.

g. Symptoms, signs, and abnormal findings listed in Chapter 18 associated with neoplasms

Symptoms, signs, and ill-defined conditions listed in Chapter 18 characteristic of, or associated with, an existing primary or secondary site malignancy cannot be used to replace the malignancy as principal or first-listed diagnosis, regardless of the number of admissions or encounters for treatment and care of the neoplasm.

See section I.C.21. Factors influencing health status and contact with health services, Encounter for prophylactic organ removal.

h. Admission/encounter for pain control/management

See Section I.C.6. for information on coding admission/encounter for pain control/management.

i. Malignancy in two or more noncontiguous sites

A patient may have more than one malignant tumor in the same organ. These tumors may represent different primaries or metastatic disease, depending on the site. Should the documentation be unclear, the provider should be queried as to the status of each tumor so that the correct codes can be assigned.

j. Disseminated malignant neoplasm, unspecified

Code C80.0, Disseminated malignant neoplasm, unspecified, is for use only in those cases where the patient has advanced metastatic disease and no known primary or secondary sites are specified. It should not be used in place of assigning codes for the primary site and all known secondary sites.

k. Malignant neoplasm without specification of site

Code C80.1, Malignant (primary) neoplasm, unspecified, equates to Cancer, unspecified. This code should only be used when no determination can be made as to the primary site of a malignancy. This code should rarely be used in the inpatient setting.

l. Sequencing of neoplasm codes

1) Encounter for treatment of primary malignancy

If the reason for the encounter is for treatment of a primary malignancy, assign the malignancy as the principal/first-listed diagnosis. The primary site is to be sequenced first, followed by any metastatic sites.

2) Encounter for treatment of secondary malignancy

When an encounter is for a primary malignancy with metastasis and treatment is directed toward the metastatic (secondary) site(s) only, the metastatic site(s) is designated as the principal/first-listed diagnosis. The primary malignancy is coded as an additional code.

3) Malignant neoplasm in a pregnant patient

When a pregnant woman has a malignant neoplasm, a code from subcategory O9A.1-, Malignant neoplasm complicating pregnancy, childbirth, and the puerperium, should be sequenced first, followed by the appropriate code from Chapter 2 to indicate the type of neoplasm.

4) Encounter for complication associated with a neoplasm

When an encounter is for management of a complication associated with a neoplasm, such as dehydration, and the treatment is only for the complication, the complication is coded first, followed by the appropriate code(s) for the neoplasm.

The exception to this guideline is anemia. When the admission/encounter is for management of an anemia associated with the malignancy, and the treatment is only for anemia, the appropriate code for the malignancy is sequenced as the principal or first-listed diagnosis followed by code D63.0, Anemia in neoplastic disease.

5) Complication from surgical procedure for treatment of a neoplasm

When an encounter is for treatment of a complication resulting from a surgical procedure performed for the treatment of the neoplasm, designate the complication as the principal/first-listed diagnosis. See the guideline regarding the coding of a current malignancy versus personal history to determine if the code for the neoplasm should also be assigned.

6) Pathologic fracture due to a neoplasm

When an encounter is for a pathological fracture due to a neoplasm, and the focus of treatment is the fracture, a code from subcategory M84.5, Pathological fracture in neoplastic disease, should be sequenced first, followed by the code for the neoplasm.

If the focus of treatment is the neoplasm with an associated pathological fracture, the neoplasm code should be sequenced first, followed by a code from M84.5 for the pathological fracture.

m. Current malignancy versus personal history of malignancy

When a primary malignancy has been excised but further treatment, such as an additional surgery for the malignancy, radiation therapy or chemotherapy is directed to that site, the primary malignancy code should be used until treatment is completed.

When a primary malignancy has been previously excised or eradicated from its site, there is no further treatment (of the malignancy) directed to that site, and there is no evidence of any existing primary malignancy at that site, a code from category Z85, Personal history of malignant neoplasm, should be used to indicate the former site of the malignancy.

Subcategories Z85.0 - Z85.7 should only be assigned for the former site of a primary malignancy, not the site of a secondary malignancy. Codes from subcategory Z85.8-, may be assigned for the former site(s) of either a primary or secondary malignancy included in this subcategory.

See Section I.C.21. Factors influencing health status and contact with health services, History (of)

n. Leukemia, Multiple Myeloma, and Malignant Plasma Cell Neoplasms in remission versus personal history

The categories for leukemia, and category C90, Multiple myeloma and malignant plasma cell neoplasms, have codes indicating whether or not the leukemia has achieved remission. There are also codes Z85.6, Personal history of leukemia, and Z85.79, Personal history of other malignant neoplasms of lymphoid, hematopoietic and related tissues. If the documentation is unclear, as to whether the leukemia has achieved remission, the provider should be queried.

See Section I.C.21. Factors influencing health status and contact with health services, History (of)

o. Aftercare following surgery for neoplasm

See Section I.C.21. Factors influencing health status and contact with health services, Aftercare

p. Follow-up care for completed treatment of a malignancy

See Section I.C.21. Factors influencing health status and contact with health services, Follow-up

q. Prophylactic organ removal for prevention of malignancy

See Section I.C. 21, Factors influencing health status and contact with health services, Prophylactic organ removal

r. Malignant neoplasm associated with transplanted organ

A malignant neoplasm of a transplanted organ should be coded as a transplant complication. Assign first the appropriate code from category T86.-, Complications of transplanted organs and tissue, followed by code C80.2, Malignant neoplasm associated with transplanted organ. Use an additional code for the specific malignancy.

Tumor Biology and Chemotherapy

Tumor heterogeneity

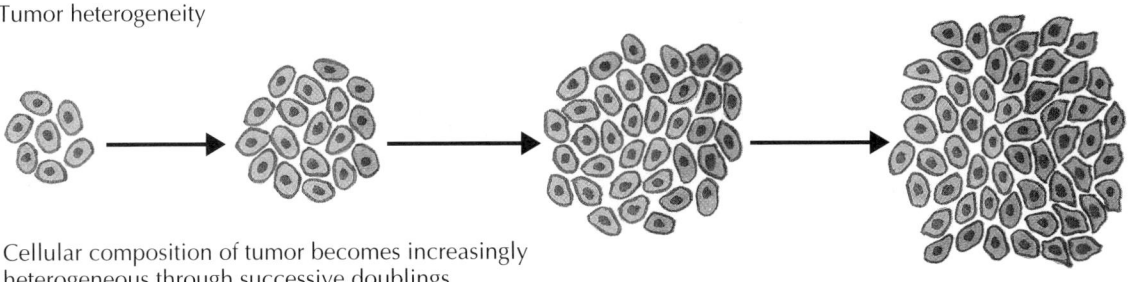

Cellular composition of tumor becomes increasingly heterogeneous through successive doublings

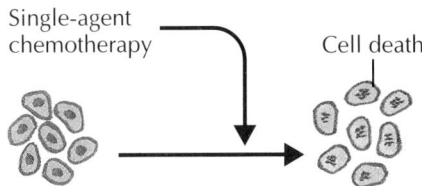

Single-agent chemotherapy

Cell death

Single-agent chemotherapy *may* be successful in susceptible homogeneous tumors

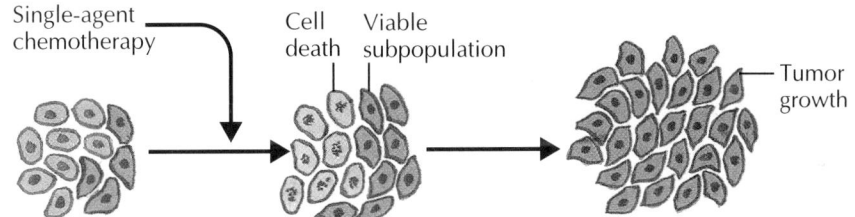

Single-agent chemotherapy

Cell death

Viable subpopulation

Tumor growth

Single-agent chemotherapy for heterogeneous tumors may result only in death of susceptible cell line, selecting nonresponsive cells for growth and spread

JOHN A.CRAIG_AD

Radiograph of lungs after multiple-agent chemotherapy

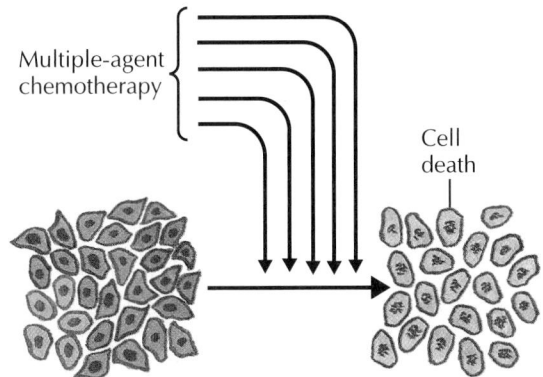

Multiple-agent chemotherapy

Cell death

Multiple-agent chemotherapy affects subpopulations of heterogeneous tumors

Chapter 2: Neoplasms

499

Malignant neoplasms (C00-C96)

Malignant neoplasms, stated or presumed to be primary (of specified sites), and certain specified histologies, except neuroendocrine, and of lymphoid, hematopoietic and related tissue (C00-C75)

Malignant neoplasms of lip, oral cavity and pharynx (C00-C14)

C00 Malignant neoplasm of lip

Use additional code to identify:
alcohol abuse and dependence (F10.-)
history of tobacco dependence (Z87.891)
tobacco dependence (F17.-)
tobacco use (Z72.0)
Excludes1: *malignant melanoma of lip (C43.0)*
Merkel cell carcinoma of lip (C4A.0)
other and unspecified malignant neoplasm of skin of lip (C44.0-)

C00.0 Malignant neoplasm of external upper lip
Malignant neoplasm of lipstick area of upper lip
Malignant neoplasm of upper lip NOS
Malignant neoplasm of vermilion border of upper lip

C00.1 Malignant neoplasm of external lower lip
Malignant neoplasm of lower lip NOS
Malignant neoplasm of lipstick area of lower lip
Malignant neoplasm of vermilion border of lower lip

C00.2 Malignant neoplasm of external lip, unspecified
Malignant neoplasm of vermilion border of lip NOS

C00.3 Malignant neoplasm of upper lip, inner aspect
Malignant neoplasm of buccal aspect of upper lip
Malignant neoplasm of frenulum of upper lip
Malignant neoplasm of mucosa of upper lip
Malignant neoplasm of oral aspect of upper lip

C00.4 Malignant neoplasm of lower lip, inner aspect
Malignant neoplasm of buccal aspect of lower lip
Malignant neoplasm of frenulum of lower lip
Malignant neoplasm of mucosa of lower lip
Malignant neoplasm of oral aspect of lower lip

C00.5 Malignant neoplasm of lip, unspecified, inner aspect
Malignant neoplasm of buccal aspect of lip, unspecified
Malignant neoplasm of frenulum of lip, unspecified
Malignant neoplasm of mucosa of lip, unspecified
Malignant neoplasm of oral aspect of lip, unspecified

C00.6 Malignant neoplasm of commissure of lip, unspecified

C00.8 Malignant neoplasm of overlapping sites of lip

C00.9 Malignant neoplasm of lip, unspecified

C01 Malignant neoplasm of base of tongue

Malignant neoplasm of dorsal surface of base of tongue
Malignant neoplasm of fixed part of tongue NOS
Malignant neoplasm of posterior third of tongue
Use additional code to identify:
alcohol abuse and dependence (F10.-)
history of tobacco dependence (Z87.891)
tobacco dependence (F17.-)
tobacco use (Z72.0)
Valid 3-character code, no further characters required

C02 Malignant neoplasm of other and unspecified parts of tongue

Use additional code to identify:
alcohol abuse and dependence (F10.-)
history of tobacco dependence (Z87.891)
tobacco dependence (F17.-)
tobacco use (Z72.0)

C02.0 Malignant neoplasm of dorsal surface of tongue
Malignant neoplasm of anterior two-thirds of tongue, dorsal surface
Excludes2: *malignant neoplasm of dorsal surface of base of tongue (C01)*

C02.1 Malignant neoplasm of border of tongue
Malignant neoplasm of tip of tongue

C02.2 Malignant neoplasm of ventral surface of tongue
Malignant neoplasm of anterior two-thirds of tongue, ventral surface
Malignant neoplasm of frenulum linguae

C02.3 Malignant neoplasm of anterior two-thirds of tongue, part unspecified
Malignant neoplasm of middle third of tongue NOS
Malignant neoplasm of mobile part of tongue NOS

C02.4 Malignant neoplasm of lingual tonsil
Excludes2: *malignant neoplasm of tonsil NOS (C09.9)*

C02.8 Malignant neoplasm of overlapping sites of tongue
Malignant neoplasm of two or more contiguous sites of tongue

C02.9 Malignant neoplasm of tongue, unspecified

C03 Malignant neoplasm of gum

Includes: malignant neoplasm of alveolar (ridge) mucosa
malignant neoplasm of gingiva
Use additional code to identify:
alcohol abuse and dependence (F10.-)
history of tobacco dependence (Z87.891)
tobacco dependence (F17.-)
tobacco use (Z72.0)
Excludes2: *malignant odontogenic neoplasms (C41.0-C41.1)*

C03.0 Malignant neoplasm of upper gum

C03.1 Malignant neoplasm of lower gum

C03.9 Malignant neoplasm of gum, unspecified

C04 Malignant neoplasm of floor of mouth

Use additional code to identify:
alcohol abuse and dependence (F10.-)
history of tobacco dependence (Z87.891)
tobacco dependence (F17.-)
tobacco use (Z72.0)

C04.0 Malignant neoplasm of anterior floor of mouth
Malignant neoplasm of anterior to the premolar-canine junction

C04.1 Malignant neoplasm of lateral floor of mouth

C04.8 Malignant neoplasm of overlapping sites of floor of mouth

C04.9 Malignant neoplasm of floor of mouth, unspecified

C05 Malignant neoplasm of palate

Use additional code to identify:
alcohol abuse and dependence (F10.-)
history of tobacco dependence (Z87.891)
tobacco dependence (F17.-)
tobacco use (Z72.0)
Excludes1: *Kaposi's sarcoma of palate (C46.2)*

C05.0 Malignant neoplasm of hard palate

C05.1 Malignant neoplasm of soft palate
Excludes2: *malignant neoplasm of nasopharyngeal surface of soft palate (C11.3)*

C05.2 Malignant neoplasm of uvula

C05.8 Malignant neoplasm of overlapping sites of palate

C05.9 Malignant neoplasm of palate, unspecified
Malignant neoplasm of roof of mouth

C06 Malignant neoplasm of other and unspecified parts of mouth

Use additional code to identify:
alcohol abuse and dependence (F10.-)
history of tobacco dependence (Z87.891)
tobacco dependence (F17.-)
tobacco use (Z72.0)

C06.0 Malignant neoplasm of cheek mucosa
Malignant neoplasm of buccal mucosa NOS
Malignant neoplasm of internal cheek

C06.1 Malignant neoplasm of vestibule of mouth
Malignant neoplasm of buccal sulcus (upper) (lower)
Malignant neoplasm of labial sulcus (upper) (lower)

C06.2 Malignant neoplasm of retromolar area

+ **C06.8 Malignant neoplasm of overlapping sites of other and unspecified parts of mouth**

C06.80 Malignant neoplasm of overlapping sites of unspecified parts of mouth

C06.89 Malignant neoplasm of overlapping sites of other parts of mouth
'book leaf' neoplasm [ventral surface of tongue and floor of mouth]

C06.9 Malignant neoplasm of mouth, unspecified
Malignant neoplasm of minor salivary gland, unspecified site
Malignant neoplasm of oral cavity NOS

C07 Malignant neoplasm of parotid gland

Use additional code to identify:
alcohol abuse and dependence (F10.-)
exposure to environmental tobacco smoke (Z77.22)
exposure to tobacco smoke in the perinatal period (P96.81)
history of tobacco dependence (Z87.891)
occupational exposure to environmental tobacco smoke (Z57.31)
tobacco dependence (F17.-)
tobacco use (Z72.0)

Valid 3-character code, no further characters required

C08 Malignant neoplasm of other and unspecified major salivary glands

Includes: malignant neoplasm of salivary ducts

Use additional code to identify:
alcohol abuse and dependence (F10.-)
exposure to environmental tobacco smoke (Z77.22)
exposure to tobacco smoke in the perinatal period (P96.81)
history of tobacco dependence (Z87.891)
occupational exposure to environmental tobacco smoke (Z57.31)
tobacco dependence (F17.-)
tobacco use (Z72.0)

Excludes1: *malignant neoplasms of specified minor salivary glands which are classified according to their anatomical location*

Excludes2: *malignant neoplasms of minor salivary glands NOS (C06.9)*
malignant neoplasm of parotid gland (C07)

C08.0 Malignant neoplasm of submandibular gland
Malignant neoplasm of submaxillary gland

C08.1 Malignant neoplasm of sublingual gland

C08.9 Malignant neoplasm of major salivary gland, unspecified
Malignant neoplasm of salivary gland (major) NOS

C09 Malignant neoplasm of tonsil

Use additional code to identify:
alcohol abuse and dependence (F10.-)
exposure to environmental tobacco smoke (Z77.22)
exposure to tobacco smoke in the perinatal period (P96.81)
history of tobacco dependence (Z87.891)
occupational exposure to environmental tobacco smoke (Z57.31)
tobacco dependence (F17.-)
tobacco use (Z72.0)

Excludes2: *malignant neoplasm of lingual tonsil (C02.4)*
malignant neoplasm of pharyngeal tonsil (C11.1)

C09.0 Malignant neoplasm of tonsillar fossa

C09.1 Malignant neoplasm of tonsillar pillar (anterior) (posterior)

C09.8 Malignant neoplasm of overlapping sites of tonsil

C09.9 Malignant neoplasm of tonsil, unspecified
Malignant neoplasm of tonsil NOS
Malignant neoplasm of faucial tonsils
Malignant neoplasm of palatine tonsils

C10 Malignant neoplasm of oropharynx

Use additional code to identify:
alcohol abuse and dependence (F10.-)
exposure to environmental tobacco smoke (Z77.22)
exposure to tobacco smoke in the perinatal period (P96.81)
history of tobacco dependence (Z87.891)
occupational exposure to environmental tobacco smoke (Z57.31)
tobacco dependence (F17.-)
tobacco use (Z72.0)

Excludes2: *malignant neoplasm of tonsil (C09.-)*

C10.0 Malignant neoplasm of vallecula

C10.1 Malignant neoplasm of anterior surface of epiglottis
Malignant neoplasm of epiglottis, free border [margin]
Malignant neoplasm of glossoepiglottic fold(s)
Excludes2: *malignant neoplasm of epiglottis (suprahyoid portion) NOS (C32.1)*

C10.2 Malignant neoplasm of lateral wall of oropharynx

C10.3 Malignant neoplasm of posterior wall of oropharynx

C10.4 Malignant neoplasm of branchial cleft
Malignant neoplasm of branchial cyst [site of neoplasm]

C10.8 Malignant neoplasm of overlapping sites of oropharynx
Malignant neoplasm of junctional region of oropharynx

C10.9 Malignant neoplasm of oropharynx, unspecified

C11 Malignant neoplasm of nasopharynx

Use additional code to identify:
exposure to environmental tobacco smoke (Z77.22)
exposure to tobacco smoke in the perinatal period (P96.81)
history of tobacco dependence (Z87.891)
occupational exposure to environmental tobacco smoke (Z57.31)
tobacco dependence (F17.-)
tobacco use (Z72.0)

C11.0 Malignant neoplasm of superior wall of nasopharynx
Malignant neoplasm of roof of nasopharynx

C11.1 Malignant neoplasm of posterior wall of nasopharynx
Malignant neoplasm of adenoid
Malignant neoplasm of pharyngeal tonsil

C11.2 Malignant neoplasm of lateral wall of nasopharynx
Malignant neoplasm of fossa of Rosenmüller
Malignant neoplasm of opening of auditory tube
Malignant neoplasm of pharyngeal recess

C11.3 Malignant neoplasm of anterior wall of nasopharynx
Malignant neoplasm of floor of nasopharynx
Malignant neoplasm of nasopharyngeal (anterior) (posterior) surface of soft palate
Malignant neoplasm of posterior margin of nasal choana
Malignant neoplasm of posterior margin of nasal septum

C11.8 Malignant neoplasm of overlapping sites of nasopharynx

C11.9 Malignant neoplasm of nasopharynx, unspecified
Malignant neoplasm of nasopharyngeal wall NOS

C12 Malignant neoplasm of pyriform sinus

Malignant neoplasm of pyriform fossa
Use additional code to identify:
exposure to environmental tobacco smoke (Z77.22)
exposure to tobacco smoke in the perinatal period (P96.81)
history of tobacco dependence (Z87.891)
occupational exposure to environmental tobacco smoke (Z57.31)
tobacco dependence (F17.-)
tobacco use (Z72.0)

Valid 3-character code, no further characters required

C13 Malignant neoplasm of hypopharynx

Use additional code to identify:
exposure to environmental tobacco smoke (Z77.22)
exposure to tobacco smoke in the perinatal period (P96.81)
history of tobacco dependence (Z87.891)
occupational exposure to environmental tobacco smoke (Z57.31)
tobacco dependence (F17.-)
tobacco use (Z72.0)

Excludes2: *malignant neoplasm of pyriform sinus (C12)*

C13.0 Malignant neoplasm of postcricoid region

C13.1 Malignant neoplasm of aryepiglottic fold, hypopharyngeal aspect
Malignant neoplasm of aryepiglottic fold NOS
Malignant neoplasm of interarytenoid fold NOS
Malignant neoplasm of aryepiglottic fold, marginal zone
Malignant neoplasm of interarytenoid fold, marginal zone
Excludes2: *malignant neoplasm of aryepiglottic fold or interarytenoid fold, laryngeal aspect (C32.1)*

C13.2 Malignant neoplasm of posterior wall of hypopharynx

C13.8 Malignant neoplasm of overlapping sites of hypopharynx

C13.9 Malignant neoplasm of hypopharynx, unspecified
Malignant neoplasm of hypopharyngeal wall NOS

C14 Malignant neoplasm of other and ill-defined sites in the lip, oral cavity and pharynx

Use additional code to identify:
alcohol abuse and dependence (F10.-)
exposure to environmental tobacco smoke (Z77.22)
exposure to tobacco smoke in the perinatal period (P96.81)
history of tobacco dependence (Z87.891)
occupational exposure to environmental tobacco smoke (Z57.31)
tobacco dependence (F17.-)
tobacco use (Z72.0)

Excludes1: *malignant neoplasm of oral cavity NOS (C06.9)*

C14.0 Malignant neoplasm of pharynx, unspecified

C14.2 Malignant neoplasm of Waldeyer's ring

C14.8 Malignant neoplasm of overlapping sites of lip, oral cavity and pharynx
Primary malignant neoplasm of two or more contiguous sites of lip, oral cavity and pharynx
Excludes1: *'book leaf' neoplasm [ventral surface of tongue and floor of mouth] (C06.89)*

Malignant neoplasms of digestive organs (C15-C26)

Excludes1: Kaposi's sarcoma of gastrointestinal sites (C46.4)

Excludes2: gastrointestinal stromal tumors (C49.A-)

C15 Malignant neoplasm of esophagus

Use additional code to identify:
alcohol abuse and dependence (F10.-)

CC **C15.3 Malignant neoplasm of upper third of esophagus**
CC **C15.4 Malignant neoplasm of middle third of esophagus**
CC **C15.5 Malignant neoplasm of lower third of esophagus**
Excludes1: malignant neoplasm of cardio-esophageal junction (C16.0)
CC **C15.8 Malignant neoplasm of overlapping sites of esophagus**
CC **C15.9 Malignant neoplasm of esophagus, unspecified**

C16 Malignant neoplasm of stomach

Use additional code to identify:
alcohol abuse and dependence (F10.-)

Excludes2: malignant carcinoid tumor of the stomach (C7A.092)

CC **C16.0 Malignant neoplasm of cardia**
Malignant neoplasm of cardiac orifice
Malignant neoplasm of cardio-esophageal junction
Malignant neoplasm of esophagus and stomach
Malignant neoplasm of gastro-esophageal junction
CC **C16.1 Malignant neoplasm of fundus of stomach**
CC **C16.2 Malignant neoplasm of body of stomach**
CC **C16.3 Malignant neoplasm of pyloric antrum**
Malignant neoplasm of gastric antrum
CC **C16.4 Malignant neoplasm of pylorus**
Malignant neoplasm of prepylorus
Malignant neoplasm of pyloric canal
CC **C16.5 Malignant neoplasm of lesser curvature of stomach, unspecified**
Malignant neoplasm of lesser curvature of stomach, not classifiable to C16.1-C16.4
CC **C16.6 Malignant neoplasm of greater curvature of stomach, unspecified**
Malignant neoplasm of greater curvature of stomach, not classifiable to C16.0-C16.4
CC **C16.8 Malignant neoplasm of overlapping sites of stomach**
CC **C16.9 Malignant neoplasm of stomach, unspecified**
Gastric cancer NOS

C17 Malignant neoplasm of small intestine

Excludes1: malignant carcinoid tumors of the small intestine (C7A.01)

CC **C17.0 Malignant neoplasm of duodenum**
CC **C17.1 Malignant neoplasm of jejunum**
CC **C17.2 Malignant neoplasm of ileum**
Excludes1: malignant neoplasm of ileocecal valve (C18.0)
CC **C17.3 Meckel's diverticulum, malignant**
Excludes1: Meckel's diverticulum, congenital (Q43.0)
CC **C17.8 Malignant neoplasm of overlapping sites of small intestine**
CC **C17.9 Malignant neoplasm of small intestine, unspecified**

C18 Malignant neoplasm of colon

Excludes1: malignant carcinoid tumors of the colon (C7A.02-)

CC **C18.0 Malignant neoplasm of cecum**
Malignant neoplasm of ileocecal valve
CC **C18.1 Malignant neoplasm of appendix**
CC **C18.2 Malignant neoplasm of ascending colon**
CC **C18.3 Malignant neoplasm of hepatic flexure**
CC **C18.4 Malignant neoplasm of transverse colon**
CC **C18.5 Malignant neoplasm of splenic flexure**
CC **C18.6 Malignant neoplasm of descending colon**
CC **C18.7 Malignant neoplasm of sigmoid colon**
Malignant neoplasm of sigmoid (flexure)
Excludes1: malignant neoplasm of rectosigmoid junction (C19)
CC **C18.8 Malignant neoplasm of overlapping sites of colon**
CC **C18.9 Malignant neoplasm of colon, unspecified**
Malignant neoplasm of large intestine NOS

CC **C19 Malignant neoplasm of rectosigmoid junction**

Malignant neoplasm of colon with rectum
Malignant neoplasm of rectosigmoid (colon)
Excludes1: malignant carcinoid tumors of the colon (C7A.02-)
Valid 3-character code, no further characters required

CC **C20 Malignant neoplasm of rectum**

Malignant neoplasm of rectal ampulla
Excludes1: malignant carcinoid tumor of the rectum (C7A.026)
Valid 3-character code, no further characters required

CC **C21 Malignant neoplasm of anus and anal canal**

Excludes2: malignant carcinoid tumors of the colon (C7A.02-)
malignant melanoma of anal margin (C43.51)
malignant melanoma of anal skin (C43.51)
malignant melanoma of perianal skin (C43.51)
other and unspecified malignant neoplasm of anal margin (C44.500, C44.510, C44.520, C44.590)
other and unspecified malignant neoplasm of anal skin (C44.500, C44.510, C44.520, C44.590)
other and unspecified malignant neoplasm of perianal skin (C44.500, C44.510, C44.520, C44.590)

CC **C21.0 Malignant neoplasm of anus, unspecified**
CC **C21.1 Malignant neoplasm of anal canal**
Malignant neoplasm of anal sphincter
CC **C21.2 Malignant neoplasm of cloacogenic zone**
CC **C21.8 Malignant neoplasm of overlapping sites of rectum, anus and anal canal**
Malignant neoplasm of anorectal junction
Malignant neoplasm of anorectum
Primary malignant neoplasm of two or more contiguous sites of rectum, anus and anal canal

C22 Malignant neoplasm of liver and intrahepatic bile ducts

Excludes1: malignant neoplasm of biliary tract NOS (C24.9)
secondary malignant neoplasm of liver and intrahepatic bile duct (C78.7)

Use additional code to identify:
alcohol abuse and dependence (F10.-)
hepatitis B (B16.-, B18.0-B18.1)
hepatitis C (B17.1-, B18.2)

CC **C22.0 Liver cell carcinoma**
Hepatocellular carcinoma
Hepatoma
AHA CC: 1Q, 2016, 18-19
CC **C22.1 Intrahepatic bile duct carcinoma**
Cholangiocarcinoma
Excludes1: malignant neoplasm of hepatic duct (C24.0)
CC **C22.2 Hepatoblastoma**
CC **C22.3 Angiosarcoma of liver**
Kupffer cell sarcoma
CC **C22.4 Other sarcomas of liver**
CC **C22.7 Other specified carcinomas of liver**
CC **C22.8 Malignant neoplasm of liver, primary, unspecified as to type**
CC **C22.9 Malignant neoplasm of liver, not specified as primary or secondary**

CC **C23 Malignant neoplasm of gallbladder**

Valid 3-character code, no further characters required

C24 Malignant neoplasm of other and unspecified parts of biliary tract

Excludes1: malignant neoplasm of intrahepatic bile duct (C22.1)
CC **C24.0 Malignant neoplasm of extrahepatic bile duct**
Malignant neoplasm of biliary duct or passage NOS
Malignant neoplasm of common bile duct
Malignant neoplasm of cystic duct
Malignant neoplasm of hepatic duct
CC **C24.1 Malignant neoplasm of ampulla of Vater**
CC **C24.8 Malignant neoplasm of overlapping sites of biliary tract**
Malignant neoplasm involving both intrahepatic and extrahepatic bile ducts
Primary malignant neoplasm of two or more contiguous sites of biliary tract
CC **C24.9 Malignant neoplasm of biliary tract, unspecified**

C25 Malignant neoplasm of pancreas

Code also exocrine pancreatic insufficiency (K86.81)

Use additional code to identify:
alcohol abuse and dependence (F10.-)

CC **C25.0 Malignant neoplasm of head of pancreas**
CC **C25.1 Malignant neoplasm of body of pancreas**
AHA CC: 4Q, 2018, 40
CC **C25.2 Malignant neoplasm of tail of pancreas**
CC **C25.3 Malignant neoplasm of pancreatic duct**
CC **C25.4 Malignant neoplasm of endocrine pancreas**
Malignant neoplasm of islets of Langerhans
Use additional code to identify any functional activity.

+, +7th, X + 7th • Newborn • Pediatric • Maternity • Adult ♀ Female ♂ Male Manifestation Unacceptable PDX HCC CC MCC HAC

CC C25.7 Malignant neoplasm of other parts of pancreas
Malignant neoplasm of neck of pancreas
CC C25.8 Malignant neoplasm of overlapping sites of pancreas
CC C25.9 Malignant neoplasm of pancreas, unspecified
C26 Malignant neoplasm of other and ill-defined digestive organs

> *Excludes1:* *malignant neoplasm of peritoneum and retroperitoneum (C48.-)*

C26.0 Malignant neoplasm of intestinal tract, part unspecified
Malignant neoplasm of intestine NOS
C26.1 Malignant neoplasm of spleen

> *Excludes1:* *Hodgkin lymphoma (C81.-)*
> *non-Hodgkin lymphoma (C82-C85)*

C26.9 Malignant neoplasm of ill-defined sites within the digestive system
Malignant neoplasm of alimentary canal or tract NOS
Malignant neoplasm of gastrointestinal tract NOS

> *Excludes1:* *malignant neoplasm of abdominal NOS (C76.2)*
> *malignant neoplasm of intra-abdominal NOS (C76.2)*

Malignant neoplasms of respiratory and intrathoracic organs (C30-C39)

Includes: malignant neoplasm of middle ear

Excludes1: *mesothelioma (C45.-)*

C30 Malignant neoplasm of nasal cavity and middle ear

C30.0 Malignant neoplasm of nasal cavity
Malignant neoplasm of cartilage of nose
Malignant neoplasm of nasal concha
Malignant neoplasm of internal nose
Malignant neoplasm of septum of nose
Malignant neoplasm of vestibule of nose

> *Excludes1:* *malignant neoplasm of nasal bone (C41.0)*
> *malignant neoplasm of nose NOS (C76.0)*
> *malignant neoplasm of olfactory bulb (C72.2-)*
> *malignant neoplasm of posterior margin of nasal septum and choana (C11.3)*
> *malignant melanoma of skin of nose (C43.31)*
> *malignant neoplasm of turbinates (C41.0)*
> *other and unspecified malignant neoplasm of skin of nose C44.301, C44.311, C44.321, C44.391)*

C30.1 Malignant neoplasm of middle ear
Malignant neoplasm of antrum tympanicum
Malignant neoplasm of auditory tube
Malignant neoplasm of eustachian tube
Malignant neoplasm of inner ear
Malignant neoplasm of mastoid air cells
Malignant neoplasm of tympanic cavity

> *Excludes1:* *malignant neoplasm of auricular canal (external) (C43.2-,C44.2-)*
> *malignant neoplasm of bone of ear (meatus) (C41.0)*
> *malignant neoplasm of cartilage of ear (C49.0)*
> *malignant melanoma of skin of (external) ear (C43.2-)*
> *other and unspecified malignant neoplasm of skin of (external) ear (C44.2-)*

C31 Malignant neoplasm of accessory sinuses

C31.0 Malignant neoplasm of maxillary sinus
Malignant neoplasm of antrum (Highmore) (maxillary)
C31.1 Malignant neoplasm of ethmoidal sinus
C31.2 Malignant neoplasm of frontal sinus
C31.3 Malignant neoplasm of sphenoid sinus
C31.8 Malignant neoplasm of overlapping sites of accessory sinuses
C31.9 Malignant neoplasm of accessory sinus, unspecified

C32 Malignant neoplasm of larynx

Use additional code to identify:
alcohol abuse and dependence (F10.-)
exposure to environmental tobacco smoke (Z77.22)
exposure to tobacco smoke in the perinatal period (P96.81)
history of tobacco dependence (Z87.891)
occupational exposure to environmental tobacco smoke (Z57.31)
tobacco dependence (F17.-)
tobacco use (Z72.0)

C32.0 Malignant neoplasm of glottis
Malignant neoplasm of intrinsic larynx
Malignant neoplasm of laryngeal commissure (anterior) (posterior)
Malignant neoplasm of vocal cord (true) NOS
C32.1 Malignant neoplasm of supraglottis
Malignant neoplasm of aryepiglottic fold or interarytenoid fold, laryngeal aspect
Malignant neoplasm of epiglottis (suprahyoid portion) NOS
Malignant neoplasm of extrinsic larynx
Malignant neoplasm of false vocal cord
Malignant neoplasm of posterior (laryngeal) surface of epiglottis
Malignant neoplasm of ventricular bands

> *Excludes2:* *malignant neoplasm of anterior surface of epiglottis (C10.1)*
> *malignant neoplasm of aryepiglottic fold or interarytenoid fold, hypopharyngeal aspect (C13.1)*
> *malignant neoplasm of aryepiglottic fold or interarytenoid fold, marginal zone (C13.1)*
> *malignant neoplasm of aryepiglottic fold or interarytenoid fold NOS (C13.1)*

C32.2 Malignant neoplasm of subglottis
C32.3 Malignant neoplasm of laryngeal cartilage
C32.8 Malignant neoplasm of overlapping sites of larynx
C32.9 Malignant neoplasm of larynx, unspecified

CC C33 Malignant neoplasm of trachea

Use additional code to identify:
exposure to environmental tobacco smoke (Z77.22)
exposure to tobacco smoke in the perinatal period (P96.81)
history of tobacco dependence (Z87.891)
occupational exposure to environmental tobacco smoke (Z57.31)
tobacco dependence (F17.-)
tobacco use (Z72.0)

Valid 3-character code, no further characters required

Lungs

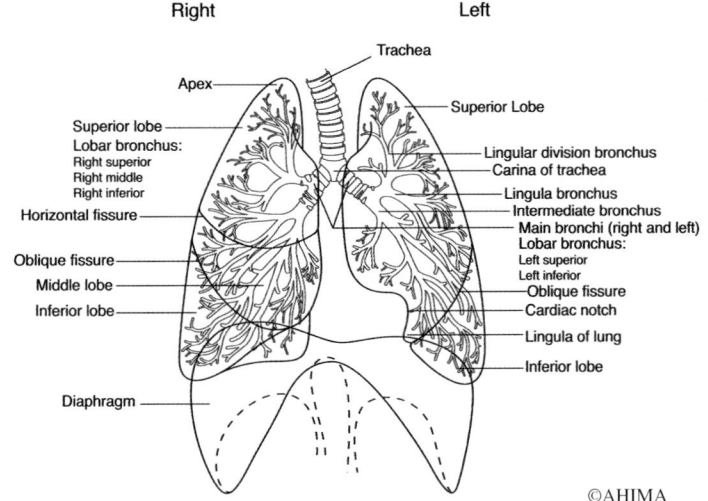

©AHIMA

C34 Malignant neoplasm of bronchus and lung

Use additional code to identify:
    exposure to environmental tobacco smoke (Z77.22)
    exposure to tobacco smoke in the perinatal period (P96.81)
    history of tobacco dependence (Z87.891)
    occupational exposure to environmental tobacco smoke (Z57.31)
    tobacco dependence (F17.-)
    tobacco use (Z72.0)
Excludes1: Kaposi's sarcoma of lung (C46.5-)
        malignant carcinoid tumor of the bronchus and lung
        (C7A.090)

+ **C34.0 Malignant neoplasm of main bronchus**
    Malignant neoplasm of carina
    Malignant neoplasm of hilus (of lung)
    CC **C34.00 Malignant neoplasm of unspecified main bronchus**
    CC **C34.01 Malignant neoplasm of right main bronchus**
    CC **C34.02 Malignant neoplasm of left main bronchus**
+ **C34.1 Malignant neoplasm of upper lobe, bronchus or lung**
    CC **C34.10 Malignant neoplasm of upper lobe, unspecified bronchus or lung**
    CC **C34.11 Malignant neoplasm of upper lobe, right bronchus or lung**
    CC **C34.12 Malignant neoplasm of upper lobe, left bronchus or lung**
CC **C34.2 Malignant neoplasm of middle lobe, bronchus or lung**
+ **C34.3 Malignant neoplasm of lower lobe, bronchus or lung**
    CC **C34.30 Malignant neoplasm of lower lobe, unspecified bronchus or lung**
    CC **C34.31 Malignant neoplasm of lower lobe, right bronchus or lung**
    CC **C34.32 Malignant neoplasm of lower lobe, left bronchus or lung**
+ **C34.8 Malignant neoplasm of overlapping sites of bronchus and lung**
    CC **C34.80 Malignant neoplasm of overlapping sites of unspecified bronchus and lung**
    CC **C34.81 Malignant neoplasm of overlapping sites of right bronchus and lung**
    CC **C34.82 Malignant neoplasm of overlapping sites of left bronchus and lung**
+ **C34.9 Malignant neoplasm of unspecified part of bronchus or lung**
    CC **C34.90 Malignant neoplasm of unspecified part of unspecified bronchus or lung**
        Lung cancer NOS
        AHA CC. 2Q, 2014, 10
    CC **C34.91 Malignant neoplasm of unspecified part of right bronchus or lung**
    CC **C34.92 Malignant neoplasm of unspecified part of left bronchus or lung**

CC **C37 Malignant neoplasm of thymus**

Excludes1: malignant carcinoid tumor of the thymus (C7A.091)
    Valid 3-character code, no further characters required

C38 Malignant neoplasm of heart, mediastinum and pleura

Excludes1: mesothelioma (C45.-)
CC **C38.0 Malignant neoplasm of heart**
    Malignant neoplasm of pericardium
    Excludes1: malignant neoplasm of great vessels (C49.3)
CC **C38.1 Malignant neoplasm of anterior mediastinum**
CC **C38.2 Malignant neoplasm of posterior mediastinum**
CC **C38.3 Malignant neoplasm of mediastinum, part unspecified**
CC **C38.4 Malignant neoplasm of pleura**
CC **C38.8 Malignant neoplasm of overlapping sites of heart, mediastinum and pleura**

C39 Malignant neoplasm of other and ill-defined sites in the respiratory system and intrathoracic organs

Use additional code to identify:
    exposure to environmental tobacco smoke (Z77.22)
    exposure to tobacco smoke in the perinatal period (P96.81)
    history of tobacco dependence (Z87.891)
    occupational exposure to environmental tobacco smoke (Z57.31)
    tobacco dependence (F17.-)
    tobacco use (Z72.0)
Excludes1: intrathoracic malignant neoplasm NOS (C76.1)
        thoracic malignant neoplasm NOS (C76.1)

C39.0 Malignant neoplasm of upper respiratory tract, part unspecified

C39.9 Malignant neoplasm of lower respiratory tract, part unspecified
    Malignant neoplasm of respiratory tract NOS

Malignant neoplasms of bone and articular cartilage (C40-C41)

Includes: malignant neoplasm of cartilage (articular) (joint)
    malignant neoplasm of periosteum

Excludes1: malignant neoplasm of bone marrow NOS (C96.9)
    malignant neoplasm of synovia (C49.-)

C40 Malignant neoplasm of bone and articular cartilage of limbs

Use additional code to identify major osseous defect, if applicable (M89.7-)

+ **C40.0 Malignant neoplasm of scapula and long bones of upper limb**
    CC **C40.00 Malignant neoplasm of scapula and long bones of unspecified upper limb**
    CC **C40.01 Malignant neoplasm of scapula and long bones of right upper limb**
    CC **C40.02 Malignant neoplasm of scapula and long bones of left upper limb**
+ **C40.1 Malignant neoplasm of short bones of upper limb**
    CC **C40.10 Malignant neoplasm of short bones of unspecified upper limb**
    CC **C40.11 Malignant neoplasm of short bones of right upper limb**
    CC **C40.12 Malignant neoplasm of short bones of left upper limb**
+ **C40.2 Malignant neoplasm of long bones of lower limb**
    CC **C40.20 Malignant neoplasm of long bones of unspecified lower limb**
    CC **C40.21 Malignant neoplasm of long bones of right lower limb**
    CC **C40.22 Malignant neoplasm of long bones of left lower limb**
+ **C40.3 Malignant neoplasm of short bones of lower limb**
    CC **C40.30 Malignant neoplasm of short bones of unspecified lower limb**
    CC **C40.31 Malignant neoplasm of short bones of right lower limb**
    CC **C40.32 Malignant neoplasm of short bones of left lower limb**
+ **C40.8 Malignant neoplasm of overlapping sites of bone and articular cartilage of limb**
    CC **C40.80 Malignant neoplasm of overlapping sites of bone and articular cartilage of unspecified limb**
    CC **C40.81 Malignant neoplasm of overlapping sites of bone and articular cartilage of right limb**
    CC **C40.82 Malignant neoplasm of overlapping sites of bone and articular cartilage of left limb**
+ **C40.9 Malignant neoplasm of unspecified bones and articular cartilage of limb**
    CC **C40.90 Malignant neoplasm of unspecified bones and articular cartilage of unspecified limb**
    CC **C40.91 Malignant neoplasm of unspecified bones and articular cartilage of right limb**
    CC **C40.92 Malignant neoplasm of unspecified bones and articular cartilage of left limb**

C41 Malignant neoplasm of bone and articular cartilage of other and unspecified sites

Excludes1: malignant neoplasm of bones of limbs (C40.-)
        malignant neoplasm of cartilage of ear (C49.0)
        malignant neoplasm of cartilage of eyelid (C49.0)
        malignant neoplasm of cartilage of larynx (C32.3)
        malignant neoplasm of cartilage of limbs (C40.-)
        malignant neoplasm of cartilage of nose (C30.0)

CC **C41.0 Malignant neoplasm of bones of skull and face**
    Malignant neoplasm of maxilla (superior)
    Malignant neoplasm of orbital bone
    Excludes2: carcinoma, any type except intraosseous or
        odontogenic of:
        maxillary sinus (C31.0)
        upper jaw (C03.0)
        malignant neoplasm of jaw bone (lower)
        (C41.1)

CC **C41.1 Malignant neoplasm of mandible**
    Malignant neoplasm of inferior maxilla
    Malignant neoplasm of lower jaw bone
    Excludes2: carcinoma, any type except intraosseous or
        odontogenic of:
        jaw NOS (C03.9)
        lower (C03.1)
        malignant neoplasm of upper jaw bone (C41.0)

CC **C41.2** Malignant neoplasm of vertebral column
      Excludes1: *malignant neoplasm of sacrum and coccyx*
            (C41.4)
CC **C41.3** Malignant neoplasm of ribs, sternum and clavicle
CC **C41.4** Malignant neoplasm of pelvic bones, sacrum and coccyx
CC **C41.9** Malignant neoplasm of bone and articular cartilage, unspecified

Melanoma and other malignant neoplasms of skin (C43-C44)

C43 Malignant melanoma of skin

    Excludes1: *melanoma in situ (D03.-)*
    Excludes2: *malignant melanoma of skin of genital organs*
            (C51-C52, C60.-, C63.-)
            Merkel cell carcinoma (C4A.-)
            sites other than skin-code to malignant neoplasm of the site

C43.0 Malignant melanoma of lip
    Excludes1: *malignant neoplasm of vermilion border of lip*
            (C00.0-C00.2)
+ **C43.1** Malignant melanoma of eyelid, including canthus
    C43.10 Malignant melanoma of unspecified eyelid, including canthus
   + **C43.11** Malignant melanoma of right eyelid, including canthus
      C43.111 Malignant melanoma of right upper eyelid, including canthus
      C43.112 Malignant melanoma of right lower eyelid, including canthus
   + **C43.12** Malignant melanoma of left eyelid, including canthus
      C43.121 Malignant melanoma of left upper eyelid, including canthus
      C43.122 Malignant melanoma of left lower eyelid, including canthus
+ **C43.2** Malignant melanoma of ear and external auricular canal
    C43.20 Malignant melanoma of unspecified ear and external auricular canal
    C43.21 Malignant melanoma of right ear and external auricular canal
    C43.22 Malignant melanoma of left ear and external auricular canal
+ **C43.3** Malignant melanoma of other and unspecified parts of face
    C43.30 Malignant melanoma of unspecified part of face
    C43.31 Malignant melanoma of nose
    C43.39 Malignant melanoma of other parts of face
C43.4 Malignant melanoma of scalp and neck
+ **C43.5** Malignant melanoma of trunk
    Excludes2: *malignant neoplasm of anus NOS (C21.0)*
            malignant neoplasm of scrotum (C63.2)
    C43.51 Malignant melanoma of anal skin
        Malignant melanoma of anal margin
        Malignant melanoma of perianal skin
    C43.52 Malignant melanoma of skin of breast
    C43.59 Malignant melanoma of other part of trunk
+ **C43.6** Malignant melanoma of upper limb, including shoulder
    C43.60 Malignant melanoma of unspecified upper limb, including shoulder
    C43.61 Malignant melanoma of right upper limb, including shoulder
    C43.62 Malignant melanoma of left upper limb, including shoulder
+ **C43.7** Malignant melanoma of lower limb, including hip
    C43.70 Malignant melanoma of unspecified lower limb, including hip
    C43.71 Malignant melanoma of right lower limb, including hip
    C43.72 Malignant melanoma of left lower limb, including hip
C43.8 Malignant melanoma of overlapping sites of skin
C43.9 Malignant melanoma of skin, unspecified
    Malignant melanoma of unspecified site of skin
    Melanoma (malignant) NOS

C4A Merkel cell carcinoma

C4A.0 Merkel cell carcinoma of lip
    Excludes1: *malignant neoplasm of vermilion border of lip*
            (C00.0-C00.2)
+ **C4A.1** Merkel cell carcinoma of eyelid, including canthus
    C4A.10 Merkel cell carcinoma of unspecified eyelid, including canthus
   + **C4A.11** Merkel cell carcinoma of right eyelid, including canthus
      C4A.111 Merkel cell carcinoma of right upper eyelid, including canthus
      C4A.112 Merkel cell carcinoma of right lower eyelid, including canthus
   + **C4A.12** Merkel cell carcinoma of left eyelid, including canthus
      C4A.121 Merkel cell carcinoma of left upper eyelid, including canthus
      C4A.122 Merkel cell carcinoma of left lower eyelid, including canthus
+ **C4A.2** Merkel cell carcinoma of ear and external auricular canal
    C4A.20 Merkel cell carcinoma of unspecified ear and external auricular canal
    C4A.21 Merkel cell carcinoma of right ear and external auricular canal
    C4A.22 Merkel cell carcinoma of left ear and external auricular canal
+ **C4A.3** Merkel cell carcinoma of other and unspecified parts of face
    C4A.30 Merkel cell carcinoma of unspecified part of face
    C4A.31 Merkel cell carcinoma of nose
    C4A.39 Merkel cell carcinoma of other parts of face
C4A.4 Merkel cell carcinoma of scalp and neck
+ **C4A.5** Merkel cell carcinoma of trunk
    Excludes2: *malignant neoplasm of anus NOS (C21.0)*
            malignant neoplasm of scrotum (C63.2)
    C4A.51 Merkel cell carcinoma of anal skin
        Merkel cell carcinoma of anal margin
        Merkel cell carcinoma of perianal skin
    C4A.52 Merkel cell carcinoma of skin of breast
    C4A.59 Merkel cell carcinoma of other part of trunk
+ **C4A.6** Merkel cell carcinoma of upper limb, including shoulder
    C4A.60 Merkel cell carcinoma of unspecified upper limb, including shoulder
    C4A.61 Merkel cell carcinoma of right upper limb, including shoulder
    C4A.62 Merkel cell carcinoma of left upper limb, including shoulder
+ **C4A.7** Merkel cell carcinoma of lower limb, including hip
    C4A.70 Merkel cell carcinoma of unspecified lower limb, including hip
    C4A.71 Merkel cell carcinoma of right lower limb, including hip
    C4A.72 Merkel cell carcinoma of left lower limb, including hip
C4A.8 Merkel cell carcinoma of overlapping sites
C4A.9 Merkel cell carcinoma, unspecified
    Merkel cell carcinoma of unspecified site
    Merkel cell carcinoma NOS

C44 Other and unspecified malignant neoplasm of skin

    Includes: malignant neoplasm of sebaceous glands
            malignant neoplasm of sweat glands
    Excludes1: *Kaposi's sarcoma of skin (C46.0)*
            malignant melanoma of skin (C43.-)
            malignant neoplasm of skin of genital organs (C51-C52, C60.-, C63.2)
            Merkel cell carcinoma (C4A.-)
+ **C44.0** Other and unspecified malignant neoplasm of skin of lip
    Excludes1: *malignant neoplasm of lip (C00.-)*
    C44.00 Unspecified malignant neoplasm of skin of lip
    C44.01 Basal cell carcinoma of skin of lip
    C44.02 Squamous cell carcinoma of skin of lip
    C44.09 Other specified malignant neoplasm of skin of lip

+ **C44.1** **Other and unspecified malignant neoplasm of skin of eyelid, including canthus**
  Excludes1: *connective tissue of eyelid (C49.0)*
  + **C44.10** **Unspecified malignant neoplasm of skin of eyelid, including canthus**
    C44.101 Unspecified malignant neoplasm of skin of unspecified eyelid, including canthus
    + **C44.102** Unspecified malignant neoplasm of skin of right eyelid, including canthus
      C44.1021 Unspecified malignant neoplasm of skin of right upper eyelid, including canthus
      C44.1022 Unspecified malignant neoplasm of skin of right lower eyelid, including canthus
    + **C44.109** Unspecified malignant neoplasm of skin of left eyelid, including canthus
      C44.1091 Unspecified malignant neoplasm of skin of left upper eyelid, including canthus
      C44.1092 Unspecified malignant neoplasm of skin of left lower eyelid, including canthus
  + **C44.11** **Basal cell carcinoma of skin of eyelid, including canthus**
    C44.111 Basal cell carcinoma of skin of unspecified eyelid, including canthus
    + **C44.112** Basal cell carcinoma of skin of right eyelid, including canthus
      C44.1121 Basal cell carcinoma of skin of right upper eyelid, including canthus
      C44.1122 Basal cell carcinoma of skin of right lower eyelid, including canthus
    + **C44.119** Basal cell carcinoma of skin of left eyelid, including canthus
      C44.1191 Basal cell carcinoma of skin of left upper eyelid, including canthus
      C44.1192 Basal cell carcinoma of skin of left lower eyelid, including canthus
  + **C44.12** **Squamous cell carcinoma of skin of eyelid, including canthus**
    C44.121 Squamous cell carcinoma of skin of unspecified eyelid, including canthus
    + **C44.122** Squamous cell carcinoma of skin of right eyelid, including canthus
      C44.1221 Squamous cell carcinoma of skin of right upper eyelid, including canthus
      C44.1222 Squamous cell carcinoma of skin of right lower eyelid, including canthus
    + **C44.129** Squamous cell carcinoma of skin of left eyelid, including canthus
      C44.1291 Squamous cell carcinoma of skin of left upper eyelid, including canthus
      C44.1292 Squamous cell carcinoma of skin of left lower eyelid, including canthus
  + **C44.13** **Sebaceous cell carcinoma of skin of eyelid, including canthus**
    C44.131 Sebaceous cell carcinoma of skin of unspecified eyelid, including canthus
    + **C44.132** Sebaceous cell carcinoma of skin of right eyelid, including canthus
      C44.1321 Sebaceous cell carcinoma of skin of right upper eyelid, including canthus
      C44.1322 Sebaceous cell carcinoma of skin of right lower eyelid, including canthus
    + **C44.139** Sebaceous cell carcinoma of skin of left eyelid, including canthus
      C44.1391 Sebaceous cell carcinoma of skin of left upper eyelid, including canthus
      C44.1392 Sebaceous cell carcinoma of skin of left lower eyelid, including canthus
  + **C44.19** **Other specified malignant neoplasm of skin of eyelid, including canthus**
    C44.191 Other specified malignant neoplasm of skin of unspecified eyelid, including canthus
    + **C44.192** Other specified malignant neoplasm of skin of right eyelid, including canthus
      C44.1921 Other specified malignant neoplasm of skin of right upper eyelid, including canthus
      C44.1922 Other specified malignant neoplasm of skin of right lower eyelid, including canthus
    + **C44.199** Other specified malignant neoplasm of skin of left eyelid, including canthus
      C44.1991 Other specified malignant neoplasm of skin of left upper eyelid, including canthus
      C44.1992 Other specified malignant neoplasm of skin of left lower eyelid, including canthus

+ **C44.2** **Other and unspecified malignant neoplasm of skin of ear and external auricular canal**
  Excludes1: *connective tissue of ear (C49.0)*
  + **C44.20** **Unspecified malignant neoplasm of skin of ear and external auricular canal**
    C44.201 Unspecified malignant neoplasm of skin of unspecified ear and external auricular canal
    C44.202 Unspecified malignant neoplasm of skin of right ear and external auricular canal
    C44.209 Unspecified malignant neoplasm of skin of left ear and external auricular canal
  + **C44.21** **Basal cell carcinoma of skin of ear and external auricular canal**
    C44.211 Basal cell carcinoma of skin of unspecified ear and external auricular canal
    C44.212 Basal cell carcinoma of skin of right ear and external auricular canal
    C44.219 Basal cell carcinoma of skin of left ear and external auricular canal
  + **C44.22** **Squamous cell carcinoma of skin of ear and external auricular canal**
    C44.221 Squamous cell carcinoma of skin of unspecified ear and external auricular canal
    C44.222 Squamous cell carcinoma of skin of right ear and external auricular canal
    C44.229 Squamous cell carcinoma of skin of left ear and external auricular canal

+, +7th, X + 7th   ● Newborn   ● Pediatric   ● Maternity   ● Adult   ♀ Female   ♂ Male   Manifestation   Unacceptable PDX   HCC   CC   MCC   HAC

+ C44.29 Other specified malignant neoplasm of skin of ear and external auricular canal
    C44.291 Other specified malignant neoplasm of skin of unspecified ear and external auricular canal
    C44.292 Other specified malignant neoplasm of skin of right ear and external auricular canal
    C44.299 Other specified malignant neoplasm of skin of left ear and external auricular canal

+ C44.3 Other and unspecified malignant neoplasm of skin of other and unspecified parts of face
  + C44.30 Unspecified malignant neoplasm of skin of other and unspecified parts of face
    C44.300 Unspecified malignant neoplasm of skin of unspecified part of face
    C44.301 Unspecified malignant neoplasm of skin of nose
    C44.309 Unspecified malignant neoplasm of skin of other parts of face
  + C44.31 Basal cell carcinoma of skin of other and unspecified parts of face
    C44.310 Basal cell carcinoma of skin of unspecified parts of face
    C44.311 Basal cell carcinoma of skin of nose
    C44.319 Basal cell carcinoma of skin of other parts of face
      AHA CC: 1Q, 2017, 4
  + C44.32 Squamous cell carcinoma of skin of other and unspecified parts of face
    C44.320 Squamous cell carcinoma of skin of unspecified parts of face
    C44.321 Squamous cell carcinoma of skin of nose
    C44.329 Squamous cell carcinoma of skin of other parts of face
  + C44.39 Other specified malignant neoplasm of skin of other and unspecified parts of face
    C44.390 Other specified malignant neoplasm of skin of unspecified parts of face
    C44.391 Other specified malignant neoplasm of skin of nose
    C44.399 Other specified malignant neoplasm of skin of other parts of face

+ C44.4 Other and unspecified malignant neoplasm of skin of scalp and neck
    C44.40 Unspecified malignant neoplasm of skin of scalp and neck
    C44.41 Basal cell carcinoma of skin of scalp and neck
    C44.42 Squamous cell carcinoma of skin of scalp and neck
    C44.49 Other specified malignant neoplasm of skin of scalp and neck

+ C44.5 Other and unspecified malignant neoplasm of skin of trunk
    Excludes1: *anus NOS (C21.0)*
             scrotum (C63.2)
  + C44.50 Unspecified malignant neoplasm of skin of trunk
    C44.500 Unspecified malignant neoplasm of anal skin
      Unspecified malignant neoplasm of anal margin
      Unspecified malignant neoplasm of perianal skin
    C44.501 Unspecified malignant neoplasm of skin of breast
    C44.509 Unspecified malignant neoplasm of skin of other part of trunk
  + C44.51 Basal cell carcinoma of skin of trunk
    C44.510 Basal cell carcinoma of anal skin
      Basal cell carcinoma of anal margin
      Basal cell carcinoma of perianal skin
    C44.511 Basal cell carcinoma of skin of breast
    C44.519 Basal cell carcinoma of skin of other part of trunk

+ C44.52 Squamous cell carcinoma of skin of trunk
    C44.520 Squamous cell carcinoma of anal skin
      Squamous cell carcinoma of anal margin
      Squamous cell carcinoma of perianal skin
    C44.521 Squamous cell carcinoma of skin of breast
    C44.529 Squamous cell carcinoma of skin of other part of trunk
+ C44.59 Other specified malignant neoplasm of skin of trunk
    C44.590 Other specified malignant neoplasm of anal skin
      Other specified malignant neoplasm of anal margin
      Other specified malignant neoplasm of perianal skin
    C44.591 Other specified malignant neoplasm of skin of breast
    C44.599 Other specified malignant neoplasm of skin of other part of trunk

+ C44.6 Other and unspecified malignant neoplasm of skin of upper limb, including shoulder
  + C44.60 Unspecified malignant neoplasm of skin of upper limb, including shoulder
    C44.601 Unspecified malignant neoplasm of skin of unspecified upper limb, including shoulder
    C44.602 Unspecified malignant neoplasm of skin of right upper limb, including shoulder
    C44.609 Unspecified malignant neoplasm of skin of left upper limb, including shoulder
  + C44.61 Basal cell carcinoma of skin of upper limb, including shoulder
    C44.611 Basal cell carcinoma of skin of unspecified upper limb, including shoulder
    C44.612 Basal cell carcinoma of skin of right upper limb, including shoulder
    C44.619 Basal cell carcinoma of skin of left upper limb, including shoulder
  + C44.62 Squamous cell carcinoma of skin of upper limb, including shoulder
    C44.621 Squamous cell carcinoma of skin of unspecified upper limb, including shoulder
    C44.622 Squamous cell carcinoma of skin of right upper limb, including shoulder
    C44.629 Squamous cell carcinoma of skin of left upper limb, including shoulder
  + C44.69 Other specified malignant neoplasm of skin of upper limb, including shoulder
    C44.691 Other specified malignant neoplasm of skin of unspecified upper limb, including shoulder
    C44.692 Other specified malignant neoplasm of skin of right upper limb, including shoulder
    C44.699 Other specified malignant neoplasm of skin of left upper limb, including shoulder

+ C44.7 Other and unspecified malignant neoplasm of skin of lower limb, including hip
  + C44.70 Unspecified malignant neoplasm of skin of lower limb, including hip
    C44.701 Unspecified malignant neoplasm of skin of unspecified lower limb, including hip
    C44.702 Unspecified malignant neoplasm of skin of right lower limb, including hip
    C44.709 Unspecified malignant neoplasm of skin of left lower limb, including hip
  + C44.71 Basal cell carcinoma of skin of lower limb, including hip
    C44.711 Basal cell carcinoma of skin of unspecified lower limb, including hip
    C44.712 Basal cell carcinoma of skin of right lower limb, including hip
    C44.719 Basal cell carcinoma of skin of left lower limb, including hip

+, +7th, X + 7th   ● Newborn   ● Pediatric   ● Maternity   ● Adult   ♀ Female   ♂ Male   Manifestation   Unacceptable PDX   HCC   CC   MCC   HAC

+ **C44.72 Squamous cell carcinoma of skin of lower limb, including hip**
    C44.721 Squamous cell carcinoma of skin of unspecified lower limb, including hip
    C44.722 Squamous cell carcinoma of skin of right lower limb, including hip
    C44.729 Squamous cell carcinoma of skin of left lower limb, including hip
+ **C44.79 Other specified malignant neoplasm of skin of lower limb, including hip**
    C44.791 Other specified malignant neoplasm of skin of unspecified lower limb, including hip
    C44.792 Other specified malignant neoplasm of skin of right lower limb, including hip
    C44.799 Other specified malignant neoplasm of skin of left lower limb, including hip
+ **C44.8 Other and unspecified malignant neoplasm of overlapping sites of skin**
    C44.80 Unspecified malignant neoplasm of overlapping sites of skin
    C44.81 Basal cell carcinoma of overlapping sites of skin
    C44.82 Squamous cell carcinoma of overlapping sites of skin
    C44.89 Other specified malignant neoplasm of overlapping sites of skin
+ **C44.9 Other and unspecified malignant neoplasm of skin, unspecified**
    C44.90 Unspecified malignant neoplasm of skin, unspecified
      Malignant neoplasm of unspecified site of skin
    C44.91 Basal cell carcinoma of skin, unspecified
    C44.92 Squamous cell carcinoma of skin, unspecified
    C44.99 Other specified malignant neoplasm of skin, unspecified

Malignant neoplasms of mesothelial and soft tissue (C45-C49)

C45 Mesothelioma

CC **C45.0 Mesothelioma of pleura**
    Excludes1: other malignant neoplasm of pleura (C38.4)
    AHA CC: 2Q, 2017, 11

CC **C45.1 Mesothelioma of peritoneum**
    Mesothelioma of cul-de-sac
    Mesothelioma of mesentery
    Mesothelioma of mesocolon
    Mesothelioma of omentum
    Mesothelioma of peritoneum (parietal) (pelvic)
    Excludes1: other malignant neoplasm of soft tissue of peritoneum (C48.-)

CC **C45.2 Mesothelioma of pericardium**
    Excludes1: other malignant neoplasm of pericardium (C38.0)

    C45.7 Mesothelioma of other sites
    C45.9 Mesothelioma, unspecified

C46 Kaposi's sarcoma

    Code first any human immunodeficiency virus [HIV] disease (B20)

CC **C46.0 Kaposi's sarcoma of skin**

CC **C46.1 Kaposi's sarcoma of soft tissue**
    Kaposi's sarcoma of blood vessel
    Kaposi's sarcoma of connective tissue
    Kaposi's sarcoma of fascia
    Kaposi's sarcoma of ligament
    Kaposi's sarcoma of lymphatic(s) NEC
    Kaposi's sarcoma of muscle
    Excludes2: Kaposi's sarcoma of lymph glands and nodes (C46.3)

CC **C46.2 Kaposi's sarcoma of palate**
CC **C46.3 Kaposi's sarcoma of lymph nodes**
CC **C46.4 Kaposi's sarcoma of gastrointestinal sites**
+ **C46.5 Kaposi's sarcoma of lung**
    CC **C46.50 Kaposi's sarcoma of unspecified lung**
    CC **C46.51 Kaposi's sarcoma of right lung**
    CC **C46.52 Kaposi's sarcoma of left lung**
CC **C46.7 Kaposi's sarcoma of other sites**
CC **C46.9 Kaposi's sarcoma, unspecified**
    Kaposi's sarcoma of unspecified site

C47 Malignant neoplasm of peripheral nerves and autonomic nervous system

    Includes: malignant neoplasm of sympathetic and parasympathetic nerves and ganglia
    Excludes1: Kaposi's sarcoma of soft tissue (C46.1)

CC **C47.0 Malignant neoplasm of peripheral nerves of head, face and neck**
    Excludes1: malignant neoplasm of peripheral nerves of orbit (C69.6-)

+ **C47.1 Malignant neoplasm of peripheral nerves of upper limb, including shoulder**
    CC **C47.10 Malignant neoplasm of peripheral nerves of unspecified upper limb, including shoulder**
    CC **C47.11 Malignant neoplasm of peripheral nerves of right upper limb, including shoulder**
    CC **C47.12 Malignant neoplasm of peripheral nerves of left upper limb, including shoulder**

+ **C47.2 Malignant neoplasm of peripheral nerves of lower limb, including hip**
    CC **C47.20 Malignant neoplasm of peripheral nerves of unspecified lower limb, including hip**
    CC **C47.21 Malignant neoplasm of peripheral nerves of right lower limb, including hip**
    CC **C47.22 Malignant neoplasm of peripheral nerves of left lower limb, including hip**

CC **C47.3 Malignant neoplasm of peripheral nerves of thorax**
CC **C47.4 Malignant neoplasm of peripheral nerves of abdomen**
CC **C47.5 Malignant neoplasm of peripheral nerves of pelvis**
CC **C47.6 Malignant neoplasm of peripheral nerves of trunk, unspecified**
    Malignant neoplasm of peripheral nerves of unspecified part of trunk
CC **C47.8 Malignant neoplasm of overlapping sites of peripheral nerves and autonomic nervous system**
CC **C47.9 Malignant neoplasm of peripheral nerves and autonomic nervous system, unspecified**
    Malignant neoplasm of unspecified site of peripheral nerves and autonomic nervous system

C48 Malignant neoplasm of retroperitoneum and peritoneum

    Excludes1: Kaposi's sarcoma of connective tissue (C46.1)
      mesothelioma (C45.-)

CC **C48.0 Malignant neoplasm of retroperitoneum**
CC **C48.1 Malignant neoplasm of specified parts of peritoneum**
    Malignant neoplasm of cul-de-sac
    Malignant neoplasm of mesentery
    Malignant neoplasm of mesocolon
    Malignant neoplasm of omentum
    Malignant neoplasm of parietal peritoneum
    Malignant neoplasm of pelvic peritoneum
CC **C48.2 Malignant neoplasm of peritoneum, unspecified**
CC **C48.8 Malignant neoplasm of overlapping sites of retroperitoneum and peritoneum**

C49 Malignant neoplasm of other connective and soft tissue

    Includes: malignant neoplasm of blood vessel
      malignant neoplasm of bursa
      malignant neoplasm of cartilage
      malignant neoplasm of fascia
      malignant neoplasm of fat
      malignant neoplasm of ligament, except uterine
      malignant neoplasm of lymphatic vessel
      malignant neoplasm of muscle
      malignant neoplasm of synovia
      malignant neoplasm of tendon (sheath)
    Excludes1: malignant neoplasm of cartilage (of):
      articular (C40-C41)
      larynx (C32.3)
      nose (C30.0)
      malignant neoplasm of connective tissue of breast (C50.-)
    Excludes2: Kaposi's sarcoma of soft tissue (C46.1)
      malignant neoplasm of heart (C38.0)
      malignant neoplasm of peripheral nerves and autonomic nervous system (C47.-)
      malignant neoplasm of peritoneum (C48.2)
      malignant neoplasm of retroperitoneum (C48.0)
      malignant neoplasm of uterine ligament (C57.3)
      mesothelioma (C45.-)

CC **C49.0** Malignant neoplasm of connective and soft tissue of head, face and neck
   Malignant neoplasm of connective tissue of ear
   Malignant neoplasm of connective tissue of eyelid
   Excludes1: *connective tissue of orbit (C69.6-)*

+ **C49.1** Malignant neoplasm of connective and soft tissue of upper limb, including shoulder
   CC **C49.10** Malignant neoplasm of connective and soft tissue of unspecified upper limb, including shoulder
   CC **C49.11** Malignant neoplasm of connective and soft tissue of right upper limb, including shoulder
   CC **C49.12** Malignant neoplasm of connective and soft tissue of left upper limb, including shoulder

+ **C49.2** Malignant neoplasm of connective and soft tissue of lower limb, including hip
   CC **C49.20** Malignant neoplasm of connective and soft tissue of unspecified lower limb, including hip
   CC **C49.21** Malignant neoplasm of connective and soft tissue of right lower limb, including hip
   CC **C49.22** Malignant neoplasm of connective and soft tissue of left lower limb, including hip

CC **C49.3** Malignant neoplasm of connective and soft tissue of thorax
   Malignant neoplasm of axilla
   Malignant neoplasm of diaphragm
   Malignant neoplasm of great vessels
   Excludes1: *malignant neoplasm of breast (C50.-)*
   malignant neoplasm of heart (C38.0)
   malignant neoplasm of mediastinum (C38.1-C38.3)
   malignant neoplasm of thymus (C37)
   AHA CC: 3Q, 2015, 19-20

CC **C49.4** Malignant neoplasm of connective and soft tissue of abdomen
   Malignant neoplasm of abdominal wall
   Malignant neoplasm of hypochondrium

CC **C49.5** Malignant neoplasm of connective and soft tissue of pelvis
   Malignant neoplasm of buttock
   Malignant neoplasm of groin
   Malignant neoplasm of perineum

CC **C49.6** Malignant neoplasm of connective and soft tissue of trunk, unspecified
   Malignant neoplasm of back NOS

CC **C49.8** Malignant neoplasm of overlapping sites of connective and soft tissue
   Primary malignant neoplasm of two or more contiguous sites of connective and soft tissue

CC **C49.9** Malignant neoplasm of connective and soft tissue, unspecified

+ **C49.A** Gastrointestinal stromal tumor
   AHA CC: 4Q, 2016, 8
   CC **C49.A0** Gastrointestinal stromal tumor, unspecified site
   CC **C49.A1** Gastrointestinal stromal tumor of esophagus
   CC **C49.A2** Gastrointestinal stromal tumor of stomach
   CC **C49.A3** Gastrointestinal stromal tumor of small intestine
   CC **C49.A4** Gastrointestinal stromal tumor of large intestine
   CC **C49.A5** Gastrointestinal stromal tumor of rectum
   CC **C49.A9** Gastrointestinal stromal tumor of other sites

Malignant neoplasms of breast (C50)

C50 Malignant neoplasm of breast
   Includes: connective tissue of breast
   Paget's disease of breast
   Paget's disease of nipple
   Use additional code to identify estrogen receptor status (Z17.0, Z17.1)
   Excludes1: *skin of breast (C44.501, C44.511, C44.521, C44.591)*

+ **C50.0** Malignant neoplasm of nipple and areola
   + **C50.01** Malignant neoplasm of nipple and areola, female
      ♀ **C50.011** Malignant neoplasm of nipple and areola, right female breast
      ♀ **C50.012** Malignant neoplasm of nipple and areola, left female breast
      ♀ **C50.019** Malignant neoplasm of nipple and areola, unspecified female breast

   + **C50.02** Malignant neoplasm of nipple and areola, male
      ♂ **C50.021** Malignant neoplasm of nipple and areola, right male breast
      ♂ **C50.022** Malignant neoplasm of nipple and areola, left male breast
      ♂ **C50.029** Malignant neoplasm of nipple and areola, unspecified male breast

+ **C50.1** Malignant neoplasm of central portion of breast
   + **C50.11** Malignant neoplasm of central portion of breast, female
      ♀ **C50.111** Malignant neoplasm of central portion of right female breast
      ♀ **C50.112** Malignant neoplasm of central portion of left female breast
      ♀ **C50.119** Malignant neoplasm of central portion of unspecified female breast
   + **C50.12** Malignant neoplasm of central portion of breast, male
      ♂ **C50.121** Malignant neoplasm of central portion of right male breast
      ♂ **C50.122** Malignant neoplasm of central portion of left male breast
      ♂ **C50.129** Malignant neoplasm of central portion of unspecified male breast

+ **C50.2** Malignant neoplasm of upper-inner quadrant of breast
   + **C50.21** Malignant neoplasm of upper-inner quadrant of breast, female
      ♀ **C50.211** Malignant neoplasm of upper-inner quadrant of right female breast
      ♀ **C50.212** Malignant neoplasm of upper-inner quadrant of left female breast
      ♀ **C50.219** Malignant neoplasm of upper-inner quadrant of unspecified female breast
   + **C50.22** Malignant neoplasm of upper-inner quadrant of breast, male
      ♂ **C50.221** Malignant neoplasm of upper-inner quadrant of right male breast
      ♂ **C50.222** Malignant neoplasm of upper-inner quadrant of left male breast
      ♂ **C50.229** Malignant neoplasm of upper-inner quadrant of unspecified male breast

+ **C50.3** Malignant neoplasm of lower-inner quadrant of breast
   + **C50.31** Malignant neoplasm of lower-inner quadrant of breast, female
      ♀ **C50.311** Malignant neoplasm of lower-inner quadrant of right female breast
      ♀ **C50.312** Malignant neoplasm of lower-inner quadrant of left female breast
      ♀ **C50.319** Malignant neoplasm of lower-inner quadrant of unspecified female breast
   + **C50.32** Malignant neoplasm of lower-inner quadrant of breast, male
      ♂ **C50.321** Malignant neoplasm of lower-inner quadrant of right male breast
      ♂ **C50.322** Malignant neoplasm of lower-inner quadrant of left male breast
      ♂ **C50.329** Malignant neoplasm of lower-inner quadrant of unspecified male breast

+ **C50.4** Malignant neoplasm of upper-outer quadrant of breast
   + **C50.41** Malignant neoplasm of upper-outer quadrant of breast, female
      ♀ **C50.411** Malignant neoplasm of upper-outer quadrant of right female breast
      ♀ **C50.412** Malignant neoplasm of upper-outer quadrant of left female breast
      ♀ **C50.419** Malignant neoplasm of upper-outer quadrant of unspecified female breast
   + **C50.42** Malignant neoplasm of upper-outer quadrant of breast, male
      ♂ **C50.421** Malignant neoplasm of upper-outer quadrant of right male breast
      ♂ **C50.422** Malignant neoplasm of upper-outer quadrant of left male breast
      ♂ **C50.429** Malignant neoplasm of upper-outer quadrant of unspecified male breast

+ **C50.5 Malignant neoplasm of lower-outer quadrant of breast**
  + **C50.51 Malignant neoplasm of lower-outer quadrant of breast, female**
    - ♀ **C50.511 Malignant neoplasm of lower-outer quadrant of right female breast**
    - ♀ **C50.512 Malignant neoplasm of lower-outer quadrant of left female breast**
    - ♀ **C50.519 Malignant neoplasm of lower-outer quadrant of unspecified female breast**
  + **C50.52 Malignant neoplasm of lower-outer quadrant of breast, male**
    - ♂ **C50.521 Malignant neoplasm of lower-outer quadrant of right male breast**
    - ♂ **C50.522 Malignant neoplasm of lower-outer quadrant of left male breast**
    - ♂ **C50.529 Malignant neoplasm of lower-outer quadrant of unspecified male breast**
+ **C50.6 Malignant neoplasm of axillary tail of breast**
  + **C50.61 Malignant neoplasm of axillary tail of breast, female**
    - ♀ **C50.611 Malignant neoplasm of axillary tail of right female breast**
    - ♀ **C50.612 Malignant neoplasm of axillary tail of left female breast**
    - ♀ **C50.619 Malignant neoplasm of axillary tail of unspecified female breast**
  + **C50.62 Malignant neoplasm of axillary tail of breast, male**
    - ♂ **C50.621 Malignant neoplasm of axillary tail of right male breast**
    - ♂ **C50.622 Malignant neoplasm of axillary tail of left male breast**
    - ♂ **C50.629 Malignant neoplasm of axillary tail of unspecified male breast**
+ **C50.8 Malignant neoplasm of overlapping sites of breast**
  + **C50.81 Malignant neoplasm of overlapping sites of breast, female**
    - ♀ **C50.811 Malignant neoplasm of overlapping sites of right female breast**
    - ♀ **C50.812 Malignant neoplasm of overlapping sites of left female breast**
    - ♀ **C50.819 Malignant neoplasm of overlapping sites of unspecified female breast**
  + **C50.82 Malignant neoplasm of overlapping sites of breast, male**
    - ♂ **C50.821 Malignant neoplasm of overlapping sites of right male breast**
    - ♂ **C50.822 Malignant neoplasm of overlapping sites of left male breast**
    - ♂ **C50.829 Malignant neoplasm of overlapping sites of unspecified male breast**
+ **C50.9 Malignant neoplasm of breast of unspecified site**
  + **C50.91 Malignant neoplasm of breast of unspecified site, female**
    - ♀ **C50.911 Malignant neoplasm of unspecified site of right female breast**
    - ♀ **C50.912 Malignant neoplasm of unspecified site of left female breast**
    - ♀ **C50.919 Malignant neoplasm of unspecified site of unspecified female breast**
  + **C50.92 Malignant neoplasm of breast of unspecified site, male**
    - ♂ **C50.921 Malignant neoplasm of unspecified site of right male breast**
    - ♂ **C50.922 Malignant neoplasm of unspecified site of left male breast**
    - ♂ **C50.929 Malignant neoplasm of unspecified site of unspecified male breast**

Malignant neoplasms of female genital organs (C51-C58)

Includes: malignant neoplasm of skin of female genital organs

C51 Malignant neoplasm of vulva

> **Excludes1:** *carcinoma in situ of vulva (D07.1)*

- ♀ **C51.0 Malignant neoplasm of labium majus**
  Malignant neoplasm of Bartholin's [greater vestibular] gland
- ♀ **C51.1 Malignant neoplasm of labium minus**
- ♀ **C51.2 Malignant neoplasm of clitoris**

- ♀ **C51.8 Malignant neoplasm of overlapping sites of vulva**
- ♀ **C51.9 Malignant neoplasm of vulva, unspecified**
  Malignant neoplasm of external female genitalia NOS
  Malignant neoplasm of pudendum

♀ **C52 Malignant neoplasm of vagina**

> **Excludes1:** *carcinoma in situ of vagina (D07.2)*
> **Valid 3-character code, no further characters required**

C53 Malignant neoplasm of cervix uteri

> **Excludes1:** *carcinoma in situ of cervix uteri (D06.-)*

- ♀ **C53.0 Malignant neoplasm of endocervix**
- ♀ **C53.1 Malignant neoplasm of exocervix**
- ♀ **C53.8 Malignant neoplasm of overlapping sites of cervix uteri**
- ♀ **C53.9 Malignant neoplasm of cervix uteri, unspecified**
  AHA CC: 4Q, 2017, 103-104

C54 Malignant neoplasm of corpus uteri

- ♀ **C54.0 Malignant neoplasm of isthmus uteri**
  Malignant neoplasm of lower uterine segment
- ♀ **C54.1 Malignant neoplasm of endometrium**
- ♀ **C54.2 Malignant neoplasm of myometrium**
- ♀ **C54.3 Malignant neoplasm of fundus uteri**
- ♀ **C54.8 Malignant neoplasm of overlapping sites of corpus uteri**
- ♀ **C54.9 Malignant neoplasm of corpus uteri, unspecified**

♀ **C55 Malignant neoplasm of uterus, part unspecified**

> **Valid 3-character code, no further characters required**

C56 Malignant neoplasm of ovary

> Use additional code to identify any functional activity

- ♀ CC **C56.1 Malignant neoplasm of right ovary**
- ♀ CC **C56.2 Malignant neoplasm of left ovary**
- ♀ CC **C56.9 Malignant neoplasm of unspecified ovary**

C57 Malignant neoplasm of other and unspecified female genital organs

+ **C57.0 Malignant neoplasm of fallopian tube**
  Malignant neoplasm of oviduct
  Malignant neoplasm of uterine tube
  - ♀ **C57.00 Malignant neoplasm of unspecified fallopian tube**
  - ♀ **C57.01 Malignant neoplasm of right fallopian tube**
  - ♀ **C57.02 Malignant neoplasm of left fallopian tube**
+ **C57.1 Malignant neoplasm of broad ligament**
  - ♀ **C57.10 Malignant neoplasm of unspecified broad ligament**
  - ♀ **C57.11 Malignant neoplasm of right broad ligament**
  - ♀ **C57.12 Malignant neoplasm of left broad ligament**
+ **C57.2 Malignant neoplasm of round ligament**
  - ♀ **C57.20 Malignant neoplasm of unspecified round ligament**
  - ♀ **C57.21 Malignant neoplasm of right round ligament**
  - ♀ **C57.22 Malignant neoplasm of left round ligament**
- ♀ **C57.3 Malignant neoplasm of parametrium**
  Malignant neoplasm of uterine ligament NOS
- ♀ **C57.4 Malignant neoplasm of uterine adnexa, unspecified**
- ♀ **C57.7 Malignant neoplasm of other specified female genital organs**
  Malignant neoplasm of wolffian body or duct
- ♀ **C57.8 Malignant neoplasm of overlapping sites of female genital organs**
  Primary malignant neoplasm of two or more contiguous sites of the female genital organs whose point of origin cannot be determined
  Primary tubo-ovarian malignant neoplasm whose point of origin cannot be determined
  Primary utero-ovarian malignant neoplasm whose point of origin cannot be determined
- ♀ **C57.9 Malignant neoplasm of female genital organ, unspecified**
  Malignant neoplasm of female genitourinary tract NOS

♀ **C58 Malignant neoplasm of placenta**

> **Includes:** choriocarcinoma NOS
> chorionepithelioma NOS
> **Excludes1:** *chorioadenoma (destruens) (D39.2)*
> *hydatidiform mole NOS (O01.9)*
> *invasive hydatidiform mole (D39.2)*
> *male choriocarcinoma NOS (C62.9-)*
> *malignant hydatidiform mole (D39.2)*
> **Valid 3-character code, no further characters required**

Malignant neoplasms of male genital organs (C60-C63)

Includes: malignant neoplasm of skin of male genital organs

C60 **Malignant neoplasm of penis**

♂ **C60.0** **Malignant neoplasm of prepuce**
Malignant neoplasm of foreskin

♂ **C60.1** **Malignant neoplasm of glans penis**

♂ **C60.2** **Malignant neoplasm of body of penis**
Malignant neoplasm of corpus cavernosum

♂ **C60.8** **Malignant neoplasm of overlapping sites of penis**

♂ **C60.9** **Malignant neoplasm of penis, unspecified**
Malignant neoplasm of skin of penis NOS

♂ **C61** **Malignant neoplasm of prostate**

Use additional code to identify:
hormone sensitivity status (Z19.1-Z19.2)
rising PSA following treatment for malignant neoplasm of prostate (R97.21)
Excludes1: *malignant neoplasm of seminal vesicle (C63.7)*
AHA CC: 1Q, 2017, 17-18
Valid 3-character code, no further characters required

C62 **Malignant neoplasm of testis**

Use additional code to identify any functional activity

+ C62.0 **Malignant neoplasm of undescended testis**
Malignant neoplasm of ectopic testis
Malignant neoplasm of retained testis

♂ **C62.00** **Malignant neoplasm of unspecified undescended testis**

♂ **C62.01** **Malignant neoplasm of undescended right testis**

♂ **C62.02** **Malignant neoplasm of undescended left testis**

+ C62.1 **Malignant neoplasm of descended testis**
Malignant neoplasm of scrotal testis

♂ **C62.10** **Malignant neoplasm of unspecified descended testis**

♂ **C62.11** **Malignant neoplasm of descended right testis**

♂ **C62.12** **Malignant neoplasm of descended left testis**

+ C62.9 **Malignant neoplasm of testis, unspecified whether descended or undescended**

♂ **C62.90** **Malignant neoplasm of unspecified testis, unspecified whether descended or undescended**
Malignant neoplasm of testis NOS

♂ **C62.91** **Malignant neoplasm of right testis, unspecified whether descended or undescended**

♂ **C62.92** **Malignant neoplasm of left testis, unspecified whether descended or undescended**

C63 **Malignant neoplasm of other and unspecified male genital organs**

+ C63.0 **Malignant neoplasm of epididymis**

♂ **C63.00** **Malignant neoplasm of unspecified epididymis**

♂ **C63.01** **Malignant neoplasm of right epididymis**

♂ **C63.02** **Malignant neoplasm of left epididymis**

+ C63.1 **Malignant neoplasm of spermatic cord**

♂ **C63.10** **Malignant neoplasm of unspecified spermatic cord**

♂ **C63.11** **Malignant neoplasm of right spermatic cord**

♂ **C63.12** **Malignant neoplasm of left spermatic cord**

♂ **C63.2** **Malignant neoplasm of scrotum**
Malignant neoplasm of skin of scrotum

♂ **C63.7** **Malignant neoplasm of other specified male genital organs**
Malignant neoplasm of seminal vesicle
Malignant neoplasm of tunica vaginalis

♂ **C63.8** **Malignant neoplasm of overlapping sites of male genital organs**
Primary malignant neoplasm of two or more contiguous sites of male genital organs whose point of origin cannot be determined

♂ **C63.9** **Malignant neoplasm of male genital organ, unspecified**
Malignant neoplasm of male genitourinary tract NOS

Malignant neoplasms of urinary tract (C64-C68)

C64 **Malignant neoplasm of kidney, except renal pelvis**

Excludes1: *malignant carcinoid tumor of the kidney (C7A.093)*
malignant neoplasm of renal calyces (C65.-)
malignant neoplasm of renal pelvis (C65.-)

CC **C64.1** **Malignant neoplasm of right kidney, except renal pelvis**

CC **C64.2** **Malignant neoplasm of left kidney, except renal pelvis**

CC **C64.9** **Malignant neoplasm of unspecified kidney, except renal pelvis**

C65 **Malignant neoplasm of renal pelvis**

Includes: malignant neoplasm of pelviureteric junction
malignant neoplasm of renal calyces

CC **C65.1** **Malignant neoplasm of right renal pelvis**

CC **C65.2** **Malignant neoplasm of left renal pelvis**

CC **C65.9** **Malignant neoplasm of unspecified renal pelvis**

C66 **Malignant neoplasm of ureter**

Excludes1: *malignant neoplasm of ureteric orifice of bladder (C67.6)*

CC **C66.1** **Malignant neoplasm of right ureter**

CC **C66.2** **Malignant neoplasm of left ureter**

CC **C66.9** **Malignant neoplasm of unspecified ureter**

C67 **Malignant neoplasm of bladder**

C67.0 **Malignant neoplasm of trigone of bladder**

C67.1 **Malignant neoplasm of dome of bladder**

C67.2 **Malignant neoplasm of lateral wall of bladder**

C67.3 **Malignant neoplasm of anterior wall of bladder**

C67.4 **Malignant neoplasm of posterior wall of bladder**

C67.5 **Malignant neoplasm of bladder neck**
Malignant neoplasm of internal urethral orifice

C67.6 **Malignant neoplasm of ureteric orifice**

C67.7 **Malignant neoplasm of urachus**

C67.8 **Malignant neoplasm of overlapping sites of bladder**

C67.9 **Malignant neoplasm of bladder, unspecified**
AHA CC: 1Q, 2016, 19; 1Q, 2017, 6

C68 **Malignant neoplasm of other and unspecified urinary organs**

Excludes1: *malignant neoplasm of female genitourinary tract NOS (C57.9)*
malignant neoplasm of male genitourinary tract NOS (C63.9)

CC **C68.0** **Malignant neoplasm of urethra**
Excludes1: *malignant neoplasm of urethral orifice of bladder (C67.5)*

CC **C68.1** **Malignant neoplasm of paraurethral glands**

CC **C68.8** **Malignant neoplasm of overlapping sites of urinary organs**
Primary malignant neoplasm of two or more contiguous sites of urinary organs whose point of origin cannot be determined

CC **C68.9** **Malignant neoplasm of urinary organ, unspecified**
Malignant neoplasm of urinary system NOS

Malignant neoplasms of eye, brain and other parts of central nervous system (C69-C72)

C69 **Malignant neoplasm of eye and adnexa**

Excludes1: *malignant neoplasm of connective tissue of eyelid (C49.0)*
malignant neoplasm of eyelid (skin) (C43.1-, C44.1-)
malignant neoplasm of optic nerve (C72.3-)

+ C69.0 **Malignant neoplasm of conjunctiva**

C69.00 **Malignant neoplasm of unspecified conjunctiva**

C69.01 **Malignant neoplasm of right conjunctiva**

C69.02 **Malignant neoplasm of left conjunctiva**

+ C69.1 **Malignant neoplasm of cornea**

C69.10 **Malignant neoplasm of unspecified cornea**

C69.11 **Malignant neoplasm of right cornea**

C69.12 **Malignant neoplasm of left cornea**

+ C69.2 **Malignant neoplasm of retina**

Excludes1: *dark area on retina (D49.81)*
neoplasm of unspecified behavior of retina and choroid (D49.81)
retinal freckle (D49.81)

C69.20 **Malignant neoplasm of unspecified retina**

C69.21 **Malignant neoplasm of right retina**

C69.22 **Malignant neoplasm of left retina**

+ C69.3 **Malignant neoplasm of choroid**

C69.30 **Malignant neoplasm of unspecified choroid**

C69.31 **Malignant neoplasm of right choroid**

C69.32 **Malignant neoplasm of left choroid**

+ C69.4 **Malignant neoplasm of ciliary body**

C69.40 **Malignant neoplasm of unspecified ciliary body**

C69.41 **Malignant neoplasm of right ciliary body**

C69.42 **Malignant neoplasm of left ciliary body**

+ C69.5 **Malignant neoplasm of lacrimal gland and duct**
Malignant neoplasm of lacrimal sac
Malignant neoplasm of nasolacrimal duct

+, +7th, X + 7th ● Newborn ● Pediatric ● Maternity ● Adult ♀ Female ♂ Male Manifestation Unacceptable PDX HCC CC MCC HAC

C69.50 Malignant neoplasm of unspecified lacrimal gland and duct
C69.51 Malignant neoplasm of right lacrimal gland and duct
C69.52 Malignant neoplasm of left lacrimal gland and duct
+ **C69.6** Malignant neoplasm of orbit
Malignant neoplasm of connective tissue of orbit
Malignant neoplasm of extraocular muscle
Malignant neoplasm of peripheral nerves of orbit
Malignant neoplasm of retrobulbar tissue
Malignant neoplasm of retro-ocular tissue
Excludes1: malignant neoplasm of orbital bone (C41.0)
C69.60 Malignant neoplasm of unspecified orbit
C69.61 Malignant neoplasm of right orbit
C69.62 Malignant neoplasm of left orbit
+ **C69.8** Malignant neoplasm of overlapping sites of eye and adnexa
C69.80 Malignant neoplasm of overlapping sites of unspecified eye and adnexa
C69.81 Malignant neoplasm of overlapping sites of right eye and adnexa
C69.82 Malignant neoplasm of overlapping sites of left eye and adnexa
+ **C69.9** Malignant neoplasm of unspecified site of eye
Malignant neoplasm of eyeball
C69.90 Malignant neoplasm of unspecified site of unspecified eye
C69.91 Malignant neoplasm of unspecified site of right eye
C69.92 Malignant neoplasm of unspecified site of left eye

C70 Malignant neoplasm of meninges
CC **C70.0** Malignant neoplasm of cerebral meninges
CC **C70.1** Malignant neoplasm of spinal meninges
CC **C70.9** Malignant neoplasm of meninges, unspecified

C71 Malignant neoplasm of brain
Excludes1: malignant neoplasm of cranial nerves (C72.2-C72.5)
retrobulbar malignant neoplasm (C69.6-)
CC **C71.0** Malignant neoplasm of cerebrum, except lobes and ventricles
Malignant neoplasm of supratentorial NOS
CC **C71.1** Malignant neoplasm of frontal lobe
CC **C71.2** Malignant neoplasm of temporal lobe
CC **C71.3** Malignant neoplasm of parietal lobe
CC **C71.4** Malignant neoplasm of occipital lobe
CC **C71.5** Malignant neoplasm of cerebral ventricle
Excludes1: malignant neoplasm of fourth cerebral ventricle (C71.7)
CC **C71.6** Malignant neoplasm of cerebellum
CC **C71.7** Malignant neoplasm of brain stem
Malignant neoplasm of fourth cerebral ventricle
Infratentorial malignant neoplasm NOS
CC **C71.8** Malignant neoplasm of overlapping sites of brain
CC **C71.9** Malignant neoplasm of brain, unspecified
AHA CC: 3Q, 2014, 3-4

C72 Malignant neoplasm of spinal cord, cranial nerves and other parts of central nervous system
Excludes1: malignant neoplasm of meninges (C70.-)
malignant neoplasm of peripheral nerves and autonomic nervous system (C47.-)
CC **C72.0** Malignant neoplasm of spinal cord
CC **C72.1** Malignant neoplasm of cauda equina
+ **C72.2** Malignant neoplasm of olfactory nerve
Malignant neoplasm of olfactory bulb
CC **C72.20** Malignant neoplasm of unspecified olfactory nerve
CC **C72.21** Malignant neoplasm of right olfactory nerve
CC **C72.22** Malignant neoplasm of left olfactory nerve
+ **C72.3** Malignant neoplasm of optic nerve
CC **C72.30** Malignant neoplasm of unspecified optic nerve
CC **C72.31** Malignant neoplasm of right optic nerve
CC **C72.32** Malignant neoplasm of left optic nerve
+ **C72.4** Malignant neoplasm of acoustic nerve
CC **C72.40** Malignant neoplasm of unspecified acoustic nerve
CC **C72.41** Malignant neoplasm of right acoustic nerve
CC **C72.42** Malignant neoplasm of left acoustic nerve
+ **C72.5** Malignant neoplasm of other and unspecified cranial nerves
CC **C72.50** Malignant neoplasm of unspecified cranial nerve
Malignant neoplasm of cranial nerve NOS
CC **C72.59** Malignant neoplasm of other cranial nerves
CC **C72.9** Malignant neoplasm of central nervous system, unspecified
Malignant neoplasm of unspecified site of central nervous system
Malignant neoplasm of nervous system NOS

Malignant neoplasms of thyroid and other endocrine glands (C73-C75)

C73 Malignant neoplasm of thyroid gland
Use additional code to identify any functional activity
Valid 3-character code, no further characters required

C74 Malignant neoplasm of adrenal gland
+ **C74.0** Malignant neoplasm of cortex of adrenal gland
CC **C74.00** Malignant neoplasm of cortex of unspecified adrenal gland
CC **C74.01** Malignant neoplasm of cortex of right adrenal gland
CC **C74.02** Malignant neoplasm of cortex of left adrenal gland
+ **C74.1** Malignant neoplasm of medulla of adrenal gland
CC **C74.10** Malignant neoplasm of medulla of unspecified adrenal gland
CC **C74.11** Malignant neoplasm of medulla of right adrenal gland
CC **C74.12** Malignant neoplasm of medulla of left adrenal gland
+ **C74.9** Malignant neoplasm of unspecified part of adrenal gland
CC **C74.90** Malignant neoplasm of unspecified part of unspecified adrenal gland
CC **C74.91** Malignant neoplasm of unspecified part of right adrenal gland
CC **C74.92** Malignant neoplasm of unspecified part of left adrenal gland

C75 Malignant neoplasm of other endocrine glands and related structures
Excludes1: malignant carcinoid tumors (C7A.0-)
malignant neoplasm of adrenal gland (C74.-)
malignant neoplasm of endocrine pancreas (C25.4)
malignant neoplasm of islets of Langerhans (C25.4)
malignant neoplasm of ovary (C56.-)
malignant neoplasm of testis (C62.-)
malignant neoplasm of thymus (C37)
malignant neoplasm of thyroid gland (C73)
malignant neuroendocrine tumors (C7A.-)
CC **C75.0** Malignant neoplasm of parathyroid gland
CC **C75.1** Malignant neoplasm of pituitary gland
CC **C75.2** Malignant neoplasm of craniopharyngeal duct
CC **C75.3** Malignant neoplasm of pineal gland
CC **C75.4** Malignant neoplasm of carotid body
CC **C75.5** Malignant neoplasm of aortic body and other paraganglia
CC **C75.8** Malignant neoplasm with pluriglandular involvement, unspecified
CC **C75.9** Malignant neoplasm of endocrine gland, unspecified

Malignant neuroendocrine tumors (C7A)

C7A Malignant neuroendocrine tumors
Code also any associated multiple endocrine neoplasia [MEN] syndromes (E31.2-)
Use additional code to identify any associated endocrine syndrome, such as:
carcinoid syndrome (E34.0)
Excludes2: malignant pancreatic islet cell tumors (C25.4)
Merkel cell carcinoma (C4A.-)
+ **C7A.0** Malignant carcinoid tumors
CC **C7A.00** Malignant carcinoid tumor of unspecified site
+ **C7A.01** Malignant carcinoid tumors of the small intestine
CC **C7A.010** Malignant carcinoid tumor of the duodenum
CC **C7A.011** Malignant carcinoid tumor of the jejunum
CC **C7A.012** Malignant carcinoid tumor of the ileum
CC **C7A.019** Malignant carcinoid tumor of the small intestine, unspecified portion
+ **C7A.02** Malignant carcinoid tumors of the appendix, large intestine, and rectum
CC **C7A.020** Malignant carcinoid tumor of the appendix
CC **C7A.021** Malignant carcinoid tumor of the cecum
CC **C7A.022** Malignant carcinoid tumor of the ascending colon
CC **C7A.023** Malignant carcinoid tumor of the transverse colon
CC **C7A.024** Malignant carcinoid tumor of the descending colon

CC **C7A.025** **Malignant carcinoid tumor of the sigmoid colon**
CC **C7A.026** **Malignant carcinoid tumor of the rectum**
CC **C7A.029** **Malignant carcinoid tumor of the large intestine, unspecified portion**
Malignant carcinoid tumor of the colon NOS
+ **C7A.09** **Malignant carcinoid tumors of other sites**
CC **C7A.090** **Malignant carcinoid tumor of the bronchus and lung**
CC **C7A.091** **Malignant carcinoid tumor of the thymus**
CC **C7A.092** **Malignant carcinoid tumor of the stomach**
CC **C7A.093** **Malignant carcinoid tumor of the kidney**
CC **C7A.094** **Malignant carcinoid tumor of the foregut, unspecified**
CC **C7A.095** **Malignant carcinoid tumor of the midgut, unspecified**
CC **C7A.096** **Malignant carcinoid tumor of the hindgut, unspecified**
CC **C7A.098** **Malignant carcinoid tumors of other sites**
CC **C7A.1** **Malignant poorly differentiated neuroendocrine tumors**
Malignant poorly differentiated neuroendocrine tumor NOS
Malignant poorly differentiated neuroendocrine carcinoma, any site
High grade neuroendocrine carcinoma, any site
CC **C7A.8** **Other malignant neuroendocrine tumors**
AHA CC: 3Q, 2019, 7-8

Secondary neuroendocrine tumors (C7B)

C7B **Secondary neuroendocrine tumors**
Use additional code to identify any functional activity
+ **C7B.0** **Secondary carcinoid tumors**
C7B.00 **Secondary carcinoid tumors, unspecified site**
CC **C7B.01** **Secondary carcinoid tumors of distant lymph nodes**
CC **C7B.02** **Secondary carcinoid tumors of liver**
CC **C7B.03** **Secondary carcinoid tumors of bone**
CC **C7B.04** **Secondary carcinoid tumors of peritoneum**
Mesentary metastasis of carcinoid tumor
CC **C7B.09** **Secondary carcinoid tumors of other sites**
C7B.1 **Secondary Merkel cell carcinoma**
Merkel cell carcinoma nodal presentation
Merkel cell carcinoma visceral metastatic presentation
CC **C7B.8** **Other secondary neuroendocrine tumors**
AHA CC: 3Q, 2019, 7-8

Malignant neoplasms of ill-defined, other secondary and unspecified sites (C76-C80)

Review coding guidelines C.2.b and C.2.l.2

C76 **Malignant neoplasm of other and ill-defined sites**
Excludes1: *malignant neoplasm of female genitourinary tract NOS (C57.9)*
malignant neoplasm of male genitourinary tract NOS (C63.9)
malignant neoplasm of lymphoid, hematopoietic and related tissue (C81-C96)
malignant neoplasm of skin (C44.-)
malignant neoplasm of unspecified site NOS (C80.1)
C76.0 **Malignant neoplasm of head, face and neck**
Malignant neoplasm of cheek NOS
Malignant neoplasm of nose NOS
C76.1 **Malignant neoplasm of thorax**
Intrathoracic malignant neoplasm NOS
Malignant neoplasm of axilla NOS
Thoracic malignant neoplasm NOS
C76.2 **Malignant neoplasm of abdomen**
C76.3 **Malignant neoplasm of pelvis**
Malignant neoplasm of groin NOS
Malignant neoplasm of sites overlapping systems within the pelvis
Rectovaginal (septum) malignant neoplasm
Rectovesical (septum) malignant neoplasm
+ **C76.4** **Malignant neoplasm of upper limb**
C76.40 **Malignant neoplasm of unspecified upper limb**
C76.41 **Malignant neoplasm of right upper limb**
C76.42 **Malignant neoplasm of left upper limb**
+ **C76.5** **Malignant neoplasm of lower limb**
C76.50 **Malignant neoplasm of unspecified lower limb**
C76.51 **Malignant neoplasm of right lower limb**
C76.52 **Malignant neoplasm of left lower limb**
C76.8 **Malignant neoplasm of other specified ill-defined sites**
Malignant neoplasm of overlapping ill-defined sites

+ **C77** **Secondary and unspecified malignant neoplasm of lymph nodes**
Excludes1: *malignant neoplasm of lymph nodes, specified as primary (C81-C86, C88, C96.-)*
mesentary metastasis of carcinoid tumor (C7B.04)
secondary carcinoid tumors of distant lymph nodes (C7B.01)
CC **C77.0** **Secondary and unspecified malignant neoplasm of lymph nodes of head, face and neck**
Secondary and unspecified malignant neoplasm of supraclavicular lymph nodes
CC **C77.1** **Secondary and unspecified malignant neoplasm of intrathoracic lymph nodes**
CC **C77.2** **Secondary and unspecified malignant neoplasm of intra-abdominal lymph nodes**
CC **C77.3** **Secondary and unspecified malignant neoplasm of axilla and upper limb lymph nodes**
Secondary and unspecified malignant neoplasm of pectoral lymph nodes
CC **C77.4** **Secondary and unspecified malignant neoplasm of inguinal and lower limb lymph nodes**
CC **C77.5** **Secondary and unspecified malignant neoplasm of intrapelvic lymph nodes**
CC **C77.8** **Secondary and unspecified malignant neoplasm of lymph nodes of multiple regions**
CC **C77.9** **Secondary and unspecified malignant neoplasm of lymph node, unspecified**

C78 **Secondary malignant neoplasm of respiratory and digestive organs**
Excludes1: *secondary carcinoid tumors of liver (C7B.02)*
secondary carcinoid tumors of peritoneum (C7B.04)
Excludes2: *lymph node metastases (C77.0)*
+ **C78.0** **Secondary malignant neoplasm of lung**
CC **C78.00** **Secondary malignant neoplasm of unspecified lung**
CC **C78.01** **Secondary malignant neoplasm of right lung**
CC **C78.02** **Secondary malignant neoplasm of left lung**
CC **C78.1** **Secondary malignant neoplasm of mediastinum**
CC **C78.2** **Secondary malignant neoplasm of pleura**
+ **C78.3** **Secondary malignant neoplasm of other and unspecified respiratory organs**
CC **C78.30** **Secondary malignant neoplasm of unspecified respiratory organ**
CC **C78.39** **Secondary malignant neoplasm of other respiratory organs**
CC **C78.4** **Secondary malignant neoplasm of small intestine**
CC **C78.5** **Secondary malignant neoplasm of large intestine and rectum**
CC **C78.6** **Secondary malignant neoplasm of retroperitoneum and peritoneum**
AHA CC: 2Q, 2017, 12
CC **C78.7** **Secondary malignant neoplasm of liver and intrahepatic bile duct**
+ **C78.8** **Secondary malignant neoplasm of other and unspecified digestive organs**
CC **C78.80** **Secondary malignant neoplasm of unspecified digestive organ**
CC **C78.89** **Secondary malignant neoplasm of other digestive organs**
Code also exocrine pancreatic insufficiency (K86.81)

C79 **Secondary malignant neoplasm of other and unspecified sites**
Excludes1: *secondary carcinoid tumors (C7B.-)*
secondary neuroendocrine tumors (C7B.-)
+ **C79.0** **Secondary malignant neoplasm of kidney and renal pelvis**
CC **C79.00** **Secondary malignant neoplasm of unspecified kidney and renal pelvis**
CC **C79.01** **Secondary malignant neoplasm of right kidney and renal pelvis**
CC **C79.02** **Secondary malignant neoplasm of left kidney and renal pelvis**

+, +7th, X + 7th   ● Newborn   ● Pediatric   ● Maternity   ● Adult   ♀ Female   ♂ Male   Manifestation   Unacceptable PDX   HCC   CC   MCC   HAC

+ **C79.1** Secondary malignant neoplasm of bladder and other and unspecified urinary organs
- CC **C79.10** Secondary malignant neoplasm of unspecified urinary organs
- CC **C79.11** Secondary malignant neoplasm of bladder
  - **Excludes2:** lymph node metastases (C77.0)
- CC **C79.19** Secondary malignant neoplasm of other urinary organs
- CC **C79.2** Secondary malignant neoplasm of skin
  - **Excludes1:** secondary Merkel cell carcinoma (C7B.1)
+ **C79.3** Secondary malignant neoplasm of brain and cerebral meninges
- CC **C79.31** Secondary malignant neoplasm of brain
- CC **C79.32** Secondary malignant neoplasm of cerebral meninges
  - *AHA CC: 1Q, 2020, 13-14*
+ **C79.4** Secondary malignant neoplasm of other and unspecified parts of nervous system
- CC **C79.40** Secondary malignant neoplasm of unspecified part of nervous system
- CC **C79.49** Secondary malignant neoplasm of other parts of nervous system
+ **C79.5** Secondary malignant neoplasm of bone and bone marrow
  - **Excludes1:** secondary carcinoid tumors of bone (C7B.03)
- CC **C79.51** Secondary malignant neoplasm of bone
- CC **C79.52** Secondary malignant neoplasm of bone marrow
+ **C79.6** Secondary malignant neoplasm of ovary
- ♀ CC **C79.60** Secondary malignant neoplasm of unspecified ovary
- ♀ CC **C79.61** Secondary malignant neoplasm of right ovary
- ♀ CC **C79.62** Secondary malignant neoplasm of left ovary
+ **C79.7** Secondary malignant neoplasm of adrenal gland
- CC **C79.70** Secondary malignant neoplasm of unspecified adrenal gland
- CC **C79.71** Secondary malignant neoplasm of right adrenal gland
- CC **C79.72** Secondary malignant neoplasm of left adrenal gland
+ **C79.8** Secondary malignant neoplasm of other specified sites
- CC **C79.81** Secondary malignant neoplasm of breast
- CC **C79.82** Secondary malignant neoplasm of genital organs
- CC **C79.89** Secondary malignant neoplasm of other specified sites
  - *AHA CC: 2Q, 2017, 11*
- CC **C79.9** Secondary malignant neoplasm of unspecified site
  - Metastatic cancer NOS
  - Metastatic disease NOS
  - **Excludes1:** carcinomatosis NOS (C80.0)
    - generalized cancer NOS (C80.0)
    - malignant (primary) neoplasm of unspecified site (C80.1)

C80 Malignant neoplasm without specification of site

Excludes1: malignant carcinoid tumor of unspecified site (C7A.00)
malignant neoplasm of specified multiple sites- code to each site

- CC **C80.0** Disseminated malignant neoplasm, unspecified
  - Carcinomatosis NOS
  - Generalized cancer, unspecified site (primary) (secondary)
  - Generalized malignancy, unspecified site (primary) (secondary)
  - Review coding guideline C.2.j
- **C80.1** Malignant (primary) neoplasm, unspecified
  - Cancer NOS
  - Cancer unspecified site (primary)
  - Carcinoma unspecified site (primary)
  - Malignancy unspecified site (primary)
  - **Excludes1:** secondary malignant neoplasm of unspecified site (C79.9)
  - Review coding guideline C.2.k
- CC **C80.2** Malignant neoplasm associated with transplanted organ
  - Code first complication of transplanted organ (T86.-)
  - Use additional code to identify the specific malignancy
  - Review coding guideline C.2.r

Malignant neoplasms of lymphoid, hematopoietic and related tissue (C81-C96)

Excludes2: Kaposi's sarcoma of lymph nodes (C46.3)
secondary and unspecified neoplasm of lymph nodes (C77.-)
secondary neoplasm of bone marrow (C79.52)
secondary neoplasm of spleen (C78.89)

C81 Hodgkin lymphoma

Excludes1: personal history of Hodgkin lymphoma (Z85.71)

+ **C81.0** Nodular lymphocyte predominant Hodgkin lymphoma
- CC **C81.00** Nodular lymphocyte predominant Hodgkin lymphoma, unspecified site
- CC **C81.01** Nodular lymphocyte predominant Hodgkin lymphoma, lymph nodes of head, face, and neck
- CC **C81.02** Nodular lymphocyte predominant Hodgkin lymphoma, intrathoracic lymph nodes
- CC **C81.03** Nodular lymphocyte predominant Hodgkin lymphoma, intra-abdominal lymph nodes
- CC **C81.04** Nodular lymphocyte predominant Hodgkin lymphoma, lymph nodes of axilla and upper limb
- CC **C81.05** Nodular lymphocyte predominant Hodgkin lymphoma, lymph nodes of inguinal region and lower limb
- CC **C81.06** Nodular lymphocyte predominant Hodgkin lymphoma, intrapelvic lymph nodes
- CC **C81.07** Nodular lymphocyte predominant Hodgkin lymphoma, spleen
- CC **C81.08** Nodular lymphocyte predominant Hodgkin lymphoma, lymph nodes of multiple sites
- CC **C81.09** Nodular lymphocyte predominant Hodgkin lymphoma, extranodal and solid organ sites
+ **C81.1** Nodular sclerosis Hodgkin lymphoma
  - Nodular sclerosis classical Hodgkin lymphoma
- CC **C81.10** Nodular sclerosis Hodgkin lymphoma, unspecified site
- CC **C81.11** Nodular sclerosis Hodgkin lymphoma, lymph nodes of head, face, and neck
- CC **C81.12** Nodular sclerosis Hodgkin lymphoma, intrathoracic lymph nodes
- CC **C81.13** Nodular sclerosis Hodgkin lymphoma, intra-abdominal lymph nodes
- CC **C81.14** Nodular sclerosis Hodgkin lymphoma, lymph nodes of axilla and upper limb
- CC **C81.15** Nodular sclerosis Hodgkin lymphoma, lymph nodes of inguinal region and lower limb
- CC **C81.16** Nodular sclerosis Hodgkin lymphoma, intrapelvic lymph nodes
- CC **C81.17** Nodular sclerosis Hodgkin lymphoma, spleen
- CC **C81.18** Nodular sclerosis Hodgkin lymphoma, lymph nodes of multiple sites
- CC **C81.19** Nodular sclerosis Hodgkin lymphoma, extranodal and solid organ sites
+ **C81.2** Mixed cellularity Hodgkin lymphoma
  - Mixed cellularity classical Hodgkin lymphoma
- CC **C81.20** Mixed cellularity Hodgkin lymphoma, unspecified site
- CC **C81.21** Mixed cellularity Hodgkin lymphoma, lymph nodes of head, face, and neck
- CC **C81.22** Mixed cellularity Hodgkin lymphoma, intrathoracic lymph nodes
- CC **C81.23** Mixed cellularity Hodgkin lymphoma, intra-abdominal lymph nodes
- CC **C81.24** Mixed cellularity Hodgkin lymphoma, lymph nodes of axilla and upper limb
- CC **C81.25** Mixed cellularity Hodgkin lymphoma, lymph nodes of inguinal region and lower limb
- CC **C81.26** Mixed cellularity Hodgkin lymphoma, intrapelvic lymph nodes
- CC **C81.27** Mixed cellularity Hodgkin lymphoma, spleen
- CC **C81.28** Mixed cellularity Hodgkin lymphoma, lymph nodes of multiple sites
- CC **C81.29** Mixed cellularity Hodgkin lymphoma, extranodal and solid organ sites
+ **C81.3** Lymphocyte depleted Hodgkin lymphoma
  - Lymphocyte depleted classical Hodgkin lymphoma
- CC **C81.30** Lymphocyte depleted Hodgkin lymphoma, unspecified site
- CC **C81.31** Lymphocyte depleted Hodgkin lymphoma, lymph nodes of head, face, and neck
- CC **C81.32** Lymphocyte depleted Hodgkin lymphoma, intrathoracic lymph nodes
- CC **C81.33** Lymphocyte depleted Hodgkin lymphoma, intra-abdominal lymph nodes
- CC **C81.34** Lymphocyte depleted Hodgkin lymphoma, lymph nodes of axilla and upper limb

+, +7th, X + 7th ● Newborn ● Pediatric ● Maternity ● Adult ♀ Female ♂ Male Manifestation Unacceptable PDX HCC CC MCC HAC

Lymphatic System

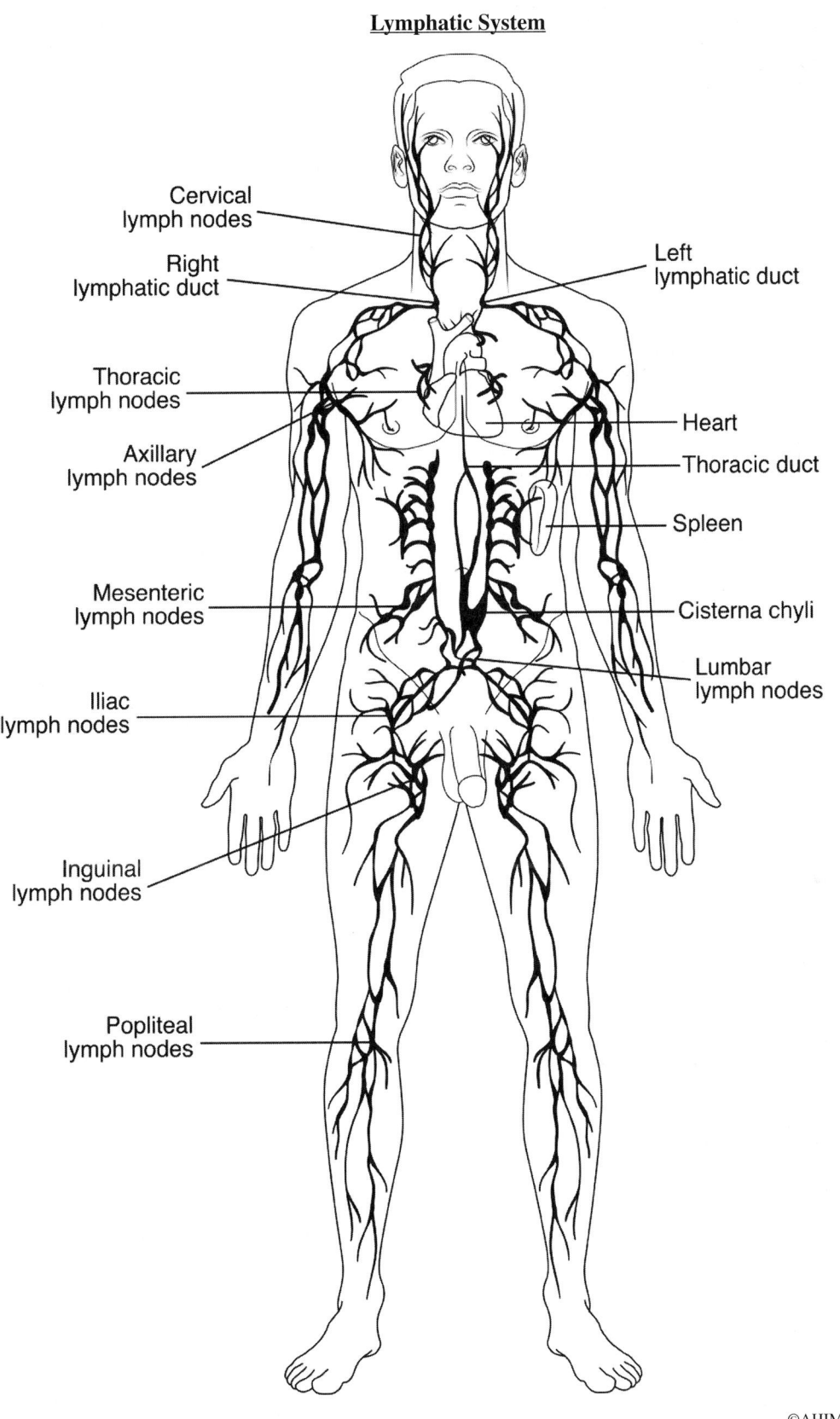

Cervical lymph nodes

Right lymphatic duct

Thoracic lymph nodes

Axillary lymph nodes

Mesenteric lymph nodes

Iliac lymph nodes

Inguinal lymph nodes

Popliteal lymph nodes

Left lymphatic duct

Heart

Thoracic duct

Spleen

Cisterna chyli

Lumbar lymph nodes

©AHIMA

CC **C81.35** Lymphocyte depleted Hodgkin lymphoma, lymph nodes of inguinal region and lower limb

CC **C81.36** Lymphocyte depleted Hodgkin lymphoma, intrapelvic lymph nodes

CC **C81.37** Lymphocyte depleted Hodgkin lymphoma, spleen

CC **C81.38** Lymphocyte depleted Hodgkin lymphoma, lymph nodes of multiple sites

CC **C81.39** Lymphocyte depleted Hodgkin lymphoma, extranodal and solid organ sites

+ **C81.4** Lymphocyte-rich Hodgkin lymphoma

Lymphocyte-rich classical Hodgkin lymphoma

Excludes1: *nodular lymphocyte predominant Hodgkin lymphoma (C81.0-)*

CC **C81.40** Lymphocyte-rich Hodgkin lymphoma, unspecified site

CC **C81.41** Lymphocyte-rich Hodgkin lymphoma, lymph nodes of head, face, and neck

CC **C81.42** Lymphocyte-rich Hodgkin lymphoma, intrathoracic lymph nodes

CC **C81.43** Lymphocyte-rich Hodgkin lymphoma, intra-abdominal lymph nodes

CC **C81.44** Lymphocyte-rich Hodgkin lymphoma, lymph nodes of axilla and upper limb

CC **C81.45** Lymphocyte-rich Hodgkin lymphoma, lymph nodes of inguinal region and lower limb

CC **C81.46** Lymphocyte-rich Hodgkin lymphoma, intrapelvic lymph nodes

CC **C81.47** Lymphocyte-rich Hodgkin lymphoma, spleen

CC **C81.48** Lymphocyte-rich Hodgkin lymphoma, lymph nodes of multiple sites

CC **C81.49** Lymphocyte-rich Hodgkin lymphoma, extranodal and solid organ sites

+ **C81.7** Other Hodgkin lymphoma

Classical Hodgkin lymphoma NOS

Other classical Hodgkin lymphoma

CC **C81.70** Other Hodgkin lymphoma, unspecified site

CC **C81.71** Other Hodgkin lymphoma, lymph nodes of head, face, and neck

CC **C81.72** Other Hodgkin lymphoma, intrathoracic lymph nodes

CC **C81.73** Other Hodgkin lymphoma, intra-abdominal lymph nodes

CC **C81.74** Other Hodgkin lymphoma, lymph nodes of axilla and upper limb

CC **C81.75** Other Hodgkin lymphoma, lymph nodes of inguinal region and lower limb

CC **C81.76** Other Hodgkin lymphoma, intrapelvic lymph nodes

CC **C81.77** Other Hodgkin lymphoma, spleen

CC **C81.78** Other Hodgkin lymphoma, lymph nodes of multiple sites

CC **C81.79** Other Hodgkin lymphoma, extranodal and solid organ sites

+ **C81.9** Hodgkin lymphoma, unspecified

CC **C81.90** Hodgkin lymphoma, unspecified, unspecified site

CC **C81.91** Hodgkin lymphoma, unspecified, lymph nodes of head, face, and neck

CC **C81.92** Hodgkin lymphoma, unspecified, intrathoracic lymph nodes

CC **C81.93** Hodgkin lymphoma, unspecified, intra-abdominal lymph nodes

CC **C81.94** Hodgkin lymphoma, unspecified, lymph nodes of axilla and upper limb

CC **C81.95** Hodgkin lymphoma, unspecified, lymph nodes of inguinal region and lower limb

CC **C81.96** Hodgkin lymphoma, unspecified, intrapelvic lymph nodes

CC **C81.97** Hodgkin lymphoma, unspecified, spleen

CC **C81.98** Hodgkin lymphoma, unspecified, lymph nodes of multiple sites

CC **C81.99** Hodgkin lymphoma, unspecified, extranodal and solid organ sites

C82 Follicular lymphoma

Includes: follicular lymphoma with or without diffuse areas

Excludes1: *mature T/NK-cell lymphomas (C84.-)*

personal history of non-Hodgkin lymphoma (Z85.72)

+ **C82.0** Follicular lymphoma grade I

CC **C82.00** Follicular lymphoma grade I, unspecified site

CC **C82.01** Follicular lymphoma grade I, lymph nodes of head, face, and neck

CC **C82.02** Follicular lymphoma grade I, intrathoracic lymph nodes

CC **C82.03** Follicular lymphoma grade I, intra-abdominal lymph nodes

CC **C82.04** Follicular lymphoma grade I, lymph nodes of axilla and upper limb

CC **C82.05** Follicular lymphoma grade I, lymph nodes of inguinal region and lower limb

CC **C82.06** Follicular lymphoma grade I, intrapelvic lymph nodes

CC **C82.07** Follicular lymphoma grade I, spleen

CC **C82.08** Follicular lymphoma grade I, lymph nodes of multiple sites

CC **C82.09** Follicular lymphoma grade I, extranodal and solid organ sites

+ **C82.1** Follicular lymphoma grade II

CC **C82.10** Follicular lymphoma grade II, unspecified site

CC **C82.11** Follicular lymphoma grade II, lymph nodes of head, face, and neck

CC **C82.12** Follicular lymphoma grade II, intrathoracic lymph nodes

CC **C82.13** Follicular lymphoma grade II, intra-abdominal lymph nodes

CC **C82.14** Follicular lymphoma grade II, lymph nodes of axilla and upper limb

CC **C82.15** Follicular lymphoma grade II, lymph nodes of inguinal region and lower limb

CC **C82.16** Follicular lymphoma grade II, intrapelvic lymph nodes

CC **C82.17** Follicular lymphoma grade II, spleen

CC **C82.18** Follicular lymphoma grade II, lymph nodes of multiple sites

CC **C82.19** Follicular lymphoma grade II, extranodal and solid organ sites

+ **C82.2** Follicular lymphoma grade III, unspecified

CC **C82.20** Follicular lymphoma grade III, unspecified, unspecified site

CC **C82.21** Follicular lymphoma grade III, unspecified, lymph nodes of head, face, and neck

CC **C82.22** Follicular lymphoma grade III, unspecified, intrathoracic lymph nodes

CC **C82.23** Follicular lymphoma grade III, unspecified, intra-abdominal lymph nodes

CC **C82.24** Follicular lymphoma grade III, unspecified, lymph nodes of axilla and upper limb

CC **C82.25** Follicular lymphoma grade III, unspecified, lymph nodes of inguinal region and lower limb

CC **C82.26** Follicular lymphoma grade III, unspecified, intrapelvic lymph nodes

CC **C82.27** Follicular lymphoma grade III, unspecified, spleen

CC **C82.28** Follicular lymphoma grade III, unspecified, lymph nodes of multiple sites

CC **C82.29** Follicular lymphoma grade III, unspecified, extranodal and solid organ sites

+ **C82.3** Follicular lymphoma grade IIIa

CC **C82.30** Follicular lymphoma grade IIIa, unspecified site

CC **C82.31** Follicular lymphoma grade IIIa, lymph nodes of head, face, and neck

CC **C82.32** Follicular lymphoma grade IIIa, intrathoracic lymph nodes

CC **C82.33** Follicular lymphoma grade IIIa, intra-abdominal lymph nodes

CC **C82.34** Follicular lymphoma grade IIIa, lymph nodes of axilla and upper limb

CC **C82.35** Follicular lymphoma grade IIIa, lymph nodes of inguinal region and lower limb

CC **C82.36** Follicular lymphoma grade IIIa, intrapelvic lymph nodes

CC **C82.37** Follicular lymphoma grade IIIa, spleen

CC **C82.38** Follicular lymphoma grade IIIa, lymph nodes of multiple sites

CC **C82.39** Follicular lymphoma grade IIIa, extranodal and solid organ sites

+ **C82.4** Follicular lymphoma grade IIIb

CC **C82.40** Follicular lymphoma grade IIIb, unspecified site

CC **C82.41** Follicular lymphoma grade IIIb, lymph nodes of head, face, and neck

CC **C82.42** Follicular lymphoma grade IIIb, intrathoracic lymph nodes

CC **C82.43** Follicular lymphoma grade IIIb, intra-abdominal lymph nodes

CC **C82.44** Follicular lymphoma grade IIIb, lymph nodes of axilla and upper limb

CC **C82.45** Follicular lymphoma grade IIIb, lymph nodes of inguinal region and lower limb

CC **C82.46** Follicular lymphoma grade IIIb, intrapelvic lymph nodes

CC **C82.47** Follicular lymphoma grade IIIb, spleen

CC **C82.48** Follicular lymphoma grade IIIb, lymph nodes of multiple sites

CC **C82.49** Follicular lymphoma grade IIIb, extranodal and solid organ sites

+ **C82.5 Diffuse follicle center lymphoma**

CC **C82.50** Diffuse follicle center lymphoma, unspecified site

CC **C82.51** Diffuse follicle center lymphoma, lymph nodes of head, face, and neck

CC **C82.52** Diffuse follicle center lymphoma, intrathoracic lymph nodes

CC **C82.53** Diffuse follicle center lymphoma, intra-abdominal lymph nodes

CC **C82.54** Diffuse follicle center lymphoma, lymph nodes of axilla and upper limb

CC **C82.55** Diffuse follicle center lymphoma, lymph nodes of inguinal region and lower limb

CC **C82.56** Diffuse follicle center lymphoma, intrapelvic lymph nodes

CC **C82.57** Diffuse follicle center lymphoma, spleen

CC **C82.58** Diffuse follicle center lymphoma, lymph nodes of multiple sites

CC **C82.59** Diffuse follicle center lymphoma, extranodal and solid organ sites

+ **C82.6 Cutaneous follicle center lymphoma**

CC **C82.60** Cutaneous follicle center lymphoma, unspecified site

CC **C82.61** Cutaneous follicle center lymphoma, lymph nodes of head, face, and neck

CC **C82.62** Cutaneous follicle center lymphoma, intrathoracic lymph nodes

CC **C82.63** Cutaneous follicle center lymphoma, intra-abdominal lymph nodes

CC **C82.64** Cutaneous follicle center lymphoma, lymph nodes of axilla and upper limb

CC **C82.65** Cutaneous follicle center lymphoma, lymph nodes of inguinal region and lower limb

CC **C82.66** Cutaneous follicle center lymphoma, intrapelvic lymph nodes

CC **C82.67** Cutaneous follicle center lymphoma, spleen

CC **C82.68** Cutaneous follicle center lymphoma, lymph nodes of multiple sites

CC **C82.69** Cutaneous follicle center lymphoma, extranodal and solid organ sites

+ **C82.8 Other types of follicular lymphoma**

CC **C82.80** Other types of follicular lymphoma, unspecified site

CC **C82.81** Other types of follicular lymphoma, lymph nodes of head, face, and neck

CC **C82.82** Other types of follicular lymphoma, intrathoracic lymph nodes

CC **C82.83** Other types of follicular lymphoma, intra-abdominal lymph nodes

CC **C82.84** Other types of follicular lymphoma, lymph nodes of axilla and upper limb

CC **C82.85** Other types of follicular lymphoma, lymph nodes of inguinal region and lower limb

CC **C82.86** Other types of follicular lymphoma, intrapelvic lymph nodes

CC **C82.87** Other types of follicular lymphoma, spleen

CC **C82.88** Other types of follicular lymphoma, lymph nodes of multiple sites

CC **C82.89** Other types of follicular lymphoma, extranodal and solid organ sites

+ **C82.9 Follicular lymphoma, unspecified**

CC **C82.90** Follicular lymphoma, unspecified, unspecified site

CC **C82.91** Follicular lymphoma, unspecified, lymph nodes of head, face, and neck

CC **C82.92** Follicular lymphoma, unspecified, intrathoracic lymph nodes

CC **C82.93** Follicular lymphoma, unspecified, intra-abdominal lymph nodes

CC **C82.94** Follicular lymphoma, unspecified, lymph nodes of axilla and upper limb

CC **C82.95** Follicular lymphoma, unspecified, lymph nodes of inguinal region and lower limb

CC **C82.96** Follicular lymphoma, unspecified, intrapelvic lymph nodes

CC **C82.97** Follicular lymphoma, unspecified, spleen

CC **C82.98** Follicular lymphoma, unspecified, lymph nodes of multiple sites

CC **C82.99** Follicular lymphoma, unspecified, extranodal and solid organ sites

C83 Non-follicular lymphoma

Excludes1: personal history of non-Hodgkin lymphoma (Z85.72)

+ **C83.0 Small cell B-cell lymphoma**

Lymphoplasmacytic lymphoma

Nodal marginal zone lymphoma

Non-leukemic variant of B-CLL

Splenic marginal zone lymphoma

Excludes1: chronic lymphocytic leukemia (C91.1)
mature T/NK-cell lymphomas (C84.-)
Waldenström macroglobulinemia (C88.0)

CC **C83.00** Small cell B-cell lymphoma, unspecified site

CC **C83.01** Small cell B-cell lymphoma, lymph nodes of head, face, and neck

CC **C83.02** Small cell B-cell lymphoma, intrathoracic lymph nodes

CC **C83.03** Small cell B-cell lymphoma, intra-abdominal lymph nodes

CC **C83.04** Small cell B-cell lymphoma, lymph nodes of axilla and upper limb

CC **C83.05** Small cell B-cell lymphoma, lymph nodes of inguinal region and lower limb

CC **C83.06** Small cell B-cell lymphoma, intrapelvic lymph nodes

CC **C83.07** Small cell B-cell lymphoma, spleen

CC **C83.08** Small cell B-cell lymphoma, lymph nodes of multiple sites

CC **C83.09** Small cell B-cell lymphoma, extranodal and solid organ sites

+ **C83.1 Mantle cell lymphoma**

Centrocytic lymphoma

Malignant lymphomatous polyposis

CC **C83.10** Mantle cell lymphoma, unspecified site

CC **C83.11** Mantle cell lymphoma, lymph nodes of head, face, and neck

CC **C83.12** Mantle cell lymphoma, intrathoracic lymph nodes

CC **C83.13** Mantle cell lymphoma, intra-abdominal lymph nodes

CC **C83.14** Mantle cell lymphoma, lymph nodes of axilla and upper limb

CC **C83.15** Mantle cell lymphoma, lymph nodes of inguinal region and lower limb

CC **C83.16** Mantle cell lymphoma, intrapelvic lymph nodes

CC **C83.17** Mantle cell lymphoma, spleen

CC **C83.18** Mantle cell lymphoma, lymph nodes of multiple sites

CC **C83.19** Mantle cell lymphoma, extranodal and solid organ sites

+ **C83.3 Diffuse large B-cell lymphoma**

Anaplastic diffuse large B-cell lymphoma

CD30-positive diffuse large B-cell lymphoma

Centroblastic diffuse large B-cell lymphoma

Diffuse large B-cell lymphoma, subtype not specified

Immunoblastic diffuse large B-cell lymphoma

Plasmablastic diffuse large B-cell lymphoma

Diffuse large B-cell lymphoma, subtype not specified

T-cell rich diffuse large B-cell lymphoma

Excludes1: mediastinal (thymic) large B-cell lymphoma (C85.2-)
mature T/NK-cell lymphomas (C84.-)

CC **C83.30** Diffuse large B-cell lymphoma, unspecified site

CC **C83.31** Diffuse large B-cell lymphoma, lymph nodes of head, face, and neck

CC **C83.32** Diffuse large B-cell lymphoma, intrathoracic lymph nodes

CC **C83.33** Diffuse large B-cell lymphoma, intra-abdominal lymph nodes

CC **C83.34** Diffuse large B-cell lymphoma, lymph nodes of axilla and upper limb

CC **C83.35** Diffuse large B-cell lymphoma, lymph nodes of inguinal region and lower limb

CC **C83.36** Diffuse large B-cell lymphoma, intrapelvic lymph nodes

CC **C83.37** Diffuse large B-cell lymphoma, spleen

+, +7th, X + 7th   ● Newborn   ● Pediatric   ● Maternity   ● Adult   ♀ Female   ♂ Male   Manifestation   Unacceptable PDX   HCC   CC   MCC   HAC

CC **C83.38** Diffuse large B-cell lymphoma, lymph nodes of multiple sites

CC **C83.39** Diffuse large B-cell lymphoma, extranodal and solid organ sites

+ **C83.5 Lymphoblastic (diffuse) lymphoma**
B-precursor lymphoma
Lymphoblastic B-cell lymphoma
Lymphoblastic lymphoma NOS
Lymphoblastic T-cell lymphoma
T-precursor lymphoma

CC **C83.50** Lymphoblastic (diffuse) lymphoma, unspecified site

CC **C83.51** Lymphoblastic (diffuse) lymphoma, lymph nodes of head, face, and neck

CC **C83.52** Lymphoblastic (diffuse) lymphoma, intrathoracic lymph nodes

CC **C83.53** Lymphoblastic (diffuse) lymphoma, intra-abdominal lymph nodes

CC **C83.54** Lymphoblastic (diffuse) lymphoma, lymph nodes of axilla and upper limb

CC **C83.55** Lymphoblastic (diffuse) lymphoma, lymph nodes of inguinal region and lower limb

CC **C83.56** Lymphoblastic (diffuse) lymphoma, intrapelvic lymph nodes

CC **C83.57** Lymphoblastic (diffuse) lymphoma, spleen

CC **C83.58** Lymphoblastic (diffuse) lymphoma, lymph nodes of multiple sites

CC **C83.59** Lymphoblastic (diffuse) lymphoma, extranodal and solid organ sites

+ **C83.7 Burkitt lymphoma**
Atypical Burkitt lymphoma
Burkitt-like lymphoma

Excludes1: *mature B-cell leukemia Burkitt type (C91.A-)*

CC **C83.70** Burkitt lymphoma, unspecified site

CC **C83.71** Burkitt lymphoma, lymph nodes of head, face, and neck

CC **C83.72** Burkitt lymphoma, intrathoracic lymph nodes

CC **C83.73** Burkitt lymphoma, intra-abdominal lymph nodes

CC **C83.74** Burkitt lymphoma, lymph nodes of axilla and upper limb

CC **C83.75** Burkitt lymphoma, lymph nodes of inguinal region and lower limb

CC **C83.76** Burkitt lymphoma, intrapelvic lymph nodes

CC **C83.77** Burkitt lymphoma, spleen

CC **C83.78** Burkitt lymphoma, lymph nodes of multiple sites

CC **C83.79** Burkitt lymphoma, extranodal and solid organ sites

+ **C83.8 Other non-follicular lymphoma**
Intravascular large B-cell lymphoma
Lymphoid granulomatosis
Primary effusion B-cell lymphoma

Excludes1: *mediastinal (thymic) large B-cell lymphoma (C85.2-)*
T-cell rich B-cell lymphoma (C83.3-)

CC **C83.80** Other non-follicular lymphoma, unspecified site

CC **C83.81** Other non-follicular lymphoma, lymph nodes of head, face, and neck

CC **C83.82** Other non-follicular lymphoma, intrathoracic lymph nodes

CC **C83.83** Other non-follicular lymphoma, intra-abdominal lymph nodes

CC **C83.84** Other non-follicular lymphoma, lymph nodes of axilla and upper limb

CC **C83.85** Other non-follicular lymphoma, lymph nodes of inguinal region and lower limb

CC **C83.86** Other non-follicular lymphoma, intrapelvic lymph nodes

CC **C83.87** Other non-follicular lymphoma, spleen

CC **C83.88** Other non-follicular lymphoma, lymph nodes of multiple sites

CC **C83.89** Other non-follicular lymphoma, extranodal and solid organ sites

+ **C83.9 Non-follicular (diffuse) lymphoma, unspecified**

CC **C83.90** Non-follicular (diffuse) lymphoma, unspecified, unspecified site

CC **C83.91** Non-follicular (diffuse) lymphoma, unspecified, lymph nodes of head, face, and neck

CC **C83.92** Non-follicular (diffuse) lymphoma, unspecified, intrathoracic lymph nodes

CC **C83.93** Non-follicular (diffuse) lymphoma, unspecified, intra-abdominal lymph nodes

CC **C83.94** Non-follicular (diffuse) lymphoma, unspecified, lymph nodes of axilla and upper limb

CC **C83.95** Non-follicular (diffuse) lymphoma, unspecified, lymph nodes of inguinal region and lower limb

CC **C83.96** Non-follicular (diffuse) lymphoma, unspecified, intrapelvic lymph nodes

CC **C83.97** Non-follicular (diffuse) lymphoma, unspecified, spleen

CC **C83.98** Non-follicular (diffuse) lymphoma, unspecified, lymph nodes of multiple sites

CC **C83.99** Non-follicular (diffuse) lymphoma, unspecified, extranodal and solid organ sites

C84 Mature T/NK-cell lymphomas

Excludes1: *personal history of non-Hodgkin lymphoma (Z85.72)*

+ **C84.0 Mycosis fungoides**

Excludes1: *peripheral T-cell lymphoma, not classified (C84.4-)*

CC **C84.00** Mycosis fungoides, unspecified site

CC **C84.01** Mycosis fungoides, lymph nodes of head, face, and neck

CC **C84.02** Mycosis fungoides, intrathoracic lymph nodes

CC **C84.03** Mycosis fungoides, intra-abdominal lymph nodes

CC **C84.04** Mycosis fungoides, lymph nodes of axilla and upper limb

CC **C84.05** Mycosis fungoides, lymph nodes of inguinal region and lower limb

CC **C84.06** Mycosis fungoides, intrapelvic lymph nodes

CC **C84.07** Mycosis fungoides, spleen

CC **C84.08** Mycosis fungoides, lymph nodes of multiple sites

CC **C84.09** Mycosis fungoides, extranodal and solid organ sites

+ **C84.1 Sézary disease**

CC **C84.10** Sézary disease, unspecified site

CC **C84.11** Sézary disease, lymph nodes of head, face, and neck

CC **C84.12** Sézary disease, intrathoracic lymph nodes

CC **C84.13** Sézary disease, intra-abdominal lymph nodes

CC **C84.14** Sézary disease, lymph nodes of axilla and upper limb

CC **C84.15** Sézary disease, lymph nodes of inguinal region and lower limb

CC **C84.16** Sézary disease, intrapelvic lymph nodes

CC **C84.17** Sézary disease, spleen

CC **C84.18** Sézary disease, lymph nodes of multiple sites

CC **C84.19** Sézary disease, extranodal and solid organ sites

+ **C84.4 Peripheral T-cell lymphoma, not classified**
Lennert's lymphoma
Lymphoepithelioid lymphoma
Mature T-cell lymphoma, not elsewhere classified

CC **C84.40** Peripheral T-cell lymphoma, not classified, unspecified site

CC **C84.41** Peripheral T-cell lymphoma, not classified, lymph nodes of head, face, and neck

CC **C84.42** Peripheral T-cell lymphoma, not classified, intrathoracic lymph nodes

CC **C84.43** Peripheral T-cell lymphoma, not classified, intra-abdominal lymph nodes

CC **C84.44** Peripheral T-cell lymphoma, not classified, lymph nodes of axilla and upper limb

CC **C84.45** Peripheral T-cell lymphoma, not classified, lymph nodes of inguinal region and lower limb

CC **C84.46** Peripheral T-cell lymphoma, not classified, intrapelvic lymph nodes

CC **C84.47** Peripheral T-cell lymphoma, not classified, spleen

CC **C84.48** Peripheral T-cell lymphoma, not classified, lymph nodes of multiple sites

CC **C84.49** Peripheral T-cell lymphoma, not classified, extranodal and solid organ sites

+ **C84.6 Anaplastic large cell lymphoma, ALK-positive**
Anaplastic large cell lymphoma, CD30-positive

CC **C84.60** Anaplastic large cell lymphoma, ALK-positive, unspecified site

CC **C84.61** Anaplastic large cell lymphoma, ALK-positive, lymph nodes of head, face, and neck

CC **C84.62** Anaplastic large cell lymphoma, ALK-positive, intrathoracic lymph nodes

CC **C84.63** Anaplastic large cell lymphoma, ALK-positive, intra-abdominal lymph nodes

CC **C84.64** Anaplastic large cell lymphoma, ALK-positive, lymph nodes of axilla and upper limb

CC **C84.65** Anaplastic large cell lymphoma, ALK-positive, lymph nodes of inguinal region and lower limb

CC **C84.66** Anaplastic large cell lymphoma, ALK-positive, intrapelvic lymph nodes

CC **C84.67** Anaplastic large cell lymphoma, ALK-positive, spleen

CC **C84.68** Anaplastic large cell lymphoma, ALK-positive, lymph nodes of multiple sites

CC **C84.69** Anaplastic large cell lymphoma, ALK-positive, extranodal and solid organ sites

\+ **C84.7 Anaplastic large cell lymphoma, ALK-negative**

　Excludes1: primary cutaneous CD30-positive T-cell proliferations (C86.6-)

CC **C84.70** Anaplastic large cell lymphoma, ALK-negative, unspecified site

CC **C84.71** Anaplastic large cell lymphoma, ALK-negative, lymph nodes of head, face, and neck

CC **C84.72** Anaplastic large cell lymphoma, ALK-negative, intrathoracic lymph nodes

CC **C84.73** Anaplastic large cell lymphoma, ALK-negative, intra-abdominal lymph nodes

CC **C84.74** Anaplastic large cell lymphoma, ALK-negative, lymph nodes of axilla and upper limb

CC **C84.75** Anaplastic large cell lymphoma, ALK-negative, lymph nodes of inguinal region and lower limb

CC **C84.76** Anaplastic large cell lymphoma, ALK-negative, intrapelvic lymph nodes

CC **C84.77** Anaplastic large cell lymphoma, ALK-negative, spleen

CC **C84.78** Anaplastic large cell lymphoma, ALK-negative, lymph nodes of multiple sites

CC **C84.79** Anaplastic large cell lymphoma, ALK-negative, extranodal and solid organ sites

\+ **C84.A Cutaneous T-cell lymphoma, unspecified**

CC **C84.A0** Cutaneous T-cell lymphoma, unspecified, unspecified site

CC **C84.A1** Cutaneous T-cell lymphoma, unspecified lymph nodes of head, face, and neck

CC **C84.A2** Cutaneous T-cell lymphoma, unspecified, intrathoracic lymph nodes

CC **C84.A3** Cutaneous T-cell lymphoma, unspecified, intra-abdominal lymph nodes

CC **C84.A4** Cutaneous T-cell lymphoma, unspecified, lymph nodes of axilla and upper limb

CC **C84.A5** Cutaneous T-cell lymphoma, unspecified, lymph nodes of inguinal region and lower limb

CC **C84.A6** Cutaneous T-cell lymphoma, unspecified, intrapelvic lymph nodes

CC **C84.A7** Cutaneous T-cell lymphoma, unspecified, spleen

CC **C84.A8** Cutaneous T-cell lymphoma, unspecified, lymph nodes of multiple sites

CC **C84.A9** Cutaneous T-cell lymphoma, unspecified, extranodal and solid organ sites

\+ **C84.Z Other mature T/NK-cell lymphomas**

　NOTE If T-cell lineage or involvement is mentioned in conjunction with a specific lymphoma, code to the more specific description.

　Excludes1: angioimmunoblastic T-cell lymphoma (C86.5) blastic NK-cell lymphoma (C86.4) enteropathy-type T-cell lymphoma (C86.2) extranodal NK-cell lymphoma, nasal type (C86.0) hepatosplenic T-cell lymphoma (C86.1) primary cutaneous CD30-positive T-cell proliferations (C86.6) subcutaneous panniculitis-like T-cell lymphoma (C86.3) T-cell leukemia (C91.1-)

CC **C84.Z0** Other mature T/NK-cell lymphomas, unspecified site

CC **C84.Z1** Other mature T/NK-cell lymphomas, lymph nodes of head, face, and neck

CC **C84.Z2** Other mature T/NK-cell lymphomas, intrathoracic lymph nodes

CC **C84.Z3** Other mature T/NK-cell lymphomas, intra-abdominal lymph nodes

CC **C84.Z4** Other mature T/NK-cell lymphomas, lymph nodes of axilla and upper limb

CC **C84.Z5** Other mature T/NK-cell lymphomas, lymph nodes of inguinal region and lower limb

CC **C84.Z6** Other mature T/NK-cell lymphomas, intrapelvic lymph nodes

CC **C84.Z7** Other mature T/NK-cell lymphomas, spleen

CC **C84.Z8** Other mature T/NK-cell lymphomas, lymph nodes of multiple sites

CC **C84.Z9** Other mature T/NK-cell lymphomas, extranodal and solid organ sites

\+ **C84.9 Mature T/NK-cell lymphomas, unspecified**

　NK/T cell lymphoma NOS

　Excludes1: mature T-cell lymphoma, not elsewhere classified (C84.4-)

CC **C84.90** Mature T/NK-cell lymphomas, unspecified, unspecified site

CC **C84.91** Mature T/NK-cell lymphomas, unspecified, lymph nodes of head, face, and neck

CC **C84.92** Mature T/NK-cell lymphomas, unspecified, intrathoracic lymph nodes

CC **C84.93** Mature T/NK-cell lymphomas, unspecified, intra-abdominal lymph nodes

CC **C84.94** Mature T/NK-cell lymphomas, unspecified, lymph nodes of axilla and upper limb

CC **C84.95** Mature T/NK-cell lymphomas, unspecified, lymph nodes of inguinal region and lower limb

CC **C84.96** Mature T/NK-cell lymphomas, unspecified, intrapelvic lymph nodes

CC **C84.97** Mature T/NK-cell lymphomas, unspecified, spleen

CC **C84.98** Mature T/NK-cell lymphomas, unspecified, lymph nodes of multiple sites

CC **C84.99** Mature T/NK-cell lymphomas, unspecified, extranodal and solid organ sites

C85 Other specified and unspecified types of non-Hodgkin lymphoma

　Excludes1: other specified types of T/NK-cell lymphoma (C86.-) personal history of non-Hodgkin lymphoma (Z85.72)

\+ **C85.1 Unspecified B-cell lymphoma**

　NOTE If B-cell lineage or involvement is mentioned in conjunction with a specific lymphoma, code to the more specific description.

CC **C85.10** Unspecified B-cell lymphoma, unspecified site

CC **C85.11** Unspecified B-cell lymphoma, lymph nodes of head, face, and neck

CC **C85.12** Unspecified B-cell lymphoma, intrathoracic lymph nodes

CC **C85.13** Unspecified B-cell lymphoma, intra-abdominal lymph nodes

CC **C85.14** Unspecified B-cell lymphoma, lymph nodes of axilla and upper limb

CC **C85.15** Unspecified B-cell lymphoma, lymph nodes of inguinal region and lower limb

CC **C85.16** Unspecified B-cell lymphoma, intrapelvic lymph nodes

CC **C85.17** Unspecified B-cell lymphoma, spleen

CC **C85.18** Unspecified B-cell lymphoma, lymph nodes of multiple sites

CC **C85.19** Unspecified B-cell lymphoma, extranodal and solid organ sites

\+ **C85.2 Mediastinal (thymic) large B-cell lymphoma**

CC **C85.20** Mediastinal (thymic) large B-cell lymphoma, unspecified site

CC **C85.21** Mediastinal (thymic) large B-cell lymphoma, lymph nodes of head, face, and neck

CC **C85.22** Mediastinal (thymic) large B-cell lymphoma, intrathoracic lymph nodes

CC **C85.23** Mediastinal (thymic) large B-cell lymphoma, intra-abdominal lymph nodes

CC **C85.24** Mediastinal (thymic) large B-cell lymphoma, lymph nodes of axilla and upper limb

CC **C85.25** Mediastinal (thymic) large B-cell lymphoma, lymph nodes of inguinal region and lower limb

CC **C85.26** Mediastinal (thymic) large B-cell lymphoma, intrapelvic lymph nodes

CC **C85.27** Mediastinal (thymic) large B-cell lymphoma, spleen

CC **C85.28** Mediastinal (thymic) large B-cell lymphoma, lymph nodes of multiple sites

CC **C85.29** Mediastinal (thymic) large B-cell lymphoma, extranodal and solid organ sites

\+ **C85.8 Other specified types of non-Hodgkin lymphoma**

CC **C85.80** Other specified types of non-Hodgkin lymphoma, unspecified site

CC **C85.81** Other specified types of non-Hodgkin lymphoma, lymph nodes of head, face, and neck

CC **C85.82** Other specified types of non-Hodgkin lymphoma, intrathoracic lymph nodes

CC **C85.83** Other specified types of non-Hodgkin lymphoma, intra-abdominal lymph nodes

CC **C85.84** Other specified types of non-Hodgkin lymphoma, lymph nodes of axilla and upper limb

CC **C85.85** Other specified types of non-Hodgkin lymphoma, lymph nodes of inguinal region and lower limb

CC **C85.86** Other specified types of non-Hodgkin lymphoma, intrapelvic lymph nodes

CC **C85.87** Other specified types of non-Hodgkin lymphoma, spleen

CC **C85.88** Other specified types of non-Hodgkin lymphoma, lymph nodes of multiple sites

CC **C85.89** Other specified types of non-Hodgkin lymphoma, extranodal and solid organ sites

+ **C85.9 Non-Hodgkin lymphoma, unspecified**
   Lymphoma NOS
   Malignant lymphoma NOS
   Non-Hodgkin lymphoma NOS

CC **C85.90** Non-Hodgkin lymphoma, unspecified, unspecified site

CC **C85.91** Non-Hodgkin lymphoma, unspecified, lymph nodes of head, face, and neck

CC **C85.92** Non-Hodgkin lymphoma, unspecified, intrathoracic lymph nodes

CC **C85.93** Non-Hodgkin lymphoma, unspecified, intra-abdominal lymph nodes

CC **C85.94** Non-Hodgkin lymphoma, unspecified, lymph nodes of axilla and upper limb

CC **C85.95** Non-Hodgkin lymphoma, unspecified, lymph nodes of inguinal region and lower limb

CC **C85.96** Non-Hodgkin lymphoma, unspecified, intrapelvic lymph nodes

CC **C85.97** Non-Hodgkin lymphoma, unspecified, spleen

CC **C85.98** Non-Hodgkin lymphoma, unspecified, lymph nodes of multiple sites

CC **C85.99** Non-Hodgkin lymphoma, unspecified, extranodal and solid organ sites

C86 Other specified types of T/NK-cell lymphoma

Excludes1: *anaplastic large cell lymphoma, ALK negative (C84.7-)*
anaplastic large cell lymphoma, ALK positive (C84.6-)
mature T/NK-cell lymphomas (C84.-)
other specified types of non-Hodgkin lymphoma (C85.8-)

CC **C86.0 Extranodal NK/T-cell lymphoma, nasal type**

CC **C86.1 Hepatosplenic T-cell lymphoma**
   Alpha-beta and gamma delta types

CC **C86.2 Enteropathy-type (intestinal) T-cell lymphoma**
   Enteropathy associated T-cell lymphoma

CC **C86.3 Subcutaneous panniculitis-like T-cell lymphoma**

CC **C86.4 Blastic NK-cell lymphoma**
   Blastic plasmacytoid dendritic cell neoplasm (BPDCN)

CC **C86.5 Angioimmunoblastic T-cell lymphoma**
   Angioimmunoblastic lymphadenopathy with dysproteinemia (AILD)

CC **C86.6 Primary cutaneous CD30-positive T-cell proliferations**
   Lymphomatoid papulosis
   Primary cutaneous anaplastic large cell lymphoma
   Primary cutaneous CD30-positive large T-cell lymphoma

C88 Malignant immunoproliferative diseases and certain other B-cell lymphomas

Excludes1: *B-cell lymphoma, unspecified (C85.1-)*
personal history of other malignant neoplasms of lymphoid, hematopoietic and related tissues (Z85.79)

C88.0 Waldenström macroglobulinemia
   Lymphoplasmacytic lymphoma with IgM-production
   Macroglobulinemia (idiopathic) (primary)
   Excludes1: *small cell B-cell lymphoma (C83.0)*

CC **C88.2 Heavy chain disease**
   Franklin disease
   Gamma heavy chain disease
   Mu heavy chain disease

CC **C88.3 Immunoproliferative small intestinal disease**
   Alpha heavy chain disease
   Mediterranean lymphoma

CC **C88.4 Extranodal marginal zone B-cell lymphoma of mucosa-associated lymphoid tissue [MALT-lymphoma]**
   Lymphoma of skin-associated lymphoid tissue [SALT-lymphoma]
   Lymphoma of bronchial-associated lymphoid tissue [BALT-lymphoma]
   Excludes1: *high malignant (diffuse large B-cell) lymphoma (C83.3-)*

CC **C88.8 Other malignant immunoproliferative diseases**

CC **C88.9 Malignant immunoproliferative disease, unspecified**
   Immunoproliferative disease NOS

C90 Multiple myeloma and malignant plasma cell neoplasms

Excludes1: *personal history of other malignant neoplasms of lymphoid, hematopoietic and related tissues (Z85.79)*

+ **C90.0 Multiple myeloma**
   Kahler's disease
   Medullary plasmacytoma
   Myelomatosis
   Plasma cell myeloma
   Excludes1: *solitary myeloma (C90.3-)*
      solitary plasmactyoma (C90.3-)

CC **C90.00 Multiple myeloma not having achieved remission**
   Multiple myeloma with failed remission
   Multiple myeloma NOS

CC **C90.01 Multiple myeloma in remission**

CC **C90.02 Multiple myeloma in relapse**

+ **C90.1 Plasma cell leukemia**
   Plasmacytic leukemia

CC **C90.10 Plasma cell leukemia not having achieved remission**
   Plasma cell leukemia with failed remission
   Plasma cell leukemia NOS
   AHA CC: 2Q, 2019, 30

CC **C90.11 Plasma cell leukemia in remission**

CC **C90.12 Plasma cell leukemia in relapse**

+ **C90.2 Extramedullary plasmacytoma**

CC **C90.20 Extramedullary plasmacytoma not having achieved remission**
   Extramedullary plasmacytoma with failed remission
   Extramedullary plasmacytoma NOS

CC **C90.21 Extramedullary plasmacytoma in remission**

CC **C90.22 Extramedullary plasmacytoma in relapse**

+ **C90.3 Solitary plasmacytoma**
   Localized malignant plasma cell tumor NOS
   Plasmacytoma NOS
   Solitary myeloma

CC **C90.30 Solitary plasmacytoma not having achieved remission**
   Solitary plasmacytoma with failed remission
   Solitary plasmacytoma NOS

CC **C90.31 Solitary plasmacytoma in remission**

CC **C90.32 Solitary plasmacytoma in relapse**

C91 Lymphoid leukemia

Excludes1: *personal history of leukemia (Z85.6)*

+ **C91.0 Acute lymphoblastic leukemia [ALL]**
   NOTE Codes in subcategory C91.0- should only be used for T-cell and B-cell precursor leukemia

CC **C91.00 Acute lymphoblastic leukemia not having achieved remission**
   Acute lymphoblastic leukemia with failed remission
   Acute lymphoblastic leukemia NOS

CC **C91.01 Acute lymphoblastic leukemia, in remission**

CC **C91.02 Acute lymphoblastic leukemia, in relapse**

+ **C91.1 Chronic lymphocytic leukemia of B-cell type**
   Lymphoplasmacytic leukemia
   Richter syndrome
   Excludes1: *lymphoplasmacytic lymphoma (C83.0-)*

CC **C91.10 Chronic lymphocytic leukemia of B-cell type not having achieved remission**
   Chronic lymphocytic leukemia of B-cell type with failed remission
   Chronic lymphocytic leukemia of B-cell type NOS

CC **C91.11** Chronic lymphocytic leukemia of B-cell type in remission

CC **C91.12** Chronic lymphocytic leukemia of B-cell type in relapse

+ **C91.3 Prolymphocytic leukemia of B-cell type**

CC **C91.30** Prolymphocytic leukemia of B-cell type not having achieved remission

Prolymphocytic leukemia of B-cell type with failed remission

Prolymphocytic leukemia of B-cell type NOS

CC **C91.31** Prolymphocytic leukemia of B-cell type, in remission

CC **C91.32** Prolymphocytic leukemia of B-cell type, in relapse

+ **C91.4 Hairy cell leukemia**

Leukemic reticuloendotheliosis

CC **C91.40** Hairy cell leukemia not having achieved remission

Hairy cell leukemia with failed remission
Hairy cell leukemia NOS

CC **C91.41** Hairy cell leukemia, in remission

CC **C91.42** Hairy cell leukemia, in relapse

+ **C91.5 Adult T-cell lymphoma/leukemia (HTLV-1-associated)**

Acute variant of adult T-cell lymphoma/leukemia (HTLV-1-associated)

Chronic variant of adult T-cell lymphoma/leukemia (HTLV-1-associated)

Lymphomatoid variant of adult T-cell lymphoma/leukemia (HTLV-1-associated)

Smouldering variant of adult T-cell lymphoma/leukemia (HTLV-1-associated)

● CC **C91.50** Adult T-cell lymphoma/leukemia (HTLV-1-associated) not having achieved remission

Adult T-cell lymphoma/leukemia (HTLV-1-associated) with failed remission

Adult T-cell lymphoma/leukemia (HTLV-1-associated) NOS

● CC **C91.51** Adult T-cell lymphoma/leukemia (HTLV-1-associated), in remission

● CC **C91.52** Adult T-cell lymphoma/leukemia (HTLV-1-associated), in relapse

+ **C91.6 Prolymphocytic leukemia of T-cell type**

CC **C91.60** Prolymphocytic leukemia of T-cell type not having achieved remission

Prolymphocytic leukemia of T-cell type with failed remission

Prolymphocytic leukemia of T-cell type NOS

CC **C91.61** Prolymphocytic leukemia of T-cell type, in remission

CC **C91.62** Prolymphocytic leukemia of T-cell type, in relapse

+ **C91.A Mature B-cell leukemia Burkitt-type**

Excludes1: *Burkitt lymphoma (C83.7-)*

CC **C91.A0** Mature B-cell leukemia Burkitt-type not having achieved remission

Mature B-cell leukemia Burkitt-type with failed remission

Mature B-cell leukemia Burkitt-type NOS

CC **C91.A1** Mature B-cell leukemia Burkitt-type, in remission

CC **C91.A2** Mature B-cell leukemia Burkitt-type, in relapse

+ **C91.Z Other lymphoid leukemia**

T-cell large granular lymphocytic leukemia (associated with rheumatoid arthritis)

CC **C91.Z0** Other lymphoid leukemia not having achieved remission

Other lymphoid leukemia with failed remission
Other lymphoid leukemia NOS

AHA CC: 2Q, 2019, 24-26

CC **C91.Z1** Other lymphoid leukemia, in remission

CC **C91.Z2** Other lymphoid leukemia, in relapse

+ **C91.9 Lymphoid leukemia, unspecified**

CC **C91.90** Lymphoid leukemia, unspecified not having achieved remission

Lymphoid leukemia with failed remission
Lymphoid leukemia NOS

CC **C91.91** Lymphoid leukemia, unspecified, in remission

CC **C91.92** Lymphoid leukemia, unspecified, in relapse

C92 Myeloid leukemia

Includes: granulocytic leukemia
myelogenous leukemia

Excludes1: *personal history of leukemia (Z85.6)*

AHA CC: 1Q, 2019, 16-17

+ **C92.0 Acute myeloblastic leukemia**

Acute myeloblastic leukemia, minimal differentiation
Acute myeloblastic leukemia (with maturation)
Acute myeloblastic leukemia 1/ETO
Acute myeloblastic leukemia M0
Acute myeloblastic leukemia M1
Acute myeloblastic leukemia M2
Acute myeloblastic leukemia with t(8;21)
Acute myeloblastic leukemia (without a FAB classification) NOS
Refractory anemia with excess blasts in transformation [RAEB T]

Excludes1: *acute exacerbation of chronic myeloid leukemia (C92.10)*

refractory anemia with excess of blasts not in transformation (D46.2-)

AHA CC: 4Q, 2018, 87

CC **C92.00** Acute myeloblastic leukemia, not having achieved remission

Acute myeloblastic leukemia with failed remission
Acute myeloblastic leukemia NOS

CC **C92.01** Acute myeloblastic leukemia, in remission

CC **C92.02** Acute myeloblastic leukemia, in relapse

+ **C92.1 Chronic myeloid leukemia, BCR/ABL-positive**

Chronic myelogenous leukemia, Philadelphia chromosome (Ph1) positive

Chronic myelogenous leukemia, t(9;22) (q34;q11)

Chronic myelogenous leukemia with crisis of blast cells

Excludes1: *atypical chronic myeloid leukemia BCR/ABL-negative (C92.2-)*

chronic myelomonocytic leukemia (C93.1-)

chronic myeloproliferative disease (D47.1)

CC **C92.10** Chronic myeloid leukemia, BCR/ABL-positive, not having achieved remission

Chronic myeloid leukemia, BCR/ABL-positive with failed remission

Chronic myeloid leukemia, BCR/ABL-positive NOS

AHA CC: 1Q, 2017, 7

CC **C92.11** Chronic myeloid leukemia, BCR/ABL-positive, in remission

CC **C92.12** Chronic myeloid leukemia, BCR/ABL-positive, in relapse

+ **C92.2 Atypical chronic myeloid leukemia, BCR/ABL-negative**

CC **C92.20** Atypical chronic myeloid leukemia, BCR/ABL-negative, not having achieved remission

Atypical chronic myeloid leukemia, BCR/ABL-negative with failed remission

Atypical chronic myeloid leukemia, BCR/ABL-negative NOS

CC **C92.21** Atypical chronic myeloid leukemia, BCR/ABL-negative, in remission

CC **C92.22** Atypical chronic myeloid leukemia, BCR/ABL-negative, in relapse

+ **C92.3 Myeloid sarcoma**

A malignant tumor of immature myeloid cells
Chloroma
Granulocytic sarcoma

CC **C92.30** Myeloid sarcoma, not having achieved remission

Myeloid sarcoma with failed remission
Myeloid sarcoma NOS

CC **C92.31** Myeloid sarcoma, in remission

CC **C92.32** Myeloid sarcoma, in relapse

+ **C92.4 Acute promyelocytic leukemia**

AML M3
AML Me with t(15;17) and variants

CC **C92.40** Acute promyelocytic leukemia, not having achieved remission

Acute promyelocytic leukemia with failed remission

Acute promyelocytic leukemia NOS

CC **C92.41** Acute promyelocytic leukemia, in remission

CC **C92.42** Acute promyelocytic leukemia, in relapse

521

+ **C92.5** **Acute myelomonocytic leukemia**
    AML M4
    AML M4 Eo with inv(16) or t(16;16)
   CC **C92.50** **Acute myelomonocytic leukemia, not having achieved remission**
       Acute myelomonocytic leukemia with failed remission
       Acute myelomonocytic leukemia NOS
   CC **C92.51** **Acute myelomonocytic leukemia, in remission**
   CC **C92.52** **Acute myelomonocytic leukemia, in relapse**
+ **C92.6** **Acute myeloid leukemia with 11q23-abnormality**
    Acute myeloid leukemia with variation of MLL-gene
   CC **C92.60** **Acute myeloid leukemia with 11q23-abnormality not having achieved remission**
       Acute myeloid leukemia with 11q23-abnormality with failed remission
       Acute myeloid leukemia with 11q23-abnormality NOS
   CC **C92.61** **Acute myeloid leukemia with 11q23-abnormality in remission**
   CC **C92.62** **Acute myeloid leukemia with 11q23-abnormality in relapse**
+ **C92.A** **Acute myeloid leukemia with multilineage dysplasia**
    Acute myeloid leukemia with dysplasia of remaining hematopoesis and/or myelodysplastic disease in its history
   CC **C92.A0** **Acute myeloid leukemia with multilineage dysplasia, not having achieved remission**
       Acute myeloid leukemia with multilineage dysplasia with failed remission
       Acute myeloid leukemia with multilineage dysplasia NOS
   CC **C92.A1** **Acute myeloid leukemia with multilineage dysplasia, in remission**
   CC **C92.A2** **Acute myeloid leukemia with multilineage dysplasia, in relapse**
+ **C92.Z** **Other myeloid leukemia**
   CC **C92.Z0** **Other myeloid leukemia not having achieved remission**
       Myeloid leukemia NEC with failed remission
       Myeloid leukemia NEC
   CC **C92.Z1** **Other myeloid leukemia, in remission**
   CC **C92.Z2** **Other myeloid leukemia, in relapse**
+ **C92.9** **Myeloid leukemia, unspecified**
   CC **C92.90** **Myeloid leukemia, unspecified, not having achieved remission**
       Myeloid leukemia, unspecified with failed remission
       Myeloid leukemia, unspecified NOS
   CC **C92.91** **Myeloid leukemia, unspecified in remission**
   CC **C92.92** **Myeloid leukemia, unspecified in relapse**

C93 **Monocytic leukemia**

   Includes: monocytoid leukemia
   Excludes1: *personal history of leukemia (Z85.6)*
+ **C93.0** **Acute monoblastic/monocytic leukemia**
    AML M5
    AML M5a
    AML M5b
   CC **C93.00** **Acute monoblastic/monocytic leukemia, not having achieved remission**
       Acute monoblastic/monocytic leukemia with failed remission
       Acute monoblastic/monocytic leukemia NOS
   CC **C93.01** **Acute monoblastic/monocytic leukemia, in remission**
   CC **C93.02** **Acute monoblastic/monocytic leukemia, in relapse**
+ **C93.1** **Chronic myelomonocytic leukemia**
    Chronic monocytic leukemia
    CMML-1
    CMML-2
    CMML with eosinophilia
    Code also, if applicable, eosinophilia (D72.18)
   CC **C93.10** **Chronic myelomonocytic leukemia not having achieved remission**
       Chronic myelomonocytic leukemia with failed remission
       Chronic myelomonocytic leukemia NOS
   CC **C93.11** **Chronic myelomonocytic leukemia, in remission**
   CC **C93.12** **Chronic myelomonocytic leukemia, in relapse**

+ **C93.3** **Juvenile myelomonocytic leukemia**
   ● CC **C93.30** **Juvenile myelomonocytic leukemia, not having achieved remission**
       Juvenile myelomonocytic leukemia with failed remission
       Juvenile myelomonocytic leukemia NOS
   ● CC **C93.31** **Juvenile myelomonocytic leukemia, in remission**
   ● CC **C93.32** **Juvenile myelomonocytic leukemia, in relapse**
+ **C93.Z** **Other monocytic leukemia**
   CC **C93.Z0** **Other monocytic leukemia, not having achieved remission**
       Other monocytic leukemia NOS
   CC **C93.Z1** **Other monocytic leukemia, in remission**
   CC **C93.Z2** **Other monocytic leukemia, in relapse**
+ **C93.9** **Monocytic leukemia, unspecified**
   CC **C93.90** **Monocytic leukemia, unspecified, not having achieved remission**
       Monocytic leukemia, unspecified with failed remission
       Monocytic leukemia, unspecified NOS
   CC **C93.91** **Monocytic leukemia, unspecified in remission**
   CC **C93.92** **Monocytic leukemia, unspecified in relapse**

C94 **Other leukemias of specified cell type**

   Excludes1: *leukemic reticuloendotheliosis (C91.4-)*
       myelodysplastic syndromes (D46.-)
       personal history of leukemia (Z85.6)
       plasma cell leukemia (C90.1-)
+ **C94.0** **Acute erythroid leukemia**
    Acute myeloid leukemia M6(a)(b)
    Erythroleukemia
   CC **C94.00** **Acute erythroid leukemia, not having achieved remission**
       Acute erythroid leukemia with failed remission
       Acute erythroid leukemia NOS
   CC **C94.01** **Acute erythroid leukemia, in remission**
   CC **C94.02** **Acute erythroid leukemia, in relapse**
+ **C94.2** **Acute megakaryoblastic leukemia**
    Acute myeloid leukemia M7
    Acute megakaryocytic leukemia
   CC **C94.20** **Acute megakaryoblastic leukemia not having achieved remission**
       Acute megakaryoblastic leukemia with failed remission
       Acute megakaryoblastic leukemia NOS
   CC **C94.21** **Acute megakaryoblastic leukemia, in remission**
   CC **C94.22** **Acute megakaryoblastic leukemia, in relapse**
+ **C94.3** **Mast cell leukemia**
    AHA CC: 4Q, 2017, 5
   CC **C94.30** **Mast cell leukemia not having achieved remission**
       Mast cell leukemia with failed remission
       Mast cell leukemia NOS
   CC **C94.31** **Mast cell leukemia, in remission**
   CC **C94.32** **Mast cell leukemia, in relapse**
+ **C94.4** **Acute panmyelosis with myelofibrosis**
    Acute myelofibrosis
   Excludes1: *myelofibrosis NOS (D75.81)*
       secondary myelofibrosis NOS (D75.81)
   CC **C94.40** **Acute panmyelosis with myelofibrosis not having achieved remission**
       Acute myelofibrosis NOS
       Acute panmyelosis with myelofibrosis with failed remission
       Acute panmyelosis NOS
   CC **C94.41** **Acute panmyelosis with myelofibrosis, in remission**
   CC **C94.42** **Acute panmyelosis with myelofibrosis, in relapse**
CC **C94.6** **Myelodysplastic disease, not classified**
    Myeloproliferative disease, not classified
+ **C94.8** **Other specified leukemias**
    Aggressive NK-cell leukemia
    Acute basophilic leukemia
   CC **C94.80** **Other specified leukemias not having achieved remission**
       Other specified leukemia with failed remission
       Other specified leukemias NOS
   CC **C94.81** **Other specified leukemias, in remission**
   CC **C94.82** **Other specified leukemias, in relapse**

+, +7th, X + 7th   ● Newborn   ● Pediatric   ● Maternity   ● Adult   ♀ Female   ♂ Male   Manifestation   Unacceptable PDX   HCC   CC   MCC   HAC

C95 **Leukemia of unspecified cell type**

Excludes1: *personal history of leukemia (Z85.6)*

+ **C95.0** **Acute leukemia of unspecified cell type**

Acute bilineal leukemia
Acute mixed lineage leukemia
Biphenotypic acute leukemia
Stem cell leukemia of unclear lineage

Excludes1: *acute exacerbation of unspecified chronic leukemia (C95.10)*

CC **C95.00** **Acute leukemia of unspecified cell type not having achieved remission**

Acute leukemia of unspecified cell type with failed remission
Acute leukemia NOS

CC **C95.01** **Acute leukemia of unspecified cell type, in remission**

CC **C95.02** **Acute leukemia of unspecified cell type, in relapse**

+ **C95.1** **Chronic leukemia of unspecified cell type**

CC **C95.10** **Chronic leukemia of unspecified cell type not having achieved remission**

Chronic leukemia of unspecified cell type with failed remission
Chronic leukemia NOS

CC **C95.11** **Chronic leukemia of unspecified cell type, in remission**

CC **C95.12** **Chronic leukemia of unspecified cell type, in relapse**

+ **C95.9** **Leukemia, unspecified**

CC **C95.90** **Leukemia, unspecified not having achieved remission**

Leukemia, unspecified with failed remission
Leukemia NOS

CC **C95.91** **Leukemia, unspecified, in remission**

CC **C95.92** **Leukemia, unspecified, in relapse**

C96 **Other and unspecified malignant neoplasms of lymphoid, hematopoietic and related tissue**

Excludes1: *personal history of other malignant neoplasms of lymphoid, hematopoietic and related tissues (Z85.79)*

CC **C96.0** **Multifocal and multisystemic (disseminated) Langerhans-cell histiocytosis**

Histiocytosis X, multisystemic
Letterer-Siwe disease

Excludes1: *adult pulmonary Langerhans cell histiocytosis (J84.82)*
multifocal and unisystemic Langerhans-cell histiocytosis (C96.5)
unifocal Langerhans-cell histiocytosis (C96.6)

+ **C96.2** **Malignant mast cell neoplasm**

Excludes1: *indolent mastocytosis (D47.02)*
mast cell leukemia (C94.30)
mastocytosis (congenital) (cutaneous) (Q82.2)

AHA CC: 4Q, 2017, 5

CC **C96.20** **Malignant mast cell neoplasm, unspecified**

CC **C96.21** **Aggressive systemic mastocytosis**

CC **C96.22** **Mast cell sarcoma**

CC **C96.29** **Other malignant mast cell neoplasm**

CC **C96.4** **Sarcoma of dendritic cells (accessory cells)**

Follicular dendritic cell sarcoma
Interdigitating dendritic cell sarcoma
Langerhans cell sarcoma

CC **C96.5** **Multifocal and unisystemic Langerhans-cell histiocytosis**

Hand-Schüller-Christian disease
Histiocytosis X, multifocal

Excludes1: *multifocal and multisystemic (disseminated) Langerhans-cell histiocytosis (C96.0)*
unifocal Langerhans-cell histiocytosis (C96.6)

CC **C96.6** **Unifocal Langerhans-cell histiocytosis**

Eosinophilic granuloma
Histiocytosis X, unifocal
Histiocytosis X NOS
Langerhans-cell histiocytosis NOS

Excludes1: *multifocal and multisysemic (disseminated) Langerhans-cell histiocytosis (C96.0)*
multifocal and unisystemic Langerhans-cell histiocytosis (C96.5)

CC **C96.A** **Histiocytic sarcoma**

Malignant histiocytosis

CC **C96.Z** **Other specified malignant neoplasms of lymphoid, hematopoietic and related tissue**

CC **C96.9** **Malignant neoplasm of lymphoid, hematopoietic and related tissue, unspecified**

In situ neoplasms (D00-D09)

Includes: Bowen's disease
erythroplasia
grade III intraepithelial neoplasia
Queyrat's erythroplasia

D00 **Carcinoma in situ of oral cavity, esophagus and stomach**

Excludes1: *melanoma in situ (D03.-)*

+ **D00.0** **Carcinoma in situ of lip, oral cavity and pharynx**

Use additional code to identify:
exposure to environmental tobacco smoke (Z77.22)
exposure to tobacco smoke in the perinatal period (P96.81)
history of tobacco dependence (Z87.891)
occupational exposure to environmental tobacco smoke (Z57.31)
tobacco dependence (F17.-)
tobacco use (Z72.0)

Excludes1: *carcinoma in situ of aryepiglottic fold or interarytenoid fold, laryngeal aspect (D02.0)*
carcinoma in situ of epiglottis NOS (D02.0)
carcinoma in situ of epiglottis suprahyoid portion (D02.0)
carcinoma in situ of skin of lip (D03.0, D04.0)

D00.00 **Carcinoma in situ of oral cavity, unspecified site**

D00.01 **Carcinoma in situ of labial mucosa and vermilion border**

D00.02 **Carcinoma in situ of buccal mucosa**

D00.03 **Carcinoma in situ of gingiva and edentulous alveolar ridge**

D00.04 **Carcinoma in situ of soft palate**

D00.05 **Carcinoma in situ of hard palate**

D00.06 **Carcinoma in situ of floor of mouth**

D00.07 **Carcinoma in situ of tongue**

D00.08 **Carcinoma in situ of pharynx**

Carcinoma in situ of aryepiglottic fold NOS
Carcinoma in situ of hypopharyngeal aspect of aryepiglottic fold
Carcinoma in situ of marginal zone of aryepiglottic fold

D00.1 **Carcinoma in situ of esophagus**

D00.2 **Carcinoma in situ of stomach**

D01 **Carcinoma in situ of other and unspecified digestive organs**

Excludes1: *melanoma in situ (D03.-)*

D01.0 **Carcinoma in situ of colon**

Excludes1: *carcinoma in situ of rectosigmoid junction (D01.1)*

D01.1 **Carcinoma in situ of rectosigmoid junction**

D01.2 **Carcinoma in situ of rectum**

D01.3 **Carcinoma in situ of anus and anal canal**

Anal intraepithelial neoplasia III [AIN III]
Severe dysplasia of anus

Excludes1: *anal intraepithelial neoplasia I and II [AIN I and AIN II] (K62.82)*
carcinoma in situ of anal margin (D04.5)
carcinoma in situ of anal skin (D04.5)
carcinoma in situ of perianal skin (D04.5)

+ **D01.4** **Carcinoma in situ of other and unspecified parts of intestine**

Excludes1: *carcinoma in situ of ampulla of Vater (D01.5)*

D01.40 **Carcinoma in situ of unspecified part of intestine**

D01.49 **Carcinoma in situ of other parts of intestine**

D01.5 **Carcinoma in situ of liver, gallbladder and bile ducts**

Carcinoma in situ of ampulla of Vater

D01.7 **Carcinoma in situ of other specified digestive organs**

Carcinoma in situ of pancreas

D01.9 **Carcinoma in situ of digestive organ, unspecified**

D02 Carcinoma in situ of middle ear and respiratory system

Use additional code to identify:
exposure to environmental tobacco smoke (Z77.22)
exposure to tobacco smoke in the perinatal period (P96.81)
history of tobacco dependence (Z87.891)
occupational exposure to environmental tobacco smoke (Z57.31)
tobacco dependence (F17.-)
tobacco use (Z72.0)

Excludes1: *melanoma in situ (D03.-)*

D02.0 Carcinoma in situ of larynx
Carcinoma in situ of aryepiglottic fold or interarytenoid fold, laryngeal aspect
Carcinoma in situ of epiglottis (suprahyoid portion)
Excludes1: *carcinoma in situ of aryepiglottic fold or interarytenoid fold NOS (D00.08)*
carcinoma in situ of hypopharyngeal aspect (D00.08)
carcinoma in situ of marginal zone (D00.08)

D02.1 Carcinoma in situ of trachea
+ D02.2 Carcinoma in situ of bronchus and lung
D02.20 Carcinoma in situ of unspecified bronchus and lung
D02.21 Carcinoma in situ of right bronchus and lung
D02.22 Carcinoma in situ of left bronchus and lung
D02.3 Carcinoma in situ of other parts of respiratory system
Carcinoma in situ of accessory sinuses
Carcinoma in situ of middle ear
Carcinoma in situ of nasal cavities
Excludes1: *carcinoma in situ of ear (external) (skin) (D04.2-)*
carcinoma in situ of nose NOS D09.8
carcinoma in situ of skin of nose (D04.3)

D02.4 Carcinoma in situ of respiratory system, unspecified

D03 Melanoma in situ

D03.0 Melanoma in situ of lip
+ D03.1 Melanoma in situ of eyelid, including canthus
D03.10 Melanoma in situ of unspecified eyelid, including canthus
+ D03.11 Melanoma in situ of right eyelid, including canthus
D03.111 Melanoma in situ of right upper eyelid, including canthus
D03.112 Melanoma in situ of right lower eyelid, including canthus
+ D03.12 Melanoma in situ of left eyelid, including canthus
D03.121 Melanoma in situ of left upper eyelid, including canthus
D03.122 Melanoma in situ of left lower eyelid, including canthus
+ D03.2 Melanoma in situ of ear and external auricular canal
D03.20 Melanoma in situ of unspecified ear and external auricular canal
D03.21 Melanoma in situ of right ear and external auricular canal
D03.22 Melanoma in situ of left ear and external auricular canal
+ D03.3 Melanoma in situ of other and unspecified parts of face
D03.30 Melanoma in situ of unspecified part of face
D03.39 Melanoma in situ of other parts of face
D03.4 Melanoma in situ of scalp and neck
+ D03.5 Melanoma in situ of trunk
D03.51 Melanoma in situ of anal skin
Melanoma in situ of anal margin
Melanoma in situ of perianal skin
D03.52 Melanoma in situ of breast (skin) (soft tissue)
D03.59 Melanoma in situ of other part of trunk
+ D03.6 Melanoma in situ of upper limb, including shoulder
D03.60 Melanoma in situ of unspecified upper limb, including shoulder
D03.61 Melanoma in situ of right upper limb, including shoulder
D03.62 Melanoma in situ of left upper limb, including shoulder
+ D03.7 Melanoma in situ of lower limb, including hip
D03.70 Melanoma in situ of unspecified lower limb, including hip
D03.71 Melanoma in situ of right lower limb, including hip
D03.72 Melanoma in situ of left lower limb, including hip

D03.8 Melanoma in situ of other sites
Melanoma in situ of scrotum
Excludes1: *carcinoma in situ of scrotum (D07.61)*
D03.9 Melanoma in situ, unspecified

D04 Carcinoma in situ of skin

Excludes1: *erythroplasia of Queyrat (penis) NOS (D07.4)*
melanoma in situ (D03.-)

D04.0 Carcinoma in situ of skin of lip
Excludes2: *carcinoma in situ of vermilion border of lip (D00.01)*
+ D04.1 Carcinoma in situ of skin of eyelid, including canthus
D04.10 Carcinoma in situ of skin of unspecified eyelid, including canthus
+ D04.11 Carcinoma in situ of skin of right eyelid, including canthus
D04.111 Carcinoma in situ of skin of right upper eyelid, including canthus
D04.112 Carcinoma in situ of skin of right lower eyelid, including canthus
+ D04.12 Carcinoma in situ of skin of left eyelid, including canthus
D04.121 Carcinoma in situ of skin of left upper eyelid, including canthus
D04.122 Carcinoma in situ of skin of left lower eyelid, including canthus
+ D04.2 Carcinoma in situ of skin of ear and external auricular canal
D04.20 Carcinoma in situ of skin of unspecified ear and external auricular canal
D04.21 Carcinoma in situ of skin of right ear and external auricular canal
D04.22 Carcinoma in situ of skin of left ear and external auricular canal
+ D04.3 Carcinoma in situ of skin of other and unspecified parts of face
D04.30 Carcinoma in situ of skin of unspecified part of face
D04.39 Carcinoma in situ of skin of other parts of face
D04.4 Carcinoma in situ of skin of scalp and neck
D04.5 Carcinoma in situ of skin of trunk
Carcinoma in situ of anal margin
Carcinoma in situ of anal skin
Carcinoma in situ of perianal skin
Carcinoma in situ of skin of breast
Excludes1: *carcinoma in situ of anus NOS (D01.3)*
carcinoma in situ of scrotum (D07.61)
carcinoma in situ of skin of genital organs (D07.-)
+ D04.6 Carcinoma in situ of skin of upper limb, including shoulder
D04.60 Carcinoma in situ of skin of unspecified upper limb, including shoulder
D04.61 Carcinoma in situ of skin of right upper limb, including shoulder
D04.62 Carcinoma in situ of skin of left upper limb, including shoulder
+ D04.7 Carcinoma in situ of skin of lower limb, including hip
D04.70 Carcinoma in situ of skin of unspecified lower limb, including hip
D04.71 Carcinoma in situ of skin of right lower limb, including hip
D04.72 Carcinoma in situ of skin of left lower limb, including hip
D04.8 Carcinoma in situ of skin of other sites
D04.9 Carcinoma in situ of skin, unspecified

D05 Carcinoma in situ of breast

Excludes1: *carcinoma in situ of skin of breast (D04.5)*
melanoma in situ of breast (skin) (D03.5)
Paget's disease of breast or nipple (C50.-)

+ D05.0 Lobular carcinoma in situ of breast
D05.00 Lobular carcinoma in situ of unspecified breast
D05.01 Lobular carcinoma in situ of right breast
D05.02 Lobular carcinoma in situ of left breast
+ D05.1 Intraductal carcinoma in situ of breast
D05.10 Intraductal carcinoma in situ of unspecified breast
D05.11 Intraductal carcinoma in situ of right breast
D05.12 Intraductal carcinoma in situ of left breast

+, +7th, X + 7th ● Newborn ● Pediatric ● Maternity ● Adult ♀ Female ♂ Male Manifestation Unacceptable PDX HCC CC MCC HAC

+ **D05.8 Other specified type of carcinoma in situ of breast**
    D05.80 Other specified type of carcinoma in situ of unspecified breast
    D05.81 Other specified type of carcinoma in situ of right breast
    D05.82 Other specified type of carcinoma in situ of left breast
+ **D05.9 Unspecified type of carcinoma in situ of breast**
    D05.90 Unspecified type of carcinoma in situ of unspecified breast
    D05.91 Unspecified type of carcinoma in situ of right breast
    D05.92 Unspecified type of carcinoma in situ of left breast

D06 Carcinoma in situ of cervix uteri

Includes: cervical adenocarcinoma in situ
    cervical intraepithelial glandular neoplasia
    cervical intraepithelial neoplasia III [CIN III]
    severe dysplasia of cervix uteri
Excludes1: *cervical intraepithelial neoplasia II [CIN II] (N87.1)*
    cytologic evidence of malignancy of cervix without histologic confirmation (R87.614)
    high grade squamous intraepithelial lesion (HGSIL) of cervix (R87.613)
    melanoma in situ of cervix (D03.5)
    moderate cervical dysplasia (N87.1)
♀ **D06.0 Carcinoma in situ of endocervix**
♀ **D06.1 Carcinoma in situ of exocervix**
♀ **D06.7 Carcinoma in situ of other parts of cervix**
♀ **D06.9 Carcinoma in situ of cervix, unspecified**

D07 Carcinoma in situ of other and unspecified genital organs

Excludes1: *melanoma in situ of trunk (D03.5)*
♀ **D07.0 Carcinoma in situ of endometrium**
♀ **D07.1 Carcinoma in situ of vulva**
    Severe dysplasia of vulva
    Vulvar intraepithelial neoplasia III [VIN III]
    Excludes1: *moderate dysplasia of vulva (N90.1)*
        vulvar intraepithelial neoplasia II [VIN II] (N90.1)
♀ **D07.2 Carcinoma in situ of vagina**
    Severe dysplasia of vagina
    Vaginal intraepithelial neoplasia III [VAIN III]
    Excludes1: *moderate dysplasia of vagina (N89.1)*
        vaginal intraepithelial neoplasia II [VIN II] (N89.1)
+ **D07.3 Carcinoma in situ of other and unspecified female genital organs**
  ♀ **D07.30 Carcinoma in situ of unspecified female genital organs**
  ♀ **D07.39 Carcinoma in situ of other female genital organs**
♂ **D07.4 Carcinoma in situ of penis**
    Erythroplasia of Queyrat NOS
♂ **D07.5 Carcinoma in situ of prostate**
    Prostatic intraepithelial neoplasia III (PIN III)
    Severe dysplasia of prostate
    Excludes1: *dysplasia (mild) (moderate) of prostate (N42.3-)*
        prostatic intraepithelial neoplasia II [PIN II] (N42.3-)
+ **D07.6 Carcinoma in situ of other and unspecified male genital organs**
  ♂ **D07.60 Carcinoma in situ of unspecified male genital organs**
  ♂ **D07.61 Carcinoma in situ of scrotum**
  ♂ **D07.69 Carcinoma in situ of other male genital organs**

D09 Carcinoma in situ of other and unspecified sites

Excludes1: *melanoma in situ (D03.-)*
D09.0 Carcinoma in situ of bladder
+ **D09.1 Carcinoma in situ of other and unspecified urinary organs**
    D09.10 Carcinoma in situ of unspecified urinary organ
    D09.19 Carcinoma in situ of other urinary organs
+ **D09.2 Carcinoma in situ of eye**
    Excludes1: *carcinoma in situ of skin of eyelid (D04.1-)*
    D09.20 Carcinoma in situ of unspecified eye
    D09.21 Carcinoma in situ of right eye
    D09.22 Carcinoma in situ of left eye
D09.3 Carcinoma in situ of thyroid and other endocrine glands
    Excludes1: *carcinoma in situ of endocrine pancreas (D01.7)*
        carcinoma in situ of ovary (D07.39)
        carcinoma in situ of testis (D07.69)
D09.8 Carcinoma in situ of other specified sites
D09.9 Carcinoma in situ, unspecified

Benign neoplasms, except benign neuroendocrine tumors (D10-D36)

D10 Benign neoplasm of mouth and pharynx
  D10.0 Benign neoplasm of lip
    Benign neoplasm of lip (frenulum) (inner aspect) (mucosa) (vermilion border)
    Excludes1: *benign neoplasm of skin of lip (D22.0, D23.0)*
  D10.1 Benign neoplasm of tongue
    Benign neoplasm of lingual tonsil
  D10.2 Benign neoplasm of floor of mouth
+ **D10.3 Benign neoplasm of other and unspecified parts of mouth**
    D10.30 Benign neoplasm of unspecified part of mouth
    D10.39 Benign neoplasm of other parts of mouth
        Benign neoplasm of minor salivary gland NOS
        Excludes1: *benign odontogenic neoplasms (D16.4-D16.5)*
            benign neoplasm of mucosa of lip (D10.0)
            benign neoplasm of nasopharyngeal surface of soft palate (D10.6)
  D10.4 Benign neoplasm of tonsil
    Benign neoplasm of tonsil (faucial) (palatine)
    Excludes1: *benign neoplasm of lingual tonsil (D10.1)*
        benign neoplasm of pharyngeal tonsil (D10.6)
        benign neoplasm of tonsillar fossa (D10.5)
        benign neoplasm of tonsillar pillars (D10.5)
  D10.5 Benign neoplasm of other parts of oropharynx
    Benign neoplasm of epiglottis, anterior aspect
    Benign neoplasm of tonsillar fossa
    Benign neoplasm of tonsillar pillars
    Benign neoplasm of vallecula
    Excludes1: *benign neoplasm of epiglottis NOS (D14.1)*
        benign neoplasm of epiglottis, suprahyoid portion (D14.1)
  D10.6 Benign neoplasm of nasopharynx
    Benign neoplasm of pharyngeal tonsil
    Benign neoplasm of posterior margin of septum and choanae
  D10.7 Benign neoplasm of hypopharynx
  D10.9 Benign neoplasm of pharynx, unspecified

D11 Benign neoplasm of major salivary glands

Excludes1: *benign neoplasms of specified minor salivary glands which are classified according to their anatomical location*
    benign neoplasms of minor salivary glands NOS (D10.39)
  D11.0 Benign neoplasm of parotid gland
  D11.7 Benign neoplasm of other major salivary glands
    Benign neoplasm of sublingual salivary gland
    Benign neoplasm of submandibular salivary gland
  D11.9 Benign neoplasm of major salivary gland, unspecified

D12 Benign neoplasm of colon, rectum, anus and anal canal

Excludes1: *benign carcinoid tumors of the large intestine, and rectum (D3A.02-)*
    polyp of colon NOS (K63.5)
  D12.0 Benign neoplasm of cecum
    Benign neoplasm of ileocecal valve
    AHA CC: 3Q, 2018, 22
  D12.1 Benign neoplasm of appendix
    Excludes1: *benign carcinoid tumor of the appendix (D3A.020)*
  D12.2 Benign neoplasm of ascending colon
    AHA CC: 2Q, 2018, 14
  D12.3 Benign neoplasm of transverse colon
    Benign neoplasm of hepatic flexure
    Benign neoplasm of splenic flexure
  D12.4 Benign neoplasm of descending colon
  D12.5 Benign neoplasm of sigmoid colon
  D12.6 Benign neoplasm of colon, unspecified
    Adenomatosis of colon
    Benign neoplasm of large intestine NOS
    Polyposis (hereditary) of colon
    Excludes1: *inflammatory polyp of colon (K51.4-)*
    AHA CC: 1Q, 2017, 8-9
  D12.7 Benign neoplasm of rectosigmoid junction
  D12.8 Benign neoplasm of rectum
    Excludes1: *benign carcinoid tumor of the rectum (D3A.026)*
    AHA CC: 1Q, 2018, 6-7

D12.9 Benign neoplasm of anus and anal canal
Benign neoplasm of anus NOS
Excludes1: *benign neoplasm of anal margin (D22.5, D23.5)*
benign neoplasm of anal skin (D22.5, D23.5)
benign neoplasm of perianal skin (D22.5, D23.5)

D13 Benign neoplasm of other and ill-defined parts of digestive system
Excludes1: *benign stromal tumors of digestive system (D21.4)*
D13.0 Benign neoplasm of esophagus
D13.1 Benign neoplasm of stomach
Excludes1: *benign carcinoid tumor of the stomach (D3A.092)*
D13.2 Benign neoplasm of duodenum
Excludes1: *benign carcinoid tumor of the duodenum (D3A.010)*
+ **D13.3 Benign neoplasm of other and unspecified parts of small intestine**
Excludes1: *benign carcinoid tumors of the small intestine (D3A.01-)*
benign neoplasm of ileocecal valve (D12.0)
D13.30 Benign neoplasm of unspecified part of small intestine
D13.39 Benign neoplasm of other parts of small intestine
D13.4 Benign neoplasm of liver
Benign neoplasm of intrahepatic bile ducts
D13.5 Benign neoplasm of extrahepatic bile ducts
D13.6 Benign neoplasm of pancreas
Excludes1: *benign neoplasm of endocrine pancreas (D13.7)*
D13.7 Benign neoplasm of endocrine pancreas
Islet cell tumor
Benign neoplasm of islets of Langerhans
Use additional code to identify any functional activity.
D13.9 Benign neoplasm of ill-defined sites within the digestive system
Benign neoplasm of digestive system NOS
Benign neoplasm of intestine NOS
Benign neoplasm of spleen

D14 Benign neoplasm of middle ear and respiratory system
D14.0 Benign neoplasm of middle ear, nasal cavity and accessory sinuses
Benign neoplasm of cartilage of nose
Excludes1: *benign neoplasm of auricular canal (external) (D22.2 , D23.2)*
benign neoplasm of bone of ear (D16.4)
benign neoplasm of bone of nose (D16.4)
benign neoplasm of cartilage of ear (D21.0)
benign neoplasm of ear (external)(skin) (D22.2-, D23.2-)
benign neoplasm of nose NOS (D36.7)
benign neoplasm of skin of nose (D22.39, D23.39)
benign neoplasm of olfactory bulb (D33.3)
benign neoplasm of posterior margin of septum and choanae (D10.6)
polyp of accessory sinus (J33.8)
polyp of ear (middle) (H74.4)
polyp of nasal (cavity) (J33.-)
D14.1 Benign neoplasm of larynx
Adenomatous polyp of larynx
Benign neoplasm of epiglottis (suprahyoid portion)
Excludes1: *benign neoplasm of epiglottis, anterior aspect (D10.5)*
polyp (nonadenomatous) of vocal cord or larynx (J38.1)
D14.2 Benign neoplasm of trachea
+ **D14.3 Benign neoplasm of bronchus and lung**
Excludes1: *benign carcinoid tumor of the bronchus and lung (D3A.090)*
D14.30 Benign neoplasm of unspecified bronchus and lung
D14.31 Benign neoplasm of right bronchus and lung
D14.32 Benign neoplasm of left bronchus and lung
D14.4 Benign neoplasm of respiratory system, unspecified

D15 Benign neoplasm of other and unspecified intrathoracic organs
Excludes1: *benign neoplasm of mesothelial tissue (D19.-)*
D15.0 Benign neoplasm of thymus
Excludes1: *benign carcinoid tumor of the thymus (D3A.091)*
D15.1 Benign neoplasm of heart
Excludes1: *benign neoplasm of great vessels (D21.3)*

D15.2 Benign neoplasm of mediastinum
D15.7 Benign neoplasm of other specified intrathoracic organs
D15.9 Benign neoplasm of intrathoracic organ, unspecified

D16 Benign neoplasm of bone and articular cartilage
Excludes1: *benign neoplasm of connective tissue of ear (D21.0)*
benign neoplasm of connective tissue of eyelid (D21.0)
benign neoplasm of connective tissue of larynx (D14.1)
benign neoplasm of connective tissue of nose (D14.0)
benign neoplasm of synovia (D21.-)
+ **D16.0 Benign neoplasm of scapula and long bones of upper limb**
D16.00 Benign neoplasm of scapula and long bones of unspecified upper limb
D16.01 Benign neoplasm of scapula and long bones of right upper limb
D16.02 Benign neoplasm of scapula and long bones of left upper limb
+ **D16.1 Benign neoplasm of short bones of upper limb**
D16.10 Benign neoplasm of short bones of unspecified upper limb
D16.11 Benign neoplasm of short bones of right upper limb
D16.12 Benign neoplasm of short bones of left upper limb
+ **D16.2 Benign neoplasm of long bones of lower limb**
D16.20 Benign neoplasm of long bones of unspecified lower limb
D16.21 Benign neoplasm of long bones of right lower limb
D16.22 Benign neoplasm of long bones of left lower limb
+ **D16.3 Benign neoplasm of short bones of lower limb**
D16.30 Benign neoplasm of short bones of unspecified lower limb
D16.31 Benign neoplasm of short bones of right lower limb
D16.32 Benign neoplasm of short bones of left lower limb
D16.4 Benign neoplasm of bones of skull and face
Benign neoplasm of maxilla (superior)
Benign neoplasm of orbital bone
Keratocyst of maxilla
Keratocystic odontogenic tumor of maxilla
Excludes2: *benign neoplasm of lower jaw bone (D16.5)*
D16.5 Benign neoplasm of lower jaw bone
Keratocyst of mandible
Keratocystic odontogenic tumor of mandible
D16.6 Benign neoplasm of vertebral column
Excludes1: *benign neoplasm of sacrum and coccyx (D16.8)*
D16.7 Benign neoplasm of ribs, sternum and clavicle
D16.8 Benign neoplasm of pelvic bones, sacrum and coccyx
D16.9 Benign neoplasm of bone and articular cartilage, unspecified

D17 Benign lipomatous neoplasm
D17.0 Benign lipomatous neoplasm of skin and subcutaneous tissue of head, face and neck
D17.1 Benign lipomatous neoplasm of skin and subcutaneous tissue of trunk
+ **D17.2 Benign lipomatous neoplasm of skin and subcutaneous tissue of limb**
D17.20 Benign lipomatous neoplasm of skin and subcutaneous tissue of unspecified limb
D17.21 Benign lipomatous neoplasm of skin and subcutaneous tissue of right arm
D17.22 Benign lipomatous neoplasm of skin and subcutaneous tissue of left arm
D17.23 Benign lipomatous neoplasm of skin and subcutaneous tissue of right leg
D17.24 Benign lipomatous neoplasm of skin and subcutaneous tissue of left leg
+ **D17.3 Benign lipomatous neoplasm of skin and subcutaneous tissue of other and unspecified sites**
D17.30 Benign lipomatous neoplasm of skin and subcutaneous tissue of unspecified sites
D17.39 Benign lipomatous neoplasm of skin and subcutaneous tissue of other sites
D17.4 Benign lipomatous neoplasm of intrathoracic organs
D17.5 Benign lipomatous neoplasm of intra-abdominal organs
Excludes1: *benign lipomatous neoplasm of peritoneum and retroperitoneum (D17.79)*
♂ **D17.6 Benign lipomatous neoplasm of spermatic cord**

+, +7th, X + 7th   ● Newborn   ● Pediatric   ● Maternity   ● Adult   ♀ Female   ♂ Male   Manifestation   Unacceptable PDX   HCC   CC   MCC   HAC

+ **D17.7** Benign lipomatous neoplasm of other sites
    D17.71 Benign lipomatous neoplasm of kidney
    D17.72 Benign lipomatous neoplasm of other genitourinary organ
    D17.79 Benign lipomatous neoplasm of other sites
        Benign lipomatous neoplasm of peritoneum
        Benign lipomatous neoplasm of retroperitoneum
D17.9 Benign lipomatous neoplasm, unspecified
    Lipoma NOS

D18 Hemangioma and lymphangioma, any site

    Excludes1: *benign neoplasm of glomus jugulare (D35.6)*
        blue or pigmented nevus (D22.-)
        nevus NOS (D22.-)
        vascular nevus (Q82.5)

+ **D18.0** Hemangioma
    Angioma NOS
    Cavernous nevus
    D18.00 Hemangioma unspecified site
    D18.01 Hemangioma of skin and subcutaneous tissue
    D18.02 Hemangioma of intracranial structures
    D18.03 Hemangioma of intra-abdominal structures
    D18.09 Hemangioma of other sites
D18.1 Lymphangioma, any site
    AHA CC: 2Q, 2018, 13; 3Q, 2018, 31

D19 Benign neoplasm of mesothelial tissue

    D19.0 Benign neoplasm of mesothelial tissue of pleura
    D19.1 Benign neoplasm of mesothelial tissue of peritoneum
    D19.7 Benign neoplasm of mesothelial tissue of other sites
    D19.9 Benign neoplasm of mesothelial tissue, unspecified
        Benign mesothelioma NOS

D20 Benign neoplasm of soft tissue of retroperitoneum and peritoneum

    Excludes1: *benign lipomatous neoplasm of peritoneum and*
        retroperitoneum (D17.79)
        benign neoplasm of mesothelial tissue (D19.-)
    D20.0 Benign neoplasm of soft tissue of retroperitoneum
    D20.1 Benign neoplasm of soft tissue of peritoneum

D21 Other benign neoplasms of connective and other soft tissue

    Includes: benign neoplasm of blood vessel
        benign neoplasm of bursa
        benign neoplasm of cartilage
        benign neoplasm of fascia
        benign neoplasm of fat
        benign neoplasm of ligament, except uterine
        benign neoplasm of lymphatic channel
        benign neoplasm of muscle
        benign neoplasm of synovia
        benign neoplasm of tendon (sheath)
        benign stromal tumors
    Excludes1: *benign neoplasm of articular cartilage (D16.-)*
        benign neoplasm of cartilage of larynx (D14.1)
        benign neoplasm of cartilage of nose (D14.0)
        benign neoplasm of connective tissue of breast (D24.-)
        benign neoplasm of peripheral nerves and autonomic
          nervous system (D36.1-)
        benign neoplasm of peritoneum (D20.1)
        benign neoplasm of retroperitoneum (D20.0)
        benign neoplasm of uterine ligament, any (D28.2)
        benign neoplasm of vascular tissue (D18.-)
        hemangioma (D18.0-)
        lipomatous neoplasm (D17.-)
        lymphangioma (D18.1)
        uterine leiomyoma (D25.-)
    D21.0 Benign neoplasm of connective and other soft tissue of head, face and neck
        Benign neoplasm of connective tissue of ear
        Benign neoplasm of connective tissue of eyelid
        Excludes1: *benign neoplasm of connective tissue of orbit*
          (D31.6-)
+ **D21.1** Benign neoplasm of connective and other soft tissue of upper limb, including shoulder
    D21.10 Benign neoplasm of connective and other soft tissue of unspecified upper limb, including shoulder
    D21.11 Benign neoplasm of connective and other soft tissue of right upper limb, including shoulder
    D21.12 Benign neoplasm of connective and other soft tissue of left upper limb, including shoulder

+ **D21.2** Benign neoplasm of connective and other soft tissue of lower limb, including hip
    D21.20 Benign neoplasm of connective and other soft tissue of unspecified lower limb, including hip
    D21.21 Benign neoplasm of connective and other soft tissue of right lower limb, including hip
    D21.22 Benign neoplasm of connective and other soft tissue of left lower limb, including hip
D21.3 Benign neoplasm of connective and other soft tissue of thorax
    Benign neoplasm of axilla
    Benign neoplasm of diaphragm
    Benign neoplasm of great vessels
    Excludes1: *benign neoplasm of heart (D15.1)*
        benign neoplasm of mediastinum (D15.2)
        benign neoplasm of thymus (D15.0)
D21.4 Benign neoplasm of connective and other soft tissue of abdomen
    Benign stromal tumors of abdomen
D21.5 Benign neoplasm of connective and other soft tissue of pelvis
    Excludes1: *benign neoplasm of any uterine ligament (D28.2)*
        uterine leiomyoma (D25.-)
D21.6 Benign neoplasm of connective and other soft tissue of trunk, unspecified
    Benign neoplasm of connective and other soft tissue of back NOS
D21.9 Benign neoplasm of connective and other soft tissue, unspecified

D22 Melanocytic nevi

    Includes: atypical nevus
        blue hairy pigmented nevus
        nevus NOS
    D22.0 Melanocytic nevi of lip
+ **D22.1** Melanocytic nevi of eyelid, including canthus
    D22.10 Melanocytic nevi of unspecified eyelid, including canthus
+   **D22.11** Melanocytic nevi of right eyelid, including canthus
        D22.111 Melanocytic nevi of right upper eyelid, including canthus
        D22.112 Melanocytic nevi of right lower eyelid, including canthus
+   **D22.12** Melanocytic nevi of left eyelid, including canthus
        D22.121 Melanocytic nevi of left upper eyelid, including canthus
        D22.122 Melanocytic nevi of left lower eyelid, including canthus
+ **D22.2** Melanocytic nevi of ear and external auricular canal
    D22.20 Melanocytic nevi of unspecified ear and external auricular canal
    D22.21 Melanocytic nevi of right ear and external auricular canal
    D22.22 Melanocytic nevi of left ear and external auricular canal
+ **D22.3** Melanocytic nevi of other and unspecified parts of face
    D22.30 Melanocytic nevi of unspecified part of face
    D22.39 Melanocytic nevi of other parts of face
D22.4 Melanocytic nevi of scalp and neck
D22.5 Melanocytic nevi of trunk
    Melanocytic nevi of anal margin
    Melanocytic nevi of anal skin
    Melanocytic nevi of perianal skin
    Melanocytic nevi of skin of breast
+ **D22.6** Melanocytic nevi of upper limb, including shoulder
    D22.60 Melanocytic nevi of unspecified upper limb, including shoulder
    D22.61 Melanocytic nevi of right upper limb, including shoulder
    D22.62 Melanocytic nevi of left upper limb, including shoulder
+ **D22.7** Melanocytic nevi of lower limb, including hip
    D22.70 Melanocytic nevi of unspecified lower limb, including hip
    D22.71 Melanocytic nevi of right lower limb, including hip
    D22.72 Melanocytic nevi of left lower limb, including hip
D22.9 Melanocytic nevi, unspecified

D23 Other benign neoplasms of skin

> **Includes:** benign neoplasm of hair follicles
>> benign neoplasm of sebaceous glands
>> benign neoplasm of sweat glands
>
> *Excludes1:* *benign lipomatous neoplasms of skin (D17.0-D17.3)*
> *Excludes2:* *melanocytic nevi (D22.-)*

D23.0 Other benign neoplasm of skin of lip

> *Excludes1:* *benign neoplasm of vermilion border of lip (D10.0)*

+ D23.1 Other benign neoplasm of skin of eyelid, including canthus

D23.10 Other benign neoplasm of skin of unspecified eyelid, including canthus

+ D23.11 Other benign neoplasm of skin of right eyelid, including canthus

D23.111 Other benign neoplasm of skin of right upper eyelid, including canthus

D23.112 Other benign neoplasm of skin of right lower eyelid, including canthus

+ D23.12 Other benign neoplasm of skin of left eyelid, including canthus

D23.121 Other benign neoplasm of skin of left upper eyelid, including canthus

D23.122 Other benign neoplasm of skin of left lower eyelid, including canthus

+ D23.2 Other benign neoplasm of skin of ear and external auricular canal

D23.20 Other benign neoplasm of skin of unspecified ear and external auricular canal

D23.21 Other benign neoplasm of skin of right ear and external auricular canal

D23.22 Other benign neoplasm of skin of left ear and external auricular canal

+ D23.3 Other benign neoplasm of skin of other and unspecified parts of face

D23.30 Other benign neoplasm of skin of unspecified part of face

D23.39 Other benign neoplasm of skin of other parts of face

D23.4 Other benign neoplasm of skin of scalp and neck

D23.5 Other benign neoplasm of skin of trunk

> Other benign neoplasm of anal margin
> Other benign neoplasm of anal skin
> Other benign neoplasm of perianal skin
> Other benign neoplasm of skin of breast
>
> *Excludes1:* *benign neoplasm of anus NOS (D12.9)*

+ D23.6 Other benign neoplasm of skin of upper limb, including shoulder

D23.60 Other benign neoplasm of skin of unspecified upper limb, including shoulder

D23.61 Other benign neoplasm of skin of right upper limb, including shoulder

D23.62 Other benign neoplasm of skin of left upper limb, including shoulder

+ D23.7 Other benign neoplasm of skin of lower limb, including hip

D23.70 Other benign neoplasm of skin of unspecified lower limb, including hip

D23.71 Other benign neoplasm of skin of right lower limb, including hip

D23.72 Other benign neoplasm of skin of left lower limb, including hip

D23.9 Other benign neoplasm of skin, unspecified

D24 Benign neoplasm of breast

> **Includes:** benign neoplasm of connective tissue of breast
>> benign neoplasm of soft parts of breast
>> fibroadenoma of breast
>
> *Excludes2:* *adenofibrosis of breast (N60.2)*
>> *benign cyst of breast (N60.-)*
>> *benign mammary dysplasia (N60.-)*
>> *benign neoplasm of skin of breast (D22.5, D23.5)*
>> *fibrocystic disease of breast (N60.-)*

D24.1 Benign neoplasm of right breast

> *AHA CC: 1Q, 2017, 5-6*

D24.2 Benign neoplasm of left breast

D24.9 Benign neoplasm of unspecified breast

D25 Leiomyoma of uterus

> **Includes:** uterine fibroid
>> uterine fibromyoma
>> uterine myoma

♀ **D25.0 Submucous leiomyoma of uterus**

♀ **D25.1 Intramural leiomyoma of uterus**

> Interstitial leiomyoma of uterus

♀ **D25.2 Subserosal leiomyoma of uterus**

> Subperitoneal leiomyoma of uterus

♀ **D25.9 Leiomyoma of uterus, unspecified**

D26 Other benign neoplasms of uterus

♀ **D26.0 Other benign neoplasm of cervix uteri**

♀ **D26.1 Other benign neoplasm of corpus uteri**

♀ **D26.7 Other benign neoplasm of other parts of uterus**

♀ **D26.9 Other benign neoplasm of uterus, unspecified**

D27 Benign neoplasm of ovary

> Use additional code to identify any functional activity.
>
> *Excludes2:* *corpus albicans cyst (N83.2-)*
>> *corpus luteum cyst (N83.1-)*
>> *endometrial cyst (N80.1)*
>> *follicular (atretic) cyst (N83.0-)*
>> *graafian follicle cyst (N83.0-)*
>> *ovarian cyst NEC (N83.2-)*
>> *ovarian retention cyst (N83.2-)*

♀ **D27.0 Benign neoplasm of right ovary**

♀ **D27.1 Benign neoplasm of left ovary**

♀ **D27.9 Benign neoplasm of unspecified ovary**

D28 Benign neoplasm of other and unspecified female genital organs

> **Includes:** adenomatous polyp
>> benign neoplasm of skin of female genital organs
>> benign teratoma
>
> *Excludes1:* *epoophoron cyst (Q50.5)*
>> *fimbrial cyst (Q50.4)*
>> *Gartner's duct cyst (Q52.4)*
>> *parovarian cyst (Q50.5)*

♀ **D28.0 Benign neoplasm of vulva**

♀ **D28.1 Benign neoplasm of vagina**

♀ **D28.2 Benign neoplasm of uterine tubes and ligaments**

> Benign neoplasm of fallopian tube
> Benign neoplasm of uterine ligament (broad) (round)

♀ **D28.7 Benign neoplasm of other specified female genital organs**

♀ **D28.9 Benign neoplasm of female genital organ, unspecified**

D29 Benign neoplasm of male genital organs

> **Includes:** benign neoplasm of skin of male genital organs

♂ **D29.0 Benign neoplasm of penis**

♂ **D29.1 Benign neoplasm of prostate**

> *Excludes1:* *enlarged prostate (N40.-)*

+ D29.2 Benign neoplasm of testis

> Use additional code to identify any functional activity.

♂ **D29.20 Benign neoplasm of unspecified testis**

♂ **D29.21 Benign neoplasm of right testis**

♂ **D29.22 Benign neoplasm of left testis**

+ D29.3 Benign neoplasm of epididymis

♂ **D29.30 Benign neoplasm of unspecified epididymis**

♂ **D29.31 Benign neoplasm of right epididymis**

♂ **D29.32 Benign neoplasm of left epididymis**

♂ **D29.4 Benign neoplasm of scrotum**

> Benign neoplasm of skin of scrotum

♂ **D29.8 Benign neoplasm of other specified male genital organs**

> Benign neoplasm of seminal vesicle
> Benign neoplasm of spermatic cord
> Benign neoplasm of tunica vaginalis

♂ **D29.9 Benign neoplasm of male genital organ, unspecified**

D30 Benign neoplasm of urinary organs

+ D30.0 Benign neoplasm of kidney

> *Excludes1:* *benign carcinoid tumor of the kidney (D3A.093)*
>> *benign neoplasm of renal calyces (D30.1-)*
>> *benign neoplasm of renal pelvis (D30.1-)*

D30.00 Benign neoplasm of unspecified kidney

D30.01 Benign neoplasm of right kidney

D30.02 Benign neoplasm of left kidney

+ **D30.1** **Benign neoplasm of renal pelvis**
  D30.10 Benign neoplasm of unspecified renal pelvis
  D30.11 Benign neoplasm of right renal pelvis
  D30.12 Benign neoplasm of left renal pelvis
+ **D30.2** **Benign neoplasm of ureter**
  Excludes1: *benign neoplasm of ureteric orifice of bladder (D30.3)*
  D30.20 Benign neoplasm of unspecified ureter
  D30.21 Benign neoplasm of right ureter
  D30.22 Benign neoplasm of left ureter
D30.3 **Benign neoplasm of bladder**
  Benign neoplasm of ureteric orifice of bladder
  Benign neoplasm of urethral orifice of bladder
D30.4 **Benign neoplasm of urethra**
  Excludes1: *benign neoplasm of urethral orifice of bladder (D30.3)*
D30.8 **Benign neoplasm of other specified urinary organs**
  Benign neoplasm of paraurethral glands
D30.9 **Benign neoplasm of urinary organ, unspecified**
  Benign neoplasm of urinary system NOS

D31 **Benign neoplasm of eye and adnexa**
  Excludes1: *benign neoplasm of connective tissue of eyelid (D21.0)*
    benign neoplasm of optic nerve (D33.3)
    benign neoplasm of skin of eyelid (D22.1-, D23.1-)
+ **D31.0** **Benign neoplasm of conjunctiva**
  D31.00 Benign neoplasm of unspecified conjunctiva
  D31.01 Benign neoplasm of right conjunctiva
  D31.02 Benign neoplasm of left conjunctiva
+ **D31.1** **Benign neoplasm of cornea**
  D31.10 Benign neoplasm of unspecified cornea
  D31.11 Benign neoplasm of right cornea
  D31.12 Benign neoplasm of left cornea
+ **D31.2** **Benign neoplasm of retina**
  Excludes1: *dark area on retina (D49.81)*
    hemangioma of retina (D49.81)
    neoplasm of unspecified behavior of retina and choroid (D49.81)
    retinal freckle (D49.81)
  D31.20 Benign neoplasm of unspecified retina
  D31.21 Benign neoplasm of right retina
  D31.22 Benign neoplasm of left retina
+ **D31.3** **Benign neoplasm of choroid**
  D31.30 Benign neoplasm of unspecified choroid
  D31.31 Benign neoplasm of right choroid
  D31.32 Benign neoplasm of left choroid
+ **D31.4** **Benign neoplasm of ciliary body**
  D31.40 Benign neoplasm of unspecified ciliary body
  D31.41 Benign neoplasm of right ciliary body
  D31.42 Benign neoplasm of left ciliary body
+ **D31.5** **Benign neoplasm of lacrimal gland and duct**
  Benign neoplasm of lacrimal sac
  Benign neoplasm of nasolacrimal duct
  D31.50 Benign neoplasm of unspecified lacrimal gland and duct
  D31.51 Benign neoplasm of right lacrimal gland and duct
  D31.52 Benign neoplasm of left lacrimal gland and duct
+ **D31.6** **Benign neoplasm of unspecified site of orbit**
  Benign neoplasm of connective tissue of orbit
  Benign neoplasm of extraocular muscle
  Benign neoplasm of peripheral nerves of orbit
  Benign neoplasm of retrobulbar tissue
  Benign neoplasm of retro-ocular tissue
  Excludes1: *benign neoplasm of orbital bone (D16.4)*
  D31.60 Benign neoplasm of unspecified site of unspecified orbit
  D31.61 Benign neoplasm of unspecified site of right orbit
  D31.62 Benign neoplasm of unspecified site of left orbit
+ **D31.9** **Benign neoplasm of unspecified part of eye**
  Benign neoplasm of eyeball
  D31.90 Benign neoplasm of unspecified part of unspecified eye
  D31.91 Benign neoplasm of unspecified part of right eye
  D31.92 Benign neoplasm of unspecified part of left eye

D32 **Benign neoplasm of meninges**
  D32.0 **Benign neoplasm of cerebral meninges**
  D32.1 **Benign neoplasm of spinal meninges**
  D32.9 **Benign neoplasm of meninges, unspecified**
    Meningioma NOS

D33 **Benign neoplasm of brain and other parts of central nervous system**
  Excludes1: *angioma (D18.0-)*
    benign neoplasm of meninges (D32.-)
    benign neoplasm of peripheral nerves and autonomic nervous system (D36.1-)
    hemangioma (D18.0-)
    neurofibromatosis (Q85.0-)
    retro-ocular benign neoplasm (D31.6-)
  D33.0 **Benign neoplasm of brain, supratentorial**
    Benign neoplasm of cerebral ventricle
    Benign neoplasm of cerebrum
    Benign neoplasm of frontal lobe
    Benign neoplasm of occipital lobe
    Benign neoplasm of parietal lobe
    Benign neoplasm of temporal lobe
    Excludes1: *benign neoplasm of fourth ventricle (D33.1)*
  D33.1 **Benign neoplasm of brain, infratentorial**
    Benign neoplasm of brain stem
    Benign neoplasm of cerebellum
    Benign neoplasm of fourth ventricle
  D33.2 **Benign neoplasm of brain, unspecified**
  D33.3 **Benign neoplasm of cranial nerves**
    Benign neoplasm of olfactory bulb
  D33.4 **Benign neoplasm of spinal cord**
  D33.7 **Benign neoplasm of other specified parts of central nervous system**
  D33.9 **Benign neoplasm of central nervous system, unspecified**
    Benign neoplasm of nervous system (central) NOS

D34 **Benign neoplasm of thyroid gland**
  Use additional code to identify any functional activity
  Valid 3-character code, no further characters required

D35 **Benign neoplasm of other and unspecified endocrine glands**
  Use additional code to identify any functional activity
  Excludes1: *benign neoplasm of endocrine pancreas (D13.7)*
    benign neoplasm of ovary (D27.-)
    benign neoplasm of testis (D29.2.-)
    benign neoplasm of thymus (D15.0)
+ **D35.0** **Benign neoplasm of adrenal gland**
  D35.00 Benign neoplasm of unspecified adrenal gland
  D35.01 Benign neoplasm of right adrenal gland
  D35.02 Benign neoplasm of left adrenal gland
D35.1 **Benign neoplasm of parathyroid gland**
D35.2 **Benign neoplasm of pituitary gland**
  AHA CC: 3Q, 2014, 22-23
D35.3 **Benign neoplasm of craniopharyngeal duct**
D35.4 **Benign neoplasm of pineal gland**
D35.5 **Benign neoplasm of carotid body**
D35.6 **Benign neoplasm of aortic body and other paraganglia**
  Benign tumor of glomus jugulare
D35.7 **Benign neoplasm of other specified endocrine glands**
D35.9 **Benign neoplasm of endocrine gland, unspecified**
  Benign neoplasm of unspecified endocrine gland

D36 **Benign neoplasm of other and unspecified sites**
  D36.0 **Benign neoplasm of lymph nodes**
    Excludes1: *lymphangioma (D18.1)*
+ **D36.1** **Benign neoplasm of peripheral nerves and autonomic nervous system**
  Excludes1: *benign neoplasm of peripheral nerves of orbit (D31.6-)*
    neurofibromatosis (Q85.0-)
  D36.10 Benign neoplasm of peripheral nerves and autonomic nervous system, unspecified
  D36.11 Benign neoplasm of peripheral nerves and autonomic nervous system of face, head, and neck
  D36.12 Benign neoplasm of peripheral nerves and autonomic nervous system, upper limb, including shoulder
  D36.13 Benign neoplasm of peripheral nerves and autonomic nervous system of lower limb, including hip
  D36.14 Benign neoplasm of peripheral nerves and autonomic nervous system of thorax
  D36.15 Benign neoplasm of peripheral nerves and autonomic nervous system of abdomen
  D36.16 Benign neoplasm of peripheral nerves and autonomic nervous system of pelvis
  D36.17 Benign neoplasm of peripheral nerves and autonomic nervous system of trunk, unspecified

D36.7 **Benign neoplasm of other specified sites**
    Benign neoplasm of nose NOS
    Benign neoplasm of back NOS
D36.9 **Benign neoplasm, unspecified site**

Benign neuroendocrine tumors (D3A)

D3A **Benign neuroendocrine tumors**

Code also any associated multiple endocrine neoplasia [MEN] syndromes (E31.2-)

Use additional code to identify any associated endocrine syndrome, such as:
carcinoid syndrome (E34.0)
Excludes2: benign pancreatic islet cell tumors (D13.7)

+ D3A.0 **Benign carcinoid tumors**
  D3A.00 **Benign carcinoid tumor of unspecified site**
    Carcinoid tumor NOS
  + D3A.01 **Benign carcinoid tumors of the small intestine**
    D3A.010 **Benign carcinoid tumor of the duodenum**
    D3A.011 **Benign carcinoid tumor of the jejunum**
    D3A.012 **Benign carcinoid tumor of the ileum**
    D3A.019 **Benign carcinoid tumor of the small intestine, unspecified portion**
  + D3A.02 **Benign carcinoid tumors of the appendix, large intestine, and rectum**
    D3A.020 **Benign carcinoid tumor of the appendix**
    D3A.021 **Benign carcinoid tumor of the cecum**
    D3A.022 **Benign carcinoid tumor of the ascending colon**
    D3A.023 **Benign carcinoid tumor of the transverse colon**
    D3A.024 **Benign carcinoid tumor of the descending colon**
    D3A.025 **Benign carcinoid tumor of the sigmoid colon**
    D3A.026 **Benign carcinoid tumor of the rectum**
    D3A.029 **Benign carcinoid tumor of the large intestine, unspecified portion**
      Benign carcinoid tumor of the colon NOS
  + D3A.09 **Benign carcinoid tumors of other sites**
    D3A.090 **Benign carcinoid tumor of the bronchus and lung**
    D3A.091 **Benign carcinoid tumor of the thymus**
    D3A.092 **Benign carcinoid tumor of the stomach**
    D3A.093 **Benign carcinoid tumor of the kidney**
    D3A.094 **Benign carcinoid tumor of the foregut, unspecified**
    D3A.095 **Benign carcinoid tumor of the midgut, unspecified**
    D3A.096 **Benign carcinoid tumor of the hindgut, unspecified**
    D3A.098 **Benign carcinoid tumors of other sites**
  D3A.8 **Other benign neuroendocrine tumors**
    Neuroendocrine tumor NOS

Neoplasms of uncertain behavior, polycythemia vera and myelodysplastic syndromes (D37-D48)

NOTE Categories D37-D44, and D48 classify by site neoplasms of uncertain behavior, i.e., histologic confirmation whether the neoplasm is malignant or benign cannot be made.

Excludes1: neoplasms of unspecified behavior (D49.-)

D37 **Neoplasm of uncertain behavior of oral cavity and digestive organs**

  Excludes1: stromal tumors of uncertain behavior of digestive system (D48.1)

+ D37.0 **Neoplasm of uncertain behavior of lip, oral cavity and pharynx**
  Excludes1: neoplasm of uncertain behavior of aryepiglottic fold or interarytenoid fold, laryngeal aspect (D38.0)
    neoplasm of uncertain behavior of epiglottis NOS (D38.0)
    neoplasm of uncertain behavior of skin of lip (D48.5)
    neoplasm of uncertain behavior of suprahyoid portion of epiglottis (D38.0)

D37.01 **Neoplasm of uncertain behavior of lip**
  Neoplasm of uncertain behavior of vermilion border of lip
D37.02 **Neoplasm of uncertain behavior of tongue**
+ D37.03 **Neoplasm of uncertain behavior of the major salivary glands**
  D37.030 **Neoplasm of uncertain behavior of the parotid salivary glands**
  D37.031 **Neoplasm of uncertain behavior of the sublingual salivary glands**
  D37.032 **Neoplasm of uncertain behavior of the submandibular salivary glands**
  D37.039 **Neoplasm of uncertain behavior of the major salivary glands, unspecified**
D37.04 **Neoplasm of uncertain behavior of the minor salivary glands**
  Neoplasm of uncertain behavior of submucosal salivary glands of lip
  Neoplasm of uncertain behavior of submucosal salivary glands of cheek
  Neoplasm of uncertain behavior of submucosal salivary glands of hard palate
  Neoplasm of uncertain behavior of submucosal salivary glands of soft palate
D37.05 **Neoplasm of uncertain behavior of pharynx**
  Neoplasm of uncertain behavior of aryepiglottic fold of pharynx NOS
  Neoplasm of uncertain behavior of hypopharyngeal aspect of aryepiglottic fold of pharynx
  Neoplasm of uncertain behavior of marginal zone of aryepiglottic fold of pharynx
D37.09 **Neoplasm of uncertain behavior of other specified sites of the oral cavity**
D37.1 **Neoplasm of uncertain behavior of stomach**
D37.2 **Neoplasm of uncertain behavior of small intestine**
D37.3 **Neoplasm of uncertain behavior of appendix**
D37.4 **Neoplasm of uncertain behavior of colon**
D37.5 **Neoplasm of uncertain behavior of rectum**
  Neoplasm of uncertain behavior of rectosigmoid junction
D37.6 **Neoplasm of uncertain behavior of liver, gallbladder and bile ducts**
  Neoplasm of uncertain behavior of ampulla of Vater
D37.8 **Neoplasm of uncertain behavior of other specified digestive organs**
  Neoplasm of uncertain behavior of anal canal
  Neoplasm of uncertain behavior of anal sphincter
  Neoplasm of uncertain behavior of anus NOS
  Neoplasm of uncertain behavior of esophagus
  Neoplasm of uncertain behavior of intestine NOS
  Neoplasm of uncertain behavior of pancreas
  Excludes1: neoplasm of uncertain behavior of anal margin (D48.5)
    neoplasm of uncertain behavior of anal skin (D48.5)
    neoplasm of uncertain behavior of perianal skin (D48.5)
D37.9 **Neoplasm of uncertain behavior of digestive organ, unspecified**

D38 **Neoplasm of uncertain behavior of middle ear and respiratory and intrathoracic organs**

  Excludes1: neoplasm of uncertain behavior of heart (D48.7)
D38.0 **Neoplasm of uncertain behavior of larynx**
  Neoplasm of uncertain behavior of aryepiglottic fold or interarytenoid fold, laryngeal aspect
  Neoplasm of uncertain behavior of epiglottis (suprahyoid portion)
  Excludes1: neoplasm of uncertain behavior of aryepiglottic fold or interarytenoid fold NOS (D37.05)
    neoplasm of uncertain behavior of hypopharyngeal aspect of aryepiglottic fold (D37.05)
    neoplasm of uncertain behavior of marginal zone of aryepiglottic fold (D37.05)
D38.1 **Neoplasm of uncertain behavior of trachea, bronchus and lung**
D38.2 **Neoplasm of uncertain behavior of pleura**
D38.3 **Neoplasm of uncertain behavior of mediastinum**
D38.4 **Neoplasm of uncertain behavior of thymus**

D38.5 **Neoplasm of uncertain behavior of other respiratory organs**
Neoplasm of uncertain behavior of accessory sinuses
Neoplasm of uncertain behavior of cartilage of nose
Neoplasm of uncertain behavior of middle ear
Neoplasm of uncertain behavior of nasal cavities
Excludes1: *neoplasm of uncertain behavior of ear (external) (skin) (D48.5)*
neoplasm of uncertain behavior of nose NOS (D48.7)
neoplasm of uncertain behavior of skin of nose (D48.5)

D38.6 **Neoplasm of uncertain behavior of respiratory organ, unspecified**

D39 **Neoplasm of uncertain behavior of female genital organs**

♀ **D39.0** **Neoplasm of uncertain behavior of uterus**
+ **D39.1** **Neoplasm of uncertain behavior of ovary**
Use additional code to identify any functional activity.

♀ **D39.10** **Neoplasm of uncertain behavior of unspecified ovary**
♀ **D39.11** **Neoplasm of uncertain behavior of right ovary**
♀ **D39.12** **Neoplasm of uncertain behavior of left ovary**
• ♀ **D39.2** **Neoplasm of uncertain behavior of placenta**
Chorioadenoma destruens
Invasive hydatidiform mole
Malignant hydatidiform mole
Excludes1: *hydatidiform mole NOS (O01.9)*
♀ **D39.8** **Neoplasm of uncertain behavior of other specified female genital organs**
Neoplasm of uncertain behavior of skin of female genital organs
♀ **D39.9** **Neoplasm of uncertain behavior of female genital organ, unspecified**

D40 **Neoplasm of uncertain behavior of male genital organs**

♂ **D40.0** **Neoplasm of uncertain behavior of prostate**
+ **D40.1** **Neoplasm of uncertain behavior of testis**
♂ **D40.10** **Neoplasm of uncertain behavior of unspecified testis**
♂ **D40.11** **Neoplasm of uncertain behavior of right testis**
♂ **D40.12** **Neoplasm of uncertain behavior of left testis**
♂ **D40.8** **Neoplasm of uncertain behavior of other specified male genital organs**
Neoplasm of uncertain behavior of skin of male genital organs
♂ **D40.9** **Neoplasm of uncertain behavior of male genital organ, unspecified**

D41 **Neoplasm of uncertain behavior of urinary organs**

+ **D41.0** **Neoplasm of uncertain behavior of kidney**
Excludes1: *neoplasm of uncertain behavior of renal pelvis (D41.1-)*
D41.00 **Neoplasm of uncertain behavior of unspecified kidney**
D41.01 **Neoplasm of uncertain behavior of right kidney**
D41.02 **Neoplasm of uncertain behavior of left kidney**
+ **D41.1** **Neoplasm of uncertain behavior of renal pelvis**
D41.10 **Neoplasm of uncertain behavior of unspecified renal pelvis**
D41.11 **Neoplasm of uncertain behavior of right renal pelvis**
D41.12 **Neoplasm of uncertain behavior of left renal pelvis**
+ **D41.2** **Neoplasm of uncertain behavior of ureter**
D41.20 **Neoplasm of uncertain behavior of unspecified ureter**
D41.21 **Neoplasm of uncertain behavior of right ureter**
D41.22 **Neoplasm of uncertain behavior of left ureter**
D41.3 **Neoplasm of uncertain behavior of urethra**
D41.4 **Neoplasm of uncertain behavior of bladder**
D41.8 **Neoplasm of uncertain behavior of other specified urinary organs**
D41.9 **Neoplasm of uncertain behavior of unspecified urinary organ**

D42 **Neoplasm of uncertain behavior of meninges**

D42.0 **Neoplasm of uncertain behavior of cerebral meninges**
D42.1 **Neoplasm of uncertain behavior of spinal meninges**
D42.9 **Neoplasm of uncertain behavior of meninges, unspecified**

D43 **Neoplasm of uncertain behavior of brain and central nervous system**

Excludes1: *neoplasm of uncertain behavior of peripheral nerves and autonomic nervous system (D48.2)*
D43.0 **Neoplasm of uncertain behavior of brain, supratentorial**
Neoplasm of uncertain behavior of cerebral ventricle
Neoplasm of uncertain behavior of cerebrum
Neoplasm of uncertain behavior of frontal lobe
Neoplasm of uncertain behavior of occipital lobe
Neoplasm of uncertain behavior of parietal lobe
Neoplasm of uncertain behavior of temporal lobe
Excludes1: *neoplasm of uncertain behavior of fourth ventricle (D43.1)*
D43.1 **Neoplasm of uncertain behavior of brain, infratentorial**
Neoplasm of uncertain behavior of brain stem
Neoplasm of uncertain behavior of cerebellum
Neoplasm of uncertain behavior of fourth ventricle
D43.2 **Neoplasm of uncertain behavior of brain, unspecified**
D43.3 **Neoplasm of uncertain behavior of cranial nerves**
D43.4 **Neoplasm of uncertain behavior of spinal cord**
D43.8 **Neoplasm of uncertain behavior of other specified parts of central nervous system**
D43.9 **Neoplasm of uncertain behavior of central nervous system, unspecified**
Neoplasm of uncertain behavior of nervous system (central) NOS

D44 **Neoplasm of uncertain behavior of endocrine glands**

Excludes1: *multiple endocrine adenomatosis (E31.2-)*
multiple endocrine neoplasia (E31.2-)
neoplasm of uncertain behavior of endocrine pancreas (D37.8)
neoplasm of uncertain behavior of ovary (D39.1-)
neoplasm of uncertain behavior of testis (D40.1-)
neoplasm of uncertain behavior of thymus (D38.4)
D44.0 **Neoplasm of uncertain behavior of thyroid gland**
+ **D44.1** **Neoplasm of uncertain behavior of adrenal gland**
Use additional code to identify any functional activity.
D44.10 **Neoplasm of uncertain behavior of unspecified adrenal gland**
D44.11 **Neoplasm of uncertain behavior of right adrenal gland**
D44.12 **Neoplasm of uncertain behavior of left adrenal gland**
D44.2 **Neoplasm of uncertain behavior of parathyroid gland**
D44.3 **Neoplasm of uncertain behavior of pituitary gland**
Use additional code to identify any functional activity.
D44.4 **Neoplasm of uncertain behavior of craniopharyngeal duct**
D44.5 **Neoplasm of uncertain behavior of pineal gland**
D44.6 **Neoplasm of uncertain behavior of carotid body**
D44.7 **Neoplasm of uncertain behavior of aortic body and other paraganglia**
AHA CC: 4Q, 2016, 26
D44.9 **Neoplasm of uncertain behavior of unspecified endocrine gland**

D45 **Polycythemia vera**

Excludes1: *familial polycythemia (D75.0)*
secondary polycythemia (D75.1)
Valid 3-character code, no further characters required

D46 **Myelodysplastic syndromes**

Use additional code for adverse effect, if applicable, to identify drug (T36-T50 with fifth or sixth character 5)
Excludes2: *drug-induced aplastic anemia (D61.1)*
D46.0 **Refractory anemia without ring sideroblasts, so stated**
Refractory anemia without sideroblasts, without excess of blasts
D46.1 **Refractory anemia with ring sideroblasts**
RARS
+ **D46.2** **Refractory anemia with excess of blasts [RAEB]**
D46.20 **Refractory anemia with excess of blasts, unspecified**
RAEB NOS
D46.21 **Refractory anemia with excess of blasts 1**
RAEB 1
CC **D46.22** **Refractory anemia with excess of blasts 2**
RAEB 2

D46.A **Refractory cytopenia with multilineage dysplasia**

D46.B **Refractory cytopenia with multilineage dysplasia and ring sideroblasts**

RCMD RS

CC **D46.C** **Myelodysplastic syndrome with isolated del(5q) chromosomal abnormality**

Myelodysplastic syndrome with 5q deletion

5q minus syndrome NOS

D46.4 **Refractory anemia, unspecified**

D46.Z **Other myelodysplastic syndromes**

Excludes1: *chronic myelomonocytic leukemia (C93.1-)*

D46.9 **Myelodysplastic syndrome, unspecified**

Myelodysplasia NOS

D47 **Other neoplasms of uncertain behavior of lymphoid, hematopoietic and related tissue**

D47.0 **Mast cell neoplasms of uncertain behavior**

Excludes1: *congenital cutaneous mastocytosis (Q82.2)*

histiocytic neoplasms of uncertain behavior (D47.Z9)

malignant mast cell neoplasm (C96.2-)

AHA CC: 4Q, 2017, 5

CC **D47.01** **Cutaneous mastocytosis**

Diffuse cutaneous mastocytosis

Maculopapular cutaneous mastocytosis

Solitary mastocytoma

Telangiectasia macularis eruptiva perstans

Urticaria pigmentosa

Excludes1: *congenital (diffuse) (maculopapular) cutaneous mastocytosis (Q82.2)*

congenital urticaria pigmentosa (Q82.2)

extracutaneous mastocytoma (D47.09)

CC **D47.02** **Systemic mastocytosis**

Indolent systemic mastocytosis

Isolated bone marrow mastocytosis

Smoldering systemic mastocytosis

Systemic mastocytosis, with an associated hematological non-mast cell lineage disease (SM-AHNMD)

Code also, if applicable, any associated hematological non-mast cell lineage disease, such as:

acute myeloid leukemia (C92.6-, C92.A-)

chronic myelomonocytic leukemia (C93.1-)

essential thrombocytosis (D47.3)

hypereosinophilic syndrome (D72.1)

myelodysplastic syndrome (D46.9)

myeloproliferative syndrome (D47.1)

non-Hodgkin lymphoma (C82-C85)

plasma cell myeloma (C90.0-)

polycythemia vera (D45)

Excludes1: *aggressive systemic mastocytosis (C96.21)*

mast cell leukemia (C94.3-)

CC **D47.09** **Other mast cell neoplasms of uncertain behavior**

Extracutaneous mastocytoma

Mast cell tumor NOS

Mastocytoma NOS

Mastocytosis NOS

Excludes1: *malignant mast cell tumor (C96.2)*

mastocytosis (congenital) (cutaneous) (Q82.2)

CC **D47.1** **Chronic myeloproliferative disease**

Chronic neutrophilic leukemia

Myeloproliferative disease, unspecified

Excludes1: *atypical chronic myeloid leukemia BCR/ABL-negative (C92.2-)*

chronic myeloid leukemia BCR/ABL-positive (C92.1-)

myelofibrosis NOS (D75.81)

myelophthisic anemia (D61.82)

myelophthisis (D61.82)

secondary myelofibrosis NOS (D75.81)

D47.2 **Monoclonal gammopathy**

Monoclonal gammopathy of undetermined significance [MGUS]

D47.3 **Essential (hemorrhagic) thrombocythemia**

Essential thrombocytosis

Idiopathic hemorrhagic thrombocythemia

D47.4 **Osteomyelofibrosis**

Chronic idiopathic myelofibrosis

Myelofibrosis (idiopathic) (with myeloid metaplasia)

Myelosclerosis (megakaryocytic) with myeloid metaplasia

Secondary myelofibrosis in myeloproliferative disease

Excludes1: *acute myelofibrosis (C94.4-)*

+ **D47.Z** **Other specified neoplasms of uncertain behavior of lymphoid, hematopoietic and related tissue**

CC **D47.Z1** **Post-transplant lymphoproliferative disorder (PTLD)**

Code first complications of transplanted organs and tissue (T86.-)

CC **D47.Z2** **Castleman disease**

Code also if applicable human herpesvirus 8 infection (B10.89)

Excludes2: *Kaposi's sarcoma (C46.-)*

AHA CC: 4Q, 2016, 8

CC **D47.Z9** **Other specified neoplasms of uncertain behavior of lymphoid, hematopoietic and related tissue**

Histiocytic tumors of uncertain behavior

CC **D47.9** **Neoplasm of uncertain behavior of lymphoid, hematopoietic and related tissue, unspecified**

Lymphoproliferative disease NOS

D48 **Neoplasm of uncertain behavior of other and unspecified sites**

Excludes1: *neurofibromatosis (nonmalignant) (Q85.0-)*

D48.0 **Neoplasm of uncertain behavior of bone and articular cartilage**

Excludes1: *neoplasm of uncertain behavior of cartilage of ear (D48.1)*

neoplasm of uncertain behavior of cartilage of larynx (D38.0)

neoplasm of uncertain behavior of cartilage of nose (D38.5)

neoplasm of uncertain behavior of connective tissue of eyelid (D48.1)

neoplasm of uncertain behavior of synovia (D48.1)

D48.1 **Neoplasm of uncertain behavior of connective and other soft tissue**

Neoplasm of uncertain behavior of connective tissue of ear

Neoplasm of uncertain behavior of connective tissue of eyelid

Stromal tumors of uncertain behavior of digestive system

Excludes1: *neoplasm of uncertain behavior of articular cartilage (D48.0)*

neoplasm of uncertain behavior of cartilage of larynx (D38.0)

neoplasm of uncertain behavior of cartilage of nose (D38.5)

neoplasm of uncertain behavior of connective tissue of breast (D48.6-)

D48.2 **Neoplasm of uncertain behavior of peripheral nerves and autonomic nervous system**

Excludes1: *neoplasm of uncertain behavior of peripheral nerves of orbit (D48.7)*

D48.3 **Neoplasm of uncertain behavior of retroperitoneum**

D48.4 **Neoplasm of uncertain behavior of peritoneum**

D48.5 **Neoplasm of uncertain behavior of skin**

Neoplasm of uncertain behavior of anal margin

Neoplasm of uncertain behavior of anal skin

Neoplasm of uncertain behavior of perianal skin

Neoplasm of uncertain behavior of skin of breast

Excludes1: *neoplasm of uncertain behavior of anus NOS (D37.8)*

neoplasm of uncertain behavior of skin of genital organs (D39.8, D40.8)

neoplasm of uncertain behavior of vermilion border of lip (D37.0)

+ **D48.6** **Neoplasm of uncertain behavior of breast**

Neoplasm of uncertain behavior of connective tissue of breast

Cystosarcoma phyllodes

Excludes1: *neoplasm of uncertain behavior of skin of breast (D48.5)*

D48.60 **Neoplasm of uncertain behavior of unspecified breast**

D48.61 **Neoplasm of uncertain behavior of right breast**

D48.62 **Neoplasm of uncertain behavior of left breast**

D48.7 Neoplasm of uncertain behavior of other specified sites
Neoplasm of uncertain behavior of eye
Neoplasm of uncertain behavior of heart
Neoplasm of uncertain behavior of peripheral nerves of orbit

Excludes1: *neoplasm of uncertain behavior of connective tissue (D48.1)*
neoplasm of uncertain behavior of skin of eyelid (D48.5)

D48.9 Neoplasm of uncertain behavior, unspecified

Neoplasms of unspecified behavior (D49)

D49 Neoplasms of unspecified behavior

NOTE Category D49 classifies by site neoplasms of unspecified morphology and behavior. The term 'mass', unless otherwise stated, is not to be regarded as a neoplastic growth.

Includes: 'growth' NOS
neoplasm NOS
new growth NOS
tumor NOS

Excludes1: *neoplasms of uncertain behavior (D37-D44, D48)*

D49.0 Neoplasm of unspecified behavior of digestive system

Excludes1: *neoplasm of unspecified behavior of margin of anus (D49.2)*
neoplasm of unspecified behavior of perianal skin (D49.2)
neoplasm of unspecified behavior of skin of anus (D49.2)

D49.1 Neoplasm of unspecified behavior of respiratory system

D49.2 Neoplasm of unspecified behavior of bone, soft tissue, and skin

Excludes1: *neoplasm of unspecified behavior of anal canal (D49.0)*
neoplasm of unspecified behavior of anus NOS (D49.0)
neoplasm of unspecified behavior of bone marrow (D49.89)
neoplasm of unspecified behavior of cartilage of larynx (D49.1)
neoplasm of unspecified behavior of cartilage of nose (D49.1)
neoplasm of unspecified behavior of connective tissue of breast (D49.3)
neoplasm of unspecified behavior of skin of genital organs (D49.59)
neoplasm of unspecified behavior of vermilion border of lip (D49.0)

D49.3 Neoplasm of unspecified behavior of breast

Excludes1: *neoplasm of unspecified behavior of skin of breast (D49.2)*

D49.4 Neoplasm of unspecified behavior of bladder

+ **D49.5 Neoplasm of unspecified behavior of other genitourinary organs**
AHA CC: 4Q, 2016, 9

+ **D49.51 Neoplasm of unspecified behavior of kidney**

D49.511 Neoplasm of unspecified behavior of right kidney

D49.512 Neoplasm of unspecified behavior of left kidney

D49.519 Neoplasm of unspecified behavior of unspecified kidney

D49.59 Neoplasm unspecified behavior of other genitourinary organ

D49.6 Neoplasm of unspecified behavior of brain

Excludes1: *neoplasm of unspecified behavior of cerebral meninges (D49.7)*
neoplasm of unspecified behavior of cranial nerves (D49.7)

D49.7 Neoplasm of unspecified behavior of endocrine glands and other parts of nervous system

Excludes1: *neoplasm of unspecified behavior of peripheral, sympathetic, and parasympathetic nerves and ganglia (D49.2)*

+ **D49.8 Neoplasm of unspecified behavior of other specified sites**

Excludes1: *neoplasm of unspecified behavior of eyelid (skin) (D49.2)*
neoplasm of unspecified behavior of eyelid cartilage (D49.2)
neoplasm of unspecified behavior of great vessels (D49.2)
neoplasm of unspecified behavior of optic nerve (D49.7)

D49.81 Neoplasm of unspecified behavior of retina and choroid
Dark area on retina
Retinal freckle

D49.89 Neoplasm of unspecified behavior of other specified sites

D49.9 Neoplasm of unspecified behavior of unspecified site

+, +7th, X + 7th   ● Newborn   ● Pediatric   ● Maternity   ● Adult   ♀ Female   ♂ Male   Manifestation   Unacceptable PDX   HCC   CC   MCC   HAC

Chapter 3: Diseases of the Blood and Blood-Forming Organs and Certain Disorders Involving the Immune Mechanism (D50-D89)

Excludes2: *autoimmune disease (systemic) NOS (M35.9)*
certain conditions originating in the perinatal period (P00-P96)
complications of pregnancy, childbirth and the puerperium (O00-O9A)
congenital malformations, deformations and chromosomal abnormalities (Q00-Q99)
endocrine, nutritional and metabolic diseases (E00-E88)
human immunodeficiency virus [HIV] disease (B20)
injury, poisoning and certain other consequences of external causes (S00-T88)
neoplasms (C00-D49)
symptoms, signs and abnormal clinical and laboratory findings, not elsewhere classified (R00-R94)

This chapter contains the following category blocks:

D50-D53 Nutritional anemias
D55-D59 Hemolytic anemias
D60-D64 Aplastic and other anemias and other bone marrow failure syndromes
D65-D69 Coagulation defects, purpura and other hemorrhagic conditions
D70-D77 Other disorders of blood and blood-forming organs
D78   Intraoperative and postprocedural complications of the spleen
D80-D89 Certain disorders involving the immune mechanism

C. Chapter-Specific Coding Guidelines

In addition to general coding guidelines, there are guidelines for specific diagnoses and/or conditions in the classification. Unless otherwise indicated, these guidelines apply to all health care settings. Please refer to Section II for guidelines on the selection of principal diagnosis.

3. Chapter 3: Diseases of the Blood and Blood-Forming Organs and Certain Disorders Involving the Immune Mechanism (D50-D89)

Reserved for future guideline expansion

Nutritional anemias (D50-D53)

D50 Iron deficiency anemia

Includes: asiderotic anemia
hypochromic anemia

D50.0 Iron deficiency anemia secondary to blood loss (chronic)
Posthemorrhagic anemia (chronic)
Excludes1: *acute posthemorrhagic anemia (D62)*
congenital anemia from fetal blood loss (P61.3)

D50.1 Sideropenic dysphagia
Kelly-Paterson syndrome
Plummer-Vinson syndrome

D50.8 Other iron deficiency anemias
Iron deficiency anemia due to inadequate dietary iron intake

D50.9 Iron deficiency anemia, unspecified

D51 Vitamin B12 deficiency anemia

Excludes1: *vitamin B12 deficiency (E53.8)*

D51.0 Vitamin B12 deficiency anemia due to intrinsic factor deficiency
Addison anemia
Biermer anemia
Pernicious (congenital) anemia
Congenital intrinsic factor deficiency

D51.1 Vitamin B12 deficiency anemia due to selective vitamin B12 malabsorption with proteinuria
Imerslund (Gräsbeck) syndrome
Megaloblastic hereditary anemia

D51.2 Transcobalamin II deficiency

D51.3 Other dietary vitamin B12 deficiency anemia
Vegan anemia

D51.8 Other vitamin B12 deficiency anemias

D51.9 Vitamin B12 deficiency anemia, unspecified

D52 Folate deficiency anemia

Excludes1: *folate deficiency without anemia (E53.8)*

D52.0 Dietary folate deficiency anemia
Nutritional megaloblastic anemia

D52.1 Drug-induced folate deficiency anemia
Use additional code for adverse effect, if applicable, to identify drug (T36-T50 with fifth or sixth character 5)

D52.8 Other folate deficiency anemias

D52.9 Folate deficiency anemia, unspecified
Folic acid deficiency anemia NOS

D53 Other nutritional anemias

Includes: megaloblastic anemia unresponsive to vitamin B12 or folate therapy

D53.0 Protein deficiency anemia
Amino-acid deficiency anemia
Orotaciduric anemia
Excludes1: *Lesch-Nyhan syndrome (E79.1)*

D53.1 Other megaloblastic anemias, not elsewhere classified
Megaloblastic anemia NOS
Excludes1: *Di Guglielmo's disease (C94.0)*

D53.2 Scorbutic anemia
Excludes1: *scurvy (E54)*

D53.8 Other specified nutritional anemias
Anemia associated with deficiency of copper
Anemia associated with deficiency of molybdenum
Anemia associated with deficiency of zinc
Excludes1: *nutritional deficiencies without anemia, such as:*
copper deficiency NOS (E61.0)
molybdenum deficiency NOS (E61.5)
zinc deficiency NOS (E60)

D53.9 Nutritional anemia, unspecified
Simple chronic anemia
Excludes1: *anemia NOS (D64.9)*
AHA CC: 4Q, 2018, 88

Hemolytic anemias (D55-D59)

D55 Anemia due to enzyme disorders

Excludes1: *drug-induced enzyme deficiency anemia (D59.2)*

D55.0 Anemia due to glucose-6-phosphate dehydrogenase [G6PD] deficiency
Favism
G6PD deficiency anemia
Excludes1: *glucose-6-phosphate dehydrogenase (G6PD) deficiency without anemia (D75.A)*

D55.1 Anemia due to other disorders of glutathione metabolism
Anemia (due to) enzyme deficiencies, except G6PD, related to the hexose monophosphate [HMP] shunt pathway
Anemia (due to) hemolytic nonspherocytic (hereditary), type I

D55.2 Anemia due to disorders of glycolytic enzymes
Hemolytic nonspherocytic (hereditary) anemia, type II
Hexokinase deficiency anemia
Pyruvate kinase [PK] deficiency anemia
Triose-phosphate isomerase deficiency anemia
Excludes1: *disorders of glycolysis not associated with anemia (E74.81-)*

D55.3 Anemia due to disorders of nucleotide metabolism

D55.8 Other anemias due to enzyme disorders

D55.9 Anemia due to enzyme disorder, unspecified

D56 Thalassemia

Excludes1: *sickle-cell thalassemia (D57.4-)*

D56.0 Alpha thalassemia
Alpha thalassemia major
Hemoglobin H Constant Spring
Hemoglobin H disease
Hydrops fetalis due to alpha thalassemia
Severe alpha thalassemia
Triple gene defect alpha thalassemia
Use additional code, if applicable, for hydrops fetalis due to alpha thalassemia (P56.99)
Excludes1: *alpha thalassemia trait or minor (D56.3)*
asymptomatic alpha thalassemia (D56.3)
hydrops fetalis due to isoimmunization (P56.0)
hydrops fetalis not due to immune hemolysis (P83.2)

D56.1 Beta thalassemia
Beta thalassemia major
Cooley's anemia
Homozygous beta thalassemia
Severe beta thalassemia
Thalassemia intermedia
Thalassemia major
Excludes1: *beta thalassemia minor (D56.3)*
beta thalassemia trait (D56.3)
delta-beta thalassemia (D56.2)
hemoglobin E-beta thalassemia (D56.5)
sickle-cell beta thalassemia (D57.4-)

+, +7th, X + 7th   ● Newborn   ● Pediatric   ● Maternity   ● Adult   ♀ Female   ♂ Male   Manifestation   Unacceptable PDX   HCC   CC   MCC   HAC

D56.2 Delta-beta thalassemia
  Homozygous delta-beta thalassemia
  Excludes1: *delta-beta thalassemia minor (D56.3)*
       delta-beta thalassemia trait (D56.3)

D56.3 Thalassemia minor
  Alpha thalassemia minor
  Alpha thalassemia silent carrier
  Alpha thalassemia trait
  Beta thalassemia minor
  Beta thalassemia trait
  Delta-beta thalassemia minor
  Delta-beta thalassemia trait
  Thalassemia trait NOS
  Excludes1: *alpha thalassemia (D56.0)*
       beta thalassemia (D56.1)
       delta-beta thalassemia (D56.2)
       hemoglobin E-beta thalassemia (D56.5)
       sickle-cell trait (D57.3)

D56.4 Hereditary persistence of fetal hemoglobin [HPFH]

D56.5 Hemoglobin E-beta thalassemia
  Excludes1: *beta thalassemia (D56.1)*
       beta thalassemia minor (D56.3)
       beta thalassemia trait (D56.3)
       delta-beta thalassemia (D56.2)
       delta-beta thalassemia trait (D56.3)
       hemoglobin E disease (D58.2)
       other hemoglobinopathies (D58.2)
       sickle-cell beta thalassemia (D57.4-)

D56.8 Other thalassemias
  Dominant thalassemia
  Hemoglobin C thalassemia
  Mixed thalassemia
  Thalassemia with other hemoglobinopathy
  Excludes1: *hemoglobin C disease (D58.2)*
       hemoglobin E disease (D58.2)
       other hemoglobinopathies (D58.2)
       sickle-cell anemia (D57.-)
       sickle-cell thalassemia (D57.4)

D56.9 Thalassemia, unspecified
  Mediterranean anemia (with other hemoglobinopathy)

D57 Sickle-cell disorders
  Use additional code for any associated fever (R50.81)
  Excludes1: *other hemoglobinopathies (D58.-)*

+ **D57.0 Hb-SS disease with crisis**
  Sickle-cell disease with crisis
  Hb-SS disease with vasoocclusive pain
  MCC **D57.00 Hb-SS disease with crisis, unspecified**
    Hb-SS disease with (painful) crisis NOS
    Hb-SS disease with vasoocclusive pain NOS
  MCC **D57.01 Hb-SS disease with acute chest syndrome**
  MCC **D57.02 Hb-SS disease with splenic sequestration**
  MCC **D57.03 Hb-SS disease with cerebral vascular involvement**
    Code also, if applicable, cerebral infarction (I63.-)
  MCC **D57.09 Hb-SS disease with crisis with other specified complication**
    Use additional code to identify complications,
      such as:
      cholelithiasis (K80.-)
      priapism (N48.32)

D57.1 Sickle-cell disease without crisis
  Hb-SS disease without crisis
  Sickle-cell anemia NOS
  Sickle-cell disease NOS
  Sickle-cell disorder NOS

+ **D57.2 Sickle-cell/Hb-C disease**
  Hb-SC disease
  Hb-S/Hb-C disease
  D57.20 Sickle-cell/Hb-C disease without crisis
  + **D57.21 Sickle-cell/Hb-C disease with crisis**
    MCC **D57.211 Sickle-cell/Hb-C disease with acute chest syndrome**
    MCC **D57.212 Sickle-cell/Hb-C disease with splenic sequestration**

MCC **D57.213 Sickle-cell/Hb-C disease with cerebral vascular involvement**
    Code also, if applicable, cerebral infarction (I63.-)
MCC **D57.218 Sickle-cell/Hb-C disease with crisis with other specified complication**
    Use additional code to identify complications, such as:
      cholelithiasis (K80.-)
      priapism (N48.32)
MCC **D57.219 Sickle-cell/Hb-C disease with crisis, unspecified**
    Sickle-cell/Hb-C disease with crisis NOS
    Sickle-cell/Hb-C disease with vasoocclusive pain NOS

D57.3 Sickle-cell trait
  Hb-S trait
  Heterozygous hemoglobin S

+ **D57.4 Sickle-cell thalassemia**
  Sickle-cell beta thalassemia
  Thalassemia Hb-S disease
  D57.40 Sickle-cell thalassemia without crisis
    Microdrepanocytosis
    Sickle-cell thalassemia NOS
  + **D57.41 Sickle-cell thalassemia, unspecified, with crisis**
    Sickle-cell thalassemia with (painful) crisis NOS
    Sickle-cell thalassemia with vasoocclusive pain NOS
    MCC **D57.411 Sickle-cell thalassemia, unspecified, with acute chest syndrome**
    MCC **D57.412 Sickle-cell thalassemia, unspecified, with splenic sequestration**
    MCC **D57.413 Sickle-cell thalassemia, unspecified, with cerebral vascular involvement**
      Code also, if applicable, cerebral infarction (I63.-)
    MCC **D57.418 Sickle-cell thalassemia, unspecified, with crisis with other specified complication**
      Use additional code to identify complications, such as:
        cholelithiasis (K80.-)
        priapism (N48.32)
    MCC **D57.419 Sickle-cell thalassemia, unspecified, with crisis**
      Sickle-cell thalassemia with (painful) crisis NOS
      Sickle-cell thalassemia with vasoocclusive pain
  D57.42 Sickle-cell thalassemia beta zero without crisis
    HbS-beta zero without crisis
    Sickle-cell beta zero without crisis
  + **D57.43 Sickle-cell thalassemia beta zero with crisis**
    HbS-beta zero with crisis
    Sickle-cell beta zero with crisis
    MCC **D57.431 Sickle-cell thalassemia beta zero with acute chest syndrome**
      HbS-beta zero with acute chest syndrome
      Sickle-cell beta zero with acute chest syndrome
    MCC **D57.432 Sickle-cell thalassemia beta zero with splenic sequestration**
      HbS-beta zero with splenic sequestration
      Sickle-cell beta zero with splenic sequestration
    MCC **D57.433 Sickle-cell thalassemia beta zero with cerebral vascular involvement**
      HbS-beta zero with cerebral vascular involvement
      Sickle-cell beta zero with cerebral vascular involvement
      Code also, if applicable, cerebral infarction (I63.-)

+, +7th, X + 7th   ● Newborn   ● Pediatric   ● Maternity   ● Adult   ♀ Female   ♂ Male   Manifestation   Unacceptable PDX   HCC   CC   MCC   HAC

MCC **D57.438** **Sickle-cell thalassemia beta zero with crisis with other specified complication**
  HbS-beta zero with other specified complication
  Sickle-cell beta zero with other specified complication
  Use additional code to identify complications, such as:
    cholelithiasis (K80.-)
    priapism (N48.32)

MCC **D57.439** **Sickle-cell thalassemia beta zero with crisis, unspecified**
  HbS-beta zero with other specified complication
  Sickle-cell beta zero with crisis unspecified
  Sickle-cell thalassemia beta zero with (painful) crisis NOS
  Sickle-cell thalassemia beta zero with vasoocclusive pain

D57.44 **Sickle-cell thalassemia beta plus without crisis**
  HbS-beta plus without crisis
  Sickle-cell beta plus without crisis

+ **D57.45** **Sickle-cell thalassemia beta plus with crisis**
  HbS-beta plus with crisis
  Sickle-cell beta plus with crisis

MCC **D57.451** **Sickle-cell thalassemia beta plus with acute chest syndrome**
  HbS-beta plus with acute chest syndrome
  Sickle-cell beta plus with acute chest syndrome

MCC **D57.452** **Sickle-cell thalassemia beta plus with splenic sequestration**
  HbS-beta plus with splenic sequestration
  Sickle-cell beta plus with splenic sequestration

MCC **D57.453** **Sickle-cell thalassemia beta plus with cerebral vascular involvement**
  HbS-beta plus with cerebral vascular involvement
  Sickle-cell beta plus with cerebral vascular involvement
  Code also, if applicable, cerebral infarction (I63.-)

MCC **D57.458** **Sickle-cell thalassemia beta plus with crisis with other specified complication**
  HbS-beta plus with crisis with other specified complication
  Sickle-cell beta plus with crisis with other specified complication
  Use additional code to identify complications, such as:
    cholelithiasis (K80.-)
    priapism (N48.32)

MCC **D57.459** **Sickle-cell thalassemia beta plus with crisis, unspecified**
  HbS-beta plus with crisis with unspecified complication
  Sickle-cell beta plus with crisis with unspecified complication
  Sickle-cell thalassemia beta plus with (painful) crisis NOS
  Sickle-cell thalassemia beta plus with vasoocclusive pain

+ **D57.8** **Other sickle-cell disorders**
  Hb-SD disease
  Hb-SE disease

  D57.80 **Other sickle-cell disorders without crisis**
+ **D57.81** **Other sickle-cell disorders with crisis**

MCC **D57.811** **Other sickle-cell disorders with acute chest syndrome**

MCC **D57.812** **Other sickle-cell disorders with splenic sequestration**

MCC **D57.813** **Other sickle-cell disorders with cerebral vascular involvement**
  Code also, if applicable, cerebral infarction (I63.-)

MCC **D57.818** **Other sickle-cell disorders with crisis with other specified complication**
  Use additional code to identify complications, such as:
    cholelithiasis (K80.-)
    priapism (N48.32)

MCC **D57.819** **Other sickle-cell disorders with crisis, unspecified**
  Other sickle-cell disorders with crisis NOS
  Other sickle-cell disorders with vasoocclusive pain NOS

D58 **Other hereditary hemolytic anemias**

  Excludes1: hemolytic anemia of the newborn (P55.-)

D58.0 **Hereditary spherocytosis**
  Acholuric (familial) jaundice
  Congenital (spherocytic) hemolytic icterus
  Minkowski-Chauffard syndrome

D58.1 **Hereditary elliptocytosis**
  Elliptocytosis (congenital)
  Ovalocytosis (congenital) (hereditary)

D58.2 **Other hemoglobinopathies**
  Abnormal hemoglobin NOS
  Congenital Heinz body anemia
  Hb-C disease
  Hb-D disease
  Hb-E disease
  Hemoglobinopathy NOS
  Unstable hemoglobin hemolytic disease
  Excludes1: familial polycythemia (D75.0)
    Hb-M disease (D74.0)
    hemoglobin E-beta thalassemia (D56.5)
    hereditary persistence of fetal hemoglobin [HPFH] (D56.4)
    high-altitude polycythemia (D75.1)
    methemoglobinemia (D74.-)
    other hemoglobinopathies with thalassemia (D56.8)

CC **D58.8** **Other specified hereditary hemolytic anemias**
  Stomatocytosis

CC **D58.9** **Hereditary hemolytic anemia, unspecified**

D59 **Acquired hemolytic anemia**

CC **D59.0** **Drug-induced autoimmune hemolytic anemia**
  Use additional code for adverse effect, if applicable, to identify drug (T36-T50 with fifth or sixth character 5)

+ **D59.1** **Other autoimmune hemolytic anemias**
  Excludes2: Evans syndrome (D69.41)
    hemolytic disease of newborn (P55.-)
    paroxysmal cold hemoglobinuria (D59.6)

CC **D59.10** **Autoimmune hemolytic anemia, unspecified**

CC **D59.11** **Warm autoimmune hemolytic anemia**
  Warm type (primary) (secondary) (symptomatic) autoimmune hemolytic anemia
  Warm type autoimmune hemolytic disease

CC **D59.12** **Cold autoimmune hemolytic anemia**
  Chronic cold hemagglutinin disease
  Cold agglutinin disease
  Cold agglutinin hemoglobinuria
  Cold type (primary) (secondary) (symptomatic) autoimmune hemolytic anemia
  Cold type autoimmune hemolytic disease

CC **D59.13** **Mixed type autoimmune hemolytic anemia**
  Mixed type autoimmune hemolytic disease
  Mixed type, cold and warm, (primary) (secondary) (symptomatic) autoimmune hemolytic anemia

CC **D59.19** **Other autoimmune hemolytic anemia**

CC **D59.2** **Drug-induced nonautoimmune hemolytic anemia**
Drug-induced enzyme deficiency anemia
Use additional code for adverse effect, if applicable, to identify drug (T36-T50 with fifth or sixth character 5)

MCC **D59.3** **Hemolytic-uremic syndrome**
Use additional code to identify associated:
E. coli infection (B96.2-)
Pneumococcal pneumonia (J13)
Shigella dysenteriae (A03.9)

CC **D59.4** **Other nonautoimmune hemolytic anemias**
Mechanical hemolytic anemia
Microangiopathic hemolytic anemia
Toxic hemolytic anemia

D59.5 **Paroxysmal nocturnal hemoglobinuria [Marchiafava-Micheli]**
Excludes1: *hemoglobinuria NOS (R82.3)*

D59.6 **Hemoglobinuria due to hemolysis from other external causes**
Hemoglobinuria from exertion
March hemoglobinuria
Paroxysmal cold hemoglobinuria
Use additional code (Chapter 20) to identify external cause
Excludes1: *hemoglobinuria NOS (R82.3)*

D59.8 **Other acquired hemolytic anemias**

CC **D59.9** **Acquired hemolytic anemia, unspecified**
Idiopathic hemolytic anemia, chronic

Aplastic and other anemias and other bone marrow failure syndromes (D60-D64)

D60 **Acquired pure red cell aplasia [erythroblastopenia]**
Includes: red cell aplasia (acquired) (adult) (with thymoma)
Excludes1: *congenital red cell aplasia (D61.01)*

MCC **D60.0** **Chronic acquired pure red cell aplasia**

MCC **D60.1** **Transient acquired pure red cell aplasia**

MCC **D60.8** **Other acquired pure red cell aplasias**

MCC **D60.9** **Acquired pure red cell aplasia, unspecified**

D61 **Other aplastic anemias and other bone marrow failure syndromes**
Excludes2: *neutropenia (D70.-)*

+ **D61.0** **Constitutional aplastic anemia**

CC **D61.01** **Constitutional (pure) red blood cell aplasia**
Blackfan-Diamond syndrome
Congenital (pure) red cell aplasia
Familial hypoplastic anemia
Primary (pure) red cell aplasia
Red cell (pure) aplasia of infants
Excludes1: *acquired red cell aplasia (D60.9)*

CC **D61.09** **Other constitutional aplastic anemia**
Fanconi's anemia
Pancytopenia with malformations

MCC **D61.1** **Drug-induced aplastic anemia**
Use additional code for adverse effect, if applicable, to identify drug (T36-T50 with fifth or sixth character 5)

MCC **D61.2** **Aplastic anemia due to other external agents**
Code first, if applicable, toxic effects of substances chiefly nonmedicinal as to source (T51-T65)

MCC **D61.3** **Idiopathic aplastic anemia**

+ **D61.8** **Other specified aplastic anemias and other bone marrow failure syndromes**

+ **D61.81** **Pancytopenia**
Excludes1: *pancytopenia (due to) (with) aplastic anemia (D61.9)*
pancytopenia (due to) (with) bone marrow infiltration (D61.82)
pancytopenia (due to) (with) congenital (pure) red cell aplasia (D61.01)
pancytopenia (due to) (with) hairy cell leukemia (C91.4-)
pancytopenia (due to) (with) human immunodeficiency virus disease (B20.-)
pancytopenia (due to) (with) leukoerythroblastic anemia (D61.82)
pancytopenia (due to) (with) myeloproliferative disease (D47.1)
Excludes2: *pancytopenia (due to) (with) myelodysplastic syndromes (D46.-)*

MCC **D61.810** **Antineoplastic chemotherapy induced pancytopenia**
Excludes2: *aplastic anemia due to antineoplastic chemotherapy (D61.1)*

MCC **D61.811** **Other drug-induced pancytopenia**
Excludes2: *aplastic anemia due to drugs (D61.1)*

CC **D61.818** **Other pancytopenia**
AHA CC: 1Q, 2019, 16-17

CC **D61.82** **Myelophthisis**
Leukoerythroblastic anemia
Myelophthisic anemia
Panmyelophthisis
Code also the underlying disorder, such as:
malignant neoplasm of breast (C50.-)
tuberculosis (A15.-)
Excludes1: *idiopathic myelofibrosis (D47.1)*
myelofibrosis NOS (D75.81)
myelofibrosis with myeloid metaplasia (D47.4)
primary myelofibrosis (D47.1)
secondary myelofibrosis (D75.81)

MCC **D61.89** **Other specified aplastic anemias and other bone marrow failure syndromes**

CC **D61.9** **Aplastic anemia, unspecified**
Hypoplastic anemia NOS
Medullary hypoplasia

CC **D62** **Acute posthemorrhagic anemia**
Excludes1: *anemia due to chronic blood loss (D50.0)*
blood loss anemia NOS (D50.0)
congenital anemia from fetal blood loss (P61.3)
AHA CC: 3Q, 2019, 11-12, 17
Valid 3-character code, no further characters required

D63 **Anemia in chronic diseases classified elsewhere**

D63.0 **Anemia in neoplastic disease**
Code first neoplasm (C00-D49)
Excludes1: *aplastic anemia due to antineoplastic chemotherapy (D61.1)*
Excludes2: *anemia due to antineoplastic chemotherapy (D64.81)*
Review coding guidelines C.2.c.1, C.2.c.2 and C.2.1.4

D63.1 **Anemia in chronic kidney disease**
Erythropoietin resistant anemia (EPO resistant anemia)
Code first underlying chronic kidney disease (CKD) (N18.-)

D63.8 **Anemia in other chronic diseases classified elsewhere**
Code first underlying disease, such as:
diphyllobothriasis (B70.0)
hookworm disease (B76.0-B76.9)
hypothyroidism (E00.0-E03.9)
malaria (B50.0-B54)
symptomatic late syphilis (A52.79)
tuberculosis (A18.89)

D64 **Other anemias**
Excludes1: *refractory anemia (D46.-)*
refractory anemia with excess blasts in transformation [RAEB T] (C92.0-)

D64.0 **Hereditary sideroblastic anemia**
Sex-linked hypochromic sideroblastic anemia

D64.1 **Secondary sideroblastic anemia due to disease**
Code first underlying disease

D64.2 **Secondary sideroblastic anemia due to drugs and toxins**
Code first poisoning due to drug or toxin, if applicable (T36-T65 with fifth or sixth character 1-4 or 6)

Use additional code for adverse effect, if applicable, to identify drug (T36-T50 with fifth or sixth character 5)

D64.3 **Other sideroblastic anemias**
Sideroblastic anemia NOS
Pyridoxine-responsive sideroblastic anemia NEC

D64.4 **Congenital dyserythropoietic anemia**
Dyshematopoietic anemia (congenital)
Excludes1: *Blackfan-Diamond syndrome (D61.01)*
Di Guglielmo's disease (C94.0)

+, +7th, X + 7th   ● Newborn   ● Pediatric   ● Maternity   ● Adult   ♀ Female   ♂ Male   Manifestation   Unacceptable PDX   HCC   CC   MCC   HAC

+ **D64.8 Other specified anemias**

  D64.81 Anemia due to antineoplastic chemotherapy
    Antineoplastic chemotherapy induced anemia
    Excludes1: aplastic anemia due to antineoplastic chemotherapy (D61.1)
    Excludes2: anemia in neoplastic disease (D63.0)
    AHA CC: 4Q, 2014, 22-23

  D64.89 Other specified anemias
    Infantile pseudoleukemia

D64.9 Anemia, unspecified
  AHA CC: 4Q, 2018, 88

Coagulation defects, purpura and other hemorrhagic conditions (D65-D69)

MCC **D65 Disseminated intravascular coagulation [defibrination syndrome]**
  Afibrinogenemia, acquired
  Consumption coagulopathy
  Diffuse or disseminated intravascular coagulation [DIC]
  Fibrinolytic hemorrhage, acquired
  Fibrinolytic purpura
  Purpura fulminans
  Excludes1: disseminated intravascular coagulation (complicating):
    abortion or ectopic or molar pregnancy (O00-O07, O08.1)
    in newborn (P60)
    pregnancy, childbirth and the puerperium (O45.0, O46.0, O67.0, O72.3)
  Valid 3-character code, no further characters required

MCC **D66 Hereditary factor VIII deficiency**
  Classical hemophilia
  Deficiency factor VIII (with functional defect)
  Hemophilia NOS
  Hemophilia A
  Excludes1: factor VIII deficiency with vascular defect (D68.0)
  Valid 3-character code, no further characters required

MCC **D67 Hereditary factor IX deficiency**
  Christmas disease
  Factor IX deficiency (with functional defect)
  Hemophilia B
  Plasma thromboplastin component [PTC] deficiency
  Valid 3-character code, no further characters required

D68 Other coagulation defects
  Excludes1: abnormal coagulation profile (R79.1)
    coagulation defects complicating abortion or ectopic or molar pregnancy (O00-O07, O08.1)
    coagulation defects complicating pregnancy, childbirth and the puerperium (O45.0, O46.0, O67.0, O72.3)

CC **D68.0 Von Willebrand's disease**
  Angiohemophilia
  Factor VIII deficiency with vascular defect
  Vascular hemophilia
  Excludes1: capillary fragility (hereditary) (D69.8)
    factor VIII deficiency NOS (D66)
    factor VIII deficiency with functional defect (D66)

CC **D68.1 Hereditary factor XI deficiency**
  Hemophilia C
  Plasma thromboplastin antecedent [PTA] deficiency
  Rosenthal's disease

CC **D68.2 Hereditary deficiency of other clotting factors**
  AC globulin deficiency
  Congenital afibrinogenemia
  Deficiency of factor I [fibrinogen]
  Deficiency of factor II [prothrombin]
  Deficiency of factor V [labile]
  Deficiency of factor VII [stable]
  Deficiency of factor X [Stuart-Prower]
  Deficiency of factor XII [Hageman]
  Deficiency of factor XIII [fibrin stabilizing]
  Dysfibrinogenemia (congenital)
  Hypoproconvertinemia
  Owren's disease
  Proaccelerin deficiency

+ **D68.3 Hemorrhagic disorder due to circulating anticoagulants**
+ **D68.31 Hemorrhagic disorder due to intrinsic circulating anticoagulants, antibodies, or inhibitors**

CC **D68.311 Acquired hemophilia**
  Autoimmune hemophilia
  Autoimmune inhibitors to clotting factors
  Secondary hemophilia

CC **D68.312 Antiphospholipid antibody with hemorrhagic disorder**
  Lupus anticoagulant (LAC) with hemorrhagic disorder
  Systemic lupus erythematosus [SLE] inhibitor with hemorrhagic disorder
  Excludes1: antiphospholipid antibody, finding without diagnosis (R76.0)
    antiphospholipid antibody syndrome (D68.61)
    antiphospholipid antibody with hypercoagulable state (D68.61)
    lupus anticoagulant (LAC) finding without diagnosis (R76.0)
    lupus anticoagulant (LAC) with hypercoagulable state (D68.62)
    systemic lupus erythematosus [SLE] inhibitor finding without diagnosis (R76.0)
    systemic lupus erythematosus [SLE] inhibitor with hypercoagulable state (D68.62)

CC **D68.318 Other hemorrhagic disorder due to intrinsic circulating anticoagulants, antibodies, or inhibitors**
  Antithromboplastinemia
  Antithromboplastinogenemia
  Hemorrhagic disorder due to intrinsic increase in antithrombin
  Hemorrhagic disorder due to intrinsic increase in anti-VIIIa
  Hemorrhagic disorder due to intrinsic increase in anti-IXa
  Hemorrhagic disorder due to intrinsic increase in anti-XIa

CC **D68.32 Hemorrhagic disorder due to extrinsic circulating anticoagulants**
  Drug-induced hemorrhagic disorder
  Hemorrhagic disorder due to increase in anti-IIa
  Hemorrhagic disorder due to increase in anti-Xa
  Hyperheparinemia
  Use additional code for adverse effect, if applicable, to identify drug (T45.515, T45.525)
  AHA CC: 1Q, 2016, 14-15

CC **D68.4 Acquired coagulation factor deficiency**
  Deficiency of coagulation factor due to liver disease
  Deficiency of coagulation factor due to vitamin K deficiency
  Excludes1: vitamin K deficiency of newborn (P53)

+ **D68.5 Primary thrombophilia**
  Primary hypercoagulable states
  Excludes1: antiphospholipid syndrome (D68.61)
    lupus anticoagulant (D68.62)
    secondary activated protein C resistance (D68.69)
    secondary antiphospholipid antibody syndrome (D68.69)
    secondary lupus anticoagulant with hypercoagulable state (D68.69)
    secondary systemic lupus erythematosus [SLE] inhibitor with hypercoagulable state (D68.69)
    systemic lupus erythematosus [SLE] inhibitor finding without diagnosis (R76.0)
    systemic lupus erythematosus [SLE] inhibitor with hemorrhagic disorder (D68.312)
    thrombotic thrombocytopenic purpura (M31.1)

CC **D68.51** **Activated protein C resistance**
Factor V Leiden mutation
CC **D68.52** **Prothrombin gene mutation**
CC **D68.59** **Other primary thrombophilia**
Antithrombin III deficiency
Hypercoagulable state NOS
Primary hypercoagulable state NEC
Primary thrombophilia NEC
Protein C deficiency
Protein S deficiency
Thrombophilia NOS
+ **D68.6** **Other thrombophilia**
Other hypercoagulable states
Excludes1: *diffuse or disseminated intravascular*
coagulation [DIC] (D65)
heparin induced thrombocytopenia (HIT)
(D75.82)
hyperhomocysteinemia (E72.11)
CC **D68.61** **Antiphospholipid syndrome**
Anticardiolipin syndrome
Antiphospholipid antibody syndrome
Excludes1: *anti-phospholipid antibody, finding*
without diagnosis (R76.0)
anti-phospholipid antibody with
hemorrhagic disorder (D68.312)
lupus anticoagulant syndrome
(D68.62)
CC **D68.62** **Lupus anticoagulant syndrome**
Lupus anticoagulant
Presence of systemic lupus erythematosus [SLE]
inhibitor
Excludes1: *anticardiolipin syndrome (D68.61)*
antiphospholipid syndrome (D68.61)
lupus anticoagulant (LAC) finding
without diagnosis (R76.0)
lupus anticoagulant (LAC) with
hemorrhagic disorder (D68.312)
CC **D68.69** **Other thrombophilia**
Hypercoagulable states NEC
Secondary hypercoagulable state NOS
CC **D68.8** **Other specified coagulation defects**
Excludes1: *hemorrhagic disease of newborn (P53)*
CC **D68.9** **Coagulation defect, unspecified**

D69 **Purpura and other hemorrhagic conditions**

Excludes1: *benign hypergammaglobulinemic purpura (D89.0)*
cryoglobulinemic purpura (D89.1)
essential (hemorrhagic) thrombocythemia (D47.3)
hemorrhagic thrombocythemia (D47.3)
purpura fulminans (D65)
thrombotic thrombocytopenic purpura (M31.1)
Waldenström hypergammaglobulinemic purpura
(D89.0)
CC **D69.0** **Allergic purpura**
Allergic vasculitis
Nonthrombocytopenic hemorrhagic purpura
Nonthrombocytopenic idiopathic purpura
Purpura anaphylactoid
Purpura Henoch(-Schönlein)
Purpura rheumatica
Vascular purpura
Excludes1: *thrombocytopenic hemorrhagic purpura*
(D69.3)
CC **D69.1** **Qualitative platelet defects**
Bernard-Soulier [giant platelet] syndrome
Glanzmann's disease
Grey platelet syndrome
Thromboasthenia (hemorrhagic) (hereditary)
Thrombocytopathy
Excludes1: *von Willebrand's disease (D68.0)*
D69.2 **Other nonthrombocytopenic purpura**
Purpura NOS
Purpura simplex
Senile purpura

CC **D69.3** **Immune thrombocytopenic purpura**
Hemorrhagic (thrombocytopenic) purpura
Idiopathic thrombocytopenic purpura
Tidal platelet dysgenesis
+ **D69.4** **Other primary thrombocytopenia**
Excludes1: *transient neonatal thrombocytopenia (P61.0)*
Wiskott-Aldrich syndrome (D82.0)
CC **D69.41** **Evans syndrome**
CC **D69.42** **Congenital and hereditary thrombocytopenia**
purpura
Congenital thrombocytopenia
Hereditary thrombocytopenia
Code first congenital or hereditary disorder, such
as:
thrombocytopenia with absent radius (TAR
syndrome) (Q87.2)
D69.49 **Other primary thrombocytopenia**
Megakaryocytic hypoplasia
Primary thrombocytopenia NOS
+ **D69.5** **Secondary thrombocytopenia**
Excludes1: *heparin induced thrombocytopenia (HIT)*
(D75.82)
transient thrombocytopenia of newborn
(P61.0)
D69.51 **Posttransfusion purpura**
Posttransfusion purpura from whole blood (fresh)
or blood products PTP
D69.59 **Other secondary thrombocytopenia**
AHA CC: 4Q, 2014, 22-23
D69.6 **Thrombocytopenia, unspecified**
D69.8 **Other specified hemorrhagic conditions**
Capillary fragility (hereditary)
Vascular pseudohemophilia
D69.9 **Hemorrhagic condition, unspecified**

Other disorders of blood and blood-forming organs (D70-D77)

D70 **Neutropenia**

Includes: agranulocytosis
decreased absolute neurophile count (ANC)
Use additional code for any associated:
fever (R50.81)
mucositis (J34.81, K12.3-, K92.81, N76.81)
Excludes1: *neutropenic splenomegaly (D73.81)*
transient neonatal neutropenia (P61.5)
D70.0 **Congenital agranulocytosis**
Congenital neutropenia
Infantile genetic agranulocytosis
Kostmann's disease
D70.1 **Agranulocytosis secondary to cancer chemotherapy**
Use additional code for adverse effect, if applicable, to
identify drug (T45.1X5)

Code also underlying neoplasm
AHA CC: 4Q, 2014, 22-23
D70.2 **Other drug-induced agranulocytosis**
Use additional code for adverse effect, if applicable, to
identify drug (T36-T50 with fifth or sixth character 5)
D70.3 **Neutropenia due to infection**
D70.4 **Cyclic neutropenia**
Cyclic hematopoiesis
Periodic neutropenia
D70.8 **Other neutropenia**
D70.9 **Neutropenia, unspecified**
AHA CC: 2Q, 2019, 24-26

D71 **Functional disorders of polymorphonuclear neutrophils**

Cell membrane receptor complex [CR3] defect
Chronic (childhood) granulomatous disease
Congenital dysphagocytosis
Progressive septic granulomatosis
Valid 3-character code, no further characters required

+, +7th, X + 7th • Newborn • Pediatric ● Maternity ● Adult ♀ Female ♂ Male Manifestation Unacceptable PDX HCC CC MCC HAC

D72   Other disorders of white blood cells

> *Excludes1:*   *basophilia (D72.824)*
> *immunity disorders (D80-D89)*
> *neutropenia (D70)*
> *preleukemia (syndrome) (D46.9)*

D72.0   Genetic anomalies of leukocytes
Alder (granulation) (granulocyte) anomaly
Alder syndrome
Hereditary leukocytic hypersegmentation
Hereditary leukocytic hyposegmentation
Hereditary leukomelanopathy
May-Hegglin (granulation) (granulocyte) anomaly
May-Hegglin syndrome
Pelger-Huët (granulation) (granulocyte) anomaly
Pelger-Huët syndrome

> *Excludes1:*   *Chédiak (-Steinbrinck)-Higashi syndrome (E70.330)*

+ **D72.1   Eosinophilia**

> *Excludes2:*   *Löffler's syndrome (J82)*
> *pulmonary eosinophilia (J82)*

D72.10   Eosinophilia, unspecified

+ **D72.11   Hypereosinophilic syndrome [HES]**

D72.110   Idiopathic hypereosinophilic syndrome [IHES]

D72.111   Lymphocytic Variant Hypereosinophilic Syndrome [LHES]
Lymphocyte variant hypereosinophilia
Code also, if applicable, any associated lymphocytic neoplastic disorder

D72.118   Other hypereosinophilic syndrome
Episodic angioendema with eosinophilia
Gleich's syndrome

D72.119   Hypereosinophilic syndrome [HES], unspecified

D72.12   Drug rash with eosinophilia and systemic symptoms syndrome
DRESS syndrome
Use additional code for adverse effect, if applicable, to identify drug (T36-T50 with fifth or sixth character 5)

D72.18   Eosinophilia in diseases classified elsewhere
Code first underlying disease, such as:
chronic myelomonocytic leukemia (C93.1-)

D72.19   Other eosinophilia
Familial eosinophilia
Hereditary eosinophilia

+ **D72.8   Other specified disorders of white blood cells**

> *Excludes1: leukemia (C91-C95)*

+ **D72.81   Decreased white blood cell count**

> *Excludes1:*   *neutropenia (D70.-)*

D72.810   Lymphocytopenia
Decreased lymphocytes

D72.818   Other decreased white blood cell count
Basophilic leukopenia
Eosinophilic leukopenia
Monocytopenia
Other decreased leukocytes
Plasmacytopenia

D72.819   Decreased white blood cell count, unspecified
Decreased leukocytes, unspecified
Leukocytopenia, unspecified
Leukopenia

> *Excludes1:*   *malignant leukopenia (D70.9)*

+ **D72.82   Elevated white blood cell count**

> *Excludes1:*   *eosinophilia (D72.1)*

D72.820   Lymphocytosis (symptomatic)
Elevated lymphocytes

D72.821   Monocytosis (symptomatic)

> *Excludes1:*   *infectious mononucleosis (B27.-)*

D72.822   Plasmacytosis

D72.823   Leukemoid reaction
Basophilic leukemoid reaction
Leukemoid reaction NOS
Lymphocytic leukemoid reaction
Monocytic leukemoid reaction
Myelocytic leukemoid reaction
Neutrophilic leukemoid reaction

D72.824   Basophilia

D72.825   Bandemia
Bandemia without diagnosis of specific infection

> *Excludes1:*   *confirmed infection - code to infection*
> *leukemia (C91.-, C92.-, C93.-, C94.-, C95.-)*

D72.828   Other elevated white blood cell count

D72.829   Elevated white blood cell count, unspecified
Elevated leukocytes, unspecified
Leukocytosis, unspecified

D72.89   Other specified disorders of white blood cells
Abnormality of white blood cells NEC

D72.9   Disorder of white blood cells, unspecified
Abnormal leukocyte differential NOS

D73   Diseases of spleen

D73.0   Hyposplenism
Atrophy of spleen

> *Excludes1:*   *asplenia (congenital) (Q89.01)*
> *postsurgical absence of spleen (Z90.81)*

D73.1   Hypersplenism

> *Excludes1:*   *neutropenic splenomegaly (D73.81)*
> *primary splenic neutropenia (D73.81)*
> *splenitis, splenomegaly in late syphilis (A52.79)*
> *splenitis, splenomegaly in tuberculosis (A18.85)*
> *splenomegaly NOS (R16.1)*
> *splenomegaly congenital (Q89.0)*

D73.2   Chronic congestive splenomegaly

D73.3   Abscess of spleen

D73.4   Cyst of spleen

D73.5   Infarction of spleen
Splenic rupture, nontraumatic
Torsion of spleen

> *Excludes1:*   *rupture of spleen due to Plasmodium vivax malaria (B51.0)*
> *traumatic rupture of spleen (S36.03-)*

+ **D73.8   Other diseases of spleen**

D73.81   Neutropenic splenomegaly
Werner-Schultz disease

D73.89   Other diseases of spleen
Fibrosis of spleen NOS
Perisplenitis
Splenitis NOS

D73.9   Disease of spleen, unspecified

D74   Methemoglobinemia

CC **D74.0   Congenital methemoglobinemia**
Congenital NADH-methemoglobin reductase deficiency
Hemoglobin-M [Hb-M] disease
Methemoglobinemia, hereditary

CC **D74.8   Other methemoglobinemias**
Acquired methemoglobinemia (with sulfhemoglobinemia)
Toxic methemoglobinemia

CC **D74.9   Methemoglobinemia, unspecified**

D75   Other and unspecified diseases of blood and blood-forming organs

> *Excludes2:*   *acute lymphadenitis (L04.-)*
> *chronic lymphadenitis (I88.1)*
> *enlarged lymph nodes (R59.-)*
> *hypergammaglobulinemia NOS (D89.2)*
> *lymphadenitis NOS (I88.9)*
> *mesenteric lymphadenitis (acute) (chronic) (I88.0)*

D75.0   Familial erythrocytosis
Benign polycythemia
Familial polycythemia

> *Excludes1:*   *hereditary ovalocytosis (D58.1)*

D75.1 **Secondary polycythemia**
 Acquired polycythemia
 Emotional polycythemia
 Erythrocytosis NOS
 Hypoxemic polycythemia
 Nephrogenous polycythemia
 Polycythemia due to erythropoietin
 Polycythemia due to fall in plasma volume
 Polycythemia due to high altitude
 Polycythemia due to stress
 Polycythemia NOS
 Relative polycythemia
 Excludes1: *polycythemia neonatorum (P61.1)*
     polycythemia vera (D45)

+ **D75.8** **Other specified diseases of blood and blood-forming organs**
 CC **D75.81** **Myelofibrosis**
  Myelofibrosis NOS
  Secondary myelofibrosis NOS
  Code first the underlying disorder, such as:
   malignant neoplasm of breast (C50.-)

  Use additional code, if applicable, for associated therapy-related myelodysplastic syndrome (D46.-)

  Use additional code for adverse effect, if applicable, to identify drug (T45.1X5)
  Excludes1: *acute myelofibrosis (C94.4-)*
     idiopathic myelofibrosis (D47.1)
     leukoerythroblastic anemia (D61.82)
     myelofibrosis with myeloid metaplasia (D47.4)
     myelophthisic anemia (D61.82)
     myelophthisis (D61.82)
     primary myelofibrosis (D47.1)
 D75.82 **Heparin induced thrombocytopenia (HIT)**
 D75.89 **Other specified diseases of blood and blood-forming organs**

D75.9 **Disease of blood and blood-forming organs, unspecified**

D75.A **Glucose-6-phosphate dehydrogenase (G6PD) deficiency without anemia**
 Excludes1: *glucose-6-phosphate dehydrogenase (G6PD) deficiency with anemia (D55.0)*
 AHA CC: 4Q, 2019, 4-5

D76 **Other specified diseases with participation of lymphoreticular and reticulohistiocytic tissue**
 Excludes1: *(Abt-) Letterer-Siwe disease (C96.0)*
     eosinophilic granuloma (C96.6)
     Hand-Schüller-Christian disease (C96.5)
     histiocytic medullary reticulosis (C96.9)
     histiocytic sarcoma (C96.A)
     histiocytosis X, multifocal (C96.5)
     histiocytosis X, unifocal (C96.6)
     Langerhans-cell histiocytosis, multifocal (C96.5)
     Langerhans-cell histiocytosis NOS (C96.6)
     Langerhans-cell histiocytosis, unifocal (C96.6)
     leukemic reticuloendotheliosis (C91.4-)
     lipomelanotic reticulosis (I89.8)
     malignant histiocytosis (C96.A)
     malignant reticulosis (C86.0)
     nonlipid reticuloendotheliosis (C96.0)
 CC **D76.1** **Hemophagocytic lymphohistiocytosis**
  Familial hemophagocytic reticulosis
  Histiocytoses of mononuclear phagocytes
 CC **D76.2** **Hemophagocytic syndrome, infection-associated**
  Use additional code to identify infectious agent or disease.
 CC **D76.3** **Other histiocytosis syndromes**
  Reticulohistiocytoma (giant-cell)
  Sinus histiocytosis with massive lymphadenopathy
  Xanthogranuloma

D77 **Other disorders of blood and blood-forming organs in diseases classified elsewhere**
 Code first underlying disease, such as:
  amyloidosis (E85.-)
  congenital early syphilis (A50.0)
  echinococcosis (B67.0-B67.9)
  malaria (B50.0-B54)
  schistosomiasis [bilharziasis] (B65.0-B65.9)
  vitamin C deficiency (E54)
 Excludes1: *rupture of spleen due to Plasmodium vivax malaria (B51.0)*
     splenitis, splenomegaly in late syphilis (A52.79)
     splenitis, splenomegaly in tuberculosis (A18.85)
 Valid 3-character code, no further characters required

Intraoperative and postprocedural complications of the spleen (D78)

D78 **Intraoperative and postprocedural complications of the spleen**
 AHA CC: 4Q, 2016, 9-10
+ **D78.0** **Intraoperative hemorrhage and hematoma of the spleen complicating a procedure**
  Excludes1: *intraoperative hemorrhage and hematoma of the spleen due to accidental puncture or laceration during a procedure (D78.1-)*
 CC **D78.01** **Intraoperative hemorrhage and hematoma of the spleen complicating a procedure on the spleen**
 CC **D78.02** **Intraoperative hemorrhage and hematoma of the spleen complicating other procedure**
+ **D78.1** **Accidental puncture and laceration of the spleen during a procedure**
 CC **D78.11** **Accidental puncture and laceration of the spleen during a procedure on the spleen**
 CC **D78.12** **Accidental puncture and laceration of the spleen during other procedure**
+ **D78.2** **Postprocedural hemorrhage of the spleen following a procedure**
 CC **D78.21** **Postprocedural hemorrhage of the spleen following a procedure on the spleen**
 CC **D78.22** **Postprocedural hemorrhage of the spleen following other procedure**
+ **D78.3** **Postprocedural hematoma and seroma of the spleen following a procedure**
 CC **D78.31** **Postprocedural hematoma of the spleen following a procedure on the spleen**
 CC **D78.32** **Postprocedural hematoma of the spleen following other procedure**
 CC **D78.33** **Postprocedural seroma of the spleen following a procedure on the spleen**
 CC **D78.34** **Postprocedural seroma of the spleen following other procedure**
+ **D78.8** **Other intraoperative and postprocedural complications of the spleen**
  Use additional code, if applicable, to further specify disorder
 CC **D78.81** **Other intraoperative complications of the spleen**
 CC **D78.89** **Other postprocedural complications of the spleen**

Certain disorders involving the immune mechanism (D80-D89)

Includes: defects in the complement system
 immunodeficiency disorders, except human immunodeficiency virus [HIV] disease sarcoidosis

Excludes1: *autoimmune disease (systemic) NOS (M35.9)*
  functional disorders of polymorphonuclear neutrophils (D71)
  human immunodeficiency virus [HIV] disease (B20)

D80 **Immunodeficiency with predominantly antibody defects**
 CC **D80.0** **Hereditary hypogammaglobulinemia**
  Autosomal recessive agammaglobulinemia (Swiss type)
  X-linked agammaglobulinemia [Bruton] (with growth hormone deficiency)

CC **D80.1** **Nonfamilial hypogammaglobulinemia**
    Agammaglobulinemia with immunoglobulin-bearing
      B-lymphocytes
    Common variable agammaglobulinemia [CVAgamma]
    Hypogammaglobulinemia NOS
CC **D80.2** **Selective deficiency of immunoglobulin A [IgA]**
CC **D80.3** **Selective deficiency of immunoglobulin G [IgG] subclasses**
CC **D80.4** **Selective deficiency of immunoglobulin M [IgM]**
CC **D80.5** **Immunodeficiency with increased immunoglobulin M [IgM]**
CC **D80.6** **Antibody deficiency with near-normal immunoglobulins or with hyperimmunoglobulinemia**
CC **D80.7** **Transient hypogammaglobulinemia of infancy**
CC **D80.8** **Other immunodeficiencies with predominantly antibody defects**
    Kappa light chain deficiency
CC **D80.9** **Immunodeficiency with predominantly antibody defects, unspecified**

D81   Combined immunodeficiencies
    Excludes1: autosomal recessive agammaglobulinemia (Swiss type) (D80.0)
CC **D81.0** **Severe combined immunodeficiency [SCID] with reticular dysgenesis**
CC **D81.1** **Severe combined immunodeficiency [SCID] with low T- and B-cell numbers**
CC **D81.2** **Severe combined immunodeficiency [SCID] with low or normal B-cell numbers**
 + **D81.3** **Adenosine deaminase [ADA] deficiency**
    AHA CC: 4Q, 2019, 5-6
    CC **D81.30** **Adenosine deaminase deficiency, unspecified**
        ADA deficiency NOS
    CC **D81.31** **Severe combined immunodeficiency due to adenosine deaminase deficiency**
        ADA deficiency with SCID
        Adenosine deaminase [ADA] deficiency with
          severe combined immunodeficiency
    CC **D81.32** **Adenosine deaminase 2 deficiency**
        ADA2 deficiency
        Adenosine deaminase deficiency type 2
        Code also, if applicable, any associated
          manifestations, such as:
            polyarteritis nodosa (M30.0)
            stroke (I63.-)
    CC **D81.39** **Other adenosine deaminase deficiency**
        Adenosine deaminase [ADA] deficiency type 1, NOS
        Adenosine deaminase [ADA] deficiency type 1,
          without SCID
        Adenosine deaminase [ADA] deficiency type 1,
          without severe combined immunodeficiency
        Partial ADA deficiency (type 1)
        Partial adenosine deaminase deficiency (type 1)
CC **D81.4** **Nezelof's syndrome**
CC **D81.5** **Purine nucleoside phosphorylase [PNP] deficiency**
CC **D81.6** **Major histocompatibility complex class I deficiency**
    Bare lymphocyte syndrome
CC **D81.7** **Major histocompatibility complex class II deficiency**
 + **D81.8** **Other combined immunodeficiencies**
   + **D81.81** **Biotin-dependent carboxylase deficiency**
      Multiple carboxylase deficiency
      Excludes1: biotin-dependent carboxylase deficiency due to dietary deficiency of biotin (E53.8)
      D81.810 **Biotinidase deficiency**
      D81.818 **Other biotin-dependent carboxylase deficiency**
         Holocarboxylase synthetase deficiency
         Other multiple carboxylase deficiency
      D81.819 **Biotin-dependent carboxylase deficiency, unspecified**
         Multiple carboxylase deficiency, unspecified
    CC **D81.89** **Other combined immunodeficiencies**
CC **D81.9** **Combined immunodeficiency, unspecified**
    Severe combined immunodeficiency disorder [SCID] NOS

D82   Immunodeficiency associated with other major defects
    Excludes1: ataxia telangiectasia [Louis-Bar] (G11.3)
CC **D82.0** **Wiskott-Aldrich syndrome**
    Immunodeficiency with thrombocytopenia and eczema
CC **D82.1** **Di George's syndrome**
    Pharyngeal pouch syndrome
    Thymic alymphoplasia
    Thymic aplasia or hypoplasia with immunodeficiency
    AHA CC: 3Q, 2019, 14-15
  D82.2 **Immunodeficiency with short-limbed stature**
  D82.3 **Immunodeficiency following hereditary defective response to Epstein-Barr virus**
    X-linked lymphoproliferative disease
  D82.4 **Hyperimmunoglobulin E [IgE] syndrome**
  D82.8 **Immunodeficiency associated with other specified major defects**
  D82.9 **Immunodeficiency associated with major defect, unspecified**

D83   Common variable immunodeficiency
CC **D83.0** **Common variable immunodeficiency with predominant abnormalities of B-cell numbers and function**
CC **D83.1** **Common variable immunodeficiency with predominant immunoregulatory T-cell disorders**
CC **D83.2** **Common variable immunodeficiency with autoantibodies to B- or T-cells**
CC **D83.8** **Other common variable immunodeficiencies**
CC **D83.9** **Common variable immunodeficiency, unspecified**

D84   Other immunodeficiencies
  D84.0 **Lymphocyte function antigen-1 [LFA-1] defect**
  D84.1 **Defects in the complement system**
    C1 esterase inhibitor [C1-INH] deficiency
 + **D84.8** **Other specified immunodeficiencies**
    CC **D84.81** **Immunodeficiency due to conditions classified elsewhere**
        Code first underlying condition, such as:
          chromosomal abnormalities (Q90-Q99)
          diabetes mellitus (E08-E13)
          malignant neoplasms (C00-C96)
        Excludes1: certain disorders involving the immune mechanism (D80-D83, D84.0, D84.1, D84.9)
              human immunodeficiency virus [HIV] disease (B20)
   + **D84.82** **Immunodeficiency due to drugs and external causes**
    CC **D84.821** **Immunodeficiency due to drugs**
        Immunodeficiency due to (current or past) medication
        Use additional code for adverse effect if applicable, to identify adverse effect of drug (T36-T50 with fifth or sixth character 5)
        Use additional code, if applicable, for associated long term (current) drug therapy drug or medication such as:
          long term (current) drug therapy systemic steroids (Z79.52)
          other long term (current) drug therapy (Z79.899)
    CC **D84.822** **Immunodeficiency due to external causes**
        Code also, if applicable, radiological procedure and radiotherapy (Y84.2)
        Use additional code for external cause such as:
          exposure to ionizing radiation (W88)
    CC **D84.89** **Other immunodeficiencies**
CC **D84.9** **Immunodeficiency, unspecified**
    Immunocompromised NOS
    Immunodeficient NOS
    Immunosuppressed NOS

D86 Sarcoidosis

    D86.0 Sarcoidosis of lung

    D86.1 Sarcoidosis of lymph nodes

    D86.2 Sarcoidosis of lung with sarcoidosis of lymph nodes

    D86.3 Sarcoidosis of skin

  + **D86.8 Sarcoidosis of other sites**

        D86.81 Sarcoid meningitis

        D86.82 Multiple cranial nerve palsies in sarcoidosis

        D86.83 Sarcoid iridocyclitis

        D86.84 Sarcoid pyelonephritis

            Tubulo-interstitial nephropathy in sarcoidosis

        D86.85 Sarcoid myocarditis

        D86.86 Sarcoid arthropathy

            Polyarthritis in sarcoidosis

        D86.87 Sarcoid myositis

        D86.89 Sarcoidosis of other sites

            Hepatic granuloma

            Uveoparotid fever [Heerfordt]

    D86.9 Sarcoidosis, unspecified

D89 Other disorders involving the immune mechanism, not elsewhere classified

    Excludes1: *hyperglobulinemia NOS (R77.1)*

                 monoclonal gammopathy (of undetermined significance) (D47.2)

    Excludes2: *transplant failure and rejection (T86.-)*

    D89.0 Polyclonal hypergammaglobulinemia

        Benign hypergammaglobulinemic purpura

        Polyclonal gammopathy NOS

    D89.1 Cryoglobulinemia

        Cryoglobulinemic purpura

        Cryoglobulinemic vasculitis

        Essential cryoglobulinemia

        Idiopathic cryoglobulinemia

        Mixed cryoglobulinemia

        Primary cryoglobulinemia

        Secondary cryoglobulinemia

    D89.2 Hypergammaglobulinemia, unspecified

    D89.3 Immune reconstitution syndrome

        Immune reconstitution inflammatory syndrome [IRIS]

        Use additional code for adverse effect, if applicable, to identify drug (T36-T50 with fifth or sixth character 5)

        Add the following new codes after D89.3.

  + **D89.4 Mast cell activation syndrome and related disorders**

    Excludes1: *aggressive systemic mastocytosis (C96.21)*

              congenital cutaneous mastocytosis (Q82.2)

              (indolent) systemic mastocytosis (D47.02)

              malignant mast cell neoplasm (C96.2-)

              malignant mastocytoma (C96.29)

              mast cell sarcoma (C96.22)

              mastocytoma NOS (D47.09)

              (non-congenital) cutaneous mastocytosis (D47.01)

              other mast cell neoplasms of uncertain behavior (D47.09)

              systemic mastocytosis associated with a clonal hematologic non-mast cell lineage disease (SM-AHNMD) (D47.02)

    AHA CC: 4Q, 2016, 11

D89.40 Mast cell activation, unspecified

    Mast cell activation disorder, unspecified

    Mast cell activation syndrome, NOS

D89.41 Monoclonal mast cell activation syndrome

D89.42 Idiopathic mast cell activation syndrome

D89.43 Secondary mast cell activation

    Secondary mast cell activation syndrome

    Code also underlying etiology, if known

D89.49 Other mast cell activation disorder

    Other mast cell activation syndrome

+ **D89.8 Other specified disorders involving the immune mechanism, not elsewhere classified**

  + **D89.81 Graft-versus-host disease**

        Code first underlying cause, such as:

            complications of transplanted organs and tissues (T86.-)

            complications of blood transfusion (T80.89)

        Use additional code to identify associated manifestations, such as:

            desquamative dermatitis (L30.8)

            diarrhea (R19.7)

            elevated bilirubin (R17)

            hair loss (L65.9)

    CC **D89.810 Acute graft-versus-host disease**

    CC **D89.811 Chronic graft-versus-host disease**

    CC **D89.812 Acute on chronic graft-versus-host disease**

    CC **D89.813 Graft-versus-host disease, unspecified**

    D89.82 Autoimmune lymphoproliferative syndrome [ALPS]

  + **D89.83 Cytokine release syndrome**

        Code first underlying cause, such as:

            complications following infusion, transfusion and therapeutic injection (T80.89-)

            complications of transplanted organs and tissues (T86.-)

        Use additional code to identify associated manifestations

        D89.831 Cytokine release syndrome, grade 1

        D89.832 Cytokine release syndrome, grade 2

    CC **D89.833 Cytokine release syndrome, grade 3**

    CC **D89.834 Cytokine release syndrome, grade 4**

    CC **D89.835 Cytokine release syndrome, grade 5**

        D89.839 Cytokine release syndrome, grade unspecified

    D89.89 Other specified disorders involving the immune mechanism, not elsewhere classified

        Excludes1: *human immunodeficiency virus disease (B20)*

        AHA CC: 4Q, 2017, 109

D89.9 Disorder involving the immune mechanism, unspecified

    Immune disease NOS

    AHA CC: 3Q, 2015, 22

+, +7th, X + 7th   ● Newborn   ● Pediatric   ● Maternity   ● Adult   ♀ Female   ♂ Male   Manifestation   Unacceptable PDX   HCC   CC   MCC   HAC

Chapter 4: Endocrine, Nutritional and Metabolic Disease (E00-E89)

NOTE All neoplasms, whether functionally active or not, are classified in Chapter 2. Appropriate codes in this chapter (i.e. E05.8, E07.0, E16-E31, E34.-) may be used as additional codes to indicate either functional activity by neoplasms and ectopic endocrine tissue or hyperfunction and hypofunction of endocrine glands associated with neoplasms and other conditions classified elsewhere.

Excludes1: *transitory endocrine and metabolic disorders specific to newborn (P70-P74)*

This chapter contains the following category blocks:

E00-E07	Disorders of thyroid gland
E08-E13	Diabetes mellitus
E15-E16	Other disorders of glucose regulation and pancreatic internal secretion
E20-E35	Disorders of other endocrine glands
E36	Intraoperative complications of endocrine system
E40-E46	Malnutrition
E50-E64	Other nutritional deficiencies
E65-E68	Overweight, obesity and other hyperalimentation
E70-E88	Metabolic disorders
E89	Postprocedural endocrine and metabolic complications and disorders, not elsewhere classified

C. Chapter-Specific Coding Guidelines

In addition to general coding guidelines, there are guidelines for specific diagnoses and/or conditions in the classification. Unless otherwise indicated, these guidelines apply to all health care settings. Please refer to Section II for guidelines on the selection of principal diagnosis.

4. Chapter 4: Endocrine, Nutritional and Metabolic Diseases (E00-E89)

a. Diabetes mellitus

The diabetes mellitus codes are combination codes that include the type of diabetes mellitus, the body system affected, and the complications affecting that body system. As many codes within a particular category as are necessary to describe all of the complications of the disease may be used. They should be sequenced based on the reason for a particular encounter. Assign as many codes from categories E08 – E13 as needed to identify all of the associated conditions that the patient has.

1) Type of diabetes

The age of a patient is not the sole determining factor, though most type 1 diabetics develop the condition before reaching puberty. For this reason type 1 diabetes mellitus is also referred to as juvenile diabetes.

2) Type of diabetes mellitus not documented

If the type of diabetes mellitus is not documented in the medical record the default is E11.-, Type 2 diabetes mellitus.

3) Diabetes mellitus and the use of insulin and oral hypoglycemics

If the documentation in a medical record does not indicate the type of diabetes but does indicate that the patient uses insulin, code E11.-, Type 2 diabetes mellitus, should be assigned. An additional code should be assigned from category Z79 to identify the long-term (current) use of insulin or oral hypoglycemic drugs. If the patient is treated with both oral medications and insulin, only the code for long-term (current) use of insulin should be assigned. **If the patient is treated with both insulin and an injectable non-insulin antidiabetic drug, assign codes Z79.4, Long-term (current) use of insulin, and Z79.899, Other long term (current) drug therapy. If the patient is treated with both oral hypoglycemic drugs and an injectable non-insulin antidiabetic drug, assign codes Z79.84, Long-term (current) use of oral hypoglycemic drugs, and Z79.899, Other long-term (current) drug therapy.** Code Z79.4 should not be assigned if insulin is given temporarily to bring a type 2 patient's blood sugar under control during an encounter.

4) Diabetes mellitus in pregnancy and gestational diabetes

See Section I.C.15. Diabetes mellitus in pregnancy.

See Section I.C.15. Gestational (pregnancy induced) diabetes

5) Complications due to insulin pump malfunction

(a) Underdose of insulin due to insulin pump failure

An underdose of insulin due to an insulin pump failure should be assigned to a code from subcategory T85.6, Mechanical complication of other specified internal and external prosthetic devices, implants and grafts, that specifies the type of pump malfunction, as the principal or first-listed code, followed by code T38.3x6-, Underdosing of insulin and oral hypoglycemic [antidiabetic] drugs. Additional codes for the type of diabetes mellitus and any associated complications due to the underdosing should also be assigned.

(b) Overdose of insulin due to insulin pump failure

The principal or first-listed code for an encounter due to an insulin pump malfunction resulting in an overdose of insulin, should also be T85.6-, Mechanical complication of other specified internal and external prosthetic devices, implants and grafts, followed by code T38.3x1-, Poisoning by insulin and oral hypoglycemic [antidiabetic] drugs, accidental (unintentional).

6) Secondary diabetes mellitus

Codes under categories E08, Diabetes mellitus due to underlying condition, E09, Drug or chemical induced diabetes mellitus, and E13, Other specified diabetes mellitus, identify complications/manifestations associated with secondary diabetes mellitus. Secondary diabetes is always caused by another condition or event (e.g., cystic fibrosis, malignant neoplasm of pancreas, pancreatectomy, adverse effect of drug, or poisoning).

(a) Secondary diabetes mellitus and the use of insulin or *oral* hypoglycemic drugs

For patients with secondary diabetes mellitus who routinely use insulin or oral hypoglycemic drugs, an additional code from category Z79 should be assigned to identify the long-term (current) use of insulin or oral hypoglycemic drugs. If the patient is treated with both oral medications and insulin, only the code for long-term (current) use of insulin should be assigned. **If the patient is treated with both insulin and an injectable non-insulin antidiabetic drug, assign codes Z79.4, Long-term (current) use of insulin, and Z79.899, Other long term (current) drug therapy. If the patient is treated with both oral hypoglycemic drugs and an injectable non-insulin antidiabetic drug, assign codes Z79.84, Long-term (current) use of oral hypoglycemic drugs, and Z79.899, Other long-term (current) drug therapy.** Code Z79.4 should not be assigned if insulin is given temporarily to bring a secondary diabetic patient's blood sugar under control during an encounter.

(b) Assigning and sequencing secondary diabetes codes and its causes

The sequencing of the secondary diabetes codes in relationship to codes for the cause of the diabetes is based on the Tabular List instructions for categories E08, E09 and E13.

(i) Secondary diabetes mellitus due to pancreatectomy

For postpancreatectomy diabetes mellitus (lack of insulin due to the surgical removal of all or part of the pancreas), assign code E89.1, Postprocedural hypoinsulinemia. Assign a code from category E13 and a code from subcategory Z90.41-, Acquired absence of pancreas, as additional codes.

(ii) Secondary diabetes due to drugs

Secondary diabetes may be caused by an adverse effect of correctly administered medications, poisoning or sequela of poisoning.

See section I.C.19.e for coding of adverse effects and poisoning, and section I.C.20 for external cause code reporting.

Disorders of thyroid gland (E00-E07)

E00 Congenital iodine-deficiency syndrome

Use additional code (F70-F79) to identify associated intellectual disabilities.

Excludes1: *subclinical iodine-deficiency hypothyroidism (E02)*

E00.0 Congenital iodine-deficiency syndrome, neurological type
Endemic cretinism, neurological type

E00.1 Congenital iodine-deficiency syndrome, myxedematous type
Endemic hypothyroid cretinism
Endemic cretinism, myxedematous type

E00.2 Congenital iodine-deficiency syndrome, mixed type
Endemic cretinism, mixed type

E00.9 Congenital iodine-deficiency syndrome, unspecified
Congenital iodine-deficiency hypothyroidism NOS
Endemic cretinism NOS

E01 Iodine-deficiency related thyroid disorders and allied conditions

Excludes1: *congenital iodine-deficiency syndrome (E00.-)*
subclinical iodine-deficiency hypothyroidism (E02)

E01.0 Iodine-deficiency related diffuse (endemic) goiter

E01.1 Iodine-deficiency related multinodular (endemic) goiter
Iodine-deficiency related nodular goiter

E01.2 Iodine-deficiency related (endemic) goiter, unspecified
Endemic goiter NOS

E01.8 Other iodine-deficiency related thyroid disorders and allied conditions
Acquired iodine-deficiency hypothyroidism NOS

E02 Subclinical iodine-deficiency hypothyroidism

Valid 3-character code, no further characters required

Endocrine System

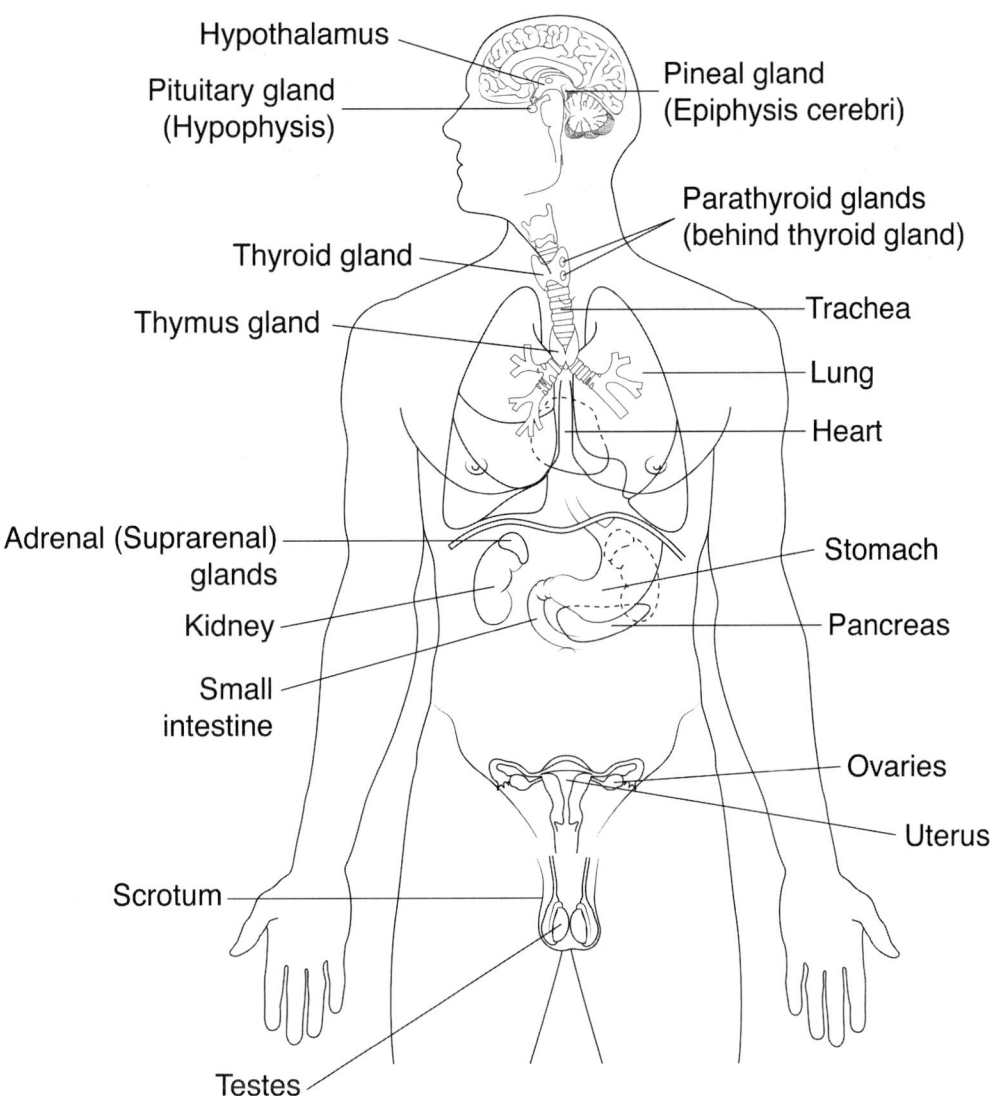

Hypothalamus

Pituitary gland
(Hypophysis)

Pineal gland
(Epiphysis cerebri)

Parathyroid glands
(behind thyroid gland)

Thyroid gland

Trachea

Thymus gland

Lung

Heart

Adrenal (Suprarenal)
glands

Stomach

Kidney

Pancreas

Small
intestine

Ovaries

Uterus

Scrotum

Testes

©AHIMA

E03 Other hypothyroidism

> ***Excludes1:*** *iodine-deficiency related hypothyroidism (E00-E02)*
> *postprocedural hypothyroidism (E89.0)*

E03.0 Congenital hypothyroidism with diffuse goiter
Congenital parenchymatous goiter (nontoxic)
Congenital goiter (nontoxic) NOS

> ***Excludes1:*** *transitory congenital goiter with normal*
> *function (P72.0)*

E03.1 Congenital hypothyroidism without goiter
Aplasia of thyroid (with myxedema)
Congenital atrophy of thyroid
Congenital hypothyroidism NOS

E03.2 Hypothyroidism due to medicaments and other exogenous substances

Code first poisoning due to drug or toxin, if applicable
(T36-T65 with fifth or sixth character 1-4 or 6)

Use additional code for adverse effect, if applicable, to
identify drug (T36-T50 with fifth or sixth character 5)

E03.3 Postinfectious hypothyroidism

E03.4 Atrophy of thyroid (acquired)

> ***Excludes1:*** *congenital atrophy of thyroid (E03.1)*

MCC **E03.5 Myxedema coma**

E03.8 Other specified hypothyroidism

E03.9 Hypothyroidism, unspecified
Myxedema NOS

E04 Other nontoxic goiter

> ***Excludes1:*** *congenital goiter (NOS) (diffuse) (parenchymatous) (E03.0)*
> *iodine-deficiency related goiter (E00-E02)*

E04.0 Nontoxic diffuse goiter
Diffuse (colloid) nontoxic goiter
Simple nontoxic goiter

E04.1 Nontoxic single thyroid nodule
Colloid nodule (cystic) (thyroid)
Nontoxic uninodular goiter
Thyroid (cystic) nodule NOS

E04.2 Nontoxic multinodular goiter
Cystic goiter NOS
Multinodular (cystic) goiter NOS

E04.8 Other specified nontoxic goiter

E04.9 Nontoxic goiter, unspecified
Goiter NOS
Nodular goiter (nontoxic) NOS

E05 Thyrotoxicosis [hyperthyroidism]

> ***Excludes1:*** *chronic thyroiditis with transient thyrotoxicosis (E06.2)*
> *neonatal thyrotoxicosis (P72.1)*

+ **E05.0 Thyrotoxicosis with diffuse goiter**
Exophthalmic or toxic goiter NOS
Graves' disease
Toxic diffuse goiter

**E05.00 Thyrotoxicosis with diffuse goiter without
thyrotoxic crisis or storm**

MCC **E05.01 Thyrotoxicosis with diffuse goiter with thyrotoxic
crisis or storm**

+ **E05.1 Thyrotoxicosis with toxic single thyroid nodule**
Thyrotoxicosis with toxic uninodular goiter

**E05.10 Thyrotoxicosis with toxic single thyroid nodule
without thyrotoxic crisis or storm**

MCC **E05.11** **Thyrotoxicosis with toxic single thyroid nodule with thyrotoxic crisis or storm**
+ **E05.2** **Thyrotoxicosis with toxic multinodular goiter**
Toxic nodular goiter NOS
E05.20 **Thyrotoxicosis with toxic multinodular goiter without thyrotoxic crisis or storm**
MCC **E05.21** **Thyrotoxicosis with toxic multinodular goiter with thyrotoxic crisis or storm**
+ **E05.3** **Thyrotoxicosis from ectopic thyroid tissue**
E05.30 **Thyrotoxicosis from ectopic thyroid tissue without thyrotoxic crisis or storm**
MCC **E05.31** **Thyrotoxicosis from ectopic thyroid tissue with thyrotoxic crisis or storm**
+ **E05.4** **Thyrotoxicosis factitia**
E05.40 **Thyrotoxicosis factitia without thyrotoxic crisis or storm**
MCC **E05.41** **Thyrotoxicosis factitia with thyrotoxic crisis or storm**
+ **E05.8** **Other thyrotoxicosis**
Overproduction of thyroid-stimulating hormone
E05.80 **Other thyrotoxicosis without thyrotoxic crisis or storm**
MCC **E05.81** **Other thyrotoxicosis with thyrotoxic crisis or storm**
+ **E05.9** **Thyrotoxicosis, unspecified**
Hyperthyroidism NOS
E05.90 **Thyrotoxicosis, unspecified without thyrotoxic crisis or storm**
MCC **E05.91** **Thyrotoxicosis, unspecified with thyrotoxic crisis or storm**

E06 **Thyroiditis**

Excludes1: postpartum thyroiditis (O90.5)
CC **E06.0** **Acute thyroiditis**
Abscess of thyroid
Pyogenic thyroiditis
Suppurative thyroiditis
Use additional code (B95-B97) to identify infectious agent.
E06.1 **Subacute thyroiditis**
de Quervain thyroiditis
Giant-cell thyroiditis
Granulomatous thyroiditis
Nonsuppurative thyroiditis
Viral thyroiditis
Excludes1: autoimmune thyroiditis (E06.3)
E06.2 **Chronic thyroiditis with transient thyrotoxicosis**
Excludes1: autoimmune thyroiditis (E06.3)
E06.3 **Autoimmune thyroiditis**
Hashimoto's thyroiditis
Hashitoxicosis (transient)
Lymphadenoid goiter
Lymphocytic thyroiditis
Struma lymphomatosa
E06.4 **Drug-induced thyroiditis**
Use additional code for adverse effect, if applicable, to identify drug (T36-T50 with fifth or sixth character 5)
E06.5 **Other chronic thyroiditis**
Chronic fibrous thyroiditis
Chronic thyroiditis NOS
Ligneous thyroiditis
Riedel thyroiditis
E06.9 **Thyroiditis, unspecified**

E07 **Other disorders of thyroid**

E07.0 **Hypersecretion of calcitonin**
C-cell hyperplasia of thyroid
Hypersecretion of thyrocalcitonin
E07.1 **Dyshormogenetic goiter**
Familial dyshormogenetic goiter
Pendred's syndrome
Excludes1: transitory congenital goiter with normal function (P72.0)
+ **E07.8** **Other specified disorders of thyroid**
E07.81 **Sick-euthyroid syndrome**
Euthyroid sick-syndrome
E07.89 **Other specified disorders of thyroid**
Abnormality of thyroid-binding globulin
Hemorrhage of thyroid
Infarction of thyroid
E07.9 **Disorder of thyroid, unspecified**

Diabetes mellitus (E08-E13)

Review coding guideline C.4.a

E08 **Diabetes mellitus due to underlying condition**

Code first the underlying condition, such as:
congenital rubella (P35.0)
Cushing's syndrome (E24.-)
cystic fibrosis (E84.-)
malignant neoplasm (C00-C96)
malnutrition (E40-E46)
pancreatitis and other diseases of the pancreas (K85-K86.-)

Use additional code to identify control using:
insulin (Z79.4)
oral antidiabetic drugs (Z79.84)
oral hypoglycemic drugs (Z79.84)
Excludes1: drug or chemical induced diabetes mellitus (E09.-)
gestational diabetes (O24.4-)
neonatal diabetes mellitus (P70.2)
postpancreatectomy diabetes mellitus (E13.-)
postprocedural diabetes mellitus (E13.-)
secondary diabetes mellitus NEC (E13.-)
type 1 diabetes mellitus (E10.-)
type 2 diabetes mellitus (E11.-)
Review coding guideline C.4.a.6.a
+ **E08.0** **Diabetes mellitus due to underlying condition with hyperosmolarity**
MCC **E08.00** **Diabetes mellitus due to underlying condition with hyperosmolarity without nonketotic hyperglycemic-hyperosmolar coma (NKHHC)**
HAC see Appendix B for HAC conditional logic
MCC **E08.01** **Diabetes mellitus due to underlying condition with hyperosmolarity with coma**
HAC see Appendix B for HAC conditional logic
+ **E08.1** **Diabetes mellitus due to underlying condition with ketoacidosis**
MCC **E08.10** **Diabetes mellitus due to underlying condition with ketoacidosis without coma**
HAC see Appendix B for HAC conditional logic
MCC **E08.11** **Diabetes mellitus due to underlying condition with ketoacidosis with coma**
+ **E08.2** **Diabetes mellitus due to underlying condition with kidney complications**
E08.21 **Diabetes mellitus due to underlying condition with diabetic nephropathy**
Diabetes mellitus due to underlying condition with intercapillary glomerulosclerosis
Diabetes mellitus due to underlying condition with intracapillary glomerulonephrosis
Diabetes mellitus due to underlying condition with Kimmelstiel-Wilson disease
E08.22 **Diabetes mellitus due to underlying condition with diabetic chronic kidney disease**
Use additional code to identify stage of chronic kidney disease (N18.1-N18.6)
E08.29 **Diabetes mellitus due to underlying condition with other diabetic kidney complication**
Renal tubular degeneration in diabetes mellitus due to underlying condition
+ **E08.3** **Diabetes mellitus due to underlying condition with ophthalmic complications**
AHA CC: 4Q, 2016, 11-13
+ **E08.31** **Diabetes mellitus due to underlying condition with unspecified diabetic retinopathy**
E08.311 **Diabetes mellitus due to underlying condition with unspecified diabetic retinopathy with macular edema**
E08.319 **Diabetes mellitus due to underlying condition with unspecified diabetic retinopathy without macular edema**

+ E08.32 Diabetes mellitus due to underlying condition with mild nonproliferative diabetic retinopathy

Diabetes mellitus due to underlying condition with nonproliferative diabetic retinopathy NOS

One of the following 7th characters is to be assigned to codes in subcategory **E08.32** to designate laterality of the disease:
1 right eye
2 left eye
3 bilateral
9 unspecified eye

+7th E08.321 Diabetes mellitus due to underlying condition with mild nonproliferative diabetic retinopathy with macular edema

+7th E08.329 Diabetes mellitus due to underlying condition with mild nonproliferative diabetic retinopathy without macular edema

+ E08.33 Diabetes mellitus due to underlying condition with moderate nonproliferative diabetic retinopathy

One of the following 7th characters is to be assigned to codes in subcategory **E08.33** to designate laterality of the disease:
1 right eye
2 left eye
3 bilateral
9 unspecified eye

+7th E08.331 Diabetes mellitus due to underlying condition with moderate nonproliferative diabetic retinopathy with macular edema

+7th E08.339 Diabetes mellitus due to underlying condition with moderate nonproliferative diabetic retinopathy without macular edema

+ E08.34 Diabetes mellitus due to underlying condition with severe nonproliferative diabetic retinopathy

One of the following 7th characters is to be assigned to codes in subcategory **E08.34** to designate laterality of the disease:
1 right eye
2 left eye
3 bilateral
9 unspecified eye

+7th E08.341 Diabetes mellitus due to underlying condition with severe nonproliferative diabetic retinopathy with macular edema

+7th E08.349 Diabetes mellitus due to underlying condition with severe nonproliferative diabetic retinopathy without macular edema

+ E08.35 Diabetes mellitus due to underlying condition with proliferative diabetic retinopathy

One of the following 7th characters is to be assigned to codes in subcategory **E08.35** to designate laterality of the disease:
1 right eye
2 left eye
3 bilateral
9 unspecified eye

+7th E08.351 Diabetes mellitus due to underlying condition with proliferative diabetic retinopathy with macular edema

+7th E08.352 Diabetes mellitus due to underlying condition with proliferative diabetic retinopathy with traction retinal detachment involving the macula

+7th E08.353 Diabetes mellitus due to underlying condition with proliferative diabetic retinopathy with traction retinal detachment not involving the macula

+7th E08.354 Diabetes mellitus due to underlying condition with proliferative diabetic retinopathy with combined traction retinal detachment and rhegmatogenous retinal detachment

+7th E08.355 Diabetes mellitus due to underlying condition with stable proliferative diabetic retinopathy

+7th E08.359 Diabetes mellitus due to underlying condition with proliferative diabetic retinopathy without macular edema

E08.36 Diabetes mellitus due to underlying condition with diabetic cataract

X+7th E08.37 Diabetes mellitus due to underlying condition with diabetic macular edema, resolved following treatment

One of the following 7th characters is to be assigned to codes in subcategory **E08.37** to designate laterality of the disease:
1 right eye
2 left eye
3 bilateral
9 unspecified eye

E08.39 Diabetes mellitus due to underlying condition with other diabetic ophthalmic complication

Use additional code to identify manifestation, such as:
diabetic glaucoma (H40-H42)

+ E08.4 Diabetes mellitus due to underlying condition with neurological complications

E08.40 Diabetes mellitus due to underlying condition with diabetic neuropathy, unspecified

E08.41 Diabetes mellitus due to underlying condition with diabetic mononeuropathy

E08.42 Diabetes mellitus due to underlying condition with diabetic polyneuropathy

Diabetes mellitus due to underlying condition with diabetic neuralgia

E08.43 Diabetes mellitus due to underlying condition with diabetic autonomic (poly)neuropathy

Diabetes mellitus due to underlying condition with diabetic gastroparesis

AHA CC: 3Q, 2013, 114-115

E08.44 Diabetes mellitus due to underlying condition with diabetic amyotrophy

E08.49 Diabetes mellitus due to underlying condition with other diabetic neurological complication

+ E08.5 Diabetes mellitus due to underlying condition with circulatory complications

E08.51 Diabetes mellitus due to underlying condition with diabetic peripheral angiopathy without gangrene

CC E08.52 Diabetes mellitus due to underlying condition with diabetic peripheral angiopathy with gangrene

Diabetes mellitus due to underlying condition with diabetic gangrene

E08.59 Diabetes mellitus due to underlying condition with other circulatory complications

+ E08.6 Diabetes mellitus due to underlying condition with other specified complications

+ E08.61 Diabetes mellitus due to underlying condition with diabetic arthropathy

E08.610 Diabetes mellitus due to underlying condition with diabetic neuropathic arthropathy

Diabetes mellitus due to underlying condition with Charcôt's joints

E08.618 Diabetes mellitus due to underlying condition with other diabetic arthropathy

+ **E08.62** Diabetes mellitus due to underlying condition with skin complications

    E08.620 Diabetes mellitus due to underlying condition with diabetic dermatitis

        Diabetes mellitus due to underlying condition with diabetic necrobiosis lipoidica

    E08.621 Diabetes mellitus due to underlying condition with foot ulcer

        Use additional code to identify site of ulcer (L97.4-, L97.5-)

    E08.622 Diabetes mellitus due to underlying condition with other skin ulcer

        Use additional code to identify site of ulcer (L97.1-L97.9, L98.41-L98.49)

    E08.628 Diabetes mellitus due to underlying condition with other skin complications

+ **E08.63** Diabetes mellitus due to underlying condition with oral complications

    E08.630 Diabetes mellitus due to underlying condition with periodontal disease

    E08.638 Diabetes mellitus due to underlying condition with other oral complications

+ **E08.64** Diabetes mellitus due to underlying condition with hypoglycemia

    MCC **E08.641** Diabetes mellitus due to underlying condition with hypoglycemia with coma

    E08.649 Diabetes mellitus due to underlying condition with hypoglycemia without coma

    E08.65 Diabetes mellitus due to underlying condition with hyperglycemia

    E08.69 Diabetes mellitus due to underlying condition with other specified complication

        Use additional code to identify complication

E08.8 Diabetes mellitus due to underlying condition with unspecified complications

E08.9 Diabetes mellitus due to underlying condition without complications

E09 Drug or chemical induced diabetes mellitus

    Code first poisoning due to drug or toxin, if applicable (T36-T65 with fifth or sixth character 1-4 or 6)

    Use additional code for adverse effect, if applicable, to identify drug (T36-T50 with fifth or sixth character 5)

    Use additional code to identify control using:
        insulin (Z79.4)
        oral antidiabetic drugs (Z79.84)
        oral hypoglycemic drugs (Z79.84)

    Excludes1: *diabetes mellitus due to underlying condition (E08.-)*
        gestational diabetes (O24.4-)
        neonatal diabetes mellitus (P70.2)
        postpancreatectomy diabetes mellitus (E13.-)
        postprocedural diabetes mellitus (E13.-)
        secondary diabetes mellitus NEC (E13.-)
        type 1 diabetes mellitus (E10.-)
        type 2 diabetes mellitus (E11.-)
    Review coding guideline C.4.a.6.a

+ **E09.0** Drug or chemical induced diabetes mellitus with hyperosmolarity

    MCC **E09.00** Drug or chemical induced diabetes mellitus with hyperosmolarity without nonketotic hyperglycemic-hyperosmolar coma (NKHHC)

        HAC see Appendix B for HAC conditional logic

    MCC **E09.01** Drug or chemical induced diabetes mellitus with hyperosmolarity with coma

        HAC see Appendix B for HAC conditional logic

+ **E09.1** Drug or chemical induced diabetes mellitus with ketoacidosis

    MCC **E09.10** Drug or chemical induced diabetes mellitus with ketoacidosis without coma

        HAC see Appendix B for HAC conditional logic

    MCC **E09.11** Drug or chemical induced diabetes mellitus with ketoacidosis with coma

+ **E09.2** Drug or chemical induced diabetes mellitus with kidney complications

    E09.21 Drug or chemical induced diabetes mellitus with diabetic nephropathy

        Drug or chemical induced diabetes mellitus with intercapillary glomerulosclerosis

        Drug or chemical induced diabetes mellitus with intracapillary glomerulonephrosis

        Drug or chemical induced diabetes mellitus with Kimmelstiel-Wilson disease

    E09.22 Drug or chemical induced diabetes mellitus with diabetic chronic kidney disease

        Use additional code to identify stage of chronic kidney disease (N18.1-N18.6)

    E09.29 Drug or chemical induced diabetes mellitus with other diabetic kidney complication

        Drug or chemical induced diabetes mellitus with renal tubular degeneration

+ **E09.3** Drug or chemical induced diabetes mellitus with ophthalmic complications

    AHA CC: 4Q, 2016, 11-13

+ **E09.31** Drug or chemical induced diabetes mellitus with unspecified diabetic retinopathy

    E09.311 Drug or chemical induced diabetes mellitus with unspecified diabetic retinopathy with macular edema

    E09.319 Drug or chemical induced diabetes mellitus with unspecified diabetic retinopathy without macular edema

+ **E09.32** Drug or chemical induced diabetes mellitus with mild nonproliferative diabetic retinopathy

    Drug or chemical induced diabetes mellitus with nonproliferative diabetic retinopathy NOS

> One of the following 7th characters is to be assigned to codes in subcategory **E09.32** to designate laterality of the disease:
> 1   right eye
> 2   left eye
> 3   bilateral
> 9   unspecified eye

    +7th **E09.321** Drug or chemical induced diabetes mellitus with mild nonproliferative diabetic retinopathy with macular edema

    +7th **E09.329** Drug or chemical induced diabetes mellitus with mild nonproliferative diabetic retinopathy without macular edema

+7th **E09.33** Drug or chemical induced diabetes mellitus with moderate nonproliferative diabetic retinopathy

> One of the following 7th characters is to be assigned to codes in subcategory **E09.33** to designate laterality of the disease:
> 1   right eye
> 2   left eye
> 3   bilateral
> 9   unspecified eye

    +7th **E09.331** Drug or chemical induced diabetes mellitus with moderate nonproliferative diabetic retinopathy with macular edema

    +7th **E09.339** Drug or chemical induced diabetes mellitus with moderate nonproliferative diabetic retinopathy without macular edema

+ **E09.34** Drug or chemical induced diabetes mellitus with severe nonproliferative diabetic retinopathy

> One of the following 7th characters is to be assigned to codes in subcategory **E09.34** to designate laterality of the disease:
> 1   right eye
> 2   left eye
> 3   bilateral
> 9   unspecified eye

+7th **E09.341** **Drug or chemical induced diabetes mellitus with severe nonproliferative diabetic retinopathy with macular edema**

+7th **E09.349** **Drug or chemical induced diabetes mellitus with severe nonproliferative diabetic retinopathy without macular edema**

+ **E09.35** **Drug or chemical induced diabetes mellitus with proliferative diabetic retinopathy**

> One of the following 7th characters is to be assigned to codes in subcategory **E09.35** to designate laterality of the disease:
> 1 right eye
> 2 left eye
> 3 bilateral
> 9 unspecified eye

+7th **E09.351** **Drug or chemical induced diabetes mellitus with proliferative diabetic retinopathy with macular edema**

+7th **E09.352** **Drug or chemical induced diabetes mellitus with proliferative diabetic retinopathy with traction retinal detachment involving the macula**

+7th **E09.353** **Drug or chemical induced diabetes mellitus with proliferative diabetic retinopathy with traction retinal detachment not involving the macula**

+7th **E09.354** **Drug or chemical induced diabetes mellitus with proliferative diabetic retinopathy with combined traction retinal detachment and rhegmatogenous retinal detachment**

+7th **E09.355** **Drug or chemical induced diabetes mellitus with stable proliferative diabetic retinopathy**

+7th **E09.359** **Drug or chemical induced diabetes mellitus with proliferative diabetic retinopathy without macular edema**

E09.36 **Drug or chemical induced diabetes mellitus with diabetic cataract**

X+7th **E09.37** **Drug or chemical induced diabetes mellitus with diabetic macular edema, resolved following treatment**

> One of the following 7th characters is to be assigned to codes in subcategory **E09.37** to designate laterality of the disease:
> 1 right eye
> 2 left eye
> 3 bilateral
> 9 unspecified eye

E09.39 **Drug or chemical induced diabetes mellitus with other diabetic ophthalmic complication**
Use additional code to identify manifestation, such as: diabetic glaucoma (H40-H42)

+ **E09.4** **Drug or chemical induced diabetes mellitus with neurological complications**

E09.40 **Drug or chemical induced diabetes mellitus with neurological complications with diabetic neuropathy, unspecified**

E09.41 **Drug or chemical induced diabetes mellitus with neurological complications with diabetic mononeuropathy**

E09.42 **Drug or chemical induced diabetes mellitus with neurological complications with diabetic polyneuropathy**
Drug or chemical induced diabetes mellitus with diabetic neuralgia

E09.43 **Drug or chemical induced diabetes mellitus with neurological complications with diabetic autonomic (poly)neuropathy**
Drug or chemical induced diabetes mellitus with diabetic gastroparesis
AHA CC: 3Q, 2013, 114-115

E09.44 **Drug or chemical induced diabetes mellitus with neurological complications with diabetic amyotrophy**

E09.49 **Drug or chemical induced diabetes mellitus with neurological complications with other diabetic neurological complication**

+ **E09.5** **Drug or chemical induced diabetes mellitus with circulatory complications**

E09.51 **Drug or chemical induced diabetes mellitus with diabetic peripheral angiopathy without gangrene**

CC **E09.52** **Drug or chemical induced diabetes mellitus with diabetic peripheral angiopathy with gangrene**
Drug or chemical induced diabetes mellitus with diabetic gangrene

E09.59 **Drug or chemical induced diabetes mellitus with other circulatory complications**

+ **E09.6** **Drug or chemical induced diabetes mellitus with other specified complications**

+ **E09.61** **Drug or chemical induced diabetes mellitus with diabetic arthropathy**

E09.610 **Drug or chemical induced diabetes mellitus with diabetic neuropathic arthropathy**
Drug or chemical induced diabetes mellitus with Charcôt's joints

E09.618 **Drug or chemical induced diabetes mellitus with other diabetic arthropathy**

+ **E09.62** **Drug or chemical induced diabetes mellitus with skin complications**

E09.620 **Drug or chemical induced diabetes mellitus with diabetic dermatitis**
Drug or chemical induced diabetes mellitus with diabetic necrobiosis lipoidica

E09.621 **Drug or chemical induced diabetes mellitus with foot ulcer**
Use additional code to identify site of ulcer (L97.4-, L97.5-)

E09.622 **Drug or chemical induced diabetes mellitus with other skin ulcer**
Use additional code to identify site of ulcer (L97.1-L97.9, L98.41-L98.49)

E09.628 **Drug or chemical induced diabetes mellitus with other skin complications**

+ **E09.63** **Drug or chemical induced diabetes mellitus with oral complications**

E09.630 **Drug or chemical induced diabetes mellitus with periodontal disease**

E09.638 **Drug or chemical induced diabetes mellitus with other oral complications**

+ **E09.64** **Drug or chemical induced diabetes mellitus with hypoglycemia**

MCC **E09.641** **Drug or chemical induced diabetes mellitus with hypoglycemia with coma**

E09.649 **Drug or chemical induced diabetes mellitus with hypoglycemia without coma**

CC **E09.65** **Drug or chemical induced diabetes mellitus with hyperglycemia**

CC **E09.69** **Drug or chemical induced diabetes mellitus with other specified complication**
Use additional code to identify complication

CC **E09.8** **Drug or chemical induced diabetes mellitus with unspecified complications**

CC **E09.9** **Drug or chemical induced diabetes mellitus without complications**

E10 **Type 1 diabetes mellitus**

Includes: brittle diabetes (mellitus)
diabetes (mellitus) due to autoimmune process
diabetes (mellitus) due to immune mediated pancreatic islet beta-cell destruction
idiopathic diabetes (mellitus)
juvenile onset diabetes (mellitus)
ketosis-prone diabetes (mellitus)

Excludes1: *diabetes mellitus due to underlying condition (E08.-)*
drug or chemical induced diabetes mellitus (E09.-)
gestational diabetes (O24.4-)
hyperglycemia NOS (R73.9)
neonatal diabetes mellitus (P70.2)
postpancreatectomy diabetes mellitus (E13.-)
postprocedural diabetes mellitus (E13.-)
secondary diabetes mellitus NEC (E13.-)
type 2 diabetes mellitus (E11.-)

Diabetes Mellitus and Its Complications: Micro and Macrovascular Complications

Diabetic retinopathy

Diabetic retinopathy can be easily detected during a dialated eye exam and is the leading cause of blindness among adults in theUnited States. Visual loss can be prevented with early recognition and treatment of retinopathy.

Nonproliferative retinopathy (early stage)

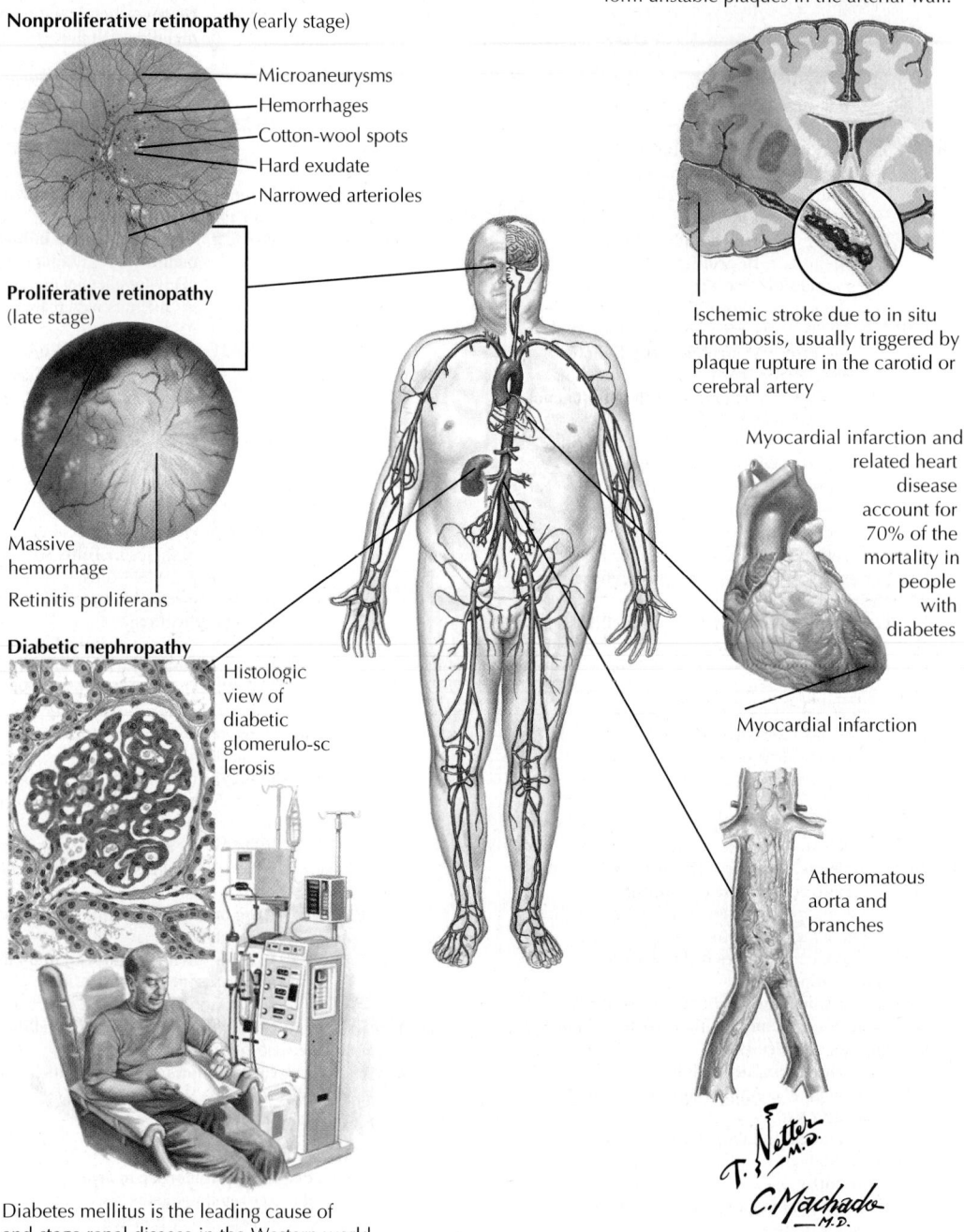

- Microaneurysms
- Hemorrhages
- Cotton-wool spots
- Hard exudate
- Narrowed arterioles

Proliferative retinopathy (late stage)

Massive hemorrhage

Retinitis proliferans

Diabetic nephropathy

Histologic view of diabetic glomerulo-sc lerosis

Diabetes mellitus is the leading cause of end-stage renal disease in the Western world

Cerebrovascular disease

The high incidence of vascular complications among patients with diabetes is related not only to blood glucose elevations, but also to the frequent association of dyslipidemia, hypertension, a procoagulant state and the tendency to form unstable plaques in the arterial wall.

Ischemic stroke due to in situ thrombosis, usually triggered by plaque rupture in the carotid or cerebral artery

Myocardial infarction and related heart disease account for 70% of the mortality in people with diabetes

Myocardial infarction

Atheromatous aorta and branches

+ **E10.1** Type 1 diabetes mellitus with ketoacidosis

MCC **E10.10** Type 1 diabetes mellitus with ketoacidosis without coma

> **HAC** see Appendix B for HAC conditional logic
> *AHA CC: 3Q, 2013, 20*

MCC **E10.11** Type 1 diabetes mellitus with ketoacidosis with coma

+ **E10.2** Type 1 diabetes mellitus with kidney complications

E10.21 Type 1 diabetes mellitus with diabetic nephropathy

> Type 1 diabetes mellitus with intercapillary glomerulosclerosis
> Type 1 diabetes mellitus with intracapillary glomerulonephrosis
> Type 1 diabetes mellitus with Kimmelstiel-Wilson disease

E10.22 Type 1 diabetes mellitus with diabetic chronic kidney disease

> Use additional code to identify stage of chronic kidney disease (N18.1-N18.6)

E10.29 Type 1 diabetes mellitus with other diabetic kidney complication

> Type 1 diabetes mellitus with renal tubular degeneration

+ **E10.3** Type 1 diabetes mellitus with ophthalmic complications

> *AHA CC: 4Q, 2016, 11-13*

+ **E10.31** Type 1 diabetes mellitus with unspecified diabetic retinopathy

E10.311 Type 1 diabetes mellitus with unspecified diabetic retinopathy with macular edema

E10.319 Type 1 diabetes mellitus with unspecified diabetic retinopathy without macular edema

+ **E10.32** Type 1 diabetes mellitus with mild nonproliferative diabetic retinopathy

> Type 1 diabetes mellitus with nonproliferative diabetic retinopathy NOS

> One of the following 7th characters is to be assigned to codes in subcategory **E10.32** to designate laterality of the disease:
> 1 right eye
> 2 left eye
> 3 bilateral
> 9 unspecified eye

+7th **E10.321** Type 1 diabetes mellitus with mild nonproliferative diabetic retinopathy with macular edema

+7th **E10.329** Type 1 diabetes mellitus with mild nonproliferative diabetic retinopathy without macular edema

+ **E10.33** Type 1 diabetes mellitus with moderate nonproliferative diabetic retinopathy

> One of the following 7th characters is to be assigned to codes in subcategory **E10.33** to designate laterality of the disease:
> 1 right eye
> 2 left eye
> 3 bilateral
> 9 unspecified eye

+7th **E10.331** Type 1 diabetes mellitus with moderate nonproliferative diabetic retinopathy with macular edema

+7th **E10.339** Type 1 diabetes mellitus with moderate nonproliferative diabetic retinopathy without macular edema

+ **E10.34** Type 1 diabetes mellitus with severe nonproliferative diabetic retinopathy

> One of the following 7th characters is to be assigned to codes in subcategory **E10.34** to designate laterality of the disease:
> 1 right eye
> 2 left eye
> 3 bilateral
> 9 unspecified eye

+7th **E10.341** Type 1 diabetes mellitus with severe nonproliferative diabetic retinopathy with macular edema

+7th **E10.349** Type 1 diabetes mellitus with severe nonproliferative diabetic retinopathy without macular edema

+ **E10.35** Type 1 diabetes mellitus with proliferative diabetic retinopathy

> One of the following 7th characters is to be assigned to codes in subcategory **E10.35** to designate laterality of the disease:
> 1 right eye
> 2 left eye
> 3 bilateral
> 9 unspecified eye

+7th **E10.351** Type 1 diabetes mellitus with proliferative diabetic retinopathy with macular edema

+7th **E10.352** Type 1 diabetes mellitus with proliferative diabetic retinopathy with traction retinal detachment involving the macula

+7th **E10.353** Type 1 diabetes mellitus with proliferative diabetic retinopathy with traction retinal detachment not involving the macula

+7th **E10.354** Type 1 diabetes mellitus with proliferative diabetic retinopathy with combined traction retinal detachment and rhegmatogenous retinal detachment

+7th **E10.355** Type 1 diabetes mellitus with stable proliferative diabetic retinopathy

+7th **E10.359** Type 1 diabetes mellitus with proliferative diabetic retinopathy without macular edema

E10.36 Type 1 diabetes mellitus with diabetic cataract

X+7th **E10.37** Type 1 diabetes mellitus with diabetic macular edema, resolved following treatment

> One of the following 7th characters is to be assigned to codes in subcategory **E10.37** to designate laterality of the disease:
> 1 right eye
> 2 left eye
> 3 bilateral
> 9 unspecified eye

E10.39 Type 1 diabetes mellitus with other diabetic ophthalmic complication

> Use additional code to identify manifestation, such as: diabetic glaucoma (H40-H42)

+ **E10.4** Type 1 diabetes mellitus with neurological complications

E10.40 Type 1 diabetes mellitus with diabetic neuropathy, unspecified

E10.41 Type 1 diabetes mellitus with diabetic mononeuropathy

E10.42 Type 1 diabetes mellitus with diabetic polyneuropathy

> Type 1 diabetes mellitus with diabetic neuralgia

E10.43 Type 1 diabetes mellitus with diabetic autonomic (poly)neuropathy

> Type 1 diabetes mellitus with diabetic gastroparesis
> *AHA CC: 3Q, 2013, 114-115*

E10.44 Type 1 diabetes mellitus with diabetic amyotrophy

E10.49 Type 1 diabetes mellitus with other diabetic neurological complication

+ **E10.5** Type 1 diabetes mellitus with circulatory complications

E10.51 Type 1 diabetes mellitus with diabetic peripheral angiopathy without gangrene

CC **E10.52** Type 1 diabetes mellitus with diabetic peripheral angiopathy with gangrene

> Type 1 diabetes mellitus with diabetic gangrene

E10.59 Type 1 diabetes mellitus with other circulatory complications

+ **E10.6** Type 1 diabetes mellitus with other specified complications

+ **E10.61** Type 1 diabetes mellitus with diabetic arthropathy

E10.610 Type 1 diabetes mellitus with diabetic neuropathic arthropathy

> Type 1 diabetes mellitus with Charcôt's joints

E10.618 Type 1 diabetes mellitus with other diabetic arthropathy

551

+ **E10.62** **Type 1 diabetes mellitus with skin complications**

    E10.620 **Type 1 diabetes mellitus with diabetic dermatitis**

        Type 1 diabetes mellitus with diabetic necrobiosis lipoidica

    E10.621 **Type 1 diabetes mellitus with foot ulcer**

        Use additional code to identify site of ulcer (L97.4-, L97.5-)

    E10.622 **Type 1 diabetes mellitus with other skin ulcer**

        Use additional code to identify site of ulcer (L97.1-L97.9, L98.41-L98.49)

    E10.628 **Type 1 diabetes mellitus with other skin complications**

+ **E10.63** **Type 1 diabetes mellitus with oral complications**

    E10.630 **Type 1 diabetes mellitus with periodontal disease**

    E10.638 **Type 1 diabetes mellitus with other oral complications**

+ **E10.64** **Type 1 diabetes mellitus with hypoglycemia**

  MCC **E10.641** **Type 1 diabetes mellitus with hypoglycemia with coma**

    E10.649 **Type 1 diabetes mellitus with hypoglycemia without coma**

        AHA CC: 1Q, 2016, 13

  E10.65 **Type 1 diabetes mellitus with hyperglycemia**

  E10.69 **Type 1 diabetes mellitus with other specified complication**

        Use additional code to identify complication

E10.8 **Type 1 diabetes mellitus with unspecified complications**

E10.9 **Type 1 diabetes mellitus without complications**

E11 **Type 2 diabetes mellitus**

  Includes: diabetes (mellitus) due to insulin secretory defect

        diabetes NOS

        insulin resistant diabetes (mellitus)

  Use additional code to identify control using:

    insulin (Z79.4)

    oral antidiabetic drugs (Z79.84)

    oral hypoglycemic drugs (Z79.84)

  Excludes1: *diabetes mellitus due to underlying condition (E08.-)*

    drug or chemical induced diabetes mellitus (E09.-)

    gestational diabetes (O24.4-)

    neonatal diabetes mellitus (P70.2)

    postpancreatectomy diabetes mellitus (E13.-)

    postprocedural diabetes mellitus (E13.-)

    secondary diabetes mellitus NEC (E13.-)

    type 1 diabetes mellitus (E10.-)

  Review coding guidelines C.4.a.2 and C.4.a.3

+ **E11.0** **Type 2 diabetes mellitus with hyperosmolarity**

    AHA CC: 4Q, 2017, 6

  MCC **E11.00** **Type 2 diabetes mellitus with hyperosmolarity without nonketotic hyperglycemic-hyperosmolar coma (NKHHC)**

        HAC see Appendix B for HAC conditional logic

  MCC **E11.01** **Type 2 diabetes mellitus with hyperosmolarity with coma**

        HAC see Appendix B for HAC conditional logic

+ **E11.1** **Type 2 diabetes mellitus with ketoacidosis**

  MCC **E11.10** **Type 2 diabetes mellitus with ketoacidosis without coma**

  MCC **E11.11** **Type 2 diabetes mellitus with ketoacidosis with coma**

        AHA CC: 4Q, 2017, 6

+ **E11.2** **Type 2 diabetes mellitus with kidney complications**

  E11.21 **Type 2 diabetes mellitus with diabetic nephropathy**

    Type 2 diabetes mellitus with intercapillary glomerulosclerosis

    Type 2 diabetes mellitus with intracapillary glomerulonephrosis

    Type 2 diabetes mellitus with Kimmelstiel-Wilson disease

  E11.22 **Type 2 diabetes mellitus with diabetic chronic kidney disease**

    Use additional code to identify stage of chronic kidney disease (N18.1-N18.6)

    AHA CC: 4Q, 2018, 88-89; 3Q, 2019, 3

  E11.29 **Type 2 diabetes mellitus with other diabetic kidney complication**

    Type 2 diabetes mellitus with renal tubular degeneration

+ **E11.3** **Type 2 diabetes mellitus with ophthalmic complications**

    AHA CC: 4Q, 2016, 11-13

+ **E11.31** **Type 2 diabetes mellitus with unspecified diabetic retinopathy**

  E11.311 **Type 2 diabetes mellitus with unspecified diabetic retinopathy with macular edema**

  E11.319 **Type 2 diabetes mellitus with unspecified diabetic retinopathy without macular edema**

    AHA CC: 3Q, 2013, 20

+ **E11.32** **Type 2 diabetes mellitus with mild nonproliferative diabetic retinopathy**

  Type 2 diabetes mellitus with nonproliferative diabetic retinopathy NOS

> One of the following 7th characters is to be assigned to codes in subcategory **E11.32** to designate laterality of the disease:
> 1 right eye
> 2 left eye
> 3 bilateral
> 9 unspecified eye

  +7th **E11.321** **Type 2 diabetes mellitus with mild nonproliferative diabetic retinopathy with macular edema**

  +7th **E11.329** **Type 2 diabetes mellitus with mild nonproliferative diabetic retinopathy without macular edema**

+ **E11.33** **Type 2 diabetes mellitus with moderate nonproliferative diabetic retinopathy**

> One of the following 7th characters is to be assigned to codes in subcategory **E11.33** to designate laterality of the disease:
> 1 right eye
> 2 left eye
> 3 bilateral
> 9 unspecified eye

  +7th **E11.331** **Type 2 diabetes mellitus with moderate nonproliferative diabetic retinopathy with macular edema**

  +7th **E11.339** **Type 2 diabetes mellitus with moderate nonproliferative diabetic retinopathy without macular edema**

+ **E11.34** **Type 2 diabetes mellitus with severe nonproliferative diabetic retinopathy**

> One of the following 7th characters is to be assigned to codes in subcategory **E11.34** to designate laterality of the disease:
> 1 right eye
> 2 left eye
> 3 bilateral
> 9 unspecified eye

  +7th **E11.341** **Type 2 diabetes mellitus with severe nonproliferative diabetic retinopathy with macular edema**

  +7th **E11.349** **Type 2 diabetes mellitus with severe nonproliferative diabetic retinopathy without macular edema**

+ **E11.35** **Type 2 diabetes mellitus with proliferative diabetic retinopathy**

> One of the following 7th characters is to be assigned to codes in subcategory **E11.35** to designate laterality of the disease:
> 1 right eye
> 2 left eye
> 3 bilateral
> 9 unspecified eye

  +7th **E11.351** **Type 2 diabetes mellitus with proliferative diabetic retinopathy with macular edema**

  +7th **E11.352** **Type 2 diabetes mellitus with proliferative diabetic retinopathy with traction retinal detachment involving the macula**

  +7th **E11.353** **Type 2 diabetes mellitus with proliferative diabetic retinopathy with traction retinal detachment not involving the macula**

+7th **E11.354** **Type 2 diabetes mellitus with proliferative diabetic retinopathy with combined traction retinal detachment and rhegmatogenous retinal detachment**

+7th **E11.355** **Type 2 diabetes mellitus with stable proliferative diabetic retinopathy**

+7th **E11.359** **Type 2 diabetes mellitus with proliferative diabetic retinopathy without macular edema**

E11.36 **Type 2 diabetes mellitus with diabetic cataract**
AHA CC: 2Q, 2019, 30-31

X+7th **E11.37** **Type 2 diabetes mellitus with diabetic macular edema, resolved following treatment**

> One of the following 7th characters is to be assigned to codes in subcategory **E11.37** to designate laterality of the disease:
> 1   right eye
> 2   left eye
> 3   bilateral
> 9   unspecified eye

E11.39 **Type 2 diabetes mellitus with other diabetic ophthalmic complication**
Use additional code to identify manifestation, such as: diabetic glaucoma (H40-H42)

+ E11.4 **Type 2 diabetes mellitus with neurological complications**

E11.40 **Type 2 diabetes mellitus with diabetic neuropathy, unspecified**
AHA CC: 4Q, 2013, 129; 3Q, 2018, 3-4

E11.41 **Type 2 diabetes mellitus with diabetic mononeuropathy**

E11.42 **Type 2 diabetes mellitus with diabetic polyneuropathy**
Type 2 diabetes mellitus with diabetic neuralgia
AHA CC: 1Q, 2020, 12

E11.43 **Type 2 diabetes mellitus with diabetic autonomic (poly)neuropathy**
Type 2 diabetes mellitus with diabetic gastroparesis
AHA CC: 4Q, 2013, 114-115

E11.44 **Type 2 diabetes mellitus with diabetic amyotrophy**

E11.49 **Type 2 diabetes mellitus with other diabetic neurological complication**

+ E11.5 **Type 2 diabetes mellitus with circulatory complications**

E11.51 **Type 2 diabetes mellitus with diabetic peripheral angiopathy without gangrene**
AHA CC: 3Q, 2018, 3-4

CC **E11.52** **Type 2 diabetes mellitus with diabetic peripheral angiopathy with gangrene**
Type 2 diabetes mellitus with diabetic gangrene
AHA CC: 4Q, 2017, 102

E11.59 **Type 2 diabetes mellitus with other circulatory complications**

+ E11.6 **Type 2 diabetes mellitus with other specified complications**

+ E11.61 **Type 2 diabetes mellitus with diabetic arthropathy**

E11.610 **Type 2 diabetes mellitus with diabetic neuropathic arthropathy**
Type 2 diabetes mellitus with Charcôt's joints

E11.618 **Type 2 diabetes mellitus with other diabetic arthropathy**

+ E11.62 **Type 2 diabetes mellitus with skin complications**

E11.620 **Type 2 diabetes mellitus with diabetic dermatitis**
Type 2 diabetes mellitus with diabetic necrobiosis lipoidica

E11.621 **Type 2 diabetes mellitus with foot ulcer**
Use additional code to identify site of ulcer (L97.4-, L97.5-)
AHA CC: 1Q, 2016, 12-13; 1Q, 2020, 12; 2Q, 2020, 19

E11.622 **Type 2 diabetes mellitus with other skin ulcer**
Use additional code to identify site of ulcer (L97.1-L97.9, L98.41-L98.49)
AHA CC: 4Q, 2017, 17

E11.628 **Type 2 diabetes mellitus with other skin complications**

+ E11.63 **Type 2 diabetes mellitus with oral complications**

E11.630 **Type 2 diabetes mellitus with periodontal disease**

E11.638 **Type 2 diabetes mellitus with other oral complications**

+ E11.64 **Type 2 diabetes mellitus with hypoglycemia**

MCC **E11.641** **Type 2 diabetes mellitus with hypoglycemia with coma**

E11.649 **Type 2 diabetes mellitus with hypoglycemia without coma**
AHA CC: 3Q, 2015, 21; 3Q, 2016, 42

E11.65 **Type 2 diabetes mellitus with hyperglycemia**
AHA CC: 3Q, 2013, 20

E11.69 **Type 2 diabetes mellitus with other specified complication**
Use additional code to identify complication
AHA CC: 4Q, 2016, 141-142; 1Q, 2020, 12

E11.8 **Type 2 diabetes mellitus with unspecified complications**

E11.9 **Type 2 diabetes mellitus without complications**
AHA CC: 4Q, 2013, 128; 2Q, 2020, 18

E13 **Other specified diabetes mellitus**

Includes: diabetes mellitus due to genetic defects of beta-cell function diabetes mellitus due to genetic defects in insulin action postpancreatectomy diabetes mellitus postprocedural diabetes mellitus secondary diabetes mellitus NEC

Use additional code to identify control using:
insulin (Z79.4)
oral antidiabetic drugs (Z79.84)
oral hypoglycemic drugs (Z79.84)

Excludes1: *diabetes (mellitus) due to autoimmune process (E10.-)*
diabetes (mellitus) due to immune mediated pancreatic islet beta-cell destruction (E10.-)
diabetes mellitus due to underlying condition (E08.-)
drug or chemical induced diabetes mellitus (E09.-)
gestational diabetes (O24.4-)
neonatal diabetes mellitus (P70.2)
type 1 diabetes mellitus (E10.-)

AHA CC: 3Q, 2018, 4-5
Review coding guidelines C.4.a.6.a and C.4.a.6.b.i

+ E13.0 **Other specified diabetes mellitus with hyperosmolarity**

MCC **E13.00** **Other specified diabetes mellitus with hyperosmolarity without nonketotic hyperglycemic-hyperosmolar coma (NKHHC)**
Excludes2: *type 2 diabetes mellitus (E11.-)*
HAC see Appendix B for HAC conditional logic

MCC **E13.01** **Other specified diabetes mellitus with hyperosmolarity with coma**
HAC see Appendix B for HAC conditional logic

+ E13.1 **Other specified diabetes mellitus with ketoacidosis**

MCC **E13.10** **Other specified diabetes mellitus with ketoacidosis without coma**
HAC see Appendix B for HAC conditional logic
AHA CC: 1Q, 2013, 26-27; 2Q, 2016,10

MCC **E13.11** **Other specified diabetes mellitus with ketoacidosis with coma**

+ E13.2 **Other specified diabetes mellitus with kidney complications**

E13.21 **Other specified diabetes mellitus with diabetic nephropathy**
Other specified diabetes mellitus with intercapillary glomerulosclerosis
Other specified diabetes mellitus with intracapillary glomerulonephrosis
Other specified diabetes mellitus with Kimmelstiel-Wilson disease

E13.22 **Other specified diabetes mellitus with diabetic chronic kidney disease**
Use additional code to identify stage of chronic kidney disease (N18.1-N18.6)

E13.29 **Other specified diabetes mellitus with other diabetic kidney complication**
Other specified diabetes mellitus with renal tubular degeneration

+ E13.3 **Other specified diabetes mellitus with ophthalmic complications**
AHA CC: 4Q, 2016, 11-13

+ **E13.31** Other specified diabetes mellitus with unspecified diabetic retinopathy

    E13.311 Other specified diabetes mellitus with unspecified diabetic retinopathy with macular edema

    E13.319 Other specified diabetes mellitus with unspecified diabetic retinopathy without macular edema

+ **E13.32** Other specified diabetes mellitus with mild nonproliferative diabetic retinopathy

    Other specified diabetes mellitus with nonproliferative diabetic retinopathy NOS

> One of the following 7th characters is to be assigned to codes in subcategory **E13.32** to designate laterality of the disease:
> 1 right eye
> 2 left eye
> 3 bilateral
> 9 unspecified eye

  +7th **E13.321** Other specified diabetes mellitus with mild nonproliferative diabetic retinopathy with macular edema

  +7th **E13.329** Other specified diabetes mellitus with mild nonproliferative diabetic retinopathy without macular edema

+ **E13.33** Other specified diabetes mellitus with moderate nonproliferative diabetic retinopathy

> One of the following 7th characters is to be assigned to codes in subcategory **E13.33** to designate laterality of the disease:
> 1 right eye
> 2 left eye
> 3 bilateral
> 9 unspecified eye

  +7th **E13.331** Other specified diabetes mellitus with moderate nonproliferative diabetic retinopathy with macular edema

  +7th **E13.339** Other specified diabetes mellitus with moderate nonproliferative diabetic retinopathy without macular edema

+ **E13.34** Other specified diabetes mellitus with severe nonproliferative diabetic retinopathy

> One of the following 7th characters is to be assigned to codes in subcategory **E13.34** to designate laterality of the disease:
> 1 right eye
> 2 left eye
> 3 bilateral
> 9 unspecified eye

  +7th **E13.341** Other specified diabetes mellitus with severe nonproliferative diabetic retinopathy with macular edema

  +7th **E13.349** Other specified diabetes mellitus with severe nonproliferative diabetic retinopathy without macular edema

+ **E13.35** Other specified diabetes mellitus with proliferative diabetic retinopathy

> One of the following 7th characters is to be assigned to codes in subcategory **E13.35** to designate laterality of the disease:
> 1 right eye
> 2 left eye
> 3 bilateral
> 9 unspecified eye

  +7th **E13.351** Other specified diabetes mellitus with proliferative diabetic retinopathy with macular edema

  +7th **E13.352** Other specified diabetes mellitus with proliferative diabetic retinopathy with traction retinal detachment involving the macula

  +7th **E13.353** Other specified diabetes mellitus with proliferative diabetic retinopathy with traction retinal detachment not involving the macula

  +7th **E13.354** Other specified diabetes mellitus with proliferative diabetic retinopathy with combined traction retinal detachment and rhegmatogenous retinal detachment

  +7th **E13.355** Other specified diabetes mellitus with stable proliferative diabetic retinopathy

  +7th **E13.359** Other specified diabetes mellitus with proliferative diabetic retinopathy without macular edema

E13.36 Other specified diabetes mellitus with diabetic cataract

X+7th **E13.37** Other specified diabetes mellitus with diabetic macular edema, resolved following treatment

> One of the following 7th characters is to be assigned to codes in subcategory **E13.37** to designate laterality of the disease:
> 1 right eye
> 2 left eye
> 3 bilateral
> 9 unspecified eye

E13.39 Other specified diabetes mellitus with other diabetic ophthalmic complication

    Use additional code to identify manifestation, such as: diabetic glaucoma (H40-H42)

+ **E13.4** Other specified diabetes mellitus with neurological complications

E13.40 Other specified diabetes mellitus with diabetic neuropathy, unspecified

    AHA CC: 4Q, 2013, 129

E13.41 Other specified diabetes mellitus with diabetic mononeuropathy

E13.42 Other specified diabetes mellitus with diabetic polyneuropathy

    Other specified diabetes mellitus with diabetic neuralgia

E13.43 Other specified diabetes mellitus with diabetic autonomic (poly)neuropathy

    Other specified diabetes mellitus with diabetic gastroparesis

    AHA CC: 4Q, 2013, 114-115

E13.44 Other specified diabetes mellitus with diabetic amyotrophy

E13.49 Other specified diabetes mellitus with other diabetic neurological complication

+ **E13.5** Other specified diabetes mellitus with circulatory complications

E13.51 Other specified diabetes mellitus with diabetic peripheral angiopathy without gangrene

CC **E13.52** Other specified diabetes mellitus with diabetic peripheral angiopathy with gangrene

    Other specified diabetes mellitus with diabetic gangrene

E13.59 Other specified diabetes mellitus with other circulatory complications

+ **E13.6** Other specified diabetes mellitus with other specified complications

  + **E13.61** Other specified diabetes mellitus with diabetic arthropathy

    E13.610 Other specified diabetes mellitus with diabetic neuropathic arthropathy

        Other specified diabetes mellitus with Charcôt's joints

    E13.618 Other specified diabetes mellitus with other diabetic arthropathy

+ **E13.62** **Other specified diabetes mellitus with skin complications**
    E13.620 **Other specified diabetes mellitus with diabetic dermatitis**
      Other specified diabetes mellitus with diabetic necrobiosis lipoidica
    E13.621 **Other specified diabetes mellitus with foot ulcer**
      Use additional code to identify site of ulcer (L97.4-, L97.5-)
    E13.622 **Other specified diabetes mellitus with other skin ulcer**
      Use additional code to identify site of ulcer (L97.1-L97.9, L98.41-L98.49)
    E13.628 **Other specified diabetes mellitus with other skin complications**

+ **E13.63** **Other specified diabetes mellitus with oral complications**
    E13.630 **Other specified diabetes mellitus with periodontal disease**
    E13.638 **Other specified diabetes mellitus with other oral complications**

+ **E13.64** **Other specified diabetes mellitus with hypoglycemia**
    MCC **E13.641** **Other specified diabetes mellitus with hypoglycemia with coma**
    E13.649 **Other specified diabetes mellitus with hypoglycemia without coma**
  E13.65 **Other specified diabetes mellitus with hyperglycemia**
    AHA CC: 3Q, 2018, 4-5
  E13.69 **Other specified diabetes mellitus with other specified complication**
    Use additional code to identify complication
E13.8 **Other specified diabetes mellitus with unspecified complications**
E13.9 **Other specified diabetes mellitus without complications**

Other disorders of glucose regulation and pancreatic internal secretion (E15-E16)

CC **E15** **Nondiabetic hypoglycemic coma**

  Includes: drug-induced insulin coma in nondiabetic
    hyperinsulinism with hypoglycemic coma
    hypoglycemic coma NOS

  HAC see Appendix B for HAC conditional logic
  Valid 3-character code, no further characters required

E16 **Other disorders of pancreatic internal secretion**

  E16.0 **Drug-induced hypoglycemia without coma**
    Use additional code for adverse effect, if applicable, to identify drug (T36-T50 with fifth or sixth character 5)
    Excludes1: *diabetes with hypoglycemia without coma (E09.649)*

  E16.1 **Other hypoglycemia**
    Functional hyperinsulinism
    Functional nonhyperinsulinemic hypoglycemia
    Hyperinsulinism NOS
    Hyperplasia of pancreatic islet beta cells NOS
    Excludes1: *diabetes with hypoglycemia (E08.649, E10.649, E11.649, E13.649)*
      hypoglycemia in infant of diabetic mother (P70.1)
      neonatal hypoglycemia (P70.4)

  E16.2 **Hypoglycemia, unspecified**
    Excludes1: *diabetes with hypoglycemia (E08.649, E10.649, E11.649, E13.649)*

  E16.3 **Increased secretion of glucagon**
    Hyperplasia of pancreatic endocrine cells with glucagon excess

  E16.4 **Increased secretion of gastrin**
    Hypergastrinemia
    Hyperplasia of pancreatic endocrine cells with gastrin excess
    Zollinger-Ellison syndrome

  E16.8 **Other specified disorders of pancreatic internal secretion**
    Increased secretion from endocrine pancreas of growth hormone-releasing hormone
    Increased secretion from endocrine pancreas of pancreatic polypeptide
    Increased secretion from endocrine pancreas of somatostatin
    Increased secretion from endocrine pancreas of vasoactive-intestinal polypeptide

  E16.9 **Disorder of pancreatic internal secretion, unspecified**
    Islet-cell hyperplasia NOS
    Pancreatic endocrine cell hyperplasia NOS

Disorders of other endocrine glands (E20-E35)

  Excludes1: *galactorrhea (N64.3)*
    gynecomastia (N62)

E20 **Hypoparathyroidism**

  Excludes1: *Di George's syndrome (D82.1)*
    postprocedural hypoparathyroidism (E89.2)
    tetany NOS (R29.0)
    transitory neonatal hypoparathyroidism (P71.4)

  E20.0 **Idiopathic hypoparathyroidism**
  E20.1 **Pseudohypoparathyroidism**
  E20.8 **Other hypoparathyroidism**
  E20.9 **Hypoparathyroidism, unspecified**
    Parathyroid tetany

E21 **Hyperparathyroidism and other disorders of parathyroid gland**

  Excludes1: *adult osteomalacia (M83.-)*
    ectopic hyperparathyroidism (E34.2)
    familial hypocalciuric hypercalcemia (E83.52)
    hungry bone syndrome (E83.81)
    infantile and juvenile osteomalacia (E55.0)

  E21.0 **Primary hyperparathyroidism**
    Hyperplasia of parathyroid
    Osteitis fibrosa cystica generalisata [von Recklinghausen's disease of bone]

  E21.1 **Secondary hyperparathyroidism, not elsewhere classified**
    Excludes1: *secondary hyperparathyroidism of renal origin (N25.81)*

  E21.2 **Other hyperparathyroidism**
    Tertiary hyperparathyroidism
    Excludes1: *familial hypocalciuric hypercalcemia (E83.52)*

  E21.3 **Hyperparathyroidism, unspecified**
  E21.4 **Other specified disorders of parathyroid gland**
  E21.5 **Disorder of parathyroid gland, unspecified**

E22 **Hyperfunction of pituitary gland**

  Excludes1: *Cushing's syndrome (E24.-)*
    Nelson's syndrome (E24.1)
    overproduction of ACTH not associated with Cushing's disease (E27.0)
    overproduction of pituitary ACTH (E24.0)
    overproduction of thyroid-stimulating hormone (E05.8-)

  E22.0 **Acromegaly and pituitary gigantism**
    Overproduction of growth hormone
    Excludes1: *constitutional gigantism (E34.4)*
      constitutional tall stature (E34.4)
      increased secretion from endocrine pancreas of growth hormone-releasing hormone (E16.8)

  CC **E22.1** **Hyperprolactinemia**
    Use additional code for adverse effect, if applicable, to identify drug (T36-T50 with fifth or sixth character 5)

  CC **E22.2** **Syndrome of inappropriate secretion of antidiuretic hormone**

  CC **E22.8** **Other hyperfunction of pituitary gland**
    Central precocious puberty

  CC **E22.9** **Hyperfunction of pituitary gland, unspecified**

+, +7th, X + 7th   ● Newborn   ● Pediatric   ● Maternity   ● Adult   ♀ Female   ♂ Male   Manifestation   Unacceptable PDX   HCC   CC   MCC   HAC

E23   Hypofunction and other disorders of the pituitary gland

> **Includes:** the listed conditions whether the disorder is in the pituitary or the hypothalamus
>
> *Excludes1: postprocedural hypopituitarism (E89.3)*

CC **E23.0   Hypopituitarism**
- Fertile eunuch syndrome
- Hypogonadotropic hypogonadism
- Idiopathic growth hormone deficiency
- Isolated deficiency of gonadotropin
- Isolated deficiency of growth hormone
- Isolated deficiency of pituitary hormone
- Kallmann's syndrome
- Lorain-Levi short stature
- Necrosis of pituitary gland (postpartum)
- Panhypopituitarism
- Pituitary cachexia
- Pituitary insufficiency NOS
- Pituitary short stature
- Sheehan's syndrome
- Simmonds' disease

E23.1   Drug-induced hypopituitarism
> Use additional code for adverse effect, if applicable, to identify drug (T36-T50 with fifth or sixth character 5)

CC **E23.2   Diabetes insipidus**
> *Excludes1: nephrogenic diabetes insipidus (N25.1)*

E23.3   Hypothalamic dysfunction, not elsewhere classified
> *Excludes1: Prader-Willi syndrome (Q87.11)*
> *Russell-Silver syndrome (Q87.19)*

E23.6   Other disorders of pituitary gland
- Abscess of pituitary
- Adiposogenital dystrophy

E23.7   Disorder of pituitary gland, unspecified

E24   Cushing's syndrome

> *Excludes1: congenital adrenal hyperplasia (E25.0)*

CC **E24.0   Pituitary-dependent Cushing's disease**
- Overproduction of pituitary ACTH
- Pituitary-dependent hypercorticalism

E24.1   Nelson's syndrome

CC **E24.2   Drug-induced Cushing's syndrome**
> Use additional code for adverse effect, if applicable, to identify drug (T36-T50 with fifth or sixth character 5)

CC **E24.3   Ectopic ACTH syndrome**

CC **E24.4   Alcohol-induced pseudo-Cushing's syndrome**

CC **E24.8   Other Cushing's syndrome**

CC **E24.9   Cushing's syndrome, unspecified**

E25   Adrenogenital disorders

> **Includes:** adrenogenital syndromes, virilizing or feminizing, whether acquired or due to adrenal hyperplasia consequent on inborn enzyme defects in hormone synthesis
> - Female adrenal pseudohermaphroditism
> - Female heterosexual precocious pseudopuberty
> - Male isosexual precocious pseudopuberty
> - Male macrogenitosomia praecox
> - Male sexual precocity with adrenal hyperplasia
> - Male virilization (female)
>
> *Excludes1: indeterminate sex and pseudohermaphroditism (Q56)*
> *chromosomal abnormalities (Q90-Q99)*

E25.0   Congenital adrenogenital disorders associated with enzyme deficiency
- Congenital adrenal hyperplasia
- 21-Hydroxylase deficiency
- Salt-losing congenital adrenal hyperplasia

E25.8   Other adrenogenital disorders
- Idiopathic adrenogenital disorder
> Use additional code for adverse effect, if applicable, to identify drug (T36-T50 with fifth or sixth character 5)

E25.9   Adrenogenital disorder, unspecified
- Adrenogenital syndrome NOS

E26   Hyperaldosteronism

+ **E26.0   Primary hyperaldosteronism**
- **E26.01   Conn's syndrome**
  > Code also adrenal adenoma (D35.0-)
- **E26.02   Glucocorticoid-remediable aldosteronism**
  - Familial aldosteronism type I
- **E26.09   Other primary hyperaldosteronism**
  - Primary aldosteronism due to adrenal hyperplasia (bilateral)

E26.1   Secondary hyperaldosteronism

+ **E26.8   Other hyperaldosteronism**
- **E26.81   Bartter's syndrome**
- **E26.89   Other hyperaldosteronism**

E26.9   Hyperaldosteronism, unspecified
- Aldosteronism NOS
- Hyperaldosteronism NOS

E27   Other disorders of adrenal gland

CC **E27.0   Other adrenocortical overactivity**
- Overproduction of ACTH, not associated with Cushing's disease
- Premature adrenarche
> *Excludes1: Cushing's syndrome (E24.-)*

CC **E27.1   Primary adrenocortical insufficiency**
- Addison's disease
- Autoimmune adrenalitis
> *Excludes1: Addison only phenotype adrenoleukodystrophy (E71.528)*
> *amyloidosis (E85.-)*
> *tuberculous Addison's disease (A18.7)*
> *Waterhouse-Friderichsen syndrome (A39.1)*

CC **E27.2   Addisonian crisis**
- Adrenal crisis
- Adrenocortical crisis

CC **E27.3   Drug-induced adrenocortical insufficiency**
> Use additional code for adverse effect, if applicable, to identify drug (T36-T50 with fifth or sixth character 5)

+ **E27.4   Other and unspecified adrenocortical insufficiency**
> *Excludes1: adrenoleukodystrophy [Addison-Schilder] (E71.528)*
> *Waterhouse-Friderichsen syndrome (A39.1)*

CC **E27.40   Unspecified adrenocortical insufficiency**
- Adrenocortical insufficiency NOS
- Hypoaldosteronism

CC **E27.49   Other adrenocortical insufficiency**
- Adrenal hemorrhage
- Adrenal infarction

CC **E27.5   Adrenomedullary hyperfunction**
- Adrenomedullary hyperplasia
- Catecholamine hypersecretion

E27.8   Other specified disorders of adrenal gland
- Abnormality of cortisol-binding globulin

E27.9   Disorder of adrenal gland, unspecified

E28   Ovarian dysfunction

> *Excludes1: isolated gonadotropin deficiency (E23.0)*
> *postprocedural ovarian failure (E89.4-)*

♀ **E28.0   Estrogen excess**
> Use additional code for adverse effect, if applicable, to identify drug (T36-T50 with fifth or sixth character 5)

♀ **E28.1   Androgen excess**
- Hypersecretion of ovarian androgens
> Use additional code for adverse effect, if applicable, to identify drug (T36-T50 with fifth or sixth character 5)

♀ **E28.2   Polycystic ovarian syndrome**
- Sclerocystic ovary syndrome
- Stein-Leventhal syndrome

+ **E28.3   Primary ovarian failure**
> *Excludes1: pure gonadal dysgenesis (Q99.1)*
> *Turner's syndrome (Q96.-)*

+ **E28.31   Premature menopause**
- ● ♀ **E28.310   Symptomatic premature menopause**
  - Symptoms such as flushing, sleeplessness, headache, lack of concentration, associated with premature menopause
- ● ♀ **E28.319   Asymptomatic premature menopause**
  - Premature menopause NOS

♀ **E28.39   Other primary ovarian failure**
- Decreased estrogen
- Resistant ovary syndrome

♀ **E28.8   Other ovarian dysfunction**
- Ovarian hyperfunction NOS
> *Excludes1: postprocedural ovarian failure (E89.4-)*

♀ **E28.9   Ovarian dysfunction, unspecified**

E29   Testicular dysfunction

    Excludes1:   *androgen insensitivity syndrome (E34.5-)*
              azoospermia or oligospermia NOS (N46.0-N46.1)
              isolated gonadotropin deficiency (E23.0)
              Klinefelter's syndrome (Q98.0-Q98.1, Q98.4)

  ♂ **E29.0   Testicular hyperfunction**
      Hypersecretion of testicular hormones

  ♂ **E29.1   Testicular hypofunction**
      Defective biosynthesis of testicular androgen NOS
      5-delta-Reductase deficiency (with male
         pseudohermaphroditism)
      Testicular hypogonadism NOS
      Use additional code for adverse effect, if applicable, to
         identify drug (T36-T50 with fifth or sixth character 5)
      Excludes1:   *postprocedural testicular hypofunction (E89.5)*

  ♂ **E29.8   Other testicular dysfunction**
  ♂ **E29.9   Testicular dysfunction, unspecified**

E30   Disorders of puberty, not elsewhere classified

  E30.0   Delayed puberty
      Constitutional delay of puberty
      Delayed sexual development

  ● **E30.1   Precocious puberty**
      Precocious menstruation
      Excludes1:   *Albright (-McCune) (-Sternberg) syndrome*
               (Q78.1)
              central precocious puberty (E22.8)
              congenital adrenal hyperplasia (E25.0)
              female heterosexual precocious pseudopuberty
               (E25.-)
              male isosexual precocious pseudopuberty (E25.-)

  ● **E30.8   Other disorders of puberty**
      Premature thelarche
  E30.9   Disorder of puberty, unspecified

E31   Polyglandular dysfunction

    Excludes1:   *ataxia telangiectasia [Louis-Bar] (G11.3)*
              dystrophia myotonica [Steinert] (G71.11)
              pseudohypoparathyroidism (E20.1)

  E31.0   Autoimmune polyglandular failure
      Schmidt's syndrome

  E31.1   Polyglandular hyperfunction
      Excludes1:   *multiple endocrine adenomatosis (E31.2-)*
               multiple endocrine neoplasia (E31.2-)

  + **E31.2   Multiple endocrine neoplasia [MEN] syndromes**
      Multiple endocrine adenomatosis
      Code also any associated malignancies and other conditions
         associated with the syndromes

    E31.20   Multiple endocrine neoplasia [MEN] syndrome,
         unspecified
         Multiple endocrine adenomatosis NOS
         Multiple endocrine neoplasia [MEN]
            syndrome NOS

    E31.21   Multiple endocrine neoplasia [MEN] type I
         Wermer's syndrome

    E31.22   Multiple endocrine neoplasia [MEN] type IIA
         Sipple's syndrome

    E31.23   Multiple endocrine neoplasia [MEN] type IIB
  E31.8   Other polyglandular dysfunction
  E31.9   Polyglandular dysfunction, unspecified

E32   Diseases of thymus

    Excludes1:   *aplasia or hypoplasia of thymus with immunodeficiency*
              (D82.1)
              myasthenia gravis (G70.0)

  E32.0   Persistent hyperplasia of thymus
      Hypertrophy of thymus

  CC **E32.1   Abscess of thymus**
  E32.8   Other diseases of thymus
      Excludes1:   *aplasia or hypoplasia with immunodeficiency*
               (D82.1)
               thymoma (D15.0)
  E32.9   Disease of thymus, unspecified

E34   Other endocrine disorders

    Excludes1:   *pseudohypoparathyroidism (E20.1)*

  CC **E34.0   Carcinoid syndrome**
      NOTE   May be used as an additional code to identify
         functional activity associated with a carcinoid tumor.

  E34.1   Other hypersecretion of intestinal hormones
  E34.2   Ectopic hormone secretion, not elsewhere classified
      Excludes1:   *ectopic ACTH syndrome (E24.3)*

  E34.3   Short stature due to endocrine disorder
      Constitutional short stature
      Laron-type short stature
      Excludes1:   *achondroplastic short stature (Q77.4)*
               hypochondroplastic short stature (Q77.4)
              nutritional short stature (E45)
              pituitary short stature (E23.0)
              progeria (E34.8)
              renal short stature (N25.0)
              Russell-Silver syndrome (Q87.19)
              short-limbed stature with immunodeficiency
               (D82.2)
              short stature in specific dysmorphic syndromes -
               code to syndrome - see Alphabetical Index
              short stature NOS (R62.52)

  E34.4   Constitutional tall stature
      Constitutional gigantism

  + **E34.5   Androgen insensitivity syndrome**
    E34.50   Androgen insensitivity syndrome, unspecified
         Androgen insensitivity NOS

    E34.51   Complete androgen insensitivity syndrome
         Complete androgen insensitivity
         de Quervain syndrome
         Goldberg-Maxwell syndrome

    E34.52   Partial androgen insensitivity syndrome
         Partial androgen insensitivity
         Reifenstein syndrome

  E34.8   Other specified endocrine disorders
      Pineal gland dysfunction
      Progeria
      Excludes2:   *pseudohypoparathyroidism (E20.1)*

  E34.9   Endocrine disorder, unspecified
      Endocrine disturbance NOS
      Hormone disturbance NOS

E35   Disorders of endocrine glands in diseases classified elsewhere

    Code first underlying disease, such as:
      late congenital syphilis of thymus gland [Dubois disease] (A50.5)

    Use additional code, if applicable, to identify:
      sequelae of tuberculosis of other organs (B90.8)

    Excludes1:   *Echinococcus granulosus infection of thyroid gland*
              (B67.3)
              meningococcal hemorrhagic adrenalitis (A39.1)
              syphilis of endocrine gland (A52.79)
              tuberculosis of adrenal gland, except calcification
               (A18.7)
              tuberculosis of endocrine gland NEC (A18.82)
              tuberculosis of thyroid gland (A18.81)
              Waterhouse-Friderichsen syndrome (A39.1)
    Valid 3-character code, no further characters required

Intraoperative complications of endocrine system (E36)

E36   Intraoperative complications of endocrine system

    Excludes2:   *postprocedural endocrine and metabolic*
              complications and disorders, not elsewhere
              classified (E89.-)

  + **E36.0   Intraoperative hemorrhage and hematoma of an**
         endocrine system organ or structure complicating a
         procedure
      Excludes1:   *intraoperative hemorrhage and hematoma of*
              an endocrine system organ or structure due
              to accidental puncture or laceration during
              a procedure (E36.1-)

    CC **E36.01   Intraoperative hemorrhage and hematoma of an**
         endocrine system organ or structure complicating
          an endocrine system procedure
          AHA CC: 1Q, 2020, 19

    CC **E36.02   Intraoperative hemorrhage and hematoma of an**
         endocrine system organ or structure complicating
          other procedure

+ E36.1 **Accidental puncture and laceration of an endocrine system organ or structure during a procedure**

CC E36.11 **Accidental puncture and laceration of an endocrine system organ or structure during an endocrine system procedure**

CC E36.12 **Accidental puncture and laceration of an endocrine system organ or structure during other procedure**

E36.8 **Other intraoperative complications of endocrine system**
Use additional code, if applicable, to further specify disorder

Malnutrition (E40-E46)

Excludes1: *intestinal malabsorption (K90.-)*
sequelae of protein-calorie malnutrition (E64.0)
Excludes2: *nutritional anemias (D50-D53)*
starvation (T73.0)

MCC E40 **Kwashiorkor**

Severe malnutrition with nutritional edema with dyspigmentation of skin and hair
Excludes1: *marasmic kwashiorkor (E42)*
AHA CC: 3Q, 2017, 25-26
Valid 3-character code, no further characters required

MCC E41 **Nutritional marasmus**

Severe malnutrition with marasmus
Excludes1: *marasmic kwashiorkor (E42)*
AHA CC: 3Q, 2017, 24-25
Valid 3-character code, no further characters required

MCC E42 **Marasmic kwashiorkor**

Intermediate form severe protein-calorie malnutrition
Severe protein-calorie malnutrition with signs of both kwashiorkor and marasmus
AHA CC: 3Q, 2017, 25-26
Valid 3-character code, no further characters required

MCC E43 **Unspecified severe protein-calorie malnutrition**

Starvation edema
AHA CC: 3Q, 2017, 25-26; 4Q, 2017, 108-109; 1Q, 2020, 4-7
Valid 3-character code, no further characters required

E44 **Protein-calorie malnutrition of moderate and mild degree**

CC E44.0 **Moderate protein-calorie malnutrition**
CC E44.1 **Mild protein-calorie malnutrition**

CC E45 **Retarded development following protein-calorie malnutrition**

Nutritional short stature
Nutritional stunting
Physical retardation due to malnutrition
Valid 3-character code, no further characters required

CC E46 **Unspecified protein-calorie malnutrition**

Malnutrition NOS
Protein-calorie imbalance NOS
Excludes1: *nutritional deficiency NOS (E63.9)*
Valid 3-character code, no further characters required

Other nutritional deficiencies (E50-E64)

Excludes2: *nutritional anemias (D50-D53)*

E50 **Vitamin A deficiency**

Excludes1: *sequelae of vitamin A deficiency (E64.1)*
E50.0 **Vitamin A deficiency with conjunctival xerosis**
E50.1 **Vitamin A deficiency with Bitot's spot and conjunctival xerosis**
Bitot's spot in the young child
E50.2 **Vitamin A deficiency with corneal xerosis**
E50.3 **Vitamin A deficiency with corneal ulceration and xerosis**
E50.4 **Vitamin A deficiency with keratomalacia**
E50.5 **Vitamin A deficiency with night blindness**
E50.6 **Vitamin A deficiency with xerophthalmic scars of cornea**
E50.7 **Other ocular manifestations of vitamin A deficiency**
Xerophthalmia NOS
E50.8 **Other manifestations of vitamin A deficiency**
Follicular keratosis
Xeroderma
E50.9 **Vitamin A deficiency, unspecified**
Hypovitaminosis A NOS

E51 **Thiamine deficiency**

Excludes1: *sequelae of thiamine deficiency (E64.8)*
+ E51.1 **Beriberi**

CC E51.11 **Dry beriberi**
Beriberi NOS
Beriberi with polyneuropathy
CC E51.12 **Wet beriberi**
Beriberi with cardiovascular manifestations
Cardiovascular beriberi
Shoshin disease
CC E51.2 **Wernicke's encephalopathy**
CC E51.8 **Other manifestations of thiamine deficiency**
CC E51.9 **Thiamine deficiency, unspecified**

E52 **Niacin deficiency [pellagra]**

Niacin (-tryptophan) deficiency
Nicotinamide deficiency
Pellagra (alcoholic)
Excludes1: *sequelae of niacin deficiency (E64.8)*
Valid 3-character code, no further characters required

E53 **Deficiency of other B group vitamins**

Excludes1: *sequelae of vitamin B deficiency (E64.8)*
CC E53.0 **Riboflavin deficiency**
Ariboflavinosis
Vitamin B2 deficiency
E53.1 **Pyridoxine deficiency**
Vitamin B6 deficiency
Excludes1: *pyridoxine-responsive sideroblastic anemia (D64.3)*
E53.8 **Deficiency of other specified B group vitamins**
Biotin deficiency
Cyanocobalamin deficiency
Folate deficiency
Folic acid deficiency
Pantothenic acid deficiency
Vitamin B12 deficiency
Excludes1: *folate deficiency anemia (D52.-)*
vitamin B12 deficiency anemia (D51.-)
E53.9 **Vitamin B deficiency, unspecified**

E54 **Ascorbic acid deficiency**

Deficiency of vitamin C
Scurvy
Excludes1: *scorbutic anemia (D53.2)*
sequelae of vitamin C deficiency (E64.2)
Valid 3-character code, no further characters required

E55 **Vitamin D deficiency**

Excludes1: *adult osteomalacia (M83.-)*
osteoporosis (M80.-)
sequelae of rickets (E64.3)
CC E55.0 **Rickets, active**
Infantile osteomalacia
Juvenile osteomalacia
Excludes1: *celiac rickets (K90.0)*
Crohn's rickets (K50.-)
hereditary vitamin D-dependent rickets (E83.32)
inactive rickets (E64.3)
renal rickets (N25.0)
sequelae of rickets (E64.3)
vitamin D-resistant rickets (E83.31)
E55.9 **Vitamin D deficiency, unspecified**
Avitaminosis D

E56 **Other vitamin deficiencies**

Excludes1: *sequelae of other vitamin deficiencies (E64.8)*
E56.0 **Deficiency of vitamin E**
E56.1 **Deficiency of vitamin K**
Excludes1: *deficiency of coagulation factor due to vitamin K deficiency (D68.4)*
vitamin K deficiency of newborn (P53)
E56.8 **Deficiency of other vitamins**
E56.9 **Vitamin deficiency, unspecified**

E58 **Dietary calcium deficiency**

Excludes1: *disorders of calcium metabolism (E83.5-)*
sequelae of calcium deficiency (E64.8)
Valid 3-character code, no further characters required

E59 **Dietary selenium deficiency**

Keshan disease
Excludes1: *sequelae of selenium deficiency (E64.8)*
Valid 3-character code, no further characters required

E60 **Dietary zinc deficiency**

Valid 3-character code, no further characters required

E61 **Deficiency of other nutrient elements**

Use additional code for adverse effect, if applicable, to identify drug (T36-T50 with fifth or sixth character 5)

Excludes1: *disorders of mineral metabolism (E83.-)*
iodine deficiency related thyroid disorders (E00-E02)
sequelae of malnutrition and other nutritional deficiencies (E64.-)

E61.0 **Copper deficiency**
E61.1 **Iron deficiency**
    Excludes1: *iron deficiency anemia (D50.-)*
E61.2 **Magnesium deficiency**
E61.3 **Manganese deficiency**
E61.4 **Chromium deficiency**
E61.5 **Molybdenum deficiency**
E61.6 **Vanadium deficiency**
E61.7 **Deficiency of multiple nutrient elements**
E61.8 **Deficiency of other specified nutrient elements**
E61.9 **Deficiency of nutrient element, unspecified**

E63 **Other nutritional deficiencies**

Excludes1: *dehydration (E86.0)*
failure to thrive, adult (R62.7)
failure to thrive, child (R62.51)
feeding problems in newborn (P92.-)
sequelae of malnutrition and other nutritional deficiencies (E64.-)

E63.0 **Essential fatty acid [EFA] deficiency**
E63.1 **Imbalance of constituents of food intake**
E63.8 **Other specified nutritional deficiencies**
E63.9 **Nutritional deficiency, unspecified**

E64 **Sequelae of malnutrition and other nutritional deficiencies**

NOTE This category is to be used to indicate conditions in categories E43, E44, E46, E50-E63 as the cause of sequelae, which are themselves classified elsewhere. The 'sequelae' include conditions specified as such; they also include the late effects of diseases classifiable to the above categories if the disease itself is no longer present

Code first condition resulting from (sequela) of malnutrition and other nutritional deficiencies

CC E64.0 **Sequelae of protein-calorie malnutrition**
    Excludes2: *retarded development following protein-calorie malnutrition (E45)*
E64.1 **Sequelae of vitamin A deficiency**
E64.2 **Sequelae of vitamin C deficiency**
E64.3 **Sequelae of rickets**
E64.8 **Sequelae of other nutritional deficiencies**
E64.9 **Sequelae of unspecified nutritional deficiency**

Overweight, obesity and other hyperalimentation (E65-E68)

E65 **Localized adiposity**

Fat pad
Valid 3-character code, no further characters required

E66 **Overweight and obesity**

Code first obesity complicating pregnancy, childbirth and the puerperium, if applicable (O99.21-)

Use additional code to identify body mass index (BMI), if known (Z68.-)

Excludes1: *adiposogenital dystrophy (E23.6)*
lipomatosis NOS (E88.2)
lipomatosis dolorosa [Dercum] (E88.2)
Prader-Willi syndrome (Q87.11)

AHA CC: 4Q, 2018, 80

+ E66.0 **Obesity due to excess calories**
    E66.01 **Morbid (severe) obesity due to excess calories**
        Excludes1: *morbid (severe) obesity with alveolar hypoventilation (E66.2)*
        AHA CC: 4Q, 2018, 79
        HAC see Appendix B for HAC conditional logic
    E66.09 **Other obesity due to excess calories**
E66.1 **Drug-induced obesity**
    Use additional code for adverse effect, if applicable, to identify drug (T36-T50 with fifth or sixth character 5)
CC E66.2 **Morbid (severe) obesity with alveolar hypoventilation**
    Obesity hypoventilation syndrome (OHS)
    Pickwickian syndrome

E66.3 **Overweight**
E66.8 **Other obesity**
E66.9 **Obesity, unspecified**
    Obesity NOS
    AHA CC: 4Q, 2013, 129

E67 **Other hyperalimentation**

Excludes1: *hyperalimentation NOS (R63.2)*
sequelae of hyperalimentation (E68)

E67.0 **Hypervitaminosis A**
E67.1 **Hypercarotenemia**
E67.2 **Megavitamin-B6 syndrome**
E67.3 **Hypervitaminosis D**
E67.8 **Other specified hyperalimentation**

E68 **Sequelae of hyperalimentation**

Code first condition resulting from (sequela) of hyperalimentation
Valid 3-character code, no further characters required

Metabolic disorders (E70-E88)

Excludes1: *androgen insensitivity syndrome (E34.5-)*
congenital adrenal hyperplasia (E25.0)
Ehlers-Danlos syndromes (Q79.6-)
hemolytic anemias attributable to enzyme disorders (D55.-)
Marfan's syndrome (Q87.4)
5-alpha-reductase deficiency (E29.1)

E70 **Disorders of aromatic amino-acid metabolism**

CC E70.0 **Classical phenylketonuria**
CC E70.1 **Other hyperphenylalaninemias**
+ E70.2 **Disorders of tyrosine metabolism**
    Excludes1: *transitory tyrosinemia of newborn (P74.5)*
  CC E70.20 **Disorder of tyrosine metabolism, unspecified**
  CC E70.21 **Tyrosinemia**
    Hypertyrosinemia
  CC E70.29 **Other disorders of tyrosine metabolism**
    Alkaptonuria
    Ochronosis
+ E70.3 **Albinism**
  CC E70.30 **Albinism, unspecified**
  + E70.31 **Ocular albinism**
    CC E70.310 **X-linked ocular albinism**
    CC E70.311 **Autosomal recessive ocular albinism**
    CC E70.318 **Other ocular albinism**
    CC E70.319 **Ocular albinism, unspecified**
  + E70.32 **Oculocutaneous albinism**
    Excludes1: *Chediak-Higashi syndrome (E70.330)*
             Hermansky-Pudlak syndrome (E70.331)
    CC E70.320 **Tyrosinase negative oculocutaneous albinism**
        Albinism I
        Oculocutaneous albinism ty-neg
    CC E70.321 **Tyrosinase positive oculocutaneous albinism**
        Albinism II
        Oculocutaneous albinism ty-pos
    CC E70.328 **Other oculocutaneous albinism**
        Cross syndrome
    CC E70.329 **Oculocutaneous albinism, unspecified**
  + E70.33 **Albinism with hematologic abnormality**
    CC E70.330 **Chediak-Higashi syndrome**
    CC E70.331 **Hermansky-Pudlak syndrome**
    CC E70.338 **Other albinism with hematologic abnormality**
    CC E70.339 **Albinism with hematologic abnormality, unspecified**
  CC E70.39 **Other specified albinism**
    Piebaldism
+ E70.4 **Disorders of histidine metabolism**
  CC E70.40 **Disorders of histidine metabolism, unspecified**
  CC E70.41 **Histidinemia**
  CC E70.49 **Other disorders of histidine metabolism**
CC E70.5 **Disorders of tryptophan metabolism**
+ E70.8 **Other disorders of aromatic amino-acid metabolism**
  CC E70.81 **Aromatic L-amino acid decarboxylase deficiency**
    AADC deficiency
  CC E70.89 **Other disorders of aromatic amino-acid metabolism**
+ E70.9 **Disorder of aromatic amino-acid metabolism, unspecified**

+, +7th, X + 7th   ● Newborn   ● Pediatric   ● Maternity   ● Adult   ♀ Female   ♂ Male   Manifestation   Unacceptable PDX   HCC   CC   MCC   **HAC**

E71 **Disorders of branched-chain amino-acid metabolism and fatty-acid metabolism**

CC **E71.0** **Maple-syrup-urine disease**
+ **E71.1** **Other disorders of branched-chain amino-acid metabolism**
  + **E71.11** **Branched-chain organic acidurias**
    CC **E71.110** **Isovaleric acidemia**
    CC **E71.111** **3-methylglutaconic aciduria**
    CC **E71.118** **Other branched-chain organic acidurias**
  + **E71.12** **Disorders of propionate metabolism**
    CC **E71.120** **Methylmalonic acidemia**
    CC **E71.121** **Propionic acidemia**
    CC **E71.128** **Other disorders of propionate metabolism**
  CC **E71.19** **Other disorders of branched-chain amino-acid metabolism**
  Hyperleucine-isoleucinemia
  Hypervalinemia

CC **E71.2** **Disorder of branched-chain amino-acid metabolism, unspecified**
+ **E71.3** **Disorders of fatty-acid metabolism**
  Excludes1: *peroxisomal disorders (E71.5)*
  Refsum's disease (G60.1)
  Schilder's disease (G37.0)
  Excludes2: *carnitine deficiency due to inborn error of metabolism (E71.42)*
  E71.30 **Disorder of fatty-acid metabolism, unspecified**
  + **E71.31** **Disorders of fatty-acid oxidation**
    CC **E71.310** **Long chain/very long chain acyl CoA dehydrogenase deficiency**
    LCAD
    VLCAD
    CC **E71.311** **Medium chain acyl CoA dehydrogenase deficiency**
    MCAD
    CC **E71.312** **Short chain acyl CoA dehydrogenase deficiency**
    SCAD
    CC **E71.313** **Glutaric aciduria type II**
    Glutaric aciduria type II A
    Glutaric aciduria type II B
    Glutaric aciduria type II C
    Excludes1: *glutaric aciduria (type 1) NOS (E72.3)*
    CC **E71.314** **Muscle carnitine palmitoyltransferase deficiency**
    CC **E71.318** **Other disorders of fatty-acid oxidation**
  CC **E71.32** **Disorders of ketone metabolism**
  CC **E71.39** **Other disorders of fatty-acid metabolism**
+ **E71.4** **Disorders of carnitine metabolism**
  Excludes1: *Muscle carnitine palmitoyltransferase deficiency (E71.314)*
  E71.40 **Disorder of carnitine metabolism, unspecified**
  E71.41 **Primary carnitine deficiency**
  E71.42 **Carnitine deficiency due to inborn errors of metabolism**
  Code also associated inborn error or metabolism
  E71.43 **Iatrogenic carnitine deficiency**
  Carnitine deficiency due to hemodialysis
  Carnitine deficiency due to Valproic acid therapy
  + **E71.44** **Other secondary carnitine deficiency**
    E71.440 **Ruvalcaba-Myhre-Smith syndrome**
    E71.448 **Other secondary carnitine deficiency**
+ **E71.5** **Peroxisomal disorders**
  Excludes1: *Schilder's disease (G37.0)*
  CC **E71.50** **Peroxisomal disorder, unspecified**
  + **E71.51** **Disorders of peroxisome biogenesis**
    Group 1 peroxisomal disorders
    Excludes1: *Refsum's disease (G60.1)*
    CC **E71.510** **Zellweger syndrome**
    CC **E71.511** **Neonatal adrenoleukodystrophy**
    Excludes1: *X-linked adrenoleu-kodystrophy (E71.42-)*
    CC **E71.518** **Other disorders of peroxisome biogenesis**

+ **E71.52** **X-linked adrenoleukodystrophy**
  CC **E71.520** **Childhood cerebral X-linked adrenoleukodystrophy**
  CC **E71.521** **Adolescent X-linked adrenoleukodystrophy**
  CC **E71.522** **Adrenomyeloneuropathy**
  CC **E71.528** **Other X-linked adrenoleukodystrophy**
  Addison only phenotype adrenoleukodystrophy
  Addison-Schilder adrenoleukodystrophy
  CC **E71.529** **X-linked adrenoleukodystrophy, unspecified type**
CC **E71.53** **Other group 2 peroxisomal disorders**
+ **E71.54** **Other peroxisomal disorders**
  CC **E71.540** **Rhizomelic chondrodysplasia punctata**
  Excludes1: *chondrodysplasia punctata NOS (Q77.3)*
  CC **E71.541** **Zellweger-like syndrome**
  CC **E71.542** **Other group 3 peroxisomal disorders**
  CC **E71.548** **Other peroxisomal disorders**

E72 **Other disorders of amino-acid metabolism**
Excludes1: *disorders of:*
aromatic amino-acid metabolism (E70.-)
branched-chain amino-acid metabolism (E71.0-E71.2)
fatty-acid metabolism (E71.3)
purine and pyrimidine metabolism (E79.-)
gout (M1A.-, M10.-)
+ **E72.0** **Disorders of amino-acid transport**
  Excludes1: *disorders of tryptophan metabolism (E70.5)*
  CC **E72.00** **Disorders of amino-acid transport, unspecified**
  CC **E72.01** **Cystinuria**
  CC **E72.02** **Hartnup's disease**
  CC **E72.03** **Lowe's syndrome**
  Use additional code for associated glaucoma (H42)
  CC **E72.04** **Cystinosis**
  Fanconi (-de Toni) (-Debré) syndrome with cystinosis
  Excludes1: *Fanconi (-de Toni) (-Debré) syndrome without cystinosis (E72.09)*
  CC **E72.09** **Other disorders of amino-acid transport**
  Fanconi (-de Toni) (-Debré) syndrome, unspecified
+ **E72.1** **Disorders of sulfur-bearing amino-acid metabolism**
  Excludes1: *cystinosis (E72.04)*
  cystinuria (E72.01)
  transcobalamin II deficiency (D51.2)
  CC **E72.10** **Disorders of sulfur-bearing amino-acid metabolism, unspecified**
  CC **E72.11** **Homocystinuria**
  Cystathionine synthase deficiency
  CC **E72.12** **Methylenetetrahydrofolate reductase deficiency**
  CC **E72.19** **Other disorders of sulfur-bearing amino-acid metabolism**
  Cystathioninuria
  Methioninemia
  Sulfite oxidase deficiency
+ **E72.2** **Disorders of urea cycle metabolism**
  Excludes1: *disorders of ornithine metabolism (E72.4)*
  CC **E72.20** **Disorder of urea cycle metabolism, unspecified**
  Hyperammonemia
  Excludes1: *hyperammonemia-hyperornithinemia-homocitrullinemia syndrome E72.4*
  transient hyperammonemia of newborn (P74.6)
  CC **E72.21** **Argininemia**
  CC **E72.22** **Arginosuccinic aciduria**
  CC **E72.23** **Citrullinemia**
  CC **E72.29** **Other disorders of urea cycle metabolism**
CC **E72.3** **Disorders of lysine and hydroxylysine metabolism**
  Glutaric aciduria NOS
  Glutaric aciduria (type I)
  Hydroxylysinemia
  Hyperlysinemia
  Excludes1: *glutaric aciduria type II (E71.313)*
  Refsum's disease (G60.1)
  Zellweger syndrome (E71.510)

CC **E72.4** **Disorders of ornithine metabolism**
　　Hyperammonemia-Hyperornithinemia-Homocitrullinemia syndrome
　　Ornithinemia (types I, II)
　　Ornithine transcarbamylase deficiency
　　Excludes1: *hereditary choroidal dystrophy (H31.2-)*
+ **E72.5** **Disorders of glycine metabolism**
　CC **E72.50** **Disorder of glycine metabolism, unspecified**
　CC **E72.51** **Non-ketotic hyperglycinemia**
　CC **E72.52** **Trimethylaminuria**
　CC **E72.53** **Primary hyperoxaluria**
　　　Oxalosis
　　　Oxaluria
　　　AHA CC: 4Q, 2018, 29
　CC **E72.59** **Other disorders of glycine metabolism**
　　　D-glycericacidemia
　　　Hyperhydroxyprolinemia
　　　Hyperprolinemia (types I, II)
　　　Sarcosinemia
+ **E72.8** **Other specified disorders of amino-acid metabolism**
　CC **E72.81** **Disorders of gamma aminobutyric acid metabolism**
　　　4-hydroxybutyric aciduria
　　　Disorders of GABA metabolism
　　　GABA metabolic defect
　　　GABA transaminase deficiency
　　　GABA-T deficiency
　　　Gamma-hydroxybutyric aciduria
　　　SSADHA
　　　Succinic semialdehyde dehydrogenase deficiency
　　　AHA CC: 4Q, 2018, 5
　CC **E72.89** **Other specified disorders of amino-acid metabolism**
　　　Disorders of beta-amino-acid metabolism
　　　Disorders of gamma-glutamyl cycle
CC **E72.9** **Disorder of amino-acid metabolism, unspecified**

E73 **Lactose intolerance**
　E73.0 **Congenital lactase deficiency**
　E73.1 **Secondary lactase deficiency**
　E73.8 **Other lactose intolerance**
　E73.9 **Lactose intolerance, unspecified**

E74 **Other disorders of carbohydrate metabolism**
　Excludes1: *diabetes mellitus (E08-E13)*
　　　　　　　NOS (E16.2)
　　　　　　　increased secretion of glucagon (E16.3)
　　　　　　　mucopolysaccharidosis (E76.0-E76.3)
+ **E74.0** **Glycogen storage disease**
　CC **E74.00** **Glycogen storage disease, unspecified**
　CC **E74.01** **von Gierke disease**
　　　Type I glycogen storage disease
　CC **E74.02** **Pompe disease**
　　　Cardiac glycogenosis
　　　Type II glycogen storage disease
　CC **E74.03** **Cori disease**
　　　Forbes disease
　　　Type III glycogen storage disease
　CC **E74.04** **McArdle disease**
　　　Type V glycogen storage disease
　CC **E74.09** **Other glycogen storage disease**
　　　Andersen disease
　　　Hers disease
　　　Tauri disease
　　　Glycogen storage disease, types 0, IV, VI-XI
　　　Liver phosphorylase deficiency
　　　Muscle phosphofructokinase deficiency
+ **E74.1** **Disorders of fructose metabolism**
　　Excludes1: *muscle phosphofructokinase deficiency (E74.09)*
　　E74.10 **Disorder of fructose metabolism, unspecified**
　　E74.11 **Essential fructosuria**
　　　　Fructokinase deficiency
　　E74.12 **Hereditary fructose intolerance**
　　　　Fructosemia
　　E74.19 **Other disorders of fructose metabolism**
　　　　Fructose-1, 6-diphosphatase deficiency
+ **E74.2** **Disorders of galactose metabolism**
　CC **E74.20** **Disorders of galactose metabolism, unspecified**
　CC **E74.21** **Galactosemia**
　CC **E74.29** **Other disorders of galactose metabolism**
　　　Galactokinase deficiency

+ **E74.3** **Other disorders of intestinal carbohydrate absorption**
　　Excludes2: *lactose intolerance (E73.-)*
　　E74.31 **Sucrase-isomaltase deficiency**
　　E74.39 **Other disorders of intestinal carbohydrate absorption**
　　　　Disorder of intestinal carbohydrate absorption NOS
　　　　Glucose-galactose malabsorption
　　　　Sucrase deficiency
CC **E74.4** **Disorders of pyruvate metabolism and gluconeogenesis**
　　Deficiency of phosphoenolpyruvate carboxykinase
　　Deficiency of pyruvate carboxylase
　　Deficiency of pyruvate dehydrogenase
　　Excludes1: *disorders of pyruvate metabolism and gluconeogenesis with anemia (D55.-)*
　　　　　　　Leigh's syndrome (G31.82)
+ **E74.8** **Other specified disorders of carbohydrate metabolism**
　+ **E74.81** **Disorders of glucose transport, not elsewhere classified**
　　CC **E74.810** **Glucose transporter protein type 1 deficiency**
　　　　De Vivo syndrome
　　　　Glucose transport defect, blood-brain barrier
　　　　Glut1 deficiency
　　　　GLUT1 deficiency syndrome 1, infantile onset
　　　　GLUT1 deficiency syndrome 2, childhood onset
　　CC **E74.818** **Other disorders of glucose transport**
　　　　(Familial) renal glycosuria
　　CC **E74.819** **Disorders of glucose transport, unspecified**
　CC **E74.89** **Other specified disorders of carbohydrate metabolism**
　　　Essential pentosuria
　E74.9 **Disorder of carbohydrate metabolism, unspecified**
E75 **Disorders of sphingolipid metabolism and other lipid storage disorders**
　Excludes1: *mucolipidosis, types I-III (E77.0-E77.1)*
　　　　　　　Refsum's disease (G60.1)
+ **E75.0** **GM2 gangliosidosis**
　CC **E75.00** **GM2 gangliosidosis, unspecified**
　CC **E75.01** **Sandhoff disease**
　CC **E75.02** **Tay-Sachs disease**
　CC **E75.09** **Other GM2 gangliosidosis**
　　　Adult GM2 gangliosidosis
　　　Juvenile GM2 gangliosidosis
+ **E75.1** **Other and unspecified gangliosidosis**
　CC **E75.10** **Unspecified gangliosidosis**
　　　Gangliosidosis NOS
　CC **E75.11** **Mucolipidosis IV**
　CC **E75.19** **Other gangliosidosis**
　　　GM1 gangliosidosis
　　　GM3 gangliosidosis
+ **E75.2** **Other sphingolipidosis**
　　Excludes1: *adrenoleukodystrophy [Addison-Schilder] (E71.528)*
　　E75.21 **Fabry (-Anderson) disease**
　　E75.22 **Gaucher disease**
　CC **E75.23** **Krabbe disease**
　+ **E75.24** **Niemann-Pick disease**
　　　E75.240 **Niemann-Pick disease type A**
　　　E75.241 **Niemann-Pick disease type B**
　　　E75.242 **Niemann-Pick disease type C**
　　　E75.243 **Niemann-Pick disease type D**
　　　E75.248 **Other Niemann-Pick disease**
　　　E75.249 **Niemann-Pick disease, unspecified**
　CC **E75.25** **Metachromatic leukodystrophy**
　CC **E75.26** **Sulfatase deficiency**
　　　Multiple sulfatase deficiency (MSD)
　　　AHA CC: 4Q, 2018, 5-6
　CC **E75.29** **Other sphingolipidosis**
　　　Farber's syndrome
　　　Sulfatide lipidosis
　E75.3 **Sphingolipidosis, unspecified**
CC **E75.4** **Neuronal ceroid lipofuscinosis**
　　Batten disease
　　Bielschowsky-Jansky disease
　　Kufs disease
　　Spielmeyer-Vogt disease
　E75.5 **Other lipid storage disorders**
　　Cerebrotendinous cholesterosis [van Bogaert-Scherer-Epstein]
　　Wolman's disease
E75.6 **Lipid storage disorder, unspecified**

+, +7th, X + 7th　● Newborn　● Pediatric　● Maternity　● Adult　♀ Female　♂ Male　Manifestation　Unacceptable PDX　HCC　CC　MCC　HAC

E76　Disorders of glycosaminoglycan metabolism

+ **E76.0　Mucopolysaccharidosis, type I**
　　CC **E76.01　Hurler's syndrome**
　　CC **E76.02　Hurler-Scheie syndrome**
　　CC **E76.03　Scheie's syndrome**
　CC **E76.1　Mucopolysaccharidosis, type II**
　　　　Hunter's syndrome
+ **E76.2　Other mucopolysaccharidoses**
　+ **E76.21　Morquio mucopolysaccharidoses**
　　CC **E76.210　Morquio A mucopolysaccharidoses**
　　　　　Classic Morquio syndrome
　　　　　Morquio syndrome A
　　　　　Mucopolysaccharidosis, type IVA
　　CC **E76.211　Morquio B mucopolysaccharidoses**
　　　　　Morquio-like mucopolysaccharidoses
　　　　　Morquio-like syndrome
　　　　　Morquio syndrome B
　　　　　Mucopolysaccharidosis, type IVB
　　CC **E76.219　Morquio mucopolysaccharidoses,**
　　　　　　unspecified
　　　　　Morquio syndrome
　　　　　Mucopolysaccharidosis, type IV
　CC **E76.22　Sanfilippo mucopolysaccharidoses**
　　　　　Mucopolysaccharidosis, type III (A) (B) (C) (D)
　　　　　Sanfilippo A syndrome
　　　　　Sanfilippo B syndrome
　　　　　Sanfilippo C syndrome
　　　　　Sanfilippo D syndrome
　CC **E76.29　Other mucopolysaccharidoses**
　　　　　beta-Glucuronidase deficiency
　　　　　Maroteaux-Lamy (mild) (severe) syndrome
　　　　　Mucopolysaccharidosis, types VI, VII
　CC **E76.3　Mucopolysaccharidosis, unspecified**
　CC **E76.8　Other disorders of glucosaminoglycan metabolism**
　CC **E76.9　Glucosaminoglycan metabolism disorder, unspecified**

E77　Disorders of glycoprotein metabolism

　E77.0　Defects in post-translational modification of lysosomal enzymes
　　　　Mucolipidosis II [I-cell disease]
　　　　Mucolipidosis III [pseudo-Hurler polydystrophy]
　E77.1　Defects in glycoprotein degradation
　　　　Aspartylglucosaminuria
　　　　Fucosidosis
　　　　Mannosidosis
　　　　Sialidosis [mucolipidosis I]
　E77.8　Other disorders of glycoprotein metabolism
　E77.9　Disorder of glycoprotein metabolism, unspecified

E78　Disorders of lipoprotein metabolism and other lipidemias

　Excludes1: sphingolipidosis (E75.0-E75.3)
+ **E78.0　Pure hypercholesterolemia**
　　E78.00　Pure hypercholesterolemia, unspecified
　　　　　Fedrickson's hyperlipoproteinemia, type IIa
　　　　　Hyperbetalipoproteinemia
　　　　　Low-density-lipoprotein-type [LDL]
　　　　　　hyperlipoproteinemia
　　　　　(Pure) hypercholesterolemia, NOS
　　　　　AHA CC: 4Q, 2016, 13-14
　　E78.01　Familial hypercholesterolemia
　E78.1　Pure hyperglyceridemia
　　　　Elevated fasting triglycerides
　　　　Endogenous hyperglyceridemia
　　　　Fredrickson's hyperlipoproteinemia, type IV
　　　　Hyperlipidemia, group B
　　　　Hyperprebetalipoproteinemia
　　　　Very-low-density-lipoprotein-type [VLDL]
　　　　　hyperlipoproteinemia
　E78.2　Mixed hyperlipidemia
　　　　Broad- or floating-betalipoproteinemia
　　　　Combined hyperlipidemia NOS
　　　　Elevated cholesterol with elevated triglycerides NEC
　　　　Fredrickson's hyperlipoproteinemia, type IIb or III
　　　　Hyperbetalipoproteinemia with prebetalipoproteinemia
　　　　Hypercholesteremia with endogenous hyperglyceridemia
　　　　Hyperlipidemia, group C
　　　　Tubo-eruptive xanthoma
　　　　Xanthoma tuberosum
　　　　Excludes1: cerebrotendinous cholesterosis
　　　　　　[van Bogaert-Scherer-Epstein] (E75.5)
　　　　　　familial combined hyperlipidemia (E78.49)

E78.3　Hyperchylomicronemia
　　　Chylomicron retention disease
　　　Fredrickson's hyperlipoproteinemia, type I or V
　　　Hyperlipidemia, group D
　　　Mixed hyperglyceridemia
+ **E78.4　Other hyperlipidemia**
　　　AHA CC: 4Q, 2018, 6
　　E78.41　Elevated Lipoprotein(a)
　　　　　Elevated Lp(a)
　　E78.49　Other hyperlipidemia
　　　　　Familial combined hyperlipidemia
E78.5　Hyperlipidemia, unspecified
E78.6　Lipoprotein deficiency
　　　Abetalipoproteinemia
　　　Depressed HDL cholesterol
　　　High-density lipoprotein deficiency
　　　Hypoalphalipoproteinemia
　　　Hypobetalipoproteinemia (familial)
　　　Lecithin cholesterol acyltransferase deficiency
　　　Tangier disease
+ **E78.7　Disorders of bile acid and cholesterol metabolism**
　　　Excludes1: Niemann-Pick disease type C (E75.242)
　　E78.70　Disorder of bile acid and cholesterol metabolism, unspecified
　　CC **E78.71　Barth syndrome**
　　CC **E78.72　Smith-Lemli-Opitz syndrome**
　　E78.79　Other disorders of bile acid and cholesterol metabolism
+ **E78.8　Other disorders of lipoprotein metabolism**
　　E78.81　Lipoid dermatoarthritis
　　E78.89　Other lipoprotein metabolism disorders
E78.9　Disorder of lipoprotein metabolism, unspecified

E79　Disorders of purine and pyrimidine metabolism

　Excludes1: Ataxia-telangiectasia (Q87.19)
　　　Bloom's syndrome (Q82.8)
　　　Cockayne's syndrome (Q87.19)
　　　calculus of kidney (N20.0)
　　　combined immunodeficiency disorders (D81.-)
　　　Fanconi's anemia (D61.09)
　　　gout (M1A.-, M10.-)
　　　orotaciduric anemia (D53.0)
　　　progeria (E34.8)
　　　Werner's syndrome (E34.8)
　　　xeroderma pigmentosum (Q82.1)
　E79.0　Hyperuricemia without signs of inflammatory arthritis and tophaceous disease
　　　Asymptomatic hyperuricemia
　CC **E79.1　Lesch-Nyhan syndrome**
　　　HGPRT deficiency
　CC **E79.2　Myoadenylate deaminase deficiency**
　CC **E79.8　Other disorders of purine and pyrimidine metabolism**
　　　Hereditary xanthinuria
　CC **E79.9　Disorder of purine and pyrimidine metabolism, unspecified**

E80　Disorders of porphyrin and bilirubin metabolism

　Includes: defects of catalase and peroxidase
　CC **E80.0　Hereditary erythropoietic porphyria**
　　　Congenital erythropoietic porphyria
　　　Erythropoietic protoporphyria
　CC **E80.1　Porphyria cutanea tarda**
　+ **E80.2　Other and unspecified porphyria**
　　CC **E80.20　Unspecified porphyria**
　　　　　Porphyria NOS
　　CC **E80.21　Acute intermittent (hepatic) porphyria**
　　CC **E80.29　Other porphyria**
　　　　　Hereditary coproporphyria
　CC **E80.3　Defects of catalase and peroxidase**
　　　　Acatalasia [Takahara]
　E80.4　Gilbert syndrome
　E80.5　Crigler-Najjar syndrome
　E80.6　Other disorders of bilirubin metabolism
　　　Dubin-Johnson syndrome
　　　Rotor's syndrome
　E80.7　Disorder of bilirubin metabolism, unspecified

E83 **Disorders of mineral metabolism**

Excludes1: *dietary mineral deficiency (E58-E61)*
parathyroid disorders (E20-E21)
vitamin D deficiency (E55.-)

+ **E83.0** **Disorders of copper metabolism**

E83.00 **Disorder of copper metabolism, unspecified**

E83.01 **Wilson's disease**
Code also associated Kayser Fleischer ring (H18.04-)

E83.09 **Other disorders of copper metabolism**
Menkes' (kinky hair) (steely hair) disease

+ **E83.1** **Disorders of iron metabolism**

Excludes1: *iron deficiency anemia (D50.-)*
sideroblastic anemia (D64.0-D64.3)

E83.10 **Disorder of iron metabolism, unspecified**

+ **E83.11** **Hemochromatosis**

Excludes1: *GALD (P78.84)*
Gestational alloimmune liver disease (P78.84)
Neonatal hemochromatosis (P78.84)

E83.110 **Hereditary hemochromatosis**
Bronzed diabetes
Pigmentary cirrhosis (of liver)
Primary (hereditary) hemochromatosis

E83.111 **Hemochromatosis due to repeated red blood cell transfusions**
Iron overload due to repeated red blood cell transfusions
Transfusion (red blood cell) associated hemochromatosis

E83.118 **Other hemochromatosis**

E83.119 **Hemochromatosis, unspecified**

E83.19 **Other disorders of iron metabolism**
Use additional code, if applicable, for idiopathic pulmonary hemosiderosis (J84.03)

E83.2 **Disorders of zinc metabolism**
Acrodermatitis enteropathica

+ **E83.3** **Disorders of phosphorus metabolism and phosphatases**

Excludes1: *adult osteomalacia (M83.-)*
osteoporosis (M80.-)

E83.30 **Disorder of phosphorus metabolism, unspecified**

E83.31 **Familial hypophosphatemia**
Vitamin D-resistant osteomalacia
Vitamin D-resistant rickets

Excludes1: *vitamin D-deficiency rickets (E55.0)*

E83.32 **Hereditary vitamin D-dependent rickets (type 1) (type 2)**
25-hydroxyvitamin D 1-alpha-hydroxylase deficiency
Pseudovitamin D deficiency
Vitamin D receptor defect

E83.39 **Other disorders of phosphorus metabolism**
Acid phosphatase deficiency
Hypophosphatasia

+ **E83.4** **Disorders of magnesium metabolism**

E83.40 **Disorders of magnesium metabolism, unspecified**

E83.41 **Hypermagnesemia**
AHA CC: 4Q, 2016, 54-55

E83.42 **Hypomagnesemia**

E83.49 **Other disorders of magnesium metabolism**

+ **E83.5** **Disorders of calcium metabolism**

Excludes1: *chondrocalcinosis (M11.1-M11.2)*
hungry bone syndrome (E83.81)
hyperparathyroidism (E21.0-E21.3)

E83.50 **Unspecified disorder of calcium metabolism**

E83.51 **Hypocalcemia**

E83.52 **Hypercalcemia**
Familial hypocalciuric hypercalcemia

E83.59 **Other disorders of calcium metabolism**

+ **E83.8** **Other disorders of mineral metabolism**

E83.81 **Hungry bone syndrome**

E83.89 **Other disorders of mineral metabolism**

E83.9 **Disorder of mineral metabolism, unspecified**

E84 **Cystic fibrosis**
Code also exocrine pancreatic insufficiency (K86.81)
Includes: mucoviscidosis

MCC **E84.0** **Cystic fibrosis with pulmonary manifestations**
Use additional code to identify any infectious organism present, such as:
Pseudomonas (B96.5)

+ **E84.1** **Cystic fibrosis with intestinal manifestations**

• MCC **E84.11** **Meconium ileus in cystic fibrosis**
Excludes1: *meconium ileus not due to cystic fibrosis (P76.0)*

CC **E84.19** **Cystic fibrosis with other intestinal manifestations**
Distal intestinal obstruction syndrome

CC **E84.8** **Cystic fibrosis with other manifestations**

CC **E84.9** **Cystic fibrosis, unspecified**

E85 **Amyloidosis**

Excludes2: *Alzheimer's disease (G30.0-)*

CC **E85.0** **Non-neuropathic heredofamilial amyloidosis**
Hereditary amyloid nephropathy
Code also associated disorders, such as:
autoinflammatory syndromes (M04.-)

Excludes2: *Transthyretin-related (ATTR) familial amyloid cardiomyopathy (E85.4)*

CC **E85.1** **Neuropathic heredofamilial amyloidosis**
Amyloid polyneuropathy (Portuguese)
Transthyretin-related (ATTR) familial amyloid polyneuropathy
AHA CC: 4Q, 2012, 99-101

CC **E85.2** **Heredofamilial amyloidosis, unspecified**

CC **E85.3** **Secondary systemic amyloidosis**
Hemodialysis-associated amyloidosis

CC **E85.4** **Organ-limited amyloidosis**
Localized amyloidosis
Transthyretin-related (ATTR) familial amyloid cardiomyopathy

+ **E85.8** **Other amyloidosis**
AHA CC: 4Q, 2017, 7

CC **E85.81** **Light chain (AL) amyloidosis**

CC **E85.82** **Wild-type transthyretin-related (ATTR) amyloidosis**
Senile systemic amyloidosis (SSA)

CC **E85.89** **Other amyloidosis**

CC **E85.9** **Amyloidosis, unspecified**

E86 **Volume depletion**
Use Additional code(s) for any associated disorders of electrolyte and acid-base balance (E87.-)

Excludes1: *dehydration of newborn (P74.1)*
postprocedural hypovolemic shock (T81.19)
traumatic hypovolemic shock (T79.4)

Excludes2: *hypovolemic shock NOS (R57.1)*

E86.0 **Dehydration**
Review coding guidelines C.2.c.3
AHA CC: 1Q, 2014, 7; 2Q, 2019, 7-8

E86.1 **Hypovolemia**
Depletion of volume of plasma

E86.9 **Volume depletion, unspecified**
AHA CC: 2Q, 2019, 7-8

E87 **Other disorders of fluid, electrolyte and acid-base balance**

Excludes1: *diabetes insipidus (E23.2)*
electrolyte imbalance associated with hyperemesis gravidarum (O21.1)
electrolyte imbalance following ectopic or molar pregnancy (O08.5)
familial periodic paralysis (G72.3)

CC **E87.0** **Hyperosmolality and hypernatremia**
Sodium [Na] excess
Sodium [Na] overload
AHA CC: 1Q, 2014, 7

CC **E87.1** **Hypo-osmolality and hyponatremia**
Sodium [Na] deficiency

Excludes1: *syndrome of inappropriate secretion of antidiuretic hormone (E22.2)*

AHA CC: 1Q, 2014, 7

+, +7th, X + 7th   ● Newborn   ● Pediatric   ● Maternity   ● Adult   ♀ Female   ♂ Male   Manifestation   Unacceptable PDX   HCC   CC   MCC   HAC

CC E87.2 Acidosis
  Acidosis NOS
  Lactic acidosis
  Metabolic acidosis
  Respiratory acidosis
  Excludes1: diabetic acidosis - see categories E08-E10, E13
      with ketoacidosis

CC E87.3 Alkalosis
  Alkalosis NOS
  Metabolic alkalosis
  Respiratory alkalosis

CC E87.4 Mixed disorder of acid-base balance

E87.5 Hyperkalemia
  Potassium [K] excess
  Potassium [K] overload

E87.6 Hypokalemia
  Potassium [K] deficiency

+ E87.7 Fluid overload
  Excludes1: edema NOS (R60.9)
      fluid retention (R60.9)
  E87.70 Fluid overload, unspecified
  E87.71 Transfusion associated circulatory overload
    Fluid overload due to transfusion (blood)
        (blood components)
    TACO
  E87.79 Other fluid overload
  E87.8 Other disorders of electrolyte and fluid balance, not elsewhere classified
    Electrolyte imbalance NOS
    Hyperchloremia
    Hypochloremia

E88 Other and unspecified metabolic disorders
  Use additional codes for associated conditions
  Excludes1: histiocytosis X (chronic) (C96.6)

+ E88.0 Disorders of plasma-protein metabolism, not elsewhere classified
  Excludes1: monoclonal gammopathy (of undetermined
        significance) (D47.2)
      polyclonal hypergammaglobulinemia (D89.0)
      Waldenström macroglobulinemia (C88.0)
  Excludes2: disorder of lipoprotein metabolism (E78.-)
  E88.01 Alpha-1-antitrypsin deficiency
    AAT deficiency
  CC E88.02 Plasminogen deficiency
    Dysplasminogenemia
    Hypoplasminogenemia
    Type 1 plasminogen deficiency
    Type 2 plasminogen deficiency
    Code also, if applicable, ligneous conjunctivitis
        (H10.51)

    Use additional code for associated findings, such as:
      hydrocephalus (G91.4)
      otitis media (H67.-)
      respiratory disorder related to plasminogen
          deficiency (J99)
    AHA CC: 4Q, 2018, 6-7
  E88.09 Other disorders of plasma-protein metabolism, not elsewhere classified
    Bisalbuminemia

E88.1 Lipodystrophy, not elsewhere classified
  Lipodystrophy NOS
  Excludes1: Whipple's disease (K90.81)

E88.2 Lipomatosis, not elsewhere classified
  Lipomatosis NOS
  Lipomatosis (Check) dolorosa [Dercum]

MCC E88.3 Tumor lysis syndrome
  Tumor lysis syndrome (spontaneous)
  Tumor lysis syndrome following antineoplastic drug
      chemotherapy
  Use additional code for adverse effect, if applicable, to
      identify drug (T45.1X5)
  AHA CC: 2Q, 2019, 24-26

+ E88.4 Mitochondrial metabolism disorders
  Excludes1: disorders of pyruvate metabolism (E74.4)
      Kearns-Sayre syndrome (H49.81)
      Leber's disease (H47.22)
      Leigh's encephalopathy (G31.82)
      Mitochondrial myopathy, NEC (G71.3)
      Reye's syndrome (G93.7)
  CC E88.40 Mitochondrial metabolism disorder, unspecified

CC E88.41 MELAS syndrome
  Mitochondrial myopathy, encephalopathy, lactic
      acidosis and stroke-like episodes
CC E88.42 MERRF syndrome
  Myoclonic epilepsy associated with ragged-red fibers
  Code also progressive myoclonic epilepsy (G40.3-)
CC E88.49 Other mitochondrial metabolism disorders
+ E88.8 Other specified metabolic disorders
  E88.81 Metabolic syndrome
    Dysmetabolic syndrome X
    Use additional codes for associated manifestations,
        such as:
      obesity (E66.-)
  E88.89 Other specified metabolic disorders
    Launois-Bensaude adenolipomatosis
    Excludes1: adult pulmonary Langerhans cell
        histiocytosis (J84.82)

E88.9 Metabolic disorder, unspecified

Postprocedural endocrine and metabolic complications and disorders, not elsewhere classified (E89)

E89 Postprocedural endocrine and metabolic complications and disorders, not elsewhere classified
  Excludes2: intraoperative complications of endocrine system organ
      or structure (E36.0-, E36.1-, E36.8)
E89.0 Postprocedural hypothyroidism
  Postirradiation hypothyroidism
  Postsurgical hypothyroidism
CC E89.1 Postprocedural hypoinsulinemia
  Postpancreatectomy hyperglycemia
  Postsurgical hypoinsulinemia
  Use additional code, if applicable, to identify:
    acquired absence of pancreas (Z90.41-)
    diabetes mellitus (postpancreatectomy) (postprocedural)
        (E13.-)
    insulin use (Z79.4)
  Excludes1: transient postprocedural hyperglycemia (R73.9)
      transient postprocedural hypoglycemia (E16.2)
  Review coding guideline C.4.a.6.b.i
E89.2 Postprocedural hypoparathyroidism
  Parathyroprival tetany
E89.3 Postprocedural hypopituitarism
  Postirradiation hypopituitarism
+ E89.4 Postprocedural ovarian failure
  ♀ **E89.40 Asymptomatic postprocedural ovarian failure**
    Postprocedural ovarian failure NOS
  ♀ **E89.41 Symptomatic postprocedural ovarian failure**
    Symptoms such as flushing, sleeplessness,
        headache, lack of concentration, associated with
        postprocedural menopause
♂ **E89.5 Postprocedural testicular hypofunction**
CC E89.6 Postprocedural adrenocortical (-medullary) hypofunction
+ E89.8 Other postprocedural endocrine and metabolic complications and disorders
  AHA CC: 4Q, 2016, 9-10
  + E89.81 Postprocedural hemorrhage of an endocrine system organ or structure following a procedure
    CC E89.810 Postprocedural hemorrhage of an endocrine system organ or structure following an endocrine system procedure
    CC E89.811 Postprocedural hemorrhage of an endocrine system organ or structure following other procedure
  + E89.82 Postprocedural hematoma and seroma of an endocrine system organ or structre
    CC E89.820 Postprocedural hematoma of an endocrine system organ or structure following an endocrine system procedure
    CC E89.821 Postprocedural hematoma of an endocrine system organ or structure following other procedure
    CC E89.822 Postprocedural seroma of an endocrine system organ or structure following an endocrine system procedure
    CC E89.823 Postprocedural seroma of an endocrine system organ or structure following other procedure
  CC E89.89 Other postprocedural endocrine and metabolic complications and disorders
    Use additional code, if applicable, to further specify
        disorder

Chapter 5: Mental, Behavioral and Neurodevelopmental Disorders (F01-F99)

Includes: disorders of psychological development

Excludes2: *symptoms, signs and abnormal clinical laboratory findings, not elsewhere classified (R00-R99)*

This chapter contains the following category blocks:

F01-F09 Mental disorders due to known physiological conditions
F10-F19 Mental and behavioral disorders due to psychoactive substance use
F20-F29 Schizophrenia, schizotypal, delusional, and other non-mood psychotic disorders
F30-F39 Mood [affective] disorders
F40-F48 Anxiety, dissociative, stress-related, somatoform and other nonpsychotic mental disorders
F50-F59 Behavioral syndromes associated with physiological disturbances and physical factors
F60-F69 Disorders of adult personality and behavior
F70-F79 Intellectual disabilities
F80-F89 Pervasive and specific developmental disorders
F90-F98 Behavioral and emotional disorders with onset usually occurring in childhood and adolescence
F99 Unspecified mental disorder

C. Chapter-Specific Coding Guidelines

In addition to general coding guidelines, there are guidelines for specific diagnoses and/or conditions in the classification. Unless otherwise indicated, these guidelines apply to all health care settings. Please refer to Section II for guidelines on the selection of principal diagnosis.

5. Chapter 5: Mental, Behavioral and Neurodevelopmental Disorders (F01-F99)

a. Pain disorders related to psychological factors

Assign code F45.41, for pain that is exclusively related to psychological disorders. As indicated by the Excludes 1 note under category G89, a code from category G89 should not be assigned with code F45.41

Code F45.42, Pain disorders with related psychological factors, should be used with a code from category G89, Pain, not elsewhere classified, if there is documentation of a psychological component for a patient with acute or chronic pain.

See Section I.C.6. Pain

b. Mental and behavioral disorders due to psychoactive substance use

1) In Remission

Selection of codes for "in remission" for categories F10-F19, Mental and behavioral disorders due to psychoactive substance use (categories F10-F19 with -.11, -.21) requires the provider's clinical judgment. The appropriate codes for "in remission" are assigned only on the basis of provider documentation (as defined in the Official Guidelines for Coding and Reporting), unless otherwise instructed by the classification.

Mild substance use disorders in early or sustained remission are classified to the appropriate codes for substance abuse in remission, and moderate or severe substance use disorders in early or sustained remission are classified to the appropriate codes for substance dependence in remission.

2) Psychoactive Substance Use, Abuse And Dependence

When the provider documentation refers to use, abuse and dependence of the same substance (e.g. alcohol, opioid, cannabis, etc.), only one code should be assigned to identify the pattern of use based on the following hierarchy:

- If both use and abuse are documented, assign only the code for abuse
- If both abuse and dependence are documented, assign only the code for dependence
- If use, abuse and dependence are all documented, assign only the code for dependence
- If both use and dependence are documented, assign only the code for dependence.

3) Psychoactive Substance Use Unspecified

As with all other unspecified diagnoses, the codes for unspecified psychoactive substance use disorders (F10.9-, F11.9-, F12.9-, F13.9-, F14.9-, F15.9-, F16.9-, F18.9-, F19.9-) should only be assigned based on provider documentation and when they meet the definition of a reportable diagnosis (see Section III, Reporting Additional Diagnoses). These codes are to be used only when the psychoactive substance use is associated with a physical **disorder included in chapter 5 (such as sexual dysfunction and sleep disorder),** mental or behavioral disorder, and such a relationship is documented by the provider.

c. Factitious Disorder

Factitious disorder imposed on self or Munchausen's syndrome is a disorder in which a person falsely reports or causes his or her own physical or psychological signs or symptoms. For patients with documented factitious disorder on self or Munchausen's syndrome, assign the appropriate code from subcategory F68.1-, Factitious disorder imposed on self.

Munchausen's syndrome by proxy (MSBP) is a disorder in which a caregiver (perpetrator) falsely reports or causes an illness or injury in another person (victim) under his or her care, such as a child, an elderly adult, or a person who has a disability. The conditions is also referred to as "factitious disorder imposed on another" or "factitious disorder by proxy." The perpetrator, not the victim, receives this diagnosis. Assign code F68.A, Factitious disorder imposed on another, to the perpetrator's record. For the victim of a patient suffering from MSBP, assign the appropriate code from categories T74, Adult and child abuse, neglect and other maltreatment, confirmed, or T76, Adult and child abuse, neglect and other maltreatment, suspected.

See Section I.C.19.f. Adult and child abuse, neglect and other maltreatment

Mental disorders due to known physiological conditions (F01-F09)

NOTE This block comprises a range of mental disorders grouped together on the basis of their having in common a demonstrable etiology in cerebral disease, brain injury, or other insult leading to cerebral dysfunction. The dysfunction may be primary, as in diseases, injuries, and insults that affect the brain directly and selectively; or secondary, as in systemic diseases and disorders that attack the brain only as one of the multiple organs or systems of the body that are involved.

F01 **Vascular dementia**

Vascular dementia as a result of infarction of the brain due to vascular disease, including hypertensive cerebrovascular disease.
Includes: arteriosclerotic dementia
Code first the underlying physiological condition or sequelae of cerebrovascular disease.

+ **F01.5** **Vascular dementia**
- **F01.50** **Vascular dementia without behavioral disturbance**
Major neurocognitive disorder without behavioral disturbance
- CC **F01.51** **Vascular dementia with behavioral disturbance**
Major neurocognitive disorder due to vascular disease, with behavioral disturbance
Major neurocognitive disorder with aggressive behavior
Major neurocognitive disorder with combative behavior
Major neurocognitive disorder with violent behavior
Vascular dementia with aggressive behavior
Vascular dementia with combative behavior
Vascular dementia with violent behavior
Use additional code, if applicable, to identify wandering in vascular dementia (Z91.83)

+, +7th, X + 7th ● Newborn ● Pediatric ● Maternity ● Adult ♀ Female ♂ Male Manifestation Unacceptable PDX HCC CC MCC HAC

F02   Dementia in other diseases classified elsewhere

> **Includes:** Major neurocognitive disorder in other diseases classified elsewhere
>
> Code first the underlying physiological condition, such as:
>> Alzheimer's (G30.-)
>> cerebral lipidosis (E75.4)
>> Creutzfeldt-Jakob disease (A81.0-)
>> dementia with Lewy bodies (G31.83)
>> dementia with Parkinsonism (G31.83)
>> epilepsy and recurrent seizures (G40.-)
>> frontotemporal dementia (G31.09)
>> hepatolenticular degeneration (E83.0)
>> human immunodeficiency virus [HIV] disease (B20)
>> Huntington's disease (G10)
>> hypercalcemia (E83.52)
>> hypothyroidism, acquired (E00-E03.-)
>> intoxications (T36-T65)
>> Jakob-Creutzfeldt disease (A81.0-)
>> multiple sclerosis (G35)
>> neurosyphilis (A52.17)
>> niacin deficiency [pellagra] (E52)
>> Parkinson's disease (G20)
>> Pick's disease (G31.01)
>> polyarteritis nodosa (M30.0)
>> prion disease (A81.9)
>> systemic lupus erythematosus (M32.-)
>> traumatic brain injury (S06.-)
>> trypanosomiasis (B56.-, B57.-)
>> vitamin B deficiency (E53.8)
>
> *Excludes2:* *dementia in alcohol and psychoactive substance*
>>> *disorders (F10-F19, with .17, .27, .97)*
>>> *vascular dementia (F01.5-)*

+ **F02.8   Dementia in other diseases classified elsewhere**

> **F02.80   Dementia in other diseases classified elsewhere without behavioral disturbance**
>> Dementia in other diseases classified elsewhere NOS
>> Major neurocognitive disorder in other diseases classified elsewhere
>> *AHA CC: 2Q, 2016, 6; 4Q, 2016, 141; 1Q, 2017, 43-44*

> CC **F02.81   Dementia in other diseases classified elsewhere with behavioral disturbance**
>> Dementia in other diseases classified elsewhere with aggressive behavior
>> Dementia in other diseases classified elsewhere with combative behavior
>> Dementia in other diseases classified elsewhere with violent behavior
>> Major neurocognitive disorder in other diseases classified elsewhere with aggressive behavior
>> Major neurocognitive disorder in other diseases classified elsewhere with combative behavior
>> Major neurocognitive disorder in other diseases classified elsewhere with violent behavior
>> Use additional code, if applicable, to identify wandering in dementia in conditions classified elsewhere (Z91.83)
>> *AHA CC: 2Q, 2017, 7-8*

F03   Unspecified dementia

> Presenile dementia NOS
> Presenile psychosis NOS
> Primary degenerative dementia NOS
> Senile dementia NOS
> Senile dementia depressed or paranoid type
> Senile psychosis NOS
> *Excludes1:* *senility NOS (R41.81)*
> *Excludes2:* *mild memory disturbance due to known physiological*
>>> *condition (F06.8)*
>>> *senile dementia with delirium or acute confusional state (F05)*

+ **F03.9   Unspecified dementia**

> • **F03.90   Unspecified dementia without behavioral disturbance**
>> Dementia NOS
>> *AHA CC: 4Q, 2012, 92-93*

> • CC **F03.91   Unspecified dementia with behavioral disturbance**
>> Unspecified dementia with aggressive behavior
>> Unspecified dementia with combative behavior
>> Unspecified dementia with violent behavior
>> Use additional code, if applicable, to identify wandering in unspecified dementia (Z91.83)

F04   Amnestic disorder due to known physiological condition

> Korsakov's psychosis or syndrome, nonalcoholic
> Code first the underlying physiological condition
> *Excludes1:* *amnesia NOS (R41.3)*
>>> *anterograde amnesia (R41.1)*
>>> *dissociative amnesia (F44.0)*
>>> *retrograde amnesia (R41.2)*
> *Excludes2:* *alcohol-induced or unspecified Korsakov's syndrome*
>>> *(F10.26, F10.96)*
>>> *Korsakov's syndrome induced by other psychoactive substances (F13.26, F13.96, F19.16, F19.26, F19.96)*
> **Valid 3-character code, no further characters required**

CC **F05   Delirium due to known physiological condition**

> Acute or subacute brain syndrome
> Acute or subacute confusional state (nonalcoholic)
> Acute or subacute infective psychosis
> Acute or subacute organic reaction
> Acute or subacute psycho-organic syndrome
> Delirium of mixed etiology
> Delirium superimposed on dementia
> Sundowning
> Code first the underlying physiological condition
> *Excludes1:* *delirium NOS (R41.0)*
> *Excludes2:* *delirium tremens alcohol-induced or unspecified*
>>> *(F10.231, F10.921)*
> *AHA CC: 2Q, 2019, 34*
> **Valid 3-character code, no further characters required**

F06   Other mental disorders due to known physiological condition

> **Includes:** mental disorders due to endocrine disorder
>> mental disorders due to exogenous hormone
>> mental disorders due to exogenous toxic substance
>> mental disorders due to primary cerebral disease
>> mental disorders due to somatic illness
>> mental disorders due to systemic disease affecting the brain
>
> Code first the underlying physiological condition
> *Excludes1:* *unspecified dementia (F03)*
> *Excludes2:* *delirium due to known physiological condition (F05)*
>>> *dementia as classified in F01-F02*
>>> *other mental disorders associated with alcohol and other psychoactive substances (F10-F19)*

CC **F06.0   Psychotic disorder with hallucinations due to known physiological condition**
>> Organic hallucinatory state (nonalcoholic)
>> *Excludes2:* *hallucinations and perceptual disturbance*
>>>> *induced by alcohol and other psychoactive substances (F10-F19 with .151, .251, .951)*
>>>> *schizophrenia (F20.-)*

F06.1   Catatonic disorder due to known physiological condition
>> Catatonia associated with another mental disorder
>> Catatonia NOS
>> *Excludes1:* *catatonic stupor (R40.1)*
>>>> *stupor NOS (R40.1)*
>> *Excludes2:* *catatonic schizophrenia (F20.2)*
>>>> *dissociative stupor (F44.2)*

CC **F06.2   Psychotic disorder with delusions due to known physiological condition**
>> Paranoid and paranoid-hallucinatory organic states
>> Schizophrenia-like psychosis in epilepsy
>> *Excludes2:* *alcohol and drug-induced psychotic disorder*
>>>> *(F10-F19 with .150, .250, .950)*
>>>> *brief psychotic disorder (F23)*
>>>> *delusional disorder (F22)*
>>>> *schizophrenia (F20.-)*

+ **F06.3   Mood disorder due to known physiological condition**
>> *Excludes2:* *mood disorders due to alcohol and other*
>>>> *psychoactive substances (F10-F19 with .14, .24, .94)*
>>>> *mood disorders, not due to known physiological condition or unspecified (F30-F39)*

> **F06.30   Mood disorder due to known physiological condition, unspecified**

> **F06.31   Mood disorder due to known physiological condition with depressive features**
>> Depressive disorder due to known physiological condition, with depressive features

F06.32 **Mood disorder due to known physiological condition with major depressive-like episode**
Depressive disorder due to known physiological condition, with major depressive-like episode

F06.33 **Mood disorder due to known physiological condition with manic features**
Bipolar and related disorder due to a known physiological condition, with manic features
Bipolar and related disorder due to known physiological condition, with manic- or hypomanic-like episodes

F06.34 **Mood disorder due to known physiological condition with mixed features**
Bipolar and related disorder due to known physiological condition, with mixed features
Depressive disorder due to known physiological condition, with mixed features

F06.4 **Anxiety disorder due to known physiological condition**
Excludes2: anxiety disorders due to alcohol and other psychoactive substances (F10-F19 with .180, .280, .980)
anxiety disorders, not due to known physiological condition or unspecified (F40.-, F41.-)

F06.8 **Other specified mental disorders due to known physiological condition**
Epileptic psychosis NOS
Obsessive-compulsive and related disorder due to a known physiological condition
Organic dissociative disorder
Organic emotionally labile [asthenic] disorder

F07 **Personality and behavioral disorders due to known physiological condition**
Code first the underlying physiological condition

F07.0 **Personality change due to known physiological condition**
Frontal lobe syndrome
Limbic epilepsy personality syndrome
Lobotomy syndrome
Organic personality disorder
Organic pseudopsychopathic personality
Organic pseudoretarded personality
Postleucotomy syndrome
Code first underlying physiological condition
Excludes1: mild cognitive impairment (G31.84)
postconcussional syndrome (F07.81)
postencephalitic syndrome (F07.89)
signs and symptoms involving emotional state (R45.-)
Excludes2: specific personality disorder (F60.-)

+ **F07.8** **Other personality and behavioral disorders due to known physiological condition**

F07.81 **Postconcussional syndrome**
Postcontusional syndrome (encephalopathy)
Post-traumatic brain syndrome, nonpsychotic
Use additional code to identify associated post-traumatic headache, if applicable (G44.3-)
Excludes1: current concussion (brain) (S06.0-)
postencephalitic syndrome (F07.89)

F07.89 **Other personality and behavioral disorders due to known physiological condition**
Postencephalitic syndrome
Right hemispheric organic affective disorder

F07.9 **Unspecified personality and behavioral disorder due to known physiological condition**
Organic psychosyndrome

F09 **Unspecified mental disorder due to known physiological condition**
Mental disorder NOS due to known physiological condition
Organic brain syndrome NOS
Organic mental disorder NOS
Organic psychosis NOS
Symptomatic psychosis NOS
Code first the underlying physiological condition
Excludes1: psychosis NOS (F29)
Valid 3-character code, no further characters required

Mental and behavioral disorders due to psychoactive substance use (F10-F19)

Review coding guideline C.5.b
AHA CC: 4Q, 2017, 8; 1Q, 2020, 9

F10 **Alcohol related disorders**
Use additional code for blood alcohol level, if applicable (Y90.-)

+ **F10.1** **Alcohol abuse**
Excludes1: alcohol dependence (F10.2-)
alcohol use, unspecified (F10.9-)

F10.10 **Alcohol abuse, uncomplicated**
Alcohol use disorder, mild

F10.11 **Alcohol abuse, in remission**
Alcohol use disorder, mild, in early remission
Alcohol use disorder, mild, in sustained remission

+ **F10.12** **Alcohol abuse with intoxication**
F10.120 **Alcohol abuse with intoxication, uncomplicated**
CC **F10.121** **Alcohol abuse with intoxication delirium**
F10.129 **Alcohol abuse with intoxication, unspecified**

+ **F10.13** **Alcohol abuse, with withdrawal**
CC **F10.130** **Alcohol abuse with withdrawal, uncomplicated**
CC **F10.131** **Alcohol abuse with withdrawal delirium**
CC **F10.132** **Alcohol abuse with withdrawal with perceptual disturbance**
CC **F10.139** **Alcohol abuse with withdrawal, unspecified**

CC **F10.14** **Alcohol abuse with alcohol-induced mood disorder**
Alcohol use disorder, mild, with alcohol-induced bipolar or related disorder
Alcohol use disorder, mild, with alcohol-induced depressive disorder

+ **F10.15** **Alcohol abuse with alcohol-induced psychotic disorder**
F10.150 **Alcohol abuse with alcohol-induced psychotic disorder with delusions**
CC **F10.151** **Alcohol abuse with alcohol-induced psychotic disorder with hallucinations**
CC **F10.159** **Alcohol abuse with alcohol-induced psychotic disorder, unspecified**

+ **F10.18** **Alcohol abuse with other alcohol-induced disorders**
CC **F10.180** **Alcohol abuse with alcohol-induced anxiety disorder**
CC **F10.181** **Alcohol abuse with alcohol-induced sexual dysfunction**
F10.182 **Alcohol abuse with alcohol-induced sleep disorder**
CC **F10.188** **Alcohol abuse with other alcohol-induced disorder**

CC **F10.19** **Alcohol abuse with unspecified alcohol-induced disorder**

+ **F10.2** **Alcohol dependence**
Excludes1: alcohol abuse (F10.1-)
alcohol use, unspecified (F10.9-)
Excludes2: toxic effect of alcohol (T51.0-)

F10.20 **Alcohol dependence, uncomplicated**
Alcohol use disorder, moderate
Alcohol use disorder, severe
AHA CC: 1Q, 2020, 9

F10.21 **Alcohol dependence, in remission**
Alcohol use disorder, moderate, in early remission
Alcohol use disorder, moderate, in sustained remission
Alcohol use disorder, severe, in early remission
Alcohol use disorder, severe, in sustained remission

+ **F10.22** **Alcohol dependence with intoxication**
Acute drunkenness (in alcoholism)
Excludes2: alcohol dependence with withdrawal (F10.23-)
F10.220 **Alcohol dependence with intoxication, uncomplicated**
CC **F10.221** **Alcohol dependence with intoxication delirium**
F10.229 **Alcohol dependence with intoxication, unspecified**

+ F10.23 Alcohol dependence with withdrawal
> *Excludes2:* *Alcohol dependence with intoxication*
> *(F10.22-)*

CC **F10.230 Alcohol dependence with withdrawal, uncomplicated**

CC **F10.231 Alcohol dependence with withdrawal delirium**

CC **F10.232 Alcohol dependence with withdrawal with perceptual disturbance**

CC **F10.239 Alcohol dependence with withdrawal, unspecified**

CC **F10.24 Alcohol dependence with alcohol-induced mood disorder**
> Alcohol use disorder, moderate, with alcohol-induced bipolar or related disorder
> Alcohol use disorder, moderate, with alcohol-induced depressive disorder
> Alcohol use disorder, severe, with alcohol-induced bipolar or related disorder
> Alcohol use disorder, severe, with alcohol-induced depressive disorder

+ F10.25 Alcohol dependence with alcohol-induced psychotic disorder

F10.250 Alcohol dependence with alcohol-induced psychotic disorder with delusions

CC **F10.251 Alcohol dependence with alcohol-induced psychotic disorder with hallucinations**

CC **F10.259 Alcohol dependence with alcohol-induced psychotic disorder, unspecified**

F10.26 Alcohol dependence with alcohol-induced persisting amnestic disorder
> Alcohol use disorder, moderate, with alcohol-induced major neurocognitive disorder, amnestic-confabulatory type
> Alcohol use disorder, severe, with alcohol-induced major neurocognitive disorder, amnestic-confabulatory type

CC **F10.27 Alcohol dependence with alcohol-induced persisting dementia**
> Alcohol use disorder, moderate, with alcohol-induced major neurocognitive disorder, nonamnestic-confabulatory type
> Alcohol use disorder, severe, with alcohol-induced major neurocognitive disorder, nonamnestic-confabulatory type

+ F10.28 Alcohol dependence with other alcohol-induced disorders

CC **F10.280 Alcohol dependence with alcohol-induced anxiety disorder**

CC **F10.281 Alcohol dependence with alcohol-induced sexual dysfunction**

F10.282 Alcohol dependence with alcohol-induced sleep disorder

CC **F10.288 Alcohol dependence with other alcohol-induced disorder**
> Alcohol use disorder, moderate, with alcohol-induced mild neurocognitive disorder
> Alcohol use disorder, severe, with alcohol-induced mild neurocognitive disorder

CC **F10.29 Alcohol dependence with unspecified alcohol-induced disorder**

+ F10.9 Alcohol use, unspecified
> *Excludes1:* *alcohol abuse (F10.1-)*
> *alcohol dependence (F10.2-)*

+ F10.92 Alcohol use, unspecified with intoxication

F10.920 Alcohol use, unspecified with intoxication, uncomplicated

CC **F10.921 Alcohol use, unspecified with intoxication delirium**

F10.929 Alcohol use, unspecified with intoxication, unspecified

+ F10.93 Alcohol use, unspecified with withdrawal

CC **F10.930 Alcohol use, unspecified with withdrawal, uncomplicated**

CC **F10.931 Alcohol use, unspecified with withdrawal delirium**

CC **F10.932 Alcohol use, unspecified with withdrawal with perceptual disturbance**

CC **F10.939 Alcohol use, unspecified with withdrawal, unspecified**

CC **F10.94 Alcohol use, unspecified with alcohol-induced mood disorder**
> Alcohol-induced bipolar or related disorder, without use disorder
> Alcohol-induced depressive disorder, without use disorder

+ F10.95 Alcohol use, unspecified with alcohol-induced psychotic disorder

F10.950 Alcohol use, unspecified with alcohol-induced psychotic disorder with delusions

CC **F10.951 Alcohol use, unspecified with alcohol-induced psychotic disorder with hallucinations**

CC **F10.959 Alcohol use, unspecified with alcohol-induced psychotic disorder, unspecified**
> Alcohol-induced psychotic disorder without use disorder

F10.96 Alcohol use, unspecified with alcohol-induced persisting amnestic disorder
> Alcohol-induced major neurocognitive disorder, amnestic-confabulatory type, without use disorder

F10.97 Alcohol use, unspecified with alcohol-induced persisting dementia
> Alcohol-induced major neurocognitive disorder, nonamnestic-confabulatory type, without use disorder

+ F10.98 Alcohol use, unspecified with other alcohol-induced disorders

CC **F10.980 Alcohol use, unspecified with alcohol-induced anxiety disorder**
> Alcohol-induced anxiety disorder, without use disorder

CC **F10.981 Alcohol use, unspecified with alcohol-induced sexual dysfunction**
> Alcohol-induced sexual dysfunction, without use disorder

F10.982 Alcohol use, unspecified with alcohol-induced sleep disorder
> Alcohol-induced sleep disorder, without use disorder

CC **F10.988 Alcohol use, unspecified with other alcohol-induced disorder**
> Alcohol-induced mild neurocognitive disorder, without use disorder
> *AHA CC: 3Q, 2019, 8*

CC **F10.99 Alcohol use, unspecified with unspecified alcohol-induced disorder**

F11 Opioid related disorders

+ F11.1 Opioid abuse
> *Excludes1:* *opioid dependence (F11.2-)*
> *opioid use, unspecified (F11.9-)*

F11.10 Opioid abuse, uncomplicated
> Opioid use disorder, mild

F11.11 Opioid abuse, in remission
> Opioid use disorder, mild, in early remission
> Opioid use disorder, mild, in sustained remission

+ F11.12 Opioid abuse with intoxication

F11.120 Opioid abuse with intoxication, uncomplicated

CC **F11.121 Opioid abuse with intoxication delirium**

F11.122 Opioid abuse with intoxication with perceptual disturbance

F11.129 Opioid abuse with intoxication, unspecified

CC **F11.13 Opioid abuse with withdrawal**

F11.14 Opioid abuse with opioid-induced mood disorder
> Opioid use disorder, mild, with opioid-induced depressive disorder

+ **F11.15** Opioid abuse with opioid-induced psychotic disorder
   CC **F11.150** Opioid abuse with opioid-induced psychotic disorder with delusions
   CC **F11.151** Opioid abuse with opioid-induced psychotic disorder with hallucinations
   F11.159 Opioid abuse with opioid-induced psychotic disorder, unspecified
+ **F11.18** Opioid abuse with other opioid-induced disorder
   F11.181 Opioid abuse with opioid-induced sexual dysfunction
   F11.182 Opioid abuse with opioid-induced sleep disorder
   F11.188 Opioid abuse with other opioid-induced disorder
F11.19 Opioid abuse with unspecified opioid-induced disorder
+ **F11.2** Opioid dependence
   Excludes1: *opioid abuse (F11.1-)*
       opioid use, unspecified (F11.9-)
   Excludes2: *opioid poisoning (T40.0-T40.2-)*
  CC **F11.20** Opioid dependence, uncomplicated
   Opioid use disorder, moderate
   Opioid use disorder, severe
  F11.21 Opioid dependence, in remission
   Opioid use disorder, moderate, in early remission
   Opioid use disorder, moderate, in sustained remission
   Opioid use disorder, severe, in early remission
   Opioid use disorder, severe, in sustained remission
+ **F11.22** Opioid dependence with intoxication
   Excludes1: *opioid dependence with withdrawal (F11.23)*
   F11.220 Opioid dependence with intoxication, uncomplicated
  CC **F11.221** Opioid dependence with intoxication delirium
  CC **F11.222** Opioid dependence with intoxication with perceptual disturbance
   F11.229 Opioid dependence with intoxication, unspecified
CC **F11.23** Opioid dependence with withdrawal
   Excludes1: *opioid dependence with intoxication (F11.22-)*
F11.24 Opioid dependence with opioid-induced mood disorder
   Opioid use disorder, moderate, with opioid-induced depressive disorder
+ **F11.25** Opioid dependence with opioid-induced psychotic disorder
  CC **F11.250** Opioid dependence with opioid-induced psychotic disorder with delusions
  CC **F11.251** Opioid dependence with opioid-induced psychotic disorder with hallucinations
  CC **F11.259** Opioid dependence with opioid-induced psychotic disorder, unspecified
+ **F11.28** Opioid dependence with other opioid-induced disorder
  CC **F11.281** Opioid dependence with opioid-induced sexual dysfunction
  CC **F11.282** Opioid dependence with opioid-induced sleep disorder
  CC **F11.288** Opioid dependence with other opioid-induced disorder
F11.29 Opioid dependence with unspecified opioid-induced disorder
+ **F11.9** Opioid use, unspecified
   Excludes1: *opioid abuse (F11.1-)*
       opioid dependence (F11.2-)
F11.90 Opioid use, unspecified, uncomplicated
+ **F11.92** Opioid use, unspecified with intoxication
   Excludes1: *opioid use, unspecified with withdrawal (F11.93)*
   F11.920 Opioid use, unspecified with intoxication, uncomplicated
  CC **F11.921** Opioid use, unspecified with intoxication delirium
   Opioid use delirium

   F11.922 Opioid use, unspecified with intoxication with perceptual disturbance
   F11.929 Opioid use, unspecified with intoxication, unspecified
CC **F11.93** Opioid use, unspecified with withdrawal
   Excludes1: *opioid use, unspecified with intoxication (F11.92-)*
F11.94 Opioid use, unspecified with opioid-induced mood disorder
   Opioid-induced depressive disorder, without use disorder
+ **F11.95** Opioid use, unspecified with opioid-induced psychotic disorder
  CC **F11.950** Opioid use, unspecified with opioid-induced psychotic disorder with delusions
  CC **F11.951** Opioid use, unspecified with opioid-induced psychotic disorder with hallucinations
   F11.959 Opioid use, unspecified with opioid-induced psychotic disorder, unspecified
+ **F11.98** Opioid use, unspecified with other specified opioid-induced disorder
   F11.981 Opioid use, unspecified with opioid-induced sexual dysfunction
    Opioid-induced sexual dysfunction, without use disorder
   F11.982 Opioid use, unspecified with opioid-induced sleep disorder
    Opioid-induced sleep disorder, without use disorder
   F11.988 Opioid use, unspecified with other opioid-induced disorder
    Opioid-induced anxiety disorder, without use disorder
F11.99 Opioid use, unspecified with unspecified opioid-induced disorder

F12 Cannabis related disorders
   Includes: marijuana
   AHA CC: 1Q, 2020, 8
+ **F12.1** Cannabis abuse
   Excludes1: *cannabis dependence (F12.2-)*
       cannabis use, unspecified (F12.9-)
F12.10 Cannabis abuse, uncomplicated
   Cannabis use disorder, mild
F12.11 Cannabis abuse, in remission
   Cannabis use disorder, mild, in early remission
   Cannabis use disorder, mild, in sustained remission
+ **F12.12** Cannabis abuse with intoxication
   F12.120 Cannabis abuse with intoxication, uncomplicated
  CC **F12.121** Cannabis abuse with intoxication delirium
   F12.122 Cannabis abuse with intoxication with perceptual disturbance
   F12.129 Cannabis abuse with intoxication, unspecified
CC **F12.13** Cannabis abuse with withdrawal
+ **F12.15** Cannabis abuse with psychotic disorder
  CC **F12.150** Cannabis abuse with psychotic disorder with delusions
  CC **F12.151** Cannabis abuse with psychotic disorder with hallucinations
   F12.159 Cannabis abuse with psychotic disorder, unspecified
+ **F12.18** Cannabis abuse with other cannabis-induced disorder
   F12.180 Cannabis abuse with cannabis-induced anxiety disorder
   F12.188 Cannabis abuse with other cannabis-induced disorder
    Cannabis use disorder, mild, with cannabis-induced sleep disorder
F12.19 Cannabis abuse with unspecified cannabis-induced disorder

+, +7th, X + 7th   ● Newborn   ● Pediatric   ● Maternity   ● Adult   ♀ Female   ♂ Male   Manifestation   Unacceptable PDX   HCC   CC   MCC   HAC

+ **F12.2   Cannabis dependence**

Excludes1: *cannabis abuse (F12.1-)*
cannabis use, unspecified (F12.9-)

Excludes2: *cannabis poisoning (T40.7-)*

F12.20   Cannabis dependence, uncomplicated
Cannabis use disorder, moderate
Cannabis use disorder, severe

F12.21   Cannabis dependence, in remission
Cannabis use disorder, moderate, in early remission
Cannabis use disorder, moderate, in sustained remission
Cannabis use disorder, severe, in early remission
Cannabis use disorder, severe, in sustained remission

+ **F12.22   Cannabis dependence with intoxication**

F12.220   Cannabis dependence with intoxication, uncomplicated

CC **F12.221   Cannabis dependence with intoxication delirium**

F12.222   Cannabis dependence with intoxication with perceptual disturbance

F12.229   Cannabis dependence with intoxication, unspecified

F12.23   Cannabis dependence with withdrawal
AHA CC: 4Q, 2018, 7

+ **F12.25   Cannabis dependence with psychotic disorder**

CC **F12.250   Cannabis dependence with psychotic disorder with delusions**

CC **F12.251   Cannabis dependence with psychotic disorder with hallucinations**

F12.259   Cannabis dependence with psychotic disorder, unspecified

+ **F12.28   Cannabis dependence with other cannabis-induced disorder**

F12.280   Cannabis dependence with cannabis-induced anxiety disorder

F12.288   Cannabis dependence with other cannabis-induced disorder
Cannabis use disorder, moderate, with cannabis-induced sleep disorder
Cannabis use disorder, severe, with cannabis-induced sleep disorder

F12.29   Cannabis dependence with unspecified cannabis-induced disorder

+ **F12.9   Cannabis use, unspecified**

Excludes1: *cannabis abuse (F12.1-)*
cannabis dependence (F12.2-)

F12.90   Cannabis use, unspecified, uncomplicated

+ **F12.92   Cannabis use, unspecified with intoxication**

F12.920   Cannabis use, unspecified with intoxication, uncomplicated

CC **F12.921   Cannabis use, unspecified with intoxication delirium**

F12.922   Cannabis use, unspecified with intoxication with perceptual disturbance

F12.929   Cannabis use, unspecified with intoxication, unspecified

F12.93   Cannabis use, unspecified with withdrawal
AHA CC: 4Q, 2018, 7

+ **F12.95   Cannabis use, unspecified with psychotic disorder**

CC **F12.950   Cannabis use, unspecified with psychotic disorder with delusions**

CC **F12.951   Cannabis use, unspecified with psychotic disorder with hallucinations**

F12.959   Cannabis use, unspecified with psychotic disorder, unspecified
Cannabis-induced psychotic disorder, without use disorder

+ **F12.98   Cannabis use, unspecified with other cannabis-induced disorder**

F12.980   Cannabis use, unspecified with anxiety disorder
Cannabis-induced anxiety disorder, without use disorder

F12.988   Cannabis use, unspecified with other cannabis-induced disorder
Cannabis-induced sleep disorder, without use disorder

F12.99   Cannabis use, unspecified with unspecified cannabis-induced disorder

F13   Sedative, hypnotic, or anxiolytic related disorders

+ **F13.1   Sedative, hypnotic or anxiolytic-related abuse**

Excludes1: *sedative, hypnotic or anxiolytic-related dependence (F13.2-)*
sedative, hypnotic, or anxiolytic use, unspecified (F13.9-)

F13.10   Sedative, hypnotic or anxiolytic abuse, uncomplicated
Sedative, hypnotic, or anxiolytic use disorder, mild

F13.11   Sedative, hypnotic or anxiolytic abuse, in remission
Sedative, hypnotic or anxiolytic use disorder, mild, in early remission
Sedative, hypnotic or anxiolytic use disorder, mild, in sustained remission

+ **F13.12   Sedative, hypnotic or anxiolytic abuse with intoxication**

F13.120   Sedative, hypnotic or anxiolytic abuse with intoxication, uncomplicated

CC **F13.121   Sedative, hypnotic or anxiolytic abuse with intoxication delirium**

F13.129   Sedative, hypnotic or anxiolytic abuse with intoxication, unspecified

+ **F13.13   Sedative, hypnotic or anxiolytic abuse with withdrawal**

CC **F13.130   Sedative, hypnotic or anxiolytic abuse with withdrawal, uncomplicated**

CC **F13.131   Sedative, hypnotic or anxiolytic abuse with withdrawal delirium**

CC **F13.132   Sedative, hypnotic or anxiolytic abuse with withdrawal with perceptual disturbance**

CC **F13.139   Sedative, hypnotic or anxiolytic abuse with withdrawal, unspecified**

F13.14   Sedative, hypnotic or anxiolytic abuse with sedative, hypnotic or anxiolytic-induced mood disorder
Sedative, hypnotic, or anxiolytic use disorder, mild, with sedative, hypnotic, or anxiolytic-induced bipolar or related disorder
Sedative, hypnotic, or anxiolytic use disorder, mild, with sedative, hypnotic, or anxiolytic-induced depressive disorder

+ **F13.15   Sedative, hypnotic or anxiolytic abuse with sedative, hypnotic or anxiolytic-induced psychotic disorder**

CC **F13.150   Sedative, hypnotic or anxiolytic abuse with sedative, hypnotic or anxiolytic-induced psychotic disorder with delusions**

CC **F13.151   Sedative, hypnotic or anxiolytic abuse with sedative, hypnotic or anxiolytic-induced psychotic disorder with hallucinations**

F13.159   Sedative, hypnotic or anxiolytic abuse with sedative, hypnotic or anxiolytic-induced psychotic disorder, unspecified

+ **F13.18   Sedative, hypnotic or anxiolytic abuse with other sedative, hypnotic or anxiolytic-induced disorders**

F13.180   Sedative, hypnotic or anxiolytic abuse with sedative, hypnotic or anxiolytic-induced anxiety disorder

F13.181   Sedative, hypnotic or anxiolytic abuse with sedative, hypnotic or anxiolytic-induced sexual dysfunction

F13.182   Sedative, hypnotic or anxiolytic abuse with sedative, hypnotic or anxiolytic-induced sleep disorder

F13.188   Sedative, hypnotic or anxiolytic abuse with other sedative, hypnotic or anxiolytic-induced disorder

F13.19   Sedative, hypnotic or anxiolytic abuse with unspecified sedative, hypnotic or anxiolytic-induced disorder

+ **F13.2   Sedative, hypnotic or anxiolytic-related dependence**

Excludes1: *sedative, hypnotic or anxiolytic-related abuse (F13.1-)*
sedative, hypnotic, or anxiolytic use, unspecified (F13.9-)

Excludes2: *sedative, hypnotic, or anxiolytic poisoning (T42.-)*

CC **F13.20** **Sedative, hypnotic or anxiolytic dependence, uncomplicated**

F13.21 **Sedative, hypnotic or anxiolytic dependence, in remission**

Sedative, hypnotic or anxiolytic use disorder, moderate, in early remission

Sedative, hypnotic or anxiolytic use disorder, moderate, in sustained remission

Sedative, hypnotic or anxiolytic use disorder, severe, in early remission

Sedative, hypnotic or anxiolytic use disorder, severe, in sustained remission

+ **F13.22** **Sedative, hypnotic or anxiolytic dependence with intoxication**

Excludes1: *sedative, hypnotic or anxiolytic dependence with withdrawal (F13.23-)*

F13.220 **Sedative, hypnotic or anxiolytic dependence with intoxication, uncomplicated**

CC **F13.221** **Sedative, hypnotic or anxiolytic dependence with intoxication delirium**

F13.229 **Sedative, hypnotic or anxiolytic dependence with intoxication, unspecified**

+ **F13.23** **Sedative, hypnotic or anxiolytic dependence with withdrawal**

Sedative, hypnotic, or anxiolytic use disorder, moderate

Sedative, hypnotic, or anxiolytic use disorder, severe

Excludes1: *sedative, hypnotic or anxiolytic dependence with intoxication (F13.22-)*

CC **F13.230** **Sedative, hypnotic or anxiolytic dependence with withdrawal, uncomplicated**

CC **F13.231** **Sedative, hypnotic or anxiolytic dependence with withdrawal delirium**

CC **F13.232** **Sedative, hypnotic or anxiolytic dependence with withdrawal with perceptual disturbance**

Sedative, hypnotic, or anxiolytic withdrawal with perceptual disturbances

CC **F13.239** **Sedative, hypnotic or anxiolytic dependence with withdrawal, unspecified**

Sedative, hypnotic, or anxiolytic withdrawal without perceptual disturbances

F13.24 **Sedative, hypnotic or anxiolytic dependence with sedative, hypnotic or anxiolytic-induced mood disorder**

Sedative, hypnotic, or anxiolytic use disorder, moderate, with sedative, hypnotic, or anxiolytic-induced bipolar or related disorder

Sedative, hypnotic, or anxiolytic use disorder, moderate, with sedative, hypnotic, or anxiolytic-induced depressive disorder

Sedative, hypnotic, or anxiolytic use disorder, severe, with sedative, hypnotic, or anxiolytic-induced bipolar or related disorder

Sedative, hypnotic, or anxiolytic use disorder, severe, with sedative, hypnotic, or anxiolytic-induced depressive disorder

+ **F13.25** **Sedative, hypnotic or anxiolytic dependence with sedative, hypnotic or anxiolytic-induced psychotic disorder**

CC **F13.250** **Sedative, hypnotic or anxiolytic dependence with sedative, hypnotic or anxiolytic-induced psychotic disorder with delusions**

CC **F13.251** **Sedative, hypnotic or anxiolytic dependence with sedative, hypnotic or anxiolytic-induced psychotic disorder with hallucinations**

CC **F13.259** **Sedative, hypnotic or anxiolytic dependence with sedative, hypnotic or anxiolytic-induced psychotic disorder, unspecified**

CC **F13.26** **Sedative, hypnotic or anxiolytic dependence with sedative, hypnotic or anxiolytic-induced persisting amnestic disorder**

CC **F13.27** **Sedative, hypnotic or anxiolytic dependence with sedative, hypnotic or anxiolytic-induced persisting dementia**

Sedative, hypnotic, or anxiolytic use disorder, moderate, with sedative, hypnotic, or anxiolytic-induced major neurocognitive disorder

Sedative, hypnotic, or anxiolytic use disorder, severe, with sedative, hypnotic, or anxiolytic-induced major neurocognitive disorder

+ **F13.28** **Sedative, hypnotic or anxiolytic dependence with other sedative, hypnotic or anxiolytic-induced disorders**

CC **F13.280** **Sedative, hypnotic or anxiolytic dependence with sedative, hypnotic or anxiolytic-induced anxiety disorder**

CC **F13.281** **Sedative, hypnotic or anxiolytic dependence with sedative, hypnotic or anxiolytic-induced sexual dysfunction**

CC **F13.282** **Sedative, hypnotic or anxiolytic dependence with sedative, hypnotic or anxiolytic-induced sleep disorder**

CC **F13.288** **Sedative, hypnotic or anxiolytic dependence with other sedative, hypnotic or anxiolytic-induced disorder**

Sedative, hypnotic, or anxiolytic use disorder, moderate, with sedative, hypnotic, or anxiolytic-induced mild neurocognitive disorder

Sedative, hypnotic, or anxiolytic use disorder, severe, with sedative, hypnotic, or anxiolytic-induced mild neurocognitive disorder

F13.29 **Sedative, hypnotic or anxiolytic dependence with unspecified sedative, hypnotic or anxiolytic-induced disorder**

+ **F13.9** **Sedative, hypnotic or anxiolytic-related use, unspecified**

Excludes1: *sedative, hypnotic or anxiolytic-related abuse (F13.1-)*

sedative, hypnotic or anxiolytic-related dependence (F13.2-)

Review coding guideline C.5.b.3

F13.90 **Sedative, hypnotic, or anxiolytic use, unspecified, uncomplicated**

+ **F13.92** **Sedative, hypnotic or anxiolytic use, unspecified with intoxication**

Excludes1: *sedative, hypnotic or anxiolytic use, unspecified with withdrawal (F13.93-)*

F13.920 **Sedative, hypnotic or anxiolytic use, unspecified with intoxication, uncomplicated**

CC **F13.921** **Sedative, hypnotic or anxiolytic use, unspecified with intoxication delirium**

Sedative, hypnotic, or anxiolytic-induced delirium

F13.929 **Sedative, hypnotic or anxiolytic use, unspecified with intoxication, unspecified**

+ **F13.93** **Sedative, hypnotic or anxiolytic use, unspecified with withdrawal**

Excludes1: *sedative, hypnotic or anxiolytic use, unspecified with intoxication (F13.92-)*

CC **F13.930** **Sedative, hypnotic or anxiolytic use, unspecified with withdrawal, uncomplicated**

CC **F13.931** **Sedative, hypnotic or anxiolytic use, unspecified with withdrawal delirium**

CC **F13.932** **Sedative, hypnotic or anxiolytic use, unspecified with withdrawal with perceptual disturbances**

CC **F13.939** **Sedative, hypnotic or anxiolytic use, unspecified with withdrawal, unspecified**

F13.94 Sedative, hypnotic or anxiolytic use, unspecified with sedative, hypnotic or anxiolytic-induced mood disorder

Sedative, hypnotic, or anxiolytic-induced bipolar or related disorder, without use disorder

Sedative, hypnotic, or anxiolytic-induced depressive disorder, without use disorder

+ **F13.95** Sedative, hypnotic or anxiolytic use, unspecified with sedative, hypnotic or anxiolytic-induced psychotic disorder

CC **F13.950** Sedative, hypnotic or anxiolytic use, unspecified with sedative, hypnotic or anxiolytic-induced psychotic disorder with delusions

CC **F13.951** Sedative, hypnotic or anxiolytic use, unspecified with sedative, hypnotic or anxiolytic-induced psychotic disorder with hallucinations

F13.959 Sedative, hypnotic or anxiolytic use, unspecified with sedative, hypnotic or anxiolytic-induced psychotic disorder, unspecified

Sedative, hypnotic, or anxiolytic-induced psychotic disorder, without use disorder

F13.96 Sedative, hypnotic or anxiolytic use, unspecified with sedative, hypnotic or anxiolytic-induced persisting amnestic disorder

CC **F13.97** Sedative, hypnotic or anxiolytic use, unspecified with sedative, hypnotic or anxiolytic-induced persisting dementia

Sedative, hypnotic, or anxiolytic-induced major neurocognitive disorder, without use disorder

+ **F13.98** Sedative, hypnotic or anxiolytic use, unspecified with other sedative, hypnotic or anxiolytic-induced disorders

F13.980 Sedative, hypnotic or anxiolytic use, unspecified with sedative, hypnotic or anxiolytic-induced anxiety disorder

Sedative, hypnotic, or anxiolytic-induced anxiety disorder, without use disorder

F13.981 Sedative, hypnotic or anxiolytic use, unspecified with sedative, hypnotic or anxiolytic-induced sexual dysfunction

Sedative, hypnotic, or anxiolytic-induced sexual dysfunction, without use disorder

F13.982 Sedative, hypnotic or anxiolytic use, unspecified with sedative, hypnotic or anxiolytic-induced sleep disorder

Sedative, hypnotic, or anxiolytic-induced sleep, without use disorder

F13.988 Sedative, hypnotic or anxiolytic use, unspecified with other sedative, hypnotic or anxiolytic-induced disorder

Sedative, hypnotic, or anxiolytic-induced mild neurocognitive disorder

F13.99 Sedative, hypnotic or anxiolytic use, unspecified with unspecified sedative, hypnotic or anxiolytic-induced disorder

F14 Cocaine related disorders

Excludes2: other stimulant-related disorders (F15.-)

+ **F14.1** Cocaine abuse

Excludes1: cocaine dependence (F14.2-)
cocaine use, unspecified (F14.9-)

F14.10 Cocaine abuse, uncomplicated
Cocaine use disorder, mild

F14.11 Cocaine abuse, in remission
Cocaine use disorder, mild, in early remission
Cocaine use disorder, mild, in sustained remission

+ **F14.12** Cocaine abuse with intoxication

F14.120 Cocaine abuse with intoxication, uncomplicated

CC **F14.121** Cocaine abuse with intoxication with delirium

F14.122 Cocaine abuse with intoxication with perceptual disturbance

F14.129 Cocaine abuse with intoxication, unspecified

CC **F14.13** Cocaine abuse, unspecified with withdrawal

F14.14 Cocaine abuse with cocaine-induced mood disorder

Cocaine use disorder, mild, with cocaine-induced bipolar or related disorder

Cocaine use disorder, mild, with cocaine-induced depressive disorder

+ **F14.15** Cocaine abuse with cocaine-induced psychotic disorder

CC **F14.150** Cocaine abuse with cocaine-induced psychotic disorder with delusions

CC **F14.151** Cocaine abuse with cocaine-induced psychotic disorder with hallucinations

F14.159 Cocaine abuse with cocaine-induced psychotic disorder, unspecified

+ **F14.18** Cocaine abuse with other cocaine-induced disorder

F14.180 Cocaine abuse with cocaine-induced anxiety disorder

F14.181 Cocaine abuse with cocaine-induced sexual dysfunction

F14.182 Cocaine abuse with cocaine-induced sleep disorder

F14.188 Cocaine abuse with other cocaine-induced disorder

Cocaine use disorder, mild, with cocaine-induced obsessive compulsive or related disorder

F14.19 Cocaine abuse with unspecified cocaine-induced disorder

+ **F14.2** Cocaine dependence

Excludes1: cocaine abuse (F14.1-)
cocaine use, unspecified (F14.9-)

Excludes2: cocaine poisoning (T40.5-)

CC **F14.20** Cocaine dependence, uncomplicated
Cocaine use disorder, moderate
Cocaine use disorder, severe

F14.21 Cocaine dependence, in remission
Cocaine use disorder, moderate, in early remission
Cocaine use disorder, moderate, in sustained remission
Cocaine use disorder, severe, in early remission
Cocaine use disorder, severe, in sustained remission
AHA CC: 2Q, 2017, 26-28

+ **F14.22** Cocaine dependence with intoxication

Excludes1: cocaine dependence with withdrawal (F14.23)

F14.220 Cocaine dependence with intoxication, uncomplicated

CC **F14.221** Cocaine dependence with intoxication delirium

CC **F14.222** Cocaine dependence with intoxication with perceptual disturbance

CC **F14.229** Cocaine dependence with intoxication, unspecified

CC **F14.23** Cocaine dependence with withdrawal

Excludes1: cocaine dependence with intoxication (F14.22-)

F14.24 Cocaine dependence with cocaine-induced mood disorder

Cocaine use disorder, moderate, with cocaine-induced bipolar or related disorder

Cocaine use disorder, moderate, with cocaine-induced depressive disorder

Cocaine use disorder, severe, with cocaine-induced bipolar or related disorder

Cocaine use disorder, severe, with cocaine-induced depressive disorder

+ **F14.25** Cocaine dependence with cocaine-induced psychotic disorder

CC **F14.250** Cocaine dependence with cocaine-induced psychotic disorder with delusions

CC **F14.251** Cocaine dependence with cocaine-induced psychotic disorder with hallucinations

CC **F14.259** Cocaine dependence with cocaine-induced psychotic disorder, unspecified

+ **F14.28** **Cocaine dependence with other cocaine-induced disorder**
  CC **F14.280** **Cocaine dependence with cocaine-induced anxiety disorder**
  CC **F14.281** **Cocaine dependence with cocaine-induced sexual dysfunction**
  CC **F14.282** **Cocaine dependence with cocaine-induced sleep disorder**
  CC **F14.288** **Cocaine dependence with other cocaine-induced disorder**
    Cocaine use disorder, moderate, with cocaine-induced obsessive compulsive or related disorder
    Cocaine use disorder, severe, with cocaine-induced obsessive compulsive or related disorder
  F14.29 **Cocaine dependence with unspecified cocaine-induced disorder**
+ **F14.9** **Cocaine use, unspecified**
  Excludes1: *cocaine abuse (F14.1-)*
    cocaine dependence (F14.2-)
  Review coding guideline C.5.b.3
  F14.90 **Cocaine use, unspecified, uncomplicated**
    AHA CC: 2Q, 2018, 10-11
+ **F14.92** **Cocaine use, unspecified with intoxication**
  F14.920 **Cocaine use, unspecified with intoxication, uncomplicated**
  CC **F14.921** **Cocaine use, unspecified with intoxication delirium**
  F14.922 **Cocaine use, unspecified with intoxication with perceptual disturbance**
  F14.929 **Cocaine use, unspecified with intoxication, unspecified**
  CC **F14.93** **Cocaine use, unspecified with withdrawal**
  F14.94 **Cocaine use, unspecified with cocaine-induced mood disorder**
    Cocaine-induced bipolar or related disorder, without use disorder
    Cocaine-induced depressive disorder, without use disorder
+ **F14.95** **Cocaine use, unspecified with cocaine-induced psychotic disorder**
  CC **F14.950** **Cocaine use, unspecified with cocaine-induced psychotic disorder with delusions**
  CC **F14.951** **Cocaine use, unspecified with cocaine-induced psychotic disorder with hallucinations**
  F14.959 **Cocaine use, unspecified with cocaine-induced psychotic disorder, unspecified**
    Cocaine-induced psychotic disorder, without use disorder
+ **F14.98** **Cocaine use, unspecified with other specified cocaine-induced disorder**
  F14.980 **Cocaine use, unspecified with cocaine-induced anxiety disorder**
    Cocaine-induced anxiety disorder, without use disorder
  F14.981 **Cocaine use, unspecified with cocaine-induced sexual dysfunction**
    Cocaine-induced sexual dysfunction, without use disorder
  F14.982 **Cocaine use, unspecified with cocaine-induced sleep disorder**
    Cocaine-induced sleep disorder, without use disorder
  F14.988 **Cocaine use, unspecified with other cocaine-induced disorder**
    Cocaine-induced obsessive compulsive or related disorder
  F14.99 **Cocaine use, unspecified with unspecified cocaine-induced disorder**

F15 **Other stimulant related disorders**
  Includes: amphetamine-related disorders
    caffeine
  Excludes2: *cocaine-related disorders (F14.-)*

+ **F15.1** **Other stimulant abuse**
  Excludes1: *other stimulant dependence (F15.2-)*
    other stimulant use, unspecified (F15.9-)
  F15.10 **Other stimulant abuse, uncomplicated**
    Amphetamine type substance use disorder, mild
    Other or unspecified stimulant use disorder, mild
  F15.11 **Other stimulant abuse, in remission**
    Amphetamine type substance use disorder, mild, in early remission
    Amphetamine type substance use disorder, mild, in sustained remission
    Other or unspecified stimulant use disorder, mild, in early remission
    Other or unspecified stimulant use disorder, mild, in sustained remission
+ **F15.12** **Other stimulant abuse with intoxication**
  F15.120 **Other stimulant abuse with intoxication, uncomplicated**
  CC **F15.121** **Other stimulant abuse with intoxication delirium**
  F15.122 **Other stimulant abuse with intoxication with perceptual disturbance**
    Amphetamine or other stimulant use disorder, mild, with amphetamine or other stimulant intoxication, with perceptual disturbances
  F15.129 **Other stimulant abuse with intoxication, unspecified**
    Amphetamine or other stimulant use disorder, mild, with amphetamine or other stimulant intoxication, without perceptual disturbances
  CC **F15.13** **Other stimulant abuse with withdrawal**
  F15.14 **Other stimulant abuse with stimulant-induced mood disorder**
    Amphetamine or other stimulant use disorder, mild, with amphetamine or other stimulant-induced bipolar or related disorder
    Amphetamine or other stimulant use disorder, mild, with amphetamine or other stimulant-induced depressive disorder
+ **F15.15** **Other stimulant abuse with stimulant-induced psychotic disorder**
  CC **F15.150** **Other stimulant abuse with stimulant-induced psychotic disorder with delusions**
  CC **F15.151** **Other stimulant abuse with stimulant-induced psychotic disorder with hallucinations**
  F15.159 **Other stimulant abuse with stimulant-induced psychotic disorder, unspecified**
+ **F15.18** **Other stimulant abuse with other stimulant-induced disorder**
  F15.180 **Other stimulant abuse with stimulant-induced anxiety disorder**
  F15.181 **Other stimulant abuse with stimulant-induced sexual dysfunction**
  F15.182 **Other stimulant abuse with stimulant-induced sleep disorder**
  F15.188 **Other stimulant abuse with other stimulant-induced disorder**
    Amphetamine or other stimulant use disorder, mild, with amphetamine or other stimulant-induced obsessive-compulsive or related disorder
  F15.19 **Other stimulant abuse with unspecified stimulant-induced disorder**
+ **F15.2** **Other stimulant dependence**
  Excludes1: *other stimulant abuse (F15.1-)*
    other stimulant use, unspecified (F15.9-)
  CC **F15.20** **Other stimulant dependence, uncomplicated**
    Amphetamine type substance use disorder, moderate
    Amphetamine type substance use disorder, severe
    Other or unspecified stimulant use disorder, moderate
    Other or unspecified stimulant use disorder, severe

+, +7th, X + 7th   ● Newborn   ● Pediatric   ● Maternity   ● Adult   ♀ Female   ♂ Male   Manifestation   Unacceptable PDX   HCC   CC   MCC   HAC

F15.21 **Other stimulant dependence, in remission**
Amphetamine type substance use disorder, moderate, in early remission
Amphetamine type substance use disorder, moderate, in sustained remission
Amphetamine type substance use disorder, severe, in early remission
Amphetamine type substance use disorder, severe, in sustained remission
Other or unspecified stimulant use disorder, moderate, in early remission
Other or unspecified stimulant use disorder, moderate, in sustained remission
Other or unspecified stimulant use disorder, severe, in early remission
Other or unspecified stimulant use disorder, severe, in sustained remission

+ **F15.22** **Other stimulant dependence with intoxication**
Excludes1: *other stimulant dependence with withdrawal (F15.23)*

F15.220 **Other stimulant dependence with intoxication, uncomplicated**

CC **F15.221** **Other stimulant dependence with intoxication delirium**

CC **F15.222** **Other stimulant dependence with intoxication with perceptual disturbance**
Amphetamine or other stimulant use disorder, moderate, with amphetamine or other stimulant intoxication, with perceptual disturbances
Amphetamine or other stimulant use disorder, severe, with amphetamine or other stimulant intoxication, with perceptual disturbances

F15.229 **Other stimulant dependence with intoxication, unspecified**
Amphetamine or other stimulant use disorder, moderate, with amphetamine or other stimulant intoxication, without perceptual disturbances
Amphetamine or other stimulant use disorder, severe, with amphetamine or other stimulant intoxication, without perceptual disturbances

CC **F15.23** **Other stimulant dependence with withdrawal**
Amphetamine or other stimulant withdrawal
Excludes1: *other stimulant dependence with intoxication (F15.22-)*

F15.24 **Other stimulant dependence with stimulant-induced mood disorder**
Amphetamine or other stimulant use disorder, moderate, with amphetamine or other stimulant-induced bipolar or related disorder
Amphetamine or other stimulant use disorder, moderate, with amphetamine or other stimulant-induced depressive disorder
Amphetamine or other stimulant use disorder, severe, with amphetamine or other stimulant-induced bipolar or related disorder
Amphetamine or other stimulant use disorder, severe, with amphetamine or other stimulant-induced depressive disorder

+ **F15.25** **Other stimulant dependence with stimulant-induced psychotic disorder**

CC **F15.250** **Other stimulant dependence with stimulant-induced psychotic disorder with delusions**

CC **F15.251** **Other stimulant dependence with stimulant-induced psychotic disorder with hallucinations**

CC **F15.259** **Other stimulant dependence with stimulant-induced psychotic disorder, unspecified**

+ **F15.28** **Other stimulant dependence with other stimulant-induced disorder**

CC **F15.280** **Other stimulant dependence with stimulant-induced anxiety disorder**

CC **F15.281** **Other stimulant dependence with stimulant-induced sexual dysfunction**

CC **F15.282** **Other stimulant dependence with stimulant-induced sleep disorder**

CC **F15.288** **Other stimulant dependence with other stimulant-induced disorder**
Amphetamine or other stimulant use disorder, moderate, with amphetamine or other stimulant-induced obsessive-compulsive or related disorder
Amphetamine or other stimulant use disorder, severe, with amphetamine or other stimulant-induced obsessive-compulsive or related disorder

F15.29 **Other stimulant dependence with unspecified stimulant-induced disorder**

+ **F15.9** **Other stimulant use, unspecified**
Excludes1: *other stimulant abuse (F15.1-)*
other stimulant dependence (F15.2-)
Review coding guideline C.5.b.3

F15.90 **Other stimulant use, unspecified, uncomplicated**

+ **F15.92** **Other stimulant use, unspecified with intoxication**
Excludes1: *other stimulant use, unspecified with withdrawal (F15.93)*

F15.920 **Other stimulant use, unspecified with intoxication, uncomplicated**

CC **F15.921** **Other stimulant use, unspecified with intoxication delirium**
Amphetamine or other stimulant-induced delirium

F15.922 **Other stimulant use, unspecified with intoxication with perceptual disturbance**

F15.929 **Other stimulant use, unspecified with intoxication, unspecified**
Caffeine intoxication

CC **F15.93** **Other stimulant use, unspecified with withdrawal**
Caffeine withdrawal
Excludes1: *other stimulant use, unspecified with intoxication (F15.92-)*

F15.94 **Other stimulant use, unspecified with stimulant-induced mood disorder**
Amphetamine or other stimulant-induced bipolar or related disorder, without use disorder
Amphetamine or other stimulant-induced depressive disorder, without use disorder

+ **F15.95** **Other stimulant use, unspecified with stimulant-induced psychotic disorder**

CC **F15.950** **Other stimulant use, unspecified with stimulant-induced psychotic disorder with delusions**

CC **F15.951** **Other stimulant use, unspecified with stimulant-induced psychotic disorder with hallucinations**

F15.959 **Other stimulant use, unspecified with stimulant-induced psychotic disorder, unspecified**
Amphetamine or other stimulant-induced psychotic disorder, without use disorder

+ **F15.98** **Other stimulant use, unspecified with other stimulant-induced disorder**

F15.980 **Other stimulant use, unspecified with stimulant-induced anxiety disorder**
Amphetamine or other stimulant-induced anxiety disorder, without use disorder
Caffeine induced anxiety disorder, without use disorder

F15.981 **Other stimulant use, unspecified with stimulant-induced sexual dysfunction**
Amphetamine or other stimulant-induced sexual dysfunction, without use disorder

F15.982 **Other stimulant use, unspecified with stimulant-induced sleep disorder**
Amphetamine or other stimulant-induced sleep disorder, without use disorder
Caffeine induced sleep disorder, without use disorder

F15.988 **Other stimulant use, unspecified with other stimulant-induced disorder**
Amphetamine or other stimulant-induced obsessive-compulsive or related disorder, without use disorder

F15.99 **Other stimulant use, unspecified with unspecified stimulant-induced disorder**

F16 Hallucinogen related disorders

Includes: ecstasy
PCP
phencyclidine

+ **F16.1 Hallucinogen abuse**
Excludes1: *hallucinogen dependence (F16.2-)*
hallucinogen use, unspecified (F16.9-)

F16.10 Hallucinogen abuse, uncomplicated
Other hallucinogen use disorder, mild
Phencyclidine use disorder, mild
AHA CC: 4Q, 2018, 31

F16.11 Hallucinogen abuse, in remission
Other hallucinogen use disorder, mild, in early remission
Other hallucinogen use disorder, mild, in sustained remission
Phencyclidine use disorder, mild, in early remission
Phencyclidine use disorder, mild, in sustained remission

+ **F16.12 Hallucinogen abuse with intoxication**
F16.120 **Hallucinogen abuse with intoxication, uncomplicated**
CC **F16.121** **Hallucinogen abuse with intoxication with delirium**
F16.122 **Hallucinogen abuse with intoxication with perceptual disturbance**
F16.129 **Hallucinogen abuse with intoxication, unspecified**

F16.14 Hallucinogen abuse with hallucinogen-induced mood disorder
Other hallucinogen use disorder, mild, with other hallucinogen-induced bipolar or related disorder
Other hallucinogen use disorder, mild, with other hallucinogen-induced depressive disorder
Phencyclidine use disorder, mild, with other hallucinogen-induced bipolar or related disorder
Phencyclidine use disorder, mild, with other hallucinogen-induced depressive disorder

+ **F16.15 Hallucinogen abuse with hallucinogen-induced psychotic disorder**
CC **F16.150** **Hallucinogen abuse with hallucinogen-induced psychotic disorder with delusions**
CC **F16.151** **Hallucinogen abuse with hallucinogen-induced psychotic disorder with hallucinations**
F16.159 **Hallucinogen abuse with hallucinogen-induced psychotic disorder, unspecified**

+ **F16.18 Hallucinogen abuse with other hallucinogen-induced disorder**
F16.180 **Hallucinogen abuse with hallucinogen-induced anxiety disorder**
F16.183 **Hallucinogen abuse with hallucinogen persisting perception disorder (flashbacks)**
F16.188 **Hallucinogen abuse with other hallucinogen-induced disorder**

F16.19 Hallucinogen abuse with unspecified hallucinogen-induced disorder

+ **F16.2 Hallucinogen dependence**
Excludes1: *hallucinogen abuse (F16.1-)*
hallucinogen use, unspecified (F16.9-)

CC **F16.20 Hallucinogen dependence, uncomplicated**
Other hallucinogen use disorder, moderate
Other hallucinogen use disorder, severe
Phencyclidine use disorder, moderate
Phencyclidine use disorder, severe

F16.21 Hallucinogen dependence, in remission
Other hallucinogen use disorder, moderate, in early remission
Other hallucinogen use disorder, moderate, in sustained remission
Other hallucinogen use disorder, severe, in early remission
Other hallucinogen use disorder, severe, in sustained remission
Phencyclidine use disorder, moderate, in early remission
Phencyclidine use disorder, moderate, in sustained remission
Phencyclidine use disorder, severe, in early remission
Phencyclidine use disorder, severe, in sustained remission

+ **F16.22 Hallucinogen dependence with intoxication**
F16.220 **Hallucinogen dependence with intoxication, uncomplicated**
CC **F16.221** **Hallucinogen dependence with intoxication with delirium**
F16.229 **Hallucinogen dependence with intoxication, unspecified**

F16.24 Hallucinogen dependence with hallucinogen-induced mood disorder
Other hallucinogen use disorder, moderate, with other hallucinogen-induced bipolar or related disorder
Other hallucinogen use disorder, moderate, with other hallucinogen-induced depressive disorder
Other hallucinogen use disorder, severe, with other hallucinogen-induced bipolar or related disorder
Other hallucinogen use disorder, severe, with other hallucinogen-induced depressive disorder
Phencyclidine use disorder, moderate, with other phencyclidine-induced bipolar or related disorder
Phencyclidine use disorder, moderate, with other phencyclidine-induced depressive disorder
Phencyclidine use disorder, severe, with other phencyclidine-induced bipolar or related disorder
Phencyclidine use disorder, severe, with other phencyclidine-induced depressive disorder

+ **F16.25 Hallucinogen dependence with hallucinogen-induced psychotic disorder**
CC **F16.250** **Hallucinogen dependence with hallucinogen-induced psychotic disorder with delusions**
CC **F16.251** **Hallucinogen dependence with hallucinogen-induced psychotic disorder with hallucinations**
CC **F16.259** **Hallucinogen dependence with hallucinogen-induced psychotic disorder, unspecified**

+ **F16.28 Hallucinogen dependence with other hallucinogen-induced disorder**
CC **F16.280** **Hallucinogen dependence with hallucinogen-induced anxiety disorder**
CC **F16.283** **Hallucinogen dependence with hallucinogen persisting perception disorder (flashbacks)**
CC **F16.288** **Hallucinogen dependence with other hallucinogen-induced disorder**

F16.29 Hallucinogen dependence with unspecified hallucinogen-induced disorder

+ **F16.9 Hallucinogen use, unspecified**
Excludes1: *hallucinogen abuse (F16.1-)*
hallucinogen dependence (F16.2-)
Review coding guideline C.5.b.3

F16.90 Hallucinogen use, unspecified, uncomplicated

+ **F16.92 Hallucinogen use, unspecified with intoxication**
F16.920 **Hallucinogen use, unspecified with intoxication, uncomplicated**
CC **F16.921** **Hallucinogen use, unspecified with intoxication with delirium**
Other hallucinogen intoxication delirium
F16.929 **Hallucinogen use, unspecified with intoxication, unspecified**

+, +7th, X + 7th ● Newborn ● Pediatric ● Maternity ● Adult ♀ Female ♂ Male | Manifestation | Unacceptable PDX | HCC | CC | MCC | HAC

F16.94 **Hallucinogen use, unspecified with hallucinogen-induced mood disorder**

Other hallucinogen-induced bipolar or related disorder, without use disorder

Other hallucinogen-induced depressive disorder, without use disorder

Phencyclidine-induced bipolar or related disorder, without use disorder

Phencyclidine-induced depressive disorder, without use disorder

+ **F16.95** **Hallucinogen use, unspecified with hallucinogen-induced psychotic disorder**

CC **F16.950** **Hallucinogen use, unspecified with hallucinogen-induced psychotic disorder with delusions**

CC **F16.951** **Hallucinogen use, unspecified with hallucinogen-induced psychotic disorder with hallucinations**

F16.959 **Hallucinogen use, unspecified with hallucinogen-induced psychotic disorder, unspecified**

Other hallucinogen-induced psychotic disorder, without use disorder

Phencyclidine-induced psychotic disorder, without use disorder

+ **F16.98** **Hallucinogen use, unspecified with other specified hallucinogen-induced disorder**

F16.980 **Hallucinogen use, unspecified with hallucinogen-induced anxiety disorder**

Other hallucinogen-induced anxiety disorder, without use disorder

Phencyclidine-induced anxiety disorder, without use disorder

F16.983 **Hallucinogen use, unspecified with hallucinogen persisting perception disorder (flashbacks)**

F16.988 **Hallucinogen use, unspecified with other hallucinogen-induced disorder**

F16.99 **Hallucinogen use, unspecified with unspecified hallucinogen-induced disorder**

F17 **Nicotine dependence**

Excludes1: *history of tobacco dependence (Z87.891)*
tobacco use NOS (Z72.0)

Excludes2: *tobacco use (smoking) during pregnancy, childbirth and the puerperium (O99.33-)*
toxic effect of nicotine (T65.2-)

Review coding guideline C.15.1.2

+ **F17.2** **Nicotine dependence**

+ **F17.20** **Nicotine dependence, unspecified**

F17.200 **Nicotine dependence, unspecified, uncomplicated**

Tobacco use disorder, mild

Tobacco use disorder, moderate

Tobacco use disorder, severe

AHA CC: 4Q, 2013, 108; 1Q, 2016, 36-37

F17.201 **Nicotine dependence, unspecified, in remission**

Tobacco use disorder, mild, in early remission

Tobacco use disorder, mild, in sustained remission

Tobacco use disorder, moderate, in early remission

Tobacco use disorder, moderate, in sustained remission

Tobacco use disorder, severe, in early remission

Tobacco use disorder, severe, in sustained remission

CC **F17.203** **Nicotine dependence unspecified, with withdrawal**

Tobacco withdrawal

F17.208 **Nicotine dependence, unspecified, with other nicotine-induced disorders**

F17.209 **Nicotine dependence, unspecified, with unspecified nicotine-induced disorders**

+ **F17.21** **Nicotine dependence, cigarettes**

F17.210 **Nicotine dependence, cigarettes, uncomplicated**

AHA CC: 4Q, 2013, 109; 2Q, 2017, 28-29

F17.211 **Nicotine dependence, cigarettes, in remission**

Tobacco use disorder, cigarettes, mild, in early remission

Tobacco use disorder, cigarettes, mild, in sustained remission

Tobacco use disorder, cigarettes, moderate, in early remission

Tobacco use disorder, cigarettes, moderate, in sustained remission

Tobacco use disorder, cigarettes, severe, in early remission

Tobacco use disorder, cigarettes, severe, in sustained remission

CC **F17.213** **Nicotine dependence, cigarettes, with withdrawal**

F17.218 **Nicotine dependence, cigarettes, with other nicotine-induced disorders**

F17.219 **Nicotine dependence, cigarettes, with unspecified nicotine-induced disorders**

+ **F17.22** **Nicotine dependence, chewing tobacco**

F17.220 **Nicotine dependence, chewing tobacco, uncomplicated**

F17.221 **Nicotine dependence, chewing tobacco, in remission**

Tobacco use disorder, chewing tobacco, mild, in early remission

Tobacco use disorder, chewing tobacco, mild, in sustained remission

Tobacco use disorder, chewing tobacco, moderate, in early remission

Tobacco use disorder, chewing tobacco, moderate, in sustained remission

Tobacco use disorder, chewing tobacco, severe, in early remission

Tobacco use disorder, chewing tobacco, severe, in sustained remission

CC **F17.223** **Nicotine dependence, chewing tobacco, with withdrawal**

F17.228 **Nicotine dependence, chewing tobacco, with other nicotine-induced disorders**

F17.229 **Nicotine dependence, chewing tobacco, with unspecified nicotine-induced disorders**

+ **F17.29** **Nicotine dependence, other tobacco product**

F17.290 **Nicotine dependence, other tobacco product, uncomplicated**

AHA CC: 2Q, 2017, 28-29

F17.291 **Nicotine dependence, other tobacco product, in remission**

Tobacco use disorder, other tobacco product, mild, in early remission

Tobacco use disorder, other tobacco product, mild, in sustained remission

Tobacco use disorder, other tobacco product, moderate, in early remission

Tobacco use disorder, other tobacco product, moderate, in sustained remission

Tobacco use disorder, other tobacco product, severe, in early remission

Tobacco use disorder, other tobacco product, severe, in sustained remission

CC **F17.293** **Nicotine dependence, other tobacco product, with withdrawal**

F17.298 **Nicotine dependence, other tobacco product, with other nicotine-induced disorders**

F17.299 **Nicotine dependence, other tobacco product, with unspecified nicotine-induced disorders**

F18 Inhalant related disorders

Includes: volatile solvents

+ **F18.1 Inhalant abuse**

  Excludes1: inhalant dependence (F18.2-)
  inhalant use, unspecified (F18.9-)

  F18.10 Inhalant abuse, uncomplicated
  Inhalant use disorder, mild

  F18.11 Inhalant abuse, in remission
  Inhalant use disorder, mild, in early remission
  Inhalant use disorder, mild, in sustained remission

  + **F18.12 Inhalant abuse with intoxication**
    F18.120 Inhalant abuse with intoxication, uncomplicated
    CC **F18.121 Inhalant abuse with intoxication delirium**
    F18.129 Inhalant abuse with intoxication, unspecified

  F18.14 Inhalant abuse with inhalant-induced mood disorder
  Inhalant use disorder, mild, with inhalant-induced depressive disorder

  + **F18.15 Inhalant abuse with inhalant-induced psychotic disorder**
    CC **F18.150 Inhalant abuse with inhalant-induced psychotic disorder with delusions**
    CC **F18.151 Inhalant abuse with inhalant-induced psychotic disorder with hallucinations**
    F18.159 Inhalant abuse with inhalant-induced psychotic disorder, unspecified

  CC **F18.17 Inhalant abuse with inhalant-induced dementia**
  Inhalant use disorder, mild, with inhalant-induced major neurocognitive disorder

  + **F18.18 Inhalant abuse with other inhalant-induced disorders**
    F18.180 Inhalant abuse with inhalant-induced anxiety disorder
    F18.188 Inhalant abuse with other inhalant-induced disorder
    Inhalant use disorder, mild, with inhalant-induced mild neurocognitive disorder

  F18.19 Inhalant abuse with unspecified inhalant-induced disorder

+ **F18.2 Inhalant dependence**

  Excludes1: inhalant abuse (F18.1-)
  inhalant use, unspecified (F18.9-)

  CC **F18.20 Inhalant dependence, uncomplicated**
  Inhalant use disorder, moderate
  Inhalant use disorder, severe

  F18.21 Inhalant dependence, in remission
  Inhalant use disorder, moderate, in early remission
  Inhalant use disorder, moderate, in sustained remission
  Inhalant use disorder, severe, in early remission
  Inhalant use disorder, severe, in sustained remission

  + **F18.22 Inhalant dependence with intoxication**
    F18.220 Inhalant dependence with intoxication, uncomplicated
    CC **F18.221 Inhalant dependence with intoxication delirium**
    F18.229 Inhalant dependence with intoxication, unspecified

  F18.24 Inhalant dependence with inhalant-induced mood disorder
  Inhalant use disorder, moderate, with inhalant-induced depressive disorder
  Inhalant use disorder, severe, with inhalant-induced depressive disorder

  + **F18.25 Inhalant dependence with inhalant-induced psychotic disorder**
    CC **F18.250 Inhalant dependence with inhalant-induced psychotic disorder with delusions**
    CC **F18.251 Inhalant dependence with inhalant-induced psychotic disorder with hallucinations**
    CC **F18.259 Inhalant dependence with inhalant-induced psychotic disorder, unspecified**

  CC **F18.27 Inhalant dependence with inhalant-induced dementia**
  Inhalant use disorder, moderate, with inhalant-induced major neurocognitive disorder
  Inhalant use disorder, severe, with inhalant-induced major neurocognitive disorder

  + **F18.28 Inhalant dependence with other inhalant-induced disorders**
    CC **F18.280 Inhalant dependence with inhalant-induced anxiety disorder**
    CC **F18.288 Inhalant dependence with other inhalant-induced disorder**
    Inhalant use disorder, moderate, with inhalant-induced mild neurocognitive disorder
    Inhalant use disorder, severe, with inhalant-induced mild neurocognitive disorder

  F18.29 Inhalant dependence with unspecified inhalant-induced disorder

+ **F18.9 Inhalant use, unspecified**

  Excludes1: inhalant abuse (F18.1-)
  inhalant dependence (F18.2-)
  Review coding guideline C.5.b.3

  F18.90 Inhalant use, unspecified, uncomplicated

  + **F18.92 Inhalant use, unspecified with intoxication**
    F18.920 Inhalant use, unspecified with intoxication, uncomplicated
    CC **F18.921 Inhalant use, unspecified with intoxication with delirium**
    F18.929 Inhalant use, unspecified with intoxication, unspecified

  F18.94 Inhalant use, unspecified with inhalant-induced mood disorder
  Inhalant-induced depressive disorder

  + **F18.95 Inhalant use, unspecified with inhalant-induced psychotic disorder**
    CC **F18.950 Inhalant use, unspecified with inhalant-induced psychotic disorder with delusions**
    CC **F18.951 Inhalant use, unspecified with inhalant-induced psychoticdisorder with hallucinations**
    F18.959 Inhalant use, unspecified with inhalant-induced psychotic disorder, unspecified

  CC **F18.97 Inhalant use, unspecified with inhalant-induced persisting dementia**
  Inhalant-induced major neurocognitive disorder

  + **F18.98 Inhalant use, unspecified with other inhalant-induced disorders**
    F18.980 Inhalant use, unspecified with inhalant-induced anxiety disorder
    F18.988 Inhalant use, unspecified with other inhalant-induced disorder
    Inhalant-induced mild neurocognitive disorder

  F18.99 Inhalant use, unspecified with unspecified inhalant-induced disorder

F19 Other psychoactive substance related disorders

Includes: polysubstance drug use (indiscriminate drug use)

+ **F19.1 Other psychoactive substance abuse**

  Excludes1: other psychoactive substance dependence (F19.2-)
  other psychoactive substance use, unspecified (F19.9-)

  F19.10 Other psychoactive substance abuse, uncomplicated
  Other (or unknown) substance use disorder, mild

  F19.11 Other psychoactive substance abuse, in remission
  Other (or unknown) substance use disorder, mild, in early remission
  Other (or unknown) substance use disorder, mild, in sustained remission

  + **F19.12 Other psychoactive substance abuse with intoxication**
    F19.120 Other psychoactive substance abuse with intoxication, uncomplicated

+, +7th, X + 7th ● Newborn ● Pediatric ● Maternity ● Adult ♀ Female ♂ Male Manifestation Unacceptable PDX HCC CC MCC HAC

CC **F19.121 Other psychoactive substance abuse with intoxication delirium**

F19.122 Other psychoactive substance abuse with intoxication with perceptual disturbances

F19.129 Other psychoactive substance abuse with intoxication, unspecified

+ **F19.13 Other psychoactive substance abuse with withdrawal**

CC **F19.130 Other psychoactive substance abuse with withdrawal, uncomplicated**

CC **F19.131 Other psychoactive substance abuse with withdrawal delirium**

CC **F19.132 Other psychoactive substance abuse with withdrawal with perceptual disturbance**

CC **F19.139 Other psychoactive substance abuse with withdrawal, unspecified**

F19.14 Other psychoactive substance abuse with psychoactive substance-induced mood disorder

Other (or unknown) substance use disorder, mild, with other (or known) substance-induced bipolar or related disorder

Other (or unknown) substance use disorder, mild, with other (or known) substance-induced depressive disorder

+ **F19.15 Other psychoactive substance abuse with psychoactive substance-induced psychotic disorder**

CC **F19.150 Other psychoactive substance abuse with psychoactive substance-induced psychotic disorder with delusions**

CC **F19.151 Other psychoactive substance abuse with psychoactive substance-induced psychotic disorder with hallucinations**

F19.159 Other psychoactive substance abuse with psychoactive substance-induced psychotic disorder, unspecified

F19.16 Other psychoactive substance abuse with psychoactive substance-induced persisting amnestic disorder

CC **F19.17 Other psychoactive substance abuse with psychoactive substance-induced persisting dementia**

Other (or unknown) substance use disorder, mild, with other (or known) substance-induced major neurocognitive disorder

+ **F19.18 Other psychoactive substance abuse with other psychoactive substance-induced disorders**

F19.180 Other psychoactive substance abuse with psychoactive substance-induced anxiety disorder

F19.181 Other psychoactive substance abuse with psychoactive substance-induced sexual dysfunction

F19.182 Other psychoactive substance abuse with psychoactive substance-induced sleep disorder

F19.188 Other psychoactive substance abuse with other psychoactive substance-induced disorder

Other (or unknown) substance use disorder, mild, with other (or known) substance-induced mild neurocognitive disorder

Other (or unknown) substance use disorder, mild, with other (or known) substance-induced obsessive-compulsive disorder

F19.19 Other psychoactive substance abuse with unspecified psychoactive substance-induced disorder

+ **F19.2 Other psychoactive substance dependence**

Excludes1: *other psychoactive substance abuse (F19.1-)*
other psychoactive substance use, unspecified (F19.9-)

CC **F19.20 Other psychoactive substance dependence, uncomplicated**

Other (or unknown) substance use disorder, moderate

Other (or unknown) substance use disorder, severe

F19.21 Other psychoactive substance dependence, in remission

Other (or unknown) substance use disorder, moderate, in early remission

Other (or unknown) substance use disorder, moderate, in sustained remission

Other (or unknown) substance use disorder, severe, in early remission

Other (or unknown) substance use disorder, severe, in sustained remission

+ **F19.22 Other psychoactive substance dependence with intoxication**

Excludes1: *other psychoactive substance dependence with withdrawal (F19.23-)*

F19.220 Other psychoactive substance dependence with intoxication, uncomplicated

CC **F19.221 Other psychoactive substance dependence with intoxication delirium**

CC **F19.222 Other psychoactive substance dependence with intoxication with perceptual disturbance**

F19.229 Other psychoactive substance dependence with intoxication, unspecified

+ **F19.23 Other psychoactive substance dependence with withdrawal**

Excludes1: *other psychoactive substance dependence with intoxication (F19.22-)*

CC **F19.230 Other psychoactive substance dependence with withdrawal, uncomplicated**

CC **F19.231 Other psychoactive substance dependence with withdrawal delirium**

CC **F19.232 Other psychoactive substance dependence with withdrawal with perceptual disturbance**

CC **F19.239 Other psychoactive substance dependence with withdrawal, unspecified**

F19.24 Other psychoactive substance dependence with psychoactive substance-induced mood disorder

Other (or known) substance use disorder, moderate, with other (or unknown) substance-induced bipolar or related disorder

Other (or known) substance use disorder, moderate, with other (or unknown) substance-induced depressive disorder

Other (or known) substance use disorder, severe, with other (or unknown) substance-induced bipolar or related disorder

Other (or known) substance use disorder, severe, with other (or unknown) substance-induced depressive disorder

+ **F19.25 Other psychoactive substance dependence with psychoactive substance-induced psychotic disorder**

CC **F19.250 Other psychoactive substance dependence with psychoactive substance-induced psychotic disorder with delusions**

CC **F19.251 Other psychoactive substance dependence with psychoactive substance-induced psychotic disorder with hallucinations**

CC **F19.259 Other psychoactive substance dependence with psychoactive substance-induced psychotic disorder, unspecified**

CC **F19.26 Other psychoactive substance dependence with psychoactive substance-induced persisting amnestic disorder**

CC **F19.27** Other psychoactive substance dependence with psychoactive substance-induced persisting dementia
    Other (or unknown) substance use disorder, moderate, with other (or known) substance-induced major neurocognitive disorder
    Other (or unknown) substance use disorder, severe, with other (or known) substance-induced major neurocognitive disorder

+ **F19.28** Other psychoactive substance dependence with other psychoactive substance-induced disorders

    CC **F19.280** Other psychoactive substance dependence with psychoactive substance-induced anxiety disorder

    CC **F19.281** Other psychoactive substance dependence with psychoactive substance-induced sexual dysfunction

    CC **F19.282** Other psychoactive substance dependence with psychoactive substance-induced sleep disorder

    CC **F19.288** Other psychoactive substance dependence with other psychoactive substance-induced disorder
        Other (or unknown) substance use disorder, moderate, with other (or known) substance-induced mild neurocognitive disorder
        Other (or unknown) substance use disorder, moderate, with other (or known) substance-induced obsessive-compulsive disorder
        Other (or unknown) substance use disorder, severe, with other (or known) substance-induced mild neurocognitive disorder
        Other (or unknown) substance use disorder, severe, with other (or known) substance-induced obsessive-compulsive disorder

F19.29 Other psychoactive substance dependence with unspecified psychoactive substance-induced disorder

+ **F19.9** Other psychoactive substance use, unspecified
    Excludes1: *other psychoactive substance abuse (F19.1-)*
        other psychoactive substance dependence (F19.2-)
    Review coding guideline C.5.b.3

F19.90 Other psychoactive substance use, unspecified, uncomplicated

+ **F19.92** Other psychoactive substance use, unspecified with intoxication
    Excludes1: *other psychoactive substance use, unspecified with withdrawal (F19.93)*

    F19.920 Other psychoactive substance use, unspecified with intoxication, uncomplicated

    CC **F19.921** Other psychoactive substance use, unspecified with intoxication with delirium
        Other (or unknown) substance-induced delirium

    F19.922 Other psychoactive substance use, unspecified with intoxication with perceptual disturbance

    F19.929 Other psychoactive substance use, unspecified with intoxication, unspecified

+ **F19.93** Other psychoactive substance use, unspecified with withdrawal
    Excludes1: *other psychoactive substance use, unspecified with intoxication (F19.92-)*

    CC **F19.930** Other psychoactive substance use, unspecified with withdrawal, uncomplicated

    CC **F19.931** Other psychoactive substance use, unspecified with withdrawal delirium

CC **F19.932** Other psychoactive substance use, unspecified with withdrawal with perceptual disturbance

CC **F19.939** Other psychoactive substance use, unspecified with withdrawal, unspecified

F19.94 Other psychoactive substance use, unspecified with psychoactive substance-induced mood disorder
    Other (or unknown) substance-induced bipolar or related disorder, without use disorder
    Other (or unknown) substance-induced depressive disorder, without use disorder

+ **F19.95** Other psychoactive substance use, unspecified with psychoactive substance-induced psychotic disorder

    CC **F19.950** Other psychoactive substance use, unspecified with psychoactive substance-induced psychotic disorder with delusions

    CC **F19.951** Other psychoactive substance use, unspecified with psychoactive substance-induced psychotic disorder with hallucinations

    F19.959 Other psychoactive substance use, unspecified with psychoactive substance-induced psychotic disorder, unspecified
        Other (or unknown) substance-induced psychotic disorder, without use disorder

F19.96 Other psychoactive substance use, unspecified with psychoactive substance-induced persisting amnestic disorder

CC **F19.97** Other psychoactive substance use, unspecified with psychoactive substance-induced persisting dementia
    Other (or unknown) substance-induced major neurocognitive disorder, without use disorder

+ **F19.98** Other psychoactive substance use, unspecified with other psychoactive substance-induced disorders

    F19.980 Other psychoactive substance use, unspecified with psychoactive substance-induced anxiety disorder
        Other (or unknown) substance-induced anxiety disorder, without use disorder

    F19.981 Other psychoactive substance use, unspecified with psychoactive substance-induced sexual dysfunction
        Other (or unknown) substance-induced sexual dysfunction, without use disorder

    F19.982 Other psychoactive substance use, unspecified with psychoactive substance-induced sleep disorder
        Other (or unknown) substance-induced sleep disorder, without use disorder

    F19.988 Other psychoactive substance use, unspecified with other psychoactive substance-induced disorder
        Other (or unknown) substance-induced mild neurocognitive disorder, without use disorder
        Other (or unknown) substance-induced obsessive-compulsive or related disorder, without use disorder

F19.99 Other psychoactive substance use, unspecified with unspecified psychoactive substance-induced disorder

Schizophrenia, schizotypal, delusional, and other non-mood psychotic disorders (F20-F29)

F20 Schizophrenia
    Excludes1: *brief psychotic disorder (F23)*
        cyclic schizophrenia (F25.0)
        mood [affective] disorders with psychotic symptoms (F30.2, F31.2, F31.5, F31.64, F32.3, F33.3)
        schizoaffective disorder (F25.-)
        schizophrenic reaction NOS (F23)
    Excludes2: *schizophrenic reaction in:*
        alcoholism (F10.15-, F10.25-, F10.95-)
        brain disease (F06.2)
        epilepsy (F06.2)
        psychoactive drug use (F11-F19 with .15, .25, .95)
        schizotypal disorder (F21)

CC **F20.0** **Paranoid schizophrenia**
　　Paraphrenic schizophrenia
　　Excludes1: *involutional paranoid state (F22)*
　　　　　　paranoia (F22)
CC **F20.1** **Disorganized schizophrenia**
　　Hebephrenic schizophrenia
　　Hebephrenia
CC **F20.2** **Catatonic schizophrenia**
　　Schizophrenic catalepsy
　　Schizophrenic catatonia
　　Schizophrenic flexibilitas cerea
　　Excludes1: *catatonic stupor (R40.1)*
　　F20.3 **Undifferentiated schizophrenia**
　　Atypical schizophrenia
　　Excludes1: *acute schizophrenia-like psychotic disorder*
　　　　　　(F23)
　　Excludes2: *post-schizophrenic depression (F32.89)*
CC **F20.5** **Residual schizophrenia**
　　Restzustand (schizophrenic)
　　Schizophrenic residual state
+ **F20.8** **Other schizophrenia**
CC **F20.81** **Schizophreniform disorder**
　　　Schizophreniform psychosis NOS
CC **F20.89** **Other schizophrenia**
　　　Cenesthopathic schizophrenia
　　　Simple schizophrenia
　　F20.9 **Schizophrenia, unspecified**
　　　AHA CC: 2Q, 2019, 32

F21 **Schizotypal disorder**
　　Borderline schizophrenia
　　Latent schizophrenia
　　Latent schizophrenic reaction
　　Prepsychotic schizophrenia
　　Prodromal schizophrenia
　　Pseudoneurotic schizophrenia
　　Pseudopsychopathic schizophrenia
　　Schizotypal personality disorder
　　Excludes2: *Asperger's syndrome (F84.5)*
　　　　　　schizoid personality disorder (F60.1)
　　Valid 3-character code, no further characters required

F22 **Delusional disorders**
　　Delusional dysmorphophobia
　　Involutional paranoid state
　　Paranoia
　　Paranoia querulans
　　Paranoid psychosis
　　Paranoid state
　　Paraphrenia (late)
　　Sensitiver Beziehungswahn
　　Excludes1: *mood [affective] disorders with psychotic symptoms*
　　　　　　(F30.2, F31.2, F31.5, F31.64, F32.3, F33.3)
　　　　　　paranoid schizophrenia (F20.0)
　　Excludes2: *paranoid personality disorder (F60.0)*
　　　　　　paranoid psychosis, psychogenic (F23)
　　　　　　paranoid reaction (F23)
　　Valid 3-character code, no further characters required

CC **F23** **Brief psychotic disorder**
　　Paranoid reaction
　　Psychogenic paranoid psychosis
　　Excludes2: *mood [affective] disorders with psychotic symptoms*
　　　　　　(F30.2, F31.2, F31.5, F31.64, F32.3, F33.3)
　　Valid 3-character code, no further characters required

F24 **Shared psychotic disorder**
　　Folie à deux
　　Induced paranoid disorder
　　Induced psychotic disorder
　　Valid 3-character code, no further characters required

F25 **Schizoaffective disorders**
　　Excludes1: *mood [affective] disorders with psychotic symptoms*
　　　　　　(F30.2, F31.2, F31.5, F31.64, F32.3, F33.3)
　　　　　　schizophrenia (F20.-)
　　F25.0 **Schizoaffective disorder, bipolar type**
　　　Cyclic schizophrenia
　　　Schizoaffective disorder, manic type
　　　Schizoaffective disorder, mixed type
　　　Schizoaffective psychosis, bipolar type

F25.1 **Schizoaffective disorder, depressive type**
　　Schizoaffective psychosis, depressive type
F25.8 **Other schizoaffective disorders**
F25.9 **Schizoaffective disorder, unspecified**
　　Schizoaffective psychosis NOS

F28 **Other psychotic disorder not due to a substance or known physiological condition**
　　Chronic hallucinatory psychosis
　　Other specified schizophrenia spectrum and other psychotic disorder
　　Valid 3-character code, no further characters required

F29 **Unspecified psychosis not due to a substance or known physiological condition**
　　Psychosis NOS
　　Unspecified schizophrenia spectrum and other psychotic disorder
　　Excludes1: *mental disorder NOS (F99)*
　　　　　　unspecified mental disorder due to known physiological condition (F09)
　　Valid 3-character code, no further characters required

Mood [affective] disorders (F30-F39)

F30 **Manic episode**
　　Includes: bipolar disorder, single manic episode
　　　　　　mixed affective episode
　　Excludes1: *bipolar disorder (F31.-)*
　　　　　　major depressive disorder, single episode (F32.-)
　　　　　　major depressive disorder, recurrent (F33.-)
+ **F30.1** **Manic episode without psychotic symptoms**
CC **F30.10** **Manic episode without psychotic symptoms, unspecified**
CC **F30.11** **Manic episode without psychotic symptoms, mild**
CC **F30.12** **Manic episode without psychotic symptoms, moderate**
CC **F30.13** **Manic episode, severe, without psychotic symptoms**
CC **F30.2** **Manic episode, severe with psychotic symptoms**
　　Manic stupor
　　Mania with mood-congruent psychotic symptoms
　　Mania with mood-incongruent psychotic symptoms
　　F30.3 **Manic episode in partial remission**
　　F30.4 **Manic episode in full remission**
　　F30.8 **Other manic episodes**
　　　Hypomania
CC **F30.9** **Manic episode, unspecified**
　　　Mania NOS

F31 **Bipolar disorder**
　　Includes: bipolar I disorder
　　　　　　bipolar type I disorder
　　　　　　manic-depressive illness
　　　　　　manic-depressive psychosis
　　　　　　manic-depressive reaction
　　Excludes1: *bipolar disorder, single manic episode (F30.-)*
　　　　　　major depressive disorder, single episode (F32.-)
　　　　　　major depressive disorder, recurrent (F33.-)
　　Excludes2: *cyclothymia (F34.0)*
CC **F31.0** **Bipolar disorder, current episode hypomanic**
+ **F31.1** **Bipolar disorder, current episode manic without psychotic features**
CC **F31.10** **Bipolar disorder, current episode manic without psychotic features, unspecified**
CC **F31.11** **Bipolar disorder, current episode manic without psychotic features, mild**
CC **F31.12** **Bipolar disorder, current episode manic without psychotic features, moderate**
CC **F31.13** **Bipolar disorder, current episode manic without psychotic features, severe**
CC **F31.2** **Bipolar disorder, current episode manic severe with psychotic features**
　　Bipolar disorder, current episode manic with mood-congruent psychotic symptoms
　　Bipolar disorder, current episode manic with mood-incongruent psychotic symptoms
　　Bipolar I disorder, current or most recent episode manic, with psychotic features

+, +7th, X + 7th　●Newborn　●Pediatric　●Maternity　●Adult　♀Female　♂Male　Manifestation　Unacceptable PDX　HCC　CC　MCC　HAC

+ **F31.3** **Bipolar disorder, current episode depressed, mild or moderate severity**
   CC **F31.30** **Bipolar disorder, current episode depressed, mild or moderate severity, unspecified**
   CC **F31.31** **Bipolar disorder, current episode depressed, mild**
   CC **F31.32** **Bipolar disorder, current episode depressed, moderate**
CC **F31.4** **Bipolar disorder, current episode depressed, severe, without psychotic features**
CC **F31.5** **Bipolar disorder, current episode depressed, severe, with psychotic features**
   Bipolar disorder, current episode depressed with mood-incongruent psychotic symptoms
   Bipolar disorder, current episode depressed with mood-congruent psychotic symptoms
   Bipolar I disorder, current or most recent episode depressed, with psychotic features
+ **F31.6** **Bipolar disorder, current episode mixed**
   CC **F31.60** **Bipolar disorder, current episode mixed, unspecified**
   CC **F31.61** **Bipolar disorder, current episode mixed, mild**
   CC **F31.62** **Bipolar disorder, current episode mixed, moderate**
   CC **F31.63** **Bipolar disorder, current episode mixed, severe, without psychotic features**
   CC **F31.64** **Bipolar disorder, current episode mixed, severe, with psychotic features**
      Bipolar disorder, current episode mixed with mood-congruent psychotic symptoms
      Bipolar disorder, current episode mixed with mood-incongruent psychotic symptoms
+ **F31.7** **Bipolar disorder, currently in remission**
   F31.70 **Bipolar disorder, currently in remission, most recent episode unspecified**
   F31.71 **Bipolar disorder, in partial remission, most recent episode hypomanic**
   F31.72 **Bipolar disorder, in full remission, most recent episode hypomanic**
   F31.73 **Bipolar disorder, in partial remission, most recent episode manic**
   F31.74 **Bipolar disorder, in full remission, most recent episode manic**
   F31.75 **Bipolar disorder, in partial remission, most recent episode depressed**
   F31.76 **Bipolar disorder, in full remission, most recent episode depressed**
   F31.77 **Bipolar disorder, in partial remission, most recent episode mixed**
   F31.78 **Bipolar disorder, in full remission, most recent episode mixed**
+ **F31.8** **Other bipolar disorders**
   CC **F31.81** **Bipolar II disorder**
      Bipolar disorder, type 2
   CC **F31.89** **Other bipolar disorder**
      Recurrent manic episodes NOS
F31.9 **Bipolar disorder, unspecified**
   Manic depression
   AHA CC: 1Q, 2020, 23

F32 **Major depressive disorder, single episode**

   Includes: single episode of agitated depression
            single episode of depressive reaction
            single episode of major depression
            single episode of psychogenic depression
            single episode of reactive depression
            single episode of vital depression
   Excludes1: bipolar disorder (F31.-)
           manic episode (F30.-)
           recurrent depressive disorder (F33.-)
   Excludes2: adjustment disorder (F43.2)
CC **F32.0** **Major depressive disorder, single episode, mild**
CC **F32.1** **Major depressive disorder, single episode, moderate**
CC **F32.2** **Major depressive disorder, single episode, severe without psychotic features**

CC **F32.3** **Major depressive disorder, single episode, severe with psychotic features**
   Single episode of major depression with mood-congruent psychotic symptoms
   Single episode of major depression with mood-incongruent psychotic symptoms
   Single episode of major depression with psychotic symptoms
   Single episode of psychogenic depressive psychosis
   Single episode of psychotic depression
   Single episode of reactive depressive psychosis
F32.4 **Major depressive disorder, single episode, in partial remission**
F32.5 **Major depressive disorder, single episode, in full remission**
+ **F32.8** **Other depressive episodes**
   AHA CC: 4Q, 2016, 14
   ♀ **F32.81** **Premenstrual dysphoric disorder**
      Excludes1: premenstrual tension syndrome (N94.3)
   F32.89 **Other specified depressive episodes**
      Atypical depression
      Post-schizophrenic depression
      Single episode of 'masked' depression NOS
F32.9 **Major depressive disorder, single episode, unspecified**
   Depression NOS
   Depressive disorder NOS
   Major depression NOS
   AHA CC: 4Q, 2013, 107-108

F33 **Major depressive disorder, recurrent**

   Includes: recurrent episodes of depressive reaction
           recurrent episodes of endogenous depression
           recurrent episodes of major depression
           recurrent episodes of psychogenic depression
           recurrent episodes of reactive depression
           recurrent episodes of seasonal depressive disorder
           recurrent episodes of vital depression
   Excludes1: bipolar disorder (F31.-)
           manic episode (F30.-)
CC **F33.0** **Major depressive disorder, recurrent, mild**
CC **F33.1** **Major depressive disorder, recurrent, moderate**
CC **F33.2** **Major depressive disorder, recurrent severe without psychotic features**
CC **F33.3** **Major depressive disorder, recurrent, severe with psychotic symptoms**
   Endogenous depression with psychotic symptoms
   Major depressive disorder, recurrent, with psychotic features
   Recurrent severe episodes of major depression with mood-congruent psychotic symptoms
   Recurrent severe episodes of major depression with mood-incongruent psychotic symptoms
   Recurrent severe episodes of major depression with psychotic symptoms
   Recurrent severe episodes of psychogenic depressive psychosis
   Recurrent severe episodes of psychotic depression
   Recurrent severe episodes of reactive depressive psychosis
+ **F33.4** **Major depressive disorder, recurrent, in remission**
   CC **F33.40** **Major depressive disorder, recurrent, in remission, unspecified**
   F33.41 **Major depressive disorder, recurrent, in partial remission**
   F33.42 **Major depressive disorder, recurrent, in full remission**
CC **F33.8** **Other recurrent depressive disorders**
   Recurrent brief depressive episodes
CC **F33.9** **Major depressive disorder, recurrent, unspecified**
   Monopolar depression NOS

F34 **Persistent mood [affective] disorders**

   F34.0 **Cyclothymic disorder**
      Affective personality disorder
      Cycloid personality
      Cyclothymia
      Cyclothymic personality

F34.1 Dysthymic disorder
Depressive neurosis
Depressive personality disorder
Dysthymia
Neurotic depression
Persistent depressive disorder
Persistent anxiety depression
Excludes2: anxiety depression (mild or not persistent) (F41.8)

+ **F34.8 Other persistent mood [affective] disorders**
AHA CC: 4Q, 2016, 14
CC **F34.81 Disruptive mood dysregulation disorder**
CC **F34.89 Other specified persistent mood disorders**
CC **F34.9 Persistent mood [affective] disorder, unspecified**

F39 Unspecified mood [affective] disorder
Affective psychosis NOS
Valid 3-character code, no further characters required

Anxiety, dissociative, stress-related, somatoform and other nonpsychotic mental disorders (F40-F48)

F40 Phobic anxiety disorders
+ **F40.0 Agoraphobia**
F40.00 Agoraphobia, unspecified
F40.01 Agoraphobia with panic disorder
Panic disorder with agoraphobia
Excludes1: panic disorder without agoraphobia (F41.0)
F40.02 Agoraphobia without panic disorder
+ **F40.1 Social phobias**
Anthropophobia
Social anxiety disorder
Social anxiety disorder of childhood
Social neurosis
F40.10 Social phobia, unspecified
F40.11 Social phobia, generalized
+ **F40.2 Specific (isolated) phobias**
Excludes2: dysmorphophobia (nondelusional) (F45.22)
nosophobia (F45.22)
+ **F40.21 Animal type phobia**
F40.210 Arachnophobia
Fear of spiders
F40.218 Other animal type phobia
+ **F40.22 Natural environment type phobia**
F40.220 Fear of thunderstorms
F40.228 Other natural environment type phobia
+ **F40.23 Blood, injection, injury type phobia**
F40.230 Fear of blood
F40.231 Fear of injections and transfusions
F40.232 Fear of other medical care
F40.233 Fear of injury
+ **F40.24 Situational type phobia**
F40.240 Claustrophobia
F40.241 Acrophobia
F40.242 Fear of bridges
F40.243 Fear of flying
F40.248 Other situational type phobia
+ **F40.29 Other specified phobia**
F40.290 Androphobia
Fear of men
F40.291 Gynephobia
Fear of women
F40.298 Other specified phobia
F40.8 Other phobic anxiety disorders
Phobic anxiety disorder of childhood
F40.9 Phobic anxiety disorder, unspecified
Phobia NOS
Phobic state NOS

F41 Other anxiety disorders
Excludes2: anxiety in:
acute stress reaction (F43.0)
transient adjustment reaction (F43.2)
neurasthenia (F48.8)
psychophysiologic disorders (F45.-)
separation anxiety (F93.0)

F41.0 Panic disorder [episodic paroxysmal anxiety]
Panic attack
Panic state
Excludes1: panic disorder with agoraphobia (F40.01)
F41.1 Generalized anxiety disorder
Anxiety neurosis
Anxiety reaction
Anxiety state
Overanxious disorder
Excludes2: neurasthenia (F48.8)
F41.3 Other mixed anxiety disorders
F41.8 Other specified anxiety disorders
Anxiety depression (mild or not persistent)
Anxiety hysteria
Mixed anxiety and depressive disorder
F41.9 Anxiety disorder, unspecified
Anxiety NOS

F42 Obsessive-compulsive disorder
Excludes2: obsessive-compulsive personality (disorder) (F60.5)
obsessive-compulsive symptoms occurring in depression (F32-F33)
obsessive-compulsive symptoms occurring in schizophrenia (F20.-)
AHA CC: 4Q, 2016, 14-15
F42.2 Mixed obsessional thoughts and acts
F42.3 Hoarding disorder
F42.4 Excoriation (skin-picking) disorder
Excludes1: factitial dermatitis (L98.1)
other specified behavioral and emotional disorders with onset usually occurring in early childhood and adolescence (F98.8)
F42.8 Other obsessive compulsive disorder
Anancastic neurosis
Obsessive-compulsive neurosis
F42.9 Obsessive-compulsive disorder, unspecified

F43 Reaction to severe stress, and adjustment disorders
F43.0 Acute stress reaction
Acute crisis reaction
Acute reaction to stress
Combat and operational stress reaction
Combat fatigue
Crisis state
Psychic shock
+ **F43.1 Post-traumatic stress disorder (PTSD)**
Traumatic neurosis
F43.10 Post-traumatic stress disorder, unspecified
F43.11 Post-traumatic stress disorder, acute
F43.12 Post-traumatic stress disorder, chronic
+ **F43.2 Adjustment disorders**
Culture shock
Grief reaction
Hospitalism in children
Excludes2: separation anxiety disorder of childhood (F93.0)
F43.20 Adjustment disorder, unspecified
F43.21 Adjustment disorder with depressed mood
AHA CC: 1Q, 2014, 25
F43.22 Adjustment disorder with anxiety
F43.23 Adjustment disorder with mixed anxiety and depressed mood
F43.24 Adjustment disorder with disturbance of conduct
F43.25 Adjustment disorder with mixed disturbance of emotions and conduct
F43.29 Adjustment disorder with other symptoms
F43.8 Other reactions to severe stress
Other specified trauma and stressor-related disorder
F43.9 Reaction to severe stress, unspecified
Trauma and stressor-related disorder, NOS

F44 Dissociative and conversion disorders
Includes: conversion hysteria
conversion reaction
hysteria
hysterical psychosis
Excludes2: malingering [conscious simulation] (Z76.5)

F44.0   Dissociative amnesia
    Excludes1: *amnesia NOS (R41.3)*
        anterograde amnesia (R41.1)
        dissociative amnesia with dissociative fugue
          (F44.1)
        retrograde amnesia (R41.2)
    Excludes2: *alcohol-or other psychoactive substance-*
        induced amnestic disorder (F10, F13, F19
        with .26, .96)
        amnestic disorder due to known physiological
        condition (F04)
        postictal amnesia in epilepsy (G40.-)

F44.1   Dissociative fugue
    Dissociative amnesia with dissociative fugue
    Excludes2: *postictal fugue in epilepsy (G40.-)*

F44.2   Dissociative stupor
    Excludes1: *catatonic stupor (R40.1)*
        stupor NOS (R40.1)
    Excludes2: *catatonic disorder due to known physiological*
        condition (F06.1)
        depressive stupor (F32, F33)
        manic stupor (F30, F31)

F44.4   Conversion disorder with motor symptom or deficit
    Conversion disorder with abnormal movement
    Conversion disorder with speech symptoms
    Conversion disorder with swallowing symptoms
    Conversion disorder with weakness/paralysis
    Dissociative motor disorders
    Psychogenic aphonia
    Psychogenic dysphonia

F44.5   Conversion disorder with seizures or convulsions
    Conversion disorder with attacks or seizures
    Dissociative convulsions
    AHA CC: 1Q, 2019, 19

F44.6   Conversion disorder with sensory symptom or deficit
    Conversion disorder with anesthesia or sensory loss
    Conversion disorder with special sensory symptoms
    Dissociative anesthesia and sensory loss
    Psychogenic deafness

F44.7   Conversion disorder with mixed symptom presentation

+ F44.8   Other dissociative and conversion disorders
    F44.81   Dissociative identity disorder
        Multiple personality disorder
    F44.89   Other dissociative and conversion disorders
        Ganser's syndrome
        Psychogenic confusion
        Psychogenic twilight state
        Trance and possession disorders

F44.9   Dissociative and conversion disorder, unspecified
    Dissociative disorder NOS

F45   Somatoform disorders

    Excludes2: *dissociative and conversion disorders (F44.-)*
        factitious disorders (F68.1-, F68.A)
        hair-plucking (F63.3)
        lalling (F80.0)
        lisping (F80.0)
        malingering [conscious simulation] (Z76.5)
        nail-biting (F98.8)
        psychological or behavioral factors associated with
        disorders or diseases classified elsewhere (F54)
        sexual dysfunction, not due to a substance or known
        physiological condition (F52.-)
        thumb-sucking (F98.8)
        tic disorders (in childhood and adolescence) (F95.-)
        Tourette's syndrome (F95.2)
        trichotillomania (F63.3)

F45.0   Somatization disorder
    Briquet's disorder
    Multiple psychosomatic disorder

F45.1   Undifferentiated somatoform disorder
    Somatic symptom disorder
    Undifferentiated psychosomatic disorder

+ F45.2   Hypochondriacal disorders
    Excludes2: *delusional dysmorphophobia (F22)*
        fixed delusions about bodily functions or
        shape (F22)

F45.20   Hypochondriacal disorder, unspecified
F45.21   Hypochondriasis
    Hypochondriacal neurosis
    Illness anxiety disorder
F45.22   Body dysmorphic disorder
    Dysmorphophobia (nondelusional)
    Nosophobia
F45.29   Other hypochondriacal disorders

+ F45.4   Pain disorders related to psychological factors
    Excludes1: *pain NOS (R52)*
    F45.41   Pain disorder exclusively related to psychological
        factors
        Somatoform pain disorder (persistent)
        Review coding guideline C.5.a
    F45.42   Pain disorder with related psychological factors
        Code also associated acute or chronic
          pain (G89.-)
        Review coding guideline C.5.a

F45.8   Other somatoform disorders
    Psychogenic dysmenorrhea
    Psychogenic dysphagia, including 'globus hystericus'
    Psychogenic pruritus
    Psychogenic torticollis
    Somatoform autonomic dysfunction
    Teeth grinding
    Excludes1: *sleep related teeth grinding (G47.63)*

F45.9   Somatoform disorder, unspecified
    Psychosomatic disorder NOS

F48   Other nonpsychotic mental disorders

F48.1   Depersonalization-derealization syndrome
F48.2   Pseudobulbar affect
    Involuntary emotional expression disorder
    Code first underlying cause, if known, such as:
        amyotrophic lateral sclerosis (G12.21)
        multiple sclerosis (G35)
        sequelae of cerebrovascular disease (I69.-)
        sequelae of traumatic intracranial injury (S06.-)
F48.8   Other specified nonpsychotic mental disorders
    Dhat syndrome
    Neurasthenia
    Occupational neurosis, including writer's cramp
    Psychasthenia
    Psychasthenic neurosis
    Psychogenic syncope
F48.9   Nonpsychotic mental disorder, unspecified
    Neurosis NOS

Behavioral syndromes associated with physiological disturbances and physical factors (F50-F59)

F50   Eating disorders

    Excludes1: *anorexia NOS (R63.0)*
        feeding difficulties (R63.3)
        feeding problems of newborn (P92.-)
        polyphagia (R63.2)
    Excludes2: *feeding disorder in infancy or childhood (F98.2-)*

+ F50.0   Anorexia nervosa
    Excludes1: *loss of appetite (R63.0)*
        psychogenic loss of appetite (F50.89)
    CC **F50.00   Anorexia nervosa, unspecified**
    CC **F50.01   Anorexia nervosa, restricting type**
    CC **F50.02   Anorexia nervosa, binge eating/purging type**
        Excludes1: *bulimia nervosa (F50.2)*

CC **F50.2   Bulimia nervosa**
    Bulimia NOS
    Hyperorexia nervosa
    Excludes1: *anorexia nervosa, binge eating/purging type*
        (F50.02)

+ F50.8   Other eating disorders
    Excludes2: *pica of infancy and childhood (F98.3)*
    AHA CC: 4Q, 2016, 15-16
    F50.81   Binge eating disorder
    F50.82   Avoidant/restrictive food intake disorder
        AHA CC: 4Q, 2017, 9
    F50.89   Other specified eating disorder
        Pica in adults
        Psychogenic loss of appetite

F50.9   Eating disorder, unspecified
Atypical anorexia nervosa
Atypical bulimia nervosa
Feeding or eating disorder, unspecified
Other specified feeding disorder

F51   Sleep disorders not due to a substance or known physiological condition

Excludes2: organic sleep disorders (G47.-)

+ **F51.0   Insomnia not due to a substance or known physiological condition**

Excludes2: alcohol related insomnia (F10.182, F10.282, F10.982)
drug-related insomnia (F11.182, F11.282, F11.982, F13.182, F13.282, F13.982, F14.182, F14.282, F14.982, F15.182, F15.282, F15.982, F19.182, F19.282, F19.982)
insomnia NOS (G47.0-)
insomnia due to known physiological condition (G47.0-)
organic insomnia (G47.0-)
sleep deprivation (Z72.820)

F51.01   Primary insomnia
Idiopathic insomnia

F51.02   Adjustment insomnia

F51.03   Paradoxical insomnia

F51.04   Psychophysiologic insomnia

F51.05   Insomnia due to other mental disorder
Code also associated mental disorder

F51.09   Other insomnia not due to a substance or known physiological condition

+ **F51.1   Hypersomnia not due to a substance or known physiological condition**

Excludes2: alcohol related hypersomnia (F10.182, F10.282, F10.982)
drug-related hypersomnia (F11.182, F11.282, F11.982, F13.182, F13.282, F13.982, F14.182, F14.282, F14.982, F15.182, F15.282, F15.982, F19.182, F19.282, F19.982)
hypersomnia NOS (G47.10)
hypersomnia due to known physiological condition (G47.10)
idiopathic hypersomnia (G47.11, G47.12)
narcolepsy (G47.4-)

F51.11   Primary hypersomnia

F51.12   Insufficient sleep syndrome
Excludes1: sleep deprivation (Z72.820)

F51.13   Hypersomnia due to other mental disorder
Code also associated mental disorder

F51.19   Other hypersomnia not due to a substance or known physiological condition

F51.3   Sleepwalking [somnambulism]
Non-rapid eye movement sleep arousal disorders, sleepwalking type

F51.4   Sleep terrors [night terrors]
Non-rapid eye movement sleep arousal disorders, sleep terror type

F51.5   Nightmare disorder
Dream anxiety disorder

F51.8   Other sleep disorders not due to a substance or known physiological condition

F51.9   Sleep disorder not due to a substance or known physiological condition, unspecified
Emotional sleep disorder NOS

F52   Sexual dysfunction not due to a substance or known physiological condition

Excludes2: Dhat syndrome (F48.8)

F52.0   Hypoactive sexual desire disorder
Lack or loss of sexual desire
Male hypoactive sexual desire disorder
Sexual anhedonia
Excludes1: decreased libido (R68.82)

F52.1   Sexual aversion disorder
Sexual aversion and lack of sexual enjoyment

+ **F52.2   Sexual arousal disorders**
Failure of genital response

♂ **F52.21   Male erectile disorder**
Erectile disorder
Psychogenic impotence
Excludes1: impotence of organic origin (N52.-)
impotence NOS (N52.-)

♀ **F52.22   Female sexual arousal disorder**
Female sexual interest/arousal disorder

+ **F52.3   Orgasmic disorder**
Inhibited orgasm
Psychogenic anorgasmy

♀ **F52.31   Female orgasmic disorder**

♂ **F52.32   Male orgasmic disorder**
Delayed ejaculation

♂ **F52.4   Premature ejaculation**

♀ **F52.5   Vaginismus not due to a substance or known physiological condition**
Psychogenic vaginismus
Excludes2: vaginismus (due to a known physiological condition) (N94.2)

F52.6   Dyspareunia not due to a substance or known physiological condition
Genito-pelvic pain penetration disorder
Psychogenic dyspareunia
Excludes2: dyspareunia (due to a known physiological condition) (N94.1-)

F52.8   Other sexual dysfunction not due to a substance or known physiological condition
Excessive sexual drive
Nymphomania
Satyriasis

F52.9   Unspecified sexual dysfunction not due to a substance or known physiological condition
Sexual dysfunction NOS

F53   Mental and behavioral disorders associated with the puerperium, not elsewhere classified

Excludes1: mood disorders with psychotic features (F30.2, F31.2, F31.5, F31.64, F32.3, F33.3)
postpartum dysphoria (O90.6)
psychosis in schizophrenia, schizotypal, delusional, and other psychotic disorders (F20-F29)
AHA CC: 4Q, 2018, 8-9

●♀ **F53.0   Postpartum depression**
Postnatal depression, NOS
Postpartum depression, NOS

●♀ **F53.1   Puerperal psychosis**
Postpartum psychosis
Puerperal psychosis, NOS

F54   Psychological and behavioral factors associated with disorders or diseases classified elsewhere

Psychological factors affecting physical conditions
Code first the associated physical disorder, such as:
asthma (J45.-)
dermatitis (L23-L25)
gastric ulcer (K25.-)
mucous colitis (K58.-)
ulcerative colitis (K51.-)
urticaria (L50.-)
Excludes2: tension-type headache (G44.2)
Valid 3-character code, no further characters required

F55   Abuse of non-psychoactive substances

Excludes2: abuse of psychoactive substances (F10-F19)

F55.0   Abuse of antacids

F55.1   Abuse of herbal or folk remedies

F55.2   Abuse of laxatives

F55.3   Abuse of steroids or hormones

F55.4   Abuse of vitamins

F55.8   Abuse of other non-psychoactive substances

F59   Unspecified behavioral syndromes associated with physiological disturbances and physical factors

Psychogenic physiological dysfunction NOS
Valid 3-character code, no further characters required

F60 Specific personality disorders

F60.0 Paranoid personality disorder
Expansive paranoid personality (disorder)
Fanatic personality (disorder)
Querulant personality (disorder)
Paranoid personality (disorder)
Sensitive paranoid personality (disorder)
Excludes2: *paranoia (F22)*
paranoia querulans (F22)
paranoid psychosis (F22)
paranoid schizophrenia (F20.0)
paranoid state (F22)

F60.1 Schizoid personality disorder
Excludes2: *Asperger's syndrome (F84.5)*
delusional disorder (F22)
schizoid disorder of childhood (F84.5)
schizophrenia (F20.-)
schizotypal disorder (F21)

F60.2 Antisocial personality disorder
Amoral personality (disorder)
Asocial personality (disorder)
Dissocial personality disorder
Psychopathic personality (disorder)
Sociopathic personality (disorder)
Excludes1: *conduct disorders (F91.-)*
Excludes2: *borderline personality disorder (F60.3)*

F60.3 Borderline personality disorder
Aggressive personality (disorder)
Emotionally unstable personality disorder
Explosive personality (disorder)
Excludes2: *antisocial personality disorder (F60.2)*

F60.4 Histrionic personality disorder
Hysterical personality (disorder)
Psychoinfantile personality (disorder)

F60.5 Obsessive-compulsive personality disorder
Anankastic personality (disorder)
Compulsive personality (disorder)
Obsessional personality (disorder)
Excludes2: *obsessive-compulsive disorder (F42.-)*

F60.6 Avoidant personality disorder
Anxious personality disorder

F60.7 Dependent personality disorder
Asthenic personality (disorder)
Inadequate personality (disorder)
Passive personality (disorder)

+ F60.8 Other specific personality disorders
F60.81 Narcissistic personality disorder
F60.89 Other specific personality disorders
Eccentric personality disorder
'Haltlose' type personality disorder
Immature personality disorder
Passive-aggressive personality disorder
Psychoneurotic personality disorder
Self-defeating personality disorder

F60.9 Personality disorder, unspecified
Character disorder NOS
Character neurosis NOS
Pathological personality NOS

F63 Impulse disorders

Excludes2: *habitual excessive use of alcohol or psychoactive substances (F10-F19)*
impulse disorders involving sexual behavior (F65.-)

F63.0 Pathological gambling
Compulsive gambling
Gambling disorder
Excludes1: *gambling and betting NOS (Z72.6)*
Excludes2: *excessive gambling by manic patients (F30, F31)*
gambling in antisocial personality disorder (F60.2)

F63.1 Pyromania
Pathological fire-setting
Excludes2: *fire-setting (by) (in):*
adult with antisocial personality disorder (F60.2)
alcohol or psychoactive substance intoxication (F10-F19)
conduct disorders (F91.-)
mental disorders due to known physiological condition (F01-F09)
schizophrenia (F20.-)

F63.2 Kleptomania
Pathological stealing
Excludes1: *shoplifting as the reason for observation for suspected mental disorder (Z03.8)*
Excludes2: *depressive disorder with stealing (F31-F33)*
stealing due to underlying mental condition-code to mental condition
stealing in mental disorders due to known physiological condition (F01-F09)

F63.3 Trichotillomania
Hair plucking
Excludes2: *other stereotyped movement disorder (F98.4)*

+ F63.8 Other impulse disorders
F63.81 Intermittent explosive disorder
F63.89 Other impulse disorders

F63.9 Impulse disorder, unspecified
Impulse control disorder NOS

F64 Gender identity disorders

AHA CC: 4Q, 2016, 16

F64.0 Transsexualism
Gender identify disorder in adolescence and adulthood
Gender dysphoria in adolescents and adults

F64.1 Dual role transvestism
Use additional code to identify sex reassignment status (Z87.890)
Excludes1: *gender identity disorder in childhood (F64.2)*
Excludes2: *fetishistic transvestism (F65.1)*

F64.2 Gender identity disorder of childhood
Gender dysphoria in children
Excludes1: *gender identity disorder in adolescence and adulthood (F64.0)*
Excludes2: *sexual maturation disorder (F66)*

F64.8 Other gender identity disorders
Other specified gender dysphoria

F64.9 Gender identity disorder, unspecified
Gender dysphoria, unspecified
Gender-role disorder NOS

F65 Paraphilias

F65.0 Fetishism
Fetishistic disorder

F65.1 Transvestic fetishism
Fetishistic transvestism
Transvestic disorder

F65.2 Exhibitionism
Exhibitionistic disorder

F65.3 Voyeurism
Voyeuristic disorder

F65.4 Pedophilia
Pedophilic disorder

+ F65.5 Sadomasochism
F65.50 Sadomasochism, unspecified
F65.51 Sexual masochism
Sexual masochism disorder
F65.52 Sexual sadism
Sexual sadism disorder

+ F65.8 Other paraphilias
F65.81 Frotteurism
Frotteuristic disorder
F65.89 Other paraphilias
Necrophilia
Other specified paraphilic disorder

F65.9 Paraphilia, unspecified
Paraphillic disorder, unspecified
Sexual deviation NOS

F66 Other sexual disorders

Sexual maturation disorder
Sexual relationship disorder
Valid 3-character code, no further characters required

F68 Other disorders of adult personality and behavior

+ F68.1 Factitious disorder imposed on self
Compensation neurosis
Elaboration of physical symptoms for psychological reasons
Hospital hopper syndrome
Münchausen's syndrome
Peregrinating patient
Excludes2: *factitial dermatitis (L98.1)*
person feigning illness (with obvious motivation) (Z76.5)
AHA CC: 4Q, 2018, 9
Review coding guideline C.5.c

CC F68.10 Factitious disorder imposed on self, unspecified

F68.11 Factitious disorder imposed on self with predominantly psychological signs and symptoms

CC F68.12 Factitious disorder imposed on self with predominantly physical signs and symptoms

F68.13 Factitious disorder imposed on self with combined psychological and physical signs and symptoms

CC F68.A Factitious disorder imposed on another

Factitious disorder by proxy

Münchaüsen's by proxy

AHA CC: 4Q, 2018, 9

Review coding guideline C.5.c

F68.8 Other specified disorders of adult personality and behavior

● **F69** Unspecified disorder of adult personality and behavior

Valid 3-character code, no further characters required

Intellectual Disabilities (F70-F79)

Code first any associated physical or developmental disorders

Excludes1: *borderline intellectual functioning, IQ above 70 to 84 (R41.83)*

F70 Mild intellectual disabilities

IQ level 50-55 to approximately 70

Mild mental subnormality

Valid 3-character code, no further characters required

F71 Moderate intellectual disabilities

IQ level 35-40 to 50-55

Moderate mental subnormality

Valid 3-character code, no further characters required

CC F72 Severe intellectual disabilities

IQ 20-25 to 35-40

Severe mental subnormality

Valid 3-character code, no further characters required

CC F73 Profound intellectual disabilities

IQ level below 20-25

Profound mental subnormality

Valid 3-character code, no further characters required

F78 Other intellectual disabilities

Valid 3-character code, no further characters required

F79 Unspecified intellectual disabilities

Mental deficiency NOS

Mental subnormality NOS

Valid 3-character code, no further characters required

Pervasive and specific developmental disorders (F80-F89)

F80 Specific developmental disorders of speech and language

F80.0 Phonological disorder

Dyslalia

Functional speech articulation disorder

Lalling

Lisping

Phonological developmental disorder

Speech articulation developmental disorder

Speech-sound disorder

Excludes1: *speech articulation impairment due to aphasia NOS (R47.01)*

speech articulation impairment due to apraxia (R48.2)

Excludes2: *speech articulation impairment due to hearing loss (F80.4)*

speech articulation impairment due to intellectual disabilities (F70-F79)

speech articulation impairment with expressive language developmental disorder (F80.1)

speech articulation impairment with mixed receptive expressive language developmental disorder (F80.2)

F80.1 Expressive language disorder

Developmental dysphasia or aphasia, expressive type

Excludes1: *mixed receptive-expressive language disorder (F80.2)*

dysphasia and aphasia NOS (R47.-)

Excludes2: *acquired aphasia with epilepsy [Landau-Kleffner] (G40.80-)*

selective mutism (F94.0)

intellectual disabilities (F70-F79)

pervasive developmental disorders (F84.-)

F80.2 Mixed receptive-expressive language disorder

Developmental dysphasia or aphasia, receptive type

Developmental Wernicke's aphasia

Excludes1: *central auditory processing disorder (H93.25)*

dysphasia or aphasia NOS (R47.-)

expressive language disorder (F80.1)

expressive type dysphasia or aphasia (F80.1)

word deafness (H93.25)

Excludes2: *acquired aphasia with epilepsy [Landau-Kleffner] (G40.80-)*

pervasive developmental disorders (F84.-)

selective mutism (F94.0)

intellectual disabilities (F70-F79)

F80.4 Speech and language development delay due to hearing loss

Code also type of hearing loss (H90.-, H91.-)

+ **F80.8** Other developmental disorders of speech and language

F80.81 Childhood onset fluency disorder

Cluttering NOS

Stuttering NOS

Excludes1: *adult onset fluency disorder (F98.5)*

fluency disorder in conditions classified elsewhere (R47.82)

fluency disorder (stuttering) following cerebrovascular disease (I69. with final characters -23)

F80.82 Social pragmatic communication disorder

Excludes1: *Asperger's syndrome (F84.5)*

autistic disorder (F84.0)

AHA CC: 4Q, 2016, 16

F80.89 Other developmental disorders of speech and language

AHA CC: 1Q, 2017, 27-28

F80.9 Developmental disorder of speech and language, unspecified

Communication disorder NOS

Language disorder NOS

F81 Specific developmental disorders of scholastic skills

F81.0 Specific reading disorder

'Backward reading'

Developmental dyslexia

Specific learning disorder, with impairment in reading

Specific reading retardation

Excludes1: *alexia NOS (R48.0)*

dyslexia NOS (R48.0)

F81.2 Mathematics disorder

Developmental acalculia

Developmental arithmetical disorder

Developmental Gerstmann's syndrome

Specific learning disorder, with impairment in mathematics

Excludes1: *acalculia NOS (R48.8)*

Excludes2: *arithmetical difficulties associated with a reading disorder (F81.0)*

arithmetical difficulties associated with a spelling disorder (F81.81)

arithmetical difficulties due to inadequate teaching (Z55.8)

+ **F81.8** Other developmental disorders of scholastic skills

F81.81 Disorder of written expression

Specific learning disorder, with impairment in written expression

Specific spelling disorder

F81.89 Other developmental disorders of scholastic skills

F81.9 Developmental disorder of scholastic skills, unspecified

Knowledge acquisition disability NOS

Learning disability NOS

Learning disorder NOS

F82 Specific developmental disorder of motor function

Clumsy child syndrome

Developmental coordination disorder

Developmental dyspraxia

Excludes1: *abnormalities of gait and mobility (R26.-)*

lack of coordination (R27.-)

Excludes2: *lack of coordination secondary to intellectual disabilities (F70-F79)*

Valid 3-character code, no further characters required

+, +7th, X + 7th   ● Newborn   ● Pediatric   ● Maternity   ● Adult   ♀ Female   ♂ Male   Manifestation   Unacceptable PDX   HCC   CC   MCC   HAC

F84   Pervasive developmental disorders

Use additional code to identify any associated medical condition and intellectual disabilities.

CC **F84.0   Autistic disorder**

Autism spectrum disorder
Infantile autism
Infantile psychosis
Kanner's syndrome
Excludes1: *Asperger's syndrome (F84.5)*
AHA CC: 1Q, 2017, 27-28

CC **F84.2   Rett's syndrome**

Excludes1: *Asperger's syndrome (F84.5)*
Autistic disorder (F84.0)
Other childhood disintegrative disorder (F84.3)

● CC **F84.3   Other childhood disintegrative disorder**

Dementia infantilis
Disintegrative psychosis
Heller's syndrome
Symbiotic psychosis
Use additional code to identify any associated neurological condition.
Excludes1: *Asperger's syndrome (F84.5)*
Autistic disorder (F84.0)
Rett's syndrome (F84.2)

CC **F84.5   Asperger's syndrome**

Asperger's disorder
Autistic psychopathy
Schizoid disorder of childhood

CC **F84.8   Other pervasive developmental disorders**

Overactive disorder associated with intellectual disabilities and stereotyped movements

CC **F84.9   Pervasive developmental disorder, unspecified**

Atypical autism

F88   Other disorders of psychological development

Developmental agnosia
Global developmental delay
Other specified neurodevelopmental disorder
Valid 3-character code, no further characters required

F89   Unspecified disorder of psychological development

Developmental disorder NOS
Neurodevelopmental disorder NOS
Valid 3-character code, no further characters required

Behavioral and emotional disorders with onset usually occurring in childhood and adolescence (F90-F98)

NOTE   Codes within categories F90-F98 may be used regardless of the age of a patient. These disorders generally have onset within the childhood or adolescent years, but may continue throughout life or not be diagnosed until adulthood

F90   Attention-deficit hyperactivity disorders

Includes: attention deficit disorder with hyperactivity
attention deficit syndrome with hyperactivity
Excludes2: *anxiety disorders (F40.-, F41.-)*
mood [affective] disorders (F30-F39)
pervasive developmental disorders (F84.-)
schizophrenia (F20.-)

F90.0   Attention-deficit hyperactivity disorder, predominantly inattentive type

Attention-deficit/hyperactivity disorder, predominantly inattentive presentation

F90.1   Attention-deficit hyperactivity disorder, predominantly hyperactive type

Attention-deficit/hyperactivity disorder, predominantly hyperactive impulsive presentation

F90.2   Attention-deficit hyperactivity disorder, combined type

Attention-deficit/hyperactivity disorder, combined presentation

F90.8   Attention-deficit hyperactivity disorder, other type

F90.9   Attention-deficit hyperactivity disorder, unspecified type

Attention-deficit hyperactivity disorder of childhood or adolescence NOS
Attention-deficit hyperactivity disorder NOS

F91   Conduct disorders

Excludes1: *antisocial behavior (Z72.81-)*
antisocial personality disorder (F60.2)

Excludes2: *conduct problems associated with attention-deficit hyperactivity disorder (F90.-)*
mood [affective] disorders (F30-F39)
pervasive developmental disorders (F84.-)
schizophrenia (F20.-)

F91.0   Conduct disorder confined to family context

F91.1   Conduct disorder, childhood-onset type

Unsocialized conduct disorder
Conduct disorder, solitary aggressive type
Unsocialized aggressive disorder

F91.2   Conduct disorder, adolescent-onset type

Socialized conduct disorder
Conduct disorder, group type

F91.3   Oppositional defiant disorder

F91.8   Other conduct disorders

Other specified conduct disorder
Other specified disruptive disorder

F91.9   Conduct disorder, unspecified

Behavioral disorder NOS
Conduct disorder NOS
Disruptive behavior disorder NOS
Disruptive disorder NOS

F93   Emotional disorders with onset specific to childhood

F93.0   Separation anxiety disorder of childhood

Excludes2: *mood [affective] disorders (F30-F39)*
nonpsychotic mental disorders (F40-F48)
phobic anxiety disorder of childhood (F40.8)
social phobia (F40.1)

F93.8   Other childhood emotional disorders

Identity disorder
Excludes2: *gender identity disorder of childhood (F64.2)*

F93.9   Childhood emotional disorder, unspecified

F94   Disorders of social functioning with onset specific to childhood and adolescence

F94.0   Selective mutism

Elective mutism
Excludes2: *pervasive developmental disorders (F84.-)*
schizophrenia (F20.-)
specific developmental disorders of speech and language (F80.-)
transient mutism as part of separation anxiety in young children (F93.0)

F94.1   Reactive attachment disorder of childhood

Use additional code to identify any associated failure to thrive or growth retardation
Excludes1: *disinhibited attachment disorder of childhood (F94.2)*
normal variation in pattern of selective attachment
Excludes2: *Asperger's syndrome (F84.5)*
maltreatment syndromes (T74.-)
sexual or physical abuse in childhood, resulting in psychosocial problems (Z62.81-)

F94.2   Disinhibited attachment disorder of childhood

Affectionless psychopathy
Institutional syndrome
Excludes1: *reactive attachment disorder of childhood (F94.1)*
Excludes2: *Asperger's syndrome (F84.5)*
attention-deficit hyperactivity disorders (F90.-)
hospitalism in children (F43.2-)

F94.8   Other childhood disorders of social functioning

F94.9   Childhood disorder of social functioning, unspecified

F95   Tic disorder

F95.0   Transient tic disorder

Provisional tic disorder

F95.1   Chronic motor or vocal tic disorder

F95.2   Tourette's disorder

Combined vocal and multiple motor tic disorder [de la Tourette]
Tourette's syndrome

F95.8   Other tic disorders

F95.9   Tic disorder, unspecified

Tic NOS

+, +7th, X + 7th   ● Newborn   ● Pediatric   ● Maternity   ● Adult   ♀ Female   ♂ Male   Manifestation   Unacceptable PDX   HCC   CC   MCC   HAC

F98 **Other behavioral and emotional disorders with onset usually occurring in childhood and adolescence**

> *Excludes2:* breath-holding spells (R06.89)
> gender identity disorder of childhood (F64.2)
> Kleine-Levin syndrome (G47.13)
> obsessive-compulsive disorder (F42.-)
> sleep disorders not due to a substance or known
> physiological condition (F51.-)

F98.0 **Enuresis not due to a substance or known physiological condition**

Enuresis (primary) (secondary) of nonorganic origin
Functional enuresis
Psychogenic enuresis
Urinary incontinence of nonorganic origin

> *Excludes1:* enuresis NOS (R32)

F98.1 **Encopresis not due to a substance or known physiological condition**

Functional encopresis
Incontinence of feces of nonorganic origin
Psychogenic encopresis
Use additional code to identify the cause of any coexisting constipation.

> *Excludes1:* encopresis NOS (R15.-)

+ F98.2 **Other feeding disorders of infancy and childhood**

> *Excludes1:* feeding difficulties (R63.3)
> *Excludes2:* anorexia nervosa and other eating disorders
> (F50.-)
> feeding problems of newborn (P92.-)
> pica of infancy or childhood (F98.3)

F98.21 **Rumination disorder of infancy**

F98.29 **Other feeding disorders of infancy and early childhood**

F98.3 **Pica of infancy and childhood**

F98.4 **Stereotyped movement disorders**

Stereotype/habit disorder

> *Excludes1:* abnormal involuntary movements (R25.-)

> *Excludes2:* compulsions in obsessive-compulsive
> disorder (F42.-)
> hair plucking (F63.3)
> movement disorders of organic origin (G20-G25)
> nail-biting (F98.8)
> nose-picking (F98.8)
> stereotypies that are part of a broader
> psychiatric condition (F01-F95)
> thumb-sucking (F98.8)
> tic disorders (F95.-)
> trichotillomania (F63.3)

F98.5 **Adult onset fluency disorder**

> *Excludes1:* childhood onset fluency disorder (F80.81)
> dysphasia (R47.02)
> fluency disorder in conditions classified
> elsewhere (R47.82)
> fluency disorder (stuttering) following
> cerebrovascular disease (I69. with final
> characters -23)
> tic disorders (F95.-)

F98.8 **Other specified behavioral and emotional disorders with onset usually occurring in childhood and adolescence**

Excessive masturbation
Nail-biting
Nose-picking
Thumb-sucking

F98.9 **Unspecified behavioral and emotional disorders with onset usually occurring in childhood and adolescence**

Unspecified mental disorder (F99)

F99 **Mental disorder, not otherwise specified**

Mental illness NOS

> *Excludes1:* unspecified mental disorder due to known physiological
> condition (F09)

Valid 3-character code, no further characters required

+, +7th, X + 7th   ● Newborn   ● Pediatric   ● Maternity   ● Adult   ♀ Female   ♂ Male   Manifestation   Unacceptable PDX   HCC   CC   MCC   HAC

Chapter 6: Diseases of the Nervous System (G00-G99)

Excludes2: *certain conditions originating in the perinatal period (P04-P96)*
certain infectious and parasitic diseases (A00-B99)
complications of pregnancy, childbirth and the puerperium (O00-O9A)
congenital malformations, deformations, and chromosomal abnormalities (Q00-Q99)
endocrine, nutritional and metabolic diseases (E00-E88)
injury, poisoning and certain other consequences of external causes (S00-T88)
neoplasms (C00-D49)
symptoms, signs and abnormal clinical and laboratory findings, not elsewhere classified (R00-R94)

This chapter contains the following category blocks:

G00-G09	Inflammatory diseases of the central nervous system
G10-G14	Systemic atrophies primarily affecting the central nervous system
G20-G26	Extrapyramidal and movement disorders
G30-G32	Other degenerative diseases of the nervous system
G35-G37	Demyelinating diseases of the central nervous system
G40-G47	Episodic and paroxysmal disorders
G50-G59	Nerve, nerve root and plexus disorders
G60-G65	Polyneuropathies and other disorders of the peripheral nervous system
G70-G73	Diseases of myoneural junction and muscle
G80-G83	Cerebral palsy and other paralytic syndromes
G89-G99	Other disorders of the nervous system

C. Chapter-Specific Coding Guidelines

In addition to general coding guidelines, there are guidelines for specific diagnoses and/or conditions in the classification. Unless otherwise indicated, these guidelines apply to all health care settings. Please refer to Section II for guidelines on the selection of principal diagnosis.

6. Chapter 6: Diseases of the Nervous System (G00-G99)

a. Dominant/nondominant side

Codes from category G81, Hemiplegia and hemiparesis, and subcategories, G83.1, Monoplegia of lower limb, G83.2, Monoplegia of upper limb, and G83.3, Monoplegia, unspecified, identify whether the dominant or nondominant side is affected. Should the affected side be documented, but not specified as dominant or nondominant, and the classification system does not indicate a default, code selection is as follows:

- For ambidextrous patients, the default should be dominant.
- If the left side is affected, the default is non-dominant.
- If the right side is affected, the default is dominant.

b. Pain-Category G89

1) General coding information

Codes in category G89, Pain, not elsewhere classified, may be used in conjunction with codes from other categories and chapters to provide more detail about acute or chronic pain and neoplasm-related pain, unless otherwise indicated below.

If the pain is not specified as acute or chronic, post- thoracotomy, post procedural, or neoplasm-related, do not assign codes from category G89.

A code from category G89 should not be assigned if the underlying (definitive) diagnosis is known, unless the reason for the encounter is pain control/management and not management of the underlying condition.

When an admission or encounter is for a procedure aimed at treating the underlying condition (e.g., spinal fusion, kyphoplasty), a code for the underlying condition (e.g., vertebral fracture, spinal stenosis) should be assigned as the principal diagnosis. No code from category G89 should be assigned.

(a) Category G89 Codes as Principal or First-Listed Diagnosis

Category G89 codes are acceptable as principal diagnosis or the first-listed code:

- When pain control or pain management is the reason for the admission/encounter (e.g., a patient with displaced intervertebral disc, nerve impingement and severe back pain presents for injection of steroid into the spinal canal). The underlying cause of the pain should be reported as an additional diagnosis, if known.

- When a patient is admitted for the insertion of a neurostimulator for pain control, assign the appropriate pain code as the principal or first-listed diagnosis. When an admission or encounter is for a procedure aimed at treating the underlying condition and a neurostimulator is inserted for pain control during the same admission/encounter, a code for the underlying condition should be assigned as the principal diagnosis and the appropriate pain code should be assigned as a secondary diagnosis.

(b) Use of Category G89 Codes in Conjunction with Site Specific Pain Codes

(i) Assigning Category G89 and Site-Specific Pain Codes

Codes from category G89 may be used in conjunction with codes that identify the site of pain (including codes from chapter 18) if the category G89 code provides additional information. For example, if the code describes the site of the pain, but does not fully describe whether the pain is acute or chronic, then both codes should be assigned.

(ii) Sequencing of Category G89 Codes with Site- Specific Pain Codes

The sequencing of category G89 codes with site-specific pain codes (including chapter 18 codes), is dependent on the circumstances of the encounter/admission as follows:

- If the encounter is for pain control or pain management, assign the code from category G89 followed by the code identifying the specific site of pain (e.g., encounter for pain management for acute neck pain from trauma is assigned code G89.11, Acute pain due to trauma, followed by code M54.2, Cervicalgia, to identify the site of pain).

- If the encounter is for any other reason except pain control or pain management, and a related definitive diagnosis has not been established (confirmed) by the provider, assign the code for the specific site of pain first, followed by the appropriate code from category G89.

2) Pain due to devices, implants and grafts

See Section I.C.19. Pain due to medical devices

3) Postoperative Pain

The provider's documentation should be used to guide the coding of postoperative pain, as well as *Section III. Reporting Additional Diagnoses and Section IV. Diagnostic Coding* and *Reporting in the Outpatient Setting.*

The default for post-thoracotomy and other postoperative pain not specified as acute or chronic is the code for the acute form.

Routine or expected postoperative pain immediately after surgery should not be coded.

(a) Postoperative pain not associated with specific postoperative complication

Postoperative pain not associated with a specific postoperative complication is assigned to the appropriate postoperative pain code in category G89.

(b) Postoperative pain associated with specific postoperative complication

Postoperative pain associated with a specific postoperative complication (such as painful wire sutures) is assigned to the appropriate code(s) found in Chapter 19, Injury, poisoning, and certain other consequences of external causes. If appropriate, use additional code(s) from category G89 to identify acute or chronic pain (G89.18 or G89.28).

4) Chronic pain

Chronic pain is classified to subcategory G89.2. There is no time frame defining when pain becomes chronic pain. The provider's documentation should be used to guide use of these codes.

5) Neoplasm Related Pain

Code G89.3 is assigned to pain documented as being related, associated or due to cancer, primary or secondary malignancy, or tumor. This code is assigned regardless of whether the pain is acute or chronic.

This code may be assigned as the principal or first- listed code when the stated reason for the admission/encounter is documented as pain control/pain management. The underlying neoplasm should be reported as an additional diagnosis.

When the reason for the admission/encounter is management of the neoplasm and the pain associated with the neoplasm is also documented, code G89.3 may be assigned as an additional diagnosis. It is not necessary to assign an additional code for the site of the pain.

See Section I.C.2 for instructions on the sequencing of neoplasms for all other stated reasons for the admission/encounter (except for pain control/pain management).

6) Chronic pain syndrome

Central pain syndrome (G89.0) and chronic pain syndrome (G89.4) are different than the term "chronic pain," and therefore codes should only be used when the provider has specifically documented this condition.

See Section I.C.5. Pain disorders related to psychological factors

Inflammatory diseases of the central nervous system (G00-G09)

G00 Bacterial meningitis, not elsewhere classified

Includes: bacterial arachnoiditis
bacterial leptomeningitis
bacterial meningitis
bacterial pachymeningitis

Excludes1: *bacterial meningoencephalitis (G04.2)*
bacterial meningomyelitis (G04.2)

MCC **G00.0 Hemophilus meningitis**
Meningitis due to Hemophilus influenzae

MCC **G00.1 Pneumococcal meningitis**
Meningtitis due to Streptococcal pneumoniae

MCC **G00.2 Streptococcal meningitis**
Use additional code to further identify organism (B95.0-B95.5)

MCC **G00.3 Staphylococcal meningitis**
Use additional code to further identify organism (B95.61-B95.8)

MCC **G00.8 Other bacterial meningitis**
Meningitis due to Escherichia coli
Meningitis due to Friedländer's bacillus
Meningitis due to Klebsiella
Use additional code to further identify organism (B96.-)

MCC **G00.9 Bacterial meningitis, unspecified**
Meningitis due to gram-negative bacteria, unspecified
Purulent meningitis NOS
Pyogenic meningitis NOS
Suppurative meningitis NOS

MCC **G01 Meningitis in bacterial diseases classified elsewhere**
Code first underlying disease
Excludes1: *meningitis (in):*
gonococcal (A54.81)
leptospirosis (A27.81)
listeriosis (A32.11)
Lyme disease (A69.21)
meningococcal (A39.0)
neurosyphilis (A52.13)
tuberculosis (A17.0)
meningoencephalitis and meningomyelitis in bacterial diseases classified elsewhere (G05)
Valid 3-character code, no further characters required

MCC **G02 Meningitis in other infectious and parasitic diseases classified elsewhere**
Code first underlying disease, such as:
African trypanosomiasis (B56.-)
poliovirus infection (A80.-)
Excludes1: *candidal meningitis (B37.5)*
coccidioidomycosis meningitis (B38.4)
cryptococcal meningitis (B45.1)
herpesviral [herpes simplex] meningitis (B00.3)
infectious mononucleosis complicated by meningitis (B27.- with fourth character 2)
measles complicated by meningitis (B05.1)
meningoencephalitis and meningomyelitis in other infectious and parasitic diseases classified elsewhere (G05)
mumps meningitis (B26.1)
rubella meningitis (B06.02)
varicella [chickenpox] meningitis (B01.0)
zoster meningitis (B02.1)
Valid 3-character code, no further characters required

G03 Meningitis due to other and unspecified causes
Includes: arachnoiditis NOS
leptomeningitis NOS
meningitis NOS
pachymeningitis NOS
Excludes1: *meningoencephalitis (G04.-)*
meningomyelitis (G04.-)

MCC **G03.0 Nonpyogenic meningitis**
Aseptic meningitis
Nonbacterial meningitis
CC **G03.1 Chronic meningitis**
CC **G03.2 Benign recurrent meningitis [Mollaret]**
MCC **G03.8 Meningitis due to other specified causes**
MCC **G03.9 Meningitis, unspecified**
Arachnoiditis (spinal) NOS

G04 Encephalitis, myelitis and encephalomyelitis
Includes: acute ascending myelitis
meningoencephalitis
meningomyelitis
Excludes1: *encephalopathy NOS (G93.40)*
Excludes2: *acute transverse myelitis (G37.3-)*
alcoholic encephalopathy (G31.2)
benign myalgic encephalomyelitis (G93.3)
multiple sclerosis (G35)
subacute necrotizing myelitis (G37.4)
toxic encephalitis (G92)
toxic encephalopathy (G92)

+ **G04.0 Acute disseminated encephalitis and encephalomyelitis (ADEM)**
Excludes1: *acute necrotizing hemorrhagic encephalopathy (G04.3-)*
other noninfectious acute disseminated encephalomyelitis (noninfectious ADEM) (G04.81)
MCC **G04.00 Acute disseminated encephalitis and encephalomyelitis, unspecified**
MCC **G04.01 Postinfectious acute disseminated encephalitis and encephalomyelitis (postinfectious ADEM)**
Excludes1: *post chickenpox encephalitis (B01.1)*
post measles encephalitis (B05.0)
post measles myelitis (B05.1)
MCC **G04.02 Postimmunization acute disseminated encephalitis, myelitis and encephalomyelitis**
Encephalitis, post immunization
Encephalomyelitis, post immunization
Use additional code to identify the vaccine (T50.A-, T50.B-, T50.Z-)

CC **G04.1 Tropical spastic paraplegia**
MCC **G04.2 Bacterial meningoencephalitis and meningomyelitis, not elsewhere classified**
+ **G04.3 Acute necrotizing hemorrhagic encephalopathy**
Excludes1: *acute disseminated encephalitis and encephalomyelitis (G04.0-)*
MCC **G04.30 Acute necrotizing hemorrhagic encephalopathy, unspecified**
MCC **G04.31 Postinfectious acute necrotizing hemorrhagic encephalopathy**
MCC **G04.32 Postimmunization acute necrotizing hemorrhagic encephalopathy**
Use additional code to identify the vaccine (T50.A-, T50.B-, T50.Z-)
MCC **G04.39 Other acute necrotizing hemorrhagic encephalopathy**
Code also underlying etiology, if applicable
+ **G04.8 Other encephalitis, myelitis and encephalomyelitis**
Code also any associated seizure (G40.-, R56.9)
MCC **G04.81 Other encephalitis and encephalomyelitis**
Noninfectious acute disseminated encephalomyelitis (noninfectious ADEM)
MCC **G04.89 Other myelitis**
AHA CC: 1Q, 2020, 14
+ **G04.9 Encephalitis, myelitis and encephalomyelitis, unspecified**
MCC **G04.90 Encephalitis and encephalomyelitis, unspecified**
Ventriculitis (cerebral) NOS
MCC **G04.91 Myelitis, unspecified**

+, +7th, X + 7th • Newborn • Pediatric • Maternity • Adult ♀ Female ♂ Male Manifestation Unacceptable PDX HCC CC MCC HAC

G05 **Encephalitis, myelitis and encephalomyelitis in diseases classified elsewhere**

Code first underlying disease, such as:
human immunodeficiency virus [HIV] disease (B20)
poliovirus (A80.-)
suppurative otitis media (H66.01-H66.4)
trichinellosis (B75)

Excludes1: *adenoviral encephalitis, myelitis and encephalomyelitis (A85.1)*
congenital toxoplasmosis encephalitis, myelitis and encephalomyelitis (P37.1)
cytomegaloviral encephalitis, myelitis and encephalomyelitis (B25.8)
encephalitis, myelitis and encephalomyelitis (in) measles (B05.0)
encephalitis, myelitis and encephalomyelitis (in) systemic lupus erythematosus (M32.19)
enteroviral encephalitis, myelitis and encephalomyelitis (A85.0)
eosinophilic meningoencephalitis (B83.2)
herpesviral [herpes simplex] encephalitis, myelitis and encephalomyelitis (B00.4)
listerial encephalitis, myelitis and encephalomyelitis (A32.12)
meningococcal encephalitis, myelitis and encephalomyelitis (A39.81)
mumps encephalitis, myelitis and encephalomyelitis (B26.2)
postchickenpox encephalitis, myelitis and encephalomyelitis (B01.1-)
rubella encephalitis, myelitis and encephalomyelitis (B06.01)
toxoplasmosis encephalitis, myelitis and encephalomyelitis (B58.2)
zoster encephalitis, myelitis and encephalomyelitis (B02.0)

MCC **G05.3** **Encephalitis and encephalomyelitis in diseases classified elsewhere**
Meningoencephalitis in diseases classified elsewhere

MCC **G05.4** **Myelitis in diseases classified elsewhere**
Meningomyelitis in diseases classified elsewhere

G06 **Intracranial and intraspinal abscess and granuloma**
Use additional code (B95-B97) to identify infectious agent.

MCC **G06.0** **Intracranial abscess and granuloma**
Brain [any part] abscess (embolic)
Cerebellar abscess (embolic)
Cerebral abscess (embolic)
Intracranial epidural abscess or granuloma
Intracranial extradural abscess or granuloma
Intracranial subdural abscess or granuloma
Otogenic abscess (embolic)
Excludes1: *tuberculous intracranial abscess and granuloma (A17.81)*

MCC **G06.1** **Intraspinal abscess and granuloma**
Abscess (embolic) of spinal cord [any part]
Intraspinal epidural abscess or granuloma
Intraspinal extradural abscess or granuloma
Intraspinal subdural abscess or granuloma
Excludes1: *tuberculous intraspinal abscess and granuloma (A17.81)*

MCC **G06.2** **Extradural and subdural abscess, unspecified**

G07 **Intracranial and intraspinal abscess and granuloma in diseases**
MCC **classified elsewhere**

Code first underlying disease such as:
schistosomiasis granuloma of brain (B65.-)

Excludes1: *abscess of brain:*
amebic (A06.6)
chromomycotic (B43.1)
gonococcal (A54.82)
tuberculous (A17.81)
tuberculoma of meninges (A17.1)

Valid 3-character code, no further characters required

MCC **G08** **Intracranial and intraspinal phlebitis and thrombophlebitis**
Septic embolism of intracranial or intraspinal venous sinuses and veins
Septic endophlebitis of intracranial or intraspinal venous sinuses and veins
Septic phlebitis of intracranial or intraspinal venous sinuses and veins
Septic thrombophlebitis of intracranial or intraspinal venous sinuses and veins
Septic thrombosis of intracranial or intraspinal venous sinuses and veins

Excludes1: *intracranial phlebitis and thrombophlebitis complicating:*
abortion, ectopic or molar pregnancy (O00-O07, O08.7)
pregnancy, childbirth and the puerperium (O22.5, O87.3)
nonpyogenic intracranial phlebitis and thrombophlebitis (I67.6)

Excludes2: *intracranial phlebitis and thrombophlebitis complicating nonpyogenic intraspinal phlebitis and thrombophlebitis (G95.1)*

Valid 3-character code, no further characters required

G09 **Sequelae of inflammatory diseases of central nervous system**

NOTE Category G09 is to be used to indicate conditions whose primary classification is to G00-G08 as the cause of sequelae, themselves classifiable elsewhere. The 'sequelae' include conditions specified as residuals.

Code first condition resulting from (sequela) of inflammatory diseases of central nervous system

Valid 3-character code, no further characters required

Systemic atrophies primarily affecting the central nervous system (G10-G14)

CC **G10** **Huntington's disease**
Huntington's chorea
Huntington's dementia
Code also dementia in other diseases classified elsewhere without behavioral disturbance (F02.80)

Valid 3-character code, no further characters required

G11 **Hereditary ataxia**

Excludes2: *cerebral palsy (G80.-)*
hereditary and idiopathic neuropathy (G60.-)
metabolic disorders (E70-E88)

CC **G11.0** **Congenital nonprogressive ataxia**

+ **G11.1** **Early-onset cerebellar ataxia**

CC **G11.10** **Early-onset cerebellar ataxia, unspecified**

CC **G11.11** **Friedreich ataxia**
Autosomal recessive Friedreich ataxia
Friedreich ataxia with retained reflexes

CC **G11.19** **Other early-onset cerebellar ataxia**
Early-onset cerebellar ataxia with essential tremor
Early-onset cerebellar ataxia with myoclonus [Hunt's ataxia]
Early-onset cerebellar ataxia with retained tendon reflexes
X-linked recessive spinocerebellar ataxia

● CC **G11.2** **Late-onset cerebellar ataxia**

CC **G11.3** **Cerebellar ataxia with defective DNA repair**
Ataxia telangiectasia [Louis-Bar]
Excludes2: *Cockayne's syndrome (Q87.19)*
other disorders of purine and pyrimidine metabolism (E79.-)
xeroderma pigmentosum (Q82.19)

CC **G11.4** **Hereditary spastic paraplegia**

CC **G11.8** **Other hereditary ataxias**

CC **G11.9** **Hereditary ataxia, unspecified**
Hereditary cerebellar ataxia NOS
Hereditary cerebellar degeneration
Hereditary cerebellar disease
Hereditary cerebellar syndrome

G12 **Spinal muscular atrophy and related syndromes**

CC **G12.0** **Infantile spinal muscular atrophy, type I [Werdnig-Hoffman]**

CC **G12.1** **Other inherited spinal muscular atrophy**
Adult form spinal muscular atrophy
Childhood form, type II spinal muscular atrophy
Distal spinal muscular atrophy
Juvenile form, type III spinal muscular atrophy [Kugelberg-Welander]
Progressive bulbar palsy of childhood [Fazio-Londe]
Scapuloperoneal form spinal muscular atrophy

+ **G12.2** **Motor neuron disease**
CC **G12.20** **Motor neuron disease, unspecified**
● CC **G12.21** **Amyotrophic lateral sclerosis**
CC **G12.22** **Progressive bulbar palsy**
CC **G12.23** **Primary lateral sclerosis**
AHA CC: 4Q, 2017, 9-10
CC **G12.24** **Familial motor neuron disease**
AHA CC: 4Q, 2017, 9-10
CC **G12.25** **Progressive spinal muscle atrophy**
AHA CC: 4Q, 2017, 9-10
CC **G12.29** **Other motor neuron disease**

CC **G12.8** **Other spinal muscular atrophies and related syndromes**
CC **G12.9** **Spinal muscular atrophy, unspecified**

G13 **Systemic atrophies primarily affecting central nervous system in diseases classified elsewhere**

G13.0 **Paraneoplastic neuromyopathy and neuropathy**
Carcinomatous neuromyopathy
Sensorial paraneoplastic neuropathy [Denny Brown]
Code first underlying neoplasm (C00-D49)

G13.1 **Other systemic atrophy primarily affecting central nervous system in neoplastic disease**
Paraneoplastic limbic encephalopathy
Code first underlying neoplasm (C00-D49)

G13.2 **Systemic atrophy primarily affecting the central nervous system in myxedema**
Code first underlying disease, such as:
hypothyroidism (E03.-)
myxedematous congenital iodine deficiency (E00.1)

G13.8 **Systemic atrophy primarily affecting central nervous system in other diseases classified elsewhere**
Code first underlying disease

G14 **Postpolio syndrome**

Includes: postpolio myelitic syndrome
Excludes1: *sequelae of poliomyelitis (B91)*
Valid 3-character code, no further characters required

Extrapyramidal and movement disorders (G20-G26)

G20 **Parkinson's disease**
Hemiparkinsonism
Idiopathic Parkinsonism or Parkinson's disease
Paralysis agitans
Parkinsonism or Parkinson's disease NOS
Primary Parkinsonism or Parkinson's disease
Excludes1: *dementia with Parkinsonism (G31.83)*
Use additional code to identify:
dementia with behavioral disturbance (F02.81)
dementia without behavioral disturbance (F02.80)
AHA CC: 2Q, 2016, 6-7; 2Q, 2017, 7-8
Valid 3-character code, no further characters required

G21 **Secondary parkinsonism**
Excludes1: *dementia with Parkinsonism (G31.83)*
Huntington's disease (G10)
Shy-Drager syndrome (G90.3)
syphilitic Parkinsonism (A52.19)

MCC **G21.0** **Malignant neuroleptic syndrome**
Use additional code for adverse effect, if applicable, to identify drug (T43.3X5, T43.4X5, T43.505, T43.595)
Excludes1: *neuroleptic induced parkinsonism (G21.11)*

+ **G21.1** **Other drug-induced secondary parkinsonism**
CC **G21.11** **Neuroleptic induced parkinsonism**
Use additional code for adverse effect, if applicable, to identify drug (T43.3X5, T43.4X5, T43.505, T43.595)
Excludes1: *malignant neuroleptic syndrome (G21.0)*
CC **G21.19** **Other drug induced secondary parkinsonism**
Other medication-induced parkinsonism
Use additional code for adverse effect, if applicable, to identify drug (T36-T50 with fifth or sixth character 5)

CC **G21.2** **Secondary parkinsonism due to other external agents**
Code first (T51-T65) to identify external agent
CC **G21.3** **Postencephalitic parkinsonism**
G21.4 **Vascular parkinsonism**
CC **G21.8** **Other secondary parkinsonism**
CC **G21.9** **Secondary parkinsonism, unspecified**

G23 **Other degenerative diseases of basal ganglia**
Excludes2: *multi-system degeneration of the autonomic nervous system (G90.3)*
CC **G23.0** **Hallervorden-Spatz disease**
Pigmentary pallidal degeneration
CC **G23.1** **Progressive supranuclear ophthalmoplegia [Steele-Richardson-Olszewski]**
Progressive supranuclear palsy
CC **G23.2** **Striatonigral degeneration**
CC **G23.8** **Other specified degenerative diseases of basal ganglia**
Calcification of basal ganglia
CC **G23.9** **Degenerative disease of basal ganglia, unspecified**

G24 **Dystonia**
Includes: dyskinesia
Excludes2: *athetoid cerebral palsy (G80.3)*
+ **G24.0** **Drug induced dystonia**
Use additional code for adverse effect, if applicable, to identify drug (T36-T50 with fifth or sixth character 5)
G24.01 **Drug induced subacute dyskinesia**
Drug induced blepharospasm
Drug induced orofacial dyskinesia
Neuroleptic induced tardive dyskinesia
Tardive dyskinesia
CC **G24.02** **Drug induced acute dystonia**
Acute dystonic reaction to drugs
Neuroleptic induced acute dystonia
CC **G24.09** **Other drug induced dystonia**
G24.1 **Genetic torsion dystonia**
Dystonia deformans progressiva
Dystonia musculorum deformans
Familial torsion dystonia
Idiopathic familial dystonia
Idiopathic (torsion) dystonia NOS
(Schwalbe-) Ziehen-Oppenheim disease
CC **G24.2** **Idiopathic nonfamilial dystonia**
G24.3 **Spasmodic torticollis**
Excludes1: *congenital torticollis (Q68.0)*
hysterical torticollis (F44.4)
ocular torticollis (R29.891)
psychogenic torticollis (F45.8)
torticollis NOS (M43.6)
traumatic recurrent torticollis (S13.4)
G24.4 **Idiopathic orofacial dystonia**
Orofacial dyskinesia
Excludes1: *drug induced orofacial dyskinesia (G24.01)*
G24.5 **Blepharospasm**
Excludes1: *drug induced blepharospasm (G24.01)*
CC **G24.8** **Other dystonia**
Acquired torsion dystonia NOS
G24.9 **Dystonia, unspecified**
Dyskinesia NOS

+, +7th, X + 7th   ● Newborn   ● Pediatric   ● Maternity   ● Adult   ♀ Female   ♂ Male   Manifestation   Unacceptable PDX   HCC   CC   MCC   HAC

G25 Other extrapyramidal and movement disorders

> *Excludes2:* sleep related movement disorders (G47.6-)

G25.0 Essential tremor
Familial tremor
> *Excludes1:* tremor NOS (R25.1)

G25.1 Drug-induced tremor
Use additional code for adverse effect, if applicable, to identify drug (T36-T50 with fifth or sixth character 5)

G25.2 Other specified forms of tremor
Intention tremor

G25.3 Myoclonus
Drug-induced myoclonus
Palatal myoclonus
Use additional code for adverse effect, if applicable, to identify drug (T36-T50 with fifth or sixth character 5)
> *Excludes1:* facial myokymia (G51.4)
> myoclonic epilepsy (G40.-)

G25.4 Drug-induced chorea
Use additional code for adverse effect, if applicable, to identify drug (T36-T50 with fifth or sixth character 5)

G25.5 Other chorea
Chorea NOS
> *Excludes1:* chorea NOS with heart involvement (I02.0)
> Huntington's chorea (G10)
> rheumatic chorea (I02.-)
> Sydenham's chorea (I02.-)

+ **G25.6 Drug induced tics and other tics of organic origin**
G25.61 Drug induced tics
Use additional code for adverse effect, if applicable, to identify drug (T36-T50 with fifth or sixth character 5)
G25.69 Other tics of organic origin
> *Excludes1:* habit spasm (F95.9)
> tic NOS (F95.9)
> Tourette's syndrome (F95.2)

+ **G25.7 Other and unspecified drug induced movement disorders**
Use additional code for adverse effect, if applicable, to identify drug (T36-T50 with fifth or sixth character 5)
G25.70 Drug induced movement disorder, unspecified
G25.71 Drug induced akathisia
Drug induced acathisia
Neuroleptic induced acute akathisia
Tardive akathisia
G25.79 Other drug induced movement disorders

+ **G25.8 Other specified extrapyramidal and movement disorders**
G25.81 Restless legs syndrome
CC **G25.82 Stiff-man syndrome**
G25.83 Benign shuddering attacks
G25.89 Other specified extrapyramidal and movement disorders

CC **G25.9 Extrapyramidal and movement disorder, unspecified**

G26 Extrapyramidal and movement disorders in diseases classified elsewhere
Code first underlying disease
Valid 3-character code, no further characters required

Other degenerative diseases of the nervous system (G30-G32)

G30 Alzheimer's disease
Includes: Alzheimer's dementia senile and presenile forms
Use additional code to identify:
delirium, if applicable (F05)
dementia with behavioral disturbance (F02.81)
dementia without behavioral disturbance (F02.80)
> *Excludes1:* senile degeneration of brain NEC (G31.1)
> senile dementia NOS (F03)
> senility NOS (R41.81)

G30.0 Alzheimer's disease with early onset
• **G30.1 Alzheimer's disease with late onset**
G30.8 Other Alzheimer's disease
G30.9 Alzheimer's disease, unspecified
> *AHA CC: 4Q, 2012, 95-96; 2Q, 2016, 6; 1Q, 2017, 43-44*

G31 Other degenerative diseases of nervous system, not elsewhere classified
For codes G31.0-G31.83, G31.85-G31.9, use additional code to identify::
dementia with behavioral disturbance (F02.81)
dementia without behavioral disturbance (F02.80)
> *Excludes2:* Reye's syndrome (G93.7)

+ **G31.0 Frontotemporal dementia**
G31.01 Pick's disease
Primary progressive aphasia
Progressive isolated aphasia
G31.09 Other frontotemporal dementia
Frontal dementia

G31.1 Senile degeneration of brain, not elsewhere classified
> *Excludes1:* Alzheimer's disease (G30.-)
> senility NOS (R41.81)

G31.2 Degeneration of nervous system due to alcohol
Alcoholic cerebellar ataxia
Alcoholic cerebellar degeneration
Alcoholic cerebral degeneration
Alcoholic encephalopathy
Dysfunction of the autonomic nervous system due to alcohol
Code also associated alcoholism (F10.-)

+ **G31.8 Other specified degenerative diseases of nervous system**
CC **G31.81 Alpers disease**
Grey-matter degeneration
CC **G31.82 Leigh's disease**
Subacute necrotizing encephalopathy
G31.83 Dementia with Lewy bodies
Dementia with Parkinsonism
Lewy body dementia
Lewy body disease
> *AHA CC: 4Q, 2016, 141*
G31.84 Mild cognitive impairment, so stated
Mild neurocognitive disorder
> *Excludes1:* age related cognitive decline (R41.81)
> altered mental status (R41.82)
> cerebral degeneration (G31.9)
> change in mental status (R41.82)
> cognitive deficits following (sequelae of) cerebral hemorrhage or infarction (I69.01-, I69.11-, I69.21-, I69.31-, I69.81-, I69.91-)
> cognitive impairment due to intracranial or head injury (S06.-)
> dementia (F01.-, F02.-, F03)
> mild memory disturbance (F06.8)
> neurologic neglect syndrome (R41.4)
> personality change, nonpsychotic (F68.8)
G31.85 Corticobasal degeneration
G31.89 Other specified degenerative diseases of nervous system

G31.9 Degenerative disease of nervous system, unspecified

G32 Other degenerative disorders of nervous system in diseases classified elsewhere

CC **G32.0 Subacute combined degeneration of spinal cord in diseases classified elsewhere**
Dana-Putnam syndrome
Sclerosis of spinal cord (combined) (dorsolateral) (posterolateral)
Code first underlying disease, such as:
anemia (D51.9)
dietary (D51.3)
pernicious (D51.0)
vitamin B12 deficiency (E53.8)
> *Excludes1:* syphilitic combined degeneration of spinal cord (A52.11)

+ **G32.8 Other specified degenerative disorders of nervous system in diseases classified elsewhere**
Code first underlying disease, such as:
amyloidosis cerebral degeneration (E85.-)
cerebral degeneration (due to) hypothyroidism (E00.0-E03.9)
cerebral degeneration (due to) neoplasm (C00-D49)
cerebral degeneration (due to) vitamin B deficiency, except thiamine (E52-E53.-)
non-celiac gluten ataxia (M35.9)
> *Excludes1:* superior hemorrhagic polioencephalitis [Wernicke's encephalopathy] (E51.2)

+, +7th, X + 7th   • Newborn   • Pediatric   • Maternity   • Adult   ♀ Female   ♂ Male   Manifestation   Unacceptable PDX   HCC   CC   MCC   HAC

CC **G32.81 Cerebellar ataxia in diseases classified elsewhere**
Code first underlying disease, such as:
celiac disease (with gluten ataxia) (K90.0)
cerebellar ataxia (in) neoplastic disease
(paraneoplastic cerebellar degeneration)
(C00-D49)
non-celiac gluten ataxia (M35.9)
Excludes1: *systemic atrophy primarily affecting*
the central nervous system in
alcoholic cerebellar ataxia (G31.2)
systemic atrophy primarily affecting
the central nervous system in
myxedema (G13.2)

G32.89 **Other specified degenerative disorders of nervous**
system in diseases classified elsewhere
Degenerative encephalopathy in diseases classified
elsewhere

Demyelinating diseases of the central nervous system (G35-G37)

G35 Multiple sclerosis

Disseminated multiple sclerosis
Generalized multiple sclerosis
Multiple sclerosis NOS
Multiple sclerosis of brain stem
Multiple sclerosis of cord
Valid 3-character code, no further characters required

G36 **Other acute disseminated demyelination**

Excludes1: *povstinfectious encephalitis and encephalomyelitis NOS*
(G04.01)

CC **G36.0 Neuromyelitis optica [Devic]**
Demyelination in optic neuritis
Excludes1: *optic neuritis NOS (H46)*
CC **G36.1 Acute and subacute hemorrhagic leukoencephalitis [Hurst]**
CC **G36.8 Other specified acute disseminated demyelination**
CC **G36.9 Acute disseminated demyelination, unspecified**

G37 **Other demyelinating diseases of central nervous system**

CC **G37.0 Diffuse sclerosis of central nervous system**
Periaxial encephalitis
Schilder's disease
Excludes1: *X linked adrenoleukodystrophy (E71.52-)*
CC **G37.1 Central demyelination of corpus callosum**
CC **G37.2 Central pontine myelinolysis**
CC **G37.3 Acute transverse myelitis in demyelinating disease of**
central nervous system
Acute transverse myelitis NOS
Acute transverse myelopathy
Excludes1: *multiple sclerosis (G35)*
neuromyelitis optica [Devic] (G36.0)
MCC **G37.4 Subacute necrotizing myelitis of central nervous system**
CC **G37.5 Concentric sclerosis [Balo] of central nervous system**
CC **G37.8 Other specified demyelinating diseases of central nervous**
system
CC **G37.9 Demyelinating disease of central nervous system,**
unspecified

Episodic and paroxysmal disorders (G40-G47)

G40 **Epilepsy and recurrent seizures**

NOTE the following terms are to be considered equivalent
to intractable: pharmacoresistant (pharmacologically
resistant), treatment resistant, refractory (medically) and
poorly controlled
Excludes1: *conversion disorder with seizures (F44.5)*
convulsions NOS (R56.9)
post traumatic seizures (R56.1)
seizure (convulsive) NOS (R56.9)
seizure of newborn (P90)
Excludes2: *hippocampal sclerosis (G93.81)*
mesial temporal sclerosis (G93.81)
temporal sclerosis (G93.81)
Todd's paralysis (G83.84)
+ **G40.0 Localization-related (focal) (partial) idiopathic epilepsy and**
epileptic syndromes with seizures of localized onset
Benign childhood epilepsy with centrotemporal EEG spikes
Childhood epilepsy with occipital EEG paroxysms
Excludes1: *adult onset localization-related epilepsy*
(G40.1-, G40.2-)

+ **G40.00 Localization-related (focal) (partial) idiopathic**
epilepsy and epileptic syndromes with seizures of
localized onset, not intractable
Localization-related (focal) (partial) idiopathic
epilepsy and epileptic syndromes with seizures
of localized onset without intractability
CC **G40.001 Localization-related (focal) (partial)**
idiopathic epilepsy and epileptic
syndromes with seizures of localized
onset, not intractable, with status
epilepticus
CC **G40.009 Localization-related (focal) (partial)**
idiopathic epilepsy and epileptic
syndromes with seizures of localized onset,
not intractable, without status epilepticus
Localization-related (focal) (partial)
idiopathic epilepsy and epileptic
syndromes with seizures of localized
onset NOS
+ **G40.01 Localization-related (focal) (partial) idiopathic**
epilepsy and epileptic syndromes with seizures of
localized onset, intractable
CC **G40.011 Localization-related (focal) (partial)**
idiopathic epilepsy and epileptic
syndromes with seizures of localized
onset, intractable, with status
epilepticus
CC **G40.019 Localization-related (focal) (partial)**
idiopathic epilepsy and epileptic
syndromes with seizures of localized
onset, intractable, without status
epilepticus
+ **G40.1 Localization-related (focal) (partial) symptomatic epilepsy**
and epileptic syndromes with simple partial seizures
Attacks without alteration of consciousness
Epilepsia partialis continua [Kozhevnikof]
Simple partial seizures developing into secondarily
generalized seizures
+ **G40.10 Localization-related (focal) (partial) symptomatic**
epilepsy and epileptic syndromes with simple
partial seizures, not intractable
Localization-related (focal) (partial) symptomatic
epilepsy and epileptic syndromes with simple
partial seizures without intractability
CC **G40.101 Localization-related (focal) (partial)**
symptomatic epilepsy and epileptic
syndromes with simple partial seizures,
not intractable, with status epilepticus
CC **G40.109 Localization-related (focal) (partial)**
symptomatic epilepsy and epileptic
syndromes with simple partial seizures,
not intractable, without status epilepticus
Localization-related (focal) (partial)
symptomatic epilepsy and epileptic
syndromes with simple partial
seizures NOS
+ **G40.11 Localization-related (focal) (partial) symptomatic**
epilepsy and epileptic syndromes with simple
partial seizures, intractable
CC **G40.111 Localization-related (focal) (partial)**
symptomatic epilepsy and epileptic
syndromes with simple partial
seizures, intractable, with status
epilepticus
CC **G40.119 Localization-related (focal) (partial)**
symptomatic epilepsy and epileptic
syndromes with simple partial seizures,
intractable, without status epilepticus
+ **G40.2 Localization-related (focal) (partial) symptomatic epilepsy**
and epileptic syndromes with complex partial seizures
Attacks with alteration of consciousness, often with
automatisms
Complex partial seizures developing into secondarily
generalized seizures
+ **G40.20 Localization-related (focal) (partial) symptomatic**
epilepsy and epileptic syndromes with complex
partial seizures, not intractable
Localization-related (focal) (partial) symptomatic
epilepsy and epileptic syndromes with complex
partial seizures without intractability

CC **G40.201** **Localization-related (focal) (partial) symptomatic epilepsy and epileptic syndromes with complex partial seizures, not intractable, with status epilepticus**

CC **G40.209** **Localization-related (focal) (partial) symptomatic epilepsy and epileptic syndromes with complex partial seizures, not intractable, without status epilepticus**

Localization-related (focal) (partial) symptomatic epilepsy and epileptic syndromes with complex partial seizures NOS

+ **G40.21** **Localization-related (focal) (partial) symptomatic epilepsy and epileptic syndromes with complex partial seizures, intractable**

CC **G40.211** **Localization-related (focal) (partial) symptomatic epilepsy and epileptic syndromes with complex partial seizures, intractable, with status epilepticus**

CC **G40.219** **Localization-related (focal) (partial) symptomatic epilepsy and epileptic syndromes with complex partial seizures, intractable, without status epilepticus**

+ **G40.3** **Generalized idiopathic epilepsy and epileptic syndromes**
Code also MERRF syndrome, if applicable (E88.42)

+ **G40.30** **Generalized idiopathic epilepsy and epileptic syndromes, not intractable**
Generalized idiopathic epilepsy and epileptic syndromes without intractability

MCC **G40.301** **Generalized idiopathic epilepsy and epileptic syndromes, not intractable, with status epilepticus**

G40.309 **Generalized idiopathic epilepsy and epileptic syndromes, not intractable, without status epilepticus**
Generalized idiopathic epilepsy and epileptic syndromes NOS

+ **G40.31** **Generalized idiopathic epilepsy and epileptic syndromes, intractable**

MCC **G40.311** **Generalized idiopathic epilepsy and epileptic syndromes, intractable, with status epilepticus**

MCC **G40.319** **Generalized idiopathic epilepsy and epileptic syndromes, intractable, without status epilepticus**

+ **G40.A** **Absence epileptic syndrome**
Childhood absence epilepsy [pyknolepsy]
Juvenile absence epilepsy
Absence epileptic syndrome, NOS

+ **G40.A0** **Absence epileptic syndrome, not intractable**

G40.A01 **Absence epileptic syndrome, not intractable, with status epilepticus**

G40.A09 **Absence epileptic syndrome, not intractable, without status epilepticus**

+ **G40.A1** **Absence epileptic syndrome, intractable**

CC **G40.A11** **Absence epileptic syndrome, intractable, with status epilepticus**

CC **G40.A19** **Absence epileptic syndrome, intractable, without status epilepticus**

+ **G40.B** **Juvenile myoclonic epilepsy [impulsive petit mal]**

+ **G40.B0** **Juvenile myoclonic epilepsy, not intractable**

CC **G40.B01** **Juvenile myoclonic epilepsy, not intractable, with status epilepticus**

CC **G40.B09** **Juvenile myoclonic epilepsy, not intractable, without status epilepticus**

+ **G40.B1** **Juvenile myoclonic epilepsy, intractable**

CC **G40.B11** **Juvenile myoclonic epilepsy, intractable, with status epilepticus**

CC **G40.B19** **Juvenile myoclonic epilepsy, intractable, without status epilepticus**

+ **G40.4** **Other generalized epilepsy and epileptic syndromes**
Epilepsy with grand mal seizures on awakening
Epilepsy with myoclonic absences
Epilepsy with myoclonic-astatic seizures
Grand mal seizure NOS
Nonspecific atonic epileptic seizures
Nonspecific clonic epileptic seizures
Nonspecific myoclonic epileptic seizures
Nonspecific tonic epileptic seizures
Nonspecific tonic-clonic epileptic seizures
Symptomatic early myoclonic encephalopathy

+ **G40.40** **Other generalized epilepsy and epileptic syndromes, not intractable**
Other generalized epilepsy and epileptic syndromes without intractability
Other generalized epilepsy and epileptic syndromes NOS

G40.401 **Other generalized epilepsy and epileptic syndromes, not intractable, with status epilepticus**

G40.409 **Other generalized epilepsy and epileptic syndromes, not intractable, without status epilepticus**

+ **G40.41** **Other generalized epilepsy and epileptic syndromes, intractable**

CC **G40.411** **Other generalized epilepsy and epileptic syndromes, intractable, with status epilepticus**

CC **G40.419** **Other generalized epilepsy and epileptic syndromes, intractable, without status epilepticus**

G40.42 **Cyclin-Dependent Kinase-Like 5 Deficiency Disorder**
CDKL5
Use additional code, if known, to identify associated manifestations, such as:
cortical blindness (H47.61-)
global developmental delay (F88)

+ **G40.5** **Epileptic seizures related to external causes**
Epileptic seizures related to alcohol
Epileptic seizures related to drugs
Epileptic seizures related to hormonal changes
Epileptic seizures related to sleep deprivation
Epileptic seizures related to stress
Use additional code for adverse effect, if applicable, to identify drug (T36-T50 with fifth or sixth character 5)
Code also if applicable, associated epilepsy and recurrent seizures (G40.-)

+ **G40.50** **Epileptic seizures related to external causes, not intractable**

CC **G40.501** **Epileptic seizures related to external causes, not intractable, with status epilepticus**

CC **G40.509** **Epileptic seizures related to external causes, not intractable, without status epilepticus**
Epileptic seizures related to external causes, NOS

+ **G40.8** **Other epilepsy and recurrent seizures**
Epilepsies and epileptic syndromes undetermined as to whether they are focal or generalized
Landau-Kleffner syndrome

+ **G40.80** **Other epilepsy**

CC **G40.801** **Other epilepsy, not intractable, with status epilepticus**
Other epilepsy without intractability with status epilepticus

CC **G40.802** **Other epilepsy, not intractable, without status epilepticus**
Other epilepsy NOS
Other epilepsy without intractability without status epilepticus

CC **G40.803** **Other epilepsy, intractable, with status epilepticus**

CC **G40.804** **Other epilepsy, intractable, without status epilepticus**

+ **G40.81** **Lennox-Gastaut syndrome**

CC **G40.811** **Lennox-Gastaut syndrome, not intractable, with status epilepticus**

CC **G40.812** **Lennox-Gastaut syndrome, not intractable, without status epilepticus**

CC **G40.813** **Lennox-Gastaut syndrome, intractable, with status epilepticus**

CC **G40.814** **Lennox-Gastaut syndrome, intractable, without status epilepticus**

+ **G40.82** **Epileptic spasms**
Infantile spasms
Salaam attacks
West's syndrome

+, +7th, X + 7th ● Newborn ● Pediatric ● Maternity ● Adult ♀ Female ♂ Male Manifestation Unacceptable PDX HCC CC MCC HAC

CC **G40.821** Epileptic spasms, not intractable, with status epilepticus

CC **G40.822** Epileptic spasms, not intractable, without status epilepticus

CC **G40.823** Epileptic spasms, intractable, with status epilepticus

CC **G40.824** Epileptic spasms, intractable, without status epilepticus

+ **G40.83 Dravet syndrome**
Polymorphic epilepsy in infancy (PMEI)
Severe myoclonic epilepsy in infancy (SMEI)

CC **G40.833** Dravet syndrome, intractable, with status epilepticus

CC **G40.834** Dravet syndrome, intractable, without status epilepticus
Dravet syndrome NOS

CC **G40.89 Other seizures**
Excludes1: *post traumatic seizures (R56.1)*
recurrent seizures NOS (G40.909)
seizure NOS (R56.9)

+ **G40.9 Epilepsy, unspecified**

+ **G40.90 Epilepsy, unspecified, not intractable**
Epilepsy, unspecified, without intractability

G40.901 Epilepsy, unspecified, not intractable, with status epilepticus

G40.909 Epilepsy, unspecified, not intractable, without status epilepticus
Epilepsy NOS
Epileptic convulsions NOS
Epileptic fits NOS
Epileptic seizures NOS
Recurrent seizures NOS
Seizure disorder NOS

+ **G40.91 Epilepsy, unspecified, intractable**
Intractable seizure disorder NOS

CC **G40.911** Epilepsy, unspecified, intractable, with status epilepticus

CC **G40.919** Epilepsy, unspecified, intractable, without status epilepticus

G43 Migraine

NOTE The following terms are to be considered equivalent to intractable: pharmacoresistant (pharmacologically resistant), treatment resistant, refractory (medically) and poorly controlled

Use additional code for adverse effect, if applicable, to identify drug (T36-T50 with fifth or sixth character 5)

Excludes1: *headache NOS (R51.9)*
lower half migraine (G44.00)
Excludes2: *headache syndromes (G44.-)*

+ **G43.0 Migraine without aura**
Common migraine
Excludes1: *chronic migraine without aura (G43.7-)*

+ **G43.00 Migraine without aura, not intractable**
Migraine without aura without mention of refractory migraine

G43.001 Migraine without aura, not intractable, with status migrainosus

G43.009 Migraine without aura, not intractable, without status migrainosus
Migraine without aura NOS

+ **G43.01 Migraine without aura, intractable**
Migraine without aura with refractory migraine

G43.011 Migraine without aura, intractable, with status migrainosus

G43.019 Migraine without aura, intractable, without status migrainosus

+ **G43.1 Migraine with aura**
Basilar migraine
Classical migraine
Migraine equivalents
Migraine preceded or accompanied by transient focal neurological phenomena
Migraine triggered seizures
Migraine with acute-onset aura
Migraine with aura without headache (migraine equivalents)
Migraine with prolonged aura
Migraine with typical aura
Retinal migraine
Code also any associated seizure (G40.-, R56.9)
Excludes1: *persistent migraine aura (G43.5-, G43.6-)*

+ **G43.10 Migraine with aura, not intractable**
Migraine with aura without mention of refractory migraine

G43.101 Migraine with aura, not intractable, with status migrainosus

G43.109 Migraine with aura, not intractable, without status migrainosus
Migraine with aura NOS

+ **G43.11 Migraine with aura, intractable**
Migraine with aura with refractory migraine

G43.111 Migraine with aura, intractable, with status migrainosus

G43.119 Migraine with aura, intractable, without status migrainosus

+ **G43.4 Hemiplegic migraine**
Familial migraine
Sporadic migraine

+ **G43.40 Hemiplegic migraine, not intractable**
Hemiplegic migraine without refractory migraine

G43.401 Hemiplegic migraine, not intractable, with status migrainosus

G43.409 Hemiplegic migraine, not intractable, without status migrainosus
Hemiplegic migraine NOS

+ **G43.41 Hemiplegic migraine, intractable**
Hemiplegic migraine with refractory migraine

G43.411 Hemiplegic migraine, intractable, with status migrainosus

G43.419 Hemiplegic migraine, intractable, without status migrainosus

+ **G43.5 Persistent migraine aura without cerebral infarction**

+ **G43.50 Persistent migraine aura without cerebral infarction, not intractable**
Persistent migraine aura without cerebral infarction, without refractory migraine

G43.501 Persistent migraine aura without cerebral infarction, not intractable, with status migrainosus

G43.509 Persistent migraine aura without cerebral infarction, not intractable, without status migrainosus
Persistent migraine aura NOS

+ **G43.51 Persistent migraine aura without cerebral infarction, intractable**
Persistent migraine aura without cerebral infarction, with refractory migraine

G43.511 Persistent migraine aura without cerebral infarction, intractable, with status migrainosus

G43.519 Persistent migraine aura without cerebral infarction, intractable, without status migrainosus

+ **G43.6 Persistent migraine aura with cerebral infarction**
Code also the type of cerebral infarction (I63.-)

+ **G43.60 Persistent migraine aura with cerebral infarction, not intractable**
Persistent migraine aura with cerebral infarction, without refractory migraine

CC **G43.601** Persistent migraine aura with cerebral infarction, not intractable, with status migrainosus

CC **G43.609** Persistent migraine aura with cerebral infarction, not intractable, without status migrainosus

+ **G43.61 Persistent migraine aura with cerebral infarction, intractable**
Persistent migraine aura with cerebral infarction, with refractory migraine

CC **G43.611** Persistent migraine aura with cerebral infarction, intractable, with status migrainosus

CC **G43.619** Persistent migraine aura with cerebral infarction, intractable, without status migrainosus

+ **G43.7 Chronic migraine without aura**
Transformed migraine
Excludes1: *migraine without aura (G43.0-)*

Mechanisms in Migraine

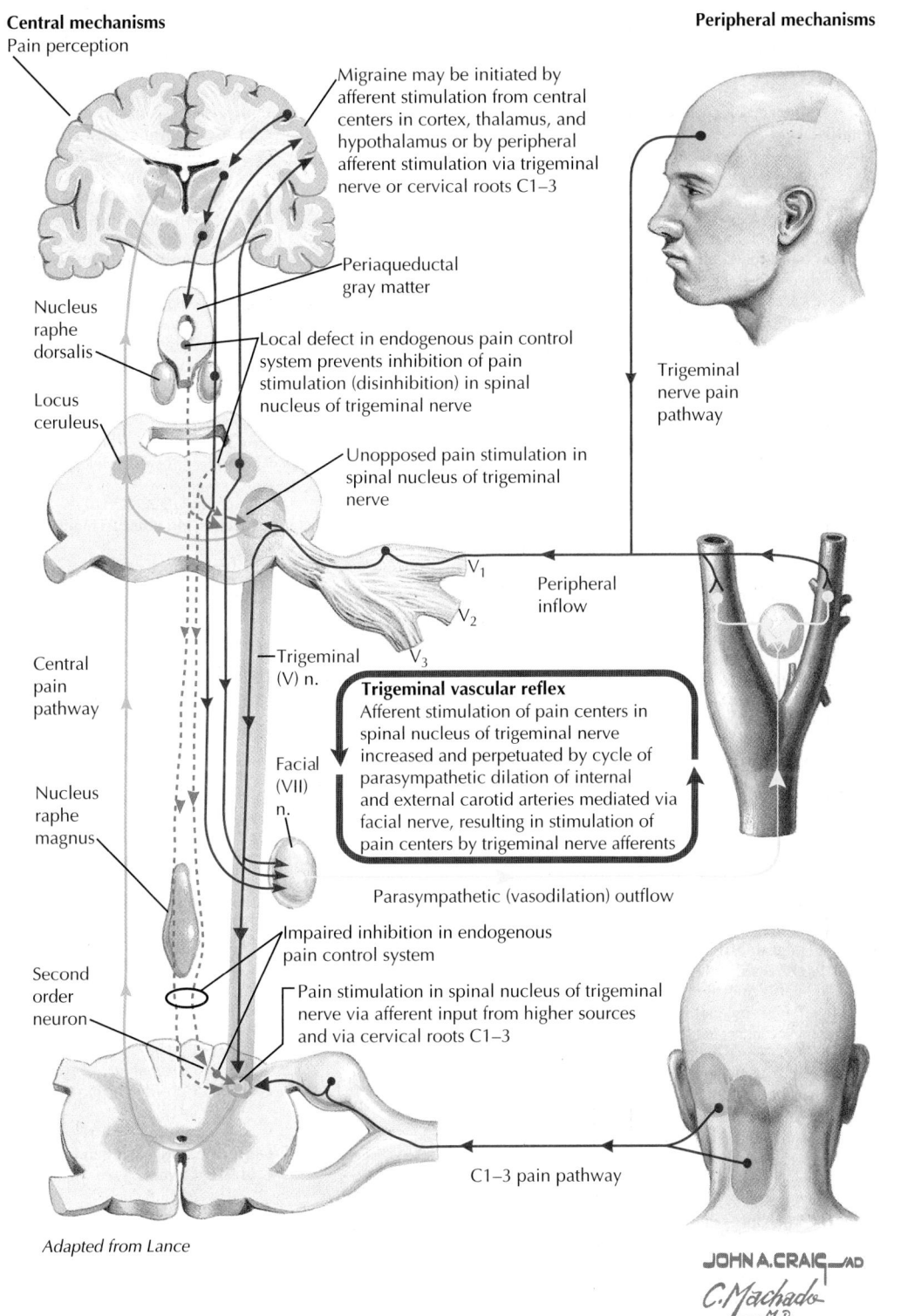

Central mechanisms

Pain perception

Migraine may be initiated by afferent stimulation from central centers in cortex, thalamus, and hypothalamus or by peripheral afferent stimulation via trigeminal nerve or cervical roots C1–3

Periaqueductal gray matter

Nucleus raphe dorsalis

Local defect in endogenous pain control system prevents inhibition of pain stimulation (disinhibition) in spinal nucleus of trigeminal nerve

Locus ceruleus

Unopposed pain stimulation in spinal nucleus of trigeminal nerve

Central pain pathway

Trigeminal (V) n.

V_1

V_2

V_3

Peripheral mechanisms

Trigeminal nerve pain pathway

Peripheral inflow

Trigeminal vascular reflex
Afferent stimulation of pain centers in spinal nucleus of trigeminal nerve increased and perpetuated by cycle of parasympathetic dilation of internal and external carotid arteries mediated via facial nerve, resulting in stimulation of pain centers by trigeminal nerve afferents

Nucleus raphe magnus

Facial (VII) n.

Parasympathetic (vasodilation) outflow

Second order neuron

Impaired inhibition in endogenous pain control system

Pain stimulation in spinal nucleus of trigeminal nerve via afferent input from higher sources and via cervical roots C1–3

C1–3 pain pathway

Adapted from Lance

JOHN A. CRAIG_AD

C. Machado
_M.D.

+ **G43.70 Chronic migraine without aura, not intractable**
Chronic migraine without aura, without refractory migraine
 G43.701 Chronic migraine without aura, not intractable, with status migrainosus
 G43.709 Chronic migraine without aura, not intractable, without status migrainosus
  Chronic migraine without aura NOS

+ **G43.71 Chronic migraine without aura, intractable**
Chronic migraine without aura, with refractory migraine
 G43.711 Chronic migraine without aura, intractable, with status migrainosus
 G43.719 Chronic migraine without aura, intractable, without status migrainosus

+ **G43.A Cyclical vomiting**
 Excludes1: cyclical vomiting syndrome unrelated to migraine (R11.15)
 AHA CC: 4Q, 2019, 15
 G43.A0 Cyclical vomiting, in migraine, not intractable
  Cyclical vomiting, without refractory migraine
 G43.A1 Cyclical vomiting, in migraine, intractable
  Cyclical vomiting, with refractory migraine

+ **G43.B Ophthalmoplegic migraine**
 G43.B0 Ophthalmoplegic migraine, not intractable
  Ophthalmoplegic migraine, without refractory migraine
 G43.B1 Ophthalmoplegic migraine, intractable
  Ophthalmoplegic migraine, with refractory migraine

+ **G43.C Periodic headache syndromes in child or adult**
 G43.C0 Periodic headache syndromes in child or adult, not intractable
  Periodic headache syndromes in child or adult, without refractory migraine
 G43.C1 Periodic headache syndromes in child or adult, intractable
  Periodic headache syndromes in child or adult, with refractory migraine

+ **G43.D Abdominal migraine**
 G43.D0 Abdominal migraine, not intractable
  Abdominal migraine, without refractory migraine
 G43.D1 Abdominal migraine, intractable
  Abdominal migraine, with refractory migraine

+ **G43.8 Other migraine**
+ **G43.80 Other migraine, not intractable**
 Other migraine, without refractory migraine
 G43.801 Other migraine, not intractable, with status migrainosus
 G43.809 Other migraine, not intractable, without status migrainosus

+ **G43.81 Other migraine, intractable**
 Other migraine, with refractory migraine
 G43.811 Other migraine, intractable, with status migrainosus
 G43.819 Other migraine, intractable, without status migrainosus

+ **G43.82 Menstrual migraine, not intractable**
Menstrual headache, not intractable
Menstrual migraine, without refractory migraine
Menstrually related migraine, not intractable
Pre-menstrual headache, not intractable
Pre-menstrual migraine, not intractable
Pure menstrual migraine, not intractable
Code also associated premenstrual tension syndrome (N94.3)
 ♀ **G43.821 Menstrual migraine, not intractable, with status migrainosus**
 ♀ **G43.829 Menstrual migraine, not intractable, without status migrainosus**
  Menstrual migraine NOS

+ **G43.83 Menstrual migraine, intractable**
Menstrual headache, intractable
Menstrual migraine, with refractory migraine
Menstrually related migraine, intractable
Pre-menstrual headache, intractable
Pre-menstrual migraine, intractable
Pure menstrual migraine, intractable
Code also associated premenstrual tension syndrome (N94.3)
 ♀ **G43.831 Menstrual migraine, intractable, with status migrainosus**
 ♀ **G43.839 Menstrual migraine, intractable, without status migrainosus**

+ **G43.9 Migraine, unspecified**
+ **G43.90 Migraine, unspecified, not intractable**
Migraine, unspecified, without refractory migraine
 G43.901 Migraine, unspecified, not intractable, with status migrainosus
  Status migrainosus NOS
 G43.909 Migraine, unspecified, not intractable, without status migrainosus
  Migraine NOS

+ **G43.91 Migraine, unspecified, intractable**
Migraine, unspecified, with refractory migraine
 G43.911 Migraine, unspecified, intractable, with status migrainosus
 G43.919 Migraine, unspecified, intractable, without status migrainosus

G44 Other headache syndromes
 Excludes1: headache NOS (R51.9)
 Excludes2: atypical facial pain (G50.1)
  headache due to lumbar puncture (G97.1)
  migraines (G43.-)
  trigeminal neuralgia (G50.0)

+ **G44.0 Cluster headaches and other trigeminal autonomic cephalgias (TAC)**
+ **G44.00 Cluster headache syndrome, unspecified**
Ciliary neuralgia
Cluster headache NOS
Histamine cephalgia
Lower half migraine
Migrainous neuralgia
 G44.001 Cluster headache syndrome, unspecified, intractable
 G44.009 Cluster headache syndrome, unspecified, not intractable
  Cluster headache syndrome NOS

+ **G44.01 Episodic cluster headache**
 G44.011 Episodic cluster headache, intractable
 G44.019 Episodic cluster headache, not intractable
  Episodic cluster headache NOS

+ **G44.02 Chronic cluster headache**
 G44.021 Chronic cluster headache, intractable
 G44.029 Chronic cluster headache, not intractable
  Chronic cluster headache NOS

+ **G44.03 Episodic paroxysmal hemicrania**
Paroxysmal hemicrania NOS
 G44.031 Episodic paroxysmal hemicrania, intractable
 G44.039 Episodic paroxysmal hemicrania, not intractable
  Episodic paroxysmal hemicrania NOS

+ **G44.04 Chronic paroxysmal hemicrania**
 G44.041 Chronic paroxysmal hemicrania, intractable
 G44.049 Chronic paroxysmal hemicrania, not intractable
  Chronic paroxysmal hemicrania NOS

+ **G44.05** **Short lasting unilateral neuralgiform headache with conjunctival injection and tearing (SUNCT)**
    G44.051 **Short lasting unilateral neuralgiform headache with conjunctival injection and tearing (SUNCT), intractable**
    G44.059 **Short lasting unilateral neuralgiform headache with conjunctival injection and tearing (SUNCT), not intractable**
        Short lasting unilateral neuralgiform headache with conjunctival injection and tearing (SUNCT) NOS

+ **G44.09** **Other trigeminal autonomic cephalgias (TAC)**
    G44.091 **Other trigeminal autonomic cephalgias (TAC), intractable**
    G44.099 **Other trigeminal autonomic cephalgias (TAC), not intractable**

G44.1 **Vascular headache, not elsewhere classified**
    Excludes2: *cluster headache (G44.0)*
        complicated headache syndromes (G44.5-)
        drug-induced headache (G44.4-)
        migraine (G43.-)
        other specified headache syndromes (G44.8-)
        post-traumatic headache (G44.3-)
        tension-type headache (G44.2-)

+ **G44.2** **Tension-type headache**
+ **G44.20** **Tension-type headache, unspecified**
    G44.201 **Tension-type headache, unspecified, intractable**
    G44.209 **Tension-type headache, unspecified, not intractable**
        Tension headache NOS

+ **G44.21** **Episodic tension-type headache**
    G44.211 **Episodic tension-type headache, intractable**
    G44.219 **Episodic tension-type headache, not intractable**
        Episodic tension-type headache NOS

+ **G44.22** **Chronic tension-type headache**
    G44.221 **Chronic tension-type headache, intractable**
    G44.229 **Chronic tension-type headache, not intractable**
        Chronic tension-type headache NOS

+ **G44.3** **Post-traumatic headache**
+ **G44.30** **Post-traumatic headache, unspecified**
    G44.301 **Post-traumatic headache, unspecified, intractable**
    G44.309 **Post-traumatic headache, unspecified, not intractable**
        Post-traumatic headache NOS

+ **G44.31** **Acute post-traumatic headache**
    G44.311 **Acute post-traumatic headache, intractable**
    G44.319 **Acute post-traumatic headache, not intractable**
        Acute post-traumatic headache NOS

+ **G44.32** **Chronic post-traumatic headache**
    G44.321 **Chronic post-traumatic headache, intractable**
    G44.329 **Chronic post-traumatic headache, not intractable**
        Chronic post-traumatic headache NOS

+ **G44.4** **Drug-induced headache, not elsewhere classified**
    Medication overuse headache
    Use additional code for adverse effect, if applicable, to identify drug (T36-T50 with fifth or sixth character 5)
    G44.40 **Drug-induced headache, not elsewhere classified, not intractable**
    G44.41 **Drug-induced headache, not elsewhere classified, intractable**

+ **G44.5** **Complicated headache syndromes**
    G44.51 **Hemicrania continua**
    G44.52 **New daily persistent headache (NDPH)**
    G44.53 **Primary thunderclap headache**
    G44.59 **Other complicated headache syndrome**

+ **G44.8** **Other specified headache syndromes**
    Excludes2: *headache with orthostatic or positional component, not elsewhere classified (R51.0)*
    G44.81 **Hypnic headache**
    G44.82 **Headache associated with sexual activity**
        Orgasmic headache
        Preorgasmic headache
    G44.83 **Primary cough headache**
    G44.84 **Primary exertional headache**
    G44.85 **Primary stabbing headache**
    G44.89 **Other headache syndrome**

G45 **Transient cerebral ischemic attacks and related syndromes**
    Excludes1: *neonatal cerebral ischemia (P91.0)*
        transient retinal artery occlusion (H34.0-)

CC **G45.0** **Vertebro-basilar artery syndrome**
CC **G45.1** **Carotid artery syndrome (hemispheric)**
CC **G45.2** **Multiple and bilateral precerebral artery syndromes**
CC **G45.3** **Amaurosis fugax**
    G45.4 **Transient global amnesia**
        Excludes1: *amnesia NOS (R41.3)*
CC **G45.8** **Other transient cerebral ischemic attacks and related syndromes**
CC **G45.9** **Transient cerebral ischemic attack, unspecified**
        Spasm of cerebral artery
        TIA
        Transient cerebral ischemia NOS

G46 **Vascular syndromes of brain in cerebrovascular diseases**
    Code first underlying cerebrovascular disease (I60-I69)
CC **G46.0** **Middle cerebral artery syndrome**
CC **G46.1** **Anterior cerebral artery syndrome**
CC **G46.2** **Posterior cerebral artery syndrome**
    G46.3 **Brain stem stroke syndrome**
        Benedikt syndrome
        Claude syndrome
        Foville syndrome
        Millard-Gubler syndrome
        Wallenberg syndrome
        Weber syndrome
    G46.4 **Cerebellar stroke syndrome**
    G46.5 **Pure motor lacunar syndrome**
    G46.6 **Pure sensory lacunar syndrome**
    G46.7 **Other lacunar syndromes**
    G46.8 **Other vascular syndromes of brain in cerebrovascular diseases**

G47 **Sleep disorders**
    Excludes2: *nightmares (F51.5)*
        nonorganic sleep disorders (F51.-)
        sleep terrors (F51.4)
        sleepwalking (F51.3)

+ **G47.0** **Insomnia**
    Excludes2: *alcohol related insomnia (F10.182, F10.282, F10.982)*
        drug-related insomnia (F11.182, F11.282, F11.982, F13.182, F13.282, F13.982, F14.182, F14.282, F14.982, F15.182, F15.282, F15.982, F19.182, F19.282, F19.982)
        idiopathic insomnia (F51.01)
        insomnia due to a mental disorder (F51.05)
        insomnia not due to a substance or known physiological condition (F51.0-)
        nonorganic insomnia (F51.0-)
        primary insomnia (F51.01)
        sleep apnea (G47.3-)
    G47.00 **Insomnia, unspecified**
        Insomnia NOS
    G47.01 **Insomnia due to medical condition**
        Code also associated medical condition
    G47.09 **Other insomnia**

+, +7th, X + 7th   ● Newborn   ● Pediatric   ● Maternity   ● Adult   ♀ Female   ♂ Male   Manifestation   Unacceptable PDX   HCC   CC   MCC   HAC

Medial Views of Cerebrum

Sagittal section of brain in situ

Cingulate gyrus
Cingulate sulcus
Medial frontal gyrus
Sulcus of corpus callosum
Fornix
Septum pellucidum
Interventricular foramen (of Monro)
Interthalamic adhesion
Thalamus and 3rd ventricle
Subcallosal (parolfactory) area
Anterior commissure
Subcallosal gyrus
Hypothalamic sulcus
Lamina terminalis
Supra-optic recess
Optic chiasm
Tuber cinereum
Hypophysis (pituitary gland)
Mammillary body
Cerebral peduncle
Pons
Cerebral aqueduct (of Sylvius)

Paracentral sulcus
Central sulcus (of Rolando)
Paracentral lobule
Marginal sulcus
Corpus callosum
Precuneus
Superior sagittal sinus
Choroid plexus of 3rd ventricle
Stria medullaris of thalamus
Parietooccipital sulcus
Cuneus
Habenular commissure
Pineal body
Posterior commissure
Calcarine sulcus
Straight sinus in tentorium cerebelli
Great cerebral vein (of Galen)
Superior colliculus
Inferior colliculus
Tectal (quadrigeminal) plate
Cerebellum
Superior medullary velum
4th ventricle and choroid plexus
Inferior medullary velum
Medulla oblongata

Medial surface of cerebral hemisphere: brainstem excised

Cingulate gyrus
Mammillothalamic fasciculus
Mammillary body
Uncus
Optic nerve (II)
Olfactory tract
Collateral sulcus
Rhinal sulcus
Medial occipitotemporal gyrus
Occipitotemporal sulcus
Lateral occipitotemporal gyrus

Genu
Rostrum
Trunk } of corpus callosum
Splenium
Isthmus of cingulate gyrus
Parietooccipital sulcus
Cuneus
Calcarine sulcus
Lingual gyrus
Crus
Body } of fornix
Column
Fimbria of hippocampus
Dentate gyrus
Parahippocampal gyrus

F. Netter M.D.

Cranial Nerves: Schema

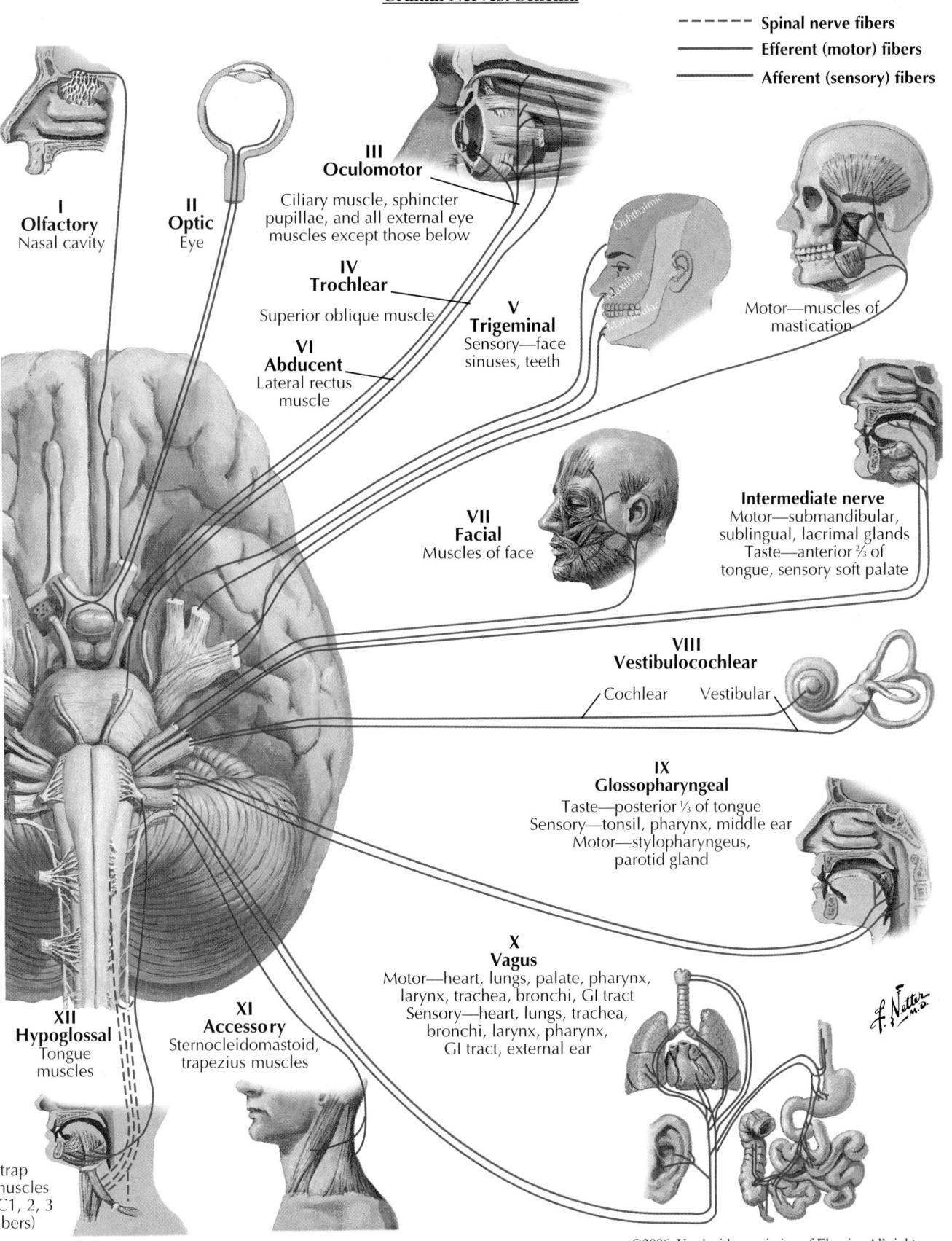

----- Spinal nerve fibers
—— Efferent (motor) fibers
—— Afferent (sensory) fibers

I Olfactory
Nasal cavity

II Optic
Eye

III Oculomotor
Ciliary muscle, sphincter pupillae, and all external eye muscles except those below

IV Trochlear
Superior oblique muscle

VI Abducent
Lateral rectus muscle

V Trigeminal
Sensory—face sinuses, teeth

Ophthalmic
Maxillary
Mandibular

Motor—muscles of mastication

VII Facial
Muscles of face

Intermediate nerve
Motor—submandibular, sublingual, lacrimal glands
Taste—anterior ⅔ of tongue, sensory soft palate

VIII Vestibulocochlear
Cochlear   Vestibular

IX Glossopharyngeal
Taste—posterior ⅓ of tongue
Sensory—tonsil, pharynx, middle ear
Motor—stylopharyngeus, parotid gland

X Vagus
Motor—heart, lungs, palate, pharynx, larynx, trachea, bronchi, GI tract
Sensory—heart, lungs, trachea, bronchi, larynx, pharynx, GI tract, external ear

XII Hypoglossal
Tongue muscles

Strap muscles (C1, 2, 3 fibers)

XI Accessory
Sternocleidomastoid, trapezius muscles

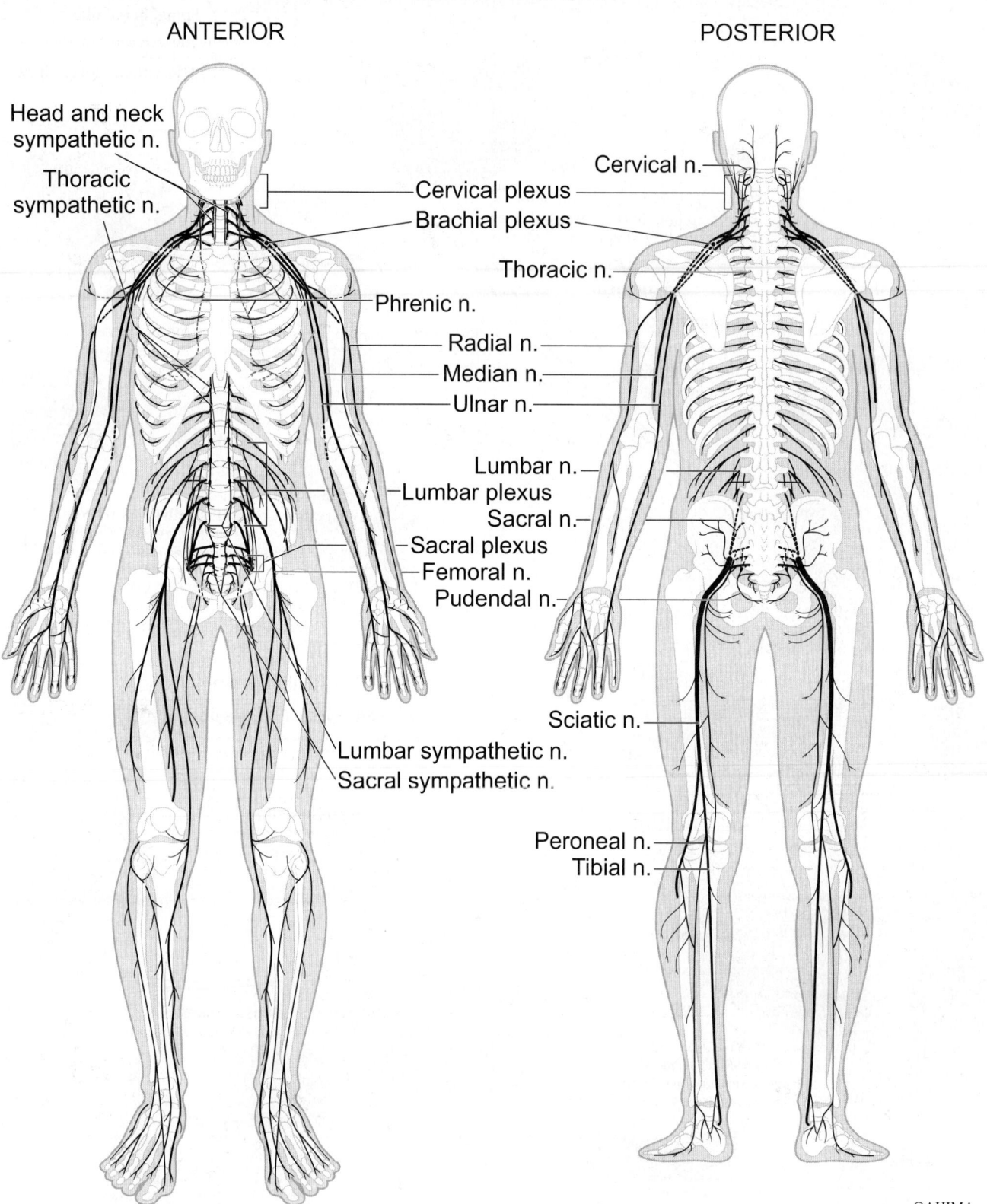

ANTERIOR

POSTERIOR

Head and neck
sympathetic n.

Thoracic
sympathetic n.

Cervical n.

Cervical plexus

Brachial plexus

Thoracic n.

Phrenic n.

Radial n.

Median n.

Ulnar n.

Lumbar n.

Lumbar plexus

Sacral n.

Sacral plexus

Femoral n.

Pudendal n.

Sciatic n.

Lumbar sympathetic n.

Sacral sympathetic n.

Peroneal n.

Tibial n.

©AHIMA

+ **G47.1 Hypersomnia**
    Excludes2: *alcohol-related hypersomnia (F10.182,*
      F10.282, F10.982)
    drug-related hypersomnia (F11.182, F11.282,
      F11.982, F13.182, F13.282, F13.982,
      F14.182, F14.282, F14.982, F15.182,
      F15.282, F15.982, F19.182, F19.282,
      F19.982)
    hypersomnia due to a mental disorder (F51.13)
    hypersomnia not due to a substance or known
      physiological condition (F51.1-)
    primary hypersomnia (F51.11)
    sleep apnea (G47.3-)

  G47.10 Hypersomnia, unspecified
    Hypersomnia NOS
  G47.11 Idiopathic hypersomnia with long sleep time
    Idiopathic hypersomnia NOS
  G47.12 Idiopathic hypersomnia without long sleep time
  G47.13 Recurrent hypersomnia
    Kleine-Levin syndrome
    Menstrual related hypersomnia
  G47.14 Hypersomnia due to medical condition
    Code also associated medical condition
  G47.19 Other hypersomnia

+ **G47.2 Circadian rhythm sleep disorders**
    Disorders of the sleep wake schedule
    Inversion of nyctohemeral rhythm
    Inversion of sleep rhythm
  G47.20 Circadian rhythm sleep disorder,
    unspecified type
    Sleep wake schedule disorder NOS
  G47.21 Circadian rhythm sleep disorder, delayed sleep
    phase type
    Delayed sleep phase syndrome
  G47.22 Circadian rhythm sleep disorder, advanced sleep
    phase type
  G47.23 Circadian rhythm sleep disorder, irregular sleep
    wake type
    Irregular sleep-wake pattern
  G47.24 Circadian rhythm sleep disorder, free
    running type
    Circadian rhythm sleep disorder, non-24-hour
      sleep-wake type
  G47.25 Circadian rhythm sleep disorder, jet lag type
  G47.26 Circadian rhythm sleep disorder, shift
    work type
  G47.27 Circadian rhythm sleep disorder in conditions
    classified elsewhere
    Code first underlying condition
  G47.29 Other circadian rhythm sleep disorder

+ **G47.3 Sleep apnea**
    Code also any associated underlying condition
    Excludes1: *apnea NOS (R06.81)*
      Cheyne-Stokes breathing (R06.3)
      pickwickian syndrome (E66.2)
      sleep apnea of newborn (P28.3)
  G47.30 Sleep apnea, unspecified
    Sleep apnea NOS
  G47.31 Primary central sleep apnea
    Idiopathic central sleep apnea
  G47.32 High altitude periodic breathing
  G47.33 Obstructive sleep apnea (adult) (pediatric)
    Obstructive sleep apnea hypopnea
    Excludes1: *obstructive sleep apnea of newborn*
      (P28.3)
  G47.34 Idiopathic sleep related nonobstructive alveolar
    hypoventilation
    Sleep related hypoxia
  G47.35 Congenital central alveolar hypoventilation
    syndrome
  G47.36 Sleep related hypoventilation in conditions
    classified elsewhere
    Sleep related hypoxemia in conditions classified
      elsewhere
    Code first underlying condition
  G47.37 Central sleep apnea in conditions classified
    elsewhere
    Code first underlying condition
  G47.39 Other sleep apnea

+ **G47.4 Narcolepsy and cataplexy**
  + **G47.41 Narcolepsy**
    G47.411 Narcolepsy with cataplexy
    G47.419 Narcolepsy without cataplexy
      Narcolepsy NOS
  + **G47.42 Narcolepsy in conditions classified elsewhere**
    Code first underlying condition
    G47.421 Narcolepsy in conditions classified
      elsewhere with cataplexy
    G47.429 Narcolepsy in conditions
      classified elsewhere without cataplexy

+ **G47.5 Parasomnia**
    Excludes1: *alcohol induced parasomnia (F10.182,*
      F10.282, F10.982)
    drug induced parasomnia (F11.182, F11.282,
      F11.982, F13.182, F13.282, F13.982,
      F14.182, F14.282, F14.982, F15.182,
      F15.282, F15.982, F19.182, F19.282,
      F19.982)
    parasomnia not due to a substance or known
      physiological condition (F51.8)
  G47.50 Parasomnia, unspecified
    Parasomnia NOS
  G47.51 Confusional arousals
  G47.52 REM sleep behavior disorder
  G47.53 Recurrent isolated sleep paralysis
  G47.54 Parasomnia in conditions classified elsewhere
    Code first underlying condition
  G47.59 Other parasomnia

+ **G47.6 Sleep related movement disorders**
    Excludes2: *restless legs syndrome (G25.81)*
  G47.61 Periodic limb movement disorder
  G47.62 Sleep related leg cramps
  G47.63 Sleep related bruxism
    Excludes1: *psychogenic bruxism (F45.8)*
  G47.69 Other sleep related movement disorders
G47.8 Other sleep disorders
    Other specified sleep-wake disorder
G47.9 Sleep disorder, unspecified
    Sleep disorder NOS
    Unspecified sleep-wake disorder

Nerve, nerve root and plexus disorders (G50-G59)

Excludes1: *current traumatic nerve, nerve root and plexus disorders - see*
    Injury, nerve by body region
    neuralgia NOS (M79.2)
    neuritis NOS (M79.2)
    peripheral neuritis in pregnancy (O26.82-)
    radiculitis NOS (M54.1-)

G50 Disorders of trigeminal nerve
  Includes: disorders of 5th cranial nerve
  G50.0 Trigeminal neuralgia
    Syndrome of paroxysmal facial pain
    Tic douloureux
  G50.1 Atypical facial pain
  G50.8 Other disorders of trigeminal nerve
  G50.9 Disorder of trigeminal nerve, unspecified

G51 Facial nerve disorders
  Includes: disorders of 7th cranial nerve
  G51.0 Bell's palsy
    Facial palsy
  G51.1 Geniculate ganglionitis
    Excludes1: *postherpetic geniculate ganglionitis*
      (B02.21)
  G51.2 Melkersson's syndrome
    Melkersson-Rosenthal syndrome
  + **G51.3 Clonic hemifacial spasm**
    AHA CC: 4Q, 2018, 10
    G51.31 Clonic hemifacial spasm, right
    G51.32 Clonic hemifacial spasm, left
      AHA CC: 4Q, 2018, 10
    G51.33 Clonic hemifacial spasm, bilateral
    G51.39 Clonic hemifacial spasm, unspecified
  G51.4 Facial myokymia
  G51.8 Other disorders of facial nerve
  G51.9 Disorder of facial nerve, unspecified

+, +7th, X + 7th   ● Newborn   ● Pediatric   ● Maternity   ● Adult   ♀ Female   ♂ Male   Manifestation   Unacceptable PDX   HCC   CC   MCC   HAC

G52   Disorders of other cranial nerves

Excludes2: *disorders of acoustic [8th] nerve (H93.3)*
disorders of optic [2nd] nerve (H46, H47.0)
paralytic strabismus due to nerve palsy
(H49.0-H49.2)

G52.0   Disorders of olfactory nerve
Disorders of 1st cranial nerve

G52.1   Disorders of glossopharyngeal nerve
Disorder of 9th cranial nerve
Glossopharyngeal neuralgia

G52.2   Disorders of vagus nerve
Disorders of pneumogastric [10th] nerve

G52.3   Disorders of hypoglossal nerve
Disorders of 12th cranial nerve

G52.7   Disorders of multiple cranial nerves
Polyneuritis cranialis

G52.8   Disorders of other specified cranial nerves
G52.9   Cranial nerve disorder, unspecified

G53   Cranial nerve disorders in diseases classified elsewhere

Code first underlying disease, such as:
neoplasm (C00-D49)

Excludes1: *multiple cranial nerve palsy in sarcoidosis (D86.82)*
multiple cranial nerve palsy in syphilis (A52.15)
postherpetic geniculate ganglionitis (B02.21)
postherpetic trigeminal neuralgia (B02.22)

Valid 3-character code, no further characters required

G54   Nerve root and plexus disorders

Excludes1: *current traumatic nerve root and plexus disorders - see*
nerve injury by body region
intervertebral disc disorders (M50-M51)
neuralgia or neuritis NOS (M79.2)
neuritis or radiculitis brachial NOS (M54.13)
neuritis or radiculitis lumbar NOS (M54.16)
neuritis or radiculitis lumbosacral NOS (M54.17)
neuritis or radiculitis thoracic NOS (M54.14)
radiculitis NOS (M54.10)
radiculopathy NOS (M54.10)
spondylosis (M47.-)

G54.0   Brachial plexus disorders
Thoracic outlet syndrome

G54.1   Lumbosacral plexus disorders
G54.2   Cervical root disorders, not elsewhere classified
G54.3   Thoracic root disorders, not elsewhere classified
G54.4   Lumbosacral root disorders, not elsewhere classified
G54.5   Neuralgic amyotrophy
Parsonage-Aldren-Turner syndrome
Shoulder-girdle neuritis

Excludes1: *neuralgic amyotrophy in diabetes mellitus*
(E08-E13 with .44)

G54.6   Phantom limb syndrome with pain
G54.7   Phantom limb syndrome without pain
Phantom limb syndrome NOS

G54.8   Other nerve root and plexus disorders
G54.9   Nerve root and plexus disorder, unspecified

G55   Nerve root and plexus compressions in diseases classified elsewhere

Code first underlying disease, such as:
neoplasm (C00-D49)

Excludes1: *nerve root compression (due to) (in) ankylosing*
spondylitis (M45.-)
nerve root compression (due to) (in) ankylosing
spondylitis (M45.-)
nerve root compression (due to) (in) dorsopathies
(M53.-, M54.-)
nerve root compression (due to) (in) intervertebral disc
disorders (M50.1.-, M51.1.-)
nerve root compression (due to) (in) spondylopathies
(M46.-, M48.-)

Valid 3-character code, no further characters required

G56   Mononeuropathies of upper limb

Excludes1: *current traumatic nerve disorder - see nerve injury by*
body region
AHA CC: 4Q, 2016, 17-18

+ **G56.0   Carpal tunnel syndrome**
G56.00   Carpal tunnel syndrome, unspecified upper limb
G56.01   Carpal tunnel syndrome, right upper limb
G56.02   Carpal tunnel syndrome, left upper limb
G56.03   Carpal tunnel syndrome, bilateral upper limbs

+ **G56.1   Other lesions of median nerve**
G56.10   Other lesions of median nerve, unspecified
upper limb
G56.11   Other lesions of median nerve, right upper limb
G56.12   Other lesions of median nerve, left upper limb
G56.13   Other lesions of median nerve, bilateral upper
limbs

+ **G56.2   Lesion of ulnar nerve**
Tardy ulnar nerve palsy
G56.20   Lesion of ulnar nerve, unspecified upper limb
G56.21   Lesion of ulnar nerve, right upper limb
G56.22   Lesion of ulnar nerve, left upper limb
G56.23   Lesion of ulnar nerve, bilateral upper limbs

+ **G56.3   Lesion of radial nerve**
G56.30   Lesion of radial nerve, unspecified upper limb
G56.31   Lesion of radial nerve, right upper limb
G56.32   Lesion of radial nerve, left upper limb
G56.33   Lesion of radial nerve, bilateral upper limbs

+ **G56.4   Causalgia of upper limb**
Complex regional pain syndrome II of upper limb

Excludes1: *complex regional pain syndrome I of lower limb*
(G90.52-)
complex regional pain syndrome I of upper limb
(G90.51-)
complex regional pain syndrome II of lower
limb (G57.7-)
reflex sympathetic dystrophy of lower limb
(G90.52-)
reflex sympathetic dystrophy of upper limb
(G90.51-)

G56.40   Causalgia of unspecified upper limb
G56.41   Causalgia of right upper limb
G56.42   Causalgia of left upper limb
G56.43   Causalgia of bilateral upper limbs

+ **G56.8   Other specified mononeuropathies of upper limb**
Interdigital neuroma of upper limb
G56.80   Other specified mononeuropathies of unspecified
upper limb
G56.81   Other specified mononeuropathies of right upper
limb
G56.82   Other specified mononeuropathies of left upper
limb
G56.83   Other specified mononeuropathies of bilateral
upper limbs

+ **G56.9   Unspecified mononeuropathy of upper limb**
G56.90   Unspecified mononeuropathy of unspecified upper
limb
G56.91   Unspecified mononeuropathy of right upper limb
G56.92   Unspecified mononeuropathy of left upper limb
G56.93   Unspecified mononeuropathy of bilateral upper
limbs

G57   Mononeuropathies of lower limb

Excludes1: *current traumatic nerve disorder - see nerve injury by*
body region
AHA CC: 4Q, 2016, 17-18

+ **G57.0   Lesion of sciatic nerve**
Excludes1: *sciatica NOS (M54.3-)*
Excludes2: *sciatica attributed to intervertebral disc*
disorder (M51.1.-)
G57.00   Lesion of sciatic nerve, unspecified lower limb
G57.01   Lesion of sciatic nerve, right lower limb
G57.02   Lesion of sciatic nerve, left lower limb
G57.03   Lesion of sciatic nerve, bilateral lower limbs

+, +7th, X + 7th   ● Newborn   ● Pediatric   ● Maternity   ● Adult   ♀ Female   ♂ Male   Manifestation   Unacceptable PDX   HCC   CC   MCC   HAC

+ **G57.1 Meralgia paresthetica**
   Lateral cutaneous nerve of thigh syndrome
  G57.10 Meralgia paresthetica, unspecified lower limb
  G57.11 Meralgia paresthetica, right lower limb
  G57.12 Meralgia paresthetica, left lower limb
  G57.13 Meralgia paresthetica, bilateral lower limbs
+ **G57.2 Lesion of femoral nerve**
  G57.20 Lesion of femoral nerve, unspecified lower limb
  G57.21 Lesion of femoral nerve, right lower limb
  G57.22 Lesion of femoral nerve, left lower limb
  G57.23 Lesion of femoral nerve, bilateral lower limbs
+ **G57.3 Lesion of lateral popliteal nerve**
   Peroneal nerve palsy
  G57.30 Lesion of lateral popliteal nerve, unspecified lower limb
  G57.31 Lesion of lateral popliteal nerve, right lower limb
  G57.32 Lesion of lateral popliteal nerve, left lower limb
  G57.33 Lesion of lateral popliteal nerve, bilateral lower limbs
+ **G57.4 Lesion of medial popliteal nerve**
  G57.40 Lesion of medial popliteal nerve, unspecified lower limb
  G57.41 Lesion of medial popliteal nerve, right lower limb
  G57.42 Lesion of medial popliteal nerve, left lower limb
  G57.43 Lesion of medial popliteal nerve, bilateral lower limbs
+ **G57.5 Tarsal tunnel syndrome**
  G57.50 Tarsal tunnel syndrome, unspecified lower limb
  G57.51 Tarsal tunnel syndrome, right lower limb
  G57.52 Tarsal tunnel syndrome, left lower limb
  G57.53 Tarsal tunnel syndrome, bilateral lower limbs
+ **G57.6 Lesion of plantar nerve**
   Morton's metatarsalgia
  G57.60 Lesion of plantar nerve, unspecified lower limb
  G57.61 Lesion of plantar nerve, right lower limb
  G57.62 Lesion of plantar nerve, left lower limb
  G57.63 Lesion of plantar nerve, bilateral lower limbs
+ **G57.7 Causalgia of lower limb**
   Complex regional pain syndrome II of lower limb
   Excludes1: *complex regional pain syndrome I of lower limb (G90.52-)*
      complex regional pain syndrome I of upper limb (G90.51-)
      complex regional pain syndrome II of upper limb (G56.4-)
      reflex sympathetic dystrophy of lower limb (G90.52-)
      reflex sympathetic dystrophy of upper limb (G90.51-)
  G57.70 Causalgia of unspecified lower limb
  G57.71 Causalgia of right lower limb
  G57.72 Causalgia of left lower limb
  G57.73 Causalgia of bilateral lower limbs
+ **G57.8 Other specified mononeuropathies of lower limb**
   Interdigital neuroma of lower limb
  G57.80 Other specified mononeuropathies of unspecified lower limb
  G57.81 Other specified mononeuropathies of right lower limb
  G57.82 Other specified mononeuropathies of left lower limb
  G57.83 Other specified mononeuropathies of bilateral lower limbs
+ **G57.9 Unspecified mononeuropathy of lower limb**
  G57.90 Unspecified mononeuropathy of unspecified lower limb
  G57.91 Unspecified mononeuropathy of right lower limb
  G57.92 Unspecified mononeuropathy of left lower limb
  G57.93 Unspecified mononeuropathy of bilateral lower limbs

G58 Other mononeuropathies

  G58.0 Intercostal neuropathy
  G58.7 Mononeuritis multiplex
  G58.8 Other specified mononeuropathies
  G58.9 Mononeuropathy, unspecified

G59 Mononeuropathy in diseases classified elsewhere

  Code first underlying disease
  Excludes1: *diabetic mononeuropathy (E08-E13 with .41)*
      syphilitic nerve paralysis (A52.19)
      syphilitic neuritis (A52.15)
      tuberculous mononeuropathy (A17.83)
  Valid 3-character code, no further characters required

Polyneuropathies and other disorders of the peripheral nervous system (G60-G65)

Excludes1: *neuralgia NOS (M79.2)*
    neuritis NOS (M79.2)
    peripheral neuritis in pregnancy (O26.82-)
    radiculitis NOS (M54.10)

G60 Hereditary and idiopathic neuropathy

  G60.0 Hereditary motor and sensory neuropathy
   Charcot-Marie-Tooth disease
   Déjérine-Sottas disease
   Hereditary motor and sensory neuropathy, types I-IV
   Hypertrophic neuropathy of infancy
   Peroneal muscular atrophy (axonal type) (hypertrophic type)
   Roussy-Levy syndrome
  CC **G60.1 Refsum's disease**
   Infantile Refsum disease
  G60.2 Neuropathy in association with hereditary ataxia
  G60.3 Idiopathic progressive neuropathy
  G60.8 Other hereditary and idiopathic neuropathies
   Dominantly inherited sensory neuropathy
   Morvan's disease
   Nelaton's syndrome
   Recessively inherited sensory neuropathy
  G60.9 Hereditary and idiopathic neuropathy, unspecified

G61 Inflammatory polyneuropathy

  CC **G61.0 Guillain-Barre syndrome**
   Acute (post-)infective polyneuritis
   Miller Fisher Syndrome
   AHA CC: 2Q, 2014, 4
  G61.1 Serum neuropathy
   Use additional code for adverse effect, if applicable, to identify serum (T50.-)
  G61.8 Other inflammatory polyneuropathies
   CC **G61.81 Chronic inflammatory demyelinating polyneuritis**
   G61.82 Multifocal motor neuropathy
    MMN
    AHA CC: 4Q, 2016, 18
   G61.89 Other inflammatory polyneuropathies
  G61.9 Inflammatory polyneuropathy, unspecified

G62 Other and unspecified polyneuropathies

  G62.0 Drug-induced polyneuropathy
   Use additional code for adverse effect, if applicable, to identify drug (T36-T50 with fifth or sixth character 5)
  G62.1 Alcoholic polyneuropathy
   AHA CC: 3Q, 2019, 8
  G62.2 Polyneuropathy due to other toxic agents
   Code first (T51-T65) to identify toxic agent
+ **G62.8 Other specified polyneuropathies**
  CC **G62.81 Critical illness polyneuropathy**
   Acute motor neuropathy
  G62.82 Radiation-induced polyneuropathy
   Use additional external cause code (W88-W90, X39.0-) to identify cause
  G62.89 Other specified polyneuropathies
   AHA CC: 2Q, 2016, 11
  G62.9 Polyneuropathy, unspecified
   Neuropathy NOS

G63 Polyneuropathy in diseases classified elsewhere

  Code first underlying disease, such as:
   amyloidosis (E85.-)
   endocrine disease, except diabetes (E00-E07, E15-E16, E20-E34)
   metabolic diseases (E70-E88)
   neoplasm (C00-D49)
   nutritional deficiency (E40-E64)
  Excludes1: *polyneuropathy (in):*
      diabetes mellitus (E08-E13 with .42)
      diphtheria (A36.83)
      infectious mononucleosis (B27.0-B27.9 with 1)
      Lyme disease (A69.22)
      mumps (B26.84)
      postherpetic (B02.23)
      rheumatoid arthritis (M05.5-)
      scleroderma (M34.83)
      systemic lupus erythematosus (M32.19)
   AHA CC: 4Q, 2012, 99-101
  Valid 3-character code, no further characters required

+, +7th, X + 7th   ● Newborn   ● Pediatric   ● Maternity   ● Adult   ♀ Female   ♂ Male   Manifestation   Unacceptable PDX   HCC   CC   MCC   HAC

G64 Other disorders of peripheral nervous system

Disorder of peripheral nervous system NOS
Valid 3-character code, no further characters required

G65 Sequelae of inflammatory and toxic polyneuropathies

Code first condition resulting from (sequela) of inflammatory and toxic polyneuropathies

G65.0 Sequelae of Guillain-Barré syndrome

G65.1 Sequelae of other inflammatory polyneuropathy

G65.2 Sequelae of toxic polyneuropathy

Diseases of myoneural junction and muscle (G70-G73)

G70 Myasthenia gravis and other myoneural disorders

Excludes1: botulism (A05.1, A48.51-A48.52)
transient neonatal myasthenia gravis (P94.0)

+ **G70.0 Myasthenia gravis**

G70.00 Myasthenia gravis without (acute) exacerbation
Myasthenia gravis NOS

MCC **G70.01 Myasthenia gravis with (acute) exacerbation**
Myasthenia gravis in crisis

G70.1 Toxic myoneural disorders
Code first (T51-T65) to identify toxic agent

G70.2 Congenital and developmental myasthenia

+ **G70.8 Other specified myoneural disorders**

CC **G70.80 Lambert-Eaton syndrome, unspecified**
Lambert-Eaton syndrome NOS

CC **G70.81 Lambert-Eaton syndrome in disease classified elsewhere**
Code first underlying disease
Excludes1: Lambert-Eaton syndrome in neoplastic disease (G73.1)

G70.89 Other specified myoneural disorders

G70.9 Myoneural disorder, unspecified

G71 Primary disorders of muscles

Excludes2: arthrogryposis multiplex congenita (Q74.3)
metabolic disorders (E70-E88)
myositis (M60.-)

+ **G71.0 Muscular dystrophy**
AHA CC: 4Q, 2018, 11

G71.00 Muscular dystrophy, unspecified

G71.01 Duchenne or Becker muscular dystrophy
Autosomal recessive, childhood type, muscular dystrophy resembling Duchenne or Becker muscular dystrophy
Benign [Becker] muscular dystrophy
Severe [Duchenne] muscular dystrophy

G71.02 Facioscapulohumeral muscular dystrophy
Scapulohumeral muscular dystrophy
AHA CC: 4Q, 2018, 12-13

G71.09 Other specified muscular dystrophies
Benign scapuloperoneal muscular dystrophy with early contractures [Emery-Dreifuss]
Congenital muscular dystrophy NOS
Congenital muscular dystrophy with specific morphological abnormalities of the muscle fiber
Distal muscular dystrophy
Limb-girdle muscular dystrophy
Ocular muscular dystrophy
Oculopharyngeal muscular dystrophy
Scapuloperoneal muscular dystrophy

+ **G71.1 Myotonic disorders**

G71.11 Myotonic muscular dystrophy
Dystrophia myotonica [Steinert]
Myotonia atrophica
Myotonic dystrophy
Proximal myotonic myopathy (PROMM)
Steinert disease

G71.12 Myotonia congenita
Acetazolamide responsive myotonia congenita
Dominant myotonia congenita [Thomsen disease]
Myotonia levior
Recessive myotonia congenita [Becker disease]

G71.13 Myotonic chondrodystrophy
Chondrodystrophic myotonia
Congenital myotonic chondrodystrophy
Schwartz-Jampel disease

G71.14 Drug induced myotonia
Use additional code for adverse effect, if applicable, to identify drug (T36-T50 with fifth or sixth character 5)

G71.19 Other specified myotonic disorders
Myotonia fluctuans
Myotonia permanens
Neuromyotonia [Isaacs]
Paramyotonia congenita (of von Eulenburg)
Pseudomyotonia
Symptomatic myotonia

+ **G71.2 Congenital myopathies**
Excludes2: arthrogryposis multiplex congenita (Q74.3)

CC **G71.20 Congenital myopathy, unspecifed**

CC **G71.21 Nemaline myopathy**

+ **G71.22 Centronuclear myopathy**

CC **G71.220 X-linked myotubular myopathy**
Myotubular (centronuclear) myopathy

CC **G71.228 Other centronuclear myopathy**
Autosomal centronuclear myopathy
Autosomal dominant centronuclear myopathy
Autosomal recessive centronuclear myopathy
Centronuclear myopathy, NOS

CC **G71.29 Other congenital myopathy**
Central core disease
Minicore disease
Multicore disease
Multiminicore disease

G71.3 Mitochondrial myopathy, not elsewhere classified
Excludes1: Kearns-Sayre syndrome (H49.81)
Leber's disease (H47.21)
Leigh's encephalopathy (G31.82)
mitochondrial metabolism disorders (E88.4.-)
Reye's syndrome (G93.7)

G71.8 Other primary disorders of muscles

G71.9 Primary disorder of muscle, unspecified
Hereditary myopathy NOS

G72 Other and unspecified myopathies

Excludes1: arthrogryposis multiplex congenita (Q74.3)
dermatopolymyositis (M33.-)
ischemic infarction of muscle (M62.2-)
myositis (M60.-)
polymyositis (M33.2.-)

CC **G72.0 Drug-induced myopathy**
Use additional code for adverse effect, if applicable, to identify drug (T36-T50 with fifth or sixth character 5)

CC **G72.1 Alcoholic myopathy**
Use additional code to identify alcoholism (F10.-)

CC **G72.2 Myopathy due to other toxic agents**
Code first (T51-T65) to identify toxic agent

G72.3 Periodic paralysis
Familial periodic paralysis
Hyperkalemic periodic paralysis (familial)
Hypokalemic periodic paralysis (familial)
Myotonic periodic paralysis (familial)
Normokalemic paralysis (familial)
Potassium sensitive periodic paralysis
Excludes1: paramyotonia congenita (of von Eulenburg) (G71.19)

+ **G72.4 Inflammatory and immune myopathies, not elsewhere classified**

G72.41 Inclusion body myositis [IBM]

G72.49 Other inflammatory and immune myopathies, not elsewhere classified
Inflammatory myopathy NOS

+ **G72.8 Other specified myopathies**

CC **G72.81 Critical illness myopathy**
Acute necrotizing myopathy
Acute quadriplegic myopathy
Intensive care (ICU) myopathy
Myopathy of critical illness

G72.89 Other specified myopathies

G72.9 Myopathy, unspecified

+, +7th, X + 7th   ● Newborn   ● Pediatric   ● Maternity   ● Adult   ♀ Female   ♂ Male   Manifestation   Unacceptable PDX   HCC   CC   MCC   HAC

G73 Disorders of myoneural junction and muscle in diseases classified elsewhere

CC **G73.1 Lambert-Eaton syndrome in neoplastic disease**
  Code first underlying neoplasm (C00-D49)
  Excludes1: Lambert-Eaton syndrome not associated with neoplasm (G70.80-G70.81)

CC **G73.3 Myasthenic syndromes in other diseases classified elsewhere**
  Code first underlying disease, such as:
    neoplasm (C00-D49)
    thyrotoxicosis (E05.-)

G73.7 Myopathy in diseases classified elsewhere
  Code first underlying disease, such as:
    hyperparathyroidism (E21.0, E21.3)
    hypoparathyroidism (E20.-)
    glycogen storage disease (E74.0)
    lipid storage disorders (E75.-)
  Excludes1: myopathy in:
    rheumatoid arthritis (M05.32)
    sarcoidosis (D86.87)
    scleroderma (M34.82)
    sicca syndrome [Sjögren] (M35.03)
    systemic lupus erythematosus (M32.19)

Cerebral palsy and other paralytic syndromes (G80-G83)

G80 Cerebral palsy
  Excludes1: hereditary spastic paraplegia (G11.4)

MCC **G80.0 Spastic quadriplegic cerebral palsy**
  Congenital spastic paralysis (cerebral)

CC **G80.1 Spastic diplegic cerebral palsy**
  Spastic cerebral palsy NOS

CC **G80.2 Spastic hemiplegic cerebral palsy**

CC **G80.3 Athetoid cerebral palsy**
  Double athetosis (syndrome)
  Dyskinetic cerebral palsy
  Dystonic cerebral palsy
  Vogt disease

G80.4 Ataxic cerebral palsy

G80.8 Other cerebral palsy
  Mixed cerebral palsy syndromes

G80.9 Cerebral palsy, unspecified
  Cerebral palsy NOS

G81 Hemiplegia and hemiparesis

NOTE This category is to be used only when hemiplegia (complete) (incomplete) is reported without further specification, or is stated to be old or longstanding but of unspecified cause. The category is also for use in multiple coding to identify these types of hemiplegia resulting from any cause.

  Excludes1: congenital cerebral palsy (G80.-)
    hemiplegia and hemiparesis due to sequela of cerebrovascular disease (I69.05-, I69.15-, I69.25-, I69.35-, I69.85-, I69.95-)
  Review coding guideline C.6.a

+ **G81.0 Flaccid hemiplegia**
  CC **G81.00 Flaccid hemiplegia affecting unspecified side**
  CC **G81.01 Flaccid hemiplegia affecting right dominant side**
  CC **G81.02 Flaccid hemiplegia affecting left dominant side**
  CC **G81.03 Flaccid hemiplegia affecting right nondominant side**
  CC **G81.04 Flaccid hemiplegia affecting left nondominant side**

+ **G81.1 Spastic hemiplegia**
  CC **G81.10 Spastic hemiplegia affecting unspecified side**
  CC **G81.11 Spastic hemiplegia affecting right dominant side**
  CC **G81.12 Spastic hemiplegia affecting left dominant side**
  CC **G81.13 Spastic hemiplegia affecting right nondominant side**
  CC **G81.14 Spastic hemiplegia affecting left nondominant side**

+ **G81.9 Hemiplegia, unspecified**
  CC **G81.90 Hemiplegia, unspecified affecting unspecified side**
  CC **G81.91 Hemiplegia, unspecified affecting right dominant side**
  CC **G81.92 Hemiplegia, unspecified affecting left dominant side**
  CC **G81.93 Hemiplegia, unspecified affecting right nondominant side**
  CC **G81.94 Hemiplegia, unspecified affecting left nondominant side**
    AHA CC: 1Q, 2015, 26

G82 Paraplegia (paraparesis) and quadriplegia (quadriparesis)

NOTE This category is to be used only when the listed conditions are reported without further specification, or are stated to be old or longstanding but of unspecified cause. The category is also for use in multiple coding to identify these conditions resulting from any cause

  Excludes1: congenital cerebral palsy (G80.-)
    functional quadriplegia (R53.2)
    hysterical paralysis (F44.4)

+ **G82.2 Paraplegia**
  Paralysis of both lower limbs NOS
  Paraparesis (lower) NOS
  Paraplegia (lower) NOS
  CC **G82.20 Paraplegia, unspecified**
    AHA CC: 3Q, 2017, 3
  CC **G82.21 Paraplegia, complete**
  CC **G82.22 Paraplegia, incomplete**

+ **G82.5 Quadriplegia**
  MCC **G82.50 Quadriplegia, unspecified**
  MCC **G82.51 Quadriplegia, C1-C4 complete**
  MCC **G82.52 Quadriplegia, C1-C4 incomplete**
  MCC **G82.53 Quadriplegia, C5-C7 complete**
  MCC **G82.54 Quadriplegia, C5-C7 incomplete**

G83 Other paralytic syndromes

NOTE This category is to be used only when the listed conditions are reported without further specification, or are stated to be old or longstanding but of unspecified cause. The category is also for use in multiple coding to identify these conditions resulting from any cause.

Includes: paralysis (complete) (incomplete), except as in G80-G82

CC **G83.0 Diplegia of upper limbs**
  Diplegia (upper)
  Paralysis of both upper limbs

+ **G83.1 Monoplegia of lower limb**
  Paralysis of lower limb
  Excludes1: monoplegia of lower limbs due to sequela of cerebrovascular disease (I69.04-, I69.14-, I69.24-, I69.34-, I69.84-, I69.94-)
  Review coding guideline C.6.a
  G83.10 Monoplegia of lower limb affecting unspecified side
  G83.11 Monoplegia of lower limb affecting right dominant side
  G83.12 Monoplegia of lower limb affecting left dominant side
  G83.13 Monoplegia of lower limb affecting right nondominant side
  G83.14 Monoplegia of lower limb affecting left nondominant side

+ **G83.2 Monoplegia of upper limb**
  Paralysis of upper limb
  Excludes1: monoplegia of upper limbs due to sequela of cerebrovascular disease (I69.03-, I69.13-, I69.23-, I69.33-, I69.83-, I69.93-)
  Review coding guideline C.6.a
  G83.20 Monoplegia of upper limb affecting unspecified side
  G83.21 Monoplegia of upper limb affecting right dominant side
  G83.22 Monoplegia of upper limb affecting left dominant side
  G83.23 Monoplegia of upper limb affecting right nondominant side
  G83.24 Monoplegia of upper limb affecting left nondominant side

+, +7th, X + 7th   • Newborn   • Pediatric   • Maternity   • Adult   ♀ Female   ♂ Male   Manifestation   Unacceptable PDX   HCC   CC   MCC   HAC

+ **G83.3 Monoplegia, unspecified**
    Review coding guideline C.6.a
    G83.30 Monoplegia, unspecified affecting unspecified side
    G83.31 Monoplegia, unspecified affecting right dominant side
    G83.32 Monoplegia, unspecified affecting left dominant side
    G83.33 Monoplegia, unspecified affecting right nondominant side
    G83.34 Monoplegia, unspecified affecting left nondominant side

CC **G83.4 Cauda equina syndrome**
    Neurogenic bladder due to cauda equina syndrome
    Excludes1: *cord bladder NOS (G95.89)*
        neurogenic bladder NOS (N31.9)

MCC **G83.5 Locked-in state**

+ **G83.8 Other specified paralytic syndromes**
    Excludes1: *paralytic syndromes due to current spinal cord injury-code to spinal cord injury (S14, S24, S34)*
    G83.81 Brown-Séquard syndrome
    G83.82 Anterior cord syndrome
    G83.83 Posterior cord syndrome
    G83.84 Todd's paralysis (postepileptic)
    G83.89 Other specified paralytic syndromes

G83.9 Paralytic syndrome, unspecified

Other disorders of the nervous system (G89-G99)

G89 Pain, not elsewhere classified

Code also related psychological factors associated with pain (F45.42)
Excludes1: *generalized pain NOS (R52)*
    pain disorders exclusively related to psychological factors (F45.41)
    pain NOS (R52)
Excludes2: *atypical face pain (G50.1)*
    headache syndromes (G44.-)
    localized pain, unspecified type - code to pain by site, such as:
      abdomen pain (R10.-)
      back pain (M54.9)
      breast pain (N64.4)
      chest pain (R07.1-R07.9)
      ear pain (H92.0-)
      eye pain (H57.1)
      headache (R51.9)
      joint pain (M25.5-)
      limb pain (M79.6-)
      lumbar region pain (M54.5)
      painful urination (R30.9)
      pelvic and perineal pain (R10.2)
      shoulder pain (M25.51-)
      spine pain (M54.-)
      throat pain (R07.0)
      tongue pain (K14.6)
      tooth pain (K08.8)
      renal colic (N23)
    migraines (G43.-)
    myalgia (M79.1-)
    pain from prosthetic devices, implants, and grafts (T82.84, T83.84, T84.84, T85.84-)
    phantom limb syndrome with pain (G54.6)
    vulvar vestibulitis (N94.810)
    vulvodynia (N94.81-)
Review coding guideline C.5.a
Review coding guidelines C.6.b.1 and C.6.b.3
Review coding guideline C.19.g.2

G89.0 Central pain syndrome
    Déjérine-Roussy syndrome
    Myelopathic pain syndrome
    Thalamic pain syndrome (hyperesthetic)
    Review coding guideline C.6.b.6

+ **G89.1 Acute pain, not elsewhere classified**
    G89.11 Acute pain due to trauma
    G89.12 Acute post-thoracotomy pain
      Post-thoracotomy pain NOS
    G89.18 Other acute postprocedural pain
      Postoperative pain NOS
      Postprocedural pain NOS

+ **G89.2 Chronic pain, not elsewhere classified**
    Excludes1: *causalgia, lower limb (G57.7-)*
      causalgia, upper limb (G56.4-)
      central pain syndrome (G89.0)
      chronic pain syndrome (G89.4)
      complex regional pain syndrome II, lower limb (G57.7-)
      complex regional pain syndrome II, upper limb (G56.4-)
      neoplasm related chronic pain (G89.3)
      reflex sympathetic dystrophy (G90.5-)
    Review coding guideline C.6.b.4
    G89.21 Chronic pain due to trauma
    G89.22 Chronic post-thoracotomy pain
    G89.28 Other chronic postprocedural pain
      Other chronic postoperative pain
    G89.29 Other chronic pain

G89.3 Neoplasm related pain (acute) (chronic)
    Cancer associated pain
    Pain due to malignancy (primary) (secondary)
    Tumor associated pain
    Review coding guideline C.6.b.5

G89.4 Chronic pain syndrome
    Chronic pain associated with significant psychosocial dysfunction
    Review coding guideline C.6.b.6

G90 Disorders of autonomic nervous system
    Excludes1: *dysfunction of the autonomic nervous system due to alcohol (G31.2)*

+ **G90.0 Idiopathic peripheral autonomic neuropathy**
    G90.01 Carotid sinus syncope
      Carotid sinus syndrome
    G90.09 Other idiopathic peripheral autonomic neuropathy
      Idiopathic peripheral autonomic neuropathy NOS

G90.1 Familial dysautonomia [Riley-Day]

G90.2 Horner's syndrome
    Bernard(-Horner) syndrome
    Cervical sympathetic dystrophy or paralysis

CC **G90.3 Multi-system degeneration of the autonomic nervous system**
    Neurogenic orthostatic hypotension [Shy-Drager]
    Excludes1: *orthostatic hypotension NOS (I95.1)*

G90.4 Autonomic dysreflexia
    Use additional code to identify the cause, such as:
      fecal impaction (K56.41)
      pressure ulcer (pressure area) (L89.-)
      urinary tract infection (N39.0)

+ **G90.5 Complex regional pain syndrome I (CRPS I)**
    Reflex sympathetic dystrophy
    Excludes1: *causalgia of lower limb (G57.7-)*
      causalgia of upper limb (G56.4-)
      complex regional pain syndrome II of lower limb (G57.7-)
      complex regional pain syndrome II of upper limb (G56.4-)
    CC **G90.50 Complex regional pain syndrome I, unspecified**
    + **G90.51 Complex regional pain syndrome I of upper limb**
      CC **G90.511 Complex regional pain syndrome I of right upper limb**
      CC **G90.512 Complex regional pain syndrome I of left upper limb**
      CC **G90.513 Complex regional pain syndrome I of upper limb, bilateral**
      CC **G90.519 Complex regional pain syndrome I of unspecified upper limb**
    + **G90.52 Complex regional pain syndrome I of lower limb**
      CC **G90.521 Complex regional pain syndrome I of right lower limb**
      CC **G90.522 Complex regional pain syndrome I of left lower limb**
      CC **G90.523 Complex regional pain syndrome I of lower limb, bilateral**
      CC **G90.529 Complex regional pain syndrome I of unspecified lower limb**
    CC **G90.59 Complex regional pain syndrome I of other specified site**

G90.8 Other disorders of autonomic nervous system

G90.9 Disorder of the autonomic nervous system, unspecified

G91 **Hydrocephalus**
    Includes: acquired hydrocephalus
    Excludes1: Arnold-Chiari syndrome with hydrocephalus (Q07.-)
         congenital hydrocephalus (Q03.-)
         spina bifida with hydrocephalus (Q05.-)
CC **G91.0** **Communicating hydrocephalus**
    Secondary normal pressure hydrocephalus
CC **G91.1** **Obstructive hydrocephalus**
CC **G91.2** **(Idiopathic) normal pressure hydrocephalus**
    Normal pressure hydrocephalus NOS
CC **G91.3** **Post-traumatic hydrocephalus, unspecified**
    G91.4 **Hydrocephalus in diseases classified elsewhere**
        Code first underlying condition, such as:
           congenital syphilis (A50.4-)
           neoplasm (C00-D49)
           plasminogen deficiency (E88.02)
        Excludes1: hydrocephalus due to congenital toxoplasmosis
           (P37.1)
        AHA CC: 3Q, 2014, 3-4
CC **G91.8** **Other hydrocephalus**
CC **G91.9** **Hydrocephalus, unspecified**
MCC **G92** **Toxic encephalopathy**
    Toxic encephalitis
    Toxic metabolic encephalopathy
    Code first, if applicable, drug induced (T36-T50) or use
        (T51-T65) to identify toxic agent
    AHA CC: 1Q, 2017, 39-40
    Valid 3-character code, no further characters required
G93 **Other disorders of brain**
    G93.0 **Cerebral cysts**
        Arachnoid cyst
        Porencephalic cyst, acquired
        Excludes1: acquired periventricular cysts of newborn (P91.1)
           congenital cerebral cysts (Q04.6)
CC **G93.1** **Anoxic brain damage, not elsewhere classified**
        Excludes1: cerebral anoxia due to anesthesia during labor
           and delivery (O74.3)
           cerebral anoxia due to anesthesia during the
           puerperium (O89.2)
           neonatal anoxia (P84)
    G93.2 **Benign intracranial hypertension**
        Pseudotumor
        Excludes1: hypertensive encephalopathy (I67.4)
           obstructive hydrocephalus (G91.1)
    G93.3 **Postviral fatigue syndrome**
        Benign myalgic encephalomyelitis
        Excludes1: chronic fatigue syndrome NOS (R53.82)
+ **G93.4** **Other and unspecified encephalopathy**
        Excludes1: alcoholic encephalopathy (G31.2)
           encephalopathy in diseases classified
           elsewhere (G94)
           hypertensive encephalopathy (I67.4)
        Excludes2: toxic (metabolic) encephalopathy (G92)
        AHA CC: 2Q, 2017, 8-9
CC **G93.40** **Encephalopathy, unspecified**
MCC **G93.41** **Metabolic encephalopathy**
        Septic encephalopathy
        AHA CC: 3Q, 2015, 21; 3Q, 2016, 42
CC **G93.49** **Other encephalopathy**
        Encephalopathy NEC
        AHA CC: 2Q, 2017, 9; 2Q, 2018, 22, 25; 4Q, 2018, 16
MCC **G93.5** **Compression of brain**
        Arnold-Chiari type 1 compression of brain
        Compression of brain (stem)
        Herniation of brain (stem)
        Excludes1: diffuse traumatic compression of brain (S06.2-)
           focal traumatic compression of brain (S06.3-)
        AHA CC: 2Q, 2020, 31
MCC **G93.6** **Cerebral edema**
        Excludes1: cerebral edema due to birth injury (P11.0)
           traumatic cerebral edema (S06.1-)
• MCC **G93.7** **Reye's syndrome**
        Code first poisoning due to salicylates, if applicable
           (T39.0-, with sixth character 1-4)
        Use additional code for adverse effect due to salicylates,
           if applicable (T39.0-, with sixth character 5)

+ **G93.8** **Other specified disorders of brain**
    G93.81 **Temporal sclerosis**
        Hippocampal sclerosis
        Mesial temporal sclerosis
MCC **G93.82** **Brain death**
    G93.89 **Other specified disorders of brain**
        Postradiation encephalopathy
        AHA CC: 4Q, 2016, 4-7; 3Q, 2019, 8-9; 2Q, 2020, 24
    G93.9 **Disorder of brain, unspecified**
G94 **Other disorders of brain in diseases classified elsewhere**
    Code first underlying disease
    Excludes1: encephalopathy in congenital syphilis (A50.49)
         encephalopathy in influenza (J09.X9, J10.81, J11.81)
         encephalopathy in syphilis (A52.19)
         hydrocephalus in diseases classified elsewhere (G91.4)
    AHA CC: 2Q, 2017, 8-9
    Valid 3-character code, no further characters required
G95 **Other and unspecified diseases of spinal cord**
    Excludes2: myelitis (G04.-)
CC **G95.0** **Syringomyelia and syringobulbia**
+ **G95.1** **Vascular myelopathies**
        Excludes2: intraspinal phlebitis and thrombophlebitis,
           except non-pyogenic (G08)
MCC **G95.11** **Acute infarction of spinal cord (embolic)**
        (nonembolic)
        Anoxia of spinal cord
        Arterial thrombosis of spinal cord
MCC **G95.19** **Other vascular myelopathies**
        Edema of spinal cord
        Hematomyelia
        Nonpyogenic intraspinal phlebitis and
           thrombophlebitis
        Subacute necrotic myelopathy
+ **G95.2** **Other and unspecified cord compression**
CC **G95.20** **Unspecified cord compression**
CC **G95.29** **Other cord compression**
+ **G95.8** **Other specified diseases of spinal cord**
        Excludes1: neurogenic bladder NOS (N31.9)
           neurogenic bladder due to cauda equina
           syndrome (G83.4)
           neuromuscular dysfunction of bladder without
           spinal cord lesion (N31.-)
CC **G95.81** **Conus medullaris syndrome**
CC **G95.89** **Other specified diseases of spinal cord**
        Cord bladder NOS
        Drug-induced myelopathy
        Radiation-induced myelopathy
        Excludes1: myelopathy NOS (G95.9)
CC **G95.9** **Disease of spinal cord, unspecified**
    Myelopathy NOS
G96 **Other disorders of central nervous system**
+ **G96.0** **Cerebrospinal fluid leak**
        Excludes1: cerebrospinal fluid leak from spinal puncture
           (G97.0)
        Code also if applicable:
           intracranial hypotension (G96.81-)
        AHA CC: 2Q, 2018, 13
CC **G96.00** **Cerebrospinal fluid leak, unspecified**
        Code also if applicable:
           head injury (S00.- to S09.-)
CC **G96.01** **Cranial cerebrospinal fluid leak, spontaneous**
        Otorrhea due to spontaneous cerebrospinal fluid
           CSF leak
        Rhinorrhea due to spontaneous cerebrospinal fluid
           CSF leak
        Spontaneous cerebrospinal fluid leak from skull base
CC **G96.02** **Spinal cerebrospinal fluid leak, spontaneous**
        Spontaneous cerebrospinal fluid leak from spine
CC **G96.08** **Other cranial cerebrospinal fluid leak**
        Postoperative cranial cerebrospinal fluid leak
        Traumatic cranial cerebrospinal fluid leak
        Code also if applicable:
           head injury (S00.- to S09.-)
CC **G96.09** **Other spinal cerebrospinal fluid leak**
        Other spinal CSF leak
        Postoperative spinal cerebrospinal fluid leak
        Traumatic spinal cerebrospinal fluid leak
        Code also if applicable:
           head injury (S00.- to S09.-)

609

+, +7th, X + 7th   ● Newborn   ● Pediatric   ● Maternity   ● Adult   ♀ Female   ♂ Male   Manifestation   Unacceptable PDX   HCC   CC   MCC   HAC

+ **G96.1 Disorders of meninges, not elsewhere classified**
  CC **G96.11 Dural tear**
      Excludes1: *accidental puncture or laceration of dura during a procedure (G97.41)*
      Code also intracranial hypotension, if applicable (G96.81-)
      AHA CC: 4Q, 2014, 24
  G96.12 Meningeal adhesions (cerebral) (spinal)
  + **G96.19 Other disorders of meninges, not elsewhere classified**
    G96.191 Perineural cyst
      Cervical nerve root cyst
      Lumbar nerve root cyst
      Sacral nerve root cyst
      Tarlov cyst
      Thoracic nerve root cyst
    G96.198 Other disorders of meninges, not elsewhere classified
+ **G96.8 Other specified disorders of central nervous system**
  + **G96.81 Intracranial hypotension**
      Code also any associated diagnoses, such as:
        Brachial amyotrophy (G54.5)
        Cerebrospinal fluid leak from spine (G96.02)
        Cranial nerve disorders in diseases classified elsewhere (G53)
        Nerve root and compressions in diseases classified elsewhere (G55)
        Nonpyogenic thrombosis of intracranial venous system (I67.6)
        Nontraumatic intracerebral hemorrhage (I61.-)
        Nontraumatic subdural hemorrhage (I62.0-)
        Other and unspecified cord compression (G95.2-)
        Other secondary parkinsonism (G21.8)
        Reversible cerebrovascular vasoconstriction syndrome (I67.841)
        Spinal cord herniation (G95.89)
        Stroke (I63.-)
        Syringomyelia (G95.0)
    G96.810 Intracranial hypotension, unspecified
    G96.811 Intracranial hypotension, spontaneous
    G96.819 Other intracranial hypotension
  G96.89 Other specified disorders of central nervous system
G96.9 Disorder of central nervous system, unspecified

G97 Intraoperative and postprocedural complications and disorders of nervous system, not elsewhere classified
  Excludes2: *intraoperative and postprocedural cerebrovascular infarction (I97.81-, I97.82-)*
  AHA CC: 4Q, 2016, 9-10
  CC **G97.0 Cerebrospinal fluid leak from spinal puncture**
      Code also any associated diagnoses or complications, such as:
        intracranial hypotension following a procedure (G97.83-G97.84)
  G97.1 Other reaction to spinal and lumbar puncture
      Headache due to lumbar puncture
      Other reaction to spinal dural puncture
      Code also, if applicable, any associated headache with orthostatic component (R51.0)
  CC **G97.2 Intracranial hypotension following ventricular shunting**
      Code also any associated diagnoses or complications
  + **G97.3 Intraoperative hemorrhage and hematoma of a nervous system organ or structure complicating a procedure**
      Excludes1: *intraoperative hemorrhage and hematoma of a nervous system organ or structure due to accidental puncture and laceration during a procedure (G97.4-)*
  CC **G97.31 Intraoperative hemorrhage and hematoma of a nervous system organ or structure complicating a nervous system procedure**
  CC **G97.32 Intraoperative hemorrhage and hematoma of a nervous system organ or structure complicating other procedure**
+ **G97.4 Accidental puncture and laceration of a nervous system organ or structure during a procedure**
  CC **G97.41 Accidental puncture or laceration of dura during a procedure**
      Incidental (inadvertent) durotomy
      Code also any associated diagnoses or complications

  CC **G97.48 Accidental puncture and laceration of other nervous system organ or structure during a nervous system procedure**
  CC **G97.49 Accidental puncture and laceration of other nervous system organ or structure during other procedure**
+ **G97.5 Postprocedural hemorrhage of a nervous system organ or structure following a procedure**
  CC **G97.51 Postprocedural hemorrhage of a nervous system organ or structure following a nervous system procedure**
  CC **G97.52 Postprocedural hemorrhage of a nervous system organ or structure following other procedure**
+ **G97.6 Postprocedural hematoma and seroma of a nervous system organ or structure following a procedure**
  CC **G97.61 Postprocedural hematoma of a nervous system organ or structure following a nervous system procedure**
  CC **G97.62 Postprocedural hematoma of a nervous system organ or structure following other procedure**
  CC **G97.63 Postprocedural seroma of a nervous system organ or structure following a nervous system procedure**
  CC **G97.64 Postprocedural seroma of a nervous system organ or structure following other procedure**
+ **G97.8 Other intraoperative and postprocedural complications and disorders of nervous system**
      Use additional code to further specify disorder
  CC **G97.81 Other intraoperative complications of nervous system**
  CC **G97.82 Other postprocedural complications and disorders of nervous system**
  CC **G97.83 Intracranial hypotension following lumbar cerebrospinal fluid shunting**
      Code also any associated diagnoses or complications
  CC **G97.84 Intracranial hypotension following other procedure**
      Code also, if applicable:
        accidental puncture or laceration of dura during a procedure (G97.41)
        cerebrospinal fluid leak from spinal puncture (G97.0)

G98 Other disorders of nervous system not elsewhere classified
  Includes: nervous system disorder NOS
  G98.0 Neurogenic arthritis, not elsewhere classified
      Nonsyphilitic neurogenic arthropathy NEC
      Nonsyphilitic neurogenic spondylopathy NEC
      Excludes1: *spondylopathy (in):*
        syringomyelia and syringobulbia (G95.0)
        tabes dorsalis (A52.11)
  G98.8 Other disorders of nervous system
      Nervous system disorder NOS

G99 Other disorders of nervous system in diseases classified elsewhere
  CC **G99.0 Autonomic neuropathy in diseases classified elsewhere**
      Code first underlying disease, such as:
        amyloidosis (E85.-)
        gout (M1A.-, M10.-)
        hyperthyroidism (E05.-)
      Excludes1: *diabetic autonomic neuropathy (E08-E13 with .43)*
  CC **G99.2 Myelopathy in diseases classified elsewhere**
      Code first underlying disease, such as:
        neoplasm (C00-D49)
      Excludes1: *myelopathy in:*
        intervertebral disease (M50.0-, M51.0-)
        spondylosis (M47.0-, M47.1-)
      AHA CC: 3Q, 2018, 18-19
  G99.8 Other specified disorders of nervous system in diseases classified elsewhere
      Code first underlying disorder, such as:
        amyloidosis (E85.-)
        avitaminosis (E56.9)
      Excludes1: *nervous system involvement in:*
        cysticercosis (B69.0)
        rubella (B06.0-)
        syphilis (A52.1-)

+, +7th, X + 7th   ● Newborn   ● Pediatric   ● Maternity   ● Adult   ♀ Female   ♂ Male   Manifestation   Unacceptable PDX   HCC   CC   MCC   HAC

Chapter 7: Diseases of the Eye and Adnexa (H00-H59)

NOTE Use an external cause code following the code for the eye condition, if applicable, to identify the cause of the eye condition

Excludes2: *certain conditions originating in the perinatal period (P04-P96)*
certain infectious and parasitic diseases (A00-B99)
complications of pregnancy, childbirth and the puerperium (O00-O9A)
congenital malformations, deformations, and chromosomal abnormalities (Q00-Q99)
diabetes mellitus related eye conditions (E09.3-, E10.3-, E11.3-, E13.3-)
endocrine, nutritional and metabolic diseases (E00-E88)
injury (trauma) of eye and orbit (S05.-)
injury, poisoning and certain other consequences of external causes (S00-T88)
neoplasms (C00-D49)
symptoms, signs and abnormal clinical and laboratory findings, not elsewhere classified (R00-R94)
syphilis related eye disorders (A50.01, A50.3-, A51.43, A52.71)

This chapter contains the following category blocks:

H00-H05 Disorders of eyelid, lacrimal system and orbit
H10-H11 Disorders of conjunctiva
H15-H22 Disorders of sclera, cornea, iris and ciliary body
H25-H28 Disorders of lens
H30-H36 Disorders of choroid and retina
H40-H42 Glaucoma
H43-H44 Disorders of vitreous body and globe
H46-H47 Disorders of optic nerve and visual pathways
H49-H52 Disorders of ocular muscles, binocular movement, accommodation and refraction
H53-H54 Visual disturbances and blindness
H55-H57 Other disorders of eye and adnexa
H59 Intraoperative and postprocedural complications and disorders of eye and adnexa, not elsewhere classified

C. Chapter-Specific Coding Guidelines

In addition to general coding guidelines, there are guidelines for specific diagnoses and/or conditions in the classification. Unless otherwise indicated, these guidelines apply to all health care settings. Please refer to Section II for guidelines on the selection of principal diagnosis.

7. Chapter 7: Diseases of the Eye and Adnexa (H00-H59)

a. Glaucoma

1) Assigning Glaucoma Codes

Assign as many codes from category H40, Glaucoma, as needed to identify the type of glaucoma, the affected eye, and the glaucoma stage.

2) Bilateral glaucoma with same type and stage

When a patient has bilateral glaucoma and both eyes are documented as being the same type and stage, and there is a code for bilateral glaucoma, report only the code for the type of glaucoma, bilateral, with the seventh character for the stage.

When a patient has bilateral glaucoma and both eyes are documented as being the same type and stage, and the classification does not provide a code for bilateral glaucoma (i.e. subcategories H40.10, H40.11 and H40.20) report only one code for the type of glaucoma with the appropriate seventh character for the stage.

3) Bilateral glaucoma stage with different types or stages

When a patient has bilateral glaucoma and each eye is documented as having a different type or stage, and the classification distinguishes laterality, assign the appropriate code for each eye rather than the code for bilateral glaucoma.

When a patient has bilateral glaucoma and each eye is documented as having a different type, and the classification does not distinguish laterality (i.e. subcategories H40.10, H40.11 and H40.20), assign one code for each type of glaucoma with the appropriate seventh character for the stage.

When a patient has bilateral glaucoma and each eye is documented as having the same type, but different stage, and the classification does not distinguish laterality (i.e. subcategories H40.10, H40.11 and H40.20), assign a code for the type of glaucoma for each eye with the seventh character for the specific glaucoma stage documented for each eye.

4) Patient admitted with glaucoma and stage evolves during the admission

If a patient is admitted with glaucoma and the stage progresses during the admission, assign the code for highest stage documented.

5) Indeterminate stage glaucoma

Assignment of the seventh character "4" for "indeterminate stage" should be based on the clinical documentation. The seventh character "4" is used for glaucomas whose stage cannot be clinically determined. This seventh character should not be confused with the seventh character "0", unspecified, which should be assigned when there is no documentation regarding the stage of the glaucoma.

b. Blindness

If "blindness" or "low vision" of both eyes is documented but the visual impairment category is not documented, assign code H54.3, Unqualified visual loss, both eyes. If "blindness" or "low vision" in one eye is documented but the visual impairment category is not documented, assign a code from H54.6-, Unqualified visual loss, one eye. If "blindness" or "visual loss" is documented without any information about whether one or both eyes are affected, assign code H54.7, Unspecified visual loss.

Disorders of eyelid, lacrimal system and orbit (H00-H05)

Excludes2: *open wound of eyelid (S01.1-)*
superficial injury of eyelid (S00.1-, S00.2-)

H00 Hordeolum and chalazion

+ H00.0 Hordeolum (externum) (internum) of eyelid
 + H00.01 Hordeolum externum
  Hordeolum NOS
  Stye
  H00.011 Hordeolum externum right upper eyelid
  H00.012 Hordeolum externum right lower eyelid
  H00.013 Hordeolum externum right eye, unspecified eyelid
  H00.014 Hordeolum externum left upper eyelid
  H00.015 Hordeolum externum left lower eyelid
  H00.016 Hordeolum externum left eye, unspecified eyelid
  H00.019 Hordeolum externum unspecified eye, unspecified eyelid
 + H00.02 Hordeolum internum
  Infection of meibomian gland
  H00.021 Hordeolum internum right upper eyelid
  H00.022 Hordeolum internum right lower eyelid
  H00.023 Hordeolum internum right eye, unspecified eyelid
  H00.024 Hordeolum internum left upper eyelid
  H00.025 Hordeolum internum left lower eyelid
  H00.026 Hordeolum internum left eye, unspecified eyelid
  H00.029 Hordeolum internum unspecified eye, unspecified eyelid
 + H00.03 Abscess of eyelid
  Furuncle of eyelid
  H00.031 Abscess of right upper eyelid
  H00.032 Abscess of right lower eyelid
  H00.033 Abscess of eyelid right eye, unspecified eyelid
  H00.034 Abscess of left upper eyelid
  H00.035 Abscess of left lower eyelid
  H00.036 Abscess of eyelid left eye, unspecified eyelid
  H00.039 Abscess of eyelid unspecified eye, unspecified eyelid
+ H00.1 Chalazion
 Meibomian (gland) cyst
 Excludes2: *infected meibomian gland (H00.02-)*
 H00.11 Chalazion right upper eyelid
 H00.12 Chalazion right lower eyelid
 H00.13 Chalazion right eye, unspecified eyelid
 H00.14 Chalazion left upper eyelid
 H00.15 Chalazion left lower eyelid
 H00.16 Chalazion left eye, unspecified eyelid
 H00.19 Chalazion unspecified eye, unspecified eyelid

H01 Other inflammation of eyelid
+ H01.0 Blepharitis
 Excludes1: *blepharoconjunctivitis (H10.5-)*
 AHA CC: 4Q, 2018, 13
 + H01.00 Unspecified blepharitis
  H01.001 Unspecified blepharitis right upper eyelid
  H01.002 Unspecified blepharitis right lower eyelid
  H01.003 Unspecified blepharitis right eye, unspecified eyelid
  H01.004 Unspecified blepharitis left upper eyelid
  H01.005 Unspecified blepharitis left lower eyelid

+, +7th, X + 7th ● Newborn ● Pediatric ● Maternity ● Adult ♀ Female ♂ Male Manifestation Unacceptable PDX HCC CC MCC HAC

Eye

©AHIMA

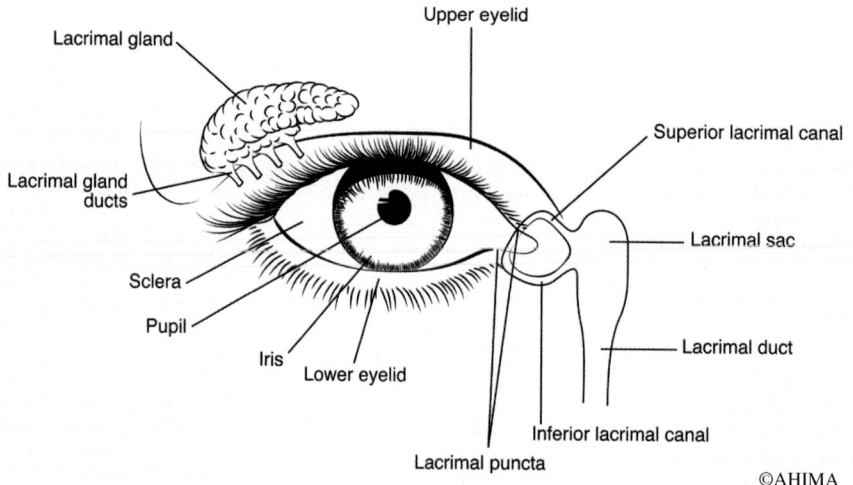

©AHIMA

Muscles of the Eye

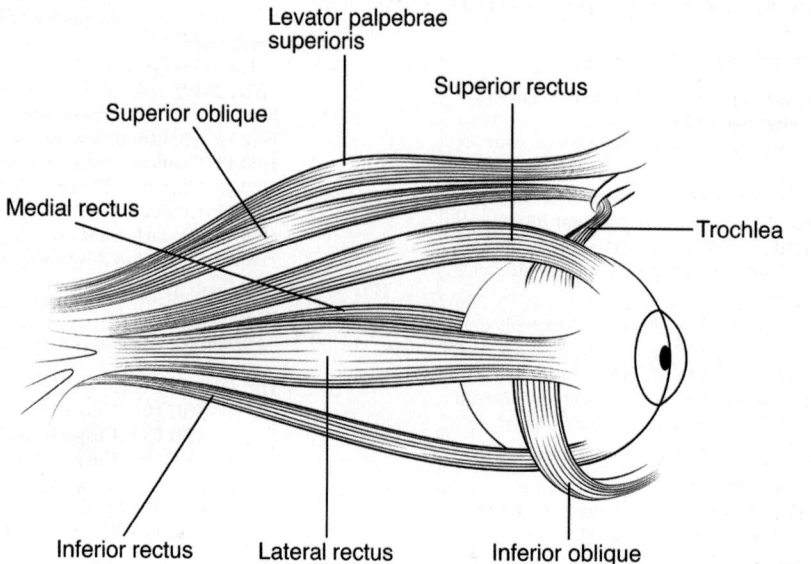

©AHIMA

H01.006 Unspecified blepharitis left eye, unspecified eyelid
H01.009 Unspecified blepharitis unspecified eye, unspecified eyelid
H01.00A Unspecified blepharitis right eye, upper and lower eyelids
H01.00B Unspecified blepharitis left eye, upper and lower eyelids
+ H01.01 Ulcerative blepharitis
H01.011 Ulcerative blepharitis right upper eyelid
H01.012 Ulcerative blepharitis right lower eyelid
H01.013 Ulcerative blepharitis right eye, unspecified eyelid
H01.014 Ulcerative blepharitis left upper eyelid
H01.015 Ulcerative blepharitis left lower eyelid
H01.016 Ulcerative blepharitis left eye, unspecified eyelid
H01.019 Ulcerative blepharitis unspecified eye, unspecified eyelid
H01.01A Ulcerative blepharitis right eye, upper and lower eyelids
H01.01B Ulcerative blepharitis left eye, upper and lower eyelids
+ H01.02 Squamous blepharitis
H01.021 Squamous blepharitis right upper eyelid
H01.022 Squamous blepharitis right lower eyelid
H01.023 Squamous blepharitis right eye, unspecified eyelid
H01.024 Squamous blepharitis left upper eyelid
H01.025 Squamous blepharitis left lower eyelid
H01.026 Squamous blepharitis left eye, unspecified eyelid
H01.029 Squamous blepharitis unspecified eye, unspecified eyelid
H01.02A Squamous blepharitis right eye, upper and lower eyelids
H01.02B Squamous blepharitis left eye, upper and lower eyelids
+ H01.1 Noninfectious dermatoses of eyelid
+ H01.11 Allergic dermatitis of eyelid
Contact dermatitis of eyelid
H01.111 Allergic dermatitis of right upper eyelid
H01.112 Allergic dermatitis of right lower eyelid
H01.113 Allergic dermatitis of right eye, unspecified eyelid
H01.114 Allergic dermatitis of left upper eyelid
H01.115 Allergic dermatitis of left lower eyelid
H01.116 Allergic dermatitis of left eye, unspecified eyelid
H01.119 Allergic dermatitis of unspecified eye, unspecified eyelid
+ H01.12 Discoid lupus erythematosus of eyelid
H01.121 Discoid lupus erythematosus of right upper eyelid
H01.122 Discoid lupus erythematosus of right lower eyelid
H01.123 Discoid lupus erythematosus of right eye, unspecified eyelid
H01.124 Discoid lupus erythematosus of left upper eyelid
H01.125 Discoid lupus erythematosus of left lower eyelid
H01.126 Discoid lupus erythematosus of left eye, unspecified eyelid
H01.129 Discoid lupus erythematosus of unspecified eye, unspecified eyelid
+ H01.13 Eczematous dermatitis of eyelid
H01.131 Eczematous dermatitis of right upper eyelid
H01.132 Eczematous dermatitis of right lower eyelid
H01.133 Eczematous dermatitis of right eye, unspecified eyelid
H01.134 Eczematous dermatitis of left upper eyelid
H01.135 Eczematous dermatitis of left lower eyelid
H01.136 Eczematous dermatitis of left eye, unspecified eyelid
H01.139 Eczematous dermatitis of unspecified eye, unspecified eyelid

+ H01.14 Xeroderma of eyelid
H01.141 Xeroderma of right upper eyelid
H01.142 Xeroderma of right lower eyelid
H01.143 Xeroderma of right eye, unspecified eyelid
H01.144 Xeroderma of left upper eyelid
H01.145 Xeroderma of left lower eyelid
H01.146 Xeroderma of left eye, unspecified eyelid
H01.149 Xeroderma of unspecified eye, unspecified eyelid
H01.8 Other specified inflammations of eyelid
H01.9 Unspecified inflammation of eyelid
Inflammation of eyelid NOS

H02 Other disorders of eyelid
Excludes1: congenital malformations of eyelid (Q10.0-Q10.3)
+ H02.0 Entropion and trichiasis of eyelid
+ H02.00 Unspecified entropion of eyelid
H02.001 Unspecified entropion of right upper eyelid
H02.002 Unspecified entropion of right lower eyelid
H02.003 Unspecified entropion of right eye, unspecified eyelid
H02.004 Unspecified entropion of left upper eyelid
H02.005 Unspecified entropion of left lower eyelid
H02.006 Unspecified entropion of left eye, unspecified eyelid
H02.009 Unspecified entropion of unspecified eye, unspecified eyelid
+ H02.01 Cicatricial entropion of eyelid
H02.011 Cicatricial entropion of right upper eyelid
H02.012 Cicatricial entropion of right lower eyelid
H02.013 Cicatricial entropion of right eye, unspecified eyelid
H02.014 Cicatricial entropion of left upper eyelid
H02.015 Cicatricial entropion of left lower eyelid
H02.016 Cicatricial entropion of left eye, unspecified eyelid
H02.019 Cicatricial entropion of unspecified eye, unspecified eyelid
+ H02.02 Mechanical entropion of eyelid
H02.021 Mechanical entropion of right upper eyelid
H02.022 Mechanical entropion of right lower eyelid
H02.023 Mechanical entropion of right eye, unspecified eyelid
H02.024 Mechanical entropion of left upper eyelid
H02.025 Mechanical entropion of left lower eyelid
H02.026 Mechanical entropion of left eye, unspecified eyelid
H02.029 Mechanical entropion of unspecified eye, unspecified eyelid
+ H02.03 Senile entropion of eyelid
● H02.031 Senile entropion of right upper eyelid
● H02.032 Senile entropion of right lower eyelid
● H02.033 Senile entropion of right eye, unspecified eyelid
● H02.034 Senile entropion of left upper eyelid
● H02.035 Senile entropion of left lower eyelid
● H02.036 Senile entropion of left eye, unspecified eyelid
● H02.039 Senile entropion of unspecified eye, unspecified eyelid
+ H02.04 Spastic entropion of eyelid
H02.041 Spastic entropion of right upper eyelid
H02.042 Spastic entropion of right lower eyelid
H02.043 Spastic entropion of right eye, unspecified eyelid
H02.044 Spastic entropion of left upper eyelid
H02.045 Spastic entropion of left lower eyelid
H02.046 Spastic entropion of left eye, unspecified eyelid
H02.049 Spastic entropion of unspecified eye, unspecified eyelid

613

+, +7th, X + 7th   ● Newborn   ● Pediatric   ● Maternity   ● Adult   ♀ Female   ♂ Male   Manifestation   Unacceptable PDX   HCC   CC   MCC   HAC

+ H02.05 Trichiasis without entropion
H02.051 Trichiasis without entropion right upper eyelid
H02.052 Trichiasis without entropion right lower eyelid
H02.053 Trichiasis without entropion right eye, unspecified eyelid
H02.054 Trichiasis without entropion left upper eyelid
H02.055 Trichiasis without entropion left lower eyelid
H02.056 Trichiasis without entropion left eye, unspecified eyelid
H02.059 Trichiasis without entropion unspecified eye, unspecified eyelid

+ H02.1 Ectropion of eyelid
+ H02.10 Unspecified ectropion of eyelid
H02.101 Unspecified ectropion of right upper eyelid
H02.102 Unspecified ectropion of right lower eyelid
H02.103 Unspecified ectropion of right eye, unspecified eyelid
H02.104 Unspecified ectropion of left upper eyelid
H02.105 Unspecified ectropion of left lower eyelid
H02.106 Unspecified ectropion of left eye, unspecified eyelid
H02.109 Unspecified ectropion of unspecified eye, unspecified eyelid

+ H02.11 Cicatricial ectropion of eyelid
H02.111 Cicatricial ectropion of right upper eyelid
H02.112 Cicatricial ectropion of right lower eyelid
H02.113 Cicatricial ectropion of right eye, unspecified eyelid
H02.114 Cicatricial ectropion of left upper eyelid
H02.115 Cicatricial ectropion of left lower eyelid
H02.116 Cicatricial ectropion of left eye, unspecified eyelid
H02.119 Cicatricial ectropion of unspecified eye, unspecified eyelid

+ H02.12 Mechanical ectropion of eyelid
H02.121 Mechanical ectropion of right upper eyelid
H02.122 Mechanical ectropion of right lower eyelid
H02.123 Mechanical ectropion of right eye, unspecified eyelid
H02.124 Mechanical ectropion of left upper eyelid
H02.125 Mechanical ectropion of left lower eyelid
H02.126 Mechanical ectropion of left eye, unspecified eyelid
H02.129 Mechanical ectropion of unspecified eye, unspecified eyelid

+ H02.13 Senile ectropion of eyelid
H02.131 Senile ectropion of right upper eyelid
H02.132 Senile ectropion of right lower eyelid
H02.133 Senile ectropion of right eye, unspecified eyelid
H02.134 Senile ectropion of left upper eyelid
H02.135 Senile ectropion of left lower eyelid
H02.136 Senile ectropion of left eye, unspecified eyelid
H02.139 Senile ectropion of unspecified eye, unspecified eyelid

+ H02.14 Spastic ectropion of eyelid
H02.141 Spastic ectropion of right upper eyelid
H02.142 Spastic ectropion of right lower eyelid
H02.143 Spastic ectropion of right eye, unspecified eyelid
H02.144 Spastic ectropion of left upper eyelid
H02.145 Spastic ectropion of left lower eyelid
H02.146 Spastic ectropion of left eye, unspecified eyelid
H02.149 Spastic ectropion of unspecified eye, unspecified eyelid

+ H02.15 Paralytic ectropion of eyelid
AHA CC: 4Q, 2018, 13
H02.151 Paralytic ectropion of right upper eyelid
H02.152 Paralytic ectropion of right lower eyelid
H02.153 Paralytic ectropion of right eye, unspecified eyelid
H02.154 Paralytic ectropion of left upper eyelid
H02.155 Paralytic ectropion of left lower eyelid
H02.156 Paralytic ectropion of left eye, unspecified eyelid
H02.159 Paralytic ectropion of unspecified eye, unspecified eyelid

+ H02.2 Lagophthalmos
AHA CC: 4Q, 2018, 14
+ H02.20 Unspecified lagophthalmos
H02.201 Unspecified lagophthalmos right upper eyelid
H02.202 Unspecified lagophthalmos right lower eyelid
H02.203 Unspecified lagophthalmos right eye, unspecified eyelid
H02.204 Unspecified lagophthalmos left upper eyelid
H02.205 Unspecified lagophthalmos left lower eyelid
H02.206 Unspecified lagophthalmos left eye, unspecified eyelid
H02.209 Unspecified lagophthalmos unspecified eye, unspecified eyelid
H02.20A Unspecified lagophthalmos right eye, upper and lower eyelids
H02.20B Unspecified lagophthalmos left eye, upper and lower eyelids
H02.20C Unspecified lagophthalmos, bilateral, upper and lower eyelids

+ H02.21 Cicatricial lagophthalmos
H02.211 Cicatricial lagophthalmos right upper eyelid
H02.212 Cicatricial lagophthalmos right lower eyelid
H02.213 Cicatricial lagophthalmos right eye, unspecified eyelid
H02.214 Cicatricial lagophthalmos left upper eyelid
H02.215 Cicatricial lagophthalmos left lower eyelid
H02.216 Cicatricial lagophthalmos left eye, unspecified eyelid
H02.219 Cicatricial lagophthalmos unspecified eye, unspecified eyelid
H02.21A Cicatricial lagophthalmos right eye, upper and lower eyelids
H02.21B Cicatricial lagophthalmos left eye, upper and lower eyelids
H02.21C Cicatricial lagophthalmos, bilateral, upper and lower eyelids

+ H02.22 Mechanical lagophthalmos
H02.221 Mechanical lagophthalmos right upper eyelid
H02.222 Mechanical lagophthalmos right lower eyelid
H02.223 Mechanical lagophthalmos right eye, unspecified eyelid
H02.224 Mechanical lagophthalmos left upper eyelid
H02.225 Mechanical lagophthalmos left lower eyelid
H02.226 Mechanical lagophthalmos left eye, unspecified eyelid
H02.229 Mechanical lagophthalmos unspecified eye, unspecified eyelid
H02.22A Mechanical lagophthalmos right eye, upper and lower eyelids
H02.22B Mechanical lagophthalmos left eye, upper and lower eyelids
H02.22C Mechanical lagophthalmos, bilateral, upper and lower eyelids

+ **H02.23** **Paralytic lagophthalmos**
    H02.231 **Paralytic lagophthalmos right upper eyelid**
    H02.232 **Paralytic lagophthalmos right lower eyelid**
    H02.233 **Paralytic lagophthalmos right eye, unspecified eyelid**
    H02.234 **Paralytic lagophthalmos left upper eyelid**
    H02.235 **Paralytic lagophthalmos left lower eyelid**
    H02.236 **Paralytic lagophthalmos left eye, unspecified eyelid**
    H02.239 **Paralytic lagophthalmos unspecified eye, unspecified eyelid**
    H02.23A **Paralytic lagophthalmos right eye, upper and lower eyelids**
    H02.23B **Paralytic lagophthalmos left eye, upper and lower eyelids**
    H02.23C **Paralytic lagophthalmos, bilateral, upper and lower eyelids**

+ **H02.3** **Blepharochalasis**
    Pseudoptosis
    H02.30 **Blepharochalasis unspecified eye, unspecified eyelid**
    H02.31 **Blepharochalasis right upper eyelid**
    H02.32 **Blepharochalasis right lower eyelid**
    H02.33 **Blepharochalasis right eye, unspecified eyelid**
    H02.34 **Blepharochalasis left upper eyelid**
    H02.35 **Blepharochalasis left lower eyelid**
    H02.36 **Blepharochalasis left eye, unspecified eyelid**

+ **H02.4** **Ptosis of eyelid**
  + **H02.40** **Unspecified ptosis of eyelid**
    H02.401 **Unspecified ptosis of right eyelid**
    H02.402 **Unspecified ptosis of left eyelid**
    H02.403 **Unspecified ptosis of bilateral eyelids**
    H02.409 **Unspecified ptosis of unspecified eyelid**
  + **H02.41** **Mechanical ptosis of eyelid**
    H02.411 **Mechanical ptosis of right eyelid**
    H02.412 **Mechanical ptosis of left eyelid**
    H02.413 **Mechanical ptosis of bilateral eyelids**
    H02.419 **Mechanical ptosis of unspecified eyelid**
  + **H02.42** **Myogenic ptosis of eyelid**
    H02.421 **Myogenic ptosis of right eyelid**
    H02.422 **Myogenic ptosis of left eyelid**
    H02.423 **Myogenic ptosis of bilateral eyelids**
    H02.429 **Myogenic ptosis of unspecified eyelid**
  + **H02.43** **Paralytic ptosis of eyelid**
    Neurogenic ptosis of eyelid
    H02.431 **Paralytic ptosis of right eyelid**
    H02.432 **Paralytic ptosis of left eyelid**
    H02.433 **Paralytic ptosis of bilateral eyelids**
    H02.439 **Paralytic ptosis unspecified eyelid**

+ **H02.5** **Other disorders affecting eyelid function**
    Excludes2: *blepharospasm (G24.5)*
        organic tic (G25.69)
        psychogenic tic (F95.-)
  + **H02.51** **Abnormal innervation syndrome**
    H02.511 **Abnormal innervation syndrome right upper eyelid**
    H02.512 **Abnormal innervation syndrome right lower eyelid**
    H02.513 **Abnormal innervation syndrome right eye, unspecified eyelid**
    H02.514 **Abnormal innervation syndrome left upper eyelid**
    H02.515 **Abnormal innervation syndrome left lower eyelid**
    H02.516 **Abnormal innervation syndrome left eye, unspecified eyelid**
    H02.519 **Abnormal innervation syndrome unspecified eye, unspecified eyelid**
  + **H02.52** **Blepharophimosis**
    Ankyloblepharon
    H02.521 **Blepharophimosis right upper eyelid**
    H02.522 **Blepharophimosis right lower eyelid**
    H02.523 **Blepharophimosis right eye, unspecified eyelid**
    H02.524 **Blepharophimosis left upper eyelid**
    H02.525 **Blepharophimosis left lower eyelid**
    H02.526 **Blepharophimosis left eye, unspecified eyelid**
    H02.529 **Blepharophimosis unspecified eye, unspecified lid**

+ **H02.53** **Eyelid retraction**
    Eyelid lag
    H02.531 **Eyelid retraction right upper eyelid**
    H02.532 **Eyelid retraction right lower eyelid**
    H02.533 **Eyelid retraction right eye, unspecified eyelid**
    H02.534 **Eyelid retraction left upper eyelid**
    H02.535 **Eyelid retraction left lower eyelid**
    H02.536 **Eyelid retraction left eye, unspecified eyelid**
    H02.539 **Eyelid retraction unspecified eye, unspecified lid**

H02.59 **Other disorders affecting eyelid function**
    Deficient blink reflex
    Sensory disorders

+ **H02.6** **Xanthelasma of eyelid**
    H02.60 **Xanthelasma of unspecified eye, unspecified eyelid**
    H02.61 **Xanthelasma of right upper eyelid**
    H02.62 **Xanthelasma of right lower eyelid**
    H02.63 **Xanthelasma of right eye, unspecified eyelid**
    H02.64 **Xanthelasma of left upper eyelid**
    H02.65 **Xanthelasma of left lower eyelid**
    H02.66 **Xanthelasma of left eye, unspecified eyelid**

+ **H02.7** **Other and unspecified degenerative disorders of eyelid and periocular area**
    H02.70 **Unspecified degenerative disorders of eyelid and periocular area**
  + **H02.71** **Chloasma of eyelid and periocular area**
    Dyspigmentation of eyelid
    Hyperpigmentation of eyelid
    H02.711 **Chloasma of right upper eyelid and periocular area**
    H02.712 **Chloasma of right lower eyelid and periocular area**
    H02.713 **Chloasma of right eye, unspecified eyelid and periocular area**
    H02.714 **Chloasma of left upper eyelid and periocular area**
    H02.715 **Chloasma of left lower eyelid and periocular area**
    H02.716 **Chloasma of left eye, unspecified eyelid and periocular area**
    H02.719 **Chloasma of unspecified eye, unspecified eyelid and periocular area**
  + **H02.72** **Madarosis of eyelid and periocular area**
    Hypotrichosis of eyelid
    H02.721 **Madarosis of right upper eyelid and periocular area**
    H02.722 **Madarosis of right lower eyelid and periocular area**
    H02.723 **Madarosis of right eye, unspecified eyelid and periocular area**
    H02.724 **Madarosis of left upper eyelid and periocular area**
    H02.725 **Madarosis of left lower eyelid and periocular area**
    H02.726 **Madarosis of left eye, unspecified eyelid and periocular area**
    H02.729 **Madarosis of unspecified eye, unspecified eyelid and periocular area**
  + **H02.73** **Vitiligo of eyelid and periocular area**
    Hypopigmentation of eyelid
    H02.731 **Vitiligo of right upper eyelid and periocular area**
    H02.732 **Vitiligo of right lower eyelid and periocular area**
    H02.733 **Vitiligo of right eye, unspecified eyelid and periocular area**
    H02.734 **Vitiligo of left upper eyelid and periocular area**
    H02.735 **Vitiligo of left lower eyelid and periocular area**
    H02.736 **Vitiligo of left eye, unspecified eyelid and periocular area**
    H02.739 **Vitiligo of unspecified eye, unspecified eyelid and periocular area**
    H02.79 **Other degenerative disorders of eyelid and periocular area**

615

+, +7th, X + 7th   ● Newborn   ● Pediatric   ● Maternity   ● Adult   ♀ Female   ♂ Male   Manifestation   Unacceptable PDX   HCC   CC   MCC   HAC

+ **H02.8 Other specified disorders of eyelid**
+ **H02.81 Retained foreign body in eyelid**

Use additional code to identify the type of retained foreign body (Z18.-)

Excludes1: *laceration of eyelid with foreign body (S01.12-)*
retained intraocular foreign body (H44.6-, H44.7-)
superficial foreign body of eyelid and periocular area (S00.25-)

H02.811 Retained foreign body in right upper eyelid
H02.812 Retained foreign body in right lower eyelid
H02.813 Retained foreign body in right eye, unspecified eyelid
H02.814 Retained foreign body in left upper eyelid
H02.815 Retained foreign body in left lower eyelid
H02.816 Retained foreign body in left eye, unspecified eyelid
H02.819 Retained foreign body in unspecified eye, unspecified eyelid

+ **H02.82 Cysts of eyelid**

Sebaceous cyst of eyelid

H02.821 Cysts of right upper eyelid
H02.822 Cysts of right lower eyelid
H02.823 Cysts of right eye, unspecified eyelid
H02.824 Cysts of left upper eyelid
H02.825 Cysts of left lower eyelid
H02.826 Cysts of left eye, unspecified eyelid
H02.829 Cysts of unspecified eye, unspecified eyelid

+ **H02.83 Dermatochalasis of eyelid**

H02.831 Dermatochalasis of right upper eyelid
H02.832 Dermatochalasis of right lower eyelid
H02.833 Dermatochalasis of right eye, unspecified eyelid
H02.834 Dermatochalasis of left upper eyelid
H02.835 Dermatochalasis of left lower eyelid
H02.836 Dermatochalasis of left eye, unspecified eyelid
H02.839 Dermatochalasis of unspecified eye, unspecified eyelid

+ **H02.84 Edema of eyelid**

Hyperemia of eyelid

H02.841 Edema of right upper eyelid
H02.842 Edema of right lower eyelid
H02.843 Edema of right eye, unspecified eyelid
H02.844 Edema of left upper eyelid
H02.845 Edema of left lower eyelid
H02.846 Edema of left eye, unspecified eyelid
H02.849 Edema of unspecified eye, unspecified eyelid

+ **H02.85 Elephantiasis of eyelid**

H02.851 Elephantiasis of right upper eyelid
H02.852 Elephantiasis of right lower eyelid
H02.853 Elephantiasis of right eye, unspecified eyelid
H02.854 Elephantiasis of left upper eyelid
H02.855 Elephantiasis of left lower eyelid
H02.856 Elephantiasis of left eye, unspecified eyelid
H02.859 Elephantiasis of unspecified eye, unspecified eyelid

+ **H02.86 Hypertrichosis of eyelid**

H02.861 Hypertrichosis of right upper eyelid
H02.862 Hypertrichosis of right lower eyelid
H02.863 Hypertrichosis of right eye, unspecified eyelid
H02.864 Hypertrichosis of left upper eyelid
H02.865 Hypertrichosis of left lower eyelid
H02.866 Hypertrichosis of left eye, unspecified eyelid
H02.869 Hypertrichosis of unspecified eye, unspecified eyelid

+ **H02.87 Vascular anomalies of eyelid**

H02.871 Vascular anomalies of right upper eyelid
H02.872 Vascular anomalies of right lower eyelid
H02.873 Vascular anomalies of right eye, unspecified eyelid
H02.874 Vascular anomalies of left upper eyelid
H02.875 Vascular anomalies of left lower eyelid
H02.876 Vascular anomalies of left eye, unspecified eyelid
H02.879 Vascular anomalies of unspecified eye, unspecified eyelid

+ **H02.88 Meibomian gland dysfunction of eyelid**

AHA CC: 4Q, 2018, 14-15

H02.881 Meibomian gland dysfunction right upper eyelid
H02.882 Meibomian gland dysfunction right lower eyelid
H02.883 Meibomian gland dysfunction of right eye, unspecified eyelid
H02.884 Meibomian gland dysfunction left upper eyelid
H02.885 Meibomian gland dysfunction left lower eyelid
H02.886 Meibomian gland dysfunction of left eye, unspecified eyelid
H02.889 Meibomian gland dysfunction of unspecified eye, unspecified eyelid
H02.88A Meibomian gland dysfunction right eye, upper and lower eyelids
H02.88B Meibomian gland dysfunction left eye, upper and lower eyelids

H02.89 Other specified disorders of eyelid

Hemorrhage of eyelid

H02.9 Unspecified disorder of eyelid

Disorder of eyelid NOS

H04 Disorders of lacrimal system

Excludes1: *congenital malformations of lacrimal system (Q10.4-Q10.6)*

+ **H04.0 Dacryoadenitis**
+ **H04.00 Unspecified dacryoadenitis**

H04.001 Unspecified dacryoadenitis, right lacrimal gland
H04.002 Unspecified dacryoadenitis, left lacrimal gland
H04.003 Unspecified dacryoadenitis, bilateral lacrimal glands
H04.009 Unspecified dacryoadenitis, unspecified lacrimal gland

+ **H04.01 Acute dacryoadenitis**

H04.011 Acute dacryoadenitis, right lacrimal gland
H04.012 Acute dacryoadenitis, left lacrimal gland
H04.013 Acute dacryoadenitis, bilateral lacrimal glands
H04.019 Acute dacryoadenitis, unspecified lacrimal gland

+ **H04.02 Chronic dacryoadenitis**

H04.021 Chronic dacryoadenitis, right lacrimal gland
H04.022 Chronic dacryoadenitis, left lacrimal gland
H04.023 Chronic dacryoadenitis, bilateral lacrimal gland
H04.029 Chronic dacryoadenitis, unspecified lacrimal gland

+ **H04.03 Chronic enlargement of lacrimal gland**

H04.031 Chronic enlargement of right lacrimal gland
H04.032 Chronic enlargement of left lacrimal gland
H04.033 Chronic enlargement of bilateral lacrimal glands
H04.039 Chronic enlargement of unspecified lacrimal gland

+ **H04.1 Other disorders of lacrimal gland**
+ **H04.11 Dacryops**

H04.111 Dacryops of right lacrimal gland
H04.112 Dacryops of left lacrimal gland
H04.113 Dacryops of bilateral lacrimal glands
H04.119 Dacryops of unspecified lacrimal gland

+ **H04.12** Dry eye syndrome
  Tear film insufficiency, NOS
   H04.121 Dry eye syndrome of right lacrimal gland
   H04.122 Dry eye syndrome of left lacrimal gland
   H04.123 Dry eye syndrome of bilateral lacrimal glands
   H04.129 Dry eye syndrome of unspecified lacrimal gland
+ **H04.13** Lacrimal cyst
  Lacrimal cystic degeneration
   H04.131 Lacrimal cyst, right lacrimal gland
   H04.132 Lacrimal cyst, left lacrimal gland
   H04.133 Lacrimal cyst, bilateral lacrimal glands
   H04.139 Lacrimal cyst, unspecified lacrimal gland
+ **H04.14** Primary lacrimal gland atrophy
   H04.141 Primary lacrimal gland atrophy, right lacrimal gland
   H04.142 Primary lacrimal gland atrophy, left lacrimal gland
   H04.143 Primary lacrimal gland atrophy, bilateral lacrimal glands
   H04.149 Primary lacrimal gland atrophy, unspecified lacrimal gland
+ **H04.15** Secondary lacrimal gland atrophy
   H04.151 Secondary lacrimal gland atrophy, right lacrimal gland
   H04.152 Secondary lacrimal gland atrophy, left lacrimal gland
   H04.153 Secondary lacrimal gland atrophy, bilateral lacrimal glands
   H04.159 Secondary lacrimal gland atrophy, unspecified lacrimal gland
+ **H04.16** Lacrimal gland dislocation
   H04.161 Lacrimal gland dislocation, right lacrimal gland
   H04.162 Lacrimal gland dislocation, left lacrimal gland
   H04.163 Lacrimal gland dislocation, bilateral lacrimal glands
   H04.169 Lacrimal gland dislocation, unspecified lacrimal gland
  H04.19 Other specified disorders of lacrimal gland
+ **H04.2** Epiphora
  + **H04.20** Unspecified epiphora
    H04.201 Unspecified epiphora, right side
    H04.202 Unspecified epiphora, left side
    H04.203 Unspecified epiphora, bilateral
    H04.209 Unspecified epiphora, unspecified side
  + **H04.21** Epiphora due to excess lacrimation
    H04.211 Epiphora due to excess lacrimation, right lacrimal gland
    H04.212 Epiphora due to excess lacrimation, left lacrimal gland
    H04.213 Epiphora due to excess lacrimation, bilateral lacrimal glands
    H04.219 Epiphora due to excess lacrimation, unspecified lacrimal gland
  + **H04.22** Epiphora due to insufficient drainage
    H04.221 Epiphora due to insufficient drainage, right side
    H04.222 Epiphora due to insufficient drainage, left side
    H04.223 Epiphora due to insufficient drainage, bilateral
    H04.229 Epiphora due to insufficient drainage, unspecified side
+ **H04.3** Acute and unspecified inflammation of lacrimal passages
  Excludes1: *neonatal dacryocystitis (P39.1)*
  + **H04.30** Unspecified dacryocystitis
    H04.301 Unspecified dacryocystitis of right lacrimal passage
    H04.302 Unspecified dacryocystitis of left lacrimal passage
    H04.303 Unspecified dacryocystitis of bilateral lacrimal passages
    H04.309 Unspecified dacryocystitis of unspecified lacrimal passage

+ **H04.31** Phlegmonous dacryocystitis
   H04.311 Phlegmonous dacryocystitis of right lacrimal passage
   H04.312 Phlegmonous dacryocystitis of left lacrimal passage
   H04.313 Phlegmonous dacryocystitis of bilateral lacrimal passages
   H04.319 Phlegmonous dacryocystitis of unspecified lacrimal passage
+ **H04.32** Acute dacryocystitis
  Acute dacryopericystitis
   H04.321 Acute dacryocystitis of right lacrimal passage
   H04.322 Acute dacryocystitis of left lacrimal passage
   H04.323 Acute dacryocystitis of bilateral lacrimal passages
   H04.329 Acute dacryocystitis of unspecified lacrimal passage
+ **H04.33** Acute lacrimal canaliculitis
   H04.331 Acute lacrimal canaliculitis of right lacrimal passage
   H04.332 Acute lacrimal canaliculitis of left lacrimal passage
   H04.333 Acute lacrimal canaliculitis of bilateral lacrimal passages
   H04.339 Acute lacrimal canaliculitis of unspecified lacrimal passage
+ **H04.4** Chronic inflammation of lacrimal passages
  + **H04.41** Chronic dacryocystitis
    H04.411 Chronic dacryocystitis of right lacrimal passage
    H04.412 Chronic dacryocystitis of left lacrimal passage
    H04.413 Chronic dacryocystitis of bilateral lacrimal passages
    H04.419 Chronic dacryocystitis of unspecified lacrimal passage
  + **H04.42** Chronic lacrimal canaliculitis
    H04.421 Chronic lacrimal canaliculitis of right lacrimal passage
    H04.422 Chronic lacrimal canaliculitis of left lacrimal passage
    H04.423 Chronic lacrimal canaliculitis of bilateral lacrimal passages
    H04.429 Chronic lacrimal canaliculitis of unspecified lacrimal passage
  + **H04.43** Chronic lacrimal mucocele
    H04.431 Chronic lacrimal mucocele of right lacrimal passage
    H04.432 Chronic lacrimal mucocele of left lacrimal passage
    H04.433 Chronic lacrimal mucocele of bilateral lacrimal passages
    H04.439 Chronic lacrimal mucocele of unspecified lacrimal passage
+ **H04.5** Stenosis and insufficiency of lacrimal passages
  + **H04.51** Dacryolith
    H04.511 Dacryolith of right lacrimal passage
    H04.512 Dacryolith of left lacrimal passage
    H04.513 Dacryolith of bilateral lacrimal passages
    H04.519 Dacryolith of unspecified lacrimal passage
  + **H04.52** Eversion of lacrimal punctum
    H04.521 Eversion of right lacrimal punctum
    H04.522 Eversion of left lacrimal punctum
    H04.523 Eversion of bilateral lacrimal punctum
    H04.529 Eversion of unspecified lacrimal punctum
  + **H04.53** Neonatal obstruction of nasolacrimal duct
    Excludes1: *congenital stenosis and stricture of lacrimal duct (Q10.5)*
    ● **H04.531** Neonatal obstruction of right nasolacrimal duct
    ● **H04.532** Neonatal obstruction of left nasolacrimal duct
    ● **H04.533** Neonatal obstruction of bilateral nasolacrimal duct
    ● **H04.539** Neonatal obstruction of unspecified nasolacrimal duct

+, +7th, X + 7th   ● Newborn   ● Pediatric   ● Maternity   ● Adult   ♀ Female   ♂ Male   Manifestation   Unacceptable PDX   HCC   CC   MCC   HAC

+ **H04.54 Stenosis of lacrimal canaliculi**
    H04.541 Stenosis of right lacrimal canaliculi
    H04.542 Stenosis of left lacrimal canaliculi
    H04.543 Stenosis of bilateral lacrimal canaliculi
    H04.549 Stenosis of unspecified lacrimal canaliculi

+ **H04.55 Acquired stenosis of nasolacrimal duct**
    H04.551 Acquired stenosis of right nasolacrimal duct
    H04.552 Acquired stenosis of left nasolacrimal duct
    H04.553 Acquired stenosis of bilateral nasolacrimal duct
    H04.559 Acquired stenosis of unspecified nasolacrimal duct

+ **H04.56 Stenosis of lacrimal punctum**
    H04.561 Stenosis of right lacrimal punctum
    H04.562 Stenosis of left lacrimal punctum
    H04.563 Stenosis of bilateral lacrimal punctum
    H04.569 Stenosis of unspecified lacrimal punctum

+ **H04.57 Stenosis of lacrimal sac**
    H04.571 Stenosis of right lacrimal sac
    H04.572 Stenosis of left lacrimal sac
    H04.573 Stenosis of bilateral lacrimal sac
    H04.579 Stenosis of unspecified lacrimal sac

+ **H04.6 Other changes of lacrimal passages**
  + **H04.61 Lacrimal fistula**
    H04.611 Lacrimal fistula right lacrimal passage
    H04.612 Lacrimal fistula left lacrimal passage
    H04.613 Lacrimal fistula bilateral lacrimal passages
    H04.619 Lacrimal fistula unspecified lacrimal passage
  H04.69 Other changes of lacrimal passages

+ **H04.8 Other disorders of lacrimal system**
  + **H04.81 Granuloma of lacrimal passages**
    H04.811 Granuloma of right lacrimal passage
    H04.812 Granuloma of left lacrimal passage
    H04.813 Granuloma of bilateral lacrimal passages
    H04.819 Granuloma of unspecified lacrimal passage
  H04.89 Other disorders of lacrimal system

H04.9 Disorder of lacrimal system, unspecified

H05 Disorders of orbit

  Excludes1: congenital malformation of orbit (Q10.7)

+ **H05.0 Acute inflammation of orbit**
  H05.00 Unspecified acute inflammation of orbit
  + **H05.01 Cellulitis of orbit**
    Abscess of orbit
    CC H05.011 Cellulitis of right orbit
    CC H05.012 Cellulitis of left orbit
    CC H05.013 Cellulitis of bilateral orbits
    CC H05.019 Cellulitis of unspecified orbit
  + **H05.02 Osteomyelitis of orbit**
    CC H05.021 Osteomyelitis of right orbit
    CC H05.022 Osteomyelitis of left orbit
    CC H05.023 Osteomyelitis of bilateral orbits
    CC H05.029 Osteomyelitis of unspecified orbit
  + **H05.03 Periostitis of orbit**
    CC H05.031 Periostitis of right orbit
    CC H05.032 Periostitis of left orbit
    CC H05.033 Periostitis of bilateral orbits
    CC H05.039 Periostitis of unspecified orbit
  + **H05.04 Tenonitis of orbit**
    H05.041 Tenonitis of right orbit
    H05.042 Tenonitis of left orbit
    H05.043 Tenonitis of bilateral orbits
    H05.049 Tenonitis of unspecified orbit

+ **H05.1 Chronic inflammatory disorders of orbit**
  H05.10 Unspecified chronic inflammatory disorders of orbit
  + **H05.11 Granuloma of orbit**
    Pseudotumor (inflammatory) of orbit
    H05.111 Granuloma of right orbit
    H05.112 Granuloma of left orbit
    H05.113 Granuloma of bilateral orbits
    H05.119 Granuloma of unspecified orbit

+ **H05.12 Orbital myositis**
    H05.121 Orbital myositis, right orbit
    H05.122 Orbital myositis, left orbit
    H05.123 Orbital myositis, bilateral
    H05.129 Orbital myositis, unspecified orbit

+ **H05.2 Exophthalmic conditions**
  H05.20 Unspecified exophthalmos
  + **H05.21 Displacement (lateral) of globe**
    H05.211 Displacement (lateral) of globe, right eye
    H05.212 Displacement (lateral) of globe, left eye
    H05.213 Displacement (lateral) of globe, bilateral
    H05.219 Displacement (lateral) of globe, unspecified eye
  + **H05.22 Edema of orbit**
    Orbital congestion
    H05.221 Edema of right orbit
    H05.222 Edema of left orbit
    H05.223 Edema of bilateral orbit
    H05.229 Edema of unspecified orbit
  + **H05.23 Hemorrhage of orbit**
    H05.231 Hemorrhage of right orbit
    H05.232 Hemorrhage of left orbit
    H05.233 Hemorrhage of bilateral orbit
    H05.239 Hemorrhage of unspecified orbit
  + **H05.24 Constant exophthalmos**
    H05.241 Constant exophthalmos, right eye
    H05.242 Constant exophthalmos, left eye
    H05.243 Constant exophthalmos, bilateral
    H05.249 Constant exophthalmos, unspecified eye
  + **H05.25 Intermittent exophthalmos**
    H05.251 Intermittent exophthalmos, right eye
    H05.252 Intermittent exophthalmos, left eye
    H05.253 Intermittent exophthalmos, bilateral
    H05.259 Intermittent exophthalmos, unspecified eye
  + **H05.26 Pulsating exophthalmos**
    H05.261 Pulsating exophthalmos, right eye
    H05.262 Pulsating exophthalmos, left eye
    H05.263 Pulsating exophthalmos, bilateral
    H05.269 Pulsating exophthalmos, unspecified eye

+ **H05.3 Deformity of orbit**
  Excludes1: congenital deformity of orbit (Q10.7)
          hypertelorism (Q75.2)
  H05.30 Unspecified deformity of orbit
  + **H05.31 Atrophy of orbit**
    H05.311 Atrophy of right orbit
    H05.312 Atrophy of left orbit
    H05.313 Atrophy of bilateral orbit
    H05.319 Atrophy of unspecified orbit
  + **H05.32 Deformity of orbit due to bone disease**
    Code also associated bone disease
    H05.321 Deformity of right orbit due to bone disease
    H05.322 Deformity of left orbit due to bone disease
    H05.323 Deformity of bilateral orbits due to bone disease
    H05.329 Deformity of unspecified orbit due to bone disease
  + **H05.33 Deformity of orbit due to trauma or surgery**
    H05.331 Deformity of right orbit due to trauma or surgery
    H05.332 Deformity of left orbit due to trauma or surgery
    H05.333 Deformity of bilateral orbits due to trauma or surgery
    H05.339 Deformity of unspecified orbit due to trauma or surgery
  + **H05.34 Enlargement of orbit**
    H05.341 Enlargement of right orbit
    H05.342 Enlargement of left orbit
    H05.343 Enlargement of bilateral orbits
    H05.349 Enlargement of unspecified orbit
  + **H05.35 Exostosis of orbit**
    H05.351 Exostosis of right orbit
    H05.352 Exostosis of left orbit
    H05.353 Exostosis of bilateral orbits
    H05.359 Exostosis of unspecified orbit

+ **H05.4 Enophthalmos**
  + **H05.40 Unspecified enophthalmos**
    H05.401 Unspecified enophthalmos, right eye
    H05.402 Unspecified enophthalmos, left eye
    H05.403 Unspecified enophthalmos, bilateral
    H05.409 Unspecified enophthalmos, unspecified eye
  + **H05.41 Enophthalmos due to atrophy of orbital tissue**
    H05.411 Enophthalmos due to atrophy of orbital tissue, right eye
    H05.412 Enophthalmos due to atrophy of orbital tissue, left eye
    H05.413 Enophthalmos due to atrophy of orbital tissue, bilateral
    H05.419 Enophthalmos due to atrophy of orbital tissue, unspecified eye
  + **H05.42 Enophthalmos due to trauma or surgery**
    H05.421 Enophthalmos due to trauma or surgery, right eye
    H05.422 Enophthalmos due to trauma or surgery, left eye
    H05.423 Enophthalmos due to trauma or surgery, bilateral
    H05.429 Enophthalmos due to trauma or surgery, unspecified eye
+ **H05.5 Retained (old) foreign body following penetrating wound of orbit**
  Retrobulbar foreign body
  Use additional code to identify the type of retained foreign body (Z18.-)
  Excludes1: *current penetrating wound of orbit (S05.4-)*
  Excludes2: *retained foreign body of eyelid (H02.81-)*
  retained intraocular foreign body (H44.6-, H44.7-)
  H05.50 Retained (old) foreign body following penetrating wound of unspecified orbit
  H05.51 Retained (old) foreign body following penetrating wound of right orbit
  H05.52 Retained (old) foreign body following penetrating wound of left orbit
  H05.53 Retained (old) foreign body following penetrating wound of bilateral orbits
+ **H05.8 Other disorders of orbit**
  + **H05.81 Cyst of orbit**
    Encephalocele of orbit
    H05.811 Cyst of right orbit
    H05.812 Cyst of left orbit
    H05.813 Cyst of bilateral orbits
    H05.819 Cyst of unspecified orbit
  + **H05.82 Myopathy of extraocular muscles**
    H05.821 Myopathy of extraocular muscles, right orbit
    H05.822 Myopathy of extraocular muscles, left orbit
    H05.823 Myopathy of extraocular muscles, bilateral
    H05.829 Myopathy of extraocular muscles, unspecified orbit
  H05.89 Other disorders of orbit
H05.9 Unspecified disorder of orbit

Disorders of conjunctiva (H10-H11)

H10 Conjunctivitis

  Excludes1: *keratoconjunctivitis (H16.2-)*
  + **H10.0 Mucopurulent conjunctivitis**
    + **H10.01 Acute follicular conjunctivitis**
      H10.011 Acute follicular conjunctivitis, right eye
      H10.012 Acute follicular conjunctivitis, left eye
      H10.013 Acute follicular conjunctivitis, bilateral
      H10.019 Acute follicular conjunctivitis, unspecified eye
    + **H10.02 Other mucopurulent conjunctivitis**
      H10.021 Other mucopurulent conjunctivitis, right eye
      H10.022 Other mucopurulent conjunctivitis, left eye
      H10.023 Other mucopurulent conjunctivitis, bilateral
      H10.029 Other mucopurulent conjunctivitis, unspecified eye

+ **H10.1 Acute atopic conjunctivitis**
  Acute papillary conjunctivitis
  H10.10 Acute atopic conjunctivitis, unspecified eye
  H10.11 Acute atopic conjunctivitis, right eye
  H10.12 Acute atopic conjunctivitis, left eye
  H10.13 Acute atopic conjunctivitis, bilateral
+ **H10.2 Other acute conjunctivitis**
  + **H10.21 Acute toxic conjunctivitis**
    Acute chemical conjunctivitis
    Code first (T51-T65) to identify chemical and intent
    Excludes1: *burn and corrosion of eye and adnexa (T26.-)*
    H10.211 Acute toxic conjunctivitis, right eye
    H10.212 Acute toxic conjunctivitis, left eye
    H10.213 Acute toxic conjunctivitis, bilateral
    H10.219 Acute toxic conjunctivitis, unspecified eye
  + **H10.22 Pseudomembranous conjunctivitis**
    H10.221 Pseudomembranous conjunctivitis, right eye
    H10.222 Pseudomembranous conjunctivitis, left eye
    H10.223 Pseudomembranous conjunctivitis, bilateral
    H10.229 Pseudomembranous conjunctivitis, unspecified eye
  + **H10.23 Serous conjunctivitis, except viral**
    Excludes1: *viral conjunctivitis (B30.-)*
    H10.231 Serous conjunctivitis, except viral, right eye
    H10.232 Serous conjunctivitis, except viral, left eye
    H10.233 Serous conjunctivitis, except viral, bilateral
    H10.239 Serous conjunctivitis, except viral, unspecified eye
+ **H10.3 Unspecified acute conjunctivitis**
  Excludes1: *ophthalmia neonatorum NOS (P39.1)*
  H10.30 Unspecified acute conjunctivitis, unspecified eye
  H10.31 Unspecified acute conjunctivitis, right eye
  H10.32 Unspecified acute conjunctivitis, left eye
  H10.33 Unspecified acute conjunctivitis, bilateral
+ **H10.4 Chronic conjunctivitis**
  + **H10.40 Unspecified chronic conjunctivitis**
    H10.401 Unspecified chronic conjunctivitis, right eye
    H10.402 Unspecified chronic conjunctivitis, left eye
    H10.403 Unspecified chronic conjunctivitis, bilateral
    H10.409 Unspecified chronic conjunctivitis, unspecified eye
  + **H10.41 Chronic giant papillary conjunctivitis**
    H10.411 Chronic giant papillary conjunctivitis, right eye
    H10.412 Chronic giant papillary conjunctivitis, left eye
    H10.413 Chronic giant papillary conjunctivitis, bilateral
    H10.419 Chronic giant papillary conjunctivitis, unspecified eye
  + **H10.42 Simple chronic conjunctivitis**
    H10.421 Simple chronic conjunctivitis, right eye
    H10.422 Simple chronic conjunctivitis, left eye
    H10.423 Simple chronic conjunctivitis, bilateral
    H10.429 Simple chronic conjunctivitis, unspecified eye
  + **H10.43 Chronic follicular conjunctivitis**
    H10.431 Chronic follicular conjunctivitis, right eye
    H10.432 Chronic follicular conjunctivitis, left eye
    H10.433 Chronic follicular conjunctivitis, bilateral
    H10.439 Chronic follicular conjunctivitis, unspecified eye
  H10.44 Vernal conjunctivitis
    Excludes1: *vernal keratoconjunctivitis with limbar and corneal involvement (H16.26-)*
  H10.45 Other chronic allergic conjunctivitis

+ **H10.5** **Blepharoconjunctivitis**
  + **H10.50** **Unspecified blepharoconjunctivitis**
    H10.501 Unspecified blepharoconjunctivitis, right eye
    H10.502 Unspecified blepharoconjunctivitis, left eye
    H10.503 Unspecified blepharoconjunctivitis, bilateral
    H10.509 Unspecified blepharoconjunctivitis, unspecified eye
  + **H10.51** **Ligneous conjunctivitis**
    Code also underlying condition if known, such as: plasminogen deficiency (E88.02)
    H10.511 Ligneous conjunctivitis, right eye
    H10.512 Ligneous conjunctivitis, left eye
    H10.513 Ligneous conjunctivitis, bilateral
    H10.519 Ligneous conjunctivitis, unspecified eye
  + **H10.52** **Angular blepharoconjunctivitis**
    H10.521 Angular blepharoconjunctivitis, right eye
    H10.522 Angular blepharoconjunctivitis, left eye
    H10.523 Angular blepharoconjunctivitis, bilateral
    H10.529 Angular blepharoconjunctivitis, unspecified eye
  + **H10.53** **Contact blepharoconjunctivitis**
    H10.531 Contact blepharoconjunctivitis, right eye
    H10.532 Contact blepharoconjunctivitis, left eye
    H10.533 Contact blepharoconjunctivitis, bilateral
    H10.539 Contact blepharoconjunctivitis, unspecified eye
+ **H10.8** **Other conjunctivitis**
    AHA CC: 4Q, 2018, 15
  + **H10.81** **Pingueculitis**
      Excludes1: pinguecula (H11.15-)
    H10.811 Pingueculitis, right eye
    H10.812 Pingueculitis, left eye
    H10.813 Pingueculitis, bilateral
    H10.819 Pingueculitis, unspecified eye
  + **H10.82** **Rosacea conjunctivitis**
      Code first underlying rosacea dermatitis (L71.-)
    H10.821 Rosacea conjunctivitis, right eye
    H10.822 Rosacea conjunctivitis, left eye
    H10.823 Rosacea conjunctivitis, bilateral
      AHA CC: 4Q, 2018, 15
    H10.829 Rosacea conjunctivitis, unspecified eye
  H10.89 **Other conjunctivitis**
  H10.9 **Unspecified conjunctivitis**

H11 **Other disorders of conjunctiva**
    Excludes1: keratoconjunctivitis (H16.2-)
+ **H11.0** **Pterygium of eye**
    Excludes1: pseudopterygium (H11.81-)
  + **H11.00** **Unspecified pterygium of eye**
    H11.001 Unspecified pterygium of right eye
    H11.002 Unspecified pterygium of left eye
    H11.003 Unspecified pterygium of eye, bilateral
    H11.009 Unspecified pterygium of unspecified eye
  + **H11.01** **Amyloid pterygium**
    H11.011 Amyloid pterygium of right eye
    H11.012 Amyloid pterygium of left eye
    H11.013 Amyloid pterygium of eye, bilateral
    H11.019 Amyloid pterygium of unspecified eye
  + **H11.02** **Central pterygium of eye**
    H11.021 Central pterygium of right eye
    H11.022 Central pterygium of left eye
    H11.023 Central pterygium of eye, bilateral
    H11.029 Central pterygium of unspecified eye
  + **H11.03** **Double pterygium of eye**
    H11.031 Double pterygium of right eye
    H11.032 Double pterygium of left eye
    H11.033 Double pterygium of eye, bilateral
    H11.039 Double pterygium of unspecified eye
  + **H11.04** **Peripheral pterygium of eye, stationary**
    H11.041 Peripheral pterygium, stationary, right eye
    H11.042 Peripheral pterygium, stationary, left eye
    H11.043 Peripheral pterygium, stationary, bilateral
    H11.049 Peripheral pterygium, stationary, unspecified eye

+ **H11.05** **Peripheral pterygium of eye, progressive**
    H11.051 Peripheral pterygium, progressive, right eye
    H11.052 Peripheral pterygium, progressive, left eye
    H11.053 Peripheral pterygium, progressive, bilateral
    H11.059 Peripheral pterygium, progressive, unspecified eye
+ **H11.06** **Recurrent pterygium of eye**
    H11.061 Recurrent pterygium of right eye
    H11.062 Recurrent pterygium of left eye
    H11.063 Recurrent pterygium of eye, bilateral
    H11.069 Recurrent pterygium of unspecified eye
+ **H11.1** **Conjunctival degenerations and deposits**
    Excludes2: pseudopterygium (H11.81)
  H11.10 **Unspecified conjunctival degenerations**
  + **H11.11** **Conjunctival deposits**
    H11.111 Conjunctival deposits, right eye
    H11.112 Conjunctival deposits, left eye
    H11.113 Conjunctival deposits, bilateral
    H11.119 Conjunctival deposits, unspecified eye
  + **H11.12** **Conjunctival concretions**
    H11.121 Conjunctival concretions, right eye
    H11.122 Conjunctival concretions, left eye
    H11.123 Conjunctival concretions, bilateral
    H11.129 Conjunctival concretions, unspecified eye
  + **H11.13** **Conjunctival pigmentations**
      Conjunctival argyrosis [argyria]
    H11.131 Conjunctival pigmentations, right eye
    H11.132 Conjunctival pigmentations, left eye
    H11.133 Conjunctival pigmentations, bilateral
    H11.139 Conjunctival pigmentations, unspecified eye
  + **H11.14** **Conjunctival xerosis, unspecified**
      Excludes1: xerosis of conjunctiva due to vitamin A deficiency (E50.0, E50.1)
    H11.141 Conjunctival xerosis, unspecified, right eye
    H11.142 Conjunctival xerosis, unspecified, left eye
    H11.143 Conjunctival xerosis, unspecified, bilateral
    H11.149 Conjunctival xerosis, unspecified, unspecified eye
  + **H11.15** **Pinguecula**
      Excludes1: pingueculitis (H10.81-)
    H11.151 Pinguecula, right eye
    H11.152 Pinguecula, left eye
    H11.153 Pinguecula, bilateral
    H11.159 Pinguecula, unspecified eye
+ **H11.2** **Conjunctival scars**
  + **H11.21** **Conjunctival adhesions and strands (localized)**
    H11.211 Conjunctival adhesions and strands (localized), right eye
    H11.212 Conjunctival adhesions and strands (localized), left eye
    H11.213 Conjunctival adhesions and strands (localized), bilateral
    H11.219 Conjunctival adhesions and strands (localized), unspecified eye
  + **H11.22** **Conjunctival granuloma**
    H11.221 Conjunctival granuloma, right eye
    H11.222 Conjunctival granuloma, left eye
    H11.223 Conjunctival granuloma, bilateral
    H11.229 Conjunctival granuloma, unspecified
  + **H11.23** **Symblepharon**
    H11.231 Symblepharon, right eye
    H11.232 Symblepharon, left eye
    H11.233 Symblepharon, bilateral
    H11.239 Symblepharon, unspecified eye
  + **H11.24** **Scarring of conjunctiva**
    H11.241 Scarring of conjunctiva, right eye
    H11.242 Scarring of conjunctiva, left eye
    H11.243 Scarring of conjunctiva, bilateral
    H11.249 Scarring of conjunctiva, unspecified eye
+ **H11.3** **Conjunctival hemorrhage**
    Subconjunctival hemorrhage
  H11.30 Conjunctival hemorrhage, unspecified eye
  H11.31 Conjunctival hemorrhage, right eye
  H11.32 Conjunctival hemorrhage, left eye
  H11.33 Conjunctival hemorrhage, bilateral

+, +7th, X + 7th   ● Newborn   ● Pediatric   ● Maternity   ● Adult   ♀ Female   ♂ Male   Manifestation   Unacceptable PDX   HCC   CC   MCC   HAC

+ **H11.4 Other conjunctival vascular disorders and cysts**
  + **H11.41 Vascular abnormalities of conjunctiva**
      Conjunctival aneurysm
      H11.411 Vascular abnormalities of conjunctiva, right eye
      H11.412 Vascular abnormalities of conjunctiva, left eye
      H11.413 Vascular abnormalities of conjunctiva, bilateral
      H11.419 Vascular abnormalities of conjunctiva, unspecified eye
  + **H11.42 Conjunctival edema**
      H11.421 Conjunctival edema, right eye
      H11.422 Conjunctival edema, left eye
      H11.423 Conjunctival edema, bilateral
      H11.429 Conjunctival edema, unspecified eye
  + **H11.43 Conjunctival hyperemia**
      H11.431 Conjunctival hyperemia, right eye
      H11.432 Conjunctival hyperemia, left eye
      H11.433 Conjunctival hyperemia, bilateral
      H11.439 Conjunctival hyperemia, unspecified eye
  + **H11.44 Conjunctival cysts**
      H11.441 Conjunctival cysts, right eye
      H11.442 Conjunctival cysts, left eye
      H11.443 Conjunctival cysts, bilateral
      H11.449 Conjunctival cysts, unspecified eye
+ **H11.8 Other specified disorders of conjunctiva**
  + **H11.81 Pseudopterygium of conjunctiva**
      H11.811 Pseudopterygium of conjunctiva, right eye
      H11.812 Pseudopterygium of conjunctiva, left eye
      H11.813 Pseudopterygium of conjunctiva, bilateral
      H11.819 Pseudopterygium of conjunctiva, unspecified eye
  + **H11.82 Conjunctivochalasis**
      H11.821 Conjunctivochalasis, right eye
      H11.822 Conjunctivochalasis, left eye
      H11.823 Conjunctivochalasis, bilateral
      H11.829 Conjunctivochalasis, unspecified eye
    H11.89 Other specified disorders of conjunctiva
  H11.9 Unspecified disorder of conjunctiva

Disorders of sclera, cornea, iris and ciliary body (H15-H22)

+ **H15 Disorders of sclera**
  + **H15.0 Scleritis**
    + **H15.00 Unspecified scleritis**
        H15.001 Unspecified scleritis, right eye
        H15.002 Unspecified scleritis, left eye
        H15.003 Unspecified scleritis, bilateral
        H15.009 Unspecified scleritis, unspecified eye
    + **H15.01 Anterior scleritis**
        H15.011 Anterior scleritis, right eye
        H15.012 Anterior scleritis, left eye
        H15.013 Anterior scleritis, bilateral
        H15.019 Anterior scleritis, unspecified eye
    + **H15.02 Brawny scleritis**
        H15.021 Brawny scleritis, right eye
        H15.022 Brawny scleritis, left eye
        H15.023 Brawny scleritis, bilateral
        H15.029 Brawny scleritis, unspecified eye
    + **H15.03 Posterior scleritis**
        Sclerotenonitis
        H15.031 Posterior scleritis, right eye
        H15.032 Posterior scleritis, left eye
        H15.033 Posterior scleritis, bilateral
        H15.039 Posterior scleritis, unspecified eye
    + **H15.04 Scleritis with corneal involvement**
        H15.041 Scleritis with corneal involvement, right eye
        H15.042 Scleritis with corneal involvement, left eye
        H15.043 Scleritis with corneal involvement, bilateral
        H15.049 Scleritis with corneal involvement, unspecified eye
    + **H15.05 Scleromalacia perforans**
        H15.051 Scleromalacia perforans, right eye
        H15.052 Scleromalacia perforans, left eye
        H15.053 Scleromalacia perforans, bilateral
        H15.059 Scleromalacia perforans, unspecified eye

+ **H15.09 Other scleritis**
    Scleral abscess
    H15.091 Other scleritis, right eye
    H15.092 Other scleritis, left eye
    H15.093 Other scleritis, bilateral
    H15.099 Other scleritis, unspecified eye
+ **H15.1 Episcleritis**
  + **H15.10 Unspecified episcleritis**
      H15.101 Unspecified episcleritis, right eye
      H15.102 Unspecified episcleritis, left eye
      H15.103 Unspecified episcleritis, bilateral
      H15.109 Unspecified episcleritis, unspecified eye
  + **H15.11 Episcleritis periodica fugax**
      H15.111 Episcleritis periodica fugax, right eye
      H15.112 Episcleritis periodica fugax, left eye
      H15.113 Episcleritis periodica fugax, bilateral
      H15.119 Episcleritis periodica fugax, unspecified eye
  + **H15.12 Nodular episcleritis**
      H15.121 Nodular episcleritis, right eye
      H15.122 Nodular episcleritis, left eye
      H15.123 Nodular episcleritis, bilateral
      H15.129 Nodular episcleritis, unspecified eye
+ **H15.8 Other disorders of sclera**
    Excludes2: *blue sclera (Q13.5)*
                degenerative myopia (H44.2-)
  + **H15.81 Equatorial staphyloma**
      H15.811 Equatorial staphyloma, right eye
      H15.812 Equatorial staphyloma, left eye
      H15.813 Equatorial staphyloma, bilateral
      H15.819 Equatorial staphyloma, unspecified eye
  + **H15.82 Localized anterior staphyloma**
      H15.821 Localized anterior staphyloma, right eye
      H15.822 Localized anterior staphyloma, left eye
      H15.823 Localized anterior staphyloma, bilateral
      H15.829 Localized anterior staphyloma, unspecified eye
  + **H15.83 Staphyloma posticum**
      H15.831 Staphyloma posticum, right eye
      H15.832 Staphyloma posticum, left eye
      H15.833 Staphyloma posticum, bilateral
      H15.839 Staphyloma posticum, unspecified eye
  + **H15.84 Scleral ectasia**
      H15.841 Scleral ectasia, right eye
      H15.842 Scleral ectasia, left eye
      H15.843 Scleral ectasia, bilateral
      H15.849 Scleral ectasia, unspecified eye
  + **H15.85 Ring staphyloma**
      H15.851 Ring staphyloma, right eye
      H15.852 Ring staphyloma, left eye
      H15.853 Ring staphyloma, bilateral
      H15.859 Ring staphyloma, unspecified eye
    H15.89 Other disorders of sclera
  H15.9 Unspecified disorder of sclera

H16 Keratitis
  + **H16.0 Corneal ulcer**
    + **H16.00 Unspecified corneal ulcer**
        H16.001 Unspecified corneal ulcer, right eye
        H16.002 Unspecified corneal ulcer, left eye
        H16.003 Unspecified corneal ulcer, bilateral
        H16.009 Unspecified corneal ulcer, unspecified eye
    + **H16.01 Central corneal ulcer**
        H16.011 Central corneal ulcer, right eye
        H16.012 Central corneal ulcer, left eye
        H16.013 Central corneal ulcer, bilateral
        H16.019 Central corneal ulcer, unspecified eye
    + **H16.02 Ring corneal ulcer**
        H16.021 Ring corneal ulcer, right eye
        H16.022 Ring corneal ulcer, left eye
        H16.023 Ring corneal ulcer, bilateral
        H16.029 Ring corneal ulcer, unspecified eye

+, +7th, X + 7th   • Newborn   • Pediatric   • Maternity   • Adult   ♀ Female   ♂ Male   Manifestation   Unacceptable PDX   HCC   CC   MCC   HAC

+ **H16.03** Corneal ulcer with hypopyon
　　H16.031 Corneal ulcer with hypopyon, right eye
　　H16.032 Corneal ulcer with hypopyon, left eye
　　H16.033 Corneal ulcer with hypopyon, bilateral
　　H16.039 Corneal ulcer with hypopyon, unspecified eye
+ **H16.04** Marginal corneal ulcer
　　H16.041 Marginal corneal ulcer, right eye
　　H16.042 Marginal corneal ulcer, left eye
　　H16.043 Marginal corneal ulcer, bilateral
　　H16.049 Marginal corneal ulcer, unspecified eye
+ **H16.05** Mooren's corneal ulcer
　　H16.051 Mooren's corneal ulcer, right eye
　　H16.052 Mooren's corneal ulcer, left eye
　　H16.053 Mooren's corneal ulcer, bilateral
　　H16.059 Mooren's corneal ulcer, unspecified eye
+ **H16.06** Mycotic corneal ulcer
　　H16.061 Mycotic corneal ulcer, right eye
　　H16.062 Mycotic corneal ulcer, left eye
　　H16.063 Mycotic corneal ulcer, bilateral
　　H16.069 Mycotic corneal ulcer, unspecified eye
+ **H16.07** Perforated corneal ulcer
　　H16.071 Perforated corneal ulcer, right eye
　　H16.072 Perforated corneal ulcer, left eye
　　H16.073 Perforated corneal ulcer, bilateral
　　H16.079 Perforated corneal ulcer, unspecified eye
+ **H16.1** Other and unspecified superficial keratitis without conjunctivitis
　+ **H16.10** Unspecified superficial keratitis
　　H16.101 Unspecified superficial keratitis, right eye
　　H16.102 Unspecified superficial keratitis, left eye
　　H16.103 Unspecified superficial keratitis, bilateral
　　H16.109 Unspecified superficial keratitis, unspecified eye
　+ **H16.11** Macular keratitis
　　　Areolar keratitis
　　　Nummular keratitis
　　　Stellate keratitis
　　　Striate keratitis
　　H16.111 Macular keratitis, right eye
　　H16.112 Macular keratitis, left eye
　　H16.113 Macular keratitis, bilateral
　　H16.119 Macular keratitis, unspecified eye
　+ **H16.12** Filamentary keratitis
　　H16.121 Filamentary keratitis, right eye
　　H16.122 Filamentary keratitis, left eye
　　H16.123 Filamentary keratitis, bilateral
　　H16.129 Filamentary keratitis, unspecified eye
　+ **H16.13** Photokeratitis
　　　Snow blindness
　　　Welders keratitis
　　H16.131 Photokeratitis, right eye
　　H16.132 Photokeratitis, left eye
　　H16.133 Photokeratitis, bilateral
　　H16.139 Photokeratitis, unspecified eye
　+ **H16.14** Punctate keratitis
　　H16.141 Punctate keratitis, right eye
　　H16.142 Punctate keratitis, left eye
　　H16.143 Punctate keratitis, bilateral
　　H16.149 Punctate keratitis, unspecified eye
+ **H16.2** Keratoconjunctivitis
　+ **H16.20** Unspecified keratoconjunctivitis
　　　Superficial keratitis with conjunctivitis NOS
　　H16.201 Unspecified keratoconjunctivitis, right eye
　　H16.202 Unspecified keratoconjunctivitis, left eye
　　H16.203 Unspecified keratoconjunctivitis, bilateral
　　H16.209 Unspecified keratoconjunctivitis, unspecified eye
　+ **H16.21** Exposure keratoconjunctivitis
　　H16.211 Exposure keratoconjunctivitis, right eye
　　H16.212 Exposure keratoconjunctivitis, left eye
　　H16.213 Exposure keratoconjunctivitis, bilateral
　　H16.219 Exposure keratoconjunctivitis, unspecified eye
　+ **H16.22** Keratoconjunctivitis sicca, not specified as Sjögren's
　　　Excludes1: Sjögren's syndrome (M35.01)

　　H16.221 Keratoconjunctivitis sicca, not specified as Sjögren's, right eye
　　H16.222 Keratoconjunctivitis sicca, not specified as Sjögren's, left eye
　　H16.223 Keratoconjunctivitis sicca, not specified as Sjögren's, bilateral
　　H16.229 Keratoconjunctivitis sicca, not specified as Sjögren's, unspecified eye
　+ **H16.23** Neurotrophic keratoconjunctivitis
　　H16.231 Neurotrophic keratoconjunctivitis, right eye
　　H16.232 Neurotrophic keratoconjunctivitis, left eye
　　H16.233 Neurotrophic keratoconjunctivitis, bilateral
　　H16.239 Neurotrophic keratoconjunctivitis, unspecified eye
　+ **H16.24** Ophthalmia nodosa
　　H16.241 Ophthalmia nodosa, right eye
　　H16.242 Ophthalmia nodosa, left eye
　　H16.243 Ophthalmia nodosa, bilateral
　　H16.249 Ophthalmia nodosa, unspecified eye
　+ **H16.25** Phlyctenular keratoconjunctivitis
　　H16.251 Phlyctenular keratoconjunctivitis, right eye
　　H16.252 Phlyctenular keratoconjunctivitis, left eye
　　H16.253 Phlyctenular keratoconjunctivitis, bilateral
　　H16.259 Phlyctenular keratoconjunctivitis, unspecified eye
　+ **H16.26** Vernal keratoconjunctivitis, with limbar and corneal involvement
　　　Excludes1: vernal conjunctivitis without limbar and corneal involvement (H10.44)
　　H16.261 Vernal keratoconjunctivitis, with limbar and corneal involvement, right eye
　　H16.262 Vernal keratoconjunctivitis, with limbar and corneal involvement, left eye
　　H16.263 Vernal keratoconjunctivitis, with limbar and corneal involvement, bilateral
　　H16.269 Vernal keratoconjunctivitis, with limbar and corneal involvement, unspecified eye
　+ **H16.29** Other keratoconjunctivitis
　　H16.291 Other keratoconjunctivitis, right eye
　　H16.292 Other keratoconjunctivitis, left eye
　　H16.293 Other keratoconjunctivitis, bilateral
　　H16.299 Other keratoconjunctivitis, unspecified eye
+ **H16.3** Interstitial and deep keratitis
　+ **H16.30** Unspecified interstitial keratitis
　　H16.301 Unspecified interstitial keratitis, right eye
　　H16.302 Unspecified interstitial keratitis, left eye
　　H16.303 Unspecified interstitial keratitis, bilateral
　　H16.309 Unspecified interstitial keratitis, unspecified eye
　+ **H16.31** Corneal abscess
　　H16.311 Corneal abscess, right eye
　　H16.312 Corneal abscess, left eye
　　H16.313 Corneal abscess, bilateral
　　H16.319 Corneal abscess, unspecified eye
　+ **H16.32** Diffuse interstitial keratitis
　　　Cogan's syndrome
　　H16.321 Diffuse interstitial keratitis, right eye
　　H16.322 Diffuse interstitial keratitis, left eye
　　H16.323 Diffuse interstitial keratitis, bilateral
　　H16.329 Diffuse interstitial keratitis, unspecified eye
　+ **H16.33** Sclerosing keratitis
　　H16.331 Sclerosing keratitis, right eye
　　H16.332 Sclerosing keratitis, left eye
　　H16.333 Sclerosing keratitis, bilateral
　　H16.339 Sclerosing keratitis, unspecified eye

+ **H16.39** Other interstitial and deep keratitis
- **H16.391** Other interstitial and deep keratitis, right eye
- **H16.392** Other interstitial and deep keratitis, left eye
- **H16.393** Other interstitial and deep keratitis, bilateral
- **H16.399** Other interstitial and deep keratitis, unspecified eye

+ **H16.4** Corneal neovascularization
- + **H16.40** Unspecified corneal neovascularization
  - **H16.401** Unspecified corneal neovascularization, right eye
  - **H16.402** Unspecified corneal neovascularization, left eye
  - **H16.403** Unspecified corneal neovascularization, bilateral
  - **H16.409** Unspecified corneal neovascularization, unspecified eye
- + **H16.41** Ghost vessels (corneal)
  - **H16.411** Ghost vessels (corneal), right eye
  - **H16.412** Ghost vessels (corneal), left eye
  - **H16.413** Ghost vessels (corneal), bilateral
  - **H16.419** Ghost vessels (corneal), unspecified eye
- + **H16.42** Pannus (corneal)
  - **H16.421** Pannus (corneal), right eye
  - **H16.422** Pannus (corneal), left eye
  - **H16.423** Pannus (corneal), bilateral
  - **H16.429** Pannus (corneal), unspecified eye
- + **H16.43** Localized vascularization of cornea
  - **H16.431** Localized vascularization of cornea, right eye
  - **H16.432** Localized vascularization of cornea, left eye
  - **H16.433** Localized vascularization of cornea, bilateral
  - **H16.439** Localized vascularization of cornea, unspecified eye
- + **H16.44** Deep vascularization of cornea
  - **H16.441** Deep vascularization of cornea, right eye
  - **H16.442** Deep vascularization of cornea, left eye
  - **H16.443** Deep vascularization of cornea, bilateral
  - **H16.449** Deep vascularization of cornea, unspecified eye

H16.8 Other keratitis
H16.9 Unspecified keratitis

H17 Corneal scars and opacities
- + **H17.0** Adherent leukoma
  - **H17.00** Adherent leukoma, unspecified eye
  - **H17.01** Adherent leukoma, right eye
  - **H17.02** Adherent leukoma, left eye
  - **H17.03** Adherent leukoma, bilateral
- + **H17.1** Central corneal opacity
  - **H17.10** Central corneal opacity, unspecified eye
  - **H17.11** Central corneal opacity, right eye
  - **H17.12** Central corneal opacity, left eye
  - **H17.13** Central corneal opacity, bilateral
- + **H17.8** Other corneal scars and opacities
  - + **H17.81** Minor opacity of cornea
    Corneal nebula
    - **H17.811** Minor opacity of cornea, right eye
    - **H17.812** Minor opacity of cornea, left eye
    - **H17.813** Minor opacity of cornea, bilateral
    - **H17.819** Minor opacity of cornea, unspecified eye
  - + **H17.82** Peripheral opacity of cornea
    - **H17.821** Peripheral opacity of cornea, right eye
    - **H17.822** Peripheral opacity of cornea, left eye
    - **H17.823** Peripheral opacity of cornea, bilateral
    - **H17.829** Peripheral opacity of cornea, unspecified eye
  - **H17.89** Other corneal scars and opacities
- **H17.9** Unspecified corneal scar and opacity

H18 Other disorders of cornea
- + **H18.0** Corneal pigmentations and deposits
  - + **H18.00** Unspecified corneal deposit
    - **H18.001** Unspecified corneal deposit, right eye
    - **H18.002** Unspecified corneal deposit, left eye
    - **H18.003** Unspecified corneal deposit, bilateral
    - **H18.009** Unspecified corneal deposit, unspecified eye
  - + **H18.01** Anterior corneal pigmentations
    Staehli's line
    - **H18.011** Anterior corneal pigmentations, right eye
    - **H18.012** Anterior corneal pigmentations, left eye
    - **H18.013** Anterior corneal pigmentations, bilateral
    - **H18.019** Anterior corneal pigmentations, unspecified eye
  - + **H18.02** Argentous corneal deposits
    - **H18.021** Argentous corneal deposits, right eye
    - **H18.022** Argentous corneal deposits, left eye
    - **H18.023** Argentous corneal deposits, bilateral
    - **H18.029** Argentous corneal deposits, unspecified eye
  - + **H18.03** Corneal deposits in metabolic disorders
    Code also associated metabolic disorder
    - **H18.031** Corneal deposits in metabolic disorders, right eye
    - **H18.032** Corneal deposits in metabolic disorders, left eye
    - **H18.033** Corneal deposits in metabolic disorders, bilateral
    - **H18.039** Corneal deposits in metabolic disorders, unspecified eye
  - + **H18.04** Kayser-Fleischer ring
    Code also associated Wilson's disease (E83.01)
    - **H18.041** Kayser-Fleischer ring, right eye
    - **H18.042** Kayser-Fleischer ring, left eye
    - **H18.043** Kayser-Fleischer ring, bilateral
    - **H18.049** Kayser-Fleischer ring, unspecified eye
  - + **H18.05** Posterior corneal pigmentations
    Krukenberg's spindle
    - **H18.051** Posterior corneal pigmentations, right eye
    - **H18.052** Posterior corneal pigmentations, left eye
    - **H18.053** Posterior corneal pigmentations, bilateral
    - **H18.059** Posterior corneal pigmentations, unspecified eye
  - + **H18.06** Stromal corneal pigmentations
    Hematocornea
    - **H18.061** Stromal corneal pigmentations, right eye
    - **H18.062** Stromal corneal pigmentations, left eye
    - **H18.063** Stromal corneal pigmentations, bilateral
    - **H18.069** Stromal corneal pigmentations, unspecified eye
- + **H18.1** Bullous keratopathy
  - **H18.10** Bullous keratopathy, unspecified eye
  - **H18.11** Bullous keratopathy, right eye
  - **H18.12** Bullous keratopathy, left eye
  - **H18.13** Bullous keratopathy, bilateral
- + **H18.2** Other and unspecified corneal edema
  - **H18.20** Unspecified corneal edema
  - + **H18.21** Corneal edema secondary to contact lens
    Excludes2: other corneal disorders due to contact lens (H18.82-)
    - **H18.211** Corneal edema secondary to contact lens, right eye
    - **H18.212** Corneal edema secondary to contact lens, left eye
    - **H18.213** Corneal edema secondary to contact lens, bilateral
    - **H18.219** Corneal edema secondary to contact lens, unspecified eye

+, +7th, X + 7th   ● Newborn   ○ Pediatric   ● Maternity   ● Adult   ♀ Female   ♂ Male   Manifestation   Unacceptable PDX   HCC   CC   MCC   HAC

+ H18.22 **Idiopathic corneal edema**
    H18.221 **Idiopathic corneal edema, right eye**
    H18.222 **Idiopathic corneal edema, left eye**
    H18.223 **Idiopathic corneal edema, bilateral**
    H18.229 **Idiopathic corneal edema, unspecified eye**
+ H18.23 **Secondary corneal edema**
    H18.231 **Secondary corneal edema, right eye**
    H18.232 **Secondary corneal edema, left eye**
    H18.233 **Secondary corneal edema, bilateral**
    H18.239 **Secondary corneal edema, unspecified eye**

+ H18.3 **Changes of corneal membranes**
    H18.30 **Unspecified corneal membrane change**
+ H18.31 **Folds and rupture in Bowman's membrane**
    H18.311 **Folds and rupture in Bowman's membrane, right eye**
    H18.312 **Folds and rupture in Bowman's membrane, left eye**
    H18.313 **Folds and rupture in Bowman's membrane, bilateral**
    H18.319 **Folds and rupture in Bowman's membrane, unspecified eye**
+ H18.32 **Folds in Descemet's membrane**
    H18.321 **Folds in Descemet's membrane, right eye**
    H18.322 **Folds in Descemet's membrane, left eye**
    H18.323 **Folds in Descemet's membrane, bilateral**
    H18.329 **Folds in Descemet's membrane, unspecified eye**
+ H18.33 **Rupture in Descemet's membrane**
    H18.331 **Rupture in Descemet's membrane, right eye**
    H18.332 **Rupture in Descemet's membrane, left eye**
    H18.333 **Rupture in Descemet's membrane, bilateral**
    H18.339 **Rupture in Descemet's membrane, unspecified eye**

+ H18.4 **Corneal degeneration**
    Excludes1: *Mooren's ulcer (H16.0-)*
        recurrent erosion of cornea (H18.83-)
    H18.40 **Unspecified corneal degeneration**
+ H18.41 **Arcus senilis**
    Senile corneal changes
    H18.411 **Arcus senilis, right eye**
    H18.412 **Arcus senilis, left eye**
    H18.413 **Arcus senilis, bilateral**
    H18.419 **Arcus senilis, unspecified eye**
+ H18.42 **Band keratopathy**
    H18.421 **Band keratopathy, right eye**
    H18.422 **Band keratopathy, left eye**
    H18.423 **Band keratopathy, bilateral**
    H18.429 **Band keratopathy, unspecified eye**
    H18.43 **Other calcerous corneal degeneration**
+ H18.44 **Keratomalacia**
    Excludes1: *keratomalacia due to vitamin A deficiency (E50.4)*
    H18.441 **Keratomalacia, right eye**
    H18.442 **Keratomalacia, left eye**
    H18.443 **Keratomalacia, bilateral**
    H18.449 **Keratomalacia, unspecified eye**
+ H18.45 **Nodular corneal degeneration**
    H18.451 **Nodular corneal degeneration, right eye**
    H18.452 **Nodular corneal degeneration, left eye**
    H18.453 **Nodular corneal degeneration, bilateral**
    H18.459 **Nodular corneal degeneration, unspecified eye**
+ H18.46 **Peripheral corneal degeneration**
    H18.461 **Peripheral corneal degeneration, right eye**
    H18.462 **Peripheral corneal degeneration, left eye**
    H18.463 **Peripheral corneal degeneration, bilateral**
    H18.469 **Peripheral corneal degeneration, unspecified eye**
    H18.49 **Other corneal degeneration**

+ H18.5 **Hereditary corneal dystrophies**
+ H18.50 **Unspecified hereditary corneal dystrophies**
    H18.501 **Unspecified hereditary corneal dystrophies, right eye**
    H18.502 **Unspecified hereditary corneal dystrophies, left eye**
    H18.503 **Unspecified hereditary corneal dystrophies, bilateral**
    H18.509 **Unspecified hereditary corneal dystrophies, unspecified eye**
+ H18.51 **Endothelial corneal dystrophy**
    Fuchs' dystrophy
    H18.511 **Endothelial corneal dystrophy, right eye**
    H18.512 **Endothelial corneal dystrophy, left eye**
    H18.513 **Endothelial corneal dystrophy, bilateral**
    H18.519 **Endothelial corneal dystrophy, unspecified eye**
+ H18.52 **Epithelial (juvenile) corneal dystrophy**
    H18.521 **Epithelial (juvenile) corneal dystrophy, right eye**
    H18.522 **Epithelial (juvenile) corneal dystrophy, left eye**
    H18.523 **Epithelial (juvenile) corneal dystrophy, bilateral**
    H18.529 **Epithelial (juvenile) corneal dystrophy, unspecified eye**
+ H18.53 **Granular corneal dystrophy**
    H18.531 **Granular corneal dystrophy, right eye**
    H18.532 **Granular corneal dystrophy, left eye**
    H18.533 **Granular corneal dystrophy, bilateral**
    H18.539 **Granular corneal dystrophy, unspecified eye**
+ H18.54 **Lattice corneal dystrophy**
    H18.541 **Lattice corneal dystrophy, right eye**
    H18.542 **Lattice corneal dystrophy, left eye**
    H18.543 **Lattice corneal dystrophy, bilateral**
    H18.549 **Lattice corneal dystrophy, unspecified eye**
+ H18.55 **Macular corneal dystrophy**
    H18.551 **Macular corneal dystrophy, right eye**
    H18.552 **Macular corneal dystrophy, left eye**
    H18.553 **Macular corneal dystrophy, bilateral**
    H18.559 **Macular corneal dystrphy, unspecified eye**
+ H18.59 **Other hereditary corneal dystrophies**
    H18.591 **Other hereditary corneal dystrophies, right eye**
    H18.592 **Other hereditary corneal dystrophies, left eye**
    H18.593 **Other hereditary corneal dystrophies, bilateral**
    H18.599 **Other hereditary corneal dystrophies, unspecified eye**

+ H18.6 **Keratoconus**
+ H18.60 **Keratoconus, unspecified**
    H18.601 **Keratoconus, unspecified, right eye**
    H18.602 **Keratoconus, unspecified, left eye**
    H18.603 **Keratoconus, unspecified, bilateral**
    H18.609 **Keratoconus, unspecified, unspecified eye**
+ H18.61 **Keratoconus, stable**
    H18.611 **Keratoconus, stable, right eye**
    H18.612 **Keratoconus, stable, left eye**
    H18.613 **Keratoconus, stable, bilateral**
    H18.619 **Keratoconus, stable, unspecified eye**
+ H18.62 **Keratoconus, unstable**
    Acute hydrops
    H18.621 **Keratoconus, unstable, right eye**
    H18.622 **Keratoconus, unstable, left eye**
    H18.623 **Keratoconus, unstable, bilateral**
    H18.629 **Keratoconus, unstable, unspecified eye**

+ H18.7 **Other and unspecified corneal deformities**
    Excludes1: *congenital malformations of cornea (Q13.3-Q13.4)*
    H18.70 **Unspecified corneal deformity**
+ H18.71 **Corneal ectasia**
    H18.711 **Corneal ectasia, right eye**
    H18.712 **Corneal ectasia, left eye**
    H18.713 **Corneal ectasia, bilateral**
    H18.719 **Corneal ectasia, unspecified eye**
+ H18.72 **Corneal staphyloma**
    H18.721 **Corneal staphyloma, right eye**
    H18.722 **Corneal staphyloma, left eye**
    H18.723 **Corneal staphyloma, bilateral**
    H18.729 **Corneal staphyloma, unspecified eye**

+, +7th, X + 7th   ● Newborn   ● Pediatric   ● Maternity   ● Adult   ♀ Female   ♂ Male   Manifestation   Unacceptable PDX   HCC   CC   MCC   HAC

+ **H18.73 Descemetocele**
    H18.731 **Descemetocele, right eye**
    H18.732 **Descemetocele, left eye**
    H18.733 **Descemetocele, bilateral**
    H18.739 **Descemetocele, unspecified eye**
+ **H18.79 Other corneal deformities**
    H18.791 **Other corneal deformities, right eye**
    H18.792 **Other corneal deformities, left eye**
    H18.793 **Other corneal deformities, bilateral**
    H18.799 **Other corneal deformities, unspecified eye**

+ **H18.8 Other specified disorders of cornea**
  + **H18.81 Anesthesia and hypoesthesia of cornea**
    H18.811 **Anesthesia and hypoesthesia of cornea, right eye**
    H18.812 **Anesthesia and hypoesthesia of cornea, left eye**
    H18.813 **Anesthesia and hypoesthesia of cornea, bilateral**
    H18.819 **Anesthesia and hypoesthesia of cornea, unspecified eye**
  + **H18.82 Corneal disorder due to contact lens**
    Excludes2: *corneal edema due to contact lens (H18.21-)*
    H18.821 **Corneal disorder due to contact lens, right eye**
    H18.822 **Corneal disorder due to contact lens, left eye**
    H18.823 **Corneal disorder due to contact lens, bilateral**
    H18.829 **Corneal disorder due to contact lens, unspecified eye**
  + **H18.83 Recurrent erosion of cornea**
    H18.831 **Recurrent erosion of cornea, right eye**
    H18.832 **Recurrent erosion of cornea, left eye**
    H18.833 **Recurrent erosion of cornea, bilateral**
    H18.839 **Recurrent erosion of cornea, unspecified eye**
  + **H18.89 Other specified disorders of cornea**
    H18.891 **Other specified disorders of cornea, right eye**
    H18.892 **Other specified disorders of cornea, left eye**
    H18.893 **Other specified disorders of cornea, bilateral**
    H18.899 **Other specified disorders of cornea, unspecified eye**

H18.9 Unspecified disorder of cornea

H20 Iridocyclitis
+ **H20.0 Acute and subacute iridocyclitis**
  Acute anterior uveitis
  Acute cyclitis
  Acute iritis
  Subacute anterior uveitis
  Subacute cyclitis
  Subacute iritis
  Excludes1: *iridocyclitis, iritis, uveitis (due to) (in) diabetes mellitus (E08-E13 with .39)*
    iridocyclitis, iritis, uveitis (due to) (in) diphtheria (A36.89)
    iridocyclitis, iritis, uveitis (due to) (in) gonococcal (A54.32)
    iridocyclitis, iritis, uveitis (due to) (in) herpes (simplex) (B00.51)
    iridocyclitis, iritis, uveitis (due to) (in) herpes zoster (B02.32)
    iridocyclitis, iritis, uveitis (due to) (in) late congenital syphilis (A50.39)
    iridocyclitis, iritis, uveitis (due to) (in) late syphilis (A52.71)
    iridocyclitis, iritis, uveitis (due to) (in) sarcoidosis (D86.83)
    iridocyclitis, iritis, uveitis (due to) (in) syphilis (A51.43)
    iridocyclitis, iritis, uveitis (due to) (in) toxoplasmosis (B58.09)
    iridocyclitis, iritis, uveitis (due to) (in) tuberculosis (A18.54)

CC **H20.00 Unspecified acute and subacute iridocyclitis**
+ **H20.01 Primary iridocyclitis**
  CC H20.011 **Primary iridocyclitis, right eye**
  CC H20.012 **Primary iridocyclitis, left eye**
  CC H20.013 **Primary iridocyclitis, bilateral**
  CC H20.019 **Primary iridocyclitis, unspecified eye**
+ **H20.02 Recurrent acute iridocyclitis**
  CC H20.021 **Recurrent acute iridocyclitis, right eye**
  CC H20.022 **Recurrent acute iridocyclitis, left eye**
  CC H20.023 **Recurrent acute iridocyclitis, bilateral**
  CC H20.029 **Recurrent acute iridocyclitis, unspecified eye**
+ **H20.03 Secondary infectious iridocyclitis**
  CC H20.031 **Secondary infectious iridocyclitis, right eye**
  CC H20.032 **Secondary infectious iridocyclitis, left eye**
  CC H20.033 **Secondary infectious iridocyclitis, bilateral**
  CC H20.039 **Secondary infectious iridocyclitis, unspecified eye**
+ **H20.04 Secondary noninfectious iridocyclitis**
  H20.041 **Secondary noninfectious iridocyclitis, right eye**
  H20.042 **Secondary noninfectious iridocyclitis, left eye**
  H20.043 **Secondary noninfectious iridocyclitis, bilateral**
  H20.049 **Secondary noninfectious iridocyclitis, unspecified eye**
+ **H20.05 Hypopyon**
  H20.051 **Hypopyon, right eye**
  H20.052 **Hypopyon, left eye**
  H20.053 **Hypopyon, bilateral**
  H20.059 **Hypopyon, unspecified eye**

+ **H20.1 Chronic iridocyclitis**
  Use additional code for any associated cataract (H26.21-)
  Excludes2: *posterior cyclitis (H30.2-)*
  H20.10 **Chronic iridocyclitis, unspecified eye**
  H20.11 **Chronic iridocyclitis, right eye**
  H20.12 **Chronic iridocyclitis, left eye**
  H20.13 **Chronic iridocyclitis, bilateral**
+ **H20.2 Lens-induced iridocyclitis**
  H20.20 **Lens-induced iridocyclitis, unspecified eye**
  H20.21 **Lens-induced iridocyclitis, right eye**
  H20.22 **Lens-induced iridocyclitis, left eye**
  H20.23 **Lens-induced iridocyclitis, bilateral**
+ **H20.8 Other iridocyclitis**
  Excludes2: *glaucomatocyclitis crises (H40.4-)*
    posterior cyclitis (H30.2-)
    sympathetic uveitis (H44.13-)
  + **H20.81 Fuchs' heterochromic cyclitis**
    H20.811 **Fuchs' heterochromic cyclitis, right eye**
    H20.812 **Fuchs' heterochromic cyclitis, left eye**
    H20.813 **Fuchs' heterochromic cyclitis, bilateral**
    H20.819 **Fuchs' heterochromic cyclitis, unspecified eye**
  + **H20.82 Vogt-Koyanagi syndrome**
    H20.821 **Vogt-Koyanagi syndrome, right eye**
    H20.822 **Vogt-Koyanagi syndrome, left eye**
    H20.823 **Vogt-Koyanagi syndrome, bilateral**
    H20.829 **Vogt-Koyanagi syndrome, unspecified eye**

CC **H20.9 Unspecified iridocyclitis**
  Uveitis NOS

H21 Other disorders of iris and ciliary body
  Excludes2: *sympathetic uveitis (H44.1-)*
+ **H21.0 Hyphema**
  Excludes1: *traumatic hyphema (S05.1-)*
  H21.00 **Hyphema, unspecified eye**
  H21.01 **Hyphema, right eye**
  H21.02 **Hyphema, left eye**
  H21.03 **Hyphema, bilateral**

+, +7th, X + 7th   ● Newborn   ● Pediatric   ● Maternity   ● Adult   ♀ Female   ♂ Male   Manifestation   Unacceptable PDX   HCC   CC   MCC   HAC

+ H21.1 Other vascular disorders of iris and ciliary body
Neovascularization of iris or ciliary body
Rubeosis iridis
Rubeosis of iris
  + H21.1X Other vascular disorders of iris and ciliary body
    H21.1X1 Other vascular disorders of iris and ciliary body, right eye
    H21.1X2 Other vascular disorders of iris and ciliary body, left eye
    H21.1X3 Other vascular disorders of iris and ciliary body, bilateral
    H21.1X9 Other vascular disorders of iris and ciliary body, unspecified eye
+ H21.2 Degeneration of iris and ciliary body
  + H21.21 Degeneration of chamber angle
    H21.211 Degeneration of chamber angle, right eye
    H21.212 Degeneration of chamber angle, left eye
    H21.213 Degeneration of chamber angle, bilateral
    H21.219 Degeneration of chamber angle, unspecified eye
  + H21.22 Degeneration of ciliary body
    H21.221 Degeneration of ciliary body, right eye
    H21.222 Degeneration of ciliary body, left eye
    H21.223 Degeneration of ciliary body, bilateral
    H21.229 Degeneration of ciliary body, unspecified eye
  + H21.23 Degeneration of iris (pigmentary)
    Translucency of iris
    H21.231 Degeneration of iris (pigmentary), right eye
    H21.232 Degeneration of iris (pigmentary), left eye
    H21.233 Degeneration of iris (pigmentary), bilateral
    H21.239 Degeneration of iris (pigmentary), unspecified eye
  + H21.24 Degeneration of pupillary margin
    H21.241 Degeneration of pupillary margin, right eye
    H21.242 Degeneration of pupillary margin, left eye
    H21.243 Degeneration of pupillary margin, bilateral
    H21.249 Degeneration of pupillary margin, unspecified eye
  + H21.25 Iridoschisis
    H21.251 Iridoschisis, right eye
    H21.252 Iridoschisis, left eye
    H21.253 Iridoschisis, bilateral
    H21.259 Iridoschisis, unspecified eye
  + H21.26 Iris atrophy (essential) (progressive)
    H21.261 Iris atrophy (essential) (progressive), right eye
    H21.262 Iris atrophy (essential) (progressive), left eye
    H21.263 Iris atrophy (essential) (progressive), bilateral
    H21.269 Iris atrophy (essential) (progressive), unspecified eye
  + H21.27 Miotic pupillary cyst
    H21.271 Miotic pupillary cyst, right eye
    H21.272 Miotic pupillary cyst, left eye
    H21.273 Miotic pupillary cyst, bilateral
    H21.279 Miotic pupillary cyst, unspecified eye
  H21.29 Other iris atrophy
+ H21.3 Cyst of iris, ciliary body and anterior chamber
  Excludes2: *miotic pupillary cyst (H21.27-)*
  + H21.30 Idiopathic cysts of iris, ciliary body or anterior chamber
    Cyst of iris, ciliary body or anterior chamber NOS
    H21.301 Idiopathic cysts of iris, ciliary body or anterior chamber, right eye
    H21.302 Idiopathic cysts of iris, ciliary body or anterior chamber, left eye
    H21.303 Idiopathic cysts of iris, ciliary body or anterior chamber, bilateral
    H21.309 Idiopathic cysts of iris, ciliary body or anterior chamber, unspecified eye

+ H21.31 Exudative cysts of iris or anterior chamber
  H21.311 Exudative cysts of iris or anterior chamber, right eye
  H21.312 Exudative cysts of iris or anterior chamber, left eye
  H21.313 Exudative cysts of iris or anterior chamber, bilateral
  H21.319 Exudative cysts of iris or anterior chamber, unspecified eye
+ H21.32 Implantation cysts of iris, ciliary body or anterior chamber
  H21.321 Implantation cysts of iris, ciliary body or anterior chamber, right eye
  H21.322 Implantation cysts of iris, ciliary body or anterior chamber, left eye
  H21.323 Implantation cysts of iris, ciliary body or anterior chamber, bilateral
  H21.329 Implantation cysts of iris, ciliary body or anterior chamber, unspecified eye
+ H21.33 Parasitic cyst of iris, ciliary body or anterior chamber
  CC H21.331 Parasitic cyst of iris, ciliary body or anterior chamber, right eye
  CC H21.332 Parasitic cyst of iris, ciliary body or anterior chamber, left eye
  CC H21.333 Parasitic cyst of iris, ciliary body or anterior chamber, bilateral
  CC H21.339 Parasitic cyst of iris, ciliary body or anterior chamber, unspecified eye
+ H21.34 Primary cyst of pars plana
  H21.341 Primary cyst of pars plana, right eye
  H21.342 Primary cyst of pars plana, left eye
  H21.343 Primary cyst of pars plana, bilateral
  H21.349 Primary cyst of pars plana, unspecified eye
+ H21.35 Exudative cyst of pars plana
  H21.351 Exudative cyst of pars plana, right eye
  H21.352 Exudative cyst of pars plana, left eye
  H21.353 Exudative cyst of pars plana, bilateral
  H21.359 Exudative cyst of pars plana, unspecified eye
+ H21.4 Pupillary membranes
  Iris bombé
  Pupillary occlusion
  Pupillary seclusion
  Excludes1: *congenital pupillary membranes (Q13.8)*
  H21.40 Pupillary membranes, unspecified eye
  H21.41 Pupillary membranes, right eye
  H21.42 Pupillary membranes, left eye
  H21.43 Pupillary membranes, bilateral
+ H21.5 Other and unspecified adhesions and disruptions of iris and ciliary body
  Excludes1: *corectopia (Q13.2)*
  + H21.50 Unspecified adhesions of iris
    Synechia (iris) NOS
    H21.501 Unspecified adhesions of iris, right eye
    H21.502 Unspecified adhesions of iris, left eye
    H21.503 Unspecified adhesions of iris, bilateral
    H21.509 Unspecified adhesions of iris and ciliary body, unspecified eye
  + H21.51 Anterior synechiae (iris)
    H21.511 Anterior synechiae (iris), right eye
    H21.512 Anterior synechiae (iris), left eye
    H21.513 Anterior synechiae (iris), bilateral
    H21.519 Anterior synechiae (iris), unspecified eye
  + H21.52 Goniosynechiae
    H21.521 Goniosynechiae, right eye
    H21.522 Goniosynechiae, left eye
    H21.523 Goniosynechiae, bilateral
    H21.529 Goniosynechiae, unspecified eye

+ **H21.53 Iridodialysis**
  - **H21.531 Iridodialysis, right eye**
  - **H21.532 Iridodialysis, left eye**
  - **H21.533 Iridodialysis, bilateral**
  - **H21.539 Iridodialysis, unspecified eye**
+ **H21.54 Posterior synechiae (iris)**
  - **H21.541 Posterior synechiae (iris), right eye**
  - **H21.542 Posterior synechiae (iris), left eye**
  - **H21.543 Posterior synechiae (iris), bilateral**
  - **H21.549 Posterior synechiae (iris), unspecified eye**
+ **H21.55 Recession of chamber angle**
  - **H21.551 Recession of chamber angle, right eye**
  - **H21.552 Recession of chamber angle, left eye**
  - **H21.553 Recession of chamber angle, bilateral**
  - **H21.559 Recession of chamber angle, unspecified eye**
+ **H21.56 Pupillary abnormalities**
  Deformed pupil
  Ectopic pupil
  Rupture of sphincter, pupil
  Excludes1: *congenital deformity of pupil (Q13.2-)*
  - **H21.561 Pupillary abnormality, right eye**
  - **H21.562 Pupillary abnormality, left eye**
  - **H21.563 Pupillary abnormality, bilateral**
  - **H21.569 Pupillary abnormality, unspecified eye**
+ **H21.8 Other specified disorders of iris and ciliary body**
  - **H21.81 Floppy iris syndrome**
    Intraoperative floppy iris syndrome (IFIS)
    Use additional code for adverse effect, if applicable, to identify drug (T36-T50 with fifth or sixth character 5)
  - **H21.82 Plateau iris syndrome (post-iridectomy) (postprocedural)**
  - **H21.89 Other specified disorders of iris and ciliary body**
- **H21.9 Unspecified disorder of iris and ciliary body**

H22 Disorders of iris and ciliary body in diseases classified elsewhere

Code first underlying disease, such as:
   gout (M1A.-, M10.-)
   leprosy (A30.-)
   parasitic disease (B89)
Valid 3-character code, no further characters required

Disorders of lens (H25-H28)

H25 Age-related cataract

Senile cataract
Excludes2: *capsular glaucoma with pseudoexfoliation of lens (H40.1-)*

+ **H25.0 Age-related incipient cataract**
  + **H25.01 Cortical age-related cataract**
    - **H25.011 Cortical age-related cataract, right eye**
    - **H25.012 Cortical age-related cataract, left eye**
    - **H25.013 Cortical age-related cataract, bilateral**
    - **H25.019 Cortical age-related cataract, unspecified eye**
  + **H25.03 Anterior subcapsular polar age-related cataract**
    - **H25.031 Anterior subcapsular polar age-related cataract, right eye**
    - **H25.032 Anterior subcapsular polar age-related cataract, left eye**
    - **H25.033 Anterior subcapsular polar age-related cataract, bilateral**
    - **H25.039 Anterior subcapsular polar age-related cataract, unspecified eye**
  + **H25.04 Posterior subcapsular polar age-related cataract**
    - **H25.041 Posterior subcapsular polar age-related cataract, right eye**
    - **H25.042 Posterior subcapsular polar age-related cataract, left eye**
    - **H25.043 Posterior subcapsular polar age-related cataract, bilateral**
    - **H25.049 Posterior subcapsular polar age-related cataract, unspecified eye**

+ **H25.09 Other age-related incipient cataract**
  Coronary age-related cataract
  Punctate age-related cataract
  Water clefts
  - **H25.091 Other age-related incipient cataract, right eye**
  - **H25.092 Other age-related incipient cataract, left eye**
  - **H25.093 Other age-related incipient cataract, bilateral**
  - **H25.099 Other age-related incipient cataract, unspecified eye**
+ **H25.1 Age-related nuclear cataract**
  Cataracta brunescens
  Nuclear sclerosis cataract
  - **H25.10 Age-related nuclear cataract, unspecified eye**
  - **H25.11 Age-related nuclear cataract, right eye**
    AHA CC: 2Q, 2019, 31
  - **H25.12 Age-related nuclear cataract, left eye**
    AHA CC: 1Q, 2016, 32-33
  - **H25.13 Age-related nuclear cataract, bilateral**
    AHA CC: 1Q, 2016, 32-33
+ **H25.2 Age-related cataract, morgagnian type**
  Age-related hypermature cataract
  - **H25.20 Age-related cataract, morgagnian type, unspecified eye**
  - **H25.21 Age-related cataract, morgagnian type, right eye**
  - **H25.22 Age-related cataract, morgagnian type, left eye**
  - **H25.23 Age-related cataract, morgagnian type, bilateral**
+ **H25.8 Other age-related cataract**
  + **H25.81 Combined forms of age-related cataract**
    - **H25.811 Combined forms of age-related cataract, right eye**
    - **H25.812 Combined forms of age-related cataract, left eye**
    - **H25.813 Combined forms of age-related cataract, bilateral**
      AHA CC: 2Q, 2019, 30
    - **H25.819 Combined forms of age-related cataract, unspecified eye**
  - **H25.89 Other age-related cataract**
- **H25.9 Unspecified age-related cataract**

H26 Other cataract

Excludes1: *congenital cataract (Q12.0)*

+ **H26.0 Infantile and juvenile cataract**
  + **H26.00 Unspecified infantile and juvenile cataract**
    - **H26.001 Unspecified infantile and juvenile cataract, right eye**
    - **H26.002 Unspecified infantile and juvenile cataract, left eye**
    - **H26.003 Unspecified infantile and juvenile cataract, bilateral**
    - **H26.009 Unspecified infantile and juvenile cataract, unspecified eye**
  + **H26.01 Infantile and juvenile cortical, lamellar, or zonular cataract**
    - **H26.011 Infantile and juvenile cortical, lamellar, or zonular cataract, right eye**
    - **H26.012 Infantile and juvenile cortical, lamellar, or zonular cataract, left eye**
    - **H26.013 Infantile and juvenile cortical, lamellar, or zonular cataract, bilateral**
    - **H26.019 Infantile and juvenile cortical, lamellar, or zonular cataract, unspecified eye**
  + **H26.03 Infantile and juvenile nuclear cataract**
    - **H26.031 Infantile and juvenile nuclear cataract, right eye**
    - **H26.032 Infantile and juvenile nuclear cataract, left eye**
    - **H26.033 Infantile and juvenile nuclear cataract, bilateral**
    - **H26.039 Infantile and juvenile nuclear cataract, unspecified eye**

+, +7th, X + 7th   ● Newborn   ● Pediatric   ● Maternity   ● Adult   ♀ Female   ♂ Male   Manifestation   Unacceptable PDX   HCC   CC   MCC   HAC

+ **H26.04 Anterior subcapsular polar infantile and juvenile cataract**
- H26.041 Anterior subcapsular polar infantile and juvenile cataract, right eye
- H26.042 Anterior subcapsular polar infantile and juvenile cataract, left eye
- H26.043 Anterior subcapsular polar infantile and juvenile cataract, bilateral
- H26.049 Anterior subcapsular polar infantile and juvenile cataract, unspecified eye

+ **H26.05 Posterior subcapsular polar infantile and juvenile cataract**
- H26.051 Posterior subcapsular polar infantile and juvenile cataract, right eye
- H26.052 Posterior subcapsular polar infantile and juvenile cataract, left eye
- H26.053 Posterior subcapsular polar infantile and juvenile cataract, bilateral
- H26.059 Posterior subcapsular polar infantile and juvenile cataract, unspecified eye

+ **H26.06 Combined forms of infantile and juvenile cataract**
- H26.061 Combined forms of infantile and juvenile cataract, right eye
- H26.062 Combined forms of infantile and juvenile cataract, left eye
- H26.063 Combined forms of infantile and juvenile cataract, bilateral
- H26.069 Combined forms of infantile and juvenile cataract, unspecified eye
- **H26.09 Other infantile and juvenile cataract**

+ **H26.1 Traumatic cataract**
    Use additional code (Chapter 20) to identify external cause

+ **H26.10 Unspecified traumatic cataract**
- H26.101 Unspecified traumatic cataract, right eye
- H26.102 Unspecified traumatic cataract, left eye
- H26.103 Unspecified traumatic cataract, bilateral
- H26.109 Unspecified traumatic cataract, unspecified eye

+ **H26.11 Localized traumatic opacities**
- H26.111 Localized traumatic opacities, right eye
- H26.112 Localized traumatic opacities, left eye
- H26.113 Localized traumatic opacities, bilateral
- H26.119 Localized traumatic opacities, unspecified eye

+ **H26.12 Partially resolved traumatic cataract**
- H26.121 Partially resolved traumatic cataract, right eye
- H26.122 Partially resolved traumatic cataract, left eye
- H26.123 Partially resolved traumatic cataract, bilateral
- H26.129 Partially resolved traumatic cataract, unspecified eye

+ **H26.13 Total traumatic cataract**
- H26.131 Total traumatic cataract, right eye
- H26.132 Total traumatic cataract, left eye
- H26.133 Total traumatic cataract, bilateral
- H26.139 Total traumatic cataract, unspecified eye

+ **H26.2 Complicated cataract**

H26.20 Unspecified complicated cataract
    Cataracta complicata NOS

+ **H26.21 Cataract with neovascularization**
    Code also associated condition, such as:
        chronic iridocyclitis (H20.1-)
- H26.211 Cataract with neovascularization, right eye
- H26.212 Cataract with neovascularization, left eye
- H26.213 Cataract with neovascularization, bilateral
- H26.219 Cataract with neovascularization, unspecified eye

+ **H26.22 Cataract secondary to ocular disorders (degenerative) (inflammatory)**
    Code also associated ocular disorder
- H26.221 Cataract secondary to ocular disorders (degenerative) (inflammatory), right eye
- H26.222 Cataract secondary to ocular disorders (degenerative) (inflammatory), left eye
- H26.223 Cataract secondary to ocular disorders (degenerative) (inflammatory), bilateral
- H26.229 Cataract secondary to ocular disorders (degenerative) (inflammatory), unspecified eye

+ **H26.23 Glaucomatous flecks (subcapsular)**
    Code first underlying glaucoma (H40-H42)
- H26.231 Glaucomatous flecks (subcapsular), right eye
- H26.232 Glaucomatous flecks (subcapsular), left eye
- H26.233 Glaucomatous flecks (subcapsular), bilateral
- H26.239 Glaucomatous flecks (subcapsular), unspecified eye

+ **H26.3 Drug-induced cataract**
    Toxic cataract
    Use additional code for adverse effect, if applicable, to identify drug (T36-T50 with fifth or sixth character 5)
- H26.30 Drug-induced cataract, unspecified eye
- H26.31 Drug-induced cataract, right eye
- H26.32 Drug-induced cataract, left eye
- H26.33 Drug-induced cataract, bilateral

+ **H26.4 Secondary cataract**
- H26.40 Unspecified secondary cataract

+ **H26.41 Soemmering's ring**
- H26.411 Soemmering's ring, right eye
- H26.412 Soemmering's ring, left eye
- H26.413 Soemmering's ring, bilateral
- H26.419 Soemmering's ring, unspecified eye

+ **H26.49 Other secondary cataract**
- H26.491 Other secondary cataract, right eye
- H26.492 Other secondary cataract, left eye
    AHA CC: 2Q, 2018, 14
- H26.493 Other secondary cataract, bilateral
- H26.499 Other secondary cataract, unspecified eye

H26.8 Other specified cataract

H26.9 Unspecified cataract

H27 Other disorders of lens

Excludes1: congenital lens malformations (Q12.-)
    mechanical complications of intraocular lens implant (T85.2)
    pseudophakia (Z96.1)

+ **H27.0 Aphakia**
    Acquired absence of lens
    Acquired aphakia
    Aphakia due to trauma
    Excludes1: cataract extraction status (Z98.4-)
        congenital absence of lens (Q12.3)
        congenital aphakia (Q12.3)
- H27.00 Aphakia, unspecified eye
- H27.01 Aphakia, right eye
- H27.02 Aphakia, left eye
- H27.03 Aphakia, bilateral

+ **H27.1 Dislocation of lens**
- H27.10 Unspecified dislocation of lens

+ **H27.11 Subluxation of lens**
- H27.111 Subluxation of lens, right eye
- H27.112 Subluxation of lens, left eye
- H27.113 Subluxation of lens, bilateral
- H27.119 Subluxation of lens, unspecified eye

+ **H27.12 Anterior dislocation of lens**
- H27.121 Anterior dislocation of lens, right eye
- H27.122 Anterior dislocation of lens, left eye
- H27.123 Anterior dislocation of lens, bilateral
- H27.129 Anterior dislocation of lens, unspecified eye

+ **H27.13 Posterior dislocation of lens**
- H27.131 Posterior dislocation of lens, right eye
- H27.132 Posterior dislocation of lens, left eye
- H27.133 Posterior dislocation of lens, bilateral
- H27.139 Posterior dislocation of lens, unspecified eye

H27.8 Other specified disorders of lens

H27.9 Unspecified disorder of lens

H28 Cataract in diseases classified elsewhere

Code first underlying disease, such as:
    hypoparathyroidism (E20.-)
    myotonia (G71.1-)
    myxedema (E03.-)
    protein-calorie malnutrition (E40-E46)
Excludes1: cataract in diabetes mellitus (E08.36, E09.36, E10.36, E11.36, E13.36)
Valid 3-character code, no further characters required

Disorders of choroid and retina (H30-H36)

H30 Chorioretinal inflammation

+ **H30.0 Focal chorioretinal inflammation**
Focal chorioretinitis
Focal choroiditis
Focal retinitis
Focal retinochoroiditis
+ **H30.00 Unspecified focal chorioretinal inflammation**
Focal chorioretinitis NOS
Focal choroiditis NOS
Focal retinitis NOS
Focal retinochoroiditis NOS
H30.001 Unspecified focal chorioretinal inflammation, right eye
H30.002 Unspecified focal chorioretinal inflammation, left eye
H30.003 Unspecified focal chorioretinal inflammation, bilateral
H30.009 Unspecified focal chorioretinal inflammation, unspecified eye
+ **H30.01 Focal chorioretinal inflammation, juxtapapillary**
H30.011 Focal chorioretinal inflammation, juxtapapillary, right eye
H30.012 Focal chorioretinal inflammation, juxtapapillary, left eye
H30.013 Focal chorioretinal inflammation, juxtapapillary, bilateral
H30.019 Focal chorioretinal inflammation, juxtapapillary, unspecified eye
+ **H30.02 Focal chorioretinal inflammation of posterior pole**
H30.021 Focal chorioretinal inflammation of posterior pole, right eye
H30.022 Focal chorioretinal inflammation of posterior pole, left eye
H30.023 Focal chorioretinal inflammation of posterior pole, bilateral
H30.029 Focal chorioretinal inflammation of posterior pole, unspecified eye
+ **H30.03 Focal chorioretinal inflammation, peripheral**
H30.031 Focal chorioretinal inflammation, peripheral, right eye
H30.032 Focal chorioretinal inflammation, peripheral, left eye
H30.033 Focal chorioretinal inflammation, peripheral, bilateral
H30.039 Focal chorioretinal inflammation, peripheral, unspecified eye
+ **H30.04 Focal chorioretinal inflammation, macular or paramacular**
H30.041 Focal chorioretinal inflammation, macular or paramacular, right eye
H30.042 Focal chorioretinal inflammation, macular or paramacular, left eye
H30.043 Focal chorioretinal inflammation, macular or paramacular, bilateral
H30.049 Focal chorioretinal inflammation, macular or paramacular, unspecified eye
+ **H30.1 Disseminated chorioretinal inflammation**
Disseminated chorioretinitis
Disseminated choroiditis
Disseminated retinitis
Disseminated retinochoroiditis
Excludes2: *exudative retinopathy (H35.02-)*
+ **H30.10 Unspecified disseminated chorioretinal inflammation**
Disseminated chorioretinitis NOS
Disseminated choroiditis NOS
Disseminated retinitis NOS
Disseminated retinochoroiditis NOS
CC **H30.101** Unspecified disseminated chorioretinal inflammation, right eye
CC **H30.102** Unspecified disseminated chorioretinal inflammation, left eye
CC **H30.103** Unspecified disseminated chorioretinal inflammation, bilateral
CC **H30.109** Unspecified disseminated chorioretinal inflammation, unspecified eye

+ **H30.11 Disseminated chorioretinal inflammation of posterior pole**
CC **H30.111** Disseminated chorioretinal inflammation of posterior pole, right eye
CC **H30.112** Disseminated chorioretinal inflammation of posterior pole, left eye
CC **H30.113** Disseminated chorioretinal inflammation of posterior pole, bilateral
CC **H30.119** Disseminated chorioretinal inflammation of posterior pole, unspecified eye
+ **H30.12 Disseminated chorioretinal inflammation, peripheral**
CC **H30.121** Disseminated chorioretinal inflammation, peripheral right eye
CC **H30.122** Disseminated chorioretinal inflammation, peripheral, left eye
CC **H30.123** Disseminated chorioretinal inflammation, peripheral, bilateral
CC **H30.129** Disseminated chorioretinal inflammation, peripheral, unspecified eye
+ **H30.13 Disseminated chorioretinal inflammation, generalized**
CC **H30.131** Disseminated chorioretinal inflammation, generalized, right eye
CC **H30.132** Disseminated chorioretinal inflammation, generalized, left eye
CC **H30.133** Disseminated chorioretinal inflammation, generalized, bilateral
CC **H30.139** Disseminated chorioretinal inflammation, generalized, unspecified eye
+ **H30.14 Acute posterior multifocal placoid pigment epitheliopathy**
CC **H30.141** Acute posterior multifocal placoid pigment epitheliopathy, right eye
CC **H30.142** Acute posterior multifocal placoid pigment epitheliopathy, left eye
CC **H30.143** Acute posterior multifocal placoid pigment epitheliopathy, bilateral
CC **H30.149** Acute posterior multifocal placoid pigment epitheliopathy, unspecified eye
+ **H30.2 Posterior cyclitis**
Pars planitis
H30.20 Posterior cyclitis, unspecified eye
H30.21 Posterior cyclitis, right eye
H30.22 Posterior cyclitis, left eye
H30.23 Posterior cyclitis, bilateral
+ **H30.8 Other chorioretinal inflammations**
+ **H30.81 Harada's disease**
H30.811 Harada's disease, right eye
H30.812 Harada's disease, left eye
H30.813 Harada's disease, bilateral
H30.819 Harada's disease, unspecified eye
+ **H30.89 Other chorioretinal inflammations**
CC **H30.891** Other chorioretinal inflammations, right eye
CC **H30.892** Other chorioretinal inflammations, left eye
CC **H30.893** Other chorioretinal inflammations, bilateral
CC **H30.899** Other chorioretinal inflammations, unspecified eye
+ **H30.9 Unspecified chorioretinal inflammation**
Chorioretinitis NOS
Choroiditis NOS
Neuroretinitis NOS
Retinitis NOS
Retinochoroiditis NOS
CC **H30.90** Unspecified chorioretinal inflammation, unspecified eye
CC **H30.91** Unspecified chorioretinal inflammation, right eye
CC **H30.92** Unspecified chorioretinal inflammation, left eye
CC **H30.93** Unspecified chorioretinal inflammation, bilateral

629

+, +7th, X + 7th ● Newborn ● Pediatric ● Maternity ● Adult ♀ Female ♂ Male Manifestation Unacceptable PDX HCC CC MCC HAC

H31 Other disorders of choroid

+ **H31.0 Chorioretinal scars**

Excludes2: *postsurgical chorioretinal scars (H59.81-)*

+ **H31.00 Unspecified chorioretinal scars**

H31.001 Unspecified chorioretinal scars, right eye

H31.002 Unspecified chorioretinal scars, left eye

H31.003 Unspecified chorioretinal scars, bilateral

H31.009 Unspecified chorioretinal scars, unspecified eye

+ **H31.01 Macula scars of posterior pole (postinflammatory) (post-traumatic)**

Excludes1: *postprocedural chorioretinal scar (H59.81-)*

H31.011 Macula scars of posterior pole (postinflammatory) (post-traumatic), right eye

H31.012 Macula scars of posterior pole (postinflammatory) (post-traumatic), left eye

H31.013 Macula scars of posterior pole (postinflammatory) (post-traumatic), bilateral

H31.019 Macula scars of posterior pole (postinflammatory) (post-traumatic), unspecified eye

+ **H31.02 Solar retinopathy**

H31.021 Solar retinopathy, right eye

H31.022 Solar retinopathy, left eye

H31.023 Solar retinopathy, bilateral

H31.029 Solar retinopathy, unspecified eye

+ **H31.09 Other chorioretinal scars**

H31.091 Other chorioretinal scars, right eye

H31.092 Other chorioretinal scars, left eye

H31.093 Other chorioretinal scars, bilateral

H31.099 Other chorioretinal scars, unspecified eye

+ **H31.1 Choroidal degeneration**

Excludes2: *angioid streaks of macula (H35.33)*

+ **H31.10 Unspecified choroidal degeneration**

Choroidal sclerosis NOS

H31.101 Choroidal degeneration, unspecified, right eye

H31.102 Choroidal degeneration, unspecified, left eye

H31.103 Choroidal degeneration, unspecified, bilateral

H31.109 Choroidal degeneration, unspecified, unspecified eye

+ **H31.11 Age-related choroidal atrophy**

• H31.111 Age-related choroidal atrophy, right eye

• H31.112 Age-related choroidal atrophy, left eye

• H31.113 Age-related choroidal atrophy, bilateral

• H31.119 Age-related choroidal atrophy, unspecified eye

+ **H31.12 Diffuse secondary atrophy of choroid**

H31.121 Diffuse secondary atrophy of choroid, right eye

H31.122 Diffuse secondary atrophy of choroid, left eye

H31.123 Diffuse secondary atrophy of choroid, bilateral

H31.129 Diffuse secondary atrophy of choroid, unspecified eye

+ **H31.2 Hereditary choroidal dystrophy**

Excludes2: *hyperornithinemia (E72.4)*
ornithinemia (E72.4)

H31.20 Hereditary choroidal dystrophy, unspecified

H31.21 Choroideremia

H31.22 Choroidal dystrophy (central areolar) (generalized) (peripapillary)

H31.23 Gyrate atrophy, choroid

H31.29 Other hereditary choroidal dystrophy

+ **H31.3 Choroidal hemorrhage and rupture**

+ **H31.30 Unspecified choroidal hemorrhage**

H31.301 Unspecified choroidal hemorrhage, right eye

H31.302 Unspecified choroidal hemorrhage, left eye

H31.303 Unspecified choroidal hemorrhage, bilateral

H31.309 Unspecified choroidal hemorrhage, unspecified eye

+ **H31.31 Expulsive choroidal hemorrhage**

H31.311 Expulsive choroidal hemorrhage, right eye

H31.312 Expulsive choroidal hemorrhage, left eye

H31.313 Expulsive choroidal hemorrhage, bilateral

H31.319 Expulsive choroidal hemorrhage, unspecified eye

+ **H31.32 Choroidal rupture**

CC H31.321 Choroidal rupture, right eye

CC H31.322 Choroidal rupture, left eye

CC H31.323 Choroidal rupture, bilateral

CC H31.329 Choroidal rupture, unspecified eye

+ **H31.4 Choroidal detachment**

+ **H31.40 Unspecified choroidal detachment**

CC H31.401 Unspecified choroidal detachment, right eye

CC H31.402 Unspecified choroidal detachment, left eye

CC H31.403 Unspecified choroidal detachment, bilateral

CC H31.409 Unspecified choroidal detachment, unspecified eye

+ **H31.41 Hemorrhagic choroidal detachment**

CC H31.411 Hemorrhagic choroidal detachment, right eye

CC H31.412 Hemorrhagic choroidal detachment, left eye

CC H31.413 Hemorrhagic choroidal detachment, bilateral

CC H31.419 Hemorrhagic choroidal detachment, unspecified eye

+ **H31.42 Serous choroidal detachment**

CC H31.421 Serous choroidal detachment, right eye

CC H31.422 Serous choroidal detachment, left eye

CC H31.423 Serous choroidal detachment, bilateral

CC H31.429 Serous choroidal detachment, unspecified eye

H31.8 Other specified disorders of choroid

H31.9 Unspecified disorder of choroid

H32 Chorioretinal disorders in diseases classified elsewhere

Code first underlying disease, such as:
congenital toxoplasmosis (P37.1)
histoplasmosis (B39.-)
leprosy (A30.-)

Excludes1: *chorioretinitis (in):*
toxoplasmosis (acquired) (B58.01)
tuberculosis (A18.53)

Valid 3-character code, no further characters required

H33 Retinal detachments and breaks

Excludes1: *detachment of retinal pigment epithelium (H35.72-, H35.73-)*

+ **H33.0 Retinal detachment with retinal break**
Rhegmatogenous retinal detachment
Excludes1: *serous retinal detachment (without retinal break) (H33.2-)*
+ **H33.00 Unspecified retinal detachment with retinal break**
H33.001 Unspecified retinal detachment with retinal break, right eye
H33.002 Unspecified retinal detachment with retinal break, left eye
H33.003 Unspecified retinal detachment with retinal break, bilateral
H33.009 Unspecified retinal detachment with retinal break, unspecified eye
+ **H33.01 Retinal detachment with single break**
H33.011 Retinal detachment with single break, right eye
H33.012 Retinal detachment with single break, left eye
H33.013 Retinal detachment with single break, bilateral
H33.019 Retinal detachment with single break, unspecified eye
+ **H33.02 Retinal detachment with multiple breaks**
H33.021 Retinal detachment with multiple breaks, right eye
H33.022 Retinal detachment with multiple breaks, left eye
H33.023 Retinal detachment with multiple breaks, bilateral
H33.029 Retinal detachment with multiple breaks, unspecified eye
+ **H33.03 Retinal detachment with giant retinal tear**
H33.031 Retinal detachment with giant retinal tear, right eye
H33.032 Retinal detachment with giant retinal tear, left eye
H33.033 Retinal detachment with giant retinal tear, bilateral
H33.039 Retinal detachment with giant retinal tear, unspecified eye
+ **H33.04 Retinal detachment with retinal dialysis**
H33.041 Retinal detachment with retinal dialysis, right eye
H33.042 Retinal detachment with retinal dialysis, left eye
H33.043 Retinal detachment with retinal dialysis, bilateral
H33.049 Retinal detachment with retinal dialysis, unspecified eye
+ **H33.05 Total retinal detachment**
H33.051 Total retinal detachment, right eye
H33.052 Total retinal detachment, left eye
H33.053 Total retinal detachment, bilateral
H33.059 Total retinal detachment, unspecified eye
+ **H33.1 Retinoschisis and retinal cysts**
Excludes1: *congenital retinoschisis (Q14.1)*
microcystoid degeneration of retina (H35.42-)
+ **H33.10 Unspecified retinoschisis**
H33.101 Unspecified retinoschisis, right eye
H33.102 Unspecified retinoschisis, left eye
H33.103 Unspecified retinoschisis, bilateral
H33.109 Unspecified retinoschisis, unspecified eye

+ **H33.11 Cyst of ora serrata**
H33.111 Cyst of ora serrata, right eye
H33.112 Cyst of ora serrata, left eye
H33.113 Cyst of ora serrata, bilateral
H33.119 Cyst of ora serrata, unspecified eye
+ **H33.12 Parasitic cyst of retina**
CC H33.121 Parasitic cyst of retina, right eye
CC H33.122 Parasitic cyst of retina, left eye
CC H33.123 Parasitic cyst of retina, bilateral
CC H33.129 Parasitic cyst of retina, unspecified eye
+ **H33.19 Other retinoschisis and retinal cysts**
Pseudocyst of retina
H33.191 Other retinoschisis and retinal cysts, right eye
H33.192 Other retinoschisis and retinal cysts, left eye
H33.193 Other retinoschisis and retinal cysts, bilateral
H33.199 Other retinoschisis and retinal cysts, unspecified eye
+ **H33.2 Serous retinal detachment**
Retinal detachment NOS
Retinal detachment without retinal break
Excludes1: *central serous chorioretinopathy (H35.71-)*
CC H33.20 Serous retinal detachment, unspecified eye
CC H33.21 Serous retinal detachment, right eye
CC H33.22 Serous retinal detachment, left eye
CC H33.23 Serous retinal detachment, bilateral
+ **H33.3 Retinal breaks without detachment**
Excludes1: *chorioretinal scars after surgery for detachment (H59.81-)*
peripheral retinal degeneration without break (H35.4-)
+ **H33.30 Unspecified retinal break**
H33.301 Unspecified retinal break, right eye
H33.302 Unspecified retinal break, left eye
H33.303 Unspecified retinal break, bilateral
H33.309 Unspecified retinal break, unspecified eye
+ **H33.31 Horseshoe tear of retina without detachment**
Operculum of retina without detachment
H33.311 Horseshoe tear of retina without detachment, right eye
H33.312 Horseshoe tear of retina without detachment, left eye
H33.313 Horseshoe tear of retina without detachment, bilateral
H33.319 Horseshoe tear of retina without detachment, unspecified eye
+ **H33.32 Round hole of retina without detachment**
H33.321 Round hole, right eye
H33.322 Round hole, left eye
H33.323 Round hole, bilateral
H33.329 Round hole, unspecified eye
+ **H33.33 Multiple defects of retina without detachment**
H33.331 Multiple defects of retina without detachment, right eye
H33.332 Multiple defects of retina without detachment, left eye
H33.333 Multiple defects of retina without detachment, bilateral
H33.339 Multiple defects of retina without detachment, unspecified eye
+ **H33.4 Traction detachment of retina**
Proliferative vitreo-retinopathy with retinal detachment
CC H33.40 Traction detachment of retina, unspecified eye
CC H33.41 Traction detachment of retina, right eye
CC H33.42 Traction detachment of retina, left eye
CC H33.43 Traction detachment of retina, bilateral
CC **H33.8 Other retinal detachments**

+, +7th, X + 7th   ● Newborn   ● Pediatric   ● Maternity   ● Adult   ♀ Female   ♂ Male   Manifestation   Unacceptable PDX   HCC   CC   MCC   HAC

H34 Retinal vascular occlusions

Excludes1: amaurosis fugax (G45.3)

+ **H34.0 Transient retinal artery occlusion**
- CC **H34.00** Transient retinal artery occlusion, unspecified eye
- CC **H34.01** Transient retinal artery occlusion, right eye
- CC **H34.02** Transient retinal artery occlusion, left eye
- CC **H34.03** Transient retinal artery occlusion, bilateral

+ **H34.1 Central retinal artery occlusion**
- CC **H34.10** Central retinal artery occlusion, unspecified eye
- CC **H34.11** Central retinal artery occlusion, right eye
- CC **H34.12** Central retinal artery occlusion, left eye
- CC **H34.13** Central retinal artery occlusion, bilateral

+ **H34.2 Other retinal artery occlusions**
- + **H34.21 Partial retinal artery occlusion**
  - Hollenhorst's plaque
  - Retinal microembolism
  - CC **H34.211** Partial retinal artery occlusion, right eye
  - CC **H34.212** Partial retinal artery occlusion, left eye
  - CC **H34.213** Partial retinal artery occlusion, bilateral
  - CC **H34.219** Partial retinal artery occlusion, unspecified eye
- + **H34.23 Retinal artery branch occlusion**
  - CC **H34.231** Retinal artery branch occlusion, right eye
  - CC **H34.232** Retinal artery branch occlusion, left eye
  - CC **H34.233** Retinal artery branch occlusion, bilateral
  - CC **H34.239** Retinal artery branch occlusion, unspecified eye

+ **H34.8 Other retinal vascular occlusions**
  - *AHA CC: 4Q, 2016, 19*
- + **H34.81 Central retinal vein occlusion**

  > One of the following 7th characters is to be assigned to codes in subcategory **H34.81** to designate the severity of the occlusion:
  > 0 with macular edema
  > 1 with retinal neovascularization
  > 2 stable
  >   Old central retinal vein occlusion

  - +7th CC **H34.811** Central retinal vein occlusion, right eye
  - +7th CC **H34.812** Central retinal vein occlusion, left eye
  - +7th CC **H34.813** Central retinal vein occlusion, bilateral
  - +7th CC **H34.819** Central retinal vein occlusion, unspecified eye
- + **H34.82 Venous engorgement**
  - Incipient retinal vein occlusion
  - Partial retinal vein occlusion
  - **H34.821** Venous engorgement, right eye
  - **H34.822** Venous engorgement, left eye
  - **H34.823** Venous engorgement, bilateral
  - **H34.829** Venous engorgement, unspecified eye
- + **H34.83 Tributary (branch) retinal vein occlusion**

  > One of the following 7th characters is to be assigned to codes in subcategory **H34.83** to designate the severity of the occlusion:
  > 0 with macular edema
  > 1 with retinal neovascularization
  > 2 stable
  >   Old central retinal vein occlusion

  - +7th **H34.831** Tributary (branch) retinal vein occlusion, right eye
  - +7th **H34.832** Tributary (branch) retinal vein occlusion, left eye
  - +7th **H34.833** Tributary (branch) retinal vein occlusion, bilateral
  - +7th **H34.839** Tributary (branch) retinal vein occlusion, unspecified eye

- CC **H34.9 Unspecified retinal vascular occlusion**

H35 Other retinal disorders

Excludes2: diabetic retinal disorders (E08.311-E08.359, E09.311-E09.359, E10.311-E10.359, E11.311-E11.359, E13.311-E13.359)

+ **H35.0 Background retinopathy and retinal vascular changes**
  - Review coding guideline C.9.a.5
  - Code also any associated hypertension (I10)
  - **H35.00** Unspecified background retinopathy
  - + **H35.01 Changes in retinal vascular appearance**
    - Retinal vascular sheathing
    - **H35.011** Changes in retinal vascular appearance, right eye
    - **H35.012** Changes in retinal vascular appearance, left eye
    - **H35.013** Changes in retinal vascular appearance, bilateral
    - **H35.019** Changes in retinal vascular appearance, unspecified eye
  - + **H35.02 Exudative retinopathy**
    - Coats retinopathy
    - **H35.021** Exudative retinopathy, right eye
    - **H35.022** Exudative retinopathy, left eye
    - **H35.023** Exudative retinopathy, bilateral
    - **H35.029** Exudative retinopathy, unspecified eye
  - + **H35.03 Hypertensive retinopathy**
    - **H35.031** Hypertensive retinopathy, right eye
    - **H35.032** Hypertensive retinopathy, left eye
    - **H35.033** Hypertensive retinopathy, bilateral
    - **H35.039** Hypertensive retinopathy, unspecified eye
  - + **H35.04 Retinal micro-aneurysms, unspecified**
    - **H35.041** Retinal micro-aneurysms, unspecified, right eye
    - **H35.042** Retinal micro-aneurysms, unspecified, left eye
    - **H35.043** Retinal micro-aneurysms, unspecified, bilateral
    - **H35.049** Retinal micro-aneurysms, unspecified, unspecified eye
  - + **H35.05 Retinal neovascularization, unspecified**
    - **H35.051** Retinal neovascularization, unspecified, right eye
    - **H35.052** Retinal neovascularization, unspecified, left eye
    - **H35.053** Retinal neovascularization, unspecified, bilateral
    - **H35.059** Retinal neovascularization, unspecified, unspecified eye
  - + **H35.06 Retinal vasculitis**
    - Eales disease
    - Retinal perivasculitis
    - **H35.061** Retinal vasculitis, right eye
    - **H35.062** Retinal vasculitis, left eye
    - **H35.063** Retinal vasculitis, bilateral
    - **H35.069** Retinal vasculitis, unspecified eye
  - + **H35.07 Retinal telangiectasis**
    - **H35.071** Retinal telangiectasis, right eye
    - **H35.072** Retinal telangiectasis, left eye
    - **H35.073** Retinal telangiectasis, bilateral
    - **H35.079** Retinal telangiectasis, unspecified eye
  - **H35.09** Other intraretinal microvascular abnormalities
    - Retinal varices

+ **H35.1 Retinopathy of prematurity**
  - + **H35.10 Retinopathy of prematurity, unspecified**
    - Retinopathy of prematurity NOS

+, +7th, X + 7th   ● Newborn   ● Pediatric   ● Maternity   ● Adult   ♀ Female   ♂ Male   Manifestation   Unacceptable PDX   HCC   CC   MCC   HAC

H35.101   **Retinopathy of prematurity, unspecified, right eye**

H35.102   **Retinopathy of prematurity, unspecified, left eye**

H35.103   **Retinopathy of prematurity, unspecified, bilateral**

H35.109   **Retinopathy of prematurity, unspecified, unspecified eye**

+ **H35.11** **Retinopathy of prematurity, stage 0**

H35.111   **Retinopathy of prematurity, stage 0, right eye**

H35.112   **Retinopathy of prematurity, stage 0, left eye**

H35.113   **Retinopathy of prematurity, stage 0, bilateral**

H35.119   **Retinopathy of prematurity, stage 0, unspecified eye**

+ **H35.12** **Retinopathy of prematurity, stage 1**

H35.121   **Retinopathy of prematurity, stage 1, right eye**

H35.122   **Retinopathy of prematurity, stage 1, left eye**

H35.123   **Retinopathy of prematurity, stage 1, bilateral**

H35.129   **Retinopathy of prematurity, stage 1, unspecified eye**

+ **H35.13** **Retinopathy of prematurity, stage 2**

H35.131   **Retinopathy of prematurity, stage 2, right eye**

H35.132   **Retinopathy of prematurity, stage 2, left eye**

H35.133   **Retinopathy of prematurity, stage 2, bilateral**

H35.139   **Retinopathy of prematurity, stage 2, unspecified eye**

+ **H35.14** **Retinopathy of prematurity, stage 3**

H35.141   **Retinopathy of prematurity, stage 3, right eye**

H35.142   **Retinopathy of prematurity, stage 3, left eye**

H35.143   **Retinopathy of prematurity, stage 3, bilateral**

H35.149   **Retinopathy of prematurity, stage 3, unspecified eye**

+ **H35.15** **Retinopathy of prematurity, stage 4**

H35.151   **Retinopathy of prematurity, stage 4, right eye**

H35.152   **Retinopathy of prematurity, stage 4, left eye**

H35.153   **Retinopathy of prematurity, stage 4, bilateral**

H35.159   **Retinopathy of prematurity, stage 4, unspecified eye**

+ **H35.16** **Retinopathy of prematurity, stage 5**

H35.161   **Retinopathy of prematurity, stage 5, right eye**

H35.162   **Retinopathy of prematurity, stage 5, left eye**

H35.163   **Retinopathy of prematurity, stage 5, bilateral**

H35.169   **Retinopathy of prematurity, stage 5, unspecified eye**

+ **H35.17** **Retrolental fibroplasia**

H35.171   **Retrolental fibroplasia, right eye**

H35.172   **Retrolental fibroplasia, left eye**

H35.173   **Retrolental fibroplasia, bilateral**

H35.179   **Retrolental fibroplasia, unspecified eye**

+ **H35.2** **Other non-diabetic proliferative retinopathy**

Proliferative vitreo-retinopathy

Excludes1: *proliferative vitreo-retinopathy with retinal detachment (H33.4-)*

H35.20   **Other non-diabetic proliferative retinopathy, unspecified eye**

H35.21   **Other non-diabetic proliferative retinopathy, right eye**

H35.22   **Other non-diabetic proliferative retinopathy, left eye**

H35.23   **Other non-diabetic proliferative retinopathy, bilateral**

+ **H35.3** **Degeneration of macula and posterior pole**

    AHA CC: 4Q, 2016, 20-21

• **H35.30** **Unspecified macular degeneration**

Age-related macular degeneration

+ **H35.31** **Nonexudative age-related macular degeneration**

Atrophic age-related macular degeneration

Dry age-related macular degeneration

> One of the following 7th characters is to be assigned to codes in subcategory **H35.31** to designate the stage of the disease:
> 0   stage unspecified
> 1   early dry stage
> 2   intermediate dry stage
> 3   advanced atrophic without subfoveal involvement advanced dry stage
> 4   advanced atrophic with sobfoveal involvement

• +7th **H35.311** **Nonexudative age-related macular degeneration, right eye**

    AHA CC: 4Q, 2016, 21

• +7th **H35.312** **Nonexudative age-related macular degeneration, left eye**

    AHA CC: 4Q, 2016, 21

• +7th **H35.313** **Nonexudative age-related macular degeneration, bilateral**

• +7th **H35.319** **Nonexudative age-related macular degeneration, unspecified eye**

+ **H35.32** **Exudative age-related macular degeneration**

Wet age-related macular degeneration

> One of the following 7th characters is to be assigned to codes in subcategory **H35.32** to designate the stage of the disease:
> 0   stage unspecified
> 1   with active choroidal neovascularization
> 2   with inactive choroidal neovascularization
>   with involuted or regressed neovascularization
> 3   with inactive scar

• +7th **H35.321** **Exudative age-related macular degeneration, right eye**

• +7th **H35.322** **Exudative age-related macular degeneration, left eye**

• +7th **H35.323** **Exudative age-related macular degeneration, bilateral**

• +7th **H35.329** **Exudative age-related macular degeneration, unspecified eye**

H35.33 **Angioid streaks of macula**

+ **H35.34** **Macular cyst, hole, or pseudohole**

H35.341   **Macular cyst, hole, or pseudohole, right eye**

H35.342   **Macular cyst, hole, or pseudohole, left eye**

H35.343   **Macular cyst, hole, or pseudohole, bilateral**

H35.349   **Macular cyst, hole, or pseudohole, unspecified eye**

+ **H35.35** **Cystoid macular degeneration**

Excludes1: *cystoid macular edema following cataract surgery (H59.03-)*

H35.351   **Cystoid macular degeneration, right eye**

H35.352   **Cystoid macular degeneration, left eye**

H35.353   **Cystoid macular degeneration, bilateral**

H35.359   **Cystoid macular degeneration, unspecified eye**

+ **H35.36 Drusen (degenerative) of macula**
  - H35.361 Drusen (degenerative) of macula, right eye
  - H35.362 Drusen (degenerative) of macula, left eye
    AHA CC: 4Q, 2016, 21
  - H35.363 Drusen (degenerative) of macula, bilateral
    AHA CC: 4Q, 2016, 21; 1Q, 2017, 51
  - H35.369 Drusen (degenerative) of macula, unspecified eye
+ **H35.37 Puckering of macula**
  - H35.371 Puckering of macula, right eye
  - H35.372 Puckering of macula, left eye
  - H35.373 Puckering of macula, bilateral
  - H35.379 Puckering of macula, unspecified eye
+ **H35.38 Toxic maculopathy**
  Code first poisoning due to drug or toxin, if applicable (T36-T65 with fifth or sixth character 1-4 or 6)

  Use additional code for adverse effect, if applicable, to identify drug (T36-T50 with fifth or sixth character 5)
  - H35.381 Toxic maculopathy, right eye
  - H35.382 Toxic maculopathy, left eye
  - H35.383 Toxic maculopathy, bilateral
  - H35.389 Toxic maculopathy, unspecified eye
+ **H35.4 Peripheral retinal degeneration**
  Excludes1: hereditary retinal degeneration (dystrophy) (H35.5-)
  peripheral retinal degeneration with retinal break (H33.3-)
  - **H35.40 Unspecified peripheral retinal degeneration**
  + **H35.41 Lattice degeneration of retina**
    Palisade degeneration of retina
    - H35.411 Lattice degeneration of retina, right eye
    - H35.412 Lattice degeneration of retina, left eye
    - H35.413 Lattice degeneration of retina, bilateral
    - H35.419 Lattice degeneration of retina, unspecified eye
  + **H35.42 Microcystoid degeneration of retina**
    - H35.421 Microcystoid degeneration of retina, right eye
    - H35.422 Microcystoid degeneration of retina, left eye
    - H35.423 Microcystoid degeneration of retina, bilateral
    - H35.429 Microcystoid degeneration of retina, unspecified eye
  + **H35.43 Paving stone degeneration of retina**
    - H35.431 Paving stone degeneration of retina, right eye
    - H35.432 Paving stone degeneration of retina, left eye
    - H35.433 Paving stone degeneration of retina, bilateral
    - H35.439 Paving stone degeneration of retina, unspecified eye
  + **H35.44 Age-related reticular degeneration of retina**
    - ● H35.441 Age-related reticular degeneration of retina, right eye
    - ● H35.442 Age-related reticular degeneration of retina, left eye
    - ● H35.443 Age-related reticular degeneration of retina, bilateral
    - ● H35.449 Age-related reticular degeneration of retina, unspecified eye
  + **H35.45 Secondary pigmentary degeneration**
    - H35.451 Secondary pigmentary degeneration, right eye
    - H35.452 Secondary pigmentary degeneration, left eye
    - H35.453 Secondary pigmentary degeneration, bilateral
    - H35.459 Secondary pigmentary degeneration, unspecified eye
+ **H35.46 Secondary vitreoretinal degeneration**
  - H35.461 Secondary vitreoretinal degeneration, right eye
  - H35.462 Secondary vitreoretinal degeneration, left eye
  - H35.463 Secondary vitreoretinal degeneration, bilateral
  - H35.469 Secondary vitreoretinal degeneration, unspecified eye
+ **H35.5 Hereditary retinal dystrophy**
  Excludes1: dystrophies primarily involving Bruch's membrane (H31.1-)
  - **H35.50 Unspecified hereditary retinal dystrophy**
  - **H35.51 Vitreoretinal dystrophy**
  - **H35.52 Pigmentary retinal dystrophy**
    Albipunctate retinal dystrophy
    Retinitis pigmentosa
    Tapetoretinal dystrophy
  - **H35.53 Other dystrophies primarily involving the sensory retina**
    Stargardt's disease
  - **H35.54 Dystrophies primarily involving the retinal pigment epithelium**
    Vitelliform retinal dystrophy
+ **H35.6 Retinal hemorrhage**
  - **H35.60 Retinal hemorrhage, unspecified eye**
  - **H35.61 Retinal hemorrhage, right eye**
  - **H35.62 Retinal hemorrhage, left eye**
  - **H35.63 Retinal hemorrhage, bilateral**
+ **H35.7 Separation of retinal layers**
  Excludes1: retinal detachment (serous) (H33.2-)
  rhegmatogenous retinal detachment (H33.0-)
  - CC **H35.70 Unspecified separation of retinal layers**
  + **H35.71 Central serous chorioretinopathy**
    - H35.711 Central serous chorioretinopathy, right eye
    - H35.712 Central serous chorioretinopathy, left eye
    - H35.713 Central serous chorioretinopathy, bilateral
    - H35.719 Central serous chorioretinopathy, unspecified eye
  + **H35.72 Serous detachment of retinal pigment epithelium**
    - CC H35.721 Serous detachment of retinal pigment epithelium, right eye
    - CC H35.722 Serous detachment of retinal pigment epithelium, left eye
    - CC H35.723 Serous detachment of retinal pigment epithelium, bilateral
    - CC H35.729 Serous detachment of retinal pigment epithelium, unspecified eye
  + **H35.73 Hemorrhagic detachment of retinal pigment epithelium**
    - CC H35.731 Hemorrhagic detachment of retinal pigment epithelium, right eye
    - CC H35.732 Hemorrhagic detachment of retinal pigment epithelium, left eye
    - CC H35.733 Hemorrhagic detachment of retinal pigment epithelium, bilateral
    - CC H35.739 Hemorrhagic detachment of retinal pigment epithelium, unspecified eye
+ **H35.8 Other specified retinal disorders**
  Excludes2: retinal hemorrhage (H35.6-)
  - **H35.81 Retinal edema**
    Retinal cotton wool spots
  - CC **H35.82 Retinal ischemia**
  - **H35.89 Other specified retinal disorders**
- **H35.9 Unspecified retinal disorder**

+, +7th, X + 7th   ● Newborn   ● Pediatric   ● Maternity   ● Adult   ♀ Female   ♂ Male   Manifestation   Unacceptable PDX   HCC   CC   MCC   HAC

H36 Retinal disorders in diseases classified elsewhere

Code first underlying disease, such as:
  lipid storage disorders (E75.-)
  sickle-cell disorders (D57.-)
Excludes1: *arteriosclerotic retinopathy (H35.0-)*
           diabetic retinopathy (E08.3-, E09.3-, E10.3-, E11.3-, E13.3-)
Valid 3-character code, no further characters required

Glaucoma (H40-H42)

H40 Glaucoma

Excludes1: *absolute glaucoma (H44.51-)*
           congenital glaucoma (Q15.0)
           traumatic glaucoma due to birth injury (P15.3)
Review coding guideline C.7.a
+ **H40.0 Glaucoma suspect**
  + **H40.00 Preglaucoma, unspecified**
      H40.001 Preglaucoma, unspecified, right eye
      H40.002 Preglaucoma, unspecified, left eye
      H40.003 Preglaucoma, unspecified, bilateral
      H40.009 Preglaucoma, unspecified, unspecified eye
  + **H40.01 Open angle with borderline findings, low risk**
      Open angle, low risk
      H40.011 Open angle with borderline findings, low risk, right eye
      H40.012 Open angle with borderline findings, low risk, left eye
      H40.013 Open angle with borderline findings, low risk, bilateral
      H40.019 Open angle with borderline findings, low risk, unspecified eye
  + **H40.02 Open angle with borderline findings, high risk**
      Open angle, high risk
      H40.021 Open angle with borderline findings, high risk, right eye
      H40.022 Open angle with borderline findings, high risk, left eye
      H40.023 Open angle with borderline findings, high risk, bilateral
      H40.029 Open angle with borderline findings, high risk, unspecified eye
  + **H40.03 Anatomical narrow angle**
      Primary angle closure suspect
      H40.031 Anatomical narrow angle, right eye
      H40.032 Anatomical narrow angle, left eye
      H40.033 Anatomical narrow angle, bilateral
      H40.039 Anatomical narrow angle, unspecified eye
  + **H40.04 Steroid responder**
      H40.041 Steroid responder, right eye
      H40.042 Steroid responder, left eye
      H40.043 Steroid responder, bilateral
      H40.049 Steroid responder, unspecified eye
  + **H40.05 Ocular hypertension**
      H40.051 Ocular hypertension, right eye
      H40.052 Ocular hypertension, left eye
      H40.053 Ocular hypertension, bilateral
      H40.059 Ocular hypertension, unspecified eye
  + **H40.06 Primary angle closure without glaucoma damage**
      H40.061 Primary angle closure without glaucoma damage, right eye
      H40.062 Primary angle closure without glaucoma damage, left eye
      H40.063 Primary angle closure without glaucoma damage, bilateral
      H40.069 Primary angle closure without glaucoma damage, unspecified eye

+ **H40.1 Open-angle glaucoma**
    AHA CC: 4Q, 2016, 22
  X+7th **H40.10 Unspecified open-angle glaucoma**

    One of the following 7th characters is to be assigned to code **H40.10** to designate the stage of glaucoma
    0 stage unspecified
    1 mild stage
    2 moderate stage
    3 severe stage
    4 indeterminate stage

  + **H40.11 Primary open-angle glaucoma**
      Chronic simple glaucoma

    One of the following 7th characters is to be assigned to each code in subcategory **H40.11** to designate the stage of glaucoma
    0 stage unspecified
    1 mild stage
    2 moderate stage
    3 severe stage
    4 indeterminate stage

    +7th **H40.111 Primary open-angle glaucoma, right eye**
        AHA CC: 2Q, 2019, 31
    +7th **H40.112 Primary open-angle glaucoma, left eye**
    +7th **H40.113 Primary open-angle glaucoma, bilateral**
    +7th **H40.119 Primary open-angle glaucoma, unspecified eye**
  + **H40.12 Low-tension glaucoma**

    One of the following 7th characters is to be assigned to each code in subcategory **H40.12** to designate the stage of glaucoma
    0 stage unspecified
    1 mild stage
    2 moderate stage
    3 severe stage
    4 indeterminate stage

    +7th **H40.121 Low-tension glaucoma, right eye**
    +7th **H40.122 Low-tension glaucoma, left eye**
    +7th **H40.123 Low-tension glaucoma, bilateral**
    +7th **H40.129 Low-tension glaucoma, unspecified eye**
  + **H40.13 Pigmentary glaucoma**

    One of the following 7th characters is to be assigned to each code in subcategory **H40.13** to designate the stage of glaucoma
    0 stage unspecified
    1 mild stage
    2 moderate stage
    3 severe stage
    4 indeterminate stage

    +7th **H40.131 Pigmentary glaucoma, right eye**
    +7th **H40.132 Pigmentary glaucoma, left eye**
    +7th **H40.133 Pigmentary glaucoma, bilateral**
    +7th **H40.139 Pigmentary glaucoma, unspecified eye**
  + **H40.14 Capsular glaucoma with pseudoexfoliation of lens**

    One of the following 7th characters is to be assigned to each code in subcategory **H40.14** to designate the stage of glaucoma
    0 stage unspecified
    1 mild stage
    2 moderate stage
    3 severe stage
    4 indeterminate stage

    +7th **H40.141 Capsular glaucoma with pseudoexfoliation of lens, right eye**
    +7th **H40.142 Capsular glaucoma with pseudoexfoliation of lens, left eye**
    +7th **H40.143 Capsular glaucoma with pseudoexfoliation of lens, bilateral**
    +7th **H40.149 Capsular glaucoma with pseudoexfoliation of lens, unspecified eye**

+, +7th, X + 7th   ● Newborn   ● Pediatric   ● Maternity   ● Adult   ♀ Female   ♂ Male   Manifestation   Unacceptable PDX   HCC   CC   MCC   HAC

+ **H40.15** **Residual stage of open-angle glaucoma**
    H40.151 **Residual stage of open-angle glaucoma, right eye**
    H40.152 **Residual stage of open-angle glaucoma, left eye**
    H40.153 **Residual stage of open-angle glaucoma, bilateral**
    H40.159 **Residual stage of open-angle glaucoma, unspecified eye**
+ **H40.2** **Primary angle-closure glaucoma**
    Excludes1: *aqueous misdirection (H40.83-)*
            malignant glaucoma (H40.83-)
X+7th **H40.20** **Unspecified primary angle-closure glaucoma**

> One of the following 7th characters is to be assigned to code **H40.20** to designate the stage of glaucoma
> 0   stage unspecified
> 1   mild stage
> 2   moderate stage
> 3   severe stage
> 4   indeterminate stage

+ **H40.21** **Acute angle-closure glaucoma**
    Acute angle-closure glaucoma attack
    Acute angle-closure glaucoma crisis
CC **H40.211** **Acute angle-closure glaucoma, right eye**
CC **H40.212** **Acute angle-closure glaucoma, left eye**
CC **H40.213** **Acute angle-closure glaucoma, bilateral**
CC **H40.219** **Acute angle-closure glaucoma, unspecified eye**
+ **H40.22** **Chronic angle-closure glaucoma**
    Chronic primary angle closure glaucoma

> One of the following 7th characters is to be assigned to each code in subcategory **H40.22** to designate the stage of glaucoma
> 0   stage unspecified
> 1   mild stage
> 2   moderate stage
> 3   severe stage
> 4   indeterminate stage

+7th **H40.221** **Chronic angle-closure glaucoma, right eye**
+7th **H40.222** **Chronic angle-closure glaucoma, left eye**
+7th **H40.223** **Chronic angle-closure glaucoma, bilateral**
+7th **H40.229** **Chronic angle-closure glaucoma, unspecified eye**
+ **H40.23** **Intermittent angle-closure glaucoma**
    H40.231 **Intermittent angle-closure glaucoma, right eye**
    H40.232 **Intermittent angle-closure glaucoma, left eye**
    H40.233 **Intermittent angle-closure glaucoma, bilateral**
    H40.239 **Intermittent angle-closure glaucoma, unspecified eye**
+ **H40.24** **Residual stage of angle-closure glaucoma**
    H40.241 **Residual stage of angle-closure glaucoma, right eye**
    H40.242 **Residual stage of angle-closure glaucoma, left eye**
    H40.243 **Residual stage of angle-closure glaucoma, bilateral**
    H40.249 **Residual stage of angle-closure glaucoma, unspecified eye**
+ **H40.3** **Glaucoma secondary to eye trauma**
    Code also underlying condition

> One of the following 7th characters is to be assigned to each code in subcategory **H40.3** to designate the stage of glaucoma
> 0   stage unspecified
> 1   mild stage
> 2   moderate stage
> 3   severe stage
> 4   indeterminate stage

X+7th **H40.30** **Glaucoma secondary to eye trauma, unspecified eye**
X+7th **H40.31** **Glaucoma secondary to eye trauma, right eye**
X+7th **H40.32** **Glaucoma secondary to eye trauma, left eye**
X+7th **H40.33** **Glaucoma secondary to eye trauma, bilateral**
+ **H40.4** **Glaucoma secondary to eye inflammation**
    Code also underlying condition

> One of the following 7th characters is to be assigned to each code in subcategory **H40.4** to designate the stage of glaucoma
> 0   stage unspecified
> 1   mild stage
> 2   moderate stage
> 3   severe stage
> 4   indeterminate stage

X+7th **H40.40** **Glaucoma secondary to eye inflammation, unspecified eye**
X+7th **H40.41** **Glaucoma secondary to eye inflammation, right eye**
X+7th **H40.42** **Glaucoma secondary to eye inflammation, left eye**
X+7th **H40.43** **Glaucoma secondary to eye inflammation, bilateral**
+ **H40.5** **Glaucoma secondary to other eye disorders**
    Code also underlying eye disorder

> One of the following 7th characters is to be assigned to each code in subcategory **H40.5** to designate the stage of glaucoma
> 0   stage unspecified
> 1   mild stage
> 2   moderate stage
> 3   severe stage
> 4   indeterminate stage

X+7th **H40.50** **Glaucoma secondary to other eye disorders, unspecified eye**
X+7th **H40.51** **Glaucoma secondary to other eye disorders, right eye**
X+7th **H40.52** **Glaucoma secondary to other eye disorders, left eye**
X+7th **H40.53** **Glaucoma secondary to other eye disorders, bilateral**
+ **H40.6** **Glaucoma secondary to drugs**
    Use additional code for adverse effect, if applicable, to identify drug (T36-T50 with fifth or sixth character 5)

> One of the following 7th characters is to be assigned to each code in subcategory **H40.6** to designate the stage of glaucoma
> 0   stage unspecified
> 1   mild stage
> 2   moderate stage
> 3   severe stage
> 4   indeterminate stage

X+7th **H40.60** **Glaucoma secondary to drugs, unspecified eye**
X+7th **H40.61** **Glaucoma secondary to drugs, right eye**
X+7th **H40.62** **Glaucoma secondary to drugs, left eye**
X+7th **H40.63** **Glaucoma secondary to drugs, bilateral**
+ **H40.8** **Other glaucoma**
  + **H40.81** **Glaucoma with increased episcleral venous pressure**
    H40.811 **Glaucoma with increased episcleral venous pressure, right eye**
    H40.812 **Glaucoma with increased episcleral venous pressure, left eye**
    H40.813 **Glaucoma with increased episcleral venous pressure, bilateral**
    H40.819 **Glaucoma with increased episcleral venous pressure, unspecified eye**
  + **H40.82** **Hypersecretion glaucoma**
    H40.821 **Hypersecretion glaucoma, right eye**
    H40.822 **Hypersecretion glaucoma, left eye**
    H40.823 **Hypersecretion glaucoma, bilateral**
    H40.829 **Hypersecretion glaucoma, unspecified eye**
  + **H40.83** **Aqueous misdirection**
    Malignant glaucoma
    H40.831 **Aqueous misdirection, right eye**
    H40.832 **Aqueous misdirection, left eye**
    H40.833 **Aqueous misdirection, bilateral**
    H40.839 **Aqueous misdirection, unspecified eye**
    H40.89 **Other specified glaucoma**
H40.9 **Unspecified glaucoma**

H42 **Glaucoma in diseases classified elsewhere**

Code first underlying condition, such as:
amyloidosis (E85.-)
aniridia (Q13.1)
glaucoma (in) diabetes mellitus (E08.39, E09.39, E10.39, E11.39, E13.39)
Lowe's syndrome (E72.03)
Reiger's anomaly (Q13.81)
specified metabolic disorder (E70-E88)

Excludes1: *glaucoma (in) onchocerciasis (B73.02)*
glaucoma (in) syphilis (A52.71)
glaucoma (in) tuberculous (A18.59)

Valid 3-character code, no further characters required

Disorders of vitreous body and globe (H43-H44)

H43 **Disorders of vitreous body**

+ **H43.0** **Vitreous prolapse**
  Excludes1: *vitreous syndrome following cataract surgery (H59.0-)*
  traumatic vitreous prolapse (S05.2-)
  H43.00 **Vitreous prolapse, unspecified eye**
  H43.01 **Vitreous prolapse, right eye**
  H43.02 **Vitreous prolapse, left eye**
  H43.03 **Vitreous prolapse, bilateral**

+ **H43.1** **Vitreous hemorrhage**
  H43.10 **Vitreous hemorrhage, unspecified eye**
  H43.11 **Vitreous hemorrhage, right eye**
  H43.12 **Vitreous hemorrhage, left eye**
  H43.13 **Vitreous hemorrhage, bilateral**

+ **H43.2** **Crystalline deposits in vitreous body**
  H43.20 **Crystalline deposits in vitreous body, unspecified eye**
  H43.21 **Crystalline deposits in vitreous body, right eye**
  H43.22 **Crystalline deposits in vitreous body, left eye**
  H43.23 **Crystalline deposits in vitreous body, bilateral**

+ **H43.3** **Other vitreous opacities**
  + **H43.31** **Vitreous membranes and strands**
    H43.311 **Vitreous membranes and strands, right eye**
    H43.312 **Vitreous membranes and strands, left eye**
    H43.313 **Vitreous membranes and strands, bilateral**
    H43.319 **Vitreous membranes and strands, unspecified eye**
  + **H43.39** **Other vitreous opacities**
    Vitreous floaters
    H43.391 **Other vitreous opacities, right eye**
    H43.392 **Other vitreous opacities, left eye**
    H43.393 **Other vitreous opacities, bilateral**
    H43.399 **Other vitreous opacities, unspecified eye**

+ **H43.8** **Other disorders of vitreous body**
  Excludes1: *proliferative vitreo-retinopathy with retinal detachment (H33.4-)*
  Excludes2: *vitreous abscess (H44.02-)*
  + **H43.81** **Vitreous degeneration**
    Vitreous detachment
    H43.811 **Vitreous degeneration, right eye**
    H43.812 **Vitreous degeneration, left eye**
    H43.813 **Vitreous degeneration, bilateral**
    H43.819 **Vitreous degeneration, unspecified eye**
  + **H43.82** **Vitreomacular adhesion**
    Vitreomacular traction
    ● **H43.821** **Vitreomacular adhesion, right eye**
    ● **H43.822** **Vitreomacular adhesion, left eye**
    ● **H43.823** **Vitreomacular adhesion, bilateral**
    ● **H43.829** **Vitreomacular adhesion, unspecified eye**
  H43.89 **Other disorders of vitreous body**
H43.9 **Unspecified disorder of vitreous body**

H44 **Disorders of globe**
Includes: disorders affecting multiple structures of eye
+ **H44.0** **Purulent endophthalmitis**
  Use additional code to identify organism
  Excludes1: *bleb associated endophthalmitis (H59.4-)*
  + **H44.00** **Unspecified purulent endophthalmitis**
    CC **H44.001** **Unspecified purulent endophthalmitis, right eye**
    CC **H44.002** **Unspecified purulent endophthalmitis, left eye**
    CC **H44.003** **Unspecified purulent endophthalmitis, bilateral**
    CC **H44.009** **Unspecified purulent endophthalmitis, unspecified eye**
  + **H44.01** **Panophthalmitis (acute)**
    CC **H44.011** **Panophthalmitis (acute), right eye**
    CC **H44.012** **Panophthalmitis (acute), left eye**
    CC **H44.013** **Panophthalmitis (acute), bilateral**
    CC **H44.019** **Panophthalmitis (acute), unspecified eye**
  + **H44.02** **Vitreous abscess (chronic)**
    CC **H44.021** **Vitreous abscess (chronic), right eye**
    CC **H44.022** **Vitreous abscess (chronic), left eye**
    CC **H44.023** **Vitreous abscess (chronic), bilateral**
    CC **H44.029** **Vitreous abscess (chronic), unspecified eye**

+ **H44.1** **Other endophthalmitis**
  Excludes1: *bleb associated endophthalmitis (H59.4-)*
  Excludes2: *ophthalmia nodosa (H16.2-)*
  + **H44.11** **Panuveitis**
    CC **H44.111** **Panuveitis, right eye**
    CC **H44.112** **Panuveitis, left eye**
    CC **H44.113** **Panuveitis, bilateral**
    CC **H44.119** **Panuveitis, unspecified eye**
  + **H44.12** **Parasitic endophthalmitis, unspecified**
    CC **H44.121** **Parasitic endophthalmitis, unspecified, right eye**
    CC **H44.122** **Parasitic endophthalmitis, unspecified, left eye**
    CC **H44.123** **Parasitic endophthalmitis, unspecified, bilateral**
    CC **H44.129** **Parasitic endophthalmitis, unspecified, unspecified eye**
  + **H44.13** **Sympathetic uveitis**
    CC **H44.131** **Sympathetic uveitis, right eye**
    CC **H44.132** **Sympathetic uveitis, left eye**
    CC **H44.133** **Sympathetic uveitis, bilateral**
    CC **H44.139** **Sympathetic uveitis, unspecified eye**
  CC **H44.19** **Other endophthalmitis**

+ **H44.2** **Degenerative myopia**
  Malignant myopia
  AHA CC: 4Q, 2017, 10-11
  H44.20 **Degenerative myopia, unspecified eye**
  H44.21 **Degenerative myopia, right eye**
  H44.22 **Degenerative myopia, left eye**
  H44.23 **Degenerative myopia, bilateral**
  + **H44.2A** **Degenerative myopia with choroidal neovascularization**
    Use additional code for any associated choroid disorders (H31.-)
    H44.2A1 **Degenerative myopia with choroidal neovascularization, right eye**
    H44.2A2 **Degenerative myopia with choroidal neovascularization, left eye**
    H44.2A3 **Degenerative myopia with choroidal neovascularization, bilateral eye**
    H44.2A9 **Degenerative myopia with choroidal neovascularization, unspecified eye**

637

+ **H44.2B** **Degenerative myopia with macular hole**
    H44.2B1 Degenerative myopia with macular hole, right eye
    H44.2B2 Degenerative myopia with macular hole, left eye
    H44.2B3 Degenerative myopia with macular hole, bilateral eye
    H44.2B9 Degenerative myopia with macular hole, unspecified eye

+ **H44.2C** **Degenerative myopia with retinal detachment**
    Use additional code to identify the retinal detachment (H33.-)
    H44.2C1 Degenerative myopia with retinal detachment, right eye
    H44.2C2 Degenerative myopia with retinal detachment, left eye
    H44.2C3 Degenerative myopia with retinal detachment, bilateral eye
    H44.2C9 Degenerative myopia with retinal detachment, unspecified eye

+ **H44.2D** **Degenerative myopia with foveoschisis**
    H44.2D1 Degenerative myopia with foveoschisis, right eye
    H44.2D2 Degenerative myopia with foveoschisis, left eye
    H44.2D3 Degenerative myopia with foveoschisis, bilateral eye
    H44.2D9 Degenerative myopia with foveoschisis, unspecified eye

+ **H44.2E** **Degenerative myopia with other maculopathy**
    H44.2E1 Degenerative myopia with other maculopathy, right eye
    H44.2E2 Degenerative myopia with other maculopathy, left eye
    H44.2E3 Degenerative myopia with other maculopathy, bilateral eye
    H44.2E9 Degenerative myopia with other maculopathy, unspecified eye

+ **H44.3** **Other and unspecified degenerative disorders of globe**
    H44.30 Unspecified degenerative disorder of globe
+ **H44.31** **Chalcosis**
    H44.311 Chalcosis, right eye
    H44.312 Chalcosis, left eye
    H44.313 Chalcosis, bilateral
    H44.319 Chalcosis, unspecified eye
+ **H44.32** **Siderosis of eye**
    H44.321 Siderosis of eye, right eye
    H44.322 Siderosis of eye, left eye
    H44.323 Siderosis of eye, bilateral
    H44.329 Siderosis of eye, unspecified eye
+ **H44.39** **Other degenerative disorders of globe**
    H44.391 Other degenerative disorders of globe, right eye
    H44.392 Other degenerative disorders of globe, left eye
    H44.393 Other degenerative disorders of globe, bilateral
    H44.399 Other degenerative disorders of globe, unspecified eye

+ **H44.4** **Hypotony of eye**
    H44.40 Unspecified hypotony of eye
+ **H44.41** **Flat anterior chamber hypotony of eye**
    H44.411 Flat anterior chamber hypotony of right eye
    H44.412 Flat anterior chamber hypotony of left eye
    H44.413 Flat anterior chamber hypotony of eye, bilateral
    H44.419 Flat anterior chamber hypotony of unspecified eye
+ **H44.42** **Hypotony of eye due to ocular fistula**
    H44.421 Hypotony of right eye due to ocular fistula
    H44.422 Hypotony of left eye due to ocular fistula
    H44.423 Hypotony of eye due to ocular fistula, bilateral
    H44.429 Hypotony of unspecified eye due to ocular fistula
+ **H44.43** **Hypotony of eye due to other ocular disorders**
    H44.431 Hypotony of eye due to other ocular disorders, right eye
    H44.432 Hypotony of eye due to other ocular disorders, left eye
    H44.433 Hypotony of eye due to other ocular disorders, bilateral
    H44.439 Hypotony of eye due to other ocular disorders, unspecified eye
+ **H44.44** **Primary hypotony of eye**
    H44.441 Primary hypotony of right eye
    H44.442 Primary hypotony of left eye
    H44.443 Primary hypotony of eye, bilateral
    H44.449 Primary hypotony of unspecified eye

+ **H44.5** **Degenerated conditions of globe**
    H44.50 Unspecified degenerated conditions of globe
+ **H44.51** **Absolute glaucoma**
    H44.511 Absolute glaucoma, right eye
    H44.512 Absolute glaucoma, left eye
    H44.513 Absolute glaucoma, bilateral
    H44.519 Absolute glaucoma, unspecified eye
+ **H44.52** **Atrophy of globe**
    Phthisis bulbi
    H44.521 Atrophy of globe, right eye
    H44.522 Atrophy of globe, left eye
    H44.523 Atrophy of globe, bilateral
    H44.529 Atrophy of globe, unspecified eye
+ **H44.53** **Leucocoria**
    H44.531 Leucocoria, right eye
    H44.532 Leucocoria, left eye
    H44.533 Leucocoria, bilateral
    H44.539 Leucocoria, unspecified eye

+ **H44.6** **Retained (old) intraocular foreign body, magnetic**
    Use additional code to identify magnetic foreign body (Z18.11)
    Excludes1: *current intraocular foreign body (S05.-)*
    Excludes2: *retained foreign body in eyelid (H02.81-)*
      retained (old) foreign body following penetrating wound of orbit (H05.5-)
      retained (old) intraocular foreign body, nonmagnetic (H44.7-)
+ **H44.60** **Unspecified retained (old) intraocular foreign body, magnetic**
    H44.601 Unspecified retained (old) intraocular foreign body, magnetic, right eye
    H44.602 Unspecified retained (old) intraocular foreign body, magnetic, left eye
    H44.603 Unspecified retained (old) intraocular foreign body, magnetic, bilateral
    H44.609 Unspecified retained (old) intraocular foreign body, magnetic, unspecified eye

+ **H44.61** Retained (old) magnetic foreign body in anterior chamber

    H44.611 Retained (old) magnetic foreign body in anterior chamber, right eye

    H44.612 Retained (old) magnetic foreign body in anterior chamber, left eye

    H44.613 Retained (old) magnetic foreign body in anterior chamber, bilateral

    H44.619 Retained (old) magnetic foreign body in anterior chamber, unspecified eye

+ **H44.62** Retained (old) magnetic foreign body in iris or ciliary body

    H44.621 Retained (old) magnetic foreign body in iris or ciliary body, right eye

    H44.622 Retained (old) magnetic foreign body in iris or ciliary body, left eye

    H44.623 Retained (old) magnetic foreign body in iris or ciliary body, bilateral

    H44.629 Retained (old) magnetic foreign body in iris or ciliary body, unspecified eye

+ **H44.63** Retained (old) magnetic foreign body in lens

    H44.631 Retained (old) magnetic foreign body in lens, right eye

    H44.632 Retained (old) magnetic foreign body in lens, left eye

    H44.633 Retained (old) magnetic foreign body in lens, bilateral

    H44.639 Retained (old) magnetic foreign body in lens, unspecified eye

+ **H44.64** Retained (old) magnetic foreign body in posterior wall of globe

    H44.641 Retained (old) magnetic foreign body in posterior wall of globe, right eye

    H44.642 Retained (old) magnetic foreign body in posterior wall of globe, left eye

    H44.643 Retained (old) magnetic foreign body in posterior wall of globe, bilateral

    H44.649 Retained (old) magnetic foreign body in posterior wall of globe, unspecified eye

+ **H44.65** Retained (old) magnetic foreign body in vitreous body

    H44.651 Retained (old) magnetic foreign body in vitreous body, right eye

    H44.652 Retained (old) magnetic foreign body in vitreous body, left eye

    H44.653 Retained (old) magnetic foreign body in vitreous body, bilateral

    H44.659 Retained (old) magnetic foreign body in vitreous body, unspecified eye

+ **H44.69** Retained (old) intraocular foreign body, magnetic, in other or multiple sites

    H44.691 Retained (old) intraocular foreign body, magnetic, in other or multiple sites, right eye

    H44.692 Retained (old) intraocular foreign body, magnetic, in other or multiple sites, left eye

    H44.693 Retained (old) intraocular foreign body, magnetic, in other or multiple sites, bilateral

    H44.699 Retained (old) intraocular foreign body, magnetic, in other or multiple sites, unspecified eye

+ **H44.7** **Retained (old) intraocular foreign body, nonmagnetic**

  Use additional code to identify nonmagnetic foreign body (Z18.01-Z18.10, Z18.12, Z18.2-Z18.9)

  Excludes1: *current intraocular foreign body (S05.-)*

  Excludes2: *retained foreign body in eyelid (H02.81-)*
    retained (old) foreign body following penetrating wound of orbit (H05.5-)
    retained (old) intraocular foreign body, magnetic (H44.6-)

+ **H44.70** Unspecified retained (old) intraocular foreign body, nonmagnetic

    H44.701 Unspecified retained (old) intraocular foreign body, nonmagnetic, right eye

    H44.702 Unspecified retained (old) intraocular foreign body, nonmagnetic, left eye

    H44.703 Unspecified retained (old) intraocular foreign body, nonmagnetic, bilateral

    H44.709 Unspecified retained (old) intraocular foreign body, nonmagnetic, unspecified eye

      Retained (old) intraocular foreign body NOS

+ **H44.71** Retained (nonmagnetic) (old) foreign body in anterior chamber

    H44.711 Retained (nonmagnetic) (old) foreign body in anterior chamber, right eye

    H44.712 Retained (nonmagnetic) (old) foreign body in anterior chamber, left eye

    H44.713 Retained (nonmagnetic) (old) foreign body in anterior chamber, bilateral

    H44.719 Retained (nonmagnetic) (old) foreign body in anterior chamber, unspecified eye

+ **H44.72** Retained (nonmagnetic) (old) foreign body in iris or ciliary body

    H44.721 Retained (nonmagnetic) (old) foreign body in iris or ciliary body, right eye

    H44.722 Retained (nonmagnetic) (old) foreign body in iris or ciliary body, left eye

    H44.723 Retained (nonmagnetic) (old) foreign body in iris or ciliary body, bilateral

    H44.729 Retained (nonmagnetic) (old) foreign body in iris or ciliary body, unspecified eye

+ **H44.73** Retained (nonmagnetic) (old) foreign body in lens

    H44.731 Retained (nonmagnetic) (old) foreign body in lens, right eye

    H44.732 Retained (nonmagnetic) (old) foreign body in lens, left eye

    H44.733 Retained (nonmagnetic) (old) foreign body in lens, bilateral

    H44.739 Retained (nonmagnetic) (old) foreign body in lens, unspecified eye

+ **H44.74** Retained (nonmagnetic) (old) foreign body in posterior wall of globe

    H44.741 Retained (nonmagnetic) (old) foreign body in posterior wall of globe, right eye

    H44.742 Retained (nonmagnetic) (old) foreign body in posterior wall of globe, left eye

    H44.743 Retained (nonmagnetic) (old) foreign body in posterior wall of globe, bilateral

    H44.749 Retained (nonmagnetic) (old) foreign body in posterior wall of globe, unspecified eye

+ **H44.75** Retained (nonmagnetic) (old) foreign body in vitreous body

    H44.751 Retained (nonmagnetic) (old) foreign body in vitreous body, right eye

    H44.752 Retained (nonmagnetic) (old) foreign body in vitreous body, left eye

    H44.753 Retained (nonmagnetic) (old) foreign body in vitreous body, bilateral

    H44.759 Retained (nonmagnetic) (old) foreign body in vitreous body, unspecified eye

+ **H44.79** Retained (old) intraocular foreign body, nonmagnetic, in other or multiple sites

    H44.791 Retained (old) intraocular foreign body, nonmagnetic, in other or multiple sites, right eye

639

H44.792 Retained (old) intraocular foreign body, nonmagnetic, in other or multiple sites, left eye

H44.793 Retained (old) intraocular foreign body, nonmagnetic, in other or multiple sites, bilateral

H44.799 Retained (old) intraocular foreign body, nonmagnetic, in other or multiple sites, unspecified eye

+ **H44.8 Other disorders of globe**

+ **H44.81 Hemophthalmos**

H44.811 Hemophthalmos, right eye

H44.812 Hemophthalmos, left eye

H44.813 Hemophthalmos, bilateral

H44.819 Hemophthalmos, unspecified eye

+ **H44.82 Luxation of globe**

H44.821 Luxation of globe, right eye

H44.822 Luxation of globe, left eye

H44.823 Luxation of globe, bilateral

H44.829 Luxation of globe, unspecified eye

H44.89 Other disorders of globe

H44.9 Unspecified disorder of globe

Disorders of optic nerve and visual pathways (H46-H47)

H46 Optic neuritis

Excludes2: *ischemic optic neuropathy (H47.01-)*
neuromyelitis optica [Devic] (G36.0)

+ **H46.0 Optic papillitis**

CC H46.00 Optic papillitis, unspecified eye

CC H46.01 Optic papillitis, right eye

CC H46.02 Optic papillitis, left eye

CC H46.03 Optic papillitis, bilateral

+ **H46.1 Retrobulbar neuritis**

Retrobulbar neuritis NOS

Excludes1: *syphilitic retrobulbar neuritis (A52.15)*

CC H46.10 Retrobulbar neuritis, unspecified eye

CC H46.11 Retrobulbar neuritis, right eye

CC H46.12 Retrobulbar neuritis, left eye

CC H46.13 Retrobulbar neuritis, bilateral

H46.2 Nutritional optic neuropathy

H46.3 Toxic optic neuropathy

Code first (T51-T65) to identify cause

CC **H46.8 Other optic neuritis**

CC **H46.9 Unspecified optic neuritis**

H47 Other disorders of optic [2nd] nerve and visual pathways

+ **H47.0 Disorders of optic nerve, not elsewhere classified**

+ **H47.01 Ischemic optic neuropathy**

H47.011 Ischemic optic neuropathy, right eye

H47.012 Ischemic optic neuropathy, left eye

H47.013 Ischemic optic neuropathy, bilateral

H47.019 Ischemic optic neuropathy, unspecified eye

+ **H47.02 Hemorrhage in optic nerve sheath**

H47.021 Hemorrhage in optic nerve sheath, right eye

H47.022 Hemorrhage in optic nerve sheath, left eye

H47.023 Hemorrhage in optic nerve sheath, bilateral

H47.029 Hemorrhage in optic nerve sheath, unspecified eye

+ **H47.03 Optic nerve hypoplasia**

H47.031 Optic nerve hypoplasia, right eye

H47.032 Optic nerve hypoplasia, left eye

H47.033 Optic nerve hypoplasia, bilateral

H47.039 Optic nerve hypoplasia, unspecified eye

+ **H47.09 Other disorders of optic nerve, not elsewhere classified**

Compression of optic nerve

H47.091 Other disorders of optic nerve, not elsewhere classified, right eye

H47.092 Other disorders of optic nerve, not elsewhere classified, left eye

H47.093 Other disorders of optic nerve, not elsewhere classified, bilateral

H47.099 Other disorders of optic nerve, not elsewhere classified, unspecified eye

+ **H47.1 Papilledema**

CC H47.10 Unspecified papilledema

CC H47.11 Papilledema associated with increased intracranial pressure

H47.12 Papilledema associated with decreased ocular pressure

H47.13 Papilledema associated with retinal disorder

+ **H47.14 Foster-Kennedy syndrome**

H47.141 Foster-Kennedy syndrome, right eye

H47.142 Foster-Kennedy syndrome, left eye

H47.143 Foster-Kennedy syndrome, bilateral

H47.149 Foster-Kennedy syndrome, unspecified eye

+ **H47.2 Optic atrophy**

H47.20 Unspecified optic atrophy

+ **H47.21 Primary optic atrophy**

H47.211 Primary optic atrophy, right eye

H47.212 Primary optic atrophy, left eye

H47.213 Primary optic atrophy, bilateral

H47.219 Primary optic atrophy, unspecified eye

H47.22 Hereditary optic atrophy

Leber's optic atrophy

+ **H47.23 Glaucomatous optic atrophy**

H47.231 Glaucomatous optic atrophy, right eye

H47.232 Glaucomatous optic atrophy, left eye

H47.233 Glaucomatous optic atrophy, bilateral

H47.239 Glaucomatous optic atrophy, unspecified eye

+ **H47.29 Other optic atrophy**

Temporal pallor of optic disc

H47.291 Other optic atrophy, right eye

H47.292 Other optic atrophy, left eye

H47.293 Other optic atrophy, bilateral

H47.299 Other optic atrophy, unspecified eye

+ **H47.3 Other disorders of optic disc**

+ **H47.31 Coloboma of optic disc**

H47.311 Coloboma of optic disc, right eye

H47.312 Coloboma of optic disc, left eye

H47.313 Coloboma of optic disc, bilateral

H47.319 Coloboma of optic disc, unspecified eye

+ **H47.32 Drusen of optic disc**

H47.321 Drusen of optic disc, right eye

H47.322 Drusen of optic disc, left eye

H47.323 Drusen of optic disc, bilateral

H47.329 Drusen of optic disc, unspecified eye

+ **H47.33 Pseudopapilledema of optic disc**

H47.331 Pseudopapilledema of optic disc, right eye

H47.332 Pseudopapilledema of optic disc, left eye

H47.333 Pseudopapilledema of optic disc, bilateral

H47.339 Pseudopapilledema of optic disc, unspecified eye

+ **H47.39 Other disorders of optic disc**

H47.391 Other disorders of optic disc, right eye

H47.392 Other disorders of optic disc, left eye

H47.393 Other disorders of optic disc, bilateral

H47.399 Other disorders of optic disc, unspecified eye

+ **H47.4 Disorders of optic chiasm**

Code also underlying condition

CC H47.41 Disorders of optic chiasm in (due to) inflammatory disorders

CC H47.42 Disorders of optic chiasm in (due to) neoplasm

CC H47.43 Disorders of optic chiasm in (due to) vascular disorders

CC H47.49 Disorders of optic chiasm in (due to) other disorders

+ **H47.5 Disorders of other visual pathways**

Disorders of optic tracts, geniculate nuclei and optic radiations

Code also underlying condition

+ **H47.51 Disorders of visual pathways in (due to) inflammatory disorders**

CC H47.511 Disorders of visual pathways in (due to) inflammatory disorders, right side

CC H47.512 Disorders of visual pathways in (due to) inflammatory disorders, left side

CC H47.519 Disorders of visual pathways in (due to) inflammatory disorders, unspecified side

+, +7th, X + 7th   ● Newborn   ● Pediatric   ● Maternity   ● Adult   ♀ Female   ♂ Male   Manifestation   Unacceptable PDX   HCC   CC   MCC   HAC

+ H47.52 Disorders of visual pathways in (due to) neoplasm
- CC **H47.521** Disorders of visual pathways in (due to) neoplasm, right side
- CC **H47.522** Disorders of visual pathways in (due to) neoplasm, left side
- CC **H47.529** Disorders of visual pathways in (due to) neoplasm, unspecified side

+ H47.53 Disorders of visual pathways in (due to) vascular disorders
- CC **H47.531** Disorders of visual pathways in (due to) vascular disorders, right side
- CC **H47.532** Disorders of visual pathways in (due to) vascular disorders, left side
- CC **H47.539** Disorders of visual pathways in (due to) vascular disorders, unspecified side

+ H47.6 Disorders of visual cortex

Code also underlying condition

Excludes1: injury to visual cortex S04.04-

+ H47.61 Cortical blindness
- **H47.611** Cortical blindness, right side of brain
- **H47.612** Cortical blindness, left side of brain
- **H47.619** Cortical blindness, unspecified side of brain

+ H47.62 Disorders of visual cortex in (due to) inflammatory disorders
- CC **H47.621** Disorders of visual cortex in (due to) inflammatory disorders, right side of brain
- CC **H47.622** Disorders of visual cortex in (due to) inflammatory disorders, left side of brain
- CC **H47.629** Disorders of visual cortex in (due to) inflammatory disorders, unspecified side of brain

+ H47.63 Disorders of visual cortex in (due to) neoplasm
- CC **H47.631** Disorders of visual cortex in (due to) neoplasm, right side of brain
- CC **H47.632** Disorders of visual cortex in (due to) neoplasm, left side of brain
- CC **H47.639** Disorders of visual cortex in (due to) neoplasm, unspecified side of brain

+ H47.64 Disorders of visual cortex in (due to) vascular disorders
- CC **H47.641** Disorders of visual cortex in (due to) vascular disorders, right side of brain
- CC **H47.642** Disorders of visual cortex in (due to) vascular disorders, left side of brain
- CC **H47.649** Disorders of visual cortex in (due to) vascular disorders, unspecified side of brain

H47.9 Unspecified disorder of visual pathways

Disorders of ocular muscles, binocular movement, accommodation and refraction (H49-H52)

Excludes2: nystagmus and other irregular eye movements (H55)

H49 Paralytic strabismus

Excludes2: internal ophthalmoplegia (H52.51-)
internuclear ophthalmoplegia (H51.2-)
progressive supranuclear ophthalmoplegia (G23.1)

+ H49.0 Third [oculomotor] nerve palsy
- **H49.00** Third [oculomotor] nerve palsy, unspecified eye
- **H49.01** Third [oculomotor] nerve palsy, right eye
- **H49.02** Third [oculomotor] nerve palsy, left eye
- **H49.03** Third [oculomotor] nerve palsy, bilateral

+ H49.1 Fourth [trochlear] nerve palsy
- **H49.10** Fourth [trochlear] nerve palsy, unspecified eye
- **H49.11** Fourth [trochlear] nerve palsy, right eye
- **H49.12** Fourth [trochlear] nerve palsy, left eye
- **H49.13** Fourth [trochlear] nerve palsy, bilateral

+ H49.2 Sixth [abducent] nerve palsy
- **H49.20** Sixth [abducent] nerve palsy, unspecified eye
- **H49.21** Sixth [abducent] nerve palsy, right eye
- **H49.22** Sixth [abducent] nerve palsy, left eye
- **H49.23** Sixth [abducent] nerve palsy, bilateral

+ H49.3 Total (external) ophthalmoplegia
- **H49.30** Total (external) ophthalmoplegia, unspecified eye
- **H49.31** Total (external) ophthalmoplegia, right eye
- **H49.32** Total (external) ophthalmoplegia, left eye
- **H49.33** Total (external) ophthalmoplegia, bilateral

+ H49.4 Progressive external ophthalmoplegia

Excludes1: Kearns-Sayre syndrome (H49.81-)
- **H49.40** Progressive external ophthalmoplegia, unspecified eye
- **H49.41** Progressive external ophthalmoplegia, right eye
- **H49.42** Progressive external ophthalmoplegia, left eye
- **H49.43** Progressive external ophthalmoplegia, bilateral

+ H49.8 Other paralytic strabismus

+ H49.81 Kearns-Sayre syndrome

Progressive external ophthalmoplegia with pigmentary retinopathy

Use additional code for other manifestation, such as: heart block (I45.9)
- CC **H49.811** Kearns-Sayre syndrome, right eye
- CC **H49.812** Kearns-Sayre syndrome, left eye
- CC **H49.813** Kearns-Sayre syndrome, bilateral
- CC **H49.819** Kearns-Sayre syndrome, unspecified eye

+ H49.88 Other paralytic strabismus

External ophthalmoplegia NOS
- **H49.881** Other paralytic strabismus, right eye
- **H49.882** Other paralytic strabismus, left eye
- **H49.883** Other paralytic strabismus, bilateral
- **H49.889** Other paralytic strabismus, unspecified eye

H49.9 Unspecified paralytic strabismus

H50 Other strabismus

+ H50.0 Esotropia

Convergent concomitant strabismus

Excludes1: intermittent esotropia (H50.31-, H50.32)
- **H50.00** Unspecified esotropia
- **+ H50.01 Monocular esotropia**
  - **H50.011** Monocular esotropia, right eye
  - **H50.012** Monocular esotropia, left eye
- **+ H50.02 Monocular esotropia with A pattern**
  - **H50.021** Monocular esotropia with A pattern, right eye
  - **H50.022** Monocular esotropia with A pattern, left eye
- **+ H50.03 Monocular esotropia with V pattern**
  - **H50.031** Monocular esotropia with V pattern, right eye
  - **H50.032** Monocular esotropia with V pattern, left eye
- **+ H50.04 Monocular esotropia with other noncomitancies**
  - **H50.041** Monocular esotropia with other noncomitancies, right eye
  - **H50.042** Monocular esotropia with other noncomitancies, left eye
- **H50.05** Alternating esotropia
- **H50.06** Alternating esotropia with A pattern
- **H50.07** Alternating esotropia with V pattern
- **H50.08** Alternating esotropia with other noncomitancies

+ H50.1 Exotropia

Divergent concomitant strabismus

Excludes1: intermittent exotropia (H50.33-, H50.34)
- **H50.10** Unspecified exotropia
- **+ H50.11 Monocular exotropia**
  - **H50.111** Monocular exotropia, right eye
  - **H50.112** Monocular exotropia, left eye
- **+ H50.12 Monocular exotropia with A pattern**
  - **H50.121** Monocular exotropia with A pattern, right eye
  - **H50.122** Monocular exotropia with A pattern, left eye
- **+ H50.13 Monocular exotropia with V pattern**
  - **H50.131** Monocular exotropia with V pattern, right eye
  - **H50.132** Monocular exotropia with V pattern, left eye
- **+ H50.14 Monocular exotropia with other noncomitancies**
  - **H50.141** Monocular exotropia with other noncomitancies, right eye
  - **H50.142** Monocular exotropia with other noncomitancies, left eye
- **H50.15** Alternating exotropia
- **H50.16** Alternating exotropia with A pattern
- **H50.17** Alternating exotropia with V pattern
- **H50.18** Alternating exotropia with other noncomitancies

+, +7th, X + 7th • Newborn • Pediatric • Maternity • Adult ♀ Female ♂ Male Manifestation Unacceptable PDX HCC CC MCC HAC

+ **H50.2** **Vertical strabismus**
Hypertropia
H50.21 Vertical strabismus, right eye
H50.22 Vertical strabismus, left eye
+ **H50.3** **Intermittent heterotropia**
H50.30 Unspecified intermittent heterotropia
+ **H50.31** Intermittent monocular esotropia
H50.311 Intermittent monocular esotropia, right eye
H50.312 Intermittent monocular esotropia, left eye
H50.32 Intermittent alternating esotropia
+ **H50.33** Intermittent monocular exotropia
H50.331 Intermittent monocular exotropia, right eye
H50.332 Intermittent monocular exotropia, left eye
H50.34 Intermittent alternating exotropia
+ **H50.4** **Other and unspecified heterotropia**
H50.40 Unspecified heterotropia
+ **H50.41** Cyclotropia
H50.411 Cyclotropia, right eye
H50.412 Cyclotropia, left eye
H50.42 Monofixation syndrome
H50.43 Accommodative component in esotropia
+ **H50.5** **Heterophoria**
H50.50 Unspecified heterophoria
H50.51 Esophoria
H50.52 Exophoria
H50.53 Vertical heterophoria
H50.54 Cyclophoria
H50.55 Alternating heterophoria
+ **H50.6** **Mechanical strabismus**
H50.60 Mechanical strabismus, unspecified
+ **H50.61** Brown's sheath syndrome
H50.611 Brown's sheath syndrome, right eye
H50.612 Brown's sheath syndrome, left eye
H50.69 Other mechanical strabismus
Strabismus due to adhesions
Traumatic limitation of duction of eye muscle
+ **H50.8** **Other specified strabismus**
+ **H50.81** Duane's syndrome
H50.811 Duane's syndrome, right eye
H50.812 Duane's syndrome, left eye
H50.89 Other specified strabismus
H50.9 **Unspecified strabismus**

H51 **Other disorders of binocular movement**

H51.0 **Palsy (spasm) of conjugate gaze**
+ **H51.1** **Convergence insufficiency and excess**
H51.11 Convergence insufficiency
H51.12 Convergence excess
+ **H51.2** **Internuclear ophthalmoplegia**
H51.20 Internuclear ophthalmoplegia, unspecified eye
H51.21 Internuclear ophthalmoplegia, right eye
H51.22 Internuclear ophthalmoplegia, left eye
H51.23 Internuclear ophthalmoplegia, bilateral
H51.8 **Other specified disorders of binocular movement**
H51.9 **Unspecified disorder of binocular movement**

H52 **Disorders of refraction and accommodation**

+ **H52.0** **Hypermetropia**
H52.00 Hypermetropia, unspecified eye
H52.01 Hypermetropia, right eye
H52.02 Hypermetropia, left eye
H52.03 Hypermetropia, bilateral
+ **H52.1** **Myopia**
Excludes1: *degenerative myopia (H44.2-)*
H52.10 Myopia, unspecified eye
H52.11 Myopia, right eye
H52.12 Myopia, left eye
H52.13 Myopia, bilateral
+ **H52.2** **Astigmatism**
+ **H52.20** Unspecified astigmatism
H52.201 Unspecified astigmatism, right eye
H52.202 Unspecified astigmatism, left eye
H52.203 Unspecified astigmatism, bilateral
H52.209 Unspecified astigmatism, unspecified eye
+ **H52.21** Irregular astigmatism
H52.211 Irregular astigmatism, right eye
H52.212 Irregular astigmatism, left eye
H52.213 Irregular astigmatism, bilateral
H52.219 Irregular astigmatism, unspecified eye

+ **H52.22** Regular astigmatism
H52.221 Regular astigmatism, right eye
H52.222 Regular astigmatism, left eye
H52.223 Regular astigmatism, bilateral
H52.229 Regular astigmatism, unspecified eye
+ **H52.3** **Anisometropia and aniseikonia**
H52.31 Anisometropia
H52.32 Aniseikonia
H52.4 **Presbyopia**
+ **H52.5** **Disorders of accommodation**
+ **H52.51** Internal ophthalmoplegia (complete) (total)
H52.511 Internal ophthalmoplegia (complete) (total), right eye
H52.512 Internal ophthalmoplegia (complete) (total), left eye
H52.513 Internal ophthalmoplegia (complete) (total), bilateral
H52.519 Internal ophthalmoplegia (complete) (total), unspecified eye
+ **H52.52** Paresis of accommodation
H52.521 Paresis of accommodation, right eye
H52.522 Paresis of accommodation, left eye
H52.523 Paresis of accommodation, bilateral
H52.529 Paresis of accommodation, unspecified eye
+ **H52.53** Spasm of accommodation
H52.531 Spasm of accommodation, right eye
H52.532 Spasm of accommodation, left eye
H52.533 Spasm of accommodation, bilateral
H52.539 Spasm of accommodation, unspecified eye
H52.6 **Other disorders of refraction**
H52.7 **Unspecified disorder of refraction**

Visual disturbances and blindness (H53-H54)

H53 **Visual disturbances**

+ **H53.0** **Amblyopia ex anopsia**
Excludes1: *amblyopia due to vitamin A deficiency (E50.5)*
+ **H53.00** Unspecified amblyopia
H53.001 Unspecified amblyopia, right eye
H53.002 Unspecified amblyopia, left eye
H53.003 Unspecified amblyopia, bilateral
H53.009 Unspecified amblyopia, unspecified eye
+ **H53.01** Deprivation amblyopia
H53.011 Deprivation amblyopia, right eye
H53.012 Deprivation amblyopia, left eye
H53.013 Deprivation amblyopia, bilateral
H53.019 Deprivation amblyopia, unspecified eye
+ **H53.02** Refractive amblyopia
H53.021 Refractive amblyopia, right eye
H53.022 Refractive amblyopia, left eye
H53.023 Refractive amblyopia, bilateral
H53.029 Refractive amblyopia, unspecified eye
+ **H53.03** Strabismic amblyopia
Excludes1: *strabismus (H50.-)*
H53.031 Strabismic amblyopia, right eye
H53.032 Strabismic amblyopia, left eye
H53.033 Strabismic amblyopia, bilateral
H53.039 Strabismic amblyopia, unspecified eye
+ **H53.04** Amblyopia suspect
AHA CC: 4Q, 2016, 22-23
H53.041 Amblyopia suspect, right eye
H53.042 Amblyopia suspect, left eye
H53.043 Amblyopia suspect, bilateral
H53.049 Amblyopia suspect, unspecified eye
+ **H53.1** **Subjective visual disturbances**
Excludes1: *subjective visual disturbances due to vitamin A deficiency (E50.5)*
visual hallucinations (R44.1)
H53.10 Unspecified subjective visual disturbances
H53.11 Day blindness
Hemeralopia
+ **H53.12** Transient visual loss
Scintillating scotoma
Excludes1: *amaurosis fugax (G45.3-)*
transient retinal artery occlusion (H34.0-)
CC **H53.121** Transient visual loss, right eye
CC **H53.122** Transient visual loss, left eye
CC **H53.123** Transient visual loss, bilateral
CC **H53.129** Transient visual loss, unspecified eye

+, +7th, X + 7th ● Newborn ● Pediatric ● Maternity ● Adult ♀ Female ♂ Male Manifestation Unacceptable PDX HCC CC MCC HAC

+ **H53.13** **Sudden visual loss**
   CC **H53.131** **Sudden visual loss, right eye**
   CC **H53.132** **Sudden visual loss, left eye**
   CC **H53.133** **Sudden visual loss, bilateral**
   CC **H53.139** **Sudden visual loss, unspecified eye**
+ **H53.14** **Visual discomfort**
   Asthenopia
   Photophobia
   H53.141 **Visual discomfort, right eye**
   H53.142 **Visual discomfort, left eye**
   H53.143 **Visual discomfort, bilateral**
   H53.149 **Visual discomfort, unspecified**
H53.15 **Visual distortions of shape and size**
   Metamorphopsia
H53.16 **Psychophysical visual disturbances**
H53.19 **Other subjective visual disturbances**
   Visual halos

H53.2 **Diplopia**
   Double vision
+ **H53.3** **Other and unspecified disorders of binocular vision**
H53.30 **Unspecified disorder of binocular vision**
H53.31 **Abnormal retinal correspondence**
H53.32 **Fusion with defective stereopsis**
H53.33 **Simultaneous visual perception without fusion**
H53.34 **Suppression of binocular vision**
+ **H53.4** **Visual field defects**
H53.40 **Unspecified visual field defects**
+ **H53.41** **Scotoma involving central area**
   Central scotoma
   H53.411 **Scotoma involving central area, right eye**
   H53.412 **Scotoma involving central area, left eye**
   H53.413 **Scotoma involving central area, bilateral**
   H53.419 **Scotoma involving central area, unspecified eye**
+ **H53.42** **Scotoma of blind spot area**
   Enlarged blind spot
   H53.421 **Scotoma of blind spot area, right eye**
   H53.422 **Scotoma of blind spot area, left eye**
   H53.423 **Scotoma of blind spot area, bilateral**
   H53.429 **Scotoma of blind spot area, unspecified eye**
+ **H53.43** **Sector or arcuate defects**
   Arcuate scotoma
   Bjerrum scotoma
   H53.431 **Sector or arcuate defects, right eye**
   H53.432 **Sector or arcuate defects, left eye**
   H53.433 **Sector or arcuate defects, bilateral**
   H53.439 **Sector or arcuate defects, unspecified eye**
+ **H53.45** **Other localized visual field defect**
   Peripheral visual field defect
   Ring scotoma NOS
   Scotoma NOS
   H53.451 **Other localized visual field defect, right eye**
   H53.452 **Other localized visual field defect, left eye**
   H53.453 **Other localized visual field defect, bilateral**
   H53.459 **Other localized visual field defect, unspecified eye**
+ **H53.46** **Homonymous bilateral field defects**
   Homonymous hemianopsia
   Quadrant anopia
   Quadrant anopsia
   H53.461 **Homonymous bilateral field defects, right side**
   H53.462 **Homonymous bilateral field defects, left side**
   H53.469 **Homonymous bilateral field defects, unspecified side**
     Homonymous bilateral field defects NOS
H53.47 **Heteronymous bilateral field defects**
   Heteronymous hemianop(s)ia
+ **H53.48** **Generalized contraction of visual field**
   H53.481 **Generalized contraction of visual field, right eye**
   H53.482 **Generalized contraction of visual field, left eye**

   H53.483 **Generalized contraction of visual field, bilateral**
   H53.489 **Generalized contraction of visual field, unspecified eye**
+ **H53.5** **Color vision deficiencies**
   Color blindness
   Excludes2: day blindness (H53.11)
H53.50 **Unspecified color vision deficiencies**
   Color blindness NOS
H53.51 **Achromatopsia**
H53.52 **Acquired color vision deficiency**
H53.53 **Deuteranomaly**
   Deuteranopia
H53.54 **Protanomaly**
   Protanopia
H53.55 **Tritanomaly**
   Tritanopia
H53.59 **Other color vision deficiencies**
+ **H53.6** **Night blindness**
   Excludes1: night blindness due to vitamin A deficiency (E50.5)
H53.60 **Unspecified night blindness**
H53.61 **Abnormal dark adaptation curve**
H53.62 **Acquired night blindness**
H53.63 **Congenital night blindness**
H53.69 **Other night blindness**
+ **H53.7** **Vision sensitivity deficiencies**
H53.71 **Glare sensitivity**
H53.72 **Impaired contrast sensitivity**
H53.8 **Other visual disturbances**
H53.9 **Unspecified visual disturbance**

H54 **Blindness and low vision**
   NOTE For definition of visual impairment categories see table below
   Code first any associated underlying cause of the blindness
   Excludes1: amaurosis fugax (G45.3)
   AHA CC: 4Q, 2017, 11-12
+ **H54.0** **Blindness, both eyes**
   Visual impairment categories 3, 4, 5 in both eyes.
   H54.0X **Blindness, both eyes, different category levels**
    + **H54.0X3** **Blindness right eye, category 3**
      H54.0X33 **Blindness right eye category 3, blindness left eye category 3**
      H54.0X34 **Blindness right eye category 3, blindness left eye category 4**
      H54.0X35 **Blindness right eye category 3, blindness left eye category 5**
    + **H54.0X4** **Blindness right eye, category 4**
      H54.0X43 **Blindness right eye category 4, blindness left eye category 3**
      H54.0X44 **Blindness right eye category 4, blindness left eye category 4**
      H54.0X45 **Blindness right eye category 4, blindness left eye category 5**
    + **H54.0X5** **Blindness right eye, category 5**
      H54.0X53 **Blindness right eye category 5, blindness left eye category 3**
      H54.0X54 **Blindness right eye category 5, blindness left eye category 4**
      H54.0X55 **Blindness right eye category 5, blindness left eye category 5**
+ **H54.1** **Blindness, one eye, low vision other eye**
   Visual impairment categories 3, 4, 5 in one eye, with categories 1 or 2 in the other eye.
   H54.10 **Blindness, one eye, low vision other eye, unspecified eyes**
   + **H54.11** **Blindness, right eye, low vision left eye**
    + **H54.113** **Blindness right eye category 3, low vision left eye**
      H54.1131 **Blindness right eye category 3, low vision left eye category 1**
      H54.1132 **Blindness right eye category 3, low vision left eye category 2**
    + **H54.114** **Blindness right eye category 4, low vision left eye**
      H54.1141 **Blindness right eye category 4, low vision left eye category 1**
      H54.1142 **Blindness right eye category 4, low vision left eye category 2**

+ **H54.115 Blindness right eye category 5, low vision left eye**
- **H54.1151 Blindness right eye category 5, low vision left eye category 1**
- **H54.1152 Blindness right eye category 5, low vision left eye category 2**

+ **H54.12 Blindness, left eye, low vision right eye**
- + **H54.121 Low vision right eye category 1, blindness left eye**
  - **H54.1213 Low vision right eye category 1, blindness left eye category 3**
  - **H54.1214 Low vision right eye category 1, blindness left eye category 4**
  - **H54.1215 Low vision right eye category 1, blindness left eye category 5**
- + **H54.122 Low vision right eye category 2, blindness left eye**
  - **H54.1223 Low vision right eye category 2, blindness left eye category 3**
  - **H54.1224 Low vision right eye category 2, blindness left eye category 4**
  - **H54.1225 Low vision right eye category 2, blindness left eye category 5**

+ **H54.2 Low vision, both eyes**
Visual impairment categories 1 or 2 in both eyes.
- + **H54.2X Low vision, both eyes, different category levels**
  - + **H54.2X1 Low vision, right eye, category 1**
    - **H54.2X11 Low vision, right eye, category 1, low vision left eye category 1**
    - **H54.2X12 Low vision, right eye, category 1, low vision left eye category 2**
  - + **H54.2X2 Low vision, right eye, category 2**
    - **H54.2X21 Low vision, right eye, category 2, low vision left eye category 1**
    - **H54.2X22 Low vision, right eye, category 2, low vision left eye category 2**

H54.3 Unqualified visual loss, both eyes
Visual impairment category 9 in both eyes.
Review coding guideline C.7.b

+ **H54.4 Blindness, one eye**
Visual impairment categories 3, 4, 5 in one eye [normal vision in other eye]
- **H54.40 Blindness, one eye, unspecified eye**
- + **H54.41 Blindness, right eye, normal vision left eye**
  - + **H54.413 Blindness, right eye, category 3**
    - **H54.413A Blindness right eye category 3, normal vision left eye**
  - + **H54.414 Blindness, right eye, category 4**
    - **H54.414A Blindness right eye category 4, normal vision left eye**
  - + **H54.415 Blindness, right eye, category 5**
    - **H54.415A Blindness right eye category 5, normal vision left eye**
- + **H54.42 Blindness, left eye, normal vision right eye**
  - + **H54.42A Blindness, left eye, category 3-5**
    - **H54.42A3 Blindness left eye category 3, normal vision right eye**
    - **H54.42A4 Blindness left eye category 4, normal vision right eye**
    - **H54.42A5 Blindness left eye category 5, normal vision right eye**

+ **H54.5 Low vision, one eye**
Visual impairment categories 1 or 2 in one eye [normal vision in other eye].

H54.50 Low vision, one eye, unspecified eye
+ **H54.51 Low vision, right eye, normal vision left eye**
- + **H54.511 Low vision, right eye, category 1-2**
  - **H54.511A Low vision right eye category 1, normal vision left eye**
  - **H54.512A Low vision right eye category 2, normal vision left eye**
+ **H54.52 Low vision, left eye, normal vision right eye**
- + **H54.52A Low vision, left eye, category 1-2**
  - **H54.52A1 Low vision left eye category 1, normal vision right eye**
  - **H54.52A2 Low vision left eye category 2, normal vision right eye**

+ **H54.6 Unqualified visual loss, one eye**
Visual impairment category 9 in one eye [normal vision in other eye].
Review coding guideline C.7.b
- **H54.60 Unqualified visual loss, one eye, unspecified**
- **H54.61 Unqualified visual loss, right eye, normal vision left eye**
- **H54.62 Unqualified visual loss, left eye, normal vision right eye**

H54.7 Unspecified visual loss
Visual impairment category 9 NOS
Review coding guideline C.7.b

H54.8 Legal blindness, as defined in USA
Blindness NOS according to USA definition
Excludes1: *legal blindness with specification of impairment level (H54.0-H54.7)*

NOTE The table below gives a classification of severity of visual impairment recommended by a WHO Study Group on the Prevention of Blindness, Geneva, 6-10 November 1972.
The term 'low vision' in category H54 comprises categories 1 and 2 of the table, the term 'blindness' categories 3, 4 and 5, and the term 'unqualified visual loss' category 9.
If the extent of the visual field is taken into account, patients with a field no greater than 10 but greater than 5 around central fixation should be placed in category 3 and patients with a field no greater than 5 around central fixation should be placed in category 4, even if the central acuity is not impaired.

Category of visual impairment	Visual acuity with best possible correction	
	Maximum less than:	**Minimum equal to or better than:**
	6/18	6/60
3/10(0.3)	1/10(0.1)	
20/70	20/200	
	6/60	3/60
1/10(0.1)	1/20(0.05)	
20/200	20/400	
	3/60	1/60(finger counting at one meter)
1/20(0.05)	1/50(0.02)	
20/400	5/300(20/1200)	
	1/60(finger counting at one meter)	Light perception
1/50(0.02)		
5/300		
	No light perception	
	Undetermined or unspecified	

Note: Document 508 compliance requires all cells in the above table to be filled.

Other disorders of eye and adnexa (H55-H57)

H55 Nystagmus and other irregular eye movements

+ **H55.0 Nystagmus**
  - H55.00 Unspecified nystagmus
  - H55.01 Congenital nystagmus
  - H55.02 Latent nystagmus
  - H55.03 Visual deprivation nystagmus
  - H55.04 Dissociated nystagmus
  - H55.09 Other forms of nystagmus
+ **H55.8 Other irregular eye movements**
  - H55.81 Deficient saccadic eye movements
  - H55.82 Deficient smooth pursuit eye movements
  - H55.89 Other irregular eye movements

H57 Other disorders of eye and adnexa

+ **H57.0 Anomalies of pupillary function**
  - H57.00 Unspecified anomaly of pupillary function
  - H57.01 Argyll Robertson pupil, atypical
      - **Excludes1:** *syphilitic Argyll Robertson pupil (A52.19)*
  - H57.02 Anisocoria
  - H57.03 Miosis
  - H57.04 Mydriasis
  + **H57.05 Tonic pupil**
      - H57.051 Tonic pupil, right eye
      - H57.052 Tonic pupil, left eye
      - H57.053 Tonic pupil, bilateral
      - H57.059 Tonic pupil, unspecified eye
  - H57.09 Other anomalies of pupillary function
+ **H57.1 Ocular pain**
  - H57.10 Ocular pain, unspecified eye
  - H57.11 Ocular pain, right eyew
  - H57.12 Ocular pain, left eye
  - H57.13 Ocular pain, bilateral
+ **H57.8 Other specified disorders of eye and adnexa**
    AHA CC: 4Q, 2018, 15-16
  + **H57.81 Brow ptosis**
      - H57.811 Brow ptosis, right
      - H57.812 Brow ptosis, left
      - H57.813 Brow ptosis, bilateral
      - H57.819 Brow ptosis, unspecified
  - H57.89 Other specified disorders of eye and adnexa
- **H57.9 Unspecified disorder of eye and adnexa**

Intraoperative and postprocedural complications and disorders of eye and adnexa, not elsewhere classified (H59)

H59 Intraoperative and postprocedural complications and disorders of eye and adnexa, not elsewhere classified

Excludes1: *mechanical complication of intraocular lens (T85.2)*
mechanical complication of other ocular prosthetic devices, implants and grafts (T85.3)
pseudophakia (Z96.1)
secondary cataracts (H26.4-)

+ **H59.0 Disorders of the eye following cataract surgery**
  + **H59.01 Keratopathy (bullous aphakic) following cataract surgery**
      - Vitreal corneal syndrome
      - Vitreous (touch) syndrome
      - CC H59.011 Keratopathy (bullous aphakic) following cataract surgery, right eye
      - CC H59.012 Keratopathy (bullous aphakic) following cataract surgery, left eye
      - CC H59.013 Keratopathy (bullous aphakic) following cataract surgery, bilateral
      - CC H59.019 Keratopathy (bullous aphakic) following cataract surgery, unspecified eye
  + **H59.02 Cataract (lens) fragments in eye following cataract surgery**
      - H59.021 Cataract (lens) fragments in eye following cataract surgery, right eye
      - H59.022 Cataract (lens) fragments in eye following cataract surgery, left eye
      - H59.023 Cataract (lens) fragments in eye following cataract surgery, bilateral
      - H59.029 Cataract (lens) fragments in eye following cataract surgery, unspecified eye
  + **H59.03 Cystoid macular edema following cataract surgery**
      - CC H59.031 Cystoid macular edema following cataract surgery, right eye
      - CC H59.032 Cystoid macular edema following cataract surgery, left eye
      - CC H59.033 Cystoid macular edema following cataract surgery, bilateral
      - CC H59.039 Cystoid macular edema following cataract surgery, unspecified eye
  + **H59.09 Other disorders of the eye following cataract surgery**
      - CC H59.091 Other disorders of the right eye following cataract surgery
      - CC H59.092 Other disorders of the left eye following cataract surgery
      - CC H59.093 Other disorders of the eye following cataract surgery, bilateral
      - CC H59.099 Other disorders of unspecified eye following cataract surgery
+ **H59.1 Intraoperative hemorrhage and hematoma of eye and adnexa complicating a procedure**
    Excludes1: *intraoperative hemorrhage and hematoma of eye and adnexa due to accidental puncture or laceration during a procedure (H59.2-)*
  + **H59.11 Intraoperative hemorrhage and hematoma of eye and adnexa complicating an ophthalmic procedure**
      - CC H59.111 Intraoperative hemorrhage and hematoma of right eye and adnexa complicating an ophthalmic procedure
      - CC H59.112 Intraoperative hemorrhage and hematoma of left eye and adnexa complicating an ophthalmic procedure
      - CC H59.113 Intraoperative hemorrhage and hematoma of eye and adnexa complicating an ophthalmic procedure, bilateral
      - CC H59.119 Intraoperative hemorrhage and hematoma of unspecified eye and adnexa complicating an ophthalmic procedure
  + **H59.12 Intraoperative hemorrhage and hematoma of eye and adnexa complicating other procedure**
      - CC H59.121 Intraoperative hemorrhage and hematoma of right eye and adnexa complicating other procedure
      - CC H59.122 Intraoperative hemorrhage and hematoma of left eye and adnexa complicating other procedure
      - CC H59.123 Intraoperative hemorrhage and hematoma of eye and adnexa complicating other procedure, bilateral
      - CC H59.129 Intraoperative hemorrhage and hematoma of unspecified eye and adnexa complicating other procedure
+ **H59.2 Accidental puncture and laceration of eye and adnexa during a procedure**
  + **H59.21 Accidental puncture and laceration of eye and adnexa during an ophthalmic procedure**
      - CC H59.211 Accidental puncture and laceration of right eye and adnexa during an ophthalmic procedure
      - CC H59.212 Accidental puncture and laceration of left eye and adnexa during an ophthalmic procedure
      - CC H59.213 Accidental puncture and laceration of eye and adnexa during an ophthalmic procedure, bilateral
      - CC H59.219 Accidental puncture and laceration of unspecified eye and adnexa during an ophthalmic procedure

+ **H59.22** **Accidental puncture and laceration of eye and adnexa during other procedure**
  - CC **H59.221** Accidental puncture and laceration of right eye and adnexa during other procedure
  - CC **H59.222** Accidental puncture and laceration of left eye and adnexa during other procedure
  - CC **H59.223** Accidental puncture and laceration of eye and adnexa during other procedure, bilateral
  - CC **H59.229** Accidental puncture and laceration of unspecified eye and adnexa during other procedure

+ **H59.3** **Postprocedural hemorrhage, hematoma and seroma of eye and adnexa following a procedure**
  AHA CC: 4Q, 2016, 9-10

  + **H59.31** **Postprocedural hemorrhage of eye and adnexa following an ophthalmic procedure**
    - CC **H59.311** Postprocedural hemorrhage of right eye and adnexa following an ophthalmic procedure
    - CC **H59.312** Postprocedural hemorrhage of left eye and adnexa following an ophthalmic procedure
    - CC **H59.313** Postprocedural hemorrhage of eye and adnexa following an ophthalmic procedure, bilateral
    - CC **H59.319** Postprocedural hemorrhage of unspecified eye and adnexa following an ophthalmic procedure

  + **H59.32** **Postprocedural hemorrhage of eye and adnexa following other procedure**
    - CC **H59.321** Postprocedural hemorrhage of right eye and adnexa following other procedure
    - CC **H59.322** Postprocedural hemorrhage of left eye and adnexa following other procedure
    - CC **H59.323** Postprocedural hemorrhage of eye and adnexa following other procedure, bilateral
    - CC **H59.329** Postprocedural hemorrhage of unspecified eye and adnexa following other procedure

  + **H59.33** **Postprocedural hematoma of eye and adnexa following an ophthalmic procedure**
    - CC **H59.331** Postprocedural hematoma of right eye and adnexa following an ophthalmic procedure
    - CC **H59.332** Postprocedural hematoma of left eye and adnexa following an ophthalmic procedure
    - CC **H59.333** Postprocedural hematoma of eye and adnexa following an ophthalmic procedure, bilateral
    - CC **H59.339** Postprocedural hematoma of unspecified eye and adnexa following an ophthalmic procedure

  + **H59.34** **Postprocedural hematoma of eye and adnexa following other procedure**
    - CC **H59.341** Postprocedural hematoma of right eye and adnexa following other procedure
    - CC **H59.342** Postprocedural hematoma of left eye and adnexa following other procedure

- CC **H59.343** Postprocedural hematoma of eye and adnexa following other procedure, bilateral
- CC **H59.349** Postprocedural hematoma of unspecified eye and adnexa following other procedure

  + **H59.35** **Postprocedural seroma of eye and adnexa following an ophthalmic procedure**
    - CC **H59.351** Postprocedural seroma of right eye and adnexa following an ophthalmic procedure
    - CC **H59.352** Postprocedural seroma of left eye and adnexa following an ophthalmic procedure
    - CC **H59.353** Postprocedural seroma of eye and adnexa following an ophthalmic procedure, bilateral
    - CC **H59.359** Postprocedural seroma of unspecified eye and adnexa following an ophthalmic procedure

  + **H59.36** **Postprocedural seroma of eye and adnexa following other procedure**
    - CC **H59.361** Postprocedural seroma of right eye and adnexa following other procedure
    - CC **H59.362** Postprocedural seroma of left eye and adnexa following other procedure
    - CC **H59.363** Postprocedural seroma of eye and adnexa following other procedure, bilateral
    - CC **H59.369** Postprocedural seroma of unspecified eye and adnexa following other procedure

+ **H59.4** **Inflammation (infection) of postprocedural bleb**
  Postprocedural blebitis
  Excludes1: *filtering (vitreous) bleb after glaucoma surgery status (Z98.83)*

  - **H59.40** Inflammation (infection) of postprocedural bleb, unspecified
  - **H59.41** Inflammation (infection) of postprocedural bleb, stage 1
  - **H59.42** Inflammation (infection) of postprocedural bleb, stage 2
  - **H59.43** Inflammation (infection) of postprocedural bleb, stage 3
    Bleb endophthalmitis

+ **H59.8** **Other intraoperative and postprocedural complications and disorders of eye and adnexa, not elsewhere classified**

  + **H59.81** **Chorioretinal scars after surgery for detachment**
    - CC **H59.811** Chorioretinal scars after surgery for detachment, right eye
    - CC **H59.812** Chorioretinal scars after surgery for detachment, left eye
    - CC **H59.813** Chorioretinal scars after surgery for detachment, bilateral
    - CC **H59.819** Chorioretinal scars after surgery for detachment, unspecified eye

  - CC **H59.88** Other intraoperative complications of eye and adnexa, not elsewhere classified
  - CC **H59.89** Other postprocedural complications and disorders of eye and adnexa, not elsewhere classified
    One of the following 7th characters is to be assigned to code H40.10 to designate the stage of glaucoma

Chapter 8: Diseases of the Ear and Mastoid Process (H60-H95)

NOTE Use an external cause code following the code for the ear condition, if applicable, to identify the cause of the ear condition

Excludes2: *certain conditions originating in the perinatal period (P04-P96)*
certain infectious and parasitic diseases (A00-B99)
complications of pregnancy, childbirth and the puerperium (O00-O9A)
congenital malformations, deformations and chromosomal abnormalities (Q00-Q99)
endocrine, nutritional and metabolic diseases (E00-E88)
injury, poisoning and certain other consequences of external causes (S00-T88)
neoplasms (C00-D49)
symptoms, signs and abnormal clinical and laboratory findings, not elsewhere classified (R00-R94)

This chapter contains the following category blocks:
H60-H62   Diseases of external ear
H65-H75   Diseases of middle ear and mastoid
H80-H83   Diseases of inner ear
H90-H94   Other disorders of ear
H95   Intraoperative and postprocedural complications and disorders of ear and mastoid process, not elsewhere classified

C. Chapter-Specific Coding Guidelines

In addition to general coding guidelines, there are guidelines for specific diagnoses and/or conditions in the classification. Unless otherwise indicated, these guidelines apply to all health care settings. Please refer to Section II for guidelines on the selection of principal diagnosis.

8. Chapter 8: Diseases of the Ear and Mastoid Process (H60-H95)

Reserved for future guideline expansion

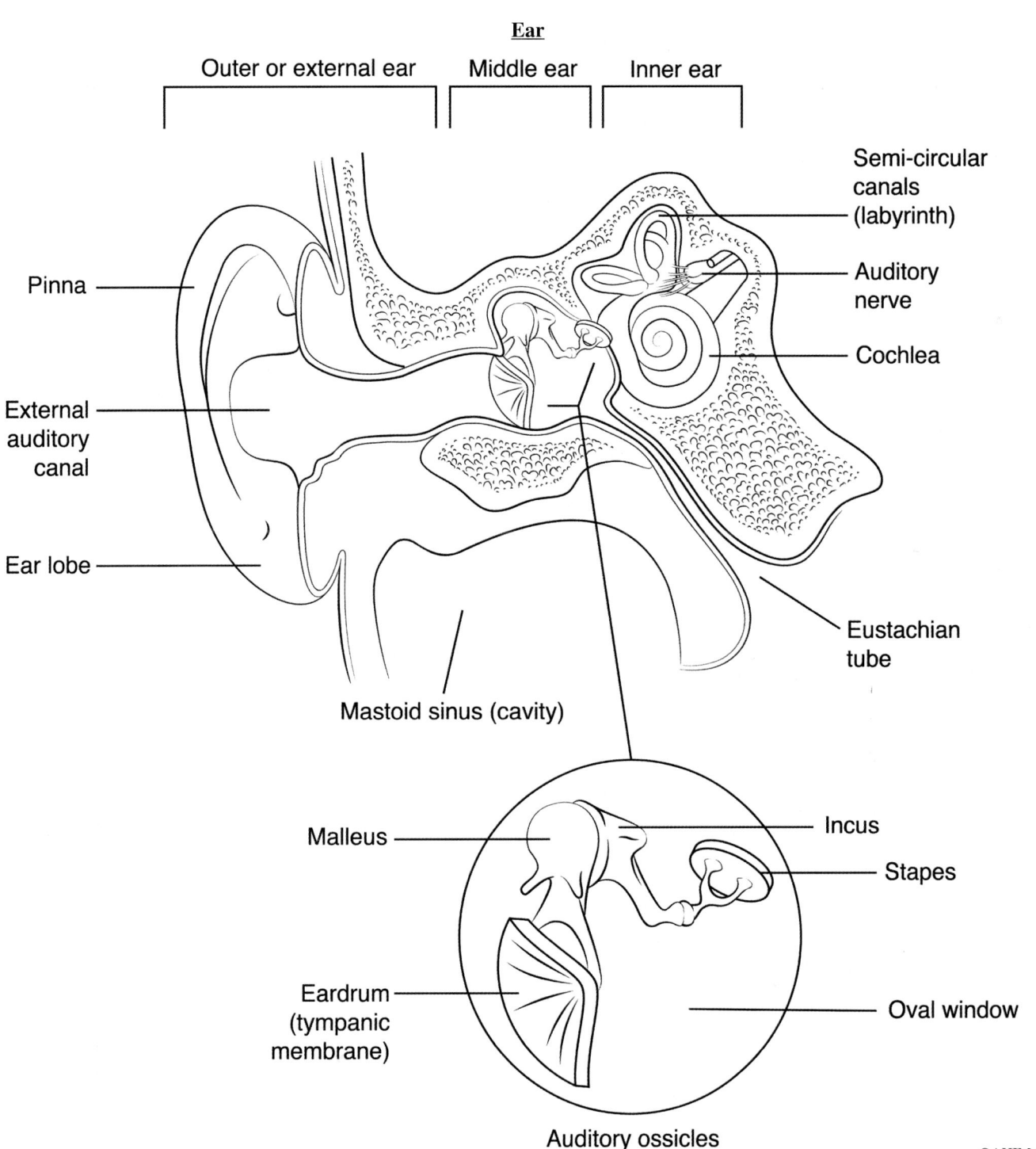

Ear

Outer or external ear — Middle ear — Inner ear

Semi-circular canals (labyrinth)
Auditory nerve
Cochlea
Pinna
External auditory canal
Ear lobe
Eustachian tube
Mastoid sinus (cavity)

Malleus — Incus
Stapes
Eardrum (tympanic membrane)
Oval window

Auditory ossicles

©AHIMA

+, +7th, X + 7th   ● Newborn   ● Pediatric   ● Maternity   ● Adult   ♀ Female   ♂ Male   Manifestation   Unacceptable PDX   HCC   CC   MCC   HAC

Diseases of external ear (H60-H62)

H60 Otitis externa

+ **H60.0 Abscess of external ear**
Boil of external ear
Carbuncle of auricle or external auditory canal
Furuncle of external ear
H60.00 Abscess of external ear, unspecified ear
H60.01 Abscess of right external ear
H60.02 Abscess of left external ear
H60.03 Abscess of external ear, bilateral

+ **H60.1 Cellulitis of external ear**
Cellulitis of auricle
Cellulitis of external auditory canal
H60.10 Cellulitis of external ear, unspecified ear
H60.11 Cellulitis of right external ear
H60.12 Cellulitis of left external ear
H60.13 Cellulitis of external ear, bilateral

+ **H60.2 Malignant otitis externa**
CC **H60.20 Malignant otitis externa, unspecified ear**
CC **H60.21 Malignant otitis externa, right ear**
CC **H60.22 Malignant otitis externa, left ear**
CC **H60.23 Malignant otitis externa, bilateral**

+ **H60.3 Other infective otitis externa**
+ **H60.31 Diffuse otitis externa**
H60.311 Diffuse otitis externa, right ear
H60.312 Diffuse otitis externa, left ear
H60.313 Diffuse otitis externa, bilateral
H60.319 Diffuse otitis externa, unspecified ear
+ **H60.32 Hemorrhagic otitis externa**
H60.321 Hemorrhagic otitis externa, right ear
H60.322 Hemorrhagic otitis externa, left ear
H60.323 Hemorrhagic otitis externa, bilateral
H60.329 Hemorrhagic otitis externa, unspecified ear
+ **H60.33 Swimmer's ear**
H60.331 Swimmer's ear, right ear
H60.332 Swimmer's ear, left ear
H60.333 Swimmer's ear, bilateral
H60.339 Swimmer's ear, unspecified ear
+ **H60.39 Other infective otitis externa**
H60.391 Other infective otitis externa, right ear
H60.392 Other infective otitis externa, left ear
H60.393 Other infective otitis externa, bilateral
H60.399 Other infective otitis externa, unspecified ear

+ **H60.4 Cholesteatoma of external ear**
Keratosis obturans of external ear (canal)
Excludes2: *cholesteatoma of middle ear (H71.-)*
recurrent cholesteatoma of postmastoidectomy cavity (H95.0-)
H60.40 Cholesteatoma of external ear, unspecified ear
H60.41 Cholesteatoma of right external ear
H60.42 Cholesteatoma of left external ear
H60.43 Cholesteatoma of external ear, bilateral

+ **H60.5 Acute noninfective otitis externa**
+ **H60.50 Unspecified acute noninfective otitis externa**
Acute otitis externa NOS
H60.501 Unspecified acute noninfective otitis externa, right ear
H60.502 Unspecified acute noninfective otitis externa, left ear
H60.503 Unspecified acute noninfective otitis externa, bilateral
H60.509 Unspecified acute noninfective otitis externa, unspecified ear
+ **H60.51 Acute actinic otitis externa**
H60.511 Acute actinic otitis externa, right ear
H60.512 Acute actinic otitis externa, left ear
H60.513 Acute actinic otitis externa, bilateral
H60.519 Acute actinic otitis externa, unspecified ear
+ **H60.52 Acute chemical otitis externa**
H60.521 Acute chemical otitis externa, right ear
H60.522 Acute chemical otitis externa, left ear
H60.523 Acute chemical otitis externa, bilateral
H60.529 Acute chemical otitis externa, unspecified ear

+ **H60.53 Acute contact otitis externa**
H60.531 Acute contact otitis externa, right ear
H60.532 Acute contact otitis externa, left ear
H60.533 Acute contact otitis externa, bilateral
H60.539 Acute contact otitis externa, unspecified ear
+ **H60.54 Acute eczematoid otitis externa**
H60.541 Acute eczematoid otitis externa, right ear
H60.542 Acute eczematoid otitis externa, left ear
H60.543 Acute eczematoid otitis externa, bilateral
H60.549 Acute eczematoid otitis externa, unspecified ear
+ **H60.55 Acute reactive otitis externa**
H60.551 Acute reactive otitis externa, right ear
H60.552 Acute reactive otitis externa, left ear
H60.553 Acute reactive otitis externa, bilateral
H60.559 Acute reactive otitis externa, unspecified ear
+ **H60.59 Other noninfective acute otitis externa**
H60.591 Other noninfective acute otitis externa, right ear
H60.592 Other noninfective acute otitis externa, left ear
H60.593 Other noninfective acute otitis externa, bilateral
H60.599 Other noninfective acute otitis externa, unspecified ear

+ **H60.6 Unspecified chronic otitis externa**
H60.60 Unspecified chronic otitis externa, unspecified ear
H60.61 Unspecified chronic otitis externa, right ear
H60.62 Unspecified chronic otitis externa, left ear
H60.63 Unspecified chronic otitis externa, bilateral

+ **H60.8 Other otitis externa**
+ **H60.8X Other otitis externa**
H60.8X1 Other otitis externa, right ear
H60.8X2 Other otitis externa, left ear
H60.8X3 Other otitis externa, bilateral
H60.8X9 Other otitis externa, unspecified ear

+ **H60.9 Unspecified otitis externa**
H60.90 Unspecified otitis externa, unspecified ear
H60.91 Unspecified otitis externa, right ear
H60.92 Unspecified otitis externa, left ear
H60.93 Unspecified otitis externa, bilateral

H61 Other disorders of external ear

+ **H61.0 Chondritis and perichondritis of external ear**
Chondrodermatitis nodularis chronica helicis
Perichondritis of auricle
Perichondritis of pinna
+ **H61.00 Unspecified perichondritis of external ear**
H61.001 Unspecified perichondritis of right external ear
H61.002 Unspecified perichondritis of left external ear
H61.003 Unspecified perichondritis of external ear, bilateral
H61.009 Unspecified perichondritis of external ear, unspecified ear
+ **H61.01 Acute perichondritis of external ear**
H61.011 Acute perichondritis of right external ear
H61.012 Acute perichondritis of left external ear
H61.013 Acute perichondritis of external ear, bilateral
H61.019 Acute perichondritis of external ear, unspecified ear
+ **H61.02 Chronic perichondritis of external ear**
H61.021 Chronic perichondritis of right external ear
H61.022 Chronic perichondritis of left external ear
H61.023 Chronic perichondritis of external ear, bilateral
H61.029 Chronic perichondritis of external ear, unspecified ear

+, +7th, X + 7th   • Newborn   • Pediatric   • Maternity   • Adult   ♀ Female   ♂ Male   Manifestation   Unacceptable PDX   HCC   CC   MCC   HAC

+ H61.03 Chondritis of external ear
Chondritis of auricle
Chondritis of pinna
H61.031 Chondritis of right external ear
H61.032 Chondritis of left external ear
AHA CC: 1Q, 2015, 18-19
H61.033 Chondritis of external ear, bilateral
H61.039 Chondritis of external ear, unspecified ear

+ H61.1 Noninfective disorders of pinna
Excludes2: cauliflower ear (M95.1-)
gouty tophi of ear (M1A.-)
+ H61.10 Unspecified noninfective disorders of pinna
Disorder of pinna NOS
H61.101 Unspecified noninfective disorders of pinna, right ear
H61.102 Unspecified noninfective disorders of pinna, left ear
H61.103 Unspecified noninfective disorders of pinna, bilateral
H61.109 Unspecified noninfective disorders of pinna, unspecified ear
+ H61.11 Acquired deformity of pinna
Acquired deformity of auricle
Excludes2: cauliflower ear (M95.1-)
H61.111 Acquired deformity of pinna, right ear
H61.112 Acquired deformity of pinna, left ear
H61.113 Acquired deformity of pinna, bilateral
H61.119 Acquired deformity of pinna, unspecified ear
+ H61.12 Hematoma of pinna
Hematoma of auricle
H61.121 Hematoma of pinna, right ear
H61.122 Hematoma of pinna, left ear
H61.123 Hematoma of pinna, bilateral
H61.129 Hematoma of pinna, unspecified ear
+ H61.19 Other noninfective disorders of pinna
H61.191 Noninfective disorders of pinna, right ear
H61.192 Noninfective disorders of pinna, left ear
H61.193 Noninfective disorders of pinna, bilateral
H61.199 Noninfective disorders of pinna, unspecified ear

+ H61.2 Impacted cerumen
Wax in ear
H61.20 Impacted cerumen, unspecified ear
H61.21 Impacted cerumen, right ear
H61.22 Impacted cerumen, left ear
H61.23 Impacted cerumen, bilateral

+ H61.3 Acquired stenosis of external ear canal
Collapse of external ear canal
Excludes1: postprocedural stenosis of external ear canal (H95.81-)
+ H61.30 Acquired stenosis of external ear canal, unspecified
H61.301 Acquired stenosis of right external ear canal, unspecified
H61.302 Acquired stenosis of left external ear canal, unspecified
H61.303 Acquired stenosis of external ear canal, unspecified, bilateral
H61.309 Acquired stenosis of external ear canal, unspecified, unspecified ear
+ H61.31 Acquired stenosis of external ear canal secondary to trauma
H61.311 Acquired stenosis of right external ear canal secondary to trauma
H61.312 Acquired stenosis of left external ear canal secondary to trauma
H61.313 Acquired stenosis of external ear canal secondary to trauma, bilateral
H61.319 Acquired stenosis of external ear canal secondary to trauma, unspecified ear

+ H61.32 Acquired stenosis of external ear canal secondary to inflammation and infection
H61.321 Acquired stenosis of right external ear canal secondary to inflammation and infection
H61.322 Acquired stenosis of left external ear canal secondary to inflammation and infection
H61.323 Acquired stenosis of external ear canal secondary to inflammation and infection, bilateral
H61.329 Acquired stenosis of external ear canal secondary to inflammation and infection, unspecified ear
+ H61.39 Other acquired stenosis of external ear canal
H61.391 Other acquired stenosis of right external ear canal
H61.392 Other acquired stenosis of left external ear canal
H61.393 Other acquired stenosis of external ear canal, bilateral
H61.399 Other acquired stenosis of external ear canal, unspecified ear

+ H61.8 Other specified disorders of external ear
+ H61.81 Exostosis of external canal
H61.811 Exostosis of right external canal
H61.812 Exostosis of left external canal
H61.813 Exostosis of external canal, bilateral
H61.819 Exostosis of external canal, unspecified ear
+ H61.89 Other specified disorders of external ear
H61.891 Other specified disorders of right external ear
H61.892 Other specified disorders of left external ear
H61.893 Other specified disorders of external ear, bilateral
H61.899 Other specified disorders of external ear, unspecified ear

+ H61.9 Disorder of external ear, unspecified
H61.90 Disorder of external ear, unspecified, unspecified ear
H61.91 Disorder of right external ear, unspecified
H61.92 Disorder of left external ear, unspecified
H61.93 Disorder of external ear, unspecified, bilateral

H62 Disorders of external ear in diseases classified elsewhere
+ H62.4 Otitis externa in other diseases classified elsewhere
Code first underlying disease, such as:
erysipelas (A46)
impetigo (L01.0)
Excludes1: otitis externa (in):
candidiasis (B37.84)
herpes viral [herpes simplex] (B00.1)
herpes zoster (B02.8)
H62.40 Otitis externa in other diseases classified elsewhere, unspecified ear
H62.41 Otitis externa in other diseases classified elsewhere, right ear
H62.42 Otitis externa in other diseases classified elsewhere, left ear
H62.43 Otitis externa in other diseases classified elsewhere, bilateral
+ H62.8 Other disorders of external ear in diseases classified elsewhere
Code first underlying disease, such as:
gout (M1A.-, M10.-)
+ H62.8X Other disorders of external ear in diseases classified elsewhere
H62.8X1 Other disorders of right external ear in diseases classified elsewhere
H62.8X2 Other disorders of left external ear in diseases classified elsewhere
H62.8X3 Other disorders of external ear in diseases classified elsewhere, bilateral
H62.8X9 Other disorders of external ear in diseases classified elsewhere, unspecified ear

+, +7th, X + 7th   • Newborn   • Pediatric   • Maternity   • Adult   ♀ Female   ♂ Male   Manifestation   Unacceptable PDX   HCC   CC   MCC   HAC

Diseases of middle ear and mastoid (H65-H75)

H65 Nonsuppurative otitis media

Includes: nonsuppurative otitis media with myringitis

Use additional code for any associated perforated tympanic membrane (H72.-)

Use additional code, if applicable, to identify:
exposure to environmental tobacco smoke (Z77.22)
exposure to tobacco smoke in the perinatal period (P96.81)
history of tobacco dependence (Z87.891)
infectious agent (B95-B97)
occupational exposure to environmental tobacco smoke (Z57.31)
tobacco dependence (F17.-)
tobacco use (Z72.0)

+ **H65.0 Acute serous otitis media**
   Acute and subacute secretory otitis
   H65.00 Acute serous otitis media, unspecified ear
   H65.01 Acute serous otitis media, right ear
   H65.02 Acute serous otitis media, left ear
   H65.03 Acute serous otitis media, bilateral
   H65.04 Acute serous otitis media, recurrent, right ear
   H65.05 Acute serous otitis media, recurrent, left ear
   H65.06 Acute serous otitis media, recurrent, bilateral
   H65.07 Acute serous otitis media, recurrent, unspecified ear

+ **H65.1 Other acute nonsuppurative otitis media**
   Excludes1: *otitic barotrauma (T70.0)*
   otitis media (acute) NOS (H66.9)
   + **H65.11 Acute and subacute allergic otitis media (mucoid) (sanguinous) (serous)**
      H65.111 Acute and subacute allergic otitis media (mucoid) (sanguinous) (serous), right ear
      H65.112 Acute and subacute allergic otitis media (mucoid) (sanguinous) (serous), left ear
      H65.113 Acute and subacute allergic otitis media (mucoid) (sanguinous) (serous), bilateral
      H65.114 Acute and subacute allergic otitis media (mucoid) (sanguinous) (serous), recurrent, right ear
      H65.115 Acute and subacute allergic otitis media (mucoid) (sanguinous) (serous), recurrent, left ear
      H65.116 Acute and subacute allergic otitis media (mucoid) (sanguinous) (serous), recurrent, bilateral
      H65.117 Acute and subacute allergic otitis media (mucoid) (sanguinous) (serous), recurrent, unspecified ear
      H65.119 Acute and subacute allergic otitis media (mucoid) (sanguinous) (serous), unspecified ear
   + **H65.19 Other acute nonsuppurative otitis media**
      Acute and subacute mucoid otitis media
      Acute and subacute nonsuppurative otitis media NOS
      Acute and subacute sanguinous otitis media
      Acute and subacute seromucinous otitis media
      H65.191 Other acute nonsuppurative otitis media, right ear
      H65.192 Other acute nonsuppurative otitis media, left ear
      H65.193 Other acute nonsuppurative otitis media, bilateral
      H65.194 Other acute nonsuppurative otitis media, recurrent, right ear
      H65.195 Other acute nonsuppurative otitis media, recurrent, left ear
      H65.196 Other acute nonsuppurative otitis media, recurrent, bilateral
      H65.197 Other acute nonsuppurative otitis media recurrent, unspecified ear
      H65.199 Other acute nonsuppurative otitis media, unspecified ear

+ **H65.2 Chronic serous otitis media**
   Chronic tubotympanal catarrh
   H65.20 Chronic serous otitis media, unspecified ear
   H65.21 Chronic serous otitis media, right ear
   H65.22 Chronic serous otitis media, left ear
   H65.23 Chronic serous otitis media, bilateral

+ **H65.3 Chronic mucoid otitis media**
   Chronic mucinous otitis media
   Chronic secretory otitis media
   Chronic transudative otitis media
   Glue ear
   Excludes1: *adhesive middle ear disease (H74.1)*
   H65.30 Chronic mucoid otitis media, unspecified ear
   H65.31 Chronic mucoid otitis media, right ear
   H65.32 Chronic mucoid otitis media, left ear
   H65.33 Chronic mucoid otitis media, bilateral

+ **H65.4 Other chronic nonsuppurative otitis media**
   + **H65.41 Chronic allergic otitis media**
      H65.411 Chronic allergic otitis media, right ear
      H65.412 Chronic allergic otitis media, left ear
      H65.413 Chronic allergic otitis media, bilateral
      H65.419 Chronic allergic otitis media, unspecified ear
   + **H65.49 Other chronic nonsuppurative otitis media**
      Chronic exudative otitis media
      Chronic nonsuppurative otitis media NOS
      Chronic otitis media with effusion (nonpurulent)
      Chronic seromucinous otitis media
      H65.491 Other chronic nonsuppurative otitis media, right ear
      H65.492 Other chronic nonsuppurative otitis media, left ear
      H65.493 Other chronic nonsuppurative otitis media, bilateral
      H65.499 Other chronic nonsuppurative otitis media, unspecified ear

+ **H65.9 Unspecified nonsuppurative otitis media**
   Allergic otitis media NOS
   Catarrhal otitis media NOS
   Exudative otitis media NOS
   Mucoid otitis media NOS
   Otitis media with effusion (nonpurulent) NOS
   Secretory otitis media NOS
   Seromucinous otitis media NOS
   Serous otitis media NOS
   Transudative otitis media NOS
   H65.90 Unspecified nonsuppurative otitis media, unspecified ear
   H65.91 Unspecified nonsuppurative otitis media, right ear
   H65.92 Unspecified nonsuppurative otitis media, left ear
   H65.93 Unspecified nonsuppurative otitis media, bilateral

H66 Suppurative and unspecified otitis media

Includes: suppurative and unspecified otitis media with myringitis
Use additional code to identify:
exposure to environmental tobacco smoke (Z77.22)
exposure to tobacco smoke in the perinatal period (P96.81)
history of tobacco dependence (Z87.891)
occupational exposure to environmental tobacco smoke (Z57.31)
tobacco dependence (F17.-)
tobacco use (Z72.0)

+ **H66.0 Acute suppurative otitis media**
   + **H66.00 Acute suppurative otitis media without spontaneous rupture of ear drum**
      H66.001 Acute suppurative otitis media without spontaneous rupture of ear drum, right ear
      H66.002 Acute suppurative otitis media without spontaneous rupture of ear drum, left ear
      H66.003 Acute suppurative otitis media without spontaneous rupture of ear drum, bilateral
      H66.004 Acute suppurative otitis media without spontaneous rupture of ear drum, recurrent, right ear
      H66.005 Acute suppurative otitis media without spontaneous rupture of ear drum, recurrent, left ear
      H66.006 Acute suppurative otitis media without spontaneous rupture of ear drum, recurrent, bilateral
      H66.007 Acute suppurative otitis media without spontaneous rupture of ear drum, recurrent, unspecified ear
      H66.009 Acute suppurative otitis media without spontaneous rupture of ear drum, unspecified ear

+, +7th, X + 7th   ● Newborn   ● Pediatric   ● Maternity   ● Adult   ♀ Female   ♂ Male   Manifestation   Unacceptable PDX   HCC   CC   MCC   HAC

+ **H66.01 Acute suppurative otitis media with spontaneous rupture of ear drum**

    H66.011 Acute suppurative otitis media with spontaneous rupture of ear drum, right ear

    H66.012 Acute suppurative otitis media with spontaneous rupture of ear drum, left ear

    H66.013 Acute suppurative otitis media with spontaneous rupture of ear drum, bilateral

    H66.014 Acute suppurative otitis media with spontaneous rupture of ear drum, recurrent, right ear

    H66.015 Acute suppurative otitis media with spontaneous rupture of ear drum, recurrent, left ear

    H66.016 Acute suppurative otitis media with spontaneous rupture of ear drum, recurrent, bilateral

    H66.017 Acute suppurative otitis media with spontaneous rupture of ear drum, recurrent, unspecified ear

    H66.019 Acute suppurative otitis media with spontaneous rupture of ear drum, unspecified ear

+ **H66.1 Chronic tubotympanic suppurative otitis media**

    Benign chronic suppurative otitis media

    Chronic tubotympanic disease

    Use additional code for any associated perforated tympanic membrane (H72.-)

    H66.10 Chronic tubotympanic suppurative otitis media, unspecified

    H66.11 Chronic tubotympanic suppurative otitis media, right ear

    H66.12 Chronic tubotympanic suppurative otitis media, left ear

    H66.13 Chronic tubotympanic suppurative otitis media, bilateral

+ **H66.2 Chronic atticoantral suppurative otitis media**

    Chronic atticoantral disease

    Use additional code for any associated perforated tympanic membrane (H72.-)

    H66.20 Chronic atticoantral suppurative otitis media, unspecified ear

    H66.21 Chronic atticoantral suppurative otitis media, right ear

    H66.22 Chronic atticoantral suppurative otitis media, left ear

    H66.23 Chronic atticoantral suppurative otitis media, bilateral

+ **H66.3 Other chronic suppurative otitis media**

    Chronic suppurative otitis media NOS

    Use additional code for any associated perforated tympanic membrane (H72.-)

    Excludes1: tuberculous otitis media (A18.6)

+ **H66.3X Other chronic suppurative otitis media**

    H66.3X1 Other chronic suppurative otitis media, right ear

    H66.3X2 Other chronic suppurative otitis media, left ear

    H66.3X3 Other chronic suppurative otitis media, bilateral

    H66.3X9 Other chronic suppurative otitis media, unspecified ear

+ **H66.4 Suppurative otitis media, unspecified**

    Purulent otitis media NOS

    Use additional code for any associated perforated tympanic membrane (H72.-)

    H66.40 Suppurative otitis media, unspecified, unspecified ear

    H66.41 Suppurative otitis media, unspecified, right ear

    H66.42 Suppurative otitis media, unspecified, left ear

    H66.43 Suppurative otitis media, unspecified, bilateral

+ **H66.9 Otitis media, unspecified**

    Otitis media NOS

    Acute otitis media NOS

    Chronic otitis media NOS

    Use additional code for any associated perforated tympanic membrane (H72.-)

    H66.90 Otitis media, unspecified, unspecified ear

    H66.91 Otitis media, unspecified, right ear

    H66.92 Otitis media, unspecified, left ear

    H66.93 Otitis media, unspecified, bilateral

H67 Otitis media in diseases classified elsewhere

    Code first underlying disease, such as:

      plasminogen deficiency (E88.02)

      viral disease NEC (B00-B34)

    Use additional code for any associated perforated tympanic membrane (H72.-)

    Excludes1: otitis media in:

      influenza (J09.X9, J10.83, J11.83)

      measles (B05.3)

      scarlet fever (A38.0)

      tuberculosis (A18.6)

H67.1 Otitis media in diseases classified elsewhere, right ear

H67.2 Otitis media in diseases classified elsewhere, left ear

H67.3 Otitis media in diseases classified elsewhere, bilateral

H67.9 Otitis media in diseases classified elsewhere, unspecified ear

H68 Eustachian salpingitis and obstruction

+ **H68.0 Eustachian salpingitis**

  + **H68.00 Unspecified Eustachian salpingitis**

    H68.001 Unspecified Eustachian salpingitis, right ear

    H68.002 Unspecified Eustachian salpingitis, left ear

    H68.003 Unspecified Eustachian salpingitis, bilateral

    H68.009 Unspecified Eustachian salpingitis, unspecified ear

  + **H68.01 Acute Eustachian salpingitis**

    H68.011 Acute Eustachian salpingitis, right ear

    H68.012 Acute Eustachian salpingitis, left ear

    H68.013 Acute Eustachian salpingitis, bilateral

    H68.019 Acute Eustachian salpingitis, unspecified ear

  + **H68.02 Chronic Eustachian salpingitis**

    H68.021 Chronic Eustachian salpingitis, right ear

    H68.022 Chronic Eustachian salpingitis, left ear

    H68.023 Chronic Eustachian salpingitis, bilateral

    H68.029 Chronic Eustachian salpingitis, unspecified ear

+ **H68.1 Obstruction of Eustachian tube**

    Stenosis of Eustachian tube

    Stricture of Eustachian tube

  + **H68.10 Unspecified obstruction of Eustachian tube**

    H68.101 Unspecified obstruction of Eustachian tube, right ear

    H68.102 Unspecified obstruction of Eustachian tube, left ear

    H68.103 Unspecified obstruction of Eustachian tube, bilateral

    H68.109 Unspecified obstruction of Eustachian tube, unspecified ear

  + **H68.11 Osseous obstruction of Eustachian tube**

    H68.111 Osseous obstruction of Eustachian tube, right ear

    H68.112 Osseous obstruction of Eustachian tube, left ear

    H68.113 Osseous obstruction of Eustachian tube, bilateral

    H68.119 Osseous obstruction of Eustachian tube, unspecified ear

  + **H68.12 Intrinsic cartilagenous obstruction of Eustachian tube**

    H68.121 Intrinsic cartilagenous obstruction of Eustachian tube, right ear

    H68.122 Intrinsic cartilagenous obstruction of Eustachian tube, left ear

    H68.123 Intrinsic cartilagenous obstruction of Eustachian tube, bilateral

    H68.129 Intrinsic cartilagenous obstruction of Eustachian tube, unspecified ear

+ **H68.13** **Extrinsic cartilagenous obstruction of Eustachian tube**
  Compression of Eustachian tube
  H68.131 **Extrinsic cartilagenous obstruction of Eustachian tube, right ear**
  H68.132 **Extrinsic cartilagenous obstruction of Eustachian tube, left ear**
  H68.133 **Extrinsic cartilagenous obstruction of Eustachian tube, bilateral**
  H68.139 **Extrinsic cartilagenous obstruction of Eustachian tube, unspecified ear**

H69 **Other and unspecified disorders of Eustachian tube**

+ **H69.0** **Patulous Eustachian tube**
 H69.00 **Patulous Eustachian tube, unspecified ear**
 H69.01 **Patulous Eustachian tube, right ear**
 H69.02 **Patulous Eustachian tube, left ear**
 H69.03 **Patulous Eustachian tube, bilateral**

+ **H69.8** **Other specified disorders of Eustachian tube**
 H69.80 **Other specified disorders of Eustachian tube, unspecified ear**
 H69.81 **Other specified disorders of Eustachian tube, right ear**
 H69.82 **Other specified disorders of Eustachian tube, left ear**
 H69.83 **Other specified disorders of Eustachian tube, bilateral**

+ **H69.9** **Unspecified Eustachian tube disorder**
 H69.90 **Unspecified Eustachian tube disorder, unspecified ear**
 H69.91 **Unspecified Eustachian tube disorder, right ear**
 H69.92 **Unspecified Eustachian tube disorder, left ear**
 H69.93 **Unspecified Eustachian tube disorder, bilateral**

H70 **Mastoiditis and related conditions**

+ **H70.0** **Acute mastoiditis**
 Abscess of mastoid
 Empyema of mastoid
 + **H70.00** **Acute mastoiditis without complications**
  CC **H70.001** **Acute mastoiditis without complications, right ear**
  CC **H70.002** **Acute mastoiditis without complications, left ear**
  CC **H70.003** **Acute mastoiditis without complications, bilateral**
  CC **H70.009** **Acute mastoiditis without complications, unspecified ear**
 + **H70.01** **Subperiosteal abscess of mastoid**
  CC **H70.011** **Subperiosteal abscess of mastoid, right ear**
  CC **H70.012** **Subperiosteal abscess of mastoid, left ear**
  CC **H70.013** **Subperiosteal abscess of mastoid, bilateral**
  CC **H70.019** **Subperiosteal abscess of mastoid, unspecified ear**
 + **H70.09** **Acute mastoiditis with other complications**
  CC **H70.091** **Acute mastoiditis with other complications, right ear**
  CC **H70.092** **Acute mastoiditis with other complications, left ear**
  CC **H70.093** **Acute mastoiditis with other complications, bilateral**
  CC **H70.099** **Acute mastoiditis with other complications, unspecified ear**

+ **H70.1** **Chronic mastoiditis**
 Caries of mastoid
 Fistula of mastoid
 Excludes1: *tuberculous mastoiditis (A18.03)*
 H70.10 **Chronic mastoiditis, unspecified ear**
 H70.11 **Chronic mastoiditis, right ear**
 H70.12 **Chronic mastoiditis, left ear**
 H70.13 **Chronic mastoiditis, bilateral**

+ **H70.2** **Petrositis**
 Inflammation of petrous bone
 + **H70.20** **Unspecified petrositis**
  H70.201 **Unspecified petrositis, right ear**
  H70.202 **Unspecified petrositis, left ear**
  H70.203 **Unspecified petrositis, bilateral**
  H70.209 **Unspecified petrositis, unspecified ear**

+ **H70.21** **Acute petrositis**
 H70.211 **Acute petrositis, right ear**
 H70.212 **Acute petrositis, left ear**
 H70.213 **Acute petrositis, bilateral**
 H70.219 **Acute petrositis, unspecified ear**

+ **H70.22** **Chronic petrositis**
 H70.221 **Chronic petrositis, right ear**
 H70.222 **Chronic petrositis, left ear**
 H70.223 **Chronic petrositis, bilateral**
 H70.229 **Chronic petrositis, unspecified ear**

+ **H70.8** **Other mastoiditis and related conditions**
 Excludes1: *preauricular sinus and cyst (Q18.1)*
     sinus, fistula, and cyst of branchial cleft (Q18.0)
 + **H70.81** **Postauricular fistula**
  H70.811 **Postauricular fistula, right ear**
  H70.812 **Postauricular fistula, left ear**
  H70.813 **Postauricular fistula, bilateral**
  H70.819 **Postauricular fistula, unspecified ear**
 + **H70.89** **Other mastoiditis and related conditions**
  H70.891 **Other mastoiditis and related conditions, right ear**
  H70.892 **Other mastoiditis and related conditions, left ear**
  H70.893 **Other mastoiditis and related conditions, bilateral**
  H70.899 **Other mastoiditis and related conditions, unspecified ear**

+ **H70.9** **Unspecified mastoiditis**
 H70.90 **Unspecified mastoiditis, unspecified ear**
 H70.91 **Unspecified mastoiditis, right ear**
 H70.92 **Unspecified mastoiditis, left ear**
 H70.93 **Unspecified mastoiditis, bilateral**

H71 **Cholesteatoma of middle ear**

 Excludes2: *cholesteatoma of external ear (H60.4-)*
     recurrent cholesteatoma of postmastoidectomy cavity (H95.0-)

+ **H71.0** **Cholesteatoma of attic**
 H71.00 **Cholesteatoma of attic, unspecified ear**
 H71.01 **Cholesteatoma of attic, right ear**
 H71.02 **Cholesteatoma of attic, left ear**
 H71.03 **Cholesteatoma of attic, bilateral**

+ **H71.1** **Cholesteatoma of tympanum**
 H71.10 **Cholesteatoma of tympanum, unspecified ear**
 H71.11 **Cholesteatoma of tympanum, right ear**
 H71.12 **Cholesteatoma of tympanum, left ear**
 H71.13 **Cholesteatoma of tympanum, bilateral**

+ **H71.2** **Cholesteatoma of mastoid**
 H71.20 **Cholesteatoma of mastoid, unspecified ear**
 H71.21 **Cholesteatoma of mastoid, right ear**
 H71.22 **Cholesteatoma of mastoid, left ear**
 H71.23 **Cholesteatoma of mastoid, bilateral**

+ **H71.3** **Diffuse cholesteatosis**
 H71.30 **Diffuse cholesteatosis, unspecified ear**
 H71.31 **Diffuse cholesteatosis, right ear**
 H71.32 **Diffuse cholesteatosis, left ear**
 H71.33 **Diffuse cholesteatosis, bilateral**

+ **H71.9** **Unspecified cholesteatoma**
 H71.90 **Unspecified cholesteatoma, unspecified ear**
 H71.91 **Unspecified cholesteatoma, right ear**
 H71.92 **Unspecified cholesteatoma, left ear**
 H71.93 **Unspecified cholesteatoma, bilateral**

H72 **Perforation of tympanic membrane**

 Includes: persistent post-traumatic perforation of ear drum
     postinflammatory perforation of ear drum
 Code first any associated otitis media (H65.-, H66.1-, H66.2-, H66.3-, H66.4-, H66.9-, H67.-)
 Excludes1: *acute suppurative otitis media with rupture of the tympanic membrane (H66.01-)*
     traumatic rupture of ear drum (S09.2-)

+ **H72.0** **Central perforation of tympanic membrane**
 H72.00 **Central perforation of tympanic membrane, unspecified ear**
 H72.01 **Central perforation of tympanic membrane, right ear**
 H72.02 **Central perforation of tympanic membrane, left ear**
 H72.03 **Central perforation of tympanic membrane, bilateral**

+ **H72.1** Attic perforation of tympanic membrane
Perforation of pars flaccida
H72.10 Attic perforation of tympanic membrane, unspecified ear
H72.11 Attic perforation of tympanic membrane, right ear
H72.12 Attic perforation of tympanic membrane, left ear
H72.13 Attic perforation of tympanic membrane, bilateral
+ **H72.2** Other marginal perforations of tympanic membrane
+ **H72.2X** Other marginal perforations of tympanic membrane
H72.2X1 Other marginal perforations of tympanic membrane, right ear
H72.2X2 Other marginal perforations of tympanic membrane, left ear
H72.2X3 Other marginal perforations of tympanic membrane, bilateral
H72.2X9 Other marginal perforations of tympanic membrane, unspecified ear
+ **H72.8** Other perforations of tympanic membrane
+ **H72.81** Multiple perforations of tympanic membrane
H72.811 Multiple perforations of tympanic membrane, right ear
H72.812 Multiple perforations of tympanic membrane, left ear
H72.813 Multiple perforations of tympanic membrane, bilateral
H72.819 Multiple perforations of tympanic membrane, unspecified ear
+ **H72.82** Total perforations of tympanic membrane
H72.821 Total perforations of tympanic membrane, right ear
H72.822 Total perforations of tympanic membrane, left ear
H72.823 Total perforations of tympanic membrane, bilateral
H72.829 Total perforations of tympanic membrane, unspecified ear
+ **H72.9** Unspecified perforation of tympanic membrane
H72.90 Unspecified perforation of tympanic membrane, unspecified ear
H72.91 Unspecified perforation of tympanic membrane, right ear
H72.92 Unspecified perforation of tympanic membrane, left ear
H72.93 Unspecified perforation of tympanic membrane, bilateral

H73 Other disorders of tympanic membrane
+ **H73.0** Acute myringitis
Excludes1: acute myringitis with otitis media (H65, H66)
+ **H73.00** Unspecified acute myringitis
Acute tympanitis NOS
H73.001 Acute myringitis, right ear
H73.002 Acute myringitis, left ear
H73.003 Acute myringitis, bilateral
H73.009 Acute myringitis, unspecified ear
+ **H73.01** Bullous myringitis
H73.011 Bullous myringitis, right ear
H73.012 Bullous myringitis, left ear
H73.013 Bullous myringitis, bilateral
H73.019 Bullous myringitis, unspecified ear
+ **H73.09** Other acute myringitis
H73.091 Other acute myringitis, right ear
H73.092 Other acute myringitis, left ear
H73.093 Other acute myringitis, bilateral
H73.099 Other acute myringitis, unspecified ear
+ **H73.1** Chronic myringitis
Chronic tympanitis
Excludes1: chronic myringitis with otitis media (H65, H66)
H73.10 Chronic myringitis, unspecified ear
H73.11 Chronic myringitis, right ear
H73.12 Chronic myringitis, left ear
H73.13 Chronic myringitis, bilateral
+ **H73.2** Unspecified myringitis
H73.20 Unspecified myringitis, unspecified ear
H73.21 Unspecified myringitis, right ear
H73.22 Unspecified myringitis, left ear
H73.23 Unspecified myringitis, bilateral
+ **H73.8** Other specified disorders of tympanic membrane

+ **H73.81** Atrophic flaccid tympanic membrane
H73.811 Atrophic flaccid tympanic membrane, right ear
H73.812 Atrophic flaccid tympanic membrane, left ear
H73.813 Atrophic flaccid tympanic membrane, bilateral
H73.819 Atrophic flaccid tympanic membrane, unspecified ear
+ **H73.82** Atrophic nonflaccid tympanic membrane
H73.821 Atrophic nonflaccid tympanic membrane, right ear
H73.822 Atrophic nonflaccid tympanic membrane, left ear
H73.823 Atrophic nonflaccid tympanic membrane, bilateral
H73.829 Atrophic nonflaccid tympanic membrane, unspecified ear
+ **H73.89** Other specified disorders of tympanic membrane
H73.891 Other specified disorders of tympanic membrane, right ear
H73.892 Other specified disorders of tympanic membrane, left ear
H73.893 Other specified disorders of tympanic membrane, bilateral
H73.899 Other specified disorders of tympanic membrane, unspecified ear
+ **H73.9** Unspecified disorder of tympanic membrane
H73.90 Unspecified disorder of tympanic membrane, unspecified ear
H73.91 Unspecified disorder of tympanic membrane, right ear
H73.92 Unspecified disorder of tympanic membrane, left ear
H73.93 Unspecified disorder of tympanic membrane, bilateral

H74 Other disorders of middle ear mastoid
Excludes2: mastoiditis (H70.-)
+ **H74.0** Tympanosclerosis
H74.01 Tympanosclerosis, right ear
H74.02 Tympanosclerosis, left ear
H74.03 Tympanosclerosis, bilateral
H74.09 Tympanosclerosis, unspecified ear
+ **H74.1** Adhesive middle ear disease
Adhesive otitis
Excludes1: glue ear (H65.3-)
H74.11 Adhesive right middle ear disease
H74.12 Adhesive left middle ear disease
H74.13 Adhesive middle ear disease, bilateral
H74.19 Adhesive middle ear disease, unspecified ear
+ **H74.2** Discontinuity and dislocation of ear ossicles
H74.20 Discontinuity and dislocation of ear ossicles, unspecified ear
H74.21 Discontinuity and dislocation of right ear ossicles
H74.22 Discontinuity and dislocation of left ear ossicles
H74.23 Discontinuity and dislocation of ear ossicles, bilateral
+ **H74.3** Other acquired abnormalities of ear ossicles
+ **H74.31** Ankylosis of ear ossicles
H74.311 Ankylosis of ear ossicles, right ear
H74.312 Ankylosis of ear ossicles, left ear
H74.313 Ankylosis of ear ossicles, bilateral
H74.319 Ankylosis of ear ossicles, unspecified ear
+ **H74.32** Partial loss of ear ossicles
H74.321 Partial loss of ear ossicles, right ear
H74.322 Partial loss of ear ossicles, left ear
H74.323 Partial loss of ear ossicles, bilateral
H74.329 Partial loss of ear ossicles, unspecified ear
+ **H74.39** Other acquired abnormalities of ear ossicles
H74.391 Other acquired abnormalities of right ear ossicles
H74.392 Other acquired abnormalities of left ear ossicles
H74.393 Other acquired abnormalities of ear ossicles, bilateral
H74.399 Other acquired abnormalities of ear ossicles, unspecified ear

+, +7th, X + 7th   ● Newborn   ● Pediatric   ● Maternity   ● Adult   ♀ Female   ♂ Male   Manifestation   Unacceptable PDX   HCC   CC   MCC   HAC

+ **H74.4 Polyp of middle ear**
    H74.40 Polyp of middle ear, unspecified ear
    H74.41 Polyp of right middle ear
    H74.42 Polyp of left middle ear
    H74.43 Polyp of middle ear, bilateral
+ **H74.8 Other specified disorders of middle ear and mastoid**
  + **H74.8X Other specified disorders of middle ear and mastoid**
    H74.8X1 Other specified disorders of right middle ear and mastoid
    H74.8X2 Other specified disorders of left middle ear and mastoid
    H74.8X3 Other specified disorders of middle ear and mastoid, bilateral
    H74.8X9 Other specified disorders of middle ear and mastoid, unspecified ear
+ **H74.9 Unspecified disorder of middle ear and mastoid**
    H74.90 Unspecified disorder of middle ear and mastoid, unspecified ear
    H74.91 Unspecified disorder of right middle ear and mastoid
    H74.92 Unspecified disorder of left middle ear and mastoid
    H74.93 Unspecified disorder of middle ear and mastoid, bilateral

H75 Other disorders of middle ear and mastoid in diseases classified elsewhere
  Code first underlying disease
+ **H75.0 Mastoiditis in infectious and parasitic diseases classified elsewhere**
    Excludes1: *mastoiditis (in):*
        syphilis (A52.77)
        tuberculosis (A18.03)
    H75.00 Mastoiditis in infectious and parasitic diseases classified elsewhere, unspecified ear
    H75.01 Mastoiditis in infectious and parasitic diseases classified elsewhere, right ear
    H75.02 Mastoiditis in infectious and parasitic diseases classified elsewhere, left ear
    H75.03 Mastoiditis in infectious and parasitic diseases classified elsewhere, bilateral
+ **H75.8 Other specified disorders of middle ear and mastoid in diseases classified elsewhere**
    H75.80 Other specified disorders of middle ear and mastoid in diseases classified elsewhere, unspecified ear
    H75.81 Other specified disorders of right middle ear and mastoid in diseases classified elsewhere
    H75.82 Other specified disorders of left middle ear and mastoid in diseases classified elsewhere
    H75.83 Other specified disorders of middle ear and mastoid in diseases classified elsewhere, bilateral

Diseases of inner ear (H80-H83)

H80 Otosclerosis
  Includes: Otospongiosis
+ **H80.0 Otosclerosis involving oval window, nonobliterative**
    H80.00 Otosclerosis involving oval window, nonobliterative, unspecified ear
    H80.01 Otosclerosis involving oval window, nonobliterative, right ear
    H80.02 Otosclerosis involving oval window, nonobliterative, left ear
    H80.03 Otosclerosis involving oval window, nonobliterative, bilateral
+ **H80.1 Otosclerosis involving oval window, obliterative**
    H80.10 Otosclerosis involving oval window, obliterative, unspecified ear
    H80.11 Otosclerosis involving oval window, obliterative, right ear
    H80.12 Otosclerosis involving oval window, obliterative, left ear
    H80.13 Otosclerosis involving oval window, obliterative, bilateral

+ **H80.2 Cochlear otosclerosis**
  Otosclerosis involving otic capsule
  Otosclerosis involving round window
    H80.20 Cochlear otosclerosis, unspecified ear
    H80.21 Cochlear otosclerosis, right ear
    H80.22 Cochlear otosclerosis, left ear
    H80.23 Cochlear otosclerosis, bilateral
+ **H80.8 Other otosclerosis**
    H80.80 Other otosclerosis, unspecified ear
    H80.81 Other otosclerosis, right ear
    H80.82 Other otosclerosis, left ear
    H80.83 Other otosclerosis, bilateral
+ **H80.9 Unspecified otosclerosis**
    H80.90 Unspecified otosclerosis, unspecified ear
    H80.91 Unspecified otosclerosis, right ear
    H80.92 Unspecified otosclerosis, left ear
    H80.93 Unspecified otosclerosis, bilateral

H81 Disorders of vestibular function
  Excludes1: *epidemic vertigo (A88.1)*
        vertigo NOS (R42)
+ **H81.0 Ménière's disease**
  Labyrinthine hydrops
  Ménière's syndrome or vertigo
    H81.01 Ménière's disease, right ear
    H81.02 Ménière's disease, left ear
    H81.03 Ménière's disease, bilateral
    H81.09 Ménière's disease, unspecified ear
+ **H81.1 Benign paroxysmal vertigo**
    H81.10 Benign paroxysmal vertigo, unspecified ear
    H81.11 Benign paroxysmal vertigo, right ear
    H81.12 Benign paroxysmal vertigo, left ear
    H81.13 Benign paroxysmal vertigo, bilateral
+ **H81.2 Vestibular neuronitis**
    H81.20 Vestibular neuronitis, unspecified ear
    H81.21 Vestibular neuronitis, right ear
    H81.22 Vestibular neuronitis, left ear
    H81.23 Vestibular neuronitis, bilateral
+ **H81.3 Other peripheral vertigo**
  + **H81.31 Aural vertigo**
    H81.311 Aural vertigo, right ear
    H81.312 Aural vertigo, left ear
    H81.313 Aural vertigo, bilateral
    H81.319 Aural vertigo, unspecified ear
  + **H81.39 Other peripheral vertigo**
    Lermoyez' syndrome
    Otogenic vertigo
    Peripheral vertigo NOS
    H81.391 Other peripheral vertigo, right ear
    H81.392 Other peripheral vertigo, left ear
    H81.393 Other peripheral vertigo, bilateral
    H81.399 Other peripheral vertigo, unspecified ear
H81.4 Vertigo of central origin
  Central positional nystagmus
  AHA CC: 4Q, 2019, 4
+ **H81.8 Other disorders of vestibular function**
  + **H81.8X Other disorders of vestibular function**
    H81.8X1 Other disorders of vestibular function, right ear
    H81.8X2 Other disorders of vestibular function, left ear
    H81.8X3 Other disorders of vestibular function, bilateral
    H81.8X9 Other disorders of vestibular function, unspecified ear
+ **H81.9 Unspecified disorder of vestibular function**
  Vertiginous syndrome NOS
    H81.90 Unspecified disorder of vestibular function, unspecified ear
    H81.91 Unspecified disorder of vestibular function, right ear
    H81.92 Unspecified disorder of vestibular function, left ear
    H81.93 Unspecified disorder of vestibular function, bilateral

H82 Vertiginous syndromes in diseases classified elsewhere

Code first underlying disease

Excludes1: epidemic vertigo (A88.1)

H82.1 Vertiginous syndromes in diseases classified elsewhere, right ear

H82.2 Vertiginous syndromes in diseases classified elsewhere, left ear

H82.3 Vertiginous syndromes in diseases classified elsewhere, bilateral

H82.9 Vertiginous syndromes in diseases classified elsewhere, unspecified ear

H83 Other diseases of inner ear

+ H83.0 **Labyrinthitis**

H83.01 Labyrinthitis, right ear

H83.02 Labyrinthitis, left ear

H83.03 Labyrinthitis, bilateral

H83.09 Labyrinthitis, unspecified ear

+ H83.1 **Labyrinthine fistula**

H83.11 Labyrinthine fistula, right ear

H83.12 Labyrinthine fistula, left ear

H83.13 Labyrinthine fistula, bilateral

H83.19 Labyrinthine fistula, unspecified ear

+ H83.2 **Labyrinthine dysfunction**

Labyrinthine hypersensitivity

Labyrinthine hypofunction

Labyrinthine loss of function

+ H83.2X **Labyrinthine dysfunction**

H83.2X1 Labyrinthine dysfunction, right ear

H83.2X2 Labyrinthine dysfunction, left ear

H83.2X3 Labyrinthine dysfunction, bilateral

H83.2X9 Labyrinthine dysfunction, unspecified ear

+ H83.3 **Noise effects on inner ear**

Acoustic trauma of inner ear

Noise-induced hearing loss of inner ear

+ H83.3X **Noise effects on inner ear**

H83.3X1 Noise effects on right inner ear

H83.3X2 Noise effects on left inner ear

H83.3X3 Noise effects on inner ear, bilateral

H83.3X9 Noise effects on inner ear, unspecified ear

+ H83.8 **Other specified diseases of inner ear**

+ H83.8X **Other specified diseases of inner ear**

H83.8X1 Other specified diseases of right inner ear

H83.8X2 Other specified diseases of left inner ear

H83.8X3 Other specified diseases of inner ear, bilateral

H83.8X9 Other specified diseases of inner ear, unspecified ear

+ H83.9 **Unspecified disease of inner ear**

H83.90 Unspecified disease of inner ear, unspecified ear

H83.91 Unspecified disease of right inner ear

H83.92 Unspecified disease of left inner ear

H83.93 Unspecified disease of inner ear, bilateral

Other disorders of ear (H90-H94)

H90 Conductive and sensorineural hearing loss

Excludes1: deaf nonspeaking NEC (H91.3)

deafness NOS (H91.9-)

hearing loss NOS (H91.9-)

noise-induced hearing loss (H83.3-)

ototoxic hearing loss (H91.0-)

sudden (idiopathic) hearing loss (H91.2-)

H90.0 Conductive hearing loss, bilateral

+ H90.1 **Conductive hearing loss, unilateral with unrestricted hearing on the contralateral side**

H90.11 Conductive hearing loss, unilateral, right ear, with unrestricted hearing on the contralateral side

H90.12 Conductive hearing loss, unilateral, left ear, with unrestricted hearing on the contralateral side

H90.2 Conductive hearing loss, unspecified

Conductive deafness NOS

H90.3 Sensorineural hearing loss, bilateral

+ H90.4 **Sensorineural hearing loss, unilateral with unrestricted hearing on the contralateral side**

H90.41 Sensorineural hearing loss, unilateral, right ear, with unrestricted hearing on the contralateral side

H90.42 Sensorineural hearing loss, unilateral, left ear, with unrestricted hearing on the contralateral side

H90.5 Unspecified sensorineural hearing loss

Central hearing loss NOS

Congenital deafness NOS

Neural hearing loss NOS

Perceptive hearing loss NOS

Sensorineural deafness NOS

Sensory hearing loss NOS

Excludes1: abnormal auditory perception (H93.2-)

psychogenic deafness (F44.6)

H90.6 Mixed conductive and sensorineural hearing loss, bilateral

AHA CC: 2Q, 2015, 7

+ H90.7 **Mixed conductive and sensorineural hearing loss, unilateral with unrestricted hearing on the contralateral side**

H90.71 Mixed conductive and sensorineural hearing loss, unilateral, right ear, with unrestricted hearing on the contralateral side

H90.72 Mixed conductive and sensorineural hearing loss, unilateral, left ear, with unrestricted hearing on the contralateral side

H90.8 Mixed conductive and sensorineural hearing loss, unspecified

+ H90.A **Conductive and sensorineural hearing loss with restricted hearing on the contralateral side**

AHA CC: 4Q, 2016, 23-24

+ H90.A1 **Conductive hearing loss, unilateral, with restricted hearing on the contralateral side**

H90.A11 Conductive hearing loss, unilateral, right ear with restricted hearing on the contralateral side

H90.A12 Conductive hearing loss, unilateral, left ear with restricted hearing on the contralateral side

AHA CC: 4Q, 2016, 24-25

+ H90.A2 **Sensorineural hearing loss, unilateral, with restricted hearing on the contralateral side**

H90.A21 Sensorineural hearing loss, unilateral, right ear, with restricted hearing on the contralateral side

AHA CC: 4Q, 2016, 24-25

H90.A22 Sensorineural hearing loss, unilateral, left ear, with restricted hearing on the contralateral side

+ H90.A3 **Mixed conductive and sensorineural hearing loss, unilateral with restricted hearing on the contralateral side**

H90.A31 Mixed conductive and sensorineural hearing loss, unilateral, right ear with restricted hearing on the contralateral side

H90.A32 Mixed conductive and sensorineural hearing, unilateral, left ear with restricted hearing on the contralateral side

H91 Other and unspecified hearing loss

Excludes1: abnormal auditory perception (H93.2-)

hearing loss as classified in H90.-

impacted cerumen (H61.2-)

noise-induced hearing loss (H83.3-)

psychogenic deafness (F44.6)

transient ischemic deafness (H93.01-)

+, +7th, X + 7th   ● Newborn   ● Pediatric   ● Maternity   ● Adult   ♀ Female   ♂ Male   Manifestation   Unacceptable PDX   HCC   CC   MCC   HAC

+ **H91.0** **Ototoxic hearing loss**

    Code first poisoning due to drug or toxin, if applicable
(T36-T65 with fifth or sixth character 1-4 or 6)

    Use additional code for adverse effect, if applicable, to
identify drug (T36-T50 with fifth or sixth character 5)

    H91.01 **Ototoxic hearing loss, right ear**
    H91.02 **Ototoxic hearing loss, left ear**
    H91.03 **Ototoxic hearing loss, bilateral**
    H91.09 **Ototoxic hearing loss, unspecified ear**

+ **H91.1** **Presbycusis**
    Presbyacusia
    H91.10 **Presbycusis, unspecified ear**
    H91.11 **Presbycusis, right ear**
    H91.12 **Presbycusis, left ear**
    H91.13 **Presbycusis, bilateral**

+ **H91.2** **Sudden idiopathic hearing loss**
    Sudden hearing loss NOS
    H91.20 **Sudden idiopathic hearing loss, unspecified ear**
    H91.21 **Sudden idiopathic hearing loss, right ear**
    H91.22 **Sudden idiopathic hearing loss, left ear**
    H91.23 **Sudden idiopathic hearing loss, bilateral**

H91.3 **Deaf nonspeaking, not elsewhere classified**

+ **H91.8** **Other specified hearing loss**
  + **H91.8X** **Other specified hearing loss**
    H91.8X1 **Other specified hearing loss, right ear**
    H91.8X2 **Other specified hearing loss, left ear**
    H91.8X3 **Other specified hearing loss, bilateral**
    H91.8X9 **Other specified hearing loss, unspecified ear**

+ **H91.9** **Unspecified hearing loss**
    Deafness NOS
    High frequency deafness
    Low frequency deafness
    H91.90 **Unspecified hearing loss, unspecified ear**
    H91.91 **Unspecified hearing loss, right ear**
    H91.92 **Unspecified hearing loss, left ear**
    H91.93 **Unspecified hearing loss, bilateral**

H92 **Otalgia and effusion of ear**

+ **H92.0** **Otalgia**
    H92.01 **Otalgia, right ear**
    H92.02 **Otalgia, left ear**
    H92.03 **Otalgia, bilateral**
    H92.09 **Otalgia, unspecified ear**

+ **H92.1** **Otorrhea**
    Excludes1: *leakage of cerebrospinal fluid through ear
(G96.0)*
    H92.10 **Otorrhea, unspecified ear**
    H92.11 **Otorrhea, right ear**
    H92.12 **Otorrhea, left ear**
    H92.13 **Otorrhea, bilateral**

+ **H92.2** **Otorrhagia**
    Excludes1: *traumatic otorrhagia - code to injury*
    H92.20 **Otorrhagia, unspecified ear**
    H92.21 **Otorrhagia, right ear**
    H92.22 **Otorrhagia, left ear**
    H92.23 **Otorrhagia, bilateral**

H93 **Other disorders of ear, not elsewhere classified**

+ **H93.0** **Degenerative and vascular disorders of ear**
    Excludes1: presbycusis (H91.1)
  + **H93.01** **Transient ischemic deafness**
    H93.011 **Transient ischemic deafness, right ear**
    H93.012 **Transient ischemic deafness, left ear**
    H93.013 **Transient ischemic deafness, bilateral**
    H93.019 **Transient ischemic deafness, unspecified ear**
  + **H93.09** **Unspecified degenerative and vascular disorders of ear**
    H93.091 **Unspecified degenerative and vascular disorders of right ear**
    H93.092 **Unspecified degenerative and vascular disorders of left ear**
    H93.093 **Unspecified degenerative and vascular disorders of ear, bilateral**
    H93.099 **Unspecified degenerative and vascular disorders of unspecified ear**

+ **H93.1** **Tinnitus**
    H93.11 **Tinnitus, right ear**
    H93.12 **Tinnitus, left ear**
    H93.13 **Tinnitus, bilateral**
    H93.19 **Tinnitus, unspecified ear**

+ **H93.A** **Pulsatile tinnitus**
    AHA CC: 4Q, 2016, 25-26
    H93.A1 **Pulsatile tinnitus, right ear**
    AHA CC: 4Q, 2016, 26
    H93.A2 **Pulsatile tinnitus, left ear**
    H93.A3 **Pulsatile tinnitus, bilateral**
    H93.A9 **Pulsatile tinnitus, unspecified ear**

+ **H93.2** **Other abnormal auditory perceptions**
    Excludes2: *auditory hallucinations (R44.0)*
  + **H93.21** **Auditory recruitment**
    H93.211 **Auditory recruitment, right ear**
    H93.212 **Auditory recruitment, left ear**
    H93.213 **Auditory recruitment, bilateral**
    H93.219 **Auditory recruitment, unspecified ear**
  + **H93.22** **Diplacusis**
    H93.221 **Diplacusis, right ear**
    H93.222 **Diplacusis, left ear**
    H93.223 **Diplacusis, bilateral**
    H93.229 **Diplacusis, unspecified ear**
  + **H93.23** **Hyperacusis**
    H93.231 **Hyperacusis, right ear**
    H93.232 **Hyperacusis, left ear**
    H93.233 **Hyperacusis, bilateral**
    H93.239 **Hyperacusis, unspecified ear**
  + **H93.24** **Temporary auditory threshold shift**
    H93.241 **Temporary auditory threshold shift, right ear**
    H93.242 **Temporary auditory threshold shift, left ear**
    H93.243 **Temporary auditory threshold shift, bilateral**
    H93.249 **Temporary auditory threshold shift, unspecified ear**
  H93.25 **Central auditory processing disorder**
    Congenital auditory imperception
    Word deafness
    Excludes1: *mixed receptive-expressive language disorder (F80.2)*
  + **H93.29** **Other abnormal auditory perceptions**
    H93.291 **Other abnormal auditory perceptions, right ear**
    H93.292 **Other abnormal auditory perceptions, left ear**
    H93.293 **Other abnormal auditory perceptions, bilateral**
    H93.299 **Other abnormal auditory perceptions, unspecified ear**

+ **H93.3** **Disorders of acoustic nerve**
    Disorder of 8th cranial nerve
    Excludes1: *acoustic neuroma (D33.3)*
    syphilitic acoustic neuritis (A52.15)
  + **H93.3X** **Disorders of acoustic nerve**
    H93.3X1 **Disorders of right acoustic nerve**
    H93.3X2 **Disorders of left acoustic nerve**
    H93.3X3 **Disorders of bilateral acoustic nerves**
    H93.3X9 **Disorders of unspecified acoustic nerve**

+ **H93.8** **Other specified disorders of ear**
  + **H93.8X** **Other specified disorders of ear**
    H93.8X1 **Other specified disorders of right ear**
    H93.8X2 **Other specified disorders of left ear**
    H93.8X3 **Other specified disorders of ear, bilateral**
    H93.8X9 **Other specified disorders of ear, unspecified ear**

+ **H93.9** **Unspecified disorder of ear**
    H93.90 **Unspecified disorder of ear, unspecified ear**
    H93.91 **Unspecified disorder of right ear**
    H93.92 **Unspecified disorder of left ear**
    H93.93 **Unspecified disorder of ear, bilateral**

+, +7th, X + 7th   ● Newborn   ● Pediatric   ● Maternity   ● Adult   ♀ Female   ♂ Male   Manifestation   Unacceptable PDX   HCC   CC   MCC   HAC

H94 Other disorders of ear in diseases classified elsewhere

+ **H94.0 Acoustic neuritis in infectious and parasitic diseases classified elsewhere**

Code first underlying disease, such as:
parasitic disease (B65-B89)

Excludes1: *acoustic neuritis (in):*
herpes zoster (B02.29)
syphilis (A52.15)

H94.00 Acoustic neuritis in infectious and parasitic diseases classified elsewhere, unspecified ear

H94.01 Acoustic neuritis in infectious and parasitic diseases classified elsewhere, right ear

H94.02 Acoustic neuritis in infectious and parasitic diseases classified elsewhere, left ear

H94.03 Acoustic neuritis in infectious and parasitic diseases classified elsewhere, bilateral

+ **H94.8 Other specified disorders of ear in diseases classified elsewhere**

Code first underlying disease, such as:
congenital syphilis (A50.0)

Excludes1: *aural myiasis (B87.4)*
syphilitic labyrinthitis (A52.79)

H94.80 Other specified disorders of ear in diseases classified elsewhere, unspecified ear

H94.81 Other specified disorders of right ear in diseases classified elsewhere

H94.82 Other specified disorders of left ear in diseases classified elsewhere

H94.83 Other specified disorders of ear in diseases classified elsewhere, bilateral

Intraoperative and postprocedural complications and disorders of ear and mastoid process, not elsewhere classified (H95)

H95 Intraoperative and postprocedural complications and disorders of ear and mastoid process, not elsewhere classified

AHA CC: 4Q, 2016, 9-10

+ **H95.0 Recurrent cholesteatoma of postmastoidectomy cavity**

H95.00 Recurrent cholesteatoma of postmastoidectomy cavity, unspecified ear

H95.01 Recurrent cholesteatoma of postmastoidectomy cavity, right ear

H95.02 Recurrent cholesteatoma of postmastoidectomy cavity, left ear

H95.03 Recurrent cholesteatoma of postmastoidectomy cavity, bilateral ears

+ **H95.1 Other disorders of ear and mastoid process following mastoidectomy**

+ **H95.11 Chronic inflammation of postmastoidectomy cavity**

H95.111 Chronic inflammation of postmastoidectomy cavity, right ear

H95.112 Chronic inflammation of postmastoidectomy cavity, left ear

H95.113 Chronic inflammation of postmastoidectomy cavity, bilateral ears

H95.119 Chronic inflammation of postmastoidectomy cavity, unspecified ear

+ **H95.12 Granulation of postmastoidectomy cavity**

H95.121 Granulation of postmastoidectomy cavity, right ear

H95.122 Granulation of postmastoidectomy cavity, left ear

H95.123 Granulation of postmastoidectomy cavity, bilateral ears

H95.129 Granulation of postmastoidectomy cavity, unspecified ear

+ **H95.13 Mucosal cyst of postmastoidectomy cavity**

H95.131 Mucosal cyst of postmastoidectomy cavity, right ear

H95.132 Mucosal cyst of postmastoidectomy cavity, left ear

H95.133 Mucosal cyst of postmastoidectomy cavity, bilateral ears

H95.139 Mucosal cyst of postmastoidectomy cavity, unspecified ear

+ **H95.19 Other disorders following mastoidectomy**

H95.191 Other disorders following mastoidectomy, right ear

H95.192 Other disorders following mastoidectomy, left ear

H95.193 Other disorders following mastoidectomy, bilateral ears

H95.199 Other disorders following mastoidectomy, unspecified ear

+ **H95.2 Intraoperative hemorrhage and hematoma of ear and mastoid process complicating a procedure**

Excludes1: *intraoperative hemorrhage and hematoma of ear and mastoid process due to accidental puncture or laceration during a procedure (H95.3-)*

CC **H95.21 Intraoperative hemorrhage and hematoma of ear and mastoid process complicating a procedure on the ear and mastoid process**

CC **H95.22 Intraoperative hemorrhage and hematoma of ear and mastoid process complicating other procedure**

+ **H95.3 Accidental puncture and laceration of ear and mastoid process during a procedure**

CC **H95.31 Accidental puncture and laceration of the ear and mastoid process during a procedure on the ear and mastoid process**

CC **H95.32 Accidental puncture and laceration of the ear and mastoid process during other procedure**

+ **H95.4 Postprocedural hemorrhage of ear and mastoid process following a procedure**

CC **H95.41 Postprocedural hemorrhage of ear and mastoid process following a procedure on the ear and mastoid process**

CC **H95.42 Postprocedural hemorrhage of ear and mastoid process following other procedure**

+ **H95.5 Postprocedural hematoma and seroma of ear and mastoid process following a procedure**

CC **H95.51 Postprocedural hematoma of ear and mastoid process following a procedure on the ear and mastoid process**

CC **H95.52 Postprocedural hematoma of ear and mastoid process following other procedure**

CC **H95.53 Postprocedureal seroma of ear and mastoid process following a procedure on the ear and mastoid process**

CC **H95.54 Postprocedureal seroma of ear and mastoid process following other procedure**

+ **H95.8 Other intraoperative and postprocedural complications and disorders of the ear and mastoid process, not elsewhere classified**

Excludes2: *postprocedural complications and disorders following mastoidectomy (H95.0-, H95.1-)*

+ **H95.81 Postprocedural stenosis of external ear canal**

CC **H95.811 Postprocedural stenosis of right external ear canal**

CC **H95.812 Postprocedural stenosis of left external ear canal**

CC **H95.813 Postprocedural stenosis of external ear canal, bilateral**

CC **H95.819 Postprocedural stenosis of unspecified external ear canal**

CC **H95.88 Other intraoperative complications and disorders of the ear and mastoid process, not elsewhere classified**

Use additional code, if applicable, to further specify disorder

CC **H95.89 Other postprocedural complications and disorders of the ear and mastoid process, not elsewhere classified**

Use additional code, if applicable, to further specify disorder

+, +7th, X + 7th ● Newborn ● Pediatric ● Maternity ● Adult ♀ Female ♂ Male Manifestation Unacceptable PDX HCC CC MCC HAC

Chapter 9: Diseases of the Circulatory System (I00-I99)

Excludes2: *certain conditions originating in the perinatal period (P04-P96)*
certain infectious and parasitic diseases (A00-B99)
complications of pregnancy, childbirth and the puerperium (O00-O9A)
congenital malformations, deformations, and chromosomal abnormalities (Q00-Q99)
endocrine, nutritional and metabolic diseases (E00-E88)
injury, poisoning and certain other consequences of external causes (S00-T88)
neoplasms (C00-D49)
symptoms, signs and abnormal clinical and laboratory findings, not elsewhere classified (R00-R94)
systemic connective tissue disorders (M30-M36)
transient cerebral ischemic attacks and related syndromes (G45.-)

This chapter contains the following category blocks:

I00-I02 Acute rheumatic fever
I05-I09 Chronic rheumatic heart diseases
I10-I16 Hypertensive diseases
I20-I25 Ischemic heart diseases
I26-I28 Pulmonary heart disease and diseases of pulmonary circulation
I30-I52 Other forms of heart disease
I60-I69 Cerebrovascular diseases
I70-I79 Diseases of arteries, arterioles and capillaries
I80-I89 Diseases of veins, lymphatic vessels and lymph nodes, not elsewhere classified
I95-I99 Other and unspecified disorders of the circulatory system

C. Chapter-Specific Coding Guidelines

In addition to general coding guidelines, there are guidelines for specific diagnoses and/or conditions in the classification. Unless otherwise indicated, these guidelines apply to all health care settings. Please refer to Section II for guidelines on the selection of principal diagnosis.

9. Chapter 9: Diseases of the Circulatory System (I00-I99)

a. Hypertension

The classification presumes a causal relationship between hypertension and heart involvement and between hypertension and kidney involvement, as the two conditions are linked by the term "with" in the Alphabetic Index. These conditions should be coded as related even in the absence of provider documentation explicitly linking them, unless the documentation clearly states the conditions are unrelated.

For hypertension and conditions not specifically linked by relational terms such as "with," "associated with" or "due to" in the classification, provider documentation must link the conditions in order to code them as related.

1) Hypertension with Heart Disease

Hypertension with heart conditions classified to I50.- or I51.4-I51.7, I51.89, I51.9, are assigned to, a code from category I11, Hypertensive heart disease. Use an additional code(s) from category I50, Heart failure, to identify the type(s) of heart failure in those patients with heart failure.

The same heart conditions (I50.-, I51.4-I51.7, I51.89, I51.9) with hypertension are coded separately if the provider has documented they are unrelated to the hypertension. Sequence according to the circumstances of the admission/encounter.

2) Hypertensive Chronic Kidney Disease

Assign codes from category I12, Hypertensive chronic kidney disease, when both hypertension and a condition classifiable to category N18, Chronic kidney disease (CKD), are present. CKD should not be coded as hypertensive if the provider indicates the CKD is not related to the hypertension.

The appropriate code from category N18 should be used as a secondary code with a code from category I12 to identify the stage of chronic kidney disease.

See Section I.C.14. Chronic kidney disease.

If a patient has hypertensive chronic kidney disease and acute renal failure, **the acute renal failure should also be coded. Sequence according to the circumstances of the admission/encounter.**

3) Hypertensive Heart and Chronic Kidney Disease

Assign codes from combination category I13, Hypertensive heart and chronic kidney disease, when there is hypertension with both heart and kidney involvement. If heart failure is present, assign an additional code from category I50 to identify the type of heart failure.

The appropriate code from category N18, Chronic kidney disease, should be used as a secondary code with a code from category I13 to identify the stage of chronic kidney disease.

See Section I.C.14. Chronic kidney disease.

The codes in category I13, Hypertensive heart and chronic kidney disease, are combination codes that include hypertension, heart disease and chronic kidney disease. The Includes note at I13 specifies that the conditions included at I11 and I12 are included together in I13. If a patient has hypertension, heart disease and chronic kidney disease then a code from I13 should be used, not individual codes for hypertension, heart disease and chronic kidney disease, or codes from I11 or I12.

For patients with both acute renal failure and chronic kidney disease **the acute renal failure should also be coded. Sequence according to the circumstances of the admission/encounter.**

4) Hypertensive Cerebrovascular Disease

For hypertensive cerebrovascular disease, first assign the appropriate code from categories I60-I69, followed by the appropriate hypertension code.

5) Hypertensive Retinopathy

Subcategory H35.0, Background retinopathy and retinal vascular changes, should be used with a code from category I10 – I15, Hypertensive disease to include the systemic hypertension. The sequencing is based on the reason for the encounter.

6) Hypertension, Secondary

Secondary hypertension is due to an underlying condition. Two codes are required: one to identify the underlying etiology and one from category I15 to identify the hypertension. Sequencing of codes is determined by the reason for admission/encounter.

7) Hypertension, Transient

Assign code R03.0, Elevated blood pressure reading without diagnosis of hypertension, unless patient has an established diagnosis of hypertension. Assign code O13.-, Gestational [pregnancy-induced] hypertension without significant proteinuria, or O14.-, Pre-eclampsia, for transient hypertension of pregnancy.

8) Hypertension, Controlled

This diagnostic statement usually refers to an existing state of hypertension under control by therapy. Assign the appropriate code from categories I10-I15, Hypertensive diseases.

9) Hypertension, Uncontrolled

Uncontrolled hypertension may refer to untreated hypertension or hypertension not responding to current therapeutic regimen. In either case, assign the appropriate code from categories I10-I15, Hypertensive diseases.

10) Hypertensive Crisis

Assign a code from category I16, Hypertensive crisis, for documented hypertensive urgency, hypertensive emergency or unspecified hypertensive crisis. Code also any identified hypertensive disease (I10-I15). The sequencing is based on the reason for the encounter.

11) Pulmonary Hypertension

Pulmonary hypertension is classified to category I27, Other pulmonary heart diseases. For secondary pulmonary hypertension (I27.1, I27.2-), code also any associated conditions or adverse effects of drugs or toxins. The sequencing is based on the reason for the encounter, except for adverse effects of drugs (See Section I.C.19.e).

b. Atherosclerotic Coronary Artery Disease and Angina

ICD-10-CM has combination codes for atherosclerotic heart disease with angina pectoris. The subcategories for these codes are I25.11, Atherosclerotic heart disease of native coronary artery with angina pectoris and I25.7, Atherosclerosis of coronary artery bypass graft(s) and coronary artery of transplanted heart with angina pectoris.

When using one of these combination codes it is not necessary to use an additional code for angina pectoris. A causal relationship can be assumed in a patient with both atherosclerosis and angina pectoris, unless the documentation indicates the angina is due to something other than the atherosclerosis.

If a patient with coronary artery disease is admitted due to an acute myocardial infarction (AMI), the AMI should be sequenced before the coronary artery disease.

See Section I.C.9. Acute myocardial infarction (AMI)

c. Intraoperative and Postprocedural Cerebrovascular Accident

Medical record documentation should clearly specify the cause- and-effect relationship between the medical intervention and the cerebrovascular accident in order to assign a code for intraoperative or postprocedural cerebrovascular accident.

Proper code assignment depends on whether it was an infarction or hemorrhage and whether it occurred intraoperatively or postoperatively. If it was a cerebral hemorrhage, code assignment depends on the type of procedure performed.

d. Sequelae of Cerebrovascular Disease

1) Category I69, Sequelae of Cerebrovascular disease

Category I69 is used to indicate conditions classifiable to categories I60-I67 as the causes of sequela (neurologic deficits), themselves classified elsewhere. These "late effects" include neurologic deficits that persist after initial onset of conditions classifiable to categories I60-I67. The neurologic deficits caused by cerebrovascular disease may be present from the onset or may arise at any time after the onset of the condition classifiable to categories I60-I67.

Codes from category I69, Sequelae of cerebrovascular disease, that specify hemiplegia, hemiparesis and monoplegia identify whether the dominant or nondominant side is affected. Should the affected side be documented, but not specified as dominant or nondominant, and the classification system does not indicate a default, code selection is as follows:

- For ambidextrous patients, the default should be dominant.
- If the left side is affected, the default is non-dominant.
- If the right side is affected, the default is dominant.

2) Codes from category I69 with codes from I60-I67

Codes from category I69 may be assigned on a health care record with codes from I60-I67, if the patient has a current cerebrovascular disease and deficits from an old cerebrovascular disease.

3) Codes from category I69 and Personal history of transient ischemic attack (TIA) and cerebral infarction (Z86.73)

Codes from category I69 should not be assigned if the patient does not have neurologic deficits.

See Section I.C.21. 4. History (of) for use of personal history codes

e. Acute myocardial infarction (AMI)

1) ST elevation myocardial infarction (STEMI) and non ST elevation myocardial infarction (NSTEMI)

The ICD-10-CM codes for type 1 acute myocardial infarction (AMI) identify the site, such as anterolateral wall or true posterior wall. Subcategories I21.0-I21.2 and code I21.3 are used for type 1 ST elevation myocardial infarction (STEMI). Code I21.4, Non-ST elevation (NSTEMI) myocardial infarction, is used for type 1 non ST elevation myocardial infarction (NSTEMI) and nontransmural MIs.

If a type 1 NSTEMI evolves to STEMI, assign the STEMI code. If a type 1 STEMI converts to NSTEMI due to thrombolytic therapy, it is still coded as STEMI.

For encounters occurring while the myocardial infarction is equal to, or less than, four weeks old, including transfers to another acute setting or a postacute setting, and the myocardial infarction meets the definition for "other diagnoses" (see Section III, Reporting Additional Diagnoses), codes from category I21 may continue to be reported. For encounters after the 4 week time frame and the patient is still receiving care related to the myocardial infarction, the appropriate aftercare code should be assigned, rather than a code from category I21. For old or healed myocardial infarctions not requiring further care, code I25.2, Old myocardial infarction, may be assigned.

2) Acute myocardial infarction, unspecified

Code I21.9, Acute myocardial infarction, unspecified, is the default for unspecified acute myocardial infarction or unspecified type. If only type 1 STEMI or transmural MI without the site is documented, assign code I21.3, ST elevation (STEMI) myocardial infarction of unspecified site.

3) AMI documented as nontransmural or subendocardial but site provided

If an AMI is documented as nontransmural or subendocardial, but the site is provided, it is still coded as a subendocardial AMI.

See Section I.C.21.3 for information on coding status post administration of tPA in a different facility within the last 24 hours.

4) Subsequent acute myocardial infarction

A code from category I22, Subsequent ST elevation (STEMI) and non-ST elevation (NSTEMI) myocardial infarction, is to be used when a patient who has suffered a type 1 or unspecified AMI has a new AMI within the 4 week time frame of the initial AMI. A code from category I22 must be used in conjunction with a code from category I21. The sequencing of the I22 and I21 codes depends on the circumstances of the encounter.

Do not assign code I22 for subsequent myocardial infarctions other than type 1 or unspecified. For subsequent type 2 AMI assign only code I21. A1. For subsequent type 4 or type 5 AMI, assign only code I21.A9.

If a subsequent myocardial infarction of one type occurs within 4 weeks of a myocardial infarction of a different type, assign the appropriate codes from category I21 to identify each type. Do not assign a code from I22. Codes from category I22 should only be assigned if both the initial and subsequent myocardial infarctions are type 1 or unspecified.

5) Other Types of Myocardial Infarction

The ICD-10-CM provides codes for different types of myocardial infarction. Type 1 myocardial infarctions are assigned to codes I21.0-I21.4.

Type 2 myocardial infarction (myocardial infarction due to demand ischemia or secondary to ischemic imbalance) is assigned to code I21. A1, Myocardial infarction type 2 with the underlying cause coded first. Do not assign code I24.8, Other forms of acute ischemic heart disease, for the demand ischemia. If a type 2 AMI is described as NSTEMI or STEMI, only assign code I21.A1. Codes I21.0-I21.4 should only be assigned for type 1 AMIs.

Acute myocardial infarctions type 3, 4a, 4b, 4c and 5 are assigned to code I21.A9, Other myocardial infarction type.

The "Code also" and "Code first" notes should be followed related to complications, and for coding of postprocedural myocardial infarctions during or following cardiac surgery.

Acute rheumatic fever (I00-I02)

I00 Rheumatic fever without heart involvement

> **Includes:** arthritis, rheumatic, acute or subacute
> ***Excludes1:*** *rheumatic fever with heart involvement (I01.0-I01.9)*
> Valid 3-character code, no further characters required

I01 Rheumatic fever with heart involvement

> ***Excludes1:*** *chronic diseases of rheumatic origin (I05-I09) unless rheumatic fever is also present or there is evidence of reactivation or activity of the rheumatic process.*

CC I01.0 Acute rheumatic pericarditis
> Any condition in I00 with pericarditis
> Rheumatic pericarditis (acute)
> ***Excludes1:*** *acute pericarditis not specified as rheumatic (I30.-)*

CC I01.1 Acute rheumatic endocarditis
> Any condition in I00 with endocarditis or valvulitis
> Acute rheumatic valvulitis

CC I01.2 Acute rheumatic myocarditis
> Any condition in I00 with myocarditis

CC I01.8 Other acute rheumatic heart disease
> Any condition in I00 with other or multiple types of heart involvement
> Acute rheumatic pancarditis

CC I01.9 Acute rheumatic heart disease, unspecified
> Any condition in I00 with unspecified type of heart involvement
> Rheumatic carditis, acute
> Rheumatic heart disease, active or acute

I02 Rheumatic chorea

> **Includes:** Sydenham's chorea
> ***Excludes1:*** *chorea NOS (G25.5)*
> *Huntington's chorea (G10)*

CC I02.0 Rheumatic chorea with heart involvement
> Chorea NOS with heart involvement
> Rheumatic chorea with heart involvement of any type classifiable under I01.-

CC I02.9 Rheumatic chorea without heart involvement
> Rheumatic chorea NOS

+, +7th, X + 7th   ● Newborn   ● Pediatric   ● Maternity   ● Adult   ♀ Female   ♂ Male   Manifestation   Unacceptable PDX   HCC   CC   MCC   HAC

Atria, Ventricles, and Interventricular Septum

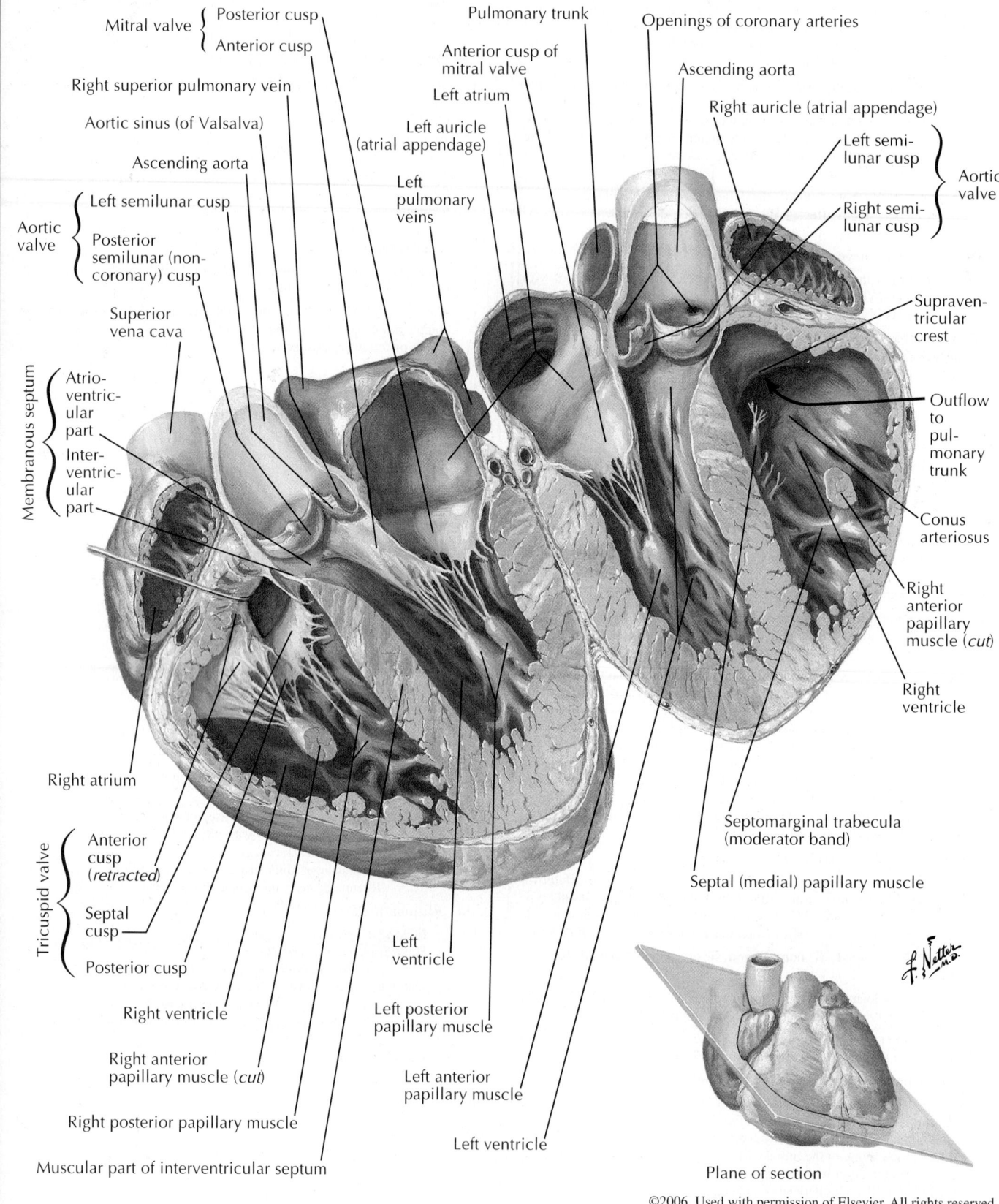

Mitral valve { Posterior cusp / Anterior cusp

Right superior pulmonary vein

Aortic sinus (of Valsalva)

Ascending aorta

Aortic valve { Left semilunar cusp / Posterior semilunar (non-coronary) cusp

Superior vena cava

Membranous septum { Atrio-ventricular part / Inter-ventricular part

Right atrium

Tricuspid valve { Anterior cusp (retracted) / Septal cusp / Posterior cusp

Right ventricle

Right anterior papillary muscle (cut)

Right posterior papillary muscle

Muscular part of interventricular septum

Pulmonary trunk

Anterior cusp of mitral valve

Left atrium

Left auricle (atrial appendage)

Left pulmonary veins

Left ventricle

Left posterior papillary muscle

Left anterior papillary muscle

Left ventricle

Openings of coronary arteries

Ascending aorta

Right auricle (atrial appendage)

Left semilunar cusp / Right semilunar cusp } Aortic valve

Supraventricular crest

Outflow to pulmonary trunk

Conus arteriosus

Right anterior papillary muscle (cut)

Right ventricle

Septomarginal trabecula (moderator band)

Septal (medial) papillary muscle

Plane of section

Veins

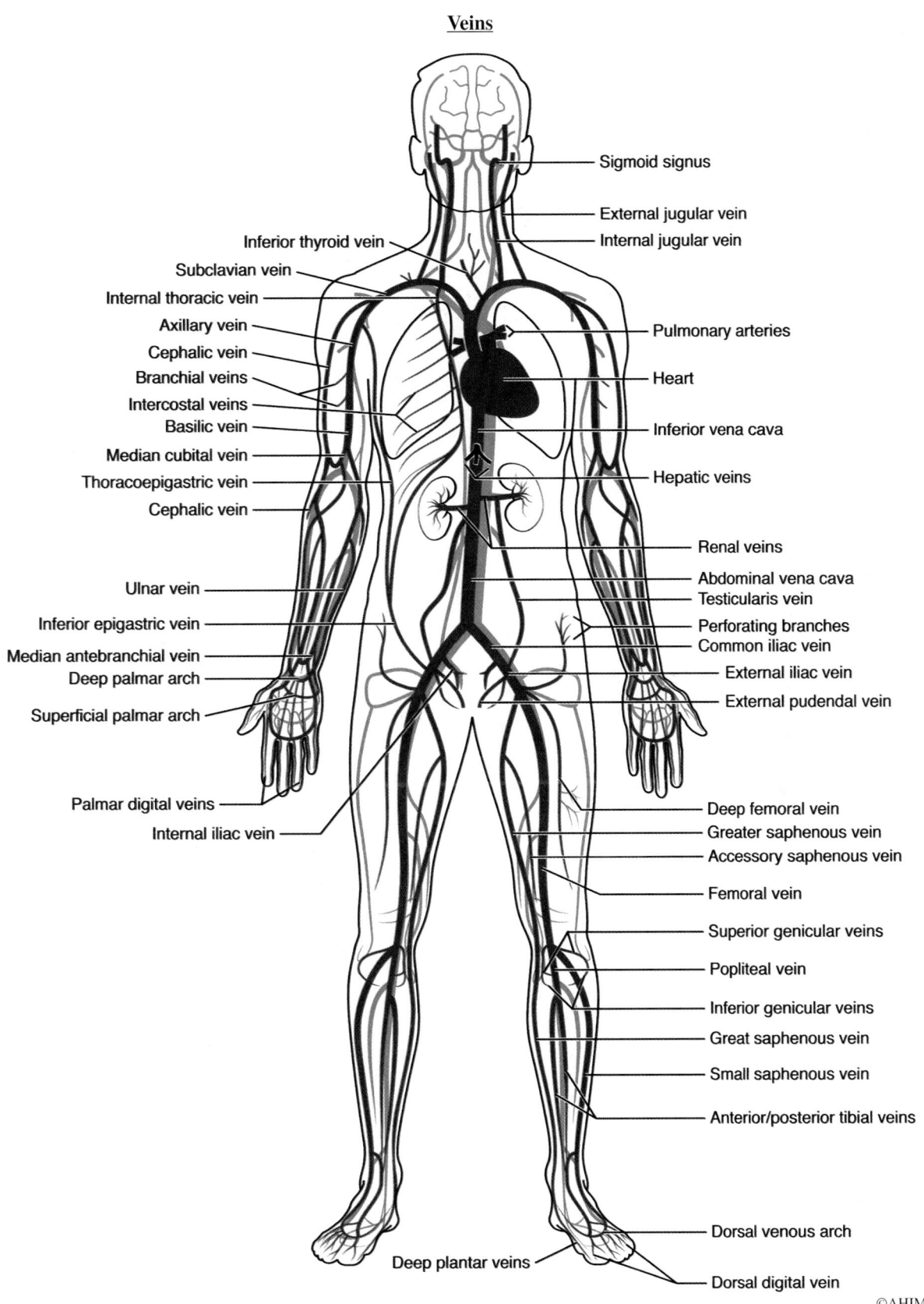

Sigmoid signus

External jugular vein

Internal jugular vein

Inferior thyroid vein

Subclavian vein

Internal thoracic vein

Axillary vein

Cephalic vein

Branchial veins

Intercostal veins

Basilic vein

Median cubital vein

Thoracoepigastric vein

Cephalic vein

Pulmonary arteries

Heart

Inferior vena cava

Hepatic veins

Renal veins

Abdominal vena cava

Testicularis vein

Perforating branches

Common iliac vein

External iliac vein

External pudendal vein

Ulnar vein

Inferior epigastric vein

Median antebranchial vein

Deep palmar arch

Superficial palmar arch

Palmar digital veins

Internal iliac vein

Deep femoral vein

Greater saphenous vein

Accessory saphenous vein

Femoral vein

Superior genicular veins

Popliteal vein

Inferior genicular veins

Great saphenous vein

Small saphenous vein

Anterior/posterior tibial veins

Dorsal venous arch

Deep plantar veins

Dorsal digital vein

©AHIMA

Anterior cerebral artery

Right middle cerebral artery

Basilar artery

Posterior cerebral artery

External carotid artery

Internal carotid artery

Vertebral arteries

Common carotid arteries

Aortic arch

Subclavian artery

Axillary artery

Pulmonary veins

Internal thoracic artery

Intercostal arteries

Branchial artery

Heart

Deep branchial artery

Left gastric artery

Radial recurrent artery

Celiac trunk

Common hepatic artery

Splenic artery

Right gastric artery

Superior mesenteric artery

Superior epigastric artery

Renal artery

Descending aorta

Interosseous artery

Radial artery

Inferior mesenteric artery

Inferior epigastric artery

Testicularis artery

Ulnar artery

Common iliac artery

Palmar carpal arch

External iliac artery

Dorsal carpal arch

Internal iliac artery

Superficial/Deep palmar arches

Femoral circumflex artery

Digital artery

Descending branch of the femoral circumflex artery

Perforating branches

Descending genicular artery

Deep femoral artery

Superior genicular arteries

Femoral artery

Popliteal artery

Inferior genicular arteries

Anterior tibial artery

Peroneal artery

Posterior tibial artery

Deep plantar arch

Dorsal metatarsal artery

Arcuate artery

Dorsal digital arteries

©AHIMA

Chronic rheumatic heart diseases (I05-I09)

I05   **Rheumatic mitral valve diseases**

     Includes: conditions classifiable to both I05.0 and I05.2-I05.9, whether specified as rheumatic or not

     Excludes1: *mitral valve disease specified as nonrheumatic (I34.-)*
         mitral valve disease with aortic and/or tricuspid valve involvement (I08.-)

   I05.0   **Rheumatic mitral stenosis**
       Mitral (valve) obstruction (rheumatic)

   I05.1   **Rheumatic mitral insufficiency**
       Rheumatic mitral incompetence
       Rheumatic mitral regurgitation
       Excludes1: *mitral insufficiency not specified as rheumatic (I34.0)*

   I05.2   **Rheumatic mitral stenosis with insufficiency**
       Rheumatic mitral stenosis with incompetence or regurgitation

   I05.8   **Other rheumatic mitral valve diseases**
       Rheumatic mitral (valve) failure

   I05.9   **Rheumatic mitral valve disease, unspecified**
       Rheumatic mitral (valve) disorder (chronic) NOS

I06   **Rheumatic aortic valve diseases**

     Excludes1: *aortic valve disease not specified as rheumatic (I35.-)*
         aortic valve disease with mitral and/or tricuspid valve involvement (I08.-)

   I06.0   **Rheumatic aortic stenosis**
       Rheumatic aortic (valve) obstruction

   I06.1   **Rheumatic aortic insufficiency**
       Rheumatic aortic incompetence
       Rheumatic aortic regurgitation

   I06.2   **Rheumatic aortic stenosis with insufficiency**
       Rheumatic aortic stenosis with incompetence or regurgitation

   I06.8   **Other rheumatic aortic valve diseases**

   I06.9   **Rheumatic aortic valve disease, unspecified**
       Rheumatic aortic (valve) disease NOS

I07   **Rheumatic tricuspid valve diseases**

     Includes: rheumatic tricuspid valve diseases specified as rheumatic or unspecified

     Excludes1: *tricuspid valve disease specified as nonrheumatic (I36.-)*
         tricuspid valve disease with aortic and/or mitral valve involvement (I08.-)

   I07.0   **Rheumatic tricuspid stenosis**
       Tricuspid (valve) stenosis (rheumatic)

   I07.1   **Rheumatic tricuspid insufficiency**
       Tricuspid (valve) insufficiency (rheumatic)

   I07.2   **Rheumatic tricuspid stenosis and insufficiency**

   I07.8   **Other rheumatic tricuspid valve diseases**

   I07.9   **Rheumatic tricuspid valve disease, unspecified**
       Rheumatic tricuspid valve disorder NOS

I08   **Multiple valve diseases**

     Includes: multiple valve diseases specified as rheumatic or unspecified

     Excludes1: *endocarditis, valve unspecified (I38)*
         multiple valve disease specified a nonrheumatic (I34.-, I35.-, I36.-, I37.-, I38.-, Q22.-, Q23.-, Q24.8-)
         rheumatic valve disease NOS (I09.1)

   I08.0   **Rheumatic disorders of both mitral and aortic valves**
       Involvement of both mitral and aortic valves specified as rheumatic or unspecified
       AHA CC: 2Q, 2019, 5

   I08.1   **Rheumatic disorders of both mitral and tricuspid valves**

   I08.2   **Rheumatic disorders of both aortic and tricuspid valves**

   I08.3   **Combined rheumatic disorders of mitral, aortic and tricuspid valves**

   I08.8   **Other rheumatic multiple valve diseases**

   I08.9   **Rheumatic multiple valve disease, unspecified**

I09   **Other rheumatic heart diseases**

CC **I09.0**   **Rheumatic myocarditis**
       Excludes1: *myocarditis not specified as rheumatic (I51.4)*

   I09.1   **Rheumatic diseases of endocardium, valve unspecified**
       Rheumatic endocarditis (chronic)
       Rheumatic valvulitis (chronic)
       Excludes1: *endocarditis, valve unspecified (I38)*

CC **I09.2**   **Chronic rheumatic pericarditis**
       Adherent pericardium, rheumatic
       Chronic rheumatic mediastinopericarditis
       Chronic rheumatic myopericarditis
       Excludes1: *chronic pericarditis not specified as rheumatic (I31.-)*

\+ **I09.8**   **Other specified rheumatic heart diseases**

     CC **I09.81**   **Rheumatic heart failure**
         Use additional code to identify type of heart failure (I50.-)

     I09.89   **Other specified rheumatic heart diseases**
         Rheumatic disease of pulmonary valve

   I09.9   **Rheumatic heart disease, unspecified**
       Rheumatic carditis
       Excludes1: *rheumatoid carditis (M05.31)*

Hypertensive diseases (I10-I16)

Use additional code to identify:
   exposure to environmental tobacco smoke (Z77.22)
   history of tobacco dependence (Z87.891)
   occupational exposure to environmental tobacco smoke (Z57.31)
   tobacco dependence (F17.-)
   tobacco use (Z72.0)

Excludes1: *neonatal hypertension (P29.2)*
         primary pulmonary hypertension (I27.0)

Excludes2: *hypertensive disease complicating pregnancy, childbirth and the puerperium (O10-O11, O13-O16)*

Review coding guidelines C.9, C.9.a.5, C.9.a.8 and C.9.a.9

   I10   **Essential (primary) hypertension**

       Includes: high blood pressure
                  hypertension (arterial) (benign) (essential) (malignant) (primary) (systemic)

       Excludes1: *hypertensive disease complicating pregnancy, childbirth and the puerperium (O10-O11, O13-O16)*

       Excludes2: *essential (primary) hypertension involving vessels of brain (I60-I69)*
             essential (primary) hypertension involving vessels of eye (H35.0-)

       AHA CC: 4Q, 2013, 128; 4Q, 2016, 27-28; 2Q, 2018, 9-10
       Valid 3-character code, no further characters required

   I11   **Hypertensive heart disease**

       Includes: any condition in I50.-or I51.4-I51.7, I51.89, I51.9 due to hypertension

       Review coding guidelines C.9.a.1 and C.9.a.3

     I11.0   **Hypertensive heart disease with heart failure**
         Hypertensive heart failure
         Use additional code to identify type of heart failure (I50.-)
         AHA CC: 1Q, 2017, 47

     I11.9   **Hypertensive heart disease without heart failure**
         Hypertensive heart disease NOS

   I12   **Hypertensive chronic kidney disease**

       Includes: any condition in N18 and N26 - due to hypertension
                  arteriosclerosis of kidney
                  arteriosclerotic nephritis (chronic) (interstitial)
                  hypertensive nephropathy
                  nephrosclerosis

       Excludes1: *hypertension due to kidney disease (I15.0, I15.1)*
             renovascular hypertension (I15.0)
             secondary hypertension (I15.-)

       Excludes2: *acute kidney failure (N17.-)*
       Review coding guidelines C.9.a.2 and C.9.a.3

   CC **I12.0**   **Hypertensive chronic kidney disease with stage 5 chronic kidney disease or end stage renal disease**
         Use additional code to identify the stage of chronic kidney disease (N18.5, N18.6)

+, +7th, X + 7th   ● Newborn   ● Pediatric   ● Maternity   ● Adult   ♀ Female   ♂ Male   Manifestation   Unacceptable PDX   HCC   CC   MCC   HAC

Hypertension and CHF

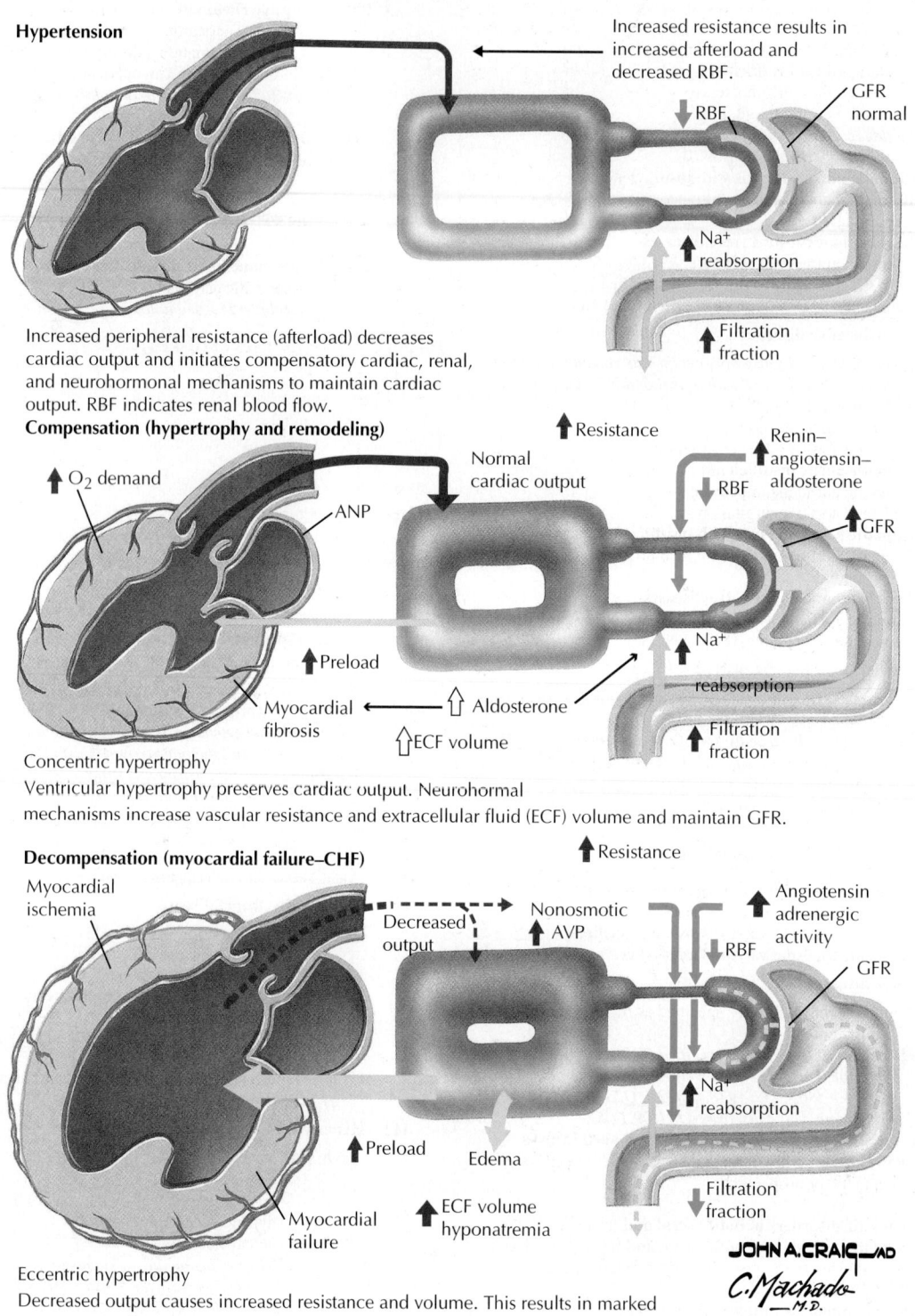

Hypertension

Increased resistance results in increased afterload and decreased RBF.

RBF

GFR normal

Na⁺ reabsorption

Filtration fraction

Increased peripheral resistance (afterload) decreases cardiac output and initiates compensatory cardiac, renal, and neurohormonal mechanisms to maintain cardiac output. RBF indicates renal blood flow.

Compensation (hypertrophy and remodeling)

↑O₂ demand

ANP

Normal cardiac output

↑Resistance

Renin–angiotensin–aldosterone

↓RBF

↑GFR

↑Preload

Myocardial fibrosis

⇧Aldosterone

⇧ECF volume

Na⁺ reabsorption

Filtration fraction

Concentric hypertrophy

Ventricular hypertrophy preserves cardiac output. Neurohormal mechanisms increase vascular resistance and extracellular fluid (ECF) volume and maintain GFR.

Decompensation (myocardial failure–CHF)

Myocardial ischemia

Decreased output

Nonosmotic ↑AVP

↑Resistance

↑Angiotensin adrenergic activity

↓RBF

GFR

↑Preload

Edema

Na⁺ reabsorption

Myocardial failure

↑ECF volume hyponatremia

Filtration fraction

Eccentric hypertrophy

Decreased output causes increased resistance and volume. This results in marked decrease in cardiac output, renal perfusion, and GFR.

JOHN A. CRAIG ᴍᴅ
C. Machado
ᴍ.ᴅ.

The Kidneys in Congestive Heart Failure (CHF)

EFFECTS OF LEFT HEART FAILURE ON RENAL BLOOD FLOW AND TUBULAR FUNCTION

Distribution of renal blood flow in CHF

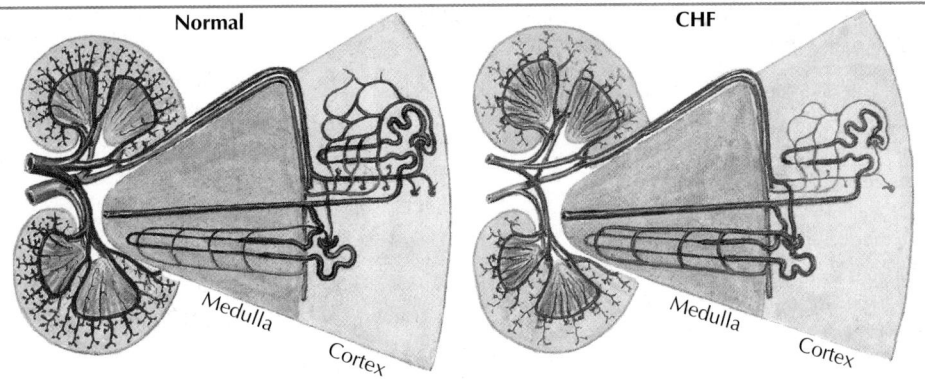

Normal

CHF

20% to 25% of cardiac output flows through kidneys: blood flows largely through cortical glomeruli, partially through juxtamedullary glomeruli

<10% of cardiac output flows through kidneys: redistribution of blood flow from cortical to juxtamedullary glomeruli

Tubular function in CHF

Low perfusion pressure activates tubuloglomerular feedback and renin release, causing afferent arteriole dilation and efferent arteriole constriction in order to maintain GFR. If hypoperfusion is severe, GFR may decline.

Marked increase in Na^+ and water reabsorption resulting from increase in filtration fraction, as well as input from angiotensin II, aldosterone, and other hormones.

As a result, serum BUN rises out of proportion to serum creatinine, and fractional excretion of sodium declines (<1%).

H_2O
Na^+

$\{ Na^+ \\ H_2O \}$

Na^+
H_2O

Capillary

Tubule cells

Intercellular space

Interstitial space

I12.9   **Hypertensive chronic kidney disease with stage 1 through stage 4 chronic kidney disease, or unspecified chronic kidney disease**

Hypertensive chronic kidney disease NOS
Hypertensive renal disease NOS
Use additional code to identify the stage of chronic kidney disease (N18.1-N18.4, N18.9)
AHA CC: 4Q, 2018, 88-89

I13   **Hypertensive heart and chronic kidney disease**

Includes: any condition in I11.- with any condition in I12.-
cardiorenal disease
cardiovascular renal disease
Review coding guideline C.9.a.3

CC **I13.0**   **Hypertensive heart and chronic kidney disease with heart failure and stage 1 through stage 4 chronic kidney disease, or unspecified chronic kidney disease**

Use additional code to identify type of heart failure (I50.-)

Use additional code to identify stage of chronic kidney disease (N18.1-N18.4, N18.9)

+ **I13.1**   **Hypertensive heart and chronic kidney disease without heart failure**

I13.10   **Hypertensive heart and chronic kidney disease without heart failure, with stage 1 through stage 4 chronic kidney disease, or unspecified chronic kidney disease**

Hypertensive heart disease and hypertensive chronic kidney disease NOS
Use additional code to identify the stage of chronic kidney disease (N18.1-N18.4, N18.9)

+, +7th, X + 7th   ● Newborn   ● Pediatric   ● Maternity   ● Adult   ♀ Female   ♂ Male   Manifestation   Unacceptable PDX   HCC   CC   MCC   HAC

CC **I13.11** **Hypertensive heart and chronic kidney disease without heart failure, with stage 5 chronic kidney disease, or end stage renal disease**
Use additional code to identify the stage of chronic kidney disease (N18.5, N18.6)

CC **I13.2** **Hypertensive heart and chronic kidney disease with heart failure and with stage 5 chronic kidney disease, or end stage renal disease**
Use additional code to identify type of heart failure (I50.-)

Use additional code to identify the stage of chronic kidney disease (N18.5, N18.6)

I15 **Secondary hypertension**
Code also underlying condition
Excludes1: *postprocedural hypertension (I97.3)*
Excludes2: *secondary hypertension involving vessels of brain (I60-I69)*
secondary hypertension involving vessels of eye (H35.0-)
Review coding guideline C.9.a.6

I15.0 **Renovascular hypertension**
I15.1 **Hypertension secondary to other renal disorders**
AHA CC: 3Q, 2016, 22-23
I15.2 **Hypertension secondary to endocrine disorders**
I15.8 **Other secondary hypertension**
I15.9 **Secondary hypertension, unspecified**

I16 **Hypertensive crisis**
Code also any identified hypertensive disease (I10-I15)
Review coding guideline C.9.a.10
AHA CC: 4Q, 2016, 26-28

I16.0 **Hypertensive urgency**
AHA CC: 4Q, 2016, 27-28
CC **I16.1** **Hypertensive emergency**
AHA CC: 4Q, 2016, 27-28
CC **I16.9** **Hypertensive crisis, unspecified**

Ischemic heart diseases (I20-I25)

Use additional code to identify presence of hypertension (I10-I16)

I20 **Angina pectoris**
Use additional code to identify:
exposure to environmental tobacco smoke (Z77.22)
history of tobacco dependence (Z87.891)
occupational exposure to environmental tobacco smoke (Z57.31)
tobacco dependence (F17.-)
tobacco use (Z72.0)
Excludes1: *angina pectoris with atherosclerotic heart disease of native coronary arteries (I25.1-)*
atherosclerosis of coronary artery bypass graft(s) and coronary artery of transplanted heart with angina pectoris (I25.7-)
postinfarction angina (I23.7)

CC **I20.0** **Unstable angina**
Accelerated angina
Crescendo angina
De novo effort angina
Intermediate coronary syndrome
Preinfarction syndrome
Worsening effort angina

CC **I20.1** **Angina pectoris with documented spasm**
Angiospastic angina
Prinzmetal angina
Spasm-induced angina
Variant angina

I20.8 **Other forms of angina pectoris**
Angina equivalent
Angina of effort
Coronary slow flow syndrome
Stable angina
Stenocardia
Use additional code(s) for symptoms associated with angina equivalent

I20.9 **Angina pectoris, unspecified**
Angina NOS
Anginal syndrome
Cardiac angina
Ischemic chest pain

I21 **Acute myocardial infarction**
Includes: cardiac infarction
coronary (artery) embolism
coronary (artery) occlusion
coronary (artery) rupture
coronary (artery) thrombosis
infarction of heart, myocardium, or ventricle
myocardial infarction specified as acute or with a stated duration of 4 weeks (28 days) or less from onset
Use additional code, if applicable, to identify:
exposure to environmental tobacco smoke (Z77.22)
history of tobacco dependence (Z87.891)
occupational exposure to environmental tobacco smoke (Z57.31)
status post administration of tPA (rtPA) in a different facility within the last 24 hours prior to admission to current facility (Z92.82)
tobacco dependence (F17.-)
tobacco use (Z72.0)
Excludes2: *old myocardial infarction (I25.2)*
postmyocardial infarction syndrome (I24.1)
subsequent type 1 myocardial infarction (I22.-)
AHA CC: 1Q, 2013, 25; 4Q, 2016, 140

+ **I21.0** **ST elevation (STEMI) myocardial infarction of anterior wall**
Type 1 ST elevation myocardial infarction of anterior wall
Review coding guideline C.9.e.1

MCC **I21.01** **ST elevation (STEMI) myocardial infarction involving left main coronary artery**
MCC **I21.02** **ST elevation (STEMI) myocardial infarction involving left anterior descending coronary artery**
ST elevation (STEMI) myocardial infarction involving diagonal coronary artery
AHA CC: 1Q, 2013, 25-26

MCC **I21.09** **ST elevation (STEMI) myocardial infarction involving other coronary artery of anterior wall**
Acute transmural myocardial infarction of anterior wall
Anteroapical transmural (Q wave) infarction (acute)
Anterolateral transmural (Q wave) infarction (acute)
Anteroseptal transmural (Q wave) infarction (acute)
Transmural (Q wave) infarction (acute) (of) anterior (wall) NOS
AHA CC: 4Q, 2012, 102-104

+ **I21.1** **ST elevation (STEMI) myocardial infarction of inferior wall**
Type 1 ST elevation myocardial infarction of inferior wall
Review coding guideline C.9.e.1

MCC **I21.11** **ST elevation (STEMI) myocardial infarction involving right coronary artery**
Inferoposterior transmural (Q wave) infarction (acute)

MCC **I21.19** **ST elevation (STEMI) myocardial infarction involving other coronary artery of inferior wall**
Acute transmural myocardial infarction of inferior wall
Inferolateral transmural (Q wave) infarction (acute)
Transmural (Q wave) infarction (acute) (of) diaphragmatic wall
Transmural (Q wave) infarction (acute) (of) inferior (wall) NOS
Excludes2: *ST elevation (STEMI) myocardial infarction involving left circumflex coronary artery (I21.21)*
AHA CC: 4Q, 2012, 97

+ **I21.2** **ST elevation (STEMI) myocardial infarction of other sites**
Type 1 ST elevation myocardial infarction of other sites
Review coding guideline C.9.e.1

MCC **I21.21** **ST elevation (STEMI) myocardial infarction involving left circumflex coronary artery**
ST elevation (STEMI) myocardial infarction involving oblique marginal coronary artery

Localization of Anterior and Posterior Infarcts

Localization of Posterior Infarcts

Occlusion of posterior interventricular branch of R. coronary artery

Postero-inferior infarct

Occlusion of R. coronary artery or its posterior interventricular branch

Strictly posterior (posteroseptal) infarct

Occlusion of circumflex branch of L. coronary artery

Postero-lateral infarct

Occlusion of circumflex branch of L. coronary artery (note variations in vessel distribution)

Postero-basal infarct

Localization of Anterior Infarcts

Occlusion of anterior interventricular branch of left coronary artery

Anterolateral infarct

Occlusion of R. division of anterior interventricular branch of L. coronary artery

Small, strictly anterior (anteroseptal) infarct

Occlusion of terminal portion of anterior interventricular branch of left coronary artery

Small apical infarct

Occlusion of branch of circumflex branch of L. coronary artery

Antero-basal infarct

MCC **I21.29** **ST elevation (STEMI) myocardial infarction involving other sites**
   Acute transmural myocardial infarction of other sites
   Apical-lateral transmural (Q wave) infarction (acute)
   Basal-lateral transmural (Q wave) infarction (acute)
   High lateral transmural (Q wave) infarction (acute)
   Lateral (wall) NOS transmural (Q wave) infarction (acute)
   Posterior (true) transmural (Q wave) infarction (acute)
   Posterobasal transmural (Q wave) infarction (acute)
   Posterolateral transmural (Q wave) infarction (acute)
   Posteroseptal transmural (Q wave) infarction (acute)
   Septal transmural (Q wave) infarction (acute) NOS

MCC **I21.3** **ST elevation (STEMI) myocardial infarction of unspecified site**
   Acute transmural myocardial infarction of unspecified site
   Transmural (Q wave) myocardial infarction NOS
   Type 1 ST elevation myocardial infarction of unspecified site
   Review coding guidelines C.9.e.1 and C.9.e.2

MCC **I21.4** **Non-ST elevation (NSTEMI) myocardial infarction**
   Acute subendocardial myocardial infarction
   Non-Q wave myocardial infarction NOS
   Nontransmural myocardial infarction NOS
   Type 1 non-ST elevation myocardial infarction
   Review coding guideline C.9.e.1
   AHA CC: 2Q, 2015, 16-17; 1Q, 2017, 44-45

MCC **I21.9** **Acute myocardial infarction, unspecified**
   Myocardial infarction (acute) NOS
   Review coding guideline C.9.e.5

+ **I21.A** **Other type of myocardial infarction**
   AHA CC: 4Q, 2017, 12-14

MCC **I21.A1** **Myocardial infarction type 2**
   Myocardial infarction due to demand ischemia
   Myocardial infarction secondary to ischemic imbalance
   Code first the underlying cause, such as:
   anemia (D50.0-D64.9)
   chronic obstructive pulmonary disease (J44.-)
   paroxysmal tachycardia (I47.0-I47.9)
   shock (R57.0-R57.9)

MCC **I21.A9** **Other myocardial infarction type**
   Myocardial infarction associated with revascularization procedure
   Myocardial infarction type 3
   Myocardial infarction type 4a
   Myocardial infarction type 4b
   Myocardial infarction type 4c
   Myocardial infarction type 5
   Code first, if applicable, postprocedural myocardial infarction following cardiac surgery (I97.190), or postprocedural myocardial infarction during cardiac surgery (I97.790)
   Code also complication, if known and applicable, such as:
   (acute) stent occlusion (T82.897-)
   (acute) stent stenosis (T82.855-)
   (acute) stent thrombosis (T82.867-)
   cardiac arrest due to underlying cardiac condition (I46.2)
   complication of percutaneous coronary intervention (PCI) (I97.89)
   occlusion of coronary artery bypass graft (T82.218-)
   AHA CC: 2Q, 2019, 32-33

I22 **Subsequent ST elevation (STEMI) and non-ST elevation (NSTEMI) myocardial infarction**
   Includes: acute myocardial infarction occurring within four weeks (28 days) of a previous acute myocardial infarction, regardless of site
   cardiac infarction
   coronary (artery) embolism
   coronary (artery) occlusion
   coronary (artery) rupture
   coronary (artery) thrombosis
   infarction of heart, myocardium, or ventricle
   recurrent myocardial infarction
   reinfarction of myocardium
   rupture of heart, myocardium, or ventricle
   subsequent type 1 myocardial infarction
   Use additional code, if applicable, to identify:
   exposure to environmental tobacco smoke (Z77.22)
   history of tobacco dependence (Z87.891)
   occupational exposure to environmental tobacco smoke (Z57.31)
   status post administration of tPA (rtPA) in a different facility within the last 24 hours prior to admission to current facility (Z92.82)
   tobacco dependence (F17.-)
   tobacco use (Z72.0)
   Excludes1: subsequent myocardial infarction, type 2 (I21.A1)
   subsequent myocardial infarction of other type (type 3) (type 4) (type 5) (I21.A9)
   Review coding guideline C.9.e.4
   AHA CC: 1Q, 2013, 25

MCC **I22.0** **Subsequent ST elevation (STEMI) myocardial infarction of anterior wall**
   Subsequent acute transmural myocardial infarction of anterior wall
   Subsequent transmural (Q wave) infarction (acute)(of) anterior (wall) NOS
   Subsequent anteroapical transmural (Q wave) infarction (acute)
   Subsequent anterolateral transmural (Q wave) infarction (acute)
   Subsequent anteroseptal transmural (Q wave) infarction (acute)

MCC **I22.1** **Subsequent ST elevation (STEMI) myocardial infarction of inferior wall**
   Subsequent acute transmural myocardial infarction of inferior wall
   Subsequent transmural (Q wave) infarction (acute)(of) diaphragmatic wall
   Subsequent transmural (Q wave) infarction (acute)(of) inferior (wall) NOS
   Subsequent inferolateral transmural (Q wave) infarction (acute)
   Subsequent inferoposterior transmural (Q wave) infarction (acute)
   AHA CC: 4Q, 2012, 102-104

MCC **I22.2** **Subsequent non-ST elevation (NSTEMI) myocardial infarction**
   Subsequent acute subendocardial myocardial infarction
   Subsequent non-Q wave myocardial infarction NOS
   Subsequent nontransmural myocardial infarction NOS

MCC **I22.8** **Subsequent ST elevation (STEMI) myocardial infarction of other sites**
   Subsequent acute transmural myocardial infarction of other sites
   Subsequent apical-lateral transmural (Q wave) myocardial infarction (acute)
   Subsequent basal-lateral transmural (Q wave) myocardial infarction (acute)
   Subsequent high lateral transmural (Q wave) myocardial infarction (acute)
   Subsequent transmural (Q wave) myocardial infarction (acute)(of) lateral (wall) NOS
   Subsequent posterior (true) transmural (Q wave) myocardial infarction (acute)
   Subsequent posterobasal transmural (Q wave) myocardial infarction (acute)
   Subsequent posterolateral transmural (Q wave) myocardial infarction (acute)
   Subsequent posteroseptal transmural (Q wave) myocardial infarction (acute)
   Subsequent septal NOS transmural (Q wave) myocardial infarction (acute)

+, +7th, X + 7th   • Newborn   • Pediatric   • Maternity   • Adult   ♀ Female   ♂ Male   Manifestation   Unacceptable PDX   HCC   CC   MCC   HAC

MCC **I22.9** **Subsequent ST elevation (STEMI) myocardial infarction of unspecified site**
Subsequent acute myocardial infarction of unspecified site
Subsequent myocardial infarction (acute) NOS

I23 **Certain current complications following ST elevation (STEMI) and non-ST elevation (NSTEMI) myocardial infarction (within the 28 day period)**

• CC **I23.0** **Hemopericardium as current complication following acute myocardial infarction**
Excludes1: *hemopericardium not specified as current complication following acute myocardial infarction (I31.2)*

• CC **I23.1** **Atrial septal defect as current complication following acute myocardial infarction**
Excludes1: *acquired atrial septal defect not specified as current complication following acute myocardial infarction (I51.0)*

• CC **I23.2** **Ventricular septal defect as current complication following acute myocardial infarction**
Excludes1: *acquired ventricular septal defect not specified as current complication following acute myocardial infarction (I51.0)*

• CC **I23.3** **Rupture of cardiac wall without hemopericardium as current complication following acute myocardial infarction**
AHA CC: 2Q, 2017, 11-12

MCC **I23.4** **Rupture of chordae tendineae as current complication following acute myocardial infarction**
Excludes1: *rupture of chordae tendineae not specified as current complication following acute myocardial infarction (I51.1)*

MCC **I23.5** **Rupture of papillary muscle as current complication following acute myocardial infarction**
Excludes1: *rupture of papillary muscle not specified as current complication following acute myocardial infarction (I51.2)*

• CC **I23.6** **Thrombosis of atrium, auricular appendage, and ventricle as current complications following acute myocardial infarction**
Excludes1: *thrombosis of atrium, auricular appendage, and ventricle not specified as current complication following acute myocardial infarction (I51.3)*

• CC **I23.7** **Postinfarction angina**
AHA CC: 2Q, 2015, 16-17

• CC **I23.8** **Other current complications following acute myocardial infarction**

I24 **Other acute ischemic heart diseases**
Excludes1: *angina pectoris (I20.-)*
transient myocardial ischemia in newborn (P29.4)

CC **I24.0** **Acute coronary thrombosis not resulting in myocardial infarction**
Acute coronary (artery) (vein) embolism not resulting in myocardial infarction
Acute coronary (artery) (vein) occlusion not resulting in myocardial infarction
Acute coronary (artery) (vein) thromboembolism not resulting in myocardial infarction
Excludes1: *atherosclerotic heart disease (I25.1-)*

CC **I24.1** **Dressler's syndrome**
Postmyocardial infarction syndrome
Excludes1: *postinfarction angina (I23.7)*

CC **I24.8** **Other forms of acute ischemic heart disease**
Excludes1: *myocardial infarction due to demand ischemia (I21.A1)*

CC **I24.9** **Acute ischemic heart disease, unspecified**
Excludes1: *ischemic heart disease (chronic) NOS (I25.9)*

I25 **Chronic ischemic heart disease**
Use additional code to identify:
chronic total occlusion of coronary artery (I25.82)
exposure to environmental tobacco smoke (Z77.22)
history of tobacco dependence (Z87.891)
occupational exposure to environmental tobacco smoke (Z57.31)
tobacco dependence (F17.-)
tobacco use (Z72.0)

I25.1 **Atherosclerotic heart disease of native coronary artery**
Atherosclerotic cardiovascular disease
Coronary (artery) atheroma
Coronary (artery) atherosclerosis
Coronary (artery) disease
Coronary (artery) sclerosis
Use additional code, if applicable, to identify:
coronary atherosclerosis due to calcified coronary lesion (I25.84)
coronary atherosclerosis due to lipid rich plaque (I25.83)
Excludes2: *atheroembolism (I75.-)*
atherosclerosis of coronary artery bypass graft(s) and transplanted heart (I25.7-)

• **I25.10** **Atherosclerotic heart disease of native coronary artery without angina pectoris**
Atherosclerotic heart disease NOS
AHA CC: 4Q, 2012, 92-92; 4Q, 2013, 128

+ **I25.11** **Atherosclerotic heart disease of native coronary artery with angina pectoris**
Review coding guideline C.9.b

Great Vessels of the Heart

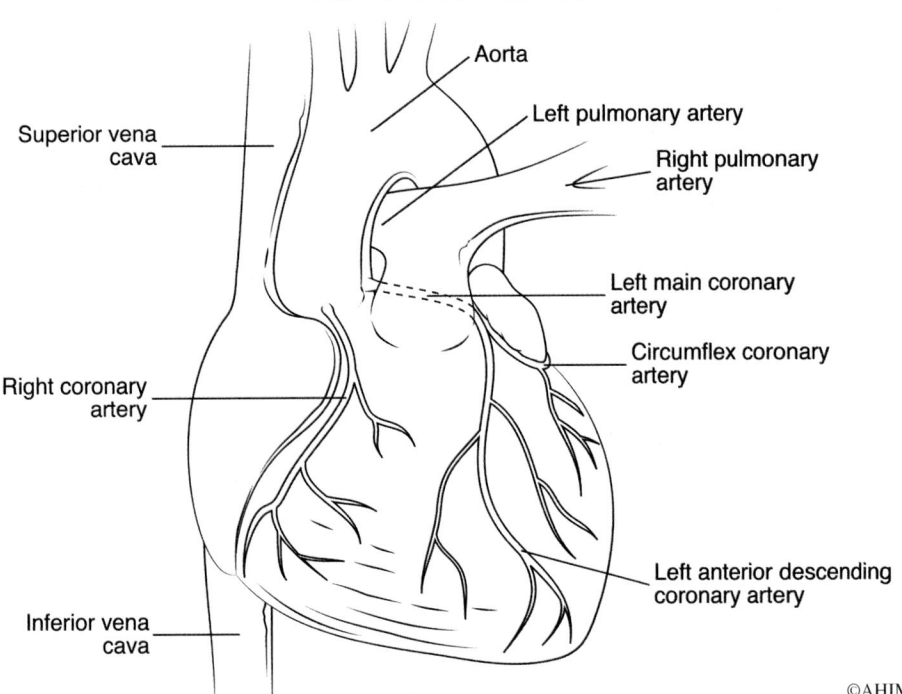

Aorta
Left pulmonary artery
Right pulmonary artery
Superior vena cava
Left main coronary artery
Circumflex coronary artery
Right coronary artery
Left anterior descending coronary artery
Inferior vena cava

©AHIMA

+, +7th, X + 7th • Newborn • Pediatric • Maternity • Adult ♀ Female ♂ Male Manifestation Unacceptable PDX HCC CC MCC HAC

● CC **I25.110** **Atherosclerotic heart disease of native coronary artery with unstable angina pectoris**
    Excludes1: *unstable angina without atherosclerotic heart disease (I20.0)*

● **I25.111** **Atherosclerotic heart disease of native coronary artery with angina pectoris with documented spasm**
    Excludes1: *angina pectoris with documented spasm without atherosclerotic heart disease (I20.1)*

● **I25.118** **Atherosclerotic heart disease of native coronary artery with other forms of angina pectoris**
    Excludes1: *other forms of angina pectoris without atherosclerotic heart disease (I20.8)*
    AHA CC: 2Q, 2015, 16-17

● **I25.119** **Atherosclerotic heart disease of native coronary artery with unspecified angina pectoris**
    Atherosclerotic heart disease with angina NOS
    Atherosclerotic heart disease with ischemic chest pain
    Excludes1: *unspecified angina pectoris without atherosclerotic heart disease (I20.9)*

I25.2 **Old myocardial infarction**
  Healed myocardial infarction
  Past myocardial infarction diagnosed by ECG or other investigation, but currently presenting no symptoms

CC **I25.3** **Aneurysm of heart**
  Mural aneurysm
  Ventricular aneurysm

+ **I25.4** **Coronary artery aneurysm and dissection**
  I25.41 **Coronary artery aneurysm**
    Coronary arteriovenous fistula, acquired
    Excludes1: *congenital coronary (artery) aneurysm (Q24.5)*
  MCC **I25.42** **Coronary artery dissection**

I25.5 **Ischemic cardiomyopathy**
  Excludes2: *coronary atherosclerosis (I25.1-, I25.7-)*

I25.6 **Silent myocardial ischemia**

+ **I25.7** **Atherosclerosis of coronary artery bypass graft(s) and coronary artery of transplanted heart with angina pectoris**
  Use additional code, if applicable, to identify:
    coronary atherosclerosis due to calcified coronary lesion (I25.84)
    coronary atherosclerosis due to lipid rich plaque (I25.83)
  Excludes1: *atherosclerosis of bypass graft(s) of transplanted heart without angina pectoris (I25.812)*
    atherosclerosis of coronary artery bypass graft(s) without angina pectoris (I25.810)
    atherosclerosis of native coronary artery of transplanted heart without angina pectoris (I25.811)
  Review coding guideline C.9.b

+ **I25.70** **Atherosclerosis of coronary artery bypass graft(s), unspecified, with angina pectoris**
  ● CC **I25.700** **Atherosclerosis of coronary artery bypass graft(s), unspecified, with unstable angina pectoris**
    Excludes1: *unstable angina pectoris without atherosclerosis of coronary artery bypass graft (I20.0)*

  ● **I25.701** **Atherosclerosis of coronary artery bypass graft(s), unspecified, with angina pectoris with documented spasm**
    Excludes1: *angina pectoris with documented spasm without atherosclerosis of coronary artery bypass graft (I20.1)*

● **I25.708** **Atherosclerosis of coronary artery bypass graft(s), unspecified, with other forms of angina pectoris**
    Excludes1: *other forms of angina pectoris without atherosclerosis of coronary artery bypass graft (I20.8)*

● **I25.709** **Atherosclerosis of coronary artery bypass graft(s), unspecified, with unspecified angina pectoris**
    Excludes1: *unspecified angina pectoris without atherosclerosis of coronary artery bypass graft (I20.9)*

+ **I25.71** **Atherosclerosis of autologous vein coronary artery bypass graft(s) with angina pectoris**
  ● CC **I25.710** **Atherosclerosis of autologous vein coronary artery bypass graft(s) with unstable angina pectoris**
    Excludes1: *unstable angina without atherosclerosis of autologous vein coronary artery bypass graft(s) (I20.0)*
    Excludes2: *embolism or thrombus of coronary artery bypass graft(s) (T82.8-)*

  ● CC **I25.711** **Atherosclerosis of autologous vein coronary artery bypass graft(s) with angina pectoris with documented spasm**
    Excludes1: *angina pectoris with documented spasm without atherosclerosis of autologous vein coronary artery bypass graft(s) (I20.1)*

  ● CC **I25.718** **Atherosclerosis of autologous vein coronary artery bypass graft(s) with other forms of angina pectoris**
    Excludes1: *other forms of angina pectoris without atherosclerosis of autologous vein coronary artery bypass graft(s) (I20.8)*

  ● CC **I25.719** **Atherosclerosis of autologous vein coronary artery bypass graft(s) with unspecified angina pectoris**
    Excludes1: *unspecified angina pectoris without atherosclerosis of autologous vein coronary artery bypass graft(s) (I20.9)*

+ **I25.72** **Atherosclerosis of autologous artery coronary artery bypass graft(s) with angina pectoris**
  Atherosclerosis of internal mammary artery graft with angina pectoris
  ● CC **I25.720** **Atherosclerosis of autologous artery coronary artery bypass graft(s) with unstable angina pectoris**
    Excludes1: *unstable angina without atherosclerosis of autologous artery coronary artery bypass graft(s) (I20.0)*

  ● CC **I25.721** **Atherosclerosis of autologous artery coronary artery bypass graft(s) with angina pectoris with documented spasm**
    Excludes1: *angina pectoris with documented spasm without atherosclerosis of autologous artery coronary artery bypass graft(s) (I20.1)*

Pathologic Changes in CAD; Types and Degrees of Coronary Atherosclerotic Narrowing or Occlusion

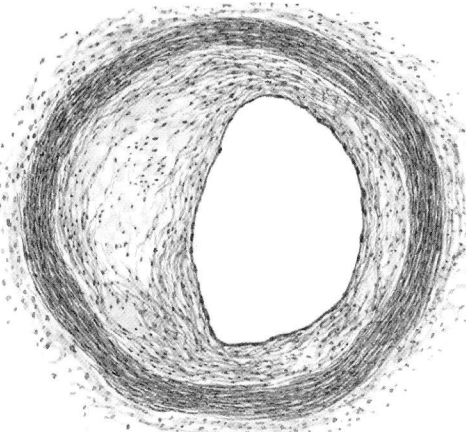

Moderate atherosclerotic narrowing of lumen

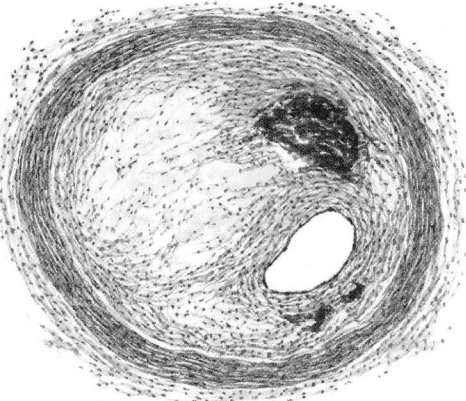

Almost complete occlusion by intimal atherosclerosis with calcium deposition

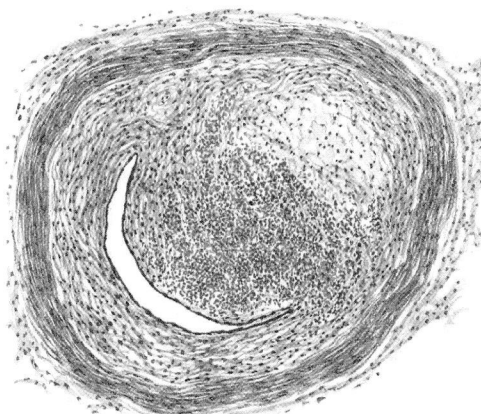

Hemorrhage into atheroma, leaving only a slit-like lumen

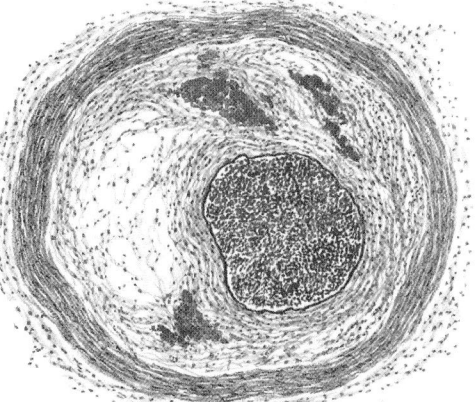

Complete occlusion by thrombus in lumen greatly narrowed by atheroma

Organization of thrombus

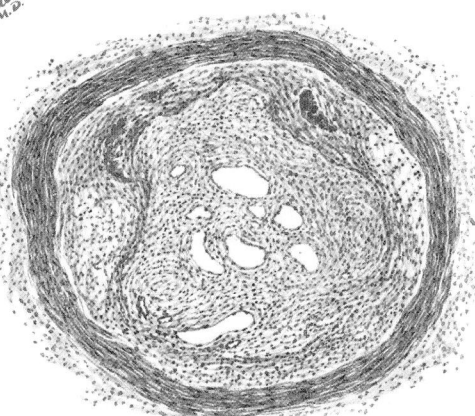

Organization with recanalization may occur

- CC **I25.728** Atherosclerosis of autologous artery coronary artery bypass graft(s) with other forms of angina pectoris

  Excludes1: *other forms of angina pectoris without atherosclerosis of autologous artery coronary artery bypass graft(s) (I20.8)*

- CC **I25.729** Atherosclerosis of autologous artery coronary artery bypass graft(s) with unspecified angina pectoris

  Excludes1: *unspecified angina pectoris without atherosclerosis of autologous artery coronary artery bypass graft(s) (I20.9)*

+ **I25.73** Atherosclerosis of nonautologous biological coronary artery bypass graft(s) with angina pectoris

- CC **I25.730** Atherosclerosis of nonautologous biological coronary artery bypass graft(s) with unstable angina pectoris

  Excludes1: *unstable angina without atherosclerosis of nonautologousbiological coronary artery bypass graft(s) (I20.0)*

- CC **I25.731** Atherosclerosis of nonautologous biological coronary artery bypass graft(s) with angina pectoris with documented spasm

  Excludes1: *angina pectoris with documented spasm withoutatherosclerosisof nonautologousbiological coronary artery bypass graft(s) (I20.1)*

- CC **I25.738** Atherosclerosis of nonautologous biological coronary artery bypass graft(s) with other forms of angina pectoris

  Excludes1: *other forms of angina pectoris without atherosclerosis of nonautologousbiological coronary artery bypass graft(s) (I20.8)*

- CC **I25.739** Atherosclerosis of nonautologous biological coronary artery bypass graft(s) with unspecified angina pectoris

  Excludes1: *unspecified angina pectoris withoutatherosclerosisof nonautologousbiological coronary artery bypass graft(s) (I20.9)*

+ **I25.75** Atherosclerosis of native coronary artery of transplanted heart with angina pectoris

  Excludes1: *atherosclerosis of native coronary arteryoftransplantedheartwithout angina pectoris (I25.811)*

  CC **I25.750** Atherosclerosis of native coronary artery of transplanted heart with unstable angina

  CC **I25.751** Atherosclerosis of native coronary artery of transplanted heart with angina pectoris with documented spasm

  CC **I25.758** Atherosclerosis of native coronary artery of transplanted heart with other forms of angina pectoris

  CC **I25.759** Atherosclerosis of native coronary artery of transplanted heart with unspecified angina pectoris

+ **I25.76** Atherosclerosis of bypass graft of coronary artery of transplanted heart with angina pectoris

  Excludes1: *atherosclerosis of bypass graft of coronary artery of transplanted heart without angina pectoris (I25.812)*

- CC **I25.760** Atherosclerosis of bypass graft of coronary artery of transplanted heart with unstable angina

- CC **I25.761** Atherosclerosis of bypass graft of coronary artery of transplanted heart with angina pectoris with documented spasm

- CC **I25.768** Atherosclerosis of bypass graft of coronary artery of transplanted heart with other forms of angina pectoris

- CC **I25.769** Atherosclerosis of bypass graft of coronary artery of transplanted heart with unspecified angina pectoris

+ **I25.79** Atherosclerosis of other coronary artery bypass graft(s) with angina pectoris

- CC **I25.790** Atherosclerosis of other coronary artery bypass graft(s) with unstable angina pectoris

  Excludes1: *unstable angina without atherosclerosis of other coronary artery bypass graft(s) (I20.0)*

- CC **I25.791** Atherosclerosis of other coronary artery bypass graft(s) with angina pectoris with documented spasm

  Excludes1: *angina pectoris with documented spasm without atherosclerosis of other coronary artery bypass graft(s) (I20.1)*

- CC **I25.798** Atherosclerosis of other coronary artery bypass graft(s) with other forms of angina pectoris

  Excludes1: *other forms of angina pectoris without atherosclerosis of other coronary artery bypass graft(s) (I20.8)*

- CC **I25.799** Atherosclerosis of other coronary artery bypass graft(s) with unspecified angina pectoris

  Excludes1: *unspecified angina pectoris without atherosclerosis of other coronary artery bypass graft(s) (I20.9)*

+ **I25.8** Other forms of chronic ischemic heart disease

+ **I25.81** Atherosclerosis of other coronary vessels without angina pectoris

  Use additional code, if applicable, to identify: coronary atherosclerosis due to calcified coronary lesion (I25.84) coronary atherosclerosis due to lipid rich plaque (I25.83)

  Excludes2: *atherosclerotic heart disease of native coronary artery without angina pectoris (I25.10)*

- CC **I25.810** Atherosclerosis of coronary artery bypass graft(s) without angina pectoris

  Atherosclerosis of coronary artery bypass graft NOS

  Excludes1: *atherosclerosis of coronary bypassgraft(s)withangina pectoris (I25.70-I25.73-, I25.79-)*

  CC **I25.811** Atherosclerosis of native coronary artery of transplanted heart without angina pectoris

  Atherosclerosis of native coronary artery of transplanted heart NOS

  Excludes1: *atherosclerosis of native coronary artery of transplanted heart with angina pectoris (I25.75-)*

- CC **I25.812** **Atherosclerosis of bypass graft of coronary artery of transplanted heart without angina pectoris**
  Atherosclerosis of bypass graft of transplanted heart NOS
  Excludes1: atherosclerosis of bypass graft of transplanted heart with angina pectoris (I25.76)

I25.82 **Chronic total occlusion of coronary artery**
  Complete occlusion of coronary artery
  Total occlusion of coronary artery
  Code first coronary atherosclerosis (I25.1-, I25.7-, I25.81-)
  Excludes1: acute coronary occlusion with myocardial infarction (I21.0-I21.9, I22.-)
  acute coronary occlusion without myocardial infarction (I24.0)
  AHA CC: 3Q, 2018, 5-6

- **I25.83** **Coronary atherosclerosis due to lipid rich plaque**
  Code first coronary atherosclerosis (I25.1-, I25.7-, I25.81-)

I25.84 **Coronary atherosclerosis due to calcified coronary lesion**
  Coronary atherosclerosis due to severely calcified coronary lesion
  Code first coronary atherosclerosis (I25.1-, I25.7-, I25.81-)

I25.89 **Other forms of chronic ischemic heart disease**

I25.9 **Chronic ischemic heart disease, unspecified**
  Ischemic heart disease (chronic) NOS

Pulmonary heart disease and diseases of pulmonary circulation (I26-I28)

I26 **Pulmonary embolism**
  Includes: pulmonary (acute) (artery)(vein) infarction
  pulmonary (acute) (artery)(vein) thromboembolism
  pulmonary (acute) (artery)(vein) thrombosis
  Excludes2: *chronic pulmonary embolism (I27.82)*
  personal history of pulmonary embolism (Z86.711)
  pulmonary embolism due to trauma (T79.0, T79.1)
  pulmonary embolism due to complications of surgical and medical care (T80.0, T81.7-, T82.8-)
  pulmonary embolism complicating abortion, ectopic or molar pregnancy (O00-O07, O08.2)
  pulmonary embolism complicating pregnancy, childbirth and the puerperium (O88.-)
  septic (non-pulmonary) arterial embolism (I76)

+ **I26.0** **Pulmonary embolism with acute cor pulmonale**
  MCC **I26.01** **Septic pulmonary embolism with acute cor pulmonale**
  Code first underlying infection

  MCC **I26.02** **Saddle embolus of pulmonary artery with acute cor pulmonale**
  HAC *see Appendix B for HAC conditional logic*

  MCC **I26.09** **Other pulmonary embolism with acute cor pulmonale**
  HAC *see Appendix B for HAC conditional logic*

+ **I26.9** **Pulmonary embolism without acute cor pulmonale**
  MCC **I26.90** **Septic pulmonary embolism without acute cor pulmonale**
  Code first underlying infection

  MCC **I26.92** **Saddle embolus of pulmonary artery without acute cor pulmonale**
  HAC *see Appendix B for HAC conditional logic*

  MCC **I26.93** **Single subsegmental pulmonary embolism without acute cor pulmonale**
  Subsegmental pulmonary embolism NOS
  AHA CC: 4Q, 2019, 6-7
  HAC *see Appendix B for HAC conditional logic*

  MCC **I26.94** **Multiple subsegmental pulmonary emboli without acute cor pulmonale**
  AHA CC: 4Q, 2019, 6-7
  HAC *see Appendix B for HAC conditional logic*

  MCC **I26.99** **Other pulmonary embolism without acute cor pulmonale**
  Acute pulmonary embolism NOS
  Pulmonary embolism NOS
  AHA CC: 2Q, 2019, 22-23
  HAC *see Appendix B for HAC conditional logic*

I27 **Other pulmonary heart diseases**
  Review coding guideline C.9.a.11

CC **I27.0** **Primary pulmonary hypertension**
  Heritable pulmonary arterial hypertension
  Idiopathic pulmonary arterial hypertension
  Primary group 1 pulmonary hypertension
  Primary pulmonary arterial hypertension
  Excludes1: persistent pulmonary hypertension of newborn (P29.30)
  pulmonary hypertension NOS (I27.20)
  secondary pulmonary arterial hypertension (I27.21)
  secondary pulmonary hypertension (I27.29)
  AHA CC: 4Q, 2017, 14-15

CC **I27.1** **Kyphoscoliotic heart disease**

+ **I27.2** **Other secondary pulmonary hypertension**
  Code also associated underlying condition
  Excludes1: Eisenmenger's syndrome (I27.83)
  AHA CC: 4Q, 2014, 21-22; 2Q, 2016, 8; 4Q, 2017, 14-15

I27.20 **Pulmonary hypertension, unspecified**
  Pulmonary hypertension NOS

I27.21 **Secondary pulmonary arterial hypertension**
  (Associated) (drug-induced) (toxin-induced) pulmonary arterial hypertension NOS
  (Associated) (drug-induced) (toxin-induced) (secondary) group 1 pulmonary hypertension
  Code also associated conditions if applicable, or adverse effects of drugs or toxins, such as:
  adverse effect of appetite depressants (T50.5X5)
  congenital heart disease (Q20-Q28)
  human immunodeficiency virus [HIV] disease (B20)
  polymyositis (M33.2-)
  portal hypertension (K76.6)
  rheumatoid arthritis (M05.-)
  schistosomiasis (B65.-)
  Sjögren syndrome (M35.0-)
  systemic sclerosis (M34.-)

I27.22 **Pulmonary hypertension due to left heart disease**
  Group 2 pulmonary hypertension
  Code also associated left heart disease, if known, such as:
  multiple valve disease (I08.-)
  rheumatic mitral valve diseases (I05.-)
  rheumatic aortic valve diseases (I06.-)

I27.23 **Pulmonary hypertension due to lung diseases and hypoxia**
  Group 3 pulmonary hypertension
  Code also associated lung disease, if known, such as:
  bronchiectasis (J47.-)
  cystic fibrosis with pulmonary manifestations (E84.0)
  interstitial lung disease (J84.-)
  pleural effusion (J90)
  sleep apnea (G47.3-)

I27.24 **Chronic thromboembolic pulmonary hypertension**
  Group 4 pulmonary hypertension
  Code also associated pulmonary embolism, if applicable (I26.-, I27.82)

I27.29 **Other secondary pulmonary hypertension**
  Group 5 pulmonary hypertension
  Pulmonary hypertension with unclear multifactorial mechanisms
  Pulmonary hypertension due to hematologic disorders
  Pulmonary hypertension due to metabolic disorders
  Pulmonary hypertension due to other systemic disorders
  Code also other associated disorders, if known, such as:
  chronic myeloid leukemia (C92.10-C92.22)
  essential thrombocythemia (D47.3)
  Gaucher disease (E75.22)
  hypertensive chronic kidney disease with end stage renal disease (I12.0, I13.11, I13.2)
  hyperthyroidism (E05.-)
  hypothyroidism (E00-E03)
  polycythemia vera (D45)
  sarcoidosis (D86.-)

+, +7th, X + 7th   ● Newborn   ● Pediatric   ● Maternity   ● Adult   ♀ Female   ♂ Male   Manifestation   Unacceptable PDX   HCC   CC   MCC   **HAC**

+ **127.8** **Other specified pulmonary heart diseases**
  I27.81 **Cor pulmonale (chronic)**
  Cor pulmonale NOS
  Excludes1: acute cor pulmonale (I26.0-)
  AHA CC: 4Q, 2014, 21-22

CC **I27.82** **Chronic pulmonary embolism**
  Use additional code, if applicable, for associated
    long-term (current) use of anticoagulants
    (Z79.01)
  Excludes1: personal history of pulmonary
    embolism (Z86.711)

  I27.83 **Eisenmenger's syndrome**
  Eisenmenger's complex
  (Irreversible) Eisenmenger's disease
  Pulmonary hypertension with right to left shunt
    related to congential heart disease
  Code also underlying heart defect, if known, such
    as:
      atrial septal defect (Q21.1)
      Eisenmenger's defect (Q21.8)
      patent ductus arteriosus (Q25.0)
      ventricular septal defect (Q21.0)

  I27.89 **Other specified pulmonary heart diseases**

I27.9 **Pulmonary heart disease, unspecified**
  Chronic cardiopulmonary disease

I28 **Other diseases of pulmonary vessels**

CC **I28.0** **Arteriovenous fistula of pulmonary vessels**
  Excludes1: congenital arteriovenous fistula (Q25.72)

CC **I28.1** **Aneurysm of pulmonary artery**
  Excludes1: congenital aneurysm (Q25.79)
    congenital arteriovenous aneurysm (Q25.72)

I28.8 **Other diseases of pulmonary vessels**
  Pulmonary arteritis
  Pulmonary endarteritis
  Rupture of pulmonary vessels
  Stenosis of pulmonary vessels
  Stricture of pulmonary vessels

I28.9 **Disease of pulmonary vessels, unspecified**

Other forms of heart disease (I30-I52)

I30 **Acute pericarditis**

  Includes: acute mediastinopericarditis
    acute myopericarditis
    acute pericardial effusion
    acute pleuropericarditis
    acute pneumopericarditis

  Excludes1: Dressler's syndrome (I24.1)
    rheumatic pericarditis (acute) (I01.0)
    viral pericarditis due to Coxsakie virus (B33.23)

CC **I30.0** **Acute nonspecific idiopathic pericarditis**

CC **I30.1** **Infective pericarditis**
  Pneumococcal pericarditis
  Pneumopyopericardium
  Purulent pericarditis
  Pyopericarditis
  Pyopericardium
  Pyopneumopericardium
  Staphylococcal pericarditis
  Streptococcal pericarditis
  Suppurative pericarditis
  Viral pericarditis
  Use additional code (B95-B97) to identify infectious agent

CC **I30.8** **Other forms of acute pericarditis**

CC **I30.9** **Acute pericarditis, unspecified**

I31 **Other diseases of pericardium**

  Excludes1: diseases of pericardium specified as rheumatic (I09.2)
    postcardiotomy syndrome (I97.0)
    traumatic injury to pericardium (S26.-)

CC **I31.0** **Chronic adhesive pericarditis**
  Accretio cordis
  Adherent pericardium
  Adhesive mediastinopericarditis

CC **I31.1** **Chronic constrictive pericarditis**
  Concretio cordis
  Pericardial calcification

CC **I31.2** **Hemopericardium, not elsewhere classified**
  Excludes1: hemopericardium as current complication
    following acute myocardial
    infarction (I23.0)

CC **I31.3** **Pericardial effusion (noninflammatory)**
  Chylopericardium
  Excludes1: acute pericardial effusion (I30.9)
  AHA CC: 1Q, 2019, 16

CC **I31.4** **Cardiac tamponade**
  Code first underlying cause

CC **I31.8** **Other specified diseases of pericardium**
  Epicardial plaques
  Focal pericardial adhesions

CC **I31.9** **Disease of pericardium, unspecified**
  Pericarditis (chronic) NOS

CC **I32** **Pericarditis in diseases classified elsewhere**
  Code first underlying disease
  Excludes1: pericarditis (in):
    coxsackie (virus) (B33.23)
    gonococcal (A54.83)
    meningococcal (A39.53)
    rheumatoid (arthritis) (M05.31)
    syphilitic (A52.06)
    systemic lupus erythematosus (M32.12)
    tuberculosis (A18.84)
  Valid 3-character code, no further characters required

I33 **Acute and subacute endocarditis**
  Excludes1: acute rheumatic endocarditis (I01.1)
    endocarditis NOS (I38)

MCC **I33.0** **Acute and subacute infective endocarditis**
  Bacterial endocarditis (acute) (subacute)
  Infective endocarditis (acute) (subacute) NOS
  Endocarditis lenta (acute) (subacute)
  Malignant endocarditis (acute) (subacute)
  Purulent endocarditis (acute) (subacute)
  Septic endocarditis (acute) (subacute)
  Ulcerative endocarditis (acute) (subacute)
  Vegetative endocarditis (acute) (subacute)
  Use additional code (B95-B97) to identify infectious agent

MCC **I33.9** **Acute and subacute endocarditis, unspecified**
  Acute endocarditis NOS
  Acute myoendocarditis NOS
  Acute periendocarditis NOS
  Subacute endocarditis NOS
  Subacute myoendocarditis NOS
  Subacute periendocarditis NOS

I34 **Nonrheumatic mitral valve disorders**
  Excludes1: mitral valve disease (I05.9)
    mitral valve failure (I05.8)
    mitral valve stenosis (I05.0)
    mitral valve disorder of unspecified cause with diseases
      of aortic and/or tricuspid valve(s) (I08.-)
    mitral valve disorder of unspecified cause with mitral
      stenosis or obstruction (I05.0)
    mitral valve disorder specified as congenital (Q23.2, Q23.9)
    mitral valve disorder specified as rheumatic (I05.-)

I34.0 **Nonrheumatic mitral (valve) insufficiency**
  Nonrheumatic mitral (valve) incompetence NOS
  Nonrheumatic mitral (valve) regurgitation NOS

I34.1 **Nonrheumatic mitral (valve) prolapse**
  Floppy nonrheumatic mitral valve syndrome
  Excludes1: Marfan's syndrome (Q87.4-)

I34.2 **Nonrheumatic mitral (valve) stenosis**

I34.8 **Other nonrheumatic mitral valve disorders**

I34.9 **Nonrheumatic mitral valve disorder, unspecified**

I35 **Nonrheumatic aortic valve disorders**
  Excludes1: aortic valve disorder of unspecified cause but with
      diseases of mitral and/or tricuspid valve(s) (I08.-)
    aortic valve disorder specified as congenital (Q23.0,
      Q23.1)
    aortic valve disorder specified as rheumatic (I06.-)
    hypertrophic subaortic stenosis (I42.1)

I35.0 **Nonrheumatic aortic (valve) stenosis**

I35.1 **Nonrheumatic aortic (valve) insufficiency**
  Nonrheumatic aortic (valve) incompetence NOS
  Nonrheumatic aortic (valve) regurgitation NOS

I35.2 **Nonrheumatic aortic (valve) stenosis with insufficiency**

I35.8 **Other nonrheumatic aortic valve disorders**

I35.9 **Nonrheumatic aortic valve disorder, unspecified**

+, +7th, X + 7th   ● Newborn   ● Pediatric   ● Maternity   ● Adult   ♀ Female   ♂ Male   Manifestation   Unacceptable PDX   HCC   CC   MCC   HAC

I36 Nonrheumatic tricuspid valve disorders

Excludes1: *tricuspid valve disorders of unspecified cause (I07.-)*
tricuspid valve disorders specified as congenital (Q22.4, Q22.8, Q22.9)
tricuspid valve disorders specified as rheumatic (I07.-)
tricuspid valve disorders with aortic and/or mitral valve involvement (I08.-)

I36.0 **Nonrheumatic tricuspid (valve) stenosis**

I36.1 **Nonrheumatic tricuspid (valve) insufficiency**
Nonrheumatic tricuspid (valve) incompetence
Nonrheumatic tricuspid (valve) regurgitation

I36.2 **Nonrheumatic tricuspid (valve) stenosis with insufficiency**

I36.8 **Other nonrheumatic tricuspid valve disorders**

I36.9 **Nonrheumatic tricuspid valve disorder, unspecified**

I37 Nonrheumatic pulmonary valve disorders

Excludes1: *pulmonary valve disorder specified as congenital (Q22.1, Q22.2, Q22.3)*
pulmonary valve disorder specified as rheumatic (I09.89)

I37.0 **Nonrheumatic pulmonary valve stenosis**

I37.1 **Nonrheumatic pulmonary valve insufficiency**
Nonrheumatic pulmonary valve incompetence
Nonrheumatic pulmonary valve regurgitation

I37.2 **Nonrheumatic pulmonary valve stenosis with insufficiency**

I37.8 **Other nonrheumatic pulmonary valve disorders**

I37.9 **Nonrheumatic pulmonary valve disorder, unspecified**

CC I38 Endocarditis, valve unspecified

Includes: endocarditis (chronic) NOS
valvular incompetence NOS
valvular insufficiency NOS
valvular regurgitation NOS
valvular stenosis NOS
valvulitis (chronic) NOS

Excludes1: *congenital insufficiency of cardiac valve NOS (Q24.8)*
congenital stenosis of cardiac valve NOS (Q24.8)
endocardial fibroelastosis (I42.4)
endocarditis specified as rheumatic (I09.1)

Valid 3-character code, no further characters required

CC I39 Endocarditis and heart valve disorders in diseases classified elsewhere

Code first underlying disease, such as:
Q fever (A78)

Excludes1: *endocardial involvement in:*
candidiasis (B37.6)
gonococcal infection (A54.83)
Libman-Sacks disease (M32.11)
listerosis (A32.82)
meningococcal infection (A39.51)
rheumatoid arthritis (M05.31)
syphilis (A52.03)
tuberculosis (A18.84)
typhoid fever (A01.02)

Valid 3-character code, no further characters required

I40 Acute myocarditis

Includes: subacute myocarditis

Excludes1: *acute rheumatic myocarditis (I01.2)*

MCC I40.0 **Infective myocarditis**
Septic myocarditis
Use additional code (B95-B97) to identify infectious agent

MCC I40.1 **Isolated myocarditis**
Fiedler's myocarditis
Giant cell myocarditis
Idiopathic myocarditis

MCC I40.8 **Other acute myocarditis**

MCC I40.9 **Acute myocarditis, unspecified**

MCC I41 Myocarditis in diseases classified elsewhere

Code first underlying disease, such as:
typhus (A75.0-A75.9)

Excludes1: *myocarditis (in):*
Chagas' disease (chronic) (B57.2)
acute (B57.0)
coxsackie (virus) infection (B33.22)
diphtheritic (A36.81)
gonococcal (A54.83)
influenzal (J09.X9, J10.82, J11.82)
meningococcal (A39.52)
mumps (B26.82)

rheumatoid arthritis (M05.31)
sarcoid (D86.85)
syphilis (A52.06)
toxoplasmosis (B58.81)
tuberculous (A18.84)

Valid 3-character code, no further characters required

I42 Cardiomyopathy

Includes: myocardiopathy

Code first pre-existing cardiomyopathy complicating pregnancy and puerperium (O99.4)

Excludes2: *ischemic cardiomyopathy (I25.5)*
peripartum cardiomyopathy (O90.3)
ventricular hypertrophy (I51.7)

CC I42.0 **Dilated cardiomyopathy**
Congestive cardiomyopathy

CC I42.1 **Obstructive hypertrophic cardiomyopathy**
Hypertrophic subaortic stenosis (idiopathic)

CC I42.2 **Other hypertrophic cardiomyopathy**
Nonobstructive hypertrophic cardiomyopathy

CC I42.3 **Endomyocardial (eosinophilic) disease**
Endomyocardial (tropical) fibrosis
Löffler's endocarditis

CC I42.4 **Endocardial fibroelastosis**
Congenital cardiomyopathy
Elastomyofibrosis

CC I42.5 **Other restrictive cardiomyopathy**
Constrictive cardiomyopathy NOS

CC I42.6 **Alcoholic cardiomyopathy**
Code also presence of alcoholism (F10.-)

CC I42.7 **Cardiomyopathy due to drug and external agent**
Code first poisoning due to drug or toxin, if applicable (T36-T65 with fifth or sixth character 1-4 or 6)

Use additional code for adverse effect, if appv licable, to identify drug (T36-T50 with fifth or sixth character 5)

CC I42.8 **Other cardiomyopathies**

CC I42.9 **Cardiomyopathy, unspecified**
Cardiomyopathy (primary) (secondary) NOS

CC I43 Cardiomyopathy in diseases classified elsewhere

Code first underlying disease, such as:
amyloidosis (E85.-)
glycogen storage disease (E74.0)
gout (M10.0-)
thyrotoxicosis (E05.0-E05.9-)

Excludes1: *cardiomyopathy (in):*
coxsackie (virus) (B33.24)
diphtheria (A36.81)
sarcoidosis (D86.85)
tuberculosis (A18.84)

Valid 3-character code, no further characters required

I44 Atrioventricular and left bundle-branch block

I44.0 **Atrioventricular block, first degree**

I44.1 **Atrioventricular block, second degree**
Atrioventricular block, type I and II
Möbitz block, type I and II
Second degree block, type I and II
Wenckebach's block

CC I44.2 **Atrioventricular block, complete**
Complete heart block NOS
Third degree block
AHA CC: 2Q, 2019, 4

+ I44.3 **Other and unspecified atrioventricular block**
Atrioventricular block NOS

I44.30 **Unspecified atrioventricular block**

I44.39 **Other atrioventricular block**

I44.4 **Left anterior fascicular block**

I44.5 **Left posterior fascicular block**

+ I44.6 **Other and unspecified fascicular block**

I44.60 **Unspecified fascicular block**
Left bundle-branch hemiblock NOS

I44.69 **Other fascicular block**

I44.7 **Left bundle-branch block, unspecified**

I45 Other conduction disorders

I45.0 **Right fascicular block**

+ I45.1 **Other and unspecified right bundle-branch block**

I45.10 **Unspecified right bundle-branch block**
Right bundle-branch block NOS

I45.19 **Other right bundle-branch block**

CC I45.2 **Bifascicular block**

675

CC I45.3 Trifascicular block

I45.4 Nonspecific intraventricular block
Bundle-branch block NOS

I45.5 Other specified heart block
Sinoatrial block
Sinoauricular block
Excludes1: *heart block NOS (I45.9)*

I45.6 Pre-excitation syndrome
Accelerated atrioventricular conduction
Accessory atrioventricular conduction
Anomalous atrioventricular excitation
Lown-Ganong-Levine syndrome
Pre-excitation atrioventricular conduction
Wolff-Parkinson-White syndrome

+ I45.8 Other specified conduction disorders
I45.81 Long QT syndrome
CC I45.89 Other specified conduction disorders
Atrioventricular [AV] dissociation
Interference dissociation
Isorhythmic dissociation
Nonparoxysmal AV nodal tachycardia
AHA CC: 2Q, 2013, 31-32

I45.9 Conduction disorder, unspecified
Heart block NOS
Stokes-Adams syndrome

I46 Cardiac arrest
Excludes2: *cardiogenic shock (R57.0)*

MCC I46.2 Cardiac arrest due to underlying cardiac condition
Code first underlying cardiac condition

MCC I46.8 Cardiac arrest due to other underlying condition
Code first underlying condition

MCC I46.9 Cardiac arrest, cause unspecified

I47 Paroxysmal tachycardia
Code first tachycardia complicating:
abortion or ectopic or molar pregnancy (O00-O07, O08.8)
obstetric surgery and procedures (O75.4)
Excludes1: *tachycardia NOS (R00.0)*
sinoauricular tachycardia NOS (R00.0)
sinus [sinusal] tachycardia NOS (R00.0)

CC I47.0 Re-entry ventricular arrhythmia
CC I47.1 Supraventricular tachycardia
Atrial (paroxysmal) tachycardia
Atrioventricular [AV] (paroxysmal) tachycardia
Atrioventricular re-entrant (nodal) tachycardia [AVNRT] [AVRT]
Junctional (paroxysmal) tachycardia
Nodal (paroxysmal) tachycardia

CC I47.2 Ventricular tachycardia
AHA CC: 3Q, 2013, 23-24

I47.9 Paroxysmal tachycardia, unspecified
Bouveret (-Hoffman) syndrome

I48 Atrial fibrillation and flutter
AHA CC: 4Q, 2019, 7

I48.0 Paroxysmal atrial fibrillation
+ I48.1 Persistent atrial fibrillation
Excludes1: *Permanent atrial fibrillation (I48.21)*
AHA CC: 2Q, 2019, 3-4

CC I48.11 Longstanding persistent atrial fibrillation
CC I48.19 Other persistent atrial fibrillation
Chronic persistent atrial fibrillation
Persistent atrial fibrillation, NOS

+ I48.2 Chronic atrial fibrillation
AHA CC: 4Q, 2013, 128; 3Q, 2018, 6

CC I48.20 Chronic atrial fibrillation, unspecified
Excludes1: *Chronic persistent atrial fibrillation (I48.19)*
CC I48.21 Permanent atrial fibrillation

I48.3 Typical atrial flutter
Type I atrial flutter

CC I48.4 Atypical atrial flutter
Type II atrial flutter

+ I48.9 Unspecified atrial fibrillation and atrial flutter
I48.91 Unspecified atrial fibrillation
CC I48.92 Unspecified atrial flutter

I49 Other cardiac arrhythmias
Code first cardiac arrhythmia complicating:
abortion or ectopic or molar pregnancy (O00-O07, O08.8)
obstetric surgery and procedures (O75.4)

Excludes1: *neonatal dysrhythmia (P29.1-)*
sinoatrial bradycardia (R00.1)
sinus bradycardia (R00.1)
vagal bradycardia (R00.1)
Excludes2: *bradycardia NOS (R00.1)*

+ I49.0 Ventricular fibrillation and flutter
MCC I49.01 Ventricular fibrillation
MCC I49.02 Ventricular flutter

I49.1 Atrial premature depolarization
Atrial premature beats

CC I49.2 Junctional premature depolarization
I49.3 Ventricular premature depolarization
AHA CC: 2Q, 2020, 23-24

+ I49.4 Other and unspecified premature depolarization
I49.40 Unspecified premature depolarization
Premature beats NOS
I49.49 Other premature depolarization
Ectopic beats
Extrasystoles
Extrasystolic arrhythmias
Premature contractions

I49.5 Sick sinus syndrome
Tachycardia-bradycardia syndrome
AHA CC: 1Q, 2019, 33-34

I49.8 Other specified cardiac arrhythmias
Brugada syndrome
Coronary sinus rhythm disorder
Ectopic rhythm disorder
Nodal rhythm disorder

I49.9 Cardiac arrhythmia, unspecified
Arrhythmia (cardiac) NOS

I50 Heart failure
Code first:
heart failure complicating abortion or ectopic or molar pregnancy O00-O07, O08.8)
heart failure following surgery (I97.13-)
heart failure due to hypertension (I11.0)
heart failure due to hypertension with chronic kidney disease (I13.-)
obstetric surgery and procedures (O75.4)
rheumatic heart failure (I09.81)
Excludes1: *neonatal cardiac failure (P29.0)*
Excludes2: *cardiac arrest (I46.-)t*
Review coding guidelines C.9.a.1 and C.9.a.3
AHA CC: 1Q, 2017, 47

CC I50.1 Left ventricular failure, unspecified
Cardiac asthma
Edema of lung with heart disease NOS
Edema of lung with heart failure
Left heart failure
Pulmonary edema with heart disease NOS
Pulmonary edema with heart failure
Excludes1: *edema of lung without heart disease or heart failure (J81.-)*
pulmonary edema without heart disease or failure (J81.-)

+ I50.2 Systolic (congestive) heart failure
Heart failure with reduced ejection fraction [HFrEF]
Systolic left ventricular heart failure
Code also end stage heart failure, if applicable (I50.84)
Excludes1: *combined systolic (congestive) and diastolic (congestive) heart failure (I50.4-)*
CC I50.20 Unspecified systolic (congestive) heart failure
MCC I50.21 Acute systolic (congestive) heart failure
CC I50.22 Chronic systolic (congestive) heart failure
MCC I50.23 Acute on chronic systolic (congestive) heart failure
AHA CC: 2Q, 2013, 33

+ I50.3 Diastolic (congestive) heart failure
Diastolic left ventricular heart failure
Heart failure with normal ejection fraction
Heart failure with preserved ejection fraction [HFpEF]
Code also end stage heart failure, if applicable (I50.84)
Excludes1: *combined systolic (congestive) and diastolic (congestive) heart failure (I50.4-)*
CC I50.30 Unspecified diastolic (congestive) heart failure
MCC I50.31 Acute diastolic (congestive) heart failure
AHA CC: 1Q, 2017, 46
CC I50.32 Chronic diastolic (congestive) heart failure
MCC I50.33 Acute on chronic diastolic (congestive) heart failure

+, +7th, X + 7th   ● Newborn   ● Pediatric   ● Maternity   ● Adult   ♀ Female   ♂ Male   Manifestation   Unacceptable PDX   HCC   CC   MCC   HAC

+ I50.4 Combined systolic (congestive) and diastolic (congestive) heart failure
    Combined systolic and diastolic left ventricular heart failure
    Heart failure with reduced ejection fraction and diastolic dysfunction
    Code also end stage heart failure, if applicable (I50.84)

CC I50.40 Unspecified combined systolic (congestive) and diastolic (congestive) heart failure

MCC I50.41 Acute combined systolic (congestive) and diastolic (congestive) heart failure

CC I50.42 Chronic combined systolic (congestive) and diastolic (congestive) heart failure

MCC I50.43 Acute on chronic combined systolic (congestive) and diastolic (congestive) heart failure

+ I50.8 Other heart failure
    AHA CC: 4Q, 2017, 15-16

+ I50.81 Right heart failure
    Right ventricular failure

I50.810 Right heart failure, unspecified
    Right heart failure without mention of left heart failure
    Right ventricular failure NOS

I50.811 Acute right heart failure
    Acute isolated right heart failure
    Acute (isolated) right ventricular failure

I50.812 Chronic right heart failure
    Chronic isolated right heart failure
    Chronic (isolated) right ventricular failure

I50.813 Acute on chronic right heart failure
    Acute on chronic isolated right heart failure
    Acute on chronic (isolated) right ventricular failure
    Acute decompensation of chronic (isolated) right ventricular failure
    Acute exacerbation of chronic (isolated) right ventricular failure

I50.814 Right heart failure, unspecified
    Right ventricular failure secondary to left ventricular failure
    Code also the type of left ventricular failure, if known (I50.2-I50.43)
    Excludes1: *right heart failure with but not due to left heart failure (I50.82)*

I50.82 Biventricular heart failure
    Code also the type of left ventricular failure as systolic, diastolic, or combined, if known (I50.2-I50.43)

I50.83 High output heart failure

I50.84 End stage heart failure
    Stage D heart failure
    Code also the type of heart failure as systolic, diastolic, or combined, if known (I50.2-I50.43)

I50.89 Heart failure, unspecified

I50.9 Heart failure, unspecified
    Cardiac, heart or myocardial failure NOS
    Congestive heart disease
    Congestive heart failure NOS
    Excludes2: *fluid overload unrelated to congestive heart failure (E87.70)*
    AHA CC: 4Q, 2012, 92-93; 4Q, 2014, 21-22; 1Q, 2017, 46

I51 Complications and ill-defined descriptions of heart disease
    Excludes1: *any condition in I51.4-I51.9 due to hypertension (I11.-)*
    any condition in I51.4-I51.9 due to hypertension and chronic kidney disease (I13.-)
    heart disease specified as rheumatic (I00-I09)

● CC I51.0 Cardiac septal defect, acquired
    Acquired septal atrial defect (old)
    Acquired septal auricular defect (old)
    Acquired septal ventricular defect (old)
    Excludes1: *cardiac septal defect as current complication following acute myocardial infarction (I23.1, I23.2)*

MCC I51.1 Rupture of chordae tendineae, not elsewhere classified
    Excludes1: *rupture of chordae tendineae as current complication following acute myocardial infarction (I23.4)*

MCC I51.2 Rupture of papillary muscle, not elsewhere classified
    Excludes1: *rupture of papillary muscle as current complication following acute myocardial infarction (I23.5)*

I51.3 Intracardiac thrombosis, not elsewhere classified
    Apical thrombosis (old)
    Atrial thrombosis (old)
    Auricular thrombosis (old)
    Mural thrombosis (old)
    Ventricular thrombosis (old)
    Excludes1: *intracardiac thrombosis as current complication following acute myocardial infarction (I23.6)*
    AHA CC: 1Q, 2013, 24

I51.4 Myocarditis, unspecified
    Chronic (interstitial) myocarditis
    Myocardial fibrosis
    Myocarditis NOS
    Excludes1: *acute or subacute myocarditis (I40.-)*
    Review coding guideline C.9.a.1

I51.5 Myocardial degeneration
    Fatty degeneration of heart or myocardium
    Myocardial disease
    Senile degeneration of heart or myocardium
    Review coding guideline C.9.a.1

I51.7 Cardiomegaly
    Cardiac dilatation
    Cardiac hypertrophy
    Ventricular dilatation
    Review coding guideline C.9.a.1

+ I51.8 Other ill-defined heart diseases
    Review coding guideline C.9.a.1

CC I51.81 Takotsubo syndrome
    Reversible left ventricular dysfunction following sudden emotional stress
    Stress induced cardiomyopathy
    Takotsubo cardiomyopathy
    Transient left ventricular apical ballooning syndrome
    AHA CC: 2Q, 2018, 9-10

I51.89 Other ill-defined heart diseases
    Carditis (acute)(chronic)
    Pancarditis (acute)(chronic)
    AHA CC: 2Q, 2019, 5-6

I51.9 Heart disease, unspecified
    Review coding guideline C.9.a.1

I52 Other heart disorders in diseases classified elsewhere
    Code first underlying disease, such as:
    congenital syphilis (A50.5)
    mucopolysaccharidosis (E76.3)
    schistosomiasis (B65.0-B65.9)
    Excludes1: *heart disease (in):*
    gonococcal infection (A54.83)
    meningococcal infection (A39.50)
    rheumatoid arthritis (M05.31)
    syphilis (A52.06)
    Valid 3-character code, no further characters required

Cerebrovascular diseases (I60-I69)

Use additional code to identify presence of:
    alcohol abuse and dependence (F10.-)
    exposure to environmental tobacco smoke (Z77.22)
    history of tobacco dependence (Z87.891)
    hypertension (I10-I16)
    occupational exposure to environmental tobacco smoke (Z57.31)
    tobacco dependence (F17.-)
    tobacco use (Z72.0)

Excludes1: *traumatic intracranial hemorrhage (S06.-)*
Review coding guidelines C.9.a.4 and C.9.d

I60 Nontraumatic subarachnoid hemorrhage
    Excludes1: *syphilitic ruptured cerebral aneurysm (A52.05)*
    Excludes2: *sequelae of subarachnoid hemorrhage (I69.0-)*

+ I60.0 Nontraumatic subarachnoid hemorrhage from carotid siphon and bifurcation

MCC I60.00 Nontraumatic subarachnoid hemorrhage from unspecified carotid siphon and bifurcation

MCC I60.01 Nontraumatic subarachnoid hemorrhage from right carotid siphon and bifurcation

+, +7th, X + 7th   ● Newborn   ● Pediatric   ● Maternity   ● Adult   ♀ Female   ♂ Male   Manifestation   Unacceptable PDX   HCC   CC   MCC   HAC

MCC **I60.02** Nontraumatic subarachnoid hemorrhage from left carotid siphon and bifurcation

+ **I60.1** Nontraumatic subarachnoid hemorrhage from middle cerebral artery

MCC **I60.10** Nontraumatic subarachnoid hemorrhage from unspecified middle cerebral artery

MCC **I60.11** Nontraumatic subarachnoid hemorrhage from right middle cerebral artery

MCC **I60.12** Nontraumatic subarachnoid hemorrhage from left middle cerebral artery

MCC **I60.2** Nontraumatic subarachnoid hemorrhage from anterior communicating artery

+ **I60.3** Nontraumatic subarachnoid hemorrhage from posterior communicating artery

MCC **I60.30** Nontraumatic subarachnoid hemorrhage from unspecified posterior communicating artery

MCC **I60.31** Nontraumatic subarachnoid hemorrhage from right posterior communicating artery

MCC **I60.32** Nontraumatic subarachnoid hemorrhage from left posterior communicating artery

MCC **I60.4** Nontraumatic subarachnoid hemorrhage from basilar artery

+ **I60.5** Nontraumatic subarachnoid hemorrhage from vertebral artery

MCC **I60.50** Nontraumatic subarachnoid hemorrhage from unspecified vertebral artery

MCC **I60.51** Nontraumatic subarachnoid hemorrhage from right vertebral artery

MCC **I60.52** Nontraumatic subarachnoid hemorrhage from left vertebral artery

MCC **I60.6** Nontraumatic subarachnoid hemorrhage from other intracranial arteries

MCC **I60.7** Nontraumatic subarachnoid hemorrhage from unspecified intracranial artery

Ruptured (congenital) berry aneurysm
Ruptured (congenital) cerebral aneurysm
Subarachnoid hemorrhage (nontraumatic) from cerebral artery NOS
Subarachnoid hemorrhage (nontraumatic) from communicating artery NOS

Excludes1: *berry aneurysm, nonruptured (I67.1)*

MCC **I60.8** Other nontraumatic subarachnoid hemorrhage

Meningeal hemorrhage
Rupture of cerebral arteriovenous malformation

MCC **I60.9** Nontraumatic subarachnoid hemorrhage, unspecified

I61 Nontraumatic intracerebral hemorrhage

Excludes2: *sequelae of intracerebral hemorrhage (I69.1-)*
AHA CC: 2Q, 2017, 10

MCC **I61.0** Nontraumatic intracerebral hemorrhage in hemisphere, subcortical

Deep intracerebral hemorrhage (nontraumatic)

MCC **I61.1** Nontraumatic intracerebral hemorrhage in hemisphere, cortical

Cerebral lobe hemorrhage (nontraumatic)
Superficial intracerebral hemorrhage (nontraumatic)

MCC **I61.2** Nontraumatic intracerebral hemorrhage in hemisphere, unspecified

MCC **I61.3** Nontraumatic intracerebral hemorrhage in brain stem

MCC **I61.4** Nontraumatic intracerebral hemorrhage in cerebellum

MCC **I61.5** Nontraumatic intracerebral hemorrhage, intraventricular

MCC **I61.6** Nontraumatic intracerebral hemorrhage, multiple localized

MCC **I61.8** Other nontraumatic intracerebral hemorrhage

MCC **I61.9** Nontraumatic intracerebral hemorrhage, unspecified

I62 Other and unspecified nontraumatic intracranial hemorrhage

Excludes2: *sequelae of intracranial hemorrhage (I69.2)*

+ **I62.0** Nontraumatic subdural hemorrhage

MCC **I62.00** Nontraumatic subdural hemorrhage, unspecified

MCC **I62.01** Nontraumatic acute subdural hemorrhage

MCC **I62.02** Nontraumatic subacute subdural hemorrhage

MCC **I62.03** Nontraumatic chronic subdural hemorrhage

MCC **I62.1** Nontraumatic extradural hemorrhage

Nontraumatic epidural hemorrhage

CC **I62.9** Nontraumatic intracranial hemorrhage, unspecified

I63 Cerebral infarction

Includes: occlusion and stenosis of cerebral and precerebral arteries, resulting in cerebral infarction

Use additional code, if applicable, to identify status post administration of tPA (rtPA) in a different facility within the last 24 hours prior to admission to current facility (Z92.82)

Use additional code, if known, to indicate National Institutes of Health Stroke Scale (NIHSS) score (R29.7-)

Excludes1: *neonatal cerebral infarction (P91.82-)*
Excludes2: *sequelae of cerebral infarction (I69.3-)*
AHA CC: 4Q, 2016, 28

+ **I63.0** Cerebral infarction due to thrombosis of precerebral arteries

MCC **I63.00** Cerebral infarction due to thrombosis of unspecified precerebral artery

+ **I63.01** Cerebral infarction due to thrombosis of vertebral artery

MCC **I63.011** Cerebral infarction due to thrombosis of right vertebral artery

MCC **I63.012** Cerebral infarction due to thrombosis of left vertebral artery

MCC **I63.013** Cerebral infarction due to thrombosis of bilateral vertebral arteries

MCC **I63.019** Cerebral infarction due to thrombosis of unspecified vertebral artery

MCC **I63.02** Cerebral infarction due to thrombosis of basilar artery

+ **I63.03** Cerebral infarction due to thrombosis of carotid artery

MCC **I63.031** Cerebral infarction due to thrombosis of right carotid artery

MCC **I63.032** Cerebral infarction due to thrombosis of left carotid artery

MCC **I63.033** Cerebral infarction due to thrombosis of bilateral carotid arteries

MCC **I63.039** Cerebral infarction due to thrombosis of unspecified carotid artery

MCC **I63.09** Cerebral infarction due to thrombosis of other precerebral artery

+ **I63.1** Cerebral infarction due to embolism of precerebral arteries

MCC **I63.10** Cerebral infarction due to embolism of unspecified precerebral artery

+ **I63.11** Cerebral infarction due to embolism of vertebral artery

MCC **I63.111** Cerebral infarction due to embolism of right vertebral artery

MCC **I63.112** Cerebral infarction due to embolism of left vertebral artery

MCC **I63.113** Cerebral infarction due to embolism of bilateral vertebral arteries

MCC **I63.119** Cerebral infarction due to embolism of unspecified vertebral artery

MCC **I63.12** Cerebral infarction due to embolism of basilar artery

+ **I63.13** Cerebral infarction due to embolism of carotid artery

MCC **I63.131** Cerebral infarction due to embolism of right carotid artery

MCC **I63.132** Cerebral infarction due to embolism of left carotid artery

MCC **I63.133** Cerebral infarction due to embolism of bilateral carotid arteries

MCC **I63.139** Cerebral infarction due to embolism of unspecified carotid artery

MCC **I63.19** Cerebral infarction due to embolism of other precerebral artery

+, +7th, X + 7th　●Newborn　●Pediatric　●Maternity　●Adult　♀Female　♂Male　Manifestation　Unacceptable PDX　HCC　CC　MCC　HAC

+ I63.2 **Cerebral infarction due to unspecified occlusion or stenosis of precerebral arteries**

MCC **I63.20** Cerebral infarction due to unspecified occlusion or stenosis of unspecified precerebral arteries

+ I63.21 Cerebral infarction due to unspecified occlusion or stenosis of vertebral arteries

MCC **I63.211** Cerebral infarction due to unspecified occlusion or stenosis of right vertebral artery

MCC **I63.212** Cerebral infarction due to unspecified occlusion or stenosis of left vertebral artery

MCC **I63.213** Cerebral infarction due to unspecified occlusion or stenosis of bilateral vertebral arteries

MCC **I63.219** Cerebral infarction due to unspecified occlusion or stenosis of unspecified vertebral artery

MCC **I63.22** Cerebral infarction due to unspecified occlusion or stenosis of basilar artery

+ I63.23 Cerebral infarction due to unspecified occlusion or stenosis of carotid arteries

MCC **I63.231** Cerebral infarction due to unspecified occlusion or stenosis of right carotid arteries

MCC **I63.232** Cerebral infarction due to unspecified occlusion or stenosis of left carotid arteries

MCC **I63.233** Cerebral infarction due to unspecified occlusion or stenosis of bilateral carotid arteries

MCC **I63.239** Cerebral infarction due to unspecified occlusion or stenosis of unspecified carotid artery

MCC **I63.29** Cerebral infarction due to unspecified occlusion or stenosis of other precerebral arteries

+ I63.3 **Cerebral infarction due to thrombosis of cerebral arteries**

MCC **I63.30** Cerebral infarction due to thrombosis of unspecified cerebral artery

+ I63.31 Cerebral infarction due to thrombosis of middle cerebral artery

MCC **I63.311** Cerebral infarction due to thrombosis of right middle cerebral artery

MCC **I63.312** Cerebral infarction due to thrombosis of left middle cerebral artery

MCC **I63.313** Cerebral infarction due to thrombosis of bilateral middle cerebral arteries

MCC **I63.319** Cerebral infarction due to thrombosis of unspecified middle cerebral artery

+ I63.32 Cerebral infarction due to thrombosis of anterior cerebral artery

MCC **I63.321** Cerebral infarction due to thrombosis of right anterior cerebral artery

MCC **I63.322** Cerebral infarction due to thrombosis of left anterior cerebral artery

MCC **I63.323** Cerebral infarction due to thrombosis of bilateral anterior cerebral arteries

MCC **I63.329** Cerebral infarction due to thrombosis of unspecified anterior cerebral artery

+ I63.33 Cerebral infarction due to thrombosis of posterior cerebral artery

MCC **I63.331** Cerebral infarction due to thrombosis of right posterior cerebral artery

MCC **I63.332** Cerebral infarction due to thrombosis of left posterior cerebral artery

MCC **I63.333** Cerebral infarction due to thrombosis of bilateral posterior cerebral arteries

MCC **I63.339** Cerebral infarction due to thrombosis of unspecified posterior cerebral artery

+ I63.34 Cerebral infarction due to thrombosis of cerebellar artery

MCC **I63.341** Cerebral infarction due to thrombosis of right cerebellar artery

MCC **I63.342** Cerebral infarction due to thrombosis of left cerebellar artery

MCC **I63.343** Cerebral infarction due to thrombosis of bilateral cerebellar arteries

MCC **I63.349** Cerebral infarction due to thrombosis of unspecified cerebellar artery

MCC **I63.39** Cerebral infarction due to thrombosis of other cerebral artery

+ I63.4 **Cerebral infarction due to embolism of cerebral arteries**

MCC **I63.40** Cerebral infarction due to embolism of unspecified cerebral artery

+ I63.41 Cerebral infarction due to embolism of middle cerebral artery

MCC **I63.411** Cerebral infarction due to embolism of right middle cerebral artery

MCC **I63.412** Cerebral infarction due to embolism of left middle cerebral artery

MCC **I63.413** Cerebral infarction due to embolism of bilateral middle cerebral arteries

MCC **I63.419** Cerebral infarction due to embolism of unspecified middle cerebral artery

+ I63.42 Cerebral infarction due to embolism of anterior cerebral artery

MCC **I63.421** Cerebral infarction due to embolism of right anterior cerebral artery

MCC **I63.422** Cerebral infarction due to embolism of left anterior cerebral artery

MCC **I63.423** Cerebral infarction due to embolism of bilateral anterior cerebral arteries

MCC **I63.429** Cerebral infarction due to embolism of unspecified anterior cerebral artery

+ I63.43 Cerebral infarction due to embolism of posterior cerebral artery

MCC **I63.431** Cerebral infarction due to embolism of right posterior cerebral artery

MCC **I63.432** Cerebral infarction due to embolism of left posterior cerebral artery

MCC **I63.433** Cerebral infarction due to embolism of bilateral posterior cerebral arteries

MCC **I63.439** Cerebral infarction due to embolism of unspecified posterior cerebral artery

+ I63.44 Cerebral infarction due to embolism of cerebellar artery

MCC **I63.441** Cerebral infarction due to embolism of right cerebellar artery

MCC **I63.442** Cerebral infarction due to embolism of left cerebellar artery

MCC **I64.443** Cerebral infarction due to embolism of bilateral cerebellar arteries

MCC **I63.449** Cerebral infarction due to embolism of unspecified cerebellar artery

MCC **I63.49** Cerebral infarction due to embolism of other cerebral artery

+ I63.5 **Cerebral infarction due to unspecified occlusion or stenosis of cerebral arteries**

MCC **I63.50** Cerebral infarction due to unspecified occlusion or stenosis of unspecified cerebral artery

+ I63.51 Cerebral infarction due to unspecified occlusion or stenosis of middle cerebral artery

MCC **I63.511** Cerebral infarction due to unspecified occlusion or stenosis of right middle cerebral artery

MCC **I63.512** Cerebral infarction due to unspecified occlusion or stenosis of left middle cerebral artery

MCC **I63.513** Cerebral infarction due to unspecified occlusion or stenosis of bilateral middle cerebral arteries

MCC **I63.519** Cerebral infarction due to unspecified occlusion or stenosis of unspecified middle cerebral artery

+ I63.52 Cerebral infarction due to unspecified occlusion or stenosis of anterior cerebral artery

MCC **I63.521** Cerebral infarction due to unspecified occlusion or stenosis of right anterior cerebral artery

MCC **I63.522** Cerebral infarction due to unspecified occlusion or stenosis of left anterior cerebral artery

MCC **I63.523** Cerebral infarction due to unspecified occlusion or stenosis of bilateral anterior cerebral arteries

MCC **I63.529** Cerebral infarction due to unspecified occlusion or stenosis of unspecified anterior cerebral artery

679

+, +7th, X + 7th　● Newborn　● Pediatric　● Maternity　● Adult　♀ Female　♂ Male　Manifestation　Unacceptable PDX　HCC　CC　MCC　HAC

+ **I63.53** Cerebral infarction due to unspecified occlusion or stenosis of posterior cerebral artery

MCC **I63.531** Cerebral infarction due to unspecified occlusion or stenosis of right posterior cerebral artery

MCC **I63.532** Cerebral infarction due to unspecified occlusion or stenosis of left posterior cerebral artery
AHA CC: 2Q, 2017, 10

MCC **I63.533** Cerebral infarction due to unspecified occlusion or stenosis of bilateral posterior cerebral arteries

MCC **I63.539** Cerebral infarction due to unspecified occlusion or stenosis of unspecified posterior cerebral artery

+ **I63.54** Cerebral infarction due to unspecified occlusion or stenosis of cerebellar artery

MCC **I63.541** Cerebral infarction due to unspecified occlusion or stenosis of right cerebellar artery

MCC **I63.542** Cerebral infarction due to unspecified occlusion or stenosis of left cerebellar artery

MCC **I63.543** Cerebral infarction due to unspecified occlusion or stenosis of bilateral cerebellar arteries

MCC **I63.549** Cerebral infarction due to unspecified occlusion or stenosis of unspecified cerebellar artery

MCC **I63.59** Cerebral infarction due to unspecified occlusion or stenosis of other cerebral artery

MCC **I63.6** Cerebral infarction due to cerebral venous thrombosis, nonpyogenic

+ **I63.8** Other cerebral infarction
AHA CC: 2Q, 2017, 9-10; 4Q, 2018, 16

MCC **I63.81** Other cerebral infarction due to occlusion or stenosis of small artery
Lacunar infarction
AHA CC: 4Q, 2018, 16

MCC **I63.89** Other cerebral infarction

MCC **I63.9** Cerebral infarction, unspecified
Stroke NOS
Excludes2: transient cerebral ischemic attacks and related syndromes (G45.-)
AHA CC: 1Q, 2015, 26; 4Q, 2016, 61 62

I65 Occlusion and stenosis of precerebral arteries, not resulting in cerebral infarction

Includes: embolism of precerebral artery
narrowing of precerebral artery
obstruction (complete) (partial) of precerebral artery
thrombosis of precerebral artery
Excludes1: insufficiency, NOS, of precerebral artery (G45.-)
insufficiency of precerebral arteries causing cerebral infarction (I63.0-I63.2)

+ **I65.0** Occlusion and stenosis of vertebral artery

I65.01 Occlusion and stenosis of right vertebral artery

I65.02 Occlusion and stenosis of left vertebral artery

I65.03 Occlusion and stenosis of bilateral vertebral arteries

I65.09 Occlusion and stenosis of unspecified vertebral artery

I65.1 Occlusion and stenosis of basilar artery

+ **I65.2** Occlusion and stenosis of carotid artery

I65.21 Occlusion and stenosis of right carotid artery

I65.22 Occlusion and stenosis of left carotid artery

I65.23 Occlusion and stenosis of bilateral carotid arteries
AHA CC: 2Q, 2018, 9

I65.29 Occlusion and stenosis of unspecified carotid artery

I65.8 Occlusion and stenosis of other precerebral arteries

I65.9 Occlusion and stenosis of unspecified precerebral artery
Occlusion and stenosis of precerebral artery NOS

I66 Occlusion and stenosis of cerebral arteries, not resulting in cerebral infarction

Includes: embolism of cerebral artery
narrowing of cerebral artery
obstruction (complete) (partial) of cerebral artery
thrombosis of cerebral artery
Excludes1: Occlusion and stenosis of cerebral artery causing cerebral infarction (I63.3-I63.5)

+ **I66.0** Occlusion and stenosis of middle cerebral artery

I66.01 Occlusion and stenosis of right middle cerebral artery

I66.02 Occlusion and stenosis of left middle cerebral artery

I66.03 Occlusion and stenosis of bilateral middle cerebral arteries

I66.09 Occlusion and stenosis of unspecified middle cerebral artery

+ **I66.1** Occlusion and stenosis of anterior cerebral artery

I66.11 Occlusion and stenosis of right anterior cerebral artery

I66.12 Occlusion and stenosis of left anterior cerebral artery

I66.13 Occlusion and stenosis of bilateral anterior cerebral arteries

I66.19 Occlusion and stenosis of unspecified anterior cerebral artery

+ **I66.2** Occlusion and stenosis of posterior cerebral artery

I66.21 Occlusion and stenosis of right posterior cerebral artery

I66.22 Occlusion and stenosis of left posterior cerebral artery

I66.23 Occlusion and stenosis of bilateral posterior cerebral arteries

I66.29 Occlusion and stenosis of unspecified posterior cerebral artery

I66.3 Occlusion and stenosis of cerebellar arteries

I66.8 Occlusion and stenosis of other cerebral arteries
Occlusion and stenosis of perforating arteries

I66.9 Occlusion and stenosis of unspecified cerebral artery

I67 Other cerebrovascular diseases
Excludes2: sequelae of the listed conditions (I69.8)

MCC **I67.0** Dissection of cerebral arteries, nonruptured
Excludes1: ruptured cerebral arteries (I60.7)

I67.1 Cerebral aneurysm, nonruptured
Cerebral aneurysm NOS
Cerebral arteriovenous fistula, acquired
Internal carotid artery aneurysm, intracranial portion
Internal carotid artery aneurysm, NOS
Excludes1: congenital cerebral aneurysm, nonruptured (Q28.-)
ruptured cerebral aneurysm (I60.7)

● **I67.2** Cerebral atherosclerosis
Atheroma of cerebral and precerebral arteries

CC **I67.3** Progressive vascular leukoencephalopathy
Binswanger's disease

CC **I67.4** Hypertensive encephalopathy
Excludes2: insufficiency, NOS, of precerebral arteries (G45.2)

CC **I67.5** Moyamoya disease

CC **I67.6** Nonpyogenic thrombosis of intracranial venous system
Nonpyogenic thrombosis of cerebral vein
Nonpyogenic thrombosis of intracranial venous sinus
Excludes1: nonpyogenic thrombosis of intracranial venous system causing infarction (I63.6)

CC **I67.7** Cerebral arteritis, not elsewhere classified
Granulomatous angiitis of the nervous system
Excludes1: allergic granulomatous angiitis (M30.1)

+ **I67.8** Other specified cerebrovascular diseases
AHA CC: 4Q, 2018, 17

CC **I67.81** Acute cerebrovascular insufficiency
Acute cerebrovascular insufficiency unspecified as to location or reversibility

CC **I67.82** Cerebral ischemia
Chronic cerebral ischemia

MCC **I67.83** Posterior reversible encephalopathy syndrome
PRES

+ **I67.84** Cerebral vasospasm and vasoconstriction

CC **I67.841** Reversible cerebrovascular vasoconstriction syndrome
Call-Fleming syndrome
Code first underlying condition, if applicable, such as eclampsia (O15.00-O15.9)

CC **I67.848** Other cerebrovascular vasospasm and vasoconstriction

+ **I67.85** Hereditary cerebrovascular diseases

+, +7th, X + 7th ● Newborn ● Pediatric ● Maternity ● Adult ♀ Female ♂ Male Manifestation Unacceptable PDX HCC CC MCC HAC

CC I67.850 **Cerebral autosomal dominant arteriopathy with subcortical infarcts and leukoencephalopathy**
CADASIL
Code also any associated diagnoses, such as:
epilepsy (G40.-)
stroke (I63.-)
vascular dementia (F01.-)

CC I67.858 **Other hereditary cerebrovascular disease**

CC I67.89 **Other cerebrovascular disease**

I67.9 **Cerebrovascular disease, unspecified**

I68 **Cerebrovascular disorders in diseases classified elsewhere**

I68.0 **Cerebral amyloid angiopathy**
Code first underlying amyloidosis (E85.-)

CC I68.2 **Cerebral arteritis in other diseases classified elsewhere**
Code first underlying disease
Excludes1: *cerebral arteritis (in):*
listerosis (A32.89)
systemic lupus erythematosus (M32.19)
syphilis (A52.04)
tuberculosis (A18.89)

I68.8 **Other cerebrovascular disorders in diseases classified elsewhere**
Code first underlying disease
Excludes1: *syphilitic cerebral aneurysm (A52.05)*

I69 **Sequelae of cerebrovascular disease**

NOTE Category I69 is to be used to indicate conditions in I60-I67 as the cause of sequelae. The 'sequelae' include conditions specified as such or as residuals which may occur at any time after the onset of the causal condition

Excludes1: *personal history of cerebral infarction without residual deficit (Z86.73)*
personal history of prolonged reversible ischemic neurologic deficit (PRIND) (Z86.73)
personal history of reversible ischemic neurologcial deficit (RIND) (Z86.73)
sequelae of traumatic intracranial injury (S06.-)
Review coding guideline C.9.d
AHA CC: 4Q, 2016, 28

+ I69.0 **Sequelae of nontraumatic subarachnoid hemorrhage**

I69.00 **Unspecified sequelae of nontraumatic subarachnoid hemorrhage**

+ I69.01 **Cognitive deficits following nontraumatic subarachnoid hemorrhage**

I69.010 **Attention and concentration deficit following nontraumatic subarachnoid hemorrhage**

I69.011 **Memory deficit following nontraumatic subarachnoid hemorrhage**

I69.012 **Visuospatial deficit and spatial neglect following nontraumatic subarachnoid hemorrhage**

I69.013 **Psychomotor deficit following nontraumatic subarachnoid hemorrhage**

I69.014 **Frontal lobe and executive function deficit following nontraumatic subarachnoid hemorrhage**

I69.015 **Cognitive social or emotional deficit following nontraumatic subarachnoid hemorrhage**

I69.018 **Other symptoms and signs involving cognitive functions following nontraumatic subarachnoid hemorrhage**

I69.019 **Unspecified symptoms and signs involving cognitive functions following nontraumatic subarachnoid hemorrhage**

+ I69.02 **Speech and language deficits following nontraumatic subarachnoid hemorrhage**

I69.020 **Aphasia following nontraumatic subarachnoid hemorrhage**

I69.021 **Dysphasia following nontraumatic subarachnoid hemorrhage**

I69.022 **Dysarthria following nontraumatic subarachnoid hemorrhage**

I69.023 **Fluency disorder following nontraumatic subarachnoid hemorrhage**
Stuttering following nontraumatic subarachnoid hemorrhage

I69.028 **Other speech and language deficits following nontraumatic subarachnoid hemorrhage**

+ I69.03 **Monoplegia of upper limb following nontraumatic subarachnoid hemorrhage**

I69.031 **Monoplegia of upper limb following nontraumatic subarachnoid hemorrhage affecting right dominant side**

I69.032 **Monoplegia of upper limb following nontraumatic subarachnoid hemorrhage affecting left dominant side**

I69.033 **Monoplegia of upper limb following nontraumatic subarachnoid hemorrhage affecting right non-dominant side**

I69.034 **Monoplegia of upper limb following nontraumatic subarachnoid hemorrhage affecting left non-dominant side**

I69.039 **Monoplegia of upper limb following nontraumatic subarachnoid hemorrhage affecting unspecified side**

+ I69.04 **Monoplegia of lower limb following nontraumatic subarachnoid hemorrhage**

I69.041 **Monoplegia of lower limb following nontraumatic subarachnoid hemorrhage affecting right dominant side**

I69.042 **Monoplegia of lower limb following nontraumatic subarachnoid hemorrhage affecting left dominant side**

I69.043 **Monoplegia of lower limb following nontraumatic subarachnoid hemorrhage affecting right non-dominant side**

I69.044 **Monoplegia of lower limb following nontraumatic subarachnoid hemorrhage affecting left non-dominant side**

I69.049 **Monoplegia of lower limb following nontraumatic subarachnoid hemorrhage affecting unspecified side**

+ I69.05 **Hemiplegia and hemiparesis following nontraumatic subarachnoid hemorrhage**

CC I69.051 **Hemiplegia and hemiparesis following nontraumatic subarachnoid hemorrhage affecting right dominant side**

CC I69.052 **Hemiplegia and hemiparesis following nontraumatic subarachnoid hemorrhage affecting left dominant side**

CC I69.053 **Hemiplegia and hemiparesis following nontraumatic subarachnoid hemorrhage affecting right non-dominant side**

CC I69.054 **Hemiplegia and hemiparesis following nontraumatic subarachnoid hemorrhage affecting left non-dominant side**

CC I69.059 **Hemiplegia and hemiparesis following nontraumatic subarachnoid hemorrhage affecting unspecified side**

+ I69.06 **Other paralytic syndrome following nontraumatic subarachnoid hemorrhage**
Use additional code to identify type of paralytic syndrome, such as:
locked-in state (G83.5)
quadriplegia (G82.5-)
Excludes1: *hemiplegia/hemiparesis following nontraumatic subarachnoid hemorrhage (I69.05-)*
monoplegia of lower limb following nontraumatic subarachnoid hemorrhage (I69.04-)
monoplegia of upper limb following nontraumatic subarachnoid hemorrhage (I69.03-)

681

I69.061   Other paralytic syndrome following nontraumatic subarachnoid hemorrhage affecting right dominant side

I69.062   Other paralytic syndrome following nontraumatic subarachnoid hemorrhage affecting left dominant side

I69.063   Other paralytic syndrome following nontraumatic subarachnoid hemorrhage affecting right non-dominant side

I69.064   Other paralytic syndrome following nontraumatic subarachnoid hemorrhage affecting left non-dominant side

I69.065   Other paralytic syndrome following nontraumatic subarachnoid hemorrhage, bilateral

I69.069   Other paralytic syndrome following nontraumatic subarachnoid hemorrhage affecting unspecified side

+ **I69.09**   Other sequelae of nontraumatic subarachnoid hemorrhage

I69.090   Apraxia following nontraumatic subarachnoid hemorrhage

I69.091   Dysphagia following nontraumatic subarachnoid hemorrhage

   Use additional code to identify the type of dysphagia, if known (R13.1-)

I69.092   Facial weakness following nontraumatic subarachnoid hemorrhage

   Facial droop following nontraumatic subarachnoid hemorrhage

I69.093   Ataxia following nontraumatic subarachnoid hemorrhage

I69.098   Other sequelae following nontraumatic subarachnoid hemorrhage

   Alterations of sensation following nontraumatic subarachnoid hemorrhage

   Disturbance of vision following nontraumatic subarachnoid hemorrhage

   Use additional code to identify the sequelae

+ **I69.1**   Sequelae of nontraumatic intracerebral hemorrhage

I69.10   Unspecified sequelae of nontraumatic intracerebral hemorrhage

+ **I69.11**   Cognitive deficits following nontraumatic intracerebral hemorrhage

I69.110   Attention and concentration deficit following nontraumatic intracerebral hemorrhage

I69.111   Memory deficit following nontraumatic intracerebral hemorrhage

I69.112   Visuospatial deficit and spatial neglect following nontraumatic intracerebral hemorrhage

I69.113   Psychomotor deficit following nontraumatic intracerebral hemorrhage

I69.114   Frontal lobe and executive function deficit following nontraumatic intracerebral hemorrhage

I69.115   Cognitive social or emotional deficit following nontraumatic intracerebral hemorrhage

I69.118   Other symptoms and signs involving cognitive functions following nontraumatic intracerebral hemorrhage

I69.119   Unspecified symptoms and signs involving cognitive functions following nontraumatic intracerebral hemorrhage

+ **I69.12**   Speech and language deficits following nontraumatic intracerebral hemorrhage

I69.120   Aphasia following nontraumatic intracerebral hemorrhage

I69.121   Dysphasia following nontraumatic intracerebral hemorrhage

I69.122   Dysarthria following nontraumatic intracerebral hemorrhage

I69.123   Fluency disorder following nontraumatic intracerebral hemorrhage

   Stuttering following nontraumatic intracerebral hemorrhage

I69.128   Other speech and language deficits following nontraumatic intracerebral hemorrhage

+ **I69.13**   Monoplegia of upper limb following nontraumatic intracerebral hemorrhage

I69.131   Monoplegia of upper limb following nontraumatic intracerebral hemorrhage affecting right dominant side

I69.132   Monoplegia of upper limb following nontraumatic intracerebral hemorrhage affecting left dominant side

I69.133   Monoplegia of upper limb following nontraumatic intracerebral hemorrhage affecting right non-dominant side

I69.134   Monoplegia of upper limb following nontraumatic intracerebral hemorrhage affecting left non-dominant side

I69.139   Monoplegia of upper limb following nontraumatic intracerebral hemorrhage affecting unspecified side

+ **I69.14**   Monoplegia of lower limb following nontraumatic intracerebral hemorrhage

I69.141   Monoplegia of lower limb following nontraumatic intracerebral hemorrhage affecting right dominant side

I69.142   Monoplegia of lower limb following nontraumatic intracerebral hemorrhage affecting left dominant side

I69.143   Monoplegia of lower limb following nontraumatic intracerebral hemorrhage affecting right non-dominant side

I69.144   Monoplegia of lower limb following nontraumatic intracerebral hemorrhage affecting left non-dominant side

I69.149   Monoplegia of lower limb following nontraumatic intracerebral hemorrhage affecting unspecified side

+ **I69.15**   Hemiplegia and hemiparesis following nontraumatic intracerebral hemorrhage

CC **I69.151**   Hemiplegia and hemiparesis following nontraumatic intracerebral hemorrhage affecting right dominant side

CC **I69.152**   Hemiplegia and hemiparesis following nontraumatic intracerebral hemorrhage affecting left dominant side

CC **I69.153**   Hemiplegia and hemiparesis following nontraumatic intracerebral hemorrhage affecting right non-dominant side

CC **I69.154**   Hemiplegia and hemiparesis following nontraumatic intracerebral hemorrhage affecting left non-dominant side

CC **I69.159**   Hemiplegia and hemiparesis following nontraumatic intracerebral hemorrhage affecting unspecified side

+ **I69.16**   Other paralytic syndrome following nontraumatic intracerebral hemorrhage

   Use additional code to identify type of paralytic syndrome, such as:

   locked-in state (G83.5)

   quadriplegia (G82.5-)

   Excludes1:   *hemiplegia/hemiparesis following nontraumatic intracerebral hemorrhage (I69.15-)*

      monoplegia of lower limb following nontraumatic intracerebral hemorrhage (I69.14-)

      monoplegia of upper limb following nontraumatic intracerebral hemorrhage (I69.13-)

I69.161   Other paralytic syndrome following nontraumatic intracerebral hemorrhage affecting right dominant side

I69.162   Other paralytic syndrome following nontraumatic intracerebral hemorrhage affecting left dominant side

I69.163 Other paralytic syndrome following nontraumatic intracerebral hemorrhage affecting right non-dominant side

I69.164 Other paralytic syndrome following nontraumatic intracerebral hemorrhage affecting left non-dominant side

I69.165 Other paralytic syndrome following nontraumatic intracerebral hemorrhage, bilateral

I69.169 Other paralytic syndrome following nontraumatic intracerebral hemorrhage affecting unspecified side

+ **I69.19** Other sequelae of nontraumatic intracerebral hemorrhage

I69.190 Apraxia following nontraumatic intracerebral hemorrhage

I69.191 Dysphagia following nontraumatic intracerebral hemorrhage

Use additional code to identify the type of dysphagia, if known (R13.1-)

I69.192 Facial weakness following nontraumatic intracerebral hemorrhage

Facial droop following nontraumatic intracerebral hemorrhage

I69.193 Ataxia following nontraumatic intracerebral hemorrhage

I69.198 Other sequelae of nontraumatic intracerebral hemorrhage

Alteration of sensations following nontraumatic intracerebral hemorrhage

Disturbance of vision following nontraumatic intracerebral hemorrhage

Use additional code to identify the sequelae

+ **I69.2** Sequelae of other nontraumatic intracranial hemorrhage

I69.20 Unspecified sequelae of other nontraumatic intracranial hemorrhage

+ **I69.21** Cognitive deficits following other nontraumatic intracranial hemorrhage

I69.210 Attention and concentration deficit following other nontraumatic intracranial hemorrhage

I69.211 Memory deficit following other nontraumatic intracranial hemorrhage

I69.212 Visuospatial deficit and spatial neglect following other nontraumatic intracranial hemorrhage

I69.213 Psychomotor deficit following other nontraumatic intracranial hemorrhage

I69.214 Frontal lobe and executive function deficit following other nontraumatic intracranial hemorrhage

I69.215 Cognitive social or emotional deficit following other nontraumatic intracranial hemorrhage

I69.218 Other symptoms and signs involving cognitive functions following other nontraumatic intracranial hemorrhage

I69.219 Unspecified symptoms and signs involving cognitive functions following other nontraumatic intracranial hemorrhage

+ **I69.22** Speech and language deficits following other nontraumatic intracranial hemorrhage

I69.220 Aphasia following other nontraumatic intracranial hemorrhage

I69.221 Dysphasia following other nontraumatic intracranial hemorrhage

I69.222 Dysarthria following other nontraumatic intracranial hemorrhage

I69.223 Fluency disorder following other nontraumatic intracranial hemorrhage

Stuttering following other nontraumatic intracranial hemorrhage

I69.228 Other speech and language deficits following other nontraumatic intracranial hemorrhage

+ **I69.23** Monoplegia of upper limb following other nontraumatic intracranial hemorrhage

I69.231 Monoplegia of upper limb following other nontraumatic intracranial hemorrhage affecting right dominant side

I69.232 Monoplegia of upper limb following other nontraumatic intracranial hemorrhage affecting left dominant side

I69.233 Monoplegia of upper limb following other nontraumatic intracranial hemorrhage affecting right non-dominant side

I69.234 Monoplegia of upper limb following other nontraumatic intracranial hemorrhage affecting left non-dominant side

I69.239 Monoplegia of upper limb following other nontraumatic intracranial hemorrhage affecting unspecified side

+ **I69.24** Monoplegia of lower limb following other nontraumatic intracranial hemorrhage

I69.241 Monoplegia of lower limb following other nontraumatic intracranial hemorrhage affecting right dominant side

I69.242 Monoplegia of lower limb following other nontraumatic intracranial hemorrhage affecting left dominant side

I69.243 Monoplegia of lower limb following other nontraumatic intracranial hemorrhage affecting right non-dominant side

I69.244 Monoplegia of lower limb following other nontraumatic intracranial hemorrhage affecting left non-dominant side

I69.249 Monoplegia of lower limb following other nontraumatic intracranial hemorrhage affecting unspecified side

+ **I69.25** Hemiplegia and hemiparesis following other nontraumatic intracranial hemorrhage

CC **I69.251** Hemiplegia and hemiparesis following other nontraumatic intracranial hemorrhage affecting right dominant side

CC **I69.252** Hemiplegia and hemiparesis following other nontraumatic intracranial hemorrhage affecting left dominant side

CC **I69.253** Hemiplegia and hemiparesis following other nontraumatic intracranial hemorrhage affecting right non-dominant side

CC **I69.254** Hemiplegia and hemiparesis following other nontraumatic intracranial hemorrhage affecting left non-dominant side

CC **I69.259** Hemiplegia and hemiparesis following other nontraumatic intracranial hemorrhage affecting unspecified side

+ **I69.26** Other paralytic syndrome following other nontraumatic intracranial hemorrhage

Use additional code to identify type of paralytic syndrome, such as:
locked-in state (G83.5)
quadriplegia (G82.5-)

Excludes1: *hemiplegia/hemiparesis following other nontraumatic intracranial hemorrhage (I69.25-)*
monoplegia of lower limb following other nontraumatic intracranial hemorrhage (I69.24-)
monoplegia of upper limb following other nontraumatic intracranial hemorrhage (I69.23-)

+, +7th, X + 7th • Newborn • Pediatric • Maternity • Adult ♀ Female ♂ Male Manifestation Unacceptable PDX HCC CC MCC HAC

I69.261 Other paralytic syndrome following other nontraumatic intracranial hemorrhage affecting right dominant side

I69.262 Other paralytic syndrome following other nontraumatic intracranial hemorrhage affecting left dominant side

I69.263 Other paralytic syndrome following other nontraumatic intracranial hemorrhage affecting right non-dominant side

I69.264 Other paralytic syndrome following other nontraumatic intracranial hemorrhage affecting left non-dominant side

I69.265 Other paralytic syndrome following other nontraumatic intracranial hemorrhage, bilateral

I69.269 Other paralytic syndrome following other nontraumatic intracranial hemorrhage affecting unspecified side

+ **I69.29** Other sequelae of other nontraumatic intracranial hemorrhage

I69.290 Apraxia following other nontraumatic intracranial hemorrhage

I69.291 Dysphagia following other nontraumatic intracranial hemorrhage

Use additional code to identify the type of dysphagia, if known (R13.1-)

I69.292 Facial weakness following other nontraumatic intracranial hemorrhage

Facial droop following other nontraumatic intracranial hemorrhage

I69.293 Ataxia following other nontraumatic intracranial hemorrhage

I69.298 Other sequelae of other nontraumatic intracranial hemorrhage

Alteration of sensation following other nontraumatic intracranial hemorrhage

Disturbance of vision following other nontraumatic intracranial hemorrhage

Use additional code to identify the sequelae

+ **I69.3** Sequelae of cerebral infarction

Sequelae of stroke NOS

AHA CC: 4Q, 2012, 95; 4Q, 2013, 127-128

I69.30 Unspecified sequelae of cerebral infarction

+ **I69.31** Cognitive deficits following cerebral infarction

I69.310 Attention and concentration deficit following cerebral infarction

I69.311 Memory deficit following cerebral infarction

I69.312 Visuospatial deficit and spatial neglect following cerebral infarction

I69.313 Psychomotor deficit following cerebral infarction

I69.314 Frontal lobe and executive function deficit following cerebral infarction

I69.315 Cognitive social or emotional deficit following cerebral infarction

I69.318 Other symptoms and signs involving cognitive functions following cerebral infarction

I69.319 Unspecified symptoms and signs involving cognitive functions following cerebral infarction

+ **I69.32** Speech and language deficits following cerebral infarction

I69.320 Aphasia following cerebral infarction

AHA CC: 4Q, 2013, 128

I69.321 Dysphasia following cerebral infarction

AHA CC: 4Q, 2012, 91

I69.322 Dysarthria following cerebral infarction

Excludes2: *transient ischemic attach (TIA) (G45.9)*

I69.323 Fluency disorder following cerebral infarction

Stuttering following cerebral hemorrhage

I69.328 Other speech and language deficits following cerebral infarction

+ **I69.33** Monoplegia of upper limb following cerebral infarction

AHA CC: 1Q, 2017, 47-48

I69.331 Monoplegia of upper limb following cerebral infarction affecting right dominant side

I69.332 Monoplegia of upper limb following cerebral infarction affecting left dominant side

I69.333 Monoplegia of upper limb following cerebral infarction affecting right non-dominant side

I69.334 Monoplegia of upper limb following cerebral infarction affecting left non-dominant side

I69.339 Monoplegia of upper limb following cerebral infarction affecting unspecified side

+ **I69.34** Monoplegia of lower limb following cerebral infarction

AHA CC: 1Q, 2017, 47-48

I69.341 Monoplegia of lower limb following cerebral infarction affecting right dominant side

I69.342 Monoplegia of lower limb following cerebral infarction affecting left dominant side

I69.343 Monoplegia of lower limb following cerebral infarction affecting right non-dominant side

I69.344 Monoplegia of lower limb following cerebral infarction affecting left non-dominant side

I69.349 Monoplegia of lower limb following cerebral infarction affecting unspecified side

+ **I69.35** Hemiplegia and hemiparesis following cerebral infarction

CC **I69.351** Hemiplegia and hemiparesis following cerebral infarction affecting right dominant side

Excludes2: *transient ischemic attach (TIA) (G45.9)*

AHA CC: 4Q, 2013, 128; 1Q, 2015, 25

CC **I69.352** Hemiplegia and hemiparesis following cerebral infarction affecting left dominant side

CC **I69.353** Hemiplegia and hemiparesis following cerebral infarction affecting right non-dominant side

CC **I69.354** Hemiplegia and hemiparesis following cerebral infarction affecting left non-dominant side

AHA CC: 4Q, 2012, 91

CC **I69.359** Hemiplegia and hemiparesis following cerebral infarction affecting unspecified side

+ **I69.36** Other paralytic syndrome following cerebral infarction

Use additional code to identify type of paralytic syndrome, such as:

locked-in state (G83.5)

quadriplegia (G82.5-)

Excludes1: *hemiplegia/hemiparesis following cerebral infarction (I69.35-)*
monoplegia of lower limb following cerebral infarction (I69.34-)
monoplegia of upper limb following cerebral infarction (I69.33-)

I69.361 Other paralytic syndrome following cerebral infarction affecting right dominant side

I69.362 Other paralytic syndrome following cerebral infarction affecting left dominant side

I69.363 Other paralytic syndrome following cerebral infarction affecting right non-dominant side

I69.364 Other paralytic syndrome following cerebral infarction affecting left non-dominant side

I69.365 Other paralytic syndrome following cerebral infarction, bilateral

I69.369 Other paralytic syndrome following cerebral infarction affecting unspecified side

+ **I69.39** Other sequelae of cerebral infarction

I69.390 Apraxia following cerebral infarction

I69.391 Dysphagia following cerebral infarction

Use additional code to identify the type of dysphagia, if known (R13.1-)

I69.392 Facial weakness following cerebral infarction

Facial droop following cerebral infarction

I69.393 Ataxia following cerebral infarction

I69.398 Other sequelae of cerebral infarction

Alteration of sensation following cerebral infarction

Disturbance of vision following cerebral infarction

Use additional code to identify the sequelae

AHA CC: 2Q, 2020, 29

+ **I69.8** Sequelae of other cerebrovascular diseases

Excludes1: *sequelae of traumatic intracranial injury (S06.-)*

I69.80 Unspecified sequelae of other cerebrovascular disease

+ **I69.81** Cognitive deficits following other cerebrovascular disease

I69.810 Attention and concentration deficit following other cerebrovascular disease

I69.811 Memory deficit following other cerebrovascular disease

I69.812 Visuospatial deficit and spatial neglect following other cerebrovascular disease

I69.813 Psychomotor deficit following other cerebrovascular disease

I69.814 Frontal lobe and executive function deficit following other cerebrovascular disease

I69.815 Cognitive social or emotional deficit following other cerebrovascular disease

I69.818 Other symptoms and signs involving cognitive functions following other cerebrovascular disease

I69.819 Unspecified symptoms and signs involving cognitive functions following other cerebrovascular disease

+ **I69.82** Speech and language deficits following other cerebrovascular disease

I69.820 Aphasia following other cerebrovascular disease

I69.821 Dysphasia following other cerebrovascular disease

I69.822 Dysarthria following other cerebrovascular disease

I69.823 Fluency disorder following other cerebrovascular disease

Stuttering following other cerebrovascular disease hemorrhage

I69.828 Other speech and language deficits following other cerebrovascular disease

AHA CC: 3Q, 2019, 8-9

+ **I69.83** Monoplegia of upper limb following other cerebrovascular disease

I69.831 Monoplegia of upper limb following other cerebrovascular disease affecting right dominant side

I69.832 Monoplegia of upper limb following other cerebrovascular disease affecting left dominant side

I69.833 Monoplegia of upper limb following other cerebrovascular disease affecting right non-dominant side

I69.834 Monoplegia of upper limb following other cerebrovascular disease affecting left non-dominant side

I69.839 Monoplegia of upper limb following other cerebrovascular disease affecting unspecified side

+ **I69.84** Monoplegia of lower limb following other cerebrovascular disease

I69.841 Monoplegia of lower limb following other cerebrovascular disease affecting right dominant side

I69.842 Monoplegia of lower limb following other cerebrovascular disease affecting left dominant side

I69.843 Monoplegia of lower limb following other cerebrovascular disease affecting right non-dominant side

I69.844 Monoplegia of lower limb following other cerebrovascular disease affecting left non-dominant side

I69.849 Monoplegia of lower limb following other cerebrovascular disease affecting unspecified side

+ **I69.85** Hemiplegia and hemiparesis following other cerebrovascular disease

CC **I69.851** Hemiplegia and hemiparesis following other cerebrovascular disease affecting right dominant side

CC **I69.852** Hemiplegia and hemiparesis following other cerebrovascular disease affecting left dominant side

CC **I69.853** Hemiplegia and hemiparesis following other cerebrovascular disease affecting right non-dominant side

CC **I69.854** Hemiplegia and hemiparesis following other cerebrovascular disease affecting left non-dominant side

CC **I69.859** Hemiplegia and hemiparesis following other cerebrovascular disease affecting unspecified side

+ **I69.86** Other paralytic syndrome following other cerebrovascular disease

Use additional code to identify type of paralytic syndrome, such as:

locked-in state (G83.5)

quadriplegia (G82.5-)

Excludes1: *hemiplegia/hemiparesis following other cerebrovascular disease (I69.85-)*

monoplegia of lower limb following other cerebrovascular disease (I69.84-)

monoplegia of upper limb following other cerebrovascular disease (I69.83-)

I69.861 Other paralytic syndrome following other cerebrovascular disease affecting right dominant side

I69.862 Other paralytic syndrome following other cerebrovascular disease affecting left dominant side

I69.863 Other paralytic syndrome following other cerebrovascular disease affecting right non-dominant side

I69.864 Other paralytic syndrome following other cerebrovascular disease affecting left non-dominant side

I69.865 Other paralytic syndrome following other cerebrovascular disease, bilateral

I69.869 Other paralytic syndrome following other cerebrovascular disease affecting unspecified side

+ **I69.89** Other sequelae of other cerebrovascular disease

I69.890 Apraxia following other cerebrovascular disease

I69.891 Dysphagia following other cerebrovascular disease

Use additional code to identify the type of dysphagia, if known (R13.1-)

I69.892 Facial weakness following other cerebrovascular disease

Facial droop following other cerebrovascular disease

I69.893 **Ataxia following other cerebrovascular disease**

I69.898 **Other sequelae of other cerebrovascular disease**

Alteration of sensation following other cerebrovascular disease

Disturbance of vision following other cerebrovascular disease

Use additional code to identify the sequelae

+ **I69.9 Sequelae of unspecified cerebrovascular diseases**

Excludes1: *sequelae of stroke (I69.3)*
sequelae of traumatic intracranial injury (S06.-)

I69.90 **Unspecified sequelae of unspecified cerebrovascular disease**

+ I69.91 **Cognitive deficits following unspecified cerebrovascular disease**

I69.910 **Attention and concentration deficit following unspecified cerebrovascular disease**

I69.911 **Memory deficit following unspecified cerebrovascular disease**

I69.912 **Visuospatial deficit and spatial neglect following unspecified cerebrovascular disease**

I69.913 **Psychomotor deficit following unspecified cerebrovascular disease**

I69.914 **Frontal lobe and executive function deficit following unspecified cerebrovascular disease**

I69.915 **Cognitive social or emotional deficit following unspecified cerebrovascular disease**

I69.918 **Other symptoms and signs involving cognitive functions following unspecified cerebrovascular disease**

I69.919 **Unspecified symptoms and signs involving cognitive functions following unspecified cerebrovascular disease**

+ I69.92 **Speech and language deficits following unspecified cerebrovascular disease**

I69.920 **Aphasia following unspecified cerebrovascular disease**

I69.921 **Dysphasia following unspecified cerebrovascular disease**

I69.922 **Dysarthria following unspecified cerebrovascular disease**

I69.923 **Fluency disorder following unspecified cerebrovascular disease**

Stuttering following unspecified cerebrovascular disease

I69.928 **Other speech and language deficits following unspecified cerebrovascular disease**

+ I69.93 **Monoplegia of upper limb following unspecified cerebrovascular disease**

I69.931 **Monoplegia of upper limb following unspecified cerebrovascular disease affecting right dominant side**

I69.932 **Monoplegia of upper limb following unspecified cerebrovascular disease affecting left dominant side**

I69.933 **Monoplegia of upper limb following unspecified cerebrovascular disease affecting right non-dominant side**

I69.934 **Monoplegia of upper limb following unspecified cerebrovascular disease affecting left non-dominant side**

I69.939 **Monoplegia of upper limb following unspecified cerebrovascular disease affecting unspecified side**

+ I69.94 **Monoplegia of lower limb following unspecified cerebrovascular disease**

I69.941 **Monoplegia of lower limb following unspecified cerebrovascular disease affecting right dominant side**

I69.942 **Monoplegia of lower limb following unspecified cerebrovascular disease affecting left dominant side**

I69.943 **Monoplegia of lower limb following unspecified cerebrovascular disease affecting right non-dominant side**

I69.944 **Monoplegia of lower limb following unspecified cerebrovascular disease affecting left non-dominant side**

I69.949 **Monoplegia of lower limb following unspecified cerebrovascular disease affecting unspecified side**

+ I69.95 **Hemiplegia and hemiparesis following unspecified cerebrovascular disease**

CC I69.951 **Hemiplegia and hemiparesis following unspecified cerebrovascular disease affecting right dominant side**

CC I69.952 **Hemiplegia and hemiparesis following unspecified cerebrovascular disease affecting left dominant side**

CC I69.953 **Hemiplegia and hemiparesis following unspecified cerebrovascular disease affecting right non-dominant side**

CC I69.954 **Hemiplegia and hemiparesis following unspecified cerebrovascular disease affecting left non-dominant side**

CC I69.959 **Hemiplegia and hemiparesis following unspecified cerebrovascular disease affecting unspecified side**

+ I69.96 **Other paralytic syndrome following unspecified cerebrovascular disease**

Use additional code to identify type of paralytic syndrome, such as:
locked-in state (G83.5)
quadriplegia (G82.5-)

Excludes1: *hemiplegia/hemiparesis following unspecifiedcerebrovasculardisease (I69.95-)*
monoplegia of lower limb following unspecified cerebrovascular disease (I69.94-)
monoplegia of upper limb following unspecified cerebrovascular disease (I69.93-)

I69.961 **Other paralytic syndrome following unspecified cerebrovascular disease affecting right dominant side**

I69.962 **Other paralytic syndrome following unspecified cerebrovascular disease affecting left dominant side**

I69.963 **Other paralytic syndrome following unspecified cerebrovascular disease affecting right non-dominant side**

I69.964 **Other paralytic syndrome following unspecified cerebrovascular disease affecting left non-dominant side**

I69.965 **Other paralytic syndrome following unspecified cerebrovascular disease, bilateral**

I69.969 **Other paralytic syndrome following unspecified cerebrovascular disease affecting unspecified side**

+ I69.99 **Other sequelae of unspecified cerebrovascular disease**

I69.990 **Apraxia following unspecified cerebrovascular disease**

I69.991 **Dysphagia following unspecified cerebrovascular disease**

Use additional code to identify the type of dysphagia, if known (R13.1-)

I69.992 **Facial weakness following unspecified cerebrovascular disease**

Facial droop following unspecified cerebrovascular disease

I69.993 **Ataxia following unspecified cerebrovascular disease**

I69.998 **Other sequelae following unspecified cerebrovascular disease**

Alteration in sensation following unspecified cerebrovascular disease

Disturbance of vision following unspecified cerebrovascular disease

Use additional code to identify the sequelae

+, +7th, X + 7th • Newborn • Pediatric • Maternity • Adult ♀ Female ♂ Male Manifestation Unacceptable PDX HCC CC MCC HAC

Diseases of arteries, arterioles and capillaries (I70-I79)

I70   Atherosclerosis

Includes: arteriolosclerosis
arterial degeneration
arteriosclerosis
arteriosclerotic vascular disease
arteriovascular degeneration
atheroma
endarteritis deformans or obliterans
senile arteritis
senile endarteritis
vascular degeneration

Use additional code to identify:
exposure to environmental tobacco smoke (Z77.22)
history of tobacco dependence (Z87.891)
occupational exposure to environmental tobacco smoke (Z57.31)
tobacco dependence (F17.-)
tobacco use (Z72.0)

Excludes2: *arteriosclerotic cardiovascular disease (I25.1-)*
arteriosclerotic heart disease (I25.1-)
atheroembolism (I75.-)
cerebral atherosclerosis (I67.2)
coronary atherosclerosis (I25.1-)
mesenteric atherosclerosis (K55.1)
precerebral atherosclerosis (I67.2)
primary pulmonary atherosclerosis (I27.0)

● **I70.0   Atherosclerosis of aorta**

● **I70.1   Atherosclerosis of renal artery**
Goldblatt's kidney
Excludes2: *atherosclerosis of renal arterioles (I12.-)*

+ **I70.2   Atherosclerosis of native arteries of the extremities**
Mönckeberg's (medial) sclerosis
Use additional code, if applicable, to identify chronic total occlusion of artery of extremity (I70.92)
Excludes2: *atherosclerosis of bypass graft of extremities (I70.30-I70.79)*
AHA CC: 3Q, 2018, 4

+ **I70.20   Unspecified atherosclerosis of native arteries of extremities**

● **I70.201   Unspecified atherosclerosis of native arteries of extremities, right leg**

● **I70.202   Unspecified atherosclerosis of native arteries of extremities, left leg**

● **I70.203   Unspecified atherosclerosis of native arteries of extremities, bilateral legs**

● **I70.208   Unspecified atherosclerosis of native arteries of extremities, other extremity**

● **I70.209   Unspecified atherosclerosis of native arteries of extremities, unspecified extremity**

+ **I70.21   Atherosclerosis of native arteries of extremities with intermittent claudication**

● **I70.211   Atherosclerosis of native arteries of extremities with intermittent claudication, right leg**

● **I70.212   Atherosclerosis of native arteries of extremities with intermittent claudication, left leg**

● **I70.213   Atherosclerosis of native arteries of extremities with intermittent claudication, bilateral legs**

● **I70.218   Atherosclerosis of native arteries of extremities with intermittent claudication, other extremity**

● **I70.219   Atherosclerosis of native arteries of extremities with intermittent claudication, unspecified extremity**

+ **I70.22   Atherosclerosis of native arteries of extremities with rest pain**
Includes: any condition classifiable to I70.21-
chronic limb-threatening ischemia NOS of native arteries of the extremities
chronic limb-threatening ischemia of native arteries of the extremities with rest pain
critical limb ischemia NOS of native arteries of the extremities
critical limb ischemia of native arteries of the extremities with rest pain

● **I70.221   Atherosclerosis of native arteries of extremities with rest pain, right leg**

● **I70.222   Atherosclerosis of native arteries of extremities with rest pain, left leg**

● **I70.223   Atherosclerosis of native arteries of extremities with rest pain, bilateral legs**

● **I70.228   Atherosclerosis of native arteries of extremities with rest pain, other extremity**

● **I70.229   Atherosclerosis of native arteries of extremities with rest pain, unspecified extremity**

+ **I70.23   Atherosclerosis of native arteries of right leg with ulceration**
Includes: any condition classifiable to I70.211 and I70.221
chronic limb-threatening ischemia of native arteries of right leg with ulceration
critical limb ischemia of native arteries of right leg with ulceration
Use additional code to identify severity of ulcer (L97.-)

● **I70.231   Atherosclerosis of native arteries of right leg with ulceration of thigh**

● **I70.232   Atherosclerosis of native arteries of right leg with ulceration of calf**

● **I70.233   Atherosclerosis of native arteries of right leg with ulceration of ankle**

● **I70.234   Atherosclerosis of native arteries of right leg with ulceration of heel and midfoot**
Atherosclerosis of native arteries of right leg with ulceration of plantar surface of midfoot

● **I70.235   Atherosclerosis of native arteries of right leg with ulceration of other part of foot**
Atherosclerosis of native arteries of right leg extremities with ulceration of toe

● **I70.238   Atherosclerosis of native arteries of right leg with ulceration of other part of lower leg**

● **I70.239   Atherosclerosis of native arteries of right leg with ulceration of unspecified site**

+ **I70.24   Atherosclerosis of native arteries of left leg with ulceration**
Includes: any condition classifiable to I70.212 and I70.222
chronic limb-threatening ischemia of native arteries of left leg with ulceration
critical limb ischemia of native arteries of left leg with ulceration
Use additional code to identify severity of ulcer (L97.-)

● **I70.241   Atherosclerosis of native arteries of left leg with ulceration of thigh**

● **I70.242   Atherosclerosis of native arteries of left leg with ulceration of calf**

● **I70.243   Atherosclerosis of native arteries of left leg with ulceration of ankle**

● **I70.244   Atherosclerosis of native arteries of left leg with ulceration of heel and midfoot**
Atherosclerosis of native arteries of left leg with ulceration of plantar surface of midfoot

● **I70.245   Atherosclerosis of native arteries of left leg with ulceration of other part of foot**
Atherosclerosis of native arteries of left leg extremities with ulceration of toe

● **I70.248   Atherosclerosis of native arteries of left leg with ulceration of other part of lower leg**

● **I70.249   Atherosclerosis of native arteries of left leg with ulceration of unspecified site**

● **I70.25   Atherosclerosis of native arteries of other extremities with ulceration**
Includes: any condition classifiable to I70.218 and I70.228
Use additional code to identify the severity of the ulcer (L98.49-)

687

+, +7th, X + 7th   ● Newborn   ● Pediatric   ● Maternity   ● Adult   ♀ Female   ♂ Male   Manifestation   Unacceptable PDX   HCC   CC   MCC   HAC

+ **I70.26** **Atherosclerosis of native arteries of extremities with gangrene**
  Includes: any condition classifiable to I70.21-, I70.22-, I70.23-, I70.24-, and I70.25-
  chronic limb-threatening ischemia of native arteries of extremities with gangrene
  critical limb ischemia of native arteries of extremities with gangrene
  Use additional code to identify the severity of any ulcer (L97.-, L98.49-), if applicable
  - CC **I70.261** Atherosclerosis of native arteries of extremities with gangrene, right leg
  - CC **I70.262** Atherosclerosis of native arteries of extremities with gangrene, left leg
  - CC **I70.263** Atherosclerosis of native arteries of extremities with gangrene, bilateral legs
  - CC **I70.268** Atherosclerosis of native arteries of extremities with gangrene, other extremity
  - CC **I70.269** Atherosclerosis of native arteries of extremities with gangrene, unspecified extremity

+ **I70.29** **Other atherosclerosis of native arteries of extremities**
  - **I70.291** Other atherosclerosis of native arteries of extremities, right leg
  - **I70.292** Other atherosclerosis of native arteries of extremities, left leg
  - **I70.293** Other atherosclerosis of native arteries of extremities, bilateral legs
  - **I70.298** Other atherosclerosis of native arteries of extremities, other extremity
  - **I70.299** Other atherosclerosis of native arteries of extremities, unspecified extremity

+ **I70.3** **Atherosclerosis of unspecified type of bypass graft(s) of the extremities**
  Use additional code, if applicable, to identify chronic total occlusion of artery of extremity (I70.92)
  Excludes1: embolism or thrombus of bypass graft(s) of extremities (T82.8-)

+ **I70.30** **Unspecified atherosclerosis of unspecified type of bypass graft(s) of the extremities**
  - **I70.301** Unspecified atherosclerosis of unspecified type of bypass graft(s) of the extremities, right leg
  - **I70.302** Unspecified atherosclerosis of unspecified type of bypass graft(s) of the extremities, left leg
  - **I70.303** Unspecified atherosclerosis of unspecified type of bypass graft(s) of the extremities, bilateral legs
  - **I70.308** Unspecified atherosclerosis of unspecified type of bypass graft(s) of the extremities, other extremity
  - **I70.309** Unspecified atherosclerosis of unspecified type of bypass graft(s) of the extremities, unspecified extremity

+ **I70.31** **Atherosclerosis of unspecified type of bypass graft(s) of the extremities with intermittent claudication**
  - **I70.311** Atherosclerosis of unspecified type of bypass graft(s) of the extremities with intermittent claudication, right leg
  - **I70.312** Atherosclerosis of unspecified type of bypass graft(s) of the extremities with intermittent claudication, left leg
  - **I70.313** Atherosclerosis of unspecified type of bypass graft(s) of the extremities with intermittent claudication, bilateral legs
  - **I70.318** Atherosclerosis of unspecified type of bypass graft(s) of the extremities with intermittent claudication, other extremity
  - **I70.319** Atherosclerosis of unspecified type of bypass graft(s) of the extremities with intermittent claudication, unspecified extremity

+ **I70.32** **Atherosclerosis of unspecified type of bypass graft(s) of the extremities with rest pain**
  Includes: any condition classifiable to I70.31-
  chronic limb-threatening ischemia NOS of unspecified type of bypass graft(s) of the extremities
  chronic limb-threatening ischemia of unspecified type of bypass graft(s) of the extremities with rest pain
  critical limb ischemia NOS of unspecified type of bypass graft(s) of the extremities
  critical limb ischemia of unspecified type of bypass graft(s) of the extremities with rest pain
  - **I70.321** Atherosclerosis of unspecified type of bypass graft(s) of the extremities with rest pain, right leg
  - **I70.322** Atherosclerosis of unspecified type of bypass graft(s) of the extremities with rest pain, left leg
  - **I70.323** Atherosclerosis of unspecified type of bypass graft(s) of the extremities with rest pain, bilateral legs
  - **I70.328** Atherosclerosis of unspecified type of bypass graft(s) of the extremities with rest pain, other extremity
  - **I70.329** Atherosclerosis of unspecified type of bypass graft(s) of the extremities with rest pain, unspecified extremity

+ **I70.33** **Atherosclerosis of unspecified type of bypass graft(s) of the right leg with ulceration**
  Includes: any condition classifiable to I70.311 and I70.321
  chronic limb-threatening ischemia of unspecified type of bypass graft(s) of right leg with ulceration
  critical limb ischemia of unspecified type of bypass graft(s) of right leg with ulceration
  Use additional code to identify severity of ulcer (L97.-)
  - CC **I70.331** Atherosclerosis of unspecified type of bypass graft(s) of the right leg with ulceration of thigh
  - CC **I70.332** Atherosclerosis of unspecified type of bypass graft(s) of the right leg with ulceration of calf
  - CC **I70.333** Atherosclerosis of unspecified type of bypass graft(s) of the right leg with ulceration of ankle
  - CC **I70.334** Atherosclerosis of unspecified type of bypass graft(s) of the right leg with ulceration of heel and midfoot
    Atherosclerosis of unspecified type of bypass graft(s) of right leg with ulceration of plantar surface of midfoot
  - **I70.335** Atherosclerosis of unspecified type of bypass graft(s) of the right leg with ulceration of other part of foot
    Atherosclerosis of unspecified type of bypass graft(s) of the right leg with ulceration of toe
  - CC **I70.338** Atherosclerosis of unspecified type of bypass graft(s) of the right leg with ulceration of other part of lower leg
  - CC **I70.339** Atherosclerosis of unspecified type of bypass graft(s) of the right leg with ulceration of unspecified site

+ **I70.34** **Atherosclerosis of unspecified type of bypass graft(s) of the left leg with ulceration**
  Includes: any condition classifiable to I70.312 and I70.322
  chronic limb-threatening ischemia of unspecified type of bypass graft(s) of left leg with ulceration
  critical limb ischemia of unspecified type of bypass graft(s) of left leg with ulceration
  Use additional code to identify severity of ulcer (L97.-)

- CC **I70.341** Atherosclerosis of unspecified type of bypass graft(s) of the left leg with ulceration of thigh
- CC **I70.342** Atherosclerosis of unspecified type of bypass graft(s) of the left leg with ulceration of calf
- CC **I70.343** Atherosclerosis of unspecified type of bypass graft(s) of the left leg with ulceration of ankle
- CC **I70.344** Atherosclerosis of unspecified type of bypass graft(s) of the left leg with ulceration of heel and midfoot

  Atherosclerosis of unspecified type of bypass graft(s) of left leg with ulceration of plantar surface of midfoot

- **I70.345** Atherosclerosis of unspecified type of bypass graft(s) of the left leg with ulceration of other part of foot

  Atherosclerosis of unspecified type of bypass graft(s) of the left leg with ulceration of toe

- CC **I70.348** Atherosclerosis of unspecified type of bypass graft(s) of the left leg with ulceration of other part of lower leg
- CC **I70.349** Atherosclerosis of unspecified type of bypass graft(s) of the left leg with ulceration of unspecified site
- **I70.35** Atherosclerosis of unspecified type of bypass graft(s) of other extremity with ulceration

  Includes: any condition classifiable to I70.318 and I70.328

  Use additional code to identify severity of ulcer (L98.49-)

+ **I70.36** Atherosclerosis of unspecified type of bypass graft(s) of the extremities with gangrene

  Includes: any condition classifiable to I70.31-, I70.32-, I70.33-, I70.34-, I70.35

  chronic limb-threatening ischemia of unspecified type of bypass graft(s) of the extremities with gangrene

  critical limb ischemia of unspecified type of bypass graft(s) of the extremities with gangrene

  Use additional code to identify the severity of any ulcer (L97.-, L98.49-), if applicable

- CC **I70.361** Atherosclerosis of unspecified type of bypass graft(s) of the extremities with gangrene, right leg
- CC **I70.362** Atherosclerosis of unspecified type of bypass graft(s) of the extremities with gangrene, left leg
- CC **I70.363** Atherosclerosis of unspecified type of bypass graft(s) of the extremities with gangrene, bilateral legs
- CC **I70.368** Atherosclerosis of unspecified type of bypass graft(s) of the extremities with gangrene, other extremity
- CC **I70.369** Atherosclerosis of unspecified type of bypass graft(s) of the extremities with gangrene, unspecified extremity

+ **I70.39** Other atherosclerosis of unspecified type of bypass graft(s) of the extremities
- **I70.391** Other atherosclerosis of unspecified type of bypass graft(s) of the extremities, right leg
- **I70.392** Other atherosclerosis of unspecified type of bypass graft(s) of the extremities, left leg
- **I70.393** Other atherosclerosis of unspecified type of bypass graft(s) of the extremities, bilateral legs
- **I70.398** Other atherosclerosis of unspecified type of bypass graft(s) of the extremities, other extremity
- **I70.399** Other atherosclerosis of unspecified type of bypass graft(s) of the extremities, unspecified extremity

+ **I70.4** Atherosclerosis of autologous vein bypass graft(s) of the extremities

  Use additional code, if applicable, to identify chronic total occlusion of artery of extremity (I70.92)

+ **I70.40** Unspecified atherosclerosis of autologous vein bypass graft(s) of the extremities
- **I70.401** Unspecified atherosclerosis of autologous vein bypass graft(s) of the extremities, right leg
- **I70.402** Unspecified atherosclerosis of autologous vein bypass graft(s) of the extremities, left leg
- **I70.403** Unspecified atherosclerosis of autologous vein bypass graft(s) of the extremities, bilateral legs
- **I70.408** Unspecified atherosclerosis of autologous vein bypass graft(s) of the extremities, other extremity
- **I70.409** Unspecified atherosclerosis of autologous vein bypass graft(s) of the extremities, unspecified extremity

+ **I70.41** Atherosclerosis of autologous vein bypass graft(s) of the extremities with intermittent claudication
- **I70.411** Atherosclerosis of autologous vein bypass graft(s) of the extremities with intermittent claudication, right leg
- **I70.412** Atherosclerosis of autologous vein bypass graft(s) of the extremities with intermittent claudication, left leg
- **I70.413** Atherosclerosis of autologous vein bypass graft(s) of the extremities with intermittent claudication, bilateral legs
- **I70.418** Atherosclerosis of autologous vein bypass graft(s) of the extremities with intermittent claudication, other extremity
- **I70.419** Atherosclerosis of autologous vein bypass graft(s) of the extremities with intermittent claudication, unspecified extremity

+ **I70.42** Atherosclerosis of autologous vein bypass graft(s) of the extremities with rest pain

  Includes: any condition classifiable to I70.41-

  chronic limb-threatening ischemia NOS of autologous vein bypass graft(s) of the extremities

  chronic limb-threatening ischemia of autologous vein bypass graft(s) of the extremities with rest pain

  critical limb ischemia NOS of autologous vein bypass graft(s) of the extremities

  critical limb ischemia of autologous vein bypass graft(s) of the extremities with rest pain

- **I70.421** Atherosclerosis of autologous vein bypass graft(s) of the extremities with rest pain, right leg
- **I70.422** Atherosclerosis of autologous vein bypass graft(s) of the extremities with rest pain, left leg
- **I70.423** Atherosclerosis of autologous vein bypass graft(s) of the extremities with rest pain, bilateral legs
- **I70.428** Atherosclerosis of autologous vein bypass graft(s) of the extremities with rest pain, other extremity
- **I70.429** Atherosclerosis of autologous vein bypass graft(s) of the extremities with rest pain, unspecified extremity

+ **I70.43** Atherosclerosis of autologous vein bypass graft(s) of the right leg with ulceration

  Includes: any condition classifiable to I70.411 and I70.421

  chronic limb-threatening ischemia of autologous vein bypass graft(s) of right leg with ulceration

  critical limb ischemia of autologous vein bypass graft(s) of right leg with ulceration

  Use additional code to identify severity of ulcer (L97.-)

+, +7th, X + 7th ● Newborn ● Pediatric ● Maternity ● Adult ♀ Female ♂ Male Manifestation Unacceptable PDX HCC CC MCC HAC

- CC **I70.431** Atherosclerosis of autologous vein bypass graft(s) of the right leg with ulceration of thigh
- CC **I70.432** Atherosclerosis of autologous vein bypass graft(s) of the right leg with ulceration of calf
- CC **I70.433** Atherosclerosis of autologous vein bypass graft(s) of the right leg with ulceration of ankle
- CC **I70.434** Atherosclerosis of autologous vein bypass graft(s) of the right leg with ulceration of heel and midfoot

  Atherosclerosis of autologous vein bypass graft(s) of right leg with ulceration of plantar surface of midfoot

- **I70.435** Atherosclerosis of autologous vein bypass graft(s) of the right leg with ulceration of other part of foot

  Atherosclerosis of autologous vein bypass graft(s) of right leg with ulceration of toe

- CC **I70.438** Atherosclerosis of autologous vein bypass graft(s) of the right leg with ulceration of other part of lower leg
- CC **I70.439** Atherosclerosis of autologous vein bypass graft(s) of the right leg with ulceration of unspecified site

+ **I70.44** Atherosclerosis of autologous vein bypass graft(s) of the left leg with ulceration

  Includes: any condition classifiable to I70.412 and I70.422

  chronic limb-threatening ischemia of autologous vein bypass graft(s) of left leg with ulceration

  critical limb ischemia of autologous vein bypass graft(s) of left leg with ulceration

  Use additional code to identify severity of ulcer (L97.-)

- CC **I70.441** Atherosclerosis of autologous vein bypass graft(s) of the left leg with ulceration of thigh
- CC **I70.442** Atherosclerosis of autologous vein bypass graft(s) of the left leg with ulceration of calf
- CC **I70.443** Atherosclerosis of autologous vein bypass graft(s) of the left leg with ulceration of ankle
- CC **I70.444** Atherosclerosis of autologous vein bypass graft(s) of the left leg with ulceration of heel and midfoot

  Atherosclerosis of autologous vein bypass graft(s) of left leg with ulceration of plantar surface of midfoot

- **I70.445** Atherosclerosis of autologous vein bypass graft(s) of the left leg with ulceration of other part of foot

  Atherosclerosis of autologous vein bypass graft(s) of left leg with ulceration of toe

- CC **I70.448** Atherosclerosis of autologous vein bypass graft(s) of the left leg with ulceration of other part of lower leg
- CC **I70.449** Atherosclerosis of autologous vein bypass graft(s) of the left leg with ulceration of unspecified site

- **I70.45** Atherosclerosis of autologous vein bypass graft(s) of other extremity with ulceration

  Includes: any condition classifiable to I70.418, I70.428, and I70.438

  Use additional code to identify severity of ulcer (L98.49)

+ **I70.46** Atherosclerosis of autologous vein bypass graft(s) of the extremities with gangrene

  Includes: any condition classifiable to I70.41-, I70.42-, and I70.43-, I70.44-, I70.45

  chronic limb-threatening ischemia of autologous vein bypass graft(s) of the extremities with gangrene

  critical limb ischemia of autologous vein bypass graft(s) of the extremities with gangrene

  Use additional code to identify the severity of any ulcer (L97.-, L98.49-), if applicable

- CC **I70.461** Atherosclerosis of autologous vein bypass graft(s) of the extremities with gangrene, right leg
- CC **I70.462** Atherosclerosis of autologous vein bypass graft(s) of the extremities with gangrene, left leg
- CC **I70.463** Atherosclerosis of autologous vein bypass graft(s) of the extremities with gangrene, bilateral legs
- CC **I70.468** Atherosclerosis of autologous vein bypass graft(s) of the extremities with gangrene, other extremity
- CC **I70.469** Atherosclerosis of autologous vein bypass graft(s) of the extremities with gangrene, unspecified extremity

+ **I70.49** Other atherosclerosis of autologous vein bypass graft(s) of the extremities

- **I70.491** Other atherosclerosis of autologous vein bypass graft(s) of the extremities, right leg
- **I70.492** Other atherosclerosis of autologous vein bypass graft(s) of the extremities, left leg
- **I70.493** Other atherosclerosis of autologous vein bypass graft(s) of the extremities, bilateral legs
- **I70.498** Other atherosclerosis of autologous vein bypass graft(s) of the extremities, other extremity
- **I70.499** Other atherosclerosis of autologous vein bypass graft(s) of the extremities, unspecified extremity

+ **I70.5** Atherosclerosis of nonautologous biological bypass graft(s) of the extremities

  Use additional code, if applicable, to identify chronic total occlusion of artery of extremity (I70.92)

+ **I70.50** Unspecified atherosclerosis of nonautologous biological bypass graft(s) of the extremities

- **I70.501** Unspecified atherosclerosis of nonautologous biological bypass graft(s) of the extremities, right leg
- **I70.502** Unspecified atherosclerosis of nonautologous biological bypass graft(s) of the extremities, left leg
- **I70.503** Unspecified atherosclerosis of nonautologous biological bypass graft(s) of the extremities, bilateral legs
- **I70.508** Unspecified atherosclerosis of nonautologous biological bypass graft(s) of the extremities, other extremity
- **I70.509** Unspecified atherosclerosis of nonautologous biological bypass graft(s) of the extremities, unspecified extremity

+ **I70.51** Atherosclerosis of nonautologous biological bypass graft(s) of the extremities intermittent claudication

- **I70.511** Atherosclerosis of nonautologous biological bypass graft(s) of the extremities with intermittent claudication, right leg
- **I70.512** Atherosclerosis of nonautologous biological bypass graft(s) of the extremities with intermittent claudication, left leg
- **I70.513** Atherosclerosis of nonautologous biological bypass graft(s) of the extremities with intermittent claudication, bilateral legs
- **I70.518** Atherosclerosis of nonautologous biological bypass graft(s) of the extremities with intermittent claudication, other extremity
- **I70.519** Atherosclerosis of nonautologous biological bypass graft(s) of the extremities with intermittent claudication, unspecified extremity

+ **I70.52** Atherosclerosis of nonautologous biological bypass graft(s) of the extremities with rest pain

  Includes: any condition classifiable to I70.51-

  chronic limb-threatening ischemia NOS of nonautologous vein bypass graft(s) of the extremities

+, +7th, X + 7th • Newborn • Pediatric • Maternity • Adult ♀ Female ♂ Male Manifestation Unacceptable PDX HCC CC MCC HAC

chronic limb-threatening ischemia of
nonautologous vein bypass graft(s) of
the extremities with rest pain
critical limb ischemia NOS of
nonautologous vein bypass graft(s) of
the extremities
critical limb ischemia of nonautologous
vein bypass graft(s) of the extremities
with rest pain

- **I70.521 Atherosclerosis of nonautologous
biological bypass graft(s) of the
extremities with rest pain, right leg**
- **I70.522 Atherosclerosis of nonautologous
biological bypass graft(s) of the
extremities with rest pain, left leg**
- **I70.523 Atherosclerosis of nonautologous
biological bypass graft(s) of the
extremities with rest pain, bilateral legs**
- **I70.528 Atherosclerosis of nonautologous
biological bypass graft(s) of the
extremities with rest pain, other
extremity**
- **I70.529 Atherosclerosis of nonautologous
biological bypass graft(s) of the
extremities with rest pain, unspecified
extremity**

+ **I70.53 Atherosclerosis of nonautologous biological
bypass graft(s) of the right leg with ulceration**
  Includes: any condition classifiable to I70.511
  and I70.521
  chronic limb-threatening ischemia of
  nonautologous vein bypass graft(s)
  of right leg with ulceration
  critical limb ischemia of
  nonautologous vein bypass graft(s)
  of right leg with ulceration
  Use additional code to identify severity of ulcer
  (L97.-)

- CC **I70.531 Atherosclerosis of nonautologous
biological bypass graft(s) of the right leg
with ulceration of thigh**
- CC **I70.532 Atherosclerosis of nonautologous
biological bypass graft(s) of the right leg
with ulceration of calf**
- CC **I70.533 Atherosclerosis of nonautologous
biological bypass graft(s) of the right leg
with ulceration of ankle**
- CC **I70.534 Atherosclerosis of nonautologous
biological bypass graft(s) of the right leg
with ulceration of heel and midfoot**
  Atherosclerosis of nonautologous
  biological bypass graft(s) of right leg
  with ulceration of plantar surface of
  midfoot
- **I70.535 Atherosclerosis of nonautologous
biological bypass graft(s) of the right
leg with ulceration of other part
of foot**
  Atherosclerosis of nonautologous
  biological bypass graft(s) of the right
  leg with ulceration of toe
- CC **I70.538 Atherosclerosis of nonautologous
biological bypass graft(s) of the right
leg with ulceration of other part of
lower leg**
- CC **I70.539 Atherosclerosis of nonautologous
biological bypass graft(s) of the right leg
with ulceration of unspecified site**

+ **I70.54 Atherosclerosis of nonautologous biological
bypass graft(s) of the left leg with ulceration**
  Includes: any condition classifiable to I70.512 and
  I70.522
  chronic limb-threatening ischemia of
  nonautologous vein bypass graft(s) of
  left leg with ulceration
  critical limb ischemia of nonautologous
  vein bypass graft(s) of left leg with
  ulceration
  Use additional code to identify severity of ulcer
  (L97.-)

- CC **I70.541 Atherosclerosis of nonautologous
biological bypass graft(s) of the left leg
with ulceration of thigh**
- CC **I70.542 Atherosclerosis of nonautologous
biological bypass graft(s) of the left leg
with ulceration of calf**
- CC **I70.543 Atherosclerosis of nonautologous
biological bypass graft(s) of the left leg
with ulceration of ankle**
- CC **I70.544 Atherosclerosis of nonautologous
biological bypass graft(s) of the left leg
with ulceration of heel and midfoot**
  Atherosclerosis of nonautologous
  biological bypass graft(s) of left leg
  with ulceration of plantar surface of
  midfoot
- **I70.545 Atherosclerosis of nonautologous
biological bypass graft(s) of the left leg
with ulceration of other part of foot**
  Atherosclerosis of nonautologous
  biological bypass graft(s) of the left
  leg with ulceration of toe
- CC **I70.548 Atherosclerosis of nonautologous
biological bypass graft(s) of the left
leg with ulceration of other part of
lower leg**
- CC **I70.549 Atherosclerosis of nonautologous
biological bypass graft(s) of the left leg
with ulceration of unspecified site**

- **I70.55 Atherosclerosis of nonautologous biological
bypass graft(s) of other extremity with ulceration**
  Includes: any condition classifiable to I70.518,
  I70.528, and I70.538
  Use additional code to identify severity of ulcer
  (L98.49)

+ **I70.56 Atherosclerosis of nonautologous biological
bypass graft(s) of the extremities with gangrene**
  Includes: any condition classifiable to I70.51-,
  I70.52-, and I70.53-, I70.54-, I70.55
  chronic limb-threatening ischemia of
  nonautologous vein bypass graft(s) of
  the extremities with gangrene
  critical limb ischemia of nonautologous
  vein bypass graft(s) of the extremities
  with gangrene
  Use additional code to identify the severity of any
  ulcer (L97.-, L98.49-), if applicable

- CC **I70.561 Atherosclerosis of nonautologous
biological bypass graft(s) of the
extremities with gangrene, right leg**
- CC **I70.562 Atherosclerosis of nonautologous
biological bypass graft(s) of the
extremities with gangrene, left leg**
- CC **I70.563 Atherosclerosis of nonautologous
biological bypass graft(s) of the
extremities with gangrene, bilateral legs**
- CC **I70.568 Atherosclerosis of nonautologous
biological bypass graft(s) of the
extremities with gangrene, other
extremity**
- CC **I70.569 Atherosclerosis of nonautologous
biological bypass graft(s) of the
extremities with gangrene, unspecified
extremity**

+ **I70.59 Other atherosclerosis of nonautologous biological
bypass graft(s) of the extremities**

- **I70.591 Other atherosclerosis of nonautologous
biological bypass graft(s) of the
extremities, right leg**
- **I70.592 Other atherosclerosis of nonautologous
biological bypass graft(s) of the
extremities, left leg**
- **I70.593 Other atherosclerosis of nonautologous
biological bypass graft(s) of the
extremities, bilateral legs**
- **I70.598 Other atherosclerosis of
nonautologous biological bypass graft(s)
of the extremities, other extremity**
- **I70.599 Other atherosclerosis of nonautologous
biological bypass graft(s) of the
extremities, unspecified extremity**

+, +7th, X + 7th   ● Newborn   ● Pediatric   ● Maternity   ● Adult   ♀ Female   ♂ Male   Manifestation   Unacceptable PDX   HCC   CC   MCC   HAC

+ I70.6 Atherosclerosis of nonbiological bypass graft(s) of the extremities

Use additional code, if applicable, to identify chronic total occlusion of artery of extremity (I70.92)

+ I70.60 Unspecified atherosclerosis of nonbiological bypass graft(s) of the extremities

● **I70.601 Unspecified atherosclerosis of nonbiological bypass graft(s) of the extremities, right leg**

● **I70.602 Unspecified atherosclerosis of nonbiological bypass graft(s) of the extremities, left leg**

● **I70.603 Unspecified atherosclerosis of nonbiological bypass graft(s) of the extremities, bilateral legs**

● **I70.608 Unspecified atherosclerosis of nonbiological bypass graft(s) of the extremities, other extremity**

● **I70.609 Unspecified atherosclerosis of nonbiological bypass graft(s) of the extremities, unspecified extremity**

+ I70.61 Atherosclerosis of nonbiological bypass graft(s) of the extremities with intermittent claudication

● **I70.611 Atherosclerosis of nonbiological bypass graft(s) of the extremities with intermittent claudication, right leg**

● **I70.612 Atherosclerosis of nonbiological bypass graft(s) of the extremities with intermittent claudication, left leg**

● **I70.613 Atherosclerosis of nonbiological bypass graft(s) of the extremities with intermittent claudication, bilateral legs**

● **I70.618 Atherosclerosis of nonbiological bypass graft(s) of the extremities with intermittent claudication, other extremity**

● **I70.619 Atherosclerosis of nonbiological bypass graft(s) of the extremities with intermittent claudication, unspecified extremity**

+ I70.62 Atherosclerosis of nonbiological bypass graft(s) of the extremities with rest pain

Includes: any condition classifiable to I70.61-
chronic limb-threatening ischemia NOS of nonbiological bypass graft(s) of the extremities
chronic limb-threatening ischemia of nonbiological bypass graft(s) of the extremities with rest pain
critical limb ischemia NOS of nonbiological bypass graft(s) of the extremities
critical limb ischemia of nonbiological bypass graft(s) of the extremities with rest pain

● **I70.621 Atherosclerosis of nonbiological bypass graft(s) of the extremities with rest pain, right leg**

● **I70.622 Atherosclerosis of nonbiological bypass graft(s) of the extremities with rest pain, left leg**

● **I70.623 Atherosclerosis of nonbiological bypass graft(s) of the extremities with rest pain, bilateral legs**

● **I70.628 Atherosclerosis of nonbiological bypass graft(s) of the extremities with rest pain, other extremity**

● **I70.629 Atherosclerosis of nonbiological bypass graft(s) of the extremities with rest pain, unspecified extremity**

+ I70.63 Atherosclerosis of nonbiological bypass graft(s) of the right leg with ulceration

Includes: any condition classifiable to I70.611 and I70.621
chronic limb-threatening ischemia of nonbiological bypass graft(s) of the right leg with ulceration
critical limb ischemia of nonbiological bypass graft(s) of the right leg with ulceration

Use additional code to identify severity of ulcer (L97.-)

● CC **I70.631 Atherosclerosis of nonbiological bypass graft(s) of the right leg with ulceration of thigh**

● CC **I70.632 Atherosclerosis of nonbiological bypass graft(s) of the right leg with ulceration of calf**

● CC **I70.633 Atherosclerosis of nonbiological bypass graft(s) of the right leg with ulceration of ankle**

● CC **I70.634 Atherosclerosis of nonbiological bypass graft(s) of the right leg with ulceration of heel and midfoot**

Atherosclerosis of nonbiological bypass graft(s) of right leg with ulceration of plantar surface of midfoot

● **I70.635 Atherosclerosis of nonbiological bypass graft(s) of the right leg with ulceration of other part of foot**

Atherosclerosis of nonbiological bypass graft(s) of the right leg with ulceration of toe

● CC **I70.638 Atherosclerosis of nonbiological bypass graft(s) of the right leg with ulceration of other part of lower leg**

● CC **I70.639 Atherosclerosis of nonbiological bypass graft(s) of the right leg with ulceration of unspecified site**

+ I70.64 Atherosclerosis of nonbiological bypass graft(s) of the left leg with ulceration

Includes: any condition classifiable to I70.612 and I70.622
chronic limb-threatening ischemia of nonbiological bypass graft(s) of the left leg with ulceration
critical limb ischemia of nonbiological bypass graft(s) of the left leg with ulceration

Use additional code to identify severity of ulcer (L97.-)

● CC **I70.641 Atherosclerosis of nonbiological bypass graft(s) of the left leg with ulceration of thigh**

● CC **I70.642 Atherosclerosis of nonbiological bypass graft(s) of the left leg with ulceration of calf**

● CC **I70.643 Atherosclerosis of nonbiological bypass graft(s) of the left leg with ulceration of ankle**

● CC **I70.644 Atherosclerosis of nonbiological bypass graft(s) of the left leg with ulceration of heel and midfoot**

Atherosclerosis of nonbiological bypass graft(s) of left leg with ulceration of plantar surface of midfoot

● **I70.645 Atherosclerosis of nonbiological bypass graft(s) of the left leg with ulceration of other part of foot**

Atherosclerosis of nonbiological bypass graft(s) of the left leg with ulceration of toe

● CC **I70.648 Atherosclerosis of nonbiological bypass graft(s) of the left leg with ulceration of other part of lower leg**

● CC **I70.649 Atherosclerosis of nonbiological bypass graft(s) of the left leg with ulceration of unspecified site**

● **I70.65 Atherosclerosis of nonbiological bypass graft(s) of other extremity with ulceration**

Includes: any condition classifiable to I70.618 and I70.628

Use additional code to identify severity of ulcer (L98.49)

+ **I70.66** **Atherosclerosis of nonbiological bypass graft(s) of the extremities with gangrene**
  Includes: any condition classifiable to I70.61-, I70.62-, I70.63-, I70.64-, I70.65
  chronic limb-threatening ischemia of nonbiological bypass graft(s) of the extremities with gangrene
  critical limb ischemia of nonbiological bypass graft(s) of the extremities with gangrene
  Use additional code to identify the severity of any ulcer (L97.-, L98.49-), if applicable
  ● CC **I70.661** **Atherosclerosis of nonbiological bypass graft(s) of the extremities with gangrene, right leg**
  ● CC **I70.662** **Atherosclerosis of nonbiological bypass graft(s) of the extremities with gangrene, left leg**
  ● CC **I70.663** **Atherosclerosis of nonbiological bypass graft(s) of the extremities with gangrene, bilateral legs**
  ● CC **I70.668** **Atherosclerosis of nonbiological bypass graft(s) of the extremities with gangrene, other extremity**
  ● CC **I70.669** **Atherosclerosis of nonbiological bypass graft(s) of the extremities with gangrene, unspecified extremity**

+ **I70.69** **Other atherosclerosis of nonbiological bypass graft(s) of the extremities**
  ● **I70.691** **Other atherosclerosis of nonbiological bypass graft(s) of the extremities, right leg**
  ● **I70.692** **Other atherosclerosis of nonbiological bypass graft(s) of the extremities, left leg**
  ● **I70.693** **Other atherosclerosis of nonbiological bypass graft(s) of the extremities, bilateral legs**
  ● **I70.698** **Other atherosclerosis of nonbiological bypass graft(s) of the extremities, other extremity**
  ● **I70.699** **Other atherosclerosis of nonbiological bypass graft(s) of the extremities, unspecified extremity**

+ **I70.7** **Atherosclerosis of other type of bypass graft(s) of the extremities**
  Use additional code, if applicable, to identify chronic total occlusion of artery of extremity (I70.92)
  + **I70.70** **Unspecified atherosclerosis of other type of bypass graft(s) of the extremities**
    ● **I70.701** **Unspecified atherosclerosis of other type of bypass graft(s) of the extremities, right leg**
    ● **I70.702** **Unspecified atherosclerosis of other type of bypass graft(s) of the extremities, left leg**
    ● **I70.703** **Unspecified atherosclerosis of other type of bypass graft(s) of the extremities, bilateral legs**
    ● **I70.708** **Unspecified atherosclerosis of other type of bypass graft(s) of the extremities, other extremity**
    ● **I70.709** **Unspecified atherosclerosis of other type of bypass graft(s) of the extremities, unspecified extremity**
  + **I70.71** **Atherosclerosis of other type of bypass graft(s) of the extremities with intermittent claudication**
    ● **I70.711** **Atherosclerosis of other type of bypass graft(s) of the extremities with intermittent claudication, right leg**
    ● **I70.712** **Atherosclerosis of other type of bypass graft(s) of the extremities with intermittent claudication, left leg**
    ● **I70.713** **Atherosclerosis of other type of bypass graft(s) of the extremities with intermittent claudication, bilateral legs**
    ● **I70.718** **Atherosclerosis of other type of bypass graft(s) of the extremities with intermittent claudication, other extremity**
    ● **I70.719** **Atherosclerosis of other type of bypass graft(s) of the extremities with intermittent claudication, unspecified extremity**

+ **I70.72** **Atherosclerosis of other type of bypass graft(s) of the extremities with rest pain**
  Includes: any condition classifiable to I70.71-
  chronic limb-threatening ischemia NOS of other type of bypass graft(s) of the extremities
  chronic limb-threatening ischemia of other type of bypass graft(s) of the extremities with rest pain
  critical limb ischemia NOS of other type of bypass graft(s) of the extremities
  critical limb ischemia of other type of bypass graft(s) of the extremities with rest pain
  ● **I70.721** **Atherosclerosis of other type of bypass graft(s) of the extremities with rest pain, right leg**
  ● **I70.722** **Atherosclerosis of other type of bypass graft(s) of the extremities with rest pain, left leg**
  ● **I70.723** **Atherosclerosis of other type of bypass graft(s) of the extremities with rest pain, bilateral legs**
  ● **I70.728** **Atherosclerosis of other type of bypass graft(s) of the extremities with rest pain, other extremity**
  ● **I70.729** **Atherosclerosis of other type of bypass graft(s) of the extremities with rest pain, unspecified extremity**

+ **I70.73** **Atherosclerosis of other type of bypass graft(s) of the right leg with ulceration**
  Includes: any condition classifiable to I70.711 and I70.721
  chronic limb-threatening ischemia of other type of bypass graft(s) of the right leg with ulceration
  critical limb ischemia of other type of bypass graft(s) of the right leg with ulceration
  Use additional code to identify severity of ulcer (L97.-)
  ● CC **I70.731** **Atherosclerosis of other type of bypass graft(s) of the right leg with ulceration of thigh**
  ● CC **I70.732** **Atherosclerosis of other type of bypass graft(s) of the right leg with ulceration of calf**
  ● CC **I70.733** **Atherosclerosis of other type of bypass graft(s) of the right leg with ulceration of ankle**
  ● CC **I70.734** **Atherosclerosis of other type of bypass graft(s) of the right leg with ulceration of heel and midfoot**
    Atherosclerosis of other type of bypass graft(s) of right leg with ulceration of plantar surface of midfoot
  ● **I70.735** **Atherosclerosis of other type of bypass graft(s) of the right leg with ulceration of other part of foot**
    Atherosclerosis of other type of bypass graft(s) of right leg with ulceration of toe
  ● CC **I70.738** **Atherosclerosis of other type of bypass graft(s) of the right leg with ulceration of other part of lower leg**
  ● CC **I70.739** **Atherosclerosis of other type of bypass graft(s) of the right leg with ulceration of unspecified site**

+ **I70.74** **Atherosclerosis of other type of bypass graft(s) of the left leg with ulceration**
  Includes: any condition classifiable to I70.712 and I70.722
  chronic limb-threatening ischemia of other type of bypass graft(s) of the left leg with ulceration
  critical limb ischemia of other type of bypass graft(s) of the left leg with ulceration
  Use additional code to identify severity of ulcer (L97.-)

● CC **I70.741** **Atherosclerosis of other type of bypass graft(s) of the left leg with ulceration of thigh**

● CC **I70.742** **Atherosclerosis of other type of bypass graft(s) of the left leg with ulceration of calf**

● CC **I70.743** **Atherosclerosis of other type of bypass graft(s) of the left leg with ulceration of ankle**

● CC **I70.744** **Atherosclerosis of other type of bypass graft(s) of the left leg with ulceration of heel and midfoot**

Atherosclerosis of other type of bypass graft(s) of left leg with ulceration of plantar surface of midfoot

● **I70.745** **Atherosclerosis of other type of bypass graft(s) of the left leg with ulceration of other part of foot**

Atherosclerosis of other type of bypass graft(s) of left leg with ulceration of toe

● CC **I70.748** **Atherosclerosis of other type of bypass graft(s) of the left leg with ulceration of other part of lower leg**

● CC **I70.749** **Atherosclerosis of other type of bypass graft(s) of the left leg with ulceration of unspecified site**

● **I70.75** **Atherosclerosis of other type of bypass graft(s) of other extremity with ulceration**
Includes: any condition classifiable to I70.718 and I70.728
Use additional code to identify severity of ulcer (L98.49)

+ **I70.76** **Atherosclerosis of other type of bypass graft(s) of the extremities with gangrene**
Includes: any condition classifiable to I70.71-, I70.72-, I70.73-, I70.74-, I70.75
chronic limb-threatening ischemia of other type of bypass graft(s) of the extremities with gangrene
critical limb ischemia of other type of bypass graft(s) of the extremities with gangrene
Use additional code to identify the severity of any ulcer (L97.-, L98.49-), if applicable

● CC **I70.761** **Atherosclerosis of other type of bypass graft(s) of the extremities with gangrene, right leg**

● CC **I70.762** **Atherosclerosis of other type of bypass graft(s) of the extremities with gangrene, left leg**

● CC **I70.763** **Atherosclerosis of other type of bypass graft(s) of the extremities with gangrene, bilateral legs**

● CC **I70.768** **Atherosclerosis of other type of bypass graft(s) of the extremities with gangrene, other extremity**

● CC **I70.769** **Atherosclerosis of other type of bypass graft(s) of the extremities with gangrene, unspecified extremity**

+ **I70.79** **Other atherosclerosis of other type of bypass graft(s) of the extremities**

● **I70.791** **Other atherosclerosis of other type of bypass graft(s) of the extremities, right leg**

● **I70.792** **Other atherosclerosis of other type of bypass graft(s) of the extremities, left leg**

● **I70.793** **Other atherosclerosis of other type of bypass graft(s) of the extremities, bilateral legs**

● **I70.798** **Other atherosclerosis of other type of bypass graft(s) of the extremities, other extremity**

● **I70.799** **Other atherosclerosis of other type of bypass graft(s) of the extremities, unspecified extremity**

● **I70.8** **Atherosclerosis of other arteries**

+ **I70.9** **Other and unspecified atherosclerosis**

● **I70.90** **Unspecified atherosclerosis**

● **I70.91** **Generalized atherosclerosis**

● CC **I70.92** **Chronic total occlusion of artery of the extremities**
Complete occlusion of artery of the extremities
Total occlusion of artery of the extremities
Code first atherosclerosis of arteries of the extremities (I70.2-, I70.3-, I70.4-, I70.5-, I70.6-, I70.7-)

I71 **Aortic aneurysm and dissection**
Excludes1: *aortic ectasia (I77.81-)*
syphilitic aortic aneurysm (A52.01)
traumatic aortic aneurysm (S25.09, S35.09)

+ **I71.0** **Dissection of aorta**
MCC **I71.00** **Dissection of unspecified site of aorta**
MCC **I71.01** **Dissection of thoracic aorta**
MCC **I71.02** **Dissection of abdominal aorta**
MCC **I71.03** **Dissection of thoracoabdominal aorta**

MCC **I71.1** **Thoracic aortic aneurysm, ruptured**
I71.2 **Thoracic aortic aneurysm, without rupture**
MCC **I71.3** **Abdominal aortic aneurysm, ruptured**
I71.4 **Abdominal aortic aneurysm, without rupture**
MCC **I71.5** **Thoracoabdominal aortic aneurysm, ruptured**
I71.6 **Thoracoabdominal aortic aneurysm, without rupture**
MCC **I71.8** **Aortic aneurysm of unspecified site, ruptured**
Rupture of aorta NOS
I71.9 **Aortic aneurysm of unspecified site, without rupture**
Aneurysm of aorta
Dilatation of aorta
Hyaline necrosis of aorta

I72 **Other aneurysm**
Includes: aneurysm (cirsoid) (false) (ruptured)
Excludes2: *acquired aneurysm (I77.0)*
aneurysm (of) aorta (I71.-)
aneurysm (of) arteriovenous NOS (Q27.3-)
carotid artery dissection (I77.71)
cerebral (nonruptured) aneurysm (I67.1)
coronary aneurysm (I25.4)
coronary artery dissection (I25.42)
dissection of artery NEC (I77.79)
dissection of precerebral artery, congenital (nonruptured) (Q28.1)
heart aneurysm (I25.3)
iliac artery dissection (I77.72)
precerebral artery, congenital (nonruptured) (Q28.1)
pulmonary artery aneurysm (I28.1)
renal artery dissection (I77.73)
retinal aneurysm (H35.0)
ruptured cerebral aneurysm (I60.7)
varicose aneurysm (I77.0)
vertebral artery dissection (I77.74)

I72.0 **Aneurysm of carotid artery**
Aneurysm of common carotid artery
Aneurysm of external carotid artery
Aneurysm of internal carotid artery, extracranial portion
Excludes1: *aneurysm of internal carotid artery, intracranial portion (I67.1)*
aneurysm of internal carotid artery NOS (I67.1)

I72.1 **Aneurysm of artery of upper extremity**
I72.2 **Aneurysm of renal artery**
I72.3 **Aneurysm of iliac artery**
I72.4 **Aneurysm of artery of lower extremity**
AHA CC: 2Q, 2019, 21-22

I72.5 **Aneurysm of other precerebral arteries**
Aneurysm of basilar artery (trunk)
Excludes2: *aneurysm of carotid artery (I72.0)*
aneurysm of vertebral artery (I72.6)
dissection of carotid artery (I77.71)
dissection of other precerebral arteries (I77.75)
dissection of vertebral artery (I77.74)
AHA CC: 4Q, 2016, 28-29

I72.6 **Aneurysm of vertebral artery**
Excludes2: *dissection of vertebral artery (I77.74)*
AHA CC: 4Q, 2016, 28-29

I72.8 **Aneurysm of other specified arteries**
I72.9 **Aneurysm of unspecified site**

I73 **Other peripheral vascular diseases**
Excludes2: *chilblains (T69.1)*
frostbite (T33-T34)
immersion hand or foot (T69.0-)
spasm of cerebral artery (G45.9)

+ **I73.0** **Raynaud's syndrome**
Raynaud's disease
Raynaud's phenomenon (secondary)
I73.00 **Raynaud's syndrome without gangrene**
CC **I73.01** **Raynaud's syndrome with gangrene**
I73.1 **Thromboangiitis obliterans [Buerger's disease]**
+ **I73.8** **Other specified peripheral vascular diseases**
Excludes1: *diabetic (peripheral) angiopathy (E08-E13 with .51-.52)*
I73.81 **Erythromelalgia**
I73.89 **Other specified peripheral vascular diseases**
Acrocyanosis
Erythrocyanosis
Simple acroparesthesia [Schultze's type]
Vasomotor acroparesthesia [Nothnagel's type]
I73.9 **Peripheral vascular disease, unspecified**
Intermittent claudication
Peripheral angiopathy NOS
Spasm of artery
Excludes1: *atherosclerosis of the extremities (I70.2--I70.7-)*

I74 **Arterial embolism and thrombosis**
Includes: embolic infarction
embolic occlusion
thrombotic infarction
thrombotic occlusion
Code first embolism and thrombosis complicating abortion or ectopic or molar pregnancy (O00-O07, O08.2)
embolism and thrombosis complicating pregnancy, childbirth and the puerperium (O88.-)
Excludes2: *atheroembolism (I75.-)*
basilar embolism and thrombosis (I63.0-I63.2, I65.1)
carotid embolism and thrombosis (I63.0-I63.2, I65.2)
cerebral embolism and thrombosis (I63.3-I63.5, I66.-)
coronary embolism and thrombosis (I21-I25)
mesenteric embolism and thrombosis (K55.0-)
ophthalmic embolism and thrombosis (H34.-)
precerebral embolism and thrombosis NOS (I63.0-I63.2, I65.9)
pulmonary embolism and thrombosis (I26.-)
renal embolism and thrombosis (N28.0)
retinal embolism and thrombosis (H34.-)
septic embolism and thrombosis (I76)
vertebral embolism and thrombosis (I63.0-I63.2, I65.0)
+ **I74.0** **Embolism and thrombosis of abdominal aorta**
MCC **I74.01** **Saddle embolus of abdominal aorta**
CC **I74.09** **Other arterial embolism and thrombosis of abdominal aorta**
Aortic bifurcation syndrome
Aortoiliac obstruction
Leriche's syndrome
+ **I74.1** **Embolism and thrombosis of other and unspecified parts of aorta**
CC **I74.10** **Embolism and thrombosis of unspecified parts of aorta**
CC **I74.11** **Embolism and thrombosis of thoracic aorta**
CC **I74.19** **Embolism and thrombosis of other parts of aorta**
CC **I74.2** **Embolism and thrombosis of arteries of the upper extremities**
CC **I74.3** **Embolism and thrombosis of arteries of the lower extremities**
CC **I74.4** **Embolism and thrombosis of arteries of extremities, unspecified**
Peripheral arterial embolism NOS
CC **I74.5** **Embolism and thrombosis of iliac artery**
CC **I74.8** **Embolism and thrombosis of other arteries**
CC **I74.9** **Embolism and thrombosis of unspecified artery**

I75 **Atheroembolism**
Includes: atherothrombotic microembolism
cholesterol embolism
+ **I75.0** **Atheroembolism of extremities**
+ **I75.01** **Atheroembolism of upper extremity**
CC **I75.011** **Atheroembolism of right upper extremity**
CC **I75.012** **Atheroembolism of left upper extremity**
CC **I75.013** **Atheroembolism of bilateral upper extremities**
CC **I75.019** **Atheroembolism of unspecified upper extremity**
+ **I75.02** **Atheroembolism of lower extremity**

CC **I75.021** **Atheroembolism of right lower extremity**
CC **I75.022** **Atheroembolism of left lower extremity**
CC **I75.023** **Atheroembolism of bilateral lower extremities**
CC **I75.029** **Atheroembolism of unspecified lower extremity**
+ **I75.8** **Atheroembolism of other sites**
CC **I75.81** **Atheroembolism of kidney**
Use additional code for any associated acute kidney failure and chronic kidney disease (N17.-, N18.-)
CC **I75.89** **Atheroembolism of other site**

CC **I76** **Septic arterial embolism**
Code first underlying infection, such as:
infective endocarditis (I33.0)
lung abscess (J85.-)
Use additional code to identify the site of the embolism (I74.-)
Excludes2: *septic pulmonary embolism (I26.01, I26.90)*
Valid 3-character code, no further characters required

I77 **Other disorders of arteries and arterioles**
Excludes2: *collagen (vascular) diseases (M30-M36)*
hypersensitivity angiitis (M31.0)
pulmonary artery (I28.-)
I77.0 **Arteriovenous fistula, acquired**
Aneurysmal varix
Arteriovenous aneurysm, acquired
Excludes1: *arteriovenous aneurysm NOS (Q27.3-)*
presence of arteriovenous shunt (fistula) for dialysis (Z99.2)
traumatic - see injury of blood vessel by body region
Excludes2: *cerebral (I67.1)*
coronary (I25.4)
I77.1 **Stricture of artery**
Narrowing of artery
CC **I77.2** **Rupture of artery**
Erosion of artery
Fistula of artery
Ulcer of artery
Excludes1: *traumatic rupture of artery - see injury of blood vessel by body region*
I77.3 **Arterial fibromuscular dysplasia**
Fibromuscular hyperplasia (of) carotid artery
Fibromuscular hyperplasia (of) renal artery
CC **I77.4** **Celiac artery compression syndrome**
CC **I77.5** **Necrosis of artery**
I77.6 **Arteritis, unspecified**
Aortitis NOS
Endarteritis NOS
Excludes1: *arteritis or endarteritis:*
aortic arch (M31.4)
cerebral NEC (I67.7)
coronary (I25.89)
deformans (I70.-)
giant cell (M31.5, M31.6)
obliterans (I70.-)
senile (I70.-)
+ **I77.7** **Other arterial dissection**
Excludes2: *dissection of aorta (I71.0-)*
dissection of coronary artery (I25.42)
MCC **I77.70** **Dissection of unspecified artery**
AHA CC: 4Q, 2016, 28-29
MCC **I77.71** **Dissection of carotid artery**
MCC **I77.72** **Dissection of iliac artery**
MCC **I77.73** **Dissection of renal artery**
MCC **I77.74** **Dissection of vertebral artery**
Excludes2: *aneurysm of vertebral artery (I72.6)*
MCC **I77.75** **Dissection of other precerebral arteries**
Dissection of basilar artery (trunk)
Excludes2: *aneurysm of carotid artery (I72.0)*
aneurysm of other precerebral arteries (I72.5)
aneurysm of vertebral artery (I72.6)
dissection of carotid artery (I77.71)
dissection of vertebral artery (I77.74)
AHA CC: 4Q, 2016, 28-29
MCC **I77.76** **Dissection of artery of upper extremity**
AHA CC: 4Q, 2016, 28-29

+, +7th, X + 7th   ● Newborn   ● Pediatric   ● Maternity   ● Adult   ♀ Female   ♂ Male   Manifestation   Unacceptable PDX   HCC   CC   MCC   HAC

MCC **I77.77** **Dissection of artery of lower extremity**
AHA CC: 4Q, 2016, 28-29

MCC **I77.79** **Dissection of other specified artery**

+ **I77.8** **Other specified disorders of arteries and arterioles**

  + **I77.81** **Aortic ectasia**
    Ectasis aorta
    Excludes1: aortic aneurysm and dissection (I71.0-)
    I77.810 **Thoracic aortic ectasia**
    I77.811 **Abdominal aortic ectasia**
    I77.812 **Thoracoabdominal aortic ectasia**
    I77.819 **Aortic ectasia, unspecified site**

  I77.89 **Other specified disorders of arteries and arterioles**

I77.9 **Disorder of arteries and arterioles, unspecified**

I78 **Diseases of capillaries**

  I78.0 **Hereditary hemorrhagic telangiectasia**
    Rendu-Osler-Weber disease

  I78.1 **Nevus, non-neoplastic**
    Araneus nevus
    Senile nevus
    Spider nevus
    Stellar nevus
    Excludes1: nevus NOS (D22.-)
            vascular NOS (Q82.5)
    Excludes2: blue nevus (D22.-)
            flammeus nevus (Q82.5)
            hairy nevus (D22.-)
            melanocytic nevus (D22.-)
            pigmented nevus (D22.-)
            portwine nevus (Q82.5)
            sanguineous nevus (Q82.5)
            strawberry nevus (Q82.5)
            verrucous nevus (Q82.5)

  I78.8 **Other diseases of capillaries**
  I78.9 **Disease of capillaries, unspecified**

I79 **Disorders of arteries, arterioles and capillaries in diseases classified elsewhere**

  I79.0 **Aneurysm of aorta in diseases classified elsewhere**
    Code first underlying disease
    Excludes1: syphilitic aneurysm (A52.01)

  I79.1 **Aortitis in diseases classified elsewhere**
    Code first underlying disease
    Excludes1: syphilitic aortitis (A52.02)

  I79.8 **Other disorders of arteries, arterioles and capillaries in diseases classified elsewhere**
    Code first underlying disease, such as:
      amyloidosis (E85.-)
    Excludes1: diabetic (peripheral) angiopathy (E08-E13 with .51-.52)
            syphilitic endarteritis (A52.09)
            tuberculous endarteritis (A18.89)

Diseases of veins, lymphatic vessels and lymph nodes, not elsewhere classified (I80-I89)

I80 **Phlebitis and thrombophlebitis**

  Includes: endophlebitis
            inflammation, vein
            periphlebitis
            suppurative phlebitis
  Code first phlebitis and thrombophlebitis complicating abortion, ectopic or molar pregnancy (O00-O07, O08.7)
  phlebitis and thrombophlebitis complicating pregnancy, childbirth and the puerperium (O22.-, O87.-)
  Excludes1: venous embolism and thrombosis of lower extremities (I82.4-, I82.5-, I82.81-)

+ **I80.0** **Phlebitis and thrombophlebitis of superficial vessels of lower extremities**
  Phlebitis and thrombophlebitis of femoropopliteal vein
  I80.00 **Phlebitis and thrombophlebitis of superficial vessels of unspecified lower extremity**
  I80.01 **Phlebitis and thrombophlebitis of superficial vessels of right lower extremity**
  I80.02 **Phlebitis and thrombophlebitis of superficial vessels of left lower extremity**
  I80.03 **Phlebitis and thrombophlebitis of superficial vessels of lower extremities, bilateral**

+ **I80.1** **Phlebitis and thrombophlebitis of femoral vein**
  Phlebitis and thrombophlebitis of common femoral vein
  Phlebitis and thrombophlebitis of deep femoral vein

CC **I80.10** **Phlebitis and thrombophlebitis of unspecified femoral vein**
CC **I80.11** **Phlebitis and thrombophlebitis of right femoral vein**
CC **I80.12** **Phlebitis and thrombophlebitis of left femoral vein**
CC **I80.13** **Phlebitis and thrombophlebitis of femoral vein, bilateral**

+ **I80.2** **Phlebitis and thrombophlebitis of other and unspecified deep vessels of lower extremities**

  + **I80.20** **Phlebitis and thrombophlebitis of unspecified deep vessels of lower extremities**
    CC **I80.201** **Phlebitis and thrombophlebitis of unspecified deep vessels of right lower extremity**
    CC **I80.202** **Phlebitis and thrombophlebitis of unspecified deep vessels of left lower extremity**
    CC **I80.203** **Phlebitis and thrombophlebitis of unspecified deep vessels of lower extremities, bilateral**
    CC **I80.209** **Phlebitis and thrombophlebitis of unspecified deep vessels of unspecified lower extremity**

  + **I80.21** **Phlebitis and thrombophlebitis of iliac vein**
    Phlebitis and thrombophlebitis of common iliac vein
    Phlebitis and thrombophlebitis of external iliac vein
    Phlebitis and thrombophlebitis of internal iliac vein
    CC **I80.211** **Phlebitis and thrombophlebitis of right iliac vein**
    CC **I80.212** **Phlebitis and thrombophlebitis of left iliac vein**
    CC **I80.213** **Phlebitis and thrombophlebitis of iliac vein, bilateral**
    CC **I80.219** **Phlebitis and thrombophlebitis of unspecified iliac vein**

  + **I80.22** **Phlebitis and thrombophlebitis of popliteal vein**
    CC **I80.221** **Phlebitis and thrombophlebitis of right popliteal vein**
    CC **I80.222** **Phlebitis and thrombophlebitis of left popliteal vein**
    CC **I80.223** **Phlebitis and thrombophlebitis of popliteal vein, bilateral**
    CC **I80.229** **Phlebitis and thrombophlebitis of unspecified popliteal vein**

  + **I80.23** **Phlebitis and thrombophlebitis of tibial vein**
    Phlebitis and thrombophlebitis of anterior tibial vein
    Phlebitis and thrombophlebitis of posterior tibial vein
    CC **I80.231** **Phlebitis and thrombophlebitis of right tibial vein**
    CC **I80.232** **Phlebitis and thrombophlebitis of left tibial vein**
    CC **I80.233** **Phlebitis and thrombophlebitis of tibial vein, bilateral**
    CC **I80.239** **Phlebitis and thrombophlebitis of unspecified tibial vein**

  + **I80.24** **Phlebitis and thrombophlebitis of peroneal vein**
    AHA CC: 4Q, 2019, 8
    CC **I80.241** **Phlebitis and thrombophlebitis of right peroneal vein**
    CC **I80.242** **Phlebitis and thrombophlebitis of left peroneal vein**
    CC **I80.243** **Phlebitis and thrombophlebitis of peroneal vein, bilateral**
    CC **I80.249** **Phlebitis and thrombophlebitis of unspecified peroneal vein**

  + **I80.25** **Phlebitis and thrombophlebitis of calf muscular vein**
    Phlebitis and thrombophlebitis of calf muscular vein, NOS
    Phlebitis and thrombophlebitis of gastocnemial vein
    Phlebitis and thrombophlebitis of soleal vein
    AHA CC: 4Q, 2019, 8
    I80.251 **Phlebitis and thrombophlebitis of right calf muscular vein**
    I80.252 **Phlebitis and thrombophlebitis of left calf muscular vein**
    I80.253 **Phlebitis and thrombophlebitis of calf muscular vein, bilateral**
    I80.259 **Phlebitis and thrombophlebitis of unspecified calf muscular vein**

+, +7th, X + 7th   ● Newborn   ● Pediatric   ● Maternity   ● Adult   ♀ Female   ♂ Male   Manifestation   Unacceptable PDX   HCC   CC   MCC   HAC

+ **I80.29** Phlebitis and thrombophlebitis of other deep vessels of lower extremities

  CC **I80.291** Phlebitis and thrombophlebitis of other deep vessels of right lower extremity

  CC **I80.292** Phlebitis and thrombophlebitis of other deep vessels of left lower extremity

  CC **I80.293** Phlebitis and thrombophlebitis of other deep vessels of lower extremity, bilateral

  CC **I80.299** Phlebitis and thrombophlebitis of other deep vessels of unspecified lower extremity

I80.3 Phlebitis and thrombophlebitis of lower extremities, unspecified

I80.8 Phlebitis and thrombophlebitis of other sites

I80.9 Phlebitis and thrombophlebitis of unspecified site

MCC **I81** **Portal vein thrombosis**

Portal (vein) obstruction

Excludes2: *hepatic vein thrombosis (I82.0)*
phlebitis of portal vein (K75.1)

Valid 3-character code, no further characters required

I82 **Other venous embolism and thrombosis**

Code first venous embolism and thrombosis complicating:
abortion, ectopic or molar pregnancy (O00-O07, O08.7)
pregnancy, childbirth and the puerperium (O22.-, O87.-)

Excludes2: *venous embolism and thrombosis (of):*
    cerebral (I63.6, I67.6)
    coronary (I21-I25)
    intracranial and intraspinal, septic or NOS (G08)
    intracranial, nonpyogenic (I67.6)
    intraspinal, nonpyogenic (G95.1)
    mesenteric (K55.0-)
    portal (I81)
    pulmonary (I26.-)

MCC **I82.0** **Budd-Chiari syndrome**

Hepatic vein thrombosis

CC **I82.1** **Thrombophlebitis migrans**

+ **I82.2** **Embolism and thrombosis of vena cava and other thoracic veins**

  + **I82.21** **Embolism and thrombosis of superior vena cava**

    CC **I82.210** Acute embolism and thrombosis of superior vena cava

      Embolism and thrombosis of superior vena cava NOS

    CC **I82.211** Chronic embolism and thrombosis of superior vena cava

  + **I82.22** **Embolism and thrombosis of inferior vena cava**

    MCC **I82.220** Acute embolism and thrombosis of inferior vena cava

      Embolism and thrombosis of inferior vena cava NOS

    MCC **I82.221** Chronic embolism and thrombosis of inferior vena cava

  + **I82.29** **Embolism and thrombosis of other thoracic veins**

    Embolism and thrombosis of brachiocephalic (innominate) vein

    CC **I82.290** Acute embolism and thrombosis of other thoracic veins

    CC **I82.291** Chronic embolism and thrombosis of other thoracic veins

CC **I82.3** **Embolism and thrombosis of renal vein**

+ **I82.4** **Acute embolism and thrombosis of deep veins of lower extremity**

AHA CC: 4Q, 2019, 8-10

  + **I82.40** **Acute embolism and thrombosis of unspecified deep veins of lower extremity**

    Deep vein thrombosis NOS
    DVT NOS

    Excludes1: *acute embolism and thrombosis of unspecified deep veins of distal lower extremity (I82.4Z-)*
acute embolism and thrombosis of unspecified deep veins of proximal lower extremity (I82.4Y-)

    CC **I82.401** Acute embolism and thrombosis of unspecified deep veins of right lower extremity

      HAC see Appendix B for HAC conditional logic

  CC **I82.402** Acute embolism and thrombosis of unspecified deep veins of left lower extremity

    HAC see Appendix B for HAC conditional logic

  CC **I82.403** Acute embolism and thrombosis of unspecified deep veins of lower extremity, bilateral

    HAC see Appendix B for HAC conditional logic

  CC **I82.409** Acute embolism and thrombosis of unspecified deep veins of unspecified lower extremity

    HAC see Appendix B for HAC conditional logic

+ **I82.41** **Acute embolism and thrombosis of femoral vein**

Acute embolism and thrombosis of common femoral vein
Acute embolism and thrombosis of deep femoral vein

  CC **I82.411** Acute embolism and thrombosis of right femoral vein

    HAC see Appendix B for HAC conditional logic

  CC **I82.412** Acute embolism and thrombosis of left femoral vein

    HAC see Appendix B for HAC conditional logic

  CC **I82.413** Acute embolism and thrombosis of femoral vein, bilateral

    HAC see Appendix B for HAC conditional logic

  CC **I82.419** Acute embolism and thrombosis of unspecified femoral vein

    HAC see Appendix B for HAC conditional logic

+ **I82.42** **Acute embolism and thrombosis of iliac vein**

Acute embolism and thrombosis of common iliac vein
Acute embolism and thrombosis of external iliac vein
Acute embolism and thrombosis of internal iliac vein

  CC **I82.421** Acute embolism and thrombosis of right iliac vein

    HAC see Appendix B for HAC conditional logic

  CC **I82.422** Acute embolism and thrombosis of left iliac vein

    HAC see Appendix B for HAC conditional logic

  CC **I82.423** Acute embolism and thrombosis of iliac vein, bilateral

    HAC see Appendix B for HAC conditional logic

  CC **I82.429** Acute embolism and thrombosis of unspecified iliac vein

    HAC see Appendix B for HAC conditional logic

+ **I82.43** **Acute embolism and thrombosis of popliteal vein**

  CC **I82.431** Acute embolism and thrombosis of right popliteal vein

    HAC see Appendix B for HAC conditional logic

  CC **I82.432** Acute embolism and thrombosis of left popliteal vein

    HAC see Appendix B for HAC conditional logic

  CC **I82.433** Acute embolism and thrombosis of popliteal vein, bilateral

    HAC see Appendix B for HAC conditional logic

  CC **I82.439** Acute embolism and thrombosis of unspecified popliteal vein

    HAC see Appendix B for HAC conditional logic

+ **I82.44** **Acute embolism and thrombosis of tibial vein**

Acute embolism and thrombosis of anterior tibial vein
Acute embolism and thrombosis of posterior tibial vein

  CC **I82.441** Acute embolism and thrombosis of right tibial vein

    HAC see Appendix B for HAC conditional logic

697

+, +7th, X + 7th   ● Newborn   ● Pediatric   ● Maternity   ● Adult   ♀ Female   ♂ Male   Manifestation   Unacceptable PDX   HCC   CC   MCC   HAC

CC I82.442 **Acute embolism and thrombosis of left tibial vein**
HAC see Appendix B for HAC conditional logic

CC I82.443 **Acute embolism and thrombosis of tibial vein, bilateral**
HAC see Appendix B for HAC conditional logic

CC I82.449 **Acute embolism and thrombosis of unspecified tibial vein**
HAC see Appendix B for HAC conditional logic

+ **I82.45** **Acute embolism and thrombosis of peroneal vein**

CC I82.451 **Acute embolism and thrombosis of right peroneal vein**
HAC see Appendix B for HAC conditional logic

CC I82.452 **Acute embolism and thrombosis of left peroneal vein**
HAC see Appendix B for HAC conditional logic

CC I82.453 **Acute embolism and thrombosis of peroneal vein, bilateral**
HAC see Appendix B for HAC conditional logic

CC I82.459 **Acute embolism and thrombosis of unspecified peroneal vein**
HAC see Appendix B for HAC conditional logic

+ **I82.46** **Acute embolism and thrombosis of calf muscular vein**
Acute embolism and thrombosis of calf muscular vein, NOS
Acute embolism and thrombosis of gastocnemial vein
Acute embolism and thrombosis of soleal vein

I82.461 **Acute embolism and thrombosis of right calf muscular vein**

I82.462 **Acute embolism and thrombosis of left calf muscular vein**

I82.463 **Acute embolism and thrombosis of calf muscular vein, bilateral**

I82.469 **Acute embolism and thrombosis of unspecified calf muscular vein**

+ **I82.49** **Acute embolism and thrombosis of other specified deep vein of lower extremity**

CC I82.491 **Acute embolism and thrombosis of other specified deep vein of right lower extremity**
HAC see Appendix B for HAC conditional logic

CC I82.492 **Acute embolism and thrombosis of other specified deep vein of left lower extremity**
HAC see Appendix B for HAC conditional logic

CC I82.493 **Acute embolism and thrombosis of other specified deep vein of lower extremity, bilateral**
HAC see Appendix B for HAC conditional logic

CC I82.499 **Acute embolism and thrombosis of other specified deep vein of unspecified lower extremity**
HAC see Appendix B for HAC conditional logic

+ **I82.4Y** **Acute embolism and thrombosis of unspecified deep veins of proximal lower extremity**
Acute embolism and thrombosis of deep vein of thigh NOS
Acute embolism and thrombosis of deep vein of upper leg NOS

CC I82.4Y1 **Acute embolism and thrombosis of unspecified deep veins of right proximal lower extremity**
HAC see Appendix B for HAC conditional logic

CC I82.4Y2 **Acute embolism and thrombosis of unspecified deep veins of left proximal lower extremity**
HAC see Appendix B for HAC conditional logic

CC I82.4Y3 **Acute embolism and thrombosis of unspecified deep veins of proximal lower extremity, bilateral**
HAC see Appendix B for HAC conditional logic

CC I82.4Y9 **Acute embolism and thrombosis of unspecified deep veins of unspecified proximal lower extremity**
HAC see Appendix B for HAC conditional logic

+ **I82.4Z** **Acute embolism and thrombosis of unspecified deep veins of distal lower extremity**
Acute embolism and thrombosis of deep vein of calf NOS
Acute embolism and thrombosis of deep vein of lower leg NOS

CC I82.4Z1 **Acute embolism and thrombosis of unspecified deep veins of right distal lower extremity**
HAC see Appendix B for HAC conditional logic

CC I82.4Z2 **Acute embolism and thrombosis of unspecified deep veins of left distal lower extremity**
HAC see Appendix B for HAC conditional logic

CC I82.4Z3 **Acute embolism and thrombosis of unspecified deep veins of distal lower extremity, bilateral**
HAC see Appendix B for HAC conditional logic

CC I82.4Z9 **Acute embolism and thrombosis of unspecified deep veins of unspecified distal lower extremity**
HAC see Appendix B for HAC conditional logic

+ **I82.5** **Chronic embolism and thrombosis of deep veins of lower extremity**
Use additional code, if applicable, for associated long-term (current) use of anticoagulants (Z79.01)
Excludes1: *personal history of venous embolism and thrombosis (Z86.718)*
AHA CC: 4Q, 2019, 8-10

+ **I82.50** **Chronic embolism and thrombosis of unspecified deep veins of lower extremity**
Excludes1: *chronic embolism and thrombosis of unspecified deep veins of distal lower extremity (I82.5Z-)*
chronic embolism and thrombosis of unspecified deep veins of proximal lower extremity (I82.5Y-)

CC I82.501 **Chronic embolism and thrombosis of unspecified deep veins of right lower extremity**

CC I82.502 **Chronic embolism and thrombosis of unspecified deep veins of left lower extremity**

CC I82.503 **Chronic embolism and thrombosis of unspecified deep veins of lower extremity, bilateral**

CC I82.509 **Chronic embolism and thrombosis of unspecified deep veins of unspecified lower extremity**

+ **I82.51** **Chronic embolism and thrombosis of femoral vein**
Chronic embolism and thrombosis of common femoral vein
Chronic embolism and thrombosis of deep femoral vein

CC I82.511 **Chronic embolism and thrombosis of right femoral vein**

CC I82.512 **Chronic embolism and thrombosis of left femoral vein**

CC I82.513 **Chronic embolism and thrombosis of femoral vein, bilateral**

CC I82.519 **Chronic embolism and thrombosis of unspecified femoral vein**

+ **I82.52** **Chronic embolism and thrombosis of iliac vein**
Chronic embolism and thrombosis of common iliac vein
Chronic embolism and thrombosis of external iliac vein
Chronic embolism and thrombosis of internal iliac vein

+, +7th, X + 7th   ● Newborn   ● Pediatric   ● Maternity   ● Adult   ♀ Female   ♂ Male   Manifestation   Unacceptable PDX   HCC   CC   MCC   HAC

CC **I82.521** Chronic embolism and thrombosis of right iliac vein

CC **I82.522** Chronic embolism and thrombosis of left iliac vein

CC **I82.523** Chronic embolism and thrombosis of iliac vein, bilateral

CC **I82.529** Chronic embolism and thrombosis of unspecified iliac vein

+ **I82.53** Chronic embolism and thrombosis of popliteal vein

CC **I82.531** Chronic embolism and thrombosis of right popliteal vein

CC **I82.532** Chronic embolism and thrombosis of left popliteal vein

CC **I82.533** Chronic embolism and thrombosis of popliteal vein, bilateral

CC **I82.539** Chronic embolism and thrombosis of unspecified popliteal vein

+ **I82.54** Chronic embolism and thrombosis of tibial vein
　Chronic embolism and thrombosis of anterior tibial vein
　Chronic embolism and thrombosis of posterior tibial vein

CC **I82.541** Chronic embolism and thrombosis of right tibial vein

CC **I82.542** Chronic embolism and thrombosis of left tibial vein

CC **I82.543** Chronic embolism and thrombosis of tibial vein, bilateral

CC **I82.549** Chronic embolism and thrombosis of unspecified tibial vein

+ **I82.55** Acute embolism and thrombosis of peroneal vein

CC **I82.551** Chronic embolism and thrombosis of right peroneal vein

CC **I82.552** Chronic embolism and thrombosis of left peroneal vein

CC **I82.553** Chronic embolism and thrombosis of peroneal vein, bilateral

CC **I82.559** Chronic embolism and thrombosis of unspecified peroneal vein

+ **I82.56** Acute embolism and thrombosis of calf muscular vein
　Acute embolism and thrombosis of calf muscular vein, NOS
　Acute embolism and thrombosis of gastocnemial vein
　Acute embolism and thrombosis of soleal vein

I82.561 Chronic embolism and thrombosis of right calf muscular vein

I82.562 Chronic embolism and thrombosis of left calf muscular vein

I82.563 Chronic embolism and thrombosis of calf muscular vein, bilateral

I82.569 Chronic embolism and thrombosis of unspecified calf muscular vein

+ **I82.59** Chronic embolism and thrombosis of other specified deep vein of lower extremity

CC **I82.591** Chronic embolism and thrombosis of other specified deep vein of right lower extremity

CC **I82.592** Chronic embolism and thrombosis of other specified deep vein of left lower extremity

CC **I82.593** Chronic embolism and thrombosis of other specified deep vein of lower extremity, bilateral

CC **I82.599** Chronic embolism and thrombosis of other specified deep vein of unspecified lower extremity

+ **I82.5Y** Chronic embolism and thrombosis of unspecified deep veins of proximal lower extremity
　Chronic embolism and thrombosis of deep veins of thigh NOS
　Chronic embolism and thrombosis of deep veins of upper leg NOS

CC **I82.5Y1** Chronic embolism and thrombosis of unspecified deep veins of right proximal lower extremity

CC **I82.5Y2** Chronic embolism and thrombosis of unspecified deep veins of left proximal lower extremity

CC **I82.5Y3** Chronic embolism and thrombosis of unspecified deep veins of proximal lower extremity, bilateral

CC **I82.5Y9** Chronic embolism and thrombosis of unspecified deep veins of unspecified proximal lower extremity

+ **I82.5Z** Chronic embolism and thrombosis of unspecified deep veins of distal lower extremity
　Chronic embolism and thrombosis of deep veins of calf NOS
　Chronic embolism and thrombosis of deep veins of lower leg NOS

CC **I82.5Z1** Chronic embolism and thrombosis of unspecified deep veins of right distal lower extremity

CC **I82.5Z2** Chronic embolism and thrombosis of unspecified deep veins of left distal lower extremity

CC **I82.5Z3** Chronic embolism and thrombosis of unspecified deep veins of distal lower extremity, bilateral

CC **I82.5Z9** Chronic embolism and thrombosis of unspecified deep veins of unspecified distal lower extremity

+ **I82.6** Acute embolism and thrombosis of veins of upper extremity

+ **I82.60** Acute embolism and thrombosis of unspecified veins of upper extremity

CC I82.601 Acute embolism and thrombosis of unspecified veins of right upper extremity

CC I82.602 Acute embolism and thrombosis of unspecified veins of left upper extremity

CC I82.603 Acute embolism and thrombosis of unspecified veins of upper extremity, bilateral

CC I82.609 Acute embolism and thrombosis of unspecified veins of unspecified upper extremity

+ **I82.61** Acute embolism and thrombosis of superficial veins of upper extremity
　Acute embolism and thrombosis of antecubital vein
　Acute embolism and thrombosis of basilic vein
　Acute embolism and thrombosis of cephalic vein

CC I82.611 Acute embolism and thrombosis of superficial veins of right upper extremity

CC I82.612 Acute embolism and thrombosis of superficial veins of left upper extremity

CC I82.613 Acute embolism and thrombosis of superficial veins of upper extremity, bilateral

CC I82.619 Acute embolism and thrombosis of superficial veins of unspecified upper extremity

+ **I82.62** Acute embolism and thrombosis of deep veins of upper extremity
　Acute embolism and thrombosis of brachial vein
　Acute embolism and thrombosis of radial vein
　Acute embolism and thrombosis of ulnar vein

CC **I82.621** Acute embolism and thrombosis of deep veins of right upper extremity

CC **I82.622** Acute embolism and thrombosis of deep veins of left upper extremity

CC **I82.623** Acute embolism and thrombosis of deep veins of upper extremity, bilateral

CC **I82.629** Acute embolism and thrombosis of deep veins of unspecified upper extremity

+ **I82.7** Chronic embolism and thrombosis of veins of upper extremity
　Use additional code, if applicable, for associated long-term (current) use of anticoagulants (Z79.01)
　Excludes1: *personal history of venous embolism and thrombosis (Z86.718)*

+ **I82.70** Chronic embolism and thrombosis of unspecified veins of upper extremity

CC I82.701 Chronic embolism and thrombosis of unspecified veins of right upper extremity

CC I82.702 Chronic embolism and thrombosis of unspecified veins of left upper extremity

+, +7th, X + 7th　● Newborn　● Pediatric　● Maternity　● Adult　♀ Female　♂ Male　Manifestation　Unacceptable PDX　HCC　CC　MCC　HAC

CC **I82.703** Chronic embolism and thrombosis of unspecified veins of upper extremity, bilateral

CC **I82.709** Chronic embolism and thrombosis of unspecified veins of unspecified upper extremity

+ **I82.71** Chronic embolism and thrombosis of superficial veins of upper extremity

Chronic embolism and thrombosis of antecubital vein

Chronic embolism and thrombosis of basilic vein

Chronic embolism and thrombosis of cephalic vein

CC **I82.711** Chronic embolism and thrombosis of superficial veins of right upper extremity

CC **I82.712** Chronic embolism and thrombosis of superficial veins of left upper extremity

CC **I82.713** Chronic embolism and thrombosis of superficial veins of upper extremity, bilateral

CC **I82.719** Chronic embolism and thrombosis of superficial veins of unspecified upper extremity

+ **I82.72** Chronic embolism and thrombosis of deep veins of upper extremity

Chronic embolism and thrombosis of brachial vein

Chronic embolism and thrombosis of radial vein

Chronic embolism and thrombosis of ulnar vein

CC **I82.721** Chronic embolism and thrombosis of deep veins of right upper extremity

CC **I82.722** Chronic embolism and thrombosis of deep veins of left upper extremity

CC **I82.723** Chronic embolism and thrombosis of deep veins of upper extremity, bilateral

CC **I82.729** Chronic embolism and thrombosis of deep veins of unspecified upper extremity

+ **I82.A** Embolism and thrombosis of axillary vein

+ **I82.A1** Acute embolism and thrombosis of axillary vein

CC **I82.A11** Acute embolism and thrombosis of right axillary vein

CC **I82.A12** Acute embolism and thrombosis of left axillary vein

CC **I82.A13** Acute embolism and thrombosis of axillary vein, bilateral

CC **I82.A19** Acute embolism and thrombosis of unspecified axillary vein

+ **I82.A2** Chronic embolism and thrombosis of axillary vein

CC **I82.A21** Chronic embolism and thrombosis of right axillary vein

CC **I82.A22** Chronic embolism and thrombosis of left axillary vein

CC **I82.A23** Chronic embolism and thrombosis of axillary vein, bilateral

CC **I82.A29** Chronic embolism and thrombosis of unspecified axillary vein

+ **I82.B** Embolism and thrombosis of subclavian vein

+ **I82.B1** Acute embolism and thrombosis of subclavian≈vein

CC **I82.B11** Acute embolism and thrombosis of right subclavian vein

CC **I82.B12** Acute embolism and thrombosis of left subclavian vein

CC **I82.B13** Acute embolism and thrombosis of subclavian vein, bilateral

CC **I82.B19** Acute embolism and thrombosis of unspecified subclavian vein

+ **I82.B2** Chronic embolism and thrombosis of subclavian vein

CC **I82.B21** Chronic embolism and thrombosis of right subclavian vein

CC **I82.B22** Chronic embolism and thrombosis of left subclavian vein

CC **I82.B23** Chronic embolism and thrombosis of subclavian vein, bilateral

CC **I82.B29** Chronic embolism and thrombosis of unspecified subclavian vein

+ **I82.C** Embolism and thrombosis of internal jugular vein

+ **I82.C1** Acute embolism and thrombosis of internal jugular vein

CC **I82.C11** Acute embolism and thrombosis of right internal jugular vein

CC **I82.C12** Acute embolism and thrombosis of left internal jugular vein

CC **I82.C13** Acute embolism and thrombosis of internal jugular vein, bilateral

CC **I82.C19** Acute embolism and thrombosis of unspecified internal jugular vein

+ **I82.C2** Chronic embolism and thrombosis of internal jugular vein

CC **I82.C21** Chronic embolism and thrombosis of right internal jugular vein

CC **I82.C22** Chronic embolism and thrombosis of left internal jugular vein

CC **I82.C23** Chronic embolism and thrombosis of internal jugular vein, bilateral

CC **I82.C29** Chronic embolism and thrombosis of unspecified internal jugular vein

+ **I82.8** Embolism and thrombosis of other specified veins

Use additional code, if applicable, for associated long-term (current) use of anticoagulants (Z79.01)

+ **I82.81** Embolism and thrombosis of superficial veins of lower extremities

Embolism and thrombosis of saphenous vein (greater) (lesser)

CC **I82.811** Embolism and thrombosis of superficial veins of right lower extremity

CC **I82.812** Embolism and thrombosis of superficial veins of left lower extremity

CC **I82.813** Embolism and thrombosis of superficial veins of lower extremities, bilateral

CC **I82.819** Embolism and thrombosis of superficial veins of unspecified lower extremity

+ **I82.89** Embolism and thrombosis of other specified veins

CC **I82.890** Acute embolism and thrombosis of other specified veins

CC **I82.891** Chronic embolism and thrombosis of other specified veins

+ **I82.9** Embolism and thrombosis of unspecified vein

CC **I82.90** Acute embolism and thrombosis of unspecified vein

Embolism of vein NOS

Thrombosis (vein) NOS

CC **I82.91** Chronic embolism and thrombosis of unspecified vein

I83 Varicose veins of lower extremities

Excludes1: *varicose veins complicating pregnancy (O22.0-)*

varicose veins complicating the puerperium (O87.4)

+ **I83.0** Varicose veins of lower extremities with ulcer

Use additional code to identify severity of ulcer (L97.-)

+ **I83.00** Varicose veins of unspecified lower extremity with ulcer

• **I83.001** Varicose veins of unspecified lower extremity with ulcer of thigh

• **I83.002** Varicose veins of unspecified lower extremity with ulcer of calf

• **I83.003** Varicose veins of unspecified lower extremity with ulcer of ankle

• **I83.004** Varicose veins of unspecified lower extremity with ulcer of heel and midfoot

Varicose veins of unspecified lower extremity with ulcer of plantar surface of midfoot

• **I83.005** Varicose veins of unspecified lower extremity with ulcer other part of foot

Varicose veins of unspecified lower extremity with ulcer of toe

• **I83.008** Varicose veins of unspecified lower extremity with ulcer other part of lower leg

• **I83.009** Varicose veins of unspecified lower extremity with ulcer of unspecified site

+ **I83.01** Varicose veins of right lower extremity with ulcer

• **I83.011** Varicose veins of right lower extremity with ulcer of thigh

• **I83.012** Varicose veins of right lower extremity with ulcer of calf

• **I83.013** Varicose veins of right lower extremity with ulcer of ankle

• **I83.014** Varicose veins of right lower extremity with ulcer of heel and midfoot

Varicose veins of right lower extremity with ulcer of plantar surface of midfoot

- I83.015 **Varicose veins of right lower extremity with ulcer other part of foot**
  Varicose veins of right lower extremity with ulcer of toe
- I83.018 **Varicose veins of right lower extremity with ulcer other part of lower leg**
- I83.019 **Varicose veins of right lower extremity with ulcer of unspecified site**

+ I83.02 **Varicose veins of left lower extremity with ulcer**
- I83.021 **Varicose veins of left lower extremity with ulcer of thigh**
- I83.022 **Varicose veins of left lower extremity with ulcer of calf**
- I83.023 **Varicose veins of left lower extremity with ulcer of ankle**
- I83.024 **Varicose veins of left lower extremity with ulcer of heel and midfoot**
  Varicose veins of left lower extremity with ulcer of plantar surface of midfoot
- I83.025 **Varicose veins of left lower extremity with ulcer other part of foot**
  Varicose veins of left lower extremity with ulcer of toe
- I83.028 **Varicose veins of left lower extremity with ulcer other part of lower leg**
- I83.029 **Varicose veins of left lower extremity with ulcer of unspecified site**

+ I83.1 **Varicose veins of lower extremities with inflammation**
- I83.10 **Varicose veins of unspecified lower extremity with inflammation**
- I83.11 **Varicose veins of right lower extremity with inflammation**
- I83.12 **Varicose veins of left lower extremity with inflammation**

+ I83.2 **Varicose veins of lower extremities with both ulcer and inflammation**
  Use additional code to identify severity of ulcer (L97.-)
  + I83.20 **Varicose veins of unspecified lower extremity with both ulcer and inflammation**
  - CC I83.201 **Varicose veins of unspecified lower extremity with both ulcer of thigh and inflammation**
  - CC I83.202 **Varicose veins of unspecified lower extremity with both ulcer of calf and inflammation**
  - CC I83.203 **Varicose veins of unspecified lower extremity with both ulcer of ankle and inflammation**
  - CC I83.204 **Varicose veins of unspecified lower extremity with both ulcer of heel and midfoot and inflammation**
    Varicose veins of unspecified lower extremity with both ulcer of plantar surface of midfoot and inflammation
  - CC I83.205 **Varicose veins of unspecified lower extremity with both ulcer other part of foot and inflammation**
    Varicose veins of unspecified lower extremity with both ulcer of toe and inflammation
  - CC I83.208 **Varicose veins of unspecified lower extremity with both ulcer of other part of lower extremity and inflammation**
  - CC I83.209 **Varicose veins of unspecified lower extremity with both ulcer of unspecified site and inflammation**
  + I83.21 **Varicose veins of right lower extremity with both ulcer and inflammation**
  - CC I83.211 **Varicose veins of right lower extremity with both ulcer of thigh and inflammation**
  - CC I83.212 **Varicose veins of right lower extremity with both ulcer of calf and inflammation**
  - CC I83.213 **Varicose veins of right lower extremity with both ulcer of ankle and inflammation**

- CC I83.214 **Varicose veins of right lower extremity with both ulcer of heel and midfoot and inflammation**
  Varicose veins of right lower extremity with both ulcer of plantar surface of midfoot and inflammation
- CC I83.215 **Varicose veins of right lower extremity with both ulcer other part of foot and inflammation**
  Varicose veins of right lower extremity with both ulcer of toe and inflammation
- CC I83.218 **Varicose veins of right lower extremity with both ulcer of other part of lower extremity and inflammation**
- CC I83.219 **Varicose veins of right lower extremity with both ulcer of unspecified site and inflammation**

+ I83.22 **Varicose veins of left lower extremity with both ulcer and inflammation**
- CC I83.221 **Varicose veins of left lower extremity with both ulcer of thigh and inflammation**
- CC I83.222 **Varicose veins of left lower extremity with both ulcer of calf and inflammation**
- CC I83.223 **Varicose veins of left lower extremity with both ulcer of ankle and inflammation**
- CC I83.224 **Varicose veins of left lower extremity with both ulcer of heel and midfoot and inflammation**
  Varicose veins of left lower extremity with both ulcer of plantar surface of midfoot and inflammation
- CC I83.225 **Varicose veins of left lower extremity with both ulcer other part of foot and inflammation**
  Varicose veins of left lower extremity with both ulcer of toe and inflammation
- CC I83.228 **Varicose veins of left lower extremity with both ulcer of other part of lower extremity and inflammation**
- CC I83.229 **Varicose veins of left lower extremity with both ulcer of unspecified site and inflammation**

+ I83.8 **Varicose veins of lower extremities with other complications**
  + I83.81 **Varicose veins of lower extremities with pain**
  - I83.811 **Varicose veins of right lower extremity with pain**
  - I83.812 **Varicose veins of left lower extremity with pain**
  - I83.813 **Varicose veins of bilateral lower extremities with pain**
  - I83.819 **Varicose veins of unspecified lower extremity with pain**
  + I83.89 **Varicose veins of lower extremities with other complications**
    Varicose veins of lower extremities with edema
    Varicose veins of lower extremities with swelling
  - I83.891 **Varicose veins of right lower extremity with other complications**
  - I83.892 **Varicose veins of left lower extremity with other complications**
  - I83.893 **Varicose veins of bilateral lower extremities with other complications**
  - I83.899 **Varicose veins of unspecified lower extremity with other complications**

+ I83.9 **Asymptomatic varicose veins of lower extremities**
  Phlebectasia of lower extremities
  Varicose veins of lower extremities
  Varix of lower extremities
- I83.90 **Asymptomatic varicose veins of unspecified lower extremity**
  Varicose veins NOS
- I83.91 **Asymptomatic varicose veins of right lower extremity**
- I83.92 **Asymptomatic varicose veins of left lower extremity**
- I83.93 **Asymptomatic varicose veins of bilateral lower extremities**

+, +7th, X + 7th   ● Newborn   ● Pediatric   ● Maternity   ● Adult   ♀ Female   ♂ Male   Manifestation   Unacceptable PDX   HCC   CC   MCC   HAC

I85 Esophageal varices

Use additional code to identify:
alcohol abuse and dependence (F10.-)

+ **I85.0 Esophageal varices**
Idiopathic esophageal varices
Primary esophageal varices

CC **I85.00 Esophageal varices without bleeding**
Esophageal varices NOS

MCC **I85.01 Esophageal varices with bleeding**

+ **I85.1 Secondary esophageal varices**
Esophageal varices secondary to alcoholic liver disease
Esophageal varices secondary to cirrhosis of liver
Esophageal varices secondary to schistosomiasis
Esophageal varices secondary to toxic liver disease
Code first underlying disease

CC **I85.10 Secondary esophageal varices without bleeding**

MCC **I85.11 Secondary esophageal varices with bleeding**

I86 Varicose veins of other sites

Excludes1: varicose veins of unspecified site (I83.9-)
Excludes2: retinal varices (H35.0-)

I86.0 Sublingual varices

♂ **I86.1 Scrotal varices**
Varicocele

I86.2 Pelvic varices

♀ **I86.3 Vulval varices**
Excludes1: vulval varices complicating childbirth and the
puerperium (O87.8)
vulval varices complicating pregnancy (O22.1-)

I86.4 Gastric varices

• **I86.8 Varicose veins of other specified sites**
Varicose ulcer of nasal septum

I87 Other disorders of veins

+ **I87.0 Postthrombotic syndrome**
Chronic venous hypertension due to deep vein thrombosis
Postphlebitic syndrome
Excludes1: chronic venous hypertension without deep vein
thrombosis (I87.3-)

+ **I87.00 Postthrombotic syndrome without complications**
Asymptomatic Postthrombotic syndrome

**I87.001 Postthrombotic syndrome without
complications of right lower extremity**

**I87.002 Postthrombotic syndrome without
complications of left lower extremity**

**I87.003 Postthrombotic syndrome without
complications of bilateral lower extremity**

**I87.009 Postthrombotic syndrome without
complications of unspecified extremity**
Postthrombotic syndrome NOS

+ **I87.01 Postthrombotic syndrome with ulcer**
Use additional code to specify site and severity of
ulcer (L97.-)

CC **I87.011 Postthrombotic syndrome with ulcer of
right lower extremity**

CC **I87.012 Postthrombotic syndrome with ulcer of
left lower extremity**

CC **I87.013 Postthrombotic syndrome with ulcer of
bilateral lower extremity**

CC **I87.019 Postthrombotic syndrome with ulcer of
unspecified lower extremity**

+ **I87.02 Postthrombotic syndrome with inflammation**

**I87.021 Postthrombotic syndrome with
inflammation of right lower extremity**

**I87.022 Postthrombotic syndrome with
inflammation of left lower extremity**

**I87.023 Postthrombotic syndrome with
inflammation of bilateral lower extremity**

**I87.029 Postthrombotic syndrome with
inflammation of unspecified lower
extremity**

+ **I87.03 Postthrombotic syndrome with ulcer and
inflammation**
Use additional code to specify site and severity of
ulcer (L97.-)

CC **I87.031 Postthrombotic syndrome with ulcer
and inflammation of right lower
extremity**

CC **I87.032 Postthrombotic syndrome with
ulcer and inflammation of left lower
extremity**

CC **I87.033 Postthrombotic syndrome with ulcer
and inflammation of bilateral lower
extremity**

CC **I87.039 Postthrombotic syndrome with ulcer
and inflammation of unspecified lower
extremity**

+ **I87.09 Postthrombotic syndrome with other
complications**

**I87.091 Postthrombotic syndrome with other
complications of right lower extremity**

**I87.092 Postthrombotic syndrome with other
complications of left lower extremity**

**I87.093 Postthrombotic syndrome with other
complications of bilateral lower extremity**

**I87.099 Postthrombotic syndrome with other
complications of unspecified lower
extremity**

CC **I87.1 Compression of vein**
Stricture of vein
Vena cava syndrome (inferior) (superior)
Excludes2: compression of pulmonary vein (I28.8)

I87.2 Venous insufficiency (chronic) (peripheral)
Stasis dermatitis
Excludes1: stasis dermatitis with varicose veins of lower
extremities (I83.1-, I83.2-)

+ **I87.3 Chronic venous hypertension (idiopathic)**
Stasis edema
Excludes1: chronic venous hypertension due to deep vein
thrombosis (I87.0-)
varicose veins of lower extremities (I83.-)

+ **I87.30 Chronic venous hypertension (idiopathic) without
complications**
Asymptomatic chronic venous hypertension
(idiopathic)

**I87.301 Chronic venous hypertension
(idiopathic) without complications of
right lower extremity**

**I87.302 Chronic venous hypertension
(idiopathic) without complications of
left lower extremity**

**I87.303 Chronic venous hypertension
(idiopathic) without complications of
bilateral lower extremity**

**I87.309 Chronic venous hypertension
(idiopathic) without complications of
unspecified lower extremity**
Chronic venous hypertension NOS

+ **I87.31 Chronic venous hypertension (idiopathic) with ulcer**
Use additional code to specify site and severity of
ulcer (L97.-)

CC **I87.311 Chronic venous hypertension
(idiopathic) with ulcer of right lower
extremity**

CC **I87.312 Chronic venous hypertension
(idiopathic) with ulcer of left lower
extremity**

CC **I87.313 Chronic venous hypertension (idiopathic)
with ulcer of bilateral lower extremity**

CC **I87.319 Chronic venous hypertension
(idiopathic) with ulcer of unspecified
lower extremity**

+ **I87.32 Chronic venous hypertension (idiopathic) with
inflammation**

**I87.321 Chronic venous hypertension
(idiopathic) with inflammation of right
lower extremity**

**I87.322 Chronic venous hypertension
(idiopathic) with inflammation of left
lower extremity**

**I87.323 Chronic venous hypertension
(idiopathic) with inflammation of
bilateral lower extremity**

**I87.329 Chronic venous hypertension
(idiopathic) with inflammation of
unspecified lower extremity**

+ **I87.33 Chronic venous hypertension (idiopathic) with
ulcer and inflammation**
Use additional code to specify site and severity of
ulcer (L97.-)

CC **I87.331** **Chronic venous hypertension (idiopathic) with ulcer and inflammation of right lower extremity**

CC **I87.332** **Chronic venous hypertension (idiopathic) with ulcer and inflammation of left lower extremity**

CC **I87.333** **Chronic venous hypertension (idiopathic) with ulcer and inflammation of bilateral lower extremity**

CC **I87.339** **Chronic venous hypertension (idiopathic) with ulcer and inflammation of unspecified lower extremity**

+ **I87.39** **Chronic venous hypertension (idiopathic) with other complications**

I87.391 **Chronic venous hypertension (idiopathic) with other complications of right lower extremity**

I87.392 **Chronic venous hypertension (idiopathic) with other complications of left lower extremity**

I87.393 **Chronic venous hypertension (idiopathic) with other complications of bilateral lower extremity**

I87.399 **Chronic venous hypertension (idiopathic) with other complications of unspecified lower extremity**

I87.8 **Other specified disorders of veins**
Phlebosclerosis
Venofibrosis

I87.9 **Disorder of vein, unspecified**

I88 **Nonspecific lymphadenitis**

Excludes1: *acute lymphadenitis, except mesenteric (L04.-)*
enlarged lymph nodes NOS (R59.-)
human immunodeficiency virus [HIV] disease resulting in generalized lymphadenopathy (B20)

I88.0 **Nonspecific mesenteric lymphadenitis**
Mesenteric lymphadenitis (acute)(chronic)

I88.1 **Chronic lymphadenitis, except mesenteric**
Adenitis
Lymphadenitis

I88.8 **Other nonspecific lymphadenitis**

I88.9 **Nonspecific lymphadenitis, unspecified**
Lymphadenitis NOS

I89 **Other noninfective disorders of lymphatic vessels and lymph nodes**

Excludes1: *chylocele, tunica vaginalis (nonfilarial) NOS (N50.89)*
enlarged lymph nodes NOS (R59.-)
filarial chylocele (B74.-)
hereditary lymphedema (Q82.0)

I89.0 **Lymphedema, not elsewhere classified**
Elephantiasis (nonfilarial) NOS
Lymphangiectasis
Obliteration, lymphatic vessel
Praecox lymphedema
Secondary lymphedema
Excludes1: *postmastectomy lymphedema (I97.2)*

I89.1 **Lymphangitis**
Chronic lymphangitis
Lymphangitis NOS
Subacute lymphangitis
Excludes1: *acute lymphangitis (L03.-)*

I89.8 **Other specified noninfective disorders of lymphatic vessels and lymph nodes**
Chylocele (nonfilarial)
Chylous ascites
Chylous cyst
Lipomelanotic reticulosis
Lymph node or vessel fistula
Lymph node or vessel infarction
Lymph node or vessel rupture

I89.9 **Noninfective disorder of lymphatic vessels and lymph nodes, unspecified**
Disease of lymphatic vessels NOS

Other and unspecified disorders of the circulatory system (I95-I99)

I95 **Hypotension**

Excludes1: *cardiovascular collapse (R57.9)*
maternal hypotension syndrome (O26.5-)
nonspecific low blood pressure reading NOS (R03.1)

I95.0 **Idiopathic hypotension**

I95.1 **Orthostatic hypotension**
Hypotension, postural
Excludes1: *neurogenic orthostatic hypotension [Shy-Drager] (G90.3)*
orthostatic hypotension due to drugs (I95.2)

I95.2 **Hypotension due to drugs**
Orthostatic hypotension due to drugs
Use additional code for adverse effect, if applicable, to identify drug (T36-T50 with fifth or sixth character 5)

I95.3 **Hypotension of hemodialysis**
Intra-dialytic hypotension

I95.8 **Other hypotension**

I95.81 **Postprocedural hypotension**

I95.89 **Other hypotension**
Chronic hypotension

I95.9 **Hypotension, unspecified**

CC **I96** **Gangrene, not elsewhere classified**

Gangrenous cellulitis

Excludes1: *gangrene in atherosclerosis of native arteries of the extremities (I70.26)*
gangrene in hernia (K40.1, K40.4, K41.1, K41.4, K42.1, K43.1-, K44.1, K45.1, K46.1)
gangrene in other peripheral vascular diseases (I73.-)
gangrene of certain specified sites - see Alphabetical Index
gas gangrene (A48.0)
pyoderma gangrenosum (L88)

Excludes2: *gangrene in diabetes mellitus (E08-E13 with .52)*
AHA CC: Q2, 2013, 34-35; 3Q, 2017, 6; 3Q, 2018, 3-4
Valid 3-character code, no further characters required

I97 **Intraoperative and postprocedural complications and disorders of circulatory system, not elsewhere classified**

Excludes2: *postprocedural shock (T81.1-)*

I97.0 **Postcardiotomy syndrome**

+ **I97.1** **Other postprocedural cardiac functional disturbances**
Excludes2: *acute pulmonary insufficiency following thoracic surgery (J95.1)*
intraoperative cardiac functional disturbances (I97.7-)

+ **I97.11** **Postprocedural cardiac insufficiency**

CC **I97.110** **Postprocedural cardiac insufficiency following cardiac surgery**

CC **I97.111** **Postprocedural cardiac insufficiency following other surgery**

+ **I97.12** **Postprocedural cardiac arrest**

CC **I97.120** **Postprocedural cardiac arrest following cardiac surgery**

CC **I97.121** **Postprocedural cardiac arrest following other surgery**

+ **I97.13** **Postprocedural heart failure**
Use additional code to identify the heart failure (I50.-)

CC **I97.130** **Postprocedural heart failure following cardiac surgery**

CC **I97.131** **Postprocedural heart failure following other surgery**

+ **I97.19** **Other postprocedural cardiac functional disturbances**
Use additional code, if applicable, to further specify disorder

CC **I97.190** **Other postprocedural cardiac functional disturbances following cardiac surgery**
Use additional code, if applicable, for type 4 or type 5 myocardial infarction, to further specify disorder
AHA CC: 2Q, 2019, 32-33

CC **I97.191** **Other postprocedural cardiac functional disturbances following other surgery**

- I97.2 **Postmastectomy lymphedema syndrome**
  Elephantiasis due to mastectomy
  Obliteration of lymphatic vessels
- I97.3 **Postprocedural hypertension**
+ I97.4 **Intraoperative hemorrhage and hematoma of a circulatory system organ or structure complicating a procedure**
  Excludes1: intraoperative hemorrhage and hematoma of a circulatory system organ or structure due to accidental puncture and laceration during a procedure (I97.5-)
  Excludes2: intraoperative cerebrovascular hemorrhage complicating a procedure (G97.3-)
  + I97.41 **Intraoperative hemorrhage and hematoma of a circulatory system organ or structure complicating a circulatory system procedure**
    CC I97.410 **Intraoperative hemorrhage and hematoma of a circulatory system organ or structure complicating a cardiac catheterization**
    CC I97.411 **Intraoperative hemorrhage and hematoma of a circulatory system organ or structure complicating a cardiac bypass**
    CC I97.418 **Intraoperative hemorrhage and hematoma of a circulatory system organ or structure complicating other circulatory system procedure**
  CC I97.42 **Intraoperative hemorrhage and hematoma of a circulatory system organ or structure complicating other procedure**
    AHA CC: 4Q, 2016, 100-101
+ I97.5 **Accidental puncture and laceration of a circulatory system organ or structure during a procedure**
  Excludes2: accidental puncture and laceration of brain during a procedure (G97.4-)
  CC I97.51 **Accidental puncture and laceration of a circulatory system organ or structure during a circulatory system procedure**
    AHA CC: 2Q, 2019, 24
  CC I97.52 **Accidental puncture and laceration of a circulatory system organ or structure during other procedure**
+ I97.6 **Postprocedural hemorrhage, hematoma and seroma of a circulatory system organ or structure following a procedure**
  Excludes2: postprocedural cerebrovascular hemorrhage complicating a procedure (G97.5-)
    AHA CC: 4Q, 2016, 9-10
  + I97.61 **Postprocedural hemorrhage of a circulatory system organ or structure following a circulatory system procedure**
    CC I97.610 **Postprocedural hemorrhage of a circulatory system organ or structure following a cardiac catheterization**
    CC I97.611 **Postprocedural hemorrhage of a circulatory system organ or structure following cardiac bypass**
    CC I97.618 **Postprocedural hemorrhage of a circulatory system organ or structure following other circulatory system procedure**
  + I97.62 **Postprocedural hemorrhage, hematoma and seroma of a circulatory system organ or structure following other procedure**
    CC I97.620 **Postprocedural hemorrhage of a circulatory system organ or structure following other procedure**
    CC I97.621 **Postprocedural hematoma of a circulatory system organ or structure following other procedure**

CC I97.622 **Postprocedural seroma of a circulatory system organ or structure following other procedure**
+ I97.63 **Postprocedural hematoma of a circulatory system organ or structure following a circulatory system procedure**
  CC I97.630 **Postprocedural hematoma of a circulatory system organ or structure following a cardiac catheterization**
  CC I97.631 **Postprocedural hematoma of a circulatory system organ or structure following cardiac bypass**
  CC I97.638 **Postprocedural hematoma of a circulatory system organ or structure following other circulatory system procedure**
I97.64 **Postprocedural seroma of a circulatory system organ or structure following a circulatory system procedure**
  CC I97.640 **Postprocedural seroma of a circulatory system organ or structure following a cardiac catheterization**
  CC I97.641 **Postprocedural seroma of a circulatory system organ or structure following cardiac bypass**
  CC I97.648 **Postprocedural seroma of a circulatory system organ or structure following other circulatory system procedure**
+ I97.7 **Intraoperative cardiac functional disturbances**
  Excludes2: acute pulmonary insufficiency following thoracic surgery (J95.1)
    postprocedural cardiac functional disturbances (I97.1-)
  + I97.71 **Intraoperative cardiac arrest**
    CC I97.710 **Intraoperative cardiac arrest during cardiac surgery**
    CC I97.711 **Intraoperative cardiac arrest during other surgery**
  + I97.79 **Other intraoperative cardiac functional disturbances**
    Use additional code, if applicable, to further specify disorder
    CC I97.790 **Other intraoperative cardiac functional disturbances during cardiac surgery**
    CC I97.791 **Other intraoperative cardiac functional disturbances during other surgery**
+ I97.8 **Other intraoperative and postprocedural complications and disorders of the circulatory system, not elsewhere classified**
  Use additional code, if applicable, to further specify disorder
  + I97.81 **Intraoperative cerebrovascular infarction**
    CC I97.810 **Intraoperative cerebrovascular infarction cardiac surgery**
    CC I97.811 **Intraoperative cerebrovascular infarction during other surgery**
  + I97.82 **Postprocedural cerebrovascular infarction**
    CC I97.820 **Postprocedural cerebrovascular infarction following cardiac surgery**
    CC I97.821 **Postprocedural cerebrovascular infarction following other surgery**
  CC I97.88 **Other intraoperative complications of the circulatory system, not elsewhere classified**
  CC I97.89 **Other postprocedural complications and disorders of the circulatory system, not elsewhere classified**

I99 **Other and unspecified disorders of circulatory system**

I99.8 **Other disorder of circulatory system**
I99.9 **Unspecified disorder of circulatory system**

+, +7th, X + 7th　• Newborn　• Pediatric　• Maternity　• Adult　♀ Female　♂ Male　Manifestation　Unacceptable PDX　HCC　CC　MCC　HAC

Chapter 10: Diseases of the Respiratory System (J00-J99)

NOTE When a respiratory condition is described as occurring in more than one site and is not specifically indexed, it should be classified to the lower anatomic site (e.g. tracheobronchitis to bronchitis in J40).

Use additional code, where applicable, to identify:
exposure to environmental tobacco smoke (Z77.22)
exposure to tobacco smoke in the perinatal period (P96.81)
history of tobacco dependence (Z87.891)
occupational exposure to environmental tobacco smoke (Z57.31)
tobacco dependence (F17.-)
tobacco use (Z72.0)

Excludes2: *certain conditions originating in the perinatal period (P04-P96)*
certain infectious and parasitic diseases (A00-B99)
complications of pregnancy, childbirth and the puerperium (O00-O9A)
congenital malformations, deformations and chromosomal abnormalities (Q00-Q99)
endocrine, nutritional and metabolic diseases (E00-E88)
injury, poisoning and certain other consequences of external causes (S00-T88)
neoplasms (C00-D49)
smoke inhalation (T59.81-)
symptoms, signs and abnormal clinical and laboratory findings, not elsewhere classified (R00-R94)

This chapter contains the following category blocks:

J00-J06	Acute upper respiratory infections
J09-J18	Influenza and pneumonia
J20-J22	Other acute lower respiratory infections
J30-J39	Other diseases of upper respiratory tract
J40-J47	Chronic lower respiratory diseases
J60-J70	Lung diseases due to external agents
J80-J84	Other respiratory diseases principally affecting the interstitium
J85-J86	Suppurative and necrotic conditions of the lower respiratory tract
J90-J94	Other diseases of the pleura
J95	Intraoperative and postprocedural complications and disorders of respiratory system, not elsewhere classified
J96-J99	Other diseases of the respiratory system

C. Chapter-Specific Coding Guidelines

In addition to general coding guidelines, there are guidelines for specific diagnoses and/or conditions in the classification. Unless otherwise indicated, these guidelines apply to all health care settings. Please refer to Section II for guidelines on the selection of principal diagnosis.

10. Chapter 10: Diseases of the Respiratory System (J00-J99), *U07.0*

a. Chronic Obstructive Pulmonary Disease [COPD] and Asthma

1) Acute exacerbation of chronic obstructive bronchitis and asthma

The codes in categories J44 and J45 distinguish between uncomplicated cases and those in acute exacerbation. An acute exacerbation is a worsening or a decompensation of a chronic condition. An acute exacerbation is not equivalent to an infection superimposed on a chronic condition, though an exacerbation may be triggered by an infection.

b. Acute Respiratory Failure

1) Acute respiratory failure as principal diagnosis

A code from subcategory J96.0, Acute respiratory failure, or subcategory J96.2, Acute and chronic respiratory failure, may be assigned as a principal diagnosis when it is the condition established after study to be chiefly responsible for occasioning the admission to the hospital, and the selection is supported by the Alphabetic Index and Tabular List. However, chapter-specific coding guidelines (such as obstetrics, poisoning, HIV, newborn) that provide sequencing direction take precedence.

2) Acute respiratory failure as secondary diagnosis

Respiratory failure may be listed as a secondary diagnosis if it occurs after admission, or if it is present on admission, but does not meet the definition of principal diagnosis.

3) Sequencing of acute respiratory failure and another acute condition

When a patient is admitted with respiratory failure and another acute condition, (e.g., myocardial infarction, cerebrovascular accident, aspiration pneumonia), the principal diagnosis will not be the same in every situation. This applies whether the other acute condition is a respiratory or nonrespiratory condition. Selection of the principal diagnosis will be dependent on the circumstances of admission. If both the respiratory failure and the other acute condition are equally responsible for occasioning the admission to the hospital, and there are no chapter-specific sequencing rules, the guideline regarding two or more diagnoses that equally meet the definition for principal diagnosis (*Section II, C.*) may be applied in these situations.

If the documentation is not clear as to whether acute respiratory failure and another condition are equally responsible for occasioning the admission, query the provider for clarification.

c. Influenza due to certain identified influenza viruses

Code only confirmed cases of influenza due to certain identified influenza viruses (category J09), and due to other identified influenza virus (category J10). This is an exception to the hospital inpatient guideline Section II, H. (Uncertain Diagnosis).

In this context, "confirmation" does not require documentation of positive laboratory testing specific for avian or other novel influenza A or other identified influenza virus. However, coding should be based on the provider's diagnostic statement that the patient has avian influenza, or other novel influenza A, for category J09, or has another particular identified strain of influenza, such as H1N1 or H3N2, but not identified as novel or variant, for category J10.

If the provider records "suspected" or "possible" or "probable" avian influenza, or novel influenza, or other identified influenza, then the appropriate influenza code from category J11, Influenza due to unidentified influenza virus, should be assigned. A code from category J09, Influenza due to certain identified influenza viruses, should not be assigned nor should a code from category J10, Influenza due to other identified influenza virus.

d. Ventilator associated Pneumonia

1) Documentation of Ventilator associated Pneumonia

As with all procedural or postprocedural complications, code assignment is based on the provider's documentation of the relationship between the condition and the procedure.

Code J95.851, Ventilator associated pneumonia, should be assigned only when the provider has documented ventilator associated pneumonia (VAP). An additional code to identify the organism (e.g., Pseudomonas aeruginosa, code B96.5) should also be assigned. Do not assign an additional code from categories J12-J18 to identify the type of pneumonia.

Code J95.851 should not be assigned for cases where the patient has pneumonia and is on a mechanical ventilator and the provider has not specifically stated that the pneumonia is ventilator-associated pneumonia. If the documentation is unclear as to whether the patient has a pneumonia that is a complication attributable to the mechanical ventilator, query the provider.

2) Ventilator associated Pneumonia Develops after Admission

A patient may be admitted with one type of pneumonia (e.g., code J13, Pneumonia due to Streptococcus pneumonia) and subsequently develop VAP. In this instance, the principal diagnosis would be the appropriate code from categories J12- J18 for the pneumonia diagnosed at the time of admission. Code J95.851, Ventilator associated pneumonia, would be assigned as an additional diagnosis when the provider has also documented the presence of ventilator associated pneumonia.

e. Vaping-related disorders

For patients presenting with condition(s) related to vaping, assign code U07.0, Vaping-related disorder, as the principal diagnosis. For lung injury due to vaping, assign only code U07.0. Assign additional codes for other manifestations, such as acute respiratory failure (subcategory J96.0-) or pneumonitis (code J68.0)

Associated respiratory signs and symptoms due to vaping, such as cough, shortness of breath, etc., are not coded separately, when a definitive diagnosis has been established. However, it would be appropriate to code separately any gastrointestinal symptoms, such as diarrhea and abdominal pain.

Acute upper respiratory infections (J00-J06)

Excludes1: *chronic obstructive pulmonary disease with acute lower respiratory infection (J44.0)*

J00 Acute nasopharyngitis [common cold]

Acute rhinitis
Coryza (acute)
Infective nasopharyngitis NOS
Infective rhinitis
Nasal catarrh, acute
Nasopharyngitis NOS
> **Excludes1:** *acute pharyngitis (J02.-)*
> *acute sore throat NOS (J02.9)*
> *influenza virus with other respiratory manifestations (J09.X2, J10.1, J11.1)*
> *pharyngitis NOS (J02.9)*
> *rhinitis NOS (J31.0)*
> *sore throat NOS (J02.9)*

+, +7th, X + 7th   ● Newborn   ● Pediatric   ● Maternity   ● Adult   ♀ Female   ♂ Male   Manifestation   Unacceptable PDX   HCC   CC   MCC   HAC

Nose and Sinuses

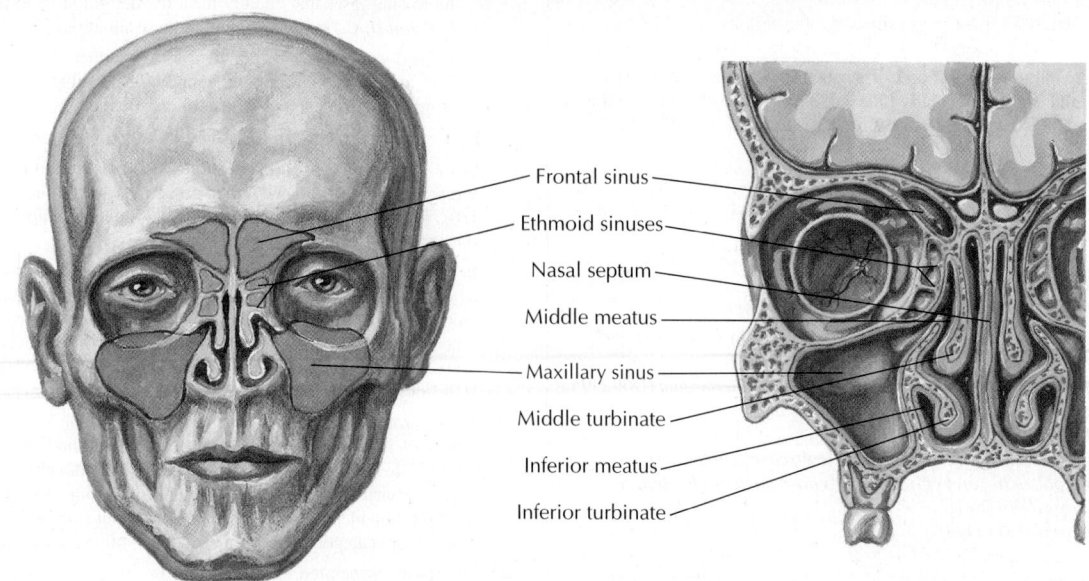

Frontal view

Coronal section

Anatomy of nasal cavity and sinuses

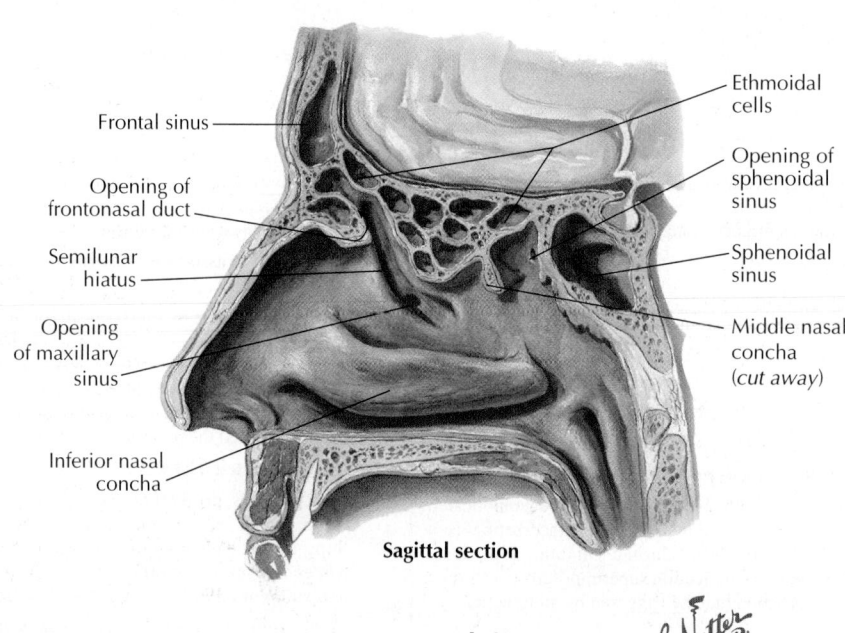

Paranasal sinuses

Excludes2: *allergic rhinitis (J30.1-J30.9)*
chronic pharyngitis (J31.2)
chronic rhinitis (J31.0)
chronic sore throat (J31.2)
nasopharyngitis, chronic (J31.1)
vasomotor rhinitis (J30.0)
Valid 3-character code, no further characters required

J01 **Acute sinusitis**

Includes: acute abscess of sinus
acute empyema of sinus
acute infection of sinus
acute inflammation of sinus
acute suppuration of sinus
Use additional code (B95-B97) to identify infectious agent
Excludes1: *sinusitis NOS (J32.9)*

Excludes2: *chronic sinusitis (J32.0-J32.8)*
+ **J01.0** **Acute maxillary sinusitis**
Acute antritis
J01.00 Acute maxillary sinusitis, unspecified
J01.01 Acute recurrent maxillary sinusitis
+ **J01.1** **Acute frontal sinusitis**
J01.10 Acute frontal sinusitis, unspecified
J01.11 Acute recurrent frontal sinusitis
+ **J01.2** **Acute ethmoidal sinusitis**
J01.20 Acute ethmoidal sinusitis, unspecified
J01.21 Acute recurrent ethmoidal sinusitis
+ **J01.3** **Acute sphenoidal sinusitis**
J01.30 Acute sphenoidal sinusitis, unspecified
J01.31 Acute recurrent sphenoidal sinusitis
+ **J01.4** **Acute pansinusitis**
J01.40 Acute pansinusitis, unspecified

+, +7th, X + 7th   ● Newborn   ● Pediatric   ● Maternity   ● Adult   ♀ Female   ♂ Male   Manifestation   Unacceptable PDX   HCC   CC   MCC   HAC

J01.41   **Acute recurrent pansinusitis**

+ J01.8   **Other acute sinusitis**

    J01.80   **Other acute sinusitis**

        Acute sinusitis involving more than one sinus but not pansinusitis

    J01.81   **Other acute recurrent sinusitis**

        Acute recurrent sinusitis involving more than one sinus but not pansinusitis

+ J01.9   **Acute sinusitis, unspecified**

    J01.90   **Acute sinusitis, unspecified**

    J01.91   **Acute recurrent sinusitis, unspecified**

J02   **Acute pharyngitis**

    Includes: acute sore throat

    Excludes1: *acute laryngopharyngitis (J06.0)*
            peritonsillar abscess (J36)
            pharyngeal abscess (J39.1)
            retropharyngeal abscess (J39.0)

    Excludes2: *chronic pharyngitis (J31.2)*

    J02.0   **Streptococcal pharyngitis**

      Septic pharyngitis
      Streptococcal sore throat

      Excludes2: *scarlet fever (A38.-)*

    J02.8   **Acute pharyngitis due to other specified organisms**

      Use additional code (B95-B97) to identify infectious agent

      Excludes1: *acute pharyngitis due to coxsackie virus (B08.5)*
             acute pharyngitis due to gonococcus (A54.5)
             acute pharyngitis due to herpes [simplex] virus (B00.2)
             acute pharyngitis due to infectious mononucleosis (B27.-)
             enteroviral vesicular pharyngitis (B08.5)

    J02.9   **Acute pharyngitis, unspecified**

      Gangrenous pharyngitis (acute)
      Infective pharyngitis (acute) NOS
      Pharyngitis (acute) NOS
      Sore throat (acute) NOS
      Suppurative pharyngitis (acute)
      Ulcerative pharyngitis (acute)

      Excludes1: *influenza virus with other respiratory manifestations (J09.X2, J10.1, J11.1)*

J03   **Acute tonsillitis**

    Excludes1: *acute sore throat (J02.-)*
            hypertrophy of tonsils (J35.1)
            peritonsillar abscess (J36)
            sore throat NOS (J02.9)
            streptococcal sore throat (J02.0)

    Excludes2: *chronic tonsillitis (J35.0)*

+ J03.0   **Streptococcal tonsillitis**

    J03.00   **Acute streptococcal tonsillitis, unspecified**

    J03.01   **Acute recurrent streptococcal tonsillitis**

+ J03.8   **Acute tonsillitis due to other specified organisms**

    Use additional code (B95-B97) to identify infectious agent

    Excludes1: *diphtheritic tonsillitis (A36.0)*
            herpesviral pharyngotonsillitis (B00.2)
            streptococcal tonsillitis (J03.0)
            tuberculous tonsillitis (A15.8)
            Vincent's tonsillitis (A69.1)

    J03.80   **Acute tonsillitis due to other specified organisms**

    J03.81   **Acute recurrent tonsillitis due to other specified organisms**

+ J03.9   **Acute tonsillitis, unspecified**

      Follicular tonsillitis (acute)
      Gangrenous tonsillitis (acute)
      Infective tonsillitis (acute)
      Tonsillitis (acute) NOS
      Ulcerative tonsillitis (acute)

      Excludes1: *influenza virus with other respiratory manifestations (J09.X2, J10.1, J11.1)*

    J03.90   **Acute tonsillitis, unspecified**

    J03.91   **Acute recurrent tonsillitis, unspecified**

J04   **Acute laryngitis and tracheitis**

    Code also influenza, if present, such as:
    influenza due to identified novel influenza A virus with other respiratory manifestations (J09.X2)
    influenza due to other identified influenza virus with other respiratory manifestations (J10.1)
    influenza due to unidentified influenza virus with other respiratory manifestations (J11.1)

    Use additional code (B95-B97) to identify infectious agent

    Excludes1: *acute obstructive laryngitis [croup] and epiglottitis (J05.-)*

    Excludes2: *laryngismus (stridulus) (J38.5)*

    J04.0   **Acute laryngitis**

      Edematous laryngitis (acute)
      Laryngitis (acute) NOS
      Subglottic laryngitis (acute)
      Suppurative laryngitis (acute)
      Ulcerative laryngitis (acute)

      Excludes1: *acute obstructive laryngitis (J05.0)*

      Excludes2: *chronic laryngitis (J37.0)*

+ J04.1   **Acute tracheitis**

      Acute viral tracheitis
      Catarrhal tracheitis (acute)
      Tracheitis (acute) NOS

      Excludes2: *chronic tracheitis (J42)*

    J04.10   **Acute tracheitis without obstruction**

    MCC **J04.11**   **Acute tracheitis with obstruction**

    J04.2   **Acute laryngotracheitis**

      Laryngotracheitis NOS
      Tracheitis (acute) with laryngitis (acute)

      Excludes1: *acute obstructive laryngotracheitis (J05.0)*

      Excludes2: *chronic laryngotracheitis (J37.1)*

+ J04.3   **Supraglottitis, unspecified**

    J04.30   **Supraglottitis, unspecified, without obstruction**

    MCC **J04.31**   **Supraglottitis, unspecified, with obstruction**

J05   **Acute obstructive laryngitis [croup] and epiglottitis**

    Code also influenza, if present, such as:
    influenza due to identified novel influenza A virus with other respiratory manifestations (J09.X2)
    influenza due to other identified influenza virus with other respiratory manifestations (J10.1)
    influenza due to unidentified influenza virus with other respiratory manifestations (J11.1)

    Use additional code (B95-B97) to identify infectious agent

    J05.0   **Acute obstructive laryngitis [croup]**

      Obstructive laryngitis (acute) NOS
      Obstructive laryngotracheitis NOS

+ J05.1   **Acute epiglottitis**

      Excludes2: *epiglottitis, chronic (J37.0)*

    CC **J05.10**   **Acute epiglottitis without obstruction**

      Epiglottitis NOS

    MCC **J05.11**   **Acute epiglottitis with obstruction**

J06   **Acute upper respiratory infections of multiple and unspecified sites**

    Excludes1: *acute respiratory infection NOS (J22)*
            influenza virus with other respiratory manifestations (J09.X2, J10.1, J11.1)
            streptococcal pharyngitis (J02.0)

    J06.0   **Acute laryngopharyngitis**

    J06.9   **Acute upper respiratory infection, unspecified**

      Upper respiratory disease, acute
      Upper respiratory infection NOS

      Use additional code (B95-B97) to identify infectious agent, if known, such as:
      respiratory syncytial virus (RSV) (B97.4)

Influenza and pneumonia (J09-J18)

Excludes2: *allergic or eosinophilic pneumonia (J82)*
            aspiration pneumonia NOS (J69.0)
            meconium pneumonia (P24.01)
            neonatal aspiration pneumonia (P24.-)
            pneumonia due to solids and liquids (J69-)
            congenital pneumonia (P23.9)
            lipid pneumonia (J69.1)
            rheumatic pneumonia (I00)
            ventilator associated pneumonia (J95.851)

J09   **Influenza due to certain identified influenza viruses**

    Excludes1: *influenza A/H1N1 (J10.-)*
            influenza due to other identified influenza virus (J10.-)
            influenza due to unidentified influenza virus (J11.-)
            seasonal influenza due to other identified influenza virus (J10.-)
            seasonal influenza due to unidentified influenza virus (J11.-)

    Review coding guideline C.10.c

+ J09.X   **Influenza due to identified novel influenza A virus**

      Avian influenza
      Bird influenza

Lungs

Right

Left

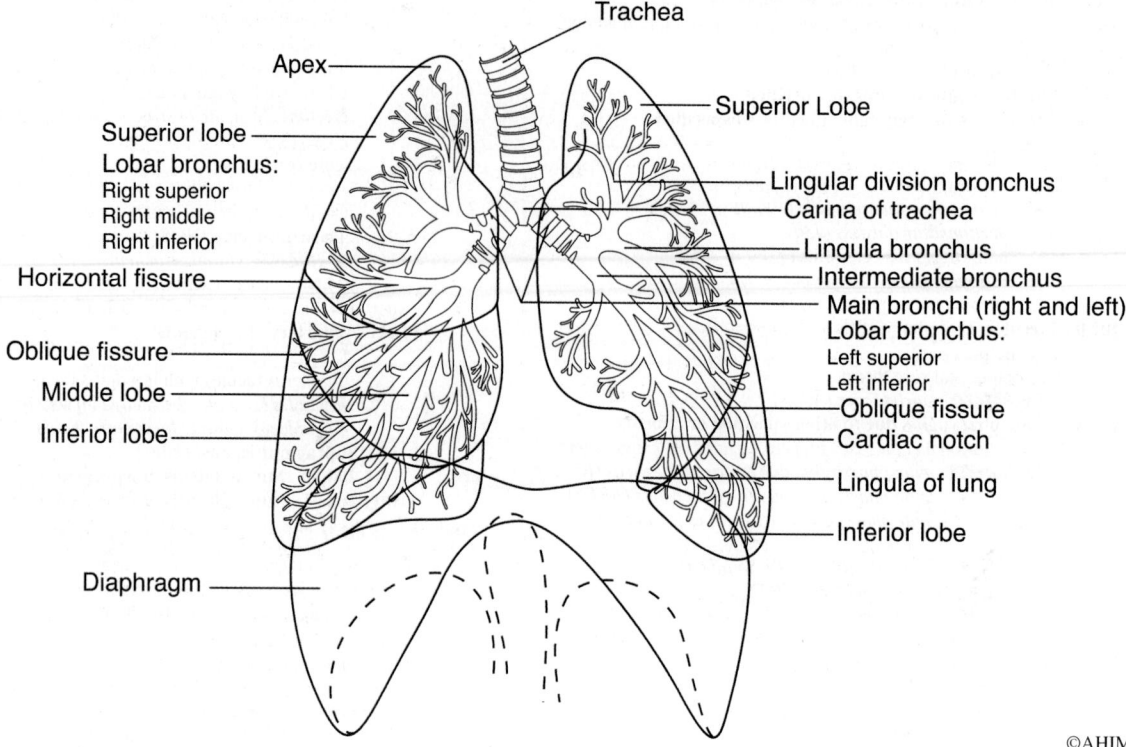

©AHIMA

Influenza A/H5N1

Influenza of other animal origin, not bird or swine

Swine influenza virus (viruses that normally cause infections in pigs)

MCC J09.X1 Influenza due to identified novel influenza A virus with pneumonia

Code also if applicable, associated:
lung abscess (J85.1)
other specified type of pneumonia

J09.X2 Influenza due to identified novel influenza A virus with other respiratory manifestations

Influenza due to identified novel influenza A virus NOS

Influenza due to identified novel influenza A virus with laryngitis

Influenza due to identified novel influenza A virus with pharyngitis

Influenza due to identified novel influenza A virus with upper respiratory symptoms

Use additional code, if applicable, for associated:
pleural effusion (J91.8)
sinusitis (J01.-)

J09.X3 Influenza due to identified novel influenza A virus with gastrointestinal manifestations

Influenza due to identified novel influenza A virus gastroenteritis

Excludes1: '*intestinal flu*' *[viral gastroenteritis] (A08.-)*

J09.X9 Influenza due to identified novel influenza A virus with other manifestations

Influenza due to identified novel influenza A virus with encephalopathy

Influenza due to identified novel influenza A virus with myocarditis

Influenza due to identified novel influenza A virus with otitis media

Use additional code to identify manifestation

J10 Influenza due to other identified influenza virus

Includes: *influenza A (non-novel)*
influenza B
influenza C

Excludes1: *influenza due to avian influenza virus (J09.X-)*
influenza due to swine flu (J09.X-)
influenza due to unidentifed influenza virus (J11.-)

Review coding guideline C.10.c

+ J10.0 Influenza due to other identified influenza virus with pneumonia

Code also associated lung abscess, if applicable (J85.1)

MCC J10.00 Influenza due to other identified influenza virus with unspecified type of pneumonia

MCC J10.01 Influenza due to other identified influenza virus with the same other identified influenza virus pneumonia

MCC J10.08 Influenza due to other identified influenza virus with other specified pneumonia

Code also other specified type of pneumonia
AHA CC: 4Q, 2017, 96

J10.1 Influenza due to other identified influenza virus with other respiratory manifestations

Influenza due to other identified influenza virus NOS

Influenza due to other identified influenza virus with laryngitis

Influenza due to other identified influenza virus with pharyngitis

Influenza due to other identified influenza virus with upper respiratory symptoms

Use additional code for associated pleural effusion, if applicable (J91.8)

Use additional code for associated sinusitis, if applicable (J01.-)

AHA CC: 3Q, 2016, 10-11

J10.2 Influenza due to other identified influenza virus with gastrointestinal manifestations

Influenza due to other identified influenza virus gastroenteritis

Excludes1: '*intestinal flu*' *[viral gastroenteritis] (A08.-)*

+ J10.8 Influenza due to other identified influenza virus with other manifestations

J10.81 Influenza due to other identified influenza virus with encephalopathy

J10.82 Influenza due to other identified influenza virus with myocarditis

J10.83 **Influenza due to other identified influenza virus with otitis media**
Use additional code for any associated perforated tympanic membrane (H72.-)

J10.89 **Influenza due to other identified influenza virus with other manifestations**
Use additional codes to identify the manifestations

J11 **Influenza due to unidentified influenza virus**

+ **J11.0** **Influenza due to unidentified influenza virus with pneumonia**
Code also associated lung abscess, if applicable (J85.1)

MCC **J11.00** **Influenza due to unidentified influenza virus with unspecified type of pneumonia**
Influenza with pneumonia NOS
AHA CC: 3Q, 2016, 11-12

MCC **J11.08** **Influenza due to unidentified influenza virus with specified pneumonia**
Code also other specified type of pneumonia

J11.1 **Influenza due to unidentified influenza virus with other respiratory manifestations**
Influenza NOS
Influenzal laryngitis NOS
Influenzal pharyngitis NOS
Influenza with upper respiratory symptoms NOS
Use additional code for associated pleural effusion, if applicable (J91.8)

Use additional code for associated sinusitis, if applicable (J01.-)

J11.2 **Influenza due to unidentified influenza virus with gastrointestinal manifestations**
Influenza gastroenteritis NOS
Excludes1: *'intestinal flu' [viral gastroenteritis] (A08.-)*

+ **J11.8** **Influenza due to unidentified influenza virus with other manifestations**

J11.81 **Influenza due to unidentified influenza virus with encephalopathy**
Influenzal encephalopathy NOS

J11.82 **Influenza due to unidentified influenza virus with myocarditis**
Influenzal myocarditis NOS

J11.83 **Influenza due to unidentified influenza virus with otitis media**
Influenzal otitis media NOS
Use additional code for any associated perforated tympanic membrane (H72.-)

J11.89 **Influenza due to unidentified influenza virus with other manifestations**
Use additional codes to identify the manifestations

J12 **Viral pneumonia, not elsewhere classified**

Includes: bronchopneumonia due to viruses other than influenza viruses
Code first associated influenza, if applicable (J09.X1, J10.0-, J11.0-)

Code also associated abscess, if applicable (J85.1)
Excludes1: *aspiration pneumonia due to anesthesia during labor and delivery (O74.0)*
aspiration pneumonia due to anesthesia during pregnancy (O29)
aspiration pneumonia due to anesthesia during puerperium (O89.0)
aspiration pneumonia due to solids and liquids (J69.-)
aspiration pneumonia NOS (J69.0)
congenital pneumonia (P23.0)
congenital rubella pneumonitis (P35.0)
interstitial pneumonia NOS (J84.9)
lipid pneumonia (J69.1)
neonatal aspiration pneumonia (P24.-)

MCC **J12.0** **Adenoviral pneumonia**

MCC **J12.1** **Respiratory syncytial virus pneumonia**
RSV pneumonia

MCC **J12.2** **Parainfluenza virus pneumonia**

MCC **J12.3** **Human metapneumovirus pneumonia**

+ **J12.8** **Other viral pneumonia**

MCC **J12.81** **Pneumonia due to SARS-associated coronavirus**
Severe acute respiratory syndrome NOS

MCC **J12.89** **Other viral pneumonia**
AHA CC: 1Q, 2020, 34-36; 2Q, 2020, 8,11
Review coding guideline C.1.g.1.c.i

MCC **J12.9** **Viral pneumonia, unspecified**

MCC **J13** **Pneumonia due to Streptococcus pneumoniae**
Bronchopneumonia due to S. pneumoniae
Code first associated influenza, if applicable (J09.X1, J10.0-, J11.0-)

Code also associated abscess, if applicable (J85.1)
Excludes1: *congenital pneumonia due to S. pneumoniae (P23.6)*
lobar pneumonia, unspecified organism (J18.1)
pneumonia due to other streptococci (J15.3-J15.4)
Valid 3-character code, no further characters required

MCC **J14** **Pneumonia due to Hemophilus influenzae**
Bronchopneumonia due to H. influenzae
Code first associated influenza, if applicable (J09.X1, J10.0-, J11.0-)

Code also associated abscess, if applicable (J85.1)
Excludes1: *congenital pneumonia due to H. influenzae (P23.6)*
Valid 3-character code, no further characters required

J15 **Bacterial pneumonia, not elsewhere classified**

Includes: bronchopneumonia due to bacteria other than S. pneumoniae and H. influenzae
Code first associated influenza, if applicable (J09.X1, J10.0-, J11.0-)

Code also associated abscess, if applicable (J85.1)
Excludes1: *chlamydial pneumonia (J16.0)*
congenital pneumonia (P23.-)
Legionnaires' disease (A48.1)
spirochetal pneumonia (A69.8)

MCC **J15.0** **Pneumonia due to Klebsiella pneumoniae**

MCC **J15.1** **Pneumonia due to Pseudomonas**

+ **J15.2** **Pneumonia due to staphylococcus**

MCC **J15.20** **Pneumonia due to staphylococcus, unspecified**

+ **J15.21** **Pneumonia due to staphylococcus aureus**

MCC **J15.211** **Pneumonia due to Methicillin susceptible Staphylococcus aureus**
MSSA pneumonia
Pneumonia due to Staphylococcus aureus NOS

MCC **J15.212** **Pneumonia due to Methicillin resistant Staphylococcus aureus**
Review coding guideline C.1.e.1.a

MCC **J15.29** **Pneumonia due to other staphylococcus**

MCC **J15.3** **Pneumonia due to streptococcus, group B**

MCC **J15.4** **Pneumonia due to other streptococci**
Excludes1: *pneumonia due to streptococcus, group B (J15.3)*
pneumonia due to Streptococcus pneumoniae (J13)

MCC **J15.5** **Pneumonia due to Escherichia coli**

MCC **J15.6** **Pneumonia due to other Gram-negative bacteria**
Pneumonia due to other aerobic Gram-negative bacteria
Pneumonia due to Serratia marcescens
AHA CC: 2Q, 2020, 29

MCC **J15.7** **Pneumonia due to Mycoplasma pneumoniae**

MCC **J15.8** **Pneumonia due to other specified bacteria**

MCC **J15.9** **Unspecified bacterial pneumonia**
Pneumonia due to gram-positive bacteria
AHA CC: 4Q, 2017, 96

J16 **Pneumonia due to other infectious organisms, not elsewhere classified**
Code first associated influenza, if applicable (J09.X1, J10.0-, J11.0-)

Code also associated abscess, if applicable (J85.1)
Excludes1: *congenital pneumonia (P23.-)*
ornithosis (A70)
pneumocystosis (B59)
pneumonia NOS (J18.9)

MCC **J16.0** **Chlamydial pneumonia**

MCC **J16.8** **Pneumonia due to other specified infectious organisms**

MCC J17 **Pneumonia in diseases classified elsewhere**

Code first underlying disease, such as:
Q fever (A78)
rheumatic fever (I00)
schistosomiasis (B65.0-B65.9)

Excludes1: *candidial pneumonia (B37.1)*
chlamydial pneumonia (J16.0)
gonorrheal pneumonia (A54.84)
histoplasmosis pneumonia (B39.0-B39.2)
measles pneumonia (B05.2)
nocardiosis pneumonia (A43.0)
pneumocystosis (B59)
pneumonia due to Pneumocystis carinii (B59)
pneumonia due to Pneumocystis jiroveci (B59)
pneumonia in actinomycosis (A42.0)
pneumonia in anthrax (A22.1)
pneumonia in ascariasis (B77.81)
pneumonia in aspergillosis (B44.0-B44.1)
pneumonia in coccidioidomycosis (B38.0-B38.2)
pneumonia in cytomegalovirus disease(B25.0)
pneumonia in toxoplasmosis (B58.3)
rubella pneumonia (B06.81)
salmonella pneumonia (A02.22)
spirochetal infection NEC with pneumonia (A69.8)
tularemia pneumonia (A21.2)
typhoid fever with pneumonia (A01.03)
varicella pneumonia (B01.2)
whooping cough with pneumonia (A37 with fifth-character 1)

Valid 3-character code, no further characters required

J18 **Pneumonia, unspecified organism**

Code first associated influenza, if applicable (J09.X1, J10.0-, J11.0-)

Excludes1: *abscess of lung with pneumonia (J85.1)*
aspiration pneumonia due to anesthesia during labor and delivery (O74.0)
aspiration pneumonia due to anesthesia during pregnancy (O29)
aspiration pneumonia due to anesthesia during puerperium (O89.0)
aspiration pneumonia due to solids and liquids (J69.-)
aspiration pneumonia NOS (J69.0)
congenital pneumonia (P23.0)
drug-induced interstitial lung disorder (J70.2-J70.4)
interstitial pneumonia NOS (J84.9)
lipid pneumonia (J69.1)
neonatal aspiration pneumonia (P24.-)
pneumonitis due to external agents (J67-J70)
pneumonitis due to fumes and vapors (J68.0)
usual interstitial pneumonia (J84.178)

MCC J18.0 **Bronchopneumonia, unspecified organism**

Excludes1: *hypostatic bronchopneumonia (J18.2)*
lipid pneumonia (J69.1)
Excludes2: *acute bronchiolitis (J21.-)*
chronic bronchiolitis (J44.9)

MCC J18.1 **Lobar pneumonia, unspecified organism**
AHA CC: 3Q, 2016, 15

CC J18.2 **Hypostatic pneumonia, unspecified organism**
Hypostatic bronchopneumonia
Passive pneumonia

MCC J18.8 **Other pneumonia, unspecified organism**

MCC J18.9 **Pneumonia, unspecified organism**
AHA CC: 4Q, 2012, 94; 3Q, 2014, 4; 3Q, 2016, 15-16; 1Q, 2019, 35-36; 3Q, 2019, 15; 2Q, 2020, 28

Other acute lower respiratory infections (J20-J22)

Excludes2: *chronic obstructive pulmonary disease with acute lower respiratory infection (J44.0)*

J20 **Acute bronchitis**

Includes: acute and subacute bronchitis (with) bronchospasm
acute and subacute bronchitis (with) tracheitis
acute and subacute bronchitis (with) tracheobronchitis, acute
acute and subacute fibrinous bronchitis
acute and subacute membranous bronchitis
acute and subacute purulent bronchitis
acute and subacute septic bronchitis

Excludes1: *bronchitis NOS (J40)*
tracheobronchitis NOS (J40)
Excludes2: *acute bronchitis with bronchiectasis (J47.0)*
acute bronchitis with chronic obstructive asthma (J44.0)
acute bronchitis with chronic obstructive pulmonary disease (J44.0)
allergic bronchitis NOS (J45.909-)
bronchitis due to chemicals, fumes and vapors (J68.0)
chronic bronchitis NOS (J42)
chronic mucopurulent bronchitis (J41.1)
chronic obstructive bronchitis (J44.-)
chronic obstructive tracheobronchitis (J44.-)
chronic simple bronchitis (J41.0)
chronic tracheobronchitis (J42)

J20.0 **Acute bronchitis due to Mycoplasma pneumoniae**
J20.1 **Acute bronchitis due to Hemophilus influenzae**
J20.2 **Acute bronchitis due to streptococcus**
J20.3 **Acute bronchitis due to coxsackievirus**
J20.4 **Acute bronchitis due to parainfluenza virus**
J20.5 **Acute bronchitis due to respiratory syncytial virus**
Acute bronchitis due to RSV
J20.6 **Acute bronchitis due to rhinovirus**
AHA CC: 3Q, 2016, 10
J20.7 **Acute bronchitis due to echovirus**
J20.8 **Acute bronchitis due to other specified organisms**
AHA CC: 3Q, 2016, 10-11; 1Q, 2020, 34-36
Review coding guideline C.1.g.1.c.ii
J20.9 **Acute bronchitis, unspecified**
AHA CC: 3Q, 2016, 16; 1Q, 2019, 35

J21 **Acute bronchiolitis**

Includes: *acute bronchiolitis with bronchospasm*
Excludes2: *respiratory bronchiolitis interstitial lung disease (J84.115)*

CC J21.0 **Acute bronchiolitis due to respiratory syncytial virus**
Acute bronchiolitis due to RSV
CC J21.1 **Acute bronchiolitis due to human metapneumovirus**
CC J21.8 **Acute bronchiolitis due to other specified organisms**
CC J21.9 **Acute bronchiolitis, unspecified**
Bronchiolitis (acute)
Excludes1: *chronic bronchiolitis (J44.-)*

J22 **Unspecified acute lower respiratory infection**

Acute (lower) respiratory (tract) infection NOS
Excludes1: *upper respiratory infection (acute) (J06.9)*
AHA CC: 1Q, 2020, 22-23, 34-36
Review coding guideline C.1.g.1.c.iii
Valid 3-character code, no further characters required

Other diseases of upper respiratory tract (J30-J39)

J30 **Vasomotor and allergic rhinitis**

Includes: spasmodic rhinorrhea
Excludes1: *allergic rhinitis with asthma (bronchial) (J45.909)*
rhinitis NOS (J31.0)
J30.0 **Vasomotor rhinitis**
J30.1 **Allergic rhinitis due to pollen**
Allergy NOS due to pollen
Hay fever
Pollinosis
J30.2 **Other seasonal allergic rhinitis**
J30.5 **Allergic rhinitis due to food**
+ J30.8 **Other allergic rhinitis**
J30.81 **Allergic rhinitis due to animal (cat) (dog) hair and dander**
J30.89 **Other allergic rhinitis**
Perennial allergic rhinitis
J30.9 **Allergic rhinitis, unspecified**

J31 **Chronic rhinitis, nasopharyngitis and pharyngitis**

Use additional code to identify:
exposure to environmental tobacco smoke (Z77.22)
exposure to tobacco smoke in the perinatal period (P96.81)
history of tobacco dependence (Z87.891)
occupational exposure to environmental tobacco smoke (Z57.31)
tobacco dependence (F17.-)
tobacco use (Z72.0)

J31.0 Chronic rhinitis
> Atrophic rhinitis (chronic)
> Granulomatous rhinitis (chronic)
> Hypertrophic rhinitis (chronic)
> Obstructive rhinitis (chronic)
> Ozena
> Purulent rhinitis (chronic)
> Rhinitis (chronic) NOS
> Ulcerative rhinitis (chronic)
> ***Excludes1:*** *allergic rhinitis (J30.1-J30.9)*
>   *vasomotor rhinitis (J30.0)*

J31.1 Chronic nasopharyngitis
> ***Excludes2:*** *acute nasopharyngitis (J00)*

J31.2 Chronic pharyngitis
> Chronic sore throat
> Atrophic pharyngitis (chronic)
> Granular pharyngitis (chronic)
> Hypertrophic pharyngitis (chronic)
> ***Excludes2:*** *acute pharyngitis (J02.9)*

J32 Chronic sinusitis

> **Includes:** sinus abscess
>   sinus empyema
>   sinus infection
>   sinus suppuration
> Use additional code to identify:
>   exposure to environmental tobacco smoke (Z77.22)
>   exposure to tobacco smoke in the perinatal period (P96.81)
>   history of tobacco dependence (Z87.891)
>   infectious agent (B95-B97)
>   occupational exposure to environmental tobacco smoke (Z57.31)
>   tobacco dependence (F17.-)
>   tobacco use (Z72.0)
> ***Excludes2:*** *acute sinusitis (J01.-)*

J32.0 Chronic maxillary sinusitis
> Antritis (chronic)
> Maxillary sinusitis NOS

J32.1 Chronic frontal sinusitis
> Frontal sinusitis NOS

J32.2 Chronic ethmoidal sinusitis
> Ethmoidal sinusitis NOS
> ***Excludes1:*** *Woakes' ethmoiditis (J33.1)*

J32.3 Chronic sphenoidal sinusitis
> Sphenoidal sinusitis NOS

J32.4 Chronic pansinusitis
> Pansinusitis NOS

J32.8 Other chronic sinusitis
> Sinusitis (chronic) involving more than one sinus but not
>   pansinusitis

J32.9 Chronic sinusitis, unspecified
> Sinusitis (chronic) NOS

J33 Nasal polyp

> Use additional code to identify:
>   exposure to environmental tobacco smoke (Z77.22)
>   exposure to tobacco smoke in the perinatal period (P96.81)
>   history of tobacco dependence (Z87.891)
>   occupational exposure to environmental tobacco smoke (Z57.31)
>   tobacco dependence (F17.-)
>   tobacco use (Z72.0)
> ***Excludes1:*** *adenomatous polyps (D14.0)*

J33.0 Polyp of nasal cavity
> Choanal polyp
> Nasopharyngeal polyp

J33.1 Polypoid sinus degeneration
> Woakes' syndrome or ethmoiditis

J33.8 Other polyp of sinus
> Accessory polyp of sinus
> Ethmoidal polyp of sinus
> Maxillary polyp of sinus
> Sphenoidal polyp of sinus

J33.9 Nasal polyp, unspecified

J34 Other and unspecified disorders of nose and nasal sinuses

> ***Excludes2:*** *varicose ulcer of nasal septum (I86.8)*

J34.0 Abscess, furuncle and carbuncle of nose
> Cellulitis of nose
> Necrosis of nose
> Ulceration of nose

J34.1 Cyst and mucocele of nose and nasal sinus

J34.2 Deviated nasal septum
> Deflection or deviation of septum (nasal) (acquired)
> ***Excludes1:*** *congenital deviated nasal septum (Q67.4)*

J34.3 Hypertrophy of nasal turbinates

+ J34.8 Other specified disorders of nose and nasal sinuses

> **J34.81 Nasal mucositis (ulcerative)**
>> Code also type of associated therapy, such as:
>>   antineoplastic and immunosuppressive drugs
>>   (T45.1X-)
>>   radiological procedure and radiotherapy (Y84.2)
>> ***Excludes2:*** *gastrointestinal mucositis (ulcerative)*
>>   *(K92.81)*
>>   *mucositis (ulcerative) of vagina and*
>>   *vulva (N76.81)*
>>   *oral mucositis (ulcerative) (K12.3-)*

> **J34.89 Other specified disorders of nose and nasal sinuses**
>> Perforation of nasal septum NOS
>> Rhinolith

J34.9 Unspecified disorder of nose and nasal sinuses

J35 Chronic diseases of tonsils and adenoids

> Use additional code to identify:
>   exposure to environmental tobacco smoke (Z77.22)
>   exposure to tobacco smoke in the perinatal period (P96.81)
>   history of tobacco dependence (Z87.891)
>   occupational exposure to environmental tobacco smoke (Z57.31)
>   tobacco dependence (F17.-)
>   tobacco use (Z72.0)

+ J35.0 Chronic tonsillitis and adenoiditis
> ***Excludes2:*** *acute tonsillitis (J03.-)*
> **J35.01 Chronic tonsillitis**
> **J35.02 Chronic adenoiditis**
> **J35.03 Chronic tonsillitis and adenoiditis**

J35.1 Hypertrophy of tonsils
> Enlargement of tonsils
> ***Excludes1:*** *hypertrophy of tonsils with tonsillitis (J35.0-)*

J35.2 Hypertrophy of adenoids
> Enlargement of adenoids
> ***Excludes1:*** *hypertrophy of adenoids with adenoiditis*
>   *(J35.0-)*

J35.3 Hypertrophy of tonsils with hypertrophy of adenoids
> ***Excludes1:*** *hypertrophy of tonsils and adenoids with*
>   *tonsillitis and adenoiditis (J35.03)*

J35.8 Other chronic diseases of tonsils and adenoids
> Adenoid vegetations
> Amygdalolith
> Calculus, tonsil
> Cicatrix of tonsil (and adenoid)
> Tonsillar tag
> Ulcer of tonsil

J35.9 Chronic disease of tonsils and adenoids, unspecified
> Disease (chronic) of tonsils and adenoids NOS

CC J36 Peritonsillar abscess

> **Includes:** abscess of tonsil
>   peritonsillar cellulitis
>   quinsy
> Use additional code (B95-B97) to identify infectious agent
> ***Excludes1:*** *acute tonsillitis (J03.-)*
>   *chronic tonsillitis (J35.0)*
>   *retropharyngeal abscess (J39.0)*
>   *tonsillitis NOS (J03.9-)*
> Valid 3-character code, no further characters required

J37 Chronic laryngitis and laryngotracheitis

> Use additional code to identify:
>   exposure to environmental tobacco smoke (Z77.22)
>   exposure to tobacco smoke in the perinatal period (P96.81)
>   history of tobacco dependence (Z87.891)
>   infectious agent (B95-B97)
>   occupational exposure to environmental tobacco smoke (Z57.31)
>   tobacco dependence (F17.-)
>   tobacco use (Z72.0)

J37.0 Chronic laryngitis
> Catarrhal laryngitis
> Hypertrophic laryngitis
> Sicca laryngitis
> ***Excludes2:*** *acute laryngitis (J04.0)*
>   *obstructive (acute) laryngitis (J05.0)*

711

J37.1 Chronic laryngotracheitis
Laryngitis, chronic, with tracheitis (chronic)
Tracheitis, chronic, with laryngitis
Excludes1: chronic tracheitis (J42)
Excludes2: acute laryngotracheitis (J04.2)
acute tracheitis (J04.1)

J38 Diseases of vocal cords and larynx, not elsewhere classified
Use additional code to identify:
exposure to environmental tobacco smoke (Z77.22)
exposure to tobacco smoke in the perinatal period (P96.81)
history of tobacco dependence (Z87.891)
occupational exposure to environmental tobacco smoke (Z57.31)
tobacco dependence (F17.-)
tobacco use (Z72.0)
Excludes1: congenital laryngeal stridor (P28.89)
obstructive laryngitis (acute) (J05.0)
postprocedural subglottic stenosis (J95.5)
stridor (R06.1)
ulcerative laryngitis (J04.0)

+ J38.0 Paralysis of vocal cords and larynx
Laryngoplegia
Paralysis of glottis
J38.00 Paralysis of vocal cords and larynx, unspecified
J38.01 Paralysis of vocal cords and larynx, unilateral
J38.02 Paralysis of vocal cords and larynx, bilateral
J38.1 Polyp of vocal cord and larynx
Excludes1: adenomatous polyps (D14.1)
J38.2 Nodules of vocal cords
Chorditis (fibrinous)(nodosa)(tuberosa)
Singer's nodes
Teacher's nodes
J38.3 Other diseases of vocal cords
Abscess of vocal cords
Cellulitis of vocal cords
Granuloma of vocal cords
Leukokeratosis of vocal cords
Leukoplakia of vocal cords
J38.4 Edema of larynx
Edema (of) glottis
Subglottic edema
Supraglottic edema
Excludes1: acute obstructive laryngitis [croup] (J05.0)
edematous laryngitis (J04.0)
J38.5 Laryngeal spasm
Laryngismus (stridulus)
J38.6 Stenosis of larynx
J38.7 Other diseases of larynx
Abscess of larynx
Cellulitis of larynx
Disease of larynx NOS
Necrosis of larynx
Pachyderma of larynx
Perichondritis of larynx
Ulcer of larynx

J39 Other diseases of upper respiratory tract
Excludes1: acute respiratory infection NOS (J22)
acute upper respiratory infection (J06.9)
upper respiratory inflammation due to chemicals, gases, fumes or vapors (J68.2)
CC J39.0 Retropharyngeal and parapharyngeal abscess
Peripharyngeal abscess
Excludes1: peritonsillar abscess (J36)
CC J39.1 Other abscess of pharynx
Cellulitis of pharynx
Nasopharyngeal abscess
J39.2 Other diseases of pharynx
Cyst of pharynx
Edema of pharynx
Excludes2: chronic pharyngitis (J31.2)
ulcerative pharyngitis (J02.9)
J39.3 Upper respiratory tract hypersensitivity reaction, site unspecified
Excludes1: hypersensitivity reaction of upper respiratory tract, such as:
extrinsic allergic alveolitis (J67.9)
pneumoconiosis (J60-J67.9)
J39.8 Other specified diseases of upper respiratory tract
J39.9 Disease of upper respiratory tract, unspecified

Chronic lower respiratory diseases (J40-J47)

Excludes1: bronchitis due to chemicals, gases, fumes and vapors (J68.0)
Excludes2: cystic fibrosis (E84.-)

J40 Bronchitis, not specified as acute or chronic
Bronchitis NOS
Bronchitis with tracheitis NOS
Catarrhal bronchitis
Tracheobronchitis NOS
Use additional code to identify:
exposure to environmental tobacco smoke (Z77.22)
exposure to tobacco smoke in the perinatal period (P96.81)
history of tobacco dependence (Z87.891)
occupational exposure to environmental tobacco smoke (Z57.31)
tobacco dependence (F17.-)
tobacco use (Z72.0)
Excludes1: allergic bronchitis NOS (J45.909-)
asthmatic bronchitis NOS (J45.9-)
acute bronchitis (J20.-)
bronchitis due to chemicals, gases, fumes and vapors (J68.0)
AHA CC: 1Q, 2020 34-36
Review coding guideline C.1.g.1.c.ii
Valid 3-character code, no further characters required

J41 Simple and mucopurulent chronic bronchitis
Use additional code to identify:
exposure to environmental tobacco smoke (Z77.22)
exposure to tobacco smoke in the perinatal period (P96.81)
history of tobacco dependence (Z87.891)
occupational exposure to environmental tobacco smoke (Z57.31)
tobacco dependence (F17.-)
tobacco use (Z72.0)
Excludes1: chronic bronchitis NOS (J42)
chronic obstructive bronchitis (J44.-)
J41.0 Simple chronic bronchitis
J41.1 Mucopurulent chronic bronchitis
J41.8 Mixed simple and mucopurulent chronic bronchitis

J42 Unspecified chronic bronchitis
Chronic bronchitis NOS
Chronic tracheitis
Chronic tracheobronchitis
Use additional code to identify:
exposure to environmental tobacco smoke (Z77.22)
exposure to tobacco smoke in the perinatal period (P96.81)
history of tobacco dependence (Z87.891)
occupational exposure to environmental tobacco smoke (Z57.31)
tobacco dependence (F17.-)
tobacco use (Z72.0)
Excludes1: chronic asthmatic bronchitis (J44.-)
chronic bronchitis with airways obstruction (J44.-)
chronic emphysematous bronchitis (J44.-)
chronic obstructive pulmonary disease NOS (J44.9)
simple and mucopurulent chronic bronchitis (J41.-)
Valid 3-character code, no further characters required

J43 Emphysema
Use additional code to identify:
exposure to environmental tobacco smoke (Z77.22)
history of tobacco dependence (Z87.891)
occupational exposure to environmental tobacco smoke (Z57.31)
tobacco dependence (F17.-)
tobacco use (Z72.0)
Excludes1: compensatory emphysema (J98.3)
emphysema due to inhalation of chemicals, gases, fumes or vapors (J68.4)
emphysema with chronic (obstructive) bronchitis (J44.-)
emphysematous (obstructive) bronchitis (J44.-)
interstitial emphysema (J98.2)
mediastinal emphysema (J98.2)
neonatal interstitial emphysema (P25.0)
surgical (subcutaneous) emphysema (T81.82)
Excludes2: traumatic subcutaneous emphysema (T79.7)
J43.0 Unilateral pulmonary emphysema [MacLeod's syndrome]
Swyer-James syndrome
Unilateral emphysema
Unilateral hyperlucent lung
Unilateral pulmonary artery functional hypoplasia
Unilateral transparency of lung
J43.1 Panlobular emphysema
Panacinar emphysema

| +, +7th, X + 7th | ● Newborn | ● Pediatric | ● Maternity | ● Adult | ♀ Female | ♂ Male | Manifestation | Unacceptable PDX | HCC | CC | MCC | HAC |

Chronic Obstructive Pulmonary Disease

Chronic bronchitis

Large cartilaginous airways

Mucous gland hyperplasia (elevated Reid index)

Dilated duct of gland

Thickened basement membrane

Squamous metaplasia

Inflammatory infiltrate

Hyperemia

Edema

Fibrosis

Epithelial desquamation

Profuse exudate in lumen

Cartilage intact

Airways partially or completely blocked or "one-way" valve effect by mucoid or mucopurulent secretions, with impaired or non-uniform distribution of ventilation

Small airways

Goblet cell hyperplasia

Thickened basement membrane

Hyperemia

Inflammatory infiltrate

Exudate in lumen

Edema

Squamous metaplasia

Fibrosis

J43.2 **Centrilobular emphysema**

J43.8 **Other emphysema**

J43.9 **Emphysema, unspecified**
Bullous emphysema (lung)(pulmonary)
Emphysema (lung)(pulmonary) NOS
Emphysematous bleb
Vesicular emphysema (lung)(pulmonary)
AHA CC: 4Q, 2017, 97-98; 1Q, 2019, 34-37

J44 **Other chronic obstructive pulmonary disease**

Includes: asthma with chronic obstructive pulmonary disease
chronic asthmatic (obstructive) bronchitis
chronic bronchitis with airways obstruction
chronic bronchitis with emphysema
chronic emphysematous bronchitis
chronic obstructive asthma
chronic obstructive bronchitis
chronic obstructive tracheobronchitis
Code also type of asthma, if applicable (J45.-)

Use additional code to identify:
exposure to environmental tobacco smoke (Z77.22)
history of tobacco dependence (Z87.891)
occupational exposure to environmental tobacco smoke (Z57.31)
tobacco dependence (F17.-)
tobacco use (Z72.0)

Excludes1: *bronchiectasis (J47.-)*
chronic bronchitis NOS (J42)
chronic simple and mucopurulent bronchitis (J41.-)
chronic tracheitis (J42)
chronic tracheobronchitis (J42)
emphysema without chronic bronchitis (J43.-)
Review coding guideline C.10.a.1

CC **J44.0** **Chronic obstructive pulmonary disease with (acute) lower respiratory infection**
Code also to identify the infection
AHA CC: 3Q, 2016, 15-16; 4Q, 2017, 96

CC **J44.1** **Chronic obstructive pulmonary disease with (acute) exacerbation**
Decompensated COPD
Decompensated COPD with (acute) exacerbation
Excludes2: *chronic obstructive pulmonary disease [COPD] with acute bronchitis (J44.0)*
lung diseases due to external agents (J60-J70)
AHA CC: 1Q, 2016, 36; 3Q, 2016, 15-16; 1Q, 2017, 26; 4Q, 2017, 96

J44.9 **Chronic obstructive pulmonary disease, unspecified**
Chronic obstructive airway disease NOS
Chronic obstructive lung disease NOS
Excludes2: *lung diseases due to external agents (J60-J70)*
AHA CC: 4Q, 2013, 109, 129; 4Q, 2014, 21-22; 1Q, 2016, 36-37;
1Q, 2017, 24-25; 4Q, 2017, 96-97

Pathology of Asthma

Gross

Tenacious, viscid mucous plugs in airways

Foci of atelectasis

Blocked airway–"mucus plug"
Muscle hypertrophy
Thickened basement membrane

Obstructed asthmatic airway*

Microscopic

PAS-positive matrix
Polymorphonuclear neutrophils
Eosinophils
Charcot-Leyden crystals
Curschmann's spirals
Cluster of epithelial cells (Creola body)
Bacteria and/or viruses
Epithelial denudation
Hyaline thickening of basement membrane
Hypertrophy of smooth muscle, mucous glands, and goblet cells
Inflammatory exudate with eosinophils and edema
Engorged blood vessels

Mucous plug

Regional or diffuse hyperinflation

Microscopy of Airway

A

B

Lumen
Epithelium
Basement membrane

(**A**) Normal airway. (**B**) Asthmatic airway before therapy with high-dose inhaled steroids demonstrating remodeling.

+, +7th, X + 7th   • Newborn   • Pediatric   • Maternity   • Adult   ♀ Female   ♂ Male   Manifestation   Unacceptable PDX   HCC   CC   MCC   HAC

J45   Asthma

Includes: allergic (predominantly) asthma
allergic bronchitis NOS
allergic rhinitis with asthma
atopic asthma
extrinsic allergic asthma
hay fever with asthma
idiosyncratic asthma
intrinsic nonallergic asthma
nonallergic asthma

Use additional code to identify:
eosinophilic asthma (J82.83)
exposure to environmental tobacco smoke (Z77.22)
exposure to tobacco smoke in the perinatal period (P96.81)
history of tobacco dependence (Z87.891)
occupational exposure to environmental tobacco smoke (Z57.31)
tobacco dependence (F17.-)
tobacco use (Z72.0)

Excludes1:   *detergent asthma (J69.8)*
eosinophilic asthma (J82)
miner's asthma (J60)
wheezing NOS (R06.2)
wood asthma (J67.8)

Excludes2:   *asthma with chronic obstructive pulmonary disease (J44.9)*
chronic asthmatic (obstructive) bronchitis (J44.9)
chronic obstructive asthma (J44.9)

AHA CC: 1Q, 2019, 36-37

Review coding guideline C.10.a.1

+ **J45.2   Mild intermittent asthma**

J45.20   Mild intermittent asthma, uncomplicated
Mild intermittent asthma NOS

CC **J45.21   Mild intermittent asthma with (acute) exacerbation**

CC **J45.22   Mild intermittent asthma with status asthmaticus**

+ **J45.3   Mild persistent asthma**

J45.30   Mild persistent asthma, uncomplicated
Mild persistent asthma NOS

CC **J45.31   Mild persistent asthma with (acute) exacerbation**
AHA CC: 1Q, 2016, 35

CC **J45.32   Mild persistent asthma with status asthmaticus**

+ **J45.4   Moderate persistent asthma**

J45.40   Moderate persistent asthma, uncomplicated
Moderate persistent asthma NOS

CC **J45.41   Moderate persistent asthma with (acute) exacerbation**
AHA CC: 1Q, 2017, 26

CC **J45.42   Moderate persistent asthma with status asthmaticus**

+ **J45.5   Severe persistent asthma**

J45.50   Severe persistent asthma, uncomplicated
Severe persistent asthma NOS

CC **J45.51   Severe persistent asthma with (acute) exacerbation**

CC **J45.52   Severe persistent asthma with status asthmaticus**

+ **J45.9   Other and unspecified asthma**

+ **J45.90   Unspecified asthma**
Asthmatic bronchitis NOS
Childhood asthma NOS
Late onset asthma

CC **J45.901   Unspecified asthma with (acute) exacerbation**
AHA CC: 4Q, 2017, 96-97

CC **J45.902   Unspecified asthma with status asthmaticus**

J45.909   Unspecified asthma, uncomplicated
Asthma NOS
Excludes2:   *lung diseases due to external agents (J60-J70)*

+ **J45.99   Other asthma**

J45.990   Exercise induced bronchospasm
J45.991   Cough variant asthma
J45.998   Other asthma

J47   Bronchiectasis

Includes: bronchiolectasis

Use additional code to identify:
exposure to environmental tobacco smoke (Z77.22)
exposure to tobacco smoke in the perinatal period (P96.81)
history of tobacco dependence (Z87.891)
occupational exposure to environmental tobacco smoke (Z57.31)
tobacco dependence (F17.-)
tobacco use (Z72.0)

Excludes1:   *congenital bronchiectasis (Q33.4)*
tuberculous bronchiectasis (current disease) (A15.0)

CC **J47.0   Bronchiectasis with acute lower respiratory infection**
Bronchiectasis with acute bronchitis
Use additional code to identify the infection

CC **J47.1   Bronchiectasis with (acute) exacerbation**

J47.9   Bronchiectasis, uncomplicated
Bronchiectasis NOS

Lung diseases due to external agents (J60-J70)

Excludes2:   *asthma (J45.-)*
malignant neoplasm of bronchus and lung (C34.-)

● **J60**   Coalworker's pneumoconiosis

Anthracosilicosis
Anthracosis
Black lung disease
Coalworker's lung
Excludes1:   *coalworker pneumoconiosis with tuberculosis, any type in A15 (J65)*
Valid 3-character code, no further characters required

● **J61**   Pneumoconiosis due to asbestos and other mineral fibers

Asbestosis
Excludes1:   *pleural plaque with asbestosis (J92.0)*
pneumoconiosis with tuberculosis, any type in A15 (J65)
Valid 3-character code, no further characters required

J62   Pneumoconiosis due to dust containing silica

Includes: silicotic fibrosis (massive) of lung
Excludes1:   *pneumoconiosis with tuberculosis, any type in A15 (J65)*
J62.0   Pneumoconiosis due to talc dust
J62.8   Pneumoconiosis due to other dust containing silica
Silicosis NOS

J63   Pneumoconiosis due to other inorganic dusts

Excludes1:   *pneumoconiosis with tuberculosis, any type in A15 (J65)*
J63.0   Aluminosis (of lung)
J63.1   Bauxite fibrosis (of lung)
J63.2   Berylliosis
J63.3   Graphite fibrosis (of lung)
J63.4   Siderosis
J63.5   Stannosis
J63.6   Pneumoconiosis due to other specified inorganic dusts

J64   Unspecified pneumoconiosis

Excludes1:   *pneumonoconiosis with tuberculosis, any type in A15 (J65)*
Valid 3-character code, no further characters required

J65   Pneumoconiosis associated with tuberculosis

Any condition in J60-J64 with tuberculosis, any type in A15
Silicotuberculosis
Valid 3-character code, no further characters required

J66   Airway disease due to specific organic dust

Excludes2:   *allergic alveolitis (J67.-)*
asbestosis (J61)
bagassosis (J67.1)
farmer's lung (J67.0)
hypersensitivity pneumonitis due to organic dust (J67.-)
reactive airways dysfunction syndrome (J68.3)
J66.0   Byssinosis
Airway disease due to cotton dust
J66.1   Flax-dressers' disease
J66.2   Cannabinosis
J66.8   Airway disease due to other specific organic dusts

+, +7th, X + 7th   ● Newborn   ● Pediatric   ● Maternity   ● Adult   ♀ Female   ♂ Male   Manifestation   Unacceptable PDX   HCC   CC   MCC   HAC

J67 **Hypersensitivity pneumonitis due to organic dust**

Includes: allergic alveolitis and pneumonitis due to inhaled organic dust and particles of fungal, actinomycetic or other origin

Excludes1: *pneumonitis due to inhalation of chemicals, gases, fumes or vapors (J68.0)*

J67.0 **Farmer's lung**
Harvester's lung
Haymaker's lung
Moldy hay disease

J67.1 **Bagassosis**
Bagasse disease
Bagasse pneumonitis

J67.2 **Bird fancier's lung**
Budgerigar fancier's disease or lung
Pigeon fancier's disease or lung

J67.3 **Suberosis**
Corkhandler's disease or lung
Corkworker's disease or lung

J67.4 **Maltworker's lung**
Alveolitis due to Aspergillus clavatus

J67.5 **Mushroom-worker's lung**

J67.6 **Maple-bark-stripper's lung**
Alveolitis due to Cryptostroma corticale
Cryptostromosis

CC **J67.7** **Air conditioner and humidifier lung**
Allergic alveolitis due to fungal, thermophilic actinomycetes and other organisms growing in ventilation [air conditioning] systems

CC **J67.8** **Hypersensitivity pneumonitis due to other organic dusts**
Cheese-washer's lung
Coffee-worker's lung
Fish-meal worker's lung
Furrier's lung
Sequoiosis

CC **J67.9** **Hypersensitivity pneumonitis due to unspecified organic dust**
Allergic alveolitis (extrinsic) NOS
Hypersensitivity pneumonitis NOS

J68 **Respiratory conditions due to inhalation of chemicals, gases, fumes and vapors**

Code first (T51-T65) to identify cause

Use additional code to identify associated respiratory conditions, such as: acute respiratory failure (J96.0-)

CC **J68.0** **Bronchitis and pneumonitis due to chemicals, gases, fumes and vapors**
Chemical bronchitis (acute)
AHA CC: 2Q, 2019, 31-32
Review coding guideline C.11.e

MCC **J68.1** **Pulmonary edema due to chemicals, gases, fumes and vapors**
Chemical pulmonary edema (acute) (chronic)
Excludes1: *pulmonary edema (acute) (chronic) NOS (J81.-)*

J68.2 **Upper respiratory inflammation due to chemicals, gases, fumes and vapors, not elsewhere classified**

J68.3 **Other acute and subacute respiratory conditions due to chemicals, gases, fumes and vapors**
Reactive airways dysfunction syndrome

J68.4 **Chronic respiratory conditions due to chemicals, gases, fumes and vapors**
Emphysema (diffuse) (chronic) due to inhalation of chemicals, gases, fumes and vapors
Obliterative bronchiolitis (chronic) (subacute) due to inhalation of chemicals, gases, fumes and vapors
Pulmonary fibrosis (chronic) due to inhalation of chemicals, gases, fumes and vapors
Excludes1: *chronic pulmonary edema due to chemicals, gases, fumes and vapors (J68.1)*

J68.8 **Other respiratory conditions due to chemicals, gases, fumes and vapors**

J68.9 **Unspecified respiratory condition due to chemicals, gases, fumes and vapors**

J69 **Pneumonitis due to solids and liquids**
Excludes1: *neonatal aspiration syndromes (P24.-)*
postprocedural pneumonitis (J95.4)
AHA CC: 2Q, 2020, 11, 28-29

MCC **J69.0** **Pneumonitis due to inhalation of food and vomit**
Aspiration pneumonia NOS
Aspiration pneumonia (due to) food (regurgitated)
Aspiration pneumonia (due to) gastric secretions
Aspiration pneumonia (due to) milk
Aspiration pneumonia (due to) vomit
Code also any associated foreign body in respiratory tract (T17.-)
Excludes1: *chemical pneumonitis due to anesthesia (J95.4)*
obstetric aspiration pneumonitis (O74.0)
AHA CC: 1Q, 2017, 24; 2Q, 2019, 6-7, 31-32

MCC **J69.1** **Pneumonitis due to inhalation of oils and essences**
Exogenous lipoid pneumonia
Lipid pneumonia NOS
Code first (T51-T65) to identify substance
Excludes1: *endogenous lipoid pneumonia (J84.89)*

MCC **J69.8** **Pneumonitis due to inhalation of other solids and liquids**
Pneumonitis due to aspiration of blood
Pneumonitis due to aspiration of detergent
Code first (T51-T65) to identify substance

J70 **Respiratory conditions due to other external agents**

CC **J70.0** **Acute pulmonary manifestations due to radiation**
Radiation pneumonitis
Use additional code (W88-W90, X39.0-) to identify the external cause

CC **J70.1** **Chronic and other pulmonary manifestations due to radiation**
Fibrosis of lung following radiation
Use additional code (W88-W90, X39.0-) to identify the external cause

J70.2 **Acute drug-induced interstitial lung disorders**
Use additional code for adverse effect, if applicable, to identify drug (T36-T50 with fifth or sixth character 5)
AHA CC: 2Q, 2019, 28
Excludes1: *interstitial pneumonia NOS (J84.9)*
lymphoid interstitial pneumonia (J84.2)

J70.3 **Chronic drug-induced interstitial lung disorders**
Use additional code for adverse effect, if applicable, to identify drug (T36-T50 with fifth or sixth character 5)
Excludes1: *interstitial pneumonia NOS (J84.9)*
lymphoid interstitial pneumonia (J84.2)

J70.4 **Drug-induced interstitial lung disorders, unspecified**
Use additional code for adverse effect, if applicable, to identify drug (T36-T50 with fifth or sixth character 5)
AHA CC: 2Q, 2019, 28
Excludes1: *interstitial pneumonia NOS (J84.9)*
lymphoid interstitial pneumonia (J84.2)

J70.5 **Respiratory conditions due to smoke inhalation**
Code first smoke inhalation (T59.81-)
Excludes2: *smoke inhalation due to chemicals, gases, fumes and vapors (J68.9)*

J70.8 **Respiratory conditions due to other specified external agents**
Code first (T51-T65) to identify the external agent

J70.9 **Respiratory conditions due to unspecified external agent**
Code first (T51-T65) to identify the external agent

Other respiratory diseases principally affecting the interstitium (J80-J84)

MCC **J80** **Acute respiratory distress syndrome**

Acute respiratory distress syndrome in adult or child
Adult hyaline membrane disease
Excludes1: *respiratory distress syndrome in newborn (perinatal) (P22.0)*
AHA CC: 1Q, 2017, 26-27; 1Q, 2020, 34-36
Review coding guideline C.1.g.1.c.iv
Valid 3-character code, no further characters required

J81 **Pulmonary edema**

Use additional code to identify:
exposure to environmental tobacco smoke (Z77.22)
history of tobacco dependence (Z87.891)
occupational exposure to environmental tobacco smoke (Z57.31)
tobacco dependence (F17.-)
tobacco use (Z72.0)
Excludes1: *chemical (acute) pulmonary edema (J68.1)*
hypostatic pneumonia (J18.2)
passive pneumonia (J18.2)
pulmonary edema due to external agents (J60-J70)
pulmonary edema with heart disease NOS (I50.1)
pulmonary edema with heart failure (I50.1)

+, +7th, X + 7th ● Newborn ● Pediatric ● Maternity ● Adult ♀ Female ♂ Male Manifestation Unacceptable PDX HCC CC MCC HAC

MCC **J81.0** **Acute pulmonary edema**
Acute edema of lung
CC **J81.1** **Chronic pulmonary edema**
Pulmonary congestion (chronic) (passive)
Pulmonary edema NOS

J82 **Pulmonary eosinophilia, not elsewhere classified**
Excludes2: *pulmonary eosinophilia due to aspergillosis (B44.-)*
pulmonary eosinophilia due to drugs (J70.2-J70.4)
pulmonary eosinophilia due to specified parasitic
infection (B50-B83)
pulmonary eosinophilia due to systemic connective
tissue disorders (M30-M36)
pulmonary infiltrate NOS (R91.8)
+ **J82.8** **Pulmonary eosinophilia, not elsewhere classified**
CC **J82.81** **Chronic eosinophilic pneumonia**
Eosinophilic pneumonia, NOS
CC **J82.82** **Acute eosinophilic pneumonia**
CC **J82.83** **Eosinophilic asthma**
Code first asthma, by type, such as:
mild intermittent asthma (J45.2-)
mild persistent asthma (J45.3-)
moderate persistent asthma (J45.4-)
severe persistent asthma (J45.5-)
CC **J82.89** **Other pulmonary eosinophilia, not elsewhere classified**
Allergic pneumonia
Löffler's pneumonia
Tropical (pulmonary) eosinophilia NOS

J84 **Other interstitial pulmonary diseases**
Excludes1: *drug-induced interstitial lung disorders (J70.2-J70.4)*
interstitial emphysema (J98.2)
Excludes2: *lung diseases due to external agents (J60-J70)*
+ **J84.0** **Alveolar and parieto-alveolar conditions**
CC **J84.01** **Alveolar proteinosis**
CC **J84.02** **Pulmonary alveolar microlithiasis**
CC **J84.03** **Idiopathic pulmonary hemosiderosis**
Essential brown induration of lung
Code first underlying disease, such as:
disorders of iron metabolism (E83.1-)
Excludes1: *acute idiopathic pulmonary*
hemorrhage in infants [AIPHI]
(R04.81)
CC **J84.09** **Other alveolar and parieto-alveolar conditions**
+ **J84.1** **Other interstitial pulmonary diseases with fibrosis**
Excludes1: *pulmonary fibrosis (chronic) due to inhalation*
of chemicals, gases, fumes or vapors (J68.4)
pulmonary fibrosis (chronic) following
radiation (J70.1)
J84.10 **Pulmonary fibrosis, unspecified**
Capillary fibrosis of lung
Cirrhosis of lung (chronic) NOS
Fibrosis of lung (atrophic) (chronic) (confluent)
(massive) (perialveolar) (peribronchial) NOS
Induration of lung (chronic) NOS
Postinflammatory pulmonary fibrosis
+ **J84.11** **Idiopathic interstitial pneumonia**
Excludes1: *lymphoid interstitial pneumonia (J84.2)*
pneumocystis pneumonia (B59)
J84.111 **Idiopathic interstitial pneumonia, not otherwise specified**
J84.112 **Idiopathic pulmonary fibrosis**
Cryptogenic fibrosing alveolitis
Idiopathic fibrosing alveolitis
J84.113 **Idiopathic non-specific interstitial pneumonitis**
Excludes1: *non-specific interstitial*
pneumonia NOS, or due to
known underlying cause
(J84.89)
CC **J84.114** **Acute interstitial pneumonitis**
Hamman-Rich syndrome
Excludes1: *pneumocystis*
pneumonia (B59)
J84.115 **Respiratory bronchiolitis interstitial lung disease**
CC **J84.116** **Cryptogenic organizing pneumonia**
Excludes1: *organizing pneumonia*
NOS, or due to known
underlying cause (J84.89)
CC **J84.117** **Desquamative interstitial pneumonia**

J84.17 **Other interstitial pulmonary diseases with fibrosis in diseases classified elsewhere**
J84.170 **Interstitial lung disease with progressive fibrotic phenotype in diseases classified elsewhere**
Progressive fibrotic interstitial lung disease
Code first underlying disease, such as:
lung diseases due to external agents (J60-J70)
rheumatoid arthritis (M05.00-M06.9)
sarcoidosis (D86)
systemic connective tissue disorders (M30-M36)
J84.178 **Other interstitial pulmonary diseases with fibrosis in diseases classified elsewhere**
Interstitial pneumonia (nonspecific) (usual) due to collagen vascular disease
Interstitial pneumonia (nonspecific) (usual) in diseases classified elsewhere
Organizing pneumonia due to collagen vascular disease
Organizing pneumonia in diseases classified elsewhere
Code first underlying diseases, such as:
progressive systemic sclerosis (M34.0)
rheumatoid arthritis (M05.00-M06.9)
systemic lupus erythematosis (M32.0-M32.9)
CC **J84.2** **Lymphoid interstitial pneumonia**
Lymphoid interstitial pneumonitis
+ **J84.8** **Other specified interstitial pulmonary diseases**
Excludes1: *exogenous lipoid pneumonia (J69.1)*
unspecified lipoid pneumonia (J69.1)
MCC **J84.81** **Lymphangioleiomyomatosis**
Lymphangiomyomatosis
● CC **J84.82** **Adult pulmonary Langerhans cell histiocytosis**
Adult PLCH
MCC **J84.83** **Surfactant mutations of the lung**
+ **J84.84** **Other interstitial lung diseases of childhood**
MCC **J84.841** **Neuroendocrine cell hyperplasia of infancy**
MCC **J84.842** **Pulmonary interstitial glycogenosis**
MCC **J84.843** **Alveolar capillary dysplasia with vein misalignment**
MCC **J84.848** **Other interstitial lung diseases of childhood**
J84.89 **Other specified interstitial pulmonary diseases**
Endogenous lipoid pneumonia
Interstitial pneumonitis
Non-specific interstitial pneumonitis NOS
Organizing pneumonia NOS
Code first if applicable:
poisoning due to drug or toxin (T51-T65 with fifth or sixth character to indicate intent), for toxic pneumonopathy
underlying cause of pneumonopathy, if known

Use additional code, for adverse effect, to identify drug (T36-T50 with fifth or sixth character 5), if drug-induced
Excludes1: *cryptogenic organizing pneumonia*
(J84.116)
idiopathic non-specific interstitial
pneumonitis (J84.113)
lipoid pneumonia, exogenous or
unspecified (J69.1)
lymphoid interstitial pneumonia (J84.2)
AHA CC: 2Q, 2019, 28
CC **J84.9** **Interstitial pulmonary disease, unspecified**
Interstitial pneumonia NOS

Suppurative and necrotic conditions of the lower respiratory tract (J85-J86)

J85 **Abscess of lung and mediastinum**
Use additional code (B95-B97) to identify infectious agent
MCC **J85.0** **Gangrene and necrosis of lung**
MCC **J85.1** **Abscess of lung with pneumonia**
Code also the type of pneumonia

717

+, +7th, X + 7th ● Newborn ● Pediatric ● Maternity ● Adult ♀ Female ♂ Male Manifestation Unacceptable PDX HCC CC MCC HAC

MCC **J85.2** **Abscess of lung without pneumonia**
Abscess of lung NOS
MCC **J85.3** **Abscess of mediastinum**
J86 **Pyothorax**
Use additional code (B95-B97) to identify infectious agent
Excludes1: *abscess of lung (J85.-)*
pyothorax due to tuberculosis (A15.6)
MCC **J86.0** **Pyothorax with fistula**
Bronchocutaneous fistula
Bronchopleural fistula
Hepatopleural fistula
Mediastinal fistula
Pleural fistula
Thoracic fistula
Any condition classifiable to J86.9 with fistula
MCC **J86.9** **Pyothorax without fistula**
Abscess of pleura
Abscess of thorax
Empyema (chest) (lung) (pleura)
Fibrinopurulent pleurisy
Purulent pleurisy
Pyopneumothorax
Septic pleurisy
Seropurulent pleurisy
Suppurative pleurisy

Other diseases of the pleura (J90-J94)

CC **J90** **Pleural effusion, not elsewhere classified**
Encysted pleurisy
Pleural effusion NOS
Pleurisy with effusion (exudative) (serous)
Excludes1: *chylous (pleural) effusion (J94.0)*
malignant pleural effusion (J91.0)
pleurisy NOS (R09.1)
tuberculous pleural effusion (A15.6)
Valid 3-character code, no further characters required
J91 **Pleural effusion in conditions classified elsewhere**
Excludes2: *pleural effusion in heart failure (I50.-)*
pleural effusion in systemic lupus erythematosus
(M32.13)
CC **J91.0** **Malignant pleural effusion**
Code first underlying neoplasm
CC **J91.8** **Pleural effusion in other conditions classified elsewhere**
Code first underlying disease, such as:
filariasis (B74.0-B74.9)
influenza (J09.X2, J10.1, J11.1)
AHA CC: 2Q, 2015, 15-16
J92 **Pleural plaque**
Includes: pleural thickening
J92.0 **Pleural plaque with presence of asbestos**
J92.9 **Pleural plaque without asbestos**
Pleural plaque NOS
J93 **Pneumothorax and air leak**
Excludes1: *congenital or perinatal pneumothorax (P25.1)*
postprocedural air leak (J95.812)
postprocedural pneumothorax (J95.811)
traumatic pneumothorax (S27.0)
tuberculous (current disease) pneumothorax (A15.-)
pyopneumothorax (J86.-)
MCC **J93.0** **Spontaneous tension pneumothorax**
+ **J93.1** **Other spontaneous pneumothorax**
CC **J93.11** **Primary spontaneous pneumothorax**
CC **J93.12** **Secondary spontaneous pneumothorax**
Code first underlying condition, such as:
catamenial pneumothorax due to endometriosis
(N80.8)
cystic fibrosis (E84.-)
eosinophilic pneumonia (J82)
lymphangioleiomyomatosis (J84.81)
malignant neoplasm of bronchus and lung (C34.-)
Marfan's syndrome (Q87.4)
pneumonia due to Pneumocystis carinii (B59)
secondary malignant neoplasm of lung (C78.0-)
spontaneous rupture of the esophagus (K22.3)
+ **J93.8** **Other pneumothorax and air leak**
CC **J93.81** **Chronic pneumothorax**
CC **J93.82** **Other air leak**
Persistent air leak

CC **J93.83** **Other pneumothorax**
Acute pneumothorax
Spontaneous pneumothorax NOS
CC **J93.9** **Pneumothorax, unspecified**
Pneumothorax NOS
J94 **Other pleural conditions**
Excludes1: *pleurisy NOS (R09.1)*
traumatic hemopneumothorax (S27.2)
traumatic hemothorax (S27.1)
tuberculous pleural conditions (current disease) (A15.-)
CC **J94.0** **Chylous effusion**
Chyliform effusion
J94.1 **Fibrothorax**
CC **J94.2** **Hemothorax**
Hemopneumothorax
CC **J94.8** **Other specified pleural conditions**
Hydropneumothorax
Hydrothorax
J94.9 **Pleural condition, unspecified**

Intraoperative and postprocedural complications and disorders of respiratory system, not elsewhere classified (J95)

J95 **Intraoperative and postprocedural complications and disorders of respiratory system, not elsewhere classified**
Excludes2: *aspiration pneumonia (J69.-)*
emphysema (subcutaneous) resulting from a procedure (T81.82)
hypostatic pneumonia (J18.2)
pulmonary manifestations due to radiation (J70.0-J70.1)
+ **J95.0** **Tracheostomy complications**
CC **J95.00** **Unspecified tracheostomy complication**
CC **J95.01** **Hemorrhage from tracheostomy stoma**
CC **J95.02** **Infection of tracheostomy stoma**
Use additional code to identify type of infection, such as:
cellulitis of neck (L03.221)
sepsis (A40, A41.-)
CC **J95.03** **Malfunction of tracheostomy stoma**
Mechanical complication of tracheostomy stoma
Obstruction of tracheostomy airway
Tracheal stenosis due to tracheostomy
CC **J95.04** **Tracheo-esophageal fistula following tracheostomy**
CC **J95.09** **Other tracheostomy complication**
MCC **J95.1** **Acute pulmonary insufficiency following thoracic surgery**
Excludes2: *Functional disturbances following cardiac surgery (I97.0, I97.1-)*
MCC **J95.2** **Acute pulmonary insufficiency following nonthoracic surgery**
Excludes2: *Functional disturbances following cardiac surgery (I97.0, I97.1-)*
MCC **J95.3** **Chronic pulmonary insufficiency following surgery**
Excludes2: *Functional disturbances following cardiac surgery (I97.0, I97.1-)*
CC **J95.4** **Chemical pneumonitis due to anesthesia**
Mendelson's syndrome
Postprocedural aspiration pneumonia
Use additional code for adverse effect, if applicable, to identify drug (T41.- with fifth or sixth character 5)
Excludes1: *aspiration pneumonitis due to anesthesia complicating labor and delivery (O74.0)*
aspiration pneumonitis due to anesthesia complicating pregnancy (O29)
aspiration pneumonitis due to anesthesia complicating the puerperium (O89.01)
CC **J95.5** **Postprocedural subglottic stenosis**
+ **J95.6** **Intraoperative hemorrhage and hematoma of a respiratory system organ or structure complicating a procedure**
Excludes1: *intraoperative hemorrhage and hematoma of a respiratory system organ or structure due to accidental puncture and laceration during procedure (J95.7-)*
CC **J95.61** **Intraoperative hemorrhage and hematoma of a respiratory system organ or structure complicating a respiratory system procedure**

+, +7th, X + 7th   ● Newborn   ● Pediatric   ● Maternity   ● Adult   ♀ Female   ♂ Male   Manifestation   Unacceptable PDX   HCC   CC   MCC   HAC

CC **J95.62** **Intraoperative hemorrhage and hematoma of a respiratory system organ or structure complicating other procedure**

+ **J95.7** **Accidental puncture and laceration of a respiratory system organ or structure during a procedure**
   Excludes2: *postprocedural pneumothorax (J95.811)*

CC **J95.71** **Accidental puncture and laceration of a respiratory system organ or structure during a respiratory system procedure**

CC **J95.72** **Accidental puncture and laceration of a respiratory system organ or structure during other procedure**

+ **J95.8** **Other intraoperative and postprocedural complications and disorders of respiratory system, not elsewhere classified**
   AHA CC: 4Q, 2016, 9-10

   + **J95.81** **Postprocedural pneumothorax and air leak**

   CC **J95.811** **Postprocedural pneumothorax**
      HAC see Appendix B for HAC conditional logic

   CC **J95.812** **Postprocedural air leak**

   + **J95.82** **Postprocedural respiratory failure**
      Excludes1: *Respiratory failure in other conditions (J96.-)*

   MCC **J95.821** **Acute postprocedural respiratory failure**
      Postprocedural respiratory failure NOS

   MCC **J95.822** **Acute and chronic postprocedural respiratory failure**

   + **J95.83** **Postprocedural hemorrhage of a respiratory system organ or structure following a procedure**

   CC **J95.830** **Postprocedural hemorrhage of a respiratory system organ or structure following a respiratory system procedure**

   CC **J95.831** **Postprocedural hemorrhage of a respiratory system organ or structure following other procedure**

CC **J95.84** **Transfusion-related acute lung injury (TRALI)**

   + **J95.85** **Complication of respirator [ventilator]**

   CC **J95.850** **Mechanical complication of respirator**
      Excludes1: *encounter for respirator [ventilator] dependence during power failure (Z99.12)*

   CC **J95.851** **Ventilator associated pneumonia**
      Ventilator associated pneumonitis
      Use additional code to identify the organism, if known (B95.-, B96.-, B97.-)
      Excludes1: *ventilator lung in newborn (P27.8)*
      Review coding guideline C.10.d.1
      AHA CC: 1Q, 2017, 25; 2Q, 2020, 17-18

   CC **J95.859** **Other complication of respirator [ventilator]**

   + **J95.86** **Postprocedural hematoma and seroma of a respiratory system organ or structure following a procedure**

   CC **J95.860** **Postprocedural hematoma of a respiratory system organ or structure following a respiratory system procedure**

   CC **J95.861** **Postprocedural hematoma of a respiratory system organ or structure following other procedure**

   CC **J95.862** **Postprocedural seroma of a respiratory system organ or structure following a respiratory system procedure**

   CC **J95.863** **Postprocedural seroma of a respiratory system organ or structure following other procedure**

CC **J95.88** **Other intraoperative complications of respiratory system, not elsewhere classified**

CC **J95.89** **Other postprocedural complications and disorders of respiratory system, not elsewhere classified**
   Use additional code to identify disorder, such as:
      aspiration pneumonia (J69.-)
      bacterial or viral pneumonia (J12-J18)
   Excludes2: *acute pulmonary insufficiency following thoracic surgery (J95.1)*
      postprocedural subglottic stenosis (J95.5)

Other diseases of the respiratory system (J96-J99)

J96 **Respiratory failure, not elsewhere classified**
   Excludes1: *acute respiratory distress syndrome (J80)*
      cardiorespiratory failure (R09.2)
      newborn respiratory distress syndrome (P22.0)
      postprocedural respiratory failure (J95.82-)
      respiratory arrest (R09.2)
      respiratory arrest of newborn (P28.81)
      respiratory failure of newborn (P28.5)

   + **J96.0** **Acute respiratory failure**
      Review coding guideline C.10.b and C.11.e

   MCC **J96.00** **Acute respiratory failure, unspecified whether with hypoxia or hypercapnia**
      AHA CC: 4Q, 2013, 121; 3Q, 2016, 14

   MCC **J96.01** **Acute respiratory failure with hypoxia**
   MCC **J96.02** **Acute respiratory failure with hypercapnia**

   + **J96.1** **Chronic respiratory failure**

   CC **J96.10** **Chronic respiratory failure, unspecified whether with hypoxia or hypercapnia**
      AHA CC: 1Q, 2015, 21

   CC **J96.11** **Chronic respiratory failure with hypoxia**
      AHA CC: 4Q, 2013, 129

   CC **J96.12** **Chronic respiratory failure with hypercapnia**

   + **J96.2** **Acute and chronic respiratory failure**
      Acute on chronic respiratory failure
      Review coding guideline C.10.b

   MCC **J96.20** **Acute and chronic respiratory failure, unspecified whether with hypoxia or hypercapnia**

   MCC **J96.21** **Acute and chronic respiratory failure with hypoxia**

   MCC **J96.22** **Acute and chronic respiratory failure with hypercapnia**

   + **J96.9** **Respiratory failure, unspecified**

   MCC **J96.90** **Respiratory failure, unspecified, unspecified whether with hypoxia or hypercapnia**

   MCC **J96.91** **Respiratory failure, unspecified with hypoxia**

   MCC **J96.92** **Respiratory failure, unspecified with hypercapnia**

J98 **Other respiratory disorders**
   Use additional code to identify:
      exposure to environmental tobacco smoke (Z77.22)
      exposure to tobacco smoke in the perinatal period (P96.81)
      history of tobacco dependence (Z87.891)
      occupational exposure to environmental tobacco smoke (Z57.31)
      tobacco dependence (F17.-)
      tobacco use (Z72.0)
   Excludes1: *newborn apnea (P28.4)*
      newborn sleep apnea (P28.3)
   Excludes2: *apnea NOS (R06.81)*
      sleep apnea (G47.3-)

   + **J98.0** **Diseases of bronchus, not elsewhere classified**

   J98.01 **Acute bronchospasm**
      Excludes1: *acute bronchiolitis with bronchospasm (J21.-)*
         acute bronchitis with bronchospasm (J20.-)
         asthma (J45.-)
         exercise induced bronchospasm (J45.990)

   J98.09 **Other diseases of bronchus, not elsewhere classified**
      Broncholithiasis
      Calcification of bronchus
      Stenosis of bronchus
      Tracheobronchial collapse
      Tracheobronchial dyskinesia
      Ulcer of bronchus

   + **J98.1** **Pulmonary collapse**
      Excludes1: *therapeutic collapse of lung status (Z98.3)*

   CC **J98.11** **Atelectasis**
      Excludes1: *newborn atelectasis tuberculous atelectasis (current disease) (A15)*

   CC **J98.19** **Other pulmonary collapse**

   J98.2 **Interstitial emphysema**
      Mediastinal emphysema
      Excludes1: *emphysema NOS (J43.9)*
         emphysema in newborn (P25.0)
         surgical emphysema (subcutaneous) (T81.82)
         traumatic subcutaneous emphysema (T79.7)

+, +7th, X + 7th   ● Newborn   ● Pediatric   ● Maternity   ● Adult   ♀ Female   ♂ Male   Manifestation   Unacceptable PDX   HCC   CC   MCC   HAC

J98.3 **Compensatory emphysema**

J98.4 **Other disorders of lung**

Calcification of lung

Cystic lung disease (acquired)

Lung disease NOS

Pulmolithiasis

Excludes1: *acute interstitial pneumonitis (J84.114)*

pulmonary insufficiency following surgery

(J95.1-J95.2)

+ **J98.5** **Diseases of mediastinum, not elsewhere classified**

Excludes2: *abscess of mediastinum (J85.3)*

AHA CC: 4Q, 2016, 29

MCC **J98.51** **Mediastinitis**

Code first underlying condition, if applicable, such

as postoperative mediastinitis (T81.-)

MCC **J98.59** **Other diseases of mediastinum, not elsewhere**

classified

Fibrosis of mediastinum

Hernia of mediastinum

Retraction of mediastinum

J98.6 **Disorders of diaphragm**

Diaphragmatitis

Paralysis of diaphragm

Relaxation of diaphragm

Excludes1: *congenital malformation of diaphragm NEC*

(Q79.1)

congenital diaphragmatic hernia (Q79.0)

Excludes2: *diaphragmatic hernia (K44.-)*

J98.8 **Other specified respiratory disorders**

AHA CC: 1Q, 2020, 34-36

Review coding guideline C.1.g.1.c.iii

J98.9 **Respiratory disorder, unspecified**

Respiratory disease (chronic) NOS

J99 **Respiratory disorders in diseases classified elsewhere**

Code first underlying disease, such as:

amyloidosis (E85.-)

ankylosing spondylitis (M45)

congenital syphilis (A50.5)

cryoglobulinemia (D89.1)

early congenital syphilis (A50.0)

plasminogen deficiency (E88.02)

schistosomiasis (B65.0-B65.9)

Excludes1: *respiratory disorders in:*

amebiasis (A06.5)

blastomycosis (B40.0-B40.2)

candidiasis (B37.1)

coccidioidomycosis (B38.0-B38.2)

cystic fibrosis with pulmonary manifestations (E84.0)

dermatomyositis (M33.01, M33.11)

histoplasmosis (B39.0-B39.2)

late syphilis (A52.72, A52.73)

polymyositis (M33.21)

sicca syndrome (M35.02)

systemic lupus erythematosus (M32.13)

systemic sclerosis (M34.81)

Wegener's granulomatosis (M31.30-M31.31)

Valid 3-character code, no further characters required

+, +7th, X + 7th ● Newborn ● Pediatric ● Maternity ● Adult ♀ Female ♂ Male Manifestation Unacceptable PDX HCC CC MCC HAC

Chapter 11: Diseases of the Digestive System (K00-K95)

Excludes2: *certain conditions originating in the perinatal period (P04-P96)*
certain infectious and parasitic diseases (A00-B99)
complications of pregnancy, childbirth and the puerperium (O00-O9A)
congenital malformations, deformations and chromosomal abnormalities (Q00-Q99)
endocrine, nutritional and metabolic diseases (E00-E88)
injury, poisoning and certain other consequences of external causes (S00-T88)
neoplasms (C00-D49)
symptoms, signs and abnormal clinical and laboratory findings, not elsewhere classified (R00-R94)

This chapter contains the following category blocks:

K00-K14   Diseases of oral cavity and salivary glands
K20-K31   Diseases of esophagus, stomach and duodenum
K35-K38   Diseases of appendix
K40-K46   Hernia
K50-K52   Noninfective enteritis and colitis
K55-K64   Other diseases of intestines
K65-K68   Diseases of peritoneum and retroperitoneum
K70-K77   Diseases of liver
K80-K87   Disorders of gallbladder, biliary tract and pancreas
K90-K95   Other diseases of the digestive system

C. Chapter-Specific Coding Guidelines

In addition to general coding guidelines, there are guidelines for specific diagnoses and/or conditions in the classification. Unless otherwise indicated, these guidelines apply to all health care settings. Please refer to Section II for guidelines on the selection of principal diagnosis.

11. **Chapter 11: Diseases of the Digestive System (K00-K95)**

Reserved for future guideline expansion

Diseases of oral cavity and salivary glands (K00-K14)

K00   Disorders of tooth development and eruption

> ***Excludes2:*** *embedded and impacted teeth (K01.-)*
>
> **K00.0   Anodontia**
> Hypodontia
> Oligodontia
> ***Excludes1:*** *acquired absence of teeth (K08.1-)*

K00.1   Supernumerary teeth
Distomolar
Fourth molar
Mesiodens
Paramolar
Supplementary teeth
Excludes2: *supernumerary roots (K00.2)*

K00.2   Abnormalities of size and form of teeth
Concrescence of teeth
Fusion of teeth
Gemination of teeth
Dens evaginatus
Dens in dente
Dens invaginatus
Enamel pearls
Macrodontia
Microdontia
Peg-shaped [conical] teeth
Supernumerary roots
Taurodontism
Tuberculum paramolare
Excludes1: *abnormalities of teeth due to congenital syphilis (A50.5)*
tuberculum Carabelli, which is regarded as a normal variation and should not be coded

K00.3   Mottled teeth
Dental fluorosis
Mottling of enamel
Nonfluoride enamel opacities
Excludes2: *deposits [accretions] on teeth (K03.6)*

K00.4   Disturbances in tooth formation
Aplasia and hypoplasia of cementum
Dilaceration of tooth
Enamel hypoplasia (neonatal) (postnatal) (prenatal)
Regional odontodysplasia
Turner's tooth
Excludes1: *Hutchinson's teeth and mulberry molars in congenital syphilis (A50.5)*
Excludes2: *mottled teeth (K00.3)*

K00.5   Hereditary disturbances in tooth structure, not elsewhere classified
Amelogenesis imperfecta
Dentinogenesis imperfecta
Odontogenesis imperfecta
Dentinal dysplasia
Shell teeth

Oral Cavity

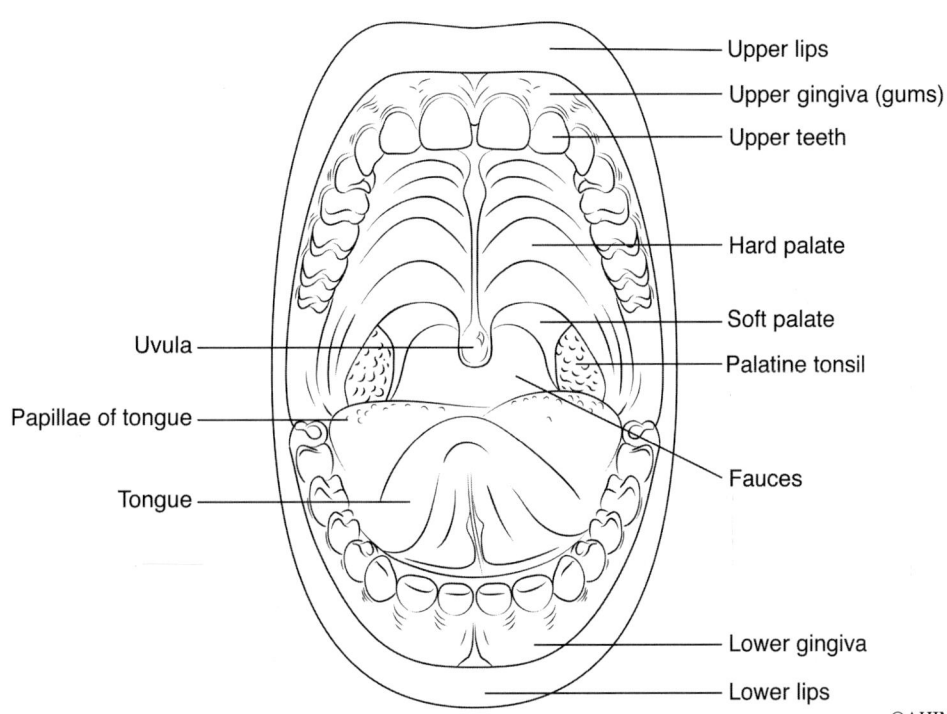

- Upper lips
- Upper gingiva (gums)
- Upper teeth
- Hard palate
- Soft palate
- Palatine tonsil
- Fauces
- Lower gingiva
- Lower lips
- Uvula
- Papillae of tongue
- Tongue

©AHIMA

+, +7th, X + 7th   • Newborn   • Pediatric   • Maternity   • Adult   ♀ Female   ♂ Male   Manifestation   Unacceptable PDX   HCC   CC   MCC   HAC

Glands of the Oral Cavity

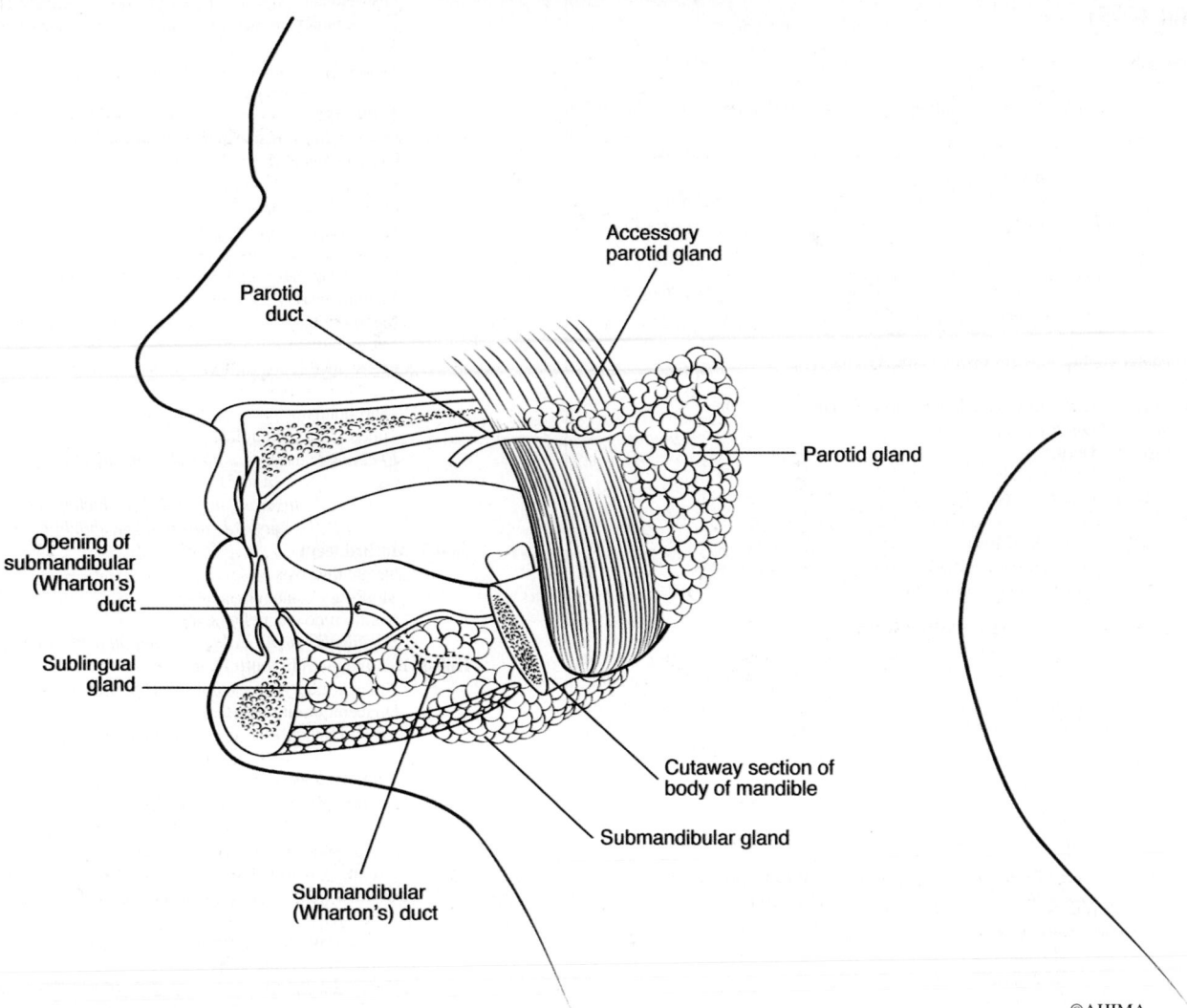

Accessory parotid gland

Parotid duct

Parotid gland

Opening of submandibular (Wharton's) duct

Sublingual gland

Cutaway section of body of mandible

Submandibular gland

Submandibular (Wharton's) duct

©AHIMA

K00.6 Disturbances in tooth eruption
Dentia praecox
Natal tooth
Neonatal tooth
Premature eruption of tooth
Premature shedding of primary [deciduous] tooth
Prenatal teeth
Retained [persistent] primary tooth
Excludes2: embedded and impacted teeth (K01.-)

K00.7 Teething syndrome

K00.8 Other disorders of tooth development
Color changes during tooth formation
Intrinsic staining of teeth NOS
Excludes2: posteruptive color changes (K03.7)

K00.9 Disorder of tooth development, unspecified
Disorder of odontogenesis NOS

K01 Embedded and impacted teeth

Excludes1: abnormal position of fully erupted teeth (M26.3-)

K01.0 Embedded teeth
K01.1 Impacted teeth

K02 Dental caries
Includes: caries of dentine
dental cavities
early childhood caries
pre-eruptive caries
recurrent caries (dentino enamel junction) (enamel) (to the pulp) tooth decay

K02.3 Arrested dental caries
Arrested coronal and root caries

+ K02.5 Dental caries on pit and fissure surface
Dental caries on chewing surface of tooth

K02.51 Dental caries on pit and fissure surface limited to enamel
White spot lesions [initial caries] on pit and fissure surface of tooth

K02.52 Dental caries on pit and fissure surface penetrating into dentin
Primary dental caries, cervical origin

K02.53 Dental caries on pit and fissure surface penetrating into pulp

+ K02.6 Dental caries on smooth surface

K02.61 Dental caries on smooth surface limited to enamel
White spot lesions [initial caries] on smooth surface of tooth

K02.62 Dental caries on smooth surface penetrating into dentin

K02.63 Dental caries on smooth surface penetrating into pulp

K02.7 Dental root caries
K02.9 Dental caries, unspecified

K03 Other diseases of hard tissues of teeth

Excludes2: bruxism (F45.8)
dental caries (K02.-)
teeth-grinding NOS (F45.8)

K03.0 Excessive attrition of teeth
Approximal wear of teeth
Occlusal wear of teeth

K03.1 Abrasion of teeth
Dentifrice abrasion of teeth
Habitual abrasion of teeth
Occupational abrasion of teeth
Ritual abrasion of teeth
Traditional abrasion of teeth
Wedge defect NOS

K03.2 Erosion of teeth
  Erosion of teeth due to diet
  Erosion of teeth due to drugs and medicaments
  Erosion of teeth due to persistent vomiting
  Erosion of teeth NOS
  Idiopathic erosion of teeth
  Occupational erosion of teeth
K03.3 Pathological resorption of teeth
  Internal granuloma of pulp
  Resorption of teeth (external)
K03.4 Hypercementosis
  Cementation hyperplasia
K03.5 Ankylosis of teeth
K03.6 Deposits [accretions] on teeth
  Betel deposits [accretions] on teeth
  Black deposits [accretions] on teeth
  Extrinsic staining of teeth NOS
  Green deposits [accretions] on teeth
  Materia alba deposits [accretions] on teeth
  Orange deposits [accretions] on teeth
  Staining of teeth NOS
  Subgingival dental calculus
  Supragingival dental calculus
  Tobacco deposits [accretions] on teeth
K03.7 Posteruptive color changes of dental hard tissues
  Excludes2: deposits [accretions] on teeth (K03.6)
+ **K03.8 Other specified diseases of hard tissues of teeth**
  K03.81 Cracked tooth
    Excludes1: asymptomatic craze lines in enamel -
        omit code
      broken or fractured tooth due to
        trauma (S02.5)
  K03.89 Other specified diseases of hard tissues of teeth
K03.9 Disease of hard tissues of teeth, unspecified

K04 Diseases of pulp and periapical tissues
  AHA CC: 4Q, 2016, 29-30
+ **K04.0 Pulpitis**
  Acute pulpitis
  Chronic (hyperplastic) (ulcerative) pulpitis
  CC **K04.01 Reversible pulpitis**
  CC **K04.02 Irreversible pulpitis**
K04.1 Necrosis of pulp
  Pulpal gangrene
K04.2 Pulp degeneration
  Denticles
  Pulpal calcifications
  Pulpal stones
K04.3 Abnormal hard tissue formation in pulp
  Secondary or irregular dentine
CC **K04.4 Acute apical periodontitis of pulpal origin**
  Acute apical periodontitis NOS
  Excludes1: acute periodontitis (K05.2-)
K04.5 Chronic apical periodontitis
  Apical or periapical granuloma
  Apical periodontitis NOS
  Excludes1: chronic periodontitis (K05.3-)
K04.6 Periapical abscess with sinus
  Dental abscess with sinus
  Dentoalveolar abscess with sinus
K04.7 Periapical abscess without sinus
  Dental abscess without sinus
  Dentoalveolar abscess without sinus
K04.8 Radicular cyst
  Apical (periodontal) cyst
  Periapical cyst
  Residual radicular cyst
  Excludes2: lateral periodontal cyst (K09.0)
+ **K04.9 Other and unspecified diseases of pulp and periapical tissues**
  K04.90 Unspecified diseases of pulp and periapical tissues
  K04.99 Other diseases of pulp and periapical tissues

K05 Gingivitis and periodontal diseases
  Use additional code to identify:
    alcohol abuse and dependence (F10.-)
    exposure to environmental tobacco smoke (Z77.22)
    exposure to tobacco smoke in the perinatal period (P96.81)
    history of tobacco dependence (Z87.891)
    occupational exposure to environmental tobacco smoke (Z57.31)
    tobacco dependence (F17.-)
    tobacco use (Z72.0)
  AHA CC: 4Q, 2016, 29-30

+ **K05.0 Acute gingivitis**
  Excludes1: acute necrotizing ulcerative gingivitis (A69.1)
    herpesviral [herpes simplex] gingivostomatitis
      (B00.2)
  K05.00 Acute gingivitis, plaque induced
    Acute gingivitis NOS
    Plaque induced gingival disease
  K05.01 Acute gingivitis, non-plaque induced
+ **K05.1 Chronic gingivitis**
  Desquamative gingivitis (chronic)
  Gingivitis (chronic) NOS
  Hyperplastic gingivitis (chronic)
  Pregnancy associated gingivitis
  Simple marginal gingivitis (chronic)
  Ulcerative gingivitis (chronic)
  Code first, if applicable, diseases of the digestive system
    complicating pregnancy (O99.61-)
  K05.10 Chronic gingivitis, plaque induced
    Chronic gingivitis NOS
    Gingivitis NOS
  K05.11 Chronic gingivitis, non-plaque induced
+ **K05.2 Aggressive periodontitis**
  Acute pericoronitis
  Excludes1: acute apical periodontitis (K04.4)
    periapical abscess (K04.7)
    periapical abscess with sinus (K04.6)
  K05.20 Aggressive periodontitis, unspecified
  + **K05.21 Aggressive periodontitis, localized**
    Periodontal abscess
    **K05.211 Aggressive periodontitis, localized,
        slight**
    **K05.212 Aggressive periodontitis, localized,
        moderate**
    **K05.213 Aggressive periodontitis, localized,
        severe**
    **K05.219 Aggressive periodontitis, localized,
        unspecified severity**
  + **K05.22 Aggressive periodontitis, generalized**
    **K05.221 Aggressive periodontitis, generalized,
        slight**
    **K05.222 Aggressive periodontitis, generalized,
        moderate**
    **K05.223 Aggressive periodontitis, generalized,
        severe**
    **K05.229 Aggressive periodontitis, generalized,
        unspecified severity**
+ **K05.3 Chronic periodontitis**
  Chronic pericoronitis
  Complex periodontitis
  Periodontitis NOS
  Simplex periodontitis
  Excludes1: chronic apical periodontitis (K04.5)
  K05.30 Chronic periodontitis, unspecified
  + **K05.31 Chronic periodontitis, localized**
    K05.311 Chronic periodontitis, localized, slight
    **K05.312 Chronic periodontitis, localized,
        moderate**
    **K05.313 Chronic periodontitis, localized,
        severe**
    **K05.319 Chronic periodontitis, localized,
        unspecified severity**
  + **K05.32 Chronic periodontitis, generalized**
    **K05.321 Chronic periodontitis, generalized,
        slight**
    **K05.322 Chronic periodontitis, generalized,
        moderate**
    **K05.323 Chronic periodontitis, generalized,
        severe**
    **K05.329 Chronic periodontitis, generalized,
        unspecified severity**
K05.4 Periodontosis
  Juvenile periodontosis
K05.5 Other periodontal diseases
  Combined periodontic-endodontic lesion
  Narrow gingival width (of periodontal soft tissue)
  Excludes2: leukoplakia of gingiva (K13.21)
K05.6 Periodontal disease, unspecified

K06 **Other disorders of gingiva and edentulous alveolar ridge**

Excludes2: *acute gingivitis (K05.0)*
atrophy of edentulous alveolar ridge (K08.2)
chronic gingivitis (K05.1)
gingivitis NOS (K05.1)
AHA CC: 4Q, 2016, 29-30

K06.0 **Gingival recession**
Gingival recession (postinfective) (postprocedural)
AHA CC: 4Q, 2017, 16

+ **K06.01** **Gingival recession, localized**
K06.010 **Localized gingival recession, unspecified**
Localized gingival recession, NOS
K06.011 **Localized gingival recession, minimal**
K06.012 **Localized gingival recession, moderate**
K06.013 **Localized gingival recession, severe**

+ **K06.02** **Gingival recession, generalized**
K06.020 **Generalized gingival recession, unspecified**
Generalized gingival recession, NOS
K06.021 **Generalized gingival recession, minimal**
K06.022 **Generalized gingival recession, moderate**
K06.023 **Generalized gingival recession, severe**

K06.1 **Gingival enlargement**
Gingival fibromatosis

K06.2 **Gingival and edentulous alveolar ridge lesions associated with trauma**
Irritative hyperplasia of edentulous ridge [denture hyperplasia]
Use additional code (Chapter 20) to identify external cause or denture status (Z97.2)

K06.3 **Horizontal alveolar bone loss**

K06.8 **Other specified disorders of gingiva and edentulous alveolar ridge**
Fibrous epulis
Flabby alveolar ridge
Giant cell epulis
Peripheral giant cell granuloma of gingiva
Pyogenic granuloma of gingiva
Vertical ridge deficiency
Excludes2: *gingival cyst (K09.0)*

K06.9 **Disorder of gingiva and edentulous alveolar ridge, unspecified**

K08 **Other disorders of teeth and supporting structures**

Excludes2: *dentofacial anomalies [including malocclusion] (M26.-)*
disorders of jaw (M27.-)
AHA CC: 4Q, 2016, 29-30

K08.0 **Exfoliation of teeth due to systemic causes**
Code also underlying systemic condition

+ **K08.1** **Complete loss of teeth**
Acquired loss of teeth, complete
Excludes1: *congenital absence of teeth (K00.0)*
exfoliation of teeth due to systemic causes (K08.0)
partial loss of teeth (K08.4-)

+ **K08.10** **Complete loss of teeth, unspecified cause**
K08.101 **Complete loss of teeth, unspecified cause, class I**
K08.102 **Complete loss of teeth, unspecified cause, class II**
K08.103 **Complete loss of teeth, unspecified cause, class III**
K08.104 **Complete loss of teeth, unspecified cause, class IV**
K08.109 **Complete loss of teeth, unspecified cause, unspecified class**
Edentulism NOS

+ **K08.11** **Complete loss of teeth due to trauma**
K08.111 **Complete loss of teeth due to trauma, class I**
K08.112 **Complete loss of teeth due to trauma, class II**
K08.113 **Complete loss of teeth due to trauma, class III**
K08.114 **Complete loss of teeth due to trauma, class IV**
K08.119 **Complete loss of teeth due to trauma, unspecified class**

+ **K08.12** **Complete loss of teeth due to periodontal diseases**
K08.121 **Complete loss of teeth due to periodontal diseases, class I**
K08.122 **Complete loss of teeth due to periodontal diseases, class II**
K08.123 **Complete loss of teeth due to periodontal diseases, class III**
K08.124 **Complete loss of teeth due to periodontal diseases, class IV**
K08.129 **Complete loss of teeth due to periodontal diseases, unspecified class**

+ **K08.13** **Complete loss of teeth due to caries**
K08.131 **Complete loss of teeth due to caries, class I**
K08.132 **Complete loss of teeth due to caries, class II**
K08.133 **Complete loss of teeth due to caries, class III**
K08.134 **Complete loss of teeth due to caries, class IV**
K08.139 **Complete loss of teeth due to caries, unspecified class**

+ **K08.19** **Complete loss of teeth due to other specified cause**
K08.191 **Complete loss of teeth due to other specified cause, class I**
K08.192 **Complete loss of teeth due to other specified cause, class II**
K08.193 **Complete loss of teeth due to other specified cause, class III**
K08.194 **Complete loss of teeth due to other specified cause, class IV**
K08.199 **Complete loss of teeth due to other specified cause, unspecified class**

+ **K08.2** **Atrophy of edentulous alveolar ridge**
K08.20 **Unspecified atrophy of edentulous alveolar ridge**
Atrophy of the mandible NOS
Atrophy of the maxilla NOS
K08.21 **Minimal atrophy of the mandible**
Minimal atrophy of the edentulous mandible
K08.22 **Moderate atrophy of the mandible**
Moderate atrophy of the edentulous mandible
K08.23 **Severe atrophy of the mandible**
Severe atrophy of the edentulous mandible
K08.24 **Minimal atrophy of maxilla**
Minimal atrophy of the edentulous maxilla
K08.25 **Moderate atrophy of the maxilla**
Moderate atrophy of the edentulous maxilla
K08.26 **Severe atrophy of the maxilla**
Severe atrophy of the edentulous maxilla

K08.3 **Retained dental root**

+ **K08.4** **Partial loss of teeth**
Acquired loss of teeth, partial
Excludes1: *complete loss of teeth (K08.1-)*
congenital absence of teeth (K00.0)
Excludes2: *exfoliation of teeth due to systemic causes (K08.0)*

+ **K08.40** **Partial loss of teeth, unspecified cause**
K08.401 **Partial loss of teeth, unspecified cause, class I**
K08.402 **Partial loss of teeth, unspecified cause, class II**
K08.403 **Partial loss of teeth, unspecified cause, class III**
K08.404 **Partial loss of teeth, unspecified cause, class IV**
K08.409 **Partial loss of teeth, unspecified cause, unspecified class**
Tooth extraction status NOS

+ **K08.41** **Partial loss of teeth due to trauma**
K08.411 **Partial loss of teeth due to trauma, class I**
K08.412 **Partial loss of teeth due to trauma, class II**
K08.413 **Partial loss of teeth due to trauma, class III**
K08.414 **Partial loss of teeth due to trauma, class IV**
K08.419 **Partial loss of teeth due to trauma, unspecified class**

+, +7th, X + 7th ● Newborn ● Pediatric ● Maternity ● Adult ♀ Female ♂ Male Manifestation Unacceptable PDX HCC CC MCC HAC

+ **K08.42 Partial loss of teeth due to periodontal diseases**
  K08.421 Partial loss of teeth due to periodontal diseases, class I
  K08.422 Partial loss of teeth due to periodontal diseases, class II
  K08.423 Partial loss of teeth due to periodontal diseases, class III
  K08.424 Partial loss of teeth due to periodontal diseases, class IV
  K08.429 Partial loss of teeth due to periodontal diseases, unspecified class

+ **K08.43 Partial loss of teeth due to caries**
  K08.431 Partial loss of teeth due to caries, class I
  K08.432 Partial loss of teeth due to caries, class II
  K08.433 Partial loss of teeth due to caries, class III
  K08.434 Partial loss of teeth due to caries, class IV
  K08.439 Partial loss of teeth due to caries, unspecified class

+ **K08.49 Partial loss of teeth due to other specified cause**
  K08.491 Partial loss of teeth due to other specified cause, class I
  K08.492 Partial loss of teeth due to other specified cause, class II
  K08.493 Partial loss of teeth due to other specified cause, class III
  K08.494 Partial loss of teeth due to other specified cause, class IV
  K08.499 Partial loss of teeth due to other specified cause, unspecified class

+ **K08.5 Unsatisfactory restoration of tooth**
Defective bridge, crown, filling
Defective dental restoration
Excludes1: dental restoration status (Z98.811)
Excludes2: endosseous dental implant failure (M27.6-)
  unsatisfactory endodontic treatment (M27.5-)

K08.50 Unsatisfactory restoration of tooth, unspecified
Defective dental restoration NOS

K08.51 Open restoration margins of tooth
Dental restoration failure of marginal integrity
Open margin on tooth restoration
Poor gingival margin to tooth restoration

K08.52 Unrepairable overhanging of dental restorative materials
Overhanging of tooth restoration

+ **K08.53 Fractured dental restorative material**
Excludes1: cracked tooth (K03.81)
  traumatic fracture of tooth (S02.5)

  K08.530 Fractured dental restorative material without loss of material
  K08.531 Fractured dental restorative material with loss of material
  K08.539 Fractured dental restorative material, unspecified

K08.54 Contour of existing restoration of tooth biologically incompatible with oral health
Dental restoration failure of periodontal anatomical integrity
Unacceptable contours of existing restoration of tooth
Unacceptable morphology of existing restoration of tooth

K08.55 Allergy to existing dental restorative material
Use additional code to identify the specific type of allergy

K08.56 Poor aesthetic of existing restoration of tooth
Dental restoration aesthetically inadequate or displeasing

K08.59 Other unsatisfactory restoration of tooth
Other defective dental restoration

+ **K08.8 Other specified disorders of teeth and supporting structures**
K08.81 Primary occlusal trauma
K08.82 Secondary occlusal trauma
K08.89 Other specified disorders of teeth and supporting structures
Enlargement of alveolar ridge NOS
Insufficient anatomic crown height
Insufficient clinical crown length
Irregular alveolar process
Toothache NOS

K08.9 Disorder of teeth and supporting structures, unspecified

K09 Cysts of oral region, not elsewhere classified
Includes: lesions showing histological features both of aneurysmal cyst and of another fibro-osseous lesion
Excludes2: cysts of jaw (M27.0-, M27.4-)
  radicular cyst (K04.8)

K09.0 Developmental odontogenic cysts
Dentigerous cyst
Eruption cyst
Follicular cyst
Gingival cyst
Lateral periodontal cyst
Primordial cyst
Excludes2: keratocysts (D16.4, D16.5)
  odontogenic keratocystic tumors (D16.4, D16.5)

K09.1 Developmental (nonodontogenic) cysts of oral region
Cyst (of) incisive canal
Cyst (of) palatine of papilla
Globulomaxillary cyst
Median palatal cyst
Nasoalveolar cyst
Nasolabial cyst
Nasopalatine duct cyst

K09.8 Other cysts of oral region, not elsewhere classified
Dermoid cyst
Epidermoid cyst
Lymphoepithelial cyst
Epstein's pearl

K09.9 Cyst of oral region, unspecified

K11 Diseases of salivary glands
Use additional code to identify:
  alcohol abuse and dependence (F10.-)
  exposure to environmental tobacco smoke (Z77.22)
  exposure to tobacco smoke in the perinatal period (P96.81)
  history of tobacco dependence (Z87.891)
  occupational exposure to environmental tobacco smoke (Z57.31)
  tobacco dependence (F17.-)
  tobacco use (Z72.0)

K11.0 Atrophy of salivary gland
K11.1 Hypertrophy of salivary gland
+ **K11.2 Sialoadenitis**
Parotitis
Excludes1: epidemic parotitis (B26.-)
  mumps (B26.-)
  uveoparotid fever [Heerfordt] (D86.89)

  K11.20 Sialoadenitis, unspecified
  K11.21 Acute sialoadenitis
    Excludes1: acute recurrent sialoadenitis (K11.22)
  K11.22 Acute recurrent sialoadenitis
  K11.23 Chronic sialoadenitis

CC **K11.3 Abscess of salivary gland**
CC **K11.4 Fistula of salivary gland**
Excludes1: congenital fistula of salivary gland (Q38.4)

K11.5 Sialolithiasis
Calculus of salivary gland or duct
Stone of salivary gland or duct

K11.6 Mucocele of salivary gland
Mucous extravasation cyst of salivary gland
Mucous retention cyst of salivary gland
Ranula

K11.7 Disturbances of salivary secretion
Hypoptyalism
Ptyalism
Xerostomia
Excludes2: dry mouth NOS (R68.2)

K11.8 Other diseases of salivary glands
Benign lymphoepithelial lesion of salivary gland
Mikulicz' disease
Necrotizing sialometaplasia
Sialectasia
Stenosis of salivary duct
Stricture of salivary duct
Excludes1: sicca syndrome [Sjögren] (M35.0-)

K11.9 Disease of salivary gland, unspecified
Sialoadenopathy NOS

K12 **Stomatitis and related lesions**

Use additional code to identify:
    alcohol abuse and dependence (F10.-)
    exposure to environmental tobacco smoke (Z77.22)
    exposure to tobacco smoke in the perinatal period (P96.81)
    history of tobacco dependence (Z87.891)
    occupational exposure to environmental tobacco smoke (Z57.31)
    tobacco dependence (F17.-)
    tobacco use (Z72.0)

Excludes1: *cancrum oris (A69.0)*
    cheilitis (K13.0)
    gangrenous stomatitis (A69.0)
    herpesviral [herpes simplex] gingivostomatitis (B00.2)
    noma (A69.0)

K12.0 **Recurrent oral aphthae**
    Aphthous stomatitis (major) (minor)
    Bednar's aphthae
    Periadenitis mucosa necrotica recurrens
    Recurrent aphthous ulcer
    Stomatitis herpetiformis

K12.1 **Other forms of stomatitis**
    Stomatitis NOS
    Denture stomatitis
    Ulcerative stomatitis
    Vesicular stomatitis

Excludes1: *acute necrotizing ulcerative stomatitis (A69.1)*
    Vincent's stomatitis (A69.1)

CC **K12.2** **Cellulitis and abscess of mouth**
    Cellulitis of mouth (floor)
    Submandibular abscess

Excludes2: *abscess of salivary gland (K11.3)*
    abscess of tongue (K14.0)
    periapical abscess (K04.6-K04.7)
    periodontal abscess (K05.21)
    peritonsillar abscess (J36)

+ **K12.3** **Oral mucositis (ulcerative)**
    Mucositis (oral) (oropharyneal)

Excludes2: *gastrointestinal mucositis (ulcerative) (K92.81)*
    mucositis (ulcerative) of vagina and vulva (N76.81)
    nasal mucositis (ulcerative) (J34.81)

K12.30 **Oral mucositis (ulcerative), unspecified**

K12.31 **Oral mucositis (ulcerative) due to antineoplastic therapy**
    Use additional code for adverse effect, if applicable, to identify antineoplastic and immunosuppressive drugs (T45.1X5)

    Use additional code for other antineoplastic therapy, such as: radiological procedure and radiotherapy (Y84.2)

K12.32 **Oral mucositis (ulcerative) due to other drugs**
    Use additional code for adverse effect, if applicable, to identify drug (T36-T50 with fifth or sixth character 5)

K12.33 **Oral mucositis (ulcerative) due to radiation**
    Use additional external cause code (W88-W90, X39.0-) to identify cause

K12.39 **Other oral mucositis (ulcerative)**
    Viral oral mucositis (ulcerative)

K13 **Other diseases of lip and oral mucosa**

Includes: epithelial disturbances of tongue

Use additional code to identify:
    alcohol abuse and dependence (F10.-)
    exposure to environmental tobacco smoke (Z77.22)
    exposure to tobacco smoke in the perinatal period (P96.81)
    history of tobacco dependence (Z87.891)
    occupational exposure to environmental tobacco smoke (Z57.31)
    tobacco dependence (F17.-)
    tobacco use (Z72.0)

Excludes2: *certain disorders of gingiva and edentulous alveolar ridge (K05-K06)*
    cysts of oral region (K09.-)
    diseases of tongue (K14.-)
    stomatitis and related lesions (K12.-)

K13.0 **Diseases of lips**
    Abscess of lips
    Angular cheilitis
    Cellulitis of lips
    Cheilitis NOS
    Cheilodynia
    Cheilosis
    Exfoliative cheilitis
    Fistula of lips
    Glandular cheilitis
    Hypertrophy of lips
    Perlèche NEC

Excludes1: *ariboflavinosis (E53.0)*
    cheilitis due to radiation-related disorders (L55-L59)
    congenital fistula of lips (Q38.0)
    congenital hypertrophy of lips (Q18.6)
    Perlèche due to candidiasis (B37.83)
    Perlèche due to riboflavin deficiency (E53.0)

K13.1 **Cheek and lip biting**

+ **K13.2** **Leukoplakia and other disturbances of oral epithelium, including tongue**

Excludes1: *carcinoma in situ of oral epithelium (D00.0-)*
    hairy leukoplakia (K13.3)

K13.21 **Leukoplakia of oral mucosa, including tongue**
    Leukokeratosis of oral mucosa
    Leukoplakia of gingiva, lips, tongue

Excludes1: *hairy leukoplakia (K13.3)*
    leukokeratosis nicotina palati (K13.24)

K13.22 **Minimal keratinized residual ridge mucosa**
    Minimal keratinization of alveolar ridge mucosa

K13.23 **Excessive keratinized residual ridge mucosa**
    Excessive keratinization of alveolar ridge mucosa

K13.24 **Leukokeratosis nicotina palati**
    Smoker's palate

K13.29 **Other disturbances of oral epithelium, including tongue**
    Erythroplakia of mouth or tongue
    Focal epithelial hyperplasia of mouth or tongue
    Leukoedema of mouth or tongue
    Other oral epithelium disturbances

K13.3 **Hairy leukoplakia**

K13.4 **Granuloma and granuloma-like lesions of oral mucosa**
    Eosinophilic granuloma
    Granuloma pyogenicum
    Verrucous xanthoma

K13.5 **Oral submucous fibrosis**
    Submucous fibrosis of tongue

K13.6 **Irritative hyperplasia of oral mucosa**
Excludes2: *irritative hyperplasia of edentulous ridge [denture hyperplasia] (K06.2)*

+ **K13.7** **Other and unspecified lesions of oral mucosa**
K13.70 **Unspecified lesions of oral mucosa**
K13.79 **Other lesions of oral mucosa**
    Focal oral mucinosis

K14 **Diseases of tongue**

Use additional code to identify:
    alcohol abuse and dependence (F10.-)
    exposure to environmental tobacco smoke (Z77.22)
    history of tobacco dependence (Z87.891)
    occupational exposure to environmental tobacco smoke (Z57.31)
    tobacco dependence (F17.-)
    tobacco use (Z72.0)

Excludes2: *erythroplakia (K13.29)*
    focal epithelial hyperplasia (K13.29)
    leukedema of tongue (K13.29)
    leukoplakia of tongue (K13.21)
    hairy leukoplakia (K13.3)
    macroglossia (congenital) (Q38.2)
    submucous fibrosis of tongue (K13.5)

K14.0 **Glossitis**
    Abscess of tongue
    Ulceration (traumatic) of tongue
Excludes1: *atrophic glossitis (K14.4)*

K14.1 Geographic tongue
Benign migratory glossitis
Glossitis areata exfoliativa
K14.2 Median rhomboid glossitis
K14.3 Hypertrophy of tongue papillae
Black hairy tongue
Coated tongue
Hypertrophy of foliate papillae
Lingua villosa nigra
K14.4 Atrophy of tongue papillae
Atrophic glossitis
K14.5 Plicated tongue
Fissured tongue
Furrowed tongue
Scrotal tongue
Excludes1: *fissured tongue, congenital (Q38.3)*
K14.6 Glossodynia
Glossopyrosis
Painful tongue
K14.8 Other diseases of tongue
Atrophy of tongue
Crenated tongue
Enlargement of tongue
Glossocele
Glossoptosis
Hypertrophy of tongue
K14.9 Disease of tongue, unspecified
Glossopathy NOS

Diseases of esophagus, stomach and duodenum (K20-K31)

Excludes2: *hiatus hernia (K44.-)*

K20 Esophagitis
Use additional code to identify:
alcohol abuse and dependence (F10.-)
Excludes1: *erosion of esophagus (K22.1-)*
esophagitis with gastro-esophageal reflux disease (K21.0-)
reflux esophagitis (K21.0-)
ulcerative esophagitis (K22.1-)
Excludes2: *eosinophilic gastritis or gastroenteritis (K52.81)*
K20.0 Eosinophilic esophagitis
+ **K20.8 Other esophagitis**
K20.80 Other esophagitis without bleeding
Abscess of esophagus
Other esophagitis NOS
MCC **K20.81 Other esophagitis with bleeding**
+ **K20.9 Esophagitis, unspecified**
K20.90 Esophagitis, unspecified without bleeding
Esophagitis NOS
MCC **K20.91 Esophagitis, unspecified with bleeding**
K21 Gastro-esophageal reflux disease
Excludes1: *newborn esophageal reflux (P78.83)*
+ **K21.0 Gastro-esophageal reflux disease with esophagitis**
K21.00 Gastro-esophageal reflux disease with esophagitis, without bleeding
Reflux esophagitis
MCC **K21.01 Gastro-esophageal reflux disease with esophagitis, with bleeding**
K21.9 Gastro-esophageal reflux disease without esophagitis
Esophageal reflux NOS
CC AHA: 1Q, 2016, 18

Gastroesophageal Reflux Disease

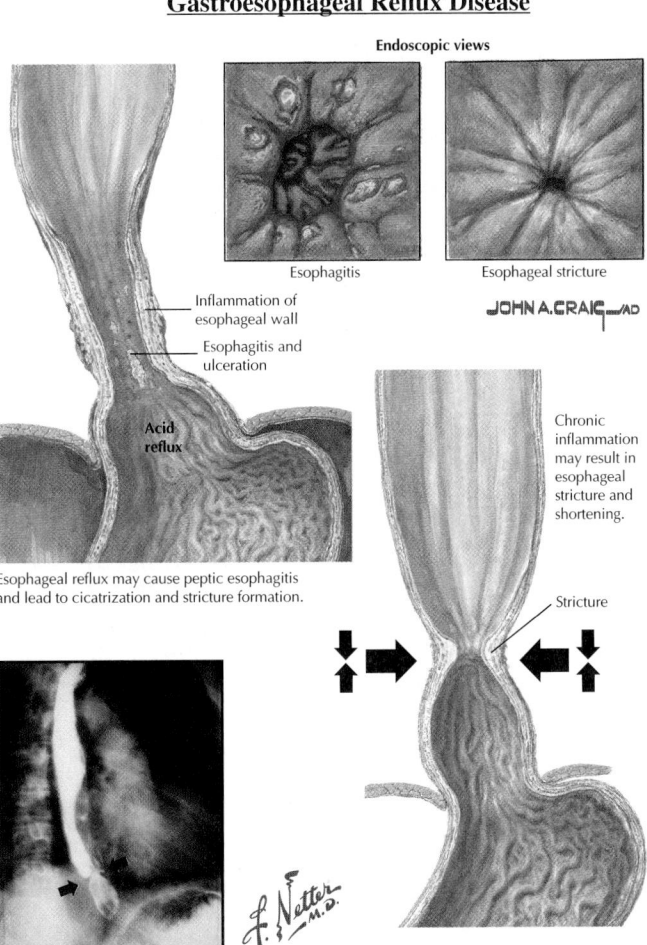

Endoscopic views

Esophagitis

Esophageal stricture

JOHN A. CRAIG _AD

Inflammation of esophageal wall

Esophagitis and ulceration

Acid reflux

Esophageal reflux may cause peptic esophagitis and lead to cicatrization and stricture formation.

Chronic inflammation may result in esophageal stricture and shortening.

Stricture

Barium study shows esophageal stricture.

+, +7th, X + 7th   ● Newborn   ● Pediatric   ● Maternity   ● Adult   ♀ Female   ♂ Male   Manifestation   Unacceptable PDX   HCC   CC   MCC   HAC

Gastrointestinal System Side View

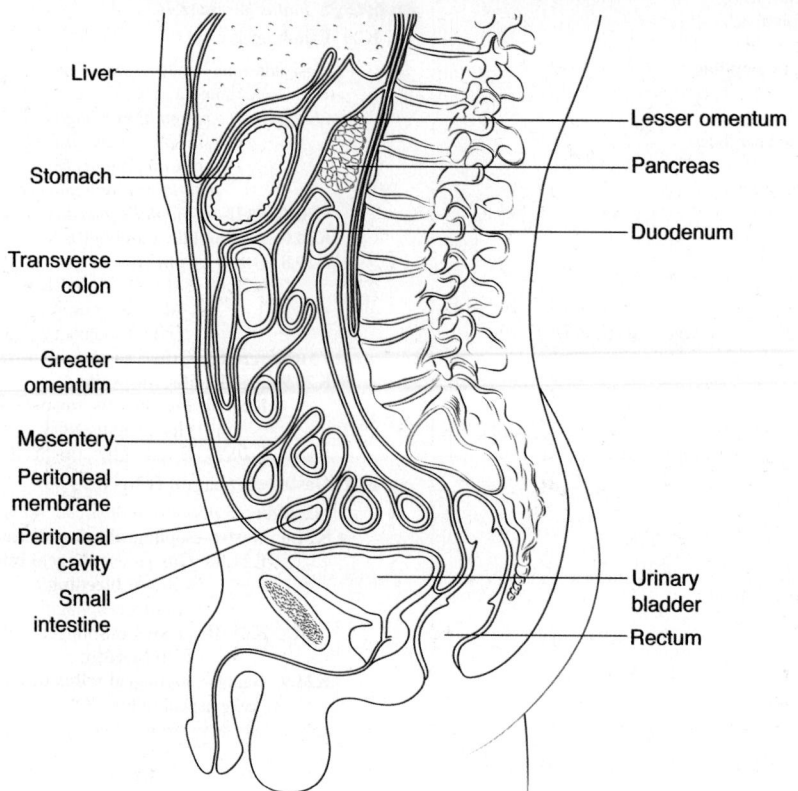

Liver

Stomach

Transverse colon

Greater omentum

Mesentery

Peritoneal membrane

Peritoneal cavity

Small intestine

Lesser omentum

Pancreas

Duodenum

Urinary bladder

Rectum

©AHIMA

Gastrointestinal System Front View

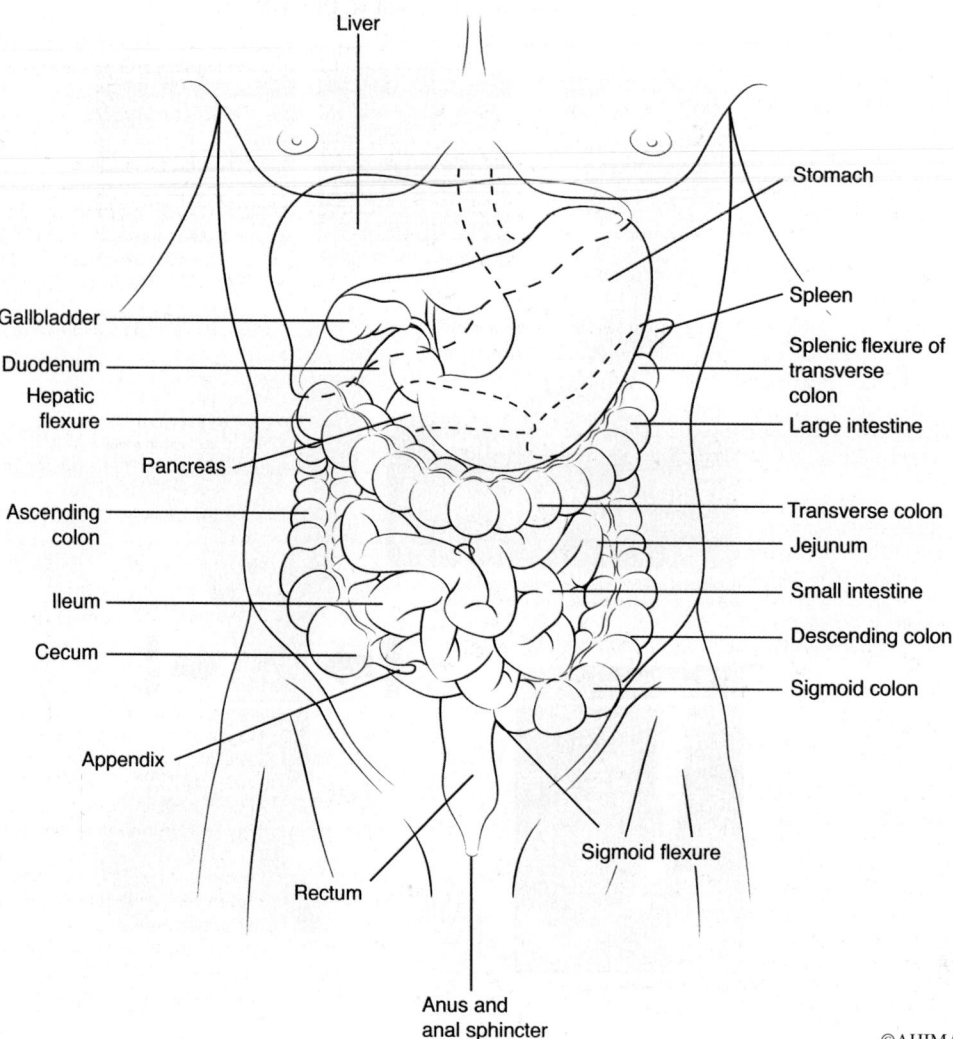

Liver

Gallbladder

Duodenum

Hepatic flexure

Pancreas

Ascending colon

Ileum

Cecum

Appendix

Rectum

Stomach

Spleen

Splenic flexure of transverse colon

Large intestine

Transverse colon

Jejunum

Small intestine

Descending colon

Sigmoid colon

Sigmoid flexure

Anus and anal sphincter

©AHIMA

Upper Gastrointestinal System

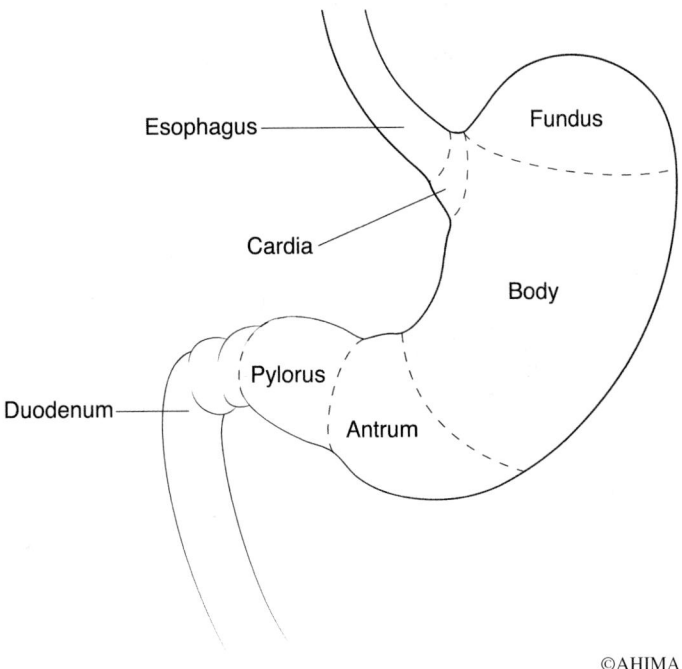

©AHIMA

K22 Other diseases of esophagus

Excludes2: esophageal varices (I85.-)

K22.0 Achalasia of cardia
Achalasia NOS
Cardiospasm
Excludes1: congenital cardiospasm (Q39.5)

+ **K22.1 Ulcer of esophagus**
Barrett's ulcer
Erosion of esophagus
Fungal ulcer of esophagus
Peptic ulcer of esophagus
Ulcer of esophagus due to ingestion of chemicals
Ulcer of esophagus due to ingestion of drugs and medicaments
Ulcerative esophagitis
Code first poisoning due to drug or toxin, if applicable (T36-T65 with fifth or sixth character 1-4 or 6)

Use additional code for adverse effect, if applicable, to identify drug (T36-T50 with fifth or sixth character 5)
Excludes1: Barrett's esophagus (K22.7-)

CC **K22.10 Ulcer of esophagus without bleeding**
Ulcer of esophagus NOS

MCC **K22.11 Ulcer of esophagus with bleeding**
Excludes2: bleeding esophageal varices (I85.01, I85.11)
AHA CC: 3Q, 2018, 22-23

K22.2 Esophageal obstruction
Compression of esophagus
Constriction of esophagus
Stenosis of esophagus
Stricture of esophagus
Excludes1: congenital stenosis or stricture of esophagus (Q39.3)

MCC **K22.3 Perforation of esophagus**
Rupture of esophagus
Excludes1: traumatic perforation of (thoracic) esophagus (S27.8-)

K22.4 Dyskinesia of esophagus
Corkscrew esophagus
Diffuse esophageal spasm
Spasm of esophagus
Excludes1: cardiospasm (K22.0)

K22.5 Diverticulum of esophagus, acquired
Esophageal pouch, acquired
Excludes1: diverticulum of esophagus (congenital) (Q39.6)

MCC **K22.6 Gastro-esophageal laceration-hemorrhage syndrome**
Mallory-Weiss syndrome

+ **K22.7 Barrett's esophagus**
Barrett's disease
Barrett's syndrome
Excludes1: Barrett's ulcer (K22.1)
malignant neoplasm of esophagus (C15.-)

K22.70 Barrett's esophagus without dysplasia
Barrett's esophagus NOS

+ **K22.71 Barrett's esophagus with dysplasia**

K22.710 Barrett's esophagus with low grade dysplasia

K22.711 Barrett's esophagus with high grade dysplasia

K22.719 Barrett's esophagus with dysplasia, unspecified

K22.8 Other specified diseases of esophagus
Hemorrhage of esophagus NOS
Excludes2: esophageal varices (I85.-)
Paterson-Kelly syndrome (D50.1)
AHA CC: 1Q, 2020, 16

K22.9 Disease of esophagus, unspecified

K23 Disorders of esophagus in diseases classified elsewhere

Code first underlying disease, such as:
congenital syphilis (A50.5)
Excludes1: late syphilis (A52.79)
megaesophagus due to Chagas' disease (B57.31)
tuberculosis (A18.83)
Valid 3-character code, no further characters required

K25 Gastric ulcer

Includes: erosion (acute) of stomach
pylorus ulcer (peptic)
stomach ulcer (peptic)
Use additional code to identify:
alcohol abuse and dependence (F10.-)
Excludes1: acute gastritis (K29.0-)
peptic ulcer NOS (K27.-)

MCC **K25.0 Acute gastric ulcer with hemorrhage**
MCC **K25.1 Acute gastric ulcer with perforation**
MCC **K25.2 Acute gastric ulcer with both hemorrhage and perforation**
CC **K25.3 Acute gastric ulcer without hemorrhage or perforation**
MCC **K25.4 Chronic or unspecified gastric ulcer with hemorrhage**
AHA CC: 3Q, 2017, 27
MCC **K25.5 Chronic or unspecified gastric ulcer with perforation**
MCC **K25.6 Chronic or unspecified gastric ulcer with both hemorrhage and perforation**
K25.7 Chronic gastric ulcer without hemorrhage or perforation
K25.9 Gastric ulcer, unspecified as acute or chronic, without hemorrhage or perforation

+, +7th, X + 7th • Newborn • Pediatric • Maternity • Adult ♀ Female ♂ Male Manifestation Unacceptable PDX HCC CC MCC HAC

Ulcers: Gastric, Duodena, Jejunal

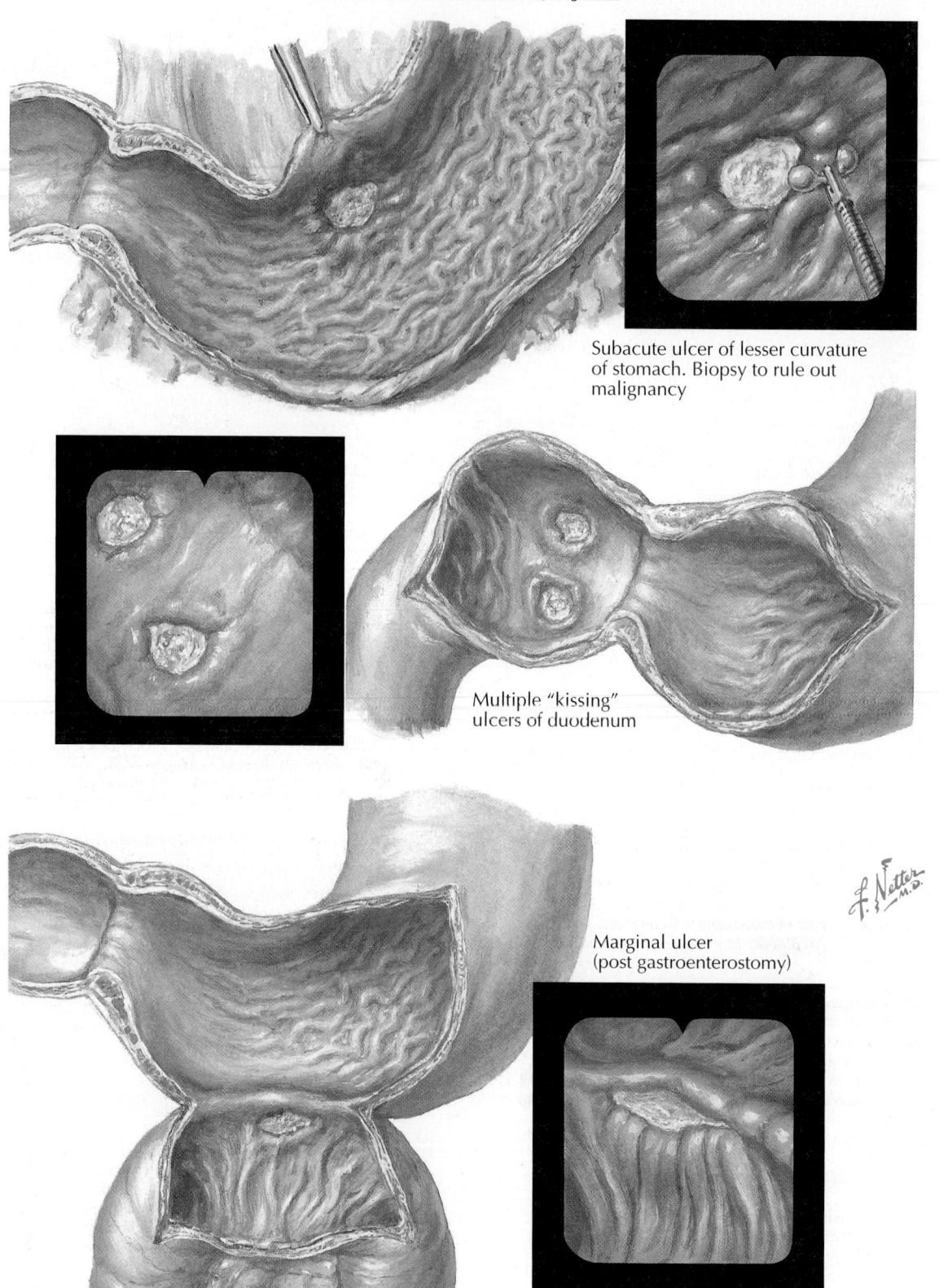

Subacute ulcer of lesser curvature of stomach. Biopsy to rule out malignancy

Multiple "kissing" ulcers of duodenum

Marginal ulcer (post gastroenterostomy)

K26 Duodenal ulcer

Includes: erosion (acute) of duodenum
duodenum ulcer (peptic)
postpyloric ulcer (peptic)
Use additional code to identify:
alcohol abuse and dependence (F10.-)
Excludes1: peptic ulcer NOS (K27.-)

MCC **K26.0 Acute duodenal ulcer with hemorrhage**
K26.1 Acute duodenal ulcer with perforation
K26.2 Acute duodenal ulcer with both hemorrhage and perforation
CC **K26.3 Acute duodenal ulcer without hemorrhage or perforation**
MCC **K26.4 Chronic or unspecified duodenal ulcer with hemorrhage**
CC AHA: 1Q, 2016, 14
MCC **K26.5 Chronic or unspecified duodenal ulcer with perforation**
MCC **K26.6 Chronic or unspecified duodenal ulcer with both hemorrhage and perforation**
K26.7 Chronic duodenal ulcer without hemorrhage or perforation
K26.9 Duodenal ulcer, unspecified as acute or chronic, without hemorrhage or perforation

K27 Peptic ulcer, site unspecified

Includes: gastroduodenal ulcer NOS
peptic ulcer NOS
Use additional code to identify:
alcohol abuse and dependence (F10.-)
Excludes1: peptic ulcer of newborn (P78.82)

MCC **K27.0 Acute peptic ulcer, site unspecified, with hemorrhage**
MCC **K27.1 Acute peptic ulcer, site unspecified, with perforation**
K27.2 Acute peptic ulcer, site unspecified, with both hemorrhage and perforation
CC **K27.3 Acute peptic ulcer, site unspecified, without hemorrhage or perforation**
MCC **K27.4 Chronic or unspecified peptic ulcer, site unspecified, with hemorrhage**
MCC **K27.5 Chronic or unspecified peptic ulcer, site unspecified, with perforation**
MCC **K27.6 Chronic or unspecified peptic ulcer, site unspecified, with both hemorrhage and perforation**
K27.7 Chronic peptic ulcer, site unspecified, without hemorrhage or perforation
K27.9 Peptic ulcer, site unspecified, unspecified as acute or chronic, without hemorrhage or perforation

K28 Gastrojejunal ulcer

Includes: anastomotic ulcer (peptic) or erosion
gastrocolic ulcer (peptic) or erosion
gastrointestinal ulcer (peptic) or erosion
gastrojejunal ulcer (peptic) or erosion
jejunal ulcer (peptic) or erosion
marginal ulcer (peptic) or erosion
stomal ulcer (peptic) or erosion
Use additional code to identify:
alcohol abuse and dependence (F10.-)
Excludes1: primary ulcer of small intestine (K63.3)

MCC **K28.0 Acute gastrojejunal ulcer with hemorrhage**
MCC **K28.1 Acute gastrojejunal ulcer with perforation**
MCC **K28.2 Acute gastrojejunal ulcer with both hemorrhage and perforation**
CC **K28.3 Acute gastrojejunal ulcer without hemorrhage or perforation**
MCC **K28.4 Chronic or unspecified gastrojejunal ulcer with hemorrhage**
MCC **K28.5 Chronic or unspecified gastrojejunal ulcer with perforation**
MCC **K28.6 Chronic or unspecified gastrojejunal ulcer with both hemorrhage and perforation**
K28.7 Chronic gastrojejunal ulcer without hemorrhage or perforation
K28.9 Gastrojejunal ulcer, unspecified as acute or chronic, without hemorrhage or perforation

K29 Gastritis and duodenitis

Excludes1: eosinophilic gastritis or gastroenteritis (K52.81)
Zollinger-Ellison syndrome (E16.4)

+ **K29.0 Acute gastritis**
Use additional code to identify:
alcohol abuse and dependence (F10.-)
Excludes1: erosion (acute) of stomach (K25.-)
K29.00 Acute gastritis without bleeding
MCC **K29.01 Acute gastritis with bleeding**

+ **K29.2 Alcoholic gastritis**
Use additional code to identify:
alcohol abuse and dependence (F10.-)
K29.20 Alcoholic gastritis without bleeding
MCC **K29.21 Alcoholic gastritis with bleeding**
+ **K29.3 Chronic superficial gastritis**
K29.30 Chronic superficial gastritis without bleeding
MCC **K29.31 Chronic superficial gastritis with bleeding**
+ **K29.4 Chronic atrophic gastritis**
Gastric atrophy
K29.40 Chronic atrophic gastritis without bleeding
MCC **K29.41 Chronic atrophic gastritis with bleeding**
+ **K29.5 Unspecified chronic gastritis**
Chronic antral gastritis
Chronic fundal gastritis
K29.50 Unspecified chronic gastritis without bleeding
MCC **K29.51 Unspecified chronic gastritis with bleeding**
+ **K29.6 Other gastritis**
Giant hypertrophic gastritis
Granulomatous gastritis
Ménétrier's disease
K29.60 Other gastritis without bleeding
MCC **K29.61 Other gastritis with bleeding**
+ **K29.7 Gastritis, unspecified**
K29.70 Gastritis, unspecified, without bleeding
MCC **K29.71 Gastritis, unspecified, with bleeding**
+ **K29.8 Duodenitis**
K29.80 Duodenitis without bleeding
MCC **K29.81 Duodenitis with bleeding**
AHA CC: 3Q, 2018, 22-23
+ **K29.9 Gastroduodenitis, unspecified**
K29.90 Gastroduodenitis, unspecified, without bleeding
MCC **K29.91 Gastroduodenitis, unspecified, with bleeding**

K30 Functional dyspepsia

Indigestion
Excludes1: dyspepsia NOS (R10.13)
heartburn (R12)
nervous dyspepsia (F45.8)
neurotic dyspepsia (F45.8)
psychogenic dyspepsia (F45.8)
Valid 3-character code, no further characters required

K31 Other diseases of stomach and duodenum

Includes: functional disorders of stomach
Excludes2: diabetic gastroparesis (E08.43, E09.43, E10.43, E11.43, E13.43)
diverticulum of duodenum (K57.00-K57.13)

K31.0 Acute dilatation of stomach
Acute distention of stomach
● **K31.1 Adult hypertrophic pyloric stenosis**
Pyloric stenosis NOS
Excludes1: congenital or infantile pyloric stenosis (Q40.0)
K31.2 Hourglass stricture and stenosis of stomach
Excludes1: congenital hourglass stomach (Q40.2)
hourglass contraction of stomach (K31.89)
K31.3 Pylorospasm, not elsewhere classified
Excludes1: congenital or infantile pylorospasm (Q40.0)
neurotic pylorospasm (F45.8)
psychogenic pylorospasm (F45.8)v
K31.4 Gastric diverticulum
Excludes1: congenital diverticulum of stomach (Q40.2)
CC **K31.5 Obstruction of duodenum**
Constriction of duodenum
Duodenal ileus (chronic)
Stenosis of duodenum
Stricture of duodenum
Volvulus of duodenum
Excludes1: congenital stenosis of duodenum (Q41.0)
CC **K31.6 Fistula of stomach and duodenum**
Gastrocolic fistula
Gastrojejunocolic fistula
K31.7 Polyp of stomach and duodenum
Excludes1: adenomatous polyp of stomach (D13.1)
AHA CC: 1Q, 2020, 16
+ **K31.8 Other specified diseases of stomach and duodenum**
+ **K31.81 Angiodysplasia of stomach and duodenum**
MCC **K31.811 Angiodysplasia of stomach and duodenum with bleeding**

+, +7th, X + 7th   ● Newborn   ● Pediatric   ● Maternity   ● Adult   ♀ Female   ♂ Male   Manifestation   Unacceptable PDX   HCC   CC   MCC   HAC

K31.819 Angiodysplasia of stomach and duodenum without bleeding
Angiodysplasia of stomach and duodenum NOS

MCC **K31.82 Dieulafoy lesion (hemorrhagic) of stomach and duodenum**
Excludes2: Dieulafoy lesion of intestine (K63.81)

K31.83 Achlorhydria

K31.84 Gastroparesis
Gastroparalysis
Code first underlying disease, if known, such as:
anorexia nervosa (F50.0-)
diabetes mellitus (E08.43, E09.43, E10.43, E11.43, E13.43)
scleroderma (M34.-)
AHA CC: 4Q, 2013, 114-115

K31.89 Other diseases of stomach and duodenum
AHA CC: 1Q, 2017, 28; 1Q, 2020, 15

K31.9 Disease of stomach and duodenum, unspecified

Diseases of appendix (K35-K38)

K35 Acute appendicitis

+ **K35.2 Acute appendicitis with generalized peritonitis**
Appendicitis (acute) with generalized (diffuse) peritonitis following rupture or perforation of appendix
AHA CC: 4Q, 2018, 17-18

CC **K35.20 Acute appendicitis with generalized peritonitis, without abscess**
(Acute) appendicitis with generalized peritonitis NOS
AHA CC: 4Q, 2018, 18

MCC **K35.21 Acute appendicitis with generalized peritonitis, with abscess**

+ **K35.3 Acute appendicitis with localized peritonitis**
AHA CC: 4Q, 2018, 17-18

CC **K35.30 Acute appendicitis with localized peritonitis, without perforation or gangrene**
Acute appendicitis with localized peritonitis NOS

CC **K35.31 Acute appendicitis with localized peritonitis and gangrene, without perforation**

MCC **K35.32 Acute appendicitis with perforation and localized peritonitis, without abscess**
(Acute) appendicitis with perforation NOS
Perforated appendix NOS
Ruptured appendix (with localized peritonitis) NOS
AHA CC: 4Q, 2018, 18; 1Q, 2020, 16

MCC **K35.33 Acute appendicitis with perforation and localized peritonitis, with abscess**
(Acute) appendicitis with (peritoneal) abscess NOS
Ruptured appendix with localized peritonitis and abscess

+ **K35.8 Other and unspecified acute appendicitis**
CC **K35.80 Unspecified acute appendicitis**
Acute appendicitis NOS
Acute appendicitis without (localized) (generalized) peritonitis

+ **K35.89 Other acute appendicitis**
AHA CC: 4Q, 2018, 17-18

CC **K35.890 Other acute appendicitis without perforation or gangrene**

CC **K35.891 Other acute appendicitis without perforation, with gangrene**
(Acute) appendicitis with gangrene NOS

K36 Other appendicitis
Chronic appendicitis
Recurrent appendicitis
Valid 3-character code, no further characters required

K37 Unspecified appendicitis
Excludes1: -unspecified appendicitis with peritonitis (K35.2-, K35.3-)
Valid 3-character code, no further characters required

K38 Other diseases of appendix

K38.0 Hyperplasia of appendix

K38.1 Appendicular concretions
Fecalith of appendix
Stercolith of appendix

K38.2 Diverticulum of appendix

K38.3 Fistula of appendix

K38.8 Other specified diseases of appendix
Intussusception of appendix

K38.9 Disease of appendix, unspecified

Hernia (K40-K46)

NOTE Hernia with both gangrene and obstruction is classified to hernia with gangrene.

Includes: acquired hernia
congenital [except diaphragmatic or hiatus] hernia
recurrent hernia

K40 Inguinal hernia

Includes: bubonocele
direct inguinal hernia
double inguinal hernia
indirect inguinal hernia
inguinal hernia NOS
oblique inguinal hernia
scrotal hernia

+ **K40.0 Bilateral inguinal hernia, with obstruction, without gangrene**
Inguinal hernia (bilateral) causing obstruction without gangrene
Incarcerated inguinal hernia (bilateral) without gangrene
Irreducible inguinal hernia (bilateral) without gangrene
Strangulated inguinal hernia (bilateral) without gangrene

CC **K40.00 Bilateral inguinal hernia, with obstruction, without gangrene, not specified as recurrent**
Bilateral inguinal hernia, with obstruction, without gangrene NOS

CC **K40.01 Bilateral inguinal hernia, with obstruction, without gangrene, recurrent**

+ **K40.1 Bilateral inguinal hernia, with gangrene**
MCC **K40.10 Bilateral inguinal hernia, with gangrene, not specified as recurrent**
Bilateral inguinal hernia, with gangrene NOS

MCC **K40.11 Bilateral inguinal hernia, with gangrene, recurrent**

Abdominal Wall: Inguinal Hernia

Peritoneum
Vas deferens
Obliterated processus vaginalis
Tunica vaginalis
Normally obliterated processus vaginalis
Completely patent processus vaginalis
Partially patent processus vaginalis (small congenital hernia)

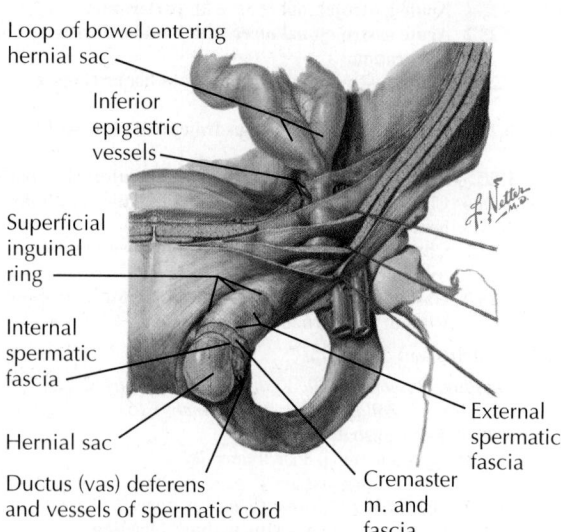

Loop of bowel entering hernial sac
Inferior epigastric vessels
Superficial inguinal ring
Internal spermatic fascia
Hernial sac
Ductus (vas) deferens and vessels of spermatic cord
External spermatic fascia
Cremaster m. and fascia

+, +7th, X + 7th   ● Newborn   ● Pediatric   ● Maternity   ● Adult   ♀ Female   ♂ Male   Manifestation   Unacceptable PDX   HCC   CC   MCC   HAC

+ **K40.2** **Bilateral inguinal hernia, without obstruction or gangrene**
    K40.20 **Bilateral inguinal hernia, without obstruction or gangrene, not specified as recurrent**
        Bilateral inguinal hernia NOS
    K40.21 **Bilateral inguinal hernia, without obstruction or gangrene, recurrent**

+ **K40.3** **Unilateral inguinal hernia, with obstruction, without gangrene**
    Inguinal hernia (unilateral) causing obstruction without gangrene
    Incarcerated inguinal hernia (unilateral) without gangrene
    Irreducible inguinal hernia (unilateral) without gangrene
    Strangulated inguinal hernia (unilateral) without gangrene
  CC **K40.30** **Unilateral inguinal hernia, with obstruction, without gangrene, not specified as recurrent**
        Inguinal hernia, with obstruction NOS
        Unilateral inguinal hernia, with obstruction, without gangrene NOS
  CC **K40.31** **Unilateral inguinal hernia, with obstruction, without gangrene, recurrent**

+ **K40.4** **Unilateral inguinal hernia, with gangrene**
  MCC **K40.40** **Unilateral inguinal hernia, with gangrene, not specified as recurrent**
        Inguinal hernia with gangrene NOS
        Unilateral inguinal hernia with gangrene NOS
  MCC **K40.41** **Unilateral inguinal hernia, with gangrene, recurrent**

+ **K40.9** **Unilateral inguinal hernia, without obstruction or gangrene**
    K40.90 **Unilateral inguinal hernia, without obstruction or gangrene, not specified as recurrent**
        Inguinal hernia NOS
        Unilateral inguinal hernia NOS
    K40.91 **Unilateral inguinal hernia, without obstruction or gangrene, recurrent**

K41 **Femoral hernia**

+ **K41.0** **Bilateral femoral hernia, with obstruction, without gangrene**
    Femoral hernia (bilateral) causing obstruction, without gangrene
    Incarcerated femoral hernia (bilateral), without gangrene
    Irreducible femoral hernia (bilateral), without gangrene
    Strangulated femoral hernia (bilateral), without gangrene
  CC **K41.00** **Bilateral femoral hernia, with obstruction, without gangrene, not specified as recurrent**
        Bilateral femoral hernia, with obstruction, without gangrene NOS
  CC **K41.01** **Bilateral femoral hernia, with obstruction, without gangrene, recurrent**

+ **K41.1** **Bilateral femoral hernia, with gangrene**
  MCC **K41.10** **Bilateral femoral hernia, with gangrene, not specified as recurrent**
        Bilateral femoral hernia, with gangrene NOS
  MCC **K41.11** **Bilateral femoral hernia, with gangrene, recurrent**

+ **K41.2** **Bilateral femoral hernia, without obstruction or gangrene**
    K41.20 **Bilateral femoral hernia, without obstruction or gangrene, not specified as recurrent**
        Bilateral femoral hernia NOS
    K41.21 **Bilateral femoral hernia, without obstruction or gangrene, recurrent**

+ **K41.3** **Unilateral femoral hernia, with obstruction, without gangrene**
    Femoral hernia (unilateral) causing obstruction, without gangrene
    Incarcerated femoral hernia (unilateral), without gangrene
    Irreducible femoral hernia (unilateral), without gangrene
    Strangulated femoral hernia (unilateral), without gangrene
  CC **K41.30** **Unilateral femoral hernia, with obstruction, without gangrene, not specified as recurrent**
        Femoral hernia, with obstruction NOS
        Unilateral femoral hernia, with obstruction NOS
  CC **K41.31** **Unilateral femoral hernia, with obstruction, without gangrene, recurrent**

+ **K41.4** **Unilateral femoral hernia, with gangrene**
  CC **K41.40** **Unilateral femoral hernia, with gangrene, not specified as recurrent**
        Femoral hernia, with gangrene NOS
        Unilateral femoral hernia, with gangrene NOS
  CC **K41.41** **Unilateral femoral hernia, with gangrene, recurrent**

+ **K41.9** **Unilateral femoral hernia, without obstruction or gangrene**
    K41.90 **Unilateral femoral hernia, without obstruction or gangrene, not specified as recurrent**
        Femoral hernia NOS
        Unilateral femoral hernia NOS
    K41.91 **Unilateral femoral hernia, without obstruction or gangrene, recurrent**

K42 **Umbilical hernia**
  Includes: paraumbilical hernia
  Excludes1: *omphalocele (Q79.2)*

  K42.0 **Umbilical hernia with obstruction, without gangrene**
    Umbilical hernia causing obstruction, without gangrene
    Incarcerated umbilical hernia, without gangrene
    Irreducible umbilical hernia, without gangrene
    Strangulated umbilical hernia, without gangrene

  K42.1 **Umbilical hernia with gangrene**
    Gangrenous umbilical hernia

  K42.9 **Umbilical hernia without obstruction or gangrene**
    Umbilical hernia NOS

K43 **Ventral hernia**

  K43.0 **Incisional hernia with obstruction, without gangrene**
    Incisional hernia causing obstruction, without gangrene
    Incarcerated incisional hernia, without gangrene
    Irreducible incisional hernia, without gangrene
    Strangulated incisional hernia, without gangrene

  K43.1 **Incisional hernia with gangrene**
    Gangrenous incisional hernia
    AHA CC: 2Q, 2020, 22

  K43.2 **Incisional hernia without obstruction or gangrene**
    Incisional hernia NOS

  K43.3 **Parastomal hernia with obstruction, without gangrene**
    Incarcerated parastomal hernia, without gangrene
    Irreducible parastomal hernia, without gangrene
    Parastomal hernia causing obstruction, without gangrene
    Strangulated parastomal hernia, without gangrene

  K43.4 **Parastomal hernia with gangrene**
    Gangrenous parastomal hernia

  K43.5 **Parastomal hernia without obstruction or gangrene**
    Parastomal hernia NOS

  K43.6 **Other and unspecified ventral hernia with obstruction, without gangrene**
    Epigastric hernia causing obstruction, without gangrene
    Hypogastric hernia causing obstruction, without gangrene
    Incarcerated epigastric hernia without gangrene
    Incarcerated hypogastric hernia without gangrene
    Incarcerated midline hernia without gangrene
    Incarcerated spigelian hernia without gangrene
    Incarcerated subxiphoid hernia without gangrene
    Irreducible epigastric hernia without gangrene
    Irreducible hypogastric hernia without gangrene
    Irreducible midline hernia without gangrene
    Irreducible spigelian hernia without gangrene
    Irreducible subxiphoid hernia without gangrene
    Midline hernia causing obstruction, without gangrene
    Spigelian hernia causing obstruction, without gangrene
    Strangulated epigastric hernia without gangrene
    Strangulated hypogastric hernia without gangrene
    Strangulated midline hernia without gangrene
    Strangulated spigelian hernia without gangrene
    Strangulated subxiphoid hernia without gangrene
    Subxiphoid hernia causing obstruction, without gangrene

  K43.7 **Other and unspecified ventral hernia with gangrene**
    Any condition listed under K43.6 specified as gangrenous

  K43.9 **Ventral hernia without obstruction or gangrene**
    Epigastric hernia
    Ventral hernia NOS

+, +7th, X + 7th   ● Newborn   ● Pediatric   ● Maternity   ● Adult   ♀ Female   ♂ Male   Manifestation   Unacceptable PDX   HCC   CC   MCC   HAC

K44 Diaphragmatic hernia

Includes: hiatus hernia (esophageal) (sliding)
paraesophageal hernia

Excludes1: *congenital diaphragmatic hernia (Q79.0)*
congenital hiatus hernia (Q40.1)

K44.0 Diaphragmatic hernia with obstruction, without gangrene
Diaphragmatic hernia causing obstruction
Incarcerated diaphragmatic hernia
Irreducible diaphragmatic hernia
Strangulated diaphragmatic hernia

K44.1 Diaphragmatic hernia with gangrene
Gangrenous diaphragmatic hernia

K44.9 Diaphragmatic hernia without obstruction or gangrene
Diaphragmatic hernia NOS

K45 Other abdominal hernia

Includes: abdominal hernia, specified site NEC
lumbar hernia
obturator hernia
pudendal hernia
retroperitoneal hernia
sciatic hernia

K45.0 Other specified abdominal hernia with obstruction, without gangrene
Other specified abdominal hernia causing obstruction
Other specified incarcerated abdominal hernia
Other specified irreducible abdominal hernia
Other specified strangulated abdominal hernia

K45.1 Other specified abdominal hernia with gangrene
Any condition listed under K45 specified as gangrenous

K45.8 Other specified abdominal hernia without obstruction or gangrene

K46 Unspecified abdominal hernia

Includes: enterocele
epiplocele
hernia NOS
interstitial hernia
intestinal hernia
intra-abdominal hernia

Excludes1: *vaginal enterocele (N81.5)*

K46.0 Unspecified abdominal hernia with obstruction, without gangrene
Unspecified abdominal hernia causing obstruction
Unspecified incarcerated abdominal hernia
Unspecified irreducible abdominal hernia
Unspecified strangulated abdominal hernia

K46.1 Unspecified abdominal hernia with gangrene
Any condition listed under K46 specified as gangrenous

K46.9 Unspecified abdominal hernia without obstruction or gangrene
Abdominal hernia NOS

Noninfective enteritis and colitis (K50-K52)

Includes: noninfective inflammatory bowel disease

Excludes1: *irritable bowel syndrome (K58.-)*
megacolon (K59.3-)

K50 Crohn's disease [regional enteritis]

Includes: granulomatous enteritis
Use additional code to identify manifestations, such as:
pyoderma gangrenosum (L88)

Excludes1: *ulcerative colitis (K51.-)*

+ **K50.0 Crohn's disease of small intestine**
Crohn's disease [regional enteritis] of duodenum
Crohn's disease [regional enteritis] of ileum
Crohn's disease [regional enteritis] of jejunum
Regional ileitis
Terminal ileitis

Excludes1: *Crohn's disease of both small and large*
intestine (K50.8-)

CC **K50.00 Crohn's disease of small intestine without complications**

+ **K50.01 Crohn's disease of small intestine with complications**

CC **K50.011 Crohn's disease of small intestine with rectal bleeding**

CC **K50.012 Crohn's disease of small intestine with intestinal obstruction**

CC **K50.013 Crohn's disease of small intestine with fistula**

CC **K50.014 Crohn's disease of small intestine with abscess**
AHA CC: 4Q, 2012, 104

CC **K50.018 Crohn's disease of small intestine with other complication**

CC **K50.019 Crohn's disease of small intestine with unspecified complications**

+ **K50.1 Crohn's disease of large intestine**
Crohn's disease [regional enteritis] of colon
Crohn's disease [regional enteritis] of large bowel
Crohn's disease [regional enteritis] of rectum
Granulomatous colitis
Regional colitis

Excludes1: *Crohn's disease of both small and large*
intestine (K50.8)

CC **K50.10 Crohn's disease of large intestine without complications**

+ **K50.11 Crohn's disease of large intestine with complications**

CC **K50.111 Crohn's disease of large intestine with rectal bleeding**

CC **K50.112 Crohn's disease of large intestine with intestinal obstruction**

CC **K50.113 Crohn's disease of large intestine with fistula**

CC **K50.114 Crohn's disease of large intestine with abscess**
AHA CC: 4Q, 2012, 104

CC **K50.118 Crohn's disease of large intestine with other complication**

CC **K50.119 Crohn's disease of large intestine with unspecified complications**

+ **K50.8 Crohn's disease of both small and large intestine**

CC **K50.80 Crohn's disease of both small and large intestine without complications**

+ **K50.81 Crohn's disease of both small and large intestine with complications**

CC **K50.811 Crohn's disease of both small and large intestine with rectal bleeding**

CC **K50.812 Crohn's disease of both small and large intestine with intestinal obstruction**

CC **K50.813 Crohn's disease of both small and large intestine with fistula**

CC **K50.814 Crohn's disease of both small and large intestine with abscess**

CC **K50.818 Crohn's disease of both small and large intestine with other complication**

CC **K50.819 Crohn's disease of both small and large intestine with unspecified complications**

+, +7th, X + 7th • Newborn • Pediatric • Maternity • Adult ♀ Female ♂ Male Manifestation Unacceptable PDX HCC CC MCC HAC

Inflammatory Bowel Disease: Progression of Inflammatory Process in Chron's Disease

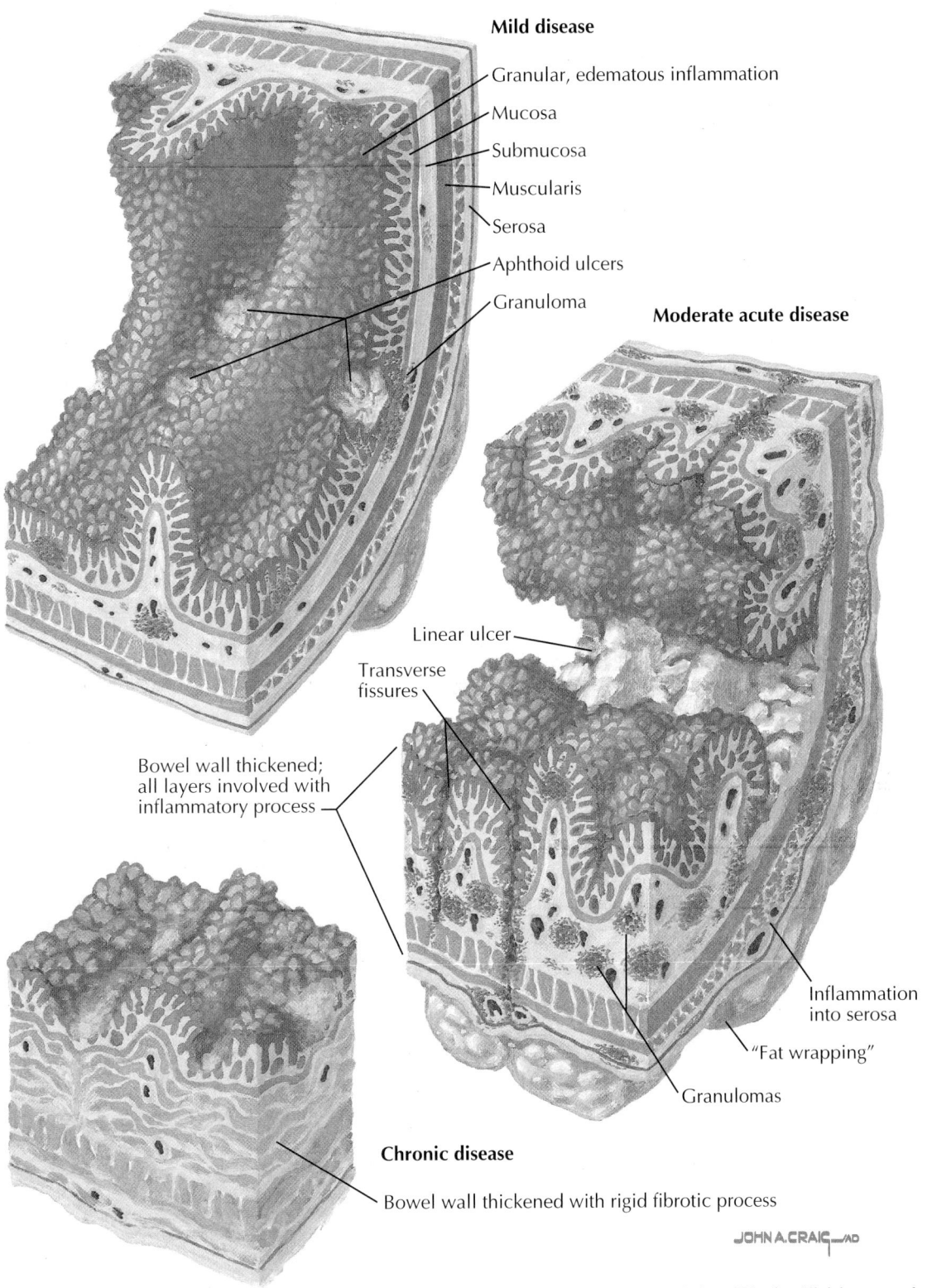

Mild disease

Granular, edematous inflammation

Mucosa

Submucosa

Muscularis

Serosa

Aphthoid ulcers

Granuloma

Moderate acute disease

Linear ulcer

Transverse fissures

Bowel wall thickened; all layers involved with inflammatory process

Inflammation into serosa

"Fat wrapping"

Granulomas

Chronic disease

Bowel wall thickened with rigid fibrotic process

JOHN A.CRAIG˷AD

+ **K50.9** **Crohn's disease, unspecified**
  CC **K50.90** **Crohn's disease, unspecified, without complications**
  Crohn's disease NOS
  Regional enteritis NOS
  + **K50.91** **Crohn's disease, unspecified, with complications**
    CC **K50.911** **Crohn's disease, unspecified, with rectal bleeding**
    CC **K50.912** **Crohn's disease, unspecified, with intestinal obstruction**
    CC **K50.913** **Crohn's disease, unspecified, with fistula**
    CC **K50.914** **Crohn's disease, unspecified, with abscess**
    CC **K50.918** **Crohn's disease, unspecified, with other complication**
    CC **K50.919** **Crohn's disease, unspecified, with unspecified complications**

K51 **Ulcerative colitis**
  Use additional code to identify manifestations, such as: pyoderma gangrenosum (L88)
  Excludes1: *Crohn's disease [regional enteritis] (K50.-)*
  + **K51.0** **Ulcerative (chronic) pancolitis**
    Backwash ileitis
    CC **K51.00** **Ulcerative (chronic) pancolitis without complications**
    Ulcerative (chronic) pancolitis NOS
    + **K51.01** **Ulcerative (chronic) pancolitis with complications**
      CC **K51.011** **Ulcerative (chronic) pancolitis with rectal bleeding**
      CC **K51.012** **Ulcerative (chronic) pancolitis with intestinal obstruction**
      CC **K51.013** **Ulcerative (chronic) pancolitis with fistula**
      CC **K51.014** **Ulcerative (chronic) pancolitis with abscess**
      CC **K51.018** **Ulcerative (chronic) pancolitis with other complication**
      CC **K51.019** **Ulcerative (chronic) pancolitis with unspecified complications**
  + **K51.2** **Ulcerative (chronic) proctitis**
    CC **K51.20** **Ulcerative (chronic) proctitis without complications**
    Ulcerative (chronic) proctitis NOS
    + **K51.21** **Ulcerative (chronic) proctitis with complications**
      CC **K51.211** **Ulcerative (chronic) proctitis with rectal bleeding**
      CC **K51.212** **Ulcerative (chronic) proctitis with intestinal obstruction**
      CC **K51.213** **Ulcerative (chronic) proctitis with fistula**
      CC **K51.214** **Ulcerative (chronic) proctitis with abscess**
      CC **K51.218** **Ulcerative (chronic) proctitis with other complication**
      CC **K51.219** **Ulcerative (chronic) proctitis with unspecified complications**
  + **K51.3** **Ulcerative (chronic) rectosigmoiditis**
    CC **K51.30** **Ulcerative (chronic) rectosigmoiditis without complications**
    Ulcerative (chronic) rectosigmoiditis NOS
    + **K51.31** **Ulcerative (chronic) rectosigmoiditis with complications**
      CC **K51.311** **Ulcerative (chronic) rectosigmoiditis with rectal bleeding**
      CC **K51.312** **Ulcerative (chronic) rectosigmoiditis with intestinal obstruction**
      CC **K51.313** **Ulcerative (chronic) rectosigmoiditis with fistula**
      CC **K51.314** **Ulcerative (chronic) rectosigmoiditis with abscess**
      CC **K51.318** **Ulcerative (chronic) rectosigmoiditis with other complication**
      CC **K51.319** **Ulcerative (chronic) rectosigmoiditis with unspecified complications**
  + **K51.4** **Inflammatory polyps of colon**
    Excludes1: *adenomatous polyp of colon (D12.6)*
    polyposis of colon (D12.6)
    polyps of colon NOS (K63.5)
    CC **K51.40** **Inflammatory polyps of colon without complications**
    Inflammatory polyps of colon NOS

+ **K51.41** **Inflammatory polyps of colon with complications**
  CC **K51.411** **Inflammatory polyps of colon with rectal bleeding**
  CC **K51.412** **Inflammatory polyps of colon with intestinal obstruction**
  CC **K51.413** **Inflammatory polyps of colon with fistula**
  CC **K51.414** **Inflammatory polyps of colon with abscess**
  CC **K51.418** **Inflammatory polyps of colon with other complication**
  CC **K51.419** **Inflammatory polyps of colon with unspecified complications**
+ **K51.5** **Left sided colitis**
  Left hemicolitis
  CC **K51.50** **Left sided colitis without complications**
  Left sided colitis NOS
  + **K51.51** **Left sided colitis with complications**
    CC **K51.511** **Left sided colitis with rectal bleeding**
    CC **K51.512** **Left sided colitis with intestinal obstruction**
    CC **K51.513** **Left sided colitis with fistula**
    CC **K51.514** **Left sided colitis with abscess**
    CC **K51.518** **Left sided colitis with other complication**
    CC **K51.519** **Left sided colitis with unspecified complications**
+ **K51.8** **Other ulcerative colitis**
  CC **K51.80** **Other ulcerative colitis without complications**
  + **K51.81** **Other ulcerative colitis with complications**
    CC **K51.811** **Other ulcerative colitis with rectal bleeding**
    CC **K51.812** **Other ulcerative colitis with intestinal obstruction**
    CC **K51.813** **Other ulcerative colitis with fistula**
    CC **K51.814** **Other ulcerative colitis with abscess**
    CC **K51.818** **Other ulcerative colitis with other complication**
    CC **K51.819** **Other ulcerative colitis with unspecified complications**
+ **K51.9** **Ulcerative colitis, unspecified**
  CC **K51.90** **Ulcerative colitis, unspecified, without complications**
  + **K51.91** **Ulcerative colitis, unspecified, with complications**
    CC **K51.911** **Ulcerative colitis, unspecified with rectal bleeding**
    CC **K51.912** **Ulcerative colitis, unspecified with intestinal obstruction**
    CC **K51.913** **Ulcerative colitis, unspecified with fistula**
    CC **K51.914** **Ulcerative colitis, unspecified with abscess**
    CC **K51.918** **Ulcerative colitis, unspecified with other complication**
    CC **K51.919** **Ulcerative colitis, unspecified with unspecified complications**

K52 **Other and unspecified noninfective gastroenteritis and colitis**
  AHA CC: 4Q, 2016, 30-31
  CC **K52.0** **Gastroenteritis and colitis due to radiation**
  CC **K52.1** **Toxic gastroenteritis and colitis**
  Drug-induced gastroenteritis and colitis
  Code first (T51-T65) to identify toxic agent
  Use additional code for adverse effect, if applicable, to identify drug (T36-T50 with fifth or sixth character 5)
  AHA CC: 1Q, 2019, 17
  + **K52.2** **Allergic and dietetic gastroenteritis and colitis**
  Food hypersensitivity gastroenteritis or colitis
  Use additional code to identify type of food allergy (Z91.01-, Z91.02-)
  Excludes2: *allergic eosinophilic colitis (K52.82)*
  allergic eosinophilic esophagitis (K20.0)
  allergic eosinophilic gastritis (K52.81)
  allergic eosinophilic gastroenteritis (K52.81)
  food protein-induced proctocolitis (K52.82)
  K52.21 **Food protein-induced enterocolitis syndrome**
  FPIES
  Use additional code for hypovolemic shock, if present (R57.1)

+, +7th, X + 7th   ● Newborn   ● Pediatric   ● Maternity   ● Adult   ♀ Female   ♂ Male   Manifestation   Unacceptable PDX   HCC   CC   MCC   HAC

K52.22 Food protein-induced enteropathy
K52.29 Other allergic and dietetic gastroenteritis and colitis
Food hypersensitivity gastroenteritis or colitis
Immediate gastrointestinal hypersensitivity
K52.3 Indeterminate colitis
Colonic inflammatory bowel disease unclassified (IBDU)
Excludes1: *unspecified colitis (K52.9)*
+ K52.8 Other specified noninfective gastroenteritis and colitis
K52.81 Eosinophilic gastritis or gastroenteritis
Eosinophilic enteritis
Excludes2: *eosinophilic esophagitis (K20.0)*
K52.82 Eosinophilic colitis
Allergic proctocolitis
Food-induced eosinophilic proctocolitis
Food protein-induced proctocolitis
Milk protein-induced proctocolitis
+ K52.83 Microscopic colitis
K52.831 Collagenous colitis
K52.832 Lymphocytic colitis
K52.838 Other microscopic colitis
K52.839 Microscopic colitis, unspecified
K52.89 Other specified noninfective gastroenteritis and colitis
AHA CC: 1Q, 2019, 20-21
K52.9 Noninfective gastroenteritis and colitis, unspecified
Colitis NOS
Enteritis NOS
Gastroenteritis NOS
Ileitis NOS
Jejunitis NOS
Sigmoiditis NOS
Excludes1: *diarrhea NOS (R19.7)*
functional diarrhea (K59.1)
infectious gastroenteritis and colitis
NOS (A09)
neonatal diarrhea (noninfective) (P78.3)
psychogenic diarrhea (F45.8)

Other diseases of intestines (K55-K64)

K55 Vascular disorders of intestine
Excludes1: *necrotizing enterocolitis of newborn (P77.-)*
AHA CC: 4Q, 2016, 32-33
+ K55.0 Acute vascular disorders of intestine
Infarction of appendices epiploicae
Mesenteric (artery) (vein) embolism
Mesenteric (artery) (vein) infarction
Mesenteric (artery) (vein) thrombosis
+ K55.01 Acute (reversible) ischemia of small intestine
MCC **K55.011** Focal (segmental) acute (reversible) ischemia of small intestine
MCC **K55.012** Diffuse acute (reversible) ischemia of small intestine
MCC **K55.019** Acute (reversible) ischemia of small intestine, extent unspecified
+ K55.02 Acute infarction of small intestine
Gangrene of small intestine
Necrosis of small intestine
MCC **K55.021** Focal (segmental) acute infarction of small intestine
MCC **K55.022** Diffuse acute infarction of small intestine
MCC **K55.029** Acute infarction of small intestine, extent unspecified
+ K55.03 Acute (reversible) ischemia of large intestine
Acute fulminant ischemic colitis
Subacute ischemic colitis
MCC **K55.031** Focal (segmental) acute (reversible) ischemia of large intestine
MCC **K55.032** Diffuse acute (reversible) ischemia of large intestine
MCC **K55.039** Acute (reversible) ischemia of large intestine, extent unspecified
AHA CC: 4Q, 2019, 68
+ K55.04 Acute infarction of large intestine
Gangrene of large intestine
Necrosis of large intestine
MCC **K55.041** Focal (segmental) acute infarction of large intestine
MCC **K55.042** Diffuse acute infarction of large intestine
MCC **K55.049** Acute infarction of large intestine, extent unspecified

+ K55.05 Acute (reversible) ischemia of intestine, part unspecified
MCC **K55.051** Focal (segmental) acute (reversible) ischemia of intestine, part unspecified
MCC **K55.052** Diffuse acute (reversible) ischemia of intestine, part unspecified
MCC **K55.059** Acute (reversible) ischemia of intestine, part and extent unspecified
+ K55.06 Acute infarction of intestine, part unspecified
Acute intestinal infarction
Gangrene of intestine
Necrosis of intestine
MCC **K55.061** Focal (segmental) acute infarction of intestine, part unspecified
MCC **K55.062** Diffuse acute infarction of intestine, part unspecified
MCC **K55.069** Acute infarction of intestine, part and extent unspecified
CC **K55.1** Chronic vascular disorders of intestine
Chronic ischemic colitis
Chronic ischemic enteritis
Chronic ischemic enterocolitis
Ischemic stricture of intestine
Mesenteric atherosclerosis
Mesenteric vascular insufficiency
+ K55.2 Angiodysplasia of colon
K55.20 Angiodysplasia of colon without hemorrhage
MCC **K55.21** Angiodysplasia of colon with hemorrhage
AHA CC: 3Q, 2018, 21
+ K55.3 Necrotizing enterocolitis
Excludes1: *necrotizing enterocolitis of newborn (P77.-)*
Excludes2: *necrotizing enterocolitis due to Clostridium difficile (A04.7-)*
MCC **K55.30** Necrotizing enterocolitis, unspecified
Necrotizing enterocolitis, NOS
MCC **K55.31** Stage 1 necrotizing enterocolitis
Necrotizing enterocolitis without pneumatosis, without perforation
MCC **K55.32** Stage 2 necrotizing enterocolitis
Necrotizing enterocolitis with pneumatosis, without perforation
MCC **K55.33** Stage 3 necrotizing enterocolitis
Necrotizing enterocolitis with perforation
Necrotizing enterocolitis with pneumatosis and perforation
CC **K55.8** Other vascular disorders of intestine
CC **K55.9** Vascular disorder of intestine, unspecified
Ischemic colitis
Ischemic enteritis
Ischemic enterocolitis

K56 Paralytic ileus and intestinal obstruction without hernia
Excludes1: *congenital stricture or stenosis of intestine (Q41-Q42)*
cystic fibrosis with meconium ileus (E84.11)
ischemic stricture of intestine (K55.1)
meconium ileus NOS (P76.0)
neonatal intestinal obstructions classifiable to P76.-
obstruction of duodenum (K31.5)
postprocedural intestinal obstruction (K91.3-)
Excludes2: *stenosis of anus or rectum (K62.4)*
CC **K56.0** Paralytic ileus
Paralysis of bowel
Paralysis of colon
Paralysis of intestine
Excludes1: *gallstone ileus (K56.3)*
ileus NOS (K56.7)
obstructive ileus NOS (K56.69-)
CC **K56.1** Intussusception
Intussusception or invagination of bowel
Intussusception or invagination of colon
Intussusception or invagination of intestine
Intussusception or invagination of rectum
Excludes2: *intussusception of appendix (K38.8)*
MCC **K56.2** Volvulus
Strangulation of colon or intestine
Torsion of colon or intestine
Twist of colon or intestine
Excludes2: *volvulus of duodenum (K31.5)*
K56.3 Gallstone ileus
Obstruction of intestine by gallstone

+ **K56.4 Other impaction of intestine**
    K56.41 Fecal impaction
      Excludes1: constipation (K59.0-)
            incomplete defecation (R15.0)
  CC **K56.49 Other impaction of intestine**
+ **K56.5 Intestinal adhesions [bands] with obstruction (postinfection)**
    Abdominal hernia due to adhesions with obstruction
    Peritoneal adhesions [bands] with intestinal obstruction (postinfection)
    AHA CC: 4Q, 2017, 16-17
  CC **K56.50 Intestinal adhesions [bands], unspecified as to partial versus complete obstruction**
    Intestinal adhesions with obstruction NOS
  CC **K56.51 Intestinal adhesions [bands], with partial obstruction**
    Intestinal adhesions with incomplete obstruction
  CC **K56.52 Intestinal adhesions [bands] with complete obstruction**
+ **K56.6 Other and unspecified intestinal obstruction**
    AHA CC: 4Q, 2017, 16-17
  + **K56.60 Unspecified intestinal obstruction**
    CC **K56.600 Partial intestinal obstruction, unspecified as to cause**
      Incomplete intestinal obstruction, NOS
    CC **K56.601 Complete intestinal obstruction, unspecified as to cause**
    CC **K56.609 Unspecified intestinal obstruction, unspecified as to partial versus complete obstruction**
      Intestinal obstruction NOS
  + **K56.69 Other intestinal obstruction**
    Enterostenosis NOS
    Obstructive ileus NOS
    Occlusion of colon or intestine NOS
    Stenosis of colon or intestine NOS
    Stricture of colon or intestine NOS
    Excludes1: intestinal obstruction due to specified condition-code to condition
    CC **K56.690 Other partial intestinal obstruction**
      Other incomplete intestinal obstruction
    CC **K56.691 Other complete intestinal obstruction**
    CC **K56.699 Other intestinal obstruction unspecified as to partial versus complete obstruction**
      Other intestinal obstruction, NEC
CC **K56.7 Ileus, unspecified**
    Excludes1: obstructive ileus (K56.69-)
    Excludes2: intestinal obstruction with hernia (K40-K46)
    AHA CC: 1Q, 2017, 40-41

K57 Diverticular disease of intestine

  Excludes1: congenital diverticulum of intestine (Q43.8)
      Meckel's diverticulum (Q43.0)
  Excludes2: diverticulum of appendix (K38.2)
  Code also if applicable peritonitis K65.-
+ **K57.0 Diverticulitis of small intestine with perforation and abscess**
    Excludes1: diverticulitis of both small and large intestine with perforation and abscess (K57.4-)
  CC **K57.00 Diverticulitis of small intestine with perforation and abscess without bleeding**
  MCC **K57.01 Diverticulitis of small intestine with perforation and abscess with bleeding**
+ **K57.1 Diverticular disease of small intestine without perforation or abscess**
    Excludes1: diverticular disease of both small and large intestine without perforation or abscess (K57.5-)
  K57.10 Diverticulosis of small intestine without perforation or abscess without bleeding
    Diverticular disease of small intestine NOS
  MCC **K57.11 Diverticulosis of small intestine without perforation or abscess with bleeding**
  CC **K57.12 Diverticulitis of small intestine without perforation or abscess without bleeding**
  MCC **K57.13 Diverticulitis of small intestine without perforation or abscess with bleeding**

+ **K57.2 Diverticulitis of large intestine with perforation and abscess**
    Excludes1: diverticulitis of both small and large intestine with perforation and abscess (K57.4-)
  CC **K57.20 Diverticulitis of large intestine with perforation and abscess without bleeding**
  MCC **K57.21 Diverticulitis of large intestine with perforation and abscess with bleeding**
+ **K57.3 Diverticular disease of large intestine without perforation or abscess**
    Excludes1: diverticular disease of both small and large intestine without perforation or abscess (K57.5-)
  K57.30 Diverticulosis of large intestine without perforation or abscess without bleeding
    Diverticular disease of colon NOS
  MCC **K57.31 Diverticulosis of large intestine without perforation or abscess with bleeding**
    AHA CC: 3Q, 2018, 21-22
  CC **K57.32 Diverticulitis of large intestine without perforation or abscess without bleeding**
  MCC **K57.33 Diverticulitis of large intestine without perforation or abscess with bleeding**
+ **K57.4 Diverticulitis of both small and large intestine with perforation and abscess**
  CC **K57.40 Diverticulitis of both small and large intestine with perforation and abscess without bleeding**
  MCC **K57.41 Diverticulitis of both small and large intestine with perforation and abscess with bleeding**
+ **K57.5 Diverticular disease of both small and large intestine without perforation or abscess**
  K57.50 Diverticulosis of both small and large intestine without perforation or abscess without bleeding
    Diverticular disease of both small and large intestine NOS
  MCC **K57.51 Diverticulosis of both small and large intestine without perforation or abscess with bleeding**
  CC **K57.52 Diverticulitis of both small and large intestine without perforation or abscess without bleeding**
  MCC **K57.53 Diverticulitis of both small and large intestine without perforation or abscess with bleeding**
+ **K57.8 Diverticulitis of intestine, part unspecified, with perforation and abscess**
  CC **K57.80 Diverticulitis of intestine, part unspecified, with perforation and abscess without bleeding**
  MCC **K57.81 Diverticulitis of intestine, part unspecified, with perforation and abscess with bleeding**
+ **K57.9 Diverticular disease of intestine, part unspecified, without perforation or abscess**
  K57.90 Diverticulosis of intestine, part unspecified, without perforation or abscess without bleeding
    Diverticular disease of intestine NOS
  MCC **K57.91 Diverticulosis of intestine, part unspecified, without perforation or abscess with bleeding**
  CC **K57.92 Diverticulitis of intestine, part unspecified, without perforation or abscess without bleeding**
  MCC **K57.93 Diverticulitis of intestine, part unspecified, without perforation or abscess with bleeding**

K58 Irritable bowel syndrome

  Includes: irritable colon
      spastic colon
  K58.0 Irritable bowel syndrome with diarrhea
  K58.1 Irritable bowel syndrome with constipation
    AHA CC: 4Q, 2016, 32-33
  K58.2 Mixed irritable bowel syndrome
    AHA CC: 4Q, 2016, 32-33
  K58.8 Other irritable bowel syndrome
    AHA CC: 4Q, 2016, 32-33
  K58.9 Irritable bowel syndrome without diarrhea
    Irritable bowel syndrome NOS

K59 Other functional intestinal disorders

  Excludes1: change in bowel habit NOS (R19.4)
      intestinal malabsorption (K90.-)
      psychogenic intestinal disorders (F45.8)
  Excludes2: functional disorders of stomach (K31.-)

+, +7th, X + 7th   ● Newborn   ● Pediatric   ● Maternity   ● Adult   ♀ Female   ♂ Male   Manifestation   Unacceptable PDX   HCC   CC   MCC   HAC

+ **K59.0** **Constipation**
  Excludes1: *fecal impaction (K56.41)*
       incomplete defecation (R15.0)
  K59.00 **Constipation, unspecified**
  K59.01 **Slow transit constipation**
  K59.02 **Outlet dysfunction constipation**
  K59.03 **Drug induced constipation**
    Use additional code for adverse effect, if applicable, to identify drug (T36-T50 with fifth or sixth character 5)
    AHA CC: 4Q, 2016, 33
  K59.04 **Chronic idiopathic constipation**
    Functional constipation
    AHA CC: 4Q, 2016, 33
  K59.09 **Other constipation**
    Chronic constipation

K59.1 **Functional diarrhea**
  Excludes1: *diarrhea NOS (R19.7)*
    irritable bowel syndrome with diarrhea (K58.0)

CC **K59.2** **Neurogenic bowel, not elsewhere classified**

+ **K59.3** **Megacolon, not elsewhere classified**
  Dilatation of colon
  Code first, if applicable (T51-T65) to identify toxic agent
  Excludes1: *congenital megacolon (aganglionic) (Q43.1)*
    megacolon (due to) (in) Chagas' disease (B57.32)
    megacolon (due to) (in) Clostridium difficile (A04.7-)
    megacolon (due to) (in) Hirschsprung's disease (Q43.1)
  AHA CC: 4Q, 2016, 33-34

  CC **K59.31** **Toxic megacolon**
  CC **K59.39** **Other megacolon**
    Megacolon NOS

K59.4 **Anal spasm**
  Proctalgia fugax

+ **K59.8** **Other specified functional intestinal disorders**
  K59.81 **Ogilvie syndrome**
    Acute colonic pseudo-obstruction (ACPO)
  K59.89 **Other specified functional intestinal disorders**
    Atony of colon
    Pseudo-obstruction (acute) (chronic) of intestine

K59.9 **Functional intestinal disorder, unspecified**

K60 **Fissure and fistula of anal and rectal regions**

  Excludes1: *fissure and fistula of anal and rectal regions with abscess or cellulitis (K61.-)*
  Excludes2: *anal sphincter tear (healed) (nontraumatic) (old) (K62.81)*
K60.0 **Acute anal fissure**
K60.1 **Chronic anal fissure**
K60.2 **Anal fissure, unspecified**
K60.3 **Anal fistula**
K60.4 **Rectal fistula**
  Fistula of rectum to skin
  Excludes1: *rectovaginal fistula (N82.3)*
    vesicorectal fistual (N32.1)
K60.5 **Anorectal fistula**

K61 **Abscess of anal and rectal regions**
  Includes: abscess of anal and rectal regions
    cellulitis of anal and rectal regions
CC **K61.0** **Anal abscess**
  Perianal abscess
  Excludes2: *intrasphincteric abscess (K61.4)*
CC **K61.1** **Rectal abscess**
  Perirectal abscess
  Excludes1: *ischiorectal abscess (K61.39)*
CC **K61.2** **Anorectal abscess**
+ **K61.3** **Ischiorectal abscess**
  AHA CC: 4Q, 2018, 19
  CC **K61.31** **Horseshoe abscess**
  CC **K61.32** **Ischiorectal abscess, NOS**
  K61.39 **Other ischiorectal abscess**
    Abscess of ischiorectal fossa
    Ischiorectal abscess, NOS
CC **K61.4** **Intrasphincteric abscess**
  Intersphincteric abscess
  AHA CC: 4Q, 2018, 19
CC **K61.5** **Supralevator abscess**
  AHA CC: 4Q, 2018, 19

K62 **Other diseases of anus and rectum**
  Includes: anal canal
  Excludes2: *colostomy and enterostomy malfunction (K94.0-, K94.1-)*
    fecal incontinence (R15.-)
    hemorrhoids (K64.-)
K62.0 **Anal polyp**
K62.1 **Rectal polyp**
  Excludes1: *adenomatous polyp (D12.8)*
K62.2 **Anal prolapse**
  Prolapse of anal canal
K62.3 **Rectal prolapse**
  Prolapse of rectal mucosa
K62.4 **Stenosis of anus and rectum**
  Stricture of anus (sphincter)
  AHA CC: 2Q, 2019, 13
CC **K62.5** **Hemorrhage of anus and rectum**
  Excludes1: *gastrointestinal bleeding NOS (K92.2)*
    melena (K92.1)
    neonatal rectal hemorrhage (P54.2)
  AHA CC: 1Q, 2019, 21
CC **K62.6** **Ulcer of anus and rectum**
  Solitary ulcer of anus and rectum
  Stercoral ulcer of anus and rectum
  Excludes1: *fissure and fistula of anus and rectum (K60.-)*
    ulcerative colitis (K51.-)
K62.7 **Radiation proctitis**
  Use additional code to identify the type of radiation (W88.-) or radiation therapy (Y84.2)
  AHA CC: 1Q, 2019, 21
+ **K62.8** **Other specified diseases of anus and rectum**
  Excludes2: *ulcerative proctitis (K51.2)*
  K62.81 **Anal sphincter tear (healed) (nontraumatic) (old)**
    Tear of anus, nontraumatic
    Use additional code for any associated fecal incontinence (R15.-)
    Excludes2: *anal fissure (K60.-)*
      anal sphincter tear (healed) (old) complicating delivery (O34.7-)
      traumatic tear of anal sphincter (S31.831)
  K62.82 **Dysplasia of anus**
    Anal intraepithelial neoplasia I and II (AIN I and II) (histologically confirmed)
    Dysplasia of anus NOS
    Mild and moderate dysplasia of anus (histologically confirmed)
    Excludes1: *abnormal results from anal cytologic examination without histologic confirmation (R85.61-)*
      anal intraepithelial neoplasia III (D01.3)
      carcinoma in situ of anus (D01.3)
      HGSIL of anus (R85.613)
      severe dysplasia of anus (D01.3)
  K62.89 **Other specified diseases of anus and rectum**
    Proctitis NOS
    Use additional code for any associated fecal incontinence (R15.-)
K62.9 **Disease of anus and rectum, unspecified**

K63 **Other diseases of intestine**

CC **K63.0** **Abscess of intestine**
  Excludes1: *abscess of intestine with Crohn's disease (K50.014, K50.114, K50.814, K50.914,)*
    abscess of intestine with diverticular disease (K57.0, K57.2, K57.4, K57.8)
    abscess of intestine with ulcerative colitis (K51.014, K51.214, K51.314, K51.414, K51.514, K51.814, K51.914)
  Excludes2: *abscess of anal and rectal regions (K61.-)*
    abscess of appendix (K35.3-)
MCC **K63.1** **Perforation of intestine (nontraumatic)**
  Perforation (nontraumatic) of rectum
  Excludes1: *perforation (nontraumatic) of duodenum (K26.-)*
    perforation (nontraumatic) of intestine with diverticular disease (K57.0, K57.2, K57.4, K57.8)
  Excludes2: *perforation (nontraumatic) of appendix (K35.2-, K35.3-)*
  AHA CC: 2Q, 2020, 22

CC **K63.2** **Fistula of intestine**
Excludes1: *fistula of duodenum (K31.6)*
fistula of intestine with Crohn's disease
(K50.013, K50.113, K50.813, K50.913,)
fistula of intestine with ulcerative colitis
(K51.013, K51.213, K51.313, K51.413,
K51.513, K51.813, K51.913)
Excludes2: *fistula of anal and rectal regions (K60.-)*
fistula of appendix (K38.3)
intestinal-genital fistula, female (N82.2-N82.4)
vesicointestinal fistula (N32.1)
AHA CC: 3Q, 2017, 4-5

CC **K63.3** **Ulcer of intestine**
Primary ulcer of small intestine
Excludes1: *duodenal ulcer (K26.-)*
gastrointestinal ulcer (K28.-)
gastrojejunal ulcer (K28.-)
jejunal ulcer (K28.-)
peptic ulcer, site unspecified (K27.-)
ulcer of intestine with perforation (K63.1)
ulcer of anus or rectum (K62.6)
ulcerative colitis (K51.-)

CC **K63.4** **Enteroptosis**
K63.5 **Polyp of colon**
Excludes1: *adenomatous polyp of colon (D12.-)*
inflammatory polyp of colon (K51.4-)
polyposis of colon (D12.6)
AHA CC: 2Q, 2015, 14; 1Q, 2017, 15-16; 1Q, 2019, 33

+ **K63.8** **Other specified diseases of intestine**
MCC **K63.81** **Dieulafoy lesion of intestine**
Excludes2: *Dieulafoy lesion of stomach and*
duodenum (K31.82)
K63.89 **Other specified diseases of intestine**
K63.9 **Disease of intestine, unspecified**

K64 **Hemorrhoids and perianal venous thrombosis**
Includes: piles
Excludes1: *hemorrhoids complicating childbirth and the*
puerperium (O87.2)
hemorrhoids complicating pregnancy (O22.4)
K64.0 **First degree hemorrhoids**
Grade/stage I hemorrhoids
Hemorrhoids (bleeding) without prolapse outside of anal
canal
K64.1 **Second degree hemorrhoids**
Grade/stage II hemorrhoids
Hemorrhoids (bleeding) that prolapse with straining, but
retract spontaneously
K64.2 **Third degree hemorrhoids**
Grade/stage III hemorrhoids
Hemorrhoids (bleeding) that prolapse with straining and
require manual replacement back inside anal canal
K64.3 **Fourth degree hemorrhoids**
Grade/stage IV hemorrhoids
Hemorrhoids (bleeding) with prolapsed tissue that cannot be
manually replaced
K64.4 **Residual hemorrhoidal skin tags**
External hemorrhoids, NOS
Skin tags of anus
K64.5 **Perianal venous thrombosis**
External hemorrhoids with thrombosis
Perianal hematoma
Thrombosed hemorrhoids NOS
K64.8 **Other hemorrhoids**
Internal hemorrhoids, without mention of degree
Prolapsed hemorrhoids, degree not specified
AHA CC: 3Q, 2018, 22
K64.9 **Unspecified hemorrhoids**
Hemorrhoids (bleeding) NOS
Hemorrhoids (bleeding) without mention of degree

Diseases of peritoneum and retroperitoneum (K65-K68)

K65 **Peritonitis**
Use additional code (B95-B97), to identify infectious agent, if
known

Code also if applicable diverticular disease of intestine (K57.-)
Excludes1: *acute appendicitis with generalized peritonitis (K35.2-)*
aseptic peritonitis (T81.6)
benign paroxysmal peritonitis (E85.0)
chemical peritonitis (T81.6)
gonococcal peritonitis (A54.85)
neonatal peritonitis (P78.0-P78.1)
pelvic peritonitis, female (N73.3-N73.5)
periodic familial peritonitis (E85.0)
peritonitis due to talc or other foreign substance (T81.6)
peritonitis in chlamydia (A74.81)
peritonitis in diphtheria (A36.89)
peritonitis in syphilis (late) (A52.74)
peritonitis in tuberculosis (A18.31)
peritonitis with or following abortion or ectopic or
molar pregnancy (O00-O07, O08.0)
peritonitis with or following appendicitis (K35.-)
puerperal peritonitis (O85)
retroperitoneal infections (K68.-)
MCC **K65.0** **Generalized (acute) peritonitis**
Pelvic peritonitis (acute), male
Subphrenic peritonitis (acute)
Suppurative peritonitis (acute)
MCC **K65.1** **Peritoneal abscess**
Abdominopelvic abscess
Abscess (of) omentum
Abscess (of) peritoneum
Mesenteric abscess
Retrocecal abscess
Subdiaphragmatic abscess
Subhepatic abscess
Subphrenic abscess
AHA CC: 1Q, 2019, 15-16
MCC **K65.2** **Spontaneous bacterial peritonitis**
Excludes1: *bacterial peritonitis NOS (K65.9)*
MCC **K65.3** **Choleperitonitis**
Peritonitis due to bile
CC **K65.4** **Sclerosing mesenteritis**
Fat necrosis of peritoneum
(Idiopathic) sclerosing mesenteric fibrosis
Mesenteric lipodystrophy
Mesenteric panniculitis
Retractile mesenteritis
MCC **K65.8** **Other peritonitis**
Chronic proliferative peritonitis
Peritonitis due to urine
MCC **K65.9** **Peritonitis, unspecified**
Bacterial peritonitis NOS
AHA CC: 2Q, 2013, 31

K66 **Other disorders of peritoneum**
Excludes2: *ascites (R18.-)*
peritoneal effusion (chronic) (R18.8)
K66.0 **Peritoneal adhesions (postprocedural) (postinfection)**
Adhesions (of) abdominal (wall)
Adhesions (of) diaphragm
Adhesions (of) intestine
Adhesions (of) male pelvis
Adhesions (of) omentum
Adhesions (of) stomach
Adhesive bands
Mesenteric adhesions
Excludes1: *female pelvic adhesions [bands] (N73.6)*
peritoneal adhesions with intestinal obstruction
(K56.5-)
MCC **K66.1** **Hemoperitoneum**
Excludes1: *traumatic hemoperitoneum (S36.8-)*
K66.8 **Other specified disorders of peritoneum**
K66.9 **Disorder of peritoneum, unspecified**

+, +7th, X + 7th   ● Newborn   ● Pediatric   ● Maternity   ● Adult   ♀ Female   ♂ Male   Manifestation   Unacceptable PDX   HCC   CC   MCC   HAC

MCC **K67** **Disorders of peritoneum in infectious diseases classified elsewhere**

Code first underlying disease, such as:
congenital syphilis (A50.0)
helminthiasis (B65.0-B83.9)
Excludes1: *peritonitis in chlamydia (A74.81)*
peritonitis in diphtheria (A36.89)
peritonitis in gonococcal (A54.85)
peritonitis in syphilis (late) (A52.74)
peritonitis in tuberculosis (A18.31)
Valid 3-character code, no further characters required

K68 **Disorders of retroperitoneum**

+ **K68.1** **Retroperitoneal abscess**
CC **K68.11** **Postprocedural retroperitoneal abscess**
Excludes2: *infection following procedure (T81.4-)*
HAC see Appendix B for HAC conditional logic
MCC **K68.12** **Psoas muscle abscess**
MCC **K68.19** **Other retroperitoneal abscess**
AHA CC: 1Q, 2019, 15-16
MCC **K68.9** **Other disorders of retroperitoneum**

Diseases of liver (K70-K77)

Excludes1: *jaundice NOS (R17)*

Excludes2: *hemochromatosis (E83.11-)*
Reye's syndrome (G93.7)
viral hepatitis (B15-B19)
Wilson's disease (E83.0)

K70 **Alcoholic liver disease**

Use additional code to identify:
alcohol abuse and dependence (F10.-)
● **K70.0** **Alcoholic fatty liver**
+ **K70.1** **Alcoholic hepatitis**
● **K70.10** **Alcoholic hepatitis without ascites**
● **K70.11** **Alcoholic hepatitis with ascites**
● **K70.2** **Alcoholic fibrosis and sclerosis of liver**
+ **K70.3** **Alcoholic cirrhosis of liver**
Alcoholic cirrhosis NOS
● **K70.30** **Alcoholic cirrhosis of liver without ascites**
● **K70.31** **Alcoholic cirrhosis of liver with ascites**
+ **K70.4** **Alcoholic hepatic failure**
Acute alcoholic hepatic failure
Alcoholic hepatic failure NOS
Chronic alcoholic hepatic failure
Subacute alcoholic hepatic failure
● **K70.40** **Alcoholic hepatic failure without coma**
● MCC **K70.41** **Alcoholic hepatic failure with coma**
● **K70.9** **Alcoholic liver disease, unspecified**

K71 **Toxic liver disease**

Includes: drug-induced idiosyncratic (unpredictable) liver disease
drug-induced toxic (predictable) liver disease
Code first poisoning due to drug or toxin, if applicable (T36-T65
with fifth or sixth character 1-4 or 6)

Use additional code for adverse effect, if applicable, to identify drug
(T36-T50 with fifth or sixth character 5)
Excludes2: *alcoholic liver disease (K70.-)*
Budd-Chiari syndrome (I82.0)
K71.0 **Toxic liver disease with cholestasis**
Cholestasis with hepatocyte injury
'Pure' cholestasis
+ **K71.1** **Toxic liver disease with hepatic necrosis**
Hepatic failure (acute) (chronic) due to drugs
K71.10 **Toxic liver disease with hepatic necrosis, without coma**
MCC **K71.11** **Toxic liver disease with hepatic necrosis, with coma**
K71.2 **Toxic liver disease with acute hepatitis**
K71.3 **Toxic liver disease with chronic persistent hepatitis**
K71.4 **Toxic liver disease with chronic lobular hepatitis**
+ **K71.5** **Toxic liver disease with chronic active hepatitis**
Toxic liver disease with lupoid hepatitis
K71.50 **Toxic liver disease with chronic active hepatitis without ascites**
K71.51 **Toxic liver disease with chronic active hepatitis with ascites**
K71.6 **Toxic liver disease with hepatitis, not elsewhere classified**
K71.7 **Toxic liver disease with fibrosis and cirrhosis of liver**

K71.8 **Toxic liver disease with other disorders of liver**
Toxic liver disease with focal nodular hyperplasia
Toxic liver disease with hepatic granulomas
Toxic liver disease with peliosis hepatis
Toxic liver disease with veno-occlusive disease of liver
K71.9 **Toxic liver disease, unspecified**

K72 **Hepatic failure, not elsewhere classified**

Includes: fulminant hepatitis NEC, with hepatic failure
hepatic encephalopathy NOS
liver (cell) necrosis with hepatic failure
malignant hepatitis NEC, with hepatic failure
yellow liver atrophy or dystrophy
Excludes1: *alcoholic hepatic failure (K70.4)*
hepatic failure with toxic liver disease (K71.1-)
icterus of newborn (P55-P59)
postprocedural hepatic failure (K91.82)
Excludes2: *hepatic failure complicating abortion or ectopic or molar pregnancy (O00-O07, O08.8)*
hepatic failure complicating pregnancy, childbirth and the puerperium (O26.6-)
viral hepatitis with hepatic coma (B15-B19)
+ **K72.0** **Acute and subacute hepatic failure**
Acute non-viral hepatitis NOS
AHA CC: 2Q, 2014, 13
MCC **K72.00** **Acute and subacute hepatic failure without coma**
MCC **K72.01** **Acute and subacute hepatic failure with coma**
+ **K72.1** **Chronic hepatic failure**
K72.10 **Chronic hepatic failure without coma**
AHA CC: 1Q, 2017, 41
MCC **K72.11** **Chronic hepatic failure with coma**
+ **K72.9** **Hepatic failure, unspecified**
K72.90 **Hepatic failure, unspecified without coma**
AHA CC: 2Q, 2016, 35; 4Q, 2018, 21
MCC **K72.91** **Hepatic failure, unspecified with coma**
Hepatic coma NOS

K73 **Chronic hepatitis, not elsewhere classified**

Excludes1: *alcoholic hepatitis (chronic) (K70.1-)*
drug-induced hepatitis (chronic) (K71.-)
granulomatous hepatitis (chronic) NEC (K75.3)
reactive, nonspecific hepatitis (chronic) (K75.2)
viral hepatitis (chronic) (B15-B19)
K73.0 **Chronic persistent hepatitis, not elsewhere classified**
K73.1 **Chronic lobular hepatitis, not elsewhere classified**
K73.2 **Chronic active hepatitis, not elsewhere classified**
K73.8 **Other chronic hepatitis, not elsewhere classified**
K73.9 **Chronic hepatitis, unspecified**

K74 **Fibrosis and cirrhosis of liver**

Code also, if applicable, viral hepatitis (acute) (chronic) (B15-B19)
Excludes1: *alcoholic cirrhosis (of liver) (K70.3)*
alcoholic fibrosis of liver (K70.2)
cardiac sclerosis of liver (K76.1)
cirrhosis (of liver) with toxic liver disease (K71.7)
congenital cirrhosis (of liver) (P78.81)
pigmentary cirrhosis (of liver) (E83.110)
+ **K74.0** **Hepatic fibrosis**
Code first underlying liver disease such as:
nonalcoholic steatohepatitis (NASH) (K57.81)
K74.00 **Hepatic fibrosis, unspecified**
K74.01 **Hepatic fibrosis, early fibrosis**
Hepatic fibrosis, stage F1 or stage F2
K74.02 **Hepatic fibrosis, advanced fibrosis**
Hepatic fibrosis, stage 3
Excludes1: *cirrhosis of liver (K74.6-)*
hepatic fibrosis, stage F4 (K74.6-)
K74.1 **Hepatic sclerosis**
K74.2 **Hepatic fibrosis with hepatic sclerosis**
K74.3 **Primary biliary cirrhosis**
Chronic nonsuppurative destructive cholangitis
Primary biliary cholangitis
Excludes2: *primary sclerosing cholangitis (K83.01)*
K74.4 **Secondary biliary cirrhosis**
K74.5 **Biliary cirrhosis, unspecified**
+ **K74.6** **Other and unspecified cirrhosis of liver**
K74.60 **Unspecified cirrhosis of liver**
Cirrhosis (of liver) NOS
AHA CC: 1Q, 2018, 4-5

+, +7th, X + 7th   ● Newborn   ● Pediatric   ● Maternity   ● Adult   ♀ Female   ♂ Male   Manifestation   Unacceptable PDX   HCC   CC   MCC   HAC

Surfaces and Bed of Liver

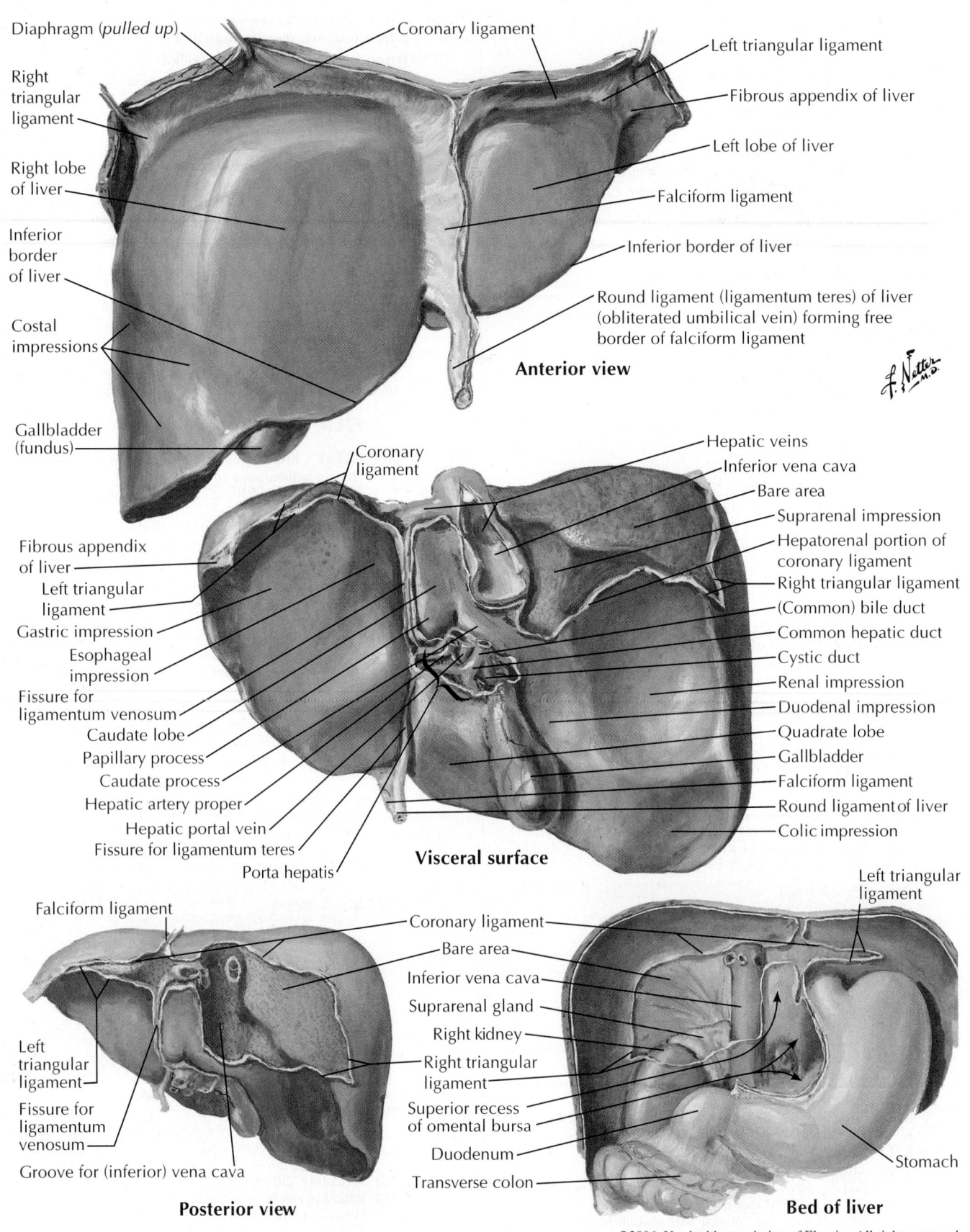

Diaphragm (*pulled up*)

Coronary ligament

Left triangular ligament

Right triangular ligament

Fibrous appendix of liver

Left lobe of liver

Right lobe of liver

Falciform ligament

Inferior border of liver

Inferior border of liver

Costal impressions

Round ligament (ligamentum teres) of liver (obliterated umbilical vein) forming free border of falciform ligament

Anterior view

Gallblader (fundus)

Coronary ligament

Hepatic veins

Inferior vena cava

Bare area

Suprarenal impression

Fibrous appendix of liver

Hepatorenal portion of coronary ligament

Left triangular ligament

Right triangular ligament

Gastric impression

(Common) bile duct

Esophageal impression

Common hepatic duct

Fissure for ligamentum venosum

Cystic duct

Caudate lobe

Renal impression

Papillary process

Duodenal impression

Caudate process

Quadrate lobe

Hepatic artery proper

Gallbladder

Hepatic portal vein

Falciform ligament

Fissure for ligamentum teres

Round ligament of liver

Porta hepatis

Colic impression

Visceral surface

Falciform ligament

Coronary ligament

Left triangular ligament

Bare area

Inferior vena cava

Suprarenal gland

Right kidney

Left triangular ligament

Right triangular ligament

Fissure for ligamentum venosum

Superior recess of omental bursa

Groove for (inferior) vena cava

Duodenum

Stomach

Transverse colon

Posterior view

Bed of liver

K74.69 Other cirrhosis of liver
Cryptogenic cirrhosis (of liver)
Macronodular cirrhosis (of liver)
Micronodular cirrhosis (of liver)
Mixed type cirrhosis (of liver)
Portal cirrhosis (of liver)
Postnecrotic cirrhosis (of liver)

K75 Other inflammatory liver diseases

Excludes2: toxic liver disease (K71.-)

MCC **K75.0 Abscess of liver**
Cholangitic hepatic abscess
Hematogenic hepatic abscess
Hepatic abscess NOS
Lymphogenic hepatic abscess
Pylephlebitic hepatic abscess
Excludes1: amebic liver abscess (A06.4)
cholangitis without liver abscess (K83.09)
pylephlebitis without liver abscess (K75.1)
Excludes2: acute or subacute hepatitis NOS (B17.9)
acute or subacute non-viral hepatitis (K72.0)
chronic hepatitis NEC (K73.8)

MCC **K75.1 Phlebitis of portal vein**
Pylephlebitis
Excludes1: pylephlebitic liver abscess (K75.0)

K75.2 Nonspecific reactive hepatitis
Excludes1: acute or subacute hepatitis (K72.0-)
chronic hepatitis NEC (K73.-)
viral hepatitis (B15-B19)

K75.3 Granulomatous hepatitis, not elsewhere classified
Excludes1: acute or subacute hepatitis (K72.0-)
chronic hepatitis NEC (K73.-)
viral hepatitis (B15-B19)

K75.4 Autoimmune hepatitis
Lupoid hepatitis NEC

+ **K75.8 Other specified inflammatory liver diseases**
K75.81 Nonalcoholic steatohepatitis (NASH)
Use additional code, if applicable, hepatic fibrosis (K74.0-)
K75.89 Other specified inflammatory liver diseases
K75.9 Inflammatory liver disease, unspecified
Hepatitis NOS
Excludes1: acute or subacute hepatitis (K72.0-)
chronic hepatitis NEC (K73.-)
viral hepatitis (B15-B19)

K76 Other diseases of liver

Excludes2: alcoholic liver disease (K70.-)
amyloid degeneration of liver (E85.-)
cystic disease of liver (congenital) (Q44.6)
hepatic vein thrombosis (I82.0)
hepatomegaly NOS (R16.0)
pigmentary cirrhosis (of liver) (E83.110)
portal vein thrombosis (I81)
toxic liver disease (K71.-)

K76.0 Fatty (change of) liver, not elsewhere classified
Nonalcoholic fatty liver disease (NAFLD)
Excludes1: nonalcoholic steatohepatitis (NASH) (K75.81)

K76.1 Chronic passive congestion of liver
Cardiac cirrhosis
Cardiac sclerosis

MCC **K76.2 Central hemorrhagic necrosis of liver**
Excludes1: liver necrosis with hepatic failure (K72.-)

MCC **K76.3 Infarction of liver**

K76.4 Peliosis hepatis
Hepatic angiomatosis

K76.5 Hepatic veno-occlusive disease
Excludes1: Budd-Chiari syndrome (I82.0)

CC **K76.6 Portal hypertension**
Use additional code for any associated complications, such as:
portal hypertensive gastropathy (K31.89)
AHA CC: 1Q, 2020, 15

MCC **K76.7 Hepatorenal syndrome**
Excludes1: hepatorenal syndrome following labor and delivery (O90.4)
postprocedural hepatorenal syndrome (K91.83)

+ **K76.8 Other specified diseases of liver**
K76.81 Hepatopulmonary syndrome
Code first underlying liver disease, such as:
alcoholic cirrhosis of liver (K70.3-)
cirrhosis of liver without mention of alcohol (K74.6-)

K76.89 Other specified diseases of liver
Cyst (simple) of liver
Focal nodular hyperplasia of liver
Hepatoptosis
K76.9 Liver disease, unspecified

CC **K77 Liver disorders in diseases classified elsewhere**
Code first underlying disease, such as:
amyloidosis (E85.-)
congenital syphilis (A50.0, A50.5)
congenital toxoplasmosis (P37.1)
schistosomiasis (B65.0-B65.9)
Excludes1: alcoholic hepatitis (K70.1-)
alcoholic liver disease (K70.-)
cytomegaloviral hepatitis (B25.1)
herpesviral [herpes simplex] hepatitis (B00.81)
infectious mononucleosis with liver disease (B27.0-B27.9 with .9)
mumps hepatitis (B26.81)
sarcoidosis with liver disease (D86.89)
secondary syphilis with liver disease (A51.45)
syphilis (late) with liver disease (A52.74)
toxoplasmosis (acquired) hepatitis (B58.1)
tuberculosis with liver disease (A18.83)
Valid 3-character code, no further characters required

Disorders of gallbladder, biliary tract and pancreas (K80-K87)

K80 Cholelithiasis

Excludes1: retained cholelithiasis following cholecystectomy (K91.86)

+ **K80.0 Calculus of gallbladder with acute cholecystitis**
Any condition listed in K80.2 with acute cholecystitis
Use additional code if applicable for associated gangrene of gallbladder (K82.A1), or perforation of gallbladder (K82.A2)
CC **K80.00 Calculus of gallbladder with acute cholecystitis without obstruction**
AHA CC: 4Q, 2018, 20
CC **K80.01 Calculus of gallbladder with acute cholecystitis with obstruction**

+ **K80.1 Calculus of gallbladder with other cholecystitis**
Use additional code if applicable for associated gangrene of gallbladder (K82.A1), or perforation of gallbladder (K82.A2)
CC **K80.10 Calculus of gallbladder with chronic cholecystitis without obstruction**
Cholelithiasis with cholecystitis NOS
CC **K80.11 Calculus of gallbladder with chronic cholecystitis with obstruction**
CC **K80.12 Calculus of gallbladder with acute and chronic cholecystitis without obstruction**
CC **K80.13 Calculus of gallbladder with acute and chronic cholecystitis with obstruction**
CC **K80.18 Calculus of gallbladder with other cholecystitis without obstruction**
CC **K80.19 Calculus of gallbladder with other cholecystitis with obstruction**

+ **K80.2 Calculus of gallbladder without cholecystitis**
Cholecystolithiasis without cholecystitis
Cholelithiasis (without cholecystitis)
Colic (recurrent) of gallbladder (without cholecystitis)
Gallstone (impacted) of cystic duct (without cholecystitis)
Gallstone (impacted) of gallbladder (without cholecystitis)
K80.20 Calculus of gallbladder without cholecystitis without obstruction
CC **K80.21 Calculus of gallbladder without cholecystitis with obstruction**

+ **K80.3 Calculus of bile duct with cholangitis**
Any condition listed in K80.5 with cholangitis
CC **K80.30 Calculus of bile duct with cholangitis, unspecified, without obstruction**
CC **K80.31 Calculus of bile duct with cholangitis, unspecified, with obstruction**
CC **K80.32 Calculus of bile duct with acute cholangitis without obstruction**
CC **K80.33 Calculus of bile duct with acute cholangitis with obstruction**
CC **K80.34 Calculus of bile duct with chronic cholangitis without obstruction**
CC **K80.35 Calculus of bile duct with chronic cholangitis with obstruction**

Cholelithiasis (Gallstones)

Sudden obstruction (biliary colic)

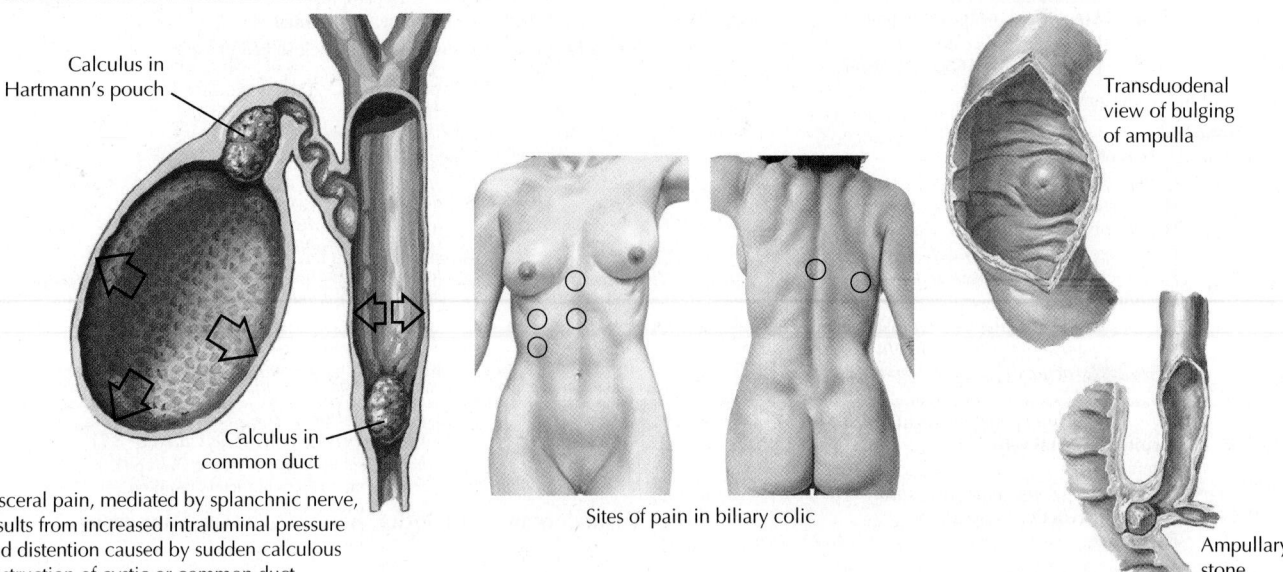

Calculus in Hartmann's pouch

Calculus in common duct

Transduodenal view of bulging of ampulla

Ampullary stone

Sites of pain in biliary colic

Visceral pain, mediated by splanchnic nerve, results from increased intraluminal pressure and distention caused by sudden calculous obstruction of cystic or common duct.

Persistent obstruction (acute cholecystitis)

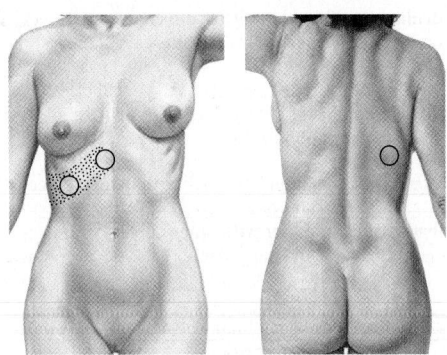

Sites of pain and hyperesthesia in acute cholecystitis

Patient lies motionless because jarring or respiration increases pain. Nausea is common.

Edema, ischemia, and transmural inflammation

Parietal epigastric or right upper quadrant pain results from ischemia and inflammation of gallbladder wall caused by persistent calculous obstruction of cystic duct. Prostaglandins are released.

CC **K80.36** **Calculus of bile duct with acute and chronic cholangitis without obstruction**

CC **K80.37** **Calculus of bile duct with acute and chronic cholangitis with obstruction**

+ **K80.4** **Calculus of bile duct with cholecystitis**
Any condition listed in K80.5 with cholecystitis (with cholangitis)
Code also fistula of bile duct (K83.3)

Use additional code if applicable for associated gangrene of gallbladder (K82.A1), or perforation of gallbladder (K82.A2)

CC **K80.40** **Calculus of bile duct with cholecystitis, unspecified, without obstruction**

CC **K80.41** **Calculus of bile duct with cholecystitis, unspecified, with obstruction**
AHA CC: 1Q, 2019, 17-18

CC **K80.42** **Calculus of bile duct with acute cholecystitis without obstruction**

CC **K80.43** **Calculus of bile duct with acute cholecystitis with obstruction**

CC **K80.44** **Calculus of bile duct with chronic cholecystitis without obstruction**

CC **K80.45** **Calculus of bile duct with chronic cholecystitis with obstruction**

CC **K80.46** **Calculus of bile duct with acute and chronic cholecystitis without obstruction**

CC **K80.47** **Calculus of bile duct with acute and chronic cholecystitis with obstruction**

+, +7th, X + 7th ● Newborn ● Pediatric ● Maternity ● Adult ♀ Female ♂ Male Manifestation Unacceptable PDX HCC CC MCC HAC

+ **K80.5** **Calculus of bile duct without cholangitis or cholecystitis**
Choledocholithiasis (without cholangitis or cholecystitis)
Gallstone (impacted) of bile duct NOS (without cholangitis
or cholecystitis)
Gallstone (impacted) of common duct (without cholangitis
or cholecystitis)
Gallstone (impacted) of hepatic duct (without cholangitis or
cholecystitis)
Hepatic cholelithiasis (without cholangitis or cholecystitis)
Hepatic colic (recurrent) (without cholangitis or
cholecystitis)

  K80.50 **Calculus of bile duct without cholangitis or
cholecystitis without obstruction**
CC **K80.51** **Calculus of bile duct without cholangitis or
cholecystitis with obstruction**

+ **K80.6** **Calculus of gallbladder and bile duct with cholecystitis**
Use additional code if applicable for associated gangrene of
gallbladder (K82.A1), or perforation of gallbladder (K82.A2)

CC **K80.60** **Calculus of gallbladder and bile duct with
cholecystitis, unspecified, without obstruction**
CC **K80.61** **Calculus of gallbladder and bile duct with
cholecystitis, unspecified, with obstruction**
CC **K80.62** **Calculus of gallbladder and bile duct with acute
cholecystitis without obstruction**
CC **K80.63** **Calculus of gallbladder and bile duct with acute
cholecystitis with obstruction**
CC **K80.64** **Calculus of gallbladder and bile duct with chronic
cholecystitis without obstruction**
CC **K80.65** **Calculus of gallbladder and bile duct with chronic
cholecystitis with obstruction**
CC **K80.66** **Calculus of gallbladder and bile duct with acute
and chronic cholecystitis without obstruction**
MCC **K80.67** **Calculus of gallbladder and bile duct with acute
and chronic cholecystitis with obstruction**

+ **K80.7** **Calculus of gallbladder and bile duct without cholecystitis**
  K80.70 **Calculus of gallbladder and bile duct without
cholecystitis without obstruction**
CC **K80.71** **Calculus of gallbladder and bile duct without
cholecystitis with obstruction**

+ **K80.8** **Other cholelithiasis**
  K80.80 **Other cholelithiasis without obstruction**
CC **K80.81** **Other cholelithiasis with obstruction**

K81 **Cholecystitis**

Excludes1: *cholecystitis with cholelithiasis (K80.-)*
Use additional code if applicable for associated gangrene of
gallbladder (K82.A1), or perforation of gallbladder (K82.A2)

  K81.0 **Acute cholecystitis**
Abscess of gallbladder
Angiocholecystitis
Emphysematous (acute) cholecystitis
Empyema of gallbladder
Gangrene of gallbladder
Gangrenous cholecystitis
Suppurative cholecystitis
  K81.1 **Chronic cholecystitis**
CC **K81.2** **Acute cholecystitis with chronic cholecystitis**
  K81.9 **Cholecystitis, unspecified**

K82 **Other diseases of gallbladder**

Excludes1: *nonvisualization of gallbladder (R93.2)*
postcholecystectomy syndrome (K91.5)

CC **K82.0** **Obstruction of gallbladder**
Occlusion of cystic duct or gallbladder without cholelithiasis
Stenosis of cystic duct or gallbladder without cholelithiasis
Stricture of cystic duct or gallbladder without cholelithiasis
Excludes1: *obstruction of gallbladder with cholelithiasis
(K80.-)*
CC **K82.1** **Hydrops of gallbladder**
Mucocele of gallbladder
MCC **K82.2** **Perforation of gallbladder**
Rupture of cystic duct or gallbladder
Exlcudes1: *Perforation of gallbladder in cholecystitis (K82.
A2)*
CC **K82.3** **Fistula of gallbladder**
Cholecystocolic fistula
Cholecystoduodenal fistula

K82.4 **Cholesterolosis of gallbladder**
Strawberry gallbladder
Excludes1: *cholesterolosis of gallbladder with cholecystitis
(K81.-)*
*cholesterolosis of gallbladder with
cholelithiasis (K80.-)*
K82.8 **Other specified diseases of gallbladder**
Adhesions of cystic duct or gallbladder
Atrophy of cystic duct or gallbladder
Cyst of cystic duct or gallbladder
Dyskinesia of cystic duct or gallbladder
Hypertrophy of cystic duct or gallbladder
Nonfunctioning of cystic duct or gallbladder
Ulcer of cystic duct or gallbladder
K82.9 **Disease of gallbladder, unspecified**

+ **K82.A** **Disorders of gallbladder in diseases classified elsewhere**
Code first the type of cholecystitis (K81.-), or cholelithiasis
with cholecystitis (K80.00-K80.19, K80.40-K80.47,
K80.60-K80.67)

  K82.A1 **Gangrene of gallbladder in cholecystitis**
AHA CC: 4Q, 2018, 19-20
CC **K82.A2** **Perforation of gallbladder in cholecystitis**
AHA CC: 4Q, 2018, 19-20

K83 **Other diseases of biliary tract**

Excludes1: *postcholecystectomy syndrome (K91.5)*
Excludes2: *conditions involving the gallbladder (K81-K82)*
conditions involving the cystic duct (K81-K82)

+ **K83.0** **Cholangitis**
Excludes1: *cholangitic liver abscess (K75.0)*
*cholangitis with choledocholithiasis (K80.3-,
K80.4-)*
Excludes2: *chronic nonsuppurative destructive cholangitis
(K74.3)*
primary biliary cholangitis (K74.3)
primary biliary cirrhosis (K74.3)
AHA CC: 4Q, 2018, 20
CC **K83.01** **Primary sclerosing cholangitis**
AHA CC: 4Q, 2018, 21
CC **K83.09** **Other cholangitis**
Ascending cholangitis
Cholangitis NOS
Primary cholangitis
Recurrent cholangitis
Sclerosing cholangitis
Secondary cholangitis
Stenosing cholangitis
Suppurative cholangitis
MCC **K83.1** **Obstruction of bile duct**
Occlusion of bile duct without cholelithiasis
Stenosis of bile duct without cholelithiasis
Stricture of bile duct without cholelithiasis
Excludes1: *congenital obstruction of bile duct (Q44.3)*
*obstruction of bile duct with cholelithiasis
(K80.-)*
CC AHA: 1Q, 2016, 18-19
MCC **K83.2** **Perforation of bile duct**
Rupture of bile duct
CC **K83.3** **Fistula of bile duct**
Choledochoduodenal fistula
AHA CC: 1Q, 2019, 17-18
K83.4 **Spasm of sphincter of Oddi**
K83.5 **Biliary cyst**
K83.8 **Other specified diseases of biliary tract**
Adhesions of biliary tract
Atrophy of biliary tract
Hypertrophy of biliary tract
Ulcer of biliary tract
K83.9 **Disease of biliary tract, unspecified**

K85 **Acute pancreatitis**

Includes: acute (recurrent) pancreatitis
subacute pancreatitis
AHA CC: 4Q, 2016, 34

+ **K85.0** **Idiopathic acute pancreatitis**
MCC **K85.00** **Idiopathic acute pancreatitis without necrosis or
infection**
MCC **K85.01** **Idiopathic acute pancreatitis with uninfected
necrosis**
MCC **K85.02** **Idiopathic acute pancreatitis with infected
necrosis**

+, +7th, X + 7th   ● Newborn   ● Pediatric   ● Maternity   ● Adult   ♀ Female   ♂ Male   Manifestation   Unacceptable PDX   HCC   CC   MCC   HAC

Acute Pancreatitis

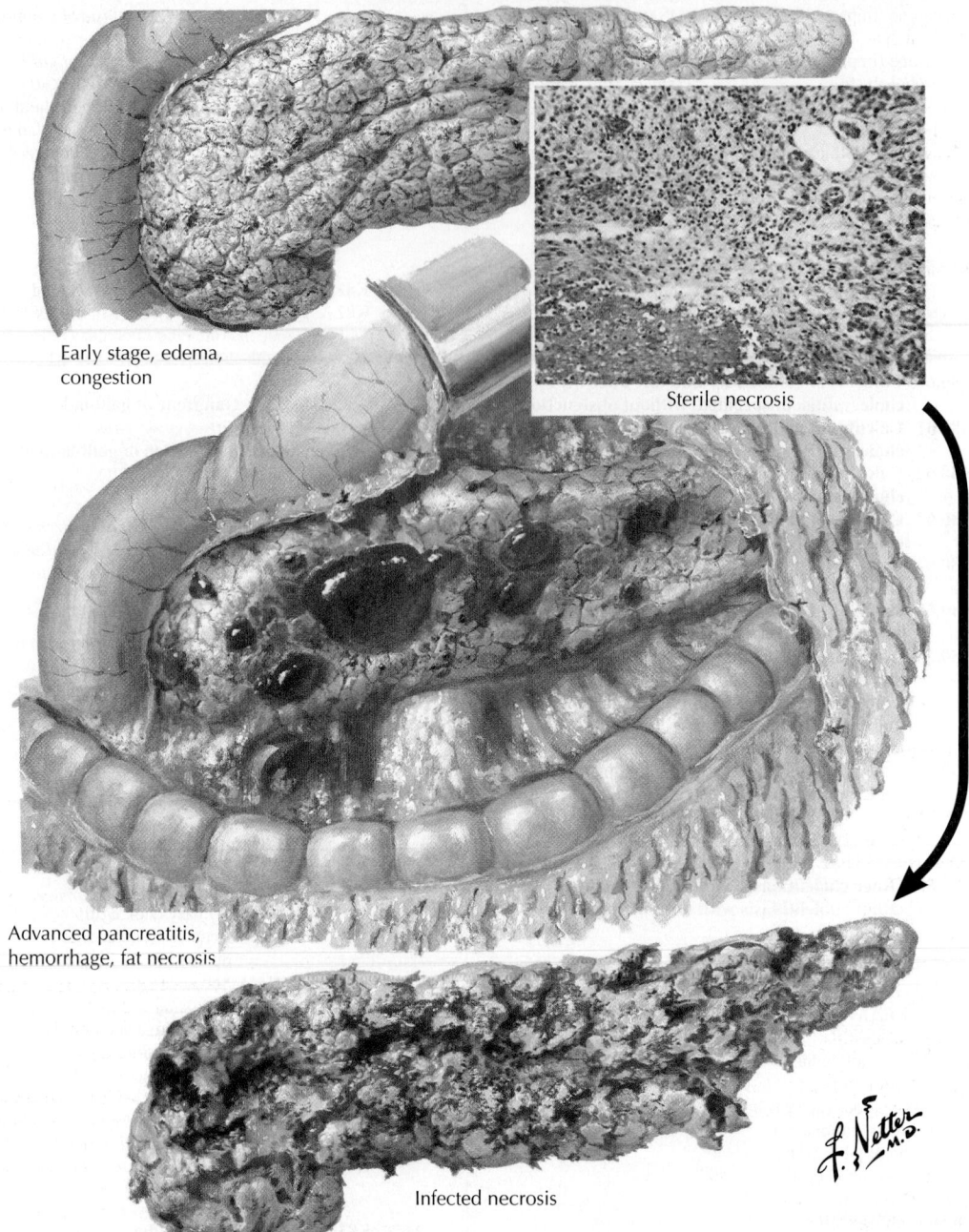

Early stage, edema, congestion

Sterile necrosis

Advanced pancreatitis, hemorrhage, fat necrosis

Infected necrosis

+ **K85.1** **Biliary acute pancreatitis**
    Gallstone pancreatitis
  MCC **K85.10** **Biliary acute pancreatitis without necrosis or infection**
  MCC **K85.11** **Biliary acute pancreatitis with uninfected necrosis**
  MCC **K85.12** **Biliary acute pancreatitis with infected necrosis**
+ **K85.2** **Alcohol induced acute pancreatitis**
    Excludes2: *alcohol induced chronic pancreatitis (K86.0)*
  MCC **K85.20** **Alcohol induced acute pancreatitis without necrosis or infection**
      AHA CC: 1Q, 2020, 9
  MCC **K85.21** **Alcohol induced acute pancreatitis with uninfected necrosis**
  MCC **K85.22** **Alcohol induced acute pancreatitis with infected necrosis**
+ **K85.3** **Drug induced acute pancreatitis**
    Use additional code for adverse effect, if applicable, to identify drug (T36-T50 with fifth or sixth character 5)

    Use additional code to identify drug abuse and dependence (F11.-F17.-)

  MCC **K85.30** **Drug induced acute pancreatitis without necrosis or infection**
  MCC **K85.31** **Drug induced acute pancreatitis with uninfected necrosis**
  MCC **K85.32** **Drug induced acute pancreatitis with infected necrosis**
+ **K85.8** **Other acute pancreatitis**
  MCC **K85.80** **Other acute pancreatitis without necrosis or infection**
  MCC **K85.81** **Other acute pancreatitis with uninfected necrosis**
  MCC **K85.82** **Other acute pancreatitis with infected necrosis**
+ **K85.9** **Acute pancreatitis, unspecified**
    Pancreatitis NOS
  MCC **K85.90** **Acute pancreatitis without necrosis or infection, unspecified**
  MCC **K85.91** **Acute pancreatitis with uninfected necrosis, unspecified**
  MCC **K85.92** **Acute pancreatitis with infected necrosis, unspecified**

K86 Other diseases of pancreas

> **Excludes2:** *fibrocystic disease of pancreas (E84.-)*
> *islet cell tumor (of pancreas) (D13.7)*
> *pancreatic steatorrhea (K90.3)*

CC **K86.0 Alcohol-induced chronic pancreatitis**
Use additional code to identify:
alcohol abuse and dependence (F10.-)

Code also exocrine pancreatic insufficiency (K86.81)
> **Excludes2:** *alcohol induced acute pancreatitis (K85.2-)*

CC **K86.1 Other chronic pancreatitis**
Chronic pancreatitis NOS
Infectious chronic pancreatitis
Recurrent chronic pancreatitis
Relapsing chronic pancreatitis
Code also exocrine pancreatic insufficiency (K86.81)

CC **K86.2 Cyst of pancreas**
CC **K86.3 Pseudocyst of pancreas**
+ **K86.8 Other specified diseases of pancreas**
AHA CC: 4Q, 2016, 33

K86.81 Exocrine pancreatic insufficiency
K86.89 Other specified diseases of pancreas
Aseptic pancreatic necrosis, unrelated to acute pancreatitis
Atrophy of pancreas
Calculus of pancreas
Cirrhosis of pancreas
Fibrosis of pancreas
Pancreatic fat necrosis, unrelated to acute pancreatitis
Pancreatic infantilism
Pancreatic necrosis NOS, unrelated to acute pancreatitis

K86.9 Disease of pancreas, unspecified

K87 Disorders of gallbladder, biliary tract and pancreas in diseases classified elsewhere

Code first underlying disease
> **Excludes1:** *cytomegaloviral pancreatitis (B25.2)*
> *mumps pancreatitis (B26.3)*
> *syphilitic gallbladder (A52.74)*
> *syphilitic pancreas (A52.74)*
> *tuberculosis of gallbladder (A18.83)*
> *tuberculosis of pancreas (A18.83)*

Valid 3-character code, no further characters required

Other diseases of the digestive system (K90-K95)

K90 Intestinal malabsorption

> **Excludes1:** *intestinal malabsorption following gastrointestinal surgery (K91.2)*

K90.0 Celiac disease
Celiac disease with steatorrhea
Celiac gluten-sensitive enteropathy
Nontropical sprue
Code also exocrine pancreatic insufficiency (K86.81)

Use additional code for associated disorders including:
dermatitis herpetiformis (L13.0)
gluten ataxia (G32.81)

CC **K90.1 Tropical sprue**
Sprue NOS
Tropical steatorrhea

CC **K90.2 Blind loop syndrome, not elsewhere classified**
Blind loop syndrome NOS
> **Excludes1:** *congenital blind loop syndrome (Q43.8)*
> *postsurgical blind loop syndrome (K91.2)*

CC **K90.3 Pancreatic steatorrhea**
+ **K90.4 Other malabsorption due to intolerance**
> **Excludes2:** *celiac gluten-sensitive enteropathy (K90.0)*
> *lactose intolerance (E73.-)*

CC **K90.41 Non-celiac gluten sensitivity**
Gluten sensitivity NOS
Non-celiac gluten sensitive enteropathy
AHA CC: 4Q, 2016, 35-36

CC **K90.49 Malabsorption due to intolerance, not elsewhere classified**
Malabsorption due to intolerance to carbohydrate
Malabsorption due to intolerance to fat
Malabsorption due to intolerance to protein
Malabsorption due to intolerance to starch

+ **K90.8 Other intestinal malabsorption**
CC **K90.81 Whipple's disease**
CC **K90.89 Other intestinal malabsorption**
CC **K90.9 Intestinal malabsorption, unspecified**
AHA CC: 4Q, 2017, 108-109

K91 Intraoperative and postprocedural complications and disorders of digestive system, not elsewhere classified

> **Excludes2:** *complications of artificial opening of digestive system (K94.-)*
> *complications of bariatric procedures (K95.-)*
> *gastrojejunal ulcer (K28.-)*
> *postprocedural (radiation) retroperitoneal abscess (K68.11)*
> *radiation colitis (K52.0)*
> *radiation gastroenteritis (K52.0)*
> *radiation proctitis (K62.7)*

AHA CC: 4Q, 2016, 9-10

K91.0 Vomiting following gastrointestinal surgery
K91.1 Postgastric surgery syndromes
Dumping syndrome
Postgastrectomy syndrome
Postvagotomy syndrome

CC **K91.2 Postsurgical malabsorption, not elsewhere classified**
Postsurgical blind loop syndrome
> **Excludes1:** *malabsorption osteomalacia in adults (M83.2)*
> *malabsorption osteoporosis, postsurgical (M80.8-, M81.8)*

+ **K91.3 Postprocedural intestinal obstruction**
AHA CC: 4Q, 2017, 16-17

CC **K91.30 Postprocedural intestinal obstruction, unspecified as to partial versus complete**
Postprocedural intestinal obstruction NOS

CC **K91.31 Postprocedural partial intestinal obstruction**
Postprocedural incomplete intestinal obstruction

CC **K91.32 Postprocedural complete intestinal obstruction**
K91.5 Postcholecystectomy syndrome
+ **K91.6 Intraoperative hemorrhage and hematoma of a digestive system organ or structure complicating a procedure**
> **Excludes1:** *intraoperative hemorrhage and hematoma of a digestive system organ or structure due to accidental puncture and laceration during a procedure (K91.7-)*

CC **K91.61 Intraoperative hemorrhage and hematoma of a digestive system organ or structure complicating a digestive sytem procedure**
AHA CC: 1Q, 2020, 19-20

CC **K91.62 Intraoperative hemorrhage and hematoma of a digestive system organ or structure complicating other procedure**

+ **K91.7 Accidental puncture and laceration of a digestive system organ or structure during a procedure**
CC **K91.71 Accidental puncture and laceration of a digestive system organ or structure during a digestive system procedure**
CC **K91.72 Accidental puncture and laceration of a digestive system organ or structure during other procedure**
AHA CC: 2Q, 2019, 23-24

+ **K91.8 Other intraoperative and postprocedural complications and disorders of digestive system**
CC **K91.81 Other intraoperative complications of digestive system**
CC **K91.82 Postprocedural hepatic failure**
CC **K91.83 Postprocedural hepatorenal syndrome**
+ **K91.84 Postprocedural hemorrhage of a digestive system organ or structure following a procedure**
CC **K91.840 Postprocedural hemorrhage of a digestive system organ or structure following a digestive system procedure**
AHA CC: 1Q, 2016, 15
CC **K91.841 Postprocedural hemorrhage of a digestive system organ or structure following other procedure**
+ **K91.85 Complications of intestinal pouch**
CC **K91.850 Pouchitis**
Inflammation of internal ileoanal pouch
CC **K91.858 Other complications of intestinal pouch**
AHA CC: 2Q, 2019, 13
CC **K91.86 Retained cholelithiasis following cholecystectomy**
+ **K91.87 Postprocedural hematoma and seroma of a digestive system organ or structure following a procedure**

747

+, +7th, X + 7th   ● Newborn   ● Pediatric   ● Maternity   ● Adult   ♀ Female   ♂ Male   Manifestation   Unacceptable PDX   HCC   CC   MCC   HAC

CC **K91.870** **Postprocedural hematoma of a digestive system organ or structure following a digestive system procedure**

CC **K91.871** **Postprocedural hematoma of a digestive system organ or structure following other procedure**

CC **K91.872** **Postprocedural seroma of a digestive system organ or structure following a digestive system procedure**

CC **K91.873** **Postprocedural seroma of a digestive system organ or structure following other procedure**

CC **K91.89** **Other postprocedural complications and disorders of digestive system**

Use additional code, if applicable, to further specify disorder

Excludes2: *postprocedural retroperitoneal abscess (K68.11)*

AHA CC: 1Q, 2017, 40-41; 2Q, 2020, 22-23

K92 **Other diseases of digestive system**

Excludes1: *neonatal gastrointestinal hemorrhage (P54.0-P54.3)*

CC **K92.0** **Hematemesis**

CC **K92.1** **Melena**

Excludes1: *occult blood in feces (R19.5)*

CC **K92.2** **Gastrointestinal hemorrhage, unspecified**

Gastric hemorrhage NOS

Intestinal hemorrhage NOS

Excludes1: *acute hemorrhagic gastritis (K29.01)*
hemorrhage of anus and rectum (K62.5)
angiodysplasia of stomach with hemorrhage (K31.811)
diverticular disease with hemorrhage (K57.-)
gastritis and duodenitis with hemorrhage (K29.-)
peptic ulcer with hemorrhage (K25-K28)

+ **K92.8** **Other specified diseases of the digestive system**

CC **K92.81** **Gastrointestinal mucositis (ulcerative)**

Code also type of associated therapy, such as:
antineoplastic and immunosuppressive drugs (T45.1X-)
radiological procedure and radiotherapy (Y84.2)

Excludes2: *mucositis (ulcerative) of vagina and vulva (N76.81)*
nasal mucositis (ulcerative) (J34.81)
oral mucositis (ulcerative) (K12.3-)

K92.89 **Other specified diseases of the digestive system**

K92.9 **Disease of digestive system, unspecified**

K94 **Complications of artificial openings of the digestive system**

+ **K94.0** **Colostomy complications**

K94.00 **Colostomy complication, unspecified**

CC **K94.01** **Colostomy hemorrhage**

CC **K94.02** **Colostomy infection**

Use additional code to specify type of infection, such as:
cellulitis of abdominal wall (L03.311)
sepsis (A40.-, A41.-)

CC **K94.03** **Colostomy malfunction**

Mechanical complication of colostomy

K94.09 **Other complications of colostomy**

+ **K94.1** **Enterostomy complications**

K94.10 **Enterostomy complication, unspecified**

CC **K94.11** **Enterostomy hemorrhage**

CC **K94.12** **Enterostomy infection**

Use additional code to specify type of infection, such as:
cellulitis of abdominal wall (L03.311)
sepsis (A40.-, A41.-)

CC **K94.13** **Enterostomy malfunction**

Mechanical complication of enterostomy

CC **K94.19** **Other complications of enterostomy**

+ **K94.2** **Gastrostomy complications**

K94.20 **Gastrostomy complication, unspecified**

K94.21 **Gastrostomy hemorrhage**

CC **K94.22** **Gastrostomy infection**

Use additional code to specify type of infection, such as:
cellulitis of abdominal wall (L03.311)
sepsis (A40.-, A41.-)

CC **K94.23** **Gastrostomy malfunction**

Mechanical complication of gastrostomy

AHA CC: 1Q, 2019, 26

K94.29 **Other complications of gastrostomy**

+ **K94.3** **Esophagostomy complications**

CC **K94.30** **Esophagostomy complications, unspecified**

CC **K94.31** **Esophagostomy hemorrhage**

CC **K94.32** **Esophagostomy infection**

Use additional code to identify the infection

CC **K94.33** **Esophagostomy malfunction**

Mechanical complication of esophagostomy

CC **K94.39** **Other complications of esophagostomy**

+ **K95** **Complications of bariatric procedures**

+ **K95.0** **Complications of gastric band procedure**

CC **K95.01** **Infection due to gastric band procedure**

Use additional code to specify type of infection or organism, such as:
bacterial and viral infectious agents (B95.-, B96.-)
cellulitis of abdominal wall (L03.311)
sepsis (A40.-, A41.-)

HAC see Appendix B for HAC conditional logic

CC **K95.09** **Other complications of gastric band procedure**

Use additional code, if applicable, to further specify complication

+ **K95.8** **Complications of other bariatric procedure**

Excludes1: *complications of gastric band surgery (K95.0-)*

CC **K95.81** **Infection due to other bariatric procedure**

Use additional code to specify type of infection or organism, such as:
bacterial and viral infectious agents (B95.-, B96.-)
cellulitis of abdominal wall (L03.311)
sepsis (A40.-, A41.-)

HAC see Appendix B for HAC conditional logic

CC **K95.89** **Other complications of other bariatric procedure**

Use additional code, if applicable, to further specify complication

+, +7th, X + 7th   ● Newborn   ● Pediatric   ● Maternity   ● Adult   ♀ Female   ♂ Male   Manifestation   Unacceptable PDX   HCC   CC   MCC   HAC

Chapter 12: Diseases of the Skin and Subcutaneous Tissue (L00-L99)

Excludes2: certain conditions originating in the perinatal period (P04-P96)
certain infectious and parasitic diseases (A00-B99)
complications of pregnancy, childbirth and the puerperium (O00-O9A)
congenital malformations, deformations, and chromosomal
abnormalities (Q00-Q99)
endocrine, nutritional and metabolic diseases (E00-E88)
lipomelanotic reticulosis (I89.8)
neoplasms (C00-D49)
symptoms, signs and abnormal clinical and laboratory findings,
not elsewhere classified (R00-R94)
systemic connective tissue disorders (M30-M36)
viral warts (B07.-)

This chapter contains the following category blocks:

L00-L08	Infections of the skin and subcutaneous tissue
L10-L14	Bullous disorders
L20-L30	Dermatitis and eczema
L40-L45	Papulosquamous disorders
L49-L54	Urticaria and erythema
L55-L59	Radiation-related disorders of the skin and subcutaneous tissue
L60-L75	Disorders of skin appendages
L76	Intraoperative and postprocedural complications of skin and subcutaneous tissue
L80-L99	Other disorders of the skin and subcutaneous tissue

C. Chapter-Specific Coding Guidelines

In addition to general coding guidelines, there are guidelines for specific diagnoses and/or conditions in the classification. Unless otherwise indicated, these guidelines apply to all health care settings. Please refer to Section II for guidelines on the selection of principal diagnosis.

12. Chapter 12: Diseases of the Skin and Subcutaneous Tissue (L00-L99)

a. Pressure ulcer stage codes

1) Pressure ulcer stages

Codes in category L89, Pressure ulcer, identify the site and stage of the pressure ulcer.

The ICD-10-CM classifies pressure ulcer stages based on severity, which is designated by stages 1-4 deep tissue pressure injury, unspecified stage and unstageable.

Assign as many codes from category L89 as needed to identify all the pressure ulcers the patient has, if applicable.

See Section I.B.14 for pressure ulcer stage documentation by clinicians other than patient's provider.

2) Unstageable pressure ulcers

Assignment of the code for unstageable pressure ulcer (L89.--0) should be based on the clinical documentation. These codes are used for pressure ulcers whose stage cannot be clinically determined (e.g., the ulcer is covered by eschar or has been treated with a skin or muscle graft) and pressure ulcers that are documented as deep tissue injury but not documented as due to trauma. This code should not be confused with the codes for unspecified stage (L89.--9). When there is no documentation regarding the stage of the pressure ulcer, assign the appropriate code for unspecified stage (L89.--9).

3) Documented pressure ulcer stage

Assignment of the pressure ulcer stage code should be guided by clinical documentation of the stage or documentation of the terms found in the Alphabetic Index. For clinical terms describing the stage that are not found in the Alphabetic Index, and there is no documentation of the stage, the provider should be queried.

4) Patients admitted with pressure ulcers documented as healed

No code is assigned if the documentation states that the pressure ulcer is completely healed at the time of admission.

5) Patients admitted with pressure ulcers documented as healing

Pressure ulcers described as healing should be assigned the appropriate pressure ulcer stage code based on the documentation in the medical record. If the documentation does not provide information about the stage of the healing pressure ulcer, assign the appropriate code for unspecified stage.

If the documentation is unclear as to whether the patient has a current (new) pressure ulcer or if the patient is being treated for a healing pressure ulcer, query the provider.

For ulcers that were present on admission but healed at the time of discharge, assign the code for the site and stage of the pressure ulcer at the time of admission.

6) Patient admitted with pressure ulcer evolving into another stage during the admission

If a patient is admitted to an inpatient hospital with a pressure ulcer at one stage and it progresses to a higher stage, two separate codes should be assigned: one code for the site and stage of the ulcer on admission and a second code for the same ulcer site and the highest stage reported during the stay.

7) Pressure-induced deep tissue damage

For pressure-induced deep tissue damage or deep tissue pressure injury, assign only the appropriate code for pressure-induced deep tissue damage (L89.--6).

b. Non-Pressure Chronic Ulcers

1) Patients admitted with non-pressure ulcers documented as healed

No code is assigned if the documentation states that the non-pressure ulcer is completely healed at the time of admission.

2) Patients admitted with non-pressure ulcers documented as healing

Non-pressure ulcers described as healing should be assigned the appropriate non-pressure ulcer code based on the documentation in the medical record. If the documentation does not provide information about the severity of the healing non-pressure ulcer, assign the appropriate code unspecified severity.

If the documentation is unclear as to whether the patient has a current (new) non-pressure ulcer or if the patient is being treated for a healing non-pressure ulcer, query the provider.

For ulcers that were present on admission but healed at the time of discharge, assign the code for the site and severity of the non-pressure ulcer at the time of admission.

3) Patient admitted with non-pressure ulcer that progresses to another severity level during the admission

If a patient is admitted to an inpatient hospital with a non-pressure ulcer at one severity level and it progresses to a higher severity level, two separate codes should be assigned; one code for the site and severity level of the ulcer on admission and a second code for the same ulcer site and the highest severity level reported during the stay.

See Section I.B.14 for pressure ulcer stage documentation by clinicians other than patient's provider.

Infections of the skin and subcutaneous tissue (L00-L08)

Use additional code (B95-B97) to identify infectious agent

Excludes2: hordeolum (H00.0)
infective dermatitis (L30.3)
local infections of skin classified in Chapter 1
lupus panniculitis (L93.2)
panniculitis NOS (M79.3)
panniculitis of neck and back (M54.0-)
Perlèche NOS (K13.0)
Perlèche due to candidiasis (B37.0)
Perlèche due to riboflavin deficiency (E53.0)
pyogenic granuloma (L98.0)
relapsing panniculitis [Weber-Christian] (M35.6)
viral warts (B07.-)
zoster (B02.-)

L00 Staphylococcal scalded skin syndrome

Ritter's disease
Use additional code to identify percentage of skin exfoliation (L49.-)
Excludes1: bullous impetigo (L01.03)
pemphigus neonatorum (L01.03)
toxic epidermal necrolysis [Lyell] (L51.2)
Valid 3-character code, no further characters required

L01 Impetigo

Excludes1: impetigo herpetiformis (L40.1)
+ **L01.0 Impetigo**
Impetigo contagiosa
Impetigo vulgaris
L01.00 Impetigo, unspecified
Impetigo NOS
L01.01 Non-bullous impetigo
L01.02 Bockhart's impetigo
Impetigo follicularis
Perifolliculitis NOS
Superficial pustular perifolliculitis
L01.03 Bullous impetigo
Impetigo neonatorum
Pemphigus neonatorum

749

Cross-Section of the Skin Showing Layers and Types of Infection

Skin compartments

- Epidermis
- Dermis
- Subcutaneous tissue
- Deep fascia
- Muscle
- Bone

Vesicle
Crust
Hair follicle
Bullae
Sebaceous gland

Lymphatic vessel
Artery
Vein
Sweat gland

Infection site — **Etiologic organisms**

Staphylococcus aureus

Group A β-hemolytic Streptococcus (common)
Group C and G Streptococcus (uncommon)
Staphylococcus aureus, Streptococcus pneumoniae,
Enterococci or aerobic Gram-negative bacilli (rare)

Folliculitis furuncles — *Staphylococcus aureus*

Group A B-hemolytic Streptococcus (most common)
Group B, C and G Streptococcus (common)
Staphylococcus aureus (uncommon)
H.Influenzae (rare)
Other (rare)

Necrotizing fasciitis — *Streptococcus pyogenes*
Enterococci Gram-negative bacilli

Myositis

J. CHOVAN

L01.09 Other impetigo
Ulcerative impetigo
L01.1 Impetiginization of other dermatoses
L02 Cutaneous abscess, furuncle and carbuncle
Use additional code to identify organism (B95-B96)
Excludes2: *abscess of anus and rectal regions (K61.-)*
abscess of female genital organs (external) (N76.4)
abscess of male genital organs (external) (N48.2, N49.-)
+ L02.0 Cutaneous abscess, furuncle and carbuncle of face
Excludes2: *abscess of ear, external (H60.0)*
abscess of eyelid (H00.0)
abscess of head [any part, except face] (L02.8)
abscess of lacrimal gland (H04.0)
abscess of lacrimal passages (H04.3)
abscess of mouth (K12.2)
abscess of nose (J34.0)
abscess of orbit (H05.0)
submandibular abscess (K12.2)
CC L02.01 Cutaneous abscess of face
L02.02 Furuncle of face
Boil of face
Folliculitis of face
L02.03 Carbuncle of face
+ L02.1 Cutaneous abscess, furuncle and carbuncle of neck
CC L02.11 Cutaneous abscess of neck

L02.12 Furuncle of neck
Boil of neck
Folliculitis of neck
L02.13 Carbuncle of neck
+ L02.2 Cutaneous abscess, furuncle and carbuncle of trunk
Excludes1: *non-newborn omphalitis (L08.82)*
omphalitis of newborn (P38.-)
Excludes2: *abscess of breast (N61.1)*
abscess of buttocks (L02.3)
abscess of female external genital organs (N76.4)
abscess of male external genital organs (N48.2, N49.-)
abscess of hip (L02.4)
CC L02.21 Cutaneous abscess of trunk
CC L02.211 Cutaneous abscess of abdominal wall
CC L02.212 Cutaneous abscess of back [any part, except buttock]
CC L02.213 Cutaneous abscess of chest wall
CC L02.214 Cutaneous abscess of groin
CC L02.215 Cutaneous abscess of perineum
CC L02.216 Cutaneous abscess of umbilicus
CC L02.219 Cutaneous abscess of trunk, unspecified
+ L02.22 Furuncle of trunk
Boil of trunk
Folliculitis of trunk

L02.221 Furuncle of abdominal wall
L02.222 Furuncle of back [any part, except buttock]
L02.223 Furuncle of chest wall
L02.224 Furuncle of groin
L02.225 Furuncle of perineum
L02.226 Furuncle of umbilicus
L02.229 Furuncle of trunk, unspecified

+ L02.23 Carbuncle of trunk
L02.231 Carbuncle of abdominal wall
L02.232 Carbuncle of back [any part, except buttock]
L02.233 Carbuncle of chest wall
L02.234 Carbuncle of groin
L02.235 Carbuncle of perineum
L02.236 Carbuncle of umbilicus
L02.239 Carbuncle of trunk, unspecified

+ L02.3 Cutaneous abscess, furuncle and carbuncle of buttock
Excludes1: *pilonidal cyst with abscess (L05.01)*
CC L02.31 Cutaneous abscess of buttock
Cutaneous abscess of gluteal region
L02.32 Furuncle of buttock
Boil of buttock
Folliculitis of buttock
Furuncle of gluteal region
L02.33 Carbuncle of buttock
Carbuncle of gluteal region

+ L02.4 Cutaneous abscess, furuncle and carbuncle of limb
Excludes2: *Cutaneous abscess, furuncle and carbuncle of groin (L02.214, L02.224, L02.234)*
Cutaneous abscess, furuncle and carbuncle of hand (L02.5-)
Cutaneous abscess, furuncle and carbuncle of foot (L02.6-)
+ L02.41 Cutaneous abscess of limb
CC L02.411 Cutaneous abscess of right axilla
CC L02.412 Cutaneous abscess of left axilla
CC L02.413 Cutaneous abscess of right upper limb
CC L02.414 Cutaneous abscess of left upper limb
CC L02.415 Cutaneous abscess of right lower limb
CC L02.416 Cutaneous abscess of left lower limb
CC L02.419 Cutaneous abscess of limb, unspecified
+ L02.42 Furuncle of limb
Boil of limb
Folliculitis of limb
L02.421 Furuncle of right axilla
L02.422 Furuncle of left axilla
L02.423 Furuncle of right upper limb
L02.424 Furuncle of left upper limb
L02.425 Furuncle of right lower limb
L02.426 Furuncle of left lower limb
L02.429 Furuncle of limb, unspecified
+ L02.43 Carbuncle of limb
L02.431 Carbuncle of right axilla
L02.432 Carbuncle of left axilla
L02.433 Carbuncle of right upper limb
L02.434 Carbuncle of left upper limb
L02.435 Carbuncle of right lower limb
L02.436 Carbuncle of left lower limb
L02.439 Carbuncle of limb, unspecified

+ L02.5 Cutaneous abscess, furuncle and carbuncle of hand
+ L02.51 Cutaneous abscess of hand
CC L02.511 Cutaneous abscess of right hand
CC L02.512 Cutaneous abscess of left hand
CC L02.519 Cutaneous abscess of unspecified hand
+ L02.52 Furuncle hand
Boil of hand
Folliculitis of hand
L02.521 Furuncle right hand
L02.522 Furuncle left hand
L02.529 Furuncle unspecified hand
+ L02.53 Carbuncle of hand
L02.531 Carbuncle of right hand
L02.532 Carbuncle of left hand
L02.539 Carbuncle of unspecified hand

+ L02.6 Cutaneous abscess, furuncle and carbuncle of foot
+ L02.61 Cutaneous abscess of foot
CC L02.611 Cutaneous abscess of right foot
CC L02.612 Cutaneous abscess of left foot
CC L02.619 Cutaneous abscess of unspecified foot

+ L02.62 Furuncle of foot
Boil of foot
Folliculitis of foot
L02.621 Furuncle of right foot
L02.622 Furuncle of left foot
L02.629 Furuncle of unspecified foot
+ L02.63 Carbuncle of foot
L02.631 Carbuncle of right foot
L02.632 Carbuncle of left foot
L02.639 Carbuncle of unspecified foot

+ L02.8 Cutaneous abscess, furuncle and carbuncle of other sites
+ L02.81 Cutaneous abscess of other sites
CC L02.811 Cutaneous abscess of head [any part, except face]
CC L02.818 Cutaneous abscess of other sites
+ L02.82 Furuncle of other sites
Boil of other sites
Folliculitis of other sites
L02.821 Furuncle of head [any part, except face]
L02.828 Furuncle of other sites
+ L02.83 Carbuncle of other sites
L02.831 Carbuncle of head [any part, except face]
L02.838 Carbuncle of other sites

+ L02.9 Cutaneous abscess, furuncle and carbuncle, unspecified
CC L02.91 Cutaneous abscess, unspecified
L02.92 Furuncle, unspecified
Boil NOS
Furunculosis NOS
L02.93 Carbuncle, unspecified

L03 Cellulitis and acute lymphangitis
Excludes2: *cellulitis of anal and rectal region (K61.-)*
cellulitis of external auditory canal (H60.1)
cellulitis of eyelid (H00.0)
cellulitis of female external genital organs (N76.4)
cellulitis of lacrimal apparatus (H04.3)
cellulitis of male external genital organs (N48.2, N49.-)
cellulitis of mouth (K12.2)
cellulitis of nose (J34.0)
eosinophilic cellulitis [Wells] (L98.3)
febrile neutrophilic dermatosis [Sweet] (L98.2)
lymphangitis (chronic) (subacute) (I89.1)

+ L03.0 Cellulitis and acute lymphangitis of finger and toe
Infection of nail
Onychia
Paronychia
Perionychia
+ L03.01 Cellulitis of finger
Felon
Whitlow
Excludes1: *herpetic whitlow (B00.89)*
L03.011 Cellulitis of right finger
L03.012 Cellulitis of left finger
L03.019 Cellulitis of unspecified finger
+ L03.02 Acute lymphangitis of finger
Hangnail with lymphangitis of finger
L03.021 Acute lymphangitis of right finger
L03.022 Acute lymphangitis of left finger
L03.029 Acute lymphangitis of unspecified finger
+ L03.03 Cellulitis of toe
L03.031 Cellulitis of right toe
L03.032 Cellulitis of left toe
L03.039 Cellulitis of unspecified toe
+ L03.04 Acute lymphangitis of toe
Hangnail with lymphangitis of toe
L03.041 Acute lymphangitis of right toe
L03.042 Acute lymphangitis of left toe
L03.049 Acute lymphangitis of unspecified toe

+ L03.1 Cellulitis and acute lymphangitis of other parts of limb
+ L03.11 Cellulitis of other parts of limb
Excludes2: *cellulitis of fingers (L03.01-)*
cellulitis of toes (L03.03-)
groin (L03.314)
CC L03.111 Cellulitis of right axilla
CC L03.112 Cellulitis of left axilla
CC L03.113 Cellulitis of right upper limb
CC L03.114 Cellulitis of left upper limb
AHA CC: 1Q, 2019, 13
CC L03.115 Cellulitis of right lower limb
CC L03.116 Cellulitis of left lower limb
CC L03.119 Cellulitis of unspecified part of limb

+, +7th, X + 7th • Newborn • Pediatric • Maternity • Adult ♀ Female ♂ Male Manifestation Unacceptable PDX HCC CC MCC HAC

+ **L03.12** **Acute lymphangitis of other parts of limb**
> *Excludes2:* *acute lymphangitis of fingers (L03.2-)*
> *acute lymphangitis of toes (L03.04-)*
> *acute lymphangitis of groin (L03.324)*

CC **L03.121** **Acute lymphangitis of right axilla**
CC **L03.122** **Acute lymphangitis of left axilla**
CC **L03.123** **Acute lymphangitis of right upper limb**
CC **L03.124** **Acute lymphangitis of left upper limb**
CC **L03.125** **Acute lymphangitis of right lower limb**
CC **L03.126** **Acute lymphangitis of left lower limb**
CC **L03.129** **Acute lymphangitis of unspecified part of limb**

+ **L03.2** **Cellulitis and acute lymphangitis of face and neck**
> + **L03.21** **Cellulitis and acute lymphangitis of face**
> > CC **L03.211** **Cellulitis of face**
> > > *Excludes2:* *abscess of orbit (H05.01-)*
> > > *cellulitis of ear (H60.1-)*
> > > *cellulitis of eyelid (H00.0-)*
> > > *cellulitis of head (L03.81)*
> > > *cellulitis of lacrimal apparatus (H04.3)*
> > > *cellulitis of lip (K13.0)*
> > > *cellulitis of mouth (K12.2)*
> > > *cellulitis of nose (internal) (J34.0)*
> > > *cellulitis of orbit (H05.01-)*
> > > *cellulitis of scalp (L03.81)*
> > > *AHA CC: 4Q, 2013, 123*
> > CC **L03.212** **Acute lymphangitis of face**
> > CC **L03.213** **Periorbital cellulitis**
> > > Preseptal cellulitis
> > > *AHA CC: 4Q, 2016, 36*
> + **L03.22** **Cellulitis and acute lymphangitis of neck**
> > CC **L03.221** **Cellulitis of neck**
> > CC **L03.222** **Acute lymphangitis of neck**

+ **L03.3** **Cellulitis and acute lymphangitis of trunk**
> + **L03.31** **Cellulitis of trunk**
> > *Excludes2:* *cellulitis of anal and rectal regions (K61.-)*
> > *cellulitis of breast NOS (N61.0)*
> > *cellulitis of female external genital organs (N76.4)*
> > *cellulitis of male external genital organs (N48.2, N49.-)*
> > *omphalitis of newborn (P38.-)*
> > *puerperal cellulitis of breast (O91.2)*
> > CC **L03.311** **Cellulitis of abdominal wall**
> > > *Excludes2:* *cellulitis of umbilicus (L03.316)*
> > > *cellulitis of groin (L03.314)*
> > CC **L03.312** **Cellulitis of back [any part except buttock]**
> > CC **L03.313** **Cellulitis of chest wall**
> > CC **L03.314** **Cellulitis of groin**
> > CC **L03.315** **Cellulitis of perineum**
> > CC **L03.316** **Cellulitis of umbilicus**
> > CC **L03.317** **Cellulitis of buttock**
> > CC **L03.319** **Cellulitis of trunk, unspecified**
> + **L03.32** **Acute lymphangitis of trunk**
> > CC **L03.321** **Acute lymphangitis of abdominal wall**
> > CC **L03.322** **Acute lymphangitis of back [any part except buttock]**
> > CC **L03.323** **Acute lymphangitis of chest wall**
> > CC **L03.324** **Acute lymphangitis of groin**
> > CC **L03.325** **Acute lymphangitis of perineum**
> > CC **L03.326** **Acute lymphangitis of umbilicus**
> > CC **L03.327** **Acute lymphangitis of buttock**
> > CC **L03.329** **Acute lymphangitis of trunk, unspecified**

+ **L03.8** **Cellulitis and acute lymphangitis of other sites**
> + **L03.81** **Cellulitis of other sites**
> > CC **L03.811** **Cellulitis of head [any part, except face]**
> > > Cellulitis of scalp
> > > *Excludes2:* *cellulitis of face (L03.211)*
> > CC **L03.818** **Cellulitis of other sites**
> + **L03.89** **Acute lymphangitis of other sites**
> > CC **L03.891** **Acute lymphangitis of head [any part, except face]**
> > CC **L03.898** **Acute lymphangitis of other sites**

+ **L03.9** **Cellulitis and acute lymphangitis, unspecified**
> CC **L03.90** **Cellulitis, unspecified**
> CC **L03.91** **Acute lymphangitis, unspecified**
> > *Excludes1:* *lymphangitis NOS (I89.1)*

L04 **Acute lymphadenitis**

> **Includes:** abscess (acute) of lymph nodes, except mesenteric
> acute lymphadenitis, except mesenteric
> *Excludes1:* *chronic or subacute lymphadenitis, except mesenteric (I88.1)*
> *enlarged lymph nodes (R59.-)*
> *human immunodeficiency virus [HIV] disease resulting in generalized lymphadenopathy (B20)*
> *lymphadenitis NOS (I88.9)*
> *nonspecific mesenteric lymphadenitis (I88.0)*

L04.0 **Acute lymphadenitis of face, head and neck**
L04.1 **Acute lymphadenitis of trunk**
L04.2 **Acute lymphadenitis of upper limb**
> Acute lymphadenitis of axilla
> Acute lymphadenitis of shoulder
L04.3 **Acute lymphadenitis of lower limb**
> Acute lymphadenitis of hip
> *Excludes2:* *acute lymphadenitis of groin (L04.1)*
L04.8 **Acute lymphadenitis of other sites**
L04.9 **Acute lymphadenitis, unspecified**

L05 **Pilonidal cyst and sinus**

> + **L05.0** **Pilonidal cyst and sinus with abscess**
> > CC **L05.01** **Pilonidal cyst with abscess**
> > > Pilonidal abscess
> > > Pilonidal dimple with abscess
> > > Postanal dimple with abscess
> > > *Excludes2:* *congenital sacral dimple (Q82.6)*
> > > *parasacral dimple (Q82.6)*
> > CC **L05.02** **Pilonidal sinus with abscess**
> > > Coccygeal fistula with abscess
> > > Coccygeal sinus with abscess
> > > Pilonidal fistula with abscess
> + **L05.9** **Pilonidal cyst and sinus without abscess**
> > **L05.91** **Pilonidal cyst without abscess**
> > > Pilonidal dimple
> > > Postanal dimple
> > > Pilonidal cyst NOS
> > > *Excludes2:* *congenital sacral dimple (Q82.6)*
> > > *parasacral dimple (Q82.6)*
> > **L05.92** **Pilonidal sinus without abscess**
> > > Coccygeal fistula
> > > Coccygeal sinus without abscess
> > > Pilonidal fistula

L08 **Other local infections of skin and subcutaneous tissue**

> **L08.0** **Pyoderma**
> > Dermatitis gangrenosa
> > Purulent dermatitis
> > Septic dermatitis
> > Suppurative dermatitis
> > *Excludes1:* *pyoderma gangrenosum (L88)*
> > *pyoderma vegetans (L08.81)*
> CC **L08.1** **Erythrasma**
> + **L08.8** **Other specified local infections of the skin and subcutaneous tissue**
> > **L08.81** **Pyoderma vegetans**
> > > *Excludes1:* *pyoderma gangrenosum (L88)*
> > > *pyoderma NOS (L08.0)*
> > **L08.82** **Omphalitis not of newborn**
> > > *Excludes1:* *omphalitis of newborn (P38.-)*
> > **L08.89** **Other specified local infections of the skin and subcutaneous tissue**
> **L08.9** **Local infection of the skin and subcutaneous tissue, unspecified**

Bullous disorders (L10-L14)

Excludes1: *benign familial pemphigus [Hailey-Hailey] (Q82.8)*
staphylococcal scalded skin syndrome (L00)
toxic epidermal necrolysis [Lyell] (L51.2)

L10 **Pemphigus**

> *Excludes1:* *pemphigus neonatorum (L01.03)*
CC **L10.0** **Pemphigus vulgaris**
CC **L10.1** **Pemphigus vegetans**

CC **L10.2 Pemphigus foliaceous**

CC **L10.3 Brazilian pemphigus [fogo selvagem]**

CC **L10.4 Pemphigus erythematosus**

Senear-Usher syndrome

CC **L10.5 Drug-induced pemphigus**

Use additional code for adverse effect, if applicable, to identify drug (T36-T50 with fifth or sixth character 5)

+ **L10.8 Other pemphigus**

CC **L10.81 Paraneoplastic pemphigus**

CC **L10.89 Other pemphigus**

CC **L10.9 Pemphigus, unspecified**

L11 Other acantholytic disorders

L11.0 Acquired keratosis follicularis

Excludes1: keratosis follicularis (congenital) [Darier-White] (Q82.8)

L11.1 Transient acantholytic dermatosis [Grover]

L11.8 Other specified acantholytic disorders

L11.9 Acantholytic disorder, unspecified

L12 Pemphigoid

Excludes1: herpes gestationis (O26.4-)
impetigo herpetiformis (L40.1)

CC **L12.0 Bullous pemphigoid**

L12.1 Cicatricial pemphigoid

Benign mucous membrane pemphigoid

• **L12.2 Chronic bullous disease of childhood**

Juvenile dermatitis herpetiformis

+ **L12.3 Acquired epidermolysis bullosa**

Excludes1: epidermolysis bullosa (congenital) (Q81.-)

CC **L12.30 Acquired epidermolysis bullosa, unspecified**

CC **L12.31 Epidermolysis bullosa due to drug**

Use additional code for adverse effect, if applicable, to identify drug (T36-T50 with fifth or sixth character 5)

CC **L12.35 Other acquired epidermolysis bullosa**

CC **L12.8 Other pemphigoid**

CC **L12.9 Pemphigoid, unspecified**

L13 Other bullous disorders

L13.0 Dermatitis herpetiformis

Duhring's disease
Hydroa herpetiformis

Excludes1: juvenile dermatitis herpetiformis (L12.2)
senile dermatitis herpetiformis (L12.0)

L13.1 Subcorneal pustular dermatitis

Sneddon-Wilkinson disease

L13.8 Other specified bullous disorders

L13.9 Bullous disorder, unspecified

L14 Bullous disorders in diseases classified elsewhere

Code first underlying disease
Valid 3-character code, no further characters required

Dermatitis and eczema (L20-L30)

NOTE In this block the terms dermatitis and eczema are used synonymously and interchangeably.

Excludes2: chronic (childhood) granulomatous disease (D71)
dermatitis gangrenosa (L08.0)
dermatitis herpetiformis (L13.0)
dry skin dermatitis (L85.3)
factitial dermatitis (L98.1)
perioral dermatitis (L71.0)
radiation-related disorders of the skin and subcutaneous tissue (L55-L59)
stasis dermatitis (I87.2)

L20 Atopic dermatitis

L20.0 Besnier's prurigo

+ **L20.8 Other atopic dermatitis**

Excludes2: circumscribed neurodermatitis (L28.0)

L20.81 Atopic neurodermatitis

Diffuse neurodermatitis

L20.82 Flexural eczema

• **L20.83 Infantile (acute) (chronic) eczema**

L20.84 Intrinsic (allergic) eczema

L20.89 Other atopic dermatitis

L20.9 Atopic dermatitis, unspecified

L21 Seborrheic dermatitis

Excludes2: infective dermatitis (L30.3)
seborrheic keratosis (L82.-)

L21.0 Seborrhea capitis

Cradle cap
AHA CC: 1Q, 2018, 6

• **L21.1 Seborrheic infantile dermatitis**

L21.8 Other seborrheic dermatitis

L21.9 Seborrheic dermatitis, unspecified

Seborrhea NOS

L22 Diaper dermatitis

Diaper erythema
Diaper rash
Psoriasiform diaper rash
Valid 3-character code, no further characters required

L23 Allergic contact dermatitis

Excludes1: allergy NOS (T78.40)
contact dermatitis NOS (L25.9)
dermatitis NOS (L30.9)

Excludes2: dermatitis due to substances taken internally (L27.-)
dermatitis of eyelid (H01.1-)
diaper dermatitis (L22)
eczema of external ear (H60.5-)
irritant contact dermatitis (L24.-)
perioral dermatitis (L71.0)
radiation-related disorders of the skin and subcutaneous tissue (L55-L59)

L23.0 Allergic contact dermatitis due to metals

Allergic contact dermatitis due to chromium
Allergic contact dermatitis due to nickel

L23.1 Allergic contact dermatitis due to adhesives

L23.2 Allergic contact dermatitis due to cosmetics

L23.3 Allergic contact dermatitis due to drugs in contact with skin

Use additional code for adverse effect, if applicable, to identify drug (T36-T50 with fifth or sixth character 5)

Excludes2: dermatitis due to ingested drugs and medicaments (L27.0-L27.1)

L23.4 Allergic contact dermatitis due to dyes

L23.5 Allergic contact dermatitis due to other chemical products

Allergic contact dermatitis due to cement
Allergic contact dermatitis due to insecticide
Allergic contact dermatitis due to plastic
Allergic contact dermatitis due to rubber

L23.6 Allergic contact dermatitis due to food in contact with the skin

Excludes2: dermatitis due to ingested food (L27.2)

L23.7 Allergic contact dermatitis due to plants, except food

Excludes2: allergy NOS due to pollen (J30.1)

+ **L23.8 Allergic contact dermatitis due to other agents**

L23.81 Allergic contact dermatitis due to animal (cat) (dog) dander

Allergic contact dermatitis due to animal (cat) (dog) hair

L23.89 Allergic contact dermatitis due to other agents

L23.9 Allergic contact dermatitis, unspecified cause

Allergic contact eczema NOS

L24 Irritant contact dermatitis

Excludes1: allergy NOS (T78.40)
contact dermatitis NOS (L25.9)
dermatitis NOS (L30.9)

Excludes2: allergic contact dermatitis (L23.-)
dermatitis due to substances taken internally (L27.-)
dermatitis of eyelid (H01.1-)
diaper dermatitis (L22)
eczema of external ear (H60.5-)
perioral dermatitis (L71.0)
radiation-related disorders of the skin and subcutaneous tissue (L55-L59)

L24.0 Irritant contact dermatitis due to detergents

L24.1 Irritant contact dermatitis due to oils and greases

+, +7th, X + 7th   • Newborn   • Pediatric   • Maternity   • Adult   ♀ Female   ♂ Male   Manifestation   Unacceptable PDX   HCC   CC   MCC   HAC

L24.2 **Irritant contact dermatitis due to solvents**
Irritant contact dermatitis due to chlorocompound
Irritant contact dermatitis due to cyclohexane
Irritant contact dermatitis due to ester
Irritant contact dermatitis due to glycol
Irritant contact dermatitis due to hydrocarbon
Irritant contact dermatitis due to ketone

L24.3 **Irritant contact dermatitis due to cosmetics**

L24.4 **Irritant contact dermatitis due to drugs in contact with skin**
Use additional code for adverse effect, if applicable, to identify drug (T36-T50 with fifth or sixth character 5)

L24.5 **Irritant contact dermatitis due to other chemical products**
Irritant contact dermatitis due to cement
Irritant contact dermatitis due to insecticide
Irritant contact dermatitis due to plastic
Irritant contact dermatitis due to rubber

L24.6 **Irritant contact dermatitis due to food in contact with skin**
Excludes2: *dermatitis due to ingested food (L27.2)*

L24.7 **Irritant contact dermatitis due to plants, except food**
Excludes2: *allergy NOS to pollen (J30.1)*

+ L24.8 **Irritant contact dermatitis due to other agents**
  L24.81 **Irritant contact dermatitis due to metals**
  Irritant contact dermatitis due to chromium
  Irritant contact dermatitis due to nickel
  L24.89 **Irritant contact dermatitis due to other agents**
  Irritant contact dermatitis due to dyes

L24.9 **Irritant contact dermatitis, unspecified cause**
Irritant contact eczema NOS

L25 **Unspecified contact dermatitis**

Excludes1: *allergic contact dermatitis (L23.-)*
allergy NOS (T78.40)
dermatitis NOS (L30.9)
irritant contact dermatitis (L24.-)
Excludes2: *dermatitis due to ingested substances (L27.-)*
dermatitis of eyelid (H01.1-)
eczema of external ear (H60.5-)
perioral dermatitis (L71.0)
radiation-related disorders of the skin and subcutaneous tissue (L55-L59)

L25.0 **Unspecified contact dermatitis due to cosmetics**

L25.1 **Unspecified contact dermatitis due to drugs in contact with skin**
Use additional code for adverse effect, if applicable, to identify drug (T36-T50 with fifth or sixth character 5)
Excludes2: *dermatitis due to ingested drugs and medicaments (L27.0-L27.1)*

L25.2 **Unspecified contact dermatitis due to dyes**

L25.3 **Unspecified contact dermatitis due to other chemical products**
Unspecified contact dermatitis due to cement
Unspecified contact dermatitis due to insecticide

L25.4 **Unspecified contact dermatitis due to food in contact with skin**
Excludes2: *dermatitis due to ingested food (L27.2)*

L25.5 **Unspecified contact dermatitis due to plants, except food**
Excludes1: *nettle rash (L50.9)*
Excludes2: *allergy NOS due to pollen (J30.1)*

L25.8 **Unspecified contact dermatitis due to other agents**

L25.9 **Unspecified contact dermatitis, unspecified cause**
Contact dermatitis (occupational) NOS
Contact eczema (occupational) NOS

L26 **Exfoliative dermatitis**

Hebra's pityriasis
Excludes1: *Ritter's disease (L00)*
Valid 3-character code, no further characters required

L27 **Dermatitis due to substances taken internally**

Excludes1: *allergy NOS (T78.40)*
Excludes2: *adverse food reaction, except dermatitis (T78.0-T78.1)*
contact dermatitis (L23-L25)
drug photoallergic response (L56.1)
drug phototoxic response (L56.0)
urticaria (L50.-)

L27.0 **Generalized skin eruption due to drugs and medicaments taken internally**
Use additional code for adverse effect, if applicable, to identify drug (T36-T50 with fifth or sixth character 5)

L27.1 **Localized skin eruption due to drugs and medicaments taken internally**
Use additional code for adverse effect, if applicable, to identify drug (T36-T50 with fifth or sixth character 5)

L27.2 **Dermatitis due to ingested food**
Excludes2: *dermatitis due to food in contact with skin (L23.6, L24.6, L25.4)*

L27.8 **Dermatitis due to other substances taken internally**

L27.9 **Dermatitis due to unspecified substance taken internally**

L28 **Lichen simplex chronicus and prurigo**

L28.0 **Lichen simplex chronicus**
Circumscribed neurodermatitis
Lichen NOS

L28.1 **Prurigo nodularis**

L28.2 **Other prurigo**
Prurigo NOS
Prurigo Hebra
Prurigo mitis
Urticaria papulosa

L29 **Pruritus**

Excludes1: *neurotic excoriation (L98.1)*
psychogenic pruritus (F45.8)

L29.0 **Pruritus ani**

♂ **L29.1** **Pruritus scroti**

♀ **L29.2** **Pruritus vulvae**

L29.3 **Anogenital pruritus, unspecified**

L29.8 **Other pruritus**

L29.9 **Pruritus, unspecified**
Itch NOS

L30 **Other and unspecified dermatitis**

Excludes2: *contact dermatitis (L23-L25)*
dry skin dermatitis (L85.3)
small plaque parapsoriasis (L41.3)
stasis dermatitis (I87.2)

L30.0 **Nummular dermatitis**

L30.1 **Dyshidrosis [pompholyx]**

L30.2 **Cutaneous autosensitization**
Candidid [levurid]
Dermatophytid
Eczematid

L30.3 **Infective dermatitis**
Infectious eczematoid dermatitis

L30.4 **Erythema intertrigo**

L30.5 **Pityriasis alba**

L30.8 **Other specified dermatitis**

L30.9 **Dermatitis, unspecified**
Eczema NOS

Papulosquamous disorders (L40-L45)

L40 **Psoriasis**

L40.0 **Psoriasis vulgaris**
Nummular psoriasis
Plaque psoriasis

L40.1 **Generalized pustular psoriasis**
Impetigo herpetiformis
Von Zumbusch's disease

L40.2 **Acrodermatitis continua**

L40.3 **Pustulosis palmaris et plantaris**

L40.4 **Guttate psoriasis**

+ L40.5 **Arthropathic psoriasis**
  L40.50 **Arthropathic psoriasis, unspecified**
  L40.51 **Distal interphalangeal psoriatic arthropathy**
  L40.52 **Psoriatic arthritis mutilans**
  L40.53 **Psoriatic spondylitis**
  L40.54 **Psoriatic juvenile arthropathy**
  L40.59 **Other psoriatic arthropathy**

L40.8 **Other psoriasis**
Flexural psoriasis

L40.9 **Psoriasis, unspecified**

L41 **Parapsoriasis**

Excludes1: *poikiloderma vasculare atrophicans (L94.5)*

L41.0 **Pityriasis lichenoides et varioliformis acuta**
Mucha-Habermann disease

L41.1 **Pityriasis lichenoides chronica**

L41.3 **Small plaque parapsoriasis**

L41.4   **Large plaque parapsoriasis**
L41.5   **Retiform parapsoriasis**
L41.8   **Other parapsoriasis**
L41.9   **Parapsoriasis, unspecified**

L42   **Pityriasis rosea**

    Valid 3-character code, no further characters required

L43   **Lichen planus**

    Excludes1: *lichen planopilaris (L66.1)*

L43.0   **Hypertrophic lichen planus**
L43.1   **Bullous lichen planus**
L43.2   **Lichenoid drug reaction**
      Use additional code for adverse effect, if applicable, to identify drug (T36-T50 with fifth or sixth character 5)
L43.3   **Subacute (active) lichen planus**
      Lichen planus tropicus
L43.8   **Other lichen planus**
L43.9   **Lichen planus, unspecified**

L44   **Other papulosquamous disorders**

L44.0   **Pityriasis rubra pilaris**
L44.1   **Lichen nitidus**
L44.2   **Lichen striatus**
L44.3   **Lichen ruber moniliformis**
● L44.4   **Infantile papular acrodermatitis [Gianotti-Crosti]**
L44.8   **Other specified papulosquamous disorders**
L44.9   **Papulosquamous disorder, unspecified**

L45   **Papulosquamous disorders in diseases classified elsewhere**

    Code first underlying disease.
    Valid 3-character code, no further characters required

Urticaria and erythema (L49-L54)

Excludes1: *Lyme disease (A69.2-)*
        rosacea (L71.-)

L49   **Exfoliation due to erythematous conditions according to extent of body surface involved**

    Code first erythematous condition causing exfoliation, such as:
      Ritter's disease (L00)
      (Staphylococcal) scalded skin syndrome (L00)
      Stevens-Johnson syndrome (L51.1)
      Stevens-Johnson syndrome-toxic epidermal necrolysis
      overlap syndrome (L51.3)
      Toxic epidermal necrolysis (L51.2)

L49.0   **Exfoliation due to erythematous condition involving less than 10 percent of body surface**
      Exfoliation due to erythematous condition NOS
L49.1   **Exfoliation due to erythematous condition involving 10-19 percent of body surface**
L49.2   **Exfoliation due to erythematous condition involving 20-29 percent of body surface**
CC L49.3   **Exfoliation due to erythematous condition involving 30-39 percent of body surface**
CC L49.4   **Exfoliation due to erythematous condition involving 40-49 percent of body surface**
CC L49.5   **Exfoliation due to erythematous condition involving 50-59 percent of body surface**
CC L49.6   **Exfoliation due to erythematous condition involving 60-69 percent of body surface**
CC L49.7   **Exfoliation due to erythematous condition involving 70-79 percent of body surface**
CC L49.8   **Exfoliation due to erythematous condition involving 80-89 percent of body surface**
CC L49.9   **Exfoliation due to erythematous condition involving 90 or more percent of body surface**

L50   **Urticaria**

    Excludes1: *allergic contact dermatitis (L23.-)*
            angioneurotic edema (T78.3)
            giant urticaria (T78.3)
            hereditary angio-edema (D84.1)
            Quincke's edema (T78.3)
            serum urticaria (T80.6-)
            solar urticaria (L56.3)
            urticaria neonatorum (P83.8)
            urticaria papulosa (L28.2)
            urticaria pigmentosa (D47.01)
L50.0   **Allergic urticaria**
L50.1   **Idiopathic urticaria**

L50.2   **Urticaria due to cold and heat**
      Excludes2: *familial cold urticaria (M04.2)*
L50.3   **Dermatographic urticaria**
L50.4   **Vibratory urticaria**
L50.5   **Cholinergic urticaria**
L50.6   **Contact urticaria**
L50.8   **Other urticaria**
      Chronic urticaria
      Recurrent periodic urticaria
L50.9   **Urticaria, unspecified**

L51   **Erythema multiforme**

    Use additional code for adverse effect, if applicable, to identify drug (T36-T50 with fifth or sixth character 5)

    Use additional code to identify associated manifestations, such as:
      arthropathy associated with dermatological disorders (M14.8-)
      conjunctival edema (H11.42)
      conjunctivitis (H10.22-)
      corneal scars and opacities (H17.-)
      corneal ulcer (H16.0-)
      edema of eyelid (H02.84-)
      inflammation of eyelid (H01.8)
      keratoconjunctivitis sicca (H16.22-)
      mechanical lagophthalmos (H02.22-)
      stomatitis (K12.-)
      symblepharon (H11.23-)

    Use additional code to identify percentage of skin exfoliation (L49.-)
    Excludes1: *staphylococcal scalded skin syndrome (L00)*
            Ritter's disease (L00)

L51.0   **Nonbullous erythema multiforme**
CC L51.1   **Stevens-Johnson syndrome**
CC L51.2   **Toxic epidermal necrolysis [Lyell]**
CC L51.3   **Stevens-Johnson syndrome-toxic epidermal necrolysis overlap syndrome**
      SJS-TEN overlap syndrome
L51.8   **Other erythema multiforme**
L51.9   **Erythema multiforme, unspecified**
      Erythema iris
      Erythema multiforme major NOS
      Erythema multiforme minor NOS
      Herpes iris

L52   **Erythema nodosum**

    Excludes1: *tuberculous erythema nodosum (A18.4)*
    Valid 3-character code, no further characters required

L53   **Other erythematous conditions**

    Excludes1: *erythema ab igne (L59.0)*
            erythema due to external agents in contact with skin (L23-L25)
            erythema intertrigo (L30.4)
CC L53.0   **Toxic erythema**
      Code first poisoning due to drug or toxin, if applicable (T36-T65 with fifth or sixth character 1-4 or 6)

      Use additional code for adverse effect, if applicable, to identify drug (T36-T50 with fifth or sixth character 5)
      Excludes1: *neonatal erythema toxicum (P83.1)*
CC L53.1   **Erythema annulare centrifugum**
CC L53.2   **Erythema marginatum**
CC L53.3   **Other chronic figurate erythema**
L53.8   **Other specified erythematous conditions**
L53.9   **Erythematous condition, unspecified**
      Erythema NOS
      Erythroderma NOS

L54   **Erythema in diseases classified elsewhere**

    Code first underlying disease
    Valid 3-character code, no further characters required

Radiation-related disorders of the skin and subcutaneous tissue (L55-L59)

L55   **Sunburn**

L55.0   **Sunburn of first degree**
L55.1   **Sunburn of second degree**
L55.2   **Sunburn of third degree**
L55.9   **Sunburn, unspecified**

755

L56   Other acute skin changes due to ultraviolet radiation

> Use additional code to identify the source of the ultraviolet radiation (W89, X32)

L56.0   Drug phototoxic response

> Use additional code for adverse effect, if applicable, to identify drug (T36-T50 with fifth or sixth character 5)

L56.1   Drug photoallergic response

> Use additional code for adverse effect, if applicable, to identify drug (T36-T50 with fifth or sixth character 5)

L56.2   Photocontact dermatitis [berloque dermatitis]

L56.3   Solar urticaria

L56.4   Polymorphous light eruption

L56.5   Disseminated superficial actinic porokeratosis (DSAP)

L56.8   Other specified acute skin changes due to ultraviolet radiation

L56.9   Acute skin change due to ultraviolet radiation, unspecified

L57   Skin changes due to chronic exposure to nonionizing radiation

> Use additional code to identify the source of the ultraviolet radiation (W89), or other nonionizing radiation (W90)

L57.0   Actinic keratosis
> Keratosis NOS
> Senile keratosis
> Solar keratosis

L57.1   Actinic reticuloid

L57.2   Cutis rhomboidalis nuchae

L57.3   Poikiloderma of Civatte

L57.4   Cutis laxa senilis
> Elastosis senilis

L57.5   Actinic granuloma

L57.8   Other skin changes due to chronic exposure to nonionizing radiation
> Farmer's skin
> Sailor's skin
> Solar dermatitis

L57.9   Skin changes due to chronic exposure to nonionizing radiation, unspecified

L58   Radiodermatitis

> Use additional code to identify the source of the radiation (W88, W90)

L58.0   Acute radiodermatitis

L58.1   Chronic radiodermatitis

L58.9   Radiodermatitis, unspecified

L59   Other disorders of skin and subcutaneous tissue related to radiation

L59.0   Erythema ab igne [dermatitis ab igne]

L59.8   Other specified disorders of the skin and subcutaneous tissue related to radiation
> *AHA CC: 1Q, 2017, 33-34*

L59.9   Disorder of the skin and subcutaneous tissue related to radiation, unspecified

Disorders of skin appendages (L60-L75)

Excludes1: congenital malformations of integument (Q84.-)

L60   Nail disorders

> *Excludes2:* clubbing of nails (R68.3)
> onychia and paronychia (L03.0-)

L60.0   Ingrowing nail

L60.1   Onycholysis

L60.2   Onychogryphosis

L60.3   Nail dystrophy

L60.4   Beau's lines

L60.5   Yellow nail syndrome

L60.8   Other nail disorders

L60.9   Nail disorder, unspecified

L62   Nail disorders in diseases classified elsewhere

> Code first underlying disease, such as:
> pachydermoperiostosis (M89.4-)
> **Valid 3-character code, no further characters required**

L63   Alopecia areata

L63.0   Alopecia (capitis) totalis

L63.1   Alopecia universalis

L63.2   Ophiasis

L63.8   Other alopecia areata

L63.9   Alopecia areata, unspecified

L64   Androgenic alopecia

> **Includes:** male-pattern baldness

L64.0   Drug-induced androgenic alopecia

> Use additional code for adverse effect, if applicable, to identify drug (T36-T50 with fifth or sixth character 5)

L64.8   Other androgenic alopecia

L64.9   Androgenic alopecia, unspecified

L65   Other nonscarring hair loss

> Use additional code for adverse effect, if applicable, to identify drug (T36-T50 with fifth or sixth character 5)

> *Excludes1:* trichotillomania (F63.3)

L65.0   Telogen effluvium

L65.1   Anagen effluvium

L65.2   Alopecia mucinosa

L65.8   Other specified nonscarring hair loss

L65.9   Nonscarring hair loss, unspecified
> Alopecia NOS

L66   Cicatricial alopecia [scarring hair loss]

L66.0   Pseudopelade

L66.1   Lichen planopilaris
> Follicular lichen planus

L66.2   Folliculitis decalvans

L66.3   Perifolliculitis capitis abscedens

L66.4   Folliculitis ulerythematosa reticulata

L66.8   Other cicatricial alopecia
> *AHA CC: 1Q, 2015, 19*

L66.9   Cicatricial alopecia, unspecified

L67   Hair color and hair shaft abnormalities

> *Excludes1:* monilethrix (Q84.1)
> pili annulati (Q84.1)
> telogen effluvium (L65.0)

L67.0   Trichorrhexis nodosa

L67.1   Variations in hair color
> Canities
> Greyness, hair (premature)
> Heterochromia of hair
> Poliosis circumscripta, acquired
> Poliosis NOS

L67.8   Other hair color and hair shaft abnormalities
> Fragilitas crinium

L67.9   Hair color and hair shaft abnormality, unspecified

L68   Hypertrichosis

> **Includes:** excess hair
> *Excludes1:* congenital hypertrichosis (Q84.2)
> persistent lanugo (Q84.2)

L68.0   Hirsutism

L68.1   Acquired hypertrichosis lanuginosa

L68.2   Localized hypertrichosis

L68.3   Polytrichia

L68.8   Other hypertrichosis

L68.9   Hypertrichosis, unspecified

L70   Acne

> *Excludes2:* acne keloid (L73.0)

L70.0   Acne vulgaris

L70.1   Acne conglobata

L70.2   Acne varioliformis
> Acne necrotica miliaris

L70.3   Acne tropica

L70.4   Infantile acne

L70.5   Acné excoriée
> Acné exocoriée des jeunes filles
> Picker's acne

L70.8   Other acne

L70.9   Acne, unspecified

L71   Rosacea

> Use additional code for adverse effect, if applicable, to identify drug (T36-T50 with fifth or sixth character 5)

L71.0   Perioral dermatitis

L71.1   Rhinophyma

L71.8   Other rosacea
> *AHA CC: 4Q, 2018, 15*

L71.9   Rosacea, unspecified

+, +7th, X + 7th   ● Newborn   ● Pediatric   ● Maternity   ● Adult   ♀ Female   ♂ Male   Manifestation   Unacceptable PDX   HCC   CC   MCC   HAC

L72 Follicular cysts of skin and subcutaneous tissue

L72.0   Epidermal cyst
+ L72.1   Pilar and trichodermal cyst
     L72.11   Pilar cyst
     L72.12   Trichodermal cyst
         Trichilemmal (proliferating) cyst
L72.2   Steatocystoma multiplex
L72.3   Sebaceous cyst
     Excludes2:   *pilar cyst (L72.11)*
         trichilemmal (proliferating) cyst (L72.12)
L72.8   Other follicular cysts of the skin and subcutaneous tissue
L72.9   Follicular cyst of the skin and subcutaneous tissue, unspecified

L73 Other follicular disorders

L73.0   Acne keloid
L73.1   Pseudofolliculitis barbae
L73.2   Hidradenitis suppurativa
L73.8   Other specified follicular disorders
     Sycosis barbae
L73.9   Follicular disorder, unspecified

L74 Eccrine sweat disorders

     Excludes2:   *generalized hyperhidrosis (R61)*
L74.0   Miliaria rubra
L74.1   Miliaria crystallina
L74.2   Miliaria profunda
     Miliaria tropicalis
L74.3   Miliaria, unspecified
L74.4   Anhidrosis
     Hypohidrosis
+ L74.5   Focal hyperhidrosis
+ L74.51   Primary focal hyperhidrosis
     L74.510   Primary focal hyperhidrosis, axilla
     L74.511   Primary focal hyperhidrosis, face
     L74.512   Primary focal hyperhidrosis, palms
     L74.513   Primary focal hyperhidrosis, soles
     L74.519   Primary focal hyperhidrosis, unspecified
     L74.52   Secondary focal hyperhidrosis
         Frey's syndrome
L74.8   Other eccrine sweat disorders
L74.9   Eccrine sweat disorder, unspecified
     Sweat gland disorder NOS

L75 Apocrine sweat disorders

     Excludes1:   *dyshidrosis (L30.1)*
         hidradenitis suppurativa (L73.2)
L75.0   Bromhidrosis
L75.1   Chromhidrosis
L75.2   Apocrine miliaria
     Fox-Fordyce disease
L75.8   Other apocrine sweat disorders
L75.9   Apocrine sweat disorder, unspecified

Intraoperative and postprocedural complications of skin and subcutaneous tissue (L76)

L76 Intraoperative and postprocedural complications of skin and subcutaneous tissue

     AHA CC: 4Q, 2016, 9-10
+ L76.0   Intraoperative hemorrhage and hematoma of skin and subcutaneous tissue complicating a procedure
     Excludes1:   *intraoperative hemorrhage and hematoma of skin and subcutaneous tissue due to accidental puncture and laceration during a procedure (L76.1-)*
CC L76.01   Intraoperative hemorrhage and hematoma of skin and subcutaneous tissue complicating a dermatologic procedure
CC L76.02   Intraoperative hemorrhage and hematoma of skin and subcutaneous tissue complicating other procedure
+ L76.1   Accidental puncture and laceration of skin and subcutaneous tissue during a procedure
CC L76.11   Accidental puncture and laceration of skin and subcutaneous tissue during a dermatologic procedure
CC L76.12   Accidental puncture and laceration of skin and subcutaneous tissue during other procedure

+ L76.2   Postprocedural hemorrhage of skin and subcutaneous tissue following a procedure
CC L76.21   Postprocedural hemorrhage of skin and subcutaneous tissue following a dermatologic procedure
CC L76.22   Postprocedural hemorrhage of skin and subcutaneous tissue following other procedure
+ L76.3   Postprocedural hematoma and seroma of skin and subcutaneous issue following a procedure
CC L76.31   Postprocedural hematoma of skin and subcutaneous tissue following a dermatologic procedure
CC L76.32   Postprocedural hematoma of skin and subcutaneous tissue following other procedure
CC L76.33   Postprocedural seroma of skin and subcutaneous tissue following a dermatologic procedure
CC L76.34   Postprocedural seroma of skin and subcutaneous tissue following other procedure
+ L76.8   Other intraoperative and postprocedural complications of skin and subcutaneous tissue
     Use additional code, if applicable, to further specify disorder
     L76.81   Other intraoperative complications of skin and subcutaneous tissue
     L76.82   Other postprocedural complications of skin and subcutaneous tissue
         AHA CC: 3Q, 2017, 6

Other disorders of the skin and subcutaneous tissue (L80-L99)

L80 Vitiligo

     Excludes2:   *vitiligo of eyelids (H02.73-)*
         vitiligo of vulva (N90.89)
     Valid 3-character code, no further characters required

L81 Other disorders of pigmentation

     Excludes1:   *birthmark NOS (Q82.5)*
         Peutz-Jeghers syndrome (Q85.8)
     Excludes2:   *nevus - see Alphabetical Index*
L81.0   Postinflammatory hyperpigmentation
L81.1   Chloasma
L81.2   Freckles
L81.3   Café au lait spots
L81.4   Other melanin hyperpigmentation
     Lentigo
L81.5   Leukoderma, not elsewhere classified
L81.6   Other disorders of diminished melanin formation
L81.7   Pigmented purpuric dermatosis
     Angioma serpiginosum
L81.8   Other specified disorders of pigmentation
     Iron pigmentation
     Tattoo pigmentation
L81.9   Disorder of pigmentation, unspecified

L82 Seborrheic keratosis

     Includes: basal cell papilloma
         dermatosis papulosa nigra
         Leser-Trélat disease
     Excludes2:   *seborrheic dermatitis (L21.-)*
L82.0   Inflamed seborrheic keratosis
L82.1   Other seborrheic keratosis
     Seborrheic keratosis NOS

L83 Acanthosis nigricans

     Confluent and reticulated papillomatosis
     Valid 3-character code, no further characters required

L84 Corns and callosities

     Callus
     Clavus
     Valid 3-character code, no further characters required

L85 Other epidermal thickening

     Excludes2:   *hypertrophic disorders of the skin (L91.-)*
L85.0   Acquired ichthyosis
     Excludes1:   *congenital ichthyosis (Q80.-)*
L85.1   Acquired keratosis [keratoderma] palmaris et plantaris
     Excludes1:   *inherited keratosis palmaris et plantaris (Q82.8)*

+, +7th, X + 7th   ● Newborn   ● Pediatric   ● Maternity   ● Adult   ♀ Female   ♂ Male   Manifestation   Unacceptable PDX   HCC   CC   MCC   HAC

L85.2 **Keratosis punctata (palmaris et plantaris)**

L85.3 **Xerosis cutis**
Dry skin dermatitis

L85.8 **Other specified epidermal thickening**
Cutaneous horn

L85.9 **Epidermal thickening, unspecified**

L86 **Keratoderma in diseases classified elsewhere**

Code first underlying disease, such as:
Reiter's disease (M02.3-)
Excludes1: *gonococcal keratoderma (A54.89)*
gonococcal keratosis (A54.89)
keratoderma due to vitamin A deficiency (E50.8)
keratosis due to vitamin A deficiency (E50.8)
xeroderma due to vitamin A deficiency (E50.8)
Valid 3-character code, no further characters required

L87 **Transepidermal elimination disorders**

Excludes1: *granuloma annulare (perforating) (L92.0)*

L87.0 **Keratosis follicularis et parafollicularis in cutem penetrans**
Kyrle disease
Hyperkeratosis follicularis penetrans

L87.1 **Reactive perforating collagenosis**

L87.2 **Elastosis perforans serpiginosa**

L87.8 **Other transepidermal elimination disorders**

L87.9 **Transepidermal elimination disorder, unspecified**

CC **L88** **Pyoderma gangrenosum**

Phagedenic pyoderma
Excludes1: *dermatitis gangrenosa (L08.0)*
Valid 3-character code, no further characters required

L89 **Pressure ulcer**

Includes: bed sore
decubitus ulcer
plaster ulcer
pressure area
pressure sore

Code first any associated gangrene (I96)
Excludes2: *decubitus (trophic) ulcer of cervix (uteri) (N86)*
diabetic ulcers (E08.621, E08.622, E09.621, E09.622,
E10.621, E10.622, E11.621, E11.622, E13.621, E13.622)
non-pressure chronic ulcer of skin (L97.-)
skin infections (L00-L08)
varicose ulcer (I83.0, I83.2)
AHA CC: 2Q, 2018, 21-22; 4Q, 2019, 10-11
Review coding guidelines B.14 and C.12.a

+ **L89.0** **Pressure ulcer of elbow**

+ **L89.00** **Pressure ulcer of unspecified elbow**

L89.000 **Pressure ulcer of unspecified elbow, unstageable**

L89.001 **Pressure ulcer of unspecified elbow, stage 1**
Healing pressure ulcer of unspecified elbow, stage 1
Pressure pre-ulcer skin changes limited to persistent focal edema, unspecified elbow

L89.002 **Pressure ulcer of unspecified elbow, stage 2**
Healing pressure ulcer of unspecified elbow, stage 2
Pressure ulcer with abrasion, blister, partial thickness skin loss involving epidermis and/or dermis, unspecified elbow

MCC **L89.003** **Pressure ulcer of unspecified elbow, stage 3**
Healing pressure ulcer of unspecified elbow, stage 3
Pressure ulcer with full thickness skin loss involving damage or necrosis of subcutaneous tissue, unspecified elbow
HAC see Appendix B for HAC conditional logic

MCC **L89.004** **Pressure ulcer of unspecified elbow, stage 4**
Healing pressure ulcer of unspecified elbow, stage 4
Pressure ulcer with necrosis of soft tissues through to underlying muscle, tendon, or bone, unspecified elbow
HAC see Appendix B for HAC conditional logic

L89.006 **Pressure-induced deep tissue damage of unspecified elbow**

L89.009 **Pressure ulcer of unspecified elbow, unspecified stage**
Healing pressure ulcer of elbow NOS
Healing pressure ulcer of unspecified elbow, unspecified stage

+ **L89.01** **Pressure ulcer of right elbow**

L89.010 **Pressure ulcer of right elbow, unstageable**

L89.011 **Pressure ulcer of right elbow, stage 1**
Healing pressure ulcer of right elbow, stage 1
Pressure pre-ulcer skin changes limited to persistent focal edema, right elbow

L89.012 **Pressure ulcer of right elbow, stage 2**
Healing pressure ulcer of right elbow, stage 2
Pressure ulcer with abrasion, blister, partial thickness skin loss involving epidermis and/or dermis, right elbow

MCC **L89.013** **Pressure ulcer of right elbow, stage 3**
Healing pressure ulcer of right elbow, stage 3
Pressure ulcer with full thickness skin loss involving damage or necrosis of subcutaneous tissue, right elbow
HAC see Appendix B for HAC conditional logic

MCC **L89.014** **Pressure ulcer of right elbow, stage 4**
Healing pressure ulcer of right elbow, stage 4
Pressure ulcer with necrosis of soft tissues through to underlying muscle, tendon, or bone, right elbow
HAC see Appendix B for HAC conditional logic

L89.016 **Pressure-induced deep tissue damage of right elbow**

L89.019 **Pressure ulcer of right elbow, unspecified stage**
Healing pressure right of elbow NOS
Healing pressure ulcer of right elbow, unspecified stage

+ **L89.02** **Pressure ulcer of left elbow**

L89.020 **Pressure ulcer of left elbow, unstageable**

L89.021 **Pressure ulcer of left elbow, stage 1**
Healing pressure ulcer of left elbow, stage 1
Pressure pre-ulcer skin changes limited to persistent focal edema, left elbow

L89.022 **Pressure ulcer of left elbow, stage 2**
Healing pressure ulcer of left elbow, stage 2
Pressure ulcer with abrasion, blister, partial thickness skin loss involving epidermis and/or dermis, left elbow

MCC **L89.023** **Pressure ulcer of left elbow, stage 3**
Healing pressure ulcer of left elbow, stage 3
Pressure ulcer with full thickness skin loss involving damage or necrosis of subcutaneous tissue, left elbow
HAC see Appendix B for HAC conditional logic

MCC **L89.024** **Pressure ulcer of left elbow, stage 4**
Healing pressure ulcer of left elbow, stage 4
Pressure ulcer with necrosis of soft tissues through to underlying muscle, tendon, or bone, left elbow
HAC see Appendix B for HAC conditional logic

L89.026 **Pressure-induced deep tissue damage of left elbow**

L89.029 **Pressure ulcer of left elbow, unspecified stage**
Healing pressure ulcer of left of elbow NOS
Healing pressure ulcer of left elbow, unspecified stage

Pressure Ulcer

+ **L89.1 Pressure ulcer of back**

  + **L89.10 Pressure ulcer of unspecified part of back**

    L89.100 Pressure ulcer of unspecified part of back, unstageable

    L89.101 Pressure ulcer of unspecified part of back, stage 1

      Healing pressure ulcer of unspecified part of back, stage 1

      Pressure pre-ulcer skin changes limited to persistent focal edema, unspecified part of back

    L89.102 Pressure ulcer of unspecified part of back, stage 2

      Healing pressure ulcer of unspecified part of back, stage 2

      Pressure ulcer with abrasion, blister, partial thickness skin loss involving epidermis and/or dermis, unspecified part of back

MCC **L89.103 Pressure ulcer of unspecified part of back, stage 3**

  Healing pressure ulcer of unspecified part of back, stage 3

  Pressure ulcer with full thickness skin loss involving damage or necrosis of subcutaneous tissue, unspecified part of back

    HAC see Appendix B for HAC conditional logic

MCC **L89.104 Pressure ulcer of unspecified part of back, stage 4**

  Healing pressure ulcer of unspecified part of back, stage 4

  Pressure ulcer with necrosis of soft tissues through to underlying muscle, tendon, or bone, unspecified part of back

    HAC see Appendix B for HAC conditional logic

759

L89.106 **Pressure-induced deep tissue damage of unspecified part of back**

L89.109 **Pressure ulcer of unspecified part of back, unspecified stage**

Healing pressure ulcer of unspecified part of back NOS

Healing pressure ulcer of unspecified part of back, unspecified stage

+ **L89.11 Pressure ulcer of right upper back**

Pressure ulcer of right shoulder blade

L89.110 **Pressure ulcer of right upper back, unstageable**

L89.111 **Pressure ulcer of right upper back, stage 1**

Healing pressure ulcer of right upper back, stage 1

Pressure pre-ulcer skin changes limited to persistent focal edema, right upper back

L89.112 **Pressure ulcer of right upper back, stage 2**

Healing pressure ulcer of right upper back, stage 2

Pressure ulcer with abrasion, blister, partial thickness skin loss involving epidermis and/or dermis, right upper back

MCC L89.113 **Pressure ulcer of right upper back, stage 3**

Healing pressure ulcer of right upper back, stage 3

Pressure ulcer with full thickness skin loss involving damage or necrosis of subcutaneous tissue, right upper back

HAC see Appendix B for HAC conditional logic

MCC L89.114 **Pressure ulcer of right upper back, stage 4**

Healing pressure ulcer of right upper back, stage 4

Pressure ulcer with necrosis of soft tissues through to underlying muscle, tendon, or bone, right upper back

HAC see Appendix B for HAC conditional logic

L89.116 **Pressure-induced deep tissue damage of right upper back**

L89.119 **Pressure ulcer of right upper back, unspecified stage**

Healing pressure ulcer of right upper back NOS

Healing pressure ulcer of right upper back, unspecified stage

+ **L89.12 Pressure ulcer of left upper back**

Pressure ulcer of left shoulder blade

L89.120 **Pressure ulcer of left upper back, unstageable**

L89.121 **Pressure ulcer of left upper back, stage 1**

Healing pressure ulcer of left upper back, stage 1

Pressure pre-ulcer skin changes limited to persistent focal edema, left upper back

L89.122 **Pressure ulcer of left upper back, stage 2**

Healing pressure ulcer of left upper back, stage 2

Pressure ulcer with abrasion, blister, partial thickness skin loss involving epidermis and/or dermis, left upper back

MCC L89.123 **Pressure ulcer of left upper back, stage 3**

Healing pressure ulcer of left upper back, stage 3

Pressure ulcer with full thickness skin loss involving damage or necrosis of subcutaneous tissue, left upper back

HAC see Appendix B for HAC conditional logic

MCC L89.124 **Pressure ulcer of left upper back, stage 4**

Healing pressure ulcer of left upper back, stage 4

Pressure ulcer with necrosis of soft tissues through to underlying muscle, tendon, or bone, left upper back

HAC see Appendix B for HAC conditional logic

L89.126 **Pressure-induced deep tissue damage of left upper back**

L89.129 **Pressure ulcer of left upper back, unspecified stage**

Healing pressure ulcer of left upper back NOS

Healing pressure ulcer of left upper back, unspecified stage

+ **L89.13 Pressure ulcer of right lower back**

L89.130 **Pressure ulcer of right lower back, unstageable**

L89.131 **Pressure ulcer of right lower back, stage 1**

Healing pressure ulcer of right lower back, stage 1

Pressure pre-ulcer skin changes limited to persistent focal edema, right lower back

L89.132 **Pressure ulcer of right lower back, stage 2**

Healing pressure ulcer of right lower back, stage 2

Pressure ulcer with abrasion, blister, partial thickness skin loss involving epidermis and/or dermis, right lower back

MCC L89.133 **Pressure ulcer of right lower back, stage 3**

Healing pressure ulcer of right lower back, stage 3

Pressure ulcer with full thickness skin loss involving damage or necrosis of subcutaneous tissue, right lower back

HAC see Appendix B for HAC conditional logic

MCC L89.134 **Pressure ulcer of right lower back, stage 4**

Healing pressure ulcer of right lower back, stage 4

Pressure ulcer with necrosis of soft tissues through to underlying muscle, tendon, or bone, right lower back

HAC see Appendix B for HAC conditional logic

L89.136 **Pressure-induced deep tissue damage of right lower back**

L89.139 **Pressure ulcer of right lower back, unspecified stage**

Healing pressure ulcer of right lower back NOS

Healing pressure ulcer of right lower back, unspecified stage

+ **L89.14 Pressure ulcer of left lower back**

L89.140 **Pressure ulcer of left lower back, unstageable**

L89.141 **Pressure ulcer of left lower back, stage 1**

Healing pressure ulcer of left lower back, stage 1

Pressure pre-ulcer skin changes limited to persistent focal edema, left lower back

L89.142 **Pressure ulcer of left lower back, stage 2**

Healing pressure ulcer of left lower back, stage 2

Pressure ulcer with abrasion, blister, partial thickness skin loss involving epidermis and/or dermis, left lower back

MCC L89.143 **Pressure ulcer of left lower back, stage 3**

Healing pressure ulcer of left lower back, stage 3

Pressure ulcer with full thickness skin loss involving damage or necrosis of subcutaneous tissue, left lower back

HAC see Appendix B for HAC conditional logic

+, +7th, X + 7th   ● Newborn   ● Pediatric   ● Maternity   ● Adult   ♀ Female   ♂ Male   Manifestation   Unacceptable PDX   HCC   CC   MCC   HAC

MCC **L89.144** **Pressure ulcer of left lower back,
stage 4**

 Healing pressure ulcer of left lower back,
stage 4

 Pressure ulcer with necrosis of soft
tissues through to underlying muscle,
tendon, or bone, left lower back

  HAC see Appendix B for HAC conditional
logic

L89.146 **Pressure-induced deep tissue damage of
left lower back**

L89.149 **Pressure ulcer of left lower back,
unspecified stage**

 Healing pressure ulcer of left lower back
NOS

 Healing pressure ulcer of left lower back,
unspecified stage

+ **L89.15** **Pressure ulcer of sacral region**

 Pressure ulcer of coccyx

 Pressure ulcer of tailbone

L89.150 **Pressure ulcer of sacral region,
unstageable**

L89.151 **Pressure ulcer of sacral region, stage 1**

 Healing pressure ulcer of sacral region,
stage 1

 Pressure pre-ulcer skin changes limited
to persistent focal edema, sacral region

L89.152 **Pressure ulcer of sacral region, stage 2**

 Healing pressure ulcer of sacral region,
stage 2

 Pressure ulcer with abrasion, blister,
partial thickness skin loss involving
epidermis and/or dermis, sacral region

MCC **L89.153** **Pressure ulcer of sacral region, stage 3**

 Healing pressure ulcer of sacral region,
stage 3

 Pressure ulcer with full thickness skin
loss involving damage or necrosis of
subcutaneous tissue, sacral region

  HAC see Appendix B for HAC conditional
logic

MCC **L89.154** **Pressure ulcer of sacral region, stage 4**

 Healing pressure ulcer of sacral region,
stage 4

 Pressure ulcer with necrosis of soft tissues
through to underlying muscle, tendon,
or bone, sacral region

  HAC see Appendix B for HAC conditional
logic

L89.156 **Pressure-induced deep tissue damage of
sacral region**

L89.159 **Pressure ulcer of sacral region,
unspecified stage**

 Healing pressure ulcer of sacral
region NOS

 Healing pressure ulcer of sacral region,
unspecified stage

+ **L89.2** **Pressure ulcer of hip**

 + **L89.20** **Pressure ulcer of unspecified hip**

L89.200 **Pressure ulcer of unspecified hip,
unstageable**

L89.201 **Pressure ulcer of unspecified hip, stage 1**

 Healing pressure ulcer of unspecified hip
back, stage 1

 Pressure pre-ulcer skin changes limited to
persistent focal edema, unspecified hip

L89.202 **Pressure ulcer of unspecified hip, stage 2**

 Healing pressure ulcer of unspecified hip,
stage 2

 Pressure ulcer with abrasion, blister, partial
thickness skin loss involving epidermis
and/or dermis, unspecified hip

MCC **L89.203** **Pressure ulcer of unspecified hip, stage 3**

 Healing pressure ulcer of unspecified hip,
stage 3

 Pressure ulcer with full thickness skin
loss involving damage or necrosis of
subcutaneous tissue, unspecified hip

  HAC see Appendix B for HAC conditional
logic

MCC **L89.204** **Pressure ulcer of unspecified hip, stage 4**

 Healing pressure ulcer of unspecified hip,
stage 4

 Pressure ulcer with necrosis of soft
tissues through to underlying muscle,
tendon, or bone, unspecified hip

  HAC see Appendix B for HAC conditional
logic

L89.206 **Pressure-induced deep tissue damage of
unspecified hip**

L89.209 **Pressure ulcer of unspecified hip,
unspecified stage**

 Healing pressure ulcer of unspecified hip
NOS

 Healing pressure ulcer of unspecified hip,
unspecified stage

+ **L89.21** **Pressure ulcer of right hip**

L89.210 **Pressure ulcer of right hip, unstageable**

L89.211 **Pressure ulcer of right hip, stage 1**

 Healing pressure ulcer of right hip back,
stage 1

 Pressure pre-ulcer skin changes limited
to persistent focal edema, right hip

L89.212 **Pressure ulcer of right hip, stage 2**

 Healing pressure ulcer of right hip,
stage 2

 Pressure ulcer with abrasion, blister,
partial thickness skin loss involving
epidermis and/or dermis, right hip

MCC **L89.213** **Pressure ulcer of right hip, stage 3**

 Healing pressure ulcer of right hip,
stage 3

 Pressure ulcer with full thickness skin
loss involving damage or necrosis of
subcutaneous tissue, right hip

  HAC see Appendix B for HAC conditional
logic

MCC **L89.214** **Pressure ulcer of right hip, stage 4**

 Healing pressure ulcer of right hip,
stage 4

 Pressure ulcer with necrosis of soft
tissues through to underlying muscle,
tendon, or bone, right hip

  HAC see Appendix B for HAC conditional
logic

L89.216 **Pressure-induced deep tissue damage of
right hip**

L89.219 **Pressure ulcer of right hip, unspecified
stage**

 Healing pressure ulcer of right hip NOS

 Healing pressure ulcer of right hip,
unspecified stage

+ **L89.22** **Pressure ulcer of left hip**

L89.220 **Pressure ulcer of left hip, unstageable**

L89.221 **Pressure ulcer of left hip, stage 1**

 Healing pressure ulcer of left hip back,
stage 1

 Pressure pre-ulcer skin changes limited
to persistent focal edema, left hip

L89.222 **Pressure ulcer of left hip, stage 2**

 Healing pressure ulcer of left hip, stage 2

 Pressure ulcer with abrasion, blister,
partial thickness skin loss involving
epidermis and/or dermis, left hip

MCC **L89.223** **Pressure ulcer of left hip, stage 3**

 Healing pressure ulcer of left hip, stage 3

 Pressure ulcer with full thickness skin
loss involving damage or necrosis of
subcutaneous tissue, left hip

  HAC see Appendix B for HAC conditional
logic

MCC **L89.224** **Pressure ulcer of left hip, stage 4**

 Healing pressure ulcer of left hip, stage 4

 Pressure ulcer with necrosis of soft
tissues through to underlying muscle,
tendon, or bone, left hip

  HAC see Appendix B for HAC conditional logic

+, +7th, X + 7th   ● Newborn   ● Pediatric   ● Maternity   ● Adult   ♀ Female   ♂ Male   Manifestation   Unacceptable PDX   HCC   CC   MCC   **HAC**

L89.226 **Pressure-induced deep tissue damage of left hip**

L89.229 **Pressure ulcer of left hip, unspecified stage**

Healing pressure ulcer of left hip NOS
Healing pressure ulcer of left hip, unspecified stage

+ L89.3 **Pressure ulcer of buttock**

+ L89.30 **Pressure ulcer of unspecified buttock**

L89.300 **Pressure ulcer of unspecified buttock, unstageable**

L89.301 **Pressure ulcer of unspecified buttock, stage 1**

Healing pressure ulcer of unspecified buttock, stage 1
Pressure pre-ulcer skin changes limited to persistent focal edema, unspecified buttock

L89.302 **Pressure ulcer of unspecified buttock, stage 2**

Healing pressure ulcer of unspecified buttock, stage 2
Pressure ulcer with abrasion, blister, partial thickness skin loss involving epidermis and/or dermis, unspecified buttock

MCC L89.303 **Pressure ulcer of unspecified buttock, stage 3**

Healing pressure ulcer of unspecified buttock, stage 3
Pressure ulcer with full thickness skin loss involving damage or necrosis of subcutaneous tissue, unspecified buttock

HAC see Appendix B for HAC conditional logic

MCC L89.304 **Pressure ulcer of unspecified buttock, stage 4**

Healing pressure ulcer of unspecified buttock, stage 4
Pressure ulcer with necrosis of soft tissues through to underlying muscle, tendon, or bone, unspecified buttock

HAC see Appendix B for HAC conditional logic

L89.306 **Pressure-induced deep tissue damage of unspecified buttock**

L89.309 **Pressure ulcer of unspecified buttock, unspecified stage**

Healing pressure ulcer of unspecified buttock NOS
Healing pressure ulcer of unspecified buttock, unspecified stage

+ L89.31 **Pressure ulcer of right buttock**

L89.310 **Pressure ulcer of right buttock, unstageable**

L89.311 **Pressure ulcer of right buttock, stage 1**

Healing pressure ulcer of right buttock, stage 1
Pressure pre-ulcer skin changes limited to persistent focal edema, right buttock

L89.312 **Pressure ulcer of right buttock, stage 2**

Healing pressure ulcer of right buttock, stage 2
Pressure ulcer with abrasion, blister, partial thickness skin loss involving epidermis and/or dermis, right buttock

MCC L89.313 **Pressure ulcer of right buttock, stage 3**

Healing pressure ulcer of right buttock, stage 3
Pressure ulcer with full thickness skin loss involving damage or necrosis of subcutaneous tissue, right buttock

HAC see Appendix B for HAC conditional logic

MCC L89.314 **Pressure ulcer of right buttock, stage 4**

Healing pressure ulcer of right buttock, stage 4
Pressure ulcer with necrosis of soft tissues through to underlying muscle, tendon, or bone, right buttock

HAC see Appendix B for HAC conditional logic

L89.316 **Pressure-induced deep tissue damage of right buttock**

L89.319 **Pressure ulcer of right buttock, unspecified stage**

Healing pressure ulcer of right buttock NOS
Healing pressure ulcer of right buttock, unspecified stage

+ L89.32 **Pressure ulcer of left buttock**

L89.320 **Pressure ulcer of left buttock, unstageable**

L89.321 **Pressure ulcer of left buttock, stage 1**

Healing pressure ulcer of left buttock, stage 1
Pressure pre-ulcer skin changes limited to persistent focal edema, left buttock

L89.322 **Pressure ulcer of left buttock, stage 2**

Healing pressure ulcer of left buttock, stage 2
Pressure ulcer with abrasion, blister, partial thickness skin loss involving epidermis and/or dermis, left buttock

MCC L89.323 **Pressure ulcer of left buttock, stage 3**

Healing pressure ulcer of left buttock, stage 3
Pressure ulcer with full thickness skin loss involving damage or necrosis of subcutaneous tissue, left buttock

HAC see Appendix B for HAC conditional logic

MCC L89.324 **Pressure ulcer of left buttock, stage 4**

Healing pressure ulcer of left buttock, stage 4
Pressure ulcer with necrosis of soft tissues through to underlying muscle, tendon, or bone, left buttock

HAC see Appendix B for HAC conditional logic

L89.326 **Pressure-induced deep tissue damage of left buttock**

L89.329 **Pressure ulcer of left buttock, unspecified stage**

Healing pressure ulcer of left buttock NOS
Healing pressure ulcer of left buttock, unspecified stage

+ L89.4 **Pressure ulcer of contiguous site of back, buttock and hip**

L89.40 **Pressure ulcer of contiguous site of back, buttock and hip, unspecified stage**

Healing pressure ulcer of contiguous site of back, buttock and hip NOS
Healing pressure ulcer of contiguous site of back, buttock and hip, unspecified stage

L89.41 **Pressure ulcer of contiguous site of back, buttock and hip, stage 1**

Healing pressure ulcer of contiguous site of back, buttock and hip, stage 1
Pressure pre-ulcer skin changes limited to persistent focal edema, contiguous site of back, buttock and hip

L89.42 **Pressure ulcer of contiguous site of back, buttock and hip, stage 2**

Healing pressure ulcer of contiguous site of back, buttock and hip, stage 2
Pressure ulcer with abrasion, blister, partial thickness skin loss involving epidermis and/or dermis, contiguous site of back, buttock and hip

MCC **L89.43** **Pressure ulcer of contiguous site of back, buttock and hip, stage 3**
Healing pressure ulcer of contiguous site of back, buttock and hip, stage 3
Pressure ulcer with full thickness skin loss involving damage or necrosis of subcutaneous tissue, contiguous site of back, buttock and hip
HAC see Appendix B for HAC conditional logic

MCC **L89.44** **Pressure ulcer of contiguous site of back, buttock and hip, stage 4**
Healing pressure ulcer of contiguous site of back, buttock and hip, stage 4
Pressure ulcer with necrosis of soft tissues through to underlying muscle, tendon, or bone, contiguous site of back, buttock and hip
HAC see Appendix B for HAC conditional logic

L89.45 **Pressure ulcer of contiguous site of back, buttock and hip, unstageable**

L89.46 **Pressure-induced deep tissue damage of contiguous site of back, buttock and hip**

+ **L89.5** **Pressure ulcer of ankle**
  + **L89.50** **Pressure ulcer of unspecified ankle**

L89.500 **Pressure ulcer of unspecified ankle, unstageable**

L89.501 **Pressure ulcer of unspecified ankle, stage 1**
Healing pressure ulcer of unspecified ankle, stage 1
Pressure pre-ulcer skin changes limited to persistent focal edema, unspecified ankle

L89.502 **Pressure ulcer of unspecified ankle, stage 2**
Healing pressure ulcer of unspecified ankle, stage 2
Pressure ulcer with abrasion, blister, partial thickness skin loss involving epidermis and/or dermis, unspecified ankle

MCC **L89.503** **Pressure ulcer of unspecified ankle, stage 3**
Healing pressure ulcer of unspecified ankle, stage 3
Pressure ulcer with full thickness skin loss involving damage or necrosis of subcutaneous tissue, unspecified ankle
HAC see Appendix B for HAC conditional logic

MCC **L89.504** **Pressure ulcer of unspecified ankle, stage 4**
Healing pressure ulcer of unspecified ankle, stage 4
Pressure ulcer with necrosis of soft tissues through to underlying muscle, tendon, or bone, unspecified ankle
HAC see Appendix B for HAC conditional logic

L89.506 **Pressure-induced deep tissue damage of unspecified ankle**

L89.509 **Pressure ulcer of unspecified ankle, unspecified stage**
Healing pressure ulcer of unspecified ankle NOS
Healing pressure ulcer of unspecified ankle, unspecified stage

+ **L89.51** **Pressure ulcer of right ankle**
L89.510 **Pressure ulcer of right ankle, unstageable**

L89.511 **Pressure ulcer of right ankle, stage 1**
Healing pressure ulcer of right ankle, stage 1
Pressure pre-ulcer skin changes limited to persistent focal edema, right ankle

L89.512 **Pressure ulcer of right ankle, stage 2**
Healing pressure ulcer of right ankle, stage 2
Pressure ulcer with abrasion, blister, partial thickness skin loss involving epidermis and/or dermis, right ankle

MCC **L89.513** **Pressure ulcer of right ankle, stage 3**
Healing pressure ulcer of right ankle, stage 3
Pressure ulcer with full thickness skin loss involving damage or necrosis of subcutaneous tissue, right ankle
HAC see Appendix B for HAC conditional logic

MCC **L89.514** **Pressure ulcer of right ankle, stage 4**
Healing pressure ulcer of right ankle, stage 4
Pressure ulcer with necrosis of soft tissues through to underlying muscle, tendon, or bone, right ankle
HAC see Appendix B for HAC conditional logic

L89.516 **Pressure-induced deep tissue damage of right ankle**

L89.519 **Pressure ulcer of right ankle, unspecified stage**
Healing pressure ulcer of right ankle NOS
Healing pressure ulcer of right ankle, unspecified stage

+ **L89.52** **Pressure ulcer of left ankle**
L89.520 **Pressure ulcer of left ankle, unstageable**

L89.521 **Pressure ulcer of left ankle, stage 1**
Healing pressure ulcer of left ankle, stage 1
Pressure pre-ulcer skin changes limited to persistent focal edema, left ankle

L89.522 **Pressure ulcer of left ankle, stage 2**
Healing pressure ulcer of left ankle, stage 2
Pressure ulcer with abrasion, blister, partial thickness skin loss involving epidermis and/or dermis, left ankle

MCC **L89.523** **Pressure ulcer of left ankle, stage 3**
Healing pressure ulcer of left ankle, stage 3
Pressure ulcer with full thickness skin loss involving damage or necrosis of subcutaneous tissue, left ankle
HAC see Appendix B for HAC conditional logic

MCC **L89.524** **Pressure ulcer of left ankle, stage 4**
Healing pressure ulcer of left ankle, stage 4
Pressure ulcer with necrosis of soft tissues through to underlying muscle, tendon, or bone, left ankle
HAC see Appendix B for HAC conditional logic

L89.526 **Pressure-induced deep tissue damage of left ankle**

L89.529 **Pressure ulcer of left ankle, unspecified stage**
Healing pressure ulcer of left ankle NOS
Healing pressure ulcer of left ankle, unspecified stage

+ **L89.6** **Pressure ulcer of heel**
  + **L89.60** **Pressure ulcer of unspecified heel**
L89.600 **Pressure ulcer of unspecified heel, unstageable**

L89.601 **Pressure ulcer of unspecified heel, stage 1**
Healing pressure ulcer of unspecified heel, stage 1
Pressure pre-ulcer skin changes limited to persistent focal edema, unspecified heel

+, +7th, X + 7th ● Newborn ● Pediatric ● Maternity ● Adult ♀ Female ♂ Male Manifestation Unacceptable PDX HCC CC MCC HAC

L89.602 **Pressure ulcer of unspecified heel, stage 2**
  Healing pressure ulcer of unspecified heel, stage 2
  Pressure ulcer with abrasion, blister, partial thickness skin loss involving epidermis and/or dermis, unspecified heel

MCC **L89.603** **Pressure ulcer of unspecified heel, stage 3**
  Healing pressure ulcer of unspecified heel, stage 3
  Pressure ulcer with full thickness skin loss involving damage or necrosis of subcutaneous tissue, unspecified heel
  HAC see Appendix B for HAC conditional logic

MCC **L89.604** **Pressure ulcer of unspecified heel, stage 4**
  Healing pressure ulcer of unspecified heel, stage 4
  Pressure ulcer with necrosis of soft tissues through to underlying muscle, tendon, or bone, unspecified heel
  HAC see Appendix B for HAC conditional logic

L89.606 **Pressure-induced deep tissue damage of unspecified heel**

L89.609 **Pressure ulcer of unspecified heel, unspecified stage**
  Healing pressure ulcer of unspecified heel NOS
  Healing pressure ulcer of unspecified heel, unspecified stage

+ **L89.61** **Pressure ulcer of right heel**
  L89.610 **Pressure ulcer of right heel, unstageable**
  L89.611 **Pressure ulcer of right heel, stage 1**
    Healing pressure ulcer of right heel, stage 1
    Pressure pre-ulcer skin changes limited to persistent focal edema, right heel
  L89.612 **Pressure ulcer of right heel, stage 2**
    Healing pressure ulcer of right heel, stage 2
    Pressure ulcer with abrasion, blister, partial thickness skin loss involving epidermis and/or dermis, right heel

MCC **L89.613** **Pressure ulcer of right heel, stage 3**
    Healing pressure ulcer of right heel, stage 3
    Pressure ulcer with full thickness skin loss involving damage or necrosis of subcutaneous tissue, right heel
    HAC see Appendix B for HAC conditional logic

MCC **L89.614** **Pressure ulcer of right heel, stage 4**
    Healing pressure ulcer of right heel, stage 4
    Pressure ulcer with necrosis of soft tissues through to underlying muscle, tendon, or bone, right heel
    HAC see Appendix B for HAC conditional logic

L89.616 **Pressure-induced deep tissue damage of right heel**

L89.619 **Pressure ulcer of right heel, unspecified stage**
    Healing pressure ulcer of right heel NOS
    Healing pressure ulcer of right heel, unspecified stage

+ **L89.62** **Pressure ulcer of left heel**
  L89.620 **Pressure ulcer of left heel, unstageable**
  L89.621 **Pressure ulcer of left heel, stage 1**
    Healing pressure ulcer of left heel, stage 1
    Pressure pre-ulcer skin changes limited to persistent focal edema, left heel

L89.622 **Pressure ulcer of left heel, stage 2**
  Healing pressure ulcer of left heel, stage 2
  Pressure ulcer with abrasion, blister, partial thickness skin loss involving epidermis and/or dermis, left heel
  AHA CC: 4Q, 2016, 144

MCC **L89.623** **Pressure ulcer of left heel, stage 3**
  Healing pressure ulcer of left heel, stage 3
  Pressure ulcer with full thickness skin loss involving damage or necrosis of subcutaneous tissue, left heel
  AHA CC: 4Q, 2016, 144; 3Q, 2018, 3-4
  HAC see Appendix B for HAC conditional logic

MCC **L89.624** **Pressure ulcer of left heel, stage 4**
  Healing pressure ulcer of left heel, stage 4
  Pressure ulcer with necrosis of soft tissues through to underlying muscle, tendon, or bone, left heel
  HAC see Appendix B for HAC conditional logic

L89.626 **Pressure-induced deep tissue damage of left heel**

L89.629 **Pressure ulcer of left heel, unspecified stage**
  Healing pressure ulcer of left heel NOS
  Healing pressure ulcer of left heel, unspecified stage

+ **L89.8** **Pressure ulcer of other site**
  + **L89.81** **Pressure ulcer of head**
    Pressure ulcer of face
    L89.810 **Pressure ulcer of head, unstageable**
    L89.811 **Pressure ulcer of head, stage 1**
      Healing pressure ulcer of head, stage 1
      Pressure pre-ulcer skin changes limited to persistent focal edema, head
    L89.812 **Pressure ulcer of head, stage 2**
      Healing pressure ulcer of head, stage 2
      Pressure ulcer with abrasion, blister, partial thickness skin loss involving epidermis and/or dermis, head

MCC **L89.813** **Pressure ulcer of head, stage 3**
      Healing pressure ulcer of head, stage 3
      Pressure ulcer with full thickness skin loss involving damage or necrosis of subcutaneous tissue, head
      HAC see Appendix B for HAC conditional logic

MCC **L89.814** **Pressure ulcer of head, stage 4**
      Healing pressure ulcer of head, stage 4
      Pressure ulcer with necrosis of soft tissues through to underlying muscle, tendon, or bone, head
      HAC see Appendix B for HAC conditional logic

L89.816 **Pressure-induced deep tissue damage of head**

L89.819 **Pressure ulcer of head, unspecified stage**
      Healing pressure ulcer of head NOS
      Healing pressure ulcer of head, unspecified stage

+ **L89.89** **Pressure ulcer of other site**
  L89.890 **Pressure ulcer of other site, unstageable**
  L89.891 **Pressure ulcer of other site, stage 1**
    Healing pressure ulcer of other site, stage 1
    Pressure pre-ulcer skin changes limited to persistent focal edema, other site
  L89.892 **Pressure ulcer of other site, stage 2**
    Healing pressure ulcer of other site, stage 2
    Pressure ulcer with abrasion, blister, partial thickness skin loss involving epidermis and/or dermis, other site

MCC `L89.893` **Pressure ulcer of other site, stage 3**
Healing pressure ulcer of other site, stage 3
Pressure ulcer with full thickness skin loss involving damage or necrosis of subcutaneous tissue, other site
`HAC` see Appendix B for HAC conditional logic

MCC `L89.894` **Pressure ulcer of other site, stage 4**
Healing pressure ulcer of other site, stage 4
Pressure ulcer with necrosis of soft tissues through to underlying muscle, tendon, or bone, other site
`HAC` see Appendix B for HAC conditional logic

`L89.896` **Pressure-induced deep tissue damage of other site**

`L89.899` **Pressure ulcer of other site, unspecified stage**
Healing pressure ulcer of other site NOS
Healing pressure ulcer of other site, unspecified stage

+ **L89.9** **Pressure ulcer of unspecified site**

`L89.90` **Pressure ulcer of unspecified site, unspecified stage**
Healing pressure ulcer of unspecified site NOS
Healing pressure ulcer of unspecified site, unspecified stage

`L89.91` **Pressure ulcer of unspecified site, stage 1**
Healing pressure ulcer of unspecified site, stage 1
Pressure pre-ulcer skin changes limited to persistent focal edema, unspecified site

`L89.92` **Pressure ulcer of unspecified site, stage 2**
Healing pressure ulcer of unspecified site, stage 2
Pressure ulcer with abrasion, blister, partial thickness skin loss involving epidermis and/or dermis, unspecified site

MCC `L89.93` **Pressure ulcer of unspecified site, stage 3**
Healing pressure ulcer of unspecified site, stage 3
Pressure ulcer with full thickness skin loss involving damage or necrosis of subcutaneous tissue, unspecified site
`HAC` see Appendix B for HAC conditional logic

MCC `L89.94` **Pressure ulcer of unspecified site, stage 4**
Healing pressure ulcer of unspecified site, stage 4
Pressure ulcer with necrosis of soft tissues through to underlying muscle, tendon, or bone, unspecified site
`HAC` see Appendix B for HAC conditional logic

`L89.95` **Pressure ulcer of unspecified site, unstageable**

`L89.96` **Pressure-induced deep tissue damage of unspecified site**

L90 **Atrophic disorders of skin**

L90.0 **Lichen sclerosus et atrophicus**
Excludes2: *lichen sclerosus of external female genital organs (N90.4)*
lichen sclerosus of external male genital organs (N48.0)

L90.1 **Anetoderma of Schweninger-Buzzi**
L90.2 **Anetoderma of Jadassohn-Pellizzari**
L90.3 **Atrophoderma of Pasini and Pierini**
L90.4 **Acrodermatitis chronica atrophicans**
L90.5 **Scar conditions and fibrosis of skin**
Adherent scar (skin)
Cicatrix
Disfigurement of skin due to scar
Fibrosis of skin NOS
Scar NOS
Excludes2: *hypertrophic scar (L91.0)*
keloid scar (L91.0)
AHA CC: 1Q, 2015, 19; 2Q, 2016, 5

L90.6 **Striae atrophicae**
L90.8 **Other atrophic disorders of skin**
L90.9 **Atrophic disorder of skin, unspecified**

L91 **Hypertrophic disorders of skin**

L91.0 **Hypertrophic scar**
Keloid
Keloid scar
Excludes2: *acne keloid (L73.0)*
scar NOS (L90.5)

L91.8 **Other hypertrophic disorders of the skin**
L91.9 **Hypertrophic disorder of the skin, unspecified**

L92 **Granulomatous disorders of skin and subcutaneous tissue**

Excludes2: *actinic granuloma (L57.5)*

L92.0 **Granuloma annulare**
Perforating granuloma annulare

L92.1 **Necrobiosis lipoidica, not elsewhere classified**
Excludes1: *necrobiosis lipoidica associated with diabetes mellitus (E08-E13 with .620)*

L92.2 **Granuloma faciale [eosinophilic granuloma of skin]**
L92.3 **Foreign body granuloma of the skin and subcutaneous tissue**
Use additional code to identify the type of retained foreign body (Z18.-)

L92.8 **Other granulomatous disorders of the skin and subcutaneous tissue**
L92.9 **Granulomatous disorder of the skin and subcutaneous tissue, unspecified**
Excludes2: *umbilical granuloma (P83.81)*

L93 **Lupus erythematosus**

Use additional code for adverse effect, if applicable, to identify drug (T36-T50 with fifth or sixth character 5)
Excludes1: *lupus exedens (A18.4)*
lupus vulgaris (A18.4)
scleroderma (M34.-)
systemic lupus erythematosus (M32.-)

L93.0 **Discoid lupus erythematosus**
Lupus erythematosus NOS

L93.1 **Subacute cutaneous lupus erythematosus**
L93.2 **Other local lupus erythematosus**
Lupus erythematosus profundus
Lupus panniculitis

L94 **Other localized connective tissue disorders**

Excludes1: *systemic connective tissue disorders (M30-M36)*

L94.0 **Localized scleroderma [morphea]**
Circumscribed scleroderma

L94.1 **Linear scleroderma**
En coup de sabre lesion

L94.2 **Calcinosis cutis**
L94.3 **Sclerodactyly**
L94.4 **Gottron's papules**
L94.5 **Poikiloderma vasculare atrophicans**
L94.6 **Ainhum**
L94.8 **Other specified localized connective tissue disorders**
L94.9 **Localized connective tissue disorder, unspecified**

L95 **Vasculitis limited to skin, not elsewhere classified**

Excludes1: *angioma serpiginosum (L81.7)*
Henoch(-Schönlein) purpura (D69.0)
hypersensitivity angiitis (M31.0)
lupus panniculitis (L93.2)
panniculitis NOS (M79.3)
panniculitis of neck and back (M54.0-)
polyarteritis nodosa (M30.0)
relapsing panniculitis (M35.6)
rheumatoid vasculitis (M05.2)
serum sickness (T80.6-)
urticaria (L50.-)
Wegener's granulomatosis (M31.3-)

L95.0 **Livedoid vasculitis**
Atrophie blanche (en plaque)

L95.1 **Erythema elevatum diutinum**
L95.8 **Other vasculitis limited to the skin**
L95.9 **Vasculitis limited to the skin, unspecified**

+, +7th, X + 7th • Newborn • Pediatric • Maternity • Adult ♀ Female ♂ Male Manifestation Unacceptable PDX HCC CC MCC `HAC`

L97 Non-pressure chronic ulcer of lower limb, not elsewhere classified

Includes: chronic ulcer of skin of lower limb NOS
non-healing ulcer of skin
non-infected sinus of skin
trophic ulcer NOS
tropical ulcer NOS
ulcer of skin of lower limb NOS

Code first any associated underlying condition, such as:
any associated gangrene (I96)
atherosclerosis of the lower extremities (I70.23-, I70.24-, I70.33-, I70.34-, I70.43-, I70.44-, I70.53-, I70.54-, I70.63-, I70.64-, I70.73-, I70.74-)
chronic venous hypertension (I87.31-, I87.33-)
diabetic ulcers (E08.621, E08.622, E09.621, E09.622, E10.621, E10.622, E11.621, E11.622, E13.621, E13.622)
postphlebitic syndrome (I87.01-, I87.03-)
postthrombotic syndrome (I87.01-, I87.03-)
varicose ulcer (I83.0-, I83.2-)

Excludes2: *pressure ulcer (pressure area) (L89.-)*
skin infections (L00-L08)
specific infections classified to A00-B99

AHA CC: 4Q, 2017, 17

Review coding guidelines B.14 and C.12.b

+ L97.1 Non-pressure chronic ulcer of thigh
+ L97.10 Non-pressure chronic ulcer of unspecified thigh
CC **L97.101** Non-pressure chronic ulcer of unspecified thigh limited to breakdown of skin
CC **L97.102** Non-pressure chronic ulcer of unspecified thigh with fat layer exposed
CC **L97.103** Non-pressure chronic ulcer of unspecified thigh with necrosis of muscle
CC **L97.104** Non-pressure chronic ulcer of unspecified thigh with necrosis of bone
CC **L97.105** Non-pressure chronic ulcer of unspecified thigh with muscle involvement without evidence of necrosis
CC **L97.106** Non-pressure chronic ulcer of unspecified thigh with bone involvement without evidence of necrosis
CC **L97.108** Non-pressure chronic ulcer of unspecified thigh with other specified severity
CC **L97.109** Non-pressure chronic ulcer of unspecified thigh with unspecified severity

+ L97.11 Non-pressure chronic ulcer of right thigh
CC **L97.111** Non-pressure chronic ulcer of right thigh limited to breakdown of skin
CC **L97.112** Non-pressure chronic ulcer of right thigh with fat layer exposed
CC **L97.113** Non-pressure chronic ulcer of right thigh with necrosis of muscle
CC **L97.114** Non-pressure chronic ulcer of right thigh with necrosis of bone
CC **L97.115** Non-pressure chronic ulcer of right thigh with muscle involvement without evidence of necrosis
CC **L97.116** Non-pressure chronic ulcer of right thigh with bone involvement without evidence of necrosis
CC **L97.118** Non-pressure chronic ulcer of right thigh with other specified severity
CC **L97.119** Non-pressure chronic ulcer of right thigh with unspecified severity

+ L97.12 Non-pressure chronic ulcer of left thigh
CC **L97.121** Non-pressure chronic ulcer of left thigh limited to breakdown of skin
CC **L97.122** Non-pressure chronic ulcer of left thigh with fat layer exposed
CC **L97.123** Non-pressure chronic ulcer of left thigh with necrosis of muscle
CC **L97.124** Non-pressure chronic ulcer of left thigh with necrosis of bone
CC **L97.125** Non-pressure chronic ulcer of left thigh with muscle involvement without evidence of necrosis

CC **L97.126** Non-pressure chronic ulcer of left thigh with bone involvement without evidence of necrosis
CC **L97.128** Non-pressure chronic ulcer of left thigh with other specified severity
CC **L97.129** Non-pressure chronic ulcer of left thigh with unspecified severity

+ L97.2 Non-pressure chronic ulcer of calf
+ L97.20 Non-pressure chronic ulcer of unspecified calf
CC **L97.201** Non-pressure chronic ulcer of unspecified calf limited to breakdown of skin
CC **L97.202** Non-pressure chronic ulcer of unspecified calf with fat layer exposed
CC **L97.203** Non-pressure chronic ulcer of unspecified calf with necrosis of muscle
CC **L97.204** Non-pressure chronic ulcer of unspecified calf with necrosis of bone
CC **L97.205** Non-pressure chronic ulcer of unspecified calf with muscle involvement without evidence of necrosis
CC **L97.206** Non-pressure chronic ulcer of unspecified calf with bone involvement without evidence of necrosis
CC **L97.208** Non-pressure chronic ulcer of unspecified calf with other specified severity
CC **L97.209** Non-pressure chronic ulcer of unspecified calf with unspecified severity

+ L97.21 Non-pressure chronic ulcer of right calf
CC **L97.211** Non-pressure chronic ulcer of right calf limited to breakdown of skin
CC **L97.212** Non-pressure chronic ulcer of right calf with fat layer exposed
CC **L97.213** Non-pressure chronic ulcer of right calf with necrosis of muscle
CC **L97.214** Non-pressure chronic ulcer of right calf with necrosis of bone
CC **L97.215** Non-pressure chronic ulcer of right calf with muscle involvement without evidence of necrosis
CC **L97.216** Non-pressure chronic ulcer of right calf with bone involvement without evidence of necrosis
CC **L97.218** Non-pressure chronic ulcer of right calf with other specified severity
CC **L97.219** Non-pressure chronic ulcer of right calf with unspecified severity

+ L97.22 Non-pressure chronic ulcer of left calf
CC **L97.221** Non-pressure chronic ulcer of left calf limited to breakdown of skin
CC **L97.222** Non-pressure chronic ulcer of left calf with fat layer exposed
AHA CC: 1Q, 2016, 12-13
CC **L97.223** Non-pressure chronic ulcer of left calf with necrosis of muscle
CC **L97.224** Non-pressure chronic ulcer of left calf with necrosis of bone
CC **L97.225** Non-pressure chronic ulcer of left calf with muscle involvement without evidence of necrosis
CC **L97.226** Non-pressure chronic ulcer of left calf with bone involvement without evidence of necrosis
CC **L97.228** Non-pressure chronic ulcer of left calf with other specified severity
CC **L97.229** Non-pressure chronic ulcer of left calf with unspecified severity

+ L97.3 Non-pressure chronic ulcer of ankle
+ L97.30 Non-pressure chronic ulcer of unspecified ankle
CC **L97.301** Non-pressure chronic ulcer of unspecified ankle limited to breakdown of skin
CC **L97.302** Non-pressure chronic ulcer of unspecified ankle with fat layer exposed
CC **L97.303** Non-pressure chronic ulcer of unspecified ankle with necrosis of muscle
CC **L97.304** Non-pressure chronic ulcer of unspecified ankle with necrosis of bone

CC **L97.305** Non-pressure chronic ulcer of unspecified ankle with muscle involvement without evidence of necrosis

CC **L97.306** Non-pressure chronic ulcer of unspecified ankle with bone involvement without evidence of necrosis

CC **L97.308** Non-pressure chronic ulcer of unspecified ankle with other specified severity

CC **L97.309** Non-pressure chronic ulcer of unspecified ankle with unspecified severity

+ **L97.31** Non-pressure chronic ulcer of right ankle

CC **L97.311** Non-pressure chronic ulcer of right ankle limited to breakdown of skin

CC **L97.312** Non-pressure chronic ulcer of right ankle with fat layer exposed

CC **L97.313** Non-pressure chronic ulcer of right ankle with necrosis of muscle

CC **L97.314** Non-pressure chronic ulcer of right ankle with necrosis of bone

CC **L97.315** Non-pressure chronic ulcer of right ankle with muscle involvement without evidence of necrosis
AHA CC: 4Q, 2017, 17

CC **L97.316** Non-pressure chronic ulcer of right ankle with bone involvement without evidence of necrosis

CC **L97.318** Non-pressure chronic ulcer of right ankle with other specified severity

CC **L97.319** Non-pressure chronic ulcer of right ankle with unspecified severity

+ **L97.32** Non-pressure chronic ulcer of left ankle

CC **L97.321** Non-pressure chronic ulcer of left ankle limited to breakdown of skin

CC **L97.322** Non-pressure chronic ulcer of left ankle with fat layer exposed

CC **L97.323** Non-pressure chronic ulcer of left ankle with necrosis of muscle

CC **L97.324** Non-pressure chronic ulcer of left ankle with necrosis of bone

CC **L97.325** Non-pressure chronic ulcer of left ankle with muscle involvement without evidence of necrosis

CC **L97.326** Non-pressure chronic ulcer of left ankle with bone involvement without evidence of necrosis

CC **L97.328** Non-pressure chronic ulcer of left ankle with other specified severity

CC **L97.329** Non-pressure chronic ulcer of left ankle with unspecified severity

+ **L97.4** Non-pressure chronic ulcer of heel and midfoot
Non-pressure chronic ulcer of plantar surface of midfoot

+ **L97.40** Non-pressure chronic ulcer of unspecified heel and midfoot

CC **L97.401** Non-pressure chronic ulcer of unspecified heel and midfoot limited to breakdown of skin

CC **L97.402** Non-pressure chronic ulcer of unspecified heel and midfoot with fat layer exposed

CC **L97.403** Non-pressure chronic ulcer of unspecified heel and midfoot with necrosis of muscle

CC **L97.404** Non-pressure chronic ulcer of unspecified heel and midfoot with necrosis of bone

CC **L97.405** Non-pressure chronic ulcer of unspecified heel and midfoot with muscle involvement without evidence of necrosis

CC **L97.406** Non-pressure chronic ulcer of unspecified heel and midfoot with bone involvement without evidence of necrosis

CC **L97.408** Non-pressure chronic ulcer of unspecified heel and midfoot with other specified severity

CC **L97.409** Non-pressure chronic ulcer of unspecified heel and midfoot with unspecified severity

+ **L97.41** Non-pressure chronic ulcer of right heel and midfoot

CC **L97.411** Non-pressure chronic ulcer of right heel and midfoot limited to breakdown of skin

CC **L97.412** Non-pressure chronic ulcer of right heel and midfoot with fat layer exposed
AHA CC: 2Q, 2020, 19

CC **L97.413** Non-pressure chronic ulcer of right heel and midfoot with necrosis of muscle

CC **L97.414** Non-pressure chronic ulcer of right heel and midfoot with necrosis of bone

CC **L97.415** Non-pressure chronic ulcer of right heel and midfoot with muscle involvement without evidence of necrosis

CC **L97.416** Non-pressure chronic ulcer of right heel and midfoot with bone involvement without evidence of necrosis

CC **L97.418** Non-pressure chronic ulcer of right heel and midfoot with other specified severity

CC **L97.419** Non-pressure chronic ulcer of right heel and midfoot with unspecified severity

+ **L97.42** Non-pressure chronic ulcer of left heel and midfoot

CC **L97.421** Non-pressure chronic ulcer of left heel and midfoot limited to breakdown of skin

CC **L97.422** Non-pressure chronic ulcer of left heel and midfoot with fat layer exposed

CC **L97.423** Non-pressure chronic ulcer of left heel and midfoot with necrosis of muscle

CC **L97.424** Non-pressure chronic ulcer of left heel and midfoot with necrosis of bone

CC **L97.425** Non-pressure chronic ulcer of left heel and midfoot with muscle involvement without evidence of necrosis

CC **L97.426** Non-pressure chronic ulcer of left heel and midfoot with bone involvement without evidence of necrosis

CC **L97.428** Non-pressure chronic ulcer of left heel and midfoot with other specified severity

CC **L97.429** Non-pressure chronic ulcer of left heel and midfoot with unspecified severity

+ **L97.5** Non-pressure chronic ulcer of other part of foot
Non-pressure chronic ulcer of toe

+ **L97.50** Non-pressure chronic ulcer of other part of unspecified foot

L97.501 Non-pressure chronic ulcer of other part of unspecified foot limited to breakdown of skin

L97.502 Non-pressure chronic ulcer of other part of unspecified foot with fat layer exposed

L97.503 Non-pressure chronic ulcer of other part of unspecified foot with necrosis of muscle

L97.504 Non-pressure chronic ulcer of other part of unspecified foot with necrosis of bone

CC **L97.505** Non-pressure chronic ulcer of other part of unspecified foot with muscle involvement without evidence of necrosis

CC **L97.506** Non-pressure chronic ulcer of other part of unspecified foot with bone involvement without evidence of necrosis

CC **L97.508** Non-pressure chronic ulcer of other part of unspecified foot with other specified severity

L97.509 Non-pressure chronic ulcer of other part of unspecified foot with unspecified severity

+ **L97.51** Non-pressure chronic ulcer of other part of right foot

L97.511 Non-pressure chronic ulcer of other part of right foot limited to breakdown of skin
AHA CC: 1Q, 2020, 12

L97.512 Non-pressure chronic ulcer of other part of right foot with fat layer exposed
AHA CC: 2Q, 2020, 19-20

L97.513 Non-pressure chronic ulcer of other part of right foot with necrosis of muscle

L97.514 Non-pressure chronic ulcer of other part of right foot with necrosis of bone

CC L97.515 Non-pressure chronic ulcer of other part of right foot with muscle involvement without evidence of necrosis

CC L97.516 Non-pressure chronic ulcer of other part of right foot with bone involvement without evidence of necrosis

CC L97.518 Non-pressure chronic ulcer of other part of right foot with other specified severity

L97.519 Non-pressure chronic ulcer of other part of right foot with unspecified severity

+ L97.52 Non-pressure chronic ulcer of other part of left foot

L97.521 Non-pressure chronic ulcer of other part of left foot limited to breakdown of skin

L97.522 Non-pressure chronic ulcer of other part of left foot with fat layer exposed

L97.523 Non-pressure chronic ulcer of other part of left foot with necrosis of muscle

L97.524 Non-pressure chronic ulcer of other part of left foot with necrosis of bone

CC L97.525 Non-pressure chronic ulcer of other part of left foot with muscle involvement without evidence of necrosis

CC L97.526 Non-pressure chronic ulcer of other part of left foot with bone involvement without evidence of necrosis

CC L97.528 Non-pressure chronic ulcer of other part of left foot with other specified severity

L97.529 Non-pressure chronic ulcer of other part of left foot with unspecified severity

+ L97.8 Non-pressure chronic ulcer of other part of lower leg

+ L97.80 Non-pressure chronic ulcer of other part of unspecified lower leg

CC L97.801 Non-pressure chronic ulcer of other part of unspecified lower leg limited to breakdown of skin

CC L97.802 Non-pressure chronic ulcer of other part of unspecified lower leg with fat layer exposed

CC L97.803 Non-pressure chronic ulcer of other part of unspecified lower leg with necrosis of muscle

CC L97.804 Non-pressure chronic ulcer of other part of unspecified lower leg with necrosis of bone

CC L97.805 Non-pressure chronic ulcer of other part of unspecified lower leg with muscle involvement without evidence of necrosis

CC L97.806 Non-pressure chronic ulcer of other part of unspecified lower leg with bone involvement without evidence of necrosis

CC L97.808 Non-pressure chronic ulcer of other part of unspecified lower leg with other specified severity

CC L97.809 Non-pressure chronic ulcer of other part of unspecified lower leg with unspecified severity

+ L97.81 Non-pressure chronic ulcer of other part of right lower leg

CC L97.811 Non-pressure chronic ulcer of other part of right lower leg limited to breakdown of skin

CC L97.812 Non-pressure chronic ulcer of other part of right lower leg with fat layer exposed

CC L97.813 Non-pressure chronic ulcer of other part of right lower leg with necrosis of muscle

CC L97.814 Non-pressure chronic ulcer of other part of right lower leg with necrosis of bone

CC L97.815 Non-pressure chronic ulcer of other part of right lower leg with muscle involvement without evidence of necrosis

CC L97.816 Non-pressure chronic ulcer of other part of right lower leg with bone involvement without evidence of necrosis

CC L97.818 Non-pressure chronic ulcer of other part of right lower leg with other specified severity

CC L97.819 Non-pressure chronic ulcer of other part of right lower leg with unspecified severity

+ L97.82 Non-pressure chronic ulcer of other part of left lower leg

CC L97.821 Non-pressure chronic ulcer of other part of left lower leg limited to breakdown of skin

CC L97.822 Non-pressure chronic ulcer of other part of left lower leg with fat layer exposed

CC L97.823 Non-pressure chronic ulcer of other part of left lower leg with necrosis of muscle

CC L97.824 Non-pressure chronic ulcer of other part of left lower leg with necrosis of bone

CC L97.825 Non-pressure chronic ulcer of other part of left lower leg with muscle involvement without evidence of necrosis

CC L97.826 Non-pressure chronic ulcer of other part of left lower leg with bone involvement without evidence of necrosis

CC L97.828 Non-pressure chronic ulcer of other part of left lower leg with other specified severity

CC L97.829 Non-pressure chronic ulcer of other part of left lower leg with unspecified severity

+ L97.9 Non-pressure chronic ulcer of unspecified part of lower leg

+ L97.90 Non-pressure chronic ulcer of unspecified part of unspecified lower leg

CC L97.901 Non-pressure chronic ulcer of unspecified part of unspecified lower leg limited to breakdown of skin

CC L97.902 Non-pressure chronic ulcer of unspecified part of unspecified lower leg with fat layer exposed

CC L97.903 Non-pressure chronic ulcer of unspecified part of unspecified lower leg with necrosis of muscle

CC L97.904 Non-pressure chronic ulcer of unspecified part of unspecified lower leg with necrosis of bone

CC L97.905 Non-pressure chronic ulcer of unspecified part of unspecified lower leg with muscle involvement without evidence of necrosis

CC L97.906 Non-pressure chronic ulcer of unspecified part of unspecified lower leg with bone involvement without evidence of necrosis

CC L97.908 Non-pressure chronic ulcer of unspecified part of unspecified lower leg with other specified severity

CC L97.909 Non-pressure chronic ulcer of unspecified part of unspecified lower leg with unspecified severity

+ L97.91 Non-pressure chronic ulcer of unspecified part of right lower leg

CC L97.911 Non-pressure chronic ulcer of unspecified part of right lower leg limited to breakdown of skin

CC L97.912 Non-pressure chronic ulcer of unspecified part of right lower leg with fat layer exposed

CC **L97.913** Non-pressure chronic ulcer of unspecified part of right lower leg with necrosis of muscle

CC **L97.914** Non-pressure chronic ulcer of unspecified part of right lower leg with necrosis of bone

CC **L97.915** Non-pressure chronic ulcer of unspecified part of right lower leg with muscle involvement without evidence of necrosis

CC **L97.916** Non-pressure chronic ulcer of unspecified part of right lower leg with bone involvement without evidence of necrosis

CC **L97.918** Non-pressure chronic ulcer of unspecified part of right lower leg with other specified severity

CC **L97.919** Non-pressure chronic ulcer of unspecified part of right lower leg with unspecified severity

+ **L97.92** Non-pressure chronic ulcer of unspecified part of left lower leg

CC **L97.921** Non-pressure chronic ulcer of unspecified part of left lower leg limited to breakdown of skin

CC **L97.922** Non-pressure chronic ulcer of unspecified part of left lower leg with fat layer exposed

CC **L97.923** Non-pressure chronic ulcer of unspecified part of left lower leg with necrosis of muscle

CC **L97.924** Non-pressure chronic ulcer of unspecified part of left lower leg with necrosis of bone

CC **L97.925** Non-pressure chronic ulcer of unspecified part of left lower leg with muscle involvement without evidence of necrosis

CC **L97.926** Non-pressure chronic ulcer of unspecified part of left lower leg with bone involvement without evidence of necrosis

CC **L97.928** Non-pressure chronic ulcer of unspecified part of left lower leg with other specified severity

CC **L97.929** Non-pressure chronic ulcer of unspecified part of left lower leg with unspecified severity

L98 Other disorders of skin and subcutaneous tissue, not elsewhere classified

L98.0 Pyogenic granuloma

Excludes2: pyogenic granuloma of gingiva (K06.8)
pyogenic granuloma of maxillary alveolar ridge (K04.5)
pyogenic granuloma of oral mucosa (K13.4)

L98.1 Factitial dermatitis
Neurotic excoriation

Excludes1: Excoriation (skin-picking) disorder (F42.4)

L98.2 Febrile neutrophilic dermatosis [Sweet]

CC **L98.3** Eosinophilic cellulitis [Wells]

+ **L98.4** Non-pressure chronic ulcer of skin, not elsewhere classified
Chronic ulcer of skin NOS
Tropical ulcer NOS
Ulcer of skin NOS

Excludes2: pressure ulcer (pressure area) (L89.-)
gangrene (I96)
skin infections (L00-L08)
specific infections classified to A00-B99
ulcer of lower limb NEC (L97.-)
varicose ulcer (I83.0-I83.93)

AHA CC: 4Q, 2017, 17

+ **L98.41** Non-pressure chronic ulcer of buttock

L98.411 Non-pressure chronic ulcer of buttock limited to breakdown of skin

L98.412 Non-pressure chronic ulcer of buttock with fat layer exposed

L98.413 Non-pressure chronic ulcer of buttock with necrosis of muscle

L98.414 Non-pressure chronic ulcer of buttock with necrosis of bone

CC **L98.415** Non-pressure chronic ulcer of buttock with muscle involvement without evidence of necrosis

CC **L98.416** Non-pressure chronic ulcer of buttock with bone involvement without evidence of necrosis

CC **L98.418** Non-pressure chronic ulcer of buttock with other specified severity

L98.419 Non-pressure chronic ulcer of buttock with unspecified severity

+ **L98.42** Non-pressure chronic ulcer of back

L98.421 Non-pressure chronic ulcer of back limited to breakdown of skin

L98.422 Non-pressure chronic ulcer of back with fat layer exposed

L98.423 Non-pressure chronic ulcer of back with necrosis of muscle

L98.424 Non-pressure chronic ulcer of back with necrosis of bone

CC **L98.425** Non-pressure chronic ulcer of back with muscle involvement without evidence of necrosis

CC **L98.426** Non-pressure chronic ulcer of back with bone involvement without evidence of necrosis

CC **L98.428** Non-pressure chronic ulcer of back with other specified severity

L98.429 Non-pressure chronic ulcer of back with unspecified severity

+ **L98.49** Non-pressure chronic ulcer of skin of other sites
Non-pressure chronic ulcer of skin NOS

L98.491 Non-pressure chronic ulcer of skin of other sites limited to breakdown of skin

L98.492 Non-pressure chronic ulcer of skin of other sites with fat layer exposed

L98.493 Non-pressure chronic ulcer of skin of other sites with necrosis of muscle

L98.494 Non-pressure chronic ulcer of skin of other sites with necrosis of bone

CC **L98.495** Non-pressure chronic ulcer of skin of other sites with muscle involvement without evidence of necrosis

CC **L98.496** Non-pressure chronic ulcer of skin of other sites with bone involvement without evidence of necrosis

CC **L98.498** Non-pressure chronic ulcer of skin of other sites with other specified severity

L98.499 Non-pressure chronic ulcer of skin of other sites with unspecified severity

L98.5 Mucinosis of the skin
Focal mucinosis
Lichen myxedematosus
Reticular erythematous mucinosis

Excludes1: focal oral mucinosis (K13.79)
myxedema (E03.9)

L98.6 Other infiltrative disorders of the skin and subcutaneous tissue

Excludes1: hyalinosis cutis et mucosae (E78.89)

L98.7 Excessive and redundant skin and subcutaneous tissue
Loose or sagging skin following bariatric surgery weight loss
Loose or sagging skin following dietary weight loss
Loose or sagging skin, NOS

Excludes2: acquired excess or redundant skin of eyelid (H02.3-)
congenital excess or redundant skin or eyelid (Q10.3)
skin changes due to chronic exposure to nonionizing radiation (L57.-)

AHA CC: 4Q, 2016, 36

L98.8 Other specified disorders of the skin and subcutaneous tissue

AHA CC: 2Q, 2013, 32-33

L98.9 Disorder of the skin and subcutaneous tissue, unspecified

L99 Other disorders of skin and subcutaneous tissue in diseases classified elsewhere

Code first underlying disease, such as:
amyloidosis (E85.-)

Excludes1: skin disorders in diabetes (E08-E13 with .62)
skin disorders in gonorrhea (A54.89)
skin disorders in syphilis (A51.31, A52.79)

Valid 3-character code, no further characters required

Intervertebral Joint

©AHIMA

Shoulder Joint

©AHIMA

Elbow

©AHIMA

Wrist

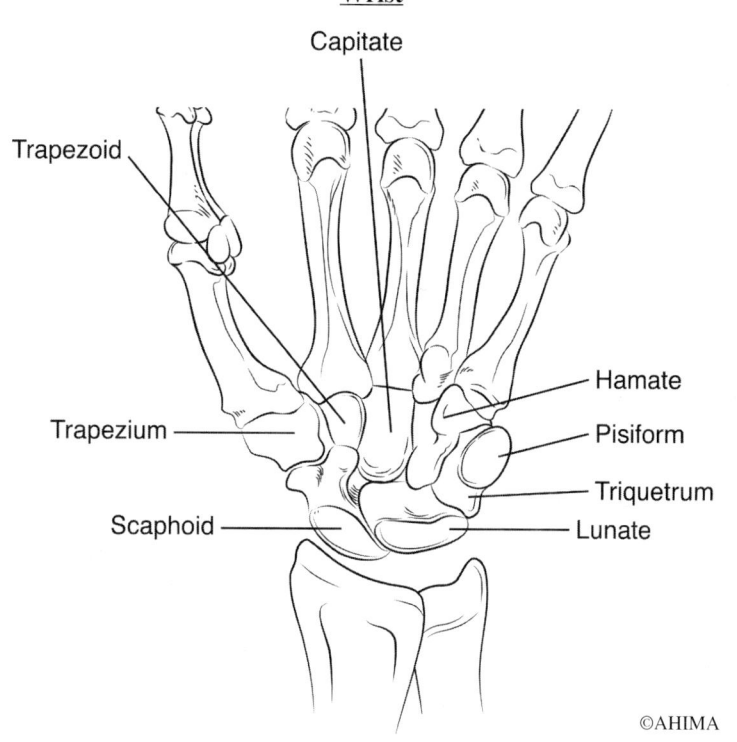

Capitate

Trapezoid

Trapezium

Scaphoid

Hamate

Pisiform

Triquetrum

Lunate

©AHIMA

Hip Joint

ANTERIOR

POSTERIOR

Anterior sacroiliac l.

Iliopectinea bursa

Pubofemoral l.

Iliofemoral l.

Greater trochanter

Lesser trochanter

Intertrochanteric line

Posterior sacroiliac ll

**Sacrospinous l.

Iliotibial band

Acetabular labrum

Iliofemoral l.

Ischiofemoral l.

Greater trochanter

Zona orbicularis

Protrusion of synovial membrane

Lesser trochanter

*Sacrotuberous l.

©AHIMA

Knee Joint

ANTERIOR

POSTERIOR

Femur

Lat. condyle of femur

Ant. cruciate l.

Fibular collateral l.

Lat. meniscus

Lat. condyle of tibia

Head of fibula

Patella

Tibia

Post. cruciate l.

Med. condyle of femur

Tibial collateral l.

Med. meniscus

Med. condyle of tibia

Transverse l. of knee

Tibial tuberosity

Femur

Tibia

Post. meniscofemoral l.

Ant. cruciate l.

Lat. condyle of femur

Fibular collateral l.

Popliteus tendon

Lat. meniscus

Head of fibula

Post. cruciate l.

©AHIMA

Ankle

Tibia

Ankle joint

Navicular

Cuneiforms

Fibula

Talus

Lateral malleolus

Calcaneus

Cuboid

©AHIMA

Chapter 13: Diseases of the Musculoskeletal System and Connective Tissue (M00-M99)

NOTE Use an external cause code following the code for the musculoskeletal condition, if applicable, to identify the cause of the musculoskeletal condition

Excludes2: *arthropathic psoriasis (L40.5-)*
certain conditions originating in the perinatal period (P04-P96)
certain infectious and parasitic diseases (A00-B99)
compartment syndrome (traumatic) (T79.A-)
complications of pregnancy, childbirth and the puerperium (O00-O9A)
congenital malformations, deformations, and chromosomal abnormalities (Q00-Q99)
endocrine, nutritional and metabolic diseases (E00-E88)
injury, poisoning and certain other consequences of external causes (S00-T88)
neoplasms (C00-D49)
symptoms, signs and abnormal clinical and laboratory findings, not elsewhere classified (R00-R94)

This chapter contains the following category blocks:

M00-M02	Infectious arthropathies
M04	Autoinflammatory syndromes
M05-M14	Inflammatory polyarthropathies
M15-M19	Osteoarthritis
M20-M25	Other joint disorders
M26-M27	Dentofacial anomalies [including malocclusion] and other disorders of jaw
M30-M36	Systemic connective tissue disorders
M40-M43	Deforming dorsopathies
M45-M49	Spondylopathies
M50-M54	Other dorsopathies
M60-M63	Disorders of muscles
M65-M67	Disorders of synovium and tendon
M70-M79	Other soft tissue disorders
M80-M85	Disorders of bone density and structure
M86-M90	Other osteopathies
M91-M94	Chondropathies
M95	Other disorders of the musculoskeletal system and connective tissue
M96	Intraoperative and postprocedural complications and disorders of musculoskeletal system, not elsewhere classified
M97	Periprosthetic fracture around internal prosthetic joint
M99	Biomechanical lesions, not elsewhere classified

C. Chapter-Specific Coding Guidelines

In addition to general coding guidelines, there are guidelines for specific diagnoses and/or conditions in the classification. Unless otherwise indicated, these guidelines apply to all health care settings. Please refer to Section II for guidelines on the selection of principal diagnosis.

13. Chapter 13: Diseases of the Musculoskeletal System and Connective Tissue (M00-M99)

a. Site and laterality

Most of the codes within Chapter 13 have site and laterality designations. The site represents the bone, joint or the muscle involved. For some conditions where more than one bone, joint or muscle is usually involved, such as osteoarthritis, there is a "multiple sites" code available. For categories where no multiple site code is provided and more than one bone, joint or muscle is involved, multiple codes should be used to indicate the different sites involved.

1) Bone versus joint

For certain conditions, the bone may be affected at the upper or lower end, (e.g., avascular necrosis of bone, M87, Osteoporosis, M80, M81). Though the portion of the bone affected may be at the joint, the site designation will be the bone, not the joint.

b. Acute traumatic versus chronic or recurrent musculoskeletal conditions

Many musculoskeletal conditions are a result of previous injury or trauma to a site, or are recurrent conditions. Bone, joint or muscle conditions that are the result of a healed injury are usually found in chapter 13. Recurrent bone, joint or muscle conditions are also usually found in chapter 13. Any current, acute injury should be coded to the appropriate injury code from chapter 19. Chronic or recurrent conditions should generally be coded with a code from chapter 13. If it is difficult to determine from the documentation in the record which code is best to describe a condition, query the provider.

c. Coding of Pathologic Fractures

7th character A is for use as long as the patient is receiving active treatment for the fracture. While the patient may be seen by a new or different provider over the course of treatment for a pathological fracture, assignment of the 7th character is based on whether the patient is undergoing active treatment and not whether the provider is seeing the patient for the first time.

7th character, D is to be used for encounters after the patient has completed active treatment for the fracture and is receiving routine care for the fracture during the healing or recovery phase. The other 7th characters, listed under each subcategory in the Tabular List, are to be used for subsequent encounters for routine care of fractures during the healing and recovery phase as well as treatment of problems associated with the healing, such as malunions, nonunions, and sequelae.

Care for complications of surgical treatment for fracture repairs during the healing or recovery phase should be coded with the appropriate complication codes.

See Section I.C.19. Coding of traumatic fractures.

d. Osteoporosis

Osteoporosis is a systemic condition, meaning that all bones of the musculoskeletal system are affected. Therefore, site is not a component of the codes under category M81, Osteoporosis without current pathological fracture. The site codes under category M80, Osteoporosis with current pathological fracture, identify the site of the fracture, not the osteoporosis.

1) Osteoporosis without pathological fracture

Category M81, Osteoporosis without current pathological fracture, is for use for patients with osteoporosis who do not currently have a pathologic fracture due to the osteoporosis, even if they have had a fracture in the past. For patients with a history of osteoporosis fractures, status code Z87.310, Personal history of (healed) osteoporosis fracture, should follow the code from M81.

2) Osteoporosis with current pathological fracture

Category M80, Osteoporosis with current pathological fracture, is for patients who have a current pathologic fracture at the time of an encounter. The codes under M80 identify the site of the fracture. A code from category M80, not a traumatic fracture code, should be used for any patient with known osteoporosis who suffers a fracture, even if the patient had a minor fall or trauma, if that fall or trauma would not usually break a normal, healthy bone.

ARTHROPATHIES (M00-M25)

Includes: Disorders affecting predominantly peripheral (limb) joints

Infectious arthropathies (M00-M02)

NOTE This block comprises arthropathies due to microbiological agents. Distinction is made between the following types of etiological relationship:
a) direct infection of joint, where organisms invade synovial tissue and microbial antigen is present in the joint;
b) indirect infection, which may be of two types: a reactive arthropathy, where microbial infection of the body is established but neither organisms nor antigens can be identified in the joint, and a postinfective arthropathy, where microbial antigen is present but recovery of an organism is inconstant and evidence of local multiplication is lacking.

M00 Pyogenic arthritis

Excludes2: *infection and inflammatory reaction due to internal joint prosthesis (T84.5-)*

+ **M00.0 Staphylococcal arthritis and polyarthritis**
Use additional code (B95.61-B95.8) to identify bacterial agent

CC **M00.00** Staphylococcal arthritis, unspecified joint
+ **M00.01** Staphylococcal arthritis, shoulder
 M00.011 Staphylococcal arthritis, right shoulder
 M00.012 Staphylococcal arthritis, left shoulder
CC **M00.019** Staphylococcal arthritis, unspecified shoulder
+ **M00.02** Staphylococcal arthritis, elbow
 M00.021 Staphylococcal arthritis, right elbow
 M00.022 Staphylococcal arthritis, left elbow
CC **M00.029** Staphylococcal arthritis, unspecified elbow
+ **M00.03** Staphylococcal arthritis, wrist
 Staphylococcal arthritis of carpal bones
 M00.031 Staphylococcal arthritis, right wrist
 M00.032 Staphylococcal arthritis, left wrist
CC **M00.039** Staphylococcal arthritis, unspecified wrist

+, +7th, X + 7th • Newborn • Pediatric • Maternity • Adult ♀ Female ♂ Male | Manifestation | Unacceptable PDX HCC CC MCC | HAC |

+ **M00.04 Staphylococcal arthritis, hand**
   Staphylococcal arthritis of metacarpus and phalanges
    M00.041 Staphylococcal arthritis, right hand
    M00.042 Staphylococcal arthritis, left hand
  CC M00.049 Staphylococcal arthritis, unspecified hand

+ **M00.05 Staphylococcal arthritis, hip**
    M00.051 Staphylococcal arthritis, right hip
    M00.052 Staphylococcal arthritis, left hip
  CC M00.059 Staphylococcal arthritis, unspecified hip

+ **M00.06 Staphylococcal arthritis, knee**
    M00.061 Staphylococcal arthritis, right knee
    M00.062 Staphylococcal arthritis, left knee
  CC M00.069 Staphylococcal arthritis, unspecified knee

+ **M00.07 Staphylococcal arthritis, ankle and foot**
   Staphylococcal arthritis, tarsus, metatarsus and phalanges
    M00.071 Staphylococcal arthritis, right ankle and foot
    M00.072 Staphylococcal arthritis, left ankle and foot
  CC M00.079 Staphylococcal arthritis, unspecified ankle and foot

CC **M00.08 Staphylococcal arthritis, vertebrae**
CC **M00.09 Staphylococcal polyarthritis**

+ **M00.1 Pneumococcal arthritis and polyarthritis**
CC **M00.10 Pneumococcal arthritis, unspecified joint**

+ **M00.11 Pneumococcal arthritis, shoulder**
  CC M00.111 Pneumococcal arthritis, right shoulder
  CC M00.112 Pneumococcal arthritis, left shoulder
  CC M00.119 Pneumococcal arthritis, unspecified shoulder

+ **M00.12 Pneumococcal arthritis, elbow**
  CC M00.121 Pneumococcal arthritis, right elbow
  CC M00.122 Pneumococcal arthritis, left elbow
  CC M00.129 Pneumococcal arthritis, unspecified elbow

+ **M00.13 Pneumococcal arthritis, wrist**
   Pneumococcal arthritis of carpal bones
  CC M00.131 Pneumococcal arthritis, right wrist
  CC M00.132 Pneumococcal arthritis, left wrist
  CC M00.139 Pneumococcal arthritis, unspecified wrist

+ **M00.14 Pneumococcal arthritis, hand**
   Pneumococcal arthritis of metacarpus and phalanges
  CC M00.141 Pneumococcal arthritis, right hand
  CC M00.142 Pneumococcal arthritis, left hand
  CC M00.149 Pneumococcal arthritis, unspecified hand

+ **M00.15 Pneumococcal arthritis, hip**
  CC M00.151 Pneumococcal arthritis, right hip
  CC M00.152 Pneumococcal arthritis, left hip
  CC M00.159 Pneumococcal arthritis, unspecified hip

+ **M00.16 Pneumococcal arthritis, knee**
  CC M00.161 Pneumococcal arthritis, right knee
  CC M00.162 Pneumococcal arthritis, left knee
  CC M00.169 Pneumococcal arthritis, unspecified knee

+ **M00.17 Pneumococcal arthritis, ankle and foot**
   Pneumococcal arthritis, tarsus, metatarsus and phalanges
  CC M00.171 Pneumococcal arthritis, right ankle and foot
  CC M00.172 Pneumococcal arthritis, left ankle and foot
  CC M00.179 Pneumococcal arthritis, unspecified ankle and foot

CC **M00.18 Pneumococcal arthritis, vertebrae**
CC **M00.19 Pneumococcal polyarthritis**

+ **M00.2 Other streptococcal arthritis and polyarthritis**
   Use additional code (B95.0-B95.2, B95.4-B95.5) to identify bacterial agent
CC **M00.20 Other streptococcal arthritis, unspecified joint**

+ **M00.21 Other streptococcal arthritis, shoulder**
  CC M00.211 Other streptococcal arthritis, right shoulder
  CC M00.212 Other streptococcal arthritis, left shoulder
  CC M00.219 Other streptococcal arthritis, unspecified shoulder

+ **M00.22 Other streptococcal arthritis, elbow**
  CC M00.221 Other streptococcal arthritis, right elbow
  CC M00.222 Other streptococcal arthritis, left elbow
  CC M00.229 Other streptococcal arthritis, unspecified elbow

+ **M00.23 Other streptococcal arthritis, wrist**
   Other streptococcal arthritis of carpal bones
  CC M00.231 Other streptococcal arthritis, right wrist
  CC M00.232 Other streptococcal arthritis, left wrist
  CC M00.239 Other streptococcal arthritis, unspecified wrist

+ **M00.24 Other streptococcal arthritis, hand**
   Other streptococcal arthritis metacarpus and phalanges
  CC M00.241 Other streptococcal arthritis, right hand
  CC M00.242 Other streptococcal arthritis, left hand
  CC M00.249 Other streptococcal arthritis, unspecified hand

+ **M00.25 Other streptococcal arthritis, hip**
  CC M00.251 Other streptococcal arthritis, right hip
  CC M00.252 Other streptococcal arthritis, left hip
  CC M00.259 Other streptococcal arthritis, unspecified hip

+ **M00.26 Other streptococcal arthritis, knee**
  CC M00.261 Other streptococcal arthritis, right knee
  CC M00.262 Other streptococcal arthritis, left knee
  CC M00.269 Other streptococcal arthritis, unspecified knee

+ **M00.27 Other streptococcal arthritis, ankle and foot**
   Other streptococcal arthritis, tarsus, metatarsus and phalanges
  CC M00.271 Other streptococcal arthritis, right ankle and foot
  CC M00.272 Other streptococcal arthritis, left ankle and foot
  CC M00.279 Other streptococcal arthritis, unspecified ankle and foot

CC **M00.28 Other streptococcal arthritis, vertebrae**
CC **M00.29 Other streptococcal polyarthritis**

+ **M00.8 Arthritis and polyarthritis due to other bacteria**
   Use additional code (B96) to identify bacteria
CC **M00.80 Arthritis due to other bacteria, unspecified joint**

+ **M00.81 Arthritis due to other bacteria, shoulder**
  CC M00.811 Arthritis due to other bacteria, right shoulder
  CC M00.812 Arthritis due to other bacteria, left shoulder
  CC M00.819 Arthritis due to other bacteria, unspecified shoulder

+ **M00.82 Arthritis due to other bacteria, elbow**
  CC M00.821 Arthritis due to other bacteria, right elbow
  CC M00.822 Arthritis due to other bacteria, left elbow
  CC M00.829 Arthritis due to other bacteria, unspecified elbow

+ **M00.83 Arthritis due to other bacteria, wrist**
   Arthritis due to other bacteria, carpal bones
  CC M00.831 Arthritis due to other bacteria, right wrist
  CC M00.832 Arthritis due to other bacteria, left wrist
  CC M00.839 Arthritis due to other bacteria, unspecified wrist

+ **M00.84 Arthritis due to other bacteria, hand**
   Arthritis due to other bacteria, metacarpus and phalanges
  CC M00.841 Arthritis due to other bacteria, right hand
  CC M00.842 Arthritis due to other bacteria, left hand
  CC M00.849 Arthritis due to other bacteria, unspecified hand

+ **M00.85 Arthritis due to other bacteria, hip**
  CC M00.851 Arthritis due to other bacteria, right hip
  CC M00.852 Arthritis due to other bacteria, left hip
  CC M00.859 Arthritis due to other bacteria, unspecified hip

+ **M00.86** Arthritis due to other bacteria, knee

CC **M00.861** Arthritis due to other bacteria, right knee

CC **M00.862** Arthritis due to other bacteria, left knee
AHA CC: 3Q, 2019, 16-17

CC **M00.869** Arthritis due to other bacteria, unspecified knee

+ **M00.87** Arthritis due to other bacteria, ankle and foot

Arthritis due to other bacteria, tarsus, metatarsus, and phalanges

CC **M00.871** Arthritis due to other bacteria, right ankle and foot

CC **M00.872** Arthritis due to other bacteria, left ankle and foot

CC **M00.879** Arthritis due to other bacteria, unspecified ankle and foot

CC **M00.88** Arthritis due to other bacteria, vertebrae

CC **M00.89** Polyarthritis due to other bacteria

CC **M00.9** Pyogenic arthritis, unspecified
Infective arthritis NOS

M01 Direct infections of joint in infectious and parasitic diseases classified elsewhere

Code first underlying disease, such as:
leprosy [Hansen's disease] (A30.-)
mycoses (B35-B49)
O'nyong-nyong fever (A92.1)
paratyphoid fever (A01.1-A01.4)

Excludes1: *arthropathy in Lyme disease (A69.23)*
gonococcal arthritis (A54.42)
meningococcal arthritis (A39.83)
mumps arthritis (B26.85)
postinfective arthropathy (M02.-)
postmeningococcal arthritis (39.84)
reactive arthritis (M02.3)
rubella arthritis (B06.82)
sarcoidosis arthritis (D86.86)
tuberculosis arthritis (A18.01-A18.02)
typhoid fever arthritis (A01.04)

+ **M01.X** Direct infection of joint in infectious and parasitic diseases classified elsewhere

CC **M01.X0** Direct infection of unspecified joint in infectious and parasitic diseases classified elsewhere

+ **M01.X1** Direct infection of shoulder joint in infectious and parasitic diseases classified elsewhere

CC **M01.X11** Direct infection of right shoulder in infectious and parasitic diseases classified elsewhere

CC **M01.X12** Direct infection of left shoulder in infectious and parasitic diseases classified elsewhere

CC **M01.X19** Direct infection of unspecified shoulder in infectious and parasitic diseases classified elsewhere

+ **M01.X2** Direct infection of elbow in infectious and parasitic diseases classified elsewhere

CC **M01.X21** Direct infection of right elbow in infectious and parasitic diseases classified elsewhere

CC **M01.X22** Direct infection of left elbow in infectious and parasitic diseases classified elsewhere

CC **M01.X29** Direct infection of unspecified elbow in infectious and parasitic diseases classified elsewhere

+ **M01.X3** Direct infection of wrist in infectious and parasitic diseases classified elsewhere

Direct infection of carpal bones in infectious and parasitic diseases classified elsewhere

CC **M01.X31** Direct infection of right wrist in infectious and parasitic diseases classified elsewhere

CC **M01.X32** Direct infection of left wrist in infectious and parasitic diseases classified elsewhere

CC **M01.X39** Direct infection of unspecified wrist in infectious and parasitic diseases classified elsewhere

+ **M01.X4** Direct infection of hand in infectious and parasitic diseases classified elsewhere

Direct infection of metacarpus and phalanges in infectious and parasitic diseases classified elsewhere

CC **M01.X41** Direct infection of right hand in infectious and parasitic diseases classified elsewhere

CC **M01.X42** Direct infection of left hand in infectious and parasitic diseases classified elsewhere

CC **M01.X49** Direct infection of unspecified hand in infectious and parasitic diseases classified elsewhere

+ **M01.X5** Direct infection of hip in infectious and parasitic diseases classified elsewhere

CC **M01.X51** Direct infection of right hip in infectious and parasitic diseases classified elsewhere

CC **M01.X52** Direct infection of left hip in infectious and parasitic diseases classified elsewhere

CC **M01.X59** Direct infection of unspecified hip in infectious and parasitic diseases classified elsewhere

+ **M01.X6** Direct infection of knee in infectious and parasitic diseases classified elsewhere

CC **M01.X61** Direct infection of right knee in infectious and parasitic diseases classified elsewhere

CC **M01.X62** Direct infection of left knee in infectious and parasitic diseases classified elsewhere

CC **M01.X69** Direct infection of unspecified knee in infectious and parasitic diseases classified elsewhere

+ **M01.X7** Direct infection of ankle and foot in infectious and parasitic diseases classified elsewhere

Direct infection of tarsus, metatarsus and phalanges in infectious and parasitic diseases classified elsewhere

CC **M01.X71** Direct infection of right ankle and foot in infectious and parasitic diseases classified elsewhere

CC **M01.X72** Direct infection of left ankle and foot in infectious and parasitic diseases classified elsewhere

CC **M01.X79** Direct infection of unspecified ankle and foot in infectious and parasitic diseases classified elsewhere

CC **M01.X8** Direct infection of vertebrae in infectious and parasitic diseases classified elsewhere

CC **M01.X9** Direct infection of multiple joints in infectious and parasitic diseases classified elsewhere

M02 Postinfective and reactive arthropathies

Code first underlying disease, such as:
congenital syphilis [Clutton's joints] (A50.5)
enteritis due to Yersinia enterocolitica (A04.6)
infective endocarditis (I33.0)
viral hepatitis (B15-B19)

Excludes1: *Behçet's disease (M35.2)*
direct infections of joint in infectious and parasitic diseases classified elsewhere (M01.-)
postmeningococcal arthritis (A39.84)
mumps arthritis (B26.85)
rubella arthritis (B06.82)
syphilis arthritis (late) (A52.77)
rheumatic fever (I00)
tabetic arthropathy [Charcôt's] (A52.16)

+ **M02.0** Arthropathy following intestinal bypass

M02.00 Arthropathy following intestinal bypass, unspecified site

+ **M02.01** Arthropathy following intestinal bypass, shoulder

M02.011 Arthropathy following intestinal bypass, right shoulder

M02.012 Arthropathy following intestinal bypass, left shoulder

M02.019 Arthropathy following intestinal bypass, unspecified shoulder

+ **M02.02** **Arthropathy following intestinal bypass, elbow**
    M02.021 **Arthropathy following intestinal bypass, right elbow**
    M02.022 **Arthropathy following intestinal bypass, left elbow**
    M02.029 **Arthropathy following intestinal bypass, unspecified elbow**
+ **M02.03** **Arthropathy following intestinal bypass, wrist**
    Arthropathy following intestinal bypass, carpal bones
    M02.031 **Arthropathy following intestinal bypass, right wrist**
    M02.032 **Arthropathy following intestinal bypass, left wrist**
    M02.039 **Arthropathy following intestinal bypass, unspecified wrist**
+ **M02.04** **Arthropathy following intestinal bypass, hand**
    Arthropathy following intestinal bypass, metacarpals and phalanges
    M02.041 **Arthropathy following intestinal bypass, right hand**
    M02.042 **Arthropathy following intestinal bypass, left hand**
    M02.049 **Arthropathy following intestinal bypass, unspecified hand**
+ **M02.05** **Arthropathy following intestinal bypass, hip**
    M02.051 **Arthropathy following intestinal bypass, right hip**
    M02.052 **Arthropathy following intestinal bypass, left hip**
    M02.059 **Arthropathy following intestinal bypass, unspecified hip**
+ **M02.06** **Arthropathy following intestinal bypass, knee**
    M02.061 **Arthropathy following intestinal bypass, right knee**
    M02.062 **Arthropathy following intestinal bypass, left knee**
    M02.069 **Arthropathy following intestinal bypass, unspecified knee**
+ **M02.07** **Arthropathy following intestinal bypass, ankle and foot**
    Arthropathy following intestinal bypass, tarsus, metatarsus and phalanges
    M02.071 **Arthropathy following intestinal bypass, right ankle and foot**
    M02.072 **Arthropathy following intestinal bypass, left ankle and foot**
    M02.079 **Arthropathy following intestinal bypass, unspecified ankle and foot**
M02.08 **Arthropathy following intestinal bypass, vertebrae**
M02.09 **Arthropathy following intestinal bypass, multiple sites**
+ **M02.1** **Postdysenteric arthropathy**
  CC **M02.10** **Postdysenteric arthropathy, unspecified site**
+ **M02.11** **Postdysenteric arthropathy, shoulder**
  CC **M02.111** **Postdysenteric arthropathy, right shoulder**
  CC **M02.112** **Postdysenteric arthropathy, left shoulder**
  CC **M02.119** **Postdysenteric arthropathy, unspecified shoulder**
+ **M02.12** **Postdysenteric arthropathy, elbow**
  CC **M02.121** **Postdysenteric arthropathy, right elbow**
  CC **M02.122** **Postdysenteric arthropathy, left elbow**
  CC **M02.129** **Postdysenteric arthropathy, unspecified elbow**
+ **M02.13** **Postdysenteric arthropathy, wrist**
    Postdysenteric arthropathy, carpal bones
  CC **M02.131** **Postdysenteric arthropathy, right wrist**
  CC **M02.132** **Postdysenteric arthropathy, left wrist**
  CC **M02.139** **Postdysenteric arthropathy, unspecified wrist**
+ **M02.14** **Postdysenteric arthropathy, hand**
    Postdysenteric arthropathy, metacarpus and phalanges
  CC **M02.141** **Postdysenteric arthropathy, right hand**
  CC **M02.142** **Postdysenteric arthropathy, left hand**
  CC **M02.149** **Postdysenteric arthropathy, unspecified hand**

+ **M02.15** **Postdysenteric arthropathy, hip**
  CC **M02.151** **Postdysenteric arthropathy, right hip**
  CC **M02.152** **Postdysenteric arthropathy, left hip**
  CC **M02.159** **Postdysenteric arthropathy, unspecified hip**
+ **M02.16** **Postdysenteric arthropathy, knee**
  CC **M02.161** **Postdysenteric arthropathy, right knee**
  CC **M02.162** **Postdysenteric arthropathy, left knee**
  CC **M02.169** **Postdysenteric arthropathy, unspecified knee**
+ **M02.17** **Postdysenteric arthropathy, ankle and foot**
    Postdysenteric arthropathy, tarsus, metatarsus and phalanges
  CC **M02.171** **Postdysenteric arthropathy, right ankle and foot**
  CC **M02.172** **Postdysenteric arthropathy, left ankle and foot**
  CC **M02.179** **Postdysenteric arthropathy, unspecified ankle and foot**
  CC **M02.18** **Postdysenteric arthropathy, vertebrae**
  CC **M02.19** **Postdysenteric arthropathy, multiple sites**
+ **M02.2** **Postimmunization arthropathy**
  M02.20 **Postimmunization arthropathy, unspecified site**
+ **M02.21** **Postimmunization arthropathy, shoulder**
    M02.211 **Postimmunization arthropathy, right shoulder**
    M02.212 **Postimmunization arthropathy, left shoulder**
    M02.219 **Postimmunization arthropathy, unspecified shoulder**
+ **M02.22** **Postimmunization arthropathy, elbow**
    M02.221 **Postimmunization arthropathy, right elbow**
    M02.222 **Postimmunization arthropathy, left elbow**
    M02.229 **Postimmunization arthropathy, unspecified elbow**
+ **M02.23** **Postimmunization arthropathy, wrist**
    Postimmunization arthropathy, carpal bones
    M02.231 **Postimmunization arthropathy, right wrist**
    M02.232 **Postimmunization arthropathy, left wrist**
    M02.239 **Postimmunization arthropathy, unspecified wrist**
+ **M02.24** **Postimmunization arthropathy, hand**
    Postimmunization arthropathy, metacarpus and phalanges
    M02.241 **Postimmunization arthropathy, right hand**
    M02.242 **Postimmunization arthropathy, left hand**
    M02.249 **Postimmunization arthropathy, unspecified hand**
+ **M02.25** **Postimmunization arthropathy, hip**
    M02.251 **Postimmunization arthropathy, right hip**
    M02.252 **Postimmunization arthropathy, left hip**
    M02.259 **Postimmunization arthropathy, unspecified hip**
+ **M02.26** **Postimmunization arthropathy, knee**
    M02.261 **Postimmunization arthropathy, right knee**
    M02.262 **Postimmunization arthropathy, left knee**
    M02.269 **Postimmunization arthropathy, unspecified knee**
+ **M02.27** **Postimmunization arthropathy, ankle and foot**
    Postimmunization arthropathy, tarsus, metatarsus and phalanges
    M02.271 **Postimmunization arthropathy, right ankle and foot**
    M02.272 **Postimmunization arthropathy, left ankle and foot**
    M02.279 **Postimmunization arthropathy, unspecified ankle and foot**
  M02.28 **Postimmunization arthropathy, vertebrae**
  M02.29 **Postimmunization arthropathy, multiple sites**

+, +7th, X + 7th   ● Newborn   ● Pediatric   ● Maternity   ● Adult   ♀ Female   ♂ Male   Manifestation   Unacceptable PDX   HCC   CC   MCC   HAC

+ **M02.3 Reiter's disease**
    Reactive arthritis
CC **M02.30** Reiter's disease, unspecified site
  + **M02.31** Reiter's disease, shoulder
    CC **M02.311** Reiter's disease, right shoulder
    CC **M02.312** Reiter's disease, left shoulder
    CC **M02.319** Reiter's disease, unspecified shoulder
  + **M02.32** Reiter's disease, elbow
    CC **M02.321** Reiter's disease, right elbow
    CC **M02.322** Reiter's disease, left elbow
    CC **M02.329** Reiter's disease, unspecified elbow
  + **M02.33** Reiter's disease, wrist
    Reiter's disease, carpal bones
    CC **M02.331** Reiter's disease, right wrist
    CC **M02.332** Reiter's disease, left wrist
    CC **M02.339** Reiter's disease, unspecified wrist
  + **M02.34** Reiter's disease, hand
    Reiter's disease, metacarpus and phalanges
    CC **M02.341** Reiter's disease, right hand
    CC **M02.342** Reiter's disease, left hand
    CC **M02.349** Reiter's disease, unspecified hand
  + **M02.35** Reiter's disease, hip
    CC **M02.351** Reiter's disease, right hip
    CC **M02.352** Reiter's disease, left hip
    CC **M02.359** Reiter's disease, unspecified hip
  + **M02.36** Reiter's disease, knee
    CC **M02.361** Reiter's disease, right knee
    CC **M02.362** Reiter's disease, left knee
    CC **M02.369** Reiter's disease, unspecified knee
  + **M02.37** Reiter's disease, ankle and foot
    Reiter's disease, tarsus, metatarsus and phalanges
    CC **M02.371** Reiter's disease, right ankle and foot
    CC **M02.372** Reiter's disease, left ankle and foot
    CC **M02.379** Reiter's disease, unspecified ankle and foot
  CC **M02.38** Reiter's disease, vertebrae
  CC **M02.39** Reiter's disease, multiple sites
+ **M02.8 Other reactive arthropathies**
CC **M02.80** Other reactive arthropathies, unspecified site
  + **M02.81** Other reactive arthropathies, shoulder
    CC **M02.811** Other reactive arthropathies, right shoulder
    CC **M02.812** Other reactive arthropathies, left shoulder
    CC **M02.819** Other reactive arthropathies, unspecified shoulder
  + **M02.82** Other reactive arthropathies, elbow
    CC **M02.821** Other reactive arthropathies, right elbow
    CC **M02.822** Other reactive arthropathies, left elbow
    CC **M02.829** Other reactive arthropathies, unspecified elbow
  + **M02.83** Other reactive arthropathies, wrist
    Other reactive arthropathies, carpal bones
    CC **M02.831** Other reactive arthropathies, right wrist
    CC **M02.832** Other reactive arthropathies, left wrist
    CC **M02.839** Other reactive arthropathies, unspecified wrist
  + **M02.84** Other reactive arthropathies, hand
    Other reactive arthropathies, metacarpus and phalanges
    CC **M02.841** Other reactive arthropathies, right hand
    CC **M02.842** Other reactive arthropathies, left hand
    CC **M02.849** Other reactive arthropathies, unspecified hand
  + **M02.85** Other reactive arthropathies, hip
    CC **M02.851** Other reactive arthropathies, right hip
    CC **M02.852** Other reactive arthropathies, left hip
    CC **M02.859** Other reactive arthropathies, unspecified hip
  + **M02.86** Other reactive arthropathies, knee
    CC **M02.861** Other reactive arthropathies, right knee
    CC **M02.862** Other reactive arthropathies, left knee
    CC **M02.869** Other reactive arthropathies, unspecified knee

  + **M02.87** Other reactive arthropathies, ankle and foot
    Other reactive arthropathies, tarsus, metatarsus and phalanges
    CC **M02.871** Other reactive arthropathies, right ankle and foot
    CC **M02.872** Other reactive arthropathies, left ankle and foot
    CC **M02.879** Other reactive arthropathies, unspecified ankle and foot
  CC **M02.88** Other reactive arthropathies, vertebrae
  CC **M02.89** Other reactive arthropathies, multiple sites
M02.9 Reactive arthropathy, unspecified

Autoinflammatory syndromes (M04)

M04 Autoinflammatory syndromes

  Excludes2: *Crohn's disease (K50.-)*
  AHA CC: 4Q, 2016, 37

M04.1 Periodic fever syndromes
  Familial Mediterranean fever
  Hyperimmunoglobin D syndrome
  Mevalonate kinase deficiency
  Tumor necrosis factor receptor associated periodic syndrome [TRAPS]

M04.2 Cryopyrin-associated periodic syndromes
  Chronic infantile neurological, cutaneous and articular syndrome [CINCA]
  Familial cold autoinflammatory syndrome
  Familial cold urticaria
  Muckle-Wells syndrome
  Neonatal onset multisystemic inflammatory disorder [NOMID]

M04.8 Other autoinflammatory syndromes
  Blau syndrome
  Deficiency of interleukin 1 receptor antagonist [DIRA]
  Majeed syndrome
  Periodic fever, aphthous stomatitis, pharyngitis, and adenopathy syndrome [PFAPA]
  Pyogenic arthritis, pyoderma gangrenosum, and acne syndrome [PAPA]

M04.9 Autoinflammatory syndrome, unspecified

Inflammatory polyarthropathies (M05-M14)

M05 Rheumatoid arthritis with rheumatoid factor

  Excludes1: *rheumatic fever (I00)*
    juvenile rheumatoid arthritis (M08.-)
    rheumatoid arthritis of spine (M45.-)

+ **M05.0 Felty's syndrome**
  Rheumatoid arthritis with splenoadenomegaly and leukopenia
  M05.00 Felty's syndrome, unspecified site
  + **M05.01** Felty's syndrome, shoulder
    M05.011 Felty's syndrome, right shoulder
    M05.012 Felty's syndrome, left shoulder
    M05.019 Felty's syndrome, unspecified shoulder
  + **M05.02** Felty's syndrome, elbow
    M05.021 Felty's syndrome, right elbow
    M05.022 Felty's syndrome, left elbow
    M05.029 Felty's syndrome, unspecified elbow
  + **M05.03** Felty's syndrome, wrist
    Felty's syndrome, carpal bones
    M05.031 Felty's syndrome, right wrist
    M05.032 Felty's syndrome, left wrist
    M05.039 Felty's syndrome, unspecified wrist
  + **M05.04** Felty's syndrome, hand
    Felty's syndrome, metacarpus and phalanges
    M05.041 Felty's syndrome, right hand
    M05.042 Felty's syndrome, left hand
    M05.049 Felty's syndrome, unspecified hand
  + **M05.05** Felty's syndrome, hip
    M05.051 Felty's syndrome, right hip
    M05.052 Felty's syndrome, left hip
    M05.059 Felty's syndrome, unspecified hip
  + **M05.06** Felty's syndrome, knee
    M05.061 Felty's syndrome, right knee
    M05.062 Felty's syndrome, left knee
    M05.069 Felty's syndrome, unspecified knee

+, +7th, X + 7th • Newborn • Pediatric • Maternity • Adult ♀ Female ♂ Male Manifestation Unacceptable PDX HCC CC MCC HAC

+ **M05.07** Felty's syndrome, ankle and foot
　Felty's syndrome, tarsus, metatarsus and phalanges
　M05.071 Felty's syndrome, right ankle and foot
　M05.072 Felty's syndrome, left ankle and foot
　M05.079 Felty's syndrome, unspecified ankle and foot
M05.09 Felty's syndrome, multiple sites
+ **M05.1** Rheumatoid lung disease with rheumatoid arthritis
M05.10 Rheumatoid lung disease with rheumatoid arthritis of unspecified site
+ **M05.11** Rheumatoid lung disease with rheumatoid arthritis of shoulder
　M05.111 Rheumatoid lung disease with rheumatoid arthritis of right shoulder
　M05.112 Rheumatoid lung disease with rheumatoid arthritis of left shoulder
　M05.119 Rheumatoid lung disease with rheumatoid arthritis of unspecified shoulder
+ **M05.12** Rheumatoid lung disease with rheumatoid arthritis of elbow
　M05.121 Rheumatoid lung disease with rheumatoid arthritis of right elbow
　M05.122 Rheumatoid lung disease with rheumatoid arthritis of left elbow
　M05.129 Rheumatoid lung disease with rheumatoid arthritis of unspecified elbow
+ **M05.13** Rheumatoid lung disease with rheumatoid arthritis of wrist
　Rheumatoid lung disease with rheumatoid arthritis, carpal bones
　M05.131 Rheumatoid lung disease with rheumatoid arthritis of right wrist
　M05.132 Rheumatoid lung disease with rheumatoid arthritis of left wrist
　M05.139 Rheumatoid lung disease with rheumatoid arthritis of unspecified wrist
+ **M05.14** Rheumatoid lung disease with rheumatoid arthritis of hand
　Rheumatoid lung disease with rheumatoid arthritis, metacarpus and phalanges
　M05.141 Rheumatoid lung disease with rheumatoid arthritis of right hand
　M05.142 Rheumatoid lung disease with rheumatoid arthritis of left hand
　M05.149 Rheumatoid lung disease with rheumatoid arthritis of unspecified hand
+ **M05.15** Rheumatoid lung disease with rheumatoid arthritis of hip
　M05.151 Rheumatoid lung disease with rheumatoid arthritis of right hip
　M05.152 Rheumatoid lung disease with rheumatoid arthritis of left hip
　M05.159 Rheumatoid lung disease with rheumatoid arthritis of unspecified hip
+ **M05.16** Rheumatoid lung disease with rheumatoid arthritis of knee
　M05.161 Rheumatoid lung disease with rheumatoid arthritis of right knee
　M05.162 Rheumatoid lung disease with rheumatoid arthritis of left knee
　M05.169 Rheumatoid lung disease with rheumatoid arthritis of unspecified knee
+ **M05.17** Rheumatoid lung disease with rheumatoid arthritis of ankle and foot
　Rheumatoid lung disease with rheumatoid arthritis, tarsus, metatarsus and phalanges
　M05.171 Rheumatoid lung disease with rheumatoid arthritis of right ankle and foot
　M05.172 Rheumatoid lung disease with rheumatoid arthritis of left ankle and foot

M05.179 Rheumatoid lung disease with rheumatoid arthritis of unspecified ankle and foot
M05.19 Rheumatoid lung disease with rheumatoid arthritis of multiple sites
+ **M05.2** Rheumatoid vasculitis with rheumatoid arthritis
M05.20 Rheumatoid vasculitis with rheumatoid arthritis of unspecified site
+ **M05.21** Rheumatoid vasculitis with rheumatoid arthritis of shoulder
　M05.211 Rheumatoid vasculitis with rheumatoid arthritis of right shoulder
　M05.212 Rheumatoid vasculitis with rheumatoid arthritis of left shoulder
　M05.219 Rheumatoid vasculitis with rheumatoid arthritis of unspecified shoulder
+ **M05.22** Rheumatoid vasculitis with rheumatoid arthritis of elbow
　M05.221 Rheumatoid vasculitis with rheumatoid arthritis of right elbow
　M05.222 Rheumatoid vasculitis with rheumatoid arthritis of left elbow
　M05.229 Rheumatoid vasculitis with rheumatoid arthritis of unspecified elbow
+ **M05.23** Rheumatoid vasculitis with rheumatoid arthritis of wrist
　Rheumatoid vasculitis with rheumatoid arthritis, carpal bones
　M05.231 Rheumatoid vasculitis with rheumatoid arthritis of right wrist
　M05.232 Rheumatoid vasculitis with rheumatoid arthritis of left wrist
　M05.239 Rheumatoid vasculitis with rheumatoid arthritis of unspecified wrist
+ **M05.24** Rheumatoid vasculitis with rheumatoid arthritis of hand
　Rheumatoid vasculitis with rheumatoid arthritis, metacarpus and phalanges
　M05.241 Rheumatoid vasculitis with rheumatoid arthritis of right hand
　M05.242 Rheumatoid vasculitis with rheumatoid arthritis of left hand
　M05.249 Rheumatoid vasculitis with rheumatoid arthritis of unspecified hand
+ **M05.25** Rheumatoid vasculitis with rheumatoid arthritis of hip
　M05.251 Rheumatoid vasculitis with rheumatoid arthritis of right hip
　M05.252 Rheumatoid vasculitis with rheumatoid arthritis of left hip
　M05.259 Rheumatoid vasculitis with rheumatoid arthritis of unspecified hip
+ **M05.26** Rheumatoid vasculitis with rheumatoid arthritis of knee
　M05.261 Rheumatoid vasculitis with rheumatoid arthritis of right knee
　M05.262 Rheumatoid vasculitis with rheumatoid arthritis of left knee
　M05.269 Rheumatoid vasculitis with rheumatoid arthritis of unspecified knee
+ **M05.27** Rheumatoid vasculitis with rheumatoid arthritis of ankle and foot
　Rheumatoid vasculitis with rheumatoid arthritis, tarsus, metatarsus and phalanges
　M05.271 Rheumatoid vasculitis with rheumatoid arthritis of right ankle and foot
　M05.272 Rheumatoid vasculitis with rheumatoid arthritis of left ankle and foot
　M05.279 Rheumatoid vasculitis with rheumatoid arthritis of unspecified ankle and foot
M05.29 Rheumatoid vasculitis with rheumatoid arthritis of multiple sites
+ **M05.3** Rheumatoid heart disease with rheumatoid arthritis
　Rheumatoid carditis
　Rheumatoid endocarditis
　Rheumatoid myocarditis
　Rheumatoid pericarditis
M05.30 Rheumatoid heart disease with rheumatoid arthritis of unspecified site

+, +7th, X + 7th　● Newborn　● Pediatric　● Maternity　● Adult　♀ Female　♂ Male　Manifestation　Unacceptable PDX　HCC　CC　MCC　HAC

+ **M05.31** **Rheumatoid heart disease with rheumatoid arthritis of shoulder**
    M05.311 **Rheumatoid heart disease with rheumatoid arthritis of right shoulder**
    M05.312 **Rheumatoid heart disease with rheumatoid arthritis of left shoulder**
    M05.319 **Rheumatoid heart disease with rheumatoid arthritis of unspecified shoulder**

+ **M05.32** **Rheumatoid heart disease with rheumatoid arthritis of elbow**
    M05.321 **Rheumatoid heart disease with rheumatoid arthritis of right elbow**
    M05.322 **Rheumatoid heart disease with rheumatoid arthritis of left elbow**
    M05.329 **Rheumatoid heart disease with rheumatoid arthritis of unspecified elbow**

+ **M05.33** **Rheumatoid heart disease with rheumatoid arthritis of wrist**
    Rheumatoid heart disease with rheumatoid arthritis, carpal bones
    M05.331 **Rheumatoid heart disease with rheumatoid arthritis of right wrist**
    M05.332 **Rheumatoid heart disease with rheumatoid arthritis of left wrist**
    M05.339 **Rheumatoid heart disease with rheumatoid arthritis of unspecified wrist**

+ **M05.34** **Rheumatoid heart disease with rheumatoid arthritis of hand**
    Rheumatoid heart disease with rheumatoid arthritis, metacarpus and phalanges
    M05.341 **Rheumatoid heart disease with rheumatoid arthritis of right hand**
    M05.342 **Rheumatoid heart disease with rheumatoid arthritis of left hand**
    M05.349 **Rheumatoid heart disease with rheumatoid arthritis of unspecified hand**

+ **M05.35** **Rheumatoid heart disease with rheumatoid arthritis of hip**
    M05.351 **Rheumatoid heart disease with rheumatoid arthritis of right hip**
    M05.352 **Rheumatoid heart disease with rheumatoid arthritis of left hip**
    M05.359 **Rheumatoid heart disease with rheumatoid arthritis of unspecified hip**

+ **M05.36** **Rheumatoid heart disease with rheumatoid arthritis of knee**
    M05.361 **Rheumatoid heart disease with rheumatoid arthritis of right knee**
    M05.362 **Rheumatoid heart disease with rheumatoid arthritis of left knee**
    M05.369 **Rheumatoid heart disease with rheumatoid arthritis of unspecified knee**

+ **M05.37** **Rheumatoid heart disease with rheumatoid arthritis of ankle and foot**
    Rheumatoid heart disease with rheumatoid arthritis, tarsus, metatarsus and phalanges
    M05.371 **Rheumatoid heart disease with rheumatoid arthritis of right ankle and foot**
    M05.372 **Rheumatoid heart disease with rheumatoid arthritis of left ankle and foot**
    M05.379 **Rheumatoid heart disease with rheumatoid arthritis of unspecified ankle and foot**

    M05.39 **Rheumatoid heart disease with rheumatoid arthritis of multiple sites**

+ **M05.4** **Rheumatoid myopathy with rheumatoid arthritis**
  CC **M05.40** **Rheumatoid myopathy with rheumatoid arthritis of unspecified site**

+ **M05.41** **Rheumatoid myopathy with rheumatoid arthritis of shoulder**
  CC **M05.411** **Rheumatoid myopathy with rheumatoid arthritis of right shoulder**
  CC **M05.412** **Rheumatoid myopathy with rheumatoid arthritis of left shoulder**
  CC **M05.419** **Rheumatoid myopathy with rheumatoid arthritis of unspecified shoulder**

+ **M05.42** **Rheumatoid myopathy with rheumatoid arthritis of elbow**
  CC **M05.421** **Rheumatoid myopathy with rheumatoid arthritis of right elbow**
  CC **M05.422** **Rheumatoid myopathy with rheumatoid arthritis of left elbow**
  CC **M05.429** **Rheumatoid myopathy with rheumatoid arthritis of unspecified elbow**

+ **M05.43** **Rheumatoid myopathy with rheumatoid arthritis of wrist**
    Rheumatoid myopathy with rheumatoid arthritis, carpal bones
  CC **M05.431** **Rheumatoid myopathy with rheumatoid arthritis of right wrist**
  CC **M05.432** **Rheumatoid myopathy with rheumatoid arthritis of left wrist**
  CC **M05.439** **Rheumatoid myopathy with rheumatoid arthritis of unspecified wrist**

+ **M05.44** **Rheumatoid myopathy with rheumatoid arthritis of hand**
    Rheumatoid myopathy with rheumatoid arthritis, metacarpus and phalanges
  CC **M05.441** **Rheumatoid myopathy with rheumatoid arthritis of right hand**
  CC **M05.442** **Rheumatoid myopathy with rheumatoid arthritis of left hand**
  CC **M05.449** **Rheumatoid myopathy with rheumatoid arthritis of unspecified hand**

+ **M05.45** **Rheumatoid myopathy with rheumatoid arthritis of hip**
  CC **M05.451** **Rheumatoid myopathy with rheumatoid arthritis of right hip**
  CC **M05.452** **Rheumatoid myopathy with rheumatoid arthritis of left hip**
  CC **M05.459** **Rheumatoid myopathy with rheumatoid arthritis of unspecified hip**

+ **M05.46** **Rheumatoid myopathy with rheumatoid arthritis of knee**
  CC **M05.461** **Rheumatoid myopathy with rheumatoid arthritis of right knee**
  CC **M05.462** **Rheumatoid myopathy with rheumatoid arthritis of left knee**
  CC **M05.469** **Rheumatoid myopathy with rheumatoid arthritis of unspecified knee**

+ **M05.47** **Rheumatoid myopathy with rheumatoid arthritis of ankle and foot**
    Rheumatoid myopathy with rheumatoid arthritis, tarsus, metatarsus and phalanges
  CC **M05.471** **Rheumatoid myopathy with rheumatoid arthritis of right ankle and foot**
  CC **M05.472** **Rheumatoid myopathy with rheumatoid arthritis of left ankle and foot**
  CC **M05.479** **Rheumatoid myopathy with rheumatoid arthritis of unspecified ankle and foot**

CC **M05.49** **Rheumatoid myopathy with rheumatoid arthritis of multiple sites**

+ **M05.5** **Rheumatoid polyneuropathy with rheumatoid arthritis**
    M05.50 **Rheumatoid polyneuropathy with rheumatoid arthritis of unspecified site**

+ **M05.51** **Rheumatoid polyneuropathy with rheumatoid arthritis of shoulder**
    M05.511 **Rheumatoid polyneuropathy with rheumatoid arthritis of right shoulder**
    M05.512 **Rheumatoid polyneuropathy with rheumatoid arthritis of left shoulder**
    M05.519 **Rheumatoid polyneuropathy with rheumatoid arthritis of unspecified shoulder**

+ **M05.52** **Rheumatoid polyneuropathy with rheumatoid arthritis of elbow**
    M05.521 **Rheumatoid polyneuropathy with rheumatoid arthritis of right elbow**
    M05.522 **Rheumatoid polyneuropathy with rheumatoid arthritis of left elbow**
    M05.529 **Rheumatoid polyneuropathy with rheumatoid arthritis of unspecified elbow**

+, +7th, X + 7th ● Newborn ● Pediatric ● Maternity ● Adult ♀ Female ♂ Male Manifestation Unacceptable PDX HCC CC MCC HAC

+ M05.53 Rheumatoid polyneuropathy with rheumatoid arthritis of wrist
  Rheumatoid polyneuropathy with rheumatoid arthritis, carpal bones
  M05.531 Rheumatoid polyneuropathy with rheumatoid arthritis of right wrist
  M05.532 Rheumatoid polyneuropathy with rheumatoid arthritis of left wrist
  M05.539 Rheumatoid polyneuropathy with rheumatoid arthritis of unspecified wrist

+ M05.54 Rheumatoid polyneuropathy with rheumatoid arthritis of hand
  Rheumatoid polyneuropathy with rheumatoid arthritis, metacarpus and phalanges
  M05.541 Rheumatoid polyneuropathy with rheumatoid arthritis of right hand
  M05.542 Rheumatoid polyneuropathy with rheumatoid arthritis of left hand
  M05.549 Rheumatoid polyneuropathy with rheumatoid arthritis of unspecified hand

+ M05.55 Rheumatoid polyneuropathy with rheumatoid arthritis of hip
  M05.551 Rheumatoid polyneuropathy with rheumatoid arthritis of right hip
  M05.552 Rheumatoid polyneuropathy with rheumatoid arthritis of left hip
  M05.559 Rheumatoid polyneuropathy with rheumatoid arthritis of unspecified hip

+ M05.56 Rheumatoid polyneuropathy with rheumatoid arthritis of knee
  M05.561 Rheumatoid polyneuropathy with rheumatoid arthritis of right knee
  M05.562 Rheumatoid polyneuropathy with rheumatoid arthritis of left knee
  M05.569 Rheumatoid polyneuropathy with rheumatoid arthritis of unspecified knee

+ M05.57 Rheumatoid polyneuropathy with rheumatoid arthritis of ankle and foot
  Rheumatoid polyneuropathy with rheumatoid arthritis, tarsus, metatarsus and phalanges
  M05.571 Rheumatoid polyneuropathy with rheumatoid arthritis of right ankle and foot
  M05.572 Rheumatoid polyneuropathy with rheumatoid arthritis of left ankle and foot
  M05.579 Rheumatoid polyneuropathy with rheumatoid arthritis of unspecified ankle and foot

M05.59 Rheumatoid polyneuropathy with rheumatoid arthritis of multiple sites

+ M05.6 Rheumatoid arthritis with involvement of other organs and systems
  M05.60 Rheumatoid arthritis of unspecified site with involvement of other organs and systems

+ M05.61 Rheumatoid arthritis of shoulder with involvement of other organs and systems
  M05.611 Rheumatoid arthritis of right shoulder with involvement of other organs and systems
  M05.612 Rheumatoid arthritis of left shoulder with involvement of other organs and systems
  M05.619 Rheumatoid arthritis of unspecified shoulder with involvement of other organs and systems

+ M05.62 Rheumatoid arthritis of elbow with involvement of other organs and systems
  M05.621 Rheumatoid arthritis of right elbow with involvement of other organs and systems
  M05.622 Rheumatoid arthritis of left elbow with involvement of other organs and systems
  M05.629 Rheumatoid arthritis of unspecified elbow with involvement of other organs and systems

+ M05.63 Rheumatoid arthritis of wrist with involvement of other organs and systems
  Rheumatoid arthritis of carpal bones with involvement of other organs and systems
  M05.631 Rheumatoid arthritis of right wrist with involvement of other organs and systems
  M05.632 Rheumatoid arthritis of left wrist with involvement of other organs and systems
  M05.639 Rheumatoid arthritis of unspecified wrist with involvement of other organs and systems

+ M05.64 Rheumatoid arthritis of hand with involvement of other organs and systems
  Rheumatoid arthritis of metacarpus and phalanges with involvement of other organs and systems
  M05.641 Rheumatoid arthritis of right hand with involvement of other organs and systems
  M05.642 Rheumatoid arthritis of left hand with involvement of other organs and systems
  M05.649 Rheumatoid arthritis of unspecified hand with involvement of other organs and systems

+ M05.65 Rheumatoid arthritis of hip with involvement of other organs and systems
  M05.651 Rheumatoid arthritis of right hip with involvement of other organs and systems
  M05.652 Rheumatoid arthritis of left hip with involvement of other organs and systems
  M05.659 Rheumatoid arthritis of unspecified hip with involvement of other organs and systems

+ M05.66 Rheumatoid arthritis of knee with involvement of other organs and systems
  M05.661 Rheumatoid arthritis of right knee with involvement of other organs and systems
  M05.662 Rheumatoid arthritis of left knee with involvement of other organs and systems
  M05.669 Rheumatoid arthritis of unspecified knee with involvement of other organs and systems

+ M05.67 Rheumatoid arthritis of ankle and foot with involvement of other organs and systems
  Rheumatoid arthritis of tarsus, metatarsus and phalanges with involvement of other organs and systems
  M05.671 Rheumatoid arthritis of right ankle and foot with involvement of other organs and systems
  M05.672 Rheumatoid arthritis of left ankle and foot with involvement of other organs and systems
  M05.679 Rheumatoid arthritis of unspecified ankle and foot with involvement of other organs and systems

M05.69 Rheumatoid arthritis of multiple sites with involvement of other organs and systems

+ M05.7 Rheumatoid arthritis with rheumatoid factor without organ or systems involvement
  M05.70 Rheumatoid arthritis with rheumatoid factor of unspecified site without organ or systems involvement

+ M05.71 Rheumatoid arthritis with rheumatoid factor of shoulder without organ or systems involvement
  M05.711 Rheumatoid arthritis with rheumatoid factor of right shoulder without organ or systems involvement
  M05.712 Rheumatoid arthritis with rheumatoid factor of left shoulder without organ or systems involvement
  M05.719 Rheumatoid arthritis with rheumatoid factor of unspecified shoulder without organ or systems involvement

+, +7th, X + 7th   • Newborn   • Pediatric   • Maternity   • Adult   ♀ Female   ♂ Male   Manifestation   Unacceptable PDX   HCC   CC   MCC   HAC

+ **M05.72** Rheumatoid arthritis with rheumatoid factor of elbow without organ or systems involvement
   M05.721 Rheumatoid arthritis with rheumatoid factor of right elbow without organ or systems involvement
   M05.722 Rheumatoid arthritis with rheumatoid factor of left elbow without organ or systems involvement
   M05.729 Rheumatoid arthritis with rheumatoid factor of unspecified elbow without organ or systems involvement

+ **M05.73** Rheumatoid arthritis with rheumatoid factor of wrist without organ or systems involvement
   M05.731 Rheumatoid arthritis with rheumatoid factor of right wrist without organ or systems involvement
   M05.732 Rheumatoid arthritis with rheumatoid factor of left wrist without organ or systems involvement
   M05.739 Rheumatoid arthritis with rheumatoid factor of unspecified wrist without organ or systems involvement

+ **M05.74** Rheumatoid arthritis with rheumatoid factor of hand without organ or systems involvement
   M05.741 Rheumatoid arthritis with rheumatoid factor of right hand without organ or systems involvement
   M05.742 Rheumatoid arthritis with rheumatoid factor of left hand without organ or systems involvement
   M05.749 Rheumatoid arthritis with rheumatoid factor of unspecified hand without organ or systems involvement

+ **M05.75** Rheumatoid arthritis with rheumatoid factor of hip without organ or systems involvement
   M05.751 Rheumatoid arthritis with rheumatoid factor of right hip without organ or systems involvement
   M05.752 Rheumatoid arthritis with rheumatoid factor of left hip without organ or systems involvement
   M05.759 Rheumatoid arthritis with rheumatoid factor of unspecified hip without organ or systems involvement

+ **M05.76** Rheumatoid arthritis with rheumatoid factor of knee without organ or systems involvement
   M05.761 Rheumatoid arthritis with rheumatoid factor of right knee without organ or systems involvement
   M05.762 Rheumatoid arthritis with rheumatoid factor of left knee without organ or systems involvement
   M05.769 Rheumatoid arthritis with rheumatoid factor of unspecified knee without organ or systems involvement

+ **M05.77** Rheumatoid arthritis with rheumatoid factor of ankle and foot without organ or systems involvement
   M05.771 Rheumatoid arthritis with rheumatoid factor of right ankle and foot without organ or systems involvement
   M05.772 Rheumatoid arthritis with rheumatoid factor of left ankle and foot without organ or systems involvement
   M05.779 Rheumatoid arthritis with rheumatoid factor of unspecified ankle and foot without organ or systems involvement

M05.79 Rheumatoid arthritis with rheumatoid factor of multiple sites without organ or systems involvement

M05.7A Rheumatoid arthritis with rheumatoid factor of other specified site without organ or systems involvement

+ **M05.8** Other rheumatoid arthritis with rheumatoid factor
  M05.80 Other rheumatoid arthritis with rheumatoid factor of unspecified site
  + **M05.81** Other rheumatoid arthritis with rheumatoid factor of shoulder
    M05.811 Other rheumatoid arthritis with rheumatoid factor of right shoulder
    M05.812 Other rheumatoid arthritis with rheumatoid factor of left shoulder
    M05.819 Other rheumatoid arthritis with rheumatoid factor of unspecified shoulder
  + **M05.82** Other rheumatoid arthritis with rheumatoid factor of elbow
    M05.821 Other rheumatoid arthritis with rheumatoid factor of right elbow
    M05.822 Other rheumatoid arthritis with rheumatoid factor of left elbow
    M05.829 Other rheumatoid arthritis with rheumatoid factor of unspecified elbow
  + **M05.83** Other rheumatoid arthritis with rheumatoid factor of wrist
    M05.831 Other rheumatoid arthritis with rheumatoid factor of right wrist
    M05.832 Other rheumatoid arthritis with rheumatoid factor of left wrist
    M05.839 Other rheumatoid arthritis with rheumatoid factor of unspecified wrist
  + **M05.84** Other rheumatoid arthritis with rheumatoid factor of hand
    M05.841 Other rheumatoid arthritis with rheumatoid factor of right hand
    M05.842 Other rheumatoid arthritis with rheumatoid factor of left hand
    M05.849 Other rheumatoid arthritis with rheumatoid factor of unspecified hand
  + **M05.85** Other rheumatoid arthritis with rheumatoid factor of hip
    M05.851 Other rheumatoid arthritis with rheumatoid factor of right hip
    M05.852 Other rheumatoid arthritis with rheumatoid factor of left hip
    M05.859 Other rheumatoid arthritis with rheumatoid factor of unspecified hip
  + **M05.86** Other rheumatoid arthritis with rheumatoid factor of knee
    M05.861 Other rheumatoid arthritis with rheumatoid factor of right knee
    M05.862 Other rheumatoid arthritis with rheumatoid factor of left knee
    M05.869 Other rheumatoid arthritis with rheumatoid factor of unspecified knee
  + **M05.87** Other rheumatoid arthritis with rheumatoid factor of ankle and foot
    M05.871 Other rheumatoid arthritis with rheumatoid factor of right ankle and foot
    M05.872 Other rheumatoid arthritis with rheumatoid factor of left ankle and foot
    M05.879 Other rheumatoid arthritis with rheumatoid factor of unspecified ankle and foot
  M05.89 Other rheumatoid arthritis with rheumatoid factor of multiple sites
  M05.8A Other rheumatoid arthritis with rheumatoid factor of other specified site

M05.9 Rheumatoid arthritis with rheumatoid factor, unspecified

M06 Other rheumatoid arthritis

+ **M06.0** Rheumatoid arthritis without rheumatoid factor
  M06.00 Rheumatoid arthritis without rheumatoid factor, unspecified site
  + **M06.01** Rheumatoid arthritis without rheumatoid factor, shoulder
    M06.011 Rheumatoid arthritis without rheumatoid factor, right shoulder
    M06.012 Rheumatoid arthritis without rheumatoid factor, left shoulder

M06.019 Rheumatoid arthritis without rheumatoid factor, unspecified shoulder

+ M06.02 Rheumatoid arthritis without rheumatoid factor, elbow

M06.021 Rheumatoid arthritis without rheumatoid factor, right elbow

M06.022 Rheumatoid arthritis without rheumatoid factor, left elbow

M06.029 Rheumatoid arthritis without rheumatoid factor, unspecified elbow

+ M06.03 Rheumatoid arthritis without rheumatoid factor, wrist

M06.031 Rheumatoid arthritis without rheumatoid factor, right wrist

M06.032 Rheumatoid arthritis without rheumatoid factor, left wrist

M06.039 Rheumatoid arthritis without rheumatoid factor, unspecified wrist

+ M06.04 Rheumatoid arthritis without rheumatoid factor, hand

M06.041 Rheumatoid arthritis without rheumatoid factor, right hand

M06.042 Rheumatoid arthritis without rheumatoid factor, left hand

M06.049 Rheumatoid arthritis without rheumatoid factor, unspecified hand

+ M06.05 Rheumatoid arthritis without rheumatoid factor, hip

M06.051 Rheumatoid arthritis without rheumatoid factor, right hip

M06.052 Rheumatoid arthritis without rheumatoid factor, left hip

M06.059 Rheumatoid arthritis without rheumatoid factor, unspecified hip

+ M06.06 Rheumatoid arthritis without rheumatoid factor, knee

M06.061 Rheumatoid arthritis without rheumatoid factor, right knee

M06.062 Rheumatoid arthritis without rheumatoid factor, left knee

M06.069 Rheumatoid arthritis without rheumatoid factor, unspecified knee

+ M06.07 Rheumatoid arthritis without rheumatoid factor, ankle and foot

M06.071 Rheumatoid arthritis without rheumatoid factor, right ankle and foot

M06.072 Rheumatoid arthritis without rheumatoid factor, left ankle and foot

M06.079 Rheumatoid arthritis without rheumatoid factor, unspecified ankle and foot

M06.08 Rheumatoid arthritis without rheumatoid factor, vertebrae

M06.09 Rheumatoid arthritis without rheumatoid factor, multiple sites

M06.0A Rheumatoid arthritis without rheumatoid factor, other specified site

• M06.1 Adult-onset Still's disease

Excludes1: Still's disease NOS (M08.2-)

+ M06.2 Rheumatoid bursitis

M06.20 Rheumatoid bursitis, unspecified site

+ M06.21 Rheumatoid bursitis, shoulder

M06.211 Rheumatoid bursitis, right shoulder

M06.212 Rheumatoid bursitis, left shoulder

M06.219 Rheumatoid bursitis, unspecified shoulder

+ M06.22 Rheumatoid bursitis, elbow

M06.221 Rheumatoid bursitis, right elbow

M06.222 Rheumatoid bursitis, left elbow

M06.229 Rheumatoid bursitis, unspecified elbow

+ M06.23 Rheumatoid bursitis, wrist

M06.231 Rheumatoid bursitis, right wrist

M06.232 Rheumatoid bursitis, left wrist

M06.239 Rheumatoid bursitis, unspecified wrist

+ M06.24 Rheumatoid bursitis, hand

M06.241 Rheumatoid bursitis, right hand

M06.242 Rheumatoid bursitis, left hand

M06.249 Rheumatoid bursitis, unspecified hand

+ M06.25 Rheumatoid bursitis, hip

M06.251 Rheumatoid bursitis, right hip

M06.252 Rheumatoid bursitis, left hip

M06.259 Rheumatoid bursitis, unspecified hip

+ M06.26 Rheumatoid bursitis, knee

M06.261 Rheumatoid bursitis, right knee

M06.262 Rheumatoid bursitis, left knee

M06.269 Rheumatoid bursitis, unspecified knee

+ M06.27 Rheumatoid bursitis, ankle and foot

M06.271 Rheumatoid bursitis, right ankle and foot

M06.272 Rheumatoid bursitis, left ankle and foot

M06.279 Rheumatoid bursitis, unspecified ankle and foot

M06.28 Rheumatoid bursitis, vertebrae

M06.29 Rheumatoid bursitis, multiple sites

+ M06.3 Rheumatoid nodule

M06.30 Rheumatoid nodule, unspecified site

+ M06.31 Rheumatoid nodule, shoulder

M06.311 Rheumatoid nodule, right shoulder

M06.312 Rheumatoid nodule, left shoulder

M06.319 Rheumatoid nodule, unspecified shoulder

+ M06.32 Rheumatoid nodule, elbow

M06.321 Rheumatoid nodule, right elbow

M06.322 Rheumatoid nodule, left elbow

M06.329 Rheumatoid nodule, unspecified elbow

+ M06.33 Rheumatoid nodule, wrist

M06.331 Rheumatoid nodule, right wrist

M06.332 Rheumatoid nodule, left wrist

M06.339 Rheumatoid nodule, unspecified wrist

+ M06.34 Rheumatoid nodule, hand

M06.341 Rheumatoid nodule, right hand

M06.342 Rheumatoid nodule, left hand

M06.349 Rheumatoid nodule, unspecified hand

+ M06.35 Rheumatoid nodule, hip

M06.351 Rheumatoid nodule, right hip

M06.352 Rheumatoid nodule, left hip

M06.359 Rheumatoid nodule, unspecified hip

+ M06.36 Rheumatoid nodule, knee

M06.361 Rheumatoid nodule, right knee

M06.362 Rheumatoid nodule, left knee

M06.369 Rheumatoid nodule, unspecified knee

+ M06.37 Rheumatoid nodule, ankle and foot

M06.371 Rheumatoid nodule, right ankle and foot

M06.372 Rheumatoid nodule, left ankle and foot

M06.379 Rheumatoid nodule, unspecified ankle and foot

M06.38 Rheumatoid nodule, vertebrae

M06.39 Rheumatoid nodule, multiple sites

M06.4 Inflammatory polyarthropathy

Excludes1: polyarthritis NOS (M13.0)

+ M06.8 Other specified rheumatoid arthritis

M06.80 Other specified rheumatoid arthritis, unspecified site

+ M06.81 Other specified rheumatoid arthritis, shoulder

M06.811 Other specified rheumatoid arthritis, right shoulder

M06.812 Other specified rheumatoid arthritis, left shoulder

M06.819 Other specified rheumatoid arthritis, unspecified shoulder

+ M06.82 Other specified rheumatoid arthritis, elbow

M06.821 Other specified rheumatoid arthritis, right elbow

M06.822 Other specified rheumatoid arthritis, left elbow

M06.829 Other specified rheumatoid arthritis, unspecified elbow

+ M06.83 Other specified rheumatoid arthritis, wrist

M06.831 Other specified rheumatoid arthritis, right wrist

M06.832 Other specified rheumatoid arthritis, left wrist

M06.839 Other specified rheumatoid arthritis, unspecified wrist

+ M06.84 Other specified rheumatoid arthritis, hand

M06.841 Other specified rheumatoid arthritis, right hand

M06.842 Other specified rheumatoid arthritis, left hand

M06.849 Other specified rheumatoid arthritis, unspecified hand

+, +7th, X + 7th   • Newborn   • Pediatric   • Maternity   • Adult   ♀ Female   ♂ Male   Manifestation   Unacceptable PDX   HCC   CC   MCC   HAC

+ M06.85 Other specified rheumatoid arthritis, hip
    M06.851 Other specified rheumatoid arthritis, right hip
    M06.852 Other specified rheumatoid arthritis, left hip
    M06.859 Other specified rheumatoid arthritis, unspecified hip
+ M06.86 Other specified rheumatoid arthritis, knee
    M06.861 Other specified rheumatoid arthritis, right knee
    M06.862 Other specified rheumatoid arthritis, left knee
    M06.869 Other specified rheumatoid arthritis, unspecified knee
+ M06.87 Other specified rheumatoid arthritis, ankle and foot
    M06.871 Other specified rheumatoid arthritis, right ankle and foot
    M06.872 Other specified rheumatoid arthritis, left ankle and foot
    M06.879 Other specified rheumatoid arthritis, unspecified ankle and foot
M06.88 Other specified rheumatoid arthritis, vertebrae
M06.89 Other specified rheumatoid arthritis, multiple sites
M06.8A Other specified rheumatoid arthritis, other specified site
M06.9 Rheumatoid arthritis, unspecified

M07 Enteropathic arthropathies

Code also associated enteropathy, such as:
  regional enteritis [Crohn's disease] (K50.-)
  ulcerative colitis (K51.-)
Excludes1: *psoriatic arthropathies (L40.5-)*

+ M07.6 Enteropathic arthropathies
M07.60 Enteropathic arthropathies, unspecified site
+ M07.61 Enteropathic arthropathies, shoulder
    M07.611 Enteropathic arthropathies, right shoulder
    M07.612 Enteropathic arthropathies, left shoulder
    M07.619 Enteropathic arthropathies, unspecified shoulder
+ M07.62 Enteropathic arthropathies, elbow
    M07.621 Enteropathic arthropathies, right elbow
    M07.622 Enteropathic arthropathies, left elbow
    M07.629 Enteropathic arthropathies, unspecified elbow
+ M07.63 Enteropathic arthropathies, wrist
    M07.631 Enteropathic arthropathies, right wrist
    M07.632 Enteropathic arthropathies, left wrist
    M07.639 Enteropathic arthropathies, unspecified wrist
+ M07.64 Enteropathic arthropathies, hand
    M07.641 Enteropathic arthropathies, right hand
    M07.642 Enteropathic arthropathies, lefthand
    M07.649 Enteropathic arthropathies, unspecified hand
+ M07.65 Enteropathic arthropathies, hip
    M07.651 Enteropathic arthropathies, right hip
    M07.652 Enteropathic arthropathies, left hip
    M07.659 Enteropathic arthropathies, unspecified hip
+ M07.66 Enteropathic arthropathies, knee
    M07.661 Enteropathic arthropathies, right knee
    M07.662 Enteropathic arthropathies, left knee
    M07.669 Enteropathic arthropathies, unspecified knee
+ M07.67 Enteropathic arthropathies, ankle and foot
    M07.671 Enteropathic arthropathies, right ankle and foot
    M07.672 Enteropathic arthropathies, left ankle and foot
    M07.679 Enteropathic arthropathies, unspecified ankle and foot
M07.68 Enteropathic arthropathies, vertebrae
M07.69 Enteropathic arthropathies, multiple sites

M08 Juvenile arthritis

Code also any associated underlying condition, such as:
  regional enteritis [Crohn's disease] (K50.-)
  ulcerative colitis (K51.-)
Excludes1: *arthropathy in Whipple's disease (M14.8)*
    Felty's syndrome (M05.0)
    juvenile dermatomyositis (M33.0-)
    psoriatic juvenile arthropathy (L40.54)

+ M08.0 Unspecified juvenile rheumatoid arthritis
Juvenile rheumatoid arthritis with or without rheumatoid factor
M08.00 Unspecified juvenile rheumatoid arthritis of unspecified site
+ M08.01 Unspecified juvenile rheumatoid arthritis, shoulder
    M08.011 Unspecified juvenile rheumatoid arthritis, right shoulder
    M08.012 Unspecified juvenile rheumatoid arthritis, left shoulder
    M08.019 Unspecified juvenile rheumatoid arthritis, unspecified shoulder
+ M08.02 Unspecified juvenile rheumatoid arthritis of elbow
    M08.021 Unspecified juvenile rheumatoid arthritis, right elbow
    M08.022 Unspecified juvenile rheumatoid arthritis, left elbow
    M08.029 Unspecified juvenile rheumatoid arthritis, unspecified elbow
+ M08.03 Unspecified juvenile rheumatoid arthritis, wrist
    M08.031 Unspecified juvenile rheumatoid arthritis, right wrist
    M08.032 Unspecified juvenile rheumatoid arthritis, left wrist
    M08.039 Unspecified juvenile rheumatoid arthritis, unspecified wrist
+ M08.04 Unspecified juvenile rheumatoid arthritis, hand
    M08.041 Unspecified juvenile rheumatoid arthritis, right hand
    M08.042 Unspecified juvenile rheumatoid arthritis, left hand
    M08.049 Unspecified juvenile rheumatoid arthritis, unspecified hand
+ M08.05 Unspecified juvenile rheumatoid arthritis, hip
    M08.051 Unspecified juvenile rheumatoid arthritis, right hip
    M08.052 Unspecified juvenile rheumatoid arthritis, left hip
    M08.059 Unspecified juvenile rheumatoid arthritis, unspecified hip
+ M08.06 Unspecified juvenile rheumatoid arthritis, knee
    M08.061 Unspecified juvenile rheumatoid arthritis, right knee
    M08.062 Unspecified juvenile rheumatoid arthritis, left knee
    M08.069 Unspecified juvenile rheumatoid arthritis, unspecified knee
+ M08.07 Unspecified juvenile rheumatoid arthritis, ankle and foot
    M08.071 Unspecified juvenile rheumatoid arthritis, right ankle and foot
    M08.072 Unspecified juvenile rheumatoid arthritis, left ankle and foot
    M08.079 Unspecified juvenile rheumatoid arthritis, unspecified ankle and foot
M08.08 Unspecified juvenile rheumatoid arthritis, vertebrae
M08.09 Unspecified juvenile rheumatoid arthritis, multiple sites
M08.0A Unspecified juvenile rheumatoid arthritis, other specified site
M08.1 Juvenile ankylosing spondylitis
  Excludes1: *ankylosing spondylitis in adults (M45.0-)*
+ M08.2 Juvenile rheumatoid arthritis with systemic onset
Still's disease NOS
  Excludes1: *adult-onset Still's disease (M06.1-)*

M08.20 Juvenile rheumatoid arthritis with systemic onset, unspecified site

+ M08.21 Juvenile rheumatoid arthritis with systemic onset, shoulder

M08.211 Juvenile rheumatoid arthritis with systemic onset, right shoulder

M08.212 Juvenile rheumatoid arthritis with systemic onset, left shoulder

M08.219 Juvenile rheumatoid arthritis with systemic onset, unspecified shoulder

+ M08.22 Juvenile rheumatoid arthritis with systemic onset, elbow

M08.221 Juvenile rheumatoid arthritis with systemic onset, right elbow

M08.222 Juvenile rheumatoid arthritis with systemic onset, left elbow

M08.229 Juvenile rheumatoid arthritis with systemic onset, unspecified elbow

+ M08.23 Juvenile rheumatoid arthritis with systemic onset, wrist

M08.231 Juvenile rheumatoid arthritis with systemic onset, right wrist

M08.232 Juvenile rheumatoid arthritis with systemic onset, left wrist

M08.239 Juvenile rheumatoid arthritis with systemic onset, unspecified wrist

+ M08.24 Juvenile rheumatoid arthritis with systemic onset, hand

M08.241 Juvenile rheumatoid arthritis with systemic onset, right hand

M08.242 Juvenile rheumatoid arthritis with systemic onset, left hand

M08.249 Juvenile rheumatoid arthritis with systemic onset, unspecified hand

+ M08.25 Juvenile rheumatoid arthritis with systemic onset, hip

M08.251 Juvenile rheumatoid arthritis with systemic onset, right hip

M08.252 Juvenile rheumatoid arthritis with systemic onset, left hip

M08.259 Juvenile rheumatoid arthritis with systemic onset, unspecified hip

+ M08.26 Juvenile rheumatoid arthritis with systemic onset, knee

M08.261 Juvenile rheumatoid arthritis with systemic onset, right knee

M08.262 Juvenile rheumatoid arthritis with systemic onset, left knee

M08.269 Juvenile rheumatoid arthritis with systemic onset, unspecified knee

+ M08.27 Juvenile rheumatoid arthritis with systemic onset, ankle and foot

M08.271 Juvenile rheumatoid arthritis with systemic onset, right ankle and foot

M08.272 Juvenile rheumatoid arthritis with systemic onset, left ankle and foot

M08.279 Juvenile rheumatoid arthritis with systemic onset, unspecified ankle and foot

M08.28 Juvenile rheumatoid arthritis with systemic onset, vertebrae

M08.29 Juvenile rheumatoid arthritis with systemic onset, multiple sites

M08.2A Juvenile rheumatoid arthritis with systemic onset, other specified site

M08.3 Juvenile rheumatoid polyarthritis (seronegative)

+ M08.4 Pauciarticular juvenile rheumatoid arthritis

M08.40 Pauciarticular juvenile rheumatoid arthritis, unspecified site

+ M08.41 Pauciarticular juvenile rheumatoid arthritis, shoulder

M08.411 Pauciarticular juvenile rheumatoid arthritis, right shoulder

M08.412 Pauciarticular juvenile rheumatoid arthritis, left shoulder

M08.419 Pauciarticular juvenile rheumatoid arthritis, unspecified shoulder

+ M08.42 Pauciarticular juvenile rheumatoid arthritis, elbow

M08.421 Pauciarticular juvenile rheumatoid arthritis, right elbow

M08.422 Pauciarticular juvenile rheumatoid arthritis, left elbow

M08.429 Pauciarticular juvenile rheumatoid arthritis, unspecified elbow

+ M08.43 Pauciarticular juvenile rheumatoid arthritis, wrist

M08.431 Pauciarticular juvenile rheumatoid arthritis, right wrist

M08.432 Pauciarticular juvenile rheumatoid arthritis, left wrist

M08.439 Pauciarticular juvenile rheumatoid arthritis, unspecified wrist

+ M08.44 Pauciarticular juvenile rheumatoid arthritis, hand

M08.441 Pauciarticular juvenile rheumatoid arthritis, right hand

M08.442 Pauciarticular juvenile rheumatoid arthritis, left hand

M08.449 Pauciarticular juvenile rheumatoid arthritis, unspecified hand

+ M08.45 Pauciarticular juvenile rheumatoid arthritis, hip

M08.451 Pauciarticular juvenile rheumatoid arthritis, right hip

M08.452 Pauciarticular juvenile rheumatoid arthritis, left hip

M08.459 Pauciarticular juvenile rheumatoid arthritis, unspecified hip

+ M08.46 Pauciarticular juvenile rheumatoid arthritis, knee

M08.461 Pauciarticular juvenile rheumatoid arthritis, right knee

M08.462 Pauciarticular juvenile rheumatoid arthritis, left knee

M08.469 Pauciarticular juvenile rheumatoid arthritis, unspecified knee

+ M08.47 Pauciarticular juvenile rheumatoid arthritis, ankle and foot

M08.471 Pauciarticular juvenile rheumatoid arthritis, right ankle and foot

M08.472 Pauciarticular juvenile rheumatoid arthritis, left ankle and foot

M08.479 Pauciarticular juvenile rheumatoid arthritis, unspecified ankle and foot

M08.48 Pauciarticular juvenile rheumatoid arthritis, vertebrae

M08.4A Pauciarticular juvenile rheumatoid arthritis, other specified site

+ M08.8 Other juvenile arthritis

M08.80 Other juvenile arthritis, unspecified site

+ M08.81 Other juvenile arthritis, shoulder

M08.811 Other juvenile arthritis, right shoulder

M08.812 Other juvenile arthritis, left shoulder

M08.819 Other juvenile arthritis, unspecified shoulder

+ M08.82 Other juvenile arthritis, elbow

M08.821 Other juvenile arthritis, right elbow

M08.822 Other juvenile arthritis, left elbow

M08.829 Other juvenile arthritis, unspecified elbow

+ M08.83 Other juvenile arthritis, wrist

M08.831 Other juvenile arthritis, right wrist

M08.832 Other juvenile arthritis, left wrist

M08.839 Other juvenile arthritis, unspecified wrist

+ M08.84 Other juvenile arthritis, hand

M08.841 Other juvenile arthritis, right hand

M08.842 Other juvenile arthritis, left hand

M08.849 Other juvenile arthritis, unspecified hand

+ M08.85 Other juvenile arthritis, hip

M08.851 Other juvenile arthritis, right hip

M08.852 Other juvenile arthritis, left hip

M08.859 Other juvenile arthritis, unspecified hip

+ M08.86 Other juvenile arthritis, knee

M08.861 Other juvenile arthritis, right knee

M08.862 Other juvenile arthritis, left knee

+, +7th, X + 7th   ● Newborn   ● Pediatric   ● Maternity   ● Adult   ♀ Female   ♂ Male   Manifestation   Unacceptable PDX   HCC   CC   MCC   HAC

M08.869 Other juvenile arthritis, unspecified knee
+ M08.87 Other juvenile arthritis, ankle and foot
　M08.871 Other juvenile arthritis, right ankle and foot
　M08.872 Other juvenile arthritis, left ankle and foot
　M08.879 Other juvenile arthritis, unspecified ankle and foot
M08.88 Other juvenile arthritis, other specified site
　Other juvenile arthritis, vertebrae
M08.89 Other juvenile arthritis, multiple sites
+ M08.9 Juvenile arthritis, unspecified
　Excludes1: *juvenile rheumatoid arthritis, unspecified (M08.0-)*
M08.90 Juvenile arthritis, unspecified, unspecified site
+ M08.91 Juvenile arthritis, unspecified, shoulder
　M08.911 Juvenile arthritis, unspecified, right shoulder
　M08.912 Juvenile arthritis, unspecified, left shoulder
　M08.919 Juvenile arthritis, unspecified, unspecified shoulder
+ M08.92 Juvenile arthritis, unspecified, elbow
　M08.921 Juvenile arthritis, unspecified, right elbow
　M08.922 Juvenile arthritis, unspecified, left elbow
　M08.929 Juvenile arthritis, unspecified, unspecified elbow
+ M08.93 Juvenile arthritis, unspecified, wrist
　M08.931 Juvenile arthritis, unspecified, right wrist
　M08.932 Juvenile arthritis, unspecified, left wrist
　M08.939 Juvenile arthritis, unspecified, unspecified wrist
+ M08.94 Juvenile arthritis, unspecified, hand
　M08.941 Juvenile arthritis, unspecified, right hand
　M08.942 Juvenile arthritis, unspecified, left hand
　M08.949 Juvenile arthritis, unspecified, unspecified hand
+ M08.95 Juvenile arthritis, unspecified, hip
　M08.951 Juvenile arthritis, unspecified, right hip
　M08.952 Juvenile arthritis, unspecified, left hip
　M08.959 Juvenile arthritis, unspecified, unspecified hip
+ M08.96 Juvenile arthritis, unspecified, knee
　M08.961 Juvenile arthritis, unspecified, right knee
　M08.962 Juvenile arthritis, unspecified, left knee
　M08.969 Juvenile arthritis, unspecified, unspecified knee
+ M08.97 Juvenile arthritis, unspecified, ankle and foot
　M08.971 Juvenile arthritis, unspecified, right ankle and foot
　M08.972 Juvenile arthritis, unspecified, left ankle and foot
　M08.979 Juvenile arthritis, unspecified, unspecified ankle and foot
M08.98 Juvenile arthritis, unspecified, vertebrae
M08.99 Juvenile arthritis, unspecified, multiple sites
M08.9A Juvenile arthritis, unspecified, other specified site

M1A Chronic gout

Use additional code to identify:
　Autonomic neuropathy in diseases classified elsewhere (G99.0)
　Calculus of urinary tract in diseases classified elsewhere (N22)
　Cardiomyopathy in diseases classified elsewhere (I43)
　Disorders of external ear in diseases classified elsewhere (H61.1-, H62.8-)
　Disorders of iris and ciliary body in diseases classified elsewhere (H22)
　Glomerular disorders in diseases classified elsewhere (N08)
Excludes1: *gout NOS (M10.-)*
Excludes2: *acute gout (M10.-)*

The appropriate 7th character is to be added to each code from category M1A

0　without tophus (tophi)
1　with tophus (tophi)

+ M1A.0 Idiopathic chronic gout
　Chronic gouty bursitis
　Primary chronic gout
X+7th M1A.00 Idiopathic chronic gout, unspecified site
+ M1A.01 Idiopathic chronic gout, shoulder
　+7th M1A.011 Idiopathic chronic gout, right shoulder
　+7th M1A.012 Idiopathic chronic gout, left shoulder
　+7th M1A.019 Idiopathic chronic gout, unspecified shoulder
+ M1A.02 Idiopathic chronic gout, elbow
　+7th M1A.021 Idiopathic chronic gout, right elbow
　+7th M1A.022 Idiopathic chronic gout, left elbow
　+7th M1A.029 Idiopathic chronic gout, unspecified elbow
+ M1A.03 Idiopathic chronic gout, wrist
　+7th M1A.031 Idiopathic chronic gout, right wrist
　+7th M1A.032 Idiopathic chronic gout, left wrist
　+7th M1A.039 Idiopathic chronic gout, unspecified wrist
+ M1A.04 Idiopathic chronic gout, hand
　+7th M1A.041 Idiopathic chronic gout, right hand
　+7th M1A.042 Idiopathic chronic gout, left hand
　+7th M1A.049 Idiopathic chronic gout, unspecified hand
+ M1A.05 Idiopathic chronic gout, hip
　+7th M1A.051 Idiopathic chronic gout, right hip
　+7th M1A.052 Idiopathic chronic gout, left hip
　+7th M1A.059 Idiopathic chronic gout, unspecified hip
+ M1A.06 Idiopathic chronic gout, knee
　+7th M1A.061 Idiopathic chronic gout, right knee
　+7th M1A.062 Idiopathic chronic gout, left knee
　+7th M1A.069 Idiopathic chronic gout, unspecified knee
+ M1A.07 Idiopathic chronic gout, ankle and foot
　+7th M1A.071 Idiopathic chronic gout, right ankle and foot
　+7th M1A.072 Idiopathic chronic gout, left ankle and foot
　+7th M1A.079 Idiopathic chronic gout, unspecified ankle and foot
X+7th M1A.08 Idiopathic chronic gout, vertebrae
M1A.09 Idiopathic chronic gout, multiple sites
+ M1A.1 Lead-induced chronic gout
　Code first toxic effects of lead and its compounds (T56.0-)
X+7th M1A.10 Lead-induced chronic gout, unspecified site
+ M1A.11 Lead-induced chronic gout, shoulder
　+7th M1A.111 Lead-induced chronic gout, right shoulder
　+7th M1A.112 Lead-induced chronic gout, left shoulder
　+7th M1A.119 Lead-induced chronic gout, unspecified shoulder
+ M1A.12 Lead-induced chronic gout, elbow
　+7th M1A.121 Lead-induced chronic gout, right elbow
　+7th M1A.122 Lead-induced chronic gout, left elbow
　+7th M1A.129 Lead-induced chronic gout, unspecified elbow
+ M1A.13 Lead-induced chronic gout, wrist
　+7th M1A.131 Lead-induced chronic gout, right wrist
　+7th M1A.132 Lead-induced chronic gout, left wrist
　+7th M1A.139 Lead-induced chronic gout, unspecified wrist
+ M1A.14 Lead-induced chronic gout, hand
　+7th M1A.141 Lead-induced chronic gout, right hand
　+7th M1A.142 Lead-induced chronic gout, left hand
　+7th M1A.149 Lead-induced chronic gout, unspecified hand
+ M1A.15 Lead-induced chronic gout, hip
　+7th M1A.151 Lead-induced chronic gout, right hip
　+7th M1A.152 Lead-induced chronic gout, left hip
　+7th M1A.159 Lead-induced chronic gout, unspecified hip
+ M1A.16 Lead-induced chronic gout, knee
　+7th M1A.161 Lead-induced chronic gout, right knee
　+7th M1A.162 Lead-induced chronic gout, left knee
　+7th M1A.169 Lead-induced chronic gout, unspecified knee
+ M1A.17 Lead-induced chronic gout, ankle and foot
　+7th M1A.171 Lead-induced chronic gout, right ankle and foot

+, +7th, X + 7th　● Newborn　● Pediatric　● Maternity　● Adult　♀ Female　♂ Male　Manifestation　Unacceptable PDX　HCC　CC　MCC　HAC

+7th **M1A.172 Lead-induced chronic gout, left ankle and foot**

+7th **M1A.179 Lead-induced chronic gout, unspecified ankle and foot**

X+7th **M1A.18 Lead-induced chronic gout, vertebrae**

X+7th **M1A.19 Lead-induced chronic gout, multiple sites**

+ **M1A.2 Drug-induced chronic gout**

Use additional code for adverse effect, if applicable, to identify drug (T36-T50 with fifth or sixth character 5)

X+7th **M1A.20 Drug-induced chronic gout, unspecified site**

+ **M1A.21 Drug-induced chronic gout, shoulder**

+7th **M1A.211 Drug-induced chronic gout, right shoulder**

+7th **M1A.212 Drug-induced chronic gout, left shoulder**

+7th **M1A.219 Drug-induced chronic gout, unspecified shoulder**

+ **M1A.22 Drug-induced chronic gout, elbow**

+7th **M1A.221 Drug-induced chronic gout, right elbow**

+7th **M1A.222 Drug-induced chronic gout, left elbow**

+7th **M1A.229 Drug-induced chronic gout, unspecified elbow**

+ **M1A.23 Drug-induced chronic gout, wrist**

+7th **M1A.231 Drug-induced chronic gout, right wrist**

+7th **M1A.232 Drug-induced chronic gout, left wrist**

+7th **M1A.239 Drug-induced chronic gout, unspecified wrist**

+ **M1A.24 Drug-induced chronic gout, hand**

+7th **M1A.241 Drug-induced chronic gout, right hand**

+7th **M1A.242 Drug-induced chronic gout, left hand**

+7th **M1A.249 Drug-induced chronic gout, unspecified hand**

+ **M1A.25 Drug-induced chronic gout, hip**

+7th **M1A.251 Drug-induced chronic gout, right hip**

+7th **M1A.252 Drug-induced chronic gout, left hip**

+7th **M1A.259 Drug-induced chronic gout, unspecified hip**

+ **M1A.26 Drug-induced chronic gout, knee**

+7th **M1A.261 Drug-induced chronic gout, right knee**

+7th **M1A.262 Drug-induced chronic gout, left knee**

+7th **M1A.269 Drug-induced chronic gout, unspecified knee**

+ **M1A.27 Drug-induced chronic gout, ankle and foot**

+7th **M1A.271 Drug-induced chronic gout, right ankle and foot**

+7th **M1A.272 Drug-induced chronic gout, left ankle and foot**

+7th **M1A.279 Drug-induced chronic gout, unspecified ankle and foot**

X+7th **M1A.28 Drug-induced chronic gout, vertebrae**

X+7th **M1A.29 Drug-induced chronic gout, multiple sites**

+ **M1A.3 Chronic gout due to renal impairment**

Code first associated renal disease

X+7th **M1A.30 Chronic gout due to renal impairment, unspecified site**

+ **M1A.31 Chronic gout due to renal impairment, shoulder**

+7th **M1A.311 Chronic gout due to renal impairment, right shoulder**

+7th **M1A.312 Chronic gout due to renal impairment, left shoulder**

+7th **M1A.319 Chronic gout due to renal impairment, unspecified shoulder**

+ **M1A.32 Chronic gout due to renal impairment, elbow**

+7th **M1A.321 Chronic gout due to renal impairment, right elbow**

+7th **M1A.322 Chronic gout due to renal impairment, left elbow**

+7th **M1A.329 Chronic gout due to renal impairment, unspecified elbow**

+ **M1A.33 Chronic gout due to renal impairment, wrist**

+7th **M1A.331 Chronic gout due to renal impairment, right wrist**

+7th **M1A.332 Chronic gout due to renal impairment, left wrist**

+7th **M1A.339 Chronic gout due to renal impairment, unspecified wrist**

+ **M1A.34 Chronic gout due to renal impairment, hand**

+7th **M1A.341 Chronic gout due to renal impairment, right hand**

+7th **M1A.342 Chronic gout due to renal impairment, left hand**

+7th **M1A.349 Chronic gout due to renal impairment, unspecified hand**

+ **M1A.35 Chronic gout due to renal impairment, hip**

+7th **M1A.351 Chronic gout due to renal impairment, right hip**

+7th **M1A.352 Chronic gout due to renal impairment, left hip**

+7th **M1A.359 Chronic gout due to renal impairment, unspecified hip**

+ **M1A.36 Chronic gout due to renal impairment, knee**

+7th **M1A.361 Chronic gout due to renal impairment, right knee**

+7th **M1A.362 Chronic gout due to renal impairment, left knee**

+7th **M1A.369 Chronic gout due to renal impairment, unspecified knee**

+ **M1A.37 Chronic gout due to renal impairment, ankle and foot**

+7th **M1A.371 Chronic gout due to renal impairment, right ankle and foot**

+7th **M1A.372 Chronic gout due to renal impairment, left ankle and foot**

+7th **M1A.379 Chronic gout due to renal impairment, unspecified ankle and foot**

X+7th **M1A.38 Chronic gout due to renal impairment, vertebrae**

X+7th **M1A.39 Chronic gout due to renal impairment, multiple sites**

+ **M1A.4 Other secondary chronic gout**

Code first associated condition

X+7th **M1A.40 Other secondary chronic gout, unspecified site**

+ **M1A.41 Other secondary chronic gout, shoulder**

+7th **M1A.411 Other secondary chronic gout, right shoulder**

+7th **M1A.412 Other secondary chronic gout, left shoulder**

+7th **M1A.419 Other secondary chronic gout, unspecified shoulder**

+ **M1A.42 Other secondary chronic gout, elbow**

+7th **M1A.421 Other secondary chronic gout, right elbow**

+7th **M1A.422 Other secondary chronic gout, left elbow**

+7th **M1A.429 Other secondary chronic gout, unspecified elbow**

+ **M1A.43 Other secondary chronic gout, wrist**

+7th **M1A.431 Other secondary chronic gout, right wrist**

+7th **M1A.432 Other secondary chronic gout, left wrist**

+7th **M1A.439 Other secondary chronic gout, unspecified wrist**

+ **M1A.44 Other secondary chronic gout, hand**

+7th **M1A.441 Other secondary chronic gout, right hand**

+7th **M1A.442 Other secondary chronic gout, left hand**

+7th **M1A.449 Other secondary chronic gout, unspecified hand**

+ **M1A.45 Other secondary chronic gout, hip**

+7th **M1A.451 Other secondary chronic gout, right hip**

+7th **M1A.452 Other secondary chronic gout, left hip**

+7th **M1A.459 Other secondary chronic gout, unspecified hip**

+ **M1A.46 Other secondary chronic gout, knee**

+7th **M1A.461 Other secondary chronic gout, right knee**

+7th **M1A.462 Other secondary chronic gout, left knee**

+7th **M1A.469 Other secondary chronic gout, unspecified knee**

+ **M1A.47 Other secondary chronic gout, ankle and foot**
+7th **M1A.471 Other secondary chronic gout, right ankle and foot**
+7th **M1A.472 Other secondary chronic gout, left ankle and foot**
+7th **M1A.479 Other secondary chronic gout, unspecified ankle and foot**
X+7th **M1A.48 Other secondary chronic gout, vertebrae**
X+7th **M1A.49 Other secondary chronic gout, multiple sites**
X+7th **M1A.9 Chronic gout, unspecified**

M10 Gout

Acute gout
Gout attack
Gout flare
Podagra
Use additional code to identify:
Autonomic neuropathy in diseases classified elsewhere (G99.0)
Calculus of urinary tract in diseases classified elsewhere (N22)
Cardiomyopathy in diseases classified elsewhere (I43)
Disorders of external ear in diseases classified elsewhere (H61.1-, H62.8-)
Disorders of iris and ciliary body in diseases classified elsewhere (H22)
Glomerular disorders in diseases classified elsewhere (N08)
Excludes2: chronic gout (M1A.-)

+ **M10.0 Idiopathic gout**
Gouty bursitis
Primary gout
M10.00 Idiopathic gout, unspecified site
+ **M10.01 Idiopathic gout, shoulder**
M10.011 Idiopathic gout, right shoulder
M10.012 Idiopathic gout, left shoulder
M10.019 Idiopathic gout, unspecified shoulder
+ **M10.02 Idiopathic gout, elbow**
M10.021 Idiopathic gout, right elbow
M10.022 Idiopathic gout, left elbow
M10.029 Idiopathic gout, unspecified elbow
+ **M10.03 Idiopathic gout, wrist**
M10.031 Idiopathic gout, right wrist
M10.032 Idiopathic gout, left wrist
M10.039 Idiopathic gout, unspecified wrist
+ **M10.04 Idiopathic gout, hand**
M10.041 Idiopathic gout, right hand
M10.042 Idiopathic gout, left hand
M10.049 Idiopathic gout, unspecified hand
+ **M10.05 Idiopathic gout, hip**
M10.051 Idiopathic gout, right hip
M10.052 Idiopathic gout, left hip
M10.059 Idiopathic gout, unspecified hip
+ **M10.06 Idiopathic gout, knee**
M10.061 Idiopathic gout, right knee
M10.062 Idiopathic gout, left knee
M10.069 Idiopathic gout, unspecified knee
+ **M10.07 Idiopathic gout, ankle and foot**
M10.071 Idiopathic gout, right ankle and foot
M10.072 Idiopathic gout, left ankle and foot
M10.079 Idiopathic gout, unspecified ankle and foot
M10.08 Idiopathic gout, vertebrae
M10.09 Idiopathic gout, multiple sites
+ **M10.1 Lead-induced gout**
Code first toxic effects of lead and its compounds (T56.0-)
M10.10 Lead-induced gout, unspecified site
+ **M10.11 Lead-induced gout, shoulder**
M10.111 Lead-induced gout, right shoulder
M10.112 Lead-induced gout, left shoulder
M10.119 Lead-induced gout, unspecified shoulder
+ **M10.12 Lead-induced gout, elbow**
M10.121 Lead-induced gout, right elbow
M10.122 Lead-induced gout, left elbow
M10.129 Lead-induced gout, unspecified elbow
+ **M10.13 Lead-induced gout, wrist**
M10.131 Lead-induced gout, right wrist
M10.132 Lead-induced gout, left wrist
M10.139 Lead-induced gout, unspecified wrist
+ **M10.14 Lead-induced gout, hand**
M10.141 Lead-induced gout, right hand
M10.142 Lead-induced gout, left hand
M10.149 Lead-induced gout, unspecified hand

+ **M10.15 Lead-induced gout, hip**
M10.151 Lead-induced gout, right hip
M10.152 Lead-induced gout, left hip
M10.159 Lead-induced gout, unspecified hip
+ **M10.16 Lead-induced gout, knee**
M10.161 Lead-induced gout, right knee
M10.162 Lead-induced gout, left knee
M10.169 Lead-induced gout, unspecified knee
+ **M10.17 Lead-induced gout, ankle and foot**
M10.171 Lead-induced gout, right ankle and foot
M10.172 Lead-induced gout, left ankle and foot
M10.179 Lead-induced gout, unspecified ankle and foot
M10.18 Lead-induced gout, vertebrae
M10.19 Lead-induced gout, multiple sites
+ **M10.2 Drug-induced gout**
Use additional code for adverse effect, if applicable, to identify drug (T36-T50 with fifth or sixth character 5)
M10.20 Drug-induced gout, unspecified site
+ **M10.21 Drug-induced gout, shoulder**
M10.211 Drug-induced gout, right shoulder
M10.212 Drug-induced gout, left shoulder
M10.219 Drug-induced gout, unspecified shoulder
+ **M10.22 Drug-induced gout, elbow**
M10.221 Drug-induced gout, right elbow
M10.222 Drug-induced gout, left elbow
M10.229 Drug-induced gout, unspecified elbow
+ **M10.23 Drug-induced gout, wrist**
M10.231 Drug-induced gout, right wrist
M10.232 Drug-induced gout, left wrist
M10.239 Drug-induced gout, unspecified wrist
+ **M10.24 Drug-induced gout, hand**
M10.241 Drug-induced gout, right hand
M10.242 Drug-induced gout, left hand
M10.249 Drug-induced gout, unspecified hand
+ **M10.25 Drug-induced gout, hip**
M10.251 Drug-induced gout, right hip
M10.252 Drug-induced gout, left hip
M10.259 Drug-induced gout, unspecified hip
+ **M10.26 Drug-induced gout, knee**
M10.261 Drug-induced gout, right knee
M10.262 Drug-induced gout, left knee
M10.269 Drug-induced gout, unspecified knee
+ **M10.27 Drug-induced gout, ankle and foot**
M10.271 Drug-induced gout, right ankle and foot
M10.272 Drug-induced gout, left ankle and foot
M10.279 Drug-induced gout, unspecified ankle and foot
M10.28 Drug-induced gout, vertebrae
M10.29 Drug-induced gout, multiple sites
+ **M10.3 Gout due to renal impairment**
Code first associated renal disease
M10.30 Gout due to renal impairment, unspecified site
+ **M10.31 Gout due to renal impairment, shoulder**
M10.311 Gout due to renal impairment, right shoulder
M10.312 Gout due to renal impairment, left shoulder
M10.319 Gout due to renal impairment, unspecified shoulder
+ **M10.32 Gout due to renal impairment, elbow**
M10.321 Gout due to renal impairment, right elbow
M10.322 Gout due to renal impairment, left elbow
M10.329 Gout due to renal impairment, unspecified elbow
+ **M10.33 Gout due to renal impairment, wrist**
M10.331 Gout due to renal impairment, right wrist
M10.332 Gout due to renal impairment, left wrist
M10.339 Gout due to renal impairment, unspecified wrist
+ **M10.34 Gout due to renal impairment, hand**
M10.341 Gout due to renal impairment, right hand
M10.342 Gout due to renal impairment, left hand
M10.349 Gout due to renal impairment, unspecified hand

+, +7th, X + 7th   ● Newborn   ● Pediatric   ● Maternity   ● Adult   ♀ Female   ♂ Male   Manifestation   Unacceptable PDX   HCC   CC   MCC   HAC

+ M10.35 Gout due to renal impairment, hip
    M10.351 Gout due to renal impairment, right hip
    M10.352 Gout due to renal impairment, left hip
    M10.359 Gout due to renal impairment, unspecified hip
+ M10.36 Gout due to renal impairment, knee
    M10.361 Gout due to renal impairment, right knee
    M10.362 Gout due to renal impairment, left knee
    M10.369 Gout due to renal impairment, unspecified knee
+ M10.37 Gout due to renal impairment, ankle and foot
    M10.371 Gout due to renal impairment, right ankle and foot
    M10.372 Gout due to renal impairment, left ankle and foot
    M10.379 Gout due to renal impairment, unspecified ankle and foot
M10.38 Gout due to renal impairment, vertebrae
M10.39 Gout due to renal impairment, multiple sites
+ M10.4 **Other secondary gout**
    Code first associated condition
M10.40 Other secondary gout, unspecified site
+ M10.41 Other secondary gout, shoulder
    M10.411 Other secondary gout, right shoulder
    M10.412 Other secondary gout, left shoulder
    M10.419 Other secondary gout, unspecified shoulder
+ M10.42 Other secondary gout, elbow
    M10.421 Other secondary gout, right elbow
    M10.422 Other secondary gout, left elbow
    M10.429 Other secondary gout, unspecified elbow
+ M10.43 Other secondary gout, wrist
    M10.431 Other secondary gout, right wrist
    M10.432 Other secondary gout, left wrist
    M10.439 Other secondary gout, unspecified wrist
+ M10.44 Other secondary gout, hand
    M10.441 Other secondary gout, right hand
    M10.442 Other secondary gout, left hand
    M10.449 Other secondary gout, unspecified hand
+ M10.45 Other secondary gout, hip
    M10.451 Other secondary gout, right hip
    M10.452 Other secondary gout, left hlp
    M10.459 Other secondary gout, unspecified hip
+ M10.46 Other secondary gout, knee
    M10.461 Other secondary gout, right knee
    M10.462 Other secondary gout, left knee
    M10.469 Other secondary gout, unspecified knee
+ M10.47 Other secondary gout, ankle and foot
    M10.471 Other secondary gout, right ankle and foot
    M10.472 Other secondary gout, left ankle and foot
    M10.479 Other secondary gout, unspecified ankle and foot
M10.48 Other secondary gout, vertebrae
M10.49 Other secondary gout, multiple sites
M10.9 **Gout, unspecified**
    Gout NOS

M11 **Other crystal arthropathies**
+ M11.0 **Hydroxyapatite deposition disease**
M11.00 Hydroxyapatite deposition disease, unspecified site
+ M11.01 Hydroxyapatite deposition disease, shoulder
    M11.011 Hydroxyapatite deposition disease, right shoulder
    M11.012 Hydroxyapatite deposition disease, left shoulder
    M11.019 Hydroxyapatite deposition disease, unspecified shoulder
+ M11.02 Hydroxyapatite deposition disease, elbow
    M11.021 Hydroxyapatite deposition disease, right elbow
    M11.022 Hydroxyapatite deposition disease, left elbow
    M11.029 Hydroxyapatite deposition disease, unspecified elbow

+ M11.03 Hydroxyapatite deposition disease, wrist
    M11.031 Hydroxyapatite deposition disease, right wrist
    M11.032 Hydroxyapatite deposition disease, left wrist
    M11.039 Hydroxyapatite deposition disease, unspecified wrist
+ M11.04 Hydroxyapatite deposition disease, hand
    M11.041 Hydroxyapatite deposition disease, right hand
    M11.042 Hydroxyapatite deposition disease, left hand
    M11.049 Hydroxyapatite deposition disease, unspecified hand
+ M11.05 Hydroxyapatite deposition disease, hip
    M11.051 Hydroxyapatite deposition disease, right hip
    M11.052 Hydroxyapatite deposition disease, left hip
    M11.059 Hydroxyapatite deposition disease, unspecified hip
+ M11.06 Hydroxyapatite deposition disease, knee
    M11.061 Hydroxyapatite deposition disease, right knee
    M11.062 Hydroxyapatite deposition disease, left knee
    M11.069 Hydroxyapatite deposition disease, unspecified knee
+ M11.07 Hydroxyapatite deposition disease, ankle and foot
    M11.071 Hydroxyapatite deposition disease, right ankle and foot
    M11.072 Hydroxyapatite deposition disease, left ankle and foot
    M11.079 Hydroxyapatite deposition disease, unspecified ankle and foot
M11.08 Hydroxyapatite deposition disease, vertebrae
M11.09 Hydroxyapatite deposition disease, multiple sites
+ M11.1 **Familial chondrocalcinosis**
M11.10 Familial chondrocalcinosis, unspecified site
+ M11.11 Familial chondrocalcinosis, shoulder
    M11.111 Familial chondrocalcinosis, right shoulder
    M11.112 Familial chondrocalcinosis, left shoulder
    M11.119 Familial chondrocalcinosis, unspecified shoulder
+ M11.12 Familial chondrocalcinosis, elbow
    M11.121 Familial chondrocalcinosis, right elbow
    M11.122 Familial chondrocalcinosis, left elbow
    M11.129 Familial chondrocalcinosis, unspecified elbow
+ M11.13 Familial chondrocalcinosis, wrist
    M11.131 Familial chondrocalcinosis, right wrist
    M11.132 Familial chondrocalcinosis, left wrist
    M11.139 Familial chondrocalcinosis, unspecified wrist
+ M11.14 Familial chondrocalcinosis, hand
    M11.141 Familial chondrocalcinosis, right hand
    M11.142 Familial chondrocalcinosis, left hand
    M11.149 Familial chondrocalcinosis, unspecified hand
+ M11.15 Familial chondrocalcinosis, hip
    M11.151 Familial chondrocalcinosis, right hip
    M11.152 Familial chondrocalcinosis, left hip
    M11.159 Familial chondrocalcinosis, unspecified hip
+ M11.16 Familial chondrocalcinosis, knee
    M11.161 Familial chondrocalcinosis, right knee
    M11.162 Familial chondrocalcinosis, left knee
    M11.169 Familial chondrocalcinosis, unspecified knee
+ M11.17 Familial chondrocalcinosis, ankle and foot
    M11.171 Familial chondrocalcinosis, right ankle and foot
    M11.172 Familial chondrocalcinosis, left ankle and foot
    M11.179 Familial chondrocalcinosis, unspecified ankle and foot
M11.18 Familial chondrocalcinosis, vertebrae
M11.19 Familial chondrocalcinosis, multiple sites

+, +7th, X + 7th   ● Newborn   ● Pediatric   ● Maternity   ● Adult   ♀ Female   ♂ Male   Manifestation   Unacceptable PDX   HCC   CC   MCC   HAC

+ **M11.2** **Other chondrocalcinosis**
  Chondrocalcinosis NOS
  M11.20 Other chondrocalcinosis, unspecified site
+ **M11.21** Other chondrocalcinosis, shoulder
    M11.211 Other chondrocalcinosis, right shoulder
    M11.212 Other chondrocalcinosis, left shoulder
    M11.219 Other chondrocalcinosis, unspecified shoulder
+ **M11.22** Other chondrocalcinosis, elbow
    M11.221 Other chondrocalcinosis, right elbow
    M11.222 Other chondrocalcinosis, left elbow
    M11.229 Other chondrocalcinosis, unspecified elbow
+ **M11.23** Other chondrocalcinosis, wrist
    M11.231 Other chondrocalcinosis, right wrist
    M11.232 Other chondrocalcinosis, left wrist
    M11.239 Other chondrocalcinosis, unspecified wrist
+ **M11.24** Other chondrocalcinosis, hand
    M11.241 Other chondrocalcinosis, right hand
    M11.242 Other chondrocalcinosis, left hand
    M11.249 Other chondrocalcinosis, unspecified hand
+ **M11.25** Other chondrocalcinosis, hip
    M11.251 Other chondrocalcinosis, right hip
    M11.252 Other chondrocalcinosis, left hip
    M11.259 Other chondrocalcinosis, unspecified hip
+ **M11.26** Other chondrocalcinosis, knee
    M11.261 Other chondrocalcinosis, right knee
    M11.262 Other chondrocalcinosis, left knee
    AHA CC: 3Q, 2018, 20
    M11.269 Other chondrocalcinosis, unspecified knee
+ **M11.27** Other chondrocalcinosis, ankle and foot
    M11.271 Other chondrocalcinosis, right ankle and foot
    M11.272 Other chondrocalcinosis, left ankle and foot
    M11.279 Other chondrocalcinosis, unspecified ankle and foot
  M11.28 Other chondrocalcinosis, vertebrae
  M11.29 Other chondrocalcinosis, multiple sites
+ **M11.8** **Other specified crystal arthropathies**
  M11.80 Other specified crystal arthropathies, unspecified site
+ **M11.81** Other specified crystal arthropathies, shoulder
    M11.811 Other specified crystal arthropathies, right shoulder
    M11.812 Other specified crystal arthropathies, left shoulder
    M11.819 Other specified crystal arthropathies, unspecified shoulder
+ **M11.82** Other specified crystal arthropathies, elbow
    M11.821 Other specified crystal arthropathies, right elbow
    M11.822 Other specified crystal arthropathies, left elbow
    M11.829 Other specified crystal arthropathies, unspecified elbow
+ **M11.83** Other specified crystal arthropathies, wrist
    M11.831 Other specified crystal arthropathies, right wrist
    M11.832 Other specified crystal arthropathies, left wrist
    M11.839 Other specified crystal arthropathies, unspecified wrist
+ **M11.84** Other specified crystal arthropathies, hand
    M11.841 Other specified crystal arthropathies, right hand
    M11.842 Other specified crystal arthropathies, left hand
    M11.849 Other specified crystal arthropathies, unspecified hand
+ **M11.85** Other specified crystal arthropathies, hip
    M11.851 Other specified crystal arthropathies, right hip
    M11.852 Other specified crystal arthropathies, left hip
    M11.859 Other specified crystal arthropathies, unspecified hip

+ **M11.86** Other specified crystal arthropathies, knee
    M11.861 Other specified crystal arthropathies, right knee
    M11.862 Other specified crystal arthropathies, left knee
    M11.869 Other specified crystal arthropathies, unspecified knee
+ **M11.87** Other specified crystal arthropathies, ankle and foot
    M11.871 Other specified crystal arthropathies, right ankle and foot
    M11.872 Other specified crystal arthropathies, left ankle and foot
    M11.879 Other specified crystal arthropathies, unspecified ankle and foot
  M11.88 Other specified crystal arthropathies, vertebrae
  M11.89 Other specified crystal arthropathies, multiple sites
  M11.9 **Crystal arthropathy, unspecified**

M12 **Other and unspecified arthropathy**

  Excludes1: *arthrosis (M15-M19)*
              cricoarytenoid arthropathy (J38.7)
+ **M12.0** **Chronic postrheumatic arthropathy [Jaccoud]**
  M12.00 Chronic postrheumatic arthropathy [Jaccoud], unspecified site
+ **M12.01** Chronic postrheumatic arthropathy [Jaccoud], shoulder
    M12.011 Chronic postrheumatic arthropathy [Jaccoud], right shoulder
    M12.012 Chronic postrheumatic arthropathy [Jaccoud], left shoulder
    M12.019 Chronic postrheumatic arthropathy [Jaccoud], unspecified shoulder
+ **M12.02** Chronic postrheumatic arthropathy [Jaccoud], elbow
    M12.021 Chronic postrheumatic arthropathy [Jaccoud], right elbow
    M12.022 Chronic postrheumatic arthropathy [Jaccoud], left elbow
    M12.029 Chronic postrheumatic arthropathy [Jaccoud], unspecified elbow
+ **M12.03** Chronic postrheumatic arthropathy [Jaccoud], wrist
    M12.031 Chronic postrheumatic arthropathy [Jaccoud], right wrist
    M12.032 Chronic postrheumatic arthropathy [Jaccoud], left wrist
    M12.039 Chronic postrheumatic arthropathy [Jaccoud], unspecified wrist
+ **M12.04** Chronic postrheumatic arthropathy [Jaccoud], hand
    M12.041 Chronic postrheumatic arthropathy [Jaccoud], right hand
    M12.042 Chronic postrheumatic arthropathy [Jaccoud], left hand
    M12.049 Chronic postrheumatic arthropathy [Jaccoud], unspecified hand
+ **M12.05** Chronic postrheumatic arthropathy [Jaccoud], hip
    M12.051 Chronic postrheumatic arthropathy [Jaccoud], right hip
    M12.052 Chronic postrheumatic arthropathy [Jaccoud], left hip
    M12.059 Chronic postrheumatic arthropathy [Jaccoud], unspecified hip
+ **M12.06** Chronic postrheumatic arthropathy [Jaccoud], knee
    M12.061 Chronic postrheumatic arthropathy [Jaccoud], right knee
    M12.062 Chronic postrheumatic arthropathy [Jaccoud], left knee
    M12.069 Chronic postrheumatic arthropathy [Jaccoud], unspecified knee
+ **M12.07** Chronic postrheumatic arthropathy [Jaccoud], ankle and foot
    M12.071 Chronic postrheumatic arthropathy [Jaccoud], right ankle and foot
    M12.072 Chronic postrheumatic arthropathy [Jaccoud], left ankle and foot
    M12.079 Chronic postrheumatic arthropathy [Jaccoud], unspecified ankle and foot

+, +7th, X + 7th   ● Newborn   ● Pediatric   ● Maternity   ● Adult   ♀ Female   ♂ Male   Manifestation   Unacceptable PDX   HCC   CC   MCC   HAC

M12.08 Chronic postrheumatic arthropathy [Jaccoud], other specified site
Chronic postrheumatic arthropathy [Jaccoud], vertebrae
M12.09 Chronic postrheumatic arthropathy [Jaccoud], multiple sites
+ **M12.1** Kaschin-Beck disease
Osteochondroarthrosis deformans endemica
M12.10 Kaschin-Beck disease, unspecified site
+ **M12.11** Kaschin-Beck disease, shoulder
M12.111 Kaschin-Beck disease, right shoulder
M12.112 Kaschin-Beck disease, left shoulder
M12.119 Kaschin-Beck disease, unspecified shoulder
+ **M12.12** Kaschin-Beck disease, elbow
M12.121 Kaschin-Beck disease, right elbow
M12.122 Kaschin-Beck disease, left elbow
M12.129 Kaschin-Beck disease, unspecified elbow
+ **M12.13** Kaschin-Beck disease, wrist
M12.131 Kaschin-Beck disease, right wrist
M12.132 Kaschin-Beck disease, left wrist
M12.139 Kaschin-Beck disease, unspecified wrist
+ **M12.14** Kaschin-Beck disease, hand
M12.141 Kaschin-Beck disease, right hand
M12.142 Kaschin-Beck disease, left hand
M12.149 Kaschin-Beck disease, unspecified hand
+ **M12.15** Kaschin-Beck disease, hip
M12.151 Kaschin-Beck disease, right hip
M12.152 Kaschin-Beck disease, left hip
M12.159 Kaschin-Beck disease, unspecified hip
+ **M12.16** Kaschin-Beck disease, knee
M12.161 Kaschin-Beck disease, right knee
M12.162 Kaschin-Beck disease, left knee
M12.169 Kaschin-Beck disease, unspecified knee
+ **M12.17** Kaschin-Beck disease, ankle and foot
M12.171 Kaschin-Beck disease, right ankle and foot
M12.172 Kaschin-Beck disease, left ankle and foot
M12.179 Kaschin-Beck disease, unspecified ankle and foot
M12.18 Kaschin-Beck disease, vertebrae
M12.19 Kaschin-Beck disease, multiple sites
+ **M12.2** Villonodular synovitis (pigmented)
M12.20 Villonodular synovitis (pigmented), unspecified site
+ **M12.21** Villonodular synovitis (pigmented), shoulder
M12.211 Villonodular synovitis (pigmented), right shoulder
M12.212 Villonodular synovitis (pigmented), left shoulder
M12.219 Villonodular synovitis (pigmented), unspecified shoulder
+ **M12.22** Villonodular synovitis (pigmented), elbow
M12.221 Villonodular synovitis (pigmented), right elbow
M12.222 Villonodular synovitis (pigmented), left elbow
M12.229 Villonodular synovitis (pigmented), unspecified elbow
+ **M12.23** Villonodular synovitis (pigmented), wrist
M12.231 Villonodular synovitis (pigmented), right wrist
M12.232 Villonodular synovitis (pigmented), left wrist
M12.239 Villonodular synovitis (pigmented), unspecified wrist
+ **M12.24** Villonodular synovitis (pigmented), hand
M12.241 Villonodular synovitis (pigmented), right hand
M12.242 Villonodular synovitis (pigmented), left hand
M12.249 Villonodular synovitis (pigmented), unspecified hand
+ **M12.25** Villonodular synovitis (pigmented), hip
M12.251 Villonodular synovitis (pigmented), right hip
M12.252 Villonodular synovitis (pigmented), left hip
M12.259 Villonodular synovitis (pigmented), unspecified hip

+ **M12.26** Villonodular synovitis (pigmented), knee
M12.261 Villonodular synovitis (pigmented), right knee
M12.262 Villonodular synovitis (pigmented), left knee
M12.269 Villonodular synovitis (pigmented), unspecified knee
+ **M12.27** Villonodular synovitis (pigmented), ankle and foot
M12.271 Villonodular synovitis (pigmented), right ankle and foot
M12.272 Villonodular synovitis (pigmented), left ankle and foot
M12.279 Villonodular synovitis (pigmented), unspecified ankle and foot
M12.28 Villonodular synovitis (pigmented), other specified site
Villonodular synovitis (pigmented), vertebrae
M12.29 Villonodular synovitis (pigmented), multiple sites
+ **M12.3** Palindromic rheumatism
M12.30 Palindromic rheumatism, unspecified site
+ **M12.31** Palindromic rheumatism, shoulder
M12.311 Palindromic rheumatism, right shoulder
M12.312 Palindromic rheumatism, left shoulder
M12.319 Palindromic rheumatism, unspecified shoulder
+ **M12.32** Palindromic rheumatism, elbow
M12.321 Palindromic rheumatism, right elbow
M12.322 Palindromic rheumatism, left elbow
M12.329 Palindromic rheumatism, unspecified elbow
+ **M12.33** Palindromic rheumatism, wrist
M12.331 Palindromic rheumatism, right wrist
M12.332 Palindromic rheumatism, left wrist
M12.339 Palindromic rheumatism, unspecified wrist
+ **M12.34** Palindromic rheumatism, hand
M12.341 Palindromic rheumatism, right hand
M12.342 Palindromic rheumatism, left hand
M12.349 Palindromic rheumatism, unspecified hand
+ **M12.35** Palindromic rheumatism, hip
M12.351 Palindromic rheumatism, right hip
M12.352 Palindromic rheumatism, left hip
M12.359 Palindromic rheumatism, unspecified hip
+ **M12.36** Palindromic rheumatism, knee
M12.361 Palindromic rheumatism, right knee
M12.362 Palindromic rheumatism, left knee
M12.369 Palindromic rheumatism, unspecified knee
+ **M12.37** Palindromic rheumatism, ankle and foot
M12.371 Palindromic rheumatism, right ankle and foot
M12.372 Palindromic rheumatism, left ankle and foot
M12.379 Palindromic rheumatism, unspecified ankle and foot
M12.38 Palindromic rheumatism, other specified site
Palindromic rheumatism, vertebrae
M12.39 Palindromic rheumatism, multiple sites
+ **M12.4** Intermittent hydrarthrosis
M12.40 Intermittent hydrarthrosis, unspecified site
+ **M12.41** Intermittent hydrarthrosis, shoulder
M12.411 Intermittent hydrarthrosis, right shoulder
M12.412 Intermittent hydrarthrosis, left shoulder
M12.419 Intermittent hydrarthrosis, unspecified shoulder
+ **M12.42** Intermittent hydrarthrosis, elbow
M12.421 Intermittent hydrarthrosis, right elbow
M12.422 Intermittent hydrarthrosis, left elbow
M12.429 Intermittent hydrarthrosis, unspecified elbow
+ **M12.43** Intermittent hydrarthrosis, wrist
M12.431 Intermittent hydrarthrosis, right wrist
M12.432 Intermittent hydrarthrosis, left wrist
M12.439 Intermittent hydrarthrosis, unspecified wrist

+ **M12.44 Intermittent hydrarthrosis, hand**
    M12.441 Intermittent hydrarthrosis, right hand
    M12.442 Intermittent hydrarthrosis, left hand
    M12.449 Intermittent hydrarthrosis, unspecified hand
+ **M12.45 Intermittent hydrarthrosis, hip**
    M12.451 Intermittent hydrarthrosis, right hip
    M12.452 Intermittent hydrarthrosis, left hip
    M12.459 Intermittent hydrarthrosis, unspecified hip
+ **M12.46 Intermittent hydrarthrosis, knee**
    M12.461 Intermittent hydrarthrosis, right knee
    M12.462 Intermittent hydrarthrosis, left knee
    M12.469 Intermittent hydrarthrosis, unspecified knee
+ **M12.47 Intermittent hydrarthrosis, ankle and foot**
    M12.471 Intermittent hydrarthrosis, right ankle and foot
    M12.472 Intermittent hydrarthrosis, left ankle and foot
    M12.479 Intermittent hydrarthrosis, unspecified ankle and foot
M12.48 Intermittent hydrarthrosis, other site
M12.49 Intermittent hydrarthrosis, multiple sites
+ **M12.5 Traumatic arthropathy**
Excludes1: current injury-see Alphabetic Index
post-traumatic osteoarthritis of first carpometacarpal joint (M18.2-M18.3)
post-traumatic osteoarthritis of hip (M16.4-M16.5)
post-traumatic osteoarthritis of knee (M17.2-M17.3)
post-traumatic osteoarthritis NOS (M19.1-)
post-traumatic osteoarthritis of other single joints (M19.1-)
M12.50 Traumatic arthropathy, unspecified site
+ **M12.51 Traumatic arthropathy, shoulder**
    M12.511 Traumatic arthropathy, right shoulder
    M12.512 Traumatic arthropathy, left shoulder
    M12.519 Traumatic arthropathy, unspecified shoulder
+ **M12.52 Traumatic arthropathy, elbow**
    M12.521 Traumatic arthropathy, right elbow
    M12.522 Traumatic arthropathy, left elbow
    M12.529 Traumatic arthropathy, unspecified elbow
+ **M12.53 Traumatic arthropathy, wrist**
    M12.531 Traumatic arthropathy, right wrist
    M12.532 Traumatic arthropathy, left wrist
    M12.539 Traumatic arthropathy, unspecified wrist
+ **M12.54 Traumatic arthropathy, hand**
    M12.541 Traumatic arthropathy, right hand
    M12.542 Traumatic arthropathy, left hand
    M12.549 Traumatic arthropathy, unspecified hand
+ **M12.55 Traumatic arthropathy, hip**
    M12.551 Traumatic arthropathy, right hip
    M12.552 Traumatic arthropathy, left hip
    AHA CC: 1Q, 2015, 17-18
    M12.559 Traumatic arthropathy, unspecified hip
+ **M12.56 Traumatic arthropathy, knee**
    M12.561 Traumatic arthropathy, right knee
    M12.562 Traumatic arthropathy, left knee
    M12.569 Traumatic arthropathy, unspecified knee
+ **M12.57 Traumatic arthropathy, ankle and foot**
    M12.571 Traumatic arthropathy, right ankle and foot
    M12.572 Traumatic arthropathy, left ankle and foot
    M12.579 Traumatic arthropathy, unspecified ankle and foot
M12.58 Traumatic arthropathy, other specified site
Traumatic arthropathy, vertebrae
M12.59 Traumatic arthropathy, multiple sites

+ **M12.8 Other specific arthropathies, not elsewhere classified**
Transient arthropathy
M12.80 Other specific arthropathies, not elsewhere classified, unspecified site
+ **M12.81 Other specific arthropathies, not elsewhere classified, shoulder**
    M12.811 Other specific arthropathies, not elsewhere classified, right shoulder
    M12.812 Other specific arthropathies, not elsewhere classified, left shoulder
    M12.819 Other specific arthropathies, not elsewhere classified, unspecified shoulder
+ **M12.82 Other specific arthropathies, not elsewhere classified, elbow**
    M12.821 Other specific arthropathies, not elsewhere classified, right elbow
    M12.822 Other specific arthropathies, not elsewhere classified, left elbow
    M12.829 Other specific arthropathies, not elsewhere classified, unspecified elbow
+ **M12.83 Other specific arthropathies, not elsewhere classified, wrist**
    M12.831 Other specific arthropathies, not elsewhere classified, right wrist
    M12.832 Other specific arthropathies, not elsewhere classified, left wrist
    M12.839 Other specific arthropathies, not elsewhere classified, unspecified wrist
+ **M12.84 Other specific arthropathies, not elsewhere classified, hand**
    M12.841 Other specific arthropathies, not elsewhere classified, right hand
    M12.842 Other specific arthropathies, not elsewhere classified, left hand
    M12.849 Other specific arthropathies, not elsewhere classified, unspecified hand
+ **M12.85 Other specific arthropathies, not elsewhere classified, hip**
    M12.851 Other specific arthropathies, not elsewhere classified, right hip
    M12.852 Other specific arthropathies, not elsewhere classified, left hip
    M12.859 Other specific arthropathies, not elsewhere classified, unspecified hip
+ **M12.86 Other specific arthropathies, not elsewhere classified, knee**
    M12.861 Other specific arthropathies, not elsewhere classified, right knee
    M12.862 Other specific arthropathies, not elsewhere classified, left knee
    M12.869 Other specific arthropathies, not elsewhere classified, unspecified knee
+ **M12.87 Other specific arthropathies, not elsewhere classified, ankle and foot**
    M12.871 Other specific arthropathies, not elsewhere classified, right ankle and foot
    M12.872 Other specific arthropathies, not elsewhere classified, left ankle and foot
    M12.879 Other specific arthropathies, not elsewhere classified, unspecified ankle and foot
M12.88 Other specific arthropathies, not elsewhere classified, other specified site
Other specific arthropathies, not elsewhere classified, vertebrae
M12.89 Other specific arthropathies, not elsewhere classified, multiple sites
M12.9 Arthropathy, unspecified

M13 Other arthritis
Excludes1: arthrosis (M15-M19)
osteoarthritis (M15-M19)
M13.0 Polyarthritis, unspecified

+, +7th, X + 7th   ● Newborn   ● Pediatric   ● Maternity   ● Adult   ♀ Female   ♂ Male   Manifestation   Unacceptable PDX   HCC   CC   MCC   HAC

+ **M13.1** Monoarthritis, not elsewhere classified
    M13.10 Monoarthritis, not elsewhere classified, unspecified site
+ **M13.11** Monoarthritis, not elsewhere classified, shoulder
    M13.111 Monoarthritis, not elsewhere classified, right shoulder
    M13.112 Monoarthritis, not elsewhere classified, left shoulder
    M13.119 Monoarthritis, not elsewhere classified, unspecified shoulder
+ **M13.12** Monoarthritis, not elsewhere classified, elbow
    M13.121 Monoarthritis, not elsewhere classified, right elbow
    M13.122 Monoarthritis, not elsewhere classified, left elbow
    M13.129 Monoarthritis, not elsewhere classified, unspecified elbow
+ **M13.13** Monoarthritis, not elsewhere classified, wrist
    M13.131 Monoarthritis, not elsewhere classified, right wrist
    M13.132 Monoarthritis, not elsewhere classified, left wrist
    M13.139 Monoarthritis, not elsewhere classified, unspecified wrist
+ **M13.14** Monoarthritis, not elsewhere classified, hand
    M13.141 Monoarthritis, not elsewhere classified, right hand
    M13.142 Monoarthritis, not elsewhere classified, left hand
    M13.149 Monoarthritis, not elsewhere classified, unspecified hand
+ **M13.15** Monoarthritis, not elsewhere classified, hip
    M13.151 Monoarthritis, not elsewhere classified, right hip
    M13.152 Monoarthritis, not elsewhere classified, left hip
    M13.159 Monoarthritis, not elsewhere classified, unspecified hip
+ **M13.16** Monoarthritis, not elsewhere classified, knee
    M13.161 Monoarthritis, not elsewhere classified, right knee
    M13.162 Monoarthritis, not elsewhere classified, left knee
    M13.169 Monoarthritis, not elsewhere classified, unspecified knee
+ **M13.17** Monoarthritis, not elsewhere classified, ankle and foot
    M13.171 Monoarthritis, not elsewhere classified, right ankle and foot
    M13.172 Monoarthritis, not elsewhere classified, left ankle and foot
    M13.179 Monoarthritis, not elsewhere classified, unspecified ankle and foot
+ **M13.8** Other specified arthritis
    Allergic arthritis
    Excludes1: *osteoarthritis (M15-M19)*
    M13.80 Other specified arthritis, unspecified site
+ **M13.81** Other specified arthritis, shoulder
    M13.811 Other specified arthritis, right shoulder
    M13.812 Other specified arthritis, left shoulder
    M13.819 Other specified arthritis, unspecified shoulder
+ **M13.82** Other specified arthritis, elbow
    M13.821 Other specified arthritis, right elbow
    M13.822 Other specified arthritis, left elbow
    M13.829 Other specified arthritis, unspecified elbow
+ **M13.83** Other specified arthritis, wrist
    M13.831 Other specified arthritis, right wrist
    M13.832 Other specified arthritis, left wrist
    M13.839 Other specified arthritis, unspecified wrist
+ **M13.84** Other specified arthritis, hand
    M13.841 Other specified arthritis, right hand
    M13.842 Other specified arthritis, left hand
    M13.849 Other specified arthritis, unspecified hand
+ **M13.85** Other specified arthritis, hip
    M13.851 Other specified arthritis, right hip
    M13.852 Other specified arthritis, left hip
    M13.859 Other specified arthritis, unspecified hip

+ **M13.86** Other specified arthritis, knee
    M13.861 Other specified arthritis, right knee
    M13.862 Other specified arthritis, left knee
    M13.869 Other specified arthritis, unspecified knee
+ **M13.87** Other specified arthritis, ankle and foot
    M13.871 Other specified arthritis, right ankle and foot
    M13.872 Other specified arthritis, left ankle and foot
    M13.879 Other specified arthritis, unspecified ankle and foot
    M13.88 Other specified arthritis, other site
    M13.89 Other specified arthritis, multiple sites

M14 Arthropathies in other diseases classified elsewhere
    Excludes1: *arthropathy in:*
      diabetes mellitus (E08-E13 with .61-)
      hematological disorders (M36.2-M36.3)
      hypersensitivity reactions (M36.4)
      neoplastic disease (M36.1)
      neurosyphillis (A52.16)
      sarcoidosis (D86.86)
      enteropathic arthropathies (M07.-)
      juvenile psoriatic arthropathy (L40.54)
      lipoid dermatoarthritis (E78.81)
+ **M14.6** Charcôt's joint
    Neuropathic arthropathy
    Excludes1: *Charcôt's joint in diabetes mellitus (E08-E13 with .610)*
      Charcôt's joint in tabes dorsalis (A52.16)
    M14.60 Charcôt's joint, unspecified site
+ **M14.61** Charcôt's joint, shoulder
    M14.611 Charcôt's joint, right shoulder
    M14.612 Charcôt's joint, left shoulder
    M14.619 Charcôt's joint, unspecified shoulder
+ **M14.62** Charcôt's joint, elbow
    M14.621 Charcôt's joint, right elbow
    M14.622 Charcôt's joint, lcft clbow
    M14.629 Charcôt's joint, unspecified elbow
+ **M14.63** Charcôt's joint, wrist
    M14.631 Charcôt's joint, right wrist
    M14.632 Charcôt's joint, left wrist
    M14.639 Charcôt's joint, unspccified wrist
+ **M14.64** Charcôt's joint, hand
    M14.641 Charcôt's joint, right hand
    M14.642 Charcôt's joint, left hand
    M14.649 Charcôt's joint, unspecified hand
+ **M14.65** Charcôt's joint, hip
    M14.651 Charcôt's joint, right hip
    M14.652 Charcôt's joint, left hip
    M14.659 Charcôt's joint, unspecified hip
+ **M14.66** Charcôt's joint, knee
    M14.661 Charcôt's joint, right knee
    M14.662 Charcôt's joint, left knee
    M14.669 Charcôt's joint, unspecified knee
+ **M14.67** Charcôt's joint, ankle and foot
    M14.671 Charcôt's joint, right ankle and foot
    M14.672 Charcôt's joint, left ankle and foot
    M14.679 Charcôt's joint, unspecified ankle and foot
    M14.68 Charcôt's joint, vertebrae
    M14.69 Charcôt's joint, multiple sites
+ **M14.8** Arthropathies in other specified diseases classified elsewhere
    Code first underlying disease, such as:
      amyloidosis (E85.-)
      erythema multiforme (L51.-)
      erythema nodosum (L52)
      hemochromatosis (E83.11-)
      hyperparathyroidism (E21.-)
      hypothyroidism (E00-E03)
      sickle-cell disorders (D57.-)
      thyrotoxicosis [hyperthyroidism] (E05.-)
      Whipple's disease (K90.81)
    M14.80 Arthropathies in other specified diseases classified elsewhere, unspecified site
+ **M14.81** Arthropathies in other specified diseases classified elsewhere, shoulder
    M14.811 Arthropathies in other specified diseases classified elsewhere, right shoulder

M14.812 Arthropathies in other specified diseases classified elsewhere, left shoulder

M14.819 Arthropathies in other specified diseases classified elsewhere, unspecified shoulder

+ **M14.82** Arthropathies in other specified diseases classified elsewhere, elbow

M14.821 Arthropathies in other specified diseases classified elsewhere, right elbow

M14.822 Arthropathies in other specified diseases classified elsewhere, left elbow

M14.829 Arthropathies in other specified diseases classified elsewhere, unspecified elbow

+ **M14.83** Arthropathies in other specified diseases classified elsewhere, wrist

M14.831 Arthropathies in other specified diseases classified elsewhere, right wrist

M14.832 Arthropathies in other specified diseases classified elsewhere, left wrist

M14.839 Arthropathies in other specified diseases classified elsewhere, unspecified wrist

+ **M14.84** Arthropathies in other specified diseases classified elsewhere, hand

M14.841 Arthropathies in other specified diseases classified elsewhere, right hand

M14.842 Arthropathies in other specified diseases classified elsewhere, left hand

M14.849 Arthropathies in other specified diseases classified elsewhere, unspecified hand

+ **M14.85** Arthropathies in other specified diseases classified elsewhere, hip

M14.851 Arthropathies in other specified diseases classified elsewhere, right hip

M14.852 Arthropathies in other specified diseases classified elsewhere, left hip

M14.859 Arthropathies in other specified diseases classified elsewhere, unspecified hip

+ **M14.86** Arthropathies in other specified diseases classified elsewhere, knee

M14.861 Arthropathies in other specified diseases classified elsewhere, right knee

M14.862 Arthropathies in other specified diseases classified elsewhere, left knee

M14.869 Arthropathies in other specified diseases classified elsewhere, unspecified knee

+ **M14.87** Arthropathies in other specified diseases classified elsewhere, ankle and foot

M14.871 Arthropathies in other specified diseases classified elsewhere, right ankle and foot

M14.872 Arthropathies in other specified diseases classified elsewhere, left ankle and foot

M14.879 Arthropathies in other specified diseases classified elsewhere, unspecified ankle and foot

M14.88 Arthropathies in other specified diseases classified elsewhere, vertebrae

M14.89 Arthropathies in other specified diseases classified elsewhere, multiple sites

Osteoarthritis (M15-M19)

Excludes2: *osteoarthritis of spine (M47.-)*

M15 Polyosteoarthritis

Includes: arthritis of multiple sites
Excludes1: *bilateral involvement of single joint (M16-M19)*

M15.0 Primary generalized (osteo)arthritis

M15.1 Heberden's nodes (with arthropathy)
Interphalangeal distal osteoarthritis

M15.2 Bouchard's nodes (with arthropathy)
Juxtaphalangeal distal osteoarthritis

M15.3 Secondary multiple arthritis
Post-traumatic polyosteoarthritis

M15.4 Erosive (osteo)arthritis

M15.8 Other polyosteoarthritis

M15.9 Polyosteoarthritis, unspecified
Generalized osteoarthritis NOS

M16 Osteoarthritis of hip

M16.0 Bilateral primary osteoarthritis of hip
AHA CC: 4Q, 2016, 146; 2Q, 2018, 15

+ **M16.1** Unilateral primary osteoarthritis of hip
Primary osteoarthritis of hip NOS

M16.10 Unilateral primary osteoarthritis, unspecified hip

M16.11 Unilateral primary osteoarthritis, right hip

M16.12 Unilateral primary osteoarthritis, left hip

M16.2 Bilateral osteoarthritis resulting from hip dysplasia

+ **M16.3** Unilateral osteoarthritis resulting from hip dysplasia
Dysplastic osteoarthritis of hip NOS

M16.30 Unilateral osteoarthritis resulting from hip dysplasia, unspecified hip

M16.31 Unilateral osteoarthritis resulting from hip dysplasia, right hip

M16.32 Unilateral osteoarthritis resulting from hip dysplasia, left hip

M16.4 Bilateral post-traumatic osteoarthritis of hip

+ **M16.5** Unilateral post-traumatic osteoarthritis of hip
Post-traumatic osteoarthritis of hip NOS

M16.50 Unilateral post-traumatic osteoarthritis, unspecified hip

M16.51 Unilateral post-traumatic osteoarthritis, right hip

M16.52 Unilateral post-traumatic osteoarthritis, left hip

M16.6 Other bilateral secondary osteoarthritis of hip

M16.7 Other unilateral secondary osteoarthritis of hip
Secondary osteoarthritis of hip NOS

M16.9 Osteoarthritis of hip, unspecified

M17 Osteoarthritis of knee

M17.0 Bilateral primary osteoarthritis of knee

+ **M17.1** Unilateral primary osteoarthritis of knee
Primary osteoarthritis of knee NOS

M17.10 Unilateral primary osteoarthritis, unspecified knee
AHA CC: 4Q, 2016, 147

M17.11 Unilateral primary osteoarthritis, right knee

M17.12 Unilateral primary osteoarthritis, left knee
AHA CC: 4Q, 2016, 146

M17.2 Bilateral post-traumatic osteoarthritis of knee

+ **M17.3** Unilateral post-traumatic osteoarthritis of knee
Post-traumatic osteoarthritis of knee NOS

M17.30 Unilateral post-traumatic osteoarthritis, unspecified knee

M17.31 Unilateral post-traumatic osteoarthritis, right knee

M17.32 Unilateral post-traumatic osteoarthritis, left knee

M17.4 Other bilateral secondary osteoarthritis of knee

M17.5 Other unilateral secondary osteoarthritis of knee
Secondary osteoarthritis of knee NOS

M17.9 Osteoarthritis of knee, unspecified

M18 Osteoarthritis of first carpometacarpal joint

M18.0 Bilateral primary osteoarthritis of first carpometacarpal joints

+ **M18.1** Unilateravl primary osteoarthritis of first carpometacarpal joint
Primary osteoarthritis of first carpometacarpal joint NOS

M18.10 Unilateral primary osteoarthritis of first carpometacarpal joint, unspecified hand

M18.11 Unilateral primary osteoarthritis of first carpometacarpal joint, right hand

M18.12 Unilateral primary osteoarthritis of first carpometacarpal joint, left hand

M18.2 Bilateral post-traumatic osteoarthritis of first carpometacarpal joints

+ **M18.3** Unilateral post-traumatic osteoarthritis of first carpometacarpal joint
Post-traumatic osteoarthritis of first carpometacarpal joint NOS

M18.30 Unilateral post-traumatic osteoarthritis of first carpometacarpal joint, unspecified hand

M18.31 Unilateral post-traumatic osteoarthritis of first carpometacarpal joint, right hand

M18.32 Unilateral post-traumatic osteoarthritis of first carpometacarpal joint, left hand

M18.4 Other bilateral secondary osteoarthritis of first carpometacarpal joints

+ **M18.5** Other unilateral secondary osteoarthritis of first carpometacarpal joint
Secondary osteoarthritis of first carpometacarpal joint NOS

Pathology in Osteoarthritis

Progressive stages in joint pathology

Early degenerative changes with surface fraying of articular cartilages

Further erosion of cartilages, pitting, and cleft formation. Hypertrophic changes of bone at joint margins.

Cartilages almost completely destroyed and joint space narrowed. Subchondral bone irregular and eburnated; spur formation at margins. Fibrosis of joint capsule.

Erosion in femur

Knee joint opened anteriorly. Reveals large erosion of articular cartilages of femur and patella with cartilaginous excrescences at intercondylar notch (arrow)

Erosion in patella

Section of articular cartilage. Fraying of surface and deep cleft. Hyaline cartilage abnormal with clumping of chondrocytes (arrows).

M18.50 Other unilateral secondary osteoarthritis of first carpometacarpal joint, unspecified hand

M18.51 Other unilateral secondary osteoarthritis of first carpometacarpal joint, right hand

M18.52 Other unilateral secondary osteoarthritis of first carpometacarpal joint, left hand

M18.9 Osteoarthritis of first carpometacarpal joint, unspecified

M19 Other and unspecified osteoarthritis

> **Excludes1:** *polyarthritis (M15.-)*
> **Excludes2:** *arthrosis of spine (M47.-)*
> *hallux rigidus (M20.2)*
> *osteoarthritis of spine (M47.-)*

+ **M19.0 Primary osteoarthritis of other joints**

+ **M19.01** Primary osteoarthritis, shoulder

M19.011 Primary osteoarthritis, right shoulder
AHA CC: 4Q, 2016, 145

M19.012 Primary osteoarthritis, left shoulder

M19.019 Primary osteoarthritis, unspecified shoulder

+ **M19.02** Primary osteoarthritis, elbow

M19.021 Primary osteoarthritis, right elbow

M19.022 Primary osteoarthritis, left elbow

M19.029 Primary osteoarthritis, unspecified elbow

+ **M19.03** Primary osteoarthritis, wrist

M19.031 Primary osteoarthritis, right wrist

M19.032 Primary osteoarthritis, left wrist

M19.039 Primary osteoarthritis, unspecified wrist

+ **M19.04** Primary osteoarthritis, hand

> **Excludes2:** *primary osteoarthritis of first carpometacarpal joint (M18.0-, M18.1-)*

M19.041 Primary osteoarthritis, right hand

M19.042 Primary osteoarthritis, left hand

M19.049 Primary osteoarthritis, unspecified hand

+ **M19.07** Primary osteoarthritis ankle and foot

M19.071 Primary osteoarthritis, right ankle and foot

M19.072 Primary osteoarthritis, left ankle and foot

M19.079 Primary osteoarthritis, unspecified ankle and foot

M19.09 Primary osteoarthritis, other specified site

+ **M19.1 Post-traumatic osteoarthritis of other joints**

+ **M19.11** Post-traumatic osteoarthritis, shoulder

M19.111 Post-traumatic osteoarthritis, right shoulder

M19.112 Post-traumatic osteoarthritis, left shoulder

M19.119 Post-traumatic osteoarthritis, unspecified shoulder

+ **M19.12** Post-traumatic osteoarthritis, elbow

M19.121 Post-traumatic osteoarthritis, right elbow

M19.122 Post-traumatic osteoarthritis, left elbow

M19.129 Post-traumatic osteoarthritis, unspecified elbow

+ **M19.13** Post-traumatic osteoarthritis, wrist

M19.131 Post-traumatic osteoarthritis, right wrist

M19.132 Post-traumatic osteoarthritis, left wrist

M19.139 Post-traumatic osteoarthritis, unspecified wrist

+ **M19.14** Post-traumatic osteoarthritis, hand

> **Excludes2:** *post-traumatic osteoarthritis of first carpometacarpal joint (M18.2-, M18.3-)*

M19.141 Post-traumatic osteoarthritis, right hand

M19.142 Post-traumatic osteoarthritis, left hand

M19.149 Post-traumatic osteoarthritis, unspecified hand

+ **M19.17** Post-traumatic osteoarthritis, ankle and foot

M19.171 Post-traumatic osteoarthritis, right ankle and foot

M19.172 Post-traumatic osteoarthritis, left ankle and foot

M19.179 Post-traumatic osteoarthritis, unspecified ankle and foot

M19.19 Post-traumatic osteoarthritis, other specified site

+ **M19.2 Secondary osteoarthritis of other joints**

+ **M19.21** Secondary osteoarthritis, shoulder

M19.211 Secondary osteoarthritis, right shoulder

M19.212 Secondary osteoarthritis, left shoulder

M19.219 Secondary osteoarthritis, unspecified shoulder

+ **M19.22** Secondary osteoarthritis, elbow

M19.221 Secondary osteoarthritis, right elbow

M19.222 Secondary osteoarthritis, left elbow

M19.229 Secondary osteoarthritis, unspecified elbow

+ **M19.23** Secondary osteoarthritis, wrist

M19.231 Secondary osteoarthritis, right wrist

M19.232 Secondary osteoarthritis, left wrist

M19.239 Secondary osteoarthritis, unspecified wrist

+ **M19.24** Secondary osteoarthritis, hand

M19.241 Secondary osteoarthritis, right hand

M19.242 Secondary osteoarthritis, left hand

M19.249 Secondary osteoarthritis, unspecified hand

+ **M19.27** Secondary osteoarthritis, ankle and foot

M19.271 Secondary osteoarthritis, right ankle and foot

M19.272 Secondary osteoarthritis, left ankle and foot

M19.279 Secondary osteoarthritis, unspecified ankle and foot

M19.29 Secondary osteoarthritis, other specified site

+ **M19.9 Osteoarthritis, unspecified site**

M19.90 Unspecified osteoarthritis, unspecified site
Arthrosis NOS
Arthritis NOS
Osteoarthritis NOS
AHA CC: 4Q, 2016, 147

M19.91 Primary osteoarthritis, unspecified site
Primary osteoarthritis NOS

M19.92 Post-traumatic osteoarthritis, unspecified site
Post-traumatic osteoarthritis NOS

M19.93 Secondary osteoarthritis, unspecified site
Secondary osteoarthritis NOS

Other joint disorders (M20-M25)

> **Excludes2:** *joints of the spine (M40-M54)*

M20 Acquired deformities of fingers and toes

> **Excludes1:** *acquired absence of fingers and toes (Z89.-)*
> *congenital absence of fingers and toes (Q71.3-, Q72.3-)*
> *congenital deformities and malformations of fingers and toes (Q66.-, Q68-Q70, Q74.-)*

+ **M20.0 Deformity of finger(s)**

> **Excludes1:** *clubbing of fingers (R68.3)*
> *palmar fascial fibromatosis [Dupuytren] (M72.0)*
> *trigger finger (M65.3)*

+ **M20.00** Unspecified deformity of finger(s)

M20.001 Unspecified deformity of right finger(s)

M20.002 Unspecified deformity of left finger(s)

M20.009 Unspecified deformity of unspecified finger(s)

+ **M20.01** Mallet finger

M20.011 Mallet finger of right finger(s)

M20.012 Mallet finger of left finger(s)

M20.019 Mallet finger of unspecified finger(s)

+ **M20.02** Boutonnière deformity

M20.021 Boutonnière deformity of right finger(s)

M20.022 Boutonnière deformity of left finger(s)

M20.029 Boutonnière deformity of unspecified finger(s)

+ **M20.03** Swan-neck deformity

M20.031 Swan-neck deformity of right finger(s)

+, +7th, X + 7th   ● Newborn   ● Pediatric   ● Maternity   ● Adult   ♀ Female   ♂ Male   Manifestation   Unacceptable PDX   HCC   CC   MCC   HAC

M20.032 Swan-neck deformity of left finger(s)
M20.039 Swan-neck deformity of unspecified finger(s)
+ M20.09 Other deformity of finger(s)
M20.091 Other deformity of right finger(s)
M20.092 Other deformity of left finger(s)
M20.099 Other deformity of finger(s), unspecified finger(s)
+ M20.1 Hallux valgus (acquired)
   Excludes2: bunion (M21.6-)
M20.10 Hallux valgus (acquired), unspecified foot
M20.11 Hallux valgus (acquired), right foot
M20.12 Hallux valgus (acquired), left foot
+ M20.2 Hallux rigidus
M20.20 Hallux rigidus, unspecified foot
M20.21 Hallux rigidus, right foot
M20.22 Hallux rigidus, left foot
+ M20.3 Hallux varus (acquired)
M20.30 Hallux varus (acquired), unspecified foot
M20.31 Hallux varus (acquired), right foot
M20.32 Hallux varus (acquired), left foot
+ M20.4 Other hammer toe(s) (acquired)
M20.40 Other hammer toe(s) (acquired), unspecified foot
M20.41 Other hammer toe(s) (acquired), right foot
M20.42 Other hammer toe(s) (acquired), left foot
+ M20.5 Other deformities of toe(s) (acquired)
   + M20.5X Other deformities of toe(s) (acquired)
M20.5X1 Other deformities of toe(s) (acquired), right foot
M20.5X2 Other deformities of toe(s) (acquired), left foot
M20.5X9 Other deformities of toe(s) (acquired), unspecified foot
+ M20.6 Acquired deformities of toe(s), unspecified
M20.60 Acquired deformities of toe(s), unspecified, unspecified foot
M20.61 Acquired deformities of toe(s), unspecified, right foot
M20.62 Acquired deformities of toe(s), unspecified, left foot

M21 Other acquired deformities of limbs

   Excludes1: acquired absence of limb (Z89.-)
      congenital absence of limbs (Q71 Q73)
      congenital deformities and malformations of limbs (Q65-Q66, Q68-Q74)
   Excludes2: acquired deformities of fingers or toes (M20.-)
      coxa plana (M91.2)
+ M21.0 Valgus deformity, not elsewhere classified
   Excludes1: metatarsus valgus (Q66.6)
      talipes calcaneovalgus (Q66.4-)
M21.00 Valgus deformity, not elsewhere classified, unspecified site
   + M21.02 Valgus deformity, not elsewhere classified, elbow
      Cubitus valgus
M21.021 Valgus deformity, not elsewhere classified, right elbow
M21.022 Valgus deformity, not elsewhere classified, left elbow
M21.029 Valgus deformity, not elsewhere classified, unspecified elbow
   + M21.05 Valgus deformity, not elsewhere classified, hip
M21.051 Valgus deformity, not elsewhere classified, right hip
M21.052 Valgus deformity, not elsewhere classified, left hip
M21.059 Valgus deformity, not elsewhere classified, unspecified hip
   + M21.06 Valgus deformity, not elsewhere classified, knee
      Genu valgum
      Knock knee
M21.061 Valgus deformity, not elsewhere classified, right knee
M21.062 Valgus deformity, not elsewhere classified, left knee
M21.069 Valgus deformity, not elsewhere classified, unspecified knee

+ M21.07 Valgus deformity, not elsewhere classified, ankle
M21.071 Valgus deformity, not elsewhere classified, right ankle
M21.072 Valgus deformity, not elsewhere classified, left ankle
M21.079 Valgus deformity, not elsewhere classified, unspecified ankle
+ M21.1 Varus deformity, not elsewhere classified
   Excludes1: metatarsus varus (Q66.22-)
      tibia vara (M92.51-)
M21.10 Varus deformity, not elsewhere classified, unspecified site
   + M21.12 Varus deformity, not elsewhere classified, elbow
      Cubitus varus, elbow
M21.121 Varus deformity, not elsewhere classified, right elbow
M21.122 Varus deformity, not elsewhere classified, left elbow
M21.129 Varus deformity, not elsewhere classified, unspecified elbow
   + M21.15 Varus deformity, not elsewhere classified, hip
M21.151 Varus deformity, not elsewhere classified, right hip
M21.152 Varus deformity, not elsewhere classified, left hip
M21.159 Varus deformity, not elsewhere classified, unspecified
   + M21.16 Varus deformity, not elsewhere classified, knee
      Bow leg
      Genu varum
M21.161 Varus deformity, not elsewhere classified, right knee
M21.162 Varus deformity, not elsewhere classified, left knee
M21.169 Varus deformity, not elsewhere classified, unspecified knee
   + M21.17 Varus deformity, not elsewhere classified, ankle
M21.171 Varus deformity, not elsewhere classified, right ankle
M21.172 Varus deformity, not elsewhere classified, left ankle
M21.179 Varus deformity, not elsewhere classified, unspecified ankle
+ M21.2 Flexion deformity
M21.20 Flexion deformity, unspecified site
   + M21.21 Flexion deformity, shoulder
M21.211 Flexion deformity, right shoulder
M21.212 Flexion deformity, left shoulder
M21.219 Flexion deformity, unspecified shoulder
   + M21.22 Flexion deformity, elbow
M21.221 Flexion deformity, right elbow
M21.222 Flexion deformity, left elbow
M21.229 Flexion deformity, unspecified elbow
   + M21.23 Flexion deformity, wrist
M21.231 Flexion deformity, right wrist
M21.232 Flexion deformity, left wrist
M21.239 Flexion deformity, unspecified wrist
   + M21.24 Flexion deformity, finger joints
M21.241 Flexion deformity, right finger joints
M21.242 Flexion deformity, left finger joints
M21.249 Flexion deformity, unspecified finger joints
   + M21.25 Flexion deformity, hip
M21.251 Flexion deformity, right hip
M21.252 Flexion deformity, left hip
M21.259 Flexion deformity, unspecified hip
   + M21.26 Flexion deformity, knee
M21.261 Flexion deformity, right knee
M21.262 Flexion deformity, left knee
M21.269 Flexion deformity, unspecified knee
   + M21.27 Flexion deformity, ankle and toes
M21.271 Flexion deformity, right ankle and toes
M21.272 Flexion deformity, left ankle and toes
M21.279 Flexion deformity, unspecified ankle and toes

+ **M21.3** **Wrist or foot drop (acquired)**
  + **M21.33** **Wrist drop (acquired)**
      M21.331 Wrist drop, right wrist
      M21.332 Wrist drop, left wrist
      M21.339 Wrist drop, unspecified wrist
  + **M21.37** **Foot drop (acquired)**
      M21.371 Foot drop, right foot
      M21.372 Foot drop, left foot
      M21.379 Foot drop, unspecified foot
+ **M21.4** **Flat foot [pes planus] (acquired)**
    Excludes1: *congenital pes planus (Q66.5-)*
    M21.40 Flat foot [pes planus] (acquired), unspecified foot
    M21.41 Flat foot [pes planus] (acquired), right foot
    M21.42 Flat foot [pes planus] (acquired), left foot
+ **M21.5** **Acquired clawhand, clubhand, clawfoot and clubfoot**
    Excludes1: *clubfoot, not specified as acquired (Q66.89)*
  + **M21.51** **Acquired clawhand**
      M21.511 Acquired clawhand, right hand
      M21.512 Acquired clawhand, left hand
      M21.519 Acquired clawhand, unspecified hand
  + **M21.52** **Acquired clubhand**
      M21.521 Acquired clubhand, right hand
      M21.522 Acquired clubhand, left hand
      M21.529 Acquired clubhand, unspecified hand
  + **M21.53** **Acquired clawfoot**
      M21.531 Acquired clawfoot, right foot
      M21.532 Acquired clawfoot, left foot
      M21.539 Acquired clawfoot, unspecified foot
  + **M21.54** **Acquired clubfoot**
      M21.541 Acquired clubfoot, right foot
      M21.542 Acquired clubfoot, left foot
      M21.549 Acquired clubfoot, unspecified foot
+ **M21.6** **Other acquired deformities of foot**
    Excludes2: *deformities of toe (acquired) (M20.1-M20.6-)*
    AHA CC: 4Q, 2016, 38
  + **M21.61** **Bunion**
      M21.611 Bunion of right foot
      M21.612 Bunion of left foot
      M21.619 Bunion of unspecified foot
  + **M21.62** **Bunionette**
      M21.621 Bunionette of right foot
      M21.622 Bunionette of left foot
      M21.629 Bunionette of unspecified foot
  + **M21.6X** **Other acquired deformities of foot**
      M21.6X1 Other acquired deformities of right foot
      M21.6X2 Other acquired deformities of left foot
      M21.6X9 Other acquired deformities of unspecified foot
+ **M21.7** **Unequal limb length (acquired)**
    NOTE The site used should correspond to the shorter limb
    M21.70 Unequal limb length (acquired), unspecified site
  + **M21.72** **Unequal limb length (acquired), humerus**
      M21.721 Unequal limb length (acquired), right humerus
      M21.722 Unequal limb length (acquired), left humerus
      M21.729 Unequal limb length (acquired), unspecified humerus
  + **M21.73** **Unequal limb length (acquired), ulna and radius**
      M21.731 Unequal limb length (acquired), right ulna
      M21.732 Unequal limb length (acquired), left ulna
      M21.733 Unequal limb length (acquired), right radius
      M21.734 Unequal limb length (acquired), left radius
      M21.739 Unequal limb length (acquired), unspecified ulna and radius
  + **M21.75** **Unequal limb length (acquired), femur**
      M21.751 Unequal limb length (acquired), right femur
      M21.752 Unequal limb length (acquired), left femur
      M21.759 Unequal limb length (acquired), unspecified femur

+ **M21.76** **Unequal limb length (acquired), tibia and fibula**
    M21.761 Unequal limb length (acquired), right tibia
    M21.762 Unequal limb length (acquired), left tibia
    M21.763 Unequal limb length (acquired), right fibula
    M21.764 Unequal limb length (acquired), left fibula
    M21.769 Unequal limb length (acquired), unspecified tibia and fibula
+ **M21.8** **Other specified acquired deformities of limbs**
    Excludes2: *coxa plana (M91.2)*
    M21.80 Other specified acquired deformities of unspecified limb
  + **M21.82** **Other specified acquired deformities of upper arm**
      M21.821 Other specified acquired deformities of right upper arm
      M21.822 Other specified acquired deformities of left upper arm
      M21.829 Other specified acquired deformities of unspecified upper arm
  + **M21.83** **Other specified acquired deformities of forearm**
      M21.831 Other specified acquired deformities of right forearm
      M21.832 Other specified acquired deformities of left forearm
      M21.839 Other specified acquired deformities of unspecified forearm
  + **M21.85** **Other specified acquired deformities of thigh**
      M21.851 Other specified acquired deformities of right thigh
      M21.852 Other specified acquired deformities of left thigh
      M21.859 Other specified acquired deformities of unspecified thigh
  + **M21.86** **Other specified acquired deformities of lower leg**
      M21.861 Other specified acquired deformities of right lower leg
      M21.862 Other specified acquired deformities of left lower leg
      M21.869 Other specified acquired deformities of unspecified lower leg
+ **M21.9** **Unspecified acquired deformity of limb and hand**
    M21.90 Unspecified acquired deformity of unspecified limb
  + **M21.92** **Unspecified acquired deformity of upper arm**
      M21.921 Unspecified acquired deformity of right upper arm
      M21.922 Unspecified acquired deformity of left upper arm
      M21.929 Unspecified acquired deformity of unspecified upper arm
  + **M21.93** **Unspecified acquired deformity of forearm**
      M21.931 Unspecified acquired deformity of right forearm
      M21.932 Unspecified acquired deformity of left forearm
      M21.939 Unspecified acquired deformity of unspecified forearm
  + **M21.94** **Unspecified acquired deformity of hand**
      M21.941 Unspecified acquired deformity of hand, right hand
      M21.942 Unspecified acquired deformity of hand, left hand
      M21.949 Unspecified acquired deformity of hand, unspecified hand
  + **M21.95** **Unspecified acquired deformity of thigh**
      M21.951 Unspecified acquired deformity of right thigh
      M21.952 Unspecified acquired deformity of left thigh
      M21.959 Unspecified acquired deformity of unspecified thigh
  + **M21.96** **Unspecified acquired deformity of lower leg**
      M21.961 Unspecified acquired deformity of right lower leg
      M21.962 Unspecified acquired deformity of left lower leg
      M21.969 Unspecified acquired deformity of unspecified lower leg

M22 Disorder of patella

> *Excludes2:* *traumatic dislocation of patella (S83.0-)*

+ **M22.0 Recurrent dislocation of patella**
> **M22.00 Recurrent dislocation of patella, unspecified knee**
> **M22.01 Recurrent dislocation of patella, right knee**
> **M22.02 Recurrent dislocation of patella, left knee**

+ **M22.1 Recurrent subluxation of patella**
> Incomplete dislocation of patella
> **M22.10 Recurrent subluxation of patella, unspecified knee**
> **M22.11 Recurrent subluxation of patella, right knee**
> **M22.12 Recurrent subluxation of patella, left knee**

+ **M22.2 Patellofemoral disorders**
> + **M22.2X Patellofemoral disorders**
>> **M22.2X1 Patellofemoral disorders, right knee**
>> **M22.2X2 Patellofemoral disorders, left knee**
>> **M22.2X9 Patellofemoral disorders, unspecified knee**

+ **M22.3 Other derangements of patella**
> + **M22.3X Other derangements of patella**
>> **M22.3X1 Other derangements of patella, right knee**
>> **M22.3X2 Other derangements of patella, left knee**
>> **M22.3X9 Other derangements of patella, unspecified knee**

+ **M22.4 Chondromalacia patellae**
> **M22.40 Chondromalacia patellae, unspecified knee**
> **M22.41 Chondromalacia patellae, right knee**
> **M22.42 Chondromalacia patellae, left knee**

+ **M22.8 Other disorders of patella**
> + **M22.8X Other disorders of patella**
>> **M22.8X1 Other disorders of patella, right knee**
>> **M22.8X2 Other disorders of patella, left knee**
>> **M22.8X9 Other disorders of patella, unspecified knee**

+ **M22.9 Unspecified disorder of patella**
> **M22.90 Unspecified disorder of patella, unspecified knee**
> **M22.91 Unspecified disorder of patella, right knee**
> **M22.92 Unspecified disorder of patella, left knee**

M23 Internal derangement of knee

> *Excludes1:* *ankylosis (M24.66)*
> *deformity of knee (M21.-)*
> *osteochondritis dissecans (M93.2)*

> *Excludes2:* *current injury - see injury of knee and lower leg (S80-S89)*
> *recurrent dislocation or subluxation of joints (M24.4)*
> *recurrent dislocation or subluxation of patella (M22.0-M22.1)*

+ **M23.0 Cystic meniscus**
> + **M23.00 Cystic meniscus, unspecified meniscus**
>> Cystic meniscus, unspecified lateral meniscus
>> Cystic meniscus, unspecified medial meniscus
>> **M23.000 Cystic meniscus, unspecified lateral meniscus, right knee**
>> **M23.001 Cystic meniscus, unspecified lateral meniscus, left knee**
>> **M23.002 Cystic meniscus, unspecified lateral meniscus, unspecified knee**
>> **M23.003 Cystic meniscus, unspecified medial meniscus, right knee**
>> **M23.004 Cystic meniscus, unspecified medial meniscus, left knee**
>> **M23.005 Cystic meniscus, unspecified medial meniscus, unspecified knee**
>> **M23.006 Cystic meniscus, unspecified meniscus, right knee**
>> **M23.007 Cystic meniscus, unspecified meniscus, left knee**
>> **M23.009 Cystic meniscus, unspecified meniscus, unspecified knee**

> + **M23.01 Cystic meniscus, anterior horn of medial meniscus**
>> **M23.011 Cystic meniscus, anterior horn of medial meniscus, right knee**
>> **M23.012 Cystic meniscus, anterior horn of medial meniscus, left knee**
>> **M23.019 Cystic meniscus, anterior horn of medial meniscus, unspecified knee**

+ **M23.02 Cystic meniscus, posterior horn of medial meniscus**
> **M23.021 Cystic meniscus, posterior horn of medial meniscus, right knee**
> **M23.022 Cystic meniscus, posterior horn of medial meniscus, left knee**
> **M23.029 Cystic meniscus, posterior horn of medial meniscus, unspecified knee**

+ **M23.03 Cystic meniscus, other medial meniscus**
> **M23.031 Cystic meniscus, other medial meniscus, right knee**
> **M23.032 Cystic meniscus, other medial meniscus, left knee**
> **M23.039 Cystic meniscus, other medial meniscus, unspecified knee**

+ **M23.04 Cystic meniscus, anterior horn of lateral meniscus**
> **M23.041 Cystic meniscus, anterior horn of lateral meniscus, right knee**
> **M23.042 Cystic meniscus, anterior horn of lateral meniscus, left knee**
> **M23.049 Cystic meniscus, anterior horn of lateral meniscus, unspecified knee**

+ **M23.05 Cystic meniscus, posterior horn of lateral meniscus**
> **M23.051 Cystic meniscus, posterior horn of lateral meniscus, right knee**
> **M23.052 Cystic meniscus, posterior horn of lateral meniscus, left knee**
> **M23.059 Cystic meniscus, posterior horn of lateral meniscus, unspecified knee**

+ **M23.06 Cystic meniscus, other lateral meniscus**
> **M23.061 Cystic meniscus, other lateral meniscus, right knee**
> **M23.062 Cystic meniscus, other lateral meniscus, left knee**
> **M23.069 Cystic meniscus, other lateral meniscus, unspecified knee**

+ **M23.2 Derangement of meniscus due to old tear or injury**
> Old bucket-handle tear
> + **M23.20 Derangement of unspecified meniscus due to old tear or injury**
>> Derangement of unspecified lateral meniscus due to old tear or injury
>> Derangement of unspecified medial meniscus due to old tear or injury
>> **M23.200 Derangement of unspecified lateral meniscus due to old tear or injury, right knee**
>> **M23.201 Derangement of unspecified lateral meniscus due to old tear or injury, left knee**
>> **M23.202 Derangement of unspecified lateral meniscus due to old tear or injury, unspecified knee**
>> **M23.203 Derangement of unspecified medial meniscus due to old tear or injury, right knee**
>> **M23.204 Derangement of unspecified medial meniscus due to old tear or injury, left knee**
>> **M23.205 Derangement of unspecified medial meniscus due to old tear or injury, unspecified knee**
>> **M23.206 Derangement of unspecified meniscus due to old tear or injury, right knee**
>> **M23.207 Derangement of unspecified meniscus due to old tear or injury, left knee**
>> **M23.209 Derangement of unspecified meniscus due to old tear or injury, unspecified knee**

> + **M23.21 Derangement of anterior horn of medial meniscus due to old tear or injury**
>> **M23.211 Derangement of anterior horn of medial meniscus due to old tear or injury, right knee**
>> **M23.212 Derangement of anterior horn of medial meniscus due to old tear or injury, left knee**
>> **M23.219 Derangement of anterior horn of medial meniscus due to old tear or injury, unspecified knee**

+, +7th, X + 7th   ● Newborn   ● Pediatric   ● Maternity   ● Adult   ♀ Female   ♂ Male   Manifestation   Unacceptable PDX   HCC   CC   MCC   HAC

+ M23.22 Derangement of posterior horn of medial meniscus due to old tear or injury
 M23.221 Derangement of posterior horn of medial meniscus due to old tear or injury, right knee
 M23.222 Derangement of posterior horn of medial meniscus due to old tear or injury, left knee
 M23.229 Derangement of posterior horn of medial meniscus due to old tear or injury, unspecified knee
+ M23.23 Derangement of other medial meniscus due to old tear or injury
 M23.231 Derangement of other medial meniscus due to old tear or injury, right knee
 M23.232 Derangement of other medial meniscus due to old tear or injury, left knee
 M23.239 Derangement of other medial meniscus due to old tear or injury, unspecified knee
+ M23.24 Derangement of anterior horn of lateral meniscus due to old tear or injury
 M23.241 Derangement of anterior horn of lateral meniscus due to old tear or injury, right knee
 M23.242 Derangement of anterior horn of lateral meniscus due to old tear or injury, left knee
 M23.249 Derangement of anterior horn of lateral meniscus due to old tear or injury, unspecified knee
+ M23.25 Derangement of posterior horn of lateral meniscus due to old tear or injury
 M23.251 Derangement of posterior horn of lateral meniscus due to old tear or injury, right knee
 M23.252 Derangement of posterior horn of lateral meniscus due to old tear or injury, left knee
 M23.259 Derangement of posterior horn of lateral meniscus due to old tear or injury, unspecified knee
+ M23.26 Derangement of other lateral meniscus due to old tear or injury
 M23.261 Derangement of other lateral meniscus due to old tear or injury, right knee
 M23.262 Derangement of other lateral meniscus due to old tear or injury, left knee
 M23.269 Derangement of other lateral meniscus due to old tear or injury, unspecified knee
+ M23.3 Other meniscus derangements
 Degenerate meniscus
 Detached meniscus
 Retained meniscus
 + M23.30 Other meniscus derangements, unspecified meniscus
  Other meniscus derangements, unspecified lateral meniscus
  Other meniscus derangements, unspecified medial meniscus
  M23.300 Other meniscus derangements, unspecified lateral meniscus, right knee
  M23.301 Other meniscus derangements, unspecified lateral meniscus, left knee
  M23.302 Other meniscus derangements, unspecified lateral meniscus, unspecified knee
  M23.303 Other meniscus derangements, unspecified medial meniscus, right knee
  M23.304 Other meniscus derangements, unspecified medial meniscus, left knee
  M23.305 Other meniscus derangements, unspecified medial meniscus, unspecified knee
  M23.306 Other meniscus derangements, unspecified meniscus, right knee
  M23.307 Other meniscus derangements, unspecified meniscus, left knee
  M23.309 Other meniscus derangements, unspecified meniscus, unspecified knee

+ M23.31 Other meniscus derangements, anterior horn of medial meniscus
 M23.311 Other meniscus derangements, anterior horn of medial meniscus, right knee
 M23.312 Other meniscus derangements, anterior horn of medial meniscus, left knee
 M23.319 Other meniscus derangements, anterior horn of medial meniscus, unspecified knee
+ M23.32 Other meniscus derangements, posterior horn of medial meniscus
 M23.321 Other meniscus derangements, posterior horn of medial meniscus, right knee
 M23.322 Other meniscus derangements, posterior horn of medial meniscus, left knee
 M23.329 Other meniscus derangements, posterior horn of medial meniscus, unspecified knee
+ M23.33 Other meniscus derangements, other medial meniscus
 M23.331 Other meniscus derangements, other medial meniscus, right knee
 M23.332 Other meniscus derangements, other medial meniscus, left knee
 M23.339 Other meniscus derangements, other medial meniscus, unspecified knee
+ M23.34 Other meniscus derangements, anterior horn of lateral meniscus
 M23.341 Other meniscus derangements, anterior horn of lateral meniscus, right knee
 M23.342 Other meniscus derangements, anterior horn of lateral meniscus, left knee
 M23.349 Other meniscus derangements, anterior horn of lateral meniscus, unspecified knee
+ M23.35 Other meniscus derangements, posterior horn of lateral meniscus
 M23.351 Other meniscus derangements, posterior horn of lateral meniscus, right knee
 M23.352 Other meniscus derangements, posterior horn of lateral meniscus, left knee
 M23.359 Other meniscus derangements, posterior horn of lateral meniscus, unspecified knee
+ M23.36 Other meniscus derangements, other lateral meniscus
 M23.361 Other meniscus derangements, other lateral meniscus, right knee
 M23.362 Other meniscus derangements, other lateral meniscus, left knee
 M23.369 Other meniscus derangements, other lateral meniscus, unspecified knee
+ M23.4 Loose body in knee
 M23.40 Loose body in knee, unspecified knee
 M23.41 Loose body in knee, right knee
 M23.42 Loose body in knee, left knee
+ M23.5 Chronic instability of knee
 M23.50 Chronic instability of knee, unspecified knee
 M23.51 Chronic instability of knee, right knee
 M23.52 Chronic instability of knee, left knee
+ M23.6 Other spontaneous disruption of ligament(s) of knee
 + M23.60 Other spontaneous disruption of unspecified ligament of knee
  M23.601 Other spontaneous disruption of unspecified ligament of right knee
  M23.602 Other spontaneous disruption of unspecified ligament of left knee
  M23.609 Other spontaneous disruption of unspecified ligament of unspecified knee

+ **M23.61 Other spontaneous disruption of anterior cruciate ligament of knee**
  - M23.611 Other spontaneous disruption of anterior cruciate ligament of right knee
  - M23.612 Other spontaneous disruption of anterior cruciate ligament of left knee
  - M23.619 Other spontaneous disruption of anterior cruciate ligament of unspecified knee
+ **M23.62 Other spontaneous disruption of posterior cruciate ligament of knee**
  - M23.621 Other spontaneous disruption of posterior cruciate ligament of right knee
  - M23.622 Other spontaneous disruption of posterior cruciate ligament of left knee
  - M23.629 Other spontaneous disruption of posterior cruciate ligament of unspecified knee
+ **M23.63 Other spontaneous disruption of medial collateral ligament of knee**
  - M23.631 Other spontaneous disruption of medial collateral ligament of right knee
  - M23.632 Other spontaneous disruption of medial collateral ligament of left knee
  - M23.639 Other spontaneous disruption of medial collateral ligament of unspecified knee
+ **M23.64 Other spontaneous disruption of lateral collateral ligament of knee**
  - M23.641 Other spontaneous disruption of lateral collateral ligament of right knee
  - M23.642 Other spontaneous disruption of lateral collateral ligament of left knee
  - M23.649 Other spontaneous disruption of lateral collateral ligament of unspecified knee
+ **M23.67 Other spontaneous disruption of capsular ligament of knee**
  - M23.671 Other spontaneous disruption of capsular ligament of right knee
  - M23.672 Other spontaneous disruption of capsular ligament of left knee
  - M23.679 Other spontaneous disruption of capsular ligament of unspecified knee
+ **M23.8 Other internal derangements of knee**
  - Laxity of ligament of knee
  - Snapping knee
  + **M23.8X Other internal derangements of knee**
    - M23.8X1 Other internal derangements of right knee
    - M23.8X2 Other internal derangements of left knee
    - M23.8X9 Other internal derangements of unspecified knee
+ **M23.9 Unspecified internal derangement of knee**
  - M23.90 Unspecified internal derangement of unspecified knee
  - M23.91 Unspecified internal derangement of right knee
  - M23.92 Unspecified internal derangement of left knee

M24 Other specific joint derangements

> **Excludes1:** *current injury - see injury of joint by body region*
> **Excludes2:** *ganglion (M67.4)*
> *snapping knee (M23.8-)*
> *temporomandibular joint disorders (M26.6-)*

+ **M24.0 Loose body in joint**
  > **Excludes2:** *loose body in knee (M23.4)*
  - M24.00 Loose body in unspecified joint
  + **M24.01 Loose body in shoulder**
    - M24.011 Loose body in right shoulder
    - M24.012 Loose body in left shoulder
    - M24.019 Loose body in unspecified shoulder
  + **M24.02 Loose body in elbow**
    - M24.021 Loose body in right elbow
    - M24.022 Loose body in left elbow
    - M24.029 Loose body in unspecified elbow
  + **M24.03 Loose body in wrist**
    - M24.031 Loose body in right wrist
    - M24.032 Loose body in left wrist
    - M24.039 Loose body in unspecified wrist

+ **M24.04 Loose body in finger joints**
  - M24.041 Loose body in right finger joint(s)
  - M24.042 Loose body in left finger joint(s)
  - M24.049 Loose body in unspecified finger joint(s)
+ **M24.05 Loose body in hip**
  - M24.051 Loose body in right hip
  - M24.052 Loose body in left hip
  - M24.059 Loose body in unspecified hip
+ **M24.07 Loose body in ankle and toe joints**
  - M24.071 Loose body in right ankle
  - M24.072 Loose body in left ankle
  - M24.073 Loose body in unspecified ankle
  - M24.074 Loose body in right toe joint(s)
  - M24.075 Loose body in left toe joint(s)
  - M24.076 Loose body in unspecified toe joints
- M24.08 Loose body, other site
+ **M24.1 Other articular cartilage disorders**
  > **Excludes2:** *chondrocalcinosis (M11.1, M11.2-)*
  > *internal derangement of knee (M23.-)*
  > *metastatic calcification (E83.5)*
  > *ochronosis (E70.2)*
  - M24.10 Other articular cartilage disorders, unspecified site
  + **M24.11 Other articular cartilage disorders, shoulder**
    - M24.111 Other articular cartilage disorders, right shoulder
    - M24.112 Other articular cartilage disorders, left shoulder
    - M24.119 Other articular cartilage disorders, unspecified shoulder
  + **M24.12 Other articular cartilage disorders, elbow**
    - M24.121 Other articular cartilage disorders, right elbow
    - M24.122 Other articular cartilage disorders, left elbow
    - M24.129 Other articular cartilage disorders, unspecified elbow
  + **M24.13 Other articular cartilage disorders, wrist**
    - M24.131 Other articular cartilage disorders, right wrist
    - M24.132 Other articular cartilage disorders, left wrist
    - M24.139 Other articular cartilage disorders, unspecified wrist
  + **M24.14 Other articular cartilage disorders, hand**
    - M24.141 Other articular cartilage disorders, right hand
    - M24.142 Other articular cartilage disorders, left hand
    - M24.149 Other articular cartilage disorders, unspecified hand
  + **M24.15 Other articular cartilage disorders, hip**
    - M24.151 Other articular cartilage disorders, right hip
    - M24.152 Other articular cartilage disorders, left hip
    - M24.159 Other articular cartilage disorders, unspecified hip
  + **M24.17 Other articular cartilage disorders, ankle and foot**
    - M24.171 Other articular cartilage disorders, right ankle
    - M24.172 Other articular cartilage disorders, left ankle
    - M24.173 Other articular cartilage disorders, unspecified ankle
    - M24.174 Other articular cartilage disorders, right foot
    - M24.175 Other articular cartilage disorders, left foot
    - M24.176 Other articular cartilage disorders, unspecified foot
  - M24.19 Other articular cartilage disorders, other specified site
+ **M24.2 Disorder of ligament**
  - Instability secondary to old ligament injury
  - Ligamentous laxity NOS
  > **Excludes1:** *familial ligamentous laxity (M35.7)*
  > **Excludes2:** *internal derangement of knee (M23.5-M23.8X9)*
  - M24.20 Disorder of ligament, unspecified site

+ **M24.21 Disorder of ligament, shoulder**
    M24.211 Disorder of ligament, right shoulder
    M24.212 Disorder of ligament, left shoulder
    M24.219 Disorder of ligament, unspecified shoulder
+ **M24.22 Disorder of ligament, elbow**
    M24.221 Disorder of ligament, right elbow
    M24.222 Disorder of ligament, left elbow
    M24.229 Disorder of ligament, unspecified elbow
+ **M24.23 Disorder of ligament, wrist**
    M24.231 Disorder of ligament, right wrist
    M24.232 Disorder of ligament, left wrist
    M24.239 Disorder of ligament, unspecified wrist
+ **M24.24 Disorder of ligament, hand**
    M24.241 Disorder of ligament, right hand
    M24.242 Disorder of ligament, left hand
    M24.249 Disorder of ligament, unspecified hand
+ **M24.25 Disorder of ligament, hip**
    M24.251 Disorder of ligament, right hip
    M24.252 Disorder of ligament, left hip
    M24.259 Disorder of ligament, unspecified hip
+ **M24.27 Disorder of ligament, ankle and foot**
    M24.271 Disorder of ligament, right ankle
    M24.272 Disorder of ligament, left ankle
    M24.273 Disorder of ligament, unspecified ankle
    M24.274 Disorder of ligament, right foot
    M24.275 Disorder of ligament, left foot
    M24.276 Disorder of ligament, unspecifiedfoot
  M24.28 Disorder of ligament, vertebrae
  M24.29 Disorder of ligament, other specified site
+ **M24.3 Pathological dislocation of joint, not elsewhere classified**
    Excludes1: *congenital dislocation or displacement of joint- see congenital malformations and deformities of the musculoskeletal system (Q65-Q79)*
        current injury - see injury of joints and ligaments by body region
        recurrent dislocation of joint (M24.4-)
  M24.30 Pathological dislocation of unspecified joint, not elsewhere classified
+ **M24.31 Pathological dislocation of shoulder, not elsewhere classified**
    M24.311 Pathological dislocation of right shoulder, not elsewhere classified
    M24.312 Pathological dislocation of left shoulder, not elsewhere classified
    M24.319 Pathological dislocation of unspecified shoulder, not elsewhere classified
+ **M24.32 Pathological dislocation of elbow, not elsewhere classified**
    M24.321 Pathological dislocation of right elbow, not elsewhere classified
    M24.322 Pathological dislocation of left elbow, not elsewhere classified
    M24.329 Pathological dislocation of unspecified elbow, not elsewhere classified
+ **M24.33 Pathological dislocation of wrist, not elsewhere classified**
    M24.331 Pathological dislocation of right wrist, not elsewhere classified
    M24.332 Pathological dislocation of left wrist, not elsewhere classified
    M24.339 Pathological dislocation of unspecified wrist, not elsewhere classified
+ **M24.34 Pathological dislocation of hand, not elsewhere classified**
    M24.341 Pathological dislocation of right hand, not elsewhere classified
    M24.342 Pathological dislocation of left hand, not elsewhere classified
    M24.349 Pathological dislocation of unspecified hand, not elsewhere classified
+ **M24.35 Pathological dislocation of hip, not elsewhere classified**
    M24.351 Pathological dislocation of right hip, not elsewhere classified
    M24.352 Pathological dislocation of left hip, not elsewhere classified
    M24.359 Pathological dislocation of unspecified hip, not elsewhere classified

+ **M24.36 Pathological dislocation of knee, not elsewhere classified**
    M24.361 Pathological dislocation of right knee, not elsewhere classified
    M24.362 Pathological dislocation of left knee, not elsewhere classified
    M24.369 Pathological dislocation of unspecified knee, not elsewhere classified
+ **M24.37 Pathological dislocation of ankle and foot, not elsewhere classified**
    M24.371 Pathological dislocation of right ankle, not elsewhere classified
    M24.372 Pathological dislocation of left ankle, not elsewhere classified
    M24.373 Pathological dislocation of unspecified ankle, not elsewhere classified
    M24.374 Pathological dislocation of right foot, not elsewhere classified
    M24.375 Pathological dislocation of left foot, not elsewhere classified
    M24.376 Pathological dislocation of unspecified foot, not elsewhere classified
  M24.39 Pathological dislocation of other specified joint, not elsewhere classified
+ **M24.4 Recurrent dislocation of joint**
    Recurrent subluxation of joint
    Excludes2: *recurrent dislocation of patella (M22.0-M22.1)*
        recurrent vertebral dislocation (M43.3-, M43.4, M43.5-)
  M24.40 Recurrent dislocation, unspecified joint
+ **M24.41 Recurrent dislocation, shoulder**
    M24.411 Recurrent dislocation, right shoulder
    M24.412 Recurrent dislocation, left shoulder
    M24.419 Recurrent dislocation, unspecified shoulder
+ **M24.42 Recurrent dislocation, elbow**
    M24.421 Recurrent dislocation, right elbow
    M24.422 Recurrent dislocation, left elbow
    M24.429 Recurrent dislocation, unspecified elbow
+ **M24.43 Recurrent dislocation, wrist**
    M24.431 Recurrent dislocation, right wrist
    M24.432 Recurrent dislocation, left wrist
    M24.439 Recurrent dislocation, unspecified wrist
+ **M24.44 Recurrent dislocation, hand and finger(s)**
    M24.441 Recurrent dislocation, right hand
    M24.442 Recurrent dislocation, left hand
    M24.443 Recurrent dislocation, unspecified hand
    M24.444 Recurrent dislocation, right finger
    M24.445 Recurrent dislocation, left finger
    M24.446 Recurrent dislocation, unspecified finger
+ **M24.45 Recurrent dislocation, hip**
    M24.451 Recurrent dislocation, right hip
    M24.452 Recurrent dislocation, left hip
    M24.459 Recurrent dislocation, unspecified hip
+ **M24.46 Recurrent dislocation, knee**
    M24.461 Recurrent dislocation, right knee
    M24.462 Recurrent dislocation, left knee
    M24.469 Recurrent dislocation, unspecified knee
+ **M24.47 Recurrent dislocation, ankle, foot and toes**
    M24.471 Recurrent dislocation, right ankle
    M24.472 Recurrent dislocation, left ankle
    M24.473 Recurrent dislocation, unspecified ankle
    M24.474 Recurrent dislocation, right foot
    M24.475 Recurrent dislocation, left foot
    M24.476 Recurrent dislocation, unspecified foot
    M24.477 Recurrent dislocation, right toe(s)
    M24.478 Recurrent dislocation, left toe(s)
    M24.479 Recurrent dislocation, unspecified toe(s)
  M24.49 Recurrent dislocation, other specified joint
+ **M24.5 Contracture of joint**
    Excludes1: *contracture of muscle without contracture of joint (M62.4-)*
        contracture of tendon (sheath) without contracture of joint (M62.4-)
        Dupuytren's contracture (M72.0)
    Excludes2: *acquired deformities of limbs (M20-M21)*
    AHA CC: 2Q, 2016. 6
  M24.50 Contracture, unspecified joint
+ **M24.51 Contracture, shoulder**

+, +7th, X + 7th   ● Newborn   ● Pediatric   ● Maternity   ● Adult   ♀ Female   ♂ Male   Manifestation   Unacceptable PDX   HCC   CC   MCC   HAC

M24.511 Contracture, right shoulder
M24.512 Contracture, left shoulder
M24.519 Contracture, unspecified shoulder
+ M24.52 Contracture, elbow
M24.521 Contracture, right elbow
M24.522 Contracture, left elbow
M24.529 Contracture, unspecified elbow
+ M24.53 Contracture, wrist
M24.531 Contracture, right wrist
M24.532 Contracture, left wrist
M24.539 Contracture, unspecified wrist
+ M24.54 Contracture, hand
M24.541 Contracture, right hand
M24.542 Contracture, left hand
M24.549 Contracture, unspecified hand
+ M24.55 Contracture, hip
M24.551 Contracture, right hip
M24.552 Contracture, left hip
M24.559 Contracture, unspecified hip
+ M24.56 Contracture, knee
M24.561 Contracture, right knee
M24.562 Contracture, left knee
M24.569 Contracture, unspecified knee
+ M24.57 Contracture, ankle and foot
M24.571 Contracture, right ankle
M24.572 Contracture, left ankle
M24.573 Contracture, unspecified ankle
M24.574 Contracture, right foot
M24.575 Contracture, left foot
M24.576 Contracture, unspecified foot
M24.59 Contracture, other specified joint
+ M24.6 Ankylosis of joint
Excludes1: *stiffness of joint without ankylosis (M25.6-)*
Excludes2: *spine (M43.2-)*
M24.60 Ankylosis, unspecified joint
+ M24.61 Ankylosis, shoulder
M24.611 Ankylosis, right shoulder
M24.612 Ankylosis, left shoulder
M24.619 Ankylosis, unspecified shoulder
+ M24.62 Ankylosis, elbow
M24.621 Ankylosis, right elbow
M24.622 Ankylosis, left elbow
M24.629 Ankylosis, unspecified elbow
+ M24.63 Ankylosis, wrist
M24.631 Ankylosis, right wrist
M24.632 Ankylosis, left wrist
M24.639 Ankylosis, unspecified wrist
+ M24.64 Ankylosis, hand
M24.641 Ankylosis, right hand
M24.642 Ankylosis, left hand
M24.649 Ankylosis, unspecified hand
+ M24.65 Ankylosis, hip
M24.651 Ankylosis, right hip
M24.652 Ankylosis, left hip
M24.659 Ankylosis, unspecified hip
+ M24.66 Ankylosis, knee
M24.661 Ankylosis, right knee
M24.662 Ankylosis, left knee
M24.669 Ankylosis, unspecified knee
+ M24.67 Ankylosis, ankle and foot
M24.671 Ankylosis, right ankle
M24.672 Ankylosis, left ankle
M24.673 Ankylosis, unspecified ankle
M24.674 Ankylosis, right foot
M24.675 Ankylosis, left foot
M24.676 Ankylosis, unspecified foot
M24.69 Ankylosis, other specified joint
M24.7 Protrusio acetabuli
+ M24.8 Other specific joint derangements, not elsewhere classified
Excludes2: *iliotibial band syndrome (M76.3)*
M24.80 Other specific joint derangements of unspecified joint, not elsewhere classified
+ M24.81 Other specific joint derangements of shoulder, not elsewhere classified
M24.811 Other specific joint derangements of right shoulder, not elsewhere classified
M24.812 Other specific joint derangements of left shoulder, not elsewhere classified
M24.819 Other specific joint derangements of unspecified shoulder, not elsewhere classified

+ M24.82 Other specific joint derangements of elbow, not elsewhere classified
M24.821 Other specific joint derangements of right elbow, not elsewhere classified
M24.822 Other specific joint derangements of left elbow, not elsewhere classified
M24.829 Other specific joint derangements of unspecified elbow, not elsewhere classified
+ M24.83 Other specific joint derangements of wrist, not elsewhere classified
M24.831 Other specific joint derangements of right wrist, not elsewhere classified
M24.832 Other specific joint derangements of left wrist, not elsewhere classified
M24.839 Other specific joint derangements of unspecified wrist, not elsewhere classified
+ M24.84 Other specific joint derangements of hand, not elsewhere classified
M24.841 Other specific joint derangements of right hand, not elsewhere classified
M24.842 Other specific joint derangements of left hand, not elsewhere classified
M24.849 Other specific joint derangements of unspecified hand, not elsewhere classified
+ M24.85 Other specific joint derangements of hip, not elsewhere classified
Irritable hip
M24.851 Other specific joint derangements of right hip, not elsewhere classified
M24.852 Other specific joint derangements of left hip, not elsewhere classified
M24.859 Other specific joint derangements of unspecified hip, not elsewhere classified
+ M24.87 Other specific joint derangements of ankle and foot, not elsewhere classified
M24.871 Other specific joint derangements of right ankle, not elsewhere classified
M24.872 Other specific joint derangements of left ankle, not elsewhere classified
M24.873 Other specific joint derangements of unspecified ankle, not elsewhere classified
M24.874 Other specific joint derangements of right foot, not elsewhere classified
M24.875 Other specific joint derangements left foot, not elsewhere classified
M24.876 Other specific joint derangements of unspecified foot, not elsewhere classified
M24.89 Other specific joint derangement of other specified joint, not elsewhere classified
M24.9 Joint derangement, unspecified

M25 Other joint disorder, not elsewhere classified
Excludes2: *abnormality of gait and mobility (R26.-)*
acquired deformities of limb (M20-M21)
calcification of bursa (M71.4-)
calcification of shoulder (joint) (M75.3)
calcification of tendon (M65.2-)
difficulty in walking (R26.2)
temporomandibular joint disorder (M26.6-)
+ M25.0 Hemarthrosis
Excludes1: *current injury - see injury of joint by body region*
hemophilic arthropathy (M36.2)
CC M25.00 Hemarthrosis, unspecified joint
+ M25.01 Hemarthrosis, shoulder
CC M25.011 Hemarthrosis, right shoulder
CC M25.012 Hemarthrosis, left shoulder
CC M25.019 Hemarthrosis, unspecified shoulder
+ M25.02 Hemarthrosis, elbow
CC M25.021 Hemarthrosis, right elbow
CC M25.022 Hemarthrosis, left elbow
CC M25.029 Hemarthrosis, unspecified elbow
+ M25.03 Hemarthrosis, wrist
CC M25.031 Hemarthrosis, right wrist
CC M25.032 Hemarthrosis, left wrist
CC M25.039 Hemarthrosis, unspecified wrist
+ M25.04 Hemarthrosis, hand
CC M25.041 Hemarthrosis, right hand
CC M25.042 Hemarthrosis, left hand
CC M25.049 Hemarthrosis, unspecified hand

+, +7th, X + 7th   ● Newborn   ● Pediatric   ● Maternity   ● Adult   ♀ Female   ♂ Male   Manifestation   Unacceptable PDX   HCC   CC   MCC   HAC

+ M25.05 Hemarthrosis, hip
    CC M25.051 Hemarthrosis, right hip
    CC M25.052 Hemarthrosis, left hip
    CC M25.059 Hemarthrosis, unspecified hip
+ M25.06 Hemarthrosis, knee
    CC M25.061 Hemarthrosis, right knee
    CC M25.062 Hemarthrosis, left knee
    CC M25.069 Hemarthrosis, unspecified knee
+ M25.07 Hemarthrosis, ankle and foot
    CC M25.071 Hemarthrosis, right ankle
    CC M25.072 Hemarthrosis, left ankle
    CC M25.073 Hemarthrosis, unspecified ankle
    CC M25.074 Hemarthrosis, right foot
    CC M25.075 Hemarthrosis, left foot
    CC M25.076 Hemarthrosis, unspecified foot
CC M25.08 Hemarthrosis, other specified site
        Hemarthrosis, vertebrae
+ M25.1 Fistula of joint
    M25.10 Fistula, unspecified joint
+ M25.11 Fistula, shoulder
    M25.111 Fistula, right shoulder
    M25.112 Fistula, left shoulder
    M25.119 Fistula, unspecified shoulder
+ M25.12 Fistula, elbow
    M25.121 Fistula, right elbow
    M25.122 Fistula, left elbow
    M25.129 Fistula, unspecified elbow
+ M25.13 Fistula, wrist
    M25.131 Fistula, right wrist
    M25.132 Fistula, left wrist
    M25.139 Fistula, unspecified wrist
+ M25.14 Fistula, hand
    M25.141 Fistula, right hand
    M25.142 Fistula, left hand
    M25.149 Fistula, unspecified hand
+ M25.15 Fistula, hip
    M25.151 Fistula, right hip
    M25.152 Fistula, left hip
    M25.159 Fistula, unspecified hip
+ M25.16 Fistula, knee
    M25.161 Fistula, right knee
    M25.162 Fistula, left knee
    M25.169 Fistula, unspecified knee
+ M25.17 Fistula, ankle and foot
    M25.171 Fistula, right ankle
    M25.172 Fistula, left ankle
    M25.173 Fistula, unspecified ankle
    M25.174 Fistula, right foot
    M25.175 Fistula, left foot
    M25.176 Fistula, unspecified foot
    M25.18 Fistula, other specified site
        Fistula, vertebrae
+ M25.2 Flail joint
    M25.20 Flail joint, unspecified joint
+ M25.21 Flail joint, shoulder
    M25.211 Flail joint, right shoulder
    M25.212 Flail joint, left shoulder
    M25.219 Flail joint, unspecified shoulder
+ M25.22 Flail joint, elbow
    M25.221 Flail joint, right elbow
    M25.222 Flail joint, left elbow
    M25.229 Flail joint, unspecified elbow
+ M25.23 Flail joint, wrist
    M25.231 Flail joint, right wrist
    M25.232 Flail joint, left wrist
    M25.239 Flail joint, unspecified wrist
+ M25.24 Flail joint, hand
    M25.241 Flail joint, right hand
    M25.242 Flail joint, left hand
    M25.249 Flail joint, unspecified hand
+ M25.25 Flail joint, hip
    M25.251 Flail joint, right hip
    M25.252 Flail joint, left hip
    M25.259 Flail joint, unspecified hip
+ M25.26 Flail joint, knee
    M25.261 Flail joint, right knee
    M25.262 Flail joint, left knee
    M25.269 Flail joint, unspecified knee

+ M25.27 Flail joint, ankle and foot
    M25.271 Flail joint, right ankle and foot
    M25.272 Flail joint, left ankle and foot
    M25.279 Flail joint, unspecified ankle and foot
    M25.28 Flail joint, other site
+ M25.3 Other instability of joint
    Excludes1: *instability of joint secondary to old ligament*
            injury (M24.2-)
            instability of joint secondary to removal of joint
            prosthesis (M96.8-)
    Excludes2: *spinal instabilities (M53.2-)*
    M25.30 Other instability, unspecified joint
+ M25.31 Other instability, shoulder
    M25.311 Other instability, right shoulder
    M25.312 Other instability, left shoulder
    M25.319 Other instability, unspecified
        shoulder
+ M25.32 Other instability, elbow
    M25.321 Other instability, right elbow
    M25.322 Other instability, left elbow
    M25.329 Other instability, unspecified elbow
+ M25.33 Other instability, wrist
    M25.331 Other instability, right wrist
    M25.332 Other instability, left wrist
    M25.339 Other instability, unspecified wrist
+ M25.34 Other instability, hand
    M25.341 Other instability, right hand
    M25.342 Other instability, left hand
    M25.349 Other instability, unspecified hand
+ M25.35 Other instability, hip
    M25.351 Other instability, right hip
    M25.352 Other instability, left hip
    M25.359 Other instability, unspecified hip
+ M25.36 Other instability, knee
    M25.361 Other instability, right knee
    M25.362 Other instability, left knee
    M25.369 Other instability, unspecified knee
+ M25.37 Other instability, ankle and foot
    M25.371 Other instability, right ankle
    M25.372 Other instability, left ankle
    M25.373 Other instability, unspecified ankle
    M25.374 Other instability, right foot
    M25.375 Other instability, left foot
    M25.376 Other instability, unspecified foot
    M25.39 Other instability, other specified joint
+ M25.4 Effusion of joint
    Excludes1: *hydrarthrosis in yaws (A66.6)*
            intermittent hydrarthrosis (M12.4-)
            other infective (teno)synovitis (M65.1-)
    M25.40 Effusion, unspecified joint
+ M25.41 Effusion, shoulder
    M25.411 Effusion, right shoulder
    M25.412 Effusion, left shoulder
    M25.419 Effusion, unspecified shoulder
+ M25.42 Effusion, elbow
    M25.421 Effusion, right elbow
    M25.422 Effusion, left elbow
    M25.429 Effusion, unspecified elbow
+ M25.43 Effusion, wrist
    M25.431 Effusion, right wrist
    M25.432 Effusion, left wrist
    M25.439 Effusion, unspecified wrist
+ M25.44 Effusion, hand
    M25.441 Effusion, right hand
    M25.442 Effusion, left hand
    M25.449 Effusion, unspecified hand
+ M25.45 Effusion, hip
    M25.451 Effusion, right hip
    M25.452 Effusion, left hip
    M25.459 Effusion, unspecified hip
+ M25.46 Effusion, knee
    M25.461 Effusion, right knee
    M25.462 Effusion, left knee
    M25.469 Effusion, unspecified knee
+ M25.47 Effusion, ankle and foot
    M25.471 Effusion, right ankle
    M25.472 Effusion, left ankle
    M25.473 Effusion, unspecified ankle
    M25.474 Effusion, right foot

M25.475 Effusion, left foot
M25.476 Effusion, unspecified foot
M25.48 Effusion, other site
+ M25.5 Pain in joint
> *Excludes2:* *pain in hand (M79.64-)*
> *pain in fingers (M79.64-)*
> *pain in foot (M79.67-)*
> *pain in limb (M79.6-)*
> *pain in toes (M79.67-)*
> *AHA CC: 4Q, 2016, 38*

M25.50 Pain in unspecified joint
+ M25.51 Pain in shoulder
M25.511 Pain in right shoulder
M25.512 Pain in left shoulder
M25.519 Pain in unspecified shoulder
+ M25.52 Pain in elbow
M25.521 Pain in right elbow
M25.522 Pain in left elbow
M25.529 Pain in unspecified elbow
+ M25.53 Pain in wrist
M25.531 Pain in right wrist
M25.532 Pain in left wrist
M25.539 Pain in unspecified wrist
+ M25.54 Pain in joints of hand
M25.541 Pain in joints of right hand
M25.542 Pain in joints of left hand
M25.549 Pain in joints of unspecified hand
> Pain in joints of hand NOS
+ M25.55 Pain in hip
M25.551 Pain in right hip
M25.552 Pain in left hip
M25.559 Pain in unspecified hip
+ M25.56 Pain in knee
M25.561 Pain in right knee
M25.562 Pain in left knee
M25.569 Pain in unspecified knee
+ M25.57 Pain in ankle and joints of foot
M25.571 Pain in right ankle and joints of right foot
M25.572 Pain in left ankle and joints of left foot
M25.579 Pain in unspecified ankle and joints of unspecified foot
M25.59 Pain in other specified joint
+ M25.6 Stiffness of joint, not elsewhere classified
> *Excludes1:* *ankylosis of joint (M24.6-)*
> *contracture of joint (M24.5-)*

M25.60 Stiffness of unspecified joint, not elsewhere classified
+ M25.61 Stiffness of shoulder, not elsewhere classified
M25.611 Stiffness of right shoulder, not elsewhere classified
M25.612 Stiffness of left shoulder, not elsewhere classified
M25.619 Stiffness of unspecified shoulder, not elsewhere classified
+ M25.62 Stiffness of elbow, not elsewhere classified
M25.621 Stiffness of right elbow, not elsewhere classified
M25.622 Stiffness of left elbow, not elsewhere classified
M25.629 Stiffness of unspecified elbow, not elsewhere classified
+ M25.63 Stiffness of wrist, not elsewhere classified
M25.631 Stiffness of right wrist, not elsewhere classified
M25.632 Stiffness of left wrist, not elsewhere classified
M25.639 Stiffness of unspecified wrist, not elsewhere classified
+ M25.64 Stiffness of hand, not elsewhere classified
M25.641 Stiffness of right hand, not elsewhere classified
M25.642 Stiffness of left hand, not elsewhere classified
M25.649 Stiffness of unspecified hand, not elsewhere classified
+ M25.65 Stiffness of hip, not elsewhere classified
M25.651 Stiffness of right hip, not elsewhere classified

M25.652 Stiffness of left hip, not elsewhere classified
M25.659 Stiffness of unspecified hip, not elsewhere classified
+ M25.66 Stiffness of knee, not elsewhere classified
M25.661 Stiffness of right knee, not elsewhere classified
M25.662 Stiffness of left knee, not elsewhere classified
M25.669 Stiffness of unspecified knee, not elsewhere classified
+ M25.67 Stiffness of ankle and foot, not elsewhere classified
M25.671 Stiffness of right ankle, not elsewhere classified
M25.672 Stiffness of left ankle, not elsewhere classified
M25.673 Stiffness of unspecified ankle, not elsewhere classified
M25.674 Stiffness of right foot, not elsewhere classified
M25.675 Stiffness of left foot, not elsewhere classified
M25.676 Stiffness of unspecified foot, not elsewhere classified
M25.69 Stiffness of other specified joint, not elsewhere classified
+ M25.7 Osteophyte
M25.70 Osteophyte, unspecified joint
+ M25.71 Osteophyte, shoulder
M25.711 Osteophyte, right shoulder
M25.712 Osteophyte, left shoulder
M25.719 Osteophyte, unspecified shoulder
+ M25.72 Osteophyte, elbow
M25.721 Osteophyte, right elbow
M25.722 Osteophyte, left elbow
M25.729 Osteophyte, unspecified elbow
+ M25.73 Osteophyte, wrist
M25.731 Osteophyte, right wrist
M25.732 Osteophyte, left wrist
M25.739 Osteophyte, unspecified wrist
+ M25.74 Osteophyte, hand
M25.741 Osteophyte, right hand
M25.742 Osteophyte, left hand
M25.749 Osteophyte, unspecified hand
+ M25.75 Osteophyte, hip
M25.751 Osteophyte, right hip
M25.752 Osteophyte, left hip
M25.759 Osteophyte, unspecified hip
+ M25.76 Osteophyte, knee
M25.761 Osteophyte, right knee
M25.762 Osteophyte, left knee
M25.769 Osteophyte, unspecified knee
+ M25.77 Osteophyte, ankle and foot
M25.771 Osteophyte, right ankle
M25.772 Osteophyte, left ankle
M25.773 Osteophyte, unspecified ankle
M25.774 Osteophyte, right foot
M25.775 Osteophyte, left foot
M25.776 Osteophyte, unspecified foot
M25.78 Osteophyte, vertebrae
+ M25.8 Other specified joint disorders
M25.80 Other specified joint disorders, unspecified joint
+ M25.81 Other specified joint disorders, shoulder
M25.811 Other specified joint disorders, right shoulder
M25.812 Other specified joint disorders, left shoulder
M25.819 Other specified joint disorders, unspecified shoulder
+ M25.82 Other specified joint disorders, elbow
M25.821 Other specified joint disorders, right elbow
M25.822 Other specified joint disorders, left elbow
M25.829 Other specified joint disorders, unspecified elbow
+ M25.83 Other specified joint disorders, wrist
M25.831 Other specified joint disorders, right wrist

M25.832 Other specified joint disorders, left wrist
M25.839 Other specified joint disorders, unspecified wrist
+ M25.84 Other specified joint disorders, hand
M25.841 Other specified joint disorders, right hand
M25.842 Other specified joint disorders, left hand
M25.849 Other specified joint disorders, unspecified hand
+ M25.85 Other specified joint disorders, hip
M25.851 Other specified joint disorders, right hip
M25.852 Other specified joint disorders, left hip
AHA CC: 4Q, 2014, 25
M25.859 Other specified joint disorders, unspecified hip
+ M25.86 Other specified joint disorders, knee
M25.861 Other specified joint disorders, right knee
M25.862 Other specified joint disorders, left knee
M25.869 Other specified joint disorders, unspecified knee
+ M25.87 Other specified joint disorders, ankle and foot
M25.871 Other specified joint disorders, right ankle and foot
M25.872 Other specified joint disorders, left ankle and foot
M25.879 Other specified joint disorders, unspecified ankle and foot
M25.9 Joint disorder, unspecified

Dentofacial anomalies [including malocclusion] and other disorders of jaw (M26-M27)

Excludes1: *hemifacial atrophy or hypertrophy (Q67.4)*
unilateral condylar hyperplasia or hypoplasia (M27.8)

M26 Dentofacial anomalies [including malocclusion]
+ M26.0 Major anomalies of jaw size
Excludes1: *acromegaly (E22.0)*
Robin's syndrome (Q87.0)
M26.00 Unspecified anomaly of jaw size
M26.01 Maxillary hyperplasia
M26.02 Maxillary hypoplasia
AHA CC: 3Q, 2014, 23-24
M26.03 Mandibular hyperplasia
M26.04 Mandibular hypoplasia
M26.05 Macrogenia
M26.06 Microgenia
M26.07 Excessive tuberosity of jaw
Entire maxillary tuberosity
M26.09 Other specified anomalies of jaw size
+ M26.1 Anomalies of jaw-cranial base relationship
M26.10 Unspecified anomaly of jaw-cranial base relationship
M26.11 Maxillary asymmetry
M26.12 Other jaw asymmetry
M26.19 Other specified anomalies of jaw-cranial base relationship
AHA CC: 1Q, 2020, 21
+ M26.2 Anomalies of dental arch relationship
M26.20 Unspecified anomaly of dental arch relationship
+ M26.21 Malocclusion, Angle's class
M26.211 Malocclusion, Angle's class I
Neutro-occlusion
M26.212 Malocclusion, Angle's class II
Disto-occlusion Division I
Disto-occlusion Division II
M26.213 Malocclusion, Angle's class III
Mesio-occlusion
M26.219 Malocclusion, Angle's class, unspecified
+ M26.22 Open occlusal relationship
M26.220 Open anterior occlusal relationship
Anterior open bite
M26.221 Open posterior occlusal relationship
Posterior open bite
M26.23 Excessive horizontal overlap
Excessive horizontal overjet
M26.24 Reverse articulation
Crossbite (anterior) (posterior)

M26.25 Anomalies of interarch distance
M26.29 Other anomalies of dental arch relationship
Midline deviation of dental arch
Overbite (excessive) deep
Overbite (excessive) horizontal
Overbite (excessive) vertical
Posterior lingual occlusion of mandibular teeth
+ M26.3 Anomalies of tooth position of fully erupted tooth or teeth
Excludes2: *embedded and impacted teeth (K01.-)*
M26.30 Unspecified anomaly of tooth position of fully erupted tooth or teeth
Abnormal spacing of fully erupted tooth or teeth NOS
Displacement of fully erupted tooth or teeth NOS
Transposition of fully erupted tooth or teeth NOS
M26.31 Crowding of fully erupted teeth
M26.32 Excessive spacing of fully erupted teeth
Diastema of fully erupted tooth or teeth NOS
M26.33 Horizontal displacement of fully erupted tooth or teeth
Tipped tooth or teeth
Tipping of fully erupted tooth
M26.34 Vertical displacement of fully erupted tooth or teeth
Extruded tooth
Infraeruption of tooth or teeth
Supraeruption of tooth or teeth
M26.35 Rotation of fully erupted tooth or teeth
M26.36 Insufficient interocclusal distance of fully erupted teeth (ridge)
Lack of adequate intermaxillary vertical dimension of fully erupted teeth
M26.37 Excessive interocclusal distance of fully erupted teeth
Excessive intermaxillary vertical dimension of fully erupted teeth
Loss of occlusal vertical dimension of fully erupted teeth
M26.39 Other anomalies of tooth position of fully erupted tooth or teeth
M26.4 Malocclusion, unspecified
+ M26.5 Dentofacial functional abnormalities
Excludes1: *bruxism (F45.8)*
teeth-grinding NOS (F45.8)
M26.50 Dentofacial functional abnormalities, unspecified
M26.51 Abnormal jaw closure
M26.52 Limited mandibular range of motion
M26.53 Deviation in opening and closing of the mandible
M26.54 Insufficient anterior guidance
Insufficient anterior occlusal guidance
M26.55 Centric occlusion maximum intercuspation discrepancy
Excludes1: *centric occlusion NOS (M26.59)*
M26.56 Non-working side interference
Balancing side interference
M26.57 Lack of posterior occlusal support
M26.59 Other dentofacial functional abnormalities
Centric occlusion (of teeth) NOS
Malocclusion due to abnormal swallowing
Malocclusion due to mouth breathing
Malocclusion due to tongue, lip or finger habits
+ M26.6 Temporomandibular joint disorders
Excludes2: *current temporomandibular joint dislocation (S03.0)*
current temporomandibular joint sprain (S03.4)
AHA CC: 4Q, 2016, 38-39
+ M26.60 Temporomandibular joint disorder, unspecified
M26.601 Right temporomandibular joint disorder, unspecified
M26.602 Left temporomandibular joint disorder, unspecified
M26.603 Bilateral temporomandibular joint disorder, unspecified
M26.609 Unspecified temporomandibular joint disorder, unspecified side
Temporomandibular joint disorder NOS
+ M26.61 Adhesions and ankylosis of temporomandibular joint
M26.611 Adhesions and ankylosis of right temporomandibular joint

+, +7th, X + 7th   ● Newborn   ● Pediatric   ● Maternity   ● Adult   ♀ Female   ♂ Male   Manifestation   Unacceptable PDX   HCC   CC   MCC   HAC

M26.612 **Adhesions and ankylosis of left temporomandibular joint**
M26.613 **Adhesions and ankylosis of bilateral temporomandibular joint**
M26.619 **Adhesions and ankylosis of temporomandibular joint, unspecified side**

+ M26.62 **Arthralgia of temporomandibular joint**
M26.621 **Arthralgia of right temporomandibular joint**
M26.622 **Arthralgia of left temporomandibular joint**
M26.623 **Arthralgia of bilateral temporomandibular joint**
M26.629 **Arthralgia of temporomandibular joint, unspecified side**

+ M26.63 **Articular disc disorder of temporomandibular joint**
M26.631 **Articular disc disorder of right temporomandibular joint**
M26.632 **Articular disc disorder of left temporomandibular joint**
M26.633 **Articular disc disorder of bilateral temporomandibular joint**
M26.639 **Articular disc disorder of temporomandibular joint, unspecified side**

+ M26.64 **Arthritis of temporomandibular joint**
M26.641 **Arthritis of right temporomandibular joint**
M26.642 **Arthritis of left temporomandibular joint**
M26.643 **Arthritis of bilateral temporomandibular joint**
M26.649 **Arthritis of unspecified temporomandibular joint**

+ M26.65 **Arthropathy of temporomandibular joing**
M26.651 **Arthropathy of right tcmporomandibular joint**
M26.652 **Arthropathy of left temporomandibular joint**
M26.653 **Arthropathy of bilateral temporomandibular joint**
M26.659 **Arthropathy of unspecified temporomandibular joint**

M26.69 **Other specified disorders of temporomandibular joint**

+ M26.7 **Dental alveolar anomalies**
M26.70 **Unspecified alveolar anomaly**
M26.71 **Alveolar maxillary hyperplasia**
M26.72 **Alveolar mandibular hyperplasia**
M26.73 **Alveolar maxillary hypoplasia**
M26.74 **Alveolar mandibular hypoplasia**
M26.79 **Other specified alveolar anomalies**

+ M26.8 **Other dentofacial anomalies**
M26.81 **Anterior soft tissue impingement**
Anterior soft tissue impingement on teeth
M26.82 **Posterior soft tissue impingement**
Posterior soft tissue impingement on teeth
M26.89 **Other dentofacial anomalies**
M26.9 **Dentofacial anomaly, unspecified**

M27 **Other diseases of jaws**

M27.0 **Developmental disorders of jaws**
Latent bone cyst of jaw
Stafne's cyst
Torus mandibularis
Torus palatinus
M27.1 **Giant cell granuloma, central**
Giant cell granuloma NOS
Excludes1: peripheral giant cell granuloma (K06.8)
M27.2 **Inflammatory conditions of jaws**
Osteitis of jaw(s)
Osteomyelitis (neonatal) jaw(s)
Osteoradionecrosis jaw(s)
Periostitis jaw(s)
Sequestrum of jaw bone
Use additional code (W88-W90, X39.0) to identify radiation, if radiation-induced
Excludes2: osteonecrosis of jaw due to drug (M87.180)

M27.3 **Alveolitis of jaws**
Alveolar osteitis
Dry socket
+ M27.4 **Other and unspecified cysts of jaw**
Excludes1: cysts of oral region (K09.-)
latent bone cyst of jaw (M27.0)
Stafne's cyst (M27.0)
M27.40 **Unspecified cyst of jaw**
Cyst of jaw NOS
M27.49 **Other cysts of jaw**
Aneurysmal cyst of jaw
Hemorrhagic cyst of jaw
Traumatic cyst of jaw
+ M27.5 **Periradicular pathology associated with previous endodontic treatment**
M27.51 **Perforation of root canal space due to endodontic treatment**
M27.52 **Endodontic overfill**
M27.53 **Endodontic underfill**
M27.59 **Other periradicular pathology associated with previous endodontic treatment**
+ M27.6 **Endosseous dental implant failure**
M27.61 **Osseointegration failure of dental implant**
Hemorrhagic complications of dental implant placement
Iatrogenic osseointegration failure of dental implant
Osseointegration failure of dental implant due to complications of systemic disease
Osseointegration failure of dental implant due to poor bone quality
Pre-integration failure of dental implant NOS
Pre-osseointegration failure of dental implant
M27.62 **Post-osseointegration biological failure of dental implant**
Failure of dental implant due to lack of attached gingiva
Failure of dental implant due to occlusal trauma (caused by poor prosthetic design)
Failure of dental implant due to parafunctional habits
Failure of dental implant due to periodontal infection (peri-implantitis)
Failure of dental implant due to poor oral hygiene
Iatrogenic post-osseointegration failure of dental implant
Post-osseointegration failure of dental implant due to complications of systemic disease
M27.63 **Post-osseointegration mechanical failure of dental implant**
Failure of dental prosthesis causing loss of dental implant
Fracture of dental implant
Excludes2: cracked tooth (K03.81)
fractured dental restorative material with loss of material (K08.531)
fractured dental restorative material without loss of material (K08.530)
fractured tooth (S02.5)
M27.69 **Other endosseous dental implant failure**
Dental implant failure NOS
M27.8 **Other specified diseases of jaws**
Cherubism
Exostosis
Fibrous dysplasia
Unilateral condylar hyperplasia
Unilateral condylar hypoplasia
Excludes1: jaw pain (R68.84)
M27.9 **Disease of jaws, unspecified**

Systemic connective tissue disorders (M30-M36)

Includes: autoimmune disease NOS
collagen (vascular) disease NOS
systemic autoimmune disease
systemic collagen (vascular) disease

Excludes1: autoimmune disease, single organ or single cell-type -code to relevant condition category

M30 **Polyarteritis nodosa and related conditions**
Excludes1: microscopic polyarteritis (M31.7)

+, +7th, X + 7th　● Newborn　● Pediatric　● Maternity　● Adult　♀ Female　♂ Male　Manifestation　Unacceptable PDX　HCC　CC　MCC　HAC

CC **M30.0** Polyarteritis nodosa
CC **M30.1** Polyarteritis with lung involvement [Churg-Strauss]
    Allergic granulomatous angiitis
    Eosinophilic granulomatosis with polyangiitis [EGPA]
CC **M30.2** Juvenile polyarteritis
CC **M30.3** Mucocutaneous lymph node syndrome [Kawasaki]
CC **M30.8** Other conditions related to polyarteritis nodosa
    Polyangiitis overlap syndrome

M31 Other necrotizing vasculopathies

CC **M31.0** Hypersensitivity angiitis
    Goodpasture's syndrome
MCC **M31.1** Thrombotic microangiopathy
    Thrombotic thrombocytopenic purpura
CC **M31.2** Lethal midline granuloma
+ **M31.3** Wegener's granulomatosis
    Granulomatosis with polyangiitis
    Necrotizing respiratory granulomatosis
    CC **M31.30** Wegener's granulomatosis without renal
        involvement
        Wegener's granulomatosis NOS
    CC **M31.31** Wegener's granulomatosis with renal
        involvement
CC **M31.4** Aortic arch syndrome [Takayasu]
M31.5 Giant cell arteritis with polymyalgia rheumatica
M31.6 Other giant cell arteritis
CC **M31.7** Microscopic polyangiitis
    Microscopic polyarteritis
    Excludes1: *polyarteritis nodosa (M30.0)*
CC **M31.8** Other specified necrotizing vasculopathies
    Hypocomplementemic vasculitis
    Septic vasculitis
CC **M31.9** Necrotizing vasculopathy, unspecified

M32 Systemic lupus erythematosus (SLE)

    Excludes1: *lupus erythematosus (discoid) (NOS) (L93.0)*
    AHA CC: 3Q, 2018, 14-15
M32.0 Drug-induced systemic lupus erythematosus
    Use additional code for adverse effect, if applicable, to
    identify drug (T36-T50 with fifth or sixth character 5)
+ **M32.1** Systemic lupus erythematosus with organ or system
    involvement
    M32.10 Systemic lupus erythematosus, organ or system
        involvement unspecified
    CC **M32.11** Endocarditis in systemic lupus erythematosus
        Libman-Sacks disease
    CC **M32.12** Pericarditis in systemic lupus erythematosus
        Lupus pericarditis
    M32.13 Lung involvement in systemic lupus
        erythematosus
        Pleural effusion due to systemic lupus
        erythematosus
    M32.14 Glomerular disease in systemic lupus
        erythematosus
        Lupus renal disease NOS
        AHA CC: 4Q, 2013, 125
    M32.15 Tubulo-interstitial nephropathy in systemic lupus
        erythematosus
    M32.19 Other organ or system involvement in systemic
        lupus erythematosus
M32.8 Other forms of systemic lupus erythematosus
M32.9 Systemic lupus erythematosus, unspecified
    SLE NOS
    Systemic lupus erythematosus NOS
    Systemic lupus erythematosus without organ involvement
    AHA CC: 3Q, 2018, 14-15

M33 Dermatopolymyositis

+ **M33.0** Juvenile dermatomyositis
    CC **M33.00** Juvenile dermatomyositis, organ involvement
        unspecified
    CC **M33.01** Juvenile dermatomyositis with respiratory
        involvement
    CC **M33.02** Juvenile dermatomyositis with myopathy
    CC **M33.03** Juvenile dermatomyositis without myopathy
        AHA CC: 4Q, 2017, 18
    CC **M33.09** Juvenile dermatomyositis with other organ
        involvement
+ **M33.1** Other dermatomyositis
    Adult dematomyositis

CC **M33.10** Other dermatomyositis, organ involvement
    unspecified
CC **M33.11** Other dermatomyositis with respiratory
    involvement
CC **M33.12** Other dermatomyositis with myopathy
CC **M33.13** Other dermatomyositis without myopathy
    Dermatomyositis NOS
    AHA CC: 4Q, 2017, 18
CC **M33.19** Other dermatomyositis with other organ
    involvement
+ **M33.2** Polymyositis
    CC **M33.20** Polymyositis, organ involvement unspecified
    CC **M33.21** Polymyositis with respiratory involvement
    CC **M33.22** Polymyositis with myopathy
    CC **M33.29** Polymyositis with other organ involvement
+ **M33.9** Dermatopolymyositis, unspecified
    CC **M33.90** Dermatopolymyositis, unspecified, organ
        involvement unspecified
    CC **M33.91** Dermatopolymyositis, unspecified with
        respiratory involvement
    CC **M33.92** Dermatopolymyositis, unspecified with myopathy
    CC **M33.93** Dermatopolymyositis, unspecified without
        myopathy
        AHA CC: 4Q, 2017, 18
    CC **M33.99** Dermatopolymyositis, unspecified with other
        organ involvement

M34 Systemic sclerosis [scleroderma]

    Excludes1: *circumscribed scleroderma (L94.0)*
    neonatal scleroderma (P83.88)
M34.0 Progressive systemic sclerosis
M34.1 CR(E)ST syndrome
    Combination of calcinosis, Raynaud's phenomenon,
    esophageal dysfunction, sclerodactyly, telangiectasia
M34.2 Systemic sclerosis induced by drug and chemical
    Code first poisoning due to drug or toxin, if applicable
    (T36-T65 with fifth or sixth character 1-4 or 6)

    Use additional code for adverse effect, if applicable, to
    identify drug (T36-T50 with fifth or sixth character 5)
+ **M34.8** Other forms of systemic sclerosis
    CC **M34.81** Systemic sclerosis with lung involvement
    CC **M34.82** Systemic sclerosis with myopathy
    M34.83 Systemic sclerosis with polyneuropathy
    M34.89 Other systemic sclerosis
M34.9 Systemic sclerosis, unspecified

M35 Other systemic involvement of connective tissue

    Excludes1: *reactive perforating collagenosis (L87.1)*
+ **M35.0** Sicca syndrome [Sjögren]
    M35.00 Sicca syndrome, unspecified
    M35.01 Sicca syndrome with keratoconjunctivitis
    M35.02 Sicca syndrome with lung involvement
    CC **M35.03** Sicca syndrome with myopathy
    M35.04 Sicca syndrome with tubulo-interstitial
        nephropathy
        Renal tubular acidosis in sicca syndrome
    M35.09 Sicca syndrome with other organ involvement
CC **M35.1** Other overlap syndromes
    Mixed connective tissue disease
    Excludes1: *polyangiitis overlap syndrome (M30.8)*
CC **M35.2** Behçet's disease
M35.3 Polymyalgia rheumatica
    Excludes1: *polymyalgia rheumatica with giant cell arteritis*
    (M31.5)
M35.4 Diffuse (eosinophilic) fasciitis
CC **M35.5** Multifocal fibrosclerosis
M35.6 Relapsing panniculitis [Weber-Christian]
    Excludes1: *lupus panniculitis (L93.2)*
    panniculitis NOS (M79.3-)
M35.7 Hypermobility syndrome
    Familial ligamentous laxity
    Excludes1: *Ehlers-Danlos syndromes (Q79.6-)*
    ligamentous laxity, NOS (M24.2-)
CC **M35.8** Other specified systemic involvement of connective tissue
M35.9 Systemic involvement of connective tissue, unspecified
    Autoimmune disease (systemic) NOS
    Collagen (vascular) disease NOS

M36 Systemic disorders of connective tissue in diseases classified
elsewhere

    Excludes2: *arthropathies in diseases classified elsewhere (M14.-)*

807

+, +7th, X + 7th   ● Newborn   ● Pediatric   ● Maternity   ● Adult   ♀ Female   ♂ Male   Manifestation   Unacceptable PDX   HCC   CC   MCC   HAC

CC M36.0 Dermato(poly)myositis in neoplastic disease
 Code first underlying neoplasm (C00-D49)

M36.1 Arthropathy in neoplastic disease
 Code first underlying neoplasm, such as:
  leukemia (C91-C95)
  malignant histiocytosis (C96.A)
  multiple myeloma (C90.0)

M36.2 Hemophilic arthropathy
 Hemarthrosis in hemophilic arthropathy
 Code first underlying disease, such as:
  factor VIII deficiency (D66)
  with vascular defect (D68.0)
  factor IX deficiency (D67)
  hemophilia (classical) (D66)
  hemophilia B (D67)
  hemophilia C (D68.1)

M36.3 Arthropathy in other blood disorders

M36.4 Arthropathy in hypersensitivity reactions classified elsewhere
 Code first underlying disease, such as:
  Henoch (-Schönlein) purpura (D69.0)
  serum sickness (T80.6-)

M36.8 Systemic disorders of connective tissue in other diseases classified elsewhere
 Code first underlying disease, such as:
  alkaptonuria (E70.2)
  hypogammaglobulinemia (D80.-)
  ochronosis (E70.2)

DORSOPATHIES (M40-M54)

Deforming dorsopathies (M40-M43)

M40 Kyphosis and lordosis

 Excludes1: congenital kyphosis and lordosis (Q76.4)
  kyphoscoliosis (M41.-)
  postprocedural kyphosis and lordosis (M96.-)

+ **M40.0 Postural kyphosis**
 Excludes1: osteochondrosis of spine (M42.-)
 M40.00 Postural kyphosis, site unspecified
 M40.03 Postural kyphosis, cervicothoracic region
 M40.04 Postural kyphosis, thoracic region
 M40.05 Postural kyphosis, thoracolumbar region

+ **M40.1 Other secondary kyphosis**
 M40.10 Other secondary kyphosis, site unspecified
 M40.12 Other secondary kyphosis, cervical region
 M40.13 Other secondary kyphosis, cervicothoracic region
 M40.14 Other secondary kyphosis, thoracic region
 M40.15 Other secondary kyphosis, thoracolumbar region

+ **M40.2 Other and unspecified kyphosis**
 + **M40.20 Unspecified kyphosis**
  M40.202 Unspecified kyphosis, cervical region
  M40.203 Unspecified kyphosis, cervicothoracic region
  M40.204 Unspecified kyphosis, thoracic region
  M40.205 Unspecified kyphosis, thoracolumbar region
  M40.209 Unspecified kyphosis, site unspecified
 + **M40.29 Other kyphosis**
  M40.292 Other kyphosis, cervical region
  M40.293 Other kyphosis, cervicothoracic region
  M40.294 Other kyphosis, thoracic region
  M40.295 Other kyphosis, thoracolumbar region
  M40.299 Other kyphosis, site unspecified

+ **M40.3 Flatback syndrome**
 M40.30 Flatback syndrome, site unspecified
 M40.35 Flatback syndrome, thoracolumbar region
 M40.36 Flatback syndrome, lumbar region
 M40.37 Flatback syndrome, lumbosacral region

+ **M40.4 Postural lordosis**
 Acquired lordosis
 M40.40 Postural lordosis, site unspecified
 M40.45 Postural lordosis, thoracolumbar region
 M40.46 Postural lordosis, lumbar region
 M40.47 Postural lordosis, lumbosacral region

+ **M40.5 Lordosis, unspecified**
 M40.50 Lordosis, unspecified, site unspecified
 M40.55 Lordosis, unspecified, thoracolumbar region
 M40.56 Lordosis, unspecified, lumbar region
 M40.57 Lordosis, unspecified, lumbosacral region

M41 Scoliosis

 Includes: kyphoscoliosis
 Excludes1: congenital scoliosis NOS (Q67.5)
  congenital scoliosis due to bony malformation (Q76.3)
  postural congenital scoliosis (Q67.5)
  kyphoscoliotic heart disease (I27.1)
  postprocedural scoliosis (M96.-)

+ **M41.0 Infantile idiopathic scoliosis**
 M41.00 Infantile idiopathic scoliosis, site unspecified
 M41.02 Infantile idiopathic scoliosis, cervical region
 M41.03 Infantile idiopathic scoliosis, cervicothoracic region
 M41.04 Infantile idiopathic scoliosis, thoracic region
  AHA CC: 4Q, 2014, 26-27
 M41.05 Infantile idiopathic scoliosis, thoracolumbar region
 M41.06 Infantile idiopathic scoliosis, lumbar region
 M41.07 Infantile idiopathic scoliosis, lumbosacral region
 M41.08 Infantile idiopathic scoliosis, sacral and sacrococcygeal region

+ **M41.1 Juvenile and adolescent idiopathic scoliosis**
 + **M41.11 Juvenile idiopathic scoliosis**
  M41.112 Juvenile idiopathic scoliosis, cervical region
  M41.113 Juvenile idiopathic scoliosis, cervicothoracic region
  M41.114 Juvenile idiopathic scoliosis, thoracic region
  M41.115 Juvenile idiopathic scoliosis, thoracolumbar region
  M41.116 Juvenile idiopathic scoliosis, lumbar region
  M41.117 Juvenile idiopathic scoliosis, lumbosacral region
  M41.119 Juvenile idiopathic scoliosis, site unspecified
   AHA CC: 4Q, 2014, 28-29
 + **M41.12 Adolescent scoliosis**
  M41.122 Adolescent idiopathic scoliosis, cervical region
  M41.123 Adolescent idiopathic scoliosis, cervicothoracic region
  M41.124 Adolescent idiopathic scoliosis, thoracic region
  M41.125 Adolescent idiopathic scoliosis, thoracolumbar region
  M41.126 Adolescent idiopathic scoliosis, lumbar region
  M41.127 Adolescent idiopathic scoliosis, lumbosacral region
  M41.129 Adolescent idiopathic scoliosis, site unspecified

+ **M41.2 Other idiopathic scoliosis**
 M41.20 Other idiopathic scoliosis, site unspecified
 M41.22 Other idiopathic scoliosis, cervical region
 M41.23 Other idiopathic scoliosis, cervicothoracic region
 M41.24 Other idiopathic scoliosis, thoracic region
 M41.25 Other idiopathic scoliosis, thoracolumbar region
 M41.26 Other idiopathic scoliosis, lumbar region
 M41.27 Other idiopathic scoliosis, lumbosacral region

+ **M41.3 Thoracogenic scoliosis**
 M41.30 Thoracogenic scoliosis, site unspecified
 M41.34 Thoracogenic scoliosis, thoracic region
 M41.35 Thoracogenic scoliosis, thoracolumbar region

+ **M41.4 Neuromuscular scoliosis**
 Scoliosis secondary to cerebral palsy, Friedreich's ataxia, poliomyelitis and other neuromuscular disorders
 Code also underlying condition
 M41.40 Neuromuscular scoliosis, site unspecified
 M41.41 Neuromuscular scoliosis, occipito-atlanto-axial region
 M41.42 Neuromuscular scoliosis, cervical region
 M41.43 Neuromuscular scoliosis, cervicothoracic region
 M41.44 Neuromuscular scoliosis, thoracic region
 M41.45 Neuromuscular scoliosis, thoracolumbar region
  AHA CC: 4Q, 2014, 27-28
 M41.46 Neuromuscular scoliosis, lumbar region
 M41.47 Neuromuscular scoliosis, lumbosacral region

+ **M41.5 Other secondary scoliosis**
  AHA CC: 1Q, 2019, 19
  - M41.50 Other secondary scoliosis, site unspecified
  - M41.52 Other secondary scoliosis, cervical region
  - M41.53 Other secondary scoliosis, cervicothoracic region
  - M41.54 Other secondary scoliosis, thoracic region
  - M41.55 Other secondary scoliosis, thoracolumbar region
  - M41.56 Other secondary scoliosis, lumbar region
  - M41.57 Other secondary scoliosis, lumbosacral region

+ **M41.8 Other forms of scoliosis**
  - M41.80 Other forms of scoliosis, site unspecified
  - M41.82 Other forms of scoliosis, cervical region
  - M41.83 Other forms of scoliosis, cervicothoracic region
  - M41.84 Other forms of scoliosis, thoracic region
  - M41.85 Other forms of scoliosis, thoracolumbar region
  - M41.86 Other forms of scoliosis, lumbar region
  - M41.87 Other forms of scoliosis, lumbosacral region

M41.9 **Scoliosis, unspecified**

M42 **Spinal osteochondrosis**

+ **M42.0 Juvenile osteochondrosis of spine**
  Calvé's disease
  Scheuermann's disease
  Excludes1: *postural kyphosis (M40.0)*
  - M42.00 Juvenile osteochondrosis of spine, site unspecified
  - M42.01 Juvenile osteochondrosis of spine, occipito-atlanto-axial region
  - M42.02 Juvenile osteochondrosis of spine, cervical region
  - M42.03 Juvenile osteochondrosis of spine, cervicothoracic region
  - M42.04 Juvenile osteochondrosis of spine, thoracic region
  - M42.05 Juvenile osteochondrosis of spine, thoracolumbar region
  - M42.06 Juvenile osteochondrosis of spine, lumbar region
  - M42.07 Juvenile osteochondrosis of spine, lumbosacral region
  - M42.08 Juvenile osteochondrosis of spine, sacral and sacrococcygeal region
  - M42.09 Juvenile osteochondrosis of spine, multiple sites in spine

+ **M42.1 Adult osteochondrosis of spine**
  - ● M42.10 Adult osteochondrosis of spine, site unspecified
  - ● M42.11 Adult osteochondrosis of spine, occipito-atlanto-axial region
  - ● M42.12 Adult osteochondrosis of spine, cervical region
  - ● M42.13 Adult osteochondrosis of spine, cervicothoracic region
  - ● M42.14 Adult osteochondrosis of spine, thoracic region
  - ● M42.15 Adult osteochondrosis of spine, thoracolumbar region
  - ● M42.16 Adult osteochondrosis of spine, lumbar region
  - ● M42.17 Adult osteochondrosis of spine, lumbosacral region
  - ● M42.18 Adult osteochondrosis of spine, sacral and sacrococcygeal region
  - ● M42.19 Adult osteochondrosis of spine, multiple sites in spine

M42.9 **Spinal osteochondrosis, unspecified**

M43 **Other deforming dorsopathies**
  Excludes1: *congenital spondylolysis and spondylolisthesis (Q76.2)*
      hemivertebra (Q76.3-Q76.4)
      Klippel-Feil syndrome (Q76.1)
      lumbarization and sacralization (Q76.4)
      platyspondylisis (Q76.4)
      spina bifida occulta (Q76.0)
      spinal curvature in osteoporosis (M80.-)
      spinal curvature in Paget's disease of bone [osteitis deformans] (M88.-)

+ **M43.0 Spondylolysis**
  Excludes1: *congenital spondylolysis (Q76.2)*
      spondylolisthesis (M43.1)
  - M43.00 Spondylolysis, site unspecified
  - M43.01 Spondylolysis, occipito-atlanto-axial region
  - M43.02 Spondylolysis, cervical region
  - M43.03 Spondylolysis, cervicothoracic region
  - M43.04 Spondylolysis, thoracic region
  - M43.05 Spondylolysis, thoracolumbar region
  - M43.06 Spondylolysis, lumbar region
  - M43.07 Spondylolysis, lumbosacral region
  - M43.08 Spondylolysis, sacral and sacrococcygeal region
  - M43.09 Spondylolysis, multiple sites in spine

+ **M43.1 Spondylolisthesis**
  Excludes1: *acute traumatic of lumbosacral region (S33.1)*
      acute traumatic of sites other than lumbosacral-code to Fracture, vertebra, by region
      congenital spondylolisthesis (Q76.2)
  AHA CC: 2Q, 2020, 21
  - M43.10 Spondylolisthesis, site unspecified
  - M43.11 Spondylolisthesis, occipito-atlanto-axial region
  - M43.12 Spondylolisthesis, cervical region
  - M43.13 Spondylolisthesis, cervicothoracic region
  - M43.14 Spondylolisthesis, thoracic region
  - M43.15 Spondylolisthesis, thoracolumbar region
  - M43.16 Spondylolisthesis, lumbar region
  AHA CC: 3Q, 2018, 18
  - M43.17 Spondylolisthesis, lumbosacral region
  - M43.18 Spondylolisthesis, sacral and sacrococcygeal region
  - M43.19 Spondylolisthesis, multiple sites in spine

+ **M43.2 Fusion of spine**
  Ankylosis of spinal joint
  Excludes1: *ankylosing spondylitis (M45.0-)*
      congenital fusion of spine (Q76.4)
  Excludes2: *arthrodesis status (Z98.1)*
      pseudoarthrosis after fusion or arthrodesis (M96.0)
  - M43.20 Fusion of spine, site unspecified
  - M43.21 Fusion of spine, occipito-atlanto-axial region
  - M43.22 Fusion of spine, cervical region
  - M43.23 Fusion of spine, cervicothoracic region
  - M43.24 Fusion of spine, thoracic region
  - M43.25 Fusion of spine, thoracolumbar region
  - M43.26 Fusion of spine, lumbar region
  - M43.27 Fusion of spine, lumbosacral region
  - M43.28 Fusion of spine, sacral and sacrococcygeal region

M43.3 **Recurrent atlantoaxial dislocation with myelopathy**

M43.4 **Other recurrent atlantoaxial dislocation**

+ **M43.5 Other recurrent vertebral dislocation**
  Excludes1: *biomechanical lesions NEC (M99.-)*
  + **M43.5X Other recurrent vertebral dislocation**
    - M43.5X2 Other recurrent vertebral dislocation, cervical region
    - M43.5X3 Other recurrent vertebral dislocation, cervicothoracic region
    - M43.5X4 Other recurrent vertebral dislocation, thoracic region
    - M43.5X5 Other recurrent vertebral dislocation, thoracolumbar region
    - M43.5X6 Other recurrent vertebral dislocation, lumbar region
    - M43.5X7 Other recurrent vertebral dislocation, lumbosacral region
    - M43.5X8 Other recurrent vertebral dislocation, sacral and sacrococcygeal region
    - M43.5X9 Other recurrent vertebral dislocation, site unspecified

M43.6 **Torticollis**
  Excludes1: *congenital (sternomastoid) torticollis (Q68.0)*
      current injury - see Injury, of spine, by body region
      ocular torticollis (R29.891)
      psychogenic torticollis (F45.8)
      spasmodic torticollis (G24.3)
      torticollis due to birth injury (P15.2)

+ **M43.8 Other specified deforming dorsopathies**
  Excludes2: *kyphosis and lordosis (M40.-)*
      scoliosis (M41.-)
  + **M43.8X Other specified deforming dorsopathies**
    - M43.8X1 Other specified deforming dorsopathies, occipito-atlanto-axial region
    - M43.8X2 Other specified deforming dorsopathies, cervical region
    - M43.8X3 Other specified deforming dorsopathies, cervicothoracic region
    - M43.8X4 Other specified deforming dorsopathies, thoracic region
    - M43.8X5 Other specified deforming dorsopathies, thoracolumbar region
    - M43.8X6 Other specified deforming dorsopathies, lumbar region
    - M43.8X7 Other specified deforming dorsopathies, lumbosacral region

M43.8X8 Other specified deforming dorsopathies, sacral and sacrococcygeal region
M43.8X9 Other specified deforming dorsopathies, site unspecified
M43.9 Deforming dorsopathy, unspecified
Curvature of spine NOS

Spondylopathies (M45-M49)

M45 Ankylosing spondylitis

Rheumatoid arthritis of spine
Excludes1: arthropathy in Reiter's disease (M02.3-)
juvenile (ankylosing) spondylitis (M08.1)
Excludes2: Behçet's disease (M35.2)
M45.0 Ankylosing spondylitis of multiple sites in spine
M45.1 Ankylosing spondylitis of occipito-atlanto-axial region
M45.2 Ankylosing spondylitis of cervical region
M45.3 Ankylosing spondylitis of cervicothoracic region
M45.4 Ankylosing spondylitis of thoracic region
M45.5 Ankylosing spondylitis of thoracolumbar region
M45.6 Ankylosing spondylitis lumbar region
M45.7 Ankylosing spondylitis of lumbosacral region
M45.8 Ankylosing spondylitis sacral and sacrococcygeal region
M45.9 Ankylosing spondylitis of unspecified sites in spine

M46 Other inflammatory spondylopathies

+ **M46.0 Spinal enthesopathy**
Disorder of ligamentous or muscular attachments of spine
M46.00 Spinal enthesopathy, site unspecified
M46.01 Spinal enthesopathy, occipito-atlanto-axial region
M46.02 Spinal enthesopathy, cervical region
M46.03 Spinal enthesopathy, cervicothoracic region
M46.04 Spinal enthesopathy, thoracic region
M46.05 Spinal enthesopathy, thoracolumbar region
M46.06 Spinal enthesopathy, lumbar region
M46.07 Spinal enthesopathy, lumbosacral region
M46.08 Spinal enthesopathy, sacral and sacrococcygeal region
M46.09 Spinal enthesopathy, multiple sites in spine
M46.1 Sacroiliitis, not elsewhere classified
AHA CC: 2Q, 2020, 14
+ **M46.2 Osteomyelitis of vertebra**
CC **M46.20** Osteomyelitis of vertebra, site unspecified
CC **M46.21** Osteomyelitis of vertebra, occipito-atlanto-axial region
CC **M46.22** Osteomyelitis of vertebra, cervical region
CC **M46.23** Osteomyelitis of vertebra, cervicothoracic region
CC **M46.24** Osteomyelitis of vertebra, thoracic region
CC **M46.25** Osteomyelitis of vertebra, thoracolumbar region
CC **M46.26** Osteomyelitis of vertebra, lumbar region
CC **M46.27** Osteomyelitis of vertebra, lumbosacral region
CC **M46.28** Osteomyelitis of vertebra, sacral and sacrococcygeal region
+ **M46.3 Infection of intervertebral disc (pyogenic)**
Use additional code (B95-B97) to identify infectious agent
CC **M46.30** Infection of intervertebral disc (pyogenic), site unspecified
CC **M46.31** Infection of intervertebral disc (pyogenic), occipito-atlanto-axial region
CC **M46.32** Infection of intervertebral disc (pyogenic), cervical region
CC **M46.33** Infection of intervertebral disc (pyogenic), cervicothoracic region
CC **M46.34** Infection of intervertebral disc (pyogenic), thoracic region
CC **M46.35** Infection of intervertebral disc (pyogenic), thoracolumbar region
CC **M46.36** Infection of intervertebral disc (pyogenic), lumbar region
CC **M46.37** Infection of intervertebral disc (pyogenic), lumbosacral region
CC **M46.38** Infection of intervertebral disc (pyogenic), sacral and sacrococcygeal region
CC **M46.39** Infection of intervertebral disc (pyogenic), multiple sites in spine
+ **M46.4 Discitis, unspecified**
M46.40 Discitis, unspecified, site unspecified
M46.41 Discitis, unspecified, occipito-atlanto-axial region
M46.42 Discitis, unspecified, cervical region
M46.43 Discitis, unspecified, cervicothoracic region

M46.44 Discitis, unspecified, thoracic region
M46.45 Discitis, unspecified, thoracolumbar region
M46.46 Discitis, unspecified, lumbar region
M46.47 Discitis, unspecified, lumbosacral region
M46.48 Discitis, unspecified, sacral and sacrococcygeal region
M46.49 Discitis, unspecified, multiple sites in spine
+ **M46.5 Other infective spondylopathies**
M46.50 Other infective spondylopathies, site unspecified
M46.51 Other infective spondylopathies, occipito-atlanto-axial region
M46.52 Other infective spondylopathies, cervical region
M46.53 Other infective spondylopathies, cervicothoracic region
M46.54 Other infective spondylopathies, thoracic region
M46.55 Other infective spondylopathies, thoracolumbar region
M46.56 Other infective spondylopathies, lumbar region
M46.57 Other infective spondylopathies, lumbosacral region
M46.58 Other infective spondylopathies, sacral and sacrococcygeal region
M46.59 Other infective spondylopathies, multiple sites in spine
+ **M46.8 Other specified inflammatory spondylopathies**
M46.80 Other specified inflammatory spondylopathies, site unspecified
M46.81 Other specified inflammatory spondylopathies, occipito-atlanto-axial region
M46.82 Other specified inflammatory spondylopathies, cervical region
M46.83 Other specified inflammatory spondylopathies, cervicothoracic region
M46.84 Other specified inflammatory spondylopathies, thoracic region
M46.85 Other specified inflammatory spondylopathies, thoracolumbar region
M46.86 Other specified inflammatory spondylopathies, lumbar region
M46.87 Other specified inflammatory spondylopathies, lumbosacral region
M46.88 Other specified inflammatory spondylopathies, sacral and sacrococcygeal region
M46.89 Other specified inflammatory spondylopathies, multiple sites in spine
+ **M46.9 Unspecified inflammatory spondylopathy**
M46.90 Unspecified inflammatory spondylopathy, site unspecified
M46.91 Unspecified inflammatory spondylopathy, occipito-atlanto-axial region
M46.92 Unspecified inflammatory spondylopathy, cervical region
M46.93 Unspecified inflammatory spondylopathy, cervicothoracic region
M46.94 Unspecified inflammatory spondylopathy, thoracic region
M46.95 Unspecified inflammatory spondylopathy, thoracolumbar region
M46.96 Unspecified inflammatory spondylopathy, lumbar region
M46.97 Unspecified inflammatory spondylopathy, lumbosacral region
M46.98 Unspecified inflammatory spondylopathy, sacral and sacrococcygeal region
M46.99 Unspecified inflammatory spondylopathy, multiple sites in spine

M47 Spondylosis

Includes: arthrosis or osteoarthritis of spine
degeneration of facet joints
+ **M47.0 Anterior spinal and vertebral artery compression syndromes**
+ **M47.01 Anterior spinal artery compression syndromes**
CC **M47.011** Anterior spinal artery compression syndromes, occipito-atlanto-axial region
CC **M47.012** Anterior spinal artery compression syndromes, cervical region
CC **M47.013** Anterior spinal artery compression syndromes, cervicothoracic region

CC M47.014 **Anterior spinal artery compression syndromes, thoracic region**
CC M47.015 **Anterior spinal artery compression syndromes, thoracolumbar region**
CC M47.016 **Anterior spinal artery compression syndromes, lumbar region**
CC M47.019 **Anterior spinal artery compression syndromes, site unspecified**
+ M47.02 **Vertebral artery compression syndromes**
CC M47.021 **Vertebral artery compression syndromes, occipito-atlanto-axial region**
CC M47.022 **Vertebral artery compression syndromes, cervical region**
CC M47.029 **Vertebral artery compression syndromes, site unspecified**
+ M47.1 **Other spondylosis with myelopathy**
Spondylogenic compression of spinal cord
Excludes1: *vertebral subluxation (M43.3-M43.5X9)*
CC M47.10 **Other spondylosis with myelopathy, site unspecified**
CC M47.11 **Other spondylosis with myelopathy, occipito-atlanto-axial region**
CC M47.12 **Other spondylosis with myelopathy, cervical region**
AHA CC: 1Q, 2020, 17
CC M47.13 **Other spondylosis with myelopathy, cervicothoracic region**
CC M47.14 **Other spondylosis with myelopathy, thoracic region**
CC M47.15 **Other spondylosis with myelopathy, thoracolumbar region**
CC M47.16 **Other spondylosis with myelopathy, lumbar region**
+ M47.2 **Other spondylosis with radiculopathy**
M47.20 **Other spondylosis with radiculopathy, site unspecified**
M47.21 **Other spondylosis with radiculopathy, occipito-atlanto-axial region**
M47.22 **Other spondylosis with radiculopathy, cervical region**
AHA CC: 1Q, 2020, 17
M47.23 **Other spondylosis with radiculopathy, cervicothoracic region**
M47.24 **Other spondylosis with radiculopathy, thoracic region**
M47.25 **Other spondylosis with radiculopathy, thoracolumbar region**
M47.26 **Other spondylosis with radiculopathy, lumbar region**
M47.27 **Other spondylosis with radiculopathy, lumbosacral region**
M47.28 **Other spondylosis with radiculopathy, sacral and sacrococcygeal region**
+ M47.8 **Other spondylosis**
+ M47.81 **Spondylosis without myelopathy or radiculopathy**
M47.811 **Spondylosis without myelopathy or radiculopathy, occipito-atlanto-axial region**
M47.812 **Spondylosis without myelopathy or radiculopathy, cervical region**
AHA CC: 2Q, 2018, 14-15; 3Q, 2019, 10-11
M47.813 **Spondylosis without myelopathy or radiculopathy, cervicothoracic region**
M47.814 **Spondylosis without myelopathy or radiculopathy, thoracic region**
M47.815 **Spondylosis without myelopathy or radiculopathy, thoracolumbar region**
M47.816 **Spondylosis without myelopathy or radiculopathy, lumbar region**
M47.817 **Spondylosis without myelopathy or radiculopathy, lumbosacral region**
M47.818 **Spondylosis without myelopathy or radiculopathy, sacral and sacrococcygeal region**
M47.819 **Spondylosis without myelopathy or radiculopathy, site unspecified**

+ M47.89 **Other spondylosis**
M47.891 **Other spondylosis, occipito-atlanto-axial region**
M47.892 **Other spondylosis, cervical region**
M47.893 **Other spondylosis, cervicothoracic region**
M47.894 **Other spondylosis, thoracic region**
M47.895 **Other spondylosis, thoracolumbar region**
M47.896 **Other spondylosis, lumbar region**
M47.897 **Other spondylosis, lumbosacral region**
M47.898 **Other spondylosis, sacral and sacrococcygeal region**
M47.899 **Other spondylosis, site unspecified**
M47.9 **Spondylosis, unspecified**
M48 **Other spondylopathies**
+ M48.0 **Spinal stenosis**
Caudal stenosis
M48.00 **Spinal stenosis, site unspecified**
M48.01 **Spinal stenosis, occipito-atlanto-axial region**
M48.02 **Spinal stenosis, cervical region**
AHA CC: 3Q, 2018, 18-19; 1Q, 2020, 17
M48.03 **Spinal stenosis, cervicothoracic region**
M48.04 **Spinal stenosis, thoracic region**
M48.05 **Spinal stenosis, thoracolumbar region**
+ M48.06 **Spinal stenosis, lumbar region**
AHA CC: 3Q, 2017, 24
M48.061 **Spinal stenosis, lumbar region without neurogenic claudication**
Spinal stenosis. lumbar region NOS
AHA CC: 4Q, 2017, 18-19; 3Q, 2018, 19-20
M48.062 **Spinal stenosis, lumbar region with neurogenic claudication**
AHA CC: 4Q, 2017, 18-19
M48.07 **Spinal stenosis, lumbosacral region**
AHA CC: 3Q, 2018, 19-20
M48.08 **Spinal stenosis, sacral and sacrococcygeal region**
+ M48.1 **Ankylosing hyperostosis [Forestier]**
Diffuse idiopathic skeletal hyperostosis [DISH]
M48.10 **Ankylosing hyperostosis [Forestier], site unspecified**
M48.11 **Ankylosing hyperostosis [Forestier], occipito-atlanto-axial region**
M48.12 **Ankylosing hyperostosis [Forestier], cervical region**
M48.13 **Ankylosing hyperostosis [Forestier], cervicothoracic region**
M48.14 **Ankylosing hyperostosis [Forestier], thoracic region**
M48.15 **Ankylosing hyperostosis [Forestier], thoracolumbar region**
M48.16 **Ankylosing hyperostosis [Forestier], lumbar region**
M48.17 **Ankylosing hyperostosis [Forestier], lumbosacral region**
M48.18 **Ankylosing hyperostosis [Forestier], sacral and sacrococcygeal region**
M48.19 **Ankylosing hyperostosis [Forestier], multiple sites in spine**
+ M48.2 **Kissing spine**
M48.20 **Kissing spine, site unspecified**
M48.21 **Kissing spine, occipito-atlanto-axial region**
M48.22 **Kissing spine, cervical region**
M48.23 **Kissing spine, cervicothoracic region**
M48.24 **Kissing spine, thoracic region**
M48.25 **Kissing spine, thoracolumbar region**
M48.26 **Kissing spine, lumbar region**
M48.27 **Kissing spine, lumbosacral region**
+ M48.3 **Traumatic spondylopathy**
CC M48.30 **Traumatic spondylopathy, site unspecified**
CC M48.31 **Traumatic spondylopathy, occipito-atlanto-axial region**
CC M48.32 **Traumatic spondylopathy, cervical region**
CC M48.33 **Traumatic spondylopathy, cervicothoracic region**
CC M48.34 **Traumatic spondylopathy, thoracic region**
CC M48.35 **Traumatic spondylopathy, thoracolumbar region**
CC M48.36 **Traumatic spondylopathy, lumbar region**
CC M48.37 **Traumatic spondylopathy, lumbosacral region**
CC M48.38 **Traumatic spondylopathy, sacral and sacrococcygeal region**

+ M48.4 Fatigue fracture of vertebra
> Stress fracture of vertebra
> ***Excludes1:*** *pathological fracture NOS (M84.4-)*
> *pathological fracture of vertebra due to neoplasm (M84.58)*
> *pathological fracture of vertebra due to other diagnosis (M84.68)*
> *pathological fracture of vertebra due to osteoporosis (M80.-)*
> *traumatic fracture of vertebrae (S12.0-S12.3-, S22.0-, S32.0-)*

> The appropriate 7th character is to be added to each code from subcategory **M48.4**:
> A   initial encounter for fracture
> D   subsequent encounter for fracture with routine healing
> G   subsequent encounter for fracture with delayed healing
> S   sequela of fracture

X+7th **M48.40 Fatigue fracture of vertebra, site unspecified**
X+7th **M48.41 Fatigue fracture of vertebra, occipito-atlanto-axial region**
X+7th **M48.42 Fatigue fracture of vertebra, cervical region**
X+7th **M48.43 Fatigue fracture of vertebra, cervicothoracic region**
X+7th **M48.44 Fatigue fracture of vertebra, thoracic region**
X+7th **M48.45 Fatigue fracture of vertebra, thoracolumbar region**
X+7th **M48.46 Fatigue fracture of vertebra, lumbar region**
X+7th **M48.47 Fatigue fracture of vertebra, lumbosacral region**
X+7th **M48.48 Fatigue fracture of vertebra, sacral and sacrococcygeal region**

+ M48.5 Collapsed vertebra, not elsewhere classified
> Collapsed vertebra NOS
> Compression fracture of vertebra NOS
> Wedging of vertebra NOS
> ***Excludes1:*** *current injury - see Injury of spine, by body region*
> *fatigue fracture of vertebra (M48.4)*
> *pathological fracture of vertebra due to neoplasm (M84.58)*
> *pathological fracture of vertebra due to other diagnosis (M84.68)*
> *pathological fracture of vertebra due to osteoporosis (M80.-)*
> *pathological fracture NOS (M84.4-)*
> *stress fracture of vertebra (M48.4-)*
> *traumatic fracture of vertebra (S12.-, S22.-, S32.-)*

> The appropriate 7th character is to be added to each code from subcategory **M48.5**:
> A   initial encounter for fracture
> D   subsequent encounter for fracture with routine healing
> G   subsequent encounter for fracture with delayed healing
> S   sequela of fracture

CC X+7th **M48.50 Collapsed vertebra, not elsewhere classified, site unspecified**
CC X+7th **M48.51 Collapsed vertebra, not elsewhere classified, occipito-atlanto-axial region**
CC X+7th **M48.52 Collapsed vertebra, not elsewhere classified, cervical region**
CC X+7th **M48.53 Collapsed vertebra, not elsewhere classified, cervicothoracic region**
CC X+7th **M48.54 Collapsed vertebra, not elsewhere classified, thoracic region**
CC X+7th **M48.55 Collapsed vertebra, not elsewhere classified, thoracolumbar region**
CC X+7th **M48.56 Collapsed vertebra, not elsewhere classified, lumbar region**
CC X+7th **M48.57 Collapsed vertebra, not elsewhere classified, lumbosacral region**
CC X+7th **M48.58 Collapsed vertebra, not elsewhere classified, sacral and sacrococcygeal region**

+ M48.8 Other specified spondylopathies
> Ossification of posterior longitudinal ligament
> **+ M48.8X Other specified spondylopathies**
>> **M48.8X1 Other specified spondylopathies, occipito-atlanto-axial region**
>> **M48.8X2 Other specified spondylopathies, cervical region**
>> **M48.8X3 Other specified spondylopathies, cervicothoracic region**
>> **M48.8X4 Other specified spondylopathies, thoracic region**
>> **M48.8X5 Other specified spondylopathies, thoracolumbar region**
>> **M48.8X6 Other specified spondylopathies, lumbar region**
>> **M48.8X7 Other specified spondylopathies, lumbosacral region**
>> **M48.8X8 Other specified spondylopathies, sacral and sacrococcygeal region**
>> **M48.8X9 Other specified spondylopathies, site unspecified**

M48.9 Spondylopathy, unspecified

M49 Spondylopathies in diseases classified elsewhere
> **Includes:** curvature of spine in diseases classified elsewhere
> deformity of spine in diseases classified elsewhere
> kyphosis in diseases classified elsewhere
> scoliosis in diseases classified elsewhere
> spondylopathy in diseases classified elsewhere
> Code first *underlying disease, such as:*
> brucellosis (A23.-)
> Charcot-Marie-Tooth disease (G60.0)
> enterobacterial infections (A01-A04)
> osteitis fibrosa cystica (E21.0)
> ***Excludes1:*** *curvature of spine in tuberculosis [Pott's] (A18.01)*
> *enteropathic arthropathies (M07.-)*
> *gonococcal spondylitis (A54.41)*
> *neuropathic [tabes dorsalis] spondylitis (A52.11)*
> *neuropathic spondylopathy in syringomyelia (G95.0)*
> *neuropathic spondylopathy in tabes dorsalis (A52.11)*
> *nonsyphilitic neuropathic spondylopathy NEC (G98.0)*
> *spondylitis in syphilis (acquired) (A52.77)*
> *tuberculous spondylitis (A18.01)*
> *typhoid fever spondylitis (A01.05)*

+ M49.8 Spondylopathy in diseases classified elsewhere
> **M49.80 Spondylopathy in diseases classified elsewhere, site unspecified**
> **M49.81 Spondylopathy in diseases classified elsewhere, occipito-atlanto-axial region**
> **M49.82 Spondylopathy in diseases classified elsewhere, cervical region**
> **M49.83 Spondylopathy in diseases classified elsewhere, cervicothoracic region**
> **M49.84 Spondylopathy in diseases classified elsewhere, thoracic region**
> **M49.85 Spondylopathy in diseases classified elsewhere, thoracolumbar region**
> **M49.86 Spondylopathy in diseases classified elsewhere, lumbar region**
> **M49.87 Spondylopathy in diseases classified elsewhere, lumbosacral region**
> **M49.88 Spondylopathy in diseases classified elsewhere, sacral and sacrococcygeal region**
> **M49.89 Spondylopathy in diseases classified elsewhere, multiple sites in spine**

Other dorsopathies (M50-M54)

Excludes1: *current injury - see injury of spine by body region*
discitis NOS (M46.4-)

M50 Cervical disc disorders
> **NOTE** code to the most superior level of disorder
> **Includes:** cervicothoracic disc disorders with cervicalgia
> cervicothoracic disc disorders
> **+ M50.0 Cervical disc disorder with myelopathy**
>> CC **M50.00 Cervical disc disorder with myelopathy, unspecified cervical region**
>> CC **M50.01 Cervical disc disorder with myelopathy, high cervical region**
>>> C2-C3 disc disorder with myelopathy
>>> C3-C4 disc disorder with myelopathy
>>> *AHA CC: 1Q, 2016, 17*
>> **+ M50.02 Cervical disc disorder with myelopathy, mid-cervical region**
>>> *AHA CC: 4Q, 2016, 39-40*
>>> CC **M50.020 Cervical disc disorder with myelopathy, mid-cervical region, unspecified level**

CC **M50.021 Cervical disc disorder at C4-C5 level with myelopathy**
C4-C5 disc disorder with myelopathy

CC **M50.022 Cervical disc disorder at C5-C6 level with myelopathy**
C5-C6 disc disorder with myelopathy
AHA CC: 3Q, 2018, 19

CC **M50.023 Cervical disc disorder at C6-C7 level with myelopathy**
C6-C7 disc disorder with myelopathy

CC **M50.03 Cervical disc disorder with myelopathy, cervicothoracic region**
C7-T1 disc disorder with myelopathy

+ **M50.1 Cervical disc disorder with radiculopathy**
Excludes2: brachial radiculitis NOS (M54.13)

M50.10 Cervical disc disorder with radiculopathy, unspecified cervical region

M50.11 Cervical disc disorder with radiculopathy, high cervical region
C2-C3 disc disorder with radiculopathy
C3 radiculopathy due to disc disorder
C3-C4 disc disorder with radiculopathy
C4 radiculopathy due to disc disorder

+ **M50.12 Cervical disc disorder with radiculopathy, mid-cervical region**
AHA CC: 4Q, 2016, 39-40

M50.120 Mid-cervical disc disorder, unspecified level

M50.121 Cervical disc disorder at C4-C5 level with radiculopathy
C4-C5 disc disorder with radiculopathy
C5 radiculopathy due to disc disorder

M50.122 Cervical disc disorder at C5-C6 level with radiculopathy
C5-C6 disc disorder with radiculopathy
C6 radiculopathy due to disc disorder
AHA CC: 3Q, 2018, 19

M50.123 Cervical disc disorder at C6-C7 level with radiculopathy
C6-C7 disc disorder with radiculopathy
C7 radiculopathy due to disc disorder

M50.13 Cervical disc disorder with radiculopathy, cervicothoracic region
C7-T1 disc disorder with radiculopathy
C8 radiculopathy due to disc disorder

+ **M50.2 Other cervical disc displacement**

M50.20 Other cervical disc displacement, unspecified cervical region

M50.21 Other cervical disc displacement, high cervical region
Other C2-C3 cervical disc displacement
Other C3-C4 cervical disc displacement

+ **M50.22 Other cervical disc displacement, mid-cervical region**

M50.220 Other cervical disc displacement, mid-cervical region, unspecified level

M50.221 Other cervical disc displacement at C4-C5 level
Other C4-C5 cervical disc displacement

M50.222 Other cervical disc displacement at C5-C6 level
Other C5-C6 cervical disc displacement

M50.223 Other cervical disc displacement at C6-C7 level
Other C6-C7 cervical disc displacement

M50.23 Other cervical disc displacement, cervicothoracic region
Other C7-T1 cervical disc displacement

+ **M50.3 Other cervical disc degeneration**

M50.30 Other cervical disc degeneration, unspecified cervical region

M50.31 Other cervical disc degeneration, high cervical region
Other C2-C3 cervical disc degeneration
Other C3-C4 cervical disc degeneration

+ **M50.32 Other cervical disc degeneration, mid-cervical region**

M50.320 Other cervical disc degeneration, mid-cervical region, unspecified level

M50.321 Other cervical disc degeneration at C4-C5 level
Other C4-C5 cervical disc degeneration

M50.322 Other cervical disc degeneration at C5-C6 level
Other C5-C6 cervical disc degeneration

M50.323 Other cervical disc degeneration at C6-C7 level
Other C6-C7 cervical disc degeneration

M50.33 Other cervical disc degeneration, cervicothoracic region
Other C7-T1 cervical disc degeneration

+ **M50.8 Other cervical disc disorders**

M50.80 Other cervical disc disorders, unspecified cervical region

M50.81 Other cervical disc disorders, high cervical region
Other C2-C3 cervical disc disorders
Other C3-C4 cervical disc disorders

+ **M50.82 Other cervical disc disorders, mid-cervical region**

M50.820 Other cervical disc disorders, mid-cervical region, unspecified level

M50.821 Other cervical disc disorders at C4-C5 level
Other C4-C5 cervical disc disorders

M50.822 Other cervical disc disorders at C5-C6 level
Other C5-C6 cervical disc disorders

M50.823 Other cervical disc disorders at C6-C7 level
Other C6-C7 cervical disc disorders

M50.83 Other cervical disc disorders, cervicothoracic region
Other C7-T1 cervical disc disorders

+ **M50.9 Cervical disc disorder, unspecified**

M50.90 Cervical disc disorder, unspecified, unspecified cervical region

M50.91 Cervical disc disorder, unspecified, high cervical region
Other C2-C3 cervical disc disorder, unspecified
Other C3-C4 cervical disc disorder, unspecified

+ **M50.92 Cervical disc disorder, unspecified, mid-cervical region**

M50.920 Unspecified cervical disc disorder, mid-cervical region, unspecified level

M50.921 Unspecified cervical disc disorder at C4-C5 level
Unspecified C4-C5 cervical disc disorder

M50.922 Unspecified cervical disc disorder at C5-C6 level
Unspecified C5-C6 cervical disc disorder

M50.923 Unspecified cervical disc disorder at C6-C7 level
Unspecified C6-C7 cervical disc disorder

M50.93 Cervical disc disorder, unspecified, cervicothoracic region
Other C7-T1 cervical disc disorder, unspecified

M51 Thoracic, thoracolumbar, and lumbosacral intervertebral disc disorders

Excludes2: cervical and cervicothoracic disc disorders (M50.-)
sacral and sacrococcygeal disorders (M53.3)

+ **M51.0 Thoracic, thoracolumbar and lumbosacral intervertebral disc disorders with myelopathy**

CC **M51.04 Intervertebral disc disorders with myelopathy, thoracic region**

CC **M51.05 Intervertebral disc disorders with myelopathy, thoracolumbar region**

CC **M51.06 Intervertebral disc disorders with myelopathy, lumbar region**

+ **M51.1 Thoracic, thoracolumbar and lumbosacral intervertebral disc disorders with radiculopathy**
Sciatica due to intervertebral disc disorder
Excludes1: lumbar radiculitis NOS (M54.16)
sciatica NOS (M54.3)

M51.14 Intervertebral disc disorders with radiculopathy, thoracic region

M51.15 Intervertebral disc disorders with radiculopathy, thoracolumbar region

M51.16 Intervertebral disc disorders with radiculopathy, lumbar region

M51.17 Intervertebral disc disorders with radiculopathy, lumbosacral region

+, +7th, X + 7th   ● Newborn   ● Pediatric   ● Maternity   ● Adult   ♀ Female   ♂ Male   Manifestation   Unacceptable PDX   HCC   CC   MCC   HAC

Lumbar Disk Herniation: Clinical Manifestation

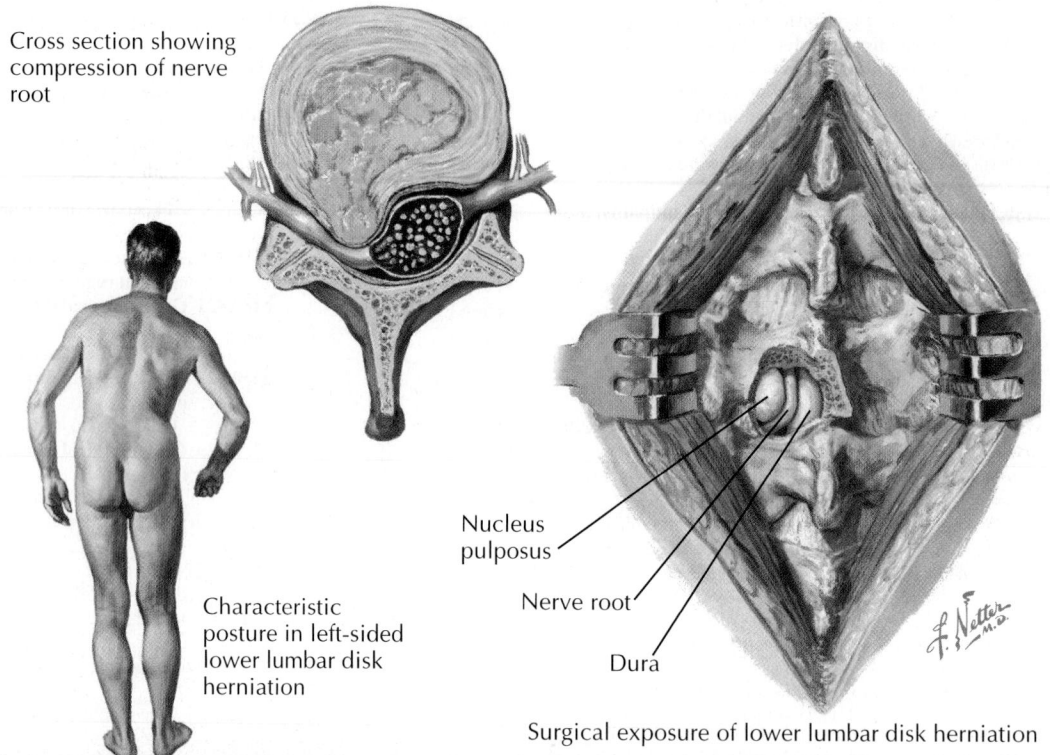

Cross section showing compression of nerve root

Characteristic posture in left-sided lower lumbar disk herniation

Nucleus pulposus

Nerve root

Dura

Surgical exposure of lower lumbar disk herniation

Clinical features of herniated lumbar nucleus pulposus					
Level of herniation	**Pain**	**Numbness**	**Weakness**	**Atrophy**	**Reflexes**
L3 L4 L5 L5 S **L4-5 disk; 5th lumbar nerve root**	Over sacro-iliac joint, hip, lateral thigh and leg	Lateral leg, first 3 toes	Dorsiflexion of great toe and foot; difficulty walking on heels; foot drop may occur	Minor	Changes uncommon in knee and ankle jerks, but internal hamstring reflex diminished or absent
L4 L5 S **L5-S1 disk; 1st sacral nerve root**	Over sacro-iliac joint, hip, postero-lateral thigh and leg to heel	Back of calf, lateral heel, foot to toe	Plantar flexion of foot and great toe may be affected; difficulty walking on toes	Gastrocnemius and soleus	Ankle jerk diminished or absent

+ **M51.2 Other thoracic, thoracolumbar and lumbosacral intervertebral disc displacement**
  Lumbago due to displacement of intervertebral disc
  - **M51.24 Other intervertebral disc displacement, thoracic region**
  - **M51.25 Other intervertebral disc displacement, thoracolumbar region**
  - **M51.26 Other intervertebral disc displacement, lumbar region**
  - **M51.27 Other intervertebral disc displacement, lumbosacral region**
+ **M51.3 Other thoracic, thoracolumbar and lumbosacral intervertebral disc degeneration**
  - **M51.34 Other intervertebral disc degeneration, thoracic region**
  - **M51.35 Other intervertebral disc degeneration, thoracolumbar region**
  - **M51.36 Other intervertebral disc degeneration, lumbar region**
    AHA CC: 2Q, 2018, 15
  - **M51.37 Other intervertebral disc degeneration, lumbosacral region**
+ **M51.4 Schmorl's nodes**
  - **M51.44 Schmorl's nodes, thoracic region**
  - **M51.45 Schmorl's nodes, thoracolumbar region**
  - **M51.46 Schmorl's nodes, lumbar region**
  - **M51.47 Schmorl's nodes, lumbosacral region**
+ **M51.8 Other thoracic, thoracolumbar and lumbosacral intervertebral disc disorders**
  - **M51.84 Other intervertebral disc disorders, thoracic region**
  - **M51.85 Other intervertebral disc disorders, thoracolumbar region**
  - **M51.86 Other intervertebral disc disorders, lumbar region**
  - **M51.87 Other intervertebral disc disorders, lumbosacral region**
  - **M51.9 Unspecified thoracic, thoracolumbar and lumbosacral intervertebral disc disorder**

M53 Other and unspecified dorsopathies, not elsewhere classified

- **M53.0 Cervicocranial syndrome**
  Posterior cervical sympathetic syndrome
- **M53.1 Cervicobrachial syndrome**
  Excludes2: *cervical disc disorder (M50.-)*
  thoracic outlet syndrome (G54.0)
+ **M53.2 Spinal instabilities**
  + **M53.2X Spinal instabilities**
    - **M53.2X1 Spinal instabilities, occipito-atlanto-axial region**
    - **M53.2X2 Spinal instabilities, cervical region**
    - **M53.2X3 Spinal instabilities, cervicothoracic region**
    - **M53.2X4 Spinal instabilities, thoracic region**
    - **M53.2X5 Spinal instabilities, thoracolumbar region**
    - **M53.2X6 Spinal instabilities, lumbar region**
    - **M53.2X7 Spinal instabilities, lumbosacral region**
    - **M53.2X8 Spinal instabilities, sacral and sacrococcygeal region**
    - **M53.2X9 Spinal instabilities, site unspecified**
- **M53.3 Sacrococcygeal disorders, not elsewhere classified**
  Coccygodynia
+ **M53.8 Other specified dorsopathies**
  - **M53.80 Other specified dorsopathies, site unspecified**
  - **M53.81 Other specified dorsopathies, occipito-atlanto-axial region**
  - **M53.82 Other specified dorsopathies, cervical region**
  - **M53.83 Other specified dorsopathies, cervicothoracic region**
  - **M53.84 Other specified dorsopathies, thoracic region**
  - **M53.85 Other specified dorsopathies, thoracolumbar region**
  - **M53.86 Other specified dorsopathies, lumbar region**
  - **M53.87 Other specified dorsopathies, lumbosacral region**
  - **M53.88 Other specified dorsopathies, sacral and sacrococcygeal region**
- **M53.9 Dorsopathy, unspecified**

M54 Dorsalgia
  Excludes1: *psychogenic dorsalgia (F45.41)*
+ **M54.0 Panniculitis affecting regions of neck and back**
  Excludes1: *lupus panniculitis (L93.2)*
  panniculitis NOS (M79.3)
  relapsing [Weber-Christian] panniculitis (M35.6)
  - **M54.00 Panniculitis affecting regions of neck and back, site unspecified**
  - **M54.01 Panniculitis affecting regions of neck and back, occipito-atlanto-axial region**
  - **M54.02 Panniculitis affecting regions of neck and back, cervical region**
  - **M54.03 Panniculitis affecting regions of neck and back, cervicothoracic region**
  - **M54.04 Panniculitis affecting regions of neck and back, thoracic region**
  - **M54.05 Panniculitis affecting regions of neck and back, thoracolumbar region**
  - **M54.06 Panniculitis affecting regions of neck and back, lumbar region**
  - **M54.07 Panniculitis affecting regions of neck and back, lumbosacral region**
  - **M54.08 Panniculitis affecting regions of neck and back, sacral and sacrococcygeal region**
  - **M54.09 Panniculitis affecting regions, neck and back, multiple sites in spine**
+ **M54.1 Radiculopathy**
  Brachial neuritis or radiculitis NOS
  Lumbar neuritis or radiculitis NOS
  Lumbosacral neuritis or radiculitis NOS
  Thoracic neuritis or radiculitis NOS
  Radiculitis NOS
  Excludes1: *neuralgia and neuritis NOS (M79.2)*
  radiculopathy with cervical disc disorder (M50.1)
  radiculopathy with lumbar and other intervertebral disc disorder (M51.1-)
  radiculopathy with spondylosis (M47.2-)
  - **M54.10 Radiculopathy, site unspecified**
  - **M54.11 Radiculopathy, occipito-atlanto-axial region**
  - **M54.12 Radiculopathy, cervical region**
    AHA CC: 3Q, 2018, 18-19
  - **M54.13 Radiculopathy, cervicothoracic region**
  - **M54.14 Radiculopathy, thoracic region**
  - **M54.15 Radiculopathy, thoracolumbar region**
  - **M54.16 Radiculopathy, lumbar region**
    AHA CC: 3Q, 2018, 18
  - **M54.17 Radiculopathy, lumbosacral region**
  - **M54.18 Radiculopathy, sacral and sacrococcygeal region**
- **M54.2 Cervicalgia**
  Excludes1: *cervicalgia due to intervertebral cervical disc disorder (M50.-)*
+ **M54.3 Sciatica**
  Excludes1: *lesion of sciatic nerve (G57.0)*
  sciatica due to intervertebral disc disorder (M51.1-)
  sciatica with lumbago (M54.4-)
  - **M54.30 Sciatica, unspecified side**
  - **M54.31 Sciatica, right side**
  - **M54.32 Sciatica, left side**
+ **M54.4 Lumbago with sciatica**
  Excludes1: *lumbago with sciatica due to intervertebral disc disorder (M51.1-)*
  - **M54.40 Lumbago with sciatica, unspecified side**
  - **M54.41 Lumbago with sciatica, right side**
  - **M54.42 Lumbago with sciatica, left side**
    AHA CC: 2Q, 2016, 7
- **M54.5 Low back pain**
  Loin pain
  Lumbago NOS
  Excludes1: *low back strain (S39.012)*
  lumbago due to intervertebral disc displacement (M51.2-)
  lumbago with sciatica (M54.4-)
- **M54.6 Pain in thoracic spine**
  Excludes1: *pain in thoracic spine due to intervertebral disc disorder (M51.-)*
+ **M54.8 Other dorsalgia**
  Excludes1: *dorsalgia in thoracic region (M54.6)*
  low back pain (M54.5)

M54.81 Occipital neuralgia
M54.89 Other dorsalgia
M54.9 Dorsalgia, unspecified
Backache NOS
Back pain NOS

SOFT TISSUE DISORDERS (M60-M79)

Disorders of muscles (M60-M63)

Excludes1: *dermatopolymyositis (M33.-)*
muscular dystrophies and myopathies (G71-G72)
myopathy in amyloidosis (E85.-)
myopathy in polyarteritis nodosa (M30.0)
myopathy in rheumatoid arthritis (M05.32)
myopathy in scleroderma (M34.-)
myopathy in Sjögren's syndrome (M35.03)
myopathy in systemic lupus erythematosus (M32.-)

M60 Myositis

Excludes2: *inclusion body myositis [IBM] (G72.41)*
+ **M60.0 Infective myositis**
Tropical pyomyositis
Use additional code (B95-B97) to identify infectious agent
+ **M60.00 Infective myositis, unspecified site**
CC **M60.000 Infective myositis, unspecified right arm**
Infective myositis, right upper limb NOS
CC **M60.001 Infective myositis, unspecified left arm**
Infective myositis, left upper limb NOS
CC **M60.002 Infective myositis, unspecified arm**
Infective myositis, upper limb NOS
CC **M60.003 Infective myositis, unspecified right leg**
Infective myositis, right lower limb NOS
CC **M60.004 Infective myositis, unspecified left leg**
Infective myositis, left lower limb NOS
CC **M60.005 Infective myositis, unspecified leg**
Infective myositis, lower limb NOS
CC **M60.009 Infective myositis, unspecified site**
+ **M60.01 Infective myositis, shoulder**
CC **M60.011 Infective myositis, right shoulder**
CC **M60.012 Infective myositis, left shoulder**
CC **M60.019 Infective myositis, unspecified shoulder**
+ **M60.02 Infective myositis, upper arm**
CC **M60.021 Infective myositis, right upper arm**
CC **M60.022 Infective myositis, left upper arm**
CC **M60.029 Infective myositis, unspecified upper arm**
+ **M60.03 Infective myositis, forearm**
CC **M60.031 Infective myositis, right forearm**
CC **M60.032 Infective myositis, left forearm**
CC **M60.039 Infective myositis, unspecified forearm**
+ **M60.04 Infective myositis, hand and fingers**
CC **M60.041 Infective myositis, right hand**
CC **M60.042 Infective myositis, left hand**
CC **M60.043 Infective myositis, unspecified hand**
CC **M60.044 Infective myositis, right finger(s)**
CC **M60.045 Infective myositis, left finger(s)**
CC **M60.046 Infective myositis, unspecified finger(s)**
+ **M60.05 Infective myositis, thigh**
CC **M60.051 Infective myositis, right thigh**
CC **M60.052 Infective myositis, left thigh**
CC **M60.059 Infective myositis, unspecified thigh**
+ **M60.06 Infective myositis, lower leg**
CC **M60.061 Infective myositis, right lower leg**
CC **M60.062 Infective myositis, left lower leg**
CC **M60.069 Infective myositis, unspecified lower leg**
+ **M60.07 Infective myositis, ankle, foot and toes**
CC **M60.070 Infective myositis, right ankle**
CC **M60.071 Infective myositis, left ankle**
CC **M60.072 Infective myositis, unspecified ankle**
CC **M60.073 Infective myositis, right foot**
CC **M60.074 Infective myositis, left foot**
CC **M60.075 Infective myositis, unspecified foot**
CC **M60.076 Infective myositis, right toe(s)**
CC **M60.077 Infective myositis, left toe(s)**
CC **M60.078 Infective myositis, unspecified toe(s)**
CC **M60.08 Infective myositis, other site**
CC **M60.09 Infective myositis, multiple sites**
+ **M60.1 Interstitial myositis**
M60.10 Interstitial myositis of unspecified site
+ **M60.11 Interstitial myositis, shoulder**
M60.111 Interstitial myositis, right shoulder

M60.112 Interstitial myositis, left shoulder
M60.119 Interstitial myositis, unspecified shoulder
+ **M60.12 Interstitial myositis, upper arm**
M60.121 Interstitial myositis, right upper arm
M60.122 Interstitial myositis, left upper arm
M60.129 Interstitial myositis, unspecified upper arm
+ **M60.13 Interstitial myositis, forearm**
M60.131 Interstitial myositis, right forearm
M60.132 Interstitial myositis, left forearm
M60.139 Interstitial myositis, unspecified forearm
+ **M60.14 Interstitial myositis, hand**
M60.141 Interstitial myositis, right hand
M60.142 Interstitial myositis, left hand
M60.149 Interstitial myositis, unspecifiedhand
+ **M60.15 Interstitial myositis, thigh**
M60.151 Interstitial myositis, right thigh
M60.152 Interstitial myositis, left thigh
M60.159 Interstitial myositis, unspecifiedthigh
+ **M60.16 Interstitial myositis, lower leg**
M60.161 Interstitial myositis, right lower leg
M60.162 Interstitial myositis, left lower leg
M60.169 Interstitial myositis, unspecified lower leg
+ **M60.17 Interstitial myositis, ankle and foot**
M60.171 Interstitial myositis, right ankle and foot
M60.172 Interstitial myositis, left ankle and foot
M60.179 Interstitial myositis, unspecified ankle and foot
M60.18 Interstitial myositis, other site
M60.19 Interstitial myositis, multiple sites
+ **M60.2 Foreign body granuloma of soft tissue, not elsewhere classified**
Use additional code to identify the type of retained foreign body (Z18.-)
Excludes1: *foreign body granuloma of skin and subcutaneous tissue (L92.3)*
M60.20 Foreign body granuloma of soft tissue, not elsewhere classified, unspecified site
+ **M60.21 Foreign body granuloma of soft tissue, not elsewhere classified, shoulder**
M60.211 Foreign body granuloma of soft tissue, not elsewhere classified, right shoulder
M60.212 Foreign body granuloma of soft tissue, not elsewhere classified, left shoulder
M60.219 Foreign body granuloma of soft tissue, not elsewhere classified, unspecified shoulder
+ **M60.22 Foreign body granuloma of soft tissue, not elsewhere classified, upper arm**
M60.221 Foreign body granuloma of soft tissue, not elsewhere classified, right upper arm
M60.222 Foreign body granuloma of soft tissue, not elsewhere classified, left upper arm
M60.229 Foreign body granuloma of soft tissue, not elsewhere classified, unspecified upper arm
+ **M60.23 Foreign body granuloma of soft tissue, not elsewhere classified, forearm**
M60.231 Foreign body granuloma of soft tissue, not elsewhere classified, right forearm
M60.232 Foreign body granuloma of soft tissue, not elsewhere classified, left forearm
M60.239 Foreign body granuloma of soft tissue, not elsewhere classified, unspecified forearm
+ **M60.24 Foreign body granuloma of soft tissue, not elsewhere classified, hand**
M60.241 Foreign body granuloma of soft tissue, not elsewhere classified, right hand
M60.242 Foreign body granuloma of soft tissue, not elsewhere classified, left hand
M60.249 Foreign body granuloma of soft tissue, not elsewhere classified, unspecified hand
+ **M60.25 Foreign body granuloma of soft tissue, not elsewhere classified, thigh**
M60.251 Foreign body granuloma of soft tissue, not elsewhere classified, right thigh

+, +7th, X + 7th • Newborn • Pediatric • Maternity • Adult ♀ Female ♂ Male Manifestation Unacceptable PDX HCC CC MCC HAC

M60.252 Foreign body granuloma of soft tissue, not elsewhere classified, left thigh

M60.259 Foreign body granuloma of soft tissue, not elsewhere classified, unspecified thigh

+ M60.26 Foreign body granuloma of soft tissue, not elsewhere classified, lower leg

M60.261 Foreign body granuloma of soft tissue, not elsewhere classified, right lower leg

M60.262 Foreign body granuloma of soft tissue, not elsewhere classified, left lower leg

M60.269 Foreign body granuloma of soft tissue, not elsewhere classified, unspecified lower leg

+ M60.27 Foreign body granuloma of soft tissue, not elsewhere classified, ankle and foot

M60.271 Foreign body granuloma of soft tissue, not elsewhere classified, right ankle and foot

M60.272 Foreign body granuloma of soft tissue, not elsewhere classified, left ankle and foot

M60.279 Foreign body granuloma of soft tissue, not elsewhere classified, unspecified ankle and foot

M60.28 Foreign body granuloma of soft tissue, not elsewhere classified, other site

+ M60.8 Other myositis

M60.80 Other myositis, unspecified site

+ M60.81 Other myositis shoulder

M60.811 Other myositis, right shoulder

M60.812 Other myositis, left shoulder

M60.819 Other myositis, unspecified shoulder

+ M60.82 Other myositis, upper arm

M60.821 Other myositis, right upper arm

M60.822 Other myositis, left upper arm

M60.829 Other myositis, unspecified upper arm

+ M60.83 Other myositis, forearm

M60.831 Other myositis, right forearm

M60.832 Other myositis, left forearm

M60.839 Other myositis, unspecified forearm

+ M60.84 Other myositis, hand

M60.841 Other myositis, right hand

M60.842 Other myositis, left hand

M60.849 Other myositis, unspecified hand

+ M60.85 Other myositis, thigh

M60.851 Other myositis, right thigh

M60.852 Other myositis, left thigh

M60.859 Other myositis, unspecified thigh

+ M60.86 Other myositis, lower leg

M60.861 Other myositis, right lower leg

M60.862 Other myositis, left lower leg

M60.869 Other myositis, unspecified lower leg

+ M60.87 Other myositis, ankle and foot

M60.871 Other myositis, right ankle and foot

M60.872 Other myositis, left ankle and foot

M60.879 Other myositis, unspecified ankle and foot

M60.88 Other myositis, other site

M60.89 Other myositis, multiple sites

M60.9 Myositis, unspecified

M61 Calcification and ossification of muscle

+ M61.0 Myositis ossificans traumatica

M61.00 Myositis ossificans traumatica, unspecified site

+ M61.01 Myositis ossificans traumatica, shoulder

M61.011 Myositis ossificans traumatica, right shoulder

M61.012 Myositis ossificans traumatica, left shoulder

M61.019 Myositis ossificans traumatica, unspecified shoulder

+ M61.02 Myositis ossificans traumatica, upper arm

M61.021 Myositis ossificans traumatica, right upper arm

M61.022 Myositis ossificans traumatica, left upper arm

M61.029 Myositis ossificans traumatica, unspecified upper arm

+ M61.03 Myositis ossificans traumatica, forearm

M61.031 Myositis ossificans traumatica, right forearm

M61.032 Myositis ossificans traumatica, left forearm

M61.039 Myositis ossificans traumatica, unspecified forearm

+ M61.04 Myositis ossificans traumatica, hand

M61.041 Myositis ossificans traumatica, right hand

M61.042 Myositis ossificans traumatica, left hand

M61.049 Myositis ossificans traumatica, unspecified hand

+ M61.05 Myositis ossificans traumatica, thigh

M61.051 Myositis ossificans traumatica, right thigh

M61.052 Myositis ossificans traumatica, left thigh

M61.059 Myositis ossificans traumatica, unspecified thigh

+ M61.06 Myositis ossificans traumatica, lower leg

M61.061 Myositis ossificans traumatica, right lower leg

M61.062 Myositis ossificans traumatica, left lower leg

M61.069 Myositis ossificans traumatica, unspecified lower leg

+ M61.07 Myositis ossificans traumatica, ankle and foot

M61.071 Myositis ossificans traumatica, right ankle and foot

M61.072 Myositis ossificans traumatica, left ankle and foot

M61.079 Myositis ossificans traumatica, unspecified ankle and foot

M61.08 Myositis ossificans traumatica, other site

M61.09 Myositis ossificans traumatica, multiple sites

+ M61.1 Myositis ossificans progressiva

Fibrodysplasia ossificans progressiva

M61.10 Myositis ossificans progressiva, unspecified site

+ M61.11 Myositis ossificans progressiva, shoulder

M61.111 Myositis ossificans progressiva, right shoulder

M61.112 Myositis ossificans progressiva, left shoulder

M61.119 Myositis ossificans progressiva, unspecified shoulder

+ M61.12 Myositis ossificans progressiva, upper arm

M61.121 Myositis ossificans progressiva, right upper arm

M61.122 Myositis ossificans progressiva, left upper arm

M61.129 Myositis ossificans progressiva, unspecified arm

+ M61.13 Myositis ossificans progressiva, forearm

M61.131 Myositis ossificans progressiva, right forearm

M61.132 Myositis ossificans progressiva, left forearm

M61.139 Myositis ossificans progressiva, unspecified forearm

+ M61.14 Myositis ossificans progressiva, hand and finger(s)

M61.141 Myositis ossificans progressiva, right hand

M61.142 Myositis ossificans progressiva, left hand

M61.143 Myositis ossificans progressiva, unspecified hand

M61.144 Myositis ossificans progressiva, right finger(s)

M61.145 Myositis ossificans progressiva, left finger(s)

M61.146 Myositis ossificans progressiva, unspecified finger(s)

+ M61.15 Myositis ossificans progressiva, thigh

M61.151 Myositis ossificans progressiva, right thigh

M61.152 Myositis ossificans progressiva, left thigh

M61.159 Myositis ossificans progressiva, unspecified thigh

+, +7th, X + 7th   ● Newborn   ● Pediatric   ● Maternity   ● Adult   ♀ Female   ♂ Male   Manifestation   Unacceptable PDX   HCC   CC   MCC   HAC

+ **M61.16** Myositis ossificans progressiva, lower leg
  - **M61.161** Myositis ossificans progressiva, right lower leg
  - **M61.162** Myositis ossificans progressiva, left lower leg
  - **M61.169** Myositis ossificans progressiva, unspecified lower leg

+ **M61.17** Myositis ossificans progressiva, ankle, foot and toe(s)
  - **M61.171** Myositis ossificans progressiva, right ankle
  - **M61.172** Myositis ossificans progressiva, left ankle
  - **M61.173** Myositis ossificans progressiva, unspecified ankle
  - **M61.174** Myositis ossificans progressiva, right foot
  - **M61.175** Myositis ossificans progressiva, left foot
  - **M61.176** Myositis ossificans progressiva, unspecified foot
  - **M61.177** Myositis ossificans progressiva, right toe(s)
  - **M61.178** Myositis ossificans progressiva, left toe(s)
  - **M61.179** Myositis ossificans progressiva, unspecified toe(s)

M61.18 Myositis ossificans progressiva, other site

M61.19 Myositis ossificans progressiva, multiple sites

+ **M61.2** Paralytic calcification and ossification of muscle

  Myositis ossificans associated with quadriplegia or paraplegia

M61.20 Paralytic calcification and ossification of muscle, unspecified site

+ **M61.21** Paralytic calcification and ossification of muscle, shoulder
  - **M61.211** Paralytic calcification and ossification of muscle, right shoulder
  - **M61.212** Paralytic calcification and ossification of muscle, left shoulder
  - **M61.219** Paralytic calcification and ossification of muscle, unspecified shoulder

+ **M61.22** Paralytic calcification and ossification of muscle, upper arm
  - **M61.221** Paralytic calcification and ossification of muscle, right upper arm
  - **M61.222** Paralytic calcification and ossification of muscle, left upper arm
  - **M61.229** Paralytic calcification and ossification of muscle, unspecified upper arm

+ **M61.23** Paralytic calcification and ossification of muscle, forearm
  - **M61.231** Paralytic calcification and ossification of muscle, right forearm
  - **M61.232** Paralytic calcification and ossification of muscle, left forearm
  - **M61.239** Paralytic calcification and ossification of muscle, unspecified forearm

+ **M61.24** Paralytic calcification and ossification of muscle, hand
  - **M61.241** Paralytic calcification and ossification of muscle, right hand
  - **M61.242** Paralytic calcification and ossification of muscle, left hand
  - **M61.249** Paralytic calcification and ossification of muscle, unspecified hand

+ **M61.25** Paralytic calcification and ossification of muscle, thigh
  - **M61.251** Paralytic calcification and ossification of muscle, right thigh
  - **M61.252** Paralytic calcification and ossification of muscle, left thigh
  - **M61.259** Paralytic calcification and ossification of muscle, unspecified thigh

+ **M61.26** Paralytic calcification and ossification of muscle, lower leg
  - **M61.261** Paralytic calcification and ossification of muscle, right lower leg
  - **M61.262** Paralytic calcification and ossification of muscle, left lower leg
  - **M61.269** Paralytic calcification and ossification of muscle, unspecified lower leg

+ **M61.27** Paralytic calcification and ossification of muscle, ankle and foot
  - **M61.271** Paralytic calcification and ossification of muscle, right ankle and foot
  - **M61.272** Paralytic calcification and ossification of muscle, left ankle and foot
  - **M61.279** Paralytic calcification and ossification of muscle, unspecified ankle and foot

M61.28 Paralytic calcification and ossification of muscle, other site

M61.29 Paralytic calcification and ossification of muscle, multiple sites

+ **M61.3** Calcification and ossification of muscles associated with burns

  Myositis ossificans associated with burns

M61.30 Calcification and ossification of muscles associated with burns, unspecified site

+ **M61.31** Calcification and ossification of muscles associated with burns, shoulder
  - **M61.311** Calcification and ossification of muscles associated with burns, right shoulder
  - **M61.312** Calcification and ossification of muscles associated with burns, left shoulder
  - **M61.319** Calcification and ossification of muscles associated with burns, unspecified shoulder

+ **M61.32** Calcification and ossification of muscles associated with burns, upper arm
  - **M61.321** Calcification and ossification of muscles associated with burns, right upper arm
  - **M61.322** Calcification and ossification of muscles associated with burns, left upper arm
  - **M61.329** Calcification and ossification of muscles associated with burns, unspecified upper arm

+ **M61.33** Calcification and ossification of muscles associated with burns, forearm
  - **M61.331** Calcification and ossification of muscles associated with burns, right forearm
  - **M61.332** Calcification and ossification of muscles associated with burns, left forearm
  - **M61.339** Calcification and ossification of muscles associated with burns, unspecified forearm

+ **M61.34** Calcification and ossification of muscles associated with burns, hand
  - **M61.341** Calcification and ossification of muscles associated with burns, right hand
  - **M61.342** Calcification and ossification of muscles associated with burns, left hand
  - **M61.349** Calcification and ossification of muscles associated with burns, unspecified hand

+ **M61.35** Calcification and ossification of muscles associated with burns, thigh
  - **M61.351** Calcification and ossification of muscles associated with burns, right thigh
  - **M61.352** Calcification and ossification of muscles associated with burns, left thigh
  - **M61.359** Calcification and ossification of muscles associated with burns, unspecified thigh

+ **M61.36** Calcification and ossification of muscles associated with burns, lower leg
  - **M61.361** Calcification and ossification of muscles associated with burns, right lower leg
  - **M61.362** Calcification and ossification of muscles associated with burns, left lower leg
  - **M61.369** Calcification and ossification of muscles associated with burns, unspecified lower leg

+ **M61.37** Calcification and ossification of muscles associated with burns, ankle and foot
  - **M61.371** Calcification and ossification of muscles associated with burns, right ankle and foot
  - **M61.372** Calcification and ossification of muscles associated with burns, left ankle and foot
  - **M61.379** Calcification and ossification of muscles associated with burns, unspecified ankle and foot

M61.38 Calcification and ossification of muscles associated with burns, other site

M61.39 Calcification and ossification of muscles associated with burns, multiple sites

+ **M61.4 Other calcification of muscle**
  Excludes1: *calcific tendinitis NOS (M65.2-)*
    calcific tendinitis of shoulder (M75.3)
  M61.40 Other calcification of muscle, unspecified site
  + **M61.41 Other calcification of muscle, shoulder**
    M61.411 Other calcification of muscle, right shoulder
    M61.412 Other calcification of muscle, left shoulder
    M61.419 Other calcification of muscle, unspecified shoulder
  + **M61.42 Other calcification of muscle, upper arm**
    M61.421 Other calcification of muscle, right upper arm
    M61.422 Other calcification of muscle, left upper arm
    M61.429 Other calcification of muscle, unspecified upper arm
  + **M61.43 Other calcification of muscle, forearm**
    M61.431 Other calcification of muscle, right forearm
    M61.432 Other calcification of muscle, left forearm
    M61.439 Other calcification of muscle, unspecified forearm
  + **M61.44 Other calcification of muscle, hand**
    M61.441 Other calcification of muscle, right hand
    M61.442 Other calcification of muscle, left hand
    M61.449 Other calcification of muscle, unspecified hand
  + **M61.45 Other calcification of muscle, thigh**
    M61.451 Other calcification of muscle, right thigh
    M61.452 Other calcification of muscle, left thigh
    M61.459 Other calcification of muscle, unspecified thigh
  + **M61.46 Other calcification of muscle, lower leg**
    M61.461 Other calcification of muscle, right lower leg
    M61.462 Other calcification of muscle, left lower leg
    M61.469 Other calcification of muscle, unspecified lower leg
  + **M61.47 Other calcification of muscle, ankle and foot**
    M61.471 Other calcification of muscle, right ankle and foot
    M61.472 Other calcification of muscle, left ankle and foot
    M61.479 Other calcification of muscle, unspecified ankle and foot
  M61.48 Other calcification of muscle, other site
  M61.49 Other calcification of muscle, multiple sites
+ **M61.5 Other ossification of muscle**
  M61.50 Other ossification of muscle, unspecified site
  + **M61.51 Other ossification of muscle, shoulder**
    M61.511 Other ossification of muscle, right shoulder
    M61.512 Other ossification of muscle, left shoulder
    M61.519 Other ossification of muscle, unspecified shoulder
  + **M61.52 Other ossification of muscle, upper arm**
    M61.521 Other ossification of muscle, right upper arm
    M61.522 Other ossification of muscle, left upper arm
    M61.529 Other ossification of muscle, unspecified upper arm
  + **M61.53 Other ossification of muscle, forearm**
    M61.531 Other ossification of muscle, right forearm
    M61.532 Other ossification of muscle, left forearm
    M61.539 Other ossification of muscle, unspecified forearm
  + **M61.54 Other ossification of muscle, hand**
    M61.541 Other ossification of muscle, right hand
    M61.542 Other ossification of muscle, left hand
    M61.549 Other ossification of muscle, unspecified hand
  + **M61.55 Other ossification of muscle, thigh**
    M61.551 Other ossification of muscle, right thigh

M61.552 Other ossification of muscle, left thigh
M61.559 Other ossification of muscle, unspecified thigh
+ **M61.56 Other ossification of muscle, lower leg**
  M61.561 Other ossification of muscle, right lower leg
  M61.562 Other ossification of muscle, left lower leg
  M61.569 Other ossification of muscle, unspecified lower leg
+ **M61.57 Other ossification of muscle, ankle and foot**
  M61.571 Other ossification of muscle, right ankle and foot
  M61.572 Other ossification of muscle, left ankle and foot
  M61.579 Other ossification of muscle, unspecified ankle and foot
M61.58 Other ossification of muscle, other site
M61.59 Other ossification of muscle, multiple sites
M61.9 Calcification and ossification of muscle, unspecified

M62 Other disorders of muscle
  Excludes1: *alcoholic myopathy (G72.1)*
    cramp and spasm (R25.2)
    drug-induced myopathy (G72.0)
    myalgia (M79.1-)
    stiff-man syndrome (G25.82)
  Excludes2: *nontraumatic hematoma of muscle (M79.81)*
  + **M62.0 Separation of muscle (nontraumatic)**
    Diastasis of muscle
    Excludes1: *diastasis recti complicating pregnancy, labor and delivery (O71.8)*
      traumatic separation of muscle- see strain of muscle by body region
    M62.00 Separation of muscle (nontraumatic), unspecified site
    + **M62.01 Separation of muscle (nontraumatic), shoulder**
      M62.011 Separation of muscle (nontraumatic), right shoulder
      M62.012 Separation of muscle (nontraumatic), left shoulder
      M62.019 Separation of muscle (nontraumatic), unspecified shoulder
    + **M62.02 Separation of muscle (nontraumatic), upper arm**
      M62.021 Separation of muscle (nontraumatic), right upper arm
      M62.022 Separation of muscle (nontraumatic), left upper arm
      M62.029 Separation of muscle (nontraumatic), unspecified upper arm
    + **M62.03 Separation of muscle (nontraumatic), forearm**
      M62.031 Separation of muscle (nontraumatic), right forearm
      M62.032 Separation of muscle (nontraumatic), left forearm
      M62.039 Separation of muscle (nontraumatic), unspecified forearm
    + **M62.04 Separation of muscle (nontraumatic), hand**
      M62.041 Separation of muscle (nontraumatic), right hand
      M62.042 Separation of muscle (nontraumatic), left hand
      M62.049 Separation of muscle (nontraumatic), unspecified hand
    + **M62.05 Separation of muscle (nontraumatic), thigh**
      M62.051 Separation of muscle (nontraumatic), right thigh
      M62.052 Separation of muscle (nontraumatic), left thigh
      M62.059 Separation of muscle (nontraumatic), unspecified thigh
    + **M62.06 Separation of muscle (nontraumatic), lower leg**
      M62.061 Separation of muscle (nontraumatic), right lower leg
      M62.062 Separation of muscle (nontraumatic), left lower leg
      M62.069 Separation of muscle (nontraumatic), unspecified lower leg

+, +7th, X + 7th   ● Newborn   ● Pediatric   ● Maternity   ● Adult   ♀ Female   ♂ Male   Manifestation   Unacceptable PDX   HCC   CC   MCC   HAC

+ **M62.07 Separation of muscle (nontraumatic), ankle and foot**
    M62.071 Separation of muscle (nontraumatic), right ankle and foot
    M62.072 Separation of muscle (nontraumatic), left ankle and foot
    M62.079 Separation of muscle (nontraumatic), unspecified ankle and foot
  M62.08 Separation of muscle (nontraumatic), other site

+ **M62.1 Other rupture of muscle (nontraumatic)**
  Excludes1: traumatic rupture of muscle - see strain of muscle by body region
  Excludes2: rupture of tendon (M66.-)
  M62.10 Other rupture of muscle (nontraumatic), unspecified site

+ **M62.11 Other rupture of muscle (nontraumatic), shoulder**
    M62.111 Other rupture of muscle (nontraumatic), right shoulder
    M62.112 Other rupture of muscle (nontraumatic), left shoulder
    M62.119 Other rupture of muscle (nontraumatic), unspecified shoulder

+ **M62.12 Other rupture of muscle (nontraumatic), upper arm**
    M62.121 Other rupture of muscle (nontraumatic), right upper arm
    M62.122 Other rupture of muscle (nontraumatic), left upper arm
    M62.129 Other rupture of muscle (nontraumatic), unspecified upper arm

+ **M62.13 Other rupture of muscle (nontraumatic), forearm**
    M62.131 Other rupture of muscle (nontraumatic), right forearm
    M62.132 Other rupture of muscle (nontraumatic), left forearm
    M62.139 Other rupture of muscle (nontraumatic), unspecified forearm

+ **M62.14 Other rupture of muscle (nontraumatic), hand**
    M62.141 Other rupture of muscle (nontraumatic), right hand
    M62.142 Other rupture of muscle (nontraumatic), left hand
    M62.149 Other rupture of muscle (nontraumatic), unspecified hand

+ **M62.15 Other rupture of muscle (nontraumatic), thigh**
    M62.151 Other rupture of muscle (nontraumatic), right thigh
    M62.152 Other rupture of muscle (nontraumatic), left thigh
    M62.159 Other rupture of muscle (nontraumatic), unspecified thigh

+ **M62.16 Other rupture of muscle (nontraumatic), lower leg**
    M62.161 Other rupture of muscle (nontraumatic), right lower leg
    M62.162 Other rupture of muscle (nontraumatic), left lower leg
    M62.169 Other rupture of muscle (nontraumatic), unspecified lower leg

+ **M62.17 Other rupture of muscle (nontraumatic), ankle and foot**
    M62.171 Other rupture of muscle (nontraumatic), right ankle and foot
    M62.172 Other rupture of muscle (nontraumatic), left ankle and foot
    M62.179 Other rupture of muscle (nontraumatic), unspecified ankle and foot
  M62.18 Other rupture of muscle (nontraumatic), other site

+ **M62.2 Nontraumatic ischemic infarction of muscle**
  Excludes1: compartment syndrome (traumatic) (T79.A-)
    nontraumatic compartment syndrome (M79.A-)
    traumatic ischemia of muscle (T79.6)
    rhabdomyolysis (M62.82)
    Volkmann's ischemic contracture (T79.6)
  M62.20 Nontraumatic ischemic infarction of muscle, unspecified site

+ **M62.21 Nontraumatic ischemic infarction of muscle, shoulder**
    M62.211 Nontraumatic ischemic infarction of muscle, right shoulder
    M62.212 Nontraumatic ischemic infarction of muscle, left shoulder
    M62.219 Nontraumatic ischemic infarction of muscle, unspecified shoulder

+ **M62.22 Nontraumatic ischemic infarction of muscle, upper arm**
    M62.221 Nontraumatic ischemic infarction of muscle, right upper arm
    M62.222 Nontraumatic ischemic infarction of muscle, left upper arm
    M62.229 Nontraumatic ischemic infarction of muscle, unspecified upper arm

+ **M62.23 Nontraumatic ischemic infarction of muscle, forearm**
    M62.231 Nontraumatic ischemic infarction of muscle, right forearm
    M62.232 Nontraumatic ischemic infarction of muscle, left forearm
    M62.239 Nontraumatic ischemic infarction of muscle, unspecified forearm

+ **M62.24 Nontraumatic ischemic infarction of muscle, hand**
    M62.241 Nontraumatic ischemic infarction of muscle, right hand
    M62.242 Nontraumatic ischemic infarction of muscle, left hand
    M62.249 Nontraumatic ischemic infarction of muscle, unspecified hand

+ **M62.25 Nontraumatic ischemic infarction of muscle, thigh**
    M62.251 Nontraumatic ischemic infarction of muscle, right thigh
    M62.252 Nontraumatic ischemic infarction of muscle, left thigh
    M62.259 Nontraumatic ischemic infarction of muscle, unspecified thigh

+ **M62.26 Nontraumatic ischemic infarction of muscle, lower leg**
    M62.261 Nontraumatic ischemic infarction of muscle, right lower leg
    M62.262 Nontraumatic ischemic infarction of muscle, left lower leg
    M62.269 Nontraumatic ischemic infarction of muscle, unspecified lower leg

+ **M62.27 Nontraumatic ischemic infarction of muscle, ankle and foot**
    M62.271 Nontraumatic ischemic infarction of muscle, right ankle and foot
    M62.272 Nontraumatic ischemic infarction of muscle, left ankle and foot
    M62.279 Nontraumatic ischemic infarction of muscle, unspecified ankle and foot
  M62.28 Nontraumatic ischemic infarction of muscle, other site

M62.3 Immobility syndrome (paraplegic)

+ **M62.4 Contracture of muscle**
  Contracture of tendon (sheath)
  Excludes1: contracture of joint (M24.5-)
  M62.40 Contracture of muscle, unspecified site

+ **M62.41 Contracture of muscle, shoulder**
    M62.411 Contracture of muscle, right shoulder
    M62.412 Contracture of muscle, left shoulder
    M62.419 Contracture of muscle, unspecified shoulder

+ **M62.42 Contracture of muscle, upper arm**
    M62.421 Contracture of muscle, right upper arm
    M62.422 Contracture of muscle, left upper arm
    M62.429 Contracture of muscle, unspecified upper arm

+ **M62.43 Contracture of muscle, forearm**
    M62.431 Contracture of muscle, right forearm
    M62.432 Contracture of muscle, left forearm
    M62.439 Contracture of muscle, unspecified forearm

+ **M62.44 Contracture of muscle, hand**
    M62.441 Contracture of muscle, right hand

M62.442 Contracture of muscle, left hand
M62.449 Contracture of muscle, unspecified hand
+ M62.45 Contracture of muscle, thigh
M62.451 Contracture of muscle, right thigh
M62.452 Contracture of muscle, left thigh
M62.459 Contracture of muscle, unspecified thigh
+ M62.46 Contracture of muscle, lower leg
M62.461 Contracture of muscle, right lower leg
M62.462 Contracture of muscle, left lower leg
M62.469 Contracture of muscle, unspecified lower leg
+ M62.47 Contracture of muscle, ankle and foot
M62.471 Contracture of muscle, right ankle and foot
M62.472 Contracture of muscle, left ankle and foot
M62.479 Contracture of muscle, unspecified ankle and foot
M62.48 Contracture of muscle, other site
M62.49 Contracture of muscle, multiple sites
+ M62.5 Muscle wasting and atrophy, not elsewhere classified
Disuse atrophy NEC
Excludes1: neuralgic amyotrophy (G54.5)
progressive muscular atrophy (G12.21)
sarcopenia (M62.84)
Excludes2: pelvic muscle wasting (N81.84)
M62.50 Muscle wasting and atrophy, not elsewhere classified, unspecified site
+ M62.51 Muscle wasting and atrophy, not elsewhere classified, shoulder
M62.511 Muscle wasting and atrophy, not elsewhere classified, right shoulder
M62.512 Muscle wasting and atrophy, not elsewhere classified, left shoulder
M62.519 Muscle wasting and atrophy, not elsewhere classified, unspecified shoulder
+ M62.52 Muscle wasting and atrophy, not elsewhere classified, upper arm
M62.521 Muscle wasting and atrophy, not elsewhere classified, right upper arm
M62.522 Muscle wasting and atrophy, not elsewhere classified, left upper arm
M62.529 Muscle wasting and atrophy, not elsewhere classified, unspecified upper arm
+ M62.53 Muscle wasting and atrophy, not elsewhere classified, forearm
M62.531 Muscle wasting and atrophy, not elsewhere classified, right forearm
M62.532 Muscle wasting and atrophy, not elsewhere classified, left forearm
M62.539 Muscle wasting and atrophy, not elsewhere classified, unspecified forearm
+ M62.54 Muscle wasting and atrophy, not elsewhere classified, hand
M62.541 Muscle wasting and atrophy, not elsewhere classified, right hand
M62.542 Muscle wasting and atrophy, not elsewhere classified, left hand
M62.549 Muscle wasting and atrophy, not elsewhere classified, unspecified hand
+ M62.55 Muscle wasting and atrophy, not elsewhere classified, thigh
M62.551 Muscle wasting and atrophy, not elsewhere classified, right thigh
M62.552 Muscle wasting and atrophy, not elsewhere classified, left thigh
M62.559 Muscle wasting and atrophy, not elsewhere classified, unspecified thigh
+ M62.56 Muscle wasting and atrophy, not elsewhere classified, lower leg
M62.561 Muscle wasting and atrophy, not elsewhere classified, right lower leg
M62.562 Muscle wasting and atrophy, not elsewhere classified, left lower leg
M62.569 Muscle wasting and atrophy, not elsewhere classified, unspecified lower leg

+ M62.57 Muscle wasting and atrophy, not elsewhere classified, ankle and foot
M62.571 Muscle wasting and atrophy, not elsewhere classified, right ankle and foot
M62.572 Muscle wasting and atrophy, not elsewhere classified, left ankle and foot
M62.579 Muscle wasting and atrophy, not elsewhere classified, unspecified ankle and foot
M62.58 Muscle wasting and atrophy, not elsewhere classified, other site
M62.59 Muscle wasting and atrophy, not elsewhere classified, multiple sites
+ M62.8 Other specified disorders of muscle
Excludes2: nontraumatic hematoma of muscle (M79.81)
M62.81 Muscle weakness (generalized)
Excludes1: muscle weakness in sarcopenia (M62.84)
CC M62.82 Rhabdomyolysis
Excludes1: traumatic rhabdomyolysis (T79.6)
AHA CC: 2Q, 2019, 12-13
+ M62.83 Muscle spasm
M62.830 Muscle spasm of back
M62.831 Muscle spasm of calf
Charley-horse
M62.838 Other muscle spasm
M62.84 Sarcopenia
Age-related sarcopenia
Code first underlying disease, if applicable, such as:
disorders of myoneural junction and muscle disease
in diseases classified elsewhere (G73.-)
other and unspecified myopathies (G72.-)
primary disorders of muscles (G71.-)
AHA CC: 4Q, 2016, 41
M62.89 Other specified disorders of muscle
Muscle (sheath) hernia
M62.9 Disorder of muscle, unspecified
M63 Disorders of muscle in diseases classified elsewhere
Code first underlying disease, such as:
leprosy (A30.-)
neoplasm (C49.-, C79.89, D21.-, D48.1)
schistosomiasis (B65.-)
trichinellosis (B75)
Excludes1: myopathy in cysticercosis (B69.81)
myopathy in endocrine diseases (G73.7)
myopathy in metabolic diseases (G73.7)
myopathy in sarcoidosis (D86.87)
myopathy in secondary syphilis (A51.49)
myopathy in syphilis (late) (A52.78)
myopathy in toxoplasmosis (B58.82)
myopathy in tuberculosis (A18.09)
+ M63.8 Disorders of muscle in diseases classified elsewhere
M63.80 Disorders of muscle in diseases classified elsewhere, unspecified site
+ M63.81 Disorders of muscle in diseases classified elsewhere, shoulder
M63.811 Disorders of muscle in diseases classified elsewhere, right shoulder
M63.812 Disorders of muscle in diseases classified elsewhere, left shoulder
M63.819 Disorders of muscle in diseases classified elsewhere, unspecified shoulder
+ M63.82 Disorders of muscle in diseases classified elsewhere, upper arm
M63.821 Disorders of muscle in diseases classified elsewhere, right upper arm
M63.822 Disorders of muscle in diseases classified elsewhere, left upper arm
M63.829 Disorders of muscle in diseases classified elsewhere, unspecified upper arm
+ M63.83 Disorders of muscle in diseases classified elsewhere, forearm
M63.831 Disorders of muscle in diseases classified elsewhere, right forearm
M63.832 Disorders of muscle in diseases classified elsewhere, left forearm
M63.839 Disorders of muscle in diseases classified elsewhere, unspecified forearm

+, +7th, X + 7th   • Newborn   • Pediatric   • Maternity   • Adult   ♀ Female   ♂ Male   Manifestation   Unacceptable PDX   HCC   CC   MCC   HAC

+ **M63.84** Disorders of muscle in diseases classified elsewhere, hand
   M63.841 Disorders of muscle in diseases classified elsewhere, right hand
   M63.842 Disorders of muscle in diseases classified elsewhere, left hand
   M63.849 Disorders of muscle in diseases classified elsewhere, unspecified hand
+ **M63.85** Disorders of muscle in diseases classified elsewhere, thigh
   M63.851 Disorders of muscle in diseases classified elsewhere, right thigh
   M63.852 Disorders of muscle in diseases classified elsewhere, left thigh
   M63.859 Disorders of muscle in diseases classified elsewhere, unspecified thigh
+ **M63.86** Disorders of muscle in diseases classified elsewhere, lower leg
   M63.861 Disorders of muscle in diseases classified elsewhere, right lower leg
   M63.862 Disorders of muscle in diseases classified elsewhere, left lower leg
   M63.869 Disorders of muscle in diseases classified elsewhere, unspecified lower leg
+ **M63.87** Disorders of muscle in diseases classified elsewhere, ankle and foot
   M63.871 Disorders of muscle in diseases classified elsewhere, right ankle and foot
   M63.872 Disorders of muscle in diseases classified elsewhere, left ankle and foot
   M63.879 Disorders of muscle in diseases classified elsewhere, unspecified ankle and foot
M63.88 Disorders of muscle in diseases classified elsewhere, other site
M63.89 Disorders of muscle in diseases classified elsewhere, multiple sites

Disorders of synovium and tendon (M65-M67)

M65 Synovitis and tenosynovitis

   Excludes1: *chronic crepitant synovitis of hand and wrist (M70.0-)*
      current injury - see injury of ligament or tendon by body region
      soft tissue disorders related to use, overuse and pressure (M70.-)

+ **M65.0** Abscess of tendon sheath
   Use additional code (B95-B96) to identify bacterial agent
   M65.00 Abscess of tendon sheath, unspecified site
+ **M65.01** Abscess of tendon sheath, shoulder
   M65.011 Abscess of tendon sheath, right shoulder
   M65.012 Abscess of tendon sheath, left shoulder
   M65.019 Abscess of tendon sheath, unspecified shoulder
+ **M65.02** Abscess of tendon sheath, upper arm
   M65.021 Abscess of tendon sheath, right upper arm
   M65.022 Abscess of tendon sheath, left upper arm
   M65.029 Abscess of tendon sheath, unspecified upper arm
+ **M65.03** Abscess of tendon sheath, forearm
   M65.031 Abscess of tendon sheath, right forearm
   M65.032 Abscess of tendon sheath, left forearm
   M65.039 Abscess of tendon sheath, unspecified forearm
+ **M65.04** Abscess of tendon sheath, hand
   M65.041 Abscess of tendon sheath, right hand
   M65.042 Abscess of tendon sheath, left hand
   M65.049 Abscess of tendon sheath, unspecified hand
+ **M65.05** Abscess of tendon sheath, thigh
   M65.051 Abscess of tendon sheath, right thigh
   M65.052 Abscess of tendon sheath, left thigh
   M65.059 Abscess of tendon sheath, unspecified thigh
+ **M65.06** Abscess of tendon sheath, lower leg
   M65.061 Abscess of tendon sheath, right lower leg
   M65.062 Abscess of tendon sheath, left lower leg
   M65.069 Abscess of tendon sheath, unspecified lower leg

+ **M65.07** Abscess of tendon sheath, ankle and foot
   M65.071 Abscess of tendon sheath, right ankle and foot
   M65.072 Abscess of tendon sheath, left ankle and foot
   M65.079 Abscess of tendon sheath, unspecified ankle and foot
M65.08 Abscess of tendon sheath, other site
+ **M65.1** Other infective (teno)synovitis
   M65.10 Other infective (teno)synovitis, unspecified site
+ **M65.11** Other infective (teno)synovitis, shoulder
   M65.111 Other infective (teno)synovitis, right shoulder
   M65.112 Other infective (teno)synovitis, left shoulder
   M65.119 Other infective (teno)synovitis, unspecified shoulder
+ **M65.12** Other infective (teno)synovitis, elbow
   M65.121 Other infective (teno)synovitis, right elbow
   M65.122 Other infective (teno)synovitis, left elbow
   M65.129 Other infective (teno)synovitis, unspecified elbow
+ **M65.13** Other infective (teno)synovitis, wrist
   M65.131 Other infective (teno)synovitis, right wrist
   M65.132 Other infective (teno)synovitis, left wrist
   M65.139 Other infective (teno)synovitis, unspecified wrist
+ **M65.14** Other infective (teno)synovitis, hand
   M65.141 Other infective (teno)synovitis, right hand
   M65.142 Other infective (teno)synovitis, left hand
   M65.149 Other infective (teno)synovitis, unspecified hand
+ **M65.15** Other infective (teno)synovitis, hip
   M65.151 Other infective (teno)synovitis, right hip
   M65.152 Other infective (teno)synovitis, left hip
   M65.159 Other infective (teno)synovitis, unspecified hip
+ **M65.16** Other infective (teno)synovitis, knee
   M65.161 Other infective (teno)synovitis, right knee
   M65.162 Other infective (teno)synovitis, left knee
   M65.169 Other infective (teno)synovitis, unspecified knee
+ **M65.17** Other infective (teno)synovitis, ankle and foot
   M65.171 Other infective (teno)synovitis, right ankle and foot
   M65.172 Other infective (teno)synovitis, left ankle and foot
   M65.179 Other infective (teno)synovitis, unspecified ankle and foot
M65.18 Other infective (teno)synovitis, other site
M65.19 Other infective (teno)synovitis, multiple sites
+ **M65.2** Calcific tendinitis
   Excludes1: *tendinitis as classified in M75-M77*
      calcified tendinitis of shoulder (M75.3)
   M65.20 Calcific tendinitis, unspecified site
+ **M65.22** Calcific tendinitis, upper arm
   M65.221 Calcific tendinitis, right upper arm
   M65.222 Calcific tendinitis, left upper arm
   M65.229 Calcific tendinitis, unspecified upper arm
+ **M65.23** Calcific tendinitis, forearm
   M65.231 Calcific tendinitis, right forearm
   M65.232 Calcific tendinitis, left forearm
   M65.239 Calcific tendinitis, unspecified forearm
+ **M65.24** Calcific tendinitis, hand
   M65.241 Calcific tendinitis, right hand
   M65.242 Calcific tendinitis, left hand
   M65.249 Calcific tendinitis, unspecified hand
+ **M65.25** Calcific tendinitis, thigh
   M65.251 Calcific tendinitis, right thigh
   M65.252 Calcific tendinitis, left thigh
   M65.259 Calcific tendinitis, unspecified thigh
+ **M65.26** Calcific tendinitis, lower leg
   M65.261 Calcific tendinitis, right lower leg
   M65.262 Calcific tendinitis, left lower leg
   M65.269 Calcific tendinitis, unspecified lower leg

+ M65.27 Calcific tendinitis, ankle and foot
    M65.271 Calcific tendinitis, right ankle and foot
    M65.272 Calcific tendinitis, left ankle and foot
    M65.279 Calcific tendinitis, unspecified ankle and foot
  M65.28 Calcific tendinitis, other site
  M65.29 Calcific tendinitis, multiple sites
+ M65.3 Trigger finger
    Nodular tendinous disease
  M65.30 Trigger finger, unspecified finger
+ M65.31 Trigger thumb
    M65.311 Trigger thumb, right thumb
    M65.312 Trigger thumb, left thumb
    M65.319 Trigger thumb, unspecified thumb
+ M65.32 Trigger finger, index finger
    M65.321 Trigger finger, right index finger
    M65.322 Trigger finger, left index finger
    M65.329 Trigger finger, unspecified index finger
+ M65.33 Trigger finger, middle finger
    M65.331 Trigger finger, right middle finger
    M65.332 Trigger finger, left middle finger
    M65.339 Trigger finger, unspecified middle finger
+ M65.34 Trigger finger, ring finger
    M65.341 Trigger finger, right ring finger
    M65.342 Trigger finger, left ring finger
    M65.349 Trigger finger, unspecified ring finger
+ M65.35 Trigger finger, little finger
    M65.351 Trigger finger, right little finger
    M65.352 Trigger finger, left little finger
    M65.359 Trigger finger, unspecified little finger
M65.4 Radial styloid tenosynovitis [de Quervain]
+ M65.8 Other synovitis and tenosynovitis
  M65.80 Other synovitis and tenosynovitis, unspecified site
+ M65.81 Other synovitis and tenosynovitis, shoulder
    M65.811 Other synovitis and tenosynovitis, right shoulder
    M65.812 Other synovitis and tenosynovitis, left shoulder
    M65.819 Other synovitis and tenosynovitis, unspecified shoulder
+ M65.82 Other synovitis and tenosynovitis, upper arm
    M65.821 Other synovitis and tenosynovitis, right upper arm
    M65.822 Other synovitis and tenosynovitis, left upper arm
    M65.829 Other synovitis and tenosynovitis, unspecified upper arm
+ M65.83 Other synovitis and tenosynovitis, forearm
    M65.831 Other synovitis and tenosynovitis, right forearm
    M65.832 Other synovitis and tenosynovitis, left forearm
    M65.839 Other synovitis and tenosynovitis, unspecified forearm
+ M65.84 Other synovitis and tenosynovitis, hand
    M65.841 Other synovitis and tenosynovitis, right hand
    M65.842 Other synovitis and tenosynovitis, left hand
    M65.849 Other synovitis and tenosynovitis, unspecified hand
+ M65.85 Other synovitis and tenosynovitis, thigh
    M65.851 Other synovitis and tenosynovitis, right thigh
    M65.852 Other synovitis and tenosynovitis, left thigh
    M65.859 Other synovitis and tenosynovitis, unspecified thigh
+ M65.86 Other synovitis and tenosynovitis, lower leg
    M65.861 Other synovitis and tenosynovitis, right lower leg
    M65.862 Other synovitis and tenosynovitis, left lower leg
    M65.869 Other synovitis and tenosynovitis, unspecified lower leg
+ M65.87 Other synovitis and tenosynovitis, ankle and foot
    M65.871 Other synovitis and tenosynovitis, right ankle and foot
    M65.872 Other synovitis and tenosynovitis, left ankle and foot

    M65.879 Other synovitis and tenosynovitis, unspecified ankle and foot
  M65.88 Other synovitis and tenosynovitis, other site
  M65.89 Other synovitis and tenosynovitis, multiple sites
M65.9 Synovitis and tenosynovitis, unspecified

M66 Spontaneous rupture of synovium and tendon

Includes: rupture that occurs when a normal force is applied to tissues that are inferred to have less than normal strength

Excludes2: rotator cuff syndrome (M75.1-)
    rupture where an abnormal force is applied to normal tissue - see injury of tendon by body region

M66.0 Rupture of popliteal cyst
+ M66.1 Rupture of synovium
    Rupture of synovial cyst
    Excludes2: *rupture of popliteal cyst (M66.0)*
  M66.10 Rupture of synovium, unspecified joint
+ M66.11 Rupture of synovium, shoulder
    M66.111 Rupture of synovium, right shoulder
    M66.112 Rupture of synovium, left shoulder
    M66.119 Rupture of synovium, unspecified shoulder
+ M66.12 Rupture of synovium, elbow
    M66.121 Rupture of synovium, right elbow
    M66.122 Rupture of synovium, left elbow
    M66.129 Rupture of synovium, unspecified elbow
+ M66.13 Rupture of synovium, wrist
    M66.131 Rupture of synovium, right wrist
    M66.132 Rupture of synovium, left wrist
    M66.139 Rupture of synovium, unspecified wrist
+ M66.14 Rupture of synovium, hand and fingers
    M66.141 Rupture of synovium, right hand
    M66.142 Rupture of synovium, left hand
    M66.143 Rupture of synovium, unspecified hand
    M66.144 Rupture of synovium, right finger(s)
    M66.145 Rupture of synovium, left finger(s)
    M66.146 Rupture of synovium, unspecified finger(s)
+ M66.15 Rupture of synovium, hip
    M66.151 Rupture of synovium, right hip
    M66.152 Rupture of synovium, left hip
    M66.159 Rupture of synovium, unspecified hip
+ M66.17 Rupture of synovium, ankle, foot and toes
    M66.171 Rupture of synovium, right ankle
    M66.172 Rupture of synovium, left ankle
    M66.173 Rupture of synovium, unspecified ankle
    M66.174 Rupture of synovium, right foot
    M66.175 Rupture of synovium, left foot
    M66.176 Rupture of synovium, unspecified foot
    M66.177 Rupture of synovium, right toe(s)
    M66.178 Rupture of synovium, left toe(s)
    M66.179 Rupture of synovium, unspecified toe(s)
  M66.18 Rupture of synovium, other site
+ M66.2 Spontaneous rupture of extensor tendons
  M66.20 Spontaneous rupture of extensor tendons, unspecified site
+ M66.21 Spontaneous rupture of extensor tendons, shoulder
    M66.211 Spontaneous rupture of extensor tendons, right shoulder
    M66.212 Spontaneous rupture of extensor tendons, left shoulder
    M66.219 Spontaneous rupture of extensor tendons, unspecified shoulder
+ M66.22 Spontaneous rupture of extensor tendons, upper arm
    M66.221 Spontaneous rupture of extensor tendons, right upper arm
    M66.222 Spontaneous rupture of extensor tendons, left upper arm
    M66.229 Spontaneous rupture of extensor tendons, unspecified upper arm
+ M66.23 Spontaneous rupture of extensor tendons, forearm
    M66.231 Spontaneous rupture of extensor tendons, right forearm
    M66.232 Spontaneous rupture of extensor tendons, left forearm
    M66.239 Spontaneous rupture of extensor tendons, unspecified forearm

+, +7th, X + 7th   ● Newborn   ● Pediatric   ● Maternity   ● Adult   ♀ Female   ♂ Male   Manifestation   Unacceptable PDX   HCC   CC   MCC   HAC

+ **M66.24** Spontaneous rupture of extensor tendons, hand
    M66.241 Spontaneous rupture of extensor tendons, right hand
    M66.242 Spontaneous rupture of extensor tendons, left hand
    M66.249 Spontaneous rupture of extensor tendons, unspecified hand
+ **M66.25** Spontaneous rupture of extensor tendons, thigh
    M66.251 Spontaneous rupture of extensor tendons, right thigh
    M66.252 Spontaneous rupture of extensor tendons, left thigh
    M66.259 Spontaneous rupture of extensor tendons, unspecified thigh
+ **M66.26** Spontaneous rupture of extensor tendons, lower leg
    M66.261 Spontaneous rupture of extensor tendons, right lower leg
    M66.262 Spontaneous rupture of extensor tendons, left lower leg
    M66.269 Spontaneous rupture of extensor tendons, unspecified lower leg
+ **M66.27** Spontaneous rupture of extensor tendons, ankle and foot
    M66.271 Spontaneous rupture of extensor tendons, right ankle and foot
    M66.272 Spontaneous rupture of extensor tendons, left ankle and foot
    M66.279 Spontaneous rupture of extensor tendons, unspecified ankle and foot
M66.28 Spontaneous rupture of extensor tendons, other site
M66.29 Spontaneous rupture of extensor tendons, multiple sites
+ **M66.3** Spontaneous rupture of flexor tendons
    M66.30 Spontaneous rupture of flexor tendons, unspecified site
+ **M66.31** Spontaneous rupture of flexor tendons, shoulder
    M66.311 Spontaneous rupture of flexor tendons, right shoulder
    M66.312 Spontaneous rupture of flexor tendons, left shoulder
    M66.319 Spontaneous rupture of flexor tendons, unspecified shoulder
+ **M66.32** Spontaneous rupture of flexor tendons, upper arm
    M66.321 Spontaneous rupture of flexor tendons, right upper arm
    M66.322 Spontaneous rupture of flexor tendons, left upper arm
    M66.329 Spontaneous rupture of flexor tendons, unspecified upper arm
+ **M66.33** Spontaneous rupture of flexor tendons, forearm
    M66.331 Spontaneous rupture of flexor tendons, right forearm
    M66.332 Spontaneous rupture of flexor tendons, left forearm
    M66.339 Spontaneous rupture of flexor tendons, unspecified forearm
+ **M66.34** Spontaneous rupture of flexor tendons, hand
    M66.341 Spontaneous rupture of flexor tendons, right hand
    M66.342 Spontaneous rupture of flexor tendons, left hand
    M66.349 Spontaneous rupture of flexor tendons, unspecified hand
+ **M66.35** Spontaneous rupture of flexor tendons, thigh
    M66.351 Spontaneous rupture of flexor tendons, right thigh
    M66.352 Spontaneous rupture of flexor tendons, left thigh
    M66.359 Spontaneous rupture of flexor tendons, unspecified thigh
+ **M66.36** Spontaneous rupture of flexor tendons, lower leg
    M66.361 Spontaneous rupture of flexor tendons, right lower leg
    M66.362 Spontaneous rupture of flexor tendons, left lower leg
    M66.369 Spontaneous rupture of flexor tendons, unspecified lower leg

+ **M66.37** Spontaneous rupture of flexor tendons, ankle and foot
    M66.371 Spontaneous rupture of flexor tendons, right ankle and foot
    M66.372 Spontaneous rupture of flexor tendons, left ankle and foot
    M66.379 Spontaneous rupture of flexor tendons, unspecified ankle and foot
M66.38 Spontaneous rupture of flexor tendons, other site
M66.39 Spontaneous rupture of flexor tendons, multiple sites
+ **M66.8** Spontaneous rupture of other tendons
    M66.80 Spontaneous rupture of other tendons, unspecified site
+ **M66.81** Spontaneous rupture of other tendons, shoulder
    M66.811 Spontaneous rupture of other tendons, right shoulder
    M66.812 Spontaneous rupture of other tendons, left shoulder
    M66.819 Spontaneous rupture of other tendons, unspecified shoulder
+ **M66.82** Spontaneous rupture of other tendons, upper arm
    M66.821 Spontaneous rupture of other tendons, right upper arm
    M66.822 Spontaneous rupture of other tendons, left upper arm
    M66.829 Spontaneous rupture of other tendons, unspecified upper arm
+ **M66.83** Spontaneous rupture of other tendons, forearm
    M66.831 Spontaneous rupture of other tendons, right forearm
    M66.832 Spontaneous rupture of other tendons, left forearm
    M66.839 Spontaneous rupture of other tendons, unspecified forearm
+ **M66.84** Spontaneous rupture of other tendons, hand
    M66.841 Spontaneous rupture of other tendons, right hand
    M66.842 Spontaneous rupture of other tendons, left hand
    M66.849 Spontaneous rupture of other tendons, unspecified hand
+ **M66.85** Spontaneous rupture of other tendons, thigh
    M66.851 Spontaneous rupture of other tendons, right thigh
    M66.852 Spontaneous rupture of other tendons, left thigh
    M66.859 Spontaneous rupture of other tendons, unspecified thigh
+ **M66.86** Spontaneous rupture of other tendons, lower leg
    M66.861 Spontaneous rupture of other tendons, right lower leg
    M66.862 Spontaneous rupture of other tendons, left lower leg
    M66.869 Spontaneous rupture of other tendons, unspecified lower leg
+ **M66.87** Spontaneous rupture of other tendons, ankle and foot
    M66.871 Spontaneous rupture of other tendons, right ankle and foot
    M66.872 Spontaneous rupture of other tendons, left ankle and foot
    M66.879 Spontaneous rupture of other tendons, unspecified ankle and foot
M66.88 Spontaneous rupture of other tendons, other sites
M66.89 Spontaneous rupture of other tendons, multiple sites
M66.9 Spontaneous rupture of unspecified tendon
    Rupture at musculotendinous junction, nontraumatic

M67 Other disorders of synovium and tendon

    Excludes1: *palmar fascial fibromatosis [Dupuytren] (M72.0)*
           tendinitis NOS (M77.9-)
           xanthomatosis localized to tendons (E78.2)
+ **M67.0** Short Achilles tendon (acquired)
    M67.00 Short Achilles tendon (acquired), unspecified ankle
    M67.01 Short Achilles tendon (acquired), right ankle
    M67.02 Short Achilles tendon (acquired), left ankle
+ **M67.2** Synovial hypertrophy, not elsewhere classified
    Excludes1: *villonodular synovitis (pigmented) (M12.2-)*

M67.20 Synovial hypertrophy, not elsewhere classified, unspecified site
+ M67.21 Synovial hypertrophy, not elsewhere classified, shoulder
　　M67.211 Synovial hypertrophy, not elsewhere classified, right shoulder
　　M67.212 Synovial hypertrophy, not elsewhere classified, left shoulder
　　M67.219 Synovial hypertrophy, not elsewhere classified, unspecified shoulder
+ M67.22 Synovial hypertrophy, not elsewhere classified, upper arm
　　M67.221 Synovial hypertrophy, not elsewhere classified, right upper arm
　　M67.222 Synovial hypertrophy, not elsewhere classified, left upper arm
　　M67.229 Synovial hypertrophy, not elsewhere classified, unspecified upper arm
+ M67.23 Synovial hypertrophy, not elsewhere classified, forearm
　　M67.231 Synovial hypertrophy, not elsewhere classified, right forearm
　　M67.232 Synovial hypertrophy, not elsewhere classified, left forearm
　　M67.239 Synovial hypertrophy, not elsewhere classified, unspecified forearm
+ M67.24 Synovial hypertrophy, not elsewhere classified, hand
　　M67.241 Synovial hypertrophy, not elsewhere classified, right hand
　　M67.242 Synovial hypertrophy, not elsewhere classified, left hand
　　M67.249 Synovial hypertrophy, not elsewhere classified, unspecified hand
+ M67.25 Synovial hypertrophy, not elsewhere classified, thigh
　　M67.251 Synovial hypertrophy, not elsewhere classified, right thigh
　　M67.252 Synovial hypertrophy, not elsewhere classified, left thigh
　　M67.259 Synovial hypertrophy, not elsewhere classified, unspecified thigh
+ M67.26 Synovial hypertrophy, not elsewhere classified, lower leg
　　M67.261 Synovial hypertrophy, not elsewhere classified, right lower leg
　　M67.262 Synovial hypertrophy, not elsewhere classified, left lower leg
　　M67.269 Synovial hypertrophy, not elsewhere classified, unspecified lower leg
+ M67.27 Synovial hypertrophy, not elsewhere classified, ankle and foot
　　M67.271 Synovial hypertrophy, not elsewhere classified, right ankle and foot
　　M67.272 Synovial hypertrophy, not elsewhere classified, left ankle and foot
　　M67.279 Synovial hypertrophy, not elsewhere classified, unspecified ankle and foot
M67.28 Synovial hypertrophy, not elsewhere classified, other site
M67.29 Synovial hypertrophy, not elsewhere classified, multiple sites
+ M67.3 Transient synovitis
　　Toxic synovitis
　　Excludes1: palindromic rheumatism (M12.3-)
M67.30 Transient synovitis, unspecified site
+ M67.31 Transient synovitis, shoulder
　　M67.311 Transient synovitis, right shoulder
　　M67.312 Transient synovitis, left shoulder
　　M67.319 Transient synovitis, unspecified shoulder
+ M67.32 Transient synovitis, elbow
　　M67.321 Transient synovitis, right elbow
　　M67.322 Transient synovitis, left elbow
　　M67.329 Transient synovitis, unspecified elbow
+ M67.33 Transient synovitis, wrist
　　M67.331 Transient synovitis, right wrist
　　M67.332 Transient synovitis, left wrist
　　M67.339 Transient synovitis, unspecified wrist
+ M67.34 Transient synovitis, hand
　　M67.341 Transient synovitis, right hand
　　M67.342 Transient synovitis, left hand
　　M67.349 Transient synovitis, unspecified hand

+ M67.35 Transient synovitis, hip
　　M67.351 Transient synovitis, right hip
　　M67.352 Transient synovitis, left hip
　　M67.359 Transient synovitis, unspecified hip
+ M67.36 Transient synovitis, knee
　　M67.361 Transient synovitis, right knee
　　M67.362 Transient synovitis, left knee
　　M67.369 Transient synovitis, unspecified knee
+ M67.37 Transient synovitis, ankle and foot
　　M67.371 Transient synovitis, right ankle and foot
　　M67.372 Transient synovitis, left ankle and foot
　　M67.379 Transient synovitis, unspecified ankle and foot
M67.38 Transient synovitis, other site
M67.39 Transient synovitis, multiple sites
+ M67.4 Ganglion
　　Ganglion of joint or tendon (sheath)
　　Excludes1: ganglion in yaws (A66.6)
　　Excludes2: cyst of bursa (M71.2-M71.3)
　　　　　　cyst of synovium (M71.2-M71.3)
M67.40 Ganglion, unspecified site
+ M67.41 Ganglion, shoulder
　　M67.411 Ganglion, right shoulder
　　M67.412 Ganglion, left shoulder
　　M67.419 Ganglion, unspecified shoulder
+ M67.42 Ganglion, elbow
　　M67.421 Ganglion, right elbow
　　M67.422 Ganglion, left elbow
　　M67.429 Ganglion, unspecified elbow
+ M67.43 Ganglion, wrist
　　M67.431 Ganglion, right wrist
　　M67.432 Ganglion, left wrist
　　M67.439 Ganglion, unspecified wrist
+ M67.44 Ganglion, hand
　　M67.441 Ganglion, right hand
　　M67.442 Ganglion, left hand
　　M67.449 Ganglion, unspecified hand
+ M67.45 Ganglion, hip
　　M67.451 Ganglion, right hip
　　M67.452 Ganglion, left hip
　　M67.459 Ganglion, unspecified hip
+ M67.46 Ganglion, knee
　　M67.461 Ganglion, right knee
　　M67.462 Ganglion, left knee
　　M67.469 Ganglion, unspecified knee
+ M67.47 Ganglion, ankle and foot
　　M67.471 Ganglion, right ankle and foot
　　M67.472 Ganglion, left ankle and foot
　　M67.479 Ganglion, unspecified ankle and foot
M67.48 Ganglion, other site
M67.49 Ganglion, multiple sites
+ M67.5 Plica syndrome
　　Plica knee
M67.50 Plica syndrome, unspecified knee
M67.51 Plica syndrome, right knee
M67.52 Plica syndrome, left knee
+ M67.8 Other specified disorders of synovium and tendon
M67.80 Other specified disorders of synovium and tendon, unspecified site
+ M67.81 Other specified disorders of synovium and tendon, shoulder
　　M67.811 Other specified disorders of synovium, right shoulder
　　M67.812 Other specified disorders of synovium, left shoulder
　　M67.813 Other specified disorders of tendon, right shoulder
　　M67.814 Other specified disorders of tendon, left shoulder
　　M67.819 Other specified disorders of synovium and tendon, unspecified shoulder
+ M67.82 Other specified disorders of synovium and tendon, elbow
　　M67.821 Other specified disorders of synovium, right elbow
　　M67.822 Other specified disorders of synovium, left elbow
　　M67.823 Other specified disorders of tendon, right elbow
　　M67.824 Other specified disorders of tendon, left elbow

+, +7th, X + 7th　　● Newborn　　● Pediatric　　● Maternity　　● Adult　　♀ Female　　♂ Male　　Manifestation　　Unacceptable PDX　　HCC　　CC　　MCC　　HAC

M67.829 Other specified disorders of synovium and tendon, unspecified elbow

+ M67.83 Other specified disorders of synovium and tendon, wrist

  M67.831 Other specified disorders of synovium, right wrist

  M67.832 Other specified disorders of synovium, left wrist

  M67.833 Other specified disorders of tendon, right wrist

  M67.834 Other specified disorders of tendon, left wrist

  M67.839 Other specified disorders of synovium and tendon, unspecified wrist

+ M67.84 Other specified disorders of synovium and tendon, hand

  M67.841 Other specified disorders of synovium, right hand

  M67.842 Other specified disorders of synovium, left hand

  M67.843 Other specified disorders of tendon, right hand

  M67.844 Other specified disorders of tendon, left hand

  M67.849 Other specified disorders of synovium and tendon, unspecified hand

+ M67.85 Other specified disorders of synovium and tendon, hip

  M67.851 Other specified disorders of synovium, right hip

  M67.852 Other specified disorders of synovium, left hip

  M67.853 Other specified disorders of tendon, right hip

  M67.854 Other specified disorders of tendon, left hip

  M67.859 Other specified disorders of synovium and tendon, unspecified hip

+ M67.86 Other specified disorders of synovium and tendon, knee

  M67.861 Other specified disorders of synovium, right knee

  M67.862 Other specified disorders of synovium, left knee

  M67.863 Other specified disorders of tendon, right knee

  M67.864 Other specified disorders of tendon, left knee

  M67.869 Other specified disorders of synovium and tendon, unspecified knee

+ M67.87 Other specified disorders of synovium and tendon, ankle and foot

  M67.871 Other specified disorders of synovium, right ankle and foot

  M67.872 Other specified disorders of synovium, left ankle and foot

  M67.873 Other specified disorders of tendon, right ankle and foot

  M67.874 Other specified disorders of tendon, left ankle and foot

  M67.879 Other specified disorders of synovium and tendon, unspecified ankle and foot

M67.88 Other specified disorders of synovium and tendon, other site

M67.89 Other specified disorders of synovium and tendon, multiple sites

+ M67.9 Unspecified disorder of synovium and tendon

  M67.90 Unspecified disorder of synovium and tendon, unspecified site

+ M67.91 Unspecified disorder of synovium and tendon, shoulder

  M67.911 Unspecified disorder of synovium and tendon, right shoulder

  M67.912 Unspecified disorder of synovium and tendon, left shoulder

  M67.919 Unspecified disorder of synovium and tendon, unspecified shoulder

+ M67.92 Unspecified disorder of synovium and tendon, upper arm

  M67.921 Unspecified disorder of synovium and tendon, right upper arm

  M67.922 Unspecified disorder of synovium and tendon, left upper arm

  M67.929 Unspecified disorder of synovium and tendon, unspecified upper arm

+ M67.93 Unspecified disorder of synovium and tendon, forearm

  M67.931 Unspecified disorder of synovium and tendon, right forearm

  M67.932 Unspecified disorder of synovium and tendon, left forearm

  M67.939 Unspecified disorder of synovium and tendon, unspecified forearm

+ M67.94 Unspecified disorder of synovium and tendon, hand

  M67.941 Unspecified disorder of synovium and tendon, right hand

  M67.942 Unspecified disorder of synovium and tendon, left hand

  M67.949 Unspecified disorder of synovium and tendon, unspecified hand

+ M67.95 Unspecified disorder of synovium and tendon, thigh

  M67.951 Unspecified disorder of synovium and tendon, right thigh

  M67.952 Unspecified disorder of synovium and tendon, left thigh

  M67.959 Unspecified disorder of synovium and tendon, unspecified thigh

+ M67.96 Unspecified disorder of synovium and tendon, lower leg

  M67.961 Unspecified disorder of synovium and tendon, right lower leg

  M67.962 Unspecified disorder of synovium and tendon, left lower leg

  M67.969 Unspecified disorder of synovium and tendon, unspecified lower leg

+ M67.97 Unspecified disorder of synovium and tendon, ankle and foot

  M67.971 Unspecified disorder of synovium and tendon, right ankle and foot

  M67.972 Unspecified disorder of synovium and tendon, left ankle and foot

  M67.979 Unspecified disorder of synovium and tendon, unspecified ankle and foot

M67.98 Unspecified disorder of synovium and tendon, other site

M67.99 Unspecified disorder of synovium and tendon, multiple sites

Other soft tissue disorders (M70-M79)

M70 Soft tissue disorders related to use, overuse and pressure

Includes: soft tissue disorders of occupational origin

Use additional external cause code to identify activity causing disorder (Y93.-)

Excludes1: bursitis NOS (M71.9-)

Excludes2: bursitis of shoulder (M75.5)

  enthesopathies (M76-M77)

  pressure ulcer (pressure area) (L89.-)

+ M70.0 Crepitant synovitis (acute) (chronic) of hand and wrist

+ M70.03 Crepitant synovitis (acute) (chronic), wrist

  M70.031 Crepitant synovitis (acute) (chronic), right wrist

  M70.032 Crepitant synovitis (acute) (chronic), left wrist

  M70.039 Crepitant synovitis (acute) (chronic), unspecified wrist

+ M70.04 Crepitant synovitis (acute) (chronic), hand

  M70.041 Crepitant synovitis (acute) (chronic), right hand

  M70.042 Crepitant synovitis (acute) (chronic), left hand

  M70.049 Crepitant synovitis (acute) (chronic), unspecified hand

+ M70.1 Bursitis of hand

  M70.10 Bursitis, unspecified hand

  M70.11 Bursitis, right hand

  M70.12 Bursitis, left hand

+ M70.2 Olecranon bursitis

  M70.20 Olecranon bursitis, unspecified elbow

  M70.21 Olecranon bursitis, right elbow

+, +7th, X + 7th   ● Newborn   ● Pediatric   ● Maternity   ● Adult   ♀ Female   ♂ Male   Manifestation   Unacceptable PDX   HCC   CC   MCC   HAC

M70.22 Olecranon bursitis, left elbow

+ M70.3 Other bursitis of elbow

   M70.30 Other bursitis of elbow, unspecified elbow

   M70.31 Other bursitis of elbow, right elbow

   M70.32 Other bursitis of elbow, left elbow

+ M70.4 Prepatellar bursitis

   M70.40 Prepatellar bursitis, unspecified knee

   M70.41 Prepatellar bursitis, right knee

   M70.42 Prepatellar bursitis, left knee

+ M70.5 Other bursitis of knee

   M70.50 Other bursitis of knee, unspecified knee

   M70.51 Other bursitis of knee, right knee

   M70.52 Other bursitis of knee, left knee

+ M70.6 Trochanteric bursitis

   Trochanteric tendinitis

   M70.60 Trochanteric bursitis, unspecified hip

   M70.61 Trochanteric bursitis, right hip

   M70.62 Trochanteric bursitis, left hip

+ M70.7 Other bursitis of hip

   Ischial bursitis

   M70.70 Other bursitis of hip, unspecified hip

   M70.71 Other bursitis of hip, right hip

   M70.72 Other bursitis of hip, left hip

+ M70.8 Other soft tissue disorders related to use, overuse and pressure

   M70.80 Other soft tissue disorders related to use, overuse and pressure of unspecified site

  + M70.81 Other soft tissue disorders related to use, overuse and pressure of shoulder

     M70.811 Other soft tissue disorders related to use, overuse and pressure, right shoulder

     M70.812 Other soft tissue disorders related to use, overuse and pressure, left shoulder

     M70.819 Other soft tissue disorders related to use, overuse and pressure, unspecified shoulder

  + M70.82 Other soft tissue disorders related to use, overuse and pressure of upper arm

     M70.821 Other soft tissue disorders related to use, overuse and pressure, right upper arm

     M70.822 Other soft tissue disorders related to use, overuse and pressure, left upper arm

     M70.829 Other soft tissue disorders related to use, overuse and pressure, unspecified upper arms

  + M70.83 Other soft tissue disorders related to use, overuse and pressure of forearm

     M70.831 Other soft tissue disorders related to use, overuse and pressure, right forearm

     M70.832 Other soft tissue disorders related to use, overuse and pressure, left forearm

     M70.839 Other soft tissue disorders related to use, overuse and pressure, unspecified forearm

  + M70.84 Other soft tissue disorders related to use, overuse and pressure of hand

     M70.841 Other soft tissue disorders related to use, overuse and pressure, right hand

     M70.842 Other soft tissue disorders related to use, overuse and pressure, left hand

     M70.849 Other soft tissue disorders related to use, overuse and pressure, unspecified hand

  + M70.85 Other soft tissue disorders related to use, overuse and pressure of thigh

     M70.851 Other soft tissue disorders related to use, overuse and pressure, right thigh

     M70.852 Other soft tissue disorders related to use, overuse and pressure, left thigh

     M70.859 Other soft tissue disorders related to use, overuse and pressure, unspecified thigh

  + M70.86 Other soft tissue disorders related to use, overuse and pressure lower leg

     M70.861 Other soft tissue disorders related to use, overuse and pressure, right lower leg

     M70.862 Other soft tissue disorders related to use, overuse and pressure, left lower leg

     M70.869 Other soft tissue disorders related to use, overuse and pressure, unspecified leg

  + M70.87 Other soft tissue disorders related to use, overuse and pressure of ankle and foot

     M70.871 Other soft tissue disorders related to use, overuse and pressure, right ankle and foot

     M70.872 Other soft tissue disorders related to use, overuse and pressure, left ankle and foot

     M70.879 Other soft tissue disorders related to use, overuse and pressure, unspecified ankle and foot

   M70.88 Other soft tissue disorders related to use, overuse and pressure other site

   M70.89 Other soft tissue disorders related to use, overuse and pressure multiple sites

+ M70.9 Unspecified soft tissue disorder related to use, overuse and pressure

   M70.90 Unspecified soft tissue disorder related to use, overuse and pressure of unspecified site

  + M70.91 Unspecified soft tissue disorder related to use, overuse and pressure of shoulder

     M70.911 Unspecified soft tissue disorder related to use, overuse and pressure, right shoulder

     M70.912 Unspecified soft tissue disorder related to use, overuse and pressure, left shoulder

     M70.919 Unspecified soft tissue disorder related to use, overuse and pressure, unspecified shoulder

  + M70.92 Unspecified soft tissue disorder related to use, overuse and pressure of upper arm

     M70.921 Unspecified soft tissue disorder related to use, overuse and pressure, right upper arm

     M70.922 Unspecified soft tissue disorder related to use, overuse and pressure, left upper arm

     M70.929 Unspecified soft tissue disorder related to use, overuse and pressure, unspecified upper arm

  + M70.93 Unspecified soft tissue disorder related to use, overuse and pressure of forearm

     M70.931 Unspecified soft tissue disorder related to use, overuse and pressure, right forearm

     M70.932 Unspecified soft tissue disorder related to use, overuse and pressure, left forearm

     M70.939 Unspecified soft tissue disorder related to use, overuse and pressure, unspecified forearm

  + M70.94 Unspecified soft tissue disorder related to use, overuse and pressure of hand

     M70.941 Unspecified soft tissue disorder related to use, overuse and pressure, right hand

     M70.942 Unspecified soft tissue disorder related to use, overuse and pressure, left hand

     M70.949 Unspecified soft tissue disorder related to use, overuse and pressure, unspecified hand

  + M70.95 Unspecified soft tissue disorder related to use, overuse and pressure of thigh

     M70.951 Unspecified soft tissue disorder related to use, overuse and pressure, right thigh

     M70.952 Unspecified soft tissue disorder related to use, overuse and pressure, left thigh

     M70.959 Unspecified soft tissue disorder related to use, overuse and pressure, unspecified thigh

  + M70.96 Unspecified soft tissue disorder related to use, overuse and pressure lower leg

     M70.961 Unspecified soft tissue disorder related to use, overuse and pressure, right lower leg

     M70.962 Unspecified soft tissue disorder related to use, overuse and pressure, left lower leg

M70.969 Unspecified soft tissue disorder related to use, overuse and pressure, unspecified lower leg

+ M70.97 Unspecified soft tissue disorder related to use, overuse and pressure of ankle and foot

    M70.971 Unspecified soft tissue disorder related to use, overuse and pressure, right ankle and foot

    M70.972 Unspecified soft tissue disorder related to use, overuse and pressure, left ankle and foot

    M70.979 Unspecified soft tissue disorder related to use, overuse and pressure, unspecified ankle and foot

M70.98 Unspecified soft tissue disorder related to use, overuse and pressure other

M70.99 Unspecified soft tissue disorder related to use, overuse and pressure multiple sites

M71 Other bursopathies

Excludes1: bunion (M20.1)
    bursitis related to use, overuse or pressure (M70.-)
    enthesopathies (M76-M77)

+ M71.0 Abscess of bursa

Use additional code (B95.-, B96.-) to identify causative organism

M71.00 Abscess of bursa, unspecified site

+ M71.01 Abscess of bursa, shoulder

    M71.011 Abscess of bursa, right shoulder
    M71.012 Abscess of bursa, left shoulder
    M71.019 Abscess of bursa, unspecified shoulder

+ M71.02 Abscess of bursa, elbow

    M71.021 Abscess of bursa, right elbow
    M71.022 Abscess of bursa, left elbow
    M71.029 Abscess of bursa, unspecified elbow

+ M71.03 Abscess of bursa, wrist

    M71.031 Abscess of bursa, right wrist
    M71.032 Abscess of bursa, left wrist
    M71.039 Abscess of bursa, unspecified wrist

+ M71.04 Abscess of bursa, hand

    M71.041 Abscess of bursa, right hand
    M71.042 Abscess of bursa, left hand
    M71.049 Abscess of bursa, unspecified hand

+ M71.05 Abscess of bursa, hip

    M71.051 Abscess of bursa, right hip
    M71.052 Abscess of bursa, left hip
    M71.059 Abscess of bursa, unspecified hip

+ M71.06 Abscess of bursa, knee

    M71.061 Abscess of bursa, right knee
    M71.062 Abscess of bursa, left knee
    M71.069 Abscess of bursa, unspecified knee

+ M71.07 Abscess of bursa, ankle and foot

    M71.071 Abscess of bursa, right ankle and foot
    M71.072 Abscess of bursa, left ankle and foot
    M71.079 Abscess of bursa, unspecified ankle and foot

M71.08 Abscess of bursa, other site

M71.09 Abscess of bursa, multiple sites

+ M71.1 Other infective bursitis

Use additional code (B95.-, B96.-) to identify causative organism

M71.10 Other infective bursitis, unspecified site

+ M71.11 Other infective bursitis, shoulder

    M71.111 Other infective bursitis, right shoulder
    M71.112 Other infective bursitis, left shoulder
    M71.119 Other infective bursitis, unspecified shoulder

+ M71.12 Other infective bursitis, elbow

    M71.121 Other infective bursitis, right elbow
    M71.122 Other infective bursitis, left elbow
    M71.129 Other infective bursitis, unspecified elbow

+ M71.13 Other infective bursitis, wrist

    M71.131 Other infective bursitis, right wrist
    M71.132 Other infective bursitis, left wrist
    M71.139 Other infective bursitis, unspecified wrist

+ M71.14 Other infective bursitis, hand

    M71.141 Other infective bursitis, right hand
    M71.142 Other infective bursitis, left hand

    M71.149 Other infective bursitis, unspecified hand

+ M71.15 Other infective bursitis, hip

    M71.151 Other infective bursitis, right hip
    M71.152 Other infective bursitis, left hip
    M71.159 Other infective bursitis, unspecified hip

+ M71.16 Other infective bursitis, knee

    M71.161 Other infective bursitis, right knee
    M71.162 Other infective bursitis, left knee
    M71.169 Other infective bursitis, unspecified knee

+ M71.17 Other infective bursitis, ankle and foot

    M71.171 Other infective bursitis, right ankle and foot
    M71.172 Other infective bursitis, left ankle and foot
    M71.179 Other infective bursitis, unspecified ankle and foot

M71.18 Other infective bursitis, other site

M71.19 Other infective bursitis, multiple sites

+ M71.2 Synovial cyst of popliteal space [Baker]

Excludes1: synovial cyst of popliteal space with rupture (M66.0)

M71.20 Synovial cyst of popliteal space [Baker], unspecified knee

M71.21 Synovial cyst of popliteal space [Baker], right knee

M71.22 Synovial cyst of popliteal space [Baker], left knee

+ M71.3 Other bursal cyst

Synovial cyst NOS

Excludes1: synovial cyst with rupture (M66.1-)

M71.30 Other bursal cyst, unspecified site

+ M71.31 Other bursal cyst, shoulder

    M71.311 Other bursal cyst, right shoulder
    M71.312 Other bursal cyst, left shoulder
    M71.319 Other bursal cyst, unspecified shoulder

+ M71.32 Other bursal cyst, elbow

    M71.321 Other bursal cyst, right elbow
    M71.322 Other bursal cyst, left elbow
    M71.329 Other bursal cyst, unspecified elbow

+ M71.33 Other bursal cyst, wrist

    M71.331 Other bursal cyst, right wrist
    M71.332 Other bursal cyst, left wrist
    M71.339 Other bursal cyst, unspecified wrist

+ M71.34 Other bursal cyst, hand

    M71.341 Other bursal cyst, right hand
    M71.342 Other bursal cyst, left hand
    M71.349 Other bursal cyst, unspecified hand

+ M71.35 Other bursal cyst, hip

    M71.351 Other bursal cyst, right hip
    M71.352 Other bursal cyst, left hip
    M71.359 Other bursal cyst, unspecified hip

+ M71.37 Other bursal cyst, ankle and foot

    M71.371 Other bursal cyst, right ankle and foot
    M71.372 Other bursal cyst, left ankle and foot
    M71.379 Other bursal cyst, unspecified ankle and foot

M71.38 Other bursal cyst, other site

M71.39 Other bursal cyst, multiple sites

+ M71.4 Calcium deposit in bursa

Excludes2: calcium deposit in bursa of shoulder (M75.3)

M71.40 Calcium deposit in bursa, unspecified site

+ M71.42 Calcium deposit in bursa, elbow

    M71.421 Calcium deposit in bursa, right elbow
    M71.422 Calcium deposit in bursa, left elbow
    M71.429 Calcium deposit in bursa, unspecified elbow

+ M71.43 Calcium deposit in bursa, wrist

    M71.431 Calcium deposit in bursa, right wrist
    M71.432 Calcium deposit in bursa, left wrist
    M71.439 Calcium deposit in bursa, unspecified wrist

+ M71.44 Calcium deposit in bursa, hand

    M71.441 Calcium deposit in bursa, right hand
    M71.442 Calcium deposit in bursa, left hand
    M71.449 Calcium deposit in bursa, unspecified hand

+ M71.45 Calcium deposit in bursa, hip

    M71.451 Calcium deposit in bursa, right hip
    M71.452 Calcium deposit in bursa, left hip
    M71.459 Calcium deposit in bursa, unspecified hip

+ M71.46 **Calcium deposit in bursa, knee**
    M71.461 **Calcium deposit in bursa, right knee**
    M71.462 **Calcium deposit in bursa, left knee**
    M71.469 **Calcium deposit in bursa, unspecified knee**
+ M71.47 **Calcium deposit in bursa, ankle and foot**
    M71.471 **Calcium deposit in bursa, right ankle and foot**
    M71.472 **Calcium deposit in bursa, left ankle and foot**
    M71.479 **Calcium deposit in bursa, unspecified ankle and foot**
  M71.48 **Calcium deposit in bursa, other site**
  M71.49 **Calcium deposit in bursa, multiple sites**
+ M71.5 **Other bursitis, not elsewhere classified**
  Excludes1: bursitis NOS (M71.9-)
  Excludes2: bursitis of shoulder (M75.5)
         bursitis of tibial collateral [Pellegrini-Stieda] (M76.4-)
  M71.50 **Other bursitis, not elsewhere classified, unspecified site**
+ M71.52 **Other bursitis, not elsewhere classified, elbow**
    M71.521 **Other bursitis, not elsewhere classified, right elbow**
    M71.522 **Other bursitis, not elsewhere classified, left elbow**
    M71.529 **Other bursitis, not elsewhere classified, unspecified elbow**
+ M71.53 **Other bursitis, not elsewhere classified, wrist**
    M71.531 **Other bursitis, not elsewhere classified, right wrist**
    M71.532 **Other bursitis, not elsewhere classified, left wrist**
    M71.539 **Other bursitis, not elsewhere classified, unspecified wrist**
+ M71.54 **Other bursitis, not elsewhere classified, hand**
    M71.541 **Other bursitis, not elsewhere classified, right hand**
    M71.542 **Other bursitis, not elsewhere classified, left hand**
    M71.549 **Other bursitis, not elsewhere classified, unspecified hand**
+ M71.55 **Other bursitis, not elsewhere classified, hip**
    M71.551 **Other bursitis, not elsewhere classified, right hip**
    M71.552 **Other bursitis, not elsewhere classified, left hip**
    M71.559 **Other bursitis, not elsewhere classified, unspecified hip**
+ M71.56 **Other bursitis, not elsewhere classified, knee**
    M71.561 **Other bursitis, not elsewhere classified, right knee**
    M71.562 **Other bursitis, not elsewhere classified, left knee**
    M71.569 **Other bursitis, not elsewhere classified, unspecified knee**
+ M71.57 **Other bursitis, not elsewhere classified, ankle and foot**
    M71.571 **Other bursitis, not elsewhere classified, right ankle and foot**
    M71.572 **Other bursitis, not elsewhere classified, left ankle and foot**
    M71.579 **Other bursitis, not elsewhere classified, unspecified ankle and foot**
  M71.58 **Other bursitis, not elsewhere classified, other site**
+ M71.8 **Other specified bursopathies**
  M71.80 **Other specified bursopathies, unspecified site**
+ M71.81 **Other specified bursopathies, shoulder**
    M71.811 **Other specified bursopathies, right shoulder**
    M71.812 **Other specified bursopathies, left shoulder**
    M71.819 **Other specified bursopathies, unspecified shoulder**
+ M71.82 **Other specified bursopathies, elbow**
    M71.821 **Other specified bursopathies, right elbow**
    M71.822 **Other specified bursopathies, left elbow**
    M71.829 **Other specified bursopathies, unspecified elbow**
+ M71.83 **Other specified bursopathies, wrist**
    M71.831 **Other specified bursopathies, right wrist**
    M71.832 **Other specified bursopathies, left wrist**
    M71.839 **Other specified bursopathies, unspecified wrist**
+ M71.84 **Other specified bursopathies, hand**
    M71.841 **Other specified bursopathies, right hand**
    M71.842 **Other specified bursopathies, left hand**
    M71.849 **Other specified bursopathies, unspecified hand**
+ M71.85 **Other specified bursopathies, hip**
    M71.851 **Other specified bursopathies, right hip**
    M71.852 **Other specified bursopathies, left hip**
    M71.859 **Other specified bursopathies, unspecified hip**
+ M71.86 **Other specified bursopathies, knee**
    M71.861 **Other specified bursopathies, right knee**
    M71.862 **Other specified bursopathies, left knee**
    M71.869 **Other specified bursopathies, unspecified knee**
+ M71.87 **Other specified bursopathies, ankle and foot**
    M71.871 **Other specified bursopathies, right ankle and foot**
    M71.872 **Other specified bursopathies, left ankle and foot**
    M71.879 **Other specified bursopathies, unspecified ankle and foot**
  M71.88 **Other specified bursopathies, other site**
  M71.89 **Other specified bursopathies, multiple sites**
M71.9 **Bursopathy, unspecified**
  Bursitis NOS

M72 Fibroblastic disorders

  Excludes2: retroperitoneal fibromatosis (D48.3)
● **M72.0 Palmar fascial fibromatosis [Dupuytren]**
M72.1 Knuckle pads
M72.2 Plantar fascial fibromatosis
  Plantar fasciitis
M72.4 Pseudosarcomatous fibromatosis
  Nodular fasciitis
MCC **M72.6 Necrotizing fasciitis**
  Use additional code (B95.-, B96.-) to identify causative organism
M72.8 Other fibroblastic disorders
  Abscess of fascia
  Fasciitis NEC
  Other infective fasciitis
  Use additional code to (B95.-, B96.-) identify causative organism
  Excludes1: diffuse (eosinophilic) fasciitis (M35.4)
        necrotizing fasciitis (M72.6)
        nodular fasciitis (M72.4)
        perirenal fasciitis NOS (N13.5)
        perirenal fasciitis with infection (N13.6)
        plantar fasciitis (M72.2)
M72.9 Fibroblastic disorder, unspecified
  Fasciitis NOS
  Fibromatosis NOS

M75 Shoulder lesions

  Excludes2: shoulder-hand syndrome (M89.0-)
+ M75.0 **Adhesive capsulitis of shoulder**
  Frozen shoulder
  Periarthritis of shoulder
  M75.00 **Adhesive capsulitis of unspecified shoulder**
  M75.01 **Adhesive capsulitis of right shoulder**
  M75.02 **Adhesive capsulitis of left shoulder**
+ M75.1 **Rotator cuff tear or rupture, not specified as traumatic**
  Rotator cuff syndrome
  Supraspinatus tear or rupture, not specified as traumatic
  Supraspinatus syndrome
  Excludes1: tear of rotator cuff, traumatic (S46.01-)
+ M75.10 **Unspecified rotator cuff tear or rupture, not specified as traumatic**
    M75.100 **Unspecified rotator cuff tear or rupture of unspecified shoulder, not specified as traumatic**
    M75.101 **Unspecified rotator cuff tear or rupture of right shoulder, not specified as traumatic**

M75.102 Unspecified rotator cuff tear or rupture of left shoulder, not specified as traumatic
+ M75.11 Incomplete rotator cuff tear or rupture not specified as traumatic
  M75.110 Incomplete rotator cuff tear or rupture of unspecified shoulder, not specified as traumatic
  M75.111 Incomplete rotator cuff tear or rupture of right shoulder, not specified as traumatic
  M75.112 Incomplete rotator cuff tear or rupture of left shoulder, not specified as traumatic
+ M75.12 Complete rotator cuff tear or rupture not specified as traumatic
  M75.120 Complete rotator cuff tear or rupture of unspecified shoulder, not specified as traumatic
  M75.121 Complete rotator cuff tear or rupture of right shoulder, not specified as traumatic
  M75.122 Complete rotator cuff tear or rupture of left shoulder, not specified as traumatic
+ M75.2 Bicipital tendinitis
  M75.20 Bicipital tendinitis, unspecified shoulder
  M75.21 Bicipital tendinitis, right shoulder
  M75.22 Bicipital tendinitis, left shoulder
+ M75.3 Calcific tendinitis of shoulder
  Calcified bursa of shoulder
  M75.30 Calcific tendinitis of unspecified shoulder
  M75.31 Calcific tendinitis of right shoulder
  M75.32 Calcific tendinitis of left shoulder
+ M75.4 Impingement syndrome of shoulder
  M75.40 Impingement syndrome of unspecified shoulder
  M75.41 Impingement syndrome of right shoulder
  M75.42 Impingement syndrome of left shoulder
+ M75.5 Bursitis of shoulder
  M75.50 Bursitis of unspecified shoulder
  M75.51 Bursitis of right shoulder
  M75.52 Bursitis of left shoulder
+ M75.8 Other shoulder lesions
  M75.80 Other shoulder lesions, unspecified shoulder
  M75.81 Other shoulder lesions, right shoulder
  M75.82 Other shoulder lesions, left shoulder
+ M75.9 Shoulder lesion, unspecified
  M75.90 Shoulder lesion, unspecified, unspecified shoulder
  M75.91 Shoulder lesion, unspecified, right shoulder
  M75.92 Shoulder lesion, unspecified, left shoulder

M76 Enthesopathies, lower limb, excluding foot

Excludes2: *bursitis due to use, overuse and pressure (M70.-)*
enthesopathies of ankle and foot (M77.5-)

+ M76.0 Gluteal tendinitis
  M76.00 Gluteal tendinitis, unspecified hip
  M76.01 Gluteal tendinitis, right hip
  M76.02 Gluteal tendinitis, left hip
+ M76.1 Psoas tendinitis
  M76.10 Psoas tendinitis, unspecified hip
  M76.11 Psoas tendinitis, right hip
  M76.12 Psoas tendinitis, left hip
+ M76.2 Iliac crest spur
  M76.20 Iliac crest spur, unspecified hip
  M76.21 Iliac crest spur, right hip
  M76.22 Iliac crest spur, left hip
+ M76.3 Iliotibial band syndrome
  M76.30 Iliotibial band syndrome, unspecified leg
  M76.31 Iliotibial band syndrome, right leg
  M76.32 Iliotibial band syndrome, left leg
+ M76.4 Tibial collateral bursitis [Pellegrini-Stieda]
  M76.40 Tibial collateral bursitis [Pellegrini-Stieda], unspecified leg
  M76.41 Tibial collateral bursitis [Pellegrini-Stieda], right leg
  M76.42 Tibial collateral bursitis [Pellegrini-Stieda], left leg
+ M76.5 Patellar tendinitis
  M76.50 Patellar tendinitis, unspecified knee
  M76.51 Patellar tendinitis, right knee
  M76.52 Patellar tendinitis, left knee

+ M76.6 Achilles tendinitis
  Achilles bursitis
  M76.60 Achilles tendinitis, unspecified leg
  M76.61 Achilles tendinitis, right leg
  M76.62 Achilles tendinitis, left leg
+ M76.7 Peroneal tendinitis
  M76.70 Peroneal tendinitis, unspecified leg
  M76.71 Peroneal tendinitis, right leg
  M76.72 Peroneal tendinitis, left leg
+ M76.8 Other specified enthesopathies of lower limb, excluding foot
  + M76.81 Anterior tibial syndrome
    M76.811 Anterior tibial syndrome, right leg
    M76.812 Anterior tibial syndrome, left leg
    M76.819 Anterior tibial syndrome, unspecified leg
  + M76.82 Posterior tibial tendinitis
    M76.821 Posterior tibial tendinitis, right leg
    M76.822 Posterior tibial tendinitis, left leg
    M76.829 Posterior tibial tendinitis, unspecified leg
  + M76.89 Other specified enthesopathies of lower limb, excluding foot
    M76.891 Other specified enthesopathies of right lower limb, excluding foot
    M76.892 Other specified enthesopathies of left lower limb, excluding foot
    M76.899 Other specified enthesopathies of unspecified lower limb, excluding foot
  M76.9 Unspecified enthesopathy, lower limb, excluding foot

M77 Other enthesopathies

Excludes1: *bursitis NOS (M71.9-)*
Excludes2: *bursitis due to use, overuse and pressure (M70.-)*
osteophyte (M25.7)
spinal enthesopathy (M46.0-)

+ M77.0 Medial epicondylitis
  M77.00 Medial epicondylitis, unspecified elbow
  M77.01 Medial epicondylitis, right elbow
  M77.02 Medial epicondylitis, left elbow
+ M77.1 Lateral epicondylitis
  Tennis elbow
  M77.10 Lateral epicondylitis, unspecified elbow
  M77.11 Lateral epicondylitis, right elbow
  M77.12 Lateral epicondylitis, left elbow
+ M77.2 Periarthritis of wrist
  M77.20 Periarthritis, unspecified wrist
  M77.21 Periarthritis, right wrist
  M77.22 Periarthritis, left wrist
+ M77.3 Calcaneal spur
  M77.30 Calcaneal spur, unspecified foot
  M77.31 Calcaneal spur, right foot
  M77.32 Calcaneal spur, left foot
+ M77.4 Metatarsalgia
  Excludes1: *Morton's metatarsalgia (G57.6)*
  M77.40 Metatarsalgia, unspecified foot
  M77.41 Metatarsalgia, right foot
  M77.42 Metatarsalgia, left foot
+ M77.5 Other enthesopathy of foot and ankle
  M77.50 Other enthesopathy of unspecified foot and ankle
  M77.51 Other enthesopathy of right foot and ankle
  M77.52 Other enthesopathy of left foot and ankle
  M77.8 Other enthesopathies, not elsewhere classified
  M77.9 Enthesopathy, unspecified
  Bone spur NOS
  Capsulitis NOS
  Periarthritis NOS
  Tendinitis NOS

M79 Other and unspecified soft tissue disorders, not elsewhere classified

Excludes1: *psychogenic rheumatism (F45.8)*
soft tissue pain, psychogenic (F45.41)

M79.0 Rheumatism, unspecified
  Excludes1: *fibromyalgia (M79.7)*
  palindromic rheumatism (M12.3-)
+ M79.1 Myalgia
  Myofascial pain syndrome
  Excludes1: *fibromyalgia (M79.7)*
  myositis (M60.-)
  AHA CC: 4Q, 2018, 21
  M79.10 Myalgia, unspecified site
  M79.11 Myalgia of mastication muscle

+, +7th, X + 7th   • Newborn   • Pediatric   • Maternity   • Adult   ♀ Female   ♂ Male   Manifestation   Unacceptable PDX   HCC   CC   MCC   HAC

M79.12 Myalgia of auxiliary muscles, head and neck
M79.18 Myalgia, other site
M79.2 Neuralgia and neuritis, unspecified
    Excludes1: *brachial radiculitis NOS (M54.1)*
        lumbosacral radiculitis NOS (M54.1)
        mononeuropathies (G56-G58)
        radiculitis NOS (M54.1)
        sciatica (M54.3-M54.4)
M79.3 Panniculitis, unspecified
    Excludes1: *lupus panniculitis (L93.2)*
        neck and back panniculitis (M54.0-)
        relapsing [Weber-Christian] panniculitis
          (M35.6)
M79.4 Hypertrophy of (infrapatellar) fat pad
M79.5 Residual foreign body in soft tissue
    Excludes1: *foreign body granuloma of skin and*
        subcutaneous tissue (L92.3)
        foreign body granuloma of soft tissue (M60.2-)
+ **M79.6** Pain in limb, hand, foot, fingers and toes
    Excludes2: *pain in joint (M25.5-)*
  + **M79.60** Pain in limb, unspecified
      M79.601 Pain in right arm
          Pain in right upper limb NOS
      M79.602 Pain in left arm
          Pain in left upper limb NOS
      M79.603 Pain in arm, unspecified
          Pain in upper limb NOS
      M79.604 Pain in right leg
          Pain in right lower limb NOS
      M79.605 Pain in left leg
          Pain in left lower limb NOS
      M79.606 Pain in leg, unspecified
          Pain in lower limb NOS
      M79.609 Pain in unspecified limb
          Pain in limb NOS
  + **M79.62** Pain in upper arm
      Pain in axillary region
      M79.621 Pain in right upper arm
      M79.622 Pain in left upper arm
      M79.629 Pain in unspecified upper arm
  + **M79.63** Pain in forearm
      M79.631 Pain in right forearm
      M79.632 Pain in left forearm
      M79.639 Pain in unspecified forearm
  + **M79.64** Pain in hand and fingers
      M79.641 Pain in right hand
      M79.642 Pain in left hand
      M79.643 Pain in unspecified hand
      M79.644 Pain in right finger(s)
      M79.645 Pain in left finger(s)
      M79.646 Pain in unspecified finger(s)
  + **M79.65** Pain in thigh
      M79.651 Pain in right thigh
      M79.652 Pain in left thigh
      M79.659 Pain in unspecified thigh
  + **M79.66** Pain in lower leg
      M79.661 Pain in right lower leg
      M79.662 Pain in left lower leg
      M79.669 Pain in unspecified lower leg
  + **M79.67** Pain in foot and toes
      M79.671 Pain in right foot
      M79.672 Pain in left foot
      M79.673 Pain in unspecified foot
      M79.674 Pain in right toe(s)
      M79.675 Pain in left toe(s)
      M79.676 Pain in unspecified toe(s)
M79.7 Fibromyalgia
    Fibromyositis
    Fibrositis
    Myofibrositis
+ **M79.A** Nontraumatic compartment syndrome
    Code first if applicable, associated postprocedural
      complication
    Excludes1: *compartment syndrome NOS (T79.A-)*
        fibromyalgia (M79.7)
        nontraumatic ischemic infarction of muscle
          (M62.2-)
        traumatic compartment syndrome (T79.A-)

+ **M79.A1** Nontraumatic compartment syndrome of upper
    extremity
      Nontraumatic compartment syndrome of shoulder,
      arm, forearm, wrist, hand, and fingers
  CC **M79.A11** Nontraumatic compartment syndrome
      of right upper extremity
  CC **M79.A12** Nontraumatic compartment syndrome
      of left upper extremity
  CC **M79.A19** Nontraumatic compartment syndrome
      of unspecified upper extremity
+ **M79.A2** Nontraumatic compartment syndrome of lower
    extremity
      Nontraumatic compartment syndrome of hip,
      buttock, thigh, leg, foot, and toes
  CC **M79.A21** Nontraumatic compartment syndrome
      of right lower extremity
  CC **M79.A22** Nontraumatic compartment syndrome
      of left lower extremity
  CC **M79.A29** Nontraumatic compartment syndrome
      of unspecified lower extremity
  CC **M79.A3** Nontraumatic compartment syndrome of
      abdomen
  CC **M79.A9** Nontraumatic compartment syndrome of
      other sites
+ **M79.8** Other specified soft tissue disorders
    M79.81 Nontraumatic hematoma of soft tissue
      Nontraumatic hematoma of muscle
      Nontraumatic seroma of muscle and soft tissue
    M79.89 Other specified soft tissue disorders
      Polyalgia
M79.9 Soft tissue disorder, unspecified

OSTEOPATHIES AND CHONDROPATHIES (M80-M94)

Disorders of bone density and structure (M80-M85)

M80 Osteoporosis with current pathological fracture
    Includes: osteoporosis with current fragility fracture
    Use additional code to identify major osseous defect, if applicable
      (M89.7-)
    Excludes1: *collapsed vertebra NOS (M48.5)*
        pathological fracture NOS (M84.4)
        wedging of vertebra NOS (M48.5)
    Excludes2: *personal history of (healed) osteoporosis fracture*
        (Z87.310)

> The appropriate 7th character is to be added to each code from
> category M80:
> A   initial encounter for fracture
> D   subsequent encounter for fracture with routine healing
> G   subsequent encounter for fracture with delayed healing
> K   subsequent encounter for fracture with nonunion
> P   subsequent encounter for fracture with malunion
> S   sequela

    Review coding guideline C.13.c
    Review coding guideline C.19.c.1
+ **M80.0** Age-related osteoporosis with current pathological
    fracture
    Involutional osteoporosis with current pathological
      fracture
    Osteoporosis NOS with current pathological fracture
    Postmenopausal osteoporosis with current pathological
      fracture
    Senile osteoporosis with current pathological fracture
● CC X+7th **M80.00** Age-related osteoporosis with current
      pathological fracture, unspecified site
  + **M80.01** Age-related osteoporosis with current
      pathological fracture, shoulder
  ● CC +7th **M80.011** Age-related osteoporosis with current
      pathological fracture, right shoulder
  ● CC +7th **M80.012** Age-related osteoporosis with current
      pathological fracture, left shoulder
  ● CC +7th **M80.019** Age-related osteoporosis with current
      pathological fracture, unspecified
      shoulder
  + **M80.02** Age-related osteoporosis with current
      pathological fracture, humerus

● CC +7th **M80.021** **Age-related osteoporosis with current pathological fracture, right humerus**
● CC +7th **M80.022** **Age-related osteoporosis with current pathological fracture, left humerus**
● CC +7th **M80.029** **Age-related osteoporosis with current pathological fracture, unspecified humerus**
+ **M80.03** **Age-related osteoporosis with current pathological fracture, forearm**
Age-related osteoporosis with current pathological fracture of wrist
● CC +7th **M80.031** **Age-related osteoporosis with current pathological fracture, right forearm**
● CC +7th **M80.032** **Age-related osteoporosis with current pathological fracture, left forearm**
● CC +7th **M80.039** **Age-related osteoporosis with current pathological fracture, unspecified forearm**
+ **M80.04** **Age-related osteoporosis with current pathological fracture, hand**
● CC +7th **M80.041** **Age-related osteoporosis with current pathological fracture, right hand**
● CC +7th **M80.042** **Age-related osteoporosis with current pathological fracture, left hand**
● CC +7th **M80.049** **Age-related osteoporosis with current pathological fracture, unspecified hand**
+ **M80.05** **Age-related osteoporosis with current pathological fracture, femur**
Age-related osteoporosis with current pathological fracture of hip
● CC +7th **M80.051** **Age-related osteoporosis with current pathological fracture, right femur**
AHA CC: 2Q, 2018, 12
● CC +7th **M80.052** **Age-related osteoporosis with current pathological fracture, left femur**
● CC +7th **M80.059** **Age-related osteoporosis with current pathological fracture, unspecified femur**
+ **M80.06** **Age-related osteoporosis with current pathological fracture, lower leg**
● CC +7th **M80.061** **Age-related osteoporosis with current pathological fracture, right lower leg**
● CC +7th **M80.062** **Age-related osteoporosis with current pathological fracture, left lower leg**
● CC +7th **M80.069** **Age-related osteoporosis with current pathological fracture, unspecified lower leg**
+ **M80.07** **Age-related osteoporosis with current pathological fracture, ankle and foot**
● CC +7th **M80.071** **Age-related osteoporosis with current pathological fracture, right ankle and foot**
● CC +7th **M80.072** **Age-related osteoporosis with current pathological fracture, left ankle and foot**
● CC +7th **M80.079** **Age-related osteoporosis with current pathological fracture, unspecified ankle and foot**
● CC X+7th **M80.08** **Age-related osteoporosis with current pathological fracture, vertebra(e)**
● CC X+7th **M80.0A** **Age-related osteoporosis with current pathological fracture, other site**
+ **M80.8** **Other osteoporosis with current pathological fracture**
Drug-induced osteoporosis with current pathological fracture
Idiopathic osteoporosis with current pathological fracture
Osteoporosis of disuse with current pathological fracture
Postoophorectomy osteoporosis with current pathological fracture
Postsurgical malabsorption osteoporosis with current pathological fracture
Post-traumatic osteoporosis with current pathological fracture
Use additional code for adverse effect, if applicable, to identify drug (T36-T50 with fifth or sixth character 5)
CC X+7th **M80.80** **Other osteoporosis with current pathological fracture, unspecified site**
+ **M80.81** **Other osteoporosis with pathological fracture, shoulder**
CC +7th **M80.811** **Other osteoporosis with current pathological fracture, right shoulder**

CC +7th **M80.812** **Other osteoporosis with current pathological fracture, left shoulder**
CC +7th **M80.819** **Other osteoporosis with current pathological fracture, unspecified shoulder**
+ **M80.82** **Other osteoporosis with current pathological fracture, humerus**
CC +7th **M80.821** **Other osteoporosis with current pathological fracture, right humerus**
CC +7th **M80.822** **Other osteoporosis with current pathological fracture, left humerus**
CC +7th **M80.829** **Other osteoporosis with current pathological fracture, unspecified humerus**
+ **M80.83** **Other osteoporosis with current pathological fracture, forearm**
Other osteoporosis with current pathological fracture of wrist
CC +7th **M80.831** **Other osteoporosis with current pathological fracture, right forearm**
CC +7th **M80.832** **Other osteoporosis with current pathological fracture, left forearm**
CC +7th **M80.839** **Other osteoporosis with current pathological fracture, unspecified forearm**
+ **M80.84** **Other osteoporosis with current pathological fracture, hand**
CC +7th **M80.841** **Other osteoporosis with current pathological fracture, right hand**
CC +7th **M80.842** **Other osteoporosis with current pathological fracture, left hand**
CC +7th **M80.849** **Other osteoporosis with current pathological fracture, unspecified hand**
+ **M80.85** **Other osteoporosis with current pathological fracture, femur**
Other osteoporosis with current pathological fracture of hip
CC +7th **M80.851** **Other osteoporosis with current pathological fracture, right femur**
CC +7th **M80.852** **Other osteoporosis with current pathological fracture, left femur**
CC +7th **M80.859** **Other osteoporosis with current pathological fracture, unspecified femur**
+ **M80.86** **Other osteoporosis with current pathological fracture, lower leg**
CC +7th **M80.861** **Other osteoporosis with current pathological fracture, right lower leg**
CC +7th **M80.862** **Other osteoporosis with current pathological fracture, left lower leg**
CC +7th **M80.869** **Other osteoporosis with current pathological fracture, unspecified lower leg**
+ **M80.87** **Other osteoporosis with current pathological fracture, ankle and foot**
CC +7th **M80.871** **Other osteoporosis with current pathological fracture, right ankle and foot**
CC +7th **M80.872** **Other osteoporosis with current pathological fracture, left ankle and foot**
CC +7th **M80.879** **Other osteoporosis with current pathological fracture, unspecified ankle and foot**
CC X+7th **M80.88** **Other osteoporosis with current pathological fracture, vertebra(e)**
CC X+7th **M80.8A** **Other osteoporosis with current pathological fracture, other site**

M81 **Osteoporosis without current pathological fracture**
Use additional code to identify:
major osseous defect, if applicable (M89.7-)
personal history of (healed) osteoporosis fracture, if applicable (Z87.310)
Excludes1: *osteoporosis with current pathological fracture (M80.-)*
Sudeck's atrophy (M89.0)
Review coding guideline C.13.d

Osteoporosis

Axial

Vertebral compression fractures cause continuous (acute) or intermittent (chronic) back pain from midthoracic to midlumbar region, occasionally to lower lumbar region.

A change in backbone strength over time

Osteoporosis is the thinning of the bones. Bones become fragile and loss of height is common as the back bones begin to collapse.

Characteristics of Osteoporosis	
Characteristic	**Description**
Etiology	Postmenopausal women, genetics, vitamin D synthesis deficiency, idiopathic
Prevalence	Approximately 10 million Americans (8 million of them women), white
Risk factors	Family history, white female, increasing age, estrogen deficiency, vitamin D deficiency, low calcium intake, smoking, excessive alcohol use, inactive lifestyle
Complications	Vertebral compression fractures, fracture of proximal femur or humerus, ribs, and distal radius (Colles' fracture)

T4
T6
T8
T10
T12
L1

Multiple compression fractures of lower thoracic and upper lumbar vertebrae in patient with severe osteoporosis

Appendicular
Fractures caused by minimal trauma

Proximal femur | Proximal humerus | Distal radius

Most common types

- **M81.0 Age-related osteoporosis without current pathological fracture**
  Involutional osteoporosis without current pathological fracture
  Osteoporosis NOS
  Postmenopausal osteoporosis without current pathological fracture
  Senile osteoporosis without current pathological fracture
M81.6 Localized osteoporosis [Lequesne]
  Excludes1: *Sudeck's atrophy (M89.0)*
M81.8 Other osteoporosis without current pathological fracture
  Drug-induced osteoporosis without current pathological fracture
  Idiopathic osteoporosis without current pathological fracture
  Osteoporosis of disuse without current pathological fracture
  Postoophorectomy osteoporosis without current pathological fracture
  Postsurgical malabsorption osteoporosis without current pathological fracture
  Post-traumatic osteoporosis without current pathological fracture
  Use additional code for adverse effect, if applicable, to identify drug (T36-T50 with fifth or sixth character 5)

M83 Adult osteomalacia

  Excludes1: *infantile and juvenile osteomalacia (E55.0)*
    renal osteodystrophy (N25.0)
    rickets (active) (E55.0)
    rickets (active) sequelae (E64.3)
    vitamin D-resistant osteomalacia (E83.3)
    vitamin D-resistant rickets (active) (E83.3)
- ♀ **M83.0 Puerperal osteomalacia**
- **M83.1 Senile osteomalacia**
- **M83.2 Adult osteomalacia due to malabsorption**
    Postsurgical malabsorption osteomalacia in adults

- **M83.3 Adult osteomalacia due to malnutrition**
  M83.4 Aluminum bone disease
- **M83.5 Other drug-induced osteomalacia in adults**
    Use additional code for adverse effect, if applicable, to identify drug (T36-T50 with fifth or sixth character 5)
- **M83.8 Other adult osteomalacia**
- **M83.9 Adult osteomalacia, unspecified**

M84 Disorder of continuity of bone

  Excludes2: *traumatic fracture of bone-see fracture, by site*
+ **M84.3 Stress fracture**
    Fatigue fracture
    March fracture
    Stress fracture NOS
    Stress reaction
    external cause code(s) to identify the cause of the stress fracture
  Excludes1: *pathological fracture NOS (M84.4.-)*
    pathological fracture due to osteoporosis (M80.-)
    traumatic fracture (S12.-, S22.-, S32.-, S42.-, S52.-, S62.-, S72.-, S82.-, S92.-)
  Excludes2: *personal history of (healed) stress (fatigue) fracture (Z87.312)*
    stress fracture of vertebra (M48.4-)

The appropriate 7th character is to be added to each code from subcategory **M84.3**:
A   initial encounter for fracture
D   subsequent encounter for fracture with routine healing
G   subsequent encounter for fracture with delayed healing
K   subsequent encounter for fracture with nonunion
P   subsequent encounter for fracture with malunion
S   sequela

+, +7th, X + 7th   ● Newborn   ● Pediatric   ● Maternity   ● Adult   ♀ Female   ♂ Male   Manifestation   Unacceptable PDX   HCC   CC   MCC   HAC

CC X+7th **M84.30 Stress fracture, unspecified site**
+ **M84.31 Stress fracture, shoulder**
CC +7th **M84.311 Stress fracture, right shoulder**
CC +7th **M84.312 Stress fracture, left shoulder**
CC +7th **M84.319 Stress fracture, unspecified shoulder**
+ **M84.32 Stress fracture, humerus**
CC +7th **M84.321 Stress fracture, right humerus**
CC +7th **M84.322 Stress fracture, left humerus**
CC +7th **M84.329 Stress fracture, unspecified humerus**
+ **M84.33 Stress fracture, ulna and radius**
CC +7th **M84.331 Stress fracture, right ulna**
CC +7th **M84.332 Stress fracture, left ulna**
CC +7th **M84.333 Stress fracture, right radius**
CC +7th **M84.334 Stress fracture, left radius**
CC +7th **M84.339 Stress fracture, unspecified ulna and radius**
+ **M84.34 Stress fracture, hand and fingers**
CC +7th **M84.341 Stress fracture, right hand**
CC +7th **M84.342 Stress fracture, left hand**
CC +7th **M84.343 Stress fracture, unspecified hand**
CC +7th **M84.344 Stress fracture, right finger(s)**
CC +7th **M84.345 Stress fracture, left finger(s)**
CC +7th **M84.346 Stress fracture, unspecified finger(s)**
+ **M84.35 Stress fracture, pelvis and femur**
Stress fracture, hip
CC +7th **M84.350 Stress fracture, pelvis**
CC +7th **M84.351 Stress fracture, right femur**
CC +7th **M84.352 Stress fracture, left femur**
CC +7th **M84.353 Stress fracture, unspecified femur**
CC +7th **M84.359 Stress fracture, hip, unspecified**
+ **M84.36 Stress fracture, tibia and fibula**
CC +7th **M84.361 Stress fracture, right tibia**
CC +7th **M84.362 Stress fracture, left tibia**
CC +7th **M84.363 Stress fracture, right fibula**
CC +7th **M84.364 Stress fracture, left fibula**
CC +7th **M84.369 Stress fracture, unspecified tibia and fibula**
+ **M84.37 Stress fracture, ankle, foot and toes**
CC +7th **M84.371 Stress fracture, right ankle**
CC +7th **M84.372 Stress fracture, left ankle**
CC +7th **M84.373 Stress fracture, unspecified ankle**
CC +7th **M84.374 Stress fracture, right foot**
CC +7th **M84.375 Stress fracture, left foot**
CC +7th **M84.376 Stress fracture, unspecified foot**
CC +7th **M84.377 Stress fracture, right toe(s)**
CC +7th **M84.378 Stress fracture, left toe(s)**
CC +7th **M84.379 Stress fracture, unspecified toe(s)**
CC X+7th **M84.38 Stress fracture, other site**

Excludes2: *stress fracture of vertebra (M48.4-)*

+ **M84.4 Pathological fracture, not elsewhere classified**
Chronic fracture
Pathological fracture NOS

Excludes1: *collapsed vertebra NEC (M48.5)*
pathological fracture in neoplastic disease (M84.5-)
pathological fracture in osteoporosis (M80.-)
pathological fracture in other disease (M84.6-)
stress fracture (M84.3-)
traumatic fracture (S12.-, S22.-, S32.-, S42.-, S52.-, S62.-, S72.-, S82.-, S92.-)

Excludes2: *personal history of (healed) pathological fracture (Z87.311)*

The appropriate 7th character is to be added to each code from subcategory **M84.4**:
A   initial encounter for fracture
D   subsequent encounter for fracture with routine healing
G   subsequent encounter for fracture with delayed healing
K   subsequent encounter for fracture with nonunion
P   subsequent encounter for fracture with malunion
S   sequela

CC X+7th **M84.40 Pathological fracture, unspecified site**
+ **M84.41 Pathological fracture, shoulder**
CC +7th **M84.411 Pathological fracture, right shoulder**
CC +7th **M84.412 Pathological fracture, left shoulder**
CC +7th **M84.419 Pathological fracture, unspecified shoulder**
+ **M84.42 Pathological fracture, humerus**
CC +7th **M84.421 Pathological fracture, right humerus**
CC +7th **M84.422 Pathological fracture, left humerus**
CC +7th **M84.429 Pathological fracture, unspecified humerus**

+ **M84.43 Pathological fracture, ulna and radius**
CC +7th **M84.431 Pathological fracture, right ulna**
CC +7th **M84.432 Pathological fracture, left ulna**
CC +7th **M84.433 Pathological fracture, right radius**
CC +7th **M84.434 Pathological fracture, left radius**
CC +7th **M84.439 Pathological fracture, unspecified ulna and radius**
+ **M84.44 Pathological fracture, hand and fingers**
CC +7th **M84.441 Pathological fracture, right hand**
CC +7th **M84.442 Pathological fracture, left hand**
CC +7th **M84.443 Pathological fracture, unspecified hand**
CC +7th **M84.444 Pathological fracture, right finger(s)**
CC +7th **M84.445 Pathological fracture, left finger(s)**
CC +7th **M84.446 Pathological fracture, unspecified finger(s)**
+ **M84.45 Pathological fracture, femur and pelvis**
CC +7th **M84.451 Pathological fracture, right femur**
CC +7th **M84.452 Pathological fracture, left femur**
CC +7th **M84.453 Pathological fracture, unspecified femur**
CC +7th **M84.454 Pathological fracture, pelvis**

AHA CC: 4Q, 2016, 42-43

CC +7th **M84.459 Pathological fracture, hip, unspecified**
+ **M84.46 Pathological fracture, tibia and fibula**
CC +7th **M84.461 Pathological fracture, right tibia**
CC +7th **M84.462 Pathological fracture, left tibia**
CC +7th **M84.463 Pathological fracture, right fibula**
CC +7th **M84.464 Pathological fracture, left fibula**
CC +7th **M84.469 Pathological fracture, unspecified tibia and fibula**
+ **M84.47 Pathological fracture, ankle, foot and toes**
CC +7th **M84.471 Pathological fracture, right ankle**
CC +7th **M84.472 Pathological fracture, left ankle**
CC +7th **M84.473 Pathological fracture, unspecified ankle**
CC +7th **M84.474 Pathological fracture, right foot**
CC +7th **M84.475 Pathological fracture, left foot**
CC +7th **M84.476 Pathological fracture, unspecified foot**
CC +7th **M84.477 Pathological fracture, right toe(s)**
CC +7th **M84.478 Pathological fracture, left toe(s)**
CC +7th **M84.479 Pathological fracture, unspecified toe(s)**
CC X+7th **M84.48 Pathological fracture, other site**
+ **M84.5 Pathological fracture in neoplastic disease**
Code also underlying neoplasm

The appropriate 7th character is to be added to each code from subcategory **M84.5**:
A   initial encounter for fracture
D   subsequent encounter for fracture with routine healing
G   subsequent encounter for fracture with delayed healing
K   subsequent encounter for fracture with nonunion
P   subsequent encounter for fracture with malunion
S   sequela

Review coding guideline C.2.l.6

CC X+7th **M84.50 Pathological fracture in neoplastic disease, unspecified site**
+ **M84.51 Pathological fracture in neoplastic disease, shoulder**
CC +7th **M84.511 Pathological fracture in neoplastic disease, right shoulder**
CC +7th **M84.512 Pathological fracture in neoplastic disease, left shoulder**
CC +7th **M84.519 Pathological fracture in neoplastic disease, unspecified shoulder**
+ **M84.52 Pathological fracture in neoplastic disease, humerus**
CC +7th **M84.521 Pathological fracture in neoplastic disease, right humerus**
CC +7th **M84.522 Pathological fracture in neoplastic disease, left humerus**
CC +7th **M84.529 Pathological fracture in neoplastic disease, unspecified humerus**
+ **M84.53 Pathological fracture in neoplastic disease, ulna and radius**
CC +7th **M84.531 Pathological fracture in neoplastic disease, right ulna**
CC +7th **M84.532 Pathological fracture in neoplastic disease, left ulna**
CC +7th **M84.533 Pathological fracture in neoplastic disease, right radius**
CC +7th **M84.534 Pathological fracture in neoplastic disease, left radius**
CC +7th **M84.539 Pathological fracture in neoplastic disease, unspecified ulna and radius**

+, +7th, X + 7th   ● Newborn   ● Pediatric   ● Maternity   ● Adult   ♀ Female   ♂ Male   Manifestation   Unacceptable PDX   HCC   CC   MCC   HAC

+ **M84.54** **Pathological fracture in neoplastic disease, hand**
CC +7th **M84.541** **Pathological fracture in neoplastic disease, right hand**
CC +7th **M84.542** **Pathological fracture in neoplastic disease, left hand**
CC +7th **M84.549** **Pathological fracture in neoplastic disease, unspecified hand**
+ **M84.55** **Pathological fracture in neoplastic disease, pelvis and femur**
CC +7th **M84.550** **Pathological fracture in neoplastic disease, pelvis**
CC +7th **M84.551** **Pathological fracture in neoplastic disease, right femur**
CC +7th **M84.552** **Pathological fracture in neoplastic disease, left femur**
CC +7th **M84.553** **Pathological fracture in neoplastic disease, unspecified femur**
CC +7th **M84.559** **Pathological fracture in neoplastic disease, hip, unspecified**
+ **M84.56** **Pathological fracture in neoplastic disease, tibia and fibula**
CC +7th **M84.561** **Pathological fracture in neoplastic disease, right tibia**
CC +7th **M84.562** **Pathological fracture in neoplastic disease, left tibia**
CC +7th **M84.563** **Pathological fracture in neoplastic disease, right fibula**
CC +7th **M84.564** **Pathological fracture in neoplastic disease, left fibula**
CC +7th **M84.569** **Pathological fracture in neoplastic disease, unspecified tibia and fibula**
+ **M84.57** **Pathological fracture in neoplastic disease, ankle and foot**
CC +7th **M84.571** **Pathological fracture in neoplastic disease, right ankle**
CC +7th **M84.572** **Pathological fracture in neoplastic disease, left ankle**
CC +7th **M84.573** **Pathological fracture in neoplastic disease, unspecified ankle**
CC +7th **M84.574** **Pathological fracture in neoplastic disease, right foot**
CC +7th **M84.575** **Pathological fracture in neoplastic disease, left foot**
CC +7th **M84.576** **Pathological fracture in neoplastic disease, unspecified foot**
CC X+7th **M84.58** **Pathological fracture in neoplastic disease, other specified site**
Pathological fracture in neoplastic disease, vertebrae
+ **M84.6** **Pathological fracture in other disease**
Code also underlying condition
Excludes1: *pathological fracture in osteoporosis (M80.-)*

The appropriate 7th character is to be added to each code from subcategory **M84.6**:
A   initial encounter for fracture
D   subsequent encounter for fracture with routine healing
G   subsequent encounter for fracture with delayed healing
K   subsequent encounter for fracture with nonunion
P   subsequent encounter for fracture with malunion
S   sequela

CC X+7th **M84.60** **Pathological fracture in other disease, unspecified site**
+ **M84.61** **Pathological fracture in other disease, shoulder**
CC +7th **M84.611** **Pathological fracture in other disease, right shoulder**
CC +7th **M84.612** **Pathological fracture in other disease, left shoulder**
CC +7th **M84.619** **Pathological fracture in other disease, unspecified shoulder**
+ **M84.62** **Pathological fracture in other disease, humerus**
CC +7th **M84.621** **Pathological fracture in other disease, right humerus**
CC +7th **M84.622** **Pathological fracture in other disease, left humerus**
CC +7th **M84.629** **Pathological fracture in other disease, unspecified humerus**

+ **M84.63** **Pathological fracture in other disease, ulna and radius**
CC +7th **M84.631** **Pathological fracture in other disease, right ulna**
CC +7th **M84.632** **Pathological fracture in other disease, left ulna**
CC +7th **M84.633** **Pathological fracture in other disease, right radius**
CC +7th **M84.634** **Pathological fracture in other disease, left radius**
CC +7th **M84.639** **Pathological fracture in other disease, unspecified ulna and radius**
+ **M84.64** **Pathological fracture in other disease, hand**
CC +7th **M84.641** **Pathological fracture in other disease, right hand**
CC +7th **M84.642** **Pathological fracture in other disease, left hand**
CC +7th **M84.649** **Pathological fracture in other disease, unspecified hand**
+ **M84.65** **Pathological fracture in other disease, pelvis and femur**
M84.650 **Pathological fracture in other disease, pelvis**
CC +7th **M84.651** **Pathological fracture in other disease, right femur**
CC +7th **M84.652** **Pathological fracture in other disease, left femur**
CC +7th **M84.653** **Pathological fracture in other disease, unspecified femur**
CC +7th **M84.659** **Pathological fracture in other disease, hip, unspecified**
+ **M84.66** **Pathological fracture in other disease, tibia and fibula**
CC +7th **M84.661** **Pathological fracture in other disease, right tibia**
CC +7th **M84.662** **Pathological fracture in other disease, left tibia**
CC +7th **M84.663** **Pathological fracture in other disease, right fibula**
CC +7th **M84.664** **Pathological fracture in other disease, left fibula**
CC +7th **M84.669** **Pathological fracture in other disease, unspecified tibia and fibula**
+ **M84.67** **Pathological fracture in other disease, ankle and foot**
CC +7th **M84.671** **Pathological fracture in other disease, right ankle**
CC +7th **M84.672** **Pathological fracture in other disease, left ankle**
CC +7th **M84.673** **Pathological fracture in other disease, unspecified ankle**
CC +7th **M84.674** **Pathological fracture in other disease, right foot**
CC +7th **M84.675** **Pathological fracture in other disease, left foot**
CC +7th **M84.676** **Pathological fracture in other disease, unspecified foot**
CC X+7th **M84.68** **Pathological fracture in other disease, other site**
+ **M84.7** **Nontraumatic fracture, not elsewhere classified**
+ **M84.75** **Atypical femoral fracture**
AHA CC: 4Q, 2016, 41-42

The appropriate 7th character is to be added to each code from subcategory **M84.75**:
A   initial encounter for fracture
D   subsequent encounter for fracture with routine healing
G   subsequent encounter for fracture with delayed healing
K   subsequent encounter for fracture with nonunion
P   subsequent encounter for fracture with malunion
S   sequela

CC +7th **M84.750** **Atypical femoral fracture, unspecified**
CC +7th **M84.751** **Incomplete atypical femoral fracture, right leg**
CC +7th **M84.752** **Incomplete atypical femoral fracture, left leg**
CC +7th **M84.753** **Incomplete atypical femoral fracture, unspecified leg**
CC +7th **M84.754** **Complete transverse atypical femoral fracture, right leg**
CC +7th **M84.755** **Complete transverse atypical femoral fracture, left leg**

+, +7th, X + 7th   ● Newborn   ● Pediatric   ● Maternity   ● Adult   ♀ Female   ♂ Male   Manifestation   Unacceptable PDX   HCC   CC   MCC   HAC

CC +7th **M84.756** **Complete transverse atypical femoral fracture, unspecified leg**

CC +7th **M84.757** **Complete oblique atypical femoral fracture, right leg**

CC +7th **M84.758** **Complete oblique atypical femoral fracture, left leg**

CC +7th **M84.759** **Complete oblique atypical femoral fracture, unspecified leg**

+ **M84.8 Other disorders of continuity of bone**

M84.80 **Other disorders of continuity of bone, unspecified site**

+ **M84.81** **Other disorders of continuity of bone, shoulder**

M84.811 **Other disorders of continuity of bone, right shoulder**

M84.812 **Other disorders of continuity of bone, left shoulder**

M84.819 **Other disorders of continuity of bone, unspecified shoulder**

+ **M84.82** **Other disorders of continuity of bone, humerus**

M84.821 **Other disorders of continuity of bone, right humerus**

M84.822 **Other disorders of continuity of bone, left humerus**

M84.829 **Other disorders of continuity of bone, unspecified humerus**

+ **M84.83** **Other disorders of continuity of bone, ulna and radius**

M84.831 **Other disorders of continuity of bone, right ulna**

M84.832 **Other disorders of continuity of bone, left ulna**

M84.833 **Other disorders of continuity of bone, right radius**

M84.834 **Other disorders of continuity of bone, left radius**

M84.839 **Other disorders of continuity of bone, unspecified ulna and radius**

+ **M84.84** **Other disorders of continuity of bone, hand**

M84.841 **Other disorders of continuity of bone, right hand**

M84.842 **Other disorders of continuity of bone, left hand**

M84.849 **Other disorders of continuity of bone, unspecified hand**

+ **M84.85** **Other disorders of continuity of bone, pelvic region and thigh**

M84.851 **Other disorders of continuity of bone, right pelvic region and thigh**

M84.852 **Other disorders of continuity of bone, left pelvic region and thigh**

M84.859 **Other disorders of continuity of bone, unspecified pelvic region and thigh**

+ **M84.86** **Other disorders of continuity of bone, tibia and fibula**

M84.861 **Other disorders of continuity of bone, right tibia**

M84.862 **Other disorders of continuity of bone, left tibia**

M84.863 **Other disorders of continuity of bone, right fibula**

M84.864 **Other disorders of continuity of bone, left fibula**

M84.869 **Other disorders of continuity of bone, unspecified tibia and fibula**

+ **M84.87** **Other disorders of continuity of bone, ankle and foot**

M84.871 **Other disorders of continuity of bone, right ankle and foot**

M84.872 **Other disorders of continuity of bone, left ankle and foot**

M84.879 **Other disorders of continuity of bone, unspecified ankle and foot**

M84.88 **Other disorders of continuity of bone, other site**

M84.9 Disorder of continuity of bone, unspecified

M85 Other disorders of bone density and structure

Excludes1: *osteogenesis imperfecta (Q78.0)*
osteopetrosis (Q78.2)
osteopoikilosis (Q78.8)
polyostotic fibrous dysplasia (Q78.1)

+ **M85.0 Fibrous dysplasia (monostotic)**

Excludes2: *fibrous dysplasia of jaw (M27.8)*

M85.00 **Fibrous dysplasia (monostotic), unspecified site**

+ **M85.01** **Fibrous dysplasia (monostotic), shoulder**

M85.011 **Fibrous dysplasia (monostotic), right shoulder**

M85.012 **Fibrous dysplasia (monostotic), left shoulder**

M85.019 **Fibrous dysplasia (monostotic), unspecified shoulder**

+ **M85.02** **Fibrous dysplasia (monostotic), upper arm**

M85.021 **Fibrous dysplasia (monostotic), right upper arm**

M85.022 **Fibrous dysplasia (monostotic), left upper arm**

M85.029 **Fibrous dysplasia (monostotic), unspecified upper arm**

+ **M85.03** **Fibrous dysplasia (monostotic), forearm**

M85.031 **Fibrous dysplasia (monostotic), right forearm**

M85.032 **Fibrous dysplasia (monostotic), left forearm**

M85.039 **Fibrous dysplasia (monostotic), unspecified forearm**

+ **M85.04** **Fibrous dysplasia (monostotic), hand**

M85.041 **Fibrous dysplasia (monostotic), right hand**

M85.042 **Fibrous dysplasia (monostotic), left hand**

M85.049 **Fibrous dysplasia (monostotic), unspecified hand**

+ **M85.05** **Fibrous dysplasia (monostotic), thigh**

M85.051 **Fibrous dysplasia (monostotic), right thigh**

M85.052 **Fibrous dysplasia (monostotic), left thigh**

M85.059 **Fibrous dysplasia (monostotic), unspecified thigh**

+ **M85.06** **Fibrous dysplasia (monostotic), lower leg**

M85.061 **Fibrous dysplasia (monostotic), right lower leg**

M85.062 **Fibrous dysplasia (monostotic), left lower leg**

M85.069 **Fibrous dysplasia (monostotic), unspecified lower leg**

+ **M85.07** **Fibrous dysplasia (monostotic), ankle and foot**

M85.071 **Fibrous dysplasia (monostotic), right ankle and foot**

M85.072 **Fibrous dysplasia (monostotic), left ankle and foot**

M85.079 **Fibrous dysplasia (monostotic), unspecified ankle and foot**

M85.08 **Fibrous dysplasia (monostotic), other site**

M85.09 **Fibrous dysplasia (monostotic), multiple sites**

+ **M85.1 Skeletal fluorosis**

M85.10 **Skeletal fluorosis, unspecified site**

+ **M85.11** **Skeletal fluorosis, shoulder**

M85.111 **Skeletal fluorosis, right shoulder**

M85.112 **Skeletal fluorosis, left shoulder**

M85.119 **Skeletal fluorosis, unspecified shoulder**

+ **M85.12** **Skeletal fluorosis, upper arm**

M85.121 **Skeletal fluorosis, right upper arm**

M85.122 **Skeletal fluorosis, left upper arm**

M85.129 **Skeletal fluorosis, unspecified upper arm**

+ **M85.13** **Skeletal fluorosis, forearm**

M85.131 **Skeletal fluorosis, right forearm**

M85.132 **Skeletal fluorosis, left forearm**

M85.139 **Skeletal fluorosis, unspecified forearm**

+ **M85.14** **Skeletal fluorosis, hand**

M85.141 **Skeletal fluorosis, right hand**

M85.142 **Skeletal fluorosis, left hand**

M85.149 **Skeletal fluorosis, unspecified hand**

+ M85.15 **Skeletal fluorosis, thigh**
    M85.151 Skeletal fluorosis, right thigh
    M85.152 Skeletal fluorosis, left thigh
    M85.159 Skeletal fluorosis, unspecified thigh
+ M85.16 **Skeletal fluorosis, lower leg**
    M85.161 Skeletal fluorosis, right lower leg
    M85.162 Skeletal fluorosis, left lower leg
    M85.169 Skeletal fluorosis, unspecified lower leg
+ M85.17 **Skeletal fluorosis, ankle and foot**
    M85.171 Skeletal fluorosis, right ankle and foot
    M85.172 Skeletal fluorosis, left ankle and foot
    M85.179 Skeletal fluorosis, unspecified ankle and foot
  M85.18 Skeletal fluorosis, other site
  M85.19 Skeletal fluorosis, multiple sites
M85.2 **Hyperostosis of skull**
+ M85.3 **Osteitis condensans**
  M85.30 Osteitis condensans, unspecified site
+ M85.31 **Osteitis condensans, shoulder**
    M85.311 Osteitis condensans, right shoulder
    M85.312 Osteitis condensans, left shoulder
    M85.319 Osteitis condensans, unspecified shoulder
+ M85.32 **Osteitis condensans, upper arm**
    M85.321 Osteitis condensans, right upper arm
    M85.322 Osteitis condensans, left upper arm
    M85.329 Osteitis condensans, unspecified upper arm
+ M85.33 **Osteitis condensans, forearm**
    M85.331 Osteitis condensans, right forearm
    M85.332 Osteitis condensans, left forearm
    M85.339 Osteitis condensans, unspecified forearm
+ M85.34 **Osteitis condensans, hand**
    M85.341 Osteitis condensans, right hand
    M85.342 Osteitis condensans, left hand
    M85.349 Osteitis condensans, unspecified hand
+ M85.35 **Osteitis condensans, thigh**
    M85.351 Osteitis condensans, right thigh
    M85.352 Osteitis condensans, left thigh
    M85.359 Osteitis condensans, unspecified thigh
+ M85.36 **Osteitis condensans, lower leg**
    M85.361 Osteitis condensans, right lower leg
    M85.362 Osteitis condensans, left lower leg
    M85.369 Osteitis condensans, unspecified lower leg
+ M85.37 **Osteitis condensans, ankle and foot**
    M85.371 Osteitis condensans, right ankle and foot
    M85.372 Osteitis condensans, left ankle and foot
    M85.379 Osteitis condensans, unspecified ankle and foot
  M85.38 Osteitis condensans, other site
  M85.39 Osteitis condensans, multiple sites
+ M85.4 **Solitary bone cyst**
    Excludes2: solitary cyst of jaw (M27.4)
  M85.40 Solitary bone cyst, unspecified site
+ M85.41 **Solitary bone cyst, shoulder**
    M85.411 Solitary bone cyst, right shoulder
    M85.412 Solitary bone cyst, left shoulder
    M85.419 Solitary bone cyst, unspecified shoulder
+ M85.42 **Solitary bone cyst, humerus**
    M85.421 Solitary bone cyst, right humerus
    M85.422 Solitary bone cyst, left humerus
    M85.429 Solitary bone cyst, unspecified humerus
+ M85.43 **Solitary bone cyst, ulna and radius**
    M85.431 Solitary bone cyst, right ulna and radius
    M85.432 Solitary bone cyst, left ulna and radius
    M85.439 Solitary bone cyst, unspecified ulna and radius
+ M85.44 **Solitary bone cyst, hand**
    M85.441 Solitary bone cyst, right hand
    M85.442 Solitary bone cyst, left hand
    M85.449 Solitary bone cyst, unspecified hand
+ M85.45 **Solitary bone cyst, pelvis**
    M85.451 Solitary bone cyst, right pelvis
    M85.452 Solitary bone cyst, left pelvis
    M85.459 Solitary bone cyst, unspecified pelvis

+ M85.46 **Solitary bone cyst, tibia and fibula**
    M85.461 Solitary bone cyst, right tibia and fibula
    M85.462 Solitary bone cyst, left tibia and fibula
    M85.469 Solitary bone cyst, unspecified tibia and fibula
+ M85.47 **Solitary bone cyst, ankle and foot**
    M85.471 Solitary bone cyst, right ankle and foot
    M85.472 Solitary bone cyst, left ankle and foot
    M85.479 Solitary bone cyst, unspecified ankle and foot
  M85.48 Solitary bone cyst, other site
+ M85.5 **Aneurysmal bone cyst**
    Excludes2: aneurysmal cyst of jaw (M27.4)
  M85.50 Aneurysmal bone cyst, unspecified site
+ M85.51 **Aneurysmal bone cyst, shoulder**
    M85.511 Aneurysmal bone cyst, right shoulder
    M85.512 Aneurysmal bone cyst, left shoulder
    M85.519 Aneurysmal bone cyst, unspecified shoulder
+ M85.52 **Aneurysmal bone cyst, upper arm**
    M85.521 Aneurysmal bone cyst, right upper arm
    M85.522 Aneurysmal bone cyst, left upper arm
    M85.529 Aneurysmal bone cyst, unspecified upper arm
+ M85.53 **Aneurysmal bone cyst, forearm**
    M85.531 Aneurysmal bone cyst, right forearm
    M85.532 Aneurysmal bone cyst, left forearm
    M85.539 Aneurysmal bone cyst, unspecified forearm
+ M85.54 **Aneurysmal bone cyst, hand**
    M85.541 Aneurysmal bone cyst, right hand
    M85.542 Aneurysmal bone cyst, left hand
    M85.549 Aneurysmal bone cyst, unspecified hand
+ M85.55 **Aneurysmal bone cyst, thigh**
    M85.551 Aneurysmal bone cyst, right thigh
    M85.552 Aneurysmal bone cyst, left thigh
    M85.559 Aneurysmal bone cyst, unspecified thigh
+ M85.56 **Aneurysmal bone cyst, lower leg**
    M85.561 Aneurysmal bone cyst, right lower leg
    M85.562 Aneurysmal bone cyst, left lower leg
    M85.569 Aneurysmal bone cyst, unspecified lower leg
+ M85.57 **Aneurysmal bone cyst, ankle and foot**
    M85.571 Aneurysmal bone cyst, right ankle and foot
    M85.572 Aneurysmal bone cyst, left ankle and foot
    M85.579 Aneurysmal bone cyst, unspecified ankle and foot
  M85.58 Aneurysmal bone cyst, other site
  M85.59 Aneurysmal bone cyst, multiple sites
+ M85.6 **Other cyst of bone**
    Excludes1: cyst of jaw NEC (M27.4)
               osteitis fibrosa cystica generalisata [von Recklinghausen's disease of bone] (E21.0)
  M85.60 Other cyst of bone, unspecified site
+ M85.61 **Other cyst of bone, shoulder**
    M85.611 Other cyst of bone, right shoulder
    M85.612 Other cyst of bone, left shoulder
    M85.619 Other cyst of bone, unspecified shoulder
+ M85.62 **Other cyst of bone, upper arm**
    M85.621 Other cyst of bone, right upper arm
    M85.622 Other cyst of bone, left upper arm
    M85.629 Other cyst of bone, unspecified upper arm
+ M85.63 **Other cyst of bone, forearm**
    M85.631 Other cyst of bone, right forearm
    M85.632 Other cyst of bone, left forearm
    M85.639 Other cyst of bone, unspecified forearm
+ M85.64 **Other cyst of bone, hand**
    M85.641 Other cyst of bone, right hand
    M85.642 Other cyst of bone, left hand
    M85.649 Other cyst of bone, unspecified hand
+ M85.65 **Other cyst of bone, thigh**
    M85.651 Other cyst of bone, right thigh
    M85.652 Other cyst of bone, left thigh
    M85.659 Other cyst of bone, unspecified thigh

+ **M85.66** Other cyst of bone, lower leg
    M85.661 Other cyst of bone, right lower leg
    M85.662 Other cyst of bone, left lower leg
    M85.669 Other cyst of bone, unspecified lower leg
+ **M85.67** Other cyst of bone, ankle and foot
    M85.671 Other cyst of bone, right ankle and foot
    M85.672 Other cyst of bone, left ankle and foot
    M85.679 Other cyst of bone, unspecified ankle and foot
    M85.68 Other cyst of bone, other site
    M85.69 Other cyst of bone, multiple sites
+ **M85.8** Other specified disorders of bone density and structure
    Hyperostosis of bones, except skull
    Osteosclerosis, acquired
    Excludes1: *diffuse idiopathic skeletal hyperostosis [DISH]*
        (M48.1)
        osteosclerosis congenita (Q77.4)
        osteosclerosis fragilitas (generalista) (Q78.2)
        osteosclerosis myelofibrosis (D75.81)
    M85.80 Other specified disorders of bone density and structure, unspecified site
+ **M85.81** Other specified disorders of bone density and structure, shoulder
    M85.811 Other specified disorders of bone density and structure, right shoulder
    M85.812 Other specified disorders of bone density and structure, left shoulder
    M85.819 Other specified disorders of bone density and structure, unspecified shoulder
+ **M85.82** Other specified disorders of bone density and structure, upper arm
    M85.821 Other specified disorders of bone density and structure, right upper arm
    M85.822 Other specified disorders of bone density and structure, left upper arm
    M85.829 Other specified disorders of bone density and structure, unspecified upper arm
+ **M85.83** Other specified disorders of bone density and structure, forearm
    M85.831 Other specified disorders of bone density and structure, right forearm
    M85.832 Other specified disorders of bone density and structure, left forearm
    M85.839 Other specified disorders of bone density and structure, unspecified forearm
+ **M85.84** Other specified disorders of bone density and structure, hand
    M85.841 Other specified disorders of bone density and structure, right hand
    M85.842 Other specified disorders of bone density and structure, left hand
    M85.849 Other specified disorders of bone density and structure, unspecified hand
+ **M85.85** Other specified disorders of bone density and structure, thigh
    M85.851 Other specified disorders of bone density and structure, right thigh
    M85.852 Other specified disorders of bone density and structure, left thigh
    M85.859 Other specified disorders of bone density and structure, unspecified thigh
+ **M85.86** Other specified disorders of bone density and structure, lower leg
    M85.861 Other specified disorders of bone density and structure, right lower leg
    M85.862 Other specified disorders of bone density and structure, left lower leg
    M85.869 Other specified disorders of bone density and structure, unspecified lower leg
+ **M85.87** Other specified disorders of bone density and structure, ankle and foot
    M85.871 Other specified disorders of bone density and structure, right ankle and foot
    M85.872 Other specified disorders of bone density and structure, left ankle and foot

    M85.879 Other specified disorders of bone density and structure, unspecified ankle and foot
    M85.88 Other specified disorders of bone density and structure, other site
    M85.89 Other specified disorders of bone density and structure, multiple sites
M85.9 Disorder of bone density and structure, unspecified

Other osteopathies (M86-M90)

Excludes1: *postprocedural osteopathies (M96.-)*

M86 Osteomyelitis

Use additional code (B95-B97) to identify infectious agent

Use additional code to identify major osseous defect, if applicable (M89.7-)

Excludes1: *osteomyelitis due to:*
    echinococcus (B67.2)
    gonococcus (A54.43)
    salmonella (A02.24)
Excludes2: *ostemyelitis of:*
    orbit (H05.0-)
    petrous bone (H70.2-)
    vertebra (M46.2-)

+ **M86.0** Acute hematogenous osteomyelitis
CC **M86.00** Acute hematogenous osteomyelitis, unspecified site
+ **M86.01** Acute hematogenous osteomyelitis, shoulder
  CC **M86.011** Acute hematogenous osteomyelitis, right shoulder
  CC **M86.012** Acute hematogenous osteomyelitis, left shoulder
  CC **M86.019** Acute hematogenous osteomyelitis, unspecified shoulder
+ **M86.02** Acute hematogenous osteomyelitis, humerus
  CC **M86.021** Acute hematogenous osteomyelitis, right humerus
  CC **M86.022** Acute hematogenous osteomyelitis, left humerus
  CC **M86.029** Acute hematogenous osteomyelitis, unspecified humerus
+ **M86.03** Acute hematogenous osteomyelitis, radius and ulna
  CC **M86.031** Acute hematogenous osteomyelitis, right radius and ulna
  CC **M86.032** Acute hematogenous osteomyelitis, left radius and ulna
  CC **M86.039** Acute hematogenous osteomyelitis, unspecified radius and ulna
+ **M86.04** Acute hematogenous osteomyelitis, hand
  CC **M86.041** Acute hematogenous osteomyelitis, right hand
  CC **M86.042** Acute hematogenous osteomyelitis, left hand
  CC **M86.049** Acute hematogenous osteomyelitis, unspecified hand
+ **M86.05** Acute hematogenous osteomyelitis, femur
  CC **M86.051** Acute hematogenous osteomyelitis, right femur
  CC **M86.052** Acute hematogenous osteomyelitis, left femur
  CC **M86.059** Acute hematogenous osteomyelitis, unspecified femur
+ **M86.06** Acute hematogenous osteomyelitis, tibia and fibula
  CC **M86.061** Acute hematogenous osteomyelitis, right tibia and fibula
  CC **M86.062** Acute hematogenous osteomyelitis, left tibia and fibula
  CC **M86.069** Acute hematogenous osteomyelitis, unspecified tibia and fibula
+ **M86.07** Acute hematogenous osteomyelitis, ankle and foot
  CC **M86.071** Acute hematogenous osteomyelitis, right ankle and foot
  CC **M86.072** Acute hematogenous osteomyelitis, left ankle and foot
  CC **M86.079** Acute hematogenous osteomyelitis, unspecified ankle and foot
CC **M86.08** Acute hematogenous osteomyelitis, other sites
CC **M86.09** Acute hematogenous osteomyelitis, multiple sites
+ **M86.1** Other acute osteomyelitis
CC **M86.10** Other acute osteomyelitis, unspecified site

+, +7th, X + 7th   ● Newborn ● Pediatric ● Maternity ● Adult ♀ Female ♂ Male Manifestation Unacceptable PDX HCC CC MCC HAC

+ M86.11 Other acute osteomyelitis, shoulder
   CC M86.111 Other acute osteomyelitis, right shoulder
   CC M86.112 Other acute osteomyelitis, left shoulder
   CC M86.119 Other acute osteomyelitis, unspecified shoulder
+ M86.12 Other acute osteomyelitis, humerus
   CC M86.121 Other acute osteomyelitis, right humerus
   CC M86.122 Other acute osteomyelitis, left humerus
   CC M86.129 Other acute osteomyelitis, unspecified humerus
+ M86.13 Other acute osteomyelitis, radius and ulna
   CC M86.131 Other acute osteomyelitis, right radius and ulna
   CC M86.132 Other acute osteomyelitis, left radius and ulna
   CC M86.139 Other acute osteomyelitis, unspecified radius and ulna
+ M86.14 Other acute osteomyelitis, hand
   CC M86.141 Other acute osteomyelitis, righthand
   CC M86.142 Other acute osteomyelitis, left hand
   CC M86.149 Other acute osteomyelitis, unspecified hand
+ M86.15 Other acute osteomyelitis, femur
   CC M86.151 Other acute osteomyelitis, right femur
   CC M86.152 Other acute osteomyelitis, left femur
   CC M86.159 Other acute osteomyelitis, unspecified femur
+ M86.16 Other acute osteomyelitis, tibia and fibula
   CC M86.161 Other acute osteomyelitis, right tibia and fibula
   CC M86.162 Other acute osteomyelitis, left tibia and fibula
   CC M86.169 Other acute osteomyelitis, unspecified tibia and fibula
+ M86.17 Other acute osteomyelitis, ankle and foot
   CC M86.171 Other acute osteomyelitis, right ankle and foot
     AHA CC: 1Q, 2020, 12
   CC M86.172 Other acute osteomyelitis, left ankle and foot
   CC M86.179 Other acute osteomyelitis, unspecified ankle and foot
CC M86.18 Other acute osteomyelitis, other site
CC M86.19 Other acute osteomyelitis, multiple sites
+ M86.2 Subacute osteomyelitis
   CC M86.20 Subacute osteomyelitis, unspecified site
   + M86.21 Subacute osteomyelitis, shoulder
      CC M86.211 Subacute osteomyelitis, right shoulder
      CC M86.212 Subacute osteomyelitis, left shoulder
      CC M86.219 Subacute osteomyelitis, unspecified shoulder
   + M86.22 Subacute osteomyelitis, humerus
      CC M86.221 Subacute osteomyelitis, right humerus
      CC M86.222 Subacute osteomyelitis, left humerus
      CC M86.229 Subacute osteomyelitis, unspecified humerus
   + M86.23 Subacute osteomyelitis, radius and ulna
      CC M86.231 Subacute osteomyelitis, right radius and ulna
      CC M86.232 Subacute osteomyelitis, left radius and ulna
      CC M86.239 Subacute osteomyelitis, unspecified radius and ulna
   + M86.24 Subacute osteomyelitis, hand
      CC M86.241 Subacute osteomyelitis, right hand
      CC M86.242 Subacute osteomyelitis, left hand
      CC M86.249 Subacute osteomyelitis, unspecified hand
   + M86.25 Subacute osteomyelitis, femur
      CC M86.251 Subacute osteomyelitis, right femur
      CC M86.252 Subacute osteomyelitis, left femur
      CC M86.259 Subacute osteomyelitis, unspecified femur
   + M86.26 Subacute osteomyelitis, tibia and fibula
      CC M86.261 Subacute osteomyelitis, right tibia and fibula
      CC M86.262 Subacute osteomyelitis, left tibia and fibula
      CC M86.269 Subacute osteomyelitis, unspecified tibia and fibula
   + M86.27 Subacute osteomyelitis, ankle and foot

      CC M86.271 Subacute osteomyelitis, right ankle and foot
      CC M86.272 Subacute osteomyelitis, left ankle and foot
      CC M86.279 Subacute osteomyelitis, unspecified ankle and foot
   CC M86.28 Subacute osteomyelitis, other site
   CC M86.29 Subacute osteomyelitis, multiple sites
+ M86.3 Chronic multifocal osteomyelitis
   CC M86.30 Chronic multifocal osteomyelitis, unspecified site
   + M86.31 Chronic multifocal osteomyelitis, shoulder
      CC M86.311 Chronic multifocal osteomyelitis, right shoulder
      CC M86.312 Chronic multifocal osteomyelitis, left shoulder
      CC M86.319 Chronic multifocal osteomyelitis, unspecified shoulder
   + M86.32 Chronic multifocal osteomyelitis, humerus
      CC M86.321 Chronic multifocal osteomyelitis, right humerus
      CC M86.322 Chronic multifocal osteomyelitis, left humerus
      CC M86.329 Chronic multifocal osteomyelitis, unspecified humerus
   + M86.33 Chronic multifocal osteomyelitis, radius and ulna
      CC M86.331 Chronic multifocal osteomyelitis, right radius and ulna
      CC M86.332 Chronic multifocal osteomyelitis, left radius and ulna
      CC M86.339 Chronic multifocal osteomyelitis, unspecified radius and ulna
   + M86.34 Chronic multifocal osteomyelitis, hand
      CC M86.341 Chronic multifocal osteomyelitis, right hand
      CC M86.342 Chronic multifocal osteomyelitis, left hand
      CC M86.349 Chronic multifocal osteomyelitis, unspecified hand
   + M86.35 Chronic multifocal osteomyelitis, femur
      CC M86.351 Chronic multifocal osteomyelitis, right femur
      CC M86.352 Chronic multifocal osteomyelitis, left femur
      CC M86.359 Chronic multifocal osteomyelitis, unspecified femur
   + M86.36 Chronic multifocal osteomyelitis, tibia and fibula
      CC M86.361 Chronic multifocal osteomyelitis, right tibia and fibula
      CC M86.362 Chronic multifocal osteomyelitis, left tibia and fibula
      CC M86.369 Chronic multifocal osteomyelitis, unspecified tibia and fibula
   + M86.37 Chronic multifocal osteomyelitis, ankle and foot
      CC M86.371 Chronic multifocal osteomyelitis, right ankle and foot
      CC M86.372 Chronic multifocal osteomyelitis, left ankle and foot
      CC M86.379 Chronic multifocal osteomyelitis, unspecified ankle and foot
   CC M86.38 Chronic multifocal osteomyelitis, other site
   CC M86.39 Chronic multifocal osteomyelitis, multiple sites
+ M86.4 Chronic osteomyelitis with draining sinus
   CC M86.40 Chronic osteomyelitis with draining sinus, unspecified site
   + M86.41 Chronic osteomyelitis with draining sinus, shoulder
      CC M86.411 Chronic osteomyelitis with draining sinus, right shoulder
      CC M86.412 Chronic osteomyelitis with draining sinus, left shoulder
      CC M86.419 Chronic osteomyelitis with draining sinus, unspecified shoulder
   + M86.42 Chronic osteomyelitis with draining sinus, humerus
      CC M86.421 Chronic osteomyelitis with draining sinus, right humerus
      CC M86.422 Chronic osteomyelitis with draining sinus, left humerus
      CC M86.429 Chronic osteomyelitis with draining sinus, unspecified humerus
   + M86.43 Chronic osteomyelitis with draining sinus, radius and ulna

+, +7th, X + 7th   ● Newborn   ● Pediatric   ● Maternity   ● Adult   ♀ Female   ♂ Male   Manifestation   Unacceptable PDX   HCC   CC   MCC   HAC

CC **M86.431** Chronic osteomyelitis with draining sinus, right radius and ulna

CC **M86.432** Chronic osteomyelitis with draining sinus, left radius and ulna

CC **M86.439** Chronic osteomyelitis with draining sinus, unspecified radius and ulna

+ **M86.44** Chronic osteomyelitis with draining sinus, hand

CC **M86.441** Chronic osteomyelitis with draining sinus, right hand

CC **M86.442** Chronic osteomyelitis with draining sinus, left hand

CC **M86.449** Chronic osteomyelitis with draining sinus, unspecified hand

+ **M86.45** Chronic osteomyelitis with draining sinus, femur

CC **M86.451** Chronic osteomyelitis with draining sinus, right femur

CC **M86.452** Chronic osteomyelitis with draining sinus, left femur

CC **M86.459** Chronic osteomyelitis with draining sinus, unspecified femur

+ **M86.46** Chronic osteomyelitis with draining sinus, tibia and fibula

CC **M86.461** Chronic osteomyelitis with draining sinus, right tibia and fibula

CC **M86.462** Chronic osteomyelitis with draining sinus, left tibia and fibula

CC **M86.469** Chronic osteomyelitis with draining sinus, unspecified tibia and fibula

+ **M86.47** Chronic osteomyelitis with draining sinus, ankle and foot

CC **M86.471** Chronic osteomyelitis with draining sinus, right ankle and foot

CC **M86.472** Chronic osteomyelitis with draining sinus, left ankle and foot

CC **M86.479** Chronic osteomyelitis with draining sinus, unspecified ankle and foot

CC **M86.48** Chronic osteomyelitis with draining sinus, other site

CC **M86.49** Chronic osteomyelitis with draining sinus, multiple sites

+ **M86.5** Other chronic hematogenous osteomyelitis

CC **M86.50** Other chronic hematogenous osteomyelitis, unspecified site

+ **M86.51** Other chronic hematogenous osteomyelitis, shoulder

CC **M86.511** Other chronic hematogenous osteomyelitis, right shoulder

CC **M86.512** Other chronic hematogenous osteomyelitis, left shoulder

CC **M86.519** Other chronic hematogenous osteomyelitis, unspecified shoulder

+ **M86.52** Other chronic hematogenous osteomyelitis, humerus

CC **M86.521** Other chronic hematogenous osteomyelitis, right humerus

CC **M86.522** Other chronic hematogenous osteomyelitis, left humerus

CC **M86.529** Other chronic hematogenous osteomyelitis, unspecified humerus

+ **M86.53** Other chronic hematogenous osteomyelitis, radius and ulna

CC **M86.531** Other chronic hematogenous osteomyelitis, right radius and ulna

CC **M86.532** Other chronic hematogenous osteomyelitis, left radius and ulna

CC **M86.539** Other chronic hematogenous osteomyelitis, unspecified radius and ulna

+ **M86.54** Other chronic hematogenous osteomyelitis, hand

CC **M86.541** Other chronic hematogenous osteomyelitis, right hand

CC **M86.542** Other chronic hematogenous osteomyelitis, left hand

CC **M86.549** Other chronic hematogenous osteomyelitis, unspecified hand

+ **M86.55** Other chronic hematogenous osteomyelitis, femur

CC **M86.551** Other chronic hematogenous osteomyelitis, right femur

CC **M86.552** Other chronic hematogenous osteomyelitis, left femur

CC **M86.559** Other chronic hematogenous osteomyelitis, unspecified femur

+ **M86.56** Other chronic hematogenous osteomyelitis, tibia and fibula

CC **M86.561** Other chronic hematogenous osteomyelitis, right tibia and fibula

CC **M86.562** Other chronic hematogenous osteomyelitis, left tibia and fibula

CC **M86.569** Other chronic hematogenous osteomyelitis, unspecified tibia and fibula

+ **M86.57** Other chronic hematogenous osteomyelitis, ankle and foot

CC **M86.571** Other chronic hematogenous osteomyelitis, right ankle and foot

CC **M86.572** Other chronic hematogenous osteomyelitis, left ankle and foot

CC **M86.579** Other chronic hematogenous osteomyelitis, unspecified ankle and foot

CC **M86.58** Other chronic hematogenous osteomyelitis, other site

CC **M86.59** Other chronic hematogenous osteomyelitis, multiple sites

+ **M86.6** Other chronic osteomyelitis

CC **M86.60** Other chronic osteomyelitis, unspecified site

+ **M86.61** Other chronic osteomyelitis, shoulder

CC **M86.611** Other chronic osteomyelitis, right shoulder

CC **M86.612** Other chronic osteomyelitis, left shoulder

CC **M86.619** Other chronic osteomyelitis, unspecified shoulder

+ **M86.62** Other chronic osteomyelitis, humerus

CC **M86.621** Other chronic osteomyelitis, right humerus

CC **M86.622** Other chronic osteomyelitis, left humerus

CC **M86.629** Other chronic osteomyelitis, unspecified humerus

+ **M86.63** Other chronic osteomyelitis, radius and ulna

CC **M86.631** Other chronic osteomyelitis, right radius and ulna

CC **M86.632** Other chronic osteomyelitis, left radius and ulna

CC **M86.639** Other chronic osteomyelitis, unspecified radius and ulna

+ **M86.64** Other chronic osteomyelitis, hand

CC **M86.641** Other chronic osteomyelitis, right hand

CC **M86.642** Other chronic osteomyelitis, left hand

CC **M86.649** Other chronic osteomyelitis, unspecified hand

+ **M86.65** Other chronic osteomyelitis, thigh

CC **M86.651** Other chronic osteomyelitis, right thigh

CC **M86.652** Other chronic osteomyelitis, left thigh

CC **M86.659** Other chronic osteomyelitis, unspecified thigh

+ **M86.66** Other chronic osteomyelitis, tibia and fibula

CC **M86.661** Other chronic osteomyelitis, right tibia and fibula

CC **M86.662** Other chronic osteomyelitis, left tibia and fibula

CC **M86.669** Other chronic osteomyelitis, unspecified tibia and fibula

+ **M86.67** Other chronic osteomyelitis, ankle and foot

CC **M86.671** Other chronic osteomyelitis, right ankle and foot

AHA CC: 1Q, 2016, 13

CC **M86.672** Other chronic osteomyelitis, left ankle and foot

CC **M86.679** Other chronic osteomyelitis, unspecified ankle and foot

CC **M86.68** Other chronic osteomyelitis, other site

CC **M86.69** Other chronic osteomyelitis, multiple sites

+ **M86.8** Other osteomyelitis

Brodie's abscess

+ **M86.8X** Other osteomyelitis

CC **M86.8X0** Other osteomyelitis, multiple sites

CC **M86.8X1** Other osteomyelitis, shoulder

CC **M86.8X2** Other osteomyelitis, upper arm

CC **M86.8X3** Other osteomyelitis, forearm

CC **M86.8X4** Other osteomyelitis, hand
CC **M86.8X5** Other osteomyelitis, thigh
CC **M86.8X6** Other osteomyelitis, lower leg
CC **M86.8X7** Other osteomyelitis, ankle and foot
CC **M86.8X8** Other osteomyelitis, other site
CC **M86.8X9** Other osteomyelitis, unspecified sites

CC **M86.9** Osteomyelitis, unspecified
Infection of bone NOS
Periostitis without osteomyelitis

M87 Osteonecrosis

Includes: avascular necrosis of bone
Use additional code to identify major osseous defect, if applicable
(M89.7-)

Excludes1: *juvenile osteonecrosis (M91-M92)*
osteochondropathies (M90-M93)

+ **M87.0 Idiopathic aseptic necrosis of bone**
CC **M87.00** Idiopathic aseptic necrosis of unspecifiedbone
+ **M87.01** Idiopathic aseptic necrosis of shoulder
Idiopathic aseptic necrosis of clavicle and scapula
CC **M87.011** Idiopathic aseptic necrosis of right shoulder
CC **M87.012** Idiopathic aseptic necrosis of left shoulder
CC **M87.019** Idiopathic aseptic necrosis of unspecified shoulder
+ **M87.02** Idiopathic aseptic necrosis of humerus
CC **M87.021** Idiopathic aseptic necrosis of right humerus
CC **M87.022** Idiopathic aseptic necrosis of left humerus
CC **M87.029** Idiopathic aseptic necrosis of unspecified humerus
+ **M87.03** Idiopathic aseptic necrosis of radius, ulna and carpus
CC **M87.031** Idiopathic aseptic necrosis of right radius
CC **M87.032** Idiopathic aseptic necrosis of left radius
CC **M87.033** Idiopathic aseptic necrosis of unspecified radius
CC **M87.034** Idiopathic aseptic necrosis of right ulna
CC **M87.035** Idiopathic aseptic necrosis of left ulna
CC **M87.036** Idiopathic aseptic necrosis of unspecified ulna
CC **M87.037** Idiopathic aseptic necrosis of right carpus
CC **M87.038** Idiopathic aseptic necrosis of left carpus
CC **M87.039** Idiopathic aseptic necrosis of unspecified carpus
+ **M87.04** Idiopathic aseptic necrosis of hand and fingers
Idiopathic aseptic necrosis of metacarpals and phalanges of hands
CC **M87.041** Idiopathic aseptic necrosis of right hand
CC **M87.042** Idiopathic aseptic necrosis of left hand
CC **M87.043** Idiopathic aseptic necrosis of unspecified hand
CC **M87.044** Idiopathic aseptic necrosis of right finger(s)
CC **M87.045** Idiopathic aseptic necrosis of left finger(s)
CC **M87.046** Idiopathic aseptic necrosis of unspecified finger(s)
+ **M87.05** Idiopathic aseptic necrosis of pelvis and femur
CC **M87.050** Idiopathic aseptic necrosis of pelvis
CC **M87.051** Idiopathic aseptic necrosis of right femur
CC **M87.052** Idiopathic aseptic necrosis of left femur
CC **M87.059** Idiopathic aseptic necrosis of unspecified femur
Idiopathic aseptic necrosis of hip NOS
+ **M87.06** Idiopathic aseptic necrosis of tibia and fibula
CC **M87.061** Idiopathic aseptic necrosis of right tibia
CC **M87.062** Idiopathic aseptic necrosis of left tibia
CC **M87.063** Idiopathic aseptic necrosis of unspecified tibia
CC **M87.064** Idiopathic aseptic necrosis of right fibula
CC **M87.065** Idiopathic aseptic necrosis of left fibula

CC **M87.066** Idiopathic aseptic necrosis of unspecified fibula
+ **M87.07** Idiopathic aseptic necrosis of ankle, foot and toes
Idiopathic aseptic necrosis of metatarsus, tarsus, and phalanges of toes
CC **M87.071** Idiopathic aseptic necrosis of right ankle
CC **M87.072** Idiopathic aseptic necrosis of left ankle
CC **M87.073** Idiopathic aseptic necrosis of unspecified ankle
CC **M87.074** Idiopathic aseptic necrosis of right foot
CC **M87.075** Idiopathic aseptic necrosis of left foot
CC **M87.076** Idiopathic aseptic necrosis of unspecified foot
CC **M87.077** Idiopathic aseptic necrosis of right toe(s)
CC **M87.078** Idiopathic aseptic necrosis of left toe(s)
CC **M87.079** Idiopathic aseptic necrosis of unspecified toe(s)
CC **M87.08** Idiopathic aseptic necrosis of bone, other site
CC **M87.09** Idiopathic aseptic necrosis of bone, multiple sites
+ **M87.1 Osteonecrosis due to drugs**
Use additional code for adverse effect, if applicable, to identify drug (T36-T50 with fifth or sixth character 5)
CC **M87.10** Osteonecrosis due to drugs, unspecified bone
+ **M87.11** Osteonecrosis due to drugs, shoulder
CC **M87.111** Osteonecrosis due to drugs, right shoulder
CC **M87.112** Osteonecrosis due to drugs, left shoulder
CC **M87.119** Osteonecrosis due to drugs, unspecified shoulder
+ **M87.12** Osteonecrosis due to drugs, humerus
CC **M87.121** Osteonecrosis due to drugs, right humerus
CC **M87.122** Osteonecrosis due to drugs, left humerus
CC **M87.129** Osteonecrosis due to drugs, unspecified humerus
+ **M87.13** Osteonecrosis due to drugs of radius, ulna and carpus
CC **M87.131** Osteonecrosis due to drugs of right radius
CC **M87.132** Osteonecrosis due to drugs of left radius
CC **M87.133** Osteonecrosis due to drugs of unspecified radius
CC **M87.134** Osteonecrosis due to drugs of right ulna
CC **M87.135** Osteonecrosis due to drugs of left ulna
CC **M87.136** Osteonecrosis due to drugs of unspecified ulna
CC **M87.137** Osteonecrosis due to drugs of right carpus
CC **M87.138** Osteonecrosis due to drugs of left carpus
CC **M87.139** Osteonecrosis due to drugs of unspecified carpus
+ **M87.14** Osteonecrosis due to drugs, hand and fingers
CC **M87.141** Osteonecrosis due to drugs, right hand
CC **M87.142** Osteonecrosis due to drugs, left hand
CC **M87.143** Osteonecrosis due to drugs, unspecified hand
CC **M87.144** Osteonecrosis due to drugs, right finger(s)
CC **M87.145** Osteonecrosis due to drugs, left finger(s)
CC **M87.146** Osteonecrosis due to drugs, unspecified finger(s)
+ **M87.15** Osteonecrosis due to drugs, pelvis and femur
CC **M87.150** Osteonecrosis due to drugs, pelvis
CC **M87.151** Osteonecrosis due to drugs, right femur
CC **M87.152** Osteonecrosis due to drugs, left femur
CC **M87.159** Osteonecrosis due to drugs, unspecified femur
+ **M87.16** Osteonecrosis due to drugs, tibia and fibula
CC **M87.161** Osteonecrosis due to drugs, right tibia
CC **M87.162** Osteonecrosis due to drugs, left tibia
CC **M87.163** Osteonecrosis due to drugs, unspecified tibia
CC **M87.164** Osteonecrosis due to drugs, right fibula
CC **M87.165** Osteonecrosis due to drugs, left fibula
CC **M87.166** Osteonecrosis due to drugs, unspecified fibula

+ **M87.17** Osteonecrosis due to drugs, ankle, foot and toes
  - CC **M87.171** Osteonecrosis due to drugs, right ankle
  - CC **M87.172** Osteonecrosis due to drugs, left ankle
  - CC **M87.173** Osteonecrosis due to drugs, unspecified ankle
  - CC **M87.174** Osteonecrosis due to drugs, right foot
  - CC **M87.175** Osteonecrosis due to drugs, left foot
  - CC **M87.176** Osteonecrosis due to drugs, unspecified foot
  - CC **M87.177** Osteonecrosis due to drugs, right toe(s)
  - CC **M87.178** Osteonecrosis due to drugs, left toe(s)
  - CC **M87.179** Osteonecrosis due to drugs, unspecified toe(s)

+ **M87.18** Osteonecrosis due to drugs, other site
  - CC **M87.180** Osteonecrosis due to drugs, jaw
  - CC **M87.188** Osteonecrosis due to drugs, other site

CC **M87.19** Osteonecrosis due to drugs, multiple sites

+ **M87.2** Osteonecrosis due to previous trauma
  - CC **M87.20** Osteonecrosis due to previous trauma, unspecified bone

+ **M87.21** Osteonecrosis due to previous trauma, shoulder
  - CC **M87.211** Osteonecrosis due to previous trauma, right shoulder
  - CC **M87.212** Osteonecrosis due to previous trauma, left shoulder
  - CC **M87.219** Osteonecrosis due to previous trauma, unspecified shoulder

+ **M87.22** Osteonecrosis due to previous trauma, humerus
  - CC **M87.221** Osteonecrosis due to previous trauma, right humerus
  - CC **M87.222** Osteonecrosis due to previous trauma, left humerus
  - CC **M87.229** Osteonecrosis due to previous trauma, unspecified humerus

+ **M87.23** Osteonecrosis due to previous trauma of radius, ulna and carpus
  - CC **M87.231** Osteonecrosis due to previous trauma of right radius
  - CC **M87.232** Osteonecrosis due to previous trauma of left radius
  - CC **M87.233** Osteonecrosis due to previous trauma of unspecified radius
  - CC **M87.234** Osteonecrosis due to previous trauma of right ulna
  - CC **M87.235** Osteonecrosis due to previous trauma of left ulna
  - CC **M87.236** Osteonecrosis due to previous trauma of unspecified ulna
  - CC **M87.237** Osteonecrosis due to previous trauma of right carpus
  - CC **M87.238** Osteonecrosis due to previous trauma of left carpus
  - CC **M87.239** Osteonecrosis due to previous trauma of unspecified carpus

+ **M87.24** Osteonecrosis due to previous trauma, hand and fingers
  - CC **M87.241** Osteonecrosis due to previous trauma, right hand
  - CC **M87.242** Osteonecrosis due to previous trauma, left hand
  - CC **M87.243** Osteonecrosis due to previous trauma, unspecified hand
  - CC **M87.244** Osteonecrosis due to previous trauma, right finger(s)
  - CC **M87.245** Osteonecrosis due to previous trauma, left finger(s)
  - CC **M87.246** Osteonecrosis due to previous trauma, unspecified finger(s)

+ **M87.25** Osteonecrosis due to previous trauma, pelvis and femur
  - CC **M87.250** Osteonecrosis due to previous trauma, pelvis
  - CC **M87.251** Osteonecrosis due to previous trauma, right femur
  - CC **M87.252** Osteonecrosis due to previous trauma, left femur
  - CC **M87.256** Osteonecrosis due to previous trauma, unspecified femur

+ **M87.26** Osteonecrosis due to previous trauma, tibia and fibula
  - CC **M87.261** Osteonecrosis due to previous trauma, right tibia
  - CC **M87.262** Osteonecrosis due to previous trauma, left tibia
  - CC **M87.263** Osteonecrosis due to previous trauma, unspecified tibia
  - CC **M87.264** Osteonecrosis due to previous trauma, right fibula
  - CC **M87.265** Osteonecrosis due to previous trauma, left fibula
  - CC **M87.266** Osteonecrosis due to previous trauma, unspecified fibula

+ **M87.27** Osteonecrosis due to previous trauma, ankle, foot and toes
  - CC **M87.271** Osteonecrosis due to previous trauma, right ankle
  - CC **M87.272** Osteonecrosis due to previous trauma, left ankle
  - CC **M87.273** Osteonecrosis due to previous trauma, unspecified ankle
  - CC **M87.274** Osteonecrosis due to previous trauma, right foot
  - CC **M87.275** Osteonecrosis due to previous trauma, left foot
  - CC **M87.276** Osteonecrosis due to previous trauma, unspecified foot
  - CC **M87.277** Osteonecrosis due to previous trauma, right toe(s)
  - CC **M87.278** Osteonecrosis due to previous trauma, left toe(s)
  - CC **M87.279** Osteonecrosis due to previous trauma, unspecified toe(s)

CC **M87.28** Osteonecrosis due to previous trauma, other site

CC **M87.29** Osteonecrosis due to previous trauma, multiple sites

+ **M87.3** Other secondary osteonecrosis
  - CC **M87.30** Other secondary osteonecrosis, unspecified bone

+ **M87.31** Other secondary osteonecrosis, shoulder
  - CC **M87.311** Other secondary osteonecrosis, right shoulder
  - CC **M87.312** Other secondary osteonecrosis, left shoulder
  - CC **M87.319** Other secondary osteonecrosis, unspecified shoulder

+ **M87.32** Other secondary osteonecrosis, humerus
  - CC **M87.321** Other secondary osteonecrosis, right humerus
  - CC **M87.322** Other secondary osteonecrosis, left humerus
  - CC **M87.329** Other secondary osteonecrosis, unspecified humerus

+ **M87.33** Other secondary osteonecrosis of radius, ulna and carpus
  - CC **M87.331** Other secondary osteonecrosis of right radius
  - CC **M87.332** Other secondary osteonecrosis of left radius
  - CC **M87.333** Other secondary osteonecrosis of unspecified radius
  - CC **M87.334** Other secondary osteonecrosis of right ulna
  - CC **M87.335** Other secondary osteonecrosis of left ulna
  - CC **M87.336** Other secondary osteonecrosis of unspecified ulna
  - CC **M87.337** Other secondary osteonecrosis of right carpus
  - CC **M87.338** Other secondary osteonecrosis of left carpus
  - CC **M87.339** Other secondary osteonecrosis of unspecified carpus

+ **M87.34** Other secondary osteonecrosis, hand and fingers
  - CC **M87.341** Other secondary osteonecrosis, right hand
  - CC **M87.342** Other secondary osteonecrosis, left hand

+, +7th, X + 7th   ● Newborn   ● Pediatric   ● Maternity   ● Adult   ♀ Female   ♂ Male   Manifestation   Unacceptable PDX   HCC   CC   MCC   HAC

CC M87.343 Other secondary osteonecrosis, unspecified hand
CC M87.344 Other secondary osteonecrosis, right finger(s)
CC M87.345 Other secondary osteonecrosis, left finger(s)
CC M87.346 Other secondary osteonecrosis, unspecified finger(s)
+ M87.35 Other secondary osteonecrosis, pelvis and femur
   CC M87.350 Other secondary osteonecrosis, pelvis
   CC M87.351 Other secondary osteonecrosis, right femur
   CC M87.352 Other secondary osteonecrosis, left femur
   CC M87.353 Other secondary osteonecrosis, unspecified femur
+ M87.36 Other secondary osteonecrosis, tibia and fibula
   CC M87.361 Other secondary osteonecrosis, right tibia
   CC M87.362 Other secondary osteonecrosis, left tibia
   CC M87.363 Other secondary osteonecrosis, unspecified tibia
   CC M87.364 Other secondary osteonecrosis, right fibula
   CC M87.365 Other secondary osteonecrosis, left fibula
   CC M87.366 Other secondary osteonecrosis, unspecified fibula
+ M87.37 Other secondary osteonecrosis, ankle and foot
   CC M87.371 Other secondary osteonecrosis, right ankle
   CC M87.372 Other secondary osteonecrosis, left ankle
   CC M87.373 Other secondary osteonecrosis, unspecified ankle
   CC M87.374 Other secondary osteonecrosis, right foot
   CC M87.375 Other secondary osteonecrosis, left foot
   CC M87.376 Other secondary osteonecrosis, unspecified foot
   CC M87.377 Other secondary osteonecrosis, right toe(s)
   CC M87.378 Other secondary osteonecrosis, left toe(s)
   CC M87.379 Other secondary osteonecrosis, unspecified toe(s)
CC M87.38 Other secondary osteonecrosis, other site
CC M87.39 Other secondary osteonecrosis, multiple sites
+ M87.8 Other osteonecrosis
   CC M87.80 Other osteonecrosis, unspecified bone
  + M87.81 Other osteonecrosis, shoulder
    CC M87.811 Other osteonecrosis, right shoulder
    CC M87.812 Other osteonecrosis, left shoulder
    CC M87.819 Other osteonecrosis, unspecified shoulder
  + M87.82 Other osteonecrosis, humerus
    CC M87.821 Other osteonecrosis, right humerus
    CC M87.822 Other osteonecrosis, left humerus
    CC M87.829 Other osteonecrosis, unspecified humerus
  + M87.83 Other osteonecrosis of radius, ulna and carpus
    CC M87.831 Other osteonecrosis of right radius
    CC M87.832 Other osteonecrosis of left radius
    CC M87.833 Other osteonecrosis of unspecified radius
    CC M87.834 Other osteonecrosis of right ulna
    CC M87.835 Other osteonecrosis of left ulna
    CC M87.836 Other osteonecrosis of unspecified ulna
    CC M87.837 Other osteonecrosis of right carpus
    CC M87.838 Other osteonecrosis of left carpus
    CC M87.839 Other osteonecrosis of unspecified carpus
  + M87.84 Other osteonecrosis, hand and fingers
    CC M87.841 Other osteonecrosis, right hand
    CC M87.842 Other osteonecrosis, left hand
    CC M87.843 Other osteonecrosis, unspecified hand
    CC M87.844 Other osteonecrosis, right finger(s)
    CC M87.845 Other osteonecrosis, left finger(s)
    CC M87.849 Other osteonecrosis, unspecified finger(s)

+ M87.85 Other osteonecrosis, pelvis and femur
   CC M87.850 Other osteonecrosis, pelvis
   CC M87.851 Other osteonecrosis, right femur
   CC M87.852 Other osteonecrosis, left femur
   CC M87.859 Other osteonecrosis, unspecified femur
+ M87.86 Other osteonecrosis, tibia and fibula
   CC M87.861 Other osteonecrosis, right tibia
   CC M87.862 Other osteonecrosis, left tibia
   CC M87.863 Other osteonecrosis, unspecified tibia
   CC M87.864 Other osteonecrosis, right fibula
   CC M87.865 Other osteonecrosis, left fibula
   CC M87.869 Other osteonecrosis, unspecified fibula
+ M87.87 Other osteonecrosis, ankle, foot and toes
   CC M87.871 Other osteonecrosis, right ankle
   CC M87.872 Other osteonecrosis, left ankle
   CC M87.873 Other osteonecrosis, unspecified ankle
   CC M87.874 Other osteonecrosis, right foot
   CC M87.875 Other osteonecrosis, left foot
   CC M87.876 Other osteonecrosis, unspecified foot
   CC M87.877 Other osteonecrosis, right toe(s)
   CC M87.878 Other osteonecrosis, left toe(s)
   CC M87.879 Other osteonecrosis, unspecified toe(s)
CC M87.88 Other osteonecrosis, other site
CC M87.89 Other osteonecrosis, multiple sites
CC M87.9 Osteonecrosis, unspecified
   Necrosis of bone NOS

M88 Osteitis deformans [Paget's disease of bone]

  Excludes1: *osteitis deformans in neoplastic disease (M90.6)*
M88.0 Osteitis deformans of skull
M88.1 Osteitis deformans of vertebrae
+ M88.8 Osteitis deformans of other bones
  + M88.81 Osteitis deformans of shoulder
    M88.811 Osteitis deformans of right shoulder
    M88.812 Osteitis deformans of left shoulder
    M88.819 Osteitis deformans of unspecified shoulder
  + M88.82 Osteitis deformans of upper arm
    M88.821 Osteitis deformans of right upper arm
    M88.822 Osteitis deformans of left upper arm
    M88.829 Osteitis deformans of unspecified upper arm
  + M88.83 Osteitis deformans of forearm
    M88.831 Osteitis deformans of right forearm
    M88.832 Osteitis deformans of left forearm
    M88.839 Osteitis deformans of unspecified forearm
  + M88.84 Osteitis deformans of hand
    M88.841 Osteitis deformans of right hand
    M88.842 Osteitis deformans of left hand
    M88.849 Osteitis deformans of unspecified hand
  + M88.85 Osteitis deformans of thigh
    M88.851 Osteitis deformans of right thigh
    M88.852 Osteitis deformans of left thigh
    M88.859 Osteitis deformans of unspecified thigh
  + M88.86 Osteitis deformans of lower leg
    M88.861 Osteitis deformans of right lower leg
    M88.862 Osteitis deformans of left lower leg
    M88.869 Osteitis deformans of unspecified lower leg
  + M88.87 Osteitis deformans of ankle and foot
    M88.871 Osteitis deformans of right ankle and foot
    M88.872 Osteitis deformans of left ankle and foot
    M88.879 Osteitis deformans of unspecified ankle and foot
    M88.88 Osteitis deformans of other bones
    Excludes2: *osteitis deformans of skull (M88.0)*
    osteitis deformans of vertebrae (M88.1)
    M88.89 Osteitis deformans of multiple sites
M88.9 Osteitis deformans of unspecified bone

M89 Other disorders of bone

  + M89.0 Algoneurodystrophy
    Shoulder-hand syndrome
    Sudeck's atrophy
    Excludes1: *causalgia, lower limb (G57.7-)*
    causalgia, upper limb (G56.4-)
    complex regional pain syndrome II, lower limb (G57.7-)
    complex regional pain syndrome II, upper limb (G56.4-)
    reflex sympathetic dystrophy (G90.5-)

+, +7th, X + 7th ● Newborn ● Pediatric ● Maternity ● Adult ♀ Female ♂ Male Manifestation Unacceptable PDX HCC CC MCC HAC

M89.00 Algoneurodystrophy, unspecified site
+ M89.01 Algoneurodystrophy, shoulder
   M89.011 Algoneurodystrophy, right shoulder
   M89.012 Algoneurodystrophy, left shoulder
   M89.019 Algoneurodystrophy, unspecified shoulder
+ M89.02 Algoneurodystrophy, upper arm
   M89.021 Algoneurodystrophy, right upper arm
   M89.022 Algoneurodystrophy, left upper arm
   M89.029 Algoneurodystrophy, unspecified upper arm
+ M89.03 Algoneurodystrophy, forearm
   M89.031 Algoneurodystrophy, right forearm
   M89.032 Algoneurodystrophy, left forearm
   M89.039 Algoneurodystrophy, unspecified forearm
+ M89.04 Algoneurodystrophy, hand
   M89.041 Algoneurodystrophy, right≈hand
   M89.042 Algoneurodystrophy, left hand
   M89.049 Algoneurodystrophy, unspecified hand
+ M89.05 Algoneurodystrophy, thigh
   M89.051 Algoneurodystrophy, right thigh
   M89.052 Algoneurodystrophy, left thigh
   M89.059 Algoneurodystrophy, unspecified thigh
+ M89.06 Algoneurodystrophy, lower leg
   M89.061 Algoneurodystrophy, right lower leg
   M89.062 Algoneurodystrophy, left lower leg
   M89.069 Algoneurodystrophy, unspecified lower leg
+ M89.07 Algoneurodystrophy, ankle and foot
   M89.071 Algoneurodystrophy, right ankle and foot
   M89.072 Algoneurodystrophy, left ankle and foot
   M89.079 Algoneurodystrophy, unspecified ankle and foot
M89.08 Algoneurodystrophy, other site
M89.09 Algoneurodystrophy, multiple sites
+ M89.1 Physeal arrest
   Arrest of growth plate
   Epiphyseal arrest
   Growth plate arrest
+ M89.12 Physeal arrest, humerus
   M89.121 Complete physeal arrest, right proximal humerus
   M89.122 Complete physeal arrest, left proximal humerus
   M89.123 Partial physeal arrest, right proximal humerus
   M89.124 Partial physeal arrest, left proximal humerus
   M89.125 Complete physeal arrest, right distal humerus
   M89.126 Complete physeal arrest, left distal humerus
   M89.127 Partial physeal arrest, right distal humerus
   M89.128 Partial physeal arrest, left distal humerus
   M89.129 Physeal arrest, humerus, unspecified
+ M89.13 Physeal arrest, forearm
   M89.131 Complete physeal arrest, right distal radius
   M89.132 Complete physeal arrest, left distal radius
   M89.133 Partial physeal arrest, right distal radius
   M89.134 Partial physeal arrest, left distal radius
   M89.138 Other physeal arrest of forearm
   M89.139 Physeal arrest, forearm, unspecified
+ M89.15 Physeal arrest, femur
   M89.151 Complete physeal arrest, right proximal femur
   M89.152 Complete physeal arrest, left proximal femur
   M89.153 Partial physeal arrest, right proximal femur
   M89.154 Partial physeal arrest, left proximal femur
   M89.155 Complete physeal arrest, right distal femur

M89.156 Complete physeal arrest, left distal femur
M89.157 Partial physeal arrest, right distal femur
M89.158 Partial physeal arrest, left distal femur
M89.159 Physeal arrest, femur, unspecified
+ M89.16 Physeal arrest, lower leg
   M89.160 Complete physeal arrest, right proximal tibia
   M89.161 Complete physeal arrest, left proximal tibia
   M89.162 Partial physeal arrest, right proximal tibia
   M89.163 Partial physeal arrest, left proximal tibia
   M89.164 Complete physeal arrest, right distal tibia
   M89.165 Complete physeal arrest, left distal tibia
   M89.166 Partial physeal arrest, right distal tibia
   M89.167 Partial physeal arrest, left distal tibia
   M89.168 Other physeal arrest of lower leg
   M89.169 Physeal arrest, lower leg, unspecified
M89.18 Physeal arrest, other site
+ M89.2 Other disorders of bone development and growth
M89.20 Other disorders of bone development and growth, unspecified site
+ M89.21 Other disorders of bone development and growth, shoulder
   M89.211 Other disorders of bone development and growth, right shoulder
   M89.212 Other disorders of bone development and growth, left shoulder
   M89.219 Other disorders of bone development and growth, unspecified shoulder
+ M89.22 Other disorders of bone development and growth, humerus
   M89.221 Other disorders of bone development and growth, right humerus
   M89.222 Other disorders of bone development and growth, left humerus
   M89.229 Other disorders of bone development and growth, unspecified humerus
+ M89.23 Other disorders of bone development and growth, ulna and radius
   M89.231 Other disorders of bone development and growth, right ulna
   M89.232 Other disorders of bone development and growth, left ulna
   M89.233 Other disorders of bone development and growth, right radius
   M89.234 Other disorders of bone development and growth, left radius
   M89.239 Other disorders of bone development and growth, unspecified ulna and radius
+ M89.24 Other disorders of bone development and growth, hand
   M89.241 Other disorders of bone development and growth, right hand
   M89.242 Other disorders of bone development and growth, left hand
   M89.249 Other disorders of bone development and growth, unspecified hand
+ M89.25 Other disorders of bone development and growth, femur
   M89.251 Other disorders of bone development and growth, right femur
   M89.252 Other disorders of bone development and growth, left femur
   M89.259 Other disorders of bone development and growth, unspecified femur
+ M89.26 Other disorders of bone development and growth, tibia and fibula
   M89.261 Other disorders of bone development and growth, right tibia
   M89.262 Other disorders of bone development and growth, left tibia
   M89.263 Other disorders of bone development and growth, right fibula
   M89.264 Other disorders of bone development and growth, left fibula
   M89.269 Other disorders of bone development and growth, unspecified lower leg

+ M89.27 Other disorders of bone development and growth, ankle and foot
 M89.271 Other disorders of bone development and growth, right ankle and foot
 M89.272 Other disorders of bone development and growth, left ankle and foot
 M89.279 Other disorders of bone development and growth, unspecified ankle and foot
M89.28 Other disorders of bone development and growth, other site
M89.29 Other disorders of bone development and growth, multiple sites
+ M89.3 Hypertrophy of bone
 M89.30 Hypertrophy of bone, unspecified site
+ M89.31 Hypertrophy of bone, shoulder
 M89.311 Hypertrophy of bone, right shoulder
 M89.312 Hypertrophy of bone, left shoulder
 M89.319 Hypertrophy of bone, unspecified shoulder
+ M89.32 Hypertrophy of bone, humerus
 M89.321 Hypertrophy of bone, right humerus
 M89.322 Hypertrophy of bone, left humerus
 M89.329 Hypertrophy of bone, unspecified humerus
+ M89.33 Hypertrophy of bone, ulna and radius
 M89.331 Hypertrophy of bone, right ulna
 M89.332 Hypertrophy of bone, left ulna
 M89.333 Hypertrophy of bone, right radius
 M89.334 Hypertrophy of bone, left radius
 M89.339 Hypertrophy of bone, unspecified ulna and radius
+ M89.34 Hypertrophy of bone, hand
 M89.341 Hypertrophy of bone, right hand
 M89.342 Hypertrophy of bone, left hand
 M89.349 Hypertrophy of bone, unspecified hand
+ M89.35 Hypertrophy of bone, femur
 M89.351 Hypertrophy of bone, right femur
 M89.352 Hypertrophy of bone, left femur
 M89.359 Hypertrophy of bone, unspecified femur
+ M89.36 Hypertrophy of bone, tibia and fibula
 M89.361 Hypertrophy of bone, right tibia
 M89.362 Hypertrophy of bone, left tibia
 M89.363 Hypertrophy of bone, right fibula
 M89.364 Hypertrophy of bone, left fibula
 M89.369 Hypertrophy of bone, unspecified tibia and fibula
+ M89.37 Hypertrophy of bone, ankle and foot
 M89.371 Hypertrophy of bone, right ankle and foot
 M89.372 Hypertrophy of bone, left ankle and foot
 M89.379 Hypertrophy of bone, unspecified ankle and foot
M89.38 Hypertrophy of bone, other site
M89.39 Hypertrophy of bone, multiple sites
+ M89.4 Other hypertrophic osteoarthropathy
 Marie-Bamberger disease
 Pachydermoperiostosis
 M89.40 Other hypertrophic osteoarthropathy, unspecified site
+ M89.41 Other hypertrophic osteoarthropathy, shoulder
 M89.411 Other hypertrophic osteoarthropathy, right shoulder
 M89.412 Other hypertrophic osteoarthropathy, left shoulder
 M89.419 Other hypertrophic osteoarthropathy, unspecified shoulder
+ M89.42 Other hypertrophic osteoarthropathy, upper arm
 M89.421 Other hypertrophic osteoarthropathy, right upper arm
 M89.422 Other hypertrophic osteoarthropathy, left upper arm
 M89.429 Other hypertrophic osteoarthropathy, unspecified upper arm
+ M89.43 Other hypertrophic osteoarthropathy, forearm
 M89.431 Other hypertrophic osteoarthropathy, right forearm
 M89.432 Other hypertrophic osteoarthropathy, left forearm
 M89.439 Other hypertrophic osteoarthropathy, unspecified forearm
+ M89.44 Other hypertrophic osteoarthropathy, hand

 M89.441 Other hypertrophic osteoarthropathy, right hand
 M89.442 Other hypertrophic osteoarthropathy, left hand
 M89.449 Other hypertrophic osteoarthropathy, unspecified hand
+ M89.45 Other hypertrophic osteoarthropathy, thigh
 M89.451 Other hypertrophic osteoarthropathy, right thigh
 M89.452 Other hypertrophic osteoarthropathy, left thigh
 M89.459 Other hypertrophic osteoarthropathy, unspecified thigh
+ M89.46 Other hypertrophic osteoarthropathy, lower leg
 M89.461 Other hypertrophic osteoarthropathy, right lower leg
 M89.462 Other hypertrophic osteoarthropathy, left lower leg
 M89.469 Other hypertrophic osteoarthropathy, unspecified lower leg
+ M89.47 Other hypertrophic osteoarthropathy, ankle and foot
 M89.471 Other hypertrophic osteoarthropathy, right ankle and foot
 M89.472 Other hypertrophic osteoarthropathy, left ankle and foot
 M89.479 Other hypertrophic osteoarthropathy, unspecified ankle and foot
M89.48 Other hypertrophic osteoarthropathy, other site
M89.49 Other hypertrophic osteoarthropathy, multiple sites
+ M89.5 Osteolysis
 Use additional code to identify major osseous defect, if applicable (M89.7-)
 Excludes2: periprosthetic osteolysis of internal prosthetic joint (T84.05-)
 M89.50 Osteolysis, unspecified site
+ M89.51 Osteolysis, shoulder
 M89.511 Osteolysis, right shoulder
 M89.512 Osteolysis, left shoulder
 M89.519 Osteolysis, unspecified shoulder
+ M89.52 Osteolysis, upper arm
 M89.521 Osteolysis, right upper arm
 M89.522 Osteolysis, left upper arm
 M89.529 Osteolysis, unspecified upper arm
+ M89.53 Osteolysis, forearm
 M89.531 Osteolysis, right forearm
 M89.532 Osteolysis, left forearm
 M89.539 Osteolysis, unspecified forearm
+ M89.54 Osteolysis, hand
 M89.541 Osteolysis, right hand
 M89.542 Osteolysis, left hand
 M89.549 Osteolysis, unspecified hand
+ M89.55 Osteolysis, thigh
 M89.551 Osteolysis, right thigh
 M89.552 Osteolysis, left thigh
 M89.559 Osteolysis, unspecified thigh
+ M89.56 Osteolysis, lower leg
 M89.561 Osteolysis, right lower leg
 M89.562 Osteolysis, left lower leg
 M89.569 Osteolysis, unspecified lower leg
+ M89.57 Osteolysis, ankle and foot
 M89.571 Osteolysis, right ankle and foot
 M89.572 Osteolysis, left ankle and foot
 M89.579 Osteolysis, unspecified ankle and foot
M89.58 Osteolysis, other site
M89.59 Osteolysis, multiple sites
+ M89.6 Osteopathy after poliomyelitis
 Use additional code (B91) to identify previous poliomyelitis
 Excludes1: postpolio syndrome (G14)
M89.60 Osteopathy after poliomyelitis, unspecified site
+ M89.61 Osteopathy after poliomyelitis, shoulder
 M89.611 Osteopathy after poliomyelitis, right shoulder
 M89.612 Osteopathy after poliomyelitis, left shoulder
 M89.619 Osteopathy after poliomyelitis, unspecified shoulder

---

+, +7th, X + 7th ● Newborn ● Pediatric ● Maternity ● Adult ♀ Female ♂ Male Manifestation Unacceptable PDX HCC CC MCC HAC

+ **M89.62** Osteopathy after poliomyelitis, upper arm
   M89.621 Osteopathy after poliomyelitis, right upper arm
   M89.622 Osteopathy after poliomyelitis, left upper arm
   M89.629 Osteopathy after poliomyelitis, unspecified upper arm

+ **M89.63** Osteopathy after poliomyelitis, forearm
   M89.631 Osteopathy after poliomyelitis, right forearm
   M89.632 Osteopathy after poliomyelitis, left forearm
   M89.639 Osteopathy after poliomyelitis, unspecified forearm

+ **M89.64** Osteopathy after poliomyelitis, hand
   M89.641 Osteopathy after poliomyelitis, right hand
   M89.642 Osteopathy after poliomyelitis, left hand
   M89.649 Osteopathy after poliomyelitis, unspecified hand

+ **M89.65** Osteopathy after poliomyelitis, thigh
   M89.651 Osteopathy after poliomyelitis, right thigh
   M89.652 Osteopathy after poliomyelitis, left thigh
   M89.659 Osteopathy after poliomyelitis, unspecified thigh

+ **M89.66** Osteopathy after poliomyelitis, lower leg
   M89.661 Osteopathy after poliomyelitis, right lower leg
   M89.662 Osteopathy after poliomyelitis, left lower leg
   M89.669 Osteopathy after poliomyelitis, unspecified lower leg

+ **M89.67** Osteopathy after poliomyelitis, ankle and foot
   M89.671 Osteopathy after poliomyelitis, right ankle and foot
   M89.672 Osteopathy after poliomyelitis, left ankle and foot
   M89.679 Osteopathy after poliomyelitis, unspecified ankle and foot

M89.68 Osteopathy after poliomyelitis, other site
M89.69 Osteopathy after poliomyelitis, multiple sites

+ **M89.7 Major osseous defect**
   Code first underlying disease, if known, such as:
    aseptic necrosis of bone (M87.-)
    malignant neoplasm of bone (C40.-)
    osteolysis (M89.5)
    osteomyelitis (M86.-)
    osteonecrosis (M87.-)
    osteoporosis (M80.-, M81.-)
    periprosthetic osteolysis (T84.05-)

M89.70 Major osseous defect, unspecified site

+ **M89.71** Major osseous defect, shoulder region
   Major osseous defect clavicle or scapula
   M89.711 Major osseous defect, right shoulder region
   M89.712 Major osseous defect, left shoulder region
   M89.719 Major osseous defect, unspecified shoulder region

+ **M89.72** Major osseous defect, humerus
   M89.721 Major osseous defect, right humerus
   M89.722 Major osseous defect, left humerus
   M89.729 Major osseous defect, unspecified humerus

+ **M89.73** Major osseous defect, forearm
   Major osseous defect of radius and ulna
   M89.731 Major osseous defect, right forearm
   M89.732 Major osseous defect, left forearm
   M89.739 Major osseous defect, unspecified forearm

+ **M89.74** Major osseous defect, hand
   Major osseous defect of carpus, fingers, metacarpus
   M89.741 Major osseous defect, right hand
   M89.742 Major osseous defect, left hand
   M89.749 Major osseous defect, unspecified hand

+ **M89.75** Major osseous defect, pelvic region and thigh
   Major osseous defect of femur and pelvis
   M89.751 Major osseous defect, right pelvic region and thigh
   M89.752 Major osseous defect, left pelvic region and thigh
   M89.759 Major osseous defect, unspecified pelvic region and thigh

+ **M89.76** Major osseous defect, lower leg
   Major osseous defect of fibula and tibia
   M89.761 Major osseous defect, right lower leg
   M89.762 Major osseous defect, left lower leg
   M89.769 Major osseous defect, unspecified lower leg

+ **M89.77** Major osseous defect, ankle and foot
   Major osseous defect of metatarsus, tarsus, toes
   M89.771 Major osseous defect, right ankle and foot
   M89.772 Major osseous defect, left ankle and foot
   M89.779 Major osseous defect, unspecified ankle and foot

M89.78 Major osseous defect, other site
M89.79 Major osseous defect, multiple sites

+ **M89.8 Other specified disorders of bone**
   Infantile cortical hyperostoses
   Post-traumatic subperiosteal ossification

+ **M89.8X Other specified disorders of bone**
   M89.8X0 Other specified disorders of bone, multiple sites
   M89.8X1 Other specified disorders of bone, shoulder
   M89.8X2 Other specified disorders of bone, upper arm
   M89.8X3 Other specified disorders of bone, forearm
    AHA CC: 3Q, 2019, 9-10
   M89.8X4 Other specified disorders of bone, hand
   M89.8X5 Other specified disorders of bone, thigh
   M89.8X6 Other specified disorders of bone, lower leg
   M89.8X7 Other specified disorders of bone, ankle and foot
   M89.8X8 Other specified disorders of bone, other site
   M89.8X9 Other specified disorders of bone, unspecified site

M89.9 Disorder of bone, unspecified

M90 Osteopathies in diseases classified elsewhere

   Excludes1: *osteochondritis, osteomyelitis, and osteopathy (in):*
    cryptococcosis (B45.3)
    diabetes mellitus (E08-E13 with .69-)
    gonococcal (A54.43)
    neurogenic syphilis (A52.11)
    renal osteodystrophy (N25.0)
    salmonellosis (A02.24)
    secondary syphilis (A51.46)
    syphilis (late) (A52.77)

+ **M90.5 Osteonecrosis in diseases classified elsewhere**
   Code first underlying disease, such as:
    caisson disease (T70.3)
    hemoglobinopathy (D50-D64)

CC **M90.50** Osteonecrosis in diseases classified elsewhere, unspecified site

+ **M90.51** Osteonecrosis in diseases classified elsewhere, shoulder
   CC **M90.511** Osteonecrosis in diseases classified elsewhere, right shoulder
   CC **M90.512** Osteonecrosis in diseases classified elsewhere, left shoulder
   CC **M90.519** Osteonecrosis in diseases classified elsewhere, unspecified shoulder

+ **M90.52** Osteonecrosis in diseases classified elsewhere, upper arm
   CC **M90.521** Osteonecrosis in diseases classified elsewhere, right upper arm
   CC **M90.522** Osteonecrosis in diseases classified elsewhere, left upper arm
   CC **M90.529** Osteonecrosis in diseases classified elsewhere, unspecified upper arm

+ **M90.53** Osteonecrosis in diseases classified elsewhere, forearm
   CC **M90.531** Osteonecrosis in diseases classified elsewhere, right forearm
   CC **M90.532** Osteonecrosis in diseases classified elsewhere, left forearm
   CC **M90.539** Osteonecrosis in diseases classified elsewhere, unspecified forearm

+ **M90.54** Osteonecrosis in diseases classified elsewhere, hand
    CC **M90.541** Osteonecrosis in diseases classified elsewhere, right hand
    CC **M90.542** Osteonecrosis in diseases classified elsewhere, left hand
    CC **M90.549** Osteonecrosis in diseases classified elsewhere, unspecified hand
+ **M90.55** Osteonecrosis in diseases classified elsewhere, thigh
    CC **M90.551** Osteonecrosis in diseases classified elsewhere, right thigh
    CC **M90.552** Osteonecrosis in diseases classified elsewhere, left thigh
    CC **M90.559** Osteonecrosis in diseases classified elsewhere, unspecified thigh
+ **M90.56** Osteonecrosis in diseases classified elsewhere, lower leg
    CC **M90.561** Osteonecrosis in diseases classified elsewhere, right lower leg
    CC **M90.562** Osteonecrosis in diseases classified elsewhere, left lower leg
    CC **M90.569** Osteonecrosis in diseases classified elsewhere, unspecified lower leg
+ **M90.57** Osteonecrosis in diseases classified elsewhere, ankle and foot
    CC **M90.571** Osteonecrosis in diseases classified elsewhere, right ankle and foot
    CC **M90.572** Osteonecrosis in diseases classified elsewhere, left ankle and foot
    CC **M90.579** Osteonecrosis in diseases classified elsewhere, unspecified ankle and foot
CC **M90.58** Osteonecrosis in diseases classified elsewhere, other site
CC **M90.59** Osteonecrosis in diseases classified elsewhere, multiple sites
+ **M90.6** Osteitis deformans in neoplastic diseases
    Osteitis deformans in malignant neoplasm of bone
    Code first the neoplasm (C40.-, C41.-)
    Excludes1: osteitis deformans [Paget's disease of bone] (M88.-)
    M90.60 Osteitis deformans in neoplastic diseases, unspecified site
    + **M90.61** Osteitis deformans in neoplastic diseases, shoulder
        M90.611 Osteitis deformans in neoplastic diseases, right shoulder
        M90.612 Osteitis deformans in neoplastic diseases, left shoulder
        M90.619 Osteitis deformans in neoplastic diseases, unspecified shoulder
    + **M90.62** Osteitis deformans in neoplastic diseases, upper arm
        M90.621 Osteitis deformans in neoplastic diseases, right upper arm
        M90.622 Osteitis deformans in neoplastic diseases, left upper arm
        M90.629 Osteitis deformans in neoplastic diseases, unspecified upper arm
    + **M90.63** Osteitis deformans in neoplastic diseases, forearm
        M90.631 Osteitis deformans in neoplastic diseases, right forearm
        M90.632 Osteitis deformans in neoplastic diseases, left forearm
        M90.639 Osteitis deformans in neoplastic diseases, unspecified forearm
    + **M90.64** Osteitis deformans in neoplastic diseases, hand
        M90.641 Osteitis deformans in neoplastic diseases, right hand
        M90.642 Osteitis deformans in neoplastic diseases, left hand
        M90.649 Osteitis deformans in neoplastic diseases, unspecified hand
    + **M90.65** Osteitis deformans in neoplastic diseases, thigh
        M90.651 Osteitis deformans in neoplastic diseases, right thigh
        M90.652 Osteitis deformans in neoplastic diseases, left thigh
        M90.659 Osteitis deformans in neoplastic diseases, unspecified thigh

+ **M90.66** Osteitis deformans in neoplastic diseases, lower leg
    M90.661 Osteitis deformans in neoplastic diseases, right lower leg
    M90.662 Osteitis deformans in neoplastic diseases, left lower leg
    M90.669 Osteitis deformans in neoplastic diseases, unspecified lower leg
+ **M90.67** Osteitis deformans in neoplastic diseases, ankle and foot
    M90.671 Osteitis deformans in neoplastic diseases, right ankle and foot
    M90.672 Osteitis deformans in neoplastic diseases, left ankle and foot
    M90.679 Osteitis deformans in neoplastic diseases, unspecified ankle and foot
M90.68 Osteitis deformans in neoplastic diseases, other site
M90.69 Osteitis deformans in neoplastic diseases, multiple sites
+ **M90.8** Osteopathy in diseases classified elsewhere
    Code first underlying disease, such as:
      rickets (E55.0)
      vitamin-D-resistant rickets (E83.3)
    M90.80 Osteopathy in diseases classified elsewhere, unspecified site
    + **M90.81** Osteopathy in diseases classified elsewhere, shoulder
        M90.811 Osteopathy in diseases classified elsewhere, right shoulder
        M90.812 Osteopathy in diseases classified elsewhere, left shoulder
        M90.819 Osteopathy in diseases classified elsewhere, unspecified shoulder
    + **M90.82** Osteopathy in diseases classified elsewhere, upper arm
        M90.821 Osteopathy in diseases classified elsewhere, right upper arm
        M90.822 Osteopathy in diseases classified elsewhere, left upper arm
        M90.829 Osteopathy in diseases classified elsewhere, unspecified upper arm
    + **M90.83** Osteopathy in diseases classified elsewhere, forearm
        M90.831 Osteopathy in diseases classified elsewhere, right forearm
        M90.832 Osteopathy in diseases classified elsewhere, left forearm
        M90.839 Osteopathy in diseases classified elsewhere, unspecified forearm
    + **M90.84** Osteopathy in diseases classified elsewhere, hand
        M90.841 Osteopathy in diseases classified elsewhere, right hand
        M90.842 Osteopathy in diseases classified elsewhere, left hand
        M90.849 Osteopathy in diseases classified elsewhere, unspecified hand
    + **M90.85** Osteopathy in diseases classified elsewhere, thigh
        M90.851 Osteopathy in diseases classified elsewhere, right thigh
        M90.852 Osteopathy in diseases classified elsewhere, left thigh
        M90.859 Osteopathy in diseases classified elsewhere, unspecified thigh
    + **M90.86** Osteopathy in diseases classified elsewhere, lower leg
        M90.861 Osteopathy in diseases classified elsewhere, right lower leg
        M90.862 Osteopathy in diseases classified elsewhere, left lower leg
        M90.869 Osteopathy in diseases classified elsewhere, unspecified lower leg
    + **M90.87** Osteopathy in diseases classified elsewhere, ankle and foot
        M90.871 Osteopathy in diseases classified elsewhere, right ankle and foot
        M90.872 Osteopathy in diseases classified elsewhere, left ankle and foot
        M90.879 Osteopathy in diseases classified elsewhere, unspecified ankle and foot

+, +7th, X + 7th   ● Newborn   ● Pediatric   ● Maternity   ● Adult   ♀ Female   ♂ Male   Manifestation   Unacceptable PDX   HCC   CC   MCC   HAC

M90.88 **Osteopathy in diseases classified elsewhere, other site**

M90.89 **Osteopathy in diseases classified elsewhere, multiple sites**

Chondropathies (M91-M94)

Excludes1: *postprocedural chondropathies (M96.-)*

M91 **Juvenile osteochondrosis of hip and pelvis**

> *Excludes1:* *slipped upper femoral epiphysis (nontraumatic) (M93.0)*

M91.0 **Juvenile osteochondrosis of pelvis**
Osteochondrosis (juvenile) of acetabulum
Osteochondrosis (juvenile) of iliac crest [Buchanan]
Osteochondrosis (juvenile) of ischiopubic synchondrosis [van Neck]
Osteochondrosis (juvenile) of symphysis pubis [Pierson]

+ M91.1 **Juvenile osteochondrosis of head of femur [Legg-Calvé-Perthes]**
M91.10 **Juvenile osteochondrosis of head of femur [Legg-Calvé-Perthes], unspecified leg**
M91.11 **Juvenile osteochondrosis of head of femur [Legg-Calvé-Perthes], right leg**
M91.12 **Juvenile osteochondrosis of head of femur [Legg-Calvé-Perthes], left leg**

+ M91.2 **Coxa plana**
Hip deformity due to previous juvenile osteochondrosis
M91.20 **Coxa plana, unspecified hip**
M91.21 **Coxa plana, right hip**
M91.22 **Coxa plana, left hip**

+ M91.3 **Pseudocoxalgia**
M91.30 **Pseudocoxalgia, unspecified hip**
M91.31 **Pseudocoxalgia, right hip**
M91.32 **Pseudocoxalgia, left hip**

+ M91.4 **Coxa magna**
M91.40 **Coxa magna, unspecified hip**
M91.41 **Coxa magna, right hip**
M91.42 **Coxa magna, left hip**

+ M91.8 **Other juvenile osteochondrosis of hip and pelvis**
Juvenile osteochondrosis after reduction of congenital dislocation of hip
M91.80 **Other juvenile osteochondrosis of hip and pelvis, unspecified leg**
M91.81 **Other juvenile osteochondrosis of hip and pelvis, right leg**
M91.82 **Other juvenile osteochondrosis of hip and pelvis, left leg**

+ M91.9 **Juvenile osteochondrosis of hip and pelvis, unspecified**
M91.90 **Juvenile osteochondrosis of hip and pelvis, unspecified, unspecified leg**
M91.91 **Juvenile osteochondrosis of hip and pelvis, unspecified, right leg**
M91.92 **Juvenile osteochondrosis of hip and pelvis, unspecified, left leg**

M92 **Other juvenile osteochondrosis**

+ M92.0 **Juvenile osteochondrosis of humerus**
Osteochondrosis (juvenile) of capitulum of humerus [Panner]
Osteochondrosis (juvenile) of head of humerus [Haas]
M92.00 **Juvenile osteochondrosis of humerus, unspecified arm**
M92.01 **Juvenile osteochondrosis of humerus, right arm**
M92.02 **Juvenile osteochondrosis of humerus, left arm**

+ M92.1 **Juvenile osteochondrosis of radius and ulna**
Osteochondrosis (juvenile) of lower ulna [Burns]
Osteochondrosis (juvenile) of radial head [Brailsford]
M92.10 **Juvenile osteochondrosis of radius and ulna, unspecified arm**
M92.11 **Juvenile osteochondrosis of radius and ulna, right arm**
M92.12 **Juvenile osteochondrosis of radius and ulna, left arm**

+ M92.2 **Juvenile osteochondrosis, hand**
+ M92.20 **Unspecified juvenile osteochondrosis, hand**
M92.201 **Unspecified juvenile osteochondrosis, right hand**
M92.202 **Unspecified juvenile osteochondrosis, left hand**
M92.209 **Unspecified juvenile osteochondrosis, unspecified hand**

+ M92.21 **Osteochondrosis (juvenile) of carpal lunate [Kienböck]**
M92.211 **Osteochondrosis (juvenile) of carpal lunate [Kienböck], right hand**
M92.212 **Osteochondrosis (juvenile) of carpal lunate [Kienböck], left hand**
M92.219 **Osteochondrosis (juvenile) of carpal lunate [Kienböck], unspecified hand**

+ M92.22 **Osteochondrosis (juvenile) of metacarpal heads [Mauclaire]**
M92.221 **Osteochondrosis (juvenile) of metacarpal heads [Mauclaire], right hand**
M92.222 **Osteochondrosis (juvenile) of metacarpal heads [Mauclaire], left hand**
M92.229 **Osteochondrosis (juvenile) of metacarpal heads [Mauclaire], unspecified hand**

+ M92.29 **Other juvenile osteochondrosis, hand**
M92.291 **Other juvenile osteochondrosis, right hand**
M92.292 **Other juvenile osteochondrosis, left hand**
M92.299 **Other juvenile osteochondrosis, unspecified hand**

+ M92.3 **Other juvenile osteochondrosis, upper limb**
M92.30 **Other juvenile osteochondrosis, unspecified upper limb**
M92.31 **Other juvenile osteochondrosis, right upper limb**
M92.32 **Other juvenile osteochondrosis, left upper limb**

+ M92.4 **Juvenile osteochondrosis of patella**
Osteochondrosis (juvenile) of primary patellar center [Köhler]
Osteochondrosis (juvenile) of secondary patellar centre [Sinding Larsen]
M92.40 **Juvenile osteochondrosis of patella, unspecified knee**
M92.41 **Juvenile osteochondrosis of patella, right knee**
M92.42 **Juvenile osteochondrosis of patella, left knee**

+ M92.5 **Juvenile osteochondrosis of tibia and fibula tubercle**
+ M92.50 **Unspecified juvenile osteochondrosis of tibia and fibula**
M92.501 **Unspecified juvenile osteochondrosis, right leg**
M92.502 **Unspecified juvenile osteochondrosis, left leg**
M92.503 **Unspecified juvenile osteochondrosis, bilateral leg**
M92.509 **Unspecified juvenile osteochondrosis, unspecified leg**

+ M92.51 **Juvenile osteochondrosis of proximal tibia**
Blount disease
Tibia vara
M92.511 **Juvenile osteochondrosis of proximal tibia, right leg**
M92.512 **Juvenile osteochondrosis of proximal tibia, left leg**
M92.513 **Juvenile osteochondrosis of proximal tibia, bilateral**
M92.519 **Juvenile osteochondrosis of proximal tibia, unspecified leg**

+ M92.52 **Juvenile osteochondrosis of tibia tubercle**
Osgood-Schlatter disease
M92.521 **Juvenile osteochondrosis of tibia tubercle, right leg**
M92.522 **Juvenile osteochondrosis of tibia tubercle, left leg**
M92.523 **Juvenile osteochondrosis of tibia tubercle, bilateral**
M92.529 **Juvenile osteochondrosis of tibia tubercle, unspecified leg**

+ M92.59 **Other juvenile osteochondrosis of tibia and fibula**
M92.591 **Other juvenile osteochondrosis of tibia and fibula, right leg**
M92.592 **Other juvenile osteochondrosis of tibia and fibula, left leg**
M92.593 **Other juvenile osteochondrosis of tibia and fibula, bilateral**
M92.599 **Other juvenile osteochondrosis of tibia and fibula, unspecified leg**

+, +7th, X + 7th   ● Newborn   ● Pediatric   ● Maternity   ● Adult   ♀ Female   ♂ Male   Manifestation   Unacceptable PDX   HCC   CC   MCC   HAC

Knee Injuries and Problems

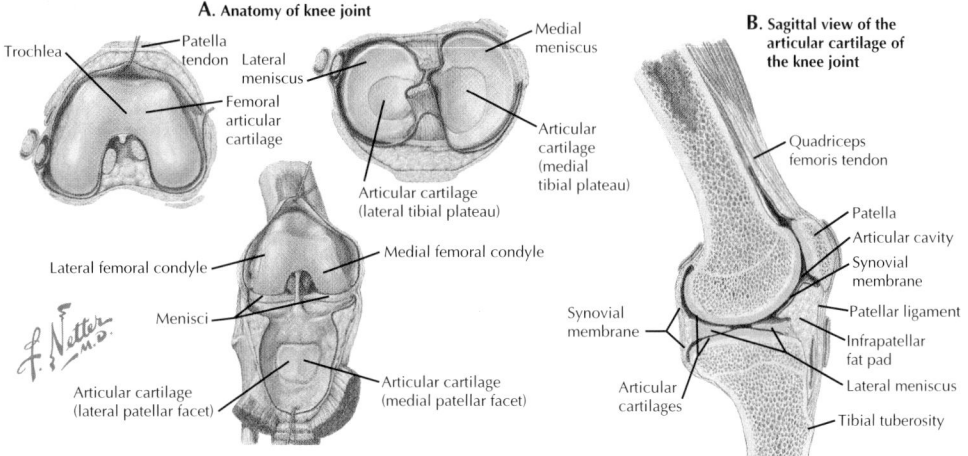

A. Anatomy of knee joint

Trochlea · Patella tendon · Lateral meniscus · Femoral articular cartilage · Medial meniscus · Articular cartilage (medial tibial plateau) · Articular cartilage (lateral tibial plateau) · Lateral femoral condyle · Medial femoral condyle · Menisci · Articular cartilage (lateral patellar facet) · Articular cartilage (medial patellar facet)

B. Sagittal view of the articular cartilage of the knee joint

Quadriceps femoris tendon · Patella · Articular cavity · Synovial membrane · Patellar ligament · Infrapatellar fat pad · Lateral meniscus · Tibial tuberosity · Synovial membrane · Articular cartilages

D. Chondromalacia

Shaving chondroplasty

Appearance immediately after shaving chondroplasty

Appearance after several months

F. Osteochondritis dissecans

Circles indicate arthroscopic view

1. Articular cartilage surface irregular but intact over defect in the subchondral bone.

2. Early separation of osteochondral defect.

3. Fragmentation and separation of osteochondral defect.

G. Radiologic appearance of OCD lesion in skeletally immature patient

Initial lesion · Healing lesion · Healed lesion

H. Treatment of OCD

1. Retrograde drilling of OCD lesion

2. Bleeding bone after drilling

3. Arthroscopic image of OCD fragment fixed in place with osteochondral plug.

I. Osgood-Schlatler disease

Classic appearance of tibial tuberosity

Initial traction at the apophysis

Resolved condition with classic enlargement of tibial tuberosity.

Fragmentation at the apophysis

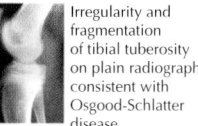

Irregularity and fragmentation of tibial tuberosity on plain radiographs consistent with Osgood-Schlatter disease.

+ **M92.6** **Juvenile osteochondrosis of tarsus**
Osteochondrosis (juvenile) of calcaneum [Sever]
Osteochondrosis (juvenile) of os tibiale externum [Haglund]
Osteochondrosis (juvenile) of talus [Diaz]
Osteochondrosis (juvenile) of tarsal navicular [Köhler]
　　M92.60 **Juvenile osteochondrosis of tarsus, unspecified ankle**
　　M92.61 **Juvenile osteochondrosis of tarsus, right ankle**
　　M92.62 **Juvenile osteochondrosis of tarsus, left ankle**
+ **M92.7** **Juvenile osteochondrosis of metatarsus**
Osteochondrosis (juvenile) of fifth metatarsus [Iselin]
Osteochondrosis (juvenile) of second metatarsus [Freiberg]
　　M92.70 **Juvenile osteochondrosis of metatarsus, unspecified foot**
　　M92.71 **Juvenile osteochondrosis of metatarsus, right foot**
　　M92.72 **Juvenile osteochondrosis of metatarsus, left foot**
M92.8 **Other specified juvenile osteochondrosis**
Calcaneal apophysitis
M92.9 **Juvenile osteochondrosis, unspecified**
Juvenile apophysitis NOS
Juvenile epiphysitis NOS
Juvenile osteochondritis NOS
Juvenile osteochondrosis NOS

M93 **Other osteochondropathies**

> *Excludes2:* osteochondrosis of spine (M42.-)

+ **M93.0** **Slipped upper femoral epiphysis (nontraumatic)**
Use additional code for associated chondrolysis (M94.3)
　+ **M93.00** **Unspecified slipped upper femoral epiphysis (nontraumatic)**
　　M93.001 **Unspecified slipped upper femoral epiphysis (nontraumatic), right hip**
　　M93.002 **Unspecified slipped upper femoral epiphysis (nontraumatic), left hip**
　　M93.003 **Unspecified slipped upper femoral epiphysis (nontraumatic), unspecified hip**
　+ **M93.01** **Acute slipped upper femoral epiphysis (nontraumatic)**
　　M93.011 **Acute slipped upper femoral epiphysis (nontraumatic), right hip**
　　M93.012 **Acute slipped upper femoral epiphysis (nontraumatic), left hip**
　　M93.013 **Acute slipped upper femoral epiphysis (nontraumatic), unspecified hip**
　+ **M93.02** **Chronic slipped upper femoral epiphysis (nontraumatic)**
　　M93.021 **Chronic slipped upper femoral epiphysis (nontraumatic), right hip**
　　M93.022 **Chronic slipped upper femoral epiphysis (nontraumatic), left hip**
　　M93.023 **Chronic slipped upper femoral epiphysis (nontraumatic), unspecified hip**
　+ **M93.03** **Acute on chronic slipped upper femoral epiphysis (nontraumatic)**
　　M93.031 **Acute on chronic slipped upper femoral epiphysis (nontraumatic), right hip**
　　M93.032 **Acute on chronic slipped upper femoral epiphysis (nontraumatic), left hip**
　　M93.033 **Acute on chronic slipped upper femoral epiphysis (nontraumatic), unspecified hip**
● **M93.1** **Kienböck's disease of adults**
Adult osteochondrosis of carpal lunates
+ **M93.2** **Osteochondritis dissecans**
M93.20 **Osteochondritis dissecans of unspecified site**
　+ **M93.21** **Osteochondritis dissecans of shoulder**
　　M93.211 **Osteochondritis dissecans, right shoulder**
　　M93.212 **Osteochondritis dissecans, left shoulder**
　　M93.219 **Osteochondritis dissecans, unspecified shoulder**
　+ **M93.22** **Osteochondritis dissecans of elbow**
　　M93.221 **Osteochondritis dissecans, right elbow**
　　M93.222 **Osteochondritis dissecans, left elbow**
　　M93.229 **Osteochondritis dissecans, unspecified elbow**
　+ **M93.23** **Osteochondritis dissecans of wrist**
　　M93.231 **Osteochondritis dissecans, right wrist**
　　M93.232 **Osteochondritis dissecans, left wrist**
　　M93.239 **Osteochondritis dissecans, unspecified wrist**

+ **M93.24** **Osteochondritis dissecans of joints of hand**
　　M93.241 **Osteochondritis dissecans, joints of right hand**
　　M93.242 **Osteochondritis dissecans, joints of left hand**
　　M93.249 **Osteochondritis dissecans, joints of unspecified hand**
+ **M93.25** **Osteochondritis dissecans of hip**
　　M93.251 **Osteochondritis dissecans, right hip**
　　M93.252 **Osteochondritis dissecans, left hip**
　　M93.259 **Osteochondritis dissecans, unspecified hip**
+ **M93.26** **Osteochondritis dissecans knee**
　　M93.261 **Osteochondritis dissecans, right knee**
　　M93.262 **Osteochondritis dissecans, left knee**
　　M93.269 **Osteochondritis dissecans, unspecified knee**
+ **M93.27** **Osteochondritis dissecans of ankle and joints of foot**
　　M93.271 **Osteochondritis dissecans, right ankle and joints of right foot**
　　M93.272 **Osteochondritis dissecans, left ankle and joints of left foot**
　　M93.279 **Osteochondritis dissecans, unspecified ankle and joints of foot**
M93.28 **Osteochondritis dissecans other site**
M93.29 **Osteochondritis dissecans multiple sites**
+ **M93.8** **Other specified osteochondropathies**
M93.80 **Other specified osteochondropathies of unspecified site**
　+ **M93.81** **Other specified osteochondropathies of shoulder**
　　M93.811 **Other specified osteochondropathies, right shoulder**
　　M93.812 **Other specified osteochondropathies, left shoulder**
　　M93.819 **Other specified osteochondropathies, unspecified shoulder**
　+ **M93.82** **Other specified osteochondropathies of upper arm**
　　M93.821 **Other specified osteochondropathies, right upper arm**
　　M93.822 **Other specified osteochondropathies, left upper arm**
　　M93.829 **Other specified osteochondropathies, unspecified upper arm**
　+ **M93.83** **Other specified osteochondropathies of forearm**
　　M93.831 **Other specified osteochondropathies, right forearm**
　　M93.832 **Other specified osteochondropathies, left forearm**
　　M93.839 **Other specified osteochondropathies, unspecified forearm**
　+ **M93.84** **Other specified osteochondropathies of hand**
　　M93.841 **Other specified osteochondropathies, right hand**
　　M93.842 **Other specified osteochondropathies, left hand**
　　M93.849 **Other specified osteochondropathies, unspecified hand**
　+ **M93.85** **Other specified osteochondropathies of thigh**
　　M93.851 **Other specified osteochondropathies, right thigh**
　　M93.852 **Other specified osteochondropathies, left thigh**
　　M93.859 **Other specified osteochondropathies, unspecified thigh**
　+ **M93.86** **Other specified osteochondropathies lower leg**
　　M93.861 **Other specified osteochondropathies, right lower leg**
　　M93.862 **Other specified osteochondropathies, left lower leg**
　　M93.869 **Other specified osteochondropathies, unspecified lower leg**
　+ **M93.87** **Other specified osteochondropathies of ankle and foot**
　　M93.871 **Other specified osteochondropathies, right ankle and foot**
　　M93.872 **Other specified osteochondropathies, left ankle and foot**
　　M93.879 **Other specified osteochondropathies, unspecified ankle and foot**
M93.88 **Other specified osteochondropathies other**

+, +7th, X + 7th　● Newborn　● Pediatric　● Maternity　● Adult　♀ Female　♂ Male　Manifestation　Unacceptable PDX　HCC　CC　MCC　HAC

M93.89 Other specified osteochondropathies multiple sites
+ **M93.9** Osteochondropathy, unspecified
Apophysitis NOS
Epiphysitis NOS
Osteochondritis NOS
Osteochondrosis NOS
M93.90 Osteochondropathy, unspecified of unspecified site
+ **M93.91** Osteochondropathy, unspecified of shoulder
M93.911 Osteochondropathy, unspecified, right shoulder
M93.912 Osteochondropathy, unspecified, left shoulder
M93.919 Osteochondropathy, unspecified, unspecified shoulder
+ **M93.92** Osteochondropathy, unspecified of upper arm
M93.921 Osteochondropathy, unspecified, right upper arm
M93.922 Osteochondropathy, unspecified, left upper arm
M93.929 Osteochondropathy, unspecified, unspecified upper arm
+ **M93.93** Osteochondropathy, unspecified of forearm
M93.931 Osteochondropathy, unspecified, right forearm
M93.932 Osteochondropathy, unspecified, left forearm
M93.939 Osteochondropathy, unspecified, unspecified forearm
+ **M93.94** Osteochondropathy, unspecified of hand
M93.941 Osteochondropathy, unspecified, right hand
M93.942 Osteochondropathy, unspecified, left hand
M93.949 Osteochondropathy, unspecified, unspecified hand
+ **M93.95** Osteochondropathy, unspecified of thigh
M93.951 Osteochondropathy, unspecified, right thigh
M93.952 Osteochondropathy, unspecified, left thigh
M93.959 Osteochondropathy, unspecified, unspecified thigh
+ **M93.96** Osteochondropathy, unspecified lower leg
M93.961 Osteochondropathy, unspecified, right lower leg
M93.962 Osteochondropathy, unspecified, left lower leg
M93.969 Osteochondropathy, unspecified, unspecified lower leg
+ **M93.97** Osteochondropathy, unspecified of ankle and foot
M93.971 Osteochondropathy, unspecified, right ankle and foot
M93.972 Osteochondropathy, unspecified, left ankle and foot
M93.979 Osteochondropathy, unspecified, unspecified ankle and foot
M93.98 Osteochondropathy, unspecified other
M93.99 Osteochondropathy, unspecified multiple sites

M94 Other disorders of cartilage

M94.0 Chondrocostal junction syndrome [Tietze]
Costochondritis
M94.1 Relapsing polychondritis
+ **M94.2** Chondromalacia
Excludes1: chondromalacia patellae (M22.4)
M94.20 Chondromalacia, unspecified site
+ **M94.21** Chondromalacia, shoulder
M94.211 Chondromalacia, right shoulder
M94.212 Chondromalacia, left shoulder
M94.219 Chondromalacia, unspecified shoulder
+ **M94.22** Chondromalacia, elbow
M94.221 Chondromalacia, right elbow
M94.222 Chondromalacia, left elbow
M94.229 Chondromalacia, unspecified elbow
+ **M94.23** Chondromalacia, wrist
M94.231 Chondromalacia, right wrist
M94.232 Chondromalacia, left wrist
M94.239 Chondromalacia, unspecified wrist

+ **M94.24** Chondromalacia, joints of hand
M94.241 Chondromalacia, joints of right hand
M94.242 Chondromalacia, joints of left hand
M94.249 Chondromalacia, joints of unspecified hand
+ **M94.25** Chondromalacia, hip
M94.251 Chondromalacia, right hip
M94.252 Chondromalacia, left hip
M94.259 Chondromalacia, unspecified hip
+ **M94.26** Chondromalacia, knee
M94.261 Chondromalacia, right knee
M94.262 Chondromalacia, left knee
M94.269 Chondromalacia, unspecified knee
+ **M94.27** Chondromalacia, ankle and joints of foot
M94.271 Chondromalacia, right ankle and joints of right foot
M94.272 Chondromalacia, left ankle and joints of left foot
M94.279 Chondromalacia, unspecified ankle and joints of foot
M94.28 Chondromalacia, other site
M94.29 Chondromalacia, multiple sites
+ **M94.3** Chondrolysis
Code first any associated slipped upper femoral epiphysis (nontraumatic) (M93.0-)
+ **M94.35** Chondrolysis, hip
M94.351 Chondrolysis, right hip
M94.352 Chondrolysis, left hip
M94.359 Chondrolysis, unspecified hip
+ **M94.8** Other specified disorders of cartilage
+ **M94.8X** Other specified disorders of cartilage
M94.8X0 Other specified disorders of cartilage, multiple sites
M94.8X1 Other specified disorders of cartilage, shoulder
M94.8X2 Other specified disorders of cartilage, upper arm
M94.8X3 Other specified disorders of cartilage, forearm
M94.8X4 Other specified disorders of cartilage, hand
M94.8X5 Other specified disorders of cartilage, thigh
M94.8X6 Other specified disorders of cartilage, lower leg
M94.8X7 Other specified disorders of cartilage, ankle and foot
M94.8X8 Other specified disorders of cartilage, other site
M94.8X9 Other specified disorders of cartilage, unspecified sites
M94.9 Disorder of cartilage, unspecified

Other disorders of the musculoskeletal system and connective tissue (M95)

M95 Other acquired deformities of musculoskeletal system and connective tissue
Excludes2: acquired absence of limbs and organs (Z89-Z90)
acquired deformities of limbs (M20-M21)
congenital malformations and deformations of the musculoskeletal system (Q65-Q79)
deforming dorsopathies (M40-M43)
dentofacial anomalies [including malocclusion] (M26.-)
postprocedural musculoskeletal disorders (M96.-)
M95.0 Acquired deformity of nose
Excludes2: deviated nasal septum (J34.2)
+ **M95.1** Cauliflower ear
Excludes2: other acquired deformities of ear (H61.1)
M95.10 Cauliflower ear, unspecified ear
M95.11 Cauliflower ear, right ear
M95.12 Cauliflower ear, left ear
M95.2 Other acquired deformity of head
M95.3 Acquired deformity of neck
M95.4 Acquired deformity of chest and rib
AHA CC: 4Q, 2014, 26-27
M95.5 Acquired deformity of pelvis
Excludes1: maternal care for known or suspected disproportion (O33.-)

+, +7th, X + 7th ● Newborn ● Pediatric ● Maternity ● Adult ♀ Female ♂ Male Manifestation Unacceptable PDX HCC CC MCC HAC

M95.8 Other specified acquired deformities of musculoskeletal system

M95.9 Acquired deformity of musculoskeletal system, unspecified

Intraoperative and postprocedural complications and disorders of musculoskeletal system, not elsewhere classified (M96)

M96 Intraoperative and postprocedural complications and disorders of musculoskeletal system, not elsewhere classified

>> *Excludes2:* *arthropathy following intestinal bypass (M02.0-)*
>> *complications of internal orthopedic prosthetic devices, implants and grafts (T84.-)*
>> *disorders associated with osteoporosis (M80)*
>> *periprosthetic fracture around internal prosthetic joint (M97.-)*
>> *presence of functional implants and other devices (Z96-Z97)*

CC M96.0 Pseudarthrosis after fusion or arthrodesis

M96.1 Postlaminectomy syndrome, not elsewhere classified

M96.2 Postradiation kyphosis

M96.3 Postlaminectomy kyphosis

M96.4 Postsurgical lordosis

M96.5 Postradiation scoliosis

+ M96.6 Fracture of bone following insertion of orthopedic implant, joint prosthesis, or bone plate

> Intraoperative fracture of bone during insertion of orthopedic implant, joint prosthesis, or bone plate

>> *Excludes2:* *complication of internal orthopedic devices, implants or grafts (T84.-)*

  + M96.62 Fracture of humerus following insertion of orthopedic implant, joint prosthesis, or bone plate

    CC M96.621 Fracture of humerus following insertion of orthopedic implant, joint prosthesis, or bone plate, right arm

    CC M96.622 Fracture of humerus following insertion of orthopedic implant, joint prosthesis, or bone plate, left arm

    CC M96.629 Fracture of humerus following insertion of orthopedic implant, joint prosthesis, or bone plate, unspecified arm

  + M96.63 Fracture of radius or ulna following insertion of orthopedic implant, joint prosthesis, or bone plate

    CC M96.631 Fracture of radius or ulna following insertion of orthopedic implant, joint prosthesis, or bone plate, right arm

    CC M96.632 Fracture of radius or ulna following insertion of orthopedic implant, joint prosthesis, or bone plate, left arm

    CC M96.639 Fracture of radius or ulna following insertion of orthopedic implant, joint prosthesis, or bone plate, unspecified arm

  CC M96.65 Fracture of pelvis following insertion of orthopedic implant, joint prosthesis, or bone plate

  + M96.66 Fracture of femur following insertion of orthopedic implant, joint prosthesis, or bone plate

    CC M96.661 Fracture of femur following insertion of orthopedic implant, joint prosthesis, or bone plate, right leg

    CC M96.662 Fracture of femur following insertion of orthopedic implant, joint prosthesis, or bone plate, left leg

    CC M96.669 Fracture of femur following insertion of orthopedic implant, joint prosthesis, or bone plate, unspecified leg

  + M96.67 Fracture of tibia or fibula following insertion of orthopedic implant, joint prosthesis, or bone plate

    CC M96.671 Fracture of tibia or fibula following insertion of orthopedic implant, joint prosthesis, or bone plate, right leg

    CC M96.672 Fracture of tibia or fibula following insertion of orthopedic implant, joint prosthesis, or bone plate, left leg

    CC M96.679 Fracture of tibia or fibula following insertion of orthopedic implant, joint prosthesis, or bone plate, unspecified leg

  CC M96.69 Fracture of other bone following insertion of orthopedic implant, joint prosthesis, or bone plate

+ M96.8 Other intraoperative and postprocedural complications and disorders of musculoskeletal system, not elsewhere classified

> *AHA CC: 4Q, 2016, 9-10*

  + M96.81 Intraoperative hemorrhage and hematoma of a musculoskeletal structure complicating a procedure

>> *Excludes1:* *intraoperative hemorrhage and hematoma of a musculoskeletal structure due to accidental puncture and laceration during a procedure (M96.82)*

    CC M96.810 Intraoperative hemorrhage and hematoma of a musculoskeletal structure complicating a musculoskeletal system procedure

    CC M96.811 Intraoperative hemorrhage and hematoma of a musculoskeletal structure complicating other procedure

  + M96.82 Accidental puncture and laceration of a musculoskeletal structure during a procedure

    CC M96.820 Accidental puncture and laceration of a musculoskeletal structure during a musculoskeletal system procedure

    CC M96.821 Accidental puncture and laceration of a musculoskeletal structure during other procedure

  + M96.83 Postprocedural hemorrhage of a musculoskeletal structure following a procedure

    CC M96.830 Postprocedural hemorrhage of a musculoskeletal structure following a musculoskeletal system procedure

    CC M96.831 Postprocedural hemorrhage of a musculoskeletal structure following other procedure

  + M96.84 Postprocedural hematoma and seroma of a musculoskeletal structure following a procedure

    CC M96.840 Postprocedural hematoma of a musculoskeletal structure following a musculoskeletal system procedure

    CC M96.841 Postprocedural hematoma of a musculoskeletal structure following other procedure

> *AHA CC: 4Q, 2016, 9-10*

    CC M96.842 Postprocedural seroma of a musculoskeletal structure following a musculoskeletal system procedure

    CC M96.843 Postprocedural seroma of a musculoskeletal structure following other procedure

> *AHA CC: 3Q, 2018, 6*

+ CC M96.89 Other intraoperative and postprocedural complications and disorders of the musculoskeletal system

> Instability of joint secondary to removal of joint prosthesis

> Use additional code, if applicable, to further specify disorder

Periprosthetic fracture around internal prosthetic joint (M97)

M97 Periprosthetic fracture around internal prosthetic joint

>> *Excludes2:* *fracture of bone following insertion of orthopedic implant, joint prosthesis or bone plate (M96.6-)*
>> *breakage (fracture) of prosthetic joint (T84.01-)*
> *AHA CC: 4Q, 2016, 42-43*

> The appropriate 7th character is to be added to each code from category M97:
> A initial encounter
> D subsequent encounter
> S sequela

+ M97.0 Periprosthetic fracture around internal prosthetic hip joint

CC X+7th M97.01 Periprosthetic fracture around internal prosthetic right hip joint

> *AHA CC: 4Q, 2016, 42-43*

CC X+7th M97.02 Periprosthetic fracture around internal prosthetic left hip joint

+ M97.1 Periprosthetic fracture around internal prosthetic knee joint

+, +7th, X + 7th ● Newborn ● Pediatric ● Maternity ● Adult ♀ Female ♂ Male Manifestation Unacceptable PDX HCC CC MCC HAC

CC X+7th **M97.11 Periprosthetic fracture around internal prosthetic right knee joint**

CC X+7th **M97.12 Periprosthetic fracture around internal prosthetic left knee joint**

+ **M97.2 Periprosthetic fracture around internal prosthetic ankle joint**

CC X+7th **M97.21 Periprosthetic fracture around internal prosthetic right ankle joint**

CC X+7th **M97.22 Periprosthetic fracture around internal prosthetic left ankle joint**

+ **M97.3 Periprosthetic fracture around internal prosthetic shoulder joint**

CC X+7th **M97.31 Periprosthetic fracture around internal prosthetic right shoulder joint**

CC X+7th **M97.32 Periprosthetic fracture around internal prosthetic left shoulder joint**

+ **M97.4 Periprosthetic fracture around internal prosthetic elbow joint**

CC X+7th **M97.41 Periprosthetic fracture around internal prosthetic right elbow joint**

CC X+7th **M97.42 Periprosthetic fracture around internal prosthetic left elbow joint**

CC X+7th **M97.8 Periprosthetic fracture around other internal prosthetic joint**

Periprosthetic fracture around internal prosthetic finger joint
Periprosthetic fracture around internal prosthetic spinal joint
Periprosthetic fracture around internal prosthetic toe joint
Periprosthetic fracture around internal prosthetic wrist joint
Use additional code to identify the joint (Z96.6-)

CC X+7th **M97.9 Periprosthetic fracture around unspecified internal prosthetic joint**

Biomechanical lesions, not elsewhere classified (M99)

M99 Biomechanical lesions, not elsewhere classified

NOTE This category should not be used if the condition can be classified elsewhere.

+ **M99.0 Segmental and somatic dysfunction**
M99.00 Segmental and somatic dysfunction of head region
M99.01 Segmental and somatic dysfunction of cervical region
M99.02 Segmental and somatic dysfunction of thoracic region
M99.03 Segmental and somatic dysfunction of lumbar region
M99.04 Segmental and somatic dysfunction of sacral region
M99.05 Segmental and somatic dysfunction of pelvic region
M99.06 Segmental and somatic dysfunction of lower extremity
M99.07 Segmental and somatic dysfunction of upper extremity
M99.08 Segmental and somatic dysfunction of rib cage
M99.09 Segmental and somatic dysfunction of abdomen and other regions

+ **M99.1 Subluxation complex (vertebral)**
CC **M99.10 Subluxation complex (vertebral) of head region**
HAC see Appendix B for HAC conditional logic
CC **M99.11 Subluxation complex (vertebral) of cervical region**
HAC see Appendix B for HAC conditional logic
M99.12 Subluxation complex (vertebral) of thoracic region
M99.13 Subluxation complex (vertebral) of lumbar region
M99.14 Subluxation complex (vertebral) of sacral region
M99.15 Subluxation complex (vertebral) of pelvic region
M99.16 Subluxation complex (vertebral) of lower extremity
M99.17 Subluxation complex (vertebral) of upper extremity
CC **M99.18 Subluxation complex (vertebral) of rib cage**
HAC see Appendix B for HAC conditional logic
M99.19 Subluxation complex (vertebral) of abdomen and other regions

+ **M99.2 Subluxation stenosis of neural canal**
M99.20 Subluxation stenosis of neural canal of head region
M99.21 Subluxation stenosis of neural canal of cervical region
M99.22 Subluxation stenosis of neural canal of thoracic region
M99.23 Subluxation stenosis of neural canal of lumbar region
M99.24 Subluxation stenosis of neural canal of sacral region
M99.25 Subluxation stenosis of neural canal of pelvic region
M99.26 Subluxation stenosis of neural canal of lower extremity
M99.27 Subluxation stenosis of neural canal of upper extremity
M99.28 Subluxation stenosis of neural canal of rib cage
M99.29 Subluxation stenosis of neural canal of abdomen and other regions

+ **M99.3 Osseous stenosis of neural canal**
M99.30 Osseous stenosis of neural canal of head region
M99.31 Osseous stenosis of neural canal of cervical region
M99.32 Osseous stenosis of neural canal of thoracic region
M99.33 Osseous stenosis of neural canal of lumbar region
M99.34 Osseous stenosis of neural canal of sacral region
M99.35 Osseous stenosis of neural canal of pelvic region
M99.36 Osseous stenosis of neural canal of lower extremity
M99.37 Osseous stenosis of neural canal of upper extremity
M99.38 Osseous stenosis of neural canal of rib cage
M99.39 Osseous stenosis of neural canal of abdomen and other regions

+ **M99.4 Connective tissue stenosis of neural canal**
M99.40 Connective tissue stenosis of neural canal of head region
M99.41 Connective tissue stenosis of neural canal of cervical region
M99.42 Connective tissue stenosis of neural canal of thoracic region
M99.43 Connective tissue stenosis of neural canal of lumbar region
M99.44 Connective tissue stenosis of neural canal of sacral region
M99.45 Connective tissue stenosis of neural canal of pelvic region
M99.46 Connective tissue stenosis of neural canal of lower extremity
M99.47 Connective tissue stenosis of neural canal of upper extremity
M99.48 Connective tissue stenosis of neural canal of rib cage
M99.49 Connective tissue stenosis of neural canal of abdomen and other regions

+ **M99.5 Intervertebral disc stenosis of neural canal**
M99.50 Intervertebral disc stenosis of neural canal of head region
M99.51 Intervertebral disc stenosis of neural canal of cervical region
M99.52 Intervertebral disc stenosis of neural canal of thoracic region
M99.53 Intervertebral disc stenosis of neural canal of lumbar region
M99.54 Intervertebral disc stenosis of neural canal of sacral region
M99.55 Intervertebral disc stenosis of neural canal of pelvic region
M99.56 Intervertebral disc stenosis of neural canal of lower extremity
M99.57 Intervertebral disc stenosis of neural canal of upper extremity
M99.58 Intervertebral disc stenosis of neural canal of rib cage
M99.59 Intervertebral disc stenosis of neural canal of abdomen and other regions

+ **M99.6 Osseous and subluxation stenosis of intervertebral foramina**
M99.60 Osseous and subluxation stenosis of intervertebral foramina of head region
M99.61 Osseous and subluxation stenosis of intervertebral foramina of cervical region
M99.62 Osseous and subluxation stenosis of intervertebral foramina of thoracic region
M99.63 Osseous and subluxation stenosis of intervertebral foramina of lumbar region

M99.64 **Osseous and subluxation stenosis of intervertebral foramina of sacral region**

M99.65 **Osseous and subluxation stenosis of intervertebral foramina of pelvic region**

M99.66 **Osseous and subluxation stenosis of intervertebral foramina of lower extremity**

M99.67 **Osseous and subluxation stenosis of intervertebral foramina of upper extremity**

M99.68 **Osseous and subluxation stenosis of intervertebral foramina of rib cage**

M99.69 **Osseous and subluxation stenosis of intervertebral foramina of abdomen and other regions**

+ M99.7 **Connective tissue and disc stenosis of intervertebral foramina**

M99.70 **Connective tissue and disc stenosis of intervertebral foramina of head region**

M99.71 **Connective tissue and disc stenosis of intervertebral foramina of cervical region**

M99.72 **Connective tissue and disc stenosis of intervertebral foramina of thoracic region**

M99.73 **Connective tissue and disc stenosis of intervertebral foramina of lumbar region**

M99.74 **Connective tissue and disc stenosis of intervertebral foramina of sacral region**

M99.75 **Connective tissue and disc stenosis of intervertebral foramina of pelvic region**

M99.76 **Connective tissue and disc stenosis of intervertebral foramina of lower extremity**

M99.77 **Connective tissue and disc stenosis of intervertebral foramina of upper extremity**

M99.78 **Connective tissue and disc stenosis of intervertebral foramina of rib cage**

M99.79 **Connective tissue and disc stenosis of intervertebral foramina of abdomen and other regions**

+ M99.8 **Other biomechanical lesions**

M99.80 **Other biomechanical lesions of head region**

M99.81 **Other biomechanical lesions of cervical region**

M99.82 **Other biomechanical lesions of thoracic region**

M99.83 **Other biomechanical lesions of lumbar region**

M99.84 **Other biomechanical lesions of sacral region**

M99.85 **Other biomechanical lesions of pelvic region**

M99.86 **Other biomechanical lesions of lower extremity**

M99.87 **Other biomechanical lesions of upper extremity**

M99.88 **Other biomechanical lesions of rib cage**

M99.89 **Other biomechanical lesions of abdomen and other regions**

M99.9 **Biomechanical lesion, unspecified**

Chapter 14: Diseases of the Genitourinary System (N00-N99)

Excludes2: *certain conditions originating in the perinatal period (P04-P96)*
certain infectious and parasitic diseases (A00-B99)
complications of pregnancy, childbirth and the puerperium (O00-O9A)
congenital malformations, deformations and chromosomal abnormalities (Q00-Q99)
endocrine, nutritional and metabolic diseases (E00-E88)
injury, poisoning and certain other consequences of external causes (S00-T88)
neoplasms (C00-D49)
symptoms, signs and abnormal clinical and laboratory findings, not elsewhere classified (R00-R94)

This chapter contains the following category blocks:
N00-N08 Glomerular diseases
N10-N16 Renal tubulo-interstitial diseases
N17-N19 Acute kidney failure and chronic kidney disease
N20-N23 Urolithiasis
N25-N29 Other disorders of kidney and ureter
N30-N39 Other diseases of the urinary system
N40-N53 Diseases of male genital organs
N60-N65 Disorders of breast
N70-N77 Inflammatory diseases of female pelvic organs
N80-N98 Noninflammatory disorders of female genital tract
N99 Intraoperative and postprocedural complications and disorders of genitourinary system, not elsewhere classified

C. Chapter-Specific Coding Guidelines

In addition to general coding guidelines, there are guidelines for specific diagnoses and/or conditions in the classification. Unless otherwise indicated, these guidelines apply to all health care settings. Please refer to Section II for guidelines on the selection of principal diagnosis.

14. Chapter 14: Diseases of the Genitourinary System (N00-N99)

a. Chronic kidney disease

1) Stages of chronic kidney disease (CKD)

The ICD-10-CM classifies CKD based on severity. The severity of CKD is designated by stages 1-5. Stage 2, code N18.2, equates to mild CKD; stage 3, code N18.3, equates to moderate CKD; and stage 4, code N18.4, equates to severe CKD. Code N18.6, End stage renal disease (ESRD), is assigned when the provider has documented end-stage-renal disease (ESRD).

If both a stage of CKD and ESRD are documented, assign code N18.6 only.

2) Chronic kidney disease and kidney transplant status

Patients who have undergone kidney transplant may still have some form of chronic kidney disease (CKD) because the kidney transplant may not fully restore kidney function. Therefore, the presence of CKD alone does not constitute a transplant complication. Assign the appropriate N18 code for the patient's stage of CKD and code Z94.0, Kidney transplant status. If a transplant complication such as failure or rejection or other transplant complication is documented, see section I.C.19.g for information on coding complications of a kidney transplant. If the documentation is unclear as to whether the patient has a complication of the transplant, query the provider.

3) Chronic kidney disease with other conditions

Patients with CKD may also suffer from other serious conditions, most commonly diabetes mellitus and hypertension. The sequencing of the CKD code in relationship to codes for other contributing conditions is based on the conventions in the Tabular List.

See I.C.9. Hypertensive chronic kidney disease.

See I.C.19. Chronic kidney disease and kidney transplant complications.

Urinary System

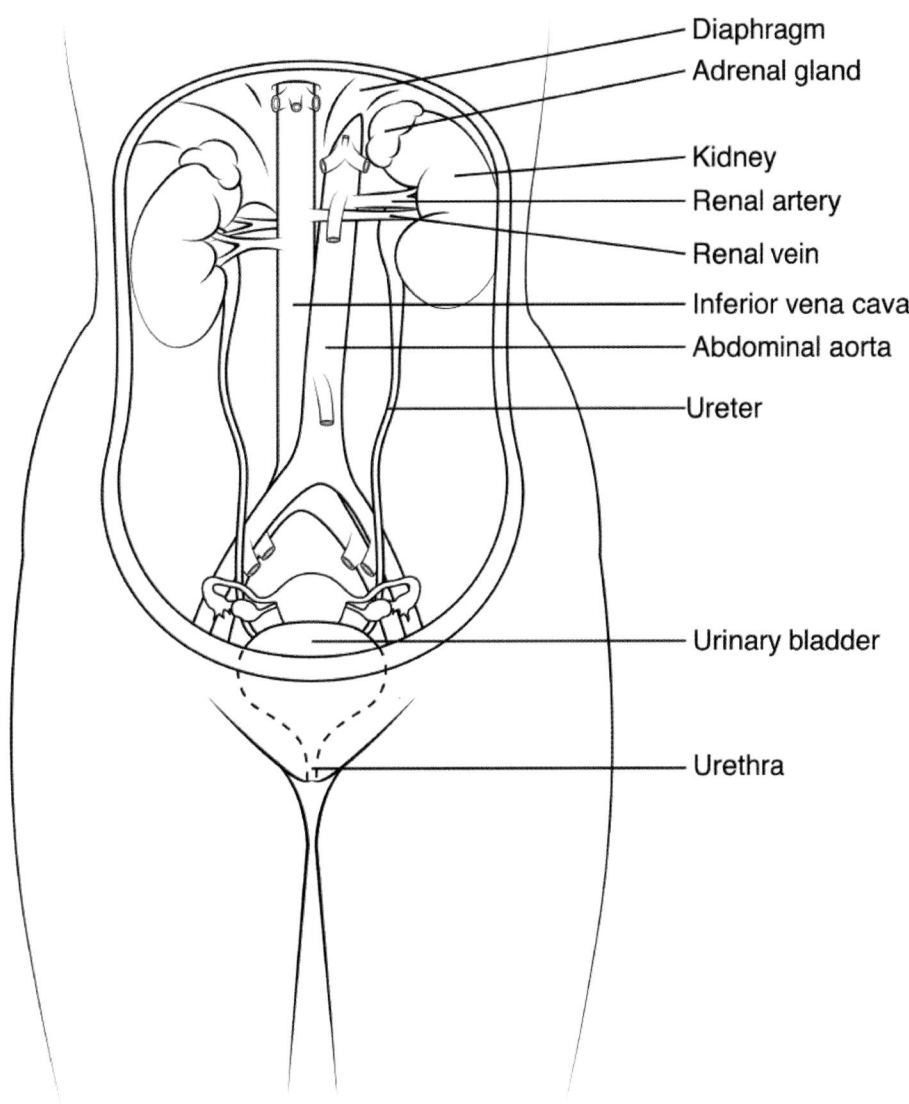

- Diaphragm
- Adrenal gland
- Kidney
- Renal artery
- Renal vein
- Inferior vena cava
- Abdominal aorta
- Ureter
- Urinary bladder
- Urethra

©AHIMA

+, +7th, X + 7th   ● Newborn   ● Pediatric   ● Maternity   ● Adult   ♀ Female   ♂ Male   Manifestation   Unacceptable PDX   HCC   CC   MCC   HAC

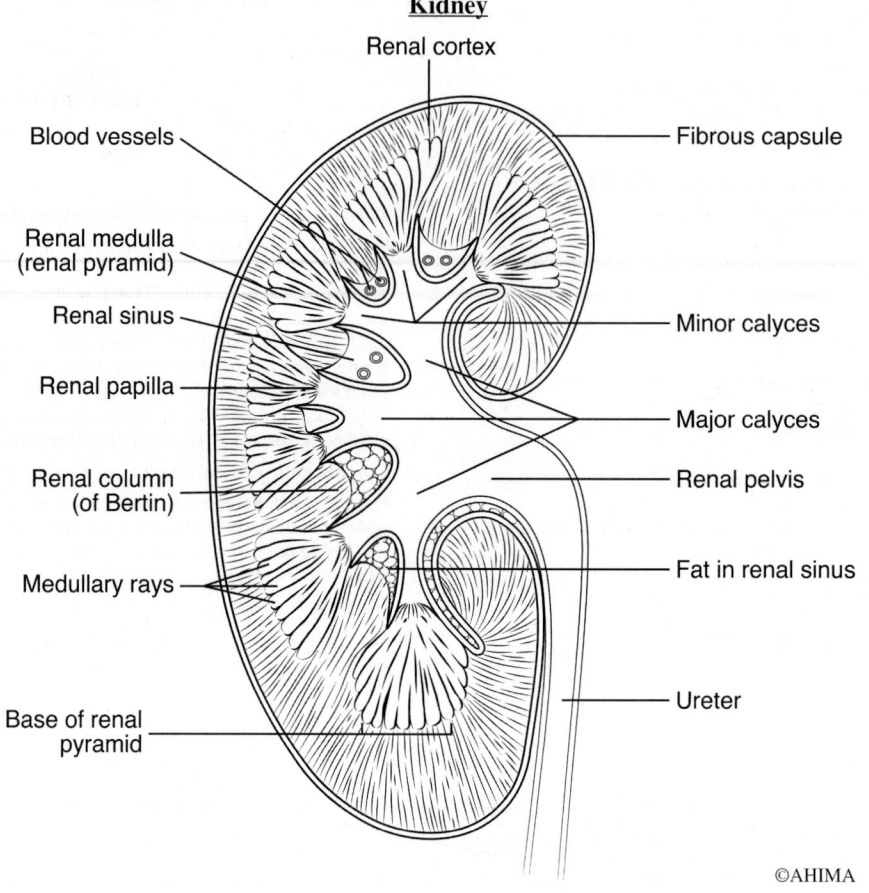

Kidney

Renal cortex

Blood vessels

Fibrous capsule

Renal medulla
(renal pyramid)

Renal sinus

Minor calyces

Renal papilla

Major calyces

Renal column
(of Bertin)

Renal pelvis

Fat in renal sinus

Medullary rays

Base of renal
pyramid

Ureter

©AHIMA

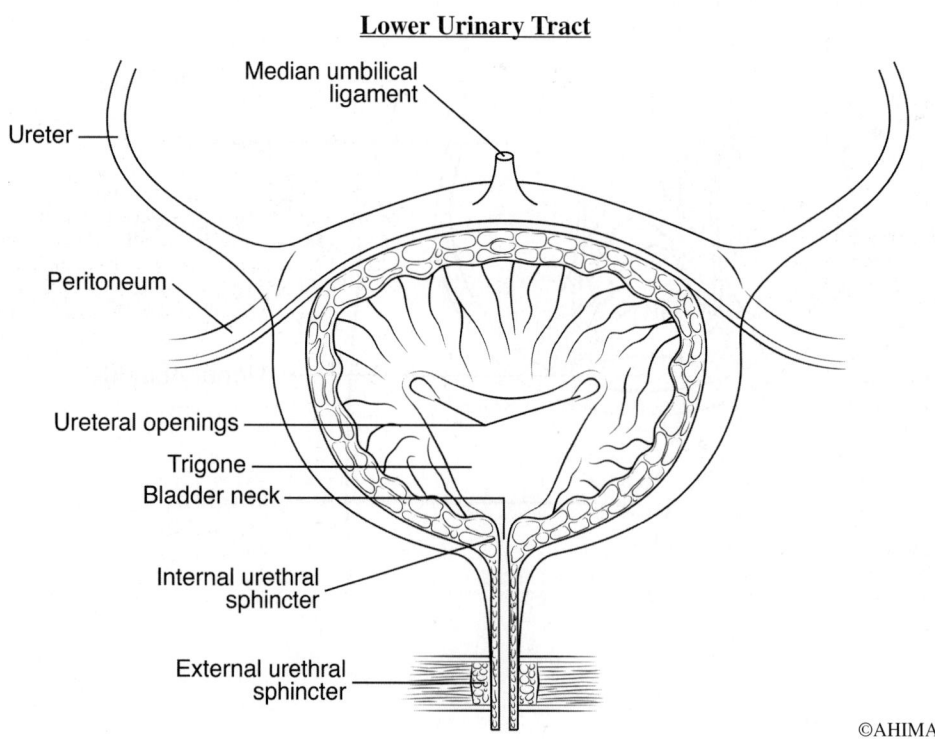

Lower Urinary Tract

Median umbilical
ligament

Ureter

Peritoneum

Ureteral openings

Trigone

Bladder neck

Internal urethral
sphincter

External urethral
sphincter

©AHIMA

Glomerular diseases (N00-N08)

Code also any associated kidney failure (N17-N19)

Excludes1: *hypertensive chronic kidney disease (I12.-)*

N00 Acute nephritic syndrome

Includes: acute glomerular disease
acute glomerulonephritis
acute nephritis

Excludes1: *acute tubulo-interstitial nephritis (N10)*
nephritic syndrome NOS (N05.-)

MCC **N00.0 Acute nephritic syndrome with minor glomerular abnormality**

Acute nephritic syndrome with minimal change lesion

MCC **N00.1 Acute nephritic syndrome with focal and segmental glomerular lesions**

Acute nephritic syndrome with focal and segmental hyalinosis
Acute nephritic syndrome with focal and segmental sclerosis
Acute nephritic syndrome with focal glomerulonephritis

MCC **N00.2 Acute nephritic syndrome with diffuse membranous glomerulonephritis**

MCC **N00.3 Acute nephritic syndrome with diffuse mesangial proliferative glomerulonephritis**

MCC **N00.4 Acute nephritic syndrome with diffuse endocapillary proliferative glomerulonephritis**

MCC **N00.5 Acute nephritic syndrome with diffuse mesangiocapillary glomerulonephritis**

Acute nephritic syndrome with membranoproliferative glomerulonephritis, types 1 and 3, or NOS

Excludes1: *Acute nephritic syndrome with C3 glomerulonephritis (N00.A)*
Acute nephritic syndrome with C3 glomerulopathy (N00.A)

MCC **N00.6 Acute nephritic syndrome with dense deposit disease**

Acute nephritic syndrome with membranoproliferative glomerulonephritis, type 2
Acute nephritic syndrome with C3 glomerulopathy with dense deposit disease

MCC **N00.7 Acute nephritic syndrome with diffuse crescentic glomerulonephritis**

Acute nephritic syndrome with extracapillary glomerulonephritis

MCC **N00.8 Acute nephritic syndrome with other morphologic changes**

Acute nephritic syndrome with proliferative glomerulonephritis NOS

MCC **N00.9 Acute nephritic syndrome with unspecified morphologic changes**

MCC **N00.A Acute nephritic syndrome with C3 glomerulonephritis**

Acute nephritic syndrome with C3 glomerulopathy, NOS

Excludes1: *Acute nephritic syndrome (with C3 glomerulopathy) with dense deposit disease (N00.6)*

N01 Rapidly progressive nephritic syndrome

Includes: rapidly progressive glomerular disease
rapidly progressive glomerulonephritis
rapidly progressive nephritis

Excludes1: *nephritic syndrome NOS (N05.-)*

MCC **N01.0 Rapidly progressive nephritic syndrome with minor glomerular abnormality**

Rapidly progressive nephritic syndrome with minimal change lesion

MCC **N01.1 Rapidly progressive nephritic syndrome with focal and segmental glomerular lesions**

Rapidly progressive nephritic syndrome with focal and segmental hyalinosis
Rapidly progressive nephritic syndrome with focal and segmental sclerosis
Rapidly progressive nephritic syndrome with focal glomerulonephritis

MCC **N01.2 Rapidly progressive nephritic syndrome with diffuse membranous glomerulonephritis**

MCC **N01.3 Rapidly progressive nephritic syndrome with diffuse mesangial proliferative glomerulonephritis**

MCC **N01.4 Rapidly progressive nephritic syndrome with diffuse endocapillary proliferative glomerulonephritis**

MCC **N01.5 Rapidly progressive nephritic syndrome with diffuse mesangiocapillary glomerulonephritis**

Rapidly progressive nephritic syndrome with membranoproliferative glomerulonephritis, types 1 and 3, or NOS

Excludes1: *Rapidly progressive nephritic syndrome with C3 glomerulonephritis (N01.A)*
Rapidly progressive nephritic syndrome with C3 glomerulopathy (N01.A)

MCC **N01.6 Rapidly progressive nephritic syndrome with dense deposit disease**

Rapidly progressive nephritic syndrome with membranoproliferative glomerulonephritis, type 2
Rapidly progressive nephritic syndrome with C3 glomerulopathy with dense deposit disease

MCC **N01.7 Rapidly progressive nephritic syndrome with diffuse crescentic glomerulonephritis**

Rapidly progressive nephritic syndrome with extracapillary glomerulonephritis

MCC **N01.8 Rapidly progressive nephritic syndrome with other morphologic changes**

Rapidly progressive nephritic syndrome with proliferative glomerulonephritis NOS

MCC **N01.9 Rapidly progressive nephritic syndrome with unspecified morphologic changes**

MCC **N01.A Rapidly progressive nephritic syndrome with C3 glomerulonephritis**

Rapidly progressive nephritic syndrome with C3 glomerulopathy, NOS

Excludes1: *Rapidly progressive nephritic syndrome (with C3 glomerulopathy) with dense deposit disease (N01.6)*

N02 Recurrent and persistent hematuria

Excludes1: *acute cystitis with hematuria (N30.01)*
hematuria NOS (R31.9)
hematuria not associated with specified morphologic lesions (R31.-)

CC **N02.0 Recurrent and persistent hematuria with minor glomerular abnormality**

Recurrent and persistent hematuria with minimal change lesion

CC **N02.1 Recurrent and persistent hematuria with focal and segmental glomerular lesions**

Recurrent and persistent hematuria with focal and segmental hyalinosis
Recurrent and persistent hematuria with focal and segmental sclerosis
Recurrent and persistent hematuria with focal glomerulonephritis

CC **N02.2 Recurrent and persistent hematuria with diffuse membranous glomerulonephritis**

CC **N02.3 Recurrent and persistent hematuria with diffuse mesangial proliferative glomerulonephritis**

CC **N02.4 Recurrent and persistent hematuria with diffuse endocapillary proliferative glomerulonephritis**

CC **N02.5 Recurrent and persistent hematuria with diffuse mesangiocapillary glomerulonephritis**

Recurrent and persistent hematuria with membranoproliferative glomerulonephritis, types 1 and 3, or NOS

Excludes1: *Recurrent and persistent hematuria with C3 glomerulonephritis (N02.A)*
Recurrent and persistent hematuria with C3 glomerulopathy (N02.A)

CC **N02.6 Recurrent and persistent hematuria with dense deposit disease**

Recurrent and persistent hematuria with membranoproliferative glomerulonephritis, type 2
Recurrent and persistent hematuria with C3 glomerulopathy with dense deposit disease

+, +7th, X + 7th ● Newborn ● Pediatric ● Maternity ● Adult ♀ Female ♂ Male Manifestation Unacceptable PDX HCC CC MCC HAC

CC N02.7 Recurrent and persistent hematuria with diffuse crescentic glomerulonephritis

Recurrent and persistent hematuria with extracapillary glomerulonephritis

CC N02.8 Recurrent and persistent hematuria with other morphologic changes

Recurrent and persistent hematuria with proliferative glomerulonephritis NOS

CC N02.9 Recurrent and persistent hematuria with unspecified morphologic changes

AHA CC: 2Q, 2017, 5

CC N02.A Recurrent and persistent hematuria with C3 glomerulonephritis

Recurrent and persistent hematuria with C3 glomerulopathy

Excludes1: *Recurrent and persistent hematuria (with C3 glomerulopathy) with dense deposit disease (N02.6)*

N03 Chronic nephritic syndrome

Includes: chronic glomerular disease
chronic glomerulonephritis
chronic nephritis

Excludes1: *chronic tubulo-interstitial nephritis (N11.-)*
diffuse sclerosing glomerulonephritis (N05.8-)
nephritic syndrome NOS (N05.-)

CC N03.0 Chronic nephritic syndrome with minor glomerular abnormality

Chronic nephritic syndrome with minimal change lesion

CC N03.1 Chronic nephritic syndrome with focal and segmental glomerular lesions

Chronic nephritic syndrome with focal and segmental hyalinosis

Chronic nephritic syndrome with focal and segmental sclerosis

Chronic nephritic syndrome with focal glomerulonephritis

CC N03.2 Chronic nephritic syndrome with diffuse membranous glomerulonephritis

CC N03.3 Chronic nephritic syndrome with diffuse mesangial proliferative glomerulonephritis

CC N03.4 Chronic nephritic syndrome with diffuse endocapillary proliferative glomerulonephritis

CC N03.5 Chronic nephritic syndrome with diffuse mesangiocapillary glomerulonephritis

Chronic nephritic syndrome with membranoproliferative glomerulonephritis, types 1 and 3, or NOS

Excludes1: *Chronic nephritic syndrome with C3 glomerulonephritis (N03.A)*
Chronic nephritic syndrome with C3 glomerulopathy (N03.A)

CC N03.6 Chronic nephritic syndrome with dense deposit disease

Chronic nephritic syndrome with membranoproliferative glomerulonephritis, type 2

Chronic nephritic syndrome with C3 glomerulopathy with dense deposit disease

CC N03.7 Chronic nephritic syndrome with diffuse crescentic glomerulonephritis

Chronic nephritic syndrome with extracapillary glomerulonephritis

CC N03.8 Chronic nephritic syndrome with other morphologic changes

Chronic nephritic syndrome with proliferative glomerulonephritis NOS

CC N03.9 Chronic nephritic syndrome with unspecified morphologic changes

CC N03.A Chronic nephritic syndrome with C3 glomerulonephritis

Chronic nephritic syndrome with C3 glomerulopathy

Excludes1: *Chronic nephritic syndrome (with C3 glomerulopathy) with dense deposit disease (N03.6)*

N04 Nephrotic syndrome

Includes: congenital nephrotic syndrome
lipoid nephrosis

CC N04.0 Nephrotic syndrome with minor glomerular abnormality

Nephrotic syndrome with minimal change lesion

CC N04.1 Nephrotic syndrome with focal and segmental glomerular lesions

Nephrotic syndrome with focal and segmental hyalinosis

Nephrotic syndrome with focal and segmental sclerosis

Nephrotic syndrome with focal glomerulonephritis

CC N04.2 Nephrotic syndrome with diffuse membranous glomerulonephritis

CC N04.3 Nephrotic syndrome with diffuse mesangial proliferative glomerulonephritis

CC N04.4 Nephrotic syndrome with diffuse endocapillary proliferative glomerulonephritis

CC N04.5 Nephrotic syndrome with diffuse mesangiocapillary glomerulonephritis

Nephrotic syndrome with membranoproliferative glomerulonephritis, types 1 and 3, or NOS

Excludes1: *Nephrotic syndrome with C3 glomerulonephritis (N04.A)*
Nephrotic syndrome with C3 glomerulopathy (N04.A)

CC N04.6 Nephrotic syndrome with dense deposit disease

Nephrotic syndrome with membranoproliferative glomerulonephritis, type 2

Nephrotic syndrome with C3 glomerulopathy with dense deposit disease

CC N04.7 Nephrotic syndrome with diffuse crescentic glomerulonephritis

Nephrotic syndrome with extracapillary glomerulonephritis

CC N04.8 Nephrotic syndrome with other morphologic changes

Nephrotic syndrome with proliferative glomerulonephritis NOS

CC N04.9 Nephrotic syndrome with unspecified morphologic changes

CC N04.A Nephrotic syndrome with C3 glomerulonephritis

Nephrotic syndrome with C3 glomerulopathy

Excludes1: *Nephrotic syndrome (with C3 glomerulopathy) with dense deposit disease (N04.6)*

N05 Unspecified nephritic syndrome

Includes: glomerular disease NOS
glomerulonephritis NOS
nephritis NOS
nephropathy NOS and renal disease NOS with morphological lesion specified in .0-.8

Excludes1: *nephropathy NOS with no stated morphological lesion (N28.9)*
renal disease NOS with no stated morphological lesion (N28.9)
tubulo-interstitial nephritis NOS (N12)

N05.0 Unspecified nephritic syndrome with minor glomerular abnormality

Unspecified nephritic syndrome with minimal change lesion

N05.1 Unspecified nephritic syndrome with focal and segmental glomerular lesions

Unspecified nephritic syndrome with focal and segmental hyalinosis

Unspecified nephritic syndrome with focal and segmental sclerosis

Unspecified nephritic syndrome with focal glomerulonephritis

CC N05.2 Unspecified nephritic syndrome with diffuse membranous glomerulonephritis

CC N05.3 Unspecified nephritic syndrome with diffuse mesangial proliferative glomerulonephritis

CC N05.4 Unspecified nephritic syndrome with diffuse endocapillary proliferative glomerulonephritis

CC N05.5 Unspecified nephritic syndrome with diffuse mesangiocapillary glomerulonephritis

Unspecified nephritic syndrome with membranoproliferative glomerulonephritis, types 1 and 3, or NOS

Excludes1: *Unspecified nephritic syndrome with C3 glomerulonephritis (N05.A)*
Unspecified nephritic syndrome with C3 glomerulopathy (N05.A)

N05.6 **Unspecified nephritic syndrome with dense deposit disease**
Unspecified nephritic syndrome with membranoproliferative glomerulonephritis, type 2
Unspecified nephritic syndrome with C3 glomerulopathy with dense deposit disease

N05.7 **Unspecified nephritic syndrome with diffuse crescentic glomerulonephritis**
Unspecified nephritic syndrome with extracapillary glomerulonephritis

N05.8 **Unspecified nephritic syndrome with other morphologic changes**
Unspecified nephritic syndrome with proliferative glomerulonephritis NOS

N05.9 **Unspecified nephritic syndrome with unspecified morphologic changes**

CC **N05.A** **Unspecified nephritic syndrome with C3 glomerulonephritis**
Unspecified nephritic syndrome with C3 glomerulopathy
> **Excludes1:** *Unspecified nephritic syndrome (with C3 glomerulopathy) with dense deposit disease (N05.6)*

N06 **Isolated proteinuria with specified morphological lesion**

> **Excludes1:** *Proteinuria not associated with specific morphologic lesions (R80.0)*

N06.0 **Isolated proteinuria with minor glomerular abnormality**
Isolated proteinuria with minimal change lesion

N06.1 **Isolated proteinuria with focal and segmental glomerular lesions**
Isolated proteinuria with focal and segmental hyalinosis
Isolated proteinuria with focal and segmental sclerosis
Isolated proteinuria with focal glomerulonephritis

CC **N06.2** **Isolated proteinuria with diffuse membranous glomerulonephritis**

CC **N06.3** **Isolated proteinuria with diffuse mesangial proliferative glomerulonephritis**

CC **N06.4** **Isolated proteinuria with diffuse endocapillary proliferative glomerulonephritis**

CC **N06.5** **Isolated proteinuria with diffuse mesangiocapillary glomerulonephritis**
Isolated proteinuria with membranoproliferative glomerulonephritis, types 1 and 3, or NOS
> **Excludes1:** *Isolated proteinuria with C3 glomerulonephritis (N06.A)*
> *Isolated proteinuria with C3 glomerulopathy (N06.A)*

N06.6 **Isolated proteinuria with dense deposit disease**
Isolated proteinuria with membranoproliferative glomerulonephritis, type 2
Isolated proteinuria with C3 glomerulopathy with dense deposit disease

N06.7 **Isolated proteinuria with diffuse crescentic glomerulonephritis**
Isolated proteinuria with extracapillary glomerulonephritis

N06.8 **Isolated proteinuria with other morphologic lesion**
Isolated proteinuria with proliferative glomerulonephritis NOS

N06.9 **Isolated proteinuria with unspecified morphologic lesion**

CC **N06.A** **Isolated proteinuria with C3 glomerulonephritis**
Isolated proteinuria with C3 glomerulopathy
> **Excludes1:** *Isolated proteinuria (with C3 glomerulopathy) with dense deposit disease (N06.6)*

N07 **Hereditary nephropathy, not elsewhere classified**

> **Excludes2:** *Alport's syndrome (Q87.81-)*
> *hereditary amyloid nephropathy (E85.-)*
> *nail patella syndrome (Q87.2)*
> *non-neuropathic heredofamilial amyloidosis (E85.-)*

N07.0 **Hereditary nephropathy, not elsewhere classified with minor glomerular abnormality**
Hereditary nephropathy, not elsewhere classified with minimal change lesion

N07.1 **Hereditary nephropathy, not elsewhere classified with focal and segmental glomerular lesions**
Hereditary nephropathy, not elsewhere classified with focal and segmental hyalinosis
Hereditary nephropathy, not elsewhere classified with focal and segmental sclerosis
Hereditary nephropathy, not elsewhere classified with focal glomerulonephritis

CC **N07.2** **Hereditary nephropathy, not elsewhere classified with diffuse membranous glomerulonephritis**

CC **N07.3** **Hereditary nephropathy, not elsewhere classified with diffuse mesangial proliferative glomerulonephritis**

CC **N07.4** **Hereditary nephropathy, not elsewhere classified with diffuse endocapillary proliferative glomerulonephritis**

CC **N07.5** **Hereditary nephropathy, not elsewhere classified with diffuse mesangiocapillary glomerulonephritis**
Hereditary nephropathy, not elsewhere classified with membranoproliferative glomerulonephritis, types 1 and 3, or NOS
> **Excludes1:** *Hereditary nephropathy, not elsewhere classified with C3 glomerulonephritis (N07.A)*
> *Hereditary nephropathy, not elsewhere classified with C3 glomerulopathy (N07.A)*

N07.6 **Hereditary nephropathy, not elsewhere classified with dense deposit disease**
Hereditary nephropathy, not elsewhere classified with membranoproliferative glomerulonephritis, type 2
Hereditary nephropathy, not elsewhere classified with C3 glomerulopathy with dense deposit disease

N07.7 **Hereditary nephropathy, not elsewhere classified with diffuse crescentic glomerulonephritis**
Hereditary nephropathy, not elsewhere classified with extracapillary glomerulonephritis

N07.8 **Hereditary nephropathy, not elsewhere classified with other morphologic lesions**
Hereditary nephropathy, not elsewhere classified with proliferative glomerulonephritis NOS

N07.9 **Hereditary nephropathy, not elsewhere classified with unspecified morphologic lesions**

CC **N07.A** **Hereditary nephropathy, not elsewhere classified with C3 glomerulonephritis**
Hereditary nephropathy, not elsewhere classified with C3 glomerulopathy
> **Excludes1:** *Hereditary nephropathy, not elsewhere classified (with C3 glomerulopathy) with dense deposit disease (N07.6)*

N08 **Glomerular disorders in diseases classified elsewhere**

Glomerulonephritis
Nephritis
Nephropathy
Code first underlying disease, such as:
    amyloidosis (E85.-)
    congenital syphilis (A50.5)
    cryoglobulinemia (D89.1)
    disseminated intravascular coagulation (D65)
    gout (M1A.-, M10.-)
    microscopic polyangiitis (M31.7)
    multiple myeloma (C90.0-)
    sepsis (A40.0-A41.9)
    sickle-cell disease (D57.0-D57.8)
> **Excludes1:** *glomerulonephritis, nephritis and nephropathy (in):*
> *antiglomerular basement membrane disease (M31.0)*
> *diabetes (E08-E13 with .21)*
> *gonococcal (A54.21)*
> *Goodpasture's syndrome (M31.0)*
> *hemolytic-uremic syndrome (D59.3)*
> *lupus (M32.14)*
> *mumps (B26.83)*
> *syphilis (A52.75)*
> *systemic lupus erythematosus (M32.14)*
> *Wegener's granulomatosis (M31.31)*
> *pyelonephritis in diseases classified elsewhere (N16)*
> *renal tubulo-interstitial disorders classified elsewhere (N16)*

Valid 3-character code, no further characters required

Renal tubulo-interstitial diseases (N10-N16)

Includes: pyelonephritis

Excludes1: *pyeloureteritis cystica (N28.85)*

CC N10 Acute pyelonephritis

> Acute infectious interstitial nephritis
> Acute pyelitis
> Acute tubulo-interstitial nephritis
> Hemoglobin nephrosis
> Myoglobin nephrosis
> Use additional code (B95-B97), to identify infectious agent
> *AHA CC: 3Q, 2019, 13-14*
> **HAC** see Appendix B for HAC conditional logic
> **Valid 3-character code, no further characters required**

N11 Chronic tubulo-interstitial nephritis

> **Includes:** chronic infectious interstitial nephritis
> chronic pyelitis
> chronic pyelonephritis
> Use additional code (B95-B97), to identify infectious agent

> **N11.0 Nonobstructive reflux-associated chronic pyelonephritis**
> > Pyelonephritis (chronic) associated with (vesicoureteral) reflux
> > ***Excludes1:*** *vesicoureteral reflux NOS (N13.70)*

> **CC N11.1 Chronic obstructive pyelonephritis**
> > Pyelonephritis (chronic) associated with anomaly of pelviureteric junction
> > Pyelonephritis (chronic) associated with anomaly of pyeloureteric junction
> > Pyelonephritis (chronic) associated with crossing of vessel
> > Pyelonephritis (chronic) associated with kinking of ureter
> > Pyelonephritis (chronic) associated with obstruction of ureter
> > Pyelonephritis (chronic) associated with stricture of pelviureteric junction
> > Pyelonephritis (chronic) associated with stricture of ureter
> > ***Excludes1:*** *calculous pyelonephritis (N20.9)*
> > *obstructive uropathy (N13.-)*

> **CC N11.8 Other chronic tubulo-interstitial nephritis**
> > Nonobstructive chronic pyelonephritis NOS

> **CC N11.9 Chronic tubulo-interstitial nephritis, unspecified**
> > Chronic interstitial nephritis NOS
> > Chronic pyelitis NOS
> > Chronic pyelonephritis NOS
> > **HAC** see Appendix B for HAC conditional logic

CC N12 Tubulo-interstitial nephritis, not specified as acute or chronic

> Interstitial nephritis NOS
> Pyelitis NOS
> Pyelonephritis NOS
> ***Excludes1:*** *calculous pyelonephritis (N20.9)*
> **HAC** see Appendix B for HAC conditional logic
> **Valid 3-character code, no further characters required**

N13 Obstructive and reflux uropathy

> ***Excludes2:*** *calculus of kidney and ureter without hydronephrosis (N20.-)*
> *congenital obstructive defects of renal pelvis and ureter (Q62.0-Q62.3)*
> *hydronephrosis with ureteropelvic junction obstruction (Q62.11)*
> *obstructive pyelonephritis (N11.1)*

> **CC N13.0 Hydronephrosis with ureteropelvic junction obstruction**
> > Hydronephrosis due to acquired occlusion of ureteropelvic junction
> > ***Excludes2:*** *Hydronephrosis with ureteropelvic junction obstruction due to calculus (N13.2)*
> > *AHA CC: 4Q, 2016, 43*

> **CC N13.1 Hydronephrosis with ureteral stricture, not elsewhere classified**
> > ***Excludes1:*** *hydronephrosis with ureteral stricture with infection (N13.6)*

> **N13.2 Hydronephrosis with renal and ureteral calculous obstruction**
> > ***Excludes1:*** *hydronephrosis with renal and ureteral calculous obstruction with infection (N13.6)*

> **+ N13.3 Other and unspecified hydronephrosis**
> > ***Excludes1:*** *hydronephrosis with infection (N13.6)*
> > **CC N13.30 Unspecified hydronephrosis**
> > **CC N13.39 Other hydronephrosis**

> **CC N13.4 Hydroureter**
> > ***Excludes1:*** *congenital hydroureter (Q62.3-)*
> > *hydroureter with infection (N13.6)*
> > *vesicoureteral-reflux with hydroureter (N13.73-)*

> **N13.5 Crossing vessel and stricture of ureter without hydronephrosis**
> > Kinking and stricture of ureter without hydronephrosis
> > ***Excludes1:*** *Crossing vessel and stricture of ureter without hydronephrosis with infection (N13.6)*

> **CC N13.6 Pyonephrosis**
> > Conditions in N13.0-N13.5 with infection
> > Obstructive uropathy with infection
> > Use additional code (B95-B97), to identify infectious agent
> > *AHA CC: 2Q, 2018, 21*
> > **HAC** see Appendix B for HAC conditional logic

> **+ N13.7 Vesicoureteral-reflux**
> > ***Excludes1:*** *reflux-associated pyelonephritis (N11.0)*
> > **N13.70 Vesicoureteral-reflux, unspecified**
> > > Vesicoureteral-reflux NOS
> > **N13.71 Vesicoureteral-reflux without reflux nephropathy**
> > **+ N13.72 Vesicoureteral-reflux with reflux nephropathy without hydroureter**
> > > **N13.721 Vesicoureteral-reflux with reflux nephropathy without hydroureter, unilateral**
> > > **N13.722 Vesicoureteral-reflux with reflux nephropathy without hydroureter, bilateral**
> > > **N13.729 Vesicoureteral-reflux with reflux nephropathy without hydroureter, unspecified**
> > **+ N13.73 Vesicoureteral-reflux with reflux nephropathy with hydroureter**
> > > **N13.731 Vesicoureteral-reflux with reflux nephropathy with hydroureter, unilateral**
> > > **N13.732 Vesicoureteral-reflux with reflux nephropathy with hydroureter, bilateral**
> > > **N13.739 Vesicoureteral-reflux with reflux nephropathy with hydroureter, unspecified**

> **CC N13.8 Other obstructive and reflux uropathy**
> > Urinary tract obstruction due to specified cause
> > Code first, if applicable, any causal condition, such as:
> > enlarged prostate (N40.1)

> **N13.9 Obstructive and reflux uropathy, unspecified**
> > Urinary tract obstruction NOS

N14 Drug- and heavy-metal-induced tubulo-interstitial and tubular conditions

> Code first poisoning due to drug or toxin, if applicable (T36-T65 with fifth or sixth character 1-4 or 6)

> Use additional code for adverse effect, if applicable, to identify drug (T36-T50 with fifth or sixth character 5)

> **N14.0 Analgesic nephropathy**
> **N14.1 Nephropathy induced by other drugs, medicaments and biological substances**
> **N14.2 Nephropathy induced by unspecified drug, medicament or biological substance**
> **N14.3 Nephropathy induced by heavy metals**
> **N14.4 Toxic nephropathy, not elsewhere classified**

N15 Other renal tubulo-interstitial diseases

> **N15.0 Balkan nephropathy**
> > Balkan endemic nephropathy
> **MCC N15.1 Renal and perinephric abscess**
> > **HAC** see Appendix B for HAC conditional logic
> **N15.8 Other specified renal tubulo-interstitial diseases**
> **N15.9 Renal tubulo-interstitial disease, unspecified**
> > Infection of kidney NOS
> > ***Excludes1:*** *urinary tract infection NOS (N39.0)*

N16 Renal tubulo-interstitial disorders in diseases classified elsewhere

> Pyelonephritis
> Tubulo-interstitial nephritis
> Code first underlying disease, such as:
> brucellosis (A23.0-A23.9)
> cryoglobulinemia (D89.1)
> glycogen storage disease (E74.0)
> leukemia (C91-C95)
> lymphoma (C81.0-C85.9, C96.0-C96.9)
> multiple myeloma (C90.0-)
> sepsis (A40.0-A41.9)
> Wilson's disease (E83.0)

Excludes1: *diphtheritic pyelonephritis and tubulo-interstitial nephritis (A36.84)*
pyelonephritis and tubulo-interstitial nephritis in candidiasis (B37.49)
pyelonephritis and tubulo-interstitial nephritis in cystinosis (E72.04)
pyelonephritis and tubulo-interstitial nephritis in salmonella infection (A02.25)
pyelonephritis and tubulo-interstitial nephritis in sarcoidosis (D86.84)
pyelonephritis and tubulo-interstitial nephritis in sicca syndrome [Sjogren's] (M35.04)
pyelonephritis and tubulo-interstitial nephritis in systemic lupus erythematosus (M32.15)
pyelonephritis and tubulo-interstitial nephritis in toxoplasmosis (B58.83)
renal tubular degeneration in diabetes (E08-E13 with .29)
syphilitic pyelonephritis and tubulo-interstitial nephritis (A52.75)
Valid 3-character code, no further characters required

Acute kidney failure and chronic kidney disease (N17-N19)

Excludes2: *congenital renal failure (P96.0)*
drug- and heavy-metal-induced tubulo-interstitial and tubular conditions (N14.-)
extrarenal uremia (R39.2)
hemolytic-uremic syndrome (D59.3)
hepatorenal syndrome (K76.7)
postpartum hepatorenal syndrome (O90.4)
posttraumatic renal failure (T79.5)
prerenal uremia (R39.2)
renal failure complicating abortion or ectopic or molar pregnancy (O00-O07, O08.4)
renal failure following labor and delivery (O90.4)
renal failure postprocedural (N99.0)

N17   Acute kidney failure
Code also associated underlying condition
Excludes1: *posttraumatic renal failure (T79.5)*

MCC N17.0   Acute kidney failure with tubular necrosis
Acute tubular necrosis
Renal tubular necrosis
Tubular necrosis NOS

MCC N17.1   Acute kidney failure with acute cortical necrosis
Acute cortical necrosis
Cortical necrosis NOS
Renal cortical necrosis

N17.2   Acute kidney failure with medullary necrosis
Medullary [papillary] necrosis NOS
Acute medullary [papillary] necrosis
Renal medullary [papillary] necrosis

CC N17.8   Other acute kidney failure

CC N17.9   Acute kidney failure, unspecified
Acute kidney injury (nontraumatic)
Excludes2: *traumatic kidney injury (S37.0-)*
AHA CC: 2Q, 2019, 7, 24-26

N18   Chronic kidney disease (CKD)
Code first any associated:
diabetic chronic kidney disease (E08.22, E09.22, E10.22, E11.22, E13.22)
hypertensive chronic kidney disease (I12.-, I13.-)

Use additional code to identify kidney transplant status, if applicable, (Z94.0)
Review coding guidelines C.9.a.2 and C.9.a.3
Review coding guidelines C.14.a.1 and C.14.a.2

N18.1   Chronic kidney disease, stage 1
N18.2   Chronic kidney disease, stage 2 (mild)
+ N18.3   Chronic kidney disease, stage 3 (moderate)
N18.30   Chronic kidney disease, stage 3 unspecified
N18.31   Chronic kidney disease, stage 3a
N18.32   Chronic kidney disease, stage 3b

CC N18.4   Chronic kidney disease, stage 4 (severe)
CC N18.5   Chronic kidney disease, stage 5
Excludes1: *chronic kidney disease, stage 5 requiring chronic dialysis (N18.6)*
MCC N18.6   End stage renal disease
Chronic kidney disease requiring chronic dialysis
Use additional code to identify dialysis status (Z99.2)
AHA CC: 4Q, 2013, 125; 3Q, 2016, 22-23

N18.9   Chronic kidney disease, unspecified
Chronic renal disease
Chronic renal failure NOS
Chronic renal insufficiency
Chronic uremia NOS
Diffuse sclerosing glomerulonephritis NOS
AHA CC: 4Q, 2018, 88-89

N19   Unspecified kidney failure
Uremia NOS
Excludes1: *acute kidney failure (N17.-)*
chronic kidney disease (N18.-)
chronic uremia (N18.9)
extrarenal uremia (R39.2)
prerenal uremia (R39.2)
renal insufficiency (acute) (N28.9)
uremia of newborn (P96.0)
Valid 3-character code, no further characters required

Urolithiasis (N20-N23)

N20   Calculus of kidney and ureter
Calculous pyelonephritis
Excludes1: *nephrocalcinosis (E83.5)*
that with hydronephrosis (N13.2)

N20.0   Calculus of kidney
Nephrolithiasis NOS
Renal calculus
Renal stone
Staghorn calculus
Stone in kidney
AHA CC: 1Q, 2017, 5; 3Q, 2019, 13-14

CC N20.1   Calculus of ureter
Calculus of the ureteropelvic junction
Ureteric stone
AHA CC: 3Q, 2016, 23-24

CC N20.2   Calculus of kidney with calculus of ureter
AHA CC: 2Q, 2015, 8-9

N20.9   Urinary calculus, unspecified

N21   Calculus of lower urinary tract
Includes: calculus of lower urinary tract with cystitis and urethritis
N21.0   Calculus in bladder
Calculus in diverticulum of bladder
Urinary bladder stone
Excludes2: *staghorn calculus (N20.0)*
N21.1   Calculus in urethra
Excludes2: *calculus of prostate (N42.0)*
N21.8   Other lower urinary tract calculus
N21.9   Calculus of lower urinary tract, unspecified
Excludes1: *calculus of urinary tract NOS (N20.9)*

N22   Calculus of urinary tract in diseases classified elsewhere
Code first underlying disease, such as:
gout (M1A.-, M10.-)
schistosomiasis (B65.0-B65.9)
Valid 3-character code, no further characters required

N23   Unspecified renal colic
Valid 3-character code, no further characters required

+, +7th, X + 7th   • Newborn   • Pediatric   • Maternity   • Adult   ♀ Female   ♂ Male   Manifestation   Unacceptable PDX   HCC   CC   MCC   HAC

Other disorders of kidney and ureter (N25-N29)

Excludes2: *disorders of kidney and ureter with urolithiasis (N20-N23)*

N25 Disorders resulting from impaired renal tubular function

N25.0 Renal osteodystrophy
Azotemic osteodystrophy
Phosphate-losing tubular disorders
Renal rickets
Renal short stature
Excludes2: metabolic disorders classifiable to E70-E88

CC **N25.1 Nephrogenic diabetes insipidus**
Excludes1: *diabetes insipidus NOS (E23.2)*

+ **N25.8 Other disorders resulting from impaired renal tubular function**

CC **N25.81 Secondary hyperparathyroidism of renal origin**
Excludes1: *secondary hyperparathyroidism, non-renal (E21.1)*
Excludes2: *metabolic disorders classifiable to E70-E88*

N25.89 Other disorders resulting from impaired renal tubular function
Hypokalemic nephropathy
Lightwood-Albright syndrome
Renal tubular acidosis NOS

N25.9 Disorder resulting from impaired renal tubular function, unspecified

N26 Unspecified contracted kidney

Excludes1: *contracted kidney due to hypertension (I12.-)*
diffuse sclerosing glomerulonephritis (N05.8.-)
hypertensive nephrosclerosis (arteriolar) (arteriosclerotic) (I12.-)
small kidney of unknown cause (N27.-)

N26.1 Atrophy of kidney (terminal)
N26.2 Page kidney
N26.9 Renal sclerosis, unspecified

N27 Small kidney of unknown cause

Includes: oligonephronia
N27.0 Small kidney, unilateral
N27.1 Small kidney, bilateral
N27.9 Small kidney, unspecified

N28 Other disorders of kidney and ureter, not elsewhere classified

CC **N28.0 Ischemia and infarction of kidney**
Renal artery embolism
Renal artery obstruction
Renal artery occlusion
Renal artery thrombosis
Renal infarct
Excludes1: *atherosclerosis of renal artery (extrarenal part) (I70.1)*
congenital stenosis of renal artery (Q27.1)
Goldblatt's kidney (I70.1)

N28.1 Cyst of kidney, acquired
Cyst (multiple) (solitary) of kidney (acquired)
Excludes1: *cystic kidney disease (congenital) (Q61.-)*

+ **N28.8 Other specified disorders of kidney and ureter**
Excludes1: *hydroureter (N13.4)*
ureteric stricture with hydronephrosis (N13.1)
ureteric stricture without hydronephrosis (N13.5)

N28.81 Hypertrophy of kidney
N28.82 Megaloureter
N28.83 Nephroptosis
CC **N28.84 Pyelitis cystica**
HAC see Appendix B for HAC conditional logic
CC **N28.85 Pyeloureteritis cystica**
HAC see Appendix B for HAC conditional logic

CC **N28.86 Ureteritis cystica**
HAC see Appendix B for HAC conditional logic
N28.89 Other specified disorders of kidney and ureter
N28.9 Disorder of kidney and ureter, unspecified
Nephropathy NOS
Renal disease (acute) NOS
Renal insufficiency (acute)
Excludes1: *chronic renal insufficiency (N18.9)*
unspecified nephritic syndrome (N05.-)
AHA CC: 1Q, 2016, 13

N29 Other disorders of kidney and ureter in diseases classified elsewhere

Code first underlying disease, such as:
amyloidosis (E85.-)
nephrocalcinosis (E83.5)
schistosomiasis (B65.0-B65.9)
Excludes1: *disorders of kidney and ureter in:*
cystinosis (E72.0)
gonorrhea (A54.21)
syphilis (A52.75)
tuberculosis (A18.11)
Valid 3-character code, no further characters required

Other diseases of the urinary system (N30-N39)

Excludes1: *urinary infection (complicating):*
abortion or ectopic or molar pregnancy (O00-O07, O08.8)
pregnancy, childbirth and the puerperium (O23.-, O75.3, O86.2-)

N30 Cystitis

Use additional code to identify infectious agent (B95-B97)
Excludes1: *prostatocystitis (N41.3)*

+ **N30.0 Acute cystitis**
Excludes1: *irradiation cystitis (N30.4-)*
trigonitis (N30.3-)
CC **N30.00 Acute cystitis without hematuria**
HAC see Appendix B for HAC conditional logic
CC **N30.01 Acute cystitis with hematuria**
HAC see Appendix B for HAC conditional logic

+ **N30.1 Interstitial cystitis (chronic)**
N30.10 Interstitial cystitis (chronic) without hematuria
N30.11 Interstitial cystitis (chronic) with hematuria

+ **N30.2 Other chronic cystitis**
N30.20 Other chronic cystitis without hematuria
N30.21 Other chronic cystitis with hematuria

+ **N30.3 Trigonitis**
Urethrotrigonitis
N30.30 Trigonitis without hematuria
N30.31 Trigonitis with hematuria

+ **N30.4 Irradiation cystitis**
CC **N30.40 Irradiation cystitis without hematuria**
CC **N30.41 Irradiation cystitis with hematuria**

+ **N30.8 Other cystitis**
Abscess of bladder
N30.80 Other cystitis without hematuria
N30.81 Other cystitis with hematuria

+ **N30.9 Cystitis, unspecified**
N30.90 Cystitis, unspecified without hematuria
N30.91 Cystitis, unspecified with hematuria

N31 Neuromuscular dysfunction of bladder, not elsewhere classified

Use additional code to identify any associated urinary incontinence (N39.3-N39.4-)
Excludes1: *cord bladder NOS (G95.89)*
neurogenic bladder due to cauda equina syndrome (G83.4)
neuromuscular dysfunction due to spinal cord lesion (G95.89)

N31.0 Uninhibited neuropathic bladder, not elsewhere classified

+, +7th, X + 7th   ● Newborn   ● Pediatric   ● Maternity   ● Adult   ♀ Female   ♂ Male   Manifestation   Unacceptable PDX   HCC   CC   MCC   HAC

Obstructive Uropathy: Etiology

Kidney
Anomalies
Ptosis
Calculus
Chronic infection
 Pyogenic
 Granulomatous
Neoplasm
Necrotizing papillitis

Ureter
Anomalies
 of number
 of termination
Aberrant vessel
Stricture stenosis
Kinks
Chronic infection
Congenital valve
Retrocaval ureter
Neoplasm
Calculus
Compression (by nodes,
 tumor, abscess,
 hematoma, bands)
Ureteritis cystica
Ovarian vein syndrome
Periureteral
 Inflammation
 (appendicitis,
 diverticulitis)
Trauma

Bladder
Ureterocele
Neoplasm
Diverticulum
Calculus
Foreign body
Congenital neck
 obstruction
Schistosomiasis

Female Urethra
Neoplasm
Stricture
Diverticulum
Papilloma
Meatal stenosis

Prostate
Benign hypertrophy
Prostatitis, abscess
Cyst
Verumontanitis
Congenital valve
Neoplasm

Male Urethra
Neoplasm
Diverticulum
Stricture
Strangulation
Papilloma
Meatal stenosis
Phimosis

N31.1 Reflex neuropathic bladder, not elsewhere classified
N31.2 Flaccid neuropathic bladder, not elsewhere classified
 Atonic (motor) (sensory) neuropathic bladder
 Autonomous neuropathic bladder
 Nonreflex neuropathic bladder
N31.8 Other neuromuscular dysfunction of bladder
N31.9 Neuromuscular dysfunction of bladder, unspecified
 Neurogenic bladder dysfunction NOS

N32 Other disorders of bladder

 Excludes2: *calculus of bladder (N21.0)*
  cystocele (N81.1-)
  hernia or prolapse of bladder, female (N81.1-)

N32.0 Bladder-neck obstruction
 Bladder-neck stenosis (acquired)
 Excludes1: *congenital bladder-neck obstruction (Q64.3-)*
CC **N32.1 Vesicointestinal fistula**
 Vesicorectal fistula
CC **N32.2 Vesical fistula, not elsewhere classified**
 Excludes1: *fistula between bladder and female genital tract*
  (N82.0-N82.1)
N32.3 Diverticulum of bladder
 Excludes1: *congenital diverticulum of bladder (Q64.6)*
  diverticulitis of bladder (N30.8-)

+ **N32.8 Other specified disorders of bladder**
 N32.81 Overactive bladder
  Detrusor muscle hyperactivity
  Excludes1: *frequent urination due to specified*
   bladdercondition-codetocondition
 N32.89 Other specified disorders of bladder
  Bladder hemorrhage
  Bladder hypertrophy
  Calcified bladder
  Contracted bladder
N32.9 Bladder disorder, unspecified

N33 Bladder disorders in diseases classified elsewhere
 Code first underlying disease, such as:
  schistosomiasis (B65.0-B65.9)
 Excludes1: *bladder disorder in syphilis (A52.76)*
  bladder disorder in tuberculosis (A18.12)
  candidal cystitis (B37.41)
  chlamydial cystitis (A56.01)
  cystitis in gonorrhea (A54.01)
  cystitis in neurogenic bladder (N31.-)
  diphtheritic cystitis (A36.85)
  syphilitic cystitis (A52.76)
  trichomonal cystitis (A59.03)
 Valid 3-character code, no further characters required

+, +7th, X + 7th • Newborn • Pediatric • Maternity • Adult ♀ Female ♂ Male Manifestation Unacceptable PDX HCC CC MCC HAC

N34 Urethritis and urethral syndrome
Use additional code (B95-B97), to identify infectious agent.
Excludes2: *Reiter's disease (M02.3-)*
urethritis in diseases with a predominantly sexual mode
of transmission (A50-A64)
urethrotrigonitis (N30.3-)

CC **N34.0 Urethral abscess**
Abscess (of) Cowper's gland
Abscess (of) Littré's gland
Abscess (of) urethral (gland)
Periurethral abscess
Excludes1: *urethral caruncle (N36.2)*
HAC see Appendix B for HAC conditional logic

N34.1 Nonspecific urethritis
Nongonococcal urethritis
Nonvenereal urethritis

N34.2 Other urethritis
Meatitis, urethral
Postmenopausal urethritis
Ulcer of urethra (meatus)
Urethritis NOS

N34.3 Urethral syndrome, unspecified

N35 Urethral stricture
Excludes1: *congenital urethral stricture (Q64.3-)*
postprocedural urethral stricture (N99.1-)

+ **N35.0 Post-traumatic urethral stricture**
Urethral stricture due to injury
Excludes1: *postprocedural urethral stricture (N99.1-)*

+ **N35.01 Post-traumatic urethral stricture, male**
♂ **N35.010 Post-traumatic urethral stricture, male, meatal**
♂ **N35.011 Post-traumatic bulbous urethral stricture**
♂ **N35.012 Post-traumatic membranous urethral stricture**
♂ **N35.013 Post-traumatic anterior urethral stricture**
♂ **N35.014 Post-traumatic urethral stricture, male, unspecified**
♂ **N35.016 Post-traumatic urethral stricture, male, overlapping sites**
AHA CC: 4Q, 2018, 21-22

+ **N35.02 Post-traumatic urethral stricture, female**
♀ **N35.021 Urethral stricture due to childbirth**
♀ **N35.028 Other post-traumatic urethral stricture, female**

+ **N35.1 Postinfective urethral stricture, not elsewhere classified**
Excludes1: *urethral stricture associated with schistosomiasis (B65.-, N29)*
gonococcal urethral stricture (A54.01)
syphilitic urethral stricture (A52.76)

+ **N35.11 Postinfective urethral stricture, not elsewhere classified, male**
♂ **N35.111 Postinfective urethral stricture, not elsewhere classified, male, meatal**
♂ **N35.112 Postinfective bulbous urethral stricture, not elsewhere classified, male**
♂ **N35.113 Postinfective membranous urethral stricture, not elsewhere classified, male**
♂ **N35.114 Postinfective anterior urethral stricture, not elsewhere classified, male**
♂ **N35.116 Postinfective urethral stricture, not elsewhere classified, male, overlapping sites**
AHA CC: 4Q, 2018, 21-22
♂ **N35.119 Postinfective urethral stricture, not elsewhere classified, male, unspecified**
♀ **N35.12 Postinfective urethral stricture, not elsewhere classified, female**

+ **N35.8 Other urethral stricture**
Excludes1: *postprocedural urethral stricture (N99.1-)*

+ **N35.81 Other urethral stricture, male**
AHA CC: 4Q, 2018, 21-22
♂ **N35.811 Other urethral stricture, male, meatal**
♂ **N35.812 Other urethral bulbous stricture, male**
♂ **N35.813 Other membranous urethral stricture, male**
♂ **N35.814 Other anterior urethral stricture, male**

♂ **N35.816 Other urethral stricture, male, overlapping sites**
♂ **N35.819 Other urethral stricture, male, unspecified site**
♀ **N35.82 Other urethral stricture, female**
AHA CC: 4Q, 2018, 21-22

+ **N35.9 Urethral stricture, unspecified**
+ **N35.91 Urethral stricture, unspecified, male**
AHA CC: 4Q, 2018, 21-22
♂ **N35.911 Unspecified urethral stricture, male, meatal**
♂ **N35.912 Unspecified bulbous urethral stricture, male**
♂ **N35.913 Unspecified membranous urethral stricture, male**
♂ **N35.914 Unspecified anterior urethral stricture, male**
♂ **N35.916 Unspecified urethral stricture, male, overlapping sites**
♂ **N35.919 Unspecified urethral stricture, male, unspecified site**
Pinhole meatus NOS
Urethral stricture NOS
♀ **N35.92 Unspecified urethral stricture, female**
AHA CC: 4Q, 2018, 21-22

N36 Other disorders of urethra

CC **N36.0 Urethral fistula**
Urethroperineal fistula
Urethrorectal fistula
Urinary fistula NOS
Excludes1: *urethroscrotal fistula (N50.89)*
urethrovaginal fistula (N82.1)
urethrovesicovaginal fistula (N82.1)

N36.1 Urethral diverticulum

N36.2 Urethral caruncle

+ **N36.4 Urethral functional and muscular disorders**
Use additional code to identify associated urinary stress incontinence (N39.3)
N36.41 Hypermobility of urethra
N36.42 Intrinsic sphincter deficiency (ISD)
N36.43 Combined hypermobility of urethra and intrinsic sphincter deficiency
N36.44 Muscular disorders of urethra
Bladder sphincter dyssynergy

N36.5 Urethral false passage

N36.8 Other specified disorders of urethra
Excludes1: *congenital urethrocele (Q64.7)*
female urethrocele (N81.0)

N36.9 Urethral disorder, unspecified

N37 Urethral disorders in diseases classified elsewhere
Code first underlying disease
Excludes1: *urethritis (in):*
candidal infection (B37.41)
chlamydial (A56.01)
gonorrhea (A54.01)
syphilis (A52.76)
trichomonal infection (A59.03)
tuberculosis (A18.13)
Valid 3-character code, no further characters required

N39 Other disorders of urinary system
Excludes2: *hematuria NOS (R31.-)*
recurrent or persistent hematuria (N02.-)
recurrent or persistent hematuria with specified morphological lesion (N02.-)
proteinuria NOS (R80.-)

CC **N39.0 Urinary tract infection, site not specified**
Use additional code (B95-B97), to identify infectious agent
Excludes1: *candidiasis of urinary tract (B37.4-)*
neonatal urinary tract infection (P39.3)
pyuria (R82.81)
urinary tract infection of specified site, such as:
cystitis (N30.-)
urethritis (N34.-)
HAC see Appendix B for HAC conditional logic
AHA CC: 4Q, 2012, 94; 1Q, 2018, 16; 2Q, 2018, 22

+, +7th, X + 7th   ● Newborn   ● Pediatric   ● Maternity   ● Adult   ♀ Female   ♂ Male   Manifestation   Unacceptable PDX   HCC   CC   MCC   HAC

N39.3 Stress incontinence (female) (male)
Code also any associated overactive bladder (N32.81)
Excludes1: *mixed incontinence (N39.46)*

+ N39.4 Other specified urinary incontinence
Code also any associated overactive bladder (N32.81)
Excludes1: *enuresis NOS (R32)*
functional urinary incontinence (R39.81)
urinary incontinence associated with cognitive
impairment (R39.81)
urinary incontinence NOS (R32)
urinary incontinence of nonorganic origin (F98.0)

    N39.41 Urge incontinence
      Excludes1: *mixed incontinence (N39.46)*

    N39.42 Incontinence without sensory awareness
      Insensible (urinary) incontinence

    N39.43 Post-void dribbling
    N39.44 Nocturnal enuresis
    N39.45 Continuous leakage
    N39.46 Mixed incontinence
      Urge and stress incontinence

  + N39.49 Other specified urinary incontinence
      AHA CC: 4Q, 2016, 44

      N39.490 Overflow incontinence
      N39.491 Coital incontinence
      N39.492 Postural (urinary) incontinence
      N39.498 Other specified urinary incontinence
        Reflex incontinence
        Total incontinence

N39.8 Other specified disorders of urinary system
N39.9 Disorder of urinary system, unspecified

Diseases of male genital organs (N40-N53)

N40 Benign prostatic hyperplasia

Includes: adenofibromatous hypertrophy of prostate
benign hypertrophy of the prostate
benign prostatic hypertrophy
BPH
enlarged prostate
nodular prostate
polyp of prostate

Excludes1: *benign neoplasms of prostate (adenoma, benign)*
(fibroadenoma) (fibroma) (myoma) (D29.1)
Excludes2: *malignant neoplasm of prostate (C61)*

● ♂ **N40.0 Benign prostatic hyperplasia without lower urinary tract symptoms**
Enlarged prostate without LUTS
Enlarged prostate NOS

● ♂ **N40.1 Benign prostatic hyperplasia with lower urinary tract symptoms**
Enlarged prostate with LUTS
Use additional code for associated symptoms, when specified:
incomplete bladder emptying (R39.14)
nocturia (R35.1)
straining on urination (R39.16)
urinary frequency (R35.0)
urinary hesitancy (R39.11)
urinary incontinence (N39.4-)
urinary obstruction (N13.8)
urinary retention (R33.8)
urinary urgency (R39.15)
weak urinary stream (R39.12)

● ♂ **N40.2 Nodular prostate without lower urinary tract symptoms**
Nodular prostate without LUTS

● ♂ **N40.3 Nodular prostate with lower urinary tract symptoms**
Use additional code for associated symptoms, when specified:
incomplete bladder emptying (R39.14)
nocturia (R35.1)
straining on urination (R39.16)
urinary frequency (R35.0)
urinary hesitancy (R39.11)
urinary incontinence (N39.4-)
urinary obstruction (N13.8)
urinary retention (R33.8)
urinary urgency (R39.15)
weak urinary stream (R39.12)

N41 Inflammatory diseases of prostate
Use additional code (B95-B97), to identify infectious agent

● ♂ CC **N41.0 Acute prostatitis**
● ♂ **N41.1 Chronic prostatitis**
● ♂ CC **N41.2 Abscess of prostate**
● ♂ **N41.3 Prostatocystitis**
● ♂ **N41.4 Granulomatous prostatitis**
● ♂ **N41.8 Other inflammatory diseases of prostate**
● ♂ **N41.9 Inflammatory disease of prostate, unspecified**
Prostatitis NOS

N42 Other and unspecified disorders of prostate

● ♂ **N42.0 Calculus of prostate**
Prostatic stone

● ♂ **N42.1 Congestion and hemorrhage of prostate**
Excludes1: *enlarged prostate (N40.-)*
hematuria (R31.-)
hyperplasia of prostate (N40.-)
inflammatory diseases of prostate (N41.-)

+ N42.3 Dysplasia of prostate
AHA CC: 4Q, 2016, 44

  ♂ **N42.30 Unspecified dysplasia of prostate**
  ♂ **N42.31 Prostatic intraepithelial neoplasia**
    PIN
    Prostatic intraepithelial neoplasia I (PIN I)
    Prostatic intraepithelial neoplasia II (PIN II)
    Exlcudes1: *prostatic intraepithelial neoplasia III*
      (PIN III) (D07.5)
  ♂ **N42.32 Atypical small acinar proliferation of prostate**
  ♂ **N42.39 Other dysplasia of prostate**

+ N42.8 Other specified disorders of prostate
● ♂ **N42.81 Prostatodynia syndrome**
    Painful prostate syndrome
● ♂ **N42.82 Prostatosis syndrome**
● ♂ **N42.83 Cyst of prostate**
● ♂ **N42.89 Other specified disorders of prostate**

● ♂ **N42.9 Disorder of prostate, unspecified**

N43 Hydrocele and spermatocele

Includes: hydrocele of spermatic cord, testis or tunica vaginalis
Excludes1: *congenital hydrocele (P83.5)*

♂ **N43.0 Encysted hydrocele**
CC ♂ **N43.1 Infected hydrocele**
Use additional code (B95-B97), to identify infectious agent
♂ **N43.2 Other hydrocele**
♂ **N43.3 Hydrocele, unspecified**

+ N43.4 Spermatocele of epididymis
Spermatic cyst
  ♂ **N43.40 Spermatocele of epididymis, unspecified**
  ♂ **N43.41 Spermatocele of epididymis, single**
  ♂ **N43.42 Spermatocele of epididymis, multiple**

N44 Noninflammatory disorders of testis

+ N44.0 Torsion of testis
  CC ♂ **N44.00 Torsion of testis, unspecified**
  CC ♂ **N44.01 Extravaginal torsion of spermatic cord**
  CC ♂ **N44.02 Intravaginal torsion of spermatic cord**
    Torsion of spermatic cord NOS
  CC ♂ **N44.03 Torsion of appendix testis**
  CC ♂ **N44.04 Torsion of appendix epididymis**
♂ **N44.1 Cyst of tunica albuginea testis**
♂ **N44.2 Benign cyst of testis**
♂ **N44.8 Other noninflammatory disorders of the testis**

N45 Orchitis and epididymitis
Use additional code (B95-B97), to identify infectious agent
♂ **N45.1 Epididymitis**
♂ **N45.2 Orchitis**
♂ **N45.3 Epididymo-orchitis**
CC ♂ **N45.4 Abscess of epididymis or testis**

N46 Male infertility

Excludes1: *vasectomy status (Z98.52)*

+ N46.0 Azoospermia
Absolute male infertility
Male infertility due to germinal (cell) aplasia
Male infertility due to spermatogenic arrest (complete)
● ♂ **N46.01 Organic azoospermia**
    Azoospermia NOS

+, +7th, X + 7th ● Newborn ● Pediatric ● Maternity ● Adult ♀ Female ♂ Male Manifestation Unacceptable PDX HCC CC MCC HAC

Male Reproductive System

Seminal vesicle

Vas deferens

Rectum

Ejaculatory duct

Prostate gland

Bulbourethral gland

Vas deferens

Bladder

Pubic bone

Erectile tissue of penis

Urethra

Testis

Epididymis

Scrotum

Glans of penis

Prepuce

Median umbilical ligament

Ureter

Ampulla of ductus deferens

Urinary bladder

Prostate gland

Prostatic portion of urethra

Bulbourethral gland

Ductus deferens

Spongy portion of urethra

Penis

Head of epididymis

Testis

Epididymis

Body of epididymis

Tail of epididymis

Glans penis

Ductus deferens

Seminal vesicle

Ejaculatory duct

Inguinal canal

Cremaster muscle

Internal spermatic fascia

Spermatic cord

Testicular artery

Genital nerve

Ductus deferens

Venous plexus

Tunica vaginalis

Dartos fascia and muscle

Scrotum

©AHIMA

+ N46.02 Azoospermia due to extratesticular causes
Code also associated cause
- ♂ **N46.021 Azoospermia due to drug therapy**
- ♂ **N46.022 Azoospermia due to infection**
- ♂ **N46.023 Azoospermia due to obstruction of efferent ducts**
- ♂ **N46.024 Azoospermia due to radiation**
- ♂ **N46.025 Azoospermia due to systemic disease**
- ♂ **N46.029 Azoospermia due to other extratesticular causes**

+ N46.1 Oligospermia
Male infertility due to germinal cell desquamation
Male infertility due to hypospermatogenesis
Male infertility due to incomplete spermatogenic arrest
- ♂ **N46.11 Organic oligospermia**
Oligospermia NOS

+ N46.12 Oligospermia due to extratesticular causes
Code also associated cause
- ♂ **N46.121 Oligospermia due to drug therapy**
- ♂ **N46.122 Oligospermia due to infection**
- ♂ **N46.123 Oligospermia due to obstruction of efferent ducts**
- ♂ **N46.124 Oligospermia due to radiation**
- ♂ **N46.125 Oligospermia due to systemic disease**
- ♂ **N46.129 Oligospermia due to other extratesticular causes**

- ♂ **N46.8 Other male infertility**
- ♂ **N46.9 Male infertility, unspecified**

N47 Disorders of prepuce

- ♂ **N47.0 Adherent prepuce, newborn**
- ♂ **N47.1 Phimosis**
- ♂ **N47.2 Paraphimosis**
- ♂ **N47.3 Deficient foreskin**
- ♂ **N47.4 Benign cyst of prepuce**
- ♂ **N47.5 Adhesions of prepuce and glans penis**
- ♂ **N47.6 Balanoposthitis**
  Use additional code (B95-B97), to identify infectious agent
  Excludes1: *balanitis (N48.1)*
- ♂ **N47.7 Other inflammatory diseases of prepuce**
  Use additional code (B95-B97), to identify infectious agent
- ♂ **N47.8 Other disorders of prepuce**

N48 Other disorders of penis

- ♂ **N48.0 Leukoplakia of penis**
  Balanitis xerotica obliterans
  Kraurosis of penis
  Lichen sclerosus of external male genital organs
  Excludes1: *carcinoma in situ of penis (D07.4)*
- ♂ **N48.1 Balanitis**
  Use additional code (B95-B97), to identify infectious agent
  Excludes1: *amebic balanitis (A06.8)*
  balanitis xerotica obliterans (N48.0)
  candidal balanitis (B37.42)
  gonococcal balanitis (A54.23)
  herpesviral [herpes simplex] balanitis (A60.01)

+ N48.2 Other inflammatory disorders of penis
Use additional code (B95-B97), to identify infectious agent
Excludes1: *balanitis (N48.1)*
balanitis xerotica obliterans (N48.0)
balanoposthitis (N47.6)
- ♂ **N48.21 Abscess of corpus cavernosum and penis**
- ♂ **N48.22 Cellulitis of corpus cavernosum and penis**
- ♂ **N48.29 Other inflammatory disorders of penis**

+ N48.3 Priapism
Painful erection
Code first underlying cause
- CC ♂ **N48.30 Priapism, unspecified**
- CC ♂ **N48.31 Priapism due to trauma**
- CC ♂ **N48.32 Priapism due to disease classified elsewhere**
- CC ♂ **N48.33 Priapism, drug-induced**
- CC ♂ **N48.39 Other priapism**
- ♂ **N48.5 Ulcer of penis**
- ♂ **N48.6 Induration penis plastica**
  Peyronie's disease
  Plastic induration of penis

+ N48.8 Other specified disorders of penis
- ♂ **N48.81 Thrombosis of superficial vein of penis**
- ♂ **N48.82 Acquired torsion of penis**
  Acquired torsion of penis NOS
  Excludes1: *congenital torsion of penis (Q55.63)*

- ♂ **N48.83 Acquired buried penis**
  Excludes1: *congenital hidden penis (Q55.64)*
- ♂ **N48.89 Other specified disorders of penis**
- ♂ **N48.9 Disorder of penis, unspecified**

N49 Inflammatory disorders of male genital organs, not elsewhere classified
Use additional code (B95-B97), to identify infectious agent
Excludes1: *inflammation of penis (N48.1, N48.2-)*
orchitis and epididymitis (N45.-)
- ♂ **N49.0 Inflammatory disorders of seminal vesicle**
  Vesiculitis NOS
- ♂ **N49.1 Inflammatory disorders of spermatic cord, tunica vaginalis and vas deferens**
  Vasitis
- ♂ **N49.2 Inflammatory disorders of scrotum**
- ♂ **N49.3 Fournier gangrene**
  AHA CC: 2Q, 2020, 18
- ♂ **N49.8 Inflammatory disorders of other specified male genital organs**
  Inflammation of multiple sites in male genital organs
- ♂ **N49.9 Inflammatory disorder of unspecified male genital organ**
  Abscess of unspecified male genital organ
  Boil of unspecified male genital organ
  Carbuncle of unspecified male genital organ
  Cellulitis of unspecified male genital organ

N50 Other and unspecified disorders of male genital organs
Excludes2: *torsion of testis (N44.0-)*
- ♂ **N50.0 Atrophy of testis**
- ♂ **N50.1 Vascular disorders of male genital organs**
  Hematocele, NOS, of male genital organs
  Hemorrhage of male genital organs
  Thrombosis of male genital organs
- ♂ **N50.3 Cyst of epididymis**

+ N50.8 Other specified disorders of male genital organs
AHA CC: 4Q, 2016, 45
+ N50.81 Testicular pain
- ♂ **N50.811 Right testicular pain**
- ♂ **N50.812 Left testicular pain**
- ♂ **N50.819 Testicular pain, unspecified**
- ♂ **N50.82 Scrotal pain**
- ♂ **N50.89 Other specified disorders of the male genital organs**
  Atrophy of scrotum, seminal vesicle, spermatic cord, tunica vaginalis and vas deferens
  Chylocele, tunica vaginalis (nonfilarial) NOS
  Edema of scrotum, seminal vesicle, spermatic cord, tunica vaginalis and vas deferens
  Hypertrophy of scrotum, seminal vesicle, spermatic cord, tunica vaginalis and vas deferens
  Stricture of spermatic cord, tunical vaginalis, and vas deferens
  Ulcer of scrotum, seminal vesicle, spermatic cord, testis, tunica vaginalis and vas deferens
  Urethroscrotal fistula
- ♂ **N50.9 Disorder of male genital organs, unspecified**

♂ **N51 Disorders of male genital organs in diseases classified elsewhere**
Code first underlying disease, such as:
filariasis (B74.0-B74.9)
Excludes1: *amebic balanitis (A06.8)*
candidal balanitis (B37.42)
gonococcal balanitis (A54.23)
gonococcal prostatitis (A54.22)
herpesviral [herpes simplex] balanitis (A60.01)
trichomonal prostatitis (A59.02)
tuberculous prostatitis (A18.14)
Valid 3-character code, no further characters required

N52 Male erectile dysfunction
Excludes1: *psychogenic impotence (F52.21)*
+ N52.0 Vasculogenic erectile dysfunction
- ♂ **N52.01 Erectile dysfunction due to arterial insufficiency**
- ♂ **N52.02 Corporo-venous occlusive erectile dysfunction**
- ♂ **N52.03 Combined arterial insufficiency and corporo-venous occlusive erectile dysfunction**
- ♂ CC **N52.1 Erectile dysfunction due to diseases classified elsewhere**
  Code first underlying disease
- ♂ CC **N52.2 Drug-induced erectile dysfunction**

+ **N52.3 Postprocedural erectile dysfunction**
  AHA CC: 4Q, 2016, 45
  - ♂ **N52.31 Erectile dysfunction following radical prostatectomy**
  - ♂ **N52.32 Erectile dysfunction following radical cystectomy**
  - ♂ **N52.33 Erectile dysfunction following urethral surgery**
  - ♂ **N52.34 Erectile dysfunction following simple prostatectomy**
  - ♂ **N52.35 Erectile dysfunction following radiation therapy**
  - ♂ **N52.36 Erectile dysfunction following interstitial seed therapy**
  - ♂ **N52.37 Erectile dysfunction following prostate ablative therapy**
    Erectile dysfunction following cryotherapy
    Erectile dysfunction following other prostate ablative therapies
    Erectile dysfunction following ultrasound ablative therapies
  - ♂ **N52.39 Other and unspecified postprocedural erectile dysfunction**
- ♂ **N52.8 Other male erectile dysfunction**
- ♂ **N52.9 Male erectile dysfunction, unspecified**
    Impotence NOS

N53 Other male sexual dysfunction

  Excludes1: psychogenic sexual dysfunction (F52.-)
+ **N53.1 Ejaculatory dysfunction**
    Excludes1: premature ejaculation (F52.4)
  - ♂ **N53.11 Retarded ejaculation**
  - ♂ **N53.12 Painful ejaculation**
  - ♂ **N53.13 Anejaculatory orgasm**
  - ♂ **N53.14 Retrograde ejaculation**
  - ♂ **N53.19 Other ejaculatory dysfunction**
      Ejaculatory dysfunction NOS
  - ♂ **N53.8 Other male sexual dysfunction**
  - ♂ **N53.9 Unspecified male sexual dysfunction**

Disorders of breast (N60-N65)

Excludes1: disorders of breast associated with childbirth (O91-O92)

N60 Benign mammary dysplasia

    Includes: fibrocystic mastopathy
+ **N60.0 Solitary cyst of breast**
    Cyst of breast
    N60.01 Solitary cyst of right breast
    N60.02 Solitary cyst of left breast
    N60.09 Solitary cyst of unspecified breast
+ **N60.1 Diffuse cystic mastopathy**
    Cystic breast
    Fibrocystic disease of breast
    Excludes1: diffuse cystic mastopathy with epithelial proliferation (N60.3-)
  - **N60.11 Diffuse cystic mastopathy of right breast**
  - **N60.12 Diffuse cystic mastopathy of left breast**
  - **N60.19 Diffuse cystic mastopathy of unspecified breast**
+ **N60.2 Fibroadenosis of breast**
    Adenofibrosis of breast
    Excludes2: fibroadenoma of breast (D24.-)
    N60.21 Fibroadenosis of right breast
    N60.22 Fibroadenosis of left breast
    N60.29 Fibroadenosis of unspecified breast
+ **N60.3 Fibrosclerosis of breast**
    Cystic mastopathy with epithelial proliferation
    N60.31 Fibrosclerosis of right breast
    N60.32 Fibrosclerosis of left breast
    N60.39 Fibrosclerosis of unspecified breast
+ **N60.4 Mammary duct ectasia**
    N60.41 Mammary duct ectasia of right breast
    N60.42 Mammary duct ectasia of left breast
    N60.49 Mammary duct ectasia of unspecified breast
+ **N60.8 Other benign mammary dysplasias**
    N60.81 Other benign mammary dysplasias of right breast
    N60.82 Other benign mammary dysplasias of left breast
    N60.89 Other benign mammary dysplasias of unspecified breast
+ **N60.9 Unspecified benign mammary dysplasia**
    N60.91 Unspecified benign mammary dysplasia of right breast

N60.92 Unspecified benign mammary dysplasia of left breast
N60.99 Unspecified benign mammary dysplasia of unspecified breast

N61 Inflammatory disorders of breast

  Excludes1: inflammatory carcinoma of breast (C50.9)
      inflammatory disorder of breast associated with childbirth (O91.-)
      neonatal infective mastitis (P39.0)
      thrombophlebitis of breast [Mondor's disease] (I80.8)
  N61.0 Mastitis without abscess
    Infective mastitis (acute) (nonpuerperal) (subacute)
    Mastitis (acute) (nonpuerperal) (subacute) NOS
    Cellulitis (acute) (nonpuerperal) (subacute) of breast NOS
    Cellulitis (acute) (nonpuerperal) (subacute) of nipple NOS
  N61.1 Abscess of the breast and nipple
    Abscess (acute) (chronic) (nonpuerperal) of areola
    Abscess (acute) (chronic) (nonpuerperal) of breast
    Carbuncle of breast
    Mastitis with abscess
+ **N61.2 Granulomatous mastitis**
    N61.20 Granulomatous mastitis, unspecified breast
    N61.21 Granulomatous mastitis, right breast
    N61.22 Granulomatous mastitis, left breast
    N61.23 Granulomatous mastitis, bilateral breast

N62 Hypertrophy of breast

    Gynecomastia
    Hypertrophy of breast NOS
    Massive pubertal hypertrophy of breast
    Excludes1: breast engorgement of newborn (P83.4)
        disproportion of reconstructed breast (N65.1)
    Valid 3-character code, no further characters required

N63 Unspecified lump in breast

    Nodule(s) NOS in breast
    AHA CC: 4Q, 2017, 19
  N63.0 Unspecified lump in unspecified breast
+ **N63.1 Unspecified lump in the right breast**
    N63.10 Unspecified lump in the right breast, unspecified quadrant
    N63.11 Unspecified lump in the right breast, upper outer quadrant
    N63.12 Unspecified lump in the right breast, upper inner quadrant
    N63.13 Unspecified lump in the right breast, lower outer quadrant
    N63.14 Unspecified lump in the right breast, lower inner quadrant
    N63.15 Unspecified lump in the right breast, overlapping quadrants
        AHA CC: 4Q, 2019, 12
+ **N63.2 Unspecified lump in the left breast**
    N63.20 Unspecified lump in the left breast, unspecified quadrant
    N63.21 Unspecified lump in the left breast, upper outer quadrant
    N63.22 Unspecified lump in the left breast, upper inner quadrant
    N63.23 Unspecified lump in the left breast, lower outer quadrant
    N63.24 Unspecified lump in the left breast, lower inner quadrant
    N63.25 Unspecified lump in the left breast, overlapping quadrants
        AHA CC: 4Q, 2019, 12
+ **N63.3 Unspecified lump in axillary tail**
    N63.31 Unspecified lump in axillary tail of the right breast
    N63.32 Unspecified lump in axillary tail of the left breast
+ **N63.4 Unspecified lump in breast, subareolar**
    N63.41 Unspecified lump in right breast, subareolar
    N63.42 Unspecified lump in left breast, subareolar

N64 Other disorders of breast

    Excludes2: mechanical complication of breast prosthesis and implant (T85.4-)
  N64.0 Fissure and fistula of nipple
  N64.1 Fat necrosis of breast
    Fat necrosis (segmental) of breast
    Code first breast necrosis due to breast graft (T85.898)

Breast

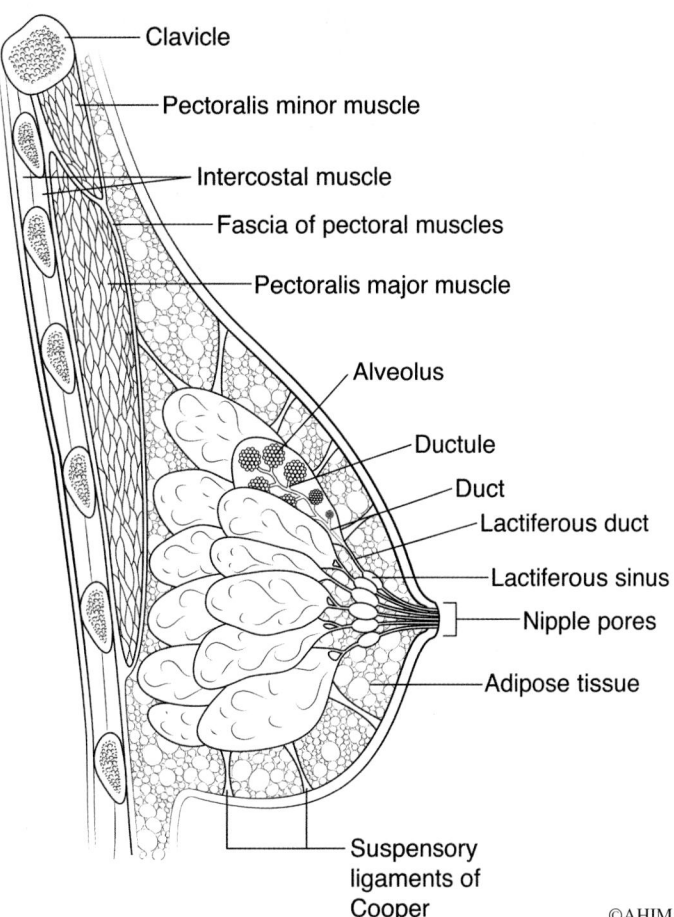

- Clavicle
- Pectoralis minor muscle
- Intercostal muscle
- Fascia of pectoral muscles
- Pectoralis major muscle
- Alveolus
- Ductule
- Duct
- Lactiferous duct
- Lactiferous sinus
- Nipple pores
- Adipose tissue
- Suspensory ligaments of Cooper

©AHIMA

N64.2 **Atrophy of breast**
N64.3 **Galactorrhea not associated with childbirth**
N64.4 **Mastodynia**
+ N64.5 **Other signs and symptoms in breast**
    Excludes2: *abnormal findings on diagnostic imaging of breast (R92.-)*
    N64.51 **Induration of breast**
    N64.52 **Nipple discharge**
    Excludes1: *abnormal findings in nipple discharge (R89.-)*
    N64.53 **Retraction of nipple**
    N64.59 **Other signs and symptoms in breast**
+ N64.8 **Other specified disorders of breast**
    • N64.81 **Ptosis of breast**
      Excludes1: *ptosis of native breast in relation to reconstructed breast (N65.1)*
    • N64.82 **Hypoplasia of breast**
      Micromastia
      Excludes1: *congenital absence of breast (Q83.0)*
                hypoplasia of native breast in relation to reconstructed breast (N65.1)
    N64.89 **Other specified disorders of breast**
      Galactocele
      Subinvolution of breast (postlactational)
      AHA CC: 1Q, 2018, 3-4; 1Q, 2019, 32
N64.9 **Disorder of breast, unspecified**

N65 **Deformity and disproportion of reconstructed breast**

• N65.0 **Deformity of reconstructed breast**
    Contour irregularity in reconstructed breast
    Excess tissue in reconstructed breast
    Misshapen reconstructed breast
• N65.1 **Disproportion of reconstructed breast**
    Breast asymmetry between native breast and reconstructed breast
    Disproportion between native breast and reconstructed breast

Inflammatory diseases of female pelvic organs (N70-N77)

Excludes1: *inflammatory diseases of female pelvic organs complicating:*
    abortion or ectopic or molar pregnancy (O00-O07, O08.0)
    pregnancy, childbirth and the puerperium (O23.-, O75.3, O85, O86.-)

N70 **Salpingitis and oophoritis**

    Includes: abscess (of) fallopian tube
      abscess (of) ovary
      pyosalpinx
      salpingo-oophoritis
      tubo-ovarian abscess
      tubo-ovarian inflammatory disease
    Use additional code (B95-B97), to identify infectious agent
    Excludes1: *gonococcal infection (A54.24)*
               tuberculous infection (A18.17)
+ N70.0 **Acute salpingitis and oophoritis**
    ♀ CC N70.01 **Acute salpingitis**
    ♀ CC N70.02 **Acute oophoritis**
    ♀ CC N70.03 **Acute salpingitis and oophoritis**
+ N70.1 **Chronic salpingitis and oophoritis**
    Hydrosalpinx
    ♀ N70.11 **Chronic salpingitis**
    ♀ N70.12 **Chronic oophoritis**
    ♀ N70.13 **Chronic salpingitis and oophoritis**
+ N70.9 **Salpingitis and oophoritis, unspecified**
    ♀ N70.91 **Salpingitis, unspecified**
    ♀ N70.92 **Oophoritis, unspecified**
    ♀ N70.93 **Salpingitis and oophoritis, unspecified**

+, +7th, X + 7th   • Newborn   • Pediatric   • Maternity   • Adult   ♀ Female   ♂ Male   Manifestation   Unacceptable PDX   HCC   CC   MCC   HAC

Female Reproductive System

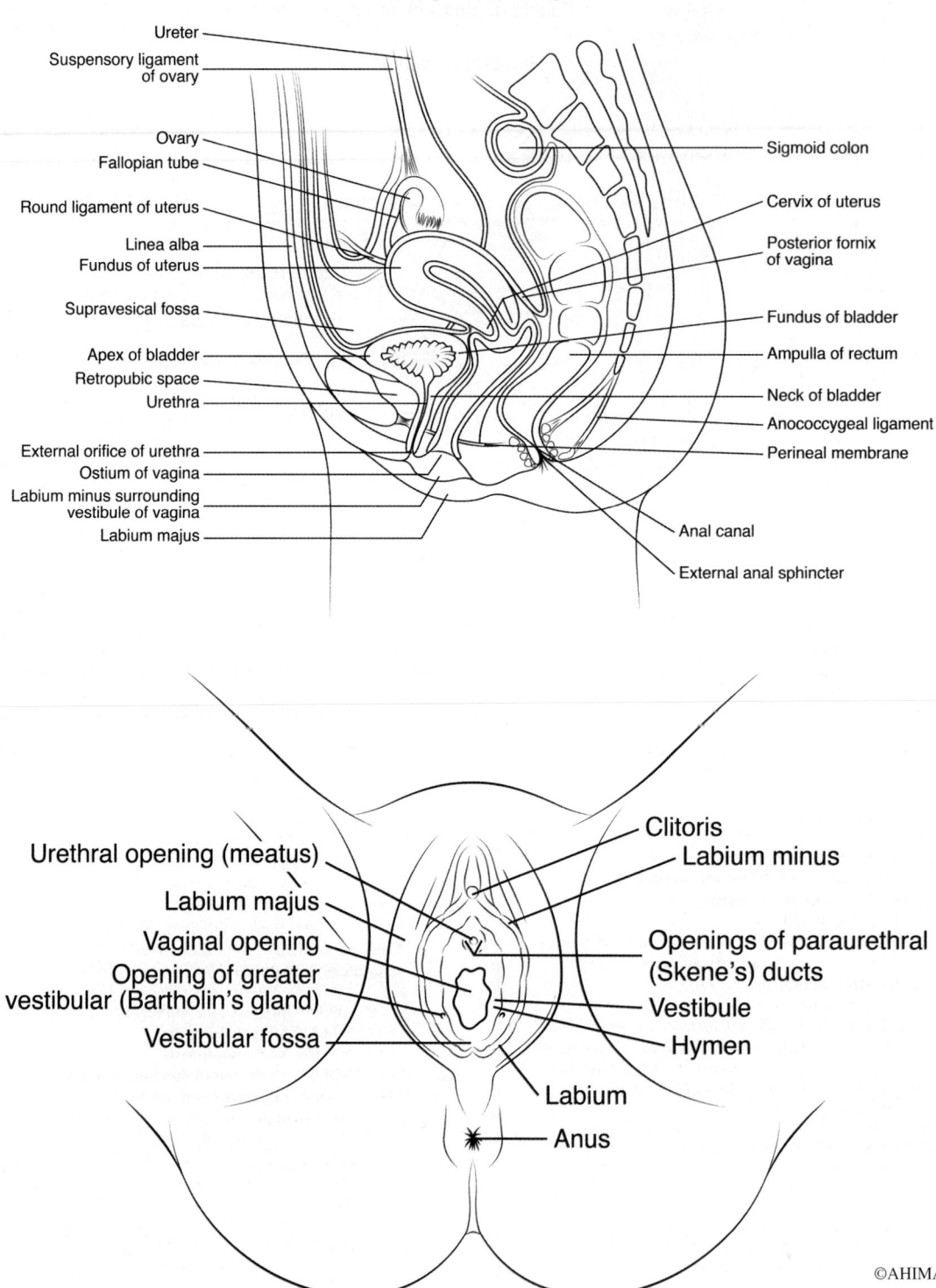

Ureter
Suspensory ligament of ovary
Ovary
Fallopian tube
Round ligament of uterus
Linea alba
Fundus of uterus
Supravesical fossa
Apex of bladder
Retropubic space
Urethra
External orifice of urethra
Ostium of vagina
Labium minus surrounding vestibule of vagina
Labium majus

Sigmoid colon
Cervix of uterus
Posterior fornix of vagina
Fundus of bladder
Ampulla of rectum
Neck of bladder
Anococcygeal ligament
Perineal membrane
Anal canal
External anal sphincter

Urethral opening (meatus)
Labium majus
Vaginal opening
Opening of greater vestibular (Bartholin's gland)
Vestibular fossa

Clitoris
Labium minus
Openings of paraurethral (Skene's) ducts
Vestibule
Hymen
Labium
Anus

©AHIMA

N71   Inflammatory disease of uterus, except cervix

> **Includes:** endo (myo) metritis
> metritis
> myometritis
> pyometra
> uterine abscess
> Use additional code (B95-B97), to identify infectious agent
> *Excludes1:* *hyperplastic endometritis (N85.0-)*
> *infection of uterus following delivery (O85, O86.-)*

♀ CC **N71.0   Acute inflammatory disease of uterus**
   ♀ **N71.1   Chronic inflammatory disease of uterus**
   ♀ **N71.9   Inflammatory disease of uterus, unspecified**

♀ **N72   Inflammatory disease of cervix uteri**

> **Includes:** cervicitis (with or without erosion or ectropion)
> endocervicitis (with or without erosion or ectropion)
> exocervicitis (with or without erosion or ectropion)
> Use additional code (B95-B97), to identify infectious agent
> *Excludes1:* *erosion and ectropion of cervix without cervicitis (N86)*
> **Valid 3-character code, no further characters required**

N73   Other female pelvic inflammatory diseases

> Use additional code (B95-B97), to identify infectious agent

♀ CC **N73.0   Acute parametritis and pelvic cellulitis**
> Abscess of broad ligament
> Abscess of parametrium
> Pelvic cellulitis, female
   ♀ **N73.1   Chronic parametritis and pelvic cellulitis**
> Any condition in N73.0 specified as chronic
> *Excludes1:* *tuberculous parametritis and pelvic cellultis*
> *(A18.17)*
   ♀ **N73.2   Unspecified parametritis and pelvic cellulitis**
> Any condition in N73.0 unspecified whether acute or chronic
♀ MCC **N73.3   Female acute pelvic peritonitis**
♀ CC **N73.4   Female chronic pelvic peritonitis**
> *Excludes1:* *tuberculous pelvic (female) peritonitis (A18.17)*
   ♀ **N73.5   Female pelvic peritonitis, unspecified**
   ♀ **N73.6   Female pelvic peritoneal adhesions (postinfective)**
> *Excludes2:* *postprocedural pelvic peritoneal adhesions*
> *(N99.4)*
> *AHA CC: 1Q, 2014, 6*
   ♀ **N73.8   Other specified female pelvic inflammatory diseases**
   ♀ **N73.9   Female pelvic inflammatory disease, unspecified**
> Female pelvic infection or inflammation NOS

♀ **N74   Female pelvic inflammatory disorders in diseases classified elsewhere**

> Code first underlying disease
> *Excludes1:* *chlamydial cervicitis (A56.02)*
> *chlamydial pelvic inflammatory disease (A56.11)*
> *gonococcal cervicitis (A54.03)*
> *gonococcal pelvic inflammatory disease (A54.24)*
> *herpesviral [herpes simplex] cervicitis (A60.03)*
> *herpesviral [herpes simplex] pelvic inflammatory*
> *disease (A60.09)*
> *syphilitic cervicitis (A52.76)*
> *syphilitic pelvic inflammatory disease (A52.76)*
> *trichomonal cervicitis (A59.09)*
> *tuberculous cervicitis (A18.16)*
> *tuberculous pelvic inflammatory disease (A18.17)*
> **Valid 3-character code, no further characters required**

N75   Diseases of Bartholin's gland

   ♀ **N75.0   Cyst of Bartholin's gland**
♀ CC **N75.1   Abscess of Bartholin's gland**
   ♀ **N75.8   Other diseases of Bartholin's gland**
> Bartholinitis
   ♀ **N75.9   Disease of Bartholin's gland, unspecified**

N76   Other inflammation of vagina and vulva

> Use additional code (B95-B97), to identify infectious agent
> *Excludes2:* *senile (atrophic) vaginitis (N95.2)*
> *vulvar vestibulitis (N94.810)*

   ♀ **N76.0   Acute vaginitis**
> Acute vulvovaginitis
> Vaginitis NOS
> Vulvovaginitis NOS

   ♀ **N76.1   Subacute and chronic vaginitis**
> Chronic vulvovaginitis
> Subacute vulvovaginitis
   ♀ **N76.2   Acute vulvitis**
> Vulvitis NOS
   ♀ **N76.3   Subacute and chronic vulvitis**
♀ CC **N76.4   Abscess of vulva**
> Furuncle of vulva
   ♀ **N76.5   Ulceration of vagina**
   ♀ **N76.6   Ulceration of vulva**
+ **N76.8   Other specified inflammation of vagina and vulva**
   ♀ CC **N76.81   Mucositis (ulcerative) of vagina and vulva**
> Code also type of associated therapy, such as:
> antineoplastic and immunosuppressive
> drugs (T45.1X-)
> radiological procedure and radiotherapy (Y84.2)
> *Excludes2:* *gastrointestinal mucositis (ulcerative)*
> *(K92.81)*
> *nasal mucositis (ulcerative) (J34.81)*
> *oral mucositis (ulcerative) (K12.3-)*
   ♀ **N76.89   Other specified inflammation of vagina and vulva**

N77   Vulvovaginal ulceration and inflammation in diseases classified elsewhere

♀ **N77.0   Ulceration of vulva in diseases classified elsewhere**
> Code first underlying disease, such as:
> Behçet's disease (M35.2)
> *Excludes1:* *ulceration of vulva in gonococcal infection*
> *(A54.02)*
> *ulceration of vulva in herpesviral [herpes*
> *simplex] infection (A60.04)*
> *ulceration of vulva in syphilis (A51.0)*
> *ulceration of vulva in tuberculosis (A18.18)*
♀ **N77.1   Vaginitis, vulvitis and vulvovaginitis in diseases classified elsewhere**
> Code first underlying disease, such as:
> pinworm (B80)
> *Excludes1:* *candidal vulvovaginitis (B37.3)*
> *chlamydial vulvovaginitis (A56.02)*
> *gonococcal vulvovaginitis (A54.02)*
> *herpesviral [herpes simplex] vulvovaginitis*
> *(A60.04)*
> *trichomonal vulvovaginitis (A59.01)*
> *tuberculous vulvovaginitis (A18.18)*
> *vulvovaginitis in early syphilis (A51.0)*
> *vulvovaginitis in late syphilis (A52.76)*

Noninflammatory disorders of female genital tract (N80-N98)

N80   Endometriosis

   ♀ **N80.0   Endometriosis of uterus**
> Adenomyosis
> *Excludes1:* *stromal endometriosis (D39.0)*
   ♀ **N80.1   Endometriosis of ovary**
   ♀ **N80.2   Endometriosis of fallopian tube**
   ♀ **N80.3   Endometriosis of pelvic peritoneum**
   ♀ **N80.4   Endometriosis of rectovaginal septum and vagina**
   ♀ **N80.5   Endometriosis of intestine**
   ♀ **N80.6   Endometriosis in cutaneous scar**
   ♀ **N80.8   Other endometriosis**
> Endometriosis of thorax
   ♀ **N80.9   Endometriosis, unspecified**

N81   Female genital prolapse
> **See page 864 for Vaginal Prolapse illustration.**

> *Excludes1:* *genital prolapse complicating pregnancy, labor or*
> *delivery (O34.5-)*
> *prolapse and hernia of ovary and fallopian tube*
> *(N83.4-)*
> *prolapse of vaginal vault after hysterectomy (N99.3)*
♀ **N81.0   Urethrocele**
> *Excludes1:* *urethrocele with cystocele (N81.1-)*
> *urethrocele with prolapse of uterus*
> *(N81.2-N81.4)*

+, +7th, X + 7th   • Newborn   • Pediatric   • Maternity   • Adult   ♀ Female   ♂ Male   Manifestation   Unacceptable PDX   HCC   CC   MCC   HAC

Vaginal Prolapse

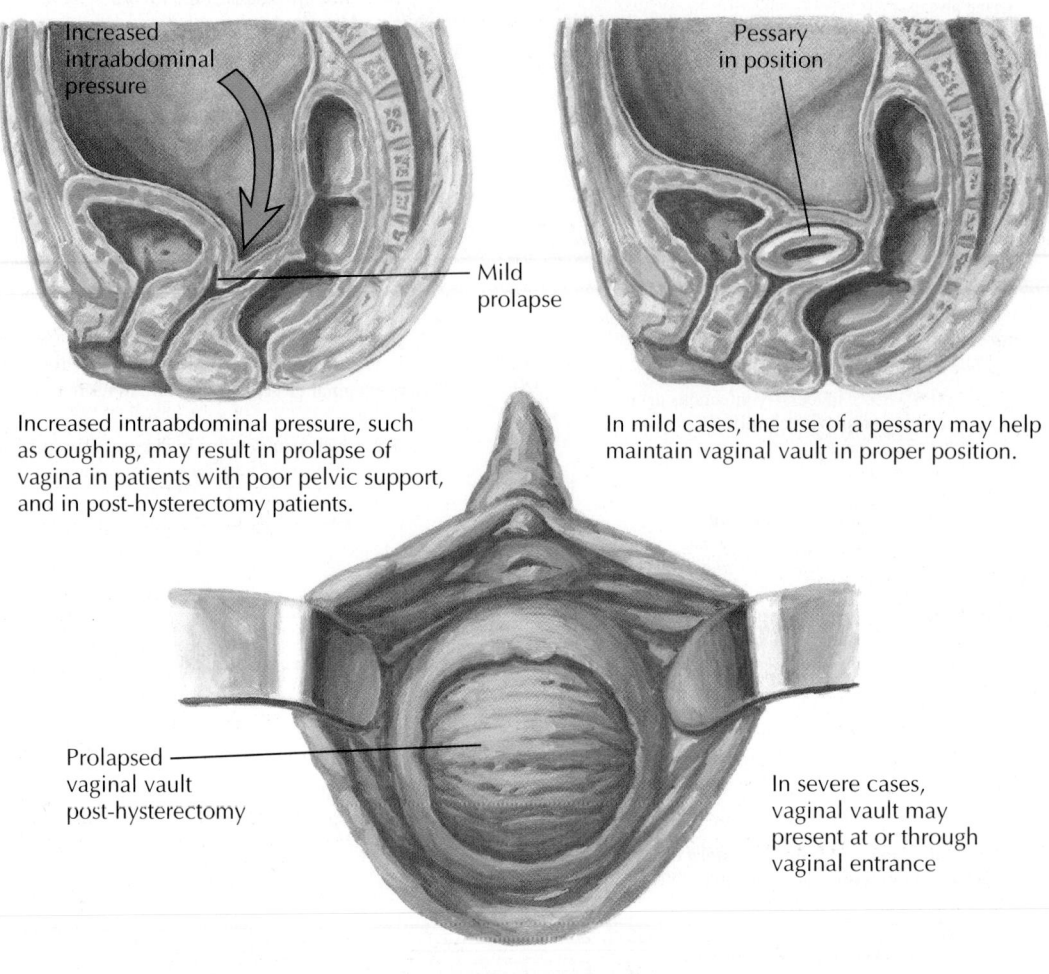

Increased intraabdominal pressure

Mild prolapse

Increased intraabdominal pressure, such as coughing, may result in prolapse of vagina in patients with poor pelvic support, and in post-hysterectomy patients.

Pessary in position

In mild cases, the use of a pessary may help maintain vaginal vault in proper position.

Prolapsed vaginal vault post-hysterectomy

In severe cases, vaginal vault may present at or through vaginal entrance

JOHN A. CRAIG—AD

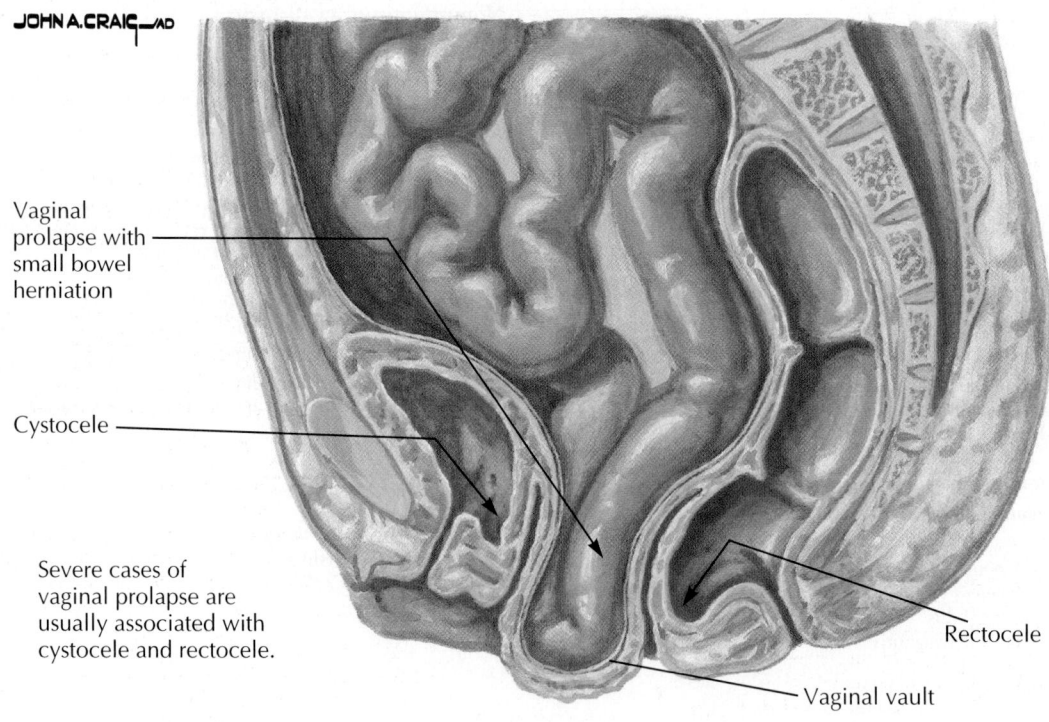

Vaginal prolapse with small bowel herniation

Cystocele

Severe cases of vaginal prolapse are usually associated with cystocele and rectocele.

Rectocele

Vaginal vault

+ **N81.1** **Cystocele**
    Cystocele with urethrocele
    Cystourethrocele
    Excludes1: cystocele with prolapse of uterus (N81.2-N81.4)
  ♀ **N81.10** **Cystocele, unspecified**
      Prolapse of (anterior) vaginal wall NOS
  ♀ **N81.11** **Cystocele, midline**
  ♀ **N81.12** **Cystocele, lateral**
      Paravaginal cystocele
♀ **N81.2** **Incomplete uterovaginal prolapse**
    First degree uterine prolapse
    Prolapse of cervix NOS
    Second degree uterine prolapse
    Excludes1: cervical stump prolapse (N81.85)
♀ **N81.3** **Complete uterovaginal prolapse**
    Procidentia (uteri) NOS
    Third degree uterine prolapse
♀ **N81.4** **Uterovaginal prolapse, unspecified**
    Prolapse of uterus NOS
♀ **N81.5** **Vaginal enterocele**
    Excludes1: enterocele with prolapse of uterus
             (N81.2-N81.4)
♀ **N81.6** **Rectocele**
    Prolapse of posterior vaginal wall
    Use additional code for any associated fecal incontinence,
      if applicable (R15.-)
    Excludes2: perineocele (N81.81)
           rectal prolapse (K62.3)
           rectocele with prolapse of uterus (N81.2-N81.4)
+ **N81.8** **Other female genital prolapse**
  ♀ **N81.81** **Perineocele**
  ♀ **N81.82** **Incompetence or weakening of pubocervical tissue**
  ♀ **N81.83** **Incompetence or weakening of rectovaginal tissue**
  ♀ **N81.84** **Pelvic muscle wasting**
      Disuse atrophy of pelvic muscles and anal sphincter
  ♀ **N81.85** **Cervical stump prolapse**
  ♀ **N81.89** **Other female genital prolapse**
      Deficient perineum
      Old laceration of muscles of pelvic floor
♀ **N81.9** **Female genital prolapse, unspecified**

N82 **Fistulae involving female genital tract**
    Excludes1: vesicointestinal fistulae (N32.1)
♀ CC **N82.0** **Vesicovaginal fistula**
♀ CC **N82.1** **Other female urinary-genital tract fistulae**
    Cervicovesical fistula
    Ureterovaginal fistula
    Urethrovaginal fistula
    Uteroureteric fistula
    Uterovesical fistula
    AHA CC: 3Q, 2017, 3-4
♀ CC **N82.2** **Fistula of vagina to small intestine**
♀ CC **N82.3** **Fistula of vagina to large intestine**
    Rectovaginal fistula
♀ CC **N82.4** **Other female intestinal-genital tract fistulae**
    Intestinouterine fistula
♀ CC **N82.5** **Female genital tract-skin fistulae**
    Uterus to abdominal wall fistula
    Vaginoperineal fistula
♀ CC **N82.8** **Other female genital tract fistulae**
♀ CC **N82.9** **Female genital tract fistula, unspecified**

N83 **Noninflammatory disorders of ovary, fallopian tube and broad ligament**
    Excludes2: hydrosalpinx (N70.1-)
    AHA CC: 4Q, 2016, 46
+ **N83.0** **Follicular cyst of ovary**
    Cyst of graafian follicle
    Hemorrhagic follicular cyst (of ovary)
  ♀ **N83.00** **Follicular cyst of ovary, unspecified side**
  ♀ **N83.01** **Follicular cyst of right ovary**
  ♀ **N83.02** **Follicular cyst of left ovary**
+ **N83.1** **Corpus luteum cyst**
    Hemorrhagic corpus luteum cyst
  ♀ **N83.10** **Corpus luteum cyst of ovary, unspecified side**
  ♀ **N83.11** **Corpus luteum cyst of right ovary**
  ♀ **N83.12** **Corpus luteum cyst of left ovary**

+ **N83.2** **Other and unspecified ovarian cysts**
    Excludes1: developmental ovarian cyst (Q50.1)
           neoplastic ovarian cyst (D27.-)
           polycystic ovarian syndrome (E28.2)
           Stein-Leventhal syndrome (E28.2)
+ **N83.20** **Unspecified ovarian cysts**
  ♀ **N83.201** **Unspecified ovarian cyst, right side**
  ♀ **N83.202** **Unspecified ovarian cyst, left side**
  ♀ **N83.209** **Unspecified ovarian cyst, unspecified side**
      Ovarian cyst, NOS
+ **N83.29** **Other ovarian cysts**
    Retention cyst of ovary
    Simple cyst of ovary
  ♀ **N83.291** **Other ovarian cyst, right side**
  ♀ **N83.292** **Other ovarian cyst, left side**
  ♀ **N83.299** **Other ovarian cyst, unspecified side**
+ **N83.3** **Acquired atrophy of ovary and fallopian tube**
  + **N83.31** **Acquired atrophy of ovary**
    ♀ **N83.311** **Acquired atrophy of right ovary**
    ♀ **N83.312** **Acquired atrophy of left ovary**
    ♀ **N83.319** **Acquired atrophy of ovary, unspecified side**
        Acquired atrophy of ovary, NOS
  + **N83.32** **Acquired atrophy of fallopian tube**
    ♀ **N83.321** **Acquired atrophy of right fallopian tube**
    ♀ **N83.322** **Acquired atrophy of left fallopian tube**
    ♀ **N83.329** **Acquired atrophy of fallopian tube, unspecified side**
        Acquired atrophy of fallopian tube, NOS
  + **N83.33** **Acquired atrophy of ovary and fallopian tube**
    ♀ **N83.331** **Acquired atrophy of right ovary and fallopian tube**
    ♀ **N83.332** **Acquired atrophy of left ovary and fallopian tube**
    ♀ **N83.339** **Acquired atrophy of ovary and fallopian tube, unspecified side**
        Acquired atrophy of ovary and fallopian tube, NOS
+ **N83.4** **Prolapse and hernia of ovary and fallopian tube**
  ♀ **N83.40** **Prolapse and hernia of ovary and fallopian tube, unspecified side**
      Prolapse and hernia of ovary and fallopian tube, NOS
  ♀ **N83.41** **Prolapse and hernia of right ovary and fallopian tube**
  ♀ **N83.42** **Prolapse and hernia of left ovary and fallopian tube**
+ **N83.5** **Torsion of ovary, ovarian pedicle and fallopian tube**
    Torsion of accessory tube
  + **N83.51** **Torsion of ovary and ovarian pedicle**
    ♀ CC **N83.511** **Torsion of right ovary and ovarian pedicle**
    ♀ CC **N83.512** **Torsion of left ovary and ovarian pedicle**
    ♀ CC **N83.519** **Torsion of ovary and ovarian pedicle, unspecified side**
        Torsion of ovary and ovarian pedicle, NOS
  + **N83.52** **Torsion of fallopian tube**
    Torsion of hydatid of Morgagni
    ♀ CC **N83.521** **Torsion of right fallopian tube**
    ♀ CC **N83.522** **Torsion of left fallopian tube**
    ♀ CC **N83.529** **Torsion of fallopian tube, unspecified side**
        Torsion of fallopian tube, NOS
  ♀ CC **N83.53** **Torsion of ovary, ovarian pedicle and fallopian tube**
♀ **N83.6** **Hematosalpinx**
    Excludes1: hematosalpinx (with) (in):
           hematocolpos (N89.7)
           hematometra (N85.7)
           tubal pregnancy (O00.1-)
♀ **N83.7** **Hematoma of broad ligament**
♀ **N83.8** **Other noninflammatory disorders of ovary, fallopian tube and broad ligament**
    Broad ligament laceration syndrome [Allen-Masters]
♀ **N83.9** **Noninflammatory disorder of ovary, fallopian tube and broad ligament, unspecified**

+, +7th, X + 7th   ● Newborn   ● Pediatric   ● Maternity   ● Adult   ♀ Female   ♂ Male   Manifestation   Unacceptable PDX   HCC   CC   MCC   HAC

N84 **Polyp of female genital tract**

> *Excludes1:* *adenomatous polyp (D28.-)*
> *placental polyp (O90.89)*

♀ **N84.0** **Polyp of corpus uteri**
Polyp of endometrium
Polyp of uterus NOS

> *Excludes1:* *polypoid endometrial hyperplasia (N85.0-)*

♀ **N84.1** **Polyp of cervix uteri**
Mucous polyp of cervix

♀ **N84.2** **Polyp of vagina**

♀ **N84.3** **Polyp of vulva**
Polyp of labia

♀ **N84.8** **Polyp of other parts of female genital tract**

♀ **N84.9** **Polyp of female genital tract, unspecified**

N85 **Other noninflammatory disorders of uterus, except cervix**

> *Excludes1:* *endometriosis (N80.-)*
> *inflammatory diseases of uterus (N71.-)*
> *noninflammatory disorders of cervix, except malposition*
> *(N86-N88)*
> *polyp of corpus uteri (N84.0)*
> *uterine prolapse (N81.-)*

+ **N85.0** **Endometrial hyperplasia**

♀ **N85.00** **Endometrial hyperplasia, unspecified**
Hyperplasia (adenomatous) (cystic) (glandular) of
endometrium
Hyperplastic endometritis

♀ **N85.01** **Benign endometrial hyperplasia**
Endometrial hyperplasia (complex) (simple)
without atypia

♀ **N85.02** **Endometrial intraepithelial neoplasia [EIN]**
Endometrial hyperplasia with atypia

> *Excludes1:* *malignant neoplasm of endometrium*
> *(with endometrial intraepithelial*
> *neoplasia [EIN]) (C54.1)*

♀ **N85.2** **Hypertrophy of uterus**
Bulky or enlarged uterus

> *Excludes1:* *puerperal hypertrophy of uterus (O90.89)*

♀ **N85.3** **Subinvolution of uterus**

> *Excludes1:* *puerperal subinvolution of uterus (O90.89)*

♀ **N85.4** **Malposition of uterus**
Anteversion of uterus
Retroflexion of uterus
Retroversion of uterus

> *Excludes1:* *malposition of uterus complicating pregnancy,*
> *labor or delivery (O34.5-, O65.5)*

♀ **N85.5** **Inversion of uterus**

> *Excludes1:* *current obstetric trauma (O71.2)*
> *postpartum inversion of uterus (O71.2)*

♀ **N85.6** **Intrauterine synechiae**

♀ **N85.7** **Hematometra**
Hematosalpinx with hematometra

> *Excludes1:* *hematometra with hematocolpos (N89.7)*

♀ **N85.8** **Other specified noninflammatory disorders of uterus**
Atrophy of uterus, acquired
Fibrosis of uterus NOS

♀ **N85.9** **Noninflammatory disorder of uterus, unspecified**
Disorder of uterus NOS

♀ **N86** **Erosion and ectropion of cervix uteri**
Decubitus (trophic) ulcer of cervix
Eversion of cervix

> *Excludes1:* *erosion and ectropion of cervix with cervicitis (N72)*
> **Valid 3-character code, no further characters required**

N87 **Dysplasia of cervix uteri**

> *Excludes1:* *abnormal results from cervical cytologic examination*
> *without histologic confirmation (R87.61-)*
> *carcinoma in situ of cervix uteri (D06.-)*
> *cervical intraepithelial neoplasia III [CIN III] (D06.-)*
> *HGSIL of cervix (R87.613)*
> *severe dysplasia of cervix uteri (D06.-)*

♀ **N87.0** **Mild cervical dysplasia**
Cervical intraepithelial neoplasia I [CIN I]

♀ **N87.1** **Moderate cervical dysplasia**
Cervical intraepithelial neoplasia II [CIN II]

♀ **N87.9** **Dysplasia of cervix uteri, unspecified**
Anaplasia of cervix
Cervical atypism
Cervical dysplasia NOS

N88 **Other noninflammatory disorders of cervix uteri**

> *Excludes2:* *inflammatory disease of cervix (N72)*
> *polyp of cervix (N84.1)*

♀ **N88.0** **Leukoplakia of cervix uteri**

♀ **N88.1** **Old laceration of cervix uteri**
Adhesions of cervix

> *Excludes1:* *current obstetric trauma (O71.3)*

♀ **N88.2** **Stricture and stenosis of cervix uteri**

> *Excludes1:* *stricture and stenosis of cervix uteri*
> *complicating labor (O65.5)*

♀ **N88.3** **Incompetence of cervix uteri**
Investigation and management of (suspected) cervical
incompetence in a nonpregnant woman

> *Excludes1:* *cervical incompetence complicating pregnancy*
> *(O34.3-)*

♀ **N88.4** **Hypertrophic elongation of cervix uteri**

♀ **N88.8** **Other specified noninflammatory disorders of cervix uteri**

> *Excludes1:* *current obstetric trauma (O71.3)*

♀ **N88.9** **Noninflammatory disorder of cervix uteri, unspecified**

N89 **Other noninflammatory disorders of vagina**

> *Excludes1:* *abnormal results from vaginal cytologic examination*
> *without histologic confirmation (R87.62-)*
> *carcinoma in situ of vagina (D07.2)*
> *HGSIL of vagina (R87.623)*
> *inflammation of vagina (N76.-)*
> *senile (atrophic) vaginitis (N95.2)*
> *severe dysplasia of vagina (D07.2)*
> *trichomonal leukorrhea (A59.00)*
> *vaginal intraepithelial neoplasia [VAIN], grade III*
> *(D07.2)*

♀ **N89.0** **Mild vaginal dysplasia**
Vaginal intraepithelial neoplasia [VAIN], grade I

♀ **N89.1** **Moderate vaginal dysplasia**
Vaginal intraepithelial neoplasia [VAIN], grade II

♀ **N89.3** **Dysplasia of vagina, unspecified**

♀ **N89.4** **Leukoplakia of vagina**

♀ **N89.5** **Stricture and atresia of vagina**
Vaginal adhesions
Vaginal stenosis

> *Excludes1:* *congenital atresia or stricture (Q52.4)*
> *postprocedural adhesions of vagina (N99.2)*

♀ **N89.6** **Tight hymenal ring**
Rigid hymen
Tight introitus

> *Excludes1:* *imperforate hymen (Q52.3)*

♀ **N89.7** **Hematocolpos**
Hematocolpos with hematometra or hematosalpinx
AHA CC: 4Q, 2016, 58-59

♀ **N89.8** **Other specified noninflammatory disorders of vagina**
Leukorrhea NOS
Old vaginal laceration
Pessary ulcer of vagina

> *Excludes1:* *current obstetric trauma (O70.-, O71.4,*
> *O71.7-O71.8)*
> *old laceration involving muscles of pelvic floor*
> *(N81.8)*

♀ **N89.9** **Noninflammatory disorder of vagina, unspecified**

N90 **Other noninflammatory disorders of vulva and perineum**

> *Excludes1:* *anogenital (venereal) warts (A63.0)*
> *carcinoma in situ of vulva (D07.1)*
> *condyloma acuminatum (A63.0)*
> *current obstetric trauma (O70.-, O71.7-O71.8)*
> *inflammation of vulva (N76.-)*
> *severe dysplasia of vulva (D07.1)*
> *vulvar intraepithelial neoplasm III [VIN III] (D07.1)*

♀ **N90.0** **Mild vulvar dysplasia**
Vulvar intraepithelial neoplasia [VIN], grade I

♀ **N90.1** **Moderate vulvar dysplasia**
Vulvar intraepithelial neoplasia [VIN], grade II

♀ **N90.3** **Dysplasia of vulva, unspecified**

♀ **N90.4** **Leukoplakia of vulva**
Dystrophy of vulva
Kraurosis of vulva
Lichen sclerosus of external female genital organs

♀ **N90.5** **Atrophy of vulva**
Stenosis of vulva

+ **N90.6 Hypertrophy of vulva**
    AHA CC: 4Q, 2016, 46
    ♀ **N90.60 Unspecified hypertrophy of vulva**
        Unspecified hypertrophy of labia
    ♀ **N90.61 Childhood asymmetric labium majus enlargement**
        CALME
    ♀ **N90.69 Other specified hypertrophy of vulva**
        Other specified hypertrophy of labia
♀ **N90.7 Vulvar cyst**
+ **N90.8 Other specified noninflammatory disorders of vulva and perineum**
    + **N90.81 Female genital mutilation status**
        Female genital cutting status
        ♀ **N90.810 Female genital mutilation status, unspecified**
            Female genital cutting status, unspecified
            Female genital mutilation status NOS
        ♀ **N90.811 Female genital mutilation Type I status**
            Clitorectomy status
            Female genital cutting Type I status
        ♀ **N90.812 Female genital mutilation Type II status**
            Clitorectomy with excision of labia minora status
            Female genital cutting Type II status
        ♀ **N90.813 Female genital mutilation Type III status**
            Female genital cutting Type III status
            Infibulation status
        ♀ **N90.818 Other female genital mutilation status**
            Female genital cutting Type IV status
            Female genital mutilation Type IV status
            Other female genital cutting status
    ♀ **N90.89 Other specified noninflammatory disorders of vulva and perineum**
        Adhesions of vulva
        Hypertrophy of clitoris
♀ **N90.9 Noninflammatory disorder of vulva and perineum, unspecified**

N91 Absent, scanty and rare menstruation
    Excludes1: ovarian dysfunction (E28.-)
♀ **N91.0 Primary amenorrhea**
♀ **N91.1 Secondary amenorrhea**
♀ **N91.2 Amenorrhea, unspecified**
♀ **N91.3 Primary oligomenorrhea**
♀ **N91.4 Secondary oligomenorrhea**
♀ **N91.5 Oligomenorrhea, unspecified**
    Hypomenorrhea NOS

N92 Excessive, frequent and irregular menstruation
    Excludes1: postmenopausal bleeding (N95.0)
                precocious puberty (menstruation) (E30.1)
♀ **N92.0 Excessive and frequent menstruation with regular cycle**
    Heavy periods NOS
    Menorrhagia NOS
    Polymenorrhea
♀ **N92.1 Excessive and frequent menstruation with irregular cycle**
    Irregular intermenstrual bleeding
    Irregular, shortened intervals between menstrual bleeding
    Menometrorrhagia
    Metrorrhagia
● ♀ **N92.2 Excessive menstruation at puberty**
    Excessive bleeding associated with onset of menstrual periods
    Pubertal menorrhagia
    Puberty bleeding
♀ **N92.3 Ovulation bleeding**
    Regular intermenstrual bleeding
♀ **N92.4 Excessive bleeding in the premenopausal period**
    Climacteric menorrhagia or metrorrhagia
    Menopausal menorrhagia or metrorrhagia
    Perimenopausal bleeding
    Perimenopausal menorrhagia or metrorrhagia
    Preclimacteric menorrhagia or metrorrhagia
    Premenopausal menorrhagia or metrorrhagia
♀ **N92.5 Other specified irregular menstruation**

♀ **N92.6 Irregular menstruation, unspecified**
    Irregular bleeding NOS
    Irregular periods NOS
    Excludes1: irregular menstruation with:
            lengthened intervals or scanty bleeding (N91.3-N91.5)
            shortened intervals or excessive bleeding (N92.1)

N93 Other abnormal uterine and vaginal bleeding
    Excludes1: neonatal vaginal hemorrhage (P54.6)
            precocious puberty (menstruation) (E30.1)
            pseudomenses (P54.6)
♀ **N93.0 Postcoital and contact bleeding**
♀ **N93.1 Pre-pubertal vaginal bleeding**
    AHA CC: 4Q, 2016, 47
♀ **N93.8 Other specified abnormal uterine and vaginal bleeding**
    Dysfunctional or functional uterine or vaginal bleeding NOS
♀ **N93.9 Abnormal uterine and vaginal bleeding, unspecified**

N94 Pain and other conditions associated with female genital organs and menstrual cycle
♀ **N94.0 Mittelschmerz**
+ **N94.1 Dyspareunia**
    Excludes1: psychogenic dyspareunia (F52.6)
    AHA CC: 4Q, 2016, 47
    ♀ **N94.10 Unspecified dyspareunia**
    ♀ **N94.11 Superficial (introital) dyspareunia**
    ♀ **N94.12 Deep dyspareunia**
    ♀ **N94.19 Other specified dyspareunia**
♀ **N94.2 Vaginismus**
    Excludes1: psychogenic vaginismus (F52.5)
♀ **N94.3 Premenstrual tension syndrome**
    Code also associated menstrual migraine (G43.82-, G43.83-)
    Excludes1: Premenstrual dysphoric disorder (F32.81)
♀ **N94.4 Primary dysmenorrhea**
♀ **N94.5 Secondary dysmenorrhea**
♀ **N94.6 Dysmenorrhea, unspecified**
    Excludes1: psychogenic dysmenorrhea (F45.8)
+ **N94.8 Other specified conditions associated with female genital organs and menstrual cycle**
    + **N94.81 Vulvodynia**
        ♀ **N94.810 Vulvar vestibulitis**
        ♀ **N94.818 Other vulvodynia**
        ♀ **N94.819 Vulvodynia, unspecified**
            Vulvodynia NOS
    ♀ **N94.89 Other specified conditions associated with female genital organs and menstrual cycle**
♀ **N94.9 Unspecified condition associated with female genital organs and menstrual cycle**

N95 Menopausal and other perimenopausal disorders
    Menopausal and other perimenopausal disorders due to naturally occurring (age-related) menopause and perimenopause
    Excludes1: excessive bleeding in the premenopausal period (N92.4)
        menopausal and perimenopausal disorders due to artificial or premature menopause (E89.4-, E28.31-)
        premature menopause (E28.31-)
    Excludes2: postmenopausal osteoporosis (M81.0-)
        postmenopausal osteoporosis with current pathological fracture (M80.0-)
        postmenopausal urethritis (N34.2)
♀ **N95.0 Postmenopausal bleeding**
♀ **N95.1 Menopausal and female climacteric states**
    Symptoms such as flushing, sleeplessness, headache, lack of concentration, associated with natural (age-related) menopause
    Use additional code for associated symptoms
    Excludes1: asymptomatic menopausal state (Z78.0)
        symptoms associated with artificial menopause (E89.41)
        symptoms associated with premature menopause (E28.310)
♀ **N95.2 Postmenopausal atrophic vaginitis**
    Senile (atrophic) vaginitis
♀ **N95.8 Other specified menopausal and perimenopausal disorders**
♀ **N95.9 Unspecified menopausal and perimenopausal disorder**

+, +7th, X + 7th   ● Newborn   ● Pediatric   ● Maternity   ● Adult   ♀ Female   ♂ Male   Manifestation   Unacceptable PDX   HCC   CC   MCC   HAC

♀ **N96 Recurrent pregnancy loss**

Investigation or care in a nonpregnant woman with history of recurrent pregnancy loss

Excludes1: recurrent pregancy loss with current pregnancy (O26.2-)

Valid 3-character code, no further characters required

N97 Female infertility

Includes: inability to achieve a pregnancy
sterility, female NOS

Excludes1: female infertility associated with:
hypopituitarism (E23.0)
Stein-Leventhal syndrome (E28.2)

Excludes2: incompetence of cervix uteri (N88.3)

♀ **N97.0 Female infertility associated with anovulation**

♀ **N97.1 Female infertility of tubal origin**

Female infertility associated with congenital anomaly of tube
Female infertility due to tubal block
Female infertility due to tubal occlusion
Female infertility due to tubal stenosis

♀ **N97.2 Female infertility of uterine origin**

Female infertility associated with congenital anomaly of uterus
Female infertility due to nonimplantation of ovum

♀ **N97.8 Female infertility of other origin**

♀ **N97.9 Female infertility, unspecified**

N98 Complications associated with artificial fertilization

♀ CC **N98.0 Infection associated with artificial insemination**

♀ CC **N98.1 Hyperstimulation of ovaries**

Hyperstimulation of ovaries NOS
Hyperstimulation of ovaries associated with induced ovulation

♀ CC **N98.2 Complications of attempted introduction of fertilized ovum following in vitro fertilization**

♀ CC **N98.3 Complications of attempted introduction of embryo in embryo transfer**

♀ CC **N98.8 Other complications associated with artificial fertilization**

♀ **N98.9 Complication associated with artificial fertilization, unspecified**

Intraoperative and postprocedural complications and disorders of genitourinary system, not elsewhere classified (N99)

N99 Intraoperative and postprocedural complications and disorders of genitourinary system, not elsewhere classified

Excludes2: irradiation cystitis (N30.4-)
postoophorectomy osteoporosis with current pathological fracture (M80.8-)
postoophorectomy osteoporosis without current pathological fracture (M81.8)

N99.0 Postprocedural (acute) (chronic) kidney failure

Use additional code to type of kidney disease

+ **N99.1 Postprocedural urethral stricture**

Postcatheterization urethral stricture

+ **N99.11 Postprocedural urethral stricture, male**

♂ **N99.110 Postprocedural urethral stricture, male, meatal**

♂ **N99.111 Postprocedural bulbous urethral stricture, male**

♂ **N99.112 Postprocedural membranous urethral stricture, male**

♂ **N99.113 Postprocedural anterior bulbous urethral stricture, male**

AHA CC: 4Q, 2016, 47-48

♂ **N99.114 Postprocedural urethral stricture, male, unspecified**

♂ **N99.115 Postprocedural fossa navicularis urethral stricture**

AHA CC: 4Q, 2016, 47-48

♂ **N99.116 Postprocedural urethral stricture, male, overlapping sites**

AHA CC: 4Q, 2018, 21-22

♀ **N99.12 Postprocedural urethral stricture, female**

♀ **N99.2 Postprocedural adhesions of vagina**

♀ **N99.3 Prolapse of vaginal vault after hysterectomy**

N99.4 Postprocedural pelvic peritoneal adhesions

Excludes2: pelvic peritoneal adhesions NOS (N73.6)
postinfective pelvic peritoneal adhesions (N73.6)

+ **N99.5 Complications of stoma of urinary tract**

Excludes2: mechanical complication of urinary catheter (T83.0-)

AHA CC: 4Q, 2016, 48

+ **N99.51 Complication of cystostomy**

CC **N99.510 Cystostomy hemorrhage**

CC **N99.511 Cystostomy infection**

CC **N99.512 Cystostomy malfunction**

CC **N99.518 Other cystostomy complication**

+ **N99.52 Complication of incontinent external stoma of urinary tract**

N99.520 Hemorrhage of incontinent external stoma of urinary tract

N99.521 Infection of incontinent external stoma of urinary tract

AHA CC: 4Q, 2016, 48

N99.522 Malfunction of incontinent external stoma of urinary tract

N99.523 Herniation of incontinent stoma of urinary tract

N99.524 Stenosis of incontinent stoma of urinary tract

N99.528 Other complication of incontinent external stoma of urinary tract

+ **N99.53 Complication of continent stoma of urinary tract**

N99.530 Hemorrhage of continent stoma of urinary tract

N99.531 Infection of continent stoma of urinary tract

N99.532 Malfunction of continent stoma of urinary tract

N99.533 Herniation of continent stoma of urinary tract

N99.534 Stenosis of continent stoma of urinary tract

N99.538 Other complication of continent stoma of urinary tract

+ **N99.6 Intraoperative hemorrhage and hematoma of a genitourinary system organ or structure complicating a procedure**

Excludes1: intraoperative hemorrhage and hematoma of a genitourinary system organ or structure due to accidental puncture or laceration during a procedure (N99.7-)

N99.61 Intraoperative hemorrhage and hematoma of a genitourinary system organ or structure complicating a genitourinary system procedure

CC **N99.62 Intraoperative hemorrhage and hematoma of a genitourinary system organ or structure complicating other procedure**

+ **N99.7 Accidental puncture and laceration of a genitourinary system organ or structure during a procedure**

CC **N99.71 Accidental puncture and laceration of a genitourinary system organ or structure during a genitourinary system procedure**

CC **N99.72 Accidental puncture and laceration of a genitourinary system organ or structure during other procedure**

+ **N99.8 Other intraoperative and postprocedural complications and disorders of genitourinary system**

AHA CC: 4Q, 2016, 9-10

N99.81 Other intraoperative complications of genitourinary system

+ **N99.82 Postprocedural hemorrhage of a genitourinary system organ or structure following a procedure**

CC **N99.820 Postprocedural hemorrhage of a genitourinary system organ or structure following a genitourinary system procedure**

CC **N99.821 Postprocedural hemorrhage of a genitourinary system organ or structure following other procedure**

♀ **N99.83 Residual ovary syndrome**

+ **N99.84 Postprocedural hematoma and seroma of a genitourinary system organ or structure following a procedure**

CC **N99.840 Postprocedural hematoma of a genitourinary system organ or structure following a genitourinary system procedure**

CC **N99.841 Postprocedural hematoma of a genitourinary system organ or structure following other procedure**

CC **N99.842 Postprocedural seroma of a genitourinary system organ or structure following a genitourinary system procedure**

CC **N99.843 Postprocedural seroma of a genitourinary system organ or structure following other procedure**

♀ **N99.85 Post endometrial ablation syndrome**
AHA CC: 4Q, 2019, 12

N99.89 Other postprocedural complications and disorders of genitourinary system

Chapter 15: Pregnancy, Childbirth and the Puerperium (O00-O9A)

NOTE Codes from this chapter are for use only on maternal records, never on newborn records

Codes from this chapter are for use for conditions related to or aggravated by the pregnancy, childbirth, or by the puerperium (maternal causes or obstetric causes)

NOTE Trimesters are counted from the first day of the last menstrual period. They are defined as follows:

1st trimester- less than 14 weeks 0 days

2nd trimester- 14 weeks 0 days to less than 28 weeks 0 days

3rd trimester- 28 weeks 0 days until delivery

Use additional code from category Z3A, Weeks of gestation, to identify the specific week of the pregnancy, if known

Excludes1: *supervision of normal pregnancy (Z34.-)*

Excludes2: *mental and behavioral disorders associated with the puerperium (F53.-)*

obstetrical tetanus (A34)

postpartum necrosis of pituitary gland (E23.0)

puerperal osteomalacia (M83.0)

This chapter contains the following category blocks:

O00-O08	Pregnancy with abortive outcome
O09	Supervision of high risk pregnancy
O10-O16	Edema, proteinuria and hypertensive disorders in pregnancy, childbirth and the puerperium
O20-O29	Other maternal disorders predominantly related to pregnancy
O30-O48	Maternal care related to the fetus and amniotic cavity and possible delivery problems
O60-O77	Complications of labor and delivery
O80-O82	Encounter for delivery
O85-O92	Complications predominantly related to the puerperium
O94-O9A	Other obstetric conditions, not elsewhere classified

C. Chapter-Specific Coding Guidelines

In addition to general coding guidelines, there are guidelines for specific diagnoses and/or conditions in the classification. Unless otherwise indicated, these guidelines apply to all health care settings. Please refer to Section II for guidelines on the selection of principal diagnosis.

15. Chapter 15: Pregnancy, Childbirth and the Puerperium (O00-O9A)

a. General Rules for Obstetric Cases

1) Codes from chapter 15 and sequencing priority

Obstetric cases require codes from chapter 15, codes in the range O00-O9A, Pregnancy, Childbirth, and the Puerperium. Chapter 15 codes have sequencing priority over codes from other chapters. Additional codes from other chapters may be used in conjunction with chapter 15 codes to further specify conditions. Should the provider document that the pregnancy is incidental to the encounter, then code Z33.1, Pregnant state, incidental, should be used in place of any chapter 15 codes. It is the provider's responsibility to state that the condition being treated is not affecting the pregnancy.

2) Chapter 15 codes used only on the maternal record

Chapter 15 codes are to be used only on the maternal record, never on the record of the newborn.

3) Final character for trimester

The majority of codes in Chapter 15 have a final character indicating the trimester of pregnancy. The timeframes for the trimesters are indicated at the beginning of the chapter. If trimester is not a component of a code it is because the condition always occurs in a specific trimester, or the concept of trimester of pregnancy is not applicable. Certain codes have characters for only certain trimesters because the condition does not occur in all trimesters, but it may occur in more than just one.

Assignment of the final character for trimester should be based on the provider's documentation of the trimester (or number of weeks) for the current admission/encounter. This applies to the assignment of trimester for pre-existing conditions as well as those that develop during or are due to the pregnancy. The provider's documentation of the number of weeks may be used to assign the appropriate code identifying the trimester.

Whenever delivery occurs during the current admission, and there is an "in childbirth" option for the obstetric complication being coded, the "in childbirth" code should be assigned.

4) Selection of trimester for inpatient admissions that encompass more than one trimester

In instances when a patient is admitted to a hospital for complications of pregnancy during one trimester and remains in the hospital into a subsequent trimester, the trimester character for the antepartum complication code should be assigned on the basis of the trimester when the complication developed, not the trimester of the discharge. If the condition developed prior to the current admission/encounter or represents a pre-existing condition, the trimester character for the trimester at the time of the admission/encounter should be assigned.

5) Unspecified trimester

Each category that includes codes for trimester has a code for "unspecified trimester." The "unspecified trimester" code should rarely be used, such as when the documentation in the record is insufficient to determine the trimester and it is not possible to obtain clarification.

6) 7th character for Fetus Identification

Where applicable, a 7th character is to be assigned for certain categories (O31, O32, O33.3 - O33.6, O35, O36, O40, O41, O60.1, O60.2, O64, and O69) to identify the fetus for which the complication code applies.

Assign 7th character "0":

- For single gestations
- When the documentation in the record is insufficient to determine the fetus affected and it is not possible to obtain clarification.
- When it is not possible to clinically determine which fetus is affected.

b. Selection of OB Principal or First-listed Diagnosis

1) Routine outpatient prenatal visits

For routine outpatient prenatal visits when no complications are present, a code from category Z34, Encounter for supervision of normal pregnancy, should be used as the first-listed diagnosis. These codes should not be used in conjunction with chapter 15 codes.

2) Supervision of High-Risk Pregnancy

Codes from category O09, Supervision of high-risk pregnancy, are intended for use only during the prenatal period. For complications during the labor or delivery episode as a result of a high-risk pregnancy, assign the applicable complication codes from Chapter 15. If there are no complications during the labor or delivery episode, assign code O80, Encounter for full-term uncomplicated delivery.

For routine prenatal outpatient visits for patients with high-risk pregnancies, a code from category O09, Supervision of high-risk pregnancy, should be used as the first-listed diagnosis. Secondary chapter 15 codes may be used in conjunction with these codes if appropriate.

3) Episodes when no delivery occurs

In episodes when no delivery occurs, the principal diagnosis should correspond to the principal complication of the pregnancy which necessitated the encounter. Should more than one complication exist, all of which are treated or monitored, any of the complications codes may be sequenced first.

4) When a delivery occurs

When an obstetric patient is admitted and delivers during that admission, the condition that prompted the admission should be sequenced as the principal diagnosis. If multiple conditions prompted the admission, sequence the one most related to the delivery as the principal diagnosis. A code for any complication of the delivery should be assigned as an additional diagnosis. In cases of cesarean delivery, if the patient was admitted with a condition that resulted in the performance of a cesarean procedure, that condition should be selected as the principal diagnosis. If the reason for the admission was unrelated to the condition resulting in the cesarean delivery, the condition related to the reason for the admission should be selected as the principal diagnosis.

5) Outcome of delivery

A code from category Z37, Outcome of delivery, should be included on every maternal record when a delivery has occurred. These codes are not to be used on subsequent records or on the newborn record.

c. Pre-existing conditions versus conditions due to the pregnancy

Certain categories in Chapter 15 distinguish between conditions of the mother that existed prior to pregnancy (pre-existing) and those that are a direct result of pregnancy. When assigning codes from Chapter 15, it is important to assess if a condition was pre-existing prior to pregnancy or developed during or due to the pregnancy in order to assign the correct code.

Categories that do not distinguish between pre-existing and pregnancy-related conditions may be used for either. It is acceptable to use codes specifically for the puerperium with codes complicating pregnancy and childbirth if a condition arises postpartum during the delivery encounter.

d. Pre-existing hypertension in pregnancy

Category O10, Pre-existing hypertension complicating pregnancy, childbirth and the puerperium, includes codes for hypertensive heart and hypertensive chronic kidney disease. When assigning one of the O10 codes that includes hypertensive heart disease or hypertensive chronic kidney disease, it is necessary to add a secondary code from the appropriate hypertension category to specify the type of heart failure or chronic kidney disease.

See Section I.C.9. Hypertension.

e. Fetal Conditions Affecting the Management of the Mother

1) Codes from categories O35 and O36

Codes from categories O35, Maternal care for known or suspected fetal abnormality and damage, and O36, Maternal care for other fetal problems, are assigned only when the fetal condition is actually responsible for modifying the management of the mother, i.e., by requiring diagnostic studies, additional observation, special care, or termination of pregnancy. The fact that the fetal condition exists does not justify assigning a code from this series to the mother's record.

2) In utero surgery

In cases when surgery is performed on the fetus, a diagnosis code from category O35, Maternal care for known or suspected fetal abnormality and damage, should be assigned identifying the fetal condition. Assign the appropriate procedure code for the procedure performed.

No code from Chapter 16, the perinatal codes, should be used on the mother's record to identify fetal conditions. Surgery performed in utero on a fetus is still to be coded as an obstetric encounter.

f. HIV Infection in Pregnancy, Childbirth and the Puerperium

During pregnancy, childbirth or the puerperium, a patient admitted because of an HIV-related illness should receive a principal diagnosis from subcategory O98.7-, Human immunodeficiency [HIV] disease complicating pregnancy, childbirth and the puerperium, followed by the code(s) for the HIV-related illness(es).

Patients with asymptomatic HIV infection status admitted during pregnancy, childbirth, or the puerperium should receive codes of O98.7- and Z21, Asymptomatic human immunodeficiency virus [HIV] infection status.

g. Diabetes mellitus in pregnancy

Diabetes mellitus is a significant complicating factor in pregnancy. Pregnant women who are diabetic should be assigned a code from category O24, Diabetes mellitus in pregnancy, childbirth, and the puerperium, first, followed by the appropriate diabetes code(s) (E08-E13) from Chapter 4.

h. Long term use of insulin and oral hypoglycemics

See section I.C.4.a.3 for information on the long term use of insulin and oral hypoglycemic.

i. Gestational (pregnancy induced) diabetes

Gestational (pregnancy induced) diabetes can occur during the second and third trimester of pregnancy in women who were not diabetic prior to pregnancy. Gestational diabetes can cause complications in the pregnancy similar to those of pre-existing diabetes mellitus. It also puts the woman at greater risk of developing diabetes after the pregnancy. Codes for gestational diabetes are in subcategory O24.4, Gestational diabetes mellitus. No other code from category O24, Diabetes mellitus in pregnancy, childbirth, and the puerperium, should be used with a code from O24.4

The codes under subcategory O24.4 include diet controlled, insulin controlled, and controlled by oral hypoglycemic drugs. If a patient with gestational diabetes is treated with both diet and insulin, only the code for insulin-controlled is required. If a patient with gestational diabetes is treated with both diet and oral hypoglycemic medications, only the code for "controlled by oral hypoglycemic drugs" is required. Code Z79.4, Long-term (current) use of insulin or code Z79.84, Long-term (current) use of oral hypoglycemic drugs, should not be assigned with codes from subcategory O24.4.

An abnormal glucose tolerance in pregnancy is assigned a code from subcategory O99.81, Abnormal glucose complicating pregnancy, childbirth, and the puerperium.

j. Sepsis and septic shock complicating abortion, pregnancy, childbirth and the puerperium

When assigning a chapter 15 code for sepsis complicating abortion, pregnancy, childbirth, and the puerperium, a code for the specific type of infection should be assigned as an additional diagnosis. If severe sepsis is present, a code from subcategory R65.2, Severe sepsis, and code(s) for associated organ dysfunction(s) should also be assigned as additional diagnoses.

k. Puerperal sepsis

Code O85, Puerperal sepsis, should be assigned with a secondary code to identify the causal organism (e.g., for a bacterial infection, assign a code from category B95-B96, Bacterial infections in conditions classified elsewhere). A code from category A40, Streptococcal sepsis, or A41, Other sepsis, should not be used for puerperal sepsis. If applicable, use additional codes to identify severe sepsis (R65.2-) and any associated acute organ dysfunction.

Code O85 should not be assigned for sepsis following an obstetrical procedure (*See Section I.C.1.d.5b., Sepsis due to a postprocedural infection*).

l. Alcohol, tobacco and drug use during pregnancy, childbirth and the puerperium

1) Alcohol use during pregnancy, childbirth and the puerperium

Codes under subcategory O99.31, Alcohol use complicating pregnancy, childbirth, and the puerperium, should be assigned for any pregnancy case when a mother uses alcohol during the pregnancy or postpartum. A secondary code from category F10, Alcohol related disorders, should also be assigned to identify manifestations of the alcohol use.

2) Tobacco use during pregnancy, childbirth and the puerperium

Codes under subcategory O99.33, Smoking (tobacco) complicating pregnancy, childbirth, and the puerperium, should be assigned for any pregnancy case when a mother uses any type of tobacco product during the pregnancy or postpartum. A secondary code from category F17, Nicotine dependence, should also be assigned to identify the type of nicotine dependence.

3) Drug use during pregnancy, childbirth and the puerperium

Codes under subcategory O99.32, Drug use complicating pregnancy, childbirth, and the puerperium, should be assigned for any pregnancy case when a mother uses drugs during the pregnancy or postpartum. This can involve illegal drugs, or inappropriate use or abuse of prescription drugs. Secondary code(s) from categories F11-F16 and F18-F19 should also be assigned to identify manifestations of the drug use.

m. Poisoning, toxic effects, adverse effects and underdosing in a pregnant patient

A code from subcategory O9A.2, Injury, poisoning and certain other consequences of external causes complicating pregnancy, childbirth, and the puerperium, should be sequenced first, followed by the appropriate injury, poisoning, toxic effect, adverse effect or underdosing code, and then the additional code(s) that specifies the condition caused by the poisoning, toxic effect, adverse effect or underdosing.

See Section I.C.19. Adverse effects, poisoning, underdosing and toxic effects.

n. Normal Delivery, Code O80

1) Encounter for full term uncomplicated delivery

Code O80 should be assigned when a woman is admitted for a full-term normal delivery and delivers a single, healthy infant without any complications antepartum, during the delivery, or postpartum during the delivery episode. Code O80 is always a principal diagnosis. It is not to be used if any other code from chapter 15 is needed to describe a current complication of the antenatal, delivery, or postnatal period. Additional codes from other chapters may be used with code O80 if they are not related to or are in any way complicating the pregnancy.

2) Uncomplicated delivery with resolved antepartum complication

Code O80 may be used if the patient had a complication at some point during the pregnancy, but the complication is not present at the time of the admission for delivery.

3) Outcome of delivery for O80

Z37.0, Single live birth, is the only outcome of delivery code appropriate for use with O80.

o. The Peripartum and Postpartum Periods

1) Peripartum and Postpartum periods

The postpartum period begins immediately after delivery and continues for six weeks following delivery. The peripartum period is defined as the last month of pregnancy to five months postpartum.

2) Peripartum and postpartum complication

A postpartum complication is any complication occurring within the six-week period.

3) Pregnancy-related complications after 6 week period

Chapter 15 codes may also be used to describe pregnancy-related complications after the peripartum or postpartum period if the provider documents that a condition is pregnancy related.

4) Admission for routine postpartum care following delivery outside hospital

When the mother delivers outside the hospital prior to admission and is admitted for routine postpartum care and no complications are noted,

+, +7th, X + 7th   ● Newborn   ● Pediatric   ● Maternity   ● Adult   ♀ Female   ♂ Male   Manifestation   Unacceptable PDX   HCC   CC   MCC   HAC

code Z39.0, Encounter for care and examination of mother immediately after delivery, should be assigned as the principal diagnosis.

5) Pregnancy associated cardiomyopathy

Pregnancy associated cardiomyopathy, code O90.3, is unique in that it may be diagnosed in the third trimester of pregnancy but may continue to progress months after delivery. For this reason, it is referred to as peripartum cardiomyopathy. Code O90.3 is only for use when the cardiomyopathy develops as a result of pregnancy in a woman who did not have pre-existing heart disease.

p. Code O94, Sequelae of complication of pregnancy, childbirth, and the puerperium

1) Code O94

Code O94, Sequelae of complication of pregnancy, childbirth, and the puerperium, is for use in those cases when an initial complication of a pregnancy develops a sequelae requiring care or treatment at a future date.

2) After the initial postpartum period

This code may be used at any time after the initial postpartum period.

3) Sequencing of Code O94

This code, like all sequela codes, is to be sequenced following the code describing the sequelae of the complication.

q. Termination of Pregnancy and Spontaneous abortions

1) Abortion with Liveborn Fetus

When an attempted termination of pregnancy results in a liveborn fetus, assign code Z33.2, Encounter for elective termination of pregnancy and a code from category Z37, Outcome of Delivery.

2) Retained Products of Conception following an abortion

Subsequent encounters for retained products of conception following a spontaneous abortion or elective termination of pregnancy, without complications are assigned O03.4, Incomplete spontaneous, abortion without complication, or codes O07.4, Failed attempted termination of pregnancy without complication. This advice is appropriate even when the patient was discharged previously with a discharge diagnosis of complete abortion. If the patient has a specific complication associated with the spontaneous abortion or elective termination of pregnancy in addition to retained products of conception, assign the appropriate complication code (e.g., O03.-, O04.-, O07.-) instead of code O03.4 or O07.4.

3) Complications leading to abortion

Codes from Chapter 15 may be used as additional codes to identify any documented complications of the pregnancy in conjunction with codes in categories in O04, O07 and O08.

r. Abuse in a pregnant patient

For suspected or confirmed cases of abuse of a pregnant patient, a code(s) from subcategories O9A.3, Physical abuse complicating pregnancy, childbirth, and the puerperium, O9A.4, Sexual abuse complicating pregnancy, childbirth, and the puerperium, and O9A.5, Psychological abuse complicating pregnancy, childbirth, and the puerperium, should be sequenced first, followed by the appropriate codes (if applicable) to identify any associated current injury due to physical abuse, sexual abuse, and the perpetrator of abuse.

See Section I.C.19. Adult and child abuse, neglect and other maltreatment.

s. COVID-19 infection in pregnancy, childbirth, and the puerperium

During pregnancy, childbirth or the puerperium, when COVID-19 is the reason for admission/encounter, code O98.5-, Other viral diseases complicating pregnancy, childbirth and the puerperium, should be sequenced as the principal/first-listed diagnosis, and code U07.1, COVID-19, and the appropriate codes for associated manifestation(s) should be assigned as additional diagnoses. Codes from Chapter 15 always take sequencing priority.

If the reason for admission/encounter is unrelated to COVID-19 but the patient tests positive for COVID-19 during the admission/encounter, the appropriate code for the reason for admission/encounter should be sequenced as the principal/first-listed diagnosis, and code O98.5- and U07.1, as well as the appropriate codes for associated COVID-19 manifestations, should be assigned as additional diagnoses.

Pregnancy with abortive outcome (O00-O08)

Excludes1: *continuing pregnancy in multiple gestation after abortion of one fetus or more (O31.1-, O31.3-)*

O00 Ectopic pregnancy

Includes: ruptured ectopic pregnancy
Use additional code from category O08 to identify any associated complication
AHA CC: 4Q, 2016, 48-50

+ **O00.0 Abdominal pregnancy**
Excludes1: *maternal care for viable fetus in abdominal pregnancy (O36.7-)*
- ♀ CC **O00.00 Abdominal pregnancy without intrauterine pregnancy**
Abdominal pregnancy NOS
- ♀ CC **O00.01 Abdominal pregnancy with intrauterine pregnancy**
+ **O00.1 Tubal pregnancy**
Fallopian pregnancy
Rupture of (fallopian) tube due to pregnancy
Tubal abortion
AHA CC: 4Q, 2017, 20
+ **O00.10 Tubal pregnancy without intrauterine pregnancy**
Tubal pregnancy NOS
- ♀ CC **O00.101 Right tubal pregnancy without intrauterine pregnancy**
- ♀ CC **O00.102 Left tubal pregnancy without intrauterine pregnancy**
- ♀ CC **O00.109 Unspecified tubal pregnancy without intrauterine pregnancy**
+ **O00.11 Tubal pregnancy with intrauterine pregnancy**
- ♀ CC **O00.111 Right tubal pregnancy with intrauterine pregnancy**
- ♀ CC **O00.112 Left tubal pregnancy with intrauterine pregnancy**
- ♀ CC **O00.119 Unspecified tubal pregnancy with intrauterine pregnancy**
+ **O00.2 Ovarian pregnancy**
AHA CC: 4Q, 2017, 20
+ **O00.20 Ovarian pregnancy without intrauterine pregnancy**
Ovarian pregnancy NOS
- ♀ CC **O00.201 Right ovarian pregnancy without intrauterine pregnancy**
- ♀ CC **O00.202 Left ovarian pregnancy without intrauterine pregnancy**
- ♀ CC **O00.209 Unspecified ovarian pregnancy without intrauterine pregnancy**
+ **O00.21 Ovarian pregnancy with intrauterine pregnancy**
- ♀ CC **O00.211 Right ovarian pregnancy with intrauterine pregnancy**
- ♀ CC **O00.212 Left ovarian pregnancy with intrauterine pregnancy**
- ♀ CC **O00.219 Unspecified ovarian pregnancy with intrauterine pregnancy**
+ **O00.8 Other ectopic pregnancy**
Cervical pregnancy
Cornual pregnancy
Intraligamentous pregnancy
Mural pregnancy
- ♀ CC **O00.80 Other ectopic pregnancy without intrauterine pregnancy**
Other ectopic pregnancy NOS
- ♀ CC **O00.81 Other ectopic pregnancy with intrauterine pregnancy**
+ **O00.9 Ectopic pregnancy, unspecified**
- ♀ CC **O00.90 Unspecified ectopic pregnancy without intrauterine pregnancy**
Ectopic pregnancy NOS
- ♀ CC **O00.91 Unspecified ectopic pregnancy with intrauterine pregnancy**

O01 Hydatidiform mole

Use additional code from category O08 to identify any associated complication
Excludes1: *chorioadenoma (destruens) (D39.2)*
malignant hydatidiform mole (D39.2)
- ♀ **O01.0 Classical hydatidiform mole**
Complete hydatidiform mole
- ♀ **O01.1 Incomplete and partial hydatidiform mole**
- ♀ **O01.9 Hydatidiform mole, unspecified**
Trophoblastic disease NOS
Vesicular mole NOS

O02 Other abnormal products of conception

Use additional code from category O08 to identify any associated complication
Excludes1: *papyraceous fetus (O31.0-)*
- ♀ **O02.0 Blighted ovum and nonhydatidiform mole**
Carneous mole
Fleshy mole
Intrauterine mole NOS
Molar pregnancy NEC
Pathological ovum

Ectopic Pregnancy I - Tubal Pregnancy

Interstitial   Tubal (isthmic)   Abdominal

Tubal (ampullar)

Infundibular (ostial)

Ovarian

Cervical

Unruptured tubal pregnancy

Section through tubal pregnancy

Villi invading tubular wall   Chorion

Hemorrhage in tubal wall   Amnion

Lumen of tube

Chorion   Amnion   Fetus

Ultrasonographic view of adnexa

- ♀ **O02.1   Missed abortion**
  Early fetal death, before completion of 20 weeks of
  gestation, with retention of dead fetus
  Excludes1: *failed induced abortion (O07.-)*
  fetal death (intrauterine) (late) (O36.4)
  missed abortion with blighted ovum (O02.0)
  missed abortion with hydatidiform mole (O01.-)
  missed abortion with nonhydatidiform (O02.0)
  missed abortion with other abnormal products
  of conception (O02.8-)
  missed delivery (O36.4)
  stillbirth (P95)
  AHA CC: 3Q, 2019, 11-12

+ **O02.8   Other specified abnormal products of conception**
  Excludes1: *abnormal products of conception with blighted*
  ovum (O02.0)
  abnormal products of conception with
  hydatidiform mole (O01.-)
  abnormal products of conception with
  nonhydatidiform mole (O02.0)

- ♀ **O02.81   Inappropriate change in quantitative human**
  chorionic gonadotropin (hCG) in early pregnancy
  Biochemical pregnancy
  Chemical pregnancy
  Inappropriate level of quantitative
  human chorionic gonadotropin
  (hCG) for gestational age in early pregnancy

- ♀ **O02.89   Other abnormal products of conception**
- ♀ **O02.9   Abnormal product of conception, unspecified**

O03   Spontaneous abortion

  NOTE   Incomplete abortion includes retained products of
  conception following spontaneous abortion
  Includes: miscarriage
  Review coding guideline C.15.q.2

- ♀ CC **O03.0   Genital tract and pelvic infection following incomplete**
  spontaneous abortion
  Endometritis following incomplete spontaneous abortion
  Oophoritis following incomplete spontaneous abortion
  Parametritis following incomplete spontaneous abortion
  Pelvic peritonitis following incomplete spontaneous abortion
  Salpingitis following incomplete spontaneous abortion
  Salpingo-oophoritis following incomplete spontaneous abortion
  Excludes1: *sepsis following incomplete spontaneous*
  abortion (O03.37)
  urinary tract infection following incomplete
  spontaneous abortion (O03.38)

- ♀ **O03.1   Delayed or excessive hemorrhage following incomplete**
  spontaneous abortion
  Afibrinogenemia following incomplete spontaneous abortion
  Defibrination syndrome following incomplete spontaneous
  abortion
  Hemolysis following incomplete spontaneous abortion
  Intravascular coagulation following incomplete spontaneous
  abortion

- ♀ MCC **O03.2   Embolism following incomplete spontaneous abortion**
  Air embolism following incomplete spontaneous abortion
  Amniotic fluid embolism following incomplete spontaneous
  abortion
  Blood-clot embolism following incomplete spontaneous
  abortion
  Embolism NOS following incomplete spontaneous abortion
  Fat embolism following incomplete spontaneous abortion
  Pulmonary embolism following incomplete spontaneous
  abortion
  Pyemic embolism following incomplete spontaneous
  abortion
  Septic or septicopyemic embolism following incomplete
  spontaneous abortion
  Soap embolism following incomplete spontaneous abortion
  Review coding guideline C.15.j

+ **O03.3   Other and unspecified complications following incomplete**
  spontaneous abortion

- ♀ CC **O03.30   Unspecified complication following incomplete**
  spontaneous abortion

- ♀ MCC **O03.31   Shock following incomplete spontaneous abortion**
  Circulatory collapse following incomplete
  spontaneous abortion
  Shock (postprocedural) following incomplete
  spontaneous abortion

  Excludes1: *shock due to infection following*
  incomplete spontaneous abortion
  (O03.37)

- ♀ MCC **O03.32   Renal failure following incomplete spontaneous**
  abortion
  Kidney failure (acute) following incomplete
  spontaneous abortion
  Oliguria following incomplete spontaneous
  abortion
  Renal shutdown following incomplete spontaneous
  abortion
  Renal tubular necrosis following incomplete
  spontaneous abortion
  Uremia following incomplete spontaneous abortion

- ♀ CC **O03.33   Metabolic disorder following incomplete**
  spontaneous abortion

- ♀ CC **O03.34   Damage to pelvic organs following incomplete**
  spontaneous abortion
  Laceration, perforation, tear or chemical damage of
  bladder following incomplete spontaneous abortion
  Laceration, perforation, tear or chemical damage
  of bowel following incomplete spontaneous
  abortion
  Laceration, perforation, tear or chemical damage
  of broad ligament following incomplete
  spontaneous abortion
  Laceration, perforation, tear or chemical damage of
  cervix following incomplete spontaneous abortion
  Laceration, perforation, tear or chemical damage
  of periurethral tissue following incomplete
  spontaneous abortion
  Laceration, perforation, tear or chemical damage
  of uterus following incomplete spontaneous
  abortion
  Laceration, perforation, tear or chemical damage
  of vagina following incomplete spontaneous
  abortion

- ♀ CC **O03.35   Other venous complications following incomplete**
  spontaneous abortion

- ♀ CC **O03.36   Cardiac arrest following incomplete spontaneous**
  abortion

- ♀ CC **O03.37   Sepsis following incomplete spontaneous abortion**
  Use additional code to identify infectious agent
  (B95-B97)
  Use additional code to identify severe sepsis, if
  applicable (R65.2-)
  Excludes1: *septic or septicopyemic embolism*
  following incomplete spontaneous
  abortion (O03.2)
  Review coding guideline C.15.j

- ♀ CC **O03.38   Urinary tract infection following incomplete**
  spontaneous abortion
  Cystitis following incomplete spontaneous abortion

- ♀ CC **O03.39   Incomplete spontaneous abortion with other**
  complications

- ♀ **O03.4   Incomplete spontaneous abortion without complication**

- ♀ CC **O03.5   Genital tract and pelvic infection following complete or**
  unspecified spontaneous abortion
  Endometritis following complete or unspecified spontaneous
  abortion
  Oophoritis following complete or unspecified spontaneous
  abortion
  Parametritis following complete or unspecified spontaneous
  abortion
  Pelvic peritonitis following complete or unspecified
  spontaneous abortion
  Salpingitis following complete or unspecified spontaneous
  abortion
  Salpingo-oophoritis following complete or unspecified
  spontaneous abortion
  Excludes1: *sepsis following complete or unspecified*
  spontaneous abortion (O03.87)
  urinary tract infection following complete or
  unspecified spontaneous abortion (O03.88)

+, +7th, X + 7th   ● Newborn   ● Pediatric   ● Maternity   ● Adult   ♀ Female   ♂ Male   Manifestation   Unacceptable PDX   HCC   CC   MCC   HAC

- ♀ **O03.6 Delayed or excessive hemorrhage following complete or unspecified spontaneous abortion**
  - Afibrinogenemia following complete or unspecified spontaneous abortion
  - Defibrination syndrome following complete or unspecified spontaneous abortion
  - Hemolysis following complete or unspecified spontaneous abortion
  - Intravascular coagulation following complete or unspecified spontaneous abortion
- ♀ CC **O03.7 Embolism following complete or unspecified spontaneous abortion**
  - Air embolism following complete or unspecified spontaneous abortion
  - Amniotic fluid embolism following complete or unspecified spontaneous abortion
  - Blood-clot embolism following complete or unspecified spontaneous abortion
  - Embolism NOS following complete or unspecified spontaneous abortion
  - Fat embolism following complete or unspecified spontaneous abortion
  - Pulmonary embolism following complete or unspecified spontaneous abortion
  - Pyemic embolism following complete or unspecified spontaneous abortion
  - Septic or septicopyemic embolism following complete or unspecified spontaneous abortion
  - Soap embolism following complete or unspecified spontaneous abortion
- + **O03.8 Other and unspecified complications following complete or unspecified spontaneous abortion**
  - ♀ CC **O03.80 Unspecified complication following complete or unspecified spontaneous abortion**
  - ♀ MCC **O03.81 Shock following complete or unspecified spontaneous abortion**
    - Circulatory collapse following complete or unspecified spontaneous abortion
    - Shock (postprocedural) following complete or unspecified spontaneous abortion
    - *Excludes1:* shock due to infection following complete or unspecified spontaneous abortion (O03.87)
  - ♀ MCC **O03.82 Renal failure following complete or unspecified spontaneous abortion**
    - Kidney failure (acute) following complete or unspecified spontaneous abortion
    - Oliguria following complete or unspecified spontaneous abortion
    - Renal shutdown following complete or unspecified spontaneous abortion
    - Renal tubular necrosis following complete or unspecified spontaneous abortion
    - Uremia following complete or unspecified spontaneous abortion
  - ♀ CC **O03.83 Metabolic disorder following complete or unspecified spontaneous abortion**
  - ♀ CC **O03.84 Damage to pelvic organs following complete or unspecified spontaneous abortion**
    - Laceration, perforation, tear or chemical damage of bladder following complete or unspecified spontaneous abortion
    - Laceration, perforation, tear or chemical damage of bowel following complete or unspecified spontaneous abortion
    - Laceration, perforation, tear or chemical damage of broad ligament following complete or unspecified spontaneous abortion
    - Laceration, perforation, tear or chemical damage of cervix following complete or unspecified spontaneous abortion
    - Laceration, perforation, tear or chemical damage of periurethral tissue following complete or unspecified spontaneous abortion
    - Laceration, perforation, tear or chemical damage of uterus following complete or unspecified spontaneous abortion
    - Laceration, perforation, tear or chemical damage of vagina following complete or unspecified spontaneous abortion

- ♀ CC **O03.85 Other venous complications following complete or unspecified spontaneous abortion**
- ♀ CC **O03.86 Cardiac arrest following complete or unspecified spontaneous abortion**
- ♀ CC **O03.87 Sepsis following complete or unspecified spontaneous abortion**
  - Use additional code to identify infectious agent (B95-B97)
  - Use additional code to identify severe sepsis, if applicable (R65.2-)
  - *Excludes1:* septic or septicopyemic embolism following complete or unspecified spontaneous abortion (O03.7)
  - Review coding guideline C.15.j
- ♀ CC **O03.88 Urinary tract infection following complete or unspecified spontaneous abortion**
  - Cystitis following complete or unspecified spontaneous abortion
- ♀ CC **O03.89 Complete or unspecified spontaneous abortion with other complications**
- ♀ **O03.9 Complete or unspecified spontaneous abortion without complication**
  - Miscarriage NOS
  - Spontaneous abortion NOS

O04 Complications following (induced) termination of pregnancy
- **Includes:** complications following (induced) termination of pregnancy
- *Excludes1:* encounter for elective termination of pregnancy, uncomplicated (Z33.2)
  - failed attempted termination of pregnancy (O07.-)
- ♀ CC **O04.5 Genital tract and pelvic infection following (induced) termination of pregnancy**
  - Endometritis following (induced) termination of pregnancy
  - Oophoritis following (induced) termination of pregnancy
  - Parametritis following (induced) termination of pregnancy
  - Pelvic peritonitis following (induced) termination of pregnancy
  - Salpingitis following (induced) termination of pregnancy
  - Salpingo-oophoritis following (induced) termination of pregnancy
  - *Excludes1:* sepsis following (induced) termination of pregnancy (O04.87)
    - urinary tract infection following (induced) termination of pregnancy (O04.88)
- ♀ **O04.6 Delayed or excessive hemorrhage following (induced) termination of pregnancy**
  - Afibrinogenemia following (induced) termination of pregnancy
  - Defibrination syndrome following (induced) termination of pregnancy
  - Hemolysis following (induced) termination of pregnancy
  - Intravascular coagulation following (induced) termination of pregnancy
  - *AHA CC: 3Q, 2019, 11-12*
- ♀ MCC **O04.7 Embolism following (induced) termination of pregnancy**
  - Air embolism following (induced) termination of pregnancy
  - Amniotic fluid embolism following (induced) termination of pregnancy
  - Blood-clot embolism following (induced) termination of pregnancy
  - Embolism NOS following (induced) termination of pregnancy
  - Fat embolism following (induced) termination of pregnancy
  - Pulmonary embolism following (induced) termination of pregnancy
  - Pyemic embolism following (induced) termination of pregnancy
  - Septic or septicopyemic embolism following (induced) termination of pregnancy
  - Soap embolism following (induced) termination of pregnancy
- + **O04.8 (Induced) termination of pregnancy with other and unspecified complications**
  - ♀ CC **O04.80 (Induced) termination of pregnancy with unspecified complications**
  - ♀ MCC **O04.81 Shock following (induced) termination of pregnancy**
    - Circulatory collapse following (induced) termination of pregnancy
    - Shock (postprocedural) following (induced) termination of pregnancy
    - *Excludes1:* shock due to infection following (induced) termination of pregnancy (O04.87)

- ♀ MCC **O04.82** **Renal failure following (induced) termination of pregnancy**
  - Kidney failure (acute) following (induced) termination of pregnancy
  - Oliguria following (induced) termination of pregnancy
  - Renal shutdown following (induced) termination of pregnancy
  - Renal tubular necrosis following (induced) termination of pregnancy
  - Uremia following (induced) termination of pregnancy
- ♀ CC **O04.83** **Metabolic disorder following (induced) termination of pregnancy**
- ♀ CC **O04.84** **Damage to pelvic organs following (induced) termination of pregnancy**
  - Laceration, perforation, tear or chemical damage of bladder following (induced) termination of pregnancy
  - Laceration, perforation, tear or chemical damage of bowel following (induced) termination of pregnancy
  - Laceration, perforation, tear or chemical damage of broad ligament following (induced) termination of pregnancy
  - Laceration, perforation, tear or chemical damage of cervix following (induced) termination of pregnancy
  - Laceration, perforation, tear or chemical damage of periurethral tissue following (induced) termination of pregnancy
  - Laceration, perforation, tear or chemical damage of uterus following (induced) termination of pregnancy
  - Laceration, perforation, tear or chemical damage of vagina following (induced) termination of pregnancy
- ♀ CC **O04.85** **Other venous complications following (induced) termination of pregnancy**
- ♀ CC **O04.86** **Cardiac arrest following (induced) termination of pregnancy**
- ♀ CC **O04.87** **Sepsis following (induced) termination of pregnancy**
  - Use additional code to identify infectious agent (B95-B97)

  - Use additional code to identify severe sepsis, if applicable (R65.2-)
  - **Excludes1:** *septic or septicopyemic embolism following (induced) termination of pregnancy (O04.7)*
  - Review coding guideline C.15.j
- ♀ CC **O04.88** **Urinary tract infection following (induced) termination of pregnancy**
  - Cystitis following (induced) termination of pregnancy
- ♀ CC **O04.89** **(Induced) termination of pregnancy with other complications**

O07 **Failed attempted termination of pregnancy**
  - **Includes:** failure of attempted induction of termination of pregnancy
    - incomplete elective abortion
  - **Excludes1:** *incomplete spontaneous abortion (O03.0-)*
- ♀ CC **O07.0** **Genital tract and pelvic infection following failed attempted termination of pregnancy**
  - Endometritis following failed attempted termination of pregnancy
  - Oophoritis following failed attempted termination of pregnancy
  - Parametritis following failed attempted termination of pregnancy
  - Pelvic peritonitis following failed attempted termination of pregnancy
  - Salpingitis following failed attempted termination of pregnancy
  - Salpingo-oophoritis following failed attempted termination of pregnancy
  - **Excludes1:** *sepsis following failed attempted termination of pregnancy (O07.37)*
    - *urinary tract infection following failed attempted termination of pregnancy (O07.38)*

- ♀ CC **O07.1** **Delayed or excessive hemorrhage following failed attempted termination of pregnancy**
  - Afibrinogenemia following failed attempted termination of pregnancy
  - Defibrination syndrome following failed attempted termination of pregnancy
  - Hemolysis following failed attempted termination of pregnancy
  - Intravascular coagulation following failed attempted termination of pregnancy
- ♀ MCC **O07.2** **Embolism following failed attempted termination of pregnancy**
  - Air embolism following failed attempted termination of pregnancy
  - Amniotic fluid embolism following failed attempted termination of pregnancy
  - Blood-clot embolism following failed attempted termination of pregnancy
  - Embolism NOS following failed attempted termination of pregnancy
  - Fat embolism following failed attempted termination of pregnancy
  - Pulmonary embolism following failed attempted termination of pregnancy
  - Pyemic embolism following failed attempted termination of pregnancy
  - Septic or septicopyemic embolism following failed attempted termination of pregnancy
  - Soap embolism following failed attempted termination of pregnancy
- + **O07.3** **Failed attempted termination of pregnancy with other and unspecified complications**
- ♀ CC **O07.30** **Failed attempted termination of pregnancy with unspecified complications**
- ♀ MCC **O07.31** **Shock following failed attempted termination of pregnancy**
  - Circulatory collapse following failed attempted termination of pregnancy
  - Shock (postprocedural) following failed attempted termination of pregnancy
  - **Excludes1:** *shock due to infection following failed attempted termination of pregnancy (O07.37)*
- ♀ MCC **O07.32** **Renal failure following failed attempted termination of pregnancy**
  - Kidney failure (acute) following failed attempted termination of pregnancy
  - Oliguria following failed attempted termination of pregnancy
  - Renal shutdown following failed attempted termination of pregnancy
  - Renal tubular necrosis following failed attempted termination of pregnancy
  - Uremia following failed attempted termination of pregnancy
- ♀ CC **O07.33** **Metabolic disorder following failed attempted termination of pregnancy**
- ♀ CC **O07.34** **Damage to pelvic organs following failed attempted termination of pregnancy**
  - Laceration, perforation, tear or chemical damage of bladder following failed attempted termination of pregnancy
  - Laceration, perforation, tear or chemical damage of bowel following failed attempted termination of pregnancy
  - Laceration, perforation, tear or chemical damage of broad ligament following failed attempted termination of pregnancy
  - Laceration, perforation, tear or chemical damage of cervix following failed attempted termination of pregnancy
  - Laceration, perforation, tear or chemical damage of periurethral tissue following failed attempted termination of pregnancy
  - Laceration, perforation, tear or chemical damage of uterus following failed attempted termination of pregnancy
  - Laceration, perforation, tear or chemical damage of vagina following failed attempted termination of pregnancy

- ♀ CC **O07.35 Other venous complications following failed attempted termination of pregnancy**
- ♀ CC **O07.36 Cardiac arrest following failed attempted termination of pregnancy**
- ♀ CC **O07.37 Sepsis following failed attempted termination of pregnancy**

  Use additional code (B95-B97), to identify infectious agent

  Use additional code (R65.2-) to identify severe sepsis, if applicable

  Excludes1: *septic or septicopyemic embolism following failed attempted termination of pregnancy (O07.2)*

  Review coding guideline C.15.j

- ♀ CC **O07.38 Urinary tract infection following failed attempted termination of pregnancy**

  Cystitis following failed attempted termination of pregnancy

- ♀ CC **O07.39 Failed attempted termination of pregnancy with other complications**
- ♀ CC **O07.4 Failed attempted termination of pregnancy without complication**

  Review coding guideline C.15.q.2

O08 Complications following ectopic and molar pregnancy

  This category is for use with categories O00-O02 to identify any associated complications

- ♀ CC **O08.0 Genital tract and pelvic infection following ectopic and molar pregnancy**

  Endometritis following ectopic and molar pregnancy
  Oophoritis following ectopic and molar pregnancy
  Parametritis following ectopic and molar pregnancy
  Pelvic peritonitis following ectopic and molar pregnancy
  Salpingitis following ectopic and molar pregnancy
  Salpingo-oophoritis following ectopic and molar pregnancy

  Excludes1: *sepsis following ectopic and molar pregnancy (O08.82)*
  urinary tract infection (O08.83)

- ♀ CC **O08.1 Delayed or excessive hemorrhage following ectopic and molar pregnancy**

  Afibrinogenemia following ectopic and molar pregnancy
  Defibrination syndrome following ectopic and molar pregnancy
  Hemolysis following ectopic and molar pregnancy
  Intravascular coagulation following ectopic and molar pregnancy

  Excludes1: *delayed or excessive hemorrhage due to incomplete abortion (O03.1)*

- ♀ MCC **O08.2 Embolism following ectopic and molar pregnancy**

  Air embolism following ectopic and molar pregnancy
  Amniotic fluid embolism following ectopic and molar pregnancy
  Blood-clot embolism following ectopic and molar pregnancy
  Embolism NOS following ectopic and molar pregnancy
  Fat embolism following ectopic and molar pregnancy
  Pulmonary embolism following ectopic and molar pregnancy
  Pyemic embolism following ectopic and molar pregnancy
  Septic or septicopyemic embolism following ectopic and molar pregnancy
  Soap embolism following ectopic and molar pregnancy

- ♀ MCC **O08.3 Shock following ectopic and molar pregnancy**

  Circulatory collapse following ectopic and molar pregnancy
  Shock (postprocedural) following ectopic and molar pregnancy

  Excludes1: *shock due to infection following ectopic and molar pregnancy (O08.82)*

- ♀ MCC **O08.4 Renal failure following ectopic and molar pregnancy**

  Kidney failure (acute) following ectopic and molar pregnancy
  Oliguria following ectopic and molar pregnancy
  Renal shutdown following ectopic and molar pregnancy
  Renal tubular necrosis following ectopic and molar pregnancy
  Uremia following ectopic and molar pregnancy

- ♀ CC **O08.5 Metabolic disorders following an ectopic and molar pregnancy**
- ♀ CC **O08.6 Damage to pelvic organs and tissues following an ectopic and molar pregnancy**

  Laceration, perforation, tear or chemical damage of bladder following an ectopic and molar pregnancy
  Laceration, perforation, tear or chemical damage of bowel following an ectopic and molar pregnancy
  Laceration, perforation, tear or chemical damage of broad ligament following an ectopic and molar pregnancy
  Laceration, perforation, tear or chemical damage of cervix following an ectopic and molar pregnancy
  Laceration, perforation, tear or chemical damage of periurethral tissue following an ectopic and molar pregnancy
  Laceration, perforation, tear or chemical damage of uterus following an ectopic and molar pregnancy
  Laceration, perforation, tear or chemical damage of vagina following an ectopic and molar pregnancy

- ♀ CC **O08.7 Other venous complications following an ectopic and molar pregnancy**
- + **O08.8 Other complications following an ectopic and molar pregnancy**
  - ♀ CC **O08.81 Cardiac arrest following an ectopic and molar pregnancy**
  - ♀ CC **O08.82 Sepsis following ectopic and molar pregnancy**

    Use additional code (B95-B97), to identify infectious agent

    Use additional code (R65.2-) to identify severe sepsis, if applicable

    Excludes1: *septic or septicopyemic embolism following ectopic and molar pregnancy (O08.2)*

    Review coding guideline C.15.j

  - ♀ CC **O08.83 Urinary tract infection following an ectopic and molar pregnancy**

    Cystitis following an ectopic and molar pregnancy

  - ♀ CC **O08.89 Other complications following an ectopic and molar pregnancy**
- ♀ CC **O08.9 Unspecified complication following an ectopic and molar pregnancy**

Supervision of high risk pregnancy (O09)

O09 Supervision of high risk pregnancy

  Review coding guideline C.15.b.2
  AHA CC: 4Q, 2016, 48-50

- + **O09.0 Supervision of pregnancy with history of infertility**
  - ♀ **O09.00 Supervision of pregnancy with history of infertility, unspecified trimester**
  - ♀ **O09.01 Supervision of pregnancy with history of infertility, first trimester**
  - ♀ **O09.02 Supervision of pregnancy with history of infertility, second trimester**
  - ♀ **O09.03 Supervision of pregnancy with history of infertility, third trimester**
- + **O09.1 Supervision of pregnancy with history of ectopic pregnancy**
  - ♀ **O09.10 Supervision of pregnancy with history of ectopic pregnancy, unspecified trimester**
  - ♀ **O09.11 Supervision of pregnancy with history of ectopic pregnancy, first trimester**
  - ♀ **O09.12 Supervision of pregnancy with history of ectopic pregnancy, second trimester**
  - ♀ **O09.13 Supervision of pregnancy with history of ectopic pregnancy, third trimester**
- + **O09.A Supervision of pregnancy with history of molar pregnancy**
  - ♀ **O09.A0 Supervision of pregnancy with history of molar pregnancy, unspecified trimester**
  - ♀ **O09.A1 Supervision of pregnancy with history of molar pregnancy, first trimester**
  - ♀ **O09.A2 Supervision of pregnancy with history of molar pregnancy, second trimester**
  - ♀ **O09.A3 Supervision of pregnancy with history of molar pregnancy, third trimester**

+ O09.2 **Supervision of pregnancy with other poor reproductive or obstetric history**

> **Excludes2:** *pregnancy care for patient with history of recurrent pregnancy loss (O26.2-)*

+ O09.21 **Supervision of pregnancy with history of pre-term labor**

- ♀ **O09.211** **Supervision of pregnancy with history of pre-term labor, first trimester**
- ♀ **O09.212** **Supervision of pregnancy with history of pre-term labor, second trimester**
- ♀ **O09.213** **Supervision of pregnancy with history of pre-term labor, third trimester**
- ♀ **O09.219** **Supervision of pregnancy with history of pre-term labor, unspecified trimester**

+ O09.29 **Supervision of pregnancy with other poor reproductive or obstetric history**

> Supervision of pregnancy with history of neonatal death
>
> Supervision of pregnancy with history of stillbirth

- ♀ **O09.291** **Supervision of pregnancy with other poor reproductive or obstetric history, first trimester**
- ♀ **O09.292** **Supervision of pregnancy with other poor reproductive or obstetric history, second trimester**
- ♀ **O09.293** **Supervision of pregnancy with other poor reproductive or obstetric history, third trimester**
- ♀ **O09.299** **Supervision of pregnancy with other poor reproductive or obstetric history, unspecified trimester**

+ O09.3 **Supervision of pregnancy with insufficient antenatal care**

> Supervision of concealed pregnancy
>
> Supervision of hidden pregnancy

- ♀ **O09.30** **Supervision of pregnancy with insufficient antenatal care, unspecified trimester**
- ♀ **O09.31** **Supervision of pregnancy with insufficient antenatal care, first trimester**
- ♀ **O09.32** **Supervision of pregnancy with insufficient antenatal care, second trimester**
- ♀ **O09.33** **Supervision of pregnancy with insufficient antenatal care, third trimester**

+ O09.4 **Supervision of pregnancy with grand multiparity**

- ♀ **O09.40** **Supervision of pregnancy with grand multiparity, unspecified trimester**
- ♀ **O09.41** **Supervision of pregnancy with grand multiparity, first trimester**
- ♀ **O09.42** **Supervision of pregnancy with grand multiparity, second trimester**
- ♀ **O09.43** **Supervision of pregnancy with grand multiparity, third trimester**

+ O09.5 **Supervision of elderly primigravida and multigravida**

> Pregnancy for a female 35 years and older at expected date of delivery

+ O09.51 **Supervision of elderly primigravida**

- ♀ **O09.511** **Supervision of elderly primigravida, first trimester**
- ♀ **O09.512** **Supervision of elderly primigravida, second trimester**
- ♀ **O09.513** **Supervision of elderly primigravida, third trimester**
- ♀ **O09.519** **Supervision of elderly primigravida, unspecified trimester**

+ O09.52 **Supervision of elderly multigravida**

- ♀ **O09.521** **Supervision of elderly multigravida, first trimester**
- ♀ **O09.522** **Supervision of elderly multigravida, second trimester**
- ♀ **O09.523** **Supervision of elderly multigravida, third trimester**
- ♀ **O09.529** **Supervision of elderly multigravida, unspecified trimester**

+ O09.6 **Supervision of young primigravida and multigravida**

> Supervision of pregnancy for a female less than 16 years old at expected date of delivery

+ O09.61 **Supervision of young primigravida**

- ♀ **O09.611** **Supervision of young primigravida, first trimester**
- ♀ **O09.612** **Supervision of young primigravida, second trimester**
- ♀ **O09.613** **Supervision of young primigravida, third trimester**
- ♀ **O09.619** **Supervision of young primigravida, unspecified trimester**

+ O09.62 **Supervision of young multigravida**

- ♀ **O09.621** **Supervision of young multigravida, first trimester**
- ♀ **O09.622** **Supervision of young multigravida, second trimester**
- ♀ **O09.623** **Supervision of young multigravida, third trimester**
- ♀ **O09.629** **Supervision of young multigravida, unspecified trimester**

+ O09.7 **Supervision of high risk pregnancy due to social problems**

- ♀ **O09.70** **Supervision of high risk pregnancy due to social problems, unspecified trimester**
- ♀ **O09.71** **Supervision of high risk pregnancy due to social problems, first trimester**
- ♀ **O09.72** **Supervision of high risk pregnancy due to social problems, second trimester**
- ♀ **O09.73** **Supervision of high risk pregnancy due to social problems, third trimester**

+ O09.8 **Supervision of other high risk pregnancies**

+ O09.81 **Supervision of pregnancy resulting from assisted reproductive technology**

> Supervision of pregnancy resulting from in-vitro fertilization
>
> **Excludes2:** *gestational carrier status (Z33.3)*

- ♀ **O09.811** **Supervision of pregnancy resulting from assisted reproductive technology, first trimester**
- ♀ **O09.812** **Supervision of pregnancy resulting from assisted reproductive technology, second trimester**
- ♀ **O09.813** **Supervision of pregnancy resulting from assisted reproductive technology, third trimester**
- ♀ **O09.819** **Supervision of pregnancy resulting from assisted reproductive technology, unspecified trimester**

+ O09.82 **Supervision of pregnancy with history of in utero procedure during previous pregnancy**

- ♀ **O09.821** **Supervision of pregnancy with history of in utero procedure during previous pregnancy, first trimester**
- ♀ **O09.822** **Supervision of pregnancy with history of in utero procedure during previous pregnancy, second trimester**
- ♀ **O09.823** **Supervision of pregnancy with history of in utero procedure during previous pregnancy, third trimester**
- ♀ **O09.829** **Supervision of pregnancy with history of in utero procedure during previous pregnancy, unspecified trimester**

> **Excludes1:** *supervision of pregnancy affected by in utero procedure during current pregnancy (O35.7)*

+ O09.89 **Supervision of other high risk pregnancies**

- ♀ **O09.891** **Supervision of other high risk pregnancies, first trimester**
- ♀ **O09.892** **Supervision of other high risk pregnancies, second trimester**
- ♀ **O09.893** **Supervision of other high risk pregnancies, third trimester**
- ♀ **O09.899** **Supervision of other high risk pregnancies, unspecified trimester**

+ O09.9 **Supervision of high risk pregnancy, unspecified**

- ♀ **O09.90** **Supervision of high risk pregnancy, unspecified, unspecified trimester**
- ♀ **O09.91** **Supervision of high risk pregnancy, unspecified, first trimester**
- ♀ **O09.92** **Supervision of high risk pregnancy, unspecified, second trimester**
- ♀ **O09.93** **Supervision of high risk pregnancy, unspecified, third trimester**

Edema, proteinuria and hypertensive disorders in pregnancy, childbirth and the puerperium (O10-O16)

O10 Pre-existing hypertension complicating pregnancy, childbirth and the puerperium

> **Includes:** pre-existing hypertension with pre-existing proteinuria complicating pregnancy, childbirth and the puerperium
>
> **Excludes2:** *pre-existing hypertension with superimposed pre-eclampsia complicating pregnancy, childbirth and the puerperium (O11.-)*
>
> Review coding guideline C.15.d

- **+ O10.0 Pre-existing essential hypertension complicating pregnancy, childbirth and the puerperium**
  > Any condition in I10 specified as a reason for obstetric care during pregnancy, childbirth or the puerperium
  - **+ O10.01 Pre-existing essential hypertension complicating pregnancy,**
    - ● ♀ CC **O10.011 Pre-existing essential hypertension complicating pregnancy, first trimester**
    - ● ♀ CC **O10.012 Pre-existing essential hypertension complicating pregnancy, second trimester**
    - ● ♀ CC **O10.013 Pre-existing essential hypertension complicating pregnancy, third trimester**
    - ● ♀ **O10.019 Pre-existing essential hypertension complicating pregnancy, unspecified trimester**
  - ● ♀ CC **O10.02 Pre-existing essential hypertension complicating childbirth**
  - ● ♀ **O10.03 Pre-existing essential hypertension complicating the puerperium**
- **+ O10.1 Pre-existing hypertensive heart disease complicating pregnancy, childbirth and the puerperium**
  > Any condition in I11 specified as a reason for obstetric care during pregnancy, childbirth or the puerperium
  > Use additional code from I11 to identify the type of hypertensive heart disease
  - **+ O10.11 Pre-existing hypertensive heart disease complicating pregnancy**
    - ● ♀ **O10.111 Pre-existing hypertensive heart disease complicating pregnancy, first trimester**
    - ● ♀ **O10.112 Pre-existing hypertensive heart disease complicating pregnancy, second trimester**
    - ● ♀ **O10.113 Pre-existing hypertensive heart disease complicating pregnancy, third trimester**
    - ● ♀ **O10.119 Pre-existing hypertensive heart disease complicating pregnancy, unspecified trimester**
  - ● ♀ **O10.12 Pre-existing hypertensive heart disease complicating childbirth**
  - ● ♀ **O10.13 Pre-existing hypertensive heart disease complicating the puerperium**
- **+ O10.2 Pre-existing hypertensive chronic kidney disease complicating pregnancy, childbirth and the puerperium**
  > Any condition in I12 specified as a reason for obstetric care during pregnancy, childbirth or the puerperium
  > Use additional code from I12 to identify the type of hypertensive chronic kidney disease
  - **+ O10.21 Pre-existing hypertensive chronic kidney disease complicating pregnancy**
    - ● ♀ **O10.211 Pre-existing hypertensive chronic kidney disease complicating pregnancy, first trimester**
    - ● ♀ **O10.212 Pre-existing hypertensive chronic kidney disease complicating pregnancy, second trimester**
    - ● ♀ **O10.213 Pre-existing hypertensive chronic kidney disease complicating pregnancy, third trimester**
    - ● ♀ **O10.219 Pre-existing hypertensive chronic kidney disease complicating pregnancy, unspecified trimester**
  - ● ♀ **O10.22 Pre-existing hypertensive chronic kidney disease complicating childbirth**
  - ● ♀ **O10.23 Pre-existing hypertensive chronic kidney disease complicating the puerperium**

- **+ O10.3 Pre-existing hypertensive heart and chronic kidney disease complicating pregnancy, childbirth and the puerperium**
  > Any condition in I13 specified as a reason for obstetric care during pregnancy, childbirth or the puerperium
  > Use additional code from I13 to identify the type of hypertensive heart and chronic kidney disease
  - **+ O10.31 Pre-existing hypertensive heart and chronic kidney disease complicating pregnancy**
    - ● ♀ **O10.311 Pre-existing hypertensive heart and chronic kidney disease complicating pregnancy, first trimester**
    - ● ♀ **O10.312 Pre-existing hypertensive heart and chronic kidney disease complicating pregnancy, second trimester**
    - ● ♀ **O10.313 Pre-existing hypertensive heart and chronic kidney disease complicating pregnancy, third trimester**
    - ● ♀ **O10.319 Pre-existing hypertensive heart and chronic kidney disease complicating pregnancy, unspecified trimester**
  - ● ♀ **O10.32 Pre-existing hypertensive heart and chronic kidney disease complicating childbirth**
  - ● ♀ **O10.33 Pre-existing hypertensive heart and chronic kidney disease complicating the puerperium**
- **+ O10.4 Pre-existing secondary hypertension complicating pregnancy, childbirth and the puerperium**
  > Any condition in I15 specified as a reason for obstetric care during pregnancy, childbirth or the puerperium
  > Use additional code from I15 to identify the type of secondary hypertension
  - **+ O10.41 Pre-existing secondary hypertension complicating pregnancy**
    - ● ♀ CC **O10.411 Pre-existing secondary hypertension complicating pregnancy, first trimester**
    - ● ♀ CC **O10.412 Pre-existing secondary hypertension complicating pregnancy, second trimester**
    - ● ♀ CC **O10.413 Pre-existing secondary hypertension complicating pregnancy, third trimester**
    - ● ♀ **O10.419 Pre-existing secondary hypertension complicating pregnancy, unspecified trimester**
  - ● ♀ MCC **O10.42 Pre-existing secondary hypertension complicating childbirth**
  - ● ♀ CC **O10.43 Pre-existing secondary hypertension complicating the puerperium**
- **+ O10.9 Unspecified pre-existing hypertension complicating pregnancy, childbirth and the puerperium**
  - **+ O10.91 Unspecified pre-existing hypertension complicating pregnancy**
    - ● ♀ CC **O10.911 Unspecified pre-existing hypertension complicating pregnancy, first trimester**
    - ● ♀ CC **O10.912 Unspecified pre-existing hypertension complicating pregnancy, second trimester**
    - ● ♀ CC **O10.913 Unspecified pre-existing hypertension complicating pregnancy, third trimester**
    - ● ♀ **O10.919 Unspecified pre-existing hypertension complicating pregnancy, unspecified trimester**
  - ● ♀ CC **O10.92 Unspecified pre-existing hypertension complicating childbirth**
  - ● ♀ **O10.93 Unspecified pre-existing hypertension complicating the puerperium**

O11 Pre-existing hypertension with pre-eclampsia

> **Includes:** conditions in O10 complicated by pre-eclampsia
> pre-eclampsia superimposed pre-existing hypertension
> Use additional code from O10 to identify the type of hypertension
> *AHA CC: 4Q, 2016, 50*

- ● ♀ MCC **O11.1 Pre-existing hypertension with pre-eclampsia, first trimester**
- ● ♀ MCC **O11.2 Pre-existing hypertension with pre-eclampsia, second trimester**
- ● ♀ MCC **O11.3 Pre-existing hypertension with pre-eclampsia, third trimester**

+, +7th, X + 7th   ● Newborn   ● Pediatric   ● Maternity   ● Adult   ♀ Female   ♂ Male   Manifestation   Unacceptable PDX   HCC   CC   MCC   HAC

- ♀ **O11.4** **Pre-existing hypertension with pre-eclampsia, complicating childbirth**
- ♀ **O11.5** **Pre-existing hypertension with pre-eclampsia, complicating the puerperium**
- ♀ **O11.9** **Pre-existing hypertension with pre-eclampsia, unspecified trimester**

O12 **Gestational [pregnancy-induced] edema and proteinuria without hypertension**

AHA CC: 4Q, 2016, 50

+ **O12.0** **Gestational edema**
- ♀ **O12.00** **Gestational edema, unspecified trimester**
- ♀ **O12.01** **Gestational edema, first trimester**
- ♀ **O12.02** **Gestational edema, second trimester**
- ♀ **O12.03** **Gestational edema, third trimester**
- ♀ **O12.04** **Gestational edema, complicating childbirth**
- ♀ **O12.05** **Gestational edema, complicating the puerperium**

+ **O12.1** **Gestational proteinuria**
- ♀ **O12.10** **Gestational proteinuria, unspecified trimester**
- ♀ CC **O12.11** **Gestational proteinuria, first trimester**
- ♀ CC **O12.12** **Gestational proteinuria, second trimester**
- ♀ CC **O12.13** **Gestational proteinuria, third trimester**
- ♀ **O12.14** **Gestational proteinuria, complicating childbirth**
- ♀ **O12.15** **Gestational proteinuria, complicating the puerperium**

+ **O12.2** **Gestational edema with proteinuria**
- ♀ **O12.20** **Gestational edema with proteinuria, unspecified trimester**
- ♀ CC **O12.21** **Gestational edema with proteinuria, first trimester**
- ♀ CC **O12.22** **Gestational edema with proteinuria, second trimester**
- ♀ CC **O12.23** **Gestational edema with proteinuria, third trimester**
- ♀ **O12.24** **Gestational edema with proteinuria, complicating childbirth**
- ♀ **O12.25** **Gestational edema with proteinuria, complicating the puerperium**

O13 **Gestational [pregnancy-induced] hypertension without significant proteinuria**

Includes: gestational hypertension NOS
transient hypertension of pregnancy
Review coding guideline C.9.a.7
AHA CC: 4Q, 2016, 50

- ♀ **O13.1** **Gestational [pregnancy-induced] hypertension without significant proteinuria, first trimester**
- ♀ **O13.2** **Gestational [pregnancy-induced] hypertension without significant proteinuria, second trimester**
- ♀ **O13.3** **Gestational [pregnancy-induced] hypertension without significant proteinuria, third trimester**
- ♀ **O13.4** **Gestational [pregnancy-induced] hypertension without significant proteinuria, complicating childbirth**
- ♀ **O13.5** **Gestational [pregnancy-induced] hypertension without significant proteinuria, complicating the puerperium**
- ♀ **O13.9** **Gestational [pregnancy-induced] hypertension without significant proteinuria, unspecified trimester**

O14 **Pre-eclampsia**

Excludes1: *pre-existing hypertension with pre-eclampsia (O11)*
Review coding guideline C.9.a.7
AHA CC: 4Q, 2016, 50

+ **O14.0** **Mild to moderate pre-eclampsia**
- ♀ **O14.00** **Mild to moderate pre-eclampsia, unspecified trimester**
- ♀ CC **O14.02** **Mild to moderate pre-eclampsia, second trimester**
- ♀ CC **O14.03** **Mild to moderate pre-eclampsia, third trimester**
- ♀ **O14.04** **Mild to moderate pre-eclampsia, complicating childbirth**
AHA CC: 2Q, 2019, 8
- ♀ **O14.05** **Mild to moderate pre-eclampsia, complicating the puerperium**

+ **O14.1** **Severe pre-eclampsia**
Excludes1: *HELLP syndrome (O14.2-)*
AHA CC: 3Q, 2019, 12
- ♀ **O14.10** **Severe pre-eclampsia, unspecified trimester**
- ♀ MCC **O14.12** **Severe pre-eclampsia, second trimester**
- ♀ MCC **O14.13** **Severe pre-eclampsia, third trimester**
- ♀ **O14.14** **Severe pre-eclampsia complicating childbirth**
- ♀ **O14.15** **Severe pre-eclampsia, complicating the puerperium**

+ **O14.2** **HELLP syndrome**
Severe pre-eclampsia with hemolysis, elevated liver enzymes and low platelet count (HELLP)
- ♀ **O14.20** **HELLP syndrome (HELLP), unspecified trimester**
- ♀ MCC **O14.22** **HELLP syndrome (HELLP), second trimester**
- ♀ MCC **O14.23** **HELLP syndrome (HELLP), third trimester**
- ♀ **O14.24** **HELLP syndrome, complicating childbirth**
- ♀ **O14.25** **HELLP syndrome, complicating the puerperium**

+ **O14.9** **Unspecified pre-eclampsia**
- ♀ **O14.90** **Unspecified pre-eclampsia, unspecified trimester**
- ♀ CC **O14.92** **Unspecified pre-eclampsia, second trimester**
- ♀ CC **O14.93** **Unspecified pre-eclampsia, third trimester**
- ♀ **O14.94** **Unspecified pre-eclampsia, complicating childbirth**
- ♀ **O14.95** **Unspecified pre-eclampsia, complicating the puerperium**

O15 **Eclampsia**

Includes: convulsions following conditions in O10-O14 and O16

+ **O15.0** **Eclampsia complicating pregnancy**
AHA CC: 4Q, 2016, 50
- ♀ **O15.00** **Eclampsia complicating pregnancy, unspecified trimester**
- ♀ MCC **O15.02** **Eclampsia complicating pregnancy, second trimester**
- ♀ MCC **O15.03** **Eclampsia complicating pregnancy, third trimester**
- ♀ MCC **O15.1** **Eclampsia complicating labor**
- ♀ MCC **O15.2** **Eclampsia complicating the puerperium**
- ♀ **O15.9** **Eclampsia, unspecified as to time period**
Eclampsia NOS

O16 **Unspecified maternal hypertension**

AHA CC: 4Q, 2016, 50

- ♀ CC **O16.1** **Unspecified maternal hypertension, first trimester**
- ♀ CC **O16.2** **Unspecified maternal hypertension, second trimester**
- ♀ CC **O16.3** **Unspecified maternal hypertension, third trimester**
- ♀ **O16.4** **Unspecified maternal hypertension, complicating childbirth**
- ♀ **O16.5** **Unspecified maternal hypertension, complicating the puerperium**
- ♀ **O16.9** **Unspecified maternal hypertension, unspecified trimester**

Other maternal disorders predominantly related to pregnancy (O20-O29)

Excludes2: *maternal care related to the fetus and amniotic cavity and possible delivery problems (O30-O48)*
maternal diseases classifiable elsewhere but complicating pregnancy, labor and delivery, and the puerperium (O98-O99)

O20 **Hemorrhage in early pregnancy**

Includes: hemorrhage before completion of 20 weeks gestation
Excludes1: *pregnancy with abortive outcome (O00-O08)*

- ♀ CC **O20.0** **Threatened abortion**
Hemorrhage specified as due to threatened abortion
- ♀ **O20.8** **Other hemorrhage in early pregnancy**
- ♀ CC **O20.9** **Hemorrhage in early pregnancy, unspecified**

O21 **Excessive vomiting in pregnancy**

- ♀ **O21.0** **Mild hyperemesis gravidarum**
Hyperemesis gravidarum, mild or unspecified, starting before the end of the 20th week of gestation
- ♀ **O21.1** **Hyperemesis gravidarum with metabolic disturbance**
Hyperemesis gravidarum, starting before the end of the 20th week of gestation, with metabolic disturbance such as carbohydrate depletion
Hyperemesis gravidarum, starting before the end of the 20th week of gestation, with metabolic disturbance such as dehydration
Hyperemesis gravidarum, starting before the end of the 20th week of gestation, with metabolic disturbance such as electrolyte imbalance
- ♀ **O21.2** **Late vomiting of pregnancy**
Excessive vomiting starting after 20 completed weeks of gestation
- ♀ **O21.8** **Other vomiting complicating pregnancy**
Vomiting due to diseases classified elsewhere, complicating pregnancy
Use additional code, to identify cause.
- ♀ **O21.9** **Vomiting of pregnancy, unspecified**

O22 Venous complications and hemorrhoids in pregnancy

> *Excludes1:* *venous complications of:*
> > *abortion NOS (O03.9)*
> > *ectopic or molar pregnancy (O08.7)*
> > *failed attempted abortion (O07.35)*
> > *induced abortion (O04.85)*
> > *spontaneous abortion (O03.89)*
>
> *Excludes2:* *obstetric pulmonary embolism (O88.-)*
> > *venous complications and hemorrhoids of childbirth*
> > *and the puerperium (O87.-)*

+ **O22.0 Varicose veins of lower extremity in pregnancy**
> Varicose veins NOS in pregnancy
- ♀ **O22.00 Varicose veins of lower extremity in pregnancy, unspecified trimester**
- ♀ **O22.01 Varicose veins of lower extremity in pregnancy, first trimester**
- ♀ **O22.02 Varicose veins of lower extremity in pregnancy, second trimester**
- ♀ **O22.03 Varicose veins of lower extremity in pregnancy, third trimester**

+ **O22.1 Genital varices in pregnancy**
> Perineal varices in pregnancy
> Vaginal varices in pregnancy
> Vulval varices in pregnancy
- ♀ **O22.10 Genital varices in pregnancy, unspecified trimester**
- ♀ **O22.11 Genital varices in pregnancy, first trimester**
- ♀ **O22.12 Genital varices in pregnancy, second trimester**
- ♀ **O22.13 Genital varices in pregnancy, third trimester**

+ **O22.2 Superficial thrombophlebitis in pregnancy**
> Phlebitis in pregnancy NOS
> Thrombophlebitis of legs in pregnancy
> Thrombosis in pregnancy NOS
> Use additional code to identify the superficial thrombophlebitis (I80.0-)
- ♀ CC **O22.20 Superficial thrombophlebitis in pregnancy, unspecified trimester**
- ♀ CC **O22.21 Superficial thrombophlebitis in pregnancy, first trimester**
- ♀ CC **O22.22 Superficial thrombophlebitis in pregnancy, second trimester**
- ♀ CC **O22.23 Superficial thrombophlebitis in pregnancy, third trimester**

+ **O22.3 Deep phlebothrombosis in pregnancy**
> Deep vein thrombosis, antepartum
> Use additional code to identify the deep vein thrombosis (I82.4-, I82.5-, I82.62-, I82.72-)
>
> Use additional code, if applicable, for associated long-term (current) use of anticoagulants (Z79.01)
- ♀ CC **O22.30 Deep phlebothrombosis in pregnancy, unspecified trimester**
- ♀ MCC **O22.31 Deep phlebothrombosis in pregnancy, first trimester**
- ♀ MCC **O22.32 Deep phlebothrombosis in pregnancy, second trimester**
- ♀ MCC **O22.33 Deep phlebothrombosis in pregnancy, third trimester**

+ **O22.4 Hemorrhoids in pregnancy**
- ♀ CC **O22.40 Hemorrhoids in pregnancy, unspecified trimester**
- ♀ CC **O22.41 Hemorrhoids in pregnancy, first trimester**
- ♀ CC **O22.42 Hemorrhoids in pregnancy, second trimester**
- ♀ CC **O22.43 Hemorrhoids in pregnancy, third trimester**

+ **O22.5 Cerebral venous thrombosis in pregnancy**
> Cerebrovenous sinus thrombosis in pregnancy
- ♀ CC **O22.50 Cerebral venous thrombosis in pregnancy, unspecified trimester**
- ♀ CC **O22.51 Cerebral venous thrombosis in pregnancy, first trimester**
- ♀ CC **O22.52 Cerebral venous thrombosis in pregnancy, second trimester**
- ♀ CC **O22.53 Cerebral venous thrombosis in pregnancy, third trimester**

+ **O22.8 Other venous complications in pregnancy**
+ **O22.8X Other venous complications in pregnancy**
- ♀ CC **O22.8X1 Other venous complications in pregnancy, first trimester**
- ♀ CC **O22.8X2 Other venous complications in pregnancy, second trimester**
- ♀ CC **O22.8X3 Other venous complications in pregnancy, third trimester**
- ♀ CC **O22.8X9 Other venous complications in pregnancy, unspecified trimester**

+ **O22.9 Venous complication in pregnancy, unspecified**
> Gestational phlebitis NOS
> Gestational phlebopathy NOS
> Gestational thrombosis NOS
- ♀ CC **O22.90 Venous complication in pregnancy, unspecified, unspecified trimester**
- ♀ **O22.91 Venous complication in pregnancy, unspecified, first trimester**
- ♀ **O22.92 Venous complication in pregnancy, unspecified, second trimester**
- ♀ **O22.93 Venous complication in pregnancy, unspecified, third trimester**

O23 Infections of genitourinary tract in pregnancy

> Use additional code to identify organism (B95.-, B96.-)
>
> *Excludes2:* *gonococcal infections complicating pregnancy,*
> > *childbirth and the puerperium (O98.2)*
> > *infections with a predominantly sexual mode of*
> > *transmission NOS complicating pregnancy, childbirth*
> > *and the puerperium (O98.3)*
> > *syphilis complicating pregnancy, childbirth and the*
> > *puerperium (O98.1)*
> > *tuberculosis of genitourinary system complicating*
> > *pregnancy, childbirth and the puerperium (O98.0)*
> > *venereal disease NOS complicating pregnancy,*
> > *childbirth and the puerperium (O98.3)*

+ **O23.0 Infections of kidney in pregnancy**
> Pyelonephritis in pregnancy
- ♀ **O23.00 Infections of kidney in pregnancy, unspecified trimester**
- ♀ CC **O23.01 Infections of kidney in pregnancy, first trimester**
- ♀ CC **O23.02 Infections of kidney in pregnancy, second trimester**
- ♀ CC **O23.03 Infections of kidney in pregnancy, third trimester**

+ **O23.1 Infections of bladder in pregnancy**
- ♀ **O23.10 Infections of bladder in pregnancy, unspecified trimester**
- ♀ CC **O23.11 Infections of bladder in pregnancy, first trimester**
- ♀ CC **O23.12 Infections of bladder in pregnancy, second trimester**
- ♀ CC **O23.13 Infections of bladder in pregnancy, third trimester**

+ **O23.2 Infections of urethra in pregnancy**
- ♀ **O23.20 Infections of urethra in pregnancy, unspecified trimester**
- ♀ CC **O23.21 Infections of urethra in pregnancy, first trimester**
- ♀ CC **O23.22 Infections of urethra in pregnancy, second trimester**
- ♀ CC **O23.23 Infections of urethra in pregnancy, third trimester**

+ **O23.3 Infections of other parts of urinary tract in pregnancy**
- ♀ **O23.30 Infections of other parts of urinary tract in pregnancy, unspecified trimester**
- ♀ CC **O23.31 Infections of other parts of urinary tract in pregnancy, first trimester**
- ♀ CC **O23.32 Infections of other parts of urinary tract in pregnancy, second trimester**
- ♀ CC **O23.33 Infections of other parts of urinary tract in pregnancy, third trimester**

+ **O23.4 Unspecified infection of urinary tract in pregnancy**
- ♀ **O23.40 Unspecified infection of urinary tract in pregnancy, unspecified trimester**
- ♀ CC **O23.41 Unspecified infection of urinary tract in pregnancy, first trimester**
- ♀ CC **O23.42 Unspecified infection of urinary tract in pregnancy, second trimester**
- ♀ CC **O23.43 Unspecified infection of urinary tract in pregnancy, third trimester**
> *AHA CC: 2Q, 2018, 20*

+ **O23.5 Infections of the genital tract in pregnancy**
  + **O23.51 Infection of cervix in pregnancy**
    ● ♀ CC **O23.511 Infections of cervix in pregnancy, first trimester**
    ● ♀ CC **O23.512 Infections of cervix in pregnancy, second trimester**
    ● ♀ CC **O23.513 Infections of cervix in pregnancy, third trimester**
    ● ♀ **O23.519 Infections of cervix in pregnancy, unspecified trimester**
  + **O23.52 Salpingo-oophoritis in pregnancy**
    Oophoritis in pregnancy
    Salpingitis in pregnancy
    ● ♀ CC **O23.521 Salpingo-oophoritis in pregnancy, first trimester**
    ● ♀ CC **O23.522 Salpingo-oophoritis in pregnancy, second trimester**
    ● ♀ CC **O23.523 Salpingo-oophoritis in pregnancy, third trimester**
    ● ♀ **O23.529 Salpingo-oophoritis in pregnancy, unspecified trimester**
  + **O23.59 Infection of other part of genital tract in pregnancy**
    ● ♀ CC **O23.591 Infection of other part of genital tract in pregnancy, first trimester**
    ● ♀ CC **O23.592 Infection of other part of genital tract in pregnancy, second trimester**
    ● ♀ CC **O23.593 Infection of other part of genital tract in pregnancy, third trimester**
    ● ♀ **O23.599 Infection of other part of genital tract in pregnancy, unspecified trimester**
+ **O23.9 Unspecified genitourinary tract infection in pregnancy**
  Genitourinary tract infection in pregnancy NOS
  ● ♀ **O23.90 Unspecified genitourinary tract infection in pregnancy, unspecified trimester**
  ● ♀ CC **O23.91 Unspecified genitourinary tract infection in pregnancy, first trimester**
  ● ♀ CC **O23.92 Unspecified genitourinary tract infection in pregnancy, second trimester**
  ● ♀ CC **O23.93 Unspecified genitourinary tract infection in pregnancy, third trimester**

O24 Diabetes mellitus in pregnancy, childbirth, and the puerperium
  Review coding guideline C.15.g
+ **O24.0 Pre-existing type 1 diabetes mellitus, in pregnancy, childbirth and the puerperium**
  Juvenile onset diabetes mellitus, in pregnancy, childbirth and the puerperium
  Ketosis-prone diabetes mellitus in pregnancy, childbirth and the puerperium
  Use additional code from category E10 to further identify any manifestations
  + **O24.01 Pre-existing type 1 diabetes mellitus, in pregnancy**
    ● ♀ CC **O24.011 Pre-existing type 1 diabetes mellitus, in pregnancy, first trimester**
    ● ♀ CC **O24.012 Pre-existing type 1 diabetes mellitus, in pregnancy, second trimester**
    ● ♀ CC **O24.013 Pre-existing type 1 diabetes mellitus, in pregnancy, third trimester**
    ● ♀ CC **O24.019 Pre-existing type 1 diabetes mellitus, in pregnancy, unspecified trimester**
  ● ♀ MCC **O24.02 Pre-existing type 1 diabetes mellitus, in childbirth**
  ● ♀ CC **O24.03 Pre-existing type 1 diabetes mellitus, in the puerperium**
+ **O24.1 Pre-existing type 2 diabetes mellitus, in pregnancy, childbirth and the puerperium**
  Insulin-resistant diabetes mellitus in pregnancy, childbirth and the puerperium
  Use additional code (for):
    from category E11 to further identify any manifestations
    long-term (current) use of insulin (Z79.4)
  + **O24.11 Pre-existing type 2 diabetes mellitus, in pregnancy**
    ● ♀ CC **O24.111 Pre-existing type 2 diabetes mellitus, in pregnancy, first trimester**
    ● ♀ CC **O24.112 Pre-existing type 2 diabetes mellitus, in pregnancy, second trimester**
    ● ♀ CC **O24.113 Pre-existing type 2 diabetes mellitus, in pregnancy, third trimester**
    ● ♀ CC **O24.119 Pre-existing type 2 diabetes mellitus, in pregnancy, unspecified trimester**
  ● ♀ MCC **O24.12 Pre-existing type 2 diabetes mellitus, in childbirth**
  ● ♀ CC **O24.13 Pre-existing type 2 diabetes mellitus, in the puerperium**

+ **O24.3 Unspecified pre-existing diabetes mellitus in pregnancy, childbirth and the puerperium**
  Use additional code (for):
    from category E11 to further identify any manifestation
    long-term (current) use of insulin (Z79.4)
  + **O24.31 Unspecified pre-existing diabetes mellitus in pregnancy**
    ● ♀ CC **O24.311 Unspecified pre-existing diabetes mellitus in pregnancy, first trimester**
    ● ♀ CC **O24.312 Unspecified pre-existing diabetes mellitus in pregnancy, second trimester**
    ● ♀ CC **O24.313 Unspecified pre-existing diabetes mellitus in pregnancy, third trimester**
    ● ♀ CC **O24.319 Unspecified pre-existing diabetes mellitus in pregnancy, unspecified trimester**
  ● ♀ MCC **O24.32 Unspecified pre-existing diabetes mellitus in childbirth**
  ● ♀ CC **O24.33 Unspecified pre-existing diabetes mellitus in the puerperium**
+ **O24.4 Gestational diabetes mellitus**
  Diabetes mellitus arising in pregnancy
  Gestational diabetes mellitus NOS
  Review coding guideline C.15.i
  AHA CC: 4Q, 2016, 50
  + **O24.41 Gestational diabetes mellitus in pregnancy**
    ● ♀ **O24.410 Gestational diabetes mellitus in pregnancy, diet controlled**
    ● ♀ **O24.414 Gestational diabetes mellitus in pregnancy, insulin controlled**
    ● ♀ **O24.415 Gestational diabetes mellitus in pregnancy, controlled by oral hypoglycemic drugs**
      Gestational diabetes mellitus in pregnancy, controlled by oral antidiabetic drugs
    ● ♀ **O24.419 Gestational diabetes mellitus in pregnancy, unspecified control**
    AHA CC: 4Q, 2015, 34
  + **O24.42 Gestational diabetes mellitus in childbirth**
    ● ♀ **O24.420 Gestational diabetes mellitus in childbirth, diet controlled**
    ● ♀ **O24.424 Gestational diabetes mellitus in childbirth, insulin controlled**
    ● ♀ **O24.425 Gestational diabetes mellitus in childbirth, controlled by oral hypoglycemic drugs**
      Gestational diabetes mellitus in childbirth, controlled by oral antidiabetic drugs
    ● ♀ **O24.429 Gestational diabetes mellitus in childbirth, unspecified control**
  + **O24.43 Gestational diabetes mellitus in the puerperium**
    ● ♀ **O24.430 Gestational diabetes mellitus in the puerperium, diet controlled**
    ● ♀ **O24.434 Gestational diabetes mellitus in the puerperium, insulin controlled**
    ● ♀ **O24.435 Gestational diabetes mellitus in puerperium, controlled by oral hypoglycemic drugs**
      Gestational diabetes mellitus in puerperium, controlled by oral antidiabetic drugs
    ● ♀ **O24.439 Gestational diabetes mellitus in the puerperium, unspecified control**
+ **O24.8 Other pre-existing diabetes mellitus in pregnancy, childbirth, and the puerperium**
  Use additional code (for):
    from categories E08, E09 and E13 to further identify any manifestation
    long-term (current) use of insulin (Z79.4)
  + **O24.81 Other pre-existing diabetes mellitus in pregnancy**
    ● ♀ CC **O24.811 Other pre-existing diabetes mellitus in pregnancy, first trimester**
    ● ♀ CC **O24.812 Other pre-existing diabetes mellitus in pregnancy, second trimester**
    ● ♀ CC **O24.813 Other pre-existing diabetes mellitus in pregnancy, third trimester**
    ● ♀ CC **O24.819 Other pre-existing diabetes mellitus in pregnancy, unspecified trimester**
  ● ♀ MCC **O24.82 Other pre-existing diabetes mellitus in childbirth**
  ● ♀ CC **O24.83 Other pre-existing diabetes mellitus in the puerperium**

+, +7th, X + 7th ● Newborn ● Pediatric ● Maternity ● Adult ♀ Female ♂ Male Manifestation Unacceptable PDX HCC CC MCC HAC

+ **O24.9** **Unspecified diabetes mellitus in pregnancy, childbirth and the puerperium**
    Use additional code for long-term (current) use of insulin (Z79.4)
  + **O24.91** **Unspecified diabetes mellitus in pregnancy**
    • ♀ CC **O24.911** **Unspecified diabetes mellitus in pregnancy, first trimester**
    • ♀ CC **O24.912** **Unspecified diabetes mellitus in pregnancy, second trimester**
    • ♀ CC **O24.913** **Unspecified diabetes mellitus in pregnancy, third trimester**
    • ♀ CC **O24.919** **Unspecified diabetes mellitus in pregnancy, unspecified trimester**
  • ♀ **O24.92** **Unspecified diabetes mellitus in childbirth**
  • ♀ CC **O24.93** **Unspecified diabetes mellitus in the puerperium**

O25 **Malnutrition in pregnancy, childbirth and the puerperium**
  + **O25.1** **Malnutrition in pregnancy**
    • ♀ **O25.10** **Malnutrition in pregnancy, unspecified trimester**
    • ♀ **O25.11** **Malnutrition in pregnancy, first trimester**
    • ♀ **O25.12** **Malnutrition in pregnancy, second trimester**
    • ♀ **O25.13** **Malnutrition in pregnancy, third trimester**
  • ♀ **O25.2** **Malnutrition in childbirth**
  • ♀ **O25.3** **Malnutrition in the puerperium**

O26 **Maternal care for other conditions predominantly related to pregnancy**
  + **O26.0** **Excessive weight gain in pregnancy**
    Excludes2: gestational edema (O12.0, O12.2)
    • ♀ **O26.00** **Excessive weight gain in pregnancy, unspecified trimester**
    • ♀ **O26.01** **Excessive weight gain in pregnancy, first trimester**
    • ♀ **O26.02** **Excessive weight gain in pregnancy, second trimester**
    • ♀ **O26.03** **Excessive weight gain in pregnancy, third trimester**
  + **O26.1** **Low weight gain in pregnancy**
    • ♀ **O26.10** **Low weight gain in pregnancy, unspecified trimester**
    • ♀ **O26.11** **Low weight gain in pregnancy, first trimester**
    • ♀ **O26.12** **Low weight gain in pregnancy, second trimester**
    • ♀ **O26.13** **Low weight gain in pregnancy, third trimester**
  + **O26.2** **Pregnancy care for patient with recurrent pregnancy loss**
    • ♀ **O26.20** **Pregnancy care for patient with recurrent pregnancy loss, unspecified trimester**
    • ♀ **O26.21** **Pregnancy care for patient with recurrent pregnancy loss, first trimester**
    • ♀ **O26.22** **Pregnancy care for patient with recurrent pregnancy loss, second trimester**
    • ♀ **O26.23** **Pregnancy care for patient with recurrent pregnancy loss, third trimester**
  + **O26.3** **Retained intrauterine contraceptive device in pregnancy**
    • ♀ **O26.30** **Retained intrauterine contraceptive device in pregnancy, unspecified trimester**
    • ♀ **O26.31** **Retained intrauterine contraceptive device in pregnancy, first trimester**
    • ♀ **O26.32** **Retained intrauterine contraceptive device in pregnancy, second trimester**
    • ♀ **O26.33** **Retained intrauterine contraceptive device in pregnancy, third trimester**
  + **O26.4** **Herpes gestationis**
    • ♀ **O26.40** **Herpes gestationis, unspecified trimester**
    • ♀ **O26.41** **Herpes gestationis, first trimester**
    • ♀ **O26.42** **Herpes gestationis, second trimester**
    • ♀ **O26.43** **Herpes gestationis, third trimester**
  + **O26.5** **Maternal hypotension syndrome**
    Supine hypotensive syndrome
    • ♀ **O26.50** **Maternal hypotension syndrome, unspecified trimester**
    • ♀ **O26.51** **Maternal hypotension syndrome, first trimester**
    • ♀ **O26.52** **Maternal hypotension syndrome, second trimester**
    • ♀ **O26.53** **Maternal hypotension syndrome, third trimester**

+ **O26.6** **Liver and biliary tract disorders in pregnancy, childbirth and the puerperium**
    Use additional code to identify the specific disorder
    Excludes2: hepatorenal syndrome following labor and delivery (O90.4)
  + **O26.61** **Liver and biliary tract disorders in pregnancy**
    • ♀ CC **O26.611** **Liver and biliary tract disorders in pregnancy, first trimester**
    • ♀ CC **O26.612** **Liver and biliary tract disorders in pregnancy, second trimester**
    • ♀ CC **O26.613** **Liver and biliary tract disorders in pregnancy, third trimester**
    • ♀ **O26.619** **Liver and biliary tract disorders in pregnancy, unspecified trimester**
  • ♀ CC **O26.62** **Liver and biliary tract disorders in childbirth**
  • ♀ **O26.63** **Liver and biliary tract disorders in the puerperium**
+ **O26.7** **Subluxation of symphysis (pubis) in pregnancy, childbirth and the puerperium**
    Excludes1: traumatic separation of symphysis (pubis) during childbirth (O71.6)
  + **O26.71** **Subluxation of symphysis (pubis) in pregnancy**
    • ♀ **O26.711** **Subluxation of symphysis (pubis) in pregnancy, first trimester**
    • ♀ **O26.712** **Subluxation of symphysis (pubis) in pregnancy, second trimester**
    • ♀ **O26.713** **Subluxation of symphysis (pubis) in pregnancy, third trimester**
    • ♀ **O26.719** **Subluxation of symphysis (pubis) in pregnancy, unspecified trimester**
  • ♀ **O26.72** **Subluxation of symphysis (pubis) in childbirth**
  • ♀ **O26.73** **Subluxation of symphysis (pubis) in the puerperium**
+ **O26.8** **Other specified pregnancy related conditions**
  + **O26.81** **Pregnancy related exhaustion and fatigue**
    • ♀ **O26.811** **Pregnancy related exhaustion and fatigue, first trimester**
    • ♀ **O26.812** **Pregnancy related exhaustion and fatigue, second trimester**
    • ♀ **O26.813** **Pregnancy related exhaustion and fatigue, third trimester**
    • ♀ **O26.819** **Pregnancy related exhaustion and fatigue, unspecified trimester**
  + **O26.82** **Pregnancy related peripheral neuritis**
    • ♀ **O26.821** **Pregnancy related peripheral neuritis, first trimester**
    • ♀ **O26.822** **Pregnancy related peripheral neuritis, second trimester**
    • ♀ **O26.823** **Pregnancy related peripheral neuritis, third trimester**
    • ♀ **O26.829** **Pregnancy related peripheral neuritis, unspecified trimester**
  + **O26.83** **Pregnancy related renal disease**
    Use additional code to identify the specific disorder
    • ♀ CC **O26.831** **Pregnancy related renal disease, first trimester**
    • ♀ CC **O26.832** **Pregnancy related renal disease, second trimester**
    • ♀ CC **O26.833** **Pregnancy related renal disease, third trimester**
    • ♀ **O26.839** **Pregnancy related renal disease, unspecified trimester**
  + **O26.84** **Uterine size-date discrepancy complicating pregnancy**
    Excludes1: encounter for suspected problem with fetal growth ruled out (Z03.74)
    • ♀ **O26.841** **Uterine size-date discrepancy, first trimester**
    • ♀ **O26.842** **Uterine size-date discrepancy, second trimester**
    • ♀ **O26.843** **Uterine size-date discrepancy, third trimester**
    • ♀ **O26.849** **Uterine size-date discrepancy, unspecified trimester**
  + **O26.85** **Spotting complicating pregnancy**
    • ♀ **O26.851** **Spotting complicating pregnancy, first trimester**
    • ♀ **O26.852** **Spotting complicating pregnancy, second trimester**
    • ♀ **O26.853** **Spotting complicating pregnancy, third trimester**
    • ♀ **O26.859** **Spotting complicating pregnancy, unspecified trimester**

+, +7th, X + 7th   ● Newborn   ● Pediatric   ● Maternity   ● Adult   ♀ Female   ♂ Male   Manifestation   Unacceptable PDX   HCC   CC   MCC   HAC

- ● ♀ **O26.86** **Pruritic urticarial papules and plaques of pregnancy (PUPPP)**
  Polymorphic eruption of pregnancy
+ **O26.87** **Cervical shortening**
  Excludes1: *encounter for suspected cervical shortening ruled out (Z03.75)*
  - ● ♀ CC **O26.872** **Cervical shortening, second trimester**
  - ● ♀ CC **O26.873** **Cervical shortening, third trimester**
  - ● ♀ CC **O26.879** **Cervical shortening, unspecified trimester**
+ **O26.89** **Other specified pregnancy related conditions**
  - ● ♀ **O26.891** **Other specified pregnancy related conditions, first trimester**
  - ● ♀ **O26.892** **Other specified pregnancy related conditions, second trimester**
  - ● ♀ **O26.893** **Other specified pregnancy related conditions, third trimester**
    AHA CC: 3Q, 2015, 40
  - ● ♀ **O26.899** **Other specified pregnancy related conditions, unspecified trimester**
+ **O26.9** **Pregnancy related conditions, unspecified**
  - ● ♀ **O26.90** **Pregnancy related conditions, unspecified, unspecified trimester**
  - ● ♀ **O26.91** **Pregnancy related conditions, unspecified, first trimester**
  - ● ♀ **O26.92** **Pregnancy related conditions, unspecified, second trimester**
  - ● ♀ **O26.93** **Pregnancy related conditions, unspecified, third trimester**

O28 **Abnormal findings on antenatal screening of mother**

  Excludes1: *diagnostic findings classified elsewhere - see Alphabetical Index*
- ● ♀ **O28.0** **Abnormal hematological finding on antenatal screening of mother**
- ● ♀ **O28.1** **Abnormal biochemical finding on antenatal screening of mother**
- ● ♀ **O28.2** **Abnormal cytological finding on antenatal screening of mother**
- ● ♀ **O28.3** **Abnormal ultrasonic finding on antenatal screening of mother**
    AHA CC: 4Q, 2016, 4-7
- ● ♀ **O28.4** **Abnormal radiological finding on antenatal screening of mother**
- ● ♀ **O28.5** **Abnormal chromosomal and genetic finding on antenatal screening of mother**
- ● ♀ **O28.8** **Other abnormal findings on antenatal screening of mother**
- ● ♀ **O28.9** **Unspecified abnormal findings on antenatal screening of mother**

O29 **Complications of anesthesia during pregnancy**

  Includes: maternal complications arising from the administration of a general, regional or local anesthetic, analgesic or other sedation during pregnancy
  Use additional code, if necessary, to identify the complication
  Excludes2: *complications of anesthesia during labor and delivery (O74.-)*
  complications of anesthesia during the puerperium (O89.-)
+ **O29.0** **Pulmonary complications of anesthesia during pregnancy**
  + **O29.01** **Aspiration pneumonitis due to anesthesia during pregnancy**
    Inhalation of stomach contents or secretions NOS due to anesthesia during pregnancy
    Mendelson's syndrome due to anesthesia during pregnancy
    - ● ♀ **O29.011** **Aspiration pneumonitis due to anesthesia during pregnancy, first trimester**
    - ● ♀ **O29.012** **Aspiration pneumonitis due to anesthesia during pregnancy, second trimester**
    - ● ♀ **O29.013** **Aspiration pneumonitis due to anesthesia during pregnancy, third trimester**
    - ● ♀ **O29.019** **Aspiration pneumonitis due to anesthesia during pregnancy, unspecified trimester**

+ **O29.02** **Pressure collapse of lung due to anesthesia during pregnancy**
  - ● ♀ **O29.021** **Pressure collapse of lung due to anesthesia during pregnancy, first trimester**
  - ● ♀ **O29.022** **Pressure collapse of lung due to anesthesia during pregnancy, second trimester**
  - ● ♀ **O29.023** **Pressure collapse of lung due to anesthesia during pregnancy, third trimester**
  - ● ♀ **O29.029** **Pressure collapse of lung due to anesthesia during pregnancy, unspecified trimester**
+ **O29.09** **Other pulmonary complications of anesthesia during pregnancy**
  - ● ♀ **O29.091** **Other pulmonary complications of anesthesia during pregnancy, first trimester**
  - ● ♀ **O29.092** **Other pulmonary complications of anesthesia during pregnancy, second trimester**
  - ● ♀ **O29.093** **Other pulmonary complications of anesthesia during pregnancy, third trimester**
  - ● ♀ **O29.099** **Other pulmonary complications of anesthesia during pregnancy, unspecified trimester**
+ **O29.1** **Cardiac complications of anesthesia during pregnancy**
  + **O29.11** **Cardiac arrest due to anesthesia during pregnancy**
    - ● ♀ **O29.111** **Cardiac arrest due to anesthesia during pregnancy, first trimester**
    - ● ♀ **O29.112** **Cardiac arrest due to anesthesia during pregnancy, second trimester**
    - ● ♀ **O29.113** **Cardiac arrest due to anesthesia during pregnancy, third trimester**
    - ● ♀ **O29.119** **Cardiac arrest due to anesthesia during pregnancy, unspecified trimester**
  + **O29.12** **Cardiac failure due to anesthesia during pregnancy**
    - ● ♀ **O29.121** **Cardiac failure due to anesthesia during pregnancy, first trimester**
    - ● ♀ **O29.122** **Cardiac failure due to anesthesia during pregnancy, second trimester**
    - ● ♀ **O29.123** **Cardiac failure due to anesthesia during pregnancy, third trimester**
    - ● ♀ **O29.129** **Cardiac failure due to anesthesia during pregnancy, unspecified trimester**
  + **O29.19** **Other cardiac complications of anesthesia during pregnancy**
    - ● ♀ **O29.191** **Other cardiac complications of anesthesia during pregnancy, first trimester**
    - ● ♀ **O29.192** **Other cardiac complications of anesthesia during pregnancy, second trimester**
    - ● ♀ **O29.193** **Other cardiac complications of anesthesia during pregnancy, third trimester**
    - ● ♀ **O29.199** **Other cardiac complications of anesthesia during pregnancy, unspecified trimester**
+ **O29.2** **Central nervous system complications of anesthesia during pregnancy**
  + **O29.21** **Cerebral anoxia due to anesthesia during pregnancy**
    - ● ♀ **O29.211** **Cerebral anoxia due to anesthesia during pregnancy, first trimester**
    - ● ♀ **O29.212** **Cerebral anoxia due to anesthesia during pregnancy, second trimester**
    - ● ♀ **O29.213** **Cerebral anoxia due to anesthesia during pregnancy, third trimester**
    - ● ♀ **O29.219** **Cerebral anoxia due to anesthesia during pregnancy, unspecified trimester**

+ O29.29 Other central nervous system complications of anesthesia during pregnancy
- ♀ O29.291 Other central nervous system complications of anesthesia during pregnancy, first trimester
- ♀ O29.292 Other central nervous system complications of anesthesia during pregnancy, second trimester
- ♀ O29.293 Other central nervous system complications of anesthesia during pregnancy, third trimester
- ♀ O29.299 Other central nervous system complications of anesthesia during pregnancy, unspecified trimester
+ O29.3 Toxic reaction to local anesthesia during pregnancy
  + O29.3X Toxic reaction to local anesthesia during pregnancy
  - ♀ O29.3X1 Toxic reaction to local anesthesia during pregnancy, first trimester
  - ♀ O29.3X2 Toxic reaction to local anesthesia during pregnancy, second trimester
  - ♀ O29.3X3 Toxic reaction to local anesthesia during pregnancy, third trimester
  - ♀ O29.3X9 Toxic reaction to local anesthesia during pregnancy, unspecified trimester
+ O29.4 Spinal and epidural anesthesia induced headache during pregnancy
  - ♀ O29.40 Spinal and epidural anesthesia induced headache during pregnancy, unspecified trimester
  - ♀ O29.41 Spinal and epidural anesthesia induced headache during pregnancy, first trimester
  - ♀ O29.42 Spinal and epidural anesthesia induced headache during pregnancy, second trimester
  - ♀ O29.43 Spinal and epidural anesthesia induced headache during pregnancy, third trimester
+ O29.5 Other complications of spinal and epidural anesthesia during pregnancy
  + O29.5X Other complications of spinal and epidural anesthesia during pregnancy
  - ♀ O29.5X1 Other complications of spinal and epidural anesthesia during pregnancy, first trimester
  - ♀ O29.5X2 Other complications of spinal and epidural anesthesia during pregnancy, second trimester
  - ♀ O29.5X3 Other complications of spinal and epidural anesthesia during pregnancy, third trimester
  - ♀ O29.5X9 Other complications of spinal and epidural anesthesia during pregnancy, unspecified trimester
+ O29.6 Failed or difficult intubation for anesthesia during pregnancy
  - ♀ O29.60 Failed or difficult intubation for anesthesia during pregnancy, unspecified trimester
  - ♀ O29.61 Failed or difficult intubation for anesthesia during pregnancy, first trimester
  - ♀ O29.62 Failed or difficult intubation for anesthesia during pregnancy, second trimester
  - ♀ O29.63 Failed or difficult intubation for anesthesia during pregnancy, third trimester
+ O29.8 Other complications of anesthesia during pregnancy
  + O29.8X Other complications of anesthesia during pregnancy
  - ♀ O29.8X1 Other complications of anesthesia during pregnancy, first trimester
  - ♀ O29.8X2 Other complications of anesthesia during pregnancy, second trimester
  - ♀ O29.8X3 Other complications of anesthesia during pregnancy, third trimester
  - ♀ O29.8X9 Other complications of anesthesia during pregnancy, unspecified trimester
+ O29.9 Unspecified complication of anesthesia during pregnancy
  - ♀ O29.90 Unspecified complication of anesthesia during pregnancy, unspecified trimester
  - ♀ O29.91 Unspecified complication of anesthesia during pregnancy, first trimester
  - ♀ O29.92 Unspecified complication of anesthesia during pregnancy, second trimester
  - ♀ O29.93 Unspecified complication of anesthesia during pregnancy, third trimester

Maternal care related to the fetus and amniotic cavity and possible delivery problems (O30-O48)

O30 Multiple gestation

Code also any complications specific to multiple gestation

+ O30.0 Twin pregnancy
  + O30.00 Twin pregnancy, unspecified number of placenta and unspecified number of amniotic sacs
  - ♀ O30.001 Twin pregnancy, unspecified number of placenta and unspecified number of amniotic sacs, first trimester
  - ♀ O30.002 Twin pregnancy, unspecified number of placenta and unspecified number of amniotic sacs, second trimester
  - ♀ O30.003 Twin pregnancy, unspecified number of placenta and unspecified number of amniotic sacs, third trimester
  - ♀ O30.009 Twin pregnancy, unspecified number of placenta and unspecified number of amniotic sacs, unspecified trimester
  + O30.01 Twin pregnancy, monochorionic/monoamniotic
    Twin pregnancy, one placenta, one amniotic sac
    Excludes1: conjoined twins (O30.02-)
  - ♀ O30.011 Twin pregnancy, monochorionic/monoamniotic, first trimester
  - ♀ O30.012 Twin pregnancy, monochorionic/monoamniotic, second trimester
  - ♀ O30.013 Twin pregnancy, monochorionic/monoamniotic, third trimester
  - ♀ O30.019 Twin pregnancy, monochorionic/monoamniotic, unspecified trimester
  + O30.02 Conjoined twin pregnancy
  - ♀ O30.021 Conjoined twin pregnancy, first trimester
  - ♀ O30.022 Conjoined twin pregnancy, second trimester
  - ♀ O30.023 Conjoined twin pregnancy, third trimester
  - ♀ O30.029 Conjoined twin pregnancy, unspecified trimester
  + O30.03 Twin pregnancy, monochorionic/diamniotic
    Twin pregnancy, one placenta, two amniotic sacs
  - ♀ O30.031 Twin pregnancy, monochorionic/diamniotic, first trimester
  - ♀ O30.032 Twin pregnancy, monochorionic/diamniotic, second trimester
  - ♀ O30.033 Twin pregnancy, monochorionic/diamniotic, third trimester
  - ♀ O30.039 Twin pregnancy, monochorionic/diamniotic, unspecified trimester
  + O30.04 Twin pregnancy, dichorionic/diamniotic
    Twin pregnancy, two placentae, two amniotic sacs
  - ♀ O30.041 Twin pregnancy, dichorionic/diamniotic, first trimester
  - ♀ O30.042 Twin pregnancy, dichorionic/diamniotic, second trimester
  - ♀ O30.043 Twin pregnancy, dichorionic/diamniotic, third trimester
  - ♀ O30.049 Twin pregnancy, dichorionic/diamniotic, unspecified trimester
  + O30.09 Twin pregnancy, unable to determine number of placenta and number of amniotic sacs
  - ♀ O30.091 Twin pregnancy, unable to determine number of placenta and number of amniotic sacs, first trimester
  - ♀ O30.092 Twin pregnancy, unable to determine number of placenta and number of amniotic sacs, second trimester
  - ♀ O30.093 Twin pregnancy, unable to determine number of placenta and number of amniotic sacs, third trimester
  - ♀ O30.099 Twin pregnancy, unable to determine number of placenta and number of amniotic sacs, unspecified trimester

+ O30.1 **Triplet pregnancy**
  + O30.10 **Triplet pregnancy, unspecified number of placenta and unspecified number of amniotic sacs**
    ● ♀ CC **O30.101** Triplet pregnancy, unspecified number of placenta and unspecified number of amniotic sacs, first trimester
    ● ♀ CC **O30.102** Triplet pregnancy, unspecified number of placenta and unspecified number of amniotic sacs, second trimester
    ● ♀ CC **O30.103** Triplet pregnancy, unspecified number of placenta and unspecified number of amniotic sacs, third trimester
      AHA CC: 2Q, 2016, 8
    ● ♀ **O30.109** Triplet pregnancy, unspecified number of placenta and unspecified number of amniotic sacs, unspecified trimester
  + O30.11 **Triplet pregnancy with two or more monochorionic fetuses**
    ● ♀ CC **O30.111** Triplet pregnancy with two or more monochorionic fetuses, first trimester
    ● ♀ CC **O30.112** Triplet pregnancy with two or more monochorionic fetuses, second trimester
    ● ♀ CC **O30.113** Triplet pregnancy with two or more monochorionic fetuses, third trimester
    ● ♀ **O30.119** Triplet pregnancy with two or more monochorionic fetuses, unspecified trimester
  + O30.12 **Triplet pregnancy with two or more monoamniotic fetuses**
    ● ♀ CC **O30.121** Triplet pregnancy with two or more monoamniotic fetuses, first trimester
    ● ♀ CC **O30.122** Triplet pregnancy with two or more monoamniotic fetuses, second trimester
    ● ♀ CC **O30.123** Triplet pregnancy with two or more monoamniotic fetuses, third trimester
    ● ♀ **O30.129** Triplet pregnancy with two or more monoamniotic fetuses, unspecified trimester
  + O30.13 **Triplet pregnancy, trichorionic/trimniotic**
      AHA CC: 4Q, 2018, 22
    ● ♀ CC **O30.131** Triplet pregnancy, trichorionic/triamniotic, first trimester
    ● ♀ CC **O30.132** Triplet pregnancy, trichorionic/triamniotic, second trimester
    ● ♀ CC **O30.133** Triplet pregnancy, trichorionic/triamniotic, third trimester
    ● ♀ **O30.139** Triplet pregnancy, trichorionic/triamniotic, unspecified trimester
  + O30.19 **Triplet pregnancy, unable to determine number of placenta and number of amniotic sacs**
    ● ♀ CC **O30.191** Triplet pregnancy, unable to determine number of placenta and number of amniotic sacs, first trimester
    ● ♀ CC **O30.192** Triplet pregnancy, unable to determine number of placenta and number of amniotic sacs, second trimester
    ● ♀ CC **O30.193** Triplet pregnancy, unable to determine number of placenta and number of amniotic sacs, third trimester
    ● ♀ **O30.199** Triplet pregnancy, unable to determine number of placenta and number of amniotic sacs, unspecified trimester

+ O30.2 **Quadruplet pregnancy**
  + O30.20 **Quadruplet pregnancy, unspecified number of placenta and unspecified number of amniotic sacs**
    ● ♀ CC **O30.201** Quadruplet pregnancy, unspecified number of placenta and unspecified number of amniotic sacs, first trimester
    ● ♀ CC **O30.202** Quadruplet pregnancy, unspecified number of placenta and unspecified number of amniotic sacs, second trimester
    ● ♀ CC **O30.203** Quadruplet pregnancy, unspecified number of placenta and unspecified number of amniotic sacs, third trimester
    ● ♀ **O30.209** Quadruplet pregnancy, unspecified number of placenta and unspecified number of amniotic sacs, unspecified trimester

+ O30.21 **Quadruplet pregnancy with two or more monochorionic fetuses**
  ● ♀ CC **O30.211** Quadruplet pregnancy with two or more monochorionic fetuses, first trimester
  ● ♀ CC **O30.212** Quadruplet pregnancy with two or more monochorionic fetuses, second trimester
  ● ♀ CC **O30.213** Quadruplet pregnancy with two or more monochorionic fetuses, third trimester
  ● ♀ **O30.219** Quadruplet pregnancy with two or more monochorionic fetuses, unspecified trimester
+ O30.22 **Quadruplet pregnancy with two or more monoamniotic fetuses**
  ● ♀ CC **O30.221** Quadruplet pregnancy with two or more monoamniotic fetuses, first trimester
  ● ♀ CC **O30.222** Quadruplet pregnancy with two or more monoamniotic fetuses, second trimester
  ● ♀ CC **O30.223** Quadruplet pregnancy with two or more monoamniotic fetuses, third trimester
  ● ♀ **O30.229** Quadruplet pregnancy with two or more monoamniotic fetuses, unspecified trimester
+ O30.23 **Quadruplet pregnancy, quadrachorionic/quadra-amniotic**
    AHA CC: 4Q, 2018, 22
  ● ♀ CC **O30.231** Quadruplet pregnancy, quadrachorionic/quadra-amniotic, first trimester
  ● ♀ CC **O30.232** Quadruplet pregnancy, quadrachorionic/quadra-amniotic, second trimester
  ● ♀ CC **O30.233** Quadruplet pregnancy, quadrachorionic/quadra-amniotic, third trimester
  ● ♀ **O30.239** Quadruplet pregnancy, quadrachorionic/quadra-amniotic, unspecified trimester
+ O30.29 **Quadruplet pregnancy, unable to determine number of placenta and number of amniotic sacs**
  ● ♀ CC **O30.291** Quadruplet pregnancy, unable to determine number of placenta and number of amniotic sacs, first trimester
  ● ♀ CC **O30.292** Quadruplet pregnancy, unable to determine number of placenta and number of amniotic sacs, second trimester
  ● ♀ CC **O30.293** Quadruplet pregnancy, unable to determine number of placenta and number of amniotic sacs, third trimester
  ● ♀ **O30.299** Quadruplet pregnancy, unable to determine number of placenta and number of amniotic sacs, unspecified trimester

+ O30.8 **Other specified multiple gestation**
  Multiple gestation pregnancy greater then quadruplets
  + O30.80 **Other specified multiple gestation, unspecified number of placenta and unspecified number of amniotic sacs**
    ● ♀ CC **O30.801** Other specified multiple gestation, unspecified number of placenta and unspecified number of amniotic sacs, first trimester
    ● ♀ CC **O30.802** Other specified multiple gestation, unspecified number of placenta and unspecified number of amniotic sacs, second trimester
    ● ♀ CC **O30.803** Other specified multiple gestation, unspecified number of placenta and unspecified number of amniotic sacs, third trimester
    ● ♀ **O30.809** Other specified multiple gestation, unspecified number of placenta and unspecified number of amniotic sacs, unspecified trimester

+ **O30.81** **Other specified multiple gestation with two or more monochorionic fetuses**
- ♀ CC **O30.811** **Other specified multiple gestation with two or more monochorionic fetuses, first trimester**
- ♀ CC **O30.812** **Other specified multiple gestation with two or more monochorionic fetuses, second trimester**
- ♀ CC **O30.813** **Other specified multiple gestation with two or more monochorionic fetuses, third trimester**
- ♀ **O30.819** **Other specified multiple gestation with two or more monochorionic fetuses, unspecified trimester**

+ **O30.82** **Other specified multiple gestation with two or more monoamniotic fetuses**
- ♀ CC **O30.821** **Other specified multiple gestation with two or more monoamniotic fetuses, first trimester**
- ♀ CC **O30.822** **Other specified multiple gestation with two or more monoamniotic fetuses, second trimester**
- ♀ CC **O30.823** **Other specified multiple gestation with two or more monoamniotic fetuses, third trimester**
- ♀ **O30.829** **Other specified multiple gestation with two or more monoamniotic fetuses, unspecified trimester**

+ **O30.83** **Other specified multiple gestation, number of chorions and amnions are both equal to the number of fetuses**
  Pentachorionic, penta-amniotic pregnancy (quintuplets)
  Hexachorionic, hexa-amniotic pregnancy (sextuplets)
  Heptachorionic, hepta-amniotic pregnancy (septuplets)
  AHA CC: 4Q, 2018, 22
- ♀ CC **O30.831** **Other specified multiple gestation, number of chorions and amnions are both equal to the number of fetuses, first trimester**
- ♀ CC **O30.832** **Other specified multiple gestation, number of chorions and amnions are both equal to the number of fetuses, second trimester**
- ♀ CC **O30.833** **Other specified multiple gestation, number of chorions and amnions are both equal to the number of fetuses, third trimester**
- ♀ **O30.839** **Other specified multiple gestation, number of chorions and amnions are both equal to the number of fetuses, unspecified trimester**

+ **O30.89** **Other specified multiple gestation, unable to determine number of placenta and number of amniotic sacs**
- ♀ CC **O30.891** **Other specified multiple gestation, unable to determine number of placenta and number of amniotic sacs, first trimester**
- ♀ CC **O30.892** **Other specified multiple gestation, unable to determine number of placenta and number of amniotic sacs, second trimester**
- ♀ CC **O30.893** **Other specified multiple gestation, unable to determine number of placenta and number of amniotic sacs, third trimester**
- ♀ **O30.899** **Other specified multiple gestation, unable to determine number of placenta and number of amniotic sacs, unspecified trimester**

+ **O30.9** **Multiple gestation, unspecified**
  Multiple pregnancy NOS
- ♀ **O30.90** **Multiple gestation, unspecified, unspecified trimester**
- ♀ **O30.91** **Multiple gestation, unspecified, first trimester**
- ♀ **O30.92** **Multiple gestation, unspecified, second trimester**
- ♀ **O30.93** **Multiple gestation, unspecified, third trimester**

O31 **Complications specific to multiple gestation**

> **Excludes2:** *delayed delivery of second twin, triplet, etc. (O63.2)*
> *malpresentation of one fetus or more (O32.9)*
> *placental transfusion syndromes (O43.0-)*

> One of the following 7th characters is to be assigned to each code under category O31. 7th character 0 is for single gestations and multiple gestations where the fetus is unspecified. 7th characters 1 through 9 are for cases of multiple gestations to identify the fetus for which the code applies. The appropriate code from category O30, Multiple gestation, must also be assigned when assigning a code from category O31 that has a 7th character of 1 through 9.
> 0 - not applicable or unspecified
> 1 - fetus 1
> 2 - fetus 2
> 3 - fetus 3
> 4 - fetus 4
> 5 - fetus 5
> 9 - other fetus

+ **O31.0** **Papyraceous fetus**
  Fetus compressus
- ♀ X+7th **O31.00** **Papyraceous fetus, unspecified trimester**
- ♀ X+7th **O31.01** **Papyraceous fetus, first trimester**
- ♀ X+7th **O31.02** **Papyraceous fetus, second trimester**
- ♀ X+7th **O31.03** **Papyraceous fetus, third trimester**

+ **O31.1** **Continuing pregnancy after spontaneous abortion of one fetus or more**
- ♀ X+7th **O31.10** **Continuing pregnancy after spontaneous abortion of one fetus or more, unspecified trimester**
- ♀ X+7th **O31.11** **Continuing pregnancy after spontaneous abortion of one fetus or more, first trimester**
- ♀ X+7th **O31.12** **Continuing pregnancy after spontaneous abortion of one fetus or more, second trimester**
- ♀ X+7th **O31.13** **Continuing pregnancy after spontaneous abortion of one fetus or more, third trimester**

+ **O31.2** **Continuing pregnancy after intrauterine death of one fetus or more**
- ♀ X+7th **O31.20** **Continuing pregnancy after intrauterine death of one fetus or more, unspecified trimester**
- ♀ X+7th **O31.21** **Continuing pregnancy after intrauterine death of one fetus or more, first trimester**
- ♀ X+7th **O31.22** **Continuing pregnancy after intrauterine death of one fetus or more, second trimester**
- ♀ X+7th **O31.23** **Continuing pregnancy after intrauterine death of one fetus or more, third trimester**

+ **O31.3** **Continuing pregnancy after elective fetal reduction of one fetus or more**
  Continuing pregnancy after selective termination of one fetus or more
- ♀ X+7th **O31.30** **Continuing pregnancy after elective fetal reduction of one fetus or more, unspecified trimester**
- ♀ X+7th **O31.31** **Continuing pregnancy after elective fetal reduction of one fetus or more, first trimester**
- ♀ X+7th **O31.32** **Continuing pregnancy after elective fetal reduction of one fetus or more, second trimester**
- ♀ X+7th **O31.33** **Continuing pregnancy after elective fetal reduction of one fetus or more, third trimester**

+ **O31.8** **Other complications specific to multiple gestation**
  + **O31.8X** **Other complications specific to multiple gestation**
  - ♀ CC +7th **O31.8X1** **Other complications specific to multiple gestation, first trimester**
  - ♀ +7th **O31.8X2** **Other complications specific to multiple gestation, second trimester**
  - ♀ +7th **O31.8X3** **Other complications specific to multiple gestation, third trimester**
  - ♀ +7th **O31.8X9** **Other complications specific to multiple gestation, unspecified trimester**

O32 Maternal care for malpresentation of fetus

Includes: the listed conditions as a reason for observation, hospitalization or other obstetric care of the mother, or for cesarean delivery before onset of labor

Excludes1: malpresentation of fetus with obstructed labor (O64.-)

One of the following 7th characters is to be assigned to each code under category O32. 7th character 0 is for single gestations and multiple gestations where the fetus is unspecified. 7th characters 1 through 9 are for cases of multiple gestations to identify the fetus for which the code applies. The appropriate code from category O30, Multiple gestation, must also be assigned when assigning a code from category O32 that has a 7th character of 1 through 9.

0 - not applicable or unspecified
1 - fetus 1
2 - fetus 2
3 - fetus 3
4 - fetus 4
5 - fetus 5
9 - other fetus

- ♀ X+7th **O32.0 Maternal care for unstable lie**
- ♀ X+7th **O32.1 Maternal care for breech presentation**
  Maternal care for buttocks presentation
  Maternal care for complete breech
  Maternal care for frank breech
  Excludes1: footling presentation (O32.8)
  incomplete breech (O32.8)
- ♀ X+7th **O32.2 Maternal care for transverse and oblique lie**
  Maternal care for oblique presentation
  Maternal care for transverse presentation
- ♀ X+7th **O32.3 Maternal care for face, brow and chin presentation**
- ♀ X+7th **O32.4 Maternal care for high head at term**
  Maternal care for failure of head to enter pelvic brim
- ♀ X+7th **O32.6 Maternal care for compound presentation**
- ♀ X+7th **O32.8 Maternal care for other malpresentation of fetus**
  Maternal care for footling presentation
  Maternal care for incomplete breech
- ♀ X+7th **O32.9 Maternal care for malpresentation of fetus, unspecified**

O33 Maternal care for disproportion

Includes: the listed conditions as a reason for observation, hospitalization or other obstetric care of the mother, or for cesarean delivery before onset of labor

Excludes1: disproportion with obstructed labor (O65-O66)

- ♀ CC **O33.0 Maternal care for disproportion due to deformity of maternal pelvic bones**
  Maternal care for disproportion due to pelvic deformity causing disproportion NOS
- ♀ **O33.1 Maternal care for disproportion due to generally contracted pelvis**
  Maternal care for disproportion due to contracted pelvis NOS causing disproportion
- ♀ **O33.2 Maternal care for disproportion due to inlet contraction of pelvis**
  Maternal care for disproportion due to inlet contraction (pelvis) causing disproportion
- ♀ +7th **O33.3 Maternal care for disproportion due to outlet contraction of pelvis**
  Maternal care for disproportion due to mid-cavity contraction (pelvis)
  Maternal care for disproportion due to outlet contraction (pelvis)

One of the following 7th characters is to be assigned to code O33.3. 7th character 0 is for single gestations and multiple gestations where the fetus is unspecified. 7th characters 1 through 9 are for cases of multiple gestations to identify the fetus for which the code applies. The appropriate code from category O30, Multiple gestation, must also be assigned when assigning code O33.3 with a 7th character of 1 through 9.

0 - not applicable or unspecified
1 - fetus 1
2 - fetus 2
3 - fetus 3
4 - fetus 4
5 - fetus 5
9 - other fetus

- ♀ X+7th **O33.4 Maternal care for disproportion of mixed maternal and fetal origin**

One of the following 7th characters is to be assigned to code O33.4. 7th character 0 is for single gestations and multiple gestations where the fetus is unspecified. 7th characters 1 through 9 are for cases of multiple gestations to identify the fetus for which the code applies. The appropriate code from category O30, Multiple gestation, must also be assigned when assigning code O33.4 with a 7th character of 1 through 9.

0 - not applicable or unspecified
1 - fetus 1
2 - fetus 2
3 - fetus 3
4 - fetus 4
5 - fetus 5
9 - other fetus

- ♀ X+7th **O33.5 Maternal care for disproportion due to unusually large fetus**
  Maternal care for disproportion due to disproportion of fetal origin with normally formed fetus
  Maternal care for disproportion due to fetal disproportion NOS

One of the following 7th characters is to be assigned to code O33.5. 7th character 0 is for single gestations and multiple gestations where the fetus is unspecified. 7th characters 1 through 9 are for cases of multiple gestations to identify the fetus for which the code applies. The appropriate code from category O30, Multiple gestation, must also be assigned when assigning code O33.5 with a 7th character of 1 through 9.

0 - not applicable or unspecified
1 - fetus 1
2 - fetus 2
3 - fetus 3
4 - fetus 4
5 - fetus 5
9 - other fetus

- ♀ X+7th **O33.6 Maternal care for disproportion due to hydrocephalic fetus**

One of the following 7th characters is to be assigned to code O33.6. 7th character 0 is for single gestations and multiple gestations where the fetus is unspecified. 7th characters 1 through 9 are for cases of multiple gestations to identify the fetus for which the code applies. The appropriate code from category O30, Multiple gestation, must also be assigned when assigning code O33.6 with a 7th character of 1 through 9.

0 - not applicable or unspecified
1 - fetus 1
2 - fetus 2
3 - fetus 3
4 - fetus 4
5 - fetus 5
9 - other fetus

- ♀ X+7th **O33.7 Maternal care for disproportion due to other fetal deformities**
  Maternal care for disproportion due to fetal ascites
  Maternal care for disproportion due to fetal hydrops
  Maternal care for disproportion due to fetal meningomyelocele
  Maternal care for disproportion due to fetal sacral teratoma
  Maternal care for disproportion due to fetal tumor
  Excludes1: obstructed labor due to other fetal deformities (O66.3)
  AHA CC: 4Q, 2016, 51

One of the following 7th characters is to be assigned to code O33.7. 7th character 0 is for single gestations and multiple gestations where the fetus is unspecified. 7th characters 1 through 9 are for cases of multiple gestations to identify the fetus for which the code applies. The appropriate code from category O30, Multiple gestation, must also be assigned when assigning code O33.7 with a 7th character of 1 through 9.

0 - not applicable or unspecified
1 - fetus 1
2 - fetus 2
3 - fetus 3
4 - fetus 4
5 - fetus 5
9 - other fetus

- ♀ **O33.8 Maternal care for disproportion of other origin**
- ♀ **O33.9 Maternal care for disproportion, unspecified**
  Maternal care for disproportion due to cephalopelvic disproportion NOS
  Maternal care for disproportion due to fetopelvic disproportion NOS

O34   Maternal care for abnormality of pelvic organs

   Includes: the listed conditions as a reason for hospitalization or
   other obstetric care of the mother, or for cesarean
   delivery before onset of labor
   Code first any associated obstructed labor (O65.5)

   Use additional code for specific condition

+ **O34.0   Maternal care for congenital malformation of uterus**
   Maternal care for double uterus
   Maternal care for uterus bicornis
   - ♀ **O34.00   Maternal care for unspecified congenital malformation of uterus, unspecified trimester**
   - ♀ **O34.01   Maternal care for unspecified congenital malformation of uterus, first trimester**
   - ♀ **O34.02   Maternal care for unspecified congenital malformation of uterus, second trimester**
   - ♀ **O34.03   Maternal care for unspecified congenital malformation of uterus, third trimester**

+ **O34.1   Maternal care for benign tumor of corpus uteri**
   Excludes2: *maternal care for benign tumor of cervix (O34.4-)*
   maternal care for malignant neoplasm of uterus (O9A.1-)
   - ♀ **O34.10   Maternal care for benign tumor of corpus uteri, unspecified trimester**
   - ♀ **O34.11   Maternal care for benign tumor of corpus uteri, first trimester**
   - ♀ **O34.12   Maternal care for benign tumor of corpus uteri, second trimester**
   - ♀ **O34.13   Maternal care for benign tumor of corpus uteri, third trimester**

+ **O34.2   Maternal care due to uterine scar from previous surgery**
   + **O34.21   Maternal care for scar from previous cesarean delivery**
      AHA CC: 4Q, 2016, 51-52
      - ♀ **O34.211   Maternal care for low transverse scar from previous cesarean delivery**
         AHA CC: 3Q, 2018, 23-24
      - ♀ **O34.212   Maternal care for vertical scar from previous cesarean delivery**
         Maternal care for classical scar from previous cesarean delivery
      - ♀ **O34.218   Maternal care for other type scar from previous cesarean delivery**
         Mid-transverse T incision
      - ♀ **O34.219   Maternal care for unspecified type scar from previous cesarean delivery**
         AHA CC: 3Q, 2018, 23
   - ♀ **O34.22   Maternal care for cesarean scar defect (isthmocele)**
   - ♀ **O34.29   Maternal care due to uterine scar from other previous surgery**
      Maternal care due to uterine scar from other transmural uterine

+ **O34.3   Maternal care for cervical incompetence**
   Maternal care for cerclage with or without cervical incompetence
   Maternal care for Shirodkar suture with or without cervical incompetence
   - ♀ **O34.30   Maternal care for cervical incompetence, unspecified trimester**
   - ♀ MCC **O34.31   Maternal care for cervical incompetence, first trimester**
   - ♀ MCC **O34.32   Maternal care for cervical incompetence, second trimester**
   - ♀ MCC **O34.33   Maternal care for cervical incompetence, third trimester**

+ **O34.4   Maternal care for other abnormalities of cervix**
   - ♀ **O34.40   Maternal care for other abnormalities of cervix, unspecified trimester**
   - ♀ **O34.41   Maternal care for other abnormalities of cervix, first trimester**
   - ♀ **O34.42   Maternal care for other abnormalities of cervix, second trimester**

   - ♀ **O34.43   Maternal care for other abnormalities of cervix, third trimester**

+ **O34.5   Maternal care for other abnormalities of gravid uterus**
   + **O34.51   Maternal care for incarceration of gravid uterus**
      - ♀ **O34.511   Maternal care for incarceration of gravid uterus, first trimester**
      - ♀ **O34.512   Maternal care for incarceration of gravid uterus, second trimester**
      - ♀ **O34.513   Maternal care for incarceration of gravid uterus, third trimester**
      - ♀ **O34.519   Maternal care for incarceration of gravid uterus, unspecified trimester**
   + **O34.52   Maternal care for prolapse of gravid uterus**
      - ♀ **O34.521   Maternal care for prolapse of gravid uterus, first trimester**
      - ♀ **O34.522   Maternal care for prolapse of gravid uterus, second trimester**
      - ♀ **O34.523   Maternal care for prolapse of gravid uterus, third trimester**
      - ♀ **O34.529   Maternal care for prolapse of gravid uterus, unspecified trimester**
   + **O34.53   Maternal care for retroversion of gravid uterus**
      - ♀ **O34.531   Maternal care for retroversion of gravid uterus, first trimester**
      - ♀ **O34.532   Maternal care for retroversion of gravid uterus, second trimester**
      - ♀ **O34.533   Maternal care for retroversion of gravid uterus, third trimester**
      - ♀ **O34.539   Maternal care for retroversion of gravid uterus, unspecified trimester**
   + **O34.59   Maternal care for other abnormalities of gravid uterus**
      - ♀ **O34.591   Maternal care for other abnormalities of gravid uterus, first trimester**
      - ♀ **O34.592   Maternal care for other abnormalities of gravid uterus, second trimester**
      - ♀ **O34.593   Maternal care for other abnormalities of gravid uterus, third trimester**
      - ♀ **O34.599   Maternal care for other abnormalities of gravid uterus, unspecified trimester**

O34.6   Maternal care for abnormality of vagina
   Excludes2: *maternal care for vaginal varices in pregnancy (O22.1-)*
   - ♀ **O34.60   Maternal care for abnormality of vagina, unspecified trimester**
   - ♀ **O34.61   Maternal care for abnormality of vagina, first trimester**
   - ♀ **O34.62   Maternal care for abnormality of vagina, second trimester**
   - ♀ **O34.63   Maternal care for abnormality of vagina, third trimester**

+ **O34.7   Maternal care for abnormality of vulva and perineum**
   Excludes2: *maternal care for perineal and vulval varices in pregnancy (O22.1-)*
   - ♀ **O34.70   Maternal care for abnormality of vulva and perineum, unspecified trimester**
   - ♀ **O34.71   Maternal care for abnormality of vulva and perineum, first trimester**
   - ♀ **O34.72   Maternal care for abnormality of vulva and perineum, second trimester**
   - ♀ **O34.73   Maternal care for abnormality of vulva and perineum, third trimester**

+ **O34.8   Maternal care for other abnormalities of pelvic organs**
   - ♀ **O34.80   Maternal care for other abnormalities of pelvic organs, unspecified trimester**
   - ♀ **O34.81   Maternal care for other abnormalities of pelvic organs, first trimester**
   - ♀ **O34.82   Maternal care for other abnormalities of pelvic organs, second trimester**
   - ♀ **O34.83   Maternal care for other abnormalities of pelvic organs, third trimester**

+, +7th, X + 7th   • Newborn   • Pediatric   • Maternity   • Adult   ♀ Female   ♂ Male   Manifestation   Unacceptable PDX   HCC   CC   MCC   HAC

+ **O34.9 Maternal care for abnormality of pelvic organ, unspecified**
- ♀ **O34.90 Maternal care for abnormality of pelvic organ, unspecified, unspecified trimester**
- ♀ **O34.91 Maternal care for abnormality of pelvic organ, unspecified, first trimester**
- ♀ **O34.92 Maternal care for abnormality of pelvic organ, unspecified, second trimester**
- ♀ **O34.93 Maternal care for abnormality of pelvic organ, unspecified, third trimester**

O35 Maternal care for known or suspected fetal abnormality and damage

Includes: the listed conditions in the fetus as a reason for hospitalization or other obstetric care to the mother, or for termination of pregnancy

Code also any associated maternal condition

Excludes1: *encounter for suspected maternal and fetal conditions ruled out (Z03.7-)*

One of the following 7th characters is to be assigned to each code under category O35. 7th character 0 is for single gestations and multiple gestations where the fetus is unspecified. 7th characters 1 through 9 are for cases of multiple gestations to identify the fetus for which the code applies. The appropriate code from category O30, Multiple gestation, must also be assigned when assigning a code from category O35 that has a 7th character of 1 through 9.

0 - not applicable or unspecified
1 - fetus 1
2 - fetus 2
3 - fetus 3
4 - fetus 4
5 - fetus 5
9 - other fetus

Review coding guideline C.15.e

- ♀ X+7th **O35.0 Maternal care for (suspected) central nervous system malformation in fetus**
  Maternal care for fetal anencephaly
  Maternal care for fetal hydrocephalus
  Maternal care for fetal spina bifida
  Excludes2: *chromosomal abnormality in fetus (O35.1)*
- ♀ X+7th **O35.1 Maternal care for (suspected) chromosomal abnormality in fetus**
- ♀ X+7th **O35.2 Maternal care for (suspected) hereditary disease in fetus**
  Excludes2: *chromosomal abnormality in fetus (O35.1)*
- ♀ X+7th **O35.3 Maternal care for (suspected) damage to fetus from viral disease in mother**
  Maternal care for damage to fetus from maternal cytomegalovirus infection
  Maternal care for damage to fetus from maternal rubella
  AHA CC: 4Q, 2016, 4-7
- ♀ X+7th **O35.4 Maternal care for (suspected) damage to fetus from alcohol**
- ♀ X+7th **O35.5 Maternal care for (suspected) damage to fetus by drugs**
  Maternal care for damage to fetus from drug addiction
- ♀ X+7th **O35.6 Maternal care for (suspected) damage to fetus by radiation**
- ♀ X+7th **O35.7 Maternal care for (suspected) damage to fetus by other medical procedures**
  Maternal care for damage to fetus by amniocentesis
  Maternal care for damage to fetus by biopsy procedures
  Maternal care for damage to fetus by hematological investigation
  Maternal care for damage to fetus by intrauterine contraceptive device
  Maternal care for damage to fetus by intrauterine surgery
- ♀ X+7th **O35.8 Maternal care for other (suspected) fetal abnormality and damage**
  Maternal care for damage to fetus from maternal listeriosis
  Maternal care for damage to fetus from maternal toxoplasmosis
- ♀ X+7th **O35.9 Maternal care for (suspected) fetal abnormality and damage, unspecified**

O36 Maternal care for other fetal problems

Includes: the listed conditions in the fetus as a reason for hospitalization or other obstetric care of the mother, or for termination of pregnancy

Excludes1: *encounter for suspected maternal and fetal conditions ruled out (Z03.7-)*
placental transfusion syndromes (O43.0-)

Excludes2: *labor and delivery complicated by fetal stress (O77.-)*

One of the following 7th characters is to be assigned to each code under category O36. 7th character 0 is for single gestations and multiple gestations where the fetus is unspecified. 7th characters 1 through 9 are for cases of multiple gestations to identify the fetus for which the code applies. The appropriate code from category O30, Multiple gestation, must also be assigned when assigning a code from category O36 that has a 7th character of 1 through 9.

0 - not applicable or unspecified
1 - fetus 1
2 - fetus 2
3 - fetus 3
4 - fetus 4
5 - fetus 5
9 - other fetus

Review coding guideline C.15.e

+ **O36.0 Maternal care for rhesus isoimmunization**
  Maternal care for Rh incompatibility (with hydrops fetalis)
  + **O36.01 Maternal care for anti-D [Rh] antibodies**
  - ♀ CC +7th **O36.011 Maternal care for anti-D [Rh] antibodies, first trimester**
  - ♀ CC +7th **O36.012 Maternal care for anti-D [Rh] antibodies, second trimester**
  - ♀ CC +7th **O36.013 Maternal care for anti-D [Rh] antibodies, third trimester**
    AHA CC: 4Q, 2014, 17-18
  - ♀ +7th **O36.019 Maternal care for anti-D [Rh] antibodies, unspecified trimester**
  + **O36.09 Maternal care for other rhesus isoimmunization**
  - ♀ CC +7th **O36.091 Maternal care for other rhesus isoimmunization, first trimester**
  - ♀ CC +7th **O36.092 Maternal care for other rhesus isoimmunization, second trimester**
  - ♀ CC +7th **O36.093 Maternal care for other rhesus isoimmunization, third trimester**
  - ♀ +7th **O36.099 Maternal care for other rhesus isoimmunization, unspecified trimester**

+ **O36.1 Maternal care for other isoimmunization**
  Maternal care for ABO isoimmunization
  + **O36.11 Maternal care for Anti-A sensitization**
    Maternal care for isoimmunization NOS (with hydrops fetalis)
  - ♀ +7th **O36.111 Maternal care for Anti-A sensitization, first trimester**
  - ♀ +7th **O36.112 Maternal care for Anti-A sensitization, second trimester**
  - ♀ +7th **O36.113 Maternal care for Anti-A sensitization, third trimester**
  - ♀ +7th **O36.119 Maternal care for Anti-A sensitization, unspecified trimester**
  + **O36.19 Maternal care for other isoimmunization**
    Maternal care for Anti-B sensitization
  - ♀ +7th **O36.191 Maternal care for other isoimmunization, first trimester**
  - ♀ +7th **O36.192 Maternal care for other isoimmunization, second trimester**
  - ♀ +7th **O36.193 Maternal care for other isoimmunization, third trimester**
  - ♀ +7th **O36.199 Maternal care for other isoimmunization, unspecified trimester**

+ O36.2 Maternal care for hydrops fetalis
Maternal care for hydrops fetalis NOS
Maternal care for hydrops fetalis not associated with isoimmunization
Excludes1: *hydrops fetalis associated with ABO isoimmunization (O36.1-)*
hydrops fetalis associated with rhesus isoimmunization (O36.0-)
- ♀ X+7th **O36.20 Maternal care for hydrops fetalis, unspecified trimester**
- ♀ X+7th **O36.21 Maternal care for hydrops fetalis, first trimester**
- ♀ X+7th **O36.22 Maternal care for hydrops fetalis, second trimester**
- ♀ X+7th **O36.23 Maternal care for hydrops fetalis, third trimester**

- ♀ CC **O36.4 Maternal care for intrauterine death**
  X+7th
Maternal care for intrauterine fetal death NOS
Maternal care for intrauterine fetal death after completion of 20 weeks of gestation
Maternal care for late fetal death
Maternal care for missed delivery
Excludes1: *missed abortion (O02.1) stillbirth (P95)*

+ O36.5 Maternal care for known or suspected poor fetal growth
+ O36.51 Maternal care for known or suspected placental insufficiency
- ♀ +7th **O36.511 Maternal care for known or suspected placental insufficiency, first trimester**
- ♀ +7th **O36.512 Maternal care for known or suspected placental insufficiency, second trimester**
- ♀ +7th **O36.513 Maternal care for known or suspected placental insufficiency, third trimester**
- ♀ +7th **O36.519 Maternal care for known or suspected placental insufficiency, unspecified trimester**
+ O36.59 Maternal care for other known or suspected poor fetal growth
Maternal care for known or suspected light-for-dates NOS
Maternal care for known or suspected small-for-dates NOS
- ♀ +7th **O36.591 Maternal care for other known or suspected poor fetal growth, first trimester**
- ♀ +7th **O36.592 Maternal care for other known or suspected poor fetal growth, second trimester**
- ♀ +7th **O36.593 Maternal care for other known or suspected poor fetal growth, third trimester**
- ♀ +7th **O36.599 Maternal care for other known or suspected poor fetal growth, unspecified trimester**

+ O36.6 Maternal care for excessive fetal growth
Maternal care for known or suspected large-for-dates
- ♀ X+7th **O36.60 Maternal care for excessive fetal growth, unspecified trimester**
- ♀ X+7th **O36.61 Maternal care for excessive fetal growth, first trimester**
- ♀ X+7th **O36.62 Maternal care for excessive fetal growth, second trimester**
- ♀ X+7th **O36.63 Maternal care for excessive fetal growth, third trimester**

+ O36.7 Maternal care for viable fetus in abdominal pregnancy
- ♀ X+7th **O36.70 Maternal care for viable fetus in abdominal pregnancy, unspecified trimester**
- ♀ X+7th **O36.71 Maternal care for viable fetus in abdominal pregnancy, first trimester**
- ♀ X+7th **O36.72 Maternal care for viable fetus in abdominal pregnancy, second trimester**
- ♀ X+7th **O36.73 Maternal care for viable fetus in abdominal pregnancy, third trimester**

+ O36.8 Maternal care for other specified fetal problems
- ♀ X+7th **O36.80 Pregnancy with inconclusive fetal viability**
Encounter to determine fetal viability of pregnancy
AHA CC: 2Q, 2019, 29
+ O36.81 Decreased fetal movements
- ♀ +7th **O36.812 Decreased fetal movements, second trimester**
- ♀ +7th **O36.813 Decreased fetal movements, third trimester**

- ♀ +7th **O36.819 Decreased fetal movements, unspecified trimester**
+ O36.82 Fetal anemia and thrombocytopenia
- ♀ +7th **O36.821 Fetal anemia and thrombocytopenia, first trimester**
- ♀ +7th **O36.822 Fetal anemia and thrombocytopenia, second trimester**
- ♀ +7th **O36.823 Fetal anemia and thrombocytopenia, third trimester**
- ♀ +7th **O36.829 Fetal anemia and thrombocytopenia, unspecified trimester**
+ O36.83 Maternal care for abnormalities of the fetal heart rate or rhythm
Maternal care for depressed fetal heart rate tones
Maternal care for fetal bradycardia
Maternal care for fetal heart rate abnormal variability
Maternal care for fetal heart rate decelerations
Maternal care for fetal heart rate irregularity
Maternal care for fetal tachycardia
Maternal care for non-reassuring fetal heart rate or rhythm
AHA CC: 4Q, 2017, 20
- ♀ +7th **O36.831 Maternal care for abnormalities of the fetal heart rate or rhythm, first trimester**
- ♀ +7th **O36.832 Maternal care for abnormalities of the fetal heart rate or rhythm, second trimester**
- ♀ +7th **O36.833 Maternal care for abnormalities of the fetal heart rate or rhythm, third trimester**
- ♀ +7th **O36.839 Maternal care for abnormalities of the fetal heart rate or rhythm, unspecified trimester**
+ O36.89 Maternal care for other specified fetal problems
- ♀ +7th **O36.891 Maternal care for other specified fetal problems, first trimester**
- ♀ +7th **O36.892 Maternal care for other specified fetal problems, second trimester**
- ♀ +7th **O36.893 Maternal care for other specified fetal problems, third trimester**
- ♀ +7th **O36.899 Maternal care for other specified fetal problems, unspecified trimester**

+ O36.9 Maternal care for fetal problem, unspecified
- ♀ X+7th **O36.90 Maternal care for fetal problem, unspecified, unspecified trimester**
- ♀ X+7th **O36.91 Maternal care for fetal problem, unspecified, first trimester**
- ♀ X+7th **O36.92 Maternal care for fetal problem, unspecified, second trimester**
- ♀ X+7th **O36.93 Maternal care for fetal problem, unspecified, third trimester**

O40 Polyhydramnios

Includes: hydramnios
Excludes1: *encounter for suspected maternal and fetal conditions ruled out (Z03.7-)*

One of the following 7th characters is to be assigned to each code under category O40. 7th character 0 is for single gestations and multiple gestations where the fetus is unspecified. 7th characters 1 through 9 are for cases of multiple gestations to identify the fetus for which the code applies. The appropriate code from category O30, Multiple gestation, must also be assigned when assigning a code from category O40 that has a 7th character of 1 through 9.
0 - not applicable or unspecified
1 - fetus 1
2 - fetus 2
3 - fetus 3
4 - fetus 4
5 - fetus 5
9 - other fetus

- ♀ X+7th **O40.1 Polyhydramnios, first trimester**
- ♀ X+7th **O40.2 Polyhydramnios, second trimester**
- ♀ X+7th **O40.3 Polyhydramnios, third trimester**
- ♀ X+7th **O40.9 Polyhydramnios, unspecified trimester**

+, +7th, X + 7th   ● Newborn   ● Pediatric   ● Maternity   ● Adult   ♀ Female   ♂ Male   Manifestation   Unacceptable PDX   HCC   CC   MCC   HAC

O41 Other disorders of amniotic fluid and membranes

> **Excludes1:** *encounter for suspected maternal and fetal conditions ruled out (Z03.7-)*

One of the following 7th characters is to be assigned to each code under category O41. 7th character 0 is for single gestations and multiple gestations where the fetus is unspecified. 7th characters 1 through 9 are for cases of multiple gestations to identify the fetus for which the code applies. The appropriate code from category O30, Multiple gestation, must also be assigned when assigning a code from category O41 that has a 7th character of 1 through 9.

0 - not applicable or unspecified
1 - fetus 1
2 - fetus 2
3 - fetus 3
4 - fetus 4
5 - fetus 5
9 - other fetus

+ **O41.0 Oligohydramnios**
Oligohydramnios without rupture of membranes
- ♀ X+7th **O41.00 Oligohydramnios, unspecified trimester**
- ♀ CC X+7th **O41.01 Oligohydramnios, first trimester**
- ♀ CC X+7th **O41.02 Oligohydramnios, second trimester**
- ♀ CC X+7th **O41.03 Oligohydramnios, third trimester**
+ **O41.1 Infection of amniotic sac and membranes**
+ **O41.10 Infection of amniotic sac and membranes, unspecified**
- ♀ MCC +7th **O41.101 Infection of amniotic sac and membranes, unspecified, first trimester**
- ♀ MCC +7th **O41.102 Infection of amniotic sac and membranes, unspecified, second trimester**
- ♀ MCC +7th **O41.103 Infection of amniotic sac and membranes, unspecified, third trimester**
- ♀ +7th **O41.109 Infection of amniotic sac and membranes, unspecified, unspecified trimester**
+ **O41.12 Chorioamnionitis**
AHA CC: 2Q, 2019, 34-35
- ♀ MCC +7th **O41.121 Chorioamnionitis, first trimester**
- ♀ MCC +7th **O41.122 Chorioamnionitis, second trimester**
- ♀ MCC +7th **O41.123 Chorioamnionitis, third trimester**
- ♀ +7th **O41.129 Chorioamnionitis, unspecified trimester**
+ **O41.14 Placentitis**
- ♀ MCC +7th **O41.141 Placentitis, first trimester**
- ♀ MCC +7th **O41.142 Placentitis, second trimester**
- ♀ MCC +7th **O41.143 Placentitis, third trimester**
- ♀ +7th **O41.149 Placentitis, unspecified trimester**
+ **O41.8 Other specified disorders of amniotic fluid and membranes**
+ **O41.8X Other specified disorders of amniotic fluid and membranes**
- ♀ +7th **O41.8X1 Other specified disorders of amniotic fluid and membranes, first trimester**
- ♀ +7th **O41.8X2 Other specified disorders of amniotic fluid and membranes, second trimester**
- ♀ +7th **O41.8X3 Other specified disorders of amniotic fluid and membranes, third trimester**
- ♀ +7th **O41.8X9 Other specified disorders of amniotic fluid and membranes, unspecified trimester**
+ **O41.9 Disorder of amniotic fluid and membranes, unspecified**
- ♀ X+7th **O41.90 Disorder of amniotic fluid and membranes, unspecified, unspecified trimester**
- ♀ X+7th **O41.91 Disorder of amniotic fluid and membranes, unspecified, first trimester**
- ♀ X+7th **O41.92 Disorder of amniotic fluid and membranes, unspecified, second trimester**
- ♀ X+7th **O41.93 Disorder of amniotic fluid and membranes, unspecified, third trimester**

O42 Premature rupture of membranes

+ **O42.0 Premature rupture of membranes, onset of labor within 24 hours of rupture**
- ♀ **O42.00 Premature rupture of membranes, onset of labor within 24 hours of rupture, unspecified weeks of gestation**
+ **O42.01 Preterm premature rupture of membranes, onset of labor within 24 hours of rupture**
Premature rupture of membranes before 37 completed weeks of gestation, onset of labor within 24 hours of rupture
- ♀ **O42.011 Preterm premature rupture of membranes, onset of labor within 24 hours of rupture, first trimester**
- ♀ **O42.012 Preterm premature rupture of membranes, onset of labor within 24 hours of rupture, second trimester**
- ♀ **O42.013 Preterm premature rupture of membranes, onset of labor within 24 hours of rupture, third trimester**
- ♀ **O42.019 Preterm premature rupture of membranes, onset of labor within 24 hours of rupture, unspecified trimester**
- ♀ **O42.02 Full-term premature rupture of membranes, onset of labor within 24 hours of rupture**
Premature rupture of membranes at or after 37 completed weeks of gestation, onset of labor within 24 hours of rupture
+ **O42.1 Premature rupture of membranes, onset of labor more than 24 hours following rupture**
- ♀ **O42.10 Premature rupture of membranes, onset of labor more than 24 hours following rupture, unspecified weeks of gestation**
+ **O42.11 Preterm premature rupture of membranes, onset of labor more than 24 hours following rupture**
Premature rupture of membranes before 37 completed weeks of gestation
- ♀ **O42.111 Preterm premature rupture of membranes, onset of labor more than 24 hours following rupture, first trimester**
- ♀ **O42.112 Preterm premature rupture of membranes, onset of labor more than 24 hours following rupture, second trimester**
- ♀ **O42.113 Preterm premature rupture of membranes, onset of labor more than 24 hours following rupture, third trimester**
- ♀ **O42.119 Preterm premature rupture of membranes, onset of labor more than 24 hours following rupture, unspecified trimester**
- ♀ **O42.12 Full-term premature rupture of membranes, onset of labor more than 24 hours following rupture**
Premature rupture of membranes at or after 37 completed weeks of gestation, onset of labor more than 24 hours following rupture
+ **O42.9 Premature rupture of membranes, unspecified as to length of time between rupture and onset of labor**
- ♀ **O42.90 Premature rupture of membranes, unspecified as to length of time between rupture and onset of labor, unspecified weeks of gestation**
+ **O42.91 Preterm premature rupture of membranes, unspecified as to length of time between rupture and onset of labor**
Premature rupture of membranes before 37 completed weeks of gestation
- ♀ **O42.911 Preterm premature rupture of membranes, unspecified as to length of time between rupture and onset of labor, first trimester**
- ♀ **O42.912 Preterm premature rupture of membranes, unspecified as to length of time between rupture and onset of labor, second trimester**
- ♀ **O42.913 Preterm premature rupture of membranes, unspecified as to length of time between rupture and onset of labor, third trimester**
- ♀ **O42.919 Preterm premature rupture of membranes, unspecified as to length of time between rupture and onset of labor, unspecified trimester**

+, +7th, X + 7th   ● Newborn   ● Pediatric   ● Maternity   ● Adult   ♀ Female   ♂ Male   Manifestation   Unacceptable PDX   HCC   CC   MCC   HAC

- ♀ **O42.92 Full-term premature rupture of membranes, unspecified as to length of time between rupture and onset of labor**
    Premature rupture of membranes at or after 37 completed weeks of gestation, unspecified as to length of time between rupture and onset of labor

O43 Placental disorders

Excludes2: *maternal care for poor fetal growth due to placental insufficiency (O36.5-)*
placenta previa (O44.-)
placental polyp (O90.89)
placentitis (O41.14-)
premature separation of placenta [abruptio placentae] (O45.-)

+ **O43.0 Placental transfusion syndromes**
    + **O43.01 Fetomaternal placental transfusion syndrome**
        Maternofetal placental transfusion syndrome
        - ♀ **O43.011 Fetomaternal placental transfusion syndrome, first trimester**
        - ♀ **O43.012 Fetomaternal placental transfusion syndrome, second trimester**
        - ♀ **O43.013 Fetomaternal placental transfusion syndrome, third trimester**
        - ♀ **O43.019 Fetomaternal placental transfusion syndrome, unspecified trimester**
    + **O43.02 Fetus-to-fetus placental transfusion syndrome**
        - ♀ **O43.021 Fetus-to-fetus placental transfusion syndrome, first trimester**
        - ♀ **O43.022 Fetus-to-fetus placental transfusion syndrome, second trimester**
        - ♀ **O43.023 Fetus-to-fetus placental transfusion syndrome, third trimester**
        - ♀ **O43.029 Fetus-to-fetus placental transfusion syndrome, unspecified trimester**

+ **O43.1 Malformation of placenta**
    + **O43.10 Malformation of placenta, unspecified**
        Abnormal placenta NOS
        - ♀ **O43.101 Malformation of placenta, unspecified, first trimester**
        - ♀ **O43.102 Malformation of placenta, unspecified, second trimester**
        - ♀ **O43.103 Malformation of placenta, unspecified, third trimester**
        - ♀ **O43.109 Malformation of placenta, unspecified, unspecified trimester**
    + **O43.11 Circumvallate placenta**
        - ♀ **O43.111 Circumvallate placenta, first trimester**
        - ♀ **O43.112 Circumvallate placenta, second trimester**
        - ♀ **O43.113 Circumvallate placenta, third trimester**
        - ♀ **O43.119 Circumvallate placenta, unspecified trimester**
    + **O43.12 Velamentous insertion of umbilical cord**
        - ♀ **O43.121 Velamentous insertion of umbilical cord, first trimester**
        - ♀ **O43.122 Velamentous insertion of umbilical cord, second trimester**
        - ♀ **O43.123 Velamentous insertion of umbilical cord, third trimester**
        - ♀ **O43.129 Velamentous insertion of umbilical cord, unspecified trimester**
    + **O43.19 Other malformation of placenta**
        - ♀ **O43.191 Other malformation of placenta, first trimester**
        - ♀ **O43.192 Other malformation of placenta, second trimester**
        - ♀ **O43.193 Other malformation of placenta, third trimester**
        - ♀ **O43.199 Other malformation of placenta, unspecified trimester**

+ **O43.2 Morbidly adherent placenta**
    Code also associated third stage postpartum hemorrhage, if applicable (O72.0)
    Excludes1: *retained placenta (O73.-)*
    MCC + **O43.21 Placenta accreta**
        - ♀ **O43.211 Placenta accreta, first trimester**
        - ♀ **O43.212 Placenta accreta, second trimester**
        - ♀ **O43.213 Placenta accreta, third trimester**
        - ♀ **O43.219 accreta, unspecified trimester**

+ **O43.22 Placenta increta**
    - ♀ **O43.221 Placenta increta, first trimester**
    - ♀ **O43.222 Placenta increta, second trimester**
    - ♀ **O43.223 Placenta increta, third trimester**
    - ♀ **O43.229 Placenta increta, unspecified trimester**
+ **O43.23 Placenta percreta**
    - ♀ **O43.231 Placenta percreta, first trimester**
    - ♀ **O43.232 Placenta percreta, second trimester**
    - ♀ **O43.233 Placenta percreta, third trimester**
    - ♀ **O43.239 Placenta percreta, unspecified trimester**

+ **O43.8 Other placental disorders**
    + **O43.81 Placental infarction**
        - ♀ **O43.811 Placental infarction, first trimester**
        - ♀ **O43.812 Placental infarction, second trimester**
        - ♀ **O43.813 Placental infarction, third trimester**
        - ♀ **O43.819 Placental infarction, unspecified trimester**
    + **O43.89 Other placental disorders**
        Placental dysfunction
        - ♀ **O43.891 Other placental disorders, first trimester**
        - ♀ **O43.892 Other placental disorders, second trimester**
        - ♀ **O43.893 Other placental disorders, third trimester**
        - ♀ **O43.899 Other placental disorders, unspecified trimester**

+ **O43.9 Unspecified placental disorder**
    - ♀ **O43.90 Unspecified placental disorder, unspecified trimester**
    - ♀ **O43.91 Unspecified placental disorder, first trimester**
    - ♀ **O43.92 Unspecified placental disorder, second trimester**
    - ♀ **O43.93 Unspecified placental disorder, third trimester**

O44 Placenta previa

AHA CC: 4Q, 2016, 52-53

+ **O44.0 Complete placenta previa NOS or without hemorrhage**
    Placenta previa NOS
    - ♀ **O44.00 Complete placenta previa NOS or without hemorrhage, unspecified trimester**
    - ♀ CC **O44.01 Complete placenta previa NOS or without hemorrhage, first trimester**
    - ♀ CC **O44.02 Complete placenta previa NOS or without hemorrhage, second trimester**
    - ♀ CC **O44.03 Complete placenta previa NOS or without hemorrhage, third trimester**
+ **O44.1 Complete placenta previa with hemorrhage**
    Excludes1: *labor and delivery complicated by hemorrhage from vasa previa (O69.4)*
    - ♀ **O44.10 Complete placenta previa with hemorrhage, unspecified trimester**
    - ♀ MCC **O44.11 Complete placenta previa with hemorrhage, first trimester**
    - ♀ MCC **O44.12 Complete placenta previa with hemorrhage, second trimester**
    - ♀ MCC **O44.13 Complete placenta previa with hemorrhage, third trimester**
+ **O44.2 Partial placenta previa without hemorrhage**
    Marginal placenta previa, NOS or without hemorrhage
    - ♀ **O44.20 Partial placenta previa NOS or without hemorrhage, unspecified trimester**
    - ♀ CC **O44.21 Partial placenta previa NOS or without hemorrhage, first trimester**
    - ♀ CC **O44.22 Partial placenta previa NOS or without hemorrhage, second trimester**
    - ♀ CC **O44.23 Partial placenta previa NOS or without hemorrhage, third trimester**
+ **O44.3 Partial placenta previa with hemorrhage**
    Marginal placenta previa with hemorrhage
    - ♀ **O44.30 Partial placenta previa with hemorrhage, unspecified trimester**
    - ♀ MCC **O44.31 Partial placenta previa with hemorrhage, first trimester**
    - ♀ MCC **O44.32 Partial placenta previa with hemorrhage, second trimester**
    - ♀ MCC **O44.33 Partial placenta previa with hemorrhage, third trimester**
+ **O44.4 Low lying placenta NOS or without hemorrhage**
    MCC Low implantation of placenta NOS or without hemorrhage
    - ♀ **O44.40 Low lying placenta NOS or without hemorrhage, unspecified trimester**

+, +7th, X + 7th • Newborn • Pediatric • Maternity • Adult ♀ Female ♂ Male Manifestation Unacceptable PDX HCC CC MCC HAC

- ♀ CC **O44.41** **Low lying placenta NOS or without hemorrhage, first trimester**
- ♀ CC **O44.42** **Low lying placenta NOS or without hemorrhage, second trimester**
- ♀ CC **O44.43** **Low lying placenta NOS or without hemorrhage, third trimester**
+ **O44.5** **Low lying placenta with hemorrhage**
  Low implantation of placenta with hemorrhage
  - ♀ **O44.50** **Low lying placenta with hemorrhage, unspecified trimester**
  - ♀ MCC **O44.51** **Low lying placenta with hemorrhage, first trimester**
  - ♀ MCC **O44.52** **Low lying placenta with hemorrhage, second trimester**
  - ♀ MCC **O44.53** **Low lying placenta with hemorrhage, third trimester**

O45 **Premature separation of placenta [abruptio placentae]**

+ **O45.0** **Premature separation of placenta with coagulation defect**
  + **O45.00** **Premature separation of placenta with coagulation defect, unspecified**
  - ♀ MCC **O45.001** **Premature separation of placenta with coagulation defect, unspecified, first trimester**
  - ♀ MCC **O45.002** **Premature separation of placenta with coagulation defect, unspecified, second trimester**
  - ♀ MCC **O45.003** **Premature separation of placenta with coagulation defect, unspecified, third trimester**
  - ♀ **O45.009** **Premature separation of placenta with coagulation defect, unspecified, unspecified trimester**
  + **O45.01** **Premature separation of placenta with afibrinogenemia**
    Premature separation of placenta with hypofibrinogenemia
  - ♀ MCC **O45.011** **Premature separation of placenta with afibrinogenemia, first trimester**
  - ♀ MCC **O45.012** **Premature separation of placenta with afibrinogenemia, second trimester**
  - ♀ MCC **O45.013** **Premature separation of placenta with afibrinogenemia, third trimester**
  - ♀ **O45.019** **Premature separation of placenta with afibrinogenemia, unspecified trimester**
  + **O45.02** **Premature separation of placenta with disseminated intravascular coagulation**
  - ♀ MCC **O45.021** **Premature separation of placenta with disseminated intravascular coagulation, first trimester**
  - ♀ MCC **O45.022** **Premature separation of placenta with disseminated intravascular coagulation, second trimester**
  - ♀ MCC **O45.023** **Premature separation of placenta with disseminated intravascular coagulation, third trimester**
  - ♀ **O45.029** **Premature separation of placenta with disseminated intravascular coagulation, unspecified trimester**
  O45.09 **Premature separation of placenta with other coagulation defect**
  - ♀ MCC **O45.091** **Premature separation of placenta with other coagulation defect, first trimester**
  - ♀ MCC **O45.092** **Premature separation of placenta with other coagulation defect, second trimester**
  - ♀ MCC **O45.093** **Premature separation of placenta with other coagulation defect, third trimester**
  - ♀ **O45.099** **Premature separation of placenta with other coagulation defect, unspecified trimester**

+ **O45.8** **Other premature separation of placenta**
  + **O45.8X** **Other premature separation of placenta**
  - ♀ MCC **O45.8X1** **Other premature separation of placenta, first trimester**
  - ♀ MCC **O45.8X2** **Other premature separation of placenta, second trimester**
  - ♀ MCC **O45.8X3** **Other premature separation of placenta, third trimester**
  - ♀ **O45.8X9** **Other premature separation of placenta, unspecified trimester**
+ **O45.9** **Premature separation of placenta, unspecified**
  Abruptio placentae NOS
  - ♀ **O45.90** **Premature separation of placenta, unspecified, unspecified trimester**
  - ♀ MCC **O45.91** **Premature separation of placenta, unspecified, first trimester**
  - ♀ MCC **O45.92** **Premature separation of placenta, unspecified, second trimester**
  - ♀ MCC **O45.93** **Premature separation of placenta, unspecified, third trimester**

O46 **Antepartum hemorrhage, not elsewhere classified**

> *Excludes1:* *hemorrhage in early pregnancy (O20.-)*
> *intrapartum hemorrhage NEC (O67.-)*
> *placenta previa (O44.-)*
> *premature separation of placenta [abruptio placentae] (O45.-)*

+ **O46.0** **Antepartum hemorrhage with coagulation defect**
  + **O46.00** **Antepartum hemorrhage with coagulation defect, unspecified**
  - ♀ MCC **O46.001** **Antepartum hemorrhage with coagulation defect, unspecified, first trimester**
  - ♀ MCC **O46.002** **Antepartum hemorrhage with coagulation defect, unspecified, second trimester**
  - ♀ MCC **O46.003** **Antepartum hemorrhage with coagulation defect, unspecified, third trimester**
  - ♀ **O46.009** **Antepartum hemorrhage with coagulation defect, unspecified, unspecified trimester**
  + **O46.01** **Antepartum hemorrhage with afibrinogenemia**
    Antepartum hemorrhage with hypofibrinogenemia
  - ♀ MCC **O46.011** **Antepartum hemorrhage with afibrinogenemia, first trimester**
  - ♀ MCC **O46.012** **Antepartum hemorrhage with afibrinogenemia, second trimester**
  - ♀ MCC **O46.013** **Antepartum hemorrhage with afibrinogenemia, third trimester**
  - ♀ **O46.019** **Antepartum hemorrhage with afibrinogenemia, unspecified trimester**
  + **O46.02** **Antepartum hemorrhage with disseminated intravascular coagulation**
  - ♀ MCC **O46.021** **Antepartum hemorrhage with disseminated intravascular coagulation, first trimester**
  - ♀ MCC **O46.022** **Antepartum hemorrhage with disseminated intravascular coagulation, second trimester**
  - ♀ MCC **O46.023** **Antepartum hemorrhage with disseminated intravascular coagulation, third trimester**
  - ♀ **O46.029** **Antepartum hemorrhage with disseminated intravascular coagulation, unspecified trimester**
  + **O46.09** **Antepartum hemorrhage with other coagulation defect**
  - ♀ MCC **O46.091** **Antepartum hemorrhage with other coagulation defect, first trimester**
  - ♀ MCC **O46.092** **Antepartum hemorrhage with other coagulation defect, second trimester**
  - ♀ MCC **O46.093** **Antepartum hemorrhage with other coagulation defect, third trimester**
  - ♀ **O46.099** **Antepartum hemorrhage with other coagulation defect, unspecified trimester**

+, +7th, X + 7th   ● Newborn   ● Pediatric   ● Maternity   ● Adult   ♀ Female   ♂ Male   Manifestation   Unacceptable PDX   HCC   CC   MCC   HAC

+ **O46.8** Other antepartum hemorrhage
  + **O46.8X** Other antepartum hemorrhage
    • ♀ **O46.8X1** Other antepartum hemorrhage, first trimester
    • ♀ **O46.8X2** Other antepartum hemorrhage, second trimester
    • ♀ **O46.8X3** Other antepartum hemorrhage, third trimester
    • ♀ **O46.8X9** Other antepartum hemorrhage, unspecified trimester
+ **O46.9** Antepartum hemorrhage, unspecified
  • ♀ **O46.90** Antepartum hemorrhage, unspecified, unspecified trimester
  • ♀ **O46.91** Antepartum hemorrhage, unspecified, first trimester
  • ♀ **O46.92** Antepartum hemorrhage, unspecified, second trimester
  • ♀ **O46.93** Antepartum hemorrhage, unspecified, third trimester

O47 False labor

  Includes: Braxton Hicks contractions
    threatened labor
  Excludes1: *preterm labor (O60.-)*
+ **O47.0** False labor before 37 completed weeks of gestation
  • ♀ **O47.00** False labor before 37 completed weeks of gestation, unspecified trimester
  • ♀ CC **O47.02** False labor before 37 completed weeks of gestation, second trimester
  • ♀ CC **O47.03** False labor before 37 completed weeks of gestation, third trimester
• ♀ CC **O47.1** False labor at or after 37 completed weeks of gestation
• ♀ **O47.9** False labor, unspecified

O48 Late pregnancy

  • ♀ **O48.0** Post-term pregnancy
    Pregnancy over 40 completed weeks to 42 completed weeks gestation
  • ♀ **O48.1** Prolonged pregnancy
    Pregnancy which has advanced beyond 42 completed weeks gestation

Complications of labor and delivery (O60-O77)

O60 Preterm labor

  Includes: onset (spontaneous) of labor before 37 completed weeks of gestation
  Excludes1: *false labor (O47.0-)*
    threatened labor NOS (O47.0-)
+ **O60.0** Preterm labor without delivery
  • ♀ **O60.00** Preterm labor without delivery, unspecified trimester
• ♀ MCC **O60.02** Preterm labor without delivery, second trimester
• ♀ MCC **O60.03** Preterm labor without delivery, third trimester
+ **O60.1** Preterm labor with preterm delivery

One of the following 7th characters is to be assigned to each code under subcategory **O60.1.** 7th character 0 is for single gestations and multiple gestations where the fetus is unspecified. 7th characters 1 through 9 are for cases of multiple gestations to identify the fetus for which the code applies. The appropriate code from category O30, Multiple gestation, must also be assigned when assigning a code from subcategory O60.1 that has a 7th character of 1 through 9.
0 - not applicable or unspecified
1 - fetus 1
2 - fetus 2
3 - fetus 3
4 - fetus 4
5 - fetus 5
9 - other fetus

• ♀ CC X+7th **O60.10** Preterm labor with preterm delivery, unspecified trimester
    Preterm labor with delivery NOS
• ♀ MCC X+7th **O60.12** Preterm labor second trimester with preterm delivery second trimester
• ♀ MCC X+7th **O60.13** Preterm labor second trimester with preterm delivery third trimester
• ♀ MCC X+7th **O60.14** Preterm labor third trimester with preterm delivery third trimester
    AHA CC: 2Q, 2016, 10-11

+ **O60.2** Term delivery with preterm labor

One of the following 7th characters is to be assigned to each code under subcategory **O60.2.** 7th character 0 is for single gestations and multiple gestations where the fetus is unspecified. 7th characters 1 through 9 are for cases of multiple gestations to identify the fetus for which the code applies. The appropriate code from category O30, Multiple gestation, must also be assigned when assigning a code from subcategory O60.2 that has a 7th character of 1 through 9.
0 - not applicable or unspecified
1 - fetus 1
2 - fetus 2
3 - fetus 3
4 - fetus 4
5 - fetus 5
9 - other fetus

• ♀ CC X+7th **O60.20** Term delivery with preterm labor, unspecified trimester
• ♀ MCC X+7th **O60.22** Term delivery with preterm labor, second trimester
• ♀ MCC X+7th **O60.23** Term delivery with preterm labor, third trimester

O61 Failed induction of labor

  • ♀ **O61.0** Failed medical induction of labor
    Failed induction (of labor) by oxytocin
    Failed induction (of labor) by prostaglandins
  • ♀ **O61.1** Failed instrumental induction of labor
    Failed mechanical induction (of labor)
    Failed surgical induction (of labor)
  • ♀ **O61.8** Other failed induction of labor
  • ♀ **O61.9** Failed induction of labor, unspecified

O62 Abnormalities of forces of labor

  • ♀ **O62.0** Primary inadequate contractions
    Failure of cervical dilatation
    Primary hypotonic uterine dysfunction
    Uterine inertia during latent phase of labor
  • ♀ **O62.1** Secondary uterine inertia
    Arrested active phase of labor
    Secondary hypotonic uterine dysfunction
  • ♀ **O62.2** Other uterine inertia
    Atony of uterus without hemorrhage
    Atony of uterus NOS
    Desultory labor
    Hypotonic uterine dysfunction NOS
    Irregular labor
    Poor contractions
    Slow slope active phase of labor
    Uterine inertia NOS
    Excludes1: *atony of uterus with hemorrhage (postpartum) (O72.1)*
      postpartum atony of uterus without hemorrhage (O75.89)
  • ♀ **O62.3** Precipitate labor
  • ♀ **O62.4** Hypertonic, incoordinate, and prolonged uterine contractions
    Cervical spasm
    Contraction ring dystocia
    Dyscoordinate labor
    Hour-glass contraction of uterus
    Hypertonic uterine dysfunction
    Incoordinate uterine action
    Tetanic contractions
    Uterine dystocia NOS
    Uterine spasm
    Excludes1: *dystocia (fetal) (maternal) NOS (O66.9)*
  • ♀ **O62.8** Other abnormalities of forces of labor
  • ♀ **O62.9** Abnormality of forces of labor, unspecified

O63 Long labor

  • ♀ **O63.0** Prolonged first stage (of labor)
  • ♀ **O63.1** Prolonged second stage (of labor)
  • ♀ **O63.2** Delayed delivery of second twin, triplet, etc.
  • ♀ CC **O63.9** Long labor, unspecified
    Prolonged labor NOS

+, +7th, X + 7th   • Newborn   • Pediatric   • Maternity   • Adult   ♀ Female   ♂ Male   Manifestation   Unacceptable PDX   HCC   CC   MCC   HAC

O64 Obstructed labor due to malposition and malpresentation of fetus

> One of the following 7th characters is to be assigned to each code
> under category O64. 7th character 0 is for single gestations and
> multiple gestations where the fetus is unspecified. 7th characters
> 1 through 9 are for cases of multiple gestations to identify the
> fetus for which the code applies. The appropriate code from category
> O30, Multiple gestation, must also be assigned when assigning a code
> from category O64 that has a 7th character of 1 through 9.
>
> 0 - not applicable or unspecified
>
> 1 - fetus 1
>
> 2 - fetus 2
>
> 3 - fetus 3
>
> 4 - fetus 4
>
> 5 - fetus 5
>
> 9 - other fetus

● ♀ X+7th **O64.0 Obstructed labor due to incomplete rotation of fetal head**
Deep transverse arrest
Obstructed labor due to persistent occipitoiliac (position)
Obstructed labor due to persistent occipitoposterior
  (position)
Obstructed labor due to persistent occipitosacral (position)
Obstructed labor due to persistent occipitotransverse
  (position)

● ♀ X+7th **O64.1 Obstructed labor due to breech presentation**
Obstructed labor due to buttocks presentation
Obstructed labor due to complete breech presentation
Obstructed labor due to frank breech presentation

● ♀ X+7th **O64.2 Obstructed labor due to face presentation**
Obstructed labor due to chin presentation

● ♀ X+7th **O64.3 Obstructed labor due to brow presentation**

● ♀ X+7th **O64.4 Obstructed labor due to shoulder presentation**
Prolapsed arm
Excludes1: *impacted shoulders (O66.0)*
  shoulder dystocia (O66.0)

● ♀ X+7th **O64.5 Obstructed labor due to compound presentation**

● ♀ X+7th **O64.8 Obstructed labor due to other malposition and
malpresentation**
Obstructed labor due to footling presentation
Obstructed labor due to incomplete breech presentation

● ♀ X+7th **O64.9 Obstructed labor due to malposition and malpresentation,
unspecified**

O65 Obstructed labor due to maternal pelvic abnormality

● ♀ **O65.0 Obstructed labor due to deformed pelvis**

● ♀ **O65.1 Obstructed labor due to generally contracted pelvis**

● ♀ **O65.2 Obstructed labor due to pelvic inlet contraction**

● ♀ **O65.3 Obstructed labor due to pelvic outlet and mid-cavity
contraction**

● ♀ **O65.4 Obstructed labor due to fetopelvic disproportion,
unspecified**
Excludes1: *dystocia due to abnormality of fetus
  (O66.2-O66.3)*

● ♀ **O65.5 Obstructed labor due to abnormality of maternal pelvic
organs**
Obstructed labor due to conditions listed in O34.-
Use additional code to identify abnormality of pelvic organs
  O34.-

● ♀ **O65.8 Obstructed labor due to other maternal pelvic
abnormalities**

● ♀ **O65.9 Obstructed labor due to maternal pelvic abnormality,
unspecified**

O66 Other obstructed labor

● ♀ **O66.0 Obstructed labor due to shoulder dystocia**
Impacted shoulders

● ♀ **O66.1 Obstructed labor due to locked twins**

● ♀ **O66.2 Obstructed labor due to unusually large fetus**

● ♀ **O66.3 Obstructed labor due to other abnormalities of fetus**
Dystocia due to fetal ascites
Dystocia due to fetal hydrops
Dystocia due to fetal meningomyelocele
Dystocia due to fetal sacral teratoma
Dystocia due to fetal tumor
Dystocia due to hydrocephalic fetus
Use additional code to identify cause of obstruction

+ **O66.4 Failed trial of labor**
● ♀ **O66.40 Failed trial of labor, unspecified**
● ♀ **O66.41 Failed attempted vaginal birth after previous
cesarean delivery**
Code first rupture of uterus, if applicable (O71.0-,
  O71.1)

● ♀ **O66.5 Attempted application of vacuum extractor and forceps**
Attempted application of vacuum or forceps,
  with subsequent delivery by forceps or cesarean delivery

● ♀ **O66.6 Obstructed labor due to other multiple fetuses**

● ♀ **O66.8 Other specified obstructed labor**
Use additional code to identify cause of obstruction

● ♀ **O66.9 Obstructed labor, unspecified**
Dystocia NOS
Fetal dystocia NOS
Maternal dystocia NOS

**O67 Labor and delivery complicated by intrapartum hemorrhage, not
elsewhere classified**

> ***Excludes1:*** *antepartum hemorrhage NEC (O46.-)*
>   *placenta previa (O44.-)*
>   *premature separation of placenta [abruptio
>   placentae] (O45.-)*
> ***Excludes2:*** *postpartum hemorrhage (O72.-)*

● ♀ MCC **O67.0 Intrapartum hemorrhage with coagulation defect**
Intrapartum hemorrhage (excessive) associated with
  afibrinogenemia
Intrapartum hemorrhage (excessive) associated with
  disseminated intravascular coagulation
Intrapartum hemorrhage (excessive) associated with
  hyperfibrinolysis
Intrapartum hemorrhage (excessive) associated with
  hypofibrinogenemia

● ♀ **O67.8 Other intrapartum hemorrhage**
Excessive intrapartum hemorrhage

● ♀ **O67.9 Intrapartum hemorrhage, unspecified**

● ♀ CC **O68 Labor and delivery complicated by abnormality of fetal acid-
base balance**

Fetal acidemia complicating labor and delivery
Fetal acidosis complicating labor and delivery
Fetal alkalosis complicating labor and delivery
Fetal metabolic acidemia complicating labor and delivery
Excludes1: *fetal stress NOS (O77.9)*
  *labor and delivery complicated by electrocardiographic
    evidence of fetal stress (O77.8)*
  *labor and delivery complicated by ultrasonic evidence
    of fetal stress (O77.8)*
Excludes2: *abnormality in fetal heart rate or rhythm (O76)*
  *labor and delivery complicated by meconium in
    amniotic fluid (O77.0)*
Valid 3-character code, no further characters required

O69 Labor and delivery complicated by umbilical cord complications

> One of the following 7th characters is to be assigned to each code
> under category O69. 7th character 0 is for single gestations and
> multiple gestations where the fetus is unspecified. 7th characters
> 1 through 9 are for cases of multiple gestations to identify the fetus
> for which the code applies. The appropriate code from category
> O30, Multiple gestation, must also be assigned when assigning a
> code from category O69 that has a 7th character of 1 through 9.
>
> 0 - not applicable or unspecified
>
> 1 - fetus 1
>
> 2 - fetus 2
>
> 3 - fetus 3
>
> 4 - fetus 4
>
> 5 - fetus 5
>
> 9 - other fetus

● ♀ X+7th **O69.0 Labor and delivery complicated by prolapse of cord**

● ♀ X+7th **O69.1 Labor and delivery complicated by cord around neck, with
compression**
Excludes1: *labor and delivery complicated by cord around
  neck, without compression (O69.81)*

● ♀ X+7th **O69.2 Labor and delivery complicated by other cord
entanglement, with compression**
Labor and delivery complicated by compression of cord NOS
Labor and delivery complicated by entanglement of cords of
  twins in monoamniotic sac
Labor and delivery complicated by knot in cord
Excludes1: *labor and delivery complicated by other cord
  entanglement, without compression (O69.82)*

- ♀ X+7th **O69.3** **Labor and delivery complicated by short cord**
- ♀ X+7th **O69.4** **Labor and delivery complicated by vasa previa**
  Labor and delivery complicated by hemorrhage from vasa previa
- ♀ X+7th **O69.5** **Labor and delivery complicated by vascular lesion of cord**
  Labor and delivery complicated by cord bruising
  Labor and delivery complicated by cord hematoma
  Labor and delivery complicated by thrombosis of umbilical vessels
- X+7th **O69.8** **Labor and delivery complicated by other cord complications**
  - ♀ X+7th **O69.81** **Labor and delivery complicated by cord around neck, without compression**
  - ♀ X+7th **O69.82** **Labor and delivery complicated by other cord entanglement, without compression**
  - ♀ X+7th **O69.89** **Labor and delivery complicated by other cord complications**
- ♀ X+7th **O69.9** **Labor and delivery complicated by cord complication, unspecified**

O70 **Perineal laceration during delivery**

  Includes: episiotomy extended by laceration
  Excludes1: *obstetric high vaginal laceration alone (O71.4)*

- ♀ **O70.0** **First degree perineal laceration during delivery**
  Perineal laceration, rupture or tear involving fourchette during delivery
  Perineal laceration, rupture or tear involving labia during delivery
  Perineal laceration, rupture or tear involving skin during delivery
  Perineal laceration, rupture or tear involving vagina during delivery
  Perineal laceration, rupture or tear involving vulva during delivery
  Slight perineal laceration, rupture or tear during delivery

- ♀ **O70.1** **Second degree perineal laceration during delivery**
  Perineal laceration, rupture or tear during delivery as in O70.0, also involving pelvic floor
  Perineal laceration, rupture or tear during delivery as in O70.0, also involving perineal muscles
  Perineal laceration, rupture or tear during delivery as in O70.0, also involving vaginal muscles
  Excludes1: *perineal laceration involving anal sphincter (O70.2)*
  AHA CC: 2Q, 2016, 34

+ **O70.2** **Third degree perineal laceration during delivery**
  Perineal laceration, rupture or tear during delivery as in O70.1, also involving anal sphincter
  Perineal laceration, rupture or tear during delivery as in O70.1, also involving rectovaginal septum
  Perineal laceration, rupture or tear during delivery as in O70.1, also involving sphincter NOS
  Excludes1: *anal sphincter tear during delivery without third degree perineal laceration (O70.4)*
  perineal laceration involving anal or rectal mucosa (O70.3)
  AHA CC: 4Q, 2016, 53-54

  - ♀ CC **O70.20** **Third degree perineal laceration during delivery, unspecified**
  - ♀ CC **O70.21** **Third degree perineal laceration during delivery, IIIa**
    Third degree perineal laceration during delivery with less than 50% of external anal sphincter (EAS) thickness torn
  - ♀ CC **O70.22** **Third degree perineal laceration during delivery, IIIb**
    Third degree perineal laceration during delivery with more than 50% of external anal sphincter (EAS) thickness torn
  - ♀ CC **O70.23** **Third degree perineal laceration during delivery, IIIc**
    Third degree perineal laceration during delivery with both external anal sphincter (EAS) and internal anal sphincter (IAS) torn

- ♀ CC **O70.3** **Fourth degree perineal laceration during delivery**
  Perineal laceration, rupture or tear during delivery as in O70.2, also involving anal mucosa
  Perineal laceration, rupture or tear during delivery as in O70.2, also involving rectal mucosa

- ♀ CC **O70.4** **Anal sphincter tear complicating delivery, not associated with third degree laceration**
  Excludes1: *anal sphincter tear with third degree perineal laceration (O70.2)*
- ♀ **O70.9** **Perineal laceration during delivery, unspecified**

O71 **Other obstetric trauma**

  Includes: obstetric damage from instruments
  + **O71.0** **Rupture of uterus (spontaneous) before onset of labor**
    Excludes1: *disruption of (current) cesarean delivery wound (O90.0)*
    laceration of uterus, NEC (O71.81)
    - ♀ **O71.00** **Rupture of uterus before onset of labor, unspecified trimester**
    - ♀ MCC **O71.02** **Rupture of uterus before onset of labor, second trimester**
    - ♀ MCC **O71.03** **Rupture of uterus before onset of labor, third trimester**
- ♀ MCC **O71.1** **Rupture of uterus during labor**
  Rupture of uterus not stated as occurring before onset of labor
  Excludes1: *disruption of cesarean delivery wound (O90.0)*
  laceration of uterus, NEC (O71.81)
- ♀ CC **O71.2** **Postpartum inversion of uterus**
- ♀ CC **O71.3** **Obstetric laceration of cervix**
  Annular detachment of cervix
- ♀ CC **O71.4** **Obstetric high vaginal laceration alone**
  Laceration of vaginal wall without perineal laceration
  Excludes1: *obstetric high vaginal laceration with perineal laceration (O70.-)*
- ♀ CC **O71.5** **Other obstetric injury to pelvic organs**
  Obstetric injury to bladder
  Obstetric injury to urethra
  Excludes2: *obstetric periurethral trauma (O71.82)*
- ♀ CC **O71.6** **Obstetric damage to pelvic joints and ligaments**
  Obstetric avulsion of inner symphyseal cartilage
  Obstetric damage to coccyx
  Obstetric traumatic separation of symphysis (pubis)
- ♀ CC **O71.7** **Obstetric hematoma of pelvis**
  Obstetric hematoma of perineum
  Obstetric hematoma of vagina
  Obstetric hematoma of vulva
  + **O71.8** **Other specified obstetric trauma**
    - ♀ **O71.81** **Laceration of uterus, not elsewhere classified**
    - ♀ **O71.82** **Other specified trauma to perineum and vulva**
      Obstetric periurethral trauma
      AHA CC: 4Q, 2014, 18-19
    - ♀ **O71.89** **Other specified obstetric trauma**
- ♀ **O71.9** **Obstetric trauma, unspecified**

O72 **Postpartum hemorrhage**

  Includes: hemorrhage after delivery of fetus or infant
- ♀ CC **O72.0** **Third-stage hemorrhage**
  Hemorrhage associated with retained, trapped or adherent placenta
  Retained placenta NOS
  Code also type of adherent placenta (O43.2-)
- ♀ CC **O72.1** **Other immediate postpartum hemorrhage**
  Hemorrhage following delivery of placenta
  Postpartum hemorrhage (atonic) NOS
  Uterine atony with hemorrhage
  Excludes1: *uterine atony NOS (O62.2)*
  uterine atony without hemorrhage (O62.2)
  postpartum atony of uterus without hemorrhage (O75.89)
- ♀ CC **O72.2** **Delayed and secondary postpartum hemorrhage**
  Hemorrhage associated with retained portions of placenta or membranes after the first 24 hours following delivery of placenta
  Retained products of conception NOS, following delivery
- ♀ **O72.3** **Postpartum coagulation defects**
  Postpartum afibrinogenemia
  Postpartum fibrinolysis

O73 **Retained placenta and membranes, without hemorrhage**

  Excludes1: *placenta accreta (O43.21-)*
  placenta increta (O43.22-)
  placenta percreta (O43.23-)
- ♀ **O73.0** **Retained placenta without hemorrhage**
  Adherent placenta, without hemorrhage
  Trapped placenta without hemorrhage

- ♀ **O73.1** **Retained portions of placenta and membranes, without hemorrhage**

  Retained products of conception following delivery, without hemorrhage

O74 **Complications of anesthesia during labor and delivery**

Includes: maternal complications arising from the administration of a general, regional or local anesthetic, analgesic or other sedation during labor and delivery

Use additional code, if applicable, to identify specific complication

- ● ♀ **O74.0** **Aspiration pneumonitis due to anesthesia during labor and delivery**

  Inhalation of stomach contents or secretions NOS due to anesthesia during labor and delivery

  Mendelson's syndrome due to anesthesia during labor and delivery

- ● ♀ **O74.1** **Other pulmonary complications of anesthesia during labor and delivery**
- ● ♀ **O74.2** **Cardiac complications of anesthesia during labor and delivery**
- ● ♀ **O74.3** **Central nervous system complications of anesthesia during labor and delivery**
- ● ♀ **O74.4** **Toxic reaction to local anesthesia during labor and delivery**
- ● ♀ **O74.5** **Spinal and epidural anesthesia-induced headache during labor and delivery**
- ● ♀ **O74.6** **Other complications of spinal and epidural anesthesia during labor and delivery**
- ● ♀ **O74.7** **Failed or difficult intubation for anesthesia during labor and delivery**
- ● ♀ **O74.8** **Other complications of anesthesia during labor and delivery**
- ● ♀ **O74.9** **Complication of anesthesia during labor and delivery, unspecified**

O75 **Other complications of labor and delivery, not elsewhere classified**

Excludes2: *puerperal (postpartum) infection (O86.-)*
puerperal (postpartum) sepsis (O85)

- ● ♀ **O75.0** **Maternal distress during labor and delivery**
- ● ♀ MCC **O75.1** **Shock during or following labor and delivery**
  Obstetric shock following labor and delivery
- ● ♀ CC **O75.2** **Pyrexia during labor, not elsewhere classified**
- ● ♀ MCC **O75.3** **Other infection during labor**
  Sepsis during labor
  Use additional code (B95-B97), to identify infectious agent
  Review coding guideline C.15.j
- ● ♀ **O75.4** **Other complications of obstetric surgery and procedures**
  Cardiac arrest following obstetric surgery or procedures
  Cardiac failure following obstetric surgery or procedures
  Cerebral anoxia following obstetric surgery or procedures
  Pulmonary edema following obstetric surgery or procedures
  Use additional code to identify specific complication
  Excludes2: *complications of anesthesia during labor and delivery (O74.-)*
  disruption of obstetrical (surgical) wound (O90.0-O90.1)
  hematoma of obstetrical (surgical) wound (O90.2)
  infection of obstetrical (surgical) wound (O86.0-)
- ● ♀ **O75.5** **Delayed delivery after artificial rupture of membranes**
- + **O75.8** **Other specified complications of labor and delivery**
  - ● ♀ **O75.81** **Maternal exhaustion complicating labor and delivery**
  - ● ♀ **O75.82** **Onset (spontaneous) of labor after 37 completed weeks of gestation but before 39 completed weeks gestation, with delivery by (planned) cesarean section**
    Delivery by (planned) cesarean section occurring after 37 completed weeks of gestation but before 39 completed weeks gestation due to (spontaneous) onset of labor
    Code first to specify reason for planned cesarean section such as:
    cephalopelvic disproportion (normally formed fetus) (O33.9)
    previous cesarean delivery (O34.21)
  - ● ♀ **O75.89** **Other specified complications of labor and delivery**
- ● ♀ **O75.9** **Complication of labor and delivery, unspecified**

- ● ♀ **O76** **Abnormality in fetal heart rate and rhythm complicating labor and delivery**

  Depressed fetal heart rate tones complicating labor and delivery
  Fetal bradycardia complicating labor and delivery
  Fetal heart rate decelerations complicating labor and delivery
  Fetal heart rate irregularity complicating labor and delivery
  Fetal heart rate abnormal variability complicating labor and delivery
  Fetal tachycardia complicating labor and delivery
  Non-reassuring fetal heart rate or rhythm complicating labor and delivery
  Excludes1: *fetal stress NOS (O77.9)*
  labor and delivery complicated by electrocardiographic evidence of fetal stress (O77.8)
  labor and delivery complicated by ultrasonic evidence of fetal stress (O77.8)
  Excludes2: *fetal metabolic acidemia (O68)*
  other fetal stress (O77.0-O77.1)
  AHA CC: 4Q, 2013, 118
  Valid 3-character code, no further characters required

O77 **Other fetal stress complicating labor and delivery**

- ● ♀ **O77.0** **Labor and delivery complicated by meconium in amniotic fluid**
  AHA CC: 4Q, 2013, 118
- ● ♀ **O77.1** **Fetal stress in labor or delivery due to drug administration**
- ● ♀ **O77.8** **Labor and delivery complicated by other evidence of fetal stress**
  Labor and delivery complicated by electrocardiographic evidence of fetal stress
  Labor and delivery complicated by ultrasonic evidence of fetal stress
  Excludes1: *abnormality of fetal acid-base balance (O68)*
  abnormality in fetal heart rate or rhythm (O76)
  fetal metabolic acidemia (O68)
- ● ♀ **O77.9** **Labor and delivery complicated by fetal stress, unspecified**
  Excludes1: *abnormality of fetal acid-base balance (O68)*
  abnormality in fetal heart rate or rhythm (O76)
  fetal metabolic acidemia (O68)

Encounter for delivery (O80-O82)

- ● ♀ **O80** **Encounter for full-term uncomplicated delivery**

  Delivery requiring minimal or no assistance, with or without episiotomy, without fetal manipulation [e.g., rotation version] or instrumentation [forceps] of a spontaneous, cephalic, vaginal, full-term, single, live-born infant. This code is for use as a single diagnosis code and is not to be used with any other code from chapter 15.
  Use additional code to indicate outcome of delivery (Z37.0)
  AHA CC: 2Q, 2014, 9; 4Q, 2016, 150
  Review coding guideline C.15.n
  Valid 3-character code, no further characters required

- ● ♀ **O82** **Encounter for cesarean delivery without indication**

  Use additional code to indicate outcome of delivery (Z37.0)
  Valid 3-character code, no further characters required

Complications predominantly related to the puerperium (O85-O92)

Excludes2: *mental and behavioral disorders associated with the puerperium (F53.-)*
obstetrical tetanus (A34)
puerperal osteomalacia (M83.0)

O85 **Puerperal sepsis**
MCC
- ● ♀ Postpartum sepsis
  Puerperal peritonitis
  Puerperal pyemia
  Use additional code (B95-B97), to identify infectious agent

  Use additional code (R65.2-) to identify severe sepsis, if applicable
  Excludes1: *fever of unknown origin following delivery (O86.4)*
  genital tract infection following delivery (O86.1-)
  obstetric pyemic and septic embolism (O88.3-)
  puerperal septic thrombophlebitis (O86.81)
  urinary tract infection following delivery (O86.2-)
  Excludes2: *sepsis during labor (O75.3)*
  Review coding guideline C.15.k
  Valid 3-character code, no further characters required

O86 Other puerperal infections

Use additional code (B95-B97), to identify infectious agent

Excludes2: *infection during labor (O75.3)*
  obstetrical tetanus (A34)

+ **O86.0 Infection of obstetric surgical wound**

Infected cesarean delivery wound following delivery
Infected perineal repair following delivery

Excludes1: *complications of procedures, not elsewhere*
  classified (T81.4-)
  postprocedural fever NOS (R50.82)
  postprocedural retroperitoneal abscess (K68.11)

AHA CC: 4Q, 2018, 22-23
Review coding guideline C.1.d.5

- ♀ **O86.00 Infection of obstetric surgical wound, unspecified**
- ♀ **O86.01 Infection of obstetric surgical wound, superficial incisional site**

Subcutaneous abscess following an obstetrical procedure
Stitch abscess following an obstetrical procedure

- ♀ **O86.02 Infection of obstetric surgical wound, deep incisional site**

Intramuscular abscess following an obstetrical procedure
Sub-fascial abscess following an obstetrical procedure

AHA CC: 4Q, 2018, 23; 2Q, 2020, 32-33

- ♀ **O86.03 Infection of obstetric surgical wound, organ and space site**

Intraabdominal abscess following an obstetrical procedure
Subphrenic abscess following an obstetrical procedure

- ♀ MCC **O86.04 Sepsis following an obstetrical procedure**

Use additional code to identify the sepsis

AHA CC: 4Q, 2018, 23; 2Q, 2019, 39; 2Q, 2020, 32-33

- ♀ **O86.09 Infection of obstetric surgical wound, other surgical site**

+ **O86.1 Other infection of genital tract following delivery**

- ♀ CC **O86.11 Cervicitis following delivery**
- ♀ CC **O86.12 Endometritis following delivery**
- ♀ CC **O86.13 Vaginitis following delivery**
- ♀ CC **O86.19 Other infection of genital tract following delivery**

+ **O86.2 Urinary tract infection following delivery**

- ♀ CC **O86.20 Urinary tract infection following delivery, unspecified**

Puerperal urinary tract infection NOS

- ♀ CC **O86.21 Infection of kidney following delivery**
- ♀ CC **O86.22 Infection of bladder following delivery**

Infection of urethra following delivery

- ♀ CC **O86.29 Other urinary tract infection following delivery**

- ♀ CC **O86.4 Pyrexia of unknown origin following delivery**

Puerperal infection NOS following delivery
Puerperal pyrexia NOS following delivery

Excludes2: *pyrexia during labor (O75.2)*

+ **O86.8 Other specified puerperal infections**

- ♀ MCC **O86.81 Puerperal septic thrombophlebitis**
- ♀ MCC **O86.89 Other specified puerperal infections**

O87 Venous complications and hemorrhoids in the puerperium

Includes: venous complications in labor, delivery and the puerperium

Excludes2: *obstetric embolism (O88.-)*
  puerperal septic thrombophlebitis (O86.81)
  venous complications in pregnancy (O22.-)

- ♀ CC **O87.0 Superficial thrombophlebitis in the puerperium**

Puerperal phlebitis NOS
Puerperal thrombosis NOS

- ♀ MCC **O87.1 Deep phlebothrombosis in the puerperium**

Deep vein thrombosis, postpartum
Pelvic thrombophlebitis, postpartum

Use additional code to identify the deep vein thrombosis (I82.4-, I82.5-, I82.62-. I82.72-)

Use additional code, if applicable, for associated long-term (current) use of anticoagulants (Z79.01)

- ♀ CC **O87.2 Hemorrhoids in the puerperium**
- ♀ CC **O87.3 Cerebral venous thrombosis in the puerperium**

Cerebrovenous sinus thrombosis in the puerperium

- ♀ **O87.4 Varicose veins of lower extremity in the puerperium**
- ♀ CC **O87.8 Other venous complications in the puerperium**

Genital varices in the puerperium

- ♀ **O87.9 Venous complication in the puerperium, unspecified**

Puerperal phlebopathy NOS

O88 Obstetric embolism

Excludes1: *embolism complicating abortion NOS (O03.2)*
  embolism complicating ectopic or molar pregnancy (O08.2)
  embolism complicating failed attempted abortion (O07.2)
  embolism complicating induced abortion (O04.7)
  embolism complicating spontaneous abortion (O03.2, O03.7)

+ **O88.0 Obstetric air embolism**

+ **O88.01 Obstetric air embolism in pregnancy**

- ♀ MCC **O88.011 Air embolism in pregnancy, first trimester**
- ♀ MCC **O88.012 Air embolism in pregnancy, second trimester**
- ♀ MCC **O88.013 Air embolism in pregnancy, third trimester**
- ♀ **O88.019 Air embolism in pregnancy, unspecified trimester**

- ♀ MCC **O88.02 Air embolism in childbirth**
- ♀ MCC **O88.03 Air embolism in the puerperium**

+ **O88.1 Amniotic fluid embolism**

Anaphylactoid syndrome in pregnancy

+ **O88.11 Amniotic fluid embolism in pregnancy**

- ♀ MCC **O88.111 Amniotic fluid embolism in pregnancy, first trimester**
- ♀ MCC **O88.112 Amniotic fluid embolism in pregnancy, second trimester**
- ♀ MCC **O88.113 Amniotic fluid embolism in pregnancy, third trimester**
- ♀ **O88.119 Amniotic fluid embolism in pregnancy, unspecified trimester**

- ♀ MCC **O88.12 Amniotic fluid embolism in childbirth**
- ♀ MCC **O88.13 Amniotic fluid embolism in the puerperium**

+ **O88.2 Obstetric thromboembolism**

+ **O88.21 Thromboembolism in pregnancy**

Obstetric (pulmonary) embolism NOS

- ♀ MCC **O88.211 Thromboembolism in pregnancy, first trimester**
- ♀ MCC **O88.212 Thromboembolism in pregnancy, second trimester**
- ♀ MCC **O88.213 Thromboembolism in pregnancy, third trimester**
- ♀ **O88.219 Thromboembolism in pregnancy, unspecified trimester**

- ♀ MCC **O88.22 Thromboembolism in childbirth**
- ♀ MCC **O88.23 Thromboembolism in the puerperium**

Puerperal (pulmonary) embolism NOS

+ **O88.3 Obstetric pyemic and septic embolism**

+ **O88.31 Pyemic and septic embolism in pregnancy**

- ♀ MCC **O88.311 Pyemic and septic embolism in pregnancy, first trimester**
- ♀ MCC **O88.312 Pyemic and septic embolism in pregnancy, second trimester**
- ♀ MCC **O88.313 Pyemic and septic embolism in pregnancy, third trimester**
- ♀ **O88.319 Pyemic and septic embolism in pregnancy, unspecified trimester**

- ♀ MCC **O88.32 Pyemic and septic embolism in childbirth**
- ♀ MCC **O88.33 Pyemic and septic embolism in the puerperium**

+ **O88.8 Other obstetric embolism**

Obstetric fat embolism

+ **O88.81 Other embolism in pregnancy**

- ♀ MCC **O88.811 Other embolism in pregnancy, first trimester**
- ♀ MCC **O88.812 Other embolism in pregnancy, second trimester**
- ♀ MCC **O88.813 Other embolism in pregnancy, third trimester**
- ♀ CC **O88.819 Other embolism in pregnancy, unspecified trimester**

- ♀ MCC **O88.82 Other embolism in childbirth**
- ♀ MCC **O88.83 Other embolism in the puerperium**

O89 Complications of anesthesia during the puerperium

Includes: maternal complications arising from the administration of a general, regional or local anesthetic, analgesic or other sedation during the puerperium

Use additional code, if applicable, to identify specific complication

+, +7th, X + 7th   ● Newborn   ● Pediatric   ● Maternity   ● Adult   ♀ Female   ♂ Male   Manifestation   Unacceptable PDX   HCC   CC   MCC   HAC

+ **O89.0** **Pulmonary complications of anesthesia during the puerperium**
- ♀ **O89.01** **Aspiration pneumonitis due to anesthesia during the puerperium**
  Inhalation of stomach contents or secretions NOS due to anesthesia during the puerperium
  Mendelson's syndrome due to anesthesia during the puerperium
- ♀ **O89.09** **Other pulmonary complications of anesthesia during the puerperium**
- ♀ **O89.1** **Cardiac complications of anesthesia during the puerperium**
- ♀ **O89.2** **Central nervous system complications of anesthesia during the puerperium**
- ♀ **O89.3** **Toxic reaction to local anesthesia during the puerperium**
- ♀ **O89.4** **Spinal and epidural anesthesia-induced headache during the puerperium**
- ♀ **O89.5** **Other complications of spinal and epidural anesthesia during the puerperium**
- ♀ **O89.6** **Failed or difficult intubation for anesthesia during the puerperium**
- ♀ **O89.8** **Other complications of anesthesia during the puerperium**
- ♀ **O89.9** **Complication of anesthesia during the puerperium, unspecified**

O90 **Complications of the puerperium, not elsewhere classified**
- ♀ **O90.0** **Disruption of cesarean delivery wound**
  Dehiscence of cesarean delivery wound
  Excludes1: *rupture of uterus (spontaneous) before onset of labor (O71.0-)*
  rupture of uterus during labor (O71.1)
- ♀ **O90.1** **Disruption of perineal obstetric wound**
  Disruption of wound of episiotomy
  Disruption of wound of perineal laceration
  Secondary perineal tear
- ♀ **O90.2** **Hematoma of obstetric wound**
- ♀ MCC **O90.3** **Peripartum cardiomyopathy**
  Conditions in I42.- arising during pregnancy and the puerperium
  Excludes1: *pre-existing heart disease complicating pregnancy and the puerperium (O99.4-)*
  Review coding guideline C.15.o.5
- ♀ MCC **O90.4** **Postpartum acute kidney failure**
  Hepatorenal syndrome following labor and delivery
- ♀ **O90.5** **Postpartum thyroiditis**
- ♀ **O90.6** **Postpartum mood disturbance**
  Postpartum blues
  Postpartum dysphoria
  Postpartum sadness
  Excludes1: *postpartum depression (F53.0)*
  puerperal psychosis (F53.1)
+ **O90.8** **Other complications of the puerperium, not elsewhere classified**
  - ♀ **O90.81** **Anemia of the puerperium**
    Postpartum anemia NOS
    Excludes1: *pre-existing anemia complicating the puerperium (O99.03)*
  - ♀ **O90.89** **Other complications of the puerperium, not elsewhere classified**
    Placental polyp
- ♀ **O90.9** **Complication of the puerperium, unspecified**

O91 **Infections of breast associated with pregnancy, the puerperium and lactation**
  Use additional code to identify infection
+ **O91.0** **Infection of nipple associated with pregnancy, the puerperium and lactation**
  + **O91.01** **Infection of nipple associated with pregnancy**
    Gestational abscess of nipple
    - ♀ **O91.011** **Infection of nipple associated with pregnancy, first trimester**
    - ♀ **O91.012** **Infection of nipple associated with pregnancy, second trimester**
    - ♀ **O91.013** **Infection of nipple associated with pregnancy, third trimester**
    - ♀ **O91.019** **Infection of nipple associated with pregnancy, unspecified trimester**
  - ♀ **O91.02** **Infection of nipple associated with the puerperium**
    Puerperal abscess of nipple
  - ♀ **O91.03** **Infection of nipple associated with lactation**
    Abscess of nipple associated with lactation

+ **O91.1** **Abscess of breast associated with pregnancy, the puerperium and lactation**
  + **O91.11** **Abscess of breast associated with pregnancy**
    Gestational mammary abscess
    Gestational purulent mastitis
    Gestational subareolar abscess
    - ♀ **O91.111** **Abscess of breast associated with pregnancy, first trimester**
    - ♀ **O91.112** **Abscess of breast associated with pregnancy, second trimester**
    - ♀ **O91.113** **Abscess of breast associated with pregnancy, third trimester**
    - ♀ **O91.119** **Abscess of breast associated with pregnancy, unspecified trimester**
  - ♀ **O91.12** **Abscess of breast associated with the puerperium**
    Puerperal mammary abscess
    Puerperal purulent mastitis
    Puerperal subareolar abscess
  - ♀ **O91.13** **Abscess of breast associated with lactation**
    Mammary abscess associated with lactation
    Purulent mastitis associated with lactation
    Subareolar abscess associated with lactation
+ **O91.2** **Nonpurulent mastitis associated with pregnancy, the puerperium and lactation**
  + **O91.21** **Nonpurulent mastitis associated with pregnancy**
    Gestational interstitial mastitis
    Gestational lymphangitis of breast
    Gestational mastitis NOS
    Gestational parenchymatous mastitis
    - ♀ **O91.211** **Nonpurulent mastitis associated with pregnancy, first trimester**
    - ♀ **O91.212** **Nonpurulent mastitis associated with pregnancy, second trimester**
    - ♀ **O91.213** **Nonpurulent mastitis associated with pregnancy, third trimester**
    - ♀ **O91.219** **Nonpurulent mastitis associated with pregnancy, unspecified trimester**
  - ♀ **O91.22** **Nonpurulent mastitis associated with the puerperium**
    Puerperal interstitial mastitis
    Puerperal lymphangitis of breast
    Puerperal mastitis NOS
    Puerperal parenchymatous mastitis
  - ♀ **O91.23** **Nonpurulent mastitis associated with lactation**
    Interstitial mastitis associated with lactation
    Lymphangitis of breast associated with lactation
    Mastitis NOS associated with lactation
    Parenchymatous mastitis associated with lactation

O92 **Other disorders of breast and disorders of lactation associated with pregnancy and the puerperium**
+ **O92.0** **Retracted nipple associated with pregnancy, the puerperium, and lactation**
  + **O92.01** **Retracted nipple associated with pregnancy**
    - ♀ **O92.011** **Retracted nipple associated with pregnancy, first trimester**
    - ♀ **O92.012** **Retracted nipple associated with pregnancy, second trimester**
    - ♀ **O92.013** **Retracted nipple associated with pregnancy, third trimester**
    - ♀ **O92.019** **Retracted nipple associated with pregnancy, unspecified trimester**
  - ♀ **O92.02** **Retracted nipple associated with the puerperium**
  - ♀ **O92.03** **Retracted nipple associated with lactation**
+ **O92.1** **Cracked nipple associated with pregnancy, the puerperium, and lactation**
  Fissure of nipple, gestational or puerperal
  + **O92.11** **Cracked nipple associated with pregnancy**
    - ♀ **O92.111** **Cracked nipple associated with pregnancy, first trimester**
    - ♀ **O92.112** **Cracked nipple associated with pregnancy, second trimester**
    - ♀ **O92.113** **Cracked nipple associated with pregnancy, third trimester**
    - ♀ **O92.119** **Cracked nipple associated with pregnancy, unspecified trimester**
  - ♀ **O92.12** **Cracked nipple associated with the puerperium**
  - ♀ **O92.13** **Cracked nipple associated with lactation**

+ **O92.2** **Other and unspecified disorders of breast associated with pregnancy and the puerperium**
- ♀ **O92.20** **Unspecified disorder of breast associated with pregnancy and the puerperium**
- ♀ **O92.29** **Other disorders of breast associated with pregnancy and the puerperium**
- ♀ **O92.3** **Agalactia**
Primary agalactia
Excludes1: *Elective agalactia (O92.5)*
Secondary agalactia (O92.5)
Therapeutic agalactia (O92.5)
- ♀ **O92.4** **Hypogalactia**
- ♀ **O92.5** **Suppressed lactation**
Elective agalactia
Secondary agalactia
Therapeutic agalactia
Excludes1: *primary agalactia (O92.3)*
- ♀ **O92.6** **Galactorrhea**
+ **O92.7** **Other and unspecified disorders of lactation**
- ♀ **O92.70** **Unspecified disorders of lactation**
- ♀ **O92.79** **Other disorders of lactation**
Puerperal galactocele

Other obstetric conditions, not elsewhere classified (O94-O9A)

- ♀ **O94** **Sequelae of complication of pregnancy, childbirth, and the puerperium**

NOTE This category is to be used to indicate conditions in O00-O77.-, O85-O94 and O98-O9A.- as the cause of late effects. The sequelae include conditions specified as such, or as late effects, which may occur at any time after the puerperium

Code first condition resulting from (sequela) of complication of pregnancy, childbirth, and the puerperium
Review coding guideline C.15.p
Valid 3-character code, no further characters required

O98 **Maternal infectious and parasitic diseases classifiable elsewhere but complicating pregnancy, childbirth and the puerperium**

Includes: the listed conditions when complicating the pregnant state, when aggravated by the pregnancy, or as a reason for obstetric care

Use additional code (Chapter 1), to identify specific infectious or parasitic disease

Excludes2: *herpes gestationis (O26.4-)*
infectious carrier state (O99.82-, O99.83-)
obstetrical tetanus (A34)
puerperal infection (O86.-)
puerperal sepsis (O85)
when the reason for maternal care is that the disease is known or suspected to have affected the fetus (O35-O36)

+ **O98.0** **Tuberculosis complicating pregnancy, childbirth and the puerperium**
Conditions in A15-A19
+ **O98.01** **Tuberculosis complicating pregnancy**
- ♀ CC **O98.011** **Tuberculosis complicating pregnancy, first trimester**
- ♀ CC **O98.012** **Tuberculosis complicating pregnancy, second trimester**
- ♀ CC **O98.013** **Tuberculosis complicating pregnancy, third trimester**
- ♀ **O98.019** **Tuberculosis complicating pregnancy, unspecified trimester**
- ♀ CC **O98.02** **Tuberculosis complicating childbirth**
- ♀ CC **O98.03** **Tuberculosis complicating the puerperium**
+ **O98.1** **Syphilis complicating pregnancy, childbirth and the puerperium**
Conditions in A50-A53
+ **O98.11** **Syphilis complicating pregnancy**
- ♀ CC **O98.111** **Syphilis complicating pregnancy, first trimester**
- ♀ CC **O98.112** **Syphilis complicating pregnancy, second trimester**
- ♀ CC **O98.113** **Syphilis complicating pregnancy, third trimester**
- ♀ **O98.119** **Syphilis complicating pregnancy, unspecified trimester**
- ♀ CC **O98.12** **Syphilis complicating childbirth**
- ♀ CC **O98.13** **Syphilis complicating the puerperium**

+ **O98.2** **Gonorrhea complicating pregnancy, childbirth and the puerperium**
Conditions in A54.-
+ **O98.21** **Gonorrhea complicating pregnancy**
- ♀ CC **O98.211** **Gonorrhea complicating pregnancy, first trimester**
- ♀ CC **O98.212** **Gonorrhea complicating pregnancy, second trimester**
- ♀ CC **O98.213** **Gonorrhea complicating pregnancy, third trimester**
- ♀ **O98.219** **Gonorrhea complicating pregnancy, unspecified trimester**
- ♀ CC **O98.22** **Gonorrhea complicating childbirth**
- ♀ CC **O98.23** **Gonorrhea complicating the puerperium**
+ **O98.3** **Other infections with a predominantly sexual mode of transmission complicating pregnancy, childbirth and the puerperium**
Conditions in A55-A64
+ **O98.31** **Other infections with a predominantly sexual mode of transmission complicating pregnancy**
- ♀ CC **O98.311** **Other infections with a predominantly sexual mode of transmission complicating pregnancy, first trimester**
- ♀ CC **O98.312** **Other infections with a predominantly sexual mode of transmission complicating pregnancy, second trimester**
- ♀ CC **O98.313** **Other infections with a predominantly sexual mode of transmission complicating pregnancy, third trimester**
- ♀ **O98.319** **Other infections with a predominantly sexual mode of transmission complicating pregnancy, unspecified trimester**
- ♀ CC **O98.32** **Other infections with a predominantly sexual mode of transmission complicating childbirth**
AHA CC: 1Q, 2020, 20
- ♀ CC **O98.33** **Other infections with a predominantly sexual mode of transmission complicating the puerperium**
+ **O98.4** **Viral hepatitis complicating pregnancy, childbirth and the puerperium**
Conditions in B15-B19
+ **O98.41** **Viral hepatitis complicating pregnancy**
- ♀ CC **O98.411** **Viral hepatitis complicating pregnancy, first trimester**
- ♀ CC **O98.412** **Viral hepatitis complicating pregnancy, second trimester**
- ♀ CC **O98.413** **Viral hepatitis complicating pregnancy, third trimester**
- ♀ **O98.419** **Viral hepatitis complicating pregnancy, unspecified trimester**
- ♀ CC **O98.42** **Viral hepatitis complicating childbirth**
- ♀ CC **O98.43** **Viral hepatitis complicating the puerperium**
+ **O98.5** **Other viral diseases complicating pregnancy, childbirth and the puerperium**
Conditions in A80-B09, B25-B34, R87.81-, R87.82-
Excludes1: *human immunodeficiency virus [HIV] disease complicating pregnancy, childbirth and the puerperium (O98.7-)*
Review coding guideline C.15.s
+ **O98.51** **Other viral diseases complicating pregnancy**
- ♀ CC **O98.511** **Other viral diseases complicating pregnancy, first trimester**
- ♀ CC **O98.512** **Other viral diseases complicating pregnancy, second trimester**
AHA CC: 4Q, 2016, 4-7
- ♀ CC **O98.513** **Other viral diseases complicating pregnancy, third trimester**
AHA CC: 4Q, 2016, 4-7
- ♀ **O98.519** **Other viral diseases complicating pregnancy, unspecified trimester**
- ♀ CC **O98.52** **Other viral diseases complicating childbirth**
- ♀ CC **O98.53** **Other viral diseases complicating the puerperium**
+ **O98.6** **Protozoal diseases complicating pregnancy, childbirth and the puerperium**
Conditions in B50-B64
+ **O98.61** **Protozoal diseases complicating pregnancy**
- ♀ CC **O98.611** **Protozoal diseases complicating pregnancy, first trimester**
- ♀ CC **O98.612** **Protozoal diseases complicating pregnancy, second trimester**
- ♀ CC **O98.613** **Protozoal diseases complicating pregnancy, third trimester**

+, +7th, X + 7th ● Newborn ● Pediatric ● Maternity ● Adult ♀ Female ♂ Male Manifestation Unacceptable PDX HCC CC MCC HAC

- ● ♀ **O98.619** **Protozoal diseases complicating pregnancy, unspecified trimester**
- ● ♀ CC **O98.62** **Protozoal diseases complicating childbirth**
- ● ♀ CC **O98.63** **Protozoal diseases complicating the puerperium**
- + **O98.7** **Human immunodeficiency virus [HIV] disease complicating pregnancy, childbirth and the puerperium**
  Use additional code to identify the type of HIV disease:
  Acquired immune deficiency syndrome (AIDS) (B20)
  Asymptomatic HIV status (Z21)
  HIV positive NOS (Z21)
  Symptomatic HIV disease (B20)
  Review coding guideline C.1.a.2.g
  Review coding guideline C.15.f
  - + **O98.71** **Human immunodeficiency virus [HIV] disease complicating pregnancy**
    - ● ♀ CC **O98.711** **Human immunodeficiency virus [HIV] disease complicating pregnancy, first trimester**
    - ● ♀ CC **O98.712** **Human immunodeficiency virus [HIV] disease complicating pregnancy, second trimester**
    - ● ♀ CC **O98.713** **Human immunodeficiency virus [HIV] disease complicating pregnancy, third trimester**
      - ● ♀ **O98.719** **Human immunodeficiency virus [HIV] disease complicating pregnancy, unspecified trimester**
  - ● ♀ CC **O98.72** **Human immunodeficiency virus [HIV] disease complicating childbirth**
  - ● ♀ CC **O98.73** **Human immunodeficiency virus [HIV] disease complicating the puerperium**
- + **O98.8** **Other maternal infectious and parasitic diseases complicating pregnancy, childbirth and the puerperium**
  - + **O98.81** **Other maternal infectious and parasitic diseases complicating pregnancy**
    - ● ♀ CC **O98.811** **Other maternal infectious and parasitic diseases complicating pregnancy, first trimester**
    - ● ♀ CC **O98.812** **Other maternal infectious and parasitic diseases complicating pregnancy, second trimester**
    - ● ♀ CC **O98.813** **Other maternal infectious and parasitic diseases complicating pregnancy, third trimester**
      - ● ♀ **O98.819** **Other maternal infectious and parasitic diseases complicating pregnancy, unspecified trimester**
  - ● ♀ CC **O98.82** **Other maternal infectious and parasitic diseases complicating childbirth**
    AHA CC: 1Q, 2020, 10
  - ● ♀ CC **O98.83** **Other maternal infectious and parasitic diseases complicating the puerperium**
- + **O98.9** **Unspecified maternal infectious and parasitic disease complicating pregnancy, childbirth and the puerperium**
  - + **O98.91** **Unspecified maternal infectious and parasitic disease complicating pregnancy**
    - ● ♀ CC **O98.911** **Unspecified maternal infectious and parasitic disease complicating pregnancy, first trimester**
    - ● ♀ CC **O98.912** **Unspecified maternal infectious and parasitic disease complicating pregnancy, second trimester**
    - ● ♀ CC **O98.913** **Unspecified maternal infectious and parasitic disease complicating pregnancy, third trimester**
      - ● ♀ **O98.919** **Unspecified maternal infectious and parasitic disease complicating pregnancy, unspecified trimester**
  - ● ♀ CC **O98.92** **Unspecified maternal infectious and parasitic disease complicating childbirth**
  - ● ♀ CC **O98.93** **Unspecified maternal infectious and parasitic disease complicating the puerperium**

O99 **Other maternal diseases classifiable elsewhere but complicating pregnancy, childbirth and the puerperium**
  Includes: conditions which complicate the pregnant state, are aggravated by the pregnancy or are a main reason for obstetric care
  Use additional code to identify specific condition

Excludes2: *when the reason for maternal care is that the condition is known or suspected to have affected the fetus (O35-O36)*
- + **O99.0** **Anemia complicating pregnancy, childbirth and the puerperium**
  Conditions in D50-D64
  Excludes1: *anemia arising in the puerperium (O90.81) postpartum anemia NOS (O90.81)*
  - + **O99.01** **Anemia complicating pregnancy**
    - ● ♀ **O99.011** **Anemia complicating pregnancy, first trimester**
    - ● ♀ **O99.012** **Anemia complicating pregnancy, second trimester**
    - ● ♀ **O99.013** **Anemia complicating pregnancy, third trimester**
    - ● ♀ **O99.019** **Anemia complicating pregnancy, unspecified trimester**
  - ● ♀ **O99.02** **Anemia complicating childbirth**
  - ● ♀ **O99.03** **Anemia complicating the puerperium**
    Excludes1: *postpartum anemia not pre-existing prior to delivery (O90.81)*
- + **O99.1** **Other diseases of the blood and blood-forming organs and certain disorders involving the immune mechanism complicating pregnancy, childbirth and the puerperium**
  Conditions in D65-D89
  Excludes1: *hemorrhage with coagulation defects (O45.-, O46.0-, O67.0, O72.3)*
  - + **O99.11** **Other diseases of the blood and blood-forming organs and certain disorders involving the immune mechanism complicating pregnancy**
    - ● ♀ CC **O99.111** **Other diseases of the blood and blood-forming organs and certain disorders involving the immune mechanism complicating pregnancy, first trimester**
    - ● ♀ CC **O99.112** **Other diseases of the blood and blood-forming organs and certain disorders involving the immune mechanism complicating pregnancy, second trimester**
    - ● ♀ CC **O99.113** **Other diseases of the blood and blood-forming organs and certain disorders involving the immune mechanism complicating pregnancy, third trimester**
    - ● ♀ CC **O99.119** **Other diseases of the blood and blood-forming organs and certain disorders involving the immune mechanism complicating pregnancy, unspecified trimester**
  - ● ♀ CC **O99.12** **Other diseases of the blood and blood-forming organs and certain disorders involving the immune mechanism complicating childbirth**
  - ● ♀ CC **O99.13** **Other diseases of the blood and blood-forming organs and certain disorders involving the immune mechanism complicating the puerperium**
- + **O99.2** **Endocrine, nutritional and metabolic diseases complicating pregnancy, childbirth and the puerperium**
  Conditions in E00-E89
  Excludes2: *diabetes mellitus (O24.-) malnutrition (O25.-) postpartum thyroiditis (O90.5)*
  - + **O99.21** **Obesity complicating pregnancy, childbirth, and the puerperium**
    Use additional code to identify the type of obesity (E66.-)
    - ● ♀ **O99.210** **Obesity complicating pregnancy, unspecified trimester**
    - ● ♀ **O99.211** **Obesity complicating pregnancy, first trimester**
    - ● ♀ **O99.212** **Obesity complicating pregnancy, second trimester**
    - ● ♀ **O99.213** **Obesity complicating pregnancy, third trimester**
    - ● ♀ **O99.214** **Obesity complicating childbirth**
      AHA CC: 4Q, 2018, 80
    - ● ♀ **O99.215** **Obesity complicating the puerperium**

+ **O99.28** **Other endocrine, nutritional and metabolic diseases complicating pregnancy, childbirth and the puerperium**
- ♀ **O99.280** Endocrine, nutritional and metabolic diseases complicating pregnancy, unspecified trimester
- ♀ **O99.281** Endocrine, nutritional and metabolic diseases complicating pregnancy, first trimester
- ♀ **O99.282** Endocrine, nutritional and metabolic diseases complicating pregnancy, second trimester
- ♀ **O99.283** Endocrine, nutritional and metabolic diseases complicating pregnancy, third trimester
- ♀ **O99.284** Endocrine, nutritional and metabolic diseases complicating childbirth
- ♀ **O99.285** Endocrine, nutritional and metabolic diseases complicating the puerperium

+ **O99.3** **Mental disorders and diseases of the nervous system complicating pregnancy, childbirth and the puerperium**

+ **O99.31** **Alcohol use complicating pregnancy, childbirth, and the puerperium**
  Use additional code(s) from F10 to identify manifestations of the alcohol use
  Review coding guideline C.15.l.1
- ♀ **O99.310** Alcohol use complicating pregnancy, unspecified trimester
- ♀ **O99.311** Alcohol use complicating pregnancy, first trimester
- ♀ **O99.312** Alcohol use complicating pregnancy, second trimester
- ♀ **O99.313** Alcohol use complicating pregnancy, third trimester
- ♀ **O99.314** Alcohol use complicating childbirth
- ♀ **O99.315** Alcohol use complicating the puerperium

+ **O99.32** **Drug use complicating pregnancy, childbirth, and the puerperium**
  Use additional code(s) from F11-F16 and F18-F19 to identify manifestations of the drug use
  AHA CC: 2Q, 2018, 10-11
  Review coding guideline C.15.l.3
- ♀ **O99.320** Drug use complicating pregnancy, unspecified trimester
- ♀ CC **O99.321** Drug use complicating pregnancy, first trimester
- ♀ CC **O99.322** Drug use complicating pregnancy, second trimester
- ♀ CC **O99.323** Drug use complicating pregnancy, third trimester
- ♀ CC **O99.324** Drug use complicating childbirth
- ♀ CC **O99.325** Drug use complicating the puerperium

+ **O99.33** **Tobacco use disorder complicating pregnancy, childbirth, and the puerperium**
  Smoking complicating pregnancy, childbirth, and the puerperium
  Use additional code from category F17 to identify type of tobacco nicotine dependence
  Review coding guideline C.15.l.2
- ♀ **O99.330** Smoking (tobacco) complicating pregnancy, unspecified trimester
- ♀ **O99.331** Smoking (tobacco) complicating pregnancy, first trimester
- ♀ **O99.332** Smoking (tobacco) complicating pregnancy, second trimester
- ♀ **O99.333** Smoking (tobacco) complicating pregnancy, third trimester
- ♀ **O99.334** Smoking (tobacco) complicating childbirth
- ♀ **O99.335** Smoking (tobacco) complicating the puerperium

+ **O99.34** **Other mental disorders complicating pregnancy, childbirth, and the puerperium**
  Conditions in F01-F09, F20-F52 and F54-F99
  Excludes2: *postpartum mood disturbance (O90.6)*
      postnatal psychosis (F53.1)
      puerperal psychosis (F53.1)
- ♀ **O99.340** Other mental disorders complicating pregnancy, unspecified trimester
- ♀ **O99.341** Other mental disorders complicating pregnancy, first trimester
- ♀ **O99.342** Other mental disorders complicating pregnancy, second trimester
- ♀ **O99.343** Other mental disorders complicating pregnancy, third trimester
- ♀ **O99.344** Other mental disorders complicating childbirth
- ♀ **O99.345** Other mental disorders complicating the puerperium
  AHA CC: 4Q, 2018, 8-9

+ **O99.35** **Diseases of the nervous system complicating pregnancy, childbirth, and the puerperium**
  Conditions in G00-G99
  Excludes2: *pregnancy related peripheral neuritis (O26.8-)*
- ♀ **O99.350** Diseases of the nervous system complicating pregnancy, unspecified trimester
- ♀ **O99.351** Diseases of the nervous system complicating pregnancy, first trimester
- ♀ **O99.352** Diseases of the nervous system complicating pregnancy, second trimester
- ♀ **O99.353** Diseases of the nervous system complicating pregnancy, third trimester
- ♀ CC **O99.354** Diseases of the nervous system complicating childbirth
- ♀ CC **O99.355** Diseases of the nervous system complicating the puerperium

+ **O99.4** **Diseases of the circulatory system complicating pregnancy, childbirth and the puerperium**
  Conditions in I00-I99
  Excludes1: *peripartum cardiomyopathy (O90.3)*
  Excludes2: *hypertensive disorders (O10-O16)*
      obstetric embolism (O88.-)
      venous complications and cerebrovenous sinus thrombosis in labor, childbirth and the puerperium (O87.-)
      venous complications and cerebrovenous sinus thrombosis in pregnancy (O22.-)

+ **O99.41** **Diseases of the circulatory system complicating pregnancy**
  AHA CC: 2Q, 2016, 8
- ♀ CC **O99.411** Diseases of the circulatory system complicating pregnancy, first trimester
- ♀ CC **O99.412** Diseases of the circulatory system complicating pregnancy, second trimester
- ♀ CC **O99.413** Diseases of the circulatory system complicating pregnancy, third trimester
- ♀ **O99.419** Diseases of the circulatory system complicating pregnancy, unspecified trimester
- ♀ MCC **O99.42** Diseases of the circulatory system complicating childbirth
- ♀ CC **O99.43** Diseases of the circulatory system complicating the puerperium

+ **O99.5** **Diseases of the respiratory system complicating pregnancy, childbirth and the puerperium**
  Conditions in J00-J99

+ **O99.51** **Diseases of the respiratory system complicating pregnancy**
- ♀ **O99.511** Diseases of the respiratory system complicating pregnancy, first trimester
- ♀ **O99.512** Diseases of the respiratory system complicating pregnancy, second trimester
- ♀ **O99.513** Diseases of the respiratory system complicating pregnancy, third trimester
- ♀ **O99.519** Diseases of the respiratory system complicating pregnancy, unspecified trimester

911

- ♀ **O99.52** **Diseases of the respiratory system complicating childbirth**
- ♀ **O99.53** **Diseases of the respiratory system complicating the puerperium**
+ **O99.6** **Diseases of the digestive system complicating pregnancy, childbirth and the puerperium**
  Conditions in K00-K93
  Excludes2: *liver and biliary tract disorders in pregnancy, childbirth and the puerperium (O26.6-)*
  hemorrhoids in pregnancy (O22.4-)
  + **O99.61** **Diseases of the digestive system complicating pregnancy**
    - ♀ **O99.611** **Diseases of the digestive system complicating pregnancy, first trimester**
    - ♀ **O99.612** **Diseases of the digestive system complicating pregnancy, second trimester**
    - ♀ **O99.613** **Diseases of the digestive system complicating pregnancy, third trimester**
    - ♀ **O99.619** **Diseases of the digestive system complicating pregnancy, unspecified trimester**
  - ♀ **O99.62** **Diseases of the digestive system complicating childbirth**
  - ♀ **O99.63** **Diseases of the digestive system complicating the puerperium**
+ **O99.7** **Diseases of the skin and subcutaneous tissue complicating pregnancy, childbirth and the puerperium**
  Conditions in L00-L99
  Excludes2: *herpes gestationis (O26.4)*
  pruritic urticarial papules and plaques of pregnancy (PUPPP) (O26.86)
  + **O99.71** **Diseases of the skin and subcutaneous tissue complicating pregnancy**
    - ♀ **O99.711** **Diseases of the skin and subcutaneous tissue complicating pregnancy, first trimester**
    - ♀ **O99.712** **Diseases of the skin and subcutaneous tissue complicating pregnancy, second trimester**
    - ♀ **O99.713** **Diseases of the skin and subcutaneous tissue complicating pregnancy, third trimester**
    - ♀ **O99.719** **Diseases of the skin and subcutaneous tissue complicating pregnancy, unspecified trimester**
  - ♀ **O99.72** **Diseases of the skin and subcutaneous tissue complicating childbirth**
  - ♀ **O99.73** **Diseases of the skin and subcutaneous tissue complicating the puerperium**
+ **O99.8** **Other specified diseases and conditions complicating pregnancy, childbirth and the puerperium**
  Conditions in D00-D48, H00-H95, M00-N99, and Q00-Q99
  Use additional code to identify condition
  Excludes2: *genitourinary infections in pregnancy (O23.-)*
  infection of genitourinary tract following delivery (O86.1-O86.4)
  malignant neoplasm complicating pregnancy, childbirth and the puerperium (O9A.1-)
  maternal care for known or suspected abnormality of maternal pelvic organs (O34.-)
  postpartum acute kidney failure (O90.4)
  traumatic injuries in pregnancy (O9A.2-)
  + **O99.81** **Abnormal glucose complicating pregnancy, childbirth and the puerperium**
    Excludes1: *gestational diabetes (O24.4-)*
    Review coding guideline C.15.i
    - ♀ **O99.810** **Abnormal glucose complicating pregnancy**
    - ♀ **O99.814** **Abnormal glucose complicating childbirth**
    - ♀ **O99.815** **Abnormal glucose complicating the puerperium**
+ **O99.82** **Streptococcus B carrier state complicating pregnancy, childbirth and the puerperium**
  Excludes1: *Carrier of streptococcus group B (GBS) in a nonpregnant woman (Z22.330)*
  - ♀ **O99.820** **Streptococcus B carrier state complicating pregnancy**
  - ♀ **O99.824** **Streptococcus B carrier state complicating childbirth**
    AHA CC: 2Q, 2019, 9
  - ♀ **O99.825** **Streptococcus B carrier state complicating the puerperium**
+ **O99.83** **Other infection carrier state complicating pregnancy, childbirth and the puerperium**
  Use additional code to identify the carrier state (Z22.-)
  - ♀ CC **O99.830** **Other infection carrier state complicating pregnancy**
  - ♀ CC **O99.834** **Other infection carrier state complicating childbirth**
  - ♀ CC **O99.835** **Other infection carrier state complicating the puerperium**
+ **O99.84** **Bariatric surgery status complicating pregnancy, childbirth and the puerperium**
  Gastric banding status complicating pregnancy, childbirth and the puerperium
  Gastric bypass status for obesity complicating pregnancy, childbirth and the puerperium
  Obesity surgery status complicating pregnancy, childbirth and the puerperium
  - ♀ **O99.840** **Bariatric surgery status complicating pregnancy, unspecified trimester**
  - ♀ **O99.841** **Bariatric surgery status complicating pregnancy, first trimester**
  - ♀ **O99.842** **Bariatric surgery status complicating pregnancy, second trimester**
  - ♀ **O99.843** **Bariatric surgery status complicating pregnancy, third trimester**
  - ♀ **O99.844** **Bariatric surgery status complicating childbirth**
  - ♀ **O99.845** **Bariatric surgery status complicating the puerperium**
+ **O99.89** **Other specified diseases and conditions complicating pregnancy, childbirth and the puerperium**
  - ♀ **O99.891** **Other specified diseases and conditions complicating pregnancy**
  - ♀ **O99.892** **Other specified diseases and conditions complicating childbirth**
  - ♀ **O99.893** **Other specified diseases and conditions complicating puerperium**

O9A Maternal malignant neoplasms, traumatic injuries and abuse classifiable elsewhere but complicating pregnancy, childbirth and the puerperium
+ **O9A.1** **Malignant neoplasm complicating pregnancy, childbirth and the puerperium**
  Conditions in C00-C96
  Use additional code to identify neoplasm
  Excludes2: *maternal care for benign tumor of corpus uteri (O34.1-)*
  maternal care for benign tumor of cervix (O34.4-)
  Review coding guideline C.2.l.3
  + **O9A.11** **Malignant neoplasm complicating pregnancy**
    - ♀ **O9A.111** **Malignant neoplasm complicating pregnancy, first trimester**
    - ♀ **O9A.112** **Malignant neoplasm complicating pregnancy, second trimester**
    - ♀ **O9A.113** **Malignant neoplasm complicating pregnancy, third trimester**
    - ♀ **O9A.119** **Malignant neoplasm complicating pregnancy, unspecified trimester**
  - ♀ **O9A.12** **Malignant neoplasm complicating childbirth**
  - ♀ **O9A.13** **Malignant neoplasm complicating the puerperium**
    AHA CC: 3Q, 2015, 19-20

+, +7th, X + 7th ● Newborn ● Pediatric ● Maternity ● Adult ♀ Female ♂ Male Manifestation Unacceptable PDX HCC CC MCC HAC

+ **O9A.2 Injury, poisoning and certain other consequences of external causes complicating pregnancy, childbirth and the puerperium**
  Conditions in S00-T88, except T74 and T76
  Use additional code(s) to identify the injury or poisoning
  Excludes2: *physical, sexual and psychological abuse complicating pregnancy, childbirth and the puerperium (O9A.3-, O9A.4-, O9A.5-)*
  Review coding guideline C.15.m

  + **O9A.21 Injury, poisoning and certain other consequences of external causes complicating pregnancy**
    - ♀ **O9A.211 Injury, poisoning and certain other consequences of external causes complicating pregnancy, first trimester**
    - ♀ **O9A.212 Injury, poisoning and certain other consequences of external causes complicating pregnancy, second trimester**
    - ♀ **O9A.213 Injury, poisoning and certain other consequences of external causes complicating pregnancy, third trimester**
    - ♀ **O9A.219 Injury, poisoning and certain other consequences of external causes complicating pregnancy, unspecified trimester**
  - ♀ **O9A.22 Injury, poisoning and certain other consequences of external causes complicating childbirth**
  - ♀ **O9A.23 Injury, poisoning and certain other consequences of external causes complicating the puerperium**

+ **O9A.3 Physical abuse complicating pregnancy, childbirth and the puerperium**
  Conditions in T74.11 or T76.11
  Use additional code (if applicable):
    to identify any associated current injury due to physical abuse
    to identify the perpetrator of abuse (Y07.-)
  Excludes2: *sexual abuse complicating pregnancy, childbirth and the puerperium (O9A.4)*
  Review coding guideline C.15.r

  + **O9A.31 Physical abuse complicating pregnancy**
    - ♀ **O9A.311 Physical abuse complicating pregnancy, first trimester**
    - ♀ **O9A.312 Physical abuse complicating pregnancy, second trimester**
    - ♀ **O9A.313 Physical abuse complicating pregnancy, third trimester**
    - ♀ **O9A.319 Physical abuse complicating pregnancy, unspecified trimester**
  - ♀ **O9A.32 Physical abuse complicating childbirth**
  - ♀ **O9A.33 Physical abuse complicating the puerperium**

+ **O9A.4 Sexual abuse complicating pregnancy, childbirth and the puerperium**
  Conditions in T74.21 or T76.21
  Use additional code (if applicable):
    to identify any associated current injury due to sexual abuse
    to identify the perpetrator of abuse (Y07.-)
  Review coding guideline C.15.r

  + **O9A.41 Sexual abuse complicating pregnancy**
    - ♀ **O9A.411 Sexual abuse complicating pregnancy, first trimester**
    - ♀ **O9A.412 Sexual abuse complicating pregnancy, second trimester**
    - ♀ **O9A.413 Sexual abuse complicating pregnancy, third trimester**
    - ♀ **O9A.419 Sexual abuse complicating pregnancy, unspecified trimester**
  - ♀ **O9A.42 Sexual abuse complicating childbirth**
  - ♀ **O9A.43 Sexual abuse complicating the puerperium**

+ **O9A.5 Psychological abuse complicating pregnancy, childbirth and the puerperium**
  Conditions in T74.31 or T76.31
  Use additional code to identify the perpetrator of abuse (Y07.-)
  Review coding guideline C.15.r

  + **O9A.51 Psychological abuse complicating pregnancy**
    - ♀ **O9A.511 Psychological abuse complicating pregnancy, first trimester**
    - ♀ **O9A.512 Psychological abuse complicating pregnancy, second trimester**
    - ♀ **O9A.513 Psychological abuse complicating pregnancy, third trimester**
    - ♀ **O9A.519 Psychological abuse complicating pregnancy, unspecified trimester**
  - ♀ **O9A.52 Psychological abuse complicating childbirth**
  - ♀ **O9A.53 Psychological abuse complicating the puerperium**

+, +7th, X + 7th • Newborn • Pediatric • Maternity • Adult ♀ Female ♂ Male Manifestation Unacceptable PDX HCC CC MCC HAC

Chapter 16: Certain Conditions Originating in the Perinatal Period (P00-P96)

NOTE Codes from this chapter are for use on newborn records only, never on maternal records

Includes: conditions that have their origin in the fetal or perinatal period (before birth through the first 28 days after birth) even if morbidity occurs later

Excludes2: congenital malformations, deformations and chromosomal abnormalities (Q00-Q99)
endocrine, nutritional and metabolic diseases (E00-E88)
injury, poisoning and certain other consequences of external causes (S00-T88)
neoplasms (C00-D49)
tetanus neonatorum (A33)

This chapter contains the following category blocks:

P00-P04 Newborn affected by maternal factors and by complications of pregnancy, labor, and delivery
P05-P08 Disorders of newborn related to length of gestation and fetal growth
P09 Abnormal findings on neonatal screening
P10-P15 Birth trauma
P19-P29 Respiratory and cardiovascular disorders specific to the perinatal period
P35-P39 Infections specific to the perinatal period
P50-P61 Hemorrhagic and hematological disorders of newborn
P70-P74 Transitory endocrine and metabolic disorders specific to newborn
P76-P78 Digestive system disorders of newborn
P80-P83 Conditions involving the integument and temperature regulation of newborn
P84 Other problems with newborn
P90-P96 Other disorders originating in the perinatal period

C. Chapter-Specific Coding Guidelines

In addition to general coding guidelines, there are guidelines for specific diagnoses and/or conditions in the classification. Unless otherwise indicated, these guidelines apply to all health care settings. Please refer to Section II for guidelines on the selection of principal diagnosis.

16. Chapter 16: Certain Conditions Originating in the Perinatal Period (P00-P96)

For coding and reporting purposes the perinatal period is defined as before birth through the 28th day following birth. The following guidelines are provided for reporting purposes

a. General Perinatal Rules

1) Use of Chapter 16 Codes

Codes in this chapter are <u>never</u> for use on the maternal record. Codes from Chapter 15, the obstetric chapter, are never permitted on the newborn record. Chapter 16 codes may be used throughout the life of the patient if the condition is still present.

2) Principal Diagnosis for Birth Record

When coding the birth episode in a newborn record, assign a code from category Z38, Liveborn infants according to place of birth and type of delivery, as the principal diagnosis. A code from category Z38 is assigned only once, to a newborn at the time of birth. If a newborn is transferred to another institution, a code from category Z38 should not be used at the receiving hospital.

A code from category Z38 is used only on the newborn record, not on the mother's record.

3) Use of Codes from other Chapters with Codes from Chapter 16

Codes from other chapters may be used with codes from chapter 16 if the codes from the other chapters provide more specific detail. Codes for signs and symptoms may be assigned when a definitive diagnosis has not been established. If the reason for the encounter is a perinatal condition, the code from chapter 16 should be sequenced first.

4) Use of Chapter 16 Codes after the Perinatal Period

Should a condition originate in the perinatal period, and continue throughout the life of the patient, the perinatal code should continue to be used regardless of the patient's age.

5) Birth process or community acquired conditions

If a newborn has a condition that may be either due to the birth process or community acquired and the documentation does not indicate which it is, the default is due to the birth process and the code from Chapter 16 should be used. If the condition is community-acquired, a code from Chapter 16 should not be assigned.

For COVID-19 infection in a newborn, see guideline I.C.16.h

6) Code all clinically significant conditions

All clinically significant conditions noted on routine newborn examination should be coded. A condition is clinically significant if it requires:

- clinical evaluation; or
- therapeutic treatment; or
- diagnostic procedures; or
- extended length of hospital stay; or
- increased nursing care and/or monitoring; or
- has implications for future health care needs

Note: The perinatal guidelines listed above are the same as the general coding guidelines for "additional diagnoses", except for the final point regarding implications for future health care needs. Codes should be assigned for conditions that have been specified by the provider as having implications for future health care needs.

b. Observation and Evaluation of Newborns for Suspected Conditions not Found

1) Use of Z05 codes

Assign a code from category Z05, Observation and evaluation of newborns and infants for suspected conditions ruled out, to identify those instances when a healthy newborn is evaluated for a suspected condition that is determined after study not to be present. Do not use a code from category Z05 when the patient has identified signs or symptoms of a suspected problem; in such cases code the sign or symptom.

2) Z05 on Other than the Birth Record

A code from category Z05 may also be assigned as a principal or first-listed code for readmissions or encounters when the code from category Z38 code no longer applies. Codes from category Z05 are fur use only for healthy newborns and infants for which no condition after study is found to be present.

3) Z05 on a birth record

A code from category Z05 is to be used as a secondary code after the code from category Z38, Liveborn infants according to place of birth and type of delivery.

c. Coding Additional Perinatal Diagnoses

1) Assigning codes for conditions that require treatment

Assign codes for conditions that require treatment or further investigation, prolong the length of stay, or require resource utilization.

2) Codes for conditions specified as having implications for future health care needs

Assign codes for conditions that have been specified by the provider as having implications for future health care needs.

Note: This guideline should not be used for adult patients.

d. Prematurity and Fetal Growth Retardation

Providers utilize different criteria in determining prematurity. A code for prematurity should not be assigned unless it is documented. Assignment of codes in categories P05, Disorders of newborn related to slow fetal growth and fetal malnutrition, and P07, Disorders of newborn related to short gestation and low birth weight, not elsewhere classified, should be based on the recorded birth weight and estimated gestational age.

When both birth weight and gestational age are available, two codes from category P07 should be assigned, with the code for birth weight sequenced before the code for gestational age.

e. Low birth weight and immaturity status

Codes from category P07, Disorders of newborn related to short gestation and low birth weight, not elsewhere classified, are for use for a child or adult who was premature or had a low birth weight as a newborn and this is affecting the patient's current health status.

See Section I.C.21. Factors influencing health status and contact with health services, Status.

f. Bacterial Sepsis of Newborn

Category P36, Bacterial sepsis of newborn, includes congenital sepsis. If a perinate is documented as having sepsis without documentation of congenital or community acquired, the default is congenital and a code from category P36 should be assigned. If the P36 code includes the causal organism, an additional code from category B95, Streptococcus, Staphylococcus, and Enterococcus as the cause of diseases classified elsewhere, or B96, Other bacterial agents as the cause of diseases classified elsewhere, should not be assigned. If the P36 code does not include the causal organism, assign an additional code from category B96. If applicable, use additional codes to identify severe sepsis (R65.2-) and any associated acute organ dysfunction.

g. Stillbirth

Code P95, Stillbirth, is only for use in institutions that maintain separate records for stillbirths. No other code should be used with P95. Code P95 should not be used on the mother's record.

+, +7th, X + 7th ● Newborn ● Pediatric ● Maternity ● Adult ♀ Female ♂ Male Manifestation Unacceptable PDX HCC CC MCC **HAC**

h. COVID-19 Infection in Newborn

For a newborn that tests positive for COVID-19, assign code U07.1, COVID-19, and the appropriate codes for associated manifestation(s) in neonates/newborns in the absence of documentation indicating a specific type of transmission. For a newborn that tests positive for COVID-19 and the provider documents the condition was contracted in utero or during the birth process, assign codes P35.8, Other congenital viral diseases, and U07.1, COVID-19. When coding the birth episode in a newborn record, the appropriate code from category Z38, Liveborn infants according to place of birth and type of delivery, should be assigned as the principal diagnosis.

Newborn affected by maternal factors and by complications of pregnancy, labor, and delivery (P00-P04)

NOTE These codes are for use when the listed maternal conditions are specified as the cause of confirmed morbidity or potential morbidity which have their origin in the perinatal period (before birth through the first 28 days after birth).

AHA CC: 4Q, 2016, 54-55

P00 Newborn affected by maternal conditions that may be unrelated to present pregnancy

Code first any current condition in newborn

Excludes2: encounter for observation for newborn for suspected diseases and conditions ruled out (Z05.-)
newborn affected by maternal complications of pregnancy (P01.-)
newborn affected by maternal endocrine and metabolic disorders (P70-P74)
newborn affected by noxious substances transmitted via placenta or breast milk (P04.-)

P00.0 Newborn affected by maternal hypertensive disorders
Newborn affected by maternal conditions classifiable to O10-O11, O13-O16

P00.1 Newborn affected by maternal renal and urinary tract diseases
Newborn affected by maternal conditions classifiable to N00-N39

P00.2 Newborn affected by maternal infectious and parasitic diseases
Newborn affected by maternal infectious disease classifiable to A00-B99, J09 and J10
Excludes1: maternal genital tract or other localized infections (P00.8)
Excludes2: infections specific to the perinatal period (P35-P39)
AHA CC: 3Q, 2015, 20; 2Q, 2019, 10

P00.3 Newborn affected by other maternal circulatory and respiratory diseases
Newborn affected by maternal conditions classifiable to I00-I99, J00-J99, Q20-Q34 and not included in P00.0, P00.2

P00.4 Newborn affected by maternal nutritional disorders
Newborn affected by maternal disorders classifiable to E40-E64
Maternal malnutrition NOS

P00.5 Newborn affected by maternal injury
Newborn affected by maternal conditions classifiable to O9A.2-

P00.6 Newborn affected by surgical procedure on mother
Newborn affected by amniocentesis
Excludes1: Cesarean delivery for present delivery (P03.4)
damage to placenta from amniocentesis, Cesarean delivery or surgical induction (P02.1)
previous surgery to uterus or pelvic organs (P03.89)
Excludes2: newborn affected by complication of (fetal) intrauterine procedure (P96.5)

P00.7 Newborn affected by other medical procedures on mother, not elsewhere classified
Newborn affected by radiation to mother
Excludes1: damage to placenta from amniocentesis, cesarean delivery or surgical induction (P02.1)
newborn affected by other complications of labor and delivery (P03.-)

+ P00.8 Newborn affected by other maternal conditions
P00.81 Newborn affected by periodontal disease in mother

P00.89 Newborn affected by other maternal conditions
Newborn affected by conditions classifiable to T80-T88
Newborn affected by maternal genital tract or other localized infections
Newborn affected by maternal systemic lupus erythematosus
Use additional code to identify infectious agent, if known
AHA CC: 2Q, 2019, 9

P00.9 Newborn affected by unspecified maternal condition

P01 Newborn affected by maternal complications of pregnancy

Code first any current condition in newborn
Excludes2: encounter for observation of newborn for suspected diseases and conditions ruled out (Z05.-)

P01.0 Newborn affected by incompetent cervix
P01.1 Newborn affected by premature rupture of membranes
P01.2 Newborn affected by oligohydramnios
Excludes1: oligohydramnios due to premature rupture of membranes (P01.1)
P01.3 Newborn affected by polyhydramnios
Newborn affected by hydramnios
P01.4 Newborn affected by ectopic pregnancy
Newborn affected by abdominal pregnancy
P01.5 Newborn affected by multiple pregnancy
Newborn affected by triplet (pregnancy)
Newborn affected by twin (pregnancy)
P01.6 Newborn affected by maternal death
P01.7 Newborn affected by malpresentation before labor
Newborn affected by breech presentation before labor
Newborn affected by external version before labor
Newborn affected by face presentation before labor
Newborn affected by transverse lie before labor
Newborn affected by unstable lie before labor
P01.8 Newborn affected by other maternal complications of pregnancy
P01.9 Newborn affected by maternal complication of pregnancy, unspecified

P02 Newborn affected by complications of placenta, cord and membranes

Code first any current condition in newborn
Excludes2: encounter for observation of newborn for suspected diseases and conditions ruled out (Z05.-)

P02.0 Newborn affected by placenta previa
P02.1 Newborn affected by other forms of placental separation and hemorrhage
Newborn affected by abruptio placenta
Newborn affected by accidental hemorrhage
Newborn affected by antepartum hemorrhage
Newborn affected by damage to placenta from amniocentesis, cesarean delivery or surgical induction
Newborn affected by maternal blood loss
Newborn affected by premature separation of placenta
+ P02.2 Newborn affected by other and unspecified morphological and functional abnormalities of placenta
P02.20 Newborn affected by unspecified morphological and functional abnormalities of placenta
P02.29 Newborn affected by other morphological and functional abnormalities of placenta
Newborn affected by placental dysfunction
Newborn affected by placental infarction
Newborn affected by placental insufficiency
P02.3 Newborn affected by placental transfusion syndromes
Newborn affected by placental and cord abnormalities resulting in twin-to-twin or other transplacental transfusion
P02.4 Newborn affected by prolapsed cord
P02.5 Newborn affected by other compression of umbilical cord
Newborn affected by umbilical cord (tightly) around neck
Newborn affected by entanglement of umbilical cord
Newborn affected by knot in umbilical cord
+ P02.6 Newborn affected by other and unspecified conditions of umbilical cord
P02.60 Newborn affected by unspecified conditions of umbilical cord
P02.69 Newborn affected by other conditions of umbilical cord
Newborn affected by short umbilical cord
Newborn affected by vasa previa
Excludes1: newborn affected by single umbilical artery (Q27.0)

+ P02.7 Newborn affected by chorioamnionitis
AHA CC: 4Q, 2018, 23-24

    P02.70 Newborn affected by fetal inflammatory response syndrome
        Newborn affected by FIRS

    P02.78 Newborn affected by other conditions from chorioamnionitis
        Newborn affected by amnionitis
        Newborn affected by membranitis
        Newborn affected by placentitis

P02.8 Newborn affected by other abnormalities of membranes

P02.9 Newborn affected by abnormality of membranes, unspecified

P03 Newborn affected by other complications of labor and delivery
    Code first any current condition in newborn
    Excludes2: encounter for observation of newborn for suspected diseases and conditions ruled out (Z05.-)

P03.0 Newborn affected by breech delivery and extraction

P03.1 Newborn affected by other malpresentation, malposition and disproportion during labor and delivery
    Newborn affected by contracted pelvis
    Newborn affected by conditions classifiable to O64-O66
    Newborn affected by persistent occipitoposterior
    Newborn affected by transverse lie

P03.2 Newborn affected by forceps delivery

P03.3 Newborn affected by delivery by vacuum extractor [ventouse]

P03.4 Newborn affected by Cesarean delivery

P03.5 Newborn affected by precipitate delivery
    Newborn affected by rapid second stage

P03.6 Newborn affected by abnormal uterine contractions
    Newborn affected by conditions classifiable to O62.-, except O62.3
    Newborn affected by hypertonic labor
    Newborn affected by uterine inertia

+ P03.8 Newborn affected by other specified complications of labor and delivery

    + P03.81 Newborn affected by abnormality in fetal (intrauterine) heart rate or rhythm
        Excludes1: neonatal cardiac dysrhythmia (P29.1-)

        P03.810 Newborn affected by abnormality in fetal (intrauterine) heart rate or rhythm before the onset of labor

        P03.811 Newborn affected by abnormality in fetal (intrauterine) heart rate or rhythm during labor

        P03.819 Newborn affected by abnormality in fetal (intrauterine) heart rate or rhythm, unspecified as to time of onset

    P03.82 Meconium passage during delivery
        Excludes1: meconium aspiration (P24.00, P24.01)
            meconium staining (P96.83)

    P03.89 Newborn affected by other specified complications of labor and delivery
        Newborn affected by abnormality of maternal soft tissues
        Newborn affected by conditions classifiable to O60-O75 and by procedures used in labor and delivery not included in P02.- and P03.0-P03.6
        Newborn affected by induction of labor

P03.9 Newborn affected by complication of labor and delivery, unspecified

P04 Newborn affected by noxious substances transmitted via placenta or breast milk
    Includes: nonteratogenic effects of substances transmitted via placenta
    Excludes2: congenital malformations (Q00-Q99)
        encounter for observation of newborn for suspected diseases and conditions ruled out (Z05.-)
        neonatal jaundice from excessive hemolysis due to drugs or toxins transmitted from mother (P58.4)
        newborn in contact with and (suspected) exposures hazardous to health not transmitted via placenta or breast milk (Z77.-)
    AHA CC: 4Q, 2018, 24-25

    P04.0 Newborn affected by maternal anesthesia and analgesia in pregnancy, labor and delivery

Newborn affected by reactions and intoxications from maternal opiates and tranquilizers administered for procedures during pregnancy or labor and delivery
    Excludes2: newborn affected by other maternal medication (P04.1-)

+ P04.1 Newborn affected by other maternal medication
    Code first withdrawal symptoms from maternal use of drugs of addiction, if applicable (P96.1)
    Excludes1: dysmorphism due to warfarin (Q86.2)
            fetal hydantoin syndrome (Q86.1)
    Excludes2: maternal anesthesia and analgesia in pregnancy, labor and delivery (P04.0)
            maternal use of drugs of addition (P04.4-)
    AHA CC: 4Q, 2016, 54-55; 4Q, 2018, 24-25

    P04.11 Newborn affected by maternal antineoplastic chemotherapy

    P04.12 Newborn affected by maternal cytotoxic drugs

    P04.13 Newborn affected by maternal use of anticonvulsants

    P04.14 Newborn affected by maternal use of opiates

    P04.15 Newborn affected by maternal use of antidepressants

    P04.16 Newborn affected by maternal use of amphetamines

    P04.17 Newborn affected by maternal use of sedative-hypnotics

    P04.1A Newborn affected by maternal use of anxiolytics

    P04.18 Newborn affected by other maternal medication

    P04.19 Newborn affected by maternal use of unspecified medication

P04.2 Newborn affected by maternal use of tobacco
    Newborn affected by exposure in utero to tobacco smoke
    Excludes2: newborn exposure to environmental tobacco smoke (P96.81)

P04.3 Newborn affected by maternal use of alcohol
    Excludes1: fetal alcohol syndrome (Q86.0)

+ P04.4 Newborn affected by maternal use of drugs of addiction
    AHA CC: 4Q, 2018, 25

    P04.40 Newborn affected by maternal use of unspecified drugs of addiction

    P04.41 Newborn affected by maternal use of cocaine

    P04.42 Newborn affected by maternal use of hallucinogens
        Excludes2: newborn affected by other maternal medication (P04.1-)

    P04.49 Newborn affected by maternal use of other drugs of addiction
        Excludes2: newborn affected by maternal anesthesia and analgesia (P04.0)
            withdrawal symptoms from maternal use of drugs of addiction (P96.1)

P04.5 Newborn affected by maternal use of nutritional chemical substances

P04.6 Newborn affected by maternal exposure to environmental chemical substances

+ P04.8 Newborn affected by other maternal noxious substances
    AHA CC: 4Q, 2018, 25

    P04.81 Newborn affected by maternal use of cannabis

    P04.89 Newborn affected by other maternal noxious substances

P04.9 Newborn affected by maternal noxious substance, unspecified

Disorders of newborn related to length of gestation and fetal growth (P05-P08)

P05 Disorders of newborn related to slow fetal growth and fetal malnutrition
    Review coding guideline C.16.d

+ P05.0 Newborn light for gestational age
    Newborn light-for-dates
    Weight below but length above 10th percentile for gestational age

    P05.00 Newborn light for gestational age, unspecified weight

    P05.01 Newborn light for gestational age, less than 500 grams

    P05.02 Newborn light for gestational age, 500-749 grams

    P05.03 Newborn light for gestational age, 750-999 grams

    P05.04 Newborn light for gestational age, 1000-1249 grams

    P05.05 Newborn light for gestational age, 1250-1499 grams

    P05.06 Newborn light for gestational age, 1500-1749 grams

    P05.07 Newborn light for gestational age, 1750-1999 grams

P05.08 **Newborn light for gestational age, 2000-2499 grams**

P05.09 **Newborn light for gestational age, 2500 grams and over**

Newborn light for gestational age, other

AHA CC: 4Q, 2016, 55-56

+ **P05.1** **Newborn small for gestational age**

Newborn small-and-light-for-dates

Newborn small-for-dates

Weight and length below 10th percentile for gestational age

P05.10 **Newborn small for gestational age, unspecified weight**

P05.11 **Newborn small for gestational age, less than 500 grams**

P05.12 **Newborn small for gestational age, 500-749 grams**

P05.13 **Newborn small for gestational age, 750-999 grams**

P05.14 **Newborn small for gestational age, 1000-1249 grams**

P05.15 **Newborn small for gestational age, 1250-1499 grams**

P05.16 **Newborn small for gestational age, 1500-1749 grams**

P05.17 **Newborn small for gestational age, 1750-1999 grams**

P05.18 **Newborn small for gestational age, 2000-2499 grams**

P05.19 **Newborn small for gestational age, other**

Newborn small for gestational age, 2500 grams and over

AHA CC: 4Q, 2016, 55-56

P05.2 **Newborn affected by fetal (intrauterine) malnutrition not light or small for gestational age**

Infant, not light or small for gestational age, showing signs of fetal malnutrition, such as dry, peeling skin and loss of subcutaneous tissue

Excludes1: *newborn affected by fetal malnutrition with light for gestational age (P05.0-)*

newborn affected by fetal malnutrition with small for gestational age (P05.1-)

P05.9 **Newborn affected by slow intrauterine growth, unspecified**

Newborn affected by fetal growth retardation NOS

P07 **Disorders of newborn related to short gestation and low birth weight, not elsewhere classified**

NOTE When both birth weight and gestational age of the newborn are available, both should be coded with birth weight sequenced before gestational age

Includes: the listed conditions, without further specification, as the cause of morbidity or additional care, in newborn

Review coding guidelines C.16.d and C.16.e

+ **P07.0** **Extremely low birth weight newborn**

Newborn birth weight 999 g. or less

Excludes1: low birth weight due to slow fetal growth and fetal malnutrition (P05.-)

P07.00 **Extremely low birth weight newborn, unspecified weight**

P07.01 **Extremely low birth weight newborn, less than 500 grams**

P07.02 **Extremely low birth weight newborn, 500-749 grams**

P07.03 **Extremely low birth weight newborn, 750-999 grams**

+ **P07.1** **Other low birth weight newborn**

Newborn birth weight 1000-2499 g.

Excludes1: low birth weight due to slow fetal growth and fetal malnutrition (P05.-)

P07.10 **Other low birth weight newborn, unspecified weight**

P07.14 **Other low birth weight newborn, 1000-1249 grams**

P07.15 **Other low birth weight newborn, 1250-1499 grams**

P07.16 **Other low birth weight newborn, 1500-1749 grams**

P07.17 **Other low birth weight newborn, 1750-1999 grams**

P07.18 **Other low birth weight newborn, 2000-2499 grams**

+ **P07.2** **Extreme immaturity of newborn**

Less than 28 completed weeks (less than 196 completed days) of gestation.

P07.20 **Extreme immaturity of newborn, unspecified weeks of gestation**

Gestational age less than 28 completed weeks NOS

P07.21 **Extreme immaturity of newborn, gestational age less than 23 completed weeks**

Extreme immaturity of newborn, gestational age less than 23 weeks, 0 days

P07.22 **Extreme immaturity of newborn, gestational age 23 completed weeks**

Extreme immaturity of newborn, gestational age 23 weeks, 0 days through 23 weeks, 6 days

P07.23 **Extreme immaturity of newborn, gestational age 24 completed weeks**

Extreme immaturity of newborn, gestational age 24 weeks, 0 days through 24 weeks, 6 days

P07.24 **Extreme immaturity of newborn, gestational age 25 completed weeks**

Extreme immaturity of newborn, gestational age 25 weeks, 0 days through 25 weeks, 6 days

P07.25 **Extreme immaturity of newborn, gestational age 26 completed weeks**

Extreme immaturity of newborn, gestational age 26 weeks, 0 days through 26 weeks, 6 days

P07.26 **Extreme immaturity of newborn, gestational age 27 completed weeks**

Extreme immaturity of newborn, gestational age 27 weeks, 0 days through 27 weeks, 6 days

+ **P07.3** **Preterm [premature] newborn [other]**

28 completed weeks or more but less than 37 completed weeks (196 completed days but less than 259 completed days) of gestation.

Prematurity NOS

P07.30 **Preterm newborn, unspecified weeks of gestation**

P07.31 **Preterm newborn, gestational age 28 completed weeks**

Preterm newborn, gestational age 28 weeks, 0 days through 28 weeks, 6 days

P07.32 **Preterm newborn, gestational age 29 completed weeks**

Preterm newborn, gestational age 29 weeks, 0 days through 29 weeks, 6 days

P07.33 **Preterm newborn, gestational age 30 completed weeks**

Preterm newborn, gestational age 30 weeks, 0 days through 30 weeks, 6 days

P07.34 **Preterm newborn, gestational age 31 completed weeks**

Preterm newborn, gestational age 31 weeks, 0 days through 31 weeks, 6 days

P07.35 **Preterm newborn, gestational age 32 completed weeks**

Preterm newborn, gestational age 32 weeks, 0 days through 32 weeks, 6 days

P07.36 **Preterm newborn, gestational age 33 completed weeks**

Preterm newborn, gestational age 33 weeks, 0 days through 33 weeks, 6 days

P07.37 **Preterm newborn, gestational age 34 completed weeks**

Preterm newborn, gestational age 34 weeks, 0 days through 34 weeks, 6 days

AHA CC: 2Q, 2017, 7

P07.38 **Preterm newborn, gestational age 35 completed weeks**

Preterm newborn, gestational age 35 weeks, 0 days through 35 weeks, 6 days

P07.39 **Preterm newborn, gestational age 36 completed weeks**

Preterm newborn, gestational age 36 weeks, 0 days through 36 weeks, 6 days

AHA CC: 3Q, 2017, 26

P08 **Disorders of newborn related to long gestation and high birth weight**

NOTE When both birth weight and gestational age of the newborn are available, priority of assignment should be given to birth weight

Includes: the listed conditions, without further specification, as causes of morbidity or additional care, in newborn

P08.0 **Exceptionally large newborn baby**

Usually implies a birth weight of 4500 g. or more

Excludes1: *syndrome of infant of diabetic mother (P70.1)*

syndrome of infant of mother with gestational diabetes (P70.0)

+, +7th, X + 7th　　● Newborn　　● Pediatric　　● Maternity　　● Adult　　♀ Female　　♂ Male　　Manifestation　　Unacceptable PDX　　HCC　　CC　　MCC　　HAC

P08.1 **Other heavy for gestational age newborn**
Other newborn heavy- or large-for-dates regardless of period of gestation
Usually implies a birth weight of 4000 g. to 4499 g.
Excludes1: *newborn with a birth weight of 4500 or more (P08.0)*
syndrome of infant of diabetic mother (P70.1)
syndrome of infant of mother with gestational diabetes (P70.0).

+ **P08.2** **Late newborn, not heavy for gestational age**
P08.21 **Post-term newborn**
Newborn with gestation period over 40 completed weeks to 42 completed weeks
AHA CC: 1Q, 2014, 14

P08.22 **Prolonged gestation of newborn**
Newborn with gestation period over 42 completed weeks (294 days or more), not heavy- or large-for-dates.
Postmaturity NOS
AHA CC: 1Q, 2014, 14

Abnormal findings on neonatal screening (P09)

P09 **Abnormal findings on neonatal screening**
Use additional code to identify signs, symptoms and conditions associated with the screening
Excludes2: *nonspecific serologic evidence of human immunodeficiency virus [HIV] (R75)*
Valid 3-character code, no further characters required

Birth trauma (P10-P15)

P10 **Intracranial laceration and hemorrhage due to birth injury**
Excludes1: *intracranial hemorrhage of newborn NOS (P52.9)*
intracranial hemorrhage of newborn due to anoxia or hypoxia (P52.-)
nontraumatic intracranial hemorrhage of newborn (P52.-)

MCC **P10.0** **Subdural hemorrhage due to birth injury**
Subdural hematoma (localized) due to birth injury
Excludes1: *subdural hemorrhage accompanying tentorial tear (P10.4)*

MCC **P10.1** **Cerebral hemorrhage due to birth injury**
CC **P10.2** **Intraventricular hemorrhage due to birth injury**
MCC **P10.3** **Subarachnoid hemorrhage due to birth injury**
MCC **P10.4** **Tentorial tear due to birth injury**
MCC **P10.8** **Other intracranial lacerations and hemorrhages due to birth injury**
MCC **P10.9** **Unspecified intracranial laceration and hemorrhage due to birth injury**

P11 **Other birth injuries to central nervous system**
MCC **P11.0** **Cerebral edema due to birth injury**
P11.1 **Other specified brain damage due to birth injury**
MCC **P11.2** **Unspecified brain damage due to birth injury**
P11.3 **Birth injury to facial nerve**
Facial palsy due to birth injury
P11.4 **Birth injury to other cranial nerves**
P11.5 **Birth injury to spine and spinal cord**
Fracture of spine due to birth injury
MCC **P11.9** **Birth injury to central nervous system, unspecified**

P12 **Birth injury to scalp**
P12.0 **Cephalhematoma due to birth injury**
P12.1 **Chignon (from vacuum extraction) due to birth injury**
CC **P12.2** **Epicranial subaponeurotic hemorrhage due to birth injury**
Subgaleal hemorrhage
P12.3 **Bruising of scalp due to birth injury**
P12.4 **Injury of scalp of newborn due to monitoring equipment**
Sampling incision of scalp of newborn
Scalp clip (electrode) injury of newborn
+ **P12.8** **Other birth injuries to scalp**
P12.81 **Caput succedaneum**
P12.89 **Other birth injuries to scalp**
P12.9 **Birth injury to scalp, unspecified**

P13 **Birth injury to skeleton**
Excludes2: *birth injury to spine (P11.5)*
P13.0 **Fracture of skull due to birth injury**
P13.1 **Other birth injuries to skull**
Excludes1: *cephalhematoma (P12.0)*
P13.2 **Birth injury to femur**
P13.3 **Birth injury to other long bones**
P13.4 **Fracture of clavicle due to birth injury**
P13.8 **Birth injuries to other parts of skeleton**
P13.9 **Birth injury to skeleton, unspecified**

P14 **Birth injury to peripheral nervous system**
P14.0 **Erb's paralysis due to birth injury**
P14.1 **Klumpke's paralysis due to birth injury**
P14.2 **Phrenic nerve paralysis due to birth injury**
P14.3 **Other brachial plexus birth injuries**
P14.8 **Birth injuries to other parts of peripheral nervous system**
P14.9 **Birth injury to peripheral nervous system, unspecified**

P15 **Other birth injuries**
P15.0 **Birth injury to liver**
Rupture of liver due to birth injury
P15.1 **Birth injury to spleen**
Rupture of spleen due to birth injury
P15.2 **Sternomastoid injury due to birth injury**
P15.3 **Birth injury to eye**
Subconjunctival hemorrhage due to birth injury
Traumatic glaucoma due to birth injury
P15.4 **Birth injury to face**
Facial congestion due to birth injury
P15.5 **Birth injury to external genitalia**
P15.6 **Subcutaneous fat necrosis due to birth injury**
P15.8 **Other specified birth injuries**
P15.9 **Birth injury, unspecified**

Respiratory and cardiovascular disorders specific to the perinatal period (P19-P29)

P19 **Metabolic acidemia in newborn**
Includes: metabolic acidemia in newborn
P19.0 **Metabolic acidemia in newborn first noted before onset of labor**
P19.1 **Metabolic acidemia in newborn first noted during labor**
P19.2 **Metabolic acidemia noted at birth**
P19.9 **Metabolic acidemia, unspecified**

P22 **Respiratory distress of newborn**
MCC **P22.0** **Respiratory distress syndrome of newborn**
Cardiorespiratory distress syndrome of newborn
Hyaline membrane disease
Idiopathic respiratory distress syndrome [IRDS or RDS] of newborn
Pulmonary hypoperfusion syndrome
Respiratory distress syndrome, type I
Excludes2: *respiratory arrest of newborn (P28.81)*
respiratory failure of newborn NOS (P28.5)
AHA CC: 2Q, 2019, 29

P22.1 **Transient tachypnea of newborn**
Idiopathic tachypnea of newborn
Respiratory distress syndrome, type II
Wet lung syndrome
P22.8 **Other respiratory distress of newborn**
Excludes1: *respiratory arrest of newborn (P28.81)*
respiratory failure of newborn NOS (P28.5)
P22.9 **Respiratory distress of newborn, unspecified**
Excludes1: *respiratory arrest of newborn (P28.81)*
respiratory failure of newborn NOS (P28.5)

P23 **Congenital pneumonia**

> **Includes:** infective pneumonia acquired in utero or during birth
>
> **Excludes1:** *neonatal pneumonia resulting from aspiration (P24.-)*

MCC **P23.0** **Congenital pneumonia due to viral agent**

> Use additional code (B97) to identify organism
>
> **Excludes1:** *congenital rubella pneumonitis (P35.0)*

MCC **P23.1** **Congenital pneumonia due to Chlamydia**

MCC **P23.2** **Congenital pneumonia due to staphylococcus**

MCC **P23.3** **Congenital pneumonia due to streptococcus, group B**

MCC **P23.4** **Congenital pneumonia due to Escherichia coli**

P23.5 **Congenital pneumonia due to Pseudomonas**

MCC **P23.6** **Congenital pneumonia due to other bacterial agents**

> Congenital pneumonia due to Hemophilus influenzae
> Congenital pneumonia due to Klebsiella pneumoniae
> Congenital pneumonia due to Mycoplasma
> Congenital pneumonia due to Streptococcus, except group B
> Use additional code (B95-B96) to identify organism

MCC **P23.8** **Congenital pneumonia due to other organisms**

MCC **P23.9** **Congenital pneumonia, unspecified**

P24 **Neonatal aspiration**

> **Includes:** aspiration in utero and during delivery

+ **P24.0** **Meconium aspiration**

> **Excludes1:** *meconium passage (without aspiration) during delivery (P03.82)*
> *meconium staining (P96.83)*

P24.00 **Meconium aspiration without respiratory symptoms**

> Meconium aspiration NOS

MCC **P24.01** **Meconium aspiration with respiratory symptoms**

> Meconium aspiration pneumonia
> Meconium aspiration pneumonitis
> Meconium aspiration syndrome NOS
> Use additional code to identify any secondary pulmonary hypertension, if applicable (I27.2-)

+ **P24.1** **Neonatal aspiration of (clear) amniotic fluid and mucus**

> Neonatal aspiration of liquor (amnii)

P24.10 **Neonatal aspiration of (clear) amniotic fluid and mucus without respiratory symptoms**

> Neonatal aspiration of amniotic fluid and mucus NOS

MCC **P24.11** **Neonatal aspiration of (clear) amniotic fluid and mucus with respiratory symptoms**

> Neonatal aspiration of amniotic fluid and mucus with pneumonia
> Neonatal aspiration of amniotic fluid and mucus with pneumonitis
> Use additional code to identify any secondary pulmonary hypertension, if applicable (I27.2-)

+ **P24.2** **Neonatal aspiration of blood**

P24.20 **Neonatal aspiration of blood without respiratory symptoms**

> Neonatal aspiration of blood NOS

MCC **P24.21** **Neonatal aspiration of blood with respiratory symptoms**

> Neonatal aspiration of blood with pneumonia
> Neonatal aspiration of blood with pneumonitis
> Use additional code to identify any secondary pulmonary hypertension, if applicable (I27.2-)

+ **P24.3** **Neonatal aspiration of milk and regurgitated food**

> Neonatal aspiration of stomach contents

P24.30 **Neonatal aspiration of milk and regurgitated food without respiratory symptoms**

> Neonatal aspiration of milk and regurgitated food NOS

MCC **P24.31** **Neonatal aspiration of milk and regurgitated food with respiratory symptoms**

> Neonatal aspiration of milk and regurgitated food with pneumonia
> Neonatal aspiration of milk and regurgitated food with pneumonitis
> Use additional code to identify any secondary pulmonary hypertension, if applicable (I27.2-)

+ **P24.8** **Other neonatal aspiration**

P24.80 **Other neonatal aspiration without respiratory symptoms**

> Neonatal aspiration NEC

MCC **P24.81** **Other neonatal aspiration with respiratory symptoms**

> Neonatal aspiration pneumonia NEC
> Neonatal aspiration with pneumonitis NEC
> Neonatal aspiration with pneumonia NOS
> Neonatal aspiration with pneumonitis NOS
> Use additional code to identify any secondary pulmonary hypertension, if applicable (I27.2-)

P24.9 **Neonatal aspiration, unspecified**

P25 **Interstitial emphysema and related conditions originating in the perinatal period**

MCC **P25.0** **Interstitial emphysema originating in the perinatal period**

MCC **P25.1** **Pneumothorax originating in the perinatal period**

MCC **P25.2** **Pneumomediastinum originating in the perinatal period**

MCC **P25.3** **Pneumopericardium originating in the perinatal period**

MCC **P25.8** **Other conditions related to interstitial emphysema originating in the perinatal period**

P26 **Pulmonary hemorrhage originating in the perinatal period**

> **Excludes1:** *acute idiopathic hemorrhage in infants over 28 days old (R04.81)*

MCC **P26.0** **Tracheobronchial hemorrhage originating in the perinatal period**

MCC **P26.1** **Massive pulmonary hemorrhage originating in the perinatal period**

MCC **P26.8** **Other pulmonary hemorrhages originating in the perinatal period**

MCC **P26.9** **Unspecified pulmonary hemorrhage originating in the perinatal period**

P27 **Chronic respiratory disease originating in the perinatal period**

> **Excludes2:** *respiratory distress of newborn (P22.0-P22.9)*

MCC **P27.0** **Wilson-Mikity syndrome**

> Pulmonary dysmaturity

MCC **P27.1** **Bronchopulmonary dysplasia originating in the perinatal period**

MCC **P27.8** **Other chronic respiratory diseases originating in the perinatal period**

> Congenital pulmonary fibrosis
> Ventilator lung in newborn

MCC **P27.9** **Unspecified chronic respiratory disease originating in the perinatal period**

P28 **Other respiratory conditions originating in the perinatal period**

> **Excludes1:** *congenital malformations of the respiratory system (Q30-Q34)*

CC **P28.0** **Primary atelectasis of newborn**

> Primary failure to expand terminal respiratory units
> Pulmonary hypoplasia associated with short gestation
> Pulmonary immaturity NOS

+ **P28.1** **Other and unspecified atelectasis of newborn**

CC **P28.10** **Unspecified atelectasis of newborn**

> Atelectasis of newborn NOS

CC **P28.11** **Resorption atelectasis without respiratory distress syndrome**

> **Excludes1:** *resorption atelectasis with respiratory distress syndrome (P22.0)*

CC **P28.19** **Other atelectasis of newborn**

> Partial atelectasis of newborn
> Secondary atelectasis of newborn

CC **P28.2** **Cyanotic attacks of newborn**

> **Excludes1:** *apnea of newborn (P28.3-P28.4)*

CC **P28.3** **Primary sleep apnea of newborn**

> Central sleep apnea of newborn
> Obstructive sleep apnea of newborn
> Sleep apnea of newborn NOS

CC **P28.4** **Other apnea of newborn**

> Apnea of prematurity
> Obstructive apnea of newborn
> **Excludes1:** *obstructive sleep apnea of newborn (P28.3)*

MCC **P28.5** **Respiratory failure of newborn**

> **Excludes1:** *respiratory arrest of newborn (P28.81)*
> *respiratory distress of newborn (P22.0-)*
>
> *AHA CC: 2Q, 2019, 29*

+ **P28.8** **Other specified respiratory conditions of newborn**
MCC **P28.81** **Respiratory arrest of newborn**
AHA CC: 2Q, 2017, 6-7
P28.89 **Other specified respiratory conditions of newborn**
Congenital laryngeal stridor
Sniffles in newborn
Snuffles in newborn
Excludes1: *early congenital syphilitic rhinitis (A50.05)*

P28.9 **Respiratory condition of newborn, unspecified**
Respiratory depression in newborn

P29 **Cardiovascular disorders originating in the perinatal period**

Excludes1: *congenital malformations of the circulatory system (Q20-Q28)*

P29.0 **Neonatal cardiac failure**
+ **P29.1** **Neonatal cardiac dysrhythmia**
P29.11 **Neonatal tachycardia**
P29.12 **Neonatal bradycardia**
P29.2 **Neonatal hypertension**
+ **P29.3** **Persistent fetal circulation**
AHA CC: 4Q, 2017, 20-21
MCC **P29.30** **Pulmonary hypertension of newborn**
Persistent pulmonary hypertension of newborn
MCC **P29.38** **Other persistent fetal circulation**
Delayed closure of ductus arteriosus
P29.4 **Transient myocardial ischemia in newborn**
+ **P29.8** **Other cardiovascular disorders originating in the perinatal period**
MCC **P29.81** **Cardiac arrest of newborn**
P29.89 **Other cardiovascular disorders originating in the perinatal period**
AHA CC: 4Q, 2014, 23
P29.9 **Cardiovascular disorder originating in the perinatal period, unspecified**

Infections specific to the perinatal period (P35-P39)

Infections acquired in utero, during birth via the umbilicus, or during the first 28 days after birth

Excludes2: *asymptomatic human immunodeficiency virus [HIV] infection status (Z21)*
congenital gonococcal infection (A54.-)
congenital pneumonia (P23.-)
congenital syphilis (A50.-)
human immunodeficiency virus [HIV] disease (B20)
infant botulism (A48.51)
infectious diseases not specific to the perinatal period (A00-B99, J09, J10.-)
intestinal infectious disease (A00-A09)
laboratory evidence of human immunodeficiency virus [HIV] (R75)
tetanus neonatorum (A33)

P35 **Congenital viral diseases**

Includes: infections acquired in utero or during birth
CC **P35.0** **Congenital rubella syndrome**
Congenital rubella pneumonitis
MCC **P35.1** **Congenital cytomegalovirus infection**
MCC **P35.2** **Congenital herpesviral [herpes simplex] infection**
MCC **P35.3** **Congenital viral hepatitis**
MCC **P35.4** **Congenital Zika virus disease**
Use additional code to identify manifestations of congenital Zika virus disease
AHA CC: 4Q, 2018, 25-26
MCC **P35.8** **Other congenital viral diseases**
Congenital varicella [chickenpox]
AHA CC: 4Q, 2016, 4-7; 2Q, 2020, 13
Review coding guideline C.16.h
MCC **P35.9** **Congenital viral disease, unspecified**

P36 **Bacterial sepsis of newborn**

Includes: congenital sepsis
Use additional code(s), if applicable, to identify severe sepsis (R65.2-) and associated acute organ dysfunction(s)
Review coding guideline C.1.d and C.16.f
MCC **P36.0** **Sepsis of newborn due to streptococcus, group B**
+ **P36.1** **Sepsis of newborn due to other and unspecified streptococci**
MCC **P36.10** **Sepsis of newborn due to unspecified streptococci**
MCC **P36.19** **Sepsis of newborn due to other streptococci**
MCC **P36.2** **Sepsis of newborn due to Staphylococcus aureus**
+ **P36.3** **Sepsis of newborn due to other and unspecified staphylococci**
MCC **P36.30** **Sepsis of newborn due to unspecified staphylococci**
MCC **P36.39** **Sepsis of newborn due to other staphylococci**

MCC **P36.4** **Sepsis of newborn due to Escherichia coli**
MCC **P36.5** **Sepsis of newborn due to anaerobes**
MCC **P36.8** **Other bacterial sepsis of newborn**
Use additional code from category B96 to identify organism
MCC **P36.9** **Bacterial sepsis of newborn, unspecified**

P37 **Other congenital infectious and parasitic diseases**

Excludes2: *congenital syphilis (A50.-)*
infectious neonatal diarrhea (A00-A09)
necrotizing enterocolitis in newborn (P77.-)
noninfectious neonatal diarrhea (P78.3)
ophthalmia neonatorum due to gonococcus (A54.31)
tetanus neonatorum (A33)

MCC **P37.0** **Congenital tuberculosis**
MCC **P37.1** **Congenital toxoplasmosis**
Hydrocephalus due to congenital toxoplasmosis
MCC **P37.2** **Neonatal (disseminated) listeriosis**
MCC **P37.3** **Congenital falciparum malaria**
MCC **P37.4** **Other congenital malaria**
P37.5 **Neonatal candidiasis**
MCC **P37.8** **Other specified congenital infectious and parasitic diseases**
MCC **P37.9** **Congenital infectious or parasitic disease, unspecified**

P38 **Omphalitis of newborn**

Excludes1: *omphalitis not of newborn (L08.82)*
tetanus omphalitis (A33)
umbilical hemorrhage of newborn (P51.-)
CC **P38.1** **Omphalitis with mild hemorrhage**
CC **P38.9** **Omphalitis without hemorrhage**
Omphalitis of newborn NOS

P39 **Other infections specific to the perinatal period**

Use additional code to identify organism or specific infection
CC **P39.0** **Neonatal infective mastitis**
Excludes1: *breast engorgement of newborn (P83.4)*
noninfective mastitis of newborn (P83.4)
P39.1 **Neonatal conjunctivitis and dacryocystitis**
Neonatal chlamydial conjunctivitis
Ophthalmia neonatorum NOS
Excludes1: *gonococcal conjunctivitis (A54.31)*
CC **P39.2** **Intra-amniotic infection affecting newborn, not elsewhere classified**
CC **P39.3** **Neonatal urinary tract infection**
CC **P39.4** **Neonatal skin infection**
Neonatal pyoderma
Excludes1: *pemphigus neonatorum (L00)*
staphylococcal scalded skin syndrome (L00)
CC **P39.8** **Other specified infections specific to the perinatal period**
CC **P39.9** **Infection specific to the perinatal period, unspecified**

Hemorrhagic and hematological disorders of newborn (P50-P61)

Excludes1: *congenital stenosis and stricture of bile ducts (Q44.3)*
Crigler-Najjar syndrome (E80.5)
Dubin-Johnson syndrome (E80.6)
Gilbert syndrome (E80.4)
hereditary hemolytic anemias (D55-D58)

P50 **Newborn affected by intrauterine (fetal) blood loss**

Excludes1: *congenital anemia from intrauterine (fetal) blood loss (P61.3)*
P50.0 **Newborn affected by intrauterine (fetal) blood loss from vasa previa**
P50.1 **Newborn affected by intrauterine (fetal) blood loss from ruptured cord**
P50.2 **Newborn affected by intrauterine (fetal) blood loss from placenta**
P50.3 **Newborn affected by hemorrhage into co-twin**
P50.4 **Newborn affected by hemorrhage into maternal circulation**
P50.5 **Newborn affected by intrauterine (fetal) blood loss from cut end of co-twin's cord**
P50.8 **Newborn affected by other intrauterine (fetal) blood loss**
P50.9 **Newborn affected by intrauterine (fetal) blood loss, unspecified**
Newborn affected by fetal hemorrhage NOS

P51 **Umbilical hemorrhage of newborn**

Excludes1: *omphalitis with mild hemorrhage (P38.1)*
umbilical hemorrhage from cut end of co-twins cord (P50.5)
P51.0 **Massive umbilical hemorrhage of newborn**
P51.8 **Other umbilical hemorrhages of newborn**
Slipped umbilical ligature NOS
P51.9 **Umbilical hemorrhage of newborn, unspecified**

+, +7th, X + 7th   ● Newborn   ● Pediatric   ● Maternity   ● Adult   ♀ Female   ♂ Male   Manifestation   Unacceptable PDX   HCC   CC   MCC   HAC

P52 Intracranial nontraumatic hemorrhage of newborn

> **Includes:** intracranial hemorrhage due to anoxia or hypoxia
> ***Excludes1:*** *intracranial hemorrhage due to birth injury (P10.-)*
> *intracranial hemorrhage due to other injury (S06.-)*

CC **P52.0 Intraventricular (nontraumatic) hemorrhage, grade 1, of newborn**

> Subependymal hemorrhage (without intraventricular extension)
> Bleeding into germinal matrix

CC **P52.1 Intraventricular (nontraumatic) hemorrhage, grade 2, of newborn**

> Subependymal hemorrhage with intraventricular extension
> Bleeding into ventricle

+ **P52.2 Intraventricular (nontraumatic) hemorrhage, grade 3 and grade 4, of newborn**

MCC **P52.21 Intraventricular (nontraumatic) hemorrhage, grade 3, of newborn**

> Subependymal hemorrhage with intraventricular extension with enlargement of ventricle

MCC **P52.22 Intraventricular (nontraumatic) hemorrhage, grade 4, of newborn**

> Bleeding into cerebral cortex
> Subependymal hemorrhage with intracerebral extension

CC **P52.3 Unspecified intraventricular (nontraumatic) hemorrhage of newborn**

MCC **P52.4 Intracerebral (nontraumatic) hemorrhage of newborn**

MCC **P52.5 Subarachnoid (nontraumatic) hemorrhage of newborn**

MCC **P52.6 Cerebellar (nontraumatic) and posterior fossa hemorrhage of newborn**

MCC **P52.8 Other intracranial (nontraumatic) hemorrhages of newborn**

MCC **P52.9 Intracranial (nontraumatic) hemorrhage of newborn, unspecified**

CC **P53 Hemorrhagic disease of newborn**

> Vitamin K deficiency of newborn
> **Valid 3-character code, no further characters required**

P54 Other neonatal hemorrhages

> ***Excludes1:*** *newborn affected by (intrauterine) blood loss (P50.-)*
> *pulmonary hemorrhage originating in the perinatal period (P26.-)*

P54.0 Neonatal hematemesis

> ***Excludes1:*** *neonatal hematemesis due to swallowed maternal blood (P78.2)*

MCC **P54.1 Neonatal melena**

> ***Excludes1:*** *neonatal melena due to swallowed maternal blood (P78.2)*

MCC **P54.2 Neonatal rectal hemorrhage**

MCC **P54.3 Other neonatal gastrointestinal hemorrhage**

CC **P54.4 Neonatal adrenal hemorrhage**

P54.5 Neonatal cutaneous hemorrhage

> Neonatal bruising
> Neonatal ecchymoses
> Neonatal petechiae
> Neonatal superficial hematomata
> ***Excludes2:*** *bruising of scalp due to birth injury (P12.3)*
> *cephalhematoma due to birth injury (P12.0)*

♀ **P54.6 Neonatal vaginal hemorrhage**

> Neonatal pseudomenses

P54.8 Other specified neonatal hemorrhages

P54.9 Neonatal hemorrhage, unspecified

P55 Hemolytic disease of newborn

P55.0 Rh isoimmunization of newborn

P55.1 ABO isoimmunization of newborn

> *AHA CC: 3Q, 2015, 20*

P55.8 Other hemolytic diseases of newborn

> *AHA CC: 3Q, 2018, 24*

P55.9 Hemolytic disease of newborn, unspecified

P56 Hydrops fetalis due to hemolytic disease

> ***Excludes1:*** *hydrops fetalis NOS (P83.2)*

MCC **P56.0 Hydrops fetalis due to isoimmunization**

+ **P56.9 Hydrops fetalis due to other and unspecified hemolytic disease**

MCC **P56.90 Hydrops fetalis due to unspecified hemolytic disease**

MCC **P56.99 Hydrops fetalis due to other hemolytic disease**

P57 Kernicterus

MCC **P57.0 Kernicterus due to isoimmunization**

MCC **P57.8 Other specified kernicterus**

> ***Excludes1:*** *Crigler-Najjar syndrome (E80.5)*

MCC **P57.9 Kernicterus, unspecified**

P58 Neonatal jaundice due to other excessive hemolysis

> ***Excludes1:*** *jaundice due to isoimmunization (P55-P57)*

P58.0 Neonatal jaundice due to bruising

P58.1 Neonatal jaundice due to bleeding

P58.2 Neonatal jaundice due to infection

P58.3 Neonatal jaundice due to polycythemia

+ **P58.4 Neonatal jaundice due to drugs or toxins transmitted from mother or given to newborn**

> Code first poisoning due to drug or toxin, if applicable (T36-T65 with fifth or sixth character 1-4 or 6)
>
> Use additional code for adverse effect, if applicable, to identify drug (T36-T50 with fifth or sixth character 5)

P58.41 Neonatal jaundice due to drugs or toxins transmitted from mother

P58.42 Neonatal jaundice due to drugs or toxins given to newborn

P58.5 Neonatal jaundice due to swallowed maternal blood

P58.8 Neonatal jaundice due to other specified excessive hemolysis

P58.9 Neonatal jaundice due to excessive hemolysis, unspecified

P59 Neonatal jaundice from other and unspecified causes

> ***Excludes1:*** *jaundice due to inborn errors of metabolism (E70-E88)*
> *kernicterus (P57.-)*

P59.0 Neonatal jaundice associated with preterm delivery

> Hyperbilirubinemia of prematurity
> Jaundice due to delayed conjugation associated with preterm delivery

MCC **P59.1 Inspissated bile syndrome**

+ **P59.2 Neonatal jaundice from other and unspecified hepatocellular damage**

> ***Excludes1:*** *congenital viral hepatitis (P35.3)*

MCC **P59.20 Neonatal jaundice from unspecified hepatocellular damage**

MCC **P59.29 Neonatal jaundice from other hepatocellular damage**

> Neonatal giant cell hepatitis
> Neonatal (idiopathic) hepatitis

P59.3 Neonatal jaundice from breast milk inhibitor

P59.8 Neonatal jaundice from other specified causes

P59.9 Neonatal jaundice, unspecified

> Neonatal physiological jaundice (intense)(prolonged) NOS
> *AHA CC: 3Q, 2015, 20*

P60 Disseminated intravascular coagulation of newborn

MCC

> Defibrination syndrome of newborn
> **Valid 3-character code, no further characters required**

P61 Other perinatal hematological disorders

> ***Excludes1:*** *transient hypogammaglobulinemia of infancy (D80.7)*

MCC **P61.0 Transient neonatal thrombocytopenia**

> Neonatal thrombocytopenia due to exchange transfusion
> Neonatal thrombocytopenia due to idiopathic maternal thrombocytopenia
> Neonatal thrombocytopenia due to isoimmunization

P61.1 Polycythemia neonatorum

CC **P61.2 Anemia of prematurity**

CC **P61.3 Congenital anemia from fetal blood loss**

CC **P61.4 Other congenital anemias, not elsewhere classified**

> Congenital anemia NOS

MCC **P61.5 Transient neonatal neutropenia**

> ***Excludes1:*** *congenital neutropenia (nontransient) (D70.0)*

CC **P61.6 Other transient neonatal disorders of coagulation**

P61.8 Other specified perinatal hematological disorders

P61.9 Perinatal hematological disorder, unspecified

+, +7th, X + 7th ● Newborn ● Pediatric ● Maternity ● Adult ♀ Female ♂ Male Manifestation Unacceptable PDX HCC CC MCC HAC

Transitory endocrine and metabolic disorders specific to newborn (P70-P74)

Includes: transitory endocrine and metabolic disturbances caused by the infant's response to maternal endocrine and metabolic factors, or its adjustment to extrauterine environment

P70   Transitory disorders of carbohydrate metabolism specific to newborn

P70.0   Syndrome of infant of mother with gestational diabetes
Newborn (with hypoglycemia) affected by maternal gestational diabetes
Excludes1: newborn (with hypoglycemia) affected by maternal (pre-existing) diabetes mellitus (P70.1)
syndrome of infant of a diabetic mother (P70.1)

P70.1   Syndrome of infant of a diabetic mother
Newborn (with hypoglycemia) affected by maternal (pre-existing) diabetes mellitus
Excludes1: newborn (with hypoglycemia) affected by maternal gestational diabetes (P70.0)
syndrome of infant of mother with gestational diabetes (P70.0)

CC **P70.2   Neonatal diabetes mellitus**

P70.3   Iatrogenic neonatal hypoglycemia

P70.4   Other neonatal hypoglycemia
Transitory neonatal hypoglycemia

CC **P70.8   Other transitory disorders of carbohydrate metabolism of newborn**

P70.9   Transitory disorder of carbohydrate metabolism of newborn, unspecified

P71   Transitory neonatal disorders of calcium and magnesium metabolism

CC **P71.0   Cow's milk hypocalcemia in newborn**

CC **P71.1   Other neonatal hypocalcemia**
Excludes1: neonatal hypoparathyroidism (P71.4)

CC **P71.2   Neonatal hypomagnesemia**

CC **P71.3   Neonatal tetany without calcium or magnesium deficiency**
Neonatal tetany NOS

CC **P71.4   Transitory neonatal hypoparathyroidism**

CC **P71.8   Other transitory neonatal disorders of calcium and magnesium metabolism**
AHA CC: 4Q, 2016, 54-55

CC **P71.9   Transitory neonatal disorder of calcium and magnesium metabolism, unspecified**

P72   Other transitory neonatal endocrine disorders

Excludes1: congenital hypothyroidism with or without goiter (E03.0-E03.1)
dyshormogenetic goiter (E07.1)
Pendred's syndrome (E07.1)

CC **P72.0   Neonatal goiter, not elsewhere classified**
Transitory congenital goiter with normal functioning

CC **P72.1   Transitory neonatal hyperthyroidism**
Neonatal thyrotoxicosis

CC **P72.2   Other transitory neonatal disorders of thyroid function, not elsewhere classified**
Transitory neonatal hypothyroidism

CC **P72.8   Other specified transitory neonatal endocrine disorders**

P72.9   Transitory neonatal endocrine disorder, unspecified

P74   Other transitory neonatal electrolyte and metabolic disturbances

MCC **P74.0   Late metabolic acidosis of newborn**
Excludes1: (fetal) metabolic acidosis of newborn (P19)

P74.1   Dehydration of newborn

+ **P74.2   Disturbances of sodium balance of newborn**
AHA CC: 2Q, 2018, 6; 4Q, 2018, 27
P74.21   Hypernatremia of newborn
P74.22   Hyponatremia of newborn

+ **P74.3   Disturbances of potassium balance of newborn**
AHA CC: 4Q, 2018, 27
P74.31   Hyperkalemia of newborn
P74.32   Hypokalemia of newborn

+ **P74.4   Other transitory electrolyte disturbances of newborn**
AHA CC: 4Q, 2018, 27
CC **P74.41   Alkalosis of newborn**
Hyperbicarbonatemia
+ **P74.42   Disturbances of chlorine balance of newborn**
P74.421   Hyperchloremia of newborn
Hyperchloremic metabolic acidosis
Excludes2: late metabolic acidosis of the newborn (P74.0)
P74.422   Hypochloremia of newborn
P74.49   Other transitory electrolyte disturbance of newborn

CC **P74.5   Transitory tyrosinemia of newborn**
CC **P74.6   Transitory hyperammonemia of newborn**
CC **P74.8   Other transitory metabolic disturbances of newborn**
Amino-acid metabolic disorders described as transitory
P74.9   Transitory metabolic disturbance of newborn, unspecified

Digestive system disorders of newborn (P76-P78)

P76   Other intestinal obstruction of newborn

P76.0   Meconium plug syndrome
Meconium ileus NOS
Excludes1: meconium ileus in cystic fibrosis (E84.11)

CC **P76.1   Transitory ileus of newborn**
Excludes1: Hirschsprung's disease (Q43.1)

P76.2   Intestinal obstruction due to inspissated milk

P76.8   Other specified intestinal obstruction of newborn
Excludes1: intestinal obstruction classifiable to K56.-

P76.9   Intestinal obstruction of newborn, unspecified

P77   Necrotizing enterocolitis of newborn

MCC **P77.1   Stage 1 necrotizing enterocolitis in newborn**
Necrotizing enterocolitis without pneumatosis, without perforation

MCC **P77.2   Stage 2 necrotizing enterocolitis in newborn**
Necrotizing enterocolitis with pneumatosis, without perforation

MCC **P77.3   Stage 3 necrotizing enterocolitis in newborn**
Necrotizing enterocolitis with perforation
Necrotizing enterocolitis with pneumatosis and perforation

MCC **P77.9   Necrotizing enterocolitis in newborn, unspecified**
Necrotizing enterocolitis in newborn, NOS

P78   Other perinatal digestive system disorders

Excludes1: cystic fibrosis (E84.0-E84.9)
neonatal gastrointestinal hemorrhages (P54.0-P54.3)

MCC **P78.0   Perinatal intestinal perforation**
Meconium peritonitis

P78.1   Other neonatal peritonitis
Neonatal peritonitis NOS

P78.2   Neonatal hematemesis and melena due to swallowed maternal blood

P78.3   Noninfective neonatal diarrhea
Neonatal diarrhea NOS

+ **P78.8   Other specified perinatal digestive system disorders**
P78.81   Congenital cirrhosis (of liver)
P78.82   Peptic ulcer of newborn
P78.83   Newborn esophageal reflux
Neonatal esophageal reflux
P78.84   Gestational alloimmune liver disease
GALD
Neonatal hemochromatosis
Excludes1: hemochromatosis (E83.11-)
AHA CC: 4Q, 2017, 21
P78.89   Other specified perinatal digestive system disorders

P78.9   Perinatal digestive system disorder, unspecified

Conditions involving the integument and temperature regulation of newborn (P80-P83)

P80   Hypothermia of newborn

P80.0   Cold injury syndrome
Severe and usually chronic hypothermia associated with a pink flushed appearance, edema and neurological and biochemical abnormalities.
Excludes1: mild hypothermia of newborn (P80.8)

P80.8   Other hypothermia of newborn
Mild hypothermia of newborn

P80.9   Hypothermia of newborn, unspecified

+, +7th, X + 7th   ● Newborn   ● Pediatric   ● Maternity   ● Adult   ♀ Female   ♂ Male   Manifestation   Unacceptable PDX   HCC   CC   MCC   HAC

P81 Other disturbances of temperature regulation of newborn

P81.0 Environmental hyperthermia of newborn

P81.8 Other specified disturbances of temperature regulation of newborn

P81.9 Disturbance of temperature regulation of newborn, unspecified
Fever of newborn NOS

P83 Other conditions of integument specific to newborn

Excludes1: congenital malformations of skin and integument (Q80-Q84)
hydrops fetalis due to hemolytic disease (P56.-)
neonatal skin infection (P39.4)
staphylococcal scalded skin syndrome (L00)
Excludes2: cradle cap (L21.0)
diaper [napkin] dermatitis (L22)

CC **P83.0 Sclerema neonatorum**

P83.1 Neonatal erythema toxicum

MCC **P83.2 Hydrops fetalis not due to hemolytic disease**
Hydrops fetalis NOS

+ **P83.3 Other and unspecified edema specific to newborn**

CC **P83.30 Unspecified edema specific to newborn**

CC **P83.39 Other edema specific to newborn**

P83.4 Breast engorgement of newborn
Noninfective mastitis of newborn

♂ **P83.5 Congenital hydrocele**

P83.6 Umbilical polyp of newborn

+ **P83.8 Other specified conditions of integument specific to newborn**
AHA CC: 4Q, 2017, 21-22

P83.81 Umbilical granuloma
Excludes2: granulomatous disorder of the skin and subcutaneous tissue, unspecified (L92.9)

P83.88 Other specified conditions of integument specific to newborn
Bronze baby syndrome
Neonatal scleroderma
Urticaria neonatorum

P83.9 Condition of the integument specific to newborn, unspecified

Other problems with newborn (P84)

P84 Other problems with newborn

Acidemia of newborn
Acidosis of newborn
Anoxia of newborn NOS
Asphyxia of newborn NOS
Hypercapnia of newborn
Hypoxemia of newborn
Hypoxia of newborn NOS
Mixed metabolic and respiratory acidosis of newborn
Excludes1: intracranial hemorrhage due to anoxia or hypoxia (P52.-)
hypoxic ischemic encephalopathy [HIE] (P91.6-)
late metabolic acidosis of newborn (P74.0)
Valid 3-character code, no further characters required

Other disorders originating in the perinatal period (P90-P96)

MCC **P90 Convulsions of newborn**

Excludes1: benign myoclonic epilepsy in infancy (G40.3-)
benign neonatal convulsions (familial) (G40.3-)
Valid 3-character code, no further characters required

P91 Other disturbances of cerebral status of newborn

MCC **P91.0 Neonatal cerebral ischemia**
Excludes1: Neonatal cerebral infarction (P91.82-)

MCC **P91.1 Acquired periventricular cysts of newborn**

MCC **P91.2 Neonatal cerebral leukomalacia**
Periventricular leukomalacia

MCC **P91.3 Neonatal cerebral irritability**

MCC **P91.4 Neonatal cerebral depression**

MCC **P91.5 Neonatal coma**

+ **P91.6 Hypoxic ischemic encephalopathy [HIE]**
Excludes1: neonatal cerebral depression (P91.4)
neonatal cerebral irritability (P91.3)
neonatal coma (P91.5)
AHA CC: 4Q, 2017, 22

CC **P91.60 Hypoxic ischemic encephalopathy [HIE], unspecified**

CC **P91.61 Mild hypoxic ischemic encephalopathy [HIE]**

P91.62 Moderate hypoxic ischemic encephalopathy [HIE]

MCC **P91.63 Severe hypoxic ischemic encephalopathy [HIE]**

+ **P91.8 Other specified disturbances of cerebral status of newborn**

+ **P91.81 Neonatal encephalopathy**
AHA CC: 4Q, 2017, 22

P91.811 Neonatal encephalopathy in diseases classified elsewhere
Code first underlying condition, if known, such as:
congenital cirrhosis (of liver) (P78.81)
intracranial nontraumatic hemorrhage of newborn (P52.-)
kernicterus (P57.-)

P91.819 Neonatal encephalopathy, unspecified

+ **P91.82 Neonatal cerebral infarction**
Neonatal stroke
Perinatal arterial ischemic stroke
Perinatal cerebral infarction
Excludes1: cerebral infarction (I63.-)
Excludes2: intracranial hemorrhage of newborn (P52.-)

MCC **P91.821 Neonatal cerebral infarction, right side of brain**

MCC **P91.822 Neonatal cerebral infarction, left side of brain**

MCC **P91.823 Neonatal cerebral infarction, bilateral**

MCC **P91.829 Neonatal cerebral infarction, unspecified side**

P91.88 Other specified disturbances of cerebral status of newborn

P91.9 Disturbance of cerebral status of newborn, unspecified

P92 Feeding problems of newborn

Excludes1: eating disorders (F50.-)
feeding problems in child over 28 days old (R63.3)

+ **P92.0 Vomiting of newborn**
Excludes1: vomiting of child over 28 days old (R11.-)

MCC **P92.01 Bilious vomiting of newborn**
Excludes1: bilious vomiting in child over 28 days old (R11.14)

P92.09 Other vomiting of newborn
Excludes1: regurgitation of food in newborn (P92.1)

P92.1 Regurgitation and rumination of newborn

P92.2 Slow feeding of newborn

P92.3 Underfeeding of newborn

P92.4 Overfeeding of newborn

P92.5 Neonatal difficulty in feeding at breast
AHA CC: 3Q, 2016, 19; 1Q, 2017, 28-29

P92.6 Failure to thrive in newborn
Excludes1: failure to thrive in child over 28 days old (R62.51)

P92.8 Other feeding problems of newborn

P92.9 Feeding problem of newborn, unspecified

P93 Reactions and intoxications due to drugs administered to newborn

Includes: reactions and intoxications due to drugs administered to fetus affecting newborn
Excludes1: jaundice due to drugs or toxins transmitted from mother or given to newborn (P58.4-)
reactions and intoxications from maternal opiates, tranquilizers and other medication (P04.0-P04.1, P04.4-)
withdrawal symptoms from maternal use of drugs of addiction (P96.1)
withdrawal symptoms from therapeutic use of drugs in newborn (P96.2)

CC **P93.0 Grey baby syndrome**
Grey syndrome from chloramphenicol administration in newborn

CC **P93.8 Other reactions and intoxications due to drugs administered to newborn**
Use additional code for adverse effect, if applicable, to identify drug (T36-T50 with fifth or sixth character 5)

P94 Disorders of muscle tone of newborn

CC **P94.0 Transient neonatal myasthenia gravis**
Excludes1: myasthenia gravis (G70.0)

P94.1 Congenital hypertonia

P94.2 Congenital hypotonia
Floppy baby syndrome, unspecified

P94.8 Other disorders of muscle tone of newborn

P94.9 Disorder of muscle tone of newborn, unspecified

923

P95 Stillbirth

Deadborn fetus NOS
Fetal death of unspecified cause
Stillbirth NOS

Excludes1: maternal care for intrauterine death (O36.4)
missed abortion (O02.1)
outcome of delivery, stillbirth (Z37.1, Z37.3, Z37.4,
Z37.7)

Review coding guideline C.16.g
Valid 3-character code, no further characters required

P96 Other conditions originating in the perinatal period

P96.0 Congenital renal failure
Uremia of newborn

CC **P96.1 Neonatal withdrawal symptoms from maternal use of drugs of addiction**
Drug withdrawal syndrome in infant of dependent mother
Neonatal abstinence syndrome

Excludes1: reactions and intoxications from maternal
opiatesandtranquilizersadministeredduring
labor and delivery (P04.0)

AHA CC: 4Q, 2018, 24-25

CC **P96.2 Withdrawal symptoms from therapeutic use of drugs in newborn**

P96.3 Wide cranial sutures of newborn
Neonatal craniotabes

P96.5 Complication to newborn due to (fetal) intrauterine procedure

Excludes2: newborn affected by amniocentesis (P00.6)

+ **P96.8 Other specified conditions originating in the perinatal period**

P96.81 Exposure to (parental) (environmental) tobacco smoke in the perinatal period

Excludes2: newborn affected by in utero exposure
to tobacco (P04.2)
exposure to environmental tobacco
smoke after the perinatal period
(Z77.22)

P96.82 Delayed separation of umbilical cord

P96.83 Meconium staining

Excludes1: meconium aspiration (P24.00, P24.01)
meconium passage during delivery
(P03.82)

P96.89 Other specified conditions originating in the perinatal period
Use additional code to specify condition

P96.9 Condition originating in the perinatal period, unspecified
Congenital debility NOS

Chapter 17: Congenital Malformations, Deformations and Chromosomal Abnormalities (Q00-Q99)

NOTE Codes from this chapter are not for use on maternal records

Excludes2: *inborn errors of metabolism (E70-E88)*

This chapter contains the following category blocks:

Q00-Q07 Congenital malformations of the nervous system
Q10-Q18 Congenital malformations of eye, ear, face and neck
Q20-Q28 Congenital malformations of the circulatory system
Q30-Q34 Congenital malformations of the respiratory system
Q35-Q37 Cleft lip and cleft palate
Q38-Q45 Other congenital malformations of the digestive system
Q50-Q56 Congenital malformations of genital organs
Q60-Q64 Congenital malformations of the urinary system
Q65-Q79 Congenital malformations and deformations of the musculoskeletal system
Q80-Q89 Other congenital malformations
Q90-Q99 Chromosomal abnormalities, not elsewhere classified

C. Chapter-Specific Coding Guidelines

In addition to general coding guidelines, there are guidelines for specific diagnoses and/or conditions in the classification. Unless otherwise indicated, these guidelines apply to all health care settings. Please refer to Section II for guidelines on the selection of principal diagnosis.

17. Chapter 17: Congenital Malformations, Deformations and Chromosomal Abnormalities (Q00-Q99)

Assign an appropriate code(s) from categories Q00-Q99, Congenital malformations, deformations, and chromosomal abnormalities when a malformation/deformation or chromosomal abnormality is documented. A malformation/deformation or chromosomal abnormality may be the principal/first-listed diagnosis on a record or a secondary diagnosis.

When a malformation/deformation or chromosomal abnormality does not have a unique code assignment, assign additional code(s) for any manifestations that may be present.

When the code assignment specifically identifies the malformation/deformation/or chromosomal abnormality, manifestations that are an inherent component of the anomaly should not be coded separately. Additional codes should be assigned for manifestations that are not an inherent component.

Codes from Chapter 17 may be used throughout the life of the patient. If a congenital malformation or deformity has been corrected, a personal history code should be used to identify the history of the malformation or deformity. Although present at birth, a malformation/deformation or chromosomal abnormality may not be identified until later in life. Whenever the condition is diagnosed by the provider, it is appropriate to assign a code from codes Q00-Q99. For the birth admission, the appropriate code from category Z38, Liveborn infants, according to place of birth and type of delivery, should be sequenced as the principal diagnosis, followed by any congenital anomaly codes, Q00-Q99.

Congenital malformations of the nervous system (Q00-Q07)

Q00 **Anencephaly and similar malformations**

MCC **Q00.0** **Anencephaly**
Acephaly
Acrania
Amyelencephaly
Hemianencephaly
Hemicephaly

MCC **Q00.1** **Craniorachischisis**

MCC **Q00.2** **Iniencephaly**

Q01 **Encephalocele**

    Includes: Arnold-Chiari syndrome, type III
encephalocystocele
encephalomyelocele
hydroencephalocele
hydromeningocele, cranial
meningocele, cerebral
meningoencephalocele

    Excludes1: *Meckel-Gruber syndrome (Q61.9)*

CC **Q01.0** **Frontal encephalocele**

CC **Q01.1** **Nasofrontal encephalocele**

CC **Q01.2** **Occipital encephalocele**

CC **Q01.8** **Encephalocele of other sites**

CC **Q01.9** **Encephalocele, unspecified**

Q02 **Microcephaly**

    Includes: hydromicrocephaly
micrencephalon

    Excludes1: *Meckel-Gruber syndrome (Q61.9)*

Code first, if applicable, congenital Zika virus disease
AHA CC: 4Q, 2016, 4-7; 4Q, 2018, 26

Valid 3-character code, no further characters required

Q03 **Congenital hydrocephalus**

    Includes: hydrocephalus in newborn

    Excludes1: *Arnold-Chiari syndrome, type II (Q07.0-)*
acquired hydrocephalus (G91.-)
hydrocephalus due to congenital toxoplasmosis (P37.1)
hydrocephalus with spina bifida (Q05.0-Q05.4)

Q03.0 **Malformations of aqueduct of Sylvius**
Anomaly of aqueduct of Sylvius
Obstruction of aqueduct of Sylvius, congenital
Stenosis of aqueduct of Sylvius

Q03.1 **Atresia of foramina of Magendie and Luschka**
Dandy-Walker syndrome

Q03.8 **Other congenital hydrocephalus**

Q03.9 **Congenital hydrocephalus, unspecified**

Q04 **Other congenital malformations of brain**

    Excludes1: *cyclopia (Q87.0)*
macrocephaly (Q75.3)

MCC **Q04.0** **Congenital malformations of corpus callosum**
Agenesis of corpus callosum

MCC **Q04.1** **Arhinencephaly**

MCC **Q04.2** **Holoprosencephaly**

MCC **Q04.3** **Other reduction deformities of brain**
Absence of part of brain
Agenesis of part of brain
Agyria
Aplasia of part of brain
Hydranencephaly
Hypoplasia of part of brain
Lissencephaly
Microgyria
Pachygyria

    Excludes1: *congenital malformations of corpus callosum (Q04.0)*

CC **Q04.4** **Septo-optic dysplasia of brain**

CC **Q04.5** **Megalencephaly**

CC **Q04.6** **Congenital cerebral cysts**
Porencephaly
Schizencephaly

    Excludes1: *acquired porencephalic cyst (G93.0)*

CC **Q04.8** **Other specified congenital malformations of brain**
Arnold-Chiari syndrome, type IV
Macrogyria

Q04.9 **Congenital malformation of brain, unspecified**
Congenital anomaly NOS of brain
Congenital deformity NOS of brain
Congenital disease or lesion NOS of brain
Multiple anomalies NOS of brain, congenital

Q05 **Spina bifida**

    Includes: hydromeningocele (spinal)
meningocele (spinal)
meningomyelocele
myelocele
myelomeningocele
rachischisis
spina bifida (aperta)(cystica)
syringomyelocele

Use additional code for any associated paraplegia (paraparesis) (G82.2-)

    Excludes1: *Arnold-Chiari syndrome, type II (Q07.0-)*
spina bifida occulta (Q76.0)

CC **Q05.0** **Cervical spina bifida with hydrocephalus**

CC **Q05.1** **Thoracic spina bifida with hydrocephalus**
Dorsal spina bifida with hydrocephalus
Thoracolumbar spina bifida with hydrocephalus

CC **Q05.2** **Lumbar spina bifida with hydrocephalus**
Lumbosacral spina bifida with hydrocephalus

CC **Q05.3** **Sacral spina bifida with hydrocephalus**

CC **Q05.4** **Unspecified spina bifida with hydrocephalus**

Q05.5 **Cervical spina bifida without hydrocephalus**

Q05.6 Thoracic spina bifida without hydrocephalus
Dorsal spina bifida NOS
Thoracolumbar spina bifida NOS

Q05.7 Lumbar spina bifida without hydrocephalus
Lumbosacral spina bifida NOS

Q05.8 Sacral spina bifida without hydrocephalus

Q05.9 Spina bifida, unspecified

Q06 Other congenital malformations of spinal cord

Q06.0 Amyelia

Q06.1 Hypoplasia and dysplasia of spinal cord
Atelomyelia
Myelatelia
Myelodysplasia of spinal cord

Q06.2 Diastematomyelia

Q06.3 Other congenital cauda equina malformations

Q06.4 Hydromyelia
Hydrorachis

Q06.8 Other specified congenital malformations of spinal cord

Q06.9 Congenital malformation of spinal cord, unspecified
Congenital anomaly NOS of spinal cord
Congenital deformity NOS of spinal cord
Congenital disease or lesion NOS of spinal cord

Q07 Other congenital malformations of nervous system

Excludes2: congenital central alveolar hypoventilation syndrome
(G47.35)
familial dysautonomia [Riley-Day] (G90.1)
neurofibromatosis (nonmalignant) (Q85.0-)

+ **Q07.0 Arnold-Chiari syndrome**
Arnold-Chiari syndrome, type II
Excludes1: Arnold-Chiari syndrome, type III (Q01.-)
Arnold-Chiari syndrome, type IV (Q04.8)

Q07.00 Arnold-Chiari syndrome without spina bifida or hydrocephalus

Q07.01 Arnold-Chiari syndrome with spina bifida

CC **Q07.02 Arnold-Chiari syndrome with hydrocephalus**

CC **Q07.03 Arnold-Chiari syndrome with spina bifida and hydrocephalus**

Q07.8 Other specified congenital malformations of nervous system
Agenesis of nerve
Displacement of brachial plexus
Jaw-winking syndrome
Marcus Gunn's syndrome

Q07.9 Congenital malformation of nervous system, unspecified
Congenital anomaly NOS of nervous system
Congenital deformity NOS of nervous system
Congenital disease or lesion NOS of nervous system

Congenital malformations of eye, ear, face and neck (Q10-Q18)

Excludes2: cleft lip and cleft palate (Q35-Q37)
congenital malformation of cervical spine (Q05.0, Q05.5, Q67.5, Q76.0-Q76.4)
congenital malformation of larynx (Q31.-)
congenital malformation of lip NEC (Q38.0)
congenital malformation of nose (Q30.-)
congenital malformation of parathyroid gland (Q89.2)
congenital malformation of thyroid gland (Q89.2)

Q10 Congenital malformations of eyelid, lacrimal apparatus and orbit

Excludes1: cryptophthalmos NOS (Q11.2)
cryptophthalmos syndrome (Q87.0)

Q10.0 Congenital ptosis

Q10.1 Congenital ectropion

Q10.2 Congenital entropion

Q10.3 Other congenital malformations of eyelid
Ablepharon
Blepharophimosis, congenital
Coloboma of eyelid
Congenital absence or agenesis of cilia
Congenital absence or agenesis of eyelid
Congenital accessory eyelid
Congenital accessory eye muscle
Congenital malformation of eyelid NOS

Q10.4 Absence and agenesis of lacrimal apparatus
Congenital absence of punctum lacrimale

Q10.5 Congenital stenosis and stricture of lacrimal duct

Q10.6 Other congenital malformations of lacrimal apparatus
Congenital malformation of lacrimal apparatus NOS

Q10.7 Congenital malformation of orbit

Q11 Anophthalmos, microphthalmos and macrophthalmos

Q11.0 Cystic eyeball

Q11.1 Other anophthalmos
Anophthalmos NOS
Agenesis of eye
Aplasia of eye

Q11.2 Microphthalmos
Cryptophthalmos NOS
Dysplasia of eye
Hypoplasia of eye
Rudimentary eye
Excludes1: cryptophthalmos syndrome (Q87.0)

Q11.3 Macrophthalmos
Excludes1: macrophthalmos in congenital glaucoma
(Q15.0)

Q12 Congenital lens malformations

CC **Q12.0 Congenital cataract**

CC **Q12.1 Congenital displaced lens**

CC **Q12.2 Coloboma of lens**

Q12.3 Congenital aphakia

Q12.4 Spherophakia

Q12.8 Other congenital lens malformations
Microphakia

Q12.9 Congenital lens malformation, unspecified

Q13 Congenital malformations of anterior segment of eye

Q13.0 Coloboma of iris
Coloboma NOS

Q13.1 Absence of iris
Aniridia
Use additional code for associated glaucoma (H42)

Q13.2 Other congenital malformations of iris
Anisocoria, congenital
Atresia of pupil
Congenital malformation of iris NOS
Corectopia

Q13.3 Congenital corneal opacity

Q13.4 Other congenital corneal malformations
Congenital malformation of cornea NOS
Microcornea
Peter's anomaly

Q13.5 Blue sclera

Q13.8 Other congenital malformations of anterior segment of eye

Q13.81 Rieger's anomaly
Use additional code for associated glaucoma (H42)

Q13.89 Other congenital malformations of anterior segment of eye

Q13.9 Congenital malformation of anterior segment of eye, unspecified

Q14 Congenital malformations of posterior segment of eye

Excludes2: optic nerve hypoplasia (H47.03-)

Q14.0 Congenital malformation of vitreous humor
Congenital vitreous opacity

Q14.1 Congenital malformation of retina
Congenital retinal aneurysm

Q14.2 Congenital malformation of optic disc
Coloboma of optic disc

Q14.3 Congenital malformation of choroid

Q14.8 Other congenital malformations of posterior segment of eye
Coloboma of the fundus

Q14.9 Congenital malformation of posterior segment of eye, unspecified

Q15 Other congenital malformations of eye

Excludes1: congenital nystagmus (H55.01)
ocular albinism (E70.31-)
optic nerve hypoplasia (H47.03-)
retinitis pigmentosa (H35.52)

Q15.0 Congenital glaucoma
Axenfeld's anomaly
Buphthalmos
Glaucoma of childhood
Glaucoma of newborn
Hydrophthalmos
Keratoglobus, congenital, with glaucoma
Macrocornea with glaucoma
Macrophthalmos in congenital glaucoma
Megalocornea with glaucoma

+, +7th, X + 7th • Newborn • Pediatric • Maternity • Adult ♀ Female ♂ Male Manifestation Unacceptable PDX HCC CC MCC HAC

Q15.8 **Other specified congenital malformations of eye**
Q15.9 **Congenital malformation of eye, unspecified**
Congenital anomaly of eye
Congenital deformity of eye

Q16 **Congenital malformations of ear causing impairment of hearing**

Excludes1: *congenital deafness (H90.-)*
Q16.0 **Congenital absence of (ear) auricle**
Q16.1 **Congenital absence, atresia and stricture of auditory canal (external)**
Congenital atresia or stricture of osseous meatus
Q16.2 **Absence of eustachian tube**
Q16.3 **Congenital malformation of ear ossicles**
Congenital fusion of ear ossicles
Q16.4 **Other congenital malformations of middle ear**
Congenital malformation of middle ear NOS
Q16.5 **Congenital malformation of inner ear**
Congenital anomaly of membranous labyrinth
Congenital anomaly of organ of Corti
Q16.9 **Congenital malformation of ear causing impairment of hearing, unspecified**
Congenital absence of ear NOS

Q17 **Other congenital malformations of ear**

Excludes1: *congenital malformations of ear with impairment of hearing (Q16.0-Q16.9)*
preauricular sinus (Q18.1)
Q17.0 **Accessory auricle**
Accessory tragus
Polyotia
Preauricular appendage or tag
Supernumerary ear
Supernumerary lobule
Q17.1 **Macrotia**
Q17.2 **Microtia**
Q17.3 **Other misshapen ear**
Pointed ear
Q17.4 **Misplaced ear**
Low-set ears
Excludes1: *cervical auricle (Q18.2)*
Q17.5 **Prominent ear**
Bat ear
Q17.8 **Other specified congenital malformations of ear**
Congenital absence of lobe of ear
Q17.9 **Congenital malformation of ear, unspecified**
Congenital anomaly of ear NOS

Q18 **Other congenital malformations of face and neck**

Excludes1: *cleft lip and cleft palate (Q35-Q37)*
conditions classified to (Q67.0-Q67.4)
congenital malformations of skull and face bones (Q75.-)
cyclopia (Q87.0)
dentofacial anomalies [including malocclusion] (M26.-)
malformation syndromes affecting facial appearance (Q87.0)
persistent thyroglossal duct (Q89.2)
Q18.0 **Sinus, fistula and cyst of branchial cleft**
Branchial vestige
Q18.1 **Preauricular sinus and cyst**
Fistula of auricle, congenital
Cervicoaural fistula
Q18.2 **Other branchial cleft malformations**
Branchial cleft malformation NOS
Cervical auricle
Otocephaly
Q18.3 **Webbing of neck**
Pterygium colli
Q18.4 **Macrostomia**
Q18.5 **Microstomia**
Q18.6 **Macrocheilia**
Hypertrophy of lip, congenital
Q18.7 **Microcheilia**
Q18.8 **Other specified congenital malformations of face and neck**
Medial cyst of face and neck
Medial fistula of face and neck
Medial sinus of face and neck
Q18.9 **Congenital malformation of face and neck, unspecified**
Congenital anomaly NOS of face and neck

Congenital malformations of the circulatory system (Q20-Q28)

Q20 **Congenital malformations of cardiac chambers and connections**

Excludes1: *dextrocardia with situs inversus (Q89.3)*
mirror-image atrial arrangement with situs inversus (Q89.3)
MCC Q20.0 **Common arterial trunk**
Persistent truncus arteriosus
Excludes1: *aortic septal defect (Q21.4)*
MCC Q20.1 **Double outlet right ventricle**
Taussig-Bing syndrome
MCC Q20.2 **Double outlet left ventricle**
MCC Q20.3 **Discordant ventriculoarterial connection**
Dextrotransposition of aorta
Transposition of great vessels (complete)
MCC Q20.4 **Double inlet ventricle**
Common ventricle
Cor triloculare biatriatum
Single ventricle
CC Q20.5 **Discordant atrioventricular connection**
Corrected transposition
Levotransposition
Ventricular inversion
Q20.6 **Isomerism of atrial appendages**
Isomerism of atrial appendages with asplenia or polysplenia
Q20.8 **Other congenital malformations of cardiac chambers and connections**
Cor binoculare
Q20.9 **Congenital malformation of cardiac chambers and connections, unspecified**

Q21 **Congenital malformations of cardiac septa**

Excludes1: *acquired cardiac septal defect (I51.0)*
CC Q21.0 **Ventricular septal defect**
Roger's disease
CC Q21.1 **Atrial septal defect**
Coronary sinus defect
Patent or persistent foramen ovale
Patent or persistent ostium secundum defect (type II)
Patent or persistent sinus venosus defect
CC Q21.2 **Atrioventricular septal defect**
Common atrioventricular canal
Endocardial cushion defect
Ostium primum atrial septal defect (type I)
MCC Q21.3 **Tetralogy of Fallot**
Ventricular septal defect with pulmonary stenosis or atresia, dextroposition of aorta and hypertrophy of right ventricle.
AHA CC: 3Q, 2014, 16-17
Q21.4 **Aortopulmonary septal defect**
Aortic septal defect
Aortopulmonary window
Q21.8 **Other congenital malformations of cardiac septa**
Eisenmenger's defect
Pentalogy of Fallot
Code also if applicable:
Eisenmenger's complex (I27.83)
Eisenmenger's syndrome (I27.83)
Q21.9 **Congenital malformation of cardiac septum, unspecified**
Septal (heart) defect NOS

Q22 **Congenital malformations of pulmonary and tricuspid valves**

MCC Q22.0 **Pulmonary valve atresia**
CC Q22.1 **Congenital pulmonary valve stenosis**
CC Q22.2 **Congenital pulmonary valve insufficiency**
Congenital pulmonary valve regurgitation
CC Q22.3 **Other congenital malformations of pulmonary valve**
Congenital malformation of pulmonary valve NOS
Supernumerary cusps of pulmonary valve
MCC Q22.4 **Congenital tricuspid stenosis**
Congenital tricuspid atresia
MCC Q22.5 **Ebstein's anomaly**
MCC Q22.6 **Hypoplastic right heart syndrome**
MCC Q22.8 **Other congenital malformations of tricuspid valve**
MCC Q22.9 **Congenital malformation of tricuspid valve, unspecified**

+, +7th, X + 7th • Newborn • Pediatric • Maternity • Adult ♀ Female ♂ Male | Manifestation | Unacceptable PDX | HCC | CC | MCC | HAC

Q23 **Congenital malformations of aortic and mitral valves**

   Q23.0 **Congenital stenosis of aortic valve**
      Congenital aortic atresia
      Congenital aortic stenosis NOS
      Excludes1: congenital stenosis of aortic valve in
            hypoplastic left heart syndrome (Q23.4)
            congenital subaortic stenosis (Q24.4)
            supravalvular aortic stenosis (congenital)
               (Q25.3)

   Q23.1 **Congenital insufficiency of aortic valve**
      Bicuspid aortic valve
      Congenital aortic insufficiency

   Q23.2 **Congenital mitral stenosis**
      Congenital mitral atresia

CC Q23.3 **Congenital mitral insufficiency**

MCC Q23.4 **Hypoplastic left heart syndrome**

CC Q23.8 **Other congenital malformations of aortic and mitral valves**

CC Q23.9 **Congenital malformation of aortic and mitral valves, unspecified**

Q24 **Other congenital malformations of heart**

    Excludes1: endocardial fibroelastosis (I42.4)

CC Q24.0 **Dextrocardia**
      Excludes1: dextrocardia with situs inversus (Q89.3)
            isomerism of atrial appendages (with asplenia
               or polysplenia) (Q20.6)
            mirror-image atrial arrangement with situs
               inversus (Q89.3)

CC Q24.1 **Levocardia**

MCC Q24.2 **Cor triatriatum**

CC Q24.3 **Pulmonary infundibular stenosis**
      Subvalvular pulmonic stenosis

MCC Q24.4 **Congenital subaortic stenosis**

CC Q24.5 **Malformation of coronary vessels**
      Congenital coronary (artery) aneurysm

MCC Q24.6 **Congenital heart block**

   Q24.8 **Other specified congenital malformations of heart**
      Congenital diverticulum of left ventricle
      Congenital malformation of myocardium
      Congenital malformation of pericardium
      Malposition of heart
      Uhl's disease

   Q24.9 **Congenital malformation of heart, unspecified**
      Congenital anomaly of heart
      Congenital disease of heart

Q25 **Congenital malformations of great arteries**

CC Q25.0 **Patent ductus arteriosus**
      Patent ductus Botallo
      Persistent ductus arteriosus

CC Q25.1 **Coarctation of aorta**
      Coarctation of aorta (preductal) (postductal)
      Stenosis of aorta
      AHA CC: 4Q, 2016, 56-57

 + Q25.2 **Atresia of aorta**
      AHA CC: 4Q, 2016, 56-57

    CC Q25.21 **Interruption of aortic arch**
        Atresia of aortic arch

    CC Q25.29 **Other atresia of aorta**
        Atresia of aorta

CC Q25.3 **Supravalvular aortic stenosis**
      Excludes1: congenital aortic stenosis NOS (Q23.0)
            congenital stenosis of aortic valve (Q23.0)

 + Q25.4 **Other congenital malformations of aorta**
      Excludes1: hypoplasia of aorta in hypoplastic left heart
            syndrome (Q23.4)
      AHA CC: 4Q, 2016, 57

    CC Q25.40 **Congenital malformation of aorta unspecified**
    CC Q25.41 **Absence and aplasia of aorta**
    CC Q25.42 **Hypoplasia of aorta**
    CC Q25.43 **Congenital aneurysm of aorta**
        Congenital aneurysm of aortic root
        Congenital aneurysm of aortic sinus
    CC Q25.44 **Congenital dilation of aorta**
    CC Q25.45 **Double aortic arch**
        Vascular ring of aorta

    CC Q25.46 **Tortuous aortic arch**
        Persistent convolutions of aortic arch

    CC Q25.47 **Right aortic arch**
        Persistent right aortic arch

    CC Q25.48 **Anomalous origin of subclavian artery**

    CC Q25.49 **Other congenital malformations of aorta**
        Aortic arch
        Bovine arch

MCC Q25.5 **Atresia of pulmonary artery**

MCC Q25.6 **Stenosis of pulmonary artery**
      Supravalvular pulmonary stenosis

 + Q25.7 **Other congenital malformations of pulmonary artery**

MCC Q25.71 **Coarctation of pulmonary artery**

MCC Q25.72 **Congenital pulmonary arteriovenous malformation**
        Congenital pulmonary arteriovenous aneurysm

MCC Q25.79 **Other congenital malformations of pulmonary artery**
        Aberrant pulmonary artery
        Agenesis of pulmonary artery
        Congenital aneurysm of pulmonary artery
        Congenital anomaly of pulmonary artery
        Hypoplasia of pulmonary artery

   Q25.8 **Other congenital malformations of other great arteries**

CC Q25.9 **Congenital malformation of great arteries, unspecified**

Q26 **Congenital malformations of great veins**

CC Q26.0 **Congenital stenosis of vena cava**
      Congenital stenosis of vena cava (inferior)(superior)

CC Q26.1 **Persistent left superior vena cava**

CC Q26.2 **Total anomalous pulmonary venous connection**
      Total anomalous pulmonary venous return [TAPVR],
        subdiaphragmatic
      Total anomalous pulmonary venous return [TAPVR],
        supradiaphragmatic

CC Q26.3 **Partial anomalous pulmonary venous connection**
      Partial anomalous pulmonary venous return

CC Q26.4 **Anomalous pulmonary venous connection, unspecified**

   Q26.5 **Anomalous portal venous connection**

   Q26.6 **Portal vein-hepatic artery fistula**

CC Q26.8 **Other congenital malformations of great veins**
      Absence of vena cava (inferior) (superior)
      Azygos continuation of inferior vena cava
      Persistent left posterior cardinal vein
      Scimitar syndrome

CC Q26.9 **Congenital malformation of great vein, unspecified**
      Congenital anomaly of vena cava (inferior) (superior) NOS

Q27 **Other congenital malformations of peripheral vascular system**

    Excludes2: anomalies of cerebral and precerebral vessels
         (Q28.0-Q28.3)
        anomalies of coronary vessels (Q24.5)
        anomalies of pulmonary artery (Q25.5-Q25.7)
        congenital retinal aneurysm (Q14.1)
        hemangioma and lymphangioma (D18.-)

   Q27.0 **Congenital absence and hypoplasia of umbilical artery**
      Single umbilical artery

   Q27.1 **Congenital renal artery stenosis**

   Q27.2 **Other congenital malformations of renal artery**
      Congenital malformation of renal artery NOS
      Multiple renal arteries

 + Q27.3 **Arteriovenous malformation (peripheral)**
      Arteriovenous aneurysm
      Excludes1: acquired arteriovenous aneurysm (I77.0)
      Excludes2: arteriovenous malformation of cerebral vessels
         (Q28.2)
        arteriovenous malformation of precerebral
         vessels (Q28.0)

    CC Q27.30 **Arteriovenous malformation, site unspecified**
       Q27.31 **Arteriovenous malformation of vessel of upper limb**
       Q27.32 **Arteriovenous malformation of vessel of lower limb**
       Q27.33 **Arteriovenous malformation of digestive system vessel**
       Q27.34 **Arteriovenous malformation of renal vessel**
       Q27.39 **Arteriovenous malformation, other site**

+, +7th, X + 7th   ● Newborn   ● Pediatric   ● Maternity   ● Adult   ♀ Female   ♂ Male   Manifestation   Unacceptable PDX   HCC   CC   MCC   HAC

CC **Q27.4** **Congenital phlebectasia**

Q27.8 **Other specified congenital malformations of peripheral vascular system**
  Absence of peripheral vascular system
  Atresia of peripheral vascular system
  Congenital aneurysm (peripheral)
  Congenital stricture, artery
  Congenital varix
  Excludes1: *arteriovenous malformation (Q27.3-)*

Q27.9 **Congenital malformation of peripheral vascular system, unspecified**
  Anomaly of artery or vein NOS

Q28 **Other congenital malformations of circulatory system**

  Excludes1: *congenital aneurysm NOS (Q27.8)*
    congenital coronary aneurysm (Q24.5)
    ruptured cerebral arteriovenous malformation (I60.8)
    ruptured malformation of precerebral vessels (I72.0)
  Excludes2: *congenital peripheral aneurysm (Q27.8)*
    congenital pulmonary aneurysm (Q25.79)
    congenital retinal aneurysm (Q14.1)

CC **Q28.0** **Arteriovenous malformation of precerebral vessels**
  Congenital arteriovenous precerebral aneurysm (nonruptured)

CC **Q28.1** **Other malformations of precerebral vessels**
  Congenital malformation of precerebral vessels NOS
  Congenital precerebral aneurysm (nonruptured)

MCC **Q28.2** **Arteriovenous malformation of cerebral vessels**
  Arteriovenous malformation of brain NOS
  Congenital arteriovenous cerebral aneurysm (nonruptured)

MCC **Q28.3** **Other malformations of cerebral vessels**
  Congenital cerebral aneurysm (nonruptured)
  Congenital malformation of cerebral vessels NOS
  Developmental venous anomaly

CC **Q28.8** **Other specified congenital malformations of circulatory system**
  Congenital aneurysm, specified site NEC
  Spinal vessel anomaly

CC **Q28.9** **Congenital malformation of circulatory system, unspecified**

Congenital malformations of the respiratory system (Q30-Q34)

Q30 **Congenital malformations of nose**

  Excludes1: *congenital deviation of nasal septum (Q67.4)*

Q30.0 **Choanal atresia**
  Atresia of nares (anterior) (posterior)
  Congenital stenosis of nares (anterior) (posterior)

Q30.1 **Agenesis and underdevelopment of nose**
  Congenital absent of nose

Q30.2 **Fissured, notched and cleft nose**

Q30.3 **Congenital perforated nasal septum**

Q30.8 **Other congenital malformations of nose**
  Accessory nose
  Congenital anomaly of nasal sinus wall

Q30.9 **Congenital malformation of nose, unspecified**

Q31 **Congenital malformations of larynx**

  Excludes1: *congenital laryngeal stridor NOS (P28.89)*

Q31.0 **Web of larynx**
  Glottic web of larynx
  Subglottic web of larynx
  Web of larynx NOS

CC **Q31.1** **Congenital subglottic stenosis**

CC **Q31.2** **Laryngeal hypoplasia**

CC **Q31.3** **Laryngocele**

CC **Q31.5** **Congenital laryngomalacia**

CC **Q31.8** **Other congenital malformations of larynx**
  Absence of larynx
  Agenesis of larynx
  Atresia of larynx
  Congenital cleft thyroid cartilage
  Congenital fissure of epiglottis
  Congenital stenosis of larynx NEC
  Posterior cleft of cricoid cartilage

CC **Q31.9** **Congenital malformation of larynx, unspecified**

Q32 **Congenital malformations of trachea and bronchus**

  Excludes1: *congenital bronchiectasis (Q33.4)*

CC **Q32.0** **Congenital tracheomalacia**

CC **Q32.1** **Other congenital malformations of trachea**
  Atresia of trachea
  Congenital anomaly of tracheal cartilage
  Congenital dilatation of trachea
  Congenital malformation of trachea
  Congenital stenosis of trachea
  Congenital tracheocele

CC **Q32.2** **Congenital bronchomalacia**

CC **Q32.3** **Congenital stenosis of bronchus**

CC **Q32.4** **Other congenital malformations of bronchus**
  Absence of bronchus
  Agenesis of bronchus
  Atresia of bronchus
  Congenital diverticulum of bronchus
  Congenital malformation of bronchus NOS

Q33 **Congenital malformations of lung**

CC **Q33.0** **Congenital cystic lung**
  Congenital cystic lung disease
  Congenital honeycomb lung
  Congenital polycystic lung disease
  Excludes1: *cystic fibrosis (E84.0)*
    cystic lung disease, acquired or unspecified (J98.4)

Q33.1 **Accessory lobe of lung**
  Azygos lobe (fissured), lung

MCC **Q33.2** **Sequestration of lung**

MCC **Q33.3** **Agenesis of lung**
  Congenital absence of lung (lobe)

CC **Q33.4** **Congenital bronchiectasis**

Q33.5 **Ectopic tissue in lung**

MCC **Q33.6** **Congenital hypoplasia and dysplasia of lung**
  Excludes1: *pulmonary hypoplasia associated with short gestation (P28.0)*

Q33.8 **Other congenital malformations of lung**

Q33.9 **Congenital malformation of lung, unspecified**

Q34 **Other congenital malformations of respiratory system**

  Excludes2: *congenital central alveolar hypoventilation syndrome (G47.35)*

Q34.0 **Anomaly of pleura**

Q34.1 **Congenital cyst of mediastinum**

Q34.8 **Other specified congenital malformations of respiratory system**
  Atresia of nasopharynx

Q34.9 **Congenital malformation of respiratory system, unspecified**
  Congenital absence of respiratory system
  Congenital anomaly of respiratory system NOS

Cleft lip and cleft palate (Q35-Q37)

Use additional code to identify associated malformation of the nose (Q30.2)

Excludes2: *Robin's syndrome (Q87.0)*

Q35 **Cleft palate**

  Includes: fissure of palate
    palatoschisis
  Excludes1: *cleft palate with cleft lip (Q37.-)*

Q35.1 **Cleft hard palate**

Q35.3 **Cleft soft palate**

Q35.5 **Cleft hard palate with cleft soft palate**

Q35.7 **Cleft uvula**

Q35.9 **Cleft palate, unspecified**
  Cleft palate NOS

Q36 **Cleft lip**

  Includes: cheiloschisis
    congenital fissure of lip
    harelip
    labium leporinum
  Excludes1: *cleft lip with cleft palate (Q37.-)*

Q36.0 **Cleft lip, bilateral**

Q36.1 **Cleft lip, median**

Q36.9 **Cleft lip, unilateral**
  Cleft lip NOS

+, +7th, X + 7th • Newborn • Pediatric • Maternity • Adult ♀ Female ♂ Male | Manifestation | Unacceptable PDX | HCC | CC | MCC | HAC

Q37 **Cleft palate with cleft lip**

Includes: cheilopalatoschisis

Q37.0 **Cleft hard palate with bilateral cleft lip**

Q37.1 **Cleft hard palate with unilateral cleft lip**
Cleft hard palate with cleft lip NOS

Q37.2 **Cleft soft palate with bilateral cleft lip**

Q37.3 **Cleft soft palate with unilateral cleft lip**
Cleft soft palate with cleft lip NOS

Q37.4 **Cleft hard and soft palate with bilateral cleft lip**

Q37.5 **Cleft hard and soft palate with unilateral cleft lip**
Cleft hard and soft palate with cleft lip NOS

Q37.8 **Unspecified cleft palate with bilateral cleft lip**

Q37.9 **Unspecified cleft palate with unilateral cleft lip**
Cleft palate with cleft lip NOS

Other congenital malformations of the digestive system (Q38-Q45)

Q38 **Other congenital malformations of tongue, mouth and pharynx**

Excludes1: *dentofacial anomalies (M26.-)*
macrostomia (Q18.4)
microstomia (Q18.5)

Q38.0 **Congenital malformations of lips, not elsewhere classified**
Congenital fistula of lip
Congenital malformation of lip NOS
Van der Woude's syndrome
Excludes1: *cleft lip (Q36.-)*
cleft lip with cleft palate (Q37.-)
macrocheilia (Q18.6)
microcheilia (Q18.7)

Q38.1 **Ankyloglossia**
Tongue tie

Q38.2 **Macroglossia**
Congenital hypertrophy of tongue

Q38.3 **Other congenital malformations of tongue**
Aglossia
Bifid tongue
Congenital adhesion of tongue
Congenital fissure of tongue
Congenital malformation of tongue NOS
Double tongue
Hypoglossia
Hypoplasia of tongue
Microglossia

Q38.4 **Congenital malformations of salivary glands and ducts**
Atresia of salivary glands and ducts
Congenital absence of salivary glands and ducts
Congenital accessory salivary glands and ducts
Congenital fistula of salivary gland

Q38.5 **Congenital malformations of palate, not elsewhere classified**
Congenital absence of uvula
Congenital malformation of palate NOS
Congenital high arched palate
Excludes1: *cleft palate (Q35.-)*
cleft palate with cleft lip (Q37.-)

Q38.6 **Other congenital malformations of mouth**
Congenital malformation of mouth NOS

Q38.7 **Congenital pharyngeal pouch**
Congenital diverticulum of pharynx
Excludes1: *pharyngeal pouch syndrome (D82.1)*

Q38.8 **Other congenital malformations of pharynx**
Congenital malformation of pharynx NOS
Imperforate pharynx

Q39 **Congenital malformations of esophagus**

MCC Q39.0 **Atresia of esophagus without fistula**
Atresia of esophagus NOS

MCC Q39.1 **Atresia of esophagus with tracheo-esophageal fistula**
Atresia of esophagus with broncho-esophageal fistula

MCC Q39.2 **Congenital tracheo-esophageal fistula without atresia**
Congenital tracheo-esophageal fistula NOS

MCC Q39.3 **Congenital stenosis and stricture of esophagus**

MCC Q39.4 **Esophageal web**

CC Q39.5 **Congenital dilatation of esophagus**
Congenital cardiospasm

CC Q39.6 **Congenital diverticulum of esophagus**
Congenital esophageal pouch

CC Q39.8 **Other congenital malformations of esophagus**
Congenital absence of esophagus
Congenital displacement of esophagus
Congenital duplication of esophagus

CC Q39.9 **Congenital malformation of esophagus, unspecified**

Q40 **Other congenital malformations of upper alimentary tract**

Q40.0 **Congenital hypertrophic pyloric stenosis**
Congenital or infantile constriction
Congenital or infantile hypertrophy
Congenital or infantile spasm
Congenital or infantile stenosis
Congenital or infantile stricture

Q40.1 **Congenital hiatus hernia**
Congenital displacement of cardia through esophageal hiatus
Excludes1: *congenital diaphragmatic hernia (Q79.0)*

Q40.2 **Other specified congenital malformations of stomach**
Congenital displacement of stomach
Congenital diverticulum of stomach
Congenital hourglass stomach
Congenital duplication of stomach
Megalogastria
Microgastria

Q40.3 **Congenital malformation of stomach, unspecified**

Q40.8 **Other specified congenital malformations of upper alimentary tract**

Q40.9 **Congenital malformation of upper alimentary tract, unspecified**
Congenital anomaly of upper alimentary tract
Congenital deformity of upper alimentary tract

Q41 **Congenital absence, atresia and stenosis of small intestine**

Includes: congenital obstruction, occlusion or stricture of small intestine or intestine NOS

Excludes1: *cystic fibrosis with intestinal manifestation (E84.11)*
meconium ileus NOS (without cystic fibrosis) (P76.0)

CC Q41.0 **Congenital absence, atresia and stenosis of duodenum**

CC Q41.1 **Congenital absence, atresia and stenosis of jejunum**
Apple peel syndrome
Imperforate jejunum

CC Q41.2 **Congenital absence, atresia and stenosis of ileum**

CC Q41.8 **Congenital absence, atresia and stenosis of other specified parts of small intestine**

CC Q41.9 **Congenital absence, atresia and stenosis of small intestine, part unspecified**
Congenital absence, atresia and stenosis of intestine NOS

Q42 **Congenital absence, atresia and stenosis of large intestine**

Includes: congenital obstruction, occlusion and stricture of large intestine

CC Q42.0 **Congenital absence, atresia and stenosis of rectum with fistula**

CC Q42.1 **Congenital absence, atresia and stenosis of rectum without fistula**
Imperforate rectum

CC Q42.2 **Congenital absence, atresia and stenosis of anus with fistula**

CC Q42.3 **Congenital absence, atresia and stenosis of anus without fistula**
Imperforate anus

CC Q42.8 **Congenital absence, atresia and stenosis of other parts of large intestine**

CC Q42.9 **Congenital absence, atresia and stenosis of large intestine, part unspecified**

Q43 **Other congenital malformations of intestine**

Q43.0 **Meckel's diverticulum (displaced) (hypertrophic)**
Persistent omphalomesenteric duct
Persistent vitelline duct

CC Q43.1 **Hirschsprung's disease**
Aganglionosis
Congenital (aganglionic) megacolon

CC Q43.2 **Other congenital functional disorders of colon**
Congenital dilatation of colon

CC Q43.3 **Congenital malformations of intestinal fixation**
Congenital omental, anomalous adhesions [bands]
Congenital peritoneal adhesions [bands]
Incomplete rotation of cecum and colon
Insufficient rotation of cecum and colon
Jackson's membrane
Malrotation of colon
Rotation failure of cecum and colon
Universal mesentery

CC **Q43.4** **Duplication of intestine**

CC **Q43.5** **Ectopic anus**

CC **Q43.6** **Congenital fistula of rectum and anus**

> ***Excludes1:*** *congenital fistula of anus with absence, atresia and stenosis (Q42.2)*
> *congenital fistula of rectum with absence, atresia and stenosis (Q42.0)*
> *congenital rectovaginal fistula (Q52.2)*
> *congenital urethrorectal fistula (Q64.73)*
> *pilonidal fistula or sinus (L05.-)*

CC **Q43.7** **Persistent cloaca**

> Cloaca NOS

CC **Q43.8** **Other specified congenital malformations of intestine**

> Congenital blind loop syndrome
> Congenital diverticulitis, colon
> Congenital diverticulum, intestine
> Dolichocolon
> Megaloappendix
> Megaloduodenum
> Microcolon
> Transposition of appendix
> Transposition of colon
> Transposition of intestine
> *AHA CC: 2Q, 2013, 31*

CC **Q43.9** **Congenital malformation of intestine, unspecified**

Q44 **Congenital malformations of gallbladder, bile ducts and liver**

CC **Q44.0** **Agenesis, aplasia and hypoplasia of gallbladder**
> Congenital absence of gallbladder

CC **Q44.1** **Other congenital malformations of gallbladder**
> Congenital malformation of gallbladder NOS
> Intrahepatic gallbladder

MCC **Q44.2** **Atresia of bile ducts**

MCC **Q44.3** **Congenital stenosis and stricture of bile ducts**

CC **Q44.4** **Choledochal cyst**

CC **Q44.5** **Other congenital malformations of bile ducts**
> Accessory hepatic duct
> Biliary duct duplication
> Congenital malformation of bile duct NOS
> Cystic duct duplication

CC **Q44.6** **Cystic disease of liver**
> Fibrocystic disease of liver

CC **Q44.7** **Other congenital malformations of liver**
> Accessory liver
> Alagille's syndrome
> Congenital absence of liver
> Congenital hepatomegaly
> Congenital malformation of liver NOS

Q45 **Other congenital malformations of digestive system**

> ***Excludes2:*** *congenital diaphragmatic hernia (Q79.0)*
> *congenital hiatus hernia (Q40.1)*

CC **Q45.0** **Agenesis, aplasia and hypoplasia of pancreas**
> Congenital absence of pancreas

CC **Q45.1** **Annular pancreas**

CC **Q45.2** **Congenital pancreatic cyst**

Q45.3 **Other congenital malformations of pancreas and pancreatic duct**
> Accessory pancreas
> Congenital malformation of pancreas or pancreatic duct NOS

> ***Excludes1:*** *congenital diabetes mellitus (E10.-)*
> *cystic fibrosis (E84.0-E84.9)*
> *fibrocystic disease of pancreas (E84.-)*
> *neonatal diabetes mellitus (P70.2)*

Q45.8 **Other specified congenital malformations of digestive system**
> Absence (complete) (partial) of alimentary tract NOS
> Duplication of digestive system
> Malposition, congenital of digestive system

Q45.9 **Congenital malformation of digestive system, unspecified**
> Congenital anomaly of digestive system
> Congenital deformity of digestive system

Congenital malformations of genital organs (Q50-Q56)

> ***Excludes1:*** *androgen insensitivity syndrome (E34.5-)*
> *syndromes associated with anomalies in the number and form of chromosomes (Q90-Q99)*

Q50 **Congenital malformations of ovaries, fallopian tubes and broad ligaments**

+ **Q50.0** **Congenital absence of ovary**
> ***Excludes1:*** *Turner's syndrome (Q96.-)*
♀ **Q50.01** **Congenital absence of ovary, unilateral**
♀ **Q50.02** **Congenital absence of ovary, bilateral**

♀ **Q50.1** **Developmental ovarian cyst**

♀ **Q50.2** **Congenital torsion of ovary**

+ **Q50.3** **Other congenital malformations of ovary**
♀ **Q50.31** **Accessory ovary**
♀ **Q50.32** **Ovarian streak**
> 46, XX with streak gonads
♀ **Q50.39** **Other congenital malformation of ovary**
> Congenital malformation of ovary NOS

♀ **Q50.4** **Embryonic cyst of fallopian tube**
> Fimbrial cyst

♀ **Q50.5** **Embryonic cyst of broad ligament**
> Epoophoron cyst
> Parovarian cyst

♀ **Q50.6** **Other congenital malformations of fallopian tube and broad ligament**
> Absence of fallopian tube and broad ligament
> Accessory fallopian tube and broad ligament
> Atresia of fallopian tube and broad ligament
> Congenital malformation of fallopian tube or broad ligament NOS

Q51 **Congenital malformations of uterus and cervix**

♀ **Q51.0** **Agenesis and aplasia of uterus**
> Congenital absence of uterus

+ **Q51.1** **Doubling of uterus with doubling of cervix and vagina**
♀ **Q51.10** **Doubling of uterus with doubling of cervix and vagina without obstruction**
> Doubling of uterus with doubling of cervix and vagina NOS
♀ **Q51.11** **Doubling of uterus with doubling of cervix and vagina with obstruction**

+ **Q51.2** **Other doubling of uterus**
> Doubling of uterus NOS
> Septate uterus
> *AHA CC: 4Q, 2018, 27*
♀ **Q51.21** **Complete doubling of uterus**
> Complete septate uterus
♀ **Q51.22** **Partial doubling of uterus**
> Partial septate uterus
♀ **Q51.28** **Other and unspecified doubling of uterus**
> Septate uterus NOS

♀ **Q51.3** **Bicornate uterus**
> Bicornate uterus, complete or partial

♀ **Q51.4** **Unicornate uterus**
> Unicornate uterus with or without a separate uterine horn
> Uterus with only one functioning horn

♀ **Q51.5** **Agenesis and aplasia of cervix**
> Congenital absence of cervix

♀ **Q51.6** **Embryonic cyst of cervix**

♀ **Q51.7** **Congenital fistulae between uterus and digestive and urinary tracts**

+ **Q51.8** **Other congenital malformations of uterus and cervix**
+ **Q51.81** **Other congenital malformations of uterus**
♀ **Q51.810** **Arcuate uterus**
> Arcuatus uterus
♀ **Q51.811** **Hypoplasia of uterus**
♀ **Q51.818** **Other congenital malformations of uterus**
> Müllerian anomaly of uterus NEC
+ **Q51.82** **Other congenital malformations of cervix**
♀ **Q51.820** **Cervical duplication**
♀ **Q51.821** **Hypoplasia of cervix**
♀ **Q51.828** **Other congenital malformations of cervix**

♀ **Q51.9** **Congenital malformation of uterus and cervix, unspecified**

+, +7th, X + 7th　　● Newborn　　● Pediatric　　● Maternity　　● Adult　　♀ Female　　♂ Male　　Manifestation　　Unacceptable PDX　　HCC　　CC　　MCC　　HAC

Q52 Other congenital malformations of female genitalia

♀ **Q52.0 Congenital absence of vagina**
Vaginal agenesis, total or partial

+ **Q52.1 Doubling of vagina**
Excludes1: doubling of vagina with doubling of uterus and cervix (Q51.1-)

♀ **Q52.10 Doubling of vagina, unspecified**
Septate vagina NOS

♀ **Q52.11 Transverse vaginal septum**

+ **Q52.12 Longitudinal vaginal septum**
AHA CC: 4Q, 2016, 58-59

♀ **Q52.120 Longitudinal vaginal septum, nonobstructing**

♀ **Q52.121 Longitudinal vaginal septum, obstructing, right side**

♀ **Q52.122 Longitudinal vaginal septum, obstructing, left side**

♀ **Q52.123 Longitudinal vaginal septum, microperforate, right side**

♀ **Q52.124 Longitudinal vaginal septum, microperforate, left side**
AHA CC: 4Q, 2016, 58-59

♀ **Q52.129 Other and unspecified longitudinal vaginal septum**

♀ **Q52.2 Congenital rectovaginal fistula**
Excludes1: cloaca (Q43.7)

♀ **Q52.3 Imperforate hymen**

♀ **Q52.4 Other congenital malformations of vagina**
Canal of Nuck cyst, congenital
Congenital malformation of vagina NOS
Embryonic vaginal cyst
Gartner's duct cyst

♀ **Q52.5 Fusion of labia**

♀ **Q52.6 Congenital malformation of clitoris**

+ **Q52.7 Other and unspecified congenital malformations of vulva**

♀ **Q52.70 Unspecified congenital malformations of vulva**
Congenital malformation of vulva NOS

♀ **Q52.71 Congenital absence of vulva**

♀ **Q52.79 Other congenital malformations of vulva**
Congenital cyst of vulva

♀ **Q52.8 Other specified congenital malformations of female genitalia**

♀ **Q52.9 Congenital malformation of female genitalia, unspecified**

Q53 Undescended and ectopic testicle

AHA CC: 4Q, 2017, 22-23

+ **Q53.0 Ectopic testis**
♂ **Q53.00 Ectopic testis, unspecified**
♂ **Q53.01 Ectopic testis, unilateral**
♂ **Q53.02 Ectopic testes, bilateral**

+ **Q53.1 Undescended testicle, unilateral**
♂ **Q53.10 Unspecified undescended testicle, unilateral**

+ **Q53.11 Abdominal testis, unilateral**
♂ **Q53.111 Unilateral intraabdominal testis**
♂ **Q53.112 Unilateral inguinal testis**
♂ **Q53.12 Ectopic perineal testis, unilateral**
♂ **Q53.13 Unilateral high scrotal testis**

+ **Q53.2 Undescended testicle, bilateral**
♂ **Q53.20 Undescended testicle, unspecified, bilateral**

+ **Q53.21 Abdominal testis, bilateral**
♂ **Q53.211 Bilateral intraabdominal testes**
♂ **Q53.212 Bilateral inguinal testes**
♂ **Q53.22 Ectopic perineal testis, bilateral**
♂ **Q53.23 Bilateral high scrotal testes**

♂ **Q53.9 Undescended testicle, unspecified**
Cryptorchism NOS

Q54 Hypospadias

Excludes1: epispadias (Q64.0)

♂ **Q54.0 Hypospadias, balanic**
Hypospadias, coronal
Hypospadias, glandular

♂ **Q54.1 Hypospadias, penile**

♂ **Q54.2 Hypospadias, penoscrotal**

♂ **Q54.3 Hypospadias, perineal**

♂ **Q54.4 Congenital chordee**
Chordee without hypospadias

♂ **Q54.8 Other hypospadias**
Hypospadias with intersex state

♂ **Q54.9 Hypospadias, unspecified**

Q55 Other congenital malformations of male genital organs

Excludes1: congenital hydrocele (P83.5)
hypospadias (Q54.-)

♂ **Q55.0 Absence and aplasia of testis**
Monorchism

♂ **Q55.1 Hypoplasia of testis and scrotum**
Fusion of testes

+ **Q55.2 Other and unspecified congenital malformations of testis and scrotum**

♂ **Q55.20 Unspecified congenital malformations of testis and scrotum**
Congenital malformation of testis or scrotum NOS

♂ **Q55.21 Polyorchism**

♂ **Q55.22 Retractile testis**

♂ **Q55.23 Scrotal transposition**

♂ **Q55.29 Other congenital malformations of testis and scrotum**

♂ **Q55.3 Atresia of vas deferens**
Code first any associated cystic fibrosis (E84.-)

♂ **Q55.4 Other congenital malformations of vas deferens, epididymis, seminal vesicles and prostate**
Absence or aplasia of prostate
Absence or aplasia of spermatic cord
Congenital malformation of vas deferens, epididymis, seminal vesicles or prostate NOS

♂ **Q55.5 Congenital absence and aplasia of penis**

+ **Q55.6 Other congenital malformations of penis**
♂ **Q55.61 Curvature of penis (lateral)**
♂ **Q55.62 Hypoplasia of penis**
Micropenis

♂ **Q55.63 Congenital torsion of penis**
Excludes1: acquired torsion of penis (N48.82)

♂ **Q55.64 Hidden penis**
Buried penis
Concealed penis
Excludes1: acquired buried penis (N48.83)

♂ **Q55.69 Other congenital malformation of penis**
Congenital malformation of penis NOS

♂ **Q55.7 Congenital vasocutaneous fistula**

♂ **Q55.8 Other specified congenital malformations of male genital organs**

♂ **Q55.9 Congenital malformation of male genital organ, unspecified**
Congenital anomaly of male genital organ
Congenital deformity of male genital organ

Q56 Indeterminate sex and pseudohermaphroditism

Excludes1: 46,XX true hermaphrodite (Q99.1)
androgen insensitivity syndrome (E34.5-)
chimera 46,XX/46,XY true hermaphrodite (Q99.0)
female pseudohermaphroditism with adrenocortical disorder (E25.-)
pseudohermaphroditism with specified chromosomal anomaly (Q96-Q99)
pure gonadal dysgenesis (Q99.1)

Q56.0 Hermaphroditism, not elsewhere classified
Ovotestis

♂ **Q56.1 Male pseudohermaphroditism, not elsewhere classified**
46, XY with streak gonads
Male pseudohermaphroditism NOS

♀ **Q56.2 Female pseudohermaphroditism, not elsewhere classified**
Female pseudohermaphroditism NOS

Q56.3 Pseudohermaphroditism, unspecified

Q56.4 Indeterminate sex, unspecified
Ambiguous genitalia

Congenital malformations of the urinary system (Q60-Q64)

Q60 Renal agenesis and other reduction defects of kidney

Includes: congenital absence of kidney
congenital atrophy of kidney
infantile atrophy of kidney

CC **Q60.0 Renal agenesis, unilateral**
CC **Q60.1 Renal agenesis, bilateral**
CC **Q60.2 Renal agenesis, unspecified**
CC **Q60.3 Renal hypoplasia, unilateral**
CC **Q60.4 Renal hypoplasia, bilateral**
CC **Q60.5 Renal hypoplasia, unspecified**
CC **Q60.6 Potter's syndrome**

+, +7th, X + 7th • Newborn • Pediatric • Maternity • Adult ♀ Female ♂ Male Manifestation Unacceptable PDX HCC CC MCC HAC

Q61 Cystic kidney disease

Excludes1: *acquired cyst of kidney (N28.1)*
Potter's syndrome (Q60.6)

+ **Q61.0 Congenital renal cyst**
- CC **Q61.00 Congenital renal cyst, unspecified**
  Cyst of kidney NOS (congenital)
- CC **Q61.01 Congenital single renal cyst**
- CC **Q61.02 Congenital multiple renal cysts**
+ **Q61.1 Polycystic kidney, infantile type**
  Polycystic kidney, autosomal recessive
- CC **Q61.11 Cystic dilatation of collecting ducts**
- CC **Q61.19 Other polycystic kidney, infantile type**
- CC **Q61.2 Polycystic kidney, adult type**
  Polycystic kidney, autosomal dominant
- CC **Q61.3 Polycystic kidney, unspecified**
  AHA CC: 3Q, 2016, 22-23
- CC **Q61.4 Renal dysplasia**
  Multicystic dysplastic kidney
  Multicystic kidney (development)
  Multicystic kidney disease
  Multicystic renal dysplasia
  Excludes1: *polycystic kidney disease (Q61.11-Q61.3)*
- CC **Q61.5 Medullary cystic kidney**
  Nephronopthisis
  Sponge kidney NOS
- CC **Q61.8 Other cystic kidney diseases**
  Fibrocystic kidney
  Fibrocystic renal degeneration or disease
- CC **Q61.9 Cystic kidney disease, unspecified**
  Meckel-Gruber syndrome

Q62 Congenital obstructive defects of renal pelvis and congenital malformations of ureter

- CC **Q62.0 Congenital hydronephrosis**
+ **Q62.1 Congenital occlusion of ureter**
  Atresia and stenosis of ureter
  - CC **Q62.10 Congenital occlusion of ureter, unspecified**
  - CC **Q62.11 Congenital occlusion of ureteropelvic junction**
  - CC **Q62.12 Congenital occlusion of ureterovesical orifice**
Q62.2 Congenital megaureter
  Congenital dilatation of ureter
+ **Q62.3 Other obstructive defects of renal pelvis and ureter**
  - CC **Q62.31 Congenital ureterocele, orthotopic**
  - CC **Q62.32 Cecoureterocele**
    Ectopic ureterocele
  - CC **Q62.39 Other obstructive defects of renal pelvis and ureter**
    Ureteropelvic junction obstruction NOS
Q62.4 Agenesis of ureter
  Congenital absence ureter
Q62.5 Duplication of ureter
  Accessory ureter
  Double ureter
+ **Q62.6 Malposition of ureter**
  Q62.60 Malposition of ureter, unspecified
  Q62.61 Deviation of ureter
  Q62.62 Displacement of ureter
  Q62.63 Anomalous implantation of ureter
    Ectopia of ureter
    Ectopic ureter
  Q62.69 Other malposition of ureter
Q62.7 Congenital vesico-uretero-renal reflux
Q62.8 Other congenital malformations of ureter
  Anomaly of ureter NOS

Q63 Other congenital malformations of kidney

Excludes1: *congenital nephrotic syndrome (N04.-)*
Q63.0 Accessory kidney
Q63.1 Lobulated, fused and horseshoe kidney
Q63.2 Ectopic kidney
  Congenital displaced kidney
  Malrotation of kidney
Q63.3 Hyperplastic and giant kidney
  Compensatory hypertrophy of kidney
Q63.8 Other specified congenital malformations of kidney
  Congenital renal calculi
Q63.9 Congenital malformation of kidney, unspecified

Q64 Other congenital malformations of urinary system

Q64.0 Epispadias
  Excludes1: *hypospadias (Q54.-)*
+ **Q64.1 Exstrophy of urinary bladder**
  - CC **Q64.10 Exstrophy of urinary bladder, unspecified**
    Ectopia vesicae
  - CC **Q64.11 Supravesical fissure of urinary bladder**
  - CC **Q64.12 Cloacal exstrophy of urinary bladder**
  - CC **Q64.19 Other exstrophy of urinary bladder**
    Extroversion of bladder
- CC **Q64.2 Congenital posterior urethral valves**
+ **Q64.3 Other atresia and stenosis of urethra and bladder neck**
  - CC **Q64.31 Congenital bladder neck obstruction**
    Congenital obstruction of vesicourethral orifice
  - CC **Q64.32 Congenital stricture of urethra**
  - CC **Q64.33 Congenital stricture of urinary meatus**
  - CC **Q64.39 Other atresia and stenosis of urethra and bladder neck**
    Atresia and stenosis of urethra and bladder neck NOS
Q64.4 Malformation of urachus
  Cyst of urachus
  Patent urachus
  Prolapse of urachus
Q64.5 Congenital absence of bladder and urethra
Q64.6 Congenital diverticulum of bladder
+ **Q64.7 Other and unspecified congenital malformations of bladder and urethra**
  Excludes1: *congenital prolapse of bladder (mucosa) (Q79.4)*
  Q64.70 Unspecified congenital malformation of bladder and urethra
    Malformation of bladder or urethra NOS
  Q64.71 Congenital prolapse of urethra
  Q64.72 Congenital prolapse of urinary meatus
  Q64.73 Congenital urethrorectal fistula
  Q64.74 Double urethra
  Q64.75 Double urinary meatus
  Q64.79 Other congenital malformations of bladder and urethra
Q64.8 Other specified congenital malformations of urinary system
Q64.9 Congenital malformation of urinary system, unspecified
  Congenital anomaly NOS of urinary system
  Congenital deformity NOS of urinary system

Congenital malformations and deformations of the musculoskeletal system (Q65-Q79)

Q65 Congenital deformities of hip

Excludes1: *clicking hip (R29.4)*
+ **Q65.0 Congenital dislocation of hip, unilateral**
  Q65.00 Congenital dislocation of unspecified hip, unilateral
  Q65.01 Congenital dislocation of right hip, unilateral
  Q65.02 Congenital dislocation of left hip, unilateral
Q65.1 Congenital dislocation of hip, bilateral
Q65.2 Congenital dislocation of hip, unspecified
+ **Q65.3 Congenital partial dislocation of hip, unilateral**
  Q65.30 Congenital partial dislocation of unspecified hip, unilateral
  Q65.31 Congenital partial dislocation of right hip, unilateral
  Q65.32 Congenital partial dislocation of left hip, unilateral
Q65.4 Congenital partial dislocation of hip, bilateral
Q65.5 Congenital partial dislocation of hip, unspecified
Q65.6 Congenital unstable hip
  Congenital dislocatable hip
+ **Q65.8 Other congenital deformities of hip**
  Q65.81 Congenital coxa valga
  Q65.82 Congenital coxa vara
  Q65.89 Other specified congenital deformities of hip
    Anteversion of femoral neck
    Congenital acetabular dysplasia
Q65.9 Congenital deformity of hip, unspecified

Q66 Congenital deformities of feet

> *Excludes1:* *reduction defects of feet (Q72.-)*
> *valgus deformities (acquired) (M21.0-)*
> *varus deformities (acquired) (M21.1-)*

> AHA CC: 4Q, 2019, 13

+ **Q66.0 Congenital talipes equinovarus**
   Q66.00 Congenital talipes equinovarus, unspecified foot
   Q66.01 Congenital talipes equinovarus, right foot
   Q66.02 Congenital talipes equinovarus, left foot
+ **Q66.1 Congenital talipes calcaneovarus**
   Q66.10 Congenital talipes calcaneovarus, unspecified foot
   Q66.11 Congenital talipes calcaneovarus, right foot
   Q66.12 Congenital talipes calcaneovarus, left foot
+ **Q66.2 Congenital metatarsus (primus) varus**

> AHA CC: 4Q, 2016, 59

  + **Q66.21 Congenital metatarsus primus varus**
     Q66.211 Congenital metatarsus primus varus, right foot
     Q66.212 Congenital metatarsus primus varus, left foot
     Q66.219 Congenital metatarsus primus varus, unspecified foot
  + **Q66.22 Congenital metatarsus adductus**
    Congenital metatarsus varus
     Q66.221 Congenital metatarsus adductus, right foot
     Q66.222 Congenital metatarsus adductus, left foot
     Q66.229 Congenital metatarsus adductus, unspecified foot
+ **Q66.3 Other congenital varus deformities of feet**
   Hallux varus, congenital
   Q66.30 Other congenital varus deformities of feet, unspecified foot
   Q66.31 Other congenital varus deformities of feet, right foot
   Q66.32 Other congenital varus deformities of feet, left foot
+ **Q66.4 Congenital talipes calcaneovalgus**
   Q66.40 Congenital talipes calcaneovalgus, unspecified foot
   Q66.41 Congenital talipes calcaneovalgus, right foot
   Q66.42 Congenital talipes calcaneovalgus, left foot
+ **Q66.5 Congenital pes planus**
   Congenital flat foot
   Congenital rigid flat foot
   Congenital spastic (everted) flat foot

> *Excludes1:* *pes planus, acquired (M21.4)*

   Q66.50 Congenital pes planus, unspecified foot
   Q66.51 Congenital pes planus, right foot
   Q66.52 Congenital pes planus, left foot
Q66.6 Other congenital valgus deformities of feet
   Congenital metatarsus valgus
+ **Q66.7 Congenital pes cavus**
   Q66.70 Congenital pes cavus, unspecified foot
   Q66.71 Congenital pes cavus, right foot
   Q66.72 Congenital pes cavus, left foot
+ **Q66.8 Other congenital deformities of feet**
   Q66.80 Congenital vertical talus deformity, unspecified foot
   Q66.81 Congenital vertical talus deformity, right foot
   Q66.82 Congenital vertical talus deformity, left foot
   Q66.89 Other specified congenital deformities of feet
     Congenital asymmetric talipes
     Congenital clubfoot NOS
     Congenital talipes NOS
     Congenital tarsal coalition
     Hammer toe, congenital
+ **Q66.9 Congenital deformity of feet, unspecified**
   Q66.90 Congenital deformity of feet, unspecified, unspecified foot
   Q66.91 Congenital deformity of feet, unspecified, right foot
   Q66.92 Congenital deformity of feet, unspecified, left foot

Q67 Congenital musculoskeletal deformities of head, face, spine and chest

> *Excludes1:* *congenital malformation syndromes classified to Q87.-*
> *Potter's syndrome (Q60.6)*

Q67.0 Congenital facial asymmetry
Q67.1 Congenital compression facies
Q67.2 Dolichocephaly
Q67.3 Plagiocephaly

Q67.4 Other congenital deformities of skull, face and jaw
   Congenital depressions in skull
   Congenital hemifacial atrophy or hypertrophy
   Deviation of nasal septum, congenital
   Squashed or bent nose, congenital

> *Excludes1:* *dentofacial anomalies [including malocclusion] (M26.-)*
> *syphilitic saddle nose (A50.5)*

CC **Q67.5 Congenital deformity of spine**
   Congenital postural scoliosis
   Congenital scoliosis NOS

> *Excludes1:* *infantile idiopathic scoliosis (M41.0)*
> *scoliosis due to congenital bony malformation (Q76.3)*

> AHA CC: 4Q, 2014, 26

Q67.6 Pectus excavatum
   Congenital funnel chest
Q67.7 Pectus carinatum
   Congenital pigeon chest
CC **Q67.8 Other congenital deformities of chest**
   Congenital deformity of chest wall NOS

Q68 Other congenital musculoskeletal deformities

> *Excludes1:* *reduction defects of limb(s) (Q71-Q73)*
> *Excludes2:* *congenital myotonic chondrodystrophy (G71.13)*

Q68.0 Congenital deformity of sternocleidomastoid muscle
   Congenital contracture of sternocleidomastoid (muscle)
   Congenital (sternomastoid) torticollis
   Sternomastoid tumor (congenital)
CC **Q68.1 Congenital deformity of finger(s) and hand**
   Congenital clubfinger
   Spade-like hand (congenital)
Q68.2 Congenital deformity of knee
   Congenital dislocation of knee
   Congenital genu recurvatum
Q68.3 Congenital bowing of femur

> *Excludes1:* *anteversion of femur (neck) (Q65.89)*

Q68.4 Congenital bowing of tibia and fibula
Q68.5 Congenital bowing of long bones of leg, unspecified
Q68.6 Discoid meniscus
Q68.8 Other specified congenital musculoskeletal deformities
   Congenital deformity of clavicle
   Congenital deformity of elbow
   Congenital deformity of forearm
   Congenital deformity of scapula
   Congenital deformity of wrist
   Congenital dislocation of elbow
   Congenital dislocation of shoulder
   Congenital dislocation of wrist

Q69 Polydactyly

Q69.0 Accessory finger(s)
Q69.1 Accessory thumb(s)
Q69.2 Accessory toe(s)
   Accessory hallux
Q69.9 Polydactyly, unspecified
   Supernumerary digit(s) NOS

Q70 Syndactyly

+ **Q70.0 Fused fingers**
   Complex syndactyly of fingers with synostosis
   Q70.00 Fused fingers, unspecified hand
   Q70.01 Fused fingers, right hand
   Q70.02 Fused fingers, left hand
   Q70.03 Fused fingers, bilateral
+ **Q70.1 Webbed fingers**
   Simple syndactyly of fingers without synostosis
   Q70.10 Webbed fingers, unspecified hand
   Q70.11 Webbed fingers, right hand
   Q70.12 Webbed fingers, left hand
   Q70.13 Webbed fingers, bilateral
+ **Q70.2 Fused toes**
   Complex syndactyly of toes with synostosis
   Q70.20 Fused toes, unspecified foot
   Q70.21 Fused toes, right foot
   Q70.22 Fused toes, left foot
   Q70.23 Fused toes, bilateral

+ **Q70.3** **Webbed toes**
  Simple syndactyly of toes without synostosis
  Q70.30 **Webbed toes, unspecified foot**
  Q70.31 **Webbed toes, right foot**
  Q70.32 **Webbed toes, left foot**
  Q70.33 **Webbed toes, bilateral**
Q70.4 **Polysyndactyly, unspecified**
  Excludes1: *specified syndactyly of hand and feet - code to*
  specified conditions (Q70.0-Q70.3-)
Q70.9 **Syndactyly, unspecified**
  Symphalangy NOS

Q71 **Reduction defects of upper limb**

+ **Q71.0** **Congenital complete absence of upper limb**
  Q71.00 **Congenital complete absence of unspecified upper limb**
  Q71.01 **Congenital complete absence of right upper limb**
  Q71.02 **Congenital complete absence of left upper limb**
  Q71.03 **Congenital complete absence of upper limb, bilateral**
+ **Q71.1** **Congenital absence of upper arm and forearm with hand present**
  Q71.10 **Congenital absence of unspecified upper arm and forearm with hand present**
  Q71.11 **Congenital absence of right upper arm and forearm with hand present**
  Q71.12 **Congenital absence of left upper arm and forearm with hand present**
  Q71.13 **Congenital absence of upper arm and forearm with hand present, bilateral**
+ **Q71.2** **Congenital absence of both forearm and hand**
  Q71.20 **Congenital absence of both forearm and hand, unspecified upper limb**
  Q71.21 **Congenital absence of both forearm and hand, right upper limb**
  Q71.22 **Congenital absence of both forearm and hand, left upper limb**
  Q71.23 **Congenital absence of both forearm and hand, bilateral**
+ **Q71.3** **Congenital absence of hand and finger**
  Q71.30 **Congenital absence of unspecified hand and finger**
  Q71.31 **Congenital absence of right hand and finger**
  Q71.32 **Congenital absence of left hand and finger**
  Q71.33 **Congenital absence of hand and finger, bilateral**
+ **Q71.4** **Longitudinal reduction defect of radius**
  Clubhand (congenital)
  Radial clubhand
  Q71.40 **Longitudinal reduction defect of unspecified radius**
  Q71.41 **Longitudinal reduction defect of right radius**
  Q71.42 **Longitudinal reduction defect of left radius**
  Q71.43 **Longitudinal reduction defect of radius, bilateral**
+ **Q71.5** **Longitudinal reduction defect of ulna**
  Q71.50 **Longitudinal reduction defect of unspecified ulna**
  Q71.51 **Longitudinal reduction defect of right ulna**
  Q71.52 **Longitudinal reduction defect of left ulna**
  Q71.53 **Longitudinal reduction defect of ulna, bilateral**
+ **Q71.6** **Lobster-claw hand**
  Q71.60 **Lobster-claw hand, unspecified hand**
  Q71.61 **Lobster-claw right hand**
  Q71.62 **Lobster-claw left hand**
  Q71.63 **Lobster-claw hand, bilateral**
+ **Q71.8** **Other reduction defects of upper limb**
  + **Q71.81** **Congenital shortening of upper limb**
    Q71.811 **Congenital shortening of right upper limb**
    Q71.812 **Congenital shortening of left upper limb**
    Q71.813 **Congenital shortening of upper limb, bilateral**
    Q71.819 **Congenital shortening of unspecified upper limb**
  + **Q71.89** **Other reduction defects of upper limb**
    Q71.891 **Other reduction defects of right upper limb**
    Q71.892 **Other reduction defects of left upper limb**
    Q71.893 **Other reduction defects of upper limb, bilateral**
    Q71.899 **Other reduction defects of unspecified upper limb**

+ **Q71.9** **Unspecified reduction defect of upper limb**
  Q71.90 **Unspecified reduction defect of unspecified upper limb**
  Q71.91 **Unspecified reduction defect of right upper limb**
  Q71.92 **Unspecified reduction defect of left upper limb**
  Q71.93 **Unspecified reduction defect of upper limb, bilateral**

Q72 **Reduction defects of lower limb**

+ **Q72.0** **Congenital complete absence of lower limb**
  Q72.00 **Congenital complete absence of unspecified lower limb**
  Q72.01 **Congenital complete absence of right lower limb**
  Q72.02 **Congenital complete absence of left lower limb**
  Q72.03 **Congenital complete absence of lower limb, bilateral**
+ **Q72.1** **Congenital absence of thigh and lower leg with foot present**
  Q72.10 **Congenital absence of unspecified thigh and lower leg with foot present**
  Q72.11 **Congenital absence of right thigh and lower leg with foot present**
  Q72.12 **Congenital absence of left thigh and lower leg with foot present**
  Q72.13 **Congenital absence of thigh and lower leg with foot present, bilateral**
+ **Q72.2** **Congenital absence of both lower leg and foot**
  Q72.20 **Congenital absence of both lower leg and foot, unspecified lower limb**
  Q72.21 **Congenital absence of both lower leg and foot, right lower limb**
  Q72.22 **Congenital absence of both lower leg and foot, left lower limb**
  Q72.23 **Congenital absence of both lower leg and foot, bilateral**
+ **Q72.3** **Congenital absence of foot and toe(s)**
  Q72.30 **Congenital absence of unspecified foot and toe(s)**
  Q72.31 **Congenital absence of right foot and toe(s)**
  Q72.32 **Congenital absence of left foot and toe(s)**
  Q72.33 **Congenital absence of foot and toe(s), bilateral**
+ **Q72.4** **Longitudinal reduction defect of femur**
  Proximal femoral focal deficiency
  Q72.40 **Longitudinal reduction defect of unspecified femur**
  Q72.41 **Longitudinal reduction defect of right femur**
  Q72.42 **Longitudinal reduction defect of left femur**
  Q72.43 **Longitudinal reduction defect of femur, bilateral**
+ **Q72.5** **Longitudinal reduction defect of tibia**
  Q72.50 **Longitudinal reduction defect of unspecified tibia**
  Q72.51 **Longitudinal reduction defect of right tibia**
  Q72.52 **Longitudinal reduction defect of left tibia**
  Q72.53 **Longitudinal reduction defect of tibia, bilateral**
+ **Q72.6** **Longitudinal reduction defect of fibula**
  Q72.60 **Longitudinal reduction defect of unspecified fibula**
  Q72.61 **Longitudinal reduction defect of right fibula**
  Q72.62 **Longitudinal reduction defect of left fibula**
  Q72.63 **Longitudinal reduction defect of fibula, bilateral**
+ **Q72.7** **Split foot**
  Q72.70 **Split foot, unspecified lower limb**
  Q72.71 **Split foot, right lower limb**
  Q72.72 **Split foot, left lower limb**
  Q72.73 **Split foot, bilateral**
+ **Q72.8** **Other reduction defects of lower limb**
  + **Q72.81** **Congenital shortening of lower limb**
    Q72.811 **Congenital shortening of right lower limb**
    Q72.812 **Congenital shortening of left lower limb**
    Q72.813 **Congenital shortening of lower limb, bilateral**
    Q72.819 **Congenital shortening of unspecified lower limb**
  + **Q72.89** **Other reduction defects of lower limb**
    Q72.891 **Other reduction defects of right lower limb**
    Q72.892 **Other reduction defects of left lower limb**
    Q72.893 **Other reduction defects of lower limb, bilateral**
    Q72.899 **Other reduction defects of unspecified lower limb**

+, +7th, X + 7th • Newborn • Pediatric • Maternity • Adult ♀ Female ♂ Male Manifestation Unacceptable PDX HCC CC MCC HAC

+ **Q72.9 Unspecified reduction defect of lower limb**
  - **Q72.90 Unspecified reduction defect of unspecified lower limb**
  - **Q72.91 Unspecified reduction defect of right lower limb**
  - **Q72.92 Unspecified reduction defect of left lower limb**
  - **Q72.93 Unspecified reduction defect of lower limb, bilateral**

Q73 Reduction defects of unspecified limb

- **Q73.0 Congenital absence of unspecified limb(s)**
  - Amelia NOS
- **Q73.1 Phocomelia, unspecified limb(s)**
  - Phocomelia NOS
- **Q73.8 Other reduction defects of unspecified limb(s)**
  - Longitudinal reduction deformity of unspecified limb(s)
  - Ectromelia of limb NOS
  - Hemimelia of limb NOS
  - Reduction defect of limb NOS

Q74 Other congenital malformations of limb(s)

- **Excludes1:** *polydactyly (Q69.-)*
  - *reduction defect of limb (Q71-Q73)*
  - *syndactyly (Q70.-)*
- **Q74.0 Other congenital malformations of upper limb(s), including shoulder girdle**
  - Accessory carpal bones
  - Cleidocranial dysostosis
  - Congenital pseudarthrosis of clavicle
  - Macrodactylia (fingers)
  - Madelung's deformity
  - Radioulnar synostosis
  - Sprengel's deformity
  - Triphalangeal thumb
- **Q74.1 Congenital malformation of knee**
  - Congenital absence of patella
  - Congenital dislocation of patella
  - Congenital genu valgum
  - Congenital genu varum
  - Rudimentary patella
  - **Excludes1:** *congenital dislocation of knee (Q68.2)*
    - *congenital genu recurvatum (Q68.2)*
    - *nail patella syndrome (Q87.2)*
- **Q74.2 Other congenital malformations of lower limb(s), including pelvic girdle**
  - Congenital fusion of sacroiliac joint
  - Congenital malformation of ankle joint
  - Congenital malformation of sacroiliac joint
  - **Excludes1:** *anteversion of femur (neck) (Q65.89)*
- CC **Q74.3 Arthrogryposis multiplex congenita**
- **Q74.8 Other specified congenital malformations of limb(s)**
- **Q74.9 Unspecified congenital malformation of limb(s)**
  - Congenital anomaly of limb(s) NOS

Q75 Other congenital malformations of skull and face bones

- **Excludes1:** *congenital malformation of face NOS (Q18.-)*
  - *congenital malformation syndromes classified to (Q87.-)*
  - *dentofacial anomalies [including malocclusion] (M26.-)*
  - *musculoskeletal deformities of head and face (Q67.0-Q67.4)*
  - *skull defects associated with congenital anomalies of brain such as:*
    - *anencephaly (Q00.0)*
    - *encephalocele (Q01.-)*
    - *hydrocephalus (Q03.-)*
    - *microcephaly (Q02)*
- **Q75.0 Craniosynostosis**
  - Acrocephaly
  - Imperfect fusion of skull
  - Oxycephaly
  - Trigonocephaly
- **Q75.1 Craniofacial dysostosis**
  - Crouzon's disease
- **Q75.2 Hypertelorism**
- **Q75.3 Macrocephaly**
- **Q75.4 Mandibulofacial dysostosis**
  - Franceschetti syndrome
  - Treacher Collins syndrome
- **Q75.5 Oculomandibular dysostosis**

- **Q75.8 Other specified congenital malformations of skull and face bones**
  - Absence of skull bone, congenital
  - Congenital deformity of forehead
  - Platybasia
- **Q75.9 Congenital malformation of skull and face bones, unspecified**
  - Congenital anomaly of face bones NOS
  - Congenital anomaly of skull NOS

Q76 Congenital malformations of spine and bony thorax

- **Excludes1:** *congenital musculoskeletal deformities of spine and chest (Q67.5-Q67.8)*
- **Q76.0 Spina bifida occulta**
  - **Excludes1:** *meningocele (spinal) (Q05.-)*
    - *spina bifida (aperta) (cystica) (Q05.-)*
- **Q76.1 Klippel-Feil syndrome**
  - Cervical fusion syndrome
- **Q76.2 Congenital spondylolisthesis**
  - Congenital spondylolysis
  - **Excludes1:** *spondylolisthesis (acquired) (M43.1-)*
    - *spondylolysis (acquired) (M43.0-)*
- CC **Q76.3 Congenital scoliosis due to congenital bony malformation**
  - Hemivertebra fusion or failure of segmentation with scoliosis
+ **Q76.4 Other congenital malformations of spine, not associated with scoliosis**
  + **Q76.41 Congenital kyphosis**
    - **Q76.411 Congenital kyphosis, occipito-atlanto-axial region**
    - **Q76.412 Congenital kyphosis, cervical region**
    - **Q76.413 Congenital kyphosis, cervicothoracic region**
    - **Q76.414 Congenital kyphosis, thoracic region**
    - **Q76.415 Congenital kyphosis, thoracolumbar region**
    - **Q76.419 Congenital kyphosis, unspecified region**
  + **Q76.42 Congenital lordosis**
    - CC **Q76.425 Congenital lordosis, thoracolumbar region**
    - CC **Q76.426 Congenital lordosis, lumbar region**
    - CC **Q76.427 Congenital lordosis, lumbosacral region**
    - CC **Q76.428 Congenital lordosis, sacral and sacrococcygeal region**
    - CC **Q76.429 Congenital lordosis, unspecified region**
  - **Q76.49 Other congenital malformations of spine, not associated with scoliosis**
    - Congenital absence of vertebra NOS
    - Congenital fusion of spine NOS
    - Congenital malformation of lumbosacral (joint) (region) NOS
    - Congenital malformation of spine NOS
    - Hemivertebra NOS
    - Malformation of spine NOS
    - Platyspondylisis NOS
    - Supernumerary vertebra NOS
- **Q76.5 Cervical rib**
  - Supernumerary rib in cervical region
- CC **Q76.6 Other congenital malformations of ribs**
  - Accessory rib
  - Congenital absence of rib
  - Congenital fusion of ribs
  - Congenital malformation of ribs NOS
  - **Excludes1:** *short rib syndrome (Q77.2)*
- CC **Q76.7 Congenital malformation of sternum**
  - Congenital absence of sternum
  - Sternum bifidum
- CC **Q76.8 Other congenital malformations of bony thorax**
- CC **Q76.9 Congenital malformation of bony thorax, unspecified**

Q77 **Osteochondrodysplasia with defects of growth of tubular bones and spine**

> *Excludes1:* *mucopolysaccharidosis (E76.0-E76.3)*
> *Excludes2:* *congenital myotonic chondrodystrophy (G71.13)*

   Q77.0 **Achondrogenesis**
      Hypochondrogenesis
   Q77.1 **Thanatophoric short stature**
CC **Q77.2** **Short rib syndrome**
      Asphyxiating thoracic dysplasia [Jeune]
   Q77.3 **Chondrodysplasia punctata**
> *Excludes1:* *Rhizomelic chondrodysplasia punctata (E71.43)*

   Q77.4 **Achondroplasia**
      Hypochondroplasia
      Osteosclerosis congenita
   Q77.5 **Diastrophic dysplasia**
   Q77.6 **Chondroectodermal dysplasia**
      Ellis-van Creveld syndrome
   Q77.7 **Spondyloepiphyseal dysplasia**
   Q77.8 **Other osteochondrodysplasia with defects of growth of tubular bones and spine**
   Q77.9 **Osteochondrodysplasia with defects of growth of tubular bones and spine, unspecified**

Q78 **Other osteochondrodysplasias**

> *Excludes2:* *congenital myotonic chondrodystrophy (G71.13)*

CC **Q78.0** **Osteogenesis imperfecta**
      Fragilitas ossium
      Osteopsathyrosis
   Q78.1 **Polyostotic fibrous dysplasia**
      Albright(-McCune)(-Sternberg) syndrome
CC **Q78.2** **Osteopetrosis**
      Albers-Schönberg syndrome
      Osteosclerosis NOS
   Q78.3 **Progressive diaphyseal dysplasia**
      Camurati-Engelmann syndrome
   Q78.4 **Enchondromatosis**
      Maffucci's syndrome
      Ollier's disease
   Q78.5 **Metaphyseal dysplasia**
      Pyle's syndrome
   Q78.6 **Multiple congenital exostoses**
      Diaphyseal aclasis
   Q78.8 **Other specified osteochondrodysplasias**
      Osteopoikilosis
   Q78.9 **Osteochondrodysplasia, unspecified**
      Chondrodystrophy NOS
      Osteodystrophy NOS

Q79 **Congenital malformations of musculoskeletal system, not elsewhere classified**

> *Excludes2:* *congenital (sternomastoid) torticollis (Q68.0)*

MCC **Q79.0** **Congenital diaphragmatic hernia**
> *Excludes1:* *congenital hiatus hernia (Q40.1)*

MCC **Q79.1** **Other congenital malformations of diaphragm**
      Absence of diaphragm
      Congenital malformation of diaphragm NOS
      Eventration of diaphragm
MCC **Q79.2** **Exomphalos**
      Omphalocele
> *Excludes1:* *umbilical hernia (K42.-)*

MCC **Q79.3** **Gastroschisis**
MCC **Q79.4** **Prune belly syndrome**
      Congenital prolapse of bladder mucosa
      Eagle-Barrett syndrome
+ **Q79.5** **Other congenital malformations of abdominal wall**
> *Excludes1:* *umbilical hernia (K42.-)*

MCC **Q79.51** **Congenital hernia of bladder**
MCC **Q79.59** **Other congenital malformations of abdominal wall**
+ **Q79.6** **Ehlers-Danlos syndromes**
> *AHA CC: 4Q, 2019, 13-14*

CC **Q79.60** **Ehlers-Danlos Syndrome, unspecified**
CC **Q79.61** **Classical Ehlers-Danlos syndrome**
      Classical EDS (cEDS)
CC **Q79.62** **Hypermobile Ehlers-Danlos syndrome**
      Hypermobile EDS (hEDS)
CC **Q79.63** **Vascular Ehlers-Danlas syndrome**
      Vascular EDS (vEDS)
CC **Q79.69** **Other Ehlers-Danlos syndromes**

   Q79.8 **Other congenital malformations of musculoskeletal system**
      Absence of muscle
      Absence of tendon
      Accessory muscle
      Amyotrophia congenita
      Congenital constricting bands
      Congenital shortening of tendon
      Poland syndrome
   Q79.9 **Congenital malformation of musculoskeletal system, unspecified**
      Congenital anomaly of musculoskeletal system NOS
      Congenital deformity of musculoskeletal system NOS

Other congenital malformations (Q80-Q89)

Q80 **Congenital ichthyosis**

> *Excludes1:* *Refsum's disease (G60.1)*

   Q80.0 **Ichthyosis vulgaris**
   Q80.1 **X-linked ichthyosis**
   Q80.2 **Lamellar ichthyosis**
      Collodion baby
   Q80.3 **Congenital bullous ichthyosiform erythroderma**
   Q80.4 **Harlequin fetus**
   Q80.8 **Other congenital ichthyosis**
   Q80.9 **Congenital ichthyosis, unspecified**

Q81 **Epidermolysis bullosa**

   Q81.0 **Epidermolysis bullosa simplex**
> *Excludes1:* *Cockayne's syndrome (Q87.19)*

   Q81.1 **Epidermolysis bullosa letalis**
      Herlitz' syndrome
   Q81.2 **Epidermolysis bullosa dystrophica**
   Q81.8 **Other epidermolysis bullosa**
   Q81.9 **Epidermolysis bullosa, unspecified**

Q82 **Other congenital malformations of skin**

> *Excludes1:* *acrodermatitis enteropathica (E83.2)*
> *congenital erythropoietic porphyria (E80.0)*
> *pilonidal cyst or sinus (L05.-)*
> *Sturge-Weber (-Dimitri) syndrome (Q85.8)*

   Q82.0 **Hereditary lymphedema**
   Q82.1 **Xeroderma pigmentosum**
   Q82.2 **Congenital cutaneous mastocytosis**
      Congenital diffuse cutaneous mastocytosis
      Congenital maculopapular cutaneous mastocytosis
      Congenital urticaria pigmentosa
> *Excludes1:* *cutaneous mastocytosis NOS (D47.01)*
> *diffuse cutaneous mastocytosis (with onset after newborn period) (D47.01)*
> *malignant mastocytosis (C96.2-)*
> *systemic mastocytosis (D47.02)*
> *urticaria pigmentosa (non-congenital) (with onset after newborn period) (D47.01)*

> *AHA CC: 4Q, 2017, 5*

   Q82.3 **Incontinentia pigmenti**
   Q82.4 **Ectodermal dysplasia (anhidrotic)**
> *Excludes1:* *Ellis-van Creveld syndrome (Q77.6)*

   Q82.5 **Congenital non-neoplastic nevus**
      Birthmark NOS
      Flammeus Nevus
      Portwine Nevus
      Sanguineous Nevus
      Strawberry Nevus
      Vascular Nevus NOS
      Verrucous Nevus
> *Excludes2:* *Café au lait spots (L81.3)*
> *lentigo (L81.4)*
> *nevus NOS (D22.-)*
> *araneus nevus (I78.1)*
> *melanocytic nevus (D22.-)*
> *pigmented nevus (D22.-)*
> *spider nevus (I78.1)*
> *stellar nevus (I78.1)*

   Q82.6 **Congenital sacral dimple**
      Parasacral dimple
> *Excludes2:* *pilonidal cyst with abscess (L05.01)*
> *pilonidal cyst without abscess (L05.91)*

> *AHA CC: 4Q, 2016, 60*

Q82.8 Other specified congenital malformations of skin
Abnormal palmar creases
Accessory skin tags
Benign familial pemphigus [Hailey-Hailey]
Congenital poikiloderma
Cutis laxa (hyperelastica)
Dermatoglyphic anomalies
Inherited keratosis palmaris et plantaris
Keratosis follicularis [Darier-White]
Excludes1: *Ehlers-Danlos syndromes (Q79.6-)*
AHA CC: 1Q, 2016, 17

Q82.9 Congenital malformation of skin, unspecified

Q83 Congenital malformations of breast
Excludes2: *absence of pectoral muscle (Q79.8)*
hypoplasia of breast (N64.82)
micromastia (N64.82)

Q83.0 Congenital absence of breast with absent nipple
Q83.1 Accessory breast
Supernumerary breast
Q83.2 Absent nipple
Q83.3 Accessory nipple
Supernumerary nipple
Q83.8 Other congenital malformations of breast
Q83.9 Congenital malformation of breast, unspecified

Q84 Other congenital malformations of integument
Q84.0 Congenital alopecia
Congenital atrichosis
Q84.1 Congenital morphological disturbances of hair, not elsewhere classified
Beaded hair
Monilethrix
Pili annulati
Excludes1: *Menkes' kinky hair syndrome (E83.0)*
Q84.2 Other congenital malformations of hair
Congenital hypertrichosis
Congenital malformation of hair NOS
Persistent lanugo
Q84.3 Anonychia
Excludes1: *nail patella syndrome (Q87.2)*
Q84.4 Congenital leukonychia
Q84.5 Enlarged and hypertrophic nails
Congenital onychauxis
Pachyonychia
Q84.6 Other congenital malformations of nails
Congenital clubnail
Congenital koilonychia
Congenital malformation of nail NOS
Q84.8 Other specified congenital malformations of integument
Aplasia cutis congenita
Q84.9 Congenital malformation of integument, unspecified
Congenital anomaly of integument NOS
Congenital deformity of integument NOS

Q85 Phakomatoses, not elsewhere classified
Excludes1: *ataxia telangiectasia [Louis-Bar] (G11.3)*
familial dysautonomia [Riley-Day] (G90.1)
+ **Q85.0 Neurofibromatosis (nonmalignant)**
Q85.00 Neurofibromatosis, unspecified
Q85.01 Neurofibromatosis, type 1
Von Recklinghausen disease
Q85.02 Neurofibromatosis, type 2
Acoustic neurofibromatosis
Q85.03 Schwannomatosis
Q85.09 Other neurofibromatosis
CC **Q85.1 Tuberous sclerosis**
Bourneville's disease
Epiloia
CC **Q85.8 Other phakomatoses, not elsewhere classified**
Peutz-Jeghers Syndrome
Sturge-Weber(-Dimitri) syndrome
von Hippel-Lindau syndrome
Excludes1: *Meckel-Gruber syndrome (Q61.9)*
CC **Q85.9 Phakomatosis, unspecified**
Hamartosis NOS

Q86 Congenital malformation syndromes due to known exogenous causes, not elsewhere classified
Excludes2: *iodine-deficiency-related hypothyroidism (E00-E02)*
nonteratogenic effects of substances transmitted via placenta or breast milk (P04.-)
Q86.0 Fetal alcohol syndrome (dysmorphic)
Q86.1 Fetal hydantoin syndrome
Meadow's syndrome
Q86.2 Dysmorphism due to warfarin
Q86.8 Other congenital malformation syndromes due to known exogenous causes

Q87 Other specified congenital malformation syndromes affecting multiple systems
Use additional code(s) to identify all associated manifestations
Q87.0 Congenital malformation syndromes predominantly affecting facial appearance
Acrocephalopolysyndactyly
Acrocephalosyndactyly [Apert]
Cryptophthalmos syndrome
Cyclopia
Goldenhar syndrome
Moebius syndrome
Oro-facial-digital syndrome
Robin syndrome
Whistling face
+ **Q87.1 Congenital malformation syndromes predominantly associated with short stature**
Excludes1: *Ellis-van Creveld syndrome (Q77.6)*
Smith-Lemli-Opitz syndrome (E78.72)
AHA CC: 4Q, 2019, 14-15
CC **Q87.11 Prader-Willi syndrome**
CC **Q87.19 Other congenital malformation syndromes predominantly associated with short stature**
Aarskog syndrome
Cockayne syndrome
De Lange syndrome
Dubowitz syndrome
Noonan syndrome
Robinow-Silverman-Smith syndrome
Russell-Silver syndrome
Seckel syndrome
CC **Q87.2 Congenital malformation syndromes predominantly involving limbs**
Holt-Oram syndrome
Klippel-Trenaunay-Weber syndrome
Nail patella syndrome
Rubinstein-Taybi syndrome
Sirenomelia syndrome
Thrombocytopenia with absent radius [TAR] syndrome
VATER syndrome
CC **Q87.3 Congenital malformation syndromes involving early overgrowth**
Beckwith-Wiedemann syndrome
Sotos syndrome
Weaver syndrome
+ **Q87.4 Marfan's syndrome**
CC **Q87.40 Marfan's syndrome, unspecified**
+ **Q87.41 Marfan's syndrome with cardiovascular manifestations**
CC **Q87.410 Marfan's syndrome with aortic dilation**
CC **Q87.418 Marfan's syndrome with other cardiovascular manifestations**
CC **Q87.42 Marfan's syndrome with ocular manifestations**
CC **Q87.43 Marfan's syndrome with skeletal manifestation**
CC **Q87.5 Other congenital malformation syndromes with other skeletal changes**
+ **Q87.8 Other specified congenital malformation syndromes, not elsewhere classified**
Excludes1: *Zellweger syndrome (E71.510)*
CC **Q87.81 Alport syndrome**
Use additional code to identify stage of chronic kidney disease (N18.1-N18.6)
CC **Q87.82 Arterial tortuosity syndrome**
AHA CC: 4Q, 2016, 60-61
CC **Q87.89 Other specified congenital malformation syndromes, not elsewhere classified**
Laurence-Moon (-Bardet)-Biedl syndrome

Q89 Other congenital malformations, not elsewhere classified

+ **Q89.0 Congenital absence and malformations of spleen**
  Excludes1: isomerism of atrial appendages (with asplenia or polysplenia) (Q20.6)
  CC **Q89.01 Asplenia (congenital)**
  CC **Q89.09 Congenital malformations of spleen**
    Congenital splenomegaly

Q89.1 Congenital malformations of adrenal gland
  Excludes1: adrenogenital disorders (E25.-)
      congenital adrenal hyperplasia (E25.0)

Q89.2 Congenital malformations of other endocrine glands
  Congenital malformation of parathyroid or thyroid gland
  Persistent thyroglossal duct
  Thyroglossal cyst
  Excludes1: congenital goiter (E03.0)
      congenital hypothyroidism (E03.1)

CC **Q89.3 Situs inversus**
  Dextrocardia with situs inversus
  Mirror-image atrial arrangement with situs inversus
  Situs inversus or transversus abdominalis
  Situs inversus or transversus thoracis
  Transposition of abdominal viscera
  Transposition of thoracic viscera
  Excludes1: dextrocardia NOS (Q24.0)

MCC **Q89.4 Conjoined twins**
  Craniopagus
  Dicephaly
  Pygopagus
  Thoracopagus

CC **Q89.7 Multiple congenital malformations, not elsewhere classified**
  Multiple congenital anomalies NOS
  Multiple congenital deformities NOS
  Excludes1: congenital malformation syndromes affecting multiple systems (Q87.-)

CC **Q89.8 Other specified congenital malformations**
  Use additional code(s) to identify all associated manifestations

Q89.9 Congenital malformation, unspecified
  Congenital anomaly NOS
  Congenital deformity NOS

Chromosomal abnormalities, not elsewhere classified (Q90-Q99)

Excludes2: mitochondrial metabolic disorders (E88.4-)

Q90 Down syndrome

  Use additional code(s) to identify any associated physical conditions and degree of intellectual disabilities (F70-F79)

  Q90.0 Trisomy 21, nonmosaicism (meiotic nondisjunction)
  Q90.1 Trisomy 21, mosaicism (mitotic nondisjunction)
  Q90.2 Trisomy 21, translocation
  Q90.9 Down syndrome, unspecified
    Trisomy 21 NOS

Q91 Trisomy 18 and Trisomy 13

  CC **Q91.0 Trisomy 18, nonmosaicism (meiotic nondisjunction)**
  CC **Q91.1 Trisomy 18, mosaicism (mitotic nondisjunction)**
  CC **Q91.2 Trisomy 18, translocation**
  CC **Q91.3 Trisomy 18, unspecified**
  CC **Q91.4 Trisomy 13, nonmosaicism (meiotic nondisjunction)**
  CC **Q91.5 Trisomy 13, mosaicism (mitotic nondisjunction)**
  CC **Q91.6 Trisomy 13, translocation**
  CC **Q91.7 Trisomy 13, unspecified**

Q92 Other trisomies and partial trisomies of the autosomes, not elsewhere classified

  Includes: unbalanced translocations and insertions
  Excludes1: trisomies of chromosomes 13, 18, 21 (Q90-Q91)
  Q92.0 Whole chromosome trisomy, nonmosaicism (meiotic nondisjunction)
  Q92.1 Whole chromosome trisomy, mosaicism (mitotic nondisjunction)
  Q92.2 Partial trisomy
    Less than whole arm duplicated
    Whole arm or more duplicated
    Excludes1: partial trisomy due to unbalanced translocation (Q92.5)
  Q92.5 Duplications with other complex rearrangements
    Partial trisomy due to unbalanced translocations
    Code also any associated deletions due to unbalanced translocations, inversions and insertions (Q93.7)

+ **Q92.6 Marker chromosomes**
    Trisomies due to dicentrics
    Trisomies due to extra rings
    Trisomies due to isochromosomes
    Individual with marker heterochromatin
    Q92.61 Marker chromosomes in normal individual
    Q92.62 Marker chromosomes in abnormal individual
  Q92.7 Triploidy and polyploidy
  Q92.8 Other specified trisomies and partial trisomies of autosomes
    Duplications identified by fluorescence in situ hybridization (FISH)
    Duplications identified by in situ hybridization (ISH)
    Duplications seen only at prometaphase
  Q92.9 Trisomy and partial trisomy of autosomes, unspecified

Q93 Monosomies and deletions from the autosomes, not elsewhere classified

  Q93.0 Whole chromosome monosomy, nonmosaicism (meiotic nondisjunction)
  Q93.1 Whole chromosome monosomy, mosaicism (mitotic nondisjunction)
  Q93.2 Chromosome replaced with ring, dicentric or isochromosome
  CC **Q93.3 Deletion of short arm of chromosome 4**
    Wolff-Hirschorn syndrome
  CC **Q93.4 Deletion of short arm of chromosome 5**
    Cri-du-chat syndrome
  + **Q93.5 Other deletions of part of a chromosome**
    AHA CC: 4Q, 2018, 28
    CC **Q93.51 Angelman syndrome**
    CC **Q93.59 Other deletions of part of a chromosome**
  CC **Q93.7 Deletions with other complex rearrangements**
    Deletions due to unbalanced translocations, inversions and insertions
    Code also any associated duplications due to unbalanced translocations, inversions and insertions (Q92.5)
  + **Q93.8 Other deletions from the autosomes**
    MCC **Q93.81 Velo-cardio-facial syndrome**
      Deletion 22q11.2
      AHA CC: 3Q, 2019, 14-15
    CC **Q93.82 Williams syndrome**
      AHA CC: 4Q, 2018, 28-29
    CC **Q93.88 Other microdeletions**
      Miller-Dieker syndrome
      Smith-Magenis syndrome
    CC **Q93.89 Other deletions from the autosomes**
      Deletions identified by fluorescence in situ hybridization (FISH)
      Deletions identified by in situ hybridization (ISH)
      Deletions seen only at prometaphase
  CC **Q93.9 Deletion from autosomes, unspecified**

Q95 Balanced rearrangements and structural markers, not elsewhere classified

  Includes: Robertsonian and balanced reciprocal translocations and insertions
  Q95.0 Balanced translocation and insertion in normal individual
  Q95.1 Chromosome inversion in normal individual
  Q95.2 Balanced autosomal rearrangement in abnormal individual
  Q95.3 Balanced sex/autosomal rearrangement in abnormal individual
  Q95.5 Individual with autosomal fragile site
  Q95.8 Other balanced rearrangements and structural markers
  Q95.9 Balanced rearrangement and structural marker, unspecified

Q96 Turner's syndrome

  Excludes1: Noonan syndrome (Q87.19)
  ♀ **Q96.0 Karyotype 45, X**
  ♀ **Q96.1 Karyotype 46, X iso (Xq)**
    Karyotype 46, isochromosome Xq
  ♀ **Q96.2 Karyotype 46, X with abnormal sex chromosome, except iso (Xq)**
    Karyotype 46, X with abnormal sex chromosome, except isochromosome Xq
  ♀ **Q96.3 Mosaicism, 45, X/46, XX or XY**
  ♀ **Q96.4 Mosaicism, 45, X/other cell line(s) with abnormal sex chromosome**
  ♀ **Q96.8 Other variants of Turner's syndrome**
  ♀ **Q96.9 Turner's syndrome, unspecified**

+, +7th, X + 7th   ● Newborn   ● Pediatric   ● Maternity   ● Adult   ♀ Female   ♂ Male   Manifestation   Unacceptable PDX   HCC   CC   MCC   HAC

Q97 Other sex chromosome abnormalities, female phenotype, not elsewhere classified

   Excludes1: Turner's syndrome (Q96.-)

♀ **Q97.0 Karyotype 47, XXX**

♀ **Q97.1 Female with more than three X chromosomes**

♀ **Q97.2 Mosaicism, lines with various numbers of X chromosomes**

♀ **Q97.3 Female with 46, XY karyotype**

♀ **Q97.8 Other specified sex chromosome abnormalities, female phenotype**

♀ **Q97.9 Sex chromosome abnormality, female phenotype, unspecified**

Q98 Other sex chromosome abnormalities, male phenotype, not elsewhere classified

♂ **Q98.0 Klinefelter syndrome karyotype 47, XXY**

♂ **Q98.1 Klinefelter syndrome, male with more than two X chromosomes**

♂ **Q98.3 Other male with 46, XX karyotype**

♂ **Q98.4 Klinefelter syndrome, unspecified**

♂ **Q98.5 Karyotype 47, XYY**

♂ **Q98.6 Male with structurally abnormal sex chromosome**

♂ **Q98.7 Male with sex chromosome mosaicism**

♂ **Q98.8 Other specified sex chromosome abnormalities, male phenotype**

♂ **Q98.9 Sex chromosome abnormality, male phenotype, unspecified**

Q99 Other chromosome abnormalities, not elsewhere classified

Q99.0 Chimera 46, XX/46, XY

   Chimera 46, XX/46, XY true hermaphrodite

Q99.1 46, XX true hermaphrodite

   46, XX with streak gonads

   46, XY with streak gonads

   Pure gonadal dysgenesis

Q99.2 Fragile X chromosome

   Fragile X syndrome

Q99.8 Other specified chromosome abnormalities

Q99.9 Chromosomal abnormality, unspecified

+, +7th, X + 7th   ● Newborn   ● Pediatric   ● Maternity   ● Adult   ♀ Female   ♂ Male   Manifestation   Unacceptable PDX   HCC   CC   MCC   HAC

Chapter 18: Symptoms, Signs and Abnormal Clinical and Laboratory Findings, Not Elsewhere Classified (R00-R99)

NOTE This chapter includes symptoms, signs, abnormal results of clinical or other investigative procedures, and ill-defined conditions regarding which no diagnosis classifiable elsewhere is recorded.

Signs and symptoms that point rather definitely to a given diagnosis have been assigned to a category in other chapters of the classification. In general, categories in this chapter include the less well-defined conditions and symptoms that, without the necessary study of the case to establish a final diagnosis, point perhaps equally to two or more diseases or to two or more systems of the body. Practically all categories in the chapter could be designated 'not otherwise specified', 'unknown etiology' or 'transient'. The Alphabetical Index should be consulted to determine which symptoms and signs are to be allocated here and which to other chapters. The residual subcategories, numbered .8, are generally provided for other relevant symptoms that cannot be allocated elsewhere in the classification.

The conditions and signs or symptoms included in categories R00-R94 consist of:
(a) cases for which no more specific diagnosis can be made even after all the facts bearing on the case have been investigated;
(b) signs or symptoms existing at the time of initial encounter that proved to be transient and whose causes could not be determined;
(c) provisional diagnosis in a patient who failed to return for further investigation or care;
(d) cases referred elsewhere for investigation or treatment before the diagnosis was made;
(e) cases in which a more precise diagnosis was not available for any other reason;
(f) certain symptoms, for which supplementary information is provided, that represent important problems in medical care in their own right.

Excludes2: *abnormal findings on antenatal screening of mother (O28.-)*
certain conditions originating in the perinatal period (P04-P96)
signs and symptoms classified in the body system chapters
signs and symptoms of breast (N63, N64.5)

This chapter contains the following category blocks:

R00-R09 Symptoms and signs involving the circulatory and respiratory systems
R10-R19 Symptoms and signs involving the digestive system and abdomen
R20-R23 Symptoms and signs involving the skin and subcutaneous tissue
R25-R29 Symptoms and signs involving the nervous and musculoskeletal systems
R30-R39 Symptoms and signs involving the genitourinary system
R40-R46 Symptoms and signs involving cognition, perception, emotional state and behavior
R47-R49 Symptoms and signs involving speech and voice
R50-R69 General symptoms and signs
R70-R79 Abnormal findings on examination of blood, without diagnosis
R80-R82 Abnormal findings on examination of urine, without diagnosis
R83-R89 Abnormal findings on examination of other body fluids, substances and tissues, without diagnosis
R90-R94 Abnormal findings on diagnostic imaging and in function studies, without diagnosis
R97 Abnormal tumor markers
R99 Ill-defined and unknown cause of mortality

C. Chapter-Specific Coding Guidelines

In addition to general coding guidelines, there are guidelines for specific diagnoses and/or conditions in the classification. Unless otherwise indicated, these guidelines apply to all health care settings. Please refer to Section II for guidelines on the selection of principal diagnosis.

18. Chapter 18: Symptoms, Signs, and Abnormal Clinical and Laboratory Findings, Not Elsewhere Classified (R00-R99)

Chapter 18 includes symptoms, signs, abnormal results of clinical or other investigative procedures, and ill-defined conditions regarding which no diagnosis classifiable elsewhere is recorded. Signs and symptoms that point to a specific diagnosis have been assigned to a category in other chapters of the classification.

a. Use of symptom codes

Codes that describe symptoms and signs are acceptable for reporting purposes when a related definitive diagnosis has not been established (confirmed) by the provider.

b. Use of a symptom code with a definitive diagnosis code

Codes for signs and symptoms may be reported in addition to a related definitive diagnosis when the sign or symptom is not routinely associated with that diagnosis, such as the various signs and symptoms associated with complex syndromes. The definitive diagnosis code should be sequenced before the symptom code.

Signs or symptoms that are associated routinely with a disease process should not be assigned as additional codes, unless otherwise instructed by the classification.

c. Combination codes that include symptoms

ICD-10-CM contains a number of combination codes that identify both the definitive diagnosis and common symptoms of that diagnosis. When using one of these combination codes, an additional code should not be assigned for the symptom.

d. Repeated falls

Code R29.6, Repeated falls, is for use for encounters when a patient has recently fallen and the reason for the fall is being investigated.

Code Z91.81, History of falling, is for use when a patient has fallen in the past and is at risk for future falls. When appropriate, both codes R29.6 and Z91.81 may be assigned together.

e. Coma scale

The coma scale codes (R40.2-) can be used in conjunction with traumatic brain injury codes, acute cerebrovascular disease or sequelae of cerebrovascular disease codes. These codes are primarily for use by trauma registries, but they may be used in any setting where this information is collected. The coma scale may also be used to assess the status of the central nervous system for other non-trauma conditions, such as monitoring patients in the intensive care unit regardless of medical conditions. The coma scale codes should be sequenced after the diagnosis code(s).

These codes, one from each subcategory, are needed to complete the scale. The 7th character indicates when the scale was recorded. The 7th character should match for all three codes.

At a minimum, report the initial score documented on presentation at your facility. This may be a score from the emergency medicine technician (EMT) or in the emergency department. If desired, a facility may choose to capture multiple coma scale scores.

Assign code R40.24, Glasgow coma scale, total score, when only the total score is documented in the medical record and not the individual score(s).

Do not report codes for individual or total Glasgow coma scale scores for a patient with a medically induced coma or a sedated patient.

See Section I.B.14 for coma scale documentation by clinicians other than the patient's provider.

f. Functional quadriplegia

GUIDELINE HAS BEEN DELETED EFFECTIVE OCTOBER 1, 2017

g. SIRS due to Non-Infectious Process

The systemic inflammatory response syndrome (SIRS) can develop as a result of certain non-infectious disease processes, such as trauma, malignant neoplasm, or pancreatitis. When SIRS is documented with a noninfectious condition, and no subsequent infection is documented, the code for the underlying condition, such as an injury, should be assigned, followed by code R65.10, Systemic inflammatory response syndrome (SIRS) of non-infectious origin without acute organ dysfunction, or code R65.11, Systemic inflammatory response syndrome (SIRS) of non-infectious origin with acute organ dysfunction. If an associated acute organ dysfunction is documented, the appropriate code(s) for the specific type of organ dysfunction(s) should be assigned in addition to code R65.11. If acute organ dysfunction is documented, but it cannot be determined if the acute organ dysfunction is associated with SIRS or due to another condition (e.g., directly due to the trauma), the provider should be queried.

h. Death NOS

Code R99, Ill-defined and unknown cause of mortality, is only for use in the very limited circumstance when a patient who has already died is brought into an emergency department or other healthcare facility and is pronounced dead upon arrival. It does not represent the discharge disposition of death.

+, +7th, X + 7th ● Newborn ● Pediatric ● Maternity ● Adult ♀ Female ♂ Male Manifestation Unacceptable PDX HCC CC MCC HAC

i. NIHSS Stroke Scale

The NIH stroke scale (NIHSS) codes (R29.7--) can be used in conjunction with acute stroke codes (I63) to identify the patient's neurological status and the severity of the stroke. The stroke scale codes should be sequenced after the acute stroke diagnosis code(s).

At a minimum, report the initial score documented. If desired, a facility may choose to capture multiple stroke scale scores.

See Section I.B.14 for NIHSS stroke scale documentation by clinicians other than patient's provider.

Symptoms and signs involving the circulatory and respiratory systems (R00-R09)

R00 Abnormalities of heart beat

> *Excludes1:* abnormalities originating in the perinatal period (P29.1-)
>
> *Excludes2:* specified arrhythmias (I47-I49)

R00.0 Tachycardia, unspecified
Rapid heart beat
Sinoauricular tachycardia NOS
Sinus [sinusal] tachycardia NOS
> *Excludes1:* neonatal tachycardia (P29.11)
> paroxysmal tachycardia (I47.-)

R00.1 Bradycardia, unspecified
Sinoatrial bradycardia
Sinus bradycardia
Slow heart beat
Systolic murmur NOS
Vagal bradycardia
Use additional code for adverse effect, if applicable, to identify drug (T36-T50 with fifth or sixth character 5)
> *Excludes1:* neonatal bradycardia (P29.12)
> *AHA CC: 2Q, 2020, 23-24*

R00.2 Palpitations
Awareness of heart beat

R00.8 Other abnormalities of heart beat

R00.9 Unspecified abnormalities of heart beat

R01 Cardiac murmurs and other cardiac sounds

> *Excludes1:* cardiac murmurs and sounds originating in the perinatal period (P29.8)

R01.0 Benign and innocent cardiac murmurs
Functional cardiac murmur

R01.1 Cardiac murmur, unspecified
Cardiac bruit NOS
Heart murmur NOS
Systolic murmur NOS

R01.2 Other cardiac sounds
Cardiac dullness, increased or decreased
Precordial friction

R03 Abnormal blood-pressure reading, without diagnosis

R03.0 Elevated blood-pressure reading, without diagnosis of hypertension
> **NOTE** This category is to be used to record an episode of elevated blood pressure in a patient in whom no formal diagnosis of hypertension has been made, or as an isolated incidental finding.
> *Review coding guideline C.9.a.7*

R03.1 Nonspecific low blood-pressure reading
> *Excludes1:* hypotension (I95.-)
> maternal hypotension syndrome (O26.5-)
> neurogenic orthostatic hypotension (G90.3)

R04 Hemorrhage from respiratory passages

R04.0 Epistaxis
Hemorrhage from nose
Nosebleed
AHA CC: 4Q, 2018, 38

R04.1 Hemorrhage from throat
> *Excludes2:* hemoptysis (R04.2)

CC R04.2 Hemoptysis
Blood-stained sputum
Cough with hemorrhage
AHA CC: 4Q, 2013, 118

+ R04.8 Hemorrhage from other sites in respiratory passages

• CC R04.81 Acute idiopathic pulmonary hemorrhage in infants
AIPHI
Acute idiopathic hemorrhage in infants over 28 days old
> *Excludes1:* perinatal pulmonary hemorrhage (P26.-)
> von Willebrand's disease (D68.0)

CC R04.89 Hemorrhage from other sites in respiratory passages
Pulmonary hemorrhage NOS

CC R04.9 Hemorrhage from respiratory passages, unspecified

R05 Cough

> *Excludes1:* cough with hemorrhage (R04.2)
> smoker's cough (J41.0)
> *AHA CC: 2Q, 2016, 34; 1Q, 2020, 34-36*

Valid 3-character code, no further characters required

R06 Abnormalities of breathing

> *Excludes1:* acute respiratory distress syndrome (J80)
> respiratory arrest (R09.2)
> respiratory arrest of newborn (P28.81)
> respiratory distress syndrome of newborn (P22.-)
> respiratory failure (J96.-)
> respiratory failure of newborn (P28.5)

+ R06.0 Dyspnea
> *Excludes1:* tachypnea NOS (R06.82)
> transient tachypnea of newborn (P22.1)

R06.00 Dyspnea, unspecified
AHA CC: 1Q, 2017, 26-27

R06.01 Orthopnea

R06.02 Shortness of breath
AHA CC: 1Q, 2020, 34-36

R06.03 Acute respiratory distress
AHA CC: 4Q, 2017, 23

R06.09 Other forms of dyspnea

R06.1 Stridor
> *Excludes1:* congenital laryngeal stridor (P28.89)
> laryngismus (stridulus) (J38.5)

R06.2 Wheezing
> *Excludes1:* Asthma (J45.-)
> *AHA CC: 2Q, 2016, 34*

CC R06.3 Periodic breathing
Cheyne-Stokes breathing

R06.4 Hyperventilation
> *Excludes1:* psychogenic hyperventilation (F45.8)

R06.5 Mouth breathing
> *Excludes2:* dry mouth NOS (R68.2)

R06.6 Hiccough
> *Excludes1:* psychogenic hiccough (F45.8)

R06.7 Sneezing

+ R06.8 Other abnormalities of breathing

R06.81 Apnea, not elsewhere classified
Apnea NOS
> *Excludes1:* apnea (of) newborn (P28.4)
> sleep apnea (G47.3-)
> sleep apnea of newborn (primary) (P28.3)

R06.82 Tachypnea, not elsewhere classified
Tachypnea NOS
> *Excludes1:* transitory tachypnea of newborn (P22.1)

R06.83 Snoring

R06.89 Other abnormalities of breathing
Breath-holding (spells)
Sighing

R06.9 Unspecified abnormalities of breathing

R07 Pain in throat and chest

> *Excludes1:* epidemic myalgia (B33.0)
> *Excludes2:* jaw pain (R68.84)
> pain in breast (N64.4)

R07.0 Pain in throat
> *Excludes1:* chronic sore throat (J31.2)
> sore throat (acute) NOS (J02.9)
> *Excludes2:* dysphagia (R13.1-)
> pain in neck (M54.2)

R07.1 **Chest pain on breathing**
   Painful respiration
R07.2 **Precordial pain**
+ **R07.8** **Other chest pain**
   R07.81 **Pleurodynia**
      Pleurodynia NOS
      Excludes1: *epidemic pleurodynia (B33.0)*
   R07.82 **Intercostal pain**
   R07.89 **Other chest pain**
      Anterior chest-wall pain NOS
R07.9 **Chest pain, unspecified**

R09 **Other symptoms and signs involving the circulatory and respiratory system**

   Excludes1: *acute respiratory distress syndrome (J80)*
      respiratory arrest of newborn (P28.81)
      respiratory distress syndrome of newborn (P22.0)
      respiratory failure (J96.-)
      respiratory failure of newborn (P28.5)
+ **R09.0** **Asphyxia and hypoxemia**
   Excludes1: *asphyxia due to carbon monoxide (T58.-)*
      asphyxia due to foreign body in respiratory
         tract (T17.-)
      birth (intrauterine) asphyxia (P84)
      hyperventilation (R06.4)
      traumatic asphyxia (T71-)
   Excludes2: *hypercapnia (R06.89)*
   CC **R09.01** **Asphyxia**
   R09.02 **Hypoxemia**
      AHA CC: 3Q, 2019, 15
R09.1 **Pleurisy**
   Excludes1: *pleurisy with effusion (J90)*
MCC **R09.2** **Respiratory arrest**
   Cardiorespiratory failure
   Excludes1: *cardiac arrest (I46.-)*
      respiratory arrest of newborn (P28.81)
      respiratory distress of newborn (P22.0)
      respiratory failure (J96.-)
      respiratory failure of newborn (P28.5)
      respiratory insufficiency (R06.89)
      respiratory insufficiency of newborn (P28.5)
R09.3 **Abnormal sputum**
   Abnormal amount of sputum
   Abnormal color of sputum
   Abnormal odor of sputum
   Excessive sputum
   Excludes1: *blood-stained sputum (R04.2)*
+ **R09.8** **Other specified symptoms and signs involving the circulatory and respiratory systems**
   R09.81 **Nasal congestion**
   R09.82 **Postnasal drip**
   R09.89 **Other specified symptoms and signs involving the circulatory and respiratory systems**
      Bruit (arterial)
      Abnormal chest percussion
      Feeling of foreign body in throat
      Friction sounds in chest
      Chest tympany
      Choking sensation
      Rales
      Weak pulse
      Excludes2: *foreign body in throat (T17.2-)*
         wheezing (R06.2)

Symptoms and signs involving the digestive system and abdomen (R10-R19)

Excludes2: *congenital or infantile pylorospasm (Q40.0)*
   gastrointestinal hemorrhage (K92.0-K92.2)
   intestinal obstruction (K56.-)
   newborn gastrointestinal hemorrhage (P54.0-P54.3)
   newborn intestinal obstruction (P76.-)
   pylorospasm (K31.3)
   signs and symptoms involving the urinary system (R30-R39)
   symptoms referable to female genital organs (N94.-)
   symptoms referable to male genital organs male (N48-N50)

R10 **Abdominal and pelvic pain**

   Excludes1: *renal colic (N23)*
   Excludes2: *dorsalgia (M54.-)*
      flatulence and related conditions (R14.-)

R10.0 **Acute abdomen**
   Severe abdominal pain (generalized) (with abdominal rigidity)
   Excludes1: *abdominal rigidity NOS (R19.3)*
      generalized abdominal pain NOS (R10.84)
      localized abdominal pain (R10.1-R10.3-)
+ **R10.1** **Pain localized to upper abdomen**
   R10.10 **Upper abdominal pain, unspecified**
   R10.11 **Right upper quadrant pain**
   R10.12 **Left upper quadrant pain**
   R10.13 **Epigastric pain**
      Dyspepsia
      Excludes1: *functional dyspepsia (K30)*
R10.2 **Pelvic and perineal pain**
   Excludes1: *vulvodynia (N94.81)*
+ **R10.3** **Pain localized to other parts of lower abdomen**
   R10.30 **Lower abdominal pain, unspecified**
   R10.31 **Right lower quadrant pain**
   R10.32 **Left lower quadrant pain**
   R10.33 **Periumbilical pain**
+ **R10.8** **Other abdominal pain**
   + **R10.81** **Abdominal tenderness**
      Abdominal tenderness NOS
      R10.811 **Right upper quadrant abdominal tenderness**
      R10.812 **Left upper quadrant abdominal tenderness**
      R10.813 **Right lower quadrant abdominal tenderness**
      R10.814 **Left lower quadrant abdominal tenderness**
      R10.815 **Periumbilic abdominal tenderness**
      R10.816 **Epigastric abdominal tenderness**
      R10.817 **Generalized abdominal tenderness**
      R10.819 **Abdominal tenderness, unspecified site**
   + **R10.82** **Rebound abdominal tenderness**
      R10.821 **Right upper quadrant rebound abdominal tenderness**
      R10.822 **Left upper quadrant rebound abdominal tenderness**
      R10.823 **Right lower quadrant rebound abdominal tenderness**
      R10.824 **Left lower quadrant rebound abdominal tenderness**
      R10.825 **Periumbilic rebound abdominal tenderness**
      R10.826 **Epigastric rebound abdominal tenderness**
      R10.827 **Generalized rebound abdominal tenderness**
      R10.829 **Rebound abdominal tenderness, unspecified site**
   • **R10.83** **Colic**
      Colic NOS
      Infantile colic
      Excludes1: *colic in adult and child over 12 months old (R10.84)*
   R10.84 **Generalized abdominal pain**
      Excludes1: *generalized abdominal pain associated with acute abdomen (R10.0)*
R10.9 **Unspecified abdominal pain**

R11 **Nausea and vomiting**

   Excludes1: *cyclical vomiting associated with migraine (G43.A-)*
      excessive vomiting in pregnancy (O21.-)
      hematemesis (K92.0)
      neonatal hematemesis (P54.0)
      newborn vomiting (P92.0-)
      psychogenic vomiting (F50.89)
      vomiting associated with bulimia nervosa (F50.2)
      vomiting following gastrointestinal surgery (K91.0)
   AHA CC: 1Q, 2017, 28
R11.0 **Nausea**
   Nausea NOS
   Nausea without vomiting

+, +7th, X + 7th   ● Newborn   ● Pediatric   ● Maternity   ● Adult   ♀ Female   ♂ Male   Manifestation   Unacceptable PDX   HCC   CC   MCC   HAC

+ **R11.1 Vomiting**
  - **R11.10 Vomiting, unspecified**
    - Vomiting NOS
  - **R11.11 Vomiting without nausea**
  - **R11.12 Projectile vomiting**
  - **R11.13 Vomiting of fecal matter**
  - **R11.14 Bilious vomiting**
    - Bilious emesis
  - **R11.15 Cyclical vomiting syndrome unrelated to migraine**
    - Cyclic vomiting syndrome NOS
    - Persistent vomiting
    - *Excludes1: cyclical vomiting in migraine (G43.A-)*
    - *Excludes2: bulimia nervosa (F50.2)*
      - *diabetes mellitus due to underlying condition (E08.-)*
    - *AHA CC: 4Q, 2019, 15*
  - **R11.2 Nausea with vomiting, unspecified**
    - Persistent nausea with vomiting NOS
    - *AHA CC: 1Q, 2020, 8*

R12 Heartburn
- *Excludes1: dyspepsia NOS (R10.13)*
  - *functional dyspepsia (K30)*
- Valid 3-character code, no further characters required

R13 Aphagia and dysphagia
- **R13.0 Aphagia**
  - Inability to swallow
  - *Excludes1: psychogenic aphagia (F50.9)*
- + **R13.1 Dysphagia**
  - Code first if applicable, dysphagia following cerebrovascular disease (I69. with final characters -91)
  - *Excludes1: psychogenic dysphagia (F45.8)*
  - **R13.10 Dysphagia, unspecified**
    - Difficulty in swallowing NOS
  - **R13.11 Dysphagia, oral phase**
  - **R13.12 Dysphagia, oropharyngeal phase**
  - **R13.13 Dysphagia, pharyngeal phase**
  - **R13.14 Dysphagia, pharyngoesophageal phase**
  - **R13.19 Other dysphagia**
    - Cervical dysphagia
    - Neurogenic dysphagia

R14 Flatulence and related conditions
- *Excludes1: psychogenic aerophagy (F45.8)*
- **R14.0 Abdominal distension (gaseous)**
  - Bloating
  - Tympanites (abdominal) (intestinal)
- **R14.1 Gas pain**
- **R14.2 Eructation**
- **R14.3 Flatulence**

R15 Fecal incontinence
- Includes: encopresis NOS
- *Excludes1: fecal incontinence of nonorganic origin (F98.1)*
- **R15.0 Incomplete defecation**
  - *Excludes1: constipation (K59.0-)*
    - *fecal impaction (K56.41)*
- **R15.1 Fecal smearing**
  - Fecal soiling
- **R15.2 Fecal urgency**
- **R15.9 Full incontinence of feces**
  - Fecal incontinence NOS

R16 Hepatomegaly and splenomegaly, not elsewhere classified
- **R16.0 Hepatomegaly, not elsewhere classified**
  - Hepatomegaly NOS
- **R16.1 Splenomegaly, not elsewhere classified**
  - Splenomegaly NOS
- **R16.2 Hepatomegaly with splenomegaly, not elsewhere classified**
  - Hepatosplenomegaly NOS

R17 Unspecified jaundice
- *Excludes1: neonatal jaundice (P55, P57-P59)*
- Valid 3-character code, no further characters required

CC **R18 Ascites**
- Includes: fluid in peritoneal cavity
- *Excludes1: ascites in alcoholic cirrhosis (K70.31)*
  - *ascites in alcoholic hepatitis (K70.11)*
  - *ascites in toxic liver disease with chronic active hepatitis (K71.51)*

CC **R18.0 Malignant ascites**
- Code first malignancy, such as:
  - malignant neoplasm of ovary (C56.-)
  - secondary malignant neoplasm of retroperitoneum and peritoneum (C78.6)

CC **R18.8 Other ascites**
- Ascites NOS
- Peritoneal effusion (chronic)
- *AHA CC: 1Q, 2018, 4-5*

R19 Other symptoms and signs involving the digestive system and abdomen
- *Excludes1: acute abdomen (R10.0)*
- + **R19.0 Intra-abdominal and pelvic swelling, mass and lump**
  - *Excludes1: abdominal distension (gaseous) (R14.-)*
    - *ascites (R18.-)*
  - **R19.00 Intra-abdominal and pelvic swelling, mass and lump, unspecified site**
  - **R19.01 Right upper quadrant abdominal swelling, mass and lump**
  - **R19.02 Left upper quadrant abdominal swelling, mass and lump**
  - **R19.03 Right lower quadrant abdominal swelling, mass and lump**
  - **R19.04 Left lower quadrant abdominal swelling, mass and lump**
  - **R19.05 Periumbilic swelling, mass or lump**
    - Diffuse or generalized umbilical swelling or mass
  - **R19.06 Epigastric swelling, mass or lump**
  - **R19.07 Generalized intra-abdominal and pelvic swelling, mass and lump**
    - Diffuse or generalized intra-abdominal swelling or mass NOS
    - Diffuse or generalized pelvic swelling or mass NOS
  - **R19.09 Other intra-abdominal and pelvic swelling, mass and lump**
- + **R19.1 Abnormal bowel sounds**
  - **R19.11 Absent bowel sounds**
  - **R19.12 Hyperactive bowel sounds**
  - **R19.15 Other abnormal bowel sounds**
    - Abnormal bowel sounds NOS
- **R19.2 Visible peristalsis**
  - Hyperperistalsis
- + **R19.3 Abdominal rigidity**
  - *Excludes1: abdominal rigidity with severe abdominal pain (R10.0)*
  - **R19.30 Abdominal rigidity, unspecified site**
  - **R19.31 Right upper quadrant abdominal rigidity**
  - **R19.32 Left upper quadrant abdominal rigidity**
  - **R19.33 Right lower quadrant abdominal rigidity**
  - **R19.34 Left lower quadrant abdominal rigidity**
  - **R19.35 Periumbilic abdominal rigidity**
  - **R19.36 Epigastric abdominal rigidity**
  - **R19.37 Generalized abdominal rigidity**
- **R19.4 Change in bowel habit**
  - *Excludes1: constipation (K59.0-)*
    - *functional diarrhea (K59.1)*
- **R19.5 Other fecal abnormalities**
  - Abnormal stool color
  - Bulky stools
  - Mucus in stools
  - Occult blood in feces
  - Occult blood in stools
  - *Excludes1: melena (K92.1)*
    - *neonatal melena (P54.1)*
  - *AHA CC: 1Q, 2019, 32*
- **R19.6 Halitosis**
- **R19.7 Diarrhea, unspecified**
  - Diarrhea NOS
  - *Excludes1: functional diarrhea (K59.1)*
    - *neonatal diarrhea (P78.3)*
    - *psychogenic diarrhea (F45.8)*
- **R19.8 Other specified symptoms and signs involving the digestive system and abdomen**

+, +7th, X + 7th • Newborn • Pediatric • Maternity • Adult ♀ Female ♂ Male Manifestation Unacceptable PDX HCC CC MCC HAC

Symptoms and signs involving the skin and subcutaneous tissue (R20-R23)

Excludes2: *symptoms relating to breast (N64.4-N64.5)*

R20 **Disturbances of skin sensation**

> *Excludes1:* *dissociative anesthesia and sensory loss (F44.6)*
> *psychogenic disturbances (F45.8)*

R20.0 **Anesthesia of skin**
R20.1 **Hypoesthesia of skin**
R20.2 **Paresthesia of skin**
> Formication
> Pins and needles
> Tingling skin
> *Excludes1:* *acroparesthesia (I73.8)*

R20.3 **Hyperesthesia**
R20.8 **Other disturbances of skin sensation**
R20.9 **Unspecified disturbances of skin sensation**

R21 **Rash and other nonspecific skin eruption**

> **Includes:** rash NOS
> *Excludes1:* *specified type of rash- code to condition vesicular eruption (R23.8)*
> Valid 3-character code, no further characters required

R22 **Localized swelling, mass and lump of skin and subcutaneous tissue**

> **Includes:** subcutaneous nodules (localized)(superficial)
> *Excludes1:* *abnormal findings on diagnostic imaging (R90-R93)*
> *edema (R60.-)*
> *enlarged lymph nodes (R59.-)*
> *localized adiposity (E65)*
> *swelling of joint (M25.4-)*

R22.0 **Localized swelling, mass and lump, head**
R22.1 **Localized swelling, mass and lump, neck**
R22.2 **Localized swelling, mass and lump, trunk**
> *Excludes1:* *intra-abdominal or pelvic mass and lump (R19.0-)*
> *intra-abdominal or pelvic swelling (R19.0-)*
> *Excludes2:* *breast mass and lump (N63)*

+ R22.3 **Localized swelling, mass and lump, upper limb**
> **R22.30** **Localized swelling, mass and lump, unspecified upper limb**
> **R22.31** **Localized swelling, mass and lump, right upper limb**
> **R22.32** **Localized swelling, mass and lump, left upper limb**
> **R22.33** **Localized swelling, mass and lump, upper limb, bilateral**

+ R22.4 **Localized swelling, mass and lump, lower limb**
> **R22.40** **Localized swelling, mass and lump, unspecified lower limb**
> **R22.41** **Localized swelling, mass and lump, right lower limb**
> **R22.42** **Localized swelling, mass and lump, left lower limb**
> **R22.43** **Localized swelling, mass and lump, lower limb, bilateral**

R22.9 **Localized swelling, mass and lump, unspecified**

R23 **Other skin changes**

R23.0 **Cyanosis**
> *Excludes1:* *acrocyanosis (I73.8)*
> *cyanotic attacks of newborn (P28.2)*

R23.1 **Pallor**
> Clammy skin

R23.2 **Flushing**
> Excessive blushing
> Code first, if applicable, menopausal and female climacteric states (N95.1)

R23.3 **Spontaneous ecchymoses**
> Petechiae
> *Excludes1:* *ecchymoses of newborn (P54.5)*
> *purpura (D69.-)*

R23.4 **Changes in skin texture**
> Desquamation of skin
> Induration of skin
> Scaling of skin
> *Excludes1:* *epidermal thickening NOS (L85.9)*

R23.8 **Other skin changes**
R23.9 **Unspecified skin changes**

Symptoms and signs involving the nervous and musculoskeletal systems (R25-R29)

R25 **Abnormal involuntary movements**

> *Excludes1:* *specific movement disorders (G20-G26)*
> *stereotyped movement disorders (F98.4)*
> *tic disorders (F95.-)*

R25.0 **Abnormal head movements**
R25.1 **Tremor, unspecified**
> *Excludes1:* *chorea NOS (G25.5)*
> *essential tremor (G25.0)*
> *hysterical tremor (F44.4)*
> *intention tremor (G25.2)*

R25.2 **Cramp and spasm**
> *Excludes2:* *carpopedal spasm (R29.0)*
> *charley-horse (M62.831)*
> *infantile spasms (G40.4-)*
> *muscle spasm of back (M62.830)*
> *muscle spasm of calf (M62.831)*

R25.3 **Fasciculation**
> Twitching NOS

R25.8 **Other abnormal involuntary movements**
R25.9 **Unspecified abnormal involuntary movements**

R26 **Abnormalities of gait and mobility**

> *Excludes1:* *ataxia NOS (R27.0)*
> *hereditary ataxia (G11.-)*
> *locomotor (syphilitic) ataxia (A52.11)*
> *immobility syndrome (paraplegic) (M62.3)*

R26.0 **Ataxic gait**
> Staggering gait

R26.1 **Paralytic gait**
> Spastic gait

R26.2 **Difficulty in walking, not elsewhere classified**
> *Excludes1:* *falling (R29.6)*
> *unsteadiness on feet (R26.81)*
> *AHA CC: 2Q, 2016, 7*

R26.8 **Other abnormalities of gait and mobility**
> **R26.81** **Unsteadiness on feet**
> **R26.89** **Other abnormalities of gait and mobility**
> *AHA CC: 2Q, 2020, 29*

R26.9 **Unspecified abnormalities of gait and mobility**

R27 **Other lack of coordination**

> *Excludes1:* *ataxic gait (R26.0)*
> *hereditary ataxia (G11.-)*
> *vertigo NOS (R42)*

R27.0 **Ataxia, unspecified**
> *Excludes1:* *ataxia following cerebrovascular disease (I69. with final characters -93)*

R27.8 **Other lack of coordination**
R27.9 **Unspecified lack of coordination**

R29 **Other symptoms and signs involving the nervous and musculoskeletal systems**

CC R29.0 **Tetany**
> Carpopedal spasm
> *Excludes1:* *hysterical tetany (F44.5)*
> *neonatal tetany (P71.3)*
> *parathyroid tetany (E20.9)*
> *post-thyroidectomy tetany (E89.2)*

CC R29.1 **Meningismus**
R29.2 **Abnormal reflex**
> *Excludes2:* *abnormal pupillary reflex (H57.0)*
> *hyperactive gag reflex (J39.2)*
> *vasovagal reaction or syncope (R55)*

R29.3 **Abnormal posture**
R29.4 **Clicking hip**
> *Excludes1:* *congenital deformities of hip (Q65.-)*

CC R29.5 **Transient paralysis**
> Code first any associated spinal cord injury (S14.0, S14.1-, S24.0, S24.1-, S34.0-, S34.1-)
> *Excludes1:* *transient ischemic attack (G45.9)*

R29.6 **Repeated falls**
> Falling
> Tendency to fall
> *Excludes2:* *at risk for falling (Z91.81)*
> *history of falling (Z91.81)*
> Review coding guideline C.18.d
> *AHA CC: 2Q, 2016, 6-7*

| +, +7th, X + 7th | ● Newborn | ○ Pediatric | ● Maternity | ● Adult | ♀ Female | ♂ Male | Manifestation | Unacceptable PDX | HCC | CC | MCC | HAC |

+ **R29.7** **National Institutes of Health Stroke Scale (NIHSS) score**
Code first the type of cerebral infarction (I63.-)
Review coding guidelines B.14 and C.18.i
AHA CC: 4Q, 2016, 61-62
+ **R29.70** **NIHSS score 0-9**
R29.700 NIHSS score 0
R29.701 NIHSS score 1
R29.702 NIHSS score 2
R29.703 NIHSS score 3
R29.704 NIHSS score 4
R29.705 NIHSS score 5
R29.706 NIHSS score 6
R29.707 NIHSS score 7
R29.708 NIHSS score 8
R29.709 NIHSS score 9
+ **R29.71** **NIHSS score 10-19**
R29.710 NIHSS score 10
R29.711 NIHSS score 11
R29.712 NIHSS score 12
R29.713 NIHSS score 13
R29.714 NIHSS score 14
R29.715 NIHSS score 15
R29.716 NIHSS score 16
R29.717 NIHSS score 17
R29.718 NIHSS score 18
R29.719 NIHSS score 19
+ **R29.72** **NIHSS score 20-29**
R29.720 NIHSS score 20
R29.721 NIHSS score 21
R29.722 NIHSS score 22
R29.723 NIHSS score 23
R29.724 NIHSS score 24
R29.725 NIHSS score 25
R29.726 NIHSS score 26
R29.727 NIHSS score 27
R29.728 NIHSS score 28
R29.729 NIHSS score 29
+ **R29.73** **NIHSS score 30-39**
R29.730 NIHSS score 30
AHA CC: 4Q, 2016, 61-62
R29.731 NIHSS score 31
R29.732 NIHSS score 32
R29.733 NIHSS score 33
R29.734 NIHSS score 34
R29.735 NIIISS score 35
R29.736 NIHSS score 36
R29.737 NIHSS score 37
R29.738 NIHSS score 38
R29.739 NIHSS score 39
+ **R29.74** **NIHSS score 40-42**
R29.740 NIHSS score 40
R29.741 NIHSS score 41
R29.742 NIHSS score 42
+ **R29.8** **Other symptoms and signs involving the nervous and musculoskeletal systems**
+ **R29.81** **Other symptoms and signs involving the nervous system**
R29.810 **Facial weakness**
Facial droop
Excludes1: Bell's palsy (G51.0)
facial weakness following cerebrovascular disease (I69. with final characters -92)
R29.818 **Other symptoms and signs involving the nervous system**
+ **R29.89** **Other symptoms and signs involving the musculoskeletal system**
Excludes2: pain in limb (M79.6-)
R29.890 **Loss of height**
Excludes1: osteoporosis (M80-M81)

R29.891 **Ocular torticollis**
Excludes1: congenital (sternomastoid) torticollis (Q68.0)
psychogenic torticollis (F45.8)
spasmodic torticollis (G24.3)
torticollis due to birth injury (P15.8)
torticollis NOS (M43.6)
R29.898 **Other symptoms and signs involving the musculoskeletal system**
+ **R29.9** **Unspecified symptoms and signs involving the nervous and musculoskeletal systems**
R29.90 **Unspecified symptoms and signs involving the nervous system**
R29.91 **Unspecified symptoms and signs involving the musculoskeletal system**

Symptoms and signs involving the genitourinary system (R30-R39)

R30 **Pain associated with micturition**
Excludes1: psychogenic pain associated with micturition (F45.8)
R30.0 **Dysuria**
Strangury
R30.1 **Vesical tenesmus**
R30.9 **Painful micturition, unspecified**
Painful urination NOS

R31 **Hematuria**
Excludes1: hematuria included with underlying conditions, such as:
acute cystitis with hematuria (N30.01)
recurrent and persistent hematuria in glomerular diseases (N02.-)
R31.0 **Gross hematuria**
AHA CC: 1Q, 2017, 17-18
R31.1 **Benign essential microscopic hematuria**
+ **R31.2** **Other microscopic hematuria**
AHA CC: 4Q, 2016, 62
R31.21 **Asymptomatic microscopic hematuria**
AMH
AHA CC: 4Q, 2016, 62
R31.29 **Other microscopic hematuria**
R31.9 **Hematuria, unspecified**
AIIA CC: 1Q, 2017, 6

R32 **Unspecified urinary incontinence**
Enuresis NOS
Excludes1: functional urinary incontinence (R39.81)
nonorganic enuresis (F98.0)
stress incontinence and other specified urinary incontinence (N39.3-N39.4-)
urinary incontinence associated with cognitive impairment (R39.81)
Valid 3-character code, no further characters required

R33 **Retention of urine**
Excludes1: psychogenic retention of urine (F45.8)
R33.0 **Drug induced retention of urine**
Use additional code for adverse effect, if applicable, to identify drug (T36-T50 with fifth or sixth character 5)
R33.8 **Other retention of urine**
Code first if applicable, any causal condition, such as: enlarged prostate (N40.1)
R33.9 **Retention of urine, unspecified**

R34 **Anuria and oliguria**
Excludes1: anuria and oliguria complicating abortion or ectopic or molar pregnancy (O00-O07, O08.4)
anuria and oliguria complicating pregnancy (O26.83-)
anuria and oliguria complicating the puerperium (O90.4)
Valid 3-character code, no further characters required

+, +7th, X + 7th   ● Newborn   ● Pediatric   ● Maternity   ● Adult   ♀ Female   ♂ Male   Manifestation   Unacceptable PDX   HCC   CC   MCC   HAC

R35 Polyuria

Code first if applicable, any causal condition, such as:
enlarged prostate (N40.1)
Excludes1: *psychogenic polyuria (F45.8)*

R35.0 Frequency of micturition

R35.1 Nocturia

R35.8 Other polyuria
Polyuria NOS

R36 Urethral discharge

R36.0 Urethral discharge without blood

♂ **R36.1 Hematospermia**

R36.9 Urethral discharge, unspecified
Penile discharge NOS
Urethrorrhea

R37 Sexual dysfunction, unspecified

Valid 3-character code, no further characters required

R39 Other and unspecified symptoms and signs involving the genitourinary system

CC **R39.0 Extravasation of urine**

+ **R39.1 Other difficulties with micturition**
Code first if applicable, any causal condition, such as:
enlarged prostate (N40.1)

R39.11 Hesitancy of micturition

R39.12 Poor urinary stream
Weak urinary steam

R39.13 Splitting of urinary stream

R39.14 Feeling of incomplete bladder emptying

R39.15 Urgency of urination
Excludes1: *urge incontinence (N39.41, N39.46)*

R39.16 Straining to void

+ **R39.19 Other difficulties with micturition**
AHA CC: 4Q, 2016, 63

R39.191 Need to immediately re-void

R39.192 Position dependent micturition

R39.198 Other difficulties with micturition

R39.2 Extrarenal uremia
Prerenal uremia
Excludes1: *uremia NOS (N19)*

+ **R39.8 Other symptoms and signs involving the genitourinary system**
AHA CC: 4Q, 2016, 64

R39.81 Functional urinary incontinence
Urinary incontinence due to cognitive impairment, or severe physical disability or immobility
Excludes1: *stress incontinence and other specified urinary incontinence (N39.3-N39.4-)*
urinary incontinence NOS (R32)

R39.82 Chronic bladder pain
AHA CC: 4Q, 2016, 64

♂ **R39.83 Unilateral non-palpable testicle**
AHA CC: 4Q, 2017, 22-23

♂ **R39.84 Bilateral non-palpable testicles**
AHA CC: 4Q, 2017, 22-23

R39.89 Other symptoms and signs involving the genitourinary system

R39.9 Unspecified symptoms and signs involving the genitourinary system

Symptoms and signs involving cognition, perception, emotional state and behavior (R40-R46)

Excludes2: *symptoms and signs constituting part of a pattern of mental disorder (F01-F99)*

R40 Somnolence, stupor and coma

Excludes1: *neonatal coma (P91.5)*
somnolence, stupor and coma in diabetes (E08-E13)
somnolence, stupor and coma in hepatic failure (K72.-)
somnolence, stupor and coma in hypoglycemia (nondiabetic) (E15)

R40.0 Somnolence
Drowsiness
Excludes1: *coma (R40.2-)*

R40.1 Stupor
Catatonic stupor
Semicoma
Excludes1: *catatonic schizophrenia (F20.2)*
coma (R40.2-)
depressive stupor (F31-F33)
dissociative stupor (F44.2)
manic stupor (F30.2)

+ **R40.2 Coma**
Code first any associated:
fracture of skull (S02.-)
intracranial injury (S06.-)
NOTE One code from each subcategory, R40.21-R40.23, is required to complete the coma scale
Review coding guidelines B.14 and C.18.e
AHA CC: 1Q, 2014, 19-20; 2Q, 2015, 17-18

MCC X+7th **R40.20 Unspecified coma**
Coma NOS
Unconsciousness NOS

+ **R40.21 Coma scale, eyes open**
AHA CC: 4Q, 2017, 25

The appropriate 7th character is to be added to each code from subcategory **R40.21-**:
0   unspecified time
1   in the field [EMT or ambulance]
2   at arrival to emergency department
3   at hospital admission
4   24 hours or more after hospital admission

MCC +7th **R40.211 Coma scale, eyes open, never**
Coma scale eye opening score of 1

MCC +7th **R40.212 Coma scale, eyes open, to pain**
Coma scale eye opening score of 2

+7th **R40.213 Coma scale, eyes open, to sound**
Coma scale eye opening score of 3

+7th **R40.214 Coma scale, eyes open, spontaneous**
Coma scale eye opening score of 4

+ **R40.22 Coma scale, best verbal response**
AHA CC: 4Q, 2017, 23-25

The appropriate 7th character is to be added to each code from subcategory **R40.22-**:
0   unspecified time
1   in the field [EMT or ambulance]
2   at arrival to emergency department
3   at hospital admission
4   24 hours or more after hospital admission

MCC +7th **R40.221 Coma scale, best verbal response, none**
Coma scale verbal score of 1

MCC +7th **R40.222 Coma scale, best verbal response, incomprehensible words**
Coma scale verbal score of 2
Incomprehensible sounds (2-5 years of age)
Moans/grunts to pain (<2 years of age)

+7th **R40.223 Coma scale, best verbal response, inappropriate words**
Coma scale verbal score of 3
Inappropriate crying or screaming (<2 years of age)
Screaming (2-5 years of age)

+7th **R40.224 Coma scale, best verbal response, confused conversation**
Coma scale verbal score of 4
Inappropriate words (2-5 years of age)
Irritable cries (<2 years of age)

+7th **R40.225 Coma scale, best verbal response, oriented**
Coma scale verbal score of 5
Cooing or babbling or crying appropriately (<2 years of age)
Uses appropriate words (2-5 years of age)

+, +7th, X + 7th   ● Newborn   ● Pediatric   ● Maternity   ● Adult   ♀ Female   ♂ Male   Manifestation   Unacceptable PDX   HCC   CC   MCC   HAC

+ **R40.23** **Coma scale, best motor response**
AHA CC: 4Q, 2017, 23-25

> The appropriate 7th character is to be added to each code from subcategory **R40.23-**:
> 0   unspecified time
> 1   in the field [EMT or ambulance]
> 2   at arrival to emergency department
> 3   at hospital admission
> 4   24 hours or more after hospital admission

MCC +7th **R40.231** **Coma scale, best motor response, none**
Coma scale motor score of 1

MCC +7th **R40.232** **Coma scale, best motor response, extension**
Abnormal extensor posturing to pain or noxious stimuli (<2 years of age)
Coma scale motor score of 2
Extensor posturing to pain or noxious stimuli (2-5 years of age)

+7th **R40.233** **Coma scale, best motor response, abnormal flexion**
Abnormal flexure posturing to pain or noxious stimuli (2-5 years of age)
Coma scale motor score of 3
Flexion/decorticate posturing (<2 years of age)

MCC +7th **R40.234** **Coma scale, best motor response, flexion withdrawal**
Coma scale motor score of 4
Withdraws from pain or noxious stimuli (2-5 years of age)

+7th **R40.235** **Coma scale, best motor response, localizes pain**
Coma scale motor score of 5
Localizes pain (2-5 years of age)
Withdraws to touch (<2 years of age)

+7th **R40.236** **Coma scale, best motor response, obeys commands**
Coma scale motor score of 6
Normal or spontaneous movement (<2 years of age)
Obeys commands (2-5 years of age)

+ **R40.24** **Glasgow coma scale, total score**
NOTE   Assign a code from subcategory R40.24, when only the total coma score is documented.
AHA CC: 4Q, 2016, 64-65

> The appropriate 7th character is to be added to each code from subcategory **R40.24-**:
> 0   unspecified time
> 1   in the field [EMT or ambulance]
> 2   at arrival to emergency department
> 3   at hospital admission
> 4   24 hours or more after hospital admission

+7th **R40.241** **Glasgow coma scale score 13-15**
+7th **R40.242** **Glasgow coma scale score 9-12**
+7th **R40.243** **Glasgow coma scale score 3-8**
+7th **R40.244** **Other coma, without documented Glasgow coma scale score, or with partial score reported**

CC **R40.3** **Persistent vegetative state**
R40.4 **Transient alteration of awareness**
AHA CC: 2Q, 2020, 24

R41 **Other symptoms and signs involving cognitive functions and awareness**

Excludes1:   *dissociative [conversion] disorders (F44.-)*
mild cognitive impairment, so stated (G31.84)

R41.0 **Disorientation, unspecified**
Confusion NOS
Delirium NOS
AHA CC: 4Q, 2016, 74-76; 2Q, 2019, 34

R41.1 **Anterograde amnesia**
R41.2 **Retrograde amnesia**
R41.3 **Other amnesia**
Amnesia NOS
Memory loss NOS
Excludes1:   *amnestic disorder due to known physiologic condition (F04)*
amnestic syndrome due to psychoactive substance use (F10-F19 with 5th character .6)
mild memory disturbance due to known physiological condition (F06.8)
transient global amnesia (G45.4)

CC **R41.4** **Neurologic neglect syndrome**
Asomatognosia
Hemi-akinesia
Hemi-inattention
Hemispatial neglect
Left-sided neglect
Sensory neglect
Visuospatial neglect
Excludes1:   *visuospatial deficit (R41.842)*

+ **R41.8** **Other symptoms and signs involving cognitive functions and awareness**

• **R41.81** **Age-related cognitive decline**
Senility NOS

R41.82 **Altered mental status, unspecified**
Change in mental status NOS
Excludes1:   *altered level of consciousness (R40.-)*
altered mental status due to known condition - code to condition
delirium NOS (R41.0)
AHA CC: 4Q, 2012, 98

R41.83 **Borderline intellectual functioning**
IQ level 71 to 84
Excludes1:   *intellectual disabilities (F70-F79)*

+ **R41.84** **Other specified cognitive deficit**
Excludes1:   *cognitive deficits as sequelae of cerebrovascular disease (I69.01 , I69.11-, I19.21-, I69.31-, I59.81-, I69.91-)*

R41.840 **Attention and concentration deficit**
Excludes1:   *attention-deficit hyperactivity disorders (F90.-)*

R41.841 **Cognitive communication deficit**
R41.842 **Visuospatial deficit**
R41.843 **Psychomotor deficit**
R41.844 **Frontal lobe and executive function deficit**

R41.89 **Other symptoms and signs involving cognitive functions and awareness**
Anosognosia

R41.9 **Unspecified symptoms and signs involving cognitive functions and awareness**
Unspecified neurocognitive disorder

R42 **Dizziness and giddiness**

Light-headedness
Vertigo NOS
Excludes1:   *vertiginous syndromes (H81.-)*
vertigo from infrasound (T75.23)
Valid 3-character code, no further characters required

R43 **Disturbances of smell and taste**

R43.0 **Anosmia**
R43.1 **Parosmia**
R43.2 **Parageusia**
R43.8 **Other disturbances of smell and taste**
Mixed disturbance of smell and taste
R43.9 **Unspecified disturbances of smell and taste**

R44 Other symptoms and signs involving general sensations and perceptions

> *Excludes1:* alcoholic hallucinations (F10.151, F10.251, F10.951)
> hallucinations in drug psychosis (F11-F19 with fifth to sixth characters 51)
> hallucinations in mood disorders with psychotic symptoms (F30.2, F31.5, F32.3, F33.3)
> hallucinations in schizophrenia, schizotypal and delusional disorders (F20-F29)
>
> *Excludes2:* disturbances of skin sensation (R20.-)

CC **R44.0 Auditory hallucinations**

R44.1 Visual hallucinations

CC **R44.2 Other hallucinations**

CC **R44.3 Hallucinations, unspecified**

R44.8 Other symptoms and signs involving general sensations and perceptions

R44.9 Unspecified symptoms and signs involving general sensations and perceptions

R45 Symptoms and signs involving emotional state

R45.0 Nervousness
    Nervous tension

R45.1 Restlessness and agitation

R45.2 Unhappiness

R45.3 Demoralization and apathy
> *Excludes1:* anhedonia (R45.84)

R45.4 Irritability and anger

R45.5 Hostility

R45.6 Violent behavior

R45.7 State of emotional shock and stress, unspecified

+ **R45.8 Other symptoms and signs involving emotional state**

R45.81 Low self-esteem

R45.82 Worries

R45.83 Excessive crying of child, adolescent or adult
> *Excludes1:* excessive crying of infant (baby) (R68.11)

R45.84 Anhedonia

+ **R45.85 Homicidal and suicidal ideations**
> *Excludes1:* suicide attempt (T14.91)

R45.850 Homicidal ideations

CC **R45.851 Suicidal ideations**

R45.86 Emotional lability

R45.87 Impulsiveness

R45.89 Other symptoms and signs involving emotional state

R46 Symptoms and signs involving appearance and behavior

> *Excludes1:* appearance and behavior in schizophrenia, schizotypal and delusional disorders (F20-F29)
> mental and behavioral disorders (F01-F99)

R46.0 Very low level of personal hygiene

R46.1 Bizarre personal appearance

R46.2 Strange and inexplicable behavior

R46.3 Overactivity

R46.4 Slowness and poor responsiveness
> *Excludes1:* stupor (R40.1)

R46.5 Suspiciousness and marked evasiveness

R46.6 Undue concern and preoccupation with stressful events

R46.7 Verbosity and circumstantial detail obscuring reason for contact

+ **R46.8 Other symptoms and signs involving appearance and behavior**

R46.81 Obsessive-compulsive behavior
> *Excludes1:* obsessive-compulsive disorder (F42.-)

R46.89 Other symptoms and signs involving appearance and behavior

Symptoms and signs involving speech and voice (R47-R49)

R47 Speech disturbances, not elsewhere classified

> *Excludes1:* autism (F84.0)
> cluttering (F80.81)
> specific developmental disorders of speech and language (F80.-)
> stuttering (F80.81)

+ **R47.0 Dysphasia and aphasia**

CC **R47.01 Aphasia**
> *Excludes1:* aphasia following cerebrovascular disease (I69. with final characters -20)
> progressive isolated aphasia (G31.01)

R47.02 Dysphasia
> *Excludes1:* dysphasia following cerebrovascular disease (I69. with final characters -21)

R47.1 Dysarthria and anarthria
> *Excludes1:* dysarthria following cerebrovascular disease (I69. with final characters -22)

+ **R47.8 Other speech disturbances**
> *Excludes1:* dysarthria following cerebrovascular disease (I69. with final characters -28)

R47.81 Slurred speech

R47.82 Fluency disorder in conditions classified elsewhere
    Stuttering in conditions classified elsewhere
    Code first underlying disease or condition, such as:
    Parkinson's disease (G20)
> *Excludes1:* adult onset fluency disorder (F98.5)
> childhood onset fluency disorder (F80.81)
> fluency disorder (stuttering) following cerebrovascular disease (I69. with final characters -23)

R47.89 Other speech disturbances

R47.9 Unspecified speech disturbances

R48 Dyslexia and other symbolic dysfunctions, not elsewhere classified

> *Excludes1:* specific developmental disorders of scholastic skills (F81.-)

R48.0 Dyslexia and alexia

R48.1 Agnosia
    Astereognosia (astereognosis)
    Autotopagnosia
> *Excludes1:* visual object agnosia (R48.3)

R48.2 Apraxia
> *Excludes1:* apraxia following cerebrovascular disease (I69. with final characters -90)

R48.3 Visual agnosia
    Prosopagnosia
    Simultanagnosia (asimultagnosia)

R48.8 Other symbolic dysfunctions
    Acalculia
    Agraphia
    AHA CC: 1Q, 2017, 27-28

R48.9 Unspecified symbolic dysfunctions

R49 Voice and resonance disorders

> *Excludes1:* psychogenic voice and resonance disorders (F44.4)

R49.0 Dysphonia
    Hoarseness

R49.1 Aphonia
    Loss of voice

+ **R49.2 Hypernasality and hyponasality**

R49.21 Hypernasality

R49.22 Hyponasality

R49.8 Other voice and resonance disorders

R49.9 Unspecified voice and resonance disorder
    Change in voice NOS
    Resonance disorder NOS

General symptoms and signs (R50-R69)

R50 Fever of other and unknown origin

> *Excludes1:* chills without fever (R68.83)
> febrile convulsions (R56.0-)
> fever of unknown origin during labor (O75.2)
> fever of unknown origin in newborn (P81.9)
> hypothermia due to illness (R68.0)
> malignant hyperthermia due to anesthesia (T88.3)
> puerperal pyrexia NOS (O86.4)

R50.2 Drug induced fever
    Use additional code for adverse effect, if applicable, to identify drug (T36-T50 with fifth or sixth character 5)
> *Excludes1:* postvaccination (postimmunization) fever (R50.83)

+ **R50.8** **Other specified fever**
 R50.81 **Fever presenting with conditions classified elsewhere**
  Code first underlying condition when associated fever is present, such as with:
   leukemia (C91-C95)
   neutropenia (D70.-)
   sickle-cell disease (D57.-)
  AHA CC: 4Q, 2014, 22-23; 2Q, 2019, 24-25

 R50.82 **Postprocedural fever**
  Excludes1: *postprocedural infection (T81.4-)*
   posttransfusion fever (R50.84)
   postvaccination (postimmunization) fever (R50.83)

 R50.83 **Postvaccination fever**
  Postimmunization fever

 R50.84 **Febrile nonhemolytic transfusion reaction**
  FNHTR
  Posttransfusion fever

R50.9 **Fever, unspecified**
 Fever NOS
 Fever of unknown origin [FUO]
 Fever with chills
 Fever with rigors
 Hyperpyrexia NOS
 Persistent fever
 Pyrexia NOS
 AHA CC: 1Q, 2020, 34-36

R51 **Headache**

 Excludes2: *atypical face pain (G50.1)*
  migraine and other headache syndromes (G43-G44)
  trigeminal neuralgia (G50.0)

R51.0 **Headache with orthostatic component, not elsewhere classified**
 Headache with positional component, not elsewhere classified

R51.9 **Headache, unspecified**
 Facial pain NOS

R52 **Pain, unspecified**

 Acute pain NOS
 Generalized pain NOS
 Pain NOS
 Excludes1: *acute and chronic pain, not elsewhere classified (G89.-)*
  localized pain, unspecified type - code to pain by site, such as:
   abdomen pain (R10.-)
   back pain (M54.9)
   breast pain (N64.4)
   chest pain (R07.1-R07.9)
   ear pain (H92.0-)
   eye pain (H57.1)
   headache (R51.9)
   joint pain (M25.5-)
   limb pain (M79.6-)
   lumbar region pain (M54.5)
   pelvic and perineal pain (R10.2)
   shoulder pain (M25.51-)
   spine pain (M54.-)
   throat pain (R07.0)
   tongue pain (K14.6)
   tooth pain (K08.8)
   renal colic (N23)
   pain disorders exclusively related to psychological factors (F45.41)
 Valid 3-character code, no further characters required

R53 **Malaise and fatigue**

 R53.0 **Neoplastic (malignant) related fatigue**
  Code first associated neoplasm

 R53.1 **Weakness**
  Asthenia NOS
  Excludes1: *age-related weakness (R54)*
   muscle weakness (generalized) (M62.81)
   sarcopenia (M62.84)
   senile asthenia (R54)
  AHA CC: 1Q, 2017, 7

MCC **R53.2** **Functional quadriplegia**
 Complete immobility due to severe physical disability or frailty

  Excludes1: *frailty NOS (R54)*
   hysterical paralysis (F44.4)
   immobility syndrome (M62.3)
   neurologic quadriplegia (G82.5-)
   quadriplegia (G82.50)
  Review coding guideline C.18.f
  AHA CC: 2Q, 2016, 6

+ **R53.8** **Other malaise and fatigue**
 Excludes1: *combat exhaustion and fatigue (F43.0)*
  congenital debility (P96.9)
  exhaustion and fatigue due to excessive exertion (T73.3)
  exhaustion and fatigue due to exposure (T73.2)
  exhaustion and fatigue due to heat (T67.-)
  exhaustion and fatigue due to pregnancy (O26.8-)
  exhaustion and fatigue due to recurrent depressive episode (F33)
  exhaustion and fatigue due to senile debility (R54)

 R53.81 **Other malaise**
  Chronic debility
  Debility NOS
  General physical deterioration
  Malaise NOS
  Nervous debility
  Excludes1: *age-related physical debility (R54)*

 R53.82 **Chronic fatigue, unspecified**
  Chronic fatigue syndrome NOS
  Excludes1: *postviral fatigue syndrome (G93.3)*

 R53.83 **Other fatigue**
  Fatigue NOS
  Lack of energy
  Lethargy
  Tiredness
  Excludes2: *exhaustion and fatigue due to depressive episode (F32.-)*
  AHA CC: 1Q, 2017, 7

● **R54** **Age-related physical debility**

 Frailty
 Old age
 Senescence
 Senile asthenia
 Senile debility
 Excludes1: *age-related cognitive decline (R41.81)*
  sarcopenia (M62.84)
  senile psychosis (F03)
  senility NOS (R41.81)
 Valid 3-character code, no further characters required

R55 **Syncope and collapse**

 Blackout
 Fainting
 Vasovagal attack
 Excludes1: *cardiogenic shock (R57.0)*
  carotid sinus syncope (G90.01)
  heat syncope (T67.1)
  neurocirculatory asthenia (F45.8)
  neurogenic orthostatic hypotension (G90.3)
  orthostatic hypotension (I95.1)
  postprocedural shock (T81.1-)
  psychogenic syncope (F48.8)
  shock NOS (R57.9)
  shock complicating or following abortion or ectopic or molar pregnancy (O00-O07, O08.3)
  shock complicating or following labor and delivery (O75.1)
  Stokes-Adams attack (I45.9)
  unconsciousness NOS (R40.2-)
 Valid 3-character code, no further characters required

R56 **Convulsions, not elsewhere classified**

 Excludes1: *dissociative convulsions and seizures (F44.5)*
  epileptic convulsions and seizures (G40.-)
  newborn convulsions and seizures (P90)

+ **R56.0** **Febrile convulsions**
 CC **R56.00** **Simple febrile convulsions**
  Febrile convulsion NOS
  Febrile seizure NOS

 CC **R56.01** **Complex febrile convulsions**
  Atypical febrile seizure
  Complex febrile seizure
  Complicated febrile seizure
  Excludes1: *status epilepticus (G40.901)*

CC **R56.1** **Post traumatic seizures**
    Excludes1: post traumatic epilepsy (G40.-)
  R56.9 **Unspecified convulsions**
    Convulsion disorder
    Fit NOS
    Recurrent convulsions
    Seizure(s) (convulsive) NOS
    AHA CC: 4Q, 2019, 17-18

R57 **Shock, not elsewhere classified**

  Excludes1: anaphylactic shock NOS (T78.2)
      anaphylactic reaction or shock due to adverse food
        reaction (T78.0-)
      anaphylactic shock due to adverse effect of correct drug
        or medicament properly administered (T88.6)
      anaphylactic shock due to serum (T80.5-)
      anesthetic shock (T88.3)
      electric shock (T75.4)
      obstetric shock (O75.1)
      postprocedural shock (T81.1-)
      psychic shock (F43.0)
      shock complicating or following ectopic or molar
        pregnancy (O00-O07, O08.3)
      shock due to lightning (T75.01)
      traumatic shock (T79.4)
      toxic shock syndrome (A48.3)

MCC **R57.0** **Cardiogenic shock**
    Excludes2: septic shock (R65.21)
MCC **R57.1** **Hypovolemic shock**
    AHA CC: 2Q, 2019, 7-8
MCC **R57.8** **Other shock**
CC **R57.9** **Shock, unspecified**
    Failure of peripheral circulation NOS

R58 **Hemorrhage, not elsewhere classified**

  Hemorrhage NOS
  Excludes1: hemorrhage included with underlying conditions, such as:
      acute duodenal ulcer with hemorrhage (K26.0)
      acute gastritis with bleeding (K29.01)
      ulcerative enterocolitis with rectal bleeding (K51.01)
  Valid 3-character code, no further characters required

R59 **Enlarged lymph nodes**

  Includes: swollen glands
  Excludes1: lymphadenitis NOS (I88.9)
      acute lymphadenitis (L04.-)
      chronic lymphadenitis (I88.1)
      mesenteric (acute) (chronic) lymphadenitis (I88.0)
  R59.0 **Localized enlarged lymph nodes**
  R59.1 **Generalized enlarged lymph nodes**
    Lymphadenopathy NOS
  R59.9 **Enlarged lymph nodes, unspecified**

R60 **Edema, not elsewhere classified**

  Excludes1: angioneurotic edema (T78.3)
      ascites (R18.-)
      cerebral edema (G93.6)
      cerebral edema due to birth injury (P11.0)
      edema of larynx (J38.4)
      edema of nasopharynx (J39.2)
      edema of pharynx (J39.2)
      gestational edema (O12.0-)
      hereditary edema (Q82.0)
      hydrops fetalis NOS (P83.2)
      hydrothorax (J94.8)
      hydrops fetalis NOS (P83.2)
      newborn edema (P83.3)
      pulmonary edema (J81.-)
  R60.0 **Localized edema**
  R60.1 **Generalized edema**
    Excludes2: nutritional edema (E40-E46)
  R60.9 **Edema, unspecified**
    Fluid retention NOS

R61 **Generalized hyperhidrosis**

  Excessive sweating
  Night sweats
  Secondary hyperhidrosis
  Code first if applicable, menopausal and female climacteric states
    (N95.1)
  Excludes1: focal (primary) (secondary) hyperhidrosis (L74.5-)
      Frey's syndrome (L74.52)

      localized (primary) (secondary) hyperhidrosis (L74.5-)
  Valid 3-character code, no further characters required

R62 **Lack of expected normal physiological development in childhood and adults**

  Excludes1: delayed puberty (E30.0)
      gonadal dysgenesis (Q99.1)
      hypopituitarism (E23.0)
• **R62.0** **Delayed milestone in childhood**
    Delayed attainment of expected physiological developmental
      stage
    Late talker
    Late walker
+ **R62.5** **Other and unspecified lack of expected normal physiological development in childhood**
    Excludes1: HIV disease resulting in failure to thrive (B20)
      physical retardation due to malnutrition (E45)
  R62.50 **Unspecified lack of expected normal physiological development in childhood**
    Infantilism NOS
• **R62.51** **Failure to thrive (child)**
    Failure to gain weight
    Excludes1: failure to thrive in child under 28 days
      old (P92.6)
    AHA CC: 4Q, 2018, 82
  R62.52 **Short stature (child)**
    Lack of growth
    Physical retardation
    Short stature NOS
    Excludes1: short stature due to endocrine disorder
      (E34.3)
  R62.59 **Other lack of expected normal physiological development in childhood**
• **R62.7** **Adult failure to thrive**

R63 **Symptoms and signs concerning food and fluid intake**

  Excludes1: bulimia NOS (F50.2)
  R63.0 **Anorexia**
    Loss of appetite
    Excludes1: anorexia nervosa (F50.0-)
      loss of appetite of nonorganic origin (F50.89)
  R63.1 **Polydipsia**
    Excessive thirst
  R63.2 **Polyphagia**
    Excessive eating
    Hyperalimentation NOS
  R63.3 **Feeding difficulties**
    Feeding problem (elderly) (infant) NOS
    Picky eater
    Excludes1: eating disorders (F50.-)
      feeding problems of newborn (P92.-)
      infant feeding disorder of nonorganic origin
      (F98.2-)
  R63.4 **Abnormal weight loss**
  R63.5 **Abnormal weight gain**
    Excludes1: excessive weight gain in pregnancy (O26.0-)
      obesity (E66.-)
  R63.6 **Underweight**
    Use additional code to identify body mass index (BMI), if
      known (Z68.-)
    Excludes1: abnormal weight loss (R63.4)
      anorexia nervosa (F50.0-)
      malnutrition (E40-E46)
  R63.8 **Other symptoms and signs concerning food and fluid intake**

CC **R64** **Cachexia**

  Wasting syndrome
  Code first underlying condition, if known
  Excludes1: abnormal weight loss (R63.4)
      nutritional marasmus (E41)
  AHA CC: 3Q, 2017, 24-25
  Valid 3-character code, no further characters required

R65 **Symptoms and signs specifically associated with systemic inflammation and infection**
  See page 944 for Sepsis illustration.

+ **R65.1** **Systemic inflammatory response syndrome (SIRS) of non-infectious origin**
    Code first underlying condition, such as:
    heatstroke (T67.0-)
    injury and trauma (S00-T88)

+, +7th, X + 7th   • Newborn   • Pediatric   • Maternity   • Adult   ♀ Female   ♂ Male   Manifestation   Unacceptable PDX   HCC   CC   MCC   HAC

Sepsis

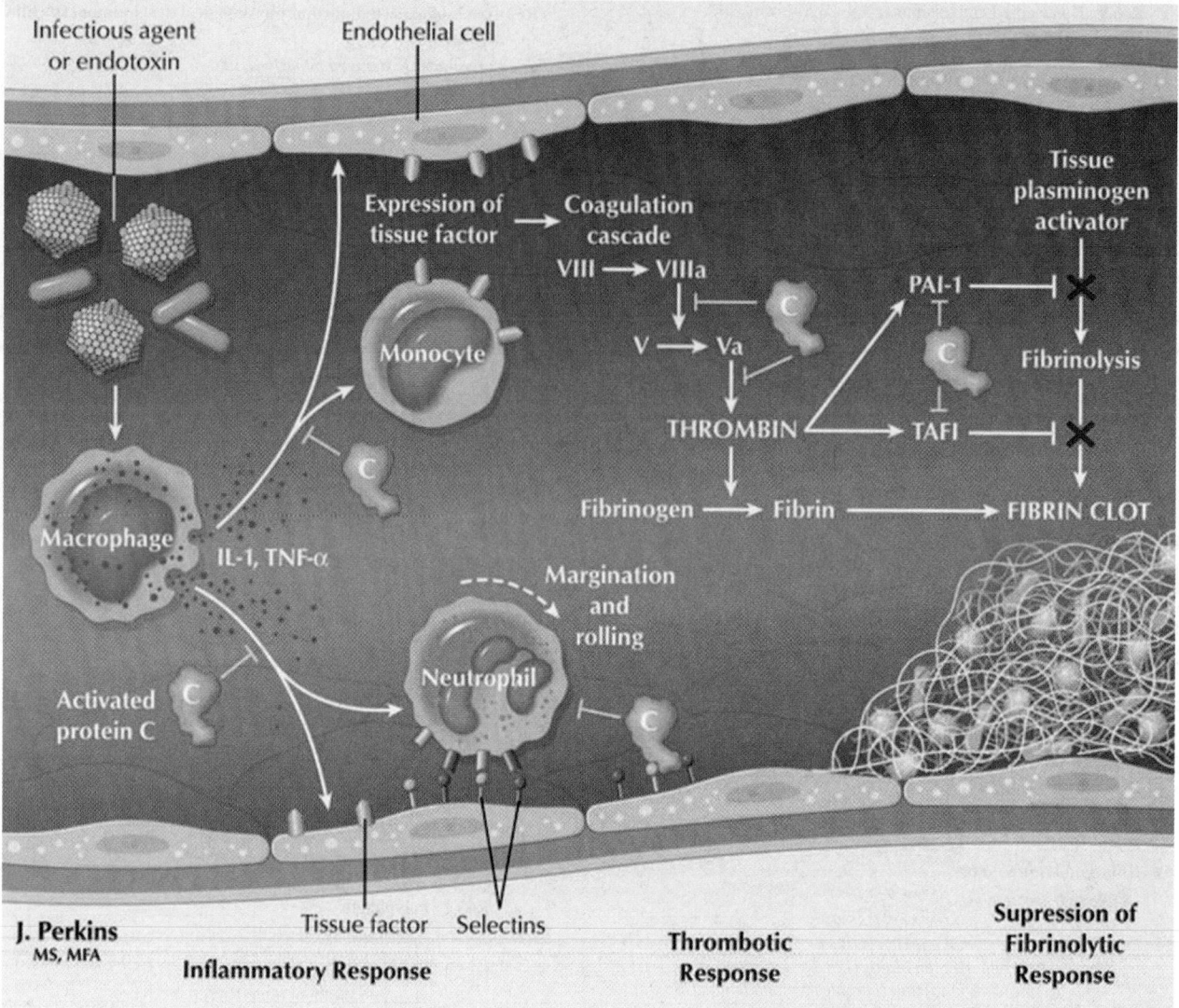

J. Perkins
MS, MFA

Tissue factor   Selectins

Inflammatory Response   **Thrombotic Response**   **Supression of Fibrinolytic Response**

Excludes1: sepsis- code to infection
severe sepsis (R65.2)

CC **R65.10** **Systemic inflammatory response syndrome (SIRS) of non-infectious origin without acute organ dysfunction**
Systemic inflammatory response syndrome (SIRS) NOS
AHA CC: 2Q, 2019, 24-26, 38
Review coding guideline C.18.g

MCC **R65.11** **Systemic inflammatory response syndrome (SIRS) of non-infectious origin with acute organ dysfunction**
Use additional code to identify specific acute organ dysfunction, such as:
acute kidney failure (N17.-)
acute respiratory failure (J96.0-)
critical illness myopathy (G72.81)
critical illness polyneuropathy (G62.81)
disseminated intravascular coagulopathy [DIC] (D65)
encephalopathy (metabolic) (septic) (G93.41)
hepatic failure (K72.0-)
Review coding guideline C.18.g

+ **R65.2** **Severe sepsis**
Infection with associated acute organ dysfunction
Sepsis with acute organ dysfunction
Sepsis with multiple organ dysfunction
Systemic inflammatory response syndrome due to infectious process with acute organ dysfunction
Code first underlying infection, such as:
infection following a procedure (T81.4-)
infections following infusion, transfusion and therapeutic injection (T80.2-)
puerperal sepsis (O85)
sepsis following complete or unspecified spontaneous abortion (O03.87)
sepsis following ectopic and molar pregnancy (O08.82)
sepsis following incomplete spontaneous abortion (O03.37)
sepsis following (induced) termination of pregnancy (O04.87)
sepsis NOS (A41.9)

Use additional code to identify specific acute organ dysfunction, such as:
acute kidney failure (N17.-)
acute respiratory failure (J96.0-)
critical illness myopathy (G72.81)
critical illness polyneuropathy (G62.81)
disseminated intravascular coagulopathy [DIC] (D65)
encephalopathy (metabolic) (septic) (G93.41)
hepatic failure (K72.0-)
AHA CC: 4Q, 2017, 98-99
Review coding guideline C.1.d

+, +7th, X + 7th   ● Newborn   ● Pediatric   ● Maternity   ● Adult   ♀ Female   ♂ Male   Manifestation   Unacceptable PDX   HCC   CC   MCC   HAC

MCC R65.20 **Severe sepsis without septic shock**
Severe sepsis NOS
AHA CC: 3Q, 2016, 14; 2Q, 2020, 17-18

MCC R65.21 **Severe sepsis with septic shock**
Review coding guideline C.1.d.2 and C.1.d.5.c

R68 **Other general symptoms and signs**

R68.0 **Hypothermia, not associated with low environmental temperature**
Excludes1: *hypothermia NOS (accidental) (T68)*
hypothermia due to anesthesia (T88.51)
hypothermia due to low environmental temperature (T68)
newborn hypothermia (P80.-)

+ **R68.1** **Nonspecific symptoms peculiar to infancy**
Excludes1: *colic, infantile (R10.83)*
neonatal cerebral irritability (P91.3)
teething syndrome (K00.7)

● **R68.11** **Excessive crying of infant (baby)**
Excludes1: *excessive crying of child, adolescent, or adult (R45.83)*

● **R68.12** **Fussy infant (baby)**
Irritable infant

● **R68.13** **Apparent life threatening event in infant (ALTE)**
Apparent life threatening event in newborn
Brief resolved unexplained event (BRUE)
Code first confirmed diagnosis, if known

Use additional code(s) for associated signs and symptoms if no confirmed diagnosis established, or if signs and symptoms are not associated routinely with confirmed diagnosis, or provide additional information for cause of ALTE

● **R68.19** **Other nonspecific symptoms peculiar to infancy**

R68.2 **Dry mouth, unspecified**
Excludes1: *dry mouth due to dehydration (E86.0)*
dry mouth due to sicca syndrome [Sjögren] (M35.0-)
salivary gland hyposecretion (K11.7)

R68.3 **Clubbing of fingers**
Clubbing of nails
Excludes1: *congenital clubfinger (Q68.1)*

+ **R68.8** **Other general symptoms and signs**
R68.81 **Early satiety**
● **R68.82** **Decreased libido**
Decreased sexual desire
R68.83 **Chills (without fever)**
Chills NOS
Excludes1: *chills with fever (R50.9)*
R68.84 **Jaw pain**
Mandibular pain
Maxilla pain
Excludes1: *temporomandibular joint arthralgia (M26.62-)*
R68.89 **Other general symptoms and signs**

R69 **Illness, unspecified**

Unknown and unspecified cases of morbidity
Valid 3-character code, no further characters required

Abnormal findings on examination of blood, without diagnosis (R70-R79)

Excludes2: *abnormal findings on antenatal screening of mother (O28.-)*
abnormalities of lipids (E78.-)
abnormalities of platelets and thrombocytes (D69.-)
abnormalities of white blood cells classified elsewhere (D70-D72)
coagulation hemorrhagic disorders (D65-D68)
diagnostic abnormal findings classified elsewhere - see Alphabetic Index
hemorrhagic and hematological disorders of newborn (P50-P61)

R70 **Elevated erythrocyte sedimentation rate and abnormality of plasma viscosity**

R70.0 **Elevated erythrocyte sedimentation rate**
R70.1 **Abnormal plasma viscosity**

R71 **Abnormality of red blood cells**

Excludes1: *anemias (D50-D64)*
anemia of premature infant (P61.2)
benign (familial) polycythemia (D75.0)
congenital anemias (P61.2-P61.4)
newborn anemia due to isoimmunization (P55.-)
polycythemia neonatorum (P61.1)
polycythemia NOS (D75.1)
polycythemia vera (D45)
secondary polycythemia (D75.1)

CC R71.0 **Precipitous drop in hematocrit**
Drop (precipitous) in hemoglobin
Drop in hematocrit

R71.8 **Other abnormality of red blood cells**
Abnormal red-cell morphology NOS
Abnormal red-cell volume NOS
Anisocytosis
Poikilocytosis

R73 **Elevated blood glucose level**

Excludes1: *diabetes mellitus (E08-E13)*
diabetes mellitus in pregnancy, childbirth and the puerperium (O24.-)
neonatal disorders (P70.0-P70.2)
postsurgical hypoinsulinemia (E89.1)

+ **R73.0** **Abnormal glucose**
Excludes1: *abnormal glucose in pregnancy (O99.81-)*
diabetes mellitus (E08-E13)
dysmetabolic syndrome X (E88.81)
gestational diabetes (O24.4-)
glycosuria (R81)
hypoglycemia (E16.2)

R73.01 **Impaired fasting glucose**
Elevated fasting glucose

R73.02 **Impaired glucose tolerance (oral)**
Elevated glucose tolerance

R73.03 **Prediabetes**
Latent diabetes
AHA CC: 4Q, 2016, 65

R73.09 **Other abnormal glucose**
Abnormal glucose NOS
Abnormal non-fasting glucose tolerance

R73.9 **Hyperglycemia, unspecified**

R74 **Abnormal serum enzyme levels**

+ **R74.0** **Nonspecific elevation of levels of transaminase and lactic acid dehydrogenase [LDH]**
R74.01 **Elevation of levels of liver transaminase levels**
Elevation of levels of alanine transaminase (ALT)
Elevation of levels of aspartate transaminase (AST)
R74.02 **Elevation of levels of lactic acid dehydrogenase [LDH]**

R74.8 **Abnormal levels of other serum enzymes**
Abnormal level of acid phosphatase
Abnormal level of alkaline phosphatase
Abnormal level of amylase
Abnormal level of lipase [triacylglycerol lipase]
AHA CC: 2Q, 2019, 6

R74.9 **Abnormal serum enzyme level, unspecified**

R75 **Inconclusive laboratory evidence of human immunodeficiency virus [HIV]**

Nonconclusive HIV-test finding in infants
Excludes1: *asymptomatic human immunodeficiency virus [HIV] infection status (Z21)*
human immunodeficiency virus [HIV] disease (B20)
Review coding guidelines C.1.a.2.e and C.1.a.2.f
Valid 3-character code, no further characters required

R76 **Other abnormal immunological findings in serum**

R76.0 **Raised antibody titer**
Excludes1: *isoimmunization in pregnancy (O36.0-O36.1)*
isoimmunization affecting newborn (P55.-)

+ **R76.1** **Nonspecific reaction to test for tuberculosis**
R76.11 **Nonspecific reaction to tuberculin skin test without active tuberculosis**
Abnormal result of Mantoux test
PPD positive
Tuberculin (skin test) positive
Tuberculin (skin test) reactor
Excludes1: *nonspecific reaction to cell mediated immunity measurement of gamma interferon antigen response without active tuberculosis (R76.12)*

R76.12 **Nonspecific reaction to cell mediated immunity measurement of gamma interferon antigen response without active tuberculosis**
  Nonspecific reaction to QuantiFERON-TB test (QFT) without active tuberculosis
    Excludes1: *nonspecific reaction to tuberculin skin test without active tuberculosis (R76.11)*
      positive tuberculin skin test (R76.11)
R76.8 **Other specified abnormal immunological findings in serum**
  Raised level of immunoglobulins NOS
R76.9 **Abnormal immunological finding in serum, unspecified**

R77 **Other abnormalities of plasma proteins**
  Excludes1: *disorders of plasma-protein metabolism (E88.0-)*
R77.0 **Abnormality of albumin**
R77.1 **Abnormality of globulin**
  Hyperglobulinemia NOS
R77.2 **Abnormality of alphafetoprotein**
R77.8 **Other specified abnormalities of plasma proteins**
R77.9 **Abnormality of plasma protein, unspecified**
  AHA CC: 2Q, 2019, 6

R78 **Findings of drugs and other substances, not normally found in blood**
  Use additional code to identify the any retained foreign body, if applicable (Z18.-)
  Excludes1: *mental or behavioral disorders due to psychoactive substance use (F10-F19)*
R78.0 **Finding of alcohol in blood**
  external cause code (Y90.-), for detail regarding alcohol level.
R78.1 **Finding of opiate drug in blood**
R78.2 **Finding of cocaine in blood**
R78.3 **Finding of hallucinogen in blood**
R78.4 **Finding of other drugs of addictive potential in blood**
R78.5 **Finding of other psychotropic drug in blood**
R78.6 **Finding of steroid agent in blood**
+ **R78.7** **Finding of abnormal level of heavy metals in blood**
  R78.71 **Abnormal lead level in blood**
    Excludes1: *lead poisoning (T56.0-)*
  R78.79 **Finding of abnormal level of heavy metals in blood**
+ **R78.8** **Finding of other specified substances, not normally found in blood**
  CC **R78.81** **Bacteremia**
    Excludes1: *sepsis-code to specified infection*
  R78.89 **Finding of other specified substances, not normally found in blood**
    Finding of abnormal level of lithium in blood
R78.9 **Finding of unspecified substance, not normally found in blood**

R79 **Other abnormal findings of blood chemistry**
  Use additional code to identify any retained foreign body, if applicable (Z18.-)
  Excludes1: *asymptomatic hyperuricemia (E79.0)*
    hyperglycemia NOS (R73.9)
    hypoglycemia NOS (E16.2)
    neonatal hypoglycemia (P70.3-P70.4)
    specific findings indicating disorder of amino-acid metabolism (E70-E72)
    specific findings indicating disorder of carbohydrate metabolism (E73-E74)
    specific findings indicating disorder of lipid metabolism (E75.-)
R79.0 **Abnormal level of blood mineral**
  Abnormal blood level of cobalt
  Abnormal blood level of copper
  Abnormal blood level of iron
  Abnormal blood level of magnesium
  Abnormal blood level of mineral NEC
  Abnormal blood level of zinc
  Excludes1: *abnormal level of lithium (R78.89)*
    disorders of mineral metabolism (E83.-)
    neonatal hypomagnesemia (P71.2)
    nutritional mineral deficiency (E58-E61)

R79.1 **Abnormal coagulation profile**
  Abnormal or prolonged bleeding time
  Abnormal or prolonged coagulation time
  Abnormal or prolonged partial thromboplastin time [PTT]
  Abnormal or prolonged prothrombin time [PT]
  Excludes2: *abnormality of fluid, electrolyte or acid-base balance (E86-E87)*
    coagulation defects (D68.-)
+ **R79.8** **Other specified abnormal findings of blood chemistry**
  R79.81 **Abnormal blood-gas level**
  R79.82 **Elevated C-reactive protein (CRP)**
  R79.89 **Other specified abnormal findings of blood chemistry**
    AHA CC: 2Q, 2019, 6
R79.9 **Abnormal finding of blood chemistry, unspecified**

Abnormal findings on examination of urine, without diagnosis (R80-R82)

Excludes1: *abnormal findings on antenatal screening of mother (O28.-)*
  diagnostic abnormal findings classified elsewhere - see Alphabetical Index
  specific findings indicating disorder of amino-acid metabolism (E70-E72)
  specific findings indicating disorder of carbohydrate metabolism (E73-E74)

R80 **Proteinuria**
  Excludes1: *gestational proteinuria (O12.1-)*
R80.0 **Isolated proteinuria**
  Idiopathic proteinuria
  Excludes1: *isolated proteinuria with specific morphological lesion (N06.-)*
R80.1 **Persistent proteinuria, unspecified**
R80.2 **Orthostatic proteinuria, unspecified**
  Postural proteinuria
R80.3 **Bence Jones proteinuria**
R80.8 **Other proteinuria**
R80.9 **Proteinuria, unspecified**
  Albuminuria NOS

R81 **Glycosuria**
  Excludes1: *renal glycosuria (E74.818)*
  Valid 3-character code, no further characters required

R82 **Other and unspecified abnormal findings in urine**
  Includes: chromoabnormalities in urine
  Use additional code to identify any retained foreign body, if applicable (Z18.-)
  Excludes2: *hematuria (R31.-)*
  CC **R82.0** **Chyluria**
    Excludes1: *filarial chyluria (B74.-)*
  CC **R82.1** **Myoglobinuria**
  R82.2 **Biliuria**
  R82.3 **Hemoglobinuria**
    Excludes1: *hemoglobinuria due to hemolysis from external causes NEC (D59.6)*
      hemoglobinuria due to paroxysmal nocturnal [Marchiafava-Micheli] (D59.5)
  R82.4 **Acetonuria**
    Ketonuria
  R82.5 **Elevated urine levels of drugs, medicaments and biological substances**
    Elevated urine levels of catecholamines
    Elevated urine levels of indoleacetic acid
    Elevated urine levels of 17-ketosteroids
    Elevated urine levels of steroids
  R82.6 **Abnormal urine levels of substances chiefly nonmedicinal as to source**
    Abnormal urine level of heavy metals
+ **R82.7** **Abnormal findings on microbiological examination of urine**
    Excludes1: *colonization status (Z22.-)*
    AHA CC: 4Q, 2016, 65
    R82.71 **Bacteriuria**
    R82.79 **Other abnormal findings on microbiological examination of urine**
      Positive culture findings of urine

+ **R82.8** **Abnormal findings on cytological and histological examination of urine**
AHA CC: 4Q, 2019, 16

    R82.81 **Pyuria**
        Sterile pyuria
        AHA CC: 4Q, 2019, 16

    R82.89 **Other abnormal findings on cytological and histological examination of urine**

+ **R82.9** **Other and unspecified abnormal findings in urine**
    R82.90 **Unspecified abnormal findings in urine**
    R82.91 **Other chromoabnormalities of urine**
        Chromoconversion (dipstick)
        Idiopathic dipstick converts positive for blood with no cellular forms in sediment
        Excludes1: *hemoglobinuria (R82.3)*
                  myoglobinuria (R82.1)

  + **R82.99** **Other abnormal findings in urine**
      AHA CC: 4Q, 2018, 29-30
    R82.991 **Hypocitraturia**
    R82.992 **Hyperoxaluria**
        Excludes1: *Primary hyperoxaluria (E72.53)*
    R82.993 **Hyperuricosuria**
    R82.994 **Hypercalciuria**
        Idiopathic hypercalciuria
    R82.998 **Other abnormal findings in urine**
        Cells and casts in urine
        Crystalluria
        Melanuria

Abnormal findings on examination of other body fluids, substances and tissues, without diagnosis (R83-R89)

Excludes1: *abnormal findings on antenatal screening of mother (O28.-)*
diagnostic abnormal findings classified elsewhere - see Alphabetical Index

Excludes2: *abnormal findings on examination of blood, without diagnosis (R70-R79)*
abnormal findings on examination of urine, without diagnosis (R80-R82)
abnormal tumor markers (R97.-)

R83 **Abnormal findings in cerebrospinal fluid**

  R83.0 **Abnormal level of enzymes in cerebrospinal fluid**
  R83.1 **Abnormal level of hormones in cerebrospinal fluid**
  R83.2 **Abnormal level of other drugs, medicaments and biological substances in cerebrospinal fluid**
  R83.3 **Abnormal level of substances chiefly nonmedicinal as to source in cerebrospinal fluid**
  R83.4 **Abnormal immunological findings in cerebrospinal fluid**
  R83.5 **Abnormal microbiological findings in cerebrospinal fluid**
    Positive culture findings in cerebrospinal fluid
    Excludes1: *colonization status (Z22.-)*
  R83.6 **Abnormal cytological findings in cerebrospinal fluid**
  R83.8 **Other abnormal findings in cerebrospinal fluid**
    Abnormal chromosomal findings in cerebrospinal fluid
  R83.9 **Unspecified abnormal finding in cerebrospinal fluid**

R84 **Abnormal findings in specimens from respiratory organs and thorax**

  Includes: abnormal findings in bronchial washings
    abnormal findings in nasal secretions
    abnormal findings in pleural fluid
    abnormal findings in sputum
    abnormal findings in throat scrapings
  Excludes1: *blood-stained sputum (R04.2)*
  R84.0 **Abnormal level of enzymes in specimens from respiratory organs and thorax**
  R84.1 **Abnormal level of hormones in specimens from respiratory organs and thorax**
  R84.2 **Abnormal level of other drugs, medicaments and biological substances in specimens from respiratory organs and thorax**
  R84.3 **Abnormal level of substances chiefly nonmedicinal as to source in specimens from respiratory organs and thorax**
  R84.4 **Abnormal immunological findings in specimens from respiratory organs and thorax**
  R84.5 **Abnormal microbiological findings in specimens from respiratory organs and thorax**
    Positive culture findings in specimens from respiratory organs and thorax
    Excludes1: *colonization status (Z22.-)*

R84.6 **Abnormal cytological findings in specimens from respiratory organs and thorax**
R84.7 **Abnormal histological findings in specimens from respiratory organs and thorax**
R84.8 **Other abnormal findings in specimens from respiratory organs and thorax**
  Abnormal chromosomal findings in specimens from respiratory organs and thorax
R84.9 **Unspecified abnormal finding in specimens from respiratory organs and thorax**

R85 **Abnormal findings in specimens from digestive organs and abdominal cavity**

  Includes: abnormal findings in peritoneal fluid
    abnormal findings in saliva
  Excludes1: *cloudy peritoneal dialysis effluent (R88.0)*
    fecal abnormalities (R19.5)
  R85.0 **Abnormal level of enzymes in specimens from digestive organs and abdominal cavity**
  R85.1 **Abnormal level of hormones in specimens from digestive organs and abdominal cavity**
  R85.2 **Abnormal level of other drugs, medicaments and biological substances in specimens from digestive organs and abdominal cavity**
  R85.3 **Abnormal level of substances chiefly nonmedicinal as to source in specimens from digestive organs and abdominal cavity**
  R85.4 **Abnormal immunological findings in specimens from digestive organs and abdominal cavity**
  R85.5 **Abnormal microbiological findings in specimens from digestive organs and abdominal cavity**
    Positive culture findings in specimens from digestive organs and abdominal cavity
    Excludes1: *colonization status (Z22.-)*
+ **R85.6** **Abnormal cytological findings in specimens from digestive organs and abdominal cavity**
  + **R85.61** **Abnormal cytologic smear of anus**
    Excludes1: *abnormal cytological findings in specimens from other digestive organs and abdominal cavity (R85.69)*
        carcinoma in situ of anus (histologically confirmed) (D01.3)
        anal intraepithelial neoplasia I [AIN I] (K62.82)
        anal intraepithelial neoplasia II [AIN II] (K62.82)
        anal intraepithelial neoplasia III [AIN III] (D01.3)
        dysplasia (mild) (moderate) of anus (histologically confirmed) (K62.82)
        severe dysplasia of anus (histologically confirmed) (D01.3)
    Excludes2: *anal high risk human papillomavirus (HPV) DNA test positive (R85.81)*
        anal low risk human papillomavirus (HPV) DNA test positive (R85.82)
    R85.610 **Atypical squamous cells of undetermined significance on cytologic smear of anus (ASC-US)**
    R85.611 **Atypical squamous cells cannot exclude high grade squamous intraepithelial lesion on cytologic smear of anus (ASC-H)**
    R85.612 **Low grade squamous intraepithelial lesion on cytologic smear of anus (LGSIL)**
    R85.613 **High grade squamous intraepithelial lesion on cytologic smear of anus (HGSIL)**
    R85.614 **Cytologic evidence of malignancy on smear of anus**

+, +7th, X + 7th ● Newborn ● Pediatric ● Maternity ● Adult ♀ Female ♂ Male Manifestation Unacceptable PDX HCC CC MCC HAC

R85.615 Unsatisfactory cytologic smear of anus
Inadequate sample of cytologic smear of anus

R85.616 Satisfactory anal smear but lacking transformation zone

R85.618 Other abnormal cytological findings on specimens from anus

R85.619 Unspecified abnormal cytological findings in specimens from anus
Abnormal anal cytology NOS
Atypical glandular cells of anus NOS

R85.69 Abnormal cytological findings in specimens from other digestive organs and abdominal cavity

R85.7 Abnormal histological findings in specimens from digestive organs and abdominal cavity

+ **R85.8 Other abnormal findings in specimens from digestive organs and abdominal cavity**

R85.81 Anal high risk human papillomavirus (HPV) DNA test positive
Excludes1: *anogenital warts due to human papillomavirus (HPV) (A63.0)*
condyloma acuminatum (A63.0)

R85.82 Anal low risk human papillomavirus (HPV) DNA test positive
Use additional code for associated human papillomavirus (B97.7)

R85.89 Other abnormal findings in specimens from digestive organs and abdominal cavity
Abnormal chromosomal findings in specimens from digestive organs and abdominal cavity

R85.9 Unspecified abnormal finding in specimens from digestive organs and abdominal cavity

R86 Abnormal findings in specimens from male genital organs

Includes: abnormal findings in prostatic secretions
abnormal findings in semen, seminal fluid
abnormal spermatozoa

Excludes1: *azoospermia (N46.0-)*
oligospermia (N46.1-)

♂ **R86.0 Abnormal level of enzymes in specimens from male genital organs**

♂ **R86.1 Abnormal level of hormones in specimens from male genital organs**

♂ **R86.2 Abnormal level of other drugs, medicaments and biological substances in specimens from male genital organs**

♂ **R86.3 Abnormal level of substances chiefly nonmedicinal as to source in specimens from male genital organs**

♂ **R86.4 Abnormal immunological findings in specimens from male genital organs**

♂ **R86.5 Abnormal microbiological findings in specimens from male genital organs**
Positive culture findings in specimens from male genital organs
Excludes1: *colonization status (Z22.-)*

♂ **R86.6 Abnormal cytological findings in specimens from male genital organs**

♂ **R86.7 Abnormal histological findings in specimens from male genital organs**

♂ **R86.8 Other abnormal findings in specimens from male genital organs**
Abnormal chromosomal findings in specimens from male genital organs

♂ **R86.9 Unspecified abnormal finding in specimens from male genital organs**

R87 Abnormal findings in specimens from female genital organs

Includes: abnormal findings in secretion and smears from cervix uteri
abnormal findings in secretion and smears from vagina
abnormal findings in secretion and smears from vulva

♀ **R87.0 Abnormal level of enzymes in specimens from female genital organs**

♀ **R87.1 Abnormal level of hormones in specimens from female genital organs**

♀ **R87.2 Abnormal level of other drugs, medicaments and biological substances in specimens from female genital organs**

♀ **R87.3 Abnormal level of substances chiefly nonmedicinal as to source in specimens from female genital organs**

♀ **R87.4 Abnormal immunological findings in specimens from female genital organs**

♀ **R87.5 Abnormal microbiological findings in specimens from female genital organs**
Positive culture findings in specimens from female genital organs
Excludes1: *colonization status (Z22.-)*

+ **R87.6 Abnormal cytological findings in specimens from female genital organs**

+ **R87.61 Abnormal cytological findings in specimens from cervix uteri**
Excludes1: *abnormal cytological findings in specimens from other female genital organs (R87.69)*
abnormal cytological findings in specimens from vagina (R87.62-)
carcinoma in situ of cervix uteri (histologically confirmed) (D06.-)
cervical intraepithelial neoplasia I [CIN I] (N87.0)
cervical intraepithelial neoplasia II [CIN II] (N87.1)
cervical intraepithelial neoplasia III [CIN III] (D06.-)
dysplasia (mild) (moderate) of cervix uteri (histologically confirmed) (N87.-)
severe dysplasia of cervix uteri (histologically confirmed) (D06.-)
Excludes2: *cervical high risk human papillomavirus (HPV) DNA test positive (R87.810)*
cervical low risk human papillomavirus (HPV) DNA test positive (R87.820)

♀ **R87.610 Atypical squamous cells of undetermined significance on cytologic smear of cervix (ASC-US)**

♀ **R87.611 Atypical squamous cells cannot exclude high grade squamous intraepithelial lesion on cytologic smear of cervix (ASC-H)**

♀ **R87.612 Low grade squamous intraepithelial lesion on cytologic smear of cervix (LGSIL)**

♀ **R87.613 High grade squamous intraepithelial lesion on cytologic smear of cervix (HGSIL)**

♀ **R87.614 Cytologic evidence of malignancy on smear of cervix**

♀ **R87.615 Unsatisfactory cytologic smear of cervix**
Inadequate sample of cytologic smear of cervix

♀ **R87.616 Satisfactory cervical smear but lacking transformation zone**

♀ **R87.618 Other abnormal cytological findings on specimens from cervix uteri**

♀ **R87.619 Unspecified abnormal cytological findings in specimens from cervix uteri**
Abnormal cervical cytology NOS
Abnormal Papanicolaou smear of cervix NOS
Abnormal thin preparation smear of cervix NOS
Atypical endocervial cells of cervix NOS
Atypical endometrial cells of cervix NOS
Atypical glandular cells of cervix NOS

+ **R87.62 Abnormal cytological findings in specimens from vagina**

Use additional code to identify acquired absence of uterus and cervix, if applicable (Z90.71-)

Excludes1: *abnormal cytological findings in specimens from cervix uteri (R87.61-)*
abnormal cytological findings in specimens from other female genital organs (R87.69)
carcinoma in situ of vagina (histologically confirmed) (D07.2)
vaginal intraepithelial neoplasia I [VAIN I] (N89.0)
vaginal intraepithelial neoplasia II [VAIN II] (N89.1)
vaginal intraepithelial neoplasia III [VAIN III] (D07.2)
dysplasia (mild) (moderate) of vagina (histologically confirmed) (N89.-)
severe dysplasia of vagina (histologically confirmed) (D07.2)

Excludes2: *vaginal high risk human papillomavirus (HPV) DNA test positive (R87.811)*
vaginal low risk human papillomavirus (HPV) DNA test positive (R87.821)

♀ **R87.620 Atypical squamous cells of undetermined significance on cytologic smear of vagina (ASC-US)**

♀ **R87.621 Atypical squamous cells cannot exclude high grade squamous intraepithelial lesion on cytologic smear of vagina (ASC-H)**

♀ **R87.622 Low grade squamous intraepithelial lesion on cytologic smear of vagina (LGSIL)**

♀ **R87.623 High grade squamous intraepithelial lesion on cytologic smear of vagina (HGSIL)**

♀ **R87.624 Cytologic evidence of malignancy on smear of vagina**

♀ **R87.625 Unsatisfactory cytologic smear of vagina**

Inadequate sample of cytologic smear of vagina

♀ **R87.628 Other abnormal cytological findings on specimens from vagina**

♀ **R87.629 Unspecified abnormal cytological findings in specimens from vagina**

Abnormal Papanicolaou smear of vagina NOS
Abnormal thin preparation smear of vagina NOS
Abnormal vaginal cytology NOS
Atypical endocervical cells of vagina NOS
Atypical endometrial cells of vagina NOS
Atypical glandular cells of vagina NOS

♀ **R87.69 Abnormal cytological findings in specimens from other female genital organs**

Abnormal cytological findings in specimens from female genital organs NOS

Excludes1: *dysplasia of vulva (histologically confirmed) (N90.0-N90.3)*

♀ **R87.7 Abnormal histological findings in specimens from female genital organs**

Excludes1: *carcinoma in situ (histologically confirmed) of female genital organs (D06-D07.3)*
cervical intraepithelial neoplasia I [CIN I] (N87.0)
cervical intraepithelial neoplasia II [CIN II] (N87.1)
cervical intraepithelial neoplasia III [CIN III] (D06.-)
dysplasia (mild) (moderate) of cervix uteri (histologically confirmed) (N87.-)
dysplasia (mild) (moderate) of vagina (histologically confirmed) (N89.-)
vaginal intraepithelial neoplasia I [VAIN I] (N89.0)
vaginal intraepithelial neoplasia II [VAIN II] (N89.1)
vaginal intraepithelial neoplasia III [VAIN III] (D07.2)
severe dysplasia of cervix uteri (histologically confirmed) (D06.-)
severe dysplasia of vagina (histologically confirmed) (D07.2)

+ **R87.8 Other abnormal findings in specimens from female genital organs**

+ **R87.81 High risk human papillomavirus (HPV) DNA test positive from female genital organs**

Excludes1: *anogenital warts due to human papillomavirus (HPV) (A63.0)*
condyloma acuminatum (A63.0)

♀ **R87.810 Cervical high risk human papillomavirus (HPV) DNA test positive**

♀ **R87.811 Vaginal high risk human papillomavirus (HPV) DNA test positive**

+ **R87.82 Low risk human papillomavirus (HPV) DNA test positive from female genital organs**

Use additional code for associated human papillomavirus (B97.7)

♀ **R87.820 Cervical low risk human papillomavirus (HPV) DNA test positive**

♀ **R87.821 Vaginal low risk human papillomavirus (HPV) DNA test positive**

♀ **R87.89 Other abnormal findings in specimens from female genital organs**

Abnormal chromosomal findings in specimens from female genital organs

♀ **R87.9 Unspecified abnormal finding in specimens from female genital organs**

R88 Abnormal findings in other body fluids and substances

R88.0 Cloudy (hemodialysis) (peritoneal) dialysis effluent

R88.8 Abnormal findings in other body fluids and substances

R89 Abnormal findings in specimens from other organs, systems and tissues

Includes: abnormal findings in nipple discharge
abnormal findings in synovial fluid
abnormal findings in wound secretions

R89.0 Abnormal level of enzymes in specimens from other organs, systems and tissues

R89.1 Abnormal level of hormones in specimens from other organs, systems and tissues

R89.2 Abnormal level of other drugs, medicaments and biological substances in specimens from other organs, systems and tissues

R89.3 Abnormal level of substances chiefly nonmedicinal as to source in specimens from other organs, systems and tissues

+, +7th, X + 7th   ● Newborn   ● Pediatric   ● Maternity   ● Adult   ♀ Female   ♂ Male   Manifestation   Unacceptable PDX   HCC   CC   MCC   HAC

R89.4 **Abnormal immunological findings in specimens from other organs, systems and tissues**

R89.5 **Abnormal microbiological findings in specimens from other organs, systems and tissues**
Positive culture findings in specimens from other organs, systems and tissues
Excludes1: colonization status (Z22.-)

R89.6 **Abnormal cytological findings in specimens from other organs, systems and tissues**

R89.7 **Abnormal histological findings in specimens from other organs, systems and tissues**

R89.8 **Other abnormal findings in specimens from other organs, systems and tissues**
Abnormal chromosomal findings in specimens from other organs, systems and tissues

R89.9 **Unspecified abnormal finding in specimens from other organs, systems and tissues**

Abnormal findings on diagnostic imaging and in function studies, without diagnosis (R90-R94)

Includes: nonspecific abnormal findings on diagnostic imaging by computerized axial tomography [CAT scan]
nonspecific abnormal findings on diagnostic imaging by magnetic resonance imaging [MRI][NMR]
nonspecific abnormal findings on diagnostic imaging by positron emission tomography [PET scan]
nonspecific abnormal findings on diagnostic imaging by thermography
nonspecific abnormal findings on diagnostic imaging by ultrasound [echogram]
nonspecific abnormal findings on diagnostic imaging by X-ray examination

Excludes1: abnormal findings on antenatal screening of mother (O28.-)
diagnostic abnormal findings classified elsewhere - see Alphabetical Index

R90 **Abnormal findings on diagnostic imaging of central nervous system**

R90.0 **Intracranial space-occupying lesion found on diagnostic imaging of central nervous system**

+ R90.8 **Other abnormal findings on diagnostic imaging of central nervous system**
R90.81 **Abnormal echoencephalogram**
R90.82 **White matter disease, unspecified**
R90.89 **Other abnormal findings on diagnostic imaging of central nervous system**
Other cerebrovascular abnormality found on diagnostic imaging of central nervous system

R91 **Abnormal findings on diagnostic imaging of lung**

R91.1 **Solitary pulmonary nodule**
Coin lesion lung
Solitary pulmonary nodule, subsegmental branch of the bronchial tree

R91.8 **Other nonspecific abnormal finding of lung field**
Lung mass NOS found on diagnostic imaging of lung
Pulmonary infiltrate NOS
Shadow, lung

R92 **Abnormal and inconclusive findings on diagnostic imaging of breast**

R92.0 **Mammographic microcalcification found on diagnostic imaging of breast**
Excludes2: mammographic calcification (calculus) found on diagnostic imaging of breast (R92.1)

R92.1 **Mammographic calcification found on diagnostic imaging of breast**
Mammographic calculus found on diagnostic imaging of breast

R92.2 **Inconclusive mammogram**
Dense breasts NOS
Inconclusive mammogram NEC
Inconclusive mammography due to dense breasts
Inconclusive mammography NEC
AHA CC: 1Q, 2015, 24

R92.8 **Other abnormal and inconclusive findings on diagnostic imaging of breast**

R93 **Abnormal findings on diagnostic imaging of other body structures**

R93.0 **Abnormal findings on diagnostic imaging of skull and head, not elsewhere classified**
Excludes1: intracranial space-occupying lesion found on diagnostic imaging (R90.0)

R93.1 **Abnormal findings on diagnostic imaging of heart and coronary circulation**
Abnormal echocardiogram NOS
Abnormal heart shadow

R93.2 **Abnormal findings on diagnostic imaging of liver and biliary tract**
Nonvisualization of gallbladder

R93.3 **Abnormal findings on diagnostic imaging of other parts of digestive tract**

+ R93.4 **Abnormal findings on diagnostic imaging of urinary organs**
Excludes2: hypertrophy of kidney (N28.81)
AHA CC: 4Q, 2016, 66
R93.41 **Abnormal radiologic findings on diagnostic imaging of of renal pelvis, ureter, or bladder**
Filling defect of bladder found on diagnostic imaging
Filling defect of renal pelvis found on diagnostic imaging
Filling defect of ureter found on diagnostic imaging

+ R93.42 **Abnormal radiologic findings on diagnostic imaging of kidney**
R93.421 **Abnormal radiologic findings on diagnostic imaging of right kidney**
R93.422 **Abnormal radiologic findings on diagnostic imaging of left kidney**
R93.429 **Abnormal radiologic findings on diagnostic imaging of unspecified kidney**

R93.49 **Abnormal radiologic findings on diagnostic imaging of other urinary organs**

R93.5 **Abnormal findings on diagnostic imaging of other abdominal regions, including retroperitoneum**

R93.6 **Abnormal findings on diagnostic imaging of limbs**
Excludes2: abnormal finding in skin and subcutaneous tissue (R93.8-)
AHA CC: 1Q, 2020, 14-15

R93.7 **Abnormal findings on diagnostic imaging of other parts of musculoskeletal system**
Excludes2: abnormal findings on diagnostic imaging of skull (R93.0)

+ R93.8 **Abnormal findings on diagnostic imaging of other specified body structures**
AHA CC: 4Q, 2018, 30
+ R93.81 **Abnormal radiologic findings on diagnostic imaging of testis**
♂ R93.811 **Abnormal radiologic findings on diagnostic imaging of right testicle**
♂ R93.812 **Abnormal radiologic findings on diagnostic imaging of left testicle**
♂ R93.813 **Abnormal radiologic findings on diagnostic imaging of testicles, bilateral**
♂ R93.819 **Abnormal radiologic findings on diagnostic imaging of unspecified testicle**

R93.89 **Abnormal findings on diagnostic imaging of other specified body structures**
Abnormal findings by radioisotope localization of placenta
Abnormal radiological finding in skin and subcutaneous tissue
Mediastinal shift

R93.9 **Diagnostic imaging inconclusive due to excess body fat of patient**

R94 **Abnormal results of function studies**

> Includes: abnormal results of radionuclide [radioisotope] uptake
> studies
> abnormal results of scintigraphy

+ **R94.0** **Abnormal results of function studies of central nervous system**

    R94.01 **Abnormal electroencephalogram [EEG]**

    R94.02 **Abnormal brain scan**

    R94.09 **Abnormal results of other function studies of central nervous system**

+ **R94.1** **Abnormal results of function studies of peripheral nervous system and special senses**

  + **R94.11** **Abnormal results of function studies of eye**

      R94.110 **Abnormal electro-oculogram [EOG]**

      R94.111 **Abnormal electroretinogram [ERG]**
        Abnormal retinal function study

      R94.112 **Abnormal visually evoked potential [VEP]**

      R94.113 **Abnormal oculomotor study**

      R94.118 **Abnormal results of other function studies of eye**

  + **R94.12** **Abnormal results of function studies of ear and other special senses**

      R94.120 **Abnormal auditory function study**
        AHA CC: 3Q, 2016, 17

      R94.121 **Abnormal vestibular function study**

      R94.128 **Abnormal results of other function studies of ear and other special senses**

  + **R94.13** **Abnormal results of function studies of peripheral nervous system**

      R94.130 **Abnormal response to nerve stimulation, unspecified**

      R94.131 **Abnormal electromyogram [EMG]**
        Excludes1: *electromyogram of eye (R94.113)*

      R94.138 **Abnormal results of other function studies of peripheral nervous system**

R94.2 **Abnormal results of pulmonary function studies**
  Reduced ventilatory capacity
  Reduced vital capacity

+ **R94.3** **Abnormal results of cardiovascular function studies**

    R94.30 **Abnormal result of cardiovascular function study, unspecified**

    R94.31 **Abnormal electrocardiogram [ECG] [EKG]**
      Excludes1: *long QT syndrome (I45.81)*

    R94.39 **Abnormal result of other cardiovascular function study**
      Abnormal electrophysiological intracardiac studies
      Abnormal phonocardiogram
      Abnormal vectorcardiogram

R94.4 **Abnormal results of kidney function studies**
  Abnormal renal function test

R94.5 **Abnormal results of liver function studies**

R94.6 **Abnormal results of thyroid function studies**

R94.7 **Abnormal results of other endocrine function studies**
  Excludes2: *abnormal glucose (R73.0-)*

R94.8 **Abnormal results of function studies of other organs and systems**
  Abnormal basal metabolic rate [BMR]
  Abnormal bladder function test
  Abnormal splenic function test

Abnormal tumor markers (R97)

R97 **Abnormal tumor markers**

  Elevated tumor associated antigens [TAA]
  Elevated tumor specific antigens [TSA]

R97.0 **Elevated carcinoembryonic antigen [CEA]**

R97.1 **Elevated cancer antigen 125 [CA 125]**

+ **R97.2** **Elevated prostate specific antigen [PSA]**
  AHA CC: 4Q, 2016, 66

  ● ♂ **R97.20** **Elevated prostate specific antigen [PSA]**

  ● ♂ **R97.21** **Rising PSA following treatment for malignant neoplasm of prostate**

R97.8 **Other abnormal tumor markers**

Ill-defined and unknown cause of mortality (R99)

R99 **Ill-defined and unknown cause of mortality**

  Death (unexplained) NOS
  Unspecified cause of mortality
  Review coding guideline C.18.h
  Valid 3-character code, no further characters required

+, +7th, X + 7th   ● Newborn   ● Pediatric   ● Maternity   ● Adult   ♀ Female   ♂ Male   Manifestation   Unacceptable PDX   HCC   CC   MCC   HAC

Muscles

Frontalis

Sternocleidomastoid

Trapezius

Deltoid

Pectoralis major

Serratus anterior

Brachioradialis

Biceps

External oblique

Adductor longus

Vastus lateralis

Vastus medialis

Peroneus longus

Extensor digitorum brevis

Flexor digitorum superficialis

Palmaris longus

Flexor carpi radialis

Rectus abdominus

Gluteus medius

Tensor faciae latae

Pectineus

Rectus femoris

Sartorius

Gracilis

Tibialis anterior

Gastrocnemius

Soleus

Extensor hallucis brevis

©AHIMA

Skeleton - Front and Side Views

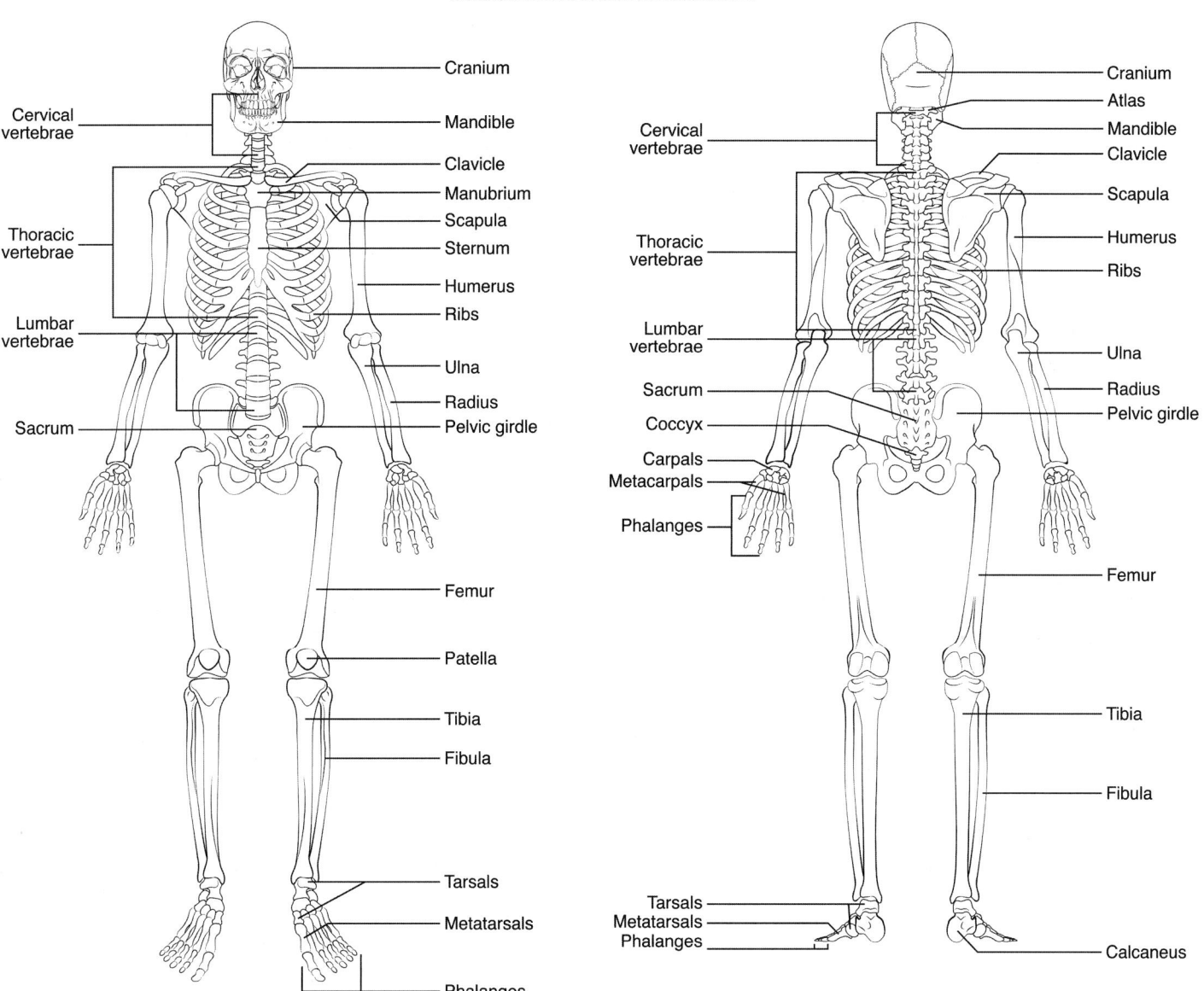

Cranium
Mandible
Clavicle
Manubrium
Scapula
Sternum
Humerus
Ribs
Ulna
Radius
Pelvic girdle

Cervical vertebrae
Thoracic vertebrae
Lumbar vertebrae
Sacrum

Femur
Patella
Tibia
Fibula
Tarsals
Metatarsals
Phalanges

Cranium
Atlas
Mandible
Clavicle
Scapula
Humerus
Ribs
Ulna
Radius
Pelvic girdle
Femur
Tibia
Fibula
Calcaneus

Cervical vertebrae
Thoracic vertebrae
Lumbar vertebrae
Sacrum
Coccyx
Carpals
Metacarpals
Phalanges
Tarsals
Metatarsals
Phalanges

©AHIMA

Chapter 19: Injury, Poisoning and Certain Other Consequences of External Causes (S00-T88)

NOTE Use secondary code(s) from Chapter 20, External causes of morbidity, to indicate cause of injury. Codes within the T-section that include the external cause do not require an additional external cause code

Use additional code to identify any retained foreign body, if applicable (Z18.-)

Excludes1: birth trauma (P10-P15)
obstetric trauma (O70-O71)

NOTE The chapter uses the S-section for coding different types of injuries related to single body regions and the T-section to cover injuries to unspecified body regions as well as poisoning and certain other consequences of external causes.
AHA CC: 1Q, 2015, 3-21

This chapter contains the following category blocks:

S00-S09 Injuries to the head
S10-S19 Injuries to the neck
S20-S29 Injuries to the thorax
S30-S39 Injuries to the abdomen, lower back, lumbar spine, pelvis and external genitals
S40-S49 Injuries to the shoulder and upper arm
S50-S59 Injuries to the elbow and forearm
S60-S69 Injuries to the wrist, hand and fingers
S70-S79 Injuries to the hip and thigh
S80-S89 Injuries to the knee and lower leg
S90-S99 Injuries to the ankle and foot
T07 Injuries involving multiple body regions
T14 Injury of unspecified body region
T15-T19 Effects of foreign body entering through natural orifice
T20-T25 Burns and corrosions of external body surface, specified by site
T26-T28 Burns and corrosions confined to eye and internal organs
T30-T32 Burns and corrosions of multiple and unspecified body regions
T33-T34 Frostbite
T36-T50 Poisoning by, adverse effect of and underdosing of drugs, medicaments and biological substances
T51-T65 Toxic effects of substances chiefly nonmedicinal as to source
T66-T78 Other and unspecified effects of external causes
T79 Certain early complications of trauma
T80-T88 Complications of surgical and medical care, not elsewhere classified

C. Chapter-Specific Coding Guidelines

In addition to general coding guidelines, there are guidelines for specific diagnoses and/or conditions in the classification. Unless otherwise indicated, these guidelines apply to all health care settings. Please refer to Section II for guidelines on the selection of principal diagnosis.

19. Chapter 19: Injury, Poisoning and Certain Other Consequences of External Causes (S00-T88)

a. Application of 7th Characters in Chapter 19

Most categories in chapter 19 have a 7th character requirement for each applicable code. Most categories in this chapter have three 7th character values (with the exception of fractures): A, initial encounter, D, subsequent encounter and S, sequela. Categories for traumatic fractures have additional 7th character values. While the patient may be seen by a new or different provider over the course of treatment for an injury, assignment of the 7th character is based on whether the patient is undergoing active treatment and not whether the provider is seeing the patient for the first time.

For complication codes, active treatment refers to treatment for the condition described by the code, even though it may be related to an earlier precipitating problem. For example, code T84.50XA, Infection and inflammatory reaction due to unspecified internal joint prosthesis, initial encounter, is used when active treatment is provided for the infection, even though the condition relates to the prosthetic device, implant or graft that was placed at a previous encounter.

7th character "A", initial encounter is used for each encounter where the patient is receiving active treatment for the condition.

7th character "D" subsequent encounter is used for encounters after the patient has completed active treatment of the condition and is receiving routine care for the condition during the healing or recovery phase.

The aftercare Z codes should not be used for aftercare for conditions such as injuries or poisonings, where 7th characters are provided to identify subsequent care. For example, for aftercare of an injury, assign the acute injury code with the 7th character "D" (subsequent encounter).

7th character "S", sequela, is for use for complications or conditions that arise as a direct result of a condition, such as scar formation after a burn. The scars are sequelae of the burn. When using 7th character "S", it is necessary to use both the injury code that precipitated the sequela and the code for the sequela itself. The "S" is added only to the injury code, not the sequela code. The 7th character "S" identifies the injury responsible for the sequela. The specific type of sequela (e.g. scar) is sequenced first, followed by the injury code.
See Section I.B.10 Sequela (Late Effects)

b. Coding of Injuries

When coding injuries, assign separate codes for each injury unless a combination code is provided, in which case the combination code is assigned. Codes from category T07, Unspecified multiple injuries should not be assigned in the inpatient setting unless information for a more specific code is not available. Traumatic injury codes (S00-T14.9) are not to be used for normal, healing surgical wounds or to identify complications of surgical wounds.

The code for the most serious injury, as determined by the provider and the focus of treatment, is sequenced first.

1) Superficial injuries

Superficial injuries such as abrasions or contusions are not coded when associated with more severe injuries of the same site.

2) Primary injury with damage to nerves/blood vessels

When a primary injury results in minor damage to peripheral nerves or blood vessels, the primary injury is sequenced first with additional code(s) for injuries to nerves and spinal cord (such as category S04), and/or injury to blood vessels (such as category S15). When the primary injury is to the blood vessels or nerves, that injury should be sequenced first.

3) Iatrogenic injuries

Injury codes from Chapter 19 should not be assigned for injuries that occur during, or as a result of, a medical intervention. Assign the appropriate complication code(s).

c. Coding of Traumatic Fractures

The principles of multiple coding of injuries should be followed in coding fractures. Fractures of specified sites are coded individually by site in accordance with both the provisions within categories S02, S12, S22, S32, S42, S49, S52, S59, S62, S72, S79, S82, S89, S92 and the level of detail furnished by medical record content.

A fracture not indicated as open or closed should be coded to closed. A fracture not indicated whether displaced or not displaced should be coded to displaced.

More specific guidelines are as follows:

1) Initial vs. Subsequent Encounter for Fractures

Traumatic fractures are coded using the appropriate 7th character for initial encounter (A, B, C) for each encounter where the patient is receiving active treatment for the fracture. The appropriate 7th character for initial encounter should also be assigned for a patient who delayed seeking treatment for the fracture or nonunion.

Fractures are coded using the appropriate 7th character for subsequent care for encounters after the patient has completed active treatment of the fracture and is receiving routine care for the fracture during the healing or recovery phase.

Care for complications of surgical treatment for fracture repairs during the healing or recovery phase should be coded with the appropriate complication codes.

Care of complications of fractures, such as malunion and nonunion, should be reported with the appropriate 7th character for subsequent care with nonunion (K, M, N,) or subsequent care with malunion (P, Q, R).

Malunion/nonunion: The appropriate 7th character for initial encounter should also be assigned for a patient who delayed seeking treatment for the fracture or nonunion.

The open fracture designations in the assignment of the 7th character for fractures of the forearm, femur and lower leg, including ankle are based on the Gustilo open fracture classification. When the Gustilo classification type is not specified for an open fracture, the 7th character for open fracture type I or II should be assigned (B, E, H, M, Q).

A code from category M80, not a traumatic fracture code, should be used for any patient with known osteoporosis who suffers a fracture, even if the patient had a minor fall or trauma, if that fall or trauma would not usually break a normal, healthy bone.
See Section I.C.13. Osteoporosis.

The aftercare Z codes should not be used for aftercare for traumatic fractures. For aftercare of a traumatic fracture, assign the acute fracture code with the appropriate 7th character.

2) Multiple fractures sequencing

Multiple fractures are sequenced in accordance with the severity of the fracture.

+, +7th, X + 7th ● Newborn ● Pediatric ● Maternity ● Adult ♀ Female ♂ Male Manifestation Unacceptable PDX HCC CC MCC HAC

3) Physeal fractures

For physeal fractures, assign only the code identifying the type of physeal fracture. Do not assign a separate code to identify the specific bone that is fractured.

d. Coding of Burns and Corrosions

The ICD-10-CM makes a distinction between burns and corrosions. The burn codes are for thermal burns, except sunburns, that come from a heat source, such as a fire or hot appliance. The burn codes are also for burns resulting from electricity and radiation. Corrosions are burns due to chemicals. The guidelines are the same for burns and corrosions.

Current burns (T20-T25) are classified by depth, extent and by agent (X code). Burns are classified by depth as first degree (erythema), second degree (blistering), and third degree (full-thickness involvement). Burns of the eye and internal organs (T26-T28) are classified by site, but not by degree.

1) Sequencing of burn and related condition codes

Sequence first the code that reflects the highest degree of burn when more than one burn is present.

a. When the reason for the admission or encounter is for treatment of external multiple burns, sequence first the code that reflects the burn of the highest degree.

b. When a patient has both internal and external burns, the circumstances of admission govern the selection of the principal diagnosis or first-listed diagnosis.

c. When a patient is admitted for burn injuries and other related conditions such as smoke inhalation and/or respiratory failure, the circumstances of admission govern the selection of the principal or first-listed diagnosis.

2) Burns of the same anatomical site

Classify burns of the same anatomical site and on the same site but of different degrees to the subcategory identifying the highest degree recorded in the diagnosis (e.g., for second and third degree burns of right thigh, assign only code T24.311-).

3) Non-healing burns

Non-healing burns are coded as acute burns.

Necrosis of burned skin should be coded as a non-healed burn.

4) Infected Burn

For any documented infected burn site, use an additional code for the infection.

5) Assign separate codes for each burn site

When coding burns, assign separate codes for each burn site. Category T30, Burn and corrosion, body region unspecified is extremely vague and should rarely be used.

Codes for burns of "multiple sites" should only be assigned when the medical record documentation does not specify the individual sites.

6) Burns and Corrosions Classified According to Extent of Body Surface Involved

Assign codes from category T31, Burns classified according to extent of body surface involved, or T32, Corrosions classified according to extent of body surface involved, when the site of the burn is not specified or when there is a need for additional data. It is advisable to use category T31 as additional coding when needed to provide data for evaluating burn mortality, such as that needed by burn units. It is also advisable to use category T31 as an additional code for reporting purposes when there is mention of a third-degree burn involving 20 percent or more of the body surface.

Categories T31 and T32 are based on the classic "rule of nines" in estimating body surface involved: head and neck are assigned nine percent, each arm nine percent, each leg 18 percent, the anterior trunk 18 percent, posterior trunk 18 percent, and genitalia one percent. Providers may change these percentage assignments where necessary to accommodate infants and children who have proportionately larger heads than adults, and patients who have large buttocks, thighs, or abdomen that involve burns.

7) Encounters for treatment of sequela of burns

Encounters for the treatment of the late effects of burns or corrosions (i.e., scars or joint contractures) should be coded with a burn or corrosion code with the 7th character "S" for sequela.

8) Sequelae with a late effect code and current burn

When appropriate, both a code for a current burn or corrosion with 7th character "A" or "D" and a burn or corrosion code with 7th character "S" may be assigned on the same record (when both a current burn and sequelae of an old burn exist). Burns and corrosions do not heal at the same rate and a current healing wound may still exist with sequela of a healed burn or corrosion. *See Section I.B.10 Sequela (Late Effects)*

9) Use of an external cause code with burns and corrosions

An external cause code should be used with burns and corrosions to identify the source and intent of the burn, as well as the place where it occurred.

e. Adverse Effects, Poisoning, Underdosing and Toxic Effects

Codes in categories T36-T65 are combination codes that include the substance that was taken as well as the intent. No additional external cause code is required for poisonings, toxic effects, adverse effects and underdosing codes.

1) Do not code directly from the Table of Drugs

Do not code directly from the Table of Drugs and Chemicals. Always refer back to the Tabular List.

2) Use as many codes as necessary to describe

Use as many codes as necessary to describe completely all drugs, medicinal or biological substances.

3) If the same code would describe the causative agent

If the same code would describe the causative agent for more than one adverse reaction, poisoning, toxic effect or underdosing, assign the code only once.

4) If two or more drugs, medicinal or biological substances

If two or more drugs, medicinal or biological substances are taken, code each individually unless a combination code is listed in the Table of Drugs and Chemicals.

If multiple unspecified drugs, medicinal or biological substances were taken, assign the appropriate code from subcategory T50.91, Poisoning by, adverse effect of and underdosing of multiple unspecified drugs, medicaments and biological substances.

5) The occurrence of drug toxicity is classified in ICD-10-CM as follows:

(a) Adverse Effect

When coding an adverse effect of a drug that has been correctly prescribed and properly administered, assign the appropriate code for the nature of the adverse effect followed by the appropriate code for the adverse effect of the drug (T36-T50). The code for the drug should have a 5th or 6th character "5" (for example T36.0X5-) Examples of the nature of an adverse effect are tachycardia, delirium, gastrointestinal hemorrhaging, vomiting, hypokalemia, hepatitis, renal failure, or respiratory failure.

(b) Poisoning

When coding a poisoning or reaction to the improper use of a medication (e.g., overdose, wrong substance given or taken in error, wrong route of administration), first assign the appropriate code from categories T36-T50. The poisoning codes have an associated intent as their 5th or 6th character (accidental, intentional self-harm, assault and undetermined.) If the intent of the poisoning is unknown or unspecified, code the intent as accidental intent. The undetermined intent is only for use if the documentation in the record specifies that the intent cannot be determined. Use additional code(s) for all manifestations of poisonings.

If there is also a diagnosis of abuse or dependence of the substance, the abuse or dependence is assigned as an additional code.

Examples of poisoning include:

(i)   Error was made in drug prescription

Errors made in drug prescription or in the administration of the drug by provider, nurse, patient, or other person.

(ii) Overdose of a drug intentionally taken

If an overdose of a drug was intentionally taken or administered and resulted in drug toxicity, it would be coded as a poisoning.

(iii) Nonprescribed drug taken with correctly prescribed and properly administered drug

If a nonprescribed drug or medicinal agent was taken in combination with a correctly prescribed and properly administered drug, any drug toxicity or other reaction resulting from the interaction of the two drugs would be classified as a poisoning.

(iv) Interaction of drug(s) and alcohol

When a reaction results from the interaction of a drug(s) and alcohol, this would be classified as poisoning.

See Section I.C.4. if poisoning is the result of insulin pump malfunctions.

(c) Underdosing

Underdosing refers to taking less of a medication than is prescribed by a provider or a manufacturer's instruction. Discontinuing the use of a prescribed medication on the patient's own initiative (not directed by the patient's provider) is also classified as an underdosing. For underdosing, assign the code from categories T36-T50 (fifth or sixth character "6").

Codes for underdosing should never be assigned as principal or first-listed codes. If a patient has a relapse or exacerbation of the medical condition for which the drug is prescribed because of the reduction in dose, then the medical condition itself should be coded.

+, +7th, X + 7th   • Newborn   • Pediatric   • Maternity   • Adult   ♀ Female   ♂ Male   Manifestation   Unacceptable PDX   HCC   CC   MCC   HAC

Noncompliance (Z91.12-, Z91.13- and Z91.14-) or complication of care (Y63.6-Y63.9) codes are to be used with an underdosing code to indicate intent, if known.

(d) Toxic Effects

When a harmful substance is ingested or comes in contact with a person, this is classified as a toxic effect. The toxic effect codes are in categories T51-T65.

Toxic effect codes have an associated intent: accidental, intentional self-harm, assault and undetermined.

f. Adult and child abuse, neglect and other maltreatment

Sequence first the appropriate code from categories T74.- (Adult and child abuse, neglect and other maltreatment, confirmed) or T76.- (Adult and child abuse, neglect and other maltreatment, suspected) for abuse, neglect and other maltreatment, followed by any accompanying mental health or injury code(s).

If the documentation in the medical record states abuse or neglect it is coded as confirmed (T74.-). It is coded as suspected if it is documented as suspected (T76.-).

For cases of confirmed abuse or neglect an external cause code from the assault section (X92-Y09) should be added to identify the cause of any physical injuries. A perpetrator code (Y07) should be added when the perpetrator of the abuse is known. For suspected cases of abuse or neglect, do not report external cause or perpetrator code.

If a suspected case of abuse, neglect or mistreatment is ruled out during an encounter code Z04.71, Encounter for examination and observation following alleged physical adult abuse, ruled out, or code Z04.72, Encounter for examination and observation following alleged child physical abuse, ruled out, should be used, not a code from T76.

If a suspected case of alleged rape or sexual abuse is ruled out during an encounter code Z04.41, Encounter for examination and observation following alleged adult rape or code Z04.42, Encounter for examination and observation following alleged child rape, should be used, not a code from T76.

If a suspected case of forced sexual exploitation or forced labor exploitation is ruled out during an encounter, code Z04.81, Encounter for examination and observation of victim following forced sexual exploitation, or code Z04.82, Encounter for examination and observation of victim following forced labor exploitation, should be used, not a code from T76.

See Section I.C.15. Abuse in a pregnant patient.

g. Complications of care

1) General guidelines for complications of care

(a) Documentation of complications of care

See Section I.B.16. for information on documentation of complications of care.

2) Pain due to medical devices

Pain associated with devices, implants or grafts left in a surgical site (for example painful hip prosthesis) is assigned to the appropriate code(s) found in Chapter 19, Injury, poisoning, and certain other consequences of external causes. Specific codes for pain due to medical devices are found in the T code section of the ICD-10-CM. Use additional code(s) from category G89 to identify acute or chronic pain due to presence of the device, implant or graft (G89.18 or G89.28).

3) Transplant complications

(a) Transplant complications other than kidney

Codes under category T86, Complications of transplanted organs and tissues, are for use for both complications and rejection of transplanted organs. A transplant complication code is only assigned if the complication affects the function of the transplanted organ. Two codes are required to fully describe a transplant complication: the appropriate code from category T86 and a secondary code that identifies the complication.

Pre-existing conditions or conditions that develop after the transplant are not coded as complications unless they affect the function of the transplanted organs.

See I.C.21. for transplant organ removal status.

See I.C.2. for malignant neoplasm associated with transplanted organ.

(b) Kidney transplant complications

Patients who have undergone kidney transplant may still have some form of chronic kidney disease (CKD) because the kidney transplant may not fully restore kidney function. Code T86.1- should be assigned for documented complications of a kidney transplant, such as transplant failure or rejection or other transplant complication. Code T86.1- should not be assigned for post kidney transplant patients who have chronic kidney (CKD) unless a transplant complication such as transplant failure or rejection is documented.

If the documentation is unclear as to whether the patient has a complication of the transplant, query the provider.

Conditions that affect the function of the transplanted kidney, other than CKD, should be assigned a code from subcategory T86.1, Complications of transplanted organ, Kidney, and a secondary code that identifies the complication.

For patients with CKD following a kidney transplant, but who do not have a complication such as failure or rejection, *see section I.C.14. Chronic kidney disease and kidney transplant status.*

4) Complication codes that include the external cause

As with certain other T codes, some of the complications of care codes have the external cause included in the code. The code includes the nature of the complication as well as the type of procedure that caused the complication. No external cause code indicating the type of procedure is necessary for these codes.

5) Complications of care codes within the body system chapters

Intraoperative and postprocedural complication codes are found within the body system chapters with codes specific to the organs and structures of that body system. These codes should be sequenced first, followed by a code(s) for the specific complication, if applicable.

Complication codes from the body system chapters should be assigned for intraoperative and postprocedural complications (e.g., the appropriate complication code from chapter 9 would be assigned for a vascular intraoperative or postprocedural complication) unless the complication is specifically indexed to a T code in chapter 19.

Injuries to the head (S00-S09)

Includes: *injuries of ear*
injuries of eye
injuries of face [any part]
injuries of gum
injuries of jaw
injuries of oral cavity
injuries of palate
injuries of periocular area
injuries of scalp
injuries of temporomandibular joint area
injuries of tongue
injuries of tooth

Code also for any associated infection

Excludes2: *burns and corrosions (T20-T32)*
effects of foreign body in ear (T16)
effects of foreign body in larynx (T17.3)
effects of foreign body in mouth NOS (T18.0)
effects of foreign body in nose (T17.0-T17.1)
effects of foreign body in pharynx (T17.2)
effects of foreign body on external eye (T15.-)
frostbite (T33-T34)
insect bite or sting, venomous (T63.4)

S00 Superficial injury of head

Excludes1: *diffuse cerebral contusion (S06.2-)*
focal cerebral contusion (S06.3-)
injury of eye and orbit (S05.-)
open wound of head (S01.-)

> The appropriate 7th character is to be added to each code from category S00
> A initial encounter
> D subsequent encounter
> S sequela

+ **S00.0 Superficial injury of scalp**
  X+7th **S00.00 Unspecified superficial injury of scalp**
  X+7th **S00.01 Abrasion of scalp**
  X+7th **S00.02 Blister (nonthermal) of scalp**
  X+7th **S00.03 Contusion of scalp**
  Bruise of scalp
  Hematoma of scalp
  X+7th **S00.04 External constriction of part of scalp**
  X+7th **S00.05 Superficial foreign body of scalp**
  Splinter in the scalp
  X+7th **S00.06 Insect bite (nonvenomous) of scalp**
  X+7th **S00.07 Other superficial bite of scalp**
  Excludes1: *open bite of scalp (S01.05)*
+ **S00.1 Contusion of eyelid and periocular area**
  Black eye
  Excludes2: *contusion of eyeball and orbital tissues (S05.1)*
  X+7th **S00.10 Contusion of unspecified eyelid and periocular area**

X+7th **S00.11** **Contusion of right eyelid and periocular area**
X+7th **S00.12** **Contusion of left eyelid and periocular area**
+ **S00.2** **Other and unspecified superficial injuries of eyelid and periocular area**
    Excludes2: *superficial injury of conjunctiva and cornea (S05.0-)*
+ **S00.20** **Unspecified superficial injury of eyelid and periocular area**
    +7th **S00.201** **Unspecified superficial injury of right eyelid and periocular area**
    +7th **S00.202** **Unspecified superficial injury of left eyelid and periocular area**
    +7th **S00.209** **Unspecified superficial injury of unspecified eyelid and periocular area**
+ **S00.21** **Abrasion of eyelid and periocular area**
    +7th **S00.211** **Abrasion of right eyelid and periocular area**
    +7th **S00.212** **Abrasion of left eyelid and periocular area**
    +7th **S00.219** **Abrasion of unspecified eyelid and periocular area**
+ **S00.22** **Blister (nonthermal) of eyelid and periocular area**
    +7th **S00.221** **Blister (nonthermal) of right eyelid and periocular area**
    +7th **S00.222** **Blister (nonthermal) of left eyelid and periocular area**
    +7th **S00.229** **Blister (nonthermal) of unspecified eyelid and periocular area**
+ **S00.24** **External constriction of eyelid and periocular area**
    +7th **S00.241** **External constriction of right eyelid and periocular area**
    +7th **S00.242** **External constriction of left eyelid and periocular area**
    +7th **S00.249** **External constriction of unspecified eyelid and periocular area**
+ **S00.25** **Superficial foreign body of eyelid and periocular area**
    Splinter of eyelid and periocular area
    Excludes2: *retained foreign body in eyelid (H02.81-)*
    +7th **S00.251** **Superficial foreign body of right eyelid and periocular area**
    +7th **S00.252** **Superficial foreign body of left eyelid and periocular area**
    +7th **S00.259** **Superficial foreign body of unspecified eyelid and periocular area**
+ **S00.26** **Insect bite (nonvenomous) of eyelid and periocular area**
    +7th **S00.261** **Insect bite (nonvenomous) of right eyelid and periocular area**
    +7th **S00.262** **Insect bite (nonvenomous) of left eyelid and periocular area**
    +7th **S00.269** **Insect bite (nonvenomous) of unspecified eyelid and periocular area**
+ **S00.27** **Other superficial bite of eyelid and periocular area**
    Excludes1: *open bite of eyelid and periocular area (S01.15)*
    +7th **S00.271** **Other superficial bite of right eyelid and periocular area**
    +7th **S00.272** **Other superficial bite of left eyelid and periocular area**
    +7th **S00.279** **Other superficial bite of unspecified eyelid and periocular area**
+ **S00.3** **Superficial injury of nose**
X+7th **S00.30** **Unspecified superficial injury of nose**
X+7th **S00.31** **Abrasion of nose**
X+7th **S00.32** **Blister (nonthermal) of nose**
X+7th **S00.33** **Contusion of nose**
    Bruise of nose
    Hematoma of nose
X+7th **S00.34** **External constriction of nose**
X+7th **S00.35** **Superficial foreign body of nose**
    Splinter in the nose
X+7th **S00.36** **Insect bite (nonvenomous) of nose**
X+7th **S00.37** **Other superficial bite of nose**
    Excludes1: *open bite of nose (S01.25)*
+ **S00.4** **Superficial injury of ear**
+ **S00.40** **Unspecified superficial injury of ear**
    +7th **S00.401** **Unspecified superficial injury of right ear**
    +7th **S00.402** **Unspecified superficial injury of left ear**

+7th **S00.409** **Unspecified superficial injury of unspecified ear**
+ **S00.41** **Abrasion of ear**
    +7th **S00.411** **Abrasion of right ear**
    +7th **S00.412** **Abrasion of left ear**
    +7th **S00.419** **Abrasion of unspecified ear**
+ **S00.42** **Blister (nonthermal) of ear**
    +7th **S00.421** **Blister (nonthermal) of right ear**
    +7th **S00.422** **Blister (nonthermal) of left ear**
    +7th **S00.429** **Blister (nonthermal) of unspecified ear**
+ **S00.43** **Contusion of ear**
    Bruise of ear
    Hematoma of ear
    +7th **S00.431** **Contusion of right ear**
    +7th **S00.432** **Contusion of left ear**
    +7th **S00.439** **Contusion of unspecified ear**
+ **S00.44** **External constriction of ear**
    +7th **S00.441** **External constriction of right ear**
    +7th **S00.442** **External constriction of left ear**
    +7th **S00.449** **External constriction of unspecified ear**
+ **S00.45** **Superficial foreign body of ear**
    Splinter in the ear
    +7th **S00.451** **Superficial foreign body of right ear**
    +7th **S00.452** **Superficial foreign body of left ear**
    +7th **S00.459** **Superficial foreign body of unspecified ear**
+ **S00.46** **Insect bite (nonvenomous) of ear**
    +7th **S00.461** **Insect bite (nonvenomous) of right ear**
    +7th **S00.462** **Insect bite (nonvenomous) of left ear**
    +7th **S00.469** **Insect bite (nonvenomous) of unspecified ear**
+ **S00.47** **Other superficial bite of ear**
    Excludes1: *open bite of ear (S01.35)*
    +7th **S00.471** **Other superficial bite of right ear**
    +7th **S00.472** **Other superficial bite of left ear**
    +7th **S00.479** **Other superficial bite of unspecified ear**
+ **S00.5** **Superficial injury of lip and oral cavity**
+ **S00.50** **Unspecified superficial injury of lip and oral cavity**
    +7th **S00.501** **Unspecified superficial injury of lip**
    +7th **S00.502** **Unspecified superficial injury of oral cavity**
+ **S00.51** **Abrasion of lip and oral cavity**
    +7th **S00.511** **Abrasion of lip**
    +7th **S00.512** **Abrasion of oral cavity**
+ **S00.52** **Blister (nonthermal) of lip and oral cavity**
    +7th **S00.521** **Blister (nonthermal) of lip**
    +7th **S00.522** **Blister (nonthermal) of oral cavity**
+ **S00.53** **Contusion of lip and oral cavity**
    +7th **S00.531** **Contusion of lip**
        Bruise of lip
        Hematoma of lip
    +7th **S00.532** **Contusion of oral cavity**
        Bruise of oral cavity
        Hematoma of oral cavity
+ **S00.54** **External constriction of lip and oral cavity**
    +7th **S00.541** **External constriction of lip**
    +7th **S00.542** **External constriction of oral cavity**
+ **S00.55** **Superficial foreign body of lip and oral cavity**
    +7th **S00.551** **Superficial foreign body of lip**
        Splinter of lip and oral cavity
    +7th **S00.552** **Superficial foreign body of oral cavity**
        Splinter of lip and oral cavity
+ **S00.56** **Insect bite (nonvenomous) of lip and oral cavity**
    +7th **S00.561** **Insect bite (nonvenomous) of lip**
    +7th **S00.562** **Insect bite (nonvenomous) of oral cavity**
+ **S00.57** **Other superficial bite of lip and oral cavity**
    +7th **S00.571** **Other superficial bite of lip**
        Excludes1: *open bite of lip (S01.551)*
    +7th **S00.572** **Other superficial bite of oral cavity**
        Excludes1: *open bite of oral cavity (S01.552)*
+ **S00.8** **Superficial injury of other parts of head**
    Superficial injuries of face [any part]
X+7th **S00.80** **Unspecified superficial injury of other part of head**
X+7th **S00.81** **Abrasion of other part of head**
X+7th **S00.82** **Blister (nonthermal) of other part of head**
X+7th **S00.83** **Contusion of other part of head**
    Bruise of other part of head
    Hematoma of other part of head

+, +7th, X + 7th   ● Newborn   ● Pediatric   ● Maternity   ● Adult   ♀ Female   ♂ Male   Manifestation   Unacceptable PDX   HCC   CC   MCC   HAC

X+7th **S00.84** **External constriction of other part of head**
X+7th **S00.85** **Superficial foreign body of other part of head**
  Splinter in other part of head
X+7th **S00.86** **Insect bite (nonvenomous) of other part of head**
X+7th **S00.87** **Other superficial bite of other part of head**
  Excludes1: *open bite of other part of head*
  (S01.85)
+ **S00.9** **Superficial injury of unspecified part of head**
X+7th **S00.90** **Unspecified superficial injury of unspecified part of head**
X+7th **S00.91** **Abrasion of unspecified part of head**
X+7th **S00.92** **Blister (nonthermal) of unspecified part of head**
X+7th **S00.93** **Contusion of unspecified part of head**
  Bruise of head
  Hematoma of head
X+7th **S00.94** **External constriction of unspecified part of head**
X+7th **S00.95** **Superficial foreign body of unspecified part of head**
  Splinter of head
X+7th **S00.96** **Insect bite (nonvenomous) of unspecified part of head**
X+7th **S00.97** **Other superficial bite of unspecified part of head**
  Excludes1: *open bite of head (S01.95)*

S01 **Open wound of head**

Code also any associated:
injury of cranial nerve (S04.-)
injury of muscle and tendon of head (S09.1-)
intracranial injury (S06.-)
wound infection
  Excludes1: *open skull fracture (S02.- with 7th character B)*
  Excludes2: *injury of eye and orbit (S05.-)*
    traumatic amputation of part of head (S08.-)

The appropriate 7th character is to be added to each code from category S01
A   initial encounter
D   subsequent encounter
S   sequela

+ **S01.0** **Open wound of scalp**
  Excludes1: *avulsion of scalp (S08.0)*
X+7th **S01.00** **Unspecified open wound of scalp**
X+7th **S01.01** **Laceration without foreign body of scalp**
X+7th **S01.02** **Laceration with foreign body of scalp**
  AHA CC: 1Q, 2015, 3-21
X+7th **S01.03** **Puncture wound without foreign body of scalp**
X+7th **S01.04** **Puncture wound with foreign body of scalp**
X+7th **S01.05** **Open bite of scalp**
  Bite of scalp NOS
  Excludes1: *superficial bite of scalp (S00.06,*
    S00.07-)
+ **S01.1** **Open wound of eyelid and periocular area**
  Open wound of eyelid and periocular area with or without involvement of lacrimal passages
  + **S01.10** **Unspecified open wound of eyelid and periocular area**
  CC +7th **S01.101** **Unspecified open wound of right eyelid and periocular area**
  CC +7th **S01.102** **Unspecified open wound of left eyelid and periocular area**
  CC +7th **S01.109** **Unspecified open wound of unspecified eyelid and periocular area**
  + **S01.11** **Laceration without foreign body of eyelid and periocular area**
    +7th **S01.111** **Laceration without foreign body of right eyelid and periocular area**
    +7th **S01.112** **Laceration without foreign body of left eyelid and periocular area**
    +7th **S01.119** **Laceration without foreign body of unspecified eyelid and periocular area**
  + **S01.12** **Laceration with foreign body of eyelid and periocular area**
    +7th **S01.121** **Laceration with foreign body of right eyelid and periocular area**
    +7th **S01.122** **Laceration with foreign body of left eyelid and periocular area**
    +7th **S01.129** **Laceration with foreign body of unspecified eyelid and periocular area**
  + **S01.13** **Puncture wound without foreign body of eyelid and periocular area**
    +7th **S01.131** **Puncture wound without foreign body of right eyelid and periocular area**

+7th **S01.132** **Puncture wound without foreign body of left eyelid and periocular area**
+7th **S01.139** **Puncture wound without foreign body of unspecified eyelid and periocular area**
+ **S01.14** **Puncture wound with foreign body of eyelid and periocular area**
  +7th **S01.141** **Puncture wound with foreign body of right eyelid and periocular area**
  +7th **S01.142** **Puncture wound with foreign body of left eyelid and periocular area**
  +7th **S01.149** **Puncture wound with foreign body of unspecified eyelid and periocular area**
+ **S01.15** **Open bite of eyelid and periocular area**
  Bite of eyelid and periocular area NOS
  Excludes1: *superficial bite of eyelid and*
    periocular area (S00.26, S00.27)
  +7th **S01.151** **Open bite of right eyelid and periocular area**
  +7th **S01.152** **Open bite of left eyelid and periocular area**
  +7th **S01.159** **Open bite of unspecified eyelid and periocular area**
+ **S01.2** **Open wound of nose**
X+7th **S01.20** **Unspecified open wound of nose**
X+7th **S01.21** **Laceration without foreign body of nose**
  AHA CC: 1Q, 2015, 3-21
X+7th **S01.22** **Laceration with foreign body of nose**
X+7th **S01.23** **Puncture wound without foreign body of nose**
X+7th **S01.24** **Puncture wound with foreign body of nose**
X+7th **S01.25** **Open bite of nose**
  Bite of nose NOS
  Excludes1: *superficial bite of nose (S00.36,*
    S00.37)
+ **S01.3** **Open wound of ear**
  + **S01.30** **Unspecified open wound of ear**
    +7th **S01.301** **Unspecified open wound of right ear**
    +7th **S01.302** **Unspecified open wound of left ear**
    +7th **S01.309** **Unspecified open wound of unspecified ear**
  + **S01.31** **Laceration without foreign body of ear**
    +7th **S01.311** **Laceration without foreign body of right ear**
    +7th **S01.312** **Laceration without foreign body of left ear**
    +7th **S01.319** **Laceration without foreign body of unspecified ear**
  + **S01.32** **Laceration with foreign body of ear**
    +7th **S01.321** **Laceration with foreign body of right ear**
    +7th **S01.322** **Laceration with foreign body of left ear**
    +7th **S01.329** **Laceration with foreign body of unspecified ear**
  + **S01.33** **Puncture wound without foreign body of ear**
    +7th **S01.331** **Puncture wound without foreign body of right ear**
    +7th **S01.332** **Puncture wound without foreign body of left ear**
    +7th **S01.339** **Puncture wound without foreign body of unspecified ear**
  + **S01.34** **Puncture wound with foreign body of ear**
    +7th **S01.341** **Puncture wound with foreign body of right ear**
    +7th **S01.342** **Puncture wound with foreign body of left ear**
    +7th **S01.349** **Puncture wound with foreign body of unspecified ear**
  + **S01.35** **Open bite of ear**
    Bite of ear NOS
    Excludes1: *superficial bite of ear (S00.46, S00.47)*
    +7th **S01.351** **Open bite of right ear**
    +7th **S01.352** **Open bite of left ear**
    +7th **S01.359** **Open bite of unspecified ear**
+ **S01.4** **Open wound of cheek and temporomandibular area**
  + **S01.40** **Unspecified open wound of cheek and temporomandibular area**
    +7th **S01.401** **Unspecified open wound of right cheek and temporomandibular area**
    +7th **S01.402** **Unspecified open wound of left cheek and temporomandibular area**
    +7th **S01.409** **Unspecified open wound of unspecified cheek and temporomandibular area**

+ **S01.41** **Laceration without foreign body of cheek and temporomandibular area**
  +7th **S01.411** **Laceration without foreign body of right cheek and temporomandibular area**
    AHA CC: 1Q, 2015, 3-21
  +7th **S01.412** **Laceration without foreign body of left cheek and temporomandibular area**
  +7th **S01.419** **Laceration without foreign body of unspecified cheek and temporomandibular area**
+ **S01.42** **Laceration with foreign body of cheek and temporomandibular area**
  +7th **S01.421** **Laceration with foreign body of right cheek and temporomandibular area**
  +7th **S01.422** **Laceration with foreign body of left cheek and temporomandibular area**
  +7th **S01.429** **Laceration with foreign body of unspecified cheek and temporomandibular area**
+ **S01.43** **Puncture wound without foreign body of cheek and temporomandibular area**
  +7th **S01.431** **Puncture wound without foreign body of right cheek and temporomandibular area**
  +7th **S01.432** **Puncture wound without foreign body of left cheek and temporomandibular area**
  +7th **S01.439** **Puncture wound without foreign body of unspecified cheek and temporomandibular area**
+ **S01.44** **Puncture wound with foreign body of cheek and temporomandibular area**
  +7th **S01.441** **Puncture wound with foreign body of right cheek and temporomandibular area**
  +7th **S01.442** **Puncture wound with foreign body of left cheek and temporomandibular area**
  +7th **S01.449** **Puncture wound with foreign body of unspecified cheek and temporomandibular area**
+ **S01.45** **Open bite of cheek and temporomandibular area**
  Bite of cheek and temporomandibular area NOS
  Excludes2: *superficial bite of cheek and temporomandibular area (S00.86, S00.87)*
  +7th **S01.451** **Open bite of right cheek and temporomandibular area**
  +7th **S01.452** **Open bite of left cheek and temporomandibular area**
  +7th **S01.459** **Open bite of unspecified cheek and temporomandibular area**
+ **S01.5** **Open wound of lip and oral cavity**
  Excludes2: *tooth dislocation (S03.2)*
  tooth fracture (S02.5)
+ **S01.50** **Unspecified open wound of lip and oral cavity**
  +7th **S01.501** **Unspecified open wound of lip**
  +7th **S01.502** **Unspecified open wound of oral cavity**
+ **S01.51** **Laceration of lip and oral cavity without foreign body**
  +7th **S01.511** **Laceration without foreign body of lip**
  +7th **S01.512** **Laceration without foreign body of oral cavity**
+ **S01.52** **Laceration of lip and oral cavity with foreign body**
  +7th **S01.521** **Laceration with foreign body of lip**
  +7th **S01.522** **Laceration with foreign body of oral cavity**
+ **S01.53** **Puncture wound of lip and oral cavity without foreign body**
  +7th **S01.531** **Puncture wound without foreign body of lip**
  +7th **S01.532** **Puncture wound without foreign body of oral cavity**
+ **S01.54** **Puncture wound of lip and oral cavity with foreign body**
  +7th **S01.541** **Puncture wound with foreign body of lip**
  +7th **S01.542** **Puncture wound with foreign body of oral cavity**

+ **S01.55** **Open bite of lip and oral cavity**
  +7th **S01.551** **Open bite of lip**
    Bite of lip NOS
    Excludes1: *superficial bite of lip (S00.571)*
  +7th **S01.552** **Open bite of oral cavity**
    Bite of oral cavity NOS
    Excludes1: *superficial bite of oral cavity (S00.572)*
+ **S01.8** **Open wound of other parts of head**
  X+7th **S01.80** **Unspecified open wound of other part of head**
  X+7th **S01.81** **Laceration without foreign body of other part of head**
  X+7th **S01.82** **Laceration with foreign body of other part of head**
  X+7th **S01.83** **Puncture wound without foreign body of other part of head**
  X+7th **S01.84** **Puncture wound with foreign body of other part of head**
  X+7th **S01.85** **Open bite of other part of head**
    Bite of other part of head NOS
    Excludes1: *superficial bite of other part of head (S00.87)*
+ **S01.9** **Open wound of unspecified part of head**
  X+7th **S01.90** **Unspecified open wound of unspecified part of head**
  X+7th **S01.91** **Laceration without foreign body of unspecified part of head**
  X+7th **S01.92** **Laceration with foreign body of unspecified part of head**
  X+7th **S01.93** **Puncture wound without foreign body of unspecified part of head**
  X+7th **S01.94** **Puncture wound with foreign body of unspecified part of head**
  X+7th **S01.95** **Open bite of unspecified part of head**
    Bite of head NOS
    Excludes1: *superficial bite of head NOS (S00.97)*

S02 **Fracture of skull and facial bones**

> **NOTE** A fracture not indicated as open or closed should be coded to closed

Code also any associated intracranial injury (S06.-)
Review coding guideline C.19.c
AHA CC: 4Q, 2016, 66-67

> The appropriate 7th character is to be added to each code from category S02
> A   initial encounter for closed fracture
> B   initial encounter for open fracture
> D   subsequent encounter for fracture with routine healing
> G   subsequent encounter for fracture with delayed healing
> K   subsequent encounter for fracture with nonunion
> S   sequela

X+7th **S02.0** **Fracture of vault of skull**
CC MCC   Fracture of frontal bone
         Fracture of parietal bone
         HAC 7th characters A & B see Appendix B for HAC conditional logic
+ **S02.1** **Fracture of base of skull**
  Excludes2: *lateral orbital wall (S02.84-)*
  medial orbital wall (S02.83-)
  orbital floor (S02.3-)
  AHA CC: 4Q, 2019, 16
  + **S02.10** **Unspecified fracture of base of skull**
  CC MCC +7th **S02.101** **Fracture of base of skull, right side**
    HAC 7th characters A & B see Appendix B for HAC conditional logic
  CC MCC +7th **S02.102** **Fracture of base of skull, left side**
    HAC 7th characters A & B see Appendix B for HAC conditional logic
  CC MCC +7th **S02.109** **Fracture of base of skull, unspecified side**
    HAC 7th characters A & B see Appendix B for HAC conditional logic
  + **S02.11** **Fracture of occiput**
  CC MCC +7th **S02.110** **Type I occipital condyle fracture, unspecified side**
    HAC 7th characters A & B see Appendix B for HAC conditional logic
  CC MCC +7th **S02.111** **Type II occipital condyle fracture, unspecified side**
    HAC 7th characters A & B see Appendix B for HAC conditional logic

Head and Facial Bones - Side View

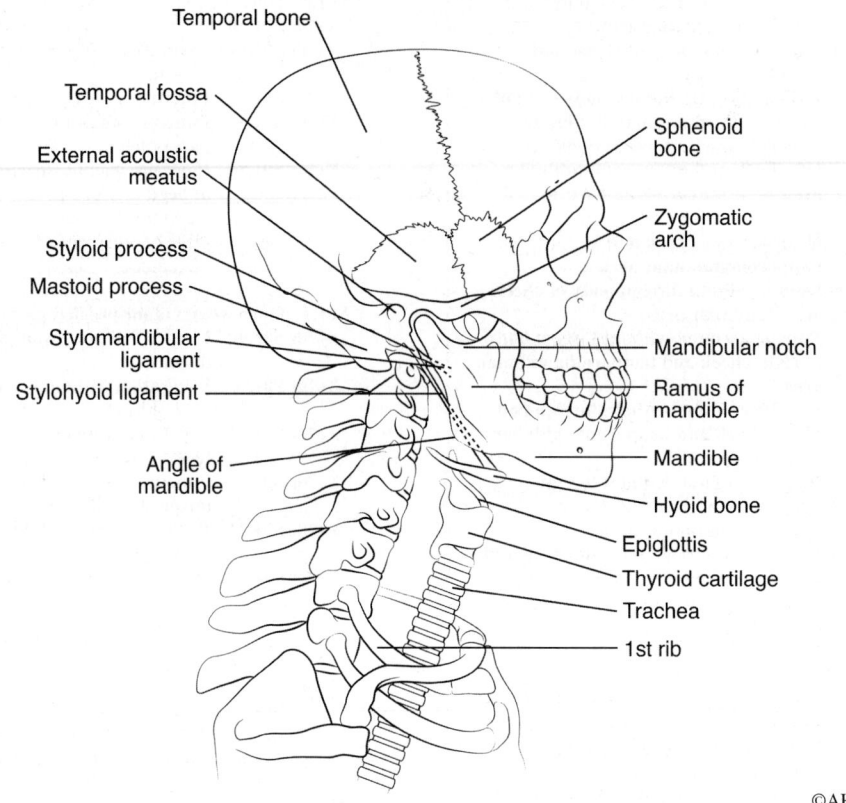

Temporal bone

Temporal fossa

External acoustic meatus

Styloid process

Mastoid process

Stylomandibular ligament

Stylohyoid ligament

Angle of mandible

Sphenoid bone

Zygomatic arch

Mandibular notch

Ramus of mandible

Mandible

Hyoid bone

Epiglottis

Thyroid cartilage

Trachea

1st rib

©AHIMA

Head and Facial Bones - Side View

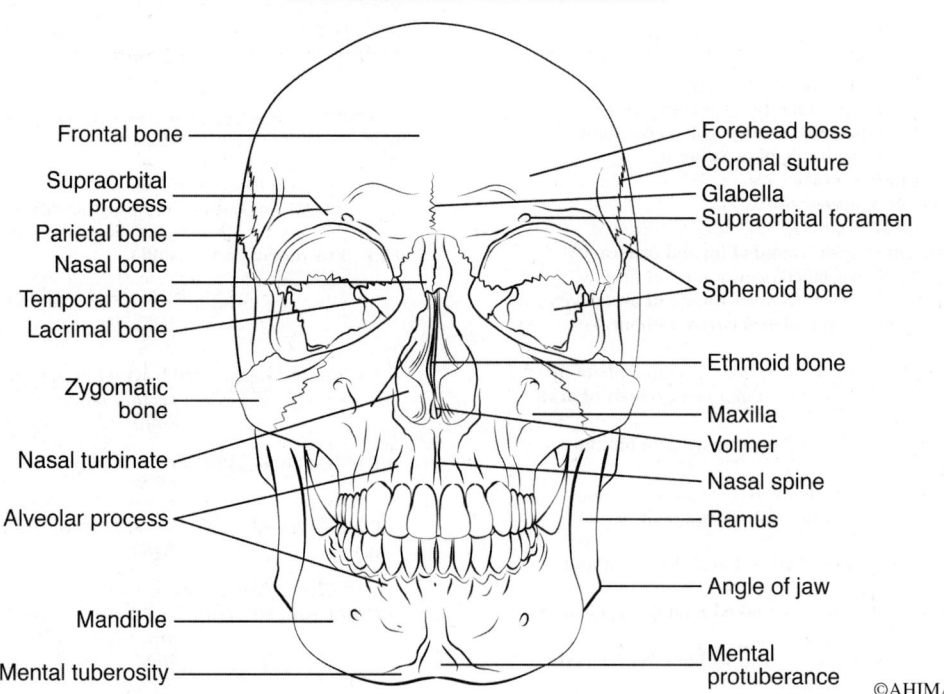

Frontal bone

Supraorbital process

Parietal bone

Nasal bone

Temporal bone

Lacrimal bone

Zygomatic bone

Nasal turbinate

Alveolar process

Mandible

Mental tuberosity

Forehead boss

Coronal suture

Glabella

Supraorbital foramen

Sphenoid bone

Ethmoid bone

Maxilla

Volmer

Nasal spine

Ramus

Angle of jaw

Mental protuberance

©AHIMA

CC MCC +7th **S02.112** **Type III occipital condyle fracture, unspecified side**
HAC 7th characters A & B see Appendix B for HAC conditional logic

CC MCC +7th **S02.113** **Unspecified occipital condyle fracture**
HAC 7th characters A & B see Appendix B for HAC conditional logic

CC MCC +7th **S02.118** **Other fracture of occiput, unspecified side**
HAC 7th characters A & B see Appendix B for HAC conditional logic

CC MCC +7th **S02.119** **Unspecified fracture of occiput**
HAC 7th characters A & B see Appendix B for HAC conditional logic

CC MCC +7th **S02.11A** **Type I occipital condyle fracture, right side**
HAC 7th characters A & B see Appendix B for HAC conditional logic

CC MCC +7th **S02.11B** **Type I occipital condyle fracture, left side**
HAC 7th characters A & B see Appendix B for HAC conditional logic

CC MCC +7th **S02.11C** **Type II occipital condyle fracture, right side**
HAC 7th characters A & B see Appendix B for HAC conditional logic

CC MCC +7th **S02.11D** **Type II occipital condyle fracture, left side**
HAC 7th characters A & B see Appendix B for HAC conditional logic

CC MCC +7th **S02.11E** **Type III occipital condyle fracture, right side**
HAC 7th characters A & B see Appendix B for HAC conditional logic

CC MCC +7th **S02.11F** **Type III occipital condyle fracture, left side**
HAC 7th characters A & B see Appendix B for HAC conditional logic

CC MCC +7th **S02.11G** **Other fracture or occiput, right side**
HAC 7th characters A & B see Appendix B for HAC conditional logic

CC MCC +7th **S02.11H** **Other fracture or occiput, left side**
HAC 7th characters A & B see Appendix B for HAC conditional logic

+ **S02.12** **Fracture of orbital roof**
CC MCC **S02.121** **Fracture of orbital roof, right side**
HAC 7th characters A & B see Appendix B for HAC conditional logic

CC MCC **S02.122** **Fracture of orbital roof, left side**
HAC 7th characters A & B see Appendix B for HAC conditional logic

CC MCC **S02.129** **Fracture of orbital roof, unspecified side**
HAC 7th characters A & B see Appendix B for HAC conditional logic

CC MCC X+7th **S02.19** **Other fracture of base of skull**
Fracture of anterior fossa of base of skull
Fracture of ethmoid sinus
Fracture of frontal sinus
Fracture of middle fossa of base of skull
Fracture of posterior fossa of base of skull
Fracture of sphenoid
Fracture of temporal bone
HAC 7th characters A & B see Appendix B for HAC conditional logic

CC X+7th **S02.2** **Fracture of nasal bones**
HAC 7th character B see Appendix B for HAC conditional logic

+ **S02.3** **Fracture of orbital floor**
Excludes1: *orbit NOS (S02.85)*
Excludes2: *lateral orbital wall (S02.84-)*
medial orbital wall (S02.83-)
orbital roof (S02.1-)

CC X+7th **S02.30** **Fracture of orbital floor, unspecified side**
HAC 7th characters A & B see Appendix B for HAC conditional logic

CC X+7th **S02.31** **Fracture of orbital floor, right side**
HAC 7th characters A & B see Appendix B for HAC conditional logic

CC X+7th **S02.32** **Fracture of orbital floor, left side**
HAC 7th characters A & B see Appendix B for HAC conditional logic

+ **S02.4** **Fracture of malar, maxillary and zygoma bones**
Fracture of superior maxilla
Fracture of upper jaw (bone)
Fracture of zygomatic process of temporal bone

+ **S02.40** **Fracture of malar, maxillary and zygoma bones, unspecified**
CC +7th **S02.400** **Malar fracture, unspecified side**
HAC 7th characters A & B see Appendix B for HAC conditional logic

CC +7th **S02.401** **Maxillary fracture, unspecified side**
HAC 7th characters A & B see Appendix B for HAC conditional logic

CC +7th **S02.402** **Zygomatic fracture, unspecified side**
HAC 7th characters A & B see Appendix B for HAC conditional logic

CC +7th **S02.40A** **Malar fracture, right side**
HAC 7th characters A & B see Appendix B for HAC conditional logic

CC +7th **S02.40B** **Malar fracture, left side**
HAC 7th characters A & B see Appendix B for HAC conditional logic

CC +7th **S02.40C** **Maxillary fracture, right side**
HAC 7th characters A & B see Appendix B for HAC conditional logic

CC +7th **S02.40D** **Maxillary fracture, left side**
HAC 7th characters A & B see Appendix B for HAC conditional logic

CC +7th **S02.40E** **Zygomatic fracture, right side**
HAC 7th characters A & B see Appendix B for HAC conditional logic

CC +7th **S02.40F** **Zygomatic fracture, left side**
HAC 7th characters A & B see Appendix B for HAC conditional logic

+ **S02.41** **LeFort fracture**
CC +7th **S02.411** **LeFort I fracture**
HAC 7th characters A & B see Appendix B for HAC conditional logic

CC +7th **S02.412** **LeFort II fracture**
HAC 7th characters A & B see Appendix B for HAC conditional logic

CC +7th **S02.413** **LeFort III fracture**
HAC 7th characters A & B see Appendix B for HAC conditional logic

CC X+7th **S02.42** **Fracture of alveolus of maxilla**
HAC 7th characters A & B see Appendix B for HAC conditional logic

CC X+7th **S02.5** **Fracture of tooth (traumatic)**
Broken tooth
Excludes1: *cracked tooth (nontraumatic) (K03.81)*

+ **S02.6** **Fracture of mandible**
Fracture of lower jaw (bone)

+ **S02.60** **Fracture of mandible, unspecified**
CC +7th **S02.600** **Fracture of unspecified part of body of mandible, unspecified side**
HAC 7th characters A & B see Appendix B for HAC conditional logic

CC +7th **S02.601** **Fracture of unspecified part of body of right mandible**
HAC 7th characters A & B see Appendix B for HAC conditional logic

CC +7th **S02.602** **Fracture of unspecified part of body of left mandible**
HAC 7th characters A & B see Appendix B for HAC conditional logic

CC X+7th **S02.609** **Fracture of mandible, unspecified**
HAC 7th characters A & B see Appendix B for HAC conditional logic

+ **S02.61** **Fracture of condylar process of mandible**
CC +7th **S02.610** **Fracture of condylar process of mandible, unspecified side**
HAC 7th characters A & B see Appendix B for HAC conditional logic

CC +7th **S02.611** **Fracture of condylar process of right mandible**
HAC 7th characters A & B see Appendix B for HAC conditional logic

CC +7th **S02.612** **Fracture of condylar process of left mandible**
HAC 7th characters A & B see Appendix B for HAC conditional logic

+ **S02.62** **Fracture of subcondylar process of mandible**
CC +7th **S02.620** **Fracture of subcondylar process of mandible, unspecified side**
HAC 7th characters A & B see Appendix B for HAC conditional logic

CC +7th **S02.621** **Fracture of subcondylar process of right mandible**
HAC 7th characters A & B see Appendix B for HAC conditional logic

CC +7th **S02.622** **Fracture of subcondylar process of left mandible**
HAC 7th characters A & B see Appendix B for HAC conditional logic

+, +7th, X + 7th   ● Newborn   ● Pediatric   ● Maternity   ● Adult   ♀ Female   ♂ Male   Manifestation   Unacceptable PDX   HCC   CC   MCC   HAC

+ **S02.63** **Fracture of coronoid process of mandible**
CC +7th **S02.630** **Fracture of coronoid process of mandible, unspecified side**
HAC 7th characters A & B see Appendix B for HAC conditional logic
CC +7th **S02.631** **Fracture of coronoid process of right mandible**
HAC 7th characters A & B see Appendix B for HAC conditional logic
CC +7th **S02.632** **Fracture of coronoid process of left mandible**
HAC 7th characters A & B see Appendix B for HAC conditional logic
+ **S02.64** **Fracture of ramus of mandible**
CC +7th **S02.640** **Fracture of ramus of mandible, unspecified side**
HAC 7th characters A & B see Appendix B for HAC conditional logic
CC +7th **S02.641** **Fracture of ramus of right mandible**
HAC 7th characters A & B see Appendix B for HAC conditional logic
CC +7th **S02.642** **Fracture of ramus of left mandible**
HAC 7th characters A & B see Appendix B for HAC conditional logic
+ **S02.65** **Fracture of angle of mandible**
CC +7th **S02.650** **Fracture of angle of mandible, unspecified side**
HAC 7th characters A & B see Appendix B for HAC conditional logic
CC +7th **S02.651** **Fracture of angle of right mandible**
HAC 7th characters A & B see Appendix B for HAC conditional logic
CC +7th **S02.652** **Fracture of angle of left mandible**
HAC 7th characters A & B see Appendix B for HAC conditional logic
CC X+7th **S02.66** **Fracture of symphysis of mandible**
HAC 7th characters A & B see Appendix B for HAC conditional logic
+ **S02.67** **Fracture of alveolus of mandible**
CC +7th **S02.670** **Fracture of alveolus of mandible, unspecified side**
HAC 7th characters A & B see Appendix B for HAC conditional logic
CC +7th **S02.671** **Fracture of alveolus of right mandible**
HAC 7th characters A & B see Appendix B for HAC conditional logic
CC +7th **S02.672** **Fracture of alveolus of left mandible**
HAC 7th characters A & B see Appendix B for HAC conditional logic
CC X+7th **S02.69** **Fracture of mandible of other specified site**
HAC 7th characters A & B see Appendix B for HAC conditional logic
+ **S02.8** **Fractures of other specified skull and facial bones**
Fracture of palate
Excludes2: *fracture of orbital floor (S02.3-)*
fracture of orbital roof (S02.12-)
AHA CC: 4Q, 2019, 16-17
CC X+7th **S02.80** **Fracture of other specified skull and facial bones, unspecified side**
HAC 7th characters A & B see Appendix B for HAC conditional logic
CC X+7th **S02.81** **Fracture of other specified skull and facial bones, right side**
HAC 7th characters A & B see Appendix B for HAC conditional logic
CC X+7th **S02.82** **Fracture of other specified skull and facial bones, left side**
HAC 7th characters A & B see Appendix B for HAC conditional logic
+ **S02.83** **Fracture of medial orbital wall**
Excludes2: *orbital floor (S02.3-)*
orbital roof (S02.12-)
CC **S02.831** **Fracture of medial orbital wall, right side**
HAC 7th characters A & B see Appendix B for HAC conditional logic
CC **S02.832** **Fracture of medical orbital wall, left side**
HAC 7th characters A & B see Appendix B for HAC conditional logic
CC **S03.839** **Fracture of medial orbital wall, unspecified side**
HAC 7th characters A & B see Appendix B for HAC conditional logic
+ **S02.84** **Fracture of lateral orbital wall**
Excludes2: *orbital floor (S02.3-)*
orbital roof (S02.12-)

CC **S02.841** **Fracture of lateral orbital wall, right side**
HAC 7th characters A & B see Appendix B for HAC conditional logic
CC **S02.842** **Fracture of lateral orbital wall, left side**
HAC 7th characters A & B see Appendix B for HAC conditional logic
CC **S02.849** **Fracture of lateral orbital wall, unspecified side**
HAC 7th characters A & B see Appendix B for HAC conditional logic
CC **S02.85** **Fracture of orbit, unspecified**
Fracture of orbit NOS
Fracture of orbit wall NOS
Excludes1: *lateral orbital wall (S02.84-)*
medial orbital wall (S02.83-)
orbital floor (S02.3-)
orbital roof (S02.12-)
HAC 7th characters A & B see Appendix B for HAC conditional logic
+ **S02.9** **Fracture of unspecified skull and facial bones**
CC MCC X+7th **S02.91** **Unspecified fracture of skull**
AHA CC: 2Q, 2020, 24
HAC 7th characters A & B see Appendix B for HAC conditional logic
CC X+7th **S02.92** **Unspecified fracture of facial bones**
HAC 7th characters A & B see Appendix B for HAC conditional logic

S03 **Dislocation and sprain of joints and ligaments of head**
Includes: avulsion of joint (capsule) or ligament of head
laceration of cartilage, joint (capsule) or ligament of head
sprain of cartilage, joint (capsule) or ligament of head
traumatic hemarthrosis of joint or ligament of head
traumatic rupture of joint or ligament of head
traumatic subluxation of joint or ligament of head
traumatic tear of joint or ligament of head
Code also any associated open wound
Excludes2: *Strain of muscle or tendon of head (S09.1)*

The appropriate 7th character is to be added to each code from category S03
A   initial encounter
D   subsequent encounter
S   sequela

+ **S03.0** **Dislocation of jaw**
Dislocation of jaw (cartilage) (meniscus)
Dislocation of mandible
Dislocation of temporomandibular (joint)
AHA CC: 4Q, 2016, 67
X+7th **S03.00** **Dislocation of jaw, unspecified side**
X+7th **S03.01** **Dislocation of jaw, right side**
X+7th **S03.02** **Dislocation of jaw, left side**
X+7th **S03.03** **Dislocation of jaw, bilateral**
X+7th **S03.1** **Dislocation of septal cartilage of nose**
X+7th **S03.2** **Dislocation of tooth**
+ **S03.4** **Sprain of jaw**
Sprain of temporomandibular (joint) (ligament)
AHA CC: 4Q, 2016, 67
X+7th **S03.40** **Sprain of jaw, unspecified side**
X+7th **S03.41** **Sprain of jaw, right side**
X+7th **S03.42** **Sprain of jaw, left side**
X+7th **S03.43** **Sprain of jaw, bilateral**
X+7th **S03.8** **Sprain of joints and ligaments of other parts of head**
X+7th **S03.9** **Sprain of joints and ligaments of unspecified parts of head**

S04 **Injury of cranial nerve**
The selection of side should be based on the side of the body being affected
Code first any associated intracranial injury (S06.-)
Code also any associated:
open wound of head (S01.-)
skull fracture (S02.-)

The appropriate 7th character is to be added to each code from category S04
A   initial encounter
D   subsequent encounter
S   sequela

+, +7th, X + 7th   ● Newborn   ● Pediatric   ● Maternity   ● Adult   ♀ Female   ♂ Male   Manifestation   Unacceptable PDX   HCC   CC   MCC   HAC

+ S04.0 Injury of optic nerve and pathways
Use additional code to identify any visual field defect or blindness (H53.4-, H54.-)
    + S04.01 Injury of optic nerve
      Injury of 2nd cranial nerve
    CC +7th **S04.011 Injury of optic nerve, right eye**
    CC +7th **S04.012 Injury of optic nerve, left eye**
    CC +7th **S04.019 Injury of optic nerve, unspecified eye**
      Injury of optic nerve NOS
  CC X+7th **S04.02 Injury of optic chiasm**
    + S04.03 Injury of optic tract and pathways
      Injury of optic radiation
    CC +7th **S04.031 Injury of optic tract and pathways, right side**
    CC +7th **S04.032 Injury of optic tract and pathways, left side**
    CC +7th **S04.039 Injury of optic tract and pathways, unspecified side**
      Injury of optic tract and pathways NOS
    + S04.04 Injury of visual cortex
    CC +7th **S04.041 Injury of visual cortex, right side**
    CC +7th **S04.042 Injury of visual cortex, left side**
    CC +7th **S04.049 Injury of visual cortex, unspecified side**
      Injury of visual cortex NOS
+ S04.1 Injury of oculomotor nerve
  Injury of 3rd cranial nerve
  CC X+7th **S04.10 Injury of oculomotor nerve, unspecified side**
  CC X+7th **S04.11 Injury of oculomotor nerve, right side**
  CC X+7th **S04.12 Injury of oculomotor nerve, left side**
+ S04.2 Injury of trochlear nerve
  Injury of 4th cranial nerve
  CC X+7th **S04.20 Injury of trochlear nerve, unspecified side**
  CC X+7th **S04.21 Injury of trochlear nerve, right side**
  CC X+7th **S04.22 Injury of trochlear nerve, left side**
+ S04.3 Injury of trigeminal nerve
  Injury of 5th cranial nerve
  CC X+7th **S04.30 Injury of trigeminal nerve, unspecified side**
  CC X+7th **S04.31 Injury of trigeminal nerve, right side**
  CC X+7th **S04.32 Injury of trigeminal nerve, left side**
+ S04.4 Injury of abducent nerve
  Injury of 6th cranial nerve
  CC X+7th **S04.40 Injury of abducent nerve, unspecified side**
  CC X+7th **S04.41 Injury of abducent nerve, right side**
  CC X+7th **S04.42 Injury of abducent nerve, left side**
+ S04.5 Injury of facial nerve
  Injury of 7th cranial nerve
  CC X+7th **S04.50 Injury of facial nerve, unspecified side**
  CC X+7th **S04.51 Injury of facial nerve, right side**
  CC X+7th **S04.52 Injury of facial nerve, left side**
+ S04.6 Injury of acoustic nerve
  Injury of auditory nerve
  Injury of 8th cranial nerve
  CC X+7th **S04.60 Injury of acoustic nerve, unspecified side**
  CC X+7th **S04.61 Injury of acoustic nerve, right side**
  CC X+7th **S04.62 Injury of acoustic nerve, left side**
+ S04.7 Injury of accessory nerve
  Injury of 11th cranial nerve
  CC X+7th **S04.70 Injury of accessory nerve, unspecified side**
  CC X+7th **S04.71 Injury of accessory nerve, right side**
  CC X+7th **S04.72 Injury of accessory nerve, left side**
+ S04.8 Injury of other cranial nerves
    + S04.81 Injury of olfactory [1st] nerve
    CC +7th **S04.811 Injury of olfactory [1st] nerve, right side**
    CC +7th **S04.812 Injury of olfactory [1st] nerve, left side**
    CC +7th **S04.819 Injury of olfactory [1st] nerve, unspecified side**
    + S04.89 Injury of other cranial nerves
      Injury of vagus [10th] nerve
    CC +7th **S04.891 Injury of other cranial nerves, right side**
    CC +7th **S04.892 Injury of other cranial nerves, left side**
    CC +7th **S04.899 Injury of other cranial nerves, unspecified side**
CC X+7th **S04.9 Injury of unspecified cranial nerve**

S05 Injury of eye and orbit
  Includes: open wound of eye and orbit
  Excludes2: *2nd cranial [optic] nerve injury (S04.0-)*
    3rd cranial [oculomotor] nerve injury (S04.1-)
    open wound of eyelid and periocular area (S01.1-)
    orbital bone fracture (S02.1-, S02.3-, S02.8-)
    superficial injury of eyelid (S00.1-S00.2)

The appropriate 7th character is to be added to each code from category S05
A initial encounter
D subsequent encounter
S sequela

+ S05.0 Injury of conjunctiva and corneal abrasion without foreign body
  Excludes1: *foreign body in conjunctival sac (T15.1)*
    foreign body in cornea (T15.0)
  X+7th **S05.00 Injury of conjunctiva and corneal abrasion without foreign body, unspecified eye**
  X+7th **S05.01 Injury of conjunctiva and corneal abrasion without foreign body, right eye**
  X+7th **S05.02 Injury of conjunctiva and corneal abrasion without foreign body, left eye**
+ S05.1 Contusion of eyeball and orbital tissues
  Traumatic hyphema
  Excludes2: *black eye NOS (S00.1)*
    contusion of eyelid and periocular area (S00.1)
  X+7th **S05.10 Contusion of eyeball and orbital tissues, unspecified eye**
  X+7th **S05.11 Contusion of eyeball and orbital tissues, right eye**
  X+7th **S05.12 Contusion of eyeball and orbital tissues, left eye**
+ S05.2 Ocular laceration and rupture with prolapse or loss of intraocular tissue
  CC X+7th **S05.20 Ocular laceration and rupture with prolapse or loss of intraocular tissue, unspecified eye**
  CC X+7th **S05.21 Ocular laceration and rupture with prolapse or loss of intraocular tissue, right eye**
  CC X+7th **S05.22 Ocular laceration and rupture with prolapse or loss of intraocular tissue, left eye**
+ S05.3 Ocular laceration without prolapse or loss of intraocular tissue
  Laceration of eye NOS
  CC X+7th **S05.30 Ocular laceration without prolapse or loss of intraocular tissue, unspecified eye**
  CC X+7th **S05.31 Ocular laceration without prolapse or loss of intraocular tissue, right eye**
  CC X+7th **S05.32 Ocular laceration without prolapse or loss of intraocular tissue, left eye**
+ S05.4 Penetrating wound of orbit with or without foreign body
  Excludes2: *retained (old) foreign body following penetrating wound in orbit (H05.5-)*
  CC X+7th **S05.40 Penetrating wound of orbit with or without foreign body, unspecified eye**
  CC X+7th **S05.41 Penetrating wound of orbit with or without foreign body, right eye**
  CC X+7th **S05.42 Penetrating wound of orbit with or without foreign body, left eye**
+ S05.5 Penetrating wound with foreign body of eyeball
  Excludes2: *retained (old) intraocular foreign body (H44.6-, H44.7)*
  CC X+7th **S05.50 Penetrating wound with foreign body of unspecified eyeball**
  CC X+7th **S05.51 Penetrating wound with foreign body of right eyeball**
  CC X+7th **S05.52 Penetrating wound with foreign body of left eyeball**
+ S05.6 Penetrating wound without foreign body of eyeball
  Ocular penetration NOS
  X+7th **S05.60 Penetrating wound without foreign body of unspecified eyeball**
  X+7th **S05.61 Penetrating wound without foreign body of right eyeball**
  X+7th **S05.62 Penetrating wound without foreign body of left eyeball**
+ S05.7 Avulsion of eye
  Traumatic enucleation
  CC X+7th **S05.70 Avulsion of unspecified eye**
  CC X+7th **S05.71 Avulsion of right eye**
  CC X+7th **S05.72 Avulsion of left eye**

+, +7th, X + 7th ● Newborn ● Pediatric ● Maternity ● Adult ♀ Female ♂ Male Manifestation Unacceptable PDX HCC CC MCC HAC

CC + **S05.8** **Other injuries of eye and orbit**
Lacrimal duct injury
 + **S05.8X** **Other injuries of eye and orbit**
  +7th **S05.8X1** **Other injuries of right eye and orbit**
  +7th **S05.8X2** **Other injuries of left eye and orbit**
  +7th **S05.8X9** **Other injuries of unspecified eye and orbit**
 + **S05.9** **Unspecified injury of eye and orbit**
Injury of eye NOS
 X+7th **S05.90** **Unspecified injury of unspecified eye and orbit**
CC X+7th **S05.91** **Unspecified injury of right eye and orbit**
CC X+7th **S05.92** **Unspecified injury of left eye and orbit**

S06 **Intracranial injury**
 Includes: traumatic brain injury
 Code also any associated:
  open wound of head (S01.-)
  skull fracture (S02.-)
 Excludes1: *head injury NOS (S09.90)*
 AHA CC: 4Q, 2017, 25

The appropriate 7th character is to be added to each code from category S06
A initial encounter
D subsequent encounter
S sequela

 NOTE 7th characters D and S do not apply to codes in category S06 with 6th character 7 - death due to brain injury prior to regaining consciousness, or 8 - death due to other cause prior to regaining consciousness.

 + **S06.0** **Concussion**
Commotio cerebri
 Excludes1: *concussion with other intracranial injuries classified in category S06.1- to S06.6-, S06.81- and S06.82- code to specified intracranial injury*
 AHA CC: 4Q, 2016, 67-68
 + **S06.0X** **Concussion**
  +7th **S06.0X0** **Concussion without loss of consciousness**
   HAC 7th character A see Appendix B for HAC conditional logic
 CC +7th **S06.0X1** **Concussion with loss of consciousness of 30 minutes or less**
   HAC 7th character A see Appendix B for HAC conditional logic
 CC +7th **S06.0X9** **Concussion with loss of consciousness of unspecified duration**
Concussion NOS
   HAC 7th character A see Appendix B for HAC conditional logic

 + **S06.1** **Traumatic cerebral edema**
Diffuse traumatic cerebral edema
Focal traumatic cerebral edema
 + **S06.1X** **Traumatic cerebral edema**
 MCC +7th **S06.1X0** **Traumatic cerebral edema without loss of consciousness**
   HAC 7th character A see Appendix B for HAC conditional logic
   AHA CC: 1Q, 2015, 3-21
 MCC +7th **S06.1X1** **Traumatic cerebral edema with loss of consciousness of 30 minutes or less**
   HAC 7th character A see Appendix B for HAC conditional logic
 MCC +7th **S06.1X2** **Traumatic cerebral edema with loss of consciousness of 31 minutes to 59 minutes**
   HAC 7th character A see Appendix B for HAC conditional logic
 MCC +7th **S06.1X3** **Traumatic cerebral edema with loss of consciousness of 1 hour to 5 hours 59 minutes**
   HAC 7th character A see Appendix B for HAC conditional logic
 MCC +7th **S06.1X4** **Traumatic cerebral edema with loss of consciousness of 6 hours to 24 hours**
   HAC 7th character A see Appendix B for HAC conditional logic

 MCC +7th **S06.1X5** **Traumatic cerebral edema with loss of consciousness greater than 24 hours with return to pre-existing conscious level**
   HAC 7th character A see Appendix B for HAC conditional logic
 MCC +7th **S06.1X6** **Traumatic cerebral edema with loss of consciousness greater than 24 hours without return to pre-existing conscious level with patient surviving**
   HAC 7th character A see Appendix B for HAC conditional logic
 MCC +7th **S06.1X7** **Traumatic cerebral edema with loss of consciousness of any duration with death due to brain injury prior to regaining consciousness**
   HAC 7th character A see Appendix B for HAC conditional logic
 MCC +7th **S06.1X8** **Traumatic cerebral edema with loss of consciousness of any duration with death due to other cause prior to regaining consciousness**
   HAC 7th character A see Appendix B for HAC conditional logic
 MCC +7th **S06.1X9** **Traumatic cerebral edema with loss of consciousness of unspecified duration**
Traumatic cerebral edema NOS
   HAC 7th character A see Appendix B for HAC conditional logic

CC + **S06.2** **Diffuse traumatic brain injury**
Diffuse axonal brain injury
 Excludes1: *traumatic diffuse cerebral edema (S06.1X-)*
 + **S06.2X** **Diffuse traumatic brain injury**
  +7th **S06.2X0** **Diffuse traumatic brain injury without loss of consciousness**
   HAC 7th character A see Appendix B for HAC conditional logic
  +7th **S06.2X1** **Diffuse traumatic brain injury with loss of consciousness of 30 minutes or less**
   HAC 7th character A see Appendix B for HAC conditional logic
  +7th **S06.2X2** **Diffuse traumatic brain injury with loss of consciousness of 31 minutes to 59 minutes**
   HAC 7th character A see Appendix B for HAC conditional logic
  +7th **S06.2X3** **Diffuse traumatic brain injury with loss of consciousness of 1 hour to 5 hours 59 minutes**
   HAC 7th character A see Appendix B for HAC conditional logic
  +7th **S06.2X4** **Diffuse traumatic brain injury with loss of consciousness of 6 hours to 24 hours**
   HAC 7th character A see Appendix B for HAC conditional logic
  +7th **S06.2X5** **Diffuse traumatic brain injury with loss of consciousness greater than 24 hours with return to pre-existing conscious levels**
   HAC 7th character A see Appendix B for HAC conditional logic
 MCC +7th **S06.2X6** **Diffuse traumatic brain injury with loss of consciousness greater than 24 hours without return to pre-existing conscious level with patient surviving**
   HAC 7th character A see Appendix B for HAC conditional logic
 MCC +7th **S06.2X7** **Diffuse traumatic brain injury with loss of consciousness of any duration with death due to brain injury prior to regaining consciousness**
   HAC 7th character A see Appendix B for HAC conditional logic
 MCC +7th **S06.2X8** **Diffuse traumatic brain injury with loss of consciousness of any duration with death due to other cause prior to regaining consciousness**
   HAC 7th character A see Appendix B for HAC conditional logic
  +7th **S06.2X9** **Diffuse traumatic brain injury with loss of consciousness of unspecified duration**
Diffuse traumatic brain injury NOS
   HAC 7th character A see Appendix B for HAC conditional logic

+ **S06.3** **Focal traumatic brain injury**
  Excludes1: *any condition classifiable to S06.4-S06.6*
  Excludes2: *focal cerebral edema (S06.1)*

+ **S06.30** **Unspecified focal traumatic brain injury**

+7th **S06.300** **Unspecified focal traumatic brain injury without loss of consciousness**

CC +7th **S06.301** **Unspecified focal traumatic brain injury with loss of consciousness of 30 minutes or less**
HAC 7th character A see Appendix B for HAC conditional logic

CC +7th **S06.302** **Unspecified focal traumatic brain injury with loss of consciousness of 31 minutes to 59 minutes**
HAC 7th character A see Appendix B for HAC conditional logic

CC +7th **S06.303** **Unspecified focal traumatic brain injury with loss of consciousness of 1 hour to 5 hours 59 minutes**
HAC 7th character A see Appendix B for HAC conditional logic

CC +7th **S06.304** **Unspecified focal traumatic brain injury with loss of consciousness of 6 hours to 24 hours**
HAC 7th character A see Appendix B for HAC conditional logic

CC +7th **S06.305** **Unspecified focal traumatic brain injury with loss of consciousness greater than 24 hours with return to pre-existing conscious level**
HAC 7th character A see Appendix B for HAC conditional logic

MCC +7th **S06.306** **Unspecified focal traumatic brain injury with loss of consciousness greater than 24 hours without return to pre-existing conscious level with patient surviving**
HAC 7th character A see Appendix B for HAC conditional logic

MCC +7th **S06.307** **Unspecified focal traumatic brain injury with loss of consciousness of any duration with death due to brain injury prior to regaining consciousness**
HAC 7th character A see Appendix B for HAC conditional logic

MCC +7th **S06.308** **Unspecified focal traumatic brain injury with loss of consciousness of any duration with death due to other cause prior to regaining consciousness**
HAC 7th character A see Appendix B for HAC conditional logic

CC +7th **S06.309** **Unspecified focal traumatic brain injury with loss of consciousness of unspecified duration**
Unspecified focal traumatic brain injury NOS
HAC 7th character A see Appendix B for HAC conditional logic

+ **S06.31** **Contusion and laceration of right cerebrum**

MCC +7th **S06.310** **Contusion and laceration of right cerebrum without loss of consciousness**
HAC 7th character A see Appendix B for HAC conditional logic

MCC +7th **S06.311** **Contusion and laceration of right cerebrum with loss of consciousness of 30 minutes or less**
HAC 7th character A see Appendix B for HAC conditional logic

MCC +7th **S06.312** **Contusion and laceration of right cerebrum with loss of consciousness of 31 minutes to 59 minutes**
HAC 7th character A see Appendix B for HAC conditional logic

MCC +7th **S06.313** **Contusion and laceration of right cerebrum with loss of consciousness of 1 hour to 5 hours 59 minutes**
HAC 7th character A see Appendix B for HAC conditional logic

MCC +7th **S06.314** **Contusion and laceration of right cerebrum with loss of consciousness of 6 hours to 24 hours**
HAC 7th character A see Appendix B for HAC conditional logic

MCC +7th **S06.315** **Contusion and laceration of right cerebrum with loss of consciousness greater than 24 hours with return to pre-existing conscious level**
HAC 7th character A see Appendix B for HAC conditional logic

MCC +7th **S06.316** **Contusion and laceration of right cerebrum with loss of consciousness greater than 24 hours without return to pre-existing conscious level with patient surviving**
HAC 7th character A see Appendix B for HAC conditional logic

MCC +7th **S06.317** **Contusion and laceration of right cerebrum with loss of consciousness of any duration with death due to brain injury prior to regaining consciousness**
HAC 7th character A see Appendix B for HAC conditional logic

MCC +7th **S06.318** **Contusion and laceration of right cerebrum with loss of consciousness of any duration with death due to other cause prior to regaining consciousness**
HAC 7th character A see Appendix B for HAC conditional logic

MCC +7th **S06.319** **Contusion and laceration of right cerebrum with loss of consciousness of unspecified duration**
Contusion and laceration of right cerebrum NOS
HAC 7th character A see Appendix B for HAC conditional logic

+ **S06.32** **Contusion and laceration of left cerebrum**

MCC +7th **S06.320** **Contusion and laceration of left cerebrum without loss of consciousness**
HAC 7th character A see Appendix B for HAC conditional logic

MCC +7th **S06.321** **Contusion and laceration of left cerebrum with loss of consciousness of 30 minutes or less**
HAC 7th character A see Appendix B for HAC conditional logic

MCC +7th **S06.322** **Contusion and laceration of left cerebrum with loss of consciousness of 31 minutes to 59 minutes**
HAC 7th character A see Appendix B for HAC conditional logic

MCC +7th **S06.323** **Contusion and laceration of left cerebrum with loss of consciousness of 1 hour to 5 hours 59 minutes**
HAC 7th character A see Appendix B for HAC conditional logic

MCC +7th **S06.324** **Contusion and laceration of left cerebrum with loss of consciousness of 6 hours to 24 hours**
HAC 7th character A see Appendix B for HAC conditional logic

MCC +7th **S06.325** **Contusion and laceration of left cerebrum with loss of consciousness greater than 24 hours with return to pre-existing conscious level**
HAC 7th character A see Appendix B for HAC conditional logic

MCC +7th **S06.326** **Contusion and laceration of left cerebrum with loss of consciousness greater than 24 hours without return to pre-existing conscious level with patient surviving**
HAC 7th character A see Appendix B for HAC conditional logic

MCC +7th **S06.327** **Contusion and laceration of left cerebrum with loss of consciousness of any duration with death due to brain injury prior to regaining consciousness**
HAC 7th character A see Appendix B for HAC conditional logic

MCC +7th **S06.328** **Contusion and laceration of left cerebrum with loss of consciousness of any duration with death due to other cause prior to regaining consciousness**
HAC 7th character A see Appendix B for HAC conditional logic

MCC +7th **S06.329** **Contusion and laceration of left cerebrum with loss of consciousness of unspecified duration**

    Contusion and laceration of left cerebrum NOS

    HAC 7th character A see Appendix B for HAC conditional logic

+ **S06.33** **Contusion and laceration of cerebrum, unspecified**

MCC +7th **S06.330** **Contusion and laceration of cerebrum, unspecified, without loss of consciousness**

    HAC 7th character A see Appendix B for HAC conditional logic

MCC +7th **S06.331** **Contusion and laceration of cerebrum, unspecified, with loss of consciousness of 30 minutes or less**

    HAC 7th character A see Appendix B for HAC conditional logic

MCC +7th **S06.332** **Contusion and laceration of cerebrum, unspecified, with loss of consciousness of 31 minutes to 59 minutes**

    HAC 7th character A see Appendix B for HAC conditional logic

MCC +7th **S06.333** **Contusion and laceration of cerebrum, unspecified, with loss of consciousness of 1 hour to 5 hours 59 minutes**

    HAC 7th character A see Appendix B for HAC conditional logic

MCC +7th **S06.334** **Contusion and laceration of cerebrum, unspecified, with loss of consciousness of 6 hours to 24 hours**

    HAC 7th character A see Appendix B for HAC conditional logic

MCC +7th **S06.335** **Contusion and laceration of cerebrum, unspecified, with loss of consciousness greater than 24 hours with return to pre-existing conscious level**

    HAC 7th character A see Appendix B for HAC conditional logic

MCC +7th **S06.336** **Contusion and laceration of cerebrum, unspecified, with loss of consciousness greater than 24 hours without return to pre-existing conscious level with patient surviving**

    HAC 7th character A see Appendix B for HAC conditional logic

MCC +7th **S06.337** **Contusion and laceration of cerebrum, unspecified, with loss of consciousness of any duration with death due to brain injury prior to regaining consciousness**

    HAC 7th character A see Appendix B for HAC conditional logic

MCC +7th **S06.338** **Contusion and laceration of cerebrum, unspecified, with loss of consciousness of any duration with death due to other cause prior to regaining consciousness**

    HAC 7th character A see Appendix B for HAC conditional logic

MCC +7th **S06.339** **Contusion and laceration of cerebrum, unspecified, with loss of consciousness of unspecified duration**

    Contusion and laceration of cerebrum NOS

    HAC 7th character A see Appendix B for HAC conditional logic

+ **S06.34** **Traumatic hemorrhage of right cerebrum**

    Traumatic intracerebral hemorrhage and hematoma of right cerebrum

MCC +7th **S06.340** **Traumatic hemorrhage of right cerebrum without loss of consciousness**

    HAC 7th character A see Appendix B for HAC conditional logic

    AHA CC: 1Q, 2015, 3-21

MCC +7th **S06.341** **Traumatic hemorrhage of right cerebrum with loss of consciousness of 30 minutes or less**

    HAC 7th character A see Appendix B for HAC conditional logic

MCC +7th **S06.342** **Traumatic hemorrhage of right cerebrum with loss of consciousness of 31 minutes to 59 minutes**

    HAC 7th character A see Appendix B for HAC conditional logic

MCC +7th **S06.343** **Traumatic hemorrhage of right cerebrum with loss of consciousness of 1 hours to 5 hours 59 minutes**

    HAC 7th character A see Appendix B for HAC conditional logic

MCC +7th **S06.344** **Traumatic hemorrhage of right cerebrum with loss of consciousness of 6 hours to 24 hours**

    HAC 7th character A see Appendix B for HAC conditional logic

MCC +7th **S06.345** **Traumatic hemorrhage of right cerebrum with loss of consciousness greater than 24 hours with return to pre-existing conscious level**

    HAC 7th character A see Appendix B for HAC conditional logic

MCC +7th **S06.346** **Traumatic hemorrhage of right cerebrum with loss of consciousness greater than 24 hours without return to pre-existing conscious level with patient surviving**

    HAC 7th character A see Appendix B for HAC conditional logic

MCC +7th **S06.347** **Traumatic hemorrhage of right cerebrum with loss of consciousness of any duration with death due to brain injury prior to regaining consciousness**

    HAC 7th character A see Appendix B for HAC conditional logic

MCC +7th **S06.348** **Traumatic hemorrhage of right cerebrum with loss of consciousness of any duration with death due to other cause prior to regaining consciousness**

    HAC 7th character A see Appendix B for HAC conditional logic

MCC +7th **S06.349** **Traumatic hemorrhage of right cerebrum with loss of consciousness of unspecified duration**

    Traumatic hemorrhage of right cerebrum NOS

    HAC 7th character A see Appendix B for HAC conditional logic

+ **S06.35** **Traumatic hemorrhage of left cerebrum**

    Traumatic intracerebral hemorrhage and hematoma of left cerebrum

MCC +7th **S06.350** **Traumatic hemorrhage of left cerebrum without loss of consciousness**

    HAC 7th character A see Appendix B for HAC conditional logic

MCC +7th **S06.351** **Traumatic hemorrhage of left cerebrum with loss of consciousness of 30 minutes or less**

    HAC 7th character A see Appendix B for HAC conditional logic

MCC +7th **S06.352** **Traumatic hemorrhage of left cerebrum with loss of consciousness of 31 minutes to 59 minutes**

    HAC 7th character A see Appendix B for HAC conditional logic

MCC +7th **S06.353** **Traumatic hemorrhage of left cerebrum with loss of consciousness of 1 hours to 5 hours 59 minutes**

    HAC 7th character A see Appendix B for HAC conditional logic

MCC +7th **S06.354** **Traumatic hemorrhage of left cerebrum with loss of consciousness of 6 hours to 24 hours**

    HAC 7th character A see Appendix B for HAC conditional logic

MCC +7th **S06.355** **Traumatic hemorrhage of left cerebrum with loss of consciousness greater than 24 hours with return to pre-existing conscious level**

    HAC 7th character A see Appendix B for HAC conditional logic

MCC +7th **S06.356** **Traumatic hemorrhage of left cerebrum with loss of consciousness greater than 24 hours without return to pre-existing conscious level with patient surviving**

    HAC 7th character A see Appendix B for HAC conditional logic

+, +7th, X + 7th   ● Newborn   ● Pediatric   ● Maternity   ● Adult   ♀ Female   ♂ Male   Manifestation   Unacceptable PDX   HCC   CC   MCC   HAC

MCC +7th **S06.357** **Traumatic hemorrhage of left cerebrum with loss of consciousness of≈any duration with death due to brain injury prior to regaining consciousness**
> HAC 7th character A see Appendix B for HAC conditional logic

MCC +7th **S06.358** **Traumatic hemorrhage of left cerebrum with loss of consciousness of any duration with death due to other cause prior to regaining consciousness**
> HAC 7th character A see Appendix B for HAC conditional logic

MCC +7th **S06.359** **Traumatic hemorrhage of left cerebrum with loss of consciousness of unspecified duration**
> Traumatic hemorrhage of left cerebrum NOS
> HAC 7th character A see Appendix B for HAC conditional logic

+ **S06.36** **Traumatic hemorrhage of cerebrum, unspecified**
> Traumatic intracerebral hemorrhage and hematoma, unspecified

MCC +7th **S06.360** **Traumatic hemorrhage of cerebrum, unspecified, without loss of consciousness**
> HAC 7th character A see Appendix B for HAC conditional logic

MCC +7th **S06.361** **Traumatic hemorrhage of cerebrum, unspecified, with loss of consciousness of 30 minutes or less**
> HAC 7th character A see Appendix B for HAC conditional logic

MCC +7th **S06.362** **Traumatic hemorrhage of cerebrum, unspecified, with loss of consciousness of 31 minutes to 59 minutes**
> HAC 7th character A see Appendix B for HAC conditional logic

MCC +7th **S06.363** **Traumatic hemorrhage of cerebrum, unspecified, with loss of consciousness of 1 hours to 5 hours 59 minutes**
> HAC 7th character A see Appendix B for HAC conditional logic

MCC +7th **S06.364** **Traumatic hemorrhage of cerebrum, unspecified, with loss of consciousness of 6 hours to 24 hours**
> HAC 7th character A see Appendix B for HAC conditional logic

MCC +7th **S06.365** **Traumatic hemorrhage of cerebrum, unspecified, with loss of consciousness greater than 24 hours with return to pre-existing conscious level**
> HAC 7th character A see Appendix B for HAC conditional logic

MCC +7th **S06.366** **Traumatic hemorrhage of cerebrum, unspecified, with loss of consciousness greater than 24 hours without return to pre-existing conscious level with patient surviving**
> HAC 7th character A see Appendix B for HAC conditional logic

MCC +7th **S06.367** **Traumatic hemorrhage of cerebrum, unspecified, with loss of consciousness of any duration with death due to brain injury prior to regaining consciousness**
> HAC 7th character A see Appendix B for HAC conditional logic

MCC +7th **S06.368** **Traumatic hemorrhage of cerebrum, unspecified, with loss of consciousness of any duration with death due to other cause prior to regaining consciousness**
> HAC 7th character A see Appendix B for HAC conditional logic

MCC +7th **S06.369** **Traumatic hemorrhage of cerebrum, unspecified, with loss of consciousness of unspecified duration**
> Traumatic hemorrhage of cerebrum NOS
> HAC 7th character A see Appendix B for HAC conditional logic

+ **S06.37** **Contusion, laceration, and hemorrhage of cerebellum**

MCC +7th **S06.370** **Contusion, laceration, and hemorrhage of cerebellum without loss of consciousness**
> HAC 7th character A see Appendix B for HAC conditional logic

CC +7th **S06.371** **Contusion, laceration, and hemorrhage of cerebellum with loss of consciousness of 30 minutes or less**
> HAC 7th character A see Appendix B for HAC conditional logic

CC +7th **S06.372** **Contusion, laceration, and hemorrhage of cerebellum with loss of consciousness of 31 minutes to 59 minutes**
> HAC 7th character A see Appendix B for HAC conditional logic

CC +7th **S06.373** **Contusion, laceration, and hemorrhage of cerebellum with loss of consciousness of 1 hour to 5 hours 59 minutes**
> HAC 7th character A see Appendix B for HAC conditional logic

CC +7th **S06.374** **Contusion, laceration, and hemorrhage of cerebellum with loss of consciousness of 6 hours to 24 hours**
> HAC 7th character A see Appendix B for HAC conditional logic

CC +7th **S06.375** **Contusion, laceration, and hemorrhage of cerebellum with loss of consciousness greater than 24 hours with return to pre-existing conscious level**
> HAC 7th character A see Appendix B for HAC conditional logic

MCC +7th **S06.376** **Contusion, laceration, and hemorrhage of cerebellum with loss of consciousness greater than 24 hours without return to pre-existing conscious level with patient surviving**
> HAC 7th character A see Appendix B for HAC conditional logic

MCC +7th **S06.377** **Contusion, laceration, and hemorrhage of cerebellum with loss of consciousness of any duration with death due to brain injury prior to regaining consciousness**
> HAC 7th character A see Appendix B for HAC conditional logic

MCC +7th **S06.378** **Contusion, laceration, and hemorrhage of cerebellum with loss of consciousness of any duration with death due to other cause prior to regaining consciousness**
> HAC 7th character A see Appendix B for HAC conditional logic

CC +7th **S06.379** **Contusion, laceration, and hemorrhage of cerebellum with loss of consciousness of unspecified duration**
> Contusion, laceration, and hemorrhage of cerebellum NOS
> HAC 7th character A see Appendix B for HAC conditional logic

+ **S06.38** **Contusion, laceration, and hemorrhage of brainstem**

MCC +7th **S06.380** **Contusion, laceration, and hemorrhage of brainstem without loss of consciousness**
> HAC 7th character A see Appendix B for HAC conditional logic

CC +7th **S06.381** **Contusion, laceration, and hemorrhage of brainstem with loss of consciousness of 30 minutes or less**
> HAC 7th character A see Appendix B for HAC conditional logic

CC +7th **S06.382** **Contusion, laceration, and hemorrhage of brainstem with loss of consciousness of 31 minutes to 59 minutes**
> HAC 7th character A see Appendix B for HAC conditional logic

CC +7th **S06.383** **Contusion, laceration, and hemorrhage of brainstem with loss of consciousness of 1 hour to 5 hours 59 minutes**
> HAC 7th character A see Appendix B for HAC conditional logic

CC +7th **S06.384** **Contusion, laceration, and hemorrhage of brainstem with loss of consciousness of 6 hours to 24 hours**
> HAC 7th character A see Appendix B for HAC conditional logic

+, +7th, X + 7th   ● Newborn   ● Pediatric   ● Maternity   ● Adult   ♀ Female   ♂ Male   Manifestation   Unacceptable PDX   HCC   CC   MCC   HAC

CC +7th **S06.385** Contusion, laceration, and hemorrhage of brainstem with loss of consciousness greater than 24 hours with return to pre-existing conscious level
> HAC 7th character A see Appendix B for HAC conditional logic

MCC +7th **S06.386** Contusion, laceration, and hemorrhage of brainstem with loss of consciousness greater than 24 hours without return to pre-existing conscious level with patient surviving
> HAC 7th character A see Appendix B for HAC conditional logic

MCC +7th **S06.387** Contusion, laceration, and hemorrhage of brainstem with loss of consciousness of any duration with death due to brain injury prior to regaining consciousness
> HAC 7th character A see Appendix B for HAC conditional logic

MCC +7th **S06.388** Contusion, laceration, and hemorrhage of brainstem with loss of consciousness of any duration with death due to other cause prior to regaining consciousness
> HAC 7th character A see Appendix B for HAC conditional logic

CC +7th **S06.389** Contusion, laceration, and hemorrhage of brainstem with loss of consciousness of unspecified duration
> Contusion, laceration, and hemorrhage of brainstem NOS
> HAC 7th character A see Appendix B for HAC conditional logic

+ **S06.4** **Epidural hemorrhage**
> Extradural hemorrhage NOS
> Extradural hemorrhage (traumatic)

+ **S06.4X** **Epidural hemorrhage**

MCC +7th **S06.4X0** Epidural hemorrhage without loss of consciousness
> HAC 7th character A see Appendix B for HAC conditional logic

MCC +7th **S06.4X1** Epidural hemorrhage with loss of consciousness of 30 minutes or less
> HAC 7th character A see Appendix B for HAC conditional logic

MCC +7th **S06.4X2** Epidural hemorrhage with loss of consciousness of 31 minutes to 59 minutes
> HAC 7th character A see Appendix B for HAC conditional logic

MCC +7th **S06.4X3** Epidural hemorrhage with loss of consciousness of 1 hour to 5 hours 59 minutes
> HAC 7th character A see Appendix B for HAC conditional logic

MCC +7th **S06.4X4** Epidural hemorrhage with loss of consciousness of 6 hours to 24 hours
> HAC 7th character A see Appendix B for HAC conditional logic

MCC +7th **S06.4X5** Epidural hemorrhage with loss of consciousness greater than 24 hours with return to pre-existing conscious level
> HAC 7th character A see Appendix B for HAC conditional logic

MCC +7th **S06.4X6** Epidural hemorrhage with loss of consciousness greater than 24 hours without return to pre-existing conscious level with patient surviving
> HAC 7th character A see Appendix B for HAC conditional logic

MCC +7th **S06.4X7** Epidural hemorrhage with loss of consciousness of any duration with death due to brain injury prior to regaining consciousness
> HAC 7th character A see Appendix B for HAC conditional logic

MCC +7th **S06.4X8** Epidural hemorrhage with loss of consciousness of any duration with death due to other causes prior to regaining consciousness
> HAC 7th character A see Appendix B for HAC conditional logic

MCC +7th **S06.4X9** Epidural hemorrhage with loss of consciousness of unspecified duration
> Epidural hemorrhage NOS
> HAC 7th character A see Appendix B for HAC conditional logic

+ **S06.5** **Traumatic subdural hemorrhage**

+ **S06.5X** **Traumatic subdural hemorrhage**

MCC +7th **S06.5X0** Traumatic subdural hemorrhage without loss of consciousness
> HAC 7th character A see Appendix B for HAC conditional logic
> *AHA CC: 3Q, 2015, 37; 2Q, 2018, 13*

MCC +7th **S06.5X1** Traumatic subdural hemorrhage with loss of consciousness of 30 minutes or less
> HAC 7th character A see Appendix B for HAC conditional logic

MCC +7th **S06.5X2** Traumatic subdural hemorrhage with loss of consciousness of 31 minutes to 59 minutes
> HAC 7th character A see Appendix B for HAC conditional logic

MCC +7th **S06.5X3** Traumatic subdural hemorrhage with loss of consciousness of 1 hour to 5 hours 59 minutes
> HAC 7th character A see Appendix B for HAC conditional logic

MCC +7th **S06.5X4** Traumatic subdural hemorrhage with loss of consciousness of 6 hours to 24 hours
> HAC 7th character A see Appendix B for HAC conditional logic

MCC +7th **S06.5X5** Traumatic subdural hemorrhage with loss of consciousness greater than 24 hours with return to pre-existing conscious level
> HAC 7th character A see Appendix B for HAC conditional logic

MCC +7th **S06.5X6** Traumatic subdural hemorrhage with loss of consciousness greater than 24 hours without return to pre-existing conscious level with patient surviving
> HAC 7th character A see Appendix B for HAC conditional logic

MCC +7th **S06.5X7** Traumatic subdural hemorrhage with loss of consciousness of any duration with death due to brain injury before regaining consciousness
> HAC 7th character A see Appendix B for HAC conditional logic

MCC +7th **S06.5X8** Traumatic subdural hemorrhage with loss of consciousness of any duration with death due to other cause before regaining consciousness
> HAC 7th character A see Appendix B for HAC conditional logic

MCC +7th **S06.5X9** Traumatic subdural hemorrhage with loss of consciousness of unspecified duration
> Traumatic subdural hemorrhage NOS
> HAC 7th character A see Appendix B for HAC conditional logic

+ **S06.6** **Traumatic subarachnoid hemorrhage**

+ **S06.6X** **Traumatic subarachnoid hemorrhage**

MCC +7th **S06.6X0** Traumatic subarachnoid hemorrhage without loss of consciousness
> HAC 7th character A see Appendix B for HAC conditional logic
> *AHA CC: 3Q, 2015, 37*

MCC +7th **S06.6X1** Traumatic subarachnoid hemorrhage with loss of consciousness of 30 minutes or less
> HAC 7th character A see Appendix B for HAC conditional logic

MCC +7th **S06.6X2** Traumatic subarachnoid hemorrhage with loss of consciousness of 31 minutes to 59 minutes
> HAC 7th character A see Appendix B for HAC conditional logic

MCC +7th **S06.6X3** Traumatic subarachnoid hemorrhage with loss of consciousness of 1 hour to 5 hours 59 minutes
> HAC 7th character A see Appendix B for HAC conditional logic

MCC +7th **S06.6X4** **Traumatic subarachnoid hemorrhage with loss of consciousness of 6 hours to 24 hours**
> HAC 7th character A see Appendix B for HAC conditional logic

MCC +7th **S06.6X5** **Traumatic subarachnoid hemorrhage with loss of consciousness greater than 24 hours with return to pre-existing conscious level**
> HAC 7th character A see Appendix B for HAC conditional logic

MCC +7th **S06.6X6** **Traumatic subarachnoid hemorrhage with loss of consciousness greater than 24 hours without return to pre-existing conscious level with patient surviving**
> HAC 7th character A see Appendix B for HAC conditional logic

MCC +7th **S06.6X7** **Traumatic subarachnoid hemorrhage with loss of consciousness of any duration with death due to brain injury prior to regaining consciousness**
> HAC 7th character A see Appendix B for HAC conditional logic

MCC +7th **S06.6X8** **Traumatic subarachnoid hemorrhage with loss of consciousness of any duration with death due to other cause prior to regaining consciousness**
> HAC 7th character A see Appendix B for HAC conditional logic

MCC +7th **S06.6X9** **Traumatic subarachnoid hemorrhage with loss of consciousness of unspecified duration**
> Traumatic subarachnoid hemorrhage NOS
> HAC 7th character A see Appendix B for HAC conditional logic

+ **S06.8** **Other specified intracranial injuries**

+ **S06.81** **Injury of right internal carotid artery, intracranial portion, not elsewhere classified**

+7th **S06.810** **Injury of right internal carotid artery, intracranial portion, not elsewhere classified without loss of consciousness**

CC +7th **S06.811** **Injury of right internal carotid artery, intracranial portion, not elsewhere classified with loss of consciousness of 30 minutes or less**
> HAC 7th character A see Appendix B for HAC conditional logic

CC +7th **S06.812** **Injury of right internal carotid artery, intracranial portion, not elsewhere classified with loss of consciousness of 31 minutes to 59 minutes**
> HAC 7th character A see Appendix B for HAC conditional logic

CC +7th **S06.813** **Injury of right internal carotid artery, intracranial portion, not elsewhere classified with loss of consciousness of 1 hour to 5 hours 59 minutes**
> HAC 7th character A see Appendix B for HAC conditional logic

CC +7th **S06.814** **Injury of right internal carotid artery, intracranial portion, not elsewhere classified with loss of consciousness of 6 hours to 24 hours**
> HAC 7th character A see Appendix B for HAC conditional logic

CC +7th **S06.815** **Injury of right internal carotid artery, intracranial portion, not elsewhere classified with loss of consciousness greater than 24 hours with return to pre-existing conscious level**
> HAC 7th character A see Appendix B for HAC conditional logic

MCC +7th **S06.816** **Injury of right internal carotid artery, intracranial portion, not elsewhere classified with loss of consciousness greater than 24 hours without return to pre-existing conscious level with patient surviving**
> HAC 7th character A see Appendix B for HAC conditional logic

MCC +7th **S06.817** **Injury of right internal carotid artery, intracranial portion, not elsewhere classified with loss of consciousness of any duration with death due to brain injury prior to regaining consciousness**
> HAC 7th character A see Appendix B for HAC conditional logic

MCC +7th **S06.818** **Injury of right internal carotid artery, intracranial portion, not elsewhere classified with loss of consciousness of any duration with death due to other cause prior to regaining consciousness**
> HAC 7th character A see Appendix B for HAC conditional logic

CC +7th **S06.819** **Injury of right internal carotid artery, intracranial portion, not elsewhere classified with loss of consciousness of unspecified duration**
> Injury of right internal carotid artery, intracranial portion, not elsewhere classified NOS
> HAC 7th character A see Appendix B for HAC conditional logic

+ **S06.82** **Injury of left internal carotid artery, intracranial portion, not elsewhere classified**

+7th **S06.820** **Injury of left internal carotid artery, intracranial portion, not elsewhere classified without loss of consciousness**

CC +7th **S06.821** **Injury of left internal carotid artery, intracranial portion, not elsewhere classified with loss of consciousness of 30 minutes or less**
> HAC 7th character A see Appendix B for HAC conditional logic

CC +7th **S06.822** **Injury of left internal carotid artery, intracranial portion, not elsewhere classified with loss of consciousness of 31 minutes to 59 minutes**
> HAC 7th character A see Appendix B for HAC conditional logic

CC +7th **S06.823** **Injury of left internal carotid artery, intracranial portion, not elsewhere classified with loss of consciousness of 1 hour to 5 hours 59 minutes**
> HAC 7th character A see Appendix B for HAC conditional logic

CC +7th **S06.824** **Injury of left internal carotid artery, intracranial portion, not elsewhere classified with loss of consciousness of 6 hours to 24 hours**
> HAC 7th character A see Appendix B for HAC conditional logic

CC +7th **S06.825** **Injury of left internal carotid artery, intracranial portion, not elsewhere classified with loss of consciousness greater than 24 hours with return to pre-existing conscious level**
> HAC 7th character A see Appendix B for HAC conditional logic

MCC +7th **S06.826** **Injury of left internal carotid artery, intracranial portion, not elsewhere classified with loss of consciousness greater than 24 hours without return to pre-existing conscious level with patient surviving**
> HAC 7th character A see Appendix B for HAC conditional logic

MCC +7th **S06.827** **Injury of left internal carotid artery, intracranial portion, not elsewhere classified with loss of consciousness of any duration with death due to brain injury prior to regaining consciousness**
> HAC 7th character A see Appendix B for HAC conditional logic

+, +7th, X + 7th ● Newborn ● Pediatric ● Maternity ● Adult ♀ Female ♂ Male Manifestation Unacceptable PDX HCC CC MCC HAC

MCC +7th **S06.828** **Injury of left internal carotid artery, intracranial portion, not elsewhere classified with loss of consciousness of any duration with death due to other cause prior to regaining consciousness**
 HAC 7th character A see Appendix B for HAC conditional logic

CC +7th **S06.829** **Injury of left internal carotid artery, intracranial portion, not elsewhere classified with loss of consciousness of unspecified duration**
 Injury of left internal carotid artery, intracranial portion, not elsewhere classified NOS
 HAC 7th character A see Appendix B for HAC conditional logic

+ **S06.89** **Other specified intracranial injury**
 Excludes1: concussion (S06.0X-)

+7th **S06.890** **Other specified intracranial injury without loss of consciousness**

CC +7th **S06.891** **Other specified intracranial injury with loss of consciousness of 30 minutes or less**
 HAC 7th character A see Appendix B for HAC conditional logic

CC +7th **S06.892** **Other specified intracranial injury with loss of consciousness of 31 minutes to 59 minutes**
 HAC 7th character A see Appendix B for HAC conditional logic

CC +7th **S06.893** **Other specified intracranial injury with loss of consciousness of 1 hour to 5 hours 59 minutes**
 HAC 7th character A see Appendix B for HAC conditional logic

CC +7th **S06.894** **Other specified intracranial injury with loss of consciousness of 6 hours to 24 hours**
 HAC 7th character A see Appendix B for HAC conditional logic

CC +7th **S06.895** **Other specified intracranial injury with loss of consciousness greater than 24 hours with return to pre-existing conscious level**
 HAC 7th character A see Appendix B for HAC conditional logic

MCC +7th **S06.896** **Other specified intracranial injury with loss of consciousness greater than 24 hours without return to pre-existing conscious level with patient surviving**
 HAC 7th character A see Appendix B for HAC conditional logic

MCC +7th **S06.897** **Other specified intracranial injury with loss of consciousness of any duration with death due to brain injury prior to regaining consciousness**
 HAC 7th character A see Appendix B for HAC conditional logic

MCC +7th **S06.898** **Other specified intracranial injury with loss of consciousness of any duration with death due to other cause prior to regaining consciousness**
 HAC 7th character A see Appendix B for HAC conditional logic

CC +7th **S06.899** **Other specified intracranial injury with loss of consciousness of unspecified duration**
 HAC 7th character A see Appendix B for HAC conditional logic

CC + **S06.9** **Unspecified intracranial injury**
 Brain injury NOS
 Head injury NOS with loss of consciousness
 Traumatic brain injury NOS
 Excludes1: conditions classifiable to S06.0- to S06.8- code to specified intracranial injury
 head injury NOS (S09.90)

+ **S06.9X** **Unspecified intracranial injury**

+7th **S06.9X0** **Unspecified intracranial injury without loss of consciousness**
 AHA CC: 2Q, 2020, 31
 HAC 7th character A see Appendix B for HAC conditional logic

+7th **S06.9X1** **Unspecified intracranial injury with loss of consciousness of 30 minutes or less**
 HAC 7th character A see Appendix B for HAC conditional logic

+7th **S06.9X2** **Unspecified intracranial injury with loss of consciousness of 31 minutes to 59 minutes**
 HAC 7th character A see Appendix B for HAC conditional logic

+7th **S06.9X3** **Unspecified intracranial injury with loss of consciousness of 1 hour to 5 hours 59 minutes**
 HAC 7th character A see Appendix B for HAC conditional logic

+7th **S06.9X4** **Unspecified intracranial injury with loss of consciousness of 6 hours to 24 hours**
 HAC 7th character A see Appendix B for HAC conditional logic

+7th **S06.9X5** **Unspecified intracranial injury with loss of consciousness greater than 24 hours with return to pre-existing conscious level**
 HAC 7th character A see Appendix B for HAC conditional logic

MCC +7th **S06.9X6** **Unspecified intracranial injury with loss of consciousness greater than 24 hours without return to pre-existing conscious level with patient surviving**
 HAC 7th character A see Appendix B for HAC conditional logic

MCC +7th **S06.9X7** **Unspecified intracranial injury with loss of consciousness of any duration with death due to brain injury prior to regaining consciousness**
 HAC 7th character A see Appendix B for HAC conditional logic

MCC +7th **S06.9X8** **Unspecified intracranial injury with loss of consciousness of any duration with death due to other cause prior to regaining consciousness**
 HAC 7th character A see Appendix B for HAC conditional logic

+7th **S06.9X9** **Unspecified intracranial injury with loss of consciousness of unspecified duration**
 HAC 7th character A see Appendix B for HAC conditional logic

S07 **Crushing injury of head**

Use additional code for all associated injuries, such as:
 intracranial injuries (S06.-)
 skull fractures (S02.-)

The appropriate 7th character is to be added to each code from category S07
A   initial encounter
D   subsequent encounter
S   sequela

CC X+7th **S07.0** **Crushing injury of face**
 HAC 7th character A see Appendix B for HAC conditional logic

CC X+7th **S07.1** **Crushing injury of skull**
 HAC 7th character A see Appendix B for HAC conditional logic

CC X+7th **S07.8** **Crushing injury of other parts of head**
 HAC 7th character A see Appendix B for HAC conditional logic

CC X+7th **S07.9** **Crushing injury of head, part unspecified**
 HAC 7th character A see Appendix B for HAC conditional logic

S08 **Avulsion and traumatic amputation of part of head**

An amputation not identified as partial or complete should be coded to complete

The appropriate 7th character is to be added to each code from category S08
A   initial encounter
D   subsequent encounter
S   sequela

+, +7th, X + 7th   ● Newborn   ● Pediatric   ● Maternity   ● Adult   ♀ Female   ♂ Male   Manifestation   Unacceptable PDX   HCC   CC   MCC   **HAC**

X+7th **S08.0** **Avulsion of scalp**
+ **S08.1** **Traumatic amputation of ear**
  + **S08.11** **Complete traumatic amputation of ear**
    +7th **S08.111** **Complete traumatic amputation of right ear**
    +7th **S08.112** **Complete traumatic amputation of left ear**
    +7th **S08.119** **Complete traumatic amputation of unspecified ear**
  + **S08.12** **Partial traumatic amputation of ear**
    +7th **S08.121** **Partial traumatic amputation of right ear**
    +7th **S08.122** **Partial traumatic amputation of left ear**
    +7th **S08.129** **Partial traumatic amputation of unspecified ear**
+ **S08.8** **Traumatic amputation of other parts of head**
  + **S08.81** **Traumatic amputation of nose**
    +7th **S08.811** **Complete traumatic amputation of nose**
    +7th **S08.812** **Partial traumatic amputation of nose**
  X+7th **S08.89** **Traumatic amputation of other parts of head**

S09 **Other and unspecified injuries of head**

> The appropriate 7th character is to be added to each code from category S09
> A initial encounter
> D subsequent encounter
> S sequela

CC X+7th **S09.0** **Injury of blood vessels of head, not elsewhere classified**
    Excludes1: *injury of cerebral blood vessels (S06.-)*
      injury of precerebral blood vessels (S15.-)
+ **S09.1** **Injury of muscle and tendon of head**
    Code also any associated open wound (S01.-)
    Excludes2: *sprain to joints and ligament of head (S03.9)*
  X+7th **S09.10** **Unspecified injury of muscle and tendon of head**
    Injury of muscle and tendon of head NOS
  X+7th **S09.11** **Strain of muscle and tendon of head**
  X+7th **S09.12** **Laceration of muscle and tendon of head**
  X+7th **S09.19** **Other specified injury of muscle and tendon of head**
+ **S09.2** **Traumatic rupture of ear drum**
    Excludes1: *traumatic rupture of ear drum due to blast injury (S09.31-)*
  CC X+7th **S09.20** **Traumatic rupture of unspecified ear drum**
  CC X+7th **S09.21** **Traumatic rupture of right ear drum**
  CC X+7th **S09.22** **Traumatic rupture of left ear drum**
+ **S09.3** **Other specified and unspecified injury of middle and inner ear**
    Excludes1: *injury to ear NOS (S09.91-)*
    Excludes2: *injury to external ear (S00.4-, S01.3-, S08.1-)*
  + **S09.30** **Unspecified injury of middle and inner ear**
    CC +7th **S09.301** **Unspecified injury of right middle and inner ear**
    CC +7th **S09.302** **Unspecified injury of left middle and inner ear**
    CC +7th **S09.309** **Unspecified injury of unspecified middle and inner ear**
  + **S09.31** **Primary blast injury of ear**
    Blast injury of ear NOS
    CC +7th **S09.311** **Primary blast injury of right ear**
    CC +7th **S09.312** **Primary blast injury of left ear**
    CC +7th **S09.313** **Primary blast injury of ear, bilateral**
    CC +7th **S09.319** **Primary blast injury of unspecified ear**
  + **S09.39** **Other specified injury of middle and inner ear**
    Secondary blast injury to ear
    CC +7th **S09.391** **Other specified injury of right middle and inner ear**
    CC +7th **S09.392** **Other specified injury of left middle and inner ear**
    CC +7th **S09.399** **Other specified injury of unspecified middle and inner ear**
X+7th **S09.8** **Other specified injuries of head**
+ **S09.9** **Unspecified injury of face and head**
  X+7th **S09.90** **Unspecified injury of head**
    Head injury NOS
    Excludes1: *brain injury NOS (S06.9-)*
      head injury NOS with loss of consciousness (S06.9-)
      intracranial injury NOS (S06.9-)

X+7th **S09.91** **Unspecified injury of ear**
    Injury of ear NOS
X+7th **S09.92** **Unspecified injury of nose**
    Injury of nose NOS
X+7th **S09.93** **Unspecified injury of face**
    Injury of face NOS

Injuries to the neck (S10-S19)

Includes: injuries of nape
      injuries of supraclavicular region
      injuries of throat

Excludes2: *burns and corrosions (T20-T32)*
    effects of foreign body in esophagus (T18.1)
    effects of foreign body in larynx (T17.3)
    effects of foreign body in pharynx (T17.2)
    effects of foreign body in trachea (T17.4)
    frostbite (T33-T34)
    insect bite or sting, venomous (T63.4)

S10 **Superficial injury of neck**

> The appropriate 7th character is to be added to each code from category S10
> A initial encounter
> D subsequent encounter
> S sequela

X+7th **S10.0** **Contusion of throat**
    Contusion of cervical esophagus
    Contusion of larynx
    Contusion of pharynx
    Contusion of trachea
+ **S10.1** **Other and unspecified superficial injuries of throat**
  X+7th **S10.10** **Unspecified superficial injuries of throat**
  X+7th **S10.11** **Abrasion of throat**
  X+7th **S10.12** **Blister (nonthermal) of throat**
  X+7th **S10.14** **External constriction of part of throat**
  X+7th **S10.15** **Superficial foreign body of throat**
    Splinter in the throat
  X+7th **S10.16** **Insect bite (nonvenomous) of throat**
  X+7th **S10.17** **Other superficial bite of throat**
    Excludes1: *open bite of throat (S11.85)*
+ **S10.8** **Superficial injury of other specified parts of neck**
  X+7th **S10.80** **Unspecified superficial injury of other specified part of neck**
  X+7th **S10.81** **Abrasion of other specified part of neck**
  X+7th **S10.82** **Blister (nonthermal) of other specified part of neck**
  X+7th **S10.83** **Contusion of other specified part of neck**
  X+7th **S10.84** **External constriction of other specified part of neck**
  X+7th **S10.85** **Superficial foreign body of other specified part of neck**
    Splinter in other specified part of neck
  X+7th **S10.86** **Insect bite of other specified part of neck**
  X+7th **S10.87** **Other superficial bite of other specified part of neck**
    Excludes1: *open bite of other specified parts of neck (S11.85)*
+ **S10.9** **Superficial injury of unspecified part of neck**
  X+7th **S10.90** **Unspecified superficial injury of unspecified part of neck**
  X+7th **S10.91** **Abrasion of unspecified part of neck**
  X+7th **S10.92** **Blister (nonthermal) of unspecified part of neck**
  X+7th **S10.93** **Contusion of unspecified part of neck**
  X+7th **S10.94** **External constriction of unspecified part of neck**
  X+7th **S10.95** **Superficial foreign body of unspecified part of neck**
  X+7th **S10.96** **Insect bite of unspecified part of neck**
  X+7th **S10.97** **Other superficial bite of unspecified part of neck**

S11 **Open wound of neck**

Code also any associated:
  spinal cord injury (S14.0, S14.1-)
  wound infection
Excludes2: *open fracture of vertebra (S12.- with 7th character B)*

> The appropriate 7th character is to be added to each code from category S11
> A initial encounter
> D subsequent encounter
> S sequela

+, +7th, X + 7th   ● Newborn   ○ Pediatric   ● Maternity   ● Adult   ♀ Female   ♂ Male   Manifestation   Unacceptable PDX   HCC   CC   MCC   HAC

Vertebrae

©AHIMA

+ **S11.0 Open wound of larynx and trachea**
    + **S11.01 Open wound of larynx**
              Excludes2: *open wound of vocal cord (S11.03)*
   MCC +7th **S11.011 Laceration without foreign body of larynx**
   MCC +7th **S11.012 Laceration with foreign body of larynx**
   MCC +7th **S11.013 Puncture wound without foreign body of larynx**
   MCC +7th **S11.014 Puncture wound with foreign body of larynx**
   MCC +7th **S11.015 Open bite of larynx**
              Bite of larynx NOS
   MCC +7th **S11.019 Unspecified open wound of larynx**
    + **S11.02 Open wound of trachea**
            Open wound of cervical trachea
            Open wound of trachea NOS
            Excludes2: *open wound of thoracic trachea (S27.5-)*
   MCC +7th **S11.021 Laceration without foreign body of trachea**
   MCC +7th **S11.022 Laceration with foreign body of trachea**
   MCC +7th **S11.023 Puncture wound without foreign body of trachea**
   MCC +7th **S11.024 Puncture wound with foreign body of trachea**
   MCC +7th **S11.025 Open bite of trachea**
              Bite of trachea NOS
   MCC +7th **S11.029 Unspecified open wound of trachea**
    + **S11.03 Open wound of vocal cord**
   MCC +7th **S11.031 Laceration without foreign body of vocal cord**
   MCC +7th **S11.032 Laceration with foreign body of vocal cord**

   MCC +7th **S11.033 Puncture wound without foreign body of vocal cord**
   MCC +7th **S11.034 Puncture wound with foreign body of vocal cord**
   MCC +7th **S11.035 Open bite of vocal cord**
              Bite of vocal cord NOS
   MCC +7th **S11.039 Unspecified open wound of vocal cord**
+ **S11.1 Open wound of thyroid gland**
   CC X+7th **S11.10 Unspecified open wound of thyroid gland**
   CC X+7th **S11.11 Laceration without foreign body of thyroid gland**
   CC X+7th **S11.12 Laceration with foreign body of thyroid gland**
   CC X+7th **S11.13 Puncture wound without foreign body of thyroid gland**
   CC X+7th **S11.14 Puncture wound with foreign body of thyroid gland**
   CC X+7th **S11.15 Open bite of thyroid gland**
              Bite of thyroid gland NOS
+ **S11.2 Open wound of pharynx and cervical esophagus**
       Excludes1: *open wound of esophagus NOS (S27.8-)*
   CC X+7th **S11.20 Unspecified open wound of pharynx and cervical esophagus**
   CC X+7th **S11.21 Laceration without foreign body of pharynx and cervical esophagus**
   CC X+7th **S11.22 Laceration with foreign body of pharynx and cervical esophagus**
   CC X+7th **S11.23 Puncture wound without foreign body of pharynx and cervical esophagus**
   CC X+7th **S11.24 Puncture wound with foreign body of pharynx and cervical esophagus**
   CC X+7th **S11.25 Open bite of pharynx and cervical esophagus**
              Bite of pharynx and cervical esophagus NOS
+ **S11.8 Open wound of other specified parts of neck**
   X+7th **S11.80 Unspecified open wound of other specified part of neck**

+, +7th, X + 7th   ● Newborn   ● Pediatric   ● Maternity   ● Adult   ♀ Female   ♂ Male   Manifestation   Unacceptable PDX   HCC   CC   MCC   HAC

X+7th **S11.81** **Laceration without foreign body of other specified part of neck**

X+7th **S11.82** **Laceration with foreign body of other specified part of neck**

X+7th **S11.83** **Puncture wound without foreign body of other specified part of neck**

X+7th **S11.84** **Puncture wound with foreign body of other specified part of neck**

X+7th **S11.85** **Open bite of other specified part of neck**
Bite of other specified part of neck NOS
Excludes1: *superficial bite of other specified part of neck (S10.87)*

X+7th **S11.89** **Other open wound of other specified part of neck**

+ **S11.9** **Open wound of unspecified part of neck**

X+7th **S11.90** **Unspecified open wound of unspecified part of neck**

X+7th **S11.91** **Laceration without foreign body of unspecified part of neck**

X+7th **S11.92** **Laceration with foreign body of unspecified part of neck**

X+7th **S11.93** **Puncture wound without foreign body of unspecified part of neck**

X+7th **S11.94** **Puncture wound with foreign body of unspecified part of neck**

X+7th **S11.95** **Open bite of unspecified part of neck**
Bite of neck NOS
Excludes1: *superficial bite of neck (S10.97)*

S12 **Fracture of cervical vertebra and other parts of neck**

NOTE A fracture not indicated as displaced or nondisplaced should be coded to displaced
A fracture not indicated as open or closed should be coded to closed

Includes: fracture of cervical neural arch
fracture of cervical spine
fracture of cervical spinous process
fracture of cervical transverse process
fracture of cervical vertebral arch
fracture of neck

Code first any associated cervical spinal cord injury (S14.0, S14.1-)

The appropriate 7th character is to be added to all codes from subcategories **S12.0-S12.6**
A initial encounter for closed fracture
B initial encounter for open fracture
D subsequent encounter for fracture with routine healing
G subsequent encounter for fracture with delayed healing
K subsequent encounter for fracture with nonunion
S sequela

Review coding guideline C.19.c

+ **S12.0** **Fracture of first cervical vertebra**
Atlas

+ **S12.00** **Unspecified fracture of first cervical vertebra**

CC MCC +7th **S12.000** **Unspecified displaced fracture of first cervical vertebra**
HAC 7th characters A & B see Appendix B for HAC conditional logic

CC MCC +7th **S12.001** **Unspecified nondisplaced fracture of first cervical vertebra**
HAC 7th characters A & B see Appendix B for HAC conditional logic

CC MCC X+7th **S12.01** **Stable burst fracture of first cervical vertebra**
HAC 7th characters A & B see Appendix B for HAC conditional logic

CC MCC X+7th **S12.02** **Unstable burst fracture of first cervical vertebra**
HAC 7th characters A & B see Appendix B for HAC conditional logic

+ **S12.03** **Posterior arch fracture of first cervical vertebra**

CC MCC +7th **S12.030** **Displaced posterior arch fracture of first cervical vertebra**
HAC 7th characters A & B see Appendix B for HAC conditional logic

CC MCC +7th **S12.031** **Nondisplaced posterior arch fracture of first cervical vertebra**
HAC 7th characters A & B see Appendix B for HAC conditional logic

+ **S12.04** **Lateral mass fracture of first cervical vertebra**

CC MCC +7th **S12.040** **Displaced lateral mass fracture of first cervical vertebra**
HAC 7th characters A & B see Appendix B for HAC conditional logic

CC MCC +7th **S12.041** **Nondisplaced lateral mass fracture of first cervical vertebra**
HAC 7th characters A & B see Appendix B for HAC conditional logic

+ **S12.09** **Other fracture of first cervical vertebra**

CC MCC +7th **S12.090** **Other displaced fracture of first cervical vertebra**
HAC 7th characters A & B see Appendix B for HAC conditional logic

CC MCC +7th **S12.091** **Other nondisplaced fracture of first cervical vertebra**
HAC 7th characters A & B see Appendix B for HAC conditional logic

+ **S12.1** **Fracture of second cervical vertebra**
Axis

+ **S12.10** **Unspecified fracture of second cervical vertebra**

CC MCC +7th **S12.100** **Unspecified displaced fracture of second cervical vertebra**
HAC 7th characters A & B see Appendix B for HAC conditional logic

CC MCC +7th **S12.101** **Unspecified nondisplaced fracture of second cervical vertebra**
HAC 7th characters A & B see Appendix B for HAC conditional logic

+ **S12.11** **Type II dens fracture**

CC MCC +7th **S12.110** **Anterior displaced Type II dens fracture**
HAC 7th characters A & B see Appendix B for HAC conditional logic

CC MCC +7th **S12.111** **Posterior displaced Type II dens fracture**
HAC 7th characters A & B see Appendix B for HAC conditional logic

CC MCC +7th **S12.112** **Nondisplaced Type II dens fracture**
HAC 7th characters A & B see Appendix B for HAC conditional logic

+ **S12.12** **Other dens fracture**

CC MCC +7th **S12.120** **Other displaced dens fracture**
HAC 7th characters A & B see Appendix B for HAC conditional logic

CC MCC +7th **S12.121** **Other nondisplaced dens fracture**
HAC 7th characters A & B see Appendix B for HAC conditional logic

+ **S12.13** **Unspecified traumatic spondylolisthesis of second cervical vertebra**

CC MCC +7th **S12.130** **Unspecified traumatic displaced spondylolisthesis of second cervical vertebra**
HAC 7th characters A & B see Appendix B for HAC conditional logic

CC MCC +7th **S12.131** **Unspecified traumatic nondisplaced spondylolisthesis of second cervical vertebra**
HAC 7th characters A & B see Appendix B for HAC conditional logic

CC MCC X+7th **S12.14** **Type III traumatic spondylolisthesis of second cervical vertebra**
HAC 7th characters A & B see Appendix B for HAC conditional logic

+ **S12.15** **Other traumatic spondylolisthesis of second cervical vertebra**

CC MCC +7th **S12.150** **Other traumatic displaced spondylolisthesis of second cervical vertebra**
HAC 7th characters A & B see Appendix B for HAC conditional logic

CC MCC +7th **S12.151** **Other traumatic nondisplaced spondylolisthesis of second cervical vertebra**
HAC 7th characters A & B see Appendix B for HAC conditional logic

+ **S12.19** **Other fracture of second cervical vertebra**

CC MCC +7th **S12.190** **Other displaced fracture of second cervical vertebra**
HAC 7th characters A & B see Appendix B for HAC conditional logic

CC MCC +7th **S12.191** **Other nondisplaced fracture of second cervical vertebra**
HAC 7th characters A & B see Appendix B for HAC conditional logic

+ **S12.2** **Fracture of third cervical vertebra**

+ **S12.20** **Unspecified fracture of third cervical vertebra**

CC MCC +7th **S12.200** **Unspecified displaced fracture of third cervical vertebra**
HAC 7th characters A & B see Appendix B for HAC conditional logic

CC MCC +7th **S12.201** **Unspecified nondisplaced fracture of third cervical vertebra**
> HAC 7th characters A & B see Appendix B for HAC conditional logic

+ **S12.23** **Unspecified traumatic spondylolisthesis of third cervical vertebra**

CC MCC +7th **S12.230** **Unspecified traumatic displaced spondylolisthesis of third cervical vertebra**
> HAC 7th characters A & B see Appendix B for HAC conditional logic

CC MCC +7th **S12.231** **Unspecified traumatic nondisplaced spondylolisthesis of third cervical vertebra**
> HAC 7th characters A & B see Appendix B for HAC conditional logic

CC MCC X+7th **S12.24** **Type III traumatic spondylolisthesis of third cervical vertebra**
> HAC 7th characters A & B see Appendix B for HAC conditional logic

+ **S12.25** **Other traumatic spondylolisthesis of third cervical vertebra**

CC MCC +7th **S12.250** **Other traumatic displaced spondylolisthesis of third cervical vertebra**
> HAC 7th characters A & B see Appendix B for HAC conditional logic

CC MCC +7th **S12.251** **Other traumatic nondisplaced spondylolisthesis of third cervical vertebra**
> HAC 7th characters A & B see Appendix B for HAC conditional logic

+ **S12.29** **Other fracture of third cervical vertebra**

CC MCC +7th **S12.290** **Other displaced fracture of third cervical vertebra**
> HAC 7th characters A & B see Appendix B for HAC conditional logic

CC MCC +7th **S12.291** **Other nondisplaced fracture of third cervical vertebra**
> HAC 7th characters A & B see Appendix B for HAC conditional logic

+ **S12.3** **Fracture of fourth cervical vertebra**

+ **S12.30** **Unspecified fracture of fourth cervical vertebra**

CC MCC +7th **S12.300** **Unspecified displaced fracture of fourth cervical vertebra**
> HAC 7th characters A & B see Appendix B for HAC conditional logic

CC MCC +7th **S12.301** **Unspecified nondisplaced fracture of fourth cervical vertebra**
> HAC 7th characters A & B see Appendix B for HAC conditional logic

+ **S12.33** **Unspecified traumatic spondylolisthesis of fourth cervical vertebra**

CC MCC +7th **S12.330** **Unspecified traumatic displaced spondylolisthesis of fourth cervical vertebra**
> HAC 7th characters A & B see Appendix B for HAC conditional logic

CC MCC +7th **S12.331** **Unspecified traumatic nondisplaced spondylolisthesis of fourth cervical vertebra**
> HAC 7th characters A & B see Appendix B for HAC conditional logic

CC MCC X+7th **S12.34** **Type III traumatic spondylolisthesis of fourth cervical vertebra**
> HAC 7th characters A & B see Appendix B for HAC conditional logic

+ **S12.35** **Other traumatic spondylolisthesis of fourth cervical vertebra**

CC MCC +7th **S12.350** **Other traumatic displaced spondylolisthesis of fourth cervical vertebra**
> HAC 7th characters A & B see Appendix B for HAC conditional logic

CC MCC +7th **S12.351** **Other traumatic nondisplaced spondylolisthesis of fourth cervical vertebra**
> HAC 7th characters A & B see Appendix B for HAC conditional logic

+ **S12.39** **Other fracture of fourth cervical vertebra**

CC MCC +7th **S12.390** **Other displaced fracture of fourth cervical vertebra**
> HAC 7th characters A & B see Appendix B for HAC conditional logic

CC MCC +7th **S12.391** **Other nondisplaced fracture of fourth cervical vertebra**
> HAC 7th characters A & B see Appendix B for HAC conditional logic

+ **S12.4** **Fracture of fifth cervical vertebra**

+ **S12.40** **Unspecified fracture of fifth cervical vertebra**

CC MCC +7th **S12.400** **Unspecified displaced fracture of fifth cervical vertebra**
> HAC 7th characters A & B see Appendix B for HAC conditional logic

CC MCC +7th **S12.401** **Unspecified nondisplaced fracture of fifth cervical vertebra**
> HAC 7th characters A & B see Appendix B for HAC conditional logic

+ **S12.43** **Unspecified traumatic spondylolisthesis of fifth cervical vertebra**

CC MCC +7th **S12.430** **Unspecified traumatic displaced spondylolisthesis of fifth cervical vertebra**
> HAC 7th characters A & B see Appendix B for HAC conditional logic

CC MCC +7th **S12.431** **Unspecified traumatic nondisplaced spondylolisthesis of fifth cervical vertebra**
> HAC 7th characters A & B see Appendix B for HAC conditional logic

CC MCC X+7th **S12.44** **Type III traumatic spondylolisthesis of fifth cervical vertebra**
> HAC 7th characters A & B see Appendix B for HAC conditional logic

+ **S12.45** **Other traumatic spondylolisthesis of fifth cervical vertebra**

CC MCC +7th **S12.450** **Other traumatic displaced spondylolisthesis of fifth cervical vertebra**
> HAC 7th characters A & B see Appendix B for HAC conditional logic

CC MCC +7th **S12.451** **Other traumatic nondisplaced spondylolisthesis of fifth cervical vertebra**
> HAC 7th characters A & B see Appendix B for HAC conditional logic

+ **S12.49** **Other fracture of fifth cervical vertebra**

CC MCC +7th **S12.490** **Other displaced fracture of fifth cervical vertebra**
> HAC 7th characters A & B see Appendix B for HAC conditional logic

CC MCC +7th **S12.491** **Other nondisplaced fracture of fifth cervical vertebra**
> HAC 7th characters A & B see Appendix B for HAC conditional logic

+ **S12.5** **Fracture of sixth cervical vertebra**

+ **S12.50** **Unspecified fracture of sixth cervical vertebra**

CC MCC +7th **S12.500** **Unspecified displaced fracture of sixth cervical vertebra**
> HAC 7th characters A & B see Appendix B for HAC conditional logic

CC MCC +7th **S12.501** **Unspecified nondisplaced fracture of sixth cervical vertebra**
> HAC 7th characters A & B see Appendix B for HAC conditional logic

+ **S12.53** **Unspecified traumatic spondylolisthesis of sixth cervical vertebra**

CC MCC +7th **S12.530** **Unspecified traumatic displaced spondylolisthesis of sixth cervical vertebra**
> HAC 7th characters A & B see Appendix B for HAC conditional logic

CC MCC +7th **S12.531** **Unspecified traumatic nondisplaced spondylolisthesis of sixth cervical vertebra**
> HAC 7th characters A & B see Appendix B for HAC conditional logic

CC MCC X+7th **S12.54** **Type III traumatic spondylolisthesis of sixth cervical vertebra**
> HAC 7th characters A & B see Appendix B for HAC conditional logic

+ **S12.55** **Other traumatic spondylolisthesis of sixth cervical vertebra**

CC MCC +7th **S12.550** **Other traumatic displaced spondylolisthesis of sixth cervical vertebra**
> HAC 7th characters A & B see Appendix B for HAC conditional logic

+, +7th, X + 7th   ● Newborn   ● Pediatric   ● Maternity   ● Adult   ♀ Female   ♂ Male   Manifestation   Unacceptable PDX   HCC   CC   MCC   HAC

CC MCC +7th **S12.551** **Other traumatic nondisplaced spondylolisthesis of sixth cervical vertebra**
   HAC 7th characters A & B see Appendix B for HAC conditional logic

+ **S12.59** **Other fracture of sixth cervical vertebra**
CC MCC +7th **S12.590** **Other displaced fracture of sixth cervical vertebra**
   HAC 7th characters A & B see Appendix B for HAC conditional logic

CC MCC +7th **S12.591** **Other nondisplaced fracture of sixth cervical vertebra**
   HAC 7th characters A & B see Appendix B for HAC conditional logic

+ **S12.6** **Fracture of seventh cervical vertebra**
   + **S12.60** **Unspecified fracture of seventh cervical vertebra**
CC MCC +7th **S12.600** **Unspecified displaced fracture of seventh cervical vertebra**
   HAC 7th characters A & B see Appendix B for HAC conditional logic

CC MCC +7th **S12.601** **Unspecified nondisplaced fracture of seventh cervical vertebra**
   HAC 7th characters A & B see Appendix B for HAC conditional logic

   + **S12.63** **Unspecified traumatic spondylolisthesis of seventh cervical vertebra**
CC MCC +7th **S12.630** **Unspecified traumatic displaced spondylolisthesis of seventh cervical vertebra**
   HAC 7th characters A & B see Appendix B for HAC conditional logic

CC MCC +7th **S12.631** **Unspecified traumatic nondisplaced spondylolisthesis of seventh cervical vertebra**
   HAC 7th characters A & B see Appendix B for HAC conditional logic

CC MCC X+7th **S12.64** **Type III traumatic spondylolisthesis of seventh cervical vertebra**
   HAC 7th characters A & B see Appendix B for HAC conditional logic

   + **S12.65** **Other traumatic spondylolisthesis of seventh cervical vertebra**
CC MCC +7th **S12.650** **Other traumatic displaced spondylolisthesis of seventh cervical vertebra**
   HAC 7th characters A & B see Appendix B for HAC conditional logic

CC MCC +7th **S12.651** **Other traumatic nondisplaced spondylolisthesis of seventh cervical vertebra**
   HAC 7th characters A & B see Appendix B for HAC conditional logic

   + **S12.69** **Other fracture of seventh cervical vertebra**
CC MCC +7th **S12.690** **Other displaced fracture of seventh cervical vertebra**
   HAC 7th characters A & B see Appendix B for HAC conditional logic

CC MCC +7th **S12.691** **Other nondisplaced fracture of seventh cervical vertebra**
   HAC 7th characters A & B see Appendix B for HAC conditional logic

X+7th **S12.8** **Fracture of other parts of neck**
MCC

The appropriate 7th character is to be added to code S12.8
A   initial encounter
D   subsequent encounter
S   sequela

Hyoid bone
Larynx
Thyroid cartilage
Trachea
HAC 7th character A see Appendix B for HAC conditional logic

CC X+7th **S12.9** **Fracture of neck, unspecified**

The appropriate 7th character is to be added to code S12.9
A   initial encounter
D   subsequent encounter
S   sequela

Fracture of neck NOS
Fracture of cervical spine NOS
Fracture of cervical vertebra NOS
HAC 7th character A see Appendix B for HAC conditional logic

S13 **Dislocation and sprain of joints and ligaments at neck level**
   Includes: avulsion of joint or ligament at neck level
      laceration of cartilage, joint or ligament at neck level
      sprain of cartilage, joint or ligament at neck level
      traumatic hemarthrosis of joint or ligament at neck level
      traumatic rupture of joint or ligament at neck level
      traumatic subluxation of joint or ligament at neck level
      traumatic tear of joint or ligament at neck level
   Code also any associated open wound
   Excludes2: *strain of muscle or tendon at neck level (S16.1)*

The appropriate 7th character is to be added to each code from category S13
A   initial encounter
D   subsequent encounter
S   sequela

CC X+7th **S13.0** **Traumatic rupture of cervical intervertebral disc**
   Excludes1: *rupture or displacement (nontraumatic) of cervical intervertebral disc NOS (M50.-)*
   HAC 7th character A see Appendix B for HAC conditional logic

+ **S13.1** **Subluxation and dislocation of cervical vertebrae**
   Code also any associated:
      open wound of neck (S11.-)
      spinal cord injury (S14.1-)
   Excludes2: *fracture of cervical vertebrae (S12.0-S12.3-)*

   + **S13.10** **Subluxation and dislocation of unspecified cervical vertebrae**
CC +7th **S13.100** **Subluxation of unspecified cervical vertebrae**
   HAC 7th character A see Appendix B for HAC conditional logic

CC +7th **S13.101** **Dislocation of unspecified cervical vertebrae**
   HAC 7th character A see Appendix B for HAC conditional logic

   + **S13.11** **Subluxation and dislocation of C0/C1 cervical vertebrae**
      Subluxation and dislocation of atlantooccipital joint
      Subluxation and dislocation of atloidooccipital joint
      Subluxation and dislocation of occipitoatloid joint
CC +7th **S13.110** **Subluxation of C0/C1 cervical vertebrae**
   HAC 7th character A see Appendix B for HAC conditional logic

CC +7th **S13.111** **Dislocation of C0/C1 cervical vertebrae**
   HAC 7th character A see Appendix B for HAC conditional logic

   + **S13.12** **Subluxation and dislocation of C1/C2 cervical vertebrae**
      Subluxation and dislocation of atlantoaxial joint
CC +7th **S13.120** **Subluxation of C1/C2 cervical vertebrae**
   HAC 7th character A see Appendix B for HAC conditional logic

CC +7th **S13.121** **Dislocation of C1/C2 cervical vertebrae**
   HAC 7th character A see Appendix B for HAC conditional logic

   + **S13.13** **Subluxation and dislocation of C2/C3 cervical vertebrae**
CC +7th **S13.130** **Subluxation of C2/C3 cervical vertebrae**
   HAC 7th character A see Appendix B for HAC conditional logic

CC +7th **S13.131** **Dislocation of C2/C3 cervical vertebrae**
   HAC 7th character A see Appendix B for HAC conditional logic

   + **S13.14** **Subluxation and dislocation of C3/C4 cervical vertebrae**
CC +7th **S13.140** **Subluxation of C3/C4 cervical vertebrae**
   HAC 7th character A see Appendix B for HAC conditional logic

CC +7th **S13.141** **Dislocation of C3/C4 cervical vertebrae**
   HAC 7th character A see Appendix B for HAC conditional logic

   + **S13.15** **Subluxation and dislocation of C4/C5 cervical vertebrae**
CC +7th **S13.150** **Subluxation of C4/C5 cervical vertebrae**
   HAC 7th character A see Appendix B for HAC conditional logic

CC +7th **S13.151** **Dislocation of C4/C5 cervical vertebrae**
   HAC 7th character A see Appendix B for HAC conditional logic

+, +7th, X + 7th   ● Newborn   ● Pediatric   ● Maternity   ● Adult   ♀ Female   ♂ Male   Manifestation   Unacceptable PDX   HCC   CC   MCC   HAC

+ S13.16 **Subluxation and dislocation of C5/C6 cervical vertebrae**

CC +7th **S13.160** **Subluxation of C5/C6 cervical vertebrae**
HAC 7th character A see Appendix B for HAC conditional logic

CC +7th **S13.161** **Dislocation of C5/C6 cervical vertebrae**
HAC 7th character A see Appendix B for HAC conditional logic

+ S13.17 **Subluxation and dislocation of C6/C7 cervical vertebrae**

CC +7th **S13.170** **Subluxation of C6/C7 cervical vertebrae**
HAC 7th character A see Appendix B for HAC conditional logic

CC +7th **S13.171** **Dislocation of C6/C7 cervical vertebrae**
HAC 7th character A see Appendix B for HAC conditional logic

+ S13.18 **Subluxation and dislocation of C7/T1 cervical vertebrae**

CC +7th **S13.180** **Subluxation of C7/T1 cervical vertebrae**
HAC 7th character A see Appendix B for HAC conditional logic

CC +7th **S13.181** **Dislocation of C7/T1 cervical vertebrae**
HAC 7th character A see Appendix B for HAC conditional logic

+ S13.2 **Dislocation of other and unspecified parts of neck**

CC X+7th **S13.20** **Dislocation of unspecified parts of neck**
HAC 7th character A see Appendix B for HAC conditional logic

CC X+7th **S13.29** **Dislocation of other parts of neck**
HAC 7th character A see Appendix B for HAC conditional logic

X+7th **S13.4** **Sprain of ligaments of cervical spine**
Sprain of anterior longitudinal (ligament), cervical
Sprain of atlanto-axial (joints)
Sprain of atlanto-occipital (joints)
Whiplash injury of cervical spine

X+7th **S13.5** **Sprain of thyroid region**
Sprain of cricoarytenoid (joint) (ligament)
Sprain of cricothyroid (joint) (ligament)
Sprain of thyroid cartilage

X+7th **S13.8** **Sprain of joints and ligaments of other parts of neck**

X+7th **S13.9** **Sprain of joints and ligaments of unspecified parts of neck**

S14 **Injury of nerves and spinal cord at neck level**

NOTE Code to highest level of cervical cord injury
Code also any associated:
fracture of cervical vertebra (S12.0--S12.6.-)
open wound of neck (S11.)
transient paralysis (R29.5)

The appropriate 7th character is to be added to each code from category S14
A initial encounter
D subsequent encounter
S sequela

MCC X+7th **S14.0** **Concussion and edema of cervical spinal cord**

+ S14.1 **Other and unspecified injuries of cervical spinal cord**

+ S14.10 **Unspecified injury of cervical spinal cord**

MCC +7th **S14.101** **Unspecified injury at C1 level of cervical spinal cord**
HAC 7th character A see Appendix B for HAC conditional logic

MCC +7th **S14.102** **Unspecified injury at C2 level of cervical spinal cord**
HAC 7th character A see Appendix B for HAC conditional logic

MCC +7th **S14.103** **Unspecified injury at C3 level of cervical spinal cord**
HAC 7th character A see Appendix B for HAC conditional logic

MCC +7th **S14.104** **Unspecified injury at C4 level of cervical spinal cord**
HAC 7th character A see Appendix B for HAC conditional logic

MCC +7th **S14.105** **Unspecified injury at C5 level of cervical spinal cord**
HAC 7th character A see Appendix B for HAC conditional logic

MCC +7th **S14.106** **Unspecified injury at C6 level of cervical spinal cord**
HAC 7th character A see Appendix B for HAC conditional logic

MCC +7th **S14.107** **Unspecified injury at C7 level of cervical spinal cord**
HAC 7th character A see Appendix B for HAC conditional logic

MCC +7th **S14.108** **Unspecified injury at C8 level of cervical spinal cord**

+7th **S14.109** **Unspecified injury at unspecified level of cervical spinal cord**
Injury of cervical spinal cord NOS
HAC 7th character A see Appendix B for HAC conditional logic

+ S14.11 **Complete lesion of cervical spinal cord**

MCC +7th **S14.111** **Complete lesion at C1 level of cervical spinal cord**
HAC 7th character A see Appendix B for HAC conditional logic

MCC +7th **S14.112** **Complete lesion at C2 level of cervical spinal cord**
HAC 7th character A see Appendix B for HAC conditional logic

MCC +7th **S14.113** **Complete lesion at C3 level of cervical spinal cord**
HAC 7th character A see Appendix B for HAC conditional logic

MCC +7th **S14.114** **Complete lesion at C4 level of cervical spinal cord**
HAC 7th character A see Appendix B for HAC conditional logic

MCC +7th **S14.115** **Complete lesion at C5 level of cervical spinal cord**
HAC 7th character A see Appendix B for HAC conditional logic

MCC +7th **S14.116** **Complete lesion at C6 level of cervical spinal cord**
HAC 7th character A see Appendix B for HAC conditional logic

MCC +7th **S14.117** **Complete lesion at C7 level of cervical spinal cord**
HAC 7th character A see Appendix B for HAC conditional logic

MCC +7th **S14.118** **Complete lesion at C8 level of cervical spinal cord**

+7th **S14.119** **Complete lesion at unspecified level of cervical spinal cord**

+ S14.12 **Central cord syndrome of cervical spinal cord**

MCC +7th **S14.121** **Central cord syndrome at C1 level of cervical spinal cord**
HAC 7th character A see Appendix B for HAC conditional logic

MCC +7th **S14.122** **Central cord syndrome at C2 level of cervical spinal cord**
HAC 7th character A see Appendix B for HAC conditional logic

MCC +7th **S14.123** **Central cord syndrome at C3 level of cervical spinal cord**
HAC 7th character A see Appendix B for HAC conditional logic

MCC +7th **S14.124** **Central cord syndrome at C4 level of cervical spinal cord**
HAC 7th character A see Appendix B for HAC conditional logic

MCC +7th **S14.125** **Central cord syndrome at C5 level of cervical spinal cord**
HAC 7th character A see Appendix B for HAC conditional logic

MCC +7th **S14.126** **Central cord syndrome at C6 level of cervical spinal cord**
HAC 7th character A see Appendix B for HAC conditional logic

MCC +7th **S14.127** **Central cord syndrome at C7 level of cervical spinal cord**
HAC 7th character A see Appendix B for HAC conditional logic

MCC +7th **S14.128** **Central cord syndrome at C8 level of cervical spinal cord**

+7th **S14.129** **Central cord syndrome at unspecified level of cervical spinal cord**

+ S14.13 **Anterior cord syndrome of cervical spinal cord**

MCC +7th **S14.131** **Anterior cord syndrome at C1 level of cervical spinal cord**
HAC 7th character A see Appendix B for HAC conditional logic

MCC +7th **S14.132** **Anterior cord syndrome at C2 level of cervical spinal cord**
HAC 7th character A see Appendix B for HAC conditional logic

+, +7th, X + 7th ● Newborn ● Pediatric ● Maternity ● Adult ♀ Female ♂ Male Manifestation Unacceptable PDX HCC CC MCC HAC

MCC +7th **S14.133** **Anterior cord syndrome at C3 level of cervical spinal cord**
> HAC 7th character A see Appendix B for HAC conditional logic

MCC +7th **S14.134** **Anterior cord syndrome at C4 level of cervical spinal cord**
> HAC 7th character A see Appendix B for HAC conditional logic

MCC +7th **S14.135** **Anterior cord syndrome at C5 level of cervical spinal cord**
> HAC 7th character A see Appendix B for HAC conditional logic

MCC +7th **S14.136** **Anterior cord syndrome at C6 level of cervical spinal cord**
> HAC 7th character A see Appendix B for HAC conditional logic

MCC +7th **S14.137** **Anterior cord syndrome at C7 level of cervical spinal cord**
> HAC 7th character A see Appendix B for HAC conditional logic

MCC +7th **S14.138** **Anterior cord syndrome at C8 level of cervical spinal cord**

+7th **S14.139** **Anterior cord syndrome at unspecified level of cervical spinal cord**

+ **S14.14** **Brown-Séquard syndrome of cervical spinal cord**

MCC +7th **S14.141** **Brown-Séquard syndrome at C1 level of cervical spinal cord**

MCC +7th **S14.142** **Brown-Séquard syndrome at C2 level of cervical spinal cord**

MCC +7th **S14.143** **Brown-Séquard syndrome at C3 level of cervical spinal cord**

MCC +7th **S14.144** **Brown-Séquard syndrome at C4 level of cervical spinal cord**

MCC +7th **S14.145** **Brown-Séquard syndrome at C5 level of cervical spinal cord**

MCC +7th **S14.146** **Brown-Séquard syndrome at C6 level of cervical spinal cord**

MCC +7th **S14.147** **Brown-Séquard syndrome at C7 level of cervical spinal cord**

MCC +7th **S14.148** **Brown-Séquard syndrome at C8 level of cervical spinal cord**

+7th **S14.149** **Brown-Séquard syndrome at unspecified level of cervical spinal cord**

+ **S14.15** **Other incomplete lesions of cervical spinal cord**
> Incomplete lesion of cervical spinal cord NOS
> Posterior cord syndrome of cervical spinal cord

MCC +7th **S14.151** **Other incomplete lesion at C1 level of cervical spinal cord**
> HAC 7th character A see Appendix B for HAC conditional logic

MCC +7th **S14.152** **Other incomplete lesion at C2 level of cervical spinal cord**
> HAC 7th character A see Appendix B for HAC conditional logic

MCC +7th **S14.153** **Other incomplete lesion at C3 level of cervical spinal cord**
> HAC 7th character A see Appendix B for HAC conditional logic

MCC +7th **S14.154** **Other incomplete lesion at C4 level of cervical spinal cord**
> HAC 7th character A see Appendix B for HAC conditional logic

MCC +7th **S14.155** **Other incomplete lesion at C5 level of cervical spinal cord**
> HAC 7th character A see Appendix B for HAC conditional logic

MCC +7th **S14.156** **Other incomplete lesion at C6 level of cervical spinal cord**
> HAC 7th character A see Appendix B for HAC conditional logic

MCC +7th **S14.157** **Other incomplete lesion at C7 level of cervical spinal cord**
> HAC 7th character A see Appendix B for HAC conditional logic

MCC +7th **S14.158** **Other incomplete lesion at C8 level of cervical spinal cord**

+7th **S14.159** **Other incomplete lesion at unspecified level of cervical spinal cord**

X+7th **S14.2** **Injury of nerve root of cervical spine**
X+7th **S14.3** **Injury of brachial plexus**
X+7th **S14.4** **Injury of peripheral nerves of neck**
X+7th **S14.5** **Injury of cervical sympathetic nerves**
X+7th **S14.8** **Injury of other specified nerves of neck**

X+7th **S14.9** **Injury of unspecified nerves of neck**

S15 **Injury of blood vessels at neck level**

> Code also any associated open wound (S11.-)

> The appropriate 7th character is to be added to each code from category S15
> A   initial encounter
> D   subsequent encounter
> S   sequela

+ **S15.0** **Injury of carotid artery of neck**
> Injury of carotid artery (common) (external) (internal, extracranial portion)
> Injury of carotid artery NOS
> **Excludes1:** *injury of internal carotid artery, intracranial portion (S06.8)*

+ **S15.00** **Unspecified injury of carotid artery**

CC +7th **S15.001** **Unspecified injury of right carotid artery**

CC +7th **S15.002** **Unspecified injury of left carotid artery**

CC +7th **S15.009** **Unspecified injury of unspecified carotid artery**

+ **S15.01** **Minor laceration of carotid artery**
> Incomplete transection of carotid artery
> Laceration of carotid artery NOS
> Superficial laceration of carotid artery

CC +7th **S15.011** **Minor laceration of right carotid artery**
CC +7th **S15.012** **Minor laceration of left carotid artery**
CC +7th **S15.019** **Minor laceration of unspecified carotid artery**

+ **S15.02** **Major laceration of carotid artery**
> Complete transection of carotid artery
> Traumatic rupture of carotid artery

CC +7th **S15.021** **Major laceration of right carotid artery**
CC +7th **S15.022** **Major laceration of left carotid artery**
CC +7th **S15.029** **Major laceration of unspecified carotid artery**

+ **S15.09** **Other specified injury of carotid artery**

CC +7th **S15.091** **Other specified injury of right carotid artery**

CC +7th **S15.092** **Other specified injury of left carotid artery**

CC +7th **S15.099** **Other specified injury of unspecified carotid artery**

+ **S15.1** **Injury of vertebral artery**

+ **S15.10** **Unspecified injury of vertebral artery**

CC +7th **S15.101** **Unspecified injury of right vertebral artery**

CC +7th **S15.102** **Unspecified injury of left vertebral artery**

CC +7th **S15.109** **Unspecified injury of unspecified vertebral artery**

+ **S15.11** **Minor laceration of vertebral artery**
> Incomplete transection of vertebral artery
> Laceration of vertebral artery NOS
> Superficial laceration of vertebral artery

CC +7th **S15.111** **Minor laceration of right vertebral artery**

CC +7th **S15.112** **Minor laceration of left vertebral artery**

CC +7th **S15.119** **Minor laceration of unspecified vertebral artery**

+ **S15.12** **Major laceration of vertebral artery**
> Complete transection of vertebral artery
> Traumatic rupture of vertebral artery

CC +7th **S15.121** **Major laceration of right vertebral artery**

CC +7th **S15.122** **Major laceration of left vertebral artery**

CC +7th **S15.129** **Major laceration of unspecified vertebral artery**

+ **S15.19** **Other specified injury of vertebral artery**

CC +7th **S15.191** **Other specified injury of right vertebral artery**

CC +7th **S15.192** **Other specified injury of left vertebral artery**

CC +7th **S15.199** **Other specified injury of unspecified vertebral artery**

+ **S15.2** **Injury of external jugular vein**

+ **S15.20** **Unspecified injury of external jugular vein**

CC +7th **S15.201** **Unspecified injury of right external jugular vein**

CC +7th **S15.202** **Unspecified injury of left external jugular vein**

CC +7th **S15.209** **Unspecified injury of unspecified external jugular vein**

+ **S15.21** **Minor laceration of external jugular vein**
Incomplete transection of external jugular vein
Laceration of external jugular vein NOS
Superficial laceration of external jugular vein

CC +7th **S15.211** **Minor laceration of right external jugular vein**

CC +7th **S15.212** **Minor laceration of left external jugular vein**

CC +7th **S15.219** **Minor laceration of unspecified external jugular vein**

+ **S15.22** **Major laceration of external jugular vein**
Complete transection of external jugular vein
Traumatic rupture of external jugular vein

CC +7th **S15.221** **Major laceration of right external jugular vein**

CC +7th **S15.222** **Major laceration of left external jugular vein**

CC +7th **S15.229** **Major laceration of unspecified external jugular vein**

+ **S15.29** **Other specified injury of external jugular vein**

CC +7th **S15.291** **Other specified injury of right external jugular vein**

CC +7th **S15.292** **Other specified injury of left external jugular vein**

CC +7th **S15.299** **Other specified injury of unspecified external jugular vein**

+ **S15.3** **Injury of internal jugular vein**

+ **S15.30** **Unspecified injury of internal jugular vein**

CC +7th **S15.301** **Unspecified injury of right internal jugular vein**

CC +7th **S15.302** **Unspecified injury of left internal jugular vein**

CC +7th **S15.309** **Unspecified injury of unspecified internal jugular vein**

+ **S15.31** **Minor laceration of internal jugular vein**
Incomplete transection of internal jugular vein
Laceration of internal jugular vein NOS
Superficial laceration of internal jugular vein

CC +7th **S15.311** **Minor laceration of right internal jugular vein**

CC +7th **S15.312** **Minor laceration of left internal jugular vein**

CC +7th **S15.319** **Minor laceration of unspecified internal jugular vein**

+ **S15.32** **Major laceration of internal jugular vein**
Complete transection of internal jugular vein
Traumatic rupture of internal jugular vein

CC +7th **S15.321** **Major laceration of right internal jugular vein**

CC +7th **S15.322** **Major laceration of left internal jugular vein**

CC +7th **S15.329** **Major laceration of unspecified internal jugular vein**

+ **S15.39** **Other specified injury of internal jugular vein**

CC +7th **S15.391** **Other specified injury of right internal jugular vein**

CC +7th **S15.392** **Other specified injury of left internal jugular vein**

CC +7th **S15.399** **Other specified injury of unspecified internal jugular vein**

CC **S15.8** **Injury of other specified blood vessels at neck level**

CC **S15.9** **Injury of unspecified blood vessel at neck level**

S16 **Injury of muscle, fascia and tendon at neck level**

Code also any associated open wound (S11.-)

Excludes2: *sprain of joint or ligament at neck level (S13.9)*

The appropriate 7th character is to be added to each code from category S16
A   initial encounter
D   subsequent encounter
S   sequela

X+7th **S16.1** **Strain of muscle, fascia and tendon at neck level**

X+7th **S16.2** **Laceration of muscle, fascia and tendon at neck level**

X+7th **S16.8** **Other specified injury of muscle, fascia and tendon at neck level**

X+7th **S16.9** **Unspecified injury of muscle, fascia and tendon at neck level**

S17 **Crushing injury of neck**

Use additional code for all associated injuries, such as:
injury of blood vessels (S15.-)
open wound of neck (S11.-)
spinal cord injury (S14.0, S14.1-)
vertebral fracture (S12.0--S12.3-)

The appropriate 7th character is to be added to each code from category S17
A   initial encounter
D   subsequent encounter
S   sequela

CC **S17.0** **Crushing injury of larynx and trachea**
X+7th   HAC 7th character A see Appendix B for HAC conditional logic

CC **S17.8** **Crushing injury of other specified parts of neck**
X+7th   HAC 7th character A see Appendix B for HAC conditional logic

CC **S17.9** **Crushing injury of neck, part unspecified**
X+7th   HAC 7th character A see Appendix B for HAC conditional logic

S19 **Other specified and unspecified injuries of neck**

The appropriate 7th character is to be added to each code from category S19
A   initial encounter
D   subsequent encounter
S   sequela

+ **S19.8** **Other specified injuries of neck**

X+7th **S19.80** **Other specified injuries of unspecified part of neck**

X+7th **S19.81** **Other specified injuries of larynx**

X+7th **S19.82** **Other specified injuries of cervical trachea**
Excludes2: *other specified injury of thoracic trachea (S27.5-)*

X+7th **S19.83** **Other specified injuries of vocal cord**

X+7th **S19.84** **Other specified injuries of thyroid gland**

X+7th **S19.85** **Other specified injuries of pharynx and cervical esophagus**

X+7th **S19.89** **Other specified injuries of other specified part of neck**

X+7th **S19.9** **Unspecified injury of neck**

Injuries to the thorax (S20-S29)

Includes: injuries of breast
injuries of chest (wall)
injuries of interscapular area

Excludes2: *burns and corrosions (T20-T32)*
effects of foreign body in bronchus (T17.5)
effects of foreign body in esophagus (T18.1)
effects of foreign body in lung (T17.8)
effects of foreign body in trachea (T17.4)
frostbite (T33-T34)
injuries of axilla
injuries of clavicle
injuries of scapular region
injuries of shoulder
insect bite or sting, venomous (T63.4)

S20 **Superficial injury of thorax**

The appropriate 7th character is to be added to each code from category S20
A   initial encounter
D   subsequent encounter
S   sequela

+ **S20.0** **Contusion of breast**

X+7th **S20.00** **Contusion of breast, unspecified breast**

X+7th **S20.01** **Contusion of right breast**

X+7th **S20.02** **Contusion of left breast**

+ **S20.1** **Other and unspecified superficial injuries of breast**

+ **S20.10** **Unspecified superficial injuries of breast**

+7th **S20.101** **Unspecified superficial injuries of breast, right breast**

+7th **S20.102** **Unspecified superficial injuries of breast, left breast**

+7th **S20.109** **Unspecified superficial injuries of breast, unspecified breast**

+ **S20.11** **Abrasion of breast**

+7th **S20.111** **Abrasion of breast, right breast**

+7th **S20.112** **Abrasion of breast, left breast**

+7th **S20.119** **Abrasion of breast, unspecified breast**

+ **S20.12** **Blister (nonthermal) of breast**

+7th **S20.121** **Blister (nonthermal) of breast, right breast**

+7th **S20.122** **Blister (nonthermal) of breast, left breast**

+7th **S20.129** **Blister (nonthermal) of breast, unspecified breast**

+, +7th, X + 7th   ● Newborn   ● Pediatric   ● Maternity   ● Adult   ♀ Female   ♂ Male   Manifestation   Unacceptable PDX   HCC   CC   MCC   HAC

+ **S20.14   External constriction of part of breast**
  +7th **S20.141   External constriction of part of breast, right breast**
  +7th **S20.142   External constriction of part of breast, left breast**
  +7th **S20.149   External constriction of part of breast, unspecified breast**
+ **S20.15   Superficial foreign body of breast**
  Splinter in the breast
  +7th **S20.151   Superficial foreign body of breast, right breast**
  +7th **S20.152   Superficial foreign body of breast, left breast**
  +7th **S20.159   Superficial foreign body of breast, unspecified breast**
+ **S20.16   Insect bite (nonvenomous) of breast**
  +7th **S20.161   Insect bite (nonvenomous) of breast, right breast**
  +7th **S20.162   Insect bite (nonvenomous) of breast, left breast**
  +7th **S20.169   Insect bite (nonvenomous) of breast, unspecified breast**
+ **S20.17   Other superficial bite of breast**
  Excludes1: open bite of breast (S21.05-)
  +7th **S20.171   Other superficial bite of breast, right breast**
  +7th **S20.172   Other superficial bite of breast, left breast**
  +7th **S20.179   Other superficial bite of breast, unspecified breast**

+ **S20.2   Contusion of thorax**
  X+7th **S20.20   Contusion of thorax, unspecified**
  + **S20.21   Contusion of front wall of thorax**
    +7th **S20.211   Contusion of right front wall of thorax**
    +7th **S20.212   Contusion of left front wall of thorax**
    +7th **S20.213   Contusion of bilateral front wall of thorax**
    +7th **S20.214   Contusion of middle front wall of thorax**
    +7th **S20.219   Contusion of unspecified front wall of thorax**
  + **S20.22   Contusion of back wall of thorax**
    +7th **S20.221   Contusion of right back wall of thorax**
    +7th **S20.222   Contusion of left back wall of thorax**
    +7th **S20.223   Contusion of bilateral back wall of thorax**
    +7th **S20.224   Contusion of middle back wall of thorax**
    +7th **S20.229   Contusion of unspecified back wall of thorax**

+ **S20.3   Other and unspecified superficial injuries of front wall of thorax**
  + **S20.30   Unspecified superficial injuries of front wall of thorax**
    +7th **S20.301   Unspecified superficial injuries of right front wall of thorax**
    +7th **S20.302   Unspecified superficial injuries of left front wall of thorax**
    +7th **S20.303   Unspecified superficial injuries of bilateral front wall of thorax**
    +7th **S20.304   Unspecified superficial injuries of middle front wall of thorax**
    +7th **S20.309   Unspecified superficial injuries of unspecified front wall of thorax**
  + **S20.31   Abrasion of front wall of thorax**
    +7th **S20.311   Abrasion of right front wall of thorax**
    +7th **S20.312   Abrasion of left front wall of thorax**
    +7th **S20.313   Abrasion of bilateral front wall of thorax**
    +7th **S20.314   Abrasion of middle front wall of thorax**
    +7th **S20.319   Abrasion of unspecified front wall of thorax**
  + **S20.32   Blister (nonthermal) of front wall of thorax**
    +7th **S20.321   Blister (nonthermal) of right front wall of thorax**
    +7th **S20.322   Blister (nonthermal) of left front wall of thorax**
    +7th **S20.323   Blister (nonthermal) of bilateral front wall of thorax**
    +7th **S20.324   Blister (nonthermal) of middle front wall of thorax**
    +7th **S20.329   Blister (nonthermal) of unspecified front wall of thorax**
  + **S20.34   External constriction of front wall of thorax**
    +7th **S20.341   External constriction of right front wall of thorax**
    +7th **S20.342   External constriction of left front wall of thorax**
    +7th **S20.343   External constriction of bilateral front wall of thorax**
    +7th **S20.344   External constriction of middle front wall of thorax**
    +7th **S20.349   External constriction of unspecified front wall of thorax**
  + **S20.35   Superficial foreign body of front wall of thorax**
    Splinter in front wall of thorax
    +7th **S20.351   Superficial foreign body of right front wall of thorax**
    +7th **S20.352   Superficial foreign body of left front wall of thorax**
    +7th **S20.353   Superficial foreign body of bilateral front wall of thorax**
    +7th **S20.354   Superficial foreign body of middle front wall of thorax**
    +7th **S20.359   Superficial foreign body of unspecified front wall of thorax**
  + **S20.36   Insect bite (nonvenomous) of front wall of thorax**
    +7th **S20.361   Insect bite (nonvenomous) of right front wall of thorax**
    +7th **S20.362   Insect bite (nonvenomous) of left front wall of thorax**
    +7th **S20.363   Insect bite (nonvenomous) of bilateral front wall of thorax**
    +7th **S20.364   Insect bite (nonvenomous) of middle front wall of thorax**
    +7th **S20.369   Insect bite (nonvenomous) of unspecified front wall of thorax**
  + **S20.37   Other superficial bite of front wall of thorax**
    Excludes1: open bite of front wall of thorax (S21.14)
    +7th **S20.371   Other superficial bite of right front wall of thorax**
    +7th **S20.372   Other superficial bite of left front wall of thorax**
    +7th **S20.373   Other superficial bite of bilateral front wall of thorax**
    +7th **S20.374   Other superficial bite of middle front wall of thorax**
    +7th **S20.379   Other superficial bite of unspecified front wall of thorax**

+ **S20.4   Other and unspecified superficial injuries of back wall of thorax**
  + **S20.40   Unspecified superficial injuries of back wall of thorax**
    +7th **S20.401   Unspecified superficial injuries of right back wall of thorax**
    +7th **S20.402   Unspecified superficial injuries of left back wall of thorax**
    +7th **S20.409   Unspecified superficial injuries of unspecified back wall of thorax**
  + **S20.41   Abrasion of back wall of thorax**
    +7th **S20.411   Abrasion of right back wall of thorax**
    +7th **S20.412   Abrasion of left back wall of thorax**
    +7th **S20.419   Abrasion of unspecified back wall of thorax**
  + **S20.42   Blister (nonthermal) of back wall of thorax**
    +7th **S20.421   Blister (nonthermal) of right back wall of thorax**
    +7th **S20.422   Blister (nonthermal) of left back wall of thorax**
    +7th **S20.429   Blister (nonthermal) of unspecified back wall of thorax**
  + **S20.44   External constriction of back wall of thorax**
    +7th **S20.441   External constriction of right back wall of thorax**
    +7th **S20.442   External constriction of left back wall of thorax**
    +7th **S20.449   External constriction of unspecified back wall of thorax**
  + **S20.45   Superficial foreign body of back wall of thorax**
    Splinter of back wall of thorax
    +7th **S20.451   Superficial foreign body of right back wall of thorax**
    +7th **S20.452   Superficial foreign body of left back wall of thorax**
    +7th **S20.459   Superficial foreign body of unspecified back wall of thorax**

+ **S20.46** Insect bite (nonvenomous) of back wall of thorax
+7th **S20.461** Insect bite (nonvenomous) of right back wall of thorax
+7th **S20.462** Insect bite (nonvenomous) of left back wall of thorax
+7th **S20.469** Insect bite (nonvenomous) of unspecified back wall of thorax
+ **S20.47** Other superficial bite of back wall of thorax
Excludes1: *open bite of back wall of thorax (S21.24)*
+7th **S20.471** Other superficial bite of right back wall of thorax
+7th **S20.472** Other superficial bite of left back wall of thorax
+7th **S20.479** Other superficial bite of unspecified back wall of thorax
+ **S20.9** Superficial injury of unspecified parts of thorax
Excludes1: *contusion of thorax NOS (S20.20)*
X+7th **S20.90** Unspecified superficial injury of unspecified parts of thorax
Superficial injury of thoracic wall NOS
X+7th **S20.91** Abrasion of unspecified parts of thorax
X+7th **S20.92** Blister (nonthermal) of unspecified parts of thorax
X+7th **S20.94** External constriction of unspecified parts of thorax
X+7th **S20.95** Superficial foreign body of unspecified parts of thorax
Splinter in thorax NOS
X+7th **S20.96** Insect bite (nonvenomous) of unspecified parts of thorax
X+7th **S20.97** Other superficial bite of unspecified parts of thorax
Excludes1: *open bite of thorax NOS (S21.95)*

S21 **Open wound of thorax**
Code also any associated injury, such as:
injury of heart (S26.-)
injury of intrathoracic organs (S27.-)
rib fracture (S22.3-, S22.4-)
spinal cord injury (S24.0-, S24.1-)
traumatic hemothorax (S27.1)
traumatic hemopneumothorax (S27.3)
traumatic pneumothorax (S27.0)
wound infection
Excludes1: *traumatic amputation (partial) of thorax (S28.1)*

The appropriate 7th character is to be added to each code from category S21
A initial encounter
D subsequent encounter
S sequela

+ **S21.0** Open wound of breast
+ **S21.00** Unspecified open wound of breast
+7th **S21.001** Unspecified open wound of right breast
+7th **S21.002** Unspecified open wound of left breast
+7th **S21.009** Unspecified open wound of unspecified breast
+ **S21.01** Laceration without foreign body of breast
+7th **S21.011** Laceration without foreign body of right breast
+7th **S21.012** Laceration without foreign body of left breast
+7th **S21.019** Laceration without foreign body of unspecified breast
+ **S21.02** Laceration with foreign body of breast
+7th **S21.021** Laceration with foreign body of right breast
+7th **S21.022** Laceration with foreign body of left breast
+7th **S21.029** Laceration with foreign body of unspecified breast
+ **S21.03** Puncture wound without foreign body of breast
+7th **S21.031** Puncture wound without foreign body of right breast
+7th **S21.032** Puncture wound without foreign body of left breast
+7th **S21.039** Puncture wound without foreign body of unspecified breast

+ **S21.04** Puncture wound with foreign body of breast
+7th **S21.041** Puncture wound with foreign body of right breast
+7th **S21.042** Puncture wound with foreign body of left breast
+7th **S21.049** Puncture wound with foreign body of unspecified breast
+ **S21.05** Open bite of breast
Bite of breast NOS
Excludes1: *superficial bite of breast (S20.17)*
S21.051 Open bite of right breast
S21.052 Open bite of left breast
S21.059 Open bite of unspecified breast
+ **S21.1** Open wound of front wall of thorax without penetration into thoracic cavity
Open wound of chest without penetration into thoracic cavity
+ **S21.10** Unspecified open wound of front wall of thorax without penetration into thoracic cavity
CC +7th **S21.101** Unspecified open wound of right front wall of thorax without penetration into thoracic cavity
CC +7th **S21.102** Unspecified open wound of left front wall of thorax without penetration into thoracic cavity
CC +7th **S21.109** Unspecified open wound of unspecified front wall of thorax without penetration into thoracic cavity
+ **S21.11** Laceration without foreign body of front wall of thorax without penetration into thoracic cavity
CC +7th **S21.111** Laceration without foreign body of right front wall of thorax without penetration into thoracic cavity
CC +7th **S21.112** Laceration without foreign body of left front wall of thorax without penetration into thoracic cavity
CC +7th **S21.119** Laceration without foreign body of unspecified front wall of thorax without penetration into thoracic cavity
+ **S21.12** Laceration with foreign body of front wall of thorax without penetration into thoracic cavity
CC +7th **S21.121** Laceration with foreign body of right front wall of thorax without penetration into thoracic cavity
CC +7th **S21.122** Laceration with foreign body of left front wall of thorax without penetration into thoracic cavity
CC +7th **S21.129** Laceration with foreign body of unspecified front wall of thorax without penetration into thoracic cavity
+ **S21.13** Puncture wound without foreign body of front wall of thorax without penetration into thoracic cavity
CC +7th **S21.131** Puncture wound without foreign body of right front wall of thorax without penetration into thoracic cavity
CC +7th **S21.132** Puncture wound without foreign body of left front wall of thorax without penetration into thoracic cavity
CC +7th **S21.139** Puncture wound without foreign body of unspecified front wall of thorax without penetration into thoracic cavity
+ **S21.14** Puncture wound with foreign body of front wall of thorax without penetration into thoracic cavity
CC +7th **S21.141** Puncture wound with foreign body of right front wall of thorax without penetration into thoracic cavity
CC +7th **S21.142** Puncture wound with foreign body of left front wall of thorax without penetration into thoracic cavity
CC +7th **S21.149** Puncture wound with foreign body of unspecified front wall of thorax without penetration into thoracic cavity
+ **S21.15** Open bite of front wall of thorax without penetration into thoracic cavity
Bite of front wall of thorax NOS
Excludes1: *superficial bite of front wall of thorax (S20.37)*
CC +7th **S21.151** Open bite of right front wall of thorax without penetration into thoracic cavity

CC +7th **S21.152** **Open bite of left front wall of thorax without penetration into thoracic cavity**

CC +7th **S21.159** **Open bite of unspecified front wall of thorax without penetration into thoracic cavity**

+ **S21.2** **Open wound of back wall of thorax without penetration into thoracic cavity**

　+ **S21.20** **Unspecified open wound of back wall of thorax without penetration into thoracic cavity**

　　+7th **S21.201** **Unspecified open wound of right back wall of thorax without penetration into thoracic cavity**

　　+7th **S21.202** **Unspecified open wound of left back wall of thorax without penetration into thoracic cavity**

　　+7th **S21.209** **Unspecified open wound of unspecified back wall of thorax without penetration into thoracic cavity**

　+ **S21.21** **Laceration without foreign body of back wall of thorax without penetration into thoracic cavity**

　　+7th **S21.211** **Laceration without foreign body of right back wall of thorax without penetration into thoracic cavity**

　　+7th **S21.212** **Laceration without foreign body of left back wall of thorax without penetration into thoracic cavity**

　　+7th **S21.219** **Laceration without foreign body of unspecified back wall of thorax without penetration into thoracic cavity**

　+ **S21.22** **Laceration with foreign body of back wall of thorax without penetration into thoracic cavity**

　　+7th **S21.221** **Laceration with foreign body of right back wall of thorax without penetration into thoracic cavity**

　　+7th **S21.222** **Laceration with foreign body of left back wall of thorax without penetration into thoracic cavity**

　　+7th **S21.229** **Laceration with foreign body of unspecified back wall of thorax without penetration into thoracic cavity**

　+ **S21.23** **Puncture wound without foreign body of back wall of thorax without penetration into thoracic cavity**

　　+7th **S21.231** **Puncture wound without foreign body of right back wall of thorax without penetration into thoracic cavity**

　　+7th **S21.232** **Puncture wound without foreign body of left back wall of thorax without penetration into thoracic cavity**

　　+7th **S21.239** **Puncture wound without foreign body of unspecified back wall of thorax without penetration into thoracic cavity**

　+ **S21.24** **Puncture wound with foreign body of back wall of thorax without penetration into thoracic cavity**

　　+7th **S21.241** **Puncture wound with foreign body of right back wall of thorax without penetration into thoracic cavity**

　　+7th **S21.242** **Puncture wound with foreign body of left back wall of thorax without penetration into thoracic cavity**

　　+7th **S21.249** **Puncture wound with foreign body of unspecified back wall of thorax without penetration into thoracic cavity**

　+ **S21.25** **Open bite of back wall of thorax without penetration into thoracic cavity**

　　Bite of back wall of thorax NOS

　　Excludes1: *superficial bite of back wall of thorax (S20.47)*

　　+7th **S21.251** **Open bite of right back wall of thorax without penetration into thoracic cavity**

　　+7th **S21.252** **Open bite of left back wall of thorax without penetration into thoracic cavity**

　　+7th **S21.259** **Open bite of unspecified back wall of thorax without penetration into thoracic cavity**

+ **S21.3** **Open wound of front wall of thorax with penetration into thoracic cavity**

　Open wound of chest with penetration into thoracic cavity

　+ **S21.30** **Unspecified open wound of front wall of thorax with penetration into thoracic cavity**

MCC +7th **S21.301** **Unspecified open wound of right front wall of thorax with penetration into thoracic cavity**

MCC +7th **S21.302** **Unspecified open wound of left front wall of thorax with penetration into thoracic cavity**

MCC +7th **S21.309** **Unspecified open wound of unspecified front wall of thorax with penetration into thoracic cavity**

　+ **S21.31** **Laceration without foreign body of front wall of thorax with penetration into thoracic cavity**

MCC +7th **S21.311** **Laceration without foreign body of right front wall of thorax with penetration into thoracic cavity**

MCC +7th **S21.312** **Laceration without foreign body of left front wall of thorax with penetration into thoracic cavity**

MCC +7th **S21.319** **Laceration without foreign body of unspecified front wall of thorax with penetration into thoracic cavity**

　+ **S21.32** **Laceration with foreign body of front wall of thorax with penetration into thoracic cavity**

MCC +7th **S21.321** **Laceration with foreign body of right front wall of thorax with penetration into thoracic cavity**

MCC +7th **S21.322** **Laceration with foreign body of left front wall of thorax with penetration into thoracic cavity**

MCC +7th **S21.329** **Laceration with foreign body of unspecified front wall of thorax with penetration into thoracic cavity**

　+ **S21.33** **Puncture wound without foreign body of front wall of thorax with penetration into thoracic cavity**

MCC +7th **S21.331** **Puncture wound without foreign body of right front wall of thorax with penetration into thoracic cavity**

MCC +7th **S21.332** **Puncture wound without foreign body of left front wall of thorax with penetration into thoracic cavity**

MCC +7th **S21.339** **Puncture wound without foreign body of unspecified front wall of thorax with penetration into thoracic cavity**

　+ **S21.34** **Puncture wound with foreign body of front wall of thorax with penetration into thoracic cavity**

MCC +7th **S21.341** **Puncture wound with foreign body of right front wall of thorax with penetration into thoracic cavity**

MCC +7th **S21.342** **Puncture wound with foreign body of left front wall of thorax with penetration into thoracic cavity**

MCC +7th **S21.349** **Puncture wound with foreign body of unspecified front wall of thorax with penetration into thoracic cavity**

　+ **S21.35** **Open bite of front wall of thorax with penetration into thoracic cavity**

　　Excludes1: *superficial bite of front wall of thorax (S20.37)*

MCC +7th **S21.351** **Open bite of right front wall of thorax with penetration into thoracic cavity**

MCC +7th **S21.352** **Open bite of left front wall of thorax with penetration into thoracic cavity**

MCC +7th **S21.359** **Open bite of unspecified front wall of thorax with penetration into thoracic cavity**

+ **S21.4** **Open wound of back wall of thorax with penetration into thoracic cavity**

　+ **S21.40** **Unspecified open wound of back wall of thorax with penetration into thoracic cavity**

MCC +7th **S21.401** **Unspecified open wound of right back wall of thorax with penetration into thoracic cavity**

MCC +7th **S21.402** **Unspecified open wound of left back wall of thorax with penetration into thoracic cavity**

MCC +7th **S21.409** **Unspecified open wound of unspecified back wall of thorax with penetration into thoracic cavity**

+ S21.41 **Laceration without foreign body of back wall of thorax with penetration into thoracic cavity**

MCC +7th **S21.411** **Laceration without foreign body of right back wall of thorax with penetration into thoracic cavity**

MCC +7th **S21.412** **Laceration without foreign body of left back wall of thorax with penetration into thoracic cavity**

MCC +7th **S21.419** **Laceration without foreign body of unspecified back wall of thorax with penetration into thoracic cavity**

+ S21.42 **Laceration with foreign body of back wall of thorax with penetration into thoracic cavity**

MCC +7th **S21.421** **Laceration with foreign body of right back wall of thorax with penetration into thoracic cavity**

MCC +7th **S21.422** **Laceration with foreign body of left back wall of thorax with penetration into thoracic cavity**

MCC +7th **S21.429** **Laceration with foreign body of unspecified back wall of thorax with penetration into thoracic cavity**

+ S21.43 **Puncture wound without foreign body of back wall of thorax with penetration into thoracic cavity**

MCC +7th **S21.431** **Puncture wound without foreign body of right back wall of thorax with penetration into thoracic cavity**

MCC +7th **S21.432** **Puncture wound without foreign body of left back wall of thorax with penetration into thoracic cavity**

MCC +7th **S21.439** **Puncture wound without foreign body of unspecified back wall of thorax with penetration into thoracic cavity**

+ S21.44 **Puncture wound with foreign body of back wall of thorax with penetration into thoracic cavity**

MCC +7th **S21.441** **Puncture wound with foreign body of right back wall of thorax with penetration into thoracic cavity**

MCC +7th **S21.442** **Puncture wound with foreign body of left back wall of thorax with penetration into thoracic cavity**

MCC +7th **S21.449** **Puncture wound with foreign body of unspecified back wall of thorax with penetration into thoracic cavity**

+ S21.45 **Open bite of back wall of thorax with penetration into thoracic cavity**

Bite of back wall of thorax NOS

Excludes1: *superficial bite of back wall of thorax (S20.47)*

MCC +7th **S21.451** **Open bite of right back wall of thorax with penetration into thoracic cavity**

MCC +7th **S21.452** **Open bite of left back wall of thorax with penetration into thoracic cavity**

MCC +7th **S21.459** **Open bite of unspecified back wall of thorax with penetration into thoracic cavity**

+ S21.9 **Open wound of unspecified part of thorax**

Open wound of thoracic wall NOS

CC X+7th **S21.90** **Unspecified open wound of unspecified part of thorax**

CC X+7th **S21.91** **Laceration without foreign body of unspecified part of thorax**

CC X+7th **S21.92** **Laceration with foreign body of unspecified part of thorax**

CC X+7th **S21.93** **Puncture wound without foreign body of unspecified part of thorax**

CC X+7th **S21.94** **Puncture wound with foreign body of unspecified part of thorax**

CC X+7th **S21.95** **Open bite of unspecified part of thorax**

Excludes1: *superficial bite of thorax (S20.97)*

See page 980 for Vertebrae Illustration.

S22 **Fracture of rib(s), sternum and thoracic spine**

NOTE A fracture not indicated as displaced or nondisplaced should be coded to displaced

A fracture not indicated as open or closed should be coded to closed

Includes: fracture of thoracic neural arch

fracture of thoracic spinous process

fracture of thoracic transverse process

fracture of thoracic vertebra

fracture of thoracic vertebral arch

Code first any associated:

injury of intrathoracic organ (S27.-)

spinal cord injury (S24.0-, S24.1-)

Excludes1: *transection of thorax (S28.1)*

Excludes2: *fracture of clavicle (S42.0-)*

fracture of scapula (S42.1-)

The appropriate 7th character is to be added to each code from category S22

A initial encounter for closed fracture

B initial encounter for open fracture

D subsequent encounter for fracture with routine healing

G subsequent encounter for fracture with delayed healing

K subsequent encounter for fracture with nonunion

S sequela

Review coding guideline C.19.c

+ S22.0 **Fracture of thoracic vertebra**

+ S22.00 **Fracture of unspecified thoracic vertebra**

CC MCC +7th **S22.000** **Wedge compression fracture of unspecified thoracic vertebra**

HAC 7th characters A & B see Appendix B for HAC conditional logic

CC MCC +7th **S22.001** **Stable burst fracture of unspecified thoracic vertebra**

HAC 7th characters A & B see Appendix B for HAC conditional logic

CC MCC +7th **S22.002** **Unstable burst fracture of unspecified thoracic vertebra**

HAC 7th characters A & B see Appendix B for HAC conditional logic

CC MCC +7th **S22.008** **Other fracture of unspecified thoracic vertebra**

HAC 7th characters A & B see Appendix B for HAC conditional logic

CC MCC +7th **S22.009** **Unspecified fracture of unspecified thoracic vertebra**

HAC 7th characters A & B see Appendix B for HAC conditional logic

+ S22.01 **Fracture of first thoracic vertebra**

CC MCC +7th **S22.010** **Wedge compression fracture of first thoracic vertebra**

HAC 7th characters A & B see Appendix B for HAC conditional logic

CC MCC +7th **S22.011** **Stable burst fracture of first thoracic vertebra**

HAC 7th characters A & B see Appendix B for HAC conditional logic

CC MCC +7th **S22.012** **Unstable burst fracture of first thoracic vertebra**

HAC 7th characters A & B see Appendix B for HAC conditional logic

CC MCC +7th **S22.018** **Other fracture of first thoracic vertebra**

HAC 7th characters A & B see Appendix B for HAC conditional logic

CC MCC +7th **S22.019** **Unspecified fracture of first thoracic vertebra**

HAC 7th characters A & B see Appendix B for HAC conditional logic

+ S22.02 **Fracture of second thoracic vertebra**

CC MCC +7th **S22.020** **Wedge compression fracture of second thoracic vertebra**

HAC 7th characters A & B see Appendix B for HAC conditional logic

CC MCC +7th **S22.021** **Stable burst fracture of second thoracic vertebra**

HAC 7th characters A & B see Appendix B for HAC conditional logic

CC MCC +7th **S22.022** **Unstable burst fracture of second thoracic vertebra**

HAC 7th characters A & B see Appendix B for HAC conditional logic

CC MCC +7th **S22.028** **Other fracture of second thoracic vertebra**
> HAC 7th characters A & B see Appendix B for HAC conditional logic

CC MCC +7th **S22.029** **Unspecified fracture of second thoracic vertebra**
> HAC 7th characters A & B see Appendix B for HAC conditional logic

+ **S22.03** **Fracture of third thoracic vertebra**

CC MCC +7th **S22.030** **Wedge compression fracture of third thoracic vertebra**
> HAC 7th characters A & B see Appendix B for HAC conditional logic

CC MCC +7th **S22.031** **Stable burst fracture of third thoracic vertebra**
> HAC 7th characters A & B see Appendix B for HAC conditional logic

CC MCC +7th **S22.032** **Unstable burst fracture of third thoracic vertebra**
> HAC 7th characters A & B see Appendix B for HAC conditional logic

CC MCC +7th **S22.038** **Other fracture of third thoracic vertebra**
> HAC 7th characters A & B see Appendix B for HAC conditional logic

CC MCC +7th **S22.039** **Unspecified fracture of third thoracic vertebra**
> HAC 7th characters A & B see Appendix B for HAC conditional logic

+ **S22.04** **Fracture of fourth thoracic vertebra**

CC MCC +7th **S22.040** **Wedge compression fracture of fourth thoracic vertebra**
> HAC 7th characters A & B see Appendix B for HAC conditional logic

CC MCC +7th **S22.041** **Stable burst fracture of fourth thoracic vertebra**
> HAC 7th characters A & B see Appendix B for HAC conditional logic

CC MCC +7th **S22.042** **Unstable burst fracture of fourth thoracic vertebra**
> HAC 7th characters A & B see Appendix B for HAC conditional logic

CC MCC +7th **S22.048** **Other fracture of fourth thoracic vertebra**
> HAC 7th characters A & B see Appendix B for HAC conditional logic

CC MCC +7th **S22.049** **Unspecified fracture of fourth thoracic vertebra**
> HAC 7th characters A & B see Appendix B for HAC conditional logic

+ **S22.05** **Fracture of T5-T6 vertebra**

CC MCC +7th **S22.050** **Wedge compression fracture of T5-T6 vertebra**
> HAC 7th characters A & B see Appendix B for HAC conditional logic

CC MCC +7th **S22.051** **Stable burst fracture of T5-T6 vertebra**
> HAC 7th characters A & B see Appendix B for HAC conditional logic

CC MCC +7th **S22.052** **Unstable burst fracture of T5-T6 vertebra**
> HAC 7th characters A & B see Appendix B for HAC conditional logic

CC MCC +7th **S22.058** **Other fracture of T5-T6 vertebra**
> HAC 7th characters A & B see Appendix B for HAC conditional logic

CC MCC +7th **S22.059** **Unspecified fracture of T5-T6 vertebra**
> HAC 7th characters A & B see Appendix B for HAC conditional logic

+ **S22.06** **Fracture of T7-T8 vertebra**

CC MCC +7th **S22.060** **Wedge compression fracture of T7-T8 vertebra**
> HAC 7th characters A & B see Appendix B for HAC conditional logic

CC MCC +7th **S22.061** **Stable burst fracture of T7-T8 vertebra**
> HAC 7th characters A & B see Appendix B for HAC conditional logic

CC MCC +7th **S22.062** **Unstable burst fracture of T7-T8 vertebra**
> HAC 7th characters A & B see Appendix B for HAC conditional logic

CC MCC +7th **S22.068** **Other fracture of T7-T8 thoracic vertebra**
> HAC 7th characters A & B see Appendix B for HAC conditional logic

CC MCC +7th **S22.069** **Unspecified fracture of T7-T8 vertebra**
> HAC 7th characters A & B see Appendix B for HAC conditional logic

+ **S22.07** **Fracture of T9-T10 vertebra**

CC MCC +7th **S22.070** **Wedge compression fracture of T9-T10 vertebra**
> HAC 7th characters A & B see Appendix B for HAC conditional logic

CC MCC +7th **S22.071** **Stable burst fracture of T9-T10 vertebra**
> HAC 7th characters A & B see Appendix B for HAC conditional logic

CC MCC +7th **S22.072** **Unstable burst fracture of T9-T10 vertebra**
> HAC 7th characters A & B see Appendix B for HAC conditional logic

CC MCC +7th **S22.078** **Other fracture of T9-T10 vertebra**
> HAC 7th characters A & B see Appendix B for HAC conditional logic

CC MCC +7th **S22.079** **Unspecified fracture of T9-T10 vertebra**
> HAC 7th characters A & B see Appendix B for HAC conditional logic

+ **S22.08** **Fracture of T11-T12 vertebra**

CC MCC +7th **S22.080** **Wedge compression fracture of T11-T12 vertebra**
> HAC 7th characters A & B see Appendix B for HAC conditional logic

CC MCC +7th **S22.081** **Stable burst fracture of T11-T12 vertebra**
> HAC 7th characters A & B see Appendix B for HAC conditional logic

CC MCC +7th **S22.082** **Unstable burst fracture of T11-T12 vertebra**
> HAC 7th characters A & B see Appendix B for HAC conditional logic

CC MCC +7th **S22.088** **Other fracture of T11-T12 vertebra**
> HAC 7th characters A & B see Appendix B for HAC conditional logic

CC MCC +7th **S22.089** **Unspecified fracture of T11-T12 vertebra**
> HAC 7th characters A & B see Appendix B for HAC conditional logic

+ **S22.2** **Fracture of sternum**

MCC X+7th **S22.20** **Unspecified fracture of sternum**
> HAC 7th characters A & B see Appendix B for HAC conditional logic

CC MCC X+7th **S22.21** **Fracture of manubrium**
> HAC 7th characters A & B see Appendix B for HAC conditional logic

CC MCC X+7th **S22.22** **Fracture of body of sternum**
> HAC 7th characters A & B see Appendix B for HAC conditional logic

CC MCC X+7th **S22.23** **Sternal manubrial dissociation**
> HAC 7th characters A & B see Appendix B for HAC conditional logic

CC MCC X+7th **S22.24** **Fracture of xiphoid process**
> HAC 7th characters A & B see Appendix B for HAC conditional logic

+ **S22.3** **Fracture of one rib**

CC MCC X+7th **S22.31** **Fracture of one rib, right side**
> HAC 7th characters A & B see Appendix B for HAC conditional logic

CC MCC X+7th **S22.32** **Fracture of one rib, left side**
> HAC 7th characters A & B see Appendix B for HAC conditional logic

CC MCC X+7th **S22.39** **Fracture of one rib, unspecified side**
> HAC 7th characters A & B see Appendix B for HAC conditional logic

+ **S22.4** **Multiple fractures of ribs**
Fractures of two or more ribs
Excludes1: flail chest (S22.5-)

CC MCC X+7th **S22.41** **Multiple fractures of ribs, right side**
> HAC 7th characters A & B see Appendix B for HAC conditional logic

CC MCC X+7th **S22.42** **Multiple fractures of ribs, left side**
> HAC 7th characters A & B see Appendix B for HAC conditional logic

+, +7th, X + 7th • Newborn • Pediatric • Maternity • Adult ♀ Female ♂ Male | Manifestation | Unacceptable PDX | HCC | CC | MCC | HAC

CC MCC X+7th **S22.43** **Multiple fractures of ribs, bilateral**
> HAC 7th characters A & B see Appendix B for HAC conditional logic

CC MCC X+7th **S22.49** **Multiple fractures of ribs, unspecified side**
> HAC 7th characters A & B see Appendix B for HAC conditional logic

X+7th **S22.5** **Flail chest**
> HAC 7th characters A & B see Appendix B for HAC conditional logic

X+7th **S22.9** **Fracture of bony thorax, part unspecified**
> HAC 7th characters A & B see Appendix B for HAC conditional logic

S23 **Dislocation and sprain of joints and ligaments of thorax**

> **Includes:** avulsion of joint or ligament of thorax
> laceration of cartilage, joint or ligament of thorax
> sprain of cartilage, joint or ligament of thorax
> traumatic hemarthrosis of joint or ligament of thorax
> traumatic rupture of joint or ligament of thorax
> traumatic subluxation of joint or ligament of thorax
> traumatic tear of joint or ligament of thorax
>
> Code also any associated open wound
>
> **Excludes2:** *dislocation, sprain of sternoclavicular joint (S43.2, S43.6)*
> *strain of muscle or tendon of thorax (S29.01-)*

> The appropriate 7th character is to be added to each code from category S23
> A initial encounter
> D subsequent encounter
> S sequela

X+7th **S23.0** **Traumatic rupture of thoracic intervertebral disc**
> **Excludes1:** *rupture or displacement (nontraumatic) of thoracic intervertebral disc NOS (M51.- with fifth character 4)*

+ **S23.1** **Subluxation and dislocation of thoracic vertebra**
> Code also any associated
> open wound of thorax (S21.-)
> spinal cord injury (S24.0-, S24.1-)
> **Excludes2:** *fracture of thoracic vertebrae (S22.0-)*

   + **S23.10** **Subluxation and dislocation of unspecified thoracic vertebra**
     +7th **S23.100** **Subluxation of unspecified thoracic vertebra**
     +7th **S23.101** **Dislocation of unspecified thoracic vertebra**

   + **S23.11** **Subluxation and dislocation of T1/T2 thoracic vertebra**
     +7th **S23.110** **Subluxation of T1/T2 thoracic vertebra**
     +7th **S23.111** **Dislocation of T1/T2 thoracic vertebra**

   + **S23.12** **Subluxation and dislocation of T2/T3-T3/T4 thoracic vertebra**
     +7th **S23.120** **Subluxation of T2/T3 thoracic vertebra**
     +7th **S23.121** **Dislocation of T2/T3 thoracic vertebra**
     +7th **S23.122** **Subluxation of T3/T4 thoracic vertebra**
     +7th **S23.123** **Dislocation of T3/T4 thoracic vertebra**

   + **S23.13** **Subluxation and dislocation of T4/T5-T5/T6 thoracic vertebra**
     +7th **S23.130** **Subluxation of T4/T5 thoracic vertebra**
     +7th **S23.131** **Dislocation of T4/T5 thoracic vertebra**
     +7th **S23.132** **Subluxation of T5/T6 thoracic vertebra**
     +7th **S23.133** **Dislocation of T5/T6 thoracic vertebra**

   + **S23.14** **Subluxation and dislocation of T6/T7-T7/T8 thoracic vertebra**
     +7th **S23.140** **Subluxation of T6/T7 thoracic vertebra**
     +7th **S23.141** **Dislocation of T6/T7 thoracic vertebra**
     +7th **S23.142** **Subluxation of T7/T8 thoracic vertebra**
     +7th **S23.143** **Dislocation of T7/T8 thoracic vertebra**

   + **S23.15** **Subluxation and dislocation of T8/T9-T9/T10 thoracic vertebra**
     +7th **S23.150** **Subluxation of T8/T9 thoracic vertebra**
     +7th **S23.151** **Dislocation of T8/T9 thoracic vertebra**
     +7th **S23.152** **Subluxation of T9/T10 thoracic vertebra**
     +7th **S23.153** **Dislocation of T9/T10 thoracic vertebra**

   + **S23.16** **Subluxation and dislocation of T10/T11-T11/T12 thoracic vertebra**
     +7th **S23.160** **Subluxation of T10/T11 thoracic vertebra**
     +7th **S23.161** **Dislocation of T10/T11 thoracic vertebra**

     +7th **S23.162** **Subluxation of T11/T12 thoracic vertebra**
     +7th **S23.163** **Dislocation of T11/T12 thoracic vertebra**

   + **S23.17** **Subluxation and dislocation of T12/L1 thoracic vertebra**
     +7th **S23.170** **Subluxation of T12/L1 thoracic vertebra**
     +7th **S23.171** **Dislocation of T12/L1 thoracic vertebra**

   + **S23.2** **Dislocation of other and unspecified parts of thorax**
   X+7th **S23.20** **Dislocation of unspecified part of thorax**
   X+7th **S23.29** **Dislocation of other parts of thorax**

X+7th **S23.3** **Sprain of ligaments of thoracic spine**

+ **S23.4** **Sprain of ribs and sternum**
   X+7th **S23.41** **Sprain of ribs**
   + **S23.42** **Sprain of sternum**
     +7th **S23.420** **Sprain of sternoclavicular (joint) (ligament)**
     +7th **S23.421** **Sprain of chondrosternal joint**
     +7th **S23.428** **Other sprain of sternum**
     +7th **S23.429** **Unspecified sprain of sternum**

X+7th **S23.8** **Sprain of other specified parts of thorax**
X+7th **S23.9** **Sprain of unspecified parts of thorax**

S24 **Injury of nerves and spinal cord at thorax level**

> **NOTE** Code to highest level of thoracic spinal cord injury
> Injuries to the spinal cord (S24.0 and S24.1) refer to the cord level and not bone level injury, and can affect nerve roots at and below the level given.
>
> Code also any associated:
> fracture of thoracic vertebra (S22.0-)
> open wound of thorax (S21.-)
> transient paralysis (R29.5)
> **Excludes2:** *injury of brachial plexus (S14.3)*

> The appropriate 7th character is to be added to each code from category S24
> A initial encounter
> D subsequent encounter
> S sequela

MCC X+7th **S24.0** **Concussion and edema of thoracic spinal cord**

+ **S24.1** **Other and unspecified injuries of thoracic spinal cord**

   + **S24.10** **Unspecified injury of thoracic spinal cord**
   MCC +7th **S24.101** **Unspecified injury at T1 level of thoracic spinal cord**
> HAC 7th character A see Appendix B for HAC conditional logic

   MCC +7th **S24.102** **Unspecified injury at T2-T6 level of thoracic spinal cord**
> HAC 7th character A see Appendix B for HAC conditional logic

   MCC +7th **S24.103** **Unspecified injury at T7-T10 level of thoracic spinal cord**
> HAC 7th character A see Appendix B for HAC conditional logic

   MCC +7th **S24.104** **Unspecified injury at T11-T12 level of thoracic spinal cord**
> HAC 7th character A see Appendix B for HAC conditional logic

     +7th **S24.109** **Unspecified injury at unspecified level of thoracic spinal cord**
> Injury of thoracic spinal cord NOS
> HAC 7th character A see Appendix B for HAC conditional logic

   + **S24.11** **Complete lesion of thoracic spinal cord**
   MCC +7th **S24.111** **Complete lesion at T1 level of thoracic spinal cord**
> HAC 7th character A see Appendix B for HAC conditional logic

   MCC +7th **S24.112** **Complete lesion at T2-T6 level of thoracic spinal cord**
> HAC 7th character A see Appendix B for HAC conditional logic

   MCC +7th **S24.113** **Complete lesion at T7-T10 level of thoracic spinal cord**
> HAC 7th character A see Appendix B for HAC conditional logic

   MCC +7th **S24.114** **Complete lesion at T11-T12 level of thoracic spinal cord**
> HAC 7th character A see Appendix B for HAC conditional logic

     +7th **S24.119** **Complete lesion at unspecified level of thoracic spinal cord**

+ **S24.13** **Anterior cord syndrome of thoracic spinal cord**
MCC +7th **S24.131** **Anterior cord syndrome at T1 level of thoracic spinal cord**
> HAC 7th character A see Appendix B for HAC conditional logic

MCC +7th **S24.132** **Anterior cord syndrome at T2-T6 level of thoracic spinal cord**
> HAC 7th character A see Appendix B for HAC conditional logic

MCC +7th **S24.133** **Anterior cord syndrome at T7-T10 level of thoracic spinal cord**
> HAC 7th character A see Appendix B for HAC conditional logic

MCC +7th **S24.134** **Anterior cord syndrome at T11-T12 level of thoracic spinal cord**
> HAC 7th character A see Appendix B for HAC conditional logic

+7th **S24.139** **Anterior cord syndrome at unspecified level of thoracic spinal cord**

+ **S24.14** **Brown-Séquard syndrome of thoracic spinal cord**
MCC +7th **S24.141** **Brown-Séquard syndrome at T1 level of thoracic spinal cord**
MCC +7th **S24.142** **Brown-Séquard syndrome at T2-T6 level of thoracic spinal cord**
MCC +7th **S24.143** **Brown-Séquard syndrome at T7-T10 level of thoracic spinal cord**
MCC +7th **S24.144** **Brown-Séquard syndrome at T11-T12 level of thoracic spinal cord**
+7th **S24.149** **Brown-Séquard syndrome at unspecified level of thoracic spinal cord**

+ **S24.15** **Other incomplete lesions of thoracic spinal cord**
Incomplete lesion of thoracic spinal cord NOS
Posterior cord syndrome of thoracic spinal cord
MCC +7th **S24.151** **Other incomplete lesion at T1 level of thoracic spinal cord**
> HAC 7th character A see Appendix B for HAC conditional logic

MCC +7th **S24.152** **Other incomplete lesion at T2-T6 level of thoracic spinal cord**
> HAC 7th character A see Appendix B for HAC conditional logic

MCC +7th **S24.153** **Other incomplete lesion at T7-T10 level of thoracic spinal cord**
> HAC 7th character A see Appendix B for HAC conditional logic

MCC +7th **S24.154** **Other incomplete lesion at T11-T12 level of thoracic spinal cord**
> HAC 7th character A see Appendix B for HAC conditional logic

+7th **S24.159** **Other incomplete lesion at unspecified level of thoracic spinal cord**

X+7th **S24.2** **Injury of nerve root of thoracic spine**
X+7th **S24.3** **Injury of peripheral nerves of thorax**
X+7th **S24.4** **Injury of thoracic sympathetic nervous system**
Injury of cardiac plexus
Injury of esophageal plexus
Injury of pulmonary plexus
Injury of stellate ganglion
Injury of thoracic sympathetic ganglion
X+7th **S24.8** **Injury of other specified nerves of thorax**
X+7th **S24.9** **Injury of unspecified nerve of thorax**

S25 **Injury of blood vessels of thorax**
Code also any associated open wound (S21.-)

The appropriate 7th character is to be added to each code from category S25
A   initial encounter
D   subsequent encounter
S   sequela

+ **S25.0** **Injury of thoracic aorta**
Injury of aorta NOS
MCC X+7th **S25.00** **Unspecified injury of thoracic aorta**
MCC X+7th **S25.01** **Minor laceration of thoracic aorta**
Incomplete transection of thoracic aorta
Laceration of thoracic aorta NOS
Superficial laceration of thoracic aorta

MCC X+7th **S25.02** **Major laceration of thoracic aorta**
Complete transection of thoracic aorta
Traumatic rupture of thoracic aorta
MCC X+7th **S25.09** **Other specified injury of thoracic aorta**
+ **S25.1** **Injury of innominate or subclavian artery**
+ **S25.10** **Unspecified injury of innominate or subclavian artery**
MCC +7th **S25.101** **Unspecified injury of right innominate or subclavian artery**
MCC +7th **S25.102** **Unspecified injury of left innominate or subclavian artery**
MCC +7th **S25.109** **Unspecified injury of unspecified innominate or subclavian artery**
+ **S25.11** **Minor laceration of innominate or subclavian artery**
Incomplete transection of innominate or subclavian artery
Laceration of innominate or subclavian artery NOS
Superficial laceration of innominate or subclavian artery
MCC +7th **S25.111** **Minor laceration of right innominate or subclavian artery**
MCC +7th **S25.112** **Minor laceration of left innominate or subclavian artery**
MCC +7th **S25.119** **Minor laceration of unspecified innominate or subclavian artery**
+ **S25.12** **Major laceration of innominate or subclavian artery**
Complete transection of innominate or subclavian artery
Traumatic rupture of innominate or subclavian artery
MCC +7th **S25.121** **Major laceration of right innominate or subclavian artery**
MCC +7th **S25.122** **Major laceration of left innominate or subclavian artery**
MCC +7th **S25.129** **Major laceration of unspecified innominate or subclavian artery**
+ **S25.19** **Other specified injury of innominate or subclavian artery**
MCC +7th **S25.191** **Other specified injury of right innominate or subclavian artery**
MCC +7th **S25.192** **Other specified injury of left innominate or subclavian artery**
MCC +7th **S25.199** **Other specified injury of unspecified innominate or subclavian artery**
+ **S25.2** **Injury of superior vena cava**
Injury of vena cava NOS
MCC X+7th **S25.20** **Unspecified injury of superior vena cava**
MCC X+7th **S25.21** **Minor laceration of superior vena cava**
Incomplete transection of superior vena cava
Laceration of superior vena cava NOS
Superficial laceration of superior vena cava
MCC X+7th **S25.22** **Major laceration of superior vena cava**
Complete transection of superior vena cava
Traumatic rupture of superior vena cava
MCC X+7th **S25.29** **Other specified injury of superior vena cava**
+ **S25.3** **Injury of innominate or subclavian vein**
+ **S25.30** **Unspecified injury of innominate or subclavian vein**
MCC +7th **S25.301** **Unspecified injury of right innominate or subclavian vein**
MCC +7th **S25.302** **Unspecified injury of left innominate or subclavian vein**
MCC +7th **S25.309** **Unspecified injury of unspecified innominate or subclavian vein**
+ **S25.31** **Minor laceration of innominate or subclavian vein**
Incomplete transection of innominate or subclavian vein
Laceration of innominate or subclavian vein NOS
Superficial laceration of innominate or subclavian vein
MCC +7th **S25.311** **Minor laceration of right innominate or subclavian vein**
MCC +7th **S25.312** **Minor laceration of left innominate or subclavian vein**
MCC +7th **S25.319** **Minor laceration of unspecified innominate or subclavian vein**

+, +7th, X + 7th   ● Newborn   ● Pediatric   ● Maternity   ● Adult   ♀ Female   ♂ Male   Manifestation   Unacceptable PDX   HCC   CC   MCC   HAC

+ S25.32 **Major laceration of innominate or subclavian vein**
Complete transection of innominate or subclavian vein
Traumatic rupture of innominate or subclavian vein
MCC +7th S25.321 **Major laceration of right innominate or subclavian vein**
MCC +7th S25.322 **Major laceration of left innominate or subclavian vein**
MCC +7th S25.329 **Major laceration of unspecified innominate or subclavian vein**
+ S25.39 **Other specified injury of innominate or subclavian vein**
MCC +7th S25.391 **Other specified injury of right innominate or subclavian vein**
MCC +7th S25.392 **Other specified injury of left innominate or subclavian vein**
MCC +7th S25.399 **Other specified injury of unspecified innominate or subclavian vein**
+ S25.4 **Injury of pulmonary blood vessels**
+ S25.40 **Unspecified injury of pulmonary blood vessels**
MCC +7th S25.401 **Unspecified injury of right pulmonary blood vessels**
MCC +7th S25.402 **Unspecified injury of left pulmonary blood vessels**
MCC +7th S25.409 **Unspecified injury of unspecified pulmonary blood vessels**
+ S25.41 **Minor laceration of pulmonary blood vessels**
Incomplete transection of pulmonary blood vessels
Laceration of pulmonary blood vessels NOS
Superficial laceration of pulmonary blood vessels
MCC +7th S25.411 **Minor laceration of right pulmonary blood vessels**
MCC +7th S25.412 **Minor laceration of left pulmonary blood vessels**
MCC +7th S25.419 **Minor laceration of unspecified pulmonary blood vessels**
+ S25.42 **Major laceration of pulmonary blood vessels**
Complete transection of pulmonary blood vessels
Traumatic rupture of pulmonary blood vessels
MCC +7th S25.421 **Major laceration of right pulmonary blood vessels**
MCC +7th S25.422 **Major laceration of left pulmonary blood vessels**
MCC +7th S25.429 **Major laceration of unspecified pulmonary blood vessels**
+ S25.49 **Other specified injury of pulmonary blood vessels**
MCC +7th S25.491 **Other specified injury of right pulmonary blood vessels**
MCC +7th S25.492 **Other specified injury of left pulmonary blood vessels**
MCC +7th S25.499 **Other specified injury of unspecified pulmonary blood vessels**
+ S25.5 **Injury of intercostal blood vessels**
+ S25.50 **Unspecified injury of intercostal blood vessels**
CC +7th S25.501 **Unspecified injury of intercostal blood vessels, right side**
CC +7th S25.502 **Unspecified injury of intercostal blood vessels, left side**
CC +7th S25.509 **Unspecified injury of intercostal blood vessels, unspecified side**
+ S25.51 **Laceration of intercostal blood vessels**
CC +7th S25.511 **Laceration of intercostal blood vessels, right side**
CC +7th S25.512 **Laceration of intercostal blood vessels, left side**
CC +7th S25.519 **Laceration of intercostal blood vessels, unspecified side**
+ S25.59 **Other specified injury of intercostal blood vessels**
CC +7th S25.591 **Other specified injury of intercostal blood vessels, right side**
CC +7th S25.592 **Other specified injury of intercostal blood vessels, left side**
CC +7th S25.599 **Other specified injury of intercostal blood vessels, unspecified side**

+ S25.8 **Injury of other blood vessels of thorax**
Injury of azygos vein
Injury of mammary artery or vein
+ S25.80 **Unspecified injury of other blood vessels of thorax**
CC +7th S25.801 **Unspecified injury of other blood vessels of thorax, right side**
CC +7th S25.802 **Unspecified injury of other blood vessels of thorax, left side**
CC +7th S25.809 **Unspecified injury of other blood vessels of thorax, unspecified side**
+ S25.81 **Laceration of other blood vessels of thorax**
CC +7th S25.811 **Laceration of other blood vessels of thorax, right side**
CC +7th S25.812 **Laceration of other blood vessels of thorax, left side**
CC +7th S25.819 **Laceration of other blood vessels of thorax, unspecified side**
+ S25.89 **Other specified injury of other blood vessels of thorax**
CC +7th S25.891 **Other specified injury of other blood vessels of thorax, right side**
CC +7th S25.892 **Other specified injury of other blood vessels of thorax, left side**
CC +7th S25.899 **Other specified injury of other blood vessels of thorax, unspecified side**
+ S25.9 **Injury of unspecified blood vessel of thorax**
CC X+7th S25.90 **Unspecified injury of unspecified blood vessel of thorax**
CC X+7th S25.91 **Laceration of unspecified blood vessel of thorax**
CC X+7th S25.99 **Other specified injury of unspecified blood vessel of thorax**

S26 **Injury of heart**
Code also any associated:
open wound of thorax (S21.-)
traumatic hemopneumothorax (S27.2)
traumatic hemothorax (S27.1)
traumatic pneumothorax (S27.0)

The appropriate 7th character is to be added to each code from category S26
A   initial encounter
D   subsequent encounter
S   sequela

+ S26.0 **Injury of heart with hemopericardium**
CC X+7th S26.00 **Unspecified injury of heart with hemopericardium**
CC X+7th S26.01 **Contusion of heart with hemopericardium**
+ S26.02 **Laceration of heart with hemopericardium**
MCC +7th S26.020 **Mild laceration of heart with hemopericardium**
Laceration of heart without penetration of heart chamber
MCC +7th S26.021 **Moderate laceration of heart with hemopericardium**
Laceration of heart with penetration of heart chamber
MCC +7th S26.022 **Major laceration of heart with hemopericardium**
Laceration of heart with penetration of multiple heart chambers
CC X+7th S26.09 **Other injury of heart with hemopericardium**
+ S26.1 **Injury of heart without hemopericardium**
CC X+7th S26.10 **Unspecified injury of heart without hemopericardium**
CC X+7th S26.11 **Contusion of heart without hemopericardium**
MCC X+7th S26.12 **Laceration of heart without hemopericardium**
CC X+7th S26.19 **Other injury of heart without hemopericardium**
+ S26.9 **Injury of heart, unspecified with or without hemopericardium**
CC X+7th S26.90 **Unspecified injury of heart, unspecified with or without hemopericardium**
CC X+7th S26.91 **Contusion of heart, unspecified with or without hemopericardium**
MCC X+7th S26.92 **Laceration of heart, unspecified with or without hemopericardium**
Laceration of heart NOS
CC X+7th S26.99 **Other injury of heart, unspecified with or without hemopericardium**

+, +7th, X + 7th   • Newborn   • Pediatric   • Maternity   • Adult   ♀ Female   ♂ Male   Manifestation   Unacceptable PDX   HCC   CC   MCC   HAC

S27 Injury of other and unspecified intrathoracic organs

Code also associated open wound of thorax (S21.-)

Excludes2: *injury of cervical esophagus (S10-S19)*
injury of trachea (cervical) (S10-S19)

The appropriate 7th character is to be added to each code from category S27
A initial encounter
D subsequent encounter
S sequela

CC **S27.0 Traumatic pneumothorax**
X+7th   **Excludes1:** *spontaneous pneumothorax (J93.-)*

MCC **S27.1 Traumatic hemothorax**

MCC **S27.2 Traumatic hemopneumothorax**

S27.3 Other and unspecified injuries of lung
+ **S27.30 Unspecified injury of lung**
CC +7th **S27.301 Unspecified injury of lung, unilateral**
CC +7th **S27.302 Unspecified injury of lung, bilateral**
CC +7th **S27.309 Unspecified injury of lung, unspecified**
+ **S27.31 Primary blast injury of lung**
    Blast injury of lung NOS
CC +7th **S27.311 Primary blast injury of lung, unilateral**
CC +7th **S27.312 Primary blast injury of lung, bilateral**
CC +7th **S27.319 Primary blast injury of lung, unspecified**
+ **S27.32 Contusion of lung**
CC +7th **S27.321 Contusion of lung, unilateral**
CC +7th **S27.322 Contusion of lung, bilateral**
CC +7th **S27.329 Contusion of lung, unspecified**
+ **S27.33 Laceration of lung**
MCC +7th **S27.331 Laceration of lung, unilateral**
MCC +7th **S27.332 Laceration of lung, bilateral**
MCC +7th **S27.339 Laceration of lung, unspecified**
+ **S27.39 Other injuries of lung**
    Secondary blast injury of lung
CC +7th **S27.391 Other injuries of lung, unilateral**
CC +7th **S27.392 Other injuries of lung, bilateral**
CC +7th **S27.399 Other injuries of lung, unspecified**

S27.4 Injury of bronchus
+ **S27.40 Unspecified injury of bronchus**
MCC +7th **S27.401 Unspecified injury of bronchus, unilateral**
MCC +7th **S27.402 Unspecified injury of bronchus, bilateral**
MCC +7th **S27.409 Unspecified injury of bronchus, unspecified**
+ **S27.41 Primary blast injury of bronchus**
    Blast injury of bronchus NOS
MCC +7th **S27.411 Primary blast injury of bronchus, unilateral**
MCC +7th **S27.412 Primary blast injury of bronchus, bilateral**
MCC +7th **S27.419 Primary blast injury of bronchus, unspecified**
+ **S27.42 Contusion of bronchus**
MCC +7th **S27.421 Contusion of bronchus, unilateral**
MCC +7th **S27.422 Contusion of bronchus, bilateral**
MCC +7th **S27.429 Contusion of bronchus, unspecified**
+ **S27.43 Laceration of bronchus**
MCC +7th **S27.431 Laceration of bronchus, unilateral**
MCC +7th **S27.432 Laceration of bronchus, bilateral**
MCC +7th **S27.439 Laceration of bronchus, unspecified**
+ **S27.49 Other injury of bronchus**
    Secondary blast injury of bronchus
MCC +7th **S27.491 Other injury of bronchus, unilateral**
MCC +7th **S27.492 Other injury of bronchus, bilateral**
MCC +7th **S27.499 Other injury of bronchus, unspecified**

+ **S27.5 Injury of thoracic trachea**
CC X+7th **S27.50 Unspecified injury of thoracic trachea**
CC X+7th **S27.51 Primary blast injury of thoracic trachea**
    Blast injury of thoracic trachea NOS
CC X+7th **S27.52 Contusion of thoracic trachea**
CC X+7th **S27.53 Laceration of thoracic trachea**
CC X+7th **S27.59 Other injury of thoracic trachea**
    Secondary blast injury of thoracic trachea
+ **S27.6 Injury of pleura**
CC X+7th **S27.60 Unspecified injury of pleura**
CC X+7th **S27.63 Laceration of pleura**
CC X+7th **S27.69 Other injury of pleura**
+ **S27.8 Injury of other specified intrathoracic organs**

+ **S27.80 Injury of diaphragm**
CC +7th **S27.802 Contusion of diaphragm**
CC +7th **S27.803 Laceration of diaphragm**
CC +7th **S27.808 Other injury of diaphragm**
CC +7th **S27.809 Unspecified injury of diaphragm**
+ **S27.81 Injury of esophagus (thoracic part)**
MCC +7th **S27.812 Contusion of esophagus (thoracic part)**
MCC +7th **S27.813 Laceration of esophagus (thoracic part)**
MCC +7th **S27.818 Other injury of esophagus (thoracic part)**
MCC +7th **S27.819 Unspecified injury of esophagus (thoracic part)**
+ **S27.89 Injury of other specified intrathoracic organs**
    Injury of lymphatic thoracic duct
    Injury of thymus gland
CC +7th **S27.892 Contusion of other specified intrathoracic organs**
CC +7th **S27.893 Laceration of other specified intrathoracic organs**
CC +7th **S27.898 Other injury of other specified intrathoracic organs**
CC +7th **S27.899 Unspecified injury of other specified intrathoracic organs**
CC X+7th **S27.9 Injury of unspecified intrathoracic organ**

S28 Crushing injury of thorax, and traumatic amputation of part of thorax

The appropriate 7th character is to be added to each code from category S28
A initial encounter
D subsequent encounter
S sequela

X+7th **S28.0 Crushed chest**
    Use additional code for all associated injuries
    Excludes1: *flail chest (S22.5)*
CC X+7th **S28.1 Traumatic amputation (partial) of part of thorax, except breast**
+ **S28.2 Traumatic amputation of breast**
+ **S28.21 Complete traumatic amputation of breast**
    Traumatic amputation of breast NOS
+7th **S28.211 Complete traumatic amputation of right breast**
+7th **S28.212 Complete traumatic amputation of left breast**
+7th **S28.219 Complete traumatic amputation of unspecified breast**
+ **S28.22 Partial traumatic amputation of breast**
+7th **S28.221 Partial traumatic amputation of right breast**
+7th **S28.222 Partial traumatic amputation of left breast**
+7th **S28.229 Partial traumatic amputation of unspecified breast**

S29 Other and unspecified injuries of thorax

Code also any associated open wound (S21.-)

The appropriate 7th character is to be added to each code from category S29
A initial encounter
D subsequent encounter
S sequela

+ **S29.0 Injury of muscle and tendon at thorax level**
+ **S29.00 Unspecified injury of muscle and tendon of thorax**
+7th **S29.001 Unspecified injury of muscle and tendon of front wall of thorax**
+7th **S29.002 Unspecified injury of muscle and tendon of back wall of thorax**
+7th **S29.009 Unspecified injury of muscle and tendon of unspecified wall of thorax**
+ **S29.01 Strain of muscle and tendon of thorax**
+7th **S29.011 Strain of muscle and tendon of front wall of thorax**
+7th **S29.012 Strain of muscle and tendon of back wall of thorax**
+7th **S29.019 Strain of muscle and tendon of unspecified wall of thorax**

+, +7th, X + 7th   ● Newborn   ● Pediatric   ● Maternity   ● Adult   ♀ Female   ♂ Male   Manifestation   Unacceptable PDX   HCC   CC   MCC   HAC

+ S29.02 **Laceration of muscle and tendon of thorax**
CC +7th S29.021 **Laceration of muscle and tendon of front wall of thorax**
+7th S29.022 **Laceration of muscle and tendon of back wall of thorax**
CC +7th S29.029 **Laceration of muscle and tendon of unspecified wall of thorax**
+ S29.09 **Other injury of muscle and tendon of thorax**
+7th S29.091 **Other injury of muscle and tendon of front wall of thorax**
+7th S29.092 **Other injury of muscle and tendon of back wall of thorax**
+7th S29.099 **Other injury of muscle and tendon of unspecified wall of thorax**
X+7th S29.8 **Other specified injuries of thorax**
X+7th S29.9 **Unspecified injury of thorax**

Injuries to the abdomen, lower back, lumbar spine, pelvis and external genitals (S30-S39)

Includes: injuries to the abdominal wall
injuries to the anus
injuries to the buttock
injuries to the external genitalia
injuries to the flank
injuries to the groin

Excludes2: *burns and corrosions (T20-T32)*
effects of foreign body in anus and rectum (T18.5)
effects of foreign body in genitourinary tract (T19.-)
effects of foreign body in stomach, small intestine and colon (T18.2-T18.4)
frostbite (T33-T34)
insect bite or sting, venomous (T63.4)

S30 **Superficial injury of abdomen, lower back, pelvis and external genitals**

Excludes2: *superficial injury of hip (S70.-)*

The appropriate 7th character is to be added to each code from category S30
A   initial encounter
D   subsequent encounter
S   sequela

X+7th S30.0 **Contusion of lower back and pelvis**
Contusion of buttock
X+7th S30.1 **Contusion of abdominal wall**
Contusion of flank
Contusion of groin
+ S30.2 **Contusion of external genital organs**
+ S30.20 **Contusion of unspecified external genital organ**
♂ +7th S30.201 **Contusion of unspecified external genital organ, male**
♀ +7th S30.202 **Contusion of unspecified external genital organ, female**
♂ X+7th S30.21 **Contusion of penis**
♂ X+7th S30.22 **Contusion of scrotum and testes**
♀ X+7th S30.23 **Contusion of vagina and vulva**
X+7th S30.3 **Contusion of anus**
+ S30.8 **Other superficial injuries of abdomen, lower back, pelvis and external genitals**
+ S30.81 **Abrasion of abdomen, lower back, pelvis and external genitals**
+7th S30.810 **Abrasion of lower back and pelvis**
+7th S30.811 **Abrasion of abdominal wall**
♂ +7th S30.812 **Abrasion of penis**
♂ +7th S30.813 **Abrasion of scrotum and testes**
♀ +7th S30.814 **Abrasion of vagina and vulva**
♂ +7th S30.815 **Abrasion of unspecified external genital organs, male**
♀ +7th S30.816 **Abrasion of unspecified external genital organs, female**
+7th S30.817 **Abrasion of anus**
+ S30.82 **Blister (nonthermal) of abdomen, lower back, pelvis and external genitals**
+7th S30.820 **Blister (nonthermal) of lower back and pelvis**
+7th S30.821 **Blister (nonthermal) of abdominal wall**
♂ +7th S30.822 **Blister (nonthermal) of penis**
♂ +7th S30.823 **Blister (nonthermal) of scrotum and testes**

♀ +7th S30.824 **Blister (nonthermal) of vagina and vulva**
♂ +7th S30.825 **Blister (nonthermal) of unspecified external genital organs, male**
♀ +7th S30.826 **Blister (nonthermal) of unspecified external genital organs, female**
+7th S30.827 **Blister (nonthermal) of anus**
+ S30.84 **External constriction of abdomen, lower back, pelvis and external genitals**
+7th S30.840 **External constriction of lower back and pelvis**
+7th S30.841 **External constriction of abdominal wall**
♂ +7th S30.842 **External constriction of penis**
Hair tourniquet syndrome of penis
Use additional cause code to identify the constricting item (W49.0-)
♂ +7th S30.843 **External constriction of scrotum and testes**
♀ +7th S30.844 **External constriction of vagina and vulva**
♂ +7th S30.845 **External constriction of unspecified external genital organs, male**
♀ +7th S30.846 **External constriction of unspecified external genital organs, female**
+ S30.85 **Superficial foreign body of abdomen, lower back, pelvis and external genitals**
Splinter in the abdomen, lower back, pelvis and external genitals
+7th S30.850 **Superficial foreign body of lower back and pelvis**
+7th S30.851 **Superficial foreign body of abdominal wall**
♂ +7th S30.852 **Superficial foreign body of penis**
♂ +7th S30.853 **Superficial foreign body of scrotum and testes**
♀ +7th S30.854 **Superficial foreign body of vagina and vulva**
♂ +7th S30.855 **Superficial foreign body of unspecified external genital organs, male**
♀ +7th S30.856 **Superficial foreign body of unspecified external genital organs, female**
+7th S30.857 **Superficial foreign body of anus**
+ S30.86 **Insect bite (nonvenomous) of abdomen, lower back, pelvis and external genitals**
+7th S30.860 **Insect bite (nonvenomous) of lower back and pelvis**
+7th S30.861 **Insect bite (nonvenomous) of abdominal wall**
♂ +7th S30.862 **Insect bite (nonvenomous) of penis**
♂ +7th S30.863 **Insect bite (nonvenomous) of scrotum and testes**
♀ +7th S30.864 **Insect bite (nonvenomous) of vagina and vulva**
♂ +7th S30.865 **Insect bite (nonvenomous) of unspecified external genital organs, male**
♀ +7th S30.866 **Insect bite (nonvenomous) of unspecified external genital organs, female**
+7th S30.867 **Insect bite (nonvenomous) of anus**
+ S30.87 **Other superficial bite of abdomen, lower back, pelvis and external genitals**
Excludes1: *open bite of abdomen, lower back, pelvis and external genitals (S31.05, S31.15, S31.25, S31.35, S31.45, S31.55)*
+7th S30.870 **Other superficial bite of lower back and pelvis**
+7th S30.871 **Other superficial bite of abdominal wall**
♂ +7th S30.872 **Other superficial bite of penis**
♂ +7th S30.873 **Other superficial bite of scrotum and testes**
♀ +7th S30.874 **Other superficial bite of vagina and vulva**
♂ +7th S30.875 **Other superficial bite of unspecified external genital organs, male**
♀ +7th S30.876 **Other superficial bite of unspecified external genital organs, female**
+7th S30.877 **Other superficial bite of anus**

+ **S30.9** **Unspecified superficial injury of abdomen, lower back, pelvis and external genitals**

X+7th **S30.91** **Unspecified superficial injury of lower back and pelvis**

X+7th **S30.92** **Unspecified superficial injury of abdominal wall**

♂ X+7th **S30.93** **Unspecified superficial injury of penis**

♂ X+7th **S30.94** **Unspecified superficial injury of scrotum and testes**

♀ X+7th **S30.95** **Unspecified superficial injury of vagina and vulva**

♂ X+7th **S30.96** **Unspecified superficial injury of unspecified external genital organs, male**

♀ X+7th **S30.97** **Unspecified superficial injury of unspecified external genital organs, female**

X+7th **S30.98** **Unspecified superficial injury of anus**

S31 **Open wound of abdomen, lower back, pelvis and external genitals**

Code also any associated:
spinal cord injury (S24.0, S24.1-, S34.0-, S34.1-)
wound infection

Excludes1: *traumatic amputation of part of abdomen, lower back and pelvis (S38.2-, S38.3)*

Excludes2: *open wound of hip (S71.00-S71.02)*
open fracture of pelvis (S32.1--S32.9 with 7th character B)

The appropriate 7th character is to be added to each code from category S31
A   initial encounter
D   subsequent encounter
S   sequela

+ **S31.0** **Open wound of lower back and pelvis**

+ **S31.00** **Unspecified open wound of lower back and pelvis**

+7th **S31.000** **Unspecified open wound of lower back and pelvis without penetration into retroperitoneum**
Unspecified open wound of lower back and pelvis NOS

MCC +7th **S31.001** **Unspecified open wound of lower back and pelvis with penetration into retroperitoneum**

+ **S31.01** **Laceration without foreign body of lower back and pelvis**

+7th **S31.010** **Laceration without foreign body of lower back and pelvis without penetration into retroperitoneum**
Laceration without foreign body of lower back and pelvis NOS

MCC +7th **S31.011** **Laceration without foreign body of lower back and pelvis with penetration into retroperitoneum**

+ **S31.02** **Laceration with foreign body of lower back and pelvis**

+7th **S31.020** **Laceration with foreign body of lower back and pelvis without penetration into retroperitoneum**
Laceration with foreign body of lower back and pelvis NOS

MCC +7th **S31.021** **Laceration with foreign body of lower back and pelvis with penetration into retroperitoneum**

+ **S31.03** **Puncture wound without foreign body of lower back and pelvis**

+7th **S31.030** **Puncture wound without foreign body of lower back and pelvis without penetration into retroperitoneum**
Puncture wound without foreign body of lower back and pelvis NOS

MCC +7th **S31.031** **Puncture wound without foreign body of lower back and pelvis with penetration into retroperitoneum**

+ **S31.04** **Puncture wound with foreign body of lower back and pelvis**

+7th **S31.040** **Puncture wound with foreign body of lower back and pelvis without penetration into retroperitoneum**
Puncture wound with foreign body of lower back and pelvis NOS

MCC +7th **S31.041** **Puncture wound with foreign body of lower back and pelvis with penetration into retroperitoneum**

+ **S31.05** **Open bite of lower back and pelvis**
Bite of lower back and pelvis NOS
Excludes1: *superficial bite of lower back and pelvis (S30.860, S30.870)*

+7th **S31.050** **Open bite of lower back and pelvis without penetration into retroperitoneum**
Open bite of lower back and pelvis NOS

MCC +7th **S31.051** **Open bite of lower back and pelvis with penetration into retroperitoneum**

+ **S31.1** **Open wound of abdominal wall without penetration into peritoneal cavity**
Open wound of abdominal wall NOS
Excludes2: *open wound of abdominal wall with penetration into peritoneal cavity (S31.6-)*

+ **S31.10** **Unspecified open wound of abdominal wall without penetration into peritoneal cavity**

+7th **S31.100** **Unspecified open wound of abdominal wall, right upper quadrant without penetration into peritoneal cavity**

+7th **S31.101** **Unspecified open wound of abdominal wall, left upper quadrant without penetration into peritoneal cavity**

+7th **S31.102** **Unspecified open wound of abdominal wall, epigastric region without penetration into peritoneal cavity**

+7th **S31.103** **Unspecified open wound of abdominal wall, right lower quadrant without penetration into peritoneal cavity**

+7th **S31.104** **Unspecified open wound of abdominal wall, left lower quadrant without penetration into peritoneal cavity**

+7th **S31.105** **Unspecified open wound of abdominal wall, periumbilic region without penetration into peritoneal cavity**

+7th **S31.109** **Unspecified open wound of abdominal wall, unspecified quadrant without penetration into peritoneal cavity**
Unspecified open wound of abdominal wall NOS

+ **S31.11** **Laceration without foreign body of abdominal wall without penetration into peritoneal cavity**

+7th **S31.110** **Laceration without foreign body of abdominal wall, right upper quadrant without penetration into peritoneal cavity**

+7th **S31.111** **Laceration without foreign body of abdominal wall, left upper quadrant without penetration into peritoneal cavity**

+7th **S31.112** **Laceration without foreign body of abdominal wall, epigastric region without penetration into peritoneal cavity**

+7th **S31.113** **Laceration without foreign body of abdominal wall, right lower quadrant without penetration into peritoneal cavity**

+7th **S31.114** **Laceration without foreign body of abdominal wall, left lower quadrant without penetration into peritoneal cavity**

+7th **S31.115** **Laceration without foreign body of abdominal wall, periumbilic region without penetration into peritoneal cavity**

+7th **S31.119** **Laceration without foreign body of abdominal wall, unspecified quadrant without penetration into peritoneal cavity**

+ **S31.12** **Laceration with foreign body of abdominal wall without penetration into peritoneal cavity**

+7th **S31.120** **Laceration of abdominal wall with foreign body, right upper quadrant without penetration into peritoneal cavity**

+7th **S31.121** **Laceration of abdominal wall with foreign body, left upper quadrant without penetration into peritoneal cavity**

+7th **S31.122** **Laceration of abdominal wall with foreign body, epigastric region without penetration into peritoneal cavity**

+7th **S31.123** **Laceration of abdominal wall with foreign body, right lower quadrant without penetration into peritoneal cavity**

+7th **S31.124** **Laceration of abdominal wall with foreign body, left lower quadrant without penetration into peritoneal cavity**

+7th **S31.125** **Laceration of abdominal wall with foreign body, periumbilic region without penetration into peritoneal cavity**

+7th **S31.129** **Laceration of abdominal wall with foreign body, unspecified quadrant without penetration into peritoneal cavity**

+ **S31.13** **Puncture wound of abdominal wall without foreign body without penetration into peritoneal cavity**

+7th **S31.130** **Puncture wound of abdominal wall without foreign body, right upper quadrant without penetration into peritoneal cavity**

+7th **S31.131** **Puncture wound of abdominal wall without foreign body, left upper quadrant without penetration into peritoneal cavity**

+7th **S31.132** **Puncture wound of abdominal wall without foreign body, epigastric region without penetration into peritoneal cavity**

+7th **S31.133** **Puncture wound of abdominal wall without foreign body, right lower quadrant without penetration into peritoneal cavity**

+7th **S31.134** **Puncture wound of abdominal wall without foreign body, left lower quadrant without penetration into peritoneal cavity**

+7th **S31.135** **Puncture wound of abdominal wall without foreign body, periumbilic region without penetration into peritoneal cavity**

+7th **S31.139** **Puncture wound of abdominal wall without foreign body, unspecified quadrant without penetration into peritoneal cavity**

+ **S31.14** **Puncture wound of abdominal wall with foreign body without penetration into peritoneal cavity**

+7th **S31.140** **Puncture wound of abdominal wall with foreign body, right upper quadrant without penetration into peritoneal cavity**

+7th **S31.141** **Puncture wound of abdominal wall with foreign body, left upper quadrant without penetration into peritoneal cavity**

+7th **S31.142** **Puncture wound of abdominal wall with foreign body, epigastric region without penetration into peritoneal cavity**

+7th **S31.143** **Puncture wound of abdominal wall with foreign body, right lower quadrant without penetration into peritoneal cavity**

+7th **S31.144** **Puncture wound of abdominal wall with foreign body, left lower quadrant without penetration into peritoneal cavity**

+7th **S31.145** **Puncture wound of abdominal wall with foreign body, periumbilic region without penetration into peritoneal cavity**

+7th **S31.149** **Puncture wound of abdominal wall with foreign body, unspecified quadrant without penetration into peritoneal cavity**

+ **S31.15** **Open bite of abdominal wall without penetration into peritoneal cavity**
Bite of abdominal wall NOS
Excludes1: *superficial bite of abdominal wall (S30.871)*

+7th **S31.150** **Open bite of abdominal wall, right upper quadrant without penetration into peritoneal cavity**

+7th **S31.151** **Open bite of abdominal wall, left upper quadrant without penetration into peritoneal cavity**

+7th **S31.152** **Open bite of abdominal wall, epigastric region without penetration into peritoneal cavity**

+7th **S31.153** **Open bite of abdominal wall, right lower quadrant without penetration into peritoneal cavity**

+7th **S31.154** **Open bite of abdominal wall, left lower quadrant without penetration into peritoneal cavity**

+7th **S31.155** **Open bite of abdominal wall, periumbilic region without penetration into peritoneal cavity**

+7th **S31.159** **Open bite of abdominal wall, unspecified quadrant without penetration into peritoneal cavity**

+ **S31.2** **Open wound of penis**
♂ X+7th **S31.20** **Unspecified open wound of penis**
♂ X+7th **S31.21** **Laceration without foreign body of penis**
♂ X+7th **S31.22** **Laceration with foreign body of penis**
♂ X+7th **S31.23** **Puncture wound without foreign body of penis**
♂ X+7th **S31.24** **Puncture wound with foreign body of penis**
♂ X+7th **S31.25** **Open bite of penis**
Bite of penis NOS
Excludes1: *superficial bite of penis (S30.862, S30.872)*

+ **S31.3** **Open wound of scrotum and testes**
♂ X+7th **S31.30** **Unspecified open wound of scrotum and testes**
♂ X+7th **S31.31** **Laceration without foreign body of scrotum and testes**
♂ X+7th **S31.32** **Laceration with foreign body of scrotum and testes**
♂ X+7th **S31.33** **Puncture wound without foreign body of scrotum and testes**
♂ X+7th **S31.34** **Puncture wound with foreign body of scrotum and testes**
♂ X+7th **S31.35** **Open bite of scrotum and testes**
Bite of scrotum and testes NOS
Excludes1: *superficial bite of scrotum and testes (S30.863, S30.873)*

+ **S31.4** **Open wound of vagina and vulva**
Excludes1: *injury to vagina and vulva during delivery (O70.-, O71.4)*
♀ X+7th **S31.40** **Unspecified open wound of vagina and vulva**
♀ X+7th **S31.41** **Laceration without foreign body of vagina and vulva**
♀ X+7th **S31.42** **Laceration with foreign body of vagina and vulva**
♀ X+7th **S31.43** **Puncture wound without foreign body of vagina and vulva**
♀ X+7th **S31.44** **Puncture wound with foreign body of vagina and vulva**
♀ X+7th **S31.45** **Open bite of vagina and vulva**
Bite of vagina and vulva NOS
Excludes1: *superficial bite of vagina and vulva (S30.864, S30.874)*

+ **S31.5** **Open wound of unspecified external genital organs**
Excludes1: *traumatic amputation of external genital organs (S38.21, S38.22)*

+ **S31.50** **Unspecified open wound of unspecified external genital organs**
♂ +7th **S31.501** **Unspecified open wound of unspecified external genital organs, male**
♀ +7th **S31.502** **Unspecified open wound of unspecified external genital organs, female**

+ **S31.51** **Laceration without foreign body of unspecified external genital organs**
♂ +7th **S31.511** **Laceration without foreign body of unspecified external genital organs, male**
♀ +7th **S31.512** **Laceration without foreign body of unspecified external genital organs, female**

+, +7th, X + 7th   ● Newborn   ● Pediatric   ● Maternity   ● Adult   ♀ Female   ♂ Male   Manifestation   Unacceptable PDX   HCC   CC   MCC   HAC

+ **S31.52** **Laceration with foreign body of unspecified external genital organs**

♂ +7th **S31.521** **Laceration with foreign body of unspecified external genital organs, male**

♀ +7th **S31.522** **Laceration with foreign body of unspecified external genital organs, female**

+ **S31.53** **Puncture wound without foreign body of unspecified external genital organs**

♂ +7th **S31.531** **Puncture wound without foreign body of unspecified external genital organs, male**

♀ +7th **S31.532** **Puncture wound without foreign body of unspecified external genital organs, female**

+ **S31.54** **Puncture wound with foreign body of unspecified external genital organs**

♂ +7th **S31.541** **Puncture wound with foreign body of unspecified external genital organs, male**

♀ +7th **S31.542** **Puncture wound with foreign body of unspecified external genital organs, female**

+ **S31.55** **Open bite of unspecified external genital organs**

Bite of unspecified external genital organs NOS

Excludes1: *superficial bite of unspecified external genital organs (S30.865, S30.866, S30.875, S30.876)*

♂ +7th **S31.551** **Open bite of unspecified external genital organs, male**

♀ +7th **S31.552** **Open bite of unspecified external genital organs, female**

+ **S31.6** **Open wound of abdominal wall with penetration into peritoneal cavity**

+ **S31.60** **Unspecified open wound of abdominal wall with penetration into peritoneal cavity**

MCC +7th **S31.600** **Unspecified open wound of abdominal wall, right upper quadrant with penetration into peritoneal cavity**

MCC +7th **S31.601** **Unspecified open wound of abdominal wall, left upper quadrant with penetration into peritoneal cavity**

MCC +7th **S31.602** **Unspecified open wound of abdominal wall, epigastric region with penetration into peritoneal cavity**

MCC +7th **S31.603** **Unspecified open wound of abdominal wall, right lower quadrant with penetration into peritoneal cavity**

MCC +7th **S31.604** **Unspecified open wound of abdominal wall, left lower quadrant with penetration into peritoneal cavity**

MCC +7th **S31.605** **Unspecified open wound of abdominal wall, periumbilic region with penetration into peritoneal cavity**

MCC +7th **S31.609** **Unspecified open wound of abdominal wall, unspecified quadrant with penetration into peritoneal cavity**

+ **S31.61** **Laceration without foreign body of abdominal wall with penetration into peritoneal cavity**

MCC +7th **S31.610** **Laceration without foreign body of abdominal wall, right upper quadrant with penetration into peritoneal cavity**

MCC +7th **S31.611** **Laceration without foreign body of abdominal wall, left upper quadrant with penetration into peritoneal cavity**

MCC +7th **S31.612** **Laceration without foreign body of abdominal wall, epigastric region with penetration into peritoneal cavity**

MCC +7th **S31.613** **Laceration without foreign body of abdominal wall, right lower quadrant with penetration into peritoneal cavity**

AHA CC: 4Q, 2015, 37-38

MCC +7th **S31.614** **Laceration without foreign body of abdominal wall, left lower quadrant with penetration into peritoneal cavity**

MCC +7th **S31.615** **Laceration without foreign body of abdominal wall, periumbilic region with penetration into peritoneal cavity**

MCC +7th **S31.619** **Laceration without foreign body of abdominal wall, unspecified quadrant with penetration into peritoneal cavity**

+ **S31.62** **Laceration with foreign body of abdominal wall with penetration into peritoneal cavity**

MCC +7th **S31.620** **Laceration with foreign body of abdominal wall, right upper quadrant with penetration into peritoneal cavity**

MCC +7th **S31.621** **Laceration with foreign body of abdominal wall, left upper quadrant with penetration into peritoneal cavity**

MCC +7th **S31.622** **Laceration with foreign body of abdominal wall, epigastric region with penetration into peritoneal cavity**

MCC +7th **S31.623** **Laceration with foreign body of abdominal wall, right lower quadrant with penetration into peritoneal cavity**

MCC +7th **S31.624** **Laceration with foreign body of abdominal wall, left lower quadrant with penetration into peritoneal cavity**

MCC +7th **S31.625** **Laceration with foreign body of abdominal wall, periumbilic region with penetration into peritoneal cavity**

MCC +7th **S31.629** **Laceration with foreign body of abdominal wall, unspecified quadrant with penetration into peritoneal cavity**

+ **S31.63** **Puncture wound without foreign body of abdominal wall with penetration into peritoneal cavity**

MCC +7th **S31.630** **Puncture wound without foreign body of abdominal wall, right upper quadrant with penetration into peritoneal cavity**

MCC +7th **S31.631** **Puncture wound without foreign body of abdominal wall, left upper quadrant with penetration into peritoneal cavity**

MCC +7th **S31.632** **Puncture wound without foreign body of abdominal wall, epigastric region with penetration into peritoneal cavity**

MCC +7th **S31.633** **Puncture wound without foreign body of abdominal wall, right lower quadrant with penetration into peritoneal cavity**

MCC +7th **S31.634** **Puncture wound without foreign body of abdominal wall, left lower quadrant with penetration into peritoneal cavity**

MCC +7th **S31.635** **Puncture wound without foreign body of abdominal wall, periumbilic region with penetration into peritoneal cavity**

MCC +7th **S31.639** **Puncture wound without foreign body of abdominal wall, unspecified quadrant with penetration into peritoneal cavity**

+ **S31.64** **Puncture wound with foreign body of abdominal wall with penetration into peritoneal cavity**

MCC +7th **S31.640** **Puncture wound with foreign body of abdominal wall, right upper quadrant with penetration into peritoneal cavity**

MCC +7th **S31.641** **Puncture wound with foreign body of abdominal wall, left upper quadrant with penetration into peritoneal cavity**

MCC +7th **S31.642** **Puncture wound with foreign body of abdominal wall, epigastric region with penetration into peritoneal cavity**

MCC +7th **S31.643** **Puncture wound with foreign body of abdominal wall, right lower quadrant with penetration into peritoneal cavity**

MCC +7th **S31.644** **Puncture wound with foreign body of abdominal wall, left lower quadrant with penetration into peritoneal cavity**

+, +7th, X + 7th   • Newborn   • Pediatric   • Maternity   • Adult   ♀ Female   ♂ Male   Manifestation   Unacceptable PDX   HCC   CC   MCC   HAC

MCC +7th **S31.645** **Puncture wound with foreign body of abdominal wall, periumbilic region with penetration into peritoneal cavity**

MCC +7th **S31.649** **Puncture wound with foreign body of abdominal wall, unspecified quadrant with penetration into peritoneal cavity**

+ **S31.65** **Open bite of abdominal wall with penetration into peritoneal cavity**
   Excludes1: *superficial bite of abdominal wall (S30.861, S30.871)*

MCC +7th **S31.650** **Open bite of abdominal wall, right upper quadrant with penetration into peritoneal cavity**

MCC +7th **S31.651** **Open bite of abdominal wall, left upper quadrant with penetration into peritoneal cavity**

MCC +7th **S31.652** **Open bite of abdominal wall, epigastric region with penetration into peritoneal cavity**

MCC +7th **S31.653** **Open bite of abdominal wall, right lower quadrant with penetration into peritoneal cavity**

MCC +7th **S31.654** **Open bite of abdominal wall, left lower quadrant with penetration into peritoneal cavity**

MCC +7th **S31.655** **Open bite of abdominal wall, periumbilic region with penetration into peritoneal cavity**

MCC +7th **S31.659** **Open bite of abdominal wall, unspecified quadrant with penetration into peritoneal cavity**

+ **S31.8** **Open wound of other parts of abdomen, lower back and pelvis**

+ **S31.80** **Open wound of unspecified buttock**
   +7th **S31.801** **Laceration without foreign body of unspecified buttock**
   +7th **S31.802** **Laceration with foreign body of unspecified buttock**
   +7th **S31.803** **Puncture wound without foreign body of unspecified buttock**
   +7th **S31.804** **Puncture wound with foreign body of unspecified buttock**
   +7th **S31.805** **Open bite of unspecified buttock**
      Bite of buttock NOS
      Excludes1: *superficial bite of buttock (S30.870)*
   +7th **S31.809** **Unspecified open wound of unspecified buttock**

+ **S31.81** **Open wound of right buttock**
   +7th **S31.811** **Laceration without foreign body of right buttock**
   +7th **S31.812** **Laceration with foreign body of right buttock**
   +7th **S31.813** **Puncture wound without foreign body of right buttock**
   +7th **S31.814** **Puncture wound with foreign body of right buttock**
   +7th **S31.815** **Open bite of right buttock**
      Bite of right buttock NOS
      Excludes1: *superficial bite of buttock (S30.870)*
   +7th **S31.819** **Unspecified open wound of right buttock**

+ **S31.82** **Open wound of left buttock**
   +7th **S31.821** **Laceration without foreign body of left buttock**
   +7th **S31.822** **Laceration with foreign body of left buttock**
   +7th **S31.823** **Puncture wound without foreign body of left buttock**
   +7th **S31.824** **Puncture wound with foreign body of left buttock**
   +7th **S31.825** **Open bite of left buttock**
      Bite of left buttock NOS
      Excludes1: *superficial bite of buttock (S30.870)*
   +7th **S31.829** **Unspecified open wound of left buttock**

+ **S31.83** **Open wound of anus**
   +7th **S31.831** **Laceration without foreign body of anus**
   +7th **S31.832** **Laceration with foreign body of anus**
   +7th **S31.833** **Puncture wound without foreign body of anus**
   +7th **S31.834** **Puncture wound with foreign body of anus**
   +7th **S31.835** **Open bite of anus**
      Bite of anus NOS
      Excludes1: *superficial bite of anus (S30.877)*
   +7th **S31.839** **Unspecified open wound of anus**

See page 972 for Vertebrae Illustration.

S32 **Fracture of lumbar spine and pelvis**

   NOTE A fracture not indicated as displaced or nondisplaced should be coded to displaced
   A fracture not indicated as opened or closed should be coded to closed

   Includes: fracture of lumbosacral neural arch
   fracture of lumbosacral spinous process
   fracture of lumbosacral transverse process
   fracture of lumbosacral vertebra
   fracture of lumbosacral vertebral arch

   Code first any associated spinal cord and spinal nerve injury (S34.-)
   Excludes1: *transection of abdomen (S38.3)*
   Excludes2: *fracture of hip NOS (S72.0-)*

   The appropriate 7th character is to be added to each code from category S32
   A initial encounter for closed fracture
   B initial encounter for open fracture
   D subsequent encounter for fracture with routine healing
   G subsequent encounter for fracture with delayed healing
   K subsequent encounter for fracture with nonunion
   S sequela

   Review coding guideline C.19.c

+ **S32.0** **Fracture of lumbar vertebra**
   Fracture of lumbar spine NOS

   + **S32.00** **Fracture of unspecified lumbar vertebra**
   CC MCC +7th **S32.000** **Wedge compression fracture of unspecified lumbar vertebra**
      HAC 7th characters A & B see Appendix B for HAC conditional logic

   CC MCC +7th **S32.001** **Stable burst fracture of unspecified lumbar vertebra**
      HAC 7th characters A & B see Appendix B for HAC conditional logic

   CC MCC +7th **S32.002** **Unstable burst fracture of unspecified lumbar vertebra**
      HAC 7th characters A & B see Appendix B for HAC conditional logic

   CC MCC +7th **S32.008** **Other fracture of unspecified lumbar vertebra**
      HAC 7th characters A & B see Appendix B for HAC conditional logic

   CC MCC +7th **S32.009** **Unspecified fracture of unspecified lumbar vertebra**
      HAC 7th characters A & B see Appendix B for HAC conditional logic

   + **S32.01** **Fracture of first lumbar vertebra**
   CC MCC +7th **S32.010** **Wedge compression fracture of first lumbar vertebra**
      HAC 7th characters A & B see Appendix B for HAC conditional logic

   CC MCC +7th **S32.011** **Stable burst fracture of first lumbar vertebra**
      HAC 7th characters A & B see Appendix B for HAC conditional logic

   CC MCC +7th **S32.012** **Unstable burst fracture of first lumbar vertebra**
      HAC 7th characters A & B see Appendix B for HAC conditional logic

   CC MCC +7th **S32.018** **Other fracture of first lumbar vertebra**
      HAC 7th characters A & B see Appendix B for HAC conditional logic

   CC MCC +7th **S32.019** **Unspecified fracture of first lumbar vertebra**
      HAC 7th characters A & B see Appendix B for HAC conditional logic

+ S32.02 Fracture of second lumbar vertebra

CC MCC +7th **S32.020 Wedge compression fracture of second lumbar vertebra**
HAC 7th characters A & B see Appendix B for HAC conditional logic

CC MCC +7th **S32.021 Stable burst fracture of second lumbar vertebra**
HAC 7th characters A & B see Appendix B for HAC conditional logic

CC MCC +7th **S32.022 Unstable burst fracture of second lumbar vertebra**
HAC 7th characters A & B see Appendix B for HAC conditional logic

CC MCC +7th **S32.028 Other fracture of second lumbar vertebra**
HAC 7th characters A & B see Appendix B for HAC conditional logic

CC MCC +7th **S32.029 Unspecified fracture of second lumbar vertebra**
HAC 7th characters A & B see Appendix B for HAC conditional logic

+ S32.03 Fracture of third lumbar vertebra

CC MCC +7th **S32.030 Wedge compression fracture of third lumbar vertebra**
HAC 7th characters A & B see Appendix B for HAC conditional logic

CC MCC +7th **S32.031 Stable burst fracture of third lumbar vertebra**
HAC 7th characters A & B see Appendix B for HAC conditional logic

CC MCC +7th **S32.032 Unstable burst fracture of third lumbar vertebra**
HAC 7th characters A & B see Appendix B for HAC conditional logic

CC MCC +7th **S32.038 Other fracture of third lumbar vertebra**
HAC 7th characters A & B see Appendix B for HAC conditional logic

CC MCC +7th **S32.039 Unspecified fracture of third lumbar vertebra**
HAC 7th characters A & B see Appendix B for HAC conditional logic

+ S32.04 Fracture of fourth lumbar vertebra

CC MCC +7th **S32.040 Wedge compression fracture of fourth lumbar vertebra**
HAC 7th characters A & B see Appendix B for HAC conditional logic

CC MCC +7th **S32.041 Stable burst fracture of fourth lumbar vertebra**
HAC 7th characters A & B see Appendix B for HAC conditional logic

CC MCC +7th **S32.042 Unstable burst fracture of fourth lumbar vertebra**
HAC 7th characters A & B see Appendix B for HAC conditional logic

CC MCC +7th **S32.048 Other fracture of fourth lumbar vertebra**
HAC 7th characters A & B see Appendix B for HAC conditional logic

CC MCC +7th **S32.049 Unspecified fracture of fourth lumbar vertebra**
HAC 7th characters A & B see Appendix B for HAC conditional logic

+ S32.05 Fracture of fifth lumbar vertebra

CC MCC +7th **S32.050 Wedge compression fracture of fifth lumbar vertebra**
HAC 7th characters A & B see Appendix B for HAC conditional logic

CC MCC +7th **S32.051 Stable burst fracture of fifth lumbar vertebra**
HAC 7th characters A & B see Appendix B for HAC conditional logic

CC MCC +7th **S32.052 Unstable burst fracture of fifth lumbar vertebra**
HAC 7th characters A & B see Appendix B for HAC conditional logic

CC MCC +7th **S32.058 Other fracture of fifth lumbar vertebra**
HAC 7th characters A & B see Appendix B for HAC conditional logic

CC MCC +7th **S32.059 Unspecified fracture of fifth lumbar vertebra**
HAC 7th characters A & B see Appendix B for HAC conditional logic

+ S32.1 Fracture of sacrum
NOTE For vertical fractures, code to most medial fracture extension
Use two codes if both a vertical and transverse fracture are present

Code also any associated fracture of pelvic ring (S32.8-)

CC MCC X+7th **S32.10 Unspecified fracture of sacrum**
HAC 7th characters A & B see Appendix B for HAC conditional logic

+ S32.11 Zone I fracture of sacrum
Vertical sacral ala fracture of sacrum

CC MCC +7th **S32.110 Nondisplaced Zone I fracture of sacrum**
HAC 7th characters A & B see Appendix B for HAC conditional logic

CC MCC +7th **S32.111 Minimally displaced Zone I fracture of sacrum**
HAC 7th characters A & B see Appendix B for HAC conditional logic

CC MCC +7th **S32.112 Severely displaced Zone I fracture of sacrum**
HAC 7th characters A & B see Appendix B for HAC conditional logic

CC MCC +7th **S32.119 Unspecified Zone I fracture of sacrum**
HAC 7th characters A & B see Appendix B for HAC conditional logic

+ S32.12 Zone II fracture of sacrum
Vertical foraminal region fracture of sacrum

CC MCC +7th **S32.120 Nondisplaced Zone II fracture of sacrum**
HAC 7th characters A & B see Appendix B for HAC conditional logic

CC MCC +7th **S32.121 Minimally displaced Zone II fracture of sacrum**
HAC 7th characters A & B see Appendix B for HAC conditional logic

CC MCC +7th **S32.122 Severely displaced Zone II fracture of sacrum**
HAC 7th characters A & B see Appendix B for HAC conditional logic

CC MCC +7th **S32.129 Unspecified Zone II fracture of sacrum**
HAC 7th characters A & B see Appendix B for HAC conditional logic

+ S32.13 Zone III fracture of sacrum
Vertical fracture into spinal canal region of sacrum

CC MCC +7th **S32.130 Nondisplaced Zone III fracture of sacrum**
HAC 7th characters A & B see Appendix B for HAC conditional logic

CC MCC +7th **S32.131 Minimally displaced Zone III fracture of sacrum**
HAC 7th characters A & B see Appendix B for HAC conditional logic

CC MCC +7th **S32.132 Severely displaced Zone III fracture of sacrum**
HAC 7th characters A & B see Appendix B for HAC conditional logic

CC MCC +7th **S32.139 Unspecified Zone III fracture of sacrum**
HAC 7th characters A & B see Appendix B for HAC conditional logic

CC MCC X+7th **S32.14 Type 1 fracture of sacrum**
Transverse flexion fracture of sacrum without displacement
HAC 7th characters A & B see Appendix B for HAC conditional logic

CC MCC X+7th **S32.15 Type 2 fracture of sacrum**
Transverse flexion fracture of sacrum with posterior displacement
HAC 7th characters A & B see Appendix B for HAC conditional logic

CC MCC X+7th **S32.16 Type 3 fracture of sacrum**
Transverse extension fracture of sacrum with anterior displacement
HAC 7th characters A & B see Appendix B for HAC conditional logic

CC MCC X+7th **S32.17 Type 4 fracture of sacrum**
Transverse segmental comminution of upper sacrum
HAC 7th characters A & B see Appendix B for HAC conditional logic

CC MCC X+7th **S32.19 Other fracture of sacrum**
HAC 7th characters A & B see Appendix B for HAC conditional logic

+, +7th, X + 7th   ● Newborn   ● Pediatric   ● Maternity   ● Adult   ♀ Female   ♂ Male   Manifestation   Unacceptable PDX   HCC   CC   MCC   HAC

X+7th **S32.2** **Fracture of coccyx**
HAC 7th characters A & B see Appendix B for HAC conditional logic

+ **S32.3** **Fracture of ilium**
Excludes1: fracture of ilium with associated disruption of pelvic ring (S32.8-)

+ **S32.30** **Unspecified fracture of ilium**
CC MCC +7th **S32.301** **Unspecified fracture of right ilium**
HAC 7th characters A & B see Appendix B for HAC conditional logic

CC MCC +7th **S32.302** **Unspecified fracture of left ilium**
HAC 7th characters A & B see Appendix B for HAC conditional logic

CC MCC +7th **S32.309** **Unspecified fracture of unspecified ilium**
HAC 7th characters A & B see Appendix B for HAC conditional logic

+ **S32.31** **Avulsion fracture of ilium**
CC MCC +7th **S32.311** **Displaced avulsion fracture of right ilium**
HAC 7th characters A & B see Appendix B for HAC conditional logic

CC MCC +7th **S32.312** **Displaced avulsion fracture of left ilium**
HAC 7th characters A & B see Appendix B for HAC conditional logic

CC MCC +7th **S32.313** **Displaced avulsion fracture of unspecified ilium**
HAC 7th characters A & B see Appendix B for HAC conditional logic

CC MCC +7th **S32.314** **Nondisplaced avulsion fracture of right ilium**
HAC 7th characters A & B see Appendix B for HAC conditional logic

CC MCC +7th **S32.315** **Nondisplaced avulsion fracture of left ilium**
HAC 7th characters A & B see Appendix B for HAC conditional logic

CC MCC +7th **S32.316** **Nondisplaced avulsion fracture of unspecified ilium**
HAC 7th characters A & B see Appendix B for HAC conditional logic

+ **S32.39** **Other fracture of ilium**
CC MCC +7th **S32.391** **Other fracture of right ilium**
HAC 7th characters A & B see Appendix B for HAC conditional logic

CC MCC +7th **S32.392** **Other fracture of left ilium**
HAC 7th characters A & B see Appendix B for HAC conditional logic

CC MCC +7th **S32.399** **Other fracture of unspecified ilium**
HAC 7th characters A & B see Appendix B for HAC conditional logic

+ **S32.4** **Fracture of acetabulum**
Code also any associated fracture of pelvic ring (S32.8-)

+ **S32.40** **Unspecified fracture of acetabulum**
CC +7th **S32.401** **Unspecified fracture of right acetabulum**
HAC 7th characters A & B see Appendix B for HAC conditional logic

CC +7th **S32.402** **Unspecified fracture of left acetabulum**
HAC 7th characters A & B see Appendix B for HAC conditional logic

CC +7th **S32.409** **Unspecified fracture of unspecified acetabulum**
HAC 7th characters A & B see Appendix B for HAC conditional logic

S32.41 **Fracture of anterior wall of acetabulum**
CC MCC +7th **S32.411** **Displaced fracture of anterior wall of right acetabulum**
HAC 7th characters A & B see Appendix B for HAC conditional logic

CC MCC +7th **S32.412** **Displaced fracture of anterior wall of left acetabulum**
HAC 7th characters A & B see Appendix B for HAC conditional logic

CC MCC +7th **S32.413** **Displaced fracture of anterior wall of unspecified acetabulum**
HAC 7th characters A & B see Appendix B for HAC conditional logic

CC MCC +7th **S32.414** **Nondisplaced fracture of anterior wall of right acetabulum**
HAC 7th characters A & B see Appendix B for HAC conditional logic

CC MCC +7th **S32.415** **Nondisplaced fracture of anterior wall of left acetabulum**
HAC 7th characters A & B see Appendix B for HAC conditional logic

CC MCC +7th **S32.416** **Nondisplaced fracture of anterior wall of unspecified acetabulum**
HAC 7th characters A & B see Appendix B for HAC conditional logic

+ **S32.42** **Fracture of posterior wall of acetabulum**
CC MCC +7th **S32.421** **Displaced fracture of posterior wall of right acetabulum**
HAC 7th characters A & B see Appendix B for HAC conditional logic

CC MCC +7th **S32.422** **Displaced fracture of posterior wall of left acetabulum**
HAC 7th characters A & B see Appendix B for HAC conditional logic

CC MCC +7th **S32.423** **Displaced fracture of posterior wall of unspecified acetabulum**
HAC 7th characters A & B see Appendix B for HAC conditional logic

CC MCC +7th **S32.424** **Nondisplaced fracture of posterior wall of right acetabulum**
HAC 7th characters A & B see Appendix B for HAC conditional logic

CC MCC +7th **S32.425** **Nondisplaced fracture of posterior wall of left acetabulum**
HAC 7th characters A & B see Appendix B for HAC conditional logic

CC MCC +7th **S32.426** **Nondisplaced fracture of posterior wall of unspecified acetabulum**
HAC 7th characters A & B see Appendix B for HAC conditional logic

+ **S32.43** **Fracture of anterior column [iliopubic] of acetabulum**
CC MCC +7th **S32.431** **Displaced fracture of anterior column [iliopubic] of right acetabulum**
HAC 7th characters A & B see Appendix B for HAC conditional logic

CC MCC +7th **S32.432** **Displaced fracture of anterior column [iliopubic] of left acetabulum**
HAC 7th characters A & B see Appendix B for HAC conditional logic

CC MCC +7th **S32.433** **Displaced fracture of anterior column [iliopubic] of unspecified acetabulum**
HAC 7th characters A & B see Appendix B for HAC conditional logic

CC MCC +7th **S32.434** **Nondisplaced fracture of anterior column [iliopubic] of right acetabulum**
HAC 7th characters A & B see Appendix B for HAC conditional logic

CC MCC +7th **S32.435** **Nondisplaced fracture of anterior column [iliopubic] of left acetabulum**
HAC 7th characters A & B see Appendix B for HAC conditional logic

CC MCC +7th **S32.436** **Nondisplaced fracture of anterior column [iliopubic] of unspecified acetabulum**
HAC 7th characters A & B see Appendix B for HAC conditional logic

+ **S32.44** **Fracture of posterior column [ilioischial] of acetabulum**
CC MCC +7th **S32.441** **Displaced fracture of posterior column [ilioischial] of right acetabulum**
HAC 7th characters A & B see Appendix B for HAC conditional logic

CC MCC +7th **S32.442** **Displaced fracture of posterior column [ilioischial] of left acetabulum**
HAC 7th characters A & B see Appendix B for HAC conditional logic

CC MCC +7th **S32.443** **Displaced fracture of posterior column [ilioischial] of unspecified acetabulum**
HAC 7th characters A & B see Appendix B for HAC conditional logic

CC MCC +7th **S32.444** **Nondisplaced fracture of posterior column [ilioischial] of right acetabulum**
HAC 7th characters A & B see Appendix B for HAC conditional logic

+, +7th, X + 7th • Newborn • Pediatric • Maternity • Adult ♀ Female ♂ Male Manifestation Unacceptable PDX HCC CC MCC HAC

CC MCC +7th **S32.445** **Nondisplaced fracture of posterior column [ilioischial] of left acetabulum**
　　HAC 7th characters A & B see Appendix B for HAC conditional logic

CC MCC +7th **S32.446** **Nondisplaced fracture of posterior column [ilioischial] of unspecified acetabulum**
　　HAC 7th characters A & B see Appendix B for HAC conditional logic

+ **S32.45** **Transverse fracture of acetabulum**

CC MCC +7th **S32.451** **Displaced transverse fracture of right acetabulum**
　　HAC 7th characters A & B see Appendix B for HAC conditional logic

CC MCC +7th **S32.452** **Displaced transverse fracture of left acetabulum**
　　HAC 7th characters A & B see Appendix B for HAC conditional logic

CC MCC +7th **S32.453** **Displaced transverse fracture of unspecified acetabulum**
　　HAC 7th characters A & B see Appendix B for HAC conditional logic

CC MCC +7th **S32.454** **Nondisplaced transverse fracture of right acetabulum**
　　HAC 7th characters A & B see Appendix B for HAC conditional logic

CC MCC +7th **S32.455** **Nondisplaced transverse fracture of left acetabulum**
　　HAC 7th characters A & B see Appendix B for HAC conditional logic

CC MCC +7th **S32.456** **Nondisplaced transverse fracture of unspecified acetabulum**
　　HAC 7th characters A & B see Appendix B for HAC conditional logic

+ **S32.46** **Associated transverse-posterior fracture of acetabulum**

CC MCC +7th **S32.461** **Displaced associated transverse-posterior fracture of right acetabulum**
　　HAC 7th characters A & B see Appendix B for HAC conditional logic

CC MCC +7th **S32.462** **Displaced associated transverse-posterior fracture of left acetabulum**
　　HAC 7th characters A & B see Appendix B for HAC conditional logic

CC MCC +7th **S32.463** **Displaced associated transverse-posterior fracture of unspecified acetabulum**
　　HAC 7th characters A & B see Appendix B for HAC conditional logic

CC MCC +7th **S32.464** **Nondisplaced associated transverse-posterior fracture of right acetabulum**
　　HAC 7th characters A & B see Appendix B for HAC conditional logic

CC MCC +7th **S32.465** **Nondisplaced associated transverse-posterior fracture of left acetabulum**
　　HAC 7th characters A & B see Appendix B for HAC conditional logic

CC MCC +7th **S32.466** **Nondisplaced associated transverse-posterior fracture of unspecified acetabulum**
　　HAC 7th characters A & B see Appendix B for HAC conditional logic

+ **S32.47** **Fracture of medial wall of acetabulum**

CC MCC +7th **S32.471** **Displaced fracture of medial wall of right acetabulum**
　　HAC 7th characters A & B see Appendix B for HAC conditional logic

CC MCC +7th **S32.472** **Displaced fracture of medial wall of left acetabulum**
　　HAC 7th characters A & B see Appendix B for HAC conditional logic

CC MCC +7th **S32.473** **Displaced fracture of medial wall of unspecified acetabulum**
　　HAC 7th characters A & B see Appendix B for HAC conditional logic

CC MCC +7th **S32.474** **Nondisplaced fracture of medial wall of right acetabulum**
　　HAC 7th characters A & B see Appendix B for HAC conditional logic

CC MCC +7th **S32.475** **Nondisplaced fracture of medial wall of left acetabulum**
　　HAC 7th characters A & B see Appendix B for HAC conditional logic

CC MCC +7th **S32.476** **Nondisplaced fracture of medial wall of unspecified acetabulum**
　　HAC 7th characters A & B see Appendix B for HAC conditional logic

+ **S32.48** **Dome fracture of acetabulum**

CC MCC +7th **S32.481** **Displaced dome fracture of right acetabulum**
　　HAC 7th characters A & B see Appendix B for HAC conditional logic

CC MCC +7th **S32.482** **Displaced dome fracture of left acetabulum**
　　HAC 7th characters A & B see Appendix B for HAC conditional logic

CC MCC +7th **S32.483** **Displaced dome fracture of unspecified acetabulum**
　　HAC 7th characters A & B see Appendix B for HAC conditional logic

CC MCC +7th **S32.484** **Nondisplaced dome fracture of right acetabulum**
　　HAC 7th characters A & B see Appendix B for HAC conditional logic

CC MCC +7th **S32.485** **Nondisplaced dome fracture of left acetabulum**
　　HAC 7th characters A & B see Appendix B for HAC conditional logic

CC MCC +7th **S32.486** **Nondisplaced dome fracture of unspecified acetabulum**
　　HAC 7th characters A & B see Appendix B for HAC conditional logic

+ **S32.49** **Other specified fracture of acetabulum**

CC MCC +7th **S32.491** **Other specified fracture of right acetabulum**
　　HAC 7th characters A & B see Appendix B for HAC conditional logic

CC MCC +7th **S32.492** **Other specified fracture of left acetabulum**
　　HAC 7th characters A & B see Appendix B for HAC conditional logic

CC MCC +7th **S32.499** **Other specified fracture of unspecified acetabulum**
　　HAC 7th characters A & B see Appendix B for HAC conditional logic

+ **S32.5** **Fracture of pubis**
　Excludes1: *fracture of pubis with associated disruption of pelvic ring (S32.8-)*

+ **S32.50** **Unspecified fracture of pubis**

CC MCC +7th **S32.501** **Unspecified fracture of right pubis**
　　HAC 7th characters A & B see Appendix B for HAC conditional logic

CC MCC +7th **S32.502** **Unspecified fracture of left pubis**
　　HAC 7th characters A & B see Appendix B for HAC conditional logic

CC MCC +7th **S32.509** **Unspecified fracture of unspecified pubis**
　　HAC 7th characters A & B see Appendix B for HAC conditional logic

+ **S32.51** **Fracture of superior rim of pubis**

CC MCC +7th **S32.511** **Fracture of superior rim of right pubis**
　　HAC 7th characters A & B see Appendix B for HAC conditional logic

CC MCC +7th **S32.512** **Fracture of superior rim of left pubis**
　　HAC 7th characters A & B see Appendix B for HAC conditional logic

CC MCC +7th **S32.519** **Fracture of superior rim of unspecified pubis**
　　HAC 7th characters A & B see Appendix B for HAC conditional logic

+ **S32.59** **Other specified fracture of pubis**

CC MCC +7th **S32.591** **Other specified fracture of right pubis**
　　HAC 7th characters A & B see Appendix B for HAC conditional logic

CC MCC +7th **S32.592** **Other specified fracture of left pubis**
　　HAC 7th characters A & B see Appendix B for HAC conditional logic

CC MCC +7th **S32.599** **Other specified fracture of unspecified pubis**
　　HAC 7th characters A & B see Appendix B for HAC conditional logic

+ **S32.6** **Fracture of ischium**
　Excludes1: *fracture of ischium with associated disruption of pelvic ring (S32.8-)*

+ **S32.60** **Unspecified fracture of ischium**

CC MCC +7th **S32.601** **Unspecified fracture of right ischium**
　　HAC 7th characters A & B see Appendix B for HAC conditional logic

+, +7th, X + 7th　● Newborn　● Pediatric　● Maternity　● Adult　♀ Female　♂ Male　Manifestation　Unacceptable PDX　HCC　CC　MCC　HAC

CC MCC +7th **S32.602** **Unspecified fracture of left ischium**
> HAC 7th characters A & B see Appendix B for HAC conditional logic

CC MCC +7th **S32.609** **Unspecified fracture of unspecified ischium**
> HAC 7th characters A & B see Appendix B for HAC conditional logic

+ **S32.61** **Avulsion fracture of ischium**

CC MCC +7th **S32.611** **Displaced avulsion fracture of right ischium**
> HAC 7th characters A & B see Appendix B for HAC conditional logic

CC MCC +7th **S32.612** **Displaced avulsion fracture of left ischium**
> HAC 7th characters A & B see Appendix B for HAC conditional logic

CC MCC +7th **S32.613** **Displaced avulsion fracture of unspecified ischium**
> HAC 7th characters A & B see Appendix B for HAC conditional logic

CC MCC +7th **S32.614** **Nondisplaced avulsion fracture of right ischium**
> HAC 7th characters A & B see Appendix B for HAC conditional logic

CC MCC +7th **S32.615** **Nondisplaced avulsion fracture of left ischium**
> HAC 7th characters A & B see Appendix B for HAC conditional logic

CC MCC +7th **S32.616** **Nondisplaced avulsion fracture of unspecified ischium**
> HAC 7th characters A & B see Appendix B for HAC conditional logic

+ **S32.69** **Other specified fracture of ischium**

CC MCC +7th **S32.691** **Other specified fracture of right ischium**
> HAC 7th characters A & B see Appendix B for HAC conditional logic

CC MCC +7th **S32.692** **Other specified fracture of left ischium**
> HAC 7th characters A & B see Appendix B for HAC conditional logic

+ **S32.8** **Fracture of other parts of pelvis**
> Code also any associated:
> fracture of acetabulum (S32.4-)
> sacral fracture (S32.1-)

+ **S32.81** **Multiple fractures of pelvis with disruption of pelvic ring**
> Multiple pelvic fractures with disruption of pelvic circle

CC MCC +7th **S32.810** **Multiple fractures of pelvis with stable disruption of pelvic ring**
> HAC 7th characters A & B see Appendix B for HAC conditional logic

CC MCC +7th **S32.811** **Multiple fractures of pelvis with unstable disruption of pelvic ring**
> HAC 7th characters A & B see Appendix B for HAC conditional logic

CC MCC X+7th **S32.82** **Multiple fractures of pelvis without disruption of pelvic ring**
> Multiple pelvic fractures without disruption of pelvic circle
> HAC 7th characters A & B see Appendix B for HAC conditional logic

CC MCC X+7th **S32.89** **Fracture of other parts of pelvis**
> HAC 7th characters A & B see Appendix B for HAC conditional logic

X+7th **S32.9** **Fracture of unspecified parts of lumbosacral spine and pelvis**
MCC
CC
> Fracture of lumbosacral spine NOS
> Fracture of pelvis NOS
> HAC 7th characters A & B see Appendix B for HAC conditional logic

S33 **Dislocation and sprain of joints and ligaments of lumbar spine and pelvis**

Includes: avulsion of joint or ligament of lumbar spine and pelvis
laceration of cartilage, joint or ligament of lumbar spine and pelvis
sprain of cartilage, joint or ligament of lumbar spine and pelvis
traumatic hemarthrosis of joint or ligament of lumbar spine and pelvis
traumatic rupture of joint or ligament of lumbar spine and pelvis
traumatic subluxation of joint or ligament of lumbar spine and pelvis
traumatic tear of joint or ligament of lumbar spine and pelvis

Code also any associated open wound

Excludes1: *nontraumatic rupture or displacement of lumbar intervertebral disc NOS (M51.-)*
obstetric damage to pelvic joints and ligaments (O71.6)

Excludes2: *dislocation and sprain of joints and ligaments of hip (S73.-)*
strain of muscle of lower back and pelvis (S39.01-)

The appropriate 7th character is to be added to each code from category S33
A   initial encounter
D   subsequent encounter
S   sequela

X+7th **S33.0** **Traumatic rupture of lumbar intervertebral disc**
> ***Excludes1:*** *rupture or displacement (nontraumatic) of lumbar intervertebral disc NOS (M51.- with fifth character 6)*

+ **S33.1** **Subluxation and dislocation of lumbar vertebra**
> Code also any associated:
> open wound of abdomen, lower back and pelvis (S31)
> spinal cord injury (S24.0, S24.1-, S34.0-, S34.1-)
> ***Excludes2:*** *fracture of lumbar vertebrae (S32.0-)*

+ **S33.10** **Subluxation and dislocation of unspecified lumbar vertebra**

+7th **S33.100** **Subluxation of unspecified lumbar vertebra**

+7th **S33.101** **Dislocation of unspecified lumbar vertebra**

+ **S33.11** **Subluxation and dislocation of L1/L2 lumbar vertebra**

+7th **S33.110** **Subluxation of L1/L2 lumbar vertebra**

+7th **S33.111** **Dislocation of L1/L2 lumbar vertebra**

+ **S33.12** **Subluxation and dislocation of L2/L3 lumbar vertebra**

+7th **S33.120** **Subluxation of L2/L3 lumbar vertebra**

+7th **S33.121** **Dislocation of L2/L3 lumbar vertebra**

+ **S33.13** **Subluxation and dislocation of L3/L4 lumbar vertebra**

+7th **S33.130** **Subluxation of L3/L4 lumbar vertebra**

+7th **S33.131** **Dislocation of L3/L4 lumbar vertebra**

+ **S33.14** **Subluxation and dislocation of L4/L5 lumbar vertebra**

+7th **S33.140** **Subluxation of L4/L5 lumbar vertebra**

+7th **S33.141** **Dislocation of L4/L5 lumbar vertebra**

X+7th **S33.2** **Dislocation of sacroiliac and sacrococcygeal joint**

+ **S33.3** **Dislocation of other and unspecified parts of lumbar spine and pelvis**

X+7th **S33.30** **Dislocation of unspecified parts of lumbar spine and pelvis**

X+7th **S33.39** **Dislocation of other parts of lumbar spine and pelvis**

X+7th **S33.4** **Traumatic rupture of symphysis pubis**

X+7th **S33.5** **Sprain of ligaments of lumbar spine**

X+7th **S33.6** **Sprain of sacroiliac joint**

X+7th **S33.8** **Sprain of other parts of lumbar spine and pelvis**

X+7th **S33.9** **Sprain of unspecified parts of lumbar spine and pelvis**

S34 **Injury of lumbar and sacral spinal cord and nerves at abdomen, lower back and pelvis level**

> **NOTE** Code to highest level of lumbar cord injury
> Injuries to the spinal cord (S34.0 and S34.1) refer to the cord level and not bone level injury, and can affect nerve roots at and below the level given.

Code also any associated:
    fracture of vertebra (S22.0-, S32.0-)
    open wound of abdomen, lower back and pelvis (S31.-)
    transient paralysis (R29.5)

> The appropriate 7th character is to be added to each code from category S34
> A   initial encounter
> D   subsequent encounter
> S   sequela

+ **S34.0** **Concussion and edema of lumbar and sacral spinal cord**
MCC X+7th **S34.01** **Concussion and edema of lumbar spinal cord**
MCC X+7th **S34.02** **Concussion and edema of sacral spinal cord**
    Concussion and edema of conus medullaris
+ **S34.1** **Other and unspecified injury of lumbar and sacral spinal cord**
  + **S34.10** **Unspecified injury to lumbar spinal cord**
  MCC +7th **S34.101** **Unspecified injury to L1 level of lumbar spinal cord**
    Unspecified injury to lumbar spinal cord level 1
    HAC 7th character A see Appendix B for HAC conditional logic
  MCC +7th **S34.102** **Unspecified injury to L2 level of lumbar spinal cord**
    Unspecified injury to lumbar spinal cord level 2
    HAC 7th character A see Appendix B for HAC conditional logic
  MCC +7th **S34.103** **Unspecified injury to L3 level of lumbar spinal cord**
    Unspecified injury to lumbar spinal cord level 3
    HAC 7th character A see Appendix B for HAC conditional logic
  MCC +7th **S34.104** **Unspecified injury to L4 level of lumbar spinal cord**
    Unspecified injury to lumbar spinal cord level 4
    HAC 7th character A see Appendix B for HAC conditional logic
  MCC +7th **S34.105** **Unspecified injury to L5 level of lumbar spinal cord**
    Unspecified injury to lumbar spinal cord level 5
    HAC 7th character A see Appendix B for HAC conditional logic
  MCC +7th **S34.109** **Unspecified injury to unspecified level of lumbar spinal cord**
    HAC 7th character A see Appendix B for HAC conditional logic
  + **S34.11** **Complete lesion of lumbar spinal cord**
  MCC +7th **S34.111** **Complete lesion of L1 level of lumbar spinal cord**
    Complete lesion of lumbar spinal cord level 1
    HAC 7th character A see Appendix B for HAC conditional logic
  MCC +7th **S34.112** **Complete lesion of L2 level of lumbar spinal cord**
    Complete lesion of lumbar spinal cord level 2
    HAC 7th character A see Appendix B for HAC conditional logic
  MCC +7th **S34.113** **Complete lesion of L3 level of lumbar spinal cord**
    Complete lesion of lumbar spinal cord level 3
    HAC 7th character A see Appendix B for HAC conditional logic
  MCC +7th **S34.114** **Complete lesion of L4 level of lumbar spinal cord**
    Complete lesion of lumbar spinal cord level 4
    HAC 7th character A see Appendix B for HAC conditional logic

MCC +7th **S34.115** **Complete lesion of L5 level of lumbar spinal cord**
    Complete lesion of lumbar spinal cord level 5
    HAC 7th character A see Appendix B for HAC conditional logic
MCC +7th **S34.119** **Complete lesion of unspecified level of lumbar spinal cord**
    HAC 7th character A see Appendix B for HAC conditional logic
+ **S34.12** **Incomplete lesion of lumbar spinal cord**
MCC +7th **S34.121** **Incomplete lesion of L1 level of lumbar spinal cord**
    Incomplete lesion of lumbar spinal cord level 1
    HAC 7th character A see Appendix B for HAC conditional logic
MCC +7th **S34.122** **Incomplete lesion of L2 level of lumbar spinal cord**
    Incomplete lesion of lumbar spinal cord level 2
    HAC 7th character A see Appendix B for HAC conditional logic
MCC +7th **S34.123** **Incomplete lesion of L3 level of lumbar spinal cord**
    Incomplete lesion of lumbar spinal cord level 3
    HAC 7th character A see Appendix B for HAC conditional logic
MCC +7th **S34.124** **Incomplete lesion of L4 level of lumbar spinal cord**
    Incomplete lesion of lumbar spinal cord level 4
    HAC 7th character A see Appendix B for HAC conditional logic
MCC +7th **S34.125** **Incomplete lesion of L5 level of lumbar spinal cord**
    Incomplete lesion of lumbar spinal cord level 5
    HAC 7th character A see Appendix B for HAC conditional logic
MCC +7th **S34.129** **Incomplete lesion of unspecified level of lumbar spinal cord**
    HAC 7th character A see Appendix B for HAC conditional logic
+ **S34.13** **Other and unspecified injury to sacral spinal cord**
    Other injury to conus medullaris
MCC +7th **S34.131** **Complete lesion of sacral spinal cord**
    Complete lesion of conus medullaris
    HAC 7th character A see Appendix B for HAC conditional logic
MCC +7th **S34.132** **Incomplete lesion of sacral spinal cord**
    Incomplete lesion of conus medullaris
    HAC 7th character A see Appendix B for HAC conditional logic
MCC +7th **S34.139** **Unspecified injury to sacral spinal cord**
    Unspecified injury of conus medullaris
    HAC 7th character A see Appendix B for HAC conditional logic
+ **S34.2** **Injury of nerve root of lumbar and sacral spine**
X+7th **S34.21** **Injury of nerve root of lumbar spine**
X+7th **S34.22** **Injury of nerve root of sacral spine**
MCC X+7th **S34.3** **Injury of cauda equina**
    HAC 7th character A see Appendix B for HAC conditional logic
X+7th **S34.4** **Injury of lumbosacral plexus**
X+7th **S34.5** **Injury of lumbar, sacral and pelvic sympathetic nerves**
    Injury of celiac ganglion or plexus
    Injury of hypogastric plexus
    Injury of mesenteric plexus (inferior) (superior)
    Injury of splanchnic nerve
X+7th **S34.6** **Injury of peripheral nerve(s) at abdomen, lower back and pelvis level**
X+7th **S34.8** **Injury of other nerves at abdomen, lower back and pelvis level**
X+7th **S34.9** **Injury of unspecified nerves at abdomen, lower back and pelvis level**

S35 **Injury of blood vessels at abdomen, lower back and pelvis level**

Code also any associated open wound (S31.-)

> The appropriate 7th character is to be added to each code from category S35
> A   initial encounter
> D   subsequent encounter
> S   sequela

+, +7th, X + 7th   ● Newborn   ● Pediatric   ● Maternity   ● Adult   ♀ Female   ♂ Male   Manifestation   Unacceptable PDX   HCC   CC   MCC   HAC

+ **S35.0   Injury of abdominal aorta**
Excludes1: injury of aorta NOS (S25.0)
MCC X+7th **S35.00   Unspecified injury of abdominal aorta**
MCC X+7th **S35.01   Minor laceration of abdominal aorta**
　　　　Incomplete transection of abdominal aorta
　　　　Laceration of abdominal aorta NOS
　　　　Superficial laceration of abdominal aorta
MCC X+7th **S35.02   Major laceration of abdominal aorta**
　　　　Complete transection of abdominal aorta
　　　　Traumatic rupture of abdominal aorta
MCC X+7th **S35.09   Other injury of abdominal aorta**
+ **S35.1   Injury of inferior vena cava**
　　Injury of hepatic vein
Excludes1: injury of vena cava NOS (S25.2)
MCC X+7th **S35.10   Unspecified injury of inferior vena cava**
MCC X+7th **S35.11   Minor laceration of inferior vena cava**
　　　　Incomplete transection of inferior vena cava
　　　　Laceration of inferior vena cava NOS
　　　　Superficial laceration of inferior vena cava
MCC X+7th **S35.12   Major laceration of inferior vena cava**
　　　　Complete transection of inferior vena cava
　　　　Traumatic rupture of inferior vena cava
MCC X+7th **S35.19   Other injury of inferior vena cava**
+ **S35.2   Injury of celiac or mesenteric artery and branches**
+ **S35.21   Injury of celiac artery**
MCC +7th **S35.211   Minor laceration of celiac artery**
　　　　Incomplete transection of celiac artery
　　　　Laceration of celiac artery NOS
　　　　Superficial laceration of celiac artery
MCC +7th **S35.212   Major laceration of celiac artery**
　　　　Complete transection of celiac artery
　　　　Traumatic rupture of celiac artery
MCC +7th **S35.218   Other injury of celiac artery**
MCC +7th **S35.219   Unspecified injury of celiac artery**
+ **S35.22   Injury of superior mesenteric artery**
MCC +7th **S35.221   Minor laceration of superior mesenteric artery**
　　　　Incomplete transection of superior mesenteric artery
　　　　Laceration of superior mesenteric artery NOS
　　　　Superficial laceration of superior mesenteric artery
MCC +7th **S35.222   Major laceration of superior mesenteric artery**
　　　　Complete transection of superior mesenteric artery
　　　　Traumatic rupture of superior mesenteric artery
MCC +7th **S35.228   Other injury of superior mesenteric artery**
MCC +7th **S35.229   Unspecified injury of superior mesenteric artery**
+ **S35.23   Injury of inferior mesenteric artery**
MCC +7th **S35.231   Minor laceration of inferior mesenteric artery**
　　　　Incomplete transection of inferior mesenteric artery
　　　　Laceration of inferior mesenteric artery NOS
　　　　Superficial laceration of inferior mesenteric artery
MCC +7th **S35.232   Major laceration of inferior mesenteric artery**
　　　　Complete transection of inferior mesenteric artery
　　　　Traumatic rupture of inferior mesenteric artery
MCC +7th **S35.238   Other injury of inferior mesenteric artery**
MCC +7th **S35.239   Unspecified injury of inferior mesenteric artery**
+ **S35.29   Injury of branches of celiac and mesenteric artery**
　　　　Injury of gastric artery
　　　　Injury of gastroduodenal artery
　　　　Injury of hepatic artery
　　　　Injury of splenic artery

MCC +7th **S35.291   Minor laceration of branches of celiac and mesenteric artery**
　　　　Incomplete transection of branches of celiac and mesenteric artery
　　　　Laceration of branches of celiac and mesenteric artery NOS
　　　　Superficial laceration of branches of celiac and mesenteric artery
MCC +7th **S35.292   Major laceration of branches of celiac and mesenteric artery**
　　　　Complete transection of branches of celiac and mesenteric artery
　　　　Traumatic rupture of branches of celiac and mesenteric artery
MCC +7th **S35.298   Other injury of branches of celiac and mesenteric artery**
MCC +7th **S35.299   Unspecified injury of branches of celiac and mesenteric artery**
+ **S35.3   Injury of portal or splenic vein and branches**
+ **S35.31   Injury of portal vein**
MCC +7th **S35.311   Laceration of portal vein**
MCC +7th **S35.318   Other specified injury of portal vein**
MCC +7th **S35.319   Unspecified injury of portal vein**
+ **S35.32   Injury of splenic vein**
MCC +7th **S35.321   Laceration of splenic vein**
MCC +7th **S35.328   Other specified injury of splenic vein**
MCC +7th **S35.329   Unspecified injury of splenic vein**
+ **S35.33   Injury of superior mesenteric vein**
MCC +7th **S35.331   Laceration of superior mesenteric vein**
MCC +7th **S35.338   Other specified injury of superior mesenteric vein**
MCC +7th **S35.339   Unspecified injury of superior mesenteric vein**
+ **S35.34   Injury of inferior mesenteric vein**
MCC +7th **S35.341   Laceration of inferior mesenteric vein**
MCC +7th **S35.348   Other specified injury of inferior mesenteric vein**
MCC +7th **S35.349   Unspecified injury of inferior mesenteric vein**
+ **S35.4   Injury of renal blood vessels**
+ **S35.40   Unspecified injury of renal blood vessel**
MCC +7th **S35.401   Unspecified injury of right renal artery**
MCC +7th **S35.402   Unspecified injury of left renal artery**
MCC +7th **S35.403   Unspecified injury of unspecified renal artery**
MCC +7th **S35.404   Unspecified injury of right renal vein**
MCC +7th **S35.405   Unspecified injury of left renal vein**
MCC +7th **S35.406   Unspecified injury of unspecified renal vein**
+ **S35.41   Laceration of renal blood vessel**
MCC +7th **S35.411   Laceration of right renal artery**
MCC +7th **S35.412   Laceration of left renal artery**
MCC +7th **S35.413   Laceration of unspecified renal artery**
MCC +7th **S35.414   Laceration of right renal vein**
MCC +7th **S35.415   Laceration of left renal vein**
MCC +7th **S35.416   Laceration of unspecified renal vein**
+ **S35.49   Other specified injury of renal blood vessel**
MCC +7th **S35.491   Other specified injury of right renal artery**
MCC +7th **S35.492   Other specified injury of left renal artery**
MCC +7th **S35.493   Other specified injury of unspecified renal artery**
MCC +7th **S35.494   Other specified injury of right renal vein**
MCC +7th **S35.495   Other specified injury of left renal vein**
MCC +7th **S35.496   Other specified injury of unspecified renal vein**
+ **S35.5   Injury of iliac blood vessels**
MCC X+7th **S35.50   Injury of unspecified iliac blood vessel(s)**
+ **S35.51   Injury of iliac artery or vein**
　　　　Injury of hypogastric artery or vein
MCC +7th **S35.511   Injury of right iliac artery**
MCC +7th **S35.512   Injury of left iliac artery**
MCC +7th **S35.513   Injury of unspecified iliac artery**
MCC +7th **S35.514   Injury of right iliac vein**
MCC +7th **S35.515   Injury of left iliac vein**
MCC +7th **S35.516   Injury of unspecified iliac vein**

+ **S35.53** **Injury of uterine artery or vein**
♀ CC +7th **S35.531** **Injury of right uterine artery**
♀ CC +7th **S35.532** **Injury of left uterine artery**
♀ CC +7th **S35.533** **Injury of unspecified uterine artery**
♀ CC +7th **S35.534** **Injury of right uterine vein**
♀ CC +7th **S35.535** **Injury of left uterine vein**
♀ CC +7th **S35.536** **Injury of unspecified uterine vein**
MCC X+7th **S35.59** **Injury of other iliac blood vessels**
CC + **S35.8** **Injury of other blood vessels at abdomen, lower back and pelvis level**
　　Injury of ovarian artery or vein
+ **S35.8X** **Injury of other blood vessels at abdomen, lower back and pelvis level**
+7th **S35.8X1** **Laceration of other blood vessels at abdomen, lower back and pelvis level**
+7th **S35.8X8** **Other specified injury of other blood vessels at abdomen, lower back and pelvis level**
+7th **S35.8X9** **Unspecified injury of other blood vessels at abdomen, lower back and pelvis level**
+ **S35.9** **Injury of unspecified blood vessel at abdomen, lower back and pelvis level**
CC X+7th **S35.90** **Unspecified injury of unspecified blood vessel at abdomen, lower back and pelvis level**
CC X+7th **S35.91** **Laceration of unspecified blood vessel at abdomen, lower back and pelvis level**
CC X+7th **S35.99** **Other specified injury of unspecified blood vessel at abdomen, lower back and pelvis level**

S36 **Injury of intra-abdominal organs**

　Code also any associated open wound (S31.-)

The appropriate 7th character is to be added to each code from category S36
A　initial encounter
D　subsequent encounter
S　sequela

+ **S36.0** **Injury of spleen**
CC X+7th **S36.00** **Unspecified injury of spleen**
+ **S36.02** **Contusion of spleen**
CC +7th **S36.020** **Minor contusion of spleen**
　　Contusion of spleen less than 2 cm
CC +7th **S36.021** **Major contusion of spleen**
　　Contusion of spleen greater than 2 cm
CC +7th **S36.029** **Unspecified contusion of spleen**
+ **S36.03** **Laceration of spleen**
CC +7th **S36.030** **Superficial (capsular) laceration of spleen**
　　Laceration of spleen less than 1 cm
　　Minor laceration of spleen
　　AHA CC: 1Q, 2015, 3-21
MCC +7th **S36.031** **Moderate laceration of spleen**
　　Laceration of spleen 1 to 3 cm
　　AHA CC: 1Q, 2015, 3-21
MCC +7th **S36.032** **Major laceration of spleen**
　　Avulsion of spleen
　　Laceration of spleen greater than 3 cm
　　Massive laceration of spleen
　　Multiple moderate lacerations of spleen
　　Stellate laceration of spleen
CC +7th **S36.039** **Unspecified laceration of spleen**
CC X+7th **S36.09** **Other injury of spleen**
+ **S36.1** **Injury of liver and gallbladder and bile duct**
+ **S36.11** **Injury of liver**
CC +7th **S36.112** **Contusion of liver**
CC +7th **S36.113** **Laceration of liver, unspecified degree**
CC +7th **S36.114** **Minor laceration of liver**
　　Laceration involving capsule only, or, without significant involvement of hepatic parenchyma [i.e., less than 1 cm deep]
MCC +7th **S36.115** **Moderate laceration of liver**
　　Laceration involving parenchyma but without major disruption of parenchyma [i.e., less than 10 cm long and less than 3 cm deep]

MCC +7th **S36.116** **Major laceration of liver**
　　Laceration with significant disruption of hepatic parenchyma [i.e., greater than 10 cm long and 3 cm deep]
　　Multiple moderate lacerations, with or without hematoma
　　Stellate laceration of liver
CC +7th **S36.118** **Other injury of liver**
CC +7th **S36.119** **Unspecified injury of liver**
+ **S36.12** **Injury of gallbladder**
CC +7th **S36.122** **Contusion of gallbladder**
CC +7th **S36.123** **Laceration of gallbladder**
CC +7th **S36.128** **Other injury of gallbladder**
CC +7th **S36.129** **Unspecified injury of gallbladder**
CC X+7th **S36.13** **Injury of bile duct**
+ **S36.2** **Injury of pancreas**
+ **S36.20** **Unspecified injury of pancreas**
CC +7th **S36.200** **Unspecified injury of head of pancreas**
CC +7th **S36.201** **Unspecified injury of body of pancreas**
CC +7th **S36.202** Unspecified injury of tail of pancreas
CC +7th **S36.209** **Unspecified injury of unspecified part of pancreas**
+ **S36.22** **Contusion of pancreas**
CC **S36.220** **Contusion of head of pancreas**
CC **S36.221** **Contusion of body of pancreas**
CC **S36.222** **Contusion of tail of pancreas**
CC **S36.229** **Contusion of unspecified part of pancreas**
+ **S36.23** **Laceration of pancreas, unspecified degree**
CC +7th **S36.230** **Laceration of head of pancreas, unspecified degree**
CC +7th **S36.231** **Laceration of body of pancreas, unspecified degree**
CC +7th **S36.232** **Laceration of tail of pancreas, unspecified degree**
CC +7th **S36.239** **Laceration of unspecified part of pancreas, unspecified degree**
+ **S36.24** **Minor laceration of pancreas**
CC +7th **S36.240** **Minor laceration of head of pancreas**
CC +7th **S36.241** **Minor laceration of body of pancreas**
CC +7th **S36.242** **Minor laceration of tail of pancreas**
CC +7th **S36.249** **Minor laceration of unspecified part of pancreas**
+ **S36.25** **Moderate laceration of pancreas**
CC +7th **S36.250** **Moderate laceration of head of pancreas**
CC +7th **S36.251** **Moderate laceration of body of pancreas**
CC +7th **S36.252** **Moderate laceration of tail of pancreas**
CC +7th **S36.259** **Moderate laceration of unspecified part of pancreas**
+ **S36.26** **Major laceration of pancreas**
CC +7th **S36.260** **Major laceration of head of pancreas**
CC +7th **S36.261** **Major laceration of body of pancreas**
CC +7th **S36.262** **Major laceration of tail of pancreas**
CC +7th **S36.269** **Major laceration of unspecified part of pancreas**
+ **S36.29** **Other injury of pancreas**
CC +7th **S36.290** **Other injury of head of pancreas**
CC +7th **S36.291** **Other injury of body of pancreas**
CC +7th **S36.292** **Other injury of tail of pancreas**
CC +7th **S36.299** **Other injury of unspecified part of pancreas**
+ **S36.3** **Injury of stomach**
CC X+7th **S36.30** **Unspecified injury of stomach**
CC X+7th **S36.32** **Contusion of stomach**
CC X+7th **S36.33** **Laceration of stomach**
CC X+7th **S36.39** **Other injury of stomach**
+ **S36.4** **Injury of small intestine**
+ **S36.40** **Unspecified injury of small intestine**
CC +7th **S36.400** **Unspecified injury of duodenum**
CC +7th **S36.408** **Unspecified injury of other part of small intestine**
CC +7th **S36.409** **Unspecified injury of unspecified part of small intestine**

+ **S36.41** **Primary blast injury of small intestine**
    Blast injury of small intestine NOS
  CC +7th **S36.410** **Primary blast injury of duodenum**
  CC +7th **S36.418** **Primary blast injury of other part of small intestine**
  CC +7th **S36.419** **Primary blast injury of unspecified part of small intestine**
+ **S36.42** **Contusion of small intestine**
  CC +7th **S36.420** **Contusion of duodenum**
  CC +7th **S36.428** **Contusion of other part of small intestine**
  CC +7th **S36.429** **Contusion of unspecified part of small intestine**
+ **S36.43** **Laceration of small intestine**
  CC +7th **S36.430** **Laceration of duodenum**
  CC +7th **S36.438** **Laceration of other part of small intestine**
  CC +7th **S36.439** **Laceration of unspecified part of small intestine**
+ **S36.49** **Other injury of small intestine**
  CC +7th **S36.490** **Other injury of duodenum**
  CC +7th **S36.498** **Other injury of other part of small intestine**
  CC +7th **S36.499** **Other injury of unspecified part of small intestine**
S36.5 **Injury of colon**
  Excludes2: injury of rectum (S36.6-)
+ **S36.50** **Unspecified injury of colon**
  CC +7th **S36.500** **Unspecified injury of ascending [right] colon**
  CC +7th **S36.501** **Unspecified injury of transverse colon**
  CC +7th **S36.502** **Unspecified injury of descending [left] colon**
  CC +7th **S36.503** **Unspecified injury of sigmoid colon**
  CC +7th **S36.508** **Unspecified injury of other part of colon**
  CC +7th **S36.509** **Unspecified injury of unspecified part of colon**
+ **S36.51** **Primary blast injury of colon**
    Blast injury of colon NOS
  CC +7th **S36.510** **Primary blast injury of ascending [right] colon**
  CC +7th **S36.511** **Primary blast injury of transverse colon**
  CC +7th **S36.512** **Primary blast injury of descending [left] colon**
  CC +7th **S36.513** **Primary blast injury of sigmoid colon**
  CC +7th **S36.518** **Primary blast injury of other part of colon**
  CC +7th **S36.519** **Primary blast injury of unspecified part of colon**
+ **S36.52** **Contusion of colon**
  CC +7th **S36.520** **Contusion of ascending [right] colon**
  CC +7th **S36.521** **Contusion of transverse colon**
  CC +7th **S36.522** **Contusion of descending [left] colon**
  CC +7th **S36.523** **Contusion of sigmoid colon**
  CC +7th **S36.528** **Contusion of other part of colon**
  CC +7th **S36.529** **Contusion of unspecified part of colon**
+ **S36.53** **Laceration of colon**
  CC +7th **S36.530** **Laceration of ascending [right] colon**
  CC +7th **S36.531** **Laceration of transverse colon**
  CC +7th **S36.532** **Laceration of descending [left] colon**
  CC +7th **S36.533** **Laceration of sigmoid colon**
  CC +7th **S36.538** **Laceration of other part of colon**
  CC +7th **S36.539** **Laceration of unspecified part of colon**
+ **S36.59** **Other injury of colon**
    Secondary blast injury of colon
  CC +7th **S36.590** **Other injury of ascending [right] colon**
  CC +7th **S36.591** **Other injury of transverse colon**
  CC +7th **S36.592** **Other injury of descending [left] colon**
  CC +7th **S36.593** **Other injury of sigmoid colon**
  CC +7th **S36.598** **Other injury of other part of colon**
  CC +7th **S36.599** **Other injury of unspecified part of colon**
+ **S36.6** **Injury of rectum**
  CC X+7th **S36.60** **Unspecified injury of rectum**
  CC X+7th **S36.61** **Primary blast injury of rectum**
    Blast injury of rectum NOS
  CC X+7th **S36.62** **Contusion of rectum**
  CC X+7th **S36.63** **Laceration of rectum**

  CC X+7th **S36.69** **Other injury of rectum**
    Secondary blast injury of rectum
+ **S36.8** **Injury of other intra-abdominal organs**
  CC X+7th **S36.81** **Injury of peritoneum**
+ **S36.89** **Injury of other intra-abdominal organs**
    Injury of retroperitoneum
  CC +7th **S36.892** **Contusion of other intra-abdominal organs**
  CC +7th **S36.893** **Laceration of other intra-abdominal organs**
  CC +7th **S36.898** **Other injury of other intra-abdominal organs**
  CC +7th **S36.899** **Unspecified injury of other intra-abdominal organs**
+ **S36.9** **Injury of unspecified intra-abdominal organ**
  CC X+7th **S36.90** **Unspecified injury of unspecified intra-abdominal organ**
  CC X+7th **S36.92** **Contusion of unspecified intra-abdominal organ**
  CC X+7th **S36.93** **Laceration of unspecified intra-abdominal organ**
  CC X+7th **S36.99** **Other injury of unspecified intra-abdominal organ**

S37 **Injury of urinary and pelvic organs**
  Code also any associated open wound (S31.-)
  Excludes1: obstetric trauma to pelvic organs (O71.-)
  Excludes2: injury of peritoneum (S36.81)
           injury of retroperitoneum (S36.89-)

> The appropriate 7th character is to be added to each code from category S37
> A   initial encounter
> D   subsequent encounter
> S   sequela

+ **S37.0** **Injury of kidney**
  Excludes2: acute kidney injury (nontraumatic) (N17.9)
+ **S37.00** **Unspecified injury of kidney**
  CC +7th **S37.001** **Unspecified injury of right kidney**
  CC +7th **S37.002** **Unspecified injury of left kidney**
  CC +7th **S37.009** **Unspecified injury of unspecified kidney**
+ **S37.01** **Minor contusion of kidney**
    Contusion of kidney less than 2 cm
    Contusion of kidney NOS
  CC +7th **S37.011** **Minor contusion of right kidney**
  CC +7th **S37.012** **Minor contusion of left kidney**
  CC +7th **S37.019** **Minor contusion of unspecified kidney**
+ **S37.02** **Major contusion of kidney**
    Contusion of kidney greater than 2 cm
  CC +7th **S37.021** **Major contusion of right kidney**
  CC +7th **S37.022** **Major contusion of left kidney**
  CC +7th **S37.029** **Major contusion of unspecified kidney**
+ **S37.03** **Laceration of kidney, unspecified degree**
  CC +7th **S37.031** **Laceration of right kidney, unspecified degree**
  CC +7th **S37.032** **Laceration of left kidney, unspecified degree**
  CC +7th **S37.039** **Laceration of unspecified kidney, unspecified degree**
+ **S37.04** **Minor laceration of kidney**
    Laceration of kidney less than 1 cm
  CC +7th **S37.041** **Minor laceration of right kidney**
  CC +7th **S37.042** **Minor laceration of left kidney**
  CC +7th **S37.049** **Minor laceration of unspecified kidney**
+ **S37.05** **Moderate laceration of kidney**
    Laceration of kidney 1 to 3 cm
  CC +7th **S37.051** **Moderate laceration of right kidney**
  CC +7th **S37.052** **Moderate laceration of left kidney**
  CC +7th **S37.059** **Moderate laceration of unspecified kidney**
+ **S37.06** **Major laceration of kidney**
    Avulsion of kidney
    Laceration of kidney greater than 3 cm
    Massive laceration of kidney
    Multiple moderate lacerations of kidney
    Stellate laceration of kidney
  MCC +7th **S37.061** **Major laceration of right kidney**
  MCC +7th **S37.062** **Major laceration of left kidney**
  MCC +7th **S37.069** **Major laceration of unspecified kidney**

+, +7th, X + 7th ● Newborn ● Pediatric ● Maternity ● Adult ♀ Female ♂ Male Manifestation Unacceptable PDX HCC CC MCC HAC

Shoulder

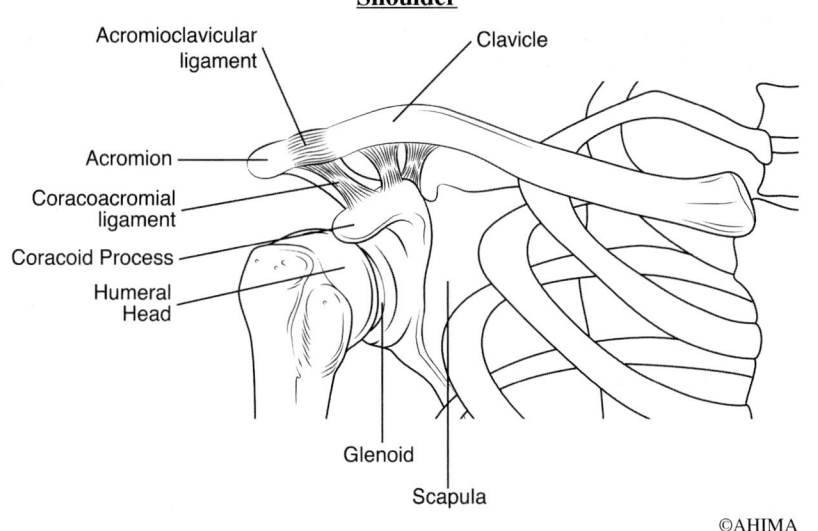

- Acromioclavicular ligament
- Clavicle
- Acromion
- Coracoacromial ligament
- Coracoid Process
- Humeral Head
- Glenoid
- Scapula

©AHIMA

Shoulder Tendons

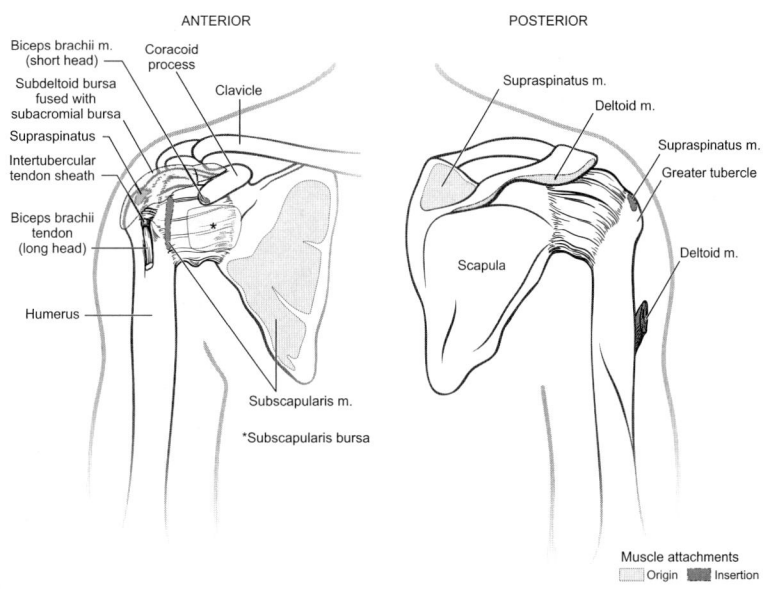

ANTERIOR

- Biceps brachii m. (short head)
- Coracoid process
- Clavicle
- Subdeltoid bursa fused with subacromial bursa
- Supraspinatus
- Intertubercular tendon sheath
- Biceps brachii tendon (long head)
- Humerus
- Subscapularis m.

*Subscapularis bursa

POSTERIOR

- Supraspinatus m.
- Deltoid m.
- Supraspinatus m.
- Greater tubercle
- Deltoid m.
- Scapula

Muscle attachments
☐ Origin ▨ Insertion

©AHIMA

Shoulder Ligaments

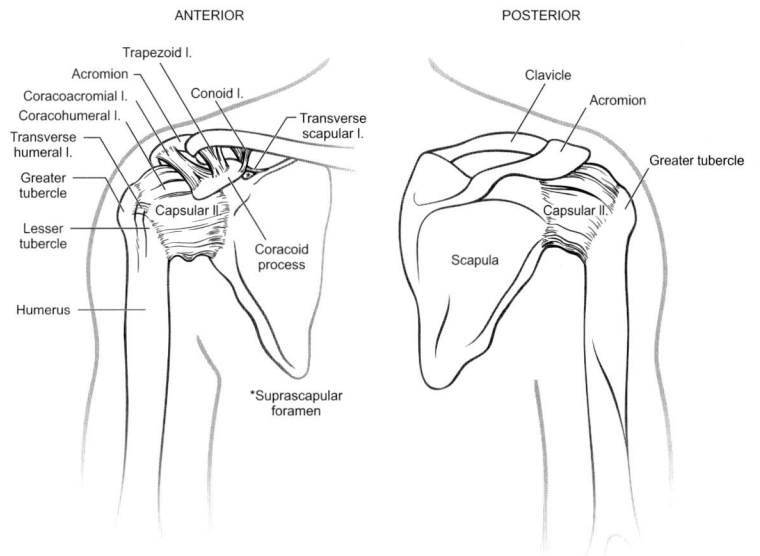

ANTERIOR

- Trapezoid l.
- Acromion
- Coracoacromial l.
- Conoid l.
- Coracohumeral l.
- Transverse scapular l.
- Transverse humeral l.
- Greater tubercle
- Capsular ll.
- Lesser tubercle
- Coracoid process
- Humerus

*Suprascapular foramen

POSTERIOR

- Clavicle
- Acromion
- Greater tubercle
- Capsular ll.
- Scapula

©AHIMA

+ **S37.09** **Other injury of kidney**
MCC +7th **S37.091** **Other injury of right kidney**
MCC +7th **S37.092** **Other injury of left kidney**
MCC +7th **S37.099** **Other injury of unspecified kidney**
+ **S37.1** **Injury of ureter**
CC X+7th **S37.10** **Unspecified injury of ureter**
CC X+7th **S37.12** **Contusion of ureter**
CC X+7th **S37.13** **Laceration of ureter**
CC X+7th **S37.19** **Other injury of ureter**
+ **S37.2** **Injury of bladder**
CC X+7th **S37.20** **Unspecified injury of bladder**
CC X+7th **S37.22** **Contusion of bladder**
CC X+7th **S37.23** **Laceration of bladder**
CC X+7th **S37.29** **Other injury of bladder**
+ **S37.3** **Injury of urethra**
CC X+7th **S37.30** **Unspecified injury of urethra**
CC X+7th **S37.32** **Contusion of urethra**
CC X+7th **S37.33** **Laceration of urethra**
CC X+7th **S37.39** **Other injury of urethra**
+ **S37.4** **Injury of ovary**
  + **S37.40** **Unspecified injury of ovary**
    ♀ +7th **S37.401** **Unspecified injury of ovary, unilateral**
    ♀ +7th **S37.402** **Unspecified injury of ovary, bilateral**
    ♀ +7th **S37.409** **Unspecified injury of ovary, unspecified**
  + **S37.42** **Contusion of ovary**
    ♀ +7th **S37.421** **Contusion of ovary, unilateral**
    ♀ +7th **S37.422** **Contusion of ovary, bilateral**
    ♀ +7th **S37.429** **Contusion of ovary, unspecified**
  + **S37.43** **Laceration of ovary**
    ♀ +7th **S37.431** **Laceration of ovary, unilateral**
    ♀ +7th **S37.432** **Laceration of ovary, bilateral**
    ♀ +7th **S37.439** **Laceration of ovary, unspecified**
  + **S37.49** **Other injury of ovary**
    ♀ +7th **S37.491** **Other injury of ovary, unilateral**
    ♀ +7th **S37.492** **Other injury of ovary, bilateral**
    ♀ +7th **S37.499** **Other injury of ovary, unspecified**
+ **S37.5** **Injury of fallopian tube**
  + **S37.50** **Unspecified injury of fallopian tube**
    ♀ +7th **S37.501** **Unspecified injury of fallopian tube, unilateral**
    ♀ +7th **S37.502** **Unspecified injury of fallopian tube, bilateral**
    ♀ +7th **S37.509** **Unspecified injury of fallopian tube, unspecified**
  + **S37.51** **Primary blast injury of fallopian tube**
    Blast injury of fallopian tube NOS
    ♀ +7th **S37.511** **Primary blast injury of fallopian tube, unilateral**
    ♀ +7th **S37.512** **Primary blast injury of fallopian tube, bilateral**
    ♀ +7th **S37.519** **Primary blast injury of fallopian tube, unspecified**
  + **S37.52** **Contusion of fallopian tube**
    ♀ +7th **S37.521** **Contusion of fallopian tube, unilateral**
    ♀ +7th **S37.522** **Contusion of fallopian tube, bilateral**
    ♀ +7th **S37.529** **Contusion of fallopian tube, unspecified**
  + **S37.53** **Laceration of fallopian tube**
    ♀ +7th **S37.531** **Laceration of fallopian tube, unilateral**
    ♀ +7th **S37.532** **Laceration of fallopian tube, bilateral**
    ♀ +7th **S37.539** **Laceration of fallopian tube, unspecified**
  + **S37.59** **Other injury of fallopian tube**
    Secondary blast injury of fallopian tube
    ♀ +7th **S37.591** **Other injury of fallopian tube, unilateral**
    ♀ +7th **S37.592** **Other injury of fallopian tube, bilateral**
    ♀ +7th **S37.599** **Other injury of fallopian tube, unspecified**
+ **S37.6** **Injury of uterus**
  Excludes1: *injury to gravid uterus (O9A.2-)*
           injury to uterus during delivery (O71.-)
♀ CC X+7th **S37.60** **Unspecified injury of uterus**
♀ CC X+7th **S37.62** **Contusion of uterus**
♀ CC X+7th **S37.63** **Laceration of uterus**
♀ CC X+7th **S37.69** **Other injury of uterus**
+ **S37.8** **Injury of other urinary and pelvic organs**
  + **S37.81** **Injury of adrenal gland**
    CC +7th **S37.812** **Contusion of adrenal gland**

CC +7th **S37.813** **Laceration of adrenal gland**
CC +7th **S37.818** **Other injury of adrenal gland**
CC +7th **S37.819** **Unspecified injury of adrenal gland**
+ **S37.82** **Injury of prostate**
  ♂ +7th **S37.822** **Contusion of prostate**
  ♂ +7th **S37.823** **Laceration of prostate**
  ♂ +7th **S37.828** **Other injury of prostate**
  ♂ +7th **S37.829** **Unspecified injury of prostate**
+ **S37.89** **Injury of other urinary and pelvic organ**
  CC +7th **S37.892** **Contusion of other urinary and pelvic organ**
  CC +7th **S37.893** **Laceration of other urinary and pelvic organ**
  CC +7th **S37.898** **Other injury of other urinary and pelvic organ**
  CC +7th **S37.899** **Unspecified injury of other urinary and pelvic organ**
+ **S37.9** **Injury of unspecified urinary and pelvic organ**
CC X+7th **S37.90** **Unspecified injury of unspecified urinary and pelvic organ**
CC X+7th **S37.92** **Contusion of unspecified urinary and pelvic organ**
CC X+7th **S37.93** **Laceration of unspecified urinary and pelvic organ**
CC X+7th **S37.99** **Other injury of unspecified urinary and pelvic organ**

S38 **Crushing injury and traumatic amputation of abdomen, lower back, pelvis and external genitals**

An amputation not identified as partial or complete should be coded to complete

The appropriate 7th character is to be added to each code from category S38
A initial encounter
D subsequent encounter
S sequela

+ **S38.0** **Crushing injury of external genital organs**
  Use additional code for any associated injuries
  + **S38.00** **Crushing injury of unspecified external genital organs**
    ♂ +7th **S38.001** **Crushing injury of unspecified external genital organs, male**
    ♀ +7th **S38.002** **Crushing injury of unspecified external genital organs, female**
  ♂ X+7th **S38.01** **Crushing injury of penis**
  ♂ X+7th **S38.02** **Crushing injury of scrotum and testis**
  ♀ X+7th **S38.03** **Crushing injury of vulva**
X+7th **S38.1** **Crushing injury of abdomen, lower back, and pelvis**
  Use additional code for all associated injuries, such as:
    fracture of thoracic or lumbar spine and pelvis (S22.0-, S32.-)
    injury to intra-abdominal organs (S36.-)
    injury to urinary and pelvic organs (S37.-)
    open wound of abdominal wall (S31.-)
    spinal cord injury (S34.0, S34.1-)
  Excludes2: *crushing injury of external genital organs (S38.0-)*
+ **S38.2** **Traumatic amputation of external genital organs**
  + **S38.21** **Traumatic amputation of female external genital organs**
    Traumatic amputation of clitoris
    Traumatic amputation of labium (majus) (minus)
    Traumatic amputation of vulva
    ♀ +7th **S38.211** **Complete traumatic amputation of female external genital organs**
    ♀ +7th **S38.212** **Partial traumatic amputation of female external genital organs**
  + **S38.22** **Traumatic amputation of penis**
    ♂ +7th **S38.221** **Complete traumatic amputation of penis**
    ♂ +7th **S38.222** **Partial traumatic amputation of penis**
  + **S38.23** **Traumatic amputation of scrotum and testis**
    ♂ +7th **S38.231** **Complete traumatic amputation of scrotum and testis**
    ♂ +7th **S38.232** **Partial traumatic amputation of scrotum and testis**
X+7th **S38.3** **Transection (partial) of abdomen**

S39 **Other and unspecified injuries of abdomen, lower back, pelvis and external genitals**

Code also any associated open wound (S31.-)

Excludes2: *sprain of joints and ligaments of lumbar spine and pelvis (S33.-)*

The appropriate 7th character is to be added to each code from category S39
A   initial encounter
D   subsequent encounter
S   sequela

+ **S39.0** **Injury of muscle, fascia and tendon of abdomen, lower back and pelvis**
  + **S39.00** **Unspecified injury of muscle, fascia and tendon of abdomen, lower back and pelvis**
    +7th **S39.001** Unspecified injury of muscle, fascia and tendon of abdomen
    +7th **S39.002** Unspecified injury of muscle, fascia and tendon of lower back
    +7th **S39.003** Unspecified injury of muscle, fascia and tendon of pelvis
  + **S39.01** **Strain of muscle, fascia and tendon of abdomen, lower back and pelvis**
    +7th **S39.011** Strain of muscle, fascia and tendon of abdomen
    +7th **S39.012** Strain of muscle, fascia and tendon of lower back
    AHA CC: 4Q, 2016, 73-74
    +7th **S39.013** Strain of muscle, fascia and tendon of pelvis
  + **S39.02** **Laceration of muscle, fascia and tendon of abdomen, lower back and pelvis**
    +7th **S39.021** Laceration of muscle, fascia and tendon of abdomen
    +7th **S39.022** Laceration of muscle, fascia and tendon of lower back
    +7th **S39.023** Laceration of muscle, fascia and tendon of pelvis
  + **S39.09** **Other injury of muscle, fascia and tendon of abdomen, lower back and pelvis**
    +7th **S39.091** Other injury of muscle, fascia and tendon of abdomen
    +7th **S39.092** Other injury of muscle, fascia and tendon of lower back
    +7th **S39.093** Other injury of muscle, fascia and tendon of pelvis
+ **S39.8** **Other specified injuries of abdomen, lower back, pelvis and external genitals**
  X+7th **S39.81** Other specified injuries of abdomen
  X+7th **S39.82** Other specified injuries of lower back
  X+7th **S39.83** Other specified injuries of pelvis
  + **S39.84** **Other specified injuries of external genitals**
    ♂ X+7th **S39.840** Fracture of corpus cavernosum penis
    X+7th **S39.848** Other specified injuries of external genitals
+ **S39.9** **Unspecified injury of abdomen, lower back, pelvis and external genitals**
  X+7th **S39.91** Unspecified injury of abdomen
  X+7th **S39.92** Unspecified injury of lower back
  X+7th **S39.93** Unspecified injury of pelvis
  X+7th **S39.94** Unspecified injury of external genitals

Injuries to the shoulder and upper arm (S40-S49)

Includes: injuries of axilla
injuries of scapular region

Excludes2: *and corrosions (T20-T32)*
frostbite (T33-T34)
injuries of elbow (S50-S59)
insect bite or sting, venomous (T63.4)

S40 **Superficial injury of shoulder and upper arm**

The appropriate 7th character is to be added to each code from category S40
A   initial encounter
D   subsequent encounter
S   sequela

+ **S40.0** **Contusion of shoulder and upper arm**
  + **S40.01** **Contusion of shoulder**
    +7th **S40.011** Contusion of right shoulder
    +7th **S40.012** Contusion of left shoulder
    +7th **S40.019** Contusion of unspecified shoulder
  + **S40.02** **Contusion of upper arm**
    +7th **S40.021** Contusion of right upper arm
    +7th **S40.022** Contusion of left upper arm
    +7th **S40.029** Contusion of unspecified upper arm
+ **S40.2** **Other superficial injuries of shoulder**
  + **S40.21** **Abrasion of shoulder**
    +7th **S40.211** Abrasion of right shoulder
    +7th **S40.212** Abrasion of left shoulder
    +7th **S40.219** Abrasion of unspecified shoulder
  + **S40.22** **Blister (nonthermal) of shoulder**
    +7th **S40.221** Blister (nonthermal) of right shoulder
    +7th **S40.222** Blister (nonthermal) of left shoulder
    +7th **S40.229** Blister (nonthermal) of unspecified shoulder
  + **S40.24** **External constriction of shoulder**
    +7th **S40.241** External constriction of right shoulder
    +7th **S40.242** External constriction of left shoulder
    +7th **S40.249** External constriction of unspecified shoulder
  + **S40.25** **Superficial foreign body of shoulder**
    Splinter in the shoulder
    +7th **S40.251** Superficial foreign body of right shoulder
    +7th **S40.252** Superficial foreign body of left shoulder
    +7th **S40.259** Superficial foreign body of unspecified shoulder
  + **S40.26** **Insect bite (nonvenomous) of shoulder**
    +7th **S40.261** Insect bite (nonvenomous) of right shoulder
    +7th **S40.262** Insect bite (nonvenomous) of left shoulder
    +7th **S40.269** Insect bite (nonvenomous) of unspecified shoulder
  + **S40.27** **Other superficial bite of shoulder**
    Excludes1: *open bite of shoulder (S41.05)*
    +7th **S40.271** Other superficial bite of right shoulder
    +7th **S40.272** Other superficial bite of left shoulder
    +7th **S40.279** Other superficial bite of unspecified shoulder
+ **S40.8** **Other superficial injuries of upper arm**
  + **S40.81** **Abrasion of upper arm**
    +7th **S40.811** Abrasion of right upper arm
    +7th **S40.812** Abrasion of left upper arm
    +7th **S40.819** Abrasion of unspecified upper arm
  + **S40.82** **Blister (nonthermal) of upper arm**
    +7th **S40.821** Blister (nonthermal) of right upper arm
    +7th **S40.822** Blister (nonthermal) of left upper arm
    +7th **S40.829** Blister (nonthermal) of unspecified upper arm
  + **S40.84** **External constriction of upper arm**
    +7th **S40.841** External constriction of right upper arm
    +7th **S40.842** External constriction of left upper arm
    +7th **S40.849** External constriction of unspecified upper arm
  + **S40.85** **Superficial foreign body of upper arm**
    Splinter in the upper arm
    +7th **S40.851** Superficial foreign body of right upper arm
    +7th **S40.852** Superficial foreign body of left upper arm
    +7th **S40.859** Superficial foreign body of unspecified upper arm

+ **S40.86 Insect bite (nonvenomous) of upper arm**
   +7th **S40.861 Insect bite (nonvenomous) of right upper arm**
   +7th **S40.862 Insect bite (nonvenomous) of left upper arm**
   +7th **S40.869 Insect bite (nonvenomous) of unspecified upper arm**
+ **S40.87 Other superficial bite of upper arm**
   Excludes1: *open bite of upper arm (S41.14)*
   Excludes2: *other superficial bite of shoulder (S40.27-)*
   +7th **S40.871 Other superficial bite of right upper arm**
   +7th **S40.872 Other superficial bite of left upper arm**
   +7th **S40.879 Other superficial bite of unspecified upper arm**
+ **S40.9 Unspecified superficial injury of shoulder and upper arm**
  + **S40.91 Unspecified superficial injury of shoulder**
   +7th **S40.911 Unspecified superficial injury of right shoulder**
   +7th **S40.912 Unspecified superficial injury of left shoulder**
   +7th **S40.919 Unspecified superficial injury of unspecified shoulder**
  + **S40.92 Unspecified superficial injury of upper arm**
   +7th **S40.921 Unspecified superficial injury of right upper arm**
   +7th **S40.922 Unspecified superficial injury of left upper arm**
   +7th **S40.929 Unspecified superficial injury of unspecified upper arm**

S41 Open wound of shoulder and upper arm

Code also any associated wound infection
Excludes1: *traumatic amputation of shoulder and upper arm (S48.-)*
Excludes2: *open fracture of shoulder and upper arm (S42.- with 7th character B or C)*

> The appropriate 7th character is to be added to each code from category S41
> A   initial encounter
> D   subsequent encounter
> S   sequela

+ **S41.0 Open wound of shoulder**
  + **S41.00 Unspecified open wound of shoulder**
   +7th **S41.001 Unspecified open wound of right shoulder**
   +7th **S41.002 Unspecified open wound of left shoulder**
   +7th **S41.009 Unspecified open wound of unspecified shoulder**
  + **S41.01 Laceration without foreign body of shoulder**
   +7th **S41.011 Laceration without foreign body of right shoulder**
   +7th **S41.012 Laceration without foreign body of left shoulder**
   +7th **S41.019 Laceration without foreign body of unspecified shoulder**
  + **S41.02 Laceration with foreign body of shoulder**
   +7th **S41.021 Laceration with foreign body of right shoulder**
   +7th **S41.022 Laceration with foreign body of left shoulder**
   +7th **S41.029 Laceration with foreign body of unspecified shoulder**
  + **S41.03 Puncture wound without foreign body of shoulder**
   +7th **S41.031 Puncture wound without foreign body of right shoulder**
   +7th **S41.032 Puncture wound without foreign body of left shoulder**
   +7th **S41.039 Puncture wound without foreign body of unspecified shoulder**
  + **S41.04 Puncture wound with foreign body of shoulder**
   +7th **S41.041 Puncture wound with foreign body of right shoulder**
   +7th **S41.042 Puncture wound with foreign body of left shoulder**
   +7th **S41.049 Puncture wound with foreign body of unspecified shoulder**

+ **S41.05 Open bite of shoulder**
  Bite of shoulder NOS
   Excludes1: *superficial bite of shoulder (S40.27)*
   +7th **S41.051 Open bite of right shoulder**
   +7th **S41.052 Open bite of left shoulder**
   +7th **S41.059 Open bite of unspecified shoulder**
+ **S41.1 Open wound of upper arm**
  + **S41.10 Unspecified open wound of upper arm**
   +7th **S41.101 Unspecified open wound of right upper arm**
   +7th **S41.102 Unspecified open wound of left upper arm**
   +7th **S41.109 Unspecified open wound of unspecified upper arm**
  + **S41.11 Laceration without foreign body of upper arm**
   S41.111 Laceration without foreign body of right upper arm
   S41.112 Laceration without foreign body of left upper arm
   S41.119 Laceration without foreign body of unspecified upper arm
  + **S41.12 Laceration with foreign body of upper arm**
   +7th **S41.121 Laceration with foreign body of right upper arm**
   +7th **S41.122 Laceration with foreign body of left upper arm**
   +7th **S41.129 Laceration with foreign body of unspecified upper arm**
  + **S41.13 Puncture wound without foreign body of upper arm**
   +7th **S41.131 Puncture wound without foreign body of right upper arm**
   +7th **S41.132 Puncture wound without foreign body of left upper arm**
   +7th **S41.139 Puncture wound without foreign body of unspecified upper arm**
  + **S41.14 Puncture wound with foreign body of upper arm**
   +7th **S41.141 Puncture wound with foreign body of right upper arm**
   +7th **S41.142 Puncture wound with foreign body of left upper arm**
   +7th **S41.149 Puncture wound with foreign body of unspecified upper arm**
  + **S41.15 Open bite of upper arm**
  Bite of upper arm NOS
   Excludes1: *superficial bite of upper arm (S40.87)*
   +7th **S41.151 Open bite of right upper arm**
   +7th **S41.152 Open bite of left upper arm**
   +7th **S41.159 Open bite of unspecified upper arm**

S42 Fracture of shoulder and upper arm

> **NOTE** A fracture not indicated as displaced or nondisplaced should be coded to displaced
> A fracture not indicated as open or closed should be coded to closed unless otherwise indicated.

Excludes1: *traumatic amputation of shoulder and upper arm (S48.-)*

> The appropriate 7th character is to be added to all codes from category S42
> A   initial encounter for closed fracture
> B   initial encounter for open fracture
> D   subsequent encounter for fracture with routine healing
> G   subsequent encounter for fracture with delayed healing
> K   subsequent encounter for fracture with nonunion
> P   subsequent encounter for fracture with malunion
> S   sequela

Review coding guideline C.19.c
+ **S42.0 Fracture of clavicle**
  + **S42.00 Fracture of unspecified part of clavicle**
  CC +7th **S42.001 Fracture of unspecified part of right clavicle**
    HAC 7th character B see Appendix B for HAC conditional logic
  CC +7th **S42.002 Fracture of unspecified part of left clavicle**
    HAC 7th character B see Appendix B for HAC conditional logic
  CC +7th **S42.009 Fracture of unspecified part of unspecified clavicle**
    HAC 7th character B see Appendix B for HAC conditional logic

+, +7th, X + 7th   ● Newborn   ● Pediatric   ● Maternity   ● Adult   ♀ Female   ♂ Male   Manifestation   Unacceptable PDX   HCC   CC   MCC   **HAC**

+ **S42.01** **Fracture of sternal end of clavicle**

CC +7th **S42.011** **Anterior displaced fracture of sternal end of right clavicle**
> HAC 7th character B see Appendix B for HAC conditional logic

CC +7th **S42.012** **Anterior displaced fracture of sternal end of left clavicle**
> HAC 7th character B see Appendix B for HAC conditional logic

CC +7th **S42.013** **Anterior displaced fracture of sternal end of unspecified clavicle**
Displaced fracture of sternal end of clavicle NOS
> HAC 7th character B see Appendix B for HAC conditional logic

CC +7th **S42.014** **Posterior displaced fracture of sternal end of right clavicle**
> HAC 7th character B see Appendix B for HAC conditional logic

CC +7th **S42.015** **Posterior displaced fracture of sternal end of left clavicle**
> HAC 7th character B see Appendix B for HAC conditional logic

CC +7th **S42.016** **Posterior displaced fracture of sternal end of unspecified clavicle**
> HAC 7th character B see Appendix B for HAC conditional logic

CC +7th **S42.017** **Nondisplaced fracture of sternal end of right clavicle**
> HAC 7th character B see Appendix B for HAC conditional logic

CC +7th **S42.018** **Nondisplaced fracture of sternal end of left clavicle**
> HAC 7th character B see Appendix B for HAC conditional logic

CC +7th **S42.019** **Nondisplaced fracture of sternal end of unspecified clavicle**
> HAC 7th character B see Appendix B for HAC conditional logic

+ **S42.02** **Fracture of shaft of clavicle**

CC +7th **S42.021** **Displaced fracture of shaft of right clavicle**
> HAC 7th character B see Appendix B for HAC conditional logic

CC +7th **S42.022** **Displaced fracture of shaft of left clavicle**
> HAC 7th character B see Appendix B for HAC conditional logic

CC +7th **S42.023** **Displaced fracture of shaft of unspecified clavicle**
> HAC 7th character B see Appendix B for HAC conditional logic

CC +7th **S42.024** **Nondisplaced fracture of shaft of right clavicle**
> HAC 7th character B see Appendix B for HAC conditional logic

CC +7th **S42.025** **Nondisplaced fracture of shaft of left clavicle**
> HAC 7th character B see Appendix B for HAC conditional logic

CC +7th **S42.026** **Nondisplaced fracture of shaft of unspecified clavicle**
> HAC 7th character B see Appendix B for HAC conditional logic

+ **S42.03** **Fracture of lateral end of clavicle**
Fracture of acromial end of clavicle

CC +7th **S42.031** **Displaced fracture of lateral end of right clavicle**
> HAC 7th character B see Appendix B for HAC conditional logic

CC +7th **S42.032** **Displaced fracture of lateral end of left clavicle**
> HAC 7th character B see Appendix B for HAC conditional logic

CC +7th **S42.033** **Displaced fracture of lateral end of unspecified clavicle**
> HAC 7th character B see Appendix B for HAC conditional logic

CC +7th **S42.034** **Nondisplaced fracture of lateral end of right clavicle**
> HAC 7th character B see Appendix B for HAC conditional logic

CC +7th **S42.035** **Nondisplaced fracture of lateral end of left clavicle**
> HAC 7th character B see Appendix B for HAC conditional logic

CC +7th **S42.036** **Nondisplaced fracture of lateral end of unspecified clavicle**
> HAC 7th character B see Appendix B for HAC conditional logic

+ **S42.1** **Fracture of scapula**

+ **S42.10** **Fracture of unspecified part of scapula**

CC +7th **S42.101** **Fracture of unspecified part of scapula, right shoulder**
> HAC 7th character B see Appendix B for HAC conditional logic

CC +7th **S42.102** **Fracture of unspecified part of scapula, left shoulder**
> HAC 7th character B see Appendix B for HAC conditional logic

CC +7th **S42.109** **Fracture of unspecified part of scapula, unspecified shoulder**
> HAC 7th character B see Appendix B for HAC conditional logic

+ **S42.11** **Fracture of body of scapula**

CC +7th **S42.111** **Displaced fracture of body of scapula, right shoulder**
> HAC 7th character B see Appendix B for HAC conditional logic

CC +7th **S42.112** **Displaced fracture of body of scapula, left shoulder**
> HAC 7th character B see Appendix B for HAC conditional logic

CC +7th **S42.113** **Displaced fracture of body of scapula, unspecified shoulder**
> HAC 7th character B see Appendix B for HAC conditional logic

CC +7th **S42.114** **Nondisplaced fracture of body of scapula, right shoulder**
> HAC 7th character B see Appendix B for HAC conditional logic

CC +7th **S42.115** **Nondisplaced fracture of body of scapula, left shoulder**
> HAC 7th character B see Appendix B for HAC conditional logic

CC +7th **S42.116** **Nondisplaced fracture of body of scapula, unspecified shoulder**
> HAC 7th character B see Appendix B for HAC conditional logic

+ **S42.12** **Fracture of acromial process**

CC +7th **S42.121** **Displaced fracture of acromial process, right shoulder**
> HAC 7th character B see Appendix B for HAC conditional logic

CC +7th **S42.122** **Displaced fracture of acromial process, left shoulder**
> HAC 7th character B see Appendix B for HAC conditional logic

CC +7th **S42.123** **Displaced fracture of acromial process, unspecified shoulder**
> HAC 7th character B see Appendix B for HAC conditional logic

CC +7th **S42.124** **Nondisplaced fracture of acromial process, right shoulder**
> HAC 7th character B see Appendix B for HAC conditional logic

CC +7th **S42.125** **Nondisplaced fracture of acromial process, left shoulder**
> HAC 7th character B see Appendix B for HAC conditional logic

CC +7th **S42.126** **Nondisplaced fracture of acromial process, unspecified shoulder**
> HAC 7th character B see Appendix B for HAC conditional logic

+ **S42.13** **Fracture of coracoid process**

CC +7th **S42.131** **Displaced fracture of coracoid process, right shoulder**
> HAC 7th character B see Appendix B for HAC conditional logic

CC +7th **S42.132** **Displaced fracture of coracoid process, left shoulder**
> HAC 7th character B see Appendix B for HAC conditional logic

CC +7th **S42.133** **Displaced fracture of coracoid process, unspecified shoulder**
> HAC 7th character B see Appendix B for HAC conditional logic

CC +7th **S42.134** **Nondisplaced fracture of coracoid process, right shoulder**
> HAC 7th character B see Appendix B for HAC conditional logic

+, +7th, X + 7th ● Newborn ● Pediatric ● Maternity ● Adult ♀ Female ♂ Male Manifestation Unacceptable PDX HCC CC MCC HAC

CC +7th **S42.135** **Nondisplaced fracture of coracoid process, left shoulder**
HAC 7th character B see Appendix B for HAC conditional logic

CC +7th **S42.136** **Nondisplaced fracture of coracoid process, unspecified shoulder**
HAC 7th character B see Appendix B for HAC conditional logic

+ **S42.14** **Fracture of glenoid cavity of scapula**

CC +7th **S42.141** **Displaced fracture of glenoid cavity of scapula, right shoulder**
HAC 7th character B see Appendix B for HAC conditional logic

CC +7th **S42.142** **Displaced fracture of glenoid cavity of scapula, left shoulder**
HAC 7th character B see Appendix B for HAC conditional logic

CC +7th **S42.143** **Displaced fracture of glenoid cavity of scapula, unspecified shoulder**
HAC 7th character B see Appendix B for HAC conditional logic

CC +7th **S42.144** **Nondisplaced fracture of glenoid cavity of scapula, right shoulder**
HAC 7th character B see Appendix B for HAC conditional logic

CC +7th **S42.145** **Nondisplaced fracture of glenoid cavity of scapula, left shoulder**
HAC 7th character B see Appendix B for HAC conditional logic

CC +7th **S42.146** **Nondisplaced fracture of glenoid cavity of scapula, unspecified shoulder**
HAC 7th character B see Appendix B for HAC conditional logic

+ **S42.15** **Fracture of neck of scapula**

CC +7th **S42.151** **Displaced fracture of neck of scapula, right shoulder**
HAC 7th character B see Appendix B for HAC conditional logic

CC +7th **S42.152** **Displaced fracture of neck of scapula, left shoulder**
HAC 7th character B see Appendix B for HAC conditional logic

CC +7th **S42.153** **Displaced fracture of neck of scapula, unspecified shoulder**
HAC 7th character B see Appendix B for HAC conditional logic

CC +7th **S42.154** **Nondisplaced fracture of neck of scapula, right shoulder**
HAC 7th character B see Appendix B for HAC conditional logic

CC +7th **S42.155** **Nondisplaced fracture of neck of scapula, left shoulder**
HAC 7th character B see Appendix B for HAC conditional logic

CC +7th **S42.156** **Nondisplaced fracture of neck of scapula, unspecified shoulder**
HAC 7th character B see Appendix B for HAC conditional logic

+ **S42.19** **Fracture of other part of scapula**

CC +7th **S42.191** **Fracture of other part of scapula, right shoulder**
HAC 7th character B see Appendix B for HAC conditional logic

CC +7th **S42.192** **Fracture of other part of scapula, left shoulder**
HAC 7th character B see Appendix B for HAC conditional logic

CC +7th **S42.199** **Fracture of other part of scapula, unspecified shoulder**
HAC 7th character B see Appendix B for HAC conditional logic

+ **S42.2** **Fracture of upper end of humerus**
Fracture of proximal end of humerus
Excludes2: *fracture of shaft of humerus (S42.3-)*
physeal fracture of upper end of humerus (S49.0-)

+ **S42.20** **Unspecified fracture of upper end of humerus**

CC MCC +7th **S42.201** **Unspecified fracture of upper end of right humerus**
HAC 7th characters A & B see Appendix B for HAC conditional logic

CC MCC +7th **S42.202** **Unspecified fracture of upper end of left humerus**
HAC 7th characters A & B see Appendix B for HAC conditional logic

CC MCC +7th **S42.209** **Unspecified fracture of upper end of unspecified humerus**
HAC 7th characters A & B see Appendix B for HAC conditional logic

+ **S42.21** **Unspecified fracture of surgical neck of humerus**
Fracture of neck of humerus NOS

CC MCC +7th **S42.211** **Unspecified displaced fracture of surgical neck of right humerus**
HAC 7th characters A & B see Appendix B for HAC conditional logic

CC MCC +7th **S42.212** **Unspecified displaced fracture of surgical neck of left humerus**

CC MCC +7th **S42.213** **Unspecified displaced fracture of surgical neck of unspecified humerus**
HAC 7th characters A & B see Appendix B for HAC conditional logic

CC MCC +7th **S42.214** **Unspecified nondisplaced fracture of surgical neck of right humerus**
HAC 7th characters A & B see Appendix B for HAC conditional logic

CC MCC +7th **S42.215** **Unspecified nondisplaced fracture of surgical neck of left humerus**
HAC 7th characters A & B see Appendix B for HAC conditional logic

CC MCC +7th **S42.216** **Unspecified nondisplaced fracture of surgical neck of unspecified humerus**
HAC 7th characters A & B see Appendix B for HAC conditional logic

+ **S42.22** **2-part fracture of surgical neck of humerus**

CC MCC +7th **S42.221** **2-part displaced fracture of surgical neck of right humerus**
HAC 7th characters A & B see Appendix B for HAC conditional logic

CC MCC +7th **S42.222** **2-part displaced fracture of surgical neck of left humerus**
HAC 7th characters A & B see Appendix B for HAC conditional logic

CC MCC +7th **S42.223** **2-part displaced fracture of surgical neck of unspecified humerus**
HAC 7th characters A & B see Appendix B for HAC conditional logic

CC MCC +7th **S42.224** **2-part nondisplaced fracture of surgical neck of right humerus**
HAC 7th characters A & B see Appendix B for HAC conditional logic

CC MCC +7th **S42.225** **2-part nondisplaced fracture of surgical neck of left humerus**
HAC 7th characters A & B see Appendix B for HAC conditional logic

CC MCC +7th **S42.226** **2-part nondisplaced fracture of surgical neck of unspecified humerus**
HAC 7th characters A & B see Appendix B for HAC conditional logic

+ **S42.23** **3-part fracture of surgical neck of humerus**

CC MCC +7th **S42.231** **3-part fracture of surgical neck of right humerus**
HAC 7th characters A & B see Appendix B for HAC conditional logic

CC MCC +7th **S42.232** **3-part fracture of surgical neck of left humerus**
HAC 7th characters A & B see Appendix B for HAC conditional logic

CC MCC +7th **S42.239** **3-part fracture of surgical neck of unspecified humerus**
HAC 7th characters A & B see Appendix B for HAC conditional logic

+ **S42.24** **4-part fracture of surgical neck of humerus**

CC MCC +7th **S42.241** **4-part fracture of surgical neck of right humerus**
HAC 7th characters A & B see Appendix B for HAC conditional logic

CC MCC +7th **S42.242** **4-part fracture of surgical neck of left humerus**
HAC 7th characters A & B see Appendix B for HAC conditional logic

CC MCC +7th **S42.249** **4-part fracture of surgical neck of unspecified humerus**
HAC 7th characters A & B see Appendix B for HAC conditional logic

+ **S42.25** **Fracture of greater tuberosity of humerus**

CC MCC +7th **S42.251** **Displaced fracture of greater tuberosity of right humerus**
HAC 7th characters A & B see Appendix B for HAC conditional logic

CC MCC +7th **S42.252** **Displaced fracture of greater tuberosity of left humerus**
> HAC 7th characters A & B see Appendix B for HAC conditional logic

CC MCC +7th **S42.253** **Displaced fracture of greater tuberosity of unspecified humerus**
> HAC 7th characters A & B see Appendix B for HAC conditional logic

CC MCC +7th **S42.254** **Nondisplaced fracture of greater tuberosity of right humerus**
> HAC 7th characters A & B see Appendix B for HAC conditional logic

CC MCC +7th **S42.255** **Nondisplaced fracture of greater tuberosity of left humerus**
> HAC 7th characters A & B see Appendix B for HAC conditional logic

CC MCC +7th **S42.256** **Nondisplaced fracture of greater tuberosity of unspecified humerus**
> HAC 7th characters A & B see Appendix B for HAC conditional logic

+ **S42.26** **Fracture of lesser tuberosity of humerus**

CC MCC +7th **S42.261** **Displaced fracture of lesser tuberosity of right humerus**
> HAC 7th characters A & B see Appendix B for HAC conditional logic

CC MCC +7th **S42.262** **Displaced fracture of lesser tuberosity of left humerus**
> HAC 7th characters A & B see Appendix B for HAC conditional logic

CC MCC +7th **S42.263** **Displaced fracture of lesser tuberosity of unspecified humerus**
> HAC 7th characters A & B see Appendix B for HAC conditional logic

CC MCC +7th **S42.264** **Nondisplaced fracture of lesser tuberosity of right humerus**
> HAC 7th characters A & B see Appendix B for HAC conditional logic

CC MCC +7th **S42.265** **Nondisplaced fracture of lesser tuberosity of left humerus**
> HAC 7th characters A & B see Appendix B for HAC conditional logic

CC MCC +7th **S42.266** **Nondisplaced fracture of lesser tuberosity of unspecified humerus**
> HAC 7th characters A & B see Appendix B for HAC conditional logic

+ **S42.27** **Torus fracture of upper end of humerus**

> The appropriate 7th character is to be added to all codes in subcategory **S42.27**
> A   initial encounter for closed fracture
> D   subsequent encounter for fracture with routine healing
> G   subsequent encounter for fracture with delayed healing
> K   subsequent encounter for fracture with nonunion
> P   subsequent encounter for fracture with malunion
> S   sequela

CC +7th **S42.271** **Torus fracture of upper end of right humerus**
> HAC 7th character A see Appendix B for HAC conditional logic

CC +7th **S42.272** **Torus fracture of upper end of left humerus**
> HAC 7th character A see Appendix B for HAC conditional logic

CC +7th **S42.279** **Torus fracture of upper end of unspecified humerus**
> HAC 7th character A see Appendix B for HAC conditional logic

+ **S42.29** **Other fracture of upper end of humerus**
Fracture of anatomical neck of humerus
Fracture of articular head of humerus

CC MCC +7th **S42.291** **Other displaced fracture of upper end of right humerus**
> HAC 7th characters A & B see Appendix B for HAC conditional logic

CC MCC +7th **S42.292** **Other displaced fracture of upper end of left humerus**
> HAC 7th characters A & B see Appendix B for HAC conditional logic

CC MCC +7th **S42.293** **Other displaced fracture of upper end of unspecified humerus**
> HAC 7th characters A & B see Appendix B for HAC conditional logic

CC MCC +7th **S42.294** **Other nondisplaced fracture of upper end of right humerus**
> HAC 7th characters A & B see Appendix B for HAC conditional logic

CC MCC +7th **S42.295** **Other nondisplaced fracture of upper end of left humerus**
> *AHA CC: 1Q, 2019, 18-19*
> HAC 7th characters A & B see Appendix B for HAC conditional logic

CC MCC +7th **S42.296** **Other nondisplaced fracture of upper end of unspecified humerus**
> HAC 7th characters A & B see Appendix B for HAC conditional logic

+ **S42.3** **Fracture of shaft of humerus**
Fracture of humerus NOS
Fracture of upper arm NOS
Excludes2: *physeal fractures of upper end of humerus (S49.0-)*
physeal fractures of lower end of humerus (S49.1-)

+ **S42.30** **Unspecified fracture of shaft of humerus**

CC MCC +7th **S42.301** **Unspecified fracture of shaft of humerus, right arm**
> HAC 7th characters A & B see Appendix B for HAC conditional logic

CC MCC +7th **S42.302** **Unspecified fracture of shaft of humerus, left arm**
> HAC 7th characters A & B see Appendix B for HAC conditional logic

CC MCC +7th **S42.309** **Unspecified fracture of shaft of humerus, unspecified arm**
> HAC 7th characters A & B see Appendix B for HAC conditional logic

+ **S42.31** **Greenstick fracture of shaft of humerus**

> The appropriate 7th character is to be added to all codes in subcategory **S42.31**
> A   initial encounter for closed fracture
> D   subsequent encounter for fracture with routine healing
> G   subsequent encounter for fracture with delayed healing
> K   subsequent encounter for fracture with nonunion
> P   subsequent encounter for fracture with malunion
> S   sequela

CC +7th **S42.311** **Greenstick fracture of shaft of humerus, right arm**
> HAC 7th character A see Appendix B for HAC conditional logic

CC +7th **S42.312** **Greenstick fracture of shaft of humerus, left arm**
> HAC 7th character A see Appendix B for HAC conditional logic

CC +7th **S42.319** **Greenstick fracture of shaft of humerus, unspecified arm**
> HAC 7th character A see Appendix B for HAC conditional logic

+ **S42.32** **Transverse fracture of shaft of humerus**

CC MCC +7th **S42.321** **Displaced transverse fracture of shaft of humerus, right arm**
> HAC 7th characters A & B see Appendix B for HAC conditional logic

CC MCC +7th **S42.322** **Displaced transverse fracture of shaft of humerus, left arm**
> HAC 7th characters A & B see Appendix B for HAC conditional logic

CC MCC +7th **S42.323** **Displaced transverse fracture of shaft of humerus, unspecified arm**
> HAC 7th characters A & B see Appendix B for HAC conditional logic

CC MCC +7th **S42.324** **Nondisplaced transverse fracture of shaft of humerus, right arm**
> HAC 7th characters A & B see Appendix B for HAC conditional logic

CC MCC +7th **S42.325** **Nondisplaced transverse fracture of shaft of humerus, left arm**
> HAC 7th characters A & B see Appendix B for HAC conditional logic

CC MCC +7th **S42.326** **Nondisplaced transverse fracture of shaft of humerus, unspecified arm**
> HAC 7th characters A & B see Appendix B for HAC conditional logic

+ **S42.33** **Oblique fracture of shaft of humerus**

CC MCC +7th **S42.331** **Displaced oblique fracture of shaft of humerus, right arm**
> HAC 7th characters A & B see Appendix B for HAC conditional logic

CC MCC +7th **S42.332** **Displaced oblique fracture of shaft of humerus, left arm**
HAC 7th characters A & B see Appendix B for HAC conditional logic

CC MCC +7th **S42.333** **Displaced oblique fracture of shaft of humerus, unspecified arm**
HAC 7th characters A & B see Appendix B for HAC conditional logic

CC MCC +7th **S42.334** **Nondisplaced oblique fracture of shaft of humerus, right arm**
HAC 7th characters A & B see Appendix B for HAC conditional logic

CC MCC +7th **S42.335** **Nondisplaced oblique fracture of shaft of humerus, left arm**
HAC 7th characters A & B see Appendix B for HAC conditional logic

CC MCC +7th **S42.336** **Nondisplaced oblique fracture of shaft of humerus, unspecified arm**
HAC 7th characters A & B see Appendix B for HAC conditional logic

+ **S42.34** **Spiral fracture of shaft of humerus**

CC MCC +7th **S42.341** **Displaced spiral fracture of shaft of humerus, right arm**
HAC 7th characters A & B see Appendix B for HAC conditional logic

CC MCC +7th **S42.342** **Displaced spiral fracture of shaft of humerus, left arm**
HAC 7th characters A & B see Appendix B for HAC conditional logic

CC MCC +7th **S42.343** **Displaced spiral fracture of shaft of humerus, unspecified arm**
HAC 7th characters A & B see Appendix B for HAC conditional logic

CC MCC +7th **S42.344** **Nondisplaced spiral fracture of shaft of humerus, right arm**
HAC 7th characters A & B see Appendix B for HAC conditional logic

CC MCC +7th **S42.345** **Nondisplaced spiral fracture of shaft of humerus, left arm**
HAC 7th characters A & B see Appendix B for HAC conditional logic

CC MCC +7th **S42.346** **Nondisplaced spiral fracture of shaft of humerus, unspecified arm**
HAC 7th characters A & B see Appendix B for HAC conditional logic

+ **S42.35** **Comminuted fracture of shaft of humerus**

CC MCC +7th **S42.351** **Displaced comminuted fracture of shaft of humerus, right arm**
HAC 7th characters A & B see Appendix B for HAC conditional logic

CC MCC +7th **S42.352** **Displaced comminuted fracture of shaft of humerus, left arm**
HAC 7th characters A & B see Appendix B for HAC conditional logic

CC MCC +7th **S42.353** **Displaced comminuted fracture of shaft of humerus, unspecified arm**
HAC 7th characters A & B see Appendix B for HAC conditional logic

CC MCC +7th **S42.354** **Nondisplaced comminuted fracture of shaft of humerus, right arm**
HAC 7th characters A & B see Appendix B for HAC conditional logic

CC MCC +7th **S42.355** **Nondisplaced comminuted fracture of shaft of humerus, left arm**
HAC 7th characters A & B see Appendix B for HAC conditional logic

CC MCC +7th **S42.356** **Nondisplaced comminuted fracture of shaft of humerus, unspecified arm**
HAC 7th characters A & B see Appendix B for HAC conditional logic

+ **S42.36** **Segmental fracture of shaft of humerus**

CC MCC +7th **S42.361** **Displaced segmental fracture of shaft of humerus, right arm**
HAC 7th characters A & B see Appendix B for HAC conditional logic

CC MCC +7th **S42.362** **Displaced segmental fracture of shaft of humerus, left arm**
HAC 7th characters A & B see Appendix B for HAC conditional logic

CC MCC +7th **S42.363** **Displaced segmental fracture of shaft of humerus, unspecified arm**
HAC 7th characters A & B see Appendix B for HAC conditional logic

CC MCC +7th **S42.364** **Nondisplaced segmental fracture of shaft of humerus, right arm**
HAC 7th characters A & B see Appendix B for HAC conditional logic

CC MCC +7th **S42.365** **Nondisplaced segmental fracture of shaft of humerus, left arm**
HAC 7th characters A & B see Appendix B for HAC conditional logic

CC MCC +7th **S42.366** **Nondisplaced segmental fracture of shaft of humerus, unspecified arm**
HAC 7th characters A & B see Appendix B for HAC conditional logic

+ **S42.39** **Other fracture of shaft of humerus**

CC MCC +7th **S42.391** **Other fracture of shaft of right humerus**
HAC 7th characters A & B see Appendix B for HAC conditional logic

CC MCC +7th **S42.392** **Other fracture of shaft of left humerus**
HAC 7th characters A & B see Appendix B for HAC conditional logic

CC MCC +7th **S42.399** **Other fracture of shaft of unspecified humerus**
HAC 7th characters A & B see Appendix B for HAC conditional logic

+ **S42.4** **Fracture of lower end of humerus**
Fracture of distal end of humerus
Excludes2: *fracture of shaft of humerus (S42.3-)*
physeal fracture of lower end of humerus (S49.1-)

+ **S42.40** **Unspecified fracture of lower end of humerus**
Fracture of elbow NOS

CC MCC +7th **S42.401** **Unspecified fracture of lower end of right humerus**
HAC 7th characters A & B see Appendix B for HAC conditional logic

CC MCC +7th **S42.402** **Unspecified fracture of lower end of left humerus**
HAC 7th characters A & B see Appendix B for HAC conditional logic

CC MCC +7th **S42.409** **Unspecified fracture of lower end of unspecified humerus**
HAC 7th characters A & B see Appendix B for HAC conditional logic

+ **S42.41** **Simple supracondylar fracture without intercondylar fracture of humerus**

CC MCC +7th **S42.411** **Displaced simple supracondylar fracture without intercondylar fracture of right humerus**
HAC 7th characters A & B see Appendix B for HAC conditional logic

CC MCC +7th **S42.412** **Displaced simple supracondylar fracture without intercondylar fracture of left humerus**
HAC 7th characters A & B see Appendix B for HAC conditional logic

CC MCC +7th **S42.413** **Displaced simple supracondylar fracture without intercondylar fracture of unspecified humerus**
HAC 7th characters A & B see Appendix B for HAC conditional logic

CC MCC +7th **S42.414** **Nondisplaced simple supracondylar fracture without intercondylar fracture of right humerus**
HAC 7th characters A & B see Appendix B for HAC conditional logic

CC MCC +7th **S42.415** **Nondisplaced simple supracondylar fracture without intercondylar fracture of left humerus**
HAC 7th characters A & B see Appendix B for HAC conditional logic

CC MCC +7th **S42.416** **Nondisplaced simple supracondylar fracture without intercondylar fracture of unspecified humerus**
HAC 7th characters A & B see Appendix B for HAC conditional logic

+ **S42.42** **Comminuted supracondylar fracture without intercondylar fracture of humerus**

CC MCC +7th **S42.421** **Displaced comminuted supracondylar fracture without intercondylar fracture of right humerus**
HAC 7th characters A & B see Appendix B for HAC conditional logic

CC MCC +7th **S42.422** **Displaced comminuted supracondylar fracture without intercondylar fracture of left humerus**
HAC 7th characters A & B see Appendix B for HAC conditional logic

+, +7th, X + 7th ● Newborn ● Pediatric ● Maternity ● Adult ♀ Female ♂ Male Manifestation Unacceptable PDX HCC CC MCC HAC

CC MCC +7th **S42.423** **Displaced comminuted supracondylar fracture without intercondylar fracture of unspecified humerus**
HAC 7th characters A & B see Appendix B for HAC conditional logic

CC MCC +7th **S42.424** **Nondisplaced comminuted supracondylar fracture without intercondylar fracture of right humerus**
HAC 7th characters A & B see Appendix B for HAC conditional logic

CC MCC +7th **S42.425** **Nondisplaced comminuted supracondylar fracture without intercondylar fracture of left humerus**
HAC 7th characters A & B see Appendix B for HAC conditional logic

CC MCC +7th **S42.426** **Nondisplaced comminuted supracondylar fracture without intercondylar fracture of unspecified humerus**
HAC 7th characters A & B see Appendix B for HAC conditional logic

+ **S42.43** **Fracture (avulsion) of lateral epicondyle of humerus**

CC MCC +7th **S42.431** **Displaced fracture (avulsion) of lateral epicondyle of right humerus**
HAC 7th characters A & B see Appendix B for HAC conditional logic

CC MCC +7th **S42.432** **Displaced fracture (avulsion) of lateral epicondyle of left humerus**
HAC 7th characters A & B see Appendix B for HAC conditional logic

CC MCC +7th **S42.433** **Displaced fracture (avulsion) of lateral epicondyle of unspecified humerus**
HAC 7th characters A & B see Appendix B for HAC conditional logic

CC MCC +7th **S42.434** **Nondisplaced fracture (avulsion) of lateral epicondyle of right humerus**
HAC 7th characters A & B see Appendix B for HAC conditional logic

CC MCC +7th **S42.435** **Nondisplaced fracture (avulsion) of lateral epicondyle of left humerus**
HAC 7th characters A & B see Appendix B for HAC conditional logic

CC MCC +7th **S42.436** **Nondisplaced fracture (avulsion) of lateral epicondyle of unspecified humerus**
HAC 7th characters A & B see Appendix B for HAC conditional logic

+ **S42.44** **Fracture (avulsion) of medial epicondyle of humerus**

CC MCC +7th **S42.441** **Displaced fracture (avulsion) of medial epicondyle of right humerus**
HAC 7th characters A & B see Appendix B for HAC conditional logic

CC MCC +7th **S42.442** **Displaced fracture (avulsion) of medial epicondyle of left humerus**
HAC 7th characters A & B see Appendix B for HAC conditional logic

CC MCC +7th **S42.443** **Displaced fracture (avulsion) of medial epicondyle of unspecified humerus**
HAC 7th characters A & B see Appendix B for HAC conditional logic

CC MCC +7th **S42.444** **Nondisplaced fracture (avulsion) of medial epicondyle of right humerus**
HAC 7th characters A & B see Appendix B for HAC conditional logic

CC MCC +7th **S42.445** **Nondisplaced fracture (avulsion) of medial epicondyle of left humerus**
HAC 7th characters A & B see Appendix B for HAC conditional logic

CC MCC +7th **S42.446** **Nondisplaced fracture (avulsion) of medial epicondyle of unspecified humerus**
HAC 7th characters A & B see Appendix B for HAC conditional logic

CC MCC +7th **S42.447** **Incarcerated fracture (avulsion) of medial epicondyle of right humerus**
HAC 7th characters A & B see Appendix B for HAC conditional logic

CC MCC +7th **S42.448** **Incarcerated fracture (avulsion) of medial epicondyle of left humerus**
HAC 7th characters A & B see Appendix B for HAC conditional logic

CC MCC +7th **S42.449** **Incarcerated fracture (avulsion) of medial epicondyle of unspecified humerus**
HAC 7th characters A & B see Appendix B for HAC conditional logic

+ **S42.45** **Fracture of lateral condyle of humerus**
Fracture of capitellum of humerus

CC MCC +7th **S42.451** **Displaced fracture of lateral condyle of right humerus**
HAC 7th characters A & B see Appendix B for HAC conditional logic

CC MCC +7th **S42.452** **Displaced fracture of lateral condyle of left humerus**
HAC 7th characters A & B see Appendix B for HAC conditional logic

CC MCC +7th **S42.453** **Displaced fracture of lateral condyle of unspecified humerus**
HAC 7th characters A & B see Appendix B for HAC conditional logic

CC MCC +7th **S42.454** **Nondisplaced fracture of lateral condyle of right humerus**
HAC 7th characters A & B see Appendix B for HAC conditional logic

CC MCC +7th **S42.455** **Nondisplaced fracture of lateral condyle of left humerus**
HAC 7th characters A & B see Appendix B for HAC conditional logic

CC MCC +7th **S42.456** **Nondisplaced fracture of lateral condyle of unspecified humerus**
HAC 7th characters A & B see Appendix B for HAC conditional logic

+ **S42.46** **Fracture of medial condyle of humerus**
Trochlea fracture of humerus

CC MCC +7th **S42.461** **Displaced fracture of medial condyle of right humerus**
HAC 7th characters A & B see Appendix B for HAC conditional logic

CC MCC +7th **S42.462** **Displaced fracture of medial condyle of left humerus**
HAC 7th characters A & B see Appendix B for HAC conditional logic

CC MCC +7th **S42.463** **Displaced fracture of medial condyle of unspecified humerus**
HAC 7th characters A & B see Appendix B for HAC conditional logic

CC MCC +7th **S42.464** **Nondisplaced fracture of medial condyle of right humerus**
HAC 7th characters A & B see Appendix B for HAC conditional logic

CC MCC +7th **S42.465** **Nondisplaced fracture of medial condyle of left humerus**
HAC 7th characters A & B see Appendix B for HAC conditional logic

CC MCC +7th **S42.466** **Nondisplaced fracture of medial condyle of unspecified humerus**
HAC 7th characters A & B see Appendix B for HAC conditional logic

+ **S42.47** **Transcondylar fracture of humerus**

CC MCC +7th **S42.471** **Displaced transcondylar fracture of right humerus**
HAC 7th characters A & B see Appendix B for HAC conditional logic

CC MCC +7th **S42.472** **Displaced transcondylar fracture of left humerus**
HAC 7th characters A & B see Appendix B for HAC conditional logic

CC MCC +7th **S42.473** **Displaced transcondylar fracture of unspecified humerus**
HAC 7th characters A & B see Appendix B for HAC conditional logic

CC MCC +7th **S42.474** **Nondisplaced transcondylar fracture of right humerus**
HAC 7th characters A & B see Appendix B for HAC conditional logic

CC MCC +7th **S42.475** **Nondisplaced transcondylar fracture of left humerus**
HAC 7th characters A & B see Appendix B for HAC conditional logic

CC MCC +7th **S42.476** **Nondisplaced transcondylar fracture of unspecified humerus**
HAC 7th characters A & B see Appendix B for HAC conditional logic

+, +7th, X + 7th ● Newborn ● Pediatric ● Maternity ● Adult ♀ Female ♂ Male Manifestation Unacceptable PDX HCC CC MCC HAC

+ S42.48 Torus fracture of lower end of humerus

> The appropriate 7th character is to be added to all codes in subcategory **S42.48**
> A initial encounter for closed fracture
> D subsequent encounter for fracture with routine healing
> G subsequent encounter for fracture with delayed healing
> K subsequent encounter for fracture with nonunion
> P subsequent encounter for fracture with malunion
> S sequela

CC +7th **S42.481 Torus fracture of lower end of right humerus**
> HAC 7th character A see Appendix B for HAC conditional logic

CC +7th **S42.482 Torus fracture of lower end of left humerus**
> HAC 7th character A see Appendix B for HAC conditional logic

CC +7th **S42.489 Torus fracture of lower end of unspecified humerus**
> HAC 7th character A see Appendix B for HAC conditional logic

+ S42.49 Other fracture of lower end of humerus

CC MCC +7th **S42.491 Other displaced fracture of lower end of right humerus**
> HAC 7th characters A & B see Appendix B for HAC conditional logic

CC MCC +7th **S42.492 Other displaced fracture of lower end of left humerus**
> HAC 7th characters A & B see Appendix B for HAC conditional logic

CC MCC +7th **S42.493 Other displaced fracture of lower end of unspecified humerus**
> HAC 7th characters A & B see Appendix B for HAC conditional logic

CC MCC +7th **S42.494 Other nondisplaced fracture of lower end of right humerus**
> HAC 7th characters A & B see Appendix B for HAC conditional logic

CC MCC +7th **S42.495 Other nondisplaced fracture of lower end of left humerus**
> HAC 7th characters A & B see Appendix B for HAC conditional logic

CC MCC +7th **S42.496 Other nondisplaced fracture of lower end of unspecified humerus**
> HAC 7th characters A & B see Appendix B for HAC conditional logic

+ S42.9 Fracture of shoulder girdle, part specified
> Fracture of shoulder NOS

CC MCC X+7th **S42.90 Fracture of unspecified shoulder girdle, part unspecified**
> HAC 7th characters A & B see Appendix B for HAC conditional logic

CC MCC X+7th **S42.91 Fracture of right shoulder girdle, part unspecified**
> HAC 7th characters A & B see Appendix B for HAC conditional logic

CC MCC X+7th **S42.92 Fracture of left shoulder girdle, part unspecified**
> HAC 7th characters A & B see Appendix B for HAC conditional logic

S43 Dislocation and sprain of joints and ligaments of shoulder girdle

> **Includes:** avulsion of joint or ligament of shoulder girdle
> laceration of cartilage, joint or ligament of shoulder girdle
> sprain of cartilage, joint or ligament of shoulder girdle
> traumatic hemarthrosis of joint or ligament of shoulder girdle
> traumatic rupture of joint or ligament of shoulder girdle
> traumatic subluxation of joint or ligament of shoulder girdle
> traumatic tear of joint or ligament of shoulder girdle

> Code also any associated open wound

> **Excludes2:** strain of muscle, fascia and tendon of shoulder and upper arm (S46.-)

> The appropriate 7th character is to be added to each code from category S43
> A initial encounter
> D subsequent encounter
> S sequela

+ S43.0 Subluxation and dislocation of shoulder joint
> Dislocation of glenohumeral joint
> Subluxation of glenohumeral joint

+ S43.00 Unspecified subluxation and dislocation of shoulder joint
> Dislocation of humerus NOS
> Subluxation of humerus NOS

+7th **S43.001 Unspecified subluxation of right shoulder joint**
+7th **S43.002 Unspecified subluxation of left shoulder joint**
+7th **S43.003 Unspecified subluxation of unspecified shoulder joint**
+7th **S43.004 Unspecified dislocation of right shoulder joint**
+7th **S43.005 Unspecified dislocation of left shoulder joint**
+7th **S43.006 Unspecified dislocation of unspecified shoulder joint**

+ S43.01 Anterior subluxation and dislocation of humerus
+7th **S43.011 Anterior subluxation of right humerus**
+7th **S43.012 Anterior subluxation of left humerus**
+7th **S43.013 Anterior subluxation of unspecified humerus**
+7th **S43.014 Anterior dislocation of right humerus**
+7th **S43.015 Anterior dislocation of left humerus**
+7th **S43.016 Anterior dislocation of unspecified humerus**

+ S43.02 Posterior subluxation and dislocation of humerus
+7th **S43.021 Posterior subluxation of right humerus**
+7th **S43.022 Posterior subluxation of left humerus**
+7th **S43.023 Posterior subluxation of unspecified humerus**
+7th **S43.024 Posterior dislocation of right humerus**
+7th **S43.025 Posterior dislocation of left humerus**
+7th **S43.026 Posterior dislocation of unspecified humerus**

+ S43.03 Inferior subluxation and dislocation of humerus
+7th **S43.031 Inferior subluxation of right humerus**
+7th **S43.032 Inferior subluxation of left humerus**
+7th **S43.033 Inferior subluxation of unspecified humerus**
+7th **S43.034 Inferior dislocation of right humerus**
+7th **S43.035 Inferior dislocation of left humerus**
+7th **S43.036 Inferior dislocation of unspecified humerus**

+ S43.08 Other subluxation and dislocation of shoulder joint
+7th **S43.081 Other subluxation of right shoulder joint**
+7th **S43.082 Other subluxation of left shoulder joint**
+7th **S43.083 Other subluxation of unspecified shoulder joint**
+7th **S43.084 Other dislocation of right shoulder joint**
+7th **S43.085 Other dislocation of left shoulder joint**
+7th **S43.086 Other dislocation of unspecified shoulder joint**

+ S43.1 Subluxation and dislocation of acromioclavicular joint

+ S43.10 Unspecified dislocation of acromioclavicular joint
+7th **S43.101 Unspecified dislocation of right acromioclavicular joint**
+7th **S43.102 Unspecified dislocation of left acromioclavicular joint**
+7th **S43.109 Unspecified dislocation of unspecified acromioclavicular joint**

+ S43.11 Subluxation of acromioclavicular joint
+7th **S43.111 Subluxation of right acromioclavicular joint**
+7th **S43.112 Subluxation of left acromioclavicular joint**
+7th **S43.119 Subluxation of unspecified acromioclavicular joint**

+ S43.12 Dislocation of acromioclavicular joint, 100%-200% displacement
+7th **S43.121 Dislocation of right acromioclavicular joint, 100%-200% displacement**
+7th **S43.122 Dislocation of left acromioclavicular joint, 100%-200% displacement**
+7th **S43.129 Dislocation of unspecified acromioclavicular joint, 100%-200% displacement**

+ **S43.13** **Dislocation of acromioclavicular joint, greater than 200% displacement**
  +7th **S43.131** Dislocation of right acromioclavicular joint, greater than 200% displacement
  +7th **S43.132** Dislocation of left acromioclavicular joint, greater than 200% displacement
  +7th **S43.139** Dislocation of unspecified acromioclavicular joint, greater than 200% displacement
+ **S43.14** **Inferior dislocation of acromioclavicular joint**
  +7th **S43.141** Inferior dislocation of right acromioclavicular joint
  +7th **S43.142** Inferior dislocation of left acromioclavicular joint
  +7th **S43.149** Inferior dislocation of unspecified acromioclavicular joint
+ **S43.15** **Posterior dislocation of acromioclavicular joint**
  +7th **S43.151** Posterior dislocation of right acromioclavicular joint
  +7th **S43.152** Posterior dislocation of left acromioclavicular joint
  +7th **S43.159** Posterior dislocation of unspecified acromioclavicular joint
+ **S43.2** **Subluxation and dislocation of sternoclavicular joint**
  + **S43.20** **Unspecified subluxation and dislocation of sternoclavicular joint**
  CC +7th **S43.201** Unspecified subluxation of right sternoclavicular joint
    HAC 7th character A see Appendix B for HAC conditional logic
  CC +7th **S43.202** Unspecified subluxation of left sternoclavicular joint
    HAC 7th character A see Appendix B for HAC conditional logic
  CC +7th **S43.203** Unspecified subluxation of unspecified sternoclavicular joint
    HAC 7th character A see Appendix B for HAC conditional logic
  CC +7th **S43.204** Unspecified dislocation of right sternoclavicular joint
    HAC 7th character A see Appendix B for HAC conditional logic
  CC +7th **S43.205** Unspecified dislocation of left sternoclavicular joint
    HAC 7th character A see Appendix B for HAC conditional logic
  CC +7th **S43.206** Unspecified dislocation of unspecified sternoclavicular joint
    HAC 7th character A see Appendix B for HAC conditional logic
  + **S43.21** **Anterior subluxation and dislocation of sternoclavicular joint**
  CC +7th **S43.211** Anterior subluxation of right sternoclavicular joint
    HAC 7th character A see Appendix B for HAC conditional logic
  CC +7th **S43.212** Anterior subluxation of left sternoclavicular joint
    HAC 7th character A see Appendix B for HAC conditional logic
  CC +7th **S43.213** Anterior subluxation of unspecified sternoclavicular joint
    HAC 7th character A see Appendix B for HAC conditional logic
  CC +7th **S43.214** Anterior dislocation of right sternoclavicular joint
    HAC 7th character A see Appendix B for HAC conditional logic
  CC +7th **S43.215** Anterior dislocation of left sternoclavicular joint
    HAC 7th character A see Appendix B for HAC conditional logic
  CC +7th **S43.216** Anterior dislocation of unspecified sternoclavicular joint
    HAC 7th character A see Appendix B for HAC conditional logic
  + **S43.22** **Posterior subluxation and dislocation of sternoclavicular joint**
  CC +7th **S43.221** Posterior subluxation of right sternoclavicular joint
    HAC 7th character A see Appendix B for HAC conditional logic
  CC +7th **S43.222** Posterior subluxation of left sternoclavicular joint
    HAC 7th character A see Appendix B for HAC conditional logic
  CC +7th **S43.223** Posterior subluxation of unspecified sternoclavicular joint
    HAC 7th character A see Appendix B for HAC conditional logic
  CC +7th **S43.224** Posterior dislocation of right sternoclavicular joint
    HAC 7th character A see Appendix B for HAC conditional logic
  CC +7th **S43.225** Posterior dislocation of left sternoclavicular joint
    HAC 7th character A see Appendix B for HAC conditional logic
  CC +7th **S43.226** Posterior dislocation of unspecified sternoclavicular joint
+ **S43.3** **Subluxation and dislocation of other and unspecified parts of shoulder girdle**
  + **S43.30** **Subluxation and dislocation of unspecified parts of shoulder girdle**
    Dislocation of shoulder girdle NOS
    Subluxation of shoulder girdle NOS
  +7th **S43.301** Subluxation of unspecified parts of right shoulder girdle
  +7th **S43.302** Subluxation of unspecified parts of left shoulder girdle
  +7th **S43.303** Subluxation of unspecified parts of unspecified shoulder girdle
  +7th **S43.304** Dislocation of unspecified parts of right shoulder girdle
  +7th **S43.305** Dislocation of unspecified parts of left shoulder girdle
  +7th **S43.306** Dislocation of unspecified parts of unspecified shoulder girdle
  + **S43.31** **Subluxation and dislocation of scapula**
  +7th **S43.311** Subluxation of right scapula
  +7th **S43.312** Subluxation of left scapula
  +7th **S43.313** Subluxation of unspecified scapula
  +7th **S43.314** Dislocation of right scapula
  +7th **S43.315** Dislocation of left scapula
  +7th **S43.316** Dislocation of unspecified scapula
  + **S43.39** **Subluxation and dislocation of other parts of shoulder girdle**
  +7th **S43.391** Subluxation of other parts of right shoulder girdle
  +7th **S43.392** Subluxation of other parts of left shoulder girdle
  +7th **S43.393** Subluxation of other parts of unspecified shoulder girdle
  +7th **S43.394** Dislocation of other parts of right shoulder girdle
  +7th **S43.395** Dislocation of other parts of left shoulder girdle
  +7th **S43.396** Dislocation of other parts of unspecified shoulder girdle
+ **S43.4** **Sprain of shoulder joint**
  + **S43.40** **Unspecified sprain of shoulder joint**
  +7th **S43.401** Unspecified sprain of right shoulder joint
  +7th **S43.402** Unspecified sprain of left shoulder joint
  +7th **S43.409** Unspecified sprain of unspecified shoulder joint
  + **S43.41** **Sprain of coracohumeral (ligament)**
  +7th **S43.411** Sprain of right coracohumeral (ligament)
  +7th **S43.412** Sprain of left coracohumeral (ligament)
  +7th **S43.419** Sprain of unspecified coracohumeral (ligament)
  + **S43.42** **Sprain of rotator cuff capsule**
    Excludes1: *rotator cuff syndrome (complete) (incomplete), not specified as traumatic (M75.1-)*
    Excludes2: *injury of tendon of rotator cuff (S46.0-)*
  +7th **S43.421** Sprain of right rotator cuff capsule
  +7th **S43.422** Sprain of left rotator cuff capsule
  +7th **S43.429** Sprain of unspecified rotator cuff capsule

+ **S43.43** **Superior glenoid labrum lesion**
SLAP lesion
AHA CC: 2Q, 2019, 26-27

+7th **S43.431** Superior glenoid labrum lesion of right shoulder

+7th **S43.432** Superior glenoid labrum lesion of left shoulder

+7th **S43.439** Superior glenoid labrum lesion of unspecified shoulder

+ **S43.49** **Other sprain of shoulder joint**

S43.491 Other sprain of right shoulder joint

S43.492 Other sprain of left shoulder joint

S43.499 Other sprain of unspecified shoulder joint

+ **S43.5** **Sprain of acromioclavicular joint**
Sprain of acromioclavicular ligament

X+7th **S43.50** Sprain of unspecified acromioclavicular joint

X+7th **S43.51** Sprain of right acromioclavicular joint

X+7th **S43.52** Sprain of left acromioclavicular joint

+ **S43.6** **Sprain of sternoclavicular joint**

X+7th **S43.60** Sprain of unspecified sternoclavicular joint

X+7th **S43.61** Sprain of right sternoclavicular joint

X+7th **S43.62** Sprain of left sternoclavicular joint

+ **S43.8** **Sprain of other specified parts of shoulder girdle**

X+7th **S43.80** Sprain of other specified parts of unspecified shoulder girdle

X+7th **S43.81** Sprain of other specified parts of right shoulder girdle

X+7th **S43.82** Sprain of other specified parts of left shoulder girdle

+ **S43.9** **Sprain of unspecified parts of shoulder girdle**

X+7th **S43.90** Sprain of unspecified parts of unspecified shoulder girdle
Sprain of shoulder girdle NOS

X+7th **S43.91** Sprain of unspecified parts of right shoulder girdle

X+7th **S43.92** Sprain of unspecified parts of left shoulder girdle

S44 **Injury of nerves at shoulder and upper arm level**

Code also any associated open wound (S41.-)
Excludes2: *injury of brachial plexus (S14.3-)*

The appropriate 7th character is to be added to each code from category S44
A   initial encounter
D   subsequent encounter
S   sequela

+ **S44.0** **Injury of ulnar nerve at upper arm level**
Excludes1: *ulnar nerve NOS (S54.0)*

X+7th **S44.00** Injury of ulnar nerve at upper arm level, unspecified arm

X+7th **S44.01** Injury of ulnar nerve at upper arm level, right arm

X+7th **S44.02** Injury of ulnar nerve at upper arm level, left arm

+ **S44.1** **Injury of median nerve at upper arm level**
Excludes1: *median nerve NOS (S54.1)*

X+7th **S44.10** Injury of median nerve at upper arm level, unspecified arm

X+7th **S44.11** Injury of median nerve at upper arm level, right arm

X+7th **S44.12** Injury of median nerve at upper arm level, left arm

+ **S44.2** **Injury of radial nerve at upper arm level**
Excludes1: *radial nerve NOS (S54.2)*

X+7th **S44.20** Injury of radial nerve at upper arm level, unspecified arm

X+7th **S44.21** Injury of radial nerve at upper arm level, right arm

X+7th **S44.22** Injury of radial nerve at upper arm level, left arm

+ **S44.3** **Injury of axillary nerve**

X+7th **S44.30** Injury of axillary nerve, unspecified arm

X+7th **S44.31** Injury of axillary nerve, right arm

X+7th **S44.32** Injury of axillary nerve, left arm

+ **S44.4** **Injury of musculocutaneous nerve**

X+7th **S44.40** Injury of musculocutaneous nerve, unspecified arm

X+7th **S44.41** Injury of musculocutaneous nerve, right arm

X+7th **S44.42** Injury of musculocutaneous nerve, left arm

+ **S44.5** **Injury of cutaneous sensory nerve at shoulder and upper arm level**

X+7th **S44.50** Injury of cutaneous sensory nerve at shoulder and upper arm level, unspecified arm

X+7th **S44.51** Injury of cutaneous sensory nerve at shoulder and upper arm level, right arm

X+7th **S44.52** Injury of cutaneous sensory nerve at shoulder and upper arm level, left arm

+ **S44.8** **Injury of other nerves at shoulder and upper arm level**

+ **S44.8X** Injury of other nerves at shoulder and upper arm level

+7th **S44.8X1** Injury of other nerves at shoulder and upper arm level, right arm

+7th **S44.8X2** Injury of other nerves at shoulder and upper arm level, left arm

+7th **S44.8X9** Injury of other nerves at shoulder and upper arm level, unspecified arm

+ **S44.9** **Injury of unspecified nerve at shoulder and upper arm level**

X+7th **S44.90** Injury of unspecified nerve at shoulder and upper arm level, unspecified arm

X+7th **S44.91** Injury of unspecified nerve at shoulder and upper arm level, right arm

X+7th **S44.92** Injury of unspecified nerve at shoulder and upper arm level, left arm

S45 **Injury of blood vessels at shoulder and upper arm level**

Code also any associated open wound (S41.-)
Excludes2: *injury of subclavian artery (S25.1)*
injury of subclavian vein (S25.3)

The appropriate 7th character is to be added to each code from category S45
A   initial encounter
D   subsequent encounter
S   sequela

+ **S45.0** **Injury of axillary artery**

+ **S45.00** Unspecified injury of axillary artery

MCC +7th **S45.001** Unspecified injury of axillary artery, right side

MCC +7th **S45.002** Unspecified injury of axillary artery, left side

MCC +7th **S45.009** Unspecified injury of axillary artery, unspecified side

+ **S45.01** Laceration of axillary artery

MCC +7th **S45.011** Laceration of axillary artery, right side

MCC +7th **S45.012** Laceration of axillary artery, left side

MCC +7th **S45.019** Laceration of axillary artery, unspecified side

+ **S45.09** Other specified injury of axillary artery

MCC +7th **S45.091** Other specified injury of axillary artery, right side

MCC +7th **S45.092** Other specified injury of axillary artery, left side

MCC +7th **S45.099** Other specified injury of axillary artery, unspecified side

+ **S45.1** **Injury of brachial artery**

+ **S45.10** Unspecified injury of brachial artery

CC +7th **S45.101** Unspecified injury of brachial artery, right side

CC +7th **S45.102** Unspecified injury of brachial artery, left side

CC +7th **S45.109** Unspecified injury of brachial artery, unspecified side

+ **S45.11** Laceration of brachial artery

CC +7th **S45.111** Laceration of brachial artery, right side

CC +7th **S45.112** Laceration of brachial artery, left side

CC +7th **S45.119** Laceration of brachial artery, unspecified side

+ **S45.19** Other specified injury of brachial artery

CC +7th **S45.191** Other specified injury of brachial artery, right side

CC +7th **S45.192** Other specified injury of brachial artery, left side

CC +7th **S45.199** Other specified injury of brachial artery, unspecified side

+ **S45.2** **Injury of axillary or brachial vein**

+ **S45.20** Unspecified injury of axillary or brachial vein

CC +7th **S45.201** Unspecified injury of axillary or brachial vein, right side

CC +7th **S45.202** Unspecified injury of axillary or brachial vein, left side

CC +7th **S45.209** Unspecified injury of axillary or brachial vein, unspecified side

+ **S45.21** Laceration of axillary or brachial vein
   CC +7th **S45.211** Laceration of axillary or brachial vein, right side
   CC +7th **S45.212** Laceration of axillary or brachial vein, left side
   CC +7th **S45.219** Laceration of axillary or brachial vein, unspecified side
  + **S45.29** Other specified injury of axillary or brachial vein
   CC +7th **S45.291** Other specified injury of axillary or brachial vein, right side
   CC +7th **S45.292** Other specified injury of axillary or brachial vein, left side
   CC +7th **S45.299** Other specified injury of axillary or brachial vein, unspecified side
+ **S45.3** Injury of superficial vein at shoulder and upper arm level
  + **S45.30** Unspecified injury of superficial vein at shoulder and upper arm level
   CC +7th **S45.301** Unspecified injury of superficial vein at shoulder and upper arm level, right arm
   CC +7th **S45.302** Unspecified injury of superficial vein at shoulder and upper arm level, left arm
   CC +7th **S45.309** Unspecified injury of superficial vein at shoulder and upper arm level, unspecified arm
  + **S45.31** Laceration of superficial vein at shoulder and upper arm level
   CC +7th **S45.311** Laceration of superficial vein at shoulder and upper arm level, right arm
   CC +7th **S45.312** Laceration of superficial vein at shoulder and upper arm level, left arm
   CC +7th **S45.319** Laceration of superficial vein at shoulder and upper arm level, unspecified arm
  + **S45.39** Other specified injury of superficial vein at shoulder and upper arm level
   CC +7th **S45.391** Other specified injury of superficial vein at shoulder and upper arm level, right arm
   CC +7th **S45.392** Other specified injury of superficial vein at shoulder and upper arm level, left arm
   CC +7th **S45.399** Other specified injury of superficial vein at shoulder and upper arm level, unspecified arm
+ **S45.8** Injury of other specified blood vessels at shoulder and upper arm level
  + **S45.80** Unspecified injury of other specified blood vessels at shoulder and upper arm level
   CC +7th **S45.801** Unspecified injury of other specified blood vessels at shoulder and upper arm level, right arm
   CC +7th **S45.802** Unspecified injury of other specified blood vessels at shoulder and upper arm level, left arm
   CC +7th **S45.809** Unspecified injury of other specified blood vessels at shoulder and upper arm level, unspecified arm
  + **S45.81** Laceration of other specified blood vessels at shoulder and upper arm level
   CC +7th **S45.811** Laceration of other specified blood vessels at shoulder and upper arm level, right arm
   CC +7th **S45.812** Laceration of other specified blood vessels at shoulder and upper arm level, left arm
   CC +7th **S45.819** Laceration of other specified blood vessels at shoulder and upper arm level, unspecified arm
  + **S45.89** Other specified injury of other specified blood vessels at shoulder and upper arm level
   CC +7th **S45.891** Other specified injury of other specified blood vessels at shoulder and upper arm level, right arm
   CC +7th **S45.892** Other specified injury of other specified blood vessels at shoulder and upper arm level, left arm
   CC +7th **S45.899** Other specified injury of other specified blood vessels at shoulder and upper arm level, unspecified arm

+ **S45.9** Injury of unspecified blood vessel at shoulder and upper arm level
  + **S45.90** Unspecified injury of unspecified blood vessel at shoulder and upper arm level
   CC +7th **S45.901** Unspecified injury of unspecified blood vessel at shoulder and upper arm level, right arm
   CC +7th **S45.902** Unspecified injury of unspecified blood vessel at shoulder and upper arm level, left arm
   CC +7th **S45.909** Unspecified injury of unspecified blood vessel at shoulder and upper arm level, unspecified arm
  + **S45.91** Laceration of unspecified blood vessel at shoulder and upper arm level
   CC +7th **S45.911** Laceration of unspecified blood vessel at shoulder and upper arm level, right arm
   CC +7th **S45.912** Laceration of unspecified blood vessel at shoulder and upper arm level, left arm
   CC +7th **S45.919** Laceration of unspecified blood vessel at shoulder and upper arm level, unspecified arm
  + **S45.99** Other specified injury of unspecified blood vessel at shoulder and upper arm level
   CC +7th **S45.991** Other specified injury of unspecified blood vessel at shoulder and upper arm level, right arm
   CC +7th **S45.992** Other specified injury of unspecified blood vessel at shoulder and upper arm level, left arm
   CC +7th **S45.999** Other specified injury of unspecified blood vessel at shoulder and upper arm level, unspecified arm

S46 Injury of muscle, fascia and tendon at shoulder and upper arm level

Code also any associated open wound (S41.-)
Excludes2: *injury of muscle, fascia and tendon at elbow (S56.-)*
     sprain of joints and ligaments of shoulder girdle (S43.9)

The appropriate 7th character is to be added to each code from category S46
A   initial encounter
D   subsequent encounter
S   sequela

+ **S46.0** Injury of muscle(s) and tendon(s) of the rotator cuff of shoulder
  + **S46.00** Unspecified injury of muscle(s) and tendon(s) of the rotator cuff of shoulder
   +7th **S46.001** Unspecified injury of muscle(s) and tendon(s) of the rotator cuff of right shoulder
   +7th **S46.002** Unspecified injury of muscle(s) and tendon(s) of the rotator cuff of left shoulder
   +7th **S46.009** Unspecified injury of muscle(s) and tendon(s) of the rotator cuff of unspecified shoulder
  + **S46.01** Strain of muscle(s) and tendon(s) of the rotator cuff of shoulder
   +7th **S46.011** Strain of muscle(s) and tendon(s) of the rotator cuff of right shoulder
   +7th **S46.012** Strain of muscle(s) and tendon(s) of the rotator cuff of left shoulder
   +7th **S46.019** Strain of muscle(s) and tendon(s) of the rotator cuff of unspecified shoulder
  + **S46.02** Laceration of muscle(s) and tendon(s) of the rotator cuff of shoulder
   CC +7th **S46.021** Laceration of muscle(s) and tendon(s) of the rotator cuff of right shoulder
   CC +7th **S46.022** Laceration of muscle(s) and tendon(s) of the rotator cuff of left shoulder
   CC +7th **S46.029** Laceration of muscle(s) and tendon(s) of the rotator cuff of unspecified shoulder
  + **S46.09** Other injury of muscle(s) and tendon(s) of the rotator cuff of shoulder
   +7th **S46.091** Other injury of muscle(s) and tendon(s) of the rotator cuff of right shoulder

+, +7th, X + 7th   ● Newborn   ● Pediatric   ● Maternity   ● Adult   ♀ Female   ♂ Male   Manifestation   Unacceptable PDX   HCC   CC   MCC   HAC

+7th **S46.092** Other injury of muscle(s) and tendon(s) of the rotator cuff of left shoulder

+7th **S46.099** Other injury of muscle(s) and tendon(s) of the rotator cuff of unspecified shoulder

+ **S46.1** Injury of muscle, fascia and tendon of long head of biceps

  + **S46.10** Unspecified injury of muscle, fascia and tendon of long head of biceps

    +7th **S46.101** Unspecified injury of muscle, fascia and tendon of long head of biceps, right arm

    +7th **S46.102** Unspecified injury of muscle, fascia and tendon of long head of biceps, left arm

    +7th **S46.109** Unspecified injury of muscle, fascia and tendon of long head of biceps, unspecified arm

  + **S46.11** Strain of muscle, fascia and tendon of long head of biceps

AHA CC: 2Q, 2019, 27

    +7th **S46.111** Strain of muscle, fascia and tendon of long head of biceps, right arm

    +7th **S46.112** Strain of muscle, fascia and tendon of long head of biceps, left arm

    +7th **S46.119** Strain of muscle, fascia and tendon of long head of biceps, unspecified arm

  + **S46.12** Laceration of muscle, fascia and tendon of long head of biceps

    CC +7th **S46.121** Laceration of muscle, fascia and tendon of long head of biceps, right arm

    CC +7th **S46.122** Laceration of muscle, fascia and tendon of long head of biceps, left arm

    CC +7th **S46.129** Laceration of muscle, fascia and tendon of long head of biceps, unspecified arm

  + **S46.19** Other injury of muscle, fascia and tendon of long head of biceps

    +7th **S46.191** Other injury of muscle, fascia and tendon of long head of biceps, right arm

    +7th **S46.192** Other injury of muscle, fascia and tendon of long head of biceps, left arm

    +7th **S46.199** Other injury of muscle, fascia and tendon of long head of biceps, unspecified arm

+ **S46.2** Injury of muscle, fascia and tendon of other parts of biceps

  + **S46.20** Unspecified injury of muscle, fascia and tendon of other parts of biceps

    +7th **S46.201** Unspecified injury of muscle, fascia and tendon of other parts of biceps, right arm

    +7th **S46.202** Unspecified injury of muscle, fascia and tendon of other parts of biceps, left arm

    +7th **S46.209** Unspecified injury of muscle, fascia and tendon of other parts of biceps, unspecified arm

  + **S46.21** Strain of muscle, fascia and tendon of other parts of biceps

    +7th **S46.211** Strain of muscle, fascia and tendon of other parts of biceps, right arm

    +7th **S46.212** Strain of muscle, fascia and tendon of other parts of biceps, left arm

    +7th **S46.219** Strain of muscle, fascia and tendon of other parts of biceps, unspecified arm

  + **S46.22** Laceration of muscle, fascia and tendon of other parts of biceps

    CC +7th **S46.221** Laceration of muscle, fascia and tendon of other parts of biceps, right arm

    CC +7th **S46.222** Laceration of muscle, fascia and tendon of other parts of biceps, left arm

    CC +7th **S46.229** Laceration of muscle, fascia and tendon of other parts of biceps, unspecified arm

  + **S46.29** Other injury of muscle, fascia and tendon of other parts of biceps

    +7th **S46.291** Other injury of muscle, fascia and tendon of other parts of biceps, right arm

    +7th **S46.292** Other injury of muscle, fascia and tendon of other parts of biceps, left arm

    +7th **S46.299** Other injury of muscle, fascia and tendon of other parts of biceps, unspecified arm

+ **S46.3** Injury of muscle, fascia and tendon of triceps

  + **S46.30** Unspecified injury of muscle, fascia and tendon of triceps

    +7th **S46.301** Unspecified injury of muscle, fascia and tendon of triceps, right arm

    +7th **S46.302** Unspecified injury of muscle, fascia and tendon of triceps, left arm

    +7th **S46.309** Unspecified injury of muscle, fascia and tendon of triceps, unspecified arm

  + **S46.31** Strain of muscle, fascia and tendon of triceps

    +7th **S46.311** Strain of muscle, fascia and tendon of triceps, right arm

    +7th **S46.312** Strain of muscle, fascia and tendon of triceps, left arm

    +7th **S46.319** Strain of muscle, fascia and tendon of triceps, unspecified arm

  + **S46.32** Laceration of muscle, fascia and tendon of triceps

    CC +7th **S46.321** Laceration of muscle, fascia and tendon of triceps, right arm

    CC +7th **S46.322** Laceration of muscle, fascia and tendon of triceps, left arm

    CC +7th **S46.329** Laceration of muscle, fascia and tendon of triceps, unspecified arm

  + **S46.39** Other injury of muscle, fascia and tendon of triceps

    +7th **S46.391** Other injury of muscle, fascia and tendon of triceps, right arm

    +7th **S46.392** Other injury of muscle, fascia and tendon of triceps, left arm

    +7th **S46.399** Other injury of muscle, fascia and tendon of triceps, unspecified arm

+ **S46.8** Injury of other muscles, fascia and tendons at shoulder and upper arm level

  + **S46.80** Unspecified injury of other muscles, fascia and tendons at shoulder and upper arm level

    +7th **S46.801** Unspecified injury of other muscles, fascia and tendons at shoulder and upper arm level, right arm

    +7th **S46.802** Unspecified injury of other muscles, fascia and tendons at shoulder and upper arm level, left arm

    +7th **S46.809** Unspecified injury of other muscles, fascia and tendons at shoulder and upper arm level, unspecified arm

  + **S46.81** Strain of other muscles, fascia and tendons at shoulder and upper arm level

    +7th **S46.811** Strain of other muscles, fascia and tendons at shoulder and upper arm level, right arm

    +7th **S46.812** Strain of other muscles, fascia and tendons at shoulder and upper arm level, left arm

    +7th **S46.819** Strain of other muscles, fascia and tendons at shoulder and upper arm level, unspecified arm

  + **S46.82** Laceration of other muscles, fascia and tendons at shoulder and upper arm level

    CC +7th **S46.821** Laceration of other muscles, fascia and tendons at shoulder and upper arm level, right arm

    CC +7th **S46.822** Laceration of other muscles, fascia and tendons at shoulder and upper arm level, left arm

    CC +7th **S46.829** Laceration of other muscles, fascia and tendons at shoulder and upper arm level, unspecified arm

  + **S46.89** Other injury of other muscles, fascia and tendons at shoulder and upper arm level

    +7th **S46.891** Other injury of other muscles, fascia and tendons at shoulder and upper arm level, right arm

    +7th **S46.892** Other injury of other muscles, fascia and tendons at shoulder and upper arm level, left arm

    +7th **S46.899** Other injury of other muscles, fascia and tendons at shoulder and upper arm level, unspecified arm

+ **S46.9** **Injury of unspecified muscle, fascia and tendon at shoulder and upper arm level**
    + **S46.90** **Unspecified injury of unspecified muscle, fascia and tendon at shoulder and upper arm level**
      +7th **S46.901** Unspecified injury of unspecified muscle, fascia and tendon at shoulder and upper arm level, right arm
      +7th **S46.902** Unspecified injury of unspecified muscle, fascia and tendon at shoulder and upper arm level, left arm
      +7th **S46.909** Unspecified injury of unspecified muscle, fascia and tendon at shoulder and upper arm level, unspecified arm
    + **S46.91** **Strain of unspecified muscle, fascia and tendon at shoulder and upper arm level**
      +7th **S46.911** Strain of unspecified muscle, fascia and tendon at shoulder and upper arm level, right arm
      +7th **S46.912** Strain of unspecified muscle, fascia and tendon at shoulder and upper arm level, left arm
      +7th **S46.919** Strain of unspecified muscle, fascia and tendon at shoulder and upper arm level, unspecified arm
    + **S46.92** **Laceration of unspecified muscle, fascia and tendon at shoulder and upper arm level**
      CC +7th **S46.921** Laceration of unspecified muscle, fascia and tendon at shoulder and upper arm level, right arm
      CC +7th **S46.922** Laceration of unspecified muscle, fascia and tendon at shoulder and upper arm level, left arm
      CC +7th **S46.929** Laceration of unspecified muscle, fascia and tendon at shoulder and upper arm level, unspecified arm
    + **S46.99** **Other injury of unspecified muscle, fascia and tendon at shoulder and upper arm level**
      +7th **S46.991** Other injury of unspecified muscle, fascia and tendon at shoulder and upper arm level, right arm
      +7th **S46.992** Other injury of unspecified muscle, fascia and tendon at shoulder and upper arm level, left arm
      +7th **S46.999** Other injury of unspecified muscle, fascia and tendon at shoulder and upper arm level, unspecified arm

S47 **Crushing injury of shoulder and upper arm**

Use additional code for all associated injuries
Excludes2: *crushing injury of elbow (S57.0-)*

The appropriate 7th character is to be added to each code from category S47
A initial encounter
D subsequent encounter
S sequela

X+7th **S47.1** **Crushing injury of right shoulder and upper arm**
X+7th **S47.2** **Crushing injury of left shoulder and upper arm**
X+7th **S47.9** **Crushing injury of shoulder and upper arm, unspecified arm**

S48 **Traumatic amputation of shoulder and upper arm**

An amputation not identified as partial or complete should be coded to complete
Excludes1: *traumatic amputation at elbow level (S58.0)*

The appropriate 7th character is to be added to each code from category S48
A initial encounter
D subsequent encounter
S sequela

+ **S48.0** **Traumatic amputation at shoulder joint**
    + **S48.01** **Complete traumatic amputation at shoulder joint**
      CC +7th **S48.011** Complete traumatic amputation at right shoulder joint
      CC +7th **S48.012** Complete traumatic amputation at left shoulder joint
      CC +7th **S48.019** Complete traumatic amputation at unspecified shoulder joint
    + **S48.02** **Partial traumatic amputation at shoulder joint**
      CC +7th **S48.021** Partial traumatic amputation at right shoulder joint
      CC +7th **S48.022** Partial traumatic amputation at left shoulder joint
      CC +7th **S48.029** Partial traumatic amputation at unspecified shoulder joint
+ **S48.1** **Traumatic amputation at level between shoulder and elbow**
    + **S48.11** **Complete traumatic amputation at level between shoulder and elbow**
      CC +7th **S48.111** Complete traumatic amputation at level between right shoulder and elbow
      CC +7th **S48.112** Complete traumatic amputation at level between left shoulder and elbow
      CC +7th **S48.119** Complete traumatic amputation at level between unspecified shoulder and elbow
    + **S48.12** **Partial traumatic amputation at level between shoulder and elbow**
      CC +7th **S48.121** Partial traumatic amputation at level between right shoulder and elbow
      CC +7th **S48.122** Partial traumatic amputation at level between left shoulder and elbow
      CC +7th **S48.129** Partial traumatic amputation at level between unspecified shoulder and elbow
+ **S48.9** **Traumatic amputation of shoulder and upper arm, level unspecified**
    + **S48.91** **Complete traumatic amputation of shoulder and upper arm, level unspecified**
      CC +7th **S48.911** Complete traumatic amputation of right shoulder and upper arm, level unspecified
      CC +7th **S48.912** Complete traumatic amputation of left shoulder and upper arm, level unspecified
      CC +7th **S48.919** Complete traumatic amputation of unspecified shoulder and upper arm, level unspecified
    + **S48.92** **Partial traumatic amputation of shoulder and upper arm, level unspecified**
      CC +7th **S48.921** Partial traumatic amputation of right shoulder and upper arm, level unspecified
      CC +7th **S48.922** Partial traumatic amputation of left shoulder and upper arm, level unspecified
      CC +7th **S48.929** Partial traumatic amputation of unspecified shoulder and upper arm, level unspecified

S49 **Other and unspecified injuries of shoulder and upper arm**

The appropriate 7th character is to be added to each code from subcategories S49.0 and S49.1
A initial encounter for closed fracture
D subsequent encounter for fracture with routine healing
G subsequent encounter for fracture with delayed healing
K subsequent encounter for fracture with nonunion
P subsequent encounter for fracture with malunion
S sequela

Review coding guideline C.19.c

+ **S49.0** **Physeal fracture of upper end of humerus**
    + **S49.00** **Unspecified physeal fracture of upper end of humerus**
      CC +7th **S49.001** Unspecified physeal fracture of upper end of humerus, right arm
        HAC 7th character A see Appendix B for HAC conditional logic
      CC +7th **S49.002** Unspecified physeal fracture of upper end of humerus, left arm
        HAC 7th character A see Appendix B for HAC conditional logic

+, +7th, X + 7th   ● Newborn   ● Pediatric   ● Maternity   ● Adult   ♀ Female   ♂ Male   Manifestation   Unacceptable PDX   HCC   CC   MCC   HAC

Injury to Growth Plate (Salter-Harris Classification, Rang Modification)

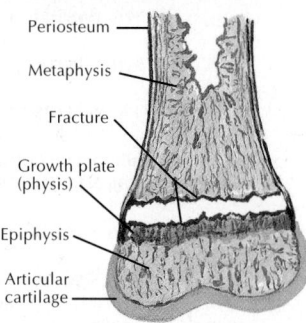

Periosteum
Metaphysis
Fracture
Growth plate (physis)
Epiphysis
Articular cartilage

Type I. Complete separation of epiphysis from shaft through calcified cartilage (growth zone) of growth plate. No bone actually fractured; periosteum may remain intact. Most common in newborns and young children

Type II. Most common. Line of separation extends partially across deep layer of growth plate and extends through metaphysis, leaving triangular portion of metaphysis attached to epiphyseal fragment

Type III. Uncommon. Intra-articular fracture throug hepiphysis, across deep zone of growth plate to periphery. Open reduction and fixation often necessary

Type IV. Fracture line extends from articular surface through epiphysis, growth plate, and metaphysis. If fractured segment not perfectly realigned with open reduction, osseous bridge across growth plate may occur, resulting in partial growth arrest and joint angulation

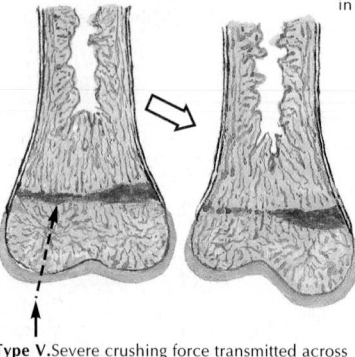

Type V. Severe crushing force transmitted across epiphysis to portion of growth plate by abduction or adduction stress or axial load. Minimal or no displacement makes radiographic diagnosis difficult; growth plate may nevertheless be damaged, resulting in partial growth arrest or shortening and angular deformity

Type VI. Portion of growth plate sheared or cut off. Raw surface heals by forming bone bridge across growth plate, limiting growth on injured side and resulting in angular deformity

CC +7th **S49.009** **Unspecified physeal fracture of upper end of humerus, unspecified arm**
HAC 7th character A see Appendix B for HAC conditional logic

+ **S49.01** **Salter-Harris Type I physeal fracture of upper end of humerus**
CC +7th **S49.011** **Salter-Harris Type I physeal fracture of upper end of humerus, right arm**
HAC 7th character A see Appendix B for HAC conditional logic
CC +7th **S49.012** **Salter-Harris Type I physeal fracture of upper end of humerus, left arm**
HAC 7th character A see Appendix B for HAC conditional logic
CC +7th **S49.019** **Salter-Harris Type I physeal fracture of upper end of humerus, unspecified arm**
HAC 7th character A see Appendix B for HAC conditional logic

+ **S49.02** **Salter-Harris Type II physeal fracture of upper end of humerus**
CC +7th **S49.021** **Salter-Harris Type II physeal fracture of upper end of humerus, right arm**
HAC 7th character A see Appendix B for HAC conditional logic
CC +7th **S49.022** **Salter-Harris Type II physeal fracture of upper end of humerus, left arm**
HAC 7th character A see Appendix B for HAC conditional logic
CC +7th **S49.029** **Salter-Harris Type II physeal fracture of upper end of humerus, unspecified arm**
HAC 7th character A see Appendix B for HAC conditional logic

+, +7th, X + 7th   ● Newborn   ● Pediatric   ● Maternity   ● Adult   ♀ Female   ♂ Male   Manifestation   Unacceptable PDX   HCC   CC   MCC   HAC

Elbow

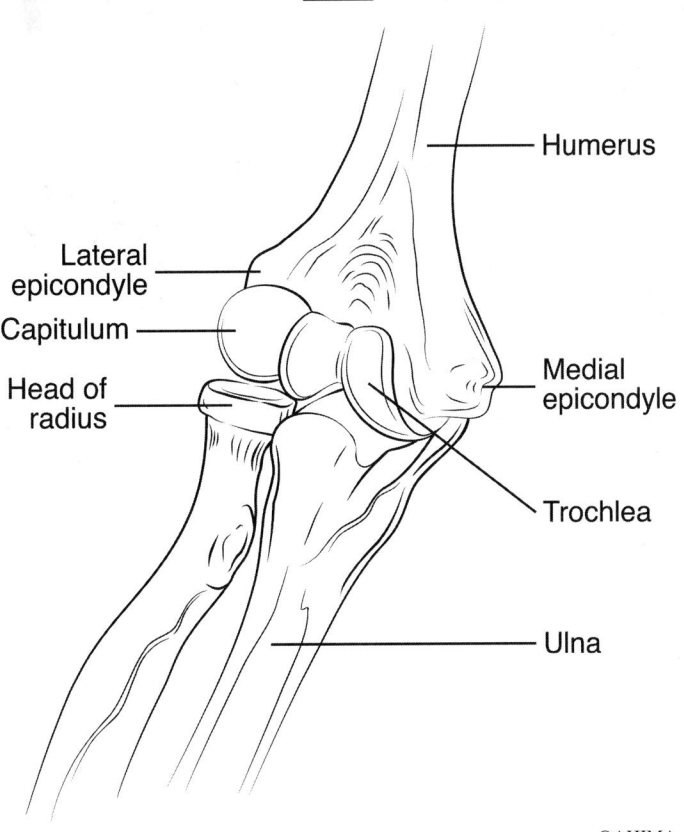

Humerus

Lateral epicondyle

Capitulum

Head of radius

Medial epicondyle

Trochlea

Ulna

©AHIMA

+ S49.03 **Salter-Harris Type III physeal fracture of upper end of humerus**
CC +7th S49.031 **Salter-Harris Type III physeal fracture of upper end of humerus, right arm**
HAC 7th character A see Appendix B for HAC conditional logic

CC +7th S49.032 **Salter-Harris Type III physeal fracture of upper end of humerus, left arm**
HAC 7th character A see Appendix B for HAC conditional logic

CC +7th S49.039 **Salter-Harris Type III physeal fracture of upper end of humerus, unspecified arm**
HAC 7th character A see Appendix B for HAC conditional logic

+ S49.04 **Salter-Harris Type IV physeal fracture of upper end of humerus**
CC +7th S49.041 **Salter-Harris Type IV physeal fracture of upper end of humerus, right arm**
HAC 7th character A see Appendix B for HAC conditional logic

CC +7th S49.042 **Salter-Harris Type IV physeal fracture of upper end of humerus, left arm**
HAC 7th character A see Appendix B for HAC conditional logic

CC +7th S49.049 **Salter-Harris Type IV physeal fracture of upper end of humerus, unspecified arm**
HAC 7th character A see Appendix B for HAC conditional logic

+ S49.09 **Other physeal fracture of upper end of humerus**
CC +7th S49.091 **Other physeal fracture of upper end of humerus, right arm**
HAC 7th character A see Appendix B for HAC conditional logic

CC +7th S49.092 **Other physeal fracture of upper end of humerus, left arm**
HAC 7th character A see Appendix B for HAC conditional logic

CC +7th S49.099 **Other physeal fracture of upper end of humerus, unspecified arm**
HAC 7th character A see Appendix B for HAC conditional logic

+ S49.1 **Physeal fracture of lower end of humerus**
+ S49.10 **Unspecified physeal fracture of lower end of humerus**
CC +7th S49.101 **Unspecified physeal fracture of lower end of humerus, right arm**
HAC 7th character A see Appendix B for HAC conditional logic

CC +7th S49.102 **Unspecified physeal fracture of lower end of humerus, left arm**
HAC 7th character A see Appendix B for HAC conditional logic

CC +7th S49.109 **Unspecified physeal fracture of lower end of humerus, unspecified arm**
HAC 7th character A see Appendix B for HAC conditional logic

+ S49.11 **Salter-Harris Type I physeal fracture of lower end of humerus**
CC +7th S49.111 **Salter-Harris Type I physeal fracture of lower end of humerus, right arm**
HAC 7th character A see Appendix B for HAC conditional logic

CC +7th S49.112 **Salter-Harris Type I physeal fracture of lower end of humerus, left arm**
HAC 7th character A see Appendix B for HAC conditional logic

CC +7th S49.119 **Salter-Harris Type I physeal fracture of lower end of humerus, unspecified arm**
HAC 7th character A see Appendix B for HAC conditional logic

+ S49.12 **Salter-Harris Type II physeal fracture of lower end of humerus**
CC +7th S49.121 **Salter-Harris Type II physeal fracture of lower end of humerus, right arm**
HAC 7th character A see Appendix B for HAC conditional logic

CC +7th S49.122 **Salter-Harris Type II physeal fracture of lower end of humerus, left arm**
HAC 7th character A see Appendix B for HAC conditional logic

1025

+, +7th, X + 7th　　● Newborn　　● Pediatric　　● Maternity　　● Adult　　♀ Female　　♂ Male　　Manifestation　　Unacceptable PDX　　HCC　　CC　　MCC　　HAC

CC +7th **S49.129** **Salter-Harris Type II physeal fracture of lower end of humerus, unspecified arm**
    HAC 7th character A see Appendix B for HAC conditional logic

+ **S49.13** **Salter-Harris Type III physeal fracture of lower end of humerus**

CC +7th **S49.131** **Salter-Harris Type III physeal fracture of lower end of humerus, right arm**
    HAC 7th character A see Appendix B for HAC conditional logic

CC +7th **S49.132** **Salter-Harris Type III physeal fracture of lower end of humerus, left arm**
    HAC 7th character A see Appendix B for HAC conditional logic

CC +7th **S49.139** **Salter-Harris Type III physeal fracture of lower end of humerus, unspecified arm**
    HAC 7th character A see Appendix B for HAC conditional logic

+ **S49.14** **Salter-Harris Type IV physeal fracture of lower end of humerus**

CC +7th **S49.141** **Salter-Harris Type IV physeal fracture of lower end of humerus, right arm**
    HAC 7th character A see Appendix B for HAC conditional logic

CC +7th **S49.142** **Salter-Harris Type IV physeal fracture of lower end of humerus, left arm**
    HAC 7th character A see Appendix B for HAC conditional logic

CC +7th **S49.149** **Salter-Harris Type IV physeal fracture of lower end of humerus, unspecified arm**
    HAC 7th character A see Appendix B for HAC conditional logic

+ **S49.19** **Other physeal fracture of lower end of humerus**

CC +7th **S49.191** **Other physeal fracture of lower end of humerus, right arm**
    HAC 7th character A see Appendix B for HAC conditional logic

CC +7th **S49.192** **Other physeal fracture of lower end of humerus, left arm**
    HAC 7th character A see Appendix B for HAC conditional logic

CC +7th **S49.199** **Other physeal fracture of lower end of humerus, unspecified arm**
    HAC 7th character A see Appendix B for HAC conditional logic

+ **S49.8** **Other specified injuries of shoulder and upper arm**

> The appropriate 7th character is to be added to each code in subcategory **S49.8**
> A initial encounter
> D subsequent encounter
> S sequela

X+7th **S49.80** **Other specified injuries of shoulder and upper arm, unspecified arm**

X+7th **S49.81** **Other specified injuries of right shoulder and upper arm**

X+7th **S49.82** **Other specified injuries of left shoulder and upper arm**

+ **S49.9** **Unspecified injury of shoulder and upper arm**

> The appropriate 7th character is to be added to each code in subcategory **S49.9**
> A initial encounter
> D subsequent encounter
> S sequela

X+7th **S49.90** **Unspecified injury of shoulder and upper arm, unspecified arm**

X+7th **S49.91** **Unspecified injury of right shoulder and upper arm**

X+7th **S49.92** **Unspecified injury of left shoulder and upper arm**

Injuries to the elbow and forearm (S50-S59)

Excludes2: *burns and corrosions (T20-T32)*
frostbite (T33-T34)
injuries of wrist and hand (S60-S69)
insect bite or sting, venomous (T63.4)

S50 **Superficial injury of elbow and forearm**

Excludes2: *superficial injury of wrist and hand (S60.-)*

> The appropriate 7th character is to be added to each code from category S50
> A initial encounter
> D subsequent encounter
> S sequela

+ **S50.0** **Contusion of elbow**
X+7th **S50.00** **Contusion of unspecified elbow**
X+7th **S50.01** **Contusion of right elbow**
X+7th **S50.02** **Contusion of left elbow**

+ **S50.1** **Contusion of forearm**
X+7th **S50.10** **Contusion of unspecified forearm**
X+7th **S50.11** **Contusion of right forearm**
X+7th **S50.12** **Contusion of left forearm**

+ **S50.3** **Other superficial injuries of elbow**
  + **S50.31** **Abrasion of elbow**
    +7th **S50.311** **Abrasion of right elbow**
    +7th **S50.312** **Abrasion of left elbow**
    +7th **S50.319** **Abrasion of unspecified elbow**
  + **S50.32** **Blister (nonthermal) of elbow**
    +7th **S50.321** **Blister (nonthermal) of right elbow**
    +7th **S50.322** **Blister (nonthermal) of left elbow**
    +7th **S50.329** **Blister (nonthermal) of unspecified elbow**
  + **S50.34** **External constriction of elbow**
    +7th **S50.341** **External constriction of right elbow**
    +7th **S50.342** **External constriction of left elbow**
    +7th **S50.349** **External constriction of unspecified elbow**
  + **S50.35** **Superficial foreign body of elbow**
    Splinter in the elbow
    +7th **S50.351** **Superficial foreign body of right elbow**
    +7th **S50.352** **Superficial foreign body of left elbow**
    +7th **S50.359** **Superficial foreign body of unspecified elbow**
  + **S50.36** **Insect bite (nonvenomous) of elbow**
    +7th **S50.361** **Insect bite (nonvenomous) of right elbow**
    +7th **S50.362** **Insect bite (nonvenomous) of left elbow**
    +7th **S50.369** **Insect bite (nonvenomous) of unspecified elbow**
  + **S50.37** **Other superficial bite of elbow**
    Excludes1: *open bite of elbow (S51.04)*
    +7th **S50.371** **Other superficial bite of right elbow**
    +7th **S50.372** **Other superficial bite of left elbow**
    +7th **S50.379** **Other superficial bite of unspecified elbow**

+ **S50.8** **Other superficial injuries of forearm**
  + **S50.81** **Abrasion of forearm**
    +7th **S50.811** **Abrasion of right forearm**
    +7th **S50.812** **Abrasion of left forearm**
    +7th **S50.819** **Abrasion of unspecified forearm**
  + **S50.82** **Blister (nonthermal) of forearm**
    +7th **S50.821** **Blister (nonthermal) of right forearm**
    +7th **S50.822** **Blister (nonthermal) of left forearm**
    +7th **S50.829** **Blister (nonthermal) of unspecified forearm**
  + **S50.84** **External constriction of forearm**
    +7th **S50.841** **External constriction of right forearm**
    +7th **S50.842** **External constriction of left forearm**
    +7th **S50.849** **External constriction of unspecified forearm**
  + **S50.85** **Superficial foreign body of forearm**
    Splinter in the forearm
    +7th **S50.851** **Superficial foreign body of right forearm**
    +7th **S50.852** **Superficial foreign body of left forearm**
    +7th **S50.859** **Superficial foreign body of unspecified forearm**

+, +7th, X + 7th ● Newborn ● Pediatric ● Maternity ● Adult ♀ Female ♂ Male Manifestation Unacceptable PDX HCC CC MCC **HAC**

+ **S50.86** **Insect bite (nonvenomous) of forearm**
    +7th **S50.861** Insect bite (nonvenomous) of right forearm
    +7th **S50.862** Insect bite (nonvenomous) of left forearm
    +7th **S50.869** Insect bite (nonvenomous) of unspecified forearm
+ **S50.87** **Other superficial bite of forearm**
    Excludes1: *open bite of forearm (S51.84)*
    +7th **S50.871** Other superficial bite of right forearm
    +7th **S50.872** Other superficial bite of left forearm
    +7th **S50.879** Other superficial bite of unspecified forearm
+ **S50.9** **Unspecified superficial injury of elbow and forearm**
  + **S50.90** **Unspecified superficial injury of elbow**
    +7th **S50.901** Unspecified superficial injury of right elbow
    +7th **S50.902** Unspecified superficial injury of left elbow
    +7th **S50.909** Unspecified superficial injury of unspecified elbow
  + **S50.91** **Unspecified superficial injury of forearm**
    S50.911 Unspecified superficial injury of right forearm
    S50.912 Unspecified superficial injury of left forearm
    S50.919 Unspecified superficial injury of unspecified forearm

S51 **Open wound of elbow and forearm**
    Code also any associated wound infection
    Excludes1: *open fracture of elbow and forearm (S52.- with open fracture 7th character)*
    traumatic amputation of elbow and forearm (S58.-)
    Excludes2: *open wound of wrist and hand (S61.-)*

> The appropriate 7th character is to be added to each code from category S51
> A initial encounter
> D subsequent encounter
> S sequela

+ **S51.0** **Open wound of elbow**
  + **S51.00** **Unspecified open wound of elbow**
    +7th **S51.001** Unspecified open wound of right elbow
      AHA CC: 4Q, 2012, 108
    +7th **S51.002** Unspecified open wound of left elbow
    +7th **S51.009** Unspecified open wound of unspecified elbow
      Open wound of elbow NOS
  + **S51.01** **Laceration without foreign body of elbow**
    +7th **S51.011** Laceration without foreign body of right elbow
    +7th **S51.012** Laceration without foreign body of left elbow
    +7th **S51.019** Laceration without foreign body of unspecified elbow
  + **S51.02** **Laceration with foreign body of elbow**
    +7th **S51.021** Laceration with foreign body of right elbow
    +7th **S51.022** Laceration with foreign body of left elbow
    +7th **S51.029** Laceration with foreign body of unspecified elbow

+ **S51.03** **Puncture wound without foreign body of elbow**
    +7th **S51.031** Puncture wound without foreign body of right elbow
    +7th **S51.032** Puncture wound without foreign body of left elbow
    +7th **S51.039** Puncture wound without foreign body of unspecified elbow
+ **S51.04** **Puncture wound with foreign body of elbow**
    +7th **S51.041** Puncture wound with foreign body of right elbow
    +7th **S51.042** Puncture wound with foreign body of left elbow
    +7th **S51.049** Puncture wound with foreign body of unspecified elbow
+ **S51.05** **Open bite of elbow**
    Bite of elbow NOS
    Excludes1: *superficial bite of elbow (S50.36, S50.37)*
    +7th **S51.051** Open bite, right elbow
    +7th **S51.052** Open bite, left elbow
    +7th **S51.059** Open bite, unspecified elbow
+ **S51.8** **Open wound of forearm**
    Excludes2: *open wound of elbow (S51.0-)*
  + **S51.80** **Unspecified open wound of forearm**
    +7th **S51.801** Unspecified open wound of right forearm
    +7th **S51.802** Unspecified open wound of left forearm
    +7th **S51.809** Unspecified open wound of unspecified forearm
      Open wound of forearm NOS
  + **S51.81** **Laceration without foreign body of forearm**
    +7th **S51.811** Laceration without foreign body of right forearm
    +7th **S51.812** Laceration without foreign body of left forearm
    +7th **S51.819** Laceration without foreign body of unspecified forearm
  + **S51.82** **Laceration with foreign body of forearm**
    +7th **S51.821** Laceration with foreign body of right forearm
    +7th **S51.822** Laceration with foreign body of left forearm
    +7th **S51.829** Laceration with foreign body of unspecified forearm
  + **S51.83** **Puncture wound without foreign body of forearm**
    +7th **S51.831** Puncture wound without foreign body of right forearm
    +7th **S51.832** Puncture wound without foreign body of left forearm
    +7th **S51.839** Puncture wound without foreign body of unspecified forearm
  + **S51.84** **Puncture wound with foreign body of forearm**
    +7th **S51.841** Puncture wound with foreign body of right forearm
    +7th **S51.842** Puncture wound with foreign body of left forearm
    +7th **S51.849** Puncture wound with foreign body of unspecified forearm
  + **S51.85** **Open bite of forearm**
    Bite of forearm NOS
    Excludes1: *superficial bite of forearm (S50.86, S50.87)*
    +7th **S51.851** Open bite of right forearm
    +7th **S51.852** Open bite of left forearm
    +7th **S51.859** Open bite of unspecified forearm

+, +7th, X + 7th   ● Newborn   ● Pediatric   ● Maternity   ● Adult   ♀ Female   ♂ Male   Manifestation   Unacceptable PDX   HCC   CC   MCC   HAC

S52   Fracture of forearm

> **NOTE**   A fracture not indicated as displaced or nondisplaced should be coded to displaced
>
> A fracture not indicated as open or closed should be coded to closed
>
> The open fracture designations are based on the Gustilo open fracture classification

Excludes1: *traumatic amputation of forearm (S58.-)*
Excludes2: *fracture at wrist and hand level (S62.-)*

The appropriate 7th character is to be added to all codes from category S52

A   initial encounter for closed fracture
B   initial encounter for open fracture type I or II initial encounter for open fracture NOS
C   initial encounter for open fracture type IIIA, IIIB, or IIIC
D   subsequent encounter for closed fracture with routine healing
E   subsequent encounter for open fracture type I or II with routine healing
F   subsequent encounter for open fracture type IIIA, IIIB, or IIIC with routine healing
G   subsequent encounter for closed fracture with delayed healing
H   subsequent encounter for open fracture type I or II with delayed healing
J   subsequent encounter for open fracture type IIIA, IIIB, or IIIC with delayed healing
K   subsequent encounter for closed fracture with nonunion
M   subsequent encounter for open fracture type I or II with nonunion
N   subsequent encounter for open fracture type IIIA, IIIB, or IIIC with nonunion
P   subsequent encounter for closed fracture with malunion
Q   subsequent encounter for open fracture type I or II with malunion
R   subsequent encounter for open fracture type IIIA, IIIB, or IIIC with malunion
S   sequela

Review coding guideline C.19.c

+ S52.0   Fracture of upper end of ulna
> Fracture of proximal end of ulna
> **Excludes2:** *fracture of elbow NOS (S42.40-)*
> *fractures of shaft of ulna (S52.2-)*

+ S52.00   Unspecified fracture of upper end of ulna
CC MCC +7th **S52.001   Unspecified fracture of upper end of right ulna**
> **HAC** 7th characters B & C see Appendix B for HAC conditional logic

CC MCC +7th **S52.002   Unspecified fracture of upper end of left ulna**
> **HAC** 7th characters B & C see Appendix B for HAC conditional logic

CC MCC +7th **S52.009   Unspecified fracture of upper end of unspecified ulna**
> **HAC** 7th characters B & C see Appendix B for HAC conditional logic

+ S52.01   Torus fracture of upper end of ulna

> The appropriate 7th character is to be added to all codes in subcategory **S52.01**
> A   initial encounter for closed fracture
> D   subsequent encounter for fracture with routine healing
> G   subsequent encounter for fracture with delayed healing
> K   subsequent encounter for fracture with nonunion
> P - subsequent encounter for fracture with malunion
> S - sequela

CC +7th **S52.011   Torus fracture of upper end of right ulna**
> **HAC** 7th character A see Appendix B for HAC conditional logic

CC +7th **S52.012   Torus fracture of upper end of left ulna**
> **HAC** 7th character A see Appendix B for HAC conditional logic

CC +7th **S52.019   Torus fracture of upper end of unspecified ulna**
> **HAC** 7th character A see Appendix B for HAC conditional logic

+ S52.02   Fracture of olecranon process without intraarticular extension of ulna
CC MCC +7th **S52.021   Displaced fracture of olecranon process without intraarticular extension of right ulna**
> **HAC** 7th characters B & C see Appendix B for HAC conditional logic

CC MCC +7th **S52.022   Displaced fracture of olecranon process without intraarticular extension of left ulna**
> **HAC** 7th characters B & C see Appendix B for HAC conditional logic

CC MCC +7th **S52.023   Displaced fracture of olecranon process without intraarticular extension of unspecified ulna**
> **HAC** 7th characters B & C see Appendix B for HAC conditional logic

CC MCC +7th **S52.024   Nondisplaced fracture of olecranon process without intraarticular extension of right ulna**
> **HAC** 7th characters B & C see Appendix B for HAC conditional logic

CC MCC +7th **S52.025   Nondisplaced fracture of olecranon process without intraarticular extension of left ulna**
> **HAC** 7th characters B & C see Appendix B for HAC conditional logic

CC MCC +7th **S52.026   Nondisplaced fracture of olecranon process without intraarticular extension of unspecified ulna**
> **HAC** 7th characters B & C see Appendix B for HAC conditional logic

+ S52.03   Fracture of olecranon process with intraarticular extension of ulna
CC MCC +7th **S52.031   Displaced fracture of olecranon process with intraarticular extension of right ulna**
> **HAC** 7th characters B & C see Appendix B for HAC conditional logic

CC MCC +7th **S52.032   Displaced fracture of olecranon process with intraarticular extension of left ulna**
> **HAC** 7th characters B & C see Appendix B for HAC conditional logic

CC MCC +7th **S52.033   Displaced fracture of olecranon process with intraarticular extension of unspecified ulna**
> **HAC** 7th characters B & C see Appendix B for HAC conditional logic

CC MCC +7th **S52.034   Nondisplaced fracture of olecranon process with intraarticular extension of right ulna**
> **HAC** 7th characters B & C see Appendix B for HAC conditional logic

CC MCC +7th **S52.035   Nondisplaced fracture of olecranon process with intraarticular extension of left ulna**
> **HAC** 7th characters B & C see Appendix B for HAC conditional logic

CC MCC +7th **S52.036   Nondisplaced fracture of olecranon process with intraarticular extension of unspecified ulna**
> **HAC** 7th characters B & C see Appendix B for HAC conditional logic

+ S52.04   Fracture of coronoid process of ulna
CC MCC +7th **S52.041   Displaced fracture of coronoid process of right ulna**
> **HAC** 7th characters B & C see Appendix B for HAC conditional logic

CC MCC +7th **S52.042   Displaced fracture of coronoid process of left ulna**
> **HAC** 7th characters B & C see Appendix B for HAC conditional logic

CC MCC +7th **S52.043   Displaced fracture of coronoid process of unspecified ulna**
> **HAC** 7th characters B & C see Appendix B for HAC conditional logic

CC MCC +7th **S52.044   Nondisplaced fracture of coronoid process of right ulna**
> **HAC** 7th characters B & C see Appendix B for HAC conditional logic

CC MCC +7th **S52.045** **Nondisplaced fracture of coronoid process of left ulna**
> HAC 7th characters B & C see Appendix B for HAC conditional logic

CC MCC +7th **S52.046** **Nondisplaced fracture of coronoid process of unspecified ulna**
> HAC 7th characters B & C see Appendix B for HAC conditional logic

+ **S52.09** **Other fracture of upper end of ulna**

CC MCC +7th **S52.091** **Other fracture of upper end of right ulna**
> HAC 7th characters B & C see Appendix B for HAC conditional logic

CC MCC +7th **S52.092** **Other fracture of upper end of left ulna**
> HAC 7th characters B & C see Appendix B for HAC conditional logic

CC MCC +7th **S52.099** **Other fracture of upper end of unspecified ulna**
> HAC 7th characters B & C see Appendix B for HAC conditional logic

+ **S52.1** **Fracture of upper end of radius**
> Fracture of proximal end of radius
> *Excludes2:* *physeal fractures of upper end of radius (S59.2-)*
> *fracture of shaft of radius (S52.3-)*

+ **S52.10** **Unspecified fracture of upper end of radius**

CC MCC +7th **S52.101** **Unspecified fracture of upper end of right radius**
> HAC 7th characters B & C see Appendix B for HAC conditional logic

CC MCC +7th **S52.102** **Unspecified fracture of upper end of left radius**
> HAC 7th characters B & C see Appendix B for HAC conditional logic

CC MCC +7th **S52.109** **Unspecified fracture of upper end of unspecified radius**
> HAC 7th characters B & C see Appendix B for HAC conditional logic

+ **S52.11** **Torus fracture of upper end of radius**

> The appropriate 7th character is to be added to all codes in subcategory **S52.11**
> A initial encounter for closed fracture
> D subsequent encounter for fracture with routine healing
> G subsequent encounter for fracture with delayed healing
> K subsequent encounter for fracture with nonunion
> P subsequent encounter for fracture with malunion
> S sequela

CC +7th **S52.111** **Torus fracture of upper end of right radius**
> HAC 7th character A see Appendix B for HAC conditional logic

CC +7th **S52.112** **Torus fracture of upper end of left radius**
> HAC 7th character A see Appendix B for HAC conditional logic

CC +7th **S52.119** **Torus fracture of upper end of unspecified radius**
> HAC 7th character A see Appendix B for HAC conditional logic

+ **S52.12** **Fracture of head of radius**

CC MCC +7th **S52.121** **Displaced fracture of head of right radius**
> HAC 7th characters B & C see Appendix B for HAC conditional logic

CC MCC +7th **S52.122** **Displaced fracture of head of left radius**
> HAC 7th characters B & C see Appendix B for HAC conditional logic

CC MCC +7th **S52.123** **Displaced fracture of head of unspecified radius**
> HAC 7th characters B & C see Appendix B for HAC conditional logic

CC MCC +7th **S52.124** **Nondisplaced fracture of head of right radius**
> HAC 7th characters B & C see Appendix B for HAC conditional logic

CC MCC +7th **S52.125** **Nondisplaced fracture of head of left radius**
> HAC 7th characters B & C see Appendix B for HAC conditional logic

CC MCC +7th **S52.126** **Nondisplaced fracture of head of unspecified radius**
> HAC 7th characters B & C see Appendix B for HAC conditional logic

+ **S52.13** **Fracture of neck of radius**

CC MCC +7th **S52.131** **Displaced fracture of neck of right radius**
> HAC 7th characters B & C see Appendix B for HAC conditional logic

CC MCC +7th **S52.132** **Displaced fracture of neck of left radius**
> HAC 7th characters B & C see Appendix B for HAC conditional logic

CC MCC +7th **S52.133** **Displaced fracture of neck of unspecified radius**
> HAC 7th characters B & C see Appendix B for HAC conditional logic

CC MCC +7th **S52.134** **Nondisplaced fracture of neck of right radius**
> HAC 7th characters B & C see Appendix B for HAC conditional logic

CC MCC +7th **S52.135** **Nondisplaced fracture of neck of left radius**
> HAC 7th characters B & C see Appendix B for HAC conditional logic

CC MCC +7th **S52.136** **Nondisplaced fracture of neck of unspecified radius**
> HAC 7th characters B & C see Appendix B for HAC conditional logic

+ **S52.18** **Other fracture of upper end of radius**

CC MCC +7th **S52.181** **Other fracture of upper end of right radius**
> HAC 7th characters B & C see Appendix B for HAC conditional logic

CC MCC +7th **S52.182** **Other fracture of upper end of left radius**
> HAC 7th characters B & C see Appendix B for HAC conditional logic

CC MCC +7th **S52.189** **Other fracture of upper end of unspecified radius**
> HAC 7th characters B & C see Appendix B for HAC conditional logic

+ **S52.2** **Fracture of shaft of ulna**

+ **S52.20** **Unspecified fracture of shaft of ulna**
> Fracture of ulna NOS

CC MCC +7th **S52.201** **Unspecified fracture of shaft of right ulna**
> HAC 7th characters A - C see Appendix B for HAC conditional logic

CC MCC +7th **S52.202** **Unspecified fracture of shaft of left ulna**
> HAC 7th characters A - C see Appendix B for HAC conditional logic

CC MCC +7th **S52.209** **Unspecified fracture of shaft of unspecified ulna**
> HAC 7th characters A - C see Appendix B for HAC conditional logic

+ **S52.21** **Greenstick fracture of shaft of ulna**

> The appropriate 7th character is to be added to all codes in subcategory **S52.21**
> A initial encounter for closed fracture
> D subsequent encounter for fracture with routine healing
> G subsequent encounter for fracture with delayed healing
> K subsequent encounter for fracture with nonunion
> P subsequent encounter for fracture with malunion
> S sequela

CC +7th **S52.211** **Greenstick fracture of shaft of right ulna**
> HAC 7th character A see Appendix B for HAC conditional logic

CC +7th **S52.212** **Greenstick fracture of shaft of left ulna**
> HAC 7th character A see Appendix B for HAC conditional logic

CC +7th **S52.219** **Greenstick fracture of shaft of unspecified ulna**
> HAC 7th character A see Appendix B for HAC conditional logic

+, +7th, X + 7th   ● Newborn   ● Pediatric   ● Maternity   ● Adult   ♀ Female   ♂ Male   Manifestation   Unacceptable PDX   HCC   CC   MCC   HAC

+ **S52.22** **Transverse fracture of shaft of ulna**

CC MCC +7th **S52.221** **Displaced transverse fracture of shaft of right ulna**
   HAC 7th characters A - C see Appendix B for HAC conditional logic

CC MCC +7th **S52.222** **Displaced transverse fracture of shaft of left ulna**
   HAC 7th characters A - C see Appendix B for HAC conditional logic

CC MCC +7th **S52.223** **Displaced transverse fracture of shaft of unspecified ulna**
   HAC 7th characters A - C see Appendix B for HAC conditional logic

CC MCC +7th **S52.224** **Nondisplaced transverse fracture of shaft of right ulna**
   HAC 7th characters A - C see Appendix B for HAC conditional logic

CC MCC +7th **S52.225** **Nondisplaced transverse fracture of shaft of left ulna**
   HAC 7th characters A - C see Appendix B for HAC conditional logic

CC MCC +7th **S52.226** **Nondisplaced transverse fracture of shaft of unspecified ulna**
   HAC 7th characters A - C see Appendix B for HAC conditional logic

+ **S52.23** **Oblique fracture of shaft of ulna**

CC MCC +7th **S52.231** **Displaced oblique fracture of shaft of right ulna**
   HAC 7th characters A - C see Appendix B for HAC conditional logic

CC MCC +7th **S52.232** **Displaced oblique fracture of shaft of left ulna**
   HAC 7th characters A - C see Appendix B for HAC conditional logic

CC MCC +7th **S52.233** **Displaced oblique fracture of shaft of unspecified ulna**
   HAC 7th characters A - C see Appendix B for HAC conditional logic

CC MCC +7th **S52.234** **Nondisplaced oblique fracture of shaft of right ulna**
   HAC 7th characters A - C see Appendix B for HAC conditional logic

CC MCC +7th **S52.235** **Nondisplaced oblique fracture of shaft of left ulna**
   HAC 7th characters A - C see Appendix B for HAC conditional logic

CC MCC +7th **S52.236** **Nondisplaced oblique fracture of shaft of unspecified ulna**
   HAC 7th characters A - C see Appendix B for HAC conditional logic

+ **S52.24** **Spiral fracture of shaft of ulna**

CC MCC +7th **S52.241** **Displaced spiral fracture of shaft of ulna, right arm**
   HAC 7th characters A - C see Appendix B for HAC conditional logic

CC MCC +7th **S52.242** **Displaced spiral fracture of shaft of ulna, left arm**
   HAC 7th characters A - C see Appendix B for HAC conditional logic

CC MCC +7th **S52.243** **Displaced spiral fracture of shaft of ulna, unspecified arm**
   HAC 7th characters A - C see Appendix B for HAC conditional logic

CC MCC +7th **S52.244** **Nondisplaced spiral fracture of shaft of ulna, right arm**
   HAC 7th characters A - C see Appendix B for HAC conditional logic

CC MCC +7th **S52.245** **Nondisplaced spiral fracture of shaft of ulna, left arm**
   HAC 7th characters A - C see Appendix B for HAC conditional logic

CC MCC +7th **S52.246** **Nondisplaced spiral fracture of shaft of ulna, unspecified arm**
   HAC 7th characters A - C see Appendix B for HAC conditional logic

+ **S52.25** **Comminuted fracture of shaft of ulna**

CC MCC +7th **S52.251** **Displaced comminuted fracture of shaft of ulna, right arm**
   HAC 7th characters A - C see Appendix B for HAC conditional logic

CC MCC +7th **S52.252** **Displaced comminuted fracture of shaft of ulna, left arm**
   HAC 7th characters A - C see Appendix B for HAC conditional logic

CC MCC +7th **S52.253** **Displaced comminuted fracture of shaft of ulna, unspecified arm**
   HAC 7th characters A - C see Appendix B for HAC conditional logic

CC MCC +7th **S52.254** **Nondisplaced comminuted fracture of shaft of ulna, right arm**
   HAC 7th characters A - C see Appendix B for HAC conditional logic

CC MCC +7th **S52.255** **Nondisplaced comminuted fracture of shaft of ulna, left arm**
   HAC 7th characters A - C see Appendix B for HAC conditional logic

CC MCC +7th **S52.256** **Nondisplaced comminuted fracture of shaft of ulna, unspecified arm**
   HAC 7th characters A - C see Appendix B for HAC conditional logic

+ **S52.26** **Segmental fracture of shaft of ulna**

CC MCC +7th **S52.261** **Displaced segmental fracture of shaft of ulna, right arm**
   HAC 7th characters A - C see Appendix B for HAC conditional logic

CC MCC +7th **S52.262** **Displaced segmental fracture of shaft of ulna, left arm**
   HAC 7th characters A - C see Appendix B for HAC conditional logic

CC MCC +7th **S52.263** **Displaced segmental fracture of shaft of ulna, unspecified arm**
   HAC 7th characters A - C see Appendix B for HAC conditional logic

CC MCC +7th **S52.264** **Nondisplaced segmental fracture of shaft of ulna, right arm**
   HAC 7th characters A - C see Appendix B for HAC conditional logic

CC MCC +7th **S52.265** **Nondisplaced segmental fracture of shaft of ulna, left arm**
   HAC 7th characters A - C see Appendix B for HAC conditional logic

CC MCC +7th **S52.266** **Nondisplaced segmental fracture of shaft of ulna, unspecified arm**
   HAC 7th characters A - C see Appendix B for HAC conditional logic

+ **S52.27** **Monteggia's fracture of ulna**
   Fracture of upper shaft of ulna with dislocation of radial head

CC MCC +7th **S52.271** **Monteggia's fracture of right ulna**
   HAC 7th characters B & C see Appendix B for HAC conditional logic

CC MCC +7th **S52.272** **Monteggia's fracture of left ulna**
   HAC 7th characters B & C see Appendix B for HAC conditional logic

CC MCC +7th **S52.279** **Monteggia's fracture of unspecified ulna**
   HAC 7th characters B & C see Appendix B for HAC conditional logic

+ **S52.28** **Bent bone of ulna**

CC MCC +7th **S52.281** **Bent bone of right ulna**
   HAC 7th characters A - C see Appendix B for HAC conditional logic

CC MCC +7th **S52.282** **Bent bone of left ulna**
   HAC 7th characters A - C see Appendix B for HAC conditional logic

CC MCC +7th **S52.283** **Bent bone of unspecified ulna**
   HAC 7th characters A - C see Appendix B for HAC conditional logic

+ **S52.29** **Other fracture of shaft of ulna**

CC MCC +7th **S52.291** **Other fracture of shaft of right ulna**
   HAC 7th characters A - C see Appendix B for HAC conditional logic

CC MCC +7th **S52.292** **Other fracture of shaft of left ulna**
   HAC 7th characters A - C see Appendix B for HAC conditional logic

CC MCC +7th **S52.299** **Other fracture of shaft of unspecified ulna**
   HAC 7th characters A - C see Appendix B for HAC conditional logic

+ **S52.3** **Fracture of shaft of radius**

+ **S52.30** **Unspecified fracture of shaft of radius**

CC MCC +7th **S52.301** **Unspecified fracture of shaft of right radius**
   HAC 7th characters A - C see Appendix B for HAC conditional logic

CC MCC +7th **S52.302** **Unspecified fracture of shaft of left radius**
   HAC 7th characters A - C see Appendix B for HAC conditional logic

CC MCC +7th **S52.309** **Unspecified fracture of shaft of unspecified radius**
   HAC 7th characters A - C see Appendix B for HAC conditional logic

+, +7th, X + 7th   ● Newborn   ● Pediatric   ● Maternity   ● Adult   ♀ Female   ♂ Male   Manifestation   Unacceptable PDX   HCC   CC   MCC   HAC

+ **S52.31** **Greenstick fracture of shaft of radius**

> The appropriate 7th character is to be added to all codes in subcategory **S52.31**
> A   initial encounter for closed fracture
> D   subsequent encounter for fracture with routine healing
> G   subsequent encounter for fracture with delayed healing
> K   subsequent encounter for fracture with nonunion
> P   subsequent encounter for fracture with malunion
> S   sequela

CC +7th **S52.311** **Greenstick fracture of shaft of radius, right arm**
HAC 7th character A see Appendix B for HAC conditional logic

CC +7th **S52.312** **Greenstick fracture of shaft of radius, left arm**
HAC 7th character A see Appendix B for HAC conditional logic

CC +7th **S52.319** **Greenstick fracture of shaft of radius, unspecified arm**
HAC 7th character A see Appendix B for HAC conditional logic

+ **S52.32** **Transverse fracture of shaft of radius**

CC MCC +7th **S52.321** **Displaced transverse fracture of shaft of right radius**
HAC 7th characters A - C see Appendix B for HAC conditional logic

CC MCC +7th **S52.322** **Displaced transverse fracture of shaft of left radius**
HAC 7th characters A - C see Appendix B for HAC conditional logic

CC MCC +7th **S52.323** **Displaced transverse fracture of shaft of unspecified radius**
HAC 7th characters A - C see Appendix B for HAC conditional logic

CC MCC +7th **S52.324** **Nondisplaced transverse fracture of shaft of right radius**
HAC 7th characters A - C see Appendix B for HAC conditional logic

CC MCC +7th **S52.325** **Nondisplaced transverse fracture of shaft of left radius**
HAC 7th characters A - C see Appendix B for HAC conditional logic

CC MCC +7th **S52.326** **Nondisplaced transverse fracture of shaft of unspecified radius**
HAC 7th characters A - C see Appendix B for HAC conditional logic

+ **S52.33** **Oblique fracture of shaft of radius**

CC MCC +7th **S52.331** **Displaced oblique fracture of shaft of right radius**
HAC 7th characters A - C see Appendix B for HAC conditional logic

CC MCC +7th **S52.332** **Displaced oblique fracture of shaft of left radius**
HAC 7th characters A - C see Appendix B for HAC conditional logic

CC MCC +7th **S52.333** **Displaced oblique fracture of shaft of unspecified radius**
HAC 7th characters A - C see Appendix B for HAC conditional logic

CC MCC +7th **S52.334** **Nondisplaced oblique fracture of shaft of right radius**
HAC 7th characters A - C see Appendix B for HAC conditional logic

CC MCC +7th **S52.335** **Nondisplaced oblique fracture of shaft of left radius**
HAC 7th characters A - C see Appendix B for HAC conditional logic

CC MCC +7th **S52.336** **Nondisplaced oblique fracture of shaft of unspecified radius**
HAC 7th characters A - C see Appendix B for HAC conditional logic

+ **S52.34** **Spiral fracture of shaft of radius**

CC MCC +7th **S52.341** **Displaced spiral fracture of shaft of radius, right arm**
HAC 7th characters A - C see Appendix B for HAC conditional logic

CC MCC +7th **S52.342** **Displaced spiral fracture of shaft of radius, left arm**
HAC 7th characters A - C see Appendix B for HAC conditional logic

CC MCC +7th **S52.343** **Displaced spiral fracture of shaft of radius, unspecified arm**
HAC 7th characters A - C see Appendix B for HAC conditional logic

CC MCC +7th **S52.344** **Nondisplaced spiral fracture of shaft of radius, right arm**
HAC 7th characters A - C see Appendix B for HAC conditional logic

CC MCC +7th **S52.345** **Nondisplaced spiral fracture of shaft of radius, left arm**
HAC 7th characters A - C see Appendix B for HAC conditional logic

CC MCC +7th **S52.346** **Nondisplaced spiral fracture of shaft of radius, unspecified arm**
HAC 7th characters A - C see Appendix B for HAC conditional logic

+ **S52.35** **Comminuted fracture of shaft of radius**

CC MCC +7th **S52.351** **Displaced comminuted fracture of shaft of radius, right arm**
HAC 7th characters A - C see Appendix B for HAC conditional logic

CC MCC +7th **S52.352** **Displaced comminuted fracture of shaft of radius, left arm**
HAC 7th characters A - C see Appendix B for HAC conditional logic

CC MCC +7th **S52.353** **Displaced comminuted fracture of shaft of radius, unspecified arm**
HAC 7th characters A - C see Appendix B for HAC conditional logic

CC MCC +7th **S52.354** **Nondisplaced comminuted fracture of shaft of radius, right arm**
HAC 7th characters A - C see Appendix B for HAC conditional logic

CC MCC +7th **S52.355** **Nondisplaced comminuted fracture of shaft of radius, left arm**
HAC 7th characters A - C see Appendix B for HAC conditional logic

CC MCC +7th **S52.356** **Nondisplaced comminuted fracture of shaft of radius, unspecified arm**
HAC 7th characters A - C see Appendix B for HAC conditional logic

+ **S52.36** **Segmental fracture of shaft of radius**

CC MCC +7th **S52.361** **Displaced segmental fracture of shaft of radius, right arm**
HAC 7th characters A - C see Appendix B for HAC conditional logic

CC MCC +7th **S52.362** **Displaced segmental fracture of shaft of radius, left arm**
HAC 7th characters A - C see Appendix B for HAC conditional logic

CC MCC +7th **S52.363** **Displaced segmental fracture of shaft of radius, unspecified arm**
HAC 7th characters A - C see Appendix B for HAC conditional logic

CC MCC +7th **S52.364** **Nondisplaced segmental fracture of shaft of radius, right arm**
HAC 7th characters A - C see Appendix B for HAC conditional logic

CC MCC +7th **S52.365** **Nondisplaced segmental fracture of shaft of radius, left arm**
HAC 7th characters A - C see Appendix B for HAC conditional logic

CC MCC +7th **S52.366** **Nondisplaced segmental fracture of shaft of radius, unspecified arm**
HAC 7th characters A - C see Appendix B for HAC conditional logic

+ **S52.37** **Galeazzi's fracture**
Fracture of lower shaft of radius with radioulnar joint dislocation

CC MCC +7th **S52.371** **Galeazzi's fracture of right radius**
HAC 7th characters A - C see Appendix B for HAC conditional logic

CC MCC +7th **S52.372** **Galeazzi's fracture of left radius**
HAC 7th characters A - C see Appendix B for HAC conditional logic

CC MCC +7th **S52.379** **Galeazzi's fracture of unspecified radius**
HAC 7th characters A - C see Appendix B for HAC conditional logic

+ **S52.38** **Bent bone of radius**

CC MCC +7th **S52.381** **Bent bone of right radius**
HAC 7th characters A - C see Appendix B for HAC conditional logic

CC MCC +7th **S52.382** **Bent bone of left radius**
HAC 7th characters A - C see Appendix B for HAC conditional logic

---

+, +7th, X + 7th   ● Newborn   ● Pediatric   ● Maternity   ● Adult   ♀ Female   ♂ Male   Manifestation   Unacceptable PDX   HCC   CC   MCC   HAC

CC MCC +7th **S52.389** **Bent bone of unspecified radius**
    HAC 7th characters A - C see Appendix B for HAC conditional logic

+ **S52.39** **Other fracture of shaft of radius**
CC MCC +7th **S52.391** **Other fracture of shaft of radius, right arm**
    HAC 7th characters A - C see Appendix B for HAC conditional logic

CC MCC +7th **S52.392** **Other fracture of shaft of radius, left arm**
    HAC 7th characters A - C see Appendix B for HAC conditional logic

CC MCC +7th **S52.399** **Other fracture of shaft of radius, unspecified arm**
    HAC 7th characters A - C see Appendix B for HAC conditional logic

+ **S52.5** **Fracture of lower end of radius**
    Fracture of distal end of radius
    Excludes2: *physeal fractures of lower end of radius (S59.2-)*

+ **S52.50** **Unspecified fracture of the lower end of radius**
CC MCC +7th **S52.501** **Unspecified fracture of the lower end of right radius**
    HAC 7th characters A - C see Appendix B for HAC conditional logic

CC MCC +7th **S52.502** **Unspecified fracture of the lower end of left radius**
    HAC 7th characters A - C see Appendix B for HAC conditional logic

CC MCC +7th **S52.509** **Unspecified fracture of the lower end of unspecified radius**
    HAC 7th characters A - C see Appendix B for HAC conditional logic

+ **S52.51** **Fracture of radial styloid process**
CC MCC +7th **S52.511** **Displaced fracture of right radial styloid process**
    HAC 7th characters A - C see Appendix B for HAC conditional logic

CC MCC +7th **S52.512** **Displaced fracture of left radial styloid process**
    HAC 7th characters A - C see Appendix B for HAC conditional logic

CC MCC +7th **S52.513** **Displaced fracture of unspecified radial styloid process**
    HAC 7th characters A - C see Appendix B for HAC conditional logic

CC MCC +7th **S52.514** **Nondisplaced fracture of right radial styloid process**
    HAC 7th characters A - C see Appendix B for HAC conditional logic

CC MCC +7th **S52.515** **Nondisplaced fracture of left radial styloid process**
    HAC 7th characters A - C see Appendix B for HAC conditional logic

CC MCC +7th **S52.516** **Nondisplaced fracture of unspecified radial styloid process**
    HAC 7th characters A - C see Appendix B for HAC conditional logic

+ **S52.52** **Torus fracture of lower end of radius**

> The appropriate 7th character is to be added to all codes in subcategory **S52.52**
> A   initial encounter for closed fracture
> D   subsequent encounter for fracture with routine healing
> G   subsequent encounter for fracture with delayed healing
> K   subsequent encounter for fracture with nonunion
> P   subsequent encounter for fracture with malunion
> S   sequela

CC +7th **S52.521** **Torus fracture of lower end of right radius**
    HAC 7th character A see Appendix B for HAC conditional logic

CC +7th **S52.522** **Torus fracture of lower end of left radius**
    HAC 7th character A see Appendix B for HAC conditional logic

CC +7th **S52.529** **Torus fracture of lower end of unspecified radius**
    HAC 7th character A see Appendix B for HAC conditional logic

+ **S52.53** **Colles' fracture**
CC MCC +7th **S52.531** **Colles' fracture of right radius**
    HAC 7th characters A - C see Appendix B for HAC conditional logic

CC MCC +7th **S52.532** **Colles' fracture of left radius**
    AHA CC: 2Q, 2016, 4-5
    HAC 7th characters A - C see Appendix B for HAC conditional logic

CC MCC +7th **S52.539** **Colles' fracture of unspecified radius**
    HAC 7th characters A - C see Appendix B for HAC conditional logic

+ **S52.54** **Smith's fracture**
CC MCC +7th **S52.541** **Smith's fracture of right radius**
    HAC 7th characters A - C see Appendix B for HAC conditional logic

CC MCC +7th **S52.542** **Smith's fracture of left radius**
    HAC 7th characters A - C see Appendix B for HAC conditional logic

CC MCC +7th **S52.549** **Smith's fracture of unspecified radius**
    HAC 7th characters A - C see Appendix B for HAC conditional logic

+ **S52.55** **Other extraarticular fracture of lower end of radius**
CC MCC +7th **S52.551** **Other extraarticular fracture of lower end of right radius**
    HAC 7th characters A - C see Appendix B for HAC conditional logic

CC MCC +7th **S52.552** **Other extraarticular fracture of lower end of left radius**
    HAC 7th characters A - C see Appendix B for HAC conditional logic

CC MCC +7th **S52.559** **Other extraarticular fracture of lower end of unspecified radius**
    HAC 7th characters A - C see Appendix B for HAC conditional logic

+ **S52.56** **Barton's fracture**
CC MCC +7th **S52.561** **Barton's fracture of right radius**
    HAC 7th characters A - C see Appendix B for HAC conditional logic

CC MCC +7th **S52.562** **Barton's fracture of left radius**
    HAC 7th characters A - C see Appendix B for HAC conditional logic

CC MCC +7th **S52.569** **Barton's fracture of unspecified radius**
    HAC 7th characters A - C see Appendix B for HAC conditional logic

+ **S52.57** **Other intraarticular fracture of lower end of radius**
CC MCC +7th **S52.571** **Other intraarticular fracture of lower end of right radius**
    HAC 7th characters A - C see Appendix B for HAC conditional logic

CC MCC +7th **S52.572** **Other intraarticular fracture of lower end of left radius**
    HAC 7th characters A - C see Appendix B for HAC conditional logic

CC MCC +7th **S52.579** **Other intraarticular fracture of lower end of unspecified radius**
    HAC 7th characters A - C see Appendix B for HAC conditional logic

+ **S52.59** **Other fractures of lower end of radius**
CC MCC +7th **S52.591** **Other fractures of lower end of right radius**
    AHA CC: 3Q, 2019, 9-10
    HAC 7th characters A - C see Appendix B for HAC conditional logic

CC MCC +7th **S52.592** **Other fractures of lower end of left radius**
    HAC 7th characters A - C see Appendix B for HAC conditional logic

CC MCC +7th **S52.599** **Other fractures of lower end of unspecified radius**
    HAC 7th characters A - C see Appendix B for HAC conditional logic

+ **S52.6** **Fracture of lower end of ulna**
+ **S52.60** **Unspecified fracture of lower end of ulna**
CC MCC +7th **S52.601** **Unspecified fracture of lower end of right ulna**
    HAC 7th characters A - C see Appendix B for HAC conditional logic

CC MCC +7th **S52.602** **Unspecified fracture of lower end of left ulna**
    HAC 7th characters A - C see Appendix B for HAC conditional logic

CC MCC +7th **S52.609** **Unspecified fracture of lower end of unspecified ulna**
    HAC 7th characters A - C see Appendix B for HAC conditional logic

+, +7th, X + 7th   ● Newborn   ● Pediatric   ● Maternity   ● Adult   ♀ Female   ♂ Male   Manifestation   Unacceptable PDX   HCC   CC   MCC   HAC

	+ S52.61		**Fracture of ulna styloid process**
CC MCC +7th	S52.611		**Displaced fracture of right ulna styloid process**
		HAC	7th characters A - C see Appendix B for HAC conditional logic
CC MCC +7th	S52.612		**Displaced fracture of left ulna styloid process**
		HAC	7th characters A - C see Appendix B for HAC conditional logic
CC MCC +7th	S52.613		**Displaced fracture of unspecified ulna styloid process**
		HAC	7th characters A - C see Appendix B for HAC conditional logic
CC MCC +7th	S52.614		**Nondisplaced fracture of right ulna styloid process**
		HAC	7th characters A - C see Appendix B for HAC conditional logic
CC MCC +7th	S52.615		**Nondisplaced fracture of left ulna styloid process**
		HAC	7th characters A - C see Appendix B for HAC conditional logic
CC MCC +7th	S52.616		**Nondisplaced fracture of unspecified ulna styloid process**
		HAC	7th characters A - C see Appendix B for HAC conditional logic

+ S52.62 Torus fracture of lower end of ulna

> The appropriate 7th character is to be added to all codes in subcategory **S52.62**
> A   initial encounter for closed fracture
> D   subsequent encounter for fracture with routine healing
> G   subsequent encounter for fracture with delayed healing
> K   subsequent encounter for fracture with nonunion
> P   subsequent encounter for fracture with malunion
> S   sequela

CC +7th	S52.621		**Torus fracture of lower end of right ulna**
		HAC	7th character A see Appendix B for HAC conditional logic
CC +7th	S52.622		**Torus fracture of lower end of left ulna**
		HAC	7th character A see Appendix B for HAC conditional logic
CC +7th	S52.629		**Torus fracture of lower end of unspecified ulna**
		HAC	7th character A see Appendix B for HAC conditional logic

+ S52.69 Other fracture of lower end of ulna

CC MCC +7th	S52.691		**Other fracture of lower end of right ulna**
			AHA CC: 3Q, 2019, 9-10
		HAC	7th characters A - C see Appendix B for HAC conditional logic
CC MCC +7th	S52.692		**Other fracture of lower end of left ulna**
		HAC	7th characters A - C see Appendix B for HAC conditional logic
CC MCC +7th	S52.699		**Other fracture of lower end of unspecified ulna**
		HAC	7th characters A - C see Appendix B for HAC conditional logic

+ S52.9 Unspecified fracture of forearm

CC MCC X+7th	S52.90		**Unspecified fracture of unspecified forearm**
		HAC	7th characters A - C see Appendix B for HAC conditional logic
CC MCC X+7th	S52.91		**Unspecified fracture of right forearm**
		HAC	7th characters A - C see Appendix B for HAC conditional logic
CC MCC X+7th	S52.92		**Unspecified fracture of left forearm**
		HAC	7th characters A - C see Appendix B for HAC conditional logic

S53 Dislocation and sprain of joints and ligaments of elbow

> **Includes:** avulsion of joint or ligament of elbow
> laceration of cartilage, joint or ligament of elbow
> sprain of cartilage, joint or ligament of elbow
> traumatic hemarthrosis of joint or ligament of elbow
> traumatic rupture of joint or ligament of elbow
> traumatic subluxation of joint or ligament of elbow
> traumatic tear of joint or ligament of elbow

Code also any associated open wound

> **Excludes2:** *strain of muscle, fascia and tendon at forearm level (S56.-)*

> The appropriate 7th character is to be added to each code from category S53
> A   initial encounter
> D   subsequent encounter
> S   sequela

+ S53.0 Subluxation and dislocation of radial head
  Dislocation of radiohumeral joint
  Subluxation of radiohumeral joint
  Excludes1: *Monteggia's fracture-dislocation (S52.27-)*

+ S53.00 Unspecified subluxation and dislocation of radial head

+7th	S53.001	**Unspecified subluxation of right radial head**
+7th	S53.002	**Unspecified subluxation of left radial head**
+7th	S53.003	**Unspecified subluxation of unspecified radial head**
+7th	S53.004	**Unspecified dislocation of right radial head**
+7th	S53.005	**Unspecified dislocation of left radial head**
+7th	S53.006	**Unspecified dislocation of unspecified radial head**

+ S53.01 Anterior subluxation and dislocation of radial head
  Anteriomedial subluxation and dislocation of radial head

+7th	S53.011	**Anterior subluxation of right radial head**
+7th	S53.012	**Anterior subluxation of left radial head**
+7th	S53.013	**Anterior subluxation of unspecified radial head**
+7th	S53.014	**Anterior dislocation of right radial head**
+7th	S53.015	**Anterior dislocation of left radial head**
+7th	S53.016	**Anterior dislocation of unspecified radial head**

+ S53.02 Posterior subluxation and dislocation of radial head
  Posteriolateral subluxation and dislocation of radial head

+7th	S53.021	**Posterior subluxation of right radial head**
+7th	S53.022	**Posterior subluxation of left radial head**
+7th	S53.023	**Posterior subluxation of unspecified radial head**
+7th	S53.024	**Posterior dislocation of right radial head**
+7th	S53.025	**Posterior dislocation of left radial head**
+7th	S53.026	**Posterior dislocation of unspecified radial head**

+ S53.03 Nursemaid's elbow

+7th	S53.031	**Nursemaid's elbow, right elbow**
		AHA CC: 1Q, 2015, 3-21
+7th	S53.032	**Nursemaid's elbow, left elbow**
+7th	S53.033	**Nursemaid's elbow, unspecified elbow**

+ S53.09 Other subluxation and dislocation of radial head

+7th	S53.091	**Other subluxation of right radial head**
+7th	S53.092	**Other subluxation of left radial head**
+7th	S53.093	**Other subluxation of unspecified radial head**
+7th	S53.094	**Other dislocation of right radial head**
+7th	S53.095	**Other dislocation of left radial head**
+7th	S53.096	**Other dislocation of unspecified radial head**

+, +7th, X + 7th	• Newborn	• Pediatric	• Maternity	• Adult	♀ Female	♂ Male	Manifestation	Unacceptable PDX	HCC	CC	MCC	HAC

+ S53.1 Subluxation and dislocation of ulnohumeral joint

Subluxation and dislocation of elbow NOS

Excludes1: dislocation of radial head alone (S53.0-)

+ S53.10 Unspecified subluxation and dislocation of ulnohumeral joint

+7th S53.101 Unspecified subluxation of right ulnohumeral joint

+7th S53.102 Unspecified subluxation of left ulnohumeral joint

+7th S53.103 Unspecified subluxation of unspecified ulnohumeral joint

+7th S53.104 Unspecified dislocation of right ulnohumeral joint

+7th S53.105 Unspecified dislocation of left ulnohumeral joint

+7th S53.106 Unspecified dislocation of unspecified ulnohumeral joint

+ S53.11 Anterior subluxation and dislocation of ulnohumeral joint

+7th S53.111 Anterior subluxation of right ulnohumeral joint

+7th S53.112 Anterior subluxation of left ulnohumeral joint

+7th S53.113 Anterior subluxation of unspecified ulnohumeral joint

+7th S53.114 Anterior dislocation of right ulnohumeral joint

AHA CC: 4Q, 2012, 108

+7th S53.115 Anterior dislocation of left ulnohumeral joint

+7th S53.116 Anterior dislocation of unspecified ulnohumeral joint

+ S53.12 Posterior subluxation and dislocation of ulnohumeral joint

+7th S53.121 Posterior subluxation of right ulnohumeral joint

+7th S53.122 Posterior subluxation of left ulnohumeral joint

+7th S53.123 Posterior subluxation of unspecified ulnohumeral joint

+7th S53.124 Posterior dislocation of right ulnohumeral joint

+7th S53.125 Posterior dislocation of left ulnohumeral joint

+7th S53.126 Posterior dislocation of unspecified ulnohumeral joint

+ S53.13 Medial subluxation and dislocation of ulnohumeral joint

+7th S53.131 Medial subluxation of right ulnohumeral joint

+7th S53.132 Medial subluxation of left ulnohumeral joint

+7th S53.133 Medial subluxation of unspecified ulnohumeral joint

+7th S53.134 Medial dislocation of right ulnohumeral joint

+7th S53.135 Medial dislocation of left ulnohumeral joint

+7th S53.136 Medial dislocation of unspecified ulnohumeral joint

+ S53.14 Lateral subluxation and dislocation of ulnohumeral joint

+7th S53.141 Lateral subluxation of right ulnohumeral joint

+7th S53.142 Lateral subluxation of left ulnohumeral joint

+7th S53.143 Lateral subluxation of unspecified ulnohumeral joint

+7th S53.144 Lateral dislocation of right ulnohumeral joint

+7th S53.145 Lateral dislocation of left ulnohumeral joint

+7th S53.146 Lateral dislocation of unspecified ulnohumeral joint

+ S53.19 Other subluxation and dislocation of ulnohumeral joint

+7th S53.191 Other subluxation of right ulnohumeral joint

+7th S53.192 Other subluxation of left ulnohumeral joint

+7th S53.193 Other subluxation of unspecified ulnohumeral joint

+7th S53.194 Other dislocation of right ulnohumeral joint

+7th S53.195 Other dislocation of left ulnohumeral joint

+7th S53.196 Other dislocation of unspecified ulnohumeral joint

+ S53.2 Traumatic rupture of radial collateral ligament

Excludes1: sprain of radial collateral ligament NOS (S53.43-)

X+7th S53.20 Traumatic rupture of unspecified radial collateral ligament

X+7th S53.21 Traumatic rupture of right radial collateral ligament

X+7th S53.22 Traumatic rupture of left radial collateral ligament

+ S53.3 Traumatic rupture of ulnar collateral ligament

Excludes1: sprain of ulnar collateral ligament (S53.44-)

X+7th S53.30 Traumatic rupture of unspecified ulnar collateral ligament

X+7th S53.31 Traumatic rupture of right ulnar collateral ligament

X+7th S53.32 Traumatic rupture of left ulnar collateral ligament

+ S53.4 Sprain of elbow

Excludes2: traumatic rupture of radial collateral ligament (S53.2-)

traumatic rupture of ulnar collateral ligament (S53.3-)

+ S53.40 Unspecified sprain of elbow

+7th S53.401 Unspecified sprain of right elbow

+7th S53.402 Unspecified sprain of left elbow

+7th S53.409 Unspecified sprain of unspecified elbow

Sprain of elbow NOS

+ S53.41 Radiohumeral (joint) sprain

+7th S53.411 Radiohumeral (joint) sprain of right elbow

+7th S53.412 Radiohumeral (joint) sprain of left elbow

+7th S53.419 Radiohumeral (joint) sprain of unspecified elbow

+ S53.42 Ulnohumeral (joint) sprain

+7th S53.421 Ulnohumeral (joint) sprain of right elbow

+7th S53.422 Ulnohumeral (joint) sprain of left elbow

+7th S53.429 Ulnohumeral (joint) sprain of unspecified elbow

+ S53.43 Radial collateral ligament sprain

+7th S53.431 Radial collateral ligament sprain of right elbow

+7th S53.432 Radial collateral ligament sprain of left elbow

+7th S53.439 Radial collateral ligament sprain of unspecified elbow

+ S53.44 Ulnar collateral ligament sprain

+7th S53.441 Ulnar collateral ligament sprain of right elbow

+7th S53.442 Ulnar collateral ligament sprain of left elbow

+7th S53.449 Ulnar collateral ligament sprain of unspecified elbow

+ S53.49 Other sprain of elbow

+7th S53.491 Other sprain of right elbow

+7th S53.492 Other sprain of left elbow

+7th S53.499 Other sprain of unspecified elbow

S54 Injury of nerves at forearm level

Code also any associated open wound (S51.-)

Excludes2: injury of nerves at wrist and hand level (S64.-)

The appropriate 7th character is to be added to each code from category S54

A initial encounter

D subsequent encounter

S sequela

+ **S54.0** **Injury of ulnar nerve at forearm level**
    Injury of ulnar nerve NOS
  X+7th **S54.00** **Injury of ulnar nerve at forearm level, unspecified arm**
  X+7th **S54.01** **Injury of ulnar nerve at forearm level, right arm**
  X+7th **S54.02** **Injury of ulnar nerve at forearm level, left arm**
+ **S54.1** **Injury of median nerve at forearm level**
    Injury of median nerve NOS
  X+7th **S54.10** **Injury of median nerve at forearm level, unspecified arm**
  X+7th **S54.11** **Injury of median nerve at forearm level, right arm**
  X+7th **S54.12** **Injury of median nerve at forearm level, left arm**
+ **S54.2** **Injury of radial nerve at forearm level**
    Injury of radial nerve NOS
  X+7th **S54.20** **Injury of radial nerve at forearm level, unspecified arm**
  X+7th **S54.21** **Injury of radial nerve at forearm level, right arm**
  X+7th **S54.22** **Injury of radial nerve at forearm level, left arm**
+ **S54.3** **Injury of cutaneous sensory nerve at forearm level**
  X+7th **S54.30** **Injury of cutaneous sensory nerve at forearm level, unspecified arm**
  X+7th **S54.31** **Injury of cutaneous sensory nerve at forearm level, right arm**
  X+7th **S54.32** **Injury of cutaneous sensory nerve at forearm level, left arm**
+ **S54.8** **Injury of other nerves at forearm level**
  + **S54.8X** **Injury of other nerves at forearm level**
    +7th **S54.8X1** **Injury of other nerves at forearm level, right arm**
    +7th **S54.8X2** **Injury of other nerves at forearm level, left arm**
    +7th **S54.8X9** **Injury of other nerves at forearm level, unspecified arm**
+ **S54.9** **Injury of unspecified nerve at forearm level**
  X+7th **S54.90** **Injury of unspecified nerve at forearm level, unspecified arm**
  X+7th **S54.91** **Injury of unspecified nerve at forearm level, right arm**
  X+7th **S54.92** **Injury of unspecified nerve at forearm level, left arm**

S55 **Injury of blood vessels at forearm level**
  Code also any associated open wound (S51.-)
  Excludes2: *injury of blood vessels at wrist and hand level (S65.-)*
               injury of brachial vessels (S45.1-S45.2)

  The appropriate 7th character is to be added to each code from category S55
  A   initial encounter
  D   subsequent encounter
  S   sequela

+ **S55.0** **Injury of ulnar artery at forearm level**
  + **S55.00** **Unspecified injury of ulnar artery at forearm level**
    CC +7th **S55.001** **Unspecified injury of ulnar artery at forearm level, right arm**
    CC +7th **S55.002** **Unspecified injury of ulnar artery at forearm level, left arm**
    CC +7th **S55.009** **Unspecified injury of ulnar artery at forearm level, unspecified arm**
  + **S55.01** **Laceration of ulnar artery at forearm level**
    CC +7th **S55.011** **Laceration of ulnar artery at forearm level, right arm**
    CC +7th **S55.012** **Laceration of ulnar artery at forearm level, left arm**
    CC +7th **S55.019** **Laceration of ulnar artery at forearm level, unspecified arm**
  + **S55.09** **Other specified injury of ulnar artery at forearm level**
    CC +7th **S55.091** **Other specified injury of ulnar artery at forearm level, right arm**
    CC +7th **S55.092** **Other specified injury of ulnar artery at forearm level, left arm**
    CC +7th **S55.099** **Other specified injury of ulnar artery at forearm level, unspecified arm**

+ **S55.1** **Injury of radial artery at forearm level**
  + **S55.10** **Unspecified injury of radial artery at forearm level**
    CC +7th **S55.101** **Unspecified injury of radial artery at forearm level, right arm**
    CC +7th **S55.102** **Unspecified injury of radial artery at forearm level, left arm**
    CC +7th **S55.109** **Unspecified injury of radial artery at forearm level, unspecified arm**
  + **S55.11** **Laceration of radial artery at forearm level**
    CC +7th **S55.111** **Laceration of radial artery at forearm level, right arm**
    CC +7th **S55.112** **Laceration of radial artery at forearm level, left arm**
    CC +7th **S55.119** **Laceration of radial artery at forearm level, unspecified arm**
  + **S55.19** **Other specified injury of radial artery at forearm level**
    CC +7th **S55.191** **Other specified injury of radial artery at forearm level, right arm**
    CC +7th **S55.192** **Other specified injury of radial artery at forearm level, left arm**
    CC +7th **S55.199** **Other specified injury of radial artery at forearm level, unspecified arm**
+ **S55.2** **Injury of vein at forearm level**
  + **S55.20** **Unspecified injury of vein at forearm level**
    CC +7th **S55.201** **Unspecified injury of vein at forearm level, right arm**
    CC +7th **S55.202** **Unspecified injury of vein at forearm level, left arm**
    CC +7th **S55.209** **Unspecified injury of vein at forearm level, unspecified arm**
  + **S55.21** **Laceration of vein at forearm level**
    CC +7th **S55.211** **Laceration of vein at forearm level, right arm**
    CC +7th **S55.212** **Laceration of vein at forearm level, left arm**
    CC +7th **S55.219** **Laceration of vein at forearm level, unspecified arm**
  + **S55.29** **Other specified injury of vein at forearm level**
    CC +7th **S55.291** **Other specified injury of vein at forearm level, right arm**
    CC +7th **S55.292** **Other specified injury of vein at forearm level, left arm**
    CC +7th **S55.299** **Other specified injury of vein at forearm level, unspecified arm**
+ **S55.8** **Injury of other blood vessels at forearm level**
  + **S55.80** **Unspecified injury of other blood vessels at forearm level**
    CC +7th **S55.801** **Unspecified injury of other blood vessels at forearm level, right arm**
    CC +7th **S55.802** **Unspecified injury of other blood vessels at forearm level, left arm**
    CC +7th **S55.809** **Unspecified injury of other blood vessels at forearm level, unspecified arm**
  + **S55.81** **Laceration of other blood vessels at forearm level**
    CC +7th **S55.811** **Laceration of other blood vessels at forearm level, right arm**
    CC +7th **S55.812** **Laceration of other blood vessels at forearm level, left arm**
    CC +7th **S55.819** **Laceration of other blood vessels at forearm level, unspecified arm**
  + **S55.89** **Other specified injury of other blood vessels at forearm level**
    CC +7th **S55.891** **Other specified injury of other blood vessels at forearm level, right arm**
    CC +7th **S55.892** **Other specified injury of other blood vessels at forearm level, left arm**
    CC +7th **S55.899** **Other specified injury of other blood vessels at forearm level, unspecified arm**
+ **S55.9** **Injury of unspecified blood vessel at forearm level**
  + **S55.90** **Unspecified injury of unspecified blood vessel at forearm level**
    CC +7th **S55.901** **Unspecified injury of unspecified blood vessel at forearm level, right arm**
    CC +7th **S55.902** **Unspecified injury of unspecified blood vessel at forearm level, left arm**
    CC +7th **S55.909** **Unspecified injury of unspecified blood vessel at forearm level, unspecified arm**

+, +7th, X + 7th   ● Newborn   ● Pediatric   ● Maternity   ● Adult   ♀ Female   ♂ Male   Manifestation   Unacceptable PDX   HCC   CC   MCC   HAC

+ S55.91 Laceration of unspecified blood vessel at forearm level

CC +7th S55.911 Laceration of unspecified blood vessel at forearm level, right arm

CC +7th S55.912 Laceration of unspecified blood vessel at forearm level, left arm

CC +7th S55.919 Laceration of unspecified blood vessel at forearm level, unspecified arm

+ S55.99 Other specified injury of unspecified blood vessel at forearm level

CC +7th S55.991 Other specified injury of unspecified blood vessel at forearm level, right arm

CC +7th S55.992 Other specified injury of unspecified blood vessel at forearm level, left arm

CC +7th S55.999 Other specified injury of unspecified blood vessel at forearm level, unspecified arm

S56 Injury of muscle, fascia and tendon at forearm level

Code also any associated open wound (S51.-)

Excludes2: *injury of muscle, fascia and tendon at or below wrist (S66.-)*

sprain of joints and ligaments of elbow (S53.4-)

The appropriate 7th character is to be added to each code from category S56
A   initial encounter
D   subsequent encounter
S   sequela

+ S56.0 Injury of flexor muscle, fascia and tendon of thumb at forearm level

+ S56.00 Unspecified injury of flexor muscle, fascia and tendon of thumb at forearm level

+7th S56.001 Unspecified injury of flexor muscle, fascia and tendon of right thumb at forearm level

+7th S56.002 Unspecified injury of flexor muscle, fascia and tendon of left thumb at forearm level

+7th S56.009 Unspecified injury of flexor muscle, fascia and tendon of unspecified thumb at forearm level

+ S56.01 Strain of flexor muscle, fascia and tendon of thumb at forearm level

+7th S56.011 Strain of flexor muscle, fascia and tendon of right thumb at forearm level

+7th S56.012 Strain of flexor muscle, fascia and tendon of left thumb at forearm level

+7th S56.019 Strain of flexor muscle, fascia and tendon of unspecified thumb at forearm level

+ S56.02 Laceration of flexor muscle, fascia and tendon of thumb at forearm level

CC +7th S56.021 Laceration of flexor muscle, fascia and tendon of right thumb at forearm level

CC +7th S56.022 Laceration of flexor muscle, fascia and tendon of left thumb at forearm level

CC +7th S56.029 Laceration of flexor muscle, fascia and tendon of unspecified thumb at forearm level

+ S56.09 Other injury of flexor muscle, fascia and tendon of thumb at forearm level

+7th S56.091 Other injury of flexor muscle, fascia and tendon of right thumb at forearm level

+7th S56.092 Other injury of flexor muscle, fascia and tendon of left thumb at forearm level

+7th S56.099 Other injury of flexor muscle, fascia and tendon of unspecified thumb at forearm level

+ S56.1 Injury of flexor muscle, fascia and tendon of other and unspecified finger at forearm level

+ S56.10 Unspecified injury of flexor muscle, fascia and tendon of other and unspecified finger at forearm level

+7th S56.101 Unspecified injury of flexor muscle, fascia and tendon of right index finger at forearm level

+7th S56.102 Unspecified injury of flexor muscle, fascia and tendon of left index finger at forearm level

+7th S56.103 Unspecified injury of flexor muscle, fascia and tendon of right middle finger at forearm level

+7th S56.104 Unspecified injury of flexor muscle, fascia and tendon of left middle finger at forearm level

+7th S56.105 Unspecified injury of flexor muscle, fascia and tendon of right ring finger at forearm level

+7th S56.106 Unspecified injury of flexor muscle, fascia and tendon of left ring finger at forearm level

+7th S56.107 Unspecified injury of flexor muscle, fascia and tendon of right little finger at forearm level

+7th S56.108 Unspecified injury of flexor muscle, fascia and tendon of left little finger at forearm level

+7th S56.109 Unspecified injury of flexor muscle, fascia and tendon of unspecified finger at forearm level

+ S56.11 Strain of flexor muscle, fascia and tendon of other and unspecified finger at forearm level

+7th S56.111 Strain of flexor muscle, fascia and tendon of right index finger at forearm level

+7th S56.112 Strain of flexor muscle, fascia and tendon of left index finger at forearm level

+7th S56.113 Strain of flexor muscle, fascia and tendon of right middle finger at forearm level

+7th S56.114 Strain of flexor muscle, fascia and tendon of left middle finger at forearm level

+7th S56.115 Strain of flexor muscle, fascia and tendon of right ring finger at forearm level

+7th S56.116 Strain of flexor muscle, fascia and tendon of left ring finger at forearm level

+7th S56.117 Strain of flexor muscle, fascia and tendon of right little finger at forearm level

+7th S56.118 Strain of flexor muscle, fascia and tendon of left little finger at forearm level

+7th S56.119 Strain of flexor muscle, fascia and tendon of finger of unspecified finger at forearm level

+ S56.12 Laceration of flexor muscle, fascia and tendon of other and unspecified finger at forearm level

CC +7th S56.121 Laceration of flexor muscle, fascia and tendon of right index finger at forearm level

CC +7th S56.122 Laceration of flexor muscle, fascia and tendon of left index finger at forearm level

CC +7th S56.123 Laceration of flexor muscle, fascia and tendon of right middle finger at forearm level

CC +7th S56.124 Laceration of flexor muscle, fascia and tendon of left middle finger at forearm level

CC +7th S56.125 Laceration of flexor muscle, fascia and tendon of right ring finger at forearm level

CC +7th S56.126 Laceration of flexor muscle, fascia and tendon of left ring finger at forearm level

CC +7th S56.127 Laceration of flexor muscle, fascia and tendon of right little finger at forearm level

CC +7th S56.128 Laceration of flexor muscle, fascia and tendon of left little finger at forearm level

CC +7th S56.129 Laceration of flexor muscle, fascia and tendon of unspecified finger at forearm level

+ **S56.19** Other injury of flexor muscle, fascia and tendon of other and unspecified finger at forearm level

 +7th **S56.191** Other injury of flexor muscle, fascia and tendon of right index finger at forearm level

 +7th **S56.192** Other injury of flexor muscle, fascia and tendon of left index finger at forearm level

 +7th **S56.193** Other injury of flexor muscle, fascia and tendon of right middle finger at forearm level

 +7th **S56.194** Other injury of flexor muscle, fascia and tendon of left middle finger at forearm level

 +7th **S56.195** Other injury of flexor muscle, fascia and tendon of right ring finger at forearm level

 +7th **S56.196** Other injury of flexor muscle, fascia and tendon of left ring finger at forearm level

 +7th **S56.197** Other injury of flexor muscle, fascia and tendon of right little finger at forearm level

 +7th **S56.198** Other injury of flexor muscle, fascia and tendon of left little finger at forearm level

 +7th **S56.199** Other injury of flexor muscle, fascia and tendon of unspecified finger at forearm level

+ **S56.2** Injury of other flexor muscle, fascia and tendon at forearm level

 + **S56.20** Unspecified injury of other flexor muscle, fascia and tendon at forearm level

  +7th **S56.201** Unspecified injury of other flexor muscle, fascia and tendon at forearm level, right arm

  +7th **S56.202** Unspecified injury of other flexor muscle, fascia and tendon at forearm level, left arm

  +7th **S56.209** Unspecified injury of other flexor muscle, fascia and tendon at forearm level, unspecified arm

 + **S56.21** Strain of other flexor muscle, fascia and tendon at forearm level

  +7th **S56.211** Strain of other flexor muscle, fascia and tendon at forearm level, right arm

  +7th **S56.212** Strain of other flexor muscle, fascia and tendon at forearm level, left arm

  +7th **S56.219** Strain of other flexor muscle, fascia and tendon at forearm level, unspecified arm

 + **S56.22** Laceration of other flexor muscle, fascia and tendon at forearm level

  CC +7th **S56.221** Laceration of other flexor muscle, fascia and tendon at forearm level, right arm

  CC +7th **S56.222** Laceration of other flexor muscle, fascia and tendon at forearm level, left arm

  CC +7th **S56.229** Laceration of other flexor muscle, fascia and tendon at forearm level, unspecified arm

 + **S56.29** Other injury of other flexor muscle, fascia and tendon at forearm level

  +7th **S56.291** Other injury of other flexor muscle, fascia and tendon at forearm level, right arm

  +7th **S56.292** Other injury of other flexor muscle, fascia and tendon at forearm level, left arm

  +7th **S56.299** Other injury of other flexor muscle, fascia and tendon at forearm level, unspecified arm

+ **S56.3** Injury of extensor or abductor muscles, fascia and tendons of thumb at forearm level

 + **S56.30** Unspecified injury of extensor or abductor muscles, fascia and tendons of thumb at forearm level

  +7th **S56.301** Unspecified injury of extensor or abductor muscles, fascia and tendons of right thumb at forearm level

  +7th **S56.302** Unspecified injury of extensor or abductor muscles, fascia and tendons of left thumb at forearm level

  +7th **S56.309** Unspecified injury of extensor or abductor muscles, fascia and tendons of unspecified thumb at forearm level

 + **S56.31** Strain of extensor or abductor muscles, fascia and tendons of thumb at forearm level

  +7th **S56.311** Strain of extensor or abductor muscles, fascia and tendons of right thumb at forearm level

  +7th **S56.312** Strain of extensor or abductor muscles, fascia and tendons of left thumb at forearm level

  +7th **S56.319** Strain of extensor or abductor muscles, fascia and tendons of unspecified thumb at forearm level

 + **S56.32** Laceration of extensor or abductor muscles, fascia and tendons of thumb at forearm level

  CC +7th **S56.321** Laceration of extensor or abductor muscles, fascia and tendons of right thumb at forearm level

  CC +7th **S56.322** Laceration of extensor or abductor muscles, fascia and tendons of left thumb at forearm level

  CC +7th **S56.329** Laceration of extensor or abductor muscles, fascia and tendons of unspecified thumb at forearm level

 + **S56.39** Other injury of extensor or abductor muscles, fascia and tendons of thumb at forearm level

  +7th **S56.391** Other injury of extensor or abductor muscles, fascia and tendons of right thumb at forearm level

  +7th **S56.392** Other injury of extensor or abductor muscles, fascia and tendons of left thumb at forearm level

  +7th **S56.399** Other injury of extensor or abductor muscles, fascia and tendons of unspecified thumb at forearm level

+ **S56.4** Injury of extensor muscle, fascia and tendon of other and unspecified finger at forearm level

 + **S56.40** Unspecified injury of extensor muscle, fascia and tendon of other and unspecified finger at forearm level

  +7th **S56.401** Unspecified injury of extensor muscle, fascia and tendon of right index finger at forearm level

  +7th **S56.402** Unspecified injury of extensor muscle, fascia and tendon of left index finger at forearm level

  +7th **S56.403** Unspecified injury of extensor muscle, fascia and tendon of right middle finger at forearm level

  +7th **S56.404** Unspecified injury of extensor muscle, fascia and tendon of left middle finger at forearm level

  +7th **S56.405** Unspecified injury of extensor muscle, fascia and tendon of right ring finger at forearm level

  +7th **S56.406** Unspecified injury of extensor muscle, fascia and tendon of left ring finger at forearm level

  +7th **S56.407** Unspecified injury of extensor muscle, fascia and tendon of right little finger at forearm level

  +7th **S56.408** Unspecified injury of extensor muscle, fascia and tendon of left little finger at forearm level

  +7th **S56.409** Unspecified injury of extensor muscle, fascia and tendon of unspecified finger at forearm level

+ **S56.41** Strain of extensor muscle, fascia and tendon of other and unspecified finger at forearm level

+7th **S56.411** Strain of extensor muscle, fascia and tendon of right index finger at forearm level

+7th **S56.412** Strain of extensor muscle, fascia and tendon of left index finger at forearm level

+7th **S56.413** Strain of extensor muscle, fascia and tendon of right middle finger at forearm level

+7th **S56.414** Strain of extensor muscle, fascia and tendon of left middle finger at forearm level

+7th **S56.415** Strain of extensor muscle, fascia and tendon of right ring finger at forearm level

+7th **S56.416** Strain of extensor muscle, fascia and tendon of left ring finger at forearm level

+7th **S56.417** Strain of extensor muscle, fascia and tendon of right little finger at forearm level

+7th **S56.418** Strain of extensor muscle, fascia and tendon of left little finger at forearm level

+7th **S56.419** Strain of extensor muscle, fascia and tendon of finger, unspecified finger at forearm level

+ **S56.42** Laceration of extensor muscle, fascia and tendon of other and unspecified finger at forearm level

CC +7th **S56.421** Laceration of extensor muscle, fascia and tendon of right index finger at forearm level

CC +7th **S56.422** Laceration of extensor muscle, fascia and tendon of left index finger at forearm level

CC +7th **S56.423** Laceration of extensor muscle, fascia and tendon of right middle finger at forearm level

CC +7th **S56.424** Laceration of extensor muscle, fascia and tendon of left middle finger at forearm level

CC +7th **S56.425** Laceration of extensor muscle, fascia and tendon of right ring finger at forearm level

CC +7th **S56.426** Laceration of extensor muscle, fascia and tendon of left ring finger at forearm level

CC +7th **S56.427** Laceration of extensor muscle, fascia and tendon of right little finger at forearm level

CC +7th **S56.428** Laceration of extensor muscle, fascia and tendon of left little finger at forearm level

CC +7th **S56.429** Laceration of extensor muscle, fascia and tendon of unspecified finger at forearm level

+ **S56.49** Other injury of extensor muscle, fascia and tendon of other and unspecified finger at forearm level

+7th **S56.491** Other injury of extensor muscle, fascia and tendon of right index finger at forearm level

+7th **S56.492** Other injury of extensor muscle, fascia and tendon of left index finger at forearm level

+7th **S56.493** Other injury of extensor muscle, fascia and tendon of right middle finger at forearm level

+7th **S56.494** Other injury of extensor muscle, fascia and tendon of left middle finger at forearm level

+7th **S56.495** Other injury of extensor muscle, fascia and tendon of right ring finger at forearm level

+7th **S56.496** Other injury of extensor muscle, fascia and tendon of left ring finger at forearm level

+7th **S56.497** Other injury of extensor muscle, fascia and tendon of right little finger at forearm level

+7th **S56.498** Other injury of extensor muscle, fascia and tendon of left little finger at forearm level

+7th **S56.499** Other injury of extensor muscle, fascia and tendon of unspecified finger at forearm level

+ **S56.5** Injury of other extensor muscle, fascia and tendon at forearm level

+ **S56.50** Unspecified injury of other extensor muscle, fascia and tendon at forearm level

+7th **S56.501** Unspecified injury of other extensor muscle, fascia and tendon at forearm level, right arm

+7th **S56.502** Unspecified injury of other extensor muscle, fascia and tendon at forearm level, left arm

+7th **S56.509** Unspecified injury of other extensor muscle, fascia and tendon at forearm level, unspecified arm

+ **S56.51** Strain of other extensor muscle, fascia and tendon at forearm level

+7th **S56.511** Strain of other extensor muscle, fascia and tendon at forearm level, right arm

+7th **S56.512** Strain of other extensor muscle, fascia≈and tendon at forearm level, left arm

+7th **S56.519** Strain of other extensor muscle, fascia and tendon at forearm level, unspecified arm

+ **S56.52** Laceration of other extensor muscle, fascia and tendon at forearm level

CC +7th **S56.521** Laceration of other extensor muscle, fascia and tendon at forearm level, right arm

CC +7th **S56.522** Laceration of other extensor muscle, fascia and tendon at forearm level, left arm

CC +7th **S56.529** Laceration of other extensor muscle, fascia and tendon at forearm level, unspecified arm

+ **S56.59** Other injury of other extensor muscle, fascia and tendon at forearm level

+7th **S56.591** Other injury of other extensor muscle, fascia and tendon at forearm level, right arm

+7th **S56.592** Other injury of other extensor muscle, fascia and tendon at forearm level, left arm

+7th **S56.599** Other injury of other extensor muscle, fascia and tendon at forearm level, unspecified arm

+ **S56.8** Injury of other muscles, fascia and tendons at forearm level

+ **S56.80** Unspecified injury of other muscles, fascia and tendons at forearm level

+7th **S56.801** Unspecified injury of other muscles, fascia and tendons at forearm level, right arm

+7th **S56.802** Unspecified injury of other muscles, fascia and tendons at forearm level, left arm

+7th **S56.809** Unspecified injury of other muscles, fascia and tendons at forearm level, unspecified arm

+ **S56.81** Strain of other muscles, fascia and tendons at forearm level

+7th **S56.811** Strain of other muscles, fascia and tendons at forearm level, right arm

+7th **S56.812** Strain of other muscles, fascia and tendons at forearm level, left arm

+7th **S56.819** Strain of other muscles, fascia and tendons at forearm level, unspecified arm

+ **S56.82** Laceration of other muscles, fascia and tendons at forearm level

CC +7th **S56.821** Laceration of other muscles, fascia and tendons at forearm level, right arm

CC +7th **S56.822** Laceration of other muscles, fascia and tendons at forearm level, left arm

CC +7th **S56.829** Laceration of other muscles, fascia and tendons at forearm level, unspecified arm

+ **S56.89** Other injury of other muscles, fascia and tendons at forearm level
  +7th **S56.891** Other injury of other muscles, fascia and tendons at forearm level, right arm
  +7th **S56.892** Other injury of other muscles, fascia and tendons at forearm level, left arm
  +7th **S56.899** Other injury of other muscles, fascia and tendons at forearm level, unspecified arm

+ **S56.9** Injury of unspecified muscles, fascia and tendons at forearm level
  + **S56.90** Unspecified injury of unspecified muscles, fascia and tendons at forearm level
    +7th **S56.901** Unspecified injury of unspecified muscles, fascia and tendons at forearm level, right arm
    +7th **S56.902** Unspecified injury of unspecified muscles, fascia and tendons at forearm level, left arm
    +7th **S56.909** Unspecified injury of unspecified muscles, fascia and tendons at forearm level, unspecified arm
  + **S56.91** Strain of unspecified muscles, fascia and tendons at forearm level
    +7th **S56.911** Strain of unspecified muscles, fascia and tendons at forearm level, right arm
    +7th **S56.912** Strain of unspecified muscles, fascia and tendons at forearm level, left arm
    +7th **S56.919** Strain of unspecified muscles, fascia and tendons at forearm level, unspecified arm
  + **S56.92** Laceration of unspecified muscles, fascia and tendons at forearm level
    CC +7th **S56.921** Laceration of unspecified muscles, fascia and tendons at forearm level, right arm
    CC +7th **S56.922** Laceration of unspecified muscles, fascia and tendons at forearm level, left arm
    CC +7th **S56.929** Laceration of unspecified muscles, fascia and tendons at forearm level, unspecified arm
  + **S56.99** Other injury of unspecified muscles, fascia and tendons at forearm level
    +7th **S56.991** Other injury of unspecified muscles, fascia and tendons at forearm level, right arm
    +7th **S56.992** Other injury of unspecified muscles, fascia and tendons at forearm level, left arm
    +7th **S56.999** Other injury of unspecified muscles, fascia and tendons at forearm level, unspecified arm

S57 Crushing injury of elbow and forearm

Use additional code(s) for all associated injuries
Excludes2: crushing injury of wrist and hand (S67.-)

The appropriate 7th character is to be added to each code from category S57
A initial encounter
D subsequent encounter
S sequela

+ **S57.0** Crushing injury of elbow
  X+7th **S57.00** Crushing injury of unspecified elbow
  X+7th **S57.01** Crushing injury of right elbow
  X+7th **S57.02** Crushing injury of left elbow
+ **S57.8** Crushing injury of forearm
  X+7th **S57.80** Crushing injury of unspecified forearm
  X+7th **S57.81** Crushing injury of right forearm
  X+7th **S57.82** Crushing injury of left forearm

S58 Traumatic amputation of elbow and forearm

An amputation not identified as partial or complete should be coded to complete
Excludes1: traumatic amputation of wrist and hand (S68.-)

The appropriate 7th character is to be added to each code from category S58
A initial encounter
D subsequent encounter
S sequela

+ **S58.0** Traumatic amputation at elbow level
  + **S58.01** Complete traumatic amputation at elbow level
    CC +7th **S58.011** Complete traumatic amputation at elbow level, right arm
    CC +7th **S58.012** Complete traumatic amputation at elbow level, left arm
    CC +7th **S58.019** Complete traumatic amputation at elbow level, unspecified arm
  + **S58.02** Partial traumatic amputation at elbow level
    CC +7th **S58.021** Partial traumatic amputation at elbow level, right arm
    CC +7th **S58.022** Partial traumatic amputation at elbow level, left arm
    CC +7th **S58.029** Partial traumatic amputation at elbow level, unspecified arm
+ **S58.1** Traumatic amputation at level between elbow and wrist
  + **S58.11** Complete traumatic amputation at level between elbow and wrist
    CC +7th **S58.111** Complete traumatic amputation at level between elbow and wrist, right arm
    CC +7th **S58.112** Complete traumatic amputation at level between elbow and wrist, left arm
    CC +7th **S58.119** Complete traumatic amputation at level between elbow and wrist, unspecified arm
  + **S58.12** Partial traumatic amputation at level between elbow and wrist
    CC +7th **S58.121** Partial traumatic amputation at level between elbow and wrist, right arm
    CC +7th **S58.122** Partial traumatic amputation at level between elbow and wrist, left arm
    CC +7th **S58.129** Partial traumatic amputation at level between elbow and wrist, unspecified arm
+ **S58.9** Traumatic amputation of forearm, level unspecified
  Excludes1: traumatic amputation of wrist (S68.-)
  + **S58.91** Complete traumatic amputation of forearm, level unspecified
    CC +7th **S58.911** Complete traumatic amputation of right forearm, level unspecified
    CC +7th **S58.912** Complete traumatic amputation of left forearm, level unspecified
    CC +7th **S58.919** Complete traumatic amputation of unspecified forearm, level unspecified
  + **S58.92** Partial traumatic amputation of forearm, level unspecified
    CC +7th **S58.921** Partial traumatic amputation of right forearm, level unspecified
    CC +7th **S58.922** Partial traumatic amputation of left forearm, level unspecified
    CC +7th **S58.929** Partial traumatic amputation of unspecified forearm, level unspecified

S59 Other and unspecified injuries of elbow and forearm

Excludes2: other and unspecified injuries of wrist and hand (S69.-)

The appropriate 7th character is to be added to each code from subcategories **S59.0**, **S59.1**, and **S59.2**
A initial encounter for closed fracture
D subsequent encounter for fracture with routine healing
G subsequent encounter for fracture with delayed healing
K subsequent encounter for fracture with nonunion
P subsequent encounter for fracture with malunion
S sequela

Review coding guideline C.19.c

+, +7th, X + 7th   ● Newborn   ● Pediatric   ● Maternity   ● Adult   ♀ Female   ♂ Male   Manifestation   Unacceptable PDX   HCC   CC   MCC   HAC

+ **S59.0** **Physeal fracture of lower end of ulna**
 + **S59.00** **Unspecified physeal fracture of lower end of ulna**
  CC +7th **S59.001** **Unspecified physeal fracture of lower end of ulna, right arm**
   HAC 7th character A see Appendix B for HAC conditional logic
  CC +7th **S59.002** **Unspecified physeal fracture of lower end of ulna, left arm**
   HAC 7th character A see Appendix B for HAC conditional logic
  CC +7th **S59.009** **Unspecified physeal fracture of lower end of ulna, unspecified arm**
   HAC 7th character A see Appendix B for HAC conditional logic
 + **S59.01** **Salter-Harris Type I physeal fracture of lower end of ulna**
  CC +7th **S59.011** **Salter-Harris Type I physeal fracture of lower end of ulna, right arm**
   HAC 7th character A see Appendix B for HAC conditional logic
  CC +7th **S59.012** **Salter-Harris Type I physeal fracture of lower end of ulna, left arm**
   HAC 7th character A see Appendix B for HAC conditional logic
  CC +7th **S59.019** **Salter-Harris Type I physeal fracture of lower end of ulna, unspecified arm**
   HAC 7th character A see Appendix B for HAC conditional logic
 + **S59.02** **Salter-Harris Type II physeal fracture of lower end of ulna**
  CC +7th **S59.021** **Salter-Harris Type II physeal fracture of lower end of ulna, right arm**
   HAC 7th character A see Appendix B for HAC conditional logic
  CC +7th **S59.022** **Salter-Harris Type II physeal fracture of lower end of ulna, left arm**
   HAC 7th character A see Appendix B for HAC conditional logic
  CC +7th **S59.029** **Salter-Harris Type II physeal fracture of lower end of ulna, unspecified arm**
   HAC 7th character A see Appendix B for HAC conditional logic
 + **S59.03** **Salter-Harris Type III physeal fracture of lower end of ulna**
  CC +7th **S59.031** **Salter-Harris Type III physeal fracture of lower end of ulna, right arm**
   HAC 7th character A see Appendix B for HAC conditional logic
  CC +7th **S59.032** **Salter-Harris Type III physeal fracture of lower end of ulna, left arm**
   HAC 7th character A see Appendix B for HAC conditional logic
  CC +7th **S59.039** **Salter-Harris Type III physeal fracture of lower end of ulna, unspecified arm**
   HAC 7th character A see Appendix B for HAC conditional logic
 + **S59.04** **Salter-Harris Type IV physeal fracture of lower end of ulna**
  CC +7th **S59.041** **Salter-Harris Type IV physeal fracture of lower end of ulna, right arm**
   HAC 7th character A see Appendix B for HAC conditional logic
  CC +7th **S59.042** **Salter-Harris Type IV physeal fracture of lower end of ulna, left arm**
   HAC 7th character A see Appendix B for HAC conditional logic
  CC +7th **S59.049** **Salter-Harris Type IV physeal fracture of lower end of ulna, unspecified arm**
   HAC 7th character A see Appendix B for HAC conditional logic
 + **S59.09** **Other physeal fracture of lower end of ulna**
  CC +7th **S59.091** **Other physeal fracture of lower end of ulna, right arm**
   HAC 7th character A see Appendix B for HAC conditional logic
  CC +7th **S59.092** **Other physeal fracture of lower end of ulna, left arm**
   HAC 7th character A see Appendix B for HAC conditional logic
  CC +7th **S59.099** **Other physeal fracture of lower end of ulna, unspecified arm**
   HAC 7th character A see Appendix B for HAC conditional logic

+ **S59.1** **Physeal fracture of upper end of radius**
 + **S59.10** **Unspecified physeal fracture of upper end of radius**
  CC +7th **S59.101** **Unspecified physeal fracture of upper end of radius, right arm**
  CC +7th **S59.102** **Unspecified physeal fracture of upper end of radius, left arm**
  CC +7th **S59.109** **Unspecified physeal fracture of upper end of radius, unspecified arm**
 + **S59.11** **Salter-Harris Type I physeal fracture of upper end of radius**
  CC +7th **S59.111** **Salter-Harris Type I physeal fracture of upper end of radius, right arm**
  CC +7th **S59.112** **Salter-Harris Type I physeal fracture of upper end of radius, left arm**
  CC +7th **S59.119** **Salter-Harris Type I physeal fracture of upper end of radius, unspecified arm**
 + **S59.12** **Salter-Harris Type II physeal fracture of upper end of radius**
  CC +7th **S59.121** **Salter-Harris Type II physeal fracture of upper end of radius, right arm**
  CC +7th **S59.122** **Salter-Harris Type II physeal fracture of upper end of radius, left arm**
  CC +7th **S59.129** **Salter-Harris Type II physeal fracture of upper end of radius, unspecified arm**
 + **S59.13** **Salter-Harris Type III physeal fracture of upper end of radius**
  CC +7th **S59.131** **Salter-Harris Type III physeal fracture of upper end of radius, right arm**
  CC +7th **S59.132** **Salter-Harris Type III physeal fracture of upper end of radius, left arm**
  CC +7th **S59.139** **Salter-Harris Type III physeal fracture of upper end of radius, unspecified arm**
 + **S59.14** **Salter-Harris Type IV physeal fracture of upper end of radius**
  CC +7th **S59.141** **Salter-Harris Type IV physeal fracture of upper end of radius, right arm**
  CC +7th **S59.142** **Salter-Harris Type IV physeal fracture of upper end of radius, left arm**
  CC +7th **S59.149** **Salter-Harris Type IV physeal fracture of upper end of radius, unspecified arm**
 + **S59.19** **Other physeal fracture of upper end of radius**
  CC +7th **S59.191** **Other physeal fracture of upper end of radius, right arm**
  CC +7th **S59.192** **Other physeal fracture of upper end of radius, left arm**
  CC +7th **S59.199** **Other physeal fracture of upper end of radius, unspecified arm**
+ **S59.2** **Physeal fracture of lower end of radius**
 + **S59.20** **Unspecified physeal fracture of lower end of radius**
  CC +7th **S59.201** **Unspecified physeal fracture of lower end of radius, right arm**
   HAC 7th character A see Appendix B for HAC conditional logic
  CC +7th **S59.202** **Unspecified physeal fracture of lower end of radius, left arm**
   HAC 7th character A see Appendix B for HAC conditional logic
  CC +7th **S59.209** **Unspecified physeal fracture of lower end of radius, unspecified arm**
   HAC 7th character A see Appendix B for HAC conditional logic
 + **S59.21** **Salter-Harris Type I physeal fracture of lower end of radius**
  CC +7th **S59.211** **Salter-Harris Type I physeal fracture of lower end of radius, right arm**
   HAC 7th character A see Appendix B for HAC conditional logic

CC +7th **S59.212** **Salter-Harris Type I physeal fracture of lower end of radius, left arm**
HAC 7th character A see Appendix B for HAC conditional logic

CC +7th **S59.219** **Salter-Harris Type I physeal fracture of lower end of radius, unspecified arm**
HAC 7th character A see Appendix B for HAC conditional logic

\+ **S59.22** **Salter-Harris Type II physeal fracture of lower end of radius**

CC +7th **S59.221** **Salter-Harris Type II physeal fracture of lower end of radius, right arm**
HAC 7th character A see Appendix B for HAC conditional logic

CC +7th **S59.222** **Salter-Harris Type II physeal fracture of lower end of radius, left arm**
HAC 7th character A see Appendix B for HAC conditional logic

CC +7th **S59.229** **Salter-Harris Type II physeal fracture of lower end of radius, unspecified arm**
HAC 7th character A see Appendix B for HAC conditional logic

\+ **S59.23** **Salter-Harris Type III physeal fracture of lower end of radius**

CC +7th **S59.231** **Salter-Harris Type III physeal fracture of lower end of radius, right arm**
HAC 7th character A see Appendix B for HAC conditional logic

CC +7th **S59.232** **Salter-Harris Type III physeal fracture of lower end of radius, left arm**
HAC 7th character A see Appendix B for HAC conditional logic

CC +7th **S59.239** **Salter-Harris Type III physeal fracture of lower end of radius, unspecified arm**
HAC 7th character A see Appendix B for HAC conditional logic

\+ **S59.24** **Salter-Harris Type IV physeal fracture of lower end of radius**

CC +7th **S59.241** **Salter-Harris Type IV physeal fracture of lower end of radius, right arm**
HAC 7th character A see Appendix B for HAC conditional logic

CC +7th **S59.242** **Salter-Harris Type IV physeal fracture of lower end of radius, left arm**
HAC 7th character A see Appendix B for HAC conditional logic

CC +7th **S59.249** **Salter-Harris Type IV physeal fracture of lower end of radius, unspecified arm**
HAC 7th character A see Appendix B for HAC conditional logic

\+ **S59.29** **Other physeal fracture of lower end of radius**

CC +7th **S59.291** **Other physeal fracture of lower end of radius, right arm**
HAC 7th character A see Appendix B for HAC conditional logic

CC +7th **S59.292** **Other physeal fracture of lower end of radius, left arm**
HAC 7th character A see Appendix B for HAC conditional logic

CC +7th **S59.299** **Other physeal fracture of lower end of radius, unspecified arm**
HAC 7th character A see Appendix B for HAC conditional logic

\+ **S59.8** **Other specified injuries of elbow and forearm**

> The appropriate 7th character is to be added to each code in subcategory **S59.8**
> A   initial encounter
> D   subsequent encounter
> S   sequela

\+ **S59.80** **Other specified injuries of elbow**
+7th **S59.801** **Other specified injuries of right elbow**
+7th **S59.802** **Other specified injuries of left elbow**
+7th **S59.809** **Other specified injuries of unspecified elbow**

\+ **S59.81** **Other specified injuries of forearm**
+7th **S59.811** **Other specified injuries right forearm**
+7th **S59.812** **Other specified injuries left forearm**
+7th **S59.819** **Other specified injuries unspecified forearm**

\+ **S59.9** **Unspecified injury of elbow and forearm**

> The appropriate 7th character is to be added to each code in subcategory **S59.9**
> A   initial encounter
> D   subsequent encounter
> S   sequela

\+ **S59.90** **Unspecified injury of elbow**
+7th **S59.901** **Unspecified injury of right elbow**
+7th **S59.902** **Unspecified injury of left elbow**
+7th **S59.909** **Unspecified injury of unspecified elbow**

\+ **S59.91** **Unspecified injury of forearm**
+7th **S59.911** **Unspecified injury of right forearm**
+7th **S59.912** **Unspecified injury of left forearm**
+7th **S59.919** **Unspecified injury of unspecified forearm**

Injuries to the wrist, hand and fingers (S60-S69)

Excludes2: *burns and corrosions (T20-T32)*
frostbite (T33-T34)
insect bite or sting, venomous (T63.4)

S60 **Superficial injury of wrist, hand and fingers**

> The appropriate 7th character is to be added to each code from category S60
> A   initial encounter
> D   subsequent encounter
> S   sequela

\+ **S60.0** **Contusion of finger without damage to nail**
Excludes1: *contusion involving nail (matrix) (S60.1)*

X+7th **S60.00** **Contusion of unspecified finger without damage to nail**
Contusion of finger(s) NOS

\+ **S60.01** **Contusion of thumb without damage to nail**
+7th **S60.011** **Contusion of right thumb without damage to nail**
+7th **S60.012** **Contusion of left thumb without damage to nail**
+7th **S60.019** **Contusion of unspecified thumb without damage to nail**

\+ **S60.02** **Contusion of index finger without damage to nail**
+7th **S60.021** **Contusion of right index finger without damage to nail**
+7th **S60.022** **Contusion of left index finger without damage to nail**
+7th **S60.029** **Contusion of unspecified index finger without damage to nail**

\+ **S60.03** **Contusion of middle finger without damage to nail**
+7th **S60.031** **Contusion of right middle finger without damage to nail**
+7th **S60.032** **Contusion of left middle finger without damage to nail**
+7th **S60.039** **Contusion of unspecified middle finger without damage to nail**

\+ **S60.04** **Contusion of ring finger without damage to nail**
+7th **S60.041** **Contusion of right ring finger without damage to nail**
+7th **S60.042** **Contusion of left ring finger without damage to nail**
+7th **S60.049** **Contusion of unspecified ring finger without damage to nail**

\+ **S60.05** **Contusion of little finger without damage to nail**
+7th **S60.051** **Contusion of right little finger without damage to nail**
+7th **S60.052** **Contusion of left little finger without damage to nail**
+7th **S60.059** **Contusion of unspecified little finger without damage to nail**

Wrist

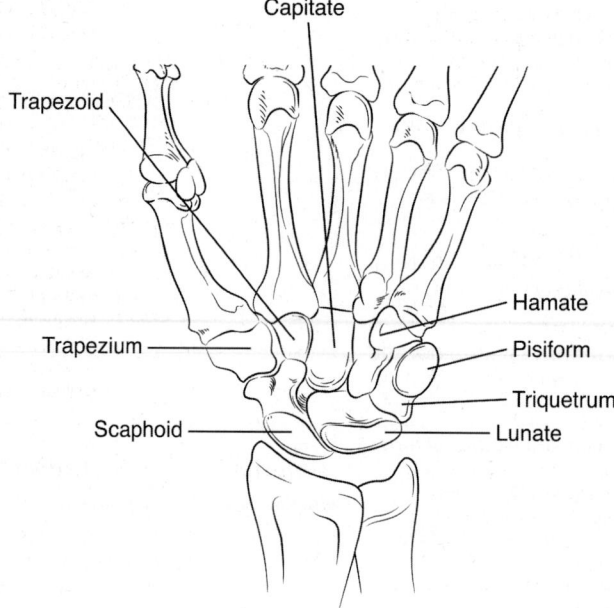

Capitate

Trapezoid

Trapezium

Scaphoid

Hamate

Pisiform

Triquetrum

Lunate

©AHIMA

Bones of the Hand

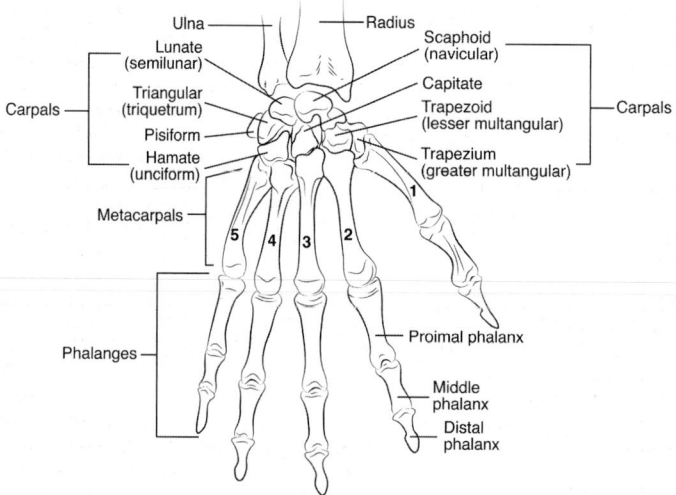

Ulna

Radius

Lunate (semilunar)

Scaphoid (navicular)

Triangular (triquetrum)

Capitate

Pisiform

Trapezoid (lesser multangular)

Hamate (unciform)

Trapezium (greater multangular)

Carpals

Carpals

Metacarpals

1

5 4 3 2

Phalanges

Proimal phalanx

Middle phalanx

Distal phalanx

©AHIMA

Muscles of the Hand

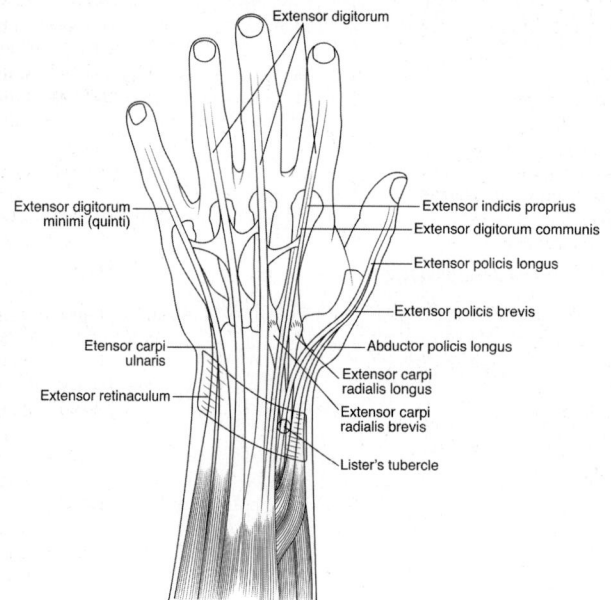

Extensor digitorum

Extensor digitorum minimi (quinti)

Extensor indicis proprius

Extensor digitorum communis

Extensor policis longus

Extensor policis brevis

Abductor policis longus

Etensor carpi ulnaris

Extensor carpi radialis longus

Extensor retinaculum

Extensor carpi radialis brevis

Lister's tubercle

©AHIMA

+ **S60.1** Contusion of finger with damage to nail
X+7th **S60.10** Contusion of unspecified finger with damage to nail
+ **S60.11** Contusion of thumb with damage to nail
+7th **S60.111** Contusion of right thumb with damage to nail
+7th **S60.112** Contusion of left thumb with damage to nail
+7th **S60.119** Contusion of unspecified thumb with damage to nail
+ **S60.12** Contusion of index finger with damage to nail
+7th **S60.121** Contusion of right index finger with damage to nail
+7th **S60.122** Contusion of left index finger with damage to nail
+7th **S60.129** Contusion of unspecified index finger with damage to nail
+ **S60.13** Contusion of middle finger with damage to nail
+7th **S60.131** Contusion of right middle finger with damage to nail
+7th **S60.132** Contusion of left middle finger with damage to nail
+7th **S60.139** Contusion of unspecified middle finger with damage to nail
+ **S60.14** Contusion of ring finger with damage to nail
+7th **S60.141** Contusion of right ring finger with damage to nail
+7th **S60.142** Contusion of left ring finger with damage to nail
+7th **S60.149** Contusion of unspecified ring finger with damage to nail
+ **S60.15** Contusion of little finger with damage to nail
+7th **S60.151** Contusion of right little finger with damage to nail
+7th **S60.152** Contusion of left little finger with damage to nail
+7th **S60.159** Contusion of unspecified little finger with damage to nail
+ **S60.2** Contusion of wrist and hand
Excludes2: contusion of fingers (S60.0-, S60.1-)
+ **S60.21** Contusion of wrist
+7th **S60.211** Contusion of right wrist
+7th **S60.212** Contusion of left wrist
+7th **S60.219** Contusion of unspecified wrist
+ **S60.22** Contusion of hand
+7th **S60.221** Contusion of right hand
+7th **S60.222** Contusion of left hand
+7th **S60.229** Contusion of unspecified hand
+ **S60.3** Other superficial injuries of thumb
+ **S60.31** Abrasion of thumb
+7th **S60.311** Abrasion of right thumb
+7th **S60.312** Abrasion of left thumb
+7th **S60.319** Abrasion of unspecified thumb
+ **S60.32** Blister (nonthermal) of thumb
+7th **S60.321** Blister (nonthermal) of right thumb
+7th **S60.322** Blister (nonthermal) of left thumb
+7th **S60.329** Blister (nonthermal) of unspecified thumb
+ **S60.34** External constriction of thumb
Hair tourniquet syndrome of thumb
Use additional cause code to identify the constricting item (W49.0-)
+7th **S60.341** External constriction of right thumb
+7th **S60.342** External constriction of left thumb
+7th **S60.349** External constriction of unspecified thumb
+ **S60.35** Superficial foreign body of thumb
Splinter in the thumb
+7th **S60.351** Superficial foreign body of right thumb
+7th **S60.352** Superficial foreign body of left thumb
+7th **S60.359** Superficial foreign body of unspecified thumb
+ **S60.36** Insect bite (nonvenomous) of thumb
+7th **S60.361** Insect bite (nonvenomous) of right thumb
+7th **S60.362** Insect bite (nonvenomous) of left thumb
+7th **S60.369** Insect bite (nonvenomous) of unspecified thumb

+ **S60.37** Other superficial bite of thumb
Excludes1: open bite of thumb (S61.05-, S61.15-)
+7th **S60.371** Other superficial bite of right thumb
+7th **S60.372** Other superficial bite of left thumb
+7th **S60.379** Other superficial bite of unspecified thumb
+ **S60.39** Other superficial injuries of thumb
+7th **S60.391** Other superficial injuries of right thumb
+7th **S60.392** Other superficial injuries of left thumb
+7th **S60.399** Other superficial injuries of unspecified thumb
+ **S60.4** Other superficial injuries of other fingers
+ **S60.41** Abrasion of fingers
+7th **S60.410** Abrasion of right index finger
+7th **S60.411** Abrasion of left index finger
+7th **S60.412** Abrasion of right middle finger
+7th **S60.413** Abrasion of left middle finger
+7th **S60.414** Abrasion of right ring finger
+7th **S60.415** Abrasion of left ring finger
+7th **S60.416** Abrasion of right little finger
+7th **S60.417** Abrasion of left little finger
+7th **S60.418** Abrasion of other finger
Abrasion of specified finger with unspecified laterality
+7th **S60.419** Abrasion of unspecified finger
+ **S60.42** Blister (nonthermal) of fingers
+7th **S60.420** Blister (nonthermal) of right index finger
+7th **S60.421** Blister (nonthermal) of left index finger
+7th **S60.422** Blister (nonthermal) of right middle finger
+7th **S60.423** Blister (nonthermal) of left middle finger
+7th **S60.424** Blister (nonthermal) of right ring finger
+7th **S60.425** Blister (nonthermal) of left ring finger
+7th **S60.426** Blister (nonthermal) of right little finger
+7th **S60.427** Blister (nonthermal) of left little finger
+7th **S60.428** Blister (nonthermal) of other finger
Blister (nonthermal) of specified finger with unspecified laterality
+7th **S60.429** Blister (nonthermal) of unspecified finger
+ **S60.44** External constriction of fingers
Hair tourniquet syndrome of finger
Use additional cause code to identify the constricting item (W49.0-)
+7th **S60.440** External constriction of right index finger
+7th **S60.441** External constriction of left index finger
+7th **S60.442** External constriction of right middle finger
+7th **S60.443** External constriction of left middle finger
+7th **S60.444** External constriction of right ring finger
+7th **S60.445** External constriction of left ring finger
+7th **S60.446** External constriction of right little finger
+7th **S60.447** External constriction of left little finger
+7th **S60.448** External constriction of other finger
External constriction of specified finger with unspecified laterality
+7th **S60.449** External constriction of unspecified finger
+ **S60.45** Superficial foreign body of fingers
Splinter in the finger(s)
+7th **S60.450** Superficial foreign body of right index finger
+7th **S60.451** Superficial foreign body of left index finger
+7th **S60.452** Superficial foreign body of right middle finger
+7th **S60.453** Superficial foreign body of left middle finger
+7th **S60.454** Superficial foreign body of right ring finger
+7th **S60.455** Superficial foreign body of left ring finger
+7th **S60.456** Superficial foreign body of right little finger

+, +7th, X + 7th ● Newborn ● Pediatric ● Maternity ● Adult ♀ Female ♂ Male Manifestation Unacceptable PDX HCC CC MCC HAC

+7th **S60.457** **Superficial foreign body of left little finger**

+7th **S60.458** **Superficial foreign body of other finger**
Superficial foreign body of specified finger with unspecified laterality

+7th **S60.459** **Superficial foreign body of unspecified finger**

+ **S60.46** **Insect bite (nonvenomous) of fingers**

+7th **S60.460** **Insect bite (nonvenomous) of right index finger**

+7th **S60.461** **Insect bite (nonvenomous) of left index finger**

+7th **S60.462** **Insect bite (nonvenomous) of right middle finger**

+7th **S60.463** **Insect bite (nonvenomous) of left middle finger**

+7th **S60.464** **Insect bite (nonvenomous) of right ring finger**

+7th **S60.465** **Insect bite (nonvenomous) of left ring finger**

+7th **S60.466** **Insect bite (nonvenomous) of right little finger**

+7th **S60.467** **Insect bite (nonvenomous) of left little finger**

+7th **S60.468** **Insect bite (nonvenomous) of other finger**
Insect bite (nonvenomous) of specified finger with unspecified laterality

+7th **S60.469** **Insect bite (nonvenomous) of unspecified finger**

+ **S60.47** **Other superficial bite of fingers**
Excludes1: open bite of fingers (S61.25-, S61.35-)

+7th **S60.470** **Other superficial bite of right index finger**

+7th **S60.471** **Other superficial bite of left index finger**

+7th **S60.472** **Other superficial bite of right middle finger**

+7th **S60.473** **Other superficial bite of left middle finger**

+7th **S60.474** **Other superficial bite of right ring finger**

+7th **S60.475** **Other superficial bite of left ring finger**

+7th **S60.476** **Other superficial bite of right little finger**

+7th **S60.477** **Other superficial bite of left little finger**

+7th **S60.478** **Other superficial bite of other finger**
Other superficial bite of specified finger with unspecified laterality

+7th **S60.479** **Other superficial bite of unspecified finger**

+ **S60.5** **Other superficial injuries of hand**
Excludes2: superficial injuries of fingers (S60.3-, S60.4-)

+ **S60.51** **Abrasion of hand**

+7th **S60.511** **Abrasion of right hand**

+7th **S60.512** **Abrasion of left hand**

+7th **S60.519** **Abrasion of unspecified hand**

+ **S60.52** **Blister (nonthermal) of hand**

+7th **S60.521** **Blister (nonthermal) of right hand**

+7th **S60.522** **Blister (nonthermal) of left hand**

+7th **S60.529** **Blister (nonthermal) of unspecified hand**

+ **S60.54** **External constriction of hand**

+7th **S60.541** **External constriction of right hand**

+7th **S60.542** **External constriction of left hand**

+7th **S60.549** **External constriction of unspecified hand**

+ **S60.55** **Superficial foreign body of hand**
Splinter in the hand

+7th **S60.551** **Superficial foreign body of right hand**

+7th **S60.552** **Superficial foreign body of left hand**

+7th **S60.559** **Superficial foreign body of unspecified hand**

+ **S60.56** **Insect bite (nonvenomous) of hand**

+7th **S60.561** **Insect bite (nonvenomous) of right hand**

+7th **S60.562** **Insect bite (nonvenomous) of left hand**

+7th **S60.569** **Insect bite (nonvenomous) of unspecified hand**

+ **S60.57** **Other superficial bite of hand**
Excludes1: open bite of hand (S61.45-)

+7th **S60.571** **Other superficial bite of hand of right hand**

+7th **S60.572** **Other superficial bite of hand of left hand**

+7th **S60.579** **Other superficial bite of hand of unspecified hand**

+ **S60.8** **Other superficial injuries of wrist**

+ **S60.81** **Abrasion of wrist**

+7th **S60.811** **Abrasion of right wrist**

+7th **S60.812** **Abrasion of left wrist**

+7th **S60.819** **Abrasion of unspecified wrist**

+ **S60.82** **Blister (nonthermal) of wrist**

+7th **S60.821** **Blister (nonthermal) of right wrist**

+7th **S60.822** **Blister (nonthermal) of left wrist**

+7th **S60.829** **Blister (nonthermal) of unspecified wrist**

+ **S60.84** **External constriction of wrist**

+7th **S60.841** **External constriction of right wrist**

+7th **S60.842** **External constriction of left wrist**

+7th **S60.849** **External constriction of unspecified wrist**

+ **S60.85** **Superficial foreign body of wrist**
Splinter in the wrist

+7th **S60.851** **Superficial foreign body of right wrist**

+7th **S60.852** **Superficial foreign body of left wrist**

+7th **S60.859** **Superficial foreign body of unspecified wrist**

+ **S60.86** **Insect bite (nonvenomous) of wrist**

+7th **S60.861** **Insect bite (nonvenomous) of right wrist**

+7th **S60.862** **Insect bite (nonvenomous) of left wrist**

+7th **S60.869** **Insect bite (nonvenomous) of unspecified wrist**

+ **S60.87** **Other superficial bite of wrist**
Excludes1: open bite of wrist (S61.55)

+7th **S60.871** **Other superficial bite of right wrist**

+7th **S60.872** **Other superficial bite of left wrist**

+7th **S60.879** **Other superficial bite of unspecified wrist**

+ **S60.9** **Unspecified superficial injury of wrist, hand and fingers**

+ **S60.91** **Unspecified superficial injury of wrist**

+7th **S60.911** **Unspecified superficial injury of right wrist**

+7th **S60.912** **Unspecified superficial injury of left wrist**

+7th **S60.919** **Unspecified superficial injury of unspecified wrist**

+ **S60.92** **Unspecified superficial injury of hand**

+7th **S60.921** **Unspecified superficial injury of right hand**

+7th **S60.922** **Unspecified superficial injury of left hand**

+7th **S60.929** **Unspecified superficial injury of unspecified hand**

+ **S60.93** **Unspecified superficial injury of thumb**

+7th **S60.931** **Unspecified superficial injury of right thumb**

+7th **S60.932** **Unspecified superficial injury of left thumb**

+7th **S60.939** **Unspecified superficial injury of unspecified thumb**

+ **S60.94** **Unspecified superficial injury of other fingers**

+7th **S60.940** **Unspecified superficial injury of right index finger**

+7th **S60.941** **Unspecified superficial injury of left index finger**

+7th **S60.942** **Unspecified superficial injury of right middle finger**

+7th **S60.943** **Unspecified superficial injury of left middle finger**

+7th **S60.944** **Unspecified superficial injury of right ring finger**

+7th **S60.945** **Unspecified superficial injury of left ring finger**

+7th **S60.946** **Unspecified superficial injury of right little finger**

+7th **S60.947** **Unspecified superficial injury of left little finger**

+7th **S60.948** **Unspecified superficial injury of other finger**
Unspecified superficial injury of specified finger with unspecified laterality

+7th **S60.949** **Unspecified superficial injury of unspecified finger**

+, +7th, X + 7th   ● Newborn   ● Pediatric   ● Maternity   ● Adult   ♀ Female   ♂ Male   Manifestation   Unacceptable PDX   HCC   CC   MCC   HAC

S61 Open wound of wrist, hand and fingers

Code also any associated wound infection

Excludes1: open fracture of wrist, hand and finger (S62.- with 7th character B)

traumatic amputation of wrist and hand (S68.-)

> The appropriate 7th character is to be added to each code from category S61
> A initial encounter
> D subsequent encounter
> S sequela

+ **S61.0 Open wound of thumb without damage to nail**

Excludes1: open wound of thumb with damage to nail (S61.1-)

+ **S61.00 Unspecified open wound of thumb without damage to nail**

+7th **S61.001** Unspecified open wound of right thumb without damage to nail

+7th **S61.002** Unspecified open wound of left thumb without damage to nail

+7th **S61.009** Unspecified open wound of unspecified thumb without damage to nail

+ **S61.01 Laceration without foreign body of thumb without damage to nail**

+7th **S61.011** Laceration without foreign body of right thumb without damage to nail

+7th **S61.012** Laceration without foreign body of left thumb without damage to nail

+7th **S61.019** Laceration without foreign body of unspecified thumb without damage to nail

+ **S61.02 Laceration with foreign body of thumb without damage to nail**

+7th **S61.021** Laceration with foreign body of right thumb without damage to nail

+7th **S61.022** Laceration with foreign body of left thumb without damage to nail

+7th **S61.029** Laceration with foreign body of unspecified thumb without damage to nail

+ **S61.03 Puncture wound without foreign body of thumb without damage to nail**

+7th **S61.031** Puncture wound without foreign body of right thumb without damage to nail

+7th **S61.032** Puncture wound without foreign body of left thumb without damage to nail

+7th **S61.039** Puncture wound without foreign body of unspecified thumb without damage to nail

+ **S61.04 Puncture wound with foreign body of thumb without damage to nail**

+7th **S61.041** Puncture wound with foreign body of right thumb without damage to nail

+7th **S61.042** Puncture wound with foreign body of left thumb without damage to nail

+7th **S61.049** Puncture wound with foreign body of unspecified thumb without damage to nail

+ **S61.05 Open bite of thumb without damage to nail**

Bite of thumb NOS

Excludes1: superficial bite of thumb (S60.36-, S60.37-)

+7th **S61.051** Open bite of right thumb without damage to nail

+7th **S61.052** Open bite of left thumb without damage to nail

+7th **S61.059** Open bite of unspecified thumb without damage to nail

+ **S61.1 Open wound of thumb with damage to nail**

+ **S61.10 Unspecified open wound of thumb with damage to nail**

+7th **S61.101** Unspecified open wound of right thumb with damage to nail

+7th **S61.102** Unspecified open wound of left thumb with damage to nail

+7th **S61.109** Unspecified open wound of unspecified thumb with damage to nail

+ **S61.11 Laceration without foreign body of thumb with damage to nail**

+7th **S61.111** Laceration without foreign body of right thumb with damage to nail

+7th **S61.112** Laceration without foreign body of left thumb with damage to nail

+7th **S61.119** Laceration without foreign body of unspecified thumb with damage to nail

+ **S61.12 Laceration with foreign body of thumb with damage to nail**

+7th **S61.121** Laceration with foreign body of right thumb with damage to nail

+7th **S61.122** Laceration with foreign body of left thumb with damage to nail

+7th **S61.129** Laceration with foreign body of unspecified thumb with damage to nail

+ **S61.13 Puncture wound without foreign body of thumb with damage to nail**

+7th **S61.131** Puncture wound without foreign body of right thumb with damage to nail

+7th **S61.132** Puncture wound without foreign body of left thumb with damage to nail

+7th **S61.139** Puncture wound without foreign body of unspecified thumb with damage to nail

+ **S61.14 Puncture wound with foreign body of thumb with damage to nail**

+7th **S61.141** Puncture wound with foreign body of right thumb with damage to nail

+7th **S61.142** Puncture wound with foreign body of left thumb with damage to nail

+7th **S61.149** Puncture wound with foreign body of unspecified thumb with damage to nail

+ **S61.15 Open bite of thumb with damage to nail**

Bite of thumb with damage to nail NOS

Excludes1: superficial bite of thumb (S60.36-, S60.37-)

+7th **S61.151** Open bite of right thumb with damage to nail

+7th **S61.152** Open bite of left thumb with damage to nail

+7th **S61.159** Open bite of unspecified thumb with damage to nail

+ **S61.2 Open wound of other finger without damage to nail**

Excludes1: open wound of finger involving nail (matrix) (S61.3-)

Excludes2: open wound of thumb without damage to nail (S61.0-)

+ **S61.20 Unspecified open wound of other finger without damage to nail**

+7th **S61.200** Unspecified open wound of right index finger without damage to nail

+7th **S61.201** Unspecified open wound of left index finger without damage to nail

+7th **S61.202** Unspecified open wound of right middle finger without damage to nail

+7th **S61.203** Unspecified open wound of left middle finger without damage to nail

+7th **S61.204** Unspecified open wound of right ring finger without damage to nail

+7th **S61.205** Unspecified open wound of left ring finger without damage to nail

+7th **S61.206** Unspecified open wound of right little finger without damage to nail

+7th **S61.207** Unspecified open wound of left little finger without damage to nail

+7th **S61.208** Unspecified open wound of other finger without damage to nail

Unspecified open wound of specified finger with unspecified laterality without damage to nail

+7th **S61.209** Unspecified open wound of unspecified finger without damage to nail

+, +7th, X + 7th ● Newborn ● Pediatric ● Maternity ● Adult ♀ Female ♂ Male Manifestation Unacceptable PDX HCC CC MCC HAC

+ **S61.21** **Laceration without foreign body of finger without damage to nail**
+7th **S61.210** **Laceration without foreign body of right index finger without damage to nail**
+7th **S61.211** **Laceration without foreign body of left index finger without damage to nail**
+7th **S61.212** **Laceration without foreign body of right middle finger without damage to nail**
+7th **S61.213** **Laceration without foreign body of left middle finger without damage to nail**
+7th **S61.214** **Laceration without foreign body of right ring finger without damage to nail**
+7th **S61.215** **Laceration without foreign body of left ring finger without damage to nail**
+7th **S61.216** **Laceration without foreign body of right little finger without damage to nail**
+7th **S61.217** **Laceration without foreign body of left little finger without damage to nail**
+7th **S61.218** **Laceration without foreign body of other finger without damage to nail**
Laceration without foreign body of specified finger with unspecified laterality without damage to nail
+7th **S61.219** **Laceration without foreign body of unspecified finger without damage to nail**

+ **S61.22** **Laceration with foreign body of finger without damage to nail**
+7th **S61.220** **Laceration with foreign body of right index finger without damage to nail**
+7th **S61.221** **Laceration with foreign body of left index finger without damage to nail**
+7th **S61.222** **Laceration with foreign body of right middle finger without damage to nail**
+7th **S61.223** **Laceration with foreign body of left middle finger without damage to nail**
+7th **S61.224** **Laceration with foreign body of right ring finger without damage to nail**
+7th **S61.225** **Laceration with foreign body of left ring finger without damage to nail**
+7th **S61.226** **Laceration with foreign body of right little finger without damage to nail**
+7th **S61.227** **Laceration with foreign body of left little finger without damage to nail**
+7th **S61.228** **Laceration with foreign body of other finger without damage to nail**
Laceration with foreign body of specified finger with unspecified laterality without damage to nail
+7th **S61.229** **Laceration with foreign body of unspecified finger without damage to nail**

+ **S61.23** **Puncture wound without foreign body of finger without damage to nail**
+7th **S61.230** **Puncture wound without foreign body of right index finger without damage to nail**
+7th **S61.231** **Puncture wound without foreign body of left index finger without damage to nail**
+7th **S61.232** **Puncture wound without foreign body of right middle finger without damage to nail**
+7th **S61.233** **Puncture wound without foreign body of left middle finger without damage to nail**
+7th **S61.234** **Puncture wound without foreign body of right ring finger without damage to nail**
+7th **S61.235** **Puncture wound without foreign body of left ring finger without damage to nail**
+7th **S61.236** **Puncture wound without foreign body of right little finger without damage to nail**

+7th **S61.237** **Puncture wound without foreign body of left little finger without damage to nail**
+7th **S61.238** **Puncture wound without foreign body of other finger without damage to nail**
Puncture wound without foreign body of specified finger with unspecified laterality without damage to nail
+7th **S61.239** **Puncture wound without foreign body of unspecified finger without damage to nail**

+ **S61.24** **Puncture wound with foreign body of finger without damage to nail**
+7th **S61.240** **Puncture wound with foreign body of right index finger without damage to nail**
+7th **S61.241** **Puncture wound with foreign body of left index finger without damage to nail**
+7th **S61.242** **Puncture wound with foreign body of right middle finger without damage to nail**
+7th **S61.243** **Puncture wound with foreign body of left middle finger without damage to nail**
+7th **S61.244** **Puncture wound with foreign body of right ring finger without damage to nail**
+7th **S61.245** **Puncture wound with foreign body of left ring finger without damage to nail**
+7th **S61.246** **Puncture wound with foreign body of right little finger without damage to nail**
+7th **S61.247** **Puncture wound with foreign body of left little finger without damage to nail**
+7th **S61.248** **Puncture wound with foreign body of other finger without damage to nail**
Puncture wound with foreign body of specified finger with unspecified laterality without damage to nail
+7th **S61.249** **Puncture wound with foreign body of unspecified finger without damage to nail**

+ **S61.25** **Open bite of finger without damage to nail**
Bite of finger without damage to nail NOS
Excludes1: *superficial bite of finger (S60.46-, S60.47-)*
+7th **S61.250** **Open bite of right index finger without damage to nail**
+7th **S61.251** **Open bite of left index finger without damage to nail**
+7th **S61.252** **Open bite of right middle finger without damage to nail**
+7th **S61.253** **Open bite of left middle finger without damage to nail**
+7th **S61.254** **Open bite of right ring finger without damage to nail**
+7th **S61.255** **Open bite of left ring finger without damage to nail**
+7th **S61.256** **Open bite of right little finger without damage to nail**
+7th **S61.257** **Open bite of left little finger without damage to nail**
+7th **S61.258** **Open bite of other finger without damage to nail**
Open bite of specified finger with unspecified laterality without damage to nail
+7th **S61.259** **Open bite of unspecified finger without damage to nail**

+ **S61.3** **Open wound of other finger with damage to nail**
+ **S61.30** **Unspecified open wound of finger with damage to nail**
+7th **S61.300** **Unspecified open wound of right index finger with damage to nail**
+7th **S61.301** **Unspecified open wound of left index finger with damage to nail**
+7th **S61.302** **Unspecified open wound of right middle finger with damage to nail**
+7th **S61.303** **Unspecified open wound of left middle finger with damage to nail**
+7th **S61.304** **Unspecified open wound of right ring finger with damage to nail**

+, +7th, X + 7th • Newborn • Pediatric • Maternity • Adult ♀ Female ♂ Male Manifestation Unacceptable PDX HCC CC MCC HAC

+7th **S61.305** **Unspecified open wound of left ring finger with damage to nail**

+7th **S61.306** **Unspecified open wound of right little finger with damage to nail**

+7th **S61.307** **Unspecified open wound of left little finger with damage to nail**

+7th **S61.308** **Unspecified open wound of other finger with damage to nail**

Unspecified open wound of specified finger with unspecified laterality with damage to nail

+7th **S61.309** **Unspecified open wound of unspecified finger with damage to nail**

+ **S61.31** **Laceration without foreign body of finger with damage to nail**

+7th **S61.310** **Laceration without foreign body of right index finger with damage to nail**

+7th **S61.311** **Laceration without foreign body of left index finger with damage to nail**

+7th **S61.312** **Laceration without foreign body of right middle finger with damage to nail**

+7th **S61.313** **Laceration without foreign body of left middle finger with damage to nail**

+7th **S61.314** **Laceration without foreign body of right ring finger with damage to nail**

+7th **S61.315** **Laceration without foreign body of left ring finger with damage to nail**

+7th **S61.316** **Laceration without foreign body of right little finger with damage to nail**

+7th **S61.317** **Laceration without foreign body of left little finger with damage to nail**

+7th **S61.318** **Laceration without foreign body of other finger with damage to nail**

Laceration without foreign body of specified finger with unspecified laterality with damage to nail

+7th **S61.319** **Laceration without foreign body of unspecified finger with damage to nail**

+ **S61.32** **Laceration with foreign body of finger with damage to nail**

+7th **S61.320** **Laceration with foreign body of right index finger with damage to nail**

+7th **S61.321** **Laceration with foreign body of left index finger with damage to nail**

+7th **S61.322** **Laceration with foreign body of right middle finger with damage to nail**

+7th **S61.323** **Laceration with foreign body of left middle finger with damage to nail**

+7th **S61.324** **Laceration with foreign body of right ring finger with damage to nail**

+7th **S61.325** **Laceration with foreign body of left ring finger with damage to nail**

+7th **S61.326** **Laceration with foreign body of right little finger with damage to nail**

+7th **S61.327** **Laceration with foreign body of left little finger with damage to nail**

+7th **S61.328** **Laceration with foreign body of other finger with damage to nail**

Laceration with foreign body of specified finger with unspecified laterality with damage to nail

+7th **S61.329** **Laceration with foreign body of unspecified finger with damage to nail**

+ **S61.33** **Puncture wound without foreign body of finger with damage to nail**

+7th **S61.330** **Puncture wound without foreign body of right index finger with damage to nail**

+7th **S61.331** **Puncture wound without foreign body of left index finger with damage to nail**

+7th **S61.332** **Puncture wound without foreign body of right middle finger with damage to nail**

+7th **S61.333** **Puncture wound without foreign body of left middle finger with damage to nail**

+7th **S61.334** **Puncture wound without foreign body of right ring finger with damage to nail**

+7th **S61.335** **Puncture wound without foreign body of left ring finger with damage to nail**

+7th **S61.336** **Puncture wound without foreign body of right little finger with damage to nail**

+7th **S61.337** **Puncture wound without foreign body of left little finger with damage to nail**

+7th **S61.338** **Puncture wound without foreign body of other finger with damage to nail**

Puncture wound without foreign body of specified finger with unspecified laterality with damage to nail

+7th **S61.339** **Puncture wound without foreign body of unspecified finger with damage to nail**

+ **S61.34** **Puncture wound with foreign body of finger with damage to nail**

+7th **S61.340** **Puncture wound with foreign body of right index finger with damage to nail**

+7th **S61.341** **Puncture wound with foreign body of left index finger with damage to nail**

+7th **S61.342** **Puncture wound with foreign body of right middle finger with damage to nail**

+7th **S61.343** **Puncture wound with foreign body of left middle finger with damage to nail**

+7th **S61.344** **Puncture wound with foreign body of right ring finger with damage to nail**

+7th **S61.345** **Puncture wound with foreign body of left ring finger with damage to nail**

+7th **S61.346** **Puncture wound with foreign body of right little finger with damage to nail**

+7th **S61.347** **Puncture wound with foreign body of left little finger with damage to nail**

+7th **S61.348** **Puncture wound with foreign body of other finger with damage to nail**

Puncture wound with foreign body of specified finger with unspecified laterality with damage to nail

+7th **S61.349** **Puncture wound with foreign body of unspecified finger with damage to nail**

+ **S61.35** **Open bite of finger with damage to nail**

Bite of finger with damage to nail NOS

Excludes1: *superficial bite of finger (S60.46-, S60.47-)*

+7th **S61.350** **Open bite of right index finger with damage to nail**

+7th **S61.351** **Open bite of left index finger with damage to nail**

+7th **S61.352** **Open bite of right middle finger with damage to nail**

+7th **S61.353** **Open bite of left middle finger with damage to nail**

+7th **S61.354** **Open bite of right ring finger with damage to nail**

+7th **S61.355** **Open bite of left ring finger with damage to nail**

+7th **S61.356** **Open bite of right little finger with damage to nail**

+7th **S61.357** **Open bite of left little finger with damage to nail**

+7th **S61.358** **Open bite of other finger with damage to nail**

Open bite of specified finger with unspecified laterality with damage to nail

+7th **S61.359** **Open bite of unspecified finger with damage to nail**

+ **S61.4** **Open wound of hand**

+ **S61.40** **Unspecified open wound of hand**

+7th **S61.401** **Unspecified open wound of right hand**

+7th **S61.402** **Unspecified open wound of left hand**

+7th **S61.409** **Unspecified open wound of unspecified hand**

+ **S61.41** **Laceration without foreign body of hand**

+7th **S61.411** **Laceration without foreign body of right hand**

+7th **S61.412** **Laceration without foreign body of left hand**

+7th **S61.419** **Laceration without foreign body of unspecified hand**

+ **S61.42** **Laceration with foreign body of hand**

+7th **S61.421** **Laceration with foreign body of right hand**

+7th **S61.422** **Laceration with foreign body of left hand**

+7th **S61.429** **Laceration with foreign body of unspecified hand**

+, +7th, X + 7th ● Newborn ● Pediatric ● Maternity ● Adult ♀ Female ♂ Male Manifestation Unacceptable PDX HCC CC MCC HAC

+ S61.43 **Puncture wound without foreign body of hand**
+7th S61.431 **Puncture wound without foreign body of right hand**
+7th S61.432 **Puncture wound without foreign body of left hand**
+7th S61.439 **Puncture wound without foreign body of unspecified hand**
+ S61.44 **Puncture wound with foreign body of hand**
+7th S61.441 **Puncture wound with foreign body of right hand**
+7th S61.442 **Puncture wound with foreign body of left hand**
+7th S61.449 **Puncture wound with foreign body of unspecified hand**
+ S61.45 **Open bite of hand**
Bite of hand NOS
Excludes1: *superficial bite of hand (S60.56-, S60.57-)*
+7th S61.451 **Open bite of right hand**
+7th S61.452 **Open bite of left hand**
+7th S61.459 **Open bite of unspecified hand**
+ S61.5 **Open wound of wrist**
+ S61.50 **Unspecified open wound of wrist**
+7th S61.501 **Unspecified open wound of right wrist**
+7th S61.502 **Unspecified open wound of left wrist**
+7th S61.509 **Unspecified open wound of unspecified wrist**
+ S61.51 **Laceration without foreign body of wrist**
+7th S61.511 **Laceration without foreign body of right wrist**
+7th S61.512 **Laceration without foreign body of left wrist**
+7th S61.519 **Laceration without foreign body of unspecified wrist**
+ S61.52 **Laceration with foreign body of wrist**
+7th S61.521 **Laceration with foreign body of right wrist**
+7th S61.522 **Laceration with foreign body of left wrist**
+7th S61.529 **Laceration with foreign body of unspecified wrist**
+ S61.53 **Puncture wound without foreign body of wrist**
+7th S61.531 **Puncture wound without foreign body of right wrist**
+7th S61.532 **Puncture wound without foreign body of left wrist**
+7th S61.539 **Puncture wound without foreign body of unspecified wrist**
+ S61.54 **Puncture wound with foreign body of wrist**
+7th S61.541 **Puncture wound with foreign body of right wrist**
+7th S61.542 **Puncture wound with foreign body of left wrist**
+7th S61.549 **Puncture wound with foreign body of unspecified wrist**
+ S61.55 **Open bite of wrist**
Bite of wrist NOS
Excludes1: *superficial bite of wrist (S60.86-, S60.87-)*
+7th S61.551 **Open bite of right wrist**
+7th S61.552 **Open bite of left wrist**
+7th S61.559 **Open bite of unspecified wrist**

S62 **Fracture at wrist and hand level**

> **NOTE** A fracture not indicated as displaced or nondisplaced should be coded to displaced
> A fracture not indicated as open or closed should be coded to closed

Excludes1: *traumatic amputation of wrist and hand (S68.-)*
Excludes2: *fracture of distal parts of ulna and radius (S52.-)*

The appropriate 7th character is to be added to each code from category S62
A initial encounter for closed fracture
B initial encounter for open fracture
D subsequent encounter for fracture with routine healing
G subsequent encounter for fracture with delayed healing
K subsequent encounter for fracture with nonunion
P subsequent encounter for fracture with malunion
S sequela

Review coding guideline C.19.c

+ S62.0 **Fracture of navicular [scaphoid] bone of wrist**
+ S62.00 **Unspecified fracture of navicular [scaphoid] bone of wrist**
CC +7th S62.001 **Unspecified fracture of navicular [scaphoid] bone of right wrist**
HAC 7th character B see Appendix B for HAC conditional logic
CC +7th S62.002 **Unspecified fracture of navicular [scaphoid] bone of left wrist**
AHA CC: 4Q, 2012, 106
HAC 7th character B see Appendix B for HAC conditional logic
CC +7th S62.009 **Unspecified fracture of navicular [scaphoid] bone of unspecified wrist**
HAC 7th character B see Appendix B for HAC conditional logic
+ S62.01 **Fracture of distal pole of navicular [scaphoid] bone of wrist**
Fracture of volar tuberosity of navicular [scaphoid] bone of wrist
CC +7th S62.011 **Displaced fracture of distal pole of navicular [scaphoid] bone of right wrist**
HAC 7th character B see Appendix B for HAC conditional logic
CC +7th S62.012 **Displaced fracture of distal pole of navicular [scaphoid] bone of left wrist**
HAC 7th character B see Appendix B for HAC conditional logic
CC +7th S62.013 **Displaced fracture of distal pole of navicular [scaphoid] bone of unspecified wrist**
HAC 7th character B see Appendix B for HAC conditional logic
CC +7th S62.014 **Nondisplaced fracture of distal pole of navicular [scaphoid] bone of right wrist**
HAC 7th character B see Appendix B for HAC conditional logic
CC +7th S62.015 **Nondisplaced fracture of distal pole of navicular [scaphoid] bone of left wrist**
HAC 7th character B see Appendix B for HAC conditional logic
CC +7th S62.016 **Nondisplaced fracture of distal pole of navicular [scaphoid] bone of unspecified wrist**
HAC 7th character B see Appendix B for HAC conditional logic
+ S62.02 **Fracture of middle third of navicular [scaphoid] bone of wrist**
CC +7th S62.021 **Displaced fracture of middle third of navicular [scaphoid] bone of right wrist**
HAC 7th character B see Appendix B for HAC conditional logic
CC +7th S62.022 **Displaced fracture of middle third of navicular [scaphoid] bone of left wrist**
HAC 7th character B see Appendix B for HAC conditional logic
CC +7th S62.023 **Displaced fracture of middle third of navicular [scaphoid] bone of unspecified wrist**
HAC 7th character B see Appendix B for HAC conditional logic
CC +7th S62.024 **Nondisplaced fracture of middle third of navicular [scaphoid] bone of right wrist**
HAC 7th character B see Appendix B for HAC conditional logic
CC +7th S62.025 **Nondisplaced fracture of middle third of navicular [scaphoid] bone of left wrist**
HAC 7th character B see Appendix B for HAC conditional logic
CC +7th S62.026 **Nondisplaced fracture of middle third of navicular [scaphoid] bone of unspecified wrist**
HAC 7th character B see Appendix B for HAC conditional logic
+ S62.03 **Fracture of proximal third of navicular [scaphoid] bone of wrist**
CC +7th S62.031 **Displaced fracture of proximal third of navicular [scaphoid] bone of right wrist**
HAC 7th character B see Appendix B for HAC conditional logic

+, +7th, X + 7th ● Newborn ● Pediatric ● Maternity ● Adult ♀ Female ♂ Male Manifestation Unacceptable PDX HCC CC MCC **HAC**

CC +7th **S62.032** **Displaced fracture of proximal third of navicular [scaphoid] bone of left wrist**
HAC 7th character B see Appendix B for HAC conditional logic

CC +7th **S62.033** **Displaced fracture of proximal third of navicular [scaphoid] bone of unspecified wrist**
HAC 7th character B see Appendix B for HAC conditional logic

CC +7th **S62.034** **Nondisplaced fracture of proximal third of navicular [scaphoid] bone of right wrist**
HAC 7th character B see Appendix B for HAC conditional logic

CC +7th **S62.035** **Nondisplaced fracture of proximal third of navicular [scaphoid] bone of left wrist**
HAC 7th character B see Appendix B for HAC conditional logic

CC +7th **S62.036** **Nondisplaced fracture of proximal third of navicular [scaphoid] bone of unspecified wrist**
HAC 7th character B see Appendix B for HAC conditional logic

+ **S62.1** **Fracture of other and unspecified carpal bone(s)**
Excludes2: *fracture of scaphoid of wrist (S62.0-)*

+ **S62.10** **Fracture of unspecified carpal bone**
Fracture of wrist NOS

CC +7th **S62.101** **Fracture of unspecified carpal bone, right wrist**
HAC 7th character B see Appendix B for HAC conditional logic

CC +7th **S62.102** **Fracture of unspecified carpal bone, left wrist**
AHA CC: 4Q, 2012, 95-96
HAC 7th character B see Appendix B for HAC conditional logic

CC +7th **S62.109** **Fracture of unspecified carpal bone, unspecified wrist**
HAC 7th character B see Appendix B for HAC conditional logic

+ **S62.11** **Fracture of triquetrum [cuneiform] bone of wrist**

CC +7th **S62.111** **Displaced fracture of triquetrum [cuneiform] bone, right wrist**
HAC 7th character B see Appendix B for HAC conditional logic

CC +7th **S62.112** **Displaced fracture of triquetrum [cuneiform] bone, left wrist**
HAC 7th character B see Appendix B for HAC conditional logic

CC +7th **S62.113** **Displaced fracture of triquetrum [cuneiform] bone, unspecified wrist**
HAC 7th character B see Appendix B for HAC conditional logic

CC +7th **S62.114** **Nondisplaced fracture of triquetrum [cuneiform] bone, right wrist**
HAC 7th character B see Appendix B for HAC conditional logic

CC +7th **S62.115** **Nondisplaced fracture of triquetrum [cuneiform] bone, left wrist**
HAC 7th character B see Appendix B for HAC conditional logic

CC +7th **S62.116** **Nondisplaced fracture of triquetrum [cuneiform] bone, unspecified wrist**
HAC 7th character B see Appendix B for HAC conditional logic

+ **S62.12** **Fracture of lunate [semilunar]**

CC +7th **S62.121** **Displaced fracture of lunate [semilunar], right wrist**
HAC 7th character B see Appendix B for HAC conditional logic

CC +7th **S62.122** **Displaced fracture of lunate [semilunar], left wrist**
HAC 7th character B see Appendix B for HAC conditional logic

CC +7th **S62.123** **Displaced fracture of lunate [semilunar], unspecified wrist**
HAC 7th character B see Appendix B for HAC conditional logic

CC +7th **S62.124** **Nondisplaced fracture of lunate [semilunar], right wrist**
HAC 7th character B see Appendix B for HAC conditional logic

CC +7th **S62.125** **Nondisplaced fracture of lunate [semilunar], left wrist**
HAC 7th character B see Appendix B for HAC conditional logic

CC +7th **S62.126** **Nondisplaced fracture of lunate [semilunar], unspecified wrist**
HAC 7th character B see Appendix B for HAC conditional logic

+ **S62.13** **Fracture of capitate [os magnum] bone**

CC +7th **S62.131** **Displaced fracture of capitate [os magnum] bone, right wrist**
HAC 7th character B see Appendix B for HAC conditional logic

CC +7th **S62.132** **Displaced fracture of capitate [os magnum] bone, left wrist**
HAC 7th character B see Appendix B for HAC conditional logic

CC +7th **S62.133** **Displaced fracture of capitate [os magnum] bone, unspecified wrist**
HAC 7th character B see Appendix B for HAC conditional logic

CC +7th **S62.134** **Nondisplaced fracture of capitate [os magnum] bone, right wrist**
HAC 7th character B see Appendix B for HAC conditional logic

CC +7th **S62.135** **Nondisplaced fracture of capitate [os magnum] bone, left wrist**
HAC 7th character B see Appendix B for HAC conditional logic

CC +7th **S62.136** **Nondisplaced fracture of capitate [os magnum] bone, unspecified wrist**
HAC 7th character B see Appendix B for HAC conditional logic

+ **S62.14** **Fracture of body of hamate [unciform] bone**
Fracture of hamate [unciform] bone NOS

CC +7th **S62.141** **Displaced fracture of body of hamate [unciform] bone, right wrist**
HAC 7th character B see Appendix B for HAC conditional logic

CC +7th **S62.142** **Displaced fracture of body of hamate [unciform] bone, left wrist**
HAC 7th character B see Appendix B for HAC conditional logic

CC +7th **S62.143** **Displaced fracture of body of hamate [unciform] bone, unspecified wrist**
HAC 7th character B see Appendix B for HAC conditional logic

CC +7th **S62.144** **Nondisplaced fracture of body of hamate [unciform] bone, right wrist**
HAC 7th character B see Appendix B for HAC conditional logic

CC +7th **S62.145** **Nondisplaced fracture of body of hamate [unciform] bone, left wrist**
HAC 7th character B see Appendix B for HAC conditional logic

CC +7th **S62.146** **Nondisplaced fracture of body of hamate [unciform] bone, unspecified wrist**
HAC 7th character B see Appendix B for HAC conditional logic

+ **S62.15** **Fracture of hook process of hamate [unciform] bone**
Fracture of unciform process of hamate [unciform] bone

CC +7th **S62.151** **Displaced fracture of hook process of hamate [unciform] bone, right wrist**
HAC 7th character B see Appendix B for HAC conditional logic

CC +7th **S62.152** **Displaced fracture of hook process of hamate [unciform] bone, left wrist**
HAC 7th character B see Appendix B for HAC conditional logic

CC +7th **S62.153** **Displaced fracture of hook process of hamate [unciform] bone, unspecified wrist**
HAC 7th character B see Appendix B for HAC conditional logic

CC +7th **S62.154** **Nondisplaced fracture of hook process of hamate [unciform] bone, right wrist**
HAC 7th character B see Appendix B for HAC conditional logic

+, +7th, X + 7th　　● Newborn　　● Pediatric　　● Maternity　　● Adult　　♀ Female　　♂ Male　　Manifestation　　Unacceptable PDX　　HCC　　CC　　MCC　　HAC

CC +7th **S62.155** **Nondisplaced fracture of hook process of hamate [unciform] bone, left wrist**
HAC 7th character B see Appendix B for HAC conditional logic

CC +7th **S62.156** **Nondisplaced fracture of hook process of hamate [unciform] bone, unspecified wrist**
HAC 7th character B see Appendix B for HAC conditional logic

+ **S62.16** **Fracture of pisiform**

CC +7th **S62.161** **Displaced fracture of pisiform, right wrist**
HAC 7th character B see Appendix B for HAC conditional logic

CC +7th **S62.162** **Displaced fracture of pisiform, left wrist**
HAC 7th character B see Appendix B for HAC conditional logic

CC +7th **S62.163** **Displaced fracture of pisiform, unspecified wrist**
HAC 7th character B see Appendix B for HAC conditional logic

CC +7th **S62.164** **Nondisplaced fracture of pisiform, right wrist**
HAC 7th character B see Appendix B for HAC conditional logic

CC +7th **S62.165** **Nondisplaced fracture of pisiform, left wrist**
HAC 7th character B see Appendix B for HAC conditional logic

CC +7th **S62.166** **Nondisplaced fracture of pisiform, unspecified wrist**
HAC 7th character B see Appendix B for HAC conditional logic

+ **S62.17** **Fracture of trapezium [larger multangular]**

CC +7th **S62.171** **Displaced fracture of trapezium [larger multangular], right wrist**
HAC 7th character B see Appendix B for HAC conditional logic

CC +7th **S62.172** **Displaced fracture of trapezium [larger multangular], left wrist**
HAC 7th character B see Appendix B for HAC conditional logic

CC +7th **S62.173** **Displaced fracture of trapezium [larger multangular], unspecified wrist**
HAC 7th character B see Appendix B for HAC conditional logic

CC +7th **S62.174** **Nondisplaced fracture of trapezium [larger multangular], right wrist**
HAC 7th character B see Appendix B for HAC conditional logic

CC +7th **S62.175** **Nondisplaced fracture of trapezium [larger multangular], left wrist**
HAC 7th character B see Appendix B for HAC conditional logic

CC +7th **S62.176** **Nondisplaced fracture of trapezium [larger multangular], unspecified wrist**
HAC 7th character B see Appendix B for HAC conditional logic

+ **S62.18** **Fracture of trapezoid [smaller multangular]**

CC +7th **S62.181** **Displaced fracture of trapezoid [smaller multangular], right wrist**
HAC 7th character B see Appendix B for HAC conditional logic

CC +7th **S62.182** **Displaced fracture of trapezoid [smaller multangular], left wrist**
HAC 7th character B see Appendix B for HAC conditional logic

CC +7th **S62.183** **Displaced fracture of trapezoid [smaller multangular], unspecified wrist**
HAC 7th character B see Appendix B for HAC conditional logic

CC +7th **S62.184** **Nondisplaced fracture of trapezoid [smaller multangular], right wrist**
HAC 7th character B see Appendix B for HAC conditional logic

CC +7th **S62.185** **Nondisplaced fracture of trapezoid [smaller multangular], left wrist**
HAC 7th character B see Appendix B for HAC conditional logic

CC +7th **S62.186** **Nondisplaced fracture of trapezoid [smaller multangular], unspecified wrist**
HAC 7th character B see Appendix B for HAC conditional logic

+ **S62.2** **Fracture of first metacarpal bone**

+ **S62.20** **Unspecified fracture of first metacarpal bone**

CC +7th **S62.201** **Unspecified fracture of first metacarpal bone, right hand**
HAC 7th character B see Appendix B for HAC conditional logic

CC +7th **S62.202** **Unspecified fracture of first metacarpal bone, left hand**
HAC 7th character B see Appendix B for HAC conditional logic

CC +7th **S62.209** **Unspecified fracture of first metacarpal bone, unspecified hand**
HAC 7th character B see Appendix B for HAC conditional logic

+ **S62.21** **Bennett's fracture**

CC +7th **S62.211** **Bennett's fracture, right hand**
HAC 7th character B see Appendix B for HAC conditional logic

CC +7th **S62.212** **Bennett's fracture, left hand**
HAC 7th character B see Appendix B for HAC conditional logic

CC +7th **S62.213** **Bennett's fracture, unspecified hand**
HAC 7th character B see Appendix B for HAC conditional logic

+ **S62.22** **Rolando's fracture**

CC +7th **S62.221** **Displaced Rolando's fracture, right hand**
HAC 7th character B see Appendix B for HAC conditional logic

CC +7th **S62.222** **Displaced Rolando's fracture, left hand**
HAC 7th character B see Appendix B for HAC conditional logic

CC +7th **S62.223** **Displaced Rolando's fracture, unspecified hand**
HAC 7th character B see Appendix B for HAC conditional logic

CC +7th **S62.224** **Nondisplaced Rolando's fracture, right hand**
HAC 7th character B see Appendix B for HAC conditional logic

CC +7th **S62.225** **Nondisplaced Rolando's fracture, left hand**
HAC 7th character B see Appendix B for HAC conditional logic

CC +7th **S62.226** **Nondisplaced Rolando's fracture, unspecified hand**
HAC 7th character B see Appendix B for HAC conditional logic

+ **S62.23** **Other fracture of base of first metacarpal bone**

CC +7th **S62.231** **Other displaced fracture of base of first metacarpal bone, right hand**
HAC 7th character B see Appendix B for HAC conditional logic

CC +7th **S62.232** **Other displaced fracture of base of first metacarpal bone, left hand**
HAC 7th character B see Appendix B for HAC conditional logic

CC +7th **S62.233** **Other displaced fracture of base of first metacarpal bone, unspecified hand**
HAC 7th character B see Appendix B for HAC conditional logic

CC +7th **S62.234** **Other nondisplaced fracture of base of first metacarpal bone, right hand**
HAC 7th character B see Appendix B for HAC conditional logic

CC +7th **S62.235** **Other nondisplaced fracture of base of first metacarpal bone, left hand**
HAC 7th character B see Appendix B for HAC conditional logic

CC +7th **S62.236** **Other nondisplaced fracture of base of first metacarpal bone, unspecified hand**
HAC 7th character B see Appendix B for HAC conditional logic

+ **S62.24** **Fracture of shaft of first metacarpal bone**

CC +7th **S62.241** **Displaced fracture of shaft of first metacarpal bone, right hand**
HAC 7th character B see Appendix B for HAC conditional logic

CC +7th **S62.242** **Displaced fracture of shaft of first metacarpal bone, left hand**
HAC 7th character B see Appendix B for HAC conditional logic

+, +7th, X + 7th ● Newborn ● Pediatric ● Maternity ● Adult ♀ Female ♂ Male Manifestation Unacceptable PDX HCC CC MCC HAC

CC +7th **S62.243** **Displaced fracture of shaft of first metacarpal bone, unspecified hand**
  HAC 7th character B see Appendix B for HAC conditional logic

CC +7th **S62.244** **Nondisplaced fracture of shaft of first metacarpal bone, right hand**
  HAC 7th character B see Appendix B for HAC conditional logic

CC +7th **S62.245** **Nondisplaced fracture of shaft of first metacarpal bone, left hand**
  HAC 7th character B see Appendix B for HAC conditional logic

CC +7th **S62.246** **Nondisplaced fracture of shaft of first metacarpal bone, unspecified hand**
  HAC 7th character B see Appendix B for HAC conditional logic

+ **S62.25** **Fracture of neck of first metacarpal bone**

CC +7th **S62.251** **Displaced fracture of neck of first metacarpal bone, right hand**
  HAC 7th character B see Appendix B for HAC conditional logic

CC +7th **S62.252** **Displaced fracture of neck of first metacarpal bone, left hand**
  HAC 7th character B see Appendix B for HAC conditional logic

CC +7th **S62.253** **Displaced fracture of neck of first metacarpal bone, unspecified hand**
  HAC 7th character B see Appendix B for HAC conditional logic

CC +7th **S62.254** **Nondisplaced fracture of neck of first metacarpal bone, right hand**
  HAC 7th character B see Appendix B for HAC conditional logic

CC +7th **S62.255** **Nondisplaced fracture of neck of first metacarpal bone, left hand**
  HAC 7th character B see Appendix B for HAC conditional logic

CC +7th **S62.256** **Nondisplaced fracture of neck of first metacarpal bone, unspecified hand**
  HAC 7th character B see Appendix B for HAC conditional logic

+ **S62.29** **Other fracture of first metacarpal bone**

CC +7th **S62.291** **Other fracture of first metacarpal bone, right hand**
  HAC 7th character B see Appendix B for HAC conditional logic

CC +7th **S62.292** **Other fracture of first metacarpal bone, left hand**
  HAC 7th character B see Appendix B for HAC conditional logic

CC +7th **S62.299** **Other fracture of first metacarpal bone, unspecified hand**
  HAC 7th character B see Appendix B for HAC conditional logic

+ **S62.3** **Fracture of other and unspecified metacarpal bone**
  Excludes2: *fracture of first metacarpal bone (S62.2-)*

+ **S62.30** **Unspecified fracture of other metacarpal bone**

CC +7th **S62.300** **Unspecified fracture of second metacarpal bone, right hand**
  HAC 7th character B see Appendix B for HAC conditional logic

CC +7th **S62.301** **Unspecified fracture of second metacarpal bone, left hand**
  HAC 7th character B see Appendix B for HAC conditional logic

CC +7th **S62.302** **Unspecified fracture of third metacarpal bone, right hand**
  HAC 7th character B see Appendix B for HAC conditional logic

CC +7th **S62.303** **Unspecified fracture of third metacarpal bone, left hand**
  HAC 7th character B see Appendix B for HAC conditional logic

CC +7th **S62.304** **Unspecified fracture of fourth metacarpal bone, right hand**
  HAC 7th character B see Appendix B for HAC conditional logic

CC +7th **S62.305** **Unspecified fracture of fourth metacarpal bone, left hand**
  HAC 7th character B see Appendix B for HAC conditional logic

CC +7th **S62.306** **Unspecified fracture of fifth metacarpal bone, right hand**
  HAC 7th character B see Appendix B for HAC conditional logic

CC +7th **S62.307** **Unspecified fracture of fifth metacarpal bone, left hand**
  HAC 7th character B see Appendix B for HAC conditional logic

CC +7th **S62.308** **Unspecified fracture of other metacarpal bone**
  Unspecified fracture of specified metacarpal bone with unspecified laterality
  HAC 7th character B see Appendix B for HAC conditional logic

CC +7th **S62.309** **Unspecified fracture of unspecified metacarpal bone**
  HAC 7th character B see Appendix B for HAC conditional logic

+ **S62.31** **Displaced fracture of base of other metacarpal bone**

CC +7th **S62.310** **Displaced fracture of base of second metacarpal bone, right hand**
  HAC 7th character B see Appendix B for HAC conditional logic

CC +7th **S62.311** **Displaced fracture of base of second metacarpal bone, left hand**
  HAC 7th character B see Appendix B for HAC conditional logic

CC +7th **S62.312** **Displaced fracture of base of third metacarpal bone, right hand**
  HAC 7th character B see Appendix B for HAC conditional logic

CC +7th **S62.313** **Displaced fracture of base of third metacarpal bone, left hand**
  HAC 7th character B see Appendix B for HAC conditional logic

CC +7th **S62.314** **Displaced fracture of base of fourth metacarpal bone, right hand**
  HAC 7th character B see Appendix B for HAC conditional logic

CC +7th **S62.315** **Displaced fracture of base of fourth metacarpal bone, left hand**
  HAC 7th character B see Appendix B for HAC conditional logic

CC +7th **S62.316** **Displaced fracture of base of fifth metacarpal bone, right hand**
  HAC 7th character B see Appendix B for HAC conditional logic

CC +7th **S62.317** **Displaced fracture of base of fifth metacarpal bone, left hand**
  HAC 7th character B see Appendix B for HAC conditional logic

CC +7th **S62.318** **Displaced fracture of base of other metacarpal bone**
  Displaced fracture of base of specified metacarpal bone with unspecified laterality
  HAC 7th character B see Appendix B for HAC conditional logic

CC +7th **S62.319** **Displaced fracture of base of unspecified metacarpal bone**
  HAC 7th character B see Appendix B for HAC conditional logic

+ **S62.32** **Displaced fracture of shaft of other metacarpal bone**

CC +7th **S62.320** **Displaced fracture of shaft of second metacarpal bone, right hand**
  HAC 7th character B see Appendix B for HAC conditional logic

CC +7th **S62.321** **Displaced fracture of shaft of second metacarpal bone, left hand**
  HAC 7th character B see Appendix B for HAC conditional logic

CC +7th **S62.322** **Displaced fracture of shaft of third metacarpal bone, right hand**
  HAC 7th character B see Appendix B for HAC conditional logic

CC +7th **S62.323** **Displaced fracture of shaft of third metacarpal bone, left hand**
  HAC 7th character B see Appendix B for HAC conditional logic

CC +7th **S62.324** **Displaced fracture of shaft of fourth metacarpal bone, right hand**
  HAC 7th character B see Appendix B for HAC conditional logic

CC +7th **S62.325** **Displaced fracture of shaft of fourth metacarpal bone, left hand**
  HAC 7th character B see Appendix B for HAC conditional logic

CC +7th **S62.326** **Displaced fracture of shaft of fifth metacarpal bone, right hand**
    HAC 7th character B see Appendix B for HAC conditional logic

CC +7th **S62.327** **Displaced fracture of shaft of fifth metacarpal bone, left hand**
    HAC 7th character B see Appendix B for HAC conditional logic

CC +7th **S62.328** **Displaced fracture of shaft of other metacarpal bone**
    Displaced fracture of shaft of specified metacarpal bone with unspecified laterality
    HAC 7th character B see Appendix B for HAC conditional logic

CC +7th **S62.329** **Displaced fracture of shaft of unspecified metacarpal bone**
    HAC 7th character B see Appendix B for HAC conditional logic

+ **S62.33** **Displaced fracture of neck of other metacarpal bone**

CC +7th **S62.330** **Displaced fracture of neck of second metacarpal bone, right hand**
    HAC 7th character B see Appendix B for HAC conditional logic

CC +7th **S62.331** **Displaced fracture of neck of second metacarpal bone, left hand**
    HAC 7th character B see Appendix B for HAC conditional logic

CC +7th **S62.332** **Displaced fracture of neck of third metacarpal bone, right hand**
    HAC 7th character B see Appendix B for HAC conditional logic

CC +7th **S62.333** **Displaced fracture of neck of third metacarpal bone, left hand**
    HAC 7th character B see Appendix B for HAC conditional logic

CC +7th **S62.334** **Displaced fracture of neck of fourth metacarpal bone, right hand**
    HAC 7th character B see Appendix B for HAC conditional logic

CC +7th **S62.335** **Displaced fracture of neck of fourth metacarpal bone, left hand**
    HAC 7th character B see Appendix B for HAC conditional logic

CC +7th **S62.336** **Displaced fracture of neck of fifth metacarpal bone, right hand**
    HAC 7th character B see Appendix B for HAC conditional logic

CC +7th **S62.337** **Displaced fracture of neck of fifth metacarpal bone, left hand**
    HAC 7th character B see Appendix B for HAC conditional logic

CC +7th **S62.338** **Displaced fracture of neck of other metacarpal bone**
    Displaced fracture of neck of specified metacarpal bone with unspecified laterality
    HAC 7th character B see Appendix B for HAC conditional logic

CC +7th **S62.339** **Displaced fracture of neck of unspecified metacarpal bone**
    HAC 7th character B see Appendix B for HAC conditional logic

+ **S62.34** **Nondisplaced fracture of base of other metacarpal bone**

CC +7th **S62.340** **Nondisplaced fracture of base of second metacarpal bone, right hand**
    HAC 7th character B see Appendix B for HAC conditional logic

CC +7th **S62.341** **Nondisplaced fracture of base of second metacarpal bone, left hand**
    HAC 7th character B see Appendix B for HAC conditional logic

CC +7th **S62.342** **Nondisplaced fracture of base of third metacarpal bone, right hand**
    HAC 7th character B see Appendix B for HAC conditional logic

CC +7th **S62.343** **Nondisplaced fracture of base of third metacarpal bone, left hand**
    HAC 7th character B see Appendix B for HAC conditional logic

CC +7th **S62.344** **Nondisplaced fracture of base of fourth metacarpal bone, right hand**
    HAC 7th character B see Appendix B for HAC conditional logic

CC +7th **S62.345** **Nondisplaced fracture of base of fourth metacarpal bone, left hand**
    HAC 7th character B see Appendix B for HAC conditional logic

CC +7th **S62.346** **Nondisplaced fracture of base of fifth metacarpal bone, right hand**
    HAC 7th character B see Appendix B for HAC conditional logic

CC +7th **S62.347** **Nondisplaced fracture of base of fifth metacarpal bone, left hand**
    HAC 7th character B see Appendix B for HAC conditional logic

CC +7th **S62.348** **Nondisplaced fracture of base of other metacarpal bone**
    Nondisplaced fracture of base of specified metacarpal bone with unspecified laterality
    HAC 7th character B see Appendix B for HAC conditional logic

CC +7th **S62.349** **Nondisplaced fracture of base of unspecified metacarpal bone**
    HAC 7th character B see Appendix B for HAC conditional logic

+ **S62.35** **Nondisplaced fracture of shaft of other metacarpal bone**

CC +7th **S62.350** **Nondisplaced fracture of shaft of second metacarpal bone, right hand**
    HAC 7th character B see Appendix B for HAC conditional logic

CC +7th **S62.351** **Nondisplaced fracture of shaft of second metacarpal bone, left hand**
    HAC 7th character B see Appendix B for HAC conditional logic

CC +7th **S62.352** **Nondisplaced fracture of shaft of third metacarpal bone, right hand**
    HAC 7th character B see Appendix B for HAC conditional logic

CC +7th **S62.353** **Nondisplaced fracture of shaft of third metacarpal bone, left hand**
    HAC 7th character B see Appendix B for HAC conditional logic

CC +7th **S62.354** **Nondisplaced fracture of shaft of fourth metacarpal bone, right hand**
    HAC 7th character B see Appendix B for HAC conditional logic

CC +7th **S62.355** **Nondisplaced fracture of shaft of fourth metacarpal bone, left hand**
    HAC 7th character B see Appendix B for HAC conditional logic

CC +7th **S62.356** **Nondisplaced fracture of shaft of fifth metacarpal bone, right hand**
    HAC 7th character B see Appendix B for HAC conditional logic

CC +7th **S62.357** **Nondisplaced fracture of shaft of fifth metacarpal bone, left hand**
    HAC 7th character B see Appendix B for HAC conditional logic

CC +7th **S62.358** **Nondisplaced fracture of shaft of other metacarpal bone**
    Nondisplaced fracture of shaft of specified metacarpal bone with unspecified laterality
    HAC 7th character B see Appendix B for HAC conditional logic

CC +7th **S62.359** **Nondisplaced fracture of shaft of unspecified metacarpal bone**
    HAC 7th character B see Appendix B for HAC conditional logic

+ **S62.36** **Nondisplaced fracture of neck of other metacarpal bone**

CC +7th **S62.360** **Nondisplaced fracture of neck of second metacarpal bone, right hand**
    HAC 7th character B see Appendix B for HAC conditional logic

CC +7th **S62.361** **Nondisplaced fracture of neck of second metacarpal bone, left hand**
    HAC 7th character B see Appendix B for HAC conditional logic

+, +7th, X + 7th   ● Newborn   ● Pediatric   ● Maternity   ● Adult   ♀ Female   ♂ Male   Manifestation   Unacceptable PDX   HCC   CC   MCC   HAC

CC +7th **S62.362** **Nondisplaced fracture of neck of third metacarpal bone, right hand**
HAC 7th character B see Appendix B for HAC conditional logic

CC +7th **S62.363** **Nondisplaced fracture of neck of third metacarpal bone, left hand**
HAC 7th character B see Appendix B for HAC conditional logic

CC +7th **S62.364** **Nondisplaced fracture of neck of fourth metacarpal bone, right hand**
HAC 7th character B see Appendix B for HAC conditional logic

CC +7th **S62.365** **Nondisplaced fracture of neck of fourth metacarpal bone, left hand**
HAC 7th character B see Appendix B for HAC conditional logic

CC +7th **S62.366** **Nondisplaced fracture of neck of fifth metacarpal bone, right hand**
HAC 7th character B see Appendix B for HAC conditional logic

CC +7th **S62.367** **Nondisplaced fracture of neck of fifth metacarpal bone, left hand**
HAC 7th character B see Appendix B for HAC conditional logic

CC +7th **S62.368** **Nondisplaced fracture of neck of other metacarpal bone**
Nondisplaced fracture of neck of specified metacarpal bone with unspecified laterality
HAC 7th character B see Appendix B for HAC conditional logic

CC +7th **S62.369** **Nondisplaced fracture of neck of unspecified metacarpal bone**
HAC 7th character B see Appendix B for HAC conditional logic

+ **S62.39** **Other fracture of other metacarpal bone**

CC +7th **S62.390** **Other fracture of second metacarpal bone, right hand**
HAC 7th character B see Appendix B for HAC conditional logic

CC +7th **S62.391** **Other fracture of second metacarpal bone, left hand**
HAC 7th character B see Appendix B for HAC conditional logic

CC +7th **S62.392** **Other fracture of third metacarpal bone, right hand**
HAC 7th character B see Appendix B for HAC conditional logic

CC +7th **S62.393** **Other fracture of third metacarpal bone, left hand**
HAC 7th character B see Appendix B for HAC conditional logic

CC +7th **S62.394** **Other fracture of fourth metacarpal bone, right hand**
HAC 7th character B see Appendix B for HAC conditional logic

CC +7th **S62.395** **Other fracture of fourth metacarpal bone, left hand**
HAC 7th character B see Appendix B for HAC conditional logic

CC +7th **S62.396** **Other fracture of fifth metacarpal bone, right hand**
HAC 7th character B see Appendix B for HAC conditional logic

CC +7th **S62.397** **Other fracture of fifth metacarpal bone, left hand**
HAC 7th character B see Appendix B for HAC conditional logic

CC +7th **S62.398** **Other fracture of other metacarpal bone**
Other fracture of specified metacarpal bone with unspecified laterality
HAC 7th character B see Appendix B for HAC conditional logic

CC +7th **S62.399** **Other fracture of unspecified metacarpal bone**
HAC 7th character B see Appendix B for HAC conditional logic

+ **S62.5** **Fracture of thumb**
+ **S62.50** **Fracture of unspecified phalanx of thumb**

CC +7th **S62.501** **Fracture of unspecified phalanx of right thumb**
HAC 7th character B see Appendix B for HAC conditional logic

CC +7th **S62.502** **Fracture of unspecified phalanx of left thumb**
HAC 7th character B see Appendix B for HAC conditional logic

CC +7th **S62.509** **Fracture of unspecified phalanx of unspecified thumb**
HAC 7th character B see Appendix B for HAC conditional logic

+ **S62.51** **Fracture of proximal phalanx of thumb**

CC +7th **S62.511** **Displaced fracture of proximal phalanx of right thumb**
HAC 7th character B see Appendix B for HAC conditional logic

CC +7th **S62.512** **Displaced fracture of proximal phalanx of left thumb**
HAC 7th character B see Appendix B for HAC conditional logic

CC +7th **S62.513** **Displaced fracture of proximal phalanx of unspecified thumb**
HAC 7th character B see Appendix B for HAC conditional logic

CC +7th **S62.514** **Nondisplaced fracture of proximal phalanx of right thumb**
HAC 7th character B see Appendix B for HAC conditional logic

CC +7th **S62.515** **Nondisplaced fracture of proximal phalanx of left thumb**
HAC 7th character B see Appendix B for HAC conditional logic

CC +7th **S62.516** **Nondisplaced fracture of proximal phalanx of unspecified thumb**
HAC 7th character B see Appendix B for HAC conditional logic

+ **S62.52** **Fracture of distal phalanx of thumb**

CC +7th **S62.521** **Displaced fracture of distal phalanx of right thumb**
HAC 7th character B see Appendix B for HAC conditional logic

CC +7th **S62.522** **Displaced fracture of distal phalanx of left thumb**
HAC 7th character B see Appendix B for HAC conditional logic

CC +7th **S62.523** **Displaced fracture of distal phalanx of unspecified thumb**
HAC 7th character B see Appendix B for HAC conditional logic

CC +7th **S62.524** **Nondisplaced fracture of distal phalanx of right thumb**
HAC 7th character B see Appendix B for HAC conditional logic

CC +7th **S62.525** **Nondisplaced fracture of distal phalanx of left thumb**
HAC 7th character B see Appendix B for HAC conditional logic

CC +7th **S62.526** **Nondisplaced fracture of distal phalanx of unspecified thumb**
HAC 7th character B see Appendix B for HAC conditional logic

+ **S62.6** **Fracture of other and unspecified finger(s)**
Excludes2: *fracture of thumb (S62.5-)*

+ **S62.60** **Fracture of unspecified phalanx of finger**

CC +7th **S62.600** **Fracture of unspecified phalanx of right index finger**
HAC 7th character B see Appendix B for HAC conditional logic

CC +7th **S62.601** **Fracture of unspecified phalanx of left index finger**
HAC 7th character B see Appendix B for HAC conditional logic

CC +7th **S62.602** **Fracture of unspecified phalanx of right middle finger**
HAC 7th character B see Appendix B for HAC conditional logic

CC +7th **S62.603** **Fracture of unspecified phalanx of left middle finger**
HAC 7th character B see Appendix B for HAC conditional logic

CC +7th **S62.604** **Fracture of unspecified phalanx of right ring finger**
HAC 7th character B see Appendix B for HAC conditional logic

CC +7th **S62.605** **Fracture of unspecified phalanx of left ring finger**
HAC 7th character B see Appendix B for HAC conditional logic

CC +7th **S62.606** **Fracture of unspecified phalanx of right little finger**
> HAC 7th character B see Appendix B for HAC conditional logic

CC +7th **S62.607** **Fracture of unspecified phalanx of left little finger**
> HAC 7th character B see Appendix B for HAC conditional logic

CC +7th **S62.608** **Fracture of unspecified phalanx of other finger**
> Fracture of unspecified phalanx of specified finger with unspecified laterality
> HAC 7th character B see Appendix B for HAC conditional logic

CC +7th **S62.609** **Fracture of unspecified phalanx of unspecified finger**
> HAC 7th character B see Appendix B for HAC conditional logic

+ **S62.61** **Displaced fracture of proximal phalanx of finger**

CC +7th **S62.610** **Displaced fracture of proximal phalanx of right index finger**
> HAC 7th character B see Appendix B for HAC conditional logic

CC +7th **S62.611** **Displaced fracture of proximal phalanx of left index finger**
> HAC 7th character B see Appendix B for HAC conditional logic

CC +7th **S62.612** **Displaced fracture of proximal phalanx of right middle finger**
> HAC 7th character B see Appendix B for HAC conditional logic

CC +7th **S62.613** **Displaced fracture of proximal phalanx of left middle finger**
> HAC 7th character B see Appendix B for HAC conditional logic

CC +7th **S62.614** **Displaced fracture of proximal phalanx of right ring finger**
> HAC 7th character B see Appendix B for HAC conditional logic

CC +7th **S62.615** **Displaced fracture of proximal phalanx of left ring finger**
> HAC 7th character B see Appendix B for HAC conditional logic

CC +7th **S62.616** **Displaced fracture of proximal phalanx of right little finger**
> HAC 7th character B see Appendix B for HAC conditional logic

CC +7th **S62.617** **Displaced fracture of proximal phalanx of left little finger**
> HAC 7th character B see Appendix B for HAC conditional logic

CC +7th **S62.618** **Displaced fracture of proximal phalanx of other finger**
> Displaced fracture of proximal phalanx of specified finger with unspecified laterality
> HAC 7th character B see Appendix B for HAC conditional logic

CC +7th **S62.619** **Displaced fracture of proximal phalanx of unspecified finger**
> HAC 7th character B see Appendix B for HAC conditional logic

+ **S62.62** **Displaced fracture of middle phalanx of finger**

CC +7th **S62.620** **Displaced fracture of middle phalanx of right index finger**
> HAC 7th character B see Appendix B for HAC conditional logic

CC +7th **S62.621** **Displaced fracture of middle phalanx of left index finger**
> HAC 7th character B see Appendix B for HAC conditional logic

CC +7th **S62.622** **Displaced fracture of middle phalanx of right middle finger**
> HAC 7th character B see Appendix B for HAC conditional logic

CC +7th **S62.623** **Displaced fracture of middle phalanx of left middle finger**
> HAC 7th character B see Appendix B for HAC conditional logic

CC +7th **S62.624** **Displaced fracture of middle phalanx of right ring finger**
> HAC 7th character B see Appendix B for HAC conditional logic

CC +7th **S62.625** **Displaced fracture of middle phalanx of left ring finger**
> HAC 7th character B see Appendix B for HAC conditional logic

CC +7th **S62.626** **Displaced fracture of middle phalanx of right little finger**
> HAC 7th character B see Appendix B for HAC conditional logic

CC +7th **S62.627** **Displaced fracture of middle phalanx of left little finger**
> HAC 7th character B see Appendix B for HAC conditional logic

CC +7th **S62.628** **Displaced fracture of middle phalanx of other finger**
> Displaced fracture of middle phalanx of specified finger with unspecified laterality
> HAC 7th character B see Appendix B for HAC conditional logic

CC +7th **S62.629** **Displaced fracture of middle phalanx of unspecified finger**
> HAC 7th character B see Appendix B for HAC conditional logic

+ **S62.63** **Displaced fracture of distal phalanx of finger**

CC +7th **S62.630** **Displaced fracture of distal phalanx of right index finger**
> HAC 7th character B see Appendix B for HAC conditional logic

CC +7th **S62.631** **Displaced fracture of distal phalanx of left index finger**
> HAC 7th character B see Appendix B for HAC conditional logic

CC +7th **S62.632** **Displaced fracture of distal phalanx of right middle finger**
> HAC 7th character B see Appendix B for HAC conditional logic

CC +7th **S62.633** **Displaced fracture of distal phalanx of left middle finger**
> HAC 7th character B see Appendix B for HAC conditional logic

CC +7th **S62.634** **Displaced fracture of distal phalanx of right ring finger**
> HAC 7th character B see Appendix B for HAC conditional logic

CC +7th **S62.635** **Displaced fracture of distal phalanx of left ring finger**
> HAC 7th character B see Appendix B for HAC conditional logic

CC +7th **S62.636** **Displaced fracture of distal phalanx of right little finger**
> HAC 7th character B see Appendix B for HAC conditional logic

CC +7th **S62.637** **Displaced fracture of distal phalanx of left little finger**
> HAC 7th character B see Appendix B for HAC conditional logic

CC +7th **S62.638** **Displaced fracture of distal phalanx of other finger**
> Displaced fracture of distal phalanx of specified finger with unspecified laterality
> HAC 7th character B see Appendix B for HAC conditional logic

CC +7th **S62.639** **Displaced fracture of distal phalanx of unspecified finger**
> HAC 7th character B see Appendix B for HAC conditional logic

+ **S62.64** **Nondisplaced fracture of proximal phalanx of finger**

CC +7th **S62.640** **Nondisplaced fracture of proximal phalanx of right index finger**
> HAC 7th character B see Appendix B for HAC conditional logic

CC +7th **S62.641** **Nondisplaced fracture of proximal phalanx of left index finger**
> HAC 7th character B see Appendix B for HAC conditional logic

CC +7th **S62.642** **Nondisplaced fracture of proximal phalanx of right middle finger**
> HAC 7th character B see Appendix B for HAC conditional logic

CC +7th **S62.643** **Nondisplaced fracture of proximal phalanx of left middle finger**
> HAC 7th character B see Appendix B for HAC conditional logic

+, +7th, X + 7th ● Newborn ● Pediatric ● Maternity ● Adult ♀ Female ♂ Male Manifestation Unacceptable PDX HCC CC MCC HAC

CC +7th **S62.644** **Nondisplaced fracture of proximal phalanx of right ring finger**
  HAC 7th character B see Appendix B for HAC conditional logic

CC +7th **S62.645** **Nondisplaced fracture of proximal phalanx of left ring finger**
  HAC 7th character B see Appendix B for HAC conditional logic

CC +7th **S62.646** **Nondisplaced fracture of proximal phalanx of right little finger**
  HAC 7th character B see Appendix B for HAC conditional logic

CC +7th **S62.647** **Nondisplaced fracture of proximal phalanx of left little finger**
  HAC 7th character B see Appendix B for HAC conditional logic

CC +7th **S62.648** **Nondisplaced fracture of proximal phalanx of other finger**
  Nondisplaced fracture of proximal phalanx of specified finger with unspecified laterality
  HAC 7th character B see Appendix B for HAC conditional logic

CC +7th **S62.649** **Nondisplaced fracture of proximal phalanx of unspecified finger**
  HAC 7th character B see Appendix B for HAC conditional logic

+ **S62.65** **Nondisplaced fracture of middle phalanx of finger**

CC +7th **S62.650** **Nondisplaced fracture of middle phalanx of right index finger**
  HAC 7th character B see Appendix B for HAC conditional logic

CC +7th **S62.651** **Nondisplaced fracture of middle phalanx of left index finger**
  HAC 7th character B see Appendix B for HAC conditional logic

CC +7th **S62.652** **Nondisplaced fracture of middle phalanx of right middle finger**
  HAC 7th character B see Appendix B for HAC conditional logic

CC +7th **S62.653** **Nondisplaced fracture of middle phalanx of left middle finger**
  HAC 7th character B see Appendix B for HAC conditional logic

CC +7th **S62.654** **Nondisplaced fracture of middle phalanx of right ring finger**
  HAC 7th character B see Appendix B for HAC conditional logic

CC +7th **S62.655** **Nondisplaced fracture of middle phalanx of left ring finger**
  HAC 7th character B see Appendix B for HAC conditional logic

CC +7th **S62.656** **Nondisplaced fracture of middle phalanx of right little finger**
  HAC 7th character B see Appendix B for HAC conditional logic

CC +7th **S62.657** **Nondisplaced fracture of middle phalanx of left little finger**
  HAC 7th character B see Appendix B for HAC conditional logic

CC +7th **S62.658** **Nondisplaced fracture of middle phalanx of other finger**
  Nondisplaced fracture of middle phalanx of specified finger with unspecified laterality
  HAC 7th character B see Appendix B for HAC conditional logic

CC +7th **S62.659** **Nondisplaced fracture of middle phalanx of unspecified finger**
  HAC 7th character B see Appendix B for HAC conditional logic

+ **S62.66** **Nondisplaced fracture of distal phalanx of finger**

CC +7th **S62.660** **Nondisplaced fracture of distal phalanx of right index finger**
  HAC 7th character B see Appendix B for HAC conditional logic

CC +7th **S62.661** **Nondisplaced fracture of distal phalanx of left index finger**
  HAC 7th character B see Appendix B for HAC conditional logic

CC +7th **S62.662** **Nondisplaced fracture of distal phalanx of right middle finger**
  HAC 7th character B see Appendix B for HAC conditional logic

CC +7th **S62.663** **Nondisplaced fracture of distal phalanx of left middle finger**
  HAC 7th character B see Appendix B for HAC conditional logic

CC +7th **S62.664** **Nondisplaced fracture of distal phalanx of right ring finger**
  HAC 7th character B see Appendix B for HAC conditional logic

CC +7th **S62.665** **Nondisplaced fracture of distal phalanx of left ring finger**
  HAC 7th character B see Appendix B for HAC conditional logic

CC +7th **S62.666** **Nondisplaced fracture of distal phalanx of right little finger**
  HAC 7th character B see Appendix B for HAC conditional logic

CC +7th **S62.667** **Nondisplaced fracture of distal phalanx of left little finger**
  HAC 7th character B see Appendix B for HAC conditional logic

CC +7th **S62.668** **Nondisplaced fracture of distal phalanx of other finger**
  Nondisplaced fracture of distal phalanx of specified finger with unspecified laterality
  HAC 7th character B see Appendix B for HAC conditional logic

CC +7th **S62.669** **Nondisplaced fracture of distal phalanx of unspecified finger**
  HAC 7th character B see Appendix B for HAC conditional logic

+ **S62.9** **Unspecified fracture of wrist and hand**

CC X+7th **S62.90** **Unspecified fracture of unspecified wrist and hand**
  HAC 7th character B see Appendix B for HAC conditional logic

CC X+7th **S62.91** **Unspecified fracture of right wrist and hand**
  HAC 7th character B see Appendix B for HAC conditional logic

CC X+7th **S62.92** **Unspecified fracture of left wrist and hand**
  HAC 7th character B see Appendix B for HAC conditional logic

S63 **Dislocation and sprain of joints and ligaments at wrist and hand level**

Includes: avulsion of joint or ligament at wrist and hand level
  laceration of cartilage, joint or ligament at wrist and hand level
  sprain of cartilage, joint or ligament at wrist and hand level
  traumatic hemarthrosis of joint or ligament at wrist and hand level
  traumatic rupture of joint or ligament at wrist and hand level
  traumatic subluxation of joint or ligament at wrist and hand level
  traumatic tear of joint or ligament at wrist and hand level

Code also any associated open wound

Excludes2: *strain of muscle, fascia and tendon of wrist and hand (S66.-)*

The appropriate 7th character is to be added to each code from category S63
A   initial encounter
D   subsequent encounter
S   sequela

+ **S63.0** **Subluxation and dislocation of wrist and hand joints**

  + **S63.00** **Unspecified subluxation and dislocation of wrist and hand**
    Dislocation of carpal bone NOS
    Dislocation of distal end of radius NOS
    Subluxation of carpal bone NOS
    Subluxation of distal end of radius NOS

    +7th **S63.001** **Unspecified subluxation of right wrist and hand**
    +7th **S63.002** **Unspecified subluxation of left wrist and hand**
    +7th **S63.003** **Unspecified subluxation of unspecified wrist and hand**
    +7th **S63.004** **Unspecified dislocation of right wrist and hand**
    +7th **S63.005** **Unspecified dislocation of left wrist and hand**
    +7th **S63.006** **Unspecified dislocation of unspecified wrist and hand**

+ S63.01 Subluxation and dislocation of distal radioulnar joint
  +7th S63.011 Subluxation of distal radioulnar joint of right wrist
  +7th S63.012 Subluxation of distal radioulnar joint of left wrist
  +7th S63.013 Subluxation of distal radioulnar joint of unspecified wrist
  +7th S63.014 Dislocation of distal radioulnar joint of right wrist
  +7th S63.015 Dislocation of distal radioulnar joint of left wrist
  +7th S63.016 Dislocation of distal radioulnar joint of unspecified wrist

+ S63.02 Subluxation and dislocation of radiocarpal joint
  +7th S63.021 Subluxation of radiocarpal joint of right wrist
  +7th S63.022 Subluxation of radiocarpal joint of left wrist
  +7th S63.023 Subluxation of radiocarpal joint of unspecified wrist
  +7th S63.024 Dislocation of radiocarpal joint of right wrist
  +7th S63.025 Dislocation of radiocarpal joint of left wrist
  +7th S63.026 Dislocation of radiocarpal joint of unspecified wrist

+ S63.03 Subluxation and dislocation of midcarpal joint
  +7th S63.031 Subluxation of midcarpal joint of right wrist
  +7th S63.032 Subluxation of midcarpal joint of left wrist
  +7th S63.033 Subluxation of midcarpal joint of unspecified wrist
  +7th S63.034 Dislocation of midcarpal joint of right wrist
  +7th S63.035 Dislocation of midcarpal joint of left wrist
  +7th S63.036 Dislocation of midcarpal joint of unspecified wrist

+ S63.04 Subluxation and dislocation of carpometacarpal joint of thumb
  Excludes2: interphalangeal subluxation and dislocation of thumb (S63.1-)
  +7th S63.041 Subluxation of carpometacarpal joint of right thumb
  +7th S63.042 Subluxation of carpometacarpal joint of left thumb
  +7th S63.043 Subluxation of carpometacarpal joint of unspecified thumb
  +7th S63.044 Dislocation of carpometacarpal joint of right thumb
  +7th S63.045 Dislocation of carpometacarpal joint of left thumb
  +7th S63.046 Dislocation of carpometacarpal joint of unspecified thumb

+ S63.05 Subluxation and dislocation of other carpometacarpal joint
  Excludes2: subluxation and dislocation of carpometacarpal joint of thumb (S63.04-)
  +7th S63.051 Subluxation of other carpometacarpal joint of right hand
  +7th S63.052 Subluxation of other carpometacarpal joint of left hand
  +7th S63.053 Subluxation of other carpometacarpal joint of unspecified hand
  +7th S63.054 Dislocation of other carpometacarpal joint of right hand
  +7th S63.055 Dislocation of other carpometacarpal joint of left hand
  +7th S63.056 Dislocation of other carpometacarpal joint of unspecified hand

+ S63.06 Subluxation and dislocation of metacarpal (bone), proximal end
  +7th S63.061 Subluxation of metacarpal (bone), proximal end of right hand
  +7th S63.062 Subluxation of metacarpal (bone), proximal end of left hand
  +7th S63.063 Subluxation of metacarpal (bone), proximal end of unspecified hand
  +7th S63.064 Dislocation of metacarpal (bone), proximal end of right hand
  +7th S63.065 Dislocation of metacarpal (bone), proximal end of left hand
  +7th S63.066 Dislocation of metacarpal (bone), proximal end of unspecified hand

+ S63.07 Subluxation and dislocation of distal end of ulna
  +7th S63.071 Subluxation of distal end of right ulna
  +7th S63.072 Subluxation of distal end of left ulna
  +7th S63.073 Subluxation of distal end of unspecified ulna
  +7th S63.074 Dislocation of distal end of right ulna
  +7th S63.075 Dislocation of distal end of left ulna
  +7th S63.076 Dislocation of distal end of unspecified ulna

+ S63.09 Other subluxation and dislocation of wrist and hand
  +7th S63.091 Other subluxation of right wrist and hand
  +7th S63.092 Other subluxation of left wrist and hand
  +7th S63.093 Other subluxation of unspecified wrist and hand
  +7th S63.094 Other dislocation of right wrist and hand
  +7th S63.095 Other dislocation of left wrist and hand
  +7th S63.096 Other dislocation of unspecified wrist and hand

+ S63.1 Subluxation and dislocation of thumb
  + S63.10 Unspecified subluxation and dislocation of thumb
    +7th S63.101 Unspecified subluxation of right thumb
    +7th S63.102 Unspecified subluxation of left thumb
    +7th S63.103 Unspecified subluxation of unspecified thumb
    +7th S63.104 Unspecified dislocation of right thumb
    +7th S63.105 Unspecified dislocation of left thumb
    +7th S63.106 Unspecified dislocation of unspecified thumb

  + S63.11 Subluxation and dislocation of metacarpophalangeal joint of thumb
    +7th S63.111 Subluxation of metacarpophalangeal joint of right thumb
    +7th S63.112 Subluxation of metacarpophalangeal joint of left thumb
    +7th S63.113 Subluxation of metacarpophalangeal joint of unspecified thumb
    +7th S63.114 Dislocation of metacarpophalangeal joint of right thumb
    +7th S63.115 Dislocation of metacarpophalangeal joint of left thumb
    +7th S63.116 Dislocation of metacarpophalangeal joint of unspecified thumb

  + S63.12 Subluxation and dislocation of interphalangeal joint of thumb
    +7th S63.121 Subluxation of interphalangeal joint of right thumb
    +7th S63.122 Subluxation of interphalangeal joint of left thumb
    +7th S63.123 Subluxation of interphalangeal joint of unspecified thumb
    +7th S63.124 Dislocation of interphalangeal joint of right thumb
    +7th S63.125 Dislocation of interphalangeal joint of left thumb
    +7th S63.126 Dislocation of interphalangeal joint of unspecified thumb

+ S63.2 Subluxation and dislocation of other finger(s)
  Excludes2: subluxation and dislocation of thumb (S63.1-)
  + S63.20 Unspecified subluxation of other finger
    +7th S63.200 Unspecified subluxation of right index finger
    +7th S63.201 Unspecified subluxation of left index finger
    +7th S63.202 Unspecified subluxation of right middle finger
    +7th S63.203 Unspecified subluxation of left middle finger
    +7th S63.204 Unspecified subluxation of right ring finger
    +7th S63.205 Unspecified subluxation of left ring finger
    +7th S63.206 Unspecified subluxation of right little finger

+7th **S63.207** **Unspecified subluxation of left little finger**

+7th **S63.208** **Unspecified subluxation of other finger**
Unspecified subluxation of specified finger with unspecified laterality

+7th **S63.209** **Unspecified subluxation of unspecified finger**

+ **S63.21** **Subluxation of metacarpophalangeal joint of finger**

+7th **S63.210** **Subluxation of metacarpophalangeal joint of right index finger**

+7th **S63.211** **Subluxation of metacarpophalangeal joint of left index finger**

+7th **S63.212** **Subluxation of metacarpophalangeal joint of right middle finger**

+7th **S63.213** **Subluxation of metacarpophalangeal joint of left middle finger**

+7th **S63.214** **Subluxation of metacarpophalangeal joint of right ring finger**

+7th **S63.215** **Subluxation of metacarpophalangeal joint of left ring finger**

+7th **S63.216** **Subluxation of metacarpophalangeal joint of right little finger**

+7th **S63.217** **Subluxation of metacarpophalangeal joint of left little finger**

+7th **S63.218** **Subluxation of metacarpophalangeal joint of other finger**
Subluxation of metacarpophalangeal joint of specified finger with unspecified laterality

+7th **S63.219** **Subluxation of metacarpophalangeal joint of unspecified finger**

+ **S63.22** **Subluxation of unspecified interphalangeal joint of finger**

+7th **S63.220** **Subluxation of unspecified interphalangeal joint of right index finger**

+7th **S63.221** **Subluxation of unspecified interphalangeal joint of left index finger**

+7th **S63.222** **Subluxation of unspecified interphalangeal joint of right middle finger**

+7th **S63.223** **Subluxation of unspecified interphalangeal joint of left middle finger**

+7th **S63.224** **Subluxation of unspecified interphalangeal joint of right ring finger**

+7th **S63.225** **Subluxation of unspecified interphalangeal joint of left ring finger**

+7th **S63.226** **Subluxation of unspecified interphalangeal joint of right little finger**

+7th **S63.227** **Subluxation of unspecified interphalangeal joint of left little finger**

+7th **S63.228** **Subluxation of unspecified interphalangeal joint of other finger**
Subluxation of unspecified interphalangeal joint of specified finger with unspecified laterality

+7th **S63.229** **Subluxation of unspecified interphalangeal joint of unspecified finger**

+ **S63.23** **Subluxation of proximal interphalangeal joint of finger**

+7th **S63.230** **Subluxation of proximal interphalangeal joint of right index finger**

+7th **S63.231** **Subluxation of proximal interphalangeal joint of left index finger**

+7th **S63.232** **Subluxation of proximal interphalangeal joint of right middle finger**

+7th **S63.233** **Subluxation of proximal interphalangeal joint of left middle finger**

+7th **S63.234** **Subluxation of proximal interphalangeal joint of right ring finger**

+7th **S63.235** **Subluxation of proximal interphalangeal joint of left ring finger**

+7th **S63.236** **Subluxation of proximal interphalangeal joint of right little finger**

+7th **S63.237** **Subluxation of proximal interphalangeal joint of left little finger**

+7th **S63.238** **Subluxation of proximal interphalangeal joint of other finger**
Subluxation of proximal interphalangeal joint of specified finger with unspecified laterality

+7th **S63.239** **Subluxation of proximal interphalangeal joint of unspecified finger**

+ **S63.24** **Subluxation of distal interphalangeal joint of finger**

+7th **S63.240** **Subluxation of distal interphalangeal joint of right index finger**

+7th **S63.241** **Subluxation of distal interphalangeal joint of left index finger**

+7th **S63.242** **Subluxation of distal interphalangeal joint of right middle finger**

+7th **S63.243** **Subluxation of distal interphalangeal joint of left middle finger**

+7th **S63.244** **Subluxation of distal interphalangeal joint of right ring finger**

+7th **S63.245** **Subluxation of distal interphalangeal joint of left ring finger**

+7th **S63.246** **Subluxation of distal interphalangeal joint of right little finger**

+7th **S63.247** **Subluxation of distal interphalangeal joint of left little finger**

+7th **S63.248** **Subluxation of distal interphalangeal joint of other finger**
Subluxation of distal interphalangeal joint of specified finger with unspecified laterality

+7th **S63.249** **Subluxation of distal interphalangeal joint of unspecified finger**

+ **S63.25** **Unspecified dislocation of other finger**

+7th **S63.250** **Unspecified dislocation of right index finger**

+7th **S63.251** **Unspecified dislocation of left index finger**

+7th **S63.252** **Unspecified dislocation of right middle finger**

+7th **S63.253** **Unspecified dislocation of left middle finger**

+7th **S63.254** **Unspecified dislocation of right ring finger**

+7th **S63.255** **Unspecified dislocation of left ring finger**

+7th **S63.256** **Unspecified dislocation of right little finger**

+7th **S63.257** **Unspecified dislocation of left little finger**

+7th **S63.258** **Unspecified dislocation of other finger**
Unspecified dislocation of specified finger with unspecified laterality

+7th **S63.259** **Unspecified dislocation of unspecified finger**
Unspecified dislocation of unspecified finger with unspecified laterality

+ **S63.26** **Dislocation of metacarpophalangeal joint of finger**

+7th **S63.260** **Dislocation of metacarpophalangeal joint of right index finger**

+7th **S63.261** **Dislocation of metacarpophalangeal joint of left index finger**

+7th **S63.262** **Dislocation of metacarpophalangeal joint of right middle finger**

+7th **S63.263** **Dislocation of metacarpophalangeal joint of left middle finger**

+7th **S63.264** **Dislocation of metacarpophalangeal joint of right ring finger**

+7th **S63.265** **Dislocation of metacarpophalangeal joint of left ring finger**

+7th **S63.266** **Dislocation of metacarpophalangeal joint of right little finger**

+, +7th, X + 7th   ● Newborn   ● Pediatric   ● Maternity   ● Adult   ♀ Female   ♂ Male   Manifestation   Unacceptable PDX   HCC   CC   MCC   HAC

+7th **S63.267** **Dislocation of metacarpophalangeal joint of left little finger**

+7th **S63.268** **Dislocation of metacarpophalangeal joint of other finger**
  Dislocation of metacarpophalangeal joint of specified finger with unspecified laterality

+7th **S63.269** **Dislocation of metacarpophalangeal joint of unspecified finger**

+ **S63.27** **Dislocation of unspecified interphalangeal joint of finger**

+7th **S63.270** **Dislocation of unspecified interphalangeal joint of right index finger**

+7th **S63.271** **Dislocation of unspecified interphalangeal joint of left index finger**

+7th **S63.272** **Dislocation of unspecified interphalangeal joint of right middle finger**

+7th **S63.273** **Dislocation of unspecified interphalangeal joint of left middle finger**

+7th **S63.274** **Dislocation of unspecified interphalangeal joint of right ring finger**

+7th **S63.275** **Dislocation of unspecified interphalangeal joint of left ring finger**

+7th **S63.276** **Dislocation of unspecified interphalangeal joint of right little finger**

+7th **S63.277** **Dislocation of unspecified interphalangeal joint of left little finger**

+7th **S63.278** **Dislocation of unspecified interphalangeal joint of other finger**
  Dislocation of unspecified interphalangeal joint of specified finger with unspecified laterality

+7th **S63.279** **Dislocation of unspecified interphalangeal joint of unspecified finger**
  Dislocation of unspecified interphalangeal joint of unspecified finger without specified laterality

+ **S63.28** **Dislocation of proximal interphalangeal joint of finger**

+7th **S63.280** **Dislocation of proximal interphalangeal joint of right index finger**

+7th **S63.281** **Dislocation of proximal interphalangeal joint of left index finger**

+7th **S63.282** **Dislocation of proximal interphalangeal joint of right middle finger**

+7th **S63.283** **Dislocation of proximal interphalangeal joint of left middle finger**

+7th **S63.284** **Dislocation of proximal interphalangeal joint of right ring finger**

+7th **S63.285** **Dislocation of proximal interphalangeal joint of left ring finger**

+7th **S63.286** **Dislocation of proximal interphalangeal joint of right little finger**

+7th **S63.287** **Dislocation of proximal interphalangeal joint of left little finger**

+7th **S63.288** **Dislocation of proximal interphalangeal joint of other finger**
  Dislocation of proximal interphalangeal joint of specified finger with unspecified laterality

+7th **S63.289** **Dislocation of proximal interphalangeal joint of unspecified finger**

+ **S63.29** **Dislocation of distal interphalangeal joint of finger**

+7th **S63.290** **Dislocation of distal interphalangeal joint of right index finger**

+7th **S63.291** **Dislocation of distal interphalangeal joint of left index finger**

+7th **S63.292** **Dislocation of distal interphalangeal joint of right middle finger**

+7th **S63.293** **Dislocation of distal interphalangeal joint of left middle finger**

+7th **S63.294** **Dislocation of distal interphalangeal joint of right ring finger**

+7th **S63.295** **Dislocation of distal interphalangeal joint of left ring finger**

+7th **S63.296** **Dislocation of distal interphalangeal joint of right little finger**

+7th **S63.297** **Dislocation of distal interphalangeal joint of left little finger**

+7th **S63.298** **Dislocation of distal interphalangeal joint of other finger**
  Dislocation of distal interphalangeal joint of specified finger with unspecified laterality

+7th **S63.299** **Dislocation of distal interphalangeal joint of unspecified finger**

+ **S63.3** **Traumatic rupture of ligament of wrist**

+ **S63.30** **Traumatic rupture of unspecified ligament of wrist**

+7th **S63.301** **Traumatic rupture of unspecified ligament of right wrist**

+7th **S63.302** **Traumatic rupture of unspecified ligament of left wrist**

+7th **S63.309** **Traumatic rupture of unspecified ligament of unspecified wrist**

+ **S63.31** **Traumatic rupture of collateral ligament of wrist**

+7th **S63.311** **Traumatic rupture of collateral ligament of right wrist**

+7th **S63.312** **Traumatic rupture of collateral ligament of left wrist**

+7th **S63.319** **Traumatic rupture of collateral ligament of unspecified wrist**

+ **S63.32** **Traumatic rupture of radiocarpal ligament**

+7th **S63.321** **Traumatic rupture of right radiocarpal ligament**

+7th **S63.322** **Traumatic rupture of left radiocarpal ligament**

+7th **S63.329** **Traumatic rupture of unspecified radiocarpal ligament**

+ **S63.33** **Traumatic rupture of ulnocarpal (palmar) ligament**

+7th **S63.331** **Traumatic rupture of right ulnocarpal (palmar) ligament**

+7th **S63.332** **Traumatic rupture of left ulnocarpal (palmar) ligament**

+7th **S63.339** **Traumatic rupture of unspecified ulnocarpal (palmar) ligament**

+ **S63.39** **Traumatic rupture of other ligament of wrist**

+7th **S63.391** **Traumatic rupture of other ligament of right wrist**

+7th **S63.392** **Traumatic rupture of other ligament of left wrist**

+7th **S63.399** **Traumatic rupture of other ligament of unspecified wrist**

+ **S63.4** **Traumatic rupture of ligament of finger at metacarpophalangeal and interphalangeal joint(s)**

+ **S63.40** **Traumatic rupture of unspecified ligament of finger at metacarpophalangeal and interphalangeal joint**

+7th **S63.400** **Traumatic rupture of unspecified ligament of right index finger at metacarpophalangeal and interphalangeal joint**

+7th **S63.401** **Traumatic rupture of unspecified ligament of left index finger at metacarpophalangeal and interphalangeal joint**

+7th **S63.402** **Traumatic rupture of unspecified ligament of right middle finger at metacarpophalangeal and interphalangeal joint**

+7th **S63.403** **Traumatic rupture of unspecified ligament of left middle finger at metacarpophalangeal and interphalangeal joint**

+7th **S63.404** **Traumatic rupture of unspecified ligament of right ring finger at metacarpophalangeal and interphalangeal joint**

+7th **S63.405** **Traumatic rupture of unspecified ligament of left ring finger at metacarpophalangeal and interphalangeal joint**

+7th **S63.406** **Traumatic rupture of unspecified ligament of right little finger at metacarpophalangeal and interphalangeal joint**

+, +7th, X + 7th　　● Newborn　　● Pediatric　　● Maternity　　● Adult　　♀ Female　　♂ Male　　Manifestation　　Unacceptable PDX　　HCC　　CC　　MCC　　HAC

+7th **S63.407** **Traumatic rupture of unspecified ligament of left little finger at metacarpophalangeal and interphalangeal joint**

+7th **S63.408** **Traumatic rupture of unspecified ligament of other finger at metacarpophalangeal and interphalangeal joint**

Traumatic rupture of unspecified ligament of specified finger with unspecified laterality at metacarpophalangeal and interphalangeal joint

+7th **S63.409** **Traumatic rupture of unspecified ligament of unspecified finger at metacarpophalangeal and interphalangeal joint**

+ **S63.41** **Traumatic rupture of collateral ligament of finger at metacarpophalangeal and interphalangeal joint**

+7th **S63.410** **Traumatic rupture of collateral ligament of right index finger at metacarpophalangeal and interphalangeal joint**

+7th **S63.411** **Traumatic rupture of collateral ligament of left index finger at metacarpophalangeal and interphalangeal joint**

+7th **S63.412** **Traumatic rupture of collateral ligament of right middle finger at metacarpophalangeal and interphalangeal joint**

+7th **S63.413** **Traumatic rupture of collateral ligament of left middle finger at metacarpophalangeal and interphalangeal joint**

+7th **S63.414** **Traumatic rupture of collateral ligament of right ring finger at metacarpophalangeal and interphalangeal joint**

+7th **S63.415** **Traumatic rupture of collateral ligament of left ring finger at metacarpophalangeal and interphalangeal joint**

+7th **S63.416** **Traumatic rupture of collateral ligament of right little finger at metacarpophalangeal and interphalangeal joint**

+7th **S63.417** **Traumatic rupture of collateral ligament of left little finger at metacarpophalangeal and interphalangeal joint**

+7th **S63.418** **Traumatic rupture of collateral ligament of other finger at metacarpophalangeal and interphalangeal joint**

Traumatic rupture of collateral ligament of specified finger with unspecified laterality at metacarpophalangeal and interphalangeal joint

+7th **S63.419** **Traumatic rupture of collateral ligament of unspecified finger at metacarpophalangeal and interphalangeal joint**

+ **S63.42** **Traumatic rupture of palmar ligament of finger at metacarpophalangeal and interphalangeal joint**

+7th **S63.420** **Traumatic rupture of palmarligament of right index finger at metacarpophalangeal and interphalangeal joint**

+7th **S63.421** **Traumatic rupture of palmar ligament of left index finger at metacarpophalangeal and interphalangeal joint**

+7th **S63.422** **Traumatic rupture of palmar ligament of right middle finger at metacarpophalangeal and interphalangeal joint**

+7th **S63.423** **Traumatic rupture of palmar ligament of left middle finger at metacarpophalangeal and interphalangeal joint**

+7th **S63.424** **Traumatic rupture of palmar ligament of right ring finger at metacarpophalangeal and interphalangeal joint**

+7th **S63.425** **Traumatic rupture of palmar ligament of left ring finger at metacarpophalangeal and interphalangeal joint**

+7th **S63.426** **Traumatic rupture of palmar ligament of right little finger at metacarpophalangeal and interphalangeal joint**

+7th **S63.427** **Traumatic rupture of palmar ligament of left little finger at metacarpophalangeal and interphalangeal joint**

+7th **S63.428** **Traumatic rupture of palmar ligament of other finger at metacarpophalangeal and interphalangeal joint**

Traumatic rupture of palmar ligament of specified finger with unspecified laterality at metacarpophalangeal and interphalangeal joint

+7th **S63.429** **Traumatic rupture of palmar ligament of unspecified finger at metacarpophalangeal and interphalangeal joint**

+ **S63.43** **Traumatic rupture of volar plate of finger at metacarpophalangeal and interphalangeal joint**

+7th **S63.430** **Traumatic rupture of volar plate of right index finger at metacarpophalangeal and interphalangeal joint**

+7th **S63.431** **Traumatic rupture of volar plate of left index finger at metacarpophalangeal and interphalangeal joint**

+7th **S63.432** **Traumatic rupture of volar plate of right middle finger at metacarpophalangeal and interphalangeal joint**

+7th **S63.433** **Traumatic rupture of volar plate of left middle finger at metacarpophalangeal and interphalangeal joint**

+7th **S63.434** **Traumatic rupture of volar plate of right ring finger at metacarpophalangeal and interphalangeal joint**

+7th **S63.435** **Traumatic rupture of volar plate of left ring finger at metacarpophalangeal and interphalangeal joint**

+7th **S63.436** **Traumatic rupture of volar plate of right little finger at metacarpophalangeal and interphalangeal joint**

+7th **S63.437** **Traumatic rupture of volar plate of left little finger at metacarpophalangeal and interphalangeal joint**

+7th **S63.438** **Traumatic rupture of volar plate of other finger at metacarpophalangeal and interphalangeal joint**

Traumatic rupture of volar plate of specified finger with unspecified laterality at metacarpophalangeal and interphalangeal joint

+7th **S63.439** **Traumatic rupture of volar plate of unspecified finger at metacarpophalangeal and interphalangeal joint**

+ **S63.49** **Traumatic rupture of other ligament of finger at metacarpophalangeal and interphalangeal joint**

+7th **S63.490** **Traumatic rupture of other ligament of right index finger at metacarpophalangeal and interphalangeal joint**

+7th **S63.491** **Traumatic rupture of other ligament of left index finger at metacarpophalangeal and interphalangeal joint**

+7th **S63.492** **Traumatic rupture of other ligament of right middle finger at metacarpophalangeal and interphalangeal joint**

+7th **S63.493** **Traumatic rupture of other ligament of left middle finger at metacarpophalangeal and interphalangeal joint**

+7th **S63.494** **Traumatic rupture of other ligament of right ring finger at metacarpophalangeal and interphalangeal joint**

+7th **S63.495** **Traumatic rupture of other ligament of left ring finger at metacarpophalangeal and interphalangeal joint**

+7th **S63.496** **Traumatic rupture of other ligament of right little finger at metacarpophalangeal and interphalangeal joint**

+7th **S63.497** **Traumatic rupture of other ligament of left little finger at metacarpophalangeal and interphalangeal joint**

+7th **S63.498** **Traumatic rupture of other ligament of other finger at metacarpophalangeal and interphalangeal joint**
  Traumatic rupture of ligament of specified finger with unspecified laterality at metacarpophalangeal and interphalangeal joint

+7th **S63.499** **Traumatic rupture of other ligament of unspecified finger at metacarpophalangeal and interphalangeal joint**

+ **S63.5** **Other and unspecified sprain of wrist**

+ **S63.50** **Unspecified sprain of wrist**

+7th **S63.501** **Unspecified sprain of right wrist**

+7th **S63.502** **Unspecified sprain of left wrist**

+7th **S63.509** **Unspecified sprain of unspecified wrist**

+ **S63.51** **Sprain of carpal (joint)**

+7th **S63.511** **Sprain of carpal joint of right wrist**

+7th **S63.512** **Sprain of carpal joint of left wrist**

+7th **S63.519** **Sprain of carpal joint of unspecified wrist**

+ **S63.52** **Sprain of radiocarpal joint**
  Excludes1: *traumatic rupture of radiocarpal ligament (S63.32-)*

+7th **S63.521** **Sprain of radiocarpal joint of right wrist**

+7th **S63.522** **Sprain of radiocarpal joint of left wrist**

+7th **S63.529** **Sprain of radiocarpal joint of unspecified wrist**

+ **S63.59** **Other specified sprain of wrist**

+7th **S63.591** **Other specified sprain of right wrist**

+7th **S63.592** **Other specified sprain of left wrist**

+7th **S63.599** **Other specified sprain of unspecified wrist**

+ **S63.6** **Other and unspecified sprain of finger(s)**
  Excludes1: *traumatic rupture of ligament of finger at metacarpophalangeal and interphalangeal joint(s) (S63.4-)*

+ **S63.60** **Unspecified sprain of thumb**

+7th **S63.601** **Unspecified sprain of right thumb**

+7th **S63.602** **Unspecified sprain of left thumb**

+7th **S63.609** **Unspecified sprain of unspecified thumb**

+ **S63.61** **Unspecified sprain of other and unspecified finger(s)**

+7th **S63.610** **Unspecified sprain of right index finger**

+7th **S63.611** **Unspecified sprain of left index finger**

+7th **S63.612** **Unspecified sprain of right middle finger**

+7th **S63.613** **Unspecified sprain of left middle finger**

+7th **S63.614** **Unspecified sprain of right ring finger**

+7th **S63.615** **Unspecified sprain of left ring finger**

+7th **S63.616** **Unspecified sprain of right little finger**

+7th **S63.617** **Unspecified sprain of left little finger**

+7th **S63.618** **Unspecified sprain of other finger**
  Unspecified sprain of specified finger with unspecified laterality

+7th **S63.619** **Unspecified sprain of unspecified finger**

+ **S63.62** **Sprain of interphalangeal joint of thumb**

+7th **S63.621** **Sprain of interphalangeal joint of right thumb**

+7th **S63.622** **Sprain of interphalangeal joint of left thumb**

+7th **S63.629** **Sprain of interphalangeal joint of unspecified thumb**

+ **S63.63** **Sprain of interphalangeal joint of other and unspecified finger(s)**

+7th **S63.630** **Sprain of interphalangeal joint of right index finger**

+7th **S63.631** **Sprain of interphalangeal joint of left index finger**

+7th **S63.632** **Sprain of interphalangeal joint of right middle finger**

+7th **S63.633** **Sprain of interphalangeal joint of left middle finger**

+7th **S63.634** **Sprain of interphalangeal joint of right ring finger**

+7th **S63.635** **Sprain of interphalangeal joint of left ring finger**

+7th **S63.636** **Sprain of interphalangeal joint of right little finger**

+7th **S63.637** **Sprain of interphalangeal joint of left little finger**

+7th **S63.638** **Sprain of interphalangeal joint of other finger**

+7th **S63.639** **Sprain of interphalangeal joint of unspecified finger**

+ **S63.64** **Sprain of metacarpophalangeal joint of thumb**

+7th **S63.641** **Sprain of metacarpophalangeal joint of right thumb**

+7th **S63.642** **Sprain of metacarpophalangeal joint of left thumb**

+7th **S63.649** **Sprain of metacarpophalangeal joint of unspecified thumb**

+ **S63.65** **Sprain of metacarpophalangeal joint of other and unspecified finger(s)**

+7th **S63.650** **Sprain of metacarpophalangeal joint of right index finger**

+7th **S63.651** **Sprain of metacarpophalangeal joint of left index finger**

+7th **S63.652** **Sprain of metacarpophalangeal joint of right middle finger**

+7th **S63.653** **Sprain of metacarpophalangeal joint of left middle finger**

+7th **S63.654** **Sprain of metacarpophalangeal joint of right ring finger**

+7th **S63.655** **Sprain of metacarpophalangeal joint of left ring finger**

+7th **S63.656** **Sprain of metacarpophalangeal joint of right little finger**

+7th **S63.657** **Sprain of metacarpophalangeal joint of left little finger**

+7th **S63.658** **Sprain of metacarpophalangeal joint of other finger**
  Sprain of metacarpophalangeal joint of specified finger with unspecified laterality

+7th **S63.659** **Sprain of metacarpophalangeal joint of unspecified finger**

+ **S63.68** **Other sprain of thumb**

+7th **S63.681** **Other sprain of right thumb**

+7th **S63.682** **Other sprain of left thumb**

+7th **S63.689** **Other sprain of unspecified thumb**

+ **S63.69** **Other sprain of other and unspecified finger(s)**

+7th **S63.690** **Other sprain of right index finger**

+7th **S63.691** **Other sprain of left index finger**

+7th **S63.692** **Other sprain of right middle finger**

+7th **S63.693** **Other sprain of left middle finger**

+7th **S63.694** **Other sprain of right ring finger**

+7th **S63.695** **Other sprain of left ring finger**

+7th **S63.696** **Other sprain of right little finger**

+7th **S63.697** **Other sprain of left little finger**

+7th **S63.698** **Other sprain of other finger**
  Other sprain of specified finger with unspecified laterality

+7th **S63.699** **Other sprain of unspecified finger**

+ **S63.8** Sprain of other part of wrist and hand
  + **S63.8X** Sprain of other part of wrist and hand
    +7th **S63.8X1** Sprain of other part of right wrist and hand
    +7th **S63.8X2** Sprain of other part of left wrist and hand
    +7th **S63.8X9** Sprain of other part of unspecified wrist and hand
+ **S63.9** Sprain of unspecified part of wrist and hand
  X+7th **S63.90** Sprain of unspecified part of unspecified wrist and hand
  X+7th **S63.91** Sprain of unspecified part of right wrist and hand
  X+7th **S63.92** Sprain of unspecified part of left wrist and hand

S64 Injury of nerves at wrist and hand level

Code also any associated open wound (S61.-)

The appropriate 7th character is to be added to each code from category S64
A initial encounter
D subsequent encounter
S sequela

+ **S64.0** Injury of ulnar nerve at wrist and hand level
  X+7th **S64.00** Injury of ulnar nerve at wrist and hand level of unspecified arm
  X+7th **S64.01** Injury of ulnar nerve at wrist and hand level of right arm
  X+7th **S64.02** Injury of ulnar nerve at wrist and hand level of left arm
+ **S64.1** Injury of median nerve at wrist and hand level
  X+7th **S64.10** Injury of median nerve at wrist and hand level of unspecified arm
  X+7th **S64.11** Injury of median nerve at wrist and hand level of right arm
  X+7th **S64.12** Injury of median nerve at wrist and hand level of left arm
+ **S64.2** Injury of radial nerve at wrist and hand level
  X+7th **S64.20** Injury of radial nerve at wrist and hand level of unspecified arm
  X+7th **S64.21** Injury of radial nerve at wrist and hand level of right arm
  X+7th **S64.22** Injury of radial nerve at wrist and hand level of left arm
+ **S64.3** Injury of digital nerve of thumb
  X+7th **S64.30** Injury of digital nerve of unspecified thumb
  X+7th **S64.31** Injury of digital nerve of right thumb
  X+7th **S64.32** Injury of digital nerve of left thumb
+ **S64.4** Injury of digital nerve of other and unspecified finger
  X+7th **S64.40** Injury of digital nerve of unspecified finger
  + **S64.49** Injury of digital nerve of other finger
    +7th **S64.490** Injury of digital nerve of right index finger
    +7th **S64.491** Injury of digital nerve of left index finger
    +7th **S64.492** Injury of digital nerve of right middle finger
    +7th **S64.493** Injury of digital nerve of left middle finger
    +7th **S64.494** Injury of digital nerve of right ring finger
    +7th **S64.495** Injury of digital nerve of left ring finger
    +7th **S64.496** Injury of digital nerve of right little finger
    +7th **S64.497** Injury of digital nerve of left little finger
    +7th **S64.498** Injury of digital nerve of other finger
      Injury of digital nerve of specified finger with unspecified laterality
+ **S64.8** Injury of other nerves at wrist and hand level
  + **S64.8X** Injury of other nerves at wrist and hand level
    +7th **S64.8X1** Injury of other nerves at wrist and hand level of right arm
    +7th **S64.8X2** Injury of other nerves at wrist and hand level of left arm
    +7th **S64.8X9** Injury of other nerves at wrist and hand level of unspecified arm

+ **S64.9** Injury of unspecified nerve at wrist and hand level
  X+7th **S64.90** Injury of unspecified nerve at wrist and hand level of unspecified arm
  X+7th **S64.91** Injury of unspecified nerve at wrist and hand level of right arm
  X+7th **S64.92** Injury of unspecified nerve at wrist and hand level of left arm

S65 Injury of blood vessels at wrist and hand level

Code also any associated open wound (S61.-)

The appropriate 7th character is to be added to each code from category S65
A initial encounter
D subsequent encounter
S sequela

+ **S65.0** Injury of ulnar artery at wrist and hand level
  + **S65.00** Unspecified injury of ulnar artery at wrist and hand level
    CC +7th **S65.001** Unspecified injury of ulnar artery at wrist and hand level of right arm
    CC +7th **S65.002** Unspecified injury of ulnar artery at wrist and hand level of left arm
    CC +7th **S65.009** Unspecified injury of ulnar artery at wrist and hand level of unspecified arm
  + **S65.01** Laceration of ulnar artery at wrist and hand level
    CC +7th **S65.011** Laceration of ulnar artery at wrist and hand level of right arm
    CC +7th **S65.012** Laceration of ulnar artery at wrist and hand level of left arm
    CC +7th **S65.019** Laceration of ulnar artery at wrist and hand level of unspecified arm
  + **S65.09** Other specified injury of ulnar artery at wrist and hand level
    CC +7th **S65.091** Other specified injury of ulnar artery at wrist and hand level of right arm
    CC +7th **S65.092** Other specified injury of ulnar artery at wrist and hand level of left arm
    CC +7th **S65.099** Other specified injury of ulnar artery at wrist and hand level of unspecified arm
+ **S65.1** Injury of radial artery at wrist and hand level
  + **S65.10** Unspecified injury of radial artery at wrist and hand level
    CC +7th **S65.101** Unspecified injury of radial artery at wrist and hand level of right arm
    CC +7th **S65.102** Unspecified injury of radial artery at wrist and hand level of left arm
    CC +7th **S65.109** Unspecified injury of radial artery at wrist and hand level of unspecified arm
  + **S65.11** Laceration of radial artery at wrist and hand level
    CC +7th **S65.111** Laceration of radial artery at wrist and hand level of right arm
    CC +7th **S65.112** Laceration of radial artery at wrist and hand level of left arm
    CC +7th **S65.119** Laceration of radial artery at wrist and hand level of unspecified arm
  + **S65.19** Other specified injury of radial artery at wrist and hand level
    CC +7th **S65.191** Other specified injury of radial artery at wrist and hand level of right arm
    CC +7th **S65.192** Other specified injury of radial artery at wrist and hand level of left arm
    CC +7th **S65.199** Other specified injury of radial artery at wrist and hand level of unspecified arm
+ **S65.2** Injury of superficial palmar arch
  + **S65.20** Unspecified injury of superficial palmar arch
    CC +7th **S65.201** Unspecified injury of superficial palmar arch of right hand
    CC +7th **S65.202** Unspecified injury of superficial palmar arch of left hand
    CC +7th **S65.209** Unspecified injury of superficial palmar arch of unspecified hand
  + **S65.21** Laceration of superficial palmar arch
    CC +7th **S65.211** Laceration of superficial palmar arch of right hand
    CC +7th **S65.212** Laceration of superficial palmar arch of left hand
    CC +7th **S65.219** Laceration of superficial palmar arch of unspecified hand

+, +7th, X + 7th   ● Newborn   ● Pediatric   ● Maternity   ● Adult   ♀ Female   ♂ Male   Manifestation   Unacceptable PDX   HCC   CC   MCC   HAC

+ **S65.29** Other specified injury of superficial palmar arch

  CC +7th **S65.291** Other specified injury of superficial palmar arch of right hand

  CC +7th **S65.292** Other specified injury of superficial palmar arch of left hand

  CC +7th **S65.299** Other specified injury of superficial palmar arch of unspecified hand

+ **S65.3** Injury of deep palmar arch

  + **S65.30** Unspecified injury of deep palmar arch

  CC +7th **S65.301** Unspecified injury of deep palmar arch of right hand

  CC +7th **S65.302** Unspecified injury of deep palmar arch of left hand

  CC +7th **S65.309** Unspecified injury of deep palmar arch of unspecified hand

  + **S65.31** Laceration of deep palmar arch

  CC +7th **S65.311** Laceration of deep palmar arch of right hand

  CC +7th **S65.312** Laceration of deep palmar arch of left hand

  CC +7th **S65.319** Laceration of deep palmar arch of unspecified hand

  + **S65.39** Other specified injury of deep palmar arch

  CC +7th **S65.391** Other specified injury of deep palmar arch of right hand

  CC +7th **S65.392** Other specified injury of deep palmar arch of left hand

  CC +7th **S65.399** Other specified injury of deep palmar arch of unspecified hand

+ **S65.4** Injury of blood vessel of thumb

  + **S65.40** Unspecified injury of blood vessel of thumb

  CC +7th **S65.401** Unspecified injury of blood vessel of right thumb

  CC +7th **S65.402** Unspecified injury of blood vessel of left thumb

  CC +7th **S65.409** Unspecified injury of blood vessel of unspecified thumb

  + **S65.41** Laceration of blood vessel of thumb

  CC +7th **S65.411** Laceration of blood vessel of right thumb

  CC +7th **S65.412** Laceration of blood vessel of left thumb

  CC +7th **S65.419** Laceration of blood vessel of unspecified thumb

  + **S65.49** Other specified injury of blood vessel of thumb

  CC +7th **S65.491** Other specified injury of blood vessel of right thumb

  CC +7th **S65.492** Other specified injury of blood vessel of left thumb

  CC +7th **S65.499** Other specified injury of blood vessel of unspecified thumb

+ **S65.5** Injury of blood vessel of other and unspecified finger

  + **S65.50** Unspecified injury of blood vessel of other and unspecified finger

  CC +7th **S65.500** Unspecified injury of blood vessel of right index finger

  CC +7th **S65.501** Unspecified injury of blood vessel of left index finger

  CC +7th **S65.502** Unspecified injury of blood vessel of right middle finger

  CC +7th **S65.503** Unspecified injury of blood vessel of left middle finger

  CC +7th **S65.504** Unspecified injury of blood vessel of right ring finger

  CC +7th **S65.505** Unspecified injury of blood vessel of left ring finger

  CC +7th **S65.506** Unspecified injury of blood vessel of right little finger

  CC +7th **S65.507** Unspecified injury of blood vessel of left little finger

  CC +7th **S65.508** Unspecified injury of blood vessel of other finger

    Unspecified injury of blood vessel of specified finger with unspecified laterality

  CC +7th **S65.509** Unspecified injury of blood vessel of unspecified finger

  + **S65.51** Laceration of blood vessel of other and unspecified finger

  CC +7th **S65.510** Laceration of blood vessel of right index finger

  CC +7th **S65.511** Laceration of blood vessel of left index finger

  CC +7th **S65.512** Laceration of blood vessel of right middle finger

  CC +7th **S65.513** Laceration of blood vessel of left middle finger

  CC +7th **S65.514** Laceration of blood vessel of right ring finger

  CC +7th **S65.515** Laceration of blood vessel of left ring finger

  CC +7th **S65.516** Laceration of blood vessel of right little finger

  CC +7th **S65.517** Laceration of blood vessel of left little finger

  CC +7th **S65.518** Laceration of blood vessel of other finger

    Laceration of blood vessel of specified finger with unspecified laterality

  CC +7th **S65.519** Laceration of blood vessel of unspecified finger

  + **S65.59** Other specified injury of blood vessel of other and unspecified finger

  CC +7th **S65.590** Other specified injury of blood vessel of right index finger

  CC +7th **S65.591** Other specified injury of blood vessel of left index finger

  CC +7th **S65.592** Other specified injury of blood vessel of right middle finger

  CC +7th **S65.593** Other specified injury of blood vessel of left middle finger

  CC +7th **S65.594** Other specified injury of blood vessel of right ring finger

  CC +7th **S65.595** Other specified injury of blood vessel of left ring finger

  CC +7th **S65.596** Other specified injury of blood vessel of right little finger

  CC +7th **S65.597** Other specified injury of blood vessel of left little finger

  CC +7th **S65.598** Other specified injury of blood vessel of other finger

    Other specified injury of blood vessel of specified finger with unspecified laterality

  CC +7th **S65.599** Other specified injury of blood vessel of unspecified finger

+ **S65.8** Injury of other blood vessels at wrist and hand level

  + **S65.80** Unspecified injury of other blood vessels at wrist and hand level

  CC +7th **S65.801** Unspecified injury of other blood vessels at wrist and hand level of right arm

  CC +7th **S65.802** Unspecified injury of other blood vessels at wrist and hand level of left arm

  CC +7th **S65.809** Unspecified injury of other blood vessels at wrist and hand level of unspecified arm

  + **S65.81** Laceration of other blood vessels at wrist and hand level

  CC +7th **S65.811** Laceration of other blood vessels at wrist and hand level of right arm

  CC +7th **S65.812** Laceration of other blood vessels at wrist and hand level of left arm

  CC +7th **S65.819** Laceration of other blood vessels at wrist and hand level of unspecified arm

  + **S65.89** Other specified injury of other blood vessels at wrist and hand level

  CC +7th **S65.891** Other specified injury of other blood vessels at wrist and hand level of right arm

  CC +7th **S65.892** Other specified injury of other blood vessels at wrist and hand level of left arm

  CC +7th **S65.899** Other specified injury of other blood vessels at wrist and hand level of unspecified arm

+ S65.9   **Injury of unspecified blood vessel at wrist and hand level**
  + S65.90   **Unspecified injury of unspecified blood vessel at wrist and hand level**
    CC +7th **S65.901**   Unspecified injury of unspecified blood vessel at wrist and hand level of right arm
    CC +7th **S65.902**   Unspecified injury of unspecified blood vessel at wrist and hand level of left arm
    CC +7th **S65.909**   Unspecified injury of unspecified blood vessel at wrist and hand level of unspecified arm
  + S65.91   **Laceration of unspecified blood vessel at wrist and hand level**
    CC +7th **S65.911**   Laceration of unspecified blood vessel at wrist and hand level of right arm
    CC +7th **S65.912**   Laceration of unspecified blood vessel at wrist and hand level of left arm
    CC +7th **S65.919**   Laceration of unspecified blood vessel at wrist and hand level of unspecified arm
  + S65.99   **Other specified injury of unspecified blood vessel at wrist and hand level**
    CC +7th **S65.991**   Other specified injury of unspecified blood vessel at wrist and hand of right arm
    CC +7th **S65.992**   Other specified injury of unspecified blood vessel at wrist and hand of left arm
    CC +7th **S65.999**   Other specified injury of unspecified blood vessel at wrist and hand of unspecified arm

S66   **Injury of muscle, fascia and tendon at wrist and hand level**

Code also any associated open wound (S61.-)

Excludes2: *sprain of joints and ligaments of wrist and hand (S63.-)*

> The appropriate 7th character is to be added to each code from category S66
> A   initial encounter
> D   subsequent encounter
> S   sequela

+ S66.0   **Injury of long flexor muscle, fascia and tendon of thumb at wrist and hand level**
  + S66.00   **Unspecified injury of long flexor muscle, fascia and tendon of thumb at wrist and hand level**
    +7th **S66.001**   Unspecified injury of long flexor muscle, fascia and tendon of right thumb at wrist and hand level
    +7th **S66.002**   Unspecified injury of long flexor muscle, fascia and tendon of left thumb at wrist and hand level
    +7th **S66.009**   Unspecified injury of long flexor muscle, fascia and tendon of unspecified thumb at wrist and hand level
  + S66.01   **Strain of long flexor muscle, fascia and tendon of thumb at wrist and hand level**
    +7th **S66.011**   Strain of long flexor muscle, fascia and tendon of right thumb at wrist and hand level
    +7th **S66.012**   Strain of long flexor muscle, fascia and tendon of left thumb at wrist and hand level
    +7th **S66.019**   Strain of long flexor muscle, fascia and tendon of unspecified thumb at wrist and hand level
  + S66.02   **Laceration of long flexor muscle, fascia and tendon of thumb at wrist and hand level**
    CC +7th **S66.021**   Laceration of long flexor muscle, fascia and tendon of right thumb at wrist and hand level
    CC +7th **S66.022**   Laceration of long flexor muscle, fascia and tendon of left thumb at wrist and hand level
    CC +7th **S66.029**   Laceration of long flexor muscle, fascia and tendon of unspecified thumb at wrist and hand level
  + S66.09   **Other specified injury of long flexor muscle, fascia and tendon of thumb at wrist and hand level**
    +7th **S66.091**   Other specified injury of long flexor muscle, fascia and tendon of right thumb at wrist and hand level

    +7th **S66.092**   Other specified injury of long flexor muscle, fascia and tendon of left thumb at wrist and hand level
    +7th **S66.099**   Other specified injury of long flexor muscle, fascia and tendon of unspecified thumb at wrist and hand level
+ S66.1   **Injury of flexor muscle, fascia and tendon of other and unspecified finger at wrist and hand level**
  Excludes2: *Injury of long flexor muscle, fascia and tendon of thumb at wrist and hand level (S66.0-)*
  + S66.10   **Unspecified injury of flexor muscle, fascia and tendon of other and unspecified finger at wrist and hand level**
    +7th **S66.100**   Unspecified injury of flexor muscle, fascia and tendon of right index finger at wrist and hand level
    +7th **S66.101**   Unspecified injury of flexor muscle, fascia and tendon of left index finger at wrist and hand level
    +7th **S66.102**   Unspecified injury of flexor muscle, fascia and tendon of right middle finger at wrist and hand level
    +7th **S66.103**   Unspecified injury of flexor muscle, fascia and tendon of left middle finger at wrist and hand level
    +7th **S66.104**   Unspecified injury of flexor muscle, fascia and tendon of right ring finger at wrist and hand level
    +7th **S66.105**   Unspecified injury of flexor muscle, fascia and tendon of left ring finger at wrist and hand level
    +7th **S66.106**   Unspecified injury of flexor muscle, fascia and tendon of right little finger at wrist and hand level
    +7th **S66.107**   Unspecified injury of flexor muscle, fascia and tendon of left little finger at wrist and hand level
    +7th **S66.108**   Unspecified injury of flexor muscle, fascia and tendon of other finger at wrist and hand level
      Unspecified injury of flexor muscle, fascia and tendon of specified finger with unspecified laterality at wrist and hand level
    +7th **S66.109**   Unspecified injury of flexor muscle, fascia and tendon of unspecified finger at wrist and hand level
  + S66.11   **Strain of flexor muscle, fascia and tendon of other and unspecified finger at wrist and hand level**
    +7th **S66.110**   Strain of flexor muscle, fascia and tendon of right index finger at wrist and hand level
    +7th **S66.111**   Strain of flexor muscle, fascia and tendon of left index finger at wrist and hand level
    +7th **S66.112**   Strain of flexor muscle, fascia and tendon of right middle finger at wrist and hand level
    +7th **S66.113**   Strain of flexor muscle, fascia and tendon of left middle finger at wrist and hand level
    +7th **S66.114**   Strain of flexor muscle, fascia and tendon of right ring finger at wrist and hand level
    +7th **S66.115**   Strain of flexor muscle, fascia and tendon of left ring finger at wrist and hand level
    +7th **S66.116**   Strain of flexor muscle, fascia and tendon of right little finger at wrist and hand level
    +7th **S66.117**   Strain of flexor muscle, fascia and tendon of left little finger at wrist and hand level
    +7th **S66.118**   Strain of flexor muscle, fascia and tendon of other finger at wrist and hand level
      Strain of flexor muscle, fascia and tendon of specified finger with unspecified laterality at wrist and hand level
    +7th **S66.119**   Strain of flexor muscle, fascia and tendon of unspecified finger at wrist and hand level

+ **S66.12** **Laceration of flexor muscle, fascia and tendon of other and unspecified finger at wrist and hand level**

CC +7th **S66.120** **Laceration of flexor muscle, fascia and tendon of right index finger at wrist and hand level**

CC +7th **S66.121** **Laceration of flexor muscle, fascia and tendon of left index finger at wrist and hand level**

CC +7th **S66.122** **Laceration of flexor muscle, fascia and tendon of right middle finger at wrist and hand level**

CC +7th **S66.123** **Laceration of flexor muscle, fascia and tendon of left middle finger at wrist and hand level**

CC +7th **S66.124** **Laceration of flexor muscle, fascia and tendon of right ring finger at wrist and hand level**

CC +7th **S66.125** **Laceration of flexor muscle, fascia and tendon of left ring finger at wrist and hand level**

CC +7th **S66.126** **Laceration of flexor muscle, fascia and tendon of right little finger at wrist and hand level**

CC +7th **S66.127** **Laceration of flexor muscle, fascia and tendon of left little finger at wrist and hand level**

CC +7th **S66.128** **Laceration of flexor muscle, fascia and tendon of other finger at wrist and hand level**

Laceration of flexor muscle, fascia and tendon of specified finger with unspecified laterality at wrist and hand level

CC +7th **S66.129** **Laceration of flexor muscle, fascia and tendon of unspecified finger at wrist and hand level**

+ **S66.19** **Other injury of flexor muscle, fascia and tendon of other and unspecified finger at wrist and hand level**

+7th **S66.190** **Other injury of flexor muscle, fascia and tendon of right index finger at wrist and hand level**

+7th **S66.191** **Other injury of flexor muscle, fascia and tendon of left index finger at wrist and hand level**

+7th **S66.192** **Other injury of flexor muscle, fascia and tendon of right middle finger at wrist and hand level**

+7th **S66.193** **Other injury of flexor muscle, fascia and tendon of left middle finger at wrist and hand level**

+7th **S66.194** **Other injury of flexor muscle, fascia and tendon of right ring finger at wrist and hand level**

+7th **S66.195** **Other injury of flexor muscle, fascia and tendon of left ring finger at wrist and hand level**

+7th **S66.196** **Other injury of flexor muscle, fascia and tendon of right little finger at wrist and hand level**

+7th **S66.197** **Other injury of flexor muscle, fascia and tendon of left little finger at wrist and hand level**

+7th **S66.198** **Other injury of flexor muscle, fascia and tendon of other finger at wrist and hand level**

Other injury of flexor muscle, fascia and tendon of specified finger with unspecified laterality at wrist and hand level

+7th **S66.199** **Other injury of flexor muscle, fascia and tendon of unspecified finger at wrist and hand level**

+ **S66.2** **Injury of extensor muscle, fascia and tendon of thumb at wrist and hand level**

+ **S66.20** **Unspecified injury of extensor muscle, fascia and tendon of thumb at wrist and hand level**

+7th **S66.201** **Unspecified injury of extensor muscle, fascia and tendon of right thumb at wrist and hand level**

+7th **S66.202** **Unspecified injury of extensor muscle, fascia and tendon of left thumb at wrist and hand level**

+7th **S66.209** **Unspecified injury of extensor muscle, fascia and tendon of unspecified thumb at wrist and hand level**

+ **S66.21** **Strain of extensor muscle, fascia and tendon of thumb at wrist and hand level**

+7th **S66.211** **Strain of extensor muscle, fascia and tendon of right thumb at wrist and hand level**

+7th **S66.212** **Strain of extensor muscle, fascia and tendon of left thumb at wrist and hand level**

+7th **S66.219** **Strain of extensor muscle, fascia and tendon of unspecified thumb at wrist and hand level**

+ **S66.22** **Laceration of extensor muscle, fascia and tendon of thumb at wrist and hand level**

CC +7th **S66.221** **Laceration of extensor muscle, fascia and tendon of right thumb at wrist and hand level**

CC +7th **S66.222** **Laceration of extensor muscle, fascia and tendon of left thumb at wrist and hand level**

CC +7th **S66.229** **Laceration of extensor muscle, fascia and tendon of unspecified thumb at wrist and hand level**

+ **S66.29** **Other specified injury of extensor muscle, fascia and tendon of thumb at wrist and hand level**

+7th **S66.291** **Other specified injury of extensor muscle, fascia and tendon of right thumb at wrist and hand level**

+7th **S66.292** **Other specified injury of extensor muscle, fascia and tendon of left thumb at wrist and hand level**

+7th **S66.299** **Other specified injury of extensor muscle, fascia and tendon of unspecified thumb at wrist and hand level**

+ **S66.3** **Injury of extensor muscle, fascia and tendon of other and unspecified finger at wrist and hand level**

Excludes2: *Injury of extensor muscle, fascia and tendon of thumb at wrist and hand level (S66.2-)*

+ **S66.30** **Unspecified injury of extensor muscle, fascia and tendon of other and unspecified finger at wrist and hand level**

+7th **S66.300** **Unspecified injury of extensor muscle, fascia and tendon of right index finger at wrist and hand level**

+7th **S66.301** **Unspecified injury of extensor muscle, fascia and tendon of left index finger at wrist and hand level**

+7th **S66.302** **Unspecified injury of extensor muscle, fascia and tendon of right middle finger at wrist and hand level**

+7th **S66.303** **Unspecified injury of extensor muscle, fascia and tendon of left middle finger at wrist and hand level**

+7th **S66.304** **Unspecified injury of extensor muscle, fascia and tendon of right ring finger at wrist and hand level**

+7th **S66.305** **Unspecified injury of extensor muscle, fascia and tendon of left ring finger at wrist and hand level**

+7th **S66.306** **Unspecified injury of extensor muscle, fascia and tendon of right little finger at wrist and hand level**

+7th **S66.307** **Unspecified injury of extensor muscle, fascia and tendon of left little finger at wrist and hand level**

+7th **S66.308** **Unspecified injury of extensor muscle, fascia and tendon of other finger at wrist and hand level**

Unspecified injury of extensor muscle, fascia and tendon of specified finger with unspecified laterality at wrist and hand level

+7th **S66.309** **Unspecified injury of extensor muscle, fascia and tendon of unspecified finger at wrist and hand level**

+ S66.31 Strain of extensor muscle, fascia and tendon of other and unspecified finger at wrist and hand level

+7th S66.310 Strain of extensor muscle, fascia and tendon of right index finger at wrist and hand level

+7th S66.311 Strain of extensor muscle, fascia and tendon of left index finger at wrist and hand level

+7th S66.312 Strain of extensor muscle, fascia and tendon of right middle finger at wrist and hand level

+7th S66.313 Strain of extensor muscle, fascia and tendon of left middle finger at wrist and hand level

+7th S66.314 Strain of extensor muscle, fascia and tendon of right ring finger at wrist and hand level

+7th S66.315 Strain of extensor muscle, fascia and tendon of left ring finger at wrist and hand level

+7th S66.316 Strain of extensor muscle, fascia and tendon of right little finger at wrist and hand level

+7th S66.317 Strain of extensor muscle, fascia and tendon of left little finger at wrist and hand level

+7th S66.318 Strain of extensor muscle, fascia and tendon of other finger at wrist and hand level

Strain of extensor muscle, fascia and tendon of specified finger with unspecified laterality at wrist and hand level

+7th S66.319 Strain of extensor muscle, fascia and tendon of unspecified finger at wrist and hand level

+ S66.32 Laceration of extensor muscle, fascia and tendon of other and unspecified finger at wrist and hand level

CC +7th S66.320 Laceration of extensor muscle, fascia and tendon of right index finger at wrist and hand level

CC +7th S66.321 Laceration of extensor muscle, fascia and tendon of left index finger at wrist and hand level

CC +7th S66.322 Laceration of extensor muscle, fascia and tendon of right middle finger at wrist and hand level

CC +7th S66.323 Laceration of extensor muscle, fascia and tendon of left middle finger at wrist and hand level

CC +7th S66.324 Laceration of extensor muscle, fascia and tendon of right ring finger at wrist and hand level

CC +7th S66.325 Laceration of extensor muscle, fascia and tendon of left ring finger at wrist and hand level

CC +7th S66.326 Laceration of extensor muscle, fascia and tendon of right little finger at wrist and hand level

CC +7th S66.327 Laceration of extensor muscle, fascia and tendon of left little finger at wrist and hand level

CC +7th S66.328 Laceration of extensor muscle, fascia and tendon of other finger at wrist and hand level

Laceration of extensor muscle, fascia and tendon of specified finger with unspecified laterality at wrist and hand level

CC +7th S66.329 Laceration of extensor muscle, fascia and tendon of unspecified finger at wrist and hand level

+ S66.39 Other injury of extensor muscle, fascia and tendon of other and unspecified finger at wrist and hand level

+7th S66.390 Other injury of extensor muscle, fascia and tendon of right index finger at wrist and hand level

+7th S66.391 Other injury of extensor muscle, fascia and tendon of left index finger at wrist and hand level

+7th S66.392 Other injury of extensor muscle, fascia and tendon of right middle finger at wrist and hand level

+7th S66.393 Other injury of extensor muscle, fascia and tendon of left middle finger at wrist and hand level

+7th S66.394 Other injury of extensor muscle, fascia and tendon of right ring finger at wrist and hand level

+7th S66.395 Other injury of extensor muscle, fascia and tendon of left ring finger at wrist and hand level

+7th S66.396 Other injury of extensor muscle, fascia and tendon of right little finger at wrist and hand level

+7th S66.397 Other injury of extensor muscle, fascia and tendon of left little finger at wrist and hand level

+7th S66.398 Other injury of extensor muscle, fascia and tendon of other finger at wrist and hand level

Other injury of extensor muscle, fascia and tendon of specified finger with unspecified laterality at wrist and hand level

+7th S66.399 Other injury of extensor muscle, fascia and tendon of unspecified finger at wrist and hand level

+ S66.4 Injury of intrinsic muscle, fascia and tendon of thumb at wrist and hand level

+ S66.40 Unspecified injury of intrinsic muscle, fascia and tendon of thumb at wrist and hand level

+7th S66.401 Unspecified injury of intrinsic muscle, fascia and tendon of right thumb at wrist and hand level

+7th S66.402 Unspecified injury of intrinsic muscle, fascia and tendon of left thumb at wrist and hand level

+7th S66.409 Unspecified injury of intrinsic muscle, fascia and tendon of unspecified thumb at wrist and hand level

+ S66.41 Strain of intrinsic muscle, fascia and tendon of thumb at wrist and hand level

+7th S66.411 Strain of intrinsic muscle, fascia and tendon of right thumb at wrist and hand level

+7th S66.412 Strain of intrinsic muscle, fascia and tendon of left thumb at wrist and hand level

+7th S66.419 Strain of intrinsic muscle, fascia and tendon of unspecified thumb at wrist and hand level

+ S66.42 Laceration of intrinsic muscle, fascia and tendon of thumb at wrist and hand level

CC +7th S66.421 Laceration of intrinsic muscle, fascia and tendon of right thumb at wrist and hand level

CC +7th S66.422 Laceration of intrinsic muscle, fascia and tendon of left thumb at wrist and hand level

CC +7th S66.429 Laceration of intrinsic muscle, fascia and tendon of unspecified thumb at wrist and hand level

+ S66.49 Other specified injury of intrinsic muscle, fascia and tendon of thumb at wrist and hand level

+7th S66.491 Other specified injury of intrinsic muscle, fascia and tendon of right thumb at wrist and hand level

+7th S66.492 Other specified injury of intrinsic muscle, fascia and tendon of left thumb at wrist and hand level

+7th S66.499 Other specified injury of intrinsic muscle, fascia and tendon of unspecified thumb at wrist and hand level

+ **S66.5** **Injury of intrinsic muscle, fascia and tendon of other and unspecified finger at wrist and hand level**
  Excludes2: *injury of intrinsic muscle, fascia and tendon of thumb at wrist and hand level (S66.4-)*

+ **S66.50** **Unspecified injury of intrinsic muscle, fascia and tendon of other and unspecified finger at wrist and hand level**

  +7th **S66.500** Unspecified injury of intrinsic muscle, fascia and tendon of right index finger at wrist and hand level

  +7th **S66.501** Unspecified injury of intrinsic muscle, fascia and tendon of left index finger at wrist and hand level

  +7th **S66.502** Unspecified injury of intrinsic muscle, fascia and tendon of right middle finger at wrist and hand level

  +7th **S66.503** Unspecified injury of intrinsic muscle, fascia and tendon of left middle finger at wrist and hand level

  +7th **S66.504** Unspecified injury of intrinsic muscle, fascia and tendon of right ring finger at wrist and hand level

  +7th **S66.505** Unspecified injury of intrinsic muscle, fascia and tendon of left ring finger at wrist and hand level

  +7th **S66.506** Unspecified injury of intrinsic muscle, fascia and tendon of right little finger at wrist and hand level

  +7th **S66.507** Unspecified injury of intrinsic muscle, fascia and tendon of left little finger at wrist and hand level

  +7th **S66.508** Unspecified injury of intrinsic muscle, fascia and tendon of other finger at wrist and hand level
    Unspecified injury of intrinsic muscle, fascia and tendon of specified finger with unspecified laterality at wrist and hand level

  +7th **S66.509** Unspecified injury of intrinsic muscle, fascia and tendon of unspecified finger at wrist and hand level

+ **S66.51** **Strain of intrinsic muscle, fascia and tendon of other and unspecified finger at wrist and hand level**

  +7th **S66.510** Strain of intrinsic muscle, fascia and tendon of right index finger at wrist and hand level

  +7th **S66.511** Strain of intrinsic muscle, fascia and tendon of left index finger at wrist and hand level

  +7th **S66.512** Strain of intrinsic muscle, fascia and tendon of right middle finger at wrist and hand level

  +7th **S66.513** Strain of intrinsic muscle, fascia and tendon of left middle finger at wrist and hand level

  +7th **S66.514** Strain of intrinsic muscle, fascia and tendon of right ring finger at wrist and hand level

  +7th **S66.515** Strain of intrinsic muscle, fascia and tendon of left ring finger at wrist and hand level

  +7th **S66.516** Strain of intrinsic muscle, fascia and tendon of right little finger at wrist and hand level

  +7th **S66.517** Strain of intrinsic muscle, fascia and tendon of left little finger at wrist and hand level

  +7th **S66.518** Strain of intrinsic muscle, fascia and tendon of other finger at wrist and hand level
    Strain of intrinsic muscle, fascia and tendon of specified finger with unspecified laterality at wrist and hand level

  +7th **S66.519** Strain of intrinsic muscle, fascia and tendon of unspecified finger at wrist and hand level

+ **S66.52** **Laceration of intrinsic muscle, fascia and tendon of other and unspecified finger at wrist and hand level**

  CC +7th **S66.520** Laceration of intrinsic muscle, fascia and tendon of right index finger at wrist and hand level

  CC +7th **S66.521** Laceration of intrinsic muscle, fascia and tendon of left index finger at wrist and hand level

  CC +7th **S66.522** Laceration of intrinsic muscle, fascia and tendon of right middle finger at wrist and hand level

  CC +7th **S66.523** Laceration of intrinsic muscle, fascia and tendon of left middle finger at wrist and hand level

  CC +7th **S66.524** Laceration of intrinsic muscle, fascia and tendon of right ring finger at wrist and hand level

  CC +7th **S66.525** Laceration of intrinsic muscle, fascia and tendon of left ring finger at wrist and hand level

  CC +7th **S66.526** Laceration of intrinsic muscle, fascia and tendon of right little finger at wrist and hand level

  CC +7th **S66.527** Laceration of intrinsic muscle, fascia and tendon of left little finger at wrist and hand level

  CC +7th **S66.528** Laceration of intrinsic muscle, fascia and tendon of other finger at wrist and hand level
    Laceration of intrinsic muscle, fascia and tendon of specified finger with unspecified laterality at wrist and hand level

  CC +7th **S66.529** Laceration of intrinsic muscle, fascia and tendon of unspecified finger at wrist and hand level

+ **S66.59** **Other injury of intrinsic muscle, fascia and tendon of other and unspecified finger at wrist and hand level**

  +7th **S66.590** Other injury of intrinsic muscle, fascia and tendon of right index finger at wrist and hand level

  +7th **S66.591** Other injury of intrinsic muscle, fascia and tendon of left index finger at wrist and hand level

  +7th **S66.592** Other injury of intrinsic muscle, fascia and tendon of right middle finger at wrist and hand level

  +7th **S66.593** Other injury of intrinsic muscle, fascia and tendon of left middle finger at wrist and hand level

  +7th **S66.594** Other injury of intrinsic muscle, fascia and tendon of right ring finger at wrist and hand level

  +7th **S66.595** Other injury of intrinsic muscle, fascia and tendon of left ring finger at wrist and hand level

  +7th **S66.596** Other injury of intrinsic muscle, fascia and tendon of right little finger at wrist and hand level

  +7th **S66.597** Other injury of intrinsic muscle, fascia and tendon of left little finger at wrist and hand level

  +7th **S66.598** Other injury of intrinsic muscle, fascia and tendon of other finger at wrist and hand level
    Other injury of intrinsic muscle, fascia and tendon of specified finger with unspecified laterality at wrist and hand level

  +7th **S66.599** Other injury of intrinsic muscle, fascia and tendon of unspecified finger at wrist and hand level

+ **S66.8** **Injury of other specified muscles, fascia and tendons at wrist and hand level**

+ **S66.80** **Unspecified injury of other specified muscles, fascia and tendons at wrist and hand level**

  +7th **S66.801** Unspecified injury of other specified muscles, fascia and tendons at wrist and hand level, right hand

  +7th **S66.802** Unspecified injury of other specified muscles, fascia and tendons at wrist and hand level, left hand

  +7th **S66.809** Unspecified injury of other specified muscles, fascia and tendons at wrist and hand level, unspecified hand

+, +7th, X + 7th　　● Newborn　● Pediatric　● Maternity　● Adult　♀ Female　♂ Male　Manifestation　Unacceptable PDX　HCC　CC　MCC　HAC

+ **S66.81** **Strain of other specified muscles, fascia and tendons at wrist and hand level**
+7th **S66.811** Strain of other specified muscles, fascia and tendons at wrist and hand level, right hand
+7th **S66.812** Strain of other specified muscles, fascia and tendons at wrist and hand level, left hand
+7th **S66.819** Strain of other specified muscles, fascia and tendons at wrist and hand level, unspecified hand

+ **S66.82** **Laceration of other specified muscles, fascia and tendons at wrist and hand level**
CC +7th **S66.821** Laceration of other specified muscles, fascia and tendons at wrist and hand level, right hand
CC +7th **S66.822** Laceration of other specified muscles, fascia and tendons at wrist and hand level, left hand
CC +7th **S66.829** Laceration of other specified muscles, fascia and tendons at wrist and hand level, unspecified hand

+ **S66.89** **Other injury of other specified muscles, fascia and tendons at wrist and hand level**
+7th **S66.891** Other injury of other specified muscles, fascia and tendons at wrist and hand level, right hand
+7th **S66.892** Other injury of other specified muscles, fascia and tendons at wrist and hand level, left hand
+7th **S66.899** Other injury of other specified muscles, fascia and tendons at wrist and hand level, unspecified hand

+ **S66.9** **Injury of unspecified muscle, fascia and tendon at wrist and hand level**
+ **S66.90** **Unspecified injury of unspecified muscle, fascia and tendon at wrist and hand level**
+7th **S66.901** Unspecified injury of unspecified muscle, fascia and tendon at wrist and hand level, right hand
+7th **S66.902** Unspecified injury of unspecified muscle, fascia and tendon at wrist and hand level, left hand
+7th **S66.909** Unspecified injury of unspecified muscle, fascia and tendon at wrist and hand level, unspecified hand

+ **S66.91** **Strain of unspecified muscle, fascia and tendon at wrist and hand level**
+7th **S66.911** Strain of unspecified muscle, fascia and tendon at wrist and hand level, right hand
+7th **S66.912** Strain of unspecified muscle, fascia and tendon at wrist and hand level, left hand
+7th **S66.919** Strain of unspecified muscle, fascia and tendon at wrist and hand level, unspecified hand

+ **S66.92** **Laceration of unspecified muscle, fascia and tendon at wrist and hand level**
CC +7th **S66.921** Laceration of unspecified muscle, fascia and tendon at wrist and hand level, right hand
CC +7th **S66.922** Laceration of unspecified muscle, fascia and tendon at wrist and hand level, left hand
CC +7th **S66.929** Laceration of unspecified muscle, fascia and tendon at wrist and hand level, unspecified hand

+ **S66.99** **Other injury of unspecified muscle, fascia and tendon at wrist and hand level**
+7th **S66.991** Other injury of unspecified muscle, fascia and tendon at wrist and hand level, right hand
+7th **S66.992** Other injury of unspecified muscle, fascia and tendon at wrist and hand level, left hand
+7th **S66.999** Other injury of unspecified muscle, fascia and tendon at wrist and hand level, unspecified hand

S67 **Crushing injury of wrist, hand and fingers**
Use additional code for all associated injuries, such as:
fracture of wrist and hand (S62.-)
open wound of wrist and hand (S61.-)

The appropriate 7th character is to be added to each code from category S67
A initial encounter
D subsequent encounter
S sequela

+ **S67.0** **Crushing injury of thumb**
X+7th **S67.00** Crushing injury of unspecified thumb
X+7th **S67.01** Crushing injury of right thumb
X+7th **S67.02** Crushing injury of left thumb

+ **S67.1** **Crushing injury of other and unspecified finger(s)**
Excludes2: *crushing injury of thumb (S67.0-)*
X+7th **S67.10** Crushing injury of unspecified finger(s)
+ **S67.19** **Crushing injury of other finger(s)**
+7th **S67.190** Crushing injury of right index finger
+7th **S67.191** Crushing injury of left index finger
+7th **S67.192** Crushing injury of right middle finger
+7th **S67.193** Crushing injury of left middle finger
+7th **S67.194** Crushing injury of right ring finger
+7th **S67.195** Crushing injury of left ring finger
+7th **S67.196** Crushing injury of right little finger
+7th **S67.197** Crushing injury of left little finger
+7th **S67.198** Crushing injury of other finger
Crushing injury of specified finger with unspecified laterality

+ **S67.2** **Crushing injury of hand**
Excludes2: *crushing injury of fingers (S67.1-)*
crushing injury of thumb (S67.0-)
X+7th **S67.20** Crushing injury of unspecified hand
X+7th **S67.21** Crushing injury of right hand
X+7th **S67.22** Crushing injury of left hand

+ **S67.3** **Crushing injury of wrist**
X+7th **S67.30** Crushing injury of unspecified wrist
X+7th **S67.31** Crushing injury of right wrist
X+7th **S67.32** Crushing injury of left wrist

+ **S67.4** **Crushing injury of wrist and hand**
Excludes1: *crushing injury of hand alone (S67.2-)*
crushing injury of wrist alone (S67.3-)
Excludes2: *crushing injury of fingers (S67.1-)*
crushing injury of thumb (S67.0-)
X+7th **S67.40** Crushing injury of unspecified wrist and hand
X+7th **S67.41** Crushing injury of right wrist and hand
X+7th **S67.42** Crushing injury of left wrist and hand

+ **S67.9** **Crushing injury of unspecified part(s) of wrist, hand and fingers**
X+7th **S67.90** Crushing injury of unspecified part(s) of unspecified wrist, hand and fingers
X+7th **S67.91** Crushing injury of unspecified part(s) of right wrist, hand and fingers
X+7th **S67.92** Crushing injury of unspecified part(s) of left wrist, hand and fingers

S68 **Traumatic amputation of wrist, hand and fingers**
An amputation not identified as partial or complete should be coded to complete

The appropriate 7th character is to be added to each code from category S68
A initial encounter
D subsequent encounter
S sequela

+ **S68.0** **Traumatic metacarpophalangeal amputation of thumb**
Traumatic amputation of thumb NOS
+ **S68.01** **Complete traumatic metacarpophalangeal amputation of thumb**
+7th **S68.011** Complete traumatic metacarpophalangeal amputation of right thumb
+7th **S68.012** Complete traumatic metacarpophalangeal amputation of left thumb
+7th **S68.019** Complete traumatic metacarpophalangeal amputation of unspecified thumb

+ **S68.02** **Partial traumatic metacarpophalangeal amputation of thumb**

  +7th **S68.021** **Partial traumatic metacarpophalangeal amputation of right thumb**

  +7th **S68.022** **Partial traumatic metacarpophalangeal amputation of left thumb**

  +7th **S68.029** **Partial traumatic metacarpophalangeal amputation of unspecified thumb**

+ **S68.1** **Traumatic metacarpophalangeal amputation of other and unspecified finger**

Traumatic amputation of finger NOS

Excludes2: *traumatic metacarpophalangeal amputation of thumb (S68.0-)*

  + **S68.11** **Complete traumatic metacarpophalangeal amputation of other and unspecified finger**

    +7th **S68.110** **Complete traumatic metacarpophalangeal amputation of right index finger**

    +7th **S68.111** **Complete traumatic metacarpophalangeal amputation of left index finger**

    +7th **S68.112** **Complete traumatic metacarpophalangeal amputation of right middle finger**

    +7th **S68.113** **Complete traumatic metacarpophalangeal amputation of left middle finger**

    +7th **S68.114** **Complete traumatic metacarpophalangeal amputation of right ring finger**

    +7th **S68.115** **Complete traumatic metacarpophalangeal amputation of left ring finger**

    +7th **S68.116** **Complete traumatic metacarpophalangeal amputation of right little finger**

    +7th **S68.117** **Complete traumatic metacarpophalangeal amputation of left little finger**

    +7th **S68.118** **Complete traumatic metacarpophalangeal amputation of other finger**

Complete traumatic metacarpophalangeal amputation of specified finger with unspecified laterality

    +7th **S68.119** **Complete traumatic metacarpophalangeal amputation of unspecified finger**

  + **S68.12** **Partial traumatic metacarpophalangeal amputation of other and unspecified finger**

    +7th **S68.120** **Partial traumatic metacarpophalangeal amputation of right index finger**

    +7th **S68.121** **Partial traumatic metacarpophalangeal amputation of left index finger**

    +7th **S68.122** **Partial traumatic metacarpophalangeal amputation of right middle finger**

    +7th **S68.123** **Partial traumatic metacarpophalangeal amputation of left middle finger**

    +7th **S68.124** **Partial traumatic metacarpophalangeal amputation of right ring finger**

    +7th **S68.125** **Partial traumatic metacarpophalangeal amputation of left ring finger**

    +7th **S68.126** **Partial traumatic metacarpophalangeal amputation of right little finger**

    +7th **S68.127** **Partial traumatic metacarpophalangeal amputation of left little finger**

    +7th **S68.128** **Partial traumatic metacarpophalangeal amputation of other finger**

Partial traumatic metacarpophalangeal amputation of specified finger with unspecified laterality

    +7th **S68.129** **Partial traumatic metacarpophalangeal amputation of unspecified finger**

+ **S68.4** **Traumatic amputation of hand at wrist level**

Traumatic amputation of hand NOS

Traumatic amputation of wrist

+ **S68.41** **Complete traumatic amputation of hand at wrist level**

  CC +7th **S68.411** **Complete traumatic amputation of right hand at wrist level**

  CC +7th **S68.412** **Complete traumatic amputation of left hand at wrist level**

  CC +7th **S68.419** **Complete traumatic amputation of unspecified hand at wrist level**

+ **S68.42** **Partial traumatic amputation of hand at wrist level**

  CC +7th **S68.421** **Partial traumatic amputation of right hand at wrist level**

  CC +7th **S68.422** **Partial traumatic amputation of left hand at wrist level**

  CC +7th **S68.429** **Partial traumatic amputation of unspecified hand at wrist level**

+ **S68.5** **Traumatic transphalangeal amputation of thumb**

Traumatic interphalangeal joint amputation of thumb

  + **S68.51** **Complete traumatic transphalangeal amputation of thumb**

    +7th **S68.511** **Complete traumatic transphalangeal amputation of right thumb**

    +7th **S68.512** **Complete traumatic transphalangeal amputation of left thumb**

    +7th **S68.519** **Complete traumatic transphalangeal amputation of unspecified thumb**

  + **S68.52** **Partial traumatic transphalangeal amputation of thumb**

    +7th **S68.521** **Partial traumatic transphalangeal amputation of right thumb**

    +7th **S68.522** **Partial traumatic transphalangeal amputation of left thumb**

    +7th **S68.529** **Partial traumatic transphalangeal amputation of unspecified thumb**

+ **S68.6** **Traumatic transphalangeal amputation of other and unspecified finger**

  + **S68.61** **Complete traumatic transphalangeal amputation of other and unspecified finger(s)**

    +7th **S68.610** **Complete traumatic transphalangeal amputation of right index finger**

    +7th **S68.611** **Complete traumatic transphalangeal amputation of left index finger**

    +7th **S68.612** **Complete traumatic transphalangeal amputation of right middle finger**

    +7th **S68.613** **Complete traumatic transphalangeal amputation of left middle finger**

    +7th **S68.614** **Complete traumatic transphalangeal amputation of right ring finger**

    +7th **S68.615** **Complete traumatic transphalangeal amputation of left ring finger**

    +7th **S68.616** **Complete traumatic transphalangeal amputation of right little finger**

    +7th **S68.617** **Complete traumatic transphalangeal amputation of left little finger**

    +7th **S68.618** **Complete traumatic transphalangeal amputation of other finger**

Complete traumatic transphalangeal amputation of specified finger with unspecified laterality

    +7th **S68.619** **Complete traumatic transphalangeal amputation of unspecified finger**

  + **S68.62** **Partial traumatic transphalangeal amputation of other and unspecified finger**

    +7th **S68.620** **Partial traumatic transphalangeal amputation of right index finger**

    +7th **S68.621** **Partial traumatic transphalangeal amputation of left index finger**

    +7th **S68.622** **Partial traumatic transphalangeal amputation of right middle finger**

    +7th **S68.623** **Partial traumatic transphalangeal amputation of left middle finger**

    +7th **S68.624** **Partial traumatic transphalangeal amputation of right ring finger**

    +7th **S68.625** **Partial traumatic transphalangeal amputation of left ring finger**

    +7th **S68.626** **Partial traumatic transphalangeal amputation of right little finger**

+7th **S68.627** **Partial traumatic transphalangeal amputation of left little finger**
+7th **S68.628** **Partial traumatic transphalangeal amputation of other finger**
Partial traumatic transphalangeal amputation of specified finger with unspecified laterality
+7th **S68.629** **Partial traumatic transphalangeal amputation of unspecified finger**
+ **S68.7** **Traumatic transmetacarpal amputation of hand**
+ **S68.71** **Complete traumatic transmetacarpal amputation of hand**
CC +7th **S68.711** **Complete traumatic transmetacarpal amputation of right hand**
CC +7th **S68.712** **Complete traumatic transmetacarpal amputation of left hand**
CC +7th **S68.719** **Complete traumatic transmetacarpal amputation of unspecified hand**
+ **S68.72** **Partial traumatic transmetacarpal amputation of hand**
CC +7th **S68.721** **Partial traumatic transmetacarpal amputation of right hand**
CC +7th **S68.722** **Partial traumatic transmetacarpal amputation of left hand**
CC +7th **S68.729** **Partial traumatic transmetacarpal amputation of unspecified hand**

S69 **Other and unspecified injuries of wrist, hand and finger(s)**

The appropriate 7th character is to be added to each code from category S69
A   initial encounter
D   subsequent encounter
S   sequela

+ **S69.8** **Other specified injuries of wrist, hand and finger(s)**
X+7th **S69.80** **Other specified injuries of unspecified wrist, hand and finger(s)**
X+7th **S69.81** **Other specified injuries of right wrist, hand and finger(s)**
X+7th **S69.82** **Other specified injuries of left wrist, hand and finger(s)**
+ **S69.9** **Unspecified injury of wrist, hand and finger(s)**
X+7th **S69.90** **Unspecified injury of unspecified wrist, hand and finger(s)**
X+7th **S69.91** **Unspecified injury of right wrist, hand and finger(s)**
X+7th **S69.92** **Unspecified injury of left wrist, hand and finger(s)**

Injuries to the hip and thigh (S70-S79)

Excludes2: *burns and corrosions (T20-T32)*
frostbite (T33-T34)
snake bite (T63.0-)
venomous insect bite or sting (T63.4-)

S70 **Superficial injury of hip and thigh**

The appropriate 7th character is to be added to each code from category S70
A   initial encounter
D   subsequent encounter
S   sequela

+ **S70.0** **Contusion of hip**
X+7th **S70.00** **Contusion of unspecified hip**
X+7th **S70.01** **Contusion of right hip**
X+7th **S70.02** **Contusion of left hip**
+ **S70.1** **Contusion of thigh**
X+7th **S70.10** **Contusion of unspecified thigh**
X+7th **S70.11** **Contusion of right thigh**
X+7th **S70.12** **Contusion of left thigh**
+ **S70.2** **Other superficial injuries of hip**
+ **S70.21** **Abrasion of hip**
+7th **S70.211** **Abrasion, right hip**
+7th **S70.212** **Abrasion, left hip**
+7th **S70.219** **Abrasion, unspecified hip**
+ **S70.22** **Blister (nonthermal) of hip**
+7th **S70.221** **Blister (nonthermal), right hip**
+7th **S70.222** **Blister (nonthermal), left hip**
+7th **S70.229** **Blister (nonthermal), unspecified hip**

+ **S70.24** **External constriction of hip**
+7th **S70.241** **External constriction, right hip**
+7th **S70.242** **External constriction, left hip**
+7th **S70.249** **External constriction, unspecified hip**
+ **S70.25** **Superficial foreign body of hip**
Splinter in the hip
+7th **S70.251** **Superficial foreign body, right hip**
+7th **S70.252** **Superficial foreign body, left hip**
+7th **S70.259** **Superficial foreign body, unspecified hip**
+ **S70.26** **Insect bite (nonvenomous) of hip**
+7th **S70.261** **Insect bite (nonvenomous), right hip**
+7th **S70.262** **Insect bite (nonvenomous), left hip**
+7th **S70.269** **Insect bite (nonvenomous), unspecified hip**
+ **S70.27** **Other superficial bite of hip**
Excludes1: *open bite of hip (S71.05-)*
+7th **S70.271** **Other superficial bite of hip, right hip**
+7th **S70.272** **Other superficial bite of hip, left hip**
+7th **S70.279** **Other superficial bite of hip, unspecified hip**
+ **S70.3** **Other superficial injuries of thigh**
+ **S70.31** **Abrasion of thigh**
+7th **S70.311** **Abrasion, right thigh**
+7th **S70.312** **Abrasion, left thigh**
+7th **S70.319** **Abrasion, unspecified thigh**
+ **S70.32** **Blister (nonthermal) of thigh**
+7th **S70.321** **Blister (nonthermal), right thigh**
+7th **S70.322** **Blister (nonthermal), left thigh**
+7th **S70.329** **Blister (nonthermal), unspecified thigh**
+ **S70.34** **External constriction of thigh**
+7th **S70.341** **External constriction, right thigh**
+7th **S70.342** **External constriction, left thigh**
+7th **S70.349** **External constriction, unspecified thigh**
+ **S70.35** **Superficial foreign body of thigh**
Splinter in the thigh
+7th **S70.351** **Superficial foreign body, right thigh**
+7th **S70.352** **Superficial foreign body, left thigh**
+7th **S70.359** **Superficial foreign body, unspecified thigh**
+ **S70.36** **Insect bite (nonvenomous) of thigh**
+7th **S70.361** **Insect bite (nonvenomous), right thigh**
+7th **S70.362** **Insect bite (nonvenomous), left thigh**
+7th **S70.369** **Insect bite (nonvenomous), unspecified thigh**
+ **S70.37** **Other superficial bite of thigh**
Excludes1: *open bite of thigh (S71.15)*
+7th **S70.371** **Other superficial bite of right thigh**
+7th **S70.372** **Other superficial bite of left thigh**
+7th **S70.379** **Other superficial bite of unspecified thigh**
+ **S70.9** **Unspecified superficial injury of hip and thigh**
+ **S70.91** **Unspecified superficial injury of hip**
+7th **S70.911** **Unspecified superficial injury of right hip**
+7th **S70.912** **Unspecified superficial injury of left hip**
+7th **S70.919** **Unspecified superficial injury of unspecified hip**
+ **S70.92** **Unspecified superficial injury of thigh**
+7th **S70.921** **Unspecified superficial injury of right thigh**
+7th **S70.922** **Unspecified superficial injury of left thigh**
+7th **S70.929** **Unspecified superficial injury of unspecified thigh**

S71 **Open wound of hip and thigh**

Code also any associated wound infection
Excludes1: *open fracture of hip and thigh (S72.-)*
traumatic amputation of hip and thigh (S78.-)
Excludes2: *bite of venomous animal (T63.-)*
open wound of ankle, foot and toes (S91.-)
open wound of knee and lower leg (S81.-)

The appropriate 7th character is to be added to each code from category S71
A   initial encounter
D   subsequent encounter
S   sequela

+, +7th, X + 7th   • Newborn   • Pediatric   ● Maternity   ● Adult   ♀ Female   ♂ Male   Manifestation   Unacceptable PDX   HCC   CC   MCC   HAC

+ **S71.0 Open wound of hip**
  + **S71.00 Unspecified open wound of hip**
    +7th **S71.001 Unspecified open wound, right hip**
    +7th **S71.002 Unspecified open wound, left hip**
    +7th **S71.009 Unspecified open wound, unspecified hip**
  + **S71.01 Laceration without foreign body of hip**
    +7th **S71.011 Laceration without foreign body, right hip**
    +7th **S71.012 Laceration without foreign body, left hip**
    +7th **S71.019 Laceration without foreign body, unspecified hip**
  + **S71.02 Laceration with foreign body of hip**
    +7th **S71.021 Laceration with foreign body, right hip**
    +7th **S71.022 Laceration with foreign body, left hip**
    +7th **S71.029 Laceration with foreign body, unspecified hip**
  + **S71.03 Puncture wound without foreign body of hip**
    +7th **S71.031 Puncture wound without foreign body, right hip**
    +7th **S71.032 Puncture wound without foreign body, left hip**
    +7th **S71.039 Puncture wound without foreign body, unspecified hip**
  + **S71.04 Puncture wound with foreign body of hip**
    +7th **S71.041 Puncture wound with foreign body, right hip**
    +7th **S71.042 Puncture wound with foreign body, left hip**
    +7th **S71.049 Puncture wound with foreign body, unspecified hip**
  + **S71.05 Open bite of hip**
    Bite of hip NOS
    Excludes1: superficial bite of hip (S70.26, S70.27)
    +7th **S71.051 Open bite, right hip**
    +7th **S71.052 Open bite, left hip**
    +7th **S71.059 Open bite, unspecified hip**
+ **S71.1 Open wound of thigh**
  + **S71.10 Unspecified open wound of thigh**
    +7th **S71.101 Unspecified open wound, right thigh**
    +7th **S71.102 Unspecified open wound, left thigh**
    +7th **S71.109 Unspecified open wound, unspecified thigh**
  + **S71.11 Laceration without foreign body of thigh**
    +7th **S71.111 Laceration without foreign body, right thigh**
    +7th **S71.112 Laceration without foreign body, left thigh**
    +7th **S71.119 Laceration without foreign body, unspecified thigh**
  + **S71.12 Laceration with foreign body of thigh**
    +7th **S71.121 Laceration with foreign body, right thigh**
    +7th **S71.122 Laceration with foreign body, left thigh**
    +7th **S71.129 Laceration with foreign body, unspecified thigh**
  + **S71.13 Puncture wound without foreign body of thigh**
    +7th **S71.131 Puncture wound without foreign body, right thigh**
    +7th **S71.132 Puncture wound without foreign body, left thigh**
    +7th **S71.139 Puncture wound without foreign body, unspecified thigh**
  + **S71.14 Puncture wound with foreign body of thigh**
    +7th **S71.141 Puncture wound with foreign body, right thigh**
    +7th **S71.142 Puncture wound with foreign body, left thigh**
    +7th **S71.149 Puncture wound with foreign body, unspecified thigh**
  + **S71.15 Open bite of thigh**
    Bite of thigh NOS
    Excludes1: superficial bite of thigh (S70.37-)
    +7th **S71.151 Open bite, right thigh**
    +7th **S71.152 Open bite, left thigh**
    +7th **S71.159 Open bite, unspecified thigh**

S72 Fracture of femur

NOTE A fracture not indicated as displaced or nondisplaced should be coded to displaced
A fracture not indicated as open or closed should be coded to closed
The open fracture designations are based on the Gustilo open fracture classification

Excludes1: traumatic amputation of hip and thigh (S78.-)
Excludes2: fracture of lower leg and ankle (S82.-)
    fracture of foot (S92.-)
    periprosthetic fracture of prosthetic implant of hip (M97.0-)

The appropriate 7th character is to be added to all codes from category S72
A initial encounter for closed fracture
B initial encounter for open fracture type I or II
    initial encounter for open fracture NOS
C initial encounter for open fracture type IIIA, IIIB, or IIIC
D subsequent encounter for closed fracture with routine healing
E subsequent encounter for open fracture type I or II with routine healing
F subsequent encounter for open fracture type IIIA, IIIB, or IIIC with routine healing
G subsequent encounter for closed fracture with delayed healing
H subsequent encounter for open fracture type I or II with delayed healing
J subsequent encounter for open fracture type IIIA, IIIB, or IIIC with delayed healing
K subsequent encounter for closed fracture with nonunion
M subsequent encounter for open fracture type I or II with nonunion
N subsequent encounter for open fracture type IIIA, IIIB, or IIIC with nonunion
P subsequent encounter for closed fracture with malunion
Q subsequent encounter for open fracture type I or II with malunion
R subsequent encounter for open fracture type IIIA, IIIB, or IIIC with malunion
S sequela

Review coding guideline C.19.c

+ **S72.0 Fracture of head and neck of femur**
  Excludes2: physeal fracture of upper end of femur (S79.0-)
  + **S72.00 Fracture of unspecified part of neck of femur**
    Fracture of hip NOS
    Fracture of neck of femur NOS
  CC MCC +7th **S72.001 Fracture of unspecified part of neck of right femur**
    HAC 7th characters A - C see Appendix B for HAC conditional logic
  CC MCC +7th **S72.002 Fracture of unspecified part of neck of left femur**
    HAC 7th characters A - C see Appendix B for HAC conditional logic
    AHA CC: 1Q, 2015, 3-21; 4Q, 2015, 36-37
  CC MCC +7th **S72.009 Fracture of unspecified part of neck of unspecified femur**
    HAC 7th characters A - C see Appendix B for HAC conditional logic
  + **S72.01 Unspecified intracapsular fracture of femur**
    Subcapital fracture of femur
  CC +7th **S72.011 Unspecified intracapsular fracture of right femur**
    HAC 7th characters A - C see Appendix B for HAC conditional logic
  CC +7th **S72.012 Unspecified intracapsular fracture of left femur**
    HAC 7th characters A - C see Appendix B for HAC conditional logic
  CC +7th **S72.019 Unspecified intracapsular fracture of unspecified femur**
    HAC 7th characters A - C see Appendix B for HAC conditional logic
  + **S72.02 Fracture of epiphysis (separation) (upper) of femur**
    Transepiphyseal fracture of femur
    Excludes1: capital femoral epiphyseal fracture (pediatric) of femur (S79.01-)
    Salter-Harris Type I physeal fracture of upper end of femur (S79.01-)

+, +7th, X + 7th   ● Newborn   ● Pediatric   ● Maternity   ● Adult   ♀ Female   ♂ Male   Manifestation   Unacceptable PDX   HCC   CC   MCC   **HAC**

CC MCC +7th **S72.021** **Displaced fracture of epiphysis (separation) (upper) of right femur**
HAC 7th characters A - C see Appendix B for HAC conditional logic

CC MCC +7th **S72.022** **Displaced fracture of epiphysis (separation) (upper) of left femur**
HAC 7th characters A - C see Appendix B for HAC conditional logic

CC MCC +7th **S72.023** **Displaced fracture of epiphysis (separation) (upper) of unspecified femur**
HAC 7th characters A - C see Appendix B for HAC conditional logic

CC MCC +7th **S72.024** **Nondisplaced fracture of epiphysis (separation) (upper) of right femur**
HAC 7th characters A - C see Appendix B for HAC conditional logic

CC MCC +7th **S72.025** **Nondisplaced fracture of epiphysis (separation) (upper) of left femur**
HAC 7th characters A - C see Appendix B for HAC conditional logic

CC MCC +7th **S72.026** **Nondisplaced fracture of epiphysis (separation) (upper) of unspecified femur**
HAC 7th characters A - C see Appendix B for HAC conditional logic

+ **S72.03** **Midcervical fracture of femur**
Transcervical fracture of femur NOS

CC MCC +7th **S72.031** **Displaced midcervical fracture of right femur**
HAC 7th characters A - C see Appendix B for HAC conditional logic

CC MCC +7th **S72.032** **Displaced midcervical fracture of left femur**
HAC 7th characters A - C see Appendix B for HAC conditional logic

CC MCC +7th **S72.033** **Displaced midcervical fracture of unspecified femur**
HAC 7th characters A - C see Appendix B for HAC conditional logic

CC MCC +7th **S72.034** **Nondisplaced midcervical fracture of right femur**
HAC 7th characters A - C see Appendix B for HAC conditional logic

CC MCC +7th **S72.035** **Nondisplaced midcervical fracture of left femur**
HAC 7th characters A - C see Appendix B for HAC conditional logic

CC MCC +7th **S72.036** **Nondisplaced midcervical fracture of unspecified femur**
HAC 7th characters A - C see Appendix B for HAC conditional logic

+ **S72.04** **Fracture of base of neck of femur**
Cervicotrochanteric fracture of femur

CC MCC +7th **S72.041** **Displaced fracture of base of neck of right femur**
HAC 7th characters A - C see Appendix B for HAC conditional logic

CC MCC +7th **S72.042** **Displaced fracture of base of neck of left femur**
HAC 7th characters A - C see Appendix B for HAC conditional logic

CC MCC +7th **S72.043** **Displaced fracture of base of neck of unspecified femur**
HAC 7th characters A - C see Appendix B for HAC conditional logic

CC MCC +7th **S72.044** **Nondisplaced fracture of base of neck of right femur**
HAC 7th characters A - C see Appendix B for HAC conditional logic

CC MCC +7th **S72.045** **Nondisplaced fracture of base of neck of left femur**
HAC 7th characters A - C see Appendix B for HAC conditional logic

CC MCC +7th **S72.046** **Nondisplaced fracture of base of neck of unspecified femur**
HAC 7th characters A - C see Appendix B for HAC conditional logic

+ **S72.05** **Unspecified fracture of head of femur**
Fracture of head of femur NOS

CC MCC +7th **S72.051** **Unspecified fracture of head of right femur**
HAC 7th characters A - C see Appendix B for HAC conditional logic

CC MCC +7th **S72.052** **Unspecified fracture of head of left femur**
HAC 7th characters A - C see Appendix B for HAC conditional logic

CC MCC +7th **S72.059** **Unspecified fracture of head of unspecified femur**
HAC 7th characters A - C see Appendix B for HAC conditional logic

+ **S72.06** **Articular fracture of head of femur**

CC MCC +7th **S72.061** **Displaced articular fracture of head of right femur**
HAC 7th characters A - C see Appendix B for HAC conditional logic

CC MCC +7th **S72.062** **Displaced articular fracture of head of left femur**
HAC 7th characters A - C see Appendix B for HAC conditional logic

CC MCC +7th **S72.063** **Displaced articular fracture of head of unspecified femur**
HAC 7th characters A - C see Appendix B for HAC conditional logic

CC MCC +7th **S72.064** **Nondisplaced articular fracture of head of right femur**
HAC 7th characters A - C see Appendix B for HAC conditional logic

CC MCC +7th **S72.065** **Nondisplaced articular fracture of head of left femur**
HAC 7th characters A - C see Appendix B for HAC conditional logic

CC MCC +7th **S72.066** **Nondisplaced articular fracture of head of unspecified femur**
HAC 7th characters A - C see Appendix B for HAC conditional logic

+ **S72.09** **Other fracture of head and neck of femur**

CC MCC +7th **S72.091** **Other fracture of head and neck of right femur**
HAC 7th characters A - C see Appendix B for HAC conditional logic

CC MCC +7th **S72.092** **Other fracture of head and neck of left femur**
HAC 7th characters A - C see Appendix B for HAC conditional logic

CC MCC +7th **S72.099** **Other fracture of head and neck of unspecified femur**
HAC 7th characters A - C see Appendix B for HAC conditional logic

+ **S72.1** **Pertrochanteric fracture**

+ **S72.10** **Unspecified trochanteric fracture of femur**
Fracture of trochanter NOS

CC MCC **S72.101** **Unspecified trochanteric fracture of right femur**
HAC 7th characters A - C see Appendix B for HAC conditional logic

CC MCC **S72.102** **Unspecified trochanteric fracture of left femur**
HAC 7th characters A - C see Appendix B for HAC conditional logic

CC MCC **S72.109** **Unspecified trochanteric fracture of unspecified femur**
HAC 7th characters A - C see Appendix B for HAC conditional logic

+ **S72.11** **Fracture of greater trochanter of femur**

CC +7th **S72.111** **Displaced fracture of greater trochanter of right femur**
HAC 7th characters A - C see Appendix B for HAC conditional logic

CC +7th **S72.112** **Displaced fracture of greater trochanter of left femur**
HAC 7th characters A - C see Appendix B for HAC conditional logic

CC +7th **S72.113** **Displaced fracture of greater trochanter of unspecified femur**
HAC 7th characters A - C see Appendix B for HAC conditional logic

CC +7th **S72.114** **Nondisplaced fracture of greater trochanter of right femur**
HAC 7th characters A - C see Appendix B for HAC conditional logic

CC +7th **S72.115** **Nondisplaced fracture of greater trochanter of left femur**
HAC 7th characters A - C see Appendix B for HAC conditional logic

CC +7th **S72.116** **Nondisplaced fracture of greater trochanter of unspecified femur**
HAC 7th characters A - C see Appendix B for HAC conditional logic

+, +7th, X + 7th   ● Newborn   ● Pediatric   ● Maternity   ● Adult   ♀ Female   ♂ Male   Manifestation   Unacceptable PDX   HCC   CC   MCC   HAC

+ S72.12 **Fracture of lesser trochanter of femur**
CC +7th **S72.121** Displaced fracture of lesser trochanter of right femur
HAC 7th characters A - C see Appendix B for HAC conditional logic
CC +7th **S72.122** Displaced fracture of lesser trochanter of left femur
HAC 7th characters A - C see Appendix B for HAC conditional logic
CC +7th **S72.123** Displaced fracture of lesser trochanter of unspecified femur
HAC 7th characters A - C see Appendix B for HAC conditional logic
CC +7th **S72.124** Nondisplaced fracture of lesser trochanter of right femur
HAC 7th characters A - C see Appendix B for HAC conditional logic
CC +7th **S72.125** Nondisplaced fracture of lesser trochanter of left femur
HAC 7th characters A - C see Appendix B for HAC conditional logic
CC +7th **S72.126** Nondisplaced fracture of lesser trochanter of unspecified femur
HAC 7th characters A - C see Appendix B for HAC conditional logic

+ S72.13 **Apophyseal fracture of femur**
Excludes1: chronic (nontraumatic) slipped upper femoral epiphysis (M93.0-)
CC +7th **S72.131** Displaced apophyseal fracture of right femur
HAC 7th characters A - C see Appendix B for HAC conditional logic
CC +7th **S72.132** Displaced apophyseal fracture of left femur
HAC 7th characters A - C see Appendix B for HAC conditional logic
CC +7th **S72.133** Displaced apophyseal fracture of unspecified femur
HAC 7th characters A - C see Appendix B for HAC conditional logic
CC +7th **S72.134** Nondisplaced apophyseal fracture of right femur
HAC 7th characters A - C see Appendix B for HAC conditional logic
CC +7th **S72.135** Nondisplaced apophyseal fracture of left femur
HAC 7th characters A - C see Appendix B for HAC conditional logic
CC +7th **S72.136** Nondisplaced apophyseal fracture of unspecified femur
HAC 7th characters A - C see Appendix B for HAC conditional logic

+ S72.14 **Intertrochanteric fracture of femur**
CC +7th **S72.141** Displaced intertrochanteric fracture of right femur
AHA CC: 4Q, 2013, 128-129; 3Q, 2016, 16-17
HAC 7th characters A - C see Appendix B for HAC conditional logic
CC +7th **S72.142** Displaced intertrochanteric fracture of left femur
HAC 7th characters A - C see Appendix B for HAC conditional logic
CC +7th **S72.143** Displaced intertrochanteric fracture of unspecified femur
HAC 7th characters A - C see Appendix B for HAC conditional logic
CC +7th **S72.144** Nondisplaced intertrochanteric fracture of right femur
HAC 7th characters A - C see Appendix B for HAC conditional logic
CC +7th **S72.145** Nondisplaced intertrochanteric fracture of left femur
HAC 7th characters A - C see Appendix B for HAC conditional logic
CC +7th **S72.146** Nondisplaced intertrochanteric fracture of unspecified femur
HAC 7th characters A - C see Appendix B for HAC conditional logic

+ S72.2 **Subtrochanteric fracture of femur**
CC X+7th **S72.21** Displaced subtrochanteric fracture of right femur
HAC 7th characters A - C see Appendix B for HAC conditional logic

CC X+7th **S72.22** Displaced subtrochanteric fracture of left femur
HAC 7th characters A - C see Appendix B for HAC conditional logic
CC X+7th **S72.23** Displaced subtrochanteric fracture of unspecified femur
HAC 7th characters A - C see Appendix B for HAC conditional logic
CC X+7th **S72.24** Nondisplaced subtrochanteric fracture of right femur
HAC 7th characters A - C see Appendix B for HAC conditional logic
CC X+7th **S72.25** Nondisplaced subtrochanteric fracture of left femur
HAC 7th characters A - C see Appendix B for HAC conditional logic
CC X+7th **S72.26** Nondisplaced subtrochanteric fracture of unspecified femur
HAC 7th characters A - C see Appendix B for HAC conditional logic

+ S72.3 **Fracture of shaft of femur**
+ S72.30 **Unspecified fracture of shaft of femur**
CC +7th **S72.301** Unspecified fracture of shaft of right femur
AHA CC: 2Q, 2018, 12
HAC 7th characters A - C see Appendix B for HAC conditional logic
CC +7th **S72.302** Unspecified fracture of shaft of left femur
HAC 7th characters A - C see Appendix B for HAC conditional logic
CC +7th **S72.309** Unspecified fracture of shaft of unspecified femur
HAC 7th characters A - C see Appendix B for HAC conditional logic

+ S72.32 **Transverse fracture of shaft of femur**
CC MCC +7th **S72.321** Displaced transverse fracture of shaft of right femur
HAC 7th characters A - C see Appendix B for HAC conditional logic
CC MCC +7th **S72.322** Displaced transverse fracture of shaft of left femur
HAC 7th characters A - C see Appendix B for HAC conditional logic
CC MCC +7th **S72.323** Displaced transverse fracture of shaft of unspecified femur
HAC 7th characters A - C see Appendix B for HAC conditional logic
CC MCC +7th **S72.324** Nondisplaced transverse fracture of shaft of right femur
HAC 7th characters A - C see Appendix B for HAC conditional logic
CC MCC +7th **S72.325** Nondisplaced transverse fracture of shaft of left femur
HAC 7th characters A - C see Appendix B for HAC conditional logic
CC MCC +7th **S72.326** Nondisplaced transverse fracture of shaft of unspecified femur
HAC 7th characters A - C see Appendix B for HAC conditional logic

+ S72.33 **Oblique fracture of shaft of femur**
CC MCC +7th **S72.331** Displaced oblique fracture of shaft of right femur
HAC 7th characters A - C see Appendix B for HAC conditional logic
CC MCC +7th **S72.332** Displaced oblique fracture of shaft of left femur
HAC 7th characters A - C see Appendix B for HAC conditional logic
CC MCC +7th **S72.333** Displaced oblique fracture of shaft of unspecified femur
HAC 7th characters A - C see Appendix B for HAC conditional logic
CC MCC +7th **S72.334** Nondisplaced oblique fracture of shaft of right femur
HAC 7th characters A - C see Appendix B for HAC conditional logic
CC MCC +7th **S72.335** Nondisplaced oblique fracture of shaft of left femur
HAC 7th characters A - C see Appendix B for HAC conditional logic
CC MCC +7th **S72.336** Nondisplaced oblique fracture of shaft of unspecified femur
HAC 7th characters A - C see Appendix B for HAC conditional logic

+ **S72.34 Spiral fracture of shaft of femur**

CC MCC +7th **S72.341** Displaced spiral fracture of shaft of right femur
> HAC 7th characters A - C see Appendix B for HAC conditional logic

CC MCC +7th **S72.342** Displaced spiral fracture of shaft of left femur
> HAC 7th characters A - C see Appendix B for HAC conditional logic

CC MCC +7th **S72.343** Displaced spiral fracture of shaft of unspecified femur
> HAC 7th characters A - C see Appendix B for HAC conditional logic

CC MCC +7th **S72.344** Nondisplaced spiral fracture of shaft of right femur
> HAC 7th characters A - C see Appendix B for HAC conditional logic

CC MCC +7th **S72.345** Nondisplaced spiral fracture of shaft of left femur
> HAC 7th characters A - C see Appendix B for HAC conditional logic

CC MCC +7th **S72.346** Nondisplaced spiral fracture of shaft of unspecified femur
> HAC 7th characters A - C see Appendix B for HAC conditional logic

+ **S72.35 Comminuted fracture of shaft of femur**

CC MCC +7th **S72.351** Displaced comminuted fracture of shaft of right femur
> HAC 7th characters A - C see Appendix B for HAC conditional logic

CC MCC +7th **S72.352** Displaced comminuted fracture of shaft of left femur
> HAC 7th characters A - C see Appendix B for HAC conditional logic

CC MCC +7th **S72.353** Displaced comminuted fracture of shaft of unspecified femur
> HAC 7th characters A - C see Appendix B for HAC conditional logic

CC MCC +7th **S72.354** Nondisplaced comminuted fracture of shaft of right femur
> HAC 7th characters A - C see Appendix B for HAC conditional logic

CC MCC +7th **S72.355** Nondisplaced comminuted fracture of shaft of left femur
> HAC 7th characters A - C see Appendix B for HAC conditional logic

CC MCC +7th **S72.356** Nondisplaced comminuted fracture of shaft of unspecified femur
> HAC 7th characters A - C see Appendix B for HAC conditional logic

+ **S72.36 Segmental fracture of shaft of femur**

CC MCC +7th **S72.361** Displaced segmental fracture of shaft of right femur
> HAC 7th characters A - C see Appendix B for HAC conditional logic

CC MCC +7th **S72.362** Displaced segmental fracture of shaft of left femur
> HAC 7th characters A - C see Appendix B for HAC conditional logic

CC MCC +7th **S72.363** Displaced segmental fracture of shaft of unspecified femur
> HAC 7th characters A - C see Appendix B for HAC conditional logic

CC MCC +7th **S72.364** Nondisplaced segmental fracture of shaft of right femur
> HAC 7th characters A - C see Appendix B for HAC conditional logic

CC MCC +7th **S72.365** Nondisplaced segmental fracture of shaft of left femur
> HAC 7th characters A - C see Appendix B for HAC conditional logic

CC MCC +7th **S72.366** Nondisplaced segmental fracture of shaft of unspecified femur
> HAC 7th characters A - C see Appendix B for HAC conditional logic

+ **S72.39 Other fracture of shaft of femur**

CC MCC +7th **S72.391** Other fracture of shaft of right femur
> HAC 7th characters A - C see Appendix B for HAC conditional logic

CC MCC +7th **S72.392** Other fracture of shaft of left femur
> HAC 7th characters A - C see Appendix B for HAC conditional logic

CC MCC +7th **S72.399** Other fracture of shaft of unspecified femur
> HAC 7th characters A - C see Appendix B for HAC conditional logic

+ **S72.4 Fracture of lower end of femur**
Fracture of distal end of femur
Excludes2: *fracture of shaft of femur (S72.3-)*
physeal fracture of lower end of femur (S79.1-)

+ **S72.40 Unspecified fracture of lower end of femur**

CC MCC +7th **S72.401** Unspecified fracture of lower end of right femur
AHA CC: 4Q, 2016, 42-43
> HAC 7th characters A - C see Appendix B for HAC conditional logic

CC MCC +7th **S72.402** Unspecified fracture of lower end of left femur
> HAC 7th characters A - C see Appendix B for HAC conditional logic

CC MCC +7th **S72.409** Unspecified fracture of lower end of unspecified femur
> HAC 7th characters A - C see Appendix B for HAC conditional logic

+ **S72.41 Unspecified condyle fracture of lower end of femur**
Condyle fracture of femur NOS

CC MCC +7th **S72.411** Displaced unspecified condyle fracture of lower end of right femur
> HAC 7th characters A - C see Appendix B for HAC conditional logic

CC MCC +7th **S72.412** Displaced unspecified condyle fracture of lower end of left femur
> HAC 7th characters A - C see Appendix B for HAC conditional logic

CC MCC +7th **S72.413** Displaced unspecified condyle fracture of lower end of unspecified femur
> HAC 7th characters A - C see Appendix B for HAC conditional logic

CC MCC +7th **S72.414** Nondisplaced unspecified condyle fracture of lower end of right femur
> HAC 7th characters A - C see Appendix B for HAC conditional logic

CC MCC +7th **S72.415** Nondisplaced unspecified condyle fracture of lower end of left femur
> HAC 7th characters A - C see Appendix B for HAC conditional logic

CC MCC +7th **S72.416** Nondisplaced unspecified condyle fracture of lower end of unspecified femur
> HAC 7th characters A - C see Appendix B for HAC conditional logic

+ **S72.42 Fracture of lateral condyle of femur**

CC MCC +7th **S72.421** Displaced fracture of lateral condyle of right femur
> HAC 7th characters A - C see Appendix B for HAC conditional logic

CC MCC +7th **S72.422** Displaced fracture of lateral condyle of left femur
> HAC 7th characters A - C see Appendix B for HAC conditional logic

CC MCC +7th **S72.423** Displaced fracture of lateral condyle of unspecified femur
> HAC 7th characters A - C see Appendix B for HAC conditional logic

CC MCC +7th **S72.424** Nondisplaced fracture of lateral condyle of right femur
> HAC 7th characters A - C see Appendix B for HAC conditional logic

---

+, +7th, X + 7th   ● Newborn   ● Pediatric   ● Maternity   ● Adult   ♀ Female   ♂ Male   Manifestation   Unacceptable PDX   HCC   CC   MCC   HAC

CC MCC +7th **S72.425** **Nondisplaced fracture of lateral condyle of left femur**
HAC 7th characters A - C see Appendix B for HAC conditional logic

CC MCC +7th **S72.426** **Nondisplaced fracture of lateral condyle of unspecified femur**
HAC 7th characters A - C see Appendix B for HAC conditional logic

+ **S72.43** **Fracture of medial condyle of femur**

CC MCC +7th **S72.431** **Displaced fracture of medial condyle of right femur**
HAC 7th characters A - C see Appendix B for HAC conditional logic

CC MCC +7th **S72.432** **Displaced fracture of medial condyle of left femur**
HAC 7th characters A - C see Appendix B for HAC conditional logic

CC MCC +7th **S72.433** **Displaced fracture of medial condyle of unspecified femur**
HAC 7th characters A - C see Appendix B for HAC conditional logic

CC MCC +7th **S72.434** **Nondisplaced fracture of medial condyle of right femur**
HAC 7th characters A - C see Appendix B for HAC conditional logic

CC MCC +7th **S72.435** **Nondisplaced fracture of medial condyle of left femur**
HAC 7th characters A - C see Appendix B for HAC conditional logic

CC MCC +7th **S72.436** **Nondisplaced fracture of medial condyle of unspecified femur**
HAC 7th characters A - C see Appendix B for HAC conditional logic

+ **S72.44** **Fracture of lower epiphysis (separation) of femur**
Excludes1: *Salter-Harris Type I physeal fracture of lower end of femur (S79.11-)*

CC MCC +7th **S72.441** **Displaced fracture of lower epiphysis (separation) of right femur**
HAC 7th characters A - C see Appendix B for HAC conditional logic

CC MCC +7th **S72.442** **Displaced fracture of lower epiphysis (separation) of left femur**
HAC 7th characters A - C see Appendix B for HAC conditional logic

CC MCC +7th **S72.443** **Displaced fracture of lower epiphysis (separation) of unspecified femur**
HAC 7th characters A - C see Appendix B for HAC conditional logic

CC MCC +7th **S72.444** **Nondisplaced fracture of lower epiphysis (separation) of right femur**
HAC 7th characters A - C see Appendix B for HAC conditional logic

CC MCC +7th **S72.445** **Nondisplaced fracture of lower epiphysis (separation) of left femur**
HAC 7th characters A - C see Appendix B for HAC conditional logic

CC MCC +7th **S72.446** **Nondisplaced fracture of lower epiphysis (separation) of unspecified femur**
HAC 7th characters A - C see Appendix B for HAC conditional logic

+ **S72.45** **Supracondylar fracture without intracondylar extension of lower end of femur**
Supracondylar fracture of lower end of femur NOS
Excludes1: *supracondylar fracture with intracondylarextensionoflowerend of femur (S72.46-)*

CC MCC +7th **S72.451** **Displaced supracondylar fracture without intracondylar extension of lower end of right femur**
HAC 7th characters A - C see Appendix B for HAC conditional logic

CC MCC +7th **S72.452** **Displaced supracondylar fracture without intracondylar extension of lower end of left femur**
HAC 7th characters A - C see Appendix B for HAC conditional logic

CC MCC +7th **S72.453** **Displaced supracondylar fracture without intracondylar extension of lower end of unspecified femur**
HAC 7th characters A - C see Appendix B for HAC conditional logic

CC MCC +7th **S72.454** **Nondisplaced supracondylar fracture without intracondylar extension of lower end of right femur**
HAC 7th characters A - C see Appendix B for HAC conditional logic

CC MCC +7th **S72.455** **Nondisplaced supracondylar fracture without intracondylar extension of lower end of left femur**
HAC 7th characters A - C see Appendix B for HAC conditional logic

CC MCC +7th **S72.456** **Nondisplaced supracondylar fracture without intracondylar extension of lower end of unspecified femur**
HAC 7th characters A - C see Appendix B for HAC conditional logic

+ **S72.46** **Supracondylar fracture with intracondylar extension of lower end of femur**
Excludes1: *supracondylar fracture without intracondylarextensionoflowerend of femur (S72.45-)*

CC MCC +7th **S72.461** **Displaced supracondylar fracture with intracondylar extension of lower end of right femur**
HAC 7th characters A - C see Appendix B for HAC conditional logic

CC MCC +7th **S72.462** **Displaced supracondylar fracture with intracondylar extension of lower end of left femur**
HAC 7th characters A - C see Appendix B for HAC conditional logic

CC MCC +7th **S72.463** **Displaced supracondylar fracture with intracondylar extension of lower end of unspecified femur**
HAC 7th characters A - C see Appendix B for HAC conditional logic

CC MCC +7th **S72.464** **Nondisplaced supracondylar fracture with intracondylar extension of lower end of right femur**
HAC 7th characters A - C see Appendix B for HAC conditional logic

CC MCC +7th **S72.465** **Nondisplaced supracondylar fracture with intracondylar extension of lower end of left femur**
HAC 7th characters A - C see Appendix B for HAC conditional logic

CC MCC +7th **S72.466** **Nondisplaced supracondylar fracture with intracondylar extension of lower end of unspecified femur**
HAC 7th characters A - C see Appendix B for HAC conditional logic

+ **S72.47** **Torus fracture of lower end of femur**

The appropriate 7th character is to be added to all codes in subcategory **S72.47**
A initial encounter for closed fracture
D subsequent encounter for fracture with routine healing
G subsequent encounter for fracture with delayed healing
K subsequent encounter for fracture with nonunion
P subsequent encounter for fracture with malunion
S sequela

CC +7th **S72.471** **Torus fracture of lower end of right femur**
HAC 7th character A see Appendix B for HAC conditional logic

CC +7th **S72.472** **Torus fracture of lower end of left femur**
HAC 7th character A see Appendix B for HAC conditional logic

CC +7th **S72.479** **Torus fracture of lower end of unspecified femur**
HAC 7th character A see Appendix B for HAC conditional logic

+ **S72.49** **Other fracture of lower end of femur**

CC MCC +7th **S72.491** **Other fracture of lower end of right femur**
HAC 7th characters A - C see Appendix B for HAC conditional logic

CC MCC +7th **S72.492** **Other fracture of lower end of left femur**
> **HAC** 7th characters A - C see Appendix B for HAC conditional logic

CC MCC +7th **S72.499** **Other fracture of lower end of unspecified femur**
> **HAC** 7th characters A - C see Appendix B for HAC conditional logic

MCC + **S72.8** **Other fracture of femur**
> **HAC** 7th characters A - C see Appendix B for HAC conditional logic

+ **S72.8X** **Other fracture of femur**
    +7th **S72.8X1** **Other fracture of right femur**
    +7th **S72.8X2** **Other fracture of left femur**
    +7th **S72.8X9** **Other fracture of unspecified femur**

+ **S72.9** **Unspecified fracture of femur**
Fracture of thigh NOS
Fracture of upper leg NOS
Excludes1: *fracture of hip NOS (S72.00-, S72.01-)*

CC MCC X+7th **S72.90** **Unspecified fracture of unspecified femur**
AHA CC: 4Q, 2012, 93-94
> **HAC** 7th characters A - C see Appendix B for HAC conditional logic

CC MCC X+7th **S72.91** **Unspecified fracture of right femur**
> **HAC** 7th characters A - C see Appendix B for HAC conditional logic

CC MCC X+7th **S72.92** **Unspecified fracture of left femur**
> **HAC** 7th characters A - C see Appendix B for HAC conditional logic

S73 **Dislocation and sprain of joint and ligaments of hip**
> **Includes:** avulsion of joint or ligament of hip
> lacervw ation of cartilage, joint or ligament of hip
> sprain of cartilage, joint or ligament of hip
> traumatic hemarthrosis of joint or ligament of hip
> traumatic rupture of joint or ligament of hip
> traumatic subluxation of joint or ligament of hip
> traumatic tear of joint or ligament of hip
> Code also any associated open wound
> ***Excludes2:*** *strain of muscle, fascia and tendon of hip and thigh (S76.-)*

> The appropriate 7th character is to be added to each code from category S73
> A   initial encounter
> D   subsequent encounter
> S   sequela

+ **S73.0** **Subluxation and dislocation of hip**
> ***Excludes2:*** *dislocation and subluxation of hip prosthesis (T84.020, T84.021)*

+ **S73.00** **Unspecified subluxation and dislocation of hip**
Dislocation of hip NOS
Subluxation of hip NOS

CC +7th **S73.001** **Unspecified subluxation of right hip**
> **HAC** 7th character A see Appendix B for HAC conditional logic

CC +7th **S73.002** **Unspecified subluxation of left hip**
> **HAC** 7th character A see Appendix B for HAC conditional logic

CC +7th **S73.003** **Unspecified subluxation of unspecified hip**
> **HAC** 7th character A see Appendix B for HAC conditional logic

CC +7th **S73.004** **Unspecified dislocation of right hip**
> **HAC** 7th character A see Appendix B for HAC conditional logic

CC +7th **S73.005** **Unspecified dislocation of left hip**
> **HAC** 7th character A see Appendix B for HAC conditional logic

CC +7th **S73.006** **Unspecified dislocation of unspecified hip**
> **HAC** 7th character A see Appendix B for HAC conditional logic

+ **S73.01** **Posterior subluxation and dislocation of hip**

CC +7th **S73.011** **Posterior subluxation of right hip**
> **HAC** 7th character A see Appendix B for HAC conditional logic

CC +7th **S73.012** **Posterior subluxation of left hip**
> **HAC** 7th character A see Appendix B for HAC conditional logic

CC +7th **S73.013** **Posterior subluxation of unspecified hip**
> **HAC** 7th character A see Appendix B for HAC conditional logic

CC +7th **S73.014** **Posterior dislocation of right hip**
> **HAC** 7th character A see Appendix B for HAC conditional logic

CC +7th **S73.015** **Posterior dislocation of left hip**
> **HAC** 7th character A see Appendix B for HAC conditional logic

CC +7th **S73.016** **Posterior dislocation of unspecified hip**
> **HAC** 7th character A see Appendix B for HAC conditional logic

+ **S73.02** **Obturator subluxation and dislocation of hip**

CC +7th **S73.021** **Obturator subluxation of right hip**
> **HAC** 7th character A see Appendix B for HAC conditional logic

CC +7th **S73.022** **Obturator subluxation of left hip**
> **HAC** 7th character A see Appendix B for HAC conditional logic

CC +7th **S73.023** **Obturator subluxation of unspecified hip**
> **HAC** 7th character A see Appendix B for HAC conditional logic

CC +7th **S73.024** **Obturator dislocation of right hip**
> **HAC** 7th character A see Appendix B for HAC conditional logic

CC +7th **S73.025** **Obturator dislocation of left hip**
> **HAC** 7th character A see Appendix B for HAC conditional logic

CC +7th **S73.026** **Obturator dislocation of unspecified hip**
> **HAC** 7th character A see Appendix B for HAC conditional logic

+ **S73.03** **Other anterior subluxation and dislocation of hip**

CC +7th **S73.031** **Other anterior subluxation of right hip**
> **HAC** 7th character A see Appendix B for HAC conditional logic

CC +7th **S73.032** **Other anterior subluxation of left hip**
> **HAC** 7th character A see Appendix B for HAC conditional logic

CC +7th **S73.033** **Other anterior subluxation of unspecified hip**
> **HAC** 7th character A see Appendix B for HAC conditional logic

CC +7th **S73.034** **Other anterior dislocation of right hip**
> **HAC** 7th character A see Appendix B for HAC conditional logic

CC +7th **S73.035** **Other anterior dislocation of left hip**
> **HAC** 7th character A see Appendix B for HAC conditional logic

CC +7th **S73.036** **Other anterior dislocation of unspecified hip**
> **HAC** 7th character A see Appendix B for HAC conditional logic

+ **S73.04** **Central subluxation and dislocation of hip**

CC +7th **S73.041** **Central subluxation of right hip**
> **HAC** 7th character A see Appendix B for HAC conditional logic

CC +7th **S73.042** **Central subluxation of left hip**
> **HAC** 7th character A see Appendix B for HAC conditional logic

CC +7th **S73.043** **Central subluxation of unspecified hip**
> **HAC** 7th character A see Appendix B for HAC conditional logic

CC +7th **S73.044** **Central dislocation of right hip**
> **HAC** 7th character A see Appendix B for HAC conditional logic

CC +7th **S73.045** **Central dislocation of left hip**
> **HAC** 7th character A see Appendix B for HAC conditional logic

CC +7th **S73.046** **Central dislocation of unspecified hip**
> **HAC** 7th character A see Appendix B for HAC conditional logic

+ **S73.1** **Sprain of hip**

+ **S73.10** **Unspecified sprain of hip**
    +7th **S73.101** **Unspecified sprain of right hip**
    +7th **S73.102** **Unspecified sprain of left hip**
    +7th **S73.109** **Unspecified sprain of unspecified hip**

+ **S73.11** **Iliofemoral ligament sprain of hip**
    +7th **S73.111** **Iliofemoral ligament sprain of right hip**
    +7th **S73.112** **Iliofemoral ligament sprain of left hip**
    +7th **S73.119** **Iliofemoral ligament sprain of unspecified hip**

+ **S73.12** **Ischiocapsular (ligament) sprain of hip**
    +7th **S73.121** **Ischiocapsular ligament sprain of right hip**
    +7th **S73.122** **Ischiocapsular ligament sprain of left hip**
    +7th **S73.129** **Ischiocapsular ligament sprain of unspecified hip**

+, +7th, X + 7th   ● Newborn   ● Pediatric   ● Maternity   ● Adult   ♀ Female   ♂ Male   Manifestation   Unacceptable PDX   HCC   CC   MCC   **HAC**

+ **S73.19** **Other sprain of hip**
   +7th **S73.191** **Other sprain of right hip**
   +7th **S73.192** **Other sprain of left hip**
         AHA CC: 4Q, 2014, 25
   +7th **S73.199** **Other sprain of unspecified hip**

S74 **Injury of nerves at hip and thigh level**
   Code also any associated open wound (S71.-)
   Excludes2: *injury of nerves at ankle and foot level (S94.-)*
      injury of nerves at lower leg level (S84.-)

   The appropriate 7th character is to be added to each code from
   category S74
   A   initial encounter
   D   subsequent encounter
   S   sequela

+ **S74.0** **Injury of sciatic nerve at hip and thigh level**
   X+7th **S74.00** **Injury of sciatic nerve at hip and thigh level,
                  unspecified leg**
   X+7th **S74.01** **Injury of sciatic nerve at hip and thigh level,
                  right leg**
   X+7th **S74.02** **Injury of sciatic nerve at hip and thigh level,
                  left leg**
+ **S74.1** **Injury of femoral nerve at hip and thigh level**
   X+7th **S74.10** **Injury of femoral nerve at hip and thigh level,
                  unspecified leg**
   X+7th **S74.11** **Injury of femoral nerve at hip and thigh level,
                  right leg**
   X+7th **S74.12** **Injury of femoral nerve at hip and thigh level,
                  left leg**
+ **S74.2** **Injury of cutaneous sensory nerve at hip and thigh level**
   X+7th **S74.20** **Injury of cutaneous sensory nerve at hip and
                  thigh level, unspecified leg**
   X+7th **S74.21** **Injury of cutaneous sensory nerve at hip and high
                  level, right leg**
   X+7th **S74.22** **Injury of cutaneous sensory nerve at hip and
                  thigh level, left leg**
+ **S74.8** **Injury of other nerves at hip and thigh level**
   + **S74.8X** **Injury of other nerves at hip and thigh level**
      +7th **S74.8X1** **Injury of other nerves at hip and thigh
                      level, right leg**
      +7th **S74.8X2** **Injury of other nerves at hip and thigh
                      level, left leg**
      +7th **S74.8X9** **Injury of other nerves at hip and thigh
                      level, unspecified leg**
+ **S74.9** **Injury of unspecified nerve at hip and thigh level**
   X+7th **S74.90** **Injury of unspecified nerve at hip and thigh level,
                  unspecified leg**
   X+7th **S74.91** **Injury of unspecified nerve at hip and thigh level,
                  right leg**
   X+7th **S74.92** **Injury of unspecified nerve at hip and thigh level,
                  left leg**

S75 **Injury of blood vessels at hip and thigh level**
   Code also any associated open wound (S71.-)
   Excludes2: *injury of blood vessels at lower leg level (S85.-)*
      injury of popliteal artery (S85.0)

   The appropriate 7th character is to be added to each code from
   category S75
   A   initial encounter
   D   subsequent encounter
   S   sequela

+ **S75.0** **Injury of femoral artery**
   + **S75.00** **Unspecified injury of femoral artery**
      MCC +7th **S75.001** **Unspecified injury of femoral artery,
                          right leg**
      MCC +7th **S75.002** **Unspecified injury of femoral artery, left
                          leg**
      MCC +7th **S75.009** **Unspecified injury of femoral artery,
                          unspecified leg**
   + **S75.01** **Minor laceration of femoral artery**
            Incomplete transection of femoral artery
            Laceration of femoral artery NOS
            Superficial laceration of femoral artery

      MCC +7th **S75.011** **Minor laceration of femoral artery,
                          right leg**
      MCC +7th **S75.012** **Minor laceration of femoral artery,
                          left leg**
      MCC +7th **S75.019** **Minor laceration of femoral artery,
                          unspecified leg**
   + **S75.02** **Major laceration of femoral artery**
            Complete transection of femoral artery
            Traumatic rupture of femoral artery
      MCC +7th **S75.021** **Major laceration of femoral artery,
                          right leg**
      MCC +7th **S75.022** **Major laceration of femoral artery,
                          left leg**
      MCC +7th **S75.029** **Major laceration of femoral artery,
                          unspecified leg**
   + **S75.09** **Other specified injury of femoral artery**
      MCC +7th **S75.091** **Other specified injury of femoral artery,
                          right leg**
      MCC +7th **S75.092** **Other specified injury of femoral artery,
                          left leg**
      MCC +7th **S75.099** **Other specified injury of femoral artery,
                          unspecified leg**
+ **S75.1** **Injury of femoral vein at hip and thigh level**
   + **S75.10** **Unspecified injury of femoral vein at hip and
                thigh level**
      MCC +7th **S75.101** **Unspecified injury of femoral vein at hip
                          and thigh level, right leg**
      MCC +7th **S75.102** **Unspecified injury of femoral vein at hip
                          and thigh level, left leg**
      MCC +7th **S75.109** **Unspecified injury of femoral vein at hip
                          and thigh level, unspecified leg**
   + **S75.11** **Minor laceration of femoral vein at hip and thigh
                level**
            Incomplete transection of femoral vein at hip and
               thigh level
            Laceration of femoral vein at hip and thigh level NOS
            Superficial laceration of femoral vein at hip and
               thigh level
      MCC +7th **S75.111** **Minor laceration of femoral vein at hip
                          and thigh level, right leg**
      MCC +7th **S75.112** **Minor laceration of femoral vein at hip
                          and thigh level, left leg**
      MCC +7th **S75.119** **Minor laceration of femoral vein at hip
                          and thigh level, unspecified leg**
   + **S75.12** **Major laceration of femoral vein at hip and thigh
                level**
            Complete transection of femoral vein at hip and
               thigh level
            Traumatic rupture of femoral vein at hip and thigh
               level
      MCC +7th **S75.121** **Major laceration of femoral vein at hip
                          and thigh level, right leg**
      MCC +7th **S75.122** **Major laceration of femoral vein at hip
                          and thigh level, left leg**
      MCC +7th **S75.129** **Major laceration of femoral vein at hip
                          and thigh level, unspecified leg**
   + **S75.19** **Other specified injury of femoral vein at hip and
                thigh level**
      MCC +7th **S75.191** **Other specified injury of femoral vein at
                          hip and thigh level, right leg**
      MCC +7th **S75.192** **Other specified injury of femoral vein at
                          hip and thigh level, left leg**
      MCC +7th **S75.199** **Other specified injury of femoral vein at
                          hip and thigh level, unspecified leg**
+ **S75.2** **Injury of greater saphenous vein at hip and thigh level**
   Excludes1: *greater saphenous vein NOS (S85.3)*
   + **S75.20** **Unspecified injury of greater saphenous vein at
                hip and thigh level**
      CC +7th **S75.201** **Unspecified injury of greater saphenous
                         vein at hip and thigh level, right leg**
      CC +7th **S75.202** **Unspecified injury of greater saphenous
                         vein at hip and thigh level, left leg**
      CC +7th **S75.209** **Unspecified injury of greater saphenous
                         vein at hip and thigh level, unspecified
                         leg**

+, +7th, X + 7th   ● Newborn   ● Pediatric   ● Maternity   ● Adult   ♀ Female   ♂ Male   Manifestation   Unacceptable PDX   HCC   CC   MCC   HAC

+ S75.21 **Minor laceration of greater saphenous vein at hip and thigh level**
  Incomplete transection of greater saphenous vein at hip and thigh level
  Laceration of greater saphenous vein at hip and thigh level NOS
  Superficial laceration of greater saphenous vein at hip and thigh level
  CC +7th S75.211 **Minor laceration of greater saphenous vein at hip and thigh level, right leg**
  CC +7th S75.212 **Minor laceration of greater saphenous vein at hip and thigh level, left leg**
  CC +7th S75.219 **Minor laceration of greater saphenous vein at hip and thigh level, unspecified leg**
+ S75.22 **Major laceration of greater saphenous vein at hip and thigh level**
  Complete transection of greater saphenous vein at hip and thigh level
  Traumatic rupture of greater saphenous vein at hip and thigh level
  CC +7th S75.221 **Major laceration of greater saphenous vein at hip and thigh level, right leg**
  CC +7th S75.222 **Major laceration of greater saphenous vein at hip and thigh level, left leg**
  CC +7th S75.229 **Major laceration of greater saphenous vein at hip and thigh level, unspecified leg**
+ S75.29 **Other specified injury of greater saphenous vein at hip and thigh level**
  CC +7th S75.291 **Other specified injury of greater saphenous vein at hip and thigh level, right leg**
  CC +7th S75.292 **Other specified injury of greater saphenous vein at hip and thigh level, left leg**
  CC +7th S75.299 **Other specified injury of greater saphenous vein at hip and thigh level, unspecified leg**
+ S75.8 **Injury of other blood vessels at hip and thigh level**
  + S75.80 **Unspecified injury of other blood vessels at hip and thigh level**
    CC +7th S75.801 **Unspecified injury of other blood vessels at hip and thigh level, right leg**
    CC +7th S75.802 **Unspecified injury of other blood vessels at hip and thigh level, left leg**
    CC +7th S75.809 **Unspecified injury of other blood vessels at hip and thigh level, unspecified leg**
  + S75.81 **Laceration of other blood vessels at hip and thigh level**
    CC +7th S75.811 **Laceration of other blood vessels at hip and thigh level, right leg**
    CC +7th S75.812 **Laceration of other blood vessels at hip and thigh level, left leg**
    CC +7th S75.819 **Laceration of other blood vessels at hip and thigh level, unspecified leg**
  + S75.89 **Other specified injury of other blood vessels at hip and thigh level**
    CC +7th S75.891 **Other specified injury of other blood vessels at hip and thigh level, right leg**
    CC +7th S75.892 **Other specified injury of other blood vessels at hip and thigh level, left leg**
    CC +7th S75.899 **Other specified injury of other blood vessels at hip and thigh level, unspecified leg**
+ S75.9 **Injury of unspecified blood vessel at hip and thigh level**
  + S75.90 **Unspecified injury of unspecified blood vessel at hip and thigh level**
    CC +7th S75.901 **Unspecified injury of unspecified blood vessel at hip and thigh level, right leg**
    CC +7th S75.902 **Unspecified injury of unspecified blood vessel at hip and thigh level, left leg**

CC +7th S75.909 **Unspecified injury of unspecified blood vessel at hip and thigh level, unspecified leg**
+ S75.91 **Laceration of unspecified blood vessel at hip and thigh level**
  CC +7th S75.911 **Laceration of unspecified blood vessel at hip and thigh level, right leg**
  CC +7th S75.912 **Laceration of unspecified blood vessel at hip and thigh level, left leg**
  CC +7th S75.919 **Laceration of unspecified blood vessel at hip and thigh level, unspecified leg**
+ S75.99 **Other specified injury of unspecified blood vessel at hip and thigh level**
  CC +7th S75.991 **Other specified injury of unspecified blood vessel at hip and thigh level, right leg**
  CC +7th S75.992 **Other specified injury of unspecified blood vessel at hip and thigh level, left leg**
  CC +7th S75.999 **Other specified injury of unspecified blood vessel at hip and thigh level, unspecified leg**

S76 **Injury of muscle, fascia and tendon at hip and thigh level**
  Code also any associated open wound (S71.-)
  Excludes2: *injury of muscle, fascia and tendon at lower leg level (S86)*
  sprain of joint and ligament of hip (S73.1)

  The appropriate 7th character is to be added to each code from category S76
  A   initial encounter
  D   subsequent encounter
  S   sequela

  + S76.0 **Injury of muscle, fascia and tendon of hip**
    + S76.00 **Unspecified injury of muscle, fascia and tendon of hip**
      +7th S76.001 **Unspecified injury of muscle, fascia and tendon of right hip**
      +7th S76.002 **Unspecified injury of muscle, fascia and tendon of left hip**
      +7th S76.009 **Unspecified injury of muscle, fascia and tendon of unspecified hip**
    + S76.01 **Strain of muscle, fascia and tendon of hip**
      +7th S76.011 **Strain of muscle, fascia and tendon of right hip**
      +7th S76.012 **Strain of muscle, fascia and tendon of left hip**
      +7th S76.019 **Strain of muscle, fascia and tendon of unspecified hip**
    + S76.02 **Laceration of muscle, fascia and tendon of hip**
      CC +7th S76.021 **Laceration of muscle, fascia and tendon of right hip**
      CC +7th S76.022 **Laceration of muscle, fascia and tendon of left hip**
      CC +7th S76.029 **Laceration of muscle, fascia and tendon of unspecified hip**
    + S76.09 **Other specified injury of muscle, fascia and tendon of hip**
      +7th S76.091 **Other specified injury of muscle, fascia and tendon of right hip**
      +7th S76.092 **Other specified injury of muscle, fascia and tendon of left hip**
      +7th S76.099 **Other specified injury of muscle, fascia and tendon of unspecified hip**
  + S76.1 **Injury of quadriceps muscle, fascia and tendon**
    Injury of patellar ligament (tendon)
    + S76.10 **Unspecified injury of quadriceps muscle, fascia and tendon**
      +7th S76.101 **Unspecified injury of right quadriceps muscle, fascia and tendon**
      +7th S76.102 **Unspecified injury of left quadriceps muscle, fascia and tendon**
      +7th S76.109 **Unspecified injury of unspecified quadriceps muscle, fascia and tendon**

+ **S76.11** Strain of quadriceps muscle, fascia and tendon
  +7th **S76.111** Strain of right quadriceps muscle, fascia and tendon
  +7th **S76.112** Strain of left quadriceps muscle, fascia and tendon
  +7th **S76.119** Strain of unspecified quadriceps muscle, fascia and tendon
+ **S76.12** Laceration of quadriceps muscle, fascia and tendon
  CC +7th **S76.121** Laceration of right quadriceps muscle, fascia and tendon
  CC +7th **S76.122** Laceration of left quadriceps muscle, fascia and tendon
  CC +7th **S76.129** Laceration of unspecified quadriceps muscle, fascia and tendon
+ **S76.19** Other specified injury of quadriceps muscle, fascia and tendon
  +7th **S76.191** Other specified injury of right quadriceps muscle, fascia and tendon
  +7th **S76.192** Other specified injury of left quadriceps muscle, fascia and tendon
  +7th **S76.199** Other specified injury of unspecified quadriceps muscle, fascia and tendon
+ **S76.2** Injury of adductor muscle, fascia and tendon of thigh
  + **S76.20** Unspecified injury of adductor muscle, fascia and tendon of thigh
    +7th **S76.201** Unspecified injury of adductor muscle, fascia and tendon of right thigh
    +7th **S76.202** Unspecified injury of adductor muscle, fascia and tendon of left thigh
    +7th **S76.209** Unspecified injury of adductor muscle, fascia and tendon of unspecified thigh
  + **S76.21** Strain of adductor muscle, fascia and tendon of thigh
    +7th **S76.211** Strain of adductor muscle, fascia and tendon of right thigh
    +7th **S76.212** Strain of adductor muscle, fascia and tendon of left thigh
    +7th **S76.219** Strain of adductor muscle, fascia and tendon of unspecified thigh
  + **S76.22** Laceration of adductor muscle, fascia and tendon of thigh
    CC +7th **S76.221** Laceration of adductor muscle, fascia and tendon of right thigh
    CC +7th **S76.222** Laceration of adductor muscle, fascia and tendon of left thigh
    CC +7th **S76.229** Laceration of adductor muscle, fascia and tendon of unspecified thigh
  + **S76.29** Other injury of adductor muscle, fascia and tendon of thigh
    +7th **S76.291** Other injury of adductor muscle, fascia and tendon of right thigh
    +7th **S76.292** Other injury of adductor muscle, fascia and tendon of left thigh
    +7th **S76.299** Other injury of adductor muscle, fascia and tendon of unspecified thigh
+ **S76.3** Injury of muscle, fascia and tendon of the posterior muscle group at thigh level
  + **S76.30** Unspecified injury of muscle, fascia and tendon of the posterior muscle group at thigh level
    +7th **S76.301** Unspecified injury of muscle, fascia and tendon of the posterior muscle group at thigh level, right thigh
    +7th **S76.302** Unspecified injury of muscle, fascia and tendon of the posterior muscle group at thigh level, left thigh
    +7th **S76.309** Unspecified injury of muscle, fascia and tendon of the posterior muscle group at thigh level, unspecified thigh
  + **S76.31** Strain of muscle, fascia and tendon of the posterior muscle group at thigh level
    +7th **S76.311** Strain of muscle, fascia and tendon of the posterior muscle group at thigh level, right thigh
    +7th **S76.312** Strain of muscle, fascia and tendon of the posterior muscle group at thigh level, left thigh
    +7th **S76.319** Strain of muscle, fascia and tendon of the posterior muscle group at thigh level, unspecified thigh
  + **S76.32** Laceration of muscle, fascia and tendon of the posterior muscle group at thigh level
    CC +7th **S76.321** Laceration of muscle, fascia and tendon of the posterior muscle group at thigh level, right thigh
    CC +7th **S76.322** Laceration of muscle, fascia and tendon of the posterior muscle group at thigh level, left thigh
    CC +7th **S76.329** Laceration of muscle, fascia and tendon of the posterior muscle group at thigh level, unspecified thigh
  + **S76.39** Other specified injury of muscle, fascia and tendon of the posterior muscle group at thigh level
    +7th **S76.391** Other specified injury of muscle, fascia and tendon of the posterior muscle group at thigh level, right thigh
    +7th **S76.392** Other specified injury of muscle, fascia and tendon of the posterior muscle group at thigh level, left thigh
    +7th **S76.399** Other specified injury of muscle, fascia and tendon of the posterior muscle group at thigh level, unspecified thigh
+ **S76.8** Injury of other specified muscles, fascia and tendons at thigh level
  + **S76.80** Unspecified injury of other specified muscles, fascia and tendons at thigh level
    +7th **S76.801** Unspecified injury of other specified muscles, fascia and tendons at thigh level, right thigh
    +7th **S76.802** Unspecified injury of other specified muscles, fascia and tendons at thigh level, left thigh
    +7th **S76.809** Unspecified injury of other specified muscles, fascia and tendons at thigh level, unspecified thigh
  + **S76.81** Strain of other specified muscles, fascia and tendons at thigh level
    +7th **S76.811** Strain of other specified muscles, fascia and tendons at thigh level, right thigh
    +7th **S76.812** Strain of other specified muscles, fascia and tendons at thigh level, left thigh
    +7th **S76.819** Strain of other specified muscles, fascia and tendons at thigh level, unspecified thigh
  + **S76.82** Laceration of other specified muscles, fascia and tendons at thigh level
    CC +7th **S76.821** Laceration of other specified muscles, fascia and tendons at thigh level, right thigh
    CC +7th **S76.822** Laceration of other specified muscles, fascia and tendons at thigh level, left thigh
    CC +7th **S76.829** Laceration of other specified muscles, fascia and tendons at thigh level, unspecified thigh
  + **S76.89** Other injury of other specified muscles, fascia and tendons at thigh level
    +7th **S76.891** Other injury of other specified muscles, fascia and tendons at thigh level, right thigh
    +7th **S76.892** Other injury of other specified muscles, fascia and tendons at thigh level, left thigh
    +7th **S76.899** Other injury of other specified muscles, fascia and tendons at thigh level, unspecified thigh

+ **S76.9** **Injury of unspecified muscles, fascia and tendons at thigh level**
  + **S76.90** Unspecified injury of unspecified muscles, fascia and tendons at thigh level
    +7th **S76.901** Unspecified injury of unspecified muscles, fascia and tendons at thigh level, right thigh
    +7th **S76.902** Unspecified injury of unspecified muscles, fascia and tendons at thigh level, left thigh
    +7th **S76.909** Unspecified injury of unspecified muscles, fascia and tendons at thigh level, unspecified thigh
  + **S76.91** Strain of unspecified muscles, fascia and tendons at thigh level
    +7th **S76.911** Strain of unspecified muscles, fascia and tendons at thigh level, right thigh
    +7th **S76.912** Strain of unspecified muscles, fascia and tendons at thigh level, left thigh
    +7th **S76.919** Strain of unspecified muscles, fascia and tendons at thigh level, unspecified thigh
  + **S76.92** Laceration of unspecified muscles, fascia and tendons at thigh level
    CC +7th **S76.921** Laceration of unspecified muscles, fascia and tendons at thigh level, right thigh
    CC +7th **S76.922** Laceration of unspecified muscles, fascia and tendons at thigh level, left thigh
    CC +7th **S76.929** Laceration of unspecified muscles, fascia and tendons at thigh level, unspecified thigh
  + **S76.99** Other specified injury of unspecified muscles, fascia and tendons at thigh level
    +7th **S76.991** Other specified injury of unspecified muscles, fascia and tendons at thigh level, right thigh
    +7th **S76.992** Other specified injury of unspecified muscles, fascia and tendons at thigh level, left thigh
    +7th **S76.999** Other specified injury of unspecified muscles, fascia and tendons at thigh level, unspecified thigh

S77 **Crushing injury of hip and thigh**

Use additional code(s) for all associated injuries

Excludes2: *crushing injury of ankle and foot (S97.-)*
crushing injury of lower leg (S87.-)

The appropriate 7th character is to be added to each code from category S77
A   initial encounter
D   subsequent encounter
S   sequela

+ **S77.0** **Crushing injury of hip**
CC X+7th **S77.00** **Crushing injury of unspecified hip**
    HAC 7th character A see Appendix B for HAC conditional logic
CC X+7th **S77.01** **Crushing injury of right hip**
    HAC 7th character A see Appendix B for HAC conditional logic
CC X+7th **S77.02** **Crushing injury of left hip**
    HAC 7th character A see Appendix B for HAC conditional logic
+ **S77.1** **Crushing injury of thigh**
CC X+7th **S77.10** **Crushing injury of unspecified thigh**
    HAC 7th character A see Appendix B for HAC conditional logic
CC X+7th **S77.11** **Crushing injury of right thigh**
    HAC 7th character A see Appendix B for HAC conditional logic
CC X+7th **S77.12** **Crushing injury of left thigh**
    HAC 7th character A see Appendix B for HAC conditional logic

+ **S77.2** **Crushing injury of hip with thigh**
X+7th **S77.20** Crushing injury of unspecified hip with thigh
X+7th **S77.21** Crushing injury of right hip with thigh
X+7th **S77.22** Crushing injury of left hip with thigh

S78 **Traumatic amputation of hip and thigh**

An amputation not identified as partial or complete should be coded to complete
Excludes1: *traumatic amputation of knee (S88.0-)*

The appropriate 7th character is to be added to each code from category S78
A   initial encounter
D   subsequent encounter
S   sequela

+ **S78.0** **Traumatic amputation at hip joint**
  + **S78.01** Complete traumatic amputation at hip joint
    CC +7th **S78.011** Complete traumatic amputation at right hip joint
    CC +7th **S78.012** Complete traumatic amputation at left hip joint
    CC +7th **S78.019** Complete traumatic amputation at unspecified hip joint
  + **S78.02** Partial traumatic amputation at hip joint
    CC +7th **S78.021** Partial traumatic amputation at right hip joint
    CC +7th **S78.022** Partial traumatic amputation at left hip joint
    CC +7th **S78.029** Partial traumatic amputation at unspecified hip joint
+ **S78.1** **Traumatic amputation at level between hip and knee**
  Excludes1: *traumatic amputation of knee (S88.0-)*
  + **S78.11** Complete traumatic amputation at level between hip and knee
    CC +7th **S78.111** Complete traumatic amputation at level between right hip and knee
    CC +7th **S78.112** Complete traumatic amputation at level between left hip and knee
    CC +7th **S78.119** Complete traumatic amputation at level between unspecified hip and knee
  + **S78.12** Partial traumatic amputation at level between hip and knee
    CC +7th **S78.121** Partial traumatic amputation at level between right hip and knee
    CC +7th **S78.122** Partial traumatic amputation at level between left hip and knee
    CC +7th **S78.129** Partial traumatic amputation at level between unspecified hip and knee
+ **S78.9** **Traumatic amputation of hip and thigh, level unspecified**
  + **S78.91** Complete traumatic amputation of hip and thigh, level unspecified
    CC +7th **S78.911** Complete traumatic amputation of right hip and thigh, level unspecified
    CC +7th **S78.912** Complete traumatic amputation of left hip and thigh, level unspecified
    CC +7th **S78.919** Complete traumatic amputation of unspecified hip and thigh, level unspecified
  + **S78.92** Partial traumatic amputation of hip and thigh, level unspecified
    CC +7th **S78.921** Partial traumatic amputation of right hip and thigh, level unspecified
    CC +7th **S78.922** Partial traumatic amputation of left hip and thigh, level unspecified
    CC +7th **S78.929** Partial traumatic amputation of unspecified hip and thigh, level unspecified

S79 Other and unspecified injuries of hip and thigh

NOTE A fracture not indicated as open or closed should be coded to closed

The appropriate 7th character is to be added to each code from subcategories **S79.0** and **S79.1**
- A initial encounter for closed fracture
- D subsequent encounter for fracture with routine healing
- G subsequent encounter for fracture with delayed healing
- K subsequent encounter for fracture with nonunion
- P subsequent encounter for fracture with malunion
- S sequela

Review coding guideline C.19.c

+ **S79.0 Physeal fracture of upper end of femur**
> **Excludes1:** apophyseal fracture of upper end of femur (S72.13-)
> nontraumatic slipped upper femoral epiphysis (M93.0-)

+ **S79.00 Unspecified physeal fracture of upper end of femur**

CC MCC +7th **S79.001 Unspecified physeal fracture of upper end of right femur**
> **HAC** 7th character A see Appendix B for HAC conditional logic

CC MCC +7th **S79.002 Unspecified physeal fracture of upper end of left femur**
> **HAC** 7th character A see Appendix B for HAC conditional logic

CC MCC +7th **S79.009 Unspecified physeal fracture of upper end of unspecified femur**
> **HAC** 7th character A see Appendix B for HAC conditional logic

+ **S79.01 Salter-Harris Type I physeal fracture of upper end of femur**
> Acute on chronic slipped capital femoral epiphysis (traumatic)
> Acute slipped capital femoral epiphysis (traumatic)
> Capital femoral epiphyseal fracture
> **Excludes1:** chronic slipped upper femoral epiphysis(nontraumatic)(M93.02-)

CC MCC +7th **S79.011 Salter-Harris Type I physeal fracture of upper end of right femur**
> **HAC** 7th character A see Appendix B for HAC conditional logic

CC MCC +7th **S79.012 Salter-Harris Type I physeal fracture of upper end of left femur**
> **HAC** 7th character A see Appendix B for HAC conditional logic

CC MCC +7th **S79.019 Salter-Harris Type I physeal fracture of upper end of unspecified femur**
> **HAC** 7th character A see Appendix B for HAC conditional logic

+ **S79.09 Other physeal fracture of upper end of femur**

CC MCC +7th **S79.091 Other physeal fracture of upper end of right femur**
> **HAC** 7th character A see Appendix B for HAC conditional logic

CC MCC +7th **S79.092 Other physeal fracture of upper end of left femur**
> **HAC** 7th character A see Appendix B for HAC conditional logic

CC MCC +7th **S79.099 Other physeal fracture of upper end of unspecified femur**
> **HAC** 7th character A see Appendix B for HAC conditional logic

+ **S79.1 Physeal fracture of lower end of femur**

+ **S79.10 Unspecified physeal fracture of lower end of femur**

CC +7th **S79.101 Unspecified physeal fracture of lower end of right femur**
> **HAC** 7th character A see Appendix B for HAC conditional logic

CC +7th **S79.102 Unspecified physeal fracture of lower end of left femur**
> **HAC** 7th character A see Appendix B for HAC conditional logic

CC +7th **S79.109 Unspecified physeal fracture of lower end of unspecified femur**
> **HAC** 7th character A see Appendix B for HAC conditional logic

+ **S79.11 Salter-Harris Type I physeal fracture of lower end of femur**

CC +7th **S79.111 Salter-Harris Type I physeal fracture of lower end of right femur**
> **HAC** 7th character A see Appendix B for HAC conditional logic

CC +7th **S79.112 Salter-Harris Type I physeal fracture of lower end of left femur**
> **HAC** 7th character A see Appendix B for HAC conditional logic

CC +7th **S79.119 Salter-Harris Type I physeal fracture of lower end of unspecified femur**
> **HAC** 7th character A see Appendix B for HAC conditional logic

+ **S79.12 Salter-Harris Type II physeal fracture of lower end of femur**

CC +7th **S79.121 Salter-Harris Type II physeal fracture of lower end of right femur**
> **HAC** 7th character A see Appendix B for HAC conditional logic

CC +7th **S79.122 Salter-Harris Type II physeal fracture of lower end of left femur**
> **HAC** 7th character A see Appendix B for HAC conditional logic

CC +7th **S79.129 Salter-Harris Type II physeal fracture of lower end of unspecified femur**
> **HAC** 7th character A see Appendix B for HAC conditional logic

+ **S79.13 Salter-Harris Type III physeal fracture of lower end of femur**

CC +7th **S79.131 Salter-Harris Type III physeal fracture of lower end of right femur**
> **HAC** 7th character A see Appendix B for HAC conditional logic

CC +7th **S79.132 Salter-Harris Type III physeal fracture of lower end of left femur**
> **HAC** 7th character A see Appendix B for HAC conditional logic

CC +7th **S79.139 Salter-Harris Type III physeal fracture of lower end of unspecified femur**
> **HAC** 7th character A see Appendix B for HAC conditional logic

+ **S79.14 Salter-Harris Type IV physeal fracture of lower end of femur**

CC +7th **S79.141 Salter-Harris Type IV physeal fracture of lower end of right femur**
> **HAC** 7th character A see Appendix B for HAC conditional logic

CC +7th **S79.142 Salter-Harris Type IV physeal fracture of lower end of left femur**
> **HAC** 7th character A see Appendix B for HAC conditional logic

CC +7th **S79.149 Salter-Harris Type IV physeal fracture of lower end of unspecified femur**
> **HAC** 7th character A see Appendix B for HAC conditional logic

+ **S79.19 Other physeal fracture of lower end of femur**

CC +7th **S79.191 Other physeal fracture of lower end of right femur**
> **HAC** 7th character A see Appendix B for HAC conditional logic

CC +7th **S79.192 Other physeal fracture of lower end of left femur**
> **HAC** 7th character A see Appendix B for HAC conditional logic

CC +7th **S79.199 Other physeal fracture of lower end of unspecified femur**
> **HAC** 7th character A see Appendix B for HAC conditional logic

+ **S79.8** **Other specified injuries of hip and thigh**

> The appropriate 7th character is to be added to each code in subcategory **S79.8**
> A   initial encounter
> D   subsequent encounter
> S   sequela

  + **S79.81** **Other specified injuries of hip**
    + 7th **S79.811** **Other specified injuries of right hip**
    + 7th **S79.812** **Other specified injuries of left hip**
    + 7th **S79.819** **Other specified injuries of unspecified hip**
  + **S79.82** **Other specified injuries of thigh**
    + 7th **S79.821** **Other specified injuries of right thigh**
    + 7th **S79.822** **Other specified injuries of left thigh**
    + 7th **S79.829** **Other specified injuries of unspecified thigh**

+ **S79.9** **Unspecified injury of hip and thigh**

> The appropriate 7th character is to be added to each code in subcategory **S79.9**
> A - initial encounter
> D - subsequent encounter
> S - sequela

  + **S79.91** **Unspecified injury of hip**
    + 7th **S79.911** **Unspecified injury of right hip**
    + 7th **S79.912** **Unspecified injury of left hip**
    + 7th **S79.919** **Unspecified injury of unspecified hip**
  + **S79.92** **Unspecified injury of thigh**
    + 7th **S79.921** **Unspecified injury of right thigh**
    + 7th **S79.922** **Unspecified injury of left thigh**
    + 7th **S79.929** **Unspecified injury of unspecified thigh**

Injuries to the knee and lower leg (S80-S89)

Excludes2: *burns and corrosions (T20-T32)*
frostbite (T33-T34)
injuries of ankle and foot, except fracture of ankle and malleolus (S90-S99)
insect bite or sting, venomous (T63.4)

S80 **Superficial injury of knee and lower leg**

> **Excludes2:** *superficial injury of ankle and foot (S90.-)*

> The appropriate 7th character is to be added to each code from category S80
> A   initial encounter
> D   subsequent encounter
> S   sequela

+ **S80.0** **Contusion of knee**
  X+7th **S80.00** **Contusion of unspecified knee**
  X+7th **S80.01** **Contusion of right knee**
  X+7th **S80.02** **Contusion of left knee**
+ **S80.1** **Contusion of lower leg**
  X+7th **S80.10** **Contusion of unspecified lower leg**
  X+7th **S80.11** **Contusion of right lower leg**
  X+7th **S80.12** **Contusion of left lower leg**
+ **S80.2** **Other superficial injuries of knee**
  + **S80.21** **Abrasion of knee**
    + 7th **S80.211** **Abrasion, right knee**
    + 7th **S80.212** **Abrasion, left knee**
    + 7th **S80.219** **Abrasion, unspecified knee**
  + **S80.22** **Blister (nonthermal) of knee**
    + 7th **S80.221** **Blister (nonthermal), right knee**
    + 7th **S80.222** **Blister (nonthermal), left knee**
    + 7th **S80.229** **Blister (nonthermal), unspecified knee**
  + **S80.24** **External constriction of knee**
    + 7th **S80.241** **External constriction, right knee**

  + 7th **S80.242** **External constriction, left knee**
  + 7th **S80.249** **External constriction, unspecified knee**
  + **S80.25** **Superficial foreign body of knee**
    Splinter in the knee
    + 7th **S80.251** **Superficial foreign body, right knee**
    + 7th **S80.252** **Superficial foreign body, left knee**
    + 7th **S80.259** **Superficial foreign body, unspecified knee**
  + **S80.26** **Insect bite (nonvenomous) of knee**
    + 7th **S80.261** **Insect bite (nonvenomous), right knee**
    + 7th **S80.262** **Insect bite (nonvenomous), left knee**
    + 7th **S80.269** **Insect bite (nonvenomous), unspecified knee**
  + **S80.27** **Other superficial bite of knee**
    > **Excludes1:** *open bite of knee (S81.05-)*
    + 7th **S80.271** **Other superficial bite of right knee**
    + 7th **S80.272** **Other superficial bite of left knee**
    + 7th **S80.279** **Other superficial bite of unspecified knee**
+ **S80.8** **Other superficial injuries of lower leg**
  + **S80.81** **Abrasion of lower leg**
    + 7th **S80.811** **Abrasion, right lower leg**
    + 7th **S80.812** **Abrasion, left lower leg**
    + 7th **S80.819** **Abrasion, unspecified lower leg**
  + **S80.82** **Blister (nonthermal) of lower leg**
    + 7th **S80.821** **Blister (nonthermal), right lower leg**
    + 7th **S80.822** **Blister (nonthermal), left lower leg**
    + 7th **S80.829** **Blister (nonthermal), unspecified lower leg**
  + **S80.84** **External constriction of lower leg**
    + 7th **S80.841** **External constriction, right lower leg**
    + 7th **S80.842** **External constriction, left lower leg**
    + 7th **S80.849** **External constriction, unspecified lower leg**
  + **S80.85** **Superficial foreign body of lower leg**
    Splinter in the lower leg
    + 7th **S80.851** **Superficial foreign body, right lower leg**
    + 7th **S80.852** **Superficial foreign body, left lower leg**
    + 7th **S80.859** **Superficial foreign body, unspecified lower leg**
  + **S80.86** **Insect bite (nonvenomous) of lower leg**
    + 7th **S80.861** **Insect bite (nonvenomous), right lower leg**
    + 7th **S80.862** **Insect bite (nonvenomous), left lower leg**
    + 7th **S80.869** **Insect bite (nonvenomous), unspecified lower leg**
  + **S80.87** **Other superficial bite of lower leg**
    > **Excludes1:** *open bite of lower leg (S81.85-)*
    + 7th **S80.871** **Other superficial bite, right lower leg**
    + 7th **S80.872** **Other superficial bite, left lower leg**
    + 7th **S80.879** **Other superficial bite, unspecified lower leg**
+ **S80.9** **Unspecified superficial injury of knee and lower leg**
  + **S80.91** **Unspecified superficial injury of knee**
    + 7th **S80.911** **Unspecified superficial injury of right knee**
    + 7th **S80.912** **Unspecified superficial injury of left knee**
    + 7th **S80.919** **Unspecified superficial injury of unspecified knee**
  + **S80.92** **Unspecified superficial injury of lower leg**
    + 7th **S80.921** **Unspecified superficial injury of right lower leg**
    + 7th **S80.922** **Unspecified superficial injury of left lower leg**
    + 7th **S80.929** **Unspecified superficial injury of unspecified lower leg**

S81   Open wound of knee and lower leg

Code also any associated wound infection

Excludes1: *open fracture of knee and lower leg (S82.-)*
traumatic amputation of lower leg (S88.-)

Excludes2: *open wound of ankle and foot (S91.-)*

The appropriate 7th character is to be added to each code from category S81
A   initial encounter
D   subsequent encounter
S   sequela

+   **S81.0   Open wound of knee**

+   **S81.00   Unspecified open wound of knee**

+7th   **S81.001   Unspecified open wound, right knee**
+7th   **S81.002   Unspecified open wound, left knee**
+7th   **S81.009   Unspecified open wound, unspecified knee**

+   **S81.01   Laceration without foreign body of knee**

+7th   **S81.011   Laceration without foreign body, right knee**
+7th   **S81.012   Laceration without foreign body, left knee**
+7th   **S81.019   Laceration without foreign body, unspecified knee**

+   **S81.02   Laceration with foreign body of knee**

+7th   **S81.021   Laceration with foreign body, right knee**
+7th   **S81.022   Laceration with foreign body, left knee**
+7th   **S81.029   Laceration with foreign body, unspecified knee**

+   **S81.03   Puncture wound without foreign body of knee**

+7th   **S81.031   Puncture wound without foreign body, right knee**
+7th   **S81.032   Puncture wound without foreign body, left knee**
+7th   **S81.039   Puncture wound without foreign body, unspecified knee**

+   **S81.04   Puncture wound with foreign body of knee**

+7th   **S81.041   Puncture wound with foreign body, right knee**
+7th   **S81.042   Puncture wound with foreign body, left knee**
+7th   **S81.049   Puncture wound with foreign body, unspecified knee**

+   **S81.05   Open bite of knee**

Bite of knee NOS

Excludes1: *superficial bite of knee (S80.27-)*

+7th   **S81.051   Open bite, right knee**
+7th   **S81.052   Open bite, left knee**
+7th   **S81.059   Open bite, unspecified knee**

+   **S81.8   Open wound of lower leg**

+   **S81.80   Unspecified open wound of lower leg**

+7th   **S81.801   Unspecified open wound, right lower leg**
+7th   **S81.802   Unspecified open wound, left lower leg**
+7th   **S81.809   Unspecified open wound, unspecified lower leg**

+   **S81.81   Laceration without foreign body of lower leg**

+7th   **S81.811   Laceration without foreign body, right lower leg**
+7th   **S81.812   Laceration without foreign body, left lower leg**
+7th   **S81.819   Laceration without foreign body, unspecified lower leg**

+   **S81.82   Laceration with foreign body of lower leg**

+7th   **S81.821   Laceration with foreign body, right lower leg**
+7th   **S81.822   Laceration with foreign body, left lower leg**
+7th   **S81.829   Laceration with foreign body, unspecified lower leg**

+   **S81.83   Puncture wound without foreign body of lower leg**

+7th   **S81.831   Puncture wound without foreign body, right lower leg**
+7th   **S81.832   Puncture wound without foreign body, left lower leg**
+7th   **S81.839   Puncture wound without foreign body, unspecified lower leg**

+   **S81.84   Puncture wound with foreign body of lower leg**

+7th   **S81.841   Puncture wound with foreign body, right lower leg**
AHA CC: 3Q, 2016, 24
+7th   **S81.842   Puncture wound with foreign body, left lower leg**
+7th   **S81.849   Puncture wound with foreign body, unspecified lower leg**

+   **S81.85   Open bite of lower leg**

Bite of lower leg NOS

Excludes1: *superficial bite of lower leg (S80.86-, S80.87-)*

+7th   **S81.851   Open bite, right lower leg**
+7th   **S81.852   Open bite, left lower leg**
+7th   **S81.859   Open bite, unspecified lower leg**

S82   Fracture of lower leg, including ankle

NOTE   A fracture not indicated as displaced or nondisplaced should be coded to displaced
A fracture not indicated as open or closed should be coded to closed
The open fracture designations are based on the Gustilo open fracture classification

Includes: fracture of malleolus

Excludes1: *traumatic amputation of lower leg (S88.-)*

Excludes2: *fracture of foot, except ankle (S92.-)*
periprosthetic fracture of prosthetic implant of knee (M97.0-)

The appropriate 7th character is to be added to all codes from category S82
A   initial encounter for closed fracture
B   initial encounter for open fracture type I or II
     initial encounter for open fracture NOS
C   initial encounter for open fracture type IIIA, IIIB, or IIIC
D   subsequent encounter for closed fracture with routine healing
E   subsequent encounter for open fracture type I or II with routine healing
F   subsequent encounter for open fracture type IIIA, IIIB, or IIIC with routine healing
G   subsequent encounter for closed fracture with delayed healing
H   subsequent encounter for open fracture type I or II with delayed healing
J   subsequent encounter for open fracture type IIIA, IIIB, or IIIC with delayed healing
K   subsequent encounter for closed fracture with nonunion
M   subsequent encounter for open fracture type I or II with nonunion
N   subsequent encounter for open fracture type IIIA, IIIB, or IIIC with nonunion
P   subsequent encounter for closed fracture with malunion
Q   subsequent encounter for open fracture type I or II with malunion
R   subsequent encounter for open fracture type IIIA, IIIB, or IIIC with malunion
S   sequela

Review coding guideline C.19.c

+   **S82.0   Fracture of patella**

Knee cap

+   **S82.00   Unspecified fracture of patella**

CC +7th   **S82.001   Unspecified fracture of right patella**
HAC 7th characters A - C see Appendix B for HAC conditional logic

CC +7th   **S82.002   Unspecified fracture of left patella**
HAC 7th characters A - C see Appendix B for HAC conditional logic

CC +7th   **S82.009   Unspecified fracture of unspecified patella**
HAC 7th characters A - C see Appendix B for HAC conditional logic

+, +7th, X + 7th   ● Newborn   ● Pediatric   ● Maternity   ● Adult   ♀ Female   ♂ Male   Manifestation   Unacceptable PDX   HCC   CC   MCC   **HAC**

+ **S82.01** **Osteochondral fracture of patella**
  - CC +7th **S82.011** **Displaced osteochondral fracture of right patella**
    - HAC 7th characters A - C see Appendix B for HAC conditional logic
  - CC +7th **S82.012** **Displaced osteochondral fracture of left patella**
    - HAC 7th characters A - C see Appendix B for HAC conditional logic
  - CC +7th **S82.013** **Displaced osteochondral fracture of unspecified patella**
    - HAC 7th characters A - C see Appendix B for HAC conditional logic
  - CC +7th **S82.014** **Nondisplaced osteochondral fracture of right patella**
    - HAC 7th characters A - C see Appendix B for HAC conditional logic
  - CC +7th **S82.015** **Nondisplaced osteochondral fracture of left patella**
    - HAC 7th characters A - C see Appendix B for HAC conditional logic
  - CC +7th **S82.016** **Nondisplaced osteochondral fracture of unspecified patella**
    - HAC 7th characters A - C see Appendix B for HAC conditional logic

+ **S82.02** **Longitudinal fracture of patella**
  - CC +7th **S82.021** **Displaced longitudinal fracture of right patella**
    - HAC 7th characters A - C see Appendix B for HAC conditional logic
  - CC +7th **S82.022** **Displaced longitudinal fracture of left patella**
    - HAC 7th characters A - C see Appendix B for HAC conditional logic
  - CC +7th **S82.023** **Displaced longitudinal fracture of unspecified patella**
    - HAC 7th characters A - C see Appendix B for HAC conditional logic
  - CC +7th **S82.024** **Nondisplaced longitudinal fracture of right patella**
    - HAC 7th characters A - C see Appendix B for HAC conditional logic
  - CC +7th **S82.025** **Nondisplaced longitudinal fracture of left patella**
    - HAC 7th characters A - C see Appendix B for HAC conditional logic
  - CC +7th **S82.026** **Nondisplaced longitudinal fracture of unspecified patella**
    - HAC 7th characters A - C see Appendix B for HAC conditional logic

+ **S82.03** **Transverse fracture of patella**
  - CC +7th **S82.031** **Displaced transverse fracture of right patella**
    - HAC 7th characters A - C see Appendix B for HAC conditional logic
  - CC +7th **S82.032** **Displaced transverse fracture of left patella**
    - HAC 7th characters A - C see Appendix B for HAC conditional logic
  - CC +7th **S82.033** **Displaced transverse fracture of unspecified patella**
    - HAC 7th characters A - C see Appendix B for HAC conditional logic
  - CC +7th **S82.034** **Nondisplaced transverse fracture of right patella**
    - HAC 7th characters A - C see Appendix B for HAC conditional logic
  - CC +7th **S82.035** **Nondisplaced transverse fracture of left patella**
    - HAC 7th characters A - C see Appendix B for HAC conditional logic
  - CC +7th **S82.036** **Nondisplaced transverse fracture of unspecified patella**
    - HAC 7th characters A - C see Appendix B for HAC conditional logic

+ **S82.04** **Comminuted fracture of patella**
  - CC +7th **S82.041** **Displaced comminuted fracture of right patella**
    - HAC 7th characters A - C see Appendix B for HAC conditional logic
  - CC +7th **S82.042** **Displaced comminuted fracture of left patella**
    - HAC 7th characters A - C see Appendix B for HAC conditional logic
  - CC +7th **S82.043** **Displaced comminuted fracture of unspecified patella**
    - HAC 7th characters A - C see Appendix B for HAC conditional logic
  - CC +7th **S82.044** **Nondisplaced comminuted fracture of right patella**
    - HAC 7th characters A - C see Appendix B for HAC conditional logic
  - CC +7th **S82.045** **Nondisplaced comminuted fracture of left patella**
    - HAC 7th characters A - C see Appendix B for HAC conditional logic
  - CC +7th **S82.046** **Nondisplaced comminuted fracture of unspecified patella**
    - HAC 7th characters A - C see Appendix B for HAC conditional logic

+ **S82.09** **Other fracture of patella**
  - CC +7th **S82.091** **Other fracture of right patella**
    - HAC 7th characters A - C see Appendix B for HAC conditional logic
  - CC +7th **S82.092** **Other fracture of left patella**
    - HAC 7th characters A - C see Appendix B for HAC conditional logic
  - CC +7th **S82.099** **Other fracture of unspecified patella**
    - HAC 7th characters A - C see Appendix B for HAC conditional logic

+ **S82.1** **Fracture of upper end of tibia**
  Fracture of proximal end of tibia
  Excludes2: *fracture of shaft of tibia (S82.2-)*
  physeal fracture of upper end of tibia (S89.0-)
  + **S82.10** **Unspecified fracture of upper end of tibia**
    - CC MCC +7th **S82.101** **Unspecified fracture of upper end of right tibia**
      - HAC 7th characters A - C see Appendix B for HAC conditional logic
    - CC MCC +7th **S82.102** **Unspecified fracture of upper end of left tibia**
      - HAC 7th characters A - C see Appendix B for HAC conditional logic
    - CC MCC +7th **S82.109** **Unspecified fracture of upper end of unspecified tibia**
      - HAC 7th characters A - C see Appendix B for HAC conditional logic
  + **S82.11** **Fracture of tibial spine**
    - CC MCC +7th **S82.111** **Displaced fracture of right tibial spine**
      - HAC 7th characters A - C see Appendix B for HAC conditional logic
    - CC MCC +7th **S82.112** **Displaced fracture of left tibial spine**
      - HAC 7th characters A - C see Appendix B for HAC conditional logic
    - CC MCC +7th **S82.113** **Displaced fracture of unspecified tibial spine**
      - HAC 7th characters A - C see Appendix B for HAC conditional logic
    - CC MCC +7th **S82.114** **Nondisplaced fracture of right tibial spine**
      - HAC 7th characters A - C see Appendix B for HAC conditional logic
    - CC MCC +7th **S82.115** **Nondisplaced fracture of left tibial spine**
      - HAC 7th characters A - C see Appendix B for HAC conditional logic
    - CC MCC +7th **S82.116** **Nondisplaced fracture of unspecified tibial spine**
      - HAC 7th characters A - C see Appendix B for HAC conditional logic

+, +7th, X + 7th   ● Newborn   ● Pediatric   ● Maternity   ● Adult   ♀ Female   ♂ Male   Manifestation   Unacceptable PDX   HCC   CC   MCC   HAC

+ **S82.12** **Fracture of lateral condyle of tibia**

CC MCC +7th **S82.121** **Displaced fracture of lateral condyle of right tibia**
HAC 7th characters A - C see Appendix B for HAC conditional logic

CC MCC +7th **S82.122** **Displaced fracture of lateral condyle of left tibia**
HAC 7th characters A - C see Appendix B for HAC conditional logic

CC MCC +7th **S82.123** **Displaced fracture of lateral condyle of unspecified tibia**
HAC 7th characters A - C see Appendix B for HAC conditional logic

CC MCC +7th **S82.124** **Nondisplaced fracture of lateral condyle of right tibia**
HAC 7th characters A - C see Appendix B for HAC conditional logic

CC MCC +7th **S82.125** **Nondisplaced fracture of lateral condyle of left tibia**
HAC 7th characters A - C see Appendix B for HAC conditional logic

CC MCC +7th **S82.126** **Nondisplaced fracture of lateral condyle of unspecified tibia**
HAC 7th characters A - C see Appendix B for HAC conditional logic

+ **S82.13** **Fracture of medial condyle of tibia**

CC MCC +7th **S82.131** **Displaced fracture of medial condyle of right tibia**
HAC 7th characters A - C see Appendix B for HAC conditional logic

CC MCC +7th **S82.132** **Displaced fracture of medial condyle of left tibia**
HAC 7th characters A - C see Appendix B for HAC conditional logic

CC MCC +7th **S82.133** **Displaced fracture of medial condyle of unspecified tibia**
HAC 7th characters A - C see Appendix B for HAC conditional logic

CC MCC +7th **S82.134** **Nondisplaced fracture of medial condyle of right tibia**
HAC 7th characters A - C see Appendix B for HAC conditional logic

CC MCC +7th **S82.135** **Nondisplaced fracture of medial condyle of left tibia**
HAC 7th characters A - C see Appendix B for HAC conditional logic

CC MCC +7th **S82.136** **Nondisplaced fracture of medial condyle of unspecified tibia**
HAC 7th characters A - C see Appendix B for HAC conditional logic

+ **S82.14** **Bicondylar fracture of tibia**
Fracture of tibial plateau NOS

CC MCC +7th **S82.141** **Displaced bicondylar fracture of right tibia**
HAC 7th characters A - C see Appendix B for HAC conditional logic

CC MCC +7th **S82.142** **Displaced bicondylar fracture of left tibia**
HAC 7th characters A - C see Appendix B for HAC conditional logic

CC MCC +7th **S82.143** **Displaced bicondylar fracture of unspecified tibia**
HAC 7th characters A - C see Appendix B for HAC conditional logic

CC MCC +7th **S82.144** **Nondisplaced bicondylar fracture of right tibia**
HAC 7th characters A - C see Appendix B for HAC conditional logic

CC MCC +7th **S82.145** **Nondisplaced bicondylar fracture of left tibia**
HAC 7th characters A - C see Appendix B for HAC conditional logic

CC MCC +7th **S82.146** **Nondisplaced bicondylar fracture of unspecified tibia**
HAC 7th characters A - C see Appendix B for HAC conditional logic

+ **S82.15** **Fracture of tibial tuberosity**

CC MCC +7th **S82.151** **Displaced fracture of right tibial tuberosity**
HAC 7th characters A - C see Appendix B for HAC conditional logic

CC MCC +7th **S82.152** **Displaced fracture of left tibial tuberosity**
HAC 7th characters A - C see Appendix B for HAC conditional logic

CC MCC +7th **S82.153** **Displaced fracture of unspecified tibial tuberosity**
HAC 7th characters A - C see Appendix B for HAC conditional logic

CC MCC +7th **S82.154** **Nondisplaced fracture of right tibial tuberosity**
HAC 7th characters A - C see Appendix B for HAC conditional logic

CC MCC +7th **S82.155** **Nondisplaced fracture of left tibial tuberosity**
HAC 7th characters A - C see Appendix B for HAC conditional logic

CC MCC +7th **S82.156** **Nondisplaced fracture of unspecified tibial tuberosity**
HAC 7th characters A - C see Appendix B for HAC conditional logic

+ **S82.16** **Torus fracture of upper end of tibia**

The appropriate 7th character is to be added to all codes in subcategory **S82.16**
A   initial encounter for closed fracture
D   subsequent encounter for fracture with routine healing
G   subsequent encounter for fracture with delayed healing
K   subsequent encounter for fracture with nonunion
P   subsequent encounter for fracture with malunion
S   sequela

CC +7th **S82.161** **Torus fracture of upper end of right tibia**
HAC 7th character A see Appendix B for HAC conditional logic

CC +7th **S82.162** **Torus fracture of upper end of left tibia**
HAC 7th character A see Appendix B for HAC conditional logic

CC +7th **S82.169** **Torus fracture of upper end of unspecified tibia**
HAC 7th character A see Appendix B for HAC conditional logic

+ **S82.19** **Other fracture of upper end of tibia**

CC MCC +7th **S82.191** **Other fracture of upper end of right tibia**
HAC 7th characters A - C see Appendix B for HAC conditional logic

CC MCC +7th **S82.192** **Other fracture of upper end of left tibia**
HAC 7th characters A - C see Appendix B for HAC conditional logic

CC MCC +7th **S82.199** **Other fracture of upper end of unspecified tibia**
HAC 7th characters A - C see Appendix B for HAC conditional logic

+ **S82.2** **Fracture of shaft of tibia**

+ **S82.20** **Unspecified fracture of shaft of tibia**
Fracture of tibia NOS

CC MCC +7th **S82.201** **Unspecified fracture of shaft of right tibia**
HAC 7th characters A - C see Appendix B for HAC conditional logic

CC MCC +7th **S82.202** **Unspecified fracture of shaft of left tibia**
HAC 7th characters A - C see Appendix B for HAC conditional logic

CC MCC +7th **S82.209** **Unspecified fracture of shaft of unspecified tibia**
HAC 7th characters A - C see Appendix B for HAC conditional logic

+ **S82.22** **Transverse fracture of shaft of tibia**

CC MCC +7th **S82.221** **Displaced transverse fracture of shaft of right tibia**
HAC 7th characters A - C see Appendix B for HAC conditional logic

+, +7th, X + 7th   ● Newborn   ● Pediatric   ● Maternity   ● Adult   ♀ Female   ♂ Male   Manifestation   Unacceptable PDX   HCC   CC   MCC   HAC

CC MCC +7th **S82.222** **Displaced transverse fracture of shaft of left tibia**
    HAC 7th characters A - C see Appendix B for HAC conditional logic

CC MCC +7th **S82.223** **Displaced transverse fracture of shaft of unspecified tibia**
    HAC 7th characters A - C see Appendix B for HAC conditional logic

CC MCC +7th **S82.224** **Nondisplaced transverse fracture of shaft of right tibia**
    HAC 7th characters A - C see Appendix B for HAC conditional logic

CC MCC +7th **S82.225** **Nondisplaced transverse fracture of shaft of left tibia**
    HAC 7th characters A - C see Appendix B for HAC conditional logic

CC MCC +7th **S82.226** **Nondisplaced transverse fracture of shaft of unspecified tibia**
    HAC 7th characters A - C see Appendix B for HAC conditional logic

+ **S82.23** **Oblique fracture of shaft of tibia**

CC MCC +7th **S82.231** **Displaced oblique fracture of shaft of right tibia**
    HAC 7th characters A - C see Appendix B for HAC conditional logic

CC MCC +7th **S82.232** **Displaced oblique fracture of shaft of left tibia**
    HAC 7th characters A - C see Appendix B for HAC conditional logic

CC MCC +7th **S82.233** **Displaced oblique fracture of shaft of unspecified tibia**
    HAC 7th characters A - C see Appendix B for HAC conditional logic

CC MCC +7th **S82.234** **Nondisplaced oblique fracture of shaft of right tibia**
    HAC 7th characters A - C see Appendix B for HAC conditional logic
    AHA CC: 1Q, 2015, 3-21

CC MCC +7th **S82.235** **Nondisplaced oblique fracture of shaft of left tibia**
    HAC 7th characters A - C see Appendix B for HAC conditional logic

CC MCC +7th **S82.236** **Nondisplaced oblique fracture of shaft of unspecified tibia**
    HAC 7th characters A - C see Appendix B for HAC conditional logic

+ **S82.24** **Spiral fracture of shaft of tibia**
    Toddler fracture

CC MCC +7th **S82.241** **Displaced spiral fracture of shaft of right tibia**
    HAC 7th characters A - C see Appendix B for HAC conditional logic

CC MCC +7th **S82.242** **Displaced spiral fracture of shaft of left tibia**
    HAC 7th characters A - C see Appendix B for HAC conditional logic

CC MCC +7th **S82.243** **Displaced spiral fracture of shaft of unspecified tibia**
    HAC 7th characters A - C see Appendix B for HAC conditional logic

CC MCC +7th **S82.244** **Nondisplaced spiral fracture of shaft of right tibia**
    HAC 7th characters A - C see Appendix B for HAC conditional logic

CC MCC +7th **S82.245** **Nondisplaced spiral fracture of shaft of left tibia**
    HAC 7th characters A - C see Appendix B for HAC conditional logic

CC MCC +7th **S82.246** **Nondisplaced spiral fracture of shaft of unspecified tibia**
    HAC 7th characters A - C see Appendix B for HAC conditional logic

+ **S82.25** **Comminuted fracture of shaft of tibia**

CC MCC +7th **S82.251** **Displaced comminuted fracture of shaft of right tibia**
    HAC 7th characters A - C see Appendix B for HAC conditional logic
    AHA CC: 2Q, 2015, 6-7

CC MCC +7th **S82.252** **Displaced comminuted fracture of shaft of left tibia**
    HAC 7th characters A - C see Appendix B for HAC conditional logic

CC MCC +7th **S82.253** **Displaced comminuted fracture of shaft of unspecified tibia**
    HAC 7th characters A - C see Appendix B for HAC conditional logic

CC MCC +7th **S82.254** **Nondisplaced comminuted fracture of shaft of right tibia**
    HAC 7th characters A - C see Appendix B for HAC conditional logic

CC MCC +7th **S82.255** **Nondisplaced comminuted fracture of shaft of left tibia**
    HAC 7th characters A - C see Appendix B for HAC conditional logic

CC MCC +7th **S82.256** **Nondisplaced comminuted fracture of shaft of unspecified tibia**
    HAC 7th characters A - C see Appendix B for HAC conditional logic

+ **S82.26** **Segmental fracture of shaft of tibia**

CC MCC +7th **S82.261** **Displaced segmental fracture of shaft of right tibia**
    HAC 7th characters A - C see Appendix B for HAC conditional logic

CC MCC +7th **S82.262** **Displaced segmental fracture of shaft of left tibia**
    HAC 7th characters A - C see Appendix B for HAC conditional logic

CC MCC +7th **S82.263** **Displaced segmental fracture of shaft of unspecified tibia**
    HAC 7th characters A - C see Appendix B for HAC conditional logic

CC MCC +7th **S82.264** **Nondisplaced segmental fracture of shaft of right tibia**
    HAC 7th characters A - C see Appendix B for HAC conditional logic

CC MCC +7th **S82.265** **Nondisplaced segmental fracture of shaft of left tibia**
    HAC 7th characters A - C see Appendix B for HAC conditional logic

CC MCC +7th **S82.266** **Nondisplaced segmental fracture of shaft of unspecified tibia**
    HAC 7th characters A - C see Appendix B for HAC conditional logic

+ **S82.29** **Other fracture of shaft of tibia**

CC MCC +7th **S82.291** **Other fracture of shaft of right tibia**
    HAC 7th characters A - C see Appendix B for HAC conditional logic

CC MCC +7th **S82.292** **Other fracture of shaft of left tibia**
    HAC 7th characters A - C see Appendix B for HAC conditional logic

CC MCC +7th **S82.299** **Other fracture of shaft of unspecified tibia**
    HAC 7th characters A - C see Appendix B for HAC conditional logic

+, +7th, X + 7th   • Newborn   • Pediatric   ● Maternity   ● Adult   ♀ Female   ♂ Male   Manifestation   Unacceptable PDX   HCC   CC   MCC   **HAC**

+ **S82.3 Fracture of lower end of tibia**

   Excludes1: *bimalleolar fracture of lower leg (S82.84-)*
      fracture of medial malleolus alone (S82.5-)
      Maisonneuve's fracture (S82.86-)
      pilon fracture of distal tibia (S82.87-)
      trimalleolar fractures of lower leg (S82.85-)

  + **S82.30 Unspecified fracture of lower end of tibia**

  CC +7th **S82.301 Unspecified fracture of lower end of right tibia**
      HAC 7th characters B & C see Appendix B for HAC conditional logic

  CC +7th **S82.302 Unspecified fracture of lower end of left tibia**
      HAC 7th characters B & C see Appendix B for HAC conditional logic

  CC +7th **S82.309 Unspecified fracture of lower end of unspecified tibia**
      HAC 7th characters B & C see Appendix B for HAC conditional logic

  + **S82.31 Torus fracture of lower end of tibia**

> The appropriate 7th character is to be added to all codes in subcategory **S82.31**
> A   initial encounter for closed fracture
> D   subsequent encounter for fracture with routine healing
> G   subsequent encounter for fracture with delayed healing
> K   subsequent encounter for fracture with nonunion
> P   subsequent encounter for fracture with malunion
> S   sequela

  CC +7th **S82.311 Torus fracture of lower end of right tibia**
      HAC 7th character A see Appendix B for HAC conditional logic

  CC +7th **S82.312 Torus fracture of lower end of left tibia**
      HAC 7th character A see Appendix B for HAC conditional logic

  CC +7th **S82.319 Torus fracture of lower end of unspecified tibia**
      HAC 7th character A see Appendix B for HAC conditional logic

  + **S82.39 Other fracture of lower end of tibia**

  CC +7th **S82.391 Other fracture of lower end of right tibia**
      HAC 7th characters B & C see Appendix B for HAC conditional logic

  CC +7th **S82.392 Other fracture of lower end of left tibia**
      HAC 7th characters B & C see Appendix B for HAC conditional logic
      AHA CC: 1Q, 2015, 25

  CC +7th **S82.399 Other fracture of lower end of unspecified tibia**
      HAC 7th characters B & C see Appendix B for HAC conditional logic

+ **S82.4 Fracture of shaft of fibula**

   Excludes2: *fracture of lateral malleolus alone (S82.6-)*

  + **S82.40 Unspecified fracture of shaft of fibula**

  CC MCC +7th **S82.401 Unspecified fracture of shaft of right fibula**
      HAC 7th characters B & C see Appendix B for HAC conditional logic

  CC MCC +7th **S82.402 Unspecified fracture of shaft of left fibula**
      HAC 7th characters B & C see Appendix B for HAC conditional logic

  CC MCC +7th **S82.409 Unspecified fracture of shaft of unspecified fibula**
      HAC 7th characters B & C see Appendix B for HAC conditional logic

  + **S82.42 Transverse fracture of shaft of fibula**

  CC MCC +7th **S82.421 Displaced transverse fracture of shaft of right fibula**
      HAC 7th characters B & C see Appendix B for HAC conditional logic

  CC MCC +7th **S82.422 Displaced transverse fracture of shaft of left fibula**
      HAC 7th characters B & C see Appendix B for HAC conditional logic

  CC MCC +7th **S82.423 Displaced transverse fracture of shaft of unspecified fibula**
      HAC 7th characters B & C see Appendix B for HAC conditional logic

  CC MCC +7th **S82.424 Nondisplaced transverse fracture of shaft of right fibula**
      HAC 7th characters B & C see Appendix B for HAC conditional logic

  CC MCC +7th **S82.425 Nondisplaced transverse fracture of shaft of left fibula**
      HAC 7th characters B & C see Appendix B for HAC conditional logic

  CC MCC +7th **S82.426 Nondisplaced transverse fracture of shaft of unspecified fibula**
      HAC 7th characters B & C see Appendix B for HAC conditional logic

  + **S82.43 Oblique fracture of shaft of fibula**

  CC MCC +7th **S82.431 Displaced oblique fracture of shaft of right fibula**
      HAC 7th characters B & C see Appendix B for HAC conditional logic

  CC MCC +7th **S82.432 Displaced oblique fracture of shaft of left fibula**
      HAC 7th characters B & C see Appendix B for HAC conditional logic

  CC MCC +7th **S82.433 Displaced oblique fracture of shaft of unspecified fibula**
      HAC 7th characters B & C see Appendix B for HAC conditional logic

  CC MCC +7th **S82.434 Nondisplaced oblique fracture of shaft of right fibula**
      HAC 7th characters B & C see Appendix B for HAC conditional logic

  CC MCC +7th **S82.435 Nondisplaced oblique fracture of shaft of left fibula**
      HAC 7th characters B & C see Appendix B for HAC conditional logic

  CC MCC +7th **S82.436 Nondisplaced oblique fracture of shaft of unspecified fibula**
      HAC 7th characters B & C see Appendix B for HAC conditional logic

  + **S82.44 Spiral fracture of shaft of fibula**

  CC MCC +7th **S82.441 Displaced spiral fracture of shaft of right fibula**
      HAC 7th characters B & C see Appendix B for HAC conditional logic

  CC MCC +7th **S82.442 Displaced spiral fracture of shaft of left fibula**
      HAC 7th characters B & C see Appendix B for HAC conditional logic

  CC MCC +7th **S82.443 Displaced spiral fracture of shaft of unspecified fibula**
      HAC 7th characters B & C see Appendix B for HAC conditional logic

  CC MCC +7th **S82.444 Nondisplaced spiral fracture of shaft of right fibula**
      HAC 7th characters B & C see Appendix B for HAC conditional logic

  CC MCC +7th **S82.445 Nondisplaced spiral fracture of shaft of left fibula**
      HAC 7th characters B & C see Appendix B for HAC conditional logic

  CC MCC +7th **S82.446 Nondisplaced spiral fracture of shaft of unspecified fibula**
      HAC 7th characters B & C see Appendix B for HAC conditional logic

  + **S82.45 Comminuted fracture of shaft of fibula**

  CC MCC +7th **S82.451 Displaced comminuted fracture of shaft of right fibula**
      HAC 7th characters B & C see Appendix B for HAC conditional logic

  CC MCC +7th **S82.452 Displaced comminuted fracture of shaft of left fibula**
      HAC 7th characters B & C see Appendix B for HAC conditional logic

  CC MCC +7th **S82.453 Displaced comminuted fracture of shaft of unspecified fibula**
      HAC 7th characters B & C see Appendix B for HAC conditional logic

  CC MCC +7th **S82.454 Nondisplaced comminuted fracture of shaft of right fibula**
      HAC 7th characters B & C see Appendix B for HAC conditional logic

CC MCC +7th **S82.455** **Nondisplaced comminuted fracture of shaft of left fibula**
HAC 7th characters B & C see Appendix B for HAC conditional logic

CC MCC +7th **S82.456** **Nondisplaced comminuted fracture of shaft of unspecified fibula**
HAC 7th characters B & C see Appendix B for HAC conditional logic

+ **S82.46** **Segmental fracture of shaft of fibula**

CC MCC +7th **S82.461** **Displaced segmental fracture of shaft of right fibula**
HAC 7th characters B & C see Appendix B for HAC conditional logic

CC MCC +7th **S82.462** **Displaced segmental fracture of shaft of left fibula**
HAC 7th characters B & C see Appendix B for HAC conditional logic

CC MCC +7th **S82.463** **Displaced segmental fracture of shaft of unspecified fibula**
HAC 7th characters B & C see Appendix B for HAC conditional logic

CC MCC +7th **S82.464** **Nondisplaced segmental fracture of shaft of right fibula**
HAC 7th characters B & C see Appendix B for HAC conditional logic

CC MCC +7th **S82.465** **Nondisplaced segmental fracture of shaft of left fibula**
HAC 7th characters B & C see Appendix B for HAC conditional logic

CC MCC +7th **S82.466** **Nondisplaced segmental fracture of shaft of unspecified fibula**
HAC 7th characters B & C see Appendix B for HAC conditional logic

+ **S82.49** **Other fracture of shaft of fibula**

CC MCC +7th **S82.491** **Other fracture of shaft of right fibula**
HAC 7th characters B & C see Appendix B for HAC conditional logic

CC MCC +7th **S82.492** **Other fracture of shaft of left fibula**
HAC 7th characters B & C see Appendix B for HAC conditional logic

CC MCC +7th **S82.499** **Other fracture of shaft of unspecified fibula**
HAC 7th characters B & C see Appendix B for HAC conditional logic

+ **S82.5** **Fracture of medial malleolus**
Excludes1: *pilon fracture of distal tibia (S82.87-)*
Salter-Harris type III of lower end of tibia (S89.13-)
Salter-Harris type IV of lower end of tibia (S89.14-)

CC X+7th **S82.51** **Displaced fracture of medial malleolus of right tibia**
HAC 7th characters B & C see Appendix B for HAC conditional logic

CC X+7th **S82.52** **Displaced fracture of medial malleolus of left tibia**
HAC 7th characters B & C see Appendix B for HAC conditional logic

CC X+7th **S82.53** **Displaced fracture of medial malleolus of unspecified tibia**
HAC 7th characters B & C see Appendix B for HAC conditional logic

CC X+7th **S82.54** **Nondisplaced fracture of medial malleolus of right tibia**
HAC 7th characters B & C see Appendix B for HAC conditional logic

CC X+7th **S82.55** **Nondisplaced fracture of medial malleolus of left tibia**
HAC 7th characters B & C see Appendix B for HAC conditional logic

CC X+7th **S82.56** **Nondisplaced fracture of medial malleolus of unspecified tibia**
HAC 7th characters B & C see Appendix B for HAC conditional logic

+ **S82.6** **Fracture of lateral malleolus**
Excludes1: *pilon fracture of distal tibia (S82.87-)*

CC X+7th **S82.61** **Displaced fracture of lateral malleolus of right fibula**
HAC 7th characters B & C see Appendix B for HAC conditional logic

CC X+7th **S82.62** **Displaced fracture of lateral malleolus of left fibula**
HAC 7th characters B & C see Appendix B for HAC conditional logic

CC X+7th **S82.63** **Displaced fracture of lateral malleolus of unspecified fibula**
HAC 7th characters B & C see Appendix B for HAC conditional logic

CC X+7th **S82.64** **Nondisplaced fracture of lateral malleolus of right fibula**
HAC 7th characters B & C see Appendix B for HAC conditional logic

CC X+7th **S82.65** **Nondisplaced fracture of lateral malleolus of left fibula**
HAC 7th characters B & C see Appendix B for HAC conditional logic

CC X+7th **S82.66** **Nondisplaced fracture of lateral malleolus of unspecified fibula**
HAC 7th characters B & C see Appendix B for HAC conditional logic

+ **S82.8** **Other fractures of lower leg**

+ **S82.81** **Torus fracture of upper end of fibula**

The appropriate 7th character is to be added to all codes in subcategory **S82.81**
A   initial encounter for closed fracture
D   subsequent encounter for fracture with routine healing
G   subsequent encounter for fracture with delayed healing
K   subsequent encounter for fracture with nonunion
P   subsequent encounter for fracture with malunion
S   sequela

CC +7th **S82.811** **Torus fracture of upper end of right fibula**

CC +7th **S82.812** **Torus fracture of upper end of left fibula**

CC +7th **S82.819** **Torus fracture of upper end of unspecified fibula**

+ **S82.82** **Torus fracture of lower end of fibula**

The appropriate 7th character is to be added to all codes in subcategory **S82.82**
A   initial encounter for closed fracture
D   subsequent encounter for fracture with routine healing
G   subsequent encounter for fracture with delayed healing
K   subsequent encounter for fracture with nonunion
P   subsequent encounter for fracture with malunion
S   sequela

CC +7th **S82.821** **Torus fracture of lower end of right fibula**

CC +7th **S82.822** **Torus fracture of lower end of left fibula**

CC +7th **S82.829** **Torus fracture of lower end of unspecified fibula**

+ **S82.83** **Other fracture of upper and lower end of fibula**

CC MCC +7th **S82.831** **Other fracture of upper and lower end of right fibula**
HAC 7th characters B & C see Appendix B for HAC conditional logic

CC MCC +7th **S82.832** **Other fracture of upper and lower end of left fibula**
HAC 7th characters B & C see Appendix B for HAC conditional logic
AHA CC: 1Q, 2015, 25

CC MCC +7th **S82.839** **Other fracture of upper and lower end of unspecified fibula**
HAC 7th characters B & C see Appendix B for HAC conditional logic

+, +7th, X + 7th   ● Newborn   ○ Pediatric   ● Maternity   ● Adult   ♀ Female   ♂ Male   Manifestation   Unacceptable PDX   HCC   CC   MCC   HAC

Tears of Meniscus

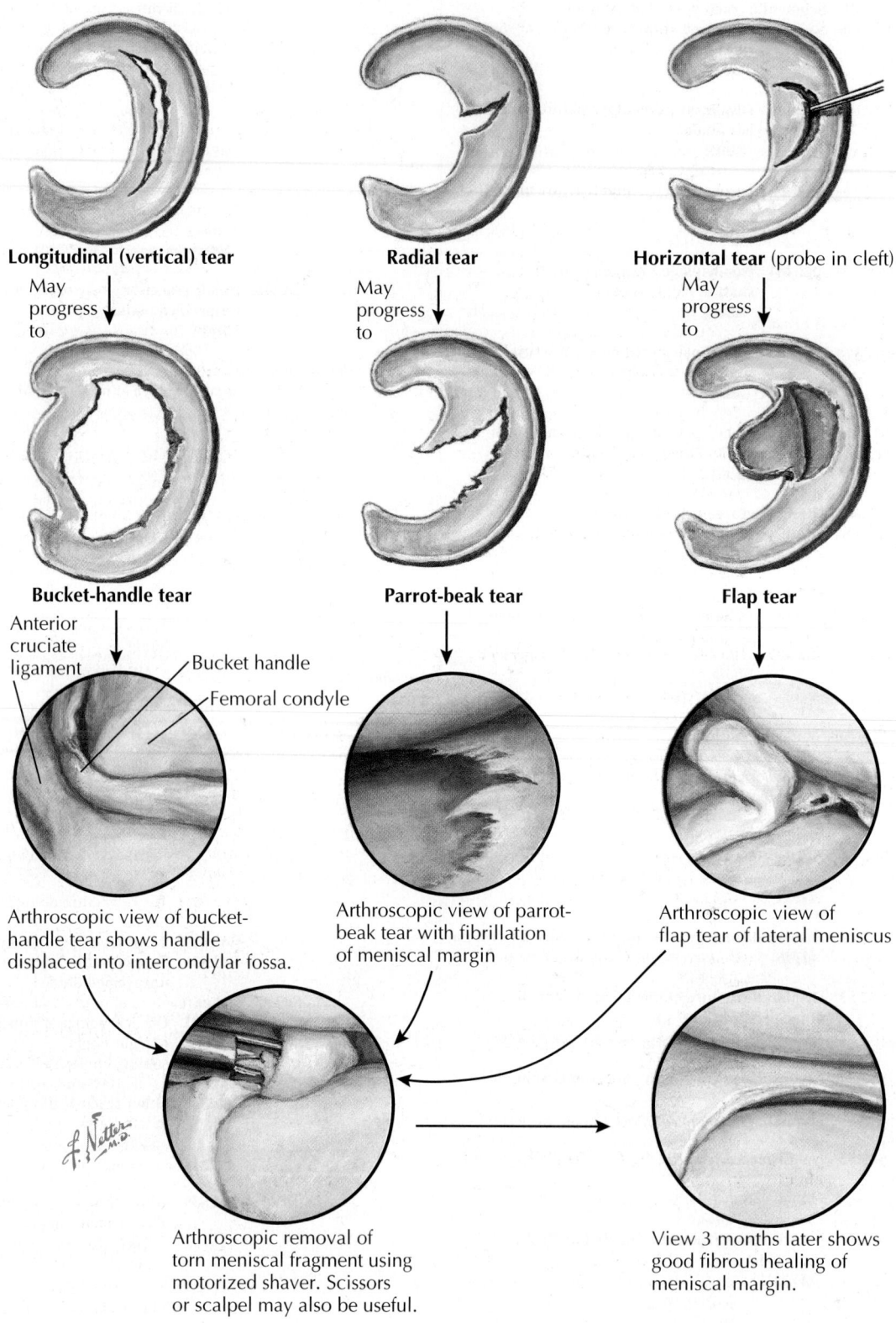

Longitudinal (vertical) tear

May
progress
to

Bucket-handle tear

Anterior
cruciate
ligament

Bucket handle
Femoral condyle

Arthroscopic view of bucket-
handle tear shows handle
displaced into intercondylar fossa.

Radial tear

May
progress
to

Parrot-beak tear

Arthroscopic view of parrot-
beak tear with fibrillation
of meniscal margin

Horizontal tear (probe in cleft)

May
progress
to

Flap tear

Arthroscopic view of
flap tear of lateral meniscus

Arthroscopic removal of
torn meniscal fragment using
motorized shaver. Scissors
or scalpel may also be useful.

View 3 months later shows
good fibrous healing of
meniscal margin.

+ **S82.84** **Bimalleolar fracture of lower leg**

CC +7th **S82.841** **Displaced bimalleolar fracture of right lower leg**

> HAC 7th characters B & C see Appendix B for HAC conditional logic

CC +7th **S82.842** **Displaced bimalleolar fracture of left lower leg**

> HAC 7th characters B & C see Appendix B for HAC conditional logic

CC +7th **S82.843** **Displaced bimalleolar fracture of unspecified lower leg**

> HAC 7th characters B & C see Appendix B for HAC conditional logic

CC +7th **S82.844** **Nondisplaced bimalleolar fracture of right lower leg**

> HAC 7th characters B & C see Appendix B for HAC conditional logic

CC +7th **S82.845** **Nondisplaced bimalleolar fracture of left lower leg**

> HAC 7th characters B & C see Appendix B for HAC conditional logic

CC +7th **S82.846** **Nondisplaced bimalleolar fracture of unspecified lower leg**

> HAC 7th characters B & C see Appendix B for HAC conditional logic

+ **S82.85** **Trimalleolar fracture of lower leg**

CC +7th **S82.851** **Displaced trimalleolar fracture of right lower leg**

> HAC 7th characters B & C see Appendix B for HAC conditional logic

CC +7th **S82.852** **Displaced trimalleolar fracture of left lower leg**

> HAC 7th characters B & C see Appendix B for HAC conditional logic

CC +7th **S82.853** **Displaced trimalleolar fracture of unspecified lower leg**

> HAC 7th characters B & C see Appendix B for HAC conditional logic

CC +7th **S82.854** **Nondisplaced trimalleolar fracture of right lower leg**

> HAC 7th characters B & C see Appendix B for HAC conditional logic

CC +7th **S82.855** **Nondisplaced trimalleolar fracture of left lower leg**

> HAC 7th characters B & C see Appendix B for HAC conditional logic

CC +7th **S82.856** **Nondisplaced trimalleolar fracture of unspecified lower leg**

> HAC 7th characters B & C see Appendix B for HAC conditional logic

+ **S82.86** **Maisonneuve's fracture**

CC MCC +7th **S82.861** **Displaced Maisonneuve's fracture of right leg**

> HAC 7th characters B & C see Appendix B for HAC conditional logic

CC MCC +7th **S82.862** **Displaced Maisonneuve's fracture of left leg**

> HAC 7th characters B & C see Appendix B for HAC conditional logic

CC MCC +7th **S82.863** **Displaced Maisonneuve's fracture of unspecified leg**

> HAC 7th characters B & C see Appendix B for HAC conditional logic

CC MCC +7th **S82.864** **Nondisplaced Maisonneuve's fracture of right leg**

> HAC 7th characters B & C see Appendix B for HAC conditional logic

CC MCC +7th **S82.865** **Nondisplaced Maisonneuve's fracture of left leg**

> HAC 7th characters B & C see Appendix B for HAC conditional logic

CC MCC +7th **S82.866** **Nondisplaced Maisonneuve's fracture of unspecified leg**

> HAC 7th characters B & C see Appendix B for HAC conditional logic

+ **S82.87** **Pilon fracture of tibia**

CC +7th **S82.871** **Displaced pilon fracture of right tibia**

> HAC 7th characters B & C see Appendix B for HAC conditional logic

CC +7th **S82.872** **Displaced pilon fracture of left tibia**

> HAC 7th characters B & C see Appendix B for HAC conditional logic

CC +7th **S82.873** **Displaced pilon fracture of unspecified tibia**

> HAC 7th characters B & C see Appendix B for HAC conditional logic

CC +7th **S82.874** **Nondisplaced pilon fracture of right tibia**

> HAC 7th characters B & C see Appendix B for HAC conditional logic

CC +7th **S82.875** **Nondisplaced pilon fracture of left tibia**

> HAC 7th characters B & C see Appendix B for HAC conditional logic

CC +7th **S82.876** **Nondisplaced pilon fracture of unspecified tibia**

> HAC 7th characters B & C see Appendix B for HAC conditional logic

+ **S82.89** **Other fractures of lower leg**

Fracture of ankle NOS

CC +7th **S82.891** **Other fracture of right lower leg**

> HAC 7th characters B & C see Appendix B for HAC conditional logic

CC +7th **S82.892** **Other fracture of left lower leg**

> HAC 7th characters B & C see Appendix B for HAC conditional logic

CC +7th **S82.899** **Other fracture of unspecified lower leg**

> HAC 7th characters B & C see Appendix B for HAC conditional logic

+ **S82.9** **Unspecified fracture of lower leg**

CC X+7th **S82.90** **Unspecified fracture of unspecified lower leg**

> HAC 7th characters B & C see Appendix B for HAC conditional logic

CC X+7th **S82.91** **Unspecified fracture of right lower leg**

> HAC 7th characters B & C see Appendix B for HAC conditional logic

CC X+7th **S82.92** **Unspecified fracture of left lower leg**

> HAC 7th characters B & C see Appendix B for HAC conditional logic

S83 **Dislocation and sprain of joints and ligaments of knee**

> **Includes:** avulsion of joint or ligament of knee
> laceration of cartilage, joint or ligament of knee
> sprain of cartilage, joint or ligament of knee
> traumatic hemarthrosis of joint or ligament of knee
> traumatic rupture of joint or ligament of knee
> traumatic subluxation of joint or ligament of knee
> traumatic tear of joint or ligament of knee

Code also any associated open wound

> *Excludes2:* *derangement of patella (M22.0-M22.3)*
> *injury of patellar ligament (tendon) (S76.1-)*
> *internal derangement of knee (M23.-)*
> *old dislocation of knee (M24.36)*
> *pathological dislocation of knee (M24.36)*
> *recurrent dislocation of knee (M22.0)*
> *strain of muscle, fascia and tendon of lower leg (S86.-)*

The appropriate 7th character is to be added to each code from category S83
A initial encounter
D subsequent encounter
S sequela

+ **S83.0** **Subluxation and dislocation of patella**

+ **S83.00** **Unspecified subluxation and dislocation of patella**

+7th **S83.001** **Unspecified subluxation of right patella**
+7th **S83.002** **Unspecified subluxation of left patella**
+7th **S83.003** **Unspecified subluxation of unspecified patella**
+7th **S83.004** **Unspecified dislocation of right patella**
+7th **S83.005** **Unspecified dislocation of left patella**
+7th **S83.006** **Unspecified dislocation of unspecified patella**

+ **S83.01** **Lateral subluxation and dislocation of patella**
+7th **S83.011** Lateral subluxation of right patella
+7th **S83.012** Lateral subluxation of left patella
+7th **S83.013** Lateral subluxation of unspecified patella
+7th **S83.014** Lateral dislocation of right patella
+7th **S83.015** Lateral dislocation of left patella
+7th **S83.016** Lateral dislocation of unspecified patella

+ **S83.09** **Other subluxation and dislocation of patella**
+7th **S83.091** Other subluxation of right patella
+7th **S83.092** Other subluxation of left patella
+7th **S83.093** Other subluxation of unspecified patella
+7th **S83.094** Other dislocation of right patella
+7th **S83.095** Other dislocation of left patella
+7th **S83.096** Other dislocation of unspecified patella

+ **S83.1** **Subluxation and dislocation of knee**
Excludes2: *instability of knee prosthesis (T84.022, T84.023)*

+ **S83.10** **Unspecified subluxation and dislocation of knee**
+7th **S83.101** Unspecified subluxation of right knee
+7th **S83.102** Unspecified subluxation of left knee
+7th **S83.103** Unspecified subluxation of unspecified knee
+7th **S83.104** Unspecified dislocation of right knee
+7th **S83.105** Unspecified dislocation of left knee
+7th **S83.106** Unspecified dislocation of unspecified knee

+ **S83.11** **Anterior subluxation and dislocation of proximal end of tibia**
Posterior subluxation and dislocation of distal end of femur
+7th **S83.111** Anterior subluxation of proximal end of tibia, right knee
+7th **S83.112** Anterior subluxation of proximal end of tibia, left knee
+7th **S83.113** Anterior subluxation of proximal end of tibia, unspecified knee
+7th **S83.114** Anterior dislocation of proximal end of tibia, right knee
+7th **S83.115** Anterior dislocation of proximal end of tibia, left knee
+7th **S83.116** Anterior dislocation of proximal end of tibia, unspecified knee

+ **S83.12** **Posterior subluxation and dislocation of proximal end of tibia**
Anterior dislocation of distal end of femur
+7th **S83.121** Posterior subluxation of proximal end of tibia, right knee
+7th **S83.122** Posterior subluxation of proximal end of tibia, left knee
+7th **S83.123** Posterior subluxation of proximal end of tibia, unspecified knee
+7th **S83.124** Posterior dislocation of proximal end of tibia, right knee
+7th **S83.125** Posterior dislocation of proximal end of tibia, left knee
+7th **S83.126** Posterior dislocation of proximal end of tibia, unspecified knee

+ **S83.13** **Medial subluxation and dislocation of proximal end of tibia**
+7th **S83.131** Medial subluxation of proximal end of tibia, right knee
+7th **S83.132** Medial subluxation of proximal end of tibia, left knee
+7th **S83.133** Medial subluxation of proximal end of tibia, unspecified knee
+7th **S83.134** Medial dislocation of proximal end of tibia, right knee
+7th **S83.135** Medial dislocation of proximal end of tibia, left knee
+7th **S83.136** Medial dislocation of proximal end of tibia, unspecified knee

+ **S83.14** **Lateral subluxation and dislocation of proximal end of tibia**
+7th **S83.141** Lateral subluxation of proximal end of tibia, right knee
+7th **S83.142** Lateral subluxation of proximal end of tibia, left knee
+7th **S83.143** Lateral subluxation of proximal end of tibia, unspecified knee
+7th **S83.144** Lateral dislocation of proximal end of tibia, right knee
+7th **S83.145** Lateral dislocation of proximal end of tibia, left knee
+7th **S83.146** Lateral dislocation of proximal end of tibia, unspecified knee

+ **S83.19** **Other subluxation and dislocation of knee**
+7th **S83.191** Other subluxation of right knee
+7th **S83.192** Other subluxation of left knee
+7th **S83.193** Other subluxation of unspecified knee
+7th **S83.194** Other dislocation of right knee
+7th **S83.195** Other dislocation of left knee
+7th **S83.196** Other dislocation of unspecified knee

+ **S83.2** **Tear of meniscus, current injury**
Excludes1: *old bucket-handle tear (M23.2)*

+ **S83.20** **Tear of unspecified meniscus, current injury**
Tear of meniscus of knee NOS
+7th **S83.200** Bucket-handle tear of unspecified meniscus, current injury, right knee
+7th **S83.201** Bucket-handle tear of unspecified meniscus, current injury, left knee
+7th **S83.202** Bucket-handle tear of unspecified meniscus, current injury, unspecified knee
+7th **S83.203** Other tear of unspecified meniscus, current injury, right knee
+7th **S83.204** Other tear of unspecified meniscus, current injury, left knee
+7th **S83.205** Other tear of unspecified meniscus, current injury, unspecified knee
+7th **S83.206** Unspecified tear of unspecified meniscus, current injury, right knee
+7th **S83.207** Unspecified tear of unspecified meniscus, current injury, left knee
+7th **S83.209** Unspecified tear of unspecified meniscus, current injury, unspecified knee

+ **S83.21** **Bucket-handle tear of medial meniscus, current injury**
+7th **S83.211** Bucket-handle tear of medial meniscus, current injury, right knee
+7th **S83.212** Bucket-handle tear of medial meniscus, current injury, left knee
+7th **S83.219** Bucket-handle tear of medial meniscus, current injury, unspecified knee

+ **S83.22** **Peripheral tear of medial meniscus, current injury**
+7th **S83.221** Peripheral tear of medial meniscus, current injury, right knee
+7th **S83.222** Peripheral tear of medial meniscus, current injury, left knee
+7th **S83.229** Peripheral tear of medial meniscus, current injury, unspecified knee

+ **S83.23** **Complex tear of medial meniscus, current injury**
+7th **S83.231** Complex tear of medial meniscus, current injury, right knee
+7th **S83.232** Complex tear of medial meniscus, current injury, left knee
AHA CC: 2Q, 2019, 26
+7th **S83.239** Complex tear of medial meniscus, current injury, unspecified knee

+ **S83.24** **Other tear of medial meniscus, current injury**
+7th **S83.241** Other tear of medial meniscus, current injury, right knee
+7th **S83.242** Other tear of medial meniscus, current injury, left knee
+7th **S83.249** Other tear of medial meniscus, current injury, unspecified knee

+, +7th, X + 7th   ● Newborn   ● Pediatric   ● Maternity   ● Adult   ♀ Female   ♂ Male   Manifestation   Unacceptable PDX   HCC   CC   MCC   HAC

+ **S83.25** **Bucket-handle tear of lateral meniscus, current injury**
- +7th **S83.251** Bucket-handle tear of lateral meniscus, current injury, right knee
- +7th **S83.252** Bucket-handle tear of lateral meniscus, current injury, left knee
- +7th **S83.259** Bucket-handle tear of lateral meniscus, current injury, unspecified knee

+ **S83.26** **Peripheral tear of lateral meniscus, current injury**
- +7th **S83.261** Peripheral tear of lateral meniscus, current injury, right knee
- +7th **S83.262** Peripheral tear of lateral meniscus, current injury, left knee
- +7th **S83.269** Peripheral tear of lateral meniscus, current injury, unspecified knee

+ **S83.27** **Complex tear of lateral meniscus, current injury**
- +7th **S83.271** Complex tear of lateral meniscus, current injury, right knee
- +7th **S83.272** Complex tear of lateral meniscus, current injury, left knee
- +7th **S83.279** Complex tear of lateral meniscus, current injury, unspecified knee

+ **S83.28** **Other tear of lateral meniscus, current injury**
- +7th **S83.281** Other tear of lateral meniscus, current injury, right knee
- +7th **S83.282** Other tear of lateral meniscus, current injury, left knee
- +7th **S83.289** Other tear of lateral meniscus, current injury, unspecified knee

+ **S83.3** **Tear of articular cartilage of knee, current**
- X+7th **S83.30** Tear of articular cartilage of unspecified knee, current
- X+7th **S83.31** Tear of articular cartilage of right knee, current
- X+7th **S83.32** Tear of articular cartilage of left knee, current

+ **S83.4** **Sprain of collateral ligament of knee**
+ **S83.40** **Sprain of unspecified collateral ligament of knee**
- +7th **S83.401** Sprain of unspecified collateral ligament of right knee
- +7th **S83.402** Sprain of unspecified collateral ligament of left knee
- +7th **S83.409** Sprain of unspecified collateral ligament of unspecified knee

+ **S83.41** **Sprain of medial collateral ligament of knee**
  Sprain of tibial collateral ligament
- +7th **S83.411** Sprain of medial collateral ligament of right knee
- +7th **S83.412** Sprain of medial collateral ligament of left knee
- +7th **S83.419** Sprain of medial collateral ligament of unspecified knee

+ **S83.42** **Sprain of lateral collateral ligament of knee**
  Sprain of fibular collateral ligament
- +7th **S83.421** Sprain of lateral collateral ligament of right knee
- +7th **S83.422** Sprain of lateral collateral ligament of left knee
- +7th **S83.429** Sprain of lateral collateral ligament of unspecified knee

+ **S83.5** **Sprain of cruciate ligament of knee**
+ **S83.50** **Sprain of unspecified cruciate ligament of knee**
- +7th **S83.501** Sprain of unspecified cruciate ligament of right knee
- +7th **S83.502** Sprain of unspecified cruciate ligament of left knee
- +7th **S83.509** Sprain of unspecified cruciate ligament of unspecified knee

+ **S83.51** **Sprain of anterior cruciate ligament of knee**
- +7th **S83.511** Sprain of anterior cruciate ligament of right knee
  AHA CC: 2Q, 2016, 3–4
- +7th **S83.512** Sprain of anterior cruciate ligament of left knee
- +7th **S83.519** Sprain of anterior cruciate ligament of unspecified knee

+ **S83.52** **Sprain of posterior cruciate ligament of knee**
- +7th **S83.521** Sprain of posterior cruciate ligament of right knee
- +7th **S83.522** Sprain of posterior cruciate ligament of left knee
- +7th **S83.529** Sprain of posterior cruciate ligament of unspecified knee

+ **S83.6** **Sprain of the superior tibiofibular joint and ligament**
- X+7th **S83.60** Sprain of the superior tibiofibular joint and ligament, unspecified knee
- X+7th **S83.61** Sprain of the superior tibiofibular joint and ligament, right knee
- X+7th **S83.62** Sprain of the superior tibiofibular joint and ligament, left knee

+ **S83.8** **Sprain of other specified parts of knee**
+ **S83.8X** **Sprain of other specified parts of knee**
- +7th **S83.8X1** Sprain of other specified parts of right knee
- +7th **S83.8X2** Sprain of other specified parts of left knee
- +7th **S83.8X9** Sprain of other specified parts of unspecified knee

+ **S83.9** **Sprain of unspecified site of knee**
- X+7th **S83.90** Sprain of unspecified site of unspecified knee
- X+7th **S83.91** Sprain of unspecified site of right knee
- X+7th **S83.92** Sprain of unspecified site of left knee

S84 **Injury of nerves at lower leg level**
Code also any associated open wound (S81.-)
Excludes2: *injury of nerves at ankle and foot level (S94.-)*

The appropriate 7th character is to be added to each code from category S84
A   initial encounter
D   subsequent encounter
S   sequela

+ **S84.0** **Injury of tibial nerve at lower leg level**
- X+7th **S84.00** Injury of tibial nerve at lower leg level, unspecified leg
- X+7th **S84.01** Injury of tibial nerve at lower leg level, right leg
- X+7th **S84.02** Injury of tibial nerve at lower leg level, left leg

+ **S84.1** **Injury of peroneal nerve at lower leg level**
- X+7th **S84.10** Injury of peroneal nerve at lower leg level, unspecified leg
- X+7th **S84.11** Injury of peroneal nerve at lower leg level, right leg
- X+7th **S84.12** Injury of peroneal nerve at lower leg level, left leg

+ **S84.2** **Injury of cutaneous sensory nerve at lower leg level**
- X+7th **S84.20** Injury of cutaneous sensory nerve at lower leg level, unspecified leg
- X+7th **S84.21** Injury of cutaneous sensory nerve at lower leg level, right leg
- X+7th **S84.22** Injury of cutaneous sensory nerve at lower leg level, left leg

+ **S84.8** **Injury of other nerves at lower leg level**
+ **S84.80** **Injury of other nerves at lower leg level**
- +7th **S84.801** Injury of other nerves at lower leg level, right leg
- +7th **S84.802** Injury of other nerves at lower leg level, left leg
- +7th **S84.809** Injury of other nerves at lower leg level, unspecified leg

+ **S84.9** **Injury of unspecified nerve at lower leg level**
- X+7th **S84.90** Injury of unspecified nerve at lower leg level, unspecified leg
- X+7th **S84.91** Injury of unspecified nerve at lower leg level, right leg
- X+7th **S84.92** Injury of unspecified nerve at lower leg level, left leg

+, +7th, X + 7th   • Newborn   • Pediatric   • Maternity   • Adult   ♀ Female   ♂ Male   Manifestation   Unacceptable PDX   HCC   CC   MCC   HAC

S85 Injury of blood vessels at lower leg level

Code also any associated open wound (S81.-)

Excludes2: *injury of blood vessels at ankle and foot level (S95.-)*

The appropriate 7th character is to be added to each code from category S85
A   initial encounter
D   subsequent encounter
S   sequela

+ **S85.0 Injury of popliteal artery**
  + **S85.00 Unspecified injury of popliteal artery**
    MCC +7th **S85.001** Unspecified injury of popliteal artery, right leg
    MCC +7th **S85.002** Unspecified injury of popliteal artery, left leg
    MCC +7th **S85.009** Unspecified injury of popliteal artery, unspecified leg
  + **S85.01 Laceration of popliteal artery**
    MCC +7th **S85.011** Laceration of popliteal artery, right leg
    MCC +7th **S85.012** Laceration of popliteal artery, left leg
    MCC +7th **S85.019** Laceration of popliteal artery, unspecified leg
  + **S85.09 Other specified injury of popliteal artery**
    MCC +7th **S85.091** Other specified injury of popliteal artery, right leg
    MCC +7th **S85.092** Other specified injury of popliteal artery, left leg
    MCC +7th **S85.099** Other specified injury of popliteal artery, unspecified leg
+ **S85.1 Injury of tibial artery**
  + **S85.10 Unspecified injury of unspecified tibial artery**
    Injury of tibial artery NOS
    CC +7th **S85.101** Unspecified injury of unspecified tibial artery, right leg
    CC +7th **S85.102** Unspecified injury of unspecified tibial artery, left leg
    CC +7th **S85.109** Unspecified injury of unspecified tibial artery, unspecified leg
  + **S85.11 Laceration of unspecified tibial artery**
    CC +7th **S85.111** Laceration of unspecified tibial artery, right leg
    CC +7th **S85.112** Laceration of unspecified tibial artery, left leg
    CC +7th **S85.119** Laceration of unspecified tibial artery, unspecified leg
  + **S85.12 Other specified injury of unspecified tibial artery**
    CC +7th **S85.121** Other specified injury of unspecified tibial artery, right leg
    CC +7th **S85.122** Other specified injury of unspecified tibial artery, left leg
    CC +7th **S85.129** Other specified injury of unspecified tibial artery, unspecified leg
  + **S85.13 Unspecified injury of anterior tibial artery**
    CC +7th **S85.131** Unspecified injury of anterior tibial artery, right leg
    CC +7th **S85.132** Unspecified injury of anterior tibial artery, left leg
    CC +7th **S85.139** Unspecified injury of anterior tibial artery, unspecified leg
  + **S85.14 Laceration of anterior tibial artery**
    CC +7th **S85.141** Laceration of anterior tibial artery, right leg
    CC +7th **S85.142** Laceration of anterior tibial artery, left leg
    CC +7th **S85.149** Laceration of anterior tibial artery, unspecified leg
  + **S85.15 Other specified injury of anterior tibial artery**
    CC +7th **S85.151** Other specified injury of anterior tibial artery, right leg
    CC +7th **S85.152** Other specified injury of anterior tibial artery, left leg
    CC +7th **S85.159** Other specified injury of anterior tibial artery, unspecified leg
  + **S85.16 Unspecified injury of posterior tibial artery**
    CC +7th **S85.161** Unspecified injury of posterior tibial artery, right leg
    CC +7th **S85.162** Unspecified injury of posterior tibial artery, left leg
    CC +7th **S85.169** Unspecified injury of posterior tibial artery, unspecified leg

+ **S85.17 Laceration of posterior tibial artery**
  CC +7th **S85.171** Laceration of posterior tibial artery, right leg
  CC +7th **S85.172** Laceration of posterior tibial artery, left leg
  CC +7th **S85.179** Laceration of posterior tibial artery, unspecified leg
+ **S85.18 Other specified injury of posterior tibial artery**
  CC +7th **S85.181** Other specified injury of posterior tibial artery, right leg
  CC +7th **S85.182** Other specified injury of posterior tibial artery, left leg
  CC +7th **S85.189** Other specified injury of posterior tibial artery, unspecified leg
+ **S85.2 Injury of peroneal artery**
  + **S85.20 Unspecified injury of peroneal artery**
    CC +7th **S85.201** Unspecified injury of peroneal artery, right leg
    CC +7th **S85.202** Unspecified injury of peroneal artery, left leg
    CC +7th **S85.209** Unspecified injury of peroneal artery, unspecified leg
  + **S85.21 Laceration of peroneal artery**
    CC +7th **S85.211** Laceration of peroneal artery, right leg
    CC +7th **S85.212** Laceration of peroneal artery, left leg
    CC +7th **S85.219** Laceration of peroneal artery, unspecified leg
  + **S85.29 Other specified injury of peroneal artery**
    CC +7th **S85.291** Other specified injury of peroneal artery, right leg
    CC +7th **S85.292** Other specified injury of peroneal artery, left leg
    CC +7th **S85.299** Other specified injury of peroneal artery, unspecified leg
+ **S85.3 Injury of greater saphenous vein at lower leg level**
  Injury of greater saphenous vein NOS
  Injury of saphenous vein NOS
  + **S85.30 Unspecified injury of greater saphenous vein at lower leg level**
    CC +7th **S85.301** Unspecified injury of greater saphenous vein at lower leg level, right leg
    CC +7th **S85.302** Unspecified injury of greater saphenous vein at lower leg level, left leg
    CC +7th **S85.309** Unspecified injury of greater saphenous vein at lower leg level, unspecified leg
  + **S85.31 Laceration of greater saphenous vein at lower leg level**
    CC +7th **S85.311** Laceration of greater saphenous vein at lower leg level, right leg
    CC +7th **S85.312** Laceration of greater saphenous vein at lower leg level, left leg
    CC +7th **S85.319** Laceration of greater saphenous vein at lower leg level, unspecified leg
  + **S85.39 Other specified injury of greater saphenous vein at lower leg level**
    CC +7th **S85.391** Other specified injury of greater saphenous vein at lower leg level, right leg
    CC +7th **S85.392** Other specified injury of greater saphenous vein at lower leg level, left leg
    CC +7th **S85.399** Other specified injury of greater saphenous vein at lower leg level, unspecified leg
+ **S85.4 Injury of lesser saphenous vein at lower leg level**
  + **S85.40 Unspecified injury of lesser saphenous vein at lower leg level**
    CC +7th **S85.401** Unspecified injury of lesser saphenous vein at lower leg level, right leg
    CC +7th **S85.402** Unspecified injury of lesser saphenous vein at lower leg level, left leg
    CC +7th **S85.409** Unspecified injury of lesser saphenous vein at lower leg level, unspecified leg
  + **S85.41 Laceration of lesser saphenous vein at lower leg level**
    CC +7th **S85.411** Laceration of lesser saphenous vein at lower leg level, right leg
    CC +7th **S85.412** Laceration of lesser saphenous vein at lower leg level, left leg
    CC +7th **S85.419** Laceration of lesser saphenous vein at lower leg level, unspecified leg

+ **S85.49** Other specified injury of lesser saphenous vein at lower leg level

CC +7th **S85.491** Other specified injury of lesser saphenous vein at lower leg level, right leg

CC +7th **S85.492** Other specified injury of lesser saphenous vein at lower leg level, left leg

CC +7th **S85.499** Other specified injury of lesser saphenous vein at lower leg level, unspecified leg

+ **S85.5** Injury of popliteal vein

+ **S85.50** Unspecified injury of popliteal vein

MCC +7th **S85.501** Unspecified injury of popliteal vein, right leg

MCC +7th **S85.502** Unspecified injury of popliteal vein, left leg

MCC +7th **S85.509** Unspecified injury of popliteal vein, unspecified leg

+ **S85.51** Laceration of popliteal vein

MCC +7th **S85.511** Laceration of popliteal vein, right leg

MCC +7th **S85.512** Laceration of popliteal vein, left leg

MCC +7th **S85.519** Laceration of popliteal vein, unspecified leg

+ **S85.59** Other specified injury of popliteal vein

MCC +7th **S85.591** Other specified injury of popliteal vein, right leg

MCC +7th **S85.592** Other specified injury of popliteal vein, left leg

MCC +7th **S85.599** Other specified injury of popliteal vein, unspecified leg

+ **S85.8** Injury of other blood vessels at lower leg level

+ **S85.80** Unspecified injury of other blood vessels at lower leg level

CC +7th **S85.801** Unspecified injury of other blood vessels at lower leg level, right leg

CC +7th **S85.802** Unspecified injury of other blood vessels at lower leg level, left leg

CC +7th **S85.809** Unspecified injury of other blood vessels at lower leg level, unspecified leg

+ **S85.81** Laceration of other blood vessels at lower leg level

CC +7th **S85.811** Laceration of other blood vessels at lower leg level, right leg

CC +7th **S85.812** Laceration of other blood vessels at lower leg level, left leg

CC +7th **S85.819** Laceration of other blood vessels at lower leg level, unspecified leg

+ **S85.89** Other specified injury of other blood vessels at lower leg level

CC +7th **S85.891** Other specified injury of other blood vessels at lower leg level, right leg

CC +7th **S85.892** Other specified injury of other blood vessels at lower leg level, left leg

CC +7th **S85.899** Other specified injury of other blood vessels at lower leg level, unspecified leg

+ **S85.9** Injury of unspecified blood vessel at lower leg level

+ **S85.90** Unspecified injury of unspecified blood vessel at lower leg level

CC +7th **S85.901** Unspecified injury of unspecified blood vessel at lower leg level, right leg

CC +7th **S85.902** Unspecified injury of unspecified blood vessel at lower leg level, left leg

CC +7th **S85.909** Unspecified injury of unspecified blood vessel at lower leg level, unspecified leg

+ **S85.91** Laceration of unspecified blood vessel at lower leg level

CC +7th **S85.911** Laceration of unspecified blood vessel at lower leg level, right leg

CC +7th **S85.912** Laceration of unspecified blood vessel at lower leg level, left leg

CC +7th **S85.919** Laceration of unspecified blood vessel at lower leg level, unspecified leg

+ **S85.99** Other specified injury of unspecified blood vessel at lower leg level

CC +7th **S85.991** Other specified injury of unspecified blood vessel at lower leg level, right leg

CC +7th **S85.992** Other specified injury of unspecified blood vessel at lower leg level, left leg

CC +7th **S85.999** Other specified injury of unspecified blood vessel at lower leg level, unspecified leg

S86 Injury of muscle, fascia and tendon at lower leg level

Code also any associated open wound (S81.-)

Excludes2: *injury of muscle, fascia and tendon at ankle (S96.-)*
injury of patellar ligament (tendon) (S76.1-)
sprain of joints and ligaments of knee (S83.-)

The appropriate 7th character is to be added to each code from category S86
A initial encounter
D subsequent encounter
S sequela

+ **S86.0** Injury of Achilles tendon

+ **S86.00** Unspecified injury of Achilles tendon

+7th **S86.001** Unspecified injury of right Achilles tendon

+7th **S86.002** Unspecified injury of left Achilles tendon

+7th **S86.009** Unspecified injury of unspecified Achilles tendon

+ **S86.01** Strain of Achilles tendon

+7th **S86.011** Strain of right Achilles tendon

+7th **S86.012** Strain of left Achilles tendon

+7th **S86.019** Strain of unspecified Achilles tendon

+ **S86.02** Laceration of Achilles tendon

CC +7th **S86.021** Laceration of right Achilles tendon

CC +7th **S86.022** Laceration of left Achilles tendon

CC +7th **S86.029** Laceration of unspecified Achilles tendon

+ **S86.09** Other specified injury of Achilles tendon

+7th **S86.091** Other specified injury of right Achilles tendon

+7th **S86.092** Other specified injury of left Achilles tendon

+7th **S86.099** Other specified injury of unspecified Achilles tendon

+ **S86.1** Injury of other muscle(s) and tendon(s) of posterior muscle group at lower leg level

+ **S86.10** Unspecified injury of other muscle(s) and tendon(s) of posterior muscle group at lower leg level

+7th **S86.101** Unspecified injury of other muscle(s) and tendon(s) of posterior muscle group at lower leg level, right leg

+7th **S86.102** Unspecified injury of other muscle(s) and tendon(s) of posterior muscle group at lower leg level, left leg

+7th **S86.109** Unspecified injury of other muscle(s) and tendon(s) of posterior muscle group at lower leg level, unspecified leg

+ **S86.11** Strain of other muscle(s) and tendon(s) of posterior muscle group at lower leg level

+7th **S86.111** Strain of other muscle(s) and tendon(s) of posterior muscle group at lower leg level, right leg

+7th **S86.112** Strain of other muscle(s) and tendon(s) of posterior muscle group at lower leg level, left leg

+7th **S86.119** Strain of other muscle(s) and tendon(s) of posterior muscle group at lower leg level, unspecified leg

+ **S86.12** Laceration of other muscle(s) and tendon(s) of posterior muscle group at lower leg level

CC +7th **S86.121** Laceration of other muscle(s) and tendon(s) of posterior muscle group at lower leg level, right leg

CC +7th **S86.122** Laceration of other muscle(s) and tendon(s) of posterior muscle group at lower leg level, left leg

CC +7th **S86.129** Laceration of other muscle(s) and tendon(s) of posterior muscle group at lower leg level, unspecified leg

+ **S86.19** Other injury of other muscle(s) and tendon(s) of posterior muscle group at lower leg level

+7th **S86.191** Other injury of other muscle(s) and tendon(s) of posterior muscle group at lower leg level, right leg

+7th **S86.192** Other injury of other muscle(s) and tendon(s) of posterior muscle group at lower leg level, left leg

+7th **S86.199** Other injury of other muscle(s) and tendon(s) of posterior muscle group at lower leg level, unspecified leg

+ **S86.2** Injury of muscle(s) and tendon(s) of anterior muscle group at lower leg level
  + **S86.20** Unspecified injury of muscle(s) and tendon(s) of anterior muscle group at lower leg level
    - +7th **S86.201** Unspecified injury of muscle(s) and tendon(s) of anterior muscle group at lower leg level, right leg
    - +7th **S86.202** Unspecified injury of muscle(s) and tendon(s) of anterior muscle group at lower leg level, left leg
    - +7th **S86.209** Unspecified injury of muscle(s) and tendon(s) of anterior muscle group at lower leg level, unspecified leg
  + **S86.21** Strain of muscle(s) and tendon(s) of anterior muscle group at lower leg level
    - +7th **S86.211** Strain of muscle(s) and tendon(s) of anterior muscle group at lower leg level, right leg
    - +7th **S86.212** Strain of muscle(s) and tendon(s) of anterior muscle group at lower leg level, left leg
    - +7th **S86.219** Strain of muscle(s) and tendon(s) of anterior muscle group at lower leg level, unspecified leg
  + **S86.22** Laceration of muscle(s) and tendon(s) of anterior muscle group at lower leg level
    - CC +7th **S86.221** Laceration of muscle(s) and tendon(s) of anterior muscle group at lower leg level, right leg
    - CC +7th **S86.222** Laceration of muscle(s) and tendon(s) of anterior muscle group at lower leg level, left leg
    - CC +7th **S86.229** Laceration of muscle(s) and tendon(s) of anterior muscle group at lower leg level, unspecified leg
  + **S86.29** Other injury of muscle(s) and tendon(s) of anterior muscle group at lower leg level
    - +7th **S86.291** Other injury of muscle(s) and tendon(s) of anterior muscle group at lower leg level, right leg
    - +7th **S86.292** Other injury of muscle(s) and tendon(s) of anterior muscle group at lower leg level, left leg
    - +7th **S86.299** Other injury of muscle(s) and tendon(s) of anterior muscle group at lower leg level, unspecified leg

+ **S86.3** Injury of muscle(s) and tendon(s) of peroneal muscle group at lower leg level
  + **S86.30** Unspecified injury of muscle(s) and tendon(s) of peroneal muscle group at lower leg level
    - +7th **S86.301** Unspecified injury of muscle(s) and tendon(s) of peroneal muscle group at lower leg level, right leg
    - +7th **S86.302** Unspecified injury of muscle(s) and tendon(s) of peroneal muscle group at lower leg level, left leg
    - +7th **S86.309** Unspecified injury of muscle(s) and tendon(s) of peroneal muscle group at lower leg level, unspecified leg
  + **S86.31** Strain of muscle(s) and tendon(s) of peroneal muscle group at lower leg level
    - +7th **S86.311** Strain of muscle(s) and tendon(s) of peroneal muscle group at lower leg level, right leg
    - +7th **S86.312** Strain of muscle(s) and tendon(s) of peroneal muscle group at lower leg level, left leg
    - +7th **S86.319** Strain of muscle(s) and tendon(s) of peroneal muscle group at lower leg level, unspecified leg
  + **S86.32** Laceration of muscle(s) and tendon(s) of peroneal muscle group at lower leg level
    - CC +7th **S86.321** Laceration of muscle(s) and tendon(s) of peroneal muscle group at lower leg level, right leg
    - CC +7th **S86.322** Laceration of muscle(s) and tendon(s) of peroneal muscle group at lower leg level, left leg
    - CC +7th **S86.329** Laceration of muscle(s) and tendon(s) of peroneal muscle group at lower leg level, unspecified leg

+ **S86.39** Other injury of muscle(s) and tendon(s) of peroneal muscle group at lower leg level
  - +7th **S86.391** Other injury of muscle(s) and tendon(s) of peroneal muscle group at lower leg level, right leg
  - +7th **S86.392** Other injury of muscle(s) and tendon(s) of peroneal muscle group at lower leg level, left leg
  - +7th **S86.399** Other injury of muscle(s) and tendon(s) of peroneal muscle group at lower leg level, unspecified leg

+ **S86.8** Injury of other muscles and tendons at lower leg level
  + **S86.80** Unspecified injury of other muscles and tendons at lower leg level
    + **S86.801** Unspecified injury of other muscle(s) and tendon(s) at lower leg level, right leg
    + **S86.802** Unspecified injury of other muscle(s) and tendon(s) at lower leg level, left leg
    + **S86.809** Unspecified injury of other muscle(s) and tendon(s) at lower leg level, unspecified leg
  + **S86.81** Strain of other muscles and tendons at lower leg level
    - +7th **S86.811** Strain of other muscle(s) and tendon(s) at lower leg level, right leg
    - +7th **S86.812** Strain of other muscle(s) and tendon(s) at lower leg level, left leg
    - +7th **S86.819** Strain of other muscle(s) and tendon(s) at lower leg level, unspecified leg
  + **S86.82** Laceration of other muscles and tendons at lower leg level
    - CC +7th **S86.821** Laceration of other muscle(s) and tendon(s) at lower leg level, right leg
    - CC +7th **S86.822** Laceration of other muscle(s) and tendon(s) at lower leg level, left leg
    - CC +7th **S86.829** Laceration of other muscle(s) and tendon(s) at lower leg level, unspecified leg
  + **S86.89** Other injury of other muscles and tendons at lower leg level
    - +7th **S86.891** Other injury of other muscle(s) and tendon(s) at lower leg level, right leg
    - +7th **S86.892** Other injury of other muscle(s) and tendon(s) at lower leg level, left leg
    - +7th **S86.899** Other injury of other muscle(s) and tendon(s) at lower leg level, unspecified leg

+ **S86.9** Injury of unspecified muscle and tendon at lower leg level
  + **S86.90** Unspecified injury of unspecified muscle and tendon at lower leg level
    - +7th **S86.901** Unspecified injury of unspecified muscle(s) and tendon(s) at lower leg level, right leg
    - +7th **S86.902** Unspecified injury of unspecified muscle(s) and tendon(s) at lower leg level, left leg
    - +7th **S86.909** Unspecified injury of unspecified muscle(s) and tendon(s) at lower leg level, unspecified leg
  + **S86.91** Strain of unspecified muscle and tendon at lower leg level
    - +7th **S86.911** Strain of unspecified muscle(s) and tendon(s) at lower leg level, right leg
    - +7th **S86.912** Strain of unspecified muscle(s) and tendon(s) at lower leg level, left leg
    - +7th **S86.919** Strain of unspecified muscle(s) and tendon(s) at lower leg level, unspecified leg
  + **S86.92** Laceration of unspecified muscle and tendon at lower leg level
    - CC +7th **S86.921** Laceration of unspecified muscle(s) and tendon(s) at lower leg level, right leg
    - CC +7th **S86.922** Laceration of unspecified muscle(s) and tendon(s) at lower leg level, left leg
    - CC +7th **S86.929** Laceration of unspecified muscle(s) and tendon(s) at lower leg level, unspecified leg

+ **S86.99** **Other injury of unspecified muscle and tendon at lower leg level**
  +7th **S86.991** Other injury of unspecified muscle(s) and tendon(s) at lower leg level, right leg
  +7th **S86.992** Other injury of unspecified muscle(s) and tendon(s) at lower leg level, left leg
  +7th **S86.999** Other injury of unspecified muscle(s) and tendon(s) at lower leg level, unspecified leg

S87 **Crushing injury of lower leg**

Use additional code(s) for all associated injuries
Excludes2: crushing injury of ankle and foot (S97.-)

The appropriate 7th character is to be added to each code from category S87
A   initial encounter
D   subsequent encounter
S   sequela

+ **S87.0** **Crushing injury of knee**
  X+7th **S87.00** Crushing injury of unspecified knee
  X+7th **S87.01** Crushing injury of right knee
  X+7th **S87.02** Crushing injury of left knee
+ **S87.8** **Crushing injury of lower leg**
  X+7th **S87.80** Crushing injury of unspecified lower leg
  X+7th **S87.81** Crushing injury of right lower leg
  X+7th **S87.82** Crushing injury of left lower leg

S88 **Traumatic amputation of lower leg**

NOTE   An amputation not identified as partial or complete should be coded to complete
Excludes1: traumatic amputation of ankle and foot (S98.-)

The appropriate 7th character is to be added to each code from category S88
A   initial encounter
D   subsequent encounter
S   sequela

+ **S88.0** **Traumatic amputation at knee level**
  + **S88.01** **Complete traumatic amputation at knee level**
    CC +7th **S88.011** Complete traumatic amputation at knee level, right lower leg
    CC +7th **S88.012** Complete traumatic amputation at knee level, left lower leg
    CC +7th **S88.019** Complete traumatic amputation at knee level, unspecified lower leg
  + **S88.02** **Partial traumatic amputation at knee level**
    CC +7th **S88.021** Partial traumatic amputation at knee level, right lower leg
    CC +7th **S88.022** Partial traumatic amputation at knee level, left lower leg
    CC +7th **S88.029** Partial traumatic amputation at knee level, unspecified lower leg
+ **S88.1** **Traumatic amputation at level between knee and ankle**
  + **S88.11** **Complete traumatic amputation at level between knee and ankle**
    CC +7th **S88.111** Complete traumatic amputation at level between knee and ankle, right lower leg
    CC +7th **S88.112** Complete traumatic amputation at level between knee and ankle, left lower leg
    CC +7th **S88.119** Complete traumatic amputation at level between knee and ankle, unspecified lower leg
  + **S88.12** **Partial traumatic amputation at level between knee and ankle**
    CC +7th **S88.121** Partial traumatic amputation at level between knee and ankle, right lower leg
    CC +7th **S88.122** Partial traumatic amputation at level between knee and ankle, left lower leg
    CC +7th **S88.129** Partial traumatic amputation at level between knee and ankle, unspecified lower leg
+ **S88.9** **Traumatic amputation of lower leg, level unspecified**
  + **S88.91** **Complete traumatic amputation of lower leg, level unspecified**
    CC +7th **S88.911** Complete traumatic amputation of right lower leg, level unspecified
    CC +7th **S88.912** Complete traumatic amputation of left lower leg, level unspecified
    CC +7th **S88.919** Complete traumatic amputation of unspecified lower leg, level unspecified

+ **S88.92** **Partial traumatic amputation of lower leg, level unspecified**
  CC +7th **S88.921** Partial traumatic amputation of right lower leg, level unspecified
  CC +7th **S88.922** Partial traumatic amputation of left lower leg, level unspecified
  CC +7th **S88.929** Partial traumatic amputation of unspecified lower leg, level unspecified

S89 **Other and unspecified injuries of lower leg**

NOTE   A fracture not indicated as open or closed should be coded to closed
Excludes2: other and unspecified injuries of ankle and foot (S99.-)

The appropriate 7th character is to be added to each code from subcategories **S89.0, S89.1, S89.2,** and **S89.3**
A   initial encounter for closed fracture
D   subsequent encounter for fracture with routine healing
G   subsequent encounter for fracture with delayed healing
K   subsequent encounter for fracture with nonunion
P   subsequent encounter for fracture with malunion
S   sequela

Review coding guideline C.19.c

+ **S89.0** **Physeal fracture of upper end of tibia**
  + **S89.00** **Unspecified physeal fracture of upper end of tibia**
    CC +7th **S89.001** Unspecified physeal fracture of upper end of right tibia
      HAC 7th character A see Appendix B for HAC conditional logic
    CC +7th **S89.002** Unspecified physeal fracture of upper end of left tibia
      HAC 7th character A see Appendix B for HAC conditional logic
    CC +7th **S89.009** Unspecified physeal fracture of upper end of unspecified tibia
      HAC 7th character A see Appendix B for HAC conditional logic
  + **S89.01** **Salter-Harris Type I physeal fracture of upper end of tibia**
    CC +7th **S89.011** Salter-Harris Type I physeal fracture of upper end of right tibia
      HAC 7th character A see Appendix B for HAC conditional logic
    CC +7th **S89.012** Salter-Harris Type I physeal fracture of upper end of left tibia
      HAC 7th character A see Appendix B for HAC conditional logic
    CC +7th **S89.019** Salter-Harris Type I physeal fracture of upper end of unspecified tibia
      HAC 7th character A see Appendix B for HAC conditional logic
  + **S89.02** **Salter-Harris Type II physeal fracture of upper end of tibia**
    CC +7th **S89.021** Salter-Harris Type II physeal fracture of upper end of right tibia
      HAC 7th character A see Appendix B for HAC conditional logic
    CC +7th **S89.022** Salter-Harris Type II physeal fracture of upper end of left tibia
      HAC 7th character A see Appendix B for HAC conditional logic
    CC +7th **S89.029** Salter-Harris Type II physeal fracture of upper end of unspecified tibia
      HAC 7th character A see Appendix B for HAC conditional logic
  + **S89.03** **Salter-Harris Type III physeal fracture of upper end of tibia**
    CC +7th **S89.031** Salter-Harris Type III physeal fracture of upper end of right tibia
      HAC 7th character A see Appendix B for HAC conditional logic
    CC +7th **S89.032** Salter-Harris Type III physeal fracture of upper end of left tibia
      HAC 7th character A see Appendix B for HAC conditional logic
    CC +7th **S89.039** Salter-Harris Type III physeal fracture of upper end of unspecified tibia
      HAC 7th character A see Appendix B for HAC conditional logic

+, +7th, X + 7th   ● Newborn   ● Pediatric   ● Maternity   ● Adult   ♀ Female   ♂ Male   Manifestation   Unacceptable PDX   HCC   CC   MCC   **HAC**

+ **S89.04** Salter-Harris Type IV physeal fracture of upper end of tibia
CC +7th **S89.041** Salter-Harris Type IV physeal fracture of upper end of right tibia
HAC 7th character A see Appendix B for HAC conditional logic
CC +7th **S89.042** Salter-Harris Type IV physeal fracture of upper end of left tibia
HAC 7th character A see Appendix B for HAC conditional logic
CC +7th **S89.049** Salter-Harris Type IV physeal fracture of upper end of unspecified tibia
HAC 7th character A see Appendix B for HAC conditional logic
+ **S89.09** Other physeal fracture of upper end of tibia
CC +7th **S89.091** Other physeal fracture of upper end of right tibia
HAC 7th character A see Appendix B for HAC conditional logic
CC +7th **S89.092** Other physeal fracture of upper end of left tibia
HAC 7th character A see Appendix B for HAC conditional logic
CC +7th **S89.099** Other physeal fracture of upper end of unspecified tibia
HAC 7th character A see Appendix B for HAC conditional logic
+ **S89.1** **Physeal fracture of lower end of tibia**
+ **S89.10** Unspecified physeal fracture of lower end of tibia
CC +7th **S89.101** Unspecified physeal fracture of lower end of right tibia
CC +7th **S89.102** Unspecified physeal fracture of lower end of left tibia
CC +7th **S89.109** Unspecified physeal fracture of lower end of unspecified tibia
+ **S89.11** Salter-Harris Type I physeal fracture of lower end of tibia
CC +7th **S89.111** Salter-Harris Type I physeal fracture of lower end of right tibia
CC +7th **S89.112** Salter-Harris Type I physeal fracture of lower end of left tibia
CC +7th **S89.119** Salter-Harris Type I physeal fracture of lower end of unspecified tibia
+ **S89.12** Salter-Harris Type II physeal fracture of lower end of tibia
CC +7th **S89.121** Salter-Harris Type II physeal fracture of lower end of right tibia
CC +7th **S89.122** Salter-Harris Type II physeal fracture of lower end of left tibia
CC +7th **S89.129** Salter-Harris Type II physeal fracture of lower end of unspecified tibia
+ **S89.13** Salter-Harris Type III physeal fracture of lower end of tibia
Excludes1: *fracture of medial malleolus (adult) (S82.5-)*
CC +7th **S89.131** Salter-Harris Type III physeal fracture of lower end of right tibia
CC +7th **S89.132** Salter-Harris Type III physeal fracture of lower end of left tibia
CC +7th **S89.139** Salter-Harris Type III physeal fracture of lower end of unspecified tibia
+ **S89.14** Salter-Harris Type IV physeal fracture of lower end of tibia
Excludes1: *fracture of medial malleolus (adult) (S82.5-)*
CC +7th **S89.141** Salter-Harris Type IV physeal fracture of lower end of right tibia
CC +7th **S89.142** Salter-Harris Type IV physeal fracture of lower end of left tibia
CC +7th **S89.149** Salter-Harris Type IV physeal fracture of lower end of unspecified tibia
+ **S89.19** Other physeal fracture of lower end of tibia
CC +7th **S89.191** Other physeal fracture of lower end of right tibia
CC +7th **S89.192** Other physeal fracture of lower end of left tibia
CC +7th **S89.199** Other physeal fracture of lower end of unspecified tibia

+ **S89.2** **Physeal fracture of upper end of fibula**
+ **S89.20** Unspecified physeal fracture of upper end of fibula
CC +7th **S89.201** Unspecified physeal fracture of upper end of right fibula
CC +7th **S89.202** Unspecified physeal fracture of upper end of left fibula
CC +7th **S89.209** Unspecified physeal fracture of upper end of unspecified fibula
+ **S89.21** Salter-Harris Type I physeal fracture of upper end of fibula
CC +7th **S89.211** Salter-Harris Type I physeal fracture of upper end of right fibula
CC +7th **S89.212** Salter-Harris Type I physeal fracture of upper end of left fibula
CC +7th **S89.219** Salter-Harris Type I physeal fracture of upper end of unspecified fibula
+ **S89.22** Salter-Harris Type II physeal fracture of upper end of fibula
CC +7th **S89.221** Salter-Harris Type II physeal fracture of upper end of right fibula
CC +7th **S89.222** Salter-Harris Type II physeal fracture of upper end of left fibula
CC +7th **S89.229** Salter-Harris Type II physeal fracture of upper end of unspecified fibula
+ **S89.29** Other physeal fracture of upper end of fibula
CC +7th **S89.291** Other physeal fracture of upper end of right fibula
CC +7th **S89.292** Other physeal fracture of upper end of left fibula
CC +7th **S89.299** Other physeal fracture of upper end of unspecified fibula
+ **S89.3** **Physeal fracture of lower end of fibula**
+ **S89.30** Unspecified physeal fracture of lower end of fibula
CC +7th **S89.301** Unspecified physeal fracture of lower end of right fibula
CC +7th **S89.302** Unspecified physeal fracture of lower end of left fibula
CC +7th **S89.309** Unspecified physeal fracture of lower end of unspecified fibula
+ **S89.31** Salter-Harris Type I physeal fracture of lower end of fibula
CC +7th **S89.311** Salter-Harris Type I physeal fracture of lower end of right fibula
CC +7th **S89.312** Salter-Harris Type I physeal fracture of lower end of left fibula
CC +7th **S89.319** Salter-Harris Type I physeal fracture of lower end of unspecified fibula
+ **S89.32** Salter-Harris Type II physeal fracture of lower end of fibula
CC +7th **S89.321** Salter-Harris Type II physeal fracture of lower end of right fibula
CC +7th **S89.322** Salter-Harris Type II physeal fracture of lower end of left fibula
CC +7th **S89.329** Salter-Harris Type II physeal fracture of lower end of unspecified fibula
+ **S89.39** Other physeal fracture of lower end of fibula
CC +7th **S89.391** Other physeal fracture of lower end of right fibula
CC +7th **S89.392** Other physeal fracture of lower end of left fibula
CC +7th **S89.399** Other physeal fracture of lower end of unspecified fibula
+ **S89.8** **Other specified injuries of lower leg**

> The appropriate 7th character is to be added to each code in subcategory **S89.8**
> A initial encounter
> D subsequent encounter
> S sequela

X+7th **S89.80** Other specified injuries of unspecified lower leg
X+7th **S89.81** Other specified injuries of right lower leg
X+7th **S89.82** Other specified injuries of left lower leg
+ **S89.9** **Unspecified injury of lower leg**

> The appropriate 7th character is to be added to each code in subcategory **S89.9**
> A initial encounter
> D subsequent encounter
> S sequela

X+7th **S89.90** Unspecified injury of unspecified lower leg
X+7th **S89.91** Unspecified injury of right lower leg
X+7th **S89.92** Unspecified injury of left lower leg

+, +7th, X + 7th ● Newborn ● Pediatric ● Maternity ● Adult ♀ Female ♂ Male Manifestation Unacceptable PDX HCC CC MCC HAC

Injuries to the ankle and foot (S90-S99)

Excludes2: *burns and corrosions (T20-T32)*
fracture of ankle and malleolus (S82.-)
frostbite (T33-T34)
insect bite or sting, venomous (T63.4)

S90 **Superficial injury of ankle, foot and toes**

> The appropriate 7th character is to be added to each code from category S90
> A   initial encounter
> D   subsequent encounter
> S   sequela

+ **S90.0** **Contusion of ankle**
  X+7th **S90.00** Contusion of unspecified ankle
  X+7th **S90.01** Contusion of right ankle
  X+7th **S90.02** Contusion of left ankle
+ **S90.1** **Contusion of toe without damage to nail**
  + **S90.11** Contusion of great toe without damage to nail
    +7th **S90.111** Contusion of right great toe without damage to nail
    +7th **S90.112** Contusion of left great toe without damage to nail
    +7th **S90.119** Contusion of unspecified great toe without damage to nail
  + **S90.12** Contusion of lesser toe without damage to nail
    +7th **S90.121** Contusion of right lesser toe(s) without damage to nail
    +7th **S90.122** Contusion of left lesser toe(s) without damage to nail
    +7th **S90.129** Contusion of unspecified lesser toe(s) without damage to nail
      Contusion of toe NOS
+ **S90.2** **Contusion of toe with damage to nail**
  + **S90.21** Contusion of great toe with damage to nail
    +7th **S90.211** Contusion of right great toe with damage to nail
    +7th **S90.212** Contusion of left great toe with damage to nail
    +7th **S90.219** Contusion of unspecified great toe with damage to nail
  + **S90.22** Contusion of lesser toe with damage to nail
    +7th **S90.221** Contusion of right lesser toe(s) with damage to nail
    +7th **S90.222** Contusion of left lesser toe(s) with damage to nail
    +7th **S90.229** Contusion of unspecified lesser toe(s) with damage to nail
+ **S90.3** **Contusion of foot**
  Excludes2: *contusion of toes (S90.1-, S90.2-)*
  X+7th **S90.30** Contusion of unspecified foot
    Contusion of foot NOS
  X+7th **S90.31** Contusion of right foot
  X+7th **S90.32** Contusion of left foot
+ **S90.4** **Other superficial injuries of toe**
  + **S90.41** Abrasion of toe
    +7th **S90.411** Abrasion, right great toe
    +7th **S90.412** Abrasion, left great toe
    +7th **S90.413** Abrasion, unspecified great toe
    +7th **S90.414** Abrasion, right lesser toe(s)
    +7th **S90.415** Abrasion, left lesser toe(s)
    +7th **S90.416** Abrasion, unspecified lesser toe(s)
  + **S90.42** Blister (nonthermal) of toe
    +7th **S90.421** Blister (nonthermal), right great toe
    +7th **S90.422** Blister (nonthermal), left great toe
    +7th **S90.423** Blister (nonthermal), unspecified great toe
    +7th **S90.424** Blister (nonthermal), right lesser toe(s)
    +7th **S90.425** Blister (nonthermal), left lesser toe(s)
    +7th **S90.426** Blister (nonthermal), unspecified lesser toe(s)
  + **S90.44** External constriction of toe
      Hair tourniquet syndrome of toe
    +7th **S90.441** External constriction, right great toe
    +7th **S90.442** External constriction, left great toe
    +7th **S90.443** External constriction, unspecified great toe
    +7th **S90.444** External constriction, right lesser toe(s)
    +7th **S90.445** External constriction, left lesser toe(s)
    +7th **S90.446** External constriction, unspecified lesser toe(s)

+ **S90.45** Superficial foreign body of toe
      Splinter in the toe
    +7th **S90.451** Superficial foreign body, right great toe
    +7th **S90.452** Superficial foreign body, left great toe
    +7th **S90.453** Superficial foreign body, unspecified great toe
    +7th **S90.454** Superficial foreign body, right lesser toe(s)
    +7th **S90.455** Superficial foreign body, left lesser toe(s)
    +7th **S90.456** Superficial foreign body, unspecified lesser toe(s)
  + **S90.46** Insect bite (nonvenomous) of toe
    +7th **S90.461** Insect bite (nonvenomous), right great toe
    +7th **S90.462** Insect bite (nonvenomous), left great toe
    +7th **S90.463** Insect bite (nonvenomous), unspecified great toe
    +7th **S90.464** Insect bite (nonvenomous), right lesser toe(s)
    +7th **S90.465** Insect bite (nonvenomous), left lesser toe(s)
    +7th **S90.466** Insect bite (nonvenomous), unspecified lesser toe(s)
  + **S90.47** Other superficial bite of toe
      Excludes1: *open bite of toe (S91.15-, S91.25-)*
    +7th **S90.471** Other superficial bite of right great toe
    +7th **S90.472** Other superficial bite of left great toe
    +7th **S90.473** Other superficial bite of unspecified great toe
    +7th **S90.474** Other superficial bite of right lesser toe(s)
    +7th **S90.475** Other superficial bite of left lesser toe(s)
    +7th **S90.476** Other superficial bite of unspecified lesser toe(s)
+ **S90.5** **Other superficial injuries of ankle**
  + **S90.51** Abrasion of ankle
    +7th **S90.511** Abrasion, right ankle
    +7th **S90.512** Abrasion, left ankle
    +7th **S90.519** Abrasion, unspecified ankle
  + **S90.52** Blister (nonthermal) of ankle
    +7th **S90.521** Blister (nonthermal), right ankle
    +7th **S90.522** Blister (nonthermal), left ankle
    +7th **S90.529** Blister (nonthermal), unspecified ankle
  + **S90.54** External constriction of ankle
    +7th **S90.541** External constriction, right ankle
    +7th **S90.542** External constriction, left ankle
    +7th **S90.549** External constriction, unspecified ankle
  + **S90.55** Superficial foreign body of ankle
      Splinter in the ankle
    +7th **S90.551** Superficial foreign body, right ankle
    +7th **S90.552** Superficial foreign body, left ankle
    +7th **S90.559** Superficial foreign body, unspecified ankle
  + **S90.56** Insect bite (nonvenomous) of ankle
    +7th **S90.561** Insect bite (nonvenomous), right ankle
    +7th **S90.562** Insect bite (nonvenomous), left ankle
    +7th **S90.569** Insect bite (nonvenomous), unspecified ankle
  + **S90.57** Other superficial bite of ankle
      Excludes1: *open bite of ankle (S91.05-)*
    +7th **S90.571** Other superficial bite of ankle, right ankle
    +7th **S90.572** Other superficial bite of ankle, left ankle
    +7th **S90.579** Other superficial bite of ankle, unspecified ankle
+ **S90.8** **Other superficial injuries of foot**
  + **S90.81** Abrasion of foot
    +7th **S90.811** Abrasion, right foot
    +7th **S90.812** Abrasion, left foot
    +7th **S90.819** Abrasion, unspecified foot
  + **S90.82** Blister (nonthermal) of foot
    +7th **S90.821** Blister (nonthermal), right foot
    +7th **S90.822** Blister (nonthermal), left foot
    +7th **S90.829** Blister (nonthermal), unspecified foot
  + **S90.84** External constriction of foot
    +7th **S90.841** External constriction, right foot
    +7th **S90.842** External constriction, left foot
    +7th **S90.849** External constriction, unspecified foot

+, +7th, X + 7th   ● Newborn   ● Pediatric   ● Maternity   ● Adult   ♀ Female   ♂ Male   Manifestation   Unacceptable PDX   HCC   CC   MCC   HAC

Ankle

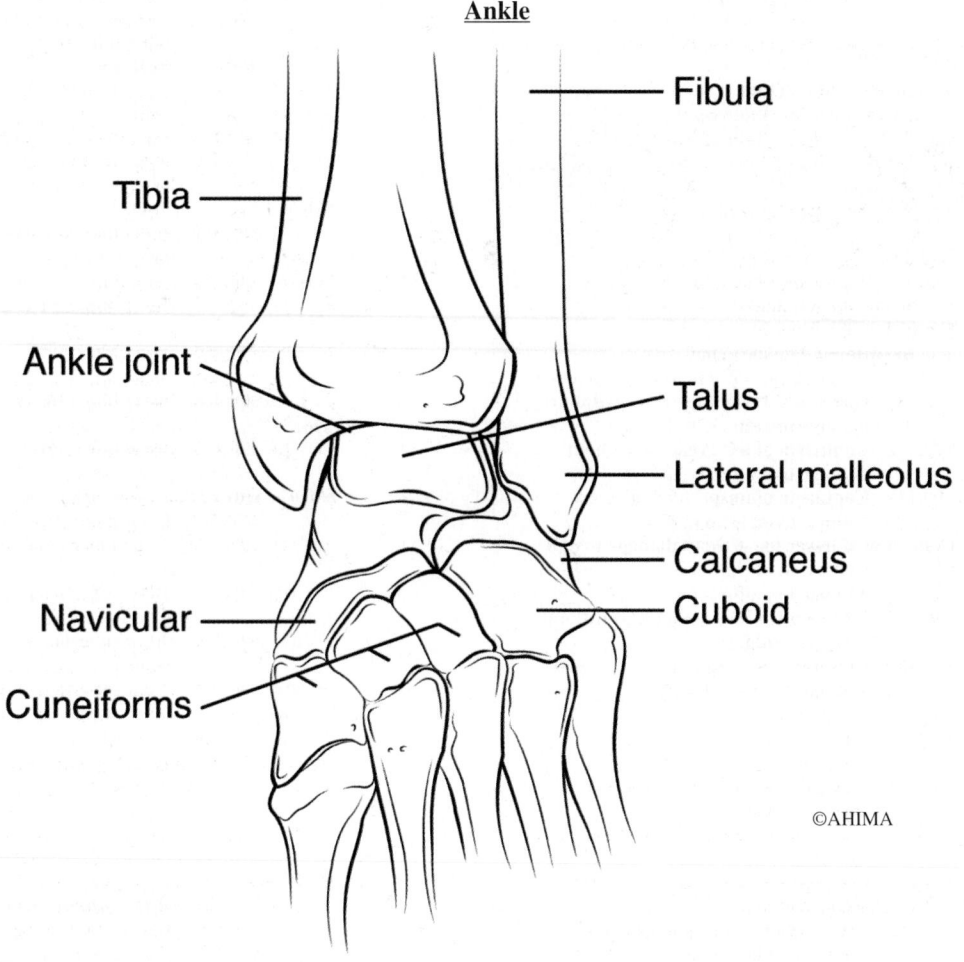

Fibula

Tibia

Ankle joint

Talus

Lateral malleolus

Calcaneus

Navicular

Cuboid

Cuneiforms

©AHIMA

Muscles of the Foot

Lateral View

Medial View

Achilles tendon

Peroneus tertius

Extensor digitorum longus

Extensor hallucis longus

Peroneus longus

Extensor hallucis brevis

Extensor digitorum brevis

Peroneus brevis

Achilles tendon

Tibialis posterior

Tibialis anterior

Flexor hallucis longus

Flexor digitorum longus

©AHIMA

+ **S90.85** **Superficial foreign body of foot**
  Splinter in the foot
  - +7th **S90.851** **Superficial foreign body, right foot**
  - +7th **S90.852** **Superficial foreign body, left foot**
  - +7th **S90.859** **Superficial foreign body, unspecified foot**
+ **S90.86** **Insect bite (nonvenomous) of foot**
  - +7th **S90.861** **Insect bite (nonvenomous), right foot**
  - +7th **S90.862** **Insect bite (nonvenomous), left foot**
  - +7th **S90.869** **Insect bite (nonvenomous), unspecified foot**
+ **S90.87** **Other superficial bite of foot**
  Excludes1: *open bite of foot (S91.35-)*
  - +7th **S90.871** **Other superficial bite of right foot**
  - +7th **S90.872** **Other superficial bite of left foot**
  - +7th **S90.879** **Other superficial bite of unspecified foot**
+ **S90.9** **Unspecified superficial injury of ankle, foot and toe**
  + **S90.91** **Unspecified superficial injury of ankle**
    - +7th **S90.911** **Unspecified superficial injury of right ankle**
    - +7th **S90.912** **Unspecified superficial injury of left ankle**
    - +7th **S90.919** **Unspecified superficial injury of unspecified ankle**
  + **S90.92** **Unspecified superficial injury of foot**
    - +7th **S90.921** **Unspecified superficial injury of right foot**
    - +7th **S90.922** **Unspecified superficial injury of left foot**
    - +7th **S90.929** **Unspecified superficial injury of unspecified foot**
  + **S90.93** **Unspecified superficial injury of toes**
    - +7th **S90.931** **Unspecified superficial injury of right great toe**
    - +7th **S90.932** **Unspecified superficial injury of left great toe**
    - +7th **S90.933** **Unspecified superficial injury of unspecified great toe**
    - +7th **S90.934** **Unspecified superficial injury of right lesser toe(s)**
    - +7th **S90.935** **Unspecified superficial injury of left lesser toe(s)**
    - +7th **S90.936** **Unspecified superficial injury of unspecified lesser toe(s)**

S91 **Open wound of ankle, foot and toes**
  Code also any associated wound infection
  Excludes1: *open fracture of ankle, foot and toes (S92.-with 7th character B)*
  traumatic amputation of ankle and foot (S98.-)

  The appropriate 7th character is to be added to each code from category S91
  A   initial encounter
  D   subsequent encounter
  S   sequela

+ **S91.0** **Open wound of ankle**
  + **S91.00** **Unspecified open wound of ankle**
    - +7th **S91.001** **Unspecified open wound, right ankle**
    - +7th **S91.002** **Unspecified open wound, left ankle**
    - +7th **S91.009** **Unspecified open wound, unspecified ankle**
  + **S91.01** **Laceration without foreign body of ankle**
    - +7th **S91.011** **Laceration without foreign body, right ankle**
    - +7th **S91.012** **Laceration without foreign body, left ankle**
    - +7th **S91.019** **Laceration without foreign body, unspecified ankle**
  + **S91.02** **Laceration with foreign body of ankle**
    - +7th **S91.021** **Laceration with foreign body, right ankle**
    - +7th **S91.022** **Laceration with foreign body, left ankle**
    - +7th **S91.029** **Laceration with foreign body, unspecified ankle**

+ **S91.03** **Puncture wound without foreign body of ankle**
  - +7th **S91.031** **Puncture wound without foreign body, right ankle**
  - +7th **S91.032** **Puncture wound without foreign body, left ankle**
  - +7th **S91.039** **Puncture wound without foreign body, unspecified ankle**
+ **S91.04** **Puncture wound with foreign body of ankle**
  - +7th **S91.041** **Puncture wound with foreign body, right ankle**
  - +7th **S91.042** **Puncture wound with foreign body, left ankle**
  - +7th **S91.049** **Puncture wound with foreign body, unspecified ankle**
+ **S91.05** **Open bite of ankle**
  Excludes1: *superficial bite of ankle (S90.56-, S90.57-)*
  - +7th **S91.051** **Open bite, right ankle**
  - +7th **S91.052** **Open bite, left ankle**
  - +7th **S91.059** **Open bite, unspecified ankle**
+ **S91.1** **Open wound of toe without damage to nail**
  + **S91.10** **Unspecified open wound of toe without damage to nail**
    - +7th **S91.101** **Unspecified open wound of right great toe without damage to nail**
    - +7th **S91.102** **Unspecified open wound of left great toe without damage to nail**
    - +7th **S91.103** **Unspecified open wound of unspecified great toe without damage to nail**
    - +7th **S91.104** **Unspecified open wound of right lesser toe(s) without damage to nail**
    - +7th **S91.105** **Unspecified open wound of left lesser toe(s) without damage to nail**
    - +7th **S91.106** **Unspecified open wound of unspecified lesser toe(s) without damage to nail**
    - +7th **S91.109** **Unspecified open wound of unspecified toe(s) without damage to nail**
  + **S91.11** **Laceration without foreign body of toe without damage to nail**
    - +7th **S91.111** **Laceration without foreign body of right great toe without damage to nail**
    - +7th **S91.112** **Laceration without foreign body of left great toe without damage to nail**
    - +7th **S91.113** **Laceration without foreign body of unspecified great toe without damage to nail**
    - +7th **S91.114** **Laceration without foreign body of right lesser toe(s) without damage to nail**
    - +7th **S91.115** **Laceration without foreign body of left lesser toe(s) without damage to nail**
    - +7th **S91.116** **Laceration without foreign body of unspecified lesser toe(s) without damage to nail**
    - +7th **S91.119** **Laceration without foreign body of unspecified toe without damage to nail**
  + **S91.12** **Laceration with foreign body of toe without damage to nail**
    - +7th **S91.121** **Laceration with foreign body of right great toe without damage to nail**
    - +7th **S91.122** **Laceration with foreign body of left great toe without damage to nail**
    - +7th **S91.123** **Laceration with foreign body of unspecified great toe without damage to nail**
    - +7th **S91.124** **Laceration with foreign body of right lesser toe(s) without damage to nail**
    - +7th **S91.125** **Laceration with foreign body of left lesser toe(s) without damage to nail**
    - +7th **S91.126** **Laceration with foreign body of unspecified lesser toe(s) without damage to nail**
    - +7th **S91.129** **Laceration with foreign body of unspecified toe(s) without damage to nail**

+ **S91.13** **Puncture wound without foreign body of toe without damage to nail**
+7th **S91.131** Puncture wound without foreign body of right great toe without damage to nail
+7th **S91.132** Puncture wound without foreign body of left great toe without damage to nail
+7th **S91.133** Puncture wound without foreign body of unspecified great toe without damage to nail
+7th **S91.134** Puncture wound without foreign body of right lesser toe(s) without damage to nail
+7th **S91.135** Puncture wound without foreign body of left lesser toe(s) without damage to nail
+7th **S91.136** Puncture wound without foreign body of unspecified lesser toe(s) without damage to nail
+7th **S91.139** Puncture wound without foreign body of unspecified toe(s) without damage to nail

+ **S91.14** **Puncture wound with foreign body of toe without damage to nail**
+7th **S91.141** Puncture wound with foreign body of right great toe without damage to nail
+7th **S91.142** Puncture wound with foreign body of left great toe without damage to nail
+7th **S91.143** Puncture wound with foreign body of unspecified great toe without damage to nail
+7th **S91.144** Puncture wound with foreign body of right lesser toe(s) without damage to nail
+7th **S91.145** Puncture wound with foreign body of left lesser toe(s) without damage to nail
+7th **S91.146** Puncture wound with foreign body of unspecified lesser toe(s) without damage to nail
+7th **S91.149** Puncture wound with foreign body of unspecified toe(s) without damage to nail

+ **S91.15** **Open bite of toe without damage to nail**
Bite of toe NOS
Excludes1: *superficial bite of toe (S90.46-,S90.47-)*
+7th **S91.151** Open bite of right great toe without damage to nail
+7th **S91.152** Open bite of left great toe without damage to nail
+7th **S91.153** Open bite of unspecified great toe without damage to nail
+7th **S91.154** Open bite of right lesser toe(s) without damage to nail
+7th **S91.155** Open bite of left lesser toe(s) without damage to nail
+7th **S91.156** Open bite of unspecified lesser toe(s) without damage to nail
+7th **S91.159** Open bite of unspecified toe(s) without damage to nail

+ **S91.2** **Open wound of toe with damage to nail**
+ **S91.20** **Unspecified open wound of toe with damage to nail**
+7th **S91.201** Unspecified open wound of right great toe with damage to nail
+7th **S91.202** Unspecified open wound of left great toe with damage to nail
+7th **S91.203** Unspecified open wound of unspecified great toe with damage to nail
+7th **S91.204** Unspecified open wound of right lesser toe(s) with damage to nail
+7th **S91.205** Unspecified open wound of left lesser toe(s) with damage to nail
+7th **S91.206** Unspecified open wound of unspecified lesser toe(s) with damage to nail
+7th **S91.209** Unspecified open wound of unspecified toe(s) with damage to nail

+ **S91.21** **Laceration without foreign body of toe with damage to nail**
+7th **S91.211** Laceration without foreign body of right great toe with damage to nail
+7th **S91.212** Laceration without foreign body of left great toe with damage to nail
+7th **S91.213** Laceration without foreign body of unspecified great toe with damage to nail
+7th **S91.214** Laceration without foreign body of right lesser toe(s) with damage to nail
+7th **S91.215** Laceration without foreign body of left lesser toe(s) with damage to nail
+7th **S91.216** Laceration without foreign body of unspecified lesser toe(s) with damage to nail
+7th **S91.219** Laceration without foreign body of unspecified toe(s) with damage to nail

+ **S91.22** **Laceration with foreign body of toe with damage to nail**
+7th **S91.221** Laceration with foreign body of right great toe with damage to nail
+7th **S91.222** Laceration with foreign body of left great toe with damage to nail
+7th **S91.223** Laceration with foreign body of unspecified great toe with damage to nail
+7th **S91.224** Laceration with foreign body of right lesser toe(s) with damage to nail
+7th **S91.225** Laceration with foreign body of left lesser toe(s) with damage to nail
+7th **S91.226** Laceration with foreign body of unspecified lesser toe(s) with damage to nail
+7th **S91.229** Laceration with foreign body of unspecified toe(s) with damage to nail

+ **S91.23** **Puncture wound without foreign body of toe with damage to nail**
+7th **S91.231** Puncture wound without foreign body of right great toe with damage to nail
+7th **S91.232** Puncture wound without foreign body of left great toe with damage to nail
+7th **S91.233** Puncture wound without foreign body of unspecified great toe with damage to nail
+7th **S91.234** Puncture wound without foreign body of right lesser toe(s) with damage to nail
+7th **S91.235** Puncture wound without foreign body of left lesser toe(s) with damage to nail
+7th **S91.236** Puncture wound without foreign body of unspecified lesser toe(s) with damage to nail
+7th **S91.239** Puncture wound without foreign body of unspecified toe(s) with damage to nail

+ **S91.24** **Puncture wound with foreign body of toe with damage to nail**
+7th **S91.241** Puncture wound with foreign body of right great toe with damage to nail
+7th **S91.242** Puncture wound with foreign body of left great toe with damage to nail
+7th **S91.243** Puncture wound with foreign body of unspecified great toe with damage to nail
+7th **S91.244** Puncture wound with foreign body of right lesser toe(s) with damage to nail
+7th **S91.245** Puncture wound with foreign body of left lesser toe(s) with damage to nail
+7th **S91.246** Puncture wound with foreign body of unspecified lesser toe(s) with damage to nail
+7th **S91.249** Puncture wound with foreign body of unspecified toe(s) with damage to nail

S91.25 **Open bite of toe with damage to nail**
Bite of toe with damage to nail NOS
Excludes1: superficial bite of toe (S90.46-, S90.47-)

+7th S91.251 **Open bite of right great toe with damage to nail**

+7th S91.252 **Open bite of left great toe with damage to nail**

+7th S91.253 **Open bite of unspecified great toe with damage to nail**

+7th S91.254 **Open bite of right lesser toe(s) with damage to nail**

+7th S91.255 **Open bite of left lesser toe(s) with damage to nail**

+7th S91.256 **Open bite of unspecified lesser toe(s) with damage to nail**

+7th S91.259 **Open bite of unspecified toe(s) with damage to nail**

+ S91.3 **Open wound of foot**

+ S91.30 **Unspecified open wound of foot**

+7th S91.301 **Unspecified open wound, right foot**

+7th S91.302 **Unspecified open wound, left foot**

+7th S91.309 **Unspecified open wound, unspecified foot**

+ S91.31 **Laceration without foreign body of foot**

+7th S91.311 **Laceration without foreign body, right foot**

+7th S91.312 **Laceration without foreign body, left foot**

+7th S91.319 **Laceration without foreign body, unspecified foot**

+ S91.32 **Laceration with foreign body of foot**

+7th S91.321 **Laceration with foreign body, right foot**

+7th S91.322 **Laceration with foreign body, left foot**

+7th S91.329 **Laceration with foreign body, unspecified foot**

+ S91.33 **Puncture wound without foreign body of foot**

+7th S91.331 **Puncture wound without foreign body, right foot**

+7th S91.332 **Puncture wound without foreign body, left foot**

+7th S91.339 **Puncture wound without foreign body, unspecified foot**

+ S91.34 **Puncture wound with foreign body of foot**

+7th S91.341 **Puncture wound with foreign body, right foot**

+7th S91.342 **Puncture wound with foreign body, left foot**

+7th S91.349 **Puncture wound with foreign body, unspecified foot**

+ S91.35 **Open bite of foot**
Excludes1: superficial bite of foot (S90.86-, S90.87-)

+7th S91.351 **Open bite, right foot**

+7th S91.352 **Open bite, left foot**

+7th S91.359 **Open bite, unspecified foot**

S92 **Fracture of foot and toe, except ankle**

NOTE A fracture not indicated as displaced or nondisplaced should be coded to displaced
A fracture not indicated as open or closed should be coded to closed

Excludes1: traumatic amputation of ankle and foot (S98.-)
Excludes2: fracture of ankle (S82.-)
fracture of malleolus (S82.-)

The appropriate 7th character is to be added to each code from category S92
A initial encounter for closed fracture
B initial encounter for open fracture
D subsequent encounter for fracture with routine healing
G subsequent encounter for fracture with delayed healing
K subsequent encounter for fracture with nonunion
P subsequent encounter for fracture with malunion
S sequela

Review coding guideline C.19.c

+ S92.0 **Fracture of calcaneus**
Heel bone
Os calcis
Excludes2: Physeal fracture of calcaneus (S99.0-)

+ S92.00 **Unspecified fracture of calcaneus**

CC +7th S92.001 **Unspecified fracture of right calcaneus**
HAC 7th character B see Appendix B for HAC conditional logic

CC +7th S92.002 **Unspecified fracture of left calcaneus**
HAC 7th character B see Appendix B for HAC conditional logic

CC +7th S92.009 **Unspecified fracture of unspecified calcaneus**
HAC 7th character B see Appendix B for HAC conditional logic

+ S92.01 **Fracture of body of calcaneus**

CC +7th S92.011 **Displaced fracture of body of right calcaneus**
HAC 7th character B see Appendix B for HAC conditional logic

CC +7th S92.012 **Displaced fracture of body of left calcaneus**
HAC 7th character B see Appendix B for HAC conditional logic

CC +7th S92.013 **Displaced fracture of body of unspecified calcaneus**
HAC 7th character B see Appendix B for HAC conditional logic

CC +7th S92.014 **Nondisplaced fracture of body of right calcaneus**
HAC 7th character B see Appendix B for HAC conditional logic

CC +7th S92.015 **Nondisplaced fracture of body of left calcaneus**
HAC 7th character B see Appendix B for HAC conditional logic

CC +7th S92.016 **Nondisplaced fracture of body of unspecified calcaneus**
HAC 7th character B see Appendix B for HAC conditional logic

+ S92.02 **Fracture of anterior process of calcaneus**

CC +7th S92.021 **Displaced fracture of anterior process of right calcaneus**
HAC 7th character B see Appendix B for HAC conditional logic

CC +7th S92.022 **Displaced fracture of anterior process of left calcaneus**
HAC 7th character B see Appendix B for HAC conditional logic

CC +7th S92.023 **Displaced fracture of anterior process of unspecified calcaneus**
HAC 7th character B see Appendix B for HAC conditional logic

CC +7th S92.024 **Nondisplaced fracture of anterior process of right calcaneus**
HAC 7th character B see Appendix B for HAC conditional logic

CC +7th S92.025 **Nondisplaced fracture of anterior process of left calcaneus**
HAC 7th character B see Appendix B for HAC conditional logic

CC +7th S92.026 **Nondisplaced fracture of anterior process of unspecified calcaneus**
HAC 7th character B see Appendix B for HAC conditional logic

+, +7th, X + 7th • Newborn • Pediatric • Maternity • Adult ♀ Female ♂ Male Manifestation Unacceptable PDX HCC CC MCC HAC

+ **S92.03   Avulsion fracture of tuberosity of calcaneus**

CC +7th **S92.031   Displaced avulsion fracture of tuberosity of right calcaneus**

   HAC 7th character B see Appendix B for HAC conditional logic

CC +7th **S92.032   Displaced avulsion fracture of tuberosity of left calcaneus**

   HAC 7th character B see Appendix B for HAC conditional logic

CC +7th **S92.033   Displaced avulsion fracture of tuberosity of unspecified calcaneus**

   HAC 7th character B see Appendix B for HAC conditional logic

CC +7th **S92.034   Nondisplaced avulsion fracture of tuberosity of right calcaneus**

   HAC 7th character B see Appendix B for HAC conditional logic

CC +7th **S92.035   Nondisplaced avulsion fracture of tuberosity of left calcaneus**

   HAC 7th character B see Appendix B for HAC conditional logic

CC +7th **S92.036   Nondisplaced avulsion fracture of tuberosity of unspecified calcaneus**

   HAC 7th character B see Appendix B for HAC conditional logic

+ **S92.04   Other fracture of tuberosity of calcaneus**

CC +7th **S92.041   Displaced other fracture of tuberosity of right calcaneus**

   HAC 7th character B see Appendix B for HAC conditional logic

CC +7th **S92.042   Displaced other fracture of tuberosity of left calcaneus**

   HAC 7th character B see Appendix B for HAC conditional logic

CC +7th **S92.043   Displaced other fracture of tuberosity of unspecified calcaneus**

   HAC 7th character B see Appendix B for HAC conditional logic

CC +7th **S92.044   Nondisplaced other fracture of tuberosity of right calcaneus**

   HAC 7th character B see Appendix B for HAC conditional logic

CC +7th **S92.045   Nondisplaced other fracture of tuberosity of left calcaneus**

   HAC 7th character B see Appendix B for HAC conditional logic

CC +7th **S92.046   Nondisplaced other fracture of tuberosity of unspecified calcaneus**

   HAC 7th character B see Appendix B for HAC conditional logic

+ **S92.05   Other extraarticular fracture of calcaneus**

CC +7th **S92.051   Displaced other extraarticular fracture of right calcaneus**

   HAC 7th character B see Appendix B for HAC conditional logic

CC +7th **S92.052   Displaced other extraarticular fracture of left calcaneus**

   HAC 7th character B see Appendix B for HAC conditional logic

CC +7th **S92.053   Displaced other extraarticular fracture of unspecified calcaneus**

   HAC 7th character B see Appendix B for HAC conditional logic

CC +7th **S92.054   Nondisplaced other extraarticular fracture of right calcaneus**

   HAC 7th character B see Appendix B for HAC conditional logic

CC +7th **S92.055   Nondisplaced other extraarticular fracture of left calcaneus**

   HAC 7th character B see Appendix B for HAC conditional logic

CC +7th **S92.056   Nondisplaced other extraarticular fracture of unspecified calcaneus**

   HAC 7th character B see Appendix B for HAC conditional logic

+ **S92.06   Intraarticular fracture of calcaneus**

CC +7th **S92.061   Displaced intraarticular fracture of right calcaneus**

   HAC 7th character B see Appendix B for HAC conditional logic

CC +7th **S92.062   Displaced intraarticular fracture of left calcaneus**

   HAC 7th character B see Appendix B for HAC conditional logic

CC +7th **S92.063   Displaced intraarticular fracture of unspecified calcaneus**

   HAC 7th character B see Appendix B for HAC conditional logic

CC +7th **S92.064   Nondisplaced intraarticular fracture of right calcaneus**

   HAC 7th character B see Appendix B for HAC conditional logic

CC +7th **S92.065   Nondisplaced intraarticular fracture of left calcaneus**

   HAC 7th character B see Appendix B for HAC conditional logic

CC +7th **S92.066   Nondisplaced intraarticular fracture of unspecified calcaneus**

   HAC 7th character B see Appendix B for HAC conditional logic

+ **S92.1   Fracture of talus**

Astragalus

+ **S92.10   Unspecified fracture of talus**

CC +7th **S92.101   Unspecified fracture of right talus**

   HAC 7th character B see Appendix B for HAC conditional logic

CC +7th **S92.102   Unspecified fracture of left talus**

   HAC 7th character B see Appendix B for HAC conditional logic

CC +7th **S92.109   Unspecified fracture of unspecified talus**

   HAC 7th character B see Appendix B for HAC conditional logic

+ **S92.11   Fracture of neck of talus**

CC +7th **S92.111   Displaced fracture of neck of right talus**

   HAC 7th character B see Appendix B for HAC conditional logic

CC +7th **S92.112   Displaced fracture of neck of left talus**

CC +7th **S92.113   Displaced fracture of neck of unspecified talus**

   HAC 7th character B see Appendix B for HAC conditional logic

CC +7th **S92.114   Nondisplaced fracture of neck of right talus**

   HAC 7th character B see Appendix B for HAC conditional logic

CC +7th **S92.115   Nondisplaced fracture of neck of left talus**

   HAC 7th character B see Appendix B for HAC conditional logic

CC +7th **S92.116   Nondisplaced fracture of neck of unspecified talus**

   HAC 7th character B see Appendix B for HAC conditional logic

+ **S92.12   Fracture of body of talus**

CC +7th **S92.121   Displaced fracture of body of right talus**

   HAC 7th character B see Appendix B for HAC conditional logic

CC +7th **S92.122   Displaced fracture of body of left talus**

   HAC 7th character B see Appendix B for HAC conditional logic

CC +7th **S92.123   Displaced fracture of body of unspecified talus**

   HAC 7th character B see Appendix B for HAC conditional logic

CC +7th **S92.124   Nondisplaced fracture of body of right talus**

   HAC 7th character B see Appendix B for HAC conditional logic

CC +7th **S92.125   Nondisplaced fracture of body of left talus**

   HAC 7th character B see Appendix B for HAC conditional logic

CC +7th **S92.126   Nondisplaced fracture of body of unspecified talus**

   HAC 7th character B see Appendix B for HAC conditional logic

+ **S92.13 Fracture of posterior process of talus**
- CC +7th **S92.131 Displaced fracture of posterior process of right talus**
  - HAC 7th character B see Appendix B for HAC conditional logic
- CC +7th **S92.132 Displaced fracture of posterior process of left talus**
  - HAC 7th character B see Appendix B for HAC conditional logic
- CC +7th **S92.133 Displaced fracture of posterior process of unspecified talus**
  - HAC 7th character B see Appendix B for HAC conditional logic
- CC +7th **S92.134 Nondisplaced fracture of posterior process of right talus**
  - HAC 7th character B see Appendix B for HAC conditional logic
- CC +7th **S92.135 Nondisplaced fracture of posterior process of left talus**
  - HAC 7th character B see Appendix B for HAC conditional logic
- CC +7th **S92.136 Nondisplaced fracture of posterior process of unspecified talus**
  - HAC 7th character B see Appendix B for HAC conditional logic

+ **S92.14 Dome fracture of talus**
- *Excludes1:* *osteochondritis dissecans (M93.2)*
- CC +7th **S92.141 Displaced dome fracture of right talus**
  - HAC 7th character B see Appendix B for HAC conditional logic
- CC +7th **S92.142 Displaced dome fracture of left talus**
  - HAC 7th character B see Appendix B for HAC conditional logic
- CC +7th **S92.143 Displaced dome fracture of unspecified talus**
  - HAC 7th character B see Appendix B for HAC conditional logic
- CC +7th **S92.144 Nondisplaced dome fracture of right talus**
  - HAC 7th character B see Appendix B for HAC conditional logic
- CC +7th **S92.145 Nondisplaced dome fracture of left talus**
  - HAC 7th character B see Appendix B for HAC conditional logic
- CC +7th **S92.146 Nondisplaced dome fracture of unspecified talus**
  - HAC 7th character B see Appendix B for HAC conditional logic

+ **S92.15 Avulsion fracture (chip fracture) of talus**
- CC +7th **S92.151 Displaced avulsion fracture (chip fracture) of right talus**
  - HAC 7th character B see Appendix B for HAC conditional logic
- CC +7th **S92.152 Displaced avulsion fracture (chip fracture) of left talus**
  - HAC 7th character B see Appendix B for HAC conditional logic
- CC +7th **S92.153 Displaced avulsion fracture (chip fracture) of unspecified talus**
  - HAC 7th character B see Appendix B for HAC conditional logic
- CC +7th **S92.154 Nondisplaced avulsion fracture (chip fracture) of right talus**
  - HAC 7th character B see Appendix B for HAC conditional logic
- CC +7th **S92.155 Nondisplaced avulsion fracture (chip fracture) of left talus**
  - HAC 7th character B see Appendix B for HAC conditional logic
- CC +7th **S92.156 Nondisplaced avulsion fracture (chip fracture) of unspecified talus**
  - HAC 7th character B see Appendix B for HAC conditional logic

+ **S92.19 Other fracture of talus**
- CC +7th **S92.191 Other fracture of right talus**
  - HAC 7th character B see Appendix B for HAC conditional logic
- CC +7th **S92.192 Other fracture of left talus**
  - HAC 7th character B see Appendix B for HAC conditional logic
- CC +7th **S92.199 Other fracture of unspecified talus**
  - HAC 7th character B see Appendix B for HAC conditional logic

+ **S92.2 Fracture of other and unspecified tarsal bone(s)**
+ **S92.20 Fracture of unspecified tarsal bone(s)**
- CC +7th **S92.201 Fracture of unspecified tarsal bone(s) of right foot**
  - HAC 7th character B see Appendix B for HAC conditional logic
- CC +7th **S92.202 Fracture of unspecified tarsal bone(s) of left foot**
  - HAC 7th character B see Appendix B for HAC conditional logic
- CC +7th **S92.209 Fracture of unspecified tarsal bone(s) of unspecified foot**
  - HAC 7th character B see Appendix B for HAC conditional logic

+ **S92.21 Fracture of cuboid bone**
- CC +7th **S92.211 Displaced fracture of cuboid bone of right foot**
  - HAC 7th character B see Appendix B for HAC conditional logic
- CC +7th **S92.212 Displaced fracture of cuboid bone of left foot**
  - HAC 7th character B see Appendix B for HAC conditional logic
- CC +7th **S92.213 Displaced fracture of cuboid bone of unspecified foot**
  - HAC 7th character B see Appendix B for HAC conditional logic
- CC +7th **S92.214 Nondisplaced fracture of cuboid bone of right foot**
  - HAC 7th character B see Appendix B for HAC conditional logic
- CC +7th **S92.215 Nondisplaced fracture of cuboid bone of left foot**
  - HAC 7th character B see Appendix B for HAC conditional logic
- CC +7th **S92.216 Nondisplaced fracture of cuboid bone of unspecified foot**
  - HAC 7th character B see Appendix B for HAC conditional logic

+ **S92.22 Fracture of lateral cuneiform**
- CC +7th **S92.221 Displaced fracture of lateral cuneiform of right foot**
  - HAC 7th character B see Appendix B for HAC conditional logic
- CC +7th **S92.222 Displaced fracture of lateral cuneiform of left foot**
  - HAC 7th character B see Appendix B for HAC conditional logic
- CC +7th **S92.223 Displaced fracture of lateral cuneiform of unspecified foot**
  - HAC 7th character B see Appendix B for HAC conditional logic
- CC +7th **S92.224 Nondisplaced fracture of lateral cuneiform of right foot**
  - HAC 7th character B see Appendix B for HAC conditional logic
- CC +7th **S92.225 Nondisplaced fracture of lateral cuneiform of left foot**
  - HAC 7th character B see Appendix B for HAC conditional logic
- CC +7th **S92.226 Nondisplaced fracture of lateral cuneiform of unspecified foot**
  - HAC 7th character B see Appendix B for HAC conditional logic

+, +7th, X + 7th   • Newborn   • Pediatric   • Maternity   • Adult   ♀ Female   ♂ Male   Manifestation   Unacceptable PDX   HCC   CC   MCC   HAC

+ **S92.23** **Fracture of intermediate cuneiform**
CC +7th **S92.231** **Displaced fracture of intermediate cuneiform of right foot**
> HAC 7th character B see Appendix B for HAC conditional logic

CC +7th **S92.232** **Displaced fracture of intermediate cuneiform of left foot**
> HAC 7th character B see Appendix B for HAC conditional logic

CC +7th **S92.233** **Displaced fracture of intermediate cuneiform of unspecified foot**
> HAC 7th character B see Appendix B for HAC conditional logic

CC +7th **S92.234** **Nondisplaced fracture of intermediate cuneiform of right foot**
> HAC 7th character B see Appendix B for HAC conditional logic

CC +7th **S92.235** **Nondisplaced fracture of intermediate cuneiform of left foot**
> HAC 7th character B see Appendix B for HAC conditional logic

CC +7th **S92.236** **Nondisplaced fracture of intermediate cuneiform of unspecified foot**
> HAC 7th character B see Appendix B for HAC conditional logic

+ **S92.24** **Fracture of medial cuneiform**
CC +7th **S92.241** **Displaced fracture of medial cuneiform of right foot**
> HAC 7th character B see Appendix B for HAC conditional logic

CC +7th **S92.242** **Displaced fracture of medial cuneiform of left foot**
> HAC 7th character B see Appendix B for HAC conditional logic

CC +7th **S92.243** **Displaced fracture of medial cuneiform of unspecified foot**
> HAC 7th character B see Appendix B for HAC conditional logic

CC +7th **S92.244** **Nondisplaced fracture of medial cuneiform of right foot**
> HAC 7th character B see Appendix B for HAC conditional logic

CC +7th **S92.245** **Nondisplaced fracture of medial cuneiform of left foot**
> HAC 7th character B see Appendix B for HAC conditional logic

CC +7th **S92.246** **Nondisplaced fracture of medial cuneiform of unspecified foot**
> HAC 7th character B see Appendix B for HAC conditional logic

+ **S92.25** **Fracture of navicular [scaphoid] of foot**
CC +7th **S92.251** **Displaced fracture of navicular [scaphoid] of right foot**
> HAC 7th character B see Appendix B for HAC conditional logic

CC +7th **S92.252** **Displaced fracture of navicular [scaphoid] of left foot**
> HAC 7th character B see Appendix B for HAC conditional logic

CC +7th **S92.253** **Displaced fracture of navicular [scaphoid] of unspecified foot**
> HAC 7th character B see Appendix B for HAC conditional logic

CC +7th **S92.254** **Nondisplaced fracture of navicular [scaphoid] of right foot**
> HAC 7th character B see Appendix B for HAC conditional logic

CC +7th **S92.255** **Nondisplaced fracture of navicular [scaphoid] of left foot**
> HAC 7th character B see Appendix B for HAC conditional logic

CC +7th **S92.256** **Nondisplaced fracture of navicular [scaphoid] of unspecified foot**
> HAC 7th character B see Appendix B for HAC conditional logic

+ **S92.3** **Fracture of metatarsal bone(s)**
> *Excludes2:* *Physeal fracture of metatarsal (S99.1-)*

+ **S92.30** **Fracture of unspecified metatarsal bone(s)**
CC +7th **S92.301** **Fracture of unspecified metatarsal bone(s), right foot**
> HAC 7th character B see Appendix B for HAC conditional logic

CC +7th **S92.302** **Fracture of unspecified metatarsal bone(s), left foot**
> HAC 7th character B see Appendix B for HAC conditional logic

CC +7th **S92.309** **Fracture of unspecified metatarsal bone(s), unspecified foot**

+ **S92.31** **Fracture of first metatarsal bone**
CC +7th **S92.311** **Displaced fracture of first metatarsal bone, right foot**
> HAC 7th character B see Appendix B for HAC conditional logic

CC +7th **S92.312** **Displaced fracture of first metatarsal bone, left foot**
> HAC 7th character B see Appendix B for HAC conditional logic

CC +7th **S92.313** **Displaced fracture of first metatarsal bone, unspecified foot**
> HAC 7th character B see Appendix B for HAC conditional logic

CC +7th **S92.314** **Nondisplaced fracture of first metatarsal bone, right foot**
> HAC 7th character B see Appendix B for HAC conditional logic

CC +7th **S92.315** **Nondisplaced fracture of first metatarsal bone, left foot**
> HAC 7th character B see Appendix B for HAC conditional logic

CC +7th **S92.316** **Nondisplaced fracture of first metatarsal bone, unspecified foot**
> HAC 7th character B see Appendix B for HAC conditional logic

+ **S92.32** **Fracture of second metatarsal bone**
CC +7th **S92.321** **Displaced fracture of second metatarsal bone, right foot**
> HAC 7th character B see Appendix B for HAC conditional logic

CC +7th **S92.322** **Displaced fracture of second metatarsal bone, left foot**
> HAC 7th character B see Appendix B for HAC conditional logic

CC +7th **S92.323** **Displaced fracture of second metatarsal bone, unspecified foot**
> HAC 7th character B see Appendix B for HAC conditional logic

CC +7th **S92.324** **Nondisplaced fracture of second metatarsal bone, right foot**
> HAC 7th character B see Appendix B for HAC conditional logic

CC +7th **S92.325** **Nondisplaced fracture of second metatarsal bone, left foot**
> HAC 7th character B see Appendix B for HAC conditional logic

CC +7th **S92.326** **Nondisplaced fracture of second metatarsal bone, unspecified foot**
> HAC 7th character B see Appendix B for HAC conditional logic

+ **S92.33** **Fracture of third metatarsal bone**
> *AHA CC: 1Q, 2018, 3*

CC +7th **S92.331** **Displaced fracture of third metatarsal bone, right foot**
> HAC 7th character B see Appendix B for HAC conditional logic

CC +7th **S92.332** **Displaced fracture of third metatarsal bone, left foot**
> HAC 7th character B see Appendix B for HAC conditional logic

CC +7th **S92.333** **Displaced fracture of third metatarsal bone, unspecified foot**
> HAC 7th character B see Appendix B for HAC conditional logic

+, +7th, X + 7th ● Newborn ● Pediatric ● Maternity ● Adult ♀ Female ♂ Male Manifestation Unacceptable PDX HCC CC MCC HAC

CC +7th **S92.334** **Nondisplaced fracture of third metatarsal bone, right foot**
> HAC 7th character B see Appendix B for HAC conditional logic

CC +7th **S92.335** **Nondisplaced fracture of third metatarsal bone, left foot**
> HAC 7th character B see Appendix B for HAC conditional logic

CC +7th **S92.336** **Nondisplaced fracture of third metatarsal bone, unspecified foot**
> HAC 7th character B see Appendix B for HAC conditional logic

+ **S92.34** **Fracture of fourth metatarsal bone**

CC +7th **S92.341** **Displaced fracture of fourth metatarsal bone, right foot**
> HAC 7th character B see Appendix B for HAC conditional logic

CC +7th **S92.342** **Displaced fracture of fourth metatarsal bone, left foot**
> HAC 7th character B see Appendix B for HAC conditional logic

CC +7th **S92.343** **Displaced fracture of fourth metatarsal bone, unspecified foot**
> HAC 7th character B see Appendix B for HAC conditional logic

CC +7th **S92.344** **Nondisplaced fracture of fourth metatarsal bone, right foot**
> HAC 7th character B see Appendix B for HAC conditional logic

CC +7th **S92.345** **Nondisplaced fracture of fourth metatarsal bone, left foot**
> HAC 7th character B see Appendix B for HAC conditional logic

CC +7th **S92.346** **Nondisplaced fracture of fourth metatarsal bone, unspecified foot**
> HAC 7th character B see Appendix B for HAC conditional logic

+ **S92.35** **Fracture of fifth metatarsal bone**

CC +7th **S92.351** **Displaced fracture of fifth metatarsal bone, right foot**
> HAC 7th character B see Appendix B for HAC conditional logic

CC +7th **S92.352** **Displaced fracture of fifth metatarsal bone, left foot**
> HAC 7th character B see Appendix B for HAC conditional logic

CC +7th **S92.353** **Displaced fracture of fifth metatarsal bone, unspecified foot**
> HAC 7th character B see Appendix B for HAC conditional logic

CC +7th **S92.354** **Nondisplaced fracture of fifth metatarsal bone, right foot**
> HAC 7th character B see Appendix B for HAC conditional logic

CC +7th **S92.355** **Nondisplaced fracture of fifth metatarsal bone, left foot**
> HAC 7th character B see Appendix B for HAC conditional logic

CC +7th **S92.356** **Nondisplaced fracture of fifth metatarsal bone, unspecified foot**
> HAC 7th character B see Appendix B for HAC conditional logic

+ **S92.4** **Fracture of great toe**
> *Excludes2:* *Physeal fracture of phalanx of toe (S99.2-)*

+ **S92.40** **Unspecified fracture of great toe**

CC +7th **S92.401** **Displaced unspecified fracture of right great toe**

CC +7th **S92.402** **Displaced unspecified fracture of left great toe**

CC +7th **S92.403** **Displaced unspecified fracture of unspecified great toe**

CC +7th **S92.404** **Nondisplaced unspecified fracture of right great toe**

CC +7th **S92.405** **Nondisplaced unspecified fracture of left great toe**

CC +7th **S92.406** **Nondisplaced unspecified fracture of unspecified great toe**

+ **S92.41** **Fracture of proximal phalanx of great toe**

CC +7th **S92.411** **Displaced fracture of proximal phalanx of right great toe**

CC +7th **S92.412** **Displaced fracture of proximal phalanx of left great toe**

CC +7th **S92.413** **Displaced fracture of proximal phalanx of unspecified great toe**

CC +7th **S92.414** **Nondisplaced fracture of proximal phalanx of right great toe**

CC +7th **S92.415** **Nondisplaced fracture of proximal phalanx of left great toe**

CC +7th **S92.416** **Nondisplaced fracture of proximal phalanx of unspecified great toe**

+ **S92.42** **Fracture of distal phalanx of great toe**

CC +7th **S92.421** **Displaced fracture of distal phalanx of right great toe**

CC +7th **S92.422** **Displaced fracture of distal phalanx of left great toe**

CC +7th **S92.423** **Displaced fracture of distal phalanx of unspecified great toe**

CC +7th **S92.424** **Nondisplaced fracture of distal phalanx of right great toe**

CC +7th **S92.425** **Nondisplaced fracture of distal phalanx of left great toe**

CC +7th **S92.426** **Nondisplaced fracture of distal phalanx of unspecified great toe**

+ **S92.49** **Other fracture of great toe**

CC +7th **S92.491** **Other fracture of right great toe**

CC +7th **S92.492** **Other fracture of left great toe**

CC +7th **S92.499** **Other fracture of unspecified great toe**

+ **S92.5** **Fracture of lesser toe(s)**
> *Excludes2:* *Physeal fracture of phalanx of toe (S99.2-)*

+ **S92.50** **Unspecified fracture of lesser toe(s)**

CC +7th **S92.501** **Displaced unspecified fracture of right lesser toe(s)**

CC +7th **S92.502** **Displaced unspecified fracture of left lesser toe(s)**

CC +7th **S92.503** **Displaced unspecified fracture of unspecified lesser toe(s)**

CC +7th **S92.504** **Nondisplaced unspecified fracture of right lesser toe(s)**

CC +7th **S92.505** **Nondisplaced unspecified fracture of left lesser toe(s)**

CC +7th **S92.506** **Nondisplaced unspecified fracture of unspecified lesser toe(s)**

+ **S92.51** **Fracture of proximal phalanx of lesser toe(s)**

CC +7th **S92.511** **Displaced fracture of proximal phalanx of right lesser toe(s)**

CC +7th **S92.512** **Displaced fracture of proximal phalanx of left lesser toe(s)**

CC +7th **S92.513** **Displaced fracture of proximal phalanx of unspecified lesser toe(s)**

CC +7th **S92.514** **Nondisplaced fracture of proximal phalanx of right lesser toe(s)**

CC +7th **S92.515** **Nondisplaced fracture of proximal phalanx of left lesser toe(s)**

CC +7th **S92.516** **Nondisplaced fracture of proximal phalanx of unspecified lesser toe(s)**

+ **S92.52** **Fracture of middle phalanx of lesser toe(s)**

CC +7th **S92.521** **Displaced fracture of middle phalanx of right lesser toe(s)**

CC +7th **S92.522** **Displaced fracture of middle phalanx of left lesser toe(s)**

CC +7th **S92.523** **Displaced fracture of middle phalanx of unspecified lesser toe(s)**

CC +7th **S92.524** **Nondisplaced fracture of middle phalanx of right lesser toe(s)**

CC +7th **S92.525** **Nondisplaced fracture of middle phalanx of left lesser toe(s)**

CC +7th **S92.526** **Nondisplaced fracture of middle phalanx of unspecified lesser toe(s)**

+, +7th, X + 7th   ● Newborn   ● Pediatric   ● Maternity   ● Adult   ♀ Female   ♂ Male   Manifestation   Unacceptable PDX   HCC   CC   MCC   HAC

+ **S92.53 Fracture of distal phalanx of lesser toe(s)**
- CC +7th **S92.531 Displaced fracture of distal phalanx of right lesser toe(s)**
- CC +7th **S92.532 Displaced fracture of distal phalanx of left lesser toe(s)**
- CC +7th **S92.533 Displaced fracture of distal phalanx of unspecified lesser toe(s)**
- CC +7th **S92.534 Nondisplaced fracture of distal phalanx of right lesser toe(s)**
- CC +7th **S92.535 Nondisplaced fracture of distal phalanx of left lesser toe(s)**
- CC +7th **S92.536 Nondisplaced fracture of distal phalanx of unspecified lesser toe(s)**

+ **S92.59 Other fracture of lesser toe(s)**
- CC +7th **S92.591 Other fracture of right lesser toe(s)**
- CC +7th **S92.592 Other fracture of left lesser toe(s)**
- CC +7th **S92.599 Other fracture of unspecified lesser toe(s)**

+ **S92.8 Other fracture of foot, except ankle**
+ **S92.81 Other fracture of foot**
  Sesamoid fracture of foot
  AHA CC: 4Q, 2016, 68
- CC +7th **S92.811 Other fracture of right foot**
  - HAC 7th character B see Appendix B for HAC conditional logic
- CC +7th **S92.812 Other fracture of left foot**
  - HAC 7th character B see Appendix B for HAC conditional logic
- CC +7th **S92.819 Other fracture of unspecified foot**
  - HAC 7th character B see Appendix B for HAC conditional logic

+ **S92.9 Unspecified fracture of foot and toe**
+ **S92.90 Unspecified fracture of foot**
- CC +7th **S92.901 Unspecified fracture of right foot**
  - HAC 7th character B see Appendix B for HAC conditional logic
- CC +7th **S92.902 Unspecified fracture of left foot**
  - HAC 7th character B see Appendix B for HAC conditional logic
- CC +7th **S92.909 Unspecified fracture of unspecified foot**
  - HAC 7th character B see Appendix B for HAC conditional logic

+ **S92.91 Unspecified fracture of toe**
- CC +7th **S92.911 Unspecified fracture of right toe(s)**
- CC +7th **S92.912 Unspecified fracture of left toe(s)**
- CC +7th **S92.919 Unspecified fracture of unspecified toe(s)**

S93 Dislocation and sprain of joints and ligaments at ankle, foot and toe level

Includes: avulsion of joint or ligament of ankle, foot and toe
laceration of cartilage, joint or ligament of ankle, foot and toe
sprain of cartilage, joint or ligament of ankle, foot and toe
traumatic hemarthrosis of joint or ligament of ankle, foot and toe
traumatic rupture of joint or ligament of ankle, foot and toe
traumatic subluxation of joint or ligament of ankle, foot and toe
traumatic tear of joint or ligament of ankle, foot and toe

Code also any associated open wound

Excludes2: *strain of muscle and tendon of ankle and foot (S96.-)*

The appropriate 7th character is to be added to each code from category S93.
A initial encounter
D subsequent encounter
S sequela

+ **S93.0 Subluxation and dislocation of ankle joint**
  Subluxation and dislocation of astragalus
  Subluxation and dislocation of fibula, lower end
  Subluxation and dislocation of talus
  Subluxation and dislocation of tibia, lower end
- X+7th **S93.01 Subluxation of right ankle joint**
- X+7th **S93.02 Subluxation of left ankle joint**
- X+7th **S93.03 Subluxation of unspecified ankle joint**
- X+7th **S93.04 Dislocation of right ankle joint**
- X+7th **S93.05 Dislocation of left ankle joint**
- X+7th **S93.06 Dislocation of unspecified ankle joint**

+ **S93.1 Subluxation and dislocation of toe**
+ **S93.10 Unspecified subluxation and dislocation of toe**
  Dislocation of toe NOS
  Subluxation of toe NOS
- +7th **S93.101 Unspecified subluxation of right toe(s)**
- +7th **S93.102 Unspecified subluxation of left toe(s)**
- +7th **S93.103 Unspecified subluxation of unspecified toe(s)**
- +7th **S93.104 Unspecified dislocation of right toe(s)**
- +7th **S93.105 Unspecified dislocation of left toe(s)**
- +7th **S93.106 Unspecified dislocation of unspecified toe(s)**

+ **S93.11 Dislocation of interphalangeal joint**
- +7th **S93.111 Dislocation of interphalangeal joint of right great toe**
- +7th **S93.112 Dislocation of interphalangeal joint of left great toe**
- +7th **S93.113 Dislocation of interphalangeal joint of unspecified great toe**
- +7th **S93.114 Dislocation of interphalangeal joint of right lesser toe(s)**
- +7th **S93.115 Dislocation of interphalangeal joint of left lesser toe(s)**
- +7th **S93.116 Dislocation of interphalangeal joint of unspecified lesser toe(s)**
- +7th **S93.119 Dislocation of interphalangeal joint of unspecified toe(s)**

+ **S93.12 Dislocation of metatarsophalangeal joint**
- +7th **S93.121 Dislocation of metatarsophalangeal joint of right great toe**
- +7th **S93.122 Dislocation of metatarsophalangeal joint of left great toe**
- +7th **S93.123 Dislocation of metatarsophalangeal joint of unspecified great toe**
- +7th **S93.124 Dislocation of metatarsophalangeal joint of right lesser toe(s)**
- +7th **S93.125 Dislocation of metatarsophalangeal joint of left lesser toe(s)**
- +7th **S93.126 Dislocation of metatarsophalangeal joint of unspecified lesser toe(s)**
- +7th **S93.129 Dislocation of metatarsophalangeal joint of unspecified toe(s)**

+ **S93.13 Subluxation of interphalangeal joint**
- +7th **S93.131 Subluxation of interphalangeal joint of right great toe**
- +7th **S93.132 Subluxation of interphalangeal joint of left great toe**
- +7th **S93.133 Subluxation of interphalangeal joint of unspecified great toe**
- +7th **S93.134 Subluxation of interphalangeal joint of right lesser toe(s)**
- +7th **S93.135 Subluxation of interphalangeal joint of left lesser toe(s)**
- +7th **S93.136 Subluxation of interphalangeal joint of unspecified lesser toe(s)**
- +7th **S93.139 Subluxation of interphalangeal joint of unspecified toe(s)**

+ **S93.14 Subluxation of metatarsophalangeal joint**
- +7th **S93.141 Subluxation of metatarsophalangeal joint of right great toe**
- +7th **S93.142 Subluxation of metatarsophalangeal joint of left great toe**
- +7th **S93.143 Subluxation of metatarsophalangeal joint of unspecified great toe**
- +7th **S93.144 Subluxation of metatarsophalangeal joint of right lesser toe(s)**
- +7th **S93.145 Subluxation of metatarsophalangeal joint of left lesser toe(s)**
- +7th **S93.146 Subluxation of metatarsophalangeal joint of unspecified lesser toe(s)**
- +7th **S93.149 Subluxation of metatarsophalangeal joint of unspecified toe(s)**

+, +7th, X + 7th   ● Newborn   ● Pediatric   ● Maternity   ● Adult   ♀ Female   ♂ Male   Manifestation   Unacceptable PDX   HCC   CC   MCC   HAC

+ **S93.3 Subluxation and dislocation of foot**
  Excludes2: *dislocation of toe (S93.1-)*
  + **S93.30 Unspecified subluxation and dislocation of foot**
    Dislocation of foot NOS
    Subluxation of foot NOS
    +7th **S93.301 Unspecified subluxation of right foot**
    +7th **S93.302 Unspecified subluxation of left foot**
    +7th **S93.303 Unspecified subluxation of unspecified foot**
    +7th **S93.304 Unspecified dislocation of right foot**
    +7th **S93.305 Unspecified dislocation of left foot**
    +7th **S93.306 Unspecified dislocation of unspecified foot**
  + **S93.31 Subluxation and dislocation of tarsal joint**
    +7th **S93.311 Subluxation of tarsal joint of right foot**
    +7th **S93.312 Subluxation of tarsal joint of left foot**
    +7th **S93.313 Subluxation of tarsal joint of unspecified foot**
    +7th **S93.314 Dislocation of tarsal joint of right foot**
    +7th **S93.315 Dislocation of tarsal joint of left foot**
    +7th **S93.316 Dislocation of tarsal joint of unspecified foot**
  + **S93.32 Subluxation and dislocation of tarsometatarsal joint**
    +7th **S93.321 Subluxation of tarsometatarsal joint of right foot**
    +7th **S93.322 Subluxation of tarsometatarsal joint of left foot**
    +7th **S93.323 Subluxation of tarsometatarsal joint of unspecified foot**
    +7th **S93.324 Dislocation of tarsometatarsal joint of right foot**
    +7th **S93.325 Dislocation of tarsometatarsal joint of left foot**
    +7th **S93.326 Dislocation of tarsometatarsal joint of unspecified foot**
  + **S93.33 Other subluxation and dislocation of foot**
    +7th **S93.331 Other subluxation of right foot**
    +7th **S93.332 Other subluxation of left foot**
    +7th **S93.333 Other subluxation of unspecified foot**
    +7th **S93.334 Other dislocation of right foot**
    +7th **S93.335 Other dislocation of left foot**
    +7th **S93.336 Other dislocation of unspecified foot**

+ **S93.4 Sprain of ankle**
  Excludes2: *injury of Achilles tendon (S86.0-)*
  + **S93.40 Sprain of unspecified ligament of ankle**
    Sprain of ankle NOS
    Sprained ankle NOS
    +7th **S93.401 Sprain of unspecified ligament of right ankle**
    +7th **S93.402 Sprain of unspecified ligament of left ankle**
    +7th **S93.409 Sprain of unspecified ligament of unspecified ankle**
  + **S93.41 Sprain of calcaneofibular ligament**
    +7th **S93.411 Sprain of calcaneofibular ligament of right ankle**
    +7th **S93.412 Sprain of calcaneofibular ligament of left ankle**
    +7th **S93.419 Sprain of calcaneofibular ligament of unspecified ankle**
  + **S93.42 Sprain of deltoid ligament**
    +7th **S93.421 Sprain of deltoid ligament of right ankle**
    +7th **S93.422 Sprain of deltoid ligament of left ankle**
    +7th **S93.429 Sprain of deltoid ligament of unspecified ankle**
  + **S93.43 Sprain of tibiofibular ligament**
    +7th **S93.431 Sprain of tibiofibular ligament of right ankle**
    +7th **S93.432 Sprain of tibiofibular ligament of left ankle**
    +7th **S93.439 Sprain of tibiofibular ligament of unspecified ankle**
  + **S93.49 Sprain of other ligament of ankle**
    Sprain of internal collateral ligament
    Sprain of talofibular ligament
    +7th **S93.491 Sprain of other ligament of right ankle**
    +7th **S93.492 Sprain of other ligament of left ankle**
    +7th **S93.499 Sprain of other ligament of unspecified ankle**

+ **S93.5 Sprain of toe**
  + **S93.50 Unspecified sprain of toe**
    +7th **S93.501 Unspecified sprain of right great toe**
    +7th **S93.502 Unspecified sprain of left great toe**
    +7th **S93.503 Unspecified sprain of unspecified great toe**
    +7th **S93.504 Unspecified sprain of right lesser toe(s)**
    +7th **S93.505 Unspecified sprain of left lesser toe(s)**
    +7th **S93.506 Unspecified sprain of unspecified lesser toe(s)**
    +7th **S93.509 Unspecified sprain of unspecified toe(s)**
  + **S93.51 Sprain of interphalangeal joint of toe**
    +7th **S93.511 Sprain of interphalangeal joint of right great toe**
    +7th **S93.512 Sprain of interphalangeal joint of left great toe**
    +7th **S93.513 Sprain of interphalangeal joint of unspecified great toe**
    +7th **S93.514 Sprain of interphalangeal joint of right lesser toe(s)**
    +7th **S93.515 Sprain of interphalangeal joint of left lesser toe(s)**
    +7th **S93.516 Sprain of interphalangeal joint of unspecified lesser toe(s)**
    +7th **S93.519 Sprain of interphalangeal joint of unspecified toe(s)**
  + **S93.52 Sprain of metatarsophalangeal joint of toe**
    +7th **S93.521 Sprain of metatarsophalangeal joint of right great toe**
    +7th **S93.522 Sprain of metatarsophalangeal joint of left great toe**
    +7th **S93.523 Sprain of metatarsophalangeal joint of unspecified great toe**
    +7th **S93.524 Sprain of metatarsophalangeal joint of right lesser toe(s)**
    +7th **S93.525 Sprain of metatarsophalangeal joint of left lesser toe(s)**
    +7th **S93.526 Sprain of metatarsophalangeal joint of unspecified lesser toe(s)**
    +7th **S93.529 Sprain of metatarsophalangeal joint of unspecified toe(s)**

+ **S93.6 Sprain of foot**
  Excludes2: *sprain of metatarsophalangeal joint of toe (S93.52-) sprain of toe (S93.5-)*
  + **S93.60 Unspecified sprain of foot**
    +7th **S93.601 Unspecified sprain of right foot**
    +7th **S93.602 Unspecified sprain of left foot**
    +7th **S93.609 Unspecified sprain of unspecified foot**
  + **S93.61 Sprain of tarsal ligament of foot**
    +7th **S93.611 Sprain of tarsal ligament of right foot**
    +7th **S93.612 Sprain of tarsal ligament of left foot**
    +7th **S93.619 Sprain of tarsal ligament of unspecified foot**
  + **S93.62 Sprain of tarsometatarsal ligament of foot**
    +7th **S93.621 Sprain of tarsometatarsal ligament of right foot**
    +7th **S93.622 Sprain of tarsometatarsal ligament of left foot**
    +7th **S93.629 Sprain of tarsometatarsal ligament of unspecified foot**
  + **S93.69 Other sprain of foot**
    +7th **S93.691 Other sprain of right foot**
    +7th **S93.692 Other sprain of left foot**
    +7th **S93.699 Other sprain of unspecified foot**

S94 Injury of nerves at ankle and foot level
  Code also any associated open wound (S91.-)

  The appropriate 7th character is to be added to each code from category S94
  A initial encounter
  D subsequent encounter
  S sequela

+ **S94.0 Injury of lateral plantar nerve**
  X+7th **S94.00 Injury of lateral plantar nerve, unspecified leg**
  X+7th **S94.01 Injury of lateral plantar nerve, right leg**
  X+7th **S94.02 Injury of lateral plantar nerve, left leg**
+ **S94.1 Injury of medial plantar nerve**
  X+7th **S94.10 Injury of medial plantar nerve, unspecified leg**
  X+7th **S94.11 Injury of medial plantar nerve, right leg**
  X+7th **S94.12 Injury of medial plantar nerve, left leg**

+ **S94.2 Injury of deep peroneal nerve at ankle and foot level**
    Injury of terminal, lateral branch of deep peroneal nerve
  X+7th **S94.20 Injury of deep peroneal nerve at ankle and foot level, unspecified leg**
  X+7th **S94.21 Injury of deep peroneal nerve at ankle and foot level, right leg**
  X+7th **S94.22 Injury of deep peroneal nerve at ankle and foot level, left leg**

+ **S94.3 Injury of cutaneous sensory nerve at ankle and foot level**
  X+7th **S94.30 Injury of cutaneous sensory nerve at ankle and foot level, unspecified leg**
  X+7th **S94.31 Injury of cutaneous sensory nerve at ankle and foot level, right leg**
  X+7th **S94.32 Injury of cutaneous sensory nerve at ankle and foot level, left leg**

+ **S94.8 Injury of other nerves at ankle and foot level**
  + **S94.8X Injury of other nerves at ankle and foot level**
    +7th **S94.8X1 Injury of other nerves at ankle and foot level, right leg**
    +7th **S94.8X2 Injury of other nerves at ankle and foot level, left leg**
    +7th **S94.8X9 Injury of other nerves at ankle and foot level, unspecified leg**

+ **S94.9 Injury of unspecified nerve at ankle and foot level**
  X+7th **S94.90 Injury of unspecified nerve at ankle and foot level, unspecified leg**
  X+7th **S94.91 Injury of unspecified nerve at ankle and foot level, right leg**
  X+7th **S94.92 Injury of unspecified nerve at ankle and foot level, left leg**

S95 Injury of blood vessels at ankle and foot level

Code also any associated open wound (S91.-)
Excludes2: *injury of posterior tibial artery and vein (S85.1-, S85.8-)*

The appropriate 7th character is to be added to each code from category S95
A initial encounter
D subsequent encounter
S sequela

+ **S95.0 Injury of dorsal artery of foot**
  + **S95.00 Unspecified injury of dorsal artery of foot**
    CC +7th **S95.001 Unspecified injury of dorsal artery of right foot**
    CC +7th **S95.002 Unspecified injury of dorsal artery of left foot**
    CC +7th **S95.009 Unspecified injury of dorsal artery of unspecified foot**
  + **S95.01 Laceration of dorsal artery of foot**
    CC +7th **S95.011 Laceration of dorsal artery of right foot**
    CC +7th **S95.012 Laceration of dorsal artery of left foot**
    CC +7th **S95.019 Laceration of dorsal artery of unspecified foot**
  + **S95.09 Other specified injury of dorsal artery of foot**
    CC +7th **S95.091 Other specified injury of dorsal artery of right foot**
    CC +7th **S95.092 Other specified injury of dorsal artery of left foot**
    CC +7th **S95.099 Other specified injury of dorsal artery of unspecified foot**

+ **S95.1 Injury of plantar artery of foot**
  + **S95.10 Unspecified injury of plantar artery of foot**
    CC +7th **S95.101 Unspecified injury of plantar artery of right foot**
    CC +7th **S95.102 Unspecified injury of plantar artery of left foot**
    CC +7th **S95.109 Unspecified injury of plantar artery of unspecified foot**
  + **S95.11 Laceration of plantar artery of foot**
    CC +7th **S95.111 Laceration of plantar artery of right foot**
    CC +7th **S95.112 Laceration of plantar artery of left foot**
    CC +7th **S95.119 Laceration of plantar artery of unspecified foot**
  + **S95.19 Other specified injury of plantar artery of foot**
    CC +7th **S95.191 Other specified injury of plantar artery of right foot**
    CC +7th **S95.192 Other specified injury of plantar artery of left foot**
    CC +7th **S95.199 Other specified injury of plantar artery of unspecified foot**

+ **S95.2 Injury of dorsal vein of foot**
  + **S95.20 Unspecified injury of dorsal vein of foot**
    CC +7th **S95.201 Unspecified injury of dorsal vein of right foot**
    CC +7th **S95.202 Unspecified injury of dorsal vein of left foot**
    CC +7th **S95.209 Unspecified injury of dorsal vein of unspecified foot**
  + **S95.21 Laceration of dorsal vein of foot**
    CC +7th **S95.211 Laceration of dorsal vein of right foot**
    CC +7th **S95.212 Laceration of dorsal vein of left foot**
    CC +7th **S95.219 Laceration of dorsal vein of unspecified foot**
  + **S95.29 Other specified injury of dorsal vein of foot**
    CC +7th **S95.291 Other specified injury of dorsal vein of right foot**
    CC +7th **S95.292 Other specified injury of dorsal vein of left foot**
    CC +7th **S95.299 Other specified injury of dorsal vein of unspecified foot**

S95.8 Injury of other blood vessels at ankle and foot level
  + **S95.80 Unspecified injury of other blood vessels at ankle and foot level**
    CC +7th **S95.801 Unspecified injury of other blood vessels at ankle and foot level, right leg**
    CC +7th **S95.802 Unspecified injury of other blood vessels at ankle and foot level, left leg**
    CC +7th **S95.809 Unspecified injury of other blood vessels at ankle and foot level, unspecified leg**
  + **S95.81 Laceration of other blood vessels at ankle and foot level**
    CC +7th **S95.811 Laceration of other blood vessels at ankle and foot level, right leg**
    CC +7th **S95.812 Laceration of other blood vessels at ankle and foot level, left leg**
    CC +7th **S95.819 Laceration of other blood vessels at ankle and foot level, unspecified leg**
  + **S95.89 Other specified injury of other blood vessels at ankle and foot level**
    CC +7th **S95.891 Other specified injury of other blood vessels at ankle and foot level, right leg**
    CC +7th **S95.892 Other specified injury of other blood vessels at ankle and foot level, left leg**
    CC +7th **S95.899 Other specified injury of other blood vessels at ankle and foot level, unspecified leg**

+ **S95.9 Injury of unspecified blood vessel at ankle and foot level**
  + **S95.90 Unspecified injury of unspecified blood vessel at ankle and foot level**
    CC +7th **S95.901 Unspecified injury of unspecified blood vessel at ankle and foot level, right leg**
    CC +7th **S95.902 Unspecified injury of unspecified blood vessel at ankle and foot level, left leg**
    CC +7th **S95.909 Unspecified injury of unspecified blood vessel at ankle and foot level, unspecified leg**
  + **S95.91 Laceration of unspecified blood vessel at ankle and foot level**
    CC +7th **S95.911 Laceration of unspecified blood vessel at ankle and foot level, right leg**
    CC +7th **S95.912 Laceration of unspecified blood vessel at ankle and foot level, left leg**
    CC +7th **S95.919 Laceration of unspecified blood vessel at ankle and foot level, unspecified leg**
  + **S95.99 Other specified injury of unspecified blood vessel at ankle and foot level**
    CC +7th **S95.991 Other specified injury of unspecified blood vessel at ankle and foot level, right leg**
    CC +7th **S95.992 Other specified injury of unspecified blood vessel at ankle and foot level, left leg**
    CC +7th **S95.999 Other specified injury of unspecified blood vessel at ankle and foot level, unspecified leg**

S96 Injury of muscle and tendon at ankle and foot level

Code also any associated open wound (S91.-)

Excludes2: *injury of Achilles tendon (S86.0-)*
sprain of joints and ligaments of ankle and foot (S93.-)

The appropriate 7th character is to be added to each code from category S96
A   initial encounter
D   subsequent encounter
S   sequela

+   **S96.0 Injury of muscle and tendon of long flexor muscle of toe at ankle and foot level**
    +   **S96.00 Unspecified injury of muscle and tendon of long flexor muscle of toe at ankle and foot level**
        +7th **S96.001** Unspecified injury of muscle and tendon of long flexor muscle of toe at ankle and foot level, right foot
        +7th **S96.002** Unspecified injury of muscle and tendon of long flexor muscle of toe at ankle and foot level, left foot
        +7th **S96.009** Unspecified injury of muscle and tendon of long flexor muscle of toe at ankle and foot level, unspecified foot
    +   **S96.01 Strain of muscle and tendon of long flexor muscle of toe at ankle and foot level**
        +7th **S96.011** Strain of muscle and tendon of long flexor muscle of toe at ankle and foot level, right foot
        +7th **S96.012** Strain of muscle and tendon of long flexor muscle of toe at ankle and foot level, left foot
        +7th **S96.019** Strain of muscle and tendon of long flexor muscle of toe at ankle and foot level, unspecified foot
    +   **S96.02 Laceration of muscle and tendon of long flexor muscle of toe at ankle and foot level**
        CC +7th **S96.021** Laceration of muscle and tendon of long flexor muscle of toe at ankle and foot level, right foot
        CC +7th **S96.022** Laceration of muscle and tendon of long flexor muscle of toe at ankle and foot level, left foot
        CC +7th **S96.029** Laceration of muscle and tendon of long flexor muscle of toe at ankle and foot level, unspecified foot
    +   **S96.09 Other injury of muscle and tendon of long flexor muscle of toe at ankle and foot level**
        +7th **S96.091** Other injury of muscle and tendon of long flexor muscle of toe at ankle and foot level, right foot
        +7th **S96.092** Other injury of muscle and tendon of long flexor muscle of toe at ankle and foot level, left foot
        +7th **S96.099** Other injury of muscle and tendon of long flexor muscle of toe at ankle and foot level, unspecified foot
+   **S96.1 Injury of muscle and tendon of long extensor muscle of toe at ankle and foot level**
    +   **S96.10 Unspecified injury of muscle and tendon of long extensor muscle of toe at ankle and foot level**
        +7th **S96.101** Unspecified injury of muscle and tendon of long extensor muscle of toe at ankle and foot level, right foot
        +7th **S96.102** Unspecified injury of muscle and tendon of long extensor muscle of toe at ankle and foot level, left foot
        +7th **S96.109** Unspecified injury of muscle and tendon of long extensor muscle of toe at ankle and foot level, unspecified foot
    +   **S96.11 Strain of muscle and tendon of long extensor muscle of toe at ankle and foot level**
        +7th **S96.111** Strain of muscle and tendon of long extensor muscle of toe at ankle and foot level, right foot
        +7th **S96.112** Strain of muscle and tendon of long extensor muscle of toe at ankle and foot level, left foot
        +7th **S96.119** Strain of muscle and tendon of long extensor muscle of toe at ankle and foot level, unspecified foot

+   **S96.12 Laceration of muscle and tendon of long extensor muscle of toe at ankle and foot level**
    CC +7th **S96.121** Laceration of muscle and tendon of long extensor muscle of toe at ankle and foot level, right foot
    CC +7th **S96.122** Laceration of muscle and tendon of long extensor muscle of toe at ankle and foot level, left foot
    CC +7th **S96.129** Laceration of muscle and tendon of long extensor muscle of toe at ankle and foot level, unspecified foot
+   **S96.19 Other specified injury of muscle and tendon of long extensor muscle of toe at ankle and foot level**
    +7th **S96.191** Other specified injury of muscle and tendon of long extensor muscle of toe at ankle and foot level, right foot
    +7th **S96.192** Other specified injury of muscle and tendon of long extensor muscle of toe at ankle and foot level, left foot
    +7th **S96.199** Other specified injury of muscle and tendon of long extensor muscle of toe at ankle and foot level, unspecified foot
+   **S96.2 Injury of intrinsic muscle and tendon at ankle and foot level**
    +   **S96.20 Unspecified injury of intrinsic muscle and tendon at ankle and foot level**
        +7th **S96.201** Unspecified injury of intrinsic muscle and tendon at ankle and foot level, right foot
        +7th **S96.202** Unspecified injury of intrinsic muscle and tendon at ankle and foot level, left foot
        +7th **S96.209** Unspecified injury of intrinsic muscle and tendon at ankle and foot level, unspecified foot
    +   **S96.21 Strain of intrinsic muscle and tendon at ankle and foot level**
        +7th **S96.211** Strain of intrinsic muscle and tendon at ankle and foot level, right foot
        +7th **S96.212** Strain of intrinsic muscle and tendon at ankle and foot level, left foot
        +7th **S96.219** Strain of intrinsic muscle and tendon at ankle and foot level, unspecified foot
    +   **S96.22 Laceration of intrinsic muscle and tendon at ankle and foot level**
        CC +7th **S96.221** Laceration of intrinsic muscle and tendon at ankle and foot level, right foot
        CC +7th **S96.222** Laceration of intrinsic muscle and tendon at ankle and foot level, left foot
        CC +7th **S96.229** Laceration of intrinsic muscle and tendon at ankle and foot level, unspecified foot
    +   **S96.29 Other specified injury of intrinsic muscle and tendon at ankle and foot level**
        +7th **S96.291** Other specified injury of intrinsic muscle and tendon at ankle and foot level, right foot
        +7th **S96.292** Other specified injury of intrinsic muscle and tendon at ankle and foot level, left foot
        +7th **S96.299** Other specified injury of intrinsic muscle and tendon at ankle and foot level, unspecified foot
+   **S96.8 Injury of other specified muscles and tendons at ankle and foot level**
    +   **S96.80 Unspecified injury of other specified muscles and tendons at ankle and foot level**
        +7th **S96.801** Unspecified injury of other specified muscles and tendons at ankle and foot level, right foot
        +7th **S96.802** Unspecified injury of other specified muscles and tendons at ankle and foot level, left foot
        +7th **S96.809** Unspecified injury of other specified muscles and tendons at ankle and foot level, unspecified foot
    +   **S96.81 Strain of other specified muscles and tendons at ankle and foot level**
        +7th **S96.811** Strain of other specified muscles and tendons at ankle and foot level, right foot
        +7th **S96.812** Strain of other specified muscles and tendons at ankle and foot level, left foot
        +7th **S96.819** Strain of other specified muscles and tendons at ankle and foot level, unspecified foot

+, +7th, X + 7th   ● Newborn   ● Pediatric   ● Maternity   ● Adult   ♀ Female   ♂ Male   Manifestation   Unacceptable PDX   HCC   CC   MCC   HAC

+ S96.82 **Laceration of other specified muscles and tendons at ankle and foot level**

CC +7th S96.821 **Laceration of other specified muscles and tendons at ankle and foot level, right foot**

CC +7th S96.822 **Laceration of other specified muscles and tendons at ankle and foot level, left foot**

CC +7th S96.829 **Laceration of other specified muscles and tendons at ankle and foot level, unspecified foot**

+ S96.89 **Other specified injury of other specified muscles and tendons at ankle and foot level**

+7th S96.891 **Other specified injury of other specified muscles and tendons at ankle and foot level, right foot**

+7th S96.892 **Other specified injury of other specified muscles and tendons at ankle and foot level, left foot**

+7th S96.899 **Other specified injury of other specified muscles and tendons at ankle and foot level, unspecified foot**

+ S96.9 **Injury of unspecified muscle and tendon at ankle and foot level**

+ S96.90 **Unspecified injury of unspecified muscle and tendon at ankle and foot level**

+7th S96.901 **Unspecified injury of unspecified muscle and tendon at ankle and foot level, right foot**

+7th S96.902 **Unspecified injury of unspecified muscle and tendon at ankle and foot level, left foot**

+7th S96.909 **Unspecified injury of unspecified muscle and tendon at ankle and foot level, unspecified foot**

+ S96.91 **Strain of unspecified muscle and tendon at ankle and foot level**

+7th S96.911 **Strain of unspecified muscle and tendon at ankle and foot level, right foot**

+7th S96.912 **Strain of unspecified muscle and tendon at ankle and foot level, left foot**

+7th S96.919 **Strain of unspecified muscle and tendon at ankle and foot level, unspecified foot**

+ S96.92 **Laceration of unspecified muscle and tendon at ankle and foot level**

CC +7th S96.921 **Laceration of unspecified muscle and tendon at ankle and foot level, right foot**

CC +7th S96.922 **Laceration of unspecified muscle and tendon at ankle and foot level, left foot**

CC +7th S96.929 **Laceration of unspecified muscle and tendon at ankle and foot level, unspecified foot**

+ S96.99 **Other specified injury of unspecified muscle and tendon at ankle and foot level**

+7th S96.991 **Other specified injury of unspecified muscle and tendon at ankle and foot level, right foot**

+7th S96.992 **Other specified injury of unspecified muscle and tendon at ankle and foot level, left foot**

+7th S96.999 **Other specified injury of unspecified muscle and tendon at ankle and foot level, unspecified foot**

S97 Crushing injury of ankle and foot

Use additional code(s) for all associated injuries

The appropriate 7th character is to be added to each code from category S97
A   initial encounter
D   subsequent encounter
S   sequela

+ S97.0 **Crushing injury of ankle**

X+7th S97.00 **Crushing injury of unspecified ankle**

X+7th S97.01 **Crushing injury of right ankle**

X+7th S97.02 **Crushing injury of left ankle**

+ S97.1 **Crushing injury of toe**

+ S97.10 **Crushing injury of unspecified toe(s)**

+7th S97.101 **Crushing injury of unspecified right toe(s)**

+7th S97.102 **Crushing injury of unspecified left toe(s)**

+7th S97.109 **Crushing injury of unspecified toe(s)**
Crushing injury of toe NOS

+ S97.11 **Crushing injury of great toe**

+7th S97.111 **Crushing injury of right great toe**

+7th S97.112 **Crushing injury of left great toe**

+7th S97.119 **Crushing injury of unspecified great toe**

+ S97.12 **Crushing injury of lesser toe(s)**

+7th S97.121 **Crushing injury of right lesser toe(s)**

+7th S97.122 **Crushing injury of left lesser toe(s)**

+7th S97.129 **Crushing injury of unspecified lesser toe(s)**

+ S97.8 **Crushing injury of foot**

X+7th S97.80 **Crushing injury of unspecified foot**
Crushing injury of foot NOS

X+7th S97.81 **Crushing injury of right foot**

X+7th S97.82 **Crushing injury of left foot**

S98 Traumatic amputation of ankle and foot

NOTE   An amputation not identified as partial or complete should be coded to complete

The appropriate 7th character is to be added to each code from category S98
A   initial encounter
D   subsequent encounter
S   sequela

+ S98.0 **Traumatic amputation of foot at ankle level**

+ S98.01 **Complete traumatic amputation of foot at ankle level**

CC +7th S98.011 **Complete traumatic amputation of right foot at ankle level**

CC +7th S98.012 **Complete traumatic amputation of left foot at ankle level**

CC +7th S98.019 **Complete traumatic amputation of unspecified foot at ankle level**

+ S98.02 **Partial traumatic amputation of foot at ankle level**

CC +7th S98.021 **Partial traumatic amputation of right foot at ankle level**

CC +7th S98.022 **Partial traumatic amputation of left foot at ankle level**

CC +7th S98.029 **Partial traumatic amputation of unspecified foot at ankle level**

+ S98.1 **Traumatic amputation of one toe**

+ S98.11 **Complete traumatic amputation of great toe**

+7th S98.111 **Complete traumatic amputation of right great toe**

+7th S98.112 **Complete traumatic amputation of left great toe**

+7th S98.119 **Complete traumatic amputation of unspecified great toe**

+ S98.12 **Partial traumatic amputation of great toe**

+7th S98.121 **Partial traumatic amputation of right great toe**

+7th S98.122 **Partial traumatic amputation of left great toe**

+7th S98.129 **Partial traumatic amputation of unspecified great toe**

+ S98.13 **Complete traumatic amputation of one lesser toe**
Traumatic amputation of toe NOS

+7th S98.131 **Complete traumatic amputation of one right lesser toe**

+7th S98.132 **Complete traumatic amputation of one left lesser toe**

+7th S98.139 **Complete traumatic amputation of one unspecified lesser toe**

+ S98.14 **Partial traumatic amputation of one lesser toe**

+7th S98.141 **Partial traumatic amputation of one right lesser toe**

+7th S98.142 **Partial traumatic amputation of one left lesser toe**

+7th S98.149 **Partial traumatic amputation of one unspecified lesser toe**

+, +7th, X + 7th   ● Newborn   ● Pediatric   ● Maternity   ● Adult   ♀ Female   ♂ Male   Manifestation   Unacceptable PDX   HCC   CC   MCC   HAC

+ **S98.2**   **Traumatic amputation of two or more lesser toes**
    + **S98.21**   **Complete traumatic amputation of two or more lesser toes**
        +7th **S98.211**   **Complete traumatic amputation of two or more right lesser toes**
        +7th **S98.212**   **Complete traumatic amputation of two or more left lesser toes**
        +7th **S98.219**   **Complete traumatic amputation of two or more unspecified lesser toes**
    + **S98.22**   **Partial traumatic amputation of two or more lesser toes**
        +7th **S98.221**   **Partial traumatic amputation of two or more right lesser toes**
        +7th **S98.222**   **Partial traumatic amputation of two or more left lesser toes**
        +7th **S98.229**   **Partial traumatic amputation of two or more unspecified lesser toes**

+ **S98.3**   **Traumatic amputation of midfoot**
    + **S98.31**   **Complete traumatic amputation of midfoot**
        CC +7th **S98.311**   **Complete traumatic amputation of right midfoot**
        CC +7th **S98.312**   **Complete traumatic amputation of left midfoot**
        CC +7th **S98.319**   **Complete traumatic amputation of unspecified midfoot**
    + **S98.32**   **Partial traumatic amputation of midfoot**
        CC +7th **S98.321**   **Partial traumatic amputation of right midfoot**
        CC +7th **S98.322**   **Partial traumatic amputation of left midfoot**
        CC +7th **S98.329**   **Partial traumatic amputation of unspecified midfoot**

+ **S98.9**   **Traumatic amputation of foot, level unspecified**
    + **S98.91**   **Complete traumatic amputation of foot, level unspecified**
        CC +7th **S98.911**   **Complete traumatic amputation of right foot, level unspecified**
        CC +7th **S98.912**   **Complete traumatic amputation of left foot, level unspecified**
        CC +7th **S98.919**   **Complete traumatic amputation of unspecified foot, level unspecified**
    + **S98.92**   **Partial traumatic amputation of foot, level unspecified**
        CC +7th **S98.921**   **Partial traumatic amputation of right foot, level unspecified**
        CC +7th **S98.922**   **Partial traumatic amputation of left foot, level unspecified**
        CC +7th **S98.929**   **Partial traumatic amputation of unspecified foot, level unspecified**

S99   **Other and unspecified injuries of ankle and foot**

+ **S99.0**   **Physeal fracture of calcaneus**
    AHA CC: 4Q, 2016, 68-69

The appropriate 7th character is to be added to each code in subcategory **S99.0**

A   initial encounter for closed fracture
B   initial encounter for open fracture
D   subsequent encounter for fracture with routine healing
G   subsequent encounter for fracture with delayed healing
K   subsequent encounter for fracture with nonunion
P   subsequent encounter for fracture with malunion
S   sequela

    + **S99.00**   **Unspecified physeal fracture of calcaneus**
        Unspecified physeal fracture of calcaneus
        +7th **S99.001**   **Unspecified physeal fracture of right calcaneus**
        +7th **S99.002**   **Unspecified physeal fracture of left calcaneus**
        +7th **S99.009**   **Unspecified physeal fracture of unspecified calcaneus**
    + **S99.01**   **Salter-Harris Type I physeal fracture of calcaneus**
        +7th **S99.011**   **Salter-Harris Type I physeal fracture of right calcaneus**
        +7th **S99.012**   **Salter-Harris Type I physeal fracture of left calcaneus**
        +7th **S99.019**   **Salter-Harris Type I physeal fracture of unspecified calcaneus**

+ **S99.02**   **Salter-Harris Type II physeal fracture of calcaneus**
    +7th **S99.021**   **Salter-Harris Type II physeal fracture of right calcaneus**
    +7th **S99.022**   **Salter-Harris Type II physeal fracture of left calcaneus**
    +7th **S99.029**   **Salter-Harris Type II physeal fracture of unspecified calcaneus**
+ **S99.03**   **Salter-Harris Type III physeal fracture of calcaneus**
    +7th **S99.031**   **Salter-Harris Type III physeal fracture of right calcaneus**
    +7th **S99.032**   **Salter-Harris Type III physeal fracture of left calcaneus**
    +7th **S99.039**   **Salter-Harris Type III physeal fracture of unspecified calcaneus**
+ **S99.04**   **Salter-Harris Type IV physeal fracture of calcaneus**
    +7th **S99.041**   **Salter-Harris Type IV physeal fracture of right calcaneus**
    +7th **S99.042**   **Salter-Harris Type IV physeal fracture of left calcaneus**
    +7th **S99.049**   **Salter-Harris Type IV physeal fracture of unspecified calcaneus**
+ **S99.09**   **Other physeal fracture of calcaneus**
    +7th **S99.091**   **Other physeal fracture of right calcaneus**
    +7th **S99.092**   **Other physeal fracture of left calcaneus**
    +7th **S99.099**   **Other physeal fracture of unspecified calcaneus**

+ **S99.1**   **Physeal fracture of metatarsal**

The appropriate 7th character is to be added to each code in subcategory **S99.1**

A   initial encounter for closed fracture
B   initial encounter for open fracture
D   subsequent encounter for fracture with routine healing
G   subsequent encounter for fracture with delayed healing
K   subsequent encounter for fracture with nonunion
P   subsequent encounter for fracture with malunion
S   sequela

    + **S99.10**   **Unspecified physeal fracture of metatarsal**
        +7th **S99.101**   **Unspecified physeal fracture of right metatarsal**
        +7th **S99.102**   **Unspecified physeal fracture of left metatarsal**
        +7th **S99.109**   **Unspecified physeal fracture of unspecified metatarsal**
    + **S99.11**   **Salter-Harris Type I physeal fracture of metatarsal**
        +7th **S99.111**   **Salter-Harris Type I physeal fracture of right metatarsal**
        +7th **S99.112**   **Salter-Harris Type I physeal fracture of left metatarsal**
        AHA CC: 1Q, 2018, 3
        +7th **S99.119**   **Salter-Harris Type I physeal fracture of unspecified metatarsal**
    + **S99.12**   **Salter-Harris Type II physeal fracture of metatarsal**
        +7th **S99.121**   **Salter-Harris Type II physeal fracture of right metatarsal**
        +7th **S99.122**   **Salter-Harris Type II physeal fracture of left metatarsal**
        +7th **S99.129**   **Salter-Harris Type II physeal fracture of unspecified metatarsal**
    + **S99.13**   **Salter-Harris Type III physeal fracture of metatarsal**
        +7th **S99.131**   **Salter-Harris Type III physeal fracture of right metatarsal**
        +7th **S99.132**   **Salter-Harris Type III physeal fracture of left metatarsal**
        +7th **S99.139**   **Salter-Harris Type III physeal fracture of unspecified metatarsal**
    + **S99.14**   **Salter-Harris Type IV physeal fracture of metatarsal**
        +7th **S99.141**   **Salter-Harris Type IV physeal fracture of right metatarsal**
        +7th **S99.142**   **Salter-Harris Type IV physeal fracture of left metatarsal**
        +7th **S99.149**   **Salter-Harris Type IV physeal fracture of unspecified metatarsal**

+, +7th, X + 7th   ● Newborn   ● Pediatric   ● Maternity   ● Adult   ♀ Female   ♂ Male   Manifestation   Unacceptable PDX   HCC   CC   MCC   HAC

+ **S99.19** Other physeal fracture of metatarsal
  - +7th **S99.191** Other physeal fracture of right metatarsal
  - +7th **S99.192** Other physeal fracture of left metatarsal
  - +7th **S99.199** Other physeal fracture of unspecified metatarsal

+ **S99.2** Phseal fracture of phalanx of toe

> The appropriate 7th character is to be added to each code in subcategory **S99.2**
>
> A initial encounter for closed fracture
> B initial encounter for open fracture
> D subsequent encounter for fracture with routine healing
> G subsequent encounter for fracture with delayed healing
> K subsequent encounter for fracture with nonunion
> P subsequent encounter for fracture with malunion
> S sequela

+ **S99.20** Unspecified physeal fracture of phalanx of toe
  - +7th **S99.201** Unspecified physeal fracture of phalanx of right toe
  - +7th **S99.202** Unspecified physeal fracture of phalanx of left toe
  - +7th **S99.209** Unspecified physeal fracture of phalanx of unspecified toe
+ **S99.21** Salter-Harris Type I physeal fracture of phalanx of toe
  - +7th **S99.211** Salter-Harris Type I physeal fracture of phalanx of right toe
  - +7th **S99.212** Salter-Harris Type I physeal fracture of phalanx of left toe
  - +7th **S99.219** Salter-Harris Type I physeal fracture of phalanx of unspecified toe
+ **S99.22** Salter-Harris Type II physeal fracture of phalanx of toe
  - +7th **S99.221** Salter-Harris Type II physeal fracture of phalanx of right toe
  - +7th **S99.222** Salter-Harris Type II physeal fracture of phalanx of left toe
  - +7th **S99.229** Salter-Harris Type II physeal fracture of phalanx of unspecified toe
+ **S99.23** Salter-Harris Type III physeal fracture of phalanx of toe
  - +7th **S99.231** Salter-Harris Type III physeal fracture of phalanx of right toe
  - +7th **S99.232** Salter-Harris Type III physeal fracture of phalanx of left toe
  - +7th **S99.239** Salter-Harris Type III physeal fracture of phalanx of unspecified toe
+ **S99.24** Salter-Harris Type IV physeal fracture of phalanx of toe
  - +7th **S99.241** Salter-Harris Type IV physeal fracture of phalanx of right toe
  - +7th **S99.242** Salter-Harris Type IV physeal fracture of phalanx of left toe
  - +7th **S99.249** Salter-Harris Type IV physeal fracture of phalanx of unspecified toe
+ **S99.29** Other physeal fracture of phalanx of toe
  - +7th **S99.291** Other physeal fracture of phalanx of right toe
  - +7th **S99.292** Other physeal fracture of phalanx of left toe
  - +7th **S99.299** Other physeal fracture of phalanx of unspecified toe

+ **S99.8** Other specified injuries of ankle and foot

> The appropriate 7th character is to be added to each code from category **S99.8**
> A initial encounter
> D subsequent encounter
> S sequela

+ **S99.81** Other specified injuries of ankle
  - +7th **S99.811** Other specified injuries of right ankle
  - +7th **S99.812** Other specified injuries of left ankle
  - +7th **S99.819** Other specified injuries of unspecified ankle
+ **S99.82** Other specified injuries of foot
  - +7th **S99.821** Other specified injuries of right foot
  - +7th **S99.822** Other specified injuries of left foot
  - +7th **S99.829** Other specified injuries of unspecified foot

+ **S99.9** Unspecified injury of ankle and foot

> The appropriate 7th character is to be added to each code from category **S99.9**
> A initial encounter
> D subsequent encounter
> S sequela

+ **S99.91** Unspecified injury of ankle
  - +7th **S99.911** Unspecified injury of right ankle
  - +7th **S99.912** Unspecified injury of left ankle
  - +7th **S99.919** Unspecified injury of unspecified ankle
+ **S99.92** Unspecified injury of foot
  - +7th **S99.921** Unspecified injury of right foot
  - +7th **S99.922** Unspecified injury of left foot
  - +7th **S99.929** Unspecified injury of unspecified foot

INJURY, POISONING AND CERTAIN OTHER CONSEQUENCES OF EXTERNAL CAUSES (T07-T88)

Injuries involving multiple body regions (T07)

Excludes1: *burns and corrosions (T20-T32)*
frostbite (T33-T34)
insect bite or sting, venomous (T63.4)
sunburn (L55.-)

T07 **Unspecified multiple injuries**

> The appropriate 7th character is to be added to each code from category T07
> A initial encounter
> D subsequent encounter
> S sequela

> **Excludes1:** *injury NOS (T14.90)*
> AHA CC: 4Q, 2017, 26
> Review coding guideline C.19.b

Injury of unspecified body region (T14)

T14 **Injury of unspecified body region**

> The appropriate 7th character is to be added to each code from category T14
> A initial encounter
> D subsequent encounter
> S sequela

> **Excludes1:** *multiple unspecified injuries (T07)*
> AHA CC: 4Q, 2017, 26

T14.8 **Other injury of unspecified body region**
Abrasion NOS
Contusion NOS
Crush injury NOS
Fracture NOS
Skin injury NOS
Vascular injury NOS
Wound NOS
+ **T14.9** **Unspecified injury**
  T14.90 **Injury, unspecified**
  Injury NOS
  T14.91 **Suicide attempt**
  Attempted suicide NOS

Effects of foreign body entering through natural orifice (T15-T19)

Excludes2: *foreign body accidentally left in operation wound (T81.5-)*
foreign body in penetrating wound - See open wound by body region
residual foreign body in soft tissue (M79.5)
splinter, without open wound - See superficial injury by body region

T15 **Foreign body on external eye**

> **Excludes2:** *foreign body in penetrating wound of orbit and eye ball (S05.4-, S05.5-)*
> *open wound of eyelid and periocular area (S01.1-)*
> *retained foreign body in eyelid (H02.8-)*
> *retained (old) foreign body in penetrating wound of orbit and eye ball (H05.5-, H44.6-, H44.7-)*
> *superficial foreign body of eyelid and periocular area (S00.25-)*

> The appropriate 7th character is to be added to each code from category T15
> A initial encounter
> D subsequent encounter
> S sequela

+ **T15.0 Foreign body in cornea**
   X+7th **T15.00** Foreign body in cornea, unspecified eye
   X+7th **T15.01** Foreign body in cornea, right eye
   X+7th **T15.02** Foreign body in cornea, left eye
+ **T15.1 Foreign body in conjunctival sac**
   X+7th **T15.10** Foreign body in conjunctival sac, unspecified eye
   X+7th **T15.11** Foreign body in conjunctival sac, right eye
   X+7th **T15.12** Foreign body in conjunctival sac, left eye
+ **T15.8 Foreign body in other and multiple parts of external eye**
     Foreign body in lacrimal punctum
   X+7th **T15.80** Foreign body in other and multiple parts of external eye, unspecified eye
   X+7th **T15.81** Foreign body in other and multiple parts of external eye, right eye
   X+7th **T15.82** Foreign body in other and multiple parts of external eye, left eye
+ **T15.9 Foreign body on external eye, part unspecified**
   X+7th **T15.90** Foreign body on external eye, part unspecified, unspecified eye
   X+7th **T15.91** Foreign body on external eye, part unspecified, right eye
   X+7th **T15.92** Foreign body on external eye, part unspecified, left eye

T16 Foreign body in ear

> **Includes:** foreign body in auditory canal

> The appropriate 7th character is to be added to each code from category T16
> A   initial encounter
> D   subsequent encounter
> S   sequela

X+7th **T16.1 Foreign body in right ear**
X+7th **T16.2 Foreign body in left ear**
X+7th **T16.9 Foreign body in ear, unspecified ear**

T17 Foreign body in respiratory tract

> The appropriate 7th character is to be added to each code from category T17
> A   initial encounter
> D   subsequent encounter
> S   sequela

X+7th **T17.0 Foreign body in nasal sinus**
X+7th **T17.1 Foreign body in nostril**
    Foreign body in nose NOS
+ **T17.2 Foreign body in pharynx**
    Foreign body in nasopharynx
    Foreign body in throat NOS
  + **T17.20 Unspecified foreign body in pharynx**
    +7th **T17.200** Unspecified foreign body in pharynx causing asphyxiation
    +7th **T17.208** Unspecified foreign body in pharynx causing other injury
  + **T17.21 Gastric contents in pharynx**
     Aspiration of gastric contents into pharynx
     Vomitus in pharynx
    +7th **T17.210** Gastric contents in pharynx causing asphyxiation
    +7th **T17.218** Gastric contents in pharynx causing other injury
  + **T17.22 Food in pharynx**
     Bones in pharynx
     Seeds in pharynx
    +7th **T17.220** Food in pharynx causing asphyxiation
    +7th **T17.228** Food in pharynx causing other injury
  + **T17.29 Other foreign object in pharynx**
    +7th **T17.290** Other foreign object in pharynx causing asphyxiation
    +7th **T17.298** Other foreign object in pharynx causing other injury

+ **T17.3 Foreign body in larynx**
  + **T17.30 Unspecified foreign body in larynx**
    +7th **T17.300** Unspecified foreign body in larynx causing asphyxiation
    +7th **T17.308** Unspecified foreign body in larynx causing other injury
  + **T17.31 Gastric contents in larynx**
     Aspiration of gastric contents into larynx
     Vomitus in larynx
    +7th **T17.310** Gastric contents in larynx causing asphyxiation
    +7th **T17.318** Gastric contents in larynx causing other injury
  + **T17.32 Food in larynx**
     Bones in larynx
     Seeds in larynx
    +7th **T17.320** Food in larynx causing asphyxiation
    +7th **T17.328** Food in larynx causing other injury
  + **T17.39 Other foreign object in larynx**
    +7th **T17.390** Other foreign object in larynx causing asphyxiation
    +7th **T17.398** Other foreign object in larynx causing other injury
+ **T17.4 Foreign body in trachea**
  + **T17.40 Unspecified foreign body in trachea**
    CC +7th **T17.400** Unspecified foreign body in trachea causing asphyxiation
    CC +7th **T17.408** Unspecified foreign body in trachea causing other injury
  + **T17.41 Gastric contents in trachea**
     Aspiration of gastric contents into trachea
     Vomitus in trachea
    CC +7th **T17.410** Gastric contents in trachea causing asphyxiation
    CC +7th **T17.418** Gastric contents in trachea causing other injury
  + **T17.42 Food in trachea**
     Bones in trachea
     Seeds in trachea
    CC +7th **T17.420** Food in trachea causing asphyxiation
    CC +7th **T17.428** Food in trachea causing other injury
  + **T17.49 Other foreign object in trachea**
    CC +7th **T17.490** Other foreign object in trachea causing asphyxiation
    CC +7th **T17.498** Other foreign object in trachea causing other injury
+ **T17.5 Foreign body in bronchus**
  + **T17.50 Unspecified foreign body in bronchus**
    CC +7th **T17.500** Unspecified foreign body in bronchus causing asphyxiation
    CC +7th **T17.508** Unspecified foreign body in bronchus causing other injury
  + **T17.51 Gastric contents in bronchus**
     Aspiration of gastric contents into bronchus
     Vomitus in bronchus
    CC +7th **T17.510** Gastric contents in bronchus causing asphyxiation
    CC +7th **T17.518** Gastric contents in bronchus causing other injury
  + **T17.52 Food in bronchus**
     Bones in bronchus
     Seeds in bronchus
    CC +7th **T17.520** Food in bronchus causing asphyxiation
    CC +7th **T17.528** Food in bronchus causing other injury
  + **T17.59 Other foreign object in bronchus**
    CC +7th **T17.590** Other foreign object in bronchus causing asphyxiation
    CC +7th **T17.598** Other foreign object in bronchus causing other injury
+ **T17.8 Foreign body in other parts of respiratory tract**
    Foreign body in bronchioles
    Foreign body in lung
  + **T17.80 Unspecified foreign body in other parts of respiratory tract**
    CC +7th **T17.800** Unspecified foreign body in other parts of respiratory tract causing asphyxiation
    CC +7th **T17.808** Unspecified foreign body in other parts of respiratory tract causing other injury

+ **T17.81** **Gastric contents in other parts of respiratory tract**
Aspiration of gastric contents into other parts of respiratory tract
Vomitus in other parts of respiratory tract
CC +7th **T17.810** **Gastric contents in other parts of respiratory tract causing asphyxiation**
CC +7th **T17.818** **Gastric contents in other parts of respiratory tract causing other injury**
+ **T17.82** **Food in other parts of respiratory tract**
Bones in other parts of respiratory tract
Seeds in other parts of respiratory tract
CC +7th **T17.820** **Food in other parts of respiratory tract causing asphyxiation**
CC +7th **T17.828** **Food in other parts of respiratory tract causing other injury**
+ **T17.89** **Other foreign object in other parts of respiratory tract**
CC +7th **T17.890** **Other foreign object in other parts of respiratory tract causing asphyxiation**
CC +7th **T17.898** **Other foreign object in other parts of respiratory tract causing other injury**
T17.9 **Foreign body in respiratory tract, part unspecified**
+ **T17.90** **Unspecified foreign body in respiratory tract, part unspecified**
+7th **T17.900** **Unspecified foreign body in respiratory tract, part unspecified causing asphyxiation**
+7th **T17.908** **Unspecified foreign body in respiratory tract, part unspecified causing other injury**
+ **T17.91** **Gastric contents in respiratory tract, part unspecified**
Aspiration of gastric contents into respiratory tract, part unspecified
Vomitus in trachea respiratory tract, part unspecified
+7th **T17.910** **Gastric contents in respiratory tract, part unspecified causing asphyxiation**
+7th **T17.918** **Gastric contents in respiratory tract, part unspecified causing other injury**
+ **T17.92** **Food in respiratory tract, part unspecified**
Bones in respiratory tract, part unspecified
Seeds in respiratory tract, part unspecified
+7th **T17.920** **Food in respiratory tract, part unspecified causing asphyxiation**
+7th **T17.928** **Food in respiratory tract, part unspecified causing other injury**
+ **T17.99** **Other foreign object in respiratory tract, part unspecified**
+7th **T17.990** **Other foreign object in respiratory tract, part unspecified in causing asphyxiation**
+7th **T17.998** **Other foreign object in respiratory tract, part unspecified causing other injury**

T18 **Foreign body in alimentary tract**

Excludes2: *foreign body in pharynx (T17.2-)*

The appropriate 7th character is to be added to each code from category T18
A   initial encounter
D   subsequent encounter
S   sequela

X+7th **T18.0** **Foreign body in mouth**
+ **T18.1** **Foreign body in esophagus**
Excludes2: *foreign body in respiratory tract (T17.-)*
+ **T18.10** **Unspecified foreign body in esophagus**
+7th **T18.100** **Unspecified foreign body in esophagus causing compression of trachea**
Unspecified foreign body in esophagus causing obstruction of respiration
+7th **T18.108** **Unspecified foreign body in esophagus causing other injury**

+ **T18.11** **Gastric contents in esophagus**
Vomitus in esophagus
+7th **T18.110** **Gastric contents in esophagus causing compression of trachea**
Gastric contents in esophagus causing obstruction of respiration
+7th **T18.118** **Gastric contents in esophagus causing other injury**
+ **T18.12** **Food in esophagus**
Bones in esophagus
Seeds in esophagus
+7th **T18.120** **Food in esophagus causing compression of trachea**
Food in esophagus causing obstruction of respiration
+7th **T18.128** **Food in esophagus causing other injury**
+ **T18.19** **Other foreign object in esophagus**
+7th **T18.190** **Other foreign object in esophagus causing compression of trachea**
Other foreign body in esophagus causing obstruction of respiration
AHA CC: 1Q, 2015, 23-24
+7th **T18.198** **Other foreign object in esophagus causing other injury**
AHA CC: 1Q, 2015, 23-24
X+7th **T18.2** **Foreign body in stomach**
X+7th **T18.3** **Foreign body in small intestine**
X+7th **T18.4** **Foreign body in colon**
X+7th **T18.5** **Foreign body in anus and rectum**
Foreign body in rectosigmoid (junction)
X+7th **T18.8** **Foreign body in other parts of alimentary tract**
X+7th **T18.9** **Foreign body of alimentary tract, part unspecified**
Foreign body in digestive system NOS
Swallowed foreign body NOS
T19 **Foreign body in genitourinary tract**
Excludes2: *complications due to implanted mesh (T83.7-)*
mechanical complications of contraceptive device (intrauterine) (vaginal) (T83.3-)
presence of contraceptive device (intrauterine) (vaginal) (Z97.5)

The appropriate 7th character is to be added to each code from category T19
A   initial encounter
D   subsequent encounter
S   sequela

X+7th **T19.0** **Foreign body in urethra**
X+7th **T19.1** **Foreign body in bladder**
♀ X+7th **T19.2** **Foreign body in vulva and vagina**
♀ X+7th **T19.3** **Foreign body in uterus**
♂ X+7th **T19.4** **Foreign body in penis**
X+7th **T19.8** **Foreign body in other parts of genitourinary tract**
X+7th **T19.9** **Foreign body in genitourinary tract, part unspecified**

BURNS AND CORROSIONS (T20-T32)

Includes: burns (thermal) from electrical heating appliances
burns (thermal) from electricity
burns (thermal) from flame
burns (thermal) from friction
burns (thermal) from hot air and hot gases
burns (thermal) from hot objects
burns (thermal) from lightning
burns (thermal) from radiation
chemical burn [corrosion] (external) (internal)
scalds

Excludes2: *erythema [dermatitis] ab igne (L59.0)*
radiation-related disorders of the skin and subcutaneous tissue (L55-L59)
sunburn (L55.-)

+, +7th, X + 7th   ● Newborn   ● Pediatric   ● Maternity   ● Adult   ♀ Female   ♂ Male   Manifestation   Unacceptable PDX   HCC   CC   MCC   HAC

Burns and corrosions of external body surface, specified by site (T20-T25)

Includes: burns and corrosions of first degree [erythema]
burns and corrosions of second degree [blisters][epidermal loss]
burns and corrosions of third degree [deep necrosis of underlying tissue] [full- thickness skin loss]

Use additional code from category T31 or T32 to identify extent of body surface involved

Review coding guideline C.19.d

T20 Burn and corrosion of head, face, and neck

> **Excludes2:** *burn and corrosion of ear drum (T28.41, T28.91)*
> *burn and corrosion of eye and adnexa (T26.-)*
> *burn and corrosion of mouth and pharynx (T28.0)*

> The appropriate 7th character is to be added to each code from category T20
> A initial encounter
> D subsequent encounter
> S sequela

+ **T20.0 Burn of unspecified degree of head, face, and neck**
Use additional external cause code to identify the source, place and intent of the burn (X00-X19, X75-X77, X96-X98, Y92)

X+7th **T20.00 Burn of unspecified degree of head, face, and neck, unspecified site**

+ **T20.01 Burn of unspecified degree of ear [any part, except ear drum]**
Excludes2: *burn of ear drum (T28.41-)*

+7th **T20.011 Burn of unspecified degree of right ear [any part, except ear drum]**

+7th **T20.012 Burn of unspecified degree of left ear [any part, except ear drum]**

+7th **T20.019 Burn of unspecified degree of unspecified ear [any part, except ear drum]**

X+7th **T20.02 Burn of unspecified degree of lip(s)**
X+7th **T20.03 Burn of unspecified degree of chin**
X+7th **T20.04 Burn of unspecified degree of nose (septum)**
X+7th **T20.05 Burn of unspecified degree of scalp [any part]**
X+7th **T20.06 Burn of unspecified degree of forehead and cheek**
X+7th **T20.07 Burn of unspecified degree of neck**
X+7th **T20.09 Burn of unspecified degree of multiple sites of head, face, and neck**

+ **T20.1 Burn of first degree of head, face, and neck**
Use additional external cause code to identify the source, place and intent of the burn (X00-X19, X75-X77, X96-X98, Y92)

X+7th **T20.10 Burn of first degree of head, face, and neck, unspecified site**

+ **T20.11 Burn of first degree of ear [any part, except ear drum]**
Excludes2: *burn of ear drum (T28.41-)*

+7th **T20.111 Burn of first degree of right ear [any part, except ear drum]**

+7th **T20.112 Burn of first degree of left ear [any part, except ear drum]**

+7th **T20.119 Burn of first degree of unspecified ear [any part, except ear drum]**

X+7th **T20.12 Burn of first degree of lip(s)**
X+7th **T20.13 Burn of first degree of chin**
X+7th **T20.14 Burn of first degree of nose (septum)**
X+7th **T20.15 Burn of first degree of scalp [any part]**
X+7th **T20.16 Burn of first degree of forehead and cheek**
X+7th **T20.17 Burn of first degree of neck**
X+7th **T20.19 Burn of first degree of multiple sites of head, face, and neck**

+ **T20.2 Burn of second degree of head, face, and neck**
Use additional external cause code to identify the source, place and intent of the burn (X00-X19, X75-X77, X96-X98, Y92)

X+7th **T20.20 Burn of second degree of head, face, and neck, unspecified site**

+ **T20.21 Burn of second degree of ear [any part, except ear drum]**
Excludes2: *burn of ear drum (T28.41-)*

+7th **T20.211 Burn of second degree of right ear [any part, except ear drum]**

+7th **T20.212 Burn of second degree of left ear [any part, except ear drum]**

+7th **T20.219 Burn of second degree of unspecified ear [any part, except ear drum]**

X+7th **T20.22 Burn of second degree of lip(s)**
X+7th **T20.23 Burn of second degree of chin**
X+7th **T20.24 Burn of second degree of nose (septum)**
X+7th **T20.25 Burn of second degree of scalp [any part]**
AHA CC: 1Q, 2015, 3-21
X+7th **T20.26 Burn of second degree of forehead and cheek**
X+7th **T20.27 Burn of second degree of neck**
X+7th **T20.29 Burn of second degree of multiple sites of head, face, and neck**

+ **T20.3 Burn of third degree of head, face, and neck**
Use additional external cause code to identify the source, place and intent of the burn (X00-X19, X75-X77, X96-X98, Y92)

CC X+7th **T20.30 Burn of third degree of head, face, and neck, unspecified site**
HAC 7th character A see Appendix B for HAC conditional logic **T20.31 Burn of third degree of ear [any part, except ear drum]**
Excludes2: *burn of ear drum (T28.41-)*

CC +7th **T20.311 Burn of third degree of right ear [any part, except ear drum]**
HAC 7th character A see Appendix B for HAC conditional logic

CC +7th **T20.312 Burn of third degree of left ear [any part, except ear drum]**
HAC 7th character A see Appendix B for HAC conditional logic
AHA CC: 1Q, 2015, 3-21

CC +7th **T20.319 Burn of third degree of unspecified ear [any part, except ear drum]**
HAC 7th character A see Appendix B for HAC conditional logic

CC X+7th **T20.32 Burn of third degree of lip(s)**
HAC 7th character A see Appendix B for HAC conditional logic

CC X+7th **T20.33 Burn of third degree of chin**
HAC 7th character A see Appendix B for HAC conditional logic

CC X+7th **T20.34 Burn of third degree of nose (septum)**
HAC 7th character A see Appendix B for HAC conditional logic

CC X+7th **T20.35 Burn of third degree of scalp [any part]**
HAC 7th character A see Appendix B for HAC conditional logic

CC X+7th **T20.36 Burn of third degree of forehead and cheek**
HAC 7th character A see Appendix B for HAC conditional logic

CC X+7th **T20.37 Burn of third degree of neck**
HAC 7th character A see Appendix B for HAC conditional logic

CC X+7th **T20.39 Burn of third degree of multiple sites of head, face, and neck**
HAC 7th character A see Appendix B for HAC conditional logic

+ **T20.4 Corrosion of unspecified degree of head, face, and neck**
Code first (T51-T65) to identify chemical and intent external cause code to identify place (Y92)

X+7th **T20.40 Corrosion of unspecified degree of head, face, and neck, unspecified site**

+, +7th, X + 7th • Newborn • Pediatric • Maternity • Adult ♀ Female ♂ Male Manifestation Unacceptable PDX HCC CC MCC HAC

+ **T20.41** **Corrosion of unspecified degree of ear [any part, except ear drum]**
> *Excludes2:* *corrosion of ear drum (T28.91-)*

+7th **T20.411** Corrosion of unspecified degree of right ear [any part, except ear drum]

+7th **T20.412** Corrosion of unspecified degree of left ear [any part, except ear drum]

+7th **T20.419** Corrosion of unspecified degree of unspecified ear [any part, except ear drum]

X+7th **T20.42** Corrosion of unspecified degree of lip(s)

X+7th **T20.43** Corrosion of unspecified degree of chin

X+7th **T20.44** Corrosion of unspecified degree of nose (septum)

X+7th **T20.45** Corrosion of unspecified degree of scalp [any part]

X+7th **T20.46** Corrosion of unspecified degree of forehead and cheek

X+7th **T20.47** Corrosion of unspecified degree of neck

X+7th **T20.49** Corrosion of unspecified degree of multiple sites of head, face, and neck

+ **T20.5** **Corrosion of first degree of head, face, and neck**
> Code first (T51-T65) to identify chemical and intent
>
> Use additional external cause code to identify place (Y92)

X+7th **T20.50** **Corrosion of first degree of head, face, and neck, unspecified site**

+ **T20.51** **Corrosion of first degree of ear [any part, except ear drum]**
> *Excludes2:* *corrosion of ear drum (T28.91-)*

+7th **T20.511** Corrosion of first degree of right ear [any part, except ear drum]

+7th **T20.512** Corrosion of first degree of left ear [any part, except ear drum]

+7th **T20.519** Corrosion of first degree of unspecified ear [any part, except ear drum]

X+7th **T20.52** Corrosion of first degree of lip(s)

X+7th **T20.53** Corrosion of first degree of chin

X+7th **T20.54** Corrosion of first degree of nose (septum)

X+7th **T20.55** Corrosion of first degree of scalp [any part]

X+7th **T20.56** Corrosion of first degree of forehead and cheek

X+7th **T20.57** Corrosion of first degree of neck

X+7th **T20.59** Corrosion of first degree of multiple sites of head, face, and neck

+ **T20.6** **Corrosion of second degree of head, face, and neck**
> Code first (T51-T65) to identify chemical and intent
>
> Use additional external cause code to identify place (Y92)

X+7th **T20.60** **Corrosion of second degree of head, face, and neck, unspecified site**

+ **T20.61** **Corrosion of second degree of ear [any part, except ear drum]**
> *Excludes2:* *corrosion of ear drum (T28.91-)*

+7th **T20.611** Corrosion of second degree of right ear [any part, except ear drum]

+7th **T20.612** Corrosion of second degree of left ear [any part, except ear drum]

+7th **T20.619** Corrosion of second degree of unspecified ear [any part, except ear drum]

X+7th **T20.62** Corrosion of second degree of lip(s)

X+7th **T20.63** Corrosion of second degree of chin

X+7th **T20.64** Corrosion of second degree of nose (septum)

X+7th **T20.65** Corrosion of second degree of scalp [any part]

X+7th **T20.66** Corrosion of second degree of forehead and cheek

X+7th **T20.67** Corrosion of second degree of neck

X+7th **T20.69** Corrosion of second degree of multiple sites of head, face, and neck

+ **T20.7** **Corrosion of third degree of head, face, and neck**
> Code first (T51-T65) to identify chemical and intent
>
> Use additional external cause code to identify place (Y92)

CC X+7th **T20.70** **Corrosion of third degree of head, face, and neck, unspecified site**
> HAC 7th character A see Appendix B for HAC conditional logic

+ **T20.71** **Corrosion of third degree of ear [any part, except ear drum]**
> *Excludes2:* *corrosion of ear drum (T28.91-)*

CC +7th **T20.711** **Corrosion of third degree of right ear [any part, except ear drum]**
> HAC 7th character A see Appendix B for HAC conditional logic

CC +7th **T20.712** **Corrosion of third degree of left ear [any part, except ear drum]**
> HAC 7th character A see Appendix B for HAC conditional logic

CC +7th **T20.719** **Corrosion of third degree of unspecified ear [any part, except ear drum]**
> HAC 7th character A see Appendix B for HAC conditional logic

CC X+7th **T20.72** **Corrosion of third degree of lip(s)**
> HAC 7th character A see Appendix B for HAC conditional logic

CC X+7th **T20.73** **Corrosion of third degree of chin**
> HAC 7th character A see Appendix B for HAC conditional logic

CC X+7th **T20.74** **Corrosion of third degree of nose (septum)**
> HAC 7th character A see Appendix B for HAC conditional logic

CC X+7th **T20.75** **Corrosion of third degree of scalp [any part]**
> HAC 7th character A see Appendix B for HAC conditional logic

CC X+7th **T20.76** **Corrosion of third degree of forehead and cheek**
> HAC 7th character A see Appendix B for HAC conditional logic

CC X+7th **T20.77** **Corrosion of third degree of neck**
> HAC 7th character A see Appendix B for HAC conditional logic

CC X+7th **T20.79** **Corrosion of third degree of multiple sites of head, face, and neck**
> HAC 7th character A see Appendix B for HAC conditional logic

T21 **Burn and corrosion of trunk**
> **Includes:** burns and corrosion of hip region
>
> *Excludes2:* *burns and corrosion of axilla (T22.- with fifth character 4)*
> *burns and corrosion of scapular region (T22.- with fifth character 6)*
> *burns and corrosion of shoulder (T22.- with fifth character 5)*

> The appropriate 7th character is to be added to each code from category T21
> A initial encounter
> D subsequent encounter
> S sequela

+ **T21.0** **Burn of unspecified degree of trunk**
> Use external cause code to identify the source, place and intent of the burn (X00-X19, X75-X77, X96-X98, Y92)

X+7th **T21.00** **Burn of unspecified degree of trunk, unspecified site**

X+7th **T21.01** **Burn of unspecified degree of chest wall**
> Burn of unspecified degree of breast

X+7th **T21.02** **Burn of unspecified degree of abdominal wall**
> Burn of unspecified degree of flank
> Burn of unspecified degree of groin

X+7th **T21.03** **Burn of unspecified degree of upper back**
> Burn of unspecified degree of interscapular region

X+7th **T21.04** **Burn of unspecified degree of lower back**

X+7th **T21.05** **Burn of unspecified degree of buttock**
> Burn of unspecified degree of anus

♂ X+7th **T21.06** **Burn of unspecified degree of male genital region**
> Burn of unspecified degree of penis
> Burn of unspecified degree of scrotum
> Burn of unspecified degree of testis

♀ X+7th **T21.07** **Burn of unspecified degree of female genital region**
> Burn of unspecified degree of labium (majus) (minus)
> Burn of unspecified degree of perineum
> Burn of unspecified degree of vulva
> *Excludes2:* *burn of vagina (T28.3)*

X+7th **T21.09** **Burn of unspecified degree of other site of trunk**

+ **T21.1** **Burn of first degree of trunk**
Use external cause code to identify the source, place and intent of the burn (X00-X19, X75-X77, X96-X98, Y92)
X+7th **T21.10** **Burn of first degree of trunk, unspecified site**
X+7th **T21.11** **Burn of first degree of chest wall**
Burn of first degree of breast
X+7th **T21.12** **Burn of first degree of abdominal wall**
Burn of first degree of flank
Burn of first degree of groin
X+7th **T21.13** **Burn of first degree of upper back**
Burn of first degree of interscapular region
X+7th **T21.14** **Burn of first degree of lower back**
X+7th **T21.15** **Burn of first degree of buttock**
Burn of first degree of anus
♂ X+7th **T21.16** **Burn of first degree of male genital region**
Burn of first degree of penis
Burn of first degree of scrotum
Burn of first degree of testis
♀ X+7th **T21.17** **Burn of first degree of female genital region**
Burn of first degree of labium (majus) (minus)
Burn of first degree of perineum
Burn of first degree of vulva
Excludes2: *burn of vagina (T28.3)*
X+7th **T21.19** **Burn of first degree of other site of trunk**

+ **T21.2** **Burn of second degree of trunk**
Use external cause code to identify the source, place and intent of the burn (X00-X19, X75-X77, X96-X98, Y92)
X+7th **T21.20** **Burn of second degree of trunk, unspecified site**
X+7th **T21.21** **Burn of second degree of chest wall**
Burn of second degree of breast
X+7th **T21.22** **Burn of second degree of abdominal wall**
Burn of second degree of flank
Burn of second degree of groin
X+7th **T21.23** **Burn of second degree of upper back**
Burn of second degree of interscapular region
X+7th **T21.24** **Burn of second degree of lower back**
X+7th **T21.25** **Burn of second degree of buttock**
Burn of second degree of anus
♂ X+7th **T21.26** **Burn of second degree of male genital region**
Burn of second degree of penis
Burn of second degree of scrotum
Burn of second degree of testis
♀ X+7th **T21.27** **Burn of second degree of female genital region**
Burn of second degree of labium (majus) (minus)
Burn of second degree of perineum
Burn of second degree of vulva
Excludes2: *burn of vagina (T28.3)*
X+7th **T21.29** **Burn of second degree of other site of trunk**

+ **T21.3** **Burn of third degree of trunk**
Use additional external cause code to identify the source, place and intent of the burn (X00-X19, X75-X77, X96-X98, Y92)
CC X+7th **T21.30** **Burn of third degree of trunk, unspecified site**
HAC 7th character A see Appendix B for HAC conditional logic
CC X+7th **T21.31** **Burn of third degree of chest wall**
Burn of third degree of breast
AHA CC: 2Q, 2016, 5-6
HAC 7th character A see Appendix B for HAC conditional logic
CC X+7th **T21.32** **Burn of third degree of abdominal wall**
Burn of third degree of flank
Burn of third degree of groin
HAC 7th character A see Appendix B for HAC conditional logic
CC X+7th **T21.33** **Burn of third degree of upper back**
Burn of third degree of interscapular region
HAC 7th character A see Appendix B for HAC conditional logic
CC X+7th **T21.34** **Burn of third degree of lower back**
HAC 7th character A see Appendix B for HAC conditional logic
CC X+7th **T21.35** **Burn of third degree of buttock**
Burn of third degree of anus
HAC 7th character A see Appendix B for HAC conditional logic

CC X+7th **T21.36** **Burn of third degree of male genital region**
Burn of third degree of penis
Burn of third degree of scrotum
Burn of third degree of testis
HAC 7th character A see Appendix B for HAC conditional logic
CC X+7th **T21.37** **Burn of third degree of female genital region**
Burn of third degree of labium (majus) (minus)
Burn of third degree of perineum
Burn of third degree of vulva
Excludes2: *burn of vagina (T28.3)*
HAC 7th character A see Appendix B for HAC conditional logic
CC X+7th **T21.39** **Burn of third degree of other site of trunk**
HAC 7th character A see Appendix B for HAC conditional logic

+ **T21.4** **Corrosion of unspecified degree of trunk**
Code first (T51-T65) to identify chemical and intent
Use additional external cause code to identify place (Y92)
X+7th **T21.40** **Corrosion of unspecified degree of trunk, unspecified site**
X+7th **T21.41** **Corrosion of unspecified degree of chest wall**
Corrosion of unspecified degree of breast
X+7th **T21.42** **Corrosion of unspecified degree of abdominal wall**
Corrosion of unspecified degree of flank
Corrosion of unspecified degree of groin
X+7th **T21.43** **Corrosion of unspecified degree of upper back**
Corrosion of unspecified degree of interscapular region
X+7th **T21.44** **Corrosion of unspecified degree of lower back**
X+7th **T21.45** **Corrosion of unspecified degree of buttock**
Corrosion of unspecified degree of anus
♂ X+7th **T21.46** **Corrosion of unspecified degree of male genital region**
Corrosion of unspecified degree of penis
Corrosion of unspecified degree of scrotum
Corrosion of unspecified degree of testis
♀ X+7th **T21.47** **Corrosion of unspecified degree of female genital region**
Corrosion of unspecified degree of labium (majus) (minus)
Corrosion of unspecified degree of perineum
Corrosion of unspecified degree of vulva
Excludes2: *corrosion of vagina (T28.8)*
X+7th **T21.49** **Corrosion of unspecified degree of other site of trunk**

+ **T21.5** **Corrosion of first degree of trunk**
Code first (T51-T65) to identify chemical and intent
Use additional external cause code to identify place (Y92)
X+7th **T21.50** **Corrosion of first degree of trunk, unspecified site**
X+7th **T21.51** **Corrosion of first degree of chest wall**
Corrosion of first degree of breast
X+7th **T21.52** **Corrosion of first degree of abdominal wall**
Corrosion of first degree of flank
Corrosion of first degree of groin
X+7th **T21.53** **Corrosion of first degree of upper back**
Corrosion of first degree of interscapular region
X+7th **T21.54** **Corrosion of first degree of lower back**
X+7th **T21.55** **Corrosion of first degree of buttock**
Corrosion of first degree of anus
♂ X+7th **T21.56** **Corrosion of first degree of male genital region**
Corrosion of first degree of penis
Corrosion of first degree of scrotum
Corrosion of first degree of testis
♀ X+7th **T21.57** **Corrosion of first degree of female genital region**
Corrosion of first degree of labium (majus) (minus)
Corrosion of first degree of perineum
Corrosion of first degree of vulva
Excludes2: *corrosion of vagina (T28.8)*
X+7th **T21.59** **Corrosion of first degree of other site of trunk**

+, +7th, X + 7th ● Newborn ● Pediatric ● Maternity ● Adult ♀ Female ♂ Male Manifestation Unacceptable PDX HCC CC MCC HAC

+ **T21.6 Corrosion of second degree of trunk**

Code first (T51-T65) to identify chemical and intent

Use additional external cause code to identify place (Y92)

X+7th **T21.60 Corrosion of second degree of trunk, unspecified site**

X+7th **T21.61 Corrosion of second degree of chest wall**
Corrosion of second degree of breast

X+7th **T21.62 Corrosion of second degree of abdominal wall**
Corrosion of second degree of flank
Corrosion of second degree of groin

X+7th **T21.63 Corrosion of second degree of upper back**
Corrosion of second degree of interscapular region

X+7th **T21.64 Corrosion of second degree of lower back**

X+7th **T21.65 Corrosion of second degree of buttock**
Corrosion of second degree of anus

♂ X+7th **T21.66 Corrosion of second degree of male genital region**
Corrosion of second degree of penis
Corrosion of second degree of scrotum
Corrosion of second degree of testis

♀ X+7th **T21.67 Corrosion of second degree of female genital region**
Corrosion of second degree of labium (majus) (minus)
Corrosion of second degree of perineum
Corrosion of second degree of vulva
Excludes2: corrosion of vagina (T28.8)

X+7th **T21.69 Corrosion of second degree of other site of trunk**

+ **T21.7 Corrosion of third degree of trunk**

Code first (T51-T65) to identify chemical and intent

Use additional external cause code to identify place (Y92)

CC X+7th **T21.70 Corrosion of third degree of trunk, unspecified site**
HAC 7th character A see Appendix B for HAC conditional logic

CC X+7th **T21.71 Corrosion of third degree of chest wall**
Corrosion of third degree of breast
HAC 7th character A see Appendix B for HAC conditional logic

CC X+7th **T21.72 Corrosion of third degree of abdominal wall**
Corrosion of third degree of flank
Corrosion of third degree of groin
HAC 7th character A see Appendix B for HAC conditional logic

CC X+7th **T21.73 Corrosion of third degree of upper back**
Corrosion of third degree of interscapular region
HAC 7th character A see Appendix B for HAC conditional logic

CC X+7th **T21.74 Corrosion of third degree of lower back**
HAC 7th character A see Appendix B for HAC conditional logic

CC X+7th **T21.75 Corrosion of third degree of buttock**
Corrosion of third degree of anus
HAC 7th character A see Appendix B for HAC conditional logic

CC X+7th **T21.76 Corrosion of third degree of male genital region**
Corrosion of third degree of penis
Corrosion of third degree of scrotum
Corrosion of third degree of testis
HAC 7th character A see Appendix B for HAC conditional logic

CC X+7th **T21.77 Corrosion of third degree of female genital region**
Corrosion of third degree of labium (majus) (minus)
Corrosion of third degree of perineum
Corrosion of third degree of vulva
Excludes2: corrosion of vagina (T28.8)
HAC 7th character A see Appendix B for HAC conditional logic

CC X+7th **T21.79 Corrosion of third degree of other site of trunk**
HAC 7th character A see Appendix B for HAC conditional logic

T22 Burn and corrosion of shoulder and upper limb, except wrist and hand

Excludes2: burn and corrosion of interscapular region (T21.-)
burn and corrosion of wrist and hand (T23.-)

The appropriate 7th character is to be added to each code from category T22
A   initial encounter
D   subsequent encounter
S   sequela

+ **T22.0 Burn of unspecified degree of shoulder and upper limb, except wrist and hand**

Use additional external cause code to identify the source, place and intent of the burn (X00-X19, X75-X77, X96-X98, Y92)

X+7th **T22.00 Burn of unspecified degree of shoulder and upper limb, except wrist and hand, unspecified site**

+ **T22.01 Burn of unspecified degree of forearm**
+7th **T22.011 Burn of unspecified degree of right forearm**
+7th **T22.012 Burn of unspecified degree of left forearm**
+7th **T22.019 Burn of unspecified degree of unspecified forearm**

+ **T22.02 Burn of unspecified degree of elbow**
+7th **T22.021 Burn of unspecified degree of right elbow**
+7th **T22.022 Burn of unspecified degree of left elbow**
+7th **T22.029 Burn of unspecified degree of unspecified elbow**

+ **T22.03 Burn of unspecified degree of upper arm**
+7th **T22.031 Burn of unspecified degree of right upper arm**
+7th **T22.032 Burn of unspecified degree of left upper arm**
+7th **T22.039 Burn of unspecified degree of unspecified upper arm**

+ **T22.04 Burn of unspecified degree of axilla**
+7th **T22.041 Burn of unspecified degree of right axilla**
+7th **T22.042 Burn of unspecified degree of left axilla**
+7th **T22.049 Burn of unspecified degree of unspecified axilla**

+ **T22.05 Burn of unspecified degree of shoulder**
+7th **T22.051 Burn of unspecified degree of right shoulder**
+7th **T22.052 Burn of unspecified degree of left shoulder**
+7th **T22.059 Burn of unspecified degree of unspecified shoulder**

+ **T22.06 Burn of unspecified degree of scapular region**
+7th **T22.061 Burn of unspecified degree of right scapular region**
+7th **T22.062 Burn of unspecified degree of left scapular region**
+7th **T22.069 Burn of unspecified degree of unspecified scapular region**

+ **T22.09 Burn of unspecified degree of multiple sites of shoulder and upper limb, except wrist and hand**
+7th **T22.091 Burn of unspecified degree of multiple sites of right shoulder and upper limb, except wrist and hand**
+7th **T22.092 Burn of unspecified degree of multiple sites of left shoulder and upper limb, except wrist and hand**
+7th **T22.099 Burn of unspecified degree of multiple sites of unspecified shoulder and upper limb, except wrist and hand**

+ **T22.1 Burn of first degree of shoulder and upper limb, except wrist and hand**

Use additional external cause code to identify the source, place and intent of the burn (X00-X19, X75-X77, X96-X98, Y92)

X+7th **T22.10 Burn of first degree of shoulder and upper limb, except wrist and hand, unspecified site**

+ **T22.11 Burn of first degree of forearm**
+7th **T22.111 Burn of first degree of right forearm**
+7th **T22.112 Burn of first degree of left forearm**
+7th **T22.119 Burn of first degree of unspecified forearm**

+ **T22.12 Burn of first degree of elbow**
+7th **T22.121 Burn of first degree of right elbow**
+7th **T22.122 Burn of first degree of left elbow**
+7th **T22.129 Burn of first degree of unspecified elbow**

+ **T22.13 Burn of first degree of upper arm**
+7th **T22.131 Burn of first degree of right upper arm**
+7th **T22.132 Burn of first degree of left upper arm**
+7th **T22.139 Burn of first degree of unspecified upper arm**

+ **T22.14** **Burn of first degree of axilla**
- +7th **T22.141** **Burn of first degree of right axilla**
- +7th **T22.142** **Burn of first degree of left axilla**
- +7th **T22.149** **Burn of first degree of unspecified axilla**

+ **T22.15** **Burn of first degree of shoulder**
- +7th **T22.151** **Burn of first degree of right shoulder**
- +7th **T22.152** **Burn of first degree of left shoulder**
- +7th **T22.159** **Burn of first degree of unspecified shoulder**

+ **T22.16** **Burn of first degree of scapular region**
- +7th **T22.161** **Burn of first degree of right scapular region**
- +7th **T22.162** **Burn of first degree of left scapular region**
- +7th **T22.169** **Burn of first degree of unspecified scapular region**

+ **T22.19** **Burn of first degree of multiple sites of shoulder and upper limb, except wrist and hand**
- +7th **T22.191** **Burn of first degree of multiple sites of right shoulder and upper limb, except wrist and hand**
- +7th **T22.192** **Burn of first degree of multiple sites of left shoulder and upper limb, except wrist and hand**
- +7th **T22.199** **Burn of first degree of multiple sites of unspecified shoulder and upper limb, except wrist and hand**

+ **T22.2** **Burn of second degree of shoulder and upper limb, except wrist and hand**

Use additional external cause code to identify the source, place and intent of the burn (X00-X19, X75-X77, X96-X98, Y92)

X+7th **T22.20** **Burn of second degree of shoulder and upper limb, except wrist and hand, unspecified site**

+ **T22.21** **Burn of second degree of forearm**
- +7th **T22.211** **Burn of second degree of right forearm**
- +7th **T22.212** **Burn of second degree of left forearm**
- +7th **T22.219** **Burn of second degree of unspecified forearm**

+ **T22.22** **Burn of second degree of elbow**
- +7th **T22.221** **Burn of second degree of right elbow**
- +7th **T22.222** **Burn of second degree of left elbow**
- +7th **T22.229** **Burn of second degree of unspecified elbow**

+ **T22.23** **Burn of second degree of upper arm**
- +7th **T22.231** **Burn of second degree of right upper arm**
- +7th **T22.232** **Burn of second degree of left upper arm**
- +7th **T22.239** **Burn of second degree of unspecified upper arm**

+ **T22.24** **Burn of second degree of axilla**
- +7th **T22.241** **Burn of second degree of right axilla**
- +7th **T22.242** **Burn of second degree of left axilla**
- +7th **T22.249** **Burn of second degree of unspecified axilla**

+ **T22.25** **Burn of second degree of shoulder**
- +7th **T22.251** **Burn of second degree of right shoulder**
- +7th **T22.252** **Burn of second degree of left shoulder**
- +7th **T22.259** **Burn of second degree of unspecified shoulder**

+ **T22.26** **Burn of second degree of scapular region**
- +7th **T22.261** **Burn of second degree of right scapular region**
- +7th **T22.262** **Burn of second degree of left scapular region**
- +7th **T22.269** **Burn of second degree of unspecified scapular region**

+ **T22.29** **Burn of second degree of multiple sites of shoulder and upper limb, except wrist and hand**
- +7th **T22.291** **Burn of second degree of multiple sites of right shoulder and upper limb, except wrist and hand**
- +7th **T22.292** **Burn of second degree of multiple sites of left shoulder and upper limb, except wrist and hand**
- +7th **T22.299** **Burn of second degree of multiple sites of unspecified shoulder and upper limb, except wrist and hand**

+ **T22.3** **Burn of third degree of shoulder and upper limb, except wrist and hand**

Use additional external cause code to identify the source, place and intent of the burn (X00-X19, X75-X77, X96-X98, Y92)

CC X+7th **T22.30** **Burn of third degree of shoulder and upper limb, except wrist and hand, unspecified site**
> HAC 7th character A see Appendix B for HAC conditional logic

+ **T22.31** **Burn of third degree of forearm**
- CC +7th **T22.311** **Burn of third degree of right forearm**
  > HAC 7th character A see Appendix B for HAC conditional logic
- CC +7th **T22.312** **Burn of third degree of left forearm**
  > HAC 7th character A see Appendix B for HAC conditional logic
- CC +7th **T22.319** **Burn of third degree of unspecified forearm**
  > HAC 7th character A see Appendix B for HAC conditional logic

+ **T22.32** **Burn of third degree of elbow**
- CC +7th **T22.321** **Burn of third degree of right elbow**
  > HAC 7th character A see Appendix B for HAC conditional logic
- CC +7th **T22.322** **Burn of third degree of left elbow**
  > HAC 7th character A see Appendix B for HAC conditional logic
- CC +7th **T22.329** **Burn of third degree of unspecified elbow**
  > HAC 7th character A see Appendix B for HAC conditional logic

+ **T22.33** **Burn of third degree of upper arm**
- CC +7th **T22.331** **Burn of third degree of right upper arm**
  > HAC 7th character A see Appendix B for HAC conditional logic
- CC +7th **T22.332** **Burn of third degree of left upper arm**
  > HAC 7th character A see Appendix B for HAC conditional logic
- CC +7th **T22.339** **Burn of third degree of unspecified upper arm**
  > HAC 7th character A see Appendix B for HAC conditional logic

+ **T22.34** **Burn of third degree of axilla**
- CC +7th **T22.341** **Burn of third degree of right axilla**
  > HAC 7th character A see Appendix B for HAC conditional logic
- CC +7th **T22.342** **Burn of third degree of left axilla**
  > HAC 7th character A see Appendix B for HAC conditional logic
- CC +7th **T22.349** **Burn of third degree of unspecified axilla**
  > HAC 7th character A see Appendix B for HAC conditional logic

+ **T22.35** **Burn of third degree of shoulder**
- CC +7th **T22.351** **Burn of third degree of right shoulder**
  > HAC 7th character A see Appendix B for HAC conditional logic
- CC +7th **T22.352** **Burn of third degree of left shoulder**
  > HAC 7th character A see Appendix B for HAC conditional logic
- CC +7th **T22.359** **Burn of third degree of unspecified shoulder**
  > HAC 7th character A see Appendix B for HAC conditional logic

+ **T22.36** **Burn of third degree of scapular region**
- CC +7th **T22.361** **Burn of third degree of right scapular region**
  > HAC 7th character A see Appendix B for HAC conditional logic
- CC +7th **T22.362** **Burn of third degree of left scapular region**
  > HAC 7th character A see Appendix B for HAC conditional logic
- CC +7th **T22.369** **Burn of third degree of unspecified scapular region**
  > HAC 7th character A see Appendix B for HAC conditional logic

+, +7th, X + 7th • Newborn • Pediatric • Maternity • Adult ♀ Female ♂ Male Manifestation Unacceptable PDX HCC CC MCC HAC

+ **T22.39** **Burn of third degree of multiple sites of shoulder and upper limb, except wrist and hand**
    CC +7th **T22.391** **Burn of third degree of multiple sites of right shoulder and upper limb, except wrist and hand**

    HAC 7th character A see Appendix B for HAC conditional logic

    CC +7th **T22.392** **Burn of third degree of multiple sites of left shoulder and upper limb, except wrist and hand**

    HAC 7th character A see Appendix B for HAC conditional logic

    CC +7th **T22.399** **Burn of third degree of multiple sites of unspecified shoulder and upper limb, except wrist and hand**

    HAC 7th character A see Appendix B for HAC conditional logic

+ **T22.4** **Corrosion of unspecified degree of shoulder and upper limb, except wrist and hand**
    Code first (T51-T65) to identify chemical and intent

    Use additional external cause code to identify place (Y92)
    X+7th **T22.40** **Corrosion of unspecified degree of shoulder and upper limb, except wrist and hand, unspecified site**
    + **T22.41** **Corrosion of unspecified degree of forearm**
        +7th **T22.411** **Corrosion of unspecified degree of right forearm**
        +7th **T22.412** **Corrosion of unspecified degree of left forearm**
        +7th **T22.419** **Corrosion of unspecified degree of unspecified forearm**
    + **T22.42** **Corrosion of unspecified degree of elbow**
        +7th **T22.421** **Corrosion of unspecified degree of right elbow**
        +7th **T22.422** **Corrosion of unspecified degree of left elbow**
        +7th **T22.429** **Corrosion of unspecified degree of unspecified elbow**
    + **T22.43** **Corrosion of unspecified degree of upper arm**
        +7th **T22.431** **Corrosion of unspecified degree of right upper arm**
        +7th **T22.432** **Corrosion of unspecified degree of left upper arm**
        +7th **T22.439** **Corrosion of unspecified degree of unspecified upper arm**
    + **T22.44** **Corrosion of unspecified degree of axilla**
        +7th **T22.441** **Corrosion of unspecified degree of right axilla**
        +7th **T22.442** **Corrosion of unspecified degree of left axilla**
        +7th **T22.449** **Corrosion of unspecified degree of unspecified axilla**
    + **T22.45** **Corrosion of unspecified degree of shoulder**
        +7th **T22.451** **Corrosion of unspecified degree of right shoulder**
        +7th **T22.452** **Corrosion of unspecified degree of left shoulder**
        +7th **T22.459** **Corrosion of unspecified degree of unspecified shoulder**
    + **T22.46** **Corrosion of unspecified degree of scapular region**
        +7th **T22.461** **Corrosion of unspecified degree of right scapular region**
        +7th **T22.462** **Corrosion of unspecified degree of left scapular region**
        +7th **T22.469** **Corrosion of unspecified degree of unspecified scapular region**
    + **T22.49** **Corrosion of unspecified degree of multiple sites of shoulder and upper limb, except wrist and hand**
        +7th **T22.491** **Corrosion of unspecified degree of multiple sites of right shoulder and upper limb, except wrist and hand**
        +7th **T22.492** **Corrosion of unspecified degree of multiple sites of left shoulder and upper limb, except wrist and hand**
        +7th **T22.499** **Corrosion of unspecified degree of multiple sites of unspecified shoulder and upper limb, except wrist and hand**

+ **T22.5** **Corrosion of first degree of shoulder and upper limb, except wrist and hand**
    Code first (T51-T65) to identify chemical and intent

    Use additional external cause code to identify place (Y92)
    X+7th **T22.50** **Corrosion of first degree of shoulder and upper limb, except wrist and hand unspecified site**
    + **T22.51** **Corrosion of first degree of forearm**
        +7th **T22.511** **Corrosion of first degree of right forearm**
        +7th **T22.512** **Corrosion of first degree of left forearm**
        +7th **T22.519** **Corrosion of first degree of unspecified forearm**
    + **T22.52** **Corrosion of first degree of elbow**
        +7th **T22.521** **Corrosion of first degree of right elbow**
        +7th **T22.522** **Corrosion of first degree of left elbow**
        +7th **T22.529** **Corrosion of first degree of unspecified elbow**
    + **T22.53** **Corrosion of first degree of upper arm**
        +7th **T22.531** **Corrosion of first degree of right upper arm**
        +7th **T22.532** **Corrosion of first degree of left upper arm**
        +7th **T22.539** **Corrosion of first degree of unspecified upper arm**
    + **T22.54** **Corrosion of first degree of axilla**
        +7th **T22.541** **Corrosion of first degree of right axilla**
        +7th **T22.542** **Corrosion of first degree of left axilla**
        +7th **T22.549** **Corrosion of first degree of unspecified axilla**
    + **T22.55** **Corrosion of first degree of shoulder**
        +7th **T22.551** **Corrosion of first degree of right shoulder**
        +7th **T22.552** **Corrosion of first degree of left shoulder**
        +7th **T22.559** **Corrosion of first degree of unspecified shoulder**
    + **T22.56** **Corrosion of first degree of scapular region**
        +7th **T22.561** **Corrosion of first degree of right scapular region**
        +7th **T22.562** **Corrosion of first degree of left scapular region**
        +7th **T22.569** **Corrosion of first degree of unspecified scapular region**
    + **T22.59** **Corrosion of first degree of multiple sites of shoulder and upper limb, except wrist and hand**
        +7th **T22.591** **Corrosion of first degree of multiple sites of right shoulder and upper limb, except wrist and hand**
        +7th **T22.592** **Corrosion of first degree of multiple sites of left shoulder and upper limb, except wrist and hand**
        +7th **T22.599** **Corrosion of first degree of multiple sites of unspecified shoulder and upper limb, except wrist and hand**
+ **T22.6** **Corrosion of second degree of shoulder and upper limb, except wrist and hand**
    Code first (T51-T65) to identify chemical and intent

    Use additional external cause code to identify place (Y92)
    X+7th **T22.60** **Corrosion of second degree of shoulder and upper limb, except wrist and hand, unspecified site**
    + **T22.61** **Corrosion of second degree of forearm**
        +7th **T22.611** **Corrosion of second degree of right forearm**
        +7th **T22.612** **Corrosion of second degree of left forearm**
        +7th **T22.619** **Corrosion of second degree of unspecified forearm**
    + **T22.62** **Corrosion of second degree of elbow**
        +7th **T22.621** **Corrosion of second degree of right elbow**
        +7th **T22.622** **Corrosion of second degree of left elbow**
        +7th **T22.629** **Corrosion of second degree of unspecified elbow**
    + **T22.63** **Corrosion of second degree of upper arm**
        +7th **T22.631** **Corrosion of second degree of right upper arm**
        +7th **T22.632** **Corrosion of second degree of left upper arm**
        +7th **T22.639** **Corrosion of second degree of unspecified upper arm**

+ **T22.64** **Corrosion of second degree of axilla**
+7th **T22.641** **Corrosion of second degree of right axilla**
+7th **T22.642** **Corrosion of second degree of left axilla**
+7th **T22.649** **Corrosion of second degree of unspecified axilla**
+ **T22.65** **Corrosion of second degree of shoulder**
+7th **T22.651** **Corrosion of second degree of right shoulder**
+7th **T22.652** **Corrosion of second degree of left shoulder**
+7th **T22.659** **Corrosion of second degree of unspecified shoulder**
+ **T22.66** **Corrosion of second degree of scapular region**
+7th **T22.661** **Corrosion of second degree of right scapular region**
+7th **T22.662** **Corrosion of second degree of left scapular region**
+7th **T22.669** **Corrosion of second degree of unspecified scapular region**
+ **T22.69** **Corrosion of second degree of multiple sites of shoulder and upper limb, except wrist and hand**
+7th **T22.691** **Corrosion of second degree of multiple sites of right shoulder and upper limb, except wrist and hand**
+7th **T22.692** **Corrosion of second degree of multiple sites of left shoulder and upper limb, except wrist and hand**
+7th **T22.699** **Corrosion of second degree of multiple sites of unspecified shoulder and upper limb, except wrist and hand**
+ **T22.7** **Corrosion of third degree of shoulder and upper limb, except wrist and hand**
Code first (T51-T65) to identify chemical and intent external cause code to identify place (Y92)
CC X+7th **T22.70** **Corrosion of third degree of shoulder and upper limb, except wrist and hand, unspecified site**
HAC 7th character A see Appendix B for HAC conditional logic
+ **T22.71** **Corrosion of third degree of forearm**
CC +7th **T22.711** **Corrosion of third degree of right forearm**
HAC 7th character A see Appendix B for HAC conditional logic
CC +7th **T22.712** **Corrosion of third degree of left forearm**
HAC 7th character A see Appendix B for HAC conditional logic
CC +7th **T22.719** **Corrosion of third degree of unspecified forearm**
HAC 7th character A see Appendix B for HAC conditional logic
+ **T22.72** **Corrosion of third degree of elbow**
CC +7th **T22.721** **Corrosion of third degree of right elbow**
HAC 7th character A see Appendix B for HAC conditional logic
CC +7th **T22.722** **Corrosion of third degree of left elbow**
HAC 7th character A see Appendix B for HAC conditional logic
CC +7th **T22.729** **Corrosion of third degree of unspecified elbow**
HAC 7th character A see Appendix B for HAC conditional logic
+ **T22.73** **Corrosion of third degree of upper arm**
CC +7th **T22.731** **Corrosion of third degree of right upper arm**
HAC 7th character A see Appendix B for HAC conditional logic
CC +7th **T22.732** **Corrosion of third degree of left upper arm**
HAC 7th character A see Appendix B for HAC conditional logic
CC +7th **T22.739** **Corrosion of third degree of unspecified upper arm**
HAC 7th character A see Appendix B for HAC conditional logic

+ **T22.74** **Corrosion of third degree of axilla**
CC +7th **T22.741** **Corrosion of third degree of right axilla**
HAC 7th character A see Appendix B for HAC conditional logic
CC +7th **T22.742** **Corrosion of third degree of left axilla**
HAC 7th character A see Appendix B for HAC conditional logic
CC +7th **T22.749** **Corrosion of third degree of unspecified axilla**
HAC 7th character A see Appendix B for HAC conditional logic
+ **T22.75** **Corrosion of third degree of shoulder**
CC +7th **T22.751** **Corrosion of third degree of right shoulder**
HAC 7th character A see Appendix B for HAC conditional logic
CC +7th **T22.752** **Corrosion of third degree of left shoulder**
HAC 7th character A see Appendix B for HAC conditional logic
CC +7th **T22.759** **Corrosion of third degree of unspecified shoulder**
HAC 7th character A see Appendix B for HAC conditional logic
+ **T22.76** **Corrosion of third degree of scapular region**
CC +7th **T22.761** **Corrosion of third degree of right scapular region**
HAC 7th character A see Appendix B for HAC conditional logic
CC +7th **T22.762** **Corrosion of third degree of left scapular region**
HAC 7th character A see Appendix B for HAC conditional logic
CC +7th **T22.769** **Corrosion of third degree of unspecified scapular region**
HAC 7th character A see Appendix B for HAC conditional logic
+ **T22.79** **Corrosion of third degree of multiple sites of shoulder and upper limb, except wrist and hand**
CC +7th **T22.791** **Corrosion of third degree of multiple sites of right shoulder and upper limb, except wrist and hand**
HAC 7th character A see Appendix B for HAC conditional logic
CC +7th **T22.792** **Corrosion of third degree of multiple sites of left shoulder and upper limb, except wrist and hand**
HAC 7th character A see Appendix B for HAC conditional logic
CC +7th **T22.799** **Corrosion of third degree of multiple sites of unspecified shoulder and upper limb, except wrist and hand**
HAC 7th character A see Appendix B for HAC conditional logic

T23 **Burn and corrosion of wrist and hand**

The appropriate 7th character is to be added to each code from category T23
A   initial encounter
D   subsequent encounter
S   sequela

+ **T23.0** **Burn of unspecified degree of wrist and hand**
Use additional external cause code to identify the source, place and intent of the burn (X00-X19, X75-X77, X96-X98, Y92)
+ **T23.00** **Burn of unspecified degree of hand, unspecified site**
+7th **T23.001** **Burn of unspecified degree of right hand, unspecified site**
+7th **T23.002** **Burn of unspecified degree of left hand, unspecified site**
+7th **T23.009** **Burn of unspecified degree of unspecified hand, unspecified site**

+ **T23.01** Burn of unspecified degree of thumb (nail)
  - +7th **T23.011** Burn of unspecified degree of right thumb (nail)
  - +7th **T23.012** Burn of unspecified degree of left thumb (nail)
  - +7th **T23.019** Burn of unspecified degree of unspecified thumb (nail)

+ **T23.02** Burn of unspecified degree of single finger (nail) except thumb
  - +7th **T23.021** Burn of unspecified degree of single right finger (nail) except thumb
  - +7th **T23.022** Burn of unspecified degree of single left finger (nail) except thumb
  - +7th **T23.029** Burn of unspecified degree of unspecified single finger (nail) except thumb

+ **T23.03** Burn of unspecified degree of multiple fingers (nail), not including thumb
  - +7th **T23.031** Burn of unspecified degree of multiple right fingers (nail), not including thumb
  - +7th **T23.032** Burn of unspecified degree of multiple left fingers (nail), not including thumb
  - +7th **T23.039** Burn of unspecified degree of unspecified multiple fingers (nail), not including thumb

+ **T23.04** Burn of unspecified degree of multiple fingers (nail), including thumb
  - +7th **T23.041** Burn of unspecified degree of multiple right fingers (nail), including thumb
  - +7th **T23.042** Burn of unspecified degree of multiple left fingers (nail), including thumb
  - +7th **T23.049** Burn of unspecified degree of unspecified multiple fingers (nail), including thumb

+ **T23.05** Burn of unspecified degree of palm
  - +7th **T23.051** Burn of unspecified degree of right palm
  - +7th **T23.052** Burn of unspecified degree of left palm
  - +7th **T23.059** Burn of unspecified degree of unspecified palm

+ **T23.06** Burn of unspecified degree of back of hand
  - +7th **T23.061** Burn of unspecified degree of back of right hand
  - +7th **T23.062** Burn of unspecified degree of back of left hand
  - +7th **T23.069** Burn of unspecified degree of back of unspecified hand

+ **T23.07** Burn of unspecified degree of wrist
  - +7th **T23.071** Burn of unspecified degree of right wrist
  - +7th **T23.072** Burn of unspecified degree of left wrist
  - +7th **T23.079** Burn of unspecified degree of unspecified wrist

+ **T23.09** Burn of unspecified degree of multiple sites of wrist and hand
  - +7th **T23.091** Burn of unspecified degree of multiple sites of right wrist and hand
  - +7th **T23.092** Burn of unspecified degree of multiple sites of left wrist and hand
  - +7th **T23.099** Burn of unspecified degree of multiple sites of unspecified wrist and hand

+ **T23.1** Burn of first degree of wrist and hand
  Use additional external cause code to identify the source, place and intent of the burn (X00-X19, X75-X77, X96-X98, Y92)

+ **T23.10** Burn of first degree of hand, unspecified site
  - +7th **T23.101** Burn of first degree of right hand, unspecified site
  - +7th **T23.102** Burn of first degree of left hand, unspecified site
  - +7th **T23.109** Burn of first degree of unspecified hand, unspecified site

+ **T23.11** Burn of first degree of thumb (nail)
  - +7th **T23.111** Burn of first degree of right thumb (nail)
  - +7th **T23.112** Burn of first degree of left thumb (nail)
  - +7th **T23.119** Burn of first degree of unspecified thumb (nail)

+ **T23.12** Burn of first degree of single finger (nail) except thumb

+ **T23.121** Burn of first degree of single right finger (nail) except thumb
  - +7th **T23.121** Burn of first degree of single right finger (nail) except thumb
  - +7th **T23.122** Burn of first degree of single left finger (nail) except thumb
  - +7th **T23.129** Burn of first degree of unspecified single finger (nail) except thumb

+ **T23.13** Burn of first degree of multiple fingers (nail), not including thumb
  - +7th **T23.131** Burn of first degree of multiple right fingers (nail), not including thumb
  - +7th **T23.132** Burn of first degree of multiple left fingers (nail), not including thumb
  - +7th **T23.139** Burn of first degree of unspecified multiple fingers (nail), not including thumb

+ **T23.14** Burn of first degree of multiple fingers (nail), including thumb
  - +7th **T23.141** Burn of first degree of multiple right fingers (nail), including thumb
  - +7th **T23.142** Burn of first degree of multiple left fingers (nail), including thumb
  - +7th **T23.149** Burn of first degree of unspecified multiple fingers (nail), including thumb

+ **T23.15** Burn of first degree of palm
  - +7th **T23.151** Burn of first degree of right palm
  - +7th **T23.152** Burn of first degree of left palm
  - +7th **T23.159** Burn of first degree of unspecified palm

+ **T23.16** Burn of first degree of back of hand
  - +7th **T23.161** Burn of first degree of back of right hand
  - +7th **T23.162** Burn of first degree of back of left hand
  - +7th **T23.169** Burn of first degree of back of unspecified hand

+ **T23.17** Burn of first degree of wrist
  - +7th **T23.171** Burn of first degree of right wrist
  - +7th **T23.172** Burn of first degree of left wrist
  - +7th **T23.179** Burn of first degree of unspecified wrist

+ **T23.19** Burn of first degree of multiple sites of wrist and hand
  - +7th **T23.191** Burn of first degree of multiple sites of right wrist and hand
  - +7th **T23.192** Burn of first degree of multiple sites of left wrist and hand
  - +7th **T23.199** Burn of first degree of multiple sites of unspecified wrist and hand

+ **T23.2** Burn of second degree of wrist and hand
  Use additional external cause code to identify the source, place and intent of the burn (X00-X19, X75-X77, X96-X98, Y92)

+ **T23.20** Burn of second degree of hand, unspecified site
  - +7th **T23.201** Burn of second degree of right hand, unspecified site
  - +7th **T23.202** Burn of second degree of left hand, unspecified site
  - +7th **T23.209** Burn of second degree of unspecified hand, unspecified site

+ **T23.21** Burn of second degree of thumb (nail)
  - +7th **T23.211** Burn of second degree of right thumb (nail)
  - +7th **T23.212** Burn of second degree of left thumb (nail)
  - +7th **T23.219** Burn of second degree of unspecified thumb (nail)

+ **T23.22** Burn of second degree of single finger (nail) except thumb
  - +7th **T23.221** Burn of second degree of single right finger (nail) except thumb
  - +7th **T23.222** Burn of second degree of single left finger (nail) except thumb
  - +7th **T23.229** Burn of second degree of unspecified single finger (nail) except thumb

+ **T23.23** Burn of second degree of multiple fingers (nail), not including thumb
  - +7th **T23.231** Burn of second degree of multiple right fingers (nail), not including thumb
  - +7th **T23.232** Burn of second degree of multiple left fingers (nail), not including thumb
  - +7th **T23.239** Burn of second degree of unspecified multiple fingers (nail), not including thumb

+ **T23.24** **Burn of second degree of multiple fingers (nail), including thumb**
  - +7th **T23.241** **Burn of second degree of multiple right fingers (nail), including thumb**
  - +7th **T23.242** **Burn of second degree of multiple left fingers (nail), including thumb**
  - +7th **T23.249** **Burn of second degree of unspecified multiple fingers (nail), including thumb**

+ **T23.25** **Burn of second degree of palm**
  - +7th **T23.251** **Burn of second degree of right palm**
  - +7th **T23.252** **Burn of second degree of left palm**
  - +7th **T23.259** **Burn of second degree of unspecified palm**

+ **T23.26** **Burn of second degree of back of hand**
  - +7th **T23.261** **Burn of second degree of back of right hand**
  - +7th **T23.262** **Burn of second degree of back of left hand**
  - +7th **T23.269** **Burn of second degree of back of unspecified hand**

+ **T23.27** **Burn of second degree of wrist**
  - +7th **T23.271** **Burn of second degree of right wrist**
  - +7th **T23.272** **Burn of second degree of left wrist**
  - +7th **T23.279** **Burn of second degree of unspecified wrist**

+ **T23.29** **Burn of second degree of multiple sites of wrist and hand**
  - +7th **T23.291** **Burn of second degree of multiple sites of right wrist and hand**
  - +7th **T23.292** **Burn of second degree of multiple sites of left wrist and hand**
  - +7th **T23.299** **Burn of second degree of multiple sites of unspecified wrist and hand**

+ **T23.3** **Burn of third degree of wrist and hand**
  Use additional external cause code to identify the source, place and intent of the burn (X00-X19, X75-X77, X96-X98, Y92)

+ **T23.30** **Burn of third degree of hand, unspecified site**
  - CC +7th **T23.301** **Burn of third degree of right hand, unspecified site**
    AHA CC: 1Q, 2015, 3-21
    HAC 7th character A see Appendix B for HAC conditional logic
  - CC +7th **T23.302** **Burn of third degree of left hand, unspecified site**
    AHA CC: 2Q, 2016, 5
    HAC 7th character A see Appendix B for HAC conditional logic
  - CC +7th **T23.309** **Burn of third degree of unspecified hand, unspecified site**
    HAC 7th character A see Appendix B for HAC conditional logic

+ **T23.31** **Burn of third degree of thumb (nail)**
  - CC +7th **T23.311** **Burn of third degree of right thumb (nail)**
    HAC 7th character A see Appendix B for HAC conditional logic
  - CC +7th **T23.312** **Burn of third degree of left thumb (nail)**
    HAC 7th character A see Appendix B for HAC conditional logic
  - CC +7th **T23.319** **Burn of third degree of unspecified thumb (nail)**
    HAC 7th character A see Appendix B for HAC conditional logic

+ **T23.32** **Burn of third degree of single finger (nail) except thumb**
  - CC +7th **T23.321** **Burn of third degree of single right finger (nail) except thumb**
    HAC 7th character A see Appendix B for HAC conditional logic
  - CC +7th **T23.322** **Burn of third degree of single left finger (nail) except thumb**
    HAC 7th character A see Appendix B for HAC conditional logic
  - CC +7th **T23.329** **Burn of third degree of unspecified single finger (nail) except thumb**
    HAC 7th character A see Appendix B for HAC conditional logic

+ **T23.33** **Burn of third degree of multiple fingers (nail), not including thumb**
  - CC +7th **T23.331** **Burn of third degree of multiple right fingers (nail), not including thumb**
    HAC 7th character A see Appendix B for HAC conditional logic
  - CC +7th **T23.332** **Burn of third degree of multiple left fingers (nail), not including thumb**
    HAC 7th character A see Appendix B for HAC conditional logic
  - CC +7th **T23.339** **Burn of third degree of unspecified multiple fingers (nail), not including thumb**

+ **T23.34** **Burn of third degree of multiple fingers (nail), including thumb**
  - CC +7th **T23.341** **Burn of third degree of multiple right fingers (nail), including thumb**
    HAC 7th character A see Appendix B for HAC conditional logic
  - CC +7th **T23.342** **Burn of third degree of multiple left fingers (nail), including thumb**
    HAC 7th character A see Appendix B for HAC conditional logic
  - CC +7th **T23.349** **Burn of third degree of unspecified multiple fingers (nail), including thumb**
    HAC 7th character A see Appendix B for HAC conditional logic

+ **T23.35** **Burn of third degree of palm**
  - CC +7th **T23.351** **Burn of third degree of right palm**
    HAC 7th character A see Appendix B for HAC conditional logic
  - CC +7th **T23.352** **Burn of third degree of left palm**
    HAC 7th character A see Appendix B for HAC conditional logic
  - CC +7th **T23.359** **Burn of third degree of unspecified palm**
    HAC 7th character A see Appendix B for HAC conditional logic

+ **T23.36** **Burn of third degree of back of hand**
  - CC +7th **T23.361** **Burn of third degree of back of right hand**
    HAC 7th character A see Appendix B for HAC conditional logic
  - CC +7th **T23.362** **Burn of third degree of back of left hand**
    HAC 7th character A see Appendix B for HAC conditional logic
  - CC +7th **T23.369** **Burn of third degree of back of unspecified hand**
    HAC 7th character A see Appendix B for HAC conditional logic

+ **T23.37** **Burn of third degree of wrist**
  - CC +7th **T23.371** **Burn of third degree of right wrist**
    HAC 7th character A see Appendix B for HAC conditional logic
  - CC +7th **T23.372** **Burn of third degree of left wrist**
    HAC 7th character A see Appendix B for HAC conditional logic
  - CC +7th **T23.379** **Burn of third degree of unspecified wrist**
    HAC 7th character A see Appendix B for HAC conditional logic

+ **T23.39** **Burn of third degree of multiple sites of wrist and hand**
  - CC +7th **T23.391** **Burn of third degree of multiple sites of right wrist and hand**
    HAC 7th character A see Appendix B for HAC conditional logic
  - CC +7th **T23.392** **Burn of third degree of multiple sites of left wrist and hand**
    HAC 7th character A see Appendix B for HAC conditional logic
  - CC +7th **T23.399** **Burn of third degree of multiple sites of unspecified wrist and hand**
    HAC 7th character A see Appendix B for HAC conditional logic

+ **T23.4** **Corrosion of unspecified degree of wrist and hand**
Code first (T51-T65) to identify chemical and intent

Use additional external cause code to identify place (Y92)

+ **T23.40** **Corrosion of unspecified degree of hand, unspecified site**
- +7th **T23.401** Corrosion of unspecified degree of right hand, unspecified site
- +7th **T23.402** Corrosion of unspecified degree of left hand, unspecified site
- +7th **T23.409** Corrosion of unspecified degree of unspecified hand, unspecified site

+ **T23.41** **Corrosion of unspecified degree of thumb (nail)**
- +7th **T23.411** Corrosion of unspecified degree of right thumb (nail)
- +7th **T23.412** Corrosion of unspecified degree of left thumb (nail)
- +7th **T23.419** Corrosion of unspecified degree of unspecified thumb (nail)

+ **T23.42** **Corrosion of unspecified degree of single finger (nail) except thumb**
- +7th **T23.421** Corrosion of unspecified degree of single right finger (nail) except thumb
- +7th **T23.422** Corrosion of unspecified degree of single left finger (nail) except thumb
- +7th **T23.429** Corrosion of unspecified degree of unspecified single finger (nail) except thumb

+ **T23.43** **Corrosion of unspecified degree of multiple fingers (nail), not including thumb**
- +7th **T23.431** Corrosion of unspecified degree of multiple right fingers (nail), not including thumb
- +7th **T23.432** Corrosion of unspecified degree of multiple left fingers (nail), not including thumb
- +7th **T23.439** Corrosion of unspecified degree of unspecified multiple fingers (nail), not including thumb

+ **T23.44** **Corrosion of unspecified degree of multiple fingers (nail), including thumb**
- +7th **T23.441** Corrosion of unspecified degree of multiple right fingers (nail), including thumb
- +7th **T23.442** Corrosion of unspecified degree of multiple left fingers (nail), including thumb
- +7th **T23.449** Corrosion of unspecified degree of unspecified multiple fingers (nail), including thumb

+ **T23.45** **Corrosion of unspecified degree of palm**
- +7th **T23.451** Corrosion of unspecified degree of right palm
- +7th **T23.452** Corrosion of unspecified degree of left palm
- +7th **T23.459** Corrosion of unspecified degree of unspecified palm

+ **T23.46** **Corrosion of unspecified degree of back of hand**
- +7th **T23.461** Corrosion of unspecified degree of back of right hand
- +7th **T23.462** Corrosion of unspecified degree of back of left hand
- +7th **T23.469** Corrosion of unspecified degree of back of unspecified hand

+ **T23.47** **Corrosion of unspecified degree of wrist**
- +7th **T23.471** Corrosion of unspecified degree of right wrist
- +7th **T23.472** Corrosion of unspecified degree of left wrist
- +7th **T23.479** Corrosion of unspecified degree of unspecified wrist

+ **T23.49** **Corrosion of unspecified degree of multiple sites of wrist and hand**
- +7th **T23.491** Corrosion of unspecified degree of multiple sites of right wrist and hand
- +7th **T23.492** Corrosion of unspecified degree of multiple sites of left wrist and hand
- +7th **T23.499** Corrosion of unspecified degree of multiple sites of unspecified wrist and hand

+ **T23.5** **Corrosion of first degree of wrist and hand**
Code first (T51-T65) to identify chemical and intent

Use additional external cause code to identify place (Y92)

+ **T23.50** **Corrosion of first degree of hand, unspecified site**
- +7th **T23.501** Corrosion of first degree of right hand, unspecified site
- +7th **T23.502** Corrosion of first degree of left hand, unspecified site
- +7th **T23.509** Corrosion of first degree of unspecified hand, unspecified site

+ **T23.51** **Corrosion of first degree of thumb (nail)**
- +7th **T23.511** Corrosion of first degree of right thumb (nail)
- +7th **T23.512** Corrosion of first degree of left thumb (nail)
- +7th **T23.519** Corrosion of first degree of unspecified thumb (nail)

+ **T23.52** **Corrosion of first degree of single finger (nail) except thumb**
- +7th **T23.521** Corrosion of first degree of single right finger (nail) except thumb
- +7th **T23.522** Corrosion of first degree of single left finger (nail) except thumb
- +7th **T23.529** Corrosion of first degree of unspecified single finger (nail) except thumb

+ **T23.53** **Corrosion of first degree of multiple fingers (nail), not including thumb**
- +7th **T23.531** Corrosion of first degree of multiple right fingers (nail), not including thumb
- +7th **T23.532** Corrosion of first degree of multiple left fingers (nail), not including thumb
- +7th **T23.539** Corrosion of first degree of unspecified multiple fingers (nail), not including thumb

+ **T23.54** **Corrosion of first degree of multiple fingers (nail), including thumb**
- +7th **T23.541** Corrosion of first degree of multiple right fingers (nail), including thumb
- +7th **T23.542** Corrosion of first degree of multiple left fingers (nail), including thumb
- +7th **T23.549** Corrosion of first degree of unspecified multiple fingers (nail), including thumb

+ **T23.55** **Corrosion of first degree of palm**
- +7th **T23.551** Corrosion of first degree of right palm
- +7th **T23.552** Corrosion of first degree of left palm
- +7th **T23.559** Corrosion of first degree of unspecified palm

+ **T23.56** **Corrosion of first degree of back of hand**
- +7th **T23.561** Corrosion of first degree of back of right hand
- +7th **T23.562** Corrosion of first degree of back of left hand
- +7th **T23.569** Corrosion of first degree of back of unspecified hand

+ **T23.57** **Corrosion of first degree of wrist**
- +7th **T23.571** Corrosion of first degree of right wrist
- +7th **T23.572** Corrosion of first degree of left wrist
- +7th **T23.579** Corrosion of first degree of unspecified wrist

+ **T23.59** **Corrosion of first degree of multiple sites of wrist and hand**
- +7th **T23.591** Corrosion of first degree of multiple sites of right wrist and hand
- +7th **T23.592** Corrosion of first degree of multiple sites of left wrist and hand
- +7th **T23.599** Corrosion of first degree of multiple sites of unspecified wrist and hand

+ **T23.6** **Corrosion of second degree of wrist and hand**
Code first (T51-T65) to identify chemical and intent

Use additionalexternal cause code to identify place (Y92)

- + **T23.60** **Corrosion of second degree of hand, unspecified site**
  - +7th **T23.601** Corrosion of second degree of right hand, unspecified site
  - +7th **T23.602** Corrosion of second degree of left hand, unspecified site
  - +7th **T23.609** Corrosion of second degree of unspecified hand, unspecified site
- + **T23.61** **Corrosion of second degree of thumb (nail)**
  - +7th **T23.611** Corrosion of second degree of right thumb (nail)
  - +7th **T23.612** Corrosion of second degree of left thumb (nail)
  - +7th **T23.619** Corrosion of second degree of unspecified thumb (nail)
- + **T23.62** **Corrosion of second degree of single finger (nail) except thumb**
  - +7th **T23.621** Corrosion of second degree of single right finger (nail) except thumb
  - +7th **T23.622** Corrosion of second degree of single left finger (nail) except thumb
  - +7th **T23.629** Corrosion of second degree of unspecified single finger (nail) except thumb
- + **T23.63** **Corrosion of second degree of multiple fingers (nail), not including thumb**
  - +7th **T23.631** Corrosion of second degree of multiple right fingers (nail), not including thumb
  - +7th **T23.632** Corrosion of second degree of multiple left fingers (nail), not including thumb
  - +7th **T23.639** Corrosion of second degree of unspecified multiple fingers (nail), not including thumb
- + **T23.64** **Corrosion of second degree of multiple fingers (nail), including thumb**
  - +7th **T23.641** Corrosion of second degree of multiple right fingers (nail), including thumb
  - +7th **T23.642** Corrosion of second degree of multiple left fingers (nail), including thumb
  - +7th **T23.649** Corrosion of second degree of unspecified multiple fingers (nail), including thumb
- + **T23.65** **Corrosion of second degree of palm**
  - +7th **T23.651** Corrosion of second degree of right palm
  - +7th **T23.652** Corrosion of second degree of left palm
  - +7th **T23.659** Corrosion of second degree of unspecified palm
- + **T23.66** **Corrosion of second degree of back of hand**
  - +7th **T23.661** Corrosion of second degree back of right hand
  - +7th **T23.662** Corrosion of second degree back of left hand
  - +7th **T23.669** Corrosion of second degree back of unspecified hand
- + **T23.67** **Corrosion of second degree of wrist**
  - +7th **T23.671** Corrosion of second degree of right wrist
  - +7th **T23.672** Corrosion of second degree of left wrist
  - +7th **T23.679** Corrosion of second degree of unspecified wrist
- + **T23.69** **Corrosion of second degree of multiple sites of wrist and hand**
  - +7th **T23.691** Corrosion of second degree of multiple sites of right wrist and hand
  - +7th **T23.692** Corrosion of second degree of multiple sites of left wrist and hand
  - +7th **T23.699** Corrosion of second degree of multiple sites of unspecified wrist and hand

+ **T23.7** **Corrosion of third degree of wrist and hand**
Code first (T51-T65) to identify chemical and intent

Use additional external cause code to identify place (Y92)

- + **T23.70** **Corrosion of third degree of hand, unspecified site**
  - CC +7th **T23.701** Corrosion of third degree of right hand, unspecified site
    - **HAC** 7th character A see Appendix B for HAC conditional logic
  - CC +7th **T23.702** Corrosion of third degree of left hand, unspecified site
    - **HAC** 7th character A see Appendix B for HAC conditional logic
  - CC +7th **T23.709** Corrosion of third degree of unspecified hand, unspecified site
    - **HAC** 7th character A see Appendix B for HAC conditional logic
- + **T23.71** **Corrosion of third degree of thumb (nail)**
  - CC +7th **T23.711** Corrosion of third degree of right thumb (nail)
    - **HAC** 7th character A see Appendix B for HAC conditional logic
  - CC +7th **T23.712** Corrosion of third degree of left thumb (nail)
    - **HAC** 7th character A see Appendix B for HAC conditional logic
  - CC +7th **T23.719** Corrosion of third degree of unspecified thumb (nail)
    - **HAC** 7th character A see Appendix B for HAC conditional logic
- + **T23.72** **Corrosion of third degree of single finger (nail) except thumb**
  - CC +7th **T23.721** Corrosion of third degree of single right finger (nail) except thumb
    - **HAC** 7th character A see Appendix B for HAC conditional logic
  - CC +7th **T23.722** Corrosion of third degree of single left finger (nail) except thumb
    - **HAC** 7th character A see Appendix B for HAC conditional logic
  - CC +7th **T23.729** Corrosion of third degree of unspecified single finger (nail) except thumb
    - **HAC** 7th character A see Appendix B for HAC conditional logic
- + **T23.73** **Corrosion of third degree of multiple fingers (nail), not including thumb**
  - CC +7th **T23.731** Corrosion of third degree of multiple right fingers (nail), not including thumb
    - **HAC** 7th character A see Appendix B for HAC conditional logic
  - CC +7th **T23.732** Corrosion of third degree of multiple left fingers (nail), not including thumb
    - **HAC** 7th character A see Appendix B for HAC conditional logic
  - CC +7th **T23.739** Corrosion of third degree of unspecified multiple fingers (nail), not including thumb
    - **HAC** 7th character A see Appendix B for HAC conditional logic
- + **T23.74** **Corrosion of third degree of multiple fingers (nail), including thumb**
  - CC +7th **T23.741** Corrosion of third degree of multiple right fingers (nail), including thumb
    - **HAC** 7th character A see Appendix B for HAC conditional logic
  - CC +7th **T23.742** Corrosion of third degree of multiple left fingers (nail), including thumb
    - **HAC** 7th character A see Appendix B for HAC conditional logic
  - CC +7th **T23.749** Corrosion of third degree of unspecified multiple fingers (nail), including thumb
    - **HAC** 7th character A see Appendix B for HAC conditional logic

1125

+ **T23.75** Corrosion of third degree of palm
CC +7th **T23.751** Corrosion of third degree of right palm
HAC 7th character A see Appendix B for HAC conditional logic
CC +7th **T23.752** Corrosion of third degree of left palm
HAC 7th character A see Appendix B for HAC conditional logic
CC +7th **T23.759** Corrosion of third degree of unspecified palm
HAC 7th character A see Appendix B for HAC conditional logic

+ **T23.76** Corrosion of third degree of back of hand
CC +7th **T23.761** Corrosion of third degree of back of right hand
HAC 7th character A see Appendix B for HAC conditional logic
CC +7th **T23.762** Corrosion of third degree of back of left hand
HAC 7th character A see Appendix B for HAC conditional logic
CC +7th **T23.769** Corrosion of third degree back of unspecified hand
HAC 7th character A see Appendix B for HAC conditional logic

+ **T23.77** Corrosion of third degree of wrist
CC +7th **T23.771** Corrosion of third degree of right wrist
HAC 7th character A see Appendix B for HAC conditional logic
CC +7th **T23.772** Corrosion of third degree of left wrist
HAC 7th character A see Appendix B for HAC conditional logic
CC +7th **T23.779** Corrosion of third degree of unspecified wrist
HAC 7th character A see Appendix B for HAC conditional logic

+ **T23.79** Corrosion of third degree of multiple sites of wrist and hand
CC +7th **T23.791** Corrosion of third degree of multiple sites of right wrist and hand
HAC 7th character A see Appendix B for HAC conditional logic
CC +7th **T23.792** Corrosion of third degree of multiple sites of left wrist and hand
HAC 7th character A see Appendix B for HAC conditional logic
CC +7th **T23.799** Corrosion of third degree of multiple sites of unspecified wrist and hand
HAC 7th character A see Appendix B for HAC conditional logic

T24 Burn and corrosion of lower limb, except ankle and foot

Excludes2: burn and corrosion of ankle and foot (T25.-)
burn and corrosion of hip region (T21.-)

The appropriate 7th character is to be added to each code from category T24
A initial encounter
D subsequent encounter
S sequela

+ **T24.0** Burn of unspecified degree of lower limb, except ankle and foot
Use additional external cause code to identify the source, place and intent of the burn (X00-X19, X75-X77, X96-X98, Y92)
+ **T24.00** Burn of unspecified degree of unspecified site of lower limb, except ankle and foot
+7th **T24.001** Burn of unspecified degree of unspecified site of right lower limb, except ankle and foot
+7th **T24.002** Burn of unspecified degree of unspecified site of left lower limb, except ankle and foot
+7th **T24.009** Burn of unspecified degree of unspecified site of unspecified lower limb, except ankle and foot

+ **T24.01** Burn of unspecified degree of thigh
+7th **T24.011** Burn of unspecified degree of right thigh
+7th **T24.012** Burn of unspecified degree of left thigh
+7th **T24.019** Burn of unspecified degree of unspecified thigh
+ **T24.02** Burn of unspecified degree of knee
+7th **T24.021** Burn of unspecified degree of right knee
+7th **T24.022** Burn of unspecified degree of left knee
+7th **T24.029** Burn of unspecified degree of unspecified knee
+ **T24.03** Burn of unspecified degree of lower leg
+7th **T24.031** Burn of unspecified degree of right lower leg
+7th **T24.032** Burn of unspecified degree of left lower leg
+7th **T24.039** Burn of unspecified degree of unspecified lower leg
+ **T24.09** Burn of unspecified degree of multiple sites of lower limb, except ankle and foot
+7th **T24.091** Burn of unspecified degree of multiple sites of right lower limb, except ankle and foot
+7th **T24.092** Burn of unspecified degree of multiple sites of left lower limb, except ankle and foot
+7th **T24.099** Burn of unspecified degree of multiple sites of unspecified lower limb, except ankle and foot

+ **T24.1** Burn of first degree of lower limb, except ankle and foot
Use additional external cause code to identify the source, place and intent of the burn (X00-X19, X75-X77, X96-X98, Y92)
+ **T24.10** Burn of first degree of unspecified site of lower limb, except ankle and foot
+7th **T24.101** Burn of first degree of unspecified site of right lower limb, except ankle and foot
+7th **T24.102** Burn of first degree of unspecified site of left lower limb, except ankle and foot
+7th **T24.109** Burn of first degree of unspecified site of unspecified lower limb, except ankle and foot
+ **T24.11** Burn of first degree of thigh
+7th **T24.111** Burn of first degree of right thigh
+7th **T24.112** Burn of first degree of left thigh
+7th **T24.119** Burn of first degree of unspecified thigh
+ **T24.12** Burn of first degree of knee
+7th **T24.121** Burn of first degree of right knee
+7th **T24.122** Burn of first degree of left knee
+7th **T24.129** Burn of first degree of unspecified knee
+ **T24.13** Burn of first degree of lower leg
+7th **T24.131** Burn of first degree of right lower leg
+7th **T24.132** Burn of first degree of left lower leg
+7th **T24.139** Burn of first degree of unspecified lower leg
+ **T24.19** Burn of first degree of multiple sites of lower limb, except ankle and foot
+7th **T24.191** Burn of first degree of multiple sites of right lower limb, except ankle and foot
+7th **T24.192** Burn of first degree of multiple sites of left lower limb, except ankle and foot
+7th **T24.199** Burn of first degree of multiple sites of unspecified lower limb, except ankle and foot

+, +7th, X + 7th   ● Newborn   ● Pediatric   ● Maternity   ● Adult   ♀ Female   ♂ Male   Manifestation   Unacceptable PDX   HCC   CC   MCC   HAC

+ **T24.2** **Burn of second degree of lower limb, except ankle and foot**
Use additional external cause code to identify the source, place and intent of the burn (X00-X19, X75-X77, X96-X98, Y92)

+ **T24.20** **Burn of second degree of unspecified site of lower limb, except ankle and foot**
+7th **T24.201** Burn of second degree of unspecified site of right lower limb, except ankle and foot
+7th **T24.202** Burn of second degree of unspecified site of left lower limb, except ankle and foot
+7th **T24.209** Burn of second degree of unspecified site of unspecified lower limb, except ankle and foot

+ **T24.21** **Burn of second degree of thigh**
+7th **T24.211** Burn of second degree of right thigh
+7th **T24.212** Burn of second degree of left thigh
+7th **T24.219** Burn of second degree of unspecified thigh

+ **T24.22** **Burn of second degree of knee**
+7th **T24.221** Burn of second degree of right knee
+7th **T24.222** Burn of second degree of left knee
+7th **T24.229** Burn of second degree of unspecified knee

+ **T24.23** **Burn of second degree of lower leg**
+7th **T24.231** Burn of second degree of right lower leg
+7th **T24.232** Burn of second degree of left lower leg
+7th **T24.239** Burn of second degree of unspecified lower leg

+ **T24.29** **Burn of second degree of multiple sites of lower limb, except ankle and foot**
+7th **T24.291** Burn of second degree of multiple sites of right lower limb, except ankle and foot
+7th **T24.292** Burn of second degree of multiple sites of left lower limb, except ankle and foot
+7th **T24.299** Burn of second degree of multiple sites of unspecified lower limb, except ankle and foot

+ **T24.3** **Burn of third degree of lower limb, except ankle and foot**
Use additional external cause code to identify the source, place and intent of the burn (X00-X19, X75-X77, X96-X98, Y92)

+ **T24.30** **Burn of third degree of unspecified site of lower limb, except ankle and foot**
CC +7th **T24.301** Burn of third degree of unspecified site of right lower limb, except ankle and foot
HAC 7th character A see Appendix B for HAC conditional logic
CC +7th **T24.302** Burn of third degree of unspecified site of left lower limb, except ankle and foot
HAC 7th character A see Appendix B for HAC conditional logic
CC +7th **T24.309** Burn of third degree of unspecified site of unspecified lower limb, except ankle and foot
HAC 7th character A see Appendix B for HAC conditional logic

+ **T24.31** **Burn of third degree of thigh**
CC +7th **T24.311** Burn of third degree of right thigh
HAC 7th character A see Appendix B for HAC conditional logic
CC +7th **T24.312** Burn of third degree of left thigh
HAC 7th character A see Appendix B for HAC conditional logic
CC +7th **T24.319** Burn of third degree of unspecified thigh
HAC 7th character A see Appendix B for HAC conditional logic

+ **T24.32** **Burn of third degree of knee**
CC +7th **T24.321** Burn of third degree of right knee
HAC 7th character A see Appendix B for HAC conditional logic
CC +7th **T24.322** Burn of third degree of left knee
HAC 7th character A see Appendix B for HAC conditional logic
CC +7th **T24.329** Burn of third degree of unspecified knee
HAC 7th character A see Appendix B for HAC conditional logic

+ **T24.33** **Burn of third degree of lower leg**
CC +7th **T24.331** Burn of third degree of right lower leg
HAC 7th character A see Appendix B for HAC conditional logic
CC +7th **T24.332** Burn of third degree of left lower leg
HAC 7th character A see Appendix B for HAC conditional logic
CC +7th **T24.339** Burn of third degree of unspecified lower leg
HAC 7th character A see Appendix B for HAC conditional logic

+ **T24.39** **Burn of third degree of multiple sites of lower limb, except ankle and foot**
CC +7th **T24.391** Burn of third degree of multiple sites of right lower limb, except ankle and foot
AHA CC: 2Q, 2016, 4
HAC 7th character A see Appendix B for HAC conditional logic
CC +7th **T24.392** Burn of third degree of multiple sites of left lower limb, except ankle and foot
AHA CC: 2Q, 2016, 4
HAC 7th character A see Appendix B for HAC conditional logic
CC +7th **T24.399** Burn of third degree of multiple sites of unspecified lower limb, except ankle and foot
HAC 7th character A see Appendix B for HAC conditional logic

+ **T24.4** **Corrosion of unspecified degree of lower limb, except ankle and foot**
Code first (T51-T65) to identify chemical and intent

Use additional external cause code to identify place (Y92)

+ **T24.40** **Corrosion of unspecified degree of unspecified site of lower limb, except ankle and foot**
+7th **T24.401** Corrosion of unspecified degree of unspecified site of right lower limb, except ankle and foot
+7th **T24.402** Corrosion of unspecified degree of unspecified site of left lower limb, except ankle and foot
+7th **T24.409** Corrosion of unspecified degree of unspecified site of unspecified lower limb, except ankle and foot

+ **T24.41** **Corrosion of unspecified degree of thigh**
+7th **T24.411** Corrosion of unspecified degree of right thigh
+7th **T24.412** Corrosion of unspecified degree of left thigh
+7th **T24.419** Corrosion of unspecified degree of unspecified thigh

+ **T24.42** **Corrosion of unspecified degree of knee**
+7th **T24.421** Corrosion of unspecified degree of right knee
+7th **T24.422** Corrosion of unspecified degree of left knee
+7th **T24.429** Corrosion of unspecified degree of unspecified knee

+ **T24.43** **Corrosion of unspecified degree of lower leg**
+7th **T24.431** Corrosion of unspecified degree of right lower leg
+7th **T24.432** Corrosion of unspecified degree of left lower leg
+7th **T24.439** Corrosion of unspecified degree of unspecified lower leg

+ **T24.49** **Corrosion of unspecified degree of multiple sites of lower limb, except ankle and foot**
+7th **T24.491** Corrosion of unspecified degree of multiple sites of right lower limb, except ankle and foot
+7th **T24.492** Corrosion of unspecified degree of multiple sites of left lower limb, except ankle and foot
+7th **T24.499** Corrosion of unspecified degree of multiple sites of unspecified lower limb, except ankle and foot

+, +7th, X + 7th ● Newborn ● Pediatric ● Maternity ● Adult ♀ Female ♂ Male **Manifestation** **Unacceptable PDX** **HCC** **CC** **MCC** **HAC**

+ T24.5 Corrosion of first degree of lower limb, except ankle and foot

Code first (T51-T65) to identify chemical and intent

Use additional external cause code to identify place (Y92)

+ T24.50 Corrosion of first degree of unspecified site of lower limb, except ankle and foot

+7th **T24.501 Corrosion of first degree of unspecified site of right lower limb, except ankle and foot**

+7th **T24.502 Corrosion of first degree of unspecified site of left lower limb, except ankle and foot**

+7th **T24.509 Corrosion of first degree of unspecified site of unspecified lower limb, except ankle and foot**

+ T24.51 Corrosion of first degree of thigh

+7th **T24.511 Corrosion of first degree of right thigh**

+7th **T24.512 Corrosion of first degree of left thigh**

+7th **T24.519 Corrosion of first degree of unspecified thigh**

+ T24.52 Corrosion of first degree of knee

+7th **T24.521 Corrosion of first degree of right knee**

+7th **T24.522 Corrosion of first degree of left knee**

+7th **T24.529 Corrosion of first degree of unspecified knee**

+ T24.53 Corrosion of first degree of lower leg

+7th **T24.531 Corrosion of first degree of right lower leg**

+7th **T24.532 Corrosion of first degree of left lower leg**

+7th **T24.539 Corrosion of first degree of unspecified lower leg**

+ T24.59 Corrosion of first degree of multiple sites of lower limb, except ankle and foot

+7th **T24.591 Corrosion of first degree of multiple sites of right lower limb, except ankle and foot**

+7th **T24.592 Corrosion of first degree of multiple sites of left lower limb, except ankle and foot**

+7th **T24.599 Corrosion of first degree of multiple sites of unspecified lower limb, except ankle and foot**

+ T24.6 Corrosion of second degree of lower limb, except ankle and foot

Code first (T51-T65) to identify chemical and intent

Use additional external cause code to identify place (Y92)

+ T24.60 Corrosion of second degree of unspecified site of lower limb, except ankle and foot

+7th **T24.601 Corrosion of second degree of unspecified site of right lower limb, except ankle and foot**

+7th **T24.602 Corrosion of second degree of unspecified site of left lower limb, except ankle and foot**

+7th **T24.609 Corrosion of second degree of unspecified site of unspecified lower limb, except ankle and foot**

+ T24.61 Corrosion of second degree of thigh

+7th **T24.611 Corrosion of second degree of right thigh**

+7th **T24.612 Corrosion of second degree of left thigh**

+7th **T24.619 Corrosion of second degree of unspecified thigh**

+ T24.62 Corrosion of second degree of knee

+7th **T24.621 Corrosion of second degree of right knee**

+7th **T24.622 Corrosion of second degree of left knee**

+7th **T24.629 Corrosion of second degree of unspecified knee**

+ T24.63 Corrosion of second degree of lower leg

+7th **T24.631 Corrosion of second degree of right lower leg**

+7th **T24.632 Corrosion of second degree of left lower leg**

+7th **T24.639 Corrosion of second degree of unspecified lower leg**

+ T24.69 Corrosion of second degree of multiple sites of lower limb, except ankle and foot

+7th **T24.691 Corrosion of second degree of multiple sites of right lower limb, except ankle and foot**

+7th **T24.692 Corrosion of second degree of multiple sites of left lower limb, except ankle and foot**

+7th **T24.699 Corrosion of second degree of multiple sites of unspecified lower limb, except ankle and foot**

+ T24.7 Corrosion of third degree of lower limb, except ankle and foot

Code first (T51-T65) to identify chemical and intent

Use additional external cause code to identify place (Y92)

+ T24.70 Corrosion of third degree of unspecified site of lower limb, except ankle and foot

CC +7th **T24.701 Corrosion of third degree of unspecified site of right lower limb, except ankle and foot**

HAC 7th character A see Appendix B for HAC conditional logic

CC +7th **T24.702 Corrosion of third degree of unspecified site of left lower limb, except ankle and foot**

HAC 7th character A see Appendix B for HAC conditional logic

CC +7th **T24.709 Corrosion of third degree of unspecified site of unspecified lower limb, except ankle and foot**

HAC 7th character A see Appendix B for HAC conditional logic

+ T24.71 Corrosion of third degree of thigh

CC +7th **T24.711 Corrosion of third degree of right thigh**

HAC 7th character A see Appendix B for HAC conditional logic

CC +7th **T24.712 Corrosion of third degree of left thigh**

HAC 7th character A see Appendix B for HAC conditional logic

CC +7th **T24.719 Corrosion of third degree of unspecified thigh**

HAC 7th character A see Appendix B for HAC conditional logic

+ T24.72 Corrosion of third degree of knee

CC +7th **T24.721 Corrosion of third degree of right knee**

HAC 7th character A see Appendix B for HAC conditional logic

CC +7th **T24.722 Corrosion of third degree of left knee**

HAC 7th character A see Appendix B for HAC conditional logic

CC +7th **T24.729 Corrosion of third degree of unspecified knee**

HAC 7th character A see Appendix B for HAC conditional logic

+ T24.73 Corrosion of third degree of lower leg

CC +7th **T24.731 Corrosion of third degree of right lower leg**

HAC 7th character A see Appendix B for HAC conditional logic

CC +7th **T24.732 Corrosion of third degree of left lower leg**

HAC 7th character A see Appendix B for HAC conditional logic

CC +7th **T24.739 Corrosion of third degree of unspecified lower leg**

HAC 7th character A see Appendix B for HAC conditional logic

+ T24.79 Corrosion of third degree of multiple sites of lower limb, except ankle and foot

CC +7th **T24.791 Corrosion of third degree of multiple sites of right lower limb, except ankle and foot**

HAC 7th character A see Appendix B for HAC conditional logic

CC +7th **T24.792** **Corrosion of third degree of multiple sites of left lower limb, except ankle and foot**

> HAC 7th character A see Appendix B for HAC conditional logic

CC +7th **T24.799** **Corrosion of third degree of multiple sites of unspecified lower limb, except ankle and foot**

> HAC 7th character A see Appendix B for HAC conditional logic

T25 **Burn and corrosion of ankle and foot**

> The appropriate 7th character is to be added to each code from category T25
> A   initial encounter
> D   subsequent encounter
> S   sequela

+ **T25.0** **Burn of unspecified degree of ankle and foot**

Use additional external cause code to identify the source, place and intent of the burn (X00-X19, X75-X77, X96-X98, Y92)

+ **T25.01** **Burn of unspecified degree of ankle**
  +7th **T25.011** **Burn of unspecified degree of right ankle**
  +7th **T25.012** **Burn of unspecified degree of left ankle**
  +7th **T25.019** **Burn of unspecified degree of unspecified ankle**

+ **T25.02** **Burn of unspecified degree of foot**
  Excludes2: *burn of unspecified degree of toe(s) (nail) (T25.03-)*
  +7th **T25.021** **Burn of unspecified degree of right foot**
  +7th **T25.022** **Burn of unspecified degree of left foot**
  +7th **T25.029** **Burn of unspecified degree of unspecified foot**

+ **T25.03** **Burn of unspecified degree of toe(s) (nail)**
  +7th **T25.031** **Burn of unspecified degree of right toe(s) (nail)**
  +7th **T25.032** **Burn of unspecified degree of left toe(s) (nail)**
  +7th **T25.039** **Burn of unspecified degree of unspecified toe(s) (nail)**

+ **T25.09** **Burn of unspecified degree of multiple sites of ankle and foot**
  +7th **T25.091** **Burn of unspecified degree of multiple sites of right ankle and foot**
  +7th **T25.092** **Burn of unspecified degree of multiple sites of left ankle and foot**
  +7th **T25.099** **Burn of unspecified degree of multiple sites of unspecified ankle and foot**

+ **T25.1** **Burn of first degree of ankle and foot**

Use additional external cause code to identify the source, place and intent of the burn (X00-X19, X75-X77, X96-X98, Y92)

+ **T25.11** **Burn of first degree of ankle**
  +7th **T25.111** **Burn of first degree of right ankle**
  +7th **T25.112** **Burn of first degree of left ankle**
  +7th **T25.119** **Burn of first degree of unspecified ankle**

+ **T25.12** **Burn of first degree of foot**
  Excludes2: *burn of first degree of toe(s) (nail) (T25.13-)*
  +7th **T25.121** **Burn of first degree of right foot**
  +7th **T25.122** **Burn of first degree of left foot**
  +7th **T25.129** **Burn of first degree of unspecified foot**

+ **T25.13** **Burn of first degree of toe(s) (nail)**
  +7th **T25.131** **Burn of first degree of right toe(s) (nail)**
  +7th **T25.132** **Burn of first degree of left toe(s) (nail)**
  +7th **T25.139** **Burn of first degree of unspecified toe(s) (nail)**

+ **T25.19** **Burn of first degree of multiple sites of ankle and foot**
  +7th **T25.191** **Burn of first degree of multiple sites of right ankle and foot**
  +7th **T25.192** **Burn of first degree of multiple sites of left ankle and foot**
  +7th **T25.199** **Burn of first degree of multiple sites of unspecified ankle and foot**

+ **T25.2** **Burn of second degree of ankle and foot**

Use additional external cause code to identify the source, place and intent of the burn (X00-X19, X75-X77, X96-X98, Y92)

+ **T25.21** **Burn of second degree of ankle**
  +7th **T25.211** **Burn of second degree of right ankle**
  +7th **T25.212** **Burn of second degree of left ankle**
  +7th **T25.219** **Burn of second degree of unspecified ankle**

+ **T25.22** **Burn of second degree of foot**
  Excludes2: *burn of second degree of toe(s) (nail) (T25.23-)*
  +7th **T25.221** **Burn of second degree of right foot**
  +7th **T25.222** **Burn of second degree of left foot**
  +7th **T25.229** **Burn of second degree of unspecified foot**

+ **T25.23** **Burn of second degree of toe(s) (nail)**
  +7th **T25.231** **Burn of second degree of right toe(s) (nail)**
  +7th **T25.232** **Burn of second degree of left toe(s) (nail)**
  +7th **T25.239** **Burn of second degree of unspecified toe(s) (nail)**

+ **T25.29** **Burn of second degree of multiple sites of ankle and foot**
  +7th **T25.291** **Burn of second degree of multiple sites of right ankle and foot**
  +7th **T25.292** **Burn of second degree of multiple sites of left ankle and foot**
  +7th **T25.299** **Burn of second degree of multiple sites of unspecified ankle and foot**

+ **T25.3** **Burn of third degree of ankle and foot**

Use external cause code to identify the source, place and intent of the burn (X00-X19, X75-X77, X96-X98, Y92)

+ **T25.31** **Burn of third degree of ankle**
  CC +7th **T25.311** **Burn of third degree of right ankle**
  > HAC 7th character A see Appendix B for HAC conditional logic
  CC +7th **T25.312** **Burn of third degree of left ankle**
  > HAC 7th character A see·Appendix B for HAC conditional logic
  CC +7th **T25.319** **Burn of third degree of unspecified ankle**
  > HAC 7th character A see Appendix B for HAC conditional logic

+ **T25.32** **Burn of third degree of foot**
  Excludes2: *burn of third degree of toe(s) (nail) (T25.33-)*
  CC +7th **T25.321** **Burn of third degree of right foot**
  > HAC 7th character A see Appendix B for HAC conditional logic
  CC +7th **T25.322** **Burn of third degree of left foot**
  > HAC 7th character A see Appendix B for HAC conditional logic
  CC +7th **T25.329** **Burn of third degree of unspecified foot**
  > HAC 7th character A see Appendix B for HAC conditional logic

+ **T25.33** **Burn of third degree of toe(s) (nail)**
  CC +7th **T25.331** **Burn of third degree of right toe(s) (nail)**
  > HAC 7th character A see Appendix B for HAC conditional logic
  CC +7th **T25.332** **Burn of third degree of left toe(s) (nail)**
  > HAC 7th character A see Appendix B for HAC conditional logic
  CC +7th **T25.339** **Burn of third degree of unspecified toe(s) (nail)**
  > HAC 7th character A see Appendix B for HAC conditional logic

+ **T25.39** **Burn of third degree of multiple sites of ankle and foot**
  CC +7th **T25.391** **Burn of third degree of multiple sites of right ankle and foot**
  > HAC 7th character A see Appendix B for HAC conditional logic
  CC +7th **T25.392** **Burn of third degree of multiple sites of left ankle and foot**
  > HAC 7th character A see Appendix B for HAC conditional logic

+, +7th, X + 7th   ● Newborn   ● Pediatric   ● Maternity   ● Adult   ♀ Female   ♂ Male   Manifestation   Unacceptable PDX   HCC   CC   MCC   HAC

CC +7th **T25.399** **Burn of third degree of multiple sites of unspecified ankle and foot**
> **HAC** 7th character A see Appendix B for HAC conditional logic

+ **T25.4** **Corrosion of unspecified of ankle and foot**
> Code first (T51-T65) to identify chemical and intent
>
> Use additional external cause code to identify place (Y92)

  + **T25.41** **Corrosion of unspecified degree of ankle**
    +7th **T25.411** **Corrosion of unspecified degree of right ankle**
    +7th **T25.412** **Corrosion of unspecified degree of left ankle**
    +7th **T25.419** **Corrosion of unspecified degree of unspecified ankle**

  + **T25.42** **Corrosion of unspecified degree of foot**
> **Excludes2:** *corrosion of unspecified degree of toe(s) (nail) (T25.43-)*

    +7th **T25.421** **Corrosion of unspecified degree of right foot**
    +7th **T25.422** **Corrosion of unspecified degree of left foot**
    +7th **T25.429** **Corrosion of unspecified degree of unspecified foot**

  + **T25.43** **Corrosion of unspecified degree of toe(s) (nail)**
    +7th **T25.431** **Corrosion of unspecified degree of right toe(s) (nail)**
    +7th **T25.432** **Corrosion of unspecified degree of left toe(s) (nail)**
    +7th **T25.439** **Corrosion of unspecified degree of unspecified toe(s) (nail)**

  + **T25.49** **Corrosion of unspecified degree of multiple sites of ankle and foot**
    +7th **T25.491** **Corrosion of unspecified degree of multiple sites of right ankle and foot**
    +7th **T25.492** **Corrosion of unspecified degree of multiple sites of left ankle and foot**
    +7th **T25.499** **Corrosion of unspecified degree of multiple sites of unspecified ankle and foot**

+ **T25.5** **Corrosion of first degree of ankle and foot**
> Code first (T51-T65) to identify chemical and intent
>
> Use additional external cause code to identify place (Y92)

  + **T25.51** **Corrosion of first degree of ankle**
    +7th **T25.511** **Corrosion of first degree of right ankle**
    +7th **T25.512** **Corrosion of first degree of left ankle**
    +7th **T25.519** **Corrosion of first degree of unspecified ankle**

  + **T25.52** **Corrosion of first degree of foot**
> **Excludes2:** *corrosion of first degree of toe(s) (nail) (T25.53-)*

    +7th **T25.521** **Corrosion of first degree of right foot**
    +7th **T25.522** **Corrosion of first degree of left foot**
    +7th **T25.529** **Corrosion of first degree of unspecified foot**

  + **T25.53** **Corrosion of first degree of toe(s) (nail)**
    +7th **T25.531** **Corrosion of first degree of right toe(s) (nail)**
    +7th **T25.532** **Corrosion of first degree of left toe(s) (nail)**
    +7th **T25.539** **Corrosion of first degree of unspecified toe(s) (nail)**

  + **T25.59** **Corrosion of first degree of multiple sites of ankle and foot**
    +7th **T25.591** **Corrosion of first degree of multiple sites of right ankle and foot**
    +7th **T25.592** **Corrosion of first degree of multiple sites of left ankle and foot**
    +7th **T25.599** **Corrosion of first degree of multiple sites of unspecified ankle and foot**

+ **T25.6** **Corrosion of second degree of ankle and foot**
> Code first (T51-T65) to identify chemical and intent
>
> Use additional external cause code to identify place (Y92)

  + **T25.61** **Corrosion of second degree of ankle**
    +7th **T25.611** **Corrosion of second degree of right ankle**
    +7th **T25.612** **Corrosion of second degree of left ankle**
    +7th **T25.619** **Corrosion of second degree of unspecified ankle**

+ **T25.62** **Corrosion of second degree of foot**
> **Excludes2:** *corrosion of second degree of toe(s) (nail) (T25.63-)*

    +7th **T25.621** **Corrosion of second degree of right foot**
    +7th **T25.622** **Corrosion of second degree of left foot**
    +7th **T25.629** **Corrosion of second degree of unspecified foot**

+ **T25.63** **Corrosion of second degree of toe(s) (nail)**
    +7th **T25.631** **Corrosion of second degree of right toe(s) (nail)**
    +7th **T25.632** **Corrosion of second degree of left toe(s) (nail)**
    +7th **T25.639** **Corrosion of second degree of unspecified toe(s) (nail)**

+ **T25.69** **Corrosion of second degree of multiple sites of ankle and foot**
    +7th **T25.691** **Corrosion of second degree of right ankle and foot**
    +7th **T25.692** **Corrosion of second degree of left ankle and foot**
    +7th **T25.699** **Corrosion of second degree of unspecified ankle and foot**

+ **T25.7** **Corrosion of third degree of ankle and foot**
> Code first (T51-T65) to identify chemical and intent
>
> Use additional external cause code to identify place (Y92)

  + **T25.71** **Corrosion of third degree of ankle**
  CC +7th **T25.711** **Corrosion of third degree of right ankle**
> **HAC** 7th character A see Appendix B for HAC conditional logic

  CC +7th **T25.712** **Corrosion of third degree of left ankle**
> **HAC** 7th character A see Appendix B for HAC conditional logic

  CC +7th **T25.719** **Corrosion of third degree of unspecified ankle**
> **HAC** 7th character A see Appendix B for HAC conditional logic

+ **T25.72** **Corrosion of third degree of foot**
> **Excludes2:** *corrosion of third degree of toe(s) (nail) (T25.73-)*

  CC +7th **T25.721** **Corrosion of third degree of right foot**
> **HAC** 7th character A see Appendix B for HAC conditional logic

  CC +7th **T25.722** **Corrosion of third degree of left foot**
> **HAC** 7th character A see Appendix B for HAC conditional logic

  CC +7th **T25.729** **Corrosion of third degree of unspecified foot**
> **HAC** 7th character A see Appendix B for HAC conditional logic

+ **T25.73** **Corrosion of third degree of toe(s) (nail)**
  CC +7th **T25.731** **Corrosion of third degree of right toe(s) (nail)**
> **HAC** 7th character A see Appendix B for HAC conditional logic

  CC +7th **T25.732** **Corrosion of third degree of left toe(s) (nail)**
> **HAC** 7th character A see Appendix B for HAC conditional logic

  CC +7th **T25.739** **Corrosion of third degree of unspecified toe(s) (nail)**
> **HAC** 7th character A see Appendix B for HAC conditional logic

+ **T25.79** **Corrosion of third degree of multiple sites of ankle and foot**
  CC +7th **T25.791** **Corrosion of third degree of multiple sites of right ankle and foot**
> **HAC** 7th character A see Appendix B for HAC conditional logic

  CC +7th **T25.792** **Corrosion of third degree of multiple sites of left ankle and foot**
> **HAC** 7th character A see Appendix B for HAC conditional logic

  CC +7th **T25.799** **Corrosion of third degree of multiple sites of unspecified ankle and foot**
> **HAC** 7th character A see Appendix B for HAC conditional logic

Burns and corrosions confined to eye and internal organs (T26-T28)

Review coding guideline C.19.d

T26 Burn and corrosion confined to eye and adnexa

> The appropriate 7th character is to be added to each code from category T26
> A initial encounter
> D subsequent encounter
> S sequela

+ **T26.0 Burn of eyelid and periocular area**

> Use additional external cause code to identify the source, place and intent of the burn (X00-X19, X75-X77, X96-X98, Y92)

X+7th **T26.00 Burn of unspecified eyelid and periocular area**
X+7th **T26.01 Burn of right eyelid and periocular area**
X+7th **T26.02 Burn of left eyelid and periocular area**

+ **T26.1 Burn of cornea and conjunctival sac**

> Use additional external cause code to identify the source, place and intent of the burn (X00-X19, X75-X77, X96-X98, Y92)

X+7th **T26.10 Burn of cornea and conjunctival sac, unspecified eye**
X+7th **T26.11 Burn of cornea and conjunctival sac, right eye**
X+7th **T26.12 Burn of cornea and conjunctival sac, left eye**

+ **T26.2 Burn with resulting rupture and destruction of eyeball**

> Use additional external cause code to identify the source, place and intent of the burn (X00-X19, X75-X77, X96-X98, Y92)

CC X+7th **T26.20 Burn with resulting rupture and destruction of unspecified eyeball**
> **HAC** 7th character A see Appendix B for HAC conditional logic

CC X+7th **T26.21 Burn with resulting rupture and destruction of right eyeball**
> **HAC** 7th character A see Appendix B for HAC conditional logic

CC X+7th **T26.22 Burn with resulting rupture and destruction of left eyeball**
> **HAC** 7th character A see Appendix B for HAC conditional logic

+ **T26.3 Burns of other specified parts of eye and adnexa**

> Use additional external cause code to identify the source, place and intent of the burn (X00-X19, X75-X77, X96-X98, Y92)

X+7th **T26.30 Burns of other specified parts of unspecified eye and adnexa**
X+7th **T26.31 Burns of other specified parts of right eye and adnexa**
X+7th **T26.32 Burns of other specified parts of left eye and adnexa**

+ **T26.4 Burn of eye and adnexa, part unspecified**

> Use additional external cause code to identify the source, place and intent of the burn (X00-X19, X75-X77, X96-X98, Y92)

X+7th **T26.40 Burn of unspecified eye and adnexa, part unspecified**
X+7th **T26.41 Burn of right eye and adnexa, part unspecified**
X+7th **T26.42 Burn of left eye and adnexa, part unspecified**

+ **T26.5 Corrosion of eyelid and periocular area**

> Code first (T51-T65) to identify chemical and intent
>
> Use additional external cause code to identify place (Y92)

X+7th **T26.50 Corrosion of unspecified eyelid and periocular area**
X+7th **T26.51 Corrosion of right eyelid and periocular area**
X+7th **T26.52 Corrosion of left eyelid and periocular area**

+ **T26.6 Corrosion of cornea and conjunctival sac**

> Code first (T51-T65) to identify chemical and intent
>
> Use additional external cause code to identify place (Y92)

X+7th **T26.60 Corrosion of cornea and conjunctival sac, unspecified eye**
X+7th **T26.61 Corrosion of cornea and conjunctival sac, right eye**
X+7th **T26.62 Corrosion of cornea and conjunctival sac, left eye**

+ **T26.7 Corrosion with resulting rupture and destruction of eyeball**

> Code first (T51-T65) to identify chemical and intent
>
> Use additional external cause code to identify place (Y92)

CC X+7th **T26.70 Corrosion with resulting rupture and destruction of unspecified eyeball**
> **HAC** 7th character A see Appendix B for HAC conditional logic

CC X+7th **T26.71 Corrosion with resulting rupture and destruction of right eyeball**
> **HAC** 7th character A see Appendix B for HAC conditional logic

CC X+7th **T26.72 Corrosion with resulting rupture and destruction of left eyeball**
> **HAC** 7th character A see Appendix B for HAC conditional logic

+ **T26.8 Corrosions of other specified parts of eye and adnexa**

> Code first (T51-T65) to identify chemical and intent
>
> Use additional external cause code to identify place (Y92)

X+7th **T26.80 Corrosions of other specified parts of unspecified eye and adnexa**
X+7th **T26.81 Corrosions of other specified parts of right eye and adnexa**
X+7th **T26.82 Corrosions of other specified parts of left eye and adnexa**

+ **T26.9 Corrosion of eye and adnexa, part unspecified**

> Code first (T51-T65) to identify chemical and intent
>
> Use additional external cause code to identify place (Y92)

X+7th **T26.90 Corrosion of unspecified eye and adnexa, part unspecified**
X+7th **T26.91 Corrosion of right eye and adnexa, part unspecified**
X+7th **T26.92 Corrosion of left eye and adnexa, part unspecified**

T27 Burn and corrosion of respiratory tract

> Use additional external cause code to identify the source and intent of the burn (X00-X19, X75-X77, X96-X98)
>
> Use external cause code to identify place (Y92)

> The appropriate 7th character is to be added to each code from category T27
> A initial encounter
> D subsequent encounter
> S sequela

CC X+7th **T27.0 Burn of larynx and trachea**
> **HAC** 7th character A see Appendix B for HAC conditional logic

CC X+7th **T27.1 Burn involving larynx and trachea with lung**
> **HAC** 7th character A see Appendix B for HAC conditional logic

CC X+7th **T27.2 Burn of other parts of respiratory tract**
> Burn of thoracic cavity
> **HAC** 7th character A see Appendix B for HAC conditional logic

CC X+7th **T27.3 Burn of respiratory tract, part unspecified**
> **HAC** 7th character A see Appendix B for HAC conditional logic

CC X+7th **T27.4 Corrosion of larynx and trachea**
> Code first (T51-T65) to identify chemical and intent
> **HAC** 7th character A see Appendix B for HAC conditional logic

CC X+7th **T27.5 Corrosion involving larynx and trachea with lung**
> Code first (T51-T65) to identify chemical and intent
> **HAC** 7th character A see Appendix B for HAC conditional logic

CC X+7th **T27.6 Corrosion of other parts of respiratory tract**
> Code first (T51-T65) to identify chemical and intent
> **HAC** 7th character A see Appendix B for HAC conditional logic

CC X+7th **T27.7 Corrosion of respiratory tract, part unspecified**
> Code first (T51-T65) to identify chemical and intent
> **HAC** 7th character A see Appendix B for HAC conditional logic

T28 Burn and corrosion of other internal organs

> Use additional external cause code to identify the source and intent of the burn (X00-X19, X75-X77, X96-X98)
>
> Use external cause code to identify place (Y92)

> The appropriate 7th character is to be added to each code from category T28
> A initial encounter
> D subsequent encounter
> S sequela

X+7th **T28.0 Burn of mouth and pharynx**
CC X+7th **T28.1 Burn of esophagus**
> **HAC** 7th character A see Appendix B for HAC conditional logic

CC X+7th **T28.2 Burn of other parts of alimentary tract**
> **HAC** 7th character A see Appendix B for HAC conditional logic

X+7th **T28.3** **Burn of internal genitourinary organs**
+ **T28.4** **Burns of other and unspecified internal organs**
X+7th **T28.40** **Burn of unspecified internal organ**
+ **T28.41** **Burn of ear drum**
+7th **T28.411** **Burn of right ear drum**
+7th **T28.412** **Burn of left ear drum**
+7th **T28.419** **Burn of unspecified ear drum**
X+7th **T28.49** **Burn of other internal organ**
X+7th **T28.5** **Corrosion of mouth and pharynx**
Code first (T51-T65) to identify chemical and intent
CC X+7th **T28.6** **Corrosion of esophagus**
Code first (T51-T65) to identify chemical and intent
HAC 7th character A see Appendix B for HAC conditional logic
CC X+7th **T28.7** **Corrosion of other parts of alimentary tract**
Code first (T51-T65) to identify chemical and intent
HAC 7th character A see Appendix B for HAC conditional logic
X+7th **T28.8** **Corrosion of internal genitourinary organs**
Code first (T51-T65) to identify chemical and intent
+ **T28.9** **Corrosions of other and unspecified internal organs**
Code first (T51-T65) to identify chemical and intent
X+7th **T28.90** **Corrosions of unspecified internal organs**
+ **T28.91** **Corrosions of ear drum**
+7th **T28.911** **Corrosions of right ear drum**
+7th **T28.912** **Corrosions of left ear drum**
+7th **T28.919** **Corrosions of unspecified ear drum**
X+7th **T28.99** **Corrosions of other internal organs**

Burns and corrosions of multiple and unspecified body regions (T30-T32)

T30 **Burn and corrosion, body region unspecified**
Review coding guideline C.19.d.5
T30.0 **Burn of unspecified body region, unspecified degree**
This code is not for inpatient use. Code to specified site and degree of burns
Burn NOS
Multiple burns NOS
T30.4 **Corrosion of unspecified body region, unspecified degree**
This code is not for inpatient use. Code to specified site and degree of corrosion
Corrosion NOS
Multiple corrosion NOS

T31 **Burns classified according to extent of body surface involved**

NOTE This category is to be used as the primary code only when the site of the burn is unspecified. It should be used as a supplementary code with categories T20-T25 when the site is specified.
Review coding guideline C.19.d.6
T31.0 **Burns involving less than 10% of body surface**
+ **T31.1** **Burns involving 10-19% of body surface**
CC **T31.10** **Burns involving 10-19% of body surface with 0% to 9% third degree burns**
Burns involving 10-19% of body surface NOS
HAC see Appendix B for HAC conditional logic
CC **T31.11** **Burns involving 10-19% of body surface with 10-19% third degree burns**
HAC see Appendix B for HAC conditional logic
+ **T31.2** **Burns involving 20-29% of body surface**
CC **T31.20** **Burns involving 20-29% of body surface with 0% to 9% third degree burns**
Burns involving 20-29% of body surface NOS
HAC see Appendix B for HAC conditional logic
MCC **T31.21** **Burns involving 20-29% of body surface with 10-19% third degree burns**
HAC see Appendix B for HAC conditional logic
MCC **T31.22** **Burns involving 20-29% of body surface with 20-29% third degree burns**
HAC see Appendix B for HAC conditional logic
+ **T31.3** **Burns involving 30-39% of body surface**
CC **T31.30** **Burns involving 30-39% of body surface with 0% to 9% third degree burns**
Burns involving 30-39% of body surface NOS
HAC see Appendix B for HAC conditional logic
MCC **T31.31** **Burns involving 30-39% of body surface with 10-19% third degree burns**
HAC see Appendix B for HAC conditional logic

MCC **T31.32** **Burns involving 30-39% of body surface with 20-29% third degree burns**
HAC see Appendix B for HAC conditional logic
MCC **T31.33** **Burns involving 30-39% of body surface with 30-39% third degree burns**
HAC see Appendix B for HAC conditional logic
+ **T31.4** **Burns involving 40-49% of body surface**
CC **T31.40** **Burns involving 40-49% of body surface with 0% to 9% third degree burns**
Burns involving 40-49% of body surface NOS
HAC see Appendix B for HAC conditional logic
MCC **T31.41** **Burns involving 40-49% of body surface with 10-19% third degree burns**
HAC see Appendix B for HAC conditional logic
MCC **T31.42** **Burns involving 40-49% of body surface with 20-29% third degree burns**
HAC see Appendix B for HAC conditional logic
MCC **T31.43** **Burns involving 40-49% of body surface with 30-39% third degree burns**
HAC see Appendix B for HAC conditional logic
MCC **T31.44** **Burns involving 40-49% of body surface with 40-49% third degree burns**
HAC see Appendix B for HAC conditional logic
+ **T31.5** **Burns involving 50-59% of body surface**
CC **T31.50** **Burns involving 50-59% of body surface with 0% to 9% third degree burns**
Burns involving 50-59% of body surface NOS
HAC see Appendix B for HAC conditional logic
MCC **T31.51** **Burns involving 50-59% of body surface with 10-19% third degree burns**
HAC see Appendix B for HAC conditional logic
MCC **T31.52** **Burns involving 50-59% of body surface with 20-29% third degree burns**
HAC see Appendix B for HAC conditional logic
MCC **T31.53** **Burns involving 50-59% of body surface with 30-39% third degree burns**
HAC see Appendix B for HAC conditional logic
MCC **T31.54** **Burns involving 50-59% of body surface with 40-49% third degree burns**
HAC see Appendix B for HAC conditional logic
MCC **T31.55** **Burns involving 50-59% of body surface with 50-59% third degree burns**
HAC see Appendix B for HAC conditional logic
+ **T31.6** **Burns involving 60-69% of body surface**
CC **T31.60** **Burns involving 60-69% of body surface with 0% to 9% third degree burns**
Burns involving 60-69% of body surface NOS
HAC see Appendix B for HAC conditional logic
MCC **T31.61** **Burns involving 60-69% of body surface with 10-19% third degree burns**
HAC see Appendix B for HAC conditional logic
MCC **T31.62** **Burns involving 60-69% of body surface with 20-29% third degree burns**
HAC see Appendix B for HAC conditional logic
MCC **T31.63** **Burns involving 60-69% of body surface with 30-39% third degree burns**
HAC see Appendix B for HAC conditional logic
MCC **T31.64** **Burns involving 60-69% of body surface with 40-49% third degree burns**
HAC see Appendix B for HAC conditional logic
MCC **T31.65** **Burns involving 60-69% of body surface with 50-59% third degree burns**
HAC see Appendix B for HAC conditional logic
MCC **T31.66** **Burns involving 60-69% of body surface with 60-69% third degree burns**
HAC see Appendix B for HAC conditional logic
+ **T31.7** **Burns involving 70-79% of body surface**
CC **T31.70** **Burns involving 70-79% of body surface with 0% to 9% third degree burns**
Burns involving 70-79% of body surface NOS
HAC see Appendix B for HAC conditional logic
MCC **T31.71** **Burns involving 70-79% of body surface with 10-19% third degree burns**
HAC see Appendix B for HAC conditional logic
MCC **T31.72** **Burns involving 70-79% of body surface with 20-29% third degree burns**
HAC see Appendix B for HAC conditional logic

+, +7th, X + 7th   ● Newborn   ● Pediatric   ● Maternity   ● Adult   ♀ Female   ♂ Male   Manifestation   Unacceptable PDX   HCC   CC   MCC   HAC

MCC **T31.73** **Burns involving 70-79% of body surface with 30-39% third degree burns**
> HAC see Appendix B for HAC conditional logic

MCC **T31.74** **Burns involving 70-79% of body surface with 40-49% third degree burns**
> HAC see Appendix B for HAC conditional logic

MCC **T31.75** **Burns involving 70-79% of body surface with 50-59% third degree burns**
> HAC see Appendix B for HAC conditional logic

MCC **T31.76** **Burns involving 70-79% of body surface with 60-69% third degree burns**
> HAC see Appendix B for HAC conditional logic

MCC **T31.77** **Burns involving 70-79% of body surface with 70-79% third degree burns**
> HAC see Appendix B for HAC conditional logic

+ **T31.8** **Burns involving 80-89% of body surface**

CC **T31.80** **Burns involving 80-89% of body surface with 0% to 9% third degree burns**
> Burns involving 80-89% of body surface NOS
> HAC see Appendix B for HAC conditional logic

MCC **T31.81** **Burns involving 80-89% of body surface with 10-19% third degree burns**
> HAC see Appendix B for HAC conditional logic

MCC **T31.82** **Burns involving 80-89% of body surface with 20-29% third degree burns**
> HAC see Appendix B for HAC conditional logic

MCC **T31.83** **Burns involving 80-89% of body surface with 30-39% third degree burns**
> HAC see Appendix B for HAC conditional logic

MCC **T31.84** **Burns involving 80-89% of body surface with 40-49% third degree burns**
> HAC see Appendix B for HAC conditional logic

MCC **T31.85** **Burns involving 80-89% of body surface with 50-59% third degree burns**
> HAC see Appendix B for HAC conditional logic

MCC **T31.86** **Burns involving 80-89% of body surface with 60-69% third degree burns**
> HAC see Appendix B for HAC conditional logic

MCC **T31.87** **Burns involving 80-89% of body surface with 70-79% third degree burns**
> HAC see Appendix B for HAC conditional logic

MCC **T31.88** **Burns involving 80-89% of body surface with 80-89% third degree burns**
> HAC see Appendix B for HAC conditional logic

+ **T31.9** **Burns involving 90% or more of body surface**

CC **T31.90** **Burns involving 90% or more of body surface with 0% to 9% third degree burns**
> Burns involving 90% or more of body surface NOS
> HAC see Appendix B for HAC conditional logic

MCC **T31.91** **Burns involving 90% or more of body surface with 10-19% third degree burns**
> HAC see Appendix B for HAC conditional logic

MCC **T31.92** **Burns involving 90% or more of body surface with 20-29% third degree burns**
> HAC see Appendix B for HAC conditional logic

MCC **T31.93** **Burns involving 90% or more of body surface with 30-39% third degree burns**
> HAC see Appendix B for HAC conditional logic

MCC **T31.94** **Burns involving 90% or more of body surface with 40-49% third degree burns**
> HAC see Appendix B for HAC conditional logic

MCC **T31.95** **Burns involving 90% or more of body surface with 50-59% third degree burns**
> HAC see Appendix B for HAC conditional logic

MCC **T31.96** **Burns involving 90% or more of body surface with 60-69% third degree burns**
> HAC see Appendix B for HAC conditional logic

MCC **T31.97** **Burns involving 90% or more of body surface with 70-79% third degree burns**
> HAC see Appendix B for HAC conditional logic

MCC **T31.98** **Burns involving 90% or more of body surface with 80-89% third degree burns**
> HAC see Appendix B for HAC conditional logic

MCC **T31.99** **Burns involving 90% or more of body surface with 90% or more third degree burns**
> HAC see Appendix B for HAC conditional logic

T32 **Corrosions classified according to extent of body surface involved**

> **NOTE** This category is to be used as the primary code only when the site of the corrosion is unspecified. It may be used as a supplementary code with categories T20-T25 when the site is specified.
> Review coding guideline C.19.d.6

T32.0 **Corrosions involving less than 10% of body surface**

+ **T32.1** **Corrosions involving 10-19% of body surface**

CC **T32.10** **Corrosions involving 10-19% of body surface with 0% to 9% third degree corrosion**
> Corrosions involving 10-19% of body surface NOS
> HAC see Appendix B for HAC conditional logic

CC **T32.11** **Corrosions involving 10-19% of body surface with 10-19% third degree corrosion**
> HAC see Appendix B for HAC conditional logic

+ **T32.2** **Corrosions involving 20-29% of body surface**

CC **T32.20** **Corrosions involving 20-29% of body surface with 0% to 9% third degree corrosion**
> HAC see Appendix B for HAC conditional logic

MCC **T32.21** **Corrosions involving 20-29% of body surface with 10-19% third degree corrosion**
> HAC see Appendix B for HAC conditional logic

MCC **T32.22** **Corrosions involving 20-29% of body surface with 20-29% third degree corrosion**
> HAC see Appendix B for HAC conditional logic

+ **T32.3** **Corrosions involving 30-39% of body surface**

CC **T32.30** **Corrosions involving 30-39% of body surface with 0% to 9% third degree corrosion**
> HAC see Appendix B for HAC conditional logic

MCC **T32.31** **Corrosions involving 30-39% of body surface with 10-19% third degree corrosion**
> HAC see Appendix B for HAC conditional logic

MCC **T32.32** **Corrosions involving 30-39% of body surface with 20-29% third degree corrosion**
> HAC see Appendix B for HAC conditional logic

MCC **T32.33** **Corrosions involving 30-39% of body surface with 30-39% third degree corrosion**
> HAC see Appendix B for HAC conditional logic

+ **T32.4** **Corrosions involving 40-49% of body surface**

CC **T32.40** **Corrosions involving 40-49% of body surface with 0% to 9% third degree corrosion**
> HAC see Appendix B for HAC conditional logic

MCC **T32.41** **Corrosions involving 40-49% of body surface with 10-19% third degree corrosion**
> HAC see Appendix B for HAC conditional logic

MCC **T32.42** **Corrosions involving 40-49% of body surface with 20-29% third degree corrosion**
> HAC see Appendix B for HAC conditional logic

MCC **T32.43** **Corrosions involving 40-49% of body surface with 30-39% third degree corrosion**
> HAC see Appendix B for HAC conditional logic

MCC **T32.44** **Corrosions involving 40-49% of body surface with 40-49% third degree corrosion**
> HAC see Appendix B for HAC conditional logic

+ **T32.5** **Corrosions involving 50-59% of body surface**

CC **T32.50** **Corrosions involving 50-59% of body surface with 0% to 9% third degree corrosion**
> HAC see Appendix B for HAC conditional logic

MCC **T32.51** **Corrosions involving 50-59% of body surface with 10-19% third degree corrosion**
> HAC see Appendix B for HAC conditional logic

MCC **T32.52** **Corrosions involving 50-59% of body surface with 20-29% third degree corrosion**
> HAC see Appendix B for HAC conditional logic

MCC **T32.53** **Corrosions involving 50-59% of body surface with 30-39% third degree corrosion**
> HAC see Appendix B for HAC conditional logic

MCC **T32.54** **Corrosions involving 50-59% of body surface with 40-49% third degree corrosion**
> HAC see Appendix B for HAC conditional logic

MCC **T32.55** **Corrosions involving 50-59% of body surface with 50-59% third degree corrosion**
> HAC see Appendix B for HAC conditional logic

+ **T32.6** Corrosions involving 60-69% of body surface

　　CC **T32.60** Corrosions involving 60-69% of body surface with 0% to 9% third degree corrosion
　　　　HAC see Appendix B for HAC conditional logic

　　MCC **T32.61** Corrosions involving 60-69% of body surface with 10-19% third degree corrosion
　　　　HAC see Appendix B for HAC conditional logic

　　MCC **T32.62** Corrosions involving 60-69% of body surface with 20-29% third degree corrosion
　　　　HAC see Appendix B for HAC conditional logic

　　MCC **T32.63** Corrosions involving 60-69% of body surface with 30-39% third degree corrosion
　　　　HAC see Appendix B for HAC conditional logic

　　MCC **T32.64** Corrosions involving 60-69% of body surface with 40-49% third degree corrosion
　　　　HAC see Appendix B for HAC conditional logic

　　MCC **T32.65** Corrosions involving 60-69% of body surface with 50-59% third degree corrosion
　　　　HAC see Appendix B for HAC conditional logic

　　MCC **T32.66** Corrosions involving 60-69% of body surface with 60-69% third degree corrosion
　　　　HAC see Appendix B for HAC conditional logic

+ **T32.7** Corrosions involving 70-79% of body surface

　　CC **T32.70** Corrosions involving 70-79% of body surface with 0% to 9% third degree corrosion
　　　　HAC see Appendix B for HAC conditional logic

　　MCC **T32.71** Corrosions involving 70-79% of body surface with 10-19% third degree corrosion
　　　　HAC see Appendix B for HAC conditional logic

　　MCC **T32.72** Corrosions involving 70-79% of body surface with 20-29% third degree corrosion
　　　　HAC see Appendix B for HAC conditional logic

　　MCC **T32.73** Corrosions involving 70-79% of body surface with 30-39% third degree corrosion
　　　　HAC see Appendix B for HAC conditional logic

　　MCC **T32.74** Corrosions involving 70-79% of body surface with 40-49% third degree corrosion
　　　　HAC see Appendix B for HAC conditional logic

　　MCC **T32.75** Corrosions involving 70-79% of body surface with 50-59% third degree corrosion
　　　　HAC see Appendix B for HAC conditional logic

　　MCC **T32.76** Corrosions involving 70-79% of body surface with 60-69% third degree corrosion
　　　　HAC see Appendix B for HAC conditional logic

　　MCC **T32.77** Corrosions involving 70-79% of body surface with 70-79% third degree corrosion
　　　　HAC see Appendix B for HAC conditional logic

+ **T32.8** Corrosions involving 80-89% of body surface

　　CC **T32.80** Corrosions involving 80-89% of body surface with 0% to 9% third degree corrosion
　　　　HAC see Appendix B for HAC conditional logic

　　MCC **T32.81** Corrosions involving 80-89% of body surface with 10-19% third degree corrosion
　　　　HAC see Appendix B for HAC conditional logic

　　MCC **T32.82** Corrosions involving 80-89% of body surface with 20-29% third degree corrosion
　　　　HAC see Appendix B for HAC conditional logic

　　MCC **T32.83** Corrosions involving 80-89% of body surface with 30-39% third degree corrosion
　　　　HAC see Appendix B for HAC conditional logic

　　MCC **T32.84** Corrosions involving 80-89% of body surface with 40-49% third degree corrosion
　　　　HAC see Appendix B for HAC conditional logic

　　MCC **T32.85** Corrosions involving 80-89% of body surface with 50-59% third degree corrosion
　　　　HAC see Appendix B for HAC conditional logic

　　MCC **T32.86** Corrosions involving 80-89% of body surface with 60-69% third degree corrosion
　　　　HAC see Appendix B for HAC conditional logic

　　MCC **T32.87** Corrosions involving 80-89% of body surface with 70-79% third degree corrosion
　　　　HAC see Appendix B for HAC conditional logic

　　MCC **T32.88** Corrosions involving 80-89% of body surface with 80-89% third degree corrosion
　　　　HAC see Appendix B for HAC conditional logic

+ **T32.9** Corrosions involving 90% or more of body surface

　　CC **T32.90** Corrosions involving 90% or more of body surface with 0% to 9% third degree corrosion
　　　　HAC see Appendix B for HAC conditional logic

　　MCC **T32.91** Corrosions involving 90% or more of body surface with 10-19% third degree corrosion
　　　　HAC see Appendix B for HAC conditional logic

　　MCC **T32.92** Corrosions involving 90% or more of body surface with 20-29% third degree corrosion
　　　　HAC see Appendix B for HAC conditional logic

　　MCC **T32.93** Corrosions involving 90% or more of body surface with 30-39% third degree corrosion
　　　　HAC see Appendix B for HAC conditional logic

　　MCC **T32.94** Corrosions involving 90% or more of body surface with 40-49% third degree corrosion
　　　　HAC see Appendix B for HAC conditional logic

　　MCC **T32.95** Corrosions involving 90% or more of body surface with 50-59% third degree corrosion

　　MCC **T32.96** Corrosions involving 90% or more of body surface with 60-69% third degree corrosion
　　　　HAC see Appendix B for HAC conditional logic

　　MCC **T32.97** Corrosions involving 90% or more of body surface with 70-79% third degree corrosion
　　　　HAC see Appendix B for HAC conditional logic

　　MCC **T32.98** Corrosions involving 90% or more of body surface with 80-89% third degree corrosion
　　　　HAC see Appendix B for HAC conditional logic

　　MCC **T32.99** Corrosions involving 90% or more of body surface with 90% or more third degree corrosion
　　　　HAC see Appendix B for HAC conditional logic

Frostbite (T33-T34)

Excludes2: *hypothermia and other effects of reduced temperature (T68, T69.-)*

T33 Superficial frostbite

　Includes: frostbite with partial thickness skin loss

> The appropriate 7th character is to be added to each code from category T33
> A　initial encounter
> D　subsequent encounter
> S　sequela

+ **T33.0** Superficial frostbite of head

　+ **T33.01** Superficial frostbite of ear

　　CC +7th **T33.011** Superficial frostbite of right ear
　　　　HAC 7th character A see Appendix B for HAC conditional logic

　　CC +7th **T33.012** Superficial frostbite of left ear
　　　　HAC 7th character A see Appendix B for HAC conditional logic

　　CC +7th **T33.019** Superficial frostbite of unspecified ear
　　　　HAC 7th character A see Appendix B for HAC conditional logic

　CC x+7th **T33.02** Superficial frostbite of nose
　　　　HAC 7th character A see Appendix B for HAC conditional logic

　CC x+7th **T33.09** Superficial frostbite of other part of head
　　　　HAC 7th character A see Appendix B for HAC conditional logic

CC x+7th **T33.1** Superficial frostbite of neck
　　　HAC 7th character A see Appendix B for HAC conditional logic

CC x+7th **T33.2** Superficial frostbite of thorax
　　　HAC 7th character A see Appendix B for HAC conditional logic

CC x+7th **T33.3** Superficial frostbite of abdominal wall, lower back and pelvis
　　　HAC 7th character A see Appendix B for HAC conditional logic

+ **T33.4** Superficial frostbite of arm
　　Excludes2: *superficial frostbite of wrist and hand (T33.5-)*

　CC x+7th **T33.40** Superficial frostbite of unspecified arm
　　　　HAC 7th character A see Appendix B for HAC conditional logic

　CC x+7th **T33.41** Superficial frostbite of right arm
　　　　HAC 7th character A see Appendix B for HAC conditional logic

　CC x+7th **T33.42** Superficial frostbite of left arm
　　　　HAC 7th character A see Appendix B for HAC conditional logic

+, +7th, X + 7th　　● Newborn　　● Pediatric　　● Maternity　　● Adult　　♀ Female　　♂ Male　　Manifestation　　Unacceptable PDX　　HCC　　CC　　MCC　　**HAC**

+ **T33.5** **Superficial frostbite of wrist, hand, and fingers**
    + **T33.51** **Superficial frostbite of wrist**
        CC +7th **T33.511** **Superficial frostbite of right wrist**
            HAC 7th character A see Appendix B for HAC conditional logic
        CC +7th **T33.512** **Superficial frostbite of left wrist**
            HAC 7th character A see Appendix B for HAC conditional logic
        CC +7th **T33.519** **Superficial frostbite of unspecified wrist**
            HAC 7th character A see Appendix B for HAC conditional logic
    + **T33.52** **Superficial frostbite of hand**
            Excludes2: *superficial frostbite of fingers (T33.53-)*
        CC +7th **T33.521** **Superficial frostbite of right hand**
            HAC 7th character A see Appendix B for HAC conditional logic
        CC +7th **T33.522** **Superficial frostbite of left hand**
            HAC 7th character A see Appendix B for HAC conditional logic
        CC +7th **T33.529** **Superficial frostbite of unspecified hand**
            HAC 7th character A see Appendix B for HAC conditional logic
    + **T33.53** **Superficial frostbite of finger(s)**
        CC +7th **T33.531** **Superficial frostbite of right finger(s)**
            HAC 7th character A see Appendix B for HAC conditional logic
        CC +7th **T33.532** **Superficial frostbite of left finger(s)**
            HAC 7th character A see Appendix B for HAC conditional logic
        CC +7th **T33.539** **Superficial frostbite of unspecified finger(s)**
            HAC 7th character A see Appendix B for HAC conditional logic
+ **T33.6** **Superficial frostbite of hip and thigh**
    CC x+7th **T33.60** **Superficial frostbite of unspecified hip and thigh**
            HAC 7th character A see Appendix B for HAC conditional logic
    CC x+7th **T33.61** **Superficial frostbite of right hip and thigh**
            HAC 7th character A see Appendix B for HAC conditional logic
    CC x+7th **T33.62** **Superficial frostbite of left hip and thigh**
            HAC 7th character A see Appendix B for HAC conditional logic
+ **T33.7** **Superficial frostbite of knee and lower leg**
            Excludes2: *superficial frostbite of ankle and foot (T33.8-)*
    CC x+7th **T33.70** **Superficial frostbite of unspecified knee and lower leg**
            HAC 7th character A see Appendix B for HAC conditional logic
    CC x+7th **T33.71** **Superficial frostbite of right knee and lower leg**
            HAC 7th character A see Appendix B for HAC conditional logic
    CC x+7th **T33.72** **Superficial frostbite of left knee and lower leg**
            HAC 7th character A see Appendix B for HAC conditional logic
+ **T33.8** **Superficial frostbite of ankle, foot, and toe(s)**
    + **T33.81** **Superficial frostbite of ankle**
        CC +7th **T33.811** **Superficial frostbite of right ankle**
            HAC 7th character A see Appendix B for HAC conditional logic
        CC +7th **T33.812** **Superficial frostbite of left ankle**
            HAC 7th character A see Appendix B for HAC conditional logic
        CC +7th **T33.819** **Superficial frostbite of unspecified ankle**
            HAC 7th character A see Appendix B for HAC conditional logic
    + **T33.82** **Superficial frostbite of foot**
        CC +7th **T33.821** **Superficial frostbite of right foot**
            HAC 7th character A see Appendix B for HAC conditional logic
        CC +7th **T33.822** **Superficial frostbite of left foot**
            HAC 7th character A see Appendix B for HAC conditional logic
        CC +7th **T33.829** **Superficial frostbite of unspecified foot**
            HAC 7th character A see Appendix B for HAC conditional logic

+ **T33.83** **Superficial frostbite of toe(s)**
        CC +7th **T33.831** **Superficial frostbite of right toe(s)**
            HAC 7th character A see Appendix B for HAC conditional logic
        CC +7th **T33.832** **Superficial frostbite of left toe(s)**
            HAC 7th character A see Appendix B for HAC conditional logic
        CC +7th **T33.839** **Superficial frostbite of unspecified toe(s)**
            HAC 7th character A see Appendix B for HAC conditional logic
+ **T33.9** **Superficial frostbite of other and unspecified sites**
    CC x+7th **T33.90** **Superficial frostbite of unspecified sites**
            Superficial frostbite NOS
            HAC 7th character A see Appendix B for HAC conditional logic
    CC x+7th **T33.99** **Superficial frostbite of other sites**
            Superficial frostbite of leg NOS
            Superficial frostbite of trunk NOS
            HAC 7th character A see Appendix B for HAC conditional logic

T34 **Frostbite with tissue necrosis**

> The appropriate 7th character is to be added to each code from category T34
> A initial encounter
> D subsequent encounter
> S sequela

+ **T34.0** **Frostbite with tissue necrosis of head**
    + **T34.01** **Frostbite with tissue necrosis of ear**
        CC +7th **T34.011** **Frostbite with tissue necrosis of right ear**
            HAC 7th character A see Appendix B for HAC conditional logic
        CC +7th **T34.012** **Frostbite with tissue necrosis of left ear**
            HAC 7th character A see Appendix B for HAC conditional logic
        CC +7th **T34.019** **Frostbite with tissue necrosis of unspecified ear**
            HAC 7th character A see Appendix B for HAC conditional logic
    CC x+7th **T34.02** **Frostbite with tissue necrosis of nose**
            HAC 7th character A see Appendix B for HAC conditional logic
    CC x+7th **T34.09** **Frostbite with tissue necrosis of other part of head**
            HAC 7th character A see Appendix B for HAC conditional logic
CC x+7th **T34.1** **Frostbite with tissue necrosis of neck**
            HAC 7th character A see Appendix B for HAC conditional logic
CC x+7th **T34.2** **Frostbite with tissue necrosis of thorax**
            HAC 7th character A see Appendix B for HAC conditional logic
CC x+7th **T34.3** **Frostbite with tissue necrosis of abdominal wall, lower back and pelvis**
            HAC 7th character A see Appendix B for HAC conditional logic
+ **T34.4** **Frostbite with tissue necrosis of arm**
            Excludes2: *frostbite with tissue necrosis of wrist and hand (T34.5-)*
    CC x+7th **T34.40** **Frostbite with tissue necrosis of unspecified arm**
            HAC 7th character A see Appendix B for HAC conditional logic
    CC x+7th **T34.41** **Frostbite with tissue necrosis of right arm**
            HAC 7th character A see Appendix B for HAC conditional logic
    CC x+7th **T34.42** **Frostbite with tissue necrosis of left arm**
            HAC 7th character A see Appendix B for HAC conditional logic
+ **T34.5** **Frostbite with tissue necrosis of wrist, hand, and finger(s)**
    + **T34.51** **Frostbite with tissue necrosis of wrist**
        CC +7th **T34.511** **Frostbite with tissue necrosis of right wrist**
            HAC 7th character A see Appendix B for HAC conditional logic
        CC +7th **T34.512** **Frostbite with tissue necrosis of left wrist**
            HAC 7th character A see Appendix B for HAC conditional logic
        CC +7th **T34.519** **Frostbite with tissue necrosis of unspecified wrist**
            HAC 7th character A see Appendix B for HAC conditional logic

+, +7th, X + 7th   ● Newborn   ● Pediatric   ● Maternity   ● Adult   ♀ Female   ♂ Male   Manifestation   Unacceptable PDX   HCC   CC   MCC   HAC

+ **T34.52** **Frostbite with tissue necrosis of hand**
　　Excludes2: *frostbite with tissue necrosis of finger(s) (T34.53-)*
CC +7th **T34.521** **Frostbite with tissue necrosis of right hand**
　　　　HAC 7th character A see Appendix B for HAC conditional logic
CC +7th **T34.522** **Frostbite with tissue necrosis of left hand**
　　　　HAC 7th character A see Appendix B for HAC conditional logic
CC +7th **T34.529** **Frostbite with tissue necrosis of unspecified hand**
　　　　HAC 7th character A see Appendix B for HAC conditional logic

+ **T34.53** **Frostbite with tissue necrosis of finger(s)**
CC +7th **T34.531** **Frostbite with tissue necrosis of right finger(s)**
　　　　HAC 7th character A see Appendix B for HAC conditional logic
CC +7th **T34.532** **Frostbite with tissue necrosis of left finger(s)**
　　　　HAC 7th character A see Appendix B for HAC conditional logic
CC +7th **T34.539** **Frostbite with tissue necrosis of unspecified finger(s)**
　　　　HAC 7th character A see Appendix B for HAC conditional logic

+ **T34.6** **Frostbite with tissue necrosis of hip and thigh**
CC X+7th **T34.60** **Frostbite with tissue necrosis of unspecified hip and thigh**
　　　　HAC 7th character A see Appendix B for HAC conditional logic
CC X+7th **T34.61** **Frostbite with tissue necrosis of right hip and thigh**
　　　　HAC 7th character A see Appendix B for HAC conditional logic
CC X+7th **T34.62** **Frostbite with tissue necrosis of left hip and thigh**
　　　　HAC 7th character A see Appendix B for HAC conditional logic

+ **T34.7** **Frostbite with tissue necrosis of knee and lower leg**
　　Excludes2: *frostbite with tissue necrosis of ankle and foot (T34.8-)*
CC X+7th **T34.70** **Frostbite with tissue necrosis of unspecified knee and lower leg**
　　　　HAC 7th character A see Appendix B for HAC conditional logic
CC X+7th **T34.71** **Frostbite with tissue necrosis of right knee and lower leg**
　　　　HAC 7th character A see Appendix B for HAC conditional logic
CC X+7th **T34.72** **Frostbite with tissue necrosis of left knee and lower leg**
　　　　HAC 7th character A see Appendix B for HAC conditional logic

+ **T34.8** **Frostbite with tissue necrosis of ankle, foot, and toe(s)**
+ **T34.81** **Frostbite with tissue necrosis of ankle**
CC +7th **T34.811** **Frostbite with tissue necrosis of right ankle**
　　　　HAC 7th character A see Appendix B for HAC conditional logic
CC +7th **T34.812** **Frostbite with tissue necrosis of left ankle**
　　　　HAC 7th character A see Appendix B for HAC conditional logic
CC +7th **T34.819** **Frostbite with tissue necrosis of unspecified ankle**
　　　　HAC 7th character A see Appendix B for HAC conditional logic

+ **T34.82** **Frostbite with tissue necrosis of foot**
CC +7th **T34.821** **Frostbite with tissue necrosis of right foot**
　　　　HAC 7th character A see Appendix B for HAC conditional logic
CC +7th **T34.822** **Frostbite with tissue necrosis of left foot**
　　　　HAC 7th character A see Appendix B for HAC conditional logic
CC +7th **T34.829** **Frostbite with tissue necrosis of unspecified foot**
　　　　HAC 7th character A see Appendix B for HAC conditional logic

+ **T34.83** **Frostbite with tissue necrosis of toe(s)**
CC +7th **T34.831** **Frostbite with tissue necrosis of right toe(s)**
　　　　HAC 7th character A see Appendix B for HAC conditional logic
CC +7th **T34.832** **Frostbite with tissue necrosis of left toe(s)**
　　　　HAC 7th character A see Appendix B for HAC conditional logic
CC +7th **T34.839** **Frostbite with tissue necrosis of unspecified toe(s)**
　　　　HAC 7th character A see Appendix B for HAC conditional logic

+ **T34.9** **Frostbite with tissue necrosis of other and unspecified sites**
CC X+7th **T34.90** **Frostbite with tissue necrosis of unspecified sites**
　　Frostbite with tissue necrosis NOS
　　　　HAC 7th character A see Appendix B for HAC conditional logic
CC X+7th **T34.99** **Frostbite with tissue necrosis of other sites**
　　Frostbite with tissue necrosis of leg NOS
　　Frostbite with tissue necrosis of trunk NOS
　　　　HAC 7th character A see Appendix B for HAC conditional logic

Poisoning by, adverse effects of and underdosing of drugs, medicaments and biological substances (T36-T50)

Includes: adverse effect of correct substance properly administered
　　poisoning by overdose of substance
　　poisoning by wrong substance given or taken in error
　　underdosing by (inadvertently) (deliberately) taking less substance than prescribed or instructed

Code first: for adverse effects, the nature of the adverse effect, such as:
　　adverse effect NOS (T88.7)
　　aspirin gastritis (K29.-)
　　blood disorders (D56-D76)
　　contact dermatitis (L23-L25)
　　dermatitis due to substances taken internally (L27.-)
　　nephropathy (N14.0-N14.2)

NOTE The drug giving rise to the adverse effect should be identified by use of codes from categories T36-T50 with fifth or sixth character 5.

Use additional: code(s) to specify:
　　manifestations of poisoning
　　underdosing or failure in dosage during medical and surgical care (Y63.6, Y63.8-Y63.9)
　　underdosing of medication regimen (Z91.12-, Z91.13-)

Excludes1: *toxic reaction to local anesthesia in pregnancy (O29.3-)*

Excludes2: *abuse and dependence of psychoactive substances (F10-F19)*
　　abuse of non-dependence-producing substances (F55.-)
　　drug reaction and poisoning affecting newborn (P00-P96)
　　immunodeficiency due to drugs (D84.821)
　　pathological drug intoxication (inebriation) (F10-F19)

Review coding guideline C.19.e

T36 **Poisoning by, adverse effect of and underdosing of systemic antibiotics**

　　Excludes1: *antineoplastic antibiotics (T45.1-)*
　　　　locally applied antibiotic NEC (T49.0)
　　　　topically used antibiotic for ear, nose and throat (T49.6)
　　　　topically used antibiotic for eye (T49.5)

> The appropriate 7th character is to be added to each code from category T36
> A initial encounter
> D subsequent encounter
> S sequela

+ **T36.0** **Poisoning by, adverse effect of and underdosing of penicillins**
+ **T36.0X** **Poisoning by, adverse effect of and underdosing of penicillins**
+7th **T36.0X1** **Poisoning by penicillins, accidental (unintentional)**
　　Poisoning by penicillins NOS
+7th **T36.0X2** **Poisoning by penicillins, intentional self-harm**
+7th **T36.0X3** **Poisoning by penicillins, assault**
+7th **T36.0X4** **Poisoning by penicillins, undetermined**
+7th **T36.0X5** **Adverse effect of penicillins**
+7th **T36.0X6** **Underdosing of penicillins**

+ **T36.1** **Poisoning by, adverse effect of and underdosing of cephalosporins and other beta-lactam antibiotics**
  + **T36.1X** **Poisoning by, adverse effect of and underdosing of cephalosporins and other beta-lactam antibiotics**
    +7th **T36.1X1** **Poisoning by cephalosporins and other beta-lactam antibiotics, accidental (unintentional)**
      Poisoning by cephalosporins and other beta-lactam antibiotics NOS
    +7th **T36.1X2** **Poisoning by cephalosporins and other beta-lactam antibiotics, intentional self-harm**
    +7th **T36.1X3** **Poisoning by cephalosporins and other beta-lactam antibiotics, assault**
    +7th **T36.1X4** **Poisoning by cephalosporins and other beta-lactam antibiotics, undetermined**
    +7th **T36.1X5** **Adverse effect of cephalosporins and other beta-lactam antibiotics**
    +7th **T36.1X6** **Underdosing of cephalosporins and other beta-lactam antibiotics**

+ **T36.2** **Poisoning by, adverse effect of and underdosing of chloramphenicol group**
  + **T36.2X** **Poisoning by, adverse effect of and underdosing of chloramphenicol group**
    +7th **T36.2X1** **Poisoning by chloramphenicol group, accidental (unintentional)**
      Poisoning by chloramphenicol group NOS
    +7th **T36.2X2** **Poisoning by chloramphenicol group, intentional self-harm**
    +7th **T36.2X3** **Poisoning by chloramphenicol group, assault**
    +7th **T36.2X4** **Poisoning by chloramphenicol group, undetermined**
    +7th **T36.2X5** **Adverse effect of chloramphenicol group**
    +7th **T36.2X6** **Underdosing of chloramphenicol group**

+ **T36.3** **Poisoning by, adverse effect of and underdosing of macrolides**
  + **T36.3X** **Poisoning by, adverse effect of and underdosing of macrolides**
    +7th **T36.3X1** **Poisoning by macrolides, accidental (unintentional)**
      Poisoning by macrolides NOS
    +7th **T36.3X2** **Poisoning by macrolides, intentional self-harm**
    +7th **T36.3X3** **Poisoning by macrolides, assault**
    +7th **T36.3X4** **Poisoning by macrolides, undetermined**
    +7th **T36.3X5** **Adverse effect of macrolides**
    +7th **T36.3X6** **Underdosing of macrolides**

+ **T36.4** **Poisoning by, adverse effect of and underdosing of tetracyclines**
  + **T36.4X** **Poisoning by, adverse effect of and underdosing of tetracyclines**
    +7th **T36.4X1** **Poisoning by tetracyclines, accidental (unintentional)**
      Poisoning by tetracyclines NOS
    +7th **T36.4X2** **Poisoning by tetracyclines, intentional self-harm**
    +7th **T36.4X3** **Poisoning by tetracyclines, assault**
    +7th **T36.4X4** **Poisoning by tetracyclines, undetermined**
    +7th **T36.4X5** **Adverse effect of tetracyclines**
    +7th **T36.4X6** **Underdosing of tetracyclines**

+ **T36.5** **Poisoning by, adverse effect of and underdosing of aminoglycosides**
  Poisoning by, adverse effect of and underdosing of streptomycin
  + **T36.5X** **Poisoning by, adverse effect of and underdosing of aminoglycosides**
    +7th **T36.5X1** **Poisoning by aminoglycosides, accidental (unintentional)**
      Poisoning by aminoglycosides NOS
    +7th **T36.5X2** **Poisoning by aminoglycosides, intentional self-harm**
    +7th **T36.5X3** **Poisoning by aminoglycosides, assault**
    +7th **T36.5X4** **Poisoning by aminoglycosides, undetermined**
    +7th **T36.5X5** **Adverse effect of aminoglycosides**
    +7th **T36.5X6** **Underdosing of aminoglycosides**

+ **T36.6** **Poisoning by, adverse effect of and underdosing of rifampicins**
  + **T36.6X** **Poisoning by, adverse effect of and underdosing of rifampicins**
    +7th **T36.6X1** **Poisoning by rifampicins, accidental (unintentional)**
      Poisoning by rifampicins NOS
    +7th **T36.6X2** **Poisoning by rifampicins, intentional self-harm**
    +7th **T36.6X3** **Poisoning by rifampicins, assault**
    +7th **T36.6X4** **Poisoning by rifampicins, undetermined**
    +7th **T36.6X5** **Adverse effect of rifampicins**
    +7th **T36.6X6** **Underdosing of rifampicins**

+ **T36.7** **Poisoning by, adverse effect of and underdosing of antifungal antibiotics, systemically used**
  + **T36.7X** **Poisoning by, adverse effect of and underdosing of antifungal antibiotics, systemically used**
    +7th **T36.7X1** **Poisoning by antifungal antibiotics, systemically used, accidental (unintentional)**
      Poisoning by antifungal antibiotics, systemically used NOS
    +7th **T36.7X2** **Poisoning by antifungal antibiotics, systemically used, intentional self-harm**
    +7th **T36.7X3** **Poisoning by antifungal antibiotics, systemically used, assault**
    +7th **T36.7X4** **Poisoning by antifungal antibiotics, systemically used, undetermined**
    +7th **T36.7X5** **Adverse effect of antifungal antibiotics, systemically used**
    +7th **T36.7X6** **Underdosing of antifungal antibiotics, systemically used**

+ **T36.8** **Poisoning by, adverse effect of and underdosing of other systemic antibiotics**
  + **T36.8X** **Poisoning by, adverse effect of and underdosing of other systemic antibiotics**
    +7th **T36.8X1** **Poisoning by other systemic antibiotics, accidental (unintentional)**
      Poisoning by other systemic antibiotics NOS
    +7th **T36.8X2** **Poisoning by other systemic antibiotics, intentional self-harm**
    +7th **T36.8X3** **Poisoning by other systemic antibiotics, assault**
    +7th **T36.8X4** **Poisoning by other systemic antibiotics, undetermined**
    +7th **T36.8X5** **Adverse effect of other systemic antibiotics**
      AHA CC: 1Q, 2017, 39
    +7th **T36.8X6** **Underdosing of other systemic antibiotics**

+ **T36.9** **Poisoning by, adverse effect of and underdosing of unspecified systemic antibiotic**
  X+7th **T36.91** **Poisoning by unspecified systemic antibiotic, accidental (unintentional)**
    Poisoning by systemic antibiotic NOS
  X+7th **T36.92** **Poisoning by unspecified systemic antibiotic, intentional self-harm**
  X+7th **T36.93** **Poisoning by unspecified systemic antibiotic, assault**
  X+7th **T36.94** **Poisoning by unspecified systemic antibiotic, undetermined**
  X+7th **T36.95** **Adverse effect of unspecified systemic antibiotic**
  X+7th **T36.96** **Underdosing of unspecified systemic antibiotic**

T37 **Poisoning by, adverse effect of and underdosing of other systemic anti-infectives and antiparasitics**

  Excludes1: *anti-infectives topically used for ear, nose and throat (T49.6-)*
    anti-infectives topically used for eye (T49.5-)
    locally applied anti-infectives NEC (T49.0-)

> The appropriate 7th character is to be added to each code from category T37
> A   initial encounter
> D   subsequent encounter
> S   sequela

+ **T37.0** Poisoning by, adverse effect of and underdosing of sulfonamides
> + **T37.0X** Poisoning by, adverse effect of and underdosing of sulfonamides
>> +7th **T37.0X1** Poisoning by sulfonamides, accidental (unintentional)
>>> Poisoning by sulfonamides NOS
>> +7th **T37.0X2** Poisoning by sulfonamides, intentional self-harm
>> +7th **T37.0X3** Poisoning by sulfonamides, assault
>> +7th **T37.0X4** Poisoning by sulfonamides, undetermined
>> +7th **T37.0X5** Adverse effect of sulfonamides
>> +7th **T37.0X6** Underdosing of sulfonamides

+ **T37.1** Poisoning by, adverse effect of and underdosing of antimycobacterial drugs
> *Excludes1:* rifampicins (T36.6-)
> streptomycin (T36.5-)
> + **T37.1X** Poisoning by, adverse effect of and underdosing of antimycobacterial drugs
>> +7th **T37.1X1** Poisoning by antimycobacterial drugs, accidental (unintentional)
>>> Poisoning by antimycobacterial drugs NOS
>> +7th **T37.1X2** Poisoning by antimycobacterial drugs, intentional self-harm
>> +7th **T37.1X3** Poisoning by antimycobacterial drugs, assault
>> +7th **T37.1X4** Poisoning by antimycobacterial drugs, undetermined
>> +7th **T37.1X5** Adverse effect of antimycobacterial drugs
>> +7th **T37.1X6** Underdosing of antimycobacterial drugs

+ **T37.2** Poisoning by, adverse effect of and underdosing of antimalarials and drugs acting on other blood protozoa
> *Excludes1:* hydroxyquinoline derivatives (T37.8-)
> + **T37.2X** Poisoning by, adverse effect of and underdosing of antimalarials and drugs acting on other blood protozoa
>> +7th **T37.2X1** Poisoning by antimalarials and drugs acting on other blood protozoa, accidental (unintentional)
>>> Poisoning by antimalarials and drugs acting on other blood protozoa NOS
>> +7th **T37.2X2** Poisoning by antimalarials and drugs acting on other blood protozoa, intentional self-harm
>> +7th **T37.2X3** Poisoning by antimalarials and drugs acting on other blood protozoa, assault
>> +7th **T37.2X4** Poisoning by antimalarials and drugs acting on other blood protozoa, undetermined
>> +7th **T37.2X5** Adverse effect of antimalarials and drugs acting on other blood protozoa
>> +7th **T37.2X6** Underdosing of antimalarials and drugs acting on other blood protozoa

+ **T37.3** Poisoning by, adverse effect of and underdosing of other antiprotozoal drugs
> + **T37.3X** Poisoning by, adverse effect of and underdosing of other antiprotozoal drugs
>> +7th **T37.3X1** Poisoning by other antiprotozoal drugs, accidental (unintentional)
>>> Poisoning by other antiprotozoal drugs NOS
>> +7th **T37.3X2** Poisoning by other antiprotozoal drugs, intentional self-harm
>> +7th **T37.3X3** Poisoning by other antiprotozoal drugs, assault
>> +7th **T37.3X4** Poisoning by other antiprotozoal drugs, undetermined
>> +7th **T37.3X5** Adverse effect of other antiprotozoal drugs
>> +7th **T37.3X6** Underdosing of other antiprotozoal drugs

+ **T37.4** Poisoning by, adverse effect of and underdosing of anthelminthics
> + **T37.4X** Poisoning by, adverse effect of and underdosing of anthelminthics
>> +7th **T37.4X1** Poisoning by anthelminthics, accidental (unintentional)
>>> Poisoning by anthelminthics NOS
>> +7th **T37.4X2** Poisoning by anthelminthics, intentional self-harm
>> +7th **T37.4X3** Poisoning by anthelminthics, assault
>> +7th **T37.4X4** Poisoning by anthelminthics, undetermined
>> +7th **T37.4X5** Adverse effect of anthelminthics
>> +7th **T37.4X6** Underdosing of anthelminthics

+ **T37.5** Poisoning by, adverse effect of and underdosing of antiviral drugs
> *Excludes1:* amantadine (T42.8-)
> cytarabine (T45.1-)
> + **T37.5X** Poisoning by, adverse effect of and underdosing of antiviral drugs
>> +7th **T37.5X1** Poisoning by antiviral drugs, accidental (unintentional)
>>> Poisoning by antiviral drugs NOS
>> +7th **T37.5X2** Poisoning by antiviral drugs, intentional self-harm
>> +7th **T37.5X3** Poisoning by antiviral drugs, assault
>> +7th **T37.5X4** Poisoning by antiviral drugs, undetermined
>> +7th **T37.5X5** Adverse effect of antiviral drugs
>> +7th **T37.5X6** Underdosing of antiviral drugs

+ **T37.8** Poisoning by, adverse effect of and underdosing of other specified systemic anti-infectives and antiparasitics
> Poisoning by, adverse effect of and underdosing of hydroxyquinoline derivatives
> *Excludes1:* antimalarial drugs (T37.2-)
> + **T37.8X** Poisoning by, adverse effect of and underdosing of other specified systemic anti-infectives and antiparasitics
>> +7th **T37.8X1** Poisoning by other specified systemic anti-infectives and antiparasitics, accidental (unintentional)
>>> Poisoning by other specified systemic anti-infectives and antiparasitics NOS
>> +7th **T37.8X2** Poisoning by other specified systemic anti-infectives and antiparasitics, intentional self-harm
>> +7th **T37.8X3** Poisoning by other specified systemic anti-infectives and antiparasitics, assault
>> +7th **T37.8X4** Poisoning by other specified systemic anti-infectives and antiparasitics, undetermined
>> +7th **T37.8X5** Adverse effect of other specified systemic anti-infectives and antiparasitics
>> +7th **T37.8X6** Underdosing of other specified systemic anti-infectives and antiparasitics

+ **T37.9** Poisoning by, adverse effect of and underdosing of unspecified systemic anti-infective and antiparasitics
> X+7th **T37.91** Poisoning by unspecified systemic anti-infective and antiparasitics, accidental (unintentional)
>> Poisoning by, adverse effect of and underdosing of systemic anti-infective and antiparasitics NOS
> X+7th **T37.92** Poisoning by unspecified systemic anti-infective and antiparasitics, intentional self-harm
> X+7th **T37.93** Poisoning by unspecified systemic anti-infective and antiparasitics, assault
> X+7th **T37.94** Poisoning by unspecified systemic anti-infective and antiparasitics, undetermined
> X+7th **T37.95** Adverse effect of unspecified systemic anti-infective and antiparasitic
> X+7th **T37.96** Underdosing of unspecified systemic anti-infectives and antiparasitics

T38 Poisoning by, adverse effect of and underdosing of hormones and their synthetic substitutes and antagonists, not elsewhere classified

> *Excludes1:* mineralocorticoids and their antagonists (T50.0-)
> oxytocic hormones (T48.0-)
> parathyroid hormones and derivatives (T50.9-)

> The appropriate 7th character is to be added to each code from category T38
> A initial encounter
> D subsequent encounter
> S sequela

+ **T38.0 Poisoning by, adverse effect of and underdosing of glucocorticoids and synthetic analogues**

> *Excludes1:* glucocorticoids, topically used (T49.-)

+ **T38.0X Poisoning by, adverse effect of and underdosing of glucocorticoids and synthetic analogues**

+7th **T38.0X1 Poisoning by glucocorticoids and synthetic analogues, accidental (unintentional)**
> Poisoning by glucocorticoids and synthetic analogues NOS

+7th **T38.0X2 Poisoning by glucocorticoids and synthetic analogues, intentional self-harm**

+7th **T38.0X3 Poisoning by glucocorticoids and synthetic analogues, assault**

+7th **T38.0X4 Poisoning by glucocorticoids and synthetic analogues, undetermined**

+7th **T38.0X5 Adverse effect of glucocorticoids and synthetic analogues**

+7th **T38.0X6 Underdosing of glucocorticoids and synthetic analogues**

+ **T38.1 Poisoning by, adverse effect of and underdosing of thyroid hormones and substitutes**

+ **T38.1X Poisoning by, adverse effect of and underdosing of thyroid hormones and substitutes**

+7th **T38.1X1 Poisoning by thyroid hormones and substitutes, accidental (unintentional)**
> Poisoning by thyroid hormones and substitutes NOS

+7th **T38.1X2 Poisoning by thyroid hormones and substitutes, intentional self-harm**

+7th **T38.1X3 Poisoning by thyroid hormones and substitutes, assault**

+7th **T38.1X4 Poisoning by thyroid hormones and substitutes, undetermined**

+7th **T38.1X5 Adverse effect of thyroid hormones and substitutes**

+7th **T38.1X6 Underdosing of thyroid hormones and substitutes**

+ **T38.2 Poisoning by, adverse effect of and underdosing of antithyroid drugs**

+ **T38.2X Poisoning by, adverse effect of and underdosing of antithyroid drugs**

+7th **T38.2X1 Poisoning by antithyroid drugs, accidental (unintentional)**
> Poisoning by antithyroid drugs NOS

+7th **T38.2X2 Poisoning by antithyroid drugs, intentional self-harm**

+7th **T38.2X3 Poisoning by antithyroid drugs, assault**

+7th **T38.2X4 Poisoning by antithyroid drugs, undetermined**

+7th **T38.2X5 Adverse effect of antithyroid drugs**

+7th **T38.2X6 Underdosing of antithyroid drugs**

+ **T38.3 Poisoning by, adverse effect of and underdosing of insulin and oral hypoglycemic [antidiabetic] drugs**

+ **T38.3X Poisoning by, adverse effect of and underdosing of insulin and oral hypoglycemic [antidiabetic] drugs**

+7th **T38.3X1 Poisoning by insulin and oral hypoglycemic [antidiabetic] drugs, accidental (unintentional)**
> Poisoning by insulin and oral hypoglycemic [antidiabetic] drugs NOS
> Review coding guideline C.4.a.5.b

+7th **T38.3X2 Poisoning by insulin and oral hypoglycemic [antidiabetic] drugs, intentional self-harm**

+7th **T38.3X3 Poisoning by insulin and oral hypoglycemic [antidiabetic] drugs, assault**

+7th **T38.3X4 Poisoning by insulin and oral hypoglycemic [antidiabetic] drugs, undetermined**

+7th **T38.3X5 Adverse effect of insulin and oral hypoglycemic [antidiabetic] drugs**

+7th **T38.3X6 Underdosing of insulin and oral hypoglycemic [antidiabetic] drugs**
> Review coding guideline C.4.a.5.a

+ **T38.4 Poisoning by, adverse effect of and underdosing of oral contraceptives**
> Poisoning by, adverse effect of and underdosing of multiple- and single-ingredient oral contraceptive preparations

+ **T38.4X Poisoning by, adverse effect of and underdosing of oral contraceptives**

+7th **T38.4X1 Poisoning by oral contraceptives, accidental (unintentional)**
> Poisoning by oral contraceptives NOS

+7th **T38.4X2 Poisoning by oral contraceptives, intentional self-harm**

+7th **T38.4X3 Poisoning by oral contraceptives, assault**

+7th **T38.4X4 Poisoning by oral contraceptives, undetermined**

+7th **T38.4X5 Adverse effect of oral contraceptives**

+7th **T38.4X6 Underdosing of oral contraceptives**

+ **T38.5 Poisoning by, adverse effect of and underdosing of other estrogens and progestogens**
> Poisoning by, adverse effect of and underdosing of estrogens and progestogens mixtures and substitutes

+ **T38.5X Poisoning by, adverse effect of and underdosing of other estrogens and progestogens**

+7th **T38.5X1 Poisoning by other estrogens and progestogens, accidental (unintentional)**
> Poisoning by other estrogens and progestogens NOS

+7th **T38.5X2 Poisoning by other estrogens and progestogens, intentional self-harm**

+7th **T38.5X3 Poisoning by other estrogens and progestogens, assault**

+7th **T38.5X4 Poisoning by other estrogens and progestogens, undetermined**

+7th **T38.5X5 Adverse effect of other estrogens and progestogens**

+7th **T38.5X6 Underdosing of other estrogens and progestogens**

+ **T38.6 Poisoning by, adverse effect of and underdosing of antigonadotrophins, antiestrogens, antiandrogens, not elsewhere classified**
> Poisoning by, adverse effect of and underdosing of tamoxifen

+ **T38.6X Poisoning by, adverse effect of and underdosing of antigonadotrophins, antiestrogens, antiandrogens, not elsewhere classified**

+7th **T38.6X1 Poisoning by antigonadotrophins, antiestrogens, antiandrogens, not elsewhere classified, accidental (unintentional)**
> Poisoning by antigonadotrophins, antiestrogens, antiandrogens, not elsewhere classified NOS

+7th **T38.6X2 Poisoning by antigonadotrophins, antiestrogens, antiandrogens, not elsewhere classified, intentional self-harm**

+7th **T38.6X3 Poisoning by antigonadotrophins, antiestrogens, antiandrogens, not elsewhere classified, assault**

+7th **T38.6X4 Poisoning by antigonadotrophins, antiestrogens, antiandrogens, not elsewhere classified, undetermined**

+7th **T38.6X5 Adverse effect of antigonadotrophins, antiestrogens, antiandrogens, not elsewhere classified**

+7th **T38.6X6 Underdosing of antigonadotrophins, antiestrogens, antiandrogens, not elsewhere classified**

+ **T38.7** Poisoning by, adverse effect of and underdosing of androgens and anabolic congeners
  + **T38.7X** Poisoning by, adverse effect of and underdosing of androgens and anabolic congeners
    +7th **T38.7X1** Poisoning by androgens and anabolic congeners, accidental (unintentional)
       Poisoning by androgens and anabolic congeners NOS
    +7th **T38.7X2** Poisoning by androgens and anabolic congeners, intentional self-harm
    +7th **T38.7X3** Poisoning by androgens and anabolic congeners, assault
    +7th **T38.7X4** Poisoning by androgens and anabolic congeners, undetermined
    +7th **T38.7X5** Adverse effect of androgens and anabolic congeners
    +7th **T38.7X6** Underdosing of androgens and anabolic congeners
+ **T38.8** Poisoning by, adverse effect of and underdosing of other and unspecified hormones and synthetic substitutes
  + **T38.80** Poisoning by, adverse effect of and underdosing of unspecified hormones and synthetic substitutes
    +7th **T38.801** Poisoning by unspecified hormones and synthetic substitutes, accidental (unintentional)
       Poisoning by unspecified hormones and synthetic substitutes NOS
    +7th **T38.802** Poisoning by unspecified hormones and synthetic substitutes, intentional self-harm
    +7th **T38.803** Poisoning by unspecified hormones and synthetic substitutes, assault
    +7th **T38.804** Poisoning by unspecified hormones and synthetic substitutes, undetermined
    +7th **T38.805** Adverse effect of unspecified hormones and synthetic substitutes
    +7th **T38.806** Underdosing of unspecified hormones and synthetic substitutes
  + **T38.81** Poisoning by, adverse effect of and underdosing of anterior pituitary [adenohypophyseal] hormones
    +7th **T38.811** Poisoning by anterior pituitary [adenohypophyseal] hormones, accidental (unintentional)
       Poisoning by anterior pituitary [adenohypophyseal] hormones NOS
    +7th **T38.812** Poisoning by anterior pituitary [adenohypophyseal] hormones, intentional self-harm
    +7th **T38.813** Poisoning by anterior pituitary [adenohypophyseal] hormones, assault
    +7th **T38.814** Poisoning by anterior pituitary [adenohypophyseal] hormones, undetermined
    +7th **T38.815** Adverse effect of anterior pituitary [adenohypophyseal] hormones
    +7th **T38.816** Underdosing of anterior pituitary [adenohypophyseal] hormones
  + **T38.89** Poisoning by, adverse effect of and underdosing of other hormones and synthetic substitutes
    +7th **T38.891** Poisoning by other hormones and synthetic substitutes, accidental (unintentional)
       Poisoning by other hormones and synthetic substitutes NOS
    +7th **T38.892** Poisoning by other hormones and synthetic substitutes, intentional self-harm
    +7th **T38.893** Poisoning by other hormones and synthetic substitutes, assault
    +7th **T38.894** Poisoning by other hormones and synthetic substitutes, undetermined
    +7th **T38.895** Adverse effect of other hormones and synthetic substitutes
    +7th **T38.896** Underdosing of other hormones and synthetic substitutes

+ **T38.9** Poisoning by, adverse effect of and underdosing of other and unspecified hormone antagonists
  + **T38.90** Poisoning by, adverse effect of and underdosing of unspecified hormone antagonists
    +7th **T38.901** Poisoning by unspecified hormone antagonists, accidental (unintentional)
       Poisoning by unspecified hormone antagonists NOS
    +7th **T38.902** Poisoning by unspecified hormone antagonists, intentional self-harm
    +7th **T38.903** Poisoning by unspecified hormone antagonists, assault
    +7th **T38.904** Poisoning by unspecified hormone antagonists, undetermined
    +7th **T38.905** Adverse effect of unspecified hormone antagonists
    +7th **T38.906** Underdosing of unspecified hormone antagonists
  + **T38.99** Poisoning by, adverse effect of and underdosing of other hormone antagonists
    +7th **T38.991** Poisoning by other hormone antagonists, accidental (unintentional)
       Poisoning by other hormone antagonists NOS
    +7th **T38.992** Poisoning by other hormone antagonists, intentional self-harm
    +7th **T38.993** Poisoning by other hormone antagonists, assault
    +7th **T38.994** Poisoning by other hormone antagonists, undetermined
    +7th **T38.995** Adverse effect of other hormone antagonists
    +7th **T38.996** Underdosing of other hormone antagonists

T39 Poisoning by, adverse effect of and underdosing of nonopioid analgesics, antipyretics and antirheumatics

> The appropriate 7th character is to be added to each code from category T39
> A   initial encounter
> D   subsequent encounter
> S   sequela

+ **T39.0** Poisoning by, adverse effect of and underdosing of salicylates
  + **T39.01** Poisoning by, adverse effect of and underdosing of aspirin
       Poisoning by, adverse effect of and underdosing of acetylsalicylic acid
    +7th **T39.011** Poisoning by aspirin, accidental (unintentional)
    +7th **T39.012** Poisoning by aspirin, intentional self-harm
    +7th **T39.013** Poisoning by aspirin, assault
    +7th **T39.014** Poisoning by aspirin, undetermined
    +7th **T39.015** Adverse effect of aspirin
       AHA CC: 1Q, 2016, 15
    +7th **T39.016** Underdosing of aspirin
  + **T39.09** Poisoning by, adverse effect of and underdosing of other salicylates
    +7th **T39.091** Poisoning by salicylates, accidental (unintentional)
       Poisoning by salicylates NOS
    +7th **T39.092** Poisoning by salicylates, intentional self-harm
    +7th **T39.093** Poisoning by salicylates, assault
    +7th **T39.094** Poisoning by salicylates, undetermined
    +7th **T39.095** Adverse effect of salicylates
    +7th **T39.096** Underdosing of salicylates
+ **T39.1** Poisoning by, adverse effect of and underdosing of 4-Aminophenol derivatives
  + **T39.1X** Poisoning by, adverse effect of and underdosing of 4-Aminophenol derivatives
    +7th **T39.1X1** Poisoning by 4-Aminophenol derivatives, accidental (unintentional)
       Poisoning by 4-Aminophenol derivatives NOS
    +7th **T39.1X2** Poisoning by 4-Aminophenol derivatives, intentional self-harm
    +7th **T39.1X3** Poisoning by 4-Aminophenol derivatives, assault

+7th **T39.1X4** Poisoning by 4-Aminophenol derivatives, undetermined

+7th **T39.1X5** Adverse effect of 4-Aminophenol derivatives

+7th **T39.1X6** Underdosing of 4-Aminophenol derivatives

+ **T39.2** Poisoning by, adverse effect of and underdosing of pyrazolone derivatives

 + **T39.2X** Poisoning by, adverse effect of and underdosing of pyrazolone derivatives

  +7th **T39.2X1** Poisoning by pyrazolone derivatives, accidental (unintentional)
   Poisoning by pyrazolone derivatives NOS

  +7th **T39.2X2** Poisoning by pyrazolone derivatives, intentional self-harm

  +7th **T39.2X3** Poisoning by pyrazolone derivatives, assault

  +7th **T39.2X4** Poisoning by pyrazolone derivatives, undetermined

  +7th **T39.2X5** Adverse effect of pyrazolone derivatives

  +7th **T39.2X6** Underdosing of pyrazolone derivatives

+ **T39.3** Poisoning by, adverse effect of and underdosing of other nonsteroidal anti-inflammatory drugs [NSAID]

 + **T39.31** Poisoning by, adverse effect of and underdosing of propionic acid derivatives
  Poisoning by, adverse effect of and underdosing of fenoprofen
  Poisoning by, adverse effect of and underdosing of flurbiprofen
  Poisoning by, adverse effect of and underdosing of ibuprofen
  Poisoning by, adverse effect of and underdosing of ketoprofen
  Poisoning by, adverse effect of and underdosing of naproxen
  Poisoning by, adverse effect of and underdosing of oxaprozin

  +7th **T39.311** Poisoning by propionic acid derivatives, accidental (unintentional)

  +7th **T39.312** Poisoning by propionic acid derivatives, intentional self-harm

  +7th **T39.313** Poisoning by propionic acid derivatives, assault

  +7th **T39.314** Poisoning by propionic acid derivatives, undetermined

  +7th **T39.315** Adverse effect of propionic acid derivatives

  +7th **T39.316** Underdosing of propionic acid derivatives

 + **T39.39** Poisoning by, adverse effect of and underdosing of other nonsteroidal anti-inflammatory drugs [NSAID]

  +7th **T39.391** Poisoning by other nonsteroidal anti-inflammatory drugs [NSAID], accidental (unintentional)
   Poisoning by other nonsteroidal anti-inflammatory drugs NOS

  +7th **T39.392** Poisoning by other nonsteroidal anti-inflammatory drugs [NSAID], intentional self-harm

  +7th **T39.393** Poisoning by other nonsteroidal anti-inflammatory drugs [NSAID], assault

  +7th **T39.394** Poisoning by other nonsteroidal anti-inflammatory drugs [NSAID], undetermined

  +7th **T39.395** Adverse effect of other nonsteroidal anti-inflammatory drugs [NSAID]

  +7th **T39.396** Underdosing of other nonsteroidal anti-inflammatory drugs [NSAID]

+ **T39.4** Poisoning by, adverse effect of and underdosing of antirheumatics, not elsewhere classified

 Excludes1: poisoning by, adverse effect of and underdosing of glucocorticoids (T38.0-)
  poisoning by, adverse effect of and underdosing of salicylates (T39.0-)

 + **T39.4X** Poisoning by, adverse effect of and underdosing of antirheumatics, not elsewhere classified

  +7th **T39.4X1** Poisoning by antirheumatics, not elsewhere classified, accidental (unintentional)
   Poisoning by antirheumatics, not elsewhere classified NOS

  +7th **T39.4X2** Poisoning by antirheumatics, not elsewhere classified, intentional self-harm

  +7th **T39.4X3** Poisoning by antirheumatics, not elsewhere classified, assault

  +7th **T39.4X4** Poisoning by antirheumatics, not elsewhere classified, undetermined

  +7th **T39.4X5** Adverse effect of antirheumatics, not elsewhere classified

  +7th **T39.4X6** Underdosing of antirheumatics, not elsewhere classified

+ **T39.8** Poisoning by, adverse effect of and underdosing of other nonopioid analgesics and antipyretics, not elsewhere classified

 + **T39.8X** Poisoning by, adverse effect of and underdosing of other nonopioid analgesics and antipyretics, not elsewhere classified

  +7th **T39.8X1** Poisoning by other nonopioid analgesics and antipyretics, not elsewhere classified, accidental (unintentional)
   Poisoning by other nonopioid analgesics and antipyretics, not elsewhere classified NOS

  +7th **T39.8X2** Poisoning by other nonopioid analgesics and antipyretics, not elsewhere classified, intentional self-harm

  +7th **T39.8X3** Poisoning by other nonopioid analgesics and antipyretics, not elsewhere classified, assault

  +7th **T39.8X4** Poisoning by other nonopioid analgesics and antipyretics, not elsewhere classified, undetermined

  +7th **T39.8X5** Adverse effect of other nonopioid analgesics and antipyretics, not elsewhere classified

  +7th **T39.8X6** Underdosing of other nonopioid analgesics and antipyretics, not elsewhere classified

+ **T39.9** Poisoning by, adverse effect of and underdosing of unspecified nonopioid analgesic, antipyretic and antirheumatic

 x+7th **T39.91** Poisoning by unspecified nonopioid analgesic, antipyretic and antirheumatic, accidental (unintentional)
  Poisoning by nonopioid analgesic, antipyretic and antirheumatic NOS

 x+7th **T39.92** Poisoning by unspecified nonopioid analgesic, antipyretic and antirheumatic, intentional self-harm

 x+7th **T39.93** Poisoning by unspecified nonopioid analgesic, antipyretic and antirheumatic, assault

 x+7th **T39.94** Poisoning by unspecified nonopioid analgesic, antipyretic and antirheumatic, undetermined

 x+7th **T39.95** Adverse effect of unspecified nonopioid analgesic, antipyretic and antirheumatic

 x+7th **T39.96** Underdosing of unspecified nonopioid analgesic, antipyretic and antirheumatic

T40 Poisoning by, adverse effect of and underdosing of narcotics and psychodysleptics [hallucinogens]

 Excludes2: drug dependence and related mental and behavioral disorders due to psychoactive substance use (F10.-F19.-)

 The appropriate 7th character is to be added to each code from category T40
 A initial encounter
 D subsequent encounter
 S sequela

+ **T40.0** Poisoning by, adverse effect of and underdosing of opium

 + **T40.0X** Poisoning by, adverse effect of and underdosing of opium

  +7th **T40.0X1** Poisoning by opium, accidental (unintentional)
   Poisoning by opium NOS

+7th **T40.0X2** Poisoning by opium, intentional self-harm

+7th **T40.0X3** Poisoning by opium, assault

+7th **T40.0X4** Poisoning by opium, undetermined

+7th **T40.0X5** Adverse effect of opium

+7th **T40.0X6** Underdosing of opium

+ **T40.1** Poisoning by and adverse effect of heroin

  + **T40.1X** Poisoning by and adverse effect of heroin

+7th **T40.1X1** Poisoning by heroin, accidental (unintentional)

    Poisoning by heroin NOS

+7th **T40.1X2** Poisoning by heroin, intentional self-harm

+7th **T40.1X3** Poisoning by heroin, assault

+7th **T40.1X4** Poisoning by heroin, undetermined

+ **T40.2** Poisoning by, adverse effect of and underdosing of other opioids

  + **T40.2X** Poisoning by, adverse effect of and underdosing of other opioids

+7th **T40.2X1** Poisoning by other opioids, accidental (unintentional)

    Poisoning by other opioids NOS

+7th **T40.2X2** Poisoning by other opioids, intentional self-harm

+7th **T40.2X3** Poisoning by other opioids, assault

+7th **T40.2X4** Poisoning by other opioids, undetermined

+7th **T40.2X5** Adverse effect of other opioids

    AHA CC: 2Q, 2020, 24

+7th **T40.2X6** Underdosing of other opioids

+ **T40.3** Poisoning by, adverse effect of and underdosing of methadone

  + **T40.3X** Poisoning by, adverse effect of and underdosing of methadone

+7th **T40.3X1** Poisoning by methadone, accidental (unintentional)

    Poisoning by methadone NOS

+7th **T40.3X2** Poisoning by methadone, intentional self-harm

+7th **T40.3X3** Poisoning by methadone, assault

+7th **T40.3X4** Poisoning by methadone, undetermined

+7th **T40.3X5** Adverse effect of methadone

+7th **T40.3X6** Underdosing of methadone

+ **T40.4** Poisoning by, adverse effect of and underdosing of other synthetic narcotics

  + **T40.41** Poisoning by, adverse effect of and underdosing of fentanyl or fentanyl analogs

+7th **T40.411** Poisoning by fentanyl or fentanyl analogs, accidental (unintentional)

+7th **T40.412** Poisoning by fentanyl or fentanyl analogs, intentional self-harm

+7th **T40.413** Poisoning by fentanyl or fentanyl analogs, assault

+7th **T40.414** Poisoning by fentanyl or fentanyl analogs, undetermined

+7th **T40.415** Adverse effect of fentanyl or fentanyl analogs

+7th **T40.416** Underdosing of fentanyl or fentanyl analogs

  + **T40.42** Poisoning by, adverse effect of and underdosing of tramadol

+7th **T40.421** Poisoning by tramadol, accidental (unintentional)

+7th **T40.422** Poisoning by tramadol, intentional self-harm

+7th **T40.423** Poisoning by tramadol, assault

+7th **T40.424** Poisoning by tramadol, undetermined

+7th **T40.425** Adverse effect of tramadol

+7th **T40.426** Underdosing of tramadol

  + **T40.49** Poisoning by, adverse effect of and underdosing of other synthetic narcotics

+7th **T40.491** Poisoning by other synthetic narcotics, accidental (unintentional)

+7th **T40.492** Poisoning by other synthetic narcotics, intentional self-harm

+7th **T40.493** Poisoning by other synthetic narcotics, assault

+7th **T40.494** Poisoning by other synthetic narcotics, undetermined

+7th **T40.495** Adverse effect of other synthetic narcotics

+7th **T40.496** Underdosing of other synthetic narcotics

+ **T40.5** Poisoning by, adverse effect of and underdosing of cocaine

  + **T40.5X** Poisoning by, adverse effect of and underdosing of cocaine

+7th **T40.5X1** Poisoning by cocaine, accidental (unintentional)

    Poisoning by cocaine NOS

    AHA CC: 2Q, 2016, 8-9

+7th **T40.5X2** Poisoning by cocaine, intentional self-harm

+7th **T40.5X3** Poisoning by cocaine, assault

+7th **T40.5X4** Poisoning by cocaine, undetermined

+7th **T40.5X5** Adverse effect of cocaine

+7th **T40.5X6** Underdosing of cocaine

+ **T40.6** Poisoning by, adverse effect of and underdosing of other and unspecified narcotics

  + **T40.60** Poisoning by, adverse effect of and underdosing of unspecified narcotics

+7th **T40.601** Poisoning by unspecified narcotics, accidental (unintentional)

    Poisoning by narcotics NOS

+7th **T40.602** Poisoning by unspecified narcotics, intentional self-harm

+7th **T40.603** Poisoning by unspecified narcotics, assault

+7th **T40.604** Poisoning by unspecified narcotics, undetermined

+7th **T40.605** Adverse effect of unspecified narcotics

+7th **T40.606** Underdosing of unspecified narcotics

  + **T40.69** Poisoning by, adverse effect of and underdosing of other narcotics

+7th **T40.691** Poisoning by other narcotics, accidental (unintentional)

    Poisoning by other narcotics NOS

+7th **T40.692** Poisoning by other narcotics, intentional self-harm

+7th **T40.693** Poisoning by other narcotics, assault

+7th **T40.694** Poisoning by other narcotics, undetermined

+7th **T40.695** Adverse effect of other narcotics

+7th **T40.696** Underdosing of other narcotics

+ **T40.7** Poisoning by, adverse effect of and underdosing of cannabis (derivatives)

  + **T40.7X** Poisoning by, adverse effect of and underdosing of cannabis (derivatives)

+7th **T40.7X1** Poisoning by cannabis (derivatives), accidental (unintentional)

    Poisoning by cannabis NOS

    AHA CC: 1Q, 2020, 8

+7th **T40.7X2** Poisoning by cannabis (derivatives), intentional self-harm

+7th **T40.7X3** Poisoning by cannabis (derivatives), assault

+7th **T40.7X4** Poisoning by cannabis (derivatives), undetermined

+7th **T40.7X5** Adverse effect of cannabis (derivatives)

+7th **T40.7X6** Underdosing of cannabis (derivatives)

+ **T40.8** Poisoning by and adverse effect of lysergide [LSD]

  + **T40.8X** Poisoning by and adverse effect of lysergide [LSD]

+7th **T40.8X1** Poisoning by lysergide [LSD], accidental (unintentional)

    Poisoning by lysergide [LSD] NOS

+7th **T40.8X2** Poisoning by lysergide [LSD], intentional self-harm

+7th **T40.8X3** Poisoning by lysergide [LSD], assault

+7th **T40.8X4** Poisoning by lysergide [LSD], undetermined

+ **T40.9** Poisoning by, adverse effect of and underdosing of other and unspecified psychodysleptics [hallucinogens]

  + **T40.90** Poisoning by, adverse effect of and underdosing of unspecified psychodysleptics [hallucinogens]

+7th **T40.901** Poisoning by unspecified psychodysleptics [hallucinogens], accidental (unintentional)

+7th **T40.902** Poisoning by unspecified psychodysleptics [hallucinogens], intentional self-harm

+, +7th, X + 7th   ● Newborn   ● Pediatric   ● Maternity   ● Adult   ♀ Female   ♂ Male   Manifestation   Unacceptable PDX   HCC   CC   MCC   HAC

+7th **T40.903** **Poisoning by unspecified psychodysleptics [hallucinogens], assault**

+7th **T40.904** **Poisoning by unspecified psychodysleptics [hallucinogens], undetermined**

+7th **T40.905** **Adverse effect of unspecified psychodysleptics [hallucinogens]**

+7th **T40.906** **Underdosing of unspecified psychodysleptics [hallucinogens]**

+ **T40.99** **Poisoning by, adverse effect of and underdosing of other psychodysleptics [hallucinogens]**

+7th **T40.991** **Poisoning by other psychodysleptics [hallucinogens], accidental (unintentional)**
Poisoning by other psychodysleptics [hallucinogens] NOS

+7th **T40.992** **Poisoning by other psychodysleptics [hallucinogens], intentional self-harm**

+7th **T40.993** **Poisoning by other psychodysleptics [hallucinogens], assault**

+7th **T40.994** **Poisoning by other psychodysleptics [hallucinogens], undetermined**

+7th **T40.995** **Adverse effect of other psychodysleptics [hallucinogens]**

+7th **T40.996** **Underdosing of other psychodysleptics [hallucinogens]**

T41 **Poisoning by, adverse effect of and underdosing of anesthetics and therapeutic gases**

Excludes1: *benzodiazepines (T42.4-)*
cocaine (T40.5-)
complications of anesthesia during pregnancy (O29.-)
complications of anesthesia during labor and delivery (O74.-)
complications of anesthesia during the puerperium (O89.-)
opioids (T40.0-T40.2-)

The appropriate 7th character is to be added to each code from category T41
A   initial encounter
D   subsequent encounter
S   sequela

+ **T41.0** **Poisoning by, adverse effect of and underdosing of inhaled anesthetics**
Excludes1: *oxygen (T41.5-)*

+ **T41.0X** **Poisoning by, adverse effect of and underdosing of inhaled anesthetics**

+7th **T41.0X1** **Poisoning by inhaled anesthetics, accidental (unintentional)**
Poisoning by inhaled anesthetics NOS

+7th **T41.0X2** **Poisoning by inhaled anesthetics, intentional self-harm**

+7th **T41.0X3** **Poisoning by inhaled anesthetics, assault**

+7th **T41.0X4** **Poisoning by inhaled anesthetics, undetermined**

+7th **T41.0X5** **Adverse effect of inhaled anesthetics**

+7th **T41.0X6** **Underdosing of inhaled anesthetics**

+ **T41.1** **Poisoning by, adverse effect of and underdosing of intravenous anesthetics**
Poisoning by, adverse effect of and underdosing of thiobarbiturates

+ **T41.1X** **Poisoning by, adverse effect of and underdosing of intravenous anesthetics**

+7th **T41.1X1** **Poisoning by intravenous anesthetics, accidental (unintentional)**
Poisoning by intravenous anesthetics NOS

+7th **T41.1X2** **Poisoning by intravenous anesthetics, intentional self-harm**

+7th **T41.1X3** **Poisoning by intravenous anesthetics, assault**

+7th **T41.1X4** **Poisoning by intravenous anesthetics, undetermined**

+7th **T41.1X5** **Adverse effect of intravenous anesthetics**

+7th **T41.1X6** **Underdosing of intravenous anesthetics**

+ **T41.2** **Poisoning by, adverse effect of and underdosing of other and unspecified general anesthetics**

+ **T41.20** **Poisoning by, adverse effect of and underdosing of unspecified general anesthetics**

+7th **T41.201** **Poisoning by unspecified general anesthetics, accidental (unintentional)**
Poisoning by general anesthetics NOS

+7th **T41.202** **Poisoning by unspecified general anesthetics, intentional self-harm**

+7th **T41.203** **Poisoning by unspecified general anesthetics, assault**

+7th **T41.204** **Poisoning by unspecified general anesthetics, undetermined**

+7th **T41.205** **Adverse effect of unspecified general anesthetics**
AHA CC: 4Q, 2016, 72-73

+7th **T41.206** **Underdosing of unspecified general anesthetics**

+ **T41.29** **Poisoning by, adverse effect of and underdosing of other general anesthetics**

+7th **T41.291** **Poisoning by other general anesthetics, accidental (unintentional)**
Poisoning by other general anesthetics NOS

+7th **T41.292** **Poisoning by other general anesthetics, intentional self-harm**

+7th **T41.293** **Poisoning by other general anesthetics, assault**

+7th **T41.294** **Poisoning by other general anesthetics, undetermined**

+7th **T41.295** **Adverse effect of other general anesthetics**

+7th **T41.296** **Underdosing of other general anesthetics**

+ **T41.3** **Poisoning by, adverse effect of and underdosing of local anesthetics**
Cocaine (topical)
Excludes2: *poisoning by cocaine used as a central nervous system stimulant (T40.5X1-T40.5X4)*

+ **T41.3X** **Poisoning by, adverse effect of and underdosing of local anesthetics**

+7th **T41.3X1** **Poisoning by local anesthetics, accidental (unintentional)**
Poisoning by local anesthetics NOS

+7th **T41.3X2** **Poisoning by local anesthetics, intentional self-harm**

+7th **T41.3X3** **Poisoning by local anesthetics, assault**

+7th **T41.3X4** **Poisoning by local anesthetics, undetermined**

+7th **T41.3X5** **Adverse effect of local anesthetics**

+7th **T41.3X6** **Underdosing of local anesthetics**

+ **T41.4** **Poisoning by, adverse effect of and underdosing of unspecified anesthetic**

X+7th **T41.41** **Poisoning by unspecified anesthetic, accidental (unintentional)**
Poisoning by anesthetic NOS

X+7th **T41.42** **Poisoning by unspecified anesthetic, intentional self-harm**

X+7th **T41.43** **Poisoning by unspecified anesthetic, assault**

X+7th **T41.44** **Poisoning by unspecified anesthetic, undetermined**

X+7th **T41.45** **Adverse effect of unspecified anesthetic**

X+7th **T41.46** **Underdosing of unspecified anesthetics**

+ **T41.5** **Poisoning by, adverse effect of and underdosing of therapeutic gases**

+ **T41.5X** **Poisoning by, adverse effect of and underdosing of therapeutic gases**

+7th **T41.5X1** **Poisoning by therapeutic gases, accidental (unintentional)**
Poisoning by therapeutic gases NOS

+7th **T41.5X2** **Poisoning by therapeutic gases, intentional self-harm**

+7th **T41.5X3** **Poisoning by therapeutic gases, assault**

+7th **T41.5X4** **Poisoning by therapeutic gases, undetermined**

+7th **T41.5X5** **Adverse effect of therapeutic gases**

+7th **T41.5X6** **Underdosing of therapeutic gases**

T42 Poisoning by, adverse effect of and underdosing of antiepileptic, sedative- hypnotic and antiparkinsonism drugs

> *Excludes2:* drug dependence and related mental and behavioral disorders due to psychoactive substance use (F10.--F19.-)

> The appropriate 7th character is to be added to each code from category T42
> A   initial encounter
> D   subsequent encounter
> S   sequela

+ **T42.0   Poisoning by, adverse effect of and underdosing of hydantoin derivatives**
> + **T42.0X   Poisoning by, adverse effect of and underdosing of hydantoin derivatives**
> > +7th **T42.0X1   Poisoning by hydantoin derivatives, accidental (unintentional)**
> > > Poisoning by hydantoin derivatives NOS
> > +7th **T42.0X2   Poisoning by hydantoin derivatives, intentional self-harm**
> > +7th **T42.0X3   Poisoning by hydantoin derivatives, assault**
> > +7th **T42.0X4   Poisoning by hydantoin derivatives, undetermined**
> > +7th **T42.0X5   Adverse effect of hydantoin derivatives**
> > +7th **T42.0X6   Underdosing of hydantoin derivatives**

+ **T42.1   Poisoning by, adverse effect of and underdosing of iminostilbenes**
> Poisoning by, adverse effect of and underdosing of carbamazepine
> + **T42.1X   Poisoning by, adverse effect of and underdosing of iminostilbenes**
> > +7th **T42.1X1   Poisoning by iminostilbenes, accidental (unintentional)**
> > > Poisoning by iminostilbenes NOS
> > +7th **T42.1X2   Poisoning by iminostilbenes, intentional self-harm**
> > +7th **T42.1X3   Poisoning by iminostilbenes, assault**
> > +7th **T42.1X4   Poisoning by iminostilbenes, undetermined**
> > +7th **T42.1X5   Adverse effect of iminostilbenes**
> > +7th **T42.1X6   Underdosing of iminostilbenes**

+ **T42.2   Poisoning by, adverse effect of and underdosing of succinimides and oxazolidinediones**
> + **T42.2X   Poisoning by, adverse effect of and underdosing of succinimides and oxazolidinediones**
> > +7th **T42.2X1   Poisoning by succinimides and oxazolidinediones, accidental (unintentional)**
> > > Poisoning by succinimides and oxazolidinediones NOS
> > +7th **T42.2X2   Poisoning by succinimides and oxazolidinediones, intentional self-harm**
> > +7th **T42.2X3   Poisoning by succinimides and oxazolidinediones, assault**
> > +7th **T42.2X4   Poisoning by succinimides and oxazolidinediones, undetermined**
> > +7th **T42.2X5   Adverse effect of succinimides and oxazolidinediones**
> > +7th **T42.2X6   Underdosing of succinimides and oxazolidinediones**

+ **T42.3   Poisoning by, adverse effect of and underdosing of barbiturates**
> *Excludes1:* poisoning by, adverse effect of and underdosing of thiobarbiturates (T41.1-)
> + **T42.3X   Poisoning by, adverse effect of and underdosing of barbiturates**
> > +7th **T42.3X1   Poisoning by barbiturates, accidental (unintentional)**
> > > Poisoning by barbiturates NOS
> > +7th **T42.3X2   Poisoning by barbiturates, intentional self-harm**
> > +7th **T42.3X3   Poisoning by barbiturates, assault**
> > +7th **T42.3X4   Poisoning by barbiturates, undetermined**
> > +7th **T42.3X5   Adverse effect of barbiturates**
> > +7th **T42.3X6   Underdosing of barbiturates**

+ **T42.4   Poisoning by, adverse effect of and underdosing of benzodiazepines**
> + **T42.4X   Poisoning by, adverse effect of and underdosing of benzodiazepines**
> > +7th **T42.4X1   Poisoning by benzodiazepines, accidental (unintentional)**
> > > Poisoning by benzodiazepines NOS
> > +7th **T42.4X2   Poisoning by benzodiazepines, intentional self-harm**
> > +7th **T42.4X3   Poisoning by benzodiazepines, assault**
> > +7th **T42.4X4   Poisoning by benzodiazepines, undetermined**
> > +7th **T42.4X5   Adverse effect of benzodiazepines**
> > +7th **T42.4X6   Underdosing of benzodiazepines**

+ **T42.5   Poisoning by, adverse effect of and underdosing of mixed antiepileptics**
> + **T42.5X   Poisoning by, adverse effect of and underdosing of antiepileptics**
> > +7th **T42.5X1   Poisoning by mixed antiepileptics, accidental (unintentional)**
> > > Poisoning by mixed antiepileptics NOS
> > +7th **T42.5X2   Poisoning by mixed antiepileptics, intentional self-harm**
> > +7th **T42.5X3   Poisoning by mixed antiepileptics, assault**
> > +7th **T42.5X4   Poisoning by mixed antiepileptics, undetermined**
> > +7th **T42.5X5   Adverse effect of mixed antiepileptics**
> > +7th **T42.5X6   Underdosing of mixed antiepileptics**

+ **T42.6   Poisoning by, adverse effect of and underdosing of other antiepileptic and sedative-hypnotic drugs**
> Poisoning by, adverse effect of and underdosing of methaqualone
> Poisoning by, adverse effect of and underdosing of valproic acid
> *Excludes1:* poisoning by, adverse effect of and underdosing of carbamazepine (T42.1-)
> + **T42.6X   Poisoning by, adverse effect of and underdosing of other antiepileptic and sedative-hypnotic drugs**
> > +7th **T42.6X1   Poisoning by other antiepileptic and sedative-hypnotic drugs, accidental (unintentional)**
> > > Poisoning by other antiepileptic and sedative-hypnotic drugs NOS
> > +7th **T42.6X2   Poisoning by other antiepileptic and sedative-hypnotic drugs, intentional self-harm**
> > +7th **T42.6X3   Poisoning by other antiepileptic and sedative-hypnotic drugs, assault**
> > +7th **T42.6X4   Poisoning by other antiepileptic and sedative-hypnotic drugs, undetermined**
> > +7th **T42.6X5   Adverse effect of other antiepileptic and sedative-hypnotic drugs**
> > +7th **T42.6X6   Underdosing of other antiepileptic and sedative-hypnotic drugs**

+ **T42.7   Poisoning by, adverse effect of and underdosing of unspecified antiepileptic and sedative-hypnotic drugs**
> X+7th **T42.71   Poisoning by unspecified antiepileptic and sedative-hypnotic drugs, accidental (unintentional)**
> > Poisoning by antiepileptic and sedative-hypnotic drugs NOS
> X+7th **T42.72   Poisoning by unspecified antiepileptic and sedative-hypnotic drugs, intentional self-harm**
> X+7th **T42.73   Poisoning by unspecified antiepileptic and sedative-hypnotic drugs, assault**
> X+7th **T42.74   Poisoning by unspecified antiepileptic and sedative-hypnotic drugs, undetermined**
> X+7th **T42.75   Adverse effect of unspecified antiepileptic and sedative-hypnotic drugs**
> X+7th **T42.76   Underdosing of unspecified antiepileptic and sedative-hypnotic drugs**

+ **T42.8** **Poisoning by, adverse effect of and underdosing of antiparkinsonism drugs and other central muscle-tone depressants**

    Poisoning by, adverse effect of and underdosing of amantadine

    + **T42.8X** **Poisoning by, adverse effect of and underdosing of antiparkinsonism drugs and other central muscle-tone depressants**

        +7th **T42.8X1** **Poisoning by antiparkinsonism drugs and other central muscle-tone depressants, accidental (unintentional)**

            Poisoning by antiparkinsonism drugs and other central muscle-tone depressants NOS

        +7th **T42.8X2** **Poisoning by antiparkinsonism drugs and other central muscle-tone depressants, intentional self-harm**

        +7th **T42.8X3** **Poisoning by antiparkinsonism drugs and other central muscle-tone depressants, assault**

        +7th **T42.8X4** **Poisoning by antiparkinsonism drugs and other central muscle-tone depressants, undetermined**

        +7th **T42.8X5** **Adverse effect of antiparkinsonism drugs and other central muscle-tone depressants**

        +7th **T42.8X6** **Underdosing of antiparkinsonism drugs and other central muscle-tone depressants**

T43 **Poisoning by, adverse effect of and underdosing of psychotropic drugs, not elsewhere classified**

    Excludes1: *appetite depressants (T50.5-)*
            barbiturates (T42.3-)
            benzodiazepines (T42.4-)
            methaqualone (T42.6-)
            psychodysleptics [hallucinogens] (T40.7-T40.9-)
    Excludes2: *drug dependence and related mental and behavioral disorders due to psychoactive substance use (F10.--F19.-)*

> The appropriate 7th character is to be added to each code from category T43
> A   initial encounter
> D   subsequent encounter
> S   sequela

+ **T43.0** **Poisoning by, adverse effect of and underdosing of tricyclic and tetracyclic antidepressants**

    + **T43.01** **Poisoning by, adverse effect of and underdosing of tricyclic antidepressants**

        +7th **T43.011** **Poisoning by tricyclic antidepressants, accidental (unintentional)**

            Poisoning by tricyclic antidepressants NOS

        +7th **T43.012** **Poisoning by tricyclic antidepressants, intentional self-harm**

        +7th **T43.013** **Poisoning by tricyclic antidepressants, assault**

        +7th **T43.014** **Poisoning by tricyclic antidepressants, undetermined**

        +7th **T43.015** **Adverse effect of tricyclic antidepressants**

        +7th **T43.016** **Underdosing of tricyclic antidepressants**

    + **T43.02** **Poisoning by, adverse effect of and underdosing of tetracyclic antidepressants**

        +7th **T43.021** **Poisoning by tetracyclic antidepressants, accidental (unintentional)**

            Poisoning by tetracyclic antidepressants NOS

        +7th **T43.022** **Poisoning by tetracyclic antidepressants, intentional self-harm**

        +7th **T43.023** **Poisoning by tetracyclic antidepressants, assault**

        +7th **T43.024** **Poisoning by tetracyclic antidepressants, undetermined**

        +7th **T43.025** **Adverse effect of tetracyclic antidepressants**

        +7th **T43.026** **Underdosing of tetracyclic antidepressants**

+ **T43.1** **Poisoning by, adverse effect of and underdosing of monoamine-oxidase-inhibitor antidepressants**

    + **T43.1X** **Poisoning by, adverse effect of and underdosing of monoamine-oxidase-inhibitor antidepressants**

        +7th **T43.1X1** **Poisoning by monoamine-oxidase-inhibitor antidepressants, accidental (unintentional)**

            Poisoning by monoamine-oxidase-inhibitor antidepressants NOS

        +7th **T43.1X2** **Poisoning by monoamine-oxidase-inhibitor antidepressants, intentional self-harm**

        +7th **T43.1X3** **Poisoning by monoamine-oxidase-inhibitor antidepressants, assault**

        +7th **T43.1X4** **Poisoning by monoamine-oxidase-inhibitor antidepressants, undetermined**

        +7th **T43.1X5** **Adverse effect of monoamine-oxidase-inhibitor antidepressants**

        +7th **T43.1X6** **Underdosing of monoamine-oxidase-inhibitor antidepressants**

+ **T43.2** **Poisoning by, adverse effect of and underdosing of other and unspecified antidepressants**

    + **T43.20** **Poisoning by, adverse effect of and underdosing of unspecified antidepressants**

        +7th **T43.201** **Poisoning by unspecified antidepressants, accidental (unintentional)**

            Poisoning by antidepressants NOS

        +7th **T43.202** **Poisoning by unspecified antidepressants, intentional self-harm**

        +7th **T43.203** **Poisoning by unspecified antidepressants, assault**

        +7th **T43.204** **Poisoning by unspecified antidepressants, undetermined**

        +7th **T43.205** **Adverse effect of unspecified antidepressants**

            Antidepressant discontinuation syndrome

        +7th **T43.206** **Underdosing of unspecified antidepressants**

    + **T43.21** **Poisoning by, adverse effect of and underdosing of selective serotonin and norepinephrine reuptake inhibitors**

        Poisoning by, adverse effect of and underdosing of SSNRI antidepressants

        +7th **T43.211** **Poisoning by selective serotonin and norepinephrine reuptake inhibitors, accidental (unintentional)**

        +7th **T43.212** **Poisoning by selective serotonin and norepinephrine reuptake inhibitors, intentional self-harm**

        +7th **T43.213** **Poisoning by selective serotonin and norepinephrine reuptake inhibitors, assault**

        +7th **T43.214** **Poisoning by selective serotonin and norepinephrine reuptake inhibitors, undetermined**

        +7th **T43.215** **Adverse effect of selective serotonin and norepinephrine reuptake inhibitors**

        +7th **T43.216** **Underdosing of selective serotonin and norepinephrine reuptake inhibitors**

    + **T43.22** **Poisoning by, adverse effect of and underdosing of selective serotonin reuptake inhibitors**

        Poisoning by, adverse effect of and underdosing of SSRI antidepressants

        +7th **T43.221** **Poisoning by selective serotonin reuptake inhibitors, accidental (unintentional)**

        +7th **T43.222** **Poisoning by selective serotonin reuptake inhibitors, intentional self-harm**

        +7th **T43.223** **Poisoning by selective serotonin reuptake inhibitors, assault**

        +7th **T43.224** **Poisoning by selective serotonin reuptake inhibitors, undetermined**

        +7th **T43.225** **Adverse effect of selective serotonin reuptake inhibitors**

        +7th **T43.226** **Underdosing of selective serotonin reuptake inhibitors**

+, +7th, X + 7th   ● Newborn   ● Pediatric   ● Maternity   ● Adult   ♀ Female   ♂ Male   Manifestation   Unacceptable PDX   HCC   CC   MCC   HAC

+ **T43.29** Poisoning by, adverse effect of and underdosing of other antidepressants

+7th **T43.291** Poisoning by other antidepressants, accidental (unintentional)

Poisoning by other antidepressants NOS

+7th **T43.292** Poisoning by other antidepressants, intentional self-harm

+7th **T43.293** Poisoning by other antidepressants, assault

+7th **T43.294** Poisoning by other antidepressants, undetermined

+7th **T43.295** Adverse effect of other antidepressants

+7th **T43.296** Underdosing of other antidepressants

+ **T43.3** Poisoning by, adverse effect of and underdosing of phenothiazine antipsychotics and neuroleptics

+ **T43.3X** Poisoning by, adverse effect of and underdosing of phenothiazine antipsychotics and neuroleptics

+7th **T43.3X1** Poisoning by phenothiazine antipsychotics and neuroleptics, accidental (unintentional)

Poisoning by phenothiazine antipsychotics and neuroleptics NOS

+7th **T43.3X2** Poisoning by phenothiazine antipsychotics and neuroleptics, intentional self-harm

+7th **T43.3X3** Poisoning by phenothiazine antipsychotics and neuroleptics, assault

+7th **T43.3X4** Poisoning by phenothiazine antipsychotics and neuroleptics, undetermined

+7th **T43.3X5** Adverse effect of phenothiazine antipsychotics and neuroleptics

+7th **T43.3X6** Underdosing of phenothiazine antipsychotics and neuroleptics

+ **T43.4** Poisoning by, adverse effect of and underdosing of butyrophenone and thiothixene neuroleptics

+ **T43.4X** Poisoning by, adverse effect of and underdosing of butyrophenone and thiothixene neuroleptics

+7th **T43.4X1** Poisoning by butyrophenone and thiothixene neuroleptics, accidental (unintentional)

Poisoning by butyrophenone and thiothixene neuroleptics NOS

+7th **T43.4X2** Poisoning by butyrophenone and thiothixene neuroleptics, intentional self-harm

+7th **T43.4X3** Poisoning by butyrophenone and thiothixene neuroleptics, assault

+7th **T43.4X4** Poisoning by butyrophenone and thiothixene neuroleptics, undetermined

+7th **T43.4X5** Adverse effect of butyrophenone and thiothixene neuroleptics

+7th **T43.4X6** Underdosing of butyrophenone and thiothixene neuroleptics

+ **T43.5** Poisoning by, adverse effect of and underdosing of other and unspecified antipsychotics and neuroleptics

Excludes1: *poisoning by, adverse effect of and underdosing of rauwolfia (T46.5-)*

+ **T43.50** Poisoning by, adverse effect of and underdosing of unspecified antipsychotics and neuroleptics

+7th **T43.501** Poisoning by unspecified antipsychotics and neuroleptics, accidental (unintentional)

Poisoning by antipsychotics and neuroleptics NOS

+7th **T43.502** Poisoning by unspecified antipsychotics and neuroleptics, intentional self-harm

+7th **T43.503** Poisoning by unspecified antipsychotics and neuroleptics, assault

+7th **T43.504** Poisoning by unspecified antipsychotics and neuroleptics, undetermined

+7th **T43.505** Adverse effect of unspecified antipsychotics and neuroleptics

+7th **T43.506** Underdosing of unspecified antipsychotics and neuroleptics

+ **T43.59** Poisoning by, adverse effect of and underdosing of other antipsychotics and neuroleptics

+7th **T43.591** Poisoning by other antipsychotics and neuroleptics, accidental (unintentional)

Poisoning by other antipsychotics and neuroleptics NOS

+7th **T43.592** Poisoning by other antipsychotics and neuroleptics, intentional self-harm

AHA CC: 1Q, 2017, 40

+7th **T43.593** Poisoning by other antipsychotics and neuroleptics, assault

+7th **T43.594** Poisoning by other antipsychotics and neuroleptics, undetermined

+7th **T43.595** Adverse effect of other antipsychotics and neuroleptics

+7th **T43.596** Underdosing of other antipsychotics and neuroleptics

+ **T43.6** Poisoning by, adverse effect of and underdosing of psychostimulants

Excludes1: *poisoning by, adverse effect of and underdosing of cocaine (T40.5-)*

+ **T43.60** Poisoning by, adverse effect of and underdosing of unspecified psychostimulant

+7th **T43.601** Poisoning by unspecified psychostimulants, accidental (unintentional)

Poisoning by psychostimulants NOS

+7th **T43.602** Poisoning by unspecified psychostimulants, intentional self-harm

+7th **T43.603** Poisoning by unspecified psychostimulants, assault

+7th **T43.604** Poisoning by unspecified psychostimulants, undetermined

+7th **T43.605** Adverse effect of unspecified psychostimulants

+7th **T43.606** Underdosing of unspecified psychostimulants

+ **T43.61** Poisoning by, adverse effect of and underdosing of caffeine

+7th **T43.611** Poisoning by caffeine, accidental (unintentional)

Poisoning by caffeine NOS

+7th **T43.612** Poisoning by caffeine, intentional self-harm

+7th **T43.613** Poisoning by caffeine, assault

+7th **T43.614** Poisoning by caffeine, undetermined

+7th **T43.615** Adverse effect of caffeine

+7th **T43.616** Underdosing of caffeine

+ **T43.62** Poisoning by, adverse effect of and underdosing of amphetamines

Poisoning by, adverse effect of and underdosing of methamphetamines

+7th **T43.621** Poisoning by amphetamines, accidental (unintentional)

Poisoning by amphetamines NOS

+7th **T43.622** Poisoning by amphetamines, intentional self-harm

+7th **T43.623** Poisoning by amphetamines, assault

+7th **T43.624** Poisoning by amphetamines, undetermined

+7th **T43.625** Adverse effect of amphetamines

+7th **T43.626** Underdosing of amphetamines

+ **T43.63** Poisoning by, adverse effect of and underdosing of methylphenidate

+7th **T43.631** Poisoning by methylphenidate, accidental (unintentional)

Poisoning by methylphenidate NOS

+7th **T43.632** Poisoning by methylphenidate, intentional self-harm

+7th **T43.633** Poisoning by methylphenidate, assault

+7th **T43.634** Poisoning by methylphenidate, undetermined

+7th **T43.635** Adverse effect of methylphenidate

+7th **T43.636** Underdosing of methylphenidate

+ **T43.64** **Poisoning by ecstasy**
Poisoning by MDMA
Poisoning by 3,4-methylenedioxymethamphetamine
AHA CC: 4Q, 2018, 30-31
+7th **T43.641** **Poisoning by ecstasy, accidental (unintentional)**
Poisoning by ecstasy NOS
AHA CC: 4Q, 2018, 31
+7th **T43.642** **Poisoning by ecstasy, intentional self-harm**
+7th **T43.643** **Poisoning by ecstasy, assault**
+7th **T43.644** **Poisoning by ecstasy, undetermined**
+ **T43.69** **Poisoning by, adverse effect of and underdosing of other psychostimulants**
+7th **T43.691** **Poisoning by other psychostimulants, accidental (unintentional)**
Poisoning by other psychostimulants NOS
+7th **T43.692** **Poisoning by other psychostimulants, intentional self-harm**
+7th **T43.693** **Poisoning by other psychostimulants, assault**
+7th **T43.694** **Poisoning by other psychostimulants, undetermined**
+7th **T43.695** **Adverse effect of other psychostimulants**
+7th **T43.696** **Underdosing of other psychostimulants**
+ **T43.8** **Poisoning by, adverse effect of and underdosing of other psychotropic drugs**
+ **T43.8X** **Poisoning by, adverse effect of and underdosing of other psychotropic drugs**
+7th **T43.8X1** **Poisoning by other psychotropic drugs, accidental (unintentional)**
Poisoning by other psychotropic drugs NOS
+7th **T43.8X2** **Poisoning by other psychotropic drugs, intentional self-harm**
+7th **T43.8X3** **Poisoning by other psychotropic drugs, assault**
+7th **T43.8X4** **Poisoning by other psychotropic drugs, undetermined**
+7th **T43.8X5** **Adverse effect of other psychotropic drugs**
+7th **T43.8X6** **Underdosing of other psychotropic drugs**
+ **T43.9** **Poisoning by, adverse effect of and underdosing of unspecified psychotropic drug**
X+7th **T43.91** **Poisoning by unspecified psychotropic drug, accidental (unintentional)**
Poisoning by psychotropic drug NOS
X+7th **T43.92** **Poisoning by unspecified psychotropic drug, intentional self-harm**
X+7th **T43.93** **Poisoning by unspecified psychotropic drug, assault**
X+7th **T43.94** **Poisoning by unspecified psychotropic drug, undetermined**
X+7th **T43.95** **Adverse effect of unspecified psychotropic drug**
X+7th **T43.96** **Underdosing of unspecified psychotropic drug**

T44 **Poisoning by, adverse effect of and underdosing of drugs primarily affecting the autonomic nervous system**

The appropriate 7th character is to be added to each code from category T44
A initial encounter
D subsequent encounter
S sequela

+ **T44.0** **Poisoning by, adverse effect of and underdosing of anticholinesterase agents**
+ **T44.0X** **Poisoning by, adverse effect of and underdosing of anticholinesterase agents**
+7th **T44.0X1** **Poisoning by anticholinesterase agents, accidental (unintentional)**
Poisoning by anticholinesterase agents NOS
+7th **T44.0X2** **Poisoning by anticholinesterase agents, intentional self-harm**
+7th **T44.0X3** **Poisoning by anticholinesterase agents, assault**
+7th **T44.0X4** **Poisoning by anticholinesterase agents, undetermined**

+7th **T44.0X5** **Adverse effect of anticholinesterase agents**
+7th **T44.0X6** **Underdosing of anticholinesterase agents**
+ **T44.1** **Poisoning by, adverse effect of and underdosing of other parasympathomimetics [cholinergics]**
+ **T44.1X** **Poisoning by, adverse effect of and underdosing of other parasympathomimetics [cholinergics]**
+7th **T44.1X1** **Poisoning by other parasympathomimetics [cholinergics], accidental (unintentional)**
Poisoning by other parasympathomimetics [cholinergics] NOS
+7th **T44.1X2** **Poisoning by other parasympathomimetics [cholinergics], intentional self-harm**
+7th **T44.1X3** **Poisoning by other parasympathomimetics [cholinergics], assault**
+7th **T44.1X4** **Poisoning by other parasympathomimetics [cholinergics], undetermined**
+7th **T44.1X5** **Adverse effect of other parasympathomimetics [cholinergics]**
+7th **T44.1X6** **Underdosing of other parasympathomimetics [cholinergics]**
+ **T44.2** **Poisoning by, adverse effect of and underdosing of ganglionic blocking drugs**
+ **T44.2X** **Poisoning by, adverse effect of and underdosing of ganglionic blocking drugs**
+7th **T44.2X1** **Poisoning by ganglionic blocking drugs, accidental (unintentional)**
Poisoning by ganglionic blocking drugs NOS
+7th **T44.2X2** **Poisoning by ganglionic blocking drugs, intentional self-harm**
+7th **T44.2X3** **Poisoning by ganglionic blocking drugs, assault**
+7th **T44.2X4** **Poisoning by ganglionic blocking drugs, undetermined**
+7th **T44.2X5** **Adverse effect of ganglionic blocking drugs**
+7th **T44.2X6** **Underdosing of ganglionic blocking drugs**
+ **T44.3** **Poisoning by, adverse effect of and underdosing of other parasympatholytics [anticholinergics and antimuscarinics] and spasmolytics**
Poisoning by, adverse effect of and underdosing of papaverine
+ **T44.3X** **Poisoning by, adverse effect of and underdosing of other parasympatholytics [anticholinergics and antimuscarinics] and spasmolytics**
+7th **T44.3X1** **Poisoning by other parasympatholytics [anticholinergics and antimuscarinics] and spasmolytics, accidental (unintentional)**
Poisoning by other parasympatholytics [anticholinergics and antimuscarinics] and spasmolytics NOS
+7th **T44.3X2** **Poisoning by other parasympatholytics [anticholinergics and antimuscarinics] and spasmolytics, intentional self-harm**
+7th **T44.3X3** **Poisoning by other parasympatholytics [anticholinergics and antimuscarinics] and spasmolytics, assault**
+7th **T44.3X4** **Poisoning by other parasympatholytics [anticholinergics and antimuscarinics] and spasmolytics, undetermined**
+7th **T44.3X5** **Adverse effect of other parasympatholytics [anticholinergics and antimuscarinics] and spasmolytics**
+7th **T44.3X6** **Underdosing of other parasympatholytics [anticholinergics and antimuscarinics] and spasmolytics**

+, +7th, X + 7th • Newborn • Pediatric • Maternity • Adult ♀ Female ♂ Male Manifestation Unacceptable PDX HCC CC MCC HAC

+ **T44.4** **Poisoning by, adverse effect of and underdosing of predominantly alpha-adrenoreceptor agonists**
　　Poisoning by, adverse effect of and underdosing of metaraminol
　+ **T44.4X** **Poisoning by, adverse effect of and underdosing of predominantly alpha-adrenoreceptor agonists**
　　+7th **T44.4X1** **Poisoning by predominantly alpha-adrenoreceptor agonists, accidental (unintentional)**
　　　　Poisoning by predominantly alpha-adrenoreceptor agonists NOS
　　+7th **T44.4X2** **Poisoning by predominantly alpha-adrenoreceptor agonists, intentional self-harm**
　　+7th **T44.4X3** **Poisoning by predominantly alpha-adrenoreceptor agonists, assault**
　　+7th **T44.4X4** **Poisoning by predominantly alpha-adrenoreceptor agonists, undetermined**
　　+7th **T44.4X5** **Adverse effect of predominantly alpha-adrenoreceptor agonists**
　　+7th **T44.4X6** **Underdosing of predominantly alpha-adrenoreceptor agonists**

+ **T44.5** **Poisoning by, adverse effect of and underdosing of predominantly beta-adrenoreceptor agonists**
　　Excludes1: *poisoning by, adverse effect of and underdosing of beta-adrenoreceptor agonists used in asthma therapy (T48.6-)*
　+ **T44.5X** **Poisoning by, adverse effect of and underdosing of predominantly beta-adrenoreceptor agonists**
　　+7th **T44.5X1** **Poisoning by predominantly beta-adrenoreceptor agonists, accidental (unintentional)**
　　　　Poisoning by predominantly beta-adrenoreceptor agonists NOS
　　+7th **T44.5X2** **Poisoning by predominantly beta-adrenoreceptor agonists, intentional self-harm**
　　+7th **T44.5X3** **Poisoning by predominantly beta-adrenoreceptor agonists, assault**
　　+7th **T44.5X4** **Poisoning by predominantly beta-adrenoreceptor agonists, undetermined**
　　+7th **T44.5X5** **Adverse effect of predominantly beta-adrenoreceptor agonists**
　　+7th **T44.5X6** **Underdosing of predominantly beta-adrenoreceptor agonists**

+ **T44.6** **Poisoning by, adverse effect of and underdosing of alpha-adrenoreceptor antagonists**
　　Excludes1: *poisoning by, adverse effect of and underdosing of ergot alkaloids (T48.0)*
　+ **T44.6X** **Poisoning by, adverse effect of and underdosing of alpha-adrenoreceptor antagonists**
　　+7th **T44.6X1** **Poisoning by alpha-adrenoreceptor antagonists, accidental (unintentional)**
　　　　Poisoning by alpha-adrenoreceptor antagonists NOS
　　+7th **T44.6X2** **Poisoning by alpha-adrenoreceptor antagonists, intentional self-harm**
　　+7th **T44.6X3** **Poisoning by alpha-adrenoreceptor antagonists, assault**
　　+7th **T44.6X4** **Poisoning by alpha-adrenoreceptor antagonists, undetermined**
　　+7th **T44.6X5** **Adverse effect of alpha-adrenoreceptor antagonists**
　　+7th **T44.6X6** **Underdosing of alpha-adrenoreceptor antagonists**

+ **T44.7** **Poisoning by, adverse effect of and underdosing of beta-adrenoreceptor antagonists**
　+ **T44.7X** **Poisoning by, adverse effect of and underdosing of beta-adrenoreceptor antagonists**
　　+7th **T44.7X1** **Poisoning by beta-adrenoreceptor antagonists, accidental (unintentional)**
　　　　Poisoning by beta-adrenoreceptor antagonists NOS
　　+7th **T44.7X2** **Poisoning by beta-adrenoreceptor antagonists, intentional self-harm**
　　+7th **T44.7X3** **Poisoning by beta-adrenoreceptor antagonists, assault**
　　+7th **T44.7X4** **Poisoning by beta-adrenoreceptor antagonists, undetermined**
　　+7th **T44.7X5** **Adverse effect of beta-adrenoreceptor antagonists**
　　+7th **T44.7X6** **Underdosing of beta-adrenoreceptor antagonists**

+ **T44.8** **Poisoning by, adverse effect of and underdosing of centrally-acting and adrenergic-neuron- blocking agents**
　　Excludes1: *poisoning by, adverse effect of and underdosing of clonidine (T46.5)*
　　　　poisoning by, adverse effect of and underdosing of guanethidine (T46.5)
　+ **T44.8X** **Poisoning by, adverse effect of and underdosing of centrally-acting and adrenergic- neuron-blocking agents**
　　+7th **T44.8X1** **Poisoning by centrally-acting and adrenergic-neuron-blocking agents, accidental (unintentional)**
　　　　Poisoning by centrally-acting and adrenergic-neuron-blocking agents NOS
　　+7th **T44.8X2** **Poisoning by centrally-acting and adrenergic-neuron-blocking agents, intentional self-harm**
　　+7th **T44.8X3** **Poisoning by centrally-acting and adrenergic-neuron-blocking agents, assault**
　　+7th **T44.8X4** **Poisoning by centrally-acting and adrenergic-neuron-blocking agents, undetermined**
　　+7th **T44.8X5** **Adverse effect of centrally-acting and adrenergic-neuron-blocking agents**
　　+7th **T44.8X6** **Underdosing of centrally-acting and adrenergic-neuron-blocking agents**

+ **T44.9** **Poisoning by, adverse effect of and underdosing of other and unspecified drugs primarily affecting the autonomic nervous system**
　　Poisoning by, adverse effect of and underdosing of drug stimulating both alpha and beta-adrenoreceptors
　+ **T44.90** **Poisoning by, adverse effect of and underdosing of unspecified drugs primarily affecting the autonomic nervous system**
　　+7th **T44.901** **Poisoning by unspecified drugs primarily affecting the autonomic nervous system, accidental (unintentional)**
　　　　Poisoning by unspecified drugs primarily affecting the autonomic nervous system NOS
　　+7th **T44.902** **Poisoning by unspecified drugs primarily affecting the autonomic nervous system, intentional self-harm**
　　+7th **T44.903** **Poisoning by unspecified drugs primarily affecting the autonomic nervous system, assault**
　　+7th **T44.904** **Poisoning by unspecified drugs primarily affecting the autonomic nervous system, undetermined**
　　+7th **T44.905** **Adverse effect of unspecified drugs primarily affecting the autonomic nervous system**
　　+7th **T44.906** **Underdosing of unspecified drugs primarily affecting the autonomic nervous system**
　+ **T44.99** **Poisoning by, adverse effect of and underdosing of other drugs primarily affecting the autonomic nervous system**
　　+7th **T44.991** **Poisoning by other drug primarily affecting the autonomic nervous system, accidental (unintentional)**
　　　　Poisoning by other drugs primarily affecting the autonomic nervous system NOS
　　+7th **T44.992** **Poisoning by other drug primarily affecting the autonomic nervous system, intentional self-harm**
　　+7th **T44.993** **Poisoning by other drug primarily affecting the autonomic nervous system, assault**
　　+7th **T44.994** **Poisoning by other drug primarily affecting the autonomic nervous system, undetermined**
　　+7th **T44.995** **Adverse effect of other drug primarily affecting the autonomic nervous system**
　　+7th **T44.996** **Underdosing of other drug primarily affecting the autonomic nervous system**

T45 Poisoning by, adverse effect of and underdosing of primarily systemic and hematological agents, not elsewhere classified

The appropriate 7th character is to be added to each code from category T45
A   initial encounter
D   subsequent encounter
S   sequela

+ **T45.0   Poisoning by, adverse effect of and underdosing of antiallergic and antiemetic drugs**
    Excludes1: *poisoning by, adverse effect of and underdosing of phenothiazine-based neuroleptics (T43.3)*

  + **T45.0X   Poisoning by, adverse effect of and underdosing of antiallergic and antiemetic drugs**
    +7th **T45.0X1   Poisoning by antiallergic and antiemetic drugs, accidental (unintentional)**
        Poisoning by antiallergic and antiemetic drugs NOS
    +7th **T45.0X2   Poisoning by antiallergic and antiemetic drugs, intentional self-harm**
    +7th **T45.0X3   Poisoning by antiallergic and antiemetic drugs, assault**
    +7th **T45.0X4   Poisoning by antiallergic and antiemetic drugs, undetermined**
    +7th **T45.0X5   Adverse effect of antiallergic and antiemetic drugs**
    +7th **T45.0X6   Underdosing of antiallergic and antiemetic drugs**

+ **T45.1   Poisoning by, adverse effect of and underdosing of antineoplastic and immunosuppressive drugs**
    Excludes1: *poisoning by, adverse effect of and underdosing of tamoxifen (T38.6)*

  + **T45.1X   Poisoning by, adverse effect of and underdosing of antineoplastic and immunosuppressive drugs**
    +7th **T45.1X1   Poisoning by antineoplastic and immunosuppressive drugs, accidental (unintentional)**
        Poisoning by antineoplastic and immunosuppressive drugs NOS
    +7th **T45.1X2   Poisoning by antineoplastic and immunosuppressive drugs, intentional self-harm**
    +7th **T45.1X3   Poisoning by antineoplastic and immunosuppressive drugs, assault**
    +7th **T45.1X4   Poisoning by antineoplastic and immunosuppressive drugs, undetermined**
    +7th **T45.1X5   Adverse effect of antineoplastic and immunosuppressive drugs**
        Review coding guideline C.2.c.2
        AHA CC: 4Q, 2014, 22-23; 1Q, 2019, 17, 20-21; 2Q, 2019, 24-26, 28
    +7th **T45.1X6   Underdosing of antineoplastic and immunosuppressive drugs**

+ **T45.2   Poisoning by, adverse effect of and underdosing of vitamins**
    Excludes2: *poisoning by, adverse effect of and underdosing of nicotinic acid (derivatives) (T46.7)*
        poisoning by, adverse effect of and underdosing of iron (T45.4)
        poisoning by, adverse effect of and underdosing of vitamin K (T45.7)

  + **T45.2X   Poisoning by, adverse effect of and underdosing of vitamins**
    +7th **T45.2X1   Poisoning by vitamins, accidental (unintentional)**
        Poisoning by vitamins NOS
    +7th **T45.2X2   Poisoning by vitamins, intentional self-harm**
    +7th **T45.2X3   Poisoning by vitamins, assault**
    +7th **T45.2X4   Poisoning by vitamins, undetermined**
    +7th **T45.2X5   Adverse effect of vitamins**
    +7th **T45.2X6   Underdosing of vitamins**
        Excludes1: *vitamin deficiencies (E50-E56)*

+ **T45.3   Poisoning by, adverse effect of and underdosing of enzymes**

+ **T45.3X   Poisoning by, adverse effect of and underdosing of enzymes**
    +7th **T45.3X1   Poisoning by enzymes, accidental (unintentional)**
        Poisoning by enzymes NOS
    +7th **T45.3X2   Poisoning by enzymes, intentional self-harm**
    +7th **T45.3X3   Poisoning by enzymes, assault**
    +7th **T45.3X4   Poisoning by enzymes, undetermined**
    +7th **T45.3X5   Adverse effect of enzymes**
    +7th **T45.3X6   Underdosing of enzymes**

+ **T45.4   Poisoning by, adverse effect of and underdosing of iron and its compounds**

  + **T45.4X   Poisoning by, adverse effect of and underdosing of iron and its compounds**
    +7th **T45.4X1   Poisoning by iron and its compounds, accidental (unintentional)**
        Poisoning by iron and its compounds NOS
    +7th **T45.4X2   Poisoning by iron and its compounds, intentional self-harm**
    +7th **T45.4X3   Poisoning by iron and its compounds, assault**
    +7th **T45.4X4   Poisoning by iron and its compounds, undetermined**
    +7th **T45.4X5   Adverse effect of iron and its compounds**
    +7th **T45.4X6   Underdosing of iron and its compounds**
        Excludes1: *iron deficiency (E61.1)*

+ **T45.5   Poisoning by, adverse effect of and underdosing of anticoagulants and antithrombotic drugs**

  + **T45.51   Poisoning by, adverse effect of and underdosing of anticoagulants**
    +7th **T45.511   Poisoning by anticoagulants, accidental (unintentional)**
        Poisoning by anticoagulants NOS
    +7th **T45.512   Poisoning by anticoagulants, intentional self-harm**
    +7th **T45.513   Poisoning by anticoagulants, assault**
    +7th **T45.514   Poisoning by anticoagulants, undetermined**
    +7th **T45.515   Adverse effect of anticoagulants**
        AHA CC: 2Q, 2013, 34-35; 1Q, 2016, 14-15
    +7th **T45.516   Underdosing of anticoagulants**

  + **T45.52   Poisoning by, adverse effect of and underdosing of antithrombotic drugs**
        Poisoning by, adverse effect of and underdosing of antiplatelet drugs
        Excludes2: *poisoning by, adverse effect of and underdosing of aspirin (T39.01-)*
            poisoning by, adverse effect of and underdosing of acetylsalicylic acid (T39.01-)
    +7th **T45.521   Poisoning by antithrombotic drugs, accidental (unintentional)**
        Poisoning by antithrombotic drug NOS
    +7th **T45.522   Poisoning by antithrombotic drugs, intentional self-harm**
    +7th **T45.523   Poisoning by antithrombotic drugs, assault**
    +7th **T45.524   Poisoning by antithrombotic drugs, undetermined**
    +7th **T45.525   Adverse effect of antithrombotic drugs**
        AHA CC: 1Q, 2016, 15
    +7th **T45.526   Underdosing of antithrombotic drugs**

+ **T45.6   Poisoning by, adverse effect of and underdosing of fibrinolysis-affecting drugs**

  + **T45.60   Poisoning by, adverse effect of and underdosing of unspecified fibrinolysis-affecting drugs**
    +7th **T45.601   Poisoning by unspecified fibrinolysis-affecting drugs, accidental (unintentional)**
        Poisoning by fibrinolysis-affecting drug NOS
    +7th **T45.602   Poisoning by unspecified fibrinolysis-affecting drugs, intentional self-harm**
    +7th **T45.603   Poisoning by unspecified fibrinolysis-affecting drugs, assault**

+7th **T45.604** **Poisoning by unspecified fibrinolysis-affecting drugs, undetermined**

+7th **T45.605** **Adverse effect of unspecified fibrinolysis-affecting drugs**

+7th **T45.606** **Underdosing of unspecified fibrinolysis-affecting drugs**

+ **T45.61** **Poisoning by, adverse effect of and underdosing of thrombolytic drugs**

  +7th **T45.611** **Poisoning by thrombolytic drug, accidental (unintentional)**
      Poisoning by thrombolytic drug NOS

  +7th **T45.612** **Poisoning by thrombolytic drug, intentional self-harm**

  +7th **T45.613** **Poisoning by thrombolytic drug, assault**

  +7th **T45.614** **Poisoning by thrombolytic drug, undetermined**

  +7th **T45.615** **Adverse effect of thrombolytic drugs**
      AHA CC: 2Q, 2017, 9-10

  +7th **T45.616** **Underdosing of thrombolytic drugs**

+ **T45.62** **Poisoning by, adverse effect of and underdosing of hemostatic drugs**

  +7th **T45.621** **Poisoning by hemostatic drug, accidental (unintentional)**
      Poisoning by hemostatic drug NOS

  +7th **T45.622** **Poisoning by hemostatic drug, intentional self-harm**

  +7th **T45.623** **Poisoning by hemostatic drug, assault**

  +7th **T45.624** **Poisoning by hemostatic drug, undetermined**

  +7th **T45.625** **Adverse effect of hemostatic drug**

  +7th **T45.626** **Underdosing of hemostatic drugs**

+ **T45.69** **Poisoning by, adverse effect of and underdosing of other fibrinolysis-affecting drugs**

  +7th **T45.691** **Poisoning by other fibrinolysis-affecting drugs, accidental (unintentional)**
      Poisoning by other fibrinolysis-affecting drug NOS

  +7th **T45.692** **Poisoning by other fibrinolysis-affecting drugs, intentional self-harm**

  +7th **T45.693** **Poisoning by other fibrinolysis-affecting drugs, assault**

  +7th **T45.694** **Poisoning by other fibrinolysis-affecting drugs, undetermined**

  +7th **T45.695** **Adverse effect of other fibrinolysis-affecting drugs**

  +7th **T45.696** **Underdosing of other fibrinolysis-affecting drugs**

+ **T45.7** **Poisoning by, adverse effect of and underdosing of anticoagulant antagonists, vitamin K and other coagulants**

+ **T45.7X** **Poisoning by, adverse effect of and underdosing of anticoagulant antagonists, vitamin K and other coagulants**

  +7th **T45.7X1** **Poisoning by anticoagulant antagonists, vitamin K and other coagulants, accidental (unintentional)**
      Poisoning by anticoagulant antagonists, vitamin K and other coagulants NOS

  +7th **T45.7X2** **Poisoning by anticoagulant antagonists, vitamin K and other coagulants, intentional self-harm**

  +7th **T45.7X3** **Poisoning by anticoagulant antagonists, vitamin K and other coagulants, assault**

  +7th **T45.7X4** **Poisoning by anticoagulant antagonists, vitamin K and other coagulants, undetermined**

  +7th **T45.7X5** **Adverse effect of anticoagulant antagonists, vitamin K and other coagulants**

  +7th **T45.7X6** **Underdosing of anticoagulant antagonist, vitamin K and other coagulants**
      Excludes1: *vitamin K deficiency (E56.1)*

+ **T45.8** **Poisoning by, adverse effect of and underdosing of other primarily systemic and hematological agents**

Poisoning by, adverse effect of and underdosing of liver preparations and other antianemic agents

Poisoning by, adverse effect of and underdosing of natural blood and blood products

Poisoning by, adverse effect of and underdosing of plasma substitute

  Excludes2: *poisoning by, adverse effect of and underdosing of immunoglobulin (T50.Z1)*
      poisoning by, adverse effect of and underdosing of iron (T45.4)
      transfusion reactions (T80.-)

+ **T45.8X** **Poisoning by, adverse effect of and underdosing of other primarily systemic and hematological agents**

  +7th **T45.8X1** **Poisoning by other primarily systemic and hematological agents, accidental (unintentional)**
      Poisoning by other primarily systemic and hematological agents NOS

  +7th **T45.8X2** **Poisoning by other primarily systemic and hematological agents, intentional self-harm**

  +7th **T45.8X3** **Poisoning by other primarily systemic and hematological agents, assault**

  +7th **T45.8X4** **Poisoning by other primarily systemic and hematological agents, undetermined**

  +7th **T45.8X5** **Adverse effect of other primarily systemic and hematological agents**
      AHA CC: 4Q, 2016, 41-42

  +7th **T45.8X6** **Underdosing of other primarily systemic and hematological agents**

+ **T45.9** **Poisoning by, adverse effect of and underdosing of unspecified primarily systemic and hematological agent**

  X+7th **T45.91** **Poisoning by unspecified primarily systemic and hematological agent, accidental (unintentional)**
      Poisoning by primarily systemic and hematological agent NOS

  X+7th **T45.92** **Poisoning by unspecified primarily systemic and hematological agent, intentional self-harm**

  X+7th **T45.93** **Poisoning by unspecified primarily systemic and hematological agent, assault**

  X+7th **T45.94** **Poisoning by unspecified primarily systemic and hematological agent, undetermined**

  X+7th **T45.95** **Adverse effect of unspecified primarily systemic and hematological agent**

  X+7th **T45.96** **Underdosing of unspecified primarily systemic and hematological agent**

T46 **Poisoning by, adverse effect of and underdosing of agents primarily affecting the cardiovascular system**

  Excludes1: *poisoning by, adverse effect of and underdosing of metaraminol (T44.4)*

> The appropriate 7th character is to be added to each code from category T46
> A   initial encounter
> D   subsequent encounter
> S   sequela

+ **T46.0** **Poisoning by, adverse effect of and underdosing of cardiac-stimulant glycosides and drugs of similar action**

+ **T46.0X** **Poisoning by, adverse effect of and underdosing of cardiac-stimulant glycosides and drugs of similar action**

  +7th **T46.0X1** **Poisoning by cardiac-stimulant glycosides and drugs of similar action, accidental (unintentional)**
      Poisoning by cardiac-stimulant glycosides and drugs of similar action NOS

  +7th **T46.0X2** **Poisoning by cardiac-stimulant glycosides and drugs of similar action, intentional self-harm**

  +7th **T46.0X3** **Poisoning by cardiac-stimulant glycosides and drugs of similar action, assault**

+7th **T46.0X4** **Poisoning by cardiac-stimulant glycosides and drugs of similar action, undetermined**

+7th **T46.0X5** **Adverse effect of cardiac-stimulant glycosides and drugs of similar action**

+7th **T46.0X6** **Underdosing of cardiac-stimulant glycosides and drugs of similar action**

+ **T46.1** **Poisoning by, adverse effect of and underdosing of calcium-channel blockers**

+ **T46.1X** **Poisoning by, adverse effect of and underdosing of calcium-channel blockers**

+7th **T46.1X1** **Poisoning by calcium-channel blockers, accidental (unintentional)**
Poisoning by calcium-channel blockers NOS

+7th **T46.1X2** **Poisoning by calcium-channel blockers, intentional self-harm**

+7th **T46.1X3** **Poisoning by calcium-channel blockers, assault**

+7th **T46.1X4** **Poisoning by calcium-channel blockers, undetermined**

+7th **T46.1X5** **Adverse effect of calcium-channel blockers**

+7th **T46.1X6** **Underdosing of calcium-channel blockers**

+ **T46.2** **Poisoning by, adverse effect of and underdosing of other antidysrhythmic drugs, not elsewhere classified**
Excludes1: *poisoning by, adverse effect of and underdosing of beta-adrenoreceptor antagonists (T44.7-)*

+ **T46.2X** **Poisoning by, adverse effect of and underdosing of other antidysrhythmic drugs**

+7th **T46.2X1** **Poisoning by other antidysrhythmic drugs, accidental (unintentional)**
Poisoning by other antidysrhythmic drugs NOS

+7th **T46.2X2** **Poisoning by other antidysrhythmic drugs, intentional self-harm**

+7th **T46.2X3** **Poisoning by other antidysrhythmic drugs, assault**

+7th **T46.2X4** **Poisoning by other antidysrhythmic drugs, undetermined**

+7th **T46.2X5** **Adverse effect of other antidysrhythmic drugs**

+7th **T46.2X6** **Underdosing of other antidysrhythmic drugs**

+ **T46.3** **Poisoning by, adverse effect of and underdosing of coronary vasodilators**
Poisoning by, adverse effect of and underdosing of dipyridamole
Excludes1: *poisoning by, adverse effect of and underdosing of calcium-channel blockers (T46.1)*

+ **T46.3X** **Poisoning by, adverse effect of and underdosing of coronary vasodilators**

+7th **T46.3X1** **Poisoning by coronary vasodilators, accidental (unintentional)**
Poisoning by coronary vasodilators NOS

+7th **T46.3X2** **Poisoning by coronary vasodilators, intentional self-harm**

+7th **T46.3X3** **Poisoning by coronary vasodilators, assault**

+7th **T46.3X4** **Poisoning by coronary vasodilators, undetermined**

+7th **T46.3X5** **Adverse effect of coronary vasodilators**

+7th **T46.3X6** **Underdosing of coronary vasodilators**

+ **T46.4** **Poisoning by, adverse effect of and underdosing of angiotensin-converting-enzyme inhibitors**

+ **T46.4X** **Poisoning by, adverse effect of and underdosing of angiotensin-converting-enzyme inhibitors**

+7th **T46.4X1** **Poisoning by angiotensin-converting-enzyme inhibitors, accidental (unintentional)**
Poisoning by angiotensin-converting-enzyme inhibitors NOS

+7th **T46.4X2** **Poisoning by angiotensin-converting-enzyme inhibitors, intentional self-harm**

+7th **T46.4X3** **Poisoning by angiotensin-converting-enzyme inhibitors, assault**

+7th **T46.4X4** **Poisoning by angiotensin-converting-enzyme inhibitors, undetermined**

+7th **T46.4X5** **Adverse effect of angiotensin-converting-enzyme inhibitors**

+7th **T46.4X6** **Underdosing of angiotensin-converting-enzyme inhibitors**

+ **T46.5** **Poisoning by, adverse effect of and underdosing of other antihypertensive drugs**
Excludes2: *poisoning by, adverse effect of and underdosing of beta-adrenoreceptor antagonists (T44.7)*
poisoning by, adverse effect of and underdosing of calcium-channel blockers (T46.1)
poisoning by, adverse effect of and underdosing of diuretics (T50.0-T50.2)

+ **T46.5X** **Poisoning by, adverse effect of and underdosing of other antihypertensive drugs**

+7th **T46.5X1** **Poisoning by other antihypertensive drugs, accidental (unintentional)**
Poisoning by other antihypertensive drugs NOS

+7th **T46.5X2** **Poisoning by other antihypertensive drugs, intentional self-harm**

+7th **T46.5X3** **Poisoning by other antihypertensive drugs, assault**

+7th **T46.5X4** **Poisoning by other antihypertensive drugs, undetermined**

+7th **T46.5X5** **Adverse effect of other antihypertensive drugs**

+7th **T46.5X6** **Underdosing of other antihypertensive drugs**

+ **T46.6** **Poisoning by, adverse effect of and underdosing of antihyperlipidemic and antiarteriosclerotic drugs**

+ **T46.6X** **Poisoning by, adverse effect of and underdosing of antihyperlipidemic and antiarteriosclerotic drugs**

+7th **T46.6X1** **Poisoning by antihyperlipidemic and antiarteriosclerotic drugs, accidental (unintentional)**
Poisoning by antihyperlipidemic and antiarteriosclerotic drugs NOS

+7th **T46.6X2** **Poisoning by antihyperlipidemic and antiarteriosclerotic drugs, intentional self-harm**

+7th **T46.6X3** **Poisoning by antihyperlipidemic and antiarteriosclerotic drugs, assault**

+7th **T46.6X4** **Poisoning by antihyperlipidemic and antiarteriosclerotic drugs, undetermined**

+7th **T46.6X5** **Adverse effect of antihyperlipidemic and antiarteriosclerotic drugs**

+7th **T46.6X6** **Underdosing of antihyperlipidemic and antiarteriosclerotic drugs**

+ **T46.7** **Poisoning by, adverse effect of and underdosing of peripheral vasodilators**
Poisoning by, adverse effect of and underdosing of nicotinic acid (derivatives)
Excludes1: *poisoning by, adverse effect of and underdosing of papaverine (T44.3)*

+ **T46.7X** **Poisoning by, adverse effect of and underdosing of peripheral vasodilators**

+7th **T46.7X1** **Poisoning by peripheral vasodilators, accidental (unintentional)**
Poisoning by peripheral vasodilators NOS

+7th **T46.7X2** **Poisoning by peripheral vasodilators, intentional self-harm**

+7th **T46.7X3** **Poisoning by peripheral vasodilators, assault**

+7th **T46.7X4** **Poisoning by peripheral vasodilators, undetermined**

+7th **T46.7X5** **Adverse effect of peripheral vasodilators**

+7th **T46.7X6** **Underdosing of peripheral vasodilators**

+ **T46.8** **Poisoning by, adverse effect of and underdosing of antivaricose drugs, including sclerosing agents**
  + **T46.8X** **Poisoning by, adverse effect of and underdosing of antivaricose drugs, including sclerosing agents**
    +7th **T46.8X1** **Poisoning by antivaricose drugs, including sclerosing agents, accidental (unintentional)**
      Poisoning by antivaricose drugs, including sclerosing agents NOS
    +7th **T46.8X2** **Poisoning by antivaricose drugs, including sclerosing agents, intentional self-harm**
    +7th **T46.8X3** **Poisoning by antivaricose drugs, including sclerosing agents, assault**
    +7th **T46.8X4** **Poisoning by antivaricose drugs, including sclerosing agents, undetermined**
    +7th **T46.8X5** **Adverse effect of antivaricose drugs, including sclerosing agents**
    +7th **T46.8X6** **Underdosing of antivaricose drugs, including sclerosing agents**
+ **T46.9** **Poisoning by, adverse effect of and underdosing of other and unspecified agents primarily affecting the cardiovascular system**
  + **T46.90** **Poisoning by, adverse effect of and underdosing of unspecified agents primarily affecting the cardiovascular system**
    +7th **T46.901** **Poisoning by unspecified agents primarily affecting the cardiovascular system, accidental (unintentional)**
    +7th **T46.902** **Poisoning by unspecified agents primarily affecting the cardiovascular system, intentional self-harm**
    +7th **T46.903** **Poisoning by unspecified agents primarily affecting the cardiovascular system, assault**
    +7th **T46.904** **Poisoning by unspecified agents primarily affecting the cardiovascular system, undetermined**
    +7th **T46.905** **Adverse effect of unspecified agents primarily affecting the cardiovascular system**
    +7th **T46.906** **Underdosing of unspecified agents primarily affecting the cardiovascular system**
  + **T46.99** **Poisoning by, adverse effect of and underdosing of other agents primarily affecting the cardiovascular system**
    +7th **T46.991** **Poisoning by other agents primarily affecting the cardiovascular system, accidental (unintentional)**
    +7th **T46.992** **Poisoning by other agents primarily affecting the cardiovascular system, intentional self-harm**
    +7th **T46.993** **Poisoning by other agents primarily affecting the cardiovascular system, assault**
    +7th **T46.994** **Poisoning by other agents primarily affecting the cardiovascular system, undetermined**
    +7th **T46.995** **Adverse effect of other agents primarily affecting the cardiovascular system**
    +7th **T46.996** **Underdosing of other agents primarily affecting the cardiovascular system**

T47 **Poisoning by, adverse effect of and underdosing of agents primarily affecting the gastrointestinal system**

> The appropriate 7th character is to be added to each code from category T47
> A initial encounter
> D subsequent encounter
> S sequela

+ **T47.0** **Poisoning by, adverse effect of and underdosing of histamine H2-receptor blockers**
  + **T47.0X** **Poisoning by, adverse effect of and underdosing of histamine H2-receptor blockers**
    +7th **T47.0X1** **Poisoning by histamine H2-receptor blockers, accidental (unintentional)**
      Poisoning by histamine H2-receptor blockers NOS
    +7th **T47.0X2** **Poisoning by histamine H2-receptor blockers, intentional self-harm**
    +7th **T47.0X3** **Poisoning by histamine H2-receptor blockers, assault**
    +7th **T47.0X4** **Poisoning by histamine H2-receptor blockers, undetermined**
    +7th **T47.0X5** **Adverse effect of histamine H2-receptor blockers**
    +7th **T47.0X6** **Underdosing of histamine H2-receptor blockers**
+ **T47.1** **Poisoning by, adverse effect of and underdosing of other antacids and anti-gastric-secretion drugs**
  + **T47.1X** **Poisoning by, adverse effect of and underdosing of other antacids and anti-gastric-secretion drugs**
    +7th **T47.1X1** **Poisoning by other antacids and anti-gastric-secretion drugs, accidental (unintentional)**
      Poisoning by other antacids and anti-gastric-secretion drugs NOS
    +7th **T47.1X2** **Poisoning by other antacids and anti-gastric-secretion drugs, intentional self-harm**
    +7th **T47.1X3** **Poisoning by other antacids and anti-gastric-secretion drugs, assault**
    +7th **T47.1X4** **Poisoning by other antacids and anti-gastric-secretion drugs, undetermined**
    +7th **T47.1X5** **Adverse effect of other antacids and anti-gastric-secretion drugs**
    +7th **T47.1X6** **Underdosing of other antacids and anti-gastric-secretion drugs**
+ **T47.2** **Poisoning by, adverse effect of and underdosing of stimulant laxatives**
  + **T47.2X** **Poisoning by, adverse effect of and underdosing of stimulant laxatives**
    +7th **T47.2X1** **Poisoning by stimulant laxatives, accidental (unintentional)**
      Poisoning by stimulant laxatives NOS
    +7th **T47.2X2** **Poisoning by stimulant laxatives, intentional self-harm**
    +7th **T47.2X3** **Poisoning by stimulant laxatives, assault**
    +7th **T47.2X4** **Poisoning by stimulant laxatives, undetermined**
    +7th **T47.2X5** **Adverse effect of stimulant laxatives**
    +7th **T47.2X6** **Underdosing of stimulant laxatives**
+ **T47.3** **Poisoning by, adverse effect of and underdosing of saline and osmotic laxatives**
  + **T47.3X** **Poisoning by and adverse effect of saline and osmotic laxatives**
    +7th **T47.3X1** **Poisoning by saline and osmotic laxatives, accidental (unintentional)**
      Poisoning by saline and osmotic laxatives NOS
    +7th **T47.3X2** **Poisoning by saline and osmotic laxatives, intentional self-harm**
    +7th **T47.3X3** **Poisoning by saline and osmotic laxatives, assault**
    +7th **T47.3X4** **Poisoning by saline and osmotic laxatives, undetermined**
    +7th **T47.3X5** **Adverse effect of saline and osmotic laxatives**
    +7th **T47.3X6** **Underdosing of saline and osmotic laxatives**

+ **T47.4** **Poisoning by, adverse effect of and underdosing of other laxatives**
  + **T47.4X** **Poisoning by, adverse effect of and underdosing of other laxatives**
    - +7th **T47.4X1** **Poisoning by other laxatives, accidental (unintentional)**
      Poisoning by other laxatives NOS
    - +7th **T47.4X2** **Poisoning by other laxatives, intentional self-harm**
    - +7th **T47.4X3** **Poisoning by other laxatives, assault**
    - +7th **T47.4X4** **Poisoning by other laxatives, undetermined**
    - +7th **T47.4X5** **Adverse effect of other l axatives**
    - +7th **T47.4X6** **Underdosing of other laxatives**
+ **T47.5** **Poisoning by, adverse effect of and underdosing of digestants**
  + **T47.5X** **Poisoning by, adverse effect of and underdosing of digestants**
    - +7th **T47.5X1** **Poisoning by digestants, accidental (unintentional)**
      Poisoning by digestants NOS
    - +7th **T47.5X2** **Poisoning by digestants, intentional self-harm**
    - +7th **T47.5X3** **Poisoning by digestants, assault**
    - +7th **T47.5X4** **Poisoning by digestants, undetermined**
    - +7th **T47.5X5** **Adverse effect of digestants**
    - +7th **T47.5X6** **Underdosing of digestants**
+ **T47.6** **Poisoning by, adverse effect of and underdosing of antidiarrheal drugs**
  Excludes2: *poisoning by, adverse effect of and underdosing of systemic antibiotics and other anti-infectives (T36-T37)*
  + **T47.6X** **Poisoning by, adverse effect of and underdosing of antidiarrheal drugs**
    - +7th **T47.6X1** **Poisoning by antidiarrheal drugs, accidental (unintentional)**
      Poisoning by antidiarrheal drugs NOS
    - +7th **T47.6X2** **Poisoning by antidiarrheal drugs, intentional self-harm**
    - +7th **T47.6X3** **Poisoning by antidiarrheal drugs, assault**
    - +7th **T47.6X4** **Poisoning by antidiarrheal drugs, undetermined**
    - +7th **T47.6X5** **Adverse effect of antidiarrheal drugs**
    - +7th **T47.6X6** **Underdosing of antidiarrheal drugs**
+ **T47.7** **Poisoning by, adverse effect of and underdosing of emetics**
  + **T47.7X** **Poisoning by, adverse effect of and underdosing of emetics**
    - +7th **T47.7X1** **Poisoning by emetics, accidental (unintentional)**
      Poisoning by emetics NOS
    - +7th **T47.7X2** **Poisoning by emetics, intentional self-harm**
    - +7th **T47.7X3** **Poisoning by emetics, assault**
    - +7th **T47.7X4** **Poisoning by emetics, undetermined**
    - +7th **T47.7X5** **Adverse effect of emetics**
    - +7th **T47.7X6** **Underdosing of emetics**
+ **T47.8** **Poisoning by, adverse effect of and underdosing of other agents primarily affecting gastrointestinal system**
  + **T47.8X** **Poisoning by, adverse effect of and underdosing of other agents primarily affecting gastrointestinal system**
    - +7th **T47.8X1** **Poisoning by other agents primarily affecting gastrointestinal system, accidental (unintentional)**
      Poisoning by other agents primarily affecting gastrointestinal system NOS
    - +7th **T47.8X2** **Poisoning by other agents primarily affecting gastrointestinal system, intentional self-harm**
    - +7th **T47.8X3** **Poisoning by other agents primarily affecting gastrointestinal system, assault**
    - +7th **T47.8X4** **Poisoning by other agents primarily affecting gastrointestinal system, undetermined**
    - +7th **T47.8X5** **Adverse effect of other agents primarily affecting gastrointestinal system**
    - +7th **T47.8X6** **Underdosing of other agents primarily affecting gastrointestinal system**

+ **T47.9** **Poisoning by, adverse effect of and underdosing of unspecified agents primarily affecting the gastrointestinal system**
  - X+7th **T47.91** **Poisoning by unspecified agents primarily affecting the gastrointestinal system, accidental (unintentional)**
    Poisoning by agents primarily affecting the gastrointestinal system NOS
  - X+7th **T47.92** **Poisoning by unspecified agents primarily affecting the gastrointestinal system, intentional self-harm**
  - X+7th **T47.93** **Poisoning by unspecified agents primarily affecting the gastrointestinal system, assault**
  - X+7th **T47.94** **Poisoning by unspecified agents primarily affecting the gastrointestinal system, undetermined**
  - X+7th **T47.95** **Adverse effect of unspecified agents primarily affecting the gastrointestinal system**
  - X+7th **T47.96** **Underdosing of unspecified agents primarily affecting the gastrointestinal system**

T48 **Poisoning by, adverse effect of and underdosing of agents primarily acting on smooth and skeletal muscles and the respiratory system**

> The appropriate 7th character is to be added to each code from category T48
> A   initial encounter
> D   subsequent encounter
> S   sequela

+ **T48.0** **Poisoning by, adverse effect of and underdosing of oxytocic drugs**
  Excludes1: *poisoning by, adverse effect of and underdosing of estrogens, progestogens and antagonists (T38.4-T38.6)*
  + **T48.0X** **Poisoning by, adverse effect of and underdosing of oxytocic drugs**
    - +7th **T48.0X1** **Poisoning by oxytocic drugs, accidental (unintentional)**
      Poisoning by oxytocic drugs NOS
    - +7th **T48.0X2** **Poisoning by oxytocic drugs, intentional self-harm**
    - +7th **T48.0X3** **Poisoning by oxytocic drugs, assault**
    - +7th **T48.0X4** **Poisoning by oxytocic drugs, undetermined**
    - +7th **T48.0X5** **Adverse effect of oxytocic drugs**
    - +7th **T48.0X6** **Underdosing of oxytocic drugs**
+ **T48.1** **Poisoning by, adverse effect of and underdosing of skeletal muscle relaxants [neuromuscular blocking agents]**
  + **T48.1X** **Poisoning by, adverse effect of and underdosing of skeletal muscle relaxants [neuromuscular blocking agents]**
    - +7th **T48.1X1** **Poisoning by skeletal muscle relaxants [neuromuscular blocking agents], accidental (unintentional)**
      Poisoning by skeletal muscle relaxants [neuromuscular blocking agents] NOS
    - +7th **T48.1X2** **Poisoning by skeletal muscle relaxants [neuromuscular blocking agents], intentional self-harm**
    - +7th **T48.1X3** **Poisoning by skeletal muscle relaxants [neuromuscular blocking agents], assault**
    - +7th **T48.1X4** **Poisoning by skeletal muscle relaxants [neuromuscular blocking agents], undetermined**
    - +7th **T48.1X5** **Adverse effect of skeletal muscle relaxants [neuromuscular blocking agents]**
    - +7th **T48.1X6** **Underdosing of skeletal muscle relaxants [neuromuscular blocking agents]**
+ **T48.2** **Poisoning by, adverse effect of and underdosing of other and unspecified drugs acting on muscles**
  + **T48.20** **Poisoning by, adverse effect of and underdosing of unspecified drugs acting on muscles**
    - +7th **T48.201** **Poisoning by unspecified drugs acting on muscles, accidental (unintentional)**
      Poisoning by unspecified drugs acting on muscles NOS
    - +7th **T48.202** **Poisoning by unspecified drugs acting on muscles, intentional self-harm**

+7th **T48.203** **Poisoning by unspecified drugs acting on muscles, assault**

+7th **T48.204** **Poisoning by unspecified drugs acting on muscles, undetermined**

+7th **T48.205** **Adverse effect of unspecified drugs acting on muscles**

+7th **T48.206** **Underdosing of unspecified drugs acting on muscles**

+ **T48.29** **Poisoning by, adverse effect of and underdosing of other drugs acting on muscles**

+7th **T48.291** **Poisoning by other drugs acting on muscles, accidental (unintentional)**
Poisoning by other drugs acting on muscles NOS

+7th **T48.292** **Poisoning by other drugs acting on muscles, intentional self-harm**

+7th **T48.293** **Poisoning by other drugs acting on muscles, assault**

+7th **T48.294** **Poisoning by other drugs acting on muscles, undetermined**

+7th **T48.295** **Adverse effect of other drugs acting on muscles**

+7th **T48.296** **Underdosing of other drugs acting on muscles**

+ **T48.3** **Poisoning by, adverse effect of and underdosing of antitussives**

+ **T48.3X** **Poisoning by, adverse effect of and underdosing of antitussives**

+7th **T48.3X1** **Poisoning by antitussives, accidental (unintentional)**
Poisoning by antitussives NOS

+7th **T48.3X2** **Poisoning by antitussives, intentional self-harm**

+7th **T48.3X3** **Poisoning by antitussives, assault**

+7th **T48.3X4** **Poisoning by antitussives, undetermined**

+7th **T48.3X5** **Adverse effect of antitussives**

+7th **T48.3X6** **Underdosing of antitussives**

+ **T48.4** **Poisoning by, adverse effect of and underdosing of expectorants**

+ **T48.4X** **Poisoning by, adverse effect of and underdosing of expectorants**

+7th **T48.4X1** **Poisoning by expectorants, accidental (unintentional)**
Poisoning by expectorants NOS

+7th **T48.4X2** **Poisoning by expectorants, intentional self-harm**

+7th **T48.4X3** **Poisoning by expectorants, assault**

+7th **T48.4X4** **Poisoning by expectorants, undetermined**

+7th **T48.4X5** **Adverse effect of expectorants**

+7th **T48.4X6** **Underdosing of expectorants**

+ **T48.5** **Poisoning by, adverse effect of and underdosing of other anti-common-cold drugs**
Poisoning by, adverse effect of and underdosing of decongestants

Excludes2: *poisoning by, adverse effect of and underdosing of antipyretics, NEC (T39.9-)*
poisoning by, adverse effect of and underdosing of non-steroidal antiinflammatory drugs (T39.3-)
poisoning by, adverse effect of and underdosing of salicylates (T39.0-)

+ **T48.5X** **Poisoning by, adverse effect of and underdosing of other anti-common-cold drugs**

+7th **T48.5X1** **Poisoning by other anti-common-cold drugs, accidental (unintentional)**
Poisoning by other anti-common-cold drugs NOS

+7th **T48.5X2** **Poisoning by other anti-common-cold drugs, intentional self-harm**

+7th **T48.5X3** **Poisoning by other anti-common-cold drugs, assault**

+7th **T48.5X4** **Poisoning by other anti-common-cold drugs, undetermined**

+7th **T48.5X5** **Adverse effect of other anti-common-cold drugs**

+7th **T48.5X6** **Underdosing of other anti-common-cold drugs**

+ **T48.6** **Poisoning by, adverse effect of and underdosing of antiasthmatics, not elsewhere classified**
Poisoning by, adverse effect of and underdosing of beta-adrenoreceptor agonists used in asthma therapy

Excludes1: *poisoning by, adverse effect of and underdosing of beta-adrenoreceptor agonists not used in asthma therapy (T44.5)*
poisoning by, adverse effect of and underdosing of anterior pituitary [adenohypophyseal] hormones (T38.8)

+ **T48.6X** **Poisoning by, adverse effect of and underdosing of antiasthmatics**

+7th **T48.6X1** **Poisoning by antiasthmatics, accidental (unintentional)**
Poisoning by antiasthmatics NOS

+7th **T48.6X2** **Poisoning by antiasthmatics, intentional self-harm**

+7th **T48.6X3** **Poisoning by antiasthmatics, assault**

+7th **T48.6X4** **Poisoning by antiasthmatics, undetermined**

+7th **T48.6X5** **Adverse effect of antiasthmatics**

+7th **T48.6X6** **Underdosing of antiasthmatics**

+ **T48.9** **Poisoning by, adverse effect of and underdosing of other and unspecified agents primarily acting on the respiratory system**

+ **T48.90** **Poisoning by, adverse effect of and underdosing of unspecified agents primarily acting on the respiratory system**

+7th **T48.901** **Poisoning by unspecified agents primarily acting on the respiratory system, accidental (unintentional)**

+7th **T48.902** **Poisoning by unspecified agents primarily acting on the respiratory system, intentional self-harm**

+7th **T48.903** **Poisoning by unspecified agents primarily acting on the respiratory system, assault**

+7th **T48.904** **Poisoning by unspecified agents primarily acting on the respiratory system, undetermined**

+7th **T48.905** **Adverse effect of unspecified agents primarily acting on the respiratory system**

+7th **T48.906** **Underdosing of unspecified agents primarily acting on the respiratory system**

+ **T48.99** **Poisoning by, adverse effect of and underdosing of other agents primarily acting on the respiratory system**

+7th **T48.991** **Poisoning by other agents primarily acting on the respiratory system, accidental (unintentional)**

+7th **T48.992** **Poisoning by other agents primarily acting on the respiratory system, intentional self-harm**

+7th **T48.993** **Poisoning by other agents primarily acting on the respiratory system, assault**

+7th **T48.994** **Poisoning by other agents primarily acting on the respiratory system, undetermined**

+7th **T48.995** **Adverse effect of other agents primarily acting on the respiratory system**

+7th **T48.996** **Underdosing of other agents primarily acting on the respiratory system**

T49 **Poisoning by, adverse effect of and underdosing of topical agents primarily affecting skin and mucous membrane and by ophthalmological, otorhinorlaryngological and dental drugs**

Includes: poisoning by, adverse effect of and underdosing of glucocorticoids, topically used

The appropriate 7th character is to be added to each code from category T49
A   initial encounter
D   subsequent encounter
S   sequela

+ **T49.0** **Poisoning by, adverse effect of and underdosing of local antifungal, anti-infective and anti-inflammatory drugs**
> + **T49.0X** **Poisoning by, adverse effect of and underdosing of local antifungal, anti-infective and anti-inflammatory drugs**
>> +7th **T49.0X1** **Poisoning by local antifungal, anti-infective and anti-inflammatory drugs, accidental (unintentional)**
>>> Poisoning by local antifungal, anti-infective and anti-inflammatory drugs NOS
>> +7th **T49.0X2** **Poisoning by local antifungal, anti-infective and anti-inflammatory drugs, intentional self-harm**
>> +7th **T49.0X3** **Poisoning by local antifungal, anti-infective and anti-inflammatory drugs, assault**
>> +7th **T49.0X4** **Poisoning by local antifungal, anti-infective and anti-inflammatory drugs, undetermined**
>> +7th **T49.0X5** **Adverse effect of local antifungal, anti-infective and anti-inflammatory drugs**
>> +7th **T49.0X6** **Underdosing of local antifungal, anti-infective and anti-inflammatory drugs**

+ **T49.1** **Poisoning by, adverse effect of and underdosing of antipruritics**
> + **T49.1X** **Poisoning by, adverse effect of and underdosing of antipruritics**
>> +7th **T49.1X1** **Poisoning by antipruritics, accidental (unintentional)**
>>> Poisoning by antipruritics NOS
>> +7th **T49.1X2** **Poisoning by antipruritics, intentional self-harm**
>> +7th **T49.1X3** **Poisoning by antipruritics, assault**
>> +7th **T49.1X4** **Poisoning by antipruritics, undetermined**
>> +7th **T49.1X5** **Adverse effect of antipruritics**
>> +7th **T49.1X6** **Underdosing of antipruritics**

+ **T49.2** **Poisoning by, adverse effect of and underdosing of local astringents and local detergents**
> + **T49.2X** **Poisoning by, adverse effect of and underdosing of local astringents and local detergents**
>> +7th **T49.2X1** **Poisoning by local astringents and local detergents, accidental (unintentional)**
>>> Poisoning by local astringents and local detergents NOS
>> +7th **T49.2X2** **Poisoning by local astringents and local detergents, intentional self-harm**
>> +7th **T49.2X3** **Poisoning by local astringents and local detergents, assault**
>> +7th **T49.2X4** **Poisoning by local astringents and local detergents, undetermined**
>> +7th **T49.2X5** **Adverse effect of local astringents and local detergents**
>> +7th **T49.2X6** **Underdosing of local astringents and local detergents**

+ **T49.3** **Poisoning by, adverse effect of and underdosing of emollients, demulcents and protectants**
> + **T49.3X** **Poisoning by, adverse effect of and underdosing of emollients, demulcents and protectants**
>> +7th **T49.3X1** **Poisoning by emollients, demulcents and protectants, accidental (unintentional)**
>>> Poisoning by emollients, demulcents and protectants NOS
>> +7th **T49.3X2** **Poisoning by emollients, demulcents and protectants, intentional self-harm**
>> +7th **T49.3X3** **Poisoning by emollients, demulcents and protectants, assault**
>> +7th **T49.3X4** **Poisoning by emollients, demulcents and protectants, undetermined**
>> +7th **T49.3X5** **Adverse effect of emollients, demulcents and protectants**
>> +7th **T49.3X6** **Underdosing of emollients, demulcents and protectants**

+ **T49.4** **Poisoning by, adverse effect of and underdosing of keratolytics, keratoplastics, and other hair treatment drugs and preparations**
> + **T49.4X** **Poisoning by, adverse effect of and underdosing of keratolytics, keratoplastics, and other hair treatment drugs and preparations**
>> +7th **T49.4X1** **Poisoning by keratolytics, keratoplastics, and other hair treatment drugs and preparations, accidental (unintentional)**
>>> Poisoning by keratolytics, keratoplastics, and other hair treatment drugs and preparations NOS
>> +7th **T49.4X2** **Poisoning by keratolytics, keratoplastics, and other hair treatment drugs and preparations, intentional self-harm**
>> +7th **T49.4X3** **Poisoning by keratolytics, keratoplastics, and other hair treatment drugs and preparations, assault**
>> +7th **T49.4X4** **Poisoning by keratolytics, keratoplastics, and other hair treatment drugs and preparations, undetermined**
>> +7th **T49.4X5** **Adverse effect of keratolytics, keratoplastics, and other hair treatment drugs and preparations**
>> +7th **T49.4X6** **Underdosing of keratolytics, keratoplastics, and other hair treatment drugs and preparations**

+ **T49.5** **Poisoning by, adverse effect of and underdosing of ophthalmological drugs and preparations**
> + **T49.5X** **Poisoning by, adverse effect of and underdosing of ophthalmological drugs and preparations**
>> +7th **T49.5X1** **Poisoning by ophthalmological drugs and preparations, accidental (unintentional)**
>>> Poisoning by ophthalmological drugs and preparations NOS
>> +7th **T49.5X2** **Poisoning by ophthalmological drugs and preparations, intentional self-harm**
>> +7th **T49.5X3** **Poisoning by ophthalmological drugs and preparations, assault**
>> +7th **T49.5X4** **Poisoning by ophthalmological drugs and preparations, undetermined**
>> +7th **T49.5X5** **Adverse effect of ophthalmological drugs and preparations**
>> +7th **T49.5X6** **Underdosing of ophthalmological drugs and preparations**

+ **T49.6** **Poisoning by, adverse effect of and underdosing of otorhinolaryngological drugs and preparations**
> + **T49.6X** **Poisoning by, adverse effect of and underdosing of otorhinolaryngological drugs and preparations**
>> +7th **T49.6X1** **Poisoning by otorhinolaryngological drugs and preparations, accidental (unintentional)**
>>> Poisoning by otorhinolaryngological drugs and preparations NOS
>> +7th **T49.6X2** **Poisoning by otorhinolaryngological drugs and preparations, intentional self-harm**
>> +7th **T49.6X3** **Poisoning by otorhinolaryngological drugs and preparations, assault**
>> +7th **T49.6X4** **Poisoning by otorhinolaryngological drugs and preparations, undetermined**
>> +7th **T49.6X5** **Adverse effect of otorhinolaryngological drugs and preparations**
>> +7th **T49.6X6** **Underdosing of otorhinolaryngological drugs and preparations**

+ **T49.7** **Poisoning by, adverse effect of and underdosing of dental drugs, topically applied**
> + **T49.7X** **Poisoning by, adverse effect of and underdosing of dental drugs, topically applied**
>> +7th **T49.7X1** **Poisoning by dental drugs, topically applied, accidental (unintentional)**
>>> Poisoning by dental drugs, topically applied NOS
>> +7th **T49.7X2** **Poisoning by dental drugs, topically applied, intentional self-harm**
>> +7th **T49.7X3** **Poisoning by dental drugs, topically applied, assault**

+, +7th, X + 7th ● Newborn ● Pediatric ● Maternity ● Adult ♀ Female ♂ Male Manifestation Unacceptable PDX HCC CC MCC HAC

+7th **T49.7X4** Poisoning by dental drugs, topically
applied, undetermined
+7th **T49.7X5** Adverse effect of dental drugs, topically
applied
+7th **T49.7X6** Underdosing of dental drugs, topically
applied
+ **T49.8** Poisoning by, adverse effect of and underdosing of other
topical agents
Poisoning by, adverse effect of and underdosing of
spermicides
+ **T49.8X** Poisoning by, adverse effect of and underdosing
of other topical agents
+7th **T49.8X1** Poisoning by other topical agents,
accidental (unintentional)
Poisoning by other topical agents NOS
+7th **T49.8X2** Poisoning by other topical agents,
intentional self-harm
+7th **T49.8X3** Poisoning by other topical agents,
assault
+7th **T49.8X4** Poisoning by other topical agents,
undetermined
+7th **T49.8X5** Adverse effect of other topical agents
+7th **T49.8X6** Underdosing of other topical agents
+ **T49.9** Poisoning by, adverse effect of and underdosing of
unspecified topical agent
X+7th **T49.91** Poisoning by unspecified topical agent, accidental
(unintentional)
X+7th **T49.92** Poisoning by unspecified topical agent, intentional
self-harm
X+7th **T49.93** Poisoning by unspecified topical agent, assault
X+7th **T49.94** Poisoning by unspecified topical agent,
undetermined
X+7th **T49.95** Adverse effect of unspecified topical agent
X+7th **T49.96** Underdosing of unspecified topical agent

T50 Poisoning by, adverse effect of and underdosing of diuretics
and other and unspecified drugs, medicaments and biological
substances

> The appropriate 7th character is to be added to each code from
> category T50
> A   initial encounter
> D   subsequent encounter
> S   sequela

+ **T50.0** Poisoning by, adverse effect of and underdosing of
mineralocorticoids and their antagonists
+ **T50.0X** Poisoning by, adverse effect of and underdosing
of mineralocorticoids and their antagonists
+7th **T50.0X1** Poisoning by mineralocorticoids
and their antagonists, accidental
(unintentional)
Poisoning by mineralocorticoids and
their antagonists NOS
+7th **T50.0X2** Poisoning by mineralocorticoids and
their antagonists, intentional self-harm
+7th **T50.0X3** Poisoning by mineralocorticoids and
their antagonists, assault
+7th **T50.0X4** Poisoning by mineralocorticoids and
their antagonists, undetermined
+7th **T50.0X5** Adverse effect of mineralocorticoids
and their antagonists
+7th **T50.0X6** Underdosing of mineralocorticoids and
their antagonists
+ **T50.1** Poisoning by, adverse effect of and underdosing of loop
[high-ceiling] diuretics
+ **T50.1X** Poisoning by, adverse effect of and underdosing
of loop [high-ceiling] diuretics
+7th **T50.1X1** Poisoning by loop [high-ceiling]
diuretics, accidental (unintentional)
Poisoning by loop [high-ceiling] diuretics
NOS
+7th **T50.1X2** Poisoning by loop [high-ceiling]
diuretics, intentional self-harm
+7th **T50.1X3** Poisoning by loop [high-ceiling]
diuretics, assault
+7th **T50.1X4** Poisoning by loop [high-ceiling]
diuretics, undetermined
+7th **T50.1X5** Adverse effect of loop [high-ceiling]
diuretics
+7th **T50.1X6** Underdosing of loop [high-ceiling]
diuretics

+ **T50.2** Poisoning by, adverse effect of and underdosing of carbonic-
anhydrase inhibitors, benzothiadiazides and other diuretics
Poisoning by, adverse effect of and underdosing of
acetazolamide
+ **T50.2X** Poisoning by, adverse effect of and underdosing of
carbonic-anhydrase inhibitors, benzothiadiazides
and other diuretics
+7th **T50.2X1** Poisoning by carbonic-anhydrase
inhibitors, benzothiadiazides and other
diuretics, accidental (unintentional)
Poisoning by carbonic-anhydrase
inhibitors, benzothiadiazides and other
diuretics NOS
+7th **T50.2X2** Poisoning by carbonic-anhydrase
inhibitors, benzothiadiazides and other
diuretics, intentional self-harm
+7th **T50.2X3** Poisoning by carbonic-anhydrase
inhibitors, benzothiadiazides and other
diuretics, assault
+7th **T50.2X4** Poisoning by carbonic-anhydrase
inhibitors, benzothiadiazides and other
diuretics, undetermined
+7th **T50.2X5** Adverse effect of carbonic-anhydrase
inhibitors, benzothiadiazides and other
diuretics
+7th **T50.2X6** Underdosing of carbonic-anhydrase
inhibitors, benzothiadiazides and other
diuretics
+ **T50.3** Poisoning by, adverse effect of and underdosing of
electrolytic, caloric and water-balance agents
Poisoning by, adverse effect of and underdosing of oral
rehydration salts
+ **T50.3X** Poisoning by, adverse effect of and underdosing of
electrolytic, caloric and water-balance agents
+7th **T50.3X1** Poisoning by electrolytic, caloric and
water-balance agents, accidental
(unintentional)
Poisoning by electrolytic, caloric and
water-balance agents NOS
+7th **T50.3X2** Poisoning by electrolytic, caloric and
water-balance agents, intentional self-harm
+7th **T50.3X3** Poisoning by electrolytic, caloric and
water-balance agents, assault
+7th **T50.3X4** Poisoning by electrolytic, caloric and
water-balance agents, undetermined
+7th **T50.3X5** Adverse effect of electrolytic, caloric
and water-balance agents
+7th **T50.3X6** Underdosing of electrolytic, caloric and
water-balance agents
+ **T50.4** Poisoning by, adverse effect of and underdosing of drugs
affecting uric acid metabolism
+ **T50.4X** Poisoning by, adverse effect of and underdosing
of drugs affecting uric acid metabolism
+7th **T50.4X1** Poisoning by drugs affecting uric acid
metabolism, accidental (unintentional)
Poisoning by drugs affecting uric acid
metabolism NOS
+7th **T50.4X2** Poisoning by drugs affecting uric
acid metabolism, intentional self-harm
+7th **T50.4X3** Poisoning by drugs affecting uric acid
metabolism, assault
+7th **T50.4X4** Poisoning by drugs affecting uric acid
metabolism, undetermined
+7th **T50.4X5** Adverse effect of drugs affecting uric
acid metabolism
+7th **T50.4X6** Underdosing of drugs affecting uric
acid metabolism
+ **T50.5** Poisoning by, adverse effect of and underdosing of appetite
depressants
+ **T50.5X** Poisoning by, adverse effect of and underdosing
of appetite depressants
+7th **T50.5X1** Poisoning by appetite depressants,
accidental (unintentional)
Poisoning by appetite depressants NOS
+7th **T50.5X2** Poisoning by appetite depressants,
intentional self-harm
+7th **T50.5X3** Poisoning by appetite depressants, assault
+7th **T50.5X4** Poisoning by appetite depressants,
undetermined
+7th **T50.5X5** Adverse effect of appetite depressants
+7th **T50.5X6** Underdosing of appetite depressants

+ **T50.6** Poisoning by, adverse effect of and underdosing of antidotes and chelating agents

    Poisoning by, adverse effect of and underdosing of alcohol deterrents

  + **T50.6X** Poisoning by, adverse effect of and underdosing of antidotes and chelating agents

    +7th **T50.6X1** Poisoning by antidotes and chelatingagents, accidental (unintentional)

      Poisoning by antidotes and chelating agents NOS

    +7th **T50.6X2** Poisoning by antidotes and chelating agents, intentional self-harm

    +7th **T50.6X3** Poisoning by antidotes and chelating agents, assault

    +7th **T50.6X4** Poisoning by antidotes and chelating agents, undetermined

    +7th **T50.6X5** Adverse effect of antidotes and chelating agents

    +7th **T50.6X6** Underdosing of antidotes and chelating agents

+ **T50.7** Poisoning by, adverse effect of and underdosing of analeptics and opioid receptor antagonists

  + **T50.7X** Poisoning by, adverse effect of and underdosing of analeptics and opioid receptor antagonists

    +7th **T50.7X1** Poisoning by analeptics and opioid receptor antagonists, accidental (unintentional)

      Poisoning by analeptics and opioid receptor antagonists NOS

    +7th **T50.7X2** Poisoning by analeptics and opioid receptor antagonists, intentional self-harm

    +7th **T50.7X3** Poisoning by analeptics and opioid receptor antagonists, assault

    +7th **T50.7X4** Poisoning by analeptics and opioid receptor antagonists, undetermined

    +7th **T50.7X5** Adverse effect of analeptics and opioid receptor antagonists

    +7th **T50.7X6** Underdosing of analeptics and opioid receptor antagonists

+ **T50.8** Poisoning by, adverse effect of and underdosing of diagnostic agents

  + **T50.8X** Poisoning by, adverse effect of and underdosing of diagnostic agents

    +7th **T50.8X1** Poisoning by diagnostic agents, accidental (unintentional)

      Poisoning by diagnostic agents NOS

    +7th **T50.8X2** Poisoning by diagnostic agents, intentional self-harm

    +7th **T50.8X3** Poisoning by diagnostic agents, assault

    +7th **T50.8X4** Poisoning by diagnostic agents, undetermined

    +7th **T50.8X5** Adverse effect of diagnostic agents

    +7th **T50.8X6** Underdosing of diagnostic agents

+ **T50.A** Poisoning by, adverse effect of and underdosing of bacterial vaccines

  + **T50.A1** Poisoning by, adverse effect of and underdosing of pertussis vaccine, including combinations with a pertussis component

    +7th **T50.A11** Poisoning by pertussis vaccine, including combinations with a pertussis component, accidental (unintentional)

    +7th **T50.A12** Poisoning by pertussis vaccine, including combinations with a pertussis component, intentional self-harm

    +7th **T50.A13** Poisoning by pertussis vaccine, including combinations with a pertussis component, assault

    +7th **T50.A14** Poisoning by pertussis vaccine, including combinations with a pertussis component, undetermined

    +7th **T50.A15** Adverse effect of pertussis vaccine, including combinations with a pertussis component

    +7th **T50.A16** Underdosing of pertussis vaccine, including combinations with a pertussis component

  + **T50.A2** Poisoning by, adverse effect of and underdosing of mixed bacterial vaccines without a pertussis component

    +7th **T50.A21** Poisoning by mixed bacterial vaccines without a pertussis component, accidental (unintentional)

    +7th **T50.A22** Poisoning by mixed bacterial vaccines without a pertussis component, intentional self-harm

    +7th **T50.A23** Poisoning by mixed bacterial vaccines without a pertussis component, assault

    +7th **T50.A24** Poisoning by mixed bacterial vaccines without a pertussis component, undetermined

    +7th **T50.A25** Adverse effect of mixed bacterial vaccines without a pertussis component

    +7th **T50.A26** Underdosing of mixed bacterial vaccines without a pertussis component

  + **T50.A9** Poisoning by, adverse effect of and underdosing of other bacterial vaccines

    +7th **T50.A91** Poisoning by other bacterial vaccines, accidental (unintentional)

    +7th **T50.A92** Poisoning by other bacterial vaccines, intentional self-harm

    +7th **T50.A93** Poisoning by other bacterial vaccines, assault

    +7th **T50.A94** Poisoning by other bacterial vaccines, undetermined

    +7th **T50.A95** Adverse effect of other bacterial vaccines

    +7th **T50.A96** Underdosing of other bacterial vaccines

+ **T50.B** Poisoning by, adverse effect of and underdosing of viral vaccines

  + **T50.B1** Poisoning by, adverse effect of and underdosing of smallpox vaccines

    +7th **T50.B11** Poisoning by smallpox vaccines, accidental (unintentional)

    +7th **T50.B12** Poisoning by smallpox vaccines, intentional self-harm

    +7th **T50.B13** Poisoning by smallpox vaccines, assault

    +7th **T50.B14** Poisoning by smallpox vaccines, undetermined

    +7th **T50.B15** Adverse effect of smallpox vaccines

    +7th **T50.B16** Underdosing of smallpox vaccines

  + **T50.B9** Poisoning by, adverse effect of and underdosing of other viral vaccines

    +7th **T50.B91** Poisoning by other viral vaccines, accidental (unintentional)

    +7th **T50.B92** Poisoning by other viral vaccines, intentional self-harm

    +7th **T50.B93** Poisoning by other viral vaccines, assault

    +7th **T50.B94** Poisoning by other viral vaccines, undetermined

    +7th **T50.B95** Adverse effect of other viral vaccines

    +7th **T50.B96** Underdosing of other viral vaccines

+ **T50.Z** Poisoning by, adverse effect of and underdosing of other vaccines and biological substances

  + **T50.Z1** Poisoning by, adverse effect of and underdosing of immunoglobulin

    +7th **T50.Z11** Poisoning by immunoglobulin, accidental (unintentional)

    +7th **T50.Z12** Poisoning by immunoglobulin, intentional self-harm

    +7th **T50.Z13** Poisoning by immunoglobulin, assault

    +7th **T50.Z14** Poisoning by immunoglobulin, undetermined

    +7th **T50.Z15** Adverse effect of immunoglobulin

    +7th **T50.Z16** Underdosing of immunoglobulin

  + **T50.Z9** Poisoning by, adverse effect of and underdosing of other vaccines and biological substances

    +7th **T50.Z91** Poisoning by other vaccines and biological substances, accidental (unintentional)

    +7th **T50.Z92** Poisoning by other vaccines and biological substances, intentional self-harm

    +7th **T50.Z93** Poisoning by other vaccines and biological substances, assault

    +7th **T50.Z94** Poisoning by other vaccines and biological substances, undetermined

    +7th **T50.Z95** Adverse effect of other vaccines and biological substances

      AHA CC: 1Q, 2020, 18-19

    +7th **T50.Z96** Underdosing of other vaccines and biological substances

---

+, +7th, X + 7th   ● Newborn   ● Pediatric   ● Maternity   ● Adult   ♀ Female   ♂ Male   Manifestation   Unacceptable PDX   HCC   CC   MCC   HAC

+ **T50.9** Poisoning by, adverse effect of and underdosing of other and unspecified drugs, medicaments and biological substances
   + **T50.90** Poisoning by, adverse effect of and underdosing of unspecified drugs, medicaments and biological substances
      +7th **T50.901** Poisoning by unspecified drugs, medicaments and biological substances, accidental (unintentional)
         AHA CC: 1Q, 2015, 3-21
      +7th **T50.902** Poisoning by unspecified drugs, medicaments and biological substances, intentional self-harm
      +7th **T50.903** Poisoning by unspecified drugs, medicaments and biological substances, assault
      +7th **T50.904** Poisoning by unspecified drugs, medicaments and biological substances, undetermined
      +7th **T50.905** Adverse effect of unspecified drugs, medicaments and biological substances
      +7th **T50.906** Underdosing of unspecified drugs, medicaments and biological substances
   + **T50.91** Poisoning by, adverse effect of and underdosing of multiple unspecified drugs, medicaments and biological substances
      Multiple drug ingestion NOS
      Code also any specific drugs, medicaments and biological substances
      AHA CC: 4Q, 2019, 17
      T50.911 Poisoning by multiple unspecified drugs, medicaments and biological substances, accidental (unintentional)
      T50.912 Poisoning by multiple unspecified drugs, medicaments and biological substances, intentional self-harm
      T50.913 Poisoning by multiple unspecified drugs, medicaments and biological substances, assault
      T50.914 Poisoning by multiple unspecified drugs, medicaments and biological substances, undetermined
      T50.915 Adverse effect of multiple unspecified drugs, medicaments and biological substances
      T50.916 Underdosing of multiple unspecified drugs, medicaments and biological substance
   + **T50.99** Poisoning by, adverse effect of and underdosing of other drugs, medicaments and biological substances
      +7th **T50.991** Poisoning by other drugs, medicaments and biological substances, accidental (unintentional)
      +7th **T50.992** Poisoning by other drugs, medicaments and biological substances, intentional self-harm
      +7th **T50.993** Poisoning by other drugs, medicaments and biological substances, assault
      +7th **T50.994** Poisoning by other drugs, medicaments and biological substances, undetermined
      +7th **T50.995** Adverse effect of other drugs, medicaments and biological substances
      +7th **T50.996** Underdosing of other drugs, medicaments and biological substances

Toxic effects of substances chiefly nonmedicinal as to source (T51-T65)

NOTE When no intent is indicated code to accidental. Undetermined intent is only for use when there is specific documentation in the record that the intent of the toxic effect cannot be determined.

Use additional code(s):
   for all associated manifestations of toxic effect, such as: respiratory conditions due to external agents (J60-J70)
   personal history of foreign body fully removed (Z87.821)
   to identify any retained foreign body, if applicable (Z18.-)

Excludes1: contact with and (suspected) exposure to toxic substances (Z77.-)

Review coding guideline C.19.e

T51 Toxic effect of alcohol

   The appropriate 7th character is to be added to each code from category T51
   A   initial encounter
   D   subsequent encounter
   S   sequela

+ **T51.0** Toxic effect of ethanol
   Toxic effect of ethyl alcohol
   Excludes2: acute alcohol intoxication or 'hangover' effects
      drunkenness (F10.129, F10.229, F10.929)
      pathological (F10.129, F10.229, F10.929)
      alcohol intoxication (F10.129, F10.229, F10.929)
   + **T51.0X** Toxic effect of ethanol
      +7th **T51.0X1** Toxic effect of ethanol, accidental (unintentional)
         Toxic effect of ethanol NOS
      +7th **T51.0X2** Toxic effect of ethanol, intentional self-harm
      +7th **T51.0X3** Toxic effect of ethanol, assault
      +7th **T51.0X4** Toxic effect of ethanol, undetermined
+ **T51.1** Toxic effect of methanol
   Toxic effect of methyl alcohol
   + **T51.1X** Toxic effect of methanol
      +7th **T51.1X1** Toxic effect of methanol, accidental (unintentional)
         Toxic effect of methanol NOS
      +7th **T51.1X2** Toxic effect of methanol, intentional self-harm
      +7th **T51.1X3** Toxic effect of methanol, assault
      +7th **T51.1X4** Toxic effect of methanol, undetermined
+ **T51.2** Toxic effect of 2-Propanol
   Toxic effect of isopropyl alcohol
   + **T51.2X** Toxic effect of 2-Propanol
      +7th **T51.2X1** Toxic effect of 2-Propanol, accidental (unintentional)
         Toxic effect of 2-Propanol NOS
      +7th **T51.2X2** Toxic effect of 2-Propanol, intentional self-harm
      +7th **T51.2X3** Toxic effect of 2-Propanol, assault
      +7th **T51.2X4** Toxic effect of 2-Propanol, undetermined
+ **T51.3** Toxic effect of fusel oil
   Toxic effect of amyl alcohol
   Toxic effect of butyl [1-butanol] alcohol
   Toxic effect of propyl [1-propanol] alcohol
   + **T51.3X** Toxic effect of fusel oil
      +7th **T51.3X1** Toxic effect of fusel oil, accidental (unintentional)
         Toxic effect of fusel oil NOS
      +7th **T51.3X2** Toxic effect of fusel oil, intentional self-harm
      +7th **T51.3X3** Toxic effect of fusel oil, assault
      +7th **T51.3X4** Toxic effect of fusel oil, undetermined
+ **T51.8** Toxic effect of other alcohols
   + **T51.8X** Toxic effect of other alcohols
      +7th **T51.8X1** Toxic effect of other alcohols, accidental (unintentional)
         Toxic effect of other alcohols NOS
      +7th **T51.8X2** Toxic effect of other alcohols, intentional self-harm
      +7th **T51.8X3** Toxic effect of other alcohols, assault
      +7th **T51.8X4** Toxic effect of other alcohols, undetermined
+ **T51.9** Toxic effect of unspecified alcohol
   X+7th **T51.91** Toxic effect of unspecified alcohol, accidental (unintentional)
   X+7th **T51.92** Toxic effect of unspecified alcohol, intentional self-harm
   X+7th **T51.93** Toxic effect of unspecified alcohol, assault
   X+7th **T51.94** Toxic effect of unspecified alcohol, undetermined

T52 Toxic effect of organic solvents

   Excludes1: halogen derivatives of aliphatic and aromatic hydrocarbons (T53.-)

   The appropriate 7th character is to be added to each code from category T52
   A   initial encounter
   D   subsequent encounter
   S   sequela

+, +7th, X + 7th   ● Newborn   ● Pediatric   ● Maternity   ● Adult   ♀ Female   ♂ Male   Manifestation   Unacceptable PDX   HCC   CC   MCC   **HAC**

+ **T52.0** **Toxic effects of petroleum products**
Toxic effects of gasoline [petrol]
Toxic effects of kerosene [paraffin oil]
Toxic effects of paraffin wax
Toxic effects of ether petroleum
Toxic effects of naphtha petroleum
Toxic effects of spirit petroleum
+ **T52.0X** **Toxic effects of petroleum products**
+7th **T52.0X1** **Toxic effect of petroleum products, accidental (unintentional)**
Toxic effects of petroleum products NOS
+7th **T52.0X2** **Toxic effect of petroleum products, intentional self-harm**
+7th **T52.0X3** **Toxic effect of petroleum products, assault**
+7th **T52.0X4** **Toxic effect of petroleum products, undetermined**
+ **T52.1** **Toxic effects of benzene**
Excludes1: homologues of benzene (T52.2)
nitroderivatives and aminoderivatives of benzene
and its homologues (T65.3)
+ **T52.1X** **Toxic effects of benzene**
+7th **T52.1X1** **Toxic effect of benzene, accidental (unintentional)**
Toxic effects of benzene NOS
+7th **T52.1X2** **Toxic effect of benzene, intentional self-harm**
+7th **T52.1X3** **Toxic effect of benzene, assault**
+7th **T52.1X4** **Toxic effect of benzene, undetermined**
+ **T52.2** **Toxic effects of homologues of benzene**
Toxic effects of toluene [methylbenzene]
Toxic effects of xylene [dimethylbenzene]
+ **T52.2X** **Toxic effects of homologues of benzene**
+7th **T52.2X1** **Toxic effect of homologues of benzene, accidental (unintentional)**
Toxic effects of homologues of benzene NOS
+7th **T52.2X2** **Toxic effect of homologues of benzene, intentional self-harm**
+7th **T52.2X3** **Toxic effect of homologues of benzene, assault**
+7th **T52.2X4** **Toxic effect of homologues of benzene, undetermined**
+ **T52.3** **Toxic effects of glycols**
+ **T52.3X** **Toxic effects of glycols**
+7th **T52.3X1** **Toxic effect of glycols, accidental (unintentional)**
Toxic effects of glycols NOS
+7th **T52.3X2** **Toxic effect of glycols, intentional self-harm**
+7th **T52.3X3** **Toxic effect of glycols, assault**
+7th **T52.3X4** **Toxic effect of glycols, undetermined**
+ **T52.4** **Toxic effects of ketones**
+ **T52.4X** **Toxic effects of ketones**
+7th **T52.4X1** **Toxic effect of ketones, accidental (unintentional)**
Toxic effects of ketones NOS
+7th **T52.4X2** **Toxic effect of ketones, intentional self-harm**
+7th **T52.4X3** **Toxic effect of ketones, assault**
+7th **T52.4X4** **Toxic effect of ketones, undetermined**

+ **T52.8** **Toxic effects of other organic solvents**
+ **T52.8X** **Toxic effects of other organic solvents**
+7th **T52.8X1** **Toxic effect of other organic solvents, accidental (unintentional)**
Toxic effects of other organic solvents NOS
+7th **T52.8X2** **Toxic effect of other organic solvents, intentional self-harm**
+7th **T52.8X3** **Toxic effect of other organic solvents, assault**
+7th **T52.8X4** **Toxic effect of other organic solvents, undetermined**
+ **T52.9** **Toxic effects of unspecified organic solvent**
X+7th **T52.91** **Toxic effect of unspecified organic solvent, accidental (unintentional)**
X+7th **T52.92** **Toxic effect of unspecified organic solvent, intentional self-harm**
X+7th **T52.93** **Toxic effect of unspecified organic solvent, assault**
X+7th **T52.94** **Toxic effect of unspecified organic solvent, undetermined**
T53 **Toxic effect of halogen derivatives of aliphatic and aromatic hydrocarbons**

> The appropriate 7th character is to be added to each code from category T53
> A   initial encounter
> D   subsequent encounter
> S   sequela

+ **T53.0** **Toxic effects of carbon tetrachloride**
Toxic effects of tetrachloromethane
+ **T53.0X** **Toxic effects of carbon tetrachloride**
+7th **T53.0X1** **Toxic effect of carbon tetrachloride, accidental (unintentional)**
Toxic effects of carbon tetrachloride NOS
+7th **T53.0X2** **Toxic effect of carbon tetrachloride, intentional self-harm**
+7th **T53.0X3** **Toxic effect of carbon tetrachloride, assault**
+7th **T53.0X4** **Toxic effect of carbon tetrachloride, undetermined**
+ **T53.1** **Toxic effects of chloroform**
Toxic effects of trichloromethane
+ **T53.1X** **Toxic effects of chloroform**
+7th **T53.1X1** **Toxic effect of chloroform, accidental (unintentional)**
Toxic effects of chloroform NOS
+7th **T53.1X2** **Toxic effect of chloroform, intentional self-harm**
+7th **T53.1X3** **Toxic effect of chloroform, assault**
+7th **T53.1X4** **Toxic effect of chloroform, undetermined**
+ **T53.2** **Toxic effects of trichloroethylene**
Toxic effects of trichloroethene
+ **T53.2X** **Toxic effects of trichloroethylene**
+7th **T53.2X1** **Toxic effect of trichloroethylene, accidental (unintentional)**
Toxic effects of trichloroethylene NOS
+7th **T53.2X2** **Toxic effect of trichloroethylene, intentional self-harm**
+7th **T53.2X3** **Toxic effect of trichloroethylene, assault**
+7th **T53.2X4** **Toxic effect of trichloroethylene, undetermined**

+, +7th, X + 7th   ● Newborn   ● Pediatric   ● Maternity   ● Adult   ♀ Female   ♂ Male   Manifestation   Unacceptable PDX   HCC   CC   MCC   HAC

+ **T53.3 Toxic effects of tetrachloroethylene**
    Toxic effects of perchloroethylene
    Toxic effect of tetrachloroethene
    + **T53.3X Toxic effects of tetrachloroethylene**
      +7th **T53.3X1 Toxic effect of tetrachloroethylene, accidental (unintentional)**
          Toxic effects of tetrachloroethylene NOS
      +7th **T53.3X2 Toxic effect of tetrachloroethylene, intentional self-harm**
      +7th **T53.3X3 Toxic effect of tetrachloroethylene, assault**
      +7th **T53.3X4 Toxic effect of tetrachloroethylene, undetermined**

+ **T53.4 Toxic effects of dichloromethane**
    Toxic effects of methylene chloride
    + **T53.4X Toxic effects of dichloromethane**
      +7th **T53.4X1 Toxic effect of dichloromethane, accidental (unintentional)**
          Toxic effects of dichloromethane NOS
      +7th **T53.4X2 Toxic effect of dichloromethane, intentional self-harm**
      +7th **T53.4X3 Toxic effect of dichloromethane, assault**
      +7th **T53.4X4 Toxic effect of dichloromethane, undetermined**

+ **T53.5 Toxic effects of chlorofluorocarbons**
    + **T53.5X Toxic effects of chlorofluorocarbons**
      +7th **T53.5X1 Toxic effect of chlorofluorocarbons, accidental (unintentional)**
          Toxic effects of chlorofluorocarbons NOS
      +7th **T53.5X2 Toxic effect of chlorofluorocarbons, intentional self-harm**
      +7th **T53.5X3 Toxic effect of chlorofluorocarbons, assault**
      +7th **T53.5X4 Toxic effect of chlorofluorocarbons, undetermined**

+ **T53.6 Toxic effects of other halogen derivatives of aliphatic hydrocarbons**
    + **T53.6X Toxic effects of other halogen derivatives of aliphatic hydrocarbons**
      +7th **T53.6X1 Toxic effect of other halogen derivatives of aliphatic hydrocarbons, accidental (unintentional)**
          Toxic effects of other halogen derivatives of aliphatic hydrocarbons NOS
      +7th **T53.6X2 Toxic effect of other halogen derivatives of aliphatic hydrocarbons, intentional self-harm**
      +7th **T53.6X3 Toxic effect of other halogen derivatives of aliphatic hydrocarbons, assault**
      +7th **T53.6X4 Toxic effect of other halogen derivatives of aliphatic hydrocarbons, undetermined**

+ **T53.7 Toxic effects of other halogen derivatives of aromatic hydrocarbons**
    + **T53.7X Toxic effects of other halogen derivatives of aromatic hydrocarbons**
      +7th **T53.7X1 Toxic effect of other halogen derivatives of aromatic hydrocarbons, accidental (unintentional)**
          Toxic effects of other halogen derivatives of aromatic hydrocarbons NOS
      +7th **T53.7X2 Toxic effect of other halogen derivatives of aromatic hydrocarbons, intentional self-harm**
      +7th **T53.7X3 Toxic effect of other halogen derivatives of aromatic hydrocarbons, assault**
      +7th **T53.7X4 Toxic effect of other halogen derivatives of aromatic hydrocarbons, undetermined**

+ **T53.9 Toxic effects of unspecified halogen derivatives of aliphatic and aromatic hydrocarbons**
    X+7th **T53.91 Toxic effect of unspecified halogen derivatives of aliphatic and aromatic hydrocarbons, accidental (unintentional)**
    X+7th **T53.92 Toxic effect of unspecified halogen derivatives of aliphatic and aromatic hydrocarbons, intentional self-harm**
    X+7th **T53.93 Toxic effect of unspecified halogen derivatives of aliphatic and aromatic hydrocarbons, assault**
    X+7th **T53.94 Toxic effect of unspecified halogen derivatives of aliphatic and aromatic hydrocarbons, undetermined**

T54 Toxic effect of corrosive substances

> The appropriate 7th character is to be added to each code from category T54
> A initial encounter
> D subsequent encounter
> S sequela

+ **T54.0 Toxic effects of phenol and phenol homologues**
    + **T54.0X Toxic effects of phenol and phenol homologues**
      +7th **T54.0X1 Toxic effect of phenol and phenol homologues, accidental (unintentional)**
          Toxic effects of phenol and phenol homologues NOS
      +7th **T54.0X2 Toxic effect of phenol and phenol homologues, intentional self-harm**
      +7th **T54.0X3 Toxic effect of phenol and phenol homologues, assault**
      +7th **T54.0X4 Toxic effect of phenol and phenol homologues, undetermined**

+ **T54.1 Toxic effects of other corrosive organic compounds**
    + **T54.1X Toxic effects of other corrosive organic compounds**
      +7th **T54.1X1 Toxic effect of other corrosive organic compounds, accidental (unintentional)**
          Toxic effects of other corrosive organic compounds NOS
      +7th **T54.1X2 Toxic effect of other corrosive organic compounds, intentional self-harm**
      +7th **T54.1X3 Toxic effect of other corrosive organic compounds, assault**
      +7th **T54.1X4 Toxic effect of other corrosive organic compounds, undetermined**

+ **T54.2 Toxic effects of corrosive acids and acid-like substances**
    Toxic effects of hydrochloric acid
    Toxic effects of sulfuric acid
    + **T54.2X Toxic effects of corrosive acids and acid-like substances**
      +7th **T54.2X1 Toxic effect of corrosive acids and acid-like substances, accidental (unintentional)**
          Toxic effects of corrosive acids and acid-like substances NOS
      +7th **T54.2X2 Toxic effect of corrosive acids and acid-like substances, intentional self-harm**
      +7th **T54.2X3 Toxic effect of corrosive acids and acid-like substances, assault**
      +7th **T54.2X4 Toxic effect of corrosive acids and acid-like substances, undetermined**

+ **T54.3 Toxic effects of corrosive alkalis and alkali-like substances**
    Toxic effects of potassium hydroxide
    Toxic effects of sodium hydroxide
    + **T54.3X Toxic effects of corrosive alkalis and alkali-like substances**
      +7th **T54.3X1 Toxic effect of corrosive alkalis and alkali-like substances, accidental (unintentional)**
          Toxic effects of corrosive alkalis and alkali-like substances NOS
      +7th **T54.3X2 Toxic effect of corrosive alkalis and alkali-like substances, intentional self-harm**
      +7th **T54.3X3 Toxic effect of corrosive alkalis and alkali-like substances, assault**
      +7th **T54.3X4 Toxic effect of corrosive alkalis and alkali-like substances, undetermined**

+ **T54.9 Toxic effects of unspecified corrosive substance**
    X+7th **T54.91 Toxic effect of unspecified corrosive substance, accidental (unintentional)**
    X+7th **T54.92 Toxic effect of unspecified corrosive substance, intentional self-harm**
    X+7th **T54.93 Toxic effect of unspecified corrosive substance, assault**
    X+7th **T54.94 Toxic effect of unspecified corrosive substance, undetermined**

T55 Toxic effect of soaps and detergents

> The appropriate 7th character is to be added to each code from category T55
> A initial encounter
> D subsequent encounter
> S sequela

+, +7th, X + 7th • Newborn • Pediatric • Maternity • Adult ♀ Female ♂ Male Manifestation Unacceptable PDX HCC CC MCC HAC

+ **T55.0** **Toxic effect of soaps**
   + **T55.0X** **Toxic effect of soaps**
     +7th **T55.0X1** **Toxic effect of soaps, accidental (unintentional)**
       Toxic effect of soaps NOS
     +7th **T55.0X2** **Toxic effect of soaps, intentional self-harm**
     +7th **T55.0X3** **Toxic effect of soaps, assault**
     +7th **T55.0X4** **Toxic effect of soaps, undetermined**
+ **T55.1** **Toxic effect of detergents**
   + **T55.1X** **Toxic effect of detergents**
     +7th **T55.1X1** **Toxic effect of detergents, accidental (unintentional)**
       Toxic effect of detergents NOS
     +7th **T55.1X2** **Toxic effect of detergents, intentional self-harm**
     +7th **T55.1X3** **Toxic effect of detergents, assault**
     +7th **T55.1X4** **Toxic effect of detergents, undetermined**

T56 **Toxic effect of metals**

> **Includes:** toxic effects of fumes and vapors of metals
> toxic effects of metals from all sources, except medicinal substances
> Use additional code to identify any retained metal foreign body, if applicable (Z18.0-, T18.1-)
> **Excludes1:** *arsenic and its compounds (T57.0)*
> *manganese and its compounds (T57.2)*

> The appropriate 7th character is to be added to each code from category T56
> A initial encounter
> D subsequent encounter
> S sequela

+ **T56.0** **Toxic effects of lead and its compounds**
   + **T56.0X** **Toxic effects of lead and its compounds**
     +7th **T56.0X1** **Toxic effect of lead and its compounds, accidental (unintentional)**
       Toxic effects of lead and its compounds NOS
     +7th **T56.0X2** **Toxic effect of lead and its compounds, intentional self-harm**
     +7th **T56.0X3** **Toxic effect of lead and its compounds, assault**
     +7th **T56.0X4** **Toxic effect of lead and its compounds, undetermined**
+ **T56.1** **Toxic effects of mercury and its compounds**
   + **T56.1X** **Toxic effects of mercury and its compounds**
     +7th **T56.1X1** **Toxic effect of mercury and its compounds, accidental (unintentional)**
       Toxic effects of mercury and its compounds NOS
     +7th **T56.1X2** **Toxic effect of mercury and its compounds, intentional self-harm**
     +7th **T56.1X3** **Toxic effect of mercury and its compounds, assault**
     +7th **T56.1X4** **Toxic effect of mercury and its compounds, undetermined**
+ **T56.2** **Toxic effects of chromium and its compounds**
   + **T56.2X** **Toxic effects of chromium and its compounds**
     +7th **T56.2X1** **Toxic effect of chromium and its compounds, accidental (unintentional)**
       Toxic effects of chromium and its compounds NOS
     +7th **T56.2X2** **Toxic effect of chromium and its compounds, intentional self-harm**
     +7th **T56.2X3** **Toxic effect of chromium and its compounds, assault**
     +7th **T56.2X4** **Toxic effect of chromium and its compounds, undetermined**
+ **T56.3** **Toxic effects of cadmium and its compounds**
   + **T56.3X** **Toxic effects of cadmium and its compounds**
     +7th **T56.3X1** **Toxic effect of cadmium and its compounds, accidental (unintentional)**
       Toxic effects of cadmium and its compounds NOS
     +7th **T56.3X2** **Toxic effect of cadmium and its compounds, intentional self-harm**
     +7th **T56.3X3** **Toxic effect of cadmium and its compounds, assault**
     +7th **T56.3X4** **Toxic effect of cadmium and its compounds, undetermined**

+ **T56.4** **Toxic effects of copper and its compounds**
   + **T56.4X** **Toxic effects of copper and its compounds**
     +7th **T56.4X1** **Toxic effect of copper and its compounds, accidental (unintentional)**
       Toxic effects of copper and its compounds NOS
     +7th **T56.4X2** **Toxic effect of copper and its compounds, intentional self-harm**
     +7th **T56.4X3** **Toxic effect of copper and its compounds, assault**
     +7th **T56.4X4** **Toxic effect of copper and its compounds, undetermined**
+ **T56.5** **Toxic effects of zinc and its compounds**
   + **T56.5X** **Toxic effects of zinc and its compounds**
     +7th **T56.5X1** **Toxic effect of zinc and its compounds, accidental (unintentional)**
       Toxic effects of zinc and its compounds NOS
     +7th **T56.5X2** **Toxic effect of zinc and its compounds, intentional self-harm**
     +7th **T56.5X3** **Toxic effect of zinc and its compounds, assault**
     +7th **T56.5X4** **Toxic effect of zinc and its compounds, undetermined**
+ **T56.6** **Toxic effects of tin and its compounds**
   + **T56.6X** **Toxic effects of tin and its compounds**
     +7th **T56.6X1** **Toxic effect of tin and its compounds, accidental (unintentional)**
       Toxic effects of tin and its compounds NOS
     +7th **T56.6X2** **Toxic effect of tin and its compounds, intentional self-harm**
     +7th **T56.6X3** **Toxic effect of tin and its compounds, assault**
     +7th **T56.6X4** **Toxic effect of tin and its compounds, undetermined**
+ **T56.7** **Toxic effects of beryllium and its compounds**
   + **T56.7X** **Toxic effects of beryllium and its compounds**
     +7th **T56.7X1** **Toxic effect of beryllium and its compounds, accidental (unintentional)**
       Toxic effects of beryllium and its compounds NOS
     +7th **T56.7X2** **Toxic effect of beryllium and its compounds, intentional self-harm**
     +7th **T56.7X3** **Toxic effect of beryllium and its compounds, assault**
     +7th **T56.7X4** **Toxic effect of beryllium and its compounds, undetermined**
+ **T56.8** **Toxic effects of other metals**
   + **T56.81** **Toxic effect of thallium**
     +7th **T56.811** **Toxic effect of thallium, accidental (unintentional)**
       Toxic effect of thallium NOS
     +7th **T56.812** **Toxic effect of thallium, intentional self-harm**
     +7th **T56.813** **Toxic effect of thallium, assault**
     +7th **T56.814** **Toxic effect of thallium, undetermined**
   + **T56.89** **Toxic effects of other metals**
     +7th **T56.891** **Toxic effect of other metals, accidental (unintentional)**
       Toxic effects of other metals NOS
     +7th **T56.892** **Toxic effect of other metals, intentional self-harm**
     +7th **T56.893** **Toxic effect of other metals, assault**
     +7th **T56.894** **Toxic effect of other metals, undetermined**
+ **T56.9** **Toxic effects of unspecified metal**
   X+7th **T56.91** **Toxic effect of unspecified metal, accidental (unintentional)**
   X+7th **T56.92** **Toxic effect of unspecified metal, intentional self-harm**
   X+7th **T56.93** **Toxic effect of unspecified metal, assault**
   X+7th **T56.94** **Toxic effect of unspecified metal, undetermined**

T57 **Toxic effect of other inorganic substances**

> The appropriate 7th character is to be added to each code from category T57
> A initial encounter
> D subsequent encounter
> S sequela

+, +7th, X + 7th ● Newborn ● Pediatric ● Maternity ● Adult ♀ Female ♂ Male Manifestation Unacceptable PDX HCC CC MCC HAC

+ **T57.0** **Toxic effect of arsenic and its compounds**
  + **T57.0X** **Toxic effect of arsenic and its compounds**
    +7th **T57.0X1** Toxic effect of arsenic and its compounds, accidental (unintentional)
      Toxic effect of arsenic and its compounds NOS
    +7th **T57.0X2** Toxic effect of arsenic and its compounds, intentional self-harm
    +7th **T57.0X3** Toxic effect of arsenic and its compounds, assault
    +7th **T57.0X4** Toxic effect of arsenic and its compounds, undetermined

+ **T57.1** **Toxic effect of phosphorus and its compounds**
    Excludes1: organophosphate insecticides (T60.0)
  + **T57.1X** **Toxic effect of phosphorus and its compounds**
    +7th **T57.1X1** Toxic effect of phosphorus and its compounds, accidental (unintentional)
      Toxic effect of phosphorus and its compounds NOS
    +7th **T57.1X2** Toxic effect of phosphorus and its compounds, intentional self-harm
    +7th **T57.1X3** Toxic effect of phosphorus and its compounds, assault
    +7th **T57.1X4** Toxic effect of phosphorus and its compounds, undetermined

+ **T57.2** **Toxic effect of manganese and its compounds**
  + **T57.2X** **Toxic effect of manganese and its compounds**
    +7th **T57.2X1** Toxic effect of manganese and its compounds, accidental (unintentional)
      Toxic effect of manganese and its compounds NOS
    +7th **T57.2X2** Toxic effect of manganese and its compounds, intentional self-harm
    +7th **T57.2X3** Toxic effect of manganese and its compounds, assault
    +7th **T57.2X4** Toxic effect of manganese and its compounds, undetermined

+ **T57.3** **Toxic effect of hydrogen cyanide**
  + **T57.3X** **Toxic effect of hydrogen cyanide**
    +7th **T57.3X1** Toxic effect of hydrogen cyanide, accidental (unintentional)
      Toxic effect of hydrogen cyanide NOS
    +7th **T57.3X2** Toxic effect of hydrogen cyanide, intentional self-harm
    +7th **T57.3X3** Toxic effect of hydrogen cyanide, assault
    +7th **T57.3X4** Toxic effect of hydrogen cyanide, undetermined

+ **T57.8** **Toxic effect of other specified inorganic substances**
  + **T57.8X** **Toxic effect of other specified inorganic substances**
    +7th **T57.8X1** Toxic effect of other specified inorganic substances, accidental (unintentional)
      Toxic effect of other specified inorganic substances NOS
    +7th **T57.8X2** Toxic effect of other specified inorganic substances, intentional self-harm
    +7th **T57.8X3** Toxic effect of other specified inorganic substances, assault
    +7th **T57.8X4** Toxic effect of other specified inorganic substances, undetermined

+ **T57.9** **Toxic effect of unspecified inorganic substance**
  X+7th **T57.91** Toxic effect of unspecified inorganic substance, accidental (unintentional)
  X+7th **T57.92** Toxic effect of unspecified inorganic substance, intentional self-harm
  X+7th **T57.93** Toxic effect of unspecified inorganic substance, assault
  X+7th **T57.94** Toxic effect of unspecified inorganic substance, undetermined

T58 **Toxic effect of carbon monoxide**

Includes: asphyxiation from carbon monoxide
  toxic effect of carbon monoxide from all sources

The appropriate 7th character is to be added to each code from category T58
A initial encounter
D subsequent encounter
S sequela

+ **T58.0** **Toxic effect of carbon monoxide from motor vehicle exhaust**
    Toxic effect of exhaust gas from gas engine
    Toxic effect of exhaust gas from motor pump
  X+7th **T58.01** Toxic effect of carbon monoxide from motor vehicle exhaust, accidental (unintentional)
  X+7th **T58.02** Toxic effect of carbon monoxide from motor vehicle exhaust, intentional self-harm
  X+7th **T58.03** Toxic effect of carbon monoxide from motor vehicle exhaust, assault
  X+7th **T58.04** Toxic effect of carbon monoxide from motor vehicle exhaust, undetermined

+ **T58.1** **Toxic effect of carbon monoxide from utility gas**
    Toxic effect of acetylene
    Toxic effect of gas NOS used for lighting, heating, cooking
    Toxic effect of water gas
  X+7th **T58.11** Toxic effect of carbon monoxide from utility gas, accidental (unintentional)
  X+7th **T58.12** Toxic effect of carbon monoxide from utility gas, intentional self-harm
  X+7th **T58.13** Toxic effect of carbon monoxide from utility gas, assault
  X+7th **T58.14** Toxic effect of carbon monoxide from utility gas, undetermined

+ **T58.2** **Toxic effect of carbon monoxide from incomplete combustion of other domestic fuels**
    Toxic effect of carbon monoxide from incomplete combustion of coal, coke, kerosene, wood
  + **T58.2X** **Toxic effect of carbon monoxide from incomplete combustion of other domestic fuels**
    +7th **T58.2X1** Toxic effect of carbon monoxide from incomplete combustion of other domestic fuels, accidental (unintentional)
    +7th **T58.2X2** Toxic effect of carbon monoxide from incomplete combustion of other domestic fuels, intentional self-harm
    +7th **T58.2X3** Toxic effect of carbon monoxide from incomplete combustion of other domestic fuels, assault
    +7th **T58.2X4** Toxic effect of carbon monoxide from incomplete combustion of other domestic fuels, undetermined

+ **T58.8** **Toxic effect of carbon monoxide from other source**
    Toxic effect of carbon monoxide from blast furnace gas
    Toxic effect of carbon monoxide from fuels in industrial use
    Toxic effect of carbon monoxide from kiln vapor
  + **T58.8X** **Toxic effect of carbon monoxide from other source**
    +7th **T58.8X1** Toxic effect of carbon monoxide from other source, accidental (unintentional)
    +7th **T58.8X2** Toxic effect of carbon monoxide from other source, intentional self-harm
    +7th **T58.8X3** Toxic effect of carbon monoxide from other source, assault
    +7th **T58.8X4** Toxic effect of carbon monoxide from other source, undetermined

+ **T58.9** **Toxic effect of carbon monoxide from unspecified source**
  X+7th **T58.91** Toxic effect of carbon monoxide from unspecified source, accidental (unintentional)
  X+7th **T58.92** Toxic effect of carbon monoxide from unspecified source, intentional self-harm
  X+7th **T58.93** Toxic effect of carbon monoxide from unspecified source, assault
  X+7th **T58.94** Toxic effect of carbon monoxide from unspecified source, undetermined

T59 **Toxic effect of other gases, fumes and vapors**

Includes: aerosol propellants
Excludes1: chlorofluorocarbons (T53.5)

The appropriate 7th character is to be added to each code from category T59
A initial encounter
D subsequent encounter
S sequela

+ **T59.0** **Toxic effect of nitrogen oxides**
+ **T59.0X** **Toxic effect of nitrogen oxides**
+7th **T59.0X1** **Toxic effect of nitrogen oxides, accidental (unintentional)**
Toxic effect of nitrogen oxides NOS
+7th **T59.0X2** **Toxic effect of nitrogen oxides, intentional self-harm**
+7th **T59.0X3** **Toxic effect of nitrogen oxides, assault**
+7th **T59.0X4** **Toxic effect of nitrogen oxides, undetermined**
+ **T59.1** **Toxic effect of sulfur dioxide**
+ **T59.1X** **Toxic effect of sulfur dioxide**
+7th **T59.1X1** **Toxic effect of sulfur dioxide, accidental (unintentional)**
Toxic effect of sulfur dioxide NOS
+7th **T59.1X2** **Toxic effect of sulfur dioxide, intentional self-harm**
+7th **T59.1X3** **Toxic effect of sulfur dioxide, assault**
+7th **T59.1X4** **Toxic effect of sulfur dioxide, undetermined**
+ **T59.2** **Toxic effect of formaldehyde**
+ **T59.2X** **Toxic effect of formaldehyde**
+7th **T59.2X1** **Toxic effect of formaldehyde, accidental (unintentional)**
Toxic effect of formaldehyde NOS
+7th **T59.2X2** **Toxic effect of formaldehyde, intentional self-harm**
+7th **T59.2X3** **Toxic effect of formaldehyde, assault**
+7th **T59.2X4** **Toxic effect of formaldehyde, undetermined**
+ **T59.3** **Toxic effect of lacrimogenic gas**
Toxic effect of tear gas
+ **T59.3X** **Toxic effect of lacrimogenic gas**
+7th **T59.3X1** **Toxic effect of lacrimogenic gas, accidental (unintentional)**
Toxic effect of lacrimogenic gas NOS
+7th **T59.3X2** **Toxic effect of lacrimogenic gas, intentional self-harm**
+7th **T59.3X3** **Toxic effect of lacrimogenic gas, assault**
+7th **T59.3X4** **Toxic effect of lacrimogenic gas, undetermined**
+ **T59.4** **Toxic effect of chlorine gas**
+ **T59.4X** **Toxic effect of chlorine gas**
+7th **T59.4X1** **Toxic effect of chlorine gas, accidental (unintentional)**
Toxic effect of chlorine gas NOS
+7th **T59.4X2** **Toxic effect of chlorine gas, intentional self-harm**
+7th **T59.4X3** **Toxic effect of chlorine gas, assault**
+7th **T59.4X4** **Toxic effect of chlorine gas, undetermined**
+ **T59.5** **Toxic effect of fluorine gas and hydrogen fluoride**
+ **T59.5X** **Toxic effect of fluorine gas and hydrogen fluoride**
+7th **T59.5X1** **Toxic effect of fluorine gas and hydrogen fluoride, accidental (unintentional)**
Toxic effect of fluorine gas and hydrogen fluoride NOS
+7th **T59.5X2** **Toxic effect of fluorine gas and hydrogen fluoride, intentional self-harm**
+7th **T59.5X3** **Toxic effect of fluorine gas and hydrogen fluoride, assault**
+7th **T59.5X4** **Toxic effect of fluorine gas and hydrogen fluoride, undetermined**
+ **T59.6** **Toxic effect of hydrogen sulfide**
+ **T59.6X** **Toxic effect of hydrogen sulfide**
+7th **T59.6X1** **Toxic effect of hydrogen sulfide, accidental (unintentional)**
Toxic effect of hydrogen sulfide NOS
+7th **T59.6X2** **Toxic effect of hydrogen sulfide, intentional self-harm**
+7th **T59.6X3** **Toxic effect of hydrogen sulfide, assault**
+7th **T59.6X4** **Toxic effect of hydrogen sulfide, undetermined**
+ **T59.7** **Toxic effect of carbon dioxide**
+ **T59.7X** **Toxic effect of carbon dioxide**
+7th **T59.7X1** **Toxic effect of carbon dioxide, accidental (unintentional)**
Toxic effect of carbon dioxide NOS
+7th **T59.7X2** **Toxic effect of carbon dioxide, intentional self-harm**
+7th **T59.7X3** **Toxic effect of carbon dioxide, assault**
+7th **T59.7X4** **Toxic effect of carbon dioxide, undetermined**

+ **T59.8** **Toxic effect of other specified gases, fumes and vapors**
+ **T59.81** **Toxic effect of smoke**
Smoke inhalation
Excludes2: *toxic effect of cigarette (tobacco) smoke (T65.22-)*
+7th **T59.811** **Toxic effect of smoke, accidental (unintentional)**
Toxic effect of smoke NOS
+7th **T59.812** **Toxic effect of smoke, intentional self-harm**
+7th **T59.813** **Toxic effect of smoke, assault**
+7th **T59.814** **Toxic effect of smoke, undetermined**
+ **T59.89** **Toxic effect of other specified gases, fumes and vapors**
+7th **T59.891** **Toxic effect of other specified gases, fumes and vapors, accidental (unintentional)**
+7th **T59.892** **Toxic effect of other specified gases, fumes and vapors, intentional self-harm**
+7th **T59.893** **Toxic effect of other specified gases, fumes and vapors, assault**
+7th **T59.894** **Toxic effect of other specified gases, fumes and vapors, undetermined**
+ **T59.9** **Toxic effect of unspecified gases, fumes and vapors**
X+7th **T59.91** **Toxic effect of unspecified gases, fumes and vapors, accidental (unintentional)**
X+7th **T59.92** **Toxic effect of unspecified gases, fumes and vapors, intentional self-harm**
X+7th **T59.93** **Toxic effect of unspecified gases, fumes and vapors, assault**
X+7th **T59.94** **Toxic effect of unspecified gases, fumes and vapors, undetermined**

T60 **Toxic effect of pesticides**

Includes: toxic effect of wood preservatives

The appropriate 7th character is to be added to each code from category T60
A   initial encounter
D   subsequent encounter
S   sequela

+ **T60.0** **Toxic effect of organophosphate and carbamate insecticides**
+ **T60.0X** **Toxic effect of organophosphate and carbamate insecticides**
+7th **T60.0X1** **Toxic effect of organophosphate and carbamate insecticides, accidental (unintentional)**
Toxic effect of organophosphate and carbamate insecticides NOS
+7th **T60.0X2** **Toxic effect of organophosphate and carbamate insecticides, intentional self-harm**
+7th **T60.0X3** **Toxic effect of organophosphate and carbamate insecticides, assault**
+7th **T60.0X4** **Toxic effect of organophosphate and carbamate insecticides, undetermined**
+ **T60.1** **Toxic effect of halogenated insecticides**
Excludes1: *chlorinated hydrocarbon (T53.-)*
+ **T60.1X** **Toxic effect of halogenated insecticides**
+7th **T60.1X1** **Toxic effect of halogenated insecticides, accidental (unintentional)**
Toxic effect of halogenated insecticides NOS
+7th **T60.1X2** **Toxic effect of halogenated insecticides, intentional self-harm**
+7th **T60.1X3** **Toxic effect of halogenated insecticides, assault**
+7th **T60.1X4** **Toxic effect of halogenated insecticides, undetermined**
+ **T60.2** **Toxic effect of other insecticides**
+ **T60.2X** **Toxic effect of other insecticides**
+7th **T60.2X1** **Toxic effect of other insecticides, accidental (unintentional)**
Toxic effect of other insecticides NOS
+7th **T60.2X2** **Toxic effect of other insecticides, intentional self-harm**
+7th **T60.2X3** **Toxic effect of other insecticides, assault**
+7th **T60.2X4** **Toxic effect of other insecticides, undetermined**

+, +7th, X + 7th   ● Newborn   ● Pediatric   ● Maternity   ● Adult   ♀ Female   ♂ Male   Manifestation   Unacceptable PDX   HCC   CC   MCC   HAC

+ **T60.3** Toxic effect of herbicides and fungicides
- + **T60.3X** Toxic effect of herbicides and fungicides
  - +7th **T60.3X1** Toxic effect of herbicides and fungicides, accidental (unintentional)
    Toxic effect of herbicides and fungicides NOS
  - +7th **T60.3X2** Toxic effect of herbicides and fungicides, intentional self-harm
  - +7th **T60.3X3** Toxic effect of herbicides and fungicides, assault
  - +7th **T60.3X4** Toxic effect of herbicides and fungicides, undetermined

+ **T60.4** Toxic effect of rodenticides
  Excludes1: strychnine and its salts (T65.1)
  thallium (T56.81-)
- + **T60.4X** Toxic effect of rodenticides
  - +7th **T60.4X1** Toxic effect of rodenticides, accidental (unintentional)
    Toxic effect of rodenticides NOS
  - +7th **T60.4X2** Toxic effect of rodenticides, intentional self-harm
  - +7th **T60.4X3** Toxic effect of rodenticides, assault
  - +7th **T60.4X4** Toxic effect of rodenticides, undetermined

+ **T60.8** Toxic effect of other pesticides
- + **T60.8X** Toxic effect of other pesticides
  - +7th **T60.8X1** Toxic effect of other pesticides, accidental (unintentional)
    Toxic effect of other pesticides NOS
  - +7th **T60.8X2** Toxic effect of other pesticides, intentional self-harm
  - +7th **T60.8X3** Toxic effect of other pesticides, assault
  - +7th **T60.8X4** Toxic effect of other pesticides, undetermined

+ **T60.9** Toxic effect of unspecified pesticide
  - X+7th **T60.91** Toxic effect of unspecified pesticide, accidental (unintentional)
  - X+7th **T60.92** Toxic effect of unspecified pesticide, intentional self-harm
  - X+7th **T60.93** Toxic effect of unspecified pesticide, assault
  - X+7th **T60.94** Toxic effect of unspecified pesticide, undetermined

T61 Toxic effect of noxious substances eaten as seafood

Excludes1: allergic reaction to food, such as:
anaphylactic reaction or shock due to adverse food reaction (T78.0-)
bacterial foodborne intoxications (A05.-)
dermatitis (L23.6, L25.4, L27.2)
food protein-induced enterocolitis syndrome (K52.21)
food protein-induced enteropathy (K52.22)
gastroenteritis (noninfective) (K52.29)
toxic effect of aflatoxin and other mycotoxins (T64)
toxic effect of cyanides (T65.0-)
toxic effect of harmful algae bloom (T65.82-)
toxic effect of hydrogen cyanide (T57.3-)
toxic effect of mercury (T56.1-)
toxic effect of red tide (T65.82-)

The appropriate 7th character is to be added to each code from category T61
A   initial encounter
D   subsequent encounter
S   sequela

+ **T61.0** Ciguatera fish poisoning
  - X+7th **T61.01** Ciguatera fish poisoning, accidental (unintentional)
  - X+7th **T61.02** Ciguatera fish poisoning, intentional self-harm
  - X+7th **T61.03** Ciguatera fish poisoning, assault
  - X+7th **T61.04** Ciguatera fish poisoning, undetermined

+ **T61.1** Scombroid fish poisoning
  Histamine-like syndrome
  - X+7th **T61.11** Scombroid fish poisoning, accidental (unintentional)
  - X+7th **T61.12** Scombroid fish poisoning, intentional self-harm
  - X+7th **T61.13** Scombroid fish poisoning, assault
  - X+7th **T61.14** Scombroid fish poisoning, undetermined

+ **T61.7** Other fish and shellfish poisoning
- + **T61.77** Other fish poisoning
  - +7th **T61.771** Other fish poisoning, accidental (unintentional)
  - +7th **T61.772** Other fish poisoning, intentional self-harm
  - +7th **T61.773** Other fish poisoning, assault
  - +7th **T61.774** Other fish poisoning, undetermined
- + **T61.78** Other shellfish poisoning
  - +7th **T61.781** Other shellfish poisoning, accidental (unintentional)
  - +7th **T61.782** Other shellfish poisoning, intentional self-harm
  - +7th **T61.783** Other shellfish poisoning, assault
  - +7th **T61.784** Other shellfish poisoning, undetermined

+ **T61.8** Toxic effect of other seafood
- + **T61.8X** Toxic effect of other seafood
  - +7th **T61.8X1** Toxic effect of other seafood, accidental (unintentional)
  - +7th **T61.8X2** Toxic effect of other seafood, intentional self-harm
  - +7th **T61.8X3** Toxic effect of other seafood, assault
  - +7th **T61.8X4** Toxic effect of other seafood, undetermined

+ **T61.9** Toxic effect of unspecified seafood
  - X+7th **T61.91** Toxic effect of unspecified seafood, accidental (unintentional)
  - X+7th **T61.92** Toxic effect of unspecified seafood, intentional self-harm
  - X+7th **T61.93** Toxic effect of unspecified seafood, assault
  - X+7th **T61.94** Toxic effect of unspecified seafood, undetermined

T62 Toxic effect of other noxious substances eaten as food

Excludes1: allergic reaction to food, such as:
anaphylactic shock (reaction) due to adverse food reaction (T78.0-)
bacterial food borne intoxications (A05.-)
dermatitis (L23.6, L25.4, L27.2)
food protein-induced enterocolitis syndrome (K52.21)
food protein-induced enteropathy (K52.22)
gastroenteritis (noninfective) (K52.29)
toxic effect of aflatoxin and other mycotoxins (T64)
toxic effect of cyanides (T65.0-)
toxic effect of hydrogen cyanide (T57.3-)
toxic effect of mercury (T56.1-)

The appropriate 7th character is to be added to each code from category T62
A   initial encounter
D   subsequent encounter
S   sequela

+ **T62.0** Toxic effect of ingested mushrooms
- + **T62.0X** Toxic effect of ingested mushrooms
  - +7th **T62.0X1** Toxic effect of ingested mushrooms, accidental (unintentional)
    Toxic effect of ingested mushrooms NOS
  - +7th **T62.0X2** Toxic effect of ingested mushrooms, intentional self-harm
  - +7th **T62.0X3** Toxic effect of ingested mushrooms, assault
  - +7th **T62.0X4** Toxic effect of ingested mushrooms, undetermined

+ **T62.1** Toxic effect of ingested berries
- + **T62.1X** Toxic effect of ingested berries
  - +7th **T62.1X1** Toxic effect of ingested berries, accidental (unintentional)
    Toxic effect of ingested berries NOS
  - +7th **T62.1X2** Toxic effect of ingested berries, intentional self-harm
  - +7th **T62.1X3** Toxic effect of ingested berries, assault
  - +7th **T62.1X4** Toxic effect of ingested berries, undetermined

+ **T62.2** **Toxic effect of other ingested (parts of) plant(s)**
  + **T62.2X** **Toxic effect of other ingested (parts of) plant(s)**
    +7th **T62.2X1** **Toxic effect of other ingested (parts of) plant(s), accidental (unintentional)**
      Toxic effect of other ingested (parts of) plant(s) NOS
    +7th **T62.2X2** **Toxic effect of other ingested (parts of) plant(s), intentional self-harm**
    +7th **T62.2X3** **Toxic effect of other ingested (parts of) plant(s), assault**
    +7th **T62.2X4** **Toxic effect of other ingested (parts of) plant(s), undetermined**
+ **T62.8** **Toxic effect of other specified noxious substances eaten as food**
  + **T62.8X** **Toxic effect of other specified noxious substances eaten as food**
    +7th **T62.8X1** **Toxic effect of other specified noxious substances eaten as food, accidental (unintentional)**
      Toxic effect of other specified noxious substances eaten as food NOS
    +7th **T62.8X2** **Toxic effect of other specified noxious substances eaten as food, intentional self-harm**
    +7th **T62.8X3** **Toxic effect of other specified noxious substances eaten as food, assault**
    +7th **T62.8X4** **Toxic effect of other specified noxious substances eaten as food, undetermined**
+ **T62.9** **Toxic effect of unspecified noxious substance eaten as food**
  X+7th **T62.91** **Toxic effect of unspecified noxious substance eaten as food, accidental (unintentional)**
    Toxic effect of unspecified noxious substance eaten as food NOS
  X+7th **T62.92** **Toxic effect of unspecified noxious substance eaten as food, intentional self-harm**
  X+7th **T62.93** **Toxic effect of unspecified noxious substance eaten as food, assault**
  X+7th **T62.94** **Toxic effect of unspecified noxious substance eaten as food, undetermined**

T63 **Toxic effect of contact with venomous animals and plants**

  Includes: bite or touch of venomous animal
      pricked or stuck by thorn or leaf
  Excludes2: *ingestion of toxic animal or plant (T61.-, T62.-)*

  The appropriate 7th character is to be added to each code from category T63
  A initial encounter
  D subsequent encounter
  S sequela

+ **T63.0** **Toxic effect of snake venom**
  + **T63.00** **Toxic effect of unspecified snake venom**
    +7th **T63.001** **Toxic effect of unspecified snake venom, accidental (unintentional)**
      Toxic effect of unspecified snake venom NOS
    +7th **T63.002** **Toxic effect of unspecified snake venom, intentional self-harm**
    +7th **T63.003** **Toxic effect of unspecified snake venom, assault**
    +7th **T63.004** **Toxic effect of unspecified snake venom, undetermined**
  + **T63.01** **Toxic effect of rattlesnake venom**
    +7th **T63.011** **Toxic effect of rattlesnake venom, accidental (unintentional)**
      Toxic effect of rattlesnake venom NOS
    +7th **T63.012** **Toxic effect of rattlesnake venom, intentional self-harm**
    +7th **T63.013** **Toxic effect of rattlesnake venom, assault**
    +7th **T63.014** **Toxic effect of rattlesnake venom, undetermined**
  + **T63.02** **Toxic effect of coral snake venom**
    +7th **T63.021** **Toxic effect of coral snake venom, accidental (unintentional)**
      Toxic effect of coral snake venom NOS
    +7th **T63.022** **Toxic effect of coral snake venom, intentional self-harm**
    +7th **T63.023** **Toxic effect of coral snake venom, assault**
    +7th **T63.024** **Toxic effect of coral snake venom, undetermined**

+ **T63.03** **Toxic effect of taipan venom**
  +7th **T63.031** **Toxic effect of taipan venom, accidental (unintentional)**
    Toxic effect of taipan venom NOS
  +7th **T63.032** **Toxic effect of taipan venom, intentional self-harm**
  +7th **T63.033** **Toxic effect of taipan venom, assault**
  +7th **T63.034** **Toxic effect of taipan venom, undetermined**
+ **T63.04** **Toxic effect of cobra venom**
  +7th **T63.041** **Toxic effect of cobra venom, accidental (unintentional)**
    Toxic effect of cobra venom NOS
  +7th **T63.042** **Toxic effect of cobra venom, intentional self-harm**
  +7th **T63.043** **Toxic effect of cobra venom, assault**
  +7th **T63.044** **Toxic effect of cobra venom, undetermined**
+ **T63.06** **Toxic effect of venom of other North and South American snake**
  +7th **T63.061** **Toxic effect of venom of other North and South American snake, accidental (unintentional)**
    Toxic effect of venom of other North and South American snake NOS
  +7th **T63.062** **Toxic effect of venom of other North and South American snake, intentional self-harm**
  +7th **T63.063** **Toxic effect of venom of other North and South American snake, assault**
  +7th **T63.064** **Toxic effect of venom of other North and South American snake, undetermined**
+ **T63.07** **Toxic effect of venom of other Australian snake**
  +7th **T63.071** **Toxic effect of venom of other Australian snake, accidental (unintentional)**
    Toxic effect of venom of other Australian snake NOS
  +7th **T63.072** **Toxic effect of venom of other Australian snake, intentional self-harm**
  +7th **T63.073** **Toxic effect of venom of other Australian snake, assault**
  +7th **T63.074** **Toxic effect of venom of other Australian snake, undetermined**
+ **T63.08** **Toxic effect of venom of other African and Asian snake**
  +7th **T63.081** **Toxic effect of venom of other African and Asian snake, accidental (unintentional)**
    Toxic effect of venom of other African and Asian snake NOS
  +7th **T63.082** **Toxic effect of venom of other African and Asian snake, intentional self-harm**
  +7th **T63.083** **Toxic effect of venom of other African and Asian snake, assault**
  +7th **T63.084** **Toxic effect of venom of other African and Asian snake, undetermined**
+ **T63.09** **Toxic effect of venom of other snake**
  +7th **T63.091** **Toxic effect of venom of other snake, accidental (unintentional)**
    Toxic effect of venom of other snake NOS
  +7th **T63.092** **Toxic effect of venom of other snake, intentional self-harm**
  +7th **T63.093** **Toxic effect of venom of other snake, assault**
  +7th **T63.094** **Toxic effect of venom of other snake, undetermined**
+ **T63.1** **Toxic effect of venom of other reptiles**
  + **T63.11** **Toxic effect of venom of gila monster**
    +7th **T63.111** **Toxic effect of venom of gila monster, accidental (unintentional)**
      Toxic effect of venom of gila monster NOS
    +7th **T63.112** **Toxic effect of venom of gila monster, intentional self-harm**
    +7th **T63.113** **Toxic effect of venom of gila monster, assault**
    +7th **T63.114** **Toxic effect of venom of gila monster, undetermined**

+, +7th, X + 7th ● Newborn ● Pediatric ● Maternity ● Adult ♀ Female ♂ Male Manifestation Unacceptable PDX HCC CC MCC HAC

+ **T63.12** **Toxic effect of venom of other venomous lizard**
  - +7th **T63.121** Toxic effect of venom of other venomous lizard, accidental (unintentional)
    - Toxic effect of venom of other venomous lizard NOS
  - +7th **T63.122** Toxic effect of venom of other venomous lizard, intentional self-harm
  - +7th **T63.123** Toxic effect of venom of other venomous lizard, assault
  - +7th **T63.124** Toxic effect of venom of other venomous lizard, undetermined

+ **T63.19** **Toxic effect of venom of other reptiles**
  - +7th **T63.191** Toxic effect of venom of other reptiles, accidental (unintentional)
    - Toxic effect of venom of other reptiles NOS
  - +7th **T63.192** Toxic effect of venom of other reptiles, intentional self-harm
  - +7th **T63.193** Toxic effect of venom of other reptiles, assault
  - +7th **T63.194** Toxic effect of venom of other reptiles, undetermined

+ **T63.2** **Toxic effect of venom of scorpion**
  + **T63.2X** **Toxic effect of venom of scorpion**
    - +7th **T63.2X1** Toxic effect of venom of scorpion, accidental (unintentional)
      - Toxic effect of venom of scorpion NOS
    - +7th **T63.2X2** Toxic effect of venom of scorpion, intentional self-harm
    - +7th **T63.2X3** Toxic effect of venom of scorpion, assault
    - +7th **T63.2X4** Toxic effect of venom of scorpion, undetermined

+ **T63.3** **Toxic effect of venom of spider**
  + **T63.30** **Toxic effect of unspecified spider venom**
    - +7th **T63.301** Toxic effect of unspecified spider venom, accidental (unintentional)
    - +7th **T63.302** Toxic effect of unspecified spider venom, intentional self-harm
    - +7th **T63.303** Toxic effect of unspecified spider venom, assault
    - +7th **T63.304** Toxic effect of unspecified spider venom, undetermined
  + **T63.31** **Toxic effect of venom of black widow spider**
    - +7th **T63.311** Toxic effect of venom of black widow spider, accidental (unintentional)
    - +7th **T63.312** Toxic effect of venom of black widow spider, intentional self-harm
    - +7th **T63.313** Toxic effect of venom of black widow spider, assault
    - +7th **T63.314** Toxic effect of venom of black widow spider, undetermined
  + **T63.32** **Toxic effect of venom of tarantula**
    - +7th **T63.321** Toxic effect of venom of tarantula, accidental (unintentional)
    - +7th **T63.322** Toxic effect of venom of tarantula, intentional self-harm
    - +7th **T63.323** Toxic effect of venom of tarantula, assault
    - +7th **T63.324** Toxic effect of venom of tarantula, undetermined
  + **T63.33** **Toxic effect of venom of brown recluse spider**
    - +7th **T63.331** Toxic effect of venom of brown recluse spider, accidental (unintentional)
    - +7th **T63.332** Toxic effect of venom of brown recluse spider, intentional self-harm
    - +7th **T63.333** Toxic effect of venom of brown recluse spider, assault
    - +7th **T63.334** Toxic effect of venom of brown recluse spider, undetermined
  + **T63.39** **Toxic effect of venom of other spider**
    - +7th **T63.391** Toxic effect of venom of other spider, accidental (unintentional)
    - +7th **T63.392** Toxic effect of venom of other spider, intentional self-harm
    - +7th **T63.393** Toxic effect of venom of other spider, assault
    - +7th **T63.394** Toxic effect of venom of other spider, undetermined

+ **T63.4** **Toxic effect of venom of other arthropods**
  + **T63.41** **Toxic effect of venom of centipedes and venomous millipedes**
    - +7th **T63.411** Toxic effect of venom of centipedes and venomous millipedes, accidental (unintentional)
    - +7th **T63.412** Toxic effect of venom of centipedes and venomous millipedes, intentional self-harm
    - +7th **T63.413** Toxic effect of venom of centipedes and venomous millipedes, assault
    - +7th **T63.414** Toxic effect of venom of centipedes and venomous millipedes, undetermined
  + **T63.42** **Toxic effect of venom of ants**
    - +7th **T63.421** Toxic effect of venom of ants, accidental (unintentional)
    - +7th **T63.422** Toxic effect of venom of ants, intentional self-harm
    - +7th **T63.423** Toxic effect of venom of ants, assault
    - +7th **T63.424** Toxic effect of venom of ants, undetermined
  + **T63.43** **Toxic effect of venom of caterpillars**
    - +7th **T63.431** Toxic effect of venom of caterpillars, accidental (unintentional)
    - +7th **T63.432** Toxic effect of venom of caterpillars, intentional self-harm
    - +7th **T63.433** Toxic effect of venom of caterpillars, assault
    - +7th **T63.434** Toxic effect of venom of caterpillars, undetermined
  + **T63.44** **Toxic effect of venom of bees**
    - +7th **T63.441** Toxic effect of venom of bees, accidental (unintentional)
    - +7th **T63.442** Toxic effect of venom of bees, intentional self-harm
    - +7th **T63.443** Toxic effect of venom of bees, assault
    - +7th **T63.444** Toxic effect of venom of bees, undetermined
  + **T63.45** **Toxic effect of venom of hornets**
    - +7th **T63.451** Toxic effect of venom of hornets, accidental (unintentional)
    - +7th **T63.452** Toxic effect of venom of hornets, intentional self-harm
    - +7th **T63.453** Toxic effect of venom of hornets, assault
    - +7th **T63.454** Toxic effect of venom of hornets, undetermined
  + **T63.46** **Toxic effect of venom of wasps**
    - Toxic effect of yellow jacket
    - +7th **T63.461** Toxic effect of venom of wasps, accidental (unintentional)
    - +7th **T63.462** Toxic effect of venom of wasps, intentional self-harm
    - +7th **T63.463** Toxic effect of venom of wasps, assault
    - +7th **T63.464** Toxic effect of venom of wasps, undetermined
  + **T63.48** **Toxic effect of venom of other arthropod**
    - +7th **T63.481** Toxic effect of venom of other arthropod, accidental (unintentional)
    - +7th **T63.482** Toxic effect of venom of other arthropod, intentional self-harm
    - +7th **T63.483** Toxic effect of venom of other arthropod, assault
    - +7th **T63.484** Toxic effect of venom of other arthropod, undetermined

+ **T63.5** **Toxic effect of contact with venomous fish**
  - *Excludes2:* *poisoning by ingestion of fish (T61.-)*
  + **T63.51** **Toxic effect of contact with stingray**
    - +7th **T63.511** Toxic effect of contact with stingray, accidental (unintentional)
    - +7th **T63.512** Toxic effect of contact with stingray, intentional self-harm
    - +7th **T63.513** Toxic effect of contact with stingray, assault
    - +7th **T63.514** Toxic effect of contact with stingray, undetermined

+ **T63.59** Toxic effect of contact with other venomous fish
+7th **T63.591** Toxic effect of contact with other venomous fish, accidental (unintentional)
+7th **T63.592** Toxic effect of contact with other venomous fish, intentional self-harm
+7th **T63.593** Toxic effect of contact with other venomous fish, assault
+7th **T63.594** Toxic effect of contact with other venomous fish, undetermined

+ **T63.6** Toxic effect of contact with other venomous marine animals
Excludes1: sea-snake venom (T63.09)
Excludes2: poisoning by ingestion of shellfish (T61.78-)

+ **T63.61** Toxic effect of contact with Portugese Man-o-war
Toxic effect of contact with bluebottle
+7th **T63.611** Toxic effect of contact with Portugese Man-o-war, accidental (unintentional)
+7th **T63.612** Toxic effect of contact with Portugese Man-o-war, intentional self-harm
+7th **T63.613** Toxic effect of contact with Portugese Man-o-war, assault
+7th **T63.614** Toxic effect of contact with Portugese Man-o-war, undetermined

+ **T63.62** Toxic effect of contact with other jellyfish
+7th **T63.621** Toxic effect of contact with other jellyfish, accidental (unintentional)
+7th **T63.622** Toxic effect of contact with other jellyfish, intentional self-harm
+7th **T63.623** Toxic effect of contact with other jellyfish, assault
+7th **T63.624** Toxic effect of contact with other jellyfish, undetermined

+ **T63.63** Toxic effect of contact with sea anemone
+7th **T63.631** Toxic effect of contact with sea anemone, accidental (unintentional)
+7th **T63.632** Toxic effect of contact with sea anemone, intentional self-harm
+7th **T63.633** Toxic effect of contact with sea anemone, assault
+7th **T63.634** Toxic effect of contact with sea anemone, undetermined

+ **T63.69** Toxic effect of contact with other venomous marine animals
+7th **T63.691** Toxic effect of contact with other venomous marine animals, accidental (unintentional)
+7th **T63.692** Toxic effect of contact with other venomous marine animals, intentional self-harm
+7th **T63.693** Toxic effect of contact with other venomous marine animals, assault
+7th **T63.694** Toxic effect of contact with other venomous marine animals, undetermined

+ **T63.7** Toxic effect of contact with venomous plant
+ **T63.71** Toxic effect of contact with venomous marine plant
+7th **T63.711** Toxic effect of contact with venomous marine plant, accidental (unintentional)
+7th **T63.712** Toxic effect of contact with venomous marine plant, intentional self-harm
+7th **T63.713** Toxic effect of contact with venomous marine plant, assault
+7th **T63.714** Toxic effect of contact with venomous marine plant, undetermined

+ **T63.79** Toxic effect of contact with other venomous plant
+7th **T63.791** Toxic effect of contact with other venomous plant, accidental (unintentional)
+7th **T63.792** Toxic effect of contact with other venomous plant, intentional self-harm
+7th **T63.793** Toxic effect of contact with other venomous plant, assault
+7th **T63.794** Toxic effect of contact with other venomous plant, undetermined

+ **T63.8** Toxic effect of contact with other venomous animals
+ **T63.81** Toxic effect of contact with venomous frog
Excludes1: contact with nonvenomous frog (W62.0)
+7th **T63.811** Toxic effect of contact with venomous frog, accidental (unintentional)
+7th **T63.812** Toxic effect of contact with venomous frog, intentional self-harm
+7th **T63.813** Toxic effect of contact with venomous frog, assault
+7th **T63.814** Toxic effect of contact with venomous frog, undetermined

+ **T63.82** Toxic effect of contact with venomous toad
Excludes1: contact with nonvenomous toad (W62.1)
+7th **T63.821** Toxic effect of contact with venomous toad, accidental (unintentional)
+7th **T63.822** Toxic effect of contact with venomous toad, intentional self-harm
+7th **T63.823** Toxic effect of contact with venomous toad, assault
+7th **T63.824** Toxic effect of contact with venomous toad, undetermined

+ **T63.83** Toxic effect of contact with other venomous amphibian
Excludes1: contact with nonvenomous amphibian (W62.9)
+7th **T63.831** Toxic effect of contact with other venomous amphibian, accidental (unintentional)
+7th **T63.832** Toxic effect of contact with other venomous amphibian, intentional self-harm
+7th **T63.833** Toxic effect of contact with other venomous amphibian, assault
+7th **T63.834** Toxic effect of contact with other venomous amphibian, undetermined

+ **T63.89** Toxic effect of contact with other venomous animals
+7th **T63.891** Toxic effect of contact with other venomous animals, accidental (unintentional)
+7th **T63.892** Toxic effect of contact with other venomous animals, intentional self-harm
+7th **T63.893** Toxic effect of contact with other venomous animals, assault
+7th **T63.894** Toxic effect of contact with other venomous animals, undetermined

+ **T63.9** Toxic effect of contact with unspecified venomous animal
X+7th **T63.91** Toxic effect of contact with unspecified venomous animal, accidental (unintentional)
X+7th **T63.92** Toxic effect of contact with unspecified venomous animal, intentional self-harm
X+7th **T63.93** Toxic effect of contact with unspecified venomous animal, assault
X+7th **T63.94** Toxic effect of contact with unspecified venomous animal, undetermined

T64 Toxic effect of aflatoxin and other mycotoxin food contaminants

> The appropriate 7th character is to be added to each code from category T64
> A   initial encounter
> D   subsequent encounter
> S   sequela

+ **T64.0** Toxic effect of aflatoxin
X+7th **T64.01** Toxic effect of aflatoxin, accidental (unintentional)
X+7th **T64.02** Toxic effect of aflatoxin, intentional self-harm
X+7th **T64.03** Toxic effect of aflatoxin, assault
X+7th **T64.04** Toxic effect of aflatoxin, undetermined

+ **T64.8** Toxic effect of other mycotoxin food contaminants
X+7th **T64.81** Toxic effect of other mycotoxin food contaminants, accidental (unintentional)
X+7th **T64.82** Toxic effect of other mycotoxin food contaminants, intentional self-harm
X+7th **T64.83** Toxic effect of other mycotoxin food contaminants, assault
X+7th **T64.84** Toxic effect of other mycotoxin food contaminants, undetermined

+, +7th, X + 7th   ● Newborn   ● Pediatric   ● Maternity   ● Adult   ♀ Female   ♂ Male   Manifestation   Unacceptable PDX   HCC   CC   MCC   HAC

T65 Toxic effect of other and unspecified substances

> The appropriate 7th character is to be added to each code from category T65
> A   initial encounter
> D   subsequent encounter
> S   sequela

+ **T65.0 Toxic effect of cyanides**
  Excludes1: hydrogen cyanide (T57.3-)
  + **T65.0X Toxic effect of cyanides**
    +7th **T65.0X1 Toxic effect of cyanides, accidental (unintentional)**
      Toxic effect of cyanides NOS
    +7th **T65.0X2 Toxic effect of cyanides, intentional self-harm**
    +7th **T65.0X3 Toxic effect of cyanides, assault**
    +7th **T65.0X4 Toxic effect of cyanides, undetermined**
+ **T65.1 Toxic effect of strychnine and its salts**
  + **T65.1X Toxic effect of strychnine and its salts**
    +7th **T65.1X1 Toxic effect of strychnine and its salts, accidental (unintentional)**
      Toxic effect of strychnine and its salts NOS
    +7th **T65.1X2 Toxic effect of strychnine and its salts, intentional self-harm**
    +7th **T65.1X3 Toxic effect of strychnine and its salts, assault**
    +7th **T65.1X4 Toxic effect of strychnine and its salts, undetermined**
+ **T65.2 Toxic effect of tobacco and nicotine**
  Excludes2: nicotine dependence (F17.-)
  + **T65.21 Toxic effect of chewing tobacco**
    +7th **T65.211 Toxic effect of chewing tobacco, accidental (unintentional)**
      Toxic effect of chewing tobacco NOS
    +7th **T65.212 Toxic effect of chewing tobacco, intentional self-harm**
    +7th **T65.213 Toxic effect of chewing tobacco, assault**
    +7th **T65.214 Toxic effect of chewing tobacco, undetermined**
  + **T65.22 Toxic effect of tobacco cigarettes**
    Toxic effect of tobacco smoke
    Use additional code for exposure to second hand tobacco smoke (Z57.31, Z77.22)
    +7th **T65.221 Toxic effect of tobacco cigarettes, accidental (unintentional)**
      Toxic effect of tobacco cigarettes NOS
    +7th **T65.222 Toxic effect of tobacco cigarettes, intentional self-harm**
    +7th **T65.223 Toxic effect of tobacco cigarettes, assault**
    +7th **T65.224 Toxic effect of tobacco cigarettes, undetermined**
  + **T65.29 Toxic effect of other tobacco and nicotine**
    +7th **T65.291 Toxic effect of other tobacco and nicotine, accidental (unintentional)**
      Toxic effect of other tobacco and nicotine NOS
    +7th **T65.292 Toxic effect of other tobacco and nicotine, intentional self-harm**
    +7th **T65.293 Toxic effect of other tobacco and nicotine, assault**
    +7th **T65.294 Toxic effect of other tobacco and nicotine, undetermined**
+ **T65.3 Toxic effect of nitroderivatives and aminoderivatives of benzene and its homologues**
  Toxic effect of anilin [benzenamine]
  Toxic effect of nitrobenzene
  Toxic effect of trinitrotoluene
  + **T65.3X Toxic effect of nitroderivatives and aminoderivatives of benzene and its homologues**
    +7th **T65.3X1 Toxic effect of nitroderivatives and aminoderivatives of benzene and its homologues, accidental (unintentional)**
      Toxic effect of nitroderivatives and aminoderivatives of benzene and its homologues NOS
    +7th **T65.3X2 Toxic effect of nitroderivatives and aminoderivatives of benzene and its homologues, intentional self-harm**

    +7th **T65.3X3 Toxic effect of nitroderivatives and aminoderivatives of benzene and its homologues, assault**
    +7th **T65.3X4 Toxic effect of nitroderivatives and aminoderivatives of benzene and its homologues, undetermined**
+ **T65.4 Toxic effect of carbon disulfide**
  + **T65.4X Toxic effect of carbon disulfide**
    +7th **T65.4X1 Toxic effect of carbon disulfide, accidental (unintentional)**
      Toxic effect of carbon disulfide NOS
    +7th **T65.4X2 Toxic effect of carbon disulfide, intentional self-harm**
    +7th **T65.4X3 Toxic effect of carbon disulfide, assault**
    +7th **T65.4X4 Toxic effect of carbon disulfide, undetermined**
+ **T65.5 Toxic effect of nitroglycerin and other nitric acids and esters**
  Toxic effect of 1,2,3-Propanetriol trinitrate
  + **T65.5X Toxic effect of nitroglycerin and other nitric acids and esters**
    +7th **T65.5X1 Toxic effect of nitroglycerin and other nitric acids and esters, accidental (unintentional)**
      Toxic effect of nitroglycerin and other nitric acids and esters NOS
    +7th **T65.5X2 Toxic effect of nitroglycerin and other nitric acids and esters, intentional self-harm**
    +7th **T65.5X3 Toxic effect of nitroglycerin and other nitric acids and esters, assault**
    +7th **T65.5X4 Toxic effect of nitroglycerin and other nitric acids and esters, undetermined**
+ **T65.6 Toxic effect of paints and dyes, not elsewhere classified**
  + **T65.6X Toxic effect of paints and dyes, not elsewhere classified**
    +7th **T65.6X1 Toxic effect of paints and dyes, not elsewhere classified, accidental (unintentional)**
      Toxic effect of paints and dyes NOS
    +7th **T65.6X2 Toxic effect of paints and dyes, not elsewhere classified, intentional self-harm**
    +7th **T65.6X3 Toxic effect of paints and dyes, not elsewhere classified, assault**
    +7th **T65.6X4 Toxic effect of paints and dyes, not elsewhere classified, undetermined**
+ **T65.8 Toxic effect of other specified substances**
  + **T65.81 Toxic effect of latex**
    +7th **T65.811 Toxic effect of latex, accidental (unintentional)**
      Toxic effect of latex NOS
    +7th **T65.812 Toxic effect of latex, intentional self-harm**
    +7th **T65.813 Toxic effect of latex, assault**
    +7th **T65.814 Toxic effect of latex, undetermined**
  + **T65.82 Toxic effect of harmful algae and algae toxins**
    Toxic effect of (harmful) algae bloom NOS
    Toxic effect of blue-green algae bloom
    Toxic effect of brown tide
    Toxic effect of cyanobacteria bloom
    Toxic effect of Florida red tide
    Toxic effect of pfiesteria piscicida
    Toxic effect of red tide
    +7th **T65.821 Toxic effect of harmful algae and algae toxins, accidental (unintentional)**
      Toxic effect of harmful algae and algae toxins NOS
    +7th **T65.822 Toxic effect of harmful algae and algae toxins, intentional self-harm**
    +7th **T65.823 Toxic effect of harmful algae and algae toxins, assault**
    +7th **T65.824 Toxic effect of harmful algae and algae toxins, undetermined**

+ **T65.83** **Toxic effect of fiberglass**
+7th **T65.831** **Toxic effect of fiberglass, accidental (unintentional)**
Toxic effect of fiberglass NOS
+7th **T65.832** **Toxic effect of fiberglass, intentional self-harm**
+7th **T65.833** **Toxic effect of fiberglass, assault**
+7th **T65.834** **Toxic effect of fiberglass, undetermined**
+ **T65.89** **Toxic effect of other specified substances**
+7th **T65.891** **Toxic effect of other specified substances, accidental (unintentional)**
Toxic effect of other specified substances NOS
AHA CC: 1Q, 2018, 5
+7th **T65.892** **Toxic effect of other specified substances, intentional self-harm**
+7th **T65.893** **Toxic effect of other specified substances, assault**
+7th **T65.894** **Toxic effect of other specified substances, undetermined**
+ **T65.9** **Toxic effect of unspecified substance**
X+7th **T65.91** **Toxic effect of unspecified substance, accidental (unintentional)**
Poisoning NOS
X+7th **T65.92** **Toxic effect of unspecified substance, intentional self-harm**
X+7th **T65.93** **Toxic effect of unspecified substance, assault**
X+7th **T65.94** **Toxic effect of unspecified substance, undetermined**

Other and unspecified effects of external causes (T66-T78)

T66 **Radiation sickness, unspecified**
X+7th
Excludes1: *specified adverse effects of radiation, such as:*
burns (T20-T31)
leukemia (C91-C95)
radiation gastroenteritis and colitis (K52.0)
radiation pneumonitis (J70.0)
radiation related disorders of the skin and subcutaneous tissue (L55-L59)
sunburn (L55.-)

The appropriate 7th character is to be added to code T66
A   initial encounter
D   subsequent encounter
S   sequela

T67 **Effects of heat and light**
Excludes1: *erythema [dermatitis] ab igne (L59.0)*
malignant hyperpyrexia due to anesthesia (T88.3)
radiation-related disorders of the skin and subcutaneous tissue (L55-L59)
Excludes2: *burns (T20-T31)*
sunburn (L55.-)
sweat disorder due to heat (L74-L75)

The appropriate 7th character is to be added to each code from category T67
A   initial encounter
D   subsequent encounter
S   sequela

+ **T67.0** **Heatstroke and sunstroke**
Use additional code(s) to identify any associated complications of heatstroke, such as:
coma and stupor (R40.-)
rhabdomyolysis (M62.82)
systemic inflammatory response syndrome (R65.1-)
AHA CC: 4Q, 2019, 17-18
HAC 7th character A see Appendix B for HAC conditional logic
CC X+7th **T67.01** **Heatstroke and sunstroke**
Heat apoplexy
Heat pyrexia
Siriasis
Thermoplegia
HAC 7th character A see Appendix B for HAC conditional logic
CC X+7th **T67.02** **Exertional heatstroke**
AHA CC: 4Q, 2019, 17-18
HAC 7th character A see Appendix B for HAC conditional logic
CC X+7th **T67.09** **Other heatstroke and sunstroke**
HAC 7th character A see Appendix B for HAC conditional logic

X+7th **T67.1** **Heat syncope**
Heat collapse
X+7th **T67.2** **Heat cramp**
X+7th **T67.3** **Heat exhaustion, anhydrotic**
Heat prostration due to water depletion
Excludes1: *heat exhaustion due to salt depletion (T67.4)*
X+7th **T67.4** **Heat exhaustion due to salt depletion**
Heat prostration due to salt (and water) depletion
X+7th **T67.5** **Heat exhaustion, unspecified**
Heat prostration NOS
X+7th **T67.6** **Heat fatigue, transient**
X+7th **T67.7** **Heat edema**
X+7th **T67.8** **Other effects of heat and light**
X+7th **T67.9** **Effect of heat and light, unspecified**

T68 **Hypothermia**
X+7th
Accidental hypothermia
Hypothermia NOS
Use additional code to identify source of exposure:
Exposure to excessive cold of man-made origin (W93)
Exposure to excessive cold of natural origin (X31)
Excludes1: *hypothermia following anesthesia (T88.51)*
hypothermia not associated with low environmental temperature (R68.0)
hypothermia of newborn (P80.-)
Excludes2: *frostbite (T33-T34)*

The appropriate 7th character is to be added to code T68
A   initial encounter
D   subsequent encounter
S   sequela

T69 **Other effects of reduced temperature**
Use additional code to identify source of exposure:
Exposure to excessive cold of man-made origin (W93)
Exposure to excessive cold of natural origin (X31)
Excludes2: *frostbite (T33-T34)*

The appropriate 7th character is to be added to each code from category T69
A   initial encounter
D   subsequent encounter
S   sequela

+ **T69.0** **Immersion hand and foot**
+ **T69.01** **Immersion hand**
+7th **T69.011** **Immersion hand, right hand**
+7th **T69.012** **Immersion hand, left hand**
+7th **T69.019** **Immersion hand, unspecified hand**
+ **T69.02** **Immersion foot**
Trench foot
CC +7th **T69.021** **Immersion foot, right foot**
HAC 7th character A see Appendix B for HAC conditional logic
CC +7th **T69.022** **Immersion foot, left foot**
HAC 7th character A see Appendix B for HAC conditional logic
CC +7th **T69.029** **Immersion foot, unspecified foot**
HAC 7th character A see Appendix B for HAC conditional logic
X+7th **T69.1** **Chilblains**
X+7th **T69.8** **Other specified effects of reduced temperature**
X+7th **T69.9** **Effect of reduced temperature, unspecified**

T70 **Effects of air pressure and water pressure**

The appropriate 7th character is to be added to each code from category T70
A   initial encounter
D   subsequent encounter
S   sequela

X+7th **T70.0** **Otitic barotrauma**
Aero-otitis media
Effects of change in ambient atmospheric pressure or water pressure on ears
X+7th **T70.1** **Sinus barotrauma**
Aerosinusitis
Effects of change in ambient atmospheric pressure on sinuses

+, +7th, X + 7th   ● Newborn   ● Pediatric   ● Maternity   ● Adult   ♀ Female   ♂ Male   Manifestation   Unacceptable PDX   HCC   CC   MCC   HAC

+ **T70.2** **Other and unspecified effects of high altitude**
  Excludes2: *polycythemia due to high altitude (D75.1)*
X+7th **T70.20** **Unspecified effects of high altitude**
X+7th **T70.29** **Other effects of high altitude**
  Alpine sickness
  Anoxia due to high altitude
  Barotrauma NOS
  Hypobaropathy
  Mountain sickness
CC X+7th **T70.3** **Caisson disease [decompression sickness]**
  Compressed-air disease
  Diver's palsy or paralysis
  HAC 7th character A see Appendix B for HAC conditional logic
X+7th **T70.4** **Effects of high-pressure fluids**
  Hydraulic jet injection (industrial)
  Pneumatic jet injection (industrial)
  Traumatic jet injection (industrial)
X+7th **T70.8** **Other effects of air pressure and water pressure**
X+7th **T70.9** **Effect of air pressure and water pressure, unspecified**

T71 **Asphyxiation**

  Mechanical suffocation
  Traumatic suffocation
  Excludes1: *acute respiratory distress (syndrome) (J80)*
    anoxia due to high altitude (T70.2)
    asphyxia NOS (R09.01)
    asphyxia from carbon monoxide (T58.-)
    asphyxia from inhalation of food or foreign body (T17.-)
    asphyxia from other gases, fumes and vapors (T59.-)
    respiratory distress (syndrome) in newborn (P22.-)

  The appropriate 7th character is to be added to each code from category T71
  A   initial encounter
  D   subsequent encounter
  S   sequela

+ **T71.1** **Asphyxiation due to mechanical threat to breathing**
  Suffocation due to mechanical threat to breathing
  + **T71.11** **Asphyxiation due to smothering under pillow**
    CC +7th **T71.111** **Asphyxiation due to smothering under pillow, accidental**
      Asphyxiation due to smothering under pillow NOS
      HAC 7th character A see Appendix B for HAC conditional logic
    CC +7th **T71.112** **Asphyxiation due to smothering under pillow, intentional self-harm**
      HAC 7th character A see Appendix B for HAC conditional logic
    CC +7th **T71.113** **Asphyxiation due to smothering under pillow, assault**
      HAC 7th character A see Appendix B for HAC conditional logic
    CC +7th **T71.114** **Asphyxiation due to smothering under pillow, undetermined**
      HAC 7th character A see Appendix B for HAC conditional logic
  + **T71.12** **Asphyxiation due to plastic bag**
    CC +7th **T71.121** **Asphyxiation due to plastic bag, accidental**
      Asphyxiation due to plastic bag NOS
      HAC 7th character A see Appendix B for HAC conditional logic
    CC +7th **T71.122** **Asphyxiation due to plastic bag, intentional self-harm**
      HAC 7th character A see Appendix B for HAC conditional logic
    CC +7th **T71.123** **Asphyxiation due to plastic bag, assault**
      HAC 7th character A see Appendix B for HAC conditional logic
    CC +7th **T71.124** **Asphyxiation due to plastic bag, undetermined**
      HAC 7th character A see Appendix B for HAC conditional logic

+ **T71.13** **Asphyxiation due to being trapped in bed linens**
  CC +7th **T71.131** **Asphyxiation due to being trapped in bed linens, accidental**
    Asphyxiation due to being trapped in bed linens NOS
    HAC 7th character A see Appendix B for HAC conditional logic
  CC +7th **T71.132** **Asphyxiation due to being trapped in bed linens, intentional self-harm**
    HAC 7th character A see Appendix B for HAC conditional logic
  CC +7th **T71.133** **Asphyxiation due to being trapped in bed linens, assault**
    HAC 7th character A see Appendix B for HAC conditional logic
  CC +7th **T71.134** **Asphyxiation due to being trapped in bed linens, undetermined**
    HAC 7th character A see Appendix B for HAC conditional logic
+ **T71.14** **Asphyxiation due to smothering under another person's body (in bed)**
  CC +7th **T71.141** **Asphyxiation due to smothering under another person's body (in bed), accidental**
    Asphyxiation due to smothering under another person's body (in bed) NOS
    HAC 7th character A see Appendix B for HAC conditional logic
  CC +7th **T71.143** **Asphyxiation due to smothering under another person's body (in bed), assault**
    HAC 7th character A see Appendix B for HAC conditional logic
  CC +7th **T71.144** **Asphyxiation due to smothering under another person's body (in bed), undetermined**
    HAC 7th character A see Appendix B for HAC conditional logic
+ **T71.15** **Asphyxiation due to smothering in furniture**
  CC +7th **T71.151** **Asphyxiation due to smothering in furniture, accidental**
    Asphyxiation due to smothering in furniture NOS
    HAC 7th character A see Appendix B for HAC conditional logic
  CC +7th **T71.152** **Asphyxiation due to smothering in furniture, intentional self-harm**
    HAC 7th character A see Appendix B for HAC conditional logic
  CC +7th **T71.153** **Asphyxiation due to smothering in furniture, assault**
    HAC 7th character A see Appendix B for HAC conditional logic
  CC +7th **T71.154** **Asphyxiation due to smothering in furniture, undetermined**
    HAC 7th character A see Appendix B for HAC conditional logic
+ **T71.16** **Asphyxiation due to hanging**
  Hanging by window shade cord
  Use additional code for any associated injuries, such as:
    crushing injury of neck (S17.-)
    fracture of cervical vertebrae (S12.0-S12.2-)
    open wound of neck (S11.-)
  CC +7th **T71.161** **Asphyxiation due to hanging, accidental**
    Asphyxiation due to hanging NOS
    Hanging NOS
    HAC 7th character A see Appendix B for HAC conditional logic
  CC +7th **T71.162** **Asphyxiation due to hanging, intentional self-harm**
    HAC 7th character A see Appendix B for HAC conditional logic
  CC +7th **T71.163** **Asphyxiation due to hanging, assault**
    HAC 7th character A see Appendix B for HAC conditional logic
  CC +7th **T71.164** **Asphyxiation due to hanging, undetermined**
    HAC 7th character A see Appendix B for HAC conditional logic

+, +7th, X + 7th   • Newborn   • Pediatric   • Maternity   • Adult   ♀ Female   ♂ Male   Manifestation   Unacceptable PDX   HCC   CC   MCC   **HAC**

+ T71.19 Asphyxiation due to mechanical threat to breathing due to other causes

CC +7th **T71.191 Asphyxiation due to mechanical threat to breathing due to other causes, accidental**

Asphyxiation due to other causes NOS

AHA CC: 4Q, 2016, 74-76

HAC 7th character A see Appendix B for HAC conditional logic

CC +7th **T71.192 Asphyxiation due to mechanical threat to breathing due to other causes, intentional self-harm**

HAC 7th character A see Appendix B for HAC conditional logic

CC +7th **T71.193 Asphyxiation due to mechanical threat to breathing due to other causes, assault**

HAC 7th character A see Appendix B for HAC conditional logic

CC +7th **T71.194 Asphyxiation due to mechanical threat to breathing due to other causes, undetermined**

HAC 7th character A see Appendix B for HAC conditional logic

+ T71.2 Asphyxiation due to systemic oxygen deficiency due to low oxygen content in ambient air

Suffocation due to systemic oxygen deficiency due to low oxygen content in ambient air

CC X+7th **T71.20 Asphyxiation due to systemic oxygen deficiency due to low oxygen content in ambient air due to unspecified cause**

HAC 7th character A see Appendix B for HAC conditional logic

CC X+7th **T71.21 Asphyxiation due to cave-in or falling earth**

Use additional code for any associated cataclysm (X34-X38)

HAC 7th character A see Appendix B for HAC conditional logic

+ T71.22 Asphyxiation due to being trapped in a car trunk

CC +7th **T71.221 Asphyxiation due to being trapped in a car trunk, accidental**

CC +7th **T71.222 Asphyxiation due to being trapped in a car trunk, intentional self-harm**

CC +7th **T71.223 Asphyxiation due to being trapped in a car trunk, assault**

CC +7th **T71.224 Asphyxiation due to being trapped in a car trunk, undetermined**

+ T71.23 Asphyxiation due to being trapped in a (discarded) refrigerator

CC +7th **T71.231 Asphyxiation due to being trapped in a (discarded) refrigerator, accidental**

CC +7th **T71.232 Asphyxiation due to being trapped in a (discarded) refrigerator, intentional self-harm**

CC +7th **T71.233 Asphyxiation due to being trapped in a (discarded) refrigerator, assault**

CC +7th **T71.234 Asphyxiation due to being trapped in a (discarded) refrigerator, undetermined**

CC X+7th **T71.29 Asphyxiation due to being trapped in other low oxygen environment**

HAC 7th character A see Appendix B for HAC conditional logic

CC X+7th **T71.9 Asphyxiation due to unspecified cause**

Suffocation (by strangulation) due to unspecified cause

Suffocation NOS

Systemic oxygen deficiency due to low oxygen content in ambient air due to unspecified cause

Systemic oxygen deficiency due to mechanical threat to breathing due to unspecified cause

Traumatic asphyxia NOS

HAC 7th character A see Appendix B for HAC conditional logic

T73 Effects of other deprivation

The appropriate 7th character is to be added to each code from category T73

A initial encounter
D subsequent encounter
S sequela

X+7th **T73.0 Starvation**

Deprivation of food

X+7th **T73.1 Deprivation of water**

X+7th **T73.2 Exhaustion due to exposure**

X+7th **T73.3 Exhaustion due to excessive exertion**

Exhaustion due to overexertion

X+7th **T73.8 Other effects of deprivation**

X+7th **T73.9 Effect of deprivation, unspecified**

T74 Adult and child abuse, neglect and other maltreatment, confirmed

Use additional code, if applicable, to identify any associated current injury.

Use additional external cause code to identify perpetrator, if known (Y07.-)

Excludes1: *abuse and maltreatment in pregnancy (O9A.3-, O9A.4-, O9A.5-)*

adult and child maltreatment, suspected (T76.-)

AHA CC: 4Q, 2018, 9

The appropriate 7th character is to be added to each code from category T74

A initial encounter
D subsequent encounter
S sequela

Review coding guidelines C.5.c and C.19.f

+ T74.0 Neglect or abandonment, confirmed

● CC X+7th **T74.01 Adult neglect or abandonment, confirmed**

● CC X+7th **T74.02 Child neglect or abandonment, confirmed**

+ T74.1 Physical abuse, confirmed

Excludes2: *sexual abuse (T74.2-)*

● CC X+7th **T74.11 Adult physical abuse, confirmed**

● CC X+7th **T74.12 Child physical abuse, confirmed**

Excludes2: *shaken infant syndrome (T74.4)*

+ T74.2 Sexual abuse, confirmed

Rape, confirmed

Sexual assault, confirmed

● CC X+7th **T74.21 Adult sexual abuse, confirmed**

● CC X+7th **T74.22 Child sexual abuse, confirmed**

+ T74.3 Psychological abuse, confirmed

Bullying and intimidation, confirmed

Intimidation through social media, confirmed

● X+7th **T74.31 Adult psychological abuse, confirmed**

● CC X+7th **T74.32 Child psychological abuse, confirmed**

● CC X+7th **T74.4 Shaken infant syndrome**

+ T74.5 Forced sexual exploitation, confirmed

AHA CC: 4Q, 2018, 32-33

● CC X+7th **T74.51 Adult forced sexual exploitation, confirmed**

● CC X+7th **T74.52 Child sexual exploitation, confirmed**

+ T74.6 Forced labor exploitation, confirmed

AHA CC: 4Q, 2018, 32-33

● CC X+7th **T74.61 Adult forced labor exploitation, confirmed**

● CC X+7th **T74.62 Child forced labor exploitation, confirmed**

+ T74.9 Unspecified maltreatment, confirmed

● CC X+7th **T74.91 Unspecified adult maltreatment, confirmed**

● CC X+7th **T74.92 Unspecified child maltreatment, confirmed**

T75 Other and unspecified effects of other external causes

Excludes1: *adverse effects NEC (T78.-)*

Excludes2: *burns (electric) (T20-T31)*

The appropriate 7th character is to be added to each code from category T75

A initial encounter
D subsequent encounter
S sequela

+ T75.0 Effects of lightning

Struck by lightning

X+7th **T75.00 Unspecified effects of lightning**

Struck by lightning NOS

X+7th **T75.01 Shock due to being struck by lightning**

X+7th **T75.09 Other effects of lightning**

Use additional code for other effects of lightning

CC X+7th **T75.1** **Unspecified effects of drowning and nonfatal submersion**
Immersion
Excludes1: *specified effects of drowning- code to effects*
HAC 7th character A see Appendix B for HAC conditional logic

+ **T75.2** **Effects of vibration**
X+7th **T75.20** **Unspecified effects of vibration**
X+7th **T75.21** **Pneumatic hammer syndrome**
X+7th **T75.22** **Traumatic vasospastic syndrome**
X+7th **T75.23** **Vertigo from infrasound**
Excludes1: *vertigo NOS (R42)*
X+7th **T75.29** **Other effects of vibration**

X+7th **T75.3** **Motion sickness**
Airsickness
Seasickness
Travel sickness
Use additional external cause code to identify vehicle or type
of motion (Y92.81-, Y93.5-)

X+7th **T75.4** **Electrocution**
Shock from electric current
Shock from electroshock gun (taser)

+ **T75.8** **Other specified effects of external causes**
X+7th **T75.81** **Effects of abnormal gravitation [G] forces**
X+7th **T75.82** **Effects of weightlessness**
X+7th **T75.89** **Other specified effects of external causes**

T76 **Adult and child abuse, neglect and other maltreatment, suspected**
Use additional code, if applicable, to identify any associated current
injury
Excludes1: *adult and child maltreatment, confirmed (T74.-)*
suspected abuse and maltreatment in pregnancy
(O9A.3-, O9A.4-, O9A.5-)
suspected adult physical abuse, ruled out (Z04.71)
suspected adult sexual abuse, ruled out (Z04.41)
suspected child physical abuse, ruled out (Z04.72)
suspected child sexual abuse, ruled out (Z04.42)
AHA CC: 4Q, 2018, 9

The appropriate 7th character is to be added to each code from
category T76
A   initial encounter
D   subsequent encounter
S   sequela

Review coding guidelines C.5.c and C.19.f

+ **T76.0** **Neglect or abandonment, suspected**
● CC X+7th **T76.01** **Adult neglect or abandonment, suspected**
● CC X+7th **T76.02** **Child neglect or abandonment, suspected**
+ **T76.1** **Physical abuse, suspected**
● CC X+7th **T76.11** **Adult physical abuse, suspected**
● CC X+7th **T76.12** **Child physical abuse, suspected**
AHA CC: 2Q, 2019, 12
+ **T76.2** **Sexual abuse, suspected**
Rape, suspected
Excludes1: *alleged abuse, ruled out (Z04.7)*
● CC X+7th **T76.21** **Adult sexual abuse, suspected**
● CC X+7th **T76.22** **Child sexual abuse, suspected**
+ **T76.3** **Psychological abuse, suspected**
Bullying and intimidation, suspected
Intimidation through social medial, suspected
● X+7th **T76.31** **Adult psychological abuse, suspected**
● CC X+7th **T76.32** **Child psychological abuse, suspected**
+ **T76.5** **Forced sexual exploitation, suspected**
AHA CC: 4Q, 2018, 32-33
● CC X+7th **T76.51** **Adult forced sexual exploitation, suspected**
● CC X+7th **T76.52** **Child sexual exploitation, suspected**
+ **T76.6** **Forced labor exploitation, suspected**
AHA CC: 4Q, 2018, 32-33
● CC X+7th **T76.61** **Adult forced labor exploitation, suspected**
● CC X+7th **T76.62** **Child forced labor exploitation, suspected**
+ **T76.9** **Unspecified maltreatment, suspected**
● CC X+7th **T76.91** **Unspecified adult maltreatment, suspected**
● CC X+7th **T76.92** **Unspecified child maltreatment, suspected**

T78 **Adverse effects, not elsewhere classified**
Excludes2: *complications of surgical and medical care NEC*
(T80-T88)

The appropriate 7th character is to be added to each code from
category T78
A   initial encounter
D   subsequent encounter
S   sequela

+ **T78.0** **Anaphylactic reaction due to food**
Anaphylactic reaction due to adverse food reaction
Anaphylactic shock or reaction due to nonpoisonous foods
Anaphylactoid reaction due to food
CC X+7th **T78.00** **Anaphylactic reaction due to unspecified food**
CC X+7th **T78.01** **Anaphylactic reaction due to peanuts**
CC X+7th **T78.02** **Anaphylactic reaction due to shellfish**
(crustaceans)
CC X+7th **T78.03** **Anaphylactic reaction due to other fish**
CC X+7th **T78.04** **Anaphylactic reaction due to fruits and vegetables**
CC X+7th **T78.05** **Anaphylactic reaction due to tree nuts and seeds**
Excludes2: *anaphylactic reaction due to peanuts*
(T78.01)
CC X+7th **T78.06** **Anaphylactic reaction due to food additives**
CC X+7th **T78.07** **Anaphylactic reaction due to milk and dairy**
products
CC X+7th **T78.08** **Anaphylactic reaction due to eggs**
CC X+7th **T78.09** **Anaphylactic reaction due to other food products**
X+7th **T78.1** **Other adverse food reactions, not elsewhere classified**
Use additional code to identify the type of reaction, if
applicable
Excludes1: *anaphylactic reaction or shock due to adverse*
food reaction (T78.0-)
anaphylactic reaction due to food (T78.0-)
bacterial food borne intoxications (A05.-)
Excludes2: *allergic and dietetic gastroenteritis and colitis*
(K52.29)
allergic rhinitis due to food (J30.5)
dermatitis due to food in contact with skin
(L23.6, L24.6, L25.4)
dermatitis due to ingested food (L27.2)
food protein-induced entercolitis syndrome
(K52.21)
food protein-induced enteropathy (K52.22)

CC X+7th **T78.2** **Anaphylactic shock, unspecified**
Allergic shock
Anaphylactic reaction
Anaphylaxis
Excludes1: *anaphylactic reaction or shock due to adverse*
effect of correct medicinal substance properly
administered (T88.6)
anaphylactic reaction or shock due to adverse
food reaction (T78.0-)
anaphylactic reaction or shock due to serum
(T80.5-)

X+7th **T78.3** **Angioneurotic edema**
Allergic angioedema
Giant urticaria
Quincke's edema
Excludes1: *serum urticaria (T80.6-)*
urticaria (L50.-)

+ **T78.4** **Other and unspecified allergy**
Excludes1: *specified types of allergic reaction such as:*
allergic diarrhea (K52.29)
allergic gastroenteritis and colitis (K52.29)
dermatitis (L23-L25, L27.-)
food protein-induced entercolitis syndrome
(K52.21)
food protein-induced enteropathy (K52.22)
hay fever (J30.1)
X+7th **T78.40** **Allergy, unspecified**
Allergic reaction NOS
Hypersensitivity NOS
X+7th **T78.41** **Arthus phenomenon**
Arthus reaction
X+7th **T78.49** **Other allergy**
X+7th **T78.8** **Other adverse effects, not elsewhere classified**

+, +7th, X + 7th   ● Newborn   ● Pediatric   ● Maternity   ● Adult   ♀ Female   ♂ Male   Manifestation   Unacceptable PDX   HCC   CC   MCC   HAC

Certain early complications of trauma (T79)

T79 **Certain early complications of trauma, not elsewhere classified**

> **Excludes2:** *acute respiratory distress syndrome (J80)*
> *complications occurring during or following medical procedures (T80-T88)*
> *complications of surgical and medical care NEC (T80-T88)*
> *newborn respiratory distress syndrome (P22.0)*

> The appropriate 7th character is to be added to each code from category T79
> A   initial encounter
> D   subsequent encounter
> S   sequela

MCC X+7th **T79.0** **Air embolism (traumatic)**
> **Excludes1:** *air embolism complicating abortion or ectopic or molar pregnancy (O00-O07, O08.2)*
> *air embolism complicating pregnancy, childbirth and the puerperium (O88.0)*
> *air embolism following infusion, transfusion, and therapeutic injection (T80.0)*
> *air embolism following procedure NEC (T81.7-)*

MCC X+7th **T79.1** **Fat embolism (traumatic)**
> **Excludes1:** *fat embolism complicating:*
> *abortion or ectopic or molar pregnancy (O00-O07, O08.2)*
> *pregnancy, childbirth and the puerperium (O88.8)*

CC X+7th **T79.2** **Traumatic secondary and recurrent hemorrhage and seroma**

MCC X+7th **T79.4** **Traumatic shock**
> Shock (immediate) (delayed) following injury
> **Excludes1:** *anaphylactic shock due to adverse food reaction (T78.0-)*
> *anaphylactic shock due to correct medicinal substance properly administered (T88.6)*
> *anaphylactic shock due to serum (T80.5-)*
> *anaphylactic shock NOS (T78.2)*
> *anesthetic shock (T88.2)*
> *electric shock (T75.4)*
> *nontraumatic shock NEC (R57.-)*
> *obstetric shock (O75.1)*
> *postprocedural shock (T81.1-)*
> *septic shock (R65.21)*
> *shock complicating abortion or ectopic or molar pregnancy (O00-O07, O08.3)*
> *shock due to lightning (T75.01)*
> *shock NOS (R57.9)*

MCC X+7th **T79.5** **Traumatic anuria**
> Crush syndrome
> Renal failure following crushing

X+7th **T79.6** **Traumatic ischemia of muscle**
> Traumatic rhabdomyolysis
> Volkmann's ischemic contracture
> **Excludes2:** *anterior tibial syndrome (M76.8)*
> *compartment syndrome (traumatic) (T79.A-)*
> *nontraumatic ischemia of muscle (M62.2-)*

CC X+7th **T79.7** **Traumatic subcutaneous emphysema**
> **Excludes2:** *emphysema NOS (J43)*
> *emphysema (subcutaneous) resulting from a procedure (T81.82)*

+ **T79.A** **Traumatic compartment syndrome**
> **Excludes1:** *fibromyalgia (M79.7)*
> *nontraumatic compartment syndrome (M79.A-)*
> **Excludes2:** *traumatic ischemic infarction of muscle (T79.6)*

CC X+7th **T79.A0** **Compartment syndrome, unspecified**
> Compartment syndrome NOS

+ **T79.A1** **Traumatic compartment syndrome of upper extremity**
> Traumatic compartment syndrome of shoulder, arm, forearm, wrist, hand, and fingers

CC +7th **T79.A11** **Traumatic compartment syndrome of right upper extremity**

CC +7th **T79.A12** **Traumatic compartment syndrome of left upper extremity**

CC +7th **T79.A19** **Traumatic compartment syndrome of unspecified upper extremity**

+ **T79.A2** **Traumatic compartment syndrome of lower extremity**
> Traumatic compartment syndrome of hip, buttock, thigh, leg, foot, and toes

CC +7th **T79.A21** **Traumatic compartment syndrome of right lower extremity**

CC +7th **T79.A22** **Traumatic compartment syndrome of left lower extremity**

CC +7th **T79.A29** **Traumatic compartment syndrome of unspecified lower extremity**

CC X+7th **T79.A3** **Traumatic compartment syndrome of abdomen**

CC X+7th **T79.A9** **Traumatic compartment syndrome of other sites**

X+7th **T79.8** **Other early complications of trauma**

X+7th **T79.9** **Unspecified early complication of trauma**

Complications of surgical and medical care, not elsewhere classified (T80-T88)

Use additional code for adverse effect, if applicable, to identify drug (T36-T50 with fifth or sixth character 5)

Use additional code(s) to identify the specified condition resulting from the complication

Use additional code to identify devices involved and details of circumstances (Y62-Y82)

> **Excludes2:** *any encounters with medical care for postprocedural conditions in which no complications are present, such as:*
> *artificial opening status (Z93.-)*
> *closure of external stoma (Z43.-)*
> *fitting and adjustment of external prosthetic device (Z44.-)*
> *burns and corrosions from local applications and irradiation (T20-T32)*
> *complications of surgical procedures during pregnancy, childbirth and the puerperium (O00-O9A)*
> *mechanical complication of respirator [ventilator] (J95.850)*
> *poisoning and toxic effects of drugs and chemicals (T36-T65 with fifth or sixth character 1-4 or 6)*
> *postprocedural fever (R50.82)*
> *specified complications classified elsewhere, such as:*
> *cerebrospinal fluid leak from spinal puncture (G97.0)*
> *colostomy malfunction (K94.0-)*
> *disorders of fluid and electrolyte imbalance (E86-E87)*
> *functional disturbances following cardiac surgery (I97.0-I97.1)*
> *intraoperative and postprocedural complications of specified body systems (D78.-, E36.-, E89.-, G97.3-, G97.4, H59.3-, H59.-, H95.2-, H95.3, I97.4-, I97.5, J95.6-, J95.7, K91.6-, L76.-, M96.-, N99.-)*
> *ostomy complications (J95.0-, K94.-, N99.5-)*
> *postgastric surgery syndromes (K91.1)*
> *postlaminectomy syndrome NEC (M96.1)*
> *postmastectomy lymphedema syndrome (I97.2)*
> *postsurgical blind-loop syndrome (K91.2)*
> *ventilator associated pneumonia (J95.851)*

T80 **Complications following infusion, transfusion and therapeutic injection**

> **Includes:** complications following perfusion
> **Excludes2:** *bone marrow transplant rejection (T86.01)*
> *febrile nonhemolytic transfusion reaction (R50.84)*
> *fluid overload due to transfusion (E87.71)*
> *posttransfusion purpura (D69.51)*
> *transfusion associated circulatory overload (TACO) (E87.71)*
> *transfusion (red blood cell) associated hemochromatosis (E83.111)*
> *transfusion related acute lung injury (TRALI) (J95.84)*

> The appropriate 7th character is to be added to each code from category T80
> A   initial encounter
> D   subsequent encounter
> S   sequela

MCC X+7th **T80.0** **Air embolism following infusion, transfusion and therapeutic injection**
> **HAC** 7th character A see Appendix B for HAC conditional logic

+, +7th, X + 7th ● Newborn ● Pediatric ● Maternity ● Adult ♀ Female ♂ Male Manifestation Unacceptable PDX HCC CC MCC HAC

CC X+7th **T80.1** **Vascular complications following infusion, transfusion and therapeutic injection**

Use additional code to identify the vascular complication

Excludes2: *extravasation of vesicant agent (T80.81-)*
infiltration of vesicant agent (T80.81-)
vascular complications specified as due to prosthetic devices, implants and grafts (T82.8-, T83.8-, T84.8-, T85.8-)
postprocedural vascular complications (T81.7-)

+ T80.2 **Infections following infusion, transfusion and therapeutic injection**

Use additional code to identify the specific infection, such as: sepsis (A41.9)

Use additional code (R65.2-) to identify severe sepsis, if applicable

Excludes2: *infections specified as due to prosthetic devices, implants and grafts (T82.6-T82.7, T83.5-T83.6, T84.5-T84.7, T85.7)*
postprocedural infections (T81.4-)

Review coding guideline C.1.d.5

+ T80.21 **Infection due to central venous catheter**

Infection due to pulmonary artery catheter (Swan-Ganz catheter)

CC +7th **T80.211** **Bloodstream infection due to central venous catheter**

Catheter-related bloodstream infection (CRBSI) NOS

Central line-associated bloodstream infection (CLABSI)

Bloodstream infection due to Hickman catheter

Bloodstream infection due to peripherally inserted central catheter (PICC)

Bloodstream infection due to portacath (port-a-cath)

Bloodstream infection due to pulmonary artery catheter

Bloodstream infection due to triple lumen catheter

Bloodstream infection due to umbilical venous catheter

AHA CC: 4Q, 2018, 89; 1Q, 2019, 14

HAC 7th character A see Appendix B for HAC conditional logic

CC +7th **T80.212** **Local infection due to central venous catheter**

Exit or insertion site infection

Local infection due to Hickman catheter

Local infection due to peripherally inserted central catheter (PICC)

Local infection due to portacath (port-a-cath)

Local infection due to pulmonary artery catheter

Local infection due to triple lumen catheter

Local infection due to umbilical venous catheter

Port or reservoir infection

Tunnel infection

HAC 7th character A see Appendix B for HAC conditional logic

CC +7th **T80.218** **Other infection due to central venous catheter**

Other central line-associated infection

Other infection due to Hickman catheter

Other infection due to peripherally inserted central catheter (PICC)

Other infection due to portacath (port-a-cath)

Other infection due to pulmonary artery catheter

Other infection due to triple lumen catheter

Other infection due to umbilical venous catheter

HAC 7th character A see Appendix B for HAC conditional logic

CC +7th **T80.219** **Unspecified infection due to central venous catheter**

Central line-associated infection NOS

Unspecified infection due to Hickman catheter

Unspecified infection due to peripherally inserted central catheter (PICC)

Unspecified infection due to portacath (port-a-cath)

Unspecified infection due to pulmonary artery catheter

Unspecified infection due to triple lumen catheter

Unspecified infection due to umbilical venous catheter

HAC 7th character A see Appendix B for HAC conditional logic

CC X+7th **T80.22** **Acute infection following transfusion, infusion, or injection of blood and blood products**

CC X+7th **T80.29** **Infection following other infusion, transfusion and therapeutic injection**

+ T80.3 **ABO incompatibility reaction due to transfusion of blood or blood products**

Excludes1: *minor blood group antigens reactions (Duffy) (E) (K) (Kell) (Kidd) (Lewis) (M) (N) (P) (S) (T80.A-)*

CC X+7th **T80.30** **ABO incompatibility reaction due to transfusion of blood or blood products, unspecified**

ABO incompatibility blood transfusion NOS

Reaction to ABO incompatibility from transfusion NOS

HAC 7th character A see Appendix B for HAC conditional logic

+ T80.31 **ABO incompatibility with hemolytic transfusion reaction**

CC +7th **T80.310** **ABO incompatibility with acute hemolytic transfusion reaction**

ABO incompatibility with hemolytic transfusion reaction less than 24 hours after transfusion

Acute hemolytic transfusion reaction (AHTR) due to ABO incompatibility

HAC 7th character A see Appendix B for HAC conditional logic

CC +7th **T80.311** **ABO incompatibility with delayed hemolytic transfusion reaction**

ABO incompatibility with hemolytic transfusion reaction 24 hours or more after transfusion

Delayed hemolytic transfusion reaction (DHTR) due to ABO incompatibility

HAC 7th character A see Appendix B for HAC conditional logic

CC +7th **T80.319** **ABO incompatibility with hemolytic transfusion reaction, unspecified**

ABO incompatibility with hemolytic transfusion reaction at unspecified time after transfusion

Hemolytic transfusion reaction (HTR) due to ABO incompatibility NOS

HAC 7th character A see Appendix B for HAC conditional logic

CC X+7th **T80.39** **Other ABO incompatibility reaction due to transfusion of blood or blood products**

Delayed serologic transfusion reaction (DSTR) from ABO incompatibility

Other ABO incompatible blood transfusion

Other reaction to ABO incompatible blood transfusion

HAC 7th character A see Appendix B for HAC conditional logic

+, +7th, X + 7th　● Newborn　● Pediatric　● Maternity　● Adult　♀ Female　♂ Male　Manifestation　Unacceptable PDX　HCC　CC　MCC　**HAC**

+ T80.4 Rh incompatibility reaction due to transfusion of blood or blood products

    Reaction due to incompatibility of Rh antigens (C) (c) (D) (E) (e)

CC X+7th **T80.40 Rh incompatibility reaction due to transfusion of blood or blood products, unspecified**

    Reaction due to Rh factor in transfusion NOS

    Rh incompatible blood transfusion NOS

    + T80.41 Rh incompatibility with hemolytic transfusion reaction

    CC +7th **T80.410 Rh incompatibility with acute hemolytic transfusion reaction**

        Acute hemolytic transfusion reaction (AHTR) due to Rh incompatibility

        Rh incompatibility with hemolytic transfusion reaction less than 24 hours after transfusion

    CC +7th **T80.411 Rh incompatibility with delayed hemolytic transfusion reaction**

        Delayed hemolytic transfusion reaction (DHTR) due to Rh incompatibility

        Rh incompatibility with hemolytic transfusion reaction 24 hours or more after transfusion

    CC +7th **T80.419 Rh incompatibility with hemolytic transfusion reaction, unspecified**

        Rh incompatibility with hemolytic transfusion reaction at unspecified time after transfusion

        Hemolytic transfusion reaction (HTR) due to Rh incompatibility NOS

CC X+7th **T80.49 Other Rh incompatibility reaction due to transfusion of blood or blood products**

    Delayed serologic transfusion reaction (DSTR) from Rh incompatibility

    Other reaction to Rh incompatible blood transfusion

+ T80.A Non-ABO incompatibility reaction due to transfusion of blood or blood products

    Reaction due to incompatibility of minor antigens (Duffy) (Kell) (Kidd) (Lewis) (M) (N) (P) (S)

CC X+7th **T80.A0 Non-ABO incompatibility reaction due to transfusion of blood or blood products, unspecified**

    Non-ABO antigen incompatibility reaction from transfusion NOS

+ T80.A1 Non-ABO incompatibility with hemolytic transfusion reaction

    CC +7th **T80.A10 Non-ABO incompatibility with acute hemolytic transfusion reaction**

        Acute hemolytic transfusion reaction (AHTR) due to non-ABO incompatibility

        Non-ABO incompatibility with hemolytic transfusion reaction less than 24 hours after transfusion

    CC +7th **T80.A11 Non-ABO incompatibility with delayed hemolytic transfusion reaction**

        Delayed hemolytic transfusion reaction (DHTR) due to non-ABO incompatibility

        Non-ABO incompatibility with hemolytic transfusion reaction 24 or more hours after transfusion

    CC +7th **T80.A19 Non-ABO incompatibility with hemolytic transfusion reaction, unspecified**

        Hemolytic transfusion reaction (HTR) due to non-ABO incompatibility NOS

        Non-ABO incompatibility with hemolytic transfusion reaction at unspecified time after transfusion

CC X+7th **T80.A9 Other non-ABO incompatibility reaction due to transfusion of blood or blood products**

    Delayed serologic transfusion reaction (DSTR) from non-ABO incompatibility

    Other reaction to non-ABO incompatible blood transfusion

+ T80.5 Anaphylactic reaction due to serum

    Allergic shock due to serum

    Anaphylactic shock due to serum

    Anaphylactoid reaction due to serum

    Anaphylaxis due to serum

    Excludes1: *ABO incompatibility reaction due to transfusion of blood or blood products (T80.3-)*

        allergic reaction or shock NOS (T78.2)

        anaphylactic reaction or shock NOS (T78.2)

        anaphylactic reaction or shock due to adverse effect of correct medicinal substance properly administered (T88.6)

        other serum reaction (T80.6-)

CC X+7th **T80.51 Anaphylactic reaction due to administration of blood and blood products**

CC X+7th **T80.52 Anaphylactic reaction due to vaccination**

CC X+7th **T80.59 Anaphylactic reaction due to other serum**

+ T80.6 Other serum reactions

    Intoxication by serum

    Protein sickness

    Serum rash

    Serum sickness

    Serum urticaria

    Excludes2: *serum hepatitis (B16-B19)*

CC X+7th **T80.61 Other serum reaction due to administration of blood and blood products**

CC X+7th **T80.62 Other serum reaction due to vaccination**

CC X+7th **T80.69 Other serum reaction due to other serum**

    Code also, if applicable, arthropathy in hypersensitivity reactions classified elsewhere (M36.4)

+ T80.8 Other complications following infusion, transfusion and therapeutic injection

    + T80.81 Extravasation of vesicant agent

        Infiltration of vesicant agent

    CC +7th **T80.810 Extravasation of vesicant antineoplastic chemotherapy**

        Infiltration of vesicant antineoplastic chemotherapy

    CC +7th **T80.818 Extravasation of other vesicant agent**

        Infiltration of other vesicant agent

    X+7th **T80.89 Other complications following infusion, transfusion and therapeutic injection**

        Delayed serologic transfusion reaction (DSTR), unspecified incompatibility

        Use additional code to identify graft-versus-host reaction, if applicable, (D89.81-)

+ T80.9 Unspecified complication following infusion, transfusion and therapeutic injection

    X+7th **T80.90 Unspecified complication following infusion and therapeutic injection**

    + T80.91 Hemolytic transfusion reaction, unspecified incompatibility

        Excludes1: *ABO incompatibility with hemolytic transfusion reaction (T80.31-)*

          Non-ABO incompatibility with hemolytic transfusion reaction (T80.A1-)

          Rh incompatibility with hemolytic transfusion reaction (T80.41-)

    CC +7th **T80.910 Acute hemolytic transfusion reaction, unspecified incompatibility**

    CC +7th **T80.911 Delayed hemolytic transfusion reaction, unspecified incompatibility**

    CC +7th **T80.919 Hemolytic transfusion reaction, unspecified incompatibility, unspecified as acute or delayed**

        Hemolytic transfusion reaction NOS

    X+7th **T80.92 Unspecified transfusion reaction**

        Transfusion reaction NOS

+, +7th, X + 7th   ● Newborn   ● Pediatric   ● Maternity   ● Adult   ♀ Female   ♂ Male   Manifestation   Unacceptable PDX   HCC   CC   MCC   HAC

T81 **Complications of procedures, not elsewhere classified**

Use additional code for adverse effect, if applicable, to identify drug (T36-T50 with fifth or sixth character 5)

Excludes2: *complications following immunization (T88.0-T88.1)*
complications following infusion, transfusion and therapeutic injection (T80.-)
complications of transplanted organs and tissue (T86.-)
specified complications classified elsewhere, such as:
complication of prosthetic devices, implants and grafts (T82-T85)
dermatitis due to drugs and medicaments (L23.3, L24.4, L25.1, L27.0-L27.1)
endosseous dental implant failure (M27.6-)
floppy iris syndrome (IFIS) (intraoperative) H21.81
intraoperative and postprocedural complications of specific body system (D78.-, E36.-, E89.-, G97.3-, G97.4, H59.3-, H59.-, H95.2-, H95.3, I97.4-, I97.5, J95, K91.-, L76.-, M96.-, N99.-)
ostomy complications (J95.0-, K94.-, N99.5-)
plateau iris syndrome (post-iridectomy) (postprocedural) (H21.82)
poisoning and toxic effects of drugs and chemicals (T36-T65 with fifth or sixth character 1-4 or 6)

> The appropriate 7th character is to be added to each code from category T81
> A   initial encounter
> D   subsequent encounter
> S   sequela

+ T81.1 **Postprocedural shock**

Shock during or resulting from a procedure, not elsewhere classified

Excludes1: *anaphylactic shock NOS (T78.2)*
anaphylactic shock due to correct substance properly administered (T88.6)
anaphylactic shock due to serum (T80.5-)
anesthetic shock (T88.2)
electric shock (T75.4)
obstetric shock (O75.1)
septic shock (R65.21)
shock following abortion or ectopic or molar pregnancy (O00-O07, O08.3)
traumatic shock (T79.4)

CC X+7th **T81.10** **Postprocedural shock unspecified**

Collapse NOS during or resulting from a procedure, not elsewhere classified
Postprocedural failure of peripheral circulation
Postprocedural shock NOS

MCC X+7th **T81.11** **Postprocedural cardiogenic shock**

MCC X+7th **T81.12** **Postprocedural septic shock**

Postprocedural endotoxic shock resulting from a procedure, not elsewhere classified
Postprocedural gram-negative shock resulting from a procedure, not elsewhere classified
Code first underlying infection

Use additional code, to identify any associated acute organ dysfunction, if applicable
Review coding guideline C.1.d.2 and C.1.d.5.c

MCC X+7th **T81.19** **Other postprocedural shock**

Postprocedural hypovolemic shock

+ T81.3 **Disruption of wound, not elsewhere classified**

Disruption of any suture materials or other closure methods
Excludes1: *breakdown (mechanical) of permanent sutures (T85.612)*
displacement of permanent sutures (T85.622)
disruption of cesarean delivery wound (O90.0)
disruption of perineal obstetric wound (O90.1)
mechanical complication of permanent sutures NEC (T85.692)
AHA CC: 1Q, 2014, 23

CC X+7th **T81.30** **Disruption of wound, unspecified**

Disruption of wound NOS

CC X+7th **T81.31** **Disruption of external operation (surgical) wound, not elsewhere classified**

Dehiscence of operation wound NOS
Disruption of operation wound NOS
Disruption or dehiscence of closure of cornea
Disruption or dehiscence of closure of mucosa
Disruption or dehiscence of closure of skin and subcutaneous tissue
Full-thickness skin disruption or dehiscence
Superficial disruption or dehiscence of operation wound
Excludes1: *dehiscence of amputation stump (T87.81)*
AHA CC: 1Q, 2015, 3-21

CC X+7th **T81.32** **Disruption of internal operation (surgical) wound, not elsewhere classified**

Deep disruption or dehiscence of operation wound NOS
Disruption or dehiscence of closure of internal organ or other internal tissue
Disruption or dehiscence of closure of muscle or muscle flap
Disruption or dehiscence of closure of ribs or rib cage
Disruption or dehiscence of closure of skull or craniotomy
Disruption or dehiscence of closure of sternum or sternotomy
Disruption or dehiscence of closure of tendon or ligament
Disruption or dehiscence of closure of superficial or muscular fascia
AHA CC: 3Q, 2017, 4; 2Q, 2020, 22-23

CC X+7th **T81.33** **Disruption of traumatic injury wound repair**

Disruption or dehiscence of closure of traumatic laceration (external) (internal)

+ T81.4 **Infection following a procedure**

Wound abscess following a procedure
Use additional code to identify infection

Use additional code (R65.2-) to identify severe sepsis, if applicable
Excludes2: *bleb associated endophthalmitis (H59.4-)*
infection due to infusion, transfusion and therapeutic injection (T80.2-)
infection due to prosthetic devices, implants and grafts (T82.6-T82.7, T83.5-T83.6, T84.5-T84.7, T85.7)
obstetric surgical wound infection (O86.0-)
postprocedural fever NOS (R50.82)
postprocedural retroperitoneal abscess (K68.11)
AHA CC: 1Q, 2014, 23; 4Q, 2015, 37; 4Q, 2018, 33-34
Review coding guidelines C.1.d.5.b and C.1.d.5

CC X+7th **T81.40** **Infection following a procedure, unspecified**

HAC 7th character A see Appendix B for HAC conditional logic

CC X+7th **T81.41** **Infection following a procedure, superficial incisional surgical site**

Subcutaneous abscess following a procedure
Stitch abscess following a procedure
HAC 7th character A see Appendix B for HAC conditional logic
AHA CC: 4Q, 2018, 34

CC X+7th **T81.42** **Infection following a procedure, deep incisional surgical site**

Intra-muscular abscess following a procedure
HAC 7th character A see Appendix B for HAC conditional logic

CC X+7th **T81.43** **Infection following a procedure, organ and space surgical site**

Intra-abdominal abscess following a procedure
Subphrenic abscess following a procedure
HAC 7th character A see Appendix B for HAC conditional logic

CC X+7th **T81.44** **Sepsis following a procedure**

Use additional code to identify the sepsis
HAC 7th character A see Appendix B for HAC conditional logic

CC X+7th **T81.49** **Infection following a procedure, other surgical site**

HAC 7th character A see Appendix B for HAC conditional logic

+, +7th, X + 7th   ● Newborn   ● Pediatric   ● Maternity   ● Adult   ♀ Female   ♂ Male   Manifestation   Unacceptable PDX   HCC   CC   MCC   HAC

+ **T81.5** **Complications of foreign body accidentally left in body following procedure**

+ **T81.50** **Unspecified complication of foreign body accidentally left in body following procedure**

CC +7th **T81.500** **Unspecified complication of foreign body accidentally left in body following surgical operation**
HAC 7th character A see Appendix B for HAC conditional logic

CC +7th **T81.501** **Unspecified complication of foreign body accidentally left in body following infusion or transfusion**
HAC 7th character A see Appendix B for HAC conditional logic

CC +7th **T81.502** **Unspecified complication of foreign body accidentally left in body following kidney dialysis**
HAC 7th character A see Appendix B for HAC conditional logic

CC +7th **T81.503** **Unspecified complication of foreign body accidentally left in body following injection or immunization**
HAC 7th character A see Appendix B for HAC conditional logic

CC +7th **T81.504** **Unspecified complication of foreign body accidentally left in body following endoscopic examination**
HAC 7th character A see Appendix B for HAC conditional logic

CC +7th **T81.505** **Unspecified complication of foreign body accidentally left in body following heart catheterization**
HAC 7th character A see Appendix B for HAC conditional logic

CC +7th **T81.506** **Unspecified complication of foreign body accidentally left in body following aspiration, puncture or other catheterization**
HAC 7th character A see Appendix B for HAC conditional logic

CC +7th **T81.507** **Unspecified complication of foreign body accidentally left in body following removal of catheter or packing**
HAC 7th character A see Appendix B for HAC conditional logic

CC +7th **T81.508** **Unspecified complication of foreign body accidentally left in body following other procedure**
HAC 7th character A see Appendix B for HAC conditional logic

CC +7th **T81.509** **Unspecified complication of foreign body accidentally left in body following unspecified procedure**
HAC 7th character A see Appendix B for HAC conditional logic

+ **T81.51** **Adhesions due to foreign body accidentally left in body following procedure**

CC +7th **T81.510** **Adhesions due to foreign body accidentally left in body following surgical operation**
HAC 7th character A see Appendix B for HAC conditional logic

CC +7th **T81.511** **Adhesions due to foreign body accidentally left in body following infusion or transfusion**
HAC 7th character A see Appendix B for HAC conditional logic

CC +7th **T81.512** **Adhesions due to foreign body accidentally left in body following kidney dialysis**
HAC 7th character A see Appendix B for HAC conditional logic

CC +7th **T81.513** **Adhesions due to foreign body accidentally left in body following injection or immunization**
HAC 7th character A see Appendix B for HAC conditional logic

CC +7th **T81.514** **Adhesions due to foreign body accidentally left in body following endoscopic examination**
HAC 7th character A see Appendix B for HAC conditional logic

CC +7th **T81.515** **Adhesions due to foreign body accidentally left in body following heart catheterization**
HAC 7th character A see Appendix B for HAC conditional logic

CC +7th **T81.516** **Adhesions due to foreign body accidentally left in body following aspiration, puncture or other catheterization**
HAC 7th character A see Appendix B for HAC conditional logic

CC +7th **T81.517** **Adhesions due to foreign body accidentally left in body following removal of catheter or packing**
HAC 7th character A see Appendix B for HAC conditional logic

CC +7th **T81.518** **Adhesions due to foreign body accidentally left in body following other procedure**
HAC 7th character A see Appendix B for HAC conditional logic

CC +7th **T81.519** **Adhesions due to foreign body accidentally left in body following unspecified procedure**
HAC 7th character A see Appendix B for HAC conditional logic

+ **T81.52** **Obstruction due to foreign body accidentally left in body following procedure**

CC +7th **T81.520** **Obstruction due to foreign body accidentally left in body following surgical operation**
HAC 7th character A see Appendix B for HAC conditional logic

CC +7th **T81.521** **Obstruction due to foreign body accidentally left in body following infusion or transfusion**
HAC 7th character A see Appendix B for HAC conditional logic

CC +7th **T81.522** **Obstruction due to foreign body accidentally left in body following kidney dialysis**
HAC 7th character A see Appendix B for HAC conditional logic

CC +7th **T81.523** **Obstruction due to foreign body accidentally left in body following injection or immunization**
HAC 7th character A see Appendix B for HAC conditional logic

CC +7th **T81.524** **Obstruction due to foreign body accidentally left in body following endoscopic examination**
HAC 7th character A see Appendix B for HAC conditional logic

CC +7th **T81.525** **Obstruction due to foreign body accidentally left in body following heart catheterization**
HAC 7th character A see Appendix B for HAC conditional logic

CC +7th **T81.526** **Obstruction due to foreign body accidentally left in body following aspiration, puncture or other catheterization**
HAC 7th character A see Appendix B for HAC conditional logic

CC +7th **T81.527** **Obstruction due to foreign body accidentally left in body following removal of catheter or packing**
HAC 7th character A see Appendix B for HAC conditional logic

CC +7th **T81.528** **Obstruction due to foreign body accidentally left in body following other procedure**
HAC 7th character A see Appendix B for HAC conditional logic

CC +7th **T81.529** **Obstruction due to foreign body accidentally left in body following unspecified procedure**
HAC 7th character A see Appendix B for HAC conditional logic

+, +7th, X + 7th   ● Newborn   ● Pediatric   ● Maternity   ● Adult   ♀ Female   ♂ Male   Manifestation   Unacceptable PDX   HCC   CC   MCC   HAC

+ T81.53 Perforation due to foreign body accidentally left in body following procedure

CC +7th **T81.530 Perforation due to foreign body accidentally left in body following surgical operation**

> HAC 7th character A see Appendix B for HAC conditional logic

CC +7th **T81.531 Perforation due to foreign body accidentally left in body following infusion or transfusion**

> HAC 7th character A see Appendix B for HAC conditional logic

+7th **T81.532 Perforation due to foreign body accidentally left in body following kidney dialysis**

> HAC 7th character A see Appendix B for HAC conditional logic

CC +7th **T81.533 Perforation due to foreign body accidentally left in body following injection or immunization**

> HAC 7th character A see Appendix B for HAC conditional logic

CC +7th **T81.534 Perforation due to foreign body accidentally left in body following endoscopic examination**

> HAC 7th character A see Appendix B for HAC conditional logic

CC +7th **T81.535 Perforation due to foreign body accidentally left in body following heart catheterization**

> HAC 7th character A see Appendix B for HAC conditional logic

CC +7th **T81.536 Perforation due to foreign body accidentally left in body following aspiration, puncture or other catheterization**

> HAC 7th character A see Appendix B for HAC conditional logic

CC +7th **T81.537 Perforation due to foreign body accidentally left in body following removal of catheter or packing**

> HAC 7th character A see Appendix B for HAC conditional logic

CC +7th **T81.538 Perforation due to foreign body accidentally left in body following other procedure**

> HAC 7th character A see Appendix B for HAC conditional logic

CC +7th **T81.539 Perforation due to foreign body accidentally left in body following unspecified procedure**

> HAC 7th character A see Appendix B for HAC conditional logic

+ T81.59 Other complications of foreign body accidentally left in body following procedure

> *Excludes2:* obstruction or perforation due to prosthetic devices and implants intentionally left in body (T82.0-T82.5, T83.0-T83.4, T83.7, T84.0-T84.4, T85.0-T85.6)

CC +7th **T81.590 Other complications of foreign body accidentally left in body following surgical operation**

> HAC 7th character A see Appendix B for HAC conditional logic
>
> *AHA CC: 4Q, 2014, 24*

CC +7th **T81.591 Other complications of foreign body accidentally left in body following infusion or transfusion**

> HAC 7th character A see Appendix B for HAC conditional logic

CC +7th **T81.592 Other complications of foreign body accidentally left in body following kidney dialysis**

> HAC 7th character A see Appendix B for HAC conditional logic

CC +7th **T81.593 Other complications of foreign body accidentally left in body following injection or immunization**

> HAC 7th character A see Appendix B for HAC conditional logic

CC +7th **T81.594 Other complications of foreign body accidentally left in body following endoscopic examination**

> HAC 7th character A see Appendix B for HAC conditional logic

CC +7th **T81.595 Other complications of foreign body accidentally left in body following heart catheterization**

> HAC 7th character A see Appendix B for HAC conditional logic

CC +7th **T81.596 Other complications of foreign body accidentally left in body following aspiration, puncture or other catheterization**

> HAC 7th character A see Appendix B for HAC conditional logic

CC +7th **T81.597 Other complications of foreign body accidentally left in body following removal of catheter or packing**

> HAC 7th character A see Appendix B for HAC conditional logic

CC +7th **T81.598 Other complications of foreign body accidentally left in body following other procedure**

> HAC 7th character A see Appendix B for HAC conditional logic

CC +7th **T81.599 Other complications of foreign body accidentally left in body following unspecified procedure**

> HAC 7th character A see Appendix B for HAC conditional logic

+ T81.6 Acute reaction to foreign substance accidentally left during a procedure

> *Excludes2:* complications of foreign body accidentally left in body cavity or operation wound following procedure (T81.5-)

CC X+7th **T81.60 Unspecified acute reaction to foreign substance accidentally left during a procedure**

> HAC 7th character A see Appendix B for HAC conditional logic

CC X+7th **T81.61 Aseptic peritonitis due to foreign substance accidentally left during a procedure**

> Chemical peritonitis
>
> HAC 7th character A see Appendix B for HAC conditional logic

CC X+7th **T81.69 Other acute reaction to foreign substance accidentally left during a procedure**

> HAC 7th character A see Appendix B for HAC conditional logic

+ T81.7 Vascular complications following a procedure, not elsewhere classified

> Air embolism following procedure NEC
>
> Phlebitis or thrombophlebitis resulting from a procedure
>
> *Excludes1:* embolism complicating abortion or ectopic or molar pregnancy (O00-O07, O08.2)
> embolism complicating pregnancy, childbirth and the puerperium (O88.-)
> traumatic embolism (T79.0)
>
> *Excludes2:* embolism due to prosthetic devices, implants and grafts (T82.8-, T83.81, T84.8-, T85.81-)
> embolism following infusion, transfusion and therapeutic injection (T80.0)

+ T81.71 Complication of artery following a procedure, not elsewhere classified

CC +7th **T81.710 Complication of mesenteric artery following a procedure, not elsewhere classified**

CC +7th **T81.711 Complication of renal artery following a procedure, not elsewhere classified**

CC +7th **T81.718 Complication of other artery following a procedure, not elsewhere classified**

> *AHA CC: 2Q, 2019, 21-23*

CC +7th **T81.719 Complication of unspecified artery following a procedure, not elsewhere classified**

CC X+7th **T81.72 Complication of vein following a procedure, not elsewhere classified**

+ **T81.8** **Other complications of procedures, not elsewhere classified**
    Excludes2: *hypothermia following anesthesia (T88.51)*
              malignant hyperpyrexia due to
              anesthesia (T88.3)

   X+7th **T81.81** **Complication of inhalation therapy**

   X+7th **T81.82** **Emphysema (subcutaneous) resulting from a procedure**

  CC X+7th **T81.83** **Persistent postprocedural fistula**
        AHA CC: 3Q, 2017, 3-5

   X+7th **T81.89** **Other complications of procedures, not elsewhere classified**
        Use additional code to specify complication,
          such as:
          postprocedural delirium (F05)
        AHA CC: 1Q, 2014, 23

 X+7th **T81.9** **Unspecified complication of procedure**

T82 **Complications of cardiac and vascular prosthetic devices, implants and grafts**

    Excludes2: *failure and rejection of transplanted organs and tissue (T86.-)*

> The appropriate 7th character is to be added to each code from category T82
> A   initial encounter
> D   subsequent encounter
> S   sequela

+ **T82.0** **Mechanical complication of heart valve prosthesis**
    Mechanical complication of artificial heart valve
    Excludes1: *mechanical complication of biological heart valve graft (T82.22-)*

  CC X+7th **T82.01** **Breakdown (mechanical) of heart valve prosthesis**

  CC X+7th **T82.02** **Displacement of heart valve prosthesis**
       Malposition of heart valve prosthesis

  CC X+7th **T82.03** **Leakage of heart valve prosthesis**

  CC X+7th **T82.09** **Other mechanical complication of heart valve prosthesis**
       Obstruction (mechanical) of heart valve prosthesis
       Perforation of heart valve prosthesis
       Protrusion of heart valve prosthesis

+ **T82.1** **Mechanical complication of cardiac electronic device**
  + **T82.11** **Breakdown (mechanical) of cardiac electronic device**

    CC +7th **T82.110** **Breakdown (mechanical) of cardiac electrode**

    CC +7th **T82.111** **Breakdown (mechanical) of cardiac pulse generator (battery)**

    CC +7th **T82.118** **Breakdown (mechanical) of other cardiac electronic device**

    CC +7th **T82.119** **Breakdown (mechanical) of unspecified cardiac electronic device**

  + **T82.12** **Displacement of cardiac electronic device**
       Malposition of cardiac electronic device

    CC +7th **T82.120** **Displacement of cardiac electrode**

    CC +7th **T82.121** **Displacement of cardiac pulse generator (battery)**

    CC +7th **T82.128** **Displacement of other cardiac electronic device**

    CC +7th **T82.129** **Displacement of unspecified cardiac electronic device**

  + **T82.19** **Other mechanical complication of cardiac electronic device**
       Leakage of cardiac electronic device
       Obstruction of cardiac electronic device
       Perforation of cardiac electronic device
       Protrusion of cardiac electronic device

    CC +7th **T82.190** **Other mechanical complication of cardiac electrode**

    CC +7th **T82.191** **Other mechanical complication of cardiac pulse generator (battery)**

    CC +7th **T82.198** **Other mechanical complication of other cardiac electronic device**

    CC +7th **T82.199** **Other mechanical complication of unspecified cardiac device**

+ **T82.2** **Mechanical complication of coronary artery bypass graft and biological heart valve graft**
    Excludes1: *mechanical complication of artificial heart valve prosthesis (T82.0-)*

  + **T82.21** **Mechanical complication of coronary artery bypass graft**

    CC +7th **T82.211** **Breakdown (mechanical) of coronary artery bypass graft**

    CC +7th **T82.212** **Displacement of coronary artery bypass graft**
       Malposition of coronary artery bypass graft

    CC +7th **T82.213** **Leakage of coronary artery bypass graft**

    CC +7th **T82.218** **Other mechanical complication of coronary artery bypass graft**
       Obstruction, mechanical of coronary artery bypass graft
       Perforation of coronary artery bypass graft
       Protrusion of coronary artery bypass graft

  + **T82.22** **Mechanical complication of biological heart valve graft**

    CC +7th **T82.221** **Breakdown (mechanical) of biological heart valve graft**

    CC +7th **T82.222** **Displacement of biological heart valve graft**
       Malposition of biological heart valve graft

    CC +7th **T82.223** **Leakage of biological heart valve graft**

    CC +7th **T82.228** **Other mechanical complication of biological heart valve graft**
       Obstruction of biological heart valve graft
       Perforation of biological heart valve graft
       Protrusion of biological heart valve graft

+ **T82.3** **Mechanical complication of other vascular grafts**
  + **T82.31** **Breakdown (mechanical) of other vascular grafts**

    CC +7th **T82.310** **Breakdown (mechanical) of aortic (bifurcation) graft (replacement)**

    CC +7th **T82.311** **Breakdown (mechanical) of carotid arterial graft (bypass)**

    CC +7th **T82.312** **Breakdown (mechanical) of femoral arterial graft (bypass)**

    CC +7th **T82.318** **Breakdown (mechanical) of other vascular grafts**

    CC +7th **T82.319** **Breakdown (mechanical) of unspecified vascular grafts**

  + **T82.32** **Displacement of other vascular grafts**
       Malposition of other vascular grafts

    CC +7th **T82.320** **Displacement of aortic (bifurcation) graft (replacement)**

    CC +7th **T82.321** **Displacement of carotid arterial graft (bypass)**

    CC +7th **T82.322** **Displacement of femoral arterial graft (bypass)**

    CC +7th **T82.328** **Displacement of other vascular grafts**

    CC +7th **T82.329** **Displacement of unspecified vascular grafts**

  + **T82.33** **Leakage of other vascular grafts**

    CC +7th **T82.330** **Leakage of aortic (bifurcation) graft (replacement)**

    CC +7th **T82.331** **Leakage of carotid arterial graft (bypass)**

    CC +7th **T82.332** **Leakage of femoral arterial graft (bypass)**

    CC +7th **T82.338** **Leakage of other vascular grafts**

    CC +7th **T82.339** **Leakage of unspecified vascular graft**

  + **T82.39** **Other mechanical complication of other vascular grafts**
       Obstruction (mechanical) of other vascular grafts
       Perforation of other vascular grafts
       Protrusion of other vascular grafts

    CC +7th **T82.390** **Other mechanical complication of aortic (bifurcation) graft (replacement)**

    CC +7th **T82.391** **Other mechanical complication of carotid arterial graft (bypass)**

    CC +7th **T82.392** **Other mechanical complication of femoral arterial graft (bypass)**

    CC +7th **T82.398** **Other mechanical complication of other vascular grafts**

    CC +7th **T82.399** **Other mechanical complication of unspecified vascular grafts**

+, +7th, X + 7th   ● Newborn   ● Pediatric   ● Maternity   ● Adult   ♀ Female   ♂ Male   Manifestation   Unacceptable PDX   HCC   CC   MCC   HAC

+ **T82.4** **Mechanical complication of vascular dialysis catheter**
Mechanical complication of hemodialysis catheter
Excludes1: *mechanical complication of intraperitoneal dialysis catheter (T85.62)*

CC X+7th **T82.41** **Breakdown (mechanical) of vascular dialysis catheter**

CC X+7th **T82.42** **Displacement of vascular dialysis catheter**
Malposition of vascular dialysis catheter

CC X+7th **T82.43** **Leakage of vascular dialysis catheter**

CC X+7th **T82.49** **Other complication of vascular dialysis catheter**
Obstruction (mechanical) of vascular dialysis catheter
Perforation of vascular dialysis catheter
Protrusion of vascular dialysis catheter

+ **T82.5** **Mechanical complication of other cardiac and vascular devices and implants**
Excludes2: *mechanical complication of epidural and subdural infusion catheter (T85.61)*

+ **T82.51** **Breakdown (mechanical) of other cardiac and vascular devices and implants**

CC +7th **T82.510** **Breakdown (mechanical) of surgically created arteriovenous fistula**

CC +7th **T82.511** **Breakdown (mechanical) of surgically created arteriovenous shunt**

CC +7th **T82.512** **Breakdown (mechanical) of artificial heart**

CC +7th **T82.513** **Breakdown (mechanical) of balloon (counterpulsation) device**

CC +7th **T82.514** **Breakdown (mechanical) of infusion catheter**

CC +7th **T82.515** **Breakdown (mechanical) of umbrella device**

CC +7th **T82.518** **Breakdown (mechanical) of other cardiac and vascular devices and implants**

CC +7th **T82.519** **Breakdown (mechanical) of unspecified cardiac and vascular devices and implants**

+ **T82.52** **Displacement of other cardiac and vascular devices and implants**
Malposition of other cardiac and vascular devices and implants

CC +7th **T82.520** **Displacement of surgically created arteriovenous fistula**

CC +7th **T82.521** **Displacement of surgically created arteriovenous shunt**

CC +7th **T82.522** **Displacement of artificial heart**

CC +7th **T82.523** **Displacement of balloon (counterpulsation) device**

CC +7th **T82.524** **Displacement of infusion catheter**
AHA CC: 3Q, 2019, 15-16; 2Q, 2020, 21-22

CC +7th **T82.525** **Displacement of umbrella device**

CC +7th **T82.528** **Displacement of other cardiac and vascular devices and implants**

CC +7th **T82.529** **Displacement of unspecified cardiac and vascular devices and implants**

+ **T82.53** **Leakage of other cardiac and vascular devices and implants**

CC +7th **T82.530** **Leakage of surgically created arteriovenous fistula**

CC +7th **T82.531** **Leakage of surgically created arteriovenous shunt**

CC +7th **T82.532** **Leakage of artificial heart**

CC +7th **T82.533** **Leakage of balloon (counterpulsation) device**

CC +7th **T82.534** **Leakage of infusion catheter**

CC +7th **T82.535** **Leakage of umbrella device**

CC +7th **T82.538** **Leakage of other cardiac and vascular devices and implants**

CC +7th **T82.539** **Leakage of unspecified cardiac and vascular devices and implants**

+ **T82.59** **Other mechanical complication of other cardiac and vascular devices and implants**
Obstruction (mechanical) of other cardiac and vascular devices and implants
Perforation of other cardiac and vascular devices and implants
Protrusion of other cardiac and vascular devices and implants

CC +7th **T82.590** **Other mechanical complication of surgically created arteriovenous fistula**

CC +7th **T82.591** **Other mechanical complication of surgically created arteriovenous shunt**

CC +7th **T82.592** **Other mechanical complication of artificial heart**

CC +7th **T82.593** **Other mechanical complication of balloon (counterpulsation) device**

CC +7th **T82.594** **Other mechanical complication of infusion catheter**

CC +7th **T82.595** **Other mechanical complication of umbrella device**

CC +7th **T82.598** **Other mechanical complication of other cardiac and vascular devices and implants**

CC +7th **T82.599** **Other mechanical complication of unspecified cardiac and vascular devices and implants**

CC X+7th **T82.6** **Infection and inflammatory reaction due to cardiac valve prosthesis**
Use additional code to identify infection
HAC 7th character A see Appendix B for HAC conditional logic

CC X+7th **T82.7** **Infection and inflammatory reaction due to other cardiac and vascular devices, implants and grafts**
Use additional code to identify infection
HAC 7th character A see Appendix B for HAC conditional logic
AHA CC: 1Q, 2015, 3-21; 4Q, 2018, 89; 1Q, 2019, 13-14

+ **T82.8** **Other specified complications due to cardiac and vascular prosthetic devices, implants and grafts**

+ **T82.81** **Embolism due to cardiac and vascular prosthetic devices, implants and grafts**

CC +7th **T82.817** **Embolism due to cardiac prosthetic devices, implants and grafts**

CC +7th **T82.818** **Embolism due to vascular prosthetic devices, implants and grafts**

+ **T82.82** **Fibrosis due to cardiac and vascular prosthetic devices, implants and grafts**

CC +7th **T82.827** **Fibrosis due to cardiac prosthetic devices, implants and grafts**

CC +7th **T82.828** **Fibrosis due to vascular prosthetic devices, implants and grafts**

+ **T82.83** **Hemorrhage due to cardiac and vascular prosthetic devices, implants and grafts**

CC +7th **T82.837** **Hemorrhage due to cardiac prosthetic devices, implants and grafts**

CC +7th **T82.838** **Hemorrhage due to vascular prosthetic devices, implants and grafts**

+ **T82.84** **Pain due to cardiac and vascular prosthetic devices, implants and grafts**

CC +7th **T82.847** **Pain due to cardiac prosthetic devices, implants and grafts**

CC +7th **T82.848** **Pain due to vascular prosthetic devices, implants and grafts**

+ **T82.85** **Stenosis due to cardiac and vascular prosthetic devices, implants and grafts**

CC +7th **T82.855** **Stenosis of coronary artery stent**
In-stent stenosis (restenosis) of coronary artery stent
Restenosis of coronary artery stent
AHA CC: 4Q, 2016, 69

CC +7th **T82.856** **Stenosis of peripheral vascular stent**
In-stent stenosis (restenosis) of peripheral vascular stent
Restenosis of peripheral vascular stent
AHA CC: 4Q, 2016, 69

CC +7th **T82.857** **Stenosis of other cardiac prosthetic devices, implants and grafts**

CC +7th **T82.858** **Stenosis of other vascular prosthetic devices, implants and grafts**

+, +7th, X + 7th ● Newborn ● Pediatric ● Maternity ● Adult ♀ Female ♂ Male Manifestation Unacceptable PDX HCC CC MCC **HAC**

+ T82.86 **Thrombosis due to cardiac and vascular prosthetic devices, implants and grafts**

CC +7th **T82.867** **Thrombosis due to cardiac prosthetic devices, implants and grafts**
  AHA CC: 2Q, 2019, 32-33

CC +7th **T82.868** **Thrombosis due to vascular prosthetic devices, implants and grafts**

+ T82.89 **Other specified complication of cardiac and vascular prosthetic devices, implants and grafts**

CC +7th **T82.897** **Other specified complication of cardiac prosthetic devices, implants and grafts**

CC +7th **T82.898** **Other specified complication of vascular prosthetic devices, implants and grafts**

CC X+7th **T82.9** **Unspecified complication of cardiac and vascular prosthetic device, implant and graft**

T83 **Complications of genitourinary prosthetic devices, implants and grafts**

> **Excludes2:** *failure and rejection of transplanted organs and tissue (T86.-)*
>
> *AHA CC: 4Q, 2016, 70-71*

> The appropriate 7th character is to be added to each code from category T83
> A initial encounter
> D subsequent encounter
> S sequela

+ T83.0 **Mechanical complication of urinary catheter**
> **Excludes2:** *complications of stoma of urinary tract (N99.5-)*

+ T83.01 **Breakdown (mechanical) of urinary catheter**

CC +7th **T83.010** **Breakdown (mechanical) of cystostomy catheter**

+7th **T83.011** **Breakdown (mechanical) of indwelling urethral catheter**

+7th **T83.012** **Breakdown (mechanical) of nephrostomy catheter**

+7th **T83.018** **Breakdown (mechanical) of other urinary catheter**
  Breakdown (mechanical) of Hopkins catheter
  Breakdown (mechanical) of ileostomy catheter
  Breakdown (mechanical) of urostomy catheter

+ T83.02 **Displacement of urinary catheter**
  Malposition of urinary catheter

CC +7th **T83.020** **Displacement of cystostomy catheter**

+7th **T83.021** **Displacement of indwelling urethral catheter**

+7th **T83.022** **Displacement of nephrostomy catheter**

+7th **T83.028** **Displacement of other urinary catheter**
  Displacement of Hopkins catheter
  Displacement of ileostomy catheter
  Displacement of urostomy catheter

+ T83.03 **Leakage of urinary catheter**

CC +7th **T83.030** **Leakage of cystostomy catheter**

+7th **T83.031** **Leakage of indwelling urethral catheter**

+7th **T83.032** **Leakage of nephrostomy catheter**

+7th **T83.038** **Leakage of other urinary catheter**
  Leakage of Hopkins catheter
  Leakage of ileostomy catheter
  Leakage of urostomy catheter

+ T83.09 **Other mechanical complication of urinary catheter**
  Obstruction (mechanical) of urinary catheter
  Perforation of urinary catheter
  Protrusion of urinary catheter

CC +7th **T83.090** **Other mechanical complication of cystostomy catheter**

+7th **T83.091** **Other mechanical complication of indwelling urethral catheter**

+7th **T83.092** **Other mechanical complication of nephrostomy catheter**

+7th **T83.098** **Other mechanical complication of other urinary catheter**
  Other mechanical complication of Hopkins catheter
  Other mechanical complication of ileostomy catheter
  Other mechanical complication of urostomy catheter

+ T83.1 **Mechanical complication of other urinary devices and implants**

+ T83.11 **Breakdown (mechanical) of other urinary devices and implants**

CC +7th **T83.110** **Breakdown (mechanical) of urinary electronic stimulator device**
> **Excludes2:** *breakdown (mechanical) of electrode (lead) for sacral nerve neurostimulator (T85.111)*
> *breakdown (mechanical) of implanted electronic sacral neurostimulator, pulse generator or receiver (T85.113)*

CC +7th **T83.111** **Breakdown (mechanical) of implanted urinary sphincter**

CC +7th **T83.112** **Breakdown (mechanical) of indwelling ureteral stent**

CC +7th **T83.113** **Breakdown (mechanical) of other urinary stents**
  Breakdown (mechanical) of ileal conduit stent
  Breakdown (mechanical) of nephroureteral stent

CC +7th **T83.118** **Breakdown (mechanical) of other urinary devices and implants**

+ T83.12 **Displacement of other urinary devices and implants**
  Malposition of other urinary devices and implants

CC +7th **T83.120** **Displacement of urinary electronic stimulator device**
> **Excludes2:** *displacement of electrode (lead) for sacral nerve neurostimulator(T85.121)*
> *displacement of implanted electronic sacral neurostimulator, pulse generator or receiver (T85.123)*

CC +7th **T83.121** **Displacement of implanted urinary sphincter**

CC +7th **T83.122** **Displacement of indwelling ureteral stent**

CC +7th **T83.123** **Displacement of other urinary stents**
  Displacement of ileal conduit stent
  Displacement of nephroureteral stent

CC +7th **T83.128** **Displacement of other urinary devices and implants**

+ T83.19 **Other mechanical complication of other urinary devices and implants**
  Leakage of other urinary devices and implants
  Obstruction (mechanical) of other urinary devices and implants
  Perforation of other urinary devices and implants
  Protrusion of other urinary devices and implants

CC +7th **T83.190** **Other mechanical complication of urinary electronic stimulator device**
> **Excludes2:** *other mechanical complication of electrode (lead) for sacral nerve neurostimulator(T85.191)*
> *other mechanical complication of implanted electronic sacral neurostimulator, pulse generator or receiver (T85.193)*

CC +7th **T83.191** **Other mechanical complication of implanted urinary sphincter**

CC +7th **T83.192** **Other mechanical complication of indwelling ureteral stent**

CC +7th **T83.193** **Other mechanical complication of other urinary stent**
  Other mechanical complication of ileal conduit stent
  Other mechanical complication of nephroureteral stent

CC +7th **T83.198** **Other mechanical complication of other urinary devices and implants**

+, +7th, X + 7th   ● Newborn   ● Pediatric   ● Maternity   ● Adult   ♀ Female   ♂ Male   Manifestation   Unacceptable PDX   HCC   CC   MCC   HAC

+ T83.2 Mechanical complication of graft of urinary organ

CC X+7th **T83.21 Breakdown (mechanical) of graft of urinary organ**

CC X+7th **T83.22 Displacement of graft of urinary organ**
> Malposition of graft of urinary organ

CC X+7th **T83.23 Leakage of graft of urinary organ**

CC X+7th **T83.24 Erosion of graft of urinary organ**

CC X+7th **T83.25 Exposure of graft of urinary organ**

CC X+7th **T83.29 Other mechanical complication of graft of urinary organ**
> Obstruction (mechanical) of graft of urinary organ
> Perforation of graft of urinary organ
> Protrusion of graft of urinary organ

+ T83.3 Mechanical complication of intrauterine contraceptive device

♀ X+7th **T83.31 Breakdown (mechanical) of intrauterine contraceptive device**

♀ X+7th **T83.32 Displacement of intrauterine contraceptive device**
> Malposition of intrauterine contraceptive device
> Missing string of intrauterine contraceptive device

♀ X+7th **T83.39 Other mechanical complication of intrauterine contraceptive device**
> Leakage of intrauterine contraceptive device
> Obstruction (mechanical) of intrauterine contraceptive device
> Perforation of intrauterine contraceptive device
> Protrusion of intrauterine contraceptive device

+ T83.4 Mechanical complication of other prosthetic devices, implants and grafts of genital tract

+ T83.41 Breakdown (mechanical) of other prosthetic devices, implants and grafts of genital tract

♂ CC +7th **T83.410 Breakdown (mechanical) of implanted penile prosthesis**
> Breakdown (mechanical) of penile prosthesis cylinder
> Breakdown (mechanical) of penile prosthesis pump
> Breakdown (mechanical) of penile prosthesis reservoir

CC +7th **T83.411 Breakdown (mechanical) of implanted testicular prosthesis**

CC +7th **T83.418 Breakdown (mechanical) of other prosthetic devices, implants and grafts of genital tract**

+ T83.42 Displacement of other prosthetic devices, implants and grafts of genital tract
> Malposition of other prosthetic devices, implants and grafts of genital tract

♂ CC +7th **T83.420 Displacement of implanted penile prosthesis**
> Displacement of penile prosthesis cylinder
> Displacement of penile prosthesis pump
> Displacement of penile prosthesis reservoir

CC +7th **T83.421 Displacement of implanted testicular prosthesis**

CC +7th **T83.428 Displacement of other prosthetic devices, implants and grafts of genital tract**
> *AHA CC: 1Q, 2018, 5-6*

+ T83.49 Other mechanical complication of other prosthetic devices, implants and grafts of genital tract
> Leakage of other prosthetic devices, implants and grafts of genital tract
> Obstruction, mechanical of other prosthetic devices, implants and grafts of genital tract
> Perforation of other prosthetic devices, implants and grafts of genital tract
> Protrusion of other prosthetic devices, implants and grafts of genital tract

♂ CC +7th **T83.490 Other mechanical complication of implanted penile prosthesis**
> Other mechanical complication of penile prosthesis cylinder
> Other mechanical complication of penile prosthesis pump
> Other mechanical complication of penile prosthesis reservoir

CC +7th **T83.491 Other mechanical complication of implanted testicular prosthesis**

CC +7th **T83.498 Other mechanical complication of other prosthetic devices, implants and grafts of genital tract**

+ T83.5 Infection and inflammatory reaction due to prosthetic device, implant and graft in urinary system
> Use additional code to identify infection

+ T83.51 Infection and inflammatory reaction due to urinary catheter
> *Excludes2:* complications of stoma of urinary tract (N99.5-)

CC +7th **T83.510 Infection and inflammatory reaction due to cystostomy catheter**

CC +7th **T83.511 Infection and inflammatory reaction due to indwelling urethral catheter**
> **HAC** 7th character A see Appendix B for HAC conditional logic

CC +7th **T83.512 Infection and inflammatory reaction due to nephrostomy catheter**

CC +7th **T83.518 Infection and inflammatory reaction due to other urinary catheter**
> Infection and inflammatory reaction due to Hopkins catheter
> Infection and inflammatory reaction due to ileostomy catheter
> Infection and inflammatory reaction due to urostomy catheter
> **HAC** 7th character A see Appendix B for HAC conditional logic

+ T83.59 Infection and inflammatory reaction due to prosthetic device, implant and graft in urinary system

CC +7th **T83.590 Infection and inflammatory reaction due to implanted urinary neurostimulation device**
> *Excludes2:* infection and inflammatory reaction due to electrode lead of sacral nerve neurostimulator (T85.732)
> infection and inflammatory reaction due to pulse generator or receiver of sacralnerveneurostimulator (T85.734)

CC +7th **T83.591 Infection and inflammatory reaction due to implanted urinary sphincter**

CC +7th **T83.592 Infection and inflammatory reaction due to indwelling ureteral stent**

CC +7th **T83.593 Infection and inflammatory reaction due to other urinary stents**
> Infection and inflammatory reaction due to ileal conduit stents
> Infection and inflammatory reaction due to nephroureteral stent

CC +7th **T83.598 Infection and inflammatory reaction due to other prosthetic device, implant and graft in urinary system**

+ T83.6 Infection and inflammatory reaction due to prosthetic device, implant and graft in genital tract
> Use additional code to identify infection

CC X+7th **T83.61 Infection and inflammatory reaction due to implanted penile prosthesis**
> Infection and inflammatory reaction due to penile prosthesis cylinder
> Infection and inflammatory reaction due to penile prosthesis pump
> Infection and inflammatory reaction due to penile prosthesis reservoir

CC X+7th **T83.62 Infection and inflammatory reaction due to implanted testicular prosthesis**

CC X+7th **T83.69 Infection and inflammatory reaction due to other prosthetic device, implant and graft in genital tract**

+ T83.7 Complications due to implanted mesh and other prosthetic materials
    + T83.71 Erosion of implanted mesh and other prosthetic materials to surrounding organ or tissue
        ♀ +7th **T83.711 Erosion of implanted vaginal mesh to surrounding organ or tissue**
            Erosion of implanted vaginal mesh into pelvic floor muscles
        CC +7th **T83.712 Erosion of implanted urethral mesh to surrounding organ or tissue**
            Erosion of implanted female urethral sling
            Erosion of implanted male urethral sling
            Erosion of implanted urethral mesh into pelvic floor muscles
        CC +7th **T83.713 Erosion of implanted urethral bulking agent to surrounding organ or tissue**
        CC +7th **T83.714 Erosion of implanted ureteral bulking agent to surrounding organ or tissue**
        CC +7th **T83.718 Erosion of other implanted mesh to organ or tissue**
        CC +7th **T83.719 Erosion of other prosthetic materials to surrounding organ or tissue**
    + T83.72 Exposure of implanted mesh and other prosthetic materials into surrounding organ or tissue
        Extrusion of implanted mesh
        ♀ +7th **T83.721 Exposure of implanted vaginal mesh into vagina**
            Exposure of implanted vaginal mesh through vaginal wall
        CC +7th **T83.722 Exposure of implanted urethral mesh into urethra**
            Exposure of implanted female urethral sling
            Exposure of implanted male urethral sling
            Exposure of implanted urethral mesh through urethral wall
        CC +7th **T83.723 Exposure of implanted urethral bulking agent into urethra**
        CC +7th **T83.724 Exposure of implanted ureteral bulking agent into ureter**
        CC +7th **T83.728 Exposure of other implanted mesh into organ or tissue**
        CC +7th **T83.729 Exposure of other prosthetic materials into organ or tissue**
  CC X+7th **T83.79 Other specified complications due to other genitourinary prosthetic materials**
+ T83.8 Other specified complications of genitourinary prosthetic devices, implants and grafts
  CC X+7th **T83.81 Embolism due to genitourinary prosthetic devices, implants and grafts**
  CC X+7th **T83.82 Fibrosis due to genitourinary prosthetic devices, implants and grafts**
  CC X+7th **T83.83 Hemorrhage due to genitourinary prosthetic devices, implants and grafts**
  CC X+7th **T83.84 Pain due to genitourinary prosthetic devices, implants and grafts**
  CC X+7th **T83.85 Stenosis due to genitourinary prosthetic devices, implants and grafts**
  CC X+7th **T83.86 Thrombosis due to genitourinary prosthetic devices, implants and grafts**
  CC X+7th **T83.89 Other specified complication of genitourinary prosthetic devices, implants and grafts**
CC X+7th **T83.9 Unspecified complication of genitourinary prosthetic device, implant and graft**

T84 Complications of internal orthopedic prosthetic devices, implants and grafts

  Excludes2: *failure and rejection of transplanted organs and tissues (T86.-)*
                fracture of bone following insertion of orthopedic implant, joint prosthesis or bone plate (M96.6)

The appropriate 7th character is to be added to each code from category T84
A   initial encounter
D   subsequent encounter
S   sequela

+ T84.0 Mechanical complication of internal joint prosthesis
    + T84.01 Broken internal joint prosthesis
        Breakage (fracture) of prosthetic joint
        Broken prosthetic joint implant
        Excludes1: *periprosthetic joint implant fracture (M97.-)*
    CC +7th **T84.010 Broken internal right hip prosthesis**
    CC +7th **T84.011 Broken internal left hip prosthesis**
    CC +7th **T84.012 Broken internal right knee prosthesis**
        AHA CC: 2Q, 2019, 27-28
    CC +7th **T84.013 Broken internal left knee prosthesis**
    CC +7th **T84.018 Broken internal joint prosthesis, other site**
        Use additional code to identify the joint (Z96.6-)
    CC +7th **T84.019 Broken internal joint prosthesis, unspecified site**
    + T84.02 Dislocation of internal joint prosthesis
        Instability of internal joint prosthesis
        Subluxation of internal joint prosthesis
    CC +7th **T84.020 Dislocation of internal right hip prosthesis**
    CC +7th **T84.021 Dislocation of internal left hip prosthesis**
    CC +7th **T84.022 Instability of internal right knee prosthesis**
    CC +7th **T84.023 Instability of internal left knee prosthesis**
    CC +7th **T84.028 Dislocation of other internal joint prosthesis**
        Use additional code to identify the joint (Z96.6-)
    CC +7th **T84.029 Dislocation of unspecified internal joint prosthesis**
    + T84.03 Mechanical loosening of internal prosthetic joint
        Aseptic loosening of prosthetic joint
    CC +7th **T84.030 Mechanical loosening of internal right hip prosthetic joint**
    CC +7th **T84.031 Mechanical loosening of internal left hip prosthetic joint**
    CC +7th **T84.032 Mechanical loosening of internal right knee prosthetic joint**
    CC +7th **T84.033 Mechanical loosening of internal left knee prosthetic joint**
    CC +7th **T84.038 Mechanical loosening of other internal prosthetic joint**
        Use additional code to identify the joint (Z96.6-)
    CC +7th **T84.039 Mechanical loosening of unspecified internal prosthetic joint**
    + T84.05 Periprosthetic osteolysis of internal prosthetic joint
        Use additional code to identify major osseous defect, if applicable (M89.7-)
    CC +7th **T84.050 Periprosthetic osteolysis of internal prosthetic right hip joint**
    CC +7th **T84.051 Periprosthetic osteolysis of internal prosthetic left hip joint**
    CC +7th **T84.052 Periprosthetic osteolysis of internal prosthetic right knee joint**
    CC +7th **T84.053 Periprosthetic osteolysis of internal prosthetic left knee joint**
    CC +7th **T84.058 Periprosthetic osteolysis of other internal prosthetic joint**
        Use additional code to identify the joint (Z96.6-)
    CC +7th **T84.059 Periprosthetic osteolysis of unspecified internal prosthetic joint**

+, +7th, X + 7th   ● Newborn   ● Pediatric   ● Maternity   ● Adult   ♀ Female   ♂ Male   Manifestation   Unacceptable PDX   HCC   CC   MCC   HAC

+ **T84.06** **Wear of articular bearing surface of internal prosthetic joint**

CC +7th **T84.060** **Wear of articular bearing surface of internal prosthetic right hip joint**

CC +7th **T84.061** **Wear of articular bearing surface of internal prosthetic left hip joint**

CC +7th **T84.062** **Wear of articular bearing surface of internal prosthetic right knee joint**

CC +7th **T84.063** **Wear of articular bearing surface of internal prosthetic left knee joint**

CC +7th **T84.068** **Wear of articular bearing surface of other internal prosthetic joint**
　　Use additional code to identify the joint (Z96.6-)

CC +7th **T84.069** **Wear of articular bearing surface of unspecified internal prosthetic joint**

+ **T84.09** **Other mechanical complication of internal joint prosthesis**
　　Prosthetic joint implant failure NOS

CC +7th **T84.090** **Other mechanical complication of internal right hip prosthesis**
　　　AHA CC: 1Q, 2019, 20

CC +7th **T84.091** **Other mechanical complication of internal left hip prosthesis**

CC +7th **T84.092** **Other mechanical complication of internal right knee prosthesis**

CC +7th **T84.093** **Other mechanical complication of internal left knee prosthesis**

CC +7th **T84.098** **Other mechanical complication of other internal joint prosthesis**
　　Use additional code to identify the joint (Z96.6-)

CC +7th **T84.099** **Other mechanical complication of unspecified internal joint prosthesis**

+ **T84.1** **Mechanical complication of internal fixation device of bones of limb**
　　Excludes2: *mechanical complication of internal fixation device of bones of feet (T84.2-)*
　　　mechanical complication of internal fixation device of bones of fingers (T84.2-)
　　　mechanical complication of internal fixation device of bones of hands (T84.2-)
　　　mechanical complication of internal fixation device of bones of toes (T84.2-)

+ **T84.11** **Breakdown (mechanical) of internal fixation device of bones of limb**

CC +7th **T84.110** **Breakdown (mechanical) of internal fixation device of right humerus**

CC +7th **T84.111** **Breakdown (mechanical) of internal fixation device of left humerus**

CC +7th **T84.112** **Breakdown (mechanical) of internal fixation device of bone of right forearm**

CC +7th **T84.113** **Breakdown (mechanical) of internal fixation device of bone of left forearm**

CC +7th **T84.114** **Breakdown (mechanical) of internal fixation device of right femur**

CC +7th **T84.115** **Breakdown (mechanical) of internal fixation device of left femur**

CC +7th **T84.116** **Breakdown (mechanical) of internal fixation device of bone of right lower leg**

CC +7th **T84.117** **Breakdown (mechanical) of internal fixation device of bone of left lower leg**

CC +7th **T84.119** **Breakdown (mechanical) of internal fixation device of unspecified bone of limb**

+ **T84.12** **Displacement of internal fixation device of bones of limb**
　　Malposition of internal fixation device of bones of limb

CC +7th **T84.120** **Displacement of internal fixation device of right humerus**

CC +7th **T84.121** **Displacement of internal fixation device of left humerus**

CC +7th **T84.122** **Displacement of internal fixation device of bone of right forearm**

CC +7th **T84.123** **Displacement of internal fixation device of bone of left forearm**

CC +7th **T84.124** **Displacement of internal fixation device of right femur**

CC +7th **T84.125** **Displacement of internal fixation device of left femur**

CC +7th **T84.126** **Displacement of internal fixation device of bone of right lower leg**

CC +7th **T84.127** **Displacement of internal fixation device of bone of left lower leg**

CC +7th **T84.129** **Displacement of internal fixation device of unspecified bone of limb**

+ **T84.19** **Other mechanical complication of internal fixation device of bones of limb**
　　Obstruction (mechanical) of internal fixation device of bones of limb
　　Perforation of internal fixation device of bones of limb
　　Protrusion of internal fixation device of bones of limb

CC +7th **T84.190** **Other mechanical complication of internal fixation device of right humerus**

CC +7th **T84.191** **Other mechanical complication of internal fixation device of left humerus**

CC +7th **T84.192** **Other mechanical complication of internal fixation device of bone of right forearm**

CC +7th **T84.193** **Other mechanical complication of internal fixation device of bone of left forearm**

CC +7th **T84.194** **Other mechanical complication of internal fixation device of right femur**

CC +7th **T84.195** **Other mechanical complication of internal fixation device of left femur**

CC +7th **T84.196** **Other mechanical complication of internal fixation device of bone of right lower leg**

CC +7th **T84.197** **Other mechanical complication of internal fixation device of bone of left lower leg**

CC +7th **T84.199** **Other mechanical complication of internal fixation device of unspecified bone of limb**

+ **T84.2** **Mechanical complication of internal fixation device of other bones**

+ **T84.21** **Breakdown (mechanical) of internal fixation device of other bones**

CC +7th **T84.210** **Breakdown (mechanical) of internal fixation device of bones of hand and fingers**

CC +7th **T84.213** **Breakdown (mechanical) of internal fixation device of bones of foot and toes**

CC +7th **T84.216** **Breakdown (mechanical) of internal fixation device of vertebrae**

CC +7th **T84.218** **Breakdown (mechanical) of internal fixation device of other bones**

+ **T84.22** **Displacement of internal fixation device of other bones**
　　Malposition of internal fixation device of other bones

CC +7th **T84.220** **Displacement of internal fixation device of bones of hand and fingers**

CC +7th **T84.223** **Displacement of internal fixation device of bones of foot and toes**

CC +7th **T84.226** **Displacement of internal fixation device of vertebrae**

CC +7th **T84.228** **Displacement of internal fixation device of other bones**

+ **T84.29** **Other mechanical complication of internal fixation device of other bones**

Obstruction (mechanical) of internal fixation device of other bones

Perforation of internal fixation device of other bones

Protrusion of internal fixation device of other bones

CC +7th **T84.290** **Other mechanical complication of internal fixation device of bones of hand and fingers**

CC +7th **T84.293** **Other mechanical complication of internal fixation device of bones of foot and toes**

CC +7th **T84.296** **Other mechanical complication of internal fixation device of vertebrae**

CC +7th **T84.298** **Other mechanical complication of internal fixation device of other bones**

+ **T84.3** **Mechanical complication of other bone devices, implants and grafts**

Excludes2: *other complications of bone graft (T86.83-)*

+ **T84.31** **Breakdown (mechanical) of other bone devices, implants and grafts**

CC +7th **T84.310** **Breakdown (mechanical) of electronic bone stimulator**

CC +7th **T84.318** **Breakdown (mechanical) of other bone devices, implants and grafts**

+ **T84.32** **Displacement of other bone devices, implants and grafts**

Malposition of other bone devices, implants and grafts

CC +7th **T84.320** **Displacement of electronic bone stimulator**

CC +7th **T84.328** **Displacement of other bone devices, implants and grafts**

AHA CC: 4Q, 2014, 28-29

+ **T84.39** **Other mechanical complication of other bone devices, implants and grafts**

Obstruction (mechanical) of other bone devices, implants and grafts

Perforation of other bone devices, implants and grafts

Protrusion of other bone devices, implants and grafts

CC +7th **T84.390** **Other mechanical complication of electronic bone stimulator**

CC +7th **T84.398** **Other mechanical complication of other bone devices, implants and grafts**

+ **T84.4** **Mechanical complication of other internal orthopedic devices, implants and grafts**

+ **T84.41** **Breakdown (mechanical) of other internal orthopedic devices, implants and grafts**

CC +7th **T84.410** **Breakdown (mechanical) of muscle and tendon graft**

CC +7th **T84.418** **Breakdown (mechanical) of other internal orthopedic devices, implants and grafts**

+ **T84.42** **Displacement of other internal orthopedic devices, implants and grafts**

Malposition of other internal orthopedic devices, implants and grafts

CC +7th **T84.420** **Displacement of muscle and tendon graft**

CC +7th **T84.428** **Displacement of other internal orthopedic devices, implants and grafts**

+ **T84.49** **Other mechanical complication of other internal orthopedic devices, implants and grafts**

Mechanical complication of other internal orthopedic devices, implants and grafts NOS

Obstruction (mechanical) of other internal orthopedic devices, implants and grafts

Perforation of other internal orthopedic devices, implants and grafts

Protrusion of other internal orthopedic devices, implants and grafts

CC +7th **T84.490** **Other mechanical complication of muscle and tendon graft**

CC +7th **T84.498** **Other mechanical complication of other internal orthopedic devices, implants and grafts**

+ **T84.5** **Infection and inflammatory reaction due to internal joint prosthesis**

Use additional code to identify infection

CC X+7th **T84.50** **Infection and inflammatory reaction due to unspecified internal joint prosthesis**

CC X+7th **T84.51** **Infection and inflammatory reaction due to internal right hip prosthesis**

AHA CC: 4Q, 2015, 36

CC X+7th **T84.52** **Infection and inflammatory reaction due to internal left hip prosthesis**

AHA CC: 1Q, 2015, 3-21

CC X+7th **T84.53** **Infection and inflammatory reaction due to internal right knee prosthesis**

CC X+7th **T84.54** **Infection and inflammatory reaction due to internal left knee prosthesis**

CC X+7th **T84.59** **Infection and inflammatory reaction due to other internal joint prosthesis**

+ **T84.6** **Infection and inflammatory reaction due to internal fixation device**

Use additional code to identify infection

CC X+7th **T84.60** **Infection and inflammatory reaction due to internal fixation device of unspecified site**

HAC 7th character A see Appendix B for HAC conditional logic

+ **T84.61** **Infection and inflammatory reaction due to internal fixation device of arm**

CC +7th **T84.610** **Infection and inflammatory reaction due to internal fixation device of right humerus**

HAC 7th character A see Appendix B for HAC conditional logic

CC +7th **T84.611** **Infection and inflammatory reaction due to internal fixation device of left humerus**

HAC 7th character A see Appendix B for HAC conditional logic

CC +7th **T84.612** **Infection and inflammatory reaction due to internal fixation device of right radius**

HAC 7th character A see Appendix B for HAC conditional logic

CC +7th **T84.613** **Infection and inflammatory reaction due to internal fixation device of left radius**

HAC 7th character A see Appendix B for HAC conditional logic

CC +7th **T84.614** **Infection and inflammatory reaction due to internal fixation device of right ulna**

HAC 7th character A see Appendix B for HAC conditional logic

CC +7th **T84.615** **Infection and inflammatory reaction due to internal fixation device of left ulna**

HAC 7th character A see Appendix B for HAC conditional logic

CC +7th **T84.619** **Infection and inflammatory reaction due to internal fixation device of unspecified bone of arm**

HAC 7th character A see Appendix B for HAC conditional logic

+ **T84.62** **Infection and inflammatory reaction due to internal fixation device of leg**

CC +7th **T84.620** **Infection and inflammatory reaction due to internal fixation device of right femur**

CC +7th **T84.621** **Infection and inflammatory reaction due to internal fixation device of left femur**

CC +7th **T84.622** **Infection and inflammatory reaction due to internal fixation device of right tibia**

CC +7th **T84.623** **Infection and inflammatory reaction due to internal fixation device of left tibia**

CC +7th **T84.624** **Infection and inflammatory reaction due to internal fixation device of right fibula**

CC +7th **T84.625** **Infection and inflammatory reaction due to internal fixation device of left fibula**

CC +7th **T84.629** **Infection and inflammatory reaction due to internal fixation device of unspecified bone of leg**

+, +7th, X + 7th   ● Newborn   ● Pediatric   ● Maternity   ● Adult   ♀ Female   ♂ Male   Manifestation   Unacceptable PDX   HCC   CC   MCC   HAC

CC X+7th **T84.63** **Infection and inflammatory reaction due to internal fixation device of spine**

> HAC 7th character A see Appendix B for HAC conditional logic

CC X+7th **T84.69** **Infection and inflammatory reaction due to internal fixation device of other site**

> HAC 7th character A see Appendix B for HAC conditional logic

CC X+7th **T84.7** **Infection and inflammatory reaction due to other internal orthopedic prosthetic devices, implants and grafts**

> Use additional code to identify infection
>
> HAC 7th character A see Appendix B for HAC conditional logic

+ **T84.8** **Other specified complications of internal orthopedic prosthetic devices, implants and grafts**

CC X+7th **T84.81** **Embolism due to internal orthopedic prosthetic devices, implants and grafts**

CC X+7th **T84.82** **Fibrosis due to internal orthopedic prosthetic devices, implants and grafts**

CC X+7th **T84.83** **Hemorrhage due to internal orthopedic prosthetic devices, implants and grafts**

CC X+7th **T84.84** **Pain due to internal orthopedic prosthetic devices, implants and grafts**

CC X+7th **T84.85** **Stenosis due to internal orthopedic prosthetic devices, implants and grafts**

CC X+7th **T84.86** **Thrombosis due to internal orthopedic prosthetic devices, implants and grafts**

CC X+7th **T84.89** **Other specified complication of internal orthopedic prosthetic devices, implants and grafts**

CC X+7th **T84.9** **Unspecified complication of internal orthopedic prosthetic device, implant and graft**

T85 **Complications of other internal prosthetic devices, implants and grafts**

> *Excludes2:* *failure and rejection of transplanted organs and tissue (T86.-)*
>
> *AHA CC: 4Q, 2016, 71-72*

> The appropriate 7th character is to be added to each code from category T85
> A   initial encounter
> D   subsequent encounter
> S   sequela

+ **T85.0** **Mechanical complication of ventricular intracranial (communicating) shunt**

CC X+7th **T85.01** **Breakdown (mechanical) of ventricular intracranial (communicating) shunt**

CC X+7th **T85.02** **Displacement of ventricular intracranial (communicating) shunt**

> Malposition of ventricular intracranial (communicating) shunt

CC X+7th **T85.03** **Leakage of ventricular intracranial (communicating) shunt**

CC X+7th **T85.09** **Other mechanical complication of ventricular intracranial (communicating) shunt**

> Obstruction (mechanical) of ventricular intracranial (communicating) shunt
> Perforation of ventricular intracranial (communicating) shunt
> Protrusion of ventricular intracranial (communicating) shunt

+ **T85.1** **Mechanical complication of implanted electronic stimulator of nervous system**

+ **T85.11** **Breakdown (mechanical) of implanted electronic stimulator of nervous system**

CC +7th **T85.110** **Breakdown (mechanical) of implanted electronic neurostimulator of brain electrode (lead)**

CC +7th **T85.111** **Breakdown (mechanical) of implanted electronic neurostimulator of peripheral nerve electrode (lead)**

> Breakdown of electrode (lead) for cranial nerve neurostimulators
> Breakdown of electrode (lead) for gastric neurostimulators
> Breakdown of electrode (lead) for sacral nerve neurostimulators
> Breakdown of electrode (lead) for vagal nerve neurostimulators

CC +7th **T85.112** **Breakdown (mechanical) of implanted electronic neurostimulator of spinal cord electrode (lead)**

CC +7th **T85.113** **Breakdown (mechanical) of implanted electronic neurostimulator, generator**

> Breakdown (mechanical) of implanted electronic neurostimulator generator, brain, peripheral, gastric, spinal
> Breakdown (mechanical) of implanted electronic sacral neurostimulator, pulse generator receiver

CC +7th **T85.118** **Breakdown (mechanical) of other implanted electronic stimulator of nervous system**

+ **T85.12** **Displacement of implanted electronic stimulator of nervous system**

> Malposition of implanted electronic stimulator of nervous system

CC +7th **T85.120** **Displacement of implanted electronic neurostimulator of brain electrode (lead)**

CC +7th **T85.121** **Displacement of implanted electronic neurostimulator of peripheral nerve electrode (lead)**

> Displacement of electrode (lead) for cranial nerve neurostimulators
> Displacement of electrode (lead) for gastric neurostimulators
> Displacement of electrode (lead) for sacral nerve neurostimulators
> Displacement of electrode (lead) for vagal nerve neurostimulators

CC +7th **T85.122** **Displacement of implanted electronic neurostimulator of spinal cord electrode (lead)**

CC +7th **T85.123** **Displacement of implanted electronic neurostimulator, generator**

> Displacement of implanted electronic neurostimulator generator, brain, peripheral, gastric, spinal
> Displacement of implanted electronic sacral neurostimulator, pulse generator receiver

CC +7th **T85.128** **Displacement of other implanted electronic stimulator of nervous system**

+ **T85.19** **Other mechanical complication of implanted electronic stimulator of nervous system**

> Leakage of implanted electronic stimulator of nervous system
> Obstruction (mechanical) of implanted electronic stimulator of nervous system
> Perforation of implanted electronic stimulator of nervous system
> Protrusion of implanted electronic stimulator of nervous system

CC +7th **T85.190** **Other mechanical complication of implanted electronic neurostimulator of brain electrode (lead)**

CC +7th **T85.191** **Other mechanical complication of implanted electronic neurostimulator of peripheral nerve electrode (lead)**

> Other mechanical complication of electrode (lead) for cranial nerve neurostimulators
> Other mechanical complication of electrode (lead) for gastric neurostimulators
> Other mechanical complication of electrode (lead) for sacral nerve neurostimulators
> Other mechanical complication of electrode (lead) for vagal nerve neurostimulators

CC +7th **T85.192** **Other mechanical complication of implanted electronic neurostimulator of spinal cord electrode (lead)**

CC +7th **T85.193** **Other mechanical complication of implanted electronic neurostimulator, generator**

Other mechanical complication of implanted electronic neurostimulator generator, brain, peripheral, gastric, spinal

Other mechanical complication of implanted electronic sacral neurostimulator, pulse generator receiver

CC +7th **T85.199** **Other mechanical complication of other implanted electronic stimulator of nervous system**

+ **T85.2** **Mechanical complication of intraocular lens**

CC X+7th **T85.21** **Breakdown (mechanical) of intraocular lens**

CC X+7th **T85.22** **Displacement of intraocular lens**

Malposition of intraocular lens

CC X+7th **T85.29** **Other mechanical complication of intraocular lens**

Obstruction (mechanical) of intraocular lens

Perforation of intraocular lens

Protrusion of intraocular lens

+ **T85.3** **Mechanical complication of other ocular prosthetic devices, implants and grafts**

Excludes2: other complications of corneal graft (T86.84-)

+ **T85.31** **Breakdown (mechanical) of other ocular prosthetic devices, implants and grafts**

CC +7th **T85.310** **Breakdown (mechanical) of prosthetic orbit of right eye**

CC +7th **T85.311** **Breakdown (mechanical) of prosthetic orbit of left eye**

+7th **T85.318** **Breakdown (mechanical) of other ocular prosthetic devices, implants and grafts**

+ **T85.32** **Displacement of other ocular prosthetic devices, implants and grafts**

Malposition of other ocular prosthetic devices, implants and grafts

CC +7th **T85.320** **Displacement of prosthetic orbit of right eye**

CC +7th **T85.321** **Displacement of prosthetic orbit of left eye**

+7th **T85.328** **Displacement of other ocular prosthetic devices, implants and grafts**

+ **T85.39** **Other mechanical complication of other ocular prosthetic devices, implants and grafts**

Obstruction (mechanical) of other ocular prosthetic devices, implants and grafts

Perforation of other ocular prosthetic devices, implants and grafts

Protrusion of other ocular prosthetic devices, implants and grafts

CC +7th **T85.390** **Other mechanical complication of prosthetic orbit of right eye**

CC +7th **T85.391** **Other mechanical complication of prosthetic orbit of left eye**

+7th **T85.398** **Other mechanical complication of other ocular prosthetic devices, implants and grafts**

+ **T85.4** **Mechanical complication of breast prosthesis and implant**

CC X+7th **T85.41** **Breakdown (mechanical) of breast prosthesis and implant**

CC X+7th **T85.42** **Displacement of breast prosthesis and implant**

Malposition of breast prosthesis and implant

CC X+7th **T85.43** **Leakage of breast prosthesis and implant**

CC X+7th **T85.44** **Capsular contracture of breast implant**

CC X+7th **T85.49** **Other mechanical complication of breast prosthesis and implant**

Obstruction (mechanical) of breast prosthesis and implant

Perforation of breast prosthesis and implant

Protrusion of breast prosthesis and implant

+ **T85.5** **Mechanical complication of gastrointestinal prosthetic devices, implants and grafts**

+ **T85.51** **Breakdown (mechanical) of gastrointestinal prosthetic devices, implants and grafts**

CC +7th **T85.510** **Breakdown (mechanical) of bile duct prosthesis**

CC +7th **T85.511** **Breakdown (mechanical) of esophageal anti-reflux device**

CC +7th **T85.518** **Breakdown (mechanical) of other gastrointestinal prosthetic devices, implants and grafts**

+ **T85.52** **Displacement of gastrointestinal prosthetic devices, implants and grafts**

Malposition of gastrointestinal prosthetic devices, implants and grafts

CC +7th **T85.520** **Displacement of bile duct prosthesis**

CC +7th **T85.521** **Displacement of esophageal anti-reflux device**

CC +7th **T85.528** **Displacement of other gastrointestinal prosthetic devices, implants and grafts**

+ **T85.59** **Other mechanical complication of gastrointestinal prosthetic devices, implants and**

Obstruction, mechanical of gastrointestinal prosthetic devices, implants and grafts

Perforation of gastrointestinal prosthetic devices, implants and grafts

Protrusion of gastrointestinal prosthetic devices, implants and grafts

CC +7th **T85.590** **Other mechanical complication of bile duct prosthesis**

CC +7th **T85.591** **Other mechanical complication of esophageal anti-reflux device**

CC +7th **T85.598** **Other mechanical complication of other gastrointestinal prosthetic devices, implants and grafts**

+ **T85.6** **Mechanical complication of other specified internal and external prosthetic devices, implants and grafts**

Review coding guidelines C.4.a.5.a and C.4.a.5.b

+ **T85.61** **Breakdown (mechanical) of other specified internal prosthetic devices, implants and grafts**

CC +7th **T85.610** **Breakdown (mechanical) of cranial or spinal infusion catheter**

Breakdown (mechanical) of epidural infusion catheter

Breakdown (mechanical) of intrathecal infusion catheter

Breakdown (mechanical) of subarachnoid infusion catheter

Breakdown (mechanical) of subdural infusion catheter

CC +7th **T85.611** **Breakdown (mechanical) of intraperitoneal dialysis catheter**

Excludes1: mechanical complication of vascular dialysis catheter (T82.4-)

CC +7th **T85.612** **Breakdown (mechanical) of permanent sutures**

Excludes1: mechanical complication of permanent (wire) suture used in bone repair (T84.1-T84.2)

CC +7th **T85.613** **Breakdown (mechanical) of artificial skin graft and decellularized allodermis**

Failure of artificial skin graft and decellularized allodermis

Non-adherence of artificial skin graft and decellularized allodermis

Poor incorporation of artificial skin graft and decellularized allodermis

Shearing of artificial skin graft and decellularized allodermis

CC +7th **T85.614** **Breakdown (mechanical) of insulin pump**

CC +7th **T85.615** **Breakdown (mechanical) of other nervous system device, implant or graft**

Breakdown (mechanical) of intrathecal infusion pump

CC +7th **T85.618** **Breakdown (mechanical) of other specified internal prosthetic devices, implants and grafts**

+ T85.62 **Displacement of other specified internal prosthetic devices, implants and grafts**
Malposition of other specified internal prosthetic devices, implants and grafts

CC +7th T85.620 **Displacement of cranial or spinal infusion catheter**
Displacement of epidural infusion catheter
Displacement of intrathecal infusion catheter
Displacement of subarachnoid infusion catheter
Displacement of subdural infusion catheter

CC +7th T85.621 **Displacement of intraperitoneal dialysis catheter**
Excludes1: *mechanical complication of vascular dialysis catheter (T82.4-)*

CC +7th T85.622 **Displacement of permanent sutures**
Excludes1: *mechanical complication of permanent (wire) suture used in bone repair (T84.1-T84.2)*

CC +7th T85.623 **Displacement of artificial skin graft and decellularized allodermis**
Dislodgement of artificial skin graft and decellularized allodermis

CC +7th T85.624 **Displacement of insulin pump**

CC +7th T85.625 **Displacement of other nervous system device, implant or graft**
Displacement of intrathecal infusion pump

CC +7th T85.628 **Displacement of other specified internal prosthetic devices, implants and grafts**
AHA CC: 1Q, 2015, 3-21

+ T85.63 **Leakage of other specified internal prosthetic devices, implants and grafts**

CC +7th T85.630 **Leakage of cranial or spinal infusion catheter**
Leakage of epidural infusion catheter
Leakage of intrathecal infusion catheter
Leakage of subarachnoid infusion catheter
Leakage of subdural infusion catheter

CC +7th T85.631 **Leakage of intraperitoneal dialysis catheter**
Excludes1: *mechanical complication of vascular dialysis catheter (T82.4)*

CC +7th T85.633 **Leakage of insulin pump**

CC +7th T85.635 **Leakage of other nervous system device, implant or graft**
Leakage of intrathecal infusion pump

CC +7th T85.638 **Leakage of other specified internal prosthetic devices, implants and grafts**

+ T85.69 **Other mechanical complication of other specified internal prosthetic devices, implants and grafts**
Obstruction, mechanical of other specified internal prosthetic devices, implants and grafts
Perforation of other specified internal prosthetic devices, implants and grafts
Protrusion of other specified internal prosthetic devices, implants and grafts

CC +7th T85.690 **Other mechanical complication of cranial or spinal infusion catheter**
Other mechanical complication of epidural infusion catheter
Other mechanical complication of intrathecal infusion catheter
Other mechanical complication of subarachnoid infusion catheter
Other mechanical complication of subdural infusion catheter

CC +7th T85.691 **Other mechanical complication of intraperitoneal dialysis catheter**
Excludes1: *mechanical complication of vascular dialysis catheter (T82.4)*

CC +7th T85.692 **Other mechanical complication of permanent sutures**
Excludes1: *mechanical complication of permanent (wire) suture used in bone repair (T84.1-T84.2)*

CC +7th T85.693 **Other mechanical complication of artificial skin graft and decellularized allodermis**

CC +7th T85.694 **Other mechanical complication of insulin pump**

CC +7th T85.695 **Other mechanical complication of other nervous system device, implant or graft**
Other mechanical complication of intrathecal infusion pump

CC +7th T85.698 **Other mechanical complication of other specified internal prosthetic devices, implants and grafts**
Mechanical complication of nonabsorbable surgical material NOS

+ T85.7 **Infection and inflammatory reaction due to other internal prosthetic devices, implants and grafts**
Use additional code to identify infection

CC X+7th T85.71 **Infection and inflammatory reaction due to peritoneal dialysis catheter**

CC X+7th T85.72 **Infection and inflammatory reaction due to insulin pump**

+ T85.73 **Infection and inflammatory reaction due to nervous system devices, implants and graft**

CC +7th T85.730 **Infection and inflammatory reaction due to ventricular intracranial (communicating) shunt**

CC +7th T85.731 **Infection and inflammatory reaction due to implanted electronic neurostimulator of brain, electrode (lead)**

CC +7th T85.732 **Infection and inflammatory reaction due to implanted electronic neurostimulator of peripheral nerve, electrode (lead)**
Infection and inflammatory reaction due to electrode (lead) for cranial nerve neurostimulators
Infection and inflammatory reaction due to electrode (lead) for gastric neurostimulators
Infection and inflammatory reaction due to electrode (lead) for sacral nerve neurostimulators
Infection and inflammatory reaction due to electrode (lead) for vagal nerve neurostimulators

CC +7th T85.733 **Infection and inflammatory reaction due to implanted electronic neurostimulator of spinal cord, electrode (lead)**

CC +7th T85.734 **Infection and inflammatory reaction due to implanted electronic neurostimulator, generator**
Generator pocket infection

CC +7th T85.735 **Infection and inflammatory reaction due to cranial or spinal infusion catheter**
Infection and inflammatory reaction due to epidural catheter
Infection and inflammatory reaction due to intrathecal infsuion catheter
Infection and inflammatory reaction due to subarachnoid catheter
Infection and inflammatory reaction due to subdural catheter

CC +7th T85.738 **Infection and inflammatory reaction due to other nervous system device, implant or graft**
Infection and inflammatory reaction due to intrathecal infusion pump

CC X+7th T85.79 **Infection and inflammatory reaction due to other internal prosthetic devices, implants and grafts**

+ **T85.8** **Other specified complications of internal prosthetic devices, implants and grafts, not elsewhere classified**
   + **T85.81** **Embolism due to internal prosthetic devices, implants and grafts, not elsewhere classified**
     CC +7th **T85.810** **Embolism due to nervous system prosthetic devices, implants and grafts**
     +7th **T85.818** **Embolism due to other internal prosthetic devices, implants and grafts**
   + **T85.82** **Fibrosis due to internal prosthetic devices, implants and grafts, not elsewhere classified**
     CC +7th **T85.820** **Fibrosis due to nervous system prosthetic devices, implants and grafts**
     +7th **T85.828** **Fibrosis due to other internal prosthetic devices, implants and grafts**
   + **T85.83** **Hemorrhage due to internal prosthetic devices, implants and grafts, not elsewhere classified**
     CC +7th **T85.830** **Hemorrhage due to nervous system prosthetic devices, implants and grafts**
     +7th **T85.838** **Hemorrhage due to other internal prosthetic devices, implants and grafts**
   + **T85.84** **Pain due to internal prosthetic devices, implants and grafts, not elsewhere classified**
     CC +7th **T85.840** **Pain due to nervous system prosthetic devices, implants and grafts**
     +7th **T85.848** **Pain due to other internal prosthetic devices, implants and grafts**
   + **T85.85** **Stenosis due to internal prosthetic devices, implants and grafts, not elsewhere classified**
     CC +7th **T85.850** **Stenosis due to nervous system prosthetic devices, implants and grafts**
     +7th **T85.858** **Stenosis due to other internal prosthetic devices, implants and grafts**
   + **T85.86** **Thrombosis due to internal prosthetic devices, implants and grafts, not elsewhere classified**
     CC +7th **T85.860** **Thrombosis due to nervous system prosthetic devices, implants and grafts**
     +7th **T85.868** **Thrombosis due to other internal prosthetic devices, implants and grafts**
   + **T85.89** **Other specified complication of internal prosthetic devices, implants and grafts, not elsewhere classified**
     Erosion or breakdown of subcutaneous device pocket
     CC +7th **T85.890** **Other specified complication of nervous system prosthetic devices, implants and grafts**
     +7th **T85.898** **Other specified complication of other internal prosthetic devices, implants and grafts**
X+7th **T85.9** **Unspecified complication of internal prosthetic device, implant and graft**
   Complication of internal prosthetic device, implant and graft NOS

T86 **Complications of transplanted organs and tissue**
   Use additional code to identify other transplant complications, such as:
   graft-versus-host disease (D89.81-)
   malignancy associated with organ transplant (C80.2)
   post-transplant lymphoproliferative disorders (PTLD) (D47.Z1)
   Review coding guideline C.2.r
   Review coding guideline C.19.g.3
+ **T86.0** **Complications of bone marrow transplant**
   CC **T86.00** **Unspecified complication of bone marrow transplant**
   CC **T86.01** **Bone marrow transplant rejection**
   CC **T86.02** **Bone marrow transplant failure**
   CC **T86.03** **Bone marrow transplant infection**
   CC **T86.09** **Other complications of bone marrow transplant**
+ **T86.1** **Complications of kidney transplant**
   Review coding guideline C.19.g.3.b
   CC **T86.10** **Unspecified complication of kidney transplant**
   CC **T86.11** **Kidney transplant rejection**
   CC **T86.12** **Kidney transplant failure**
     AHA CC: 1Q, 2014, 24
   CC **T86.13** **Kidney transplant infection**
     Use additional code to specify infection
   CC **T86.19** **Other complication of kidney transplant**
     AHA CC: 2Q, 2019, 7

+ **T86.2** **Complications of heart transplant**
   Excludes1: *complication of:*
     artificial heart device (T82.5)
     heart-lung transplant (T86.3)
   CC **T86.20** **Unspecified complication of heart transplant**
   CC **T86.21** **Heart transplant rejection**
   CC **T86.22** **Heart transplant failure**
   CC **T86.23** **Heart transplant infection**
     Use additional code to specify infection
   + **T86.29** **Other complications of heart transplant**
     CC **T86.290** **Cardiac allograft vasculopathy**
      Excludes1: *atherosclerosis of coronary arteries(I25.75-,I25.76-, I25.81-)*
     CC **T86.298** **Other complications of heart transplant**
+ **T86.3** **Complications of heart-lung transplant**
   CC **T86.30** **Unspecified complication of heart-lung transplant**
   CC **T86.31** **Heart-lung transplant rejection**
   CC **T86.32** **Heart-lung transplant failure**
   CC **T86.33** **Heart-lung transplant infection**
     Use additional code to specify infection
   CC **T86.39** **Other complications of heart-lung transplant**
+ **T86.4** **Complications of liver transplant**
   CC **T86.40** **Unspecified complication of liver transplant**
   CC **T86.41** **Liver transplant rejection**
   CC **T86.42** **Liver transplant failure**
   CC **T86.43** **Liver transplant infection**
     Use additional code to identify infection, such as:
     Cytomegalovirus (CMV) infection (B25.-)
   CC **T86.49** **Other complications of liver transplant**
CC **T86.5** **Complications of stem cell transplant**
   Complications from stem cells from peripheral blood
   Complications from stem cells from umbilical cord
+ **T86.8** **Complications of other transplanted organs and tissues**
   + **T86.81** **Complications of lung transplant**
     Excludes1: *complication of heart-lung transplant (T86.3-)*
     CC **T86.810** **Lung transplant rejection**
     CC **T86.811** **Lung transplant failure**
     CC **T86.812** **Lung transplant infection**
      Use additional code to specify infection
     CC **T86.818** **Other complications of lung transplant**
      AHA CC: 2Q, 2019, 6-7
     CC **T86.819** **Unspecified complication of lung transplant**
   + **T86.82** **Complications of skin graft (allograft) (autograft)**
     Excludes2: *complication of artificial skin graft (T85.693)*
     CC **T86.820** **Skin graft (allograft) rejection**
     CC **T86.821** **Skin graft (allograft) (autograft) failure**
     CC **T86.822** **Skin graft (allograft) (autograft) infection**
      Use additional code to specify infection
     CC **T86.828** **Other complications of skin graft (allograft) (autograft)**
     CC **T86.829** **Unspecified complication of skin graft (allograft) (autograft)**
   + **T86.83** **Complications of bone graft**
     Excludes2: *mechanical complications of bone graft (T84.3-)*
     CC **T86.830** **Bone graft rejection**
     CC **T86.831** **Bone graft failure**
     CC **T86.832** **Bone graft infection**
      Use additional code to specify infection
     CC **T86.838** **Other complications of bone graft**
     CC **T86.839** **Unspecified complication of bone graft**
   + **T86.84** **Complications of corneal transplant**
     Excludes2: *mechanical complications of corneal graft (T85.3-)*
     + **T86.840** **Corneal transplant rejection**
      CC **T86.8401** **Corneal transplant rejection, right eye**
      CC **T86.8402** **Corneal transplant rejection, left eye**
      CC **T86.8403** **Corneal transplant rejection, bilateral**
      CC **T86.8409** **Corneal transplant rejection, unspecified eye**

+ **T86.841 Corneal transplant failure**
  CC **T86.8411 Corneal transplant failure, right eye**
  CC **T86.8412 Corneal transplant failure, left eye**
  CC **T86.8413 Corneal transplant failure, bilateral**
  CC **T86.8419 Corneal transplant failure, unspecified eye**

+ **T86.842 Corneal transplant infection**
  CC **T86.8421 Corneal transplant infection, right eye**
  CC **T86.8422 Corneal transplant infection, left eye**
  CC **T86.8423 Corneal transplant infection, bilateral**
  CC **T86.8429 Corneal transplant infection, unspecified eye**
    Use additional code to specify infection

+ **T86.848 Other complications of corneal transplant**
  CC **T86.8481 Other complications of corneal transplant, right eye**
  CC **T86.8482 Other complications of corneal transplant, left eye**
  CC **T86.8483 Other complications of corneal transplant, bilateral**
  CC **T86.8489 Other complications of corneal transplant, unspecified eye**

+ **T86.849 Unspecified complication of corneal transplant**
  CC **T86.8491 Unspecified complication of corneal transplant, right eye**
  CC **T86.8492 Unspecified complication of corneal transplant, left eye**
  CC **T86.8493 Unspecified complication of corneal transplant, bilateral**
  CC **T86.8499 Unspecified complication of corneal transplant, unspecified eye**

+ **T86.85 Complication of intestine transplant**
  CC **T86.850 Intestine transplant rejection**
  CC **T86.851 Intestine transplant failure**
  CC **T86.852 Intestine transplant infection**
    Use additional code to specify infection
  CC **T86.858 Other complications of intestine transplant**
  CC **T86.859 Unspecified complication of intestine transplant**

+ **T86.89 Complications of other transplanted tissue**
  Transplant failure or rejection of pancreas
  CC **T86.890 Other transplanted tissue rejection**
  CC **T86.891 Other transplanted tissue failure**
  CC **T86.892 Other transplanted tissue infection**
    Use additional code to specify infection
  CC **T86.898 Other complications of other transplanted tissue**
  CC **T86.899 Unspecified complication of other transplanted tissue**

+ **T86.9 Complication of unspecified transplanted organ and tissue**
  CC **T86.90 Unspecified complication of unspecified transplanted organ and tissue**
  CC **T86.91 Unspecified transplanted organ and tissue rejection**
  CC **T86.92 Unspecified transplanted organ and tissue failure**
  CC **T86.93 Unspecified transplanted organ and tissue infection**
    Use additional code to specify infection
  CC **T86.99 Other complications of unspecified transplanted organ and tissue**

T87 Complications peculiar to reattachment and amputation

+ **T87.0 Complications of reattached (part of) upper extremity**
  + **T87.0X Complications of reattached (part of) upper extremity**
  CC **T87.0X1 Complications of reattached (part of) right upper extremity**
  CC **T87.0X2 Complications of reattached (part of) left upper extremity**
  CC **T87.0X9 Complications of reattached (part of) unspecified upper extremity**

+ **T87.1 Complications of reattached (part of) lower extremity**
  + **T87.1X Complications of reattached (part of) lower extremity**
  CC **T87.1X1 Complications of reattached (part of) right lower extremity**
  CC **T87.1X2 Complications of reattached (part of) left lower extremity**
  CC **T87.1X9 Complications of reattached (part of) unspecified lower extremity**

CC **T87.2 Complications of other reattached body part**

+ **T87.3 Neuroma of amputation stump**
  T87.30 Neuroma of amputation stump, unspecified extremity
  T87.31 Neuroma of amputation stump, right upper extremity
  T87.32 Neuroma of amputation stump, left upper extremity
  T87.33 Neuroma of amputation stump, right lower extremity
  T87.34 Neuroma of amputation stump, left lower extremity

+ **T87.4 Infection of amputation stump**
  CC **T87.40 Infection of amputation stump, unspecified extremity**
  CC **T87.41 Infection of amputation stump, right upper extremity**
  CC **T87.42 Infection of amputation stump, left upper extremity**
  CC **T87.43 Infection of amputation stump, right lower extremity**
  CC **T87.44 Infection of amputation stump, left lower extremity**

+ **T87.5 Necrosis of amputation stump**
  T87.50 Necrosis of amputation stump, unspecified extremity
  T87.51 Necrosis of amputation stump, right upper extremity
  T87.52 Necrosis of amputation stump, left upper extremity
  T87.53 Necrosis of amputation stump, right lower extremity
  T87.54 Necrosis of amputation stump, left lower extremity

+ **T87.8 Other complications of amputation stump**
  T87.81 Dehiscence of amputation stump
  T87.89 Other complications of amputation stump
    Amputation stump contracture
    Amputation stump contracture of next proximal joint
    Amputation stump flexion
    Amputation stump edema
    Amputation stump hematoma
    Excludes2: phantom limb syndrome (G54.6-G54.7)

T87.9 Unspecified complications of amputation stump

T88 **Other complications of surgical and medical care, not elsewhere classified**

Excludes2: *complication following infusion, transfusion and*
therapeutic injection (T80.-)
complication following procedure NEC (T81.-)
complications of anesthesia in labor and
delivery (O74.-)
complications of anesthesia in pregnancy (O29.-)
complications of anesthesia in puerperium (O89.-)
complications of devices, implants and grafts (T82-T85)
complications of obstetric surgery and procedure
(O75.4)
dermatitis due to drugs and medicaments (L23.3, L24.4,
L25.1, L27.0-L27.1)
poisoning and toxic effects of drugs and chemicals
(T36-T65 with fifth or sixth character 1-4 or 6)
specified complications classified elsewhere

AHA CC: 4Q, 2018, 89-90

The appropriate 7th character is to be added to each code from category T88
A   initial encounter
D   subsequent encounter
S   sequela

CC X+7th T88.0 **Infection following immunization**
Sepsis following immunization
Review coding guideline C.1.d.5

CC X+7th T88.1 **Other complications following immunization, not elsewhere classified**
Generalized vaccinia
Rash following immunization
Excludes1: *vaccinia not from vaccine (B08.011)*
Excludes2: *anaphylactic shock due to serum (T80.5-)*
other serum reactions (T80.6-)
postimmunization arthropathy (M02.2)
postimmunization encephalitis (G04.02)
postimmunization fever (R50.83)

CC X+7th T88.2 **Shock due to anesthesia**
Use additional code for adverse effect, if applicable,
to identify drug (T41.- with fifth or sixth character 5)
Excludes1: *complications of anesthesia (in):*
labor and delivery (O74.-)
pregnancy (O29.-)
puerperium (O89.-)
postprocedural shock NOS (T81.1-)

CC X+7th T88.3 **Malignant hyperthermia due to anesthesia**
Use additional code for adverse effect, if applicable, to
identify drug (T41.- with fifth or sixth character 5)

X+7th T88.4 **Failed or difficult intubation**

+ T88.5 **Other complications of anesthesia**
Use additional code for adverse effect, if applicable, to
identify drug (T41.- with fifth or sixth character 5)
AHA CC: 4Q, 2016, 72-73

X+7th T88.51 **Hypothermia following anesthesia**

X+7th T88.52 **Failed moderate sedation during procedure**
Failed conscious sedation during procedure
Excludes2: *personal history of failed moderate*
sedation (Z92.83)

X+7th T88.53 **Unintended awareness under general anesthesia during procedure**
Excludes2: *personal history of unintended awareness*
under general anesthesia (Z92.84)
AHA CC: 4Q, 2016, 72-73

X+7th T88.59 **Other complications of anesthesia**

CC X+7th T88.6 **Anaphylactic reaction due to adverse effect of correct drug or medicament properly administered**
Anaphylactic shock due to adverse effect of correct drug or
medicament properly administered
Anaphylactoid reaction NOS
Use additional code for adverse effect, if applicable, to
identify drug (T36-T50 with fifth or sixth character 5)
Excludes1: *anaphylactic reaction due to serum (T80.5-)*
anaphylactic shock or reaction due to adverse
food reaction (T78.0-)
AHA CC: 1Q, 2020, 18-19

X+7th T88.7 **Unspecified adverse effect of drug or medicament**
Drug hypersensitivity NOS
Drug reaction NOS
Use additional code for adverse effect, if applicable, to
identify drug (T36-T50 with fifth or sixth character 5)
Excludes1: *specified adverse effects of drugs*
and medicaments (A00-R94 and
T80-T88.6, T88.8)

X+7th T88.8 **Other specified complications of surgical and medical care, not elsewhere classified**
Use additional code to identify the complication

X+7th T88.9 **Complication of surgical and medical care, unspecified**

+, +7th, X + 7th   ● Newborn   ● Pediatric   ● Maternity   ● Adult   ♀ Female   ♂ Male   Manifestation   Unacceptable PDX   HCC   CC   MCC   HAC

Chapter 20: External Causes of Morbidity (V00–Y99)

NOTE This chapter permits the classification of environmental events and circumstances as the cause of injury, and other adverse effects. Where a code from this section is applicable, it is intended that it shall be used secondary to a code from another chapter of the Classification indicating the nature of the condition. Most often, the condition will be classifiable to Chapter 19, Injury, poisoning and certain other consequences of external causes (S00-T88). Other conditions that may be stated to be due to external causes are classified in Chapters 1 to 18. For these conditions, codes from Chapter 20 should be used to provide additional information as to the cause of the condition.

AHA CC: 1Q, 2015, 3-21

This chapter contains the following category blocks:

V00-X58	Accidents
V00-V99	Transport accidents
V00-V09	Pedestrian injured in transport accident
V10-V19	Pedal cycle rider injured in transport accident
V20-V29	Motorcycle rider injured in transport accident
V30-V39	Occupant of three-wheeled motor vehicle injured in transport accident
V40-V49	Car occupant injured in transport accident
V50-V59	Occupant of pick-up truck or van injured in transport accident
V60-V69	Occupant of heavy transport vehicle injured in transport accident
V70-V79	Bus occupant injured in transport accident
V80-V89	Other land transport accidents
V90-V94	Water transport accidents
V95-V97	Air and space transport accidents
V98-V99	Other and unspecified transport accidents
W00-X58	Other external causes of accidental injury
W00-W19	Slipping, tripping, stumbling and falls
W20-W49	Exposure to inanimate mechanical forces
W50-W64	Exposure to animate mechanical forces
W65-W74	Accidental non-transport drowning and submersion
W85-W99	Exposure to electric current, radiation and extreme ambient air temperature and pressure
X00-X08	Exposure to smoke, fire and flames
X10-X19	Contact with heat and hot substances
X30-X39	Exposure to forces of nature
X50	Overexertion and strenuous or repetitive movements
X52-X58	Accidental exposure to other specified factors
X71-X83	Intentional self-harm
X92-Y09	Assault
Y21-Y33	Event of undetermined intent
Y35-Y38	Legal intervention, operations of war, military operations, and terrorism
Y62-Y84	Complications of medical and surgical care
Y62-Y69	Misadventures to patients during surgical and medical care
Y70-Y82	Medical devices associated with adverse incidents in diagnostic and therapeutic use
Y83-Y84	Surgical and other medical procedures as the cause of abnormal reaction of the patient, or of later complication, without mention of misadventure at the time of the procedure
Y90-Y99	Supplementary factors related to causes of morbidity classified elsewhere

C. Chapter-Specific Coding Guidelines

In addition to general coding guidelines, there are guidelines for specific diagnoses and/or conditions in the classification. Unless otherwise indicated, these guidelines apply to all health care settings. Please refer to Section II for guidelines on the selection of principal diagnosis.

20. Chapter 20: External Causes of Morbidity (V00-Y99)

The external causes of morbidity codes should never be sequenced as the first-listed or principal diagnosis.

External cause codes are intended to provide data for injury research and evaluation of injury prevention strategies. These codes capture how the injury or health condition happened (cause), the intent (unintentional or accidental; or intentional, such as suicide or assault), the place where the event occurred the activity of the patient at the time of the event, and the person's status (e.g., civilian, military).

There is no national requirement for mandatory ICD-10-CM external cause code reporting. Unless a provider is subject to a state-based external cause code reporting mandate or these codes are required by a particular payer, reporting of ICD-10-CM codes in Chapter 20, External Causes of Morbidity, is not required. In the absence of a mandatory reporting requirement, providers are encouraged to voluntarily report external cause codes, as they provide valuable data for injury research and evaluation of injury prevention strategies.

a. General External Cause Coding Guidelines

1) Used with any code in the range of A00.0-T88.9, Z00-Z99

An external cause code may be used with any code in the range of A00.0-T88.9, Z00-Z99, classification that represents a health condition due to an external cause. Though they are most applicable to injuries, they are also valid for use with such things as infections or diseases due to an external source, and other health conditions, such as a heart attack that occurs during strenuous physical activity.

2) External cause code used for length of treatment

Assign the external cause code, with the appropriate 7th character (initial encounter, subsequent encounter or sequela) for each encounter for which the injury or condition is being treated.

Most categories in chapter 20 have a 7th character requirement for each applicable code. Most categories in this chapter have three 7th character values: A, initial encounter, D, subsequent encounter and S, sequela. While the patient may be seen by a new or different provider over the course of treatment for an injury or condition, assignment of the 7th character for external cause should match the 7th character of the code assigned for the associated injury or condition for the encounter.

3) Use the full range of external cause codes

Use the full range of external cause codes to completely describe the cause, the intent, the place of occurrence, and if applicable, the activity of the patient at the time of the event, and the patient's status, for all injuries, and other health conditions due to an external cause.

4) Assign as many external cause codes as necessary

Assign as many external cause codes as necessary to fully explain each cause. If only one external code can be recorded, assign the code most related to the principal diagnosis.

5) The selection of the appropriate external cause code

The selection of the appropriate external cause code is guided by the Alphabetic Index of External Causes and by Inclusion and Exclusion notes in the Tabular List.

6) External cause code can never be a principal diagnosis

An external cause code can never be a principal (first-listed) diagnosis.

7) Combination external cause codes

Certain of the external cause codes are combination codes that identify sequential events that result in an injury, such as a fall which results in striking against an object. The injury may be due to either event or both. The combination external cause code used should correspond to the sequence of events regardless of which caused the most serious injury.

8) No external cause code needed in certain circumstances

No external cause code from Chapter 20 is needed if the external cause and intent are included in a code from another chapter (e.g. T36.0X1-Poisoning by penicillins, accidental (unintentional)).

b. Place of Occurrence Guideline

Codes from category Y92, Place of occurrence of the external cause, are secondary codes for use after other external cause codes to identify the location of the patient at the time of injury or other condition.

Generally, a place of occurrent code is assigned only once, at the initial encounter for treatment. However, in the rare instance that a new injury occurs during hospitalization, an additional place of occurrence code may be assigned. No 7th characters are used for Y92.

Do not use place of occurrence code Y92.9 if the place is not stated or is not applicable.

c. Activity Code

Assign a code from category Y93, Activity code, to describe the activity of the patient at the time the injury or other health condition occurred.

An activity code is used only once, at the initial encounter for treatment. Only one code from Y93 should be recorded on a medical record.

The activity codes are not applicable to poisonings, adverse effects, misadventures or sequela.

Do not assign Y93.9, Unspecified activity, if the activity is not stated.

A code from category Y93 is appropriate for use with external cause and intent codes if identifying the activity provides additional information about the event.

d. Place of Occurrence, Activity, and Status Codes Used with other External Cause Code

When applicable, place of occurrence, activity, and external cause status codes are sequenced after the main external cause code(s). Regardless of the number of external cause codes assigned, generally there should be only one place of occurrence code, one activity code, and one external cause status code assigned to an encounter. However, in the rare instance that a new injury occurs during hospitalization, an additional place of occurrence code may be assigned.

e. If the Reporting Format Limits the Number of External Cause Codes

If the reporting format limits the number of external cause codes that can be used in reporting clinical data, report the code for the cause/intent most related to the principal diagnosis. If the format permits capture of additional external cause codes, the cause/intent, including medical misadventures, of the additional events should be reported rather than the codes for place, activity, or external status.

f. Multiple External Cause Coding Guidelines

More than one external cause code is required to fully describe the external cause of an illness or injury. The assignment of external cause codes should be sequenced in the following priority:

If two or more events cause separate injuries, an external cause code should be assigned for each cause. The first-listed external cause code will be selected in the following order:

External codes for child and adult abuse take priority over all other external cause codes.

See Section I.C.19., Child and Adult abuse guidelines.

External cause codes for terrorism events take priority over all other external cause codes except child and adult abuse.

External cause codes for cataclysmic events take priority over all other external cause codes except child and adult abuse and terrorism.

External cause codes for transport accidents take priority over all other external cause codes except cataclysmic events, child and adult abuse and terrorism.

Activity and external cause status codes are assigned following all causal (intent) external cause codes.

The first-listed external cause code should correspond to the cause of the most serious diagnosis due to an assault, accident, or self-harm, following the order of hierarchy listed above.

g. Child and Adult Abuse Guideline

Adult and child abuse, neglect and maltreatment are classified as assault. Any of the assault codes may be used to indicate the external cause of any injury resulting from the confirmed abuse.

For confirmed cases of abuse, neglect and maltreatment, when the perpetrator is known, a code from Y07, Perpetrator of maltreatment and neglect, should accompany any other assault codes.

See Section I.C.19. Adult and child abuse, neglect and other maltreatment

h. Unknown or Undetermined Intent Guideline

If the intent (accident, self-harm, assault) of the cause of an injury or other condition is unknown or unspecified, code the intent as accidental intent. All transport accident categories assume accidental intent.

1) Use of undetermined intent

External cause codes for events of undetermined intent are only for use if the documentation in the record specifies that the intent cannot be determined.

i. Sequelae (Late Effects) of External Cause Guidelines

1) Sequelae external cause codes

Sequela are reported using the external cause code with the 7th character "S" for sequela. These codes should be used with any report of a late effect or sequela resulting from a previous injury.

See Section I.B.10 Sequela (Late Effects)

2) Sequela external cause code with a related current injury

A sequela external cause code should never be used with a related current nature of injury code.

3) Use of sequela external cause codes for subsequent visits

Use a late effect external cause code for subsequent visits when a late effect of the initial injury is being treated. Do not use a late effect external cause code for subsequent visits for follow- up care (e.g., to assess healing, to receive rehabilitative therapy) of the injury when no late effect of the injury has been documented.

j. Terrorism Guidelines

1) Cause of injury identified by the Federal Government (FBI) as terrorism

When the cause of an injury is identified by the Federal Government (FBI) as terrorism, the first-listed external cause code should be a code from category Y38, Terrorism. The definition of terrorism employed by the FBI is found at the inclusion note at the beginning of category Y38. Use additional code for place of occurrence (Y92.-). More than one Y38 code may be assigned if the injury is the result of more than one mechanism of terrorism.

2) Cause of an injury is suspected to be the result of terrorism

When the cause of an injury is suspected to be the result of terrorism a code from category Y38 should not be assigned. Suspected cases should be classified as assault.

3) Code Y38.9, Terrorism, secondary effects

Assign code Y38.9, Terrorism, secondary effects, for conditions occurring subsequent to the terrorist event. This code should not be assigned for conditions that are due to the initial terrorist act.

It is acceptable to assign code Y38.9 with another code from Y38 if there is an injury due to the initial terrorist event and an injury that is a subsequent result of the terrorist event.

k. External cause status

A code from category Y99, External cause status, should be assigned whenever any other external cause code is assigned for an encounter, including an Activity code, except for the events noted below. Assign a code from category Y99, External cause status, to indicate the work status of the person at the time the event occurred. The status code indicates whether the event occurred during military activity, whether a non-military person was at work, whether an individual including a student or volunteer was involved in a non-work activity at the time of the causal event.

A code from Y99, External cause status, should be assigned, when applicable, with other external cause codes, such as transport accidents and falls. The external cause status codes are not applicable to poisonings, adverse effects, misadventures or late effects. Do not assign a code from category Y99 if no other external cause codes (cause, activity) are applicable for the encounter.

An external cause status code is used only once, at the initial encounter for treatment. Only one code from Y99 should be recorded on a medical record.

Do not assign code Y99.9, Unspecified external cause status, if the status is not stated.

Accidents (V00-X58)

Transport accidents (V00-V99)

NOTE This section is structured in 12 groups. Those relating to land transport accidents (V00-V89) reflect the victim's mode of transport and are subdivided to identify the victim's 'counterpart' or the type of event. The vehicle of which the injured person is an occupant is identified in the first two characters since it is seen as the most important factor to identify for prevention purposes. A transport accident is one in which the vehicle involved must be moving or running or in use for transport purposes at the time of the accident.

Use additional code to identify:
Airbag injury (W22.1)
Type of street or road (Y92.4-)
Use of cellular telephone and other electronic equipment at the time of the transport accident (Y93.C-)

Excludes1: *agricultural vehicles in stationary use or maintenance (W31.-)*
assault by crashing of motor vehicle (Y03.-)
automobile or motor cycle in stationary use or maintenance- code to type of accident
crashing of motor vehicle, undetermined intent (Y32)
intentional self-harm by crashing of motor vehicle (X82)

Excludes2: *transport accidents due to cataclysm (X34-X38)*

NOTE Definitions related to transport accidents:

(a) A transport accident (V00-V99) is any accident involving a device designed primarily for, or used at the time primarily for, conveying persons or goods from one place to another.

(b) A public highway [trafficway] or street is the entire width between property lines (or other boundary lines) of land open to the public as a matter of right or custom for purposes of moving persons or property from one place to another. A roadway is that part of the public highway designed, improved and customarily used for vehicular traffic.

(c) A traffic accident is any vehicle accident occurring on the public highway [i.e. originating on, terminating on, or involving a vehicle partially on the highway]. A vehicle accident is assumed to have occurred on the public highway unless another place is specified, except i the case of accidents involving only off-road motor vehicles, which are classified as nontraffic accidents unless the contrary is stated.

(d) A nontraffic accident is any vehicle accident that occurs entirely in any place other than a public highway.

(e) A pedestrian is any person involved in an accident who was not at the time of the accident riding in or on a motor vehicle, railway train, streetcar or animal-drawn or other vehicle, or on a pedal cycle or animal. This includes, a person changing a tire, working on a parked care, or a person on foot. It also includes the user of a pedestrian conveyance such as a baby stroller, ice-skates, skis, sled, roller skates, a skateboard, nonmotorized or motorized wheelchair, motorized mobility scooter, or nonmotorized scooter.

(f) A driver is an occupant of a transport vehicle who is operating or intending to operate it.

(g) A passenger is any occupant of a transport vehicle other than the driver, except a person traveling on the outside of the vehicle.

(h) A person on the outside of a vehicle is any person being transported by a vehicle but not occupying the space normally reserved for the driver or passengers, or the space intended for the transport of property. This includes a person travailing on the bodywork, bumper, fender, roof, running board or step of a vehicle, as well as, hanging on the outside of the vehicle.

(i) A pedal cycle is any land transport vehicle operated solely by nonmotorized pedals including a bicycle or tricycle.

(j) A pedal cyclist is any person riding a pedal cycle or in a sidecar or trailer attached to a pedal cycle.

(k) A motorcycle is a two-wheeled motor vehicle with one or two riding saddles and sometimes with a third wheel for the support of a sidecar. The sidecar is considered part of the motorcycle. This includes a moped, motor scooter, or motorized bicycle.

(l) A motorcycle rider is any person riding a motorcycle or in a sidecar or trailer attached to the motorcycle.

(m) A three-wheeled motor vehicle is a motorized tricycle designed primarily for on-road use. This includes a motor-driven tricycle, a motorized rickshaw, or a three-wheeled motor car.

(n) A car [automobile] is a four-wheeled motor vehicle designed primarily for carrying up to 7 persons. A trailer being towed by the car is considered par of the car. It does not include a van or minivan - see definition (o)

(o) A pick-up truck or van is a four or six-wheeled motor vehicle designed for carrying passengers as well as property or cargo weighing less than the local limit for classification as a heavy goods vehicle, and not requiring a special driver's license. this includes a minivan and a sport-utility vehicle (SUV)

(p) A heavy transport vehicle is a motor vehicle designed primarily for carrying property, meeting local criteria for classification as a heavy goods vehicle in terms of weight and requiring a special driver's license.

(q) A bus (coach) is a motor vehicle designed or adapted primarily for carrying more than 10 passengers, and requiring a special driver's license.

(r) A railway train or railway vehicle is any device, with or without freight or passenger cars couple to it, designed for traffic on a railway track. This includes subterranean (subways) or elevated trains.

(s) A streetcar, is a device designed and used primarily for transporting passengers within a municipality, running on rails, usually subject to normal traffic control signals, and operated principally on a right-of-way that forms part of the roadway. This includes a tram or trolley that runs on rails. A trailer being towed by a streetcar is considered part of the streetcar.

(t) A special vehicle mainly used on industrial premises is a motor vehicle designed primarily for use within the building and premises of industrial or commercial establishments. This includes battery-powered airport passenger vehicles or baggage/mail trucks, forklifts, coal-cars in a coal min, logging cars and trucks used in mines or quarries.

(u) A special vehicle mainly used in agriculture is a motor vehicle designed specifically for use in farming and agriculture (horticulture), to work the land, tend and harvest crops and transport materials on the farm. This includes harvesters, farm machinery and tractor and trailers.

(v) A special construction vehicle is a motor vehicle designed specifically for use on construction and demolition sites. This includes bulldozers, diggers, earth levellers, dump trucks, backhoes, front-end loaders, pavers, and mechanical shovels.

(w) A special all-terrain vehicle is a motor vehicle of special design to enable it to negotiate over rough or soft terrain, snow or sand. Examples of special design are high construction, special wheels and tires, tracks, and support on a cushion of air. This includes snow mobiles, All terrain vehicles (ATV), and dune buggies. It does not include passenger vehicle designated as Sport Utility Vehicles (SUV).

(x) A water craft is any device designed for transporting passengers or goods on water. This includes motor or sail boats, ships, and hovercraft.

(y) An aircraft is any device for transporting passengers or goods in the air. This includes hot-air balloons, gliders, helicopters and airplanes.

(z) A military vehicle is any motorized vehicle operating on a public roadway owned by the military and being operated by a member of the military.

Pedestrian injured in transport accident (V00-V09)

Includes: person changing tire on transport vehicle
person examining engine of vehicle broken down in (on side of) road

Excludes1: *fall due to non-transport collision with other person (W03)*
pedestrian on foot falling (slipping) on ice and snow (W00.-)
struck or bumped by another person (W51)

V00 Pedestrian conveyance accident

Use additional place of occurrence and activity external cause codes, if known (Y92.-, Y93.-)

Excludes1: *collision with another person without fall (W51)*
fall due to person on foot colliding with another person on foot (W03)
fall from non-moving wheelchair, nonmotorized scooter and motorized mobility scooter without collision (W05.-)
pedestrian (conveyance) collision with other land transport vehicle (V01-V09)
pedestrian on foot falling (slipping) on ice and snow (W00.-)

The appropriate 7th character is to be added to each code from category V00
A   initial encounter
D   subsequent encounter
S   sequela

+ **V00.0   Pedestrian on foot injured in collision with pedestrian conveyance**

X+7th **V00.01   Pedestrian on foot injured in collision with roller-skater**

X+7th **V00.02   Pedestrian on foot injured in collision with skateboarder**

+ **V00.03   Pedestrian on foot injured in collision with pedestrian conveyance**

+7th **V00.031   Pedestrian on foot injured in collision with rider of standing electric scooter**

+7th **V00.038   Pedestrian on foot injured in collision with rider of other standing micro-mobility pedestrian conveyance**

Pedestrian on foot injured in collision with rider of hoverboard
Pedestrian on foot injured in collision with rider of segway

X+7th **V00.09   Pedestrian on foot injured in collision with other pedestrian conveyance**

+ **V00.1   Rolling-type pedestrian conveyance accident**

Excludes1: *accident with baby stroller (V00.82-)*
accident with wheelchair (powered) (V00.81-)
accident with motorized mobility scooter (V00.83-)

+ **V00.11   In-line roller-skate accident**

+7th **V00.111   Fall from in-line roller-skates**

+7th **V00.112   In-line roller-skater colliding with stationary object**

+7th **V00.118   Other in-line roller-skate accident**

Excludes1: *roller-skater collision with other land transport vehicle(V01-V09 with 5th character 1)*

+ **V00.12   Non-in- line roller-skate accident**

+7th **V00.121   Fall from non-in-line roller-skates**

+7th **V00.122   Non-in-line roller-skater colliding with stationary object**

+7th **V00.128   Other non-in-line roller-skating accident**

Excludes1: *roller-skater collision with other land transport vehicle(V01-V09 with 5th character 1)*

+ **V00.13** **Skateboard accident**
 +7th **V00.131** **Fall from skateboard**
 +7th **V00.132** **Skateboarder colliding with stationary object**
 +7th **V00.138** **Other skateboard accident**
  Excludes1: *skateboarder collision with other land transport vehicle(V01-V09 with 5th character 2)*

+ **V00.14** **Scooter (nonmotorized) accident**
  Excludes1: *motor scooter accident (V20-V29)*
 +7th **V00.141** **Fall from scooter (nonmotorized)**
 +7th **V00.142** **Scooter (nonmotorized) colliding with stationary object**
 +7th **V00.148** **Other scooter (nonmotorized) accident**
  Excludes1: *scooter (nonmotorized) collision with other land transport vehicle (V01-V09 with fifth character 9)*

+ **V00.15** **Heelies accident**
 Rolling shoe
 Wheeled shoe
 Wheelies accident
 +7th **V00.151** **Fall from heelies**
 +7th **V00.152** **Heelies colliding with stationary object**
 +7th **V00.158** **Other heelies accident**

+ **V00.18** **Accident on other rolling-type pedestrian conveyance**
 +7th **V00.181** **Fall from other rolling-type pedestrian conveyance**
 +7th **V00.182** **Pedestrian on other rolling-type pedestrian conveyance colliding with stationary object**
 +7th **V00.188** **Other accident on other rolling-type pedestrian conveyance**

+ **V00.2** **Gliding-type pedestrian conveyance accident**
+ **V00.21** **Ice-skates accident**
 +7th **V00.211** **Fall from ice-skates**
 +7th **V00.212** **Ice-skater colliding with stationary object**
 +7th **V00.218** **Other ice-skates accident**
  Excludes1: *ice-skater collision with other land transport vehicle(V01-V09 with 5th character 9)*

+ **V00.22** **Sled accident**
 +7th **V00.221** **Fall from sled**
 +7th **V00.222** **Sledder colliding with stationary object**
 +7th **V00.228** **Other sled accident**
  Excludes1: *sled collision with other land transport vehicle (V01-V09 with 5th character 9)*

+ **V00.28** **Other gliding-type pedestrian conveyance accident**
 +7th **V00.281** **Fall from other gliding-type pedestrian conveyance**
 +7th **V00.282** **Pedestrian on other gliding-type pedestrian conveyance colliding with stationary object**
 +7th **V00.288** **Other accident on other gliding-type pedestrian conveyance**
  Excludes1: *gliding-type pedestrian conveyance collision with other land transport vehicle(V01-V09 with 5th character 9)*

+ **V00.3** **Flat-bottomed pedestrian conveyance accident**
+ **V00.31** **Snowboard accident**
 +7th **V00.311** **Fall from snowboard**
 +7th **V00.312** **Snowboarder colliding with stationary object**
 +7th **V00.318** **Other snowboard accident**
  Excludes1: *snowboarder collision with other land transport vehicle(V01-V09 with 5th character 9)*

+ **V00.32** **Snow-ski accident**
 +7th **V00.321** **Fall from snow-skis**
  AHA CC: 1Q, 2015, 3-21
 +7th **V00.322** **Snow-skier colliding with stationary object**

 +7th **V00.328** **Other snow-ski accident**
  Excludes1: *snow-skier collision with other land transport vehicle(V01-V09 with 5th character 9)*

+ **V00.38** **Other flat-bottomed pedestrian conveyance accident**
 +7th **V00.381** **Fall from other flat-bottomed pedestrian conveyance**
 +7th **V00.382** **Pedestrian on other flat-bottomed pedestrian conveyance colliding with stationary object**
 +7th **V00.388** **Other accident on other flat-bottomed pedestrian conveyance**

+ **V00.8** **Accident on other pedestrian conveyance**
+ **V00.81** **Accident with wheelchair (powered)**
 +7th **V00.811** **Fall from moving wheelchair (powered)**
  Excludes1: *fall from non-moving wheelchair (W05.0)*
 +7th **V00.812** **Wheelchair (powered) colliding with stationary object**
 +7th **V00.818** **Other accident with wheelchair (powered)**
+ **V00.82** **Accident with baby stroller**
 +7th **V00.821** **Fall from baby stroller**
 +7th **V00.822** **Baby stroller colliding with stationary object**
 +7th **V00.828** **Other accident with baby stroller**
+ **V00.83** **Accident with motorized mobility scooter**
 +7th **V00.831** **Fall from motorized mobility scooter**
  Excludes1: *fall from non-moving motorized mobility scooter (W05.2)*
 +7th **V00.832** **Motorized mobility scooter colliding with stationary object**
 +7th **V00.838** **Other accident with motorized mobility scooter**
+ **V00.84** **Accident with standing micro-mobility pedestrian conveyance**
 +7th **V00.841** **Fall from standing electric scooter**
 +7th **V00.842** **Pedestrian on standing electric scooter colliding with stationary object**
 +7th **V00.848** **Other accident with standing micro-mobility pedestrian conveyance**
  Accident with hoverboard
  Accident with segway
+ **V00.89** **Accident on other pedestrian conveyance**
 +7th **V00.891** **Fall from other pedestrian conveyance**
 +7th **V00.892** **Pedestrian on other pedestrian conveyance colliding with stationary object**
 +7th **V00.898** **Other accident on other pedestrian conveyance**
  Excludes1: *other pedestrian (conveyance) collision with other land transport vehicle(V01-V09 with 5th character 9)*

V01 **Pedestrian injured in collision with pedal cycle**

> The appropriate 7th character is to be added to each code from category V01
> A initial encounter
> D subsequent encounter
> S sequela

+ **V01.0** **Pedestrian injured in collision with pedal cycle in nontraffic accident**
 X+7th **V01.00** **Pedestrian on foot injured in collision with pedal cycle in nontraffic accident**
  Pedestrian NOS injured in collision with pedal cycle in nontraffic accident
 X+7th **V01.01** **Pedestrian on roller-skates injured in collision with pedal cycle in nontraffic accident**
 X+7th **V01.02** **Pedestrian on skateboard injured in collision with pedal cycle in nontraffic accident**
 + **V01.03** **Pedestrian on standing micro-mobility pedestrian conveyance injured in collision with pedal cycle in nontraffic accident**
 +7th **V01.031** **Pedestrian on standing electric scooter injured in collision with pedal cycle in nontraffic accident**

+, +7th, X + 7th ● Newborn ● Pediatric ● Maternity ● Adult ♀ Female ♂ Male Manifestation Unacceptable PDX HCC CC MCC HAC

+7th **V01.038** **Pedestrian on other standing micro-mobility pedestrian conveyance injured in collision with pedal cycle in nontraffic accident**

Pedestrian on hoverboard injured in collision with pedal cycle in nontraffic accident

Pedestrian on segway injured in collision with pedal cycle in nontraffic accident

X+7th **V01.09** **Pedestrian with other conveyance injured in collision with pedal cycle in nontraffic accident**

Pedestrian with baby stroller injured in collision with pedal cycle in nontraffic accident

Pedestrian on ice-skates injured in collision with pedal cycle in nontraffic accident

Pedestrian on nonmotorized scooter injured in collision with pedal cycle in nontraffic accident

Pedestrian on sled injured in collision with pedal cycle in nontraffic accident

Pedestrian on snowboard injured in collision with pedal cycle in nontraffic accident

Pedestrian on snow-skis injured in collision with pedal cycle in nontraffic accident

Pedestrian in wheelchair (powered) injured in collision with pedal cycle in nontraffic accident

Pedestrian in motorized mobility scooter injured in collision with pedal cycle in nontraffic accident

+ **V01.1** **Pedestrian injured in collision with pedal cycle in traffic accident**

X+7th **V01.10** **Pedestrian on foot injured in collision with pedal cycle in traffic accident**

Pedestrian NOS injured in collision with pedal cycle in traffic accident

X+7th **V01.11** **Pedestrian on roller-skates injured in collision with pedal cycle in traffic accident**

X+7th **V01.12** **Pedestrian on skateboard injured in collision with pedal cycle in traffic accident**

+ **V01.13** **Pedestrian on standing micro-mobility pedestrian conveyance injured in collision with pedal cycle in traffic accident**

+7th **V01.131** **Pedestrian on standing electric scooter injured in collision with pedal cycle in traffic accident**

+7th **V01.138** **Pedestrian on other standing micro-mobility pedestrian conveyance injured in collision with pedal cycle in traffic accident**

Pedestrian on hoverboard injured in collision with pedal cycle in traffic accident

Pedestrian on segway injured in collisiion with pedal cycle in traffic accident

X+7th **V01.19** **Pedestrian with other conveyance injured in collision with pedal cycle in traffic accident**

Pedestrian with baby stroller injured in collision with pedal cycle in traffic accident

Pedestrian on ice-skates injured in collision with pedal cycle in traffic accident

Pedestrian on nonmotorized scooter injured in collision with pedal cycle in traffic accident

Pedestrian on sled injured in collision with pedal cycle in traffic accident

Pedestrian on snowboard injured in collision with pedal cycle in traffic accident

Pedestrian on snow-skis injured in collision with pedal cycle in traffic accident

Pedestrian in wheelchair (powered) injured in collision with pedal cycle in traffic accident

Pedestrian in motorized mobility scooter injured in collision with pedal cycle in traffic accident

+ **V01.9** **Pedestrian injured in collision with pedal cycle, unspecified whether traffic or nontraffic accident**

X+7th **V01.90** **Pedestrian on foot injured in collision with pedal cycle, unspecified whether traffic or nontraffic accident**

Pedestrian NOS injured in collision with pedal cycle, unspecified whether traffic or nontraffic accident

X+7th **V01.91** **Pedestrian on roller-skates injured in collision with pedal cycle, unspecified whether traffic or nontraffic accident**

X+7th **V01.92** **Pedestrian on skateboard injured in collision with pedal cycle, unspecified whether traffic or nontraffic accident**

+ **V01.93** **Pedestrian on standing micro-mobility pedestrian conveyance injured in collision with pedal cycle, unspecified whether traffic or nontraffic accident**

+7th **V01.931** **Pedestrian on standing electric scooter injured in collision with pedal cycle, unspecified whether traffic or nontraffic accident**

+7th **V01.938** **Pedestrian on other standing micro-mobility pedestrian conveyance injured in collision with pedal cycle, unspecified whether traffic or nontraffic accident**

Pedestrian on hoverboard injured in collision with pedal cycle, unspecified whether traffic or nontraffic accident

Pedestrian on segway injured in collision with pedal cycle, unspecified whether traffic or nontraffic accident

X+7th **V01.99** **Pedestrian with other conveyance injured in collision with pedal cycle, unspecified whether traffic or nontraffic accident**

Pedestrian with baby stroller injured in collision with pedal cycle, unspecified whether traffic or nontraffic accident

Pedestrian on ice-skates injured in collision with pedal cycle unspecified, whether traffic or nontraffic accident

Pedestrian on nonmotorized scooter injured in collision with pedal cycle, unspecified whether traffic or nontraffic accident

Pedestrian on sled injured in collision with pedal cycle unspecified, whether traffic or nontraffic accident

Pedestrian on snowboard injured in collision with pedal cycle, unspecified whether traffic or nontraffic accident

Pedestrian on snow-skis injured in collision with pedal cycle, unspecified whether traffic or nontraffic accident

Pedestrian in wheelchair (powered) injured in collision with pedal cycle, unspecified whether traffic or nontraffic accident

Pedestrian in motorized mobility scooter injured in collision with pedal cycle, unspecified whether traffic or nontraffic accident

V02 **Pedestrian injured in collision with two- or three-wheeled motor vehicle**

The appropriate 7th character is to be added to each code from category V02
A   initial encounter
D   subsequent encounter
S   sequela

+ **V02.0** **Pedestrian injured in collision with two- or three-wheeled motor vehicle in nontraffic accident**

X+7th **V02.00** **Pedestrian on foot injured in collision with two- or three-wheeled motor vehicle in nontraffic accident**

Pedestrian NOS injured in collision with two- or three-wheeled motor vehicle in nontraffic accident

X+7th **V02.01** **Pedestrian on roller-skates injured in collision with two- or three-wheeled motor vehicle in nontraffic accident**

X+7th **V02.02** **Pedestrian on skateboard injured in collision with two- or three-wheeled motor vehicle in nontraffic accident**

+ **V02.03** **Pedestrian on standing micro-mobility pedestrian conveyance injured in collision with two- or three-wheeled motor vehicle in nontraffic accident**

+7th **V02.031** **Pedestrian on standing electric scooter injured in collision with two- or three-wheeled motor vehicle in nontraffic accident**

+, +7th, X + 7th   ● Newborn   ● Pediatric   ● Maternity   ● Adult   ♀ Female   ♂ Male   Manifestation   Unacceptable PDX   HCC   CC   MCC   HAC

+7th **V02.038** **Pedestrian on other standing micro-mobility pedestrian conveyance injured in collision with two- or three-wheeled motor vehicle in nontraffic accident**

  Pedestrian on hoverboard injured in collision with two- or three-wheeled motor vehicle in nontraffic accident

  Pedestrian on segway injured in collision with two- or three-wheeled motor vehicle in nontraffic accident

X+7th **V02.09** **Pedestrian with other conveyance injured in collision with two- or three-wheeled motor vehicle in nontraffic accident**

  Pedestrian with baby stroller injured in collision with two- or three-wheeled motor vehicle in nontraffic accident

  Pedestrian on ice-skates injured in collision with two- or three-wheeled motor vehicle in nontraffic accident

  Pedestrian on nonmotorized scooter injured in collision with two- or three-wheeled motor vehicle in nontraffic accident

  Pedestrian on sled injured in collision with two- or three-wheeled motor vehicle in nontraffic accident

  Pedestrian on snowboard injured in collision with two- or three-wheeled motor vehicle in nontraffic accident

  Pedestrian on snow-skis injured in collision with two- or three-wheeled motor vehicle in nontraffic accident

  Pedestrian in wheelchair (powered) injured in collision with two- or three-wheeled motor vehicle in nontraffic accident

  Pedestrian in motorized mobility scooter injured in collision with two- or three-wheeled motor vehicle in nontraffic accident

+ **V02.1** **Pedestrian injured in collision with two- or three-wheeled motor vehicle in traffic accident**

X+7th **V02.10** **Pedestrian on foot injured in collision with two- or three-wheeled motor vehicle in traffic accident**

  Pedestrian NOS injured in collision with two- or three-wheeled motor vehicle in traffic accident

X+7th **V02.11** **Pedestrian on roller-skates injured in collision with two- or three-wheeled motor vehicle in traffic accident**

X+7th **V02.12** **Pedestrian on skateboard injured in collision with two- or three-wheeled motor vehicle in traffic accident**

+ **V02.13** **Pedestrian on standing micro-mobility pedestrian conveyance injured in collision with two- or three-wheeled motor vehicle in traffic accident**

  X+7th **V02.131** **Pedestrian on standing electric scooter injured in collision with two- or three-wheeled motor vehicle in traffic accident**

  X+7th **V02.138** **Pedestrian on other standing micro-mobility pedestrian conveyance injured in collision with two- or three-wheeled motor vehicle in traffic accident**

    Pedestrian on hoverboard injured in collision with two- or three-wheeled motor vehicle in traffic accident

    Pedestrian on segway injured in collision with two- or three-wheeled motor vehicle in traffic accident

X+7th **V02.19** **Pedestrian with other conveyance injured in collision with two- or three-wheeled motor vehicle in traffic accident**

  Pedestrian with baby stroller injured in collision with two- or three-wheeled motor vehicle in traffic accident

  Pedestrian on ice-skates injured in collision with two- or three-wheeled motor vehicle in traffic accident

  Pedestrian on nonmotorized scooter injured in collision with two- or three-wheeled motor vehicle in traffic accident

  Pedestrian on sled injured in collision with two- or three-wheeled motor vehicle in traffic accident

---

  Pedestrian on snowboard injured in collision with two- or three-wheeled motor vehicle in traffic accident

  Pedestrian on snow-skis injured in collision with two- or three-wheeled motor vehicle in traffic accident

  Pedestrian in wheelchair (powered) injured in collision with two- or three-wheeled motor vehicle in traffic accident

  Pedestrian in motorized mobility scooter injured in collision with two- or three-wheeled motor vehicle in traffic accident

+ **V02.9** **Pedestrian injured in collision with two- or three-wheeled motor vehicle, unspecified whether traffic or nontraffic accident**

X+7th **V02.90** **Pedestrian on foot injured in collision with two- or three-wheeled motor vehicle, unspecified whether traffic or nontraffic accident**

  Pedestrian NOS injured in collision with two- or three-wheeled motor vehicle, unspecified whether traffic or nontraffic accident

X+7th **V02.91** **Pedestrian on roller-skates injured in collision with two- or three-wheeled motor vehicle, unspecified whether traffic or nontraffic accident**

X+7th **V02.92** **Pedestrian on skateboard injured in collision with two- or three-wheeled motor vehicle, unspecified whether traffic or nontraffic accident**

+ **V02.93** **Pedestrian on standing micro-mobility pedestrian conveyance injured in collision with two- or three wheeled motor vehicle, unspecified whether traffic or nontraffic accident**

  +7th **V02.931** **Pedestrian on standing electric scooter injured in collision with two- or three wheeled motor vehicle, unspecified whether traffic or nontraffic accident**

  +7th **V02.938** **Pedestrian on other standing micro-mobility pedestrian conveyance injured in collision with two- or three wheeled motor vehicle, unspecified whether traffic or nontraffic accident**

    Pedestrian on hoverbaord injured in collision with two- or three wheeled motor vehicle, unspecified whether traffic or nontraffic accident

    Pedestrian on segway injured in collision with two- or three wheeled motor vehicle, unspecified whether traffic or nontraffic accident

X+7th **V02.99** **Pedestrian with other conveyance injured in collision with two- or three-wheeled motor vehicle, unspecified whether traffic or nontraffic accident**

  Pedestrian with baby stroller injured in collision with two- or three-wheeled motor vehicle, unspecified whether traffic or nontraffic accident

  Pedestrian on ice-skates injured in collision with two- or three-wheeled motor vehicle, unspecified whether traffic or nontraffic accident

  Pedestrian on nonmotorized scooter injured in collision with two- or three-wheeled motor vehicle, unspecified whether traffic or nontraffic accident

  Pedestrian on sled injured in collision with two- or three-wheeled motor vehicle, unspecified whether traffic or nontraffic accident

  Pedestrian on snowboard injured in collision with two- or three-wheeled motor vehicle, unspecified whether traffic or nontraffic accident

  Pedestrian on snow-skis injured in collision with two- or three-wheeled motor vehicle, unspecified whether traffic or nontraffic accident

  Pedestrian in wheelchair (powered) injured in collision with two- or three-wheeled motor vehicle, unspecified whether traffic or nontraffic accident

  Pedestrian in motorized mobility scooter injured in collision with two- or three-wheeled motor vehicle, unspecified whether traffic or nontraffic accident

V03 Pedestrian injured in collision with car, pick-up truck or van

The appropriate 7th character is to be added to each code from category V03
A   initial encounter
D   subsequent encounter
S   sequela

+ **V03.0 Pedestrian injured in collision with car, pick-up truck or van in nontraffic accident**

X+7th **V03.00 Pedestrian on foot injured in collision with car, pick-up truck or van in nontraffic accident**

Pedestrian NOS injured in collision with car, pick-up truck or van in nontraffic accident

X+7th **V03.01 Pedestrian on roller-skates injured in collision with car, pick-up truck or van in nontraffic accident**

X+7th **V03.02 Pedestrian on skateboard injured in collision with car, pick-up truck or van in nontraffic accident**

+ **V03.03 Pedestrian on standing micro-mobility pedestrian conveyance injured in collision with car, pick-up or van in nontraffic accident**

+7th **V03.031 Pedestrian on standing electric scooter injured in collision with car, pick-up or van in nontraffic accident**

+7th **V03.038 Pedestrian on other standing micro-mobility pedestrian conveyance injured in collision with car, pick-up or van in nontraffic accident**

Pedestrian on hoverboard injured in collision with car, pick-up or van in nontraffic accident

Pedestrian on segway injured in collision with car, pick-up or van in nontraffic accident

X+7th **V03.09 Pedestrian with other conveyance injured in collision with car, pick-up truck or van in nontraffic accident**

Pedestrian with baby stroller injured in collision with car, pick-up truck or van in nontraffic accident

Pedestrian on ice-skates injured in collision with car, pick-up truck or van in nontraffic accident

Pedestrian on nonmotorized scooter injured in collision with car, pick-up truck or van in nontraffic accident

Pedestrian on sled injured in collision with car, pick-up truck or van in nontraffic accident

Pedestrian on snowboard injured in collision with car, pick-up truck or van in nontraffic accident

Pedestrian on snow-skis injured in collision with car, pick-up truck or van in nontraffic accident

Pedestrian in wheelchair (powered) injured in collision with car, pick-up truck or van in nontraffic accident

Pedestrian in motorized mobility scooter injured in collision with car, pick-up truck or van in nontraffic accident

+ **V03.1 Pedestrian injured in collision with car, pick-up truck or van in traffic accident**

X+7th **V03.10 Pedestrian on foot injured in collision with car, pick-up truck or van in traffic accident**

Pedestrian NOS injured in collision with car, pick-up truck or van in traffic accident

X+7th **V03.11 Pedestrian on roller-skates injured in collision with car, pick-up truck or van in traffic accident**

X+7th **V03.12 Pedestrian on skateboard injured in collision with car, pick-up truck or van in traffic accident**

+ **V03.13 Pedestrian on standing micro-mobility pedestrian conveyance injured in collision with car, pick-up or van in traffic accident**

+7th **V03.131 Pedestrian on standing electric scooter injured in collision with car, pick-up or van in traffic accident**

+7th **V03.138 Pedestrian on other standing micro-mobility pedestrian conveyance injured in collision with car, pick-up or van in traffic accident**

Pedestrian on hoverboard injured in collision with car, pick-up or van in traffic accident

Pedestrian on segway injured in collision with car, pick-up or van in traffic accident

X+7th **V03.19 Pedestrian with other conveyance injured in collision with car, pick-up truck or van in traffic accident**

Pedestrian with baby stroller injured in collision with car, pick-up truck or van in traffic accident

Pedestrian on ice-skates injured in collision with car, pick-up truck or van in traffic accident

Pedestrian on nonmotorized scooter injured in collision with car, pick-up truck or van in traffic accident

Pedestrian on sled injured in collision with car, pick-up truck or van in traffic accident

Pedestrian on snowboard injured in collision with car, pick-up truck or van in traffic accident

Pedestrian on snow-skis injured in collision with car, pick-up truck or van in traffic accident

Pedestrian in wheelchair (powered) injured in collision with car, pick-up truck or van in traffic accident

Pedestrian in motorized mobility scooter injured in collision with car, pick-up truck or van in traffic accident

+ **V03.9 Pedestrian injured in collision with car, pick-up truck or van, unspecified whether traffic or nontraffic accident**

X+7th **V03.90 Pedestrian on foot injured in collision with car, pick-up truck or van, unspecified whether traffic or nontraffic accident**

Pedestrian NOS injured in collision with car, pick-up truck or van, unspecified whether traffic or nontraffic accident

X+7th **V03.91 Pedestrian on roller-skates injured in collision with car, pick-up truck or van, unspecified whether traffic or nontraffic accident**

X+7th **V03.92 Pedestrian on skateboard injured in collision with car, pick-up truck or van, unspecified whether traffic or nontraffic accident**

+ **V03.93 Pedestrian on standing micro-mobility pedestrian conveyance injured in collision with car, pick-up or van, unspecified whether traffic or nontraffic accident**

+7th **V03.931 Pedestrian on standing electric scooter injured in collision with car, pick-up or van, unspecified whether traffic or nontraffic accident**

+7th **V03.938 Pedestrian on other standing micro-mobility pedestrian conveyance injured in collision with car, pick-up or van, unspecified whether traffic or nontraffic accident**

Pedestrian on hoverboard injured in collision with car, pick-up or van, unspecified whether traffic or nontraffic accident

Pedestrian on segway injured in collision with car, pick-up or van, unspecified whether traffic or nontraffic accident

X+7th **V03.99 Pedestrian with other conveyance injured in collision with car, pick-up truck or van, unspecified whether traffic or nontraffic accident**

Pedestrian with baby stroller injured in collision with car, pick-up truck or van, unspecified whether traffic or nontraffic accident

Pedestrian on ice-skates injured in collision with car, pick-up truck or van, unspecified whether traffic or nontraffic accident

Pedestrian on nonmotorized scooter injured in collision with car, pick-up truck or van, unspecified whether traffic or nontraffic accident

Pedestrian on sled injured in collision with car, pick-up truck or van in nontraffic accident

Pedestrian on snowboard injured in collision with car, pick-up truck or van, unspecified whether traffic or nontraffic accident

+, +7th, X + 7th   ● Newborn   ● Pediatric   ● Maternity   ● Adult   ♀ Female   ♂ Male   Manifestation   Unacceptable PDX   HCC   CC   MCC   HAC

Pedestrian on snow-skis injured in collision with car, pick-up truck or van, unspecified whether traffic or nontraffic accident

Pedestrian in wheelchair (powered) injured in collision with car, pick-up truck or van, unspecified whether traffic or nontraffic accident

Pedestrian in motorized mobility scooter injured in collision with car, pick-up truck or van, unspecified whether traffic or nontraffic accident

V04 Pedestrian injured in collision with heavy transport vehicle or bus

> *Excludes1:* *pedestrian injured in collision with military vehicle (V09.01, V09.21)*

> The appropriate 7th character is to be added to each code from category V04
> A   initial encounter
> D   subsequent encounter
> S   sequela

+ V04.0   Pedestrian injured in collision with heavy transport vehicle or bus in nontraffic accident

X+7th **V04.00   Pedestrian on foot injured in collision with heavy transport vehicle or bus in nontraffic accident**
  Pedestrian NOS injured in collision with heavy transport vehicle or bus in nontraffic accident

X+7th **V04.01   Pedestrian on roller-skates injured in collision with heavy transport vehicle or bus in nontraffic accident**

X+7th **V04.02   Pedestrian on skateboard injured in collision with heavy transport vehicle or bus in nontraffic accident**

+ **V04.03   Pedestrian on standing micro-mobility pedestrian conveyance injured in collision with heavy transport vehicle or bus in nontraffic accident**

  +7th **V04.031   Pedestrian on standing electric scooter injured in collision with heavy transport vehicle or bus in nontraffic accident**

  +7th **V04.038   Pedestrian on other standing micro-mobility pedestrian conveyance injured in collision with heavy transport vehicle or bus in nontraffic accident**
    Pedestrian on hoverboard injured in collision with heavy transport vehicle or bus in nontraffic accident
    Pedestrian on segway injured in collision with heavy transport vehicle or bus in nontraffic accident

X+7th **V04.09   Pedestrian with other conveyance injured in collision with heavy transport vehicle or bus in nontraffic accident**
  Pedestrian with baby stroller injured in collision with heavy transport vehicle or bus in nontraffic accident
  Pedestrian on ice-skates injured in collision with heavy transport vehicle or bus in nontraffic accident
  Pedestrian on nonmotorized scooter injured in collision with heavy transport vehicle or bus in nontraffic accident
  Pedestrian on sled injured in collision with heavy transport vehicle or bus in nontraffic accident
  Pedestrian on snowboard injured in collision with heavy transport vehicle or bus in nontraffic accident
  Pedestrian on snow-skis injured in collision with heavy transport vehicle or bus in nontraffic accident
  Pedestrian in wheelchair (powered) injured in collision with heavy transport vehicle or bus in nontraffic accident
  Pedestrian in motorized mobility scooter injured in collision with heavy transport vehicle or bus in nontraffic accident

+ V04.1   Pedestrian injured in collision with heavy transport vehicle or bus in traffic accident

X+7th **V04.10   Pedestrian on foot injured in collision with heavy transport vehicle or bus in traffic accident**
  Pedestrian NOS injured in collision with heavy transport vehicle or bus in traffic accident

X+7th **V04.11   Pedestrian on roller-skates injured in collision with heavy transport vehicle or bus in traffic accident**

X+7th **V04.12   Pedestrian on skateboard injured in collision with heavy transport vehicle or bus in traffic accident**

+ **V04.13   Pedestrian on standing micro-mobility pedestrian conveyance injured in collision with heavy transport vehicle or bus in traffic accident**

  +7th **V04.131   Pedestrian on standing electric scooter injured in collision with heavy transport vehicle or bus in traffic accident**

  +7th **V04.138   Pedestrian on other standing micro-mobility pedestrian conveyance injured in collision with heavy transport vehicle or bus in traffic accident**
    Pedestrian on hoverboard injured in collision with heavy transport vehicle or bus in traffic accident
    Pedestrian on segway injured in collision with heavy transport vehicle or bus in traffic accident

X+7th **V04.19   Pedestrian with other conveyance injured in collision with heavy transport vehicle or bus in traffic accident**
  Pedestrian with baby stroller injured in collision with heavy transport vehicle or bus in traffic accident
  Pedestrian on ice-skates injured in collision with heavy transport vehicle or bus in traffic accident
  Pedestrian on nonmotorized scooter injured in collision with heavy transport vehicle or bus in traffic accident
  Pedestrian on sled injured in collision with heavy transport vehicle or bus in traffic accident
  Pedestrian on snowboard injured in collision with heavy transport vehicle or bus in traffic accident
  Pedestrian on snow-skis injured in collision with heavy transport vehicle or bus in traffic accident
  Pedestrian in wheelchair (powered) injured in collision with heavy transport vehicle or bus in traffic accident
  Pedestrian in motorized mobility scooter injured in collision with heavy transport vehicle or bus in traffic accident

+ V04.9   Pedestrian injured in collision with heavy transport vehicle or bus, unspecified whether traffic or nontraffic accident

X+7th **V04.90   Pedestrian on foot injured in collision with heavy transport vehicle or bus, unspecified whether traffic or nontraffic accident**
  Pedestrian NOS injured in collision with heavy transport vehicle or bus, unspecified whether traffic or nontraffic accident

X+7th **V04.91   Pedestrian on roller-skates injured in collision with heavy transport vehicle or bus, unspecified whether traffic or nontraffic accident**

X+7th **V04.92   Pedestrian on skateboard injured in collision with heavy transport vehicle or bus, unspecified whether traffic or nontraffic accident**

+ **V04.93   Pedestrian on standing micro-mobility pedestrian conveyance injured in collision with heavy transport vehicle or bus, unspecified whether traffic or nontraffic accident**

  +7th **V04.931   Pedestrian on standing electric scooter injured in collision with heavy transport vehicle or bus, unspecified whether traffic or nontraffic accident**

  +7th **V04.938   Pedestrian on other standing micro-mobility pedestrian conveyance injured in collision with heavy transport vehicle or bus, unspecified whether traffic or nontraffic accident**
    Pedestrian on hoverboard injured in collision with heavy transport vehicle or bus, unspecified whether traffic or nontraffic accident
    Pedestrian on segway injured in collision with heavy transport vehicle or bus, unspecified whether traffic or nontraffic accident

X+7th V04.99 **Pedestrian with other conveyance injured in collision with heavy transport vehicle or bus, unspecified whether traffic or nontraffic accident**

Pedestrian with baby stroller injured in collision with heavy transport vehicle or bus, unspecified whether traffic or nontraffic accident

Pedestrian on ice-skates injured in collision with heavy transport vehicle or bus, unspecified whether traffic or nontraffic accident

Pedestrian on nonmotorized scooter injured in collision with heavy transport vehicle or bus, unspecified whether traffic or nontraffic accident

Pedestrian on sled injured in collision with heavy transport vehicle or bus, unspecified whether traffic or nontraffic accident

Pedestrian on snowboard injured in collision with heavy transport vehicle or bus, unspecified whether traffic or nontraffic accident

Pedestrian on snow-skis injured in collision with heavy transport vehicle or bus, unspecified whether traffic or nontraffic accident

Pedestrian in wheelchair (powered) injured in collision with heavy transport vehicle or bus, unspecified whether traffic or nontraffic accident

Pedestrian in motorized mobility scooter injured in collision with heavy transport vehicle or bus, unspecified whether traffic or nontraffic accident

V05 **Pedestrian injured in collision with railway train or railway vehicle**

> The appropriate 7th character is to be added to each code from category V05
> A   initial encounter
> D   subsequent encounter
> S   sequela

+ V05.0 **Pedestrian injured in collision with railway train or railway vehicle in nontraffic accident**

X+7th V05.00 **Pedestrian on foot injured in collision with railway train or railway vehicle in nontraffic accident**

Pedestrian NOS injured in collision with railway train or railway vehicle in nontraffic accident

X+7th V05.01 **Pedestrian on roller-skates injured in collision with railway train or railway vehicle in nontraffic accident**

X+7th V05.02 **Pedestrian on skateboard injured in collision with railway train or railway vehicle in nontraffic accident**

+ V05.03 **Pedestrian on standing micro-mobility pedestrian conveyance injured in collision with railway train or railway vehicle in nontraffic accident**

+7th V05.031 **Pedestrian on standing electric scooter injured in collision with railway train or railway vehicle in nontraffic accident**

+7th V05.038 **Pedestrian on other standing micro-mobility pedestrian conveyance injured in collision with railway train or railway vehicle in nontraffic accident**

Pedestrian on hoverboard injured in collision with railway train or railway vehicle in nontraffic accident

Pedestrian on segway injured in collision with railway train or railway vehicle in nontraffic accident

X+7th V05.09 **Pedestrian with other conveyance injured in collision with railway train or railway vehicle in nontraffic accident**

Pedestrian with baby stroller injured in collision with railway train or railway vehicle in nontraffic accident

Pedestrian on ice-skates injured in collision with railway train or railway vehicle in nontraffic accident

Pedestrian on nonmotorized scooter injured in collision with railway train or railway vehicle in nontraffic accident

Pedestrian on sled injured in collision with railway train or railway vehicle in nontraffic accident

Pedestrian on snowboard injured in collision with railway train or railway vehicle in nontraffic accident

Pedestrian on snow-skis injured in collision with railway train or railway vehicle in nontraffic accident

Pedestrian in wheelchair (powered) injured in collision with railway train or railway vehicle in nontraffic accident

Pedestrian in motorized mobility scooter injured in collision with railway train or railway vehicle in nontraffic accident

+ V05.1 **Pedestrian injured in collision with railway train or railway vehicle in traffic accident**

X+7th V05.10 **Pedestrian on foot injured in collision with railway train or railway vehicle in traffic accident**

Pedestrian NOS injured in collision with railway train or railway vehicle in traffic accident

X+7th V05.11 **Pedestrian on roller-skates injured in collision with railway train or railway vehicle in traffic accident**

X+7th V05.12 **Pedestrian on skateboard injured in collision with railway train or railway vehicle in traffic accident**

+ V05.13 **Pedestrian on standing micro-mobility pedestrian conveyance injured in collision with railway train or railway vehicle in traffic accident**

+7th V05.131 **Pedestrian on standing electric scooter injured in collision with railway train or railway vehicle in traffic accident**

+7th V05.138 **Pedestrian on other standing micro-mobility pedestrian conveyance injured in collision with railway train or railway vehicle in traffic accident**

Pedestrian on hoverboard injured in collision with railway train or railway vehicle in traffic accident

Pedestrian on segway injured in collision with railway train or railway vehicle in traffic accident

X+7th V05.19 **Pedestrian with other conveyance injured in collision with railway train or railway vehicle in traffic accident**

Pedestrian with baby stroller injured in collision with railway train or railway vehicle in traffic accident

Pedestrian on ice-skates injured in collision with railway train or railway vehicle in traffic accident

Pedestrian on nonmotorized scooter injured in collision with railway train or railway vehicle in traffic accident

Pedestrian on sled injured in collision with railway train or railway vehicle in traffic accident

Pedestrian on snowboard injured in collision with railway train or railway vehicle in traffic accident

Pedestrian on snow-skis injured in collision with railway train or railway vehicle in traffic accident

Pedestrian in wheelchair (powered) injured in collision with railway train or railway vehicle in traffic accident

Pedestrian in motorized mobility scooter injured in collision with railway train or railway vehicle in traffic accident

+ V05.9 **Pedestrian injured in collision with railway train or railway vehicle, unspecified whether traffic or nontraffic accident**

X+7th V05.90 **Pedestrian on foot injured in collision with railway train or railway vehicle, unspecified whether traffic or nontraffic accident**

Pedestrian NOS injured in collision with railway train or railway vehicle, unspecified whether traffic or nontraffic accident

X+7th V05.91 **Pedestrian on roller-skates injured in collision with railway train or railway vehicle, unspecified whether traffic or nontraffic accident**

X+7th V05.92 **Pedestrian on skateboard injured in collision with railway train or railway vehicle, unspecified whether traffic or nontraffic accident**

+ V05.93 **Pedestrian on standing micro-mobility pedestrian conveyance injured in collision with railway train or railway vehicle, unspecified whether traffic or nontraffic accident**

+7th V05.931 **Pedestrian on standing electric scooter injured in collision with railway train or railway vehicle, unspecified whether traffic or nontraffic accident**

+7th V05.938 Pedestrian on other standing micro-mobility pedestrian conveyance injured in collision with railway train or railway vehicle, unspecified whether traffic or nontraffic accident

Pedestrian on hoverboard injured in collision with railway train or railway vehicle, unspecified whether traffic or nontraffic accident

Pedestrian on segway injured in collision with railway train or railway vehicle, unspecified whether traffic or nontraffic accident

X+7th V05.99 Pedestrian with other conveyance injured in collision with railway train or railway vehicle, unspecified whether traffic or nontraffic accident

Pedestrian with baby stroller injured in collision with railway train or railway vehicle, unspecified whether traffic or nontraffic

Pedestrian on ice-skates injured in collision with railway train or railway vehicle, unspecified whether traffic or nontraffic

Pedestrian on nonmotorized scooter injured in collision with railway train or railway vehicle, unspecified whether traffic or nontraffic

Pedestrian on sled injured in collision with railway train or railway vehicle, unspecified whether traffic or nontraffic

Pedestrian on snowboard injured in collision with railway train or railway vehicle, unspecified whether traffic or nontraffic

Pedestrian on snow-skis injured in collision with railway train or railway vehicle, unspecified whether traffic or nontraffic

Pedestrian in wheelchair (powered) injured in collision with railway train or railway vehicle, unspecified whether traffic or nontraffic

Pedestrian in motorized mobility scooter injured in collision with railway train or railway vehicle, unspecified whether traffic or nontraffic

V06 Pedestrian injured in collision with other nonmotor vehicle

Includes: collision with animal-drawn vehicle, animal being ridden, nonpowered streetcar

Excludes1: *pedestrian injured in collision with pedestrian conveyance (V00.0-)*

The appropriate 7th character is to be added to each code from category V06
A   initial encounter
D   subsequent encounter
S   sequela

+ V06.0 Pedestrian injured in collision with other nonmotor vehicle in nontraffic accident

X+7th V06.00 Pedestrian on foot injured in collision with other nonmotor vehicle in nontraffic accident

Pedestrian NOS injured in collision with other nonmotor vehicle in nontraffic accident

X+7th V06.01 Pedestrian on roller-skates injured in collision with other nonmotor vehicle in nontraffic accident

X+7th V06.02 Pedestrian on skateboard injured in collision with other nonmotor vehicle in nontraffic accident

+ V06.03 Pedestrian on standing micro-mobility pedestrian conveyance injured in collision with other nonmotor vehicle in nontraffic accident

+7th V06.031 Pedestrian on standing electric scooter injured in collision with other nonmotor vehicle in nontraffic accident

+7th V06.038 Pedestrian on other standing micro-mobility pedestrian conveyance injured in collision with other nonmotor vehicle in nontraffic accident

Pedestrian on hoverboard injured in collision with other nonmotor vehicle in nontraffic accident

Pedestrian on segway injured in collision with other nonmotor vehicle in nontraffic accident

X+7th V06.09 Pedestrian with other conveyance injured in collision with other nonmotor vehicle in nontraffic accident

Pedestrian with baby stroller injured in collision with other nonmotor vehicle in nontraffic accident

Pedestrian on ice-skates injured in collision with other nonmotor vehicle in nontraffic accident

Pedestrian on nonmotorized scooter injured in collision with other nonmotor vehicle in nontraffic accident

Pedestrian on sled injured in collision with other nonmotor vehicle in nontraffic accident

Pedestrian on snowboard injured in collision with other nonmotor vehicle in nontraffic accident

Pedestrian on snow-skis injured in collision with other nonmotor vehicle in nontraffic accident

Pedestrian in wheelchair (powered) injured in collision with other nonmotor vehicle in nontraffic accident

Pedestrian in motorized mobility scooter injured in collision with other nonmotor vehicle in nontraffic accident

+ V06.1 Pedestrian injured in collision with other nonmotor vehicle in traffic accident

X+7th V06.10 Pedestrian on foot injured in collision with other nonmotor vehicle in traffic accident

Pedestrian NOS injured in collision with other nonmotor vehicle in traffic accident

X+7th V06.11 Pedestrian on roller-skates injured in collision with other nonmotor vehicle in traffic accident

X+7th V06.12 Pedestrian on skateboard injured in collision with other nonmotor vehicle in traffic accident

+ V06.13 Pedestrian on standing micro-mobility pedestrian conveyance injured in collision with other nonmotor vehicle in traffic accident

+7th V06.131 Pedestrian on standing electric scooter injured in collision with other nonmotor vehicle in traffic accident

+7th V06.138 Pedestrian on other standing micro-mobility pedestrian conveyance injured in collision with other nonmotor vehicle in traffic accident

Pedestrian on hoverboard injured in collision with other nonmotor vehicle in traffic accident

Pedestrian on segway injured in collision with other nonmotor vehicle in traffic accident

X+7th V06.19 Pedestrian with other conveyance injured in collision with other nonmotor vehicle in traffic accident

Pedestrian with baby stroller injured in collision with other nonmotor vehicle in nontraffic accident

Pedestrian on ice-skates injured in collision with other nonmotor vehicle in traffic accident

Pedestrian on nonmotorized scooter injured in collision with other nonmotor vehicle in traffic accident

Pedestrian on sled injured in collision with other nonmotor vehicle in traffic accident

Pedestrian on snowboard injured in collision with other nonmotor vehicle in traffic accident

Pedestrian on snow-skis injured in collision with other nonmotor vehicle in traffic accident

Pedestrian in wheelchair (powered) injured in collision with other nonmotor vehicle in traffic accident

Pedestrian in motorized mobility scooter injured in collision with other nonmotor vehicle in traffic accident

+ V06.9 Pedestrian injured in collision with other nonmotor vehicle, unspecified whether traffic or nontraffic accident

X+7th V06.90 Pedestrian on foot injured in collision with other nonmotor vehicle, unspecified whether traffic or nontraffic accident

Pedestrian NOS injured in collision with other nonmotor vehicle, unspecified whether traffic or nontraffic accident

+, +7th, X + 7th   ● Newborn   ● Pediatric   ● Maternity   ● Adult   ♀ Female   ♂ Male   Manifestation   Unacceptable PDX   HCC   CC   MCC   HAC

X+7th V06.91 Pedestrian on roller-skates injured in collision with other nonmotor vehicle, unspecified whether traffic or nontraffic accident

X+7th V06.92 Pedestrian on skateboard injured in collision with other nonmotor vehicle, unspecified whether traffic or nontraffic accident

+ V06.93 Pedestrian on standing micro-mobility pedestrian conveyance injured in collision with other nonmotor vehicle, unspecified whether traffic or nontraffic accident

+7th V06.931 Pedestrian on standing electric scooter injured in collision with other nonmotor vehicle, unspecified whether traffic or nontraffic accident

+7th V06.938 Pedestrian on other standing micro-mobility pedestrian conveyance injured in collision with other nonmotor vehicle, unspecified whether traffic or nontraffic accident

> Pedestrian on hoverboard injured in collision with other nonmotor vehicle, unspecified whether traffic or nontraffic accident
>
> Pedestrian on other segway injured in collision with other nonmotor vehicle, unspecified whether traffic or nontraffic accident

X+7th V06.99 Pedestrian with other conveyance injured in collision with other nonmotor vehicle, unspecified whether traffic or nontraffic accident

> Pedestrian with baby stroller injured in collision with other nonmotor vehicle, unspecified whether traffic or nontraffic accident
>
> Pedestrian on ice-skates injured in collision with other nonmotor vehicle, unspecified whether traffic or nontraffic accident
>
> Pedestrian on nonmotorized scooter injured in collision with other nonmotor vehicle, unspecified whether traffic or nontraffic accident
>
> Pedestrian on sled injured in collision with other nonmotor vehicle, unspecified whether traffic or nontraffic accident
>
> Pedestrian on snowboard injured in collision with other nonmotor vehicle, unspecified whether traffic or nontraffic accident
>
> Pedestrian on snow-skis injured in collision with other nonmotor vehicle, unspecified whether traffic or nontraffic accident
>
> Pedestrian in wheelchair (powered) injured in collision with other nonmotor vehicle, unspecified whether traffic or nontraffic accident
>
> Pedestrian in motorized mobility scooter injured in collision with other nonmotor vehicle, unspecified whether traffic or nontraffic accident

V09 Pedestrian injured in other and unspecified transport accidents

> The appropriate 7th character is to be added to each code from category V09
> A initial encounter
> D subsequent encounter
> S sequela

+ V09.0 Pedestrian injured in nontraffic accident involving other and unspecified motor vehicles

X+7th V09.00 Pedestrian injured in nontraffic accident involving unspecified motor vehicles

X+7th V09.01 Pedestrian injured in nontraffic accident involving military vehicle

X+7th V09.09 Pedestrian injured in nontraffic accident involving other motor vehicles

> Pedestrian injured in nontraffic accident by special vehicle

X+7th V09.1 Pedestrian injured in unspecified nontraffic accident

+ V09.2 Pedestrian injured in traffic accident involving other and unspecified motor vehicles

X+7th V09.20 Pedestrian injured in traffic accident involving unspecified motor vehicles

X+7th V09.21 Pedestrian injured in traffic accident involving military vehicle

X+7th V09.29 Pedestrian injured in traffic accident involving other motor vehicles

X+7th V09.3 Pedestrian injured in unspecified traffic accident

X+7th V09.9 Pedestrian injured in unspecified transport accident

Pedal cycle rider injured in transport accident (V10-V19)

Includes: any non-motorized vehicle, excluding an animal-drawn vehicle, or a sidecar or trailer attached to the pedal cycle

Excludes2: *rupture of pedal cycle tire (W37.0)*

V10 Pedal cycle rider injured in collision with pedestrian or animal

> **Excludes1:** *pedal cycle rider collision with animal-drawn vehicle or animal being ridden (V16.-)*

> The appropriate 7th character is to be added to each code from category V10
> A initial encounter
> D subsequent encounter
> S sequela

X+7th V10.0 Pedal cycle driver injured in collision with pedestrian or animal in nontraffic accident

X+7th V10.1 Pedal cycle passenger injured in collision with pedestrian or animal in nontraffic accident

X+7th V10.2 Unspecified pedal cyclist injured in collision with pedestrian or animal in nontraffic accident

X+7th V10.3 Person boarding or alighting a pedal cycle injured in collision with pedestrian or animal

X+7th V10.4 Pedal cycle driver injured in collision with pedestrian or animal in traffic accident

X+7th V10.5 Pedal cycle passenger injured in collision with pedestrian or animal in traffic accident

X+7th V10.9 Unspecified pedal cyclist injured in collision with pedestrian or animal in traffic accident

V11 Pedal cycle rider injured in collision with other pedal cycle

> The appropriate 7th character is to be added to each code from category V11
> A initial encounter
> D subsequent encounter
> S sequela

X+7th V11.0 Pedal cycle driver injured in collision with other pedal cycle in nontraffic accident

X+7th V11.1 Pedal cycle passenger injured in collision with other pedal cycle in nontraffic accident

X+7th V11.2 Unspecified pedal cyclist injured in collision with other pedal cycle in nontraffic accident

X+7th V11.3 Person boarding or alighting a pedal cycle injured in collision with other pedal cycle

X+7th V11.4 Pedal cycle driver injured in collision with other pedal cycle in traffic accident

X+7th V11.5 Pedal cycle passenger injured in collision with other pedal cycle in traffic accident

X+7th V11.9 Unspecified pedal cyclist injured in collision with other pedal cycle in traffic accident

V12 Pedal cycle rider injured in collision with two- or three-wheeled motor vehicle

> The appropriate 7th character is to be added to each code from category V12
> A initial encounter
> D subsequent encounter
> S sequela

X+7th V12.0 Pedal cycle driver injured in collision with two- or three-wheeled motor vehicle in nontraffic accident

X+7th V12.1 Pedal cycle passenger injured in collision with two- or three-wheeled motor vehicle in nontraffic accident

X+7th V12.2 Unspecified pedal cyclist injured in collision with two- or three-wheeled motor vehicle in nontraffic accident

X+7th V12.3 Person boarding or alighting a pedal cycle injured in collision with two- or three-wheeled motor vehicle

X+7th V12.4 Pedal cycle driver injured in collision with two- or three-wheeled motor vehicle in traffic accident

X+7th V12.5 Pedal cycle passenger injured in collision with two- or three-wheeled motor vehicle in traffic accident

X+7th V12.9 Unspecified pedal cyclist injured in collision with two- or three-wheeled motor vehicle in traffic accident

V13 **Pedal cycle rider injured in collision with car, pick-up truck or van**

> The appropriate 7th character is to be added to each code from category V13
> A   initial encounter
> D   subsequent encounter
> S   sequela

X+7th **V13.0** Pedal cycle driver injured in collision with car, pick-up truck or van in nontraffic accident

X+7th **V13.1** Pedal cycle passenger injured in collision with car, pick-up truck or van in nontraffic accident

X+7th **V13.2** Unspecified pedal cyclist injured in collision with car, pick-up truck or van in nontraffic accident

X+7th **V13.3** Person boarding or alighting a pedal cycle injured in collision with car, pick-up truck or van

X+7th **V13.4** Pedal cycle driver injured in collision with car, pick-up truck or van in traffic accident

X+7th **V13.5** Pedal cycle passenger injured in collision with car, pick-up truck or van in traffic accident

X+7th **V13.9** Unspecified pedal cyclist injured in collision with car, pick-up truck or van in traffic accident

V14 **Pedal cycle rider injured in collision with heavy transport vehicle or bus**

> **Excludes1:** *pedal cycle rider injured in collision with military vehicle (V19.81)*

> The appropriate 7th character is to be added to each code from category V14
> A   initial encounter
> D   subsequent encounter
> S   sequela

X+7th **V14.0** Pedal cycle driver injured in collision with heavy transport vehicle or bus in nontraffic accident

X+7th **V14.1** Pedal cycle passenger injured in collision with heavy transport vehicle or bus in nontraffic accident

X+7th **V14.2** Unspecified pedal cyclist injured in collision with heavy transport vehicle or bus in nontraffic accident

X+7th **V14.3** Person boarding or alighting a pedal cycle injured in collision with heavy transport vehicle or bus

X+7th **V14.4** Pedal cycle driver injured in collision with heavy transport vehicle or bus in traffic accident

X+7th **V14.5** Pedal cycle passenger injured in collision with heavy transport vehicle or bus in traffic accident

X+7th **V14.9** Unspecified pedal cyclist injured in collision with heavy transport vehicle or bus in traffic accident

V15 **Pedal cycle rider injured in collision with railway train or railway vehicle**

> The appropriate 7th character is to be added to each code from category V15
> A   initial encounter
> D   subsequent encounter
> S   sequela

X+7th **V15.0** Pedal cycle driver injured in collision with railway train or railway vehicle in nontraffic accident

X+7th **V15.1** Pedal cycle passenger injured in collision with railway train or railway vehicle in nontraffic accident

X+7th **V15.2** Unspecified pedal cyclist injured in collision with railway train or railway vehicle in nontraffic accident

X+7th **V15.3** Person boarding or alighting a pedal cycle injured in collision with railway train or railway vehicle

X+7th **V15.4** Pedal cycle driver injured in collision with railway train or railway vehicle in traffic accident

X+7th **V15.5** Pedal cycle passenger injured in collision with railway train or railway vehicle in traffic accident

X+7th **V15.9** Unspecified pedal cyclist injured in collision with railway train or railway vehicle in traffic accident

V16 **Pedal cycle rider injured in collision with other nonmotor vehicle**

> **Includes:** collision with animal-drawn vehicle, animal being ridden, streetcar

> The appropriate 7th character is to be added to each code from category V16
> A   initial encounter
> D   subsequent encounter
> S   sequela

X+7th **V16.0** Pedal cycle driver injured in collision with other nonmotor vehicle in nontraffic accident

X+7th **V16.1** Pedal cycle passenger injured in collision with other nonmotor vehicle in nontraffic accident

X+7th **V16.2** Unspecified pedal cyclist injured in collision with other nonmotor vehicle in nontraffic accident

X+7th **V16.3** Person boarding or alighting a pedal cycle injured in collision with other nonmotor vehicle in nontraffic accident

X+7th **V16.4** Pedal cycle driver injured in collision with other nonmotor vehicle in traffic accident

X+7th **V16.5** Pedal cycle passenger injured in collision with other nonmotor vehicle in traffic accident

X+7th **V16.9** Unspecified pedal cyclist injured in collision with other nonmotor vehicle in traffic accident

V17 **Pedal cycle rider injured in collision with fixed or stationary object**

> The appropriate 7th character is to be added to each code from category V17
> A   initial encounter
> D   subsequent encounter
> S   sequela

X+7th **V17.0** Pedal cycle driver injured in collision with fixed or stationary object in nontraffic accident

X+7th **V17.1** Pedal cycle passenger injured in collision with fixed or stationary object in nontraffic accident

X+7th **V17.2** Unspecified pedal cyclist injured in collision with fixed or stationary object in nontraffic accident

X+7th **V17.3** Person boarding or alighting a pedal cycle injured in collision with fixed or stationary object

X+7th **V17.4** Pedal cycle driver injured in collision with fixed or stationary object in traffic accident

X+7th **V17.5** Pedal cycle passenger injured in collision with fixed or stationary object in traffic accident

X+7th **V17.9** Unspecified pedal cyclist injured in collision with fixed or stationary object in traffic accident

V18 **Pedal cycle rider injured in noncollision transport accident**

> **Includes:** fall or thrown from pedal cycle (without antecedent collision)
> overturning pedal cycle NOS
> overturning pedal cycle without collision

> The appropriate 7th character is to be added to each code from category V18
> A   initial encounter
> D   subsequent encounter
> S   sequela

X+7th **V18.0** Pedal cycle driver injured in noncollision transport accident in nontraffic accident

X+7th **V18.1** Pedal cycle passenger injured in noncollision transport accident in nontraffic accident

X+7th **V18.2** Unspecified pedal cyclist injured in noncollision transport accident in nontraffic accident

X+7th **V18.3** Person boarding or alighting a pedal cycle injured in noncollision transport accident

X+7th **V18.4** Pedal cycle driver injured in noncollision transport accident in traffic accident

X+7th **V18.5** Pedal cycle passenger injured in noncollision transport accident in traffic accident

X+7th **V18.9** Unspecified pedal cyclist injured in noncollision transport accident in traffic accident

V19 **Pedal cycle rider injured in other and unspecified transport accidents**

> The appropriate 7th character is to be added to each code from category V19
> A   initial encounter
> D   subsequent encounter
> S   sequela

+ **V19.0** Pedal cycle driver injured in collision with other and unspecified motor vehicles in nontraffic accident

X+7th **V19.00** Pedal cycle driver injured in collision with unspecified motor vehicles in nontraffic accident

X+7th **V19.09** Pedal cycle driver injured in collision with other motor vehicles in nontraffic accident

+ **V19.1** Pedal cycle passenger injured in collision with other and unspecified motor vehicles in nontraffic accident

X+7th **V19.10** Pedal cycle passenger injured in collision with unspecified motor vehicles in nontraffic accident

X+7th **V19.19** Pedal cycle passenger injured in collision with other motor vehicles in nontraffic accident

+ V19.2 Unspecified pedal cyclist injured in collision with other and unspecified motor vehicles in nontraffic accident

X+7th **V19.20 Unspecified pedal cyclist injured in collision with unspecified motor vehicles in nontraffic accident**
Pedal cycle collision NOS, nontraffic

X+7th **V19.29 Unspecified pedal cyclist injured in collision with other motor vehicles in nontraffic accident**

X+7th **V19.3 Pedal cyclist (driver) (passenger) injured in unspecified nontraffic accident**
Pedal cycle accident NOS, nontraffic
Pedal cyclist injured in nontraffic accident NOS

+ V19.4 Pedal cycle driver injured in collision with other and unspecified motor vehicles in traffic accident

X+7th **V19.40 Pedal cycle driver injured in collision with unspecified motor vehicles in traffic accident**

X+7th **V19.49 Pedal cycle driver injured in collision with other motor vehicles in traffic accident**

+ V19.5 Pedal cycle passenger injured in collision with other and unspecified motor vehicles in traffic accident

X+7th **V19.50 Pedal cycle passenger injured in collision with unspecified motor vehicles in traffic accident**

X+7th **V19.59 Pedal cycle passenger injured in collision with other motor vehicles in traffic accident**

+ V19.6 Unspecified pedal cyclist injured in collision with other and unspecified motor vehicles in traffic accident

X+7th **V19.60 Unspecified pedal cyclist injured in collision with unspecified motor vehicles in traffic accident**
Pedal cycle collision NOS (traffic)

X+7th **V19.69 Unspecified pedal cyclist injured in collision with other motor vehicles in traffic accident**

+ V19.8 Pedal cyclist (driver) (passenger) injured in other specified transport accidents

X+7th **V19.81 Pedal cyclist (driver) (passenger) injured in transport accident with military vehicle**

X+7th **V19.88 Pedal cyclist (driver) (passenger) injured in other specified transport accidents**

X+7th **V19.9 Pedal cyclist (driver) (passenger) injured in unspecified traffic accident**
Pedal cycle accident NOS

Motorcycle rider injured in transport accident (V20-V29)

Includes: moped
motorcycle with sidecar
motorized bicycle
motor scooter

Excludes1: *three-wheeled motor vehicle (V30-V39)*

V20 Motorcycle rider injured in collision with pedestrian or animal

> ***Excludes1:*** *motorcycle rider collision with animal-drawn vehicle or animal being ridden (V26.-)*

> The appropriate 7th character is to be added to each code from category V20
> A   initial encounter
> D   subsequent encounter
> S   sequela

X+7th **V20.0 Motorcycle driver injured in collision with pedestrian or animal in nontraffic accident**

X+7th **V20.1 Motorcycle passenger injured in collision with pedestrian or animal in nontraffic accident**

X+7th **V20.2 Unspecified motorcycle rider injured in collision with pedestrian or animal in nontraffic accident**

X+7th **V20.3 Person boarding or alighting a motorcycle injured in collision with pedestrian or animal**

X+7th **V20.4 Motorcycle driver injured in collision with pedestrian or animal in traffic accident**

X+7th **V20.5 Motorcycle passenger injured in collision with pedestrian or animal in traffic accident**

X+7th **V20.9 Unspecified motorcycle rider injured in collision with pedestrian or animal in traffic accident**

V21 Motorcycle rider injured in collision with pedal cycle

> The appropriate 7th character is to be added to each code from category V21
> A   initial encounter
> D   subsequent encounter
> S   sequela

X+7th **V21.0 Motorcycle driver injured in collision with pedal cycle in nontraffic accident**

X+7th **V21.1 Motorcycle passenger injured in collision with pedal cycle in nontraffic accident**

X+7th **V21.2 Unspecified motorcycle rider injured in collision with pedal cycle in nontraffic accident**

X+7th **V21.3 Person boarding or alighting a motorcycle injured in collision with pedal cycle**

X+7th **V21.4 Motorcycle driver injured in collision with pedal cycle in traffic accident**

X+7th **V21.5 Motorcycle passenger injured in collision with pedal cycle in traffic accident**

X+7th **V21.9 Unspecified motorcycle rider injured in collision with pedal cycle in traffic accident**

V22 Motorcycle rider injured in collision with two- or three-wheeled motor vehicle

> The appropriate 7th character is to be added to each code from category V22
> A   initial encounter
> D   subsequent encounter
> S   sequela

X+7th **V22.0 Motorcycle driver injured in collision with two- or three-wheeled motor vehicle in nontraffic accident**

X+7th **V22.1 Motorcycle passenger injured in collision with two- or three-wheeled motor vehicle in nontraffic accident**

X+7th **V22.2 Unspecified motorcycle rider injured in collision with two- or three-wheeled motor vehicle in nontraffic accident**

X+7th **V22.3 Person boarding or alighting a motorcycle injured in collision with two- or three-wheeled motor vehicle**

X+7th **V22.4 Motorcycle driver injured in collision with two- or three-wheeled motor vehicle in traffic accident**

X+7th **V22.5 Motorcycle passenger injured in collision with two- or three-wheeled motor vehicle in traffic accident**

X+7th **V22.9 Unspecified motorcycle rider injured in collision with two- or three-wheeled motor vehicle in traffic accident**

V23 Motorcycle rider injured in collision with car, pick-up truck or van

> The appropriate 7th character is to be added to each code from category V23
> A   initial encounter
> D   subsequent encounter
> S   sequela

X+7th **V23.0 Motorcycle driver injured in collision with car, pick-up truck or van in nontraffic accident**

X+7th **V23.1 Motorcycle passenger injured in collision with car, pick-up truck or van in nontraffic accident**

X+7th **V23.2 Unspecified motorcycle rider injured in collision with car, pick-up truck or van in nontraffic accident**

X+7th **V23.3 Person boarding or alighting a motorcycle injured in collision with car, pick-up truck or van**

X+7th **V23.4 Motorcycle driver injured in collision with car, pick-up truck or van in traffic accident**

X+7th **V23.5 Motorcycle passenger injured in collision with car, pick-up truck or van in traffic accident**

X+7th **V23.9 Unspecified motorcycle rider injured in collision with car, pick-up truck or van in traffic accident**

V24 Motorcycle rider injured in collision with heavy transport vehicle or bus

> ***Excludes1:*** *motorcycle rider injured in collision with military vehicle (V29.81)*

> The appropriate 7th character is to be added to each code from category V24
> A   initial encounter
> D   subsequent encounter
> S   sequela

X+7th **V24.0 Motorcycle driver injured in collision with heavy transport vehicle or bus in nontraffic accident**

X+7th **V24.1 Motorcycle passenger injured in collision with heavy transport vehicle or bus in nontraffic accident**

X+7th **V24.2 Unspecified motorcycle rider injured in collision with heavy transport vehicle or bus in nontraffic accident**

X+7th **V24.3 Person boarding or alighting a motorcycle injured in collision with heavy transport vehicle or bus**

X+7th **V24.4 Motorcycle driver injured in collision with heavy transport vehicle or bus in traffic accident**

X+7th **V24.5 Motorcycle passenger injured in collision with heavy transport vehicle or bus in traffic accident**

X+7th **V24.9 Unspecified motorcycle rider injured in collision with heavy transport vehicle or bus in traffic accident**

V25 Motorcycle rider injured in collision with railway train or railway vehicle

> The appropriate 7th character is to be added to each code from category V25
> A   initial encounter
> D   subsequent encounter
> S   sequela

X+7th **V25.0 Motorcycle driver injured in collision with railway train or railway vehicle in nontraffic accident**

X+7th **V25.1 Motorcycle passenger injured in collision with railway train or railway vehicle in nontraffic accident**

X+7th **V25.2 Unspecified motorcycle rider injured in collision with railway train or railway vehicle in nontraffic accident**

X+7th **V25.3 Person boarding or alighting a motorcycle injured in collision with railway train or railway vehicle**

X+7th **V25.4 Motorcycle driver injured in collision with railway train or railway vehicle in traffic accident**

X+7th **V25.5 Motorcycle passenger injured in collision with railway train or railway vehicle in traffic accident**

X+7th **V25.9 Unspecified motorcycle rider injured in collision with railway train or railway vehicle in traffic accident**

V26 Motorcycle rider injured in collision with other nonmotor vehicle

> **Includes:** collision with animal-drawn vehicle, animal being ridden, streetcar

> The appropriate 7th character is to be added to each code from category V26
> A   initial encounter
> D   subsequent encounter
> S   sequela

X+7th **V26.0 Motorcycle driver injured in collision with other nonmotor vehicle in nontraffic accident**

X+7th **V26.1 Motorcycle passenger injured in collision with other nonmotor vehicle in nontraffic accident**

X+7th **V26.2 Unspecified motorcycle rider injured in collision with other nonmotor vehicle in nontraffic accident**

X+7th **V26.3 Person boarding or alighting a motorcycle injured in collision with other nonmotor vehicle**

X+7th **V26.4 Motorcycle driver injured in collision with other nonmotor vehicle in traffic accident**

X+7th **V26.5 Motorcycle passenger injured in collision with other nonmotor vehicle in traffic accident**

X+7th **V26.9 Unspecified motorcycle rider injured in collision with other nonmotor vehicle in traffic accident**

V27 Motorcycle rider injured in collision with fixed or stationary object

> The appropriate 7th character is to be added to each code from category V27
> A   initial encounter
> D   subsequent encounter
> S   sequela

X+7th **V27.0 Motorcycle driver injured in collision with fixed or stationary object in nontraffic accident**

X+7th **V27.1 Motorcycle passenger injured in collision with fixed or stationary object in nontraffic accident**

X+7th **V27.2 Unspecified motorcycle rider injured in collision with fixed or stationary object in nontraffic accident**

X+7th **V27.3 Person boarding or alighting a motorcycle injured in collision with fixed or stationary object**

X+7th **V27.4 Motorcycle driver injured in collision with fixed or stationary object in traffic accident**

X+7th **V27.5 Motorcycle passenger injured in collision with fixed or stationary object in traffic accident**

X+7th **V27.9 Unspecified motorcycle rider injured in collision with fixed or stationary object in traffic accident**

V28 Motorcycle rider injured in noncollision transport accident

> **Includes:** fall or thrown from motorcycle (without antecedent collision)
> overturning motorcycle NOS
> overturning motorcycle without collision

> The appropriate 7th character is to be added to each code from category V28
> A   initial encounter
> D   subsequent encounter
> S   sequela

X+7th **V28.0 Motorcycle driver injured in noncollision transport accident in nontraffic accident**

X+7th **V28.1 Motorcycle passenger injured in noncollision transport accident in nontraffic accident**

X+7th **V28.2 Unspecified motorcycle rider injured in noncollision transport accident in nontraffic accident**

X+7th **V28.3 Person boarding or alighting a motorcycle injured in noncollision transport accident**

X+7th **V28.4 Motorcycle driver injured in noncollision transport accident in traffic accident**

X+7th **V28.5 Motorcycle passenger injured in noncollision transport accident in traffic accident**

X+7th **V28.9 Unspecified motorcycle rider injured in noncollision transport accident in traffic accident**

V29 Motorcycle rider injured in other and unspecified transport accidents

> The appropriate 7th character is to be added to each code from category V29
> A   initial encounter
> D   subsequent encounter
> S   sequela

+ **V29.0 Motorcycle driver injured in collision with other and unspecified motor vehicles in nontraffic accident**

X+7th **V29.00 Motorcycle driver injured in collision with unspecified motor vehicles in nontraffic accident**

X+7th **V29.09 Motorcycle driver injured in collision with other motor vehicles in nontraffic accident**

+ **V29.1 Motorcycle passenger injured in collision with other and unspecified motor vehicles in nontraffic accident**

X+7th **V29.10 Motorcycle passenger injured in collision with unspecified motor vehicles in nontraffic accident**

X+7th **V29.19 Motorcycle passenger injured in collision with other motor vehicles in nontraffic accident**

+ **V29.2 Unspecified motorcycle rider injured in collision with other and unspecified motor vehicles in nontraffic accident**

X+7th **V29.20 Unspecified motorcycle rider injured in collision with unspecified motor vehicles in nontraffic accident**
> Motorcycle collision NOS, nontraffic

X+7th **V29.29 Unspecified motorcycle rider injured in collision with other motor vehicles in nontraffic accident**

X+7th **V29.3 Motorcycle rider (driver) (passenger) injured in unspecified nontraffic accident**
> Motorcycle accident NOS, nontraffic
> Motorcycle rider injured in nontraffic accident NOS

+ **V29.4 Motorcycle driver injured in collision with other and unspecified motor vehicles in traffic accident**

X+7th **V29.40 Motorcycle driver injured in collision with unspecified motor vehicles in traffic accident**

X+7th **V29.49 Motorcycle driver injured in collision with other motor vehicles in traffic accident**

+ **V29.5 Motorcycle passenger injured in collision with other and unspecified motor vehicles in traffic accident**

X+7th **V29.50 Motorcycle passenger injured in collision with unspecified motor vehicles in traffic accident**

X+7th **V29.59 Motorcycle passenger injured in collision with other motor vehicles in traffic accident**

+ **V29.6 Unspecified motorcycle rider injured in collision with other and unspecified motor vehicles in traffic accident**

X+7th **V29.60 Unspecified motorcycle rider injured in collision with unspecified motor vehicles in traffic accident**
> Motorcycle collision NOS (traffic)

X+7th **V29.69 Unspecified motorcycle rider injured in collision with other motor vehicles in traffic accident**

+ **V29.8 Motorcycle rider (driver) (passenger) injured in other specified transport accidents**

X+7th **V29.81 Motorcycle rider (driver) (passenger) injured in transport accident with military vehicle**

X+7th **V29.88 Motorcycle rider (driver) (passenger) injured in other specified transport accidents**

X+7th **V29.9 Motorcycle rider (driver) (passenger) injured in unspecified traffic accident**
> Motorcycle accident NOS

+, +7th, X + 7th   ● Newborn   ● Pediatric   ● Maternity   ● Adult   ♀ Female   ♂ Male   Manifestation   Unacceptable PDX   HCC   CC   MCC   HAC

Occupant of three-wheeled motor vehicle injured in transport accident (V30-V39)

Includes: motorized tricycle
motorized rickshaw
three-wheeled motor car

Excludes1: *all-terrain vehicles (V86.-)*
motorcycle with sidecar (V20-V29)
vehicle designed primarily for off-road use (V86.-)

V30 **Occupant of three-wheeled motor vehicle injured in collision with pedestrian or animal**

> **Excludes1:** *three-wheeled motor vehicle collision with animal-drawn vehicle or animal being ridden (V36.-)*

> The appropriate 7th character is to be added to each code from category V30
> A   initial encounter
> D   subsequent encounter
> S   sequela

X+7th **V30.0** **Driver of three-wheeled motor vehicle injured in collision with pedestrian or animal in nontraffic accident**

X+7th **V30.1** **Passenger in three-wheeled motor vehicle injured in collision with pedestrian or animal in nontraffic accident**

X+7th **V30.2** **Person on outside of three-wheeled motor vehicle injured in collision with pedestrian or animal in nontraffic accident**

X+7th **V30.3** **Unspecified occupant of three-wheeled motor vehicle injured in collision with pedestrian or animal in nontraffic accident**

X+7th **V30.4** **Person boarding or alighting a three-wheeled motor vehicle injured in collision with pedestrian or animal**

X+7th **V30.5** **Driver of three-wheeled motor vehicle injured in collision with pedestrian or animal in traffic accident**

X+7th **V30.6** **Passenger in three-wheeled motor vehicle injured in collision with pedestrian or animal in traffic accident**

X+7th **V30.7** **Person on outside of three-wheeled motor vehicle injured in collision with pedestrian or animal in traffic accident**

X+7th **V30.9** **Unspecified occupant of three-wheeled motor vehicle injured in collision with pedestrian or animal in traffic accident**

V31 **Occupant of three-wheeled motor vehicle injured in collision with pedal cycle**

> The appropriate 7th character is to be added to each code from category V31
> A   initial encounter
> D   subsequent encounter
> S   sequela

X+7th **V31.0** **Driver of three-wheeled motor vehicle injured in collision with pedal cycle in nontraffic accident**

X+7th **V31.1** **Passenger in three-wheeled motor vehicle injured in collision with pedal cycle in nontraffic accident**

X+7th **V31.2** **Person on outside of three-wheeled motor vehicle injured in collision with pedal cycle in nontraffic accident**

X+7th **V31.3** **Unspecified occupant of three-wheeled motor vehicle injured in collision with pedal cycle in nontraffic accident**

X+7th **V31.4** **Person boarding or alighting a three-wheeled motor vehicle injured in collision with pedal cycle**

X+7th **V31.5** **Driver of three-wheeled motor vehicle injured in collision with pedal cycle in traffic accident**

X+7th **V31.6** **Passenger in three-wheeled motor vehicle injured in collision with pedal cycle in traffic accident**

X+7th **V31.7** **Person on outside of three-wheeled motor vehicle injured in collision with pedal cycle in traffic accident**

X+7th **V31.9** **Unspecified occupant of three-wheeled motor vehicle injured in collision with pedal cycle in traffic accident**

V32 **Occupant of three-wheeled motor vehicle injured in collision with two- or three-wheeled motor vehicle**

> The appropriate 7th character is to be added to each code from category V32
> A   initial encounter
> D   subsequent encounter
> S   sequela

X+7th **V32.0** **Driver of three-wheeled motor vehicle injured in collision with two- or three-wheeled motor vehicle in nontraffic accident**

X+7th **V32.1** **Passenger in three-wheeled motor vehicle injured in collision with two- or three-wheeled motor vehicle in nontraffic accident**

X+7th **V32.2** **Person on outside of three-wheeled motor vehicle injured in collision with two- or three-wheeled motor vehicle in nontraffic accident**

X+7th **V32.3** **Unspecified occupant of three-wheeled motor vehicle injured in collision with two- or three-wheeled motor vehicle in nontraffic accident**

X+7th **V32.4** **Person boarding or alighting a three-wheeled motor vehicle injured in collision with two- or three-wheeled motor vehicle**

X+7th **V32.5** **Driver of three-wheeled motor vehicle injured in collision with two- or three-wheeled motor vehicle in traffic accident**

X+7th **V32.6** **Passenger in three-wheeled motor vehicle injured in collision with two- or three-wheeled motor vehicle in traffic accident**

X+7th **V32.7** **Person on outside of three-wheeled motor vehicle injured in collision with two- or three-wheeled motor vehicle in traffic accident**

X+7th **V32.9** **Unspecified occupant of three-wheeled motor vehicle injured in collision with two- or three-wheeled motor vehicle in traffic accident**

V33 **Occupant of three-wheeled motor vehicle injured in collision with car, pick-up truck or van**

> The appropriate 7th character is to be added to each code from category V33
> A   initial encounter
> D   subsequent encounter
> S   sequela

X+7th **V33.0** **Driver of three-wheeled motor vehicle injured in collision with car, pick-up truck or van in nontraffic accident**

X+7th **V33.1** **Passenger in three-wheeled motor vehicle injured in collision with car, pick-up truck or van in nontraffic accident**

X+7th **V33.2** **Person on outside of three-wheeled motor vehicle injured in collision with car, pick-up truck or van in nontraffic accident**

X+7th **V33.3** **Unspecified occupant of three-wheeled motor vehicle injured in collision with car, pick-up truck or van in nontraffic accident**

X+7th **V33.4** **Person boarding or alighting a three-wheeled motor vehicle injured in collision with car, pick-up truck or van**

X+7th **V33.5** **Driver of three-wheeled motor vehicle injured in collision with car, pick-up truck or van in traffic accident**

X+7th **V33.6** **Passenger in three-wheeled motor vehicle injured in collision with car, pick-up truck or van in traffic accident**

X+7th **V33.7** **Person on outside of three-wheeled motor vehicle injured in collision with car, pick-up truck or van in traffic accident**

X+7th **V33.9** **Unspecified occupant of three-wheeled motor vehicle injured in collision with car, pick-up truck or van in traffic accident**

V34 **Occupant of three-wheeled motor vehicle injured in collision with heavy transport vehicle or bus**

> **Excludes1:** *occupant of three-wheeled motor vehicle injured in collision with military vehicle (V39.81)*

> The appropriate 7th character is to be added to each code from category V34
> A   initial encounter
> D   subsequent encounter
> S   sequela

X+7th **V34.0** **Driver of three-wheeled motor vehicle injured in collision with heavy transport vehicle or bus in nontraffic accident**

X+7th **V34.1** **Passenger in three-wheeled motor vehicle injured in collision with heavy transport vehicle or bus in nontraffic accident**

X+7th **V34.2** **Person on outside of three-wheeled motor vehicle injured in collision with heavy transport vehicle or bus in nontraffic accident**

X+7th **V34.3** **Unspecified occupant of three-wheeled motor vehicle injured in collision with heavy transport vehicle or bus in nontraffic accident**

X+7th **V34.4** **Person boarding or alighting a three-wheeled motor vehicle injured in collision with heavy transport vehicle or bus**

X+7th **V34.5** **Driver of three-wheeled motor vehicle injured in collision with heavy transport vehicle or bus in traffic accident**

X+7th **V34.6** **Passenger in three-wheeled motor vehicle injured in collision with heavy transport vehicle or bus in traffic accident**

X+7th **V34.7** **Person on outside of three-wheeled motor vehicle injured in collision with heavy transport vehicle or bus in traffic accident**

X+7th **V34.9** **Unspecified occupant of three-wheeled motor vehicle injured in collision with heavy transport vehicle or bus in traffic accident**

V35 Occupant of three-wheeled motor vehicle injured in collision with railway train or railway vehicle

The appropriate 7th character is to be added to each code from category V35
A initial encounter
D subsequent encounter
S sequela

X+7th **V35.0 Driver of three-wheeled motor vehicle injured in collision with railway train or railway vehicle in nontraffic accident**

X+7th **V35.1 Passenger in three-wheeled motor vehicle injured in collision with railway train or railway vehicle in nontraffic accident**

X+7th **V35.2 Person on outside of three-wheeled motor vehicle injured in collision with railway train or railway vehicle in nontraffic accident**

X+7th **V35.3 Unspecified occupant of three-wheeled motor vehicle injured in collision with railway train or railway vehicle in nontraffic accident**

X+7th **V35.4 Person boarding or alighting a three-wheeled motor vehicle injured in collision with railway train or railway vehicle**

X+7th **V35.5 Driver of three-wheeled motor vehicle injured in collision with railway train or railway vehicle in traffic accident**

X+7th **V35.6 Passenger in three-wheeled motor vehicle injured in collision with railway train or railway vehicle in traffic accident**

X+7th **V35.7 Person on outside of three-wheeled motor vehicle injured in collision with railway train or railway vehicle in traffic accident**

X+7th **V35.9 Unspecified occupant of three-wheeled motor vehicle injured in collision with railway train or railway vehicle in traffic accident**

V36 Occupant of three-wheeled motor vehicle injured in collision with other nonmotor vehicle

Includes: collision with animal-drawn vehicle, animal being ridden, streetcar

The appropriate 7th character is to be added to each code from category V36
A initial encounter
D subsequent encounter
S sequela

X+7th **V36.0 Driver of three-wheeled motor vehicle injured in collision with other nonmotor vehicle in nontraffic accident**

X+7th **V36.1 Passenger in three-wheeled motor vehicle injured in collision with other nonmotor vehicle in nontraffic accident**

X+7th **V36.2 Person on outside of three-wheeled motor vehicle injured in collision with other nonmotor vehicle in nontraffic accident**

X+7th **V36.3 Unspecified occupant of three-wheeled motor vehicle injured in collision with other nonmotor vehicle in nontraffic accident**

X+7th **V36.4 Person boarding or alighting a three-wheeled motor vehicle injured in collision with other nonmotor vehicle**

X+7th **V36.5 Driver of three-wheeled motor vehicle injured in collision with other nonmotor vehicle in traffic accident**

X+7th **V36.6 Passenger in three-wheeled motor vehicle injured in collision with other nonmotor vehicle in traffic accident**

X+7th **V36.7 Person on outside of three-wheeled motor vehicle injured in collision with other nonmotor vehicle in traffic accident**

X+7th **V36.9 Unspecified occupant of three-wheeled motor vehicle injured in collision with other nonmotor vehicle in traffic accident**

V37 Occupant of three-wheeled motor vehicle injured in collision with fixed or stationary object

The appropriate 7th character is to be added to each code from category V37
A initial encounter
D subsequent encounter
S sequela

X+7th **V37.0 Driver of three-wheeled motor vehicle injured in collision with fixed or stationary object in nontraffic accident**

X+7th **V37.1 Passenger in three-wheeled motor vehicle injured in collision with fixed or stationary object in nontraffic accident**

X+7th **V37.2 Person on outside of three-wheeled motor vehicle injured in collision with fixed or stationary object in nontraffic accident**

X+7th **V37.3 Unspecified occupant of three-wheeled motor vehicle injured in collision with fixed or stationary object in nontraffic accident**

X+7th **V37.4 Person boarding or alighting a three-wheeled motor vehicle injured in collision with fixed or stationary object**

X+7th **V37.5 Driver of three-wheeled motor vehicle injured in collision with fixed or stationary object in traffic accident**

X+7th **V37.6 Passenger in three-wheeled motor vehicle injured in collision with fixed or stationary object in traffic accident**

X+7th **V37.7 Person on outside of three-wheeled motor vehicle injured in collision with fixed or stationary object in traffic accident**

X+7th **V37.9 Unspecified occupant of three-wheeled motor vehicle injured in collision with fixed or stationary object in traffic accident**

V38 Occupant of three-wheeled motor vehicle injured in noncollision transport accident

Includes: fall or thrown from three-wheeled motor vehicle
overturning of three-wheeled motor vehicle NOS
overturning of three-wheeled motor vehicle without collision

The appropriate 7th character is to be added to each code from category V38
A initial encounter
D subsequent encounter
S sequela

X+7th **V38.0 Driver of three-wheeled motor vehicle injured in noncollision transport accident in nontraffic accident**

X+7th **V38.1 Passenger in three-wheeled motor vehicle injured in noncollision transport accident in nontraffic accident**

X+7th **V38.2 Person on outside of three-wheeled motor vehicle injured in noncollision transport accident in nontraffic accident**

X+7th **V38.3 Unspecified occupant of three-wheeled motor vehicle injured in noncollision transport accident in nontraffic accident**

X+7th **V38.4 Person boarding or alighting a three-wheeled motor vehicle injured in noncollision transport accident**

X+7th **V38.5 Driver of three-wheeled motor vehicle injured in noncollision transport accident in traffic accident**

X+7th **V38.6 Passenger in three-wheeled motor vehicle injured in noncollision transport accident in traffic accident**

X+7th **V38.7 Person on outside of three-wheeled motor vehicle injured in noncollision transport accident in traffic accident**

X+7th **V38.9 Unspecified occupant of three-wheeled motor vehicle injured in noncollision transport accident in traffic accident**

V39 Occupant of three-wheeled motor vehicle injured in other and unspecified transport accidents

The appropriate 7th character is to be added to each code from category V39
A initial encounter
D subsequent encounter
S sequela

+ **V39.0 Driver of three-wheeled motor vehicle injured in collision with other and unspecified motor vehicles in nontraffic accident**

X+7th **V39.00 Driver of three-wheeled motor vehicle injured in collision with unspecified motor vehicles in nontraffic accident**

X+7th **V39.09 Driver of three-wheeled motor vehicle injured in collision with other motor vehicles in nontraffic accident**

+ **V39.1 Passenger in three-wheeled motor vehicle injured in collision with other and unspecified motor vehicles in nontraffic accident**

X+7th **V39.10 Passenger in three-wheeled motor vehicle injured in collision with unspecified motor vehicles in nontraffic accident**

X+7th **V39.19 Passenger in three-wheeled motor vehicle injured in collision with other motor vehicles in nontraffic accident**

+ **V39.2 Unspecified occupant of three-wheeled motor vehicle injured in collision with other and unspecified motor vehicles in nontraffic accident**

X+7th **V39.20 Unspecified occupant of three-wheeled motor vehicle injured in collision with unspecified motor vehicles in nontraffic accident**
Collision NOS involving three-wheeled motor vehicle, nontraffic

X+7th **V39.29 Unspecified occupant of three-wheeled motor vehicle injured in collision with other motor vehicles in nontraffic accident**

+, +7th, X + 7th   ● Newborn   ● Pediatric   ● Maternity   ● Adult   ♀ Female   ♂ Male   Manifestation   Unacceptable PDX   HCC   CC   MCC   HAC

X+7th V39.3 **Occupant (driver) (passenger) of three-wheeled motor vehicle injured in unspecified nontraffic accident**

> Accident NOS involving three-wheeled motor vehicle, nontraffic
>
> Occupant of three-wheeled motor vehicle injured in nontraffic accident NOS

+ V39.4 **Driver of three-wheeled motor vehicle injured in collision with other and unspecified motor vehicles in traffic accident**

X+7th V39.40 **Driver of three-wheeled motor vehicle injured in collision with unspecified motor vehicles in traffic accident**

X+7th V39.49 **Driver of three-wheeled motor vehicle injured in collision with other motor vehicles in traffic accident**

+ V39.5 **Passenger in three-wheeled motor vehicle injured in collision with other and unspecified motor vehicles in traffic accident**

X+7th V39.50 **Passenger in three-wheeled motor vehicle injured in collision with unspecified motor vehicles in traffic accident**

X+7th V39.59 **Passenger in three-wheeled motor vehicle injured in collision with other motor vehicles in traffic accident**

+ V39.6 **Unspecified occupant of three-wheeled motor vehicle injured in collision with other and unspecified motor vehicles in traffic accident**

X+7th V39.60 **Unspecified occupant of three-wheeled motor vehicle injured in collision with unspecified motor vehicles in traffic accident**

> Collision NOS involving three-wheeled motor vehicle (traffic)

X+7th V39.69 **Unspecified occupant of three-wheeled motor vehicle injured in collision with other motor vehicles in traffic accident**

+ V39.8 **Occupant (driver) (passenger) of three-wheeled motor vehicle injured in other specified transport accidents**

X+7th V39.81 **Occupant (driver) (passenger) of three-wheeled motor vehicle injured in transport accident with military vehicle**

X+7th V39.89 **Occupant (driver) (passenger) of three-wheeled motor vehicle injured in other specified transport accidents**

X+7th V39.9 **Occupant (driver) (passenger) of three-wheeled motor vehicle injured in unspecified traffic accident**

> Accident NOS involving three-wheeled motor vehicle

Car occupant injured in transport accident (V40-V49)

Includes: a four-wheeled motor vehicle designed primarily for carrying passengers
automobile (pulling a trailer or camper)

Excludes1: *bus (V50-V59)*
minibus (V50-V59)
minivan (V50-V59)
motorcoach (V70-V79)
pick-up truck (V50-V59)
sport utility vehicle (SUV) (V50-V59)

V40 **Car occupant injured in collision with pedestrian or animal**

> **Excludes1:** *car collision with animal-drawn vehicle or animal being ridden (V46.-)*

> The appropriate 7th character is to be added to each code from category V40
> A   initial encounter
> D   subsequent encounter
> S   sequela

X+7th V40.0 **Car driver injured in collision with pedestrian or animal in nontraffic accident**

X+7th V40.1 **Car passenger injured in collision with pedestrian or animal in nontraffic accident**

X+7th V40.2 **Person on outside of car injured in collision with pedestrian or animal in nontraffic accident**

X+7th V40.3 **Unspecified car occupant injured in collision with pedestrian or animal in nontraffic accident**

X+7th V40.4 **Person boarding or alighting a car injured in collision with pedestrian or animal**

X+7th V40.5 **Car driver injured in collision with pedestrian or animal in traffic accident**

X+7th V40.6 **Car passenger injured in collision with pedestrian or animal in traffic accident**

X+7th V40.7 **Person on outside of car injured in collision with pedestrian or animal in traffic accident**

X+7th V40.9 **Unspecified car occupant injured in collision with pedestrian or animal in traffic accident**

V41 **Car occupant injured in collision with pedal cycle**

> The appropriate 7th character is to be added to each code from category V41
> A   initial encounter
> D   subsequent encounter
> S   sequela

X+7th V41.0 **Car driver injured in collision with pedal cycle in nontraffic accident**

X+7th V41.1 **Car passenger injured in collision with pedal cycle in nontraffic accident**

X+7th V41.2 **Person on outside of car injured in collision with pedal cycle in nontraffic accident**

X+7th V41.3 **Unspecified car occupant injured in collision with pedal cycle in nontraffic accident**

X+7th V41.4 **Person boarding or alighting a car injured in collision with pedal cycle**

X+7th V41.5 **Car driver injured in collision with pedal cycle in traffic accident**

X+7th V41.6 **Car passenger injured in collision with pedal cycle in traffic accident**

X+7th V41.7 **Person on outside of car injured in collision with pedal cycle in traffic accident**

X+7th V41.9 **Unspecified car occupant injured in collision with pedal cycle in traffic accident**

V42 **Car occupant injured in collision with two- or three-wheeled motor vehicle**

> The appropriate 7th character is to be added to each code from category V42
> A   initial encounter
> D   subsequent encounter
> S   sequela

X+7th V42.0 **Car driver injured in collision with two- or three-wheeled motor vehicle in nontraffic accident**

X+7th V42.1 **Car passenger injured in collision with two- or three-wheeled motor vehicle in nontraffic accident**

X+7th V42.2 **Person on outside of car injured in collision with two- or three-wheeled motor vehicle in nontraffic accident**

X+7th V42.3 **Unspecified car occupant injured in collision with two- or three-wheeled motor vehicle in nontraffic accident**

X+7th V42.4 **Person boarding or alighting a car injured in collision with two- or three-wheeled motor vehicle**

X+7th V42.5 **Car driver injured in collision with two- or three-wheeled motor vehicle in traffic accident**

X+7th V42.6 **Car passenger injured in collision with two- or three-wheeled motor vehicle in traffic accident**

X+7th V42.7 **Person on outside of car injured in collision with two- or three-wheeled motor vehicle in traffic accident**

X+7th V42.9 **Unspecified car occupant injured in collision with two- or three-wheeled motor vehicle in traffic accident**

V43 **Car occupant injured in collision with car, pick-up truck or van**

> The appropriate 7th character is to be added to each code from category V43
> A   initial encounter
> D   subsequent encounter
> S   sequela

+ V43.0 **Car driver injured in collision with car, pick-up truck or van in nontraffic accident**

X+7th V43.01 **Car driver injured in collision with sport utility vehicle in nontraffic accident**

X+7th V43.02 **Car driver injured in collision with other type car in nontraffic accident**

X+7th V43.03 **Car driver injured in collision with pick-up truck in nontraffic accident**

X+7th V43.04 **Car driver injured in collision with van in nontraffic accident**

+, +7th, X + 7th   ● Newborn   ● Pediatric   ● Maternity   ● Adult   ♀ Female   ♂ Male   Manifestation   Unacceptable PDX   HCC   CC   MCC   HAC

+ V43.1 Car passenger injured in collision with car, pick-up truck or van in nontraffic accident

X+7th **V43.11 Car passenger injured in collision with sport utility vehicle in nontraffic accident**

X+7th **V43.12 Car passenger injured in collision with other type car in nontraffic accident**

X+7th **V43.13 Car passenger injured in collision with pick-up truck in nontraffic accident**

X+7th **V43.14 Car passenger injured in collision with van in nontraffic accident**

+ V43.2 Person on outside of car injured in collision with car, pick-up truck or van in nontraffic accident

X+7th **V43.21 Person on outside of car injured in collision with sport utility vehicle in nontraffic accident**

X+7th **V43.22 Person on outside of car injured in collision with other type car in nontraffic accident**

X+7th **V43.23 Person on outside of car injured in collision with pick-up truck in nontraffic accident**

X+7th **V43.24 Person on outside of car injured in collision with van in nontraffic accident**

+ V43.3 Unspecified car occupant injured in collision with car, pick-up truck or van in nontraffic accident

X+7th **V43.31 Unspecified car occupant injured in collision with sport utility vehicle in nontraffic accident**

X+7th **V43.32 Unspecified car occupant injured in collision with other type car in nontraffic accident**

X+7th **V43.33 Unspecified car occupant injured in collision with pick-up truck in nontraffic accident**

X+7th **V43.34 Unspecified car occupant injured in collision with van in nontraffic accident**

+ V43.4 Person boarding or alighting a car injured in collision with car, pick-up truck or van

X+7th **V43.41 Person boarding or alighting a car injured in collision with sport utility vehicle**

X+7th **V43.42 Person boarding or alighting a car injured in collision with other type car**

X+7th **V43.43 Person boarding or alighting a car injured in collision with pick-up truck**

X+7th **V43.44 Person boarding or alighting a car injured in collision with van**

+ V43.5 Car driver injured in collision with car, pick-up truck or van in traffic accident

X+7th **V43.51 Car driver injured in collision with sport utility vehicle in traffic accident**

X+7th **V43.52 Car driver injured in collision with other type car in traffic accident**

X+7th **V43.53 Car driver injured in collision with pick-up truck in traffic accident**

X+7th **V43.54 Car driver injured in collision with van in traffic accident**

+ V43.6 Car passenger injured in collision with car, pick-up truck or van in traffic accident

X+7th **V43.61 Car passenger injured in collision with sport utility vehicle in traffic accident**
AHA CC: 1Q, 2015, 3-21

X+7th **V43.62 Car passenger injured in collision with other type car in traffic accident**

X+7th **V43.63 Car passenger injured in collision with pick-up truck in traffic accident**

X+7th **V43.64 Car passenger injured in collision with van in traffic accident**

+ V43.7 Person on outside of car injured in collision with car, pick-up truck or van in traffic accident

X+7th **V43.71 Person on outside of car injured in collision with sport utility vehicle in traffic accident**

X+7th **V43.72 Person on outside of car injured in collision with other type car in traffic accident**

X+7th **V43.73 Person on outside of car injured in collision with pick-up truck in traffic accident**

X+7th **V43.74 Person on outside of car injured in collision with van in traffic accident**

+ V43.9 Unspecified car occupant injured in collision with car, pick-up truck or van in traffic accident

X+7th **V43.91 Unspecified car occupant injured in collision with sport utility vehicle in traffic accident**

X+7th **V43.92 Unspecified car occupant injured in collision with other type car in traffic accident**

X+7th **V43.93 Unspecified car occupant injured in collision with pick-up truck in traffic accident**

X+7th **V43.94 Unspecified car occupant injured in collision with van in traffic accident**

V44 Car occupant injured in collision with heavy transport vehicle or bus

> ***Excludes1:*** *car occupant injured in collision with military vehicle (V49.81)*

> The appropriate 7th character is to be added to each code from category V44
> A   initial encounter
> D   subsequent encounter
> S   sequela

X+7th **V44.0 Car driver injured in collision with heavy transport vehicle or bus in nontraffic accident**

X+7th **V44.1 Car passenger injured in collision with heavy transport vehicle or bus in nontraffic accident**

X+7th **V44.2 Person on outside of car injured in collision with heavy transport vehicle or bus in nontraffic accident**

X+7th **V44.3 Unspecified car occupant injured in collision with heavy transport vehicle or bus in nontraffic accident**

X+7th **V44.4 Person boarding or alighting a car injured in collision with heavy transport vehicle or bus**

X+7th **V44.5 Car driver injured in collision with heavy transport vehicle or bus in traffic accident**

X+7th **V44.6 Car passenger injured in collision with heavy transport vehicle or bus in traffic accident**

X+7th **V44.7 Person on outside of car injured in collision with heavy transport vehicle or bus in traffic accident**

X+7th **V44.9 Unspecified car occupant injured in collision with heavy transport vehicle or bus in traffic accident**

V45 Car occupant injured in collision with railway train or railway vehicle

> The appropriate 7th character is to be added to each code from category V45
> A   initial encounter
> D   subsequent encounter
> S   sequela

X+7th **V45.0 Car driver injured in collision with railway train or railway vehicle in nontraffic accident**

X+7th **V45.1 Car passenger injured in collision with railway train or railway vehicle in nontraffic accident**

X+7th **V45.2 Person on outside of car injured in collision with railway train or railway vehicle in nontraffic accident**

X+7th **V45.3 Unspecified car occupant injured in collision with railway train or railway vehicle in nontraffic accident**

X+7th **V45.4 Person boarding or alighting a car injured in collision with railway train or railway vehicle**

X+7th **V45.5 Car driver injured in collision with railway train or railway vehicle in traffic accident**

X+7th **V45.6 Car passenger injured in collision with railway train or railway vehicle in traffic accident**

X+7th **V45.7 Person on outside of car injured in collision with railway train or railway vehicle in traffic accident**

X+7th **V45.9 Unspecified car occupant injured in collision with railway train or railway vehicle in traffic accident**

V46 Car occupant injured in collision with other nonmotor vehicle

> **Includes:** collision with animal-drawn vehicle, animal being ridden, streetcar

> The appropriate 7th character is to be added to each code from category V46
> A   initial encounter
> D   subsequent encounter
> S   sequela

X+7th **V46.0 Car driver injured in collision with other nonmotor vehicle in nontraffic accident**

X+7th **V46.1 Car passenger injured in collision with other nonmotor vehicle in nontraffic accident**

X+7th **V46.2 Person on outside of car injured in collision with other nonmotor vehicle in nontraffic accident**

X+7th **V46.3 Unspecified car occupant injured in collision with other nonmotor vehicle in nontraffic accident**

X+7th **V46.4 Person boarding or alighting a car injured in collision with other nonmotor vehicle**

X+7th **V46.5 Car driver injured in collision with other nonmotor vehicle in traffic accident**

X+7th **V46.6 Car passenger injured in collision with other nonmotor vehicle in traffic accident**

X+7th **V46.7 Person on outside of car injured in collision with other nonmotor vehicle in traffic accident**

X+7th **V46.9 Unspecified car occupant injured in collision with other nonmotor vehicle in traffic accident**

V47 Car occupant injured in collision with fixed or stationary object

AHA CC: 4Q, 2016, 73

The appropriate 7th character is to be added to each code from category V47
A   initial encounter
D   subsequent encounter
S   sequela

X+7th **V47.0** **Car driver injured in collision with fixed or stationary object in nontraffic accident**

X+7th **V47.1** **Car passenger injured in collision with fixed or stationary object in nontraffic accident**

X+7th **V47.2** **Person on outside of car injured in collision with fixed or stationary object in nontraffic accident**

X+7th **V47.3** **Unspecified car occupant injured in collision with fixed or stationary object in nontraffic accident**

X+7th **V47.4** **Person boarding or alighting a car injured in collision with fixed or stationary object**

X+7th **V47.5** **Car driver injured in collision with fixed or stationary object in traffic accident**

X+7th **V47.6** **Car passenger injured in collision with fixed or stationary object in traffic accident**

X+7th **V47.7** **Person on outside of car injured in collision with fixed or stationary object in traffic accident**

X+7th **V47.9** **Unspecified car occupant injured in collision with fixed or stationary object in traffic accident**

V48 Car occupant injured in noncollision transport accident

Includes: overturning car NOS
overturning car without collision

The appropriate 7th character is to be added to each code from category V48
A   initial encounter
D   subsequent encounter
S   sequela

X+7th **V48.0** **Car driver injured in noncollision transport accident in nontraffic accident**

X+7th **V48.1** **Car passenger injured in noncollision transport accident in nontraffic accident**

X+7th **V48.2** **Person on outside of car injured in noncollision transport accident in nontraffic accident**

X+7th **V48.3** **Unspecified car occupant injured in noncollision transport accident in nontraffic accident**

X+7th **V48.4** **Person boarding or alighting a car injured in noncollision transport accident**

X+7th **V48.5** **Car driver injured in noncollision transport accident in traffic accident**

X+7th **V48.6** **Car passenger injured in noncollision transport accident in traffic accident**

X+7th **V48.7** **Person on outside of car injured in noncollision transport accident in traffic accident**

X+7th **V48.9** **Unspecified car occupant injured in noncollision transport accident in traffic accident**

V49 Car occupant injured in other and unspecified transport accidents

The appropriate 7th character is to be added to each code from category V49
A   initial encounter
D   subsequent encounter
S   sequela

+ **V49.0** **Driver injured in collision with other and unspecified motor vehicles in nontraffic accident**

X+7th **V49.00** **Driver injured in collision with unspecified motor vehicles in nontraffic accident**

X+7th **V49.09** **Driver injured in collision with other motor vehicles in nontraffic accident**

+ **V49.1** **Passenger injured in collision with other and unspecified motor vehicles in nontraffic accident**

X+7th **V49.10** **Passenger injured in collision with unspecified motor vehicles in nontraffic accident**

X+7th **V49.19** **Passenger injured in collision with other motor vehicles in nontraffic accident**

+ **V49.2** **Unspecified car occupant injured in collision with other and unspecified motor vehicles in nontraffic accident**

X+7th **V49.20** **Unspecified car occupant injured in collision with unspecified motor vehicles in nontraffic accident**
Car collision NOS, nontraffic

X+7th **V49.29** **Unspecified car occupant injured in collision with other motor vehicles in nontraffic accident**

X+7th **V49.3** **Car occupant (driver) (passenger) injured in unspecified nontraffic accident**
Car accident NOS, nontraffic
Car occupant injured in nontraffic accident NOS

+ **V49.4** **Driver injured in collision with other and unspecified motor vehicles in traffic accident**

X+7th **V49.40** **Driver injured in collision with unspecified motor vehicles in traffic accident**

X+7th **V49.49** **Driver injured in collision with other motor vehicles in traffic accident**

+ **V49.5** **Passenger injured in collision with other and unspecified motor vehicles in traffic accident**

X+7th **V49.50** **Passenger injured in collision with unspecified motor vehicles in traffic accident**

X+7th **V49.59** **Passenger injured in collision with other motor vehicles in traffic accident**

+ **V49.6** **Unspecified car occupant injured in collision with other and unspecified motor vehicles in traffic accident**

X+7th **V49.60** **Unspecified car occupant injured in collision with unspecified motor vehicles in traffic accident**
Car collision NOS (traffic)

X+7th **V49.69** **Unspecified car occupant injured in collision with other motor vehicles in traffic accident**

+ **V49.8** **Car occupant (driver) (passenger) injured in other specified transport accidents**

X+7th **V49.81** **Car occupant (driver) (passenger) injured in transport accident with military vehicle**

X+7th **V49.88** **Car occupant (driver) (passenger) injured in other specified transport accidents**

X+7th **V49.9** **Car occupant (driver) (passenger) injured in unspecified traffic accident**
Car accident NOS
AHA CC: 1Q, 2015, 3-21

Occupant of pick-up truck or van injured in transport accident (V50-V59)

Includes: a four or six wheel motor vehicle designed primarily for carrying passengers and property but weighing less than the local limit for classification as a heavy goods vehicle
minibus
minivan
sport utility vehicle (SUV)
truck
van

Excludes1: heavy transport vehicle (V60-V69)

V50 Occupant of pick-up truck or van injured in collision with pedestrian or animal

Excludes1: pick-up truck or van collision with animal-drawn vehicle or animal being ridden (V56.-)

The appropriate 7th character is to be added to each code from category V50
A   initial encounter
D   subsequent encounter
S   sequela

X+7th **V50.0** **Driver of pick-up truck or van injured in collision with pedestrian or animal in nontraffic accident**

X+7th **V50.1** **Passenger in pick-up truck or van injured in collision with pedestrian or animal in nontraffic accident**

X+7th **V50.2** **Person on outside of pick-up truck or van injured in collision with pedestrian or animal in nontraffic accident**

X+7th **V50.3** **Unspecified occupant of pick-up truck or van injured in collision with pedestrian or animal in nontraffic accident**

X+7th **V50.4** **Person boarding or alighting a pick-up truck or van injured in collision with pedestrian or animal**

X+7th **V50.5** **Driver of pick-up truck or van injured in collision with pedestrian or animal in traffic accident**

X+7th **V50.6** **Passenger in pick-up truck or van injured in collision with pedestrian or animal in traffic accident**

X+7th **V50.7** **Person on outside of pick-up truck or van injured in collision with pedestrian or animal in traffic accident**

X+7th **V50.9** **Unspecified occupant of pick-up truck or van injured in collision with pedestrian or animal in traffic accident**

V51 Occupant of pick-up truck or van injured in collision with pedal cycle

The appropriate 7th character is to be added to each code from category V51
A   initial encounter
D   subsequent encounter
S   sequela

+, +7th, X + 7th   ● Newborn   ● Pediatric   ● Maternity   ● Adult   ♀ Female   ♂ Male   Manifestation   Unacceptable PDX   HCC   CC   MCC   HAC

X+7th **V51.0** Driver of pick-up truck or van injured in collision with pedal cycle in nontraffic accident

X+7th **V51.1** Passenger in pick-up truck or van injured in collision with pedal cycle in nontraffic accident

X+7th **V51.2** Person on outside of pick-up truck or van injured in collision with pedal cycle in nontraffic accident

X+7th **V51.3** Unspecified occupant of pick-up truck or van injured in collision with pedal cycle in nontraffic accident

X+7th **V51.4** Person boarding or alighting a pick-up truck or van injured in collision with pedal cycle

X+7th **V51.5** Driver of pick-up truck or van injured in collision with pedal cycle in traffic accident

X+7th **V51.6** Passenger in pick-up truck or van injured in collision with pedal cycle in traffic accident

X+7th **V51.7** Person on outside of pick-up truck or van injured in collision with pedal cycle in traffic accident

X+7th **V51.9** Unspecified occupant of pick-up truck or van injured in collision with pedal cycle in traffic accident

V52 Occupant of pick-up truck or van injured in collision with two- or three-wheeled motor vehicle

> The appropriate 7th character is to be added to each code from category V52
> A initial encounter
> D subsequent encounter
> S sequela

X+7th **V52.0** Driver of pick-up truck or van injured in collision with two- or three-wheeled motor vehicle in nontraffic accident

X+7th **V52.1** Passenger in pick-up truck or van injured in collision with two- or three-wheeled motor vehicle in nontraffic accident

X+7th **V52.2** Person on outside of pick-up truck or van injured in collision with two- or three-wheeled motor vehicle in nontraffic accident

X+7th **V52.3** Unspecified occupant of pick-up truck or van injured in collision with two- or three-wheeled motor vehicle in nontraffic accident

X+7th **V52.4** Person boarding or alighting a pick-up truck or van injured in collision with two- or three-wheeled motor vehicle

X+7th **V52.5** Driver of pick-up truck or van injured in collision with two- or three-wheeled motor vehicle in traffic accident

X+7th **V52.6** Passenger in pick-up truck or van injured in collision with two- or three-wheeled motor vehicle in traffic accident

X+7th **V52.7** Person on outside of pick-up truck or van injured in collision with two- or three-wheeled motor vehicle in traffic accident

X+7th **V52.9** Unspecified occupant of pick-up truck or van injured in collision with two- or three-wheeled motor vehicle in traffic accident

V53 Occupant of pick-up truck or van injured in collision with car, pick-up truck or van

> The appropriate 7th character is to be added to each code from category V53
> A initial encounter
> D subsequent encounter
> S sequela

X+7th **V53.0** Driver of pick-up truck or van injured in collision with car, pick-up truck or van in nontraffic accident

X+7th **V53.1** Passenger in pick-up truck or van injured in collision with car, pick-up truck or van in nontraffic accident

X+7th **V53.2** Person on outside of pick-up truck or van injured in collision with car, pick-up truck or van in nontraffic accident

X+7th **V53.3** Unspecified occupant of pick-up truck or van injured in collision with car, pick-up truck or van in nontraffic accident

X+7th **V53.4** Person boarding or alighting a pick-up truck or van injured in collision with car, pick-up truck or van

X+7th **V53.5** Driver of pick-up truck or van injured in collision with car, pick-up truck or van in traffic accident

X+7th **V53.6** Passenger in pick-up truck or van injured in collision with car, pick-up truck or van in traffic accident

X+7th **V53.7** Person on outside of pick-up truck or van injured in collision with car, pick-up truck or van in traffic accident

X+7th **V53.9** Unspecified occupant of pick-up truck or van injured in collision with car, pick-up truck or van in traffic accident

V54 Occupant of pick-up truck or van injured in collision with heavy transport vehicle or bus

> ***Excludes1:*** *occupant of pick-up truck or van injured in collision with military vehicle (V59.81)*

> The appropriate 7th character is to be added to each code from category V54
> A initial encounter
> D subsequent encounter
> S sequela

X+7th **V54.0** Driver of pick-up truck or van injured in collision with heavy transport vehicle or bus in nontraffic accident

X+7th **V54.1** Passenger in pick-up truck or van injured in collision with heavy transport vehicle or bus in nontraffic accident

X+7th **V54.2** Person on outside of pick-up truck or van injured in collision with heavy transport vehicle or bus in nontraffic accident

X+7th **V54.3** Unspecified occupant of pick-up truck or van injured in collision with heavy transport vehicle or bus in nontraffic accident

X+7th **V54.4** Person boarding or alighting a pick-up truck or van injured in collision with heavy transport vehicle or bus

X+7th **V54.5** Driver of pick-up truck or van injured in collision with heavy transport vehicle or bus in traffic accident

X+7th **V54.6** Passenger in pick-up truck or van injured in collision with heavy transport vehicle or bus in traffic accident

X+7th **V54.7** Person on outside of pick-up truck or van injured in collision with heavy transport vehicle or bus in traffic accident

X+7th **V54.9** Unspecified occupant of pick-up truck or van injured in collision with heavy transport vehicle or bus in traffic accident

V55 Occupant of pick-up truck or van injured in collision with railway train or railway vehicle

> The appropriate 7th character is to be added to each code from category V55
> A initial encounter
> D subsequent encounter
> S sequela

X+7th **V55.0** Driver of pick-up truck or van injured in collision with railway train or railway vehicle in nontraffic accident

X+7th **V55.1** Passenger in pick-up truck or van injured in collision with railway train or railway vehicle in nontraffic accident

X+7th **V55.2** Person on outside of pick-up truck or van injured in collision with railway train or railway vehicle in nontraffic accident

X+7th **V55.3** Unspecified occupant of pick-up truck or van injured in collision with railway train or railway vehicle in nontraffic accident

X+7th **V55.4** Person boarding or alighting a pick-up truck or van injured in collision with railway train or railway vehicle

X+7th **V55.5** Driver of pick-up truck or van injured in collision with railway train or railway vehicle in traffic accident

X+7th **V55.6** Passenger in pick-up truck or van injured in collision with railway train or railway vehicle in traffic accident

X+7th **V55.7** Person on outside of pick-up truck or van injured in collision with railway train or railway vehicle in traffic accident

X+7th **V55.9** Unspecified occupant of pick-up truck or van injured in collision with railway train or railway vehicle in traffic accident

V56 Occupant of pick-up truck or van injured in collision with other nonmotor vehicle

> **Includes:** collision with animal-drawn vehicle, animal being ridden, streetcar

> The appropriate 7th character is to be added to each code from category V56
> A initial encounter
> D subsequent encounter
> S sequela

X+7th **V56.0** Driver of pick-up truck or van injured in collision with other nonmotor vehicle in nontraffic accident

X+7th **V56.1** Passenger in pick-up truck or van injured in collision with other nonmotor vehicle in nontraffic accident

X+7th **V56.2** Person on outside of pick-up truck or van injured in collision with other nonmotor vehicle in nontraffic accident

X+7th **V56.3** Unspecified occupant of pick-up truck or van injured in collision with other nonmotor vehicle in nontraffic accident

X+7th **V56.4** Person boarding or alighting a pick-up truck or van injured in collision with other nonmotor vehicle

X+7th **V56.5** Driver of pick-up truck or van injured in collision with other nonmotor vehicle in traffic accident

X+7th **V56.6** Passenger in pick-up truck or van injured in collision with other nonmotor vehicle in traffic accident

+, +7th, X + 7th ● Newborn ● Pediatric ● Maternity ● Adult ♀ Female ♂ Male Manifestation Unacceptable PDX HCC CC MCC HAC

X+7th V56.7 Person on outside of pick-up truck or van injured in collision with other nonmotor vehicle in traffic accident

X+7th V56.9 Unspecified occupant of pick-up truck or van injured in collision with other nonmotor vehicle in traffic accident

V57 Occupant of pick-up truck or van injured in collision with fixed or stationary object

> The appropriate 7th character is to be added to each code from category V57
> A   initial encounter
> D   subsequent encounter
> S   sequela

X+7th V57.0 Driver of pick-up truck or van injured in collision with fixed or stationary object in nontraffic accident

X+7th V57.1 Passenger in pick-up truck or van injured in collision with fixed or stationary object in nontraffic accident

X+7th V57.2 Person on outside of pick-up truck or van injured in collision with fixed or stationary object in nontraffic accident

X+7th V57.3 Unspecified occupant of pick-up truck or van injured in collision with fixed or stationary object in nontraffic accident

X+7th V57.4 Person boarding or alighting a pick-up truck or van injured in collision with fixed or stationary object

X+7th V57.5 Driver of pick-up truck or van injured in collision with fixed or stationary object in traffic accident

X+7th V57.6 Passenger in pick-up truck or van injured in collision with fixed or stationary object in traffic accident

X+7th V57.7 Person on outside of pick-up truck or van injured in collision with fixed or stationary object in traffic accident

X+7th V57.9 Unspecified occupant of pick-up truck or van injured in collision with fixed or stationary object in traffic accident

V58 Occupant of pick-up truck or van injured in noncollision transport accident

> **Includes:** overturning pick-up truck or van NOS
> overturning pick-up truck or van without collision

> The appropriate 7th character is to be added to each code from category V58
> A   initial encounter
> D   subsequent encounter
> S   sequela

X+7th V58.0 Driver of pick-up truck or van injured in noncollision transport accident in nontraffic accident

X+7th V58.1 Passenger in pick-up truck or van injured in noncollision transport accident in nontraffic accident

X+7th V58.2 Person on outside of pick-up truck or van injured in noncollision transport accident in nontraffic accident

X+7th V58.3 Unspecified occupant of pick-up truck or van injured in noncollision transport accident in nontraffic accident

X+7th V58.4 Person boarding or alighting a pick-up truck or van injured in noncollision transport accident

X+7th V58.5 Driver of pick-up truck or van injured in noncollision transport accident in traffic accident

X+7th V58.6 Passenger in pick-up truck or van injured in noncollision transport accident in traffic accident

X+7th V58.7 Person on outside of pick-up truck or van injured in noncollision transport accident in traffic accident

X+7th V58.9 Unspecified occupant of pick-up truck or van injured in noncollision transport accident in traffic accident

V59 Occupant of pick-up truck or van injured in other and unspecified transport accidents

> The appropriate 7th character is to be added to each code from category V59
> A   initial encounter
> D   subsequent encounter
> S   sequela

+ V59.0 Driver of pick-up truck or van injured in collision with other and unspecified motor vehicles in nontraffic accident

X+7th V59.00 Driver of pick-up truck or van injured in collision with unspecified motor vehicles in nontraffic accident

X+7th V59.09 Driver of pick-up truck or van injured in collision with other motor vehicles in nontraffic accident

+ V59.1 Passenger in pick-up truck or van injured in collision with other and unspecified motor vehicles in nontraffic accident

X+7th V59.10 Passenger in pick-up truck or van injured in collision with unspecified motor vehicles in nontraffic accident

X+7th V59.19 Passenger in pick-up truck or van injured in collision with other motor vehicles in nontraffic accident

+ V59.2 Unspecified occupant of pick-up truck or van injured in collision with other and unspecified motor vehicles in nontraffic accident

X+7th V59.20 Unspecified occupant of pick-up truck or van injured in collision with unspecified motor vehicles in nontraffic accident

Collision NOS involving pick-up truck or van, nontraffic

X+7th V59.29 Unspecified occupant of pick-up truck or van injured in collision with other motor vehicles in nontraffic accident

X+7th V59.3 Occupant (driver) (passenger) of pick-up truck or van injured in unspecified nontraffic accident

Accident NOS involving pick-up truck or van, nontraffic
Occupant of pick-up truck or van injured in nontraffic accident NOS

+ V59.4 Driver of pick-up truck or van injured in collision with other and unspecified motor vehicles in traffic accident

X+7th V59.40 Driver of pick-up truck or van injured in collision with unspecified motor vehicles in traffic accident

X+7th V59.49 Driver of pick-up truck or van injured in collision with other motor vehicles in traffic accident

+ V59.5 Passenger in pick-up truck or van injured in collision with other and unspecified motor vehicles in traffic accident

X+7th V59.50 Passenger in pick-up truck or van injured in collision with unspecified motor vehicles in traffic accident

X+7th V59.59 Passenger in pick-up truck or van injured in collision with other motor vehicles in traffic accident

+ V59.6 Unspecified occupant of pick-up truck or van injured in collision with other and unspecified motor vehicles in traffic accident

X+7th V59.60 Unspecified occupant of pick-up truck or van injured in collision with unspecified motor vehicles in traffic accident

Collision NOS involving pick-up truck or van (traffic)

X+7th V59.69 Unspecified occupant of pick-up truck or van injured in collision with other motor vehicles in traffic accident

+ V59.8 Occupant (driver) (passenger) of pick-up truck or van injured in other specified transport accidents

X+7th V59.81 Occupant (driver) (passenger) of pick-up truck or van injured in transport accident with military vehicle

X+7th V59.88 Occupant (driver) (passenger) of pick-up truck or van injured in other specified transport accidents

X+7th V59.9 Occupant (driver) (passenger) of pick-up truck or van injured in unspecified traffic accident

Accident NOS involving pick-up truck or van

Occupant of heavy transport vehicle injured in transport accident (V60-V69)

Includes: 18 wheeler
armored car
panel truck

Excludes1: bus
motorcoach

V60 Occupant of heavy transport vehicle injured in collision with pedestrian or animal

> **Excludes1:** heavy transport vehicle collision with animal-drawn vehicle or animal being ridden (V66.-)

> The appropriate 7th character is to be added to each code from category V60
> A   initial encounter
> D   subsequent encounter
> S   sequela

X+7th V60.0 Driver of heavy transport vehicle injured in collision with pedestrian or animal in nontraffic accident

X+7th V60.1 Passenger in heavy transport vehicle injured in collision with pedestrian or animal in nontraffic accident

X+7th V60.2 Person on outside of heavy transport vehicle injured in collision with pedestrian or animal in nontraffic accident

X+7th V60.3 Unspecified occupant of heavy transport vehicle injured in collision with pedestrian or animal in nontraffic accident

+, +7th, X + 7th   ● Newborn   ● Pediatric   ● Maternity   ● Adult   ♀ Female   ♂ Male   Manifestation   Unacceptable PDX   HCC   CC   MCC   HAC

X+7th **V60.4** Person boarding or alighting a heavy transport vehicle injured in collision with pedestrian or animal

X+7th **V60.5** Driver of heavy transport vehicle injured in collision with pedestrian or animal in traffic accident

X+7th **V60.6** Passenger in heavy transport vehicle injured in collision with pedestrian or animal in traffic accident

X+7th **V60.7** Person on outside of heavy transport vehicle injured in collision with pedestrian or animal in traffic accident

X+7th **V60.9** Unspecified occupant of heavy transport vehicle injured in collision with pedestrian or animal in traffic accident

V61 Occupant of heavy transport vehicle injured in collision with pedal cycle

> The appropriate 7th character is to be added to each code from category V61
> A initial encounter
> D subsequent encounter
> S sequela

X+7th **V61.0** Driver of heavy transport vehicle injured in collision with pedal cycle in nontraffic accident

X+7th **V61.1** Passenger in heavy transport vehicle injured in collision with pedal cycle in nontraffic accident

X+7th **V61.2** Person on outside of heavy transport vehicle injured in collision with pedal cycle in nontraffic accident

X+7th **V61.3** Unspecified occupant of heavy transport vehicle injured in collision with pedal cycle in nontraffic accident

X+7th **V61.4** Person boarding or alighting a heavy transport vehicle injured in collision with pedal cycle while boarding or alighting

X+7th **V61.5** Driver of heavy transport vehicle injured in collision with pedal cycle in traffic accident

X+7th **V61.6** Passenger in heavy transport vehicle injured in collision with pedal cycle in traffic accident

X+7th **V61.7** Person on outside of heavy transport vehicle injured in collision with pedal cycle in traffic accident

X+7th **V61.9** Unspecified occupant of heavy transport vehicle injured in collision with pedal cycle in traffic accident

V62 Occupant of heavy transport vehicle injured in collision with two- or three-wheeled motor vehicle

> The appropriate 7th character is to be added to each code from category V62
> A initial encounter
> D subsequent encounter
> S sequela

X+7th **V62.0** Driver of heavy transport vehicle injured in collision with two- or three-wheeled motor vehicle in nontraffic accident

X+7th **V62.1** Passenger in heavy transport vehicle injured in collision with two- or three-wheeled motor vehicle in nontraffic accident

X+7th **V62.2** Person on outside of heavy transport vehicle injured in collision with two- or three-wheeled motor vehicle in nontraffic accident

X+7th **V62.3** Unspecified occupant of heavy transport vehicle injured in collision with two- or three-wheeled motor vehicle in nontraffic accident

X+7th **V62.4** Person boarding or alighting a heavy transport vehicle injured in collision with two- or three-wheeled motor vehicle

X+7th **V62.5** Driver of heavy transport vehicle injured in collision with two- or three-wheeled motor vehicle in traffic accident

X+7th **V62.6** Passenger in heavy transport vehicle injured in collision with two- or three-wheeled motor vehicle in traffic accident

X+7th **V62.7** Person on outside of heavy transport vehicle injured in collision with two- or three-wheeled motor vehicle in traffic accident

X+7th **V62.9** Unspecified occupant of heavy transport vehicle injured in collision with two- or three-wheeled motor vehicle in traffic accident

V63 Occupant of heavy transport vehicle injured in collision with car, pick-up truck or van

> The appropriate 7th character is to be added to each code from category V63
> A initial encounter
> D subsequent encounter
> S sequela

X+7th **V63.0** Driver of heavy transport vehicle injured in collision with car, pick-up truck or van in nontraffic accident

X+7th **V63.1** Passenger in heavy transport vehicle injured in collision with car, pick-up truck or van in nontraffic accident

X+7th **V63.2** Person on outside of heavy transport vehicle injured in collision with car, pick-up truck or van in nontraffic accident

X+7th **V63.3** Unspecified occupant of heavy transport vehicle injured in collision with car, pick-up truck or van in nontraffic accident

X+7th **V63.4** Person boarding or alighting a heavy transport vehicle injured in collision with car, pick-up truck or van

X+7th **V63.5** Driver of heavy transport vehicle injured in collision with car, pick-up truck or van in traffic accident

X+7th **V63.6** Passenger in heavy transport vehicle injured in collision with car, pick-up truck or van in traffic accident

X+7th **V63.7** Person on outside of heavy transport vehicle injured in collision with car, pick-up truck or van in traffic accident

X+7th **V63.9** Unspecified occupant of heavy transport vehicle injured in collision with car, pick-up truck or van in traffic accident

V64 Occupant of heavy transport vehicle injured in collision with heavy transport vehicle or bus

> **Excludes1:** *occupant of heavy transport vehicle injured in collision with military vehicle (V69.81)*

> The appropriate 7th character is to be added to each code from category V64
> A initial encounter
> D subsequent encounter
> S sequela

X+7th **V64.0** Driver of heavy transport vehicle injured in collision with heavy transport vehicle or bus in nontraffic accident

X+7th **V64.1** Passenger in heavy transport vehicle injured in collision with heavy transport vehicle or bus in nontraffic accident

X+7th **V64.2** Person on outside of heavy transport vehicle injured in collision with heavy transport vehicle or bus in nontraffic accident

X+7th **V64.3** Unspecified occupant of heavy transport vehicle injured in collision with heavy transport vehicle or bus in nontraffic accident

X+7th **V64.4** Person boarding or alighting a heavy transport vehicle injured in collision with heavy transport vehicle or bus while boarding or alighting

X+7th **V64.5** Driver of heavy transport vehicle injured in collision with heavy transport vehicle or bus in traffic accident

X+7th **V64.6** Passenger in heavy transport vehicle injured in collision with heavy transport vehicle or bus in traffic accident

X+7th **V64.7** Person on outside of heavy transport vehicle injured in collision with heavy transport vehicle or bus in traffic accident

X+7th **V64.9** Unspecified occupant of heavy transport vehicle injured in collision with heavy transport vehicle or bus in traffic accident

V65 Occupant of heavy transport vehicle injured in collision with railway train or railway vehicle

> The appropriate 7th character is to be added to each code from category V65
> A initial encounter
> D subsequent encounter
> S sequela

X+7th **V65.0** Driver of heavy transport vehicle injured in collision with railway train or railway vehicle in nontraffic accident

X+7th **V65.1** Passenger in heavy transport vehicle injured in collision with railway train or railway vehicle in nontraffic accident

X+7th **V65.2** Person on outside of heavy transport vehicle injured in collision with railway train or railway vehicle in nontraffic accident

X+7th **V65.3** Unspecified occupant of heavy transport vehicle injured in collision with railway train or railway vehicle in nontraffic accident

X+7th **V65.4** Person boarding or alighting a heavy transport vehicle injured in collision with railway train or railway vehicle

X+7th **V65.5** Driver of heavy transport vehicle injured in collision with railway train or railway vehicle in traffic accident

X+7th **V65.6** Passenger in heavy transport vehicle injured in collision with railway train or railway vehicle in traffic accident

X+7th **V65.7** Person on outside of heavy transport vehicle injured in collision with railway train or railway vehicle in traffic accident

X+7th **V65.9** Unspecified occupant of heavy transport vehicle injured in collision with railway train or railway vehicle in traffic accident

+, +7th, X + 7th • Newborn • Pediatric • Maternity • Adult ♀ Female ♂ Male Manifestation Unacceptable PDX HCC CC MCC HAC

V66 Occupant of heavy transport vehicle injured in collision with other nonmotor vehicle

Includes: collision with animal-drawn vehicle, animal being ridden, streetcar

The appropriate 7th character is to be added to each code from category V66
A   initial encounter
D   subsequent encounter
S   sequela

X+7th **V66.0 Driver of heavy transport vehicle injured in collision with other nonmotor vehicle in nontraffic accident**

X+7th **V66.1 Passenger in heavy transport vehicle injured in collision with other nonmotor vehicle in nontraffic accident**

X+7th **V66.2 Person on outside of heavy transport vehicle injured in collision with other nonmotor vehicle in nontraffic accident**

X+7th **V66.3 Unspecified occupant of heavy transport vehicle injured in collision with other nonmotor vehicle in nontraffic accident**

X+7th **V66.4 Person boarding or alighting a heavy transport vehicle injured in collision with other nonmotor vehicle**

X+7th **V66.5 Driver of heavy transport vehicle injured in collision with other nonmotor vehicle in traffic accident**

X+7th **V66.6 Passenger in heavy transport vehicle injured in collision with other nonmotor vehicle in traffic accident**

X+7th **V66.7 Person on outside of heavy transport vehicle injured in collision with other nonmotor vehicle in traffic accident**

X+7th **V66.9 Unspecified occupant of heavy transport vehicle injured in collision with other nonmotor vehicle in traffic accident**

V67 Occupant of heavy transport vehicle injured in collision with fixed or stationary object

The appropriate 7th character is to be added to each code from category V67
A   initial encounter
D   subsequent encounter
S   sequela

X+7th **V67.0 Driver of heavy transport vehicle injured in collision with fixed or stationary object in nontraffic accident**

X+7th **V67.1 Passenger in heavy transport vehicle injured in collision with fixed or stationary object in nontraffic accident**

X+7th **V67.2 Person on outside of heavy transport vehicle injured in collision with fixed or stationary object in nontraffic accident**

X+7th **V67.3 Unspecified occupant of heavy transport vehicle injured in collision with fixed or stationary object in nontraffic accident**

X+7th **V67.4 Person boarding or alighting a heavy transport vehicle injured in collision with fixed or stationary object**

X+7th **V67.5 Driver of heavy transport vehicle injured in collision with fixed or stationary object in traffic accident**

X+7th **V67.6 Passenger in heavy transport vehicle injured in collision with fixed or stationary object in traffic accident**

X+7th **V67.7 Person on outside of heavy transport vehicle injured in collision with fixed or stationary object in traffic accident**

X+7th **V67.9 Unspecified occupant of heavy transport vehicle injured in collision with fixed or stationary object in traffic accident**

V68 Occupant of heavy transport vehicle injured in noncollision transport accident

Includes: overturning heavy transport vehicle NOS
overturning heavy transport vehicle without collision

The appropriate 7th character is to be added to each code from category V68
A   initial encounter
D   subsequent encounter
S   sequela

X+7th **V68.0 Driver of heavy transport vehicle injured in noncollision transport accident in nontraffic accident**

X+7th **V68.1 Passenger in heavy transport vehicle injured in noncollision transport accident in nontraffic accident**

X+7th **V68.2 Person on outside of heavy transport vehicle injured in noncollision transport accident in nontraffic accident**

X+7th **V68.3 Unspecified occupant of heavy transport vehicle injured in noncollision transport accident in nontraffic accident**

X+7th **V68.4 Person boarding or alighting a heavy transport vehicle injured in noncollision transport accident**

X+7th **V68.5 Driver of heavy transport vehicle injured in noncollision transport accident in traffic accident**

X+7th **V68.6 Passenger in heavy transport vehicle injured in noncollision transport accident in traffic accident**

X+7th **V68.7 Person on outside of heavy transport vehicle injured in noncollision transport accident in traffic accident**

X+7th **V68.9 Unspecified occupant of heavy transport vehicle injured in noncollision transport accident in traffic accident**

V69 Occupant of heavy transport vehicle injured in other and unspecified transport accidents

The appropriate 7th character is to be added to each code from category V69
A   initial encounter
D   subsequent encounter
S   sequela

+ **V69.0 Driver of heavy transport vehicle injured in collision with other and unspecified motor vehicles in nontraffic accident**

X+7th **V69.00 Driver of heavy transport vehicle injured in collision with unspecified motor vehicles in nontraffic accident**

X+7th **V69.09 Driver of heavy transport vehicle injured in collision with other motor vehicles in nontraffic accident**

+ **V69.1 Passenger in heavy transport vehicle injured in collision with other and unspecified motor vehicles in nontraffic accident**

X+7th **V69.10 Passenger in heavy transport vehicle injured in collision with unspecified motor vehicles in nontraffic accident**

X+7th **V69.19 Passenger in heavy transport vehicle injured in collision with other motor vehicles in nontraffic accident**

+ **V69.2 Unspecified occupant of heavy transport vehicle injured in collision with other and unspecified motor vehicles in nontraffic accident**

X+7th **V69.20 Unspecified occupant of heavy transport vehicle injured in collision with unspecified motor vehicles in nontraffic accident**
Collision NOS involving heavy transport vehicle, nontraffic

X+7th **V69.29 Unspecified occupant of heavy transport vehicle injured in collision with other motor vehicles in nontraffic accident**

X+7th **V69.3 Occupant (driver) (passenger) of heavy transport vehicle injured in unspecified nontraffic accident**
Accident NOS involving heavy transport vehicle, nontraffic
Occupant of heavy transport vehicle injured in nontraffic accident NOS

+ **V69.4 Driver of heavy transport vehicle injured in collision with other and unspecified motor vehicles in traffic accident**

X+7th **V69.40 Driver of heavy transport vehicle injured in collision with unspecified motor vehicles in traffic accident**

X+7th **V69.49 Driver of heavy transport vehicle injured in collision with other motor vehicles in traffic accident**

+ **V69.5 Passenger in heavy transport vehicle injured in collision with other and unspecified motor vehicles in traffic accident**

X+7th **V69.50 Passenger in heavy transport vehicle injured in collision with unspecified motor vehicles in traffic accident**

X+7th **V69.59 Passenger in heavy transport vehicle injured in collision with other motor vehicles in traffic accident**

+ **V69.6 Unspecified occupant of heavy transport vehicle injured in collision with other and unspecified motor vehicles in traffic accident**

X+7th **V69.60 Unspecified occupant of heavy transport vehicle injured in collision with unspecified motor vehicles in traffic accident**
Collision NOS involving heavy transport vehicle (traffic)

X+7th **V69.69 Unspecified occupant of heavy transport vehicle injured in collision with other motor vehicles in traffic accident**

+ **V69.8 Occupant (driver) (passenger) of heavy transport vehicle injured in other specified transport accidents**

X+7th **V69.81 Occupant (driver) (passenger) of heavy transport vehicle injured in transport accidents with military vehicle**

X+7th **V69.88 Occupant (driver) (passenger) of heavy transport vehicle injured in other specified transport accidents**

X+7th **V69.9 Occupant (driver) (passenger) of heavy transport vehicle injured in unspecified traffic accident**
Accident NOS involving heavy transport vehicle

+, +7th, X + 7th   ● Newborn   ● Pediatric   ● Maternity   ● Adult   ♀ Female   ♂ Male   Manifestation   Unacceptable PDX   HCC   CC   MCC   HAC

Bus occupant injured in transport accident (V70-V79)

Includes: motorcoach

Excludes1: *minibus (V50-V59)*

V70 Bus occupant injured in collision with pedestrian or animal

> The appropriate 7th character is to be added to each code from category V70
> A initial encounter
> D subsequent encounter
> S sequela

> **Excludes1:** *bus collision with animal-drawn vehicle or animal being ridden (V76.-)*

X+7th **V70.0** Driver of bus injured in collision with pedestrian or animal in nontraffic accident

X+7th **V70.1** Passenger on bus injured in collision with pedestrian or animal in nontraffic accident

X+7th **V70.2** Person on outside of bus injured in collision with pedestrian or animal in nontraffic accident

X+7th **V70.3** Unspecified occupant of bus injured in collision with pedestrian or animal in nontraffic accident

X+7th **V70.4** Person boarding or alighting from bus injured in collision with pedestrian or animal

X+7th **V70.5** Driver of bus injured in collision with pedestrian or animal in traffic accident

X+7th **V70.6** Passenger on bus injured in collision with pedestrian or animal in traffic accident

X+7th **V70.7** Person on outside of bus injured in collision with pedestrian or animal in traffic accident

X+7th **V70.9** Unspecified occupant of bus injured in collision with pedestrian or animal in traffic accident

V71 Bus occupant injured in collision with pedal cycle

> The appropriate 7th character is to be added to each code from category V71
> A initial encounter
> D subsequent encounter
> S sequela

X+7th **V71.0** Driver of bus injured in collision with pedal cycle in nontraffic accident

X+7th **V71.1** Passenger on bus injured in collision with pedal cycle in nontraffic accident

X+7th **V71.2** Person on outside of bus injured in collision with pedal cycle in nontraffic accident

X+7th **V71.3** Unspecified occupant of bus injured in collision with pedal cycle in nontraffic accident

X+7th **V71.4** Person boarding or alighting from bus injured in collision with pedal cycle

X+7th **V71.5** Driver of bus injured in collision with pedal cycle in traffic accident

X+7th **V71.6** Passenger on bus injured in collision with pedal cycle in traffic accident

X+7th **V71.7** Person on outside of bus injured in collision with pedal cycle in traffic accident

X+7th **V71.9** Unspecified occupant of bus injured in collision with pedal cycle in traffic accident

V72 Bus occupant injured in collision with two- or three-wheeled motor vehicle

> The appropriate 7th character is to be added to each code from category V72
> A initial encounter
> D subsequent encounter
> S sequela

X+7th **V72.0** Driver of bus injured in collision with two- or three-wheeled motor vehicle in nontraffic accident

X+7th **V72.1** Passenger on bus injured in collision with two- or three-wheeled motor vehicle in nontraffic accident

X+7th **V72.2** Person on outside of bus injured in collision with two- or three-wheeled motor vehicle in nontraffic accident

X+7th **V72.3** Unspecified occupant of bus injured in collision with two- or three-wheeled motor vehicle in nontraffic accident

X+7th **V72.4** Person boarding or alighting from bus injured in collision with two- or three-wheeled motor vehicle

X+7th **V72.5** Driver of bus injured in collision with two- or three-wheeled motor vehicle in traffic accident

X+7th **V72.6** Passenger on bus injured in collision with two- or three-wheeled motor vehicle in traffic accident

X+7th **V72.7** Person on outside of bus injured in collision with two- or three-wheeled motor vehicle in traffic accident

X+7th **V72.9** Unspecified occupant of bus injured in collision with two- or three-wheeled motor vehicle in traffic accident

V73 Bus occupant injured in collision with car, pick-up truck or van

> The appropriate 7th character is to be added to each code from category V73
> A initial encounter
> D subsequent encounter
> S sequela

X+7th **V73.0** Driver of bus injured in collision with car, pick-up truck or van in nontraffic accident

X+7th **V73.1** Passenger on bus injured in collision with car, pick-up truck or van in nontraffic accident

X+7th **V73.2** Person on outside of bus injured in collision with car, pick-up truck or van in nontraffic accident

X+7th **V73.3** Unspecified occupant of bus injured in collision with car, pick-up truck or van in nontraffic accident

X+7th **V73.4** Person boarding or alighting from bus injured in collision with car, pick-up truck or van

X+7th **V73.5** Driver of bus injured in collision with car, pick-up truck or van in traffic accident

X+7th **V73.6** Passenger on bus injured in collision with car, pick-up truck or van in traffic accident

X+7th **V73.7** Person on outside of bus injured in collision with car, pick-up truck or van in traffic accident

X+7th **V73.9** Unspecified occupant of bus injured in collision with car, pick-up truck or van in traffic accident

V74 Bus occupant injured in collision with heavy transport vehicle or bus

> **Excludes1:** *bus occupant injured in collision with military vehicle (V79.81)*

> The appropriate 7th character is to be added to each code from category V74
> A initial encounter
> D subsequent encounter
> S sequela

X+7th **V74.0** Driver of bus injured in collision with heavy transport vehicle or bus in nontraffic accident

X+7th **V74.1** Passenger on bus injured in collision with heavy transport vehicle or bus in nontraffic accident

X+7th **V74.2** Person on outside of bus injured in collision with heavy transport vehicle or bus in nontraffic accident

X+7th **V74.3** Unspecified occupant of bus injured in collision with heavy transport vehicle or bus in nontraffic accident

X+7th **V74.4** Person boarding or alighting from bus injured in collision with heavy transport vehicle or bus

X+7th **V74.5** Driver of bus injured in collision with heavy transport vehicle or bus in traffic accident

X+7th **V74.6** Passenger on bus injured in collision with heavy transport vehicle or bus in traffic accident

X+7th **V74.7** Person on outside of bus injured in collision with heavy transport vehicle or bus in traffic accident

X+7th **V74.9** Unspecified occupant of bus injured in collision with heavy transport vehicle or bus in traffic accident

V75 Bus occupant injured in collision with railway train or railway vehicle

> The appropriate 7th character is to be added to each code from category V75
> A initial encounter
> D subsequent encounter
> S sequela

X+7th **V75.0** Driver of bus injured in collision with railway train or railway vehicle in nontraffic accident

X+7th **V75.1** Passenger on bus injured in collision with railway train or railway vehicle in nontraffic accident

X+7th **V75.2** Person on outside of bus injured in collision with railway train or railway vehicle in nontraffic accident

X+7th **V75.3** Unspecified occupant of bus injured in collision with railway train or railway vehicle in nontraffic accident

X+7th **V75.4** Person boarding or alighting from bus injured in collision with railway train or railway vehicle

X+7th **V75.5** Driver of bus injured in collision with railway train or railway vehicle in traffic accident

X+7th **V75.6** Passenger on bus injured in collision with railway train or railway vehicle in traffic accident

X+7th **V75.7** Person on outside of bus injured in collision with railway train or railway vehicle in traffic accident

X+7th **V75.9** Unspecified occupant of bus injured in collision with railway train or railway vehicle in traffic accident

+, +7th, X + 7th   ● Newborn   ● Pediatric   ● Maternity   ● Adult   ♀ Female   ♂ Male   Manifestation   Unacceptable PDX   HCC   CC   MCC   HAC

V76 Bus occupant injured in collision with other nonmotor vehicle

Includes: collision with animal-drawn vehicle, animal being ridden, streetcar

> The appropriate 7th character is to be added to each code from category V76
> A   initial encounter
> D   subsequent encounter
> S   sequela

X+7th **V76.0 Driver of bus injured in collision with other nonmotor vehicle in nontraffic accident**

X+7th **V76.1 Passenger on bus injured in collision with other nonmotor vehicle in nontraffic accident**

X+7th **V76.2 Person on outside of bus injured in collision with other nonmotor vehicle in nontraffic accident**

X+7th **V76.3 Unspecified occupant of bus injured in collision with other nonmotor vehicle in nontraffic accident**

X+7th **V76.4 Person boarding or alighting from bus injured in collision with other nonmotor vehicle**

X+7th **V76.5 Driver of bus injured in collision with other nonmotor vehicle in traffic accident**

X+7th **V76.6 Passenger on bus injured in collision with other nonmotor vehicle in traffic accident**

X+7th **V76.7 Person on outside of bus injured in collision with other nonmotor vehicle in traffic accident**

X+7th **V76.9 Unspecified occupant of bus injured in collision with other nonmotor vehicle in traffic accident**

V77 Bus occupant injured in collision with fixed or stationary object

> The appropriate 7th character is to be added to each code from category V77
> A   initial encounter
> D   subsequent encounter
> S   sequela

X+7th **V77.0 Driver of bus injured in collision with fixed or stationary object in nontraffic accident**

X+7th **V77.1 Passenger on bus injured in collision with fixed or stationary object in nontraffic accident**

X+7th **V77.2 Person on outside of bus injured in collision with fixed or stationary object in nontraffic accident**

X+7th **V77.3 Unspecified occupant of bus injured in collision with fixed or stationary object in nontraffic accident**

X+7th **V77.4 Person boarding or alighting from bus injured in collision with fixed or stationary object**

X+7th **V77.5 Driver of bus injured in collision with fixed or stationary object in traffic accident**

X+7th **V77.6 Passenger on bus injured in collision with fixed or stationary object in traffic accident**

X+7th **V77.7 Person on outside of bus injured in collision with fixed or stationary object in traffic accident**

X+7th **V77.9 Unspecified occupant of bus injured in collision with fixed or stationary object in traffic accident**

V78 Bus occupant injured in noncollision transport accident

Includes: overturning bus NOS
overturning bus without collision

> The appropriate 7th character is to be added to each code from category V78
> A   initial encounter
> D   subsequent encounter
> S   sequela

X+7th **V78.0 Driver of bus injured in noncollision transport accident in nontraffic accident**

X+7th **V78.1 Passenger on bus injured in noncollision transport accident in nontraffic accident**

X+7th **V78.2 Person on outside of bus injured in noncollision transport accident in nontraffic accident**

X+7th **V78.3 Unspecified occupant of bus injured in noncollision transport accident in nontraffic accident**

X+7th **V78.4 Person boarding or alighting from bus injured in noncollision transport accident**

X+7th **V78.5 Driver of bus injured in noncollision transport accident in traffic accident**

X+7th **V78.6 Passenger on bus injured in noncollision transport accident in traffic accident**

X+7th **V78.7 Person on outside of bus injured in noncollision transport accident in traffic accident**

X+7th **V78.9 Unspecified occupant of bus injured in noncollision transport accident in traffic accident**

V79 Bus occupant injured in other and unspecified transport accidents

> The appropriate 7th character is to be added to each code from category V79
> A   initial encounter
> D   subsequent encounter
> S   sequela

+ **V79.0 Driver of bus injured in collision with other and unspecified motor vehicles in nontraffic accident**

X+7th **V79.00 Driver of bus injured in collision with unspecified motor vehicles in nontraffic accident**

X+7th **V79.09 Driver of bus injured in collision with other motor vehicles in nontraffic accident**

+ **V79.1 Passenger on bus injured in collision with other and unspecified motor vehicles in nontraffic accident**

X+7th **V79.10 Passenger on bus injured in collision with unspecified motor vehicles in nontraffic accident**

X+7th **V79.19 Passenger on bus injured in collision with other motor vehicles in nontraffic accident**

+ **V79.2 Unspecified bus occupant injured in collision with other and unspecified motor vehicles in nontraffic accident**

X+7th **V79.20 Unspecified bus occupant injured in collision with unspecified motor vehicles in nontraffic accident**
Bus collision NOS, nontraffic

X+7th **V79.29 Unspecified bus occupant injured in collision with other motor vehicles in nontraffic accident**

X+7th **V79.3 Bus occupant (driver) (passenger) injured in unspecified nontraffic accident**
Bus accident NOS, nontraffic
Bus occupant injured in nontraffic accident NOS

+ **V79.4 Driver of bus injured in collision with other and unspecified motor vehicles in traffic accident**

X+7th **V79.40 Driver of bus injured in collision with unspecified motor vehicles in traffic accident**

X+7th **V79.49 Driver of bus injured in collision with other motor vehicles in traffic accident**

+ **V79.5 Passenger on bus injured in collision with other and unspecified motor vehicles in traffic accident**

X+7th **V79.50 Passenger on bus injured in collision with unspecified motor vehicles in traffic accident**

X+7th **V79.59 Passenger on bus injured in collision with other motor vehicles in traffic accident**

+ **V79.6 Unspecified bus occupant injured in collision with other and unspecified motor vehicles in traffic accident**

X+7th **V79.60 Unspecified bus occupant injured in collision with unspecified motor vehicles in traffic accident**
Bus collision NOS (traffic)

X+7th **V79.69 Unspecified bus occupant injured in collision with other motor vehicles in traffic accident**

+ **V79.8 Bus occupant (driver) (passenger) injured in other specified transport accidents**

X+7th **V79.81 Bus occupant (driver) (passenger) injured in transport accidents with military vehicle**

X+7th **V79.88 Bus occupant (driver) (passenger) injured in other specified transport accidents**

X+7th **V79.9 Bus occupant (driver) (passenger) injured in unspecified traffic accident**
Bus accident NOS

Other land transport accidents (V80-V89)

V80 Animal-rider or occupant of animal-drawn vehicle injured in transport accident

> The appropriate 7th character is to be added to each code from category V80
> A   initial encounter
> D   subsequent encounter
> S   sequela

+ **V80.0 Animal-rider or occupant of animal drawn vehicle injured by fall from or being thrown from animal or animal-drawn vehicle in noncollision accident**

+ **V80.01 Animal-rider injured by fall from or being thrown from animal in noncollision accident**

+7th **V80.010 Animal-rider injured by fall from or being thrown from horse in noncollision accident**

+7th **V80.018 Animal-rider injured by fall from or being thrown from other animal in noncollision accident**

X+7th **V80.02 Occupant of animal-drawn vehicle injured by fall from or being thrown from animal-drawn vehicle in noncollision accident**
Overturning animal-drawn vehicle NOS
Overturning animal-drawn vehicle without collision

+ **V80.1 Animal-rider or occupant of animal-drawn vehicle injured in collision with pedestrian or animal**
Excludes1: *animal-rider or animal-drawn vehicle collision with animal-drawn vehicle or animal being ridden (V80.7)*

X+7th **V80.11 Animal-rider injured in collision with pedestrian or animal**

X+7th **V80.12 Occupant of animal-drawn vehicle injured in collision with pedestrian or animal**

+ **V80.2 Animal-rider or occupant of animal-drawn vehicle injured in collision with pedal cycle**

X+7th **V80.21 Animal-rider injured in collision with pedal cycle**

X+7th **V80.22 Occupant of animal-drawn vehicle injured in collision with pedal cycle**

+ **V80.3 Animal-rider or occupant of animal-drawn vehicle injured in collision with two- or three-wheeled motor vehicle**

X+7th **V80.31 Animal-rider injured in collision with two- or three-wheeled motor vehicle**

X+7th **V80.32 Occupant of animal-drawn vehicle injured in collision with two- or three-wheeled motor vehicle**

+ **V80.4 Animal-rider or occupant of animal-drawn vehicle injured in collision with car, pick-up truck, van, heavy transport vehicle or bus**
Excludes1: *animal-rider injured in collision with military vehicle (V80.910)*
occupant of animal-drawn vehicle injured in collision with military vehicle (V80.920)

X+7th **V80.41 Animal-rider injured in collision with car, pick-up truck, van, heavy transport vehicle or bus**

X+7th **V80.42 Occupant of animal-drawn vehicle injured in collision with car, pick-up truck, van, heavy transport vehicle or bus**

+ **V80.5 Animal-rider or occupant of animal-drawn vehicle injured in collision with other specified motor vehicle**

X+7th **V80.51 Animal-rider injured in collision with other specified motor vehicle**

X+7th **V80.52 Occupant of animal-drawn vehicle injured in collision with other specified motor vehicle**

+ **V80.6 Animal-rider or occupant of animal-drawn vehicle injured in collision with railway train or railway vehicle**

X+7th **V80.61 Animal-rider injured in collision with railway train or railway vehicle**

X+7th **V80.62 Occupant of animal-drawn vehicle injured in collision with railway train or railway vehicle**

+ **V80.7 Animal-rider or occupant of animal-drawn vehicle injured in collision with other nonmotor vehicles**

X+7th **V80.71 Animal-rider or occupant of animal-drawn vehicle injured in collision with animal being ridden**

X+7th **V80.710 Animal-rider injured in collision with other animal being ridden**

X+7th **V80.711 Occupant of animal-drawn vehicle injured in collision with animal being ridden**

X+7th **V80.72 Animal-rider or occupant of animal-drawn vehicle injured in collision with other animal-drawn vehicle**

X+7th **V80.720 Animal-rider injured in collision with animal-drawn vehicle**

X+7th **V80.721 Occupant of animal-drawn vehicle injured in collision with other animal-drawn vehicle**

+ **V80.73 Animal-rider or occupant of animal-drawn vehicle injured in collision with streetcar**

X+7th **V80.730 Animal-rider injured in collision with streetcar**

X+7th **V80.731 Occupant of animal-drawn vehicle injured in collision with streetcar**

X+7th **V80.79 Animal-rider or occupant of animal-drawn vehicle injured in collision with other nonmotor vehicles**

X+7th **V80.790 Animal-rider injured in collision with other nonmotor vehicles**

X+7th **V80.791 Occupant of animal-drawn vehicle injured in collision with other nonmotor vehicles**

+ **V80.8 Animal-rider or occupant of animal-drawn vehicle injured in collision with fixed or stationary object**

X+7th **V80.81 Animal-rider injured in collision with fixed or stationary object**

X+7th **V80.82 Occupant of animal-drawn vehicle injured in collision with fixed or stationary object**

+ **V80.9 Animal-rider or occupant of animal-drawn vehicle injured in other and unspecified transport accidents**

+ **V80.91 Animal-rider injured in other and unspecified transport accidents**

+7th **V80.910 Animal-rider injured in transport accident with military vehicle**

+7th **V80.918 Animal-rider injured in other transport accident**

+7th **V80.919 Animal-rider injured in unspecified transport accident**
Animal rider accident NOS

+ **V80.92 Occupant of animal-drawn vehicle injured in other and unspecified transport accidents**

+7th **V80.920 Occupant of animal-drawn vehicle injured in transport accident with military vehicle**

+7th **V80.928 Occupant of animal-drawn vehicle injured in other transport accident**

+7th **V80.929 Occupant of animal-drawn vehicle injured in unspecified transport accident**
Animal-drawn vehicle accident NOS

V81 Occupant of railway train or railway vehicle injured in transport accident
Includes: derailment of railway train or railway vehicle
person on outside of train
Excludes1: *streetcar (V82.-)*

The appropriate 7th character is to be added to each code from category V81
A   initial encounter
D   subsequent encounter
S   sequela

X+7th **V81.0 Occupant of railway train or railway vehicle injured in collision with motor vehicle in nontraffic accident**
Excludes1: *Occupant of railway train or railway vehicle injured due to collision with military vehicle (V81.83)*

X+7th **V81.1 Occupant of railway train or railway vehicle injured in collision with motor vehicle in traffic accident**
Excludes1: *Occupant of railway train or railway vehicle injured due to collision with military vehicle (V81.83)*

X+7th **V81.2 Occupant of railway train or railway vehicle injured in collision with or hit by rolling stock**

X+7th **V81.3 Occupant of railway train or railway vehicle injured in collision with other object**
Railway collision NOS

X+7th **V81.4 Person injured while boarding or alighting from railway train or railway vehicle**

X+7th **V81.5 Occupant of railway train or railway vehicle injured by fall in railway train or railway vehicle**

X+7th **V81.6 Occupant of railway train or railway vehicle injured by fall from railway train or railway vehicle**

X+7th **V81.7 Occupant of railway train or railway vehicle injured in derailment without antecedent collision**

+ **V81.8 Occupant of railway train or railway vehicle injured in other specified railway accidents**

X+7th **V81.81 Occupant of railway train or railway vehicle injured due to explosion or fire on train**

X+7th **V81.82 Occupant of railway train or railway vehicle injured due to object falling onto train**
Occupant of railway train or railway vehicle injured due to falling earth onto train
Occupant of railway train or railway vehicle injured due to falling rocks onto train
Occupant of railway train or railway vehicle injured due to falling snow onto train
Occupant of railway train or railway vehicle injured due to falling trees onto train

X+7th **V81.83 Occupant of railway train or railway vehicle injured due to collision with military vehicle**

X+7th **V81.89 Occupant of railway train or railway vehicle injured due to other specified railway accident**

X+7th **V81.9** **Occupant of railway train or railway vehicle injured in unspecified railway accident**
Railway accident NOS

V82 **Occupant of powered streetcar injured in transport accident**

Includes: interurban electric car
person on outside of streetcar
tram (car)
trolley (car)

Excludes1: *bus (V70-V79)*
motorcoach (V70-V79)
nonpowered streetcar (V76.-)
train (V81.-)

The appropriate 7th character is to be added to each code from category V82
A initial encounter
D subsequent encounter
S sequela

X+7th **V82.0** **Occupant of streetcar injured in collision with motor vehicle in nontraffic accident**
X+7th **V82.1** **Occupant of streetcar injured in collision with motor vehicle in traffic accident**
X+7th **V82.2** **Occupant of streetcar injured in collision with or hit by rolling stock**
X+7th **V82.3** **Occupant of streetcar injured in collision with other object**
Excludes1: *collision with animal-drawn vehicle or animal being ridden (V82.8)*
X+7th **V82.4** **Person injured while boarding or alighting from streetcar**
X+7th **V82.5** **Occupant of streetcar injured by fall in streetcar**
Excludes1: *fall in streetcar:*
while boarding or alighting (V82.4)
with antecedent collision (V82.0-V82.3)
X+7th **V82.6** **Occupant of streetcar injured by fall from streetcar**
Excludes1: *fall from streetcar:*
while boarding or alighting (V82.4)
with antecedent collision (V82.0-V82.3)
X+7th **V82.7** **Occupant of streetcar injured in derailment without antecedent collision**
Excludes1: *occupant of streetcar injured in derailment with antecedent collision (V82.0-V82.3)*
X+7th **V82.8** **Occupant of streetcar injured in other specified transport accidents**
Streetcar collision with military vehicle
Streetcar collision with train or nonmotor vehicles
X+7th **V82.9** **Occupant of streetcar injured in unspecified traffic accident**
Streetcar accident NOS

V83 **Occupant of special vehicle mainly used on industrial premises injured in transport accident**

Includes: battery-powered airport passenger vehicle
battery-powered truck (baggage) (mail)
coal-car in mine
forklift (truck)
logging car
self-propelled industrial truck
station baggage truck (powered)
tram, truck, or tub (powered) in mine or quarry

Excludes1: *special construction vehicles (V85.-)*
special industrial vehicle in stationary use or maintenance (W31.-)

The appropriate 7th character is to be added to each code from category V83
A initial encounter
D subsequent encounter
S sequela

X+7th **V83.0** **Driver of special industrial vehicle injured in traffic accident**
X+7th **V83.1** **Passenger of special industrial vehicle injured in traffic accident**
X+7th **V83.2** **Person on outside of special industrial vehicle injured in traffic accident**
X+7th **V83.3** **Unspecified occupant of special industrial vehicle injured in traffic accident**
X+7th **V83.4** **Person injured while boarding or alighting from special industrial vehicle**
X+7th **V83.5** **Driver of special industrial vehicle injured in nontraffic accident**

X+7th **V83.6** **Passenger of special industrial vehicle injured in nontraffic accident**
X+7th **V83.7** **Person on outside of special industrial vehicle injured in nontraffic accident**
X+7th **V83.9** **Unspecified occupant of special industrial vehicle injured in nontraffic accident**
Special-industrial-vehicle accident NOS

V84 **Occupant of special vehicle mainly used in agriculture injured in transport accident**

Includes: self-propelled farm machinery
tractor (and trailer)

Excludes1: *animal-powered farm machinery accident (W30.8-)*
contact with combine harvester (W30.0)
special agricultural vehicle in stationary use or maintenance (W30.-)

The appropriate 7th character is to be added to each code from category V84
A initial encounter
D subsequent encounter
S sequela

X+7th **V84.0** **Driver of special agricultural vehicle injured in traffic accident**
X+7th **V84.1** **Passenger of special agricultural vehicle injured in traffic accident**
X+7th **V84.2** **Person on outside of special agricultural vehicle injured in traffic accident**
X+7th **V84.3** **Unspecified occupant of special agricultural vehicle injured in traffic accident**
X+7th **V84.4** **Person injured while boarding or alighting from special agricultural vehicle**
X+7th **V84.5** **Driver of special agricultural vehicle injured in nontraffic accident**
X+7th **V84.6** **Passenger of special agricultural vehicle injured in nontraffic accident**
X+7th **V84.7** **Person on outside of special agricultural vehicle injured in nontraffic accident**
X+7th **V84.9** **Unspecified occupant of special agricultural vehicle injured in nontraffic accident**
Special-agricultural vehicle accident NOS

V85 **Occupant of special construction vehicle injured in transport accident**

Includes: bulldozer
digger
dump truck
earth-leveller
mechanical shovel
road-roller

Excludes1: *special industrial vehicle (V83.-)*
special construction vehicle in stationary use or maintenance (W31.-)

The appropriate 7th character is to be added to each code from category V85
A initial encounter
D subsequent encounter
S sequela

X+7th **V85.0** **Driver of special construction vehicle injured in traffic accident**
X+7th **V85.1** **Passenger of special construction vehicle injured in traffic accident**
X+7th **V85.2** **Person on outside of special construction vehicle injured in traffic accident**
X+7th **V85.3** **Unspecified occupant of special construction vehicle injured in traffic accident**
X+7th **V85.4** **Person injured while boarding or alighting from special construction vehicle**
X+7th **V85.5** **Driver of special construction vehicle injured in nontraffic accident**
X+7th **V85.6** **Passenger of special construction vehicle injured in nontraffic accident**
X+7th **V85.7** **Person on outside of special construction vehicle injured in nontraffic accident**
X+7th **V85.9** **Unspecified occupant of special construction vehicle injured in nontraffic accident**
Special-construction-vehicle accident NOS

V86   Occupant of special all-terrain or other off-road motor vehicle, injured in transport accident

> **Excludes1:** *special all-terrain vehicle in stationary use or maintenance (W31.-)*
> *sport-utility vehicle (V50-V59)*
> *three-wheeled motor vehicle designed for on-road use (V30-V39)*
>
> AHA CC: 4Q, 2017, 26

The appropriate 7th character is to be added to each code from category V86
A   initial encounter
D   subsequent encounter
S   sequela

+ **V86.0   Driver of special all-terrain or other off-road motor vehicle injured in traffic accident**
+7th **V86.01**   Driver of ambulance or fire engine injured in traffic accident
+7th **V86.02**   Driver of snowmobile injured in traffic accident
+7th **V86.03**   Driver of dune buggy injured in traffic accident
+7th **V86.04**   Driver of military vehicle injured in traffic accident
+7th **V86.05**   Driver of 3- or 4- wheeled all-terrain vehicle (ATV) injured in traffic accident
+7th **V86.06**   Driver of dirt bike or motor/cross bike injured in traffic accident
+7th **V86.09**   Driver of other special all-terrain or other off-road motor vehicle injured in traffic accident
> Driver of go cart injured in traffic accident
> Driver of golf cart injured in traffic accident

+ **V86.1   Passenger of special all-terrain or other off-road motor vehicle injured in traffic accident**
+7th **V86.11**   Passenger of ambulance or fire engine injured in traffic accident
+7th **V86.12**   Passenger of snowmobile injured in traffic accident
+7th **V86.13**   Passenger of dune buggy injured in traffic accident
+7th **V86.14**   Passenger of military vehicle injured in traffic accident
+7th **V86.15**   Passenger of 3- or 4- wheeled all-terrain vehicle (ATV) injured in traffic accident
+7th **V86.16**   Passenger of dirt bike or motor/cross bike injured in traffic accident
+7th **V86.19**   Passenger of other special all-terrain or other off-road motor vehicle injured in traffic accident
> Passenger of go cart injured in traffic accident
> Passenger of golf cart injured in traffic accident

+ **V86.2   Person on outside of special all-terrain or other off-road motor vehicle injured in traffic accident**
+7th **V86.21**   Person on outside of ambulance or fire engine injured in traffic accident
+7th **V86.22**   Person on outside of snowmobile injured in traffic accident
+7th **V86.23**   Person on outside of dune buggy injured in traffic accident
+7th **V86.24**   Person on outside of military vehicle injured in traffic accident
+7th **V86.25**   Person on outside of 3- or 4- wheeled all-terrain vehicle (ATV) injured in traffic accident
+7th **V86.26**   Person on outside of dirt bike or motor/cross bike injured in traffic accident
+7th **V86.29**   Person on outside of other special all-terrain or other off-road motor vehicle injured in traffic accident
> Person on outside of go cart in traffic accident
> Person on outside of golf cart injured in traffic accident

+ **V86.3   Unspecified occupant of special all-terrain or other off-road motor vehicle injured in traffic accident**
+7th **V86.31**   Unspecified occupant of ambulance or fire engine injured in traffic accident
+7th **V86.32**   Unspecified occupant of snowmobile injured in traffic accident
+7th **V86.33**   Unspecified occupant of dune buggy injured in traffic accident
+7th **V86.34**   Unspecified occupant of military vehicle injured in traffic accident
+7th **V86.35**   Unspecified occupant of 3- or 4- wheeled all-terrain vehicle (ATV) injured in traffic accident

+7th **V86.36**   Unspecified occupant of dirt bike or motor/cross bike injured in traffic accident
+7th **V86.39**   Unspecified occupant of other special all-terrain or other off-road motor vehicle injured in traffic accident
> Unspecified occupant of go cart injured in traffic accident
> Unspecified occupant of golf cart injured in traffic accident

+ **V86.4   Person injured while boarding or alighting from special all-terrain or other off-road motor vehicle**
+7th **V86.41**   Person injured while boarding or alighting from ambulance or fire engine
+7th **V86.42**   Person injured while boarding or alighting from snowmobile
+7th **V86.43**   Person injured while boarding or alighting from dune buggy
+7th **V86.44**   Person injured while boarding or alighting from military vehicle
+7th **V86.45**   Person injured while boarding or alighting from a 3- or 4- wheeled all-terrain vehicle (ATV)
+7th **V86.46**   Person injured while boarding or alighting from a dirt bike or motor/cross bike
+7th **V86.49**   Person injured while boarding or alighting from other special all-terrain or other off-road motor vehicle
> Person injured while boarding or alighting from go cart
> Person injured while boarding or alighting from golf cart

+ **V86.5   Driver of special all-terrain or other off-road motor vehicle injured in nontraffic accident**
+7th **V86.51**   Driver of ambulance or fire engine injured in nontraffic accident
+7th **V86.52**   Driver of snowmobile injured in nontraffic accident
+7th **V86.53**   Driver of dune buggy injured in nontraffic accident
+7th **V86.54**   Driver of military vehicle injured in nontraffic accident
+7th **V86.55**   Driver of 3- or 4- wheeled all-terrain vehicle (ATV) injured in nontraffic accident
+7th **V86.56**   Driver of dirt bike or motor/cross bike injured in nontraffic accident, initial encounter
+7th **V86.59**   Driver of other special all-terrain or other off-road motor vehicle injured in nontraffic accident
> Driver of go cart injured in nontraffic accident
> Driver of golf cart injured in nontraffic accident

+ **V86.6   Passenger of special all-terrain or other off-road motor vehicle injured in nontraffic accident**
+7th **V86.61**   Passenger of ambulance or fire engine injured in nontraffic accident
+7th **V86.62**   Passenger of snowmobile injured in nontraffic accident
+7th **V86.63**   Passenger of dune buggy injured in nontraffic accident
+7th **V86.64**   Passenger of military vehicle injured in nontraffic accident
+7th **V86.65**   Passenger of 3- or 4- wheeled all-terrain vehicle (ATV) injured in nontraffic accident
+7th **V86.66**   Passenger of dirt bike or motor/cross bike injured in nontraffic accident
+7th **V86.69**   Passenger of other special all-terrain or other off-road motor vehicle injured in nontraffic accident
> Passenger of go cart injured in nontraffic accident
> Passenger of golf cart injured in nontraffic accident

+ **V86.7   Person on outside of special all-terrain or other off-road motor vehicle injured in nontraffic accident**
+7th **V86.71**   Person on outside of ambulance or fire engine injured in nontraffic accident
+7th **V86.72**   Person on outside of snowmobile injured in nontraffic accident
+7th **V86.73**   Person on outside of dune buggy injured in nontraffic accident
+7th **V86.74**   Person on outside of military vehicle injured in nontraffic accident
+7th **V86.75**   Person on outside of 3- or 4- wheeled all-terrain vehicle (ATV) injured in nontraffic accident
+7th **V86.76**   Person on outside of dirt bike or motor/cross bike injured in nontraffic accident

+7th **V86.79** **Person on outside of other special all-terrain or other off-road motor vehicles injured in nontraffic accident**

> Person on outside of go cart injured in nontraffic accident
>
> Person on outside of golf cart injured in nontraffic accident

+ **V86.9** **Unspecified occupant of special all-terrain or other off-road motor vehicle injured in nontraffic accident**

+7th **V86.91** **Unspecified occupant of ambulance or fire engine injured in nontraffic accident**

+7th **V86.92** **Unspecified occupant of snowmobile injured in nontraffic accident**

+7th **V86.93** **Unspecified occupant of dune buggy injured in nontraffic accident**

+7th **V86.94** **Unspecified occupant of military vehicle injured in nontraffic accident**

+7th **V86.95** **Unspecified occupant of 3- or 4- wheeled all-terrain vehicle (ATV) injured in nontraffic accident**

+7th **V86.96** **Unspecified occupant of dirt bike or motor/cross bike injured in nontraffic accident**

+7th **V86.99** **Unspecified occupant of other special all-terrain or other off-road motor vehicle injured in nontraffic accident**

> Off-road motor-vehicle accident NOS
>
> Other motor-vehicle accident NOS
>
> Unspecified occupant of go cart injured in nontraffic accident
>
> Unspecified occupant of golf cart injured in nontraffic accident

V87 **Traffic accident of specified type but victim's mode of transport unknown**

> **Excludes1:** *collision involving:*
> *pedal cycle (V10-V19)*
> *pedestrian (V01-V09)*

> The appropriate 7th character is to be added to each code from category V87
> A   initial encounter
> D   subsequent encounter
> S   sequela

X+7th **V87.0** **Person injured in collision between car and two- or three-wheeled powered vehicle (traffic)**

X+7th **V87.1** **Person injured in collision between other motor vehicle and two- or three-wheeled motor vehicle (traffic)**

X+7th **V87.2** **Person injured in collision between car and pick-up truck or van (traffic)**

X+7th **V87.3** **Person injured in collision between car and bus (traffic)**

X+7th **V87.4** **Person injured in collision between car and heavy transport vehicle (traffic)**

X+7th **V87.5** **Person injured in collision between heavy transport vehicle and bus (traffic)**

X+7th **V87.6** **Person injured in collision between railway train or railway vehicle and car (traffic)**

X+7th **V87.7** **Person injured in collision between other specified motor vehicles (traffic)**

X+7th **V87.8** **Person injured in other specified noncollision transport accidents involving motor vehicle (traffic)**

X+7th **V87.9** **Person injured in other specified (collision) (noncollision) transport accidents involving nonmotor vehicle (traffic)**

V88 **Nontraffic accident of specified type but victim's mode of transport unknown**

> **Excludes1:** *collision involving:*
> *pedal cycle (V10-V19)*
> *pedestrian (V01-V09)*

> The appropriate 7th character is to be added to each code from category V88
> A   initial encounter
> D   subsequent encounter
> S   sequela

X+7th **V88.0** **Person injured in collision between car and two- or three-wheeled motor vehicle, nontraffic**

X+7th **V88.1** **Person injured in collision between other motor vehicle and two- or three-wheeled motor vehicle, nontraffic**

X+7th **V88.2** **Person injured in collision between car and pick-up truck or van, nontraffic**

X+7th **V88.3** **Person injured in collision between car and bus, nontraffic**

X+7th **V88.4** **Person injured in collision between car and heavy transport vehicle, nontraffic**

X+7th **V88.5** **Person injured in collision between heavy transport vehicle and bus, nontraffic**

X+7th **V88.6** **Person injured in collision between railway train or railway vehicle and car, nontraffic**

X+7th **V88.7** **Person injured in collision between other specified motor vehicle, nontraffic**

X+7th **V88.8** **Person injured in other specified noncollision transport accidents involving motor vehicle, nontraffic**

X+7th **V88.9** **Person injured in other specified (collision)(noncollision) transport accidents involving nonmotor vehicle, nontraffic**

V89 **Motor- or nonmotor-vehicle accident, type of vehicle unspecified**

> The appropriate 7th character is to be added to each code from category V89
> A   initial encounter
> D   subsequent encounter
> S   sequela

X+7th **V89.0** **Person injured in unspecified motor-vehicle accident, nontraffic**

> Motor-vehicle accident NOS, nontraffic

X+7th **V89.1** **Person injured in unspecified nonmotor-vehicle accident, nontraffic**

> Nonmotor-vehicle accident NOS (nontraffic)

X+7th **V89.2** **Person injured in unspecified motor-vehicle accident, traffic**

> Motor-vehicle accident [MVA] NOS
>
> Road (traffic) accident [RTA] NOS

X+7th **V89.3** **Person injured in unspecified nonmotor-vehicle accident, traffic**

> Nonmotor-vehicle traffic accident NOS

X+7th **V89.9** **Person injured in unspecified vehicle accident**

> Collision NOS

Water transport accidents (V90-V94)

V90 **Drowning and submersion due to accident to watercraft**

> **Excludes1:** *civilian water transport accident involving military*
> *watercraft (V94.81-)*
> *fall into water not from watercraft (W16.-)*
> *military watercraft accident in military or war*
> *operations (Y36.0-, Y37.0-)*
> *water-transport-related drowning or submersion*
> *without accident to watercraft (V92.-)*

> The appropriate 7th character is to be added to each code from category V90
> A   initial encounter
> D   subsequent encounter
> S   sequela

+ **V90.0** **Drowning and submersion due to watercraft overturning**

X+7th **V90.00** **Drowning and submersion due to merchant ship overturning**

X+7th **V90.01** **Drowning and submersion due to passenger ship overturning**

> Drowning and submersion due to Ferry-boat overturning
>
> Drowning and submersion due to Liner overturning

X+7th **V90.02** **Drowning and submersion due to fishing boat overturning**

X+7th **V90.03** **Drowning and submersion due to other powered watercraft overturning**

> Drowning and submersion due to Hovercraft (on open water) overturning
>
> Drowning and submersion due to Jet ski overturning

X+7th **V90.04** **Drowning and submersion due to sailboat overturning**

X+7th **V90.05** **Drowning and submersion due to canoe or kayak overturning**

X+7th **V90.06** **Drowning and submersion due to (nonpowered) inflatable craft overturning**

X+7th **V90.08** **Drowning and submersion due to other unpowered watercraft overturning**

> Drowning and submersion due to windsurfer overturning

X+7th **V90.09** **Drowning and submersion due to unspecified watercraft overturning**
    Drowning and submersion due to boat NOS overturning
    Drowning and submersion due to ship NOS overturning
    Drowning and submersion due to watercraft NOS overturning

+ **V90.1** **Drowning and submersion due to watercraft sinking**

X+7th **V90.10** **Drowning and submersion due to merchant ship sinking**

X+7th **V90.11** **Drowning and submersion due to passenger ship sinking**
    Drowning and submersion due to Ferry-boat sinking
    Drowning and submersion due to Liner sinking

X+7th **V90.12** **Drowning and submersion due to fishing boat sinking**

X+7th **V90.13** **Drowning and submersion due to other powered watercraft sinking**
    Drowning and submersion due to Hovercraft (on open water) sinking
    Drowning and submersion due to Jet ski sinking

X+7th **V90.14** **Drowning and submersion due to sailboat sinking**

X+7th **V90.15** **Drowning and submersion due to canoe or kayak sinking**

X+7th **V90.16** **Drowning and submersion due to (nonpowered) inflatable craft sinking**

X+7th **V90.18** **Drowning and submersion due to other unpowered watercraft sinking**

X+7th **V90.19** **Drowning and submersion due to unspecified watercraft sinking**
    Drowning and submersion due to boat NOS sinking
    Drowning and submersion due to ship NOS sinking
    Drowning and submersion due to watercraft NOS sinking

+ **V90.2** **Drowning and submersion due to falling or jumping from burning watercraft**

X+7th **V90.20** **Drowning and submersion due to falling or jumping from burning merchant ship**

X+7th **V90.21** **Drowning and submersion due to falling or jumping from burning passenger ship**
    Drowning and submersion due to falling or jumping from burning Ferry-boat
    Drowning and submersion due to falling or jumping from burning Liner

X+7th **V90.22** **Drowning and submersion due to falling or jumping from burning fishing boat**

X+7th **V90.23** **Drowning and submersion due to falling or jumping from other burning powered watercraft**
    Drowning and submersion due to falling and jumping from burning Hovercraft (on open water)
    Drowning and submersion due to falling and jumping from burning Jet ski

X+7th **V90.24** **Drowning and submersion due to falling or jumping from burning sailboat**

X+7th **V90.25** **Drowning and submersion due to falling or jumping from burning canoe or kayak**

X+7th **V90.26** **Drowning and submersion due to falling or jumping from burning (nonpowered) inflatable craft**

X+7th **V90.27** **Drowning and submersion due to falling or jumping from burning water-skis**

X+7th **V90.28** **Drowning and submersion due to falling or jumping from other burning unpowered watercraft**
    Drowning and submersion due to falling and jumping from burning surf-board
    Drowning and submersion due to falling and jumping from burning windsurfer

X+7th **V90.29** **Drowning and submersion due to falling or jumping from unspecified burning watercraft**
    Drowning and submersion due to falling or jumping from burning boat NOS
    Drowning and submersion due to falling or jumping from burning ship NOS
    Drowning and submersion due to falling or jumping from burning watercraft NOS

+ **V90.3** **Drowning and submersion due to falling or jumping from crushed watercraft**

X+7th **V90.30** **Drowning and submersion due to falling or jumping from crushed merchant ship**

X+7th **V90.31** **Drowning and submersion due to falling or jumping from crushed passenger ship**
    Drowning and submersion due to falling and jumping from crushed Ferry boat
    Drowning and submersion due to falling and jumping from crushed Liner

X+7th **V90.32** **Drowning and submersion due to falling or jumping from crushed fishing boat**

X+7th **V90.33** **Drowning and submersion due to falling or jumping from other crushed powered watercraft**
    Drowning and submersion due to falling and jumping from crushed Hovercraft
    Drowning and submersion due to falling and jumping from crushed Jet ski

X+7th **V90.34** **Drowning and submersion due to falling or jumping from crushed sailboat**

X+7th **V90.35** **Drowning and submersion due to falling or jumping from crushed canoe or kayak**

X+7th **V90.36** **Drowning and submersion due to falling or jumping from crushed (nonpowered) inflatable craft**

X+7th **V90.37** **Drowning and submersion due to falling or jumping from crushed water-skis**

X+7th **V90.38** **Drowning and submersion due to falling or jumping from other crushed unpowered watercraft**
    Drowning and submersion due to falling and jumping from crushed surf-board
    Drowning and submersion due to falling and jumping from crushed windsurfer

X+7th **V90.39** **Drowning and submersion due to falling or jumping from crushed unspecified watercraft**
    Drowning and submersion due to falling and jumping from crushed boat NOS
    Drowning and submersion due to falling and jumping from crushed ship NOS
    Drowning and submersion due to falling and jumping from crushed watercraft NOS

+ **V90.8** **Drowning and submersion due to other accident to watercraft**

X+7th **V90.80** **Drowning and submersion due to other accident to merchant ship**

X+7th **V90.81** **Drowning and submersion due to other accident to passenger ship**
    Drowning and submersion due to other accident to Ferry-boat
    Drowning and submersion due to other accident to Liner

X+7th **V90.82** **Drowning and submersion due to other accident to fishing boat**

X+7th **V90.83** **Drowning and submersion due to other accident to other powered watercraft**
    Drowning and submersion due to other accident to Hovercraft (on open water)
    Drowning and submersion due to other accident to Jet ski

X+7th **V90.84** **Drowning and submersion due to other accident to sailboat**

X+7th **V90.85** **Drowning and submersion due to other accident to canoe or kayak**

X+7th **V90.86** **Drowning and submersion due to other accident to (nonpowered) inflatable craft**

X+7th **V90.87** **Drowning and submersion due to other accident to water-skis**
X+7th **V90.88** **Drowning and submersion due to other accident to other unpowered watercraft**
> Drowning and submersion due to other accident to surf-board
> Drowning and submersion due to other accident to windsurfer

X+7th **V90.89** **Drowning and submersion due to other accident to unspecified watercraft**
> Drowning and submersion due to other accident to boat NOS
> Drowning and submersion due to other accident to ship NOS
> Drowning and submersion due to other accident to watercraft NOS

V91 **Other injury due to accident to watercraft**

> **Includes:** any injury except drowning and submersion as a result of an accident to watercraft
>
> **Excludes1:** *civilian water transport accident involving military watercraft (V94.81-)*
> *military watercraft accident in military or war operations (Y36, Y37.-)*
>
> **Excludes2:** *drowning and submersion due to accident to watercraft (V90.-)*

> The appropriate 7th character is to be added to each code from category V91
> A initial encounter
> D subsequent encounter
> S sequela

+ **V91.0** **Burn due to watercraft on fire**
> **Excludes1:** *burn from localized fire or explosion on board ship without accident to watercraft (V93.-)*

X+7th **V91.00** **Burn due to merchant ship on fire**
X+7th **V91.01** **Burn due to passenger ship on fire**
> Burn due to Ferry-boat on fire
> Burn due to Liner on fire

X+7th **V91.02** **Burn due to fishing boat on fire**
X+7th **V91.03** **Burn due to other powered watercraft on fire**
> Burn due to Hovercraft (on open water) on fire
> Burn due to Jet ski on fire

X+7th **V91.04** **Burn due to sailboat on fire**
X+7th **V91.05** **Burn due to canoe or kayak on fire**
X+7th **V91.06** **Burn due to (nonpowered) inflatable craft on fire**
X+7th **V91.07** **Burn due to water-skis on fire**
X+7th **V91.08** **Burn due to other unpowered watercraft on fire**
X+7th **V91.09** **Burn due to unspecified watercraft on fire**
> Burn due to boat NOS on fire
> Burn due to ship NOS on fire
> Burn due to watercraft NOS on fire

+ **V91.1** **Crushed between watercraft and other watercraft or other object due to collision**
> Crushed by lifeboat after abandoning ship in a collision
> **NOTE** Select the specified type of watercraft that the victim was on at the time of the collision

X+7th **V91.10** **Crushed between merchant ship and other watercraft or other object due to collision**
X+7th **V91.11** **Crushed between passenger ship and other watercraft or other object due to collision**
> Crushed between Ferry-boat and other watercraft or other object due to collision
> Crushed between Liner and other watercraft or other object due to collision

X+7th **V91.12** **Crushed between fishing boat and other watercraft or other object due to collision**
X+7th **V91.13** **Crushed between other powered watercraft and other watercraft or other object due to collision**
> Crushed between Hovercraft (on open water) and other watercraft or other object due to collision
> Crushed between Jet ski and other watercraft or other object due to collision

X+7th **V91.14** **Crushed between sailboat and other watercraft or other object due to collision**
X+7th **V91.15** **Crushed between canoe or kayak and other watercraft or other object due to collision**
X+7th **V91.16** **Crushed between (nonpowered) inflatable craft and other watercraft or other object due to collision**

X+7th **V91.18** **Crushed between other unpowered watercraft and other watercraft or other object due to collision**
> Crushed between surfboard and other watercraft or other object due to collision
> Crushed between windsurfer and other watercraft or other object due to collision

X+7th **V91.19** **Crushed between unspecified watercraft and other watercraft or other object due to collision**
> Crushed between boat NOS and other watercraft or other object due to collision
> Crushed between ship NOS and other watercraft or other object due to collision
> Crushed between watercraft NOS and other watercraft or other object due to collision

+ **V91.2** **Fall due to collision between watercraft and other watercraft or other object**
> Fall while remaining on watercraft after collision
> **NOTE** Select the specified type of watercraft that the victim was on at the time of the collision
>
> **Excludes1:** *crushed between watercraft and other watercraft and other object due to collision (V91.1-)*
> *drowning and submersion due to falling from crushed watercraft (V90.3-)*

X+7th **V91.20** **Fall due to collision between merchant ship and other watercraft or other object**
X+7th **V91.21** **Fall due to collision between passenger ship and other watercraft or other object**
> Fall due to collision between Ferry-boat and other watercraft or other object
> Fall due to collision between Liner and other watercraft or other object

X+7th **V91.22** **Fall due to collision between fishing boat and other watercraft or other object**
X+7th **V91.23** **Fall due to collision between other powered watercraft and other watercraft or other object**
> Fall due to collision between Hovercraft (on open water) and other watercraft or other object
> Fall due to collision between Jet ski and other watercraft or other object

X+7th **V91.24** **Fall due to collision between sailboat and other watercraft or other object**
X+7th **V91.25** **Fall due to collision between canoe or kayak and other watercraft or other object**
X+7th **V91.26** **Fall due to collision between (nonpowered) inflatable craft and other watercraft or other object**
X+7th **V91.29** **Fall due to collision between unspecified watercraft and other watercraft or other object**
> Fall due to collision between boat NOS and other watercraft or other object
> Fall due to collision between ship NOS and other watercraft or other object
> Fall due to collision between watercraft NOS and other watercraft or other object

+ **V91.3** **Hit or struck by falling object due to accident to watercraft**
> Hit or struck by falling object (part of damaged watercraft or other object) after falling or jumping from damaged watercraft
>
> **Excludes2:** *drowning or submersion due to fall or jumping from damaged watercraft (V90.2-, V90.3-)*

X+7th **V91.30** **Hit or struck by falling object due to accident to merchant ship**
X+7th **V91.31** **Hit or struck by falling object due to accident to passenger ship**
> Hit or struck by falling object due to accident to Ferry-boat
> Hit or struck by falling object due to accident to Liner

X+7th **V91.32** **Hit or struck by falling object due to accident to fishing boat**
X+7th **V91.33** **Hit or struck by falling object due to accident to other powered watercraft**
> Hit or struck by falling object due to accident to Hovercraft (on open water)
> Hit or struck by falling object due to accident to Jet ski

X+7th **V91.34** **Hit or struck by falling object due to accident to sailboat**

X+7th **V91.35** **Hit or struck by falling object due to accident to canoe or kayak**

X+7th **V91.36** **Hit or struck by falling object due to accident to (nonpowered) inflatable craft**

X+7th **V91.37** **Hit or struck by falling object due to accident to water-skis**

Hit by water-skis after jumping off of waterskis

X+7th **V91.38** **Hit or struck by falling object due to accident to other unpowered watercraft**

Hit or struck by surf-board after falling off damaged surf-board

Hit or struck by object after falling off damaged windsurfer

X+7th **V91.39** **Hit or struck by falling object due to accident to unspecified watercraft**

Hit or struck by falling object due to accident to boat NOS

Hit or struck by falling object due to accident to ship NOS

Hit or struck by falling object due to accident to watercraft NOS

+ **V91.8** **Other injury due to other accident to watercraft**

X+7th **V91.80** **Other injury due to other accident to merchant ship**

X+7th **V91.81** **Other injury due to other accident to passenger ship**

Other injury due to other accident to Ferry-boat

Other injury due to other accident to Liner

X+7th **V91.82** **Other injury due to other accident to fishing boat**

X+7th **V91.83** **Other injury due to other accident to other powered watercraft**

Other injury due to other accident to Hovercraft (on open water)

Other injury due to other accident to Jet ski

X+7th **V91.84** **Other injury due to other accident to sailboat**

X+7th **V91.85** **Other injury due to other accident to canoe or kayak**

X+7th **V91.86** **Other injury due to other accident to (nonpowered) inflatable craft**

X+7th **V91.87** **Other injury due to other accident to water-skis**

X+7th **V91.88** **Other injury due to other accident to other unpowered watercraft**

Other injury due to other accident to surf-board

Other injury due to other accident to windsurfer

X+7th **V91.89** **Other injury due to other accident to unspecified watercraft**

Other injury due to other accident to boat NOS

Other injury due to other accident to ship NOS

Other injury due to other accident to watercraft NOS

V92 **Drowning and submersion due to accident on board watercraft, without accident to watercraft**

Excludes1: *civilian water transport accident involving military watercraft (V94.81-)*

drowning or submersion due to accident to watercraft (V90-V91)

drowning or submersion of diver who voluntarily jumps from boat not involved in an accident (W16.711, W16.721)

fall into water without watercraft (W16.-)

military watercraft accident in military or war operations (Y36, Y37)

The appropriate 7th character is to be added to each code from category V92
A   initial encounter
D   subsequent encounter
S   sequela

+ **V92.0** **Drowning and submersion due to fall off watercraft**

Drowning and submersion due to fall from gangplank of watercraft

Drowning and submersion due to fall overboard watercraft

Excludes2: *hitting head on object or bottom of body of water due to fall from watercraft (V94.0-)*

X+7th **V92.00** **Drowning and submersion due to fall off merchant ship**

X+7th **V92.01** **Drowning and submersion due to fall off passenger ship**

Drowning and submersion due to fall off Ferry-boat

Drowning and submersion due to fall off Liner

X+7th **V92.02** **Drowning and submersion due to fall off fishing boat**

X+7th **V92.03** **Drowning and submersion due to fall off other powered watercraft**

Drowning and submersion due to fall off Hovercraft (on open water)

Drowning and submersion due to fall off Jet ski

X+7th **V92.04** **Drowning and submersion due to fall off sailboat**

X+7th **V92.05** **Drowning and submersion due to fall off canoe or kayak**

X+7th **V92.06** **Drowning and submersion due to fall off (nonpowered) inflatable craft**

X+7th **V92.07** **Drowning and submersion due to fall off water-skis**

Excludes1: *drowning and submersion due to falling off burning water-skis (V90.27)*

drowning and submersion due to falling off crushed water-skis (V90.37)

hit by boat while water-skiing NOS (V94.X)

X+7th **V92.08** **Drowning and submersion due to fall off other unpowered watercraft**

Drowning and submersion due to fall off surf-board

Drowning and submersion due to fall off windsurfer

Excludes1: *drowning and submersion due to fall off burning unpowered watercraft (V90.28)*

drowning and submersion due to fall off crushed unpowered watercraft (V90.38)

drowning and submersion due to fall off damaged unpowered watercraft (V90.88)

drowning and submersion due to rider of nonpowered watercraft being hit by other watercraft (V94.-)

other injury due to rider of nonpowered watercraft being hit by other watercraft (V94.-)

X+7th **V92.09** **Drowning and submersion due to fall off unspecified watercraft**

Drowning and submersion due to fall off boat NOS

Drowning and submersion due to fall off ship

Drowning and submersion due to fall off watercraft NOS

+ **V92.1** **Drowning and submersion due to being thrown overboard by motion of watercraft**

Excludes1: *drowning and submersion due to fall off surf-board (V92.08)*

drowning and submersion due to fall off water-skis (V92.07)

drowning and submersion due to fall off windsurfer (V92.08)

X+7th **V92.10** **Drowning and submersion due to being thrown overboard by motion of merchant ship**

X+7th **V92.11** **Drowning and submersion due to being thrown overboard by motion of passenger ship**

Drowning and submersion due to being thrown overboard by motion of Ferry-boat

Drowning and submersion due to being thrown overboard by motion of Liner

X+7th **V92.12** **Drowning and submersion due to being thrown overboard by motion of fishing boat**

X+7th **V92.13** **Drowning and submersion due to being thrown overboard by motion of other powered watercraft**

Drowning and submersion due to being thrown overboard by motion of Hovercraft

X+7th **V92.14** **Drowning and submersion due to being thrown overboard by motion of sailboat**

X+7th **V92.15** **Drowning and submersion due to being thrown overboard by motion of canoe or kayak**

X+7th **V92.16** **Drowning and submersion due to being thrown overboard by motion of (nonpowered) inflatable craft**

X+7th V92.19 Drowning and submersion due to being thrown overboard by motion of unspecified watercraft
    Drowning and submersion due to being thrown overboard by motion of boat NOS
    Drowning and submersion due to being thrown overboard by motion of ship NOS
    Drowning and submersion due to being thrown overboard by motion of watercraft NOS

+ V92.2 Drowning and submersion due to being washed overboard from watercraft
    Code first any associated cataclysm (X37.0-)

X+7th V92.20 Drowning and submersion due to being washed overboard from merchant ship

X+7th V92.21 Drowning and submersion due to being washed overboard from passenger ship
    Drowning and submersion due to being washed overboard from Ferry-boat
    Drowning and submersion due to being washed overboard from Liner

X+7th V92.22 Drowning and submersion due to being washed overboard from fishing boat

X+7th V92.23 Drowning and submersion due to being washed overboard from other powered watercraft
    Drowning and submersion due to being washed overboard from Hovercraft (on open water)
    Drowning and submersion due to being washed overboard from Jet ski

X+7th V92.24 Drowning and submersion due to being washed overboard from sailboat

X+7th V92.25 Drowning and submersion due to being washed overboard from canoe or kayak

X+7th V92.26 Drowning and submersion due to being washed overboard from (nonpowered) inflatable craft

X+7th V92.27 Drowning and submersion due to being washed overboard from water-skis
    Excludes1: drowning and submersion due to fall off water-skis (V92.07)

X+7th V92.28 Drowning and submersion due to being washed overboard from other unpowered watercraft
    Drowning and submersion due to being washed overboard from surf-board
    Drowning and submersion due to being washed overboard from windsurfer

X+7th V92.29 Drowning and submersion due to being washed overboard from unspecified watercraft
    Drowning and submersion due to being washed overboard from boat NOS
    Drowning and submersion due to being washed overboard from ship NOS
    Drowning and submersion due to being washed overboard from watercraft NOS

V93 Other injury due to accident on board watercraft, without accident to watercraft

    Excludes1: civilian water transport accident involving military watercraft (V94.81-)
        other injury due to accident to watercraft (V91.-)
        military watercraft accident in military or war operations (Y36, Y37.-)
    Excludes2: drowning and submersion due to accident on board watercraft, without accident to watercraft (V92.-)

    The appropriate 7th character is to be added to each code from category V93
    A   initial encounter
    D   subsequent encounter
    S   sequela

+ V93.0 Burn due to localized fire on board watercraft
    Excludes1: burn due to watercraft on fire (V91.0-)

X+7th V93.00 Burn due to localized fire on board merchant vessel

X+7th V93.01 Burn due to localized fire on board passenger vessel
    Burn due to localized fire on board Ferry-boat
    Burn due to localized fire on board Liner

X+7th V93.02 Burn due to localized fire on board fishing boat

X+7th V93.03 Burn due to localized fire on board other powered watercraft
    Burn due to localized fire on board Hovercraft
    Burn due to localized fire on board Jet ski

X+7th V93.04 Burn due to localized fire on board sailboat

X+7th V93.09 Burn due to localized fire on board unspecified watercraft
    Burn due to localized fire on board boat NOS
    Burn due to localized fire on board ship NOS
    Burn due to localized fire on board watercraft NOS

+ V93.1 Other burn on board watercraft
    Burn due to source other than fire on board watercraft
    Excludes1: burn due to watercraft on fire (V91.0-)

X+7th V93.10 Other burn on board merchant vessel

X+7th V93.11 Other burn on board passenger vessel
    Other burn on board Ferry-boat
    Other burn on board Liner

X+7th V93.12 Other burn on board fishing boat

X+7th V93.13 Other burn on board other powered watercraft
    Other burn on board Hovercraft
    Other burn on board Jet ski

X+7th V93.14 Other burn on board sailboat

X+7th V93.19 Other burn on board unspecified watercraft
    Other burn on board boat NOS
    Other burn on board ship NOS
    Other burn on board watercraft NOS

+ V93.2 Heat exposure on board watercraft
    Excludes1: exposure to man-made heat not aboard watercraft (W92)
        exposure to natural heat while on board watercraft (X30)
        exposure to sunlight while on board watercraft (X32)
    Excludes2: burn due to fire on board watercraft (V93.0-)

X+7th V93.20 Heat exposure on board merchant ship

X+7th V93.21 Heat exposure on board passenger ship
    Heat exposure on board Ferry-boat
    Heat exposure on board Liner

X+7th V93.22 Heat exposure on board fishing boat

X+7th V93.23 Heat exposure on board other powered watercraft
    Heat exposure on board hovercraft

X+7th V93.24 Heat exposure on board sailboat

X+7th V93.29 Heat exposure on board unspecified watercraft
    Heat exposure on board boat NOS
    Heat exposure on board ship NOS
    Heat exposure on board watercraft NOS

+ V93.3 Fall on board watercraft
    Excludes1: fall due to collision of watercraft (V91.2-)

X+7th V93.30 Fall on board merchant ship

X+7th V93.31 Fall on board passenger ship
    Fall on board Ferry-boat
    Fall on board Liner

X+7th V93.32 Fall on board fishing boat

X+7th V93.33 Fall on board other powered watercraft
    Fall on board Hovercraft (on open water)
    Fall on board Jet ski

X+7th V93.34 Fall on board sailboat

X+7th V93.35 Fall on board canoe or kayak

X+7th V93.36 Fall on board (nonpowered) inflatable craft

X+7th V93.38 Fall on board other unpowered watercraft

X+7th V93.39 Fall on board unspecified watercraft
    Fall on board boat NOS
    Fall on board ship NOS
    Fall on board watercraft NOS

+ V93.4 Struck by falling object on board watercraft
    Hit by falling object on board watercraft
    Excludes1: struck by falling object due to accident to watercraft (V91.3)

X+7th V93.40 Struck by falling object on merchant ship

X+7th V93.41 Struck by falling object on passenger ship
    Struck by falling object on Ferry-boat
    Struck by falling object on Liner

X+7th V93.42 Struck by falling object on fishing boat

X+7th V93.43 Struck by falling object on other powered watercraft
    Struck by falling object on Hovercraft

X+7th V93.44 Struck by falling object on sailboat

X+7th V93.48 Struck by falling object on other unpowered watercraft

X+7th V93.49 Struck by falling object on unspecified watercraft

+ V93.5 Explosion on board watercraft
    Boiler explosion on steamship
    Excludes2: fire on board watercraft (V93.0-)

+, +7th, X + 7th   ● Newborn   ● Pediatric   ● Maternity   ● Adult   ♀ Female   ♂ Male   Manifestation   Unacceptable PDX   HCC   CC   MCC   **HAC**

X+7th **V93.50 Explosion on board merchant ship**
X+7th **V93.51 Explosion on board passenger ship**
Explosion on board Ferry-boat
Explosion on board Liner
X+7th **V93.52 Explosion on board fishing boat**
X+7th **V93.53 Explosion on board other powered watercraft**
Explosion on board Hovercraft
Explosion on board Jet ski
X+7th **V93.54 Explosion on board sailboat**
X+7th **V93.59 Explosion on board unspecified watercraft**
Explosion on board boat NOS
Explosion on board ship NOS
Explosion on board watercraft NOS

+ **V93.6 Machinery accident on board watercraft**
Excludes1: *machinery explosion on board watercraft (V93.4-)*
machinery fire on board watercraft (V93.0-)
X+7th **V93.60 Machinery accident on board merchant ship**
X+7th **V93.61 Machinery accident on board passenger ship**
Machinery accident on board Ferry-boat
Machinery accident on board Liner
X+7th **V93.62 Machinery accident on board fishing boat**
X+7th **V93.63 Machinery accident on board other powered watercraft**
Machinery accident on board Hovercraft
X+7th **V93.64 Machinery accident on board sailboat**
X+7th **V93.69 Machinery accident on board unspecified watercraft**
Machinery accident on board boat NOS
Machinery accident on board ship NOS
Machinery accident on board watercraft NOS

+ **V93.8 Other injury due to other accident on board watercraft**
Accidental poisoning by gases or fumes on watercraft
X+7th **V93.80 Other injury due to other accident on board merchant ship**
X+7th **V93.81 Other injury due to other accident on board passenger ship**
Other injury due to other accident on board Ferry-boat
Other injury due to other accident on board Liner
X+7th **V93.82 Other injury due to other accident on board fishing boat**
X+7th **V93.83 Other injury due to other accident on board other powered watercraft**
Other injury due to other accident on board Hovercraft
Other injury due to other accident on board Jet ski
X+7th **V93.84 Other injury due to other accident on board sailboat**
X+7th **V93.85 Other injury due to other accident on board canoe or kayak**
X+7th **V93.86 Other injury due to other accident on board (nonpowered) inflatable craft**
X+7th **V93.87 Other injury due to other accident on board water-skis**
Hit or struck by object while waterskiing
X+7th **V93.88 Other injury due to other accident on board other unpowered watercraft**
Hit or struck by object while surfing
Hit or struck by object while on board windsurfer
X+7th **V93.89 Other injury due to other accident on board unspecified watercraft**
Other injury due to other accident on board boat NOS
Other injury due to other accident on board ship NOS
Other injury due to other accident on board watercraft NOS

V94 Other and unspecified water transport accidents
Excludes1: *military watercraft accidents in military or war operations (Y36, Y37)*

The appropriate 7th character is to be added to each code from category V94
A   initial encounter
D   subsequent encounter
S   sequela

X+7th **V94.0 Hitting object or bottom of body of water due to fall from watercraft**
Excludes2: *drowning and submersion due to fall from watercraft (V92.0-)*

+ **V94.1 Bather struck by watercraft**
Swimmer hit by watercraft
X+7th **V94.11 Bather struck by powered watercraft**
X+7th **V94.12 Bather struck by nonpowered watercraft**
+ **V94.2 Rider of nonpowered watercraft struck by other watercraft**
X+7th **V94.21 Rider of nonpowered watercraft struck by other nonpowered watercraft**
Canoer hit by other nonpowered watercraft
Surfer hit by other nonpowered watercraft
Windsurfer hit by other nonpowered watercraft
X+7th **V94.22 Rider of nonpowered watercraft struck by powered watercraft**
Canoer hit by motorboat
Surfer hit by motorboat
Windsurfer hit by motorboat
+ **V94.3 Injury to rider of (inflatable) watercraft being pulled behind other watercraft**
X+7th **V94.31 Injury to rider of (inflatable) recreational watercraft being pulled behind other watercraft**
Injury to rider of inner-tube pulled behind motor boat
X+7th **V94.32 Injury to rider of non-recreational watercraft being pulled behind other watercraft**
Injury to occupant of dingy being pulled behind boat or ship
Injury to occupant of life-raft being pulled behind boat or ship
X+7th **V94.4 Injury to barefoot water-skier**
Injury to person being pulled behind boat or ship
+ **V94.8 Other water transport accident**
+ **V94.81 Water transport accident involving military watercraft**
+7th **V94.810 Civilian watercraft involved in water transport accident with military watercraft**
Passenger on civilian watercraft injured due to accident with military watercraft
+7th **V94.811 Civilian in water injured by military watercraft**
+7th **V94.818 Other water transport accident involving military watercraft**
X+7th **V94.89 Other water transport accident**
X+7th **V94.9 Unspecified water transport accident**
Water transport accident NOS

Air and space transport accidents (V95-V97)

Excludes1: *military aircraft accidents in military or war operations (Y36, Y37.-)*

V95 Accident to powered aircraft causing injury to occupant

The appropriate 7th character is to be added to each code from category V95
A   initial encounter
D   subsequent encounter
S   sequela

+ **V95.0 Helicopter accident injuring occupant**
X+7th **V95.00 Unspecified helicopter accident injuring occupant**
X+7th **V95.01 Helicopter crash injuring occupant**
X+7th **V95.02 Forced landing of helicopter injuring occupant**
X+7th **V95.03 Helicopter collision injuring occupant**
Helicopter collision with any object, fixed, movable or moving
X+7th **V95.04 Helicopter fire injuring occupant**
X+7th **V95.05 Helicopter explosion injuring occupant**
X+7th **V95.09 Other helicopter accident injuring occupant**
+ **V95.1 Ultralight, microlight or powered-glider accident injuring occupant**
X+7th **V95.10 Unspecified ultralight, microlight or powered-glider accident injuring occupant**
X+7th **V95.11 Ultralight, microlight or powered-glider crash injuring occupant**
X+7th **V95.12 Forced landing of ultralight, microlight or powered-glider injuring occupant**
X+7th **V95.13 Ultralight, microlight or powered-glider collision injuring occupant**
Ultralight, microlight or powered-glider collision with any object, fixed, movable or moving
X+7th **V95.14 Ultralight, microlight or powered-glider fire injuring occupant**

X+7th **V95.15** **Ultralight, microlight or powered-glider explosion injuring occupant**

X+7th **V95.19** **Other ultralight, microlight or powered-glider accident injuring occupant**

+ **V95.2** **Other private fixed-wing aircraft accident injuring occupant**

X+7th **V95.20** **Unspecified accident to other private fixed-wing aircraft, injuring occupant**

X+7th **V95.21** **Other private fixed-wing aircraft crash injuring occupant**

X+7th **V95.22** **Forced landing of other private fixed-wing aircraft injuring occupant**

X+7th **V95.23** **Other private fixed-wing aircraft collision injuring occupant**

Other private fixed-wing aircraft collision with any object, fixed, movable or moving

X+7th **V95.24** **Other private fixed-wing aircraft fire injuring occupant**

X+7th **V95.25** **Other private fixed-wing aircraft explosion injuring occupant**

X+7th **V95.29** **Other accident to other private fixed-wing aircraft injuring occupant**

+ **V95.3** **Commercial fixed-wing aircraft accident injuring occupant**

X+7th **V95.30** **Unspecified accident to commercial fixed-wing aircraft injuring occupant**

X+7th **V95.31** **Commercial fixed-wing aircraft crash injuring occupant**

X+7th **V95.32** **Forced landing of commercial fixed-wing aircraft injuring occupant**

X+7th **V95.33** **Commercial fixed-wing aircraft collision injuring occupant**

Commercial fixed-wing aircraft collision with any object, fixed, movable or moving

X+7th **V95.34** **Commercial fixed-wing aircraft fire injuring occupant**

X+7th **V95.35** **Commercial fixed-wing aircraft explosion injuring occupant**

X+7th **V95.39** **Other accident to commercial fixed-wing aircraft injuring occupant**

+ **V95.4** **Spacecraft accident injuring occupant**

X+7th **V95.40** **Unspecified spacecraft accident injuring occupant**

X+7th **V95.41** **Spacecraft crash injuring occupant**

X+7th **V95.42** **Forced landing of spacecraft injuring occupant**

X+7th **V95.43** **Spacecraft collision injuring occupant**

Spacecraft collision with any object, fixed, moveable or moving

X+7th **V95.44** **Spacecraft fire injuring occupant**

X+7th **V95.45** **Spacecraft explosion injuring occupant**

X+7th **V95.49** **Other spacecraft accident injuring occupant**

X+7th **V95.8** **Other powered aircraft accidents injuring occupant**

X+7th **V95.9** **Unspecified aircraft accident injuring occupant**

Aircraft accident NOS

Air transport accident NOS

V96 **Accident to nonpowered aircraft causing injury to occupant**

The appropriate 7th character is to be added to each code from category V96
A   initial encounter
D   subsequent encounter
S   sequela

+ **V96.0** **Balloon accident injuring occupant**

X+7th **V96.00** **Unspecified balloon accident injuring occupant**

X+7th **V96.01** **Balloon crash injuring occupant**

X+7th **V96.02** **Forced landing of balloon injuring occupant**

X+7th **V96.03** **Balloon collision injuring occupant**

Balloon collision with any object, fixed, moveable or moving

X+7th **V96.04** **Balloon fire injuring occupant**

X+7th **V96.05** **Balloon explosion injuring occupant**

X+7th **V96.09** **Other balloon accident injuring occupant**

+ **V96.1** **Hang-glider accident injuring occupant**

X+7th **V96.10** **Unspecified hang-glider accident injuring occupant**

X+7th **V96.11** **Hang-glider crash injuring occupant**

X+7th **V96.12** **Forced landing of hang-glider injuring occupant**

X+7th **V96.13** **Hang-glider collision injuring occupant**

Hang-glider collision with any object, fixed, moveable or moving

X+7th **V96.14** **Hang-glider fire injuring occupant**

X+7th **V96.15** **Hang-glider explosion injuring occupant**

X+7th **V96.19** **Other hang-glider accident injuring occupant**

+ **V96.2** **Glider (nonpowered) accident injuring occupant**

X+7th **V96.20** **Unspecified glider (nonpowered) accident injuring occupant**

X+7th **V96.21** **Glider (nonpowered) crash injuring occupant**

X+7th **V96.22** **Forced landing of glider (nonpowered) injuring occupant**

X+7th **V96.23** **Glider (nonpowered) collision injuring occupant**

Glider (nonpowered) collision with any object, fixed, moveable or moving

X+7th **V96.24** **Glider (nonpowered) fire injuring occupant**

V96.25 **Glider (nonpowered) explosion injuring occupant**

X+7th **V96.29** **Other glider (nonpowered) accident injuring occupant**

X+7th **V96.8** **Other nonpowered-aircraft accidents injuring occupant**

Kite carrying a person accident injuring occupant

X+7th **V96.9** **Unspecified nonpowered-aircraft accident injuring occupant**

Nonpowered-aircraft accident NOS

V97 **Other specified air transport accidents**

The appropriate 7th character is to be added to each code from category V97
A   initial encounter
D   subsequent encounter
S   sequela

X+7th **V97.0** **Occupant of aircraft injured in other specified air transport accidents**

Fall in, on or from aircraft in air transport accident

Excludes1:   *accident while boarding or alighting aircraft (V97.1)*

X+7th **V97.1** **Person injured while boarding or alighting from aircraft**

+ **V97.2** **Parachutist accident**

X+7th **V97.21** **Parachutist entangled in object**

Parachutist landing in tree

X+7th **V97.22** **Parachutist injured on landing**

X+7th **V97.29** **Other parachutist accident**

+ **V97.3** **Person on ground injured in air transport accident**

X+7th **V97.31** **Hit by object falling from aircraft**

Hit by crashing aircraft

Injured by aircraft hitting house

Injured by aircraft hitting car

X+7th **V97.32** **Injured by rotating propeller**

X+7th **V97.33** **Sucked into jet engine**

X+7th **V97.39** **Other injury to person on ground due to air transport accident**

+ **V97.8** **Other air transport accidents, not elsewhere classified**

Excludes1:   *aircraft accident NOS (V95.9)*

exposure to changes in air pressure during ascent or descent (W94.-)

+ **V97.81** **Air transport accident involving military aircraft**

+7th **V97.810** **Civilian aircraft involved in air transport accident with military aircraft**

Passenger in civilian aircraft injured due to accident with military aircraft

+7th **V97.811** **Civilian injured by military aircraft**

+7th **V97.818** **Other air transport accident involving military aircraft**

X+7th **V97.89** **Other air transport accidents, not elsewhere classified**

Injury from machinery on aircraft

Other and unspecified transport accidents (V98-V99)

Excludes1:   *vehicle accident, type of vehicle unspecified (V89.-)*

V98 **Other specified transport accidents**

The appropriate 7th character is to be added to each code from category V98
A   initial encounter
D   subsequent encounter
S   sequela

X+7th **V98.0** **Accident to, on or involving cable-car, not on rails**

Caught or dragged by cable-car, not on rails

Fall or jump from cable-car, not on rails

Object thrown from or in cable-car, not on rails

X+7th **V98.1** **Accident to, on or involving land-yacht**

X+7th **V98.2** **Accident to, on or involving ice yacht**

X+7th **V98.3** **Accident to, on or involving ski lift**
      Accident to, on or involving ski chair-lift
      Accident to, on or involving ski-lift with gondola

X+7th **V98.8** **Other specified transport accidents**

V99 **Unspecified transport accident**
X+7th
  The appropriate 7th character is to be added to code V99
  A   initial encounter
  D   subsequent encounter
  S   sequela

Other external causes of accidental injury (W00–X58)

Slipping, tripping, stumbling and falls (W00–W19)

Excludes1: *assault involving a fall (Y01-Y02)*
    fall from animal (V80.-)
    fall (in) (from) machinery (in operation) (W28-W31)
    fall (in) (from) transport vehicle (V01-V99)
    intentional self-harm involving a fall (X80-X81)

Excludes2: *at risk for fall (history of fall) (Z91.81)*
    fall (in) (from) burning building (X00.-)
    fall into fire (X00-X04, X08)

W00 **Fall due to ice and snow**

  Includes: pedestrian on foot falling (slipping) on ice and snow
  Excludes1: *fall on (from) ice and snow involving pedestrian*
      conveyance (V00.-)
      fall from stairs and steps not due to ice and snow (W10.-)

  The appropriate 7th character is to be added to each code from
  category W00
  A   initial encounter
  D   subsequent encounter
  S   sequela

X+7th **W00.0** **Fall on same level due to ice and snow**
        AHA CC: 2Q, 2016, 4-5
X+7th **W00.1** **Fall from stairs and steps due to ice and snow**
X+7th **W00.2** **Other fall from one level to another due to ice and snow**
X+7th **W00.9** **Unspecified fall due to ice and snow**

W01 **Fall on same level from slipping, tripping and stumbling**

  Includes: fall on moving sidewalk
  Excludes1: *fall due to bumping (striking) against object (W18.0-)*
      fall in shower or bathtub (W18.2-)
      fall on same level NOS (W18.30)
      fall on same level from slipping, tripping and stumbling
        due to ice or snow (W00.0)
      fall off or from toilet (W18.1-)
      slipping, tripping and stumbling NOS (W18.40)
      slipping, tripping and stumbling without falling (W18.4-)

  The appropriate 7th character is to be added to each code from
  category W01
  A   initial encounter
  D   subsequent encounter
  S   sequela

X+7th **W01.0** **Fall on same level from slipping, tripping and stumbling**
      without subsequent striking against object
      Falling over animal

+ **W01.1** **Fall on same level from slipping, tripping and stumbling**
      with subsequent striking against object

  X+7th **W01.10** **Fall on same level from slipping, tripping and**
      stumbling with subsequent striking against
      unspecified object

  + **W01.11** **Fall on same level from slipping, tripping and**
      stumbling with subsequent striking against
      sharp object

    +7th **W01.110** **Fall on same level from slipping,**
      tripping and stumbling with
      subsequent striking against sharp glass

    +7th **W01.111** **Fall on same level from slipping,**
      tripping and stumbling with
      subsequent striking against power tool
      or machine

    +7th **W01.118** **Fall on same level from slipping,**
      tripping and stumbling with
      subsequent striking against other
      sharp object

+7th **W01.119** **Fall on same level from slipping,**
      tripping and stumbling with
      subsequent striking against unspecified
      sharp object

+ **W01.19** **Fall on same level from slipping, tripping and**
      stumbling with subsequent striking against other
      object

  +7th **W01.190** **Fall on same level from slipping,**
      tripping and stumbling with subsequent
      striking against furniture

  +7th **W01.198** **Fall on same level from slipping,**
      tripping and stumbling with subsequent
      striking against other object

W03 **Other fall on same level due to collision with another person**
X+7th
  Fall due to non-transport collision with other person
  Excludes1: *collision with another person without fall (W51)*
      crushed or pushed by a crowd or human stampede
        (W52)
      fall involving pedestrian conveyance (V00-V09)
      fall due to ice or snow (W00)
      fall on same level NOS (W18.30)
  AHA CC: 4Q, 2012, 108; 1Q, 2015, 3-21

  The appropriate 7th character is to be added to code W03
  A   initial encounter
  D   subsequent encounter
  S   sequela

W04 **Fall while being carried or supported by other persons**
X+7th
  Accidentally dropped while being carried

  The appropriate 7th character is to be added to code W04
  A   initial encounter
  D   subsequent encounter
  S   sequela

W05 **Fall from non-movitng wheelchair, nonmotorized scooter and**
    motorized mobility scooter

  Excludes1: *fall from moving wheelchair (powered) (V00.811)*
      fall from moving motorized mobility scooter (V00.831)
      fall from nonmotorized scooter (V00.141)
  AHA CC: 2Q, 2019, 27-28

  The appropriate 7th character is to be added to each code from
  category W05
  A   initial encounter
  D   subsequent encounter
  S   sequela

X+7th **W05.0** **Fall from non-moving wheelchair**
X+7th **W05.1** **Fall from non-moving nonmotorized scooter**
X+7th **W05.2** **Fall from non-moving motorized mobility scooter**

W06 **Fall from bed**
X+7th
  The appropriate 7th character is to be added to code W06
  A   initial encounter
  D   subsequent encounter
  S   sequela

W07 **Fall from chair**
X+7th
  The appropriate 7th character is to be added to code W07
  A   initial encounter
  D   subsequent encounter
  S   sequela

W08 **Fall from other furniture**
X+7th
  The appropriate 7th character is to be added to code W08
  A   initial encounter
  D   subsequent encounter
  S   sequela

W09 **Fall on and from playground equipment**

  Excludes1: *fall involving recreational machinery (W31)*

  The appropriate 7th character is to be added to each code from
  category W09
  A   initial encounter
  D   subsequent encounter
  S   sequela

X+7th **W09.0** **Fall on or from playground slide**
X+7th **W09.1** **Fall from playground swing**
X+7th **W09.2** **Fall on or from jungle gym**
X+7th **W09.8** **Fall on or from other playground equipment**

W10 Fall on and from stairs and steps

> *Excludes1:* *Fall from stairs and steps due to ice and snow (W00.1)*

> The appropriate 7th character is to be added to each code from category W10
> A   initial encounter
> D   subsequent encounter
> S   sequela

X+7th **W10.0 Fall (on)(from) escalator**
X+7th **W10.1 Fall (on)(from) sidewalk curb**
X+7th **W10.2 Fall (on)(from) incline**
> Fall (on) (from) ramp
X+7th **W10.8 Fall (on) (from) other stairs and steps**
X+7th **W10.9 Fall (on) (from) unspecified stairs and steps**

W11 Fall on and from ladder
X+7th
> The appropriate 7th character is to be added to code W11
> A   initial encounter
> D   subsequent encounter
> S   sequela

W12 Fall on and from scaffolding
X+7th
> The appropriate 7th character is to be added to code W12
> A   initial encounter
> D   subsequent encounter
> S   sequela

W13 Fall from, out of or through building or structure

> The appropriate 7th character is to be added to each code from category W13
> A   initial encounter
> D   subsequent encounter
> S   sequela

X+7th **W13.0 Fall from, out of or through balcony**
> Fall from, out of or through railing
X+7th **W13.1 Fall from, out of or through bridge**
X+7th **W13.2 Fall from, out of or through roof**
X+7th **W13.3 Fall through floor**
X+7th **W13.4 Fall from, out of or through window**
> *Excludes2:* *fall with subsequent striking against sharp glass (W01.110)*
X+7th **W13.8 Fall from, out of or through other building or structure**
> Fall from, out of or through viaduct
> Fall from, out of or through wall
> Fall from, out of or through flag-pole
X+7th **W13.9 Fall from, out of or through building, not otherwise specified**
> *Excludes1:* *collapse of a building or structure (W20.-)*
> *fall or jump from burning building or structure (X00.-)* ·

W14 Fall from tree
X+7th
> The appropriate 7th character is to be added to code W14
> A   initial encounter
> D   subsequent encounter
> S   sequela

W15 Fall from cliff
X+7th
> The appropriate 7th character is to be added to code W15
> A   initial encounter
> D   subsequent encounter
> S   sequela

W16 Fall, jump or diving into water

> *Excludes1:* *accidental non-watercraft drowning and submersion not involving fall (W65-W74)*
> *effects of air pressure from diving (W94.-)*
> *fall into water from watercraft (V90-V94)*
> *hitting an object or against bottom when falling from watercraft (V94.0)*
> *Excludes2:* *striking or hitting diving board (W21.4)*

> The appropriate 7th character is to be added to each code from category W16
> A   initial encounter
> D   subsequent encounter
> S   sequela

+ **W16.0 Fall into swimming pool**
> Fall into swimming pool NOS
> *Excludes1:* *fall into empty swimming pool (W17.3)*
> + **W16.01 Fall into swimming pool striking water surface**
> +7th **W16.011 Fall into swimming pool striking water surface causing drowning and submersion**
> > *Excludes1:* *drowning and submersion while in swimming pool without fall (W67)*
> +7th **W16.012 Fall into swimming pool striking water surface causing other injury**
> + **W16.02 Fall into swimming pool striking bottom**
> +7th **W16.021 Fall into swimming pool striking bottom causing drowning and submersion**
> > *Excludes1:* *drowning and submersion while in swimming pool without fall (W67)*
> +7th **W16.022 Fall into swimming pool striking bottom causing other injury**
> + **W16.03 Fall into swimming pool striking wall**
> +7th **W16.031 Fall into swimming pool striking wall causing drowning and submersion**
> > *Excludes1:* *drowning and submersion while in swimming pool without fall (W67)*
> +7th **W16.032 Fall into swimming pool striking wall causing other injury**

+ **W16.1 Fall into natural body of water**
> Fall into lake
> Fall into open sea
> Fall into river
> Fall into stream
> + **W16.11 Fall into natural body of water striking water surface**
> +7th **W16.111 Fall into natural body of water striking water surface causing drowning and submersion**
> > *Excludes1:* *drowning and submersion while in natural body of water without fall (W69)*
> +7th **W16.112 Fall into natural body of water striking water surface causing other injury**
> + **W16.12 Fall into natural body of water striking bottom**
> +7th **W16.121 Fall into natural body of water striking bottom causing drowning and submersion**
> > *Excludes1:* *drowning and submersion while in natural body of water without fall (W69)*
> +7th **W16.122 Fall into natural body of water striking bottom causing other injury**
> + **W16.13 Fall into natural body of water striking side**
> +7th **W16.131 Fall into natural body of water striking side causing drowning and submersion**
> > *Excludes1:* *drowning and submersion while in natural body of water without fall (W69)*
> +7th **W16.132 Fall into natural body of water striking side causing other injury**

+ **W16.2 Fall in (into) filled bathtub or bucket of water**
> + **W16.21 Fall in (into) filled bathtub**
> > *Excludes1:* *fall into empty bathtub (W18.2)*
> +7th **W16.211 Fall in (into) filled bathtub causing drowning and submersion**
> > *Excludes1:* *drowning and submersion while in filled bathtub without fall (W65)*
> +7th **W16.212 Fall in (into) filled bathtub causing other injury**
> + **W16.22 Fall in (into) bucket of water**
> +7th **W16.221 Fall in (into) bucket of water causing drowning and submersion**
> +7th **W16.222 Fall in (into) bucket of water causing other injury**

+ **W16.3 Fall into other water**
> Fall into fountain
> Fall into reservoir
> + **W16.31 Fall into other water striking water surface**
> +7th **W16.311 Fall into other water striking water surface causing drowning and submersion**
> > *Excludes1:* *drowning and submersion while in other water without fall (W73)*
> +7th **W16.312 Fall into other water striking water surface causing other injury**

+, +7th, X + 7th   ● Newborn   ● Pediatric   ● Maternity   ● Adult   ♀ Female   ♂ Male   Manifestation   Unacceptable PDX   HCC   CC   MCC   HAC

+ **W16.32** **Fall into other water striking bottom**
    +7th **W16.321** **Fall into other water striking bottom causing drowning and submersion**
        Excludes1: *drowning and submersion while in other water without fall (W73)*
    +7th **W16.322** **Fall into other water striking bottom causing other injury**
+ **W16.33** **Fall into other water striking wall**
    +7th **W16.331** **Fall into other water striking wall causing drowning and submersion**
        Excludes1: *drowning and submersion while in other water without fall (W73)*
    +7th **W16.332** **Fall into other water striking wall causing other injury**
+ **W16.4** **Fall into unspecified water**
  X+7th **W16.41** **Fall into unspecified water causing drowning and submersion**
  X+7th **W16.42** **Fall into unspecified water causing other injury**
+ **W16.5** **Jumping or diving into swimming pool**
  + **W16.51** **Jumping or diving into swimming pool striking water surface**
    +7th **W16.511** **Jumping or diving into swimming pool striking water surface causing drowning and submersion**
        Excludes1: *drowning and submersion while in swimming pool without jumping or diving (W67)*
    +7th **W16.512** **Jumping or diving into swimming pool striking water surface causing other injury**
  + **W16.52** **Jumping or diving into swimming pool striking bottom**
    +7th **W16.521** **Jumping or diving into swimming pool striking bottom causing drowning and submersion**
        Excludes1: *drowning and submersion while in swimming pool without jumping or diving (W67)*
    +7th **W16.522** **Jumping or diving into swimming pool striking bottom causing other injury**
  + **W16.53** **Jumping or diving into swimming pool striking wall**
    +7th **W16.531** **Jumping or diving into swimming pool striking wall causing drowning and submersion**
        Excludes1: *drowning and submersion while in swimming pool without jumping or diving (W67)*
    +7th **W16.532** **Jumping or diving into swimming pool striking wall causing other injury**
+ **W16.6** **Jumping or diving into natural body of water**
    Jumping or diving into lake
    Jumping or diving into open sea
    Jumping or diving into river
    Jumping or diving into stream
  + **W16.61** **Jumping or diving into natural body of water striking water surface**
    +7th **W16.611** **Jumping or diving into natural body of water striking water surface causing drowning and submersion**
        Excludes1: *drowning and submersion while in natural body of water without jumping or diving (W69)*
    +7th **W16.612** **Jumping or diving into natural body of water striking water surface causing other injury**

+ **W16.62** **Jumping or diving into natural body of water striking bottom**
    +7th **W16.621** **Jumping or diving into natural body of water striking bottom causing drowning and submersion**
        Excludes1: *drowning and submersion while in natural body of water without jumping or diving (W69)*
    +7th **W16.622** **Jumping or diving into natural body of water striking bottom causing other injury**
+ **W16.7** **Jumping or diving from boat**
    Excludes1: *Fall from boat into water -see watercraft accident (V90-V94)*
  + **W16.71** **Jumping or diving from boat striking water surface**
    +7th **W16.711** **Jumping or diving from boat striking water surface causing drowning and submersion**
    +7th **W16.712** **Jumping or diving from boat striking water surface causing other injury**
  + **W16.72** **Jumping or diving from boat striking bottom**
    +7th **W16.721** **Jumping or diving from boat striking bottom causing drowning and submersion**
    +7th **W16.722** **Jumping or diving from boat striking bottom causing other injury**
+ **W16.8** **Jumping or diving into other water**
    Jumping or diving into fountain
    Jumping or diving into reservoir
  + **W16.81** **Jumping or diving into other water striking water surface**
    +7th **W16.811** **Jumping or diving into other water striking water surface causing drowning and submersion**
        Excludes1: *drowning and submersion while in other water without jumping or diving (W73)*
    +7th **W16.812** **Jumping or diving into other water striking water surface causing other injury**
  + **W16.82** **Jumping or diving into other water striking bottom**
    +7th **W16.821** **Jumping or diving into other water striking bottom causing drowning and submersion**
        Excludes1: *drowning and submersion while in other water without jumping or diving (W73)*
    +7th **W16.822** **Jumping or diving into other water striking bottom causing other injury**
  + **W16.83** **Jumping or diving into other water striking wall**
    +7th **W16.831** **Jumping or diving into other water striking wall causing drowning and submersion**
        Excludes1: *drowning and submersion while in other water without jumping or diving (W73)*
    +7th **W16.832** **Jumping or diving into other water striking wall causing other injury**
+ **W16.9** **Jumping or diving into unspecified water**
  X+7th **W16.91** **Jumping or diving into unspecified water causing drowning and submersion**
  X+7th **W16.92** **Jumping or diving into unspecified water causing other injury**

W17 Other fall from one level to another

The appropriate 7th character is to be added to each code from category W17
A   initial encounter
D   subsequent encounter
S   sequela

X+7th **W17.0 Fall into well**
X+7th **W17.1 Fall into storm drain or manhole**
X+7th **W17.2 Fall into hole**
Fall into pit
X+7th **W17.3 Fall into empty swimming pool**
Excludes1: *fall into filled swimming pool (W16.0-)*
X+7th **W17.4 Fall from dock**
+ **W17.8 Other fall from one level to another**
X+7th **W17.81 Fall down embankment (hill)**
X+7th **W17.82 Fall from (out of) grocery cart**
Fall due to grocery cart tipping over
X+7th **W17.89 Other fall from one level to another**
Fall from cherry picker
Fall from lifting device
Fall from mobile elevated work platform [MEWP]
Fall from sky lift
AHA CC: 2Q, 2015, 6-7

W18 Other slipping, tripping and stumbling and falls

The appropriate 7th character is to be added to each code from category W18
A   initial encounter
D   subsequent encounter
S   sequela

+ **W18.0 Fall due to bumping against object**
Striking against object with subsequent fall
Excludes1: *fall on same level due to slipping, tripping, or stumbling with subsequent striking against object (W01.1-)*
X+7th **W18.00 Striking against unspecified object with subsequent fall**
X+7th **W18.01 Striking against sports equipment with subsequent fall**
X+7th **W18.02 Striking against glass with subsequent fall**
X+7th **W18.09 Striking against other object with subsequent fall**
+ **W18.1 Fall from or off toilet**
X+7th **W18.11 Fall from or off toilet without subsequent striking against object**
Fall from (off) toilet NOS
X+7th **W18.12 Fall from or off toilet with subsequent striking against object**
X+7th **W18.2 Fall in (into) shower or empty bathtub**
Excludes1: *fall in full bathtub causing drowning or submersion (W16.21-)*
+ **W18.3 Other and unspecified fall on same level**
X+7th **W18.30 Fall on same level, unspecified**
X+7th **W18.31 Fall on same level due to stepping on an object**
Fall on same level due to stepping on an animal
Excludes1: *slipping, tripping and stumbling without fall due to stepping on animal (W18.41)*
X+7th **W18.39 Other fall on same level**
+ **W18.4 Slipping, tripping and stumbling without falling**
Excludes1: *collision with another person without fall (W51)*
X+7th **W18.40 Slipping, tripping and stumbling without falling, unspecified**
X+7th **W18.41 Slipping, tripping and stumbling without falling due to stepping on object**
Slipping, tripping and stumbling without falling due to stepping on animal
Excludes1: *slipping, tripping and stumbling with fall due to stepping on animal (W18.31)*
X+7th **W18.42 Slipping, tripping and stumbling without falling due to stepping into hole or opening**
X+7th **W18.43 Slipping, tripping and stumbling without falling due to stepping from one level to another**
X+7th **W18.49 Other slipping, tripping and stumbling without falling**

W19 Unspecified fall
X+7th
Accidental fall NOS
AHA CC: 4Q, 2012, 95-96

The appropriate 7th character is to be added to code W19
A   initial encounter
D   subsequent encounter
S   sequela

Exposure to inanimate mechanical forces (W20-W49)

Excludes1: assault (X92-Y09)
contact or collision with animals or persons (W50-W64)
exposure to inanimate mechanical forces involving military or war operations (Y36.-, Y37.-)
intentional self-harm (X71-X83)

W20 Struck by thrown, projected or falling object

Code first any associated:
cataclysm (X34-X39)
lightning strike (T75.00)
Excludes1: *falling object in machinery accident (W24, W28-W31)*
falling object in transport accident (V01-V99)
object set in motion by explosion (W35-W40)
object set in motion by firearm (W32-W34)
struck by thrown sports equipment (W21.-)

The appropriate 7th character is to be added to each code from category W20
A   initial encounter
D   subsequent encounter
S   sequela

X+7th **W20.0 Struck by falling object in cave-in**
Excludes2: *asphyxiation due to cave-in (T71.21)*
X+7th **W20.1 Struck by object due to collapse of building**
Excludes1: *struck by object due to collapse of burning building (X00.2, X02.2)*
X+7th **W20.8 Other cause of strike by thrown, projected or falling object**
Excludes1: *struck by thrown sports equipment (W21.-)*

W21 Striking against or struck by sports equipment

Excludes1: *assault with sports equipment (Y08.0-)*
striking against or struck by sports equipment with subsequent fall (W18.01)

The appropriate 7th character is to be added to each code from category W21
A   initial encounter
D   subsequent encounter
S   sequela

+ **W21.0 Struck by hit or thrown ball**
X+7th **W21.00 Struck by hit or thrown ball, unspecified type**
X+7th **W21.01 Struck by football**
X+7th **W21.02 Struck by soccer ball**
X+7th **W21.03 Struck by baseball**
X+7th **W21.04 Struck by golf ball**
X+7th **W21.05 Struck by basketball**
X+7th **W21.06 Struck by volleyball**
X+7th **W21.07 Struck by softball**
X+7th **W21.09 Struck by other hit or thrown ball**
+ **W21.1 Struck by bat, racquet or club**
X+7th **W21.11 Struck by baseball bat**
X+7th **W21.12 Struck by tennis racquet**
X+7th **W21.13 Struck by golf club**
X+7th **W21.19 Struck by other bat, racquet or club**
+ **W21.2 Struck by hockey stick or puck**
+ **W21.21 Struck by hockey stick**
+7th **W21.210 Struck by ice hockey stick**
+7th **W21.211 Struck by field hockey stick**
+ **W21.22 Struck by hockey puck**
X+7th **W21.220 Struck by ice hockey puck**
X+7th **W21.221 Struck by field hockey puck**
+ **W21.3 Struck by sports foot wear**
X+7th **W21.31 Struck by shoe cleats**
Stepped on by shoe cleats
X+7th **W21.32 Struck by skate blades**
Skated over by skate blades
X+7th **W21.39 Struck by other sports foot wear**

X+7th **W21.4 Striking against diving board**
　　Use additional code for subsequent falling into water, if applicable (W16.-)
+ **W21.8 Striking against or struck by other sports equipment**
X+7th **W21.81 Striking against or struck by football helmet**
X+7th **W21.89 Striking against or struck by other sports equipment**
X+7th **W21.9 Striking against or struck by unspecified sports equipment**

W22 Striking against or struck by other objects

> *Excludes1:* striking against or struck by object with subsequent fall (W18.09)

The appropriate 7th character is to be added to each code from category W22
A　initial encounter
D　subsequent encounter
S　sequela

+ **W22.0 Striking against stationary object**
> *Excludes1:* striking against stationary sports equipment (W21.8)

X+7th **W22.01 Walked into wall**
X+7th **W22.02 Walked into lamppost**
X+7th **W22.03 Walked into furniture**
+ **W22.04 Striking against wall of swimming pool**
　+7th **W22.041 Striking against wall of swimming pool causing drowning and submersion**
> *Excludes1:* drowning and submersion while swimming without striking against wall (W67)

　+7th **W22.042 Striking against wall of swimming pool causing other injury**
X+7th **W22.09 Striking against other stationary object**
+ **W22.1 Striking against or struck by automobile airbag**
X+7th **W22.10 Striking against or struck by unspecified automobile airbag**
X+7th **W22.11 Striking against or struck by driver side automobile airbag**
X+7th **W22.12 Striking against or struck by front passenger side automobile airbag**
X+7th **W22.19 Striking against or struck by other automobile airbag**
X+7th **W22.8 Striking against or struck by other objects**
　　Striking against or struck by object NOS
> *Excludes1:* struck by thrown, projected or falling object (W20.-)

W23 Caught, crushed, jammed or pinched in or between objects

> *Excludes1:* injury caused by cutting or piercing instruments (W25-W27)
> injury caused by firearms malfunction (W32.1, W33.1-, W34.1-)
> injury caused by lifting and transmission devices (W24.-)
> injury caused by machinery (W28-W31)
> injury caused by nonpowered hand tools (W27.-)
> injury caused by transport vehicle being used as a means of transportation (V01-V99)
> injury caused by struck by thrown, projected or falling object (W20.-)

The appropriate 7th character is to be added to each code from category W23
A　initial encounter
D　subsequent encounter
S　sequela

X+7th **W23.0 Caught, crushed, jammed, or pinched between moving objects**
X+7th **W23.1 Caught, crushed, jammed, or pinched between stationary objects**

W24 Contact with lifting and transmission devices, not elsewhere classified

> *Excludes1:* transport accidents (V01-V99)

The appropriate 7th character is to be added to each code from category W24
A　initial encounter
D　subsequent encounter
S　sequela

X+7th **W24.0 Contact with lifting devices, not elsewhere classified**
　　Contact with chain hoist
　　Contact with drive belt
　　Contact with pulley (block)
X+7th **W24.1 Contact with transmission devices, not elsewhere classified**
　　Contact with transmission belt or cable

W25 Contact with sharp glass
X+7th
　Code first any associated:
　　injury due to flying glass from explosion or firearm discharge (W32-W40)
　　transport accident (V00-V99)
> *Excludes1:* fall on same level due to slipping, tripping and stumbling with subsequent striking against sharp glass (W01.110)
> striking against sharp glass with subsequent fall (W18.02)

> *Excludes2:* glass embedded in skin (W45)

The appropriate 7th character is to be added to code W25
A　initial encounter
D　subsequent encounter
S　sequela

W26 Contact with other sharp objects

> *Excludes2:* sharp object(s) embedded in skin (W45)
> *AHA CC: 4Q, 2016, 73*

The appropriate 7th character is to be added to each code from category W26
A　initial encounter
D　subsequent encounter
S　sequela

X+7th **W26.0 Contact with knife**
> *Excludes1:* contact with electric knife (W29.1)
X+7th **W26.1 Contact with sword or dagger**
X+7th **W26.2 Contact with edge of stiff paper**
　　Paper cut
X+7th **W26.8 Contact with other sharp object(s), not elsewhere classified**
　　Contact with tin can lid
X+7th **W26.9 Contact with unspecified sharp object(s)**

W27 Contact with nonpowered hand tool

The appropriate 7th character is to be added to each code from category W27
A　initial encounter
D　subsequent encounter
S　sequela

X+7th **W27.0 Contact with workbench tool**
　　Contact with auger
　　Contact with axe
　　Contact with chisel
　　Contact with handsaw
　　Contact with screwdriver
X+7th **W27.1 Contact with garden tool**
　　Contact with hoe
　　Contact with nonpowered lawn mower
　　Contact with pitchfork
　　Contact with rake
X+7th **W27.2 Contact with scissors**
X+7th **W27.3 Contact with needle (sewing)**
> *Excludes1:* contact with hypodermic needle (W46.-)
X+7th **W27.4 Contact with kitchen utensil**
　　Contact with fork
　　Contact with ice-pick
　　Contact with can-opener NOS

X+7th **W27.5** **Contact with paper-cutter**

X+7th **W27.8** **Contact with other nonpowered hand tool**
Contact with nonpowered sewing machine
Contact with shovel

W28 **Contact with powered lawn mower**
X+7th
Powered lawn mower (commercial) (residential)
Excludes1: *contact with nonpowered lawn mower (W27.1)*
Excludes2: *exposure to electric current (W86.-)*

The appropriate 7th character is to be added to code W28
A   initial encounter
D   subsequent encounter
S   sequela

W29 **Contact with other powered hand tools and household machinery**

Excludes1: *contact with commercial machinery (W31.82)*
contact with hot household appliance (X15)
contact with nonpowered hand tool (W27.-)
exposure to electric current (W86)

The appropriate 7th character is to be added to each code from category W29
A   initial encounter
D   subsequent encounter
S   sequela

X+7th **W29.0** **Contact with powered kitchen appliance**
Contact with blender
Contact with can-opener
Contact with garbage disposal
Contact with mixer

X+7th **W29.1** **Contact with electric knife**

X+7th **W29.2** **Contact with other powered household machinery**
Contact with electric fan
Contact with powered dryer (clothes) (powered) (spin)
Contact with washing-machine
Contact with sewing machine

X+7th **W29.3** **Contact with powered garden and outdoor hand tools and machinery**
Contact with chainsaw
Contact with edger
Contact with garden cultivator (tiller)
Contact with hedge trimmer
Contact with other powered garden tool
Excludes1: *contact with powered lawn mower (W28)*

X+7th **W29.4** **Contact with nail gun**

X+7th **W29.8** **Contact with other powered hand tools and household machinery**
Contact with do-it-yourself tool NOS

W30 **Contact with agricultural machinery**

Includes: animal-powered farm machine
Excludes1: *agricultural transport vehicle accident (V01-V99)*
explosion of grain store (W40.8)
exposure to electric current (W86.-)

The appropriate 7th character is to be added to each code from category W30
A   initial encounter
D   subsequent encounter
S   sequela

X+7th **W30.0** **Contact with combine harvester**
Contact with reaper
Contact with thresher

X+7th **W30.1** **Contact with power take-off devices (PTO)**

X+7th **W30.2** **Contact with hay derrick**

X+7th **W30.3** **Contact with grain storage elevator**
Excludes1: *explosion of grain store (W40.8)*

+ **W30.8** **Contact with other specified agricultural machinery**

X+7th **W30.81** **Contact with agricultural transport vehicle in stationary use**
Contact with agricultural transport vehicle under repair, not on public roadway
Excludes1: *agricultural transport vehicle accident (V01-V99)*

X+7th **W30.89** **Contact with other specified agricultural machinery**

X+7th **W30.9** **Contact with unspecified agricultural machinery**
Contact with farm machinery NOS

W31 **Contact with other and unspecified machinery**

Excludes1: *contact with agricultural machinery (W30.-)*
contact with machinery in transport under own power or being towed by a vehicle (V01-V99)
exposure to electric current (W86)

The appropriate 7th character is to be added to each code from category W31
A   initial encounter
D   subsequent encounter
S   sequela

X+7th **W31.0** **Contact with mining and earth-drilling machinery**
Contact with bore or drill (land) (seabed)
Contact with shaft hoist
Contact with shaft lift
Contact with undercutter

X+7th **W31.1** **Contact with metalworking machines**
Contact with abrasive wheel
Contact with forging machine
Contact with lathe
Contact with mechanical shears
Contact with metal drilling machine
Contact with milling machine
Contact with power press
Contact with rolling-mill
Contact with metal sawing machine

X+7th **W31.2** **Contact with powered woodworking and forming machines**
Contact with band saw
Contact with bench saw
Contact with circular saw
Contact with molding machine
Contact with overhead plane
Contact with powered saw
Contact with radial saw
Contact with sander
Excludes1: *nonpowered woodworking tools (W27.0)*

X+7th **W31.3** **Contact with prime movers**
Contact with gas turbine
Contact with internal combustion engine
Contact with steam engine
Contact with water driven turbine

+ **W31.8** **Contact with other specified machinery**

X+7th **W31.81** **Contact with recreational machinery**
Contact with roller coaster

X+7th **W31.82** **Contact with other commercial machinery**
Contact with commercial electric fan
Contact with commercial kitchen appliances
Contact with commercial powered dryer (clothes) (powered) (spin)
Contact with commercial washing-machine
Contact with commercial sewing machine
Excludes1: *contact with household machinery (W29.-)*
contact with powered lawn mower (W28)

X+7th **W31.83** **Contact with special construction vehicle in stationary use**
Contact with special construction vehicle under repair, not on public roadway
Excludes1: *special construction vehicle accident (V01-V99)*

X+7th **W31.89** **Contact with other specified machinery**

X+7th **W31.9** **Contact with unspecified machinery**
Contact with machinery NOS

W32 **Accidental handgun discharge and malfunction**

Includes: accidental discharge and malfunction of gun for single hand use
accidental discharge and malfunction of pistol
accidental discharge and malfunction of revolver
Handgun discharge and malfunction NOS
Excludes1: *accidental airgun discharge and malfunction (W34.010, W34.110)*
accidental BB gun discharge and malfunction (W34.010, W34.110)
accidental pellet gun discharge and malfunction (W34.010, W34.110)
accidental shotgun discharge and malfunction (W33.01, W33.11)

assault by handgun discharge (X93)
handgun discharge involving legal intervention (Y35.0-)
handgun discharge involving military or war operations (Y36.4-)
intentional self-harm by handgun discharge (X72)
Very pistol discharge and malfunction (W34.09, W34.19)

> The appropriate 7th character is to be added to each code from category W32
> A   initial encounter
> D   subsequent encounter
> S   sequela

X+7th **W32.0 Accidental handgun discharge**
X+7th **W32.1 Accidental handgun malfunction**
Injury due to explosion of handgun (parts)
Injury due to malfunction of mechanism or component of handgun
Injury due to recoil of handgun
Powder burn from handgun

W33 Accidental rifle, shotgun and larger firearm discharge and malfunction

Includes: rifle, shotgun and larger firearm discharge and malfunction NOS

Excludes1: accidental airgun discharge and malfunction (W34.010, W34.110)
accidental BB gun discharge and malfunction (W34.010, W34.110)
accidental handgun discharge and malfunction (W32.-)
accidental pellet gun discharge and malfunction (W34.010, W34.110)
assault by rifle, shotgun and larger firearm discharge (X94)
firearm discharge involving legal intervention (Y35.0-)
firearm discharge involving military or war operations (Y36.4-)
intentional self-harm by rifle, shotgun and larger firearm discharge (X73)

> The appropriate 7th character is to be added to each code from category W33
> A   initial encounter
> D   subsequent encounter
> S   sequela

\+ **W33.0 Accidental rifle, shotgun and larger firearm discharge**
X+7th **W33.00 Accidental discharge of unspecified larger firearm**
Discharge of unspecified larger firearm NOS
X+7th **W33.01 Accidental discharge of shotgun**
Discharge of shotgun NOS
X+7th **W33.02 Accidental discharge of hunting rifle**
Discharge of hunting rifle NOS
X+7th **W33.03 Accidental discharge of machine gun**
Discharge of machine gun NOS
X+7th **W33.09 Accidental discharge of other larger firearm**
Discharge of other larger firearm NOS
\+ **W33.1 Accidental rifle, shotgun and larger firearm malfunction**
Injury due to explosion of rifle, shotgun and larger firearm (parts)
Injury due to malfunction of mechanism or component of rifle, shotgun and larger firearm
Injury due to piercing, cutting, crushing or pinching due to (by) slide trigger mechanism, scope or other gun part
Injury due to recoil of rifle, shotgun and larger firearm
Powder burn from rifle, shotgun and larger firearm
X+7th **W33.10 Accidental malfunction of unspecified larger firearm**
Malfunction of unspecified larger firearm NOS
X+7th **W33.11 Accidental malfunction of shotgun**
Malfunction of shotgun NOS
X+7th **W33.12 Accidental malfunction of hunting rifle**
Malfunction of hunting rifle NOS
X+7th **W33.13 Accidental malfunction of machine gun**
Malfunction of machine gun NOS
X+7th **W33.19 Accidental malfunction of other larger firearm**
Malfunction of other larger firearm NOS

W34 Accidental discharge and malfunction from other and unspecified firearms and guns

> The appropriate 7th character is to be added to each code from category W34
> A   initial encounter
> D   subsequent encounter
> S   sequela

\+ **W34.0 Accidental discharge from other and unspecified firearms and guns**
X+7th **W34.00 Accidental discharge from unspecified firearms or gun**
Discharge from firearm NOS
Gunshot wound NOS
Shot NOS
AHA CC: 1Q, 2015, 3-21
\+ **W34.01 Accidental discharge of gas, air or spring-operated guns**
+7th **W34.010 Accidental discharge of airgun**
Accidental discharge of BB gun
Accidental discharge of pellet gun
+7th **W34.011 Accidental discharge of paintball gun**
Accidental injury due to paintball discharge
+7th **W34.018 Accidental discharge of other gas, air or spring-operated gun**
X+7th **W34.09 Accidental discharge from other specified firearms**
Accidental discharge from Very pistol [flare]
\+ **W34.1 Accidental malfunction from other and unspecified firearms and guns**
X+7th **W34.10 Accidental malfunction from unspecified firearms or gun**
Firearm malfunction NOS
\+ **W34.11 Accidental malfunction of gas, air or spring-operated guns**
+7th **W34.110 Accidental malfunction of airgun**
Accidental malfunction of BB gun
Accidental malfunction of pellet gun
+7th **W34.111 Accidental malfunction of paintball gun**
Accidental injury due to paintball gun malfunction
+7th **W34.118 Accidental malfunction of other gas, air or spring-operated gun**
X+7th **W34.19 Accidental malfunction from other specified firearms**
Accidental malfunction from Very pistol [flare]

W35 Explosion and rupture of boiler
X+7th
Excludes1: explosion and rupture of boiler on watercraft (V93.4)

> The appropriate 7th character is to be added to code W35
> A   initial encounter
> D   subsequent encounter
> S   sequela

W36 Explosion and rupture of gas cylinder

> The appropriate 7th character is to be added to each code from category W36
> A   initial encounter
> D   subsequent encounter
> S   sequela

X+7th **W36.1 Explosion and rupture of aerosol can**
X+7th **W36.2 Explosion and rupture of air tank**
X+7th **W36.3 Explosion and rupture of pressurized-gas tank**
X+7th **W36.8 Explosion and rupture of other gas cylinder**
X+7th **W36.9 Explosion and rupture of unspecified gas cylinder**

W37 Explosion and rupture of pressurized tire, pipe or hose

> The appropriate 7th character is to be added to each code from category W37
> A   initial encounter
> D   subsequent encounter
> S   sequela

X+7th **W37.0 Explosion of bicycle tire**
X+7th **W37.8 Explosion and rupture of other pressurized tire, pipe or hose**

+, +7th, X + 7th   ● Newborn   ● Pediatric   ● Maternity   ● Adult   ♀ Female   ♂ Male   Manifestation   Unacceptable PDX   HCC   CC   MCC   HAC

W38 Explosion and rupture of other specified pressurized devices
X+7th

The appropriate 7th character is to be added to code W38
A   initial encounter
D   subsequent encounter
S   sequela

W39 Discharge of firework
X+7th

The appropriate 7th character is to be added to code W39
A   initial encounter
D   subsequent encounter
S   sequela

W40 Explosion of other materials

> **Excludes1:** *assault by explosive material (X96)*
> *explosion involving legal intervention (Y35.1-)*
> *explosion involving military or war operations (Y36.0-, Y36.2-)*
> *intentional self-harm by explosive material (X75)*

The appropriate 7th character is to be added to each code from category W40
A   initial encounter
D   subsequent encounter
S   sequela

X+7th **W40.0 Explosion of blasting material**
  Explosion of blasting cap
  Explosion of detonator
  Explosion of dynamite
  Explosion of explosive (any) used in blasting operations

X+7th **W40.1 Explosion of explosive gases**
  Explosion of acetylene
  Explosion of butane
  Explosion of coal gas
  Explosion in mine NOS
  Explosion of explosive gas
  Explosion of fire damp
  Explosion of gasoline fumes
  Explosion of methane
  Explosion of propane

X+7th **W40.8 Explosion of other specified explosive materials**
  Explosion in dump NOS
  Explosion in factory NOS
  Explosion in grain store
  Explosion in munitions

> **Excludes1:** *explosion involving legal intervention (Y35.1-)*
> *explosion involving military or war operations (Y36.0-, Y36.2-)*

X+7th **W40.9 Explosion of unspecified explosive materials**
  Explosion NOS

W42 Exposure to noise

The appropriate 7th character is to be added to each code from category W42
A   initial encounter
D   subsequent encounter
S   sequela

X+7th **W42.0 Exposure to supersonic waves**
X+7th **W42.9 Exposure to other noise**
  Exposure to sound waves NOS

W45 Foreign body or object entering through skin

> **Includes:** foreign body or object embedded in skin
>   nail embedded in skin
> **Excludes2:** *contact with hand tools (nonpowered) (powered) (W27-W29)*
>   *contact with other sharp object(s) (W26.-)*
>   *contact with sharp glass (W25.-)*
>   *struck by objects (W20-W22)*

The appropriate 7th character is to be added to each code from category W45
A   initial encounter
D   subsequent encounter
S   sequela

X+7th **W45.0 Nail entering through skin**
X+7th **W45.8 Other foreign body or object entering through skin**
  Splinter in skin NOS

W46 Contact with hypodermic needle

The appropriate 7th character is to be added to each code from category W46
A   initial encounter
D   subsequent encounter
S   sequela

X+7th **W46.0 Contact with hypodermic needle**
  Hypodermic needle stick NOS
X+7th **W46.1 Contact with contaminated hypodermic needle**

W49 Exposure to other inanimate mechanical forces

> **Includes:** exposure to abnormal gravitational [G] forces
>   exposure to inanimate mechanical forces NEC
> **Excludes1:** *exposure to inanimate mechanical forces involving military or war operations (Y36.-, Y37.-)*

The appropriate 7th character is to be added to each code from category W49
A   initial encounter
D   subsequent encounter
S   sequela

  + **W49.0 Item causing external constriction**
X+7th **W49.01 Hair causing external constriction**
X+7th **W49.02 String or thread causing external constriction**
X+7th **W49.03 Rubber band causing external constriction**
X+7th **W49.04 Ring or other jewelry causing external constriction**
X+7th **W49.09 Other specified item causing external constriction**
X+7th **W49.9 Exposure to other inanimate mechanical forces**

Exposure to animate mechanical forces (W50-W64)

> **Excludes1:** *Toxic effect of contact with venomous animals and plants (T63.-)*

W50 Accidental hit, strike, kick, twist, bite or scratch by another person

> **Includes:** hit, strike, kick, twist, bite, or scratch by another person NOS
> **Excludes1:** *assault by bodily force (Y04)*
>   *struck by objects (W20-W22)*

The appropriate 7th character is to be added to each code from category W50
A   initial encounter
D   subsequent encounter
S   sequela

X+7th **W50.0 Accidental hit or strike by another person**
  Hit or strike by another person NOS
X+7th **W50.1 Accidental kick by another person**
  Kick by another person NOS
X+7th **W50.2 Accidental twist by another person**
  Twist by another person NOS
  AHA CC: 1Q, 2015, 3-21
X+7th **W50.3 Accidental bite by another person**
  Human bite
  Bite by another person NOS
X+7th **W50.4 Accidental scratch by another person**
  Scratch by another person NOS

W51 Accidental striking against or bumped into by another person
X+7th

> **Excludes1:** *assault by striking against or bumping into by another person (Y04.2)*
>   *fall due to collision with another person (W03)*

The appropriate 7th character is to be added to code W51
A   initial encounter
D   subsequent encounter
S   sequela

W52 Crushed, pushed or stepped on by crowd or human stampede
X+7th
  Crushed, pushed or stepped on by crowd or human stampede with or without fall

The appropriate 7th character is to be added to code W52
A   initial encounter
D   subsequent encounter
S   sequela

+ W53 Contact with rodent

    Includes: contact with saliva, feces or urine of rodent

    The appropriate 7th character is to be added to each code from category W53
    A   initial encounter
    D   subsequent encounter
    S   sequela

  + W53.0 Contact with mouse
    X+7th **W53.01 Bitten by mouse**
    X+7th **W53.09 Other contact with mouse**
  + W53.1 Contact with rat
    X+7th **W53.11 Bitten by rat**
    X+7th **W53.19 Other contact with rat**
  + W53.2 Contact with squirrel
    X+7th **W53.21 Bitten by squirrel**
    X+7th **W53.29 Other contact with squirrel**
  + W53.8 Contact with other rodent
    X+7th **W53.81 Bitten by other rodent**
    X+7th **W53.89 Other contact with other rodent**

W54 Contact with dog

    Includes: contact with saliva, feces or urine of dog

    The appropriate 7th character is to be added to each code from category W54
    A   initial encounter
    D   subsequent encounter
    S   sequela

X+7th **W54.0 Bitten by dog**
    AHA CC: 4Q, 2017, 112-114
    Review coding guideline B.19.c
X+7th **W54.1 Struck by dog**
    Knocked over by dog
X+7th **W54.8 Other contact with dog**

W55 Contact with other mammals

    Includes: contact with saliva, feces or urine of mammal
    Excludes1: *animal being ridden- see transport accidents*
        bitten or struck by dog (W54)
        bitten or struck by rodent (W53.-)
        contact with marine mammals (W56.-)

    The appropriate 7th character is to be added to each code from category W55
    A   initial encounter
    D   subsequent encounter
    S   sequela

  + W55.0 Contact with cat
    X+7th **W55.01 Bitten by cat**
    X+7th **W55.03 Scratched by cat**
    X+7th **W55.09 Other contact with cat**
  + W55.1 Contact with horse
    X+7th **W55.11 Bitten by horse**
    X+7th **W55.12 Struck by horse**
    X+7th **W55.19 Other contact with horse**
  + W55.2 Contact with cow
    Contact with bull
    X+7th **W55.21 Bitten by cow**
    X+7th **W55.22 Struck by cow**
    Gored by bull
    X+7th **W55.29 Other contact with cow**
  + W55.3 Contact with other hoof stock
    Contact with goats
    Contact with sheep
    X+7th **W55.31 Bitten by other hoof stock**
    X+7th **W55.32 Struck by other hoof stock**
    Gored by goat
    Gored by ram
    X+7th **W55.39 Other contact with other hoof stock**
  + W55.4 Contact with pig
    X+7th **W55.41 Bitten by pig**
    X+7th **W55.42 Struck by pig**
    X+7th **W55.49 Other contact with pig**
  + W55.5 Contact with raccoon
    X+7th **W55.51 Bitten by raccoon**
    X+7th **W55.52 Struck by raccoon**
    X+7th **W55.59 Other contact with raccoon**
  + W55.8 Contact with other mammals
    X+7th **W55.81 Bitten by other mammals**
    X+7th **W55.82 Struck by other mammals**
    X+7th **W55.89 Other contact with other mammals**

W56 Contact with nonvenomous marine animal

    Excludes1: *contact with venomous marine animal (T63.-)*

    The appropriate 7th character is to be added to each code from category W56
    A   initial encounter
    D   subsequent encounter
    S   sequela

  + W56.0 Contact with dolphin
    X+7th **W56.01 Bitten by dolphin**
    X+7th **W56.02 Struck by dolphin**
    X+7th **W56.09 Other contact with dolphin**
  + W56.1 Contact with sea lion
    X+7th **W56.11 Bitten by sea lion**
    X+7th **W56.12 Struck by sea lion**
    X+7th **W56.19 Other contact with sea lion**
  + W56.2 Contact with orca
    Contact with killer whale
    X+7th **W56.21 Bitten by orca**
    X+7th **W56.22 Struck by orca**
    X+7th **W56.29 Other contact with orca**
  + W56.3 Contact with other marine mammals
    X+7th **W56.31 Bitten by other marine mammals**
    X+7th **W56.32 Struck by other marine mammals**
    X+7th **W56.39 Other contact with other marine mammals**
  + W56.4 Contact with shark
    X+7th **W56.41 Bitten by shark**
    X+7th **W56.42 Struck by shark**
    X+7th **W56.49 Other contact with shark**
  + W56.5 Contact with other fish
    X+7th **W56.51 Bitten by other fish**
    X+7th **W56.52 Struck by other fish**
    X+7th **W56.59 Other contact with other fish**
  + W56.8 Contact with other nonvenomous marine animals
    X+7th **W56.81 Bitten by other nonvenomous marine animals**
    X+7th **W56.82 Struck by other nonvenomous marine animals**
    X+7th **W56.89 Other contact with other nonvenomous marine animals**

W57 Bitten or stung by nonvenomous insect and other nonvenomous X+7th **arthropods**

    Excludes1: *contact with venomous insects and arthropods (T63.2-, T63.3-, T63.4-)*

    The appropriate 7th character is to be added to code W57
    A   initial encounter
    D   subsequent encounter
    S   sequela

W58 Contact with crocodile or alligator

    The appropriate 7th character is to be added to each code from category W58
    A   initial encounter
    D   subsequent encounter
    S   sequela

  + W58.0 Contact with alligator
    X+7th **W58.01 Bitten by alligator**
    X+7th **W58.02 Struck by alligator**
    X+7th **W58.03 Crushed by alligator**
    X+7th **W58.09 Other contact with alligator**
  + W58.1 Contact with crocodile
    X+7th **W58.11 Bitten by crocodile**
    X+7th **W58.12 Struck by crocodile**
    X+7th **W58.13 Crushed by crocodile**
    X+7th **W58.19 Other contact with crocodile**

W59 Contact with other nonvenomous reptiles

    Excludes1: *contact with venomous reptile (T63.0-, T63.1-)*

    The appropriate 7th character is to be added to each code from category W59
    A   initial encounter
    D   subsequent encounter
    S   sequela

  + W59.0 Contact with nonvenomous lizards
    X+7th **W59.01 Bitten by nonvenomous lizards**
    X+7th **W59.02 Struck by nonvenomous lizards**
    X+7th **W59.09 Other contact with nonvenomous lizards**
    Exposure to nonvenomous lizards
  + W59.1 Contact with nonvenomous snakes
    X+7th **W59.11 Bitten by nonvenomous snake**
    X+7th **W59.12 Struck by nonvenomous snake**

X+7th W59.13 **Crushed by nonvenomous snake**
X+7th W59.19 **Other contact with nonvenomous snake**
+ W59.2 **Contact with turtles**
Excludes1: contact with tortoises (W59.8-)
X+7th W59.21 **Bitten by turtle**
X+7th W59.22 **Struck by turtle**
X+7th W59.29 **Other contact with turtle**
Exposure to turtles
+ W59.8 **Contact with other nonvenomous reptiles**
X+7th W59.81 **Bitten by other nonvenomous reptiles**
X+7th W59.82 **Struck by other nonvenomous reptiles**
X+7th W59.83 **Crushed by other nonvenomous reptiles**
X+7th W59.89 **Other contact with other nonvenomous reptiles**

W60 **Contact with nonvenomous plant thorns and spines and sharp**
X+7th **leaves**

Excludes1: Contact with venomous plants (T63.7-)

The appropriate 7th character is to be added to code W60
A   initial encounter
D   subsequent encounter
S   sequela

W61 **Contact with birds (domestic) (wild)**

Includes: contact with excreta of birds

The appropriate 7th character is to be added to each code from
category W61
A   initial encounter
D   subsequent encounter
S   sequela

+ W61.0 **Contact with parrot**
X+7th W61.01 **Bitten by parrot**
X+7th W61.02 **Struck by parrot**
X+7th W61.09 **Other contact with parrot**
Exposure to parrots
+ W61.1 **Contact with macaw**
X+7th W61.11 **Bitten by macaw**
X+7th W61.12 **Struck by macaw**
X+7th W61.19 **Other contact with macaw**
Exposure to macaws
+ W61.2 **Contact with other psittacines**
X+7th W61.21 **Bitten by other psittacines**
X+7th W61.22 **Struck by other psittacines**
X+7th W61.29 **Other contact with other psittacines**
Exposure to other psittacines
+ W61.3 **Contact with chicken**
X+7th W61.32 **Struck by chicken**
X+7th W61.33 **Pecked by chicken**
X+7th W61.39 **Other contact with chicken**
Exposure to chickens
+ W61.4 **Contact with turkey**
X+7th W61.42 **Struck by turkey**
X+7th W61.43 **Pecked by turkey**
X+7th W61.49 **Other contact with turkey**
+ W61.5 **Contact with goose**
X+7th W61.51 **Bitten by goose**
X+7th W61.52 **Struck by goose**
X+7th W61.59 **Other contact with goose**
+ W61.6 **Contact with duck**
X+7th W61.61 **Bitten by duck**
X+7th W61.62 **Struck by duck**
X+7th W61.69 **Other contact with duck**
+ W61.9 **Contact with other birds**
X+7th W61.91 **Bitten by other birds**
X+7th W61.92 **Struck by other birds**
X+7th W61.99 **Other contact with other birds**
Contact with bird NOS

W62 **Contact with nonvenomous amphibians**

Excludes1: contact with venomous amphibians (T63.81-R63.83)

The appropriate 7th character is to be added to each code from
category W62
A   initial encounter
D   subsequent encounter
S   sequela

X+7th W62.0 **Contact with nonvenomous frogs**
X+7th W62.1 **Contact with nonvenomous toads**
X+7th W62.9 **Contact with other nonvenomous amphibians**

W64 **Exposure to other animate mechanical forces**
X+7th **Includes:** exposure to nonvenomous animal NOS
Excludes1: contact with venomous animal (T63.-)

The appropriate 7th character is to be added to code W64
A   initial encounter
D   subsequent encounter
S   sequela

Accidental non-transport drowning and submersion (W65-W74)

Excludes1:   accidental drowning and submersion due to fall into water (W16.-)
accidental drowning and submersion due to water transport
accident (V90.-, V92.-)

Excludes2:   accidental drowning and submersion due to cataclysm (X34-X39)

W65 **Accidental drowning and submersion while in bath-tub**
X+7th **Excludes1:** accidental drowning and submersion due to fall in (into)
bathtub (W16.211)

The appropriate 7th character is to be added to code W65
A   initial encounter
D   subsequent encounter
S   sequela

W67 **Accidental drowning and submersion while in swimming-pool**
X+7th **Excludes1:** accidental drowning and submersion due to fall into
swimming pool (W16.011, W16.021, W16.031)
accidental drowning and submersion due to striking
into wall of swimming pool (W22.041)

The appropriate 7th character is to be added to code W67
A   initial encounter
D   subsequent encounter
S   sequela

W69 **Accidental drowning and submersion while in natural water**
X+7th Accidental drowning and submersion while in lake
Accidental drowning and submersion while in open sea
Accidental drowning and submersion while in river
Accidental drowning and submersion while in stream
Excludes1: accidental drowning and submersion due to fall
into natural body of water (W16.111, W16.121,
W16.131)

The appropriate 7th character is to be added to code W69
A   initial encounter
D   subsequent encounter
S   sequela

W73 **Other specified cause of accidental non-transport drowning and**
X+7th **submersion**

Accidental drowning and submersion while in quenching tank
Accidental drowning and submersion while in reservoir
Excludes1: accidental drowning and submersion due to fall into
other water (W16.311, W16.321, W16.331)

The appropriate 7th character is to be added to code W73
A   initial encounter
D   subsequent encounter
S   sequela

W74 **Unspecified cause of accidental drowning and submersion**
X+7th Drowning NOS

The appropriate 7th character is to be added to code W74
A   initial encounter
D   subsequent encounter
S   sequela

Exposure to electric current, radiation and extreme ambient air temperature and pressure (W85-W99)

Excludes1:   exposure to:
failure in dosage of radiation or temperature during surgical and
medical care (Y63.2-Y63.5)
lightning (T75.0-)
natural cold (X31)
natural heat (X30)
natural radiation NOS (X39)
radiological procedure and radiotherapy (Y84.2)
sunlight (X32)

W85 Exposure to electric transmission lines
X+7th
    Broken power line

> The appropriate 7th character is to be added to code W85
> A   initial encounter
> D   subsequent encounter
> S   sequela

W86 Exposure to other specified electric current

> The appropriate 7th character is to be added to each code from category W86
> A   initial encounter
> D   subsequent encounter
> S   sequela

X+7th **W86.0 Exposure to domestic wiring and appliances**
X+7th **W86.1 Exposure to industrial wiring, appliances and electrical machinery**
    Exposure to conductors
    Exposure to control apparatus
    Exposure to electrical equipment and machinery
    Exposure to transformers
X+7th **W86.8 Exposure to other electric current**
    Exposure to wiring and appliances in or on farm (not farmhouse)
    Exposure to wiring and appliances outdoors
    Exposure to wiring and appliances in or on public building
    Exposure to wiring and appliances in or on residential institutions
    Exposure to wiring and appliances in or on schools

W88 Exposure to ionizing radiation

> *Excludes1:* *exposure to sunlight (X32)*

> The appropriate 7th character is to be added to each code from category W88
> A   initial encounter
> D   subsequent encounter
> S   sequela

X+7th **W88.0 Exposure to X-rays**
X+7th **W88.1 Exposure to radioactive isotopes**
X+7th **W88.8 Exposure to other ionizing radiation**

W89 Exposure to man-made visible and ultraviolet light

> **Includes:** exposure to welding light (arc)
> *Excludes2:* *exposure to sunlight (X32)*

> The appropriate 7th character is to be added to each code from category W89
> A   initial encounter
> D   subsequent encounter
> S   sequela

X+7th **W89.0 Exposure to welding light (arc)**
X+7th **W89.1 Exposure to tanning bed**
X+7th **W89.8 Exposure to other man-made visible and ultraviolet light**
X+7th **W89.9 Exposure to unspecified man-made visible and ultraviolet light**

W90 Exposure to other nonionizing radiation

> *Excludes2:* *exposure to sunlight (X32)*

> The appropriate 7th character is to be added to each code from category W90
> A   initial encounter
> D   subsequent encounter
> S   sequela

X+7th **W90.0 Exposure to radiofrequency**
X+7th **W90.1 Exposure to infrared radiation**
X+7th **W90.2 Exposure to laser radiation**
X+7th **W90.8 Exposure to other nonionizing radiation**

W92 Exposure to excessive heat of man-made origin
X+7th
> The appropriate 7th character is to be added to code W92
> A   initial encounter
> D   subsequent encounter
> S   sequela

W93 Exposure to excessive cold of man-made origin

> The appropriate 7th character is to be added to each code from category W93
> A   initial encounter
> D   subsequent encounter
> S   sequela

+ **W93.0 Contact with or inhalation of dry ice**
  X+7th **W93.01 Contact with dry ice**
  X+7th **W93.02 Inhalation of dry ice**
+ **W93.1 Contact with or inhalation of liquid air**
  X+7th **W93.11 Contact with liquid air**
      Contact with liquid hydrogen
      Contact with liquid nitrogen
  X+7th **W93.12 Inhalation of liquid air**
      Inhalation of liquid hydrogen
      Inhalation of liquid nitrogen
X+7th **W93.2 Prolonged exposure in deep freeze unit or refrigerator**
X+7th **W93.8 Exposure to other excessive cold of man-made origin**

W94 Exposure to high and low air pressure and changes in air pressure

> The appropriate 7th character is to be added to each code from category W94
> A   initial encounter
> D   subsequent encounter
> S   sequela

X+7th **W94.0 Exposure to prolonged high air pressure**
+ **W94.1 Exposure to prolonged low air pressure**
  X+7th **W94.11 Exposure to residence or prolonged visit at high altitude**
  X+7th **W94.12 Exposure to other prolonged low air pressure**
+ **W94.2 Exposure to rapid changes in air pressure during ascent**
  X+7th **W94.21 Exposure to reduction in atmospheric pressure while surfacing from deep-water diving**
  X+7th **W94.22 Exposure to reduction in atmospheric pressure while surfacing from underground**
  X+7th **W94.23 Exposure to sudden change in air pressure in aircraft during ascent**
  X+7th **W94.29 Exposure to other rapid changes in air pressure during ascent**
+ **W94.3 Exposure to rapid changes in air pressure during descent**
  X+7th **W94.31 Exposure to sudden change in air pressure in aircraft during descent**
  X+7th **W94.32 Exposure to high air pressure from rapid descent in water**
  X+7th **W94.39 Exposure to other rapid changes in air pressure during descent**

W99 Exposure to other man-made environmental factors
X+7th
> The appropriate 7th character is to be added to code W99
> A   initial encounter
> D   subsequent encounter
> S   sequela

Exposure to smoke, fire and flames (X00-X08)

Excludes1: *arson (X97)*

Excludes2: *explosions (W35-W40)*
    lightning (T75.0-)
    transport accident (V01-V99)

X00 Exposure to uncontrolled fire in building or structure

> **Includes:** conflagration in building or structure
> Code first any associated cataclysm
> *Excludes2:* *Exposure to ignition or melting of nightwear (X05)*
>   *Exposure to ignition or melting of other clothing and apparel (X06.-)*
>   *Exposure to other specified smoke, fire and flames (X08.-)*

> The appropriate 7th character is to be added to each code from category X00
> A   initial encounter
> D   subsequent encounter
> S   sequela

X+7th **X00.0 Exposure to flames in uncontrolled fire in building or structure**
    AHA CC: 1Q, 2015, 3-21; 2Q, 2016, 5-6
X+7th **X00.1 Exposure to smoke in uncontrolled fire in building or structure**
X+7th **X00.2 Injury due to collapse of burning building or structure in uncontrolled fire**
> *Excludes1:* *injury due to collapse of building not on fire (W20.1)*
X+7th **X00.3 Fall from burning building or structure in uncontrolled fire**

+, +7th, X + 7th   ● Newborn   ● Pediatric   ● Maternity   ● Adult   ♀ Female   ♂ Male   Manifestation   Unacceptable PDX   HCC   CC   MCC   HAC

X+7th **X00.4** **Hit by object from burning building or structure in uncontrolled fire**

X+7th **X00.5** **Jump from burning building or structure in uncontrolled fire**

X+7th **X00.8** **Other exposure to uncontrolled fire in building or structure**

X01 **Exposure to uncontrolled fire, not in building or structure**

> **Includes:** exposure to forest fire

> The appropriate 7th character is to be added to each code from category X01
> A   initial encounter
> D   subsequent encounter
> S   sequela

X+7th **X01.0** **Exposure to flames in uncontrolled fire, not in building or structure**

X+7th **X01.1** **Exposure to smoke in uncontrolled fire, not in building or structure**

X+7th **X01.3** **Fall due to uncontrolled fire, not in building or structure**

X+7th **X01.4** **Hit by object due to uncontrolled fire, not in building or structure**

X+7th **X01.8** **Other exposure to uncontrolled fire, not in building or structure**

X02 **Exposure to controlled fire in building or structure**

> **Includes:** exposure to fire in fireplace
> exposure to fire in stove

> The appropriate 7th character is to be added to each code from category X02
> A   initial encounter
> D   subsequent encounter
> S   sequela

X+7th **X02.0** **Exposure to flames in controlled fire in building or structure**

X+7th **X02.1** **Exposure to smoke in controlled fire in building or structure**

X+7th **X02.2** **Injury due to collapse of burning building or structure in controlled fire**

> **Excludes1:** *injury due to collapse of building not on fire (W20.1)*

X+7th **X02.3** **Fall from burning building or structure in controlled fire**

X+7th **X02.4** **Hit by object from burning building or structure in controlled fire**

X+7th **X02.5** **Jump from burning building or structure in controlled fire**

X+7th **X02.8** **Other exposure to controlled fire in building or structure**

X03 **Exposure to controlled fire, not in building or structure**

> **Includes:** exposure to bon fire
> exposure to camp-fire
> exposure to trash fire

> The appropriate 7th character is to be added to each code from category X03
> A   initial encounter
> D   subsequent encounter
> S   sequela

X+7th **X03.0** **Exposure to flames in controlled fire, not in building or structure**
> *AHA CC: 1Q, 2015, 3-21*

X+7th **X03.1** **Exposure to smoke in controlled fire, not in building or structure**

X+7th **X03.3** **Fall due to controlled fire, not in building or structure**

X+7th **X03.4** **Hit by object due to controlled fire, not in building or structure**

X+7th **X03.8** **Other exposure to controlled fire, not in building or structure**

X04 **Exposure to ignition of highly flammable material**
X+7th
> Exposure to ignition of gasoline
> Exposure to ignition of kerosene
> Exposure to ignition of petrol
> **Excludes2:** *exposure to ignition or melting of nightwear (X05)*
> *exposure to ignition or melting of other clothing and apparel (X06)*
>
> *AHA CC: 2Q, 2016, 4*

> The appropriate 7th character is to be added to code X04
> A   initial encounter
> D   subsequent encounter
> S   sequela

X05 **Exposure to ignition or melting of nightwear**
X+7th
> **Excludes2:** *exposure to uncontrolled fire in building or structure (X00.-)*
> *exposure to uncontrolled fire, not in building or structure (X01.-)*
> *exposure to controlled fire in building or structure (X02.-)*
> *exposure to controlled fire, not in building or structure (X03.-)*
> *exposure to ignition of highly flammable materials (X04.-)*

> The appropriate 7th character is to be added to code X05
> A   initial encounter
> D   subsequent encounter
> S   sequela

X06 **Exposure to ignition or melting of other clothing and apparel**

> **Excludes2:** *exposure to uncontrolled fire in building or structure (X00.-)*
> *exposure to uncontrolled fire, not in building or structure (X01.-)*
> *exposure to controlled fire in building or structure (X02.-)*
> *exposure to controlled fire, not in building or structure (X03.-)*
> *exposure to ignition of highly flammable materials (X04.-)*

> The appropriate 7th character is to be added to each code from category X06
> A   initial encounter
> D   subsequent encounter
> S   sequela

X+7th **X06.0** **Exposure to ignition of plastic jewelry**
X+7th **X06.1** **Exposure to melting of plastic jewelry**
X+7th **X06.2** **Exposure to ignition of other clothing and apparel**
X+7th **X06.3** **Exposure to melting of other clothing and apparel**

X08 **Exposure to other specified smoke, fire and flames**

> The appropriate 7th character is to be added to each code from category X08
> A   initial encounter
> D   subsequent encounter
> S   sequela

+ **X08.0** **Exposure to bed fire**
> Exposure to mattress fire

X+7th **X08.00** **Exposure to bed fire due to unspecified burning material**

X+7th **X08.01** **Exposure to bed fire due to burning cigarette**
> *AHA CC: 1Q, 2015, 3-21*

X+7th **X08.09** **Exposure to bed fire due to other burning material**

+ **X08.1** **Exposure to sofa fire**

X+7th **X08.10** **Exposure to sofa fire due to unspecified burning material**

X+7th **X08.11** **Exposure to sofa fire due to burning cigarette**

X+7th **X08.19** **Exposure to sofa fire due to other burning material**

+ **X08.2** **Exposure to other furniture fire**

X+7th **X08.20** **Exposure to other furniture fire due to unspecified burning material**

X+7th **X08.21** **Exposure to other furniture fire due to burning cigarette**

X+7th **X08.29** **Exposure to other furniture fire due to other burning material**

X+7th **X08.8** **Exposure to other specified smoke, fire and flames**

Contact with heat and hot substances (X10-X19)

> **Excludes1:** *exposure to excessive natural heat (X30)*
> *exposure to fire and flames (X00-X08)*

X10 **Contact with hot drinks, food, fats and cooking oils**

> The appropriate 7th character is to be added to each code from category X10
> A   initial encounter
> D   subsequent encounter
> S   sequela

X+7th **X10.0** **Contact with hot drinks**
X+7th **X10.1** **Contact with hot food**
X+7th **X10.2** **Contact with fats and cooking oils**

X11 Contact with hot tap-water

> **Includes:** contact with boiling tap-water
> contact with boiling water NOS
>
> **Excludes1:** *contact with water heated on stove (X12)*

> The appropriate 7th character is to be added to each code from category X11
> A initial encounter
> D subsequent encounter
> S sequela

X+7th **X11.0 Contact with hot water in bath or tub**
> **Excludes1:** *contact with running hot water in bath or tub (X11.1)*

X+7th **X11.1 Contact with running hot water**
> Contact with hot water running out of hose
> Contact with hot water running out of tap

X+7th **X11.8 Contact with other hot tap-water**
> Contact with hot water in bucket
> Contact with hot tap-water NOS

X12 Contact with other hot fluids
X+7th
> Contact with water heated on stove
>
> **Excludes1:** *hot (liquid) metals (X18)*

> The appropriate 7th character is to be added to code X12
> A initial encounter
> D subsequent encounter
> S sequela

X13 Contact with steam and other hot vapors

> The appropriate 7th character is to be added to each code from category X13
> A initial encounter
> D subsequent encounter
> S sequela

X+7th **X13.0 Inhalation of steam and other hot vapors**
X+7th **X13.1 Other contact with steam and other hot vapors**

X14 Contact with hot air and other hot gases

> The appropriate 7th character is to be added to each code from category X14
> A initial encounter
> D subsequent encounter
> S sequela

X+7th **X14.0 Inhalation of hot air and gases**
X+7th **X14.1 Other contact with hot air and other hot gases**

X15 Contact with hot household appliances

> **Excludes1:** *contact with heating appliances (X16)*
> *contact with powered household appliances (W29.-)*
> *exposure to controlled fire in building or structure due to household appliance (X02.8)*
> *exposure to household appliances electrical current (W86.0)*

> The appropriate 7th character is to be added to each code from category X15
> A initial encounter
> D subsequent encounter
> S sequela

X+7th **X15.0 Contact with hot stove (kitchen)**
X+7th **X15.1 Contact with hot toaster**
X+7th **X15.2 Contact with hotplate**
X+7th **X15.3 Contact with hot saucepan or skillet**
X+7th **X15.8 Contact with other hot household appliances**
> Contact with cooker
> Contact with kettle
> Contact with light bulbs

X16 Contact with hot heating appliances, radiators and pipes
X+7th
> **Excludes1:** *contact with powered appliances (W29.-)*
> *exposure to controlled fire in building or structure due to appliance (X02.8)*
> *exposure to industrial appliances electrical current (W86.1)*

> The appropriate 7th character is to be added to code X16
> A initial encounter
> D subsequent encounter
> S sequela

X17 Contact with hot engines, machinery and tools
X+7th
> **Excludes1:** *contact with hot heating appliances, radiators and pipes (X16)*
> *contact with hot household appliances (X15)*

> The appropriate 7th character is to be added to code X17
> A initial encounter
> D subsequent encounter
> S sequela

X18 Contact with other hot metals
X+7th
> Contact with liquid metal

> The appropriate 7th character is to be added to code X18
> A initial encounter
> D subsequent encounter
> S sequela

X19 Contact with other heat and hot substances
X+7th
> **Excludes1:** *objects that are not normally hot, e.g., an object made hot by a house fire (X00-X08)*

> The appropriate 7th character is to be added to code X19
> A initial encounter
> D subsequent encounter
> S sequela

Exposure to forces of nature (X30-X39)

X30 Exposure to excessive natural heat
X+7th
> Exposure to excessive heat as the cause of sunstroke
> Exposure to heat NOS
>
> **Excludes1:** *excessive heat of man-made origin (W92)*
> *exposure to man-made radiation (W89)*
> *exposure to sunlight (X32)*
> *exposure to tanning bed (W89)*
>
> AHA CC: 4Q, 2017, 112-114
> Review coding guideline B.19.c

> The appropriate 7th character is to be added to code X30
> A initial encounter
> D subsequent encounter
> S sequela

X31 Exposure to excessive natural cold
X+7th
> Excessive cold as the cause of chilblains NOS
> Excessive cold as the cause of immersion foot or hand
> Exposure to cold NOS
> Exposure to weather conditions
>
> **Excludes1:** *cold of man-made origin (W93.-)*
> *contact with or inhalation of dry ice (W93.-)*
> *contact with or inhalation of liquefied gas (W93.-)*
>
> AHA CC: 4Q, 2017, 112-114
> Review coding guideline B.19.c

> The appropriate 7th character is to be added to code X31
> A initial encounter
> D subsequent encounter
> S sequela

X32 Exposure to sunlight
X+7th
> **Excludes1:** *man-made radiation (tanning bed) (W89)*
> **Excludes2:** *radiation-related disorders of the skin and subcutaneous tissue (L55-L59)*

> The appropriate 7th character is to be added to code X32
> A initial encounter
> D subsequent encounter
> S sequela

X34 Earthquake
X+7th
> **Excludes2:** *tidal wave (tsunami) due to earthquake (X37.41)*

> The appropriate 7th character is to be added to code X34
> A initial encounter
> D subsequent encounter
> S sequela

X35 Volcanic eruption
X+7th
> **Excludes2:** *tidal wave (tsunami) due to volcanic eruption (X37.41)*

> The appropriate 7th character is to be added to code X35
> A initial encounter
> D subsequent encounter
> S sequela

X36 Avalanche, landslide and other earth movements
X+7th

Includes: victim of mudslide of cataclysmic nature

Excludes1: *earthquake (X34)*

Excludes2: *transport accident involving collision with avalanche or landslide not in motion (V01-V99)*

> The appropriate 7th character is to be added to each code from category X36
> A   initial encounter
> D   subsequent encounter
> S   sequela

X36.0 Collapse of dam or man-made structure causing earth movement
AHA CC: 4Q, 2017, 112-114
Review coding guideline B.19.b

X36.1 Avalanche, landslide, or mudslide

X37 Cataclysmic storm

> The appropriate 7th character is to be added to each code from category X37
> A   initial encounter
> D   subsequent encounter
> S   sequela

X+7th **X37.0 Hurricane**
Storm surge
Typhoon
AHA CC: 4Q, 2017, 112-114
Review coding guideline B.19

X+7th **X37.1 Tornado**
Cyclone
Twister

X+7th **X37.2 Blizzard (snow)(ice)**

X+7th **X37.3 Dust storm**

+ **X37.4 Tidalwave**

X+7th **X37.41 Tidal wave due to earthquake or volcanic eruption**
Tidal wave NOS
Tsunami

X+7th **X37.42 Tidal wave due to storm**

X+7th **X37.43 Tidal wave due to landslide**

X+7th **X37.8 Other cataclysmic storms**
Cloudburst
Torrential rain
Excludes2: *flood (X38)*

X+7th **X37.9 Unspecified cataclysmic storm**
Storm NOS
Excludes1: *collapse of dam or man-made structure causing earth movement (X36.0)*

X38 Flood
X+7th

Flood arising from remote storm
Flood of cataclysmic nature arising from melting snow
Flood resulting directly from storm
Excludes1: *collapse of dam or man-made structure causing earth movement (X36.0)*
tidal wave NOS (X37.41)
tidal wave caused by storm (X37.42)
AHA CC: 4Q, 2017, 112-114
Review coding guideline B.19

> The appropriate 7th character is to be added to code X38
> A   initial encounter
> D   subsequent encounter
> S   sequela

X39 Exposure to other forces of nature

> The appropriate 7th character is to be added to each code from category X39
> A   initial encounter
> D   subsequent encounter
> S   sequela

+ **X39.0 Exposure to natural radiation**
Excludes1: *contact with and (suspected) exposure to radon and other naturally occurring radiation (Z77.123)*
exposure to man-made radiation (W88-W90)
exposure to sunlight (X32)

X+7th **X39.01 Exposure to radon**

X+7th **X39.08 Exposure to other natural radiation**

X+7th **X39.8 Other exposure to forces of nature**

Overexertion and strenuous or repetitive movements (X50)

X50 Overexertion and strenuous or repetitive movements
AHA CC: 4Q, 2016, 73-74

> The appropriate 7th character is to be added to each code from category X50
> A   initial encounter
> D   subsequent encounter
> S   sequela

X+7th **X50.0 Overexertion from strenuous movement or load**
Lifting heavy objects
Lifting weights

X+7th **X50.1 Overexertion from prolonged static or awkward postures**
Prolonged bending
Prolonged kneeling
Prolonged reaching
Prolonged sitting
Prolonged standing
Prolonged twisting
Static bending
Static kneeling
Static reaching
Static sitting
Static standing
Static twisting

X+7th **X50.3 Overexertion from repetitive movements**
Use of hand as hammer.
Excludes2: *Overuse from prolonged static or awkward postures (X50.1)*

X+7th **X50.9 Other and unspecified overexertion or strenuous movements or postures**
Contact pressure
Contact stress

Accidental exposure to other specified factors (X52-X58)

X52 Prolonged stay in weightless environment
X+7th
Weightlessness in spacecraft (simulator)

> The appropriate 7th character is to be added to code X52
> A   initial encounter
> D   subsequent encounter
> S   sequela

X58 Exposure to other specified factors
X+7th
Accident NOS
Exposure NOS

> The appropriate 7th character is to be added to code X58
> A   initial encounter
> D   subsequent encounter
> S   sequela

Intentional self-harm (X71-X83)

Purposely self-inflicted injury
Suicide (attempted)

X71 Intentional self-harm by drowning and submersion

> The appropriate 7th character is to be added to each code from category X71
> A   initial encounter
> D   subsequent encounter
> S   sequela

X+7th **X71.0 Intentional self-harm by drowning and submersion while in bathtub**

X+7th **X71.1 Intentional self-harm by drowning and submersion while in swimming pool**

X+7th **X71.2 Intentional self-harm by drowning and submersion after jump into swimming pool**

X+7th **X71.3 Intentional self-harm by drowning and submersion in natural water**

X+7th **X71.8 Other intentional self-harm by drowning and submersion**

X+7th **X71.9 Intentional self-harm by drowning and submersion, unspecified**

X72 Intentional self-harm by handgun discharge
X+7th
Intentional self-harm by gun for single hand use
Intentional self-harm by pistol
Intentional self-harm by revolver
Excludes1: *Very pistol (X74.8)*

The appropriate 7th character is to be added to code X72

- A initial encounter
- D subsequent encounter
- S sequela

X73 Intentional self-harm by rifle, shotgun and larger firearm
X+7th discharge

Excludes1: *airgun (X74.01)*

The appropriate 7th character is to be added to each code from category X73
- A initial encounter
- D subsequent encounter
- S sequela

X+7th **X73.0** Intentional self-harm by shotgun discharge
X+7th **X73.1** Intentional self-harm by hunting rifle discharge
X+7th **X73.2** Intentional self-harm by machine gun discharge
X+7th **X73.8** Intentional self-harm by other larger firearm discharge
X+7th **X73.9** Intentional self-harm by unspecified larger firearm discharge

X74 Intentional self-harm by other and unspecified firearm and gun discharge

The appropriate 7th character is to be added to each code from category X74
- A initial encounter
- D subsequent encounter
- S sequela

+ **X74.0 Intentional self-harm by gas, air or spring-operated guns**
X+7th **X74.01** Intentional self-harm by airgun
  Intentional self-harm by BB gun discharge
  Intentional self-harm by pellet gun discharge
X+7th **X74.02** Intentional self-harm by paintball gun
X+7th **X74.09** Intentional self-harm by other gas, air or spring-operated gun
X+7th **X74.8** Intentional self-harm by other firearm discharge
  Intentional self-harm by Very pistol [flare] discharge
X+7th **X74.9** Intentional self-harm by unspecified firearm discharge

X75 Intentional self-harm by explosive material
X+7th

The appropriate 7th character is to be added to code X75
- A initial encounter
- D subsequent encounter
- S sequela

X76 Intentional self-harm by smoke, fire and flames
X+7th

The appropriate 7th character is to be added to code X76
- A initial encounter
- D subsequent encounter
- S sequela

X77 Intentional self-harm by steam, hot vapors and hot objects

The appropriate 7th character is to be added to each code from category X77
- A initial encounter
- D subsequent encounter
- S sequela

X+7th **X77.0** Intentional self-harm by steam or hot vapors
X+7th **X77.1** Intentional self-harm by hot tap water
X+7th **X77.2** Intentional self-harm by other hot fluids
X+7th **X77.3** Intentional self-harm by hot household appliances
X+7th **X77.8** Intentional self-harm by other hot objects
X+7th **X77.9** Intentional self-harm by unspecified hot objects

X78 Intentional self-harm by sharp object

The appropriate 7th character is to be added to each code from category X78
- A initial encounter
- D subsequent encounter
- S sequela

X+7th **X78.0** Intentional self-harm by sharp glass
X+7th **X78.1** Intentional self-harm by knife
X+7th **X78.2** Intentional self-harm by sword or dagger
X+7th **X78.8** Intentional self-harm by other sharp object
X+7th **X78.9** Intentional self-harm by unspecified sharp object

X79 Intentional self-harm by blunt object
X+7th

The appropriate 7th character is to be added to code X79
- A initial encounter
- D subsequent encounter
- S sequela

X80 Intentional self-harm by jumping from a high place
X+7th

Intentional fall from one level to another

The appropriate 7th character is to be added to code X80
- A initial encounter
- D subsequent encounter
- S sequela

X81 Intentional self-harm by jumping or lying in front of moving object

The appropriate 7th character is to be added to each code from category X81
- A initial encounter
- D subsequent encounter
- S sequela

X+7th **X81.0** Intentional self-harm by jumping or lying in front of motor vehicle
X+7th **X81.1** Intentional self-harm by jumping or lying in front of (subway) train
X+7th **X81.8** Intentional self-harm by jumping or lying in front of other moving object

X82 Intentional self-harm by crashing of motor vehicle

The appropriate 7th character is to be added to each code from category X82
- A initial encounter
- D subsequent encounter
- S sequela

X+7th **X82.0** Intentional collision of motor vehicle with other motor vehicle
X+7th **X82.1** Intentional collision of motor vehicle with train
X+7th **X82.2** Intentional collision of motor vehicle with tree
X+7th **X82.8** Other intentional self-harm by crashing of motor vehicle

X83 Intentional self-harm by other specified means

Excludes1: *intentional self-harm by poisoning or contact with toxic substance- See Table of Drugs and Chemicals*

The appropriate 7th character is to be added to each code from category X83
- A initial encounter
- D subsequent encounter
- S sequela

X+7th **X83.0** Intentional self-harm by crashing of aircraft
X+7th **X83.1** Intentional self-harm by electrocution
X+7th **X83.2** Intentional self-harm by exposure to extremes of cold
X+7th **X83.8** Intentional self-harm by other specified means

Assault (X92-Y09)

Includes: homicide
injuries inflicted by another person with intent to injure or kill, by any means

Excludes1: *injuries due to legal intervention (Y35.-)*
injuries due to operations of war (Y36.-)
injuries due to terrorism (Y38.-)

Review coding guideline C.19.f

X92 Assault by drowning and submersion

The appropriate 7th character is to be added to each code from category X92
- A initial encounter
- D subsequent encounter
- S sequela

X+7th **X92.0** Assault by drowning and submersion while in bathtub
X+7th **X92.1** Assault by drowning and submersion while in swimming pool
X+7th **X92.2** Assault by drowning and submersion after push into swimming pool
X+7th **X92.3** Assault by drowning and submersion in natural water
X+7th **X92.8** Other assault by drowning and submersion
X+7th **X92.9** Assault by drowning and submersion, unspecified

X93 Assault by handgun discharge
X+7th

Assault by discharge of gun for single hand use
Assault by discharge of pistol
Assault by discharge of revolver
Excludes1: *Very pistol (X95.8)*

The appropriate 7th character is to be added to code X93
- A initial encounter
- D subsequent encounter
- S sequela

+, +7th, X + 7th   ● Newborn   ● Pediatric   ● Maternity   ● Adult   ♀ Female   ♂ Male   Manifestation   Unacceptable PDX   HCC   CC   MCC   **HAC**

X94 Assault by rifle, shotgun and larger firearm discharge

> *Excludes1:* *airgun (X95.01)*

> The appropriate 7th character is to be added to each code from category X94
> A   initial encounter
> D   subsequent encounter
> S   sequela

X+7th **X94.0 Assault by shotgun**
X+7th **X94.1 Assault by hunting rifle**
X+7th **X94.2 Assault by machine gun**
X+7th **X94.8 Assault by other larger firearm discharge**
X+7th **X94.9 Assault by unspecified larger firearm discharge**

X95 Assault by other and unspecified firearm and gun discharge

> The appropriate 7th character is to be added to each code from category X95
> A   initial encounter
> D   subsequent encounter
> S   sequela

+ **X95.0 Assault by gas, air or spring-operated guns**
X+7th **X95.01 Assault by airgun discharge**
> Assault by BB gun discharge
> Assault by pellet gun discharge
X+7th **X95.02 Assault by paintball gun discharge**
X+7th **X95.09 Assault by other gas, air or spring-operated gun**
X+7th **X95.8 Assault by other firearm discharge**
> Assault by very pistol [flare] discharge
X+7th **X95.9 Assault by unspecified firearm discharge**
> *AHA CC: 3Q, 2016, 24*

X96 Assault by explosive material

> *Excludes1:* *incendiary device (X97)*
> *terrorism involving explosive material (Y38.2-)*

> The appropriate 7th character is to be added to each code from category X96
> A   initial encounter
> D   subsequent encounter
> S   sequela

X+7th **X96.0 Assault by antipersonnel bomb**
> *Excludes1:* *antipersonnel bomb use in military or war (Y36.2-)*
X+7th **X96.1 Assault by gasoline bomb**
X+7th **X96.2 Assault by letter bomb**
X+7th **X96.3 Assault by fertilizer bomb**
X+7th **X96.4 Assault by pipe bomb**
X+7th **X96.8 Assault by other specified explosive**
X+7th **X96.9 Assault by unspecified explosive**

X97 Assault by smoke, fire and flames
X+7th
> Assault by arson
> Assault by cigarettes
> Assault by incendiary device

> The appropriate 7th character is to be added to code X97
> A   initial encounter
> D   subsequent encounter
> S   sequela

X98 Assault by steam, hot vapors and hot objects

> The appropriate 7th character is to be added to each code from category X98
> A   initial encounter
> D   subsequent encounter
> S   sequela

X+7th **X98.0 Assault by steam or hot vapors**
X+7th **X98.1 Assault by hot tap water**
X+7th **X98.2 Assault by hot fluids**
X+7th **X98.3 Assault by hot household appliances**
X+7th **X98.8 Assault by other hot objects**
X+7th **X98.9 Assault by unspecified hot objects**

X99 Assault by sharp object

> *Excludes1:* *assault by strike by sports equipment (Y08.0-)*

> The appropriate 7th character is to be added to each code from category X99
> A   initial encounter
> D   subsequent encounter
> S   sequela

X+7th **X99.0 Assault by sharp glass**
X+7th **X99.1 Assault by knife**
X+7th **X99.2 Assault by sword or dagger**
X+7th **X99.8 Assault by other sharp object**
X+7th **X99.9 Assault by unspecified sharp object**
> Assault by stabbing NOS

Y00 Assault by blunt object
X+7th
> *Excludes1:* *assault by strike by sports equipment (Y08.0-)*

> The appropriate 7th character is to be added to code Y00
> A   initial encounter
> D   subsequent encounter
> S   sequela

Y01 Assault by pushing from high place
X+7th
> The appropriate 7th character is to be added to code Y01
> A   initial encounter
> D   subsequent encounter
> S   sequela

Y02 Assault by pushing or placing victim in front of moving object

> The appropriate 7th character is to be added to each code from category Y02
> A   initial encounter
> D   subsequent encounter
> S   sequela

X+7th **Y02.0 Assault by pushing or placing victim in front of motor vehicle**
X+7th **Y02.1 Assault by pushing or placing victim in front of (subway) train**
X+7th **Y02.8 Assault by pushing or placing victim in front of other moving object**

Y03 Assault by crashing of motor vehicle

> The appropriate 7th character is to be added to each code from category Y03
> A   initial encounter
> D   subsequent encounter
> S   sequela

X+7th **Y03.0 Assault by being hit or run over by motor vehicle**
X+7th **Y03.8 Other assault by crashing of motor vehicle**

Y04 Assault by bodily force

> *Excludes1:* *assault by:*
> *submersion (X92.-)*
> *use of weapon (X93-X95, X99, Y00)*

> The appropriate 7th character is to be added to each code from category Y04
> A   initial encounter
> D   subsequent encounter
> S   sequela

X+7th **Y04.0 Assault by unarmed brawl or fight**
X+7th **Y04.1 Assault by human bite**
X+7th **Y04.2 Assault by strike against or bumped into by another person**
X+7th **Y04.8 Assault by other bodily force**
> Assault by bodily force NOS

Y07 Perpetrator of assault, maltreatment and neglect

> **NOTE** Codes from this category are for use only in cases of confirmed abuse (T74.-)
> Selection of the correct perpetrator code is based on the relationship between the perpetrator and the victim
> **Includes:** perpetrator of abandonment
> perpetrator of emotional neglect
> perpetrator of mental cruelty
> perpetrator of physical abuse
> perpetrator of physical neglect
> perpetrator of sexual abuse
> perpetrator of torture
> Review coding guideline C.20.g
> *AHA CC: 4Q, 2018, 32-33*

+ **Y07.0 Spouse or partner, perpetrator of maltreatment and neglect**
> Spouse or partner, perpetrator of maltreatment and neglect against spouse or partner
> **Y07.01 Husband, perpetrator of maltreatment and neglect**
> **Y07.02 Wife, perpetrator of maltreatment and neglect**

Y07.03 Male partner, perpetrator of maltreatment and neglect

Y07.04 Female partner, perpetrator of maltreatment and neglect

+ Y07.1 Parent (adoptive) (biological), perpetrator of maltreatment and neglect

Y07.11 Biological father, perpetrator of maltreatment and neglect

Y07.12 Biological mother, perpetrator of maltreatment and neglect

Y07.13 Adoptive father, perpetrator of maltreatment and neglect

Y07.14 Adoptive mother, perpetrator of maltreatment and neglect

+ Y07.4 Other family member, perpetrator of maltreatment and neglect

+ Y07.41 Sibling, perpetrator of maltreatment and neglect

Excludes1: *stepsibling, perpetrator of maltreatmentandneglect(Y07.435, Y07.436)*

Y07.410 Brother, perpetrator of maltreatment and neglect

Y07.411 Sister, perpetrator of maltreatment and neglect

+ Y07.42 Foster parent, perpetrator of maltreatment and neglect

Y07.420 Foster father, perpetrator of maltreatment and neglect

Y07.421 Foster mother, perpetrator of maltreatment and neglect

+ Y07.43 Stepparent or stepsibling, perpetrator of maltreatment and neglect

Y07.430 Stepfather, perpetrator of maltreatment and neglect

Y07.432 Male friend of parent (co-residing in household), perpetrator of maltreatment and neglect

Y07.433 Stepmother, perpetrator of maltreatment and neglect

Y07.434 Female friend of parent (co-residing in household), perpetrator of maltreatment and neglect

Y07.435 Stepbrother, perpetrator or maltreatment and neglect

Y07.436 Stepsister, perpetrator of maltreatment and neglect

+ Y07.49 Other family member, perpetrator of maltreatment and neglect

Y07.490 Male cousin, perpetrator of maltreatment and neglect

Y07.491 Female cousin, perpetrator of maltreatment and neglect

Y07.499 Other family member, perpetrator of maltreatment and neglect

+ Y07.5 Non-family member, perpetrator of maltreatment and neglect

Y07.50 Unspecified non-family member, perpetrator of maltreatment and neglect

+ Y07.51 Daycare provider, perpetrator of maltreatment and neglect

Y07.510 At-home childcare provider, perpetrator of maltreatment and neglect

Y07.511 Daycare center childcare provider, perpetrator of maltreatment and neglect

Y07.512 At-home adultcare provider, perpetrator of maltreatment and neglect

Y07.513 Adultcare center provider, perpetrator of maltreatment and neglect

Y07.519 Unspecified daycare provider, perpetrator of maltreatment and neglect

+ Y07.52 Healthcare provider, perpetrator of maltreatment and neglect

Y07.521 Mental health provider, perpetrator of maltreatment and neglect

Y07.528 Other therapist or healthcare provider, perpetrator of maltreatment and neglect

Nurse perpetrator of maltreatment and neglect

Occupational therapist perpetrator of maltreatment and neglect

Physical therapist perpetrator of maltreatment and neglect

Speech therapist perpetrator of maltreatment and neglect

Y07.529 Unspecified healthcare provider, perpetrator of maltreatment and neglect

Y07.53 Teacher or instructor, perpetrator of maltreatment and neglect

Coach, perpetrator of maltreatment and neglect

Y07.59 Other non-family member, perpetrator of maltreatment and neglect

Y07.6 Multiple perpetrators of maltreatment and neglect

AHA CC: 4Q, 2018, 32-33

Y07.9 Unspecified perpetrator of maltreatment and neglect

Y08 Assault by other specified means

The appropriate 7th character is to be added to each code from category Y08
A initial encounter
D subsequent encounter
S sequela

+ Y08.0 Assault by strike by sport equipment

X+7th Y08.01 Assault by strike by hockey stick

X+7th Y08.02 Assault by strike by baseball bat

X+7th Y08.09 Assault by strike by other specified type of sport equipment

+ Y08.8 Assault by other specified means

X+7th Y08.81 Assault by crashing of aircraft

X+7th Y08.89 Assault by other specified means

Y09 Assault by unspecified means

Assassination (attempted) NOS
Homicide (attempted) NOS
Manslaughter (attempted) NOS
Murder (attempted) NOS
Valid 3-character code, no further characters required

Event of undetermined intent (Y21-Y33)

Undetermined intent is only for use when there is specific documentation in the record that the intent of the injury cannot be determined. If no such documentation is present, code to accidental (unintentional)

Y21 Drowning and submersion, undetermined intent

The appropriate 7th character is to be added to each code from category Y21
A initial encounter
D subsequent encounter
S sequela

X+7th Y21.0 Drowning and submersion while in bathtub, undetermined intent

X+7th Y21.1 Drowning and submersion after fall into bathtub, undetermined intent

X+7th Y21.2 Drowning and submersion while in swimming pool, undetermined intent

X+7th Y21.3 Drowning and submersion after fall into swimming pool, undetermined intent

X+7th Y21.4 Drowning and submersion in natural water, undetermined intent

X+7th Y21.8 Other drowning and submersion, undetermined intent

X+7th Y21.9 Unspecified drowning and submersion, undetermined intent

X+7th Y22 Handgun discharge, undetermined intent

Discharge of gun for single hand use, undetermined intent
Discharge of pistol, undetermined intent
Discharge of revolver, undetermined intent
Excludes2: *very pistol (Y24.8)*

The appropriate 7th character is to be added to code Y22
A initial encounter
D subsequent encounter
S sequela

Y23 Rifle, shotgun and larger firearm discharge, undetermined intent

Excludes2: *airgun (Y24.0)*

The appropriate 7th character is to be added to each code from category Y23
A initial encounter
D subsequent encounter
S sequela

X+7th Y23.0 Shotgun discharge, undetermined intent
X+7th Y23.1 Hunting rifle discharge, undetermined intent
X+7th Y23.2 Military firearm discharge, undetermined intent
X+7th Y23.3 Machine gun discharge, undetermined intent
X+7th Y23.8 Other larger firearm discharge, undetermined intent
X+7th Y23.9 Unspecified larger firearm discharge, undetermined intent

Y24 Other and unspecified firearm discharge, undetermined intent

> The appropriate 7th character is to be added to each code from category Y24
> A   initial encounter
> D   subsequent encounter
> S   sequela

X+7th Y24.0 Airgun discharge, undetermined intent
BB gun discharge, undetermined intent
Pellet gun discharge, undetermined intent
X+7th Y24.8 Other firearm discharge, undetermined intent
Paintball gun discharge, undetermined intent
Very pistol [flare] discharge, undetermined intent
X+7th Y24.9 Unspecified firearm discharge, undetermined intent

Y25 Contact with explosive material, undetermined intent
X+7th

> The appropriate 7th character is to be added to code Y25
> A   initial encounter
> D   subsequent encounter
> S   sequela

Y26 Exposure to smoke, fire and flames, undetermined intent
X+7th

> The appropriate 7th character is to be added to code Y26
> A   initial encounter
> D   subsequent encounter
> S   sequela

Y27 Contact with steam, hot vapors and hot objects, undetermined intent

> The appropriate 7th character is to be added to each code from category Y27
> A   initial encounter
> D   subsequent encounter
> S   sequela

X+7th Y27.0 Contact with steam and hot vapors, undetermined intent
X+7th Y27.1 Contact with hot tap water, undetermined intent
X+7th Y27.2 Contact with hot fluids, undetermined intent
X+7th Y27.3 Contact with hot household appliance, undetermined intent
X+7th Y27.8 Contact with other hot objects, undetermined intent
X+7th Y27.9 Contact with unspecified hot objects, undetermined intent

Y28 Contact with sharp object, undetermined intent

> The appropriate 7th character is to be added to each code from category Y28
> A   initial encounter
> D   subsequent encounter
> S   sequela

X+7th Y28.0 Contact with sharp glass, undetermined intent
X+7th Y28.1 Contact with knife, undetermined intent
X+7th Y28.2 Contact with sword or dagger, undetermined intent
X+7th Y28.8 Contact with other sharp object, undetermined intent
X+7th Y28.9 Contact with unspecified sharp object, undetermined intent

Y29 Contact with blunt object, undetermined intent
X+7th

> The appropriate 7th character is to be added to code Y29
> A   initial encounter
> D   subsequent encounter
> S   sequela

Y30 Falling, jumping or pushed from a high place, undetermined
X+7th intent

> Victim falling from one level to another, undetermined intent

> The appropriate 7th character is to be added to code Y30
> A   initial encounter
> D   subsequent encounter
> S   sequela

Y31 Falling, lying or running before or into moving object,
X+7th undetermined intent

> The appropriate 7th character is to be added to code Y31
> A   initial encounter
> D   subsequent encounter
> S   sequela

Y32 Crashing of motor vehicle, undetermined intent
X+7th

> The appropriate 7th character is to be added to code Y32
> A   initial encounter
> D   subsequent encounter
> S   sequela

Y33 Other specified events, undetermined intent
X+7th

> The appropriate 7th character is to be added to code Y33
> A   initial encounter
> D   subsequent encounter
> S   sequela

Legal intervention, operations of war, military operations, and terrorism (Y35-Y38)

Y35 Legal intervention

> **Includes:** any injury sustained as a result of an encounter with any law enforcement official, serving in any capacity at the time of the encounter, whether on-duty or off-duty. Includes: a injury to law enforcement official, suspect and bystander

> The appropriate 7th character is to be added to each code from category Y35
> A   initial encounter
> D   subsequent encounter
> S   sequela

AHA CC: 4Q, 2019, 18-19

+ **Y35.0** Legal intervention involving firearm discharge
  + **Y35.00** Legal intervention involving unspecified firearm discharge
    Legal intervention involving gunshot wound
    Legal intervention involving shot NOS
    +7th **Y35.001** Legal intervention involving unspecified firearm discharge, law enforcement official injured
    +7th **Y35.002** Legal intervention involving unspecified firearm discharge, bystander injured
    +7th **Y35.003** Legal intervention involving unspecified firearm discharge, suspect injured
    +7th **Y35.009** Legal intervention involving unspecified firearm discharge, unspecified person injured
  + **Y35.01** Legal intervention involving injury by machine gun
    +7th **Y35.011** Legal intervention involving injury by machine gun, law enforcement official injured
    +7th **Y35.012** Legal intervention involving injury by machine gun, bystander injured
    +7th **Y35.013** Legal intervention involving injury by machine gun, suspect injured
    +7th **Y35.019** Legal intervention involving injury by machine gun, unspecified person injured
  + **Y35.02** Legal intervention involving injury by handgun
    +7th **Y35.021** Legal intervention involving injury by handgun, law enforcement official injured
    +7th **Y35.022** Legal intervention involving injury by handgun, bystander injured
    +7th **Y35.023** Legal intervention involving injury by handgun, suspect injured
    +7th **Y35.029** Legal intervention involving injury by handgun, unspecified person injured
  + **Y35.03** Legal intervention involving injury by rifle pellet
    +7th **Y35.031** Legal intervention involving injury by rifle pellet, law enforcement official injured
    +7th **Y35.032** Legal intervention involving injury by rifle pellet, bystander injured
    +7th **Y35.033** Legal intervention involving injury by rifle pellet, suspect injured
    +7th **Y35.039** Legal intervention involving injury by rifle pellet, unspecified person injured
  + **Y35.04** Legal intervention involving injury by rubber bullet
    +7th **Y35.041** Legal intervention involving injury by rubber bullet, law enforcement official injured

+, +7th, X + 7th   ● Newborn   ● Pediatric   ● Maternity   ● Adult   ♀ Female   ♂ Male   Manifestation   Unacceptable PDX   HCC   CC   MCC   HAC

+7th **Y35.042** Legal intervention involving injury by rubber bullet, bystander injured

+7th **Y35.043** Legal intervention involving injury by rubber bullet, suspect injured

+7th **Y35.049** Legal intervention involving injury by rubber bullet, unspecified person injured

+ **Y35.09** Legal intervention involving other firearm discharge

+7th **Y35.091** Legal intervention involving other firearm discharge, law enforcement official injured

+7th **Y35.092** Legal intervention involving other firearm discharge, bystander injured

+7th **Y35.093** Legal intervention involving other firearm discharge, suspect injured

+7th **Y35.099** Legal intervention involving injury other firearm discharge, unspecified person injured

+ **Y35.1** Legal intervention involving explosives

+ **Y35.10** Legal intervention involving unspecified explosives

+7th **Y35.101** Legal intervention involving unspecified explosives, law enforcement official injured

+7th **Y35.102** Legal intervention involving unspecified explosives, bystander injured

+7th **Y35.103** Legal intervention involving unspecified explosives, suspect injured

+7th **Y35.109** Legal intervention involving unspecified explosives, unspecified person injured

+ **Y35.11** Legal intervention involving injury by dynamite

+7th **Y35.111** Legal intervention involving injury by dynamite, law enforcement official injured

+7th **Y35.112** Legal intervention involving injury by dynamite, bystander injured

+7th **Y35.113** Legal intervention involving injury by dynamite, suspect injured

+7th **Y35.119** Legal intervention involving injury by dynamite, unspecified person injured

+ **Y35.12** Legal intervention involving injury by explosive shell

+7th **Y35.121** Legal intervention involving injury by explosive shell, law enforcement official injured

+7th **Y35.122** Legal intervention involving injury by explosive shell, bystander injured

+7th **Y35.123** Legal intervention involving injury by explosive shell, suspect injured

+7th **Y35.129** Legal intervention involving injury by explosive shell, unspecified person injured

+ **Y35.19** Legal intervention involving other explosives

Legal intervention involving injury by grenade

Legal intervention involving injury by mortar bomb

+7th **Y35.191** Legal intervention involving other explosives, law enforcement official injured

+7th **Y35.192** Legal intervention involving other explosives, bystander injured

+7th **Y35.193** Legal intervention involving other explosives, suspect injured

+7th **Y35.199** Legal intervention involving other explosives, unspecified person injured

+ **Y35.2** Legal intervention involving gas

Legal intervention involving asphyxiation by gas

Legal intervention involving poisoning by gas

+ **Y35.20** Legal intervention involving unspecified gas

+7th **Y35.201** Legal intervention involving unspecified gas, law enforcement official injured

+7th **Y35.202** Legal intervention involving unspecified gas, bystander injured

+7th **Y35.203** Legal intervention involving unspecified gas, suspect injured

+7th **Y35.209** Legal intervention involving unspecified gas, unspecified person injured

+ **Y35.21** Legal intervention involving injury by tear gas

+7th **Y35.211** Legal intervention involving injury by tear gas, law enforcement official injured

+7th **Y35.212** Legal intervention involving injury by tear gas, bystander injured

+7th **Y35.213** Legal intervention involving injury by tear gas, suspect injured

+7th **Y35.219** Legal intervention involving injury by tear gas, unspecified person injured

+ **Y35.29** Legal intervention involving other gas

+7th **Y35.291** Legal intervention involving other gas, law enforcement official injured

+7th **Y35.292** Legal intervention involving other gas, bystander injured

+7th **Y35.293** Legal intervention involving other gas, suspect injured

+7th **Y35.299** Legal intervention involving other gas, unspecified person injured

+ **Y35.3** Legal intervention involving blunt objects

Legal intervention involving being hit or struck by blunt object

+ **Y35.30** Legal intervention involving unspecified blunt objects

+7th **Y35.301** Legal intervention involving unspecified blunt objects, law enforcement official injured

+7th **Y35.302** Legal intervention involving unspecified blunt objects, bystander injured

+7th **Y35.303** Legal intervention involving unspecified blunt objects, suspect injured

+7th **Y35.309** Legal intervention involving unspecified blunt objects, unspecified person injured

+ **Y35.31** Legal intervention involving baton

+7th **Y35.311** Legal intervention involving baton, law enforcement official injured

+7th **Y35.312** Legal intervention involving baton, bystander injured

+7th **Y35.313** Legal intervention involving baton, suspect injured

+7th **Y35.319** Legal intervention involving baton, unspecified person injured

+ **Y35.39** Legal intervention involving other blunt objects

+7th **Y35.391** Legal intervention involving other blunt objects, law enforcement official injured

+7th **Y35.392** Legal intervention involving other blunt objects, bystander injured

+7th **Y35.393** Legal intervention involving other blunt objects, suspect injured

+7th **Y35.399** Legal intervention involving other blunt objects, unspecified person injured

+ **Y35.4** Legal intervention involving sharp objects

Legal intervention involving being cut by sharp objects

Legal intervention involving being stabbed by sharp objects

+ **Y35.40** Legal intervention involving unspecified sharp objects

+7th **Y35.401** Legal intervention involving unspecified sharp objects, law enforcement official injured

+7th **Y35.402** Legal intervention involving unspecified sharp objects, bystander injured

+7th **Y35.403** Legal intervention involving unspecified sharp objects, suspect injured

+7th **Y35.409** Legal intervention involving unspecified sharp objects, unspecified person injured

+ **Y35.41** Legal intervention involving bayonet

+7th **Y35.411** Legal intervention involving bayonet, law enforcement official injured

+7th **Y35.412** Legal intervention involving bayonet, bystander injured

+7th **Y35.413** Legal intervention involving bayonet, suspect injured

+7th **Y35.419** Legal intervention involving bayonet, unspecified person injured

+, +7th, X + 7th　　● Newborn　　● Pediatric　　● Maternity　　● Adult　　♀ Female　　♂ Male　　Manifestation　　Unacceptable PDX　　HCC　　CC　　MCC　　HAC

+ Y35.49 Legal intervention involving other sharp objects
+7th Y35.491 Legal intervention involving other sharp objects, law enforcement official injured
+7th Y35.492 Legal intervention involving other sharp objects, bystander injured
+7th Y35.493 Legal intervention involving other sharp objects, suspect injured
+7th Y35.499 Legal intervention involving other sharp objects, unspecified person injured
+ Y35.8 Legal intervention involving other specified means
+ Y35.81 Legal intervention involving manhandling
+7th Y35.811 Legal intervention involving manhandling, law enforcement official injured
+7th Y35.812 Legal intervention involving manhandling, bystander injured
+7th Y35.813 Legal intervention involving manhandling, suspect injured
+7th Y35.819 Legal intervention involving manhandling, unspecified person injured
+ Y35.83 Legal intervention involving a conducted energy device
Electroshock device (taser)
Stun gun
+7th Y35.831 Legal intervention involving a conducted energy device, law enforcement official injured
+7th Y35.832 Legal intervention involving a conducted energy device, bystander injured
+7th Y35.833 Legal intervention involving a conducted energy device, suspect injured
+7th Y35.839 Legal intervention involving a conducted energy device, unspecified person injured
+ Y35.89 Legal intervention involving other specified means
+7th Y35.891 Legal intervention involving other specified means, law enforcement official injured
+7th Y35.892 Legal intervention involving other specified means, bystanderinjured
+7th Y35.893 Legal intervention involving other specified means, suspect injured
AHA CC: 1Q, 2018, 5
+ Y35.9 Legal intervention, means unspecified
X+7th Y35.91 Legal intervention, means unspecified, law enforcement official injured
X+7th Y35.92 Legal intervention, means unspecified, bystander injured
X+7th Y35.93 Legal intervention, means unspecified, suspect injured
X+7th Y35.99 Legal intervention, means unspecified, unspecified person injured

Y36 Operations of war

Includes: injuries to military personnel and civilians caused by war, civil insurrection, and peacekeeping missions
Excludes1: *injury to military personnel occurring during peacetime military operations (Y37.-)*
military vehicles involved in transport accidents with non-military vehicle during peacetime (V09.01, V09.21, V19.81, V29.81, V39.81, V49.81, V59.81, V69.81, V79.81)
AHA CC: 3Q, 2014, 4-5

The appropriate 7th character is to be added to each code from category Y36
A initial encounter
D subsequent encounter
S sequela

+ Y36.0 War operations involving explosion of marine weapons
+ Y36.00 War operations involving explosion of unspecified marine weapon
War operations involving underwater blast NOS
+7th Y36.000 War operations involving explosion of unspecified marine weapon, military personnel
+7th Y36.001 War operations involving explosion of unspecified marine weapon, civilian

+ Y36.01 War operations involving explosion of depth-charge
+7th Y36.010 War operations involving explosion of depth-charge, military personnel
+7th Y36.011 War operations involving explosion of depth-charge, civilian
+ Y36.02 War operations involving explosion of marine mine
War operations involving explosion of marine mine, at sea or in harbor
+7th Y36.020 War operations involving explosion of marine mine, military personnel
+7th Y36.021 War operations involving explosion of marine mine, civilian
+ Y36.03 War operations involving explosion of sea-based artillery shell
+7th Y36.030 War operations involving explosion of sea-based artillery shell, military personnel
+7th Y36.031 War operations involving explosion of sea-based artillery shell, civilian
+ Y36.04 War operations involving explosion of torpedo
+7th Y36.040 War operations involving explosion of torpedo, military personnel
+7th Y36.041 War operations involving explosion of torpedo, civilian
+ Y36.05 War operations involving accidental detonation of onboard marine weapons
+7th Y36.050 War operations involving accidental detonation of onboard marine weapons, military personnel
+7th Y36.051 War operations involving accidental detonation of onboard marine weapons, civilian
+ Y36.09 War operations involving explosion of other marine weapons
+7th Y36.090 War operations involving explosion of other marine weapons, military personnel
+7th Y36.091 War operations involving explosion of other marine weapons, civilian
+ Y36.1 War operations involving destruction of aircraft
+ Y36.10 War operations involving unspecified destruction of aircraft
+7th Y36.100 War operations involving unspecified destruction of aircraft, military personnel
+7th Y36.101 War operations involving unspecified destruction of aircraft, civilian
+ Y36.11 War operations involving destruction of aircraft due to enemy fire or explosives
War operations involving destruction of aircraft due to air to air missile
War operations involving destruction of aircraft due to explosive placed on aircraft
War operations involving destruction of aircraft due to rocket propelled grenade [RPG]
War operations involving destruction of aircraft due to small arms fire
War operations involving destruction of aircraft due to surface to air missile
+7th Y36.110 War operations involving destruction of aircraft due to enemy fire or explosives, military personnel
+7th Y36.111 War operations involving destruction of aircraft due to enemy fire or explosives, civilian
+ Y36.12 War operations involving destruction of aircraft due to collision with other aircraft
+7th Y36.120 War operations involving destruction of aircraft due to collision with other aircraft, military personnel
+7th Y36.121 War operations involving destruction of aircraft due to collision with other aircraft, civilian
+ Y36.13 War operations involving destruction of aircraft due to onboard fire
+7th Y36.130 War operations involving destruction of aircraft due to onboard fire, military personnel
+7th Y36.131 War operations involving destruction of aircraft due to onboard fire, civilian

+ **Y36.14** **War operations involving destruction of aircraft due to accidental detonation of onboard munitions and explosives**

  +7th **Y36.140** **War operations involving destruction of aircraft due to accidental detonation of onboard munitions and explosives, military personnel**

  +7th **Y36.141** **War operations involving destruction of aircraft due to accidental detonation of onboard munitions and explosives, civilian**

+ **Y36.19** **War operations involving other destruction of aircraft**

  +7th **Y36.190** **War operations involving other destruction of aircraft, military personnel**

  +7th **Y36.191** **War operations involving other destruction of aircraft, civilian**

+ **Y36.2** **War operations involving other explosions and fragments**

   Excludes1: *war operations involving explosion of aircraft (Y36.1-)*
    war operations involving explosion of marine weapons (Y36.0-)
    war operations involving explosion of nuclear weapons (Y36.5-)
    war operations involving explosion occurring after cessation of hostilities (Y36.8-)

+ **Y36.20** **War operations involving unspecified explosion and fragments**

  War operations involving air blast NOS
  War operations involving blast NOS
  War operations involving blast fragments NOS
  War operations involving blast wave NOS
  War operations involving blast wind NOS
  War operations involving explosion NOS
  War operations involving explosion of bomb NOS

  +7th **Y36.200** **War operations involving unspecified explosion and fragments, military personnel**

  +7th **Y36.201** **War operations involving unspecified explosion and fragments, civilian**

+ **Y36.21** **War operations involving explosion of aerial bomb**

  +7th **Y36.210** **War operations involving explosion of aerial bomb, military personnel**

  +7th **Y36.211** **War operations involving explosion of aerial bomb, civilian**

+ **Y36.22** **War operations involving explosion of guided missile**

  +7th **Y36.220** **War operations involving explosion of guided missile, military personnel**

  +7th **Y36.221** **War operations involving explosion of guided missile, civilian**

+ **Y36.23** **War operations involving explosion of improvised explosive device [IED]**

  War operations involving explosion of person-borne improvised explosive device [IED]
  War operations involving explosion of vehicle-borne improvised explosive device [IED]
  War operations involving explosion of roadside improvised explosive device [IED]

  +7th **Y36.230** **War operations involving explosion of improvised explosive device [IED], military personnel**

  +7th **Y36.231** **War operations involving explosion of improvised explosive device [IED], civilian**

+ **Y36.24** **War operations involving explosion due to accidental detonation and discharge of own munitions or munitions launch device**

  +7th **Y36.240** **War operations involving explosion due to accidental detonation and discharge of own munitions or munitions launch device, military personnel**

  +7th **Y36.241** **War operations involving explosion due to accidental detonation and discharge of own munitions or munitions launch device, civilian**

+ **Y36.25** **War operations involving fragments from munitions**

  +7th **Y36.250** **War operations involving fragments from munitions, military personnel**

  +7th **Y36.251** **War operations involving fragments from munitions, civilian**

+ **Y36.26** **War operations involving fragments of improvised explosive device [IED]**

  War operations involving fragments of person-borne improvised explosive device [IED]
  War operations involving fragments of vehicle-borne improvised explosive device [IED]
  War operations involving fragments of roadside improvised explosive device [IED]

  +7th **Y36.260** **War operations involving fragments of improvised explosive device [IED], military personnel**

  +7th **Y36.261** **War operations involving fragments of improvised explosive device [IED], civilian**

+ **Y36.27** **War operations involving fragments from weapons**

  +7th **Y36.270** **War operations involving fragments from weapons, military personnel**

  +7th **Y36.271** **War operations involving fragments from weapons, civilian**

+ **Y36.29** **War operations involving other explosions and fragments**

  War operations involving explosion of grenade
  War operations involving explosions of land mine
  War operations involving shrapnel NOS

  +7th **Y36.290** **War operations involving other explosions and fragments, military personnel**

  +7th **Y36.291** **War operations involving other explosions and fragments, civilian**

+ **Y36.3** **War operations involving fires, conflagrations and hot substances**

  War operations involving smoke, fumes, and heat from fires, conflagrations and hot substances

   Excludes1: *war operations involving fires and conflagrations aboard military aircraft (Y36.1-)*
    war operations involving fires and conflagrations aboard military watercraft (Y36.0-)
    war operations involving fires and conflagrations caused indirectly by conventional weapons (Y36.2-)
    war operations involving fires and thermal effects of nuclear weapons (Y36.53-)

+ **Y36.30** **War operations involving unspecified fire, conflagration and hot substance**

  +7th **Y36.300** **War operations involving unspecified fire, conflagration and hot substance, military personnel**

  +7th **Y36.301** **War operations involving unspecified fire, conflagration and hot substance, civilian**

+ **Y36.31** **War operations involving gasoline bomb**

  War operations involving incendiary bomb
  War operations involving petrol bomb

  +7th **Y36.310** **War operations involving gasoline bomb, military personnel**

  +7th **Y36.311** **War operations involving gasoline bomb, civilian**

+ **Y36.32** **War operations involving incendiary bullet**

  +7th **Y36.320** **War operations involving incendiary bullet, military personnel**

  +7th **Y36.321** **War operations involving incendiary bullet, civilian**

+ **Y36.33** **War operations involving flamethrower**

  +7th **Y36.330** **War operations involving flamethrower, military personnel**

  +7th **Y36.331** **War operations involving flamethrower, civilian**

+, +7th, X + 7th   ● Newborn   ● Pediatric   ● Maternity   ● Adult   ♀ Female   ♂ Male   Manifestation   Unacceptable PDX   HCC   CC   MCC   HAC

+ **Y36.39** **War operations involving other fires, conflagrations and hot substances**

  +7th **Y36.390** **War operations involving other fires, conflagrations and hot substances, military personnel**

  +7th **Y36.391** **War operations involving other fires, conflagrations and hot substances, civilian**

+ **Y36.4** **War operations involving firearm discharge and other forms of conventional warfare**

  + **Y36.41** **War operations involving rubber bullets**

    +7th **Y36.410** **War operations involving rubber bullets, military personnel**

    +7th **Y36.411** **War operations involving rubber bullets, civilian**

  + **Y36.42** **War operations involving firearms pellets**

    +7th **Y36.420** **War operations involving firearms pellets, military personnel**

    +7th **Y36.421** **War operations involving firearms pellets, civilian**

  + **Y36.43** **War operations involving other firearms discharge**

    War operations involving bullets NOS

    Excludes1: *war operations involving munitions fragments (Y36.25-)*
    war operations involving incendiary bullets (Y36.32-)

    +7th **Y36.430** **War operations involving other firearms discharge, military personnel**

    +7th **Y36.431** **War operations involving other firearms discharge, civilian**

  + **Y36.44** **War operations involving unarmed hand to hand combat**

    Excludes1: *war operations involving combat using blunt or piercing object (Y36.45-)*
    war operations involving intentional restriction of air and airway (Y36.46-)
    war operations involving unintentional restriction of air and airway (Y36.47-)

    +7th **Y36.440** **War operations involving unarmed hand to hand combat, military personnel**

    +7th **Y36.441** **War operations involving unarmed hand to hand combat, civilian**

  + **Y36.45** **War operations involving combat using blunt or piercing object**

    +7th **Y36.450** **War operations involving combat using blunt or piercing object, military personnel**

    +7th **Y36.451** **War operations involving combat using blunt or piercing object, civilian**

  + **Y36.46** **War operations involving intentional restriction of air and airway**

    +7th **Y36.460** **War operations involving intentional restriction of air and airway, military personnel**

    +7th **Y36.461** **War operations involving intentional restriction of air and airway, civilian**

  + **Y36.47** **War operations involving unintentional restriction of air and airway**

    +7th **Y36.470** **War operations involving unintentional restriction of air and airway, military personnel**

    +7th **Y36.471** **War operations involving unintentional restriction of air and airway, civilian**

  + **Y36.49** **War operations involving other forms of conventional warfare**

    +7th **Y36.490** **War operations involving other forms of conventional warfare, military personnel**

    +7th **Y36.491** **War operations involving other forms of conventional warfare, civilian**

+ **Y36.5** **War operations involving nuclear weapons**

  War operations involving dirty bomb NOS

  + **Y36.50** **War operations involving unspecified effect of nuclear weapon**

    +7th **Y36.500** **War operations involving unspecified effect of nuclear weapon, military personnel**

    +7th **Y36.501** **War operations involving unspecified effect of nuclear weapon, civilian**

  + **Y36.51** **War operations involving direct blast effect of nuclear weapon**

    War operations involving blast pressure of nuclear weapon

    +7th **Y36.510** **War operations involving direct blast effect of nuclear weapon, military personnel**

    +7th **Y36.511** **War operations involving direct blast effect of nuclear weapon, civilian**

  + **Y36.52** **War operations involving indirect blast effect of nuclear weapon**

    War operations involving being thrown by blast of nuclear weapon

    War operations involving being struck or crushed by blast debris of nuclear weapon

    +7th **Y36.520** **War operations involving indirect blast effect of nuclear weapon, military personnel**

    +7th **Y36.521** **War operations involving indirect blast effect of nuclear weapon, civilian**

  + **Y36.53** **War operations involving thermal radiation effect of nuclear weapon**

    War operations involving direct heat from nuclear weapon

    War operation involving fireball effects from nuclear weapon

    +7th **Y36.530** **War operations involving thermal radiation effect of nuclear weapon, military personnel**

    +7th **Y36.531** **War operations involving thermal radiation effect of nuclear weapon, civilian**

  + **Y36.54** **War operation involving nuclear radiation effects of nuclear weapon**

    War operation involving acute radiation exposure from nuclear weapon

    War operation involving exposure to immediate ionizing radiation from nuclear weapon

    War operation involving fallout exposure from nuclear weapon

    War operation involving secondary effects of nuclear weapons

    +7th **Y36.540** **War operation involving nuclear radiation effects of nuclear weapon, military personnel**

    +7th **Y36.541** **War operation involving nuclear radiation effects of nuclear weapon, civilian**

  + **Y36.59** **War operation involving other effects of nuclear weapons**

    +7th **Y36.590** **War operation involving other effects of nuclear weapons, military personnel**

    +7th **Y36.591** **War operation involving other effects of nuclear weapons, civilian**

+ **Y36.6** **War operations involving biological weapons**

  + **Y36.6X** **War operations involving biological weapons**

    +7th **Y36.6X0** **War operations involving biological weapons, military personnel**

    +7th **Y36.6X1** **War operations involving biological weapons, civilian**

+ **Y36.7** **War operations involving chemical weapons and other forms of unconventional warfare**

  Excludes1: *war operations involving incendiary devices (Y36.3-, Y36.5-)*

+ **Y36.7X** **War operations involving chemical weapons and other forms of unconventional warfare**

+7th **Y36.7X0** **War operations involving chemical weapons and other forms of unconventional warfare, military personnel**

+7th **Y36.7X1** **War operations involving chemical weapons and other forms of unconventional warfare, civilian**

+ **Y36.8** **War operations occurring after cessation of hostilities**

War operations classifiable to categories Y36.0-Y36.8 but occurring after cessation of hostilities

+ **Y36.81** **Explosion of mine placed during war operations but exploding after cessation of hostilities**

+7th **Y36.810** **Explosion of mine placed during war operations but exploding after cessation of hostilities, military personnel**

+7th **Y36.811** **Explosion of mine placed during war operations but exploding after cessation of hostilities, civilian**

+ **Y36.82** **Explosion of bomb placed during war operations but exploding after cessation of hostilities**

+7th **Y36.820** **Explosion of bomb placed during war operations but exploding after cessation of hostilities, military personnel**

+7th **Y36.821** **Explosion of bomb placed during war operations but exploding after cessation of hostilities, civilian**

+ **Y36.88** **Other war operations occurring after cessation of hostilities**

+7th **Y36.880** **Other war operations occurring after cessation of hostilities, military personnel**

+7th **Y36.881** **Other war operations occurring after cessation of hostilities, civilian**

+ **Y36.89** **Unspecified war operations occurring after cessation of hostilities**

+7th **Y36.890** **Unspecified war operations occurring after cessation of hostilities, military personnel**

+7th **Y36.891** **Unspecified war operations occurring after cessation of hostilities, civilian**

+ **Y36.9** **Other and unspecified war operations**

X+7th **Y36.90** **War operations, unspecified**

X+7th **Y36.91** **War operations involving unspecified weapon of mass destruction [WMD]**

X+7th **Y36.92** **War operations involving friendly fire**

Y37 **Military operations**

Includes: injuries to military personnel and civilians occurring during peacetime on military property and during routine military exercises and operations

Excludes1: *military aircraft involved in aircraft accident with civilian aircraft (V97.81-)*
military vehicles involved in transport accident with civilian vehicle (V09.01, V09.21, V19.81, V29.81, V39.81, V49.81, V59.81, V69.81, V79.81)
military watercraft involved in water transport accident with civilian watercraft (V94.81-)
war operations (Y36.-)

The appropriate 7th character is to be added to each code from category Y37
A   initial encounter
D   subsequent encounter
S   sequela

+ **Y37.0** **Military operations involving explosion of marine weapons**

+ **Y37.00** **Military operations involving explosion of unspecified marine weapon**

Military operations involving underwater blast NOS

+7th **Y37.000** **Military operations involving explosion of unspecified marine weapon, military personnel**

+7th **Y37.001** **Military operations involving explosion of unspecified marine weapon, civilian**

+ **Y37.01** **Military operations involving explosion of depth-charge**

+7th **Y37.010** **Military operations involving explosion of depth-charge, military personnel**

+7th **Y37.011** **Military operations involving explosion of depth-charge, civilian**

+ **Y37.02** **Military operations involving explosion of marine mine**

Military operations involving explosion of marine mine, at sea or in harbor

+7th **Y37.020** **Military operations involving explosion of marine mine, military personnel**

+7th **Y37.021** **Military operations involving explosion of marine mine, civilian**

+ **Y37.03** **Military operations involving explosion of sea-based artillery shell**

+7th **Y37.030** **Military operations involving explosion of sea-based artillery shell, military personnel**

+7th **Y37.031** **Military operations involving explosion of sea-based artillery shell, civilian**

+ **Y37.04** **Military operations involving explosion of torpedo**

+7th **Y37.040** **Military operations involving explosion of torpedo, military personnel**

+7th **Y37.041** **Military operations involving explosion of torpedo, civilian**

+ **Y37.05** **Military operations involving accidental detonation of onboard marine weapons**

+7th **Y37.050** **Military operations involving accidental detonation of onboard marine weapons, military personnel**

+7th **Y37.051** **Military operations involving accidental detonation of onboard marine weapons, civilian**

+ **Y37.09** **Military operations involving explosion of other marine weapons**

+7th **Y37.090** **Military operations involving explosion of other marine weapons, military personnel**

+7th **Y37.091** **Military operations involving explosion of other marine weapons, civilian**

+ **Y37.1** **Military operations involving destruction of aircraft**

+ **Y37.10** **Military operations involving unspecified destruction of aircraft**

+7th **Y37.100** **Military operations involving unspecified destruction of aircraft, military personnel**

+7th **Y37.101** **Military operations involving unspecified destruction of aircraft, civilian**

+ **Y37.11** **Military operations involving destruction of aircraft due to enemy fire or explosives**

Military operations involving destruction of aircraft due to air to air missile
Military operations involving destruction of aircraft due to explosive placed on aircraft
Military operations involving destruction of aircraft due to rocket propelled grenade [RPG]
Military operations involving destruction of aircraft due to small arms fire
Military operations involving destruction of aircraft due to surface to air missile

+7th **Y37.110** **Military operations involving destruction of aircraft due to enemy fire or explosives, military personnel**

+7th **Y37.111** **Military operations involving destruction of aircraft due to enemy fire or explosives, civilian**

+ **Y37.12** **Military operations involving destruction of aircraft due to collision with other aircraft**

+7th **Y37.120** **Military operations involving destruction of aircraft due to collision with other aircraft, military personnel**

+7th **Y37.121** **Military operations involving destruction of aircraft due to collision with other aircraft, civilian**

+ **Y37.13** **Military operations involving destruction of aircraft due to onboard fire**

+7th **Y37.130** **Military operations involving destruction of aircraft due to onboard fire, military personnel**

+7th **Y37.131** **Military operations involving destruction of aircraft due to onboard fire, civilian**

+, +7th, X + 7th   ● Newborn   ● Pediatric   ● Maternity   ● Adult   ♀ Female   ♂ Male   Manifestation   Unacceptable PDX   HCC   CC   MCC   HAC

+ **Y37.14** **Military operations involving destruction of aircraft due to accidental detonation of onboard munitions and explosives**

+7th **Y37.140** **Military operations involving destruction of aircraft due to accidental detonation of onboard munitions and explosives, military personnel**

+7th **Y37.141** **Military operations involving destruction of aircraft due to accidental detonation of onboard munitions and explosives, civilian**

+ **Y37.19** **Military operations involving other destruction of aircraft**

+7th **Y37.190** **Military operations involving other destruction of aircraft, military personnel**

+7th **Y37.191** **Military operations involving other destruction of aircraft, civilian**

+ **Y37.2** **Military operations involving other explosions and fragments**

> *Excludes1:* *military operations involving explosion of aircraft (Y37.1-)*
> *military operations involving explosion of marine weapons (Y37.0-)*
> *military operations involving explosion of nuclear weapons (Y37.5-)*

+ **Y37.20** **Military operations involving unspecified explosion and fragments**

Military operations involving air blast NOS
Military operations involving blast NOS
Military operations involving blast fragments NOS
Military operations involving blast wave NOS
Military operations involving blast wind NOS
Military operations involving explosion NOS
Military operations involving explosion of bomb NOS

+7th **Y37.200** **Military operations involving unspecified explosion and fragments, military personnel**

+7th **Y37.201** **Military operations involving unspecified explosion and fragments, civilian**

+ **Y37.21** **Military operations involving explosion of aerial bomb**

+7th **Y37.210** **Military operations involving explosion of aerial bomb, military personnel**

+7th **Y37.211** **Military operations involving explosion of aerial bomb, civilian**

+ **Y37.22** **Military operations involving explosion of guided missile**

+7th **Y37.220** **Military operations involving explosion of guided missile, military personnel**

+7th **Y37.221** **Military operations involving explosion of guided missile, civilian**

+ **Y37.23** **Military operations involving explosion of improvised explosive device [IED]**

Military operations involving explosion of person-borne improvised explosive device [IED]
Military operations involving explosion of vehicle-borne improvised explosive device [IED]
Military operations involving explosion of roadside improvised explosive device [IED]

+7th **Y37.230** **Military operations involving explosion of improvised explosive device [IED], military personnel**

+7th **Y37.231** **Military operations involving explosion of improvised explosive device [IED], civilian**

+ **Y37.24** **Military operations involving explosion due to accidental detonation and discharge of own munitions or munitions launch device**

+7th **Y37.240** **Military operations involving explosion due to accidental detonation and discharge of own munitions or munitions launch device, military personnel**

+7th **Y37.241** **Military operations involving explosion due to accidental detonation and discharge of own munitions or munitions launch device, civilian**

+ **Y37.25** **Military operations involving fragments from munitions**

+7th **Y37.250** **Military operations involving fragments from munitions, military personnel**

+7th **Y37.251** **Military operations involving fragments from munitions, civilian**

+ **Y37.26** **Military operations involving fragments of improvised explosive device [IED]**

Military operations involving fragments of person-borne improvised explosive device [IED]
Military operations involving fragments of vehicle-borne improvised explosive device [IED]
Military operations involving fragments of roadside improvised explosive device [IED]

+7th **Y37.260** **Military operations involving fragments of improvised explosive device [IED], military personnel**

+7th **Y37.261** **Military operations involving fragments of improvised explosive device [IED], civilian**

+ **Y37.27** **Military operations involving fragments from weapons**

+7th **Y37.270** **Military operations involving fragments from weapons, military personnel**

+7th **Y37.271** **Military operations involving fragments from weapons, civilian**

+ **Y37.29** **Military operations involving other explosions and fragments**

Military operations involving explosion of grenade
Military operations involving explosions of land mine
Military operations involving shrapnel NOS

+7th **Y37.290** **Military operations involving other explosions and fragments, military personnel**

+7th **Y37.291** **Military operations involving other explosions and fragments, civilian**

+ **Y37.3** **Military operations involving fires, conflagrations and hot substances**

Military operations involving smoke, fumes, and heat from fires, conflagrations and hot substances

> *Excludes1:* *military operations involving fires and conflagrations aboard military aircraft (Y37.1-)*
> *military operations involving fires and conflagrations aboard military watercraft (Y37.0-)*
> *military operations involving fires and conflagrations caused indirectly by conventional weapons (Y37.2-)*
> *military operations involving fires and thermal effects of nuclear weapons (Y36.53-)*

+ **Y37.30** **Military operations involving unspecified fire, conflagration and hot substance**

+7th **Y37.300** **Military operations involving unspecified fire, conflagration and hot substance, military personnel**

+7th **Y37.301** **Military operations involving unspecified fire, conflagration and hot substance, civilian**

+ **Y37.31** **Military operations involving gasoline bomb**

Military operations involving incendiary bomb
Military operations involving petrol bomb

+7th **Y37.310** **Military operations involving gasoline bomb, military personnel**

+7th **Y37.311** **Military operations involving gasoline bomb, civilian**

+ **Y37.32** **Military operations involving incendiary bullet**

+7th **Y37.320** **Military operations involving incendiary bullet, military personnel**

+7th **Y37.321** **Military operations involving incendiary bullet, civilian**

+ **Y37.33** **Military operations involving flamethrower**

+7th **Y37.330** **Military operations involving flamethrower, military personnel**

+7th **Y37.331** **Military operations involving flamethrower, civilian**

+ **Y37.39** **Military operations involving other fires, conflagrations and hot substances**

+7th **Y37.390** **Military operations involving other fires, conflagrations and hot substances, military personnel**

+7th **Y37.391** **Military operations involving other fires, conflagrations and hot substances, civilian**

+ **Y37.4** **Military operations involving firearm discharge and other forms of conventional warfare**

+ **Y37.41** **Military operations involving rubber bullets**

+7th **Y37.410** **Military operations involving rubber bullets, military personnel**

+7th **Y37.411** **Military operations involving rubber bullets, civilian**

+ **Y37.42** **Military operations involving firearms pellets**

+7th **Y37.420** **Military operations involving firearms pellets, military personnel**

+7th **Y37.421** **Military operations involving firearms pellets, civilian**

+ **Y37.43** **Military operations involving other firearms discharge**

Military operations involving bullets NOS

Excludes1: *military operations involving munitions fragments (Y37.25-)*
military operations involving incendiary bullets (Y37.32-)

+7th **Y37.430** **Military operations involving other firearms discharge, military personnel**

+7th **Y37.431** **Military operations involving other firearms discharge, civilian**

+ **Y37.44** **Military operations involving unarmed hand to hand combat**

Excludes1: *military operations involving combat using blunt or piercing object (Y37.45-)*
military operations involving intentional restriction of air and airway (Y37.46-)
military operations involving unintentional restriction of air and airway (Y37.47-)

+7th **Y37.440** **Military operations involving unarmed hand to hand combat, military personnel**

+7th **Y37.441** **Military operations involving unarmed hand to hand combat, civilian**

+ **Y37.45** **Military operations involving combat using blunt or piercing object**

+7th **Y37.450** **Military operations involving combat using blunt or piercing object, military personnel**

+7th **Y37.451** **Military operations involving combat using blunt or piercing object, civilian**

+ **Y37.46** **Military operations involving intentional restriction of air and airway**

+7th **Y37.460** **Military operations involving intentional restriction of air and airway, military personnel**

+7th **Y37.461** **Military operations involving intentional restriction of air and airway, civilian**

+ **Y37.47** **Military operations involving unintentional restriction of air and airway**

+7th **Y37.470** **Military operations involving unintentional restriction of air and airway, military personnel**

+7th **Y37.471** **Military operations involving unintentional restriction of air and airway, civilian**

+ **Y37.49** **Military operations involving other forms of conventional warfare**

+7th **Y37.490** **Military operations involving other forms of conventional warfare, military personnel**

+7th **Y37.491** **Military operations involving other forms of conventional warfare, civilian**

+ **Y37.5** **Military operations involving nuclear weapons**

Military operation involving dirty bomb NOS

+ **Y37.50** **Military operations involving unspecified effect of nuclear weapon**

+7th **Y37.500** **Military operations involving unspecified effect of nuclear weapon, military personnel**

+7th **Y37.501** **Military operations involving unspecified effect of nuclear weapon, civilian**

+ **Y37.51** **Military operations involving direct blast effect of nuclear weapon**

Military operations involving blast pressure of nuclear weapon

+7th **Y37.510** **Military operations involving direct blast effect of nuclear weapon, military personnel**

+7th **Y37.511** **Military operations involving direct blast effect of nuclear weapon, civilian**

+ **Y37.52** **Military operations involving indirect blast effect of nuclear weapon**

Military operations involving being thrown by blast of nuclear weapon
Military operations involving being struck or crushed by blast debris of nuclear weapon

+7th **Y37.520** **Military operations involving indirect blast effect of nuclear weapon, military personnel**

+7th **Y37.521** **Military operations involving indirect blast effect of nuclear weapon, civilian**

+ **Y37.53** **Military operations involving thermal radiation effect of nuclear weapon**

Military operations involving direct heat from nuclear weapon
Military operation involving fireball effects from nuclear weapon

+7th **Y37.530** **Military operations involving thermal radiation effect of nuclear weapon, military personnel**

+7th **Y37.531** **Military operations involving thermal radiation effect of nuclear weapon, civilian**

+ **Y37.54** **Military operation involving nuclear radiation effects of nuclear weapon**

Military operation involving acute radiation exposure from nuclear weapon
Military operation involving exposure to immediate ionizing radiation from nuclear weapon
Military operation involving fallout exposure from nuclear weapon
Military operation involving secondary effects of nuclear weapons

+7th **Y37.540** **Military operation involving nuclear radiation effects of nuclear weapon, military personnel**

+7th **Y37.541** **Military operation involving nuclear radiation effects of nuclear weapon, civilian**

+ **Y37.59** **Military operation involving other effects of nuclear weapons**

+7th **Y37.590** **Military operation involving other effects of nuclear weapons, military personnel**

+7th **Y37.591** **Military operation involving other effects of nuclear weapons, civilian**

+ **Y37.6** **Military operations involving biological weapons**

+ **Y37.6X** **Military operations involving biological weapons**

+7th **Y37.6X0** **Military operations involving biological weapons, military personnel**

+7th **Y37.6X1** **Military operations involving biological weapons, civilian**

+ **Y37.7** **Military operations involving chemical weapons and other forms of unconventional warfare**

Excludes1: *military operations involving incendiary devices (Y36.3-, Y36.5-)*

+, +7th, X + 7th   ● Newborn   ● Pediatric   ● Maternity   ● Adult   ♀ Female   ♂ Male   Manifestation   Unacceptable PDX   HCC   CC   MCC   HAC

+ **Y37.7X** **Military operations involving chemical weapons and other forms of unconventional warfare**
+7th **Y37.7X0** **Military operations involving chemical weapons and other forms of unconventional warfare, military personnel**
+7th **Y37.7X1** **Military operations involving chemical weapons and other forms of unconventional warfare, civilian**

+ **Y37.9** **Other and unspecified military operations**
X+7th **Y37.90** **Military operations, unspecified**
X+7th **Y37.91** **Military operations involving unspecified weapon of mass destruction [WMD]**
X+7th **Y37.92** **Military operations involving friendly fire**

Y38 **Terrorism**

These codes are for use to identify injuries resulting from the unlawful use of force or violence against persons or property to intimidate or coerce a Government, the civilian population, or any segment thereof, in furtherance of political or social objective
Use additional code for place of occurrence (Y92.-)

The appropriate 7th character is to be added to each code from category Y38
A   initial encounter
D   subsequent encounter
S   sequela

Review coding guideline C.20.j

+ **Y38.0** **Terrorism involving explosion of marine weapons**
Terrorism involving depth-charge
Terrorism involving marine mine
Terrorism involving mine NOS, at sea or in harbor
Terrorism involving sea-based artillery shell
Terrorism involving torpedo
Terrorism involving underwater blast
+ **Y38.0X** **Terrorism involving explosion of marine weapons**
+7th **Y38.0X1** **Terrorism involving explosion of marine weapons, public safety official injured**
+7th **Y38.0X2** **Terrorism involving explosion of marine weapons, civilian injured**
+7th **Y38.0X3** **Terrorism involving explosion of marine weapons, terrorist injured**

+ **Y38.1** **Terrorism involving destruction of aircraft**
Terrorism involving aircraft burned
Terrorism involving aircraft exploded
Terrorism involving aircraft being shot down
Terrorism involving aircraft used as a weapon
+ **Y38.1X** **Terrorism involving destruction of aircraft**
+7th **Y38.1X1** **Terrorism involving destruction of aircraft, public safety official injured**
+7th **Y38.1X2** **Terrorism involving destruction of aircraft, civilian injured**
+7th **Y38.1X3** **Terrorism involving destruction of aircraft, terrorist injured**

+ **Y38.2** **Terrorism involving other explosions and fragments**
Terrorism involving antipersonnel (fragments) bomb
Terrorism involving blast NOS
Terrorism involving explosion NOS
Terrorism involving explosion of breech block
Terrorism involving explosion of cannon block
Terrorism involving explosion (fragments) of artillery shell
Terrorism involving explosion (fragments) of bomb
Terrorism involving explosion (fragments) of grenade
Terrorism involving explosion (fragments) of guided missile
Terrorism involving explosion (fragments) of land mine
Terrorism involving explosion of mortar bomb
Terrorism involving explosion of munitions
Terrorism involving explosion (fragments) of rocket
Terrorism involving explosion (fragments) of shell
Terrorism involving shrapnel
Terrorism involving mine NOS, on land
Excludes1: *terrorism involving explosion of nuclear weapon (Y38.5)*
terrorism involving suicide bomber (Y38.81)
+ **Y38.2X** **Terrorism involving other explosions and fragments**
+7th **Y38.2X1** **Terrorism involving other explosions and fragments, public safety official injured**
+7th **Y38.2X2** **Terrorism involving other explosions and fragments, civilian injured**
+7th **Y38.2X3** **Terrorism involving other explosions and fragments, terrorist injured**

+ **Y38.3** **Terrorism involving fires, conflagration and hot substances**
Terrorism involving conflagration NOS
Terrorism involving fire NOS
Terrorism involving petrol bomb
Excludes1: *terrorism involving fire or heat of nuclear weapon (Y38.5)*
+ **Y38.3X** **Terrorism involving fires, conflagration and hot substances**
+7th **Y38.3X1** **Terrorism involving fires, conflagration and hot substances, public safety official injured**
+7th **Y38.3X2** **Terrorism involving fires, conflagration and hot substances, civilian injured**
+7th **Y38.3X3** **Terrorism involving fires, conflagration and hot substances, terrorist injured**

+ **Y38.4** **Terrorism involving firearms**
Terrorism involving carbine bullet
Terrorism involving machine gun bullet
Terrorism involving pellets (shotgun)
Terrorism involving pistol bullet
Terrorism involving rifle bullet
Terrorism involving rubber (rifle) bullet
+ **Y38.4X** **Terrorism involving firearms**
+7th **Y38.4X1** **Terrorism involving firearms, public safety official injured**
+7th **Y38.4X2** **Terrorism involving firearms, civilian injured**
+7th **Y38.4X3** **Terrorism involving firearms, terrorist injured**

+ **Y38.5** **Terrorism involving nuclear weapons**
Terrorism involving blast effects of nuclear weapon
Terrorism involving exposure to ionizing radiation from nuclear weapon
Terrorism involving fireball effect of nuclear weapon
Terrorism involving heat from nuclear weapon
+ **Y38.5X** **Terrorism involving nuclear weapons**
+7th **Y38.5X1** **Terrorism involving nuclear weapons, public safety official injured**
+7th **Y38.5X2** **Terrorism involving nuclear weapons, civilian injured**
+7th **Y38.5X3** **Terrorism involving nuclear weapons, terrorist injured**

+ **Y38.6** **Terrorism involving biological weapons**
Terrorism involving anthrax
Terrorism involving cholera
Terrorism involving smallpox
+ **Y38.6X** **Terrorism involving biological weapons**
+7th **Y38.6X1** **Terrorism involving biological weapons, public safety official injured**
+7th **Y38.6X2** **Terrorism involving biological weapons, civilian injured**
+7th **Y38.6X3** **Terrorism involving biological weapons, terrorist injured**

+ **Y38.7** **Terrorism involving chemical weapons**
Terrorism involving gases, fumes, chemicals
Terrorism involving hydrogen cyanide
Terrorism involving phosgene
Terrorism involving sarin
+ **Y38.7X** **Terrorism involving chemical weapons**
+7th **Y38.7X1** **Terrorism involving chemical weapons, public safety official injured**
+7th **Y38.7X2** **Terrorism involving chemical weapons, civilian injured**
+7th **Y38.7X3** **Terrorism involving chemical weapons, terrorist injured**

+ **Y38.8** **Terrorism involving other and unspecified means**
X+7th **Y38.80** **Terrorism involving unspecified means**
Terrorism NOS
+ **Y38.81** **Terrorism involving suicide bomber**
+7th **Y38.811** **Terrorism involving suicide bomber, public safety official injured**
+7th **Y38.812** **Terrorism involving suicide bomber, civilian injured**
+ **Y38.89** **Terrorism involving other means**
Terrorism involving drowning and submersion
Terrorism involving lasers
Terrorism involving piercing or stabbing instruments
+7th **Y38.891** **Terrorism involving other means, public safety official injured**

+, +7th, X + 7th   ● Newborn   ● Pediatric   ● Maternity   ● Adult   ♀ Female   ♂ Male   Manifestation   Unacceptable PDX   HCC   CC   MCC   HAC

+7th **Y38.892** **Terrorism involving other means, civilian injured**
+7th **Y38.893** **Terrorism involving other means, terrorist injured**
+ **Y38.9** **Terrorism, secondary effects**
> **NOTE** This code is for use to identify conditions occurring subsequent to a terrorist attack not those that are due to the initial terrorist attack
+ **Y38.9X** **Terrorism, secondary effects**
+7th **Y38.9X1** **Terrorism, secondary effects, public safety official injured**
+7th **Y38.9X2** **Terrorism, secondary effects, civilian injured**

Complications of medical and surgical care (Y62-Y84)

Includes: complications of medical devices surgical and medical procedures as the cause of abnormal reaction of the patient, or of later complication, without mention of misadventure at the time of the procedure

Misadventures to patients during surgical and medical care (Y62-Y69)

Excludes1: *surgical and medical procedures as the cause of abnormal reaction of the patient, without mention of misadventure at the time of the procedure (Y83-Y84)*

Excludes2: *breakdown or malfunctioning of medical device (during procedure) (after implantation) (ongoing use) (Y70-Y82)*

Y62 **Failure of sterile precautions during surgical and medical care**

Y62.0 **Failure of sterile precautions during surgical operation**
Y62.1 **Failure of sterile precautions during infusion or transfusion**
Y62.2 **Failure of sterile precautions during kidney dialysis and other perfusion**
Y62.3 **Failure of sterile precautions during injection or immunization**
Y62.4 **Failure of sterile precautions during endoscopic examination**
Y62.5 **Failure of sterile precautions during heart catheterization**
Y62.6 **Failure of sterile precautions during aspiration, puncture and other catheterization**
Y62.8 **Failure of sterile precautions during other surgical and medical care**
Y62.9 **Failure of sterile precautions during unspecified surgical and medical care**

Y63 **Failure in dosage during surgical and medical care**

Excludes2: *accidental overdose of drug or wrong drug given in error (T36-T50)*
Y63.0 **Excessive amount of blood or other fluid given during transfusion or infusion**
Y63.1 **Incorrect dilution of fluid used during infusion**
Y63.2 **Overdose of radiation given during therapy**
Y63.3 **Inadvertent exposure of patient to radiation during medical care**
Y63.4 **Failure in dosage in electroshock or insulin-shock therapy**
Y63.5 **Inappropriate temperature in local application and packing**
Y63.6 **Underdosing and nonadministration of necessary drug, medicament or biological substance**
> Review coding guideline C.19.e.5.c
Y63.8 **Failure in dosage during other surgical and medical care**
> Review coding guideline C.19.e.5.c
Y63.9 **Failure in dosage during unspecified surgical and medical care**
> Review coding guideline C.19.e.5.c

Y64 **Contaminated medical or biological substances**

Y64.0 **Contaminated medical or biological substance, transfused or infused**
Y64.1 **Contaminated medical or biological substance, injected or used for immunization**
Y64.8 **Contaminated medical or biological substance administered by other means**
Y64.9 **Contaminated medical or biological substance administered by unspecified means**
> Administered contaminated medical or biological substance NOS

Y65 **Other misadventures during surgical and medical care**

Y65.0 **Mismatched blood in transfusion**
Y65.1 **Wrong fluid used in infusion**
Y65.2 **Failure in suture or ligature during surgical operation**

Y65.3 **Endotracheal tube wrongly placed during anesthetic procedure**
Y65.4 **Failure to introduce or to remove other tube or instrument**
+ **Y65.5** **Performance of wrong procedure (operation)**
Y65.51 **Performance of wrong procedure (operation) on correct patient**
> Wrong device implanted into correct surgical site
> **Excludes1:** *performance of correct procedure (operation) on wrong side or body part (Y65.53)*
Y65.52 **Performance of procedure (operation) on patient not scheduled for surgery**
> Performance of procedure (operation) intended for another patient
> Performance of procedure (operation) on wrong patient
Y65.53 **Performance of correct procedure (operation) on wrong side or body part**
> Performance of correct procedure (operation) on wrong side
> Performance of correct procedure (operation) on wrong site
Y65.8 **Other specified misadventures during surgical and medical care**
> *AHA CC: 2Q, 2019, 24*

Y66 **Nonadministration of surgical and medical care**

> Premature cessation of surgical and medical care
> **Excludes1:** *DNR status (Z66)*
> *palliative care (Z51.5)*
> Valid 3-character code, no further characters required

Y69 **Unspecified misadventure during surgical and medical care**

> Valid 3-character code, no further characters required

Medical devices associated with adverse incidents in diagnostic and therapeutic use (Y70-Y82)

Includes: breakdown or malfunction of medical devices (during use) (after implantation) (ongoing use)

Excludes2: *later complications following use of medical devices without breakdown or malfunctioning of device (Y83-Y84)*
misadventure to patients during surgical and medical care, classifiable to (Y62-Y69)
surgical and other medical procedures as the cause of abnormal reaction of the patient, or of later complication, without mention of misadventure at the time of the procedure (Y83-Y84)

Y70 **Anesthesiology devices associated with adverse incidents**

Y70.0 **Diagnostic and monitoring anesthesiology devices associated with adverse incidents**
Y70.1 **Therapeutic (nonsurgical) and rehabilitative anesthesiology devices associated with adverse incidents**
Y70.2 **Prosthetic and other implants, materials and accessory anesthesiology devices associated with adverse incidents**
Y70.3 **Surgical instruments, materials and anesthesiology devices (including sutures) associated with adverse incidents**
Y70.8 **Miscellaneous anesthesiology devices associated with adverse incidents, not elsewhere classified**

Y71 **Cardiovascular devices associated with adverse incidents**

Y71.0 **Diagnostic and monitoring cardiovascular devices associated with adverse incidents**
Y71.1 **Therapeutic (nonsurgical) and rehabilitative cardiovascular devices associated with adverse incidents**
Y71.2 **Prosthetic and other implants, materials and accessory cardiovascular devices associated with adverse incidents**
Y71.3 **Surgical instruments, materials and cardiovascular devices (including sutures) associated with adverse incidents**
Y71.8 **Miscellaneous cardiovascular devices associated with adverse incidents, not elsewhere classified**

Y72 **Otorhinolaryngological devices associated with adverse incidents**

Y72.0 **Diagnostic and monitoring otorhinolaryngological devices associated with adverse incidents**
Y72.1 **Therapeutic (nonsurgical) and rehabilitative otorhinolaryngological devices associated with adverse incidents**
Y72.2 **Prosthetic and other implants, materials and accessory otorhinolaryngological devices associated with adverse incidents**

Y72.3 Surgical instruments, materials and otorhinolaryngological devices (including sutures) associated with adverse incidents

Y72.8 Miscellaneous otorhinolaryngological devices associated with adverse incidents, not elsewhere classified

Y73 Gastroenterology and urology devices associated with adverse incidents

Y73.0 Diagnostic and monitoring gastroenterology and urology devices associated with adverse incidents

Y73.1 Therapeutic (nonsurgical) and rehabilitative gastroenterology and urology devices associated with adverse incidents

Y73.2 Prosthetic and other implants, materials and accessory gastroenterology and urology devices associated with adverse incidents

Y73.3 Surgical instruments, materials and gastroenterology and urology devices (including sutures) associated with adverse incidents

Y73.8 Miscellaneous gastroenterology and urology devices associated with adverse incidents, not elsewhere classified

Y74 General hospital and personal-use devices associated with adverse incidents

Y74.0 Diagnostic and monitoring general hospital and personal-use devices associated with adverse incidents

Y74.1 Therapeutic (nonsurgical) and rehabilitative general hospital and personal-use devices associated with adverse incidents

Y74.2 Prosthetic and other implants, materials and accessory general hospital and personal-use devices associated with adverse incidents

Y74.3 Surgical instruments, materials and general hospital and personal-use devices (including sutures) associated with adverse incidents

Y74.8 Miscellaneous general hospital and personal-use devices associated with adverse incidents, not elsewhere classified

Y75 Neurological devices associated with adverse incidents

Y75.0 Diagnostic and monitoring neurological devices associated with adverse incidents

Y75.1 Therapeutic (nonsurgical) and rehabilitative neurological devices associated with adverse incidents

Y75.2 Prosthetic and other implants, materials and neurological devices associated with adverse incidents

Y75.3 Surgical instruments, materials and neurological devices (including sutures) associated with adverse incidents

Y75.8 Miscellaneous neurological devices associated with adverse incidents, not elsewhere classified

Y76 Obstetric and gynecological devices associated with adverse incidents

♀ **Y76.0** Diagnostic and monitoring obstetric and gynecological devices associated with adverse incidents

♀ **Y76.1** Therapeutic (nonsurgical) and rehabilitative obstetric and gynecological devices associated with adverse incidents

♀ **Y76.2** Prosthetic and other implants, materials and accessory obstetric and gynecological devices associated with adverse incidents

♀ **Y76.3** Surgical instruments, materials and obstetric and gynecological devices (including sutures) associated with adverse incidents

♀ **Y76.8** Miscellaneous obstetric and gynecological devices associated with adverse incidents, not elsewhere classified

Y77 Ophthalmic devices associated with adverse incidents

Y77.0 Diagnostic and monitoring ophthalmic devices associated with adverse incidents

+ **Y77.1** Therapeutic (nonsurgical) and rehabilitative ophthalmic devices associated with adverse incidents

    Y77.11 Contact lens associated with adverse incidents

        Rigid gas permeable contact lens associated with adverse incidents

        Soft (hydrophilic) contact lens associated with adverse incidents

    Y77.19 Other therapeutic (nonsurgical) and rehabilitative ophthalmic devices associated with adverse incidents

Y77.2 Prosthetic and other implants, materials and accessory ophthalmic devices associated with adverse incidents

Y77.3 Surgical instruments, materials and ophthalmic devices (including sutures) associated with adverse incidents

Y77.8 Miscellaneous ophthalmic devices associated with adverse incidents, not elsewhere classified

Y78 Radiological devices associated with adverse incidents

Y78.0 Diagnostic and monitoring radiological devices associated with adverse incidents

Y78.1 Therapeutic (nonsurgical) and rehabilitative radiological devices associated with adverse incidents

Y78.2 Prosthetic and other implants, materials and accessory radiological devices associated with adverse incidents

Y78.3 Surgical instruments, materials and radiological devices (including sutures) associated with adverse incidents

Y78.8 Miscellaneous radiological devices associated with adverse incidents, not elsewhere classified

Y79 Orthopedic devices associated with adverse incidents

Y79.0 Diagnostic and monitoring orthopedic devices associated with adverse incidents

Y79.1 Therapeutic (nonsurgical) and rehabilitative orthopedic devices associated with adverse incidents

Y79.2 Prosthetic and other implants, materials and accessory orthopedic devices associated with adverse incidents

Y79.3 Surgical instruments, materials and orthopedic devices (including sutures) associated with adverse incidents

Y79.8 Miscellaneous orthopedic devices associated with adverse incidents, not elsewhere classified

Y80 Physical medicine devices associated with adverse incidents

Y80.0 Diagnostic and monitoring physical medicine devices associated with adverse incidents

Y80.1 Therapeutic (nonsurgical) and rehabilitative physical medicine devices associated with adverse incidents

Y80.2 Prosthetic and other implants, materials and accessory physical medicine devices associated with adverse incidents

Y80.3 Surgical instruments, materials and physical medicine devices (including sutures) associated with adverse incidents

Y80.8 Miscellaneous physical medicine devices associated with adverse incidents, not elsewhere classified

Y81 General- and plastic-surgery devices associated with adverse incidents

Y81.0 Diagnostic and monitoring general- and plastic-surgery devices associated with adverse incidents

Y81.1 Therapeutic (nonsurgical) and rehabilitative general- and plastic-surgery devices associated with adverse incidents

Y81.2 Prosthetic and other implants, materials and accessory general- and plastic-surgery devices associated with adverse incidents

Y81.3 Surgical instruments, materials and general- and plastic-surgery devices (including sutures) associated with adverse incidents

Y81.8 Miscellaneous general- and plastic-surgery devices associated with adverse incidents, not elsewhere classified

Y82 Other and unspecified medical devices associated with adverse incidents

Y82.8 Other medical devices associated with adverse incidents

Y82.9 Unspecified medical devices associated with adverse incidents

Surgical and other medical procedures as the cause of abnormal reaction of the patient, or of later complication, without mention of misadventure at the time of the procedure (Y83-Y84)

Excludes1: *misadventures to patients during surgical and medical care, classifiable to (Y62-Y69)*

Excludes2: *breakdown or malfunctioning of medical device (after implantation) (during procedure) (ongoing use) (Y70-Y82)*

+, +7th, X + 7th   ● Newborn   ● Pediatric   ● Maternity   ● Adult   ♀ Female   ♂ Male   Manifestation   Unacceptable PDX   HCC   CC   MCC   HAC

Y83 **Surgical operation and other surgical procedures as the cause of abnormal reaction of the patient, or of later complication, without mention of misadventure at the time of the procedure**

    Y83.0 **Surgical operation with transplant of whole organ as the cause of abnormal reaction of the patient, or of later complication, without mention of misadventure at the time of the procedure**

    Y83.1 **Surgical operation with implant of artificial internal device as the cause of abnormal reaction of the patient, or of later complication, without mention of misadventure at the time of the procedure**

    Y83.2 **Surgical operation with anastomosis, bypass or graft as the cause of abnormal reaction of the patient, or of later complication, without mention of misadventure at the time of the procedure**

    Y83.3 **Surgical operation with formation of external stoma as the cause of abnormal reaction of the patient, or of later complication, without mention of misadventure at the time of the procedure**

    Y83.4 **Other reconstructive surgery as the cause of abnormal reaction of the patient, or of later complication, without mention of misadventure at the time of the procedure**

    Y83.5 **Amputation of limb(s) as the cause of abnormal reaction of the patient, or of later complication, without mention of misadventure at the time of the procedure**

    Y83.6 **Removal of other organ (partial) (total) as the cause of abnormal reaction of the patient, or of later complication, without mention of misadventure at the time of the procedure**

    Y83.8 **Other surgical procedures as the cause of abnormal reaction of the patient, or of later complication, without mention of misadventure at the time of the procedure**

    Y83.9 **Surgical procedure, unspecified as the cause of abnormal reaction of the patient, or of later complication, without mention of misadventure at the time of the procedure**

Y84 **Other medical procedures as the cause of abnormal reaction of the patient, or of later complication, without mention of misadventure at the time of the procedure**

    Y84.0 **Cardiac catheterization as the cause of abnormal reaction of the patient, or of later complication, without mention of misadventure at the time of the procedure**

    Y84.1 **Kidney dialysis as the cause of abnormal reaction of the patient, or of later complication, without mention of misadventure at the time of the procedure**

    Y84.2 **Radiological procedure and radiotherapy as the cause of abnormal reaction of the patient, or of later complication, without mention of misadventure at the time of the procedure**
      AHA CC: 1Q, 2019, 21
      Review coding guideline C.2.c.2

    Y84.3 **Shock therapy as the cause of abnormal reaction of the patient, or of later complication, without mention of misadventure at the time of the procedure**

    Y84.4 **Aspiration of fluid as the cause of abnormal reaction of the patient, or of later complication, without mention of misadventure at the time of the procedure**

    Y84.5 **Insertion of gastric or duodenal sound as the cause of abnormal reaction of the patient, or of later complication, without mention of misadventure at the time of the procedure**

    Y84.6 **Urinary catheterization as the cause of abnormal reaction of the patient, or of later complication, without mention of misadventure at the time of the procedure**

    Y84.7 **Blood-sampling as the cause of abnormal reaction of the patient, or of later complication, without mention of misadventure at the time of the procedure**

    Y84.8 **Other medical procedures as the cause of abnormal reaction of the patient, or of later complication, without mention of misadventure at the time of the procedure**
      AHA CC: 4Q, 2014, 24

    Y84.9 **Medical procedure, unspecified as the cause of abnormal reaction of the patient, or of later complication, without mention of misadventure at the time of the procedure**

Supplementary factors related to causes of morbidity classified elsewhere (Y90-Y99)

NOTE These categories may be used to provide supplementary information concerning causes of morbidity. They are not to be used for single-condition coding.

Y90 **Evidence of alcohol involvement determined by blood alcohol level**

    Code first any associated alcohol related disorders (F10)

    Y90.0 **Blood alcohol level of less than 20 mg/100 ml**
    Y90.1 **Blood alcohol level of 20-39 mg/100 ml**
    Y90.2 **Blood alcohol level of 40-59 mg/100 ml**
    Y90.3 **Blood alcohol level of 60-79 mg/100 ml**
    Y90.4 **Blood alcohol level of 80-99 mg/100 ml**
    Y90.5 **Blood alcohol level of 100-119 mg/100 ml**
    Y90.6 **Blood alcohol level of 120-199 mg/100 ml**
    Y90.7 **Blood alcohol level of 200-239 mg/100 ml**
    Y90.8 **Blood alcohol level of 240 mg/100 ml or more**
    Y90.9 **Presence of alcohol in blood, level not specified**

Y92 **Place of occurrence of the external cause**

    The following category is for use, when relevant, to identify the place of occurrence of the external cause. Use in conjunction with an activity code.

    Place of occurrence should be recorded only at the initial encounter for treatment
    Review coding guideline C.20.b

  + Y92.0 **Non-institutional (private) residence as the place of occurrence of the external cause**
      Excludes1: *abandoned or derelict house (Y92.89)*
          home under construction but not yet occupied (Y92.6-)
          institutional place of residence (Y92.1-)

    + Y92.00 **Unspecified non-institutional (private) residence as the place of occurrence of the external cause**

      Y92.000 **Kitchen of unspecified non-institutional (private) residence as the place of occurrence of the external cause**

      Y92.001 **Dining room of unspecified non-institutional (private) residence as the place of occurrence of the external cause**

      Y92.002 **Bathroom of unspecified non-institutional (private) residence as the place of occurrence of the external cause**

      Y92.003 **Bedroom of unspecified non-institutional (private) residence as the place of occurrence of the external cause**

      Y92.007 **Garden or yard of unspecified non-institutional (private) residence as the place of occurrence of the external cause**

      Y92.008 **Other place in unspecified non-institutional (private) residence as the place of occurrence of the external cause**

      Y92.009 **Unspecified place in unspecified non-institutional (private) residence as the place of occurrence of the external cause**
        Home (NOS) as the place of occurrence of the external cause

    + Y92.01 **Single-family non-institutional (private) house as the place of occurrence of the external cause**
      Farmhouse as the place of occurrence of the external cause
      Excludes1: *barn (Y92.71)*
          chicken coop or hen house (Y92.72)
          farm field (Y92.73)
          orchard (Y92.74)
          single family mobile home or trailer (Y92.02-)
          slaughter house (Y92.86)

      Y92.010 **Kitchen of single-family (private) house as the place of occurrence of the external cause**

      Y92.011 **Dining room of single-family (private) house as the place of occurrence of the external cause**

      Y92.012 **Bathroom of single-family (private) house as the place of occurrence of the external cause**

      Y92.013 **Bedroom of single-family (private) house as the place of occurrence of the external cause**

      Y92.014 **Private driveway to single-family (private) house as the place of occurrence of the external cause**

      Y92.015 **Private garage of single-family (private) house as the place of occurrence of the external cause**

Y92.016 Swimming-pool in single-family (private) house or garden as the place of occurrence of the external cause

Y92.017 Garden or yard in single-family (private) house as the place of occurrence of the external cause

Y92.018 Other place in single-family (private) house as the place of occurrence of the external cause

Y92.019 Unspecified place in single-family (private) house as the place of occurrence of the external cause

+ Y92.02 Mobile home as the place of occurrence of the external cause

Y92.020 Kitchen in mobile home as the place of occurrence of the external cause

Y92.021 Dining room in mobile home as the place of occurrence of the external cause

Y92.022 Bathroom in mobile home as the place of occurrence of the external cause

Y92.023 Bedroom in mobile home as the place of occurrence of the external cause

Y92.024 Driveway of mobile home as the place of occurrence of the external cause

Y92.025 Garage of mobile home as the place of occurrence of the external cause

Y92.026 Swimming-pool of mobile home as the place of occurrence of the external cause

Y92.027 Garden or yard of mobile home as the place of occurrence of the external cause

Y92.028 Other place in mobile home as the place of occurrence of the external cause

Y92.029 Unspecified place in mobile home as the place of occurrence of the external cause

+ Y92.03 Apartment as the place of occurrence of the external cause

Condominium as the place of occurrence of the external cause

Co-op apartment as the place of occurrence of the external cause

Y92.030 Kitchen in apartment as the place of occurrence of the external cause

Y92.031 Bathroom in apartment as the place of occurrence of the external cause

Y92.032 Bedroom in apartment as the place of occurrence of the external cause

Y92.038 Other place in apartment as the place of occurrence of the external cause

Y92.039 Unspecified place in apartment as the place of occurrence of the external cause

+ Y92.04 Boarding-house as the place of occurrence of the external cause

Y92.040 Kitchen in boarding-house as the place of occurrence of the external cause

Y92.041 Bathroom in boarding-house as the place of occurrence of the external cause

Y92.042 Bedroom in boarding-house as the place of occurrence of the external cause

Y92.043 Driveway of boarding-house as the place of occurrence of the external cause

Y92.044 Garage of boarding-house as the place of occurrence of the external cause

Y92.045 Swimming-pool of boarding-house as the place of occurrence of the external cause

Y92.046 Garden or yard of boarding-house as the place of occurrence of the external cause

Y92.048 Other place in boarding-house as the place of occurrence of the external cause

Y92.049 Unspecified place in boarding-house as the place of occurrence of the external cause

+ Y92.09 Other non-institutional residence as the place of occurrence of the external cause

Y92.090 Kitchen in other non-institutional residence as the place of occurrence of the external cause

Y92.091 Bathroom in other non-institutional residence as the place of occurrence of the external cause

Y92.092 Bedroom in other non-institutional residence as the place of occurrence of the external cause

Y92.093 Driveway of other non-institutional residence as the place of occurrence of the external cause

Y92.094 Garage of other non-institutional residence as the place of occurrence of the external cause

Y92.095 Swimming-pool of other non-institutional residence as the place of occurrence of the external cause

Y92.096 Garden or yard of other non-institutional residence as the place of occurrence of the external cause

Y92.098 Other place in other non-institutional residence as the place of occurrence of the external cause

AHA CC: 2Q, 2017, 10-11

Y92.099 Unspecified place in other non-institutional residence as the place of occurrence of the external cause

+ Y92.1 Institutional (nonprivate) residence as the place of occurrence of the external cause

Y92.10 Unspecified residential institution as the place of occurrence of the external cause

+ Y92.11 Children's home and orphanage as the place of occurrence of the external cause

Y92.110 Kitchen in children's home and orphanage as the place of occurrence of the external cause

Y92.111 Bathroom in children's home and orphanage as the place of occurrence of the external cause

Y92.112 Bedroom in children's home and orphanage as the place of occurrence of the external cause

Y92.113 Driveway of children's home and orphanage as the place of occurrence of the external cause

Y92.114 Garage of children's home and orphanage as the place of occurrence of the external cause

Y92.115 Swimming-pool of children's home and orphanage as the place of occurrence of the external cause

Y92.116 Garden or yard of children's home and orphanage as the place of occurrence of the external cause

Y92.118 Other place in children's home and orphanage as the place of occurrence of the external cause

Y92.119 Unspecified place in children's home and orphanage as the place of occurrence of the external cause

+ Y92.12 Nursing home as the place of occurrence of the external cause

Home for the sick as the place of occurrence of the external cause

Hospice as the place of occurrence of the external cause

Y92.120 Kitchen in nursing home as the place of occurrence of the external cause

Y92.121 Bathroom in nursing home as the place of occurrence of the external cause

Y92.122 Bedroom in nursing home as the place of occurrence of the external cause

Y92.123 Driveway of nursing home as the place of occurrence of the external cause

Y92.124 Garage of nursing home as the place of occurrence of the external cause

Y92.125 Swimming-pool of nursing home as the place of occurrence of the external cause

Y92.126 Garden or yard of nursing home as the place of occurrence of the external cause

Y92.128 Other place in nursing home as the place of occurrence of the external cause

Y92.129 Unspecified place in nursing home as the place of occurrence of the external cause

+ **Y92.13** Military base as the place of occurrence of the external cause

    Excludes1: *military training grounds (Y92.83)*

    Y92.130 Kitchen on military base as the place of occurrence of the external cause

    Y92.131 Mess hall on military base as the place of occurrence of the external cause

    Y92.133 Barracks on military base as the place of occurrence of the external cause

    Y92.135 Garage on military base as the place of occurrence of the external cause

    Y92.136 Swimming-pool on military base as the place of occurrence of the external cause

    Y92.137 Garden or yard on military base as the place of occurrence of the external cause

    Y92.138 Other place on military base as the place of occurrence of the external cause

    Y92.139 Unspecified place military base as the place of occurrence of the external cause

+ **Y92.14** Prison as the place of occurrence of the external cause

    Y92.140 Kitchen in prison as the place of occurrence of the external cause

    Y92.141 Dining room in prison as the place of occurrence of the external cause

    Y92.142 Bathroom in prison as the place of occurrence of the external cause

    Y92.143 Cell of prison as the place of occurrence of the external cause

    Y92.146 Swimming-pool of prison as the place of occurrence of the external cause

    Y92.147 Courtyard of prison as the place of occurrence of the external cause

    Y92.148 Other place in prison as the place of occurrence of the external cause

    Y92.149 Unspecified place in prison as the place of occurrence of the external cause

+ **Y92.15** Reform school as the place of occurrence of the external cause

    Y92.150 Kitchen in reform school as the place of occurrence of the external cause

    Y92.151 Dining room in reform school as the place of occurrence of the external cause

    Y92.152 Bathroom in reform school as the place of occurrence of the external cause

    Y92.153 Bedroom in reform school as the place of occurrence of the external cause

    Y92.154 Driveway of reform school as the place of occurrence of the external cause

    Y92.155 Garage of reform school as the place of occurrence of the external cause

    Y92.156 Swimming-pool of reform school as the place of occurrence of the external cause

    Y92.157 Garden or yard of reform school as the place of occurrence of the external cause

    Y92.158 Other place in reform school as the place of occurrence of the external cause

    Y92.159 Unspecified place in reform school as the place of occurrence of the external cause

+ **Y92.16** School dormitory as the place of occurrence of the external cause

    Excludes1: *reform school as the place of occurrence of the external cause (Y92.15-)*

    school buildings and grounds as the place of occurrence of the external cause (Y92.2-)

    school sports and athletic areas as the place of occurrence of the external cause (Y92.3-)

    Y92.160 Kitchen in school dormitory as the place of occurrence of the external cause

    Y92.161 Dining room in school dormitory as the place of occurrence of the external cause

    Y92.162 Bathroom in school dormitory as the place of occurrence of the external cause

    Y92.163 Bedroom in school dormitory as the place of occurrence of the external cause

    Y92.168 Other place in school dormitory as the place of occurrence of the external cause

    Y92.169 Unspecified place in school dormitory as the place of occurrence of the external cause

+ **Y92.19** Other specified residential institution as the place of occurrence of the external cause

    Y92.190 Kitchen in other specified residential institution as the place of occurrence of the external cause

    Y92.191 Dining room in other specified residential institution as the place of occurrence of the external cause

    Y92.192 Bathroom in other specified residential institution as the place of occurrence of the external cause

    Y92.193 Bedroom in other specified residential institution as the place of occurrence of the external cause

    Y92.194 Driveway of other specified residential institution as the place of occurrence of the external cause

    Y92.195 Garage of other specified residential institution as the place of occurrence of the external cause

    Y92.196 Pool of other specified residential institution as the place of occurrence of the external cause

    Y92.197 Garden or yard of other specified residential institution as the place of occurrence of the external cause

    Y92.198 Other place in other specified residential institution as the place of occurrence of the external cause

    Y92.199 Unspecified place in other specified residential institution as the place of occurrence of the external cause

+ **Y92.2** School, other institution and public administrative area as the place of occurrence of the external cause

    Building and adjacent grounds used by the general public or by a particular group of the public

    Excludes1: *building under construction as the place of occurrence of the external cause (Y92.6)*

    residential institution as the place of occurrence of the external cause (Y92.1)

    school dormitory as the place of occurrence of the external cause (Y92.16-)

    sports and athletics area of schools as the place of occurrence of the external cause (Y92.3-)

+ **Y92.21** School (private) (public) (state) as the place of occurrence of the external cause

    Y92.210 Daycare center as the place of occurrence of the external cause

    Y92.211 Elementary school as the place of occurrence of the external cause

        Kindergarten as the place of occurrence of the external cause

    Y92.212 Middle school as the place of occurrence of the external cause

    Y92.213 High school as the place of occurrence of the external cause

        AHA CC: 4Q, 2012, 108

    Y92.214 College as the place of occurrence of the external cause

        University as the place of occurrence of the external cause

    Y92.215 Trade school as the place of occurrence of the external cause

    Y92.218 Other school as the place of occurrence of the external cause

    Y92.219 Unspecified school as the place of occurrence of the external cause

    Y92.22 Religious institution as the place of occurrence of the external cause

        Church as the place of occurrence of the external cause

        Mosque as the place of occurrence of the external cause

        Synagogue as the place of occurrence of the external cause

+ Y92.23 Hospital as the place of occurrence of the external cause
Excludes1: ambulatory (outpatient) health services establishments (Y92.53-)
home for the sick as the place of occurrence of the external cause (Y92.12-)
hospice as the place of occurrence of the external cause (Y92.12-)
nursing home as the place of occurrence of the external cause (Y92.12-)
  - Y92.230 Patient room in hospital as the place of occurrence of the external cause
  - Y92.231 Patient bathroom in hospital as the place of occurrence of the external cause
  - Y92.232 Corridor of hospital as the place of occurrence of the external cause
  - Y92.233 Cafeteria of hospital as the place of occurrence of the external cause
  - Y92.234 Operating room of hospital as the place of occurrence of the external cause
  - Y92.238 Other place in hospital as the place of occurrence of the external cause
  - Y92.239 Unspecified place in hospital as the place of occurrence of the external cause

+ Y92.24 Public administrative building as the place of occurrence of the external cause
  - Y92.240 Courthouse as the place of occurrence of the external cause
  - Y92.241 Library as the place of occurrence of the external cause
  - Y92.242 Post office as the place of occurrence of the external cause
  - Y92.243 City hall as the place of occurrence of the external cause
  - Y92.248 Other public administrative building as the place of occurrence of the external cause

+ Y92.25 Cultural building as the place of occurrence of the external cause
  - Y92.250 Art Gallery as the place of occurrence of the external cause
  - Y92.251 Museum as the place of occurrence of the external cause
  - Y92.252 Music hall as the place of occurrence of the external cause
  - Y92.253 Opera house as the place of occurrence of the external cause
  - Y92.254 Theater (live) as the place of occurrence of the external cause
  - Y92.258 Other cultural public building as the place of occurrence of the external cause

Y92.26 Movie house or cinema as the place of occurrence of the external cause

Y92.29 Other specified public building as the place of occurrence of the external cause
Assembly hall as the place of occurrence of the external cause
Clubhouse as the place of occurrence of the external cause

+ Y92.3 Sports and athletics area as the place of occurrence of the external cause

+ Y92.31 Athletic court as the place of occurrence of the external cause
Excludes1: tennis court in private home or garden (Y92.09)
  - Y92.310 Basketball court as the place of occurrence of the external cause
  - Y92.311 Squash court as the place of occurrence of the external cause
  - Y92.312 Tennis court as the place of occurrence of the external cause
  - Y92.318 Other athletic court as the place of occurrence of the external cause

+ Y92.32 Athletic field as the place of occurrence of the external cause
  - Y92.320 Baseball field as the place of occurrence of the external cause
  - Y92.321 Football field as the place of occurrence of the external cause
  - Y92.322 Soccer field as the place of occurrence of the external cause
  - Y92.328 Other athletic field as the place of occurrence of the external cause
Cricket field as the place of occurrence of the external cause
Hockey field as the place of occurrence of the external cause

+ Y92.33 Skating rink as the place of occurrence of the external cause
  - Y92.330 Ice skating rink (indoor) (outdoor) as the place of occurrence of the external cause
  - Y92.331 Roller skating rink as the place of occurrence of the external cause

Y92.34 Swimming pool (public) as the place of occurrence of the external cause
Excludes1: swimming pool in private home or garden (Y92.016)

Y92.39 Other specified sports and athletic area as the place of occurrence of the external cause
Golf-course as the place of occurrence of the external cause
Gymnasium as the place of occurrence of the external cause
Riding-school as the place of occurrence of the external cause
Stadium as the place of occurrence of the external cause

+ Y92.4 Street, highway and other paved roadways as the place of occurrence of the external cause
Excludes1: private driveway of residence (Y92.014, Y92.024, Y92.043, Y92.093, Y92.113, Y92.123, Y92.154, Y92.194)

+ Y92.41 Street and highway as the place of occurrence of the external cause
  - Y92.410 Unspecified street and highway as the place of occurrence of the external cause
Road NOS as the place of occurrence of the external cause
  - Y92.411 Interstate highway as the place of occurrence of the external cause
Freeway as the place of occurrence of the external cause
Motorway as the place of occurrence of the external cause
  - Y92.412 Parkway as the place of occurrence of the external cause
  - Y92.413 State road as the place of occurrence of the external cause
  - Y92.414 Local residential or business street as the place of occurrence of the external cause
  - Y92.415 Exit ramp or entrance ramp of street or highway as the place of occurrence of the external cause

+ Y92.48 Other paved roadways as the place of occurrence of the external cause
  - Y92.480 Sidewalk as the place of occurrence of the external cause
  - Y92.481 Parking lot as the place of occurrence of the external cause
  - Y92.482 Bike path as the place of occurrence of the external cause
  - Y92.488 Other paved roadways as the place of occurrence of the external cause

+ Y92.5 Trade and service area as the place of occurrence of the external cause
Excludes1: garage in private home (Y92.015)
schools and other public administration buildings (Y92.2-)

+ Y92.51 Private commercial establishments as the place of occurrence of the external cause
  - Y92.510 Bank as the place of occurrence of the external cause
  - Y92.511 Restaurant or café as the place of occurrence of the external cause
  - Y92.512 Supermarket, store or market as the place of occurrence of the external cause
  - Y92.513 Shop (commercial) as the place of occurrence of the external cause

+ **Y92.52** **Service areas as the place of occurrence of the external cause**
    Y92.520 **Airport as the place of occurrence of the external cause**
    Y92.521 **Bus station as the place of occurrence of the external cause**
    Y92.522 **Railway station as the place of occurrence of the external cause**
    Y92.523 **Highway rest stop as the place of occurrence of the external cause**
    Y92.524 **Gas station as the place of occurrence of the external cause**
        Petroleum station as the place of occurrence of the external cause
        Service station as the place of occurrence of the external cause

+ **Y92.53** **Ambulatory health services establishments as the place of occurrence of the external cause**
    Y92.530 **Ambulatory surgery center as the place of occurrence of the external cause**
        Outpatient surgery center, including that connected with a hospital as the place of occurrence of the external cause
        Same day surgery center, including that connected with a hospital as the place of occurrence of the external cause
    Y92.531 **Health care provider office as the place of occurrence of the external cause**
        Physician office as the place of occurrence of the external cause
    Y92.532 **Urgent care center as the place of occurrence of the external cause**
    Y92.538 **Other ambulatory health services establishments as the place of occurrence of the external cause**
        AHA CC: 1Q, 2019, 21

Y92.59 **Other trade areas as the place of occurrence of the external cause**
    Office building as the place of occurrence of the external cause
    Casino as the place of occurrence of the external cause
    Garage (commercial) as the place of occurrence of the external cause
    Hotel as the place of occurrence of the external cause
    Radio or television station as the place of occurrence of the external cause
    Shopping mall as the place of occurrence of the external cause
    Warehouse as the place of occurrence of the external cause

+ **Y92.6** **Industrial and construction area as the place of occurrence of the external cause**
    Y92.61 **Building [any] under construction as the place of occurrence of the external cause**
    Y92.62 **Dock or shipyard as the place of occurrence of the external cause**
        Dockyard as the place of occurrence of the external cause
        Dry dock as the place of occurrence of the external cause
        Shipyard as the place of occurrence of the external cause
    Y92.63 **Factory as the place of occurrence of the external cause**
        Factory building as the place of occurrence of the external cause
        Factory premises as the place of occurrence of the external cause
        Industrial yard as the place of occurrence of the external cause

Y92.64 **Mine or pit as the place of occurrence of the external cause**
    Mine as the place of occurrence of the external cause

Y92.65 **Oil rig as the place of occurrence of the external cause**
    Pit (coal) (gravel) (sand) as the place of occurrence of the external cause

Y92.69 **Other specified industrial and construction area as the place of occurrence of the external cause**
    Gasworks as the place of occurrence of the external cause
    Power-station (coal) (nuclear) (oil) as the place of occurrence of the external cause
    Tunnel under construction as the place of occurrence of the external cause
    Workshop as the place of occurrence of the external cause

+ **Y92.7** **Farm as the place of occurrence of the external cause**
    Ranch as the place of occurrence of the external cause
    Excludes1: *farmhouse and home premises of farm (Y92.01-)*
    Y92.71 **Barn as the place of occurrence of the external cause**
    Y92.72 **Chicken coop as the place of occurrence of the external cause**
        Hen house as the place of occurrence of the external cause
    Y92.73 **Farm field as the place of occurrence of the external cause**
    Y92.74 **Orchard as the place of occurrence of the external cause**
    Y92.79 **Other farm location as the place of occurrence of the external cause**

+ **Y92.8** **Other places as the place of occurrence of the external cause**
  + **Y92.81** **Transport vehicle as the place of occurrence of the external cause**
      Excludes1: *transport accidents (V00-V99)*
    Y92.810 **Car as the place of occurrence of the external cause**
    Y92.811 **Bus as the place of occurrence of the external cause**
    Y92.812 **Truck as the place of occurrence of the external cause**
    Y92.813 **Airplane as the place of occurrence of the external cause**
    Y92.814 **Boat as the place of occurrence of the external cause**
    Y92.815 **Train as the place of occurrence of the external cause**
    Y92.816 **Subway car as the place of occurrence of the external cause**
    Y92.818 **Other transport vehicle as the place of occurrence of the external cause**
  + **Y92.82** **Wilderness area**
    Y92.820 **Desert as the place of occurrence of the external cause**
    Y92.821 **Forest as the place of occurrence of the external cause**
    Y92.828 **Other wilderness area as the place of occurrence of the external cause**
        Swamp as the place of occurrence of the external cause
        Mountain as the place of occurrence of the external cause
        Marsh as the place of occurrence of the external cause
        Prairie as the place of occurrence of the external cause
  + **Y92.83** **Recreation area as the place of occurrence of the external cause**
    Y92.830 **Public park as the place of occurrence of the external cause**
    Y92.831 **Amusement park as the place of occurrence of the external cause**

Y92.832   **Beach as the place of occurrence of the external cause**
     Seashore as the place of occurrence of the external cause

Y92.833   **Campsite as the place of occurrence of the external cause**

Y92.834   **Zoological garden (Zoo) as the place of occurrence of the external cause**

Y92.838   **Other recreation area as the place of occurrence of the external cause**

Y92.84   **Military training ground as the place of occurrence of the external cause**

Y92.85   **Railroad track as the place of occurrence of the external cause**

Y92.86   **Slaughter house as the place of occurrence of the external cause**

Y92.89   **Other specified places as the place of occurrence of the external cause**
     Derelict house as the place of occurrence of the external cause

Y92.9   **Unspecified place or not applicable**

Y93   **Activity codes**

> **NOTE**   Category Y93 is provided for use to indicate the activity of the person seeking healthcare for an injury or health condition, such as a heart attack while shoveling snow, which resulted from, or was contributed to, by the activity. These codes are appropriate for use for both acute injuries, such as those from chapter 19, and conditions that are due to the long-term, cumulative effects of an activity, such as those from chapter 13. They are also appropriate for use with external cause codes for cause and intent if identifying the activity provides additional information on the event. These codes should be used in conjunction with codes for external cause status (Y99) and place of occurrence (Y92).
>
> This section contains the following broad activity categories:
> Y93.0 Activities involving walking and running
> Y93.1 Activities involving water and water craft
> Y93.2 Activities involving ice and snow
> Y93.3 Activities involving climbing, rappelling, and jumping off
> Y93.4 Activities involving dancing and other rhythmic movement
> Y93.5 Activities involving other sports and athletics played individually
> Y93.6 Activities involving other sports and athletics played as a team or group
> Y93.7 Activities involving other specified sports and athletics
> Y93.A Activities involving other cardiorespiratory exercise
> Y93.B Activities involving other muscle strengthening exercises
> Y93.C Activities involving computer technology and electronic devices
> Y93.D Activities involving arts and handcrafts
> Y93.E Activities involving personal hygiene and interior property and clothing maintenance
> Y93.F Activities involving caregiving
> Y93.G Activities involving food preparation, cooking and grilling
> Y93.H Activities involving exterior property and land maintenance, building and construction
> Y93.I Activities involving roller coasters and other types of external motion
> Y93.J Activities involving playing musical instrument
> Y93.K Activities involving animal care
> Y93.8 Activities, other specified
> Y93.9 Activity, unspecified

Review coding guideline C.20.c

+ **Y93.0**   **Activities involving walking and running**
> **Excludes1:**   *activity, walking an animal (Y93.K1)*
>   *activity, walking or running on a treadmill (Y93.A1)*

Y93.01   **Activity, walking, marching and hiking**
     Activity, walking, marching and hiking on level or elevated terrain
> **Excludes1:**   *activity, mountain climbing (Y93.31)*

Y93.02   **Activity, running**

+ **Y93.1**   **Activities involving water and water craft**
> **Excludes1:**   *activities involving ice (Y93.2-)*

Y93.11   **Activity, swimming**

Y93.12   **Activity, springboard and platform diving**

Y93.13   **Activity, water polo**

Y93.14   **Activity, water aerobics and water exercise**

Y93.15   **Activity, underwater diving and snorkeling**
     Activity, SCUBA diving

Y93.16   **Activity, rowing, canoeing, kayaking, rafting and tubing**
     Activity, canoeing, kayaking, rafting and tubing in calm and turbulent water

Y93.17   **Activity, water skiing and wake boarding**

Y93.18   **Activity, surfing, windsurfing and boogie boarding**
     Activity, water sliding

Y93.19   **Activity, other involving water and watercraft**
     Activity involving water NOS
     Activity, parasailing
     Activity, water survival training and testing

+ **Y93.2**   **Activities involving ice and snow**
> **Excludes1:**   *activity, shoveling ice and snow (Y93.H1)*

Y93.21   **Activity, ice skating**
     Activity, figure skating (singles) (pairs)
     Activity, ice dancing
> **Excludes1:**   *activity, ice hockey (Y93.22)*

Y93.22   **Activity, ice hockey**

Y93.23   **Activity, snow (alpine) (downhill) skiing, snowboarding, sledding, toboganing and snow tubing**
> **Excludes1:**   *activity, cross country skiing (Y93.24)*

Y93.24   **Activity, cross country skiing**
     Activity, nordic skiing

Y93.29   **Activity, other involving ice and snow**
     Activity involving ice and snow NOS

+ **Y93.3**   **Activities involving climbing, rappelling and jumping off**
> **Excludes1:**   *activity, hiking on level or elevated terrain (Y93.01)*
>   *activity, jumping rope (Y93.56)*
>   *activity, trampoline jumping (Y93.44)*

Y93.31   **Activity, mountain climbing, rock climbing and wall climbing**

Y93.32   **Activity, rappelling**

Y93.33   **Activity, BASE jumping**
     Activity, Building, Antenna, Span, Earth jumping

Y93.34   **Activity, bungee jumping**

Y93.35   **Activity, hang gliding**

Y93.39   **Activity, other involving climbing, rappelling and jumping off**

+ **Y93.4**   **Activities involving dancing and other rhythmic movement**
> **Excludes1:**   *activity, martial arts (Y93.75)*

Y93.41   **Activity, dancing**
     AHA CC: 4Q, 2012, 108

Y93.42   **Activity, yoga**

Y93.43   **Activity, gymnastics**
     Activity, rhythmic gymnastics
> **Excludes1:**   *activity, trampolining (Y93.44)*

Y93.44   **Activity, trampolining**

Y93.45   **Activity, cheerleading**

Y93.49   **Activity, other involving dancing and other rhythmic movements**

+ **Y93.5**   **Activities involving other sports and athletics played individually**
> **Excludes1:**   *activity, dancing (Y93.41)*
>   *activity, gymnastic (Y93.43)*
>   *activity, trampolining (Y93.44)*
>   *activity, yoga (Y93.42)*

Y93.51   **Activity, roller skating (inline) and skateboarding**

Y93.52   **Activity, horseback riding**

Y93.53   **Activity, golf**

Y93.54   **Activity, bowling**

Y93.55   **Activity, bike riding**

Y93.56   **Activity, jumping rope**

Y93.57   **Activity, non-running track and field events**
> **Excludes1:**   *activity, running (any form) (Y93.02)*

Y93.59 Activity, other involving other sports and athletics played individually

Excludes1: *activities involving climbing, rappelling, and jumping (Y93.3-)*
activities involving ice and snow (Y93.2-)
activities involving walking and running (Y93.0-)
activities involving water and watercraft (Y93.1-)

+ Y93.6 Activities involving other sports and athletics played as a team or group

Excludes1: *activity, ice hockey (Y93.22)*
activity, water polo (Y93.13)

Y93.61 Activity, american tackle football
Activity, football NOS

Y93.62 Activity, american flag or touch football

Y93.63 Activity, rugby

Y93.64 Activity, baseball
Activity, softball

Y93.65 Activity, lacrosse and field hockey
AHA CC: 1Q, 2015, 3-21

Y93.66 Activity, soccer

Y93.67 Activity, basketball
AHA CC: 4Q, 2019, 17-18

Y93.68 Activity, volleyball (beach) (court)

Y93.6A Activity, physical games generally associated with school recess, summer camp and children
Activity, capture the flag
Activity, dodge ball
Activity, four square
Activity, kickball

Y93.69 Activity, other involving other sports and athletics played as a team or group
Activity, cricket

+ Y93.7 Activities involving other specified sports and athletics

Y93.71 Activity, boxing

Y93.72 Activity, wrestling

Y93.73 Activity, racquet and hand sports
Activity, handball
Activity, racquetball
Activity, squash
Activity, tennis

Y93.74 Activity, frisbee
Activity, ultimate frisbee

Y93.75 Activity, martial arts
Activity, combatives

Y93.79 Activity, other specified sports and athletics
Excludes1: *sports and athletics activities specified in categories Y93.0-Y93.6*

+ Y93.A Activities involving other cardiorespiratory exercise
Activities involving physical training

Y93.A1 Activity, exercise machines primarily for cardiorespiratory conditioning
Activity, elliptical and stepper machines
Activity, stationary bike
Activity, treadmill

Y93.A2 Activity, calisthenics
Activity, jumping jacks
Activity, warm up and cool down

Y93.A3 Activity, aerobic and step exercise

Y93.A4 Activity, circuit training

Y93.A5 Activity, obstacle course
Activity, challenge course
Activity, confidence course

Y93.A6 Activity, grass drills
Activity, guerilla drills

Y93.A9 Activity, other involving cardiorespiratory exercise
Excludes1: *activities involving cardiorespiratory exercise specified in categories Y93.0-Y93.7*

+ Y93.B Activities involving other muscle strengthening exercises

Y93.B1 Activity, exercise machines primarily for muscle strengthening

Y93.B2 Activity, push-ups, pull-ups, sit-ups

Y93.B3 Activity, free weights
Activity, barbells
Activity, dumbbells

Y93.B4 Activity, pilates

Y93.B9 Activity, other involving muscle strengthening exercises
Excludes1: *activities involving muscle strengthening specified in categories Y93.0-Y93.A*

+ Y93.C Activities involving computer technology and electronic devices
Excludes1: *activity, electronic musical keyboard or instruments (Y93.J-)*

Y93.C1 Activity, computer keyboarding
Activity, electronic game playing using keyboard or other stationary device

Y93.C2 Activity, hand held interactive electronic device
Activity, cellular telephone and communication device
Activity, electronic game playing using interactive device
Excludes1: *activity, electronic game playing using keyboard or other stationary device (Y93.C1)*

Y93.C9 Activity, other involving computer technology and electronic devices

+ Y93.D Activities involving arts and handcrafts
Excludes1: *activities involving playing musical instrument (Y93.J-)*

Y93.D1 Activity, knitting and crocheting

Y93.D2 Activity, sewing

Y93.D3 Activity, furniture building and finishing
Activity, furniture repair

Y93.D9 Activity, other involving arts and handcrafts

+ Y93.E Activities involving personal hygiene and interior property and clothing maintenance
Excludes1: *activities involving cooking and grilling (Y93.G-)*
activities involving exterior property and land maintenance, building and construction (Y93.H-)
activities involving caregiving (Y93.F-)
activity, dishwashing (Y93.G1)
activity, food preparation (Y93.G1)
activity, gardening (Y93.H2)

Y93.E1 Activity, personal bathing and showering

Y93.E2 Activity, laundry

Y93.E3 Activity, vacuuming

Y93.E4 Activity, ironing

Y93.E5 Activity, floor mopping and cleaning

Y93.E6 Activity, residential relocation
Activity, packing up and unpacking involved in moving to a new residence

Y93.E8 Activity, other personal hygiene

Y93.E9 Activity, other interior property and clothing maintenance

+ Y93.F Activities involving caregiving
Activity involving the provider of caregiving

Y93.F1 Activity, caregiving, bathing

Y93.F2 Activity, caregiving, lifting
AHA CC: 4Q, 2016, 73-74

Y93.F9 Activity, other caregiving

+ Y93.G Activities involving food preparation, cooking and grilling

Y93.G1 Activity, food preparation and clean up
Activity, dishwashing

Y93.G2 Activity, grilling and smoking food

Y93.G3 Activity, cooking and baking
Activity, use of stove, oven and microwave oven

Y93.G9 Activity, other involving cooking and grilling

+ Y93.H Activities involving exterior property and land maintenance, building and construction

Y93.H1 Activity, digging, shoveling and raking
Activity, dirt digging
Activity, raking leaves
Activity, snow shoveling

Y93.H2 Activity, gardening and landscaping
Activity, pruning, trimming shrubs, weeding

Y93.H3 Activity, building and construction

Y93.H9 Activity, other involving exterior property and land maintenance, building and construction

+ **Y93.I** **Activities involving roller coasters and other types of external motion**
   Y93.I1 **Activity, roller coaster riding**
   Y93.I9 **Activity, other involving external motion**
+ **Y93.J** **Activities involving playing musical instrument**
   Activity involving playing electric musical instrument
   Y93.J1 **Activity, piano playing**
      Activity, musical keyboard (electronic) playing
   Y93.J2 **Activity, drum and other percussion instrument playing**
   Y93.J3 **Activity, string instrument playing**
   Y93.J4 **Activity, winds and brass instrument playing**
+ **Y93.K** **Activities involving animal care**
   Excludes1: *activity, horseback riding (Y93.52)*
   Y93.K1 **Activity, walking an animal**
   Y93.K2 **Activity, milking an animal**
   Y93.K3 **Activity, grooming and shearing an animal**
   Y93.K9 **Activity, other involving animal care**
+ **Y93.8** **Activities, other specified**
   Y93.81 **Activity, refereeing a sports activity**
   Y93.82 **Activity, spectator at an event**
   Y93.83 **Activity, rough housing and horseplay**
      AHA CC: 1Q, 2015, 3-21
   Y93.84 **Activity, sleeping**
   Y93.85 **Activity, choking game**
      Activity, blackout game
      Activity, fainting game
      Activity, pass out game
      AHA CC: 4Q, 2016, 74-76
   Y93.89 **Activity, other specified**
Y93.9 **Activity, unspecified**

Y95 **Nosocomial condition**
   Valid 3-character code, no further characters required
   AHA CC: 4Q, 2013, 119

Y99 **External cause status**
   NOTE A single code from category Y99 should be used in conjunction with the external cause code(s) assigned to a record to indicate the status of the person at the time the event occurred.
   Review coding guideline C.20.k
Y99.0 **Civilian activity done for income or pay**
   Civilian activity done for financial or other compensation
   Excludes1: *military activity (Y99.1)*
      volunteer activity (Y99.2)
   AHA CC: 4Q, 2016, 73-74
Y99.1 **Military activity**
   Excludes1: *activity of off duty military personnel (Y99.8)*
Y99.2 **Volunteer activity**
   Excludes1: *activity of child or other family member assisting in compensated work of other family member (Y99.8)*
Y99.8 **Other external cause status**
   Activity NEC
   Activity of child or other family member assisting in compensated work of other family member
   Hobby not done for income
   Leisure activity
   Off-duty activity of military personnel
   Recreation or sport not for income or while a student
   Student activity
   Excludes1: *civilian activity done for income or compensation (Y99.0)*
      military activity (Y99.1)
   AHA CC: 4Q, 2012, 108
Y99.9 **Unspecified external cause status**

+, +7th, X + 7th   • Newborn   • Pediatric   • Maternity   • Adult   ♀ Female   ♂ Male   Manifestation   Unacceptable PDX   HCC   CC   MCC   HAC

Chapter 21: Factors Influencing Health Status and Contact with Health Services (Z00-Z99)

NOTE Z codes represent reasons for encounters. A corresponding procedure code must accompany a Z code if a procedure is performed. Categories Z00-Z99 are provided for occasions when circumstances other than a disease, injury or external cause classifiable to categories A00-Y89 are recorded as 'diagnoses' or 'problems'. This can arise in two main ways:

(a) When a person who may or may not be sick encounters the health services for some specific purpose, such as to receive limited care or service for a current condition, to donate an organ or tissue, to receive prophylactic vaccination (immunization), or to discuss a problem which is in itself not a disease or injury.

(b) When some circumstance or problem is present which influences the person's health status but is not in itself a current illness or injury.

This chapter contains the following category blocks:

Z00-Z13	Persons encountering health services for examinations
Z14-Z15	Genetic carrier and genetic susceptibility to disease
Z16	Resistance to antimicrobial drugs
Z17	Estrogen receptor status
Z18	Retained foreign body fragments
Z19	Hormone sensitivity malignancy status
Z20-Z29	Persons with potential health hazards related to communicable diseases
Z30-Z39	Persons encountering health services in circumstances related to reproduction
Z40-Z53	Encounters for other specific health care
Z55-Z65	Persons with potential health hazards related to socioeconomic and psychosocial circumstances
Z66	Do not resuscitate status
Z67	Blood type
Z68	Body mass index (BMI)
Z69-Z76	Persons encountering health services in other circumstances
Z77-Z99	Persons with potential health hazards related to family and personal history and certain conditions influencing health status

C. Chapter-Specific Coding Guidelines

In addition to general coding guidelines, there are guidelines for specific diagnoses and/or conditions in the classification. Unless otherwise indicated, these guidelines apply to all health care settings. Please refer to Section II for guidelines on the selection of principal diagnosis.

21. Chapter 21: Factors Influencing Health Status and Contact with Health Services (Z00-Z99)

NOTE The chapter specific guidelines provide additional information about the use of Z codes for specified encounters.

a. Use of Z codes in any healthcare setting

Z codes are for use in any healthcare setting. Z codes may be used as either a first-listed (principal diagnosis code in the inpatient setting) or secondary code, depending on the circumstances of the encounter. Certain Z codes may only be used as first-listed or principal diagnosis.

b. Z Codes indicate a reason for an encounter

Z codes are not procedure codes. A corresponding procedure code must accompany a Z code to describe any procedure performed.

c. Categories of Z Codes

1) Contact/Exposure

Category Z20 indicates contact with, and suspected exposure to, communicable diseases. These codes are for patients who do not show any sign or symptom of a disease but are suspected to have been exposed to it by close personal contact with an infected individual or are in an area where a disease is epidemic.

Category Z77, Other contact with and (suspected) exposures hazardous to health, indicates contact with and suspected exposures hazardous to health.

Contact/exposure codes may be used as a first-listed code to explain an encounter for testing, or, more commonly, as a secondary code to identify a potential risk.

2) Inoculations and vaccinations

Code Z23 is for encounters for inoculations and vaccinations. It indicates that a patient is being seen to receive a prophylactic inoculation against a disease. Procedure codes are required to identify the actual administration of the injection and the type(s) of immunizations given. Code Z23 may be used as a secondary code if the inoculation is given as a routine part of preventive health care, such as a well-baby visit.

3) Status

Status codes indicate that a patient is either a carrier of a disease or has the sequelae or residual of a past disease or condition. This includes such things as the presence of prosthetic or mechanical devices resulting from past treatment. A status code is informative, because the status may affect the course of treatment and its outcome. A status code is distinct from a history code. The history code indicates that the patient no longer has the condition.

A status code should not be used with a diagnosis code from one of the body system chapters, if the diagnosis code includes the information provided by the status code. For example, code Z94.1, Heart transplant status, should not be used with a code from subcategory T86.2, Complications of heart transplant. The status code does not provide additional information. The complication code indicates that the patient is a heart transplant patient.

For encounters for weaning from a mechanical ventilator, assign a code from subcategory J96.1, Chronic respiratory failure, followed by code Z99.11, Dependence on respirator [ventilator] status.

The status Z codes/categories are:

Z14	Genetic carrier

Genetic carrier status indicates that a person carries a gene, associated with a particular disease, which may be passed to offspring who may develop that disease. The person does not have the disease and is not at risk of developing the disease.

Z15	Genetic susceptibility to disease

Genetic susceptibility indicates that a person has a gene that increases the risk of that person developing the disease.

Codes from category Z15 should not be used as principal or first-listed codes. If the patient has the condition to which he/she is susceptible, and that condition is the reason for the encounter, the code for the current condition should be sequenced first. If the patient is being seen for follow-up after completed treatment for this condition, and the condition no longer exists, a follow-up code should be sequenced first, followed by the appropriate personal history and genetic susceptibility codes. If the purpose of the encounter is genetic counseling associated with procreative management, code Z31.5, Encounter for genetic counseling, should be assigned as the first-listed code, followed by a code from category Z15. Additional codes should be assigned for any applicable family or personal history.

Z16	Resistance to antimicrobial drugs

This code indicates that a patient has a condition that is resistant to antimicrobial drug treatment. Sequence the infection code first.

Z17	Estrogen receptor status
Z18	Retained foreign body fragments
Z19	Hormone sensitivity malignancy status
Z21	Asymptomatic HIV infection status

This code indicates that a patient has tested positive for HIV but has manifested no signs or symptoms of the disease.

Z22	Carrier of infectious disease

Carrier status indicates that a person harbors the specific organisms of a disease without manifest symptoms and is capable of transmitting the infection.

Z28.3	Underimmunization status
Z33.1	Pregnant state, incidental

This code is a secondary code only for use when the pregnancy is in no way complicating the reason for visit. Otherwise, a code from the obstetric chapter is required.

Z66	Do not resuscitate

This code may be used when it is documented by the provider that a patient is on do not resuscitate status at any time during the stay.

Z67	Blood type
Z68	Body mass index (BMI)

BMI codes should only be assigned when there is an associated, reportable diagnosis (such as obesity). Do not assign BMI codes during pregnancy.

See Section I.B.14 for BMI documentation by clinicians other than the patient's provider.

Z74.01	Bed confinement status
Z76.82	Awaiting organ transplant status
Z78	Other specified health status

Code Z78.1, Physical restraint status, may be used when it is documented by the provider that a patient has been put in restraints during the current encounter. Please note that this code should not be reported when it is documented by the provider that a patient is temporarily restrained during a procedure.

Z79 Long-term (current) drug therapy

Codes from this category indicate a patient's continuous use of a prescribed drug (including such things as aspirin therapy) for the long-term treatment of a condition or for prophylactic use. It is not for use for patients who have addictions to drugs. This subcategory is not for use of medications for detoxification or maintenance programs to prevent withdrawal symptoms in patients with drug dependence (e.g., methadone maintenance for opiate dependence). Assign the appropriate code for the drug dependence instead.

Assign a code from Z79 if the patient is receiving a medication for an extended period as a prophylactic measure (such as for the prevention of deep vein thrombosis) or as treatment of a chronic condition (such as arthritis) or a disease requiring a lengthy course of treatment (such as cancer). Do not assign a code from category Z79 for medication being administered for a brief period of time to treat an acute illness or injury (such as a course of antibiotics to treat acute bronchitis).

Z88 Allergy status to drugs, medicaments and biological substances

Except: Z88.9, Allergy status to unspecified drugs, medicaments and biological substances status

Z89 Acquired absence of limb

Z90 Acquired absence of organs, not elsewhere classified

Z91.0- Allergy status, other than to drugs and biological substances

Z92.82 Status post administration of tPA (rtPA) in a different facility within the last 24 hours prior to admission to a current facility

Assign code Z92.82, Status post administration of tPA (rtPA) in a different facility within the last 24 hours prior to admission to current facility, as a secondary diagnosis when a patient is received by transfer into a facility and documentation indicates they were administered tissue plasminogen activator (tPA) within the last 24 hours prior to admission to the current facility.

This guideline applies even if the patient is still receiving the tPA at the time they are received into the current facility.

The appropriate code for the condition for which the tPA was administered (such as cerebrovascular disease or myocardial infarction) should be assigned first.

Code Z92.82 is only applicable to the receiving facility record and not to the transferring facility record.

Z93 Artificial opening status

Z94 Transplanted organ and tissue status

Z95 Presence of cardiac and vascular implants and grafts

Z96 Presence of other functional implants

Z97 Presence of other devices

Z98 Other postprocedural states

Assign code Z98.85, Transplanted organ removal status, to indicate that a transplanted organ has been previously removed. This code should not be assigned for the encounter in which the transplanted organ is removed. The complication necessitating removal of the transplant organ should be assigned for that encounter.

See section I.C19. for information on the coding of organ transplant complications.

Z99 Dependence on enabling machines and devices, not elsewhere classified

NOTE Categories Z89-Z90 and Z93-Z99 are for use only if there are no complications or malfunctions of the organ or tissue replaced, the amputation site or the equipment on which the patient is dependent.

4) History (of)

There are two types of history Z codes, personal and family. Personal history codes explain a patient's past medical condition that no longer exists and is not receiving any treatment, but that has the potential for recurrence, and therefore may require continued monitoring.

Family history codes are for use when a patient has a family member(s) who has had a particular disease that causes the patient to be at higher risk of also contracting the disease.

Personal history codes may be used in conjunction with follow- up codes and family history codes may be used in conjunction with screening codes to explain the need for a test or procedure. History codes are also acceptable on any medical record regardless of the reason for visit. A history of an illness, even if no longer present, is important information that may alter the type of treatment ordered.

The history Z code categories are:

Z80 Family history of primary malignant neoplasm

Z81 Family history of mental and behavioral disorders

Z82 Family history of certain disabilities and chronic diseases (leading to disablement)

Z83 Family history of other specific disorders

Z84 Family history of other conditions

Z85 Personal history of malignant neoplasm

Z86 Personal history of certain other diseases

Z87 Personal history of other diseases and conditions

Z91.4- Personal history of psychological trauma, not elsewhere classified

Z91.5 Personal history of self-harm

Z91.81 History of falling

Z91.82 Personal history of military deployment

Z92 Personal history of medical treatment

Except: Z92.0, Personal history of contraception Except: Z92.82, Status post administration of tPA (rtPA) in a different facility within the last 24 hours prior to admission to a current facility

5) Screening

Screening is the testing for disease or disease precursors in seemingly well individuals so that early detection and treatment can be provided for those who test positive for the disease (e.g., screening mammogram).

The testing of a person to rule out or confirm a suspected diagnosis because the patient has some sign or symptom is a diagnostic examination, not a screening. In these cases, the sign or symptom is used to explain the reason for the test.

A screening code may be a first-listed code if the reason for the visit is specifically the screening exam. It may also be used as an additional code if the screening is done during an office visit for other health problems. A screening code is not necessary if the screening is inherent to a routine examination, such as a pap smear done during a routine pelvic examination.

Should a condition be discovered during the screening then the code for the condition may be assigned as an additional diagnosis.

The Z code indicates that a screening exam is planned. A procedure code is required to confirm that the screening was performed.

The screening Z codes/categories:

Z11 Encounter for screening for infectious and parasitic diseases

Z12 Encounter for screening for malignant neoplasms

Z13 Encounter for screening for other diseases and disorders

Except: Z13.9, Encounter for screening, unspecified

Z36 Encounter for antenatal screening for mother

6) Observation

There are three observation Z code categories. They are for use in very limited circumstances when a person is being observed for a suspected condition that is ruled out. The observation codes are not for use if an injury or illness or any signs or symptoms related to the suspected condition are present. In such cases the diagnosis/symptom code is used with the corresponding external cause code.

The observation codes are **primarily to be used as principal/first-listed diagnosis. An observation code may be assigned as a secondary diagnosis code when the patient is being observed for a condition that is ruled out and is unrelated to the principal/first-listed diagnosis (e.g., patient presents for treatment following injuries sustained in a motor vehicle accident and is also observed for suspected COVID-19 infection that is subsequently ruled out). Also,** when the principal diagnosis is required to be a code from category Z38, Liveborn infants according to place of birth and type of delivery, **then** a code form category Z05, Encounter for observation and evaluation of newborn for suspected diseases and conditions ruled out, is sequenced after the Z38 code. Additional codes may be used in addition to the observation code but only if they are unrelated to the suspected condition being observed.

Codes from subcategory Z03.7, Encounter for suspected maternal and fetal conditions ruled out, may either be used as a first-listed or as an additional code assignment depending on the case. They are for use in very limited circumstances on a maternal record when an encounter is for a suspected maternal or fetal condition that is ruled out during that encounter (for example, a maternal or fetal condition may be suspected due to an abnormal test result). These codes should not be used when the condition is confirmed. In those cases, the confirmed condition should be coded. In addition, these codes are not for use if an illness or any signs or symptoms related to the suspected condition or problem are present. In such cases the diagnosis/symptom code is used.

Additional codes may be used in addition to the code from subcategory Z03.7, but only if they are unrelated to the suspected condition being evaluated.

Codes from subcategory Z03.7 may not be used for encounters for antenatal screening of mother. *See Section I.C.21. Screening.*

For encounters for suspected fetal condition that are inconclusive following testing and evaluation, assign the appropriate code from category O35, O36, O40 or O41.

The observation Z code categories:

Z03 Encounter for medical observation for suspected diseases and conditions ruled out

Z04 Encounter for examination and observation for other reasons Except: Z04.9, Encounter for examination and observation for unspecified reason

Z05 Encounter for observation and evaluation of newborn for suspected diseases and conditions ruled out

7) Aftercare

Aftercare visit codes cover situations when the initial treatment of a disease has been performed and the patient requires continued care during the healing or recovery phase, or for the long-term consequences of the disease. The aftercare Z code should not be used if treatment is directed at a current, acute disease. The diagnosis code is to be used in these cases. Exceptions to this rule are codes Z51.0, Encounter for antineoplastic radiation therapy, and codes from subcategory Z51.1, Encounter for antineoplastic chemotherapy and immunotherapy. These codes are to be first-listed, followed by the diagnosis code when a patient's encounter is solely to receive radiation therapy, chemotherapy, or immunotherapy for the treatment of a neoplasm. If the reason for the encounter is more than one type of antineoplastic therapy, code Z51.0 and a code from subcategory Z51.1 may be assigned together, in which case one of these codes would be reported as a secondary diagnosis.

The aftercare Z codes should also not be used for aftercare for injuries. For aftercare of an injury, assign the acute injury code with the appropriate 7th character (for subsequent encounter).

The aftercare codes are generally first-listed to explain the specific reason for the encounter. An aftercare code may be used as an additional code when some type of aftercare is provided in addition to the reason for admission and no diagnosis code is applicable. An example of this would be the closure of a colostomy during an encounter for treatment of another condition.

Aftercare codes should be used in conjunction with other aftercare codes or diagnosis codes to provide better detail on the specifics of an aftercare encounter visit, unless otherwise directed by the classification. Should a patient receive multiple types of antineoplastic therapy during the same encounter, code Z51.0, Encounter for antineoplastic radiation therapy, and codes from subcategory Z51.1, Encounter for antineoplastic chemotherapy and immunotherapy, may be used together on a record. The sequencing of multiple aftercare codes depends on the circumstances of the encounter.

Certain aftercare Z code categories need a secondary diagnosis code to describe the resolving condition or sequelae. For others, the condition is included in the code title.

Additional Z code aftercare category terms include fitting and adjustment, and attention to artificial openings.

Status Z codes may be used with aftercare Z codes to indicate the nature of the aftercare. For example code Z95.1, Presence of aortocoronary bypass graft, may be used with code Z48.812, Encounter for surgical aftercare following surgery on the circulatory system, to indicate the surgery for which the aftercare is being performed. A status code should not be used when the aftercare code indicates the type of status, such as using Z43.0, Encounter for attention to tracheostomy, with Z93.0, Tracheostomy status.

The aftercare Z category/codes:

Z42 Encounter for plastic and reconstructive surgery following medical procedure or healed injury

Z43 Encounter for attention to artificial openings

Z44 Encounter for fitting and adjustment of external prosthetic device

Z45 Encounter for adjustment and management of implanted device

Z46 Encounter for fitting and adjustment of other devices

Z47 Orthopedic aftercare

Z48 Encounter for other postprocedural aftercare

Z49 Encounter for care involving renal dialysis

Z51 Encounter for other aftercare and medical care

8) Follow-up

The follow-up codes are used to explain continuing surveillance following completed treatment of a disease, condition, or injury. They imply that the condition has been fully treated and no longer exists. They should not be confused with aftercare codes, or injury codes with a 7th character for subsequent encounter, that explain ongoing care of a healing condition or its sequelae. Follow-up codes may be used in conjunction with history codes to provide the full picture of the healed condition and its treatment. The follow-up code is sequenced first, followed by the history code.

A follow-up code may be used to explain multiple visits. Should a condition be found to have recurred on the follow-up visit, then the diagnosis code for the condition should be assigned in place of the follow-up code.

The follow-up Z code categories:

Z08 Encounter for follow-up examination after completed treatment for malignant neoplasm

Z09 Encounter for follow-up examination after completed treatment for conditions other than malignant neoplasm

Z39 Encounter for maternal postpartum care and examination

9) Donor

Codes in category Z52, Donors of organs and tissues, are used for living individuals who are donating blood or other body tissue. These codes are only for individuals donating for others, not for self-donations. They are not used to identify cadaveric donations.

10) Counseling

Counseling Z codes are used when a patient or family member receives assistance in the aftermath of an illness or injury, or when support is required in coping with family or social problems.

The counseling Z codes/categories:

Z30.0- Encounter for general counseling and advice on contraception

Z31.5 Encounter for procreative genetic counseling

Z31.6- Encounter for general counseling and advice on procreation

Z32.2 Encounter for childbirth instruction

Z32.3 Encounter for childcare instruction

Z69 Encounter for mental health services for victim and perpetrator of abuse

Z70 Counseling related to sexual attitude, behavior and orientation

Z71 Persons encountering health services for other counseling and medical advice, not elsewhere classified

NOTE Code Z71.84, Encounter for health counseling related to travel, is to be used for health risk and safety counseling for future travel purposes.

Z76.81 Expectant mother prebirth pediatrician visit

11) Encounters for Obstetrical and Reproductive Services

See Section I.C.15. Pregnancy, Childbirth, and the Puerperium, for further instruction on the use of these codes.

Z codes for pregnancy are for use in those circumstances when none of the problems or complications included in the codes from the Obstetrics chapter exist (a routine prenatal visit or postpartum care). Codes in category Z34, Encounter for supervision of normal pregnancy, are always first-listed and are not to be used with any other code from the OB chapter.

Codes in category Z3A, Weeks of gestation, may be assigned to provide additional information about the pregnancy. Category Z3A codes should not be assigned for pregnancies with abortive outcomes (categories O00-O08), elective termination of pregnancy (code Z33.2), nor for postpartum conditions, as category Z3A is not applicable to these conditions. The date of the admission should be used to determine weeks of gestation for inpatient admissions that encompass more than one gestational week.

The outcome of delivery, category Z37, should be included on all maternal delivery records. It is always a secondary code. Codes in category Z37 should not be used on the newborn record.

Z codes for family planning (contraceptive) or procreative management and counseling should be included on an obstetric record either during the pregnancy or the postpartum stage, if applicable.

Z codes/categories for obstetrical and reproductive services:

Z30 Encounter for contraceptive management

Z31 Encounter for procreative management

Z32.2 Encounter for childbirth instruction

Z32.3 Encounter for childcare instruction

Z33 Pregnant state

Z34 Encounter for supervision of normal pregnancy

Z36 Encounter for antenatal screening of mother

Z3A Weeks of gestation

Z37 Outcome of delivery

Z39 Encounter for maternal postpartum care and examination

Z76.81 Expectant mother prebirth pediatrician visit

12) Newborns and Infants

See Section I.C.16. Newborn (Perinatal) Guidelines, for further instruction on the use of these codes.

Newborn Z codes/categories:

Z76.1 Encounter for health supervision and care of foundling

Z00.1- Encounter for routine child health examination

Z38 Liveborn infants according to place of birth and type of delivery

13) Routine and administrative examinations

The Z codes allow for the description of encounters for routine examinations, such as, a general check-up, or, examinations for administrative purposes, such as, a pre-employment physical. The codes are not to be used if the examination is for diagnosis of a suspected condition or for treatment purposes. In such cases the diagnosis code is used. During a routine exam, should a diagnosis or condition be discovered, it should be coded as an additional code. Pre-existing and chronic conditions and history codes may also be included as additional codes as long as the examination is for administrative purposes and not focused on any particular condition.

Some of the codes for routine health examinations distinguish between "with" and "without" abnormal findings. Code assignment depends on the information that is known at the time the encounter is being coded. For example, if no abnormal findings were found during the examination, but the encounter is being coded before test results are back, it is acceptable to assign the code for "without abnormal findings." When assigning a code for "with abnormal findings," additional code(s) should be assigned to identify the specific abnormal finding(s).

Pre-operative examination and pre-procedural laboratory examination Z codes are for use only in those situations when a patient is being cleared for a procedure or surgery and no treatment is given.

The Z codes/categories for routine and administrative examinations:

Z00	Encounter for general examination without complaint, suspected or reported diagnosis
Z01	Encounter for other special examination without complaint, suspected or reported diagnosis
Z02	Encounter for administrative examination Except: Z02.9, Encounter for administrative examinations, unspecified
Z32.0-	Encounter for pregnancy test

14) Miscellaneous Z codes

The miscellaneous Z codes capture a number of other health care encounters that do not fall into one of the other categories. Certain of these codes identify the reason for the encounter; others are for use as additional codes that provide useful information on circumstances that may affect a patient's care and treatment.

Prophylactic Organ Removal

For encounters specifically for prophylactic removal of an organ (such as prophylactic removal of breasts due to a genetic susceptibility to cancer or a family history of cancer), the principal or first-listed code should be a code from category Z40, Encounter for prophylactic surgery, followed by the appropriate codes to identify the associated risk factor (such as genetic susceptibility or family history).

If the patient has a malignancy of one site and is having prophylactic removal at another site to prevent either a new primary malignancy or metastatic disease, a code for the malignancy should also be assigned in addition to a code from subcategory Z40.0, Encounter for prophylactic surgery for risk factors related to malignant neoplasms. A Z40.0 code should not be assigned if the patient is having organ removal for treatment of a malignancy, such as the removal of the testes for the treatment of prostate cancer.

Miscellaneous Z codes/categories:

Z28	Immunization not carried out
	Except: Z28.3, Underimmunization status
Z29	Encounter for other prophylactic measures
Z40	Encounter for prophylactic surgery
Z41	Encounter for procedures for purposes other than remedying health state
	Except: Z41.9, Encounter for procedure for purposes other than remedying health state, unspecified
Z53	Persons encountering health services for specific procedures and treatment, not carried out
Z55	Problems related to education and literacy
Z56	Problems related to employment and unemployment
Z57	Occupational exposure to risk factors
Z58	Problems related to physical environment
Z59	Problems related to housing and economic circumstances
Z60	Problems related to social environment
Z62	Problems related to upbringing
Z63	Other problems related to primary support group, including family circumstances
Z64	Problems related to certain psychosocial circumstances
Z65	Problems related to other psychosocial circumstances
Z72	Problems related to lifestyle
	Note: These codes should be assigned only when the documentation specifies that the patient has an associated problem.
Z73	Problems related to life management difficulty

Z74	Problems related to care provider dependency
	Except: Z74.01, Bed confinement status
Z75	Problems related to medical facilities and other health care
Z76.0	Encounter for issue of repeat prescription
Z76.3	Healthy person accompanying sick person
Z76.4	Other boarder to healthcare facility
Z76.5	Malingerer [conscious simulation]
Z91.1-	Patient's noncompliance with medical treatment and regimen
Z91.83	Wandering in diseases classified elsewhere
Z91.84-	Oral health risk factors
Z91.89	Other specified personal risk factors, not elsewhere classified

See Section I.B.14 for Z55-Z65 Persons with potential health hazards related to socioeconomic and psychosocial circumstances, documentation by clinicians other than the patient's provider.

15) Nonspecific Z codes

Certain Z codes are so non-specific, or potentially redundant with other codes in the classification, that there can be little justification for their use in the inpatient setting. Their use in the outpatient setting should be limited to those instances when there is no further documentation to permit more precise coding. Otherwise, any sign or symptom or any other reason for visit that is captured in another code should be used.

Nonspecific Z codes/categories:

Z02.9	Encounter for administrative examinations, unspecified
Z04.9	Encounter for examination and observation for unspecified reason
Z13.9	Encounter for screening, unspecified
Z41.9	Encounter for procedure for purposes other than remedying health state, unspecified
Z52.9	Donor of unspecified organ or tissue
Z86.59	Personal history of other mental and behavioral disorders
Z88.9	Allergy status to unspecified drugs, medicaments and biological substances status
Z92.0	Personal history of contraception

16) Z Codes That May Only be Principal/First-Listed Diagnosis

The following Z codes/categories may only be reported as the principal/first-listed diagnosis, except when there are multiple encounters on the same day and the medical records for the encounters are combined:

Z00	Encounter for general examination without complaint, suspected or reported diagnosis Except: Z00.6
Z01	Encounter for other special examination without complaint, suspected or reported diagnosis
Z02	Encounter for administrative examination
Z03	Encounter for medical observation for suspected diseases and conditions ruled out
Z04	Encounter for examination and observation for other reasons
Z33.2	Encounter for elective termination of pregnancy
Z31.81	Encounter for male factor infertility in female patient
Z31.83	Encounter for assisted reproductive fertility procedure cycle
Z31.84	Encounter for fertility preservation procedure
Z34	Encounter for supervision of normal pregnancy
Z39	Encounter for maternal postpartum care and examination
Z38	Liveborn infants according to place of birth and type of delivery
Z40	Encounter for prophylactic surgery
Z42	Encounter for plastic and reconstructive surgery following medical procedure or healed injury
Z51.0	Encounter for antineoplastic radiation therapy
Z51.1-	Encounter for antineoplastic chemotherapy and immunotherapy
Z52	Donors of organs and tissues
	Except: Z52.9, Donor of unspecified organ or tissue
Z76.1	Encounter for health supervision and care of foundling
Z76.2	Encounter for health supervision and care of other healthy infant and child
Z99.12	Encounter for respirator [ventilator] dependence during power failure

Persons encountering health services for examinations (Z00-Z13)

NOTE Nonspecific abnormal findings disclosed at the time of these examinations are classified to categories R70-R94.

Excludes1: *examinations related to pregnancy and reproduction (Z30-Z36, Z39.-)*

Z00 Encounter for general examination without complaint, suspected or reported diagnosis

Excludes1: *encounter for examination for administrative purposes (Z02.-)*

Excludes2: *encounter for pre-procedural examinations (Z01.81-) special screening examinations (Z11-Z13)*

Review coding guidelines C.21.c.13 and C.21.c.16

+ Z00.0 Encounter for general adult medical examination
Encounter for adult periodic examination (annual) (physical) and any associated laboratory and radiologic examinations
Excludes1: *encounter for examination of sign or symptom- code to sign or symptom*
general health check-up of infant orchild (Z00.12.-)
- **Z00.00 Encounter for general adult medical examination without abnormal findings**
Encounter for adult health check-up NOS
AHA CC: 1Q, 2016, 36-37; 4Q, 2017, 95-96
- **Z00.01 Encounter for general adult medical examination with abnormal findings**
Use additional code to identify abnormal findings
AHA CC: 1Q, 2016, 35-36

+ Z00.1 Encounter for newborn, infant and child health examinations
Review coding guideline C.21.c.12
+ Z00.11 Newborn health examination
Health check for child under 29 days old
Use additional code to identify any abnormal findings
Excludes1: *health check for child over 28 days old (Z00.12-)*
- **Z00.110 Health examination for newborn under 8 days old**
Health check for newborn under 8 days old
- **Z00.111 Health examination for newborn 8 to 28 days old**
Health check for newborn 8 to 28 days old
Newborn weight check

+ Z00.12 Encounter for routine child health examination
Health check (routine) for child over 28 days old
Immunizations appropriate for age
Routine developmental screening of infant or child
Routine vision and hearing testing
Excludes1: *health check for child under 29 days old (Z00.11-)*
health supervision of foundling or other healthy infant or child (Z76.1-Z76.2)
newborn health examination (Z00.11-)
- **Z00.121 Encounter for routine child health examination with abnormal findings**
Use additional code to identify abnormal findings
AHA CC: 1Q, 2016, 34-35; 4Q, 2017, 95-96
- **Z00.129 Encounter for routine child health examination without abnormal findings**
Encounter for routine child health examination NOS
AHA CC: 1Q, 2016, 34-35

- **Z00.2 Encounter for examination for period of rapid growth in childhood**
- **Z00.3 Encounter for examination for adolescent development state**
Encounter for puberty development state
Z00.5 Encounter for examination of potential donor of organ and tissue
Z00.6 Encounter for examination for normal comparison and control in clinical research program
Examination of participant or control in clinical research program
+ Z00.7 Encounter for examination for period of delayed growth in childhood
- **Z00.70 Encounter for examination for period of delayed growth in childhood without abnormal findings**
- **Z00.71 Encounter for examination for period of delayed growth in childhood with abnormal findings**
Use additional code to identify abnormal findings
Z00.8 Encounter for other general examination
Encounter for health examination in population surveys

Z01 Encounter for other special examination without complaint, suspected or reported diagnosis
Includes: routine examination of specific system
NOTE Codes from category Z01 represent the reason for the encounter. A separate procedure code is required to identify any examinations or procedures performed
Excludes1: *encounter for examination for administrative purposes (Z02.-)*
encounter for examination for suspected conditions, proven not to exist (Z03.-)
encounter for laboratory and radiologic examinations as a component of general medical examinations (Z00.0-)
encounter for laboratory, radiologic and imaging examinations for sign(s) and symptom(s) - code to the sign(s) or symptom(s)

Excludes2: *screening examinations (Z11-Z13)*
Review coding guidelines C.21.c.13 and C.21.c.16
+ Z01.0 Encounter for examination of eyes and vision
Excludes1: *examination for driving license (Z02.4)*
Z01.00 Encounter for examination of eyes and vision without abnormal findings
Encounter for examination of eyes and vision NOS
Z01.01 Encounter for examination of eyes and vision with abnormal findings
Use additional code to identify abnormal findings
AHA CC: 4Q, 2016, 21
+ Z01.02 Encounter for examination of eyes and vision following failed vision screening
Excludes1: *examination for examination of eyes and vision with abnormal findings (Z01.01)*
examination for examination of eyes and vision without abnormal findings (Z01.00)
AHA CC: 4Q, 2019, 20
Z01.020 Examination for examination of eyes and vision following failed vision screening without abnormal findings
Z01.021 Examination for examination of eyes and vision following failed vision screening with abnormal findings
Use additional code to identify abnormal findings

+ Z01.1 Encounter for examination of ears and hearing
Z01.10 Encounter for examination of ears and hearing without abnormal findings
Encounter for examination of ears and hearing NOS
AHA CC: 4Q, 2016, 21
+ Z01.11 Encounter for examination of ears and hearing with abnormal findings
Z01.110 Encounter for hearing examination following failed hearing screening
AHA CC: 3Q, 2016, 18-19
Z01.118 Encounter for examination of ears and hearing with other abnormal findings
Use additional code to identify abnormal findings
AHA CC: 3Q, 2016, 17
Z01.12 Encounter for hearing conservation and treatment

+ Z01.2 Encounter for dental examination and cleaning
Z01.20 Encounter for dental examination and cleaning without abnormal findings
Encounter for dental examination and cleaning NOS
Z01.21 Encounter for dental examination and cleaning with abnormal findings
Use additional code to identify abnormal findings

+ Z01.3 Encounter for examination of blood pressure
Z01.30 Encounter for examination of blood pressure without abnormal findings
Encounter for examination of blood pressure NOS
Z01.31 Encounter for examination of blood pressure with abnormal findings
Use additional code to identify abnormal findings

+ Z01.4 Encounter for gynecological examination
Excludes2: *pregnancy examination or test (Z32.0-)*
routine examination for contraceptive maintenance (Z30.4-)
+ Z01.41 Encounter for routine gynecological examination
Encounter for general gynecological examination with or without cervical smear
Encounter for gynecological examination (general) (routine) NOS
Encounter for pelvic examination (annual) (periodic)
Use additional code:
for screening for human papillomavirus, if applicable, (Z11.51)
for screening vaginal pap smear, if applicable (Z12.72)
to identify acquired absence of uterus, if applicable (Z90.71-)

+, +7th, X + 7th   • Newborn   • Pediatric   • Maternity   • Adult   ♀ Female   ♂ Male   Manifestation   Unacceptable PDX   HCC   CC   MCC   HAC

Excludes1: *gynecologic examination status-post hysterectomy for malignant condition (Z08)*
screening cervical pap smear not a part of a routine gynecological examination (Z12.4)

♀ **Z01.411** **Encounter for gynecological examination (general) (routine) with abnormal findings**

Use additional code to identify abnormal findings.

♀ **Z01.419** **Encounter for gynecological examination (general) (routine) without abnormal findings**

♀ **Z01.42** **Encounter for cervical smear to confirm findings of recent normal smear following initial abnormal smear**

+ **Z01.8** **Encounter for other specified special examinations**

+ **Z01.81** **Encounter for preprocedural examinations**

Encounter for preoperative examinations
Encounter for radiological and imaging examinations as part of preprocedural examination

Z01.810 **Encounter for preprocedural cardiovascular examination**

Z01.811 **Encounter for preprocedural respiratory examination**

Z01.812 **Encounter for preprocedural laboratory examination**

Blood and urine tests prior to treatment or procedure

Z01.818 **Encounter for other preprocedural examination**

Encounter for preprocedural examination NOS
Encounter for examinations prior to antineoplastic chemotherapy

Z01.82 **Encounter for allergy testing**

Excludes1: *encounter for antibody response examination (Z01.84)*

Z01.83 **Encounter for blood typing**

Encounter for Rh typing

Z01.84 **Encounter for antibody response examination**

Encounter for immunity status testing

Excludes1: *encounter for allergy testing (Z01.82)*
AHA CC: 2Q, 2020, 11
Review coding guideline C.1.g.1.k

Z01.89 **Encounter for other specified special examinations**

Z02 **Encounter for administrative examination**

Review coding guidelines C.21.c.13 and C.21.c.16

Z02.0 **Encounter for examination for admission to educational institution**

Encounter for examination for admission to preschool (education)
Encounter for examination for re-admission to school following illness or medical treatment

Z02.1 **Encounter for pre-employment examination**

Z02.2 **Encounter for examination for admission to residential institution**

Excludes1: *examination for admission to prison (Z02.89)*

Z02.3 **Encounter for examination for recruitment to armed forces**

Z02.4 **Encounter for examination for driving license**

Z02.5 **Encounter for examination for participation in sport**

Excludes1: *blood-alcohol and blood-drug test (Z02.83)*

Z02.6 **Encounter for examination for insurance purposes**

+ **Z02.7** **Encounter for issue of medical certificate**

Excludes1: *encounter for general medical examination (Z00-Z01, Z02.0-Z02.6, Z02.8-Z02.9)*

Z02.71 **Encounter for disability determination**

Encounter for issue of medical certificate of incapacity
Encounter for issue of medical certificate of invalidity

Z02.79 **Encounter for issue of other medical certificate**

+ **Z02.8** **Encounter for other administrative examinations**

Z02.81 **Encounter for paternity testing**

Z02.82 **Encounter for adoption services**

Z02.83 **Encounter for blood-alcohol and blood-drug test**

Use additional code for findings of alcohol or drugs in blood (R78.-)

Z02.89 **Encounter for other administrative examinations**

Encounter for examination for admission to prison
Encounter for examination for admission to summer camp
Encounter for immigration examination
Encounter for naturalization examination
Encounter for premarital examination

Excludes1: *health supervision of foundling or other healthy infant or child (Z76.1-Z76.2)*

Z02.9 **Encounter for administrative examinations, unspecified**

Z03 **Encounter for medical observation for suspected diseases and conditions ruled out**

This category is to be used when a person without a diagnosis is suspected of having an abnormal condition, without signs or symptoms, which requires study, but after examination and observation, is ruled out. This category is also for use for administrative and legal observation status.

Excludes1: *contact with and (suspected) exposures hazardous to health (Z77.-)*
encounter for observation and evaluation of newborn for suspected diseases and conditions, ruled out (Z05.-)
person with feared complaint in whom no diagnosis is made (Z71.1)
signs or symptoms under study- code to signs or symptoms
AHA CC: 4Q, 2017, 27
Review coding guidelines C.21.c.6 and C.21.c.16

Z03.6 **Encounter for observation for suspected toxic effect from ingested substance ruled out**

Encounter for observation for suspected adverse effect from drug
Encounter for observation for suspected poisoning

+ **Z03.7** **Encounter for suspected maternal and fetal conditions ruled out**

Encounter for suspected maternal and fetal conditions not found

Excludes1: *known or suspected fetal anomalies affecting management of mother, not ruled out (O26.-, O35.-, O36.-, O40.-, O41.-)*

• ♀ **Z03.71** **Encounter for suspected problem with amniotic cavity and membrane ruled out**

Encounter for suspected oligohydramnios ruled out
Encounter for suspected polyhydramnios ruled out

• ♀ **Z03.72** **Encounter for suspected placental problem ruled out**

• ♀ **Z03.73** **Encounter for suspected fetal anomaly ruled out**

AHA CC: 4Q, 2016, 4-7

• ♀ **Z03.74** **Encounter for suspected problem with fetal growth ruled out**

• ♀ **Z03.75** **Encounter for suspected cervical shortening ruled out**

• ♀ **Z03.79** **Encounter for other suspected maternal and fetal conditions ruled out**

AHA CC: 4Q, 2016, 4-7

+ **Z03.8** **Encounter for observation for other suspected diseases and conditions ruled out**

Z03.81 **Encounter for observation for suspected exposure to biological agents ruled out**

Z03.810 **Encounter for observation for suspected exposure to anthrax ruled out**

Z03.818 **Encounter for observation for suspected exposure to other biological agents ruled out**

AHA CC: 1Q, 2020, 34-36; 2Q, 2020, 8-9

+ **Z03.82** **Encounter for observation for suspected foreign body ruled out**

Excludes1: *retained foreign body (Z18.-)*
retained foreign body in eyelid (H02.81)
residual foreign body in soft tissue (M79.5)

Excludes2: *confirmed foreign body ingestion or aspiration including*
foreign body in alimentary tract (T18)
foreign body in ear (T16)
foreign body on external eye (T15)
foreign body in respiratory tract (T17)

Z03.821 **Encounter for observation for suspected ingested foreign body ruled out**

+, +7th, X + 7th   ● Newborn   ● Pediatric   ● Maternity   ● Adult   ♀ Female   ♂ Male   Manifestation   Unacceptable PDX   HCC   CC   MCC   HAC

Z03.822 Encounter for observation for suspected aspirated (inhaled) foreign body ruled out

Z03.823 Encounter for observation for suspected inserted (injected) foreign body ruled out

Encounter for observation for suspected inserted (injected) foreign body in eye ruled out

Encounter for observation for suspected inserted (injected) foreign body in orifice ruled out

Encounter for observation for suspected inserted (injected) foreign body in skin ruled out

Z03.89 Encounter for observation for other suspected diseases and conditions ruled out

Z04 Encounter for examination and observation for other reasons

Includes: encounter for examination for medicolegal reasons
This category is to be used when a person without a diagnosis is suspected of having an abnormal condition, without signs or symptoms, which requires study, but after examination and observation, is ruled-out. This category is also for use for administrative and legal observation status.
Review coding guidelines C.21.c.6 and C.21.c.16

Z04.1 Encounter for examination and observation following transport accident

Excludes1: *encounter for examination and observation following work accident (Z04.2)*
AHA CC: 2Q, 2018, 8; 2Q, 2019, 11

Z04.2 Encounter for examination and observation following work accident

Z04.3 Encounter for examination and observation following other accident
AHA CC: 2Q, 2018, 7-8

+ **Z04.4** Encounter for examination and observation following alleged rape

Encounter for examination and observation of victim following alleged rape

Encounter for examination and observation of victim following alleged sexual abuse

● **Z04.41** Encounter for examination and observation following alleged adult rape

Suspected adult rape, ruled out

Suspected adult sexual abuse, ruled out
Review coding guideline C.19.f

● **Z04.42** Encounter for examination and observation following alleged child rape

Suspected child rape, ruled out

Suspected child sexual abuse, ruled out
Review coding guideline C.19.f

Z04.6 Encounter for general psychiatric examination, requested by authority

+ **Z04.7** Encounter for examination and observation following alleged physical abuse

● **Z04.71** Encounter for examination and observation following alleged adult physical abuse

Suspected adult physical abuse, ruled out

Excludes1: *confirmed case of adult physical abuse (T74.-)*
encounter for examination and observation following alleged adult sexual abuse (Z04.41)
suspected case of adult physical abuse, not ruled out (T76.-)
Review coding guideline C.19.f

● **Z04.72** Encounter for examination and observation following alleged child physical abuse

Suspected child physical abuse, ruled out

Excludes1: *confirmed case of child physical abuse (T74.-)*
encounter for examination and observation following alleged child sexual abuse (Z04.42)
suspected case of child physical abuse, not ruled out (T76.-)
Review coding guideline C.19.f

+ **Z04.8** Encounter for examination and observation for other specified reasons

Encounter for examination and observation for request for expert evidence
Review coding guideline C.19.f

Z04.81 Encounter for examination and observation of victim following forced sexual exploitation
AHA CC: 4Q, 2018, 32-33, 35

Z04.82 Encounter for examination and observation of victim following forced labor exploitation
AHA CC: 4Q, 2018, 32-33, 35

Z04.89 Encounter for examination and observation for other specified reasons
AHA CC: 4Q, 2018, 35

Z04.9 Encounter for examination and observation for unspecified reason

Encounter for observation NOS

Z05 Encounter for observation and evaluation of newborn for suspected diseases and conditions ruled out

NOTE This category is to be used for newborns, within the neonatal period (the first 28 days of life), who are suspected of having an abnormal condition, but without signs or symptoms, and which, after examination and observation, is ruled out.
Review coding guideline C.16.b
Review coding guideline C.21.c.6
AHA CC: 4Q, 2016, 77; 4Q, 2017, 27

● **Z05.0** Observation and evaluation of newborn for suspected cardiac condition ruled out

● **Z05.1** Observation and evaluation of newborn for suspected infectious condition ruled out
AHA CC: 2Q, 2019, 10-11

● **Z05.2** Observation and evaluation of newborn for suspected neurological condition ruled out

● **Z05.3** Observation and evaluation of newborn for suspected respiratory condition ruled out

+ **Z05.4** Observation and evaluation of newborn for suspected genetic, metabolic or immunologic condition ruled out

● **Z05.41** Observation and evaluation of newborn for suspected genetic condition ruled out
AHA CC: 4Q, 2016, 54-55

● **Z05.42** Observation and evaluation of newborn for suspected metabolic condition ruled out

● **Z05.43** Observation and evaluation of newborn for suspected immunologic condition ruled out

● **Z05.5** Observation and evaluation of newborn for suspected gastrointestinal condition ruled out

● **Z05.6** Observation and evaluation of newborn for suspected genitourinary condition ruled out

+ **Z05.7** Observation and evaluation of newborn for suspected skin, subcutaneous, musculoskeletal and connective tissue condition ruled out

● **Z05.71** Observation and evaluation of newborn for suspected skin and subcutaneous tissue condition ruled out

● **Z05.72** Observation and evaluation of newborn for suspected musculoskeletal condition ruled out

● **Z05.73** Observation and evaluation of newborn for suspected connective tissue condition ruled out

● **Z05.8** Observation and evaluation of newborn for other specified suspected condition ruled out

● **Z05.9** Observation and evaluation of newborn for unspecified suspected condition ruled out

Z08 Encounter for follow-up examination after completed treatment for malignant neoplasm

Medical surveillance following completed treatment
Use additional code to identify any acquired absence of organs (Z90.-)

Use additional code to identify the personal history of malignant neoplasm (Z85.-)

Excludes1: *aftercare following medical care (Z43-Z49, Z51)*
Review coding guideline C.21.c.8
Valid 3-character code, no further characters required

Z09 Encounter for follow-up examination after completed treatment for conditions other than malignant neoplasm

Medical surveillance following completed treatment
Use additional code to identify any applicable history of disease code (Z86.-. Z87.-)

+, +7th, X + 7th   ● Newborn   ● Pediatric   ● Maternity   ● Adult   ♀ Female   ♂ Male   Manifestation   Unacceptable PDX   HCC   CC   MCC   HAC

Excludes1: *aftercare following medical care (Z43-Z49, Z51)*
surveillance of contraception (Z30.4-)
surveillance of prosthetic and other medical devices (Z44-Z46)
Review coding guideline C.1.g.1.j
Review coding guideline C.21.c.8
AHA CC: 1Q, 2017, 9; 2Q, 2020, 10-11
Valid 3-character code, no further characters required

Z11 **Encounter for screening for infectious and parasitic diseases**

Screening is the testing for disease or disease precursors in asymptomatic individuals so that early detection and treatment can be provided for those who test positive for the disease.

Excludes1: *encounter for diagnostic examination-code to sign or symptom*
Review coding guideline C.21.c.5

Z11.0 **Encounter for screening for intestinal infectious diseases**

Z11.1 **Encounter for screening for respiratory tuberculosis**
Encounter for screening for active tuberculosis disease

Z11.2 **Encounter for screening for other bacterial diseases**

Z11.3 **Encounter for screening for infections with a predominantly sexual mode of transmission**
Excludes2: *encounter for screening for human immunodeficiency virus [HIV] (Z11.4)*
encounter for screening for human papillomavirus (Z11.51)

Z11.4 **Encounter for screening for human immunodeficiency virus [HIV]**
Review coding guideline C.1.a.2.h

+ **Z11.5** **Encounter for screening for other viral diseases**
Excludes2: *encounter for screening for viral intestinal disease (Z11.0)*

Z11.51 **Encounter for screening for human papillomavirus (HPV)**

Z11.59 **Encounter for screening for other viral diseases**

Z11.6 **Encounter for screening for other protozoal diseases and helminthiases**
Excludes2: *encounter for screening for protozoal intestinal disease (Z11.0)*

Z11.7 **Encounter for testing for latent tuberculosis infection**
AHA CC: 4Q, 2019, 20

Z11.8 **Encounter for screening for other infectious and parasitic diseases**
Encounter for screening for chlamydia
Encounter for screening for rickettsial
Encounter for screening for spirochetal
Encounter for screening for mycoses

Z11.9 **Encounter for screening for infectious and parasitic diseases, unspecified**

Z12 **Encounter for screening for malignant neoplasms**

Screening is the testing for disease or disease precursors in asymptomatic individuals so that early detection and treatment can be provided for those who test positive for the disease.

Use additional code to identify any family history of malignant neoplasm (Z80.-)

Excludes1: *encounter for diagnostic examination-code to sign or symptom*
Review coding guideline C.21.c.5

Z12.0 **Encounter for screening for malignant neoplasm of stomach**

+ **Z12.1** **Encounter for screening for malignant neoplasm of intestinal tract**

Z12.10 **Encounter for screening for malignant neoplasm of intestinal tract, unspecified**

Z12.11 **Encounter for screening for malignant neoplasm of colon**
Encounter for screening colonoscopy NOS
AHA CC: 1Q, 2017, 8-9; 1Q, 2018, 6-7

Z12.12 **Encounter for screening for malignant neoplasm of rectum**

Z12.13 **Encounter for screening for malignant neoplasm of small intestine**

Z12.2 **Encounter for screening for malignant neoplasm of respiratory organs**

+ **Z12.3** **Encounter for screening for malignant neoplasm of breast**

Z12.31 **Encounter for screening mammogram for malignant neoplasm of breast**
Excludes1: *inconclusive mammogram (R92.2)*
AHA CC: 1Q, 2015, 24

Z12.39 **Encounter for other screening for malignant neoplasm of breast**

♀ **Z12.4** **Encounter for screening for malignant neoplasm of cervix**
Encounter for screening pap smear for malignant neoplasm of cervix
Excludes1: *when screening is part of general gynecological examination (Z01.4-)*
Excludes2: *encounter for screening for human papillomavirus (Z11.51)*

♂ **Z12.5** **Encounter for screening for malignant neoplasm of prostate**

Z12.6 **Encounter for screening for malignant neoplasm of bladder**

+ **Z12.7** **Encounter for screening for malignant neoplasm of other genitourinary organs**

♂ **Z12.71** **Encounter for screening for malignant neoplasm of testis**

♀ **Z12.72** **Encounter for screening for malignant neoplasm of vagina**
Vaginal pap smear status-post hysterectomy for non-malignant condition
Use additional code to identify acquired absence of uterus (Z90.71-)
Excludes1: *vaginal pap smear status-post hysterectomy for malignant conditions (Z08)*

♀ **Z12.73** **Encounter for screening for malignant neoplasm of ovary**

Z12.79 **Encounter for screening for malignant neoplasm of other genitourinary organs**

+ **Z12.8** **Encounter for screening for malignant neoplasm of other sites**

Z12.81 **Encounter for screening for malignant neoplasm of oral cavity**

Z12.82 **Encounter for screening for malignant neoplasm of nervous system**

Z12.83 **Encounter for screening for malignant neoplasm of skin**

Z12.89 **Encounter for screening for malignant neoplasm of other sites**

Z12.9 **Encounter for screening for malignant neoplasm, site unspecified**

Z13 **Encounter for screening for other diseases and disorders**

Screening is the testing for disease or disease precursors in asymptomatic individuals so that early detection and treatment can be provided for those who test positive for the disease.

Excludes1: *encounter for diagnostic examination-code to sign or symptom*
Review coding guideline C.21.c.5

Z13.0 **Encounter for screening for diseases of the blood and blood-forming organs and certain disorders involving the immune mechanism**

Z13.1 **Encounter for screening for diabetes mellitus**

+ **Z13.2** **Encounter for screening for nutritional, metabolic and other endocrine disorders**

Z13.21 **Encounter for screening for nutritional disorder**

+ **Z13.22** **Encounter for screening for metabolic disorder**

Z13.220 **Encounter for screening for lipoid disorders**
Encounter for screening for cholesterol level
Encounter for screening for hypercholesterolemia
Encounter for screening for hyperlipidemia

Z13.228 **Encounter for screening for other metabolic disorders**

Z13.29 **Encounter for screening for other suspected endocrine disorder**
Excludes1: *encounter for screening for diabetes mellitus (Z13.1)*

+ **Z13.3** **Encounter for screening examination for mental health and behavioral disorders**
AHA CC: 4Q, 2018, 35-36

Z13.30 **Encounter for screening examination for mental health and behavioral disorders, unspecified**

Z13.31 **Encounter for screening for depression**
Encounter for screening for depression, adult
Encounter for screening for depression for child or adolescent

♀ **Z13.32** **Encounter for screening for maternal depression**
Encounter for screening for perinatal depression

Z13.39 Encounter for screening examination for other mental health and behavioral disorders
Encounter for screening for alcoholism
Encounter for screening for intellectual disabilities

+ **Z13.4 Encounter for screening for certain developmental disorders in childhood**
Encounter for development testing of infant or child
Encounter for screening for developmental handicaps in early childhood
Excludes2: encounter for routine child health examination (Z00.12-)
AHA CC: 4Q, 2018, 36

Z13.40 Encounter for screening for unspecified developmental delays

Z13.41 Encounter for autism screening

Z13.42 Encounter for screening for global developmental delays (milestones)
Encounter for screening for developmental handicaps in early childhood

Z13.49 Encounter for screening for other developmental delays

Z13.5 Encounter for screening for eye and ear disorders
Excludes2: encounter for general hearing examination (Z01.1-)
encounter for general vision examination (Z01.0-)
AHA CC: 3Q, 2016, 17

Z13.6 Encounter for screening for cardiovascular disorders

+ **Z13.7 Encounter for screening for genetic and chromosomal anomalies**
Excludes1: genetic testing for procreative management (Z31.4-)

Z13.71 Encounter for nonprocreative screening for genetic disease carrier status

Z13.79 Encounter for other screening for genetic and chromosomal anomalies

+ **Z13.8 Encounter for screening for other specified diseases and disorders**
Excludes2: screening for malignant neoplasms (Z12.-)

+ **Z13.81 Encounter for screening for digestive system disorders**

Z13.810 Encounter for screening for upper gastrointestinal disorder

Z13.811 Encounter for screening for lower gastrointestinal disorder
Excludes1: encounter for screening for intestinal infectious disease (Z11.0)

Z13.818 Encounter for screening for other digestive system disorders

+ **Z13.82 Encounter for screening for musculoskeletal disorder**

Z13.820 Encounter for screening for osteoporosis

Z13.828 Encounter for screening for other musculoskeletal disorder

Z13.83 Encounter for screening for respiratory disorder NEC
Excludes1: encounter for screening for respiratory tuberculosis (Z11.1)

Z13.84 Encounter for screening for dental disorders

+ **Z13.85 Encounter for screening for nervous system disorders**

Z13.850 Encounter for screening for traumatic brain injury

Z13.858 Encounter for screening for other nervous system disorders

Z13.88 Encounter for screening for disorder due to exposure to contaminants
Excludes1: those exposed to contaminants without suspected disorders (Z57.-, Z77.-)

Z13.89 Encounter for screening for other disorder
Encounter for screening for genitourinary disorders

Z13.9 Encounter for screening, unspecified

Genetic carrier and genetic susceptibility to disease (Z14-Z15)

Z14 Genetic carrier
Review coding guideline C.21.c.3

+ **Z14.0 Hemophilia A carrier**

Z14.01 Asymptomatic hemophilia A carrier

Z14.02 Symptomatic hemophilia A carrier

Z14.1 Cystic fibrosis carrier

Z14.8 Genetic carrier of other disease

Z15 Genetic susceptibility to disease
Includes: confirmed abnormal gene
Use additional code, if applicable, for any associated family history of the disease (Z80-Z84)
Excludes1: chromosomal anomalies (Q90-Q99)
Review coding guideline C.21.c.3

+ **Z15.0 Genetic susceptibility to malignant neoplasm**
Code first , if applicable, any current malignant neoplasm (C00-C75, C81-C96)
Use additional code, if applicable, for any personal history of malignant neoplasm (Z85.-)

Z15.01 Genetic susceptibility to malignant neoplasm of breast

♀ **Z15.02 Genetic susceptibility to malignant neoplasm of ovary**

♂ **Z15.03 Genetic susceptibility to malignant neoplasm of prostate**

♀ **Z15.04 Genetic susceptibility to malignant neoplasm of endometrium**

Z15.09 Genetic susceptibility to other malignant neoplasm

+ **Z15.8 Genetic susceptibility to other disease**

Z15.81 Genetic susceptibility to multiple endocrine neoplasia [MEN]
Excludes1: multiple endocrine neoplasia [MEN] syndromes (E31.2-)

Z15.89 Genetic susceptibility to other disease

Resistance to antimicrobial drugs (Z16)

Z16 Resistance to antimicrobial drugs
NOTE The codes in this category are provided for use as additional codes to identify the resistance and non-responsiveness of a condition to antimicrobial drugs.
Code first the infection
Excludes1: Methicillin resistant Staphylococcus aureus infection (A49.02)
Methicillin resistant Staphylococcus aureus pneumonia (J15.212)
Sepsis due to Methicillin resistant Staphylococcus aureus (A41.02)
Review coding guideline C.1.c
Review coding guideline C.21.c.3

+ **Z16.1 Resistance to beta lactam antibiotics**
CC **Z16.10 Resistance to unspecified beta lactam antibiotics**
CC **Z16.11 Resistance to penicillins**
Resistance to amoxicillin
Resistance to ampicillin
Review coding guidelines C.1.e.1.a and C.1.e.1.b
CC **Z16.12 Extended spectrum beta lactamase (ESBL) resistance**
Excludes2: Methicillin resistant Staphylococcus aureus infection in diseases classified elsewhere (B95.62)
CC **Z16.19 Resistance to other specified beta lactam antibiotics**
Resistance to cephalosporins

+ **Z16.2 Resistance to other antibiotics**
CC **Z16.20 Resistance to unspecified antibiotic**
Resistance to antibiotics NOS

1271

+, +7th, X + 7th ● Newborn ● Pediatric ● Maternity ● Adult ♀ Female ♂ Male Manifestation Unacceptable PDX HCC CC MCC HAC

CC **Z16.21** **Resistance to vancomycin**
CC **Z16.22** **Resistance to vancomycin related antibiotics**
CC **Z16.23** **Resistance to quinolones and fluoroquinolones**
CC **Z16.24** **Resistance to multiple antibiotics**
CC **Z16.29** **Resistance to other single specified antibiotic**
  Resistance to aminoglycosides
  Resistance to macrolides
  Resistance to sulfonamides
  Resistance to tetracyclines
+ **Z16.3** **Resistance to other antimicrobial drugs**
  Excludes1: *resistance to antibiotics (Z16.1-, Z16.2-)*
CC **Z16.30** **Resistance to unspecified antimicrobial drugs**
  Drug resistance NOS
CC **Z16.31** **Resistance to antiparasitic drug(s)**
  Resistance to quinine and related compounds
CC **Z16.32** **Resistance to antifungal drug(s)**
CC **Z16.33** **Resistance to antiviral drug(s)**
+ **Z16.34** **Resistance to antimycobacterial drug(s)**
  Resistance to tuberculostatics
  CC **Z16.341** **Resistance to single antimycobacterial drug**
    Resistance to antimycobacterial drug NOS
  CC **Z16.342** **Resistance to multiple antimycobacterial drugs**
CC **Z16.35** **Resistance to multiple antimicrobial drugs**
  Excludes1: *Resistance to multiple antibiotics only (Z16.24)*
CC **Z16.39** **Resistance to other specified antimicrobial drug**

Estrogen receptor status (Z17)

Z17 **Estrogen receptor status**
  Code first malignant neoplasm of breast (C50.-)
  Review coding guideline C.21.c.3
  Z17.0 **Estrogen receptor positive status [ER+]**
  Z17.1 **Estrogen receptor negative status [ER-]**

Retained foreign body fragments (Z18)

Z18 **Retained foreign body fragments**
  Includes: embedded fragment (status)
    embedded splinter (status)
    retained foreign body status
  Excludes1: *artificial joint prosthesis status (Z96.6-)*
    foreign body accidentally left during a procedure (T81.5-)
    foreign body entering through orifice (T15-T19)
    in situ cardiac device (Z95.-)
    organ or tissue replaced by means other than transplant (Z96.-, Z97.-)
    organ or tissue replaced by transplant (Z94.-)
    personal history of retained foreign body fully removed (Z87.821)
    superficial foreign body (non-embedded splinter) - code to superficial foreign body, by site
  Review coding guideline C.21.c.3
+ **Z18.0** **Retained radioactive fragments**
  Z18.01 **Retained depleted uranium fragments**
  Z18.09 **Other retained radioactive fragments**
    Other retained depleted isotope fragments
    Retained nontherapeutic radioactive fragments
+ **Z18.1** **Retained metal fragments**
  Excludes1: *retained radioactive metal fragments (Z18.01-Z18.09)*
  Z18.10 **Retained metal fragments, unspecified**
    Retained metal fragment NOS
  Z18.11 **Retained magnetic metal fragments**
  Z18.12 **Retained nonmagnetic metal fragments**
  Z18.2 **Retained plastic fragments**
    Acrylics fragments
    Diethylhexyl phthalates fragments
    Isocyanate fragments
+ **Z18.3** **Retained organic fragments**
  Z18.31 **Retained animal quills or spines**
  Z18.32 **Retained tooth**
  Z18.33 **Retained wood fragments**
  Z18.39 **Other retained organic fragments**
+ **Z18.8** **Other specified retained foreign body**
  Z18.81 **Retained glass fragments**
  Z18.83 **Retained stone or crystalline fragments**
    Retained concrete or cement fragments

  Z18.89 **Other specified retained foreign body fragments**
    AHA CC: 3Q, 2016, 24
  Z18.9 **Retained foreign body fragments, unspecified material**

Hormone sensitivity malignancy status (Z19)

Z19 **Hormone sensitivity malignancy status**
  Code first malignant neoplasm - see Table of Neoplasms, by site, malignant
  Review coding guideline C.21.c.3
  AHA CC: 4Q, 2016, 76
  Z19.1 **Hormone sensitive malignancy status**
  Z19.2 **Hormone resistant malignancy status**
    Castrate resistant prostate malignancy status

Persons with potential health hazards related to communicable diseases (Z20-Z29)

Z20 **Contact with and (suspected) exposure to communicable diseases**
  Excludes1: *carrier of infectious disease (Z22.-)*
    diagnosed current infectious or parasitic disease -see Alphabetic Index
  Excludes2: *personal history of infectious and parasitic diseases (Z86.1-)*
  Review coding guideline C.21.c.1
+ **Z20.0** **Contact with and (suspected) exposure to intestinal infectious diseases**
  Z20.01 **Contact with and (suspected) exposure to intestinal infectious diseases due to Escherichia coli (E. coli)**
  Z20.09 **Contact with and (suspected) exposure to other intestinal infectious diseases**
  Z20.1 **Contact with and (suspected) exposure to tuberculosis**
  Z20.2 **Contact with and (suspected) exposure to infections with a predominantly sexual mode of transmission**
  Z20.3 **Contact with and (suspected) exposure to rabies**
  Z20.4 **Contact with and (suspected) exposure to rubella**
  Z20.5 **Contact with and (suspected) exposure to viral hepatitis**
  Z20.6 **Contact with and (suspected) exposure to human immunodeficiency virus [HIV]**
    Excludes1: *asymptomatic human immunodeficiency virus [HIV]*
      HIV infection status (Z21)
  Z20.7 **Contact with and (suspected) exposure to pediculosis, acariasis and other infestations**
+ **Z20.8** **Contact with and (suspected) exposure to other communicable diseases**
  + **Z20.81** **Contact with and (suspected) exposure to other bacterial communicable diseases**
    Z20.810 **Contact with and (suspected) exposure to anthrax**
    Z20.811 **Contact with and (suspected) exposure to meningococcus**
    Z20.818 **Contact with and (suspected) exposure to other bacterial communicable diseases**
      AHA CC: 2Q, 2019, 10-11
  + **Z20.82** **Contact with and (suspected) exposure to other viral communicable diseases**
    AHA CC: 4Q, 2018, 35
    Z20.820 **Contact with and (suspected) exposure to varicella**
    Z20.821 **Contact with and (suspected) exposure to Zika virus**
      Review coding guideline C.1.f
    Z20.828 **Contact with and (suspected) exposure to other viral communicable diseases**
      AHA CC: 4Q, 2016, 4-7; 1Q, 2020, 34-36; 2Q, 2020, 4-5, 8-9
      Review coding guidelines C.1.g.1.e and C.1.g.1.g
  Z20.89 **Contact with and (suspected) exposure to other communicable diseases**
  Z20.9 **Contact with and (suspected) exposure to unspecified communicable disease**

Z21 **Asymptomatic human immunodeficiency virus [HIV] infection status**

HIV positive NOS

Code first Human immunodeficiency virus [HIV] disease complicating pregnancy, childbirth and the puerperium, if applicable (O98.7-)

Excludes1: *acquired immunodeficiency syndrome (B20)*
contact with human immunodeficiency virus [HIV]
(Z20.6)
exposure to human immunodeficiency virus
[HIV] (Z20.6)
human immunodeficiency virus [HIV] disease (B20)
inconclusive laboratory evidence of human
immunodeficiency virus [HIV] (R75)

Review coding guidelines C.1.a.2.d, C.1.a.2.f and C.1.a.2.g
Review coding guideline C.15.f
Review coding guideline C.21.c.3
AHA CC: 1Q, 2019, 10-11
Valid 3-character code, no further characters required

Z22 **Carrier of infectious disease**

Includes: colonization status
suspected carrier

Excludes2: *carrier of viral hepatitis (B18.-)*
Review coding guideline C.21.c.3

Z22.0 **Carrier of typhoid**
Z22.1 **Carrier of other intestinal infectious diseases**
Z22.2 **Carrier of diphtheria**
+ **Z22.3** **Carrier of other specified bacterial diseases**
  Z22.31 **Carrier of bacterial disease due to meningococci**
+ **Z22.32** **Carrier of bacterial disease due to staphylococci**
  Z22.321 **Carrier or suspected carrier of Methicillin susceptible Staphylococcus aureus**
MSSA colonization
Review coding guidelines C.1.e.1.c and C.1.e.1.d
  Z22.322 **Carrier or suspected carrier of Methicillin resistant Staphylococcus aureus**
MRSA colonization
Review coding guidelines C.1.e.1.c and C.1.e.1.d
+ **Z22.33** **Carrier of bacterial disease due to streptococci**
  Z22.330 **Carrier of Group B streptococcus**
Excludes1: *carrier of streptococcus group B (GBS) complicating pregnancy, childbirth and the puerperium (O99.82-)*
  Z22.338 **Carrier of other streptococcus**
Z22.39 **Carrier of other specified bacterial diseases**
Z22.4 **Carrier of infections with a predominantly sexual mode of transmission**
Z22.6 **Carrier of human T-lymphotropic virus type-1 [HTLV-1] infection**
Z22.7 **Latent tuberculosis**
Latent tuberculosis infection (LTBI)
Excludes1: *nonspecific reaction to cell mediated immunity measurement of gamma interferon antigen response without active tuberculosis (R76.12)*
nonspecific reaction to tuberculin skin test without active tuberculosis (R76.11)
AHA CC: 4Q, 2019, 19
Z22.8 **Carrier of other infectious diseases**
Z22.9 **Carrier of infectious disease, unspecified**

Z23 **Encounter for immunization**

Code first any routine childhood examination
NOTE Procedure codes are required to identify the types of immunizations given
Review coding guideline C.21.c.2
Valid 3-character code, no further characters required

Z28 **Immunization not carried out and underimmunization status**

Includes: vaccination not carried out
+ **Z28.0** **Immunization not carried out because of contraindication**
  Z28.01 **Immunization not carried out because of acute illness of patient**
  Z28.02 **Immunization not carried out because of chronic illness or condition of patient**
  Z28.03 **Immunization not carried out because of immune compromised state of patient**
  Z28.04 **Immunization not carried out because of patient allergy to vaccine or component**
  Z28.09 **Immunization not carried out because of other contraindication**

Z28.1 **Immunization not carried out because of patient decision for reasons of belief or group pressure**
Immunization not carried out because of religious belief
+ **Z28.2** **Immunization not carried out because of patient decision for other and unspecified reason**
  Z28.20 **Immunization not carried out because of patient decision for unspecified reason**
  Z28.21 **Immunization not carried out because of patient refusal**
  Z28.29 **Immunization not carried out because of patient decision for other reason**
Z28.3 **Underimmunization status**
Delinquent immunization status
Lapsed immunization schedule status
Review coding guideline C.21.c.3
+ **Z28.8** **Immunization not carried out for other reason**
  Z28.81 **Immunization not carried out due to patient having had the disease**
  Z28.82 **Immunization not carried out because of caregiver refusal**
Immunization not carried out because of guardian refusal
Immunization not carried out because of parent refusal
Excludes1: *immunization not carried out because of caregiver refusal because of religious belief (Z28.1)*
  Z28.83 **Immunization not carried out due to unavailability of vaccine**
Delay in delivery of vaccine
Lack of availability of vaccine
Manufacturer delay of vaccine
AHA CC: 4Q, 2018, 36
  Z28.89 **Immunization not carried out for other reason**
Z28.9 **Immunization not carried out for unspecified reason**

Z29 **Encounter for other prophylactic measures**

Excludes1: *desensitization to allergens (Z51.6)*
prophylactic surgery (Z40.-)
Review coding guideline C.21.c.14
AHA CC: 4Q, 2016, 78-79
+ **Z29.1** **Encounter for prophylactic immunotherapy**
Encounter for administration of immunoglobulin
  Z29.11 **Encounter for prophylactic immunotherapy for respiratory syncytial virus (RSV)**
  Z29.12 **Encounter for prophylactic antivenin**
  Z29.13 **Encounter for prophylactic Rho(D) immune globulin**
AHA CC: 3Q, 2019,.5
  Z29.14 **Encounter for prophylactic rabies immune globin**
Z29.3 **Encounter for prophylactic fluoride administration**
Z29.8 **Encounter for other specified prophylactic measures**
Z29.9 **Encounter for prophylactic measures, unspecified**

Persons encountering health services in circumstances related to reproduction (Z30-Z39)

Z30 **Encounter for contraceptive management**

Review coding guideline C.21.c.11
AHA CC: 4Q, 2016, 78
+ **Z30.0** **Encounter for general counseling and advice on contraception**
Review coding guideline C.21.c.10
+ **Z30.01** **Encounter for initial prescription of contraceptives**
Excludes1: *encounter for surveillance of contraceptives (Z30.4-)*
♀ **Z30.011** **Encounter for initial prescription of contraceptive pills**
♀ **Z30.012** **Encounter for prescription of emergency contraception**
Encounter for postcoital contraception
♀ **Z30.013** **Encounter for initial prescription of injectable contraceptive**
♀ **Z30.014** **Encounter for initial prescription of intrauterine contraceptive device**
Excludes1: *encounter for insertion of intrauterine contraceptive device (Z30.430, Z30.432)*
♀ **Z30.015** **Encounter for initial prescription of vaginal ring hormonal contraceptive**

Z30.016 Encounter for initial prescription of transdermal patch hormonal contraceptive device

Z30.017 Encounter for initial prescription of implantable subdermal contraceptive

♀ **Z30.018** Encounter for initial prescription of other contraceptives

Encounter for initial prescription of barrier contraception

Encounter for initial prescription of diaphragm

♀ **Z30.019** Encounter for initial prescription of contraceptives, unspecified

Z30.02 Counseling and instruction in natural family planning to avoid pregnancy

Z30.09 Encounter for other general counseling and advice on contraception

Encounter for family planning advice NOS

Z30.2 Encounter for sterilization

+ **Z30.4** Encounter for surveillance of contraceptives

Z30.40 Encounter for surveillance of contraceptives, unspecified

♀ **Z30.41** Encounter for surveillance of contraceptive pills

Encounter for repeat prescription for contraceptive pill

♀ **Z30.42** Encounter for surveillance of injectable contraceptive

+ **Z30.43** Encounter for surveillance of intrauterine contraceptive device

♀ **Z30.430** Encounter for insertion of intrauterine contraceptive device

♀ **Z30.431** Encounter for routine checking of intrauterine contraceptive device

♀ **Z30.432** Encounter for removal of intrauterine contraceptive device

♀ **Z30.433** Encounter for removal and reinsertion of intrauterine contraceptive device

Encounter for replacement of intrauterine contraceptive device

♀ **Z30.44** Encounter for surveillance of vaginal ring hormonal contraceptive device

♀ **Z30.45** Encounter for surveillance of transdermal patch hormonal contraceptive device

♀ **Z30.46** Encounter for surveillance of implantable subdermal contraceptive

Encounter for checking, reinsertion or removal of implantable subdermal contraceptive

♀ **Z30.49** Encounter for surveillance of other contraceptives

Encounter for surveillance of barrier contraception

Encounter for surveillance of diaphragm

Z30.8 Encounter for other contraceptive management

Encounter for postvasectomy sperm count

Encounter for routine examination for contraceptive maintenance

Excludes1: *sperm count following sterilization reversal (Z31.42)*

sperm count for fertility testing (Z31.41)

Z30.9 Encounter for contraceptive management, unspecified

Z31 Encounter for procreative management

Excludes1: *complications associated with artificial fertilization (N98.-)*

female infertility (N97.-)

male infertility (N46.-)

Review coding guideline C.21.c.11

Z31.0 Encounter for reversal of previous sterilization

+ **Z31.4** Encounter for procreative investigation and testing

Excludes1: *postvasectomy sperm count (Z30.8)*

Z31.41 Encounter for fertility testing

Encounter for fallopian tube patency testing

Encounter for sperm count for fertility testing

Z31.42 Aftercare following sterilization reversal

Sperm count following sterilization reversal

+ **Z31.43** Encounter for genetic testing of female for procreative management

Use additional code for recurrent pregnancy loss, if applicable (N96, O26.2-)

Excludes1: *nonprocreative genetic testing (Z13.7-)*

♀ **Z31.430** Encounter of female for testing for genetic disease carrier status for procreative management

♀ **Z31.438** Encounter for other genetic testing of female for procreative management

+ **Z31.44** Encounter for genetic testing of male for procreative management

Excludes1: *nonprocreative genetic testing (Z13.7-)*

♂ **Z31.440** Encounter of male for testing for genetic disease carrier status for procreative management

● ♂ **Z31.441** Encounter for testing of male partner of patient with recurrent pregnancy loss

● ♂ **Z31.448** Encounter for other genetic testing of male for procreative management

Z31.49 Encounter for other procreative investigation and testing

Z31.5 Encounter for procreative genetic counseling

AHA CC: 4Q, 2017, 27

Review coding guideline C.21.c.10

+ **Z31.6** Encounter for general counseling and advice on procreation

Review coding guideline C.21.c.10

Z31.61 Procreative counseling and advice using natural family planning

Z31.62 Encounter for fertility preservation counseling

Encounter for fertility preservation counseling prior to cancer therapy

Encounter for fertility preservation counseling prior to surgical removal of gonads

Z31.69 Encounter for other general counseling and advice on procreation

♀ **Z31.7** Encounter for procreative management and counseling for gestational carrier

Excludes1: *pregnant state, gestational carrier (Z33.3)*

AHA CC: 4Q, 2016, 78

+ **Z31.8** Encounter for other procreative management

♀ **Z31.81** Encounter for male factor infertility in female patient

Review coding guideline C.21.c.16

♀ **Z31.82** Encounter for Rh incompatibility status

Review coding guideline C.21.c.16

AHA CC: 4Q, 2014, 17

♀ **Z31.83** Encounter for assisted reproductive fertility procedure cycle

Patient undergoing in vitro fertilization cycle

Use additional code to identify the type of infertility

Excludes1: *pre-cycle diagnosis and testing - code to reason for encounter*

Review coding guideline C.21.c.16

Z31.84 Encounter for fertility preservation procedure

Encounter for fertility preservation procedure prior to cancer therapy

Encounter for fertility preservation procedure prior to surgical removal of gonads

Review coding guideline C.21.c.16

Z31.89 Encounter for other procreative management

Z31.9 Encounter for procreative management, unspecified

Z32 Encounter for pregnancy test and childbirth and childcare instruction

+ **Z32.0** Encounter for pregnancy test

Review coding guideline C.21.c.13

♀ **Z32.00** Encounter for pregnancy test, result unknown

Encounter for pregnancy test NOS

● ♀ **Z32.01** Encounter for pregnancy test, result positive

♀ **Z32.02** Encounter for pregnancy test, result negative

Z32.2 Encounter for childbirth instruction

Review coding guidelines C.21.c.10 and C.21.c.11

Z32.3 Encounter for childcare instruction

Encounter for prenatal or postpartum childcare instruction

Review coding guidelines C.21.c.10 and C.21.c.11

Z33 Pregnant state

Review coding guideline C.21.c.11

AHA CC: 4Q, 2016, 78

● ♀ **Z33.1** Pregnant state, incidental

Pregnancy NOS

Pregnant state NOS

Excludes1: *complications of pregnancy (O00-O9A)*

pregnant state, gestational carrier (Z33.3)

Review coding guideline C.15.a.1

Review coding guidelines C.21.c.3

● ♀ **Z33.2** Encounter for elective termination of pregnancy

Excludes1: *early fetal death with retention of dead fetus (O02.1)*

late fetal death (O36.4)

spontaneous abortion (O03)

Review coding guidelines C.15.q.1 and C.15.q.2

Review coding guidelines C.21.c.16

+, +7th, X + 7th   ● Newborn   ● Pediatric   ● Maternity   ● Adult   ♀ Female   ♂ Male   Manifestation   Unacceptable PDX   HCC   CC   MCC   HAC

- ● ♀ **Z33.3** **Pregnant state, gestational carrier**
  - **Excludes1:** *encounter for procreative management and counseling for gestational carrier (Z31.7)*

Z34 **Encounter for supervision of normal pregnancy**

  - **Excludes1:** *any complication of pregnancy (O00-O9A)*
    encounter for pregnancy test (Z32.0-)
    encounter for supervision of high risk pregnancy (O09.-)
  - *Review coding guideline C.15.b.1*
  - *Review coding guidelines C.21.c.11 and C.21.c.16*
  - *AHA CC: 4Q, 2016, 4-7*
  - + **Z34.0** **Encounter for supervision of normal first pregnancy**
    - ● ♀ **Z34.00** **Encounter for supervision of normal first pregnancy, unspecified trimester**
    - ● ♀ **Z34.01** **Encounter for supervision of normal first pregnancy, first trimester**
    - ● ♀ **Z34.02** **Encounter for supervision of normal first pregnancy, second trimester**
    - ● ♀ **Z34.03** **Encounter for supervision of normal first pregnancy, third trimester**
  - + **Z34.8** **Encounter for supervision of other normal pregnancy**
    - ● ♀ **Z34.80** **Encounter for supervision of other normal pregnancy, unspecified trimester**
    - ● ♀ **Z34.81** **Encounter for supervision of other normal pregnancy, first trimester**
    - ● ♀ **Z34.82** **Encounter for supervision of other normal pregnancy, second trimester**
    - ● ♀ **Z34.83** **Encounter for supervision of other normal pregnancy, third trimester**
    - *AHA CC: 4Q, 2014, 17*
  - + **Z34.9** **Encounter for supervision of normal pregnancy, unspecified**
    - ● ♀ **Z34.90** **Encounter for supervision of normal pregnancy, unspecified, unspecified trimester**
    - ● ♀ **Z34.91** **Encounter for supervision of normal pregnancy, unspecified, first trimester**
    - ● ♀ **Z34.92** **Encounter for supervision of normal pregnancy, unspecified, second trimester**
    - ● ♀ **Z34.93** **Encounter for supervision of normal pregnancy, unspecified, third trimester**

Z36 **Encounter for antenatal screening of mother**

  - **Includes:** Encounter for placental sample (taken vaginally)
    Screening is the testing for disease or disease precursors in asymptomatic individuals so that early detection and treatment can be provided for those who test positive for the disease.
  - **Excludes1:** *diagnostic examination- code to sign or symptom*
    encounter for suspected maternal and fetal conditions ruled out (Z03.7-)
    suspected fetal condition affecting management of pregnancy - code to condition in Chapter 15
  - **Excludes2:** *abnormal findings on antenatal screening of mother (O28.-)*
    genetic counseling and testing (Z31.43-, Z31.5)
    routine prenatal care (Z34)
  - *AHA CC: 4Q, 2017, 28*
  - *Review coding guidelines C.21.c.5 and C.21.c.11*
  - ● ♀ **Z36.0** **Encounter for antenatal screening for chromosomal anomalies**
  - ● ♀ **Z36.1** **Encounter for antenatal screening for raised alphafetoprotein level**
    Encounter for antenatal screening for elevated maternal serum alphafetoprotein level
  - ● ♀ **Z36.2** **Encounter for other antenatal screening follow-up**
    Non-visualized anatomy on a previous scan
  - ● ♀ **Z36.3** **Encounter for antenatal screening for malformations**
    Screening for suspected anomaly
  - ● ♀ **Z36.4** **Encounter for antenatal screening for fetal growth retardation**
    Intrauterine growth restriction (IUGR)/small-for-dates
  - ● ♀ **Z36.5** **Encounter for antenatal screening for isoimmunization**
  - + **Z36.8** **Encounter for other antenatal screening**
    - ● ♀ **Z36.81** **Encounter for antenatal screening for hydrops fetalis**
    - ● ♀ **Z36.82** **Encounter for antenatal screening for nuchal translucency**
    - ● ♀ **Z36.83** **Encounter for antenatal screening for congenital cardiac abnormalities**
    - ● ♀ **Z36.84** **Encounter for antenatal screening for fetal lung maturity**
    - ● ♀ **Z36.85** **Encounter for antenatal screening for Streptococcus B**
    - ● ♀ **Z36.86** **Encounter for antenatal screening for for cervical length**
      Screening for risk of pre-term labor
    - ● ♀ **Z36.87** **Encounter for antenatal screening for uncertain dates**
    - ● ♀ **Z36.88** **Encounter for antenatal screening for fetal macrosomia**
      Screening for large-for-dates
    - ● ♀ **Z36.89** **Encounter for other specified antenatal screening**
    - ● ♀ **Z36.8A** **Encounter for antenatal screening for other genetic defects**
  - ● ♀ **Z36.9** **Encounter for antenatal screening, unspecified**

Z3A **Weeks of gestation**

  - **NOTE** Codes from category Z3A are for use, only on the maternal record, to indicate the weeks of gestation of the pregnancy, if known.
  - Code first complications of pregnancy, childbirth and the puerperium (O09-O9A)
  - *Review coding guideline C.21.c.11*
  - + **Z3A.0** **Weeks of gestation of pregnancy, unspecified or less than 10 weeks**
    - ● ♀ **Z3A.00** **Weeks of gestation of pregnancy not specified**
    - ● ♀ **Z3A.01** **Less than 8 weeks gestation of pregnancy**
    - ● ♀ **Z3A.08** **8 weeks gestation of pregnancy**
    - ● ♀ **Z3A.09** **9 weeks gestation of pregnancy**
  - + **Z3A.1** **Weeks of gestation of pregnancy, weeks 10-19**
    - ● ♀ **Z3A.10** **10 weeks gestation of pregnancy**
    - ● ♀ **Z3A.11** **11 weeks gestation of pregnancy**
    - ● ♀ **Z3A.12** **12 weeks gestation of pregnancy**
    - ● ♀ **Z3A.13** **13 weeks gestation of pregnancy**
    - ● ♀ **Z3A.14** **14 weeks gestation of pregnancy**
    - ● ♀ **Z3A.15** **15 weeks gestation of pregnancy**
    - ● ♀ **Z3A.16** **16 weeks gestation of pregnancy**
      AHA CC: 4Q, 2016, 4-7
    - ● ♀ **Z3A.17** **17 weeks gestation of pregnancy**
    - ● ♀ **Z3A.18** **18 weeks gestation of pregnancy**
      AHA CC: 2Q, 2019, 11
    - ● ♀ **Z3A.19** **19 weeks gestation of pregnancy**
  - + **Z3A.2** **Weeks of gestation of pregnancy, weeks 20-29**
    - ● ♀ **Z3A.20** **20 weeks gestation of pregnancy**
      AHA CC: 4Q, 2016, 4-7
    - ● ♀ **Z3A.21** **21 weeks gestation of pregnancy**
    - ● ♀ **Z3A.22** **22 weeks gestation of pregnancy**
      AHA CC: 4Q, 2016, 4-7
    - ● ♀ **Z3A.23** **23 weeks gestation of pregnancy**
    - ● ♀ **Z3A.24** **24 weeks gestation of pregnancy**
    - ● ♀ **Z3A.25** **25 weeks gestation of pregnancy**
    - ● ♀ **Z3A.26** **26 weeks gestation of pregnancy**
    - ● ♀ **Z3A.27** **27 weeks gestation of pregnancy**
    - ● ♀ **Z3A.28** **28 weeks gestation of pregnancy**
    - ● ♀ **Z3A.29** **29 weeks gestation of pregnancy**
  - + **Z3A.3** **Weeks of gestation of pregnancy, weeks 30-39**
    - ● ♀ **Z3A.30** **30 weeks gestation of pregnancy**
    - ● ♀ **Z3A.31** **31 weeks gestation of pregnancy**
    - ● ♀ **Z3A.32** **32 weeks gestation of pregnancy**
      AHA CC: 4Q, 2016, 4-7
    - ● ♀ **Z3A.33** **33 weeks gestation of pregnancy**
    - ● ♀ **Z3A.34** **34 weeks gestation of pregnancy**
    - ● ♀ **Z3A.35** **35 weeks gestation of pregnancy**
    - ● ♀ **Z3A.36** **36 weeks gestation of pregnancy**
    - ● ♀ **Z3A.37** **37 weeks gestation of pregnancy**
    - ● ♀ **Z3A.38** **38 weeks gestation of pregnancy**
      AHA CC: 2Q, 2016, 34
    - ● ♀ **Z3A.39** **39 weeks gestation of pregnancy**
  - + **Z3A.4** **Weeks of gestation of pregnancy, weeks 40 or greater**
    - ● ♀ **Z3A.40** **40 weeks gestation of pregnancy**
      AHA CC: 2Q, 2014, 9
    - ● ♀ **Z3A.41** **41 weeks gestation of pregnancy**
    - ● ♀ **Z3A.42** **42 weeks gestation of pregnancy**
      AHA CC: 4Q, 2014, 23
    - ● ♀ **Z3A.49** **Greater than 42 weeks gestation of pregnancy**

Z37 **Outcome of delivery**

  - This category is intended for use as an additional code to identify the outcome of delivery on the mother's record. It is not for use on the newborn record.
  - **Excludes1:** *stillbirth (P95)*
  - *Review coding guidelines C.15.b.5*
  - *Review coding guidelines C.15.n.3 and C.15.q.1*
  - *Review coding guidelines C.21.c.11*

+, +7th, X + 7th　● Newborn　● Pediatric　● Maternity　● Adult　♀ Female　♂ Male　Manifestation　Unacceptable PDX　HCC　CC　MCC　HAC

● ♀ **Z37.0** **Single live birth**
AHA CC: 2Q, 2014, 9; 4Q, 2014, 17-18; 2Q, 2016, 34

● ♀ **Z37.1** **Single stillbirth**

● ♀ **Z37.2** **Twins, both liveborn**

● ♀ **Z37.3** **Twins, one liveborn and one stillborn**

● ♀ **Z37.4** **Twins, both stillborn**

+ **Z37.5** **Other multiple births, all liveborn**

● ♀ **Z37.50** **Multiple births, unspecified, all liveborn**

● ♀ **Z37.51** **Triplets, all liveborn**

● ♀ **Z37.52** **Quadruplets, all liveborn**

● ♀ **Z37.53** **Quintuplets, all liveborn**

● ♀ **Z37.54** **Sextuplets, all liveborn**

● ♀ **Z37.59** **Other multiple births, all liveborn**

+ **Z37.6** **Other multiple births, some liveborn**

● ♀ **Z37.60** **Multiple births, unspecified, some liveborn**

● ♀ **Z37.61** **Triplets, some liveborn**

● ♀ **Z37.62** **Quadruplets, some liveborn**

● ♀ **Z37.63** **Quintuplets, some liveborn**

● ♀ **Z37.64** **Sextuplets, some liveborn**

● ♀ **Z37.69** **Other multiple births, some liveborn**

● ♀ **Z37.7** **Other multiple births, all stillborn**

● ♀ **Z37.9** **Outcome of delivery, unspecified**
Multiple birth NOS
Single birth NOS

Z38 **Liveborn infants according to place of birth and type of delivery**

This category is for use as the principal code on the initial record of a newborn baby. It is to be used for the initial birth record only. It is not to be used on the mother's record.
Review coding guideline C.16.a.2 and C.16.h
Review coding guideline C.17
Review coding guidelines C.21.c.6, C.21.c.12 and C.21.c.16
AHA CC: 2Q, 2015, 15; 4Q, 2016, 4-7, 54-55; 2Q, 2020, 13

+ **Z38.0** **Single liveborn infant, born in hospital**
Single liveborn infant, born in birthing center or other health care facility
AHA CC: 2Q, 2017, 5-7

● **Z38.00** **Single liveborn infant, delivered vaginally**
AHA CC: 4Q, 2018, 26

● **Z38.01** **Single liveborn infant, delivered by cesarean**
AHA CC: 3Q, 2016, 18

● **Z38.1** **Single liveborn infant, born outside hospital**

● **Z38.2** **Single liveborn infant, unspecified as to place of birth**
Single liveborn infant NOS

+ **Z38.3** **Twin liveborn infant, born in hospital**

● **Z38.30** **Twin liveborn infant, delivered vaginally**

● **Z38.31** **Twin liveborn infant, delivered by cesarean**

● **Z38.4** **Twin liveborn infant, born outside hospital**

● **Z38.5** **Twin liveborn infant, unspecified as to place of birth**

+ **Z38.6** **Other multiple liveborn infant, born in hospital**

● **Z38.61** **Triplet liveborn infant, delivered vaginally**

● **Z38.62** **Triplet liveborn infant, delivered by cesarean**

● **Z38.63** **Quadruplet liveborn infant, delivered vaginally**

● **Z38.64** **Quadruplet liveborn infant, delivered by cesarean**

● **Z38.65** **Quintuplet liveborn infant, delivered vaginally**

● **Z38.66** **Quintuplet liveborn infant, delivered by cesarean**

● **Z38.68** **Other multiple liveborn infant, delivered vaginally**

● **Z38.69** **Other multiple liveborn infant, delivered by cesarean**

● **Z38.7** **Other multiple liveborn infant, born outside hospital**

● **Z38.8** **Other multiple liveborn infant, unspecified as to place of birth**

Z39 **Encounter for maternal postpartum care and examination**
Review coding guidelines C.21.c.8, C.21.c.11 and C.21.c.16

● ♀ **Z39.0** **Encounter for care and examination of mother immediately after delivery**
Care and observation in uncomplicated cases when the delivery occurs outside a healthcare facility
Excludes1: *care for postpartum complication- see Alphabetic index*
Review coding guideline C.15.o.4

● ♀ **Z39.1** **Encounter for care and examination of lactating mother**
Encounter for supervision of lactation
Excludes1: *disorders of lactation (O92.-)*

● ♀ **Z39.2** **Encounter for routine postpartum follow-up**

Encounters for other specific health care (Z40-Z53)

Categories Z40-Z53 are intended for use to indicate a reason for care. They may be used for patients who have already been treated for a disease or injury, but who are receiving aftercare or prophylactic care, or care to consolidate the treatment, or to deal with a residual state

Excludes2: *follow-up examination for medical surveillance after treatment (Z08-Z09)*

Z40 **Encounter for prophylactic surgery**

Excludes1: *organ donations (Z52.-)*
therapeutic organ removal-code to condition
Review coding guideline C.21.c.14 and C.21.c.16

+ **Z40.0** **Encounter for prophylactic surgery for risk factors related to malignant neoplasms**
Admission for prophylactic organ removal
Use additional code to identify risk factor

Z40.00 **Encounter for prophylactic removal of unspecified organ**

Z40.01 **Encounter for prophylactic removal of breast**

♀ **Z40.02** **Encounter for prophylactic removal of ovary(s)**
Encounter for prophylactic removal of ovary(s) and fallopian tube(s)

♀ **Z40.03** **Encounter for prophylactic removal of fallopian tube(s)**
AHA CC: 4Q, 2017, 28

Z40.09 **Encounter for prophylactic removal of other organ**

Z40.8 **Encounter for other prophylactic surgery**

Z40.9 **Encounter for prophylactic surgery, unspecified**

Z41 **Encounter for procedures for purposes other than remedying health state**

Z41.1 **Encounter for cosmetic surgery**
Encounter for cosmetic breast implant
Encounter for cosmetic procedure
Excludes1: *encounter for plastic and reconstructive surgery following medical procedure or healed injury (Z42.-)*
encounter for post-mastectomy breast implantation (Z42.1)

♂ **Z41.2** **Encounter for routine and ritual male circumcision**
AHA CC: 3Q, 2018, 15

Z41.3 **Encounter for ear piercing**

Z41.8 **Encounter for other procedures for purposes other than remedying health state**

Z41.9 **Encounter for procedure for purposes other than remedying health state, unspecified**

Z42 **Encounter for plastic and reconstructive surgery following medical procedure or healed injury**

Excludes1: *encounter for cosmetic plastic surgery (Z41.1)*
encounter for plastic surgery for treatment of current injury - code to relevent injury
Review coding guidelines C.21.c.7 and C.21.c.16

● **Z42.1** **Encounter for breast reconstruction following mastectomy**
Excludes1: *deformity and disproportion of reconstructed breast (N65.1-)*

Z42.8 **Encounter for other plastic and reconstructive surgery following medical procedure or healed injury**
AHA CC: 1Q, 2017, 42-43

Z43 **Encounter for attention to artificial openings**

Includes: closure of artificial openings
passage of sounds or bougies through artificial openings
reforming artificial openings
removal of catheter from artificial openings
toilet or cleansing of artificial openings
Excludes1: *complications of external stoma (J95.0-, K94.-, N99.5-)*
Excludes2: *fitting and adjustment of prosthetic and other devices (Z44-Z46)*
Review coding guideline C.21.c.7

Z43.0 **Encounter for attention to tracheostomy**

CC **Z43.1** **Encounter for attention to gastrostomy**
Excludes2: *artificial opening status only, without need for care (Z93.-)*

Z43.2 **Encounter for attention to ileostomy**
AHA CC: 3Q, 2016, 5

Z43.3 **Encounter for attention to colostomy**

Z43.4 **Encounter for attention to other artificial openings of digestive tract**

Z43.5 Encounter for attention to cystostomy

Z43.6 Encounter for attention to other artificial openings of urinary tract

Encounter for attention to nephrostomy

Encounter for attention to ureterostomy

Encounter for attention to urethrostomy

Z43.7 Encounter for attention to artificial vagina

Z43.8 Encounter for attention to other artificial openings

Z43.9 Encounter for attention to unspecified artificial opening

Z44 **Encounter for fitting and adjustment of external prosthetic device**

Includes: removal or replacement of external prosthetic device

Excludes1: *malfunction or other complications of device - see Alphabetical Index*

presence of prosthetic device (Z97.-)

Review coding guideline C.21.c.7

+ **Z44.0** **Encounter for fitting and adjustment of artificial arm**

+ **Z44.00** Encounter for fitting and adjustment of unspecified artificial arm

Z44.001 Encounter for fitting and adjustment of unspecified right artificial arm

Z44.002 Encounter for fitting and adjustment of unspecified left artificial arm

Z44.009 Encounter for fitting and adjustment of unspecified artificial arm, unspecified arm

+ **Z44.01** Encounter for fitting and adjustment of complete artificial arm

Z44.011 Encounter for fitting and adjustment of complete right artificial arm

Z44.012 Encounter for fitting and adjustment of complete left artificial arm

Z44.019 Encounter for fitting and adjustment of complete artificial arm, unspecified arm

+ **Z44.02** Encounter for fitting and adjustment of partial artificial arm

Z44.021 Encounter for fitting and adjustment of partial artificial right arm

Z44.022 Encounter for fitting and adjustment of partial artificial left arm

Z44.029 Encounter for fitting and adjustment of partial artificial arm, unspecified arm

+ **Z44.1** **Encounter for fitting and adjustment of artificial leg**

+ **Z44.10** Encounter for fitting and adjustment of unspecified artificial leg

Z44.101 Encounter for fitting and adjustment of unspecified right artificial leg

Z44.102 Encounter for fitting and adjustment of unspecified left artificial leg

Z44.109 Encounter for fitting and adjustment of unspecified artificial leg, unspecified leg

+ **Z44.11** Encounter for fitting and adjustment of complete artificial leg

Z44.111 Encounter for fitting and adjustment of complete right artificial leg

Z44.112 Encounter for fitting and adjustment of complete left artificial leg

Z44.119 Encounter for fitting and adjustment of complete artificial leg, unspecified leg

+ **Z44.12** Encounter for fitting and adjustment of partial artificial leg

Z44.121 Encounter for fitting and adjustment of partial artificial right leg

Z44.122 Encounter for fitting and adjustment of partial artificial left leg

Z44.129 Encounter for fitting and adjustment of partial artificial leg, unspecified leg

+ **Z44.2** **Encounter for fitting and adjustment of artificial eye**

Excludes1: *mechanical complication of ocular prosthesis (T85.3)*

Z44.20 Encounter for fitting and adjustment of artificial eye, unspecified

Z44.21 Encounter for fitting and adjustment of artificial right eye

Z44.22 Encounter for fitting and adjustment of artificial left eye

+ **Z44.3** Encounter for fitting and adjustment of external breast prosthesis

Excludes1: *complications of breast implant (T85.4-)*

encounter for adjustment or removal of breast implant (Z45.81-)

encounter for initial breast implant insertion for cosmetic breast augmentation (Z41.1)

encounter for breast reconstruction following mastectomy (Z42.1)

Z44.30 Encounter for fitting and adjustment of external breast prosthesis, unspecified breast

Z44.31 Encounter for fitting and adjustment of external right breast prosthesis

Z44.32 Encounter for fitting and adjustment of external left breast prosthesis

Z44.8 Encounter for fitting and adjustment of other external prosthetic devices

Z44.9 Encounter for fitting and adjustment of unspecified external prosthetic device

Z45 **Encounter for adjustment and management of implanted device**

Includes: removal or replacement of implanted device

Excludes1: *malfunction or other complications of device - see Alphabetical Index*

Excludes2: *encounter for fitting and adjustment of non-implanted device (Z46.-)*

Review coding guideline C.21.c.7

+ **Z45.0** **Encounter for adjustment and management of cardiac device**

+ **Z45.01** Encounter for adjustment and management of cardiac pacemaker

Encounter for adjustment and management of cardiac resynchronization therapy pacemaker (CRT-P)

Excludes1: *encounter for adjustment and management of automatic implantable cardiac defibrillator with synchronous cardiac pacemaker (Z45.02)*

Z45.010 Encounter for checking and testing of cardiac pacemaker pulse generator [battery]

Encounter for replacing cardiac pacemaker pulse generator [battery]

Z45.018 Encounter for adjustment and management of other part of cardiac pacemaker

Excludes1: *presence of other part of cardiac pacemaker (Z95.0)*

Excludes2: *presence of prosthetic and other devices (Z95.1-Z95.5, Z95.811-Z97)*

Z45.02 Encounter for adjustment and management of automatic implantable cardiac defibrillator

Encounter for adjustment and management of automatic implantable cardiac defibrillator with synchronous cardiac pacemaker

Encounter for adjustment and management of cardiac resynchronization therapy defibrillator (CRT-D)

Z45.09 Encounter for adjustment and management of other cardiac device

Z45.1 Encounter for adjustment and management of infusion pump

Z45.2 Encounter for adjustment and management of vascular access device

Encounter for adjustment and management of vascular catheters

Excludes1: *encounter for adjustment and management of renal dialysis catheter (Z49.01)*

AHA CC: 3Q, 2018, 20-21; 2Q, 2020, 21-22

+ **Z45.3** **Encounter for adjustment and management of implanted devices of the special senses**
    Z45.31 **Encounter for adjustment and management of implanted visual substitution device**
+   **Z45.32** **Encounter for adjustment and management of implanted hearing device**
      Excludes1: *Encounter for fitting and adjustment of hearing aide (Z46.1)*
      Z45.320 **Encounter for adjustment and management of bone conduction device**
      Z45.321 **Encounter for adjustment and management of cochlear device**
      Z45.328 **Encounter for adjustment and management of other implanted hearing device**
+ **Z45.4** **Encounter for adjustment and management of implanted nervous system device**
    Z45.41 **Encounter for adjustment and management of cerebrospinal fluid drainage device**
      Encounter for adjustment and management of cerebral ventricular (communicating) shunt
    Z45.42 **Encounter for adjustment and management of neurostimulator**
      Encounter for adjustment and management of brain neurostimulator
      Encounter for adjustment and management of gastric neurostimulator
      Encounter for adjustment and management of peripheral nerve neurostimulator
      Encounter for adjustment and management of sacral nerve neurostimulator
      Encounter for adjustment and management of spinal cord neurostimulator
      Encounter for adjustment and management of vagus nerve neurostimulator
    Z45.49 **Encounter for adjustment and management of other implanted nervous system device**
      AHA CC: 3Q, 2014, 19-20
+ **Z45.8** **Encounter for adjustment and management of other implanted devices**
+   **Z45.81** **Encounter for adjustment or removal of breast implant**
      Encounter for elective implant exchange (different material) (different size)
      Encounter removal of tissue expander with or without synchronous insertion of permanent implant
      Excludes1: *complications of breast implant (T85.4-)*
      encounter for initial breast implant insertion for cosmetic breast augmentation (Z41.1)
      encounter for breast reconstruction following mastectomy (Z42.1)
      Z45.811 **Encounter for adjustment or removal of right breast implant**
      Z45.812 **Encounter for adjustment or removal of left breast implant**
      Z45.819 **Encounter for adjustment or removal of unspecified breast implant**
    Z45.82 **Encounter for adjustment or removal of myringotomy device (stent) (tube)**
    Z45.89 **Encounter for adjustment and management of other implanted devices**
      AHA CC: 4Q, 2014, 26-28
Z45.9 **Encounter for adjustment and management of unspecified implanted device**

Z46 **Encounter for fitting and adjustment of other devices**
    Includes: removal or replacement of other device
    Excludes1: *malfunction or other complications of device - see Alphabetical Index*
    Excludes2: *encounter for fitting and management of implanted devices (Z45.-)*
    issue of repeat prescription only (Z76.0)
    presence of prosthetic and other devices (Z95-Z97)
    Review coding guideline C.21.c.7
Z46.0 **Encounter for fitting and adjustment of spectacles and contact lenses**
Z46.1 **Encounter for fitting and adjustment of hearing aid**
    Excludes1: *encounter for adjustment and management of implanted hearing device (Z45.32-)*

Z46.2 **Encounter for fitting and adjustment of other devices related to nervous system and special senses**
    Excludes2: *encounter for adjustment and management of implanted nervous system device (Z45.4-)*
    encounter for adjustment and management of implanted visual substitution device (Z45.31)
Z46.3 **Encounter for fitting and adjustment of dental prosthetic device**
    Encounter for fitting and adjustment of dentures
Z46.4 **Encounter for fitting and adjustment of orthodontic device**
+ **Z46.5** **Encounter for fitting and adjustment of other gastrointestinal appliance and device**
    Excludes1: *encounter for attention to artificial openings of digestive tract (Z43.1-Z43.4)*
    Z46.51 **Encounter for fitting and adjustment of gastric lap band**
    Z46.59 **Encounter for fitting and adjustment of other gastrointestinal appliance and device**
Z46.6 **Encounter for fitting and adjustment of urinary device**
    Excludes2: *attention to artificial openings of urinary tract (Z43.5, Z43.6)*
+ **Z46.8** **Encounter for fitting and adjustment of other specified devices**
    Z46.81 **Encounter for fitting and adjustment of insulin pump**
      Encounter for insulin pump titration
      Encounter for insulin pump instruction and training
    Z46.82 **Encounter for fitting and adjustment of non-vascular catheter**
    Z46.89 **Encounter for fitting and adjustment of other specified devices**
      Encounter for fitting and adjustment of wheelchair
Z46.9 **Encounter for fitting and adjustment of unspecified device**

Z47 **Orthopedic aftercare**
    Excludes1: *aftercare for healing fracture-code to fracture with 7th character D*
    Review coding guideline C.21.c.7
Z47.1 **Aftercare following joint replacement surgery**
    Use additional code to identify the joint (Z96.6-)
    AHA CC: 1Q, 2020, 23-24
Z47.2 **Encounter for removal of internal fixation device**
    Excludes1: *encounter for adjustment of internal fixation device for fracture treatment- code to fracture with appropriate 7th character*
    encounter for removal of external fixation device- code to fracture with 7th character D
    infection or inflammatory reaction to internal fixation device (T84.6-)
    mechanical complication of internal fixation device (T84.1-)
+ **Z47.3** **Aftercare following explantation of joint prosthesis**
    Aftercare following explantation of joint prosthesis, staged procedure
    Encounter for joint prosthesis insertion following prior explantation of joint prosthesis
    AHA CC: 1Q, 2020, 23-24
    Z47.31 **Aftercare following explantation of shoulder joint prosthesis**
      Excludes1: *acquired absence of shoulder joint following prior explantation of shoulder joint prosthesis (Z89.23-)*
      shoulder joint prosthesis explantation status (Z89.23-)
    Z47.32 **Aftercare following explantation of hip joint prosthesis**
      Excludes1: *acquired absence of hip joint following prior explantation of hip joint prosthesis (Z89.62-)*
      hip joint prosthesis explantation status (Z89.62-)
      AHA CC: 1Q, 2015, 16-17
    Z47.33 **Aftercare following explantation of knee joint prosthesis**
      Excludes1: *acquired absence of knee joint following prior explantation of knee prosthesis (Z89.52-*
      knee joint prosthesis explantation status (Z89.52-)

+, +7th, X + 7th   ● Newborn   ● Pediatric   ● Maternity   ● Adult   ♀ Female   ♂ Male   Manifestation   Unacceptable PDX   HCC   CC   MCC   HAC

+ **Z47.8** **Encounter for other orthopedic aftercare**

    Z47.81 **Encounter for orthopedic aftercare following surgical amputation**

        Use additional code to identify the limb amputated (Z89.-)

    Z47.82 **Encounter for orthopedic aftercare following scoliosis surgery**

    Z47.89 **Encounter for other orthopedic aftercare**

Z48 **Encounter for other postprocedural aftercare**

    Excludes1: *encounter for aftercare following injury - code to Injury, by site, with appropriate 7th character for subsequent encounter*

    encounter for follow-up examination after completed treatment (Z08-Z09)

    Excludes2: *encounter for attention to artificial openings (Z43.-)*

    encounter for fitting and adjustment of prosthetic and other devices (Z44-Z46)

    Review coding guideline C.21.c.7

+ **Z48.0** **Encounter for attention to dressings, sutures and drains**

    Excludes1: *encounter for planned postprocedural wound closure (Z48.1)*

    Z48.00 **Encounter for change or removal of nonsurgical wound dressing**

        Encounter for change or removal of wound dressing NOS

    Z48.01 **Encounter for change or removal of surgical wound dressing**

        AHA CC: 4Q, 2015, 38; 2Q, 2019, 33

    Z48.02 **Encounter for removal of sutures**

        Encounter for removal of staples

    Z48.03 **Encounter for change or removal of drains**

Z48.1 **Encounter for planned postprocedural wound closure**

    Excludes1: *encounter for attention to dressings and sutures (Z48.0-)*

+ **Z48.2** **Encounter for aftercare following organ transplant**

  CC **Z48.21** **Encounter for aftercare following heart transplant**

  CC **Z48.22** **Encounter for aftercare following kidney transplant**

  CC **Z48.23** **Encounter for aftercare following liver transplant**

  CC **Z48.24** **Encounter for aftercare following lung transplant**

  + **Z48.28** **Encounter for aftercare following multiple organ transplant**

    CC **Z48.280** **Encounter for aftercare following heart-lung transplant**

    Z48.288 **Encounter for aftercare following multiple organ transplant**

  + **Z48.29** **Encounter for aftercare following other organ transplant**

    CC **Z48.290** **Encounter for aftercare following bone marrow transplant**

    Z48.298 **Encounter for aftercare following other organ transplant**

Z48.3 **Aftercare following surgery for neoplasm**

    Use additional code to identify the neoplasm

+ **Z48.8** **Encounter for other specified postprocedural aftercare**

  + **Z48.81** **Encounter for surgical aftercare following surgery on specified body systems**

    These codes identify the body system requiring aftercare. They are for use in conjunction with other aftercare codes to fully explain the aftercare encounter. The condition treated should also be coded if still present.

    Excludes1: *aftercare for injury- code the injury with 7th character D*

    aftercare following surgery for neoplasm (Z48.3)

    Excludes2: *aftercare following organ transplant (Z48.2-)*

    orthopedic aftercare (Z47.-)

    Z48.810 **Encounter for surgical aftercare following surgery on the sense organs**

    Z48.811 **Encounter for surgical aftercare following surgery on the nervous system**

        Excludes2: *encounter for surgical aftercare following surgery on the sense organs (Z48.810)*

    Z48.812 **Encounter for surgical aftercare following surgery on the circulatory system**

        AHA CC: 4Q, 2012, 96-97

    Z48.813 **Encounter for surgical aftercare following surgery on the respiratory system**

        AHA CC: 2Q, 2019, 33

    Z48.814 **Encounter for surgical aftercare following surgery on the teeth or oral cavity**

    Z48.815 **Encounter for surgical aftercare following surgery on the digestive system**

        AHA CC: 4Q, 2015, 38

    Z48.816 **Encounter for surgical aftercare following surgery on the genitourinary system**

        Excludes1: *encounter for aftercare following sterilization reversal (Z31.42)*

    Z48.817 **Encounter for surgical aftercare following surgery on the skin and subcutaneous tissue**

    Z48.89 **Encounter for other specified surgical aftercare**

Z49 **Encounter for 5 care involving renal dialysis**

    Code also associated end stage renal disease (N18.6)

    Review coding guideline C.21.c.7

+ **Z49.0** **Preparatory care for renal dialysis**

    Encounter for dialysis instruction and training

    Z49.01 **Encounter for fitting and adjustment of extracorporeal dialysis catheter**

        Removal or replacement of renal dialysis catheter

        Toilet or cleansing of renal dialysis catheter

    Z49.02 **Encounter for fitting and adjustment of peritoneal dialysis catheter**

+ **Z49.3** **Encounter for adequacy testing for dialysis**

    Z49.31 **Encounter for adequacy testing for hemodialysis**

    Z49.32 **Encounter for adequacy testing for peritoneal dialysis**

        Encounter for peritoneal equilibration test

Z51 **Encounter for other aftercare and medical care**

    Code also condition requiring care

    Excludes1: *follow-up examination after treatment (Z08-Z09)*

    Review coding guidelines C.2.a, C.2.e.2 and C.2.e.3

    Review coding guideline C.21.c.7

Z51.0 **Encounter for antineoplastic radiation therapy**

    Review coding guidelines C.21.c.7 and C.21.c.16

+ **Z51.1** **Encounter for antineoplastic chemotherapy and immunotherapy**

    Excludes2: *encounter for chemotherapy and immunotherapy for nonneoplastic condition-code to condition*

    Review coding guidelines C.21.c.7 and C21.c.16

    Z51.11 **Encounter for antineoplastic chemotherapy**

        AHA CC: 3Q, 2015, 19-20

    Z51.12 **Encounter for antineoplastic immunotherapy**

Z51.5 **Encounter for palliative care**

    AHA CC: 1Q, 2017, 48-49

Z51.6 **Encounter for desensitization to allergens**

    AHA CC: 4Q, 2016, 77

+ **Z51.8** **Encounter for other specified aftercare**

    Excludes1: *holiday relief care (Z75.5)*

    Z51.81 **Encounter for therapeutic drug level monitoring**

        Code also any long-term (current) drug therapy (Z79.-)

        Excludes1: *encounter for blood-drug test for administrative or medicolegal reasons (Z02.83)*

    Z51.89 **Encounter for other specified aftercare**

        AHA CC: 4Q, 2012, 96-97

  NOTE Z51.89 is an acceptable PDX when reported with a secondary diagnosis.

+, +7th, X + 7th   ● Newborn   ● Pediatric   ● Maternity   ● Adult   ♀ Female   ♂ Male   Manifestation   Unacceptable PDX   HCC   CC   MCC   HAC

Z52 Donors of organs and tissues

Includes: autologous and other living donors

Excludes1: *cadaveric donor - omit code*
examination of potential donor (Z00.5)

Review coding guidelines C.21.c.9 and C.21.c.16

- **+ Z52.0 Blood donor**
  - **+ Z52.00 Unspecified blood donor**
    - **Z52.000** Unspecified donor, whole blood
    - **Z52.001** Unspecified donor, stem cells
    - **Z52.008** Unspecified donor, other blood
  - **+ Z52.01 Autologous blood donor**
    - **Z52.010** Autologous donor, whole blood
    - **Z52.011** Autologous donor, stem cells
    - **Z52.018** Autologous donor, other blood
  - **+ Z52.09 Other blood donor**
    - Volunteer donor
    - **Z52.090** Other blood donor, whole blood
    - **Z52.091** Other blood donor, stem cells
    - **Z52.098** Other blood donor, other blood
- **+ Z52.1 Skin donor**
  - **Z52.10** Skin donor, unspecified
  - **Z52.11** Skin donor, autologous
  - **Z52.19** Skin donor, other
- **+ Z52.2 Bone donor**
  - **Z52.20** Bone donor, unspecified
  - **Z52.21** Bone donor, autologous
  - **Z52.29** Bone donor, other
- **Z52.3 Bone marrow donor**
- **Z52.4 Kidney donor**
- **Z52.5 Cornea donor**
- **Z52.6 Liver donor**
- **+ Z52.8 Donor of other specified organs or tissues**
  - **+ Z52.81 Egg (Oocyte) donor**
    - ♀ **Z52.810 Egg (Oocyte) donor under age 35, anonymous recipient**
      - Egg donor under age 35 NOS
    - ♀ **Z52.811 Egg (Oocyte) donor under age 35, designated recipient**
    - ♀ **Z52.812 Egg (Oocyte) donor age 35 and over, anonymous recipient**
      - Egg donor age 35 and over NOS
    - ♀ **Z52.813 Egg (Oocyte) donor age 35 and over, designated recipient**
    - ♀ **Z52.819 Egg (Oocyte) donor, unspecified**
  - **Z52.89** Donor of other specified organs or tissues
- **Z52.9 Donor of unspecified organ or tissue**
  - Donor NOS

Z53 Persons encountering health services for specific procedures and treatment, not carried out

- **+ Z53.0 Procedure and treatment not carried out because of contraindication**
  - **Z53.01** Procedure and treatment not carried out due to patient smoking
  - **Z53.09** Procedure and treatment not carried out because of other contraindication
- **Z53.1 Procedure and treatment not carried out because of patient's decision for reasons of belief and group pressure**
- **+ Z53.2 Procedure and treatment not carried out because of patient's decision for other and unspecified reasons**
  - **Z53.20** Procedure and treatment not carried out because of patient's decision for unspecified reasons
  - **Z53.21** Procedure and treatment not carried out due to patient leaving prior to being seen by health care provider
  - **Z53.29** Procedure and treatment not carried out because of patient's decision for other reasons
- **+ Z53.3 Procedure converted to open procedure**
  - *AHA CC: 4Q, 2016, 79*
  - **Z53.31 Laparoscopic surgical procedure converted to open procedure**
    - *AHA CC: 4Q, 2016, 100-101*
  - **Z53.32 Thoracoscopic surgical procedure converted to open procedure**
  - **Z53.33 Arthroscopic surgical procedure converted to open procedure**
  - **Z53.39 Other specified procedure converted to open procedure**
- **Z53.8 Procedure and treatment not carried out for other reasons**
- **Z53.9 Procedure and treatment not carried out, unspecified reason**

Persons with potential health hazards related to socioeconomic and psychosocial circumstances (Z55-Z65)

AHA CC: 1Q, 2018, 18
Review coding guideline B.14

Z55 Problems related to education and literacy

Excludes1: *disorders of psychological development (F80-F89)*

- **Z55.0** Illiteracy and low-level literacy
- **Z55.1** Schooling unavailable and unattainable
- **Z55.2** Failed school examinations
- **Z55.3** Underachievement in school
- **Z55.4** Educational maladjustment and discord with teachers and classmates
- **Z55.8** Other problems related to education and literacy
  - Problems related to inadequate teaching
- **Z55.9** Problems related to education and literacy, unspecified
  - Academic problems NOS

Z56 Problems related to employment and unemployment

Excludes2: *occupational exposure to risk factors (Z57.-)*
problems related to housing and economic circumstances (Z59.-)

- **Z56.0** Unemployment, unspecified
- **Z56.1** Change of job
- **Z56.2** Threat of job loss
- **Z56.3** Stressful work schedule
- **Z56.4** Discord with boss and workmates
- **Z56.5** Uncongenial work environment
  - Difficult conditions at work
- **Z56.6** Other physical and mental strain related to work
- **+ Z56.8 Other problems related to employment**
  - **Z56.81** Sexual harassment on the job
  - **Z56.82 Military deployment status**
    - Individual (civilian or military) currently deployed in theater or in support of military war, peacekeeping and humanitarian operations
  - **Z56.89** Other problems related to employment
- **Z56.9** Unspecified problems related to employment
  - Occupational problems NOS

Z57 Occupational exposure to risk factors

- **Z57.0** Occupational exposure to noise
- **Z57.1** Occupational exposure to radiation
- **Z57.2** Occupational exposure to dust
- **+ Z57.3 Occupational exposure to other air contaminants**
  - **Z57.31 Occupational exposure to environmental tobacco smoke**
    - **Excludes2:** *exposure to environmental tobacco smoke (Z77.22)*
  - **Z57.39 Occupational exposure to other air contaminants**
- **Z57.4** Occupational exposure to toxic agents in agriculture
  - Occupational exposure to solids, liquids, gases or vapors in agriculture
- **Z57.5** Occupational exposure to toxic agents in other industries
  - Occupational exposure to solids, liquids, gases or vapors in other industries
- **Z57.6** Occupational exposure to extreme temperature
- **Z57.7** Occupational exposure to vibration
- **Z57.8** Occupational exposure to other risk factors
- **Z57.9** Occupational exposure to unspecified risk factor

Z59 Problems related to housing and economic circumstances

Excludes2: *problems related to upbringing (Z62.-)*

- **Z59.0** Homelessness
  - *AHA CC: 4Q, 2017, 112-114*
  - **Review coding guideline B.19.d**
- **Z59.1** Inadequate housing
  - Lack of heating
  - Restriction of space
  - Technical defects in home preventing adequate care
  - Unsatisfactory surroundings
  - **Excludes1:** *problems related to the natural and physical environment (Z77.1-)*
  - *AHA CC: 4Q, 2017, 112-114*
  - **Review coding guideline B.19.d**
- **Z59.2** Discord with neighbors, lodgers and landlord
- **Z59.3** Problems related to living in residential institution
  - Boarding-school resident
  - **Excludes1:** *institutional upbringing (Z62.2)*

Z59.4 Lack of adequate food and safe drinking water
Inadequate drinking water supply
Excludes1: *effects of hunger (T73.0)*
inappropriate diet or eating habits (Z72.4)
malnutrition (E40-E46)
Z59.5 Extreme poverty
AHA CC: 4Q, 2017, 112-114
Review coding guideline B.19.d
Z59.6 Low income
Z59.7 Insufficient social insurance and welfare support
Z59.8 Other problems related to housing and economic circumstances
Foreclosure on loan
Isolated dwelling
Problems with creditors
Z59.9 Problem related to housing and economic circumstances, unspecified

Z60 Problems related to social environment

Z60.0 Problems of adjustment to life-cycle transitions
Empty nest syndrome
Phase of life problem
Problem with adjustment to retirement [pension]
Z60.2 Problems related to living alone
Z60.3 Acculturation difficulty
Problem with migration
Problem with social transplantation
Z60.4 Social exclusion and rejection
Exclusion and rejection on the basis of personal characteristics, such as unusual physical appearance, illness or behavior.
Excludes1: *target of adverse discrimination such as for racial or religious reasons (Z60.5)*
Z60.5 Target of (perceived) adverse discrimination and persecution
Excludes1: *social exclusion and rejection (Z60.4)*
Z60.8 Other problems related to social environment
Z60.9 Problem related to social environment, unspecified

Z62 Problems related to upbringing

Includes: current and past negative life events in childhood
current and past problems of a child related to upbringing
Excludes2: *maltreatment syndrome (T74.-)*
problems related to housing and economic circumstances (Z59.-)
Z62.0 Inadequate parental supervision and control
Z62.1 Parental overprotection
+ **Z62.2 Upbringing away from parents**
Excludes1: *problems with boarding school (Z59.3)*
• **Z62.21 Child in welfare custody**
Child in care of non-parental family member
Child in foster care
Excludes2: *problem for parent due to child in welfare custody (Z63.5)*
Z62.22 Institutional upbringing
Child living in orphanage or group home
Z62.29 Other upbringing away from parents
• **Z62.3 Hostility towards and scapegoating of child**
Z62.6 Inappropriate (excessive) parental pressure
+ **Z62.8 Other specified problems related to upbringing**
+ **Z62.81 Personal history of abuse in childhood**
Z62.810 Personal history of physical and sexual abuse in childhood
Excludes1: *current child physical abuse (T74.12, T76.12)*
current child sexual abuse (T74.22, T76.22)
Z62.811 Personal history of psychological abuse in childhood
Excludes1: *current child psychological abuse (T74.32, T76.32)*
Z62.812 Personal history of neglect in childhood
Excludes1: *current child neglect (T74.02, T76.02)*
Z62.813 Personal history of forced labor or sexual exploitation in childhood
AHA CC: 4Q, 2018, 32-33, 35
Z62.819 Personal history of unspecified abuse in childhood
Excludes1: *current child abuse NOS (T74.92, T76.92)*

+ **Z62.82 Parent-child conflict**
Z62.820 Parent-biological child conflict
Parent-child problem NOS
Z62.821 Parent-adopted child conflict
Z62.822 Parent-foster child conflict
+ **Z62.89 Other specified problems related to upbringing**
Z62.890 Parent-child estrangement NEC
Z62.891 Sibling rivalry
Z62.898 Other specified problems related to upbringing
Z62.9 Problem related to upbringing, unspecified

Z63 Other problems related to primary support group, including family circumstances

Excludes2: *maltreatment syndrome (T74.-, T76)*
parent-child problems (Z62.-)
problems related to negative life events in childhood (Z62.-)
problems related to upbringing (Z62.-)
Z63.0 Problems in relationship with spouse or partner
Relationship distress with spouse or intimate partner
Excludes1: *counseling for spousal or partner abuse problems (Z69.1)*
counseling related to sexual attitude, behavior, and orientation (Z70.-)
Z63.1 Problems in relationship with in-laws
+ **Z63.3 Absence of family member**
Excludes1: *absence of family member due to disappearance and death (Z63.4)*
absence of family member due to separation and divorce (Z63.5)
Z63.31 Absence of family member due to military deployment
Individual or family affected by other family member being on military deployment
Excludes1: *family disruption due to return of family member from military deployment (Z63.71)*
Z63.32 Other absence of family member
Z63.4 Disappearance and death of family member
Assumed death of family member
Bereavement
AHA CC: 1Q, 2014, 25
Z63.5 Disruption of family by separation and divorce
Marital estrangement
Z63.6 Dependent relative needing care at home
+ **Z63.7 Other stressful life events affecting family and household**
Z63.71 Stress on family due to return of family member from military deployment
Individual or family affected by family member having returned from military deployment (current or past conflict)
Z63.72 Alcoholism and drug addiction in family
Z63.79 Other stressful life events affecting family and household
Anxiety (normal) about sick person in family
Health problems within family
Ill or disturbed family member
Isolated family
Z63.8 Other specified problems related to primary support group
Family discord NOS
Family estrangement NOS
High expressed emotional level within family
Inadequate family support NOS
Inadequate or distorted communication within family
Z63.9 Problem related to primary support group, unspecified
Relationship disorder NOS

Z64 Problems related to certain psychosocial circumstances

♀ **Z64.0 Problems related to unwanted pregnancy**
♀ **Z64.1 Problems related to multiparity**
Z64.4 Discord with counselors
Discord with probation officer
Discord with social worker

Z65 Problems related to other psychosocial circumstances

Z65.0 Conviction in civil and criminal proceedings without imprisonment
Z65.1 Imprisonment and other incarceration
Z65.2 Problems related to release from prison

+, +7th, X + 7th   • Newborn   ◦ Pediatric   • Maternity   • Adult   ♀ Female   ♂ Male   Manifestation   Unacceptable PDX   HCC   CC   MCC   HAC

Z65.3 **Problems related to other legal circumstances**
Arrest
Child custody or support proceedings
Litigation
Prosecution

Z65.4 **Victim of crime and terrorism**
Victim of torture

• **Z65.5** **Exposure to disaster, war and other hostilities**
Excludes1: *target of perceived discrimination or*
persecution (Z60.5)

Z65.8 **Other specified problems related to psychosocial**
circumstances
Religious or spiritual problem

Z65.9 **Problem related to unspecified psychosocial circumstances**

Do not resuscitate status (Z66)

Z66 **Do not resuscitate**

DNR status
Review coding guideline C.21.c.3
Valid 3-character code, no further characters required

Blood type (Z67)

Z67 **Blood type**
Review coding guideline C.21.c.3
AHA CC: 3Q, 2015, 40

+ **Z67.1** **Type A blood**
Z67.10 **Type A blood, Rh positive**
Z67.11 **Type A blood, Rh negative**

+ **Z67.2** **Type B blood**
Z67.20 **Type B blood, Rh positive**
Z67.21 **Type B blood, Rh negative**

+ **Z67.3** **Type AB blood**
Z67.30 **Type AB blood, Rh positive**
Z67.31 **Type AB blood, Rh negative**

+ **Z67.4** **Type O blood**
Z67.40 **Type O blood, Rh positive**
Z67.41 **Type O blood, Rh negative**

+ **Z67.9** **Unspecified blood type**
Z67.90 **Unspecified blood type, Rh positive**
Z67.91 **Unspecified blood type, Rh negative**

Body mass index [BMI] (Z68)

Z68 **Body mass index [BMI]**
Kilograms per meters squared
NOTE BMI adult codes are for use for persons 20 years of age or
older
BMI pediatric codes are for use for persons 2-19 years
of age. These percentiles are based on the growth
charts published by the Centers for Disease Control and
Prevention (CDC)
Review coding guidelines B.14 and C.21.c.3
AHA CC: 4Q, 2018, 77-83; 4Q, 2019, 19

• CC **Z68.1** **Body mass index [BMI] 19.9 or less, adult**
AHA CC: 1Q, 2017, 39

+ **Z68.2** **Body mass index [BMI] 20-29, adult**
• **Z68.20** **Body mass index [BMI] 20.0-20.9, adult**
• **Z68.21** **Body mass index [BMI] 21.0-21.9, adult**
• **Z68.22** **Body mass index [BMI] 22.0-22.9, adult**
• **Z68.23** **Body mass index [BMI] 23.0-23.9, adult**
• **Z68.24** **Body mass index [BMI] 24.0-24.9, adult**
• **Z68.25** **Body mass index [BMI] 25.0-25.9, adult**
• **Z68.26** **Body mass index [BMI] 26.0-26.9, adult**
• **Z68.27** **Body mass index [BMI] 27.0-27.9, adult**
• **Z68.28** **Body mass index [BMI] 28.0-28.9, adult**
• **Z68.29** **Body mass index [BMI] 29.0-29.9, adult**

+ **Z68.3** **Body mass index [BMI] 30-39, adult**
• **Z68.30** **Body mass index [BMI] 30.0-30.9, adult**
• **Z68.31** **Body mass index [BMI] 31.0-31.9, adult**
• **Z68.32** **Body mass index [BMI] 32.0-32.9, adult**
• **Z68.33** **Body mass index [BMI] 33.0-33.9, adult**
• **Z68.34** **Body mass index [BMI] 34.0-34.9, adult**
• **Z68.35** **Body mass index [BMI] 35.0-35.9, adult**
• **Z68.36** **Body mass index [BMI] 36.0-36.9, adult**
• **Z68.37** **Body mass index [BMI] 37.0-37.9, adult**
• **Z68.38** **Body mass index [BMI] 38.0-38.9, adult**
• **Z68.39** **Body mass index [BMI] 39.0-39.9, adult**

+ **Z68.4** **Body mass index [BMI] 40 or greater, adult**
• CC **Z68.41** **Body mass index [BMI] 40.0-44.9, adult**
• CC **Z68.42** **Body mass index [BMI] 45.0-49.9, adult**
• CC **Z68.43** **Body mass index [BMI] 50.0-59.9, adult**
• CC **Z68.44** **Body mass index [BMI] 60.0-69.9, adult**
• CC **Z68.45** **Body mass index [BMI] 70 or greater, adult**

+ **Z68.5** **Body mass index [BMI] pediatric**
AHA CC: 4Q, 2018, 81
Z68.51 **Body mass index [BMI] pediatric, less than 5th**
percentile for age
AHA CC: 4Q, 2018, 82
Z68.52 **Body mass index [BMI] pediatric, 5th percentile**
to less than 85th percentile for age
Z68.53 **Body mass index [BMI] pediatric, 85th percentile**
to less than 95th percentile for age
Z68.54 **Body mass index [BMI] pediatric, greater than or**
equal to 95th percentile for age

Persons encountering health services in other circumstances (Z69-Z76)

Z69 **Encounter for mental health services for victim and perpetrator**
of abuse
Includes: counseling for victims and perpetrators of abuse
Review coding guideline C.21.c.10

+ **Z69.0** **Encounter for mental health services for child abuse**
problems

+ **Z69.01** **Encounter for mental health services for parental**
child abuse
• **Z69.010** **Encounter for mental health services for**
victim of parental child abuse
Encounter for mental health services for
victim of child abuse by parent
Encounter for mental health services for
victim of child neglect by parent
Encounter for mental health services for
victim of child psychological abuse
by parent
Encounter for mental health services for
victim of child sexual abuse by parent
Z69.011 **Encounter for mental health services for**
perpetrator of parental child abuse
Encounter for mental health services for
perpetrator of parental child neglect
Encounter for mental health services
for perpetrator of parental child
psychological abuse
Encounter for mental health services for
perpetrator of parental child sexual
abuse
Excludes1: *encounter for mental health*
services for non-parental
child abuse (Z69.02-)

+ **Z69.02** **Encounter for mental health services for non-**
parental child abuse
• **Z69.020** **Encounter for mental health services for**
victim of non-parental child abuse
Encounter for mental health services for
victim of non-parental child neglect
Encounter for mental health services
for victim of non-parental child
psychological abuse
Encounter for mental health services for
victim of non-parental child sexual
abuse
Z69.021 **Encounter for mental health services for**
perpetrator of non-parental child abuse
Encounter for mental health services
for perpetrator of non-parental child
neglect
Encounter for mental health services
for perpetrator of non-parental child
psychological abuse
Encounter for mental health services
for perpetrator of non-parental child
sexual abuse

+, +7th, X + 7th   • Newborn   • Pediatric   • Maternity   • Adult   ♀ Female   ♂ Male   Manifestation   Unacceptable PDX   HCC   CC   MCC   HAC

+ Z69.1 **Encounter for mental health services for spousal or partner abuse problems**

    Z69.11 **Encounter for mental health services for victim of spousal or partner abuse**

        Encounter for mental health services for victim of spouse or partner neglect

        Encounter for mental health services for victim of spouse or partner psychological abuse

        Encounter for mental health services for victim of spouse or partner violence, physical

    Z69.12 **Encounter for mental health services for perpetrator of spousal or partner abuse**

        Encounter for mental health services for perpetrator of spouse or partner neglect

        Encounter for mental health services for perpetrator of spouse or partner psychological abuse

        Encounter for mental health services for perpetrator of spouse or partner violence, physical

+ Z69.8 **Encounter for mental health services for victim or perpetrator of other abuse**

    Z69.81 **Encounter for mental health services for victim of other abuse**

        Encounter for mental health services for victim of non-spousal adult abuse

        Encounter for mental health services for victim of spouse or partner violence, sexual

        Encounter for rape victim counseling

    Z69.82 **Encounter for mental health services for perpetrator of other abuse**

        Encounter for mental health services for perpetrator of non-spousal adult abuse

Z70 **Counseling related to sexual attitude, behavior and orientation**

    Includes: encounter for mental health services for sexual attitude, behavior and orientation

    Excludes2: *contraceptive or procreative counseling (Z30-Z31)*

    Review coding guideline C.21.c.10

    Z70.0 **Counseling related to sexual attitude**

    Z70.1 **Counseling related to patient's sexual behavior and orientation**

        Patient concerned regarding impotence

        Patient concerned regarding non-responsiveness

        Patient concerned regarding promiscuity

        Patient concerned regarding sexual orientation

    Z70.2 **Counseling related to sexual behavior and orientation of third party**

        Advice sought regarding sexual behavior and orientation of child

        Advice sought regarding sexual behavior and orientation of partner

        Advice sought regarding sexual behavior and orientation of spouse

    Z70.3 **Counseling related to combined concerns regarding sexual attitude, behavior and orientation**

    Z70.8 **Other sex counseling**

        Encounter for sex education

    Z70.9 **Sex counseling, unspecified**

Z71 **Persons encountering health services for other counseling and medical advice, not elsewhere classified**

    Excludes2: *contraceptive or procreation counseling (Z30-Z31)*

        sex counseling (Z70.-)

    Review coding guideline C.21.c.10

    Z71.0 **Person encountering health services to consult on behalf of another person**

        Person encountering health services to seek advice or treatment for non-attending third party

        Excludes2: *anxiety (normal) about sick person in family (Z63.7)*

            expectant (adoptive) parent(s) pre-birth pediatrician visit (Z76.81)

    Z71.1 **Person with feared health complaint in whom no diagnosis is made**

        Person encountering health services with feared condition which was not demonstrated

        Person encountering health services in which problem was normal state

        'Worried well'

        Excludes1: *medical observation for suspected diseases and conditions proven not to exist (Z03.-)*

        AHA CC: 4Q, 2016, 4-7

Z71.2 **Person consulting for explanation of examination or test findings**

Z71.3 **Dietary counseling and surveillance**

    Use additional code for any associated underlying medical condition

    Use additional code to identify body mass index (BMI), if known (Z68.-)

+ Z71.4 **Alcohol abuse counseling and surveillance**

    Use additional code for alcohol abuse or dependence (F10.-)

    Z71.41 **Alcohol abuse counseling and surveillance of alcoholic**

    Z71.42 **Counseling for family member of alcoholic**

        Counseling for significant other, partner, or friend of alcoholic

+ Z71.5 **Drug abuse counseling and surveillance**

    Use additional code for drug abuse or dependence (F11-F16, F18-F19)

    Z71.51 **Drug abuse counseling and surveillance of drug abuser**

    Z71.52 **Counseling for family member of drug abuser**

        Counseling for significant other, partner, or friend of drug abuser

Z71.6 **Tobacco abuse counseling**

    Use additional code for nicotine dependence (F17.-)

Z71.7 **Human immunodeficiency virus [HIV] counseling**

    Review coding guideline C.1.a.2.h

+ Z71.8 **Other specified counseling**

    Excludes2: *counseling for contraception (Z30.0-)*

    Z71.81 **Spiritual or religious counseling**

    Z71.82 **Exercise counseling**

        AHA CC: 4Q, 2017, 27

    Z71.83 **Encounter for nonprocreative genetic counseling**

        Excludes1: *counseling for procreative genetics (Z31.5)*

            counseling for procreative management (Z31.6)

        AHA CC: 4Q, 2017, 27

    Z71.84 **Encounter for health counseling related to travel**

        Encounter for health risk and safety counseling for (international) travel

        Code also, if applicable, encounter for immunization (Z23)

        Excludes2: *encounter for administrative examination (Z02.-)*

            encounter for other special examination without complaint, suspected or reported diagnosis (Z01.-)

        AHA CC: 4Q, 2019, 20

    Z71.89 **Other specified counseling**

Z71.9 **Counseling, unspecified**

    Encounter for medical advice NOS

Z72 **Problems related to lifestyle**

    Excludes2: *problems related to life-management difficulty (Z73.-)*

        problems related to socioeconomic and psychosocial circumstances (Z55-Z65)

    Review coding guideline C.21.c.14

    Z72.0 **Tobacco use**

        Tobacco use NOS

        Excludes1: *history of tobacco dependence (Z87.891)*

            nicotine dependence (F17.2-)

            tobacco dependence (F17.2-)

            tobacco use during pregnancy (O99.33-)

        Review coding guideline C.15.l.2

    Z72.3 **Lack of physical exercise**

    Z72.4 **Inappropriate diet and eating habits**

        Excludes1: *behavioral eating disorders of infancy or childhood (F98.2-F98.3)*

            eating disorders (F50.-)

            lack of adequate food (Z59.4)

            malnutrition and other nutritional deficiencies (E40-E64)

+ Z72.5 **High risk sexual behavior**

        Promiscuity

        Excludes1: *paraphilias (F65)*

    Z72.51 **High risk heterosexual behavior**

    Z72.52 **High risk homosexual behavior**

    Z72.53 **High risk bisexual behavior**

    Z72.6 **Gambling and betting**

        Excludes1: *compulsive or pathological gambling (F63.0)*

+ **Z72.8** **Other problems related to lifestyle**

  + **Z72.81** **Antisocial behavior**

    Excludes1: *conduct disorders (F91.-)*

    ● **Z72.810** **Child and adolescent antisocial behavior**

      Antisocial behavior (child) (adolescent) without manifest psychiatric disorder

      Delinquency NOS

      Group delinquency

      Offenses in the context of gang membership

      Stealing in company with others

      Truancy from school

    ● **Z72.811** **Adult antisocial behavior**

      Adult antisocial behavior without manifest psychiatric disorder

  + **Z72.82** **Problems related to sleep**

    Z72.820 **Sleep deprivation**

      Lack of adequate sleep

      Excludes1: *insomnia (G47.0-)*

    Z72.821 **Inadequate sleep hygiene**

      Bad sleep habits

      Irregular sleep habits

      Unhealthy sleep wake schedule

      Excludes1: *insomnia (F51.0-, G47.0-)*

  Z72.89 **Other problems related to lifestyle**

    Self-damaging behavior

Z72.9 **Problem related to lifestyle, unspecified**

Z73 **Problems related to life management difficulty**

  Excludes2: *problems related to socioeconomic and psychosocial circumstances (Z55-Z65)*

Z73.0 **Burn-out**

Z73.1 **Type A behavior pattern**

Z73.2 **Lack of relaxation and leisure**

Z73.3 **Stress, not elsewhere classified**

  Physical and mental strain NOS

  Excludes1: *stress related to employment or unemployment (Z56.-)*

Z73.4 **Inadequate social skills, not elsewhere classified**

Z73.5 **Social role conflict, not elsewhere classified**

Z73.6 **Limitation of activities due to disability**

  Excludes1: *care-provider dependency (Z74.-)*

+ **Z73.8** **Other problems related to life management difficulty**

  + **Z73.81** **Behavioral insomnia of childhood**

    ● **Z73.810** **Behavioral insomnia of childhood, sleep-onset association type**

    ● **Z73.811** **Behavioral insomnia of childhood, limit setting type**

    ● **Z73.812** **Behavioral insomnia of childhood, combined type**

    ● **Z73.819** **Behavioral insomnia of childhood, unspecified type**

  Z73.82 **Dual sensory impairment**

  Z73.89 **Other problems related to life management difficulty**

Z73.9 **Problem related to life management difficulty, unspecified**

Z74 **Problems related to care provider dependency**

  Excludes2: *dependence on enabling machines or devices NEC (Z99.-)*

+ **Z74.0** **Reduced mobility**

  Z74.01 **Bed confinement status**

    Bedridden

    Review coding guideline C.21.c.3

  Z74.09 **Other reduced mobility**

    Chairridden

    Reduced mobility NOS

    Excludes2: *wheelchair dependence (Z99.3)*

Z74.1 **Need for assistance with personal care**

Z74.2 **Need for assistance at home and no other household member able to render care**

Z74.3 **Need for continuous supervision**

Z74.8 **Other problems related to care provider dependency**

Z74.9 **Problem related to care provider dependency, unspecified**

Z75 **Problems related to medical facilities and other health care**

Z75.0 **Medical services not available in home**

  Excludes1: *no other household member able to render care (Z74.2)*

Z75.1 **Person awaiting admission to adequate facility elsewhere**

  AHA CC: 4Q, 2017, 112-114

  Review coding guideline B.19.d

Z75.2 **Other waiting period for investigation and treatment**

Z75.3 **Unavailability and inaccessibility of health-care facilities**

  Excludes1: *bed unavailable (Z75.1)*

  AHA CC: 4Q, 2017, 112-114

  Review coding guideline B.19.d

Z75.4 **Unavailability and inaccessibility of other helping agencies**

  AHA CC: 4Q, 2017, 112-114

  Review coding guideline B.19.d

Z75.5 **Holiday relief care**

Z75.8 **Other problems related to medical facilities and other health care**

Z75.9 **Unspecified problem related to medical facilities and other health care**

Z76 **Persons encountering health services in other circumstances**

Z76.0 **Encounter for issue of repeat prescription**

  Encounter for issue of repeat prescription for appliance

  Encounter for issue of repeat prescription for medicaments

  Encounter for issue of repeat prescription for spectacles

  Excludes2: *issue of medical certificate (Z02.7)*

    repeat prescription for contraceptive (Z30.4-)

Z76.1 **Encounter for health supervision and care of foundling**

  Review coding guidelines C.21.c.12 and C.21.c.16

● **Z76.2** **Encounter for health supervision and care of other healthy infant and child**

  Encounter for medical or nursing care or supervision of healthy infant under circumstances such as adverse socioeconomic conditions at home

  Encounter for medical or nursing care or supervision of healthy infant under circumstances such as awaiting foster or adoptive placement

  Encounter for medical or nursing care or supervision of healthy infant under circumstances such as maternal illness

  Encounter for medical or nursing care or supervision of healthy infant under circumstances such as number of children at home preventing or interfering with normal care

  AHA CC: 4Q, 2017, 112-114

  Review coding guidelines B.19.d and C.21.c.16

Z76.3 **Healthy person accompanying sick person**

Z76.4 **Other boarder to healthcare facility**

  Excludes1: *homelessness (Z59.0)*

Z76.5 **Malingerer [conscious simulation]**

  Person feigning illness (with obvious motivation)

  Excludes1: *factitious disorder (F68.1-, F68.A)*

    peregrinating patient (F68.1-)

+ **Z76.8** **Persons encountering health services in other specified circumstances**

  Z76.81 **Expectant parent(s) prebirth pediatrician visit**

    Pre-adoption pediatrician visit for adoptive parent(s)

    Review coding guideline C.21.c.10

  Z76.82 **Awaiting organ transplant status**

    Patient waiting for organ availability

    Review coding guideline C.21.c.3

  Z76.89 **Persons encountering health services in other specified circumstances**

    Persons encountering health services NOS

    AHA CC: 2Q, 2014, 10

Persons with potential health hazards related to family and personal history and certain conditions influencing health status (Z77-Z99)

Code also any follow-up examination (Z08-Z09)

Z77 **Other contact with and (suspected) exposures hazardous to health**

  Includes: contact with and (suspected) exposures to potential hazards to health

  Excludes2: *contact with and (suspected) exposure to communicable diseases (Z20.-)*

    exposure to (parental) (environmental) tobacco smoke in the perinatal period (P96.81)

    newborn affected by noxious substances transmitted via placenta or breast milk (P04.-)

    occupational exposure to risk factors (Z57.-)

    retained foreign body (Z18.-)

    retained foreign body fully removed (Z87.821)

    toxic effects of substances chiefly nonmedicinal as to source (T51-T65)

  Review coding guideline C.21.c.1

+, +7th, X + 7th   ● Newborn   ● Pediatric   ● Maternity   ● Adult   ♀ Female   ♂ Male   Manifestation   Unacceptable PDX   HCC   CC   MCC   HAC

+ **Z77.0** **Contact with and (suspected) exposure to hazardous, chiefly nonmedicinal, chemicals**

  + **Z77.01** **Contact with and (suspected) exposure to hazardous metals**

    Z77.010 **Contact with and (suspected) exposure to arsenic**

    Z77.011 **Contact with and (suspected) exposure to lead**

    Z77.012 **Contact with and (suspected) exposure to uranium**

      Excludes1: *retained depleted uranium fragments (Z18.01)*

    Z77.018 **Contact with and (suspected) exposure to other hazardous metals**

      Contact with and (suspected) exposure to chromium compounds

      Contact with and (suspected) exposure to nickel dust

  + **Z77.02** **Contact with and (suspected) exposure to hazardous aromatic compounds**

    Z77.020 **Contact with and (suspected) exposure to aromatic amines**

    Z77.021 **Contact with and (suspected) exposure to benzene**

    Z77.028 **Contact with and (suspected) exposure to other hazardous aromatic compounds**

      Aromatic dyes NOS

      Polycyclic aromatic hydrocarbons

  + **Z77.09** **Contact with and (suspected) exposure to other hazardous, chiefly nonmedicinal, chemicals**

    Z77.090 **Contact with and (suspected) exposure to asbestos**

    Z77.098 **Contact with and (suspected) exposure to other hazardous, chiefly nonmedicinal, chemicals**

      Dyes NOS

+ **Z77.1** **Contact with and (suspected) exposure to environmental pollution and hazards in the physical environment**

  + **Z77.11** **Contact with and (suspected) exposure to environmental pollution**

    Z77.110 **Contact with and (suspected) exposure to air pollution**

    Z77.111 **Contact with and (suspected) exposure to water pollution**

    Z77.112 **Contact with and (suspected) exposure to soil pollution**

    Z77.118 **Contact with and (suspected) exposure to other environmental pollution**

  + **Z77.12** **Contact with and (suspected) exposure to hazards in the physical environment**

    Z77.120 **Contact with and (suspected) exposure to mold (toxic)**

    Z77.121 **Contact with and (suspected) exposure to harmful algae and algae toxins**

      Contact with and (suspected) exposure to (harmful) algae bloom NOS

      Contact with and (suspected) exposure to blue-green algae bloom

      Contact with and (suspected) exposure to brown tide

      Contact with and (suspected) exposure to cyanobacteria bloom

      Contact with and (suspected) exposure to Florida red tide

      Contact with and (suspected) exposure to pfiesteria piscicida

      Contact with and (suspected) exposure to red tide

    Z77.122 **Contact with and (suspected) exposure to noise**

    Z77.123 **Contact with and (suspected) exposure to radon and other naturally occurring radiation**

      Excludes2: *radiation exposure as the cause of a confirmed condition (W88-W90, X39.0-) radiation sickness NOS (T66)*

    Z77.128 **Contact with and (suspected) exposure to other hazards in the physical environment**

+ **Z77.2** **Contact with and (suspected) exposure to other hazardous substances**

  Z77.21 **Contact with and (suspected) exposure to potentially hazardous body fluids**

  Z77.22 **Contact with and (suspected) exposure to environmental tobacco smoke (acute) (chronic)**

    Exposure to second hand tobacco smoke (acute) (chronic)

    Passive smoking (acute) (chronic)

    Excludes1: *nicotine dependence (F17.-) tobacco use (Z72.0)*

    Excludes2: *occupational exposure to environmental tobacco smoke (Z57.31)*

  Z77.29 **Contact with and (suspected) exposure to other hazardous substances**

    AHA CC: 2Q, 2016, 34

Z77.9 **Other contact with and (suspected) exposures hazardous to health**

Z78 **Other specified health status**

  Excludes2: *asymptomatic human immunodeficiency virus [HIV] infection status (Z21) postprocedural status (Z93-Z99) sex reassignment status (Z87.890)*

  Review coding guideline C.21.c.3

● ♀ **Z78.0** **Asymptomatic menopausal state**

  Menopausal state NOS

  Postmenopausal status NOS

  Excludes2: *symptomatic menopausal state (N95.1)*

Z78.1 **Physical restraint status**

  Excludes1: *physical restraint due to a procedure - omit code*

Z78.9 **Other specified health status**

Z79 **Long term (current) drug therapy**

  Includes: long term (current) drug use for prophylactic purposes

  Code also any therapeutic drug level monitoring (Z51.81)

  Excludes2: *drug abuse and dependence (F11-F19) drug use complicating pregnancy, childbirth, and the puerperium (O99.32-)*

  Review coding guideline C.21.c.3

+ **Z79.0** **Long term (current) use of anticoagulants and antithrombotics/antiplatelets**

  Excludes2: *long term (current) use of aspirin (Z79.82)*

  Z79.01 **Long term (current) use of anticoagulants**

    AHA CC: 2Q, 2020, 20-21

  Z79.02 **Long term (current) use of antithrombotics/ antiplatelets**

Z79.1 **Long term (current) use of non-steroidal anti-inflammatories (NSAID)**

  Excludes2: *long term (current) use of aspirin (Z79.82)*

Z79.2 **Long term (current) use of antibiotics**

Z79.3 **Long term (current) use of hormonal contraceptives**

  Long term (current) use of birth control pill or patch

Z79.4 **Long term (current) use of insulin**

  Excludes1: *long term (current) use of oral antidiabetic drugs (Z79.84) long term (current) use of oral hypoglycemic drugs (Z79.84)*

  Review coding guidelines C.4.a.3 and C.4.a.6

  Review coding guidelines C.15.h and C.15.i

+ **Z79.5** **Long term (current) use of steroids**

  Z79.51 **Long term (current) use of inhaled steroids**

  Z79.52 **Long term (current) use of systemic steroids**

+ **Z79.8** **Other long term (current) drug therapy**

  + **Z79.81** **Long term (current) use of agents affecting estrogen receptors and estrogen levels**

    Code first if applicable:

    malignant neoplasm of breast (C50.-)

    malignant neoplasm of prostate (C61)

    Use additional code, if applicable, to identify:

    estrogen receptor positive status (Z17.0)

    family history of breast cancer (Z80.3)

    genetic susceptibility to malignant neoplasm (cancer) (Z15.0-)

    personal history of breast cancer (Z85.3)

    personal history of prostate cancer (Z85.46)

    postmenopausal status (Z78.0)

    Excludes1: *hormone replacement therapy (Z79.890)*

+, +7th, X + 7th   ● Newborn   ● Pediatric   ● Maternity   ● Adult   ♀ Female   ♂ Male   Manifestation   Unacceptable PDX   HCC   CC   MCC   HAC

Z79.810 **Long term (current) use of selective estrogen receptor modulators (SERMs)**
Long term (current) use of raloxifene (Evista)
Long term (current) use of tamoxifen (Nolvadex)
Long term (current) use of toremifene (Fareston)

Z79.811 **Long term (current) use of aromatase inhibitors**
Long term (current) use of anastrozole (Arimidex)
Long term (current) use of exemestane (Aromasin)
Long term (current) use of letrozole (Femara)

Z79.818 **Long term (current) use of other agents affecting estrogen receptors and estrogen levels**
Long term (current) use of estrogen receptor downregulators
Long term (current) use of fulvestrant (Faslodex)
Long term (current) use of gonadotropin-releasing hormone (GnRH) agonist
Long term (current) use of goserelin acetate (Zoladex)
Long term (current) use of leuprolide acetate (leuprorelin) (Lupron)
Long term (current) use of megestrol acetate (Megace)

Z79.82 **Long term (current) use of aspirin**

Z79.83 **Long term (current) use of bisphosphonates**
AHA CC: 4Q, 2016, 21

Z79.84 **Long term (current) use of oral hypoglycemic drugs**
Long term (current) use of oral antidiabetic drugs
Excludes2: *long term (current) use of insulin (Z79.4)*
Review coding guidelines C.4.a.e and C.4.a.6
Review coding guidelines C.15.h and C.15.i
AHA CC: 4Q, 2016, 76

+ **Z79.89** **Other long term (current) drug therapy**

Z79.890 **Hormone replacement therapy**

Z79.891 **Long term (current) use of opiate analgesic**
Long term (current) use of methadone for pain management
Excludes1: *methodone use NOS (F11.9-)*
use of methodone for treatment of heroin addiction (F11.2-)

Z79.899 **Other long term (current) drug therapy**
AHA CC: 3Q, 2015, 21-22; 4Q, 2015, 34; 2Q, 2020, 14-15
Review coding guideline C.4.a.3

Z80 **Family history of primary malignant neoplasm**
Review coding guideline C.21.c.4

Z80.0 **Family history of malignant neoplasm of digestive organs**
Conditions classifiable to C15-C26
AHA CC: 1Q, 2018, 6-7

Z80.1 **Family history of malignant neoplasm of trachea, bronchus and lung**
Conditions classifiable to C33-C34

Z80.2 **Family history of malignant neoplasm of other respiratory and intrathoracic organs**
Conditions classifiable to C30-C32, C37-C39

Z80.3 **Family history of malignant neoplasm of breast**
Conditions classifiable to C50.-

+ **Z80.4** **Family history of malignant neoplasm of genital organs**
Conditions classifiable to C51-C63

Z80.41 **Family history of malignant neoplasm of ovary**
Z80.42 **Family history of malignant neoplasm of prostate**
Z80.43 **Family history of malignant neoplasm of testis**
Z80.49 **Family history of malignant neoplasm of other genital organs**

+ **Z80.5** **Family history of malignant neoplasm of urinary tract**
Conditions classifiable to C64-C68

Z80.51 **Family history of malignant neoplasm of kidney**
Z80.52 **Family history of malignant neoplasm of bladder**
Z80.59 **Family history of malignant neoplasm of other urinary tract organ**

Z80.6 **Family history of leukemia**
Conditions classifiable to C91-C95

Z80.7 **Family history of other malignant neoplasms of lymphoid, hematopoietic and related tissues**
Conditions classifiable to C81-C90, C96.-

Z80.8 **Family history of malignant neoplasm of other organs or systems**
Conditions classifiable to C00-C14, C40-C49, C69-C79

Z80.9 **Family history of malignant neoplasm, unspecified**
Conditions classifiable to C80.1

Z81 **Family history of mental and behavioral disorders**
Review coding guideline C.21.c.4

Z81.0 **Family history of intellectual disabilities**
Conditions classifiable to F70-F79

Z81.1 **Family history of alcohol abuse and dependence**
Conditions classifiable to F10.-

Z81.2 **Family history of tobacco abuse and dependence**
Conditions classifiable to F17.-

Z81.3 **Family history of other psychoactive substance abuse and dependence**
Conditions classifiable to F11-F16, F18-F19

Z81.4 **Family history of other substance abuse and dependence**
Conditions classifiable to F55

Z81.8 **Family history of other mental and behavioral disorders**
Conditions classifiable elsewhere in F01-F99

Z82 **Family history of certain disabilities and chronic diseases (leading to disablement)**
Review coding guideline C.21.c.4

Z82.0 **Family history of epilepsy and other diseases of the nervous system**
Conditions classifiable to G00-G99

Z82.1 **Family history of blindness and visual loss**
Conditions classifiable to H54.-

Z82.2 **Family history of deafness and hearing loss**
Conditions classifiable to H90-H91

Z82.3 **Family history of stroke**
Conditions classifiable to I60-I64

+ **Z82.4** **Family history of ischemic heart disease and other diseases of the circulatory system**
Conditions classifiable to I00-I52, I65-I99

Z82.41 **Family history of sudden cardiac death**
Z82.49 **Family history of ischemic heart disease and other diseases of the circulatory system**

Z82.5 **Family history of asthma and other chronic lower respiratory diseases**
Conditions classifiable to J40-J47
Excludes2: *family history of other diseases of the respiratory system (Z83.6)*

+ **Z82.6** **Family history of arthritis and other diseases of the musculoskeletal system and connective tissue**
Conditions classifiable to M00-M99

Z82.61 **Family history of arthritis**
Z82.62 **Family history of osteoporosis**
Z82.69 **Family history of other diseases of the musculoskeletal system and connective tissue**

+ **Z82.7** **Family history of congenital malformations, deformations and chromosomal abnormalities**
Conditions classifiable to Q00-Q99

Z82.71 **Family history of polycystic kidney**
Z82.79 **Family history of other congenital malformations, deformations and chromosomal abnormalities**

Z82.8 **Family history of other disabilities and chronic diseases leading to disablement, not elsewhere classified**

Z83 **Family history of other specific disorders**
Excludes2: *contact with and (suspected) exposure to communicable disease in the family (Z20.-)*
Review coding guideline C.21.c.4

Z83.0 **Family history of human immunodeficiency virus [HIV] disease**
Conditions classifiable to B20

Z83.1 **Family history of other infectious and parasitic diseases**
Conditions classifiable to A00-B19, B25-B94, B99

Z83.2 **Family history of diseases of the blood and blood-forming organs and certain disorders involving the immune mechanism**
Conditions classifiable to D50-D89

Z83.3 **Family history of diabetes mellitus**
Conditions classifiable to E08-E13

+ **Z83.4** **Family history of other endocrine, nutritional and metabolic diseases**
Conditions classifiable to E00-E07, E15-E88
Z83.41 **Family history of multiple endocrine neoplasia [MEN] syndrome**
Z83.42 **Family history of familial hypercholesterolemia**
AHA CC: 4Q, 2016, 77
+ **Z83.43** **Family history of other disorder of lipoprotein metabolism and other lipidemias**
AHA CC: 4Q, 2018, 6
Z83.430 **Family history of elevated lipoprotein(a)**
Family history of elevated Lp(a)
Z83.438 **Family history of other disorder of lipoprotein metabolism and other lipidemia**
Family history of familial combined hyperlipidemia
Z83.49 **Family history of other endocrine, nutritional and metabolic diseases**
+ **Z83.5** **Family history of eye and ear disorders**
+ **Z83.51** **Family history of eye disorders**
Conditions classifiable to H00-H53, H55-H59
Excludes2: *family history of blindness and visual loss (Z82.1)*
Z83.511 **Family history of glaucoma**
Z83.518 **Family history of other specified eye disorder**
Z83.52 **Family history of ear disorders**
Conditions classifiable to H60-H83, H92-H95
Excludes2: *family history of deafness and hearing loss (Z82.2)*
Z83.6 **Family history of other diseases of the respiratory system**
Conditions classifiable to J00-J39, J60-J99
Excludes2: *family history of asthma and other chronic lower respiratory diseases (Z82.5)*
+ **Z83.7** **Family history of diseases of the digestive system**
Conditions classifiable to K00-K93
Z83.71 **Family history of colonic polyps**
Excludes2: *family history of malignant neoplasm of digestive organs (Z80.0)*
Z83.79 **Family history of other diseases of the digestive system**

Z84 **Family history of other conditions**
Review coding guideline C.21.c.4
Z84.0 **Family history of diseases of the skin and subcutaneous tissue**
Conditions classifiable to L00-L99
Z84.1 **Family history of disorders of kidney and ureter**
Conditions classifiable to N00-N29
Z84.2 **Family history of other diseases of the genitourinary system**
Conditions classifiable to N30-N99
Z84.3 **Family history of consanguinity**
+ **Z84.8** **Family history of other specified conditions**
Z84.81 **Family history of carrier of genetic disease**
Z84.82 **Family history of sudden infant death syndrome**
Family history of SIDS
AHA CC: 4Q, 2016, 77
Z84.89 **Family history of other specified conditions**

Z85 **Personal history of malignant neoplasm**
Code first any follow-up examination after treatment of malignant neoplasm (Z08)
Use additional code to identify:
alcohol use and dependence (F10.-)
exposure to environmental tobacco smoke (Z77.22)
history of tobacco dependence (Z87.891)
occupational exposure to environmental tobacco smoke (Z57.31)
tobacco dependence (F17.-)
tobacco use (Z72.0)
Excludes2: *personal history of benign neoplasm (Z86.01-)*
personal history of carcinoma-in-situ (Z86.00-)
Review coding guidelines C.2.d and C.2.m
Review coding guideline C.21.c.4
+ **Z85.0** **Personal history of malignant neoplasm of digestive organs**
Z85.00 **Personal history of malignant neoplasm of unspecified digestive organ**
Z85.01 **Personal history of malignant neoplasm of esophagus**
Conditions classifiable to C15

+ **Z85.02** **Personal history of malignant neoplasm of stomach**
Z85.020 **Personal history of malignant carcinoid tumor of stomach**
Conditions classifiable to C7A.092
Z85.028 **Personal history of other malignant neoplasm of stomach**
Conditions classifiable to C16
+ **Z85.03** **Personal history of malignant neoplasm of large intestine**
Z85.030 **Personal history of malignant carcinoid tumor of large intestine**
Conditions classifiable to C7A.022-C7A.025, C7A.029
Z85.038 **Personal history of other malignant neoplasm of large intestine**
Conditions classifiable to C18
+ **Z85.04** **Personal history of malignant neoplasm of rectum, rectosigmoid junction, and anus**
Z85.040 **Personal history of malignant carcinoid tumor of rectum**
Conditions classifiable to C7A.026
Z85.048 **Personal history of other malignant neoplasm of rectum, rectosigmoid junction, and anus**
Conditions classifiable to C19-C21
Z85.05 **Personal history of malignant neoplasm of liver**
Conditions classifiable to C22
+ **Z85.06** **Personal history of malignant neoplasm of small intestine**
Z85.060 **Personal history of malignant carcinoid tumor of small intestine**
Conditions classifiable to C7A.01-
Z85.068 **Personal history of other malignant neoplasm of small intestine**
Conditions classifiable to C17
Z85.07 **Personal history of malignant neoplasm of pancreas**
Conditions classifiable to C25
Z85.09 **Personal history of malignant neoplasm of other digestive organs**
+ **Z85.1** **Personal history of malignant neoplasm of trachea, bronchus and lung**
+ **Z85.11** **Personal history of malignant neoplasm of bronchus and lung**
Z85.110 **Personal history of malignant carcinoid tumor of bronchus and lung**
Conditions classifiable to C7A.090
Z85.118 **Personal history of other malignant neoplasm of bronchus and lung**
Conditions classifiable to C34
Z85.12 **Personal history of malignant neoplasm of trachea**
Conditions classifiable to C33
+ **Z85.2** **Personal history of malignant neoplasm of other respiratory and intrathoracic organs**
Z85.20 **Personal history of malignant neoplasm of unspecified respiratory organ**
Z85.21 **Personal history of malignant neoplasm of larynx**
Conditions classifiable to C32
Z85.22 **Personal history of malignant neoplasm of nasal cavities, middle ear, and accessory sinuses**
Conditions classifiable to C30-C31
+ **Z85.23** **Personal history of malignant neoplasm of thymus**
Z85.230 **Personal history of malignant carcinoid tumor of thymus**
Conditions classifiable to C7A.091
Z85.238 **Personal history of other malignant neoplasm of thymus**
Conditions classifiable to C37
Z85.29 **Personal history of malignant neoplasm of other respiratory and intrathoracic organs**
Z85.3 **Personal history of malignant neoplasm of breast**
Conditions classifiable to C50.-

+, +7th, X + 7th • Newborn • Pediatric • Maternity • Adult ♀ Female ♂ Male Manifestation Unacceptable PDX HCC CC MCC HAC

+ **Z85.4 Personal history of malignant neoplasm of genital organs**
Conditions classifiable to C51-C63

♀ **Z85.40 Personal history of malignant neoplasm of unspecified female genital organ**

♀ **Z85.41 Personal history of malignant neoplasm of cervix uteri**

♀ **Z85.42 Personal history of malignant neoplasm of other parts of uterus**

♀ **Z85.43 Personal history of malignant neoplasm of ovary**

♀ **Z85.44 Personal history of malignant neoplasm of other female genital organs**

♂ **Z85.45 Personal history of malignant neoplasm of unspecified male genital organ**

♂ **Z85.46 Personal history of malignant neoplasm of prostate**

♂ **Z85.47 Personal history of malignant neoplasm of testis**

♂ **Z85.48 Personal history of malignant neoplasm of epididymis**

♂ **Z85.49 Personal history of malignant neoplasm of other male genital organs**

+ **Z85.5 Personal history of malignant neoplasm of urinary tract**
Conditions classifiable to C64-C68

Z85.50 Personal history of malignant neoplasm of unspecified urinary tract organ

Z85.51 Personal history of malignant neoplasm of bladder

+ **Z85.52 Personal history of malignant neoplasm of kidney**
Excludes1: *personal history of malignant neoplasm of renal pelvis (Z85.53)*

Z85.520 Personal history of malignant carcinoid tumor of kidney
Conditions classifiable to C7A.093

Z85.528 Personal history of other malignant neoplasm of kidney
Conditions classifiable to C64

Z85.53 Personal history of malignant neoplasm of renal pelvis

Z85.54 Personal history of malignant neoplasm of ureter

Z85.59 Personal history of malignant neoplasm of other urinary tract organ

Z85.6 Personal history of leukemia
Conditions classifiable to C91-C95
Excludes1: *leukemia in remission C91.0-C95.9 with 5th character 1*
Review coding guideline C.2.n

+ **Z85.7 Personal history of other malignant neoplasms of lymphoid, hematopoietic and related tissues**

Z85.71 Personal history of Hodgkin lymphoma
Conditions classifiable to C81

Z85.72 Personal history of non-Hodgkin lymphomas
Conditions classifiable to C82-C85

Z85.79 Personal history of other malignant neoplasms of lymphoid, hematopoietic and related tissues
Conditions classifiable to C88-C90, C96
Excludes1: *multiple myeloma in remission (C90.01)*
plasma cell leukemia in remission (C90.11)
plasmacytoma in remission (C90.21)
Review coding guideline C.2.n

+ **Z85.8 Personal history of malignant neoplasms of other organs and systems**
Conditions classifiable to C00-C14, C40-C49, C69-C75, C7A.098, C76-C79

+ **Z85.81 Personal history of malignant neoplasm of lip, oral cavity, and pharynx**
Conditions classifiable to C00-C14

Z85.810 Personal history of malignant neoplasm of tongue

Z85.818 Personal history of malignant neoplasm of other sites of lip, oral cavity, and pharynx

Z85.819 Personal history of malignant neoplasm of unspecified site of lip, oral cavity, and pharynx

+ **Z85.82 Personal history of malignant neoplasm of skin**

Z85.820 Personal history of malignant melanoma of skin
Conditions classifiable to C43

Z85.821 Personal history of Merkel cell carcinoma
Conditions classifiable to C4A

Z85.828 Personal history of other malignant neoplasm of skin
Conditions classifiable to C44

+ **Z85.83 Personal history of malignant neoplasm of bone and soft tissue**
Conditions classifiable to C40-C41; C45-C49

Z85.830 Personal history of malignant neoplasm of bone

Z85.831 Personal history of malignant neoplasm of soft tissue
Excludes2: *personal history of malignant neoplasm of skin (Z85.82-)*

+ **Z85.84 Personal history of malignant neoplasm of eye and nervous tissue**
Conditions classifiable to C69-C72

Z85.840 Personal history of malignant neoplasm of eye

Z85.841 Personal history of malignant neoplasm of brain

Z85.848 Personal history of malignant neoplasm of other parts of nervous tissue

+ **Z85.85 Personal history of malignant neoplasm of endocrine glands**
Conditions classifiable to C73-C75

Z85.850 Personal history of malignant neoplasm of thyroid

Z85.858 Personal history of malignant neoplasm of other endocrine glands

Z85.89 Personal history of malignant neoplasm of other organs and systems
Conditions classifiable to C7A.098, C76, C77-C79

Z85.9 Personal history of malignant neoplasm, unspecified
Conditions classifiable to C7A.00, C80.1

Z86 Personal history of certain other diseases
Code first any follow-up examination after treatment (Z09)
AHA CC: 4Q, 2019, 20
Review coding guideline C.21.c.4

+ **Z86.0 Personal history of in-situ and benign neoplasms and neoplasms of uncertain behavior**
Excludes2: *personal history of malignant neoplasms (Z85.-)*

+ **Z86.00 Personal history of in-situ neoplasm**
Conditions classifiable to D00-D09

Z86.000 Personal history of in-situ neoplasm of breast
Conditions classifiable to D05

♀ **Z86.001 Personal history of in-situ neoplasm of cervix uteri**
Conditions classifiable to D06
Personal history of cervical intraepithelial neoplasia III [CINIII]

Z86.002 Personal history of in-situ neoplasm of other and unspecified genital organs
Conditions classifiable to D07
Personal history of high-grade prostatic intraepithelial neoplasia III [HGPIN III]
Personal history of vaginal intraepithelial neoplasia III [VAIN III]
Personal history of vulvar intraepithelial neoplasia III [VAN III]

Z86.003 Personal history of in-situ neoplasm of oral cavity, esophagus and stomach
Conditions classifiable to D00

Z86.004 Personal history of in-situ neoplasm of other and unspecified digestive organs
Conditions classifiable to D01
Personal history of anal intraepithelial neoplasia III [AIN III]

Z86.005 Personal history of in-situ neoplasm of middle ear and respiratory system
Conditions classifiable to D02

Z86.006 Personal history of melanoma in-situ
Conditions classifiable to D03
Excludes2: *sites other than skin - code to personal history of in-situ neoplasm of the site*

Z86.007 Personal history of in-situ neoplasm of skin
Conditions classifiable to D04
Personal history of carcinoma in-situ of skin

Z86.008 Personal history of in-situ neoplasm of other site
Conditions classifiable to D09

+ **Z86.01** **Personal history of benign neoplasm**
    Z86.010 **Personal history of colonic polyps**
        AHA CC: 1Q, 2017, 9
    Z86.011 **Personal history of benign neoplasm of the brain**
    Z86.012 **Personal history of benign carcinoid tumor**
    Z86.018 **Personal history of other benign neoplasm**
    Z86.03 **Personal history of neoplasm of uncertain behavior**

+ **Z86.1** **Personal history of infectious and parasitic diseases**
    Conditions classifiable to A00-B89, B99
    Excludes1: *personal history of infectious diseases specific to a body system*
        sequelae of infectious and parasitic diseases (B90-B94)
    AHA CC: 4Q, 2016, 4-7
    Z86.11 **Personal history of tuberculosis**
    Z86.12 **Personal history of poliomyelitis**
    Z86.13 **Personal history of malaria**
    Z86.14 **Personal history of Methicillin resistant Staphylococcus aureus infection**
        Personal history of MRSA infection
    Z86.15 **Personal history of latent tuberculosis infection**
    Z86.19 **Personal history of other infectious and parasitic diseases**
        AHA CC: 2Q, 2020, 10-12
        Review coding guideline C.1.g.1.i

Z86.2 **Personal history of diseases of the blood and blood-forming organs and certain disorders involving the immune mechanism**
    Conditions classifiable to D50-D89

+ **Z86.3** **Personal history of endocrine, nutritional and metabolic diseases**
    Conditions classifiable to E00-E88
    Z86.31 **Personal history of diabetic foot ulcer**
        Excludes2: *current diabetic foot ulcer (E08.621, E09.621, E10.621, E11.621, E13.621)*
    ♀ **Z86.32** **Personal history of gestational diabetes**
        Personal history of conditions classifiable to O24.4-
        Excludes1: *gestational diabetes mellitus in current pregnancy (O24.4-)*
    Z86.39 **Personal history of other endocrine, nutritional and metabolic disease**
        AHA CC: 1Q, 2020, 12-13

+ **Z86.5** **Personal history of mental and behavioral disorders**
    Conditions classifiable to F40-F59
    ● **Z86.51** **Personal history of combat and operational stress reaction**
    Z86.59 **Personal history of other mental and behavioral disorders**

+ **Z86.6** **Personal history of diseases of the nervous system and sense organs**
    Conditions classifiable to G00-G99, H00-H95
    Z86.61 **Personal history of infections of the central nervous system**
        Personal history of encephalitis
        Personal history of meningitis
    Z86.69 **Personal history of other diseases of the nervous system and sense organs**
        AHA CC: 4Q, 2016, 21

+ **Z86.7** **Personal history of diseases of the circulatory system**
    Conditions classifiable to I00-I99
    Excludes2: *old myocardial infarction (I25.2)*
        personal history of anaphylactic shock (Z87.892)
        postmyocardial infarction syndrome (I24.1)
+   **Z86.71** **Personal history of venous thrombosis and embolism**
    Z86.711 **Personal history of pulmonary embolism**
    Z86.718 **Personal history of other venous thrombosis and embolism**
        AHA CC: 2Q, 2020, 20-21
    Z86.72 **Personal history of thrombophlebitis**

Z86.73 **Personal history of transient ischemic attack (TIA), and cerebral infarction without residual deficits**
    Personal history of prolonged reversible ischemic neurological deficit (PRIND)
    Personal history of stroke NOS without residual deficits
    Excludes1: *personal history of traumatic brain injury (Z87.820)*
        sequelae of cerebrovascular disease (I69.-)
    Review coding guideline C.9.d.3
Z86.74 **Personal history of sudden cardiac arrest**
    Personal history of sudden cardiac death successfully resuscitated
Z86.79 **Personal history of other diseases of the circulatory system**
    AHA CC: 1Q, 2020, 12-13

Z87 **Personal history of other diseases and conditions**
    Code first any follow-up examination after treatment (Z09)
    Review coding guideline C.21.c.4
+ **Z87.0** **Personal history of diseases of the respiratory system**
    Conditions classifiable to J00-J99
    Z87.01 **Personal history of pneumonia (recurrent)**
    Z87.09 **Personal history of other diseases of the respiratory system**
+ **Z87.1** **Personal history of diseases of the digestive system**
    Conditions classifiable to K00-K93
    Z87.11 **Personal history of peptic ulcer disease**
    Z87.19 **Personal history of other diseases of the digestive system**
        AHA CC: 1Q, 2017, 14-15
Z87.2 **Personal history of diseases of the skin and subcutaneous tissue**
    Conditions classifiable to L00-L99
    Excludes2: *personal history of diabetic foot ulcer (Z86.31)*
+ **Z87.3** **Personal history of diseases of the musculoskeletal system and connective tissue**
    Conditions classifiable to M00-M99
    Excludes2: *personal history of (healed) traumatic fracture (Z87.81)*
+   **Z87.31** **Personal history of (healed) nontraumatic fracture**
    Z87.310 **Personal history of (healed) osteoporosis fracture**
        Personal history of (healed) fragility fracture
        Personal history of (healed) collapsed vertebra due to osteoporosis
        Review coding guideline C.13.d.1
    Z87.311 **Personal history of (healed) other pathological fracture**
        Personal history of (healed) collapsed vertebra NOS
        Excludes2: *personal history of osteoporosis fracture (Z87.310)*
    Z87.312 **Personal history of (healed) stress fracture**
        Personal history of (healed) fatigue fracture
    Z87.39 **Personal history of other diseases of the musculoskeletal system and connective tissue**
+ **Z87.4** **Personal history of diseases of genitourinary system**
    Conditions classifiable to N00-N99
+   **Z87.41** **Personal history of dysplasia of the female genital tract**
    Excludes1: *personal history of malignant neoplasm of female genital tract (Z85.40-Z85.44)*
        personal history of intraepithelial neoplasia III of female genital tract (Z86.001, Z86.008)

+, +7th, X + 7th   ● Newborn   ● Pediatric   ● Maternity   ● Adult   ♀ Female   ♂ Male   Manifestation   Unacceptable PDX   HCC   CC   MCC   HAC

♀ **Z87.410** **Personal history of cervical dysplasia**
♀ **Z87.411** **Personal history of vaginal dysplasia**
♀ **Z87.412** **Personal history of vulvar dysplasia**
♀ **Z87.42** **Personal history of other diseases of the female genital tract**
+ **Z87.43** **Personal history of diseases of male genital organs**
♂ **Z87.430** **Personal history of prostatic dysplasia**
Excludes1: *personal history of malignant neoplasm of prostate (Z85.46)*
♂ **Z87.438** **Personal history of other diseases of male genital organs**
+ **Z87.44** **Personal history of diseases of urinary system**
Excludes1: *personal history of malignant neoplasm of cervix uteri (Z85.41)*
Z87.440 **Personal history of urinary (tract) infections**
Z87.441 **Personal history of nephrotic syndrome**
Z87.442 **Personal history of urinary calculi**
Personal history of kidney stones
Z87.448 **Personal history of other diseases of urinary system**
+ **Z87.5** **Personal history of complications of pregnancy, childbirth and the puerperium**
Conditions classifiable to O00-O9A
Excludes2: *recurrent pregnancy loss (N96)*
♀ **Z87.51** **Personal history of pre-term labor**
Excludes1: *current pregnancy with history of pre-term labor (O09.21-)*
♀ **Z87.59** **Personal history of other complications of pregnancy, childbirth and the puerperium**
Personal history of trophoblastic disease
+ **Z87.7** **Personal history of (corrected) congenital malformations**
Conditions classifiable to Q00-Q89 that have been repaired or corrected
Excludes1: *congenital malformations that have been partially corrected or repair but which still require medical treatment - code to condition*
Excludes2: *other postprocedural states (Z98.-)*
personal history of medical treatment (Z92.-)
presence of cardiac and vascular implants and grafts (Z95.-)
presence of other devices (Z97.-)
presence of other functional implants (Z96.-)
transplanted organ and tissue status (Z94.-)
+ **Z87.71** **Personal history of (corrected) congenital malformations of genitourinary system**
♂ **Z87.710** **Personal history of (corrected) hypospadias**
Z87.718 **Personal history of other specified (corrected) congenital malformations of genitourinary system**
+ **Z87.72** **Personal history of (corrected) congenital malformations of nervous system and sense organs**
Z87.720 **Personal history of (corrected) congenital malformations of eye**
Z87.721 **Personal history of (corrected) congenital malformations of ear**
Z87.728 **Personal history of other specified (corrected) congenital malformations of nervous system and sense organs**
+ **Z87.73** **Personal history of (corrected) congenital malformations of digestive system**
Z87.730 **Personal history of (corrected) cleft lip and palate**
Z87.738 **Personal history of other specified (corrected) congenital malformations of digestive system**
Z87.74 **Personal history of (corrected) congenital malformations of heart and circulatory system**

Z87.75 **Personal history of (corrected) congenital malformations of respiratory system**
Z87.76 **Personal history of (corrected) congenital malformations of integument, limbs and musculoskeletal system**
+ **Z87.79** **Personal history of other (corrected) congenital malformations**
Z87.790 **Personal history of (corrected) congenital malformations of face and neck**
Z87.798 **Personal history of other (corrected) congenital malformations**
+ **Z87.8** **Personal history of other specified conditions**
Excludes2: *personal history of self harm (Z91.5)*
Z87.81 **Personal history of (healed) traumatic fracture**
Excludes2: *personal history of (healed) nontraumatic fracture (Z87.31-)*
+ **Z87.82** **Personal history of other (healed) physical injury and trauma**
Conditions classifiable to S00-T88, except traumatic fractures
Z87.820 **Personal history of traumatic brain injury**
Excludes1: *personal history of transient ischemic attack (TIA), and cerebral infarction without residual deficits (Z86.73)*
Z87.821 **Personal history of retained foreign body fully removed**
Z87.828 **Personal history of other (healed) physical injury and trauma**
+ **Z87.89** **Personal history of other specified conditions**
Z87.890 **Personal history of sex reassignment**
Z87.891 **Personal history of nicotine dependence**
Excludes1: *current nicotine dependence (F17.2-)*
AHA CC: 2Q, 2017, 26-28
Z87.892 **Personal history of anaphylaxis**
Code also allergy status such as:
allergy status to drugs, medicaments and biological substances (Z88.-)
allergy status, other than to drugs and biological substances (Z91.0-)
Z87.898 **Personal history of other specified conditions**
AHA CC: 1Q, 2013, 21

Z88 **Allergy status to drugs, medicaments and biological substances**
Excludes2: *Allergy status, other than to drugs and biological substances (Z91.0-)*
Review coding guideline C.21.c.3
Z88.0 **Allergy status to penicillin**
Z88.1 **Allergy status to other antibiotic agents**
Z88.2 **Allergy status to sulfonamides**
AHA CC: 3Q, 2015, 23
Z88.3 **Allergy status to other anti-infective agents**
Z88.4 **Allergy status to anesthetic agent**
Z88.5 **Allergy status to narcotic agent**
Z88.6 **Allergy status to analgesic agent**
Z88.7 **Allergy status to serum and vaccine**
Z88.8 **Allergy status to other drugs, medicaments and biological substances**
Z88.9 **Allergy status to unspecified drugs, medicaments and biological substances**

Z89 **Acquired absence of limb**
Includes: amputation status
postprocedural loss of limb
post-traumatic loss of limb
Excludes1: *acquired deformities of limbs (M20-M21)*
congenital absence of limbs (Q71-Q73)
Review coding guideline C.21.c.3

+, +7th, X + 7th   • Newborn   • Pediatric   • Maternity   • Adult   ♀ Female   ♂ Male   Manifestation   Unacceptable PDX   HCC   CC   MCC   HAC

+ **Z89.0** **Acquired absence of thumb and other finger(s)**
   + **Z89.01** **Acquired absence of thumb**
      Z89.011 **Acquired absence of right thumb**
      Z89.012 **Acquired absence of left thumb**
      Z89.019 **Acquired absence of unspecified thumb**
   + **Z89.02** **Acquired absence of other finger(s)**
      Excludes2: *acquired absence of thumb (Z89.01-)*
      Z89.021 **Acquired absence of right finger(s)**
      Z89.022 **Acquired absence of left finger(s)**
      Z89.029 **Acquired absence of unspecified finger(s)**
+ **Z89.1** **Acquired absence of hand and wrist**
   + **Z89.11** **Acquired absence of hand**
      Z89.111 **Acquired absence of right hand**
      Z89.112 **Acquired absence of left hand**
      Z89.119 **Acquired absence of unspecified hand**
   + **Z89.12** **Acquired absence of wrist**
      Disarticulation at wrist
      Z89.121 **Acquired absence of right wrist**
      Z89.122 **Acquired absence of left wrist**
      Z89.129 **Acquired absence of unspecified wrist**
+ **Z89.2** **Acquired absence of upper limb above wrist**
   + **Z89.20** **Acquired absence of upper limb, unspecified level**
      Z89.201 **Acquired absence of right upper limb, unspecified level**
      Z89.202 **Acquired absence of left upper limb, unspecified level**
      Z89.209 **Acquired absence of unspecified upper limb, unspecified level**
        Acquired absence of arm NOS
   + **Z89.21** **Acquired absence of upper limb below elbow**
      Z89.211 **Acquired absence of right upper limb below elbow**
      Z89.212 **Acquired absence of left upper limb below elbow**
      Z89.219 **Acquired absence of unspecified upper limb below elbow**
   + **Z89.22** **Acquired absence of upper limb above elbow**
      Disarticulation at elbow
      Z89.221 **Acquired absence of right upper limb above elbow**
      Z89.222 **Acquired absence of left upper limb above elbow**
      Z89.229 **Acquired absence of unspecified upper limb above elbow**
   + **Z89.23** **Acquired absence of shoulder**
      Acquired absence of shoulder joint following explantation of shoulder joint prosthesis, with or without presence of antibiotic-impregnated cement spacer
      Z89.231 **Acquired absence of right shoulder**
      Z89.232 **Acquired absence of left shoulder**
      Z89.239 **Acquired absence of unspecified shoulder**
+ **Z89.4** **Acquired absence of toe(s), foot, and ankle**
   + **Z89.41** **Acquired absence of great toe**
      Z89.411 **Acquired absence of right great toe**
      Z89.412 **Acquired absence of left great toe**
      Z89.419 **Acquired absence of unspecified great toe**
   + **Z89.42** **Acquired absence of other toe(s)**
      Excludes2: *acquired absence of great toe (Z89.41-)*
      Z89.421 **Acquired absence of other right toe(s)**
      Z89.422 **Acquired absence of other left toe(s)**
      Z89.429 **Acquired absence of other toe(s), unspecified side**
   + **Z89.43** **Acquired absence of foot**
      Z89.431 **Acquired absence of right foot**
      Z89.432 **Acquired absence of left foot**
      Z89.439 **Acquired absence of unspecified foot**
   + **Z89.44** **Acquired absence of ankle**
      Disarticulation of ankle
      Z89.441 **Acquired absence of right ankle**
      Z89.442 **Acquired absence of left ankle**
      Z89.449 **Acquired absence of unspecified ankle**

+ **Z89.5** **Acquired absence of leg below knee**
   + **Z89.51** **Acquired absence of leg below knee**
      Z89.511 **Acquired absence of right leg below knee**
      Z89.512 **Acquired absence of left leg below knee**
      Z89.519 **Acquired absence of unspecified leg below knee**
   + **Z89.52** **Acquired absence of knee**
      Acquired absence of knee joint following explantation of knee joint prosthesis, with or without presence of antibiotic-impregnated cement spacer
      Z89.521 **Acquired absence of right knee**
      Z89.522 **Acquired absence of left knee**
      Z89.529 **Acquired absence of unspecified knee**
+ **Z89.6** **Acquired absence of leg above knee**
   + **Z89.61** **Acquired absence of leg above knee**
      Acquired absence of leg NOS
      Disarticulation at knee
      Z89.611 **Acquired absence of right leg above knee**
      Z89.612 **Acquired absence of left leg above knee**
      Z89.619 **Acquired absence of unspecified leg above knee**
   + **Z89.62** **Acquired absence of hip**
      Acquired absence of hip joint following explantation of hip joint prosthesis, with or without presence of antibiotic-impregnated cement spacer
      Disarticulation at hip
      Z89.621 **Acquired absence of right hip joint**
      Z89.622 **Acquired absence of left hip joint**
      Z89.629 **Acquired absence of unspecified hip joint**
  Z89.9 **Acquired absence of limb, unspecified**

Z90 **Acquired absence of organs, not elsewhere classified**

  Includes: postprocedural or post-traumatic loss of body part NEC
  Excludes1: *congenital absence - see Alphabetical Index*
  Excludes2: *postprocedural absence of endocrine glands (E89.-)*
  Review coding guideline C.21.c.3
+ **Z90.0** **Acquired absence of part of head and neck**
      Z90.01 **Acquired absence of eye**
      Z90.02 **Acquired absence of larynx**
      Z90.09 **Acquired absence of other part of head and neck**
        Acquired absence of nose
        Excludes2: *teeth (K08.1)*
+ **Z90.1** **Acquired absence of breast and nipple**
      Z90.10 **Acquired absence of unspecified breast and nipple**
      Z90.11 **Acquired absence of right breast and nipple**
      Z90.12 **Acquired absence of left breast and nipple**
      Z90.13 **Acquired absence of bilateral breasts and nipples**
  Z90.2 **Acquired absence of lung [part of]**
  Z90.3 **Acquired absence of stomach [part of]**
+ **Z90.4** **Acquired absence of other specified parts of digestive tract**
   + **Z90.41** **Acquired absence of pancreas**
      Code also exocrine pancreatic insufficiency (K86.81)
      Use additional code to identify any associated:
        diabetes mellitus, postpancreatectomy (E13.-)
        insulin use (Z79.4)
      Review coding guideline C.4.a.6.b.i
      Z90.410 **Acquired total absence of pancreas**
        Acquired absence of pancreas NOS
      Z90.411 **Acquired partial absence of pancreas**
      Z90.49 **Acquired absence of other specified parts of digestive tract**
  Z90.5 **Acquired absence of kidney**
  Z90.6 **Acquired absence of other parts of urinary tract**
      Acquired absence of bladder
+ **Z90.7** **Acquired absence of genital organ(s)**
      Excludes1: *personal history of sex reassignment (Z87.890)*
      Excludes2: *female genital mutilation status (N90.81-)*

1291

+ **Z90.71** **Acquired absence of cervix and uterus**
  ♀ **Z90.710** **Acquired absence of both cervix and uterus**
    Acquired absence of uterus NOS
    Status post total hysterectomy
  ♀ **Z90.711** **Acquired absence of uterus with remaining cervical stump**
    Status post partial hysterectomy with remaining cervical stump
  ♀ **Z90.712** **Acquired absence of cervix with remaining uterus**
+ **Z90.72** **Acquired absence of ovaries**
  ♀ **Z90.721** **Acquired absence of ovaries, unilateral**
  ♀ **Z90.722** **Acquired absence of ovaries, bilateral**
Z90.79 **Acquired absence of other genital organ(s)**
+ **Z90.8** **Acquired absence of other organs**
Z90.81 **Acquired absence of spleen**
Z90.89 **Acquired absence of other organs**

Z91 **Personal risk factors, not elsewhere classified**

Excludes2: contact with and (suspected) exposures hazardous to health (Z77.-)
  exposure to pollution and other problems related to physical environment (Z77.1-)
  female genital mutilation status (N90.81-)
  personal history of physical injury and trauma (Z87.81, Z87.82-)
  occupational exposure to risk factors (Z57.-)

+ **Z91.0** **Allergy status, other than to drugs and biological substances**

Excludes2: Allergy status to drugs, medicaments, and biological substances (Z88.-)
Review coding guideline C.21.c.3

+ **Z91.01** **Food allergy status**
Excludes2: food additives allergy status (Z91.02)
Z91.010 **Allergy to peanuts**
Z91.011 **Allergy to milk products**
  Excludes1: lactose intolerance (E73.-)
Z91.012 **Allergy to eggs**
Z91.013 **Allergy to seafood**
  Allergy to shellfish
  Allergy to octopus or squid ink
Z91.018 **Allergy to other foods**
  Allergy to nuts other than peanuts
Z91.02 **Food additives allergy status**
+ **Z91.03** **Insect allergy status**
Z91.030 **Bee allergy status**
Z91.038 **Other insect allergy status**
+ **Z91.04** **Nonmedicinal substance allergy status**
Z91.040 **Latex allergy status**
  Latex sensitivity status
Z91.041 **Radiographic dye allergy status**
  Allergy status to contrast media used for diagnostic X-ray procedure
Z91.048 **Other nonmedicinal substance allergy status**
Z91.09 **Other allergy status, other than to drugs and biological substances**
+ **Z91.1** **Patient's noncompliance with medical treatment and regimen**
Z91.11 **Patient's noncompliance with dietary regimen**
+ **Z91.12** **Patient's intentional underdosing of medication regimen**
  Code first underdosing of medication (T36-T50) with fifth or sixth character 6
  Excludes1: adverse effect of prescribed drug taken as directed- code to adverse effect
    poisoning (overdose) -code to poisoning
  Review coding guideline C.19.e.5.c

Z91.120 **Patient's intentional underdosing of medication regimen due to financial hardship**
Z91.128 **Patient's intentional underdosing of medication regimen for other reason**
+ **Z91.13** **Patient's unintentional underdosing of medication regimen**
  Code first underdosing of medication (T36-T50) with fifth or sixth character 6
  Excludes1: adverse effect of prescribed drug taken as directed- code to adverse effect
    poisoning (overdose) -code to poisoning
  Review coding guideline C.19.e.5.c
Z91.130 **Patient's unintentional underdosing of medication regimen due to age-related debility**
Z91.138 **Patient's unintentional underdosing of medication regimen for other reason**
Z91.14 **Patient's other noncompliance with medication regimen**
  Patient's underdosing of medication NOS
  Review coding guideline C.19.e.5.c
Z91.15 **Patient's noncompliance with renal dialysis**
Z91.19 **Patient's noncompliance with other medical treatment and regimen**
  Nonadherence to medical treatment
+ **Z91.4** **Personal history of psychological trauma, not elsewhere classified**
  Review coding guideline C.21.c.4
+ **Z91.41** **Personal history of adult abuse**
  Excludes2: personal history of abuse in childhood (Z62.81-)
  • **Z91.410** **Personal history of adult physical and sexual abuse**
    Excludes1: current adult physical abuse (T74.11, T76.11)
      current adult sexual abuse (T74.21-T76.11)
  • **Z91.411** **Personal history of adult psychological abuse**
  • **Z91.412** **Personal history of adult neglect**
    Excludes1: current adult neglect (T74.01, T76.01)
  • **Z91.419** **Personal history of unspecified adult abuse**
Z91.42 **Personal history of forced labor or sexual exploitation**
  AHA CC: 4Q, 2018, 32-33, 35
Z91.49 **Other personal history of psychological trauma, not elsewhere classified**
Z91.5 **Personal history of self-harm**
  Personal history of parasuicide
  Personal history of self-poisoning
  Personal history of suicide attempt
  Review coding guideline C.21.c.4
+ **Z91.8** **Other specified personal risk factors, not elsewhere classified**
  Review coding guideline C.21.c.4
Z91.81 **History of falling**
  At risk for falling
  Review coding guideline C.18.d and C21.c.4
• **Z91.82** **Personal history of military deployment**
  Individual (civilian or military) with past history of military war, peacekeeping and humanitarian deployment (current or past conflict)
  Returned from military deployment
  Review coding guideline C.21.c.4
Z91.83 **Wandering in diseases classified elsewhere**
  Code first underlying disorder such as:
  Alzheimer's disease (G30.-)
  autism or pervasive developmental disorder (F84.-)
  intellectual disabilities (F70-F79)
  unspecified dementia with behavioral disturbance (F03.9-)

+ **Z91.84** **Oral health risk factors**
AHA CC: 4Q, 2017, 29
Review coding guideline C.21.c.14
Z91.841 **Risk for dental caries, low**
Z91.842 **Risk for dental caries, moderate**
Z91.843 **Risk for dental caries, high**
Z91.849 **Unspecified risk for dental caries**
Z91.89 **Other specified personal risk factors, not elsewhere classified**
AHA CC: 1Q, 2017, 45-46

Z92 **Personal history of medical treatment**
Excludes2: *postprocedural states (Z98.-)*
Review coding guideline C.21.c.4
Z92.0 **Personal history of contraception**
Excludes1: *counseling or management of current contraceptive practices (Z30.-)*
long term (current) use of contraception (Z79.3)
presence of (intrauterine) contraceptive device (Z97.5)
+ **Z92.2** **Personal history of drug therapy**
Excludes2: *long term (current) drug therapy (Z79.-)*
Z92.21 **Personal history of antineoplastic chemotherapy**
Z92.22 **Personal history of monoclonal drug therapy**
Z92.23 **Personal history of estrogen therapy**
+ **Z92.24** **Personal history of steroid therapy**
Z92.240 **Personal history of inhaled steroid therapy**
Z92.241 **Personal history of systemic steroid therapy**
Personal history of steroid therapy NOS
Z92.25 **Personal history of immunosupression therapy**
Excludes2: *personal history of steroid therapy (Z92.24)*
Z92.29 **Personal history of other drug therapy**
Z92.3 **Personal history of irradiation**
Personal history of exposure to therapeutic radiation
Excludes1: *exposure to radiation in the physical environment (Z77.12)*
occupational exposure to radiation (Z57.1)
+ **Z92.8** **Personal history of other medical treatment**
Z92.81 **Personal history of extracorporeal membrane oxygenation (ECMO)**
Z92.82 **Status post administration of tPA (rtPA) in a different facility within the last 24 hours prior to admission to current facility**
Code first condition requiring tPA administration, such as:
acute cerebral infarction (I63.-)
acute myocardial infarction (I21.-, I22.-)
AHA CC: 4Q, 2013, 124
Review coding guideline C.21.c.3
Z92.83 **Personal history of failed moderate sedation**
Personal history of failed conscious sedation
Excludes2: *failed moderate sedation during procedure (T88.52)*
Z92.84 **Personal history of unintended awareness under general anesthesia**
Excludes2: *unintended awareness under general anesthesia during procedure (T88.53)*
AHA CC: 4Q, 2016, 72-73, 77
Z92.89 **Personal history of other medical treatment**
AHA CC: 1Q, 2020, 18

Z93 **Artificial opening status**
Excludes1: *artificial openings requiring attention or management (Z43.-)*
complications of external stoma (J95.0-, K94.-, N99.5-)
Review coding guideline C.21.c.3
Z93.0 **Tracheostomy status**
AHA CC: 4Q, 2013, 129
Z93.1 **Gastrostomy status**
Z93.2 **Ileostomy status**
Z93.3 **Colostomy status**
Z93.4 **Other artificial openings of gastrointestinal tract status**
+ **Z93.5** **Cystostomy status**
Z93.50 **Unspecified cystostomy status**
Z93.51 **Cutaneous-vesicostomy status**

Z93.52 **Appendico-vesicostomy status**
Z93.59 **Other cystostomy status**
Z93.6 **Other artificial openings of urinary tract status**
Nephrostomy status
Ureterostomy status
Urethrostomy status
Z93.8 **Other artificial opening status**
Z93.9 **Artificial opening status, unspecified**

Z94 **Transplanted organ and tissue status**
Includes: organ or tissue replaced by heterogenous or homogenous transplant
Excludes1: *complications of transplanted organ or tissue - see Alphabetical Index*
Excludes2: *presence of vascular grafts (Z95.-)*
Review coding guideline C.21.c.3
CC **Z94.0** **Kidney transplant status**
Review coding guideline C.14.a.2
CC **Z94.1** **Heart transplant status**
Excludes1: *artificial heart status (Z95.812)*
heart-valve replacement status (Z95.2-Z95.4)
CC **Z94.2** **Lung transplant status**
CC **Z94.3** **Heart and lungs transplant status**
CC **Z94.4** **Liver transplant status**
Z94.5 **Skin transplant status**
Autogenous skin transplant status
Z94.6 **Bone transplant status**
Z94.7 **Corneal transplant status**
+ **Z94.8** **Other transplanted organ and tissue status**
CC **Z94.81** **Bone marrow transplant status**
CC **Z94.82** **Intestine transplant status**
CC **Z94.83** **Pancreas transplant status**
CC **Z94.84** **Stem cells transplant status**
Z94.89 **Other transplanted organ and tissue status**
Z94.9 **Transplanted organ and tissue status, unspecified**

Z95 **Presence of cardiac and vascular implants and grafts**
Excludes2: *complications of cardiac and vascular devices, implants and grafts (T82.-)*
Review coding guideline C.21.c.3
Z95.0 **Presence of cardiac pacemaker**
Presence of cardiac resynchronization therapy (CRT-P) pacemaker
Excludes1: *adjustment or management of cardiac device (Z45.0-)*
adjustment or management of cardiac pacemaker (Z45.0)
presence of automatic (implantable) cardiac defibrillator with synchronous cardiac pacemaker (Z95.810)
AHA CC: 1Q, 2019, 33-34
Z95.1 **Presence of aortocoronary bypass graft**
Presence of coronary artery bypass graft
Z95.2 **Presence of prosthetic heart valve**
Presence of heart valve NOS
Z95.3 **Presence of xenogenic heart valve**
Z95.4 **Presence of other heart-valve replacement**
Z95.5 **Presence of coronary angioplasty implant and graft**
Excludes1: *coronary angioplasty status without implant and graft (Z98.61)*
+ **Z95.8** **Presence of other cardiac and vascular implants and grafts**
+ **Z95.81** **Presence of other cardiac implants and grafts**
Z95.810 **Presence of automatic (implantable) cardiac defibrillator**
Presence of automatic (implantable) cardiac defibrillator with synchronous cardiac pacemaker
Presence of cardiac resynchronization therapy defibillator (CRT-D)
Present of cardioverter-defibrillator (ICD)
CC **Z95.811** **Presence of heart assist device**
CC **Z95.812** **Presence of fully implantable artificial heart**
Z95.818 **Presence of other cardiac implants and grafts**

+, +7th, X + 7th   • Newborn   • Pediatric   • Maternity   • Adult   ♀ Female   ♂ Male   Manifestation   Unacceptable PDX   HCC   CC   MCC   HAC

+ **Z95.82** **Presence of other vascular implants and grafts**
  Z95.820 Peripheral vascular angioplasty status with implants and grafts
      Excludes1: *peripheral vascular angioplasty without implantandgraft(Z98.62)*
  Z95.828 Presence of other vascular implants and grafts
      Presence of intravascular prosthesis NEC
Z95.9 **Presence of cardiac and vascular implant and graft, unspecified**

Z96 **Presence of other functional implants**

  Excludes2: *complications of internal prosthetic devices, implants and grafts (T82-T85)*
      fitting and adjustment of prosthetic and other devices (Z44-Z46)
  Review coding guideline C.21.c.3

Z96.0 **Presence of urogenital implants**
Z96.1 **Presence of intraocular lens**
    Presence of pseudophakia
+ **Z96.2** **Presence of otological and audiological implants**
  Z96.20 Presence of otological and audiological implant, unspecified
  Z96.21 Cochlear implant status
  Z96.22 Myringotomy tube(s) status
  Z96.29 Presence of other otological and audiological implants
      Presence of bone-conduction hearing device
      Presence of eustachian tube stent
      Stapes replacement
Z96.3 **Presence of artificial larynx**
+ **Z96.4** **Presence of endocrine implants**
  Z96.41 Presence of insulin pump (external) (internal)
  Z96.49 Presence of other endocrine implants
Z96.5 **Presence of tooth-root and mandibular implants**

+ **Z96.6** **Presence of orthopedic joint implants**
  Z96.60 Presence of unspecified orthopedic joint implant
  + **Z96.61** Presence of artificial shoulder joint
      Z96.611 Presence of right artificial shoulder joint
      Z96.612 Presence of left artificial shoulder joint
      Z96.619 Presence of unspecified artificial shoulder joint
  + **Z96.62** Presence of artificial elbow joint
      Z96.621 Presence of right artificial elbow joint
      Z96.622 Presence of left artificial elbow joint
      Z96.629 Presence of unspecified artificial elbow joint
  + **Z96.63** Presence of artificial wrist joint
      Z96.631 Presence of right artificial wrist joint
      Z96.632 Presence of left artificial wrist joint
      Z96.639 Presence of unspecified artificial wrist joint
  + **Z96.64** Presence of artificial hip joint
      Hip-joint replacement (partial) (total)
      Z96.641 Presence of right artificial hip joint
          AHA CC: 3Q, 2016, 16-17
      Z96.642 Presence of left artificial hip joint
          AHA CC: 1Q, 2015, 16-17
      Z96.643 Presence of artificial hip joint, bilateral
      Z96.649 Presence of unspecified artificial hip joint
  + **Z96.65** Presence of artificial knee joint
      Z96.651 Presence of right artificial knee joint
      Z96.652 Presence of left artificial knee joint
          AHA CC: 3Q, 2019, 16-17
      Z96.653 Presence of artificial knee joint, bilateral
      Z96.659 Presence of unspecified artificial knee joint

+ **Z96.66** **Presence of artificial ankle joint**
  Z96.661 Presence of right artificial ankle joint
  Z96.662 Presence of left artificial ankle joint
  Z96.669 Presence of unspecified artificial ankle joint
+ **Z96.69** **Presence of other orthopedic joint implants**
  Z96.691 Finger-joint replacement of right hand
  Z96.692 Finger-joint replacement of left hand
  Z96.693 Finger-joint replacement, bilateral
  Z96.698 Presence of other orthopedic joint implants
Z96.7 **Presence of other bone and tendon implants**
    Presence of skull plate
+ **Z96.8** **Presence of other specified functional implants**
  Z96.81 Presence of artificial skin
  Z96.82 Presence of neurostimulator
      Presence of brain neurostimulator
      Presence of gastric neurostimulator
      Presence of peripheral nerve neurostimulator
      Presence of sacral nerve neurostimulator
      Presence of spinal cord neurostimulator
      Presence of vagus nerve neurostimulator
      AHA CC: 4Q, 2019, 19
  Z96.89 Presence of other specified functional implants
Z96.9 **Presence of functional implant, unspecified**

Z97 **Presence of other devices**

  Excludes1: *complications of internal prosthetic devices, implants and grafts (T82-T85)*
  Excludes2: *fitting and adjustment of prosthetic and other devices (Z44-Z46)*
      presence of cerebrospinal fluid drainage device (Z98.2)
  Review coding guideline C.21.c.3

Z97.0 **Presence of artificial eye**
+ **Z97.1** **Presence of artificial limb (complete) (partial)**
  Z97.10 Presence of artificial limb (complete) (partial), unspecified
  Z97.11 Presence of artificial right arm (complete) (partial)
  Z97.12 Presence of artificial left arm (complete) (partial)
  Z97.13 Presence of artificial right leg (complete) (partial)
  Z97.14 Presence of artificial left leg (complete) (partial)
  Z97.15 Presence of artificial arms, bilateral (complete) (partial)
  Z97.16 Presence of artificial legs, bilateral (complete) (partial)
Z97.2 **Presence of dental prosthetic device (complete) (partial)**
    Presence of dentures (complete) (partial)
Z97.3 **Presence of spectacles and contact lenses**
Z97.4 **Presence of external hearing-aid**
♀ **Z97.5** **Presence of (intrauterine) contraceptive device**
  Excludes1: *checking, reinsertion or removal of implantable subdermal contraceptive (Z30.46)*
      checking, reinsertion or removal of intrauterine contraceptive device (Z30.43-)
Z97.8 **Presence of other specified devices**

Z98 **Other postprocedural states**

  Excludes2: *aftercare (Z43-Z49, Z51)*
      follow-up medical care (Z08-Z09)
      postprocedural complication - see Alphabetical Index
  Review coding guideline C.21.c.3

Z98.0 **Intestinal bypass and anastomosis status**
  Excludes2: *bariatric surgery status (Z98.84)*
      gastric bypass status (Z98.84)
      obesity surgery status (Z98.84)
Z98.1 **Arthrodesis status**
Z98.2 **Presence of cerebrospinal fluid drainage device**
    Presence of CSF shunt
Z98.3 **Post therapeutic collapse of lung status**
    Code first underlying disease
+ **Z98.4** **Cataract extraction status**
    Use additional code to identify intraocular lens implant status (Z96.1)
  Excludes1: *aphakia (H27.0)*

+, +7th, X + 7th   ● Newborn   ● Pediatric   ● Maternity   ● Adult   ♀ Female   ♂ Male   Manifestation   Unacceptable PDX   HCC   CC   MCC   HAC

Z98.41 **Cataract extraction status, right eye**
Z98.42 **Cataract extraction status, left eye**
Z98.49 **Cataract extraction status, unspecified eye**
+ Z98.5 **Sterilization status**
 Excludes1: *female infertility (N97.-)*
 male infertility (N46.-)
 ♀ Z98.51 **Tubal ligation status**
 ● ♂ Z98.52 **Vasectomy status**
+ Z98.6 **Angioplasty status**
 Z98.61 **Coronary angioplasty status**
 Excludes1: *coronary angioplasty status with*
 implant and graft (Z95.5)
 Z98.62 **Peripheral vascular angioplasty status**
 Excludes1: *peripheral vascular angioplasty*
 status with implant and graft
 (Z95.820)
+ Z98.8 **Other specified postprocedural states**
 AHA CC: 4Q, 2016, 76
 + Z98.81 **Dental procedure status**
 Z98.810 **Dental sealant status**
 Z98.811 **Dental restoration status**
 Dental crown status
 Dental fillings status
 Z98.818 **Other dental procedure status**
 Z98.82 **Breast implant status**
 Excludes1: *breast implant removal status (Z98.86)*
 Z98.83 **Filtering (vitreous) bleb after glaucoma surgery**
 status
 Excludes1: *Inflammation (infection) of*
 postprocedural bleb (H59.4-)
 Z98.84 **Bariatric surgery status**
 Gastric banding status
 Gastric bypass status for obesity
 Obesity surgery status
 Excludes1: *bariatric surgery status complicating*
 pregnancy, childbirth, or the
 puerperium (O99.84)
 Excludes2: *intestinal bypass and anastomosis*
 status (Z98.0)
 AHA CC: 1Q, 2020, 12
 Z98.85 **Transplanted organ removal status**
 Transplanted organ previously removed due to
 complication, failure, rejection or infection
 Excludes1: *encounter for removal of transplanted*
 organ -code to complication of
 transplanted organ (T86.-)
 Z98.86 **Personal history of breast implant removal**
 + Z98.87 **Personal history of in utero procedure**
 ♀ Z98.870 **Personal history of in utero procedure**
 during pregnancy
 Excludes2: *complications from in utero*
 procedure for current
 pregnancy (O35.7)
 supervision of current
 pregnancy with history
 of in utero procedure
 during previous pregnancy
 (O09.82-)
 Z98.871 **Personal history of in utero procedure**
 while a fetus

+ Z98.89 **Other specified postprocedural states**
 Z98.890 **Other specified postprocedural states**
 Personal history of surgery, note
 elsewhere classified
 ♀ Z98.891 **History of uterine scar from previous**
 surgery
 Excludes1: *Maternal care due to uterine*
 scar from previous surgery
 (O34.2-)
 AHA CC: 4Q, 2016, 51-52

Z99 **Dependence on enabling machines and devices, not elsewhere**
classified
 Excludes1: *cardiac pacemaker status (Z95.0)*
 AHA CC: 1Q, 2020, 11
 Review coding guideline C.21.c.3
 Z99.0 **Dependence on aspirator**
+ Z99.1 **Dependence on respirator**
 Dependence on ventilator
 CC Z99.11 **Dependence on respirator [ventilator] status**
 AHA CC: 1Q, 2015, 21
 CC Z99.12 **Encounter for respirator [ventilator] dependence**
 during power failure
 Excludes1: *mechanical complication of respirator*
 [ventilator] (J95.850)
 AHA CC: 4Q, 2017, 112-114
 Review coding guidelines B19.d and C.21.c.16
 Z99.2 **Dependence on renal dialysis**
 Hemodialysis status
 Peritoneal dialysis status
 Presence of arteriovenous shunt for dialysis
 Renal dialysis status NOS
 Excludes1: *encounter for fitting and adjustment of dialysis*
 catheter (Z49.0-)
 Excludes2: *noncompliance with renal dialysis (Z91.15)*
 Z99.3 **Dependence on wheelchair**
 Wheelchair confinement status
 Code first cause of dependence, such as:
 muscular dystrophy (G71.0-)
 obesity (E66.-)
+ Z99.8 **Dependence on other enabling machines and devices**
 Z99.81 **Dependence on supplemental oxygen**
 Dependence on long-term oxygen
 AHA CC: 4Q, 2013, 129
 Z99.89 **Dependence on other enabling machines and**
 devices
 Dependence on machine or device NOS

+, +7th, X + 7th ● Newborn ● Pediatric ● Maternity ● Adult ♀ Female ♂ Male Manifestation Unacceptable PDX HCC CC MCC HAC

Chapter 22: Codes for Special Purposes (U00-U85)

This chapter contains the following blocks:

U00-U49 Provisional assignment of new diseases of uncertain etiology or emergency use

C. Chapter-Specific Coding Guidelines

In addition to general coding guidelines, there are guidelines for specific diagnoses and/or conditions in the classification. Unless otherwise indicated, these guidelines apply to all health care settings. Please refer to Section II for guidelines on the selection of the principal diagnosis.

22. Chapter 22: Codes for Special Purposes (U00-U85)

U07.0 Vaping-related disorder (*see Section I.C.10.e, Vaping-related disorders*)

U07.1 COVID-19 (*see Section I.C.1.g.1., COVID-19 infection*)

Provisional assignment of new diseases of uncertain etiology or emergency use (U00-U49)

U07 **Emergency use of U07**

U07.0 **Vaping related disorder** (*see Section I.C.10.e, Vaping-related disorders*)

Dabbing related lung damage

Dabbing related lung injury

E-cigarette, or vaping, product use associated lung injury [EVALI]

Electronic cigarette related lung damage

Electronic cigarette related lung injury

Use additional code to identify manifestations, such as:

abdominal pain (R10.84)

acute respiratory distress syndrome (J80)

diarrhea (R19.7)

drug-induced interstitial lung disorder (J70.4)

lipoid pneumonia (J69.1)

weight loss (R63.4)

AHA CC: 1Q, 2020, 3-4

Review coding guideline C.11.3

MCC **U07.1** **COVID-19** (*see Section I.C.1.g.1., COVID-19 infection*)

Use additional code to identify pneumonia or other manifestations

Excludes1: *coronavirus infection, unspecified (B34.2)*

coronavirus as the cause of diseases classified elsewhere (B97.2-)

pneumonia due to SARS-associated coronavirus (J12.81)

AHA CC: 2Q, 2020, 3-13

Review coding guideline C.15.s

Review coding guideline C.16.h

Appendix A: CC/MCC Principal Diagnosis Collections and Exclusion Lists

Appendix A is provided online in a format suitable for spreadsheet and/or database use. Go to http://ahimapress.org/casto8109, click the "Online Resources" link, and enter case-sensitive password AHIMA2Qt9w2021 to download the files.

Appendix B: Hospital-Acquired Conditions (HAC) List

Appendix B is provided online in a format suitable for spreadsheet and/or database use. Go to http://ahimapress.org/casto8109, click the "Online Resources" link, and enter case-sensitive password AHIMA2Qt9w2021 to download the files.

Appendix C: New ICD-10-CM Codes FY2021

Appendix C is provided online in a format suitable for spreadsheet and/or database use. Go to http://ahimapress.org/casto8109, click the "Online Resources" link, and enter case sensitive password AHIMA2Qt9w2021 to download files.

Appendix D: Deleted ICD-10-CM Codes FY2021

Appendix D is provided online in a format suitable for spreadsheet and/or database use. Go to http://ahimapress.org/casto8109, click the "Online Resources" link, and enter case sensitive password AHIMA2Qt9w2021 to download files.